Cancer Incidence
in Five Continents

Volume VII

International Agency for Research on Cancer

The International Agency for Research on Cancer (IARC) was established in 1965 by the World Health Assembly, as an independently financed organization within the framework of the World Health Organization. The headquarters of the Agency are at Lyon, France.

The Agency conducts a programme of research concentrating particularly on the epidemiology of cancer and the study of potential carcinogens in the human environment. Its field studies are supplemented by biological and chemical research carried out in the Agency's laboratories in Lyon, and, through collaborative research agreements, in national research institutions in many countries. The Agency also conducts a programme for the education and training of personnel for cancer research.

The publications of the Agency are intended to contribute to the dissemination of authoritative information on different aspects of cancer research. A complete list is printed at the back of the book. Information about IARC publications and how to order them is also available via the Internet at: http://www.iarc.fr/

International Association of Cancer Registries

The International Association of Cancer Registries (IACR) was created following a decision taken during the Ninth International Cancer Congress held in Tokyo, Japan, in 1966. The Association is a voluntary non-governmental organization in official relations with WHO, representing the scientific and professional interests of cancer registries, with members interested in the development and application of cancer registration and morbidity survey techniques to studies of well-defined populations.

The constitution provides for a Governing Body composed of a President, General Secretary, Deputy Secretary and nine regional representatives. From 1973 the IARC has provided a secretariat for the Association with the primary functions of organizing meetings and coordinating scientific studies.

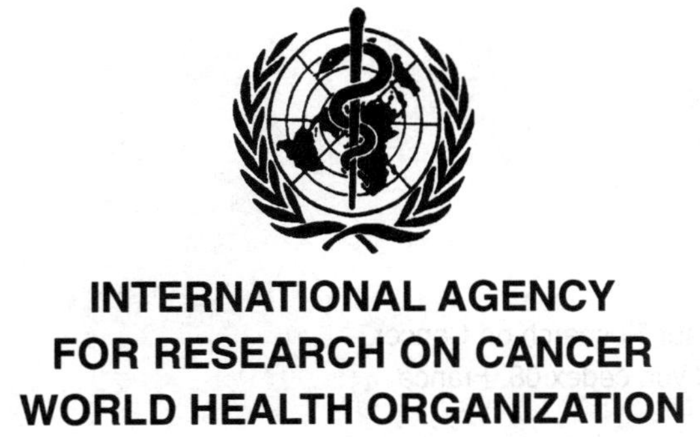

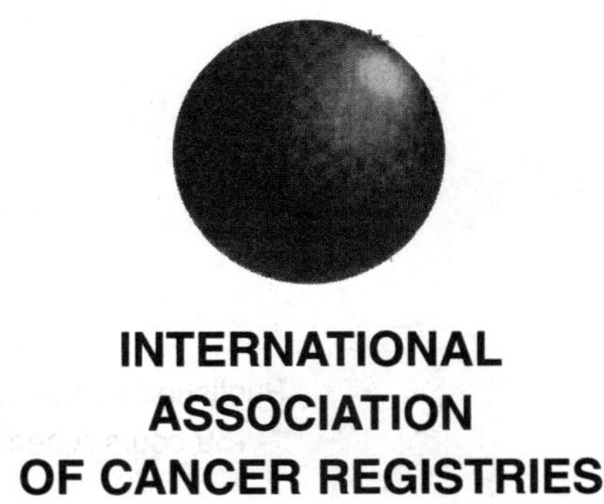

**INTERNATIONAL AGENCY
FOR RESEARCH ON CANCER
WORLD HEALTH ORGANIZATION**

**INTERNATIONAL
ASSOCIATION
OF CANCER REGISTRIES**

Cancer Incidence in Five Continents

Volume VII

**Edited by D.M. Parkin, S.L. Whelan, J. Ferlay,
L. Raymond and J. Young**

IARC Scientific Publications No. 143
Lyon, 1997

Published by the International Agency for Research on Cancer,
150 cours Albert Thomas, F-69372 Lyon cedex 08, France

Distributed by Oxford University Press, Walton Street, Oxford, UK OX2 6DP (Fax: +44 1865 267782) and in
the USA by Oxford University Press, 2001 Evans Road, Carey, NC 27513, USA (Fax: +1 919 677 1303).
All IARC publications can also be ordered directly from IARC*Press*
(Fax: +33 4 72 73 83 02; E-mail: press@iarc.fr).

IARC Library Cataloguing in Publication Data
Cancer incidence in five continents/
       editors, D. M. Parkin, S. L. Whelan, J. Ferlay,
       L. Raymond and J. Young

       (IARC Scientific Publication; 143)

       1. Neoplasms - epidemiology I. Parkin, D. M. II. Title III. Series

ISBN 92 832 2138 9   (NLM Classification: W1)
ISSN 0300–5085

Contents

Foreword

Studies of the variation in the risk of different cancers continue to provide important clues as to possible aetiology. The aim of the Cancer Incidence in Five Continents series is to present data on cancer incidence from reliable registries in a standardized way so that comparisons between geographical areas and ethnic groups may be made with confidence. Several registries have now published more than thirty years of data on cancer incidence in these volumes.

The efforts to build up cancer registration in areas of the world for which very little information on cancer occurrence is available are bearing fruit, and some of the results appear in this volume. Of particular note is the reappearance of Uganda, Kyadondo County - a registry for which data were published in Volume I but which was not able to contribute data until the period covered by the present volume. The African registries in this book are, it is hoped, the forerunners of a development in cancer registration in at least the major cities in many countries in the continent which will hopefully result in a substantially better coverage in Volume VIII. There are contributions from five new registries in Asia (including, for the first time, data from Korea and Vietnam), and from four in South America (presenting data from Argentina and Uruguay for the first time).

An innovation in Volume VII is the analysis of histological sub-types for selected sites, using data which have been checked for validity. Histological groupings appropriate for the analysis of data on cancer incidence have been established as a result of this exercise, and will be published separately. This continues the role of both the International Association of Cancer Registries and this series of publications in providing tools which facilitate the adoption of common methods and definitions by registries, so enhancing the comparability and hence value of the data.

P. Kleihues
Director, IARC

Dedication

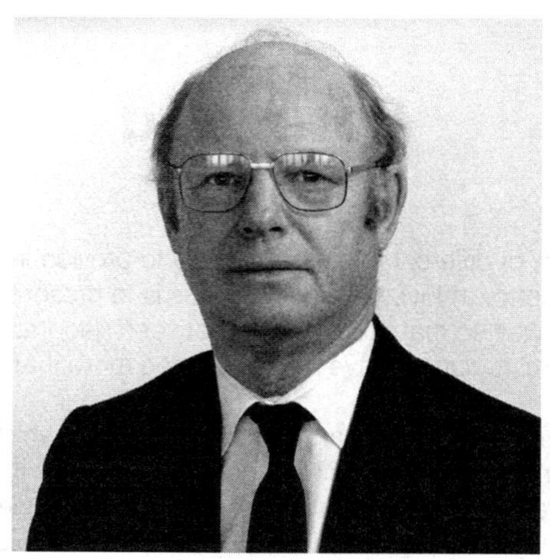

This, the seventh volume of 'Cancer Incidence in Five Continents', is dedicated to the memory of Dr Calum S. Muir.

Calum Muir began his contribution to the series with the first volume, to which he contributed data from the department of pathology in Singapore, and thereafter he became an editor of each subsequent edition. He had already begun work as an editor of this volume, when his colleagues were saddened to learn of his sudden death in June 1995. Calum Muir had a long-standing association with the International Agency for Research on Cancer (IARC), joining it in 1967 as Chief of the Unit of Epidemiology and Biostatistics, and becoming its Deputy Director in 1986. Upon his retirement from the Agency, he became the Director of Cancer Registration for Scotland. He was also instrumental in founding the International Association of Cancer Registries in 1966, and served as its Deputy Secretary from 1972 to 1990, and President from 1992 until his death.

Nearly everyone who contributed to this volume knew Calum Muir, and was influenced by his enthusiasm in collecting, analysing and presenting data, as epitomised by the 'CI5' series, which will long be associated with his name.

Contributors

AFRICA

Algeria, Sétif
Registre du Cancer de Sétif
(Cancer Registry of Sétif)
Hôpital Mère-Enfant
CHU de Sétif
Sétif 1900, Algeria
Tel: 213 (5) 911385. Fax: 213 (5) 911385

M. Hamdi-Chérif
N. Nouasria
K. Benlatreche
A. Mahnane
S. Laouamri

France, La Réunion
Registre des cancers de la Réunion
(Cancer Registry of La Réunion)
12 rue Jean Chatel
97400 - Saint Denis
La Réunion, France
Tel: 0262 203821. Fax: 0262 219323

P. Grizeau
J.Y. Vaillant
A. Begue

Mali, Bamako
Registre du cancer du Mali
(Cancer Registry of Mali)
National Institute of
Research in Public Health
P.O. Box 1771
Bamako, Mali
Tel: 223 22 42 31. Fax: 223 23 19 99

Siné Bayo
Sory Kané
Cheich Traoré
Abdel Karim Koumaré
Amadou Dolo
Tahirou Bah

Uganda, Kyadondo County
Kampala Cancer Registry
Department of Pathology
Makerere Medical school
P.O. Box 7072
Kampala, Uganda
Tel: 256 (41) 531730. Fax: 256 (41) 245580

Henry R. Wabinga
Sarah Nambooze

Zimbabwe, Harare
Zimbabwe National Cancer Registry
Parirenyatwa Hospital
P.O Box A 449, Avondale
Harare, Zimbabwe
Tel: 263 (4) 791631. Fax: 263 (4) 792020

M.T. Bassett
E. Chokunonga
L. Levy
B. Mauchaza

CENTRAL & SOUTH AMERICA

Argentina, Concordia
Registro poblacional de tumores de Concordia
(Cancer Registry of Concordia)
Mendoza 60-Concordia
C.P 3200 - Entre Rios
Argentina
Tel: 54 (45) 214988. Fax: 54 (45) 211342
e-mail: postmaster@invrof.anmat.sld.ar

Miguel Angel Prince
Dora I. Loria
Lilly Herrera
Elena L.Matos

Brazil, Belém
Registro de cancer de base
populacional de Belém
(Cancer Registry of Belém)
Rua: Presidente Pernambuco, 489
Bairro: Batista Campos
CEP: 66015-200 Belém-Parà
Tel: 55 (91) 2420077). Fax: 55 (91) 2411041

Antenor Madeira Neto
Maria Neves Costa Mùssio
Antonio Carlos Soares Leite

Brazil, Goiânia
Registro de Cancer de Base
populacional de Goiânia
(Cancer registry of Goiânia)
Associaçao de combate
ao cancer em Goiás
Rua 239 nº 206-Sector Universitário
Goiâna-Go CEP:74.605-070
Brazil
Tel: 55 (62) 2127333. Fax: 55 (62) 2245513
e-mail: saddi@aroeira.ufg.BR

Maria Paula Curado
Vera Aparecida Saddi
Sonia Martins Gonçalves
Sandra Gomes de S.Fraga
Monica Athayde
Carleane Maciel Bandeira
Elvicone Cirineu de Sousa
Elizabeth M.da Silva Arantes
Maria Inez L.Gomes

Brazil, Porto Alegre
Registro de cancer de base populacional de Porto Alegre
(Cancer registry of Porto Alegre)
Borges de Medeiros; 1501 4º Andar Ala Norte
Cidade Baixa-Porto Alegre
Rio Grande do Sul-RS
CEP 90110-150 Brazil
Tel: 55 (51)225-1859. Fax: 55 (51) 227-2798

Paulo Recena Grassi
Marieta Fátima de Brito
Carlos Eduardo Menegueti
Daniela Chiesa
Evandro de Azambuja
Mika Fukuoka
Miriam Dambros
Denise Maria Sarti de Oliveira
Luciana Sehn

Colombia, Cali
Registro Poblacional de Cancer de Cali
(Cali Cancer Registry)
Department of Pathology
School of Medicine
Universidad del Valle
Cali, Colombia, S.A.
Tel. and Fax: 90 57 (2) 5542489
e-mail:regcal@mafalda.univalle.edu.co
http://www.mafalda.edu.co/%regcal

Edwin Carrascal, MD,
Tito Collazos, Lic,
Hernan Ramirez, MD
(RIP 1946-1995)
Luis Castro
Julio Guarnizo
Juan Hernandez

Costa Rica
Registro Nacional de Tumores
(Costa Rica National Tumour Registry)
Departamento de Estadistica
Ministerio de Salud
Apartado 1253-1000
Costa Rica
Tel: (506) 2552148. Fax: (506) 2552148
e-mail:arodrigo@irazv.vna.ac.cr

Concepcion Bratti, MD
Georgina Muñoz
Ana Cecilia Rodriguez, MD
Daniel Antich

Ecuador, Quito
Registro Nacional de Tumores
(National Cancer Registry)
SOLCA
Av. de los Shyris 3307 y tomas de Berlanga
P.O. Box 17 - 11 4965 C.C.I.
Quito
Ecuador
Tel: 593 (2) 442122 Fax: 593 (2) 432859

Dr Fabían Corral Cordero
Dra Patricia Cueva Ayala
Dr José Yépez Maldonado
Sra Diana Noboa
Sra Maria Belén Morejón
Sra Mónica Galarza
Sr Galo Camacho
Sr Alfredo Dávila

Peru, Lima
Registro de Cancer de Lima Metropolitana
(Cancer Registry of Lima)
Av Angamos Este 2520
Surquillo
Lima, Peru
Tel: 51 (14) 382012. Fax: 51 (14) 483162
e-mail: postmaster@ciemh.sld.pe

Eduardo Caceres, MD
Maribel Almonte, MPH

Peru, Trujillo
Registro de Cancer de Base Poblacional de Trujillo
(Trujillo Cancer Registry)
Guillermo Charùn 279
URB, San Andres
Trujillo, Perù
Tel: 51 (44) 245281. Fax: 51 (44) 244261

P.F. Albujar

USA, Puerto Rico
Registro Central de Cancer de Puerto Rico
(Central Cancer Registry of Puerto Rico)
P.O. Box 9342
San Juan
Puerto Rico 00908-9342
Tel: 1(809) 2747865/2747866. Fax: 1(809) 2747824
e-mail: dzavala@igc.apc.org

Isidro Martinez, MD
Diego E. Zavala, PhD
Luz E. Echevarria, MPH, MPA
Nieves E. Perez Rosa, CTR
Julio E. Nevarez
Maria M. Rivera Rivera

Uruguay, Montevideo
Registro Nacional de Cancer Montevideo-Uruguay
(National Cancer Registry)
Juanicó 3265
Instituto Nacional de Oncología
11600 Montevideo-Uruguay
Tel: 598 (2) 782314. Fax:598 (2) 813625
e-mail: postmaster@urucan.org.uy

Dr Eduardo De Stefani
Dr Alvaro Ronco
Dr Juan A. Vassallo
Dr Enrique Barrios

NORTH AMERICA

Canada
Canadian Cancer Registry
18 th. Floor R.H. Coats Bldg.
Tunney's Pasture
Ottawa, Ontario Kia OT6
Canada
Tel: 1 (613) 9518571. Fax: 1 (613) 9510792

Leslie A. Gaudette
Ru-Nie Gao
Ingrid Friesen
Françoise Jean-Marie
Alice Brazeau
Diane Badger

Canada, Alberta
Alberta Cancer Registry
11560 University Avenue
Edmonton, Alberta
T6G 1Z2 Canada
Tel: 1 (403) 4928781. Fax: 1 (403) 4927039

Ms C. Russell
Mr T. Snodgrass
Ms M. Raphael

Canada, British Columbia
British Columbia Cancer Registry
600 West 10th Avenue
Vancouver, British Columbia
Canada V5Z-4E6
Tel: 1 (604) 8776000. Fax: 1 (604) 8776062

Mary McBride
Beth Tompkins

Canada, Manitoba
Manitoba Cancer Registry
Manitoba Cancer Treatment & Research Foundation
100 Olivia Street
Winnipeg, Manitoba
Canada R3E OV9
Tel: 1 (204) 7872157. Fax: 1 (204) 7836875
e-mail: cancerregistry@mctr.emb.ca

H. Whittaker
J. Kostyra, CTR
Dr N.W. Choi
Dr Erich Kliewer

Canada, New Brunswick
New Brunswick Cancer Registry
Provincial Cancer Registry
P.O Box 878
Saint John, New Brunswick,
Canada E2L 4C3
Tel: 1 (506) 6486871. Fax: 1 (506) 6486873
e-mail: chrisba@gov.nb.ca

Dr C. Balram

Canada, Newfoundland
Provincial Tumor Registry
Newfoundland Cancer Treatment & Research Foundation
The Dr H. Bliss Murphy Cancer Centre
300 Prince Philip Drive,
St. John's, Newfoundland
Canada AIB 3V6
Tel: 1 (709) 7376480. Fax: 1 (709) 7530927
e-mail: bpaulse@cancer.nf.ca

Dr T.G. Hogan
Ms Bertha Paulse
Mrs Mary Healey
Mrs Susan Ryan
Mr David Doucette

Canada, Northwest Territories
Northwest Territories Disease Registry
Department of Health
Government of the NWT
Box 1320
Yellowknife
NT Canada X1A 2L9
Tel: (403)9208946. Fax: (403) 8730266
e-mail: ian@inukshuk.gov.nt.ca

Marilyn Kenny
Carlyle Hogan
Ian Gilchrist

Canada, Nova Scotia
Nova Scotia Cancer Registry
Dickson Building
5820 University Avenue
Halifax, Nova Scotia
Canada B3H IV7
Tel: 1 (902) 4284258. Fax: 1 (902) 4284277
e-mail: ron.dewar@dal.ca

Karen Starratt
Ron Dewar
Maureen MacIntyre

Canada, Ontario
Ontario Cancer Registry
Division of Preventive Oncology
Ontario Cancer Treatment and Research Foundation
620 University Avenue, 11th Floor
Toronto, Ontario
Canada M5G 2L7
Tel: 1 (416) 9719800. Fax: 1 (416) 9716888
e-mail: eholowaty@octrf.on.ca

Eric Holowaty
Darlene Dale
Gordon Fehringer
Nelson Chong
Jill Chin

Canada, Prince Edward Island
Prince Edward Island Cancer Registry
Queen Elizabeth Hospital
P.O Box 6600
Charlottetown
Prince Edward Island C1A 8T5
Tel: 1 (902) 5666167. Fax: 1 (902) 5666187

Dr Dagny Dryer
Kim Vriends

Canada, Quebec
Fichier des tumeurs du Québec
(Quebec Cancer Registry)
Ministère de la santé et des services sociaux
Direction générale de la santé publique
Direction de l'analyse et surveillance de la santé et du bien-être
Edifice Catherine de Longpré
1075, chemin Ste-Foy, 2e étage
Québec, Canada , G1S 2M1
Tel: 1 (418) 6464745. Fax: 1 (418) 6463291

Michel Beaupré
Gaëtan Bibeau
Jeanne Bourdages
Nicole Hins

Canada, Saskatchewan
Saskatchewan Cancer Registry
Saskatchewan Cancer Foundation
400-2631 28th Avenue
Regina, Saskatchewan
Canada S4S 6X3
Tel: 1 (301) 7912767. Fax: 1 (306) 5842733

D. L. Robson
Dr D.F. White
Dr G.H. Ewing

Canada, Yukon
Yukon Cancer Registry
Yukon Bureau of Statistics
2089-2nd Avenue, Box 2703
Whitehorse, Yukon
Canada Y1A 2C6
Tel: 1 (403) 6675950. Fax:1 (403) 3936203
E-mail: jrmacgil@gov.yk.ca

Joseph MacGillivry

USA, California, Central Valley
Cancer Registry of Central California
1625 East Shaw Ave, Suite 155
Fresno, CA 93710
USA
Tel: 1 (209) 2216315. Fax: 1 (209) 2216219
e-mail: mill181w@wonder.em.cdc.gov

Paul K.Mills, PhD
Jane Breuss, CTR

USA, California, Los Angeles County
Los Angeles County Cancer Surveillance Program
University of Southern California School of Medicine
1540 Alcazar Street, CHP 204
Los Angeles, CA 90033
USA
Tel: 213 342 2300. Fax: 213 342 2301
e-mail: lbern@hsc.usc.edu

Leslie Bernstein, PhD
Judy Boone
Dennis Deapen, Dr PH
Ronald Ross, MD

USA, California, San Francisco Bay Area
Bay Area Resource for Cancer Control
Northern California Cancer Center
32960 Alvarado-Niles Road, Suite 600
Union City
CA 94587, USA
Tel: 1 (510) 4292500 Fax: 1 (510) 4292550
e-mail: dwest@nccc.org

Dee W. West, PhD
Sally Glaser, PhD
Lillia O'Connor, MBA, CTR, ART

USA, Connecticut
Connecticut Tumor Registry
State of Connecticut Department of Public Health
410 Capitol Avenue,MS# 13 TMR
P.O. Box 340308
Hartford, CT 06134-0308
USA
Tel: 1 (860) 5097163. Fax: 1 (860) 5097161

John T. Flannery
Anthony P. Polednak

USA, Georgia, Atlanta
Metropolitan Atlanta SEER Registry
Georgia Center for Cancer Statistics - Dept of Epidemiology
Rollins School of Public Health at Emory University
PhD
1518 Clifton Road NE
Atlanta, Georgia 30322, USA
Tel: 404 727 8701. Fax: 404 727 8737

Jonathan M. Liff, PhD
J. William Eley, MD, MPH
Raymond S. Greenberg, MD,

USA, Iowa
State Health Registry of Iowa
The University of Iowa
100 Westlawn Bldg. South
Iowa City
IA 52242-1100, USA
Tel: 1 (319) 335-8609. Fax: 1 (319) 335-8610
e-mail: charles-lynch@uiowa.edu

Charles F. Lynch, MD, PhD
Charles E. Platz, MD
Kathleen M. McKeen

USA, Louisiana, Central Region and New Orleans
Louisiana Tumor Registry
Louisiana State University Medical Center
Box P5-1, 1901 Perdido Street
New Orleans,
LA 70112, USA
Tel: 1 (504) 5686035. Fax: 1 (504) 5991278
e-mail: pathvwc@nomvs.lsumc.edu

Vivien W. Chen, PhD
Catherine N. Correa, MPH
Patricia A. Andrews, MPH
Xiao Cheng Wu, MD, MPH
Pelayo Correa, MD

USA, Michigan, Detroit
Metropolitan Detroit Cancer Surveillance System
Epidemiology Section
Karmanos Cancer Institute
110 E. Warren Avenue
Detroit, Michigan, USA 48201
Tel: (313) 833 07154329. Fax: (313) 8317806
e-mail: weiss@kci.wayne.edu

Linda K. Weiss, PhD
G. Marie Swanson, PhD, MPH

USA, New Mexico
New Mexico Tumor Registry
University of New Mexico Cancer Research
and Treatment Center
New Mexico Tumor Registry
900 Camino de Salud, NE
Albuquerque, New Mexico 87131-5306, USA
Tel: (505) 2773127. Fax: (505) 2778572
e-mail: amd@nmtr.unm.edu

Charles R. Key, MD, PhD
Frank Gilliland, MD, PhD
Anna Marie Davidson, CT(ASCP),
CTR

USA, Utah
Utah Cancer Registry
546 Chipeta Way
Suite 2100
Salt Lake City, Utah 84108, USA
Tel: (801) 5818407. Fax: (801) 5814560

J.L. Stanford
R. Dibble

USA, Washington, Seattle
Cancer Surveillance System of Washington State, USA
Fred Hutchinson Cancer Research Center
1124 Columbia Street, MP-826
Seattle, WA 98104
USA
Tel: 1 (206) 6674709. Fax: 1 (206) 6675530
e-mail: css@fhcrc.org

David B. Thomas, MD, DrPH
Janet Stanford, PhD
Mary Potts, RRA, CPA

USA, SEER
Surveillance Epidemiology & End Results (SEER)
Executive Plaza North, Room 343J
Bethesda, MD, 20892-7352, USA
Tel: 1 (301) 4968510. Fax: 1 (301) 4969949
e-mail connie@dcpcepn.nci.nih.gov

Constance Percy
Lynn Ries
Carol Kosary
Benjamin Hankey

ASIA

China, Qidong County
Qidong Cancer Registry
Qidong Liver Cancer Institute
57 Jianghai Bei Road
226200, Qidong, Jiangsu
People's Republic of China
Tel: 86 (513) 3312557. Fax: 86 (513) 3318224

Weng-Guang Li
Jian-Guo Chen
Zhuo-Cai Shen
Hong-Yu Yao
Jian Zhu

China, Shanghai
Shanghai Cancer Registry
Shanghai Cancer Institute
2200 Xie Tu Road
Shanghai 200032,
People's Republic of China
Tel: 86 (21) 64043057. Fax: 86 (21) 64041428

Gao Yu Tang, MD
Jin Fan, MD

China, Tianjin
Tianjin Cancer Registry
Department of Epidemiology
Tianjin Cancer Institute and Hospital
Huan Hu Xi Road
Ti Yuan Bei; Tianjin 300060
People's Republic of China
Tel: 86 (22) 3359929. Fax: 86 (22) 3359984
e-mail: tcih@v7610.tisti.ac.cn

Dr Wang, Qing-sheng
Dr Hao, Xi-shan
Dr Chen, Ke-xin
Dr Yu, Shi-bei
Dr Guo, Ce-yu
Mrs Song, Na
Mrs Dong, Shu-fen
Mrs Wang, Ji-fang

Hong Kong
Hong Kong Cancer Registry
Institute of Radiotherapy & Oncology
Queen Elizabeth Hospital
30 Gascoigne Road, Kowloon
Hong Kong
Tel: 852 2958-6021. Fax: 852 2385-1149

Dr William Foo
W. K. Mang

India, Bangalore
Population Based Cancer Registry
Kidwai Memorial Institute of Oncology
Hosur Road
Bangalore
560029 India.
Tel: 91 (80) 6632302. Fax:91 (80) 6644801

N. Anantha
A. Nandakumar

India, Barshi, Paranda and Bhum
Rural Cancer Registry: Barshi, Paranda & Bhum
Nargis, Dutt Memorial Cancer Hospital
Agalgaon Road, Barshi 413401
India
Tel: 91 (2184) 22699. Fax: 91 (2184) 23024

Kasturi Jayant
R.S. Rao
B.M. Nene
P.S. Dale

India, Bombay
Bombay Cancer Registry
Indian Cancer Society
74 Jerbai Wadia Road, Parel
Bombay 400012
India
Tel: 91 (22) 4122351

Dr D.J. Jussawalla
Mr B.B. Yeole
Mr M.V. Natekar

India, Karunagappally
Rural Cancer Registry, Karunagappally, Kerala India
Natural Background Radiation Cancer Registry
Vavvakkavu, Karunagappally
India
Tel: 91 (4756) 20609

Dr M. Krishnan Nair
Dr N. Sreedevi Amma
Mr P. Gangadharan

India, Madras
Madras Metropolitan Tumour Registry
Cancer Institute (WIA)
Adyar, Madras-600 020
India
Tel: 91 (44) 4910754/4912085. Fax: 91 (44) 4912085

Dr V. Shanta
Dr C.K. Gajalakshmi
Mr R. Swaminathan

India, Trivandrum
Population-Based Cancer Registry, Trivandrum
Regional Cancer Centre
Trivandrum - 695 011
Kerala, India
Tel: 91 0471 442541. Fax: 91 0471 447454

Dr M. Krishnan Nair
Dr Cherian Varghese
Ms Aleyamma Mathew
Mr P. Gangadharan

Israel
Israel Cancer Registry
107 Hebron Road
Jerusalem 93480
Israel
Tel: 972 (2) 6706818. Fax: 972 (2) 6706884

Micha Barchana, MD, MPH
Helena Andreev, PhD
Rachel Alon

Japan, Hiroshima
Hiroshima-Shi Ishikai Shuyo Tokei Iinkai
(Hiroshima City Medical Association Tumor
Statistics Committee)
1-1-1 Kannon Hon Machi, Nishi-Ku
Hiroshima 733, Japan
Tel: 81 (82) 2327321. Fax: 81 (82) 2925233

Kozo Sanada
Shojiro Kimura
Teruaki Fukuhara
Yasuyuki Fujita
Kiyohiko Mabuchi

Japan, Miyagi Prefecture
Miyagi Prefectural Cancer Registry
c/o Miyagi Cancer Society
Kamisugi 6-chome, Aoba-ku
Sendai, 980 Japan
Tel: 81 (22) 2330241. Fax: 81 (22) 2718686

Akira Takano, MD
Yoshi Okuno
Minoru Kurihara, MD
Sadao Okitsu, MD

Japan, Nagasaki Prefecture
Nagasaki Prefectural Cancer Registry
Midori Soda, Nagasaki Tumor Registry
Radiation Effects Research Foundation (RERF)
1-8-6 Nakagawa, Nagasaki 850
Japan
Tel: 81 (958) 231121. Fax: 81 (958) 257202
e-mail: soda@rerf.or.jp

Midori Soda
Takayoshi Ikeda
Soroku Saeki
Hisashi Ishikawa
Yoshisada Shibata

Japan, Osaka Prefecture
Osaka Cancer Registry
Department of Field Research
Medical Center for Cancer and Cardiovascular Diseases
(Center for Adult Diseases, Osaka)
1-3-3 Nakamichi, Higashinari-Ku
Osaka 537, Japan
Tel: 81 (6) 9721181. Fax; 81(6) 9727749

Aya Hanai
Wakiko Ajiki
Hideaki Tsukuma
Akira Oshima
Isaburo Fujimoto
Haruo Uematsu
Yutaka Takasugi

Japan, Saga Prefecture
Saga Prefectural Cancer Registry
Department of Community Health Science
Saga Medical School
5-1-1 Nabeshima
Saga 849, Japan
Tel: 81 0952316511. Fax: 81 0952332518
e-mail:morim3@post.saga-med.ac.jp

Mitsuru Mori
Masatoshi Ishizuka
Junichi Naramoto
Eisuke Nakazato
Ayado Maeda

Japan, Yamagata Prefecture
Yamagata Prefectural Cancer Registry
Yamagata Medical Center for Adults
7-17 Sakuracho
Yamagata City, 990, Japan
Tel: 81 (236) 234011.Fax: 81 (236) 234189

Yukio Sato
Toru Matsuda

Korea, Kangwha County
Kangwha County Cancer Registry
Dept. of Preventive Medicine and Public Health
Yonsei University College of Medicine
C.P.O. Box 8044
Seoul
Korea
Tel: 82 (2) 3922921. Fax: 82 (2) 3928133

Heechoul Ohrr
Il Soon Kim
Hee Ok Kim
Hyung Gon Kang
Il Suh
Yoon Lee
Sun Ha Jee
Byoung Soo Kim
Suk Il Kim
Kang Hee Lee
Jae Kyung Roh
Dong - Hwan Shin
June Yeon Hong

Kuwait
Kuwait Cancer Registry
Department of Community Medicine
Faculty of Medicine
Kuwait University, P.O. Box 24923
Safat 13110, Kuwait
Tel: 965 5319485. Fax: 965 5338948
e-mail: anjum@hscc.kuniv.edu.kw

Dr Anjum Memon
Mr Ali N. Al-Muhanna

Philippines, Manila
Manila Cancer Registry
Philippine Cancer Society
310 San Rafael St., San Miguel 1005
Manila, Philippines
Tel: 63 (2) 7410191. Fax: 63 (2) 7410772

Adriano V. Laudico
Divina B. Esteban,
Corazon A. Ngelangel
George Eufemio
Christopher Guzman

Singapore
Singapore Cancer Registry
c/o Dept. of Pathology
National University Hospital
Lower Kent Ridge Rd.
Singapore 119074
Tel: 65 7786783/7724310. Fax: 65 7780671

H.P Lee
K.S Chia
L.H. Seow, Adeline
K. Shanmugaratnam

Thailand, Chiang Mai
Chiang Mai Cancer Unit
Maharaj Nakorn Chiang Mai Hospital
Falculty of Medicine , Chiang Mai University
Chiang Mai
Thailand
Tel: 66 (53) 221122. Fax: 66 (53) 217144
e-mail: mdbci002@emu.chiangmai.ac.th

Nimit C. Martin
Songphol Srisukho
Maitree Suttajit
Vicharn Larvidhaya
Orathai Kunpradist
Ampai Satraruji
Udomluck Chaisaengkhum

Thailand, Khon Kaen
Khon Kaen Provincial Cancer Registry
Cancer Unit
Faculty of Medicine
Khon Kaen University
Srinagarind Hospital
Khon Kaen 40002
Thailand
Tel: 66 (43) 243088. Fax: 66 (43) 2433088/243064
e-mail: supannee@kkul.kku.ac.th

Vanchai Vatanasapt
Prasit Pengsaa
Supannee Sriamporn
Supot Kamsa-ard
Kritika Suwanrungruang
Sujinan Howrasit
Pakanant Usantia
Darunee Jintakanon Jaroensiri
Prachak Puapermpoonsiri
Jitjaroen Chaiyakum

Viet Nam, Hanoi
Hanoi Cancer Registry
Hanoi Cancer Institute
43 Quansu Street
Hanoi, Viet Nam
Tel: 84 (4) 246652. Fax: 84 (4) 253757
e-mail: anh@nci.gov.vn

Dr Pham Thi Hoang Anh
Dr Nguyen Ba Duc
Dr Hoang Xuan Khang
Dr Tran Hong Truong
Dr Nguyen Hoai Nga

EUROPE

Austria, Tyrol
Cancer Registry of Tyrol, Austria
University Hospital Innsbruck
Anichstr. 35
A-6020 Innsbruck, Austria
Tel: 43 (512) 5042310. Fax: 43 (512) 5042315
e-mail:wilhelm.oberaigner@uibk.ac.at

W. Oberaigner
H. Mühlböck
H. Leitner

Belarus
Belarusian Cancer Registry
Belarusian Center for Medical Technologies
7 A.P Brovki St.
220600 Minsk, Belarus
Tel: 375 (17) 2323080. Fax: 375 (17) 2323094
e-mail: belcmt@belcmt.belpak.minsk.by

Alexei Okeanov
Semyon Polyakov

Croatia
Croatian National Cancer Registry
Croatian National Institute of Public Health
Rockefellerova 7
HR - 10000 Zagreb
Croatia
Tel: 385 (1) 272822.Fax: 385 (1) 277307

Marija Strnad, MD, PhD
Ljubica Bubanovic
Nedeljka Vujanic
Petar Novak

Czech Republic
National Oncological Registry of the Czech Republic
Palackého NAM.4
P.O. Box 42
120 55 Praha 2
Czech Republic
Tel: 42 (2) 24972882. Fax: 42 (2) 24915982
e-mail: holubj@mzcr.cz

V. Mazánková
F. Beška
E. Geryk
J. Holub
M. Jechová

Denmark
Danish Cancer Registry
Institute of Cancer Epidemiology
Danish Cancer Society
P.O. Box 839
Strandboulevarden 49
2100 Copenhagen, Denmark
Tel: 45 35257500. Fax: 45 35257701
e-mail: hans@crg.dk

Hans H. Storm
Elli Michelsen
Jesper Pihl

Estonia
Eesti Vähiregister
(Estonian Cancer Registry)
Hiiu 44
EE 0016 Tallinn, Estonia
Tel: 372 (6) 504303. Fax: 37 (2) 6504340

Mati Rahu
Tiiu Aareleid
Taimi Vanaselja
Linda Mägi
Tiina Ristkok
Ülo Laanoja

Finland
Finnish Cancer Registry
Liisankatu 21B
00170 Helsinki, Finland
Tel: 358 (9) 135331. Fax: 358 (9) 1355378

M. Hakama
T. Hakulinen
M. Lehtonen
E. Pukkala
L. Teppo

France, Bas-Rhin
Registre Bas-Rhinois des cancers
(Cancer Registry of Bas-Rhin)
Laboratoire d'Epidémiologie et de Santé Publique
Faculté de Médecine
67085 Strasbourg Cedex
France
Tel: 33 388368597. Fax: 33 388240131

Paul Schaffer
Guy Hedelin

France, Calvados
Registre général des tumeurs du Calvados
(Calvados Cancer Registry)
Centre François Baclesse
Route de Lion sur Mer
14021 Caen Cedex, France
Tel: 33 0231455098. Fax: 33 0231455097

J. Mace-Lesech
M. Henry-Amar
V. Bastard
J.F. Héron

France, Calvados
Registre des tumeurs digestives du Calvados
(Digestive Cancer Registry)
Faculté de Médecine
CHU Côte de Nacre
14032 Caen Cedex, France
Tel: 33 231064464. Fax: 33 231064468

M.Gignoux
D. Pottier
A. Rougereau
G. Launoy

France, Doubs
Registre des tumeurs du Doubs
(Cancer Registry of Doubs)
Faculté de Médecine
C.H.U. Saint Jacques
25030 - Besançon
Tel:33 381218312. Fax: 33 3 81218311

Simon Schraub
Patrick Arveux

France, Haut-Rhin
Registre des cancers du Haut-Rhin
(Cancer Registry of Haut-Rhin)
Association pour la Recherche Epidémiologique
dans le Haut-Rhin A.R.E.R.68
9, Rue du Dr Mangeney - BP 1370
68070 Mulhouse Cedex
France
Tel: 33 389646251. Fax: 33 389646252

Antoine Buemi
Jean-Michel Halna
Mireille Grandadam

France, Hérault
Registre des tumeurs de l'Hérault
(Cancer Registry of Herault)
Epidaure Espace de Prévention
Rue des Apothicaires
BP 4111
34091 Montpellier Cedex 5
France
Tel: 33 467413417

Professor J.P. Daurès
Dr H. Mathieu-Daudé
Dr B. Tretarre
Mme A. Avon
Mme M. Boualam

France, Isère
Registre du cancer de l'Isère
(Isere Cancer Registry)
21 Chemin des Sources
38240 Meylan
France
Tel: 33 476907610. Fax: 33 476418700

F. Ménégoz
C. Exbrayat
M. Colonna
A.H. Aude
R. Schaerer

France, Somme
Registre du cancer de la Somme
(Somme Cancer Registry)
CHR Nord
Médecine 4ème Est
80054 Amiens Cedex 1 France
Tel: 33 322668226. Fax: 33 322668229

N. Raverdy-Bourdon
P. Fardellone
A. Dubreuil
A. Lorriaux
J. P. Kaufman

France, Tarn
Registre des cancers du Tarn
(Tarn Cancer Registry)
Chemin des Trois Tarn
81000 Albi
France
Tel: 33 563475951. Fax: 33 561593747

Dr Pascale Grosclaude
Dr Martine Machelard-
Roumagnac
Dr Bernard Faliu
Dr Yves Duchêne
Régine Litre-Tournier
Cécile Paillas

**Germany, Common Cancer Registry of the Federal
States of Berlin, Brandenburg, Mecklenburg-
Vorpommern, Sachsen-Anhalt and the Free States of
Sachsen and Thüringen**
Gemeinsames Krebsregister der Länder Berlin, Brandenburg,
Mecklenburg-Vorpommern, Sachsen-Anhalt und der
Freistaaten Sachsen und Thüringen (Common Cancer
Registry of the Federal States Berlin, Brandenburg,
Mecklenburg-Vorpommern, Sachsen-Anhalt and the Free
States Sachsen and Thüringen)
Brodauer Str. 16-22
D-12621 Berlin, Germany
Tel: 49 (30) 56581401. Fax: 49 (30) 56581444

Bettina Eisinger
Roland Stabenow

Germany, Saarland
Saarland Cancer Registry
Statistisches Landesamt
Postfach 10 30 44
66030 Saarbücken, Germany
Tel: 49 (681) 5015969. Fax: 49 (681) 5015998

Hartwig Ziegler
Christa Stegmaier

Iceland
Krabbameinsskra Krabbameinsfelags Islands
(Icelandic Cancer Registry)
Skogarhlid 8, Postbox 5420
125 Reykjavik
Iceland
Tel: 354 (56) 21414. Fax: 354 (56) 21417
e-mail: hrafnt@knabb.is

Hrafn Tulinius
Kristin Bjarnadóttir
Ólafur Bjarnason
Gudridur H. Ólafsdóttir

Ireland, Southern
National Cancer Registry
Elm Court
Boreenmanna Road
Cork
Ireland
Tel: 353 (21) 318014. Fax: 353 (21) 318016

Harry Comber
Mary Chambers
Patricia Duffy
Rosaleen O'Brien
Michael Crowley

Italy, Ferrara Province
Registro Tumori della Provincia di Ferrara
(Tumor Registry of Ferrara Province)
Istituto di Anatomia, Istologia e Citologia Patologica
Università di Ferrara
V.Fossato di Mortara 64 B
44100-Ferrara
Italy
Tel: 39 (532) 205701. Fax: 39 (532) 248021
e-mail: mzifeqa1@icineca.cineca.it

Stefano Ferretti
Annalisa Rasi
Giuseppe Albonico
Silvia Zago
Italo Nenci

Italy, Florence
Registro Tumori Toscano
(Tuscany Cancer Registry)
U.O. Epidemiologia - CSPO- USL 10
Via San Salvi, 12
50135 Firenze
Italy
Tel: 39 (55) 5662691. Fax: 39 (55) 679954

Eva Buiatti
Daniela Balzi
Alessandro Barchielli
Simona Carli
Emanuele Crocetti
Lucia Giovannetti

Italy, Genoa
Registro Tumori Ligure
(Ligurian Cancer Registry)
c/o Servizio Aggregato Registro Tumori-IST-
Istituto Nazionale per la Ricerca Sul Cancro
Largo Rosanna Benzi, 10
16132 Genova,
Italy
Tel: 39 (10) 5600961/963/956. Fax: 39 (10) 5600501
e-mail: envirepi@hp.380.ist.unige.it

Marina Vercelli
Maria Antonietta Orengo
Claudia Casella
Margherita Altavilla
Cinzia Orlandini
Giovanna De Lucia
Enza Marani
Flavia Di Giorgio
Luca Gogioso
Riccardo Puntoni

Italy, Latina
Registro Tumori di Populazione della Provincia di Latina
(Population Based Cancer Registry of the Latina Province)
Istituto "Regina Elena" per lo Studio e la Cura dei Tumori
Viale Regina Elena, 291
00161 Rome
Italy
Tel: 39 (6) 49852016. Fax: 39 (6) 4457086

Ettore M.S.Conti
Giuseppe Tonini
Valerio Ramazzotti
Marco Caperle
Maurilio Natali
Massimo Crespi

Italy, Macerata Province
Registro Tumori Provincia di Macerata
(Macerata Province Cancer Registry)
Università di Camerino
Via E. Betti n.3
62032 Camerino (MC)
Italy
Tel: 39 (737) 40849/40845. Fax: 39 (737) 40859

Franco Pannelli
Susanna Vitarelli
Assunta Berardi
Francesco la Rosa

Italy, Modena
Registro Tumori di Modena
(Modena Cancer Registry)
Oncologia Medica, Università di Modena
Policlinico, Via del Pozzo, 71
41100 Modena
Italy
Tel: 39 (59) 372672. Fax: 39 (59) 372672
e-mail: federico@mednw1.unimo.it

Massimo Federico
Lucia Mangone
Vittorio Silingardi

Italy, Parma Province
Registro Tumori della Provincia di Parma
(Parma Cancer Registry)
Centro di Riferimento Oncologico
Divisione Oncologia Medica
Via Gramsci, 14
43100 Parma
Italy
Tel: 39 (521) 991316/259571. Fax: 39 (521) 995448
e-mail: oncologig@ipouniv.cce.unipr.it

G. Cocconi
V. De Lisi
A. Borrini
L. Serventi
P. Zanni
P. Crafa
A. Tardini

Italy, Ragusa
Cancer Registry of Ragusa
(Registro Tumori Ragusa)
Servizio di Anatomia Patologica
Azienda Ospedaliera Ospedali Civile E M.P. Arezzo
97100 - Ragusa
Italy
Tel: 39 (932) 600681. Fax: 39 (932) 600661

Professor Lorenzo Gafà
Professor Luigi Dardanoni
Dr Rosario Tumino
Mrs Guglielmina La Rosa
Miss Giuseppina Pavone
Mrs Rosanna Spampinato
Dr Giovanni di Natale
Dr Giancarlo Gambuzza
Dr Salvatore Modica
Dr Carmela Nicita

Italy, Romagna
Cancer Registry of Romagna
Department of Medical Oncology
Hospital L. Pierantoni
Via Forlanini 11
47100 Forlì
Italy
Tel: 39 (543) 731737. Fax: 39 (543) 731736

Dino Amadori
Fabio Falcini
Patricia Vignutelli
Carlo Milandri
Monica Serafini
Carlo Cordaro
Rosa Vattiato
Stefania Giorgetti
Emanuela Montanari
Rita Danesi
Lauro Bucchi

Italy, Torino
Registro dei Tumori per il Piemonte e la Valle d'Aosta
(Piedmont Cancer Registry)
Via San Francesco da Paola, 31
10123 Torino
Italy
Tel: 39 (11) 5754006/8127354. Fax: 39 (11) 5754005

Roberto Zanetti
Stefano Rosso
Piera Vicari
Rosaria Foggetti
Silvia Patriarca
Rossana Prandi
Franca Gremo

Italy, Trieste
Registro dei Tumori della Provincia di Trieste
(Trieste Cancer Registry)
Via Pietà, 2/4
c/o Ospedale Maggiore
34125 Trieste
Italy
Tel: 39 (40) 3992376. Fax: 39 (40) 365141

G. Stanta
F. Cavallieri
L. Campagner
D. Brunetti
S. Scher
P. Peruzzo
L. Giarelli

Contributors

Italy, Varese Province
Lombardy Cancer Registry, Varese Province
Epidemiology Unit
National Cancer Institute
Via Venezian, 1
200133 Milano
Italy
Tel: 39 (2) 2390460/501/502. Fax: 39 (2) 2390762

Paolo Crosignani
Franco Berrino
Giovanna Tagliabue
Gemma Gatta
Milena Sant
Daniele Speciale
Tiziana Codazzi
Anna Maghini
Andrea Tittarelli
Clotilde Vigano'

Italy, Venetian Region
Registro Tumori del Veneto
(Venetian Cancer Registry)
ULSS 21 - Università di Padova
Via Giustiniani n°7
35100 Padova
Italy
Tel: 39 (49) 8213891. Fax: 39 (49) 8213396
e-mail: RTVØ1IPUNIVX.UNIPD.IT

Lorenzo Simonato
Stefano Guzzinati
Stefania Pacquola
Cosimo Picoco
Stefania Rodella
Stefania Sartorel
Fiorella Stocco
Sandro Tognazzo
Marcello Vettorazzi
Paola Zambon

Latvia
Latvian Cancer Registry
4 Hipokrate STR
LV 1079 Riga
Latvia
Tel: 371 (2) 539018/539209. Fax: 371 (2) 539160

Aivars Stengrevics
Aija Eglite
Irèna Rogovska
Ruta Suveizde

Malta
Malta National Cancer Registry
Department of Health Information
c/o Health Division
15, Merchants Street, Valletta
Malta
Tel: 356 234915.Fax: 356 235910

Dr Miriam Dalmas MD
Dr Hugo Agius Muscat, MD, MSc

Netherlands
The Netherlands Cancer Registry
Association of Comprehensive Cancer Centres
Catharÿnesingel 49 a
P.O Box 19001
3501 DA Utrecht
The Netherlands
Tel: 31 (302) 343780. Fax: 31 (302) 343632

O. Visser
R.A.M. Damhuis
R. Otter
J.W.W.Coebergh
M. Oostindiër
M.W.E. de Kok
C.H.F.Gimbrère
J.P. van Andel
L.J. Schouten

Netherlands, Eindhoven
Eindhoven Cancer Registry
Comprehensive Cancer Centre South
P.O Box 231
NL-5600 AE Eindhoven
The Netherlands
Tel: 31 (402) 455775. Fax: 31 (402) 457585

J.W.W. Coebergh
E. Masseling
L. H. van der Heijden
P.P. Razenberg

Netherlands, Maastricht
Comprehensive Cancer Centre (IKL)
P.O. Box 2208
6201 Ha Maastricht
The Netherlands
Tel: 31 (433) 254059. Fax: 31 (433) 252474

L.J. Schouten
P.A. Van den Brandt
J.A.M. Huveneers
J.J. Jager
A.G. Koppejan-Rensenbrink

Norway
Cancer Registry of Norway
Montebello
0310 Oslo,
Norway
Tel: 47 (22) 451300. Fax:47 (22) 451370

Aage Andersen
Eystein Glattre
Aage Johansen
Tove Dahl
Svein Hansen
Torbjørn Iversen

Poland, Cracow
Cracow Cancer Registry
Cancer Center of the Sklodowska-Curie Institute
Cracow Branch
Garncarska 11
31 115 Cracow
Poland
Tel: 48 (12) 229900 Fax: 48 (12) 226680
e-mail: zourbans@cyf.kr.edu.pl

Janusz Pawlega, MD
Alicja Urbanska
Elzbieta Podgorska

Poland, Kielce
Department of Epidemiology and Cancer Control
Regional Cancer Registry of Kielce
Jagiellonska 74 B
25-734 Kielce
P.O. Box 26
Poland
Tel: 48 (41) 662380/663454. Fax: 48 (41) 56882
e-mail: onkol-rm@srv1.tu.kielce.pl

Stanisław Góźdź
Urszula Siudowska
Ryszard Mezyk
Teresa Karpacz

Poland, Lower Silesia
Lower Silesian Cancer Registry
Dolnoslaski Rejestr Nowotworów
Dolnoslaskie Centrum Onkologii
53413 - Wroclaw
PL. Hirszfelda 12
Poland
Tel: 48 (71) 618024. Fax: 48 (71) 615561

Jerzy Blaszczyk
Marek Pudelko
Magdalena Bechtold
Elzbieta Chwieralska
Jacek Dryl
Piotr Hudziec
Helena Loboda
Malgorzata Modrzejewska
Elzbieta Polakowska
Zofia Wierzbicka

Poland, Warsaw City
Warsaw Cancer Registry
The Maria Sklodowska-Curie Memorial Cancer Centre
and Institute of Oncology
00-973 Warsaw,
Wawelska 15
Poland
Tel: 48 (2) 223447. Fax 48 (2) 222429

Zbigniew Wronkowski, MD, MPH
Maria Zwierko, MD
Marianna Romejko
Zofia Przybysz
Ewa Chorchos
Mirostawa Radlicka
Kazimiera Pieterwas
Wiktor Chmielarczyk
Andrzej Karwowski

Slovakia
Národny Onkologický Register Slovenskej Republiky
(National Cancer Registry of Slovak Republic)
Klenová I, 833 10 Bratislava,
Slovak Republic
Tel: 421 (7) 3708531/376598. Fax: 421 (7) 376598

Ivan Pleško
Adriana Obšitníková
Jozef Somogyi
Elena Manáková
Juraj Adamcík

Slovenia
Cancer Registry of Slovenia
Institute of Oncology
Zaloska c.2
61105 Ljubljana
Slovenia
Tel: 386 (61) 1324113. Fax: 386 (61) 1314180

Vera Pompe-Kirn, MD, PhD
Neva Volk, MD, MPH
Fani Škrlec
Neza Milcic
Nataša Robek
Marjeta Bukovec
Mosca Brus

Spain, Albacete
Registro de Cancer de Albacete
(Albacete Cancer Registry)
Avenida de la Guardia Civil, nº5
02005 - Albacete
Spain
Tel:34 (67) 215443. Fax: 34 (67) 211154

E. Almar Marques
A. Mateos Ramos
L.L. Gimenez Ortuño
J.A. Gomez Martinez
M. Atienzar Tobarra
A. Gonzalez Gomez

Spain, Asturias
Registro de Tumores del Principado de Asturias
(Asturias Cancer Registry)
Consejeria de Servicios Sociales
c/ General Elorza, 32
33001 Oviedo (Asturias)
Spain
Tel: 34 (98) 5106500. Fax: 34 (98) 5106520

Manuel Echeverria Rodriguez
Ramon Alonso de la Torre Lopez
Adamina Losada Garcia
Marcial Argüelles Suarez
Ana Fe Campo de la Fuente
German Meneses Castillo
Jose Antonio Alvarez Riesgo

Spain, Basque Country
Registro de Cancer de Euskadi
(Basque Country Cancer Registry)
Departamento de Sanidad
Alava 5
01006 Vitoria-Gasteiz
Spain
Tel: 34 (45) 132053. Fax: 34 (45) 145973

Isabel Izarzugaza
Elena Aldasoro
Nerea Larrañaga
Beatriz Sastre

Spain, Granada
Registro de Cáncer de Granada
(Granada Cancer Registry)
Escuela Andaluza de Salud Pública
Campus Universitario de Cartuja, s/n
Ap. Correos nº2070
18080 - Granada
Spain
Tel: 34 (58) 161044. Fax: 34 (58) 161142
e-mail: 100433.2527@compuserve.com

C. Martínez-García
Y. Fornieles-García
M. Rodríguez-Sánchez
M. J. Lamolda-Guardia
C. Ortega-Cambil
C. Ruiz-Baena
A. Calzas-Urrutia

Spain, Mallorca
Unitat d'Epidemiologia i Registre de Cancer de Mallorca
(Mallorca Cancer Registry)
Universitat de les Illes Balears
C/Miquel dels Sants Oliver, 2
07012 Palma de Mallorca
Spain
Tel: 34 (71) 172414/172715. Fax: 34 (71) 721056

I. Garau
P. Franch
E. Cabeza
J. Galceran
V. Moreno
E. Benito
M. Mulet
A. Obrador

Spain, Murcia
Registro de Cancer de Murcia
(Murcia Cancer Registry)
Servicio de Epidemíología
Consejería de Sanidad y Política Social
Ronda de Levante, 11
30008 Murcia
Spain
Tel: 34 (68) 362039. Fax: 34 (68) 201614
e-mail: carmenavarro@dgsc.sas.carm.es

Carmen Navarro
Jacinta Tortosa
Isabel Valera
Griselda Frapolli
Encarna Parraga

Spain, Navarra
Registro de Tumores de Navarra
(Navarra Cancer Registry)
Instituto de Salud Pública
S. Vigilancia y Control Epidemiológico
Calle Leyre, 15
31003 Pamplona
Spain
Tel: 34 (48) 103467. Fax: 34 (48) 103474

Eva Ardanaz
Aurelio Barricarte
Conchi Moreno
Ma. Eugenia Perez de Rada
Carmen Ezponda
Nieves Navaridas

Spain, Tarragona
Cancer Registry of Tarragona
C. Reina Maria Cristina, 54
43002 Tarragona
Spain
Tel: 34 (77) 232423 Fax: 34 (77) 211111

Jaume Galceran
Joan Borràs
Eugènia Mariné
Victor Moreno
Francesc Xavier Bosch
Josep Gumà
Jesús Muñoz
Josep Lluís Piñol
Roser Vives
Pau Viladiu

Spain, Zaragoza
Registro de Cancer de Zaragoza
(Cancer Registry of Zaragoza)
Calle Ramón y Cajal, 68
50004 - Zaragoza
Tel:34 (76) 442022. Fax: 34 (76) 446303

Alberto Vergara Ugarriza
Joaquín Guimbao Bescos
Pilar Moreo Bergada
Maria Angeles Lazaro Belanche
Pilar Muniesa Cuenca
Jose Luis Llorente

Sweden
Socialstyrelsen Cancerregister
(The Swedish Cancer Registry)
Centre for Epidemiology
The National Board of Health and Welfare
106 30 Stockholm
Sweden
Tel: 46 (8) 7833000. Fax: 46 (8) 7833327
e-mail: lotti:barlow@sos.se

Lotti Barlow
Jan Ericsson

Switzerland, Basel
Krebsregister Basel-Stadt und Basel-Landschaft
(Basel Cancer Registry)
Department of Pathology
University of Basel
Schönbeinstrasse 40
4003 Basel
Switzerland
Tel: 41 (61) 265 25 25. Fax: 41 (61) 265 31 94

J. Torhorst
R. Dougoud
V. Colaci
E. Perret

Switzerland, Geneva
Registre genevois des tumeurs
(Geneva Cancer Registry)
55, Boulevard de la Cluse
1205 Geneva
Switzerland
Tel: 41 (22) 3291011. Fax: 41 (22) 3282933
e-mail: fioretta@CIH.HCUGE.CH

Mirjana Obradovic
Gerald Fioretta
Christine Bouchardy

Switzerland, Graubünden
Krebsregister Graubünden und Glarus
(Graubünden Cancer Registry)
Department of Pathology
Kantonsspital
Loëstr 170, 7000 Chur
Switzerland
Tel: 41 (81) 266556. Fax: (81) 266544

J. Allemann
A. Abutillo
Ch. Ali

Switzerland, Neuchâtel
Registre Neuchâtelois des tumeurs
(Neuchâtel Cancer Registry)
Les Cadolles 4
2000 Neuchâtel
Switzerland
Tel: 41 (38) 243015

F. Levi
I. Portal
A.M. Mean
P. Siegenthaler
R. Choffat
L. Randimbison

Switzerland, St Gall Appenzell
Krebsregister St. Gallen Appenzell
(Cancer Registry of St. Gall Appenzell)
 Kantonsspital, Haus 22
9007 St. Gallen
Switzerland
Tel: 41 (71) 4942107. Fax: 41 (71) 4946176

T. Fisch
F. Enderlin
F. Neuweiler
E. Perret

Switzerland, Valais
Registre Valaisan des Tumeurs
(Valais Cancer Registry)
Institut Central des Hôpitaux Valaisans
Case Postale 510
1951 Sion
Tel: 41 (27) 331151. Fax: 41 (27)312976

François Joris
Fabrizio Faggiano
Daniel de Weck

Switzerland, Vaud
Registre Vaudois des Tumeurs
(Vaud Cancer Registry)
Institut Universitaire de Médecine Sociale
et Préventive, CHUV-Falaises 1
1011 Lausanne
Switzerland
Tel: 41 (21) 3147311. Fax: 41 (21) 3230303
e-mail: rvt@ulmed.unil.ch

F. Levi
V.C. Te
L. Randimbison
C. La Vecchia

Switzerland, Zürich
Kantonalzürchrisches Krebsregister
(Cancer Registry of the Canton of Zürich)
Department of Pathology and Institute of
Social and Preventive Medicine.
University Hospital, Sonneggstrasse 6
8091 Zürich
Switzerland
Tel: 41 (1) 2555634. Fax: 41 (1) 2554440

Georges Schüler, MD, MPH
Mrs Danielle Schüler
Matthias Bopp, PhD
Ph.U.Heitz, MD
Felix Gutzwiller, MD DrPH

UK, England and Wales
National Cancer Registration Bureau
Office for National Statistics
1 Drummond Gate
London SW1V 2QQ
Tel: 44(0171)5335257/5261/5266. Fax: 44(0171)5335252
e-mail: mike.quinn@ons.gov.uk

Dr M.J. Quinn

UK, England, East Anglia
East Anglian Cancer Registry
Addenbrooke's N.H.S Trust
Addenbrooke's Hospital
Hills Road, Cambridge CB2 2QQ
England
Tel:: 44 (1223) 216644. Fax: 44 (1223) 245636

Dr T.W. Davies
Dr C.H. Brown

UK, England, Merseyside and Cheshire
2nd Floor, Muspratt Building
University of Liverpool
Liverpool, L69 3BX, UK
Tel: 44 (151) 794 5691. FAX: 44 (151) 794 5700
E-mail:emiw@liv.ac.uk

E.M.I. Williams
K.M. Chester
J.E. Littler
K. Mistry

UK, England, North Western
North Western Regional Cancer Registry
Centre for Cancer Epidemiology
Kinnaird Road, Withington
Manchester, M20 4QL, UK
Tel:44(161)4463570. Fax: 44(161)3578

Ciaran Woodman
Jennifer Kennedy
Brad Donnelly

UK, England, Oxford Region
Oxford Cancer Intelligence Unit
Oxfordshire Health
Old Road, Headington
Oxford OX3 7LF
England, UK
Tel: 44 (1865) 227040. Fax: 44 (1865) 226809

Dr Monica Roche
Mr Neil Kennedy
Ms Julia Redburn
Mrs Patricia Hall

UK, England, South Thames
Thames Cancer Registry
UK England Thames Region
1st Floor, Capital House
Weston St
London SE1 3QD, UK
Tel: 44 (171) 3787688. Fax: 44 (171) 37895092
e-mail: j.hiscox@icr.ac.uk

Mrs Heather M. Bourne
Dr Janine Bell
Jason Hiscox

UK, England, South Western
South Western Cancer Registry
Cancer Epidemiology
Department of Epidemiology & Public Health Medicine
University of Bristol, Canynge Hall
Whiteladies Road, Clifton, Bristol BS8 2PR
Tel: 44 (117) 9287242. Fax: 44(117) 9287266
e-mail: D.J.Etherington@bris.ac.uk

Dr D.P.H. Pheby
Dr D.J. Etherington
Mrs A.E.Fischer
Mrs P. Thorne

UK, England, Wessex
Wessex Cancer Intelligence Unit
Romsey Road
Winchester, S022 5DH, UK
Tel: 44 (1962) 863511. Fax: 44 (1962) 877425
e-mail:j.smith@wiphm.soton.ac.uk

Dr Jenifer A.E. Smith

UK, England, West Midlands (Birmingham)
West Midlands Cancer Intelligence Unit
Queen Elizabeth Medical Centre
Birmingham B15 2TH, UK
Tel: 44 (121) 6272026. Fax: 44 (121) 627 2026
e-mail: C.I.U@hsrc.org.uk

Dr Gill Lawrence
Mrs Judith Stephenson
Mr Mike Porter
Dr Lillian Somervaille

UK, England, Yorkshire
Yorkshire Cancer Registry
Yorkshire Cancer Organisation
Arthington House, Cookridge Hospital
Hospital Lane
Leeds LS16 6QB, W. Yorkshire
England
Tel: 44 (113) 2924306. Fax: 44 (113) 2924132
e-mail: plr@yco.leeds.ac.uk

L. Rider
D. Forman
A. Smith
C. Lister
A. Ramsey
L. Wales

UK, Scotland
Scottish Cancer Registry
Information & Statistics Division
Trinity Park House
South Trinity Road
Edinburgh, Scotland EH5 3SQ
Tel: 44 (131) 5518903. Fax: 44 (131) 5511392

Ms E. Harkness
Mrs J. Crichton
Dr D. Brewster

UK, Scotland, West
West of Scotland Cancer Surveillance Unit
Ruchill Hospital
Glasgow, G20 9NB, UK
Tel: 44 (141) 946 7120. Fax: 44(141)945 2893

Dr C.R. Gillis
Mr D. Hole

Yugoslavia, Vojvodina
Cancer Registry of Vojvodina
Medical Faculty Novi Sad
Institute of Oncology
21204 Sremska Kamenica
Institutski put br. 4, Novi Sad
Yugoslavia
tel: 381 (21) 615711. Fax: 381 (21) 613741

Marica Mikov, MD, PhD
Bela Burany, MD, PhD
Nenad Vranješ, MD, MSc
Svetozar Zdravkovic, BScE

OCEANIA

Australian Capital Territory
Australian Capital Territory Cancer Registry
North Building
London Circuit, Civic, ACT, 2601
Australia
Tel: 61 (6) 2050917. Fax: 61 (6) 2050866

Dr Bruce Shadbolt
Ms Norma Briscoe
Mrs Marylon S.Coates

Australia, New South Wales
New South Wales Central Cancer Registry
LMB 1 Kings Cross
NSW 2011
Australia
Tel: 61 (2) 3341902. Fax: 61 (2) 3680843

Mrs Marylon S.Coates
Mrs Noreen Panos
Professor Richard Taylor

South Australia
South Australian Cancer Registry
Public & Environmental Health
South Australian Health Commission
P.O Box 6 Rundle Mall
Adelaide, SA. 5000
Australia
Tel: 61 (8) 2266372. Fax: 61 (8) 2266316
e-mail: laa@hc2.health.sa.gov.au

Mrs Lesley Adlam
Dr David Roder
Mr Kieren McCaul

Australia, Tasmania
Tasmanian Cancer Registry
Menzies Centre for Population Health Research
Menzies Building, 17 Liverpool Street
Hobart, 7000 Tasmania
Australia
Tel: 61 (2)-357714. Fax: 61 (2) 357704
e-mail: dace.shugg@menzies.utas.edu.au

Professor Terry Dwyer
Ms Dace Shugg

Australia, Victoria
Victorian Cancer Registry
1 Rathdowne Street
Carlton South
Victoria 3053, Australia
Tel: 61 (3) 9279 1111. Fax: 61 (3) 9279 1210
e-mail: ggg@accv.org.au

Graham Giles
Kathryn Whitfield
Vicky Thursfield

Western Australia
Western Australian Cancer Registry
Health Information Centre
1st Floor C Block
189 Royal Street, East Perth, WA 6004
Australia
Tel: 61 (9) 2224022. Fax: 61 (9) 2224236

T. J. Threlfall
J. R. Thompson
K. Garrod

French Polynesia
Registre du Cancer de Polynésie Française
(French Polynesian Cancer Registry)
Bureau d'Epidémiologie et de Statistiques Sanitaires
Direction de la Santé
BP 611, Papeete
Tahiti
French Polynesia
Tel: 689 460000. Fax: 689 430074

Dr François Laudon
Dr Laurence Gleize
Mme Laure Yen

New Zealand
New Zealand Cancer Registry
New Zealand Health Information Service
Ministry of Health
P.O. Box 5013
Wellington
New Zealand
Tel: 64 (4) 8012717. Fax: 64 (4) 8012769

James Fraser
Brenda Wordsworth

USA, Hawaii
Hawaii Tumour Registry
1236 Lauhala Street
Honolulu, HI 96813, USA
Tel: 1 (808) 5862987. Fax: 1 (808) 5862982
e-mail: htr@aloha.net

Marc T. Goodman
Laurence N. Kolonel
Marilyn C. Hurst

AFRICA

Sétif
Bamako
Kyadondo
Harare
La Réunion

ASIA

Israel
Kuwait
Tianjin
JAPAN
Kangwha
Qidong
Shanghai
Bombay
Barshi
Bangalore
Madras
Chiang Mai
Hanoi
Hong Kong
Karunagappally
Khon Kaen
Manila
Trivandrum
Singapore

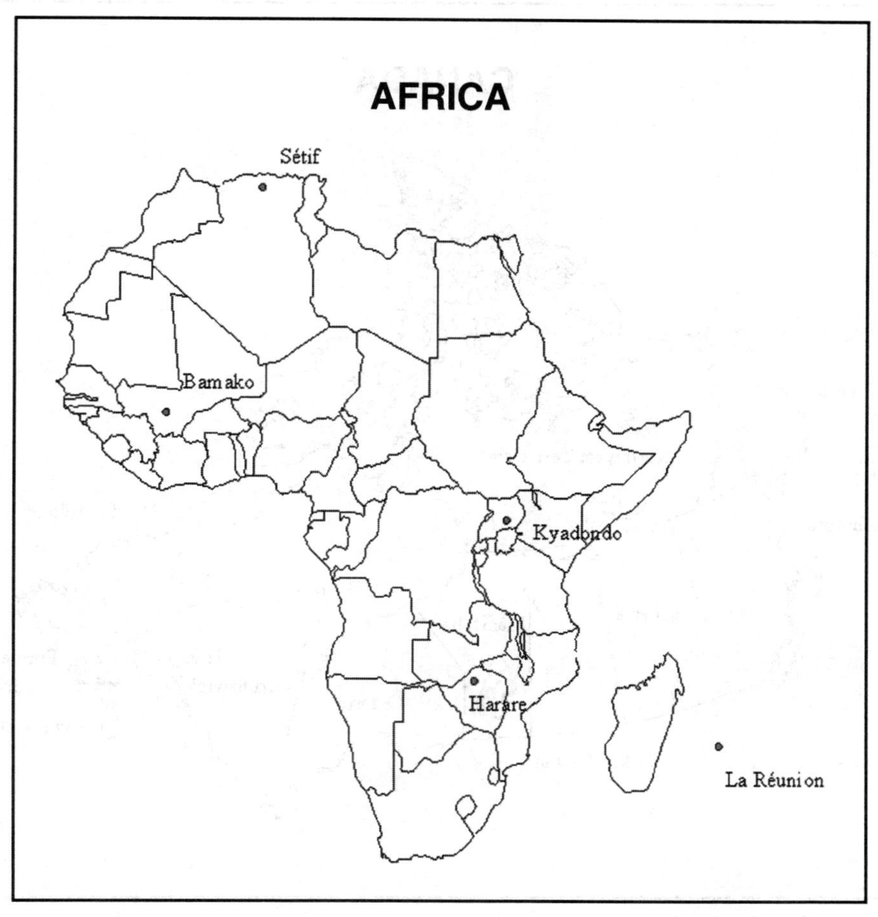

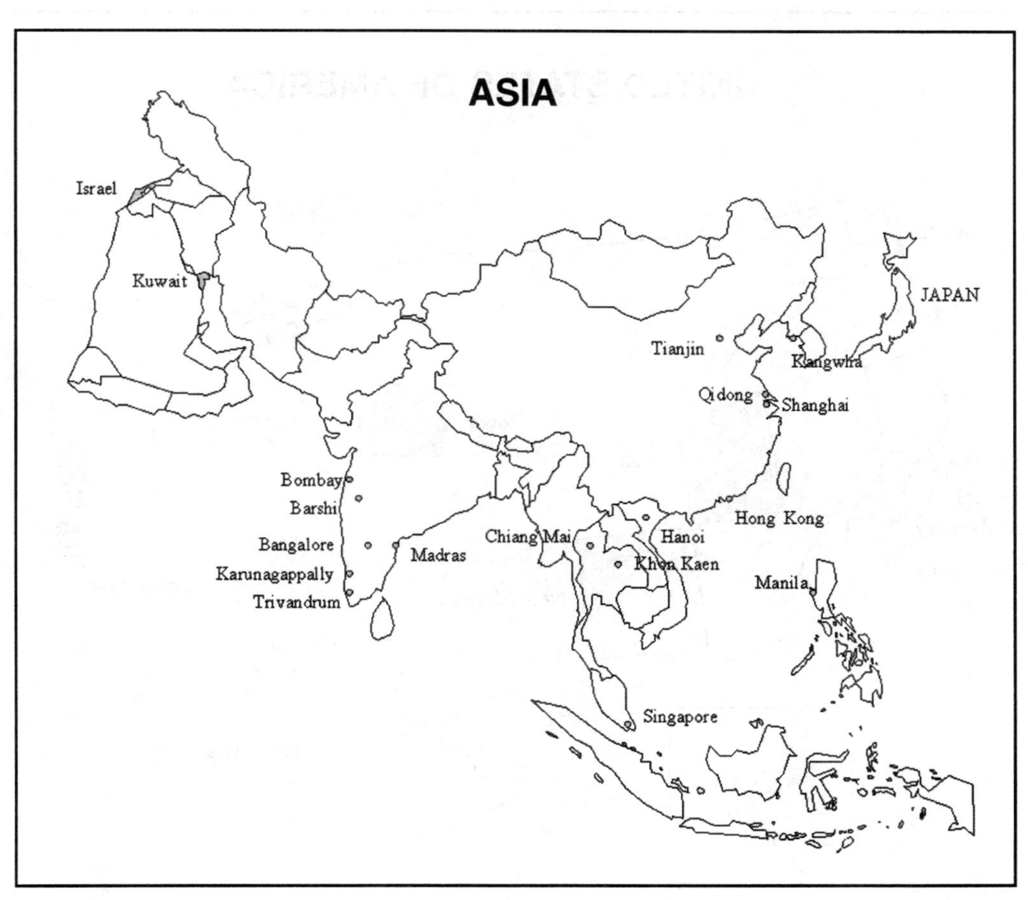

CANADA

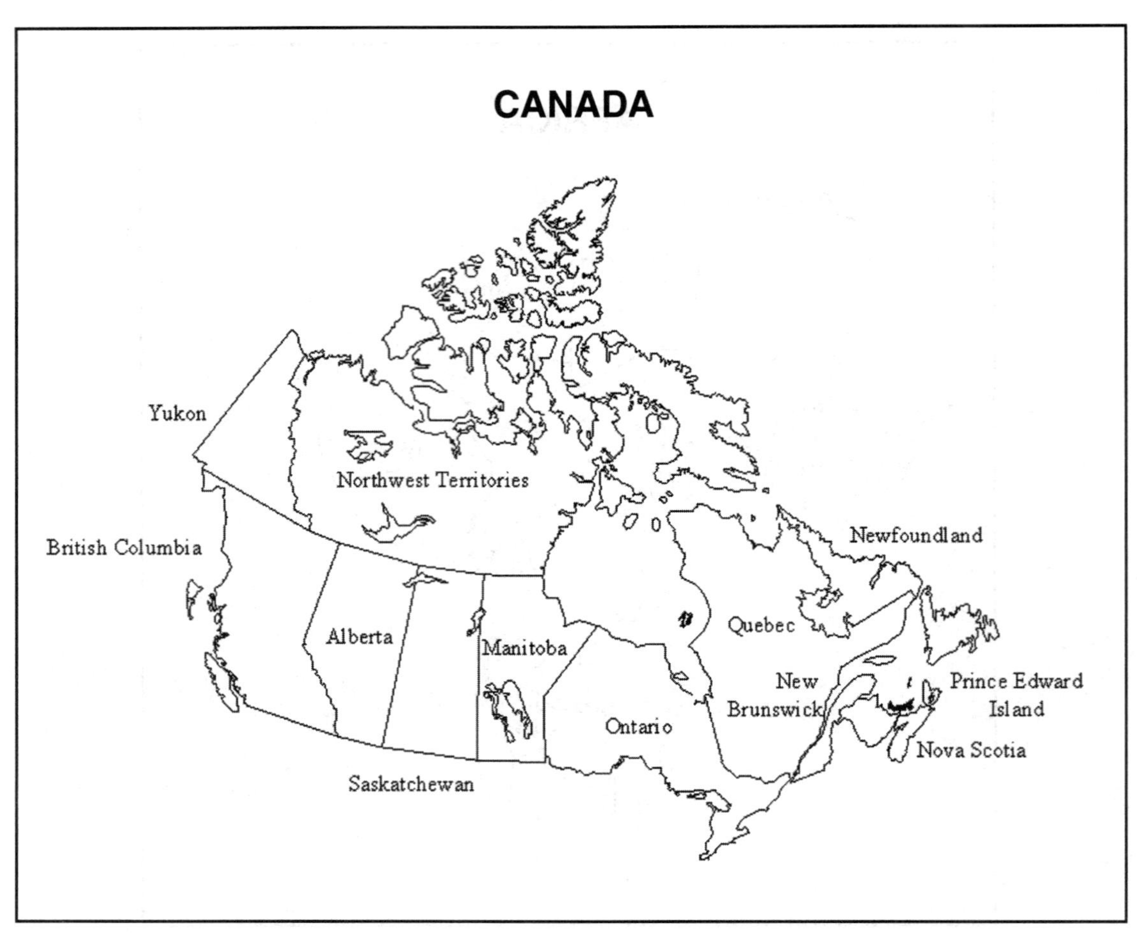

UNITED STATES OF AMERICA

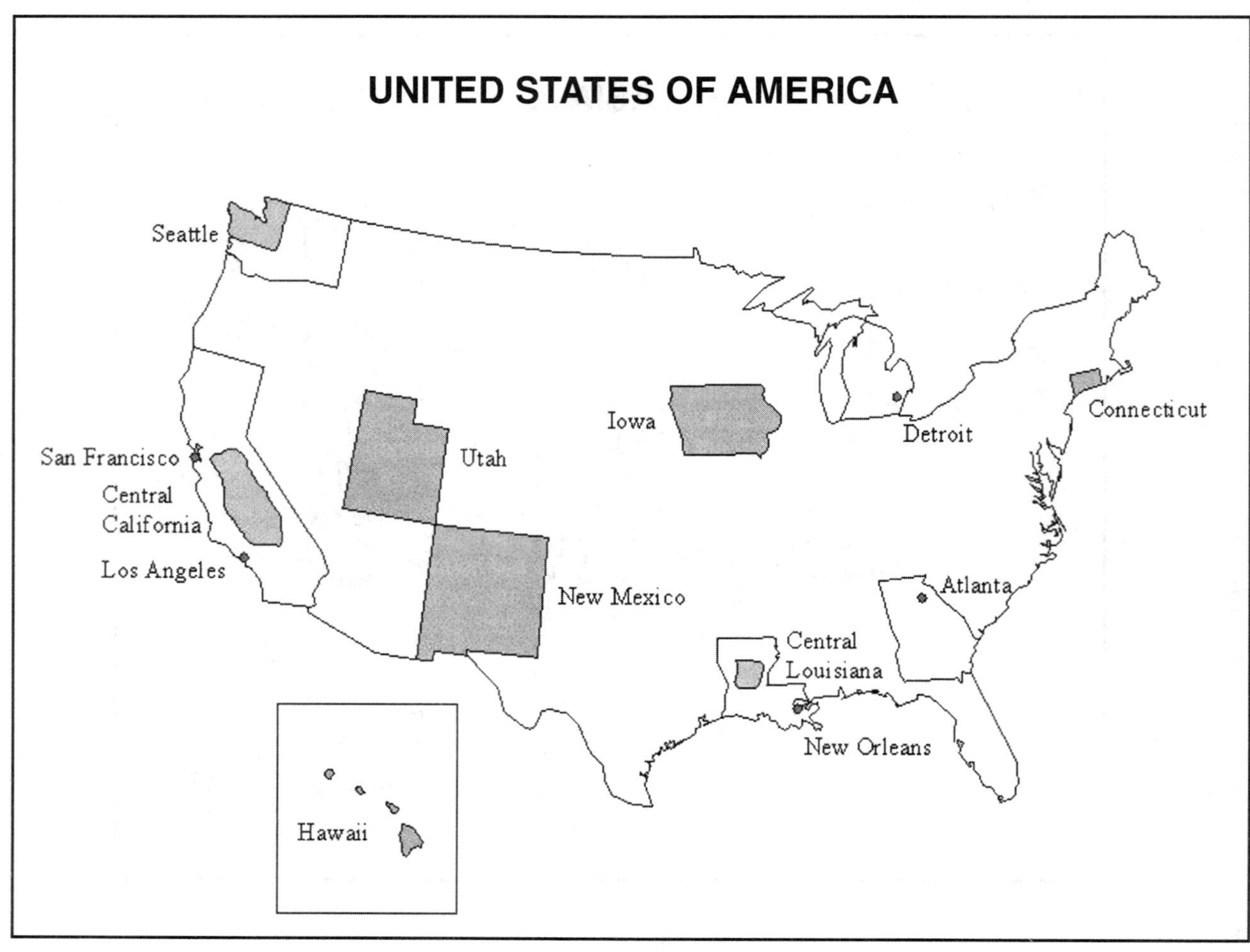

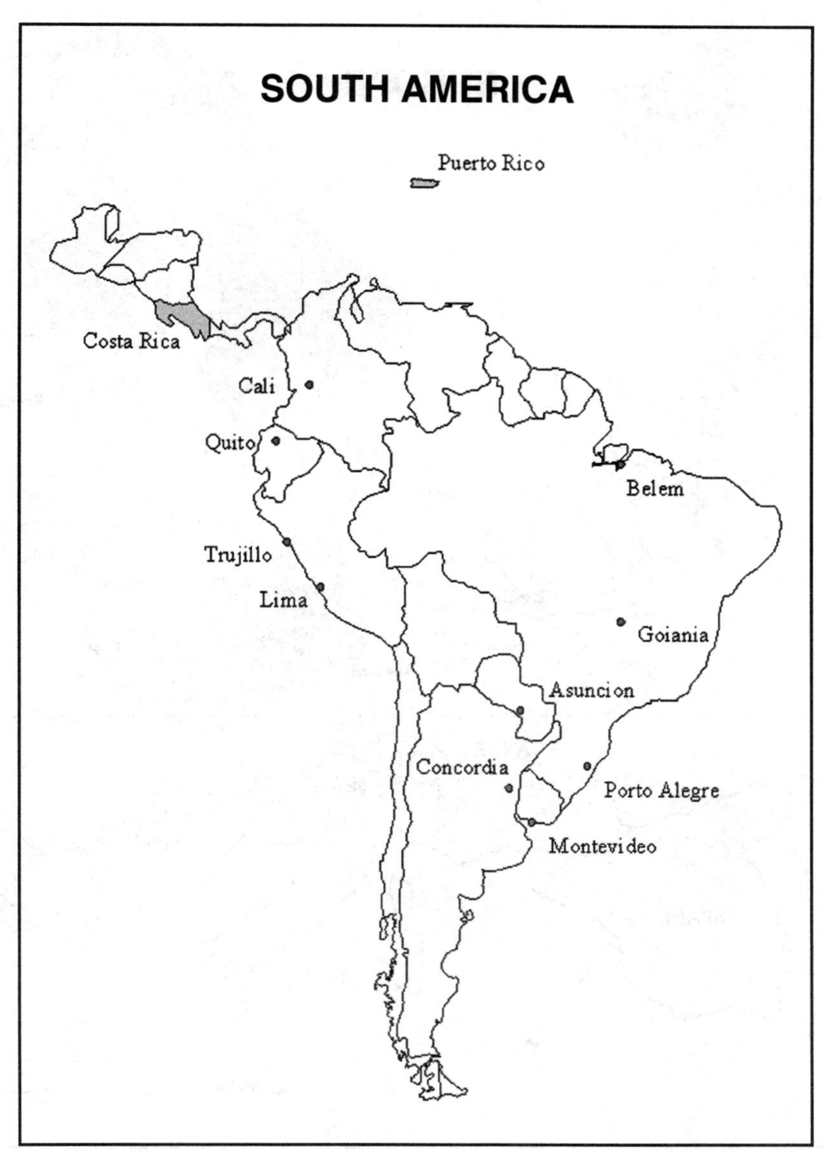

SOUTH AMERICA
Puerto Rico
Costa Rica
Cali
Quito
Belem
Trujillo
Lima
Goiania
Asuncion
Concordia
Porto Alegre
Montevideo

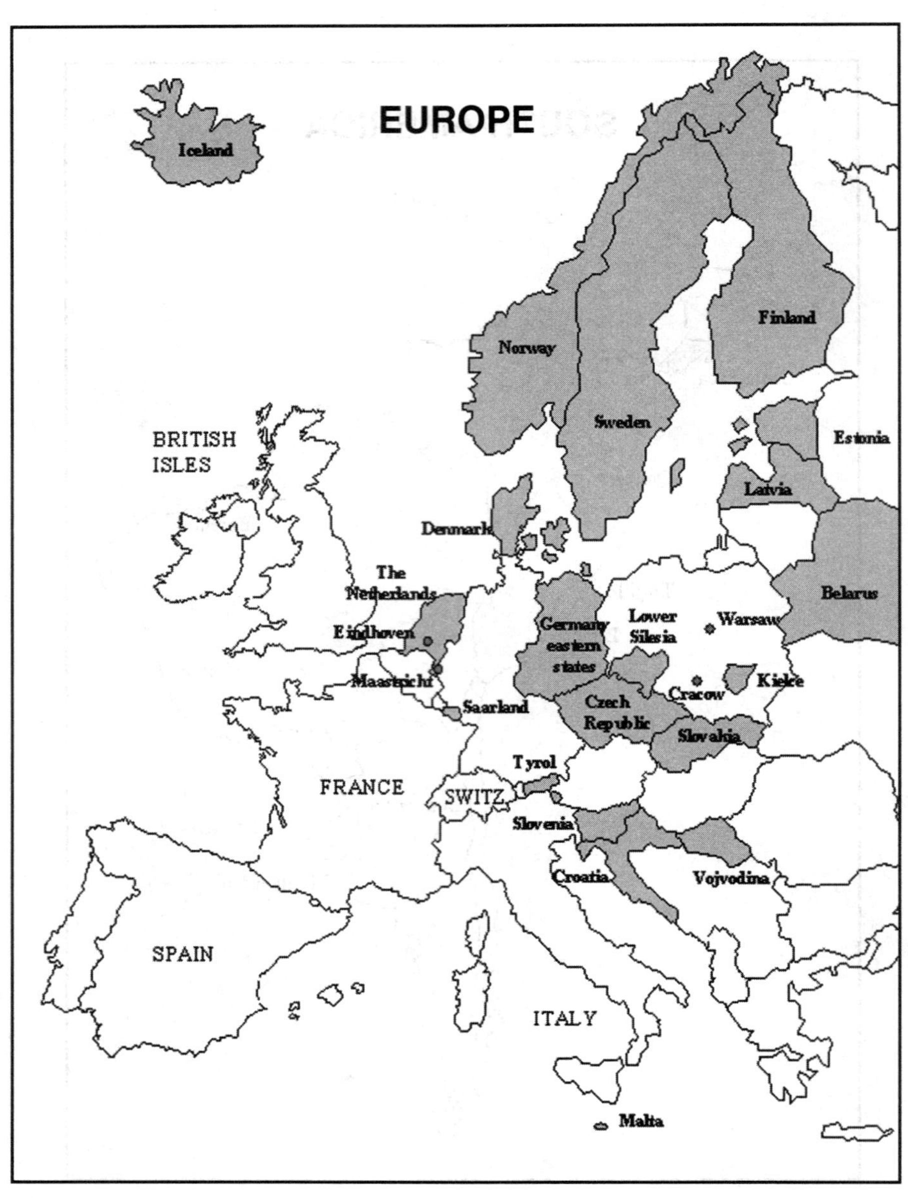

EUROPE
Iceland
Norway
Finland
Sweden
Estonia
Latvia
BRITISH
ISLES
Denmark
Belarus
The
Netherlands
Germany
eastern
states
Lower
Silesia
Warsaw
Eindhoven
Maastricht
Kielce
Saarland
Cracow
Czech
Republic
Slovakia
Tyrol
FRANCE
SWITZ.
Slovenia
Croatia
Vojvodina
SPAIN
ITALY
Malta

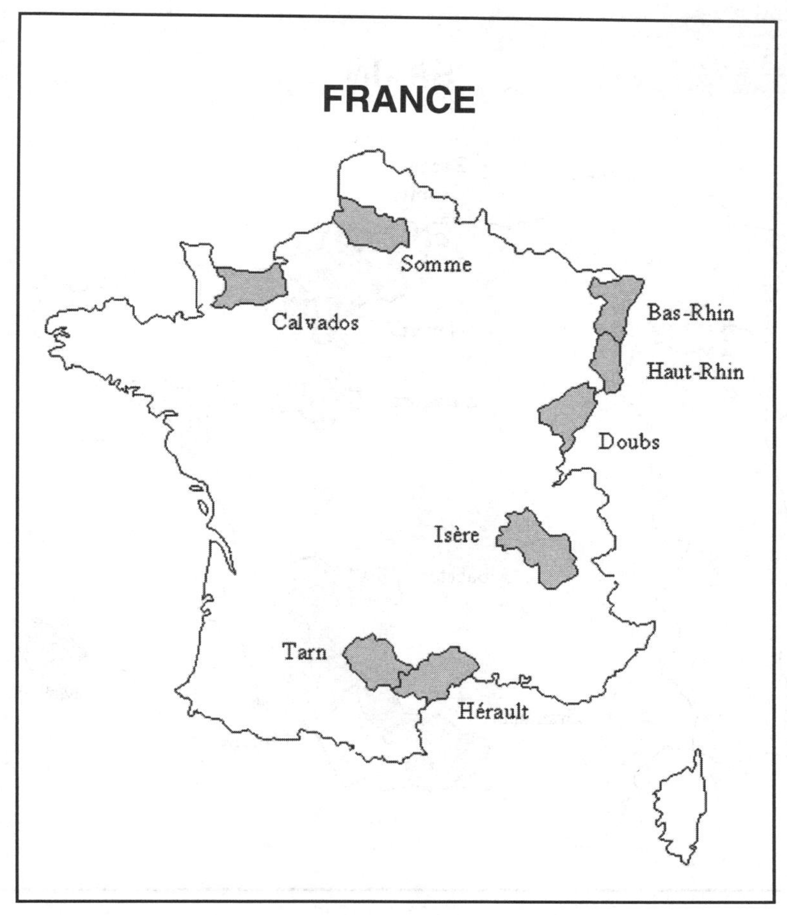

FRANCE
Somme
Calvados
Bas-Rhin
Haut-Rhin
Doubs
Isère
Tarn
Hérault

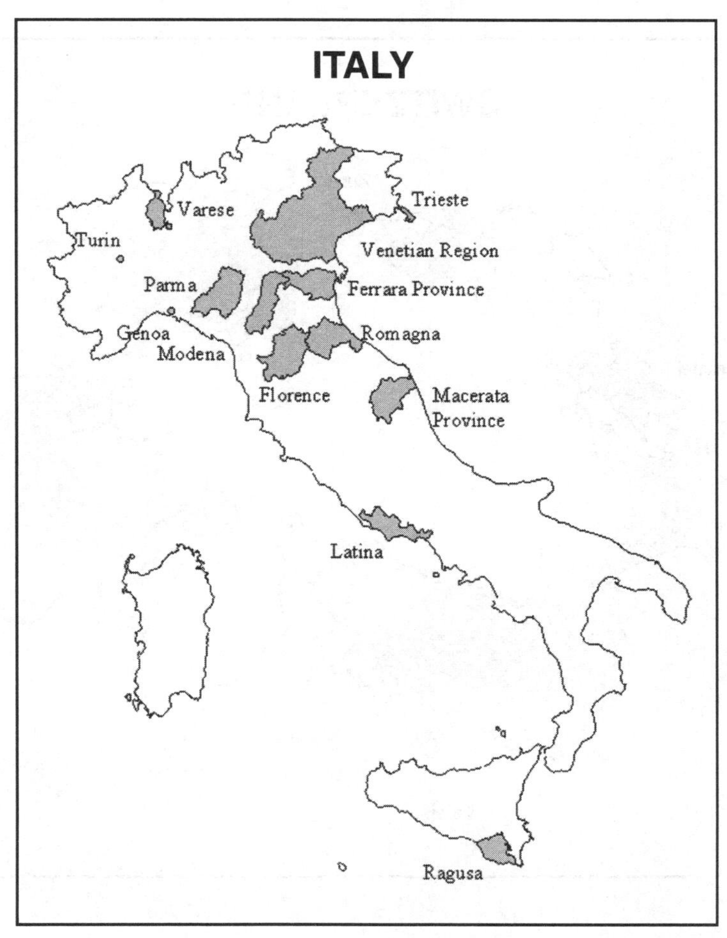

ITALY
Varese
Trieste
Turin
Venetian Region
Parma
Ferrara Province
Genoa
Romagna
Modena
Florence
Macerata
Province
Latina
Ragusa

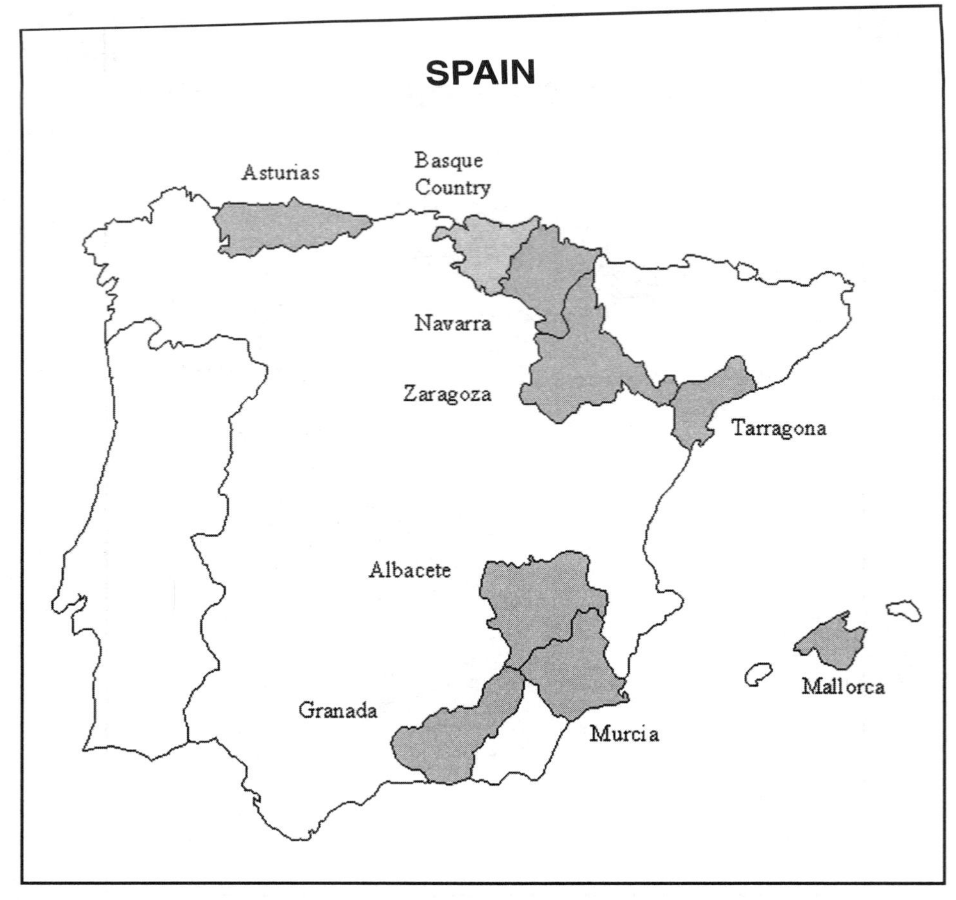

SPAIN
Asturias
Basque Country
Navarra
Zaragoza
Tarragona
Albacete
Granada
Murcia
Mallorca

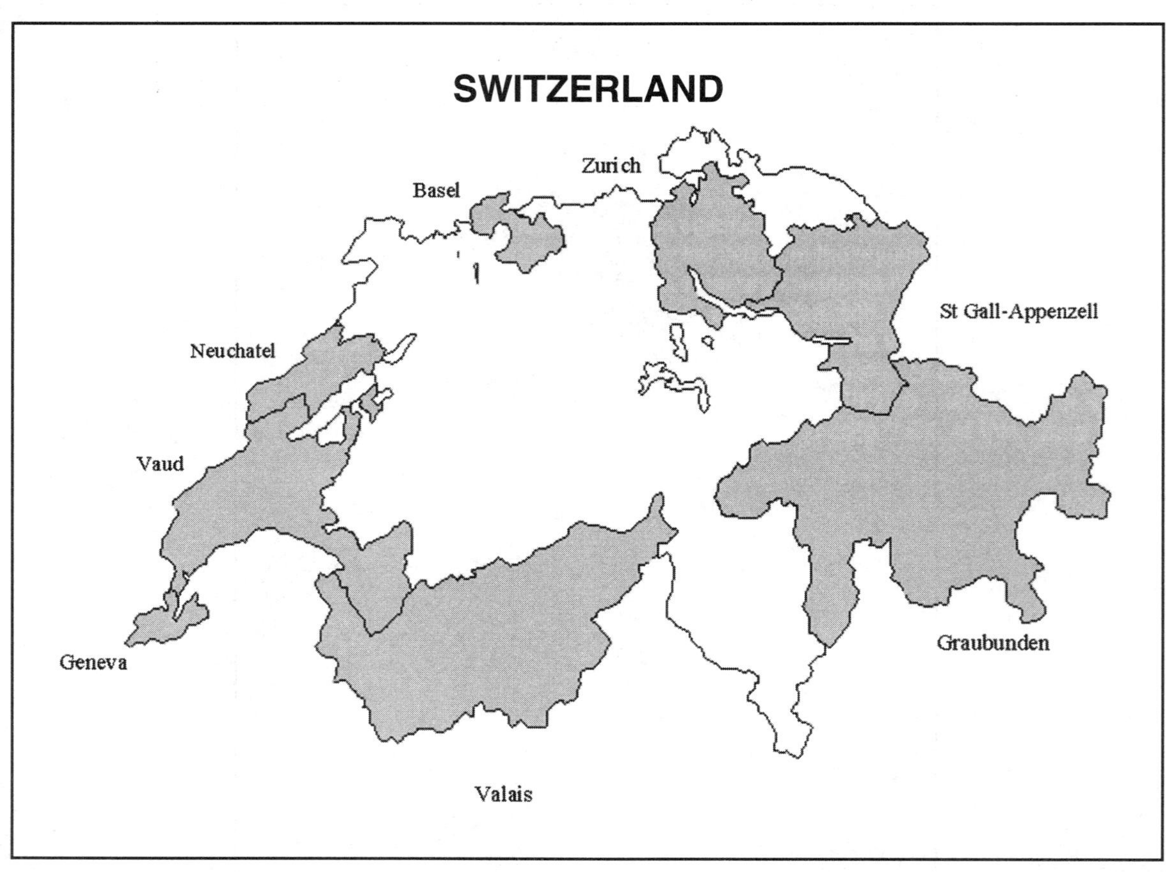

SWITZERLAND
Basel
Zurich
Neuchatel
St Gall-Appenzell
Vaud
Geneva
Graubunden
Valais

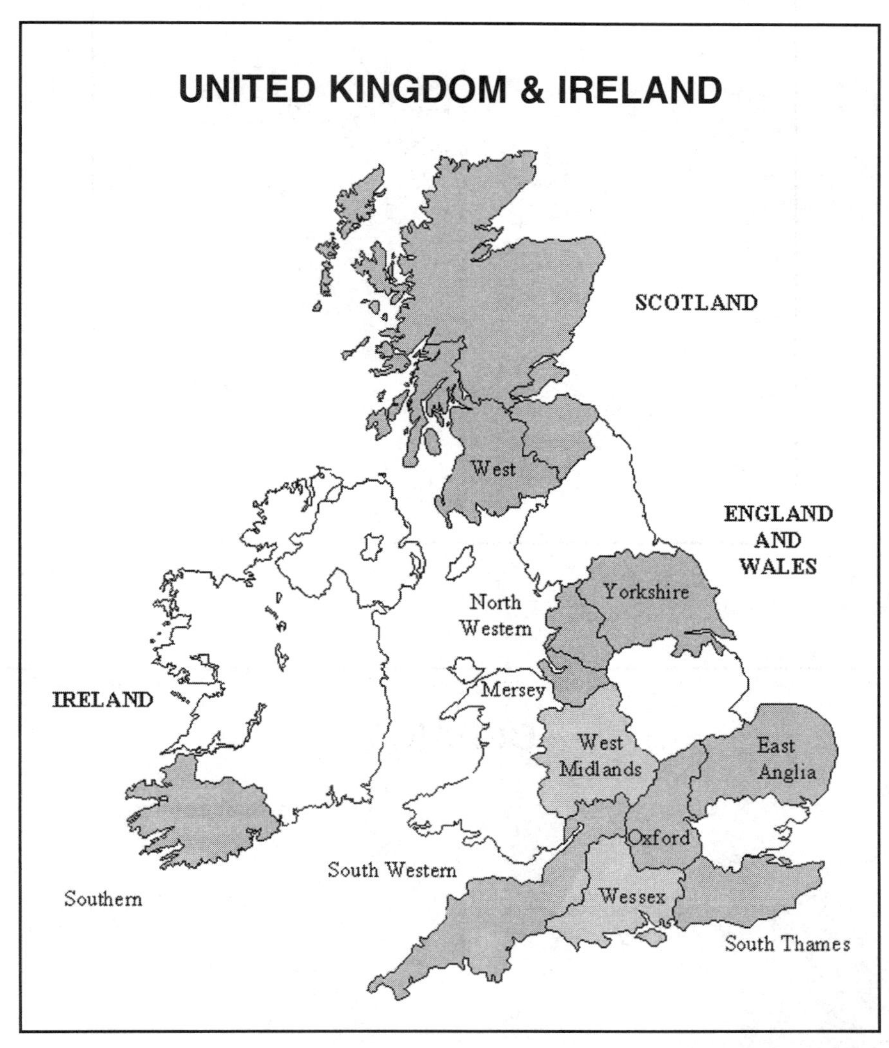

UNITED KINGDOM & IRELAND
SCOTLAND
West
ENGLAND
AND
WALES
IRELAND
North
Western
Yorkshire
Mersey
West
Midlands
East
Anglia
Oxford
South Western
Wessex
Southern
South Thames

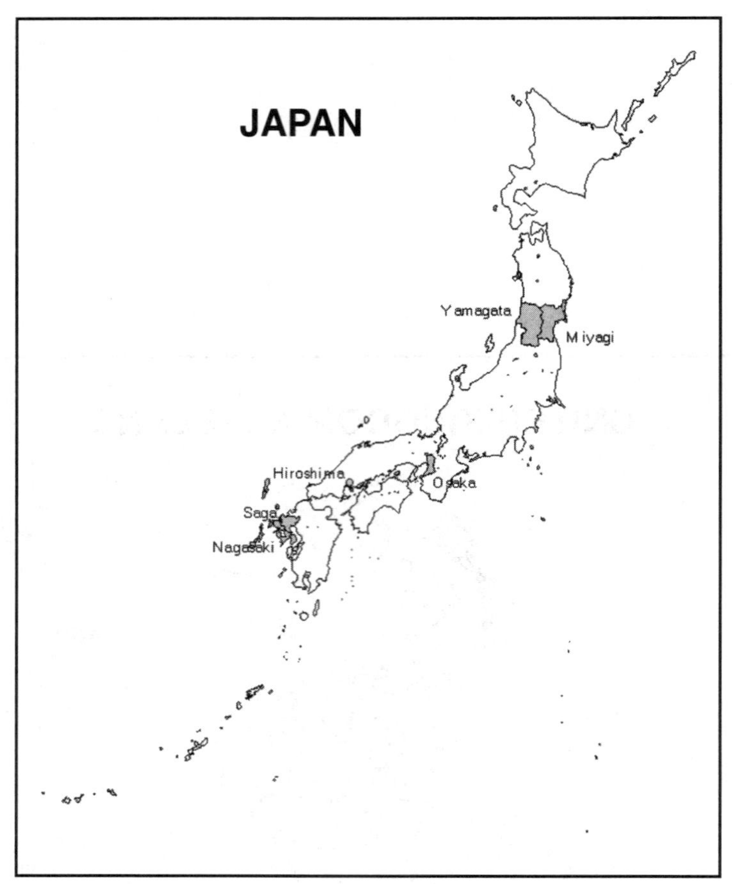

JAPAN
Yamagata
Miyagi
Hiroshima
Osaka
Saga
Nagasaki

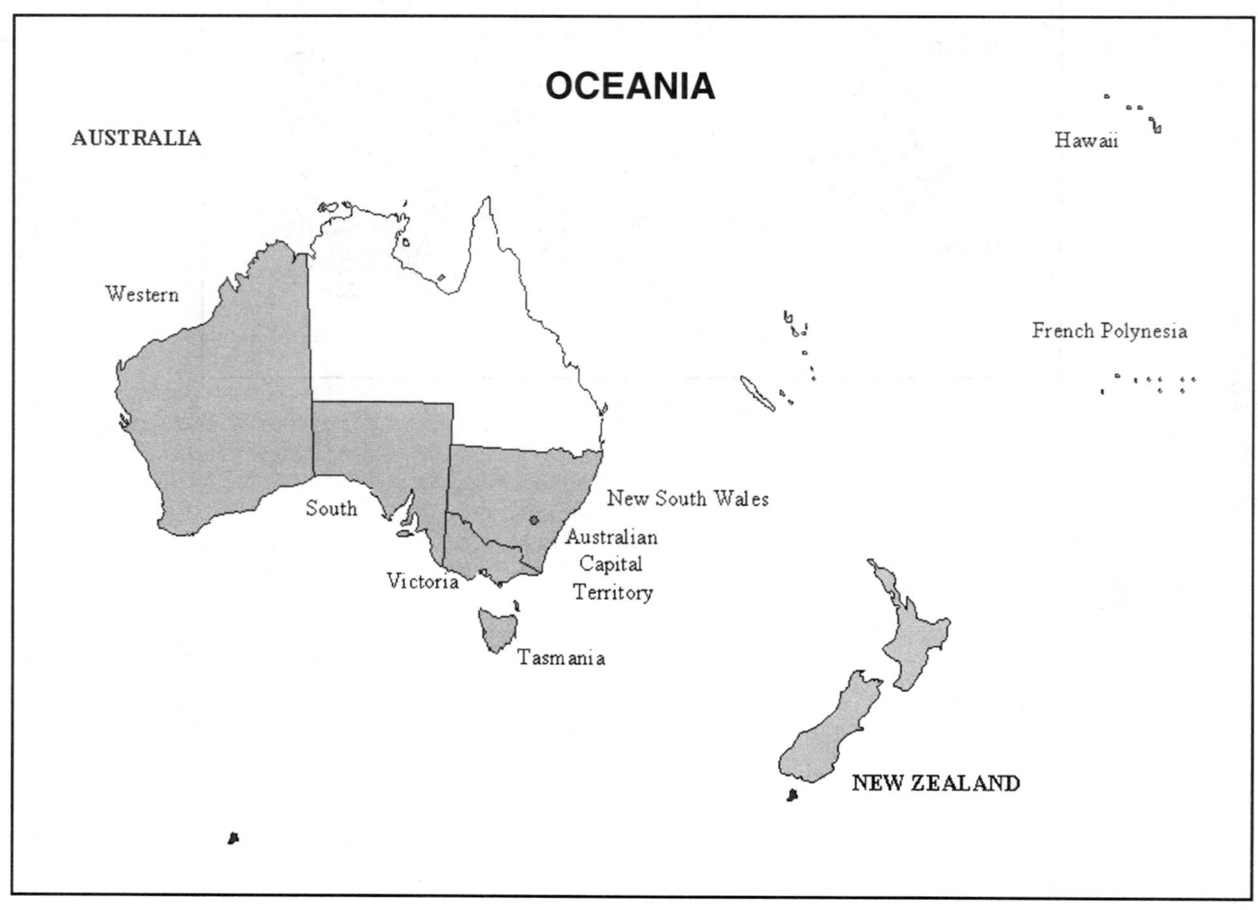

OCEANIA
AUSTRALIA
Hawaii
Western
French Polynesia
South
New South Wales
Australian
Capital
Territory
Victoria
Tasmania
NEW ZEALAND

Chapter 1. Introduction

S.L. Whelan

The objective of the 'Cancer Incidence in Five Continents' series is to provide comparable data on the incidence of cancer in different geographical locations and distinct ethnic sub-populations in these locations. Research into the causation of cancer has traditionally been based on descriptive statistics which describe the burden and patterns of the disease in diverse populations, so giving rise to hypotheses which might explain observed differences in risk.

The introduction to Volume I, published in 1966, includes the statement: 'The most valuable data are, undoubtedly, the rates obtained by recording the occurrence of every case of cancer over a specified period', a statement which has proved well founded with, more than thirty years later, recognition worldwide of the value of accurate data on cancer occurrence as derived from population-based cancer registries.

1. Geographical coverage
The last 30 years have seen a rapid growth in the development of cancer registration worldwide. In this seventh volume, data on the incidence of malignant disease are presented for 183 populations in 50 countries, and Table 1.1 below shows the scale of increase in availability of data since the publication of Volume 1. Table 1.2, Geographical coverage in the seven successive volumes of *Cancer Incidence in Five Continents*, describes precisely the populations and time periods published in each volume.

Quality of data
The steady increase in coverage of the world's population by cancer registration has been accompanied by developments in standardization of registration methodology, definitions and coding. The editors of the present volume, following the tradition laid down in the first volume, have made every effort to standardize the data presented, and where this has not been possible, to draw attention to differences which might affect comparability between registries. The task has been facilitated by computerization. Volume VII is the first in which every contributing registry has sent data in the form of a computerized case-listing, and the vast majority of these have included the coded histological diagnoses. This has enabled the editors to check the internal coherence and consistency to a greater degree than ever before. Validation procedures are described in Chapter 5, Comparability and quality, and in Chapter 6, Processing of data.

The better definition of registration methodology and increasing adherence to internationally recognized standards has also led to greater stringency in the editorial process. In the successive volumes it is clear that the editors have become more demanding about the quality of the data published in the book, and the criteria for selection of data published in the present volume, described in Chapter 5, have been more stringent than ever before. While data are published here for 150 registries covering 183 populations, data were submitted from 176 of the registries invited, covering more than 230 populations, i.e. data from 26 registries were not accepted for publication. Emphasis in the choice of registries is always on comparability and quality, not on quantity.

At the same time the editors have to accept that certain of the data sets from the developing countries are less complete than the majority from the developed countries, because of problems of under-diagnosis due to the local medical and economic background (as opposed to under-registration) and/or problems with enumeration of the population. Many such data sets have great intrinsic interest because they describe cancer incidence in populations for which little information is available, and retain unique cultural habits which might provide valuable clues to cancer etiology. An asterisk against a registry title indicates that there may be under-registration, and a note specifying the reasons for this is provided.

Table 1.1 Coverage in seven volumes of Cancer Incidence in Five Continents					
Volume	Year	Registries	Populations	Countries	Period (approx.)
I	1966	32	35	29	1960–62
II	1970	47	58	24	1963–67
III	1976	61	79	29	1968–72
IV	1982	79	103	32	1973–77
V	1987	105	137	36	1978–82
VI	1992	138	166	49	1983–87
VII	1997	150	183	50	1988–92

2. Temporal comparisons

Differences over time in completeness of coverage, registration practices and coding make it necessary to interpret trends in the data published in successive volumes of *Cancer Incidence in Five Continents* with caution. Some registries have also changed their boundaries from one volume to the next. Again, notes or the chapter texts warn the user about artefactual changes.

3. Content and layout of the book

The addresses of the contributing registries, with the names of the individuals who have collaborated in the preparation of this volume, are given in the beginning of the book. Maps showing the geographical location of each population on which data are presented are also provided. The chapter which follows this introduction, Chapter 2, describes the registries themselves, both in terms of geographical and legislative background and of registry practices.

Chapter 3 presents the system of classification used to analyse the data on incidence, and addresses the issue of comparability of coding practices within the registries. For some cancer sites, the data have been analysed by histological sub-type. Chapter 4 introduces the categorization of histology used and explains the rationale behind the groupings chosen.

The issues which can affect comparability between registries and the validity of the registry data, as well as the way in which data presented in this volume have been assessed, are discussed in Chapter 5, 'Comparability and Quality'. The following chapter, 'Processing of Data', describes the processing of the raw data received for *Cancer Incidence in Five Continents*, from validation to analysis. Chapter 7 explains the structure of the different tables of incidence in the book, and Chapter 8 introduces the summary measures of incidence used.

These chapters preface the main section of the book, the tables of cancer incidence. The bulk of these concern the age-specific and standardized incidence rates for each individual population, accompanied by a text describing the registry background, the population information and any notes on the data. The tables summarizing age-standardized rates for three-digit and four-digit rubrics and the cumulative incidence rates follow, and the third set of tables present the percentage distribution of diagnoses by histological type. The final tables give the indices of data quality, described in Chapter 5.

4. Data on diskette

Volume VI was published with two diskettes, containing the incidence data from Volumes V and VI. The data from this volume are also available on diskette, but given the amount of information now included it was decided to produce it as a separate publication, IARC CancerBase No. 2 (Ferlay, 1997).

Reference

Ferlay, J. (1997) Cancer Incidence in Five Continents VII (IARC CancerBase No. 2), Lyon, IARC

Table 1.2. Geographical coverage in the seven successive volumes of Cancer Incidence in Five Continents

	Vol. I	Vol. II	Vol. III	Vol. IV	Vol. V	Vol. VI	Vol. VII
AFRICA							
Algeria, Sétif	–	–	–	–	–	1986–89	1990–93
France, La Réunion	–	–	–	–	–	–	1988–92
The Gambia	–	–	–	–	–	1987–89	–
Mali, Bamako	–	–	–	–	–	1987–89	1988–92
Mozambique,							
Lourenço Marques	1956–60	–	–	–	–	–	–
Nigeria, Ibadan	1960–62	1960–65	1960–69	–	–	–	–
Rhodesia,							
Bulawayo: African	–	1963–67	1968–72	–	–	–	–
Senegal, Dakar	–	–	–	1969–74	–	–	–
South Africa,							
Cape Province:							
White	–	1956–59	–	–	–	–	–
Coloured	–	1956–59	–	–	–	–	–
Bantu	–	1956–59	–	–	–	–	–
South Africa,							
Johannesburg:							
Bantu	1953–55	–	–	–	–	–	–
Natal:							
African	–	1964–66	–	–	–	–	–
Indian	–	1964–66	–	–	–	–	–
Uganda,							
Kyadondo County	1954–60	–	–	–	–	–	1991–93
Zimbabwe, Harare:							
African	–	–	–	–	–	–	1990–92
European	–	–	–	–	–	–	1990–92
CENTRAL AND SOUTH AMERICA							
Argentina, Concordia	–	–	–	–	–	–	1990–94
Brazil, Belém	–	–	–	–	–	–	1989–91
Brazil, Fortaleza	–	–	–	–	1978–82	–	–
Brazil, Goiania	–	–	–	–	–	1988–89	1990–93
Brazil, Porto Alegre	–	–	–	–	1979–82	1987	1990–92
Brazil, Pernambuco, Recife	–	–	1968–71	–	1980	–	–
Brazil, Sao Paulo	–	–	1969	1973	1978	–	–
Chile	1959–61	–	–	–	–	–	–
Colombia, Cali	1962–64	1962–66	1967–71	1972–76	1977–81	1982–86	1987–91
Costa Rica	–	–	–	–	1980–82	1984–87	1988–92
Cuba	–	–	1968–72	1973–77	–	1986	–
Ecuador, Quito	–	–	–	–	–	1985–87	1988–92
Martinique	–	–	–	–	1981–82	1983–87	–
Jamaica,							
Kingston & St Andrews	1958–63	1964–66	1967–72	1973–77	–	–	–
Netherlands Antilles							
(less Aruba)	–	–	–	1973–78	1978–82	–	–
Paraguay, Asuncion	–	–	–	–	–	1988–89	–
Peru, Lima	–	–	–	–	–	–	1990–91
Peru, Trujillo	–	–	–	–	–	1984–87	1988–90
USA, Puerto Rico	1962–63	1964–66	1968–72	1973–77	1978–82	1983–87	1988–91
Uruguay, Montevideo	–	–	–	–	–	–	1990–92

Table 1.2. (Contd). Geographical coverage in the seven successive volumes of Cancer Incidence in Five Continents

	Vol. I	Vol. II	Vol. III	Vol. IV	Vol. V	Vol. VI	Vol. VII
NORTH AMERICA							
Bermuda:							
Black	–	–	–	–	–	1983–87	–
White & Other	–	–	–	–	–	1983–87	–
Canada	–	–	–	–	1978–82	1983–87	1988–92
Canada, Alberta	1960–62	1963–66	1969–72	1973–77	1978–82	1983–87	1988–92
Canada, British Columbia	–	–	1969–72	1973–77	1978–82	1983–87	1988–92
Canada, Manitoba	1960–62	1963–66	1969–72	1973–77	1978–82	1983–87	1988–92
Canada, Maritime Provinces (New Brunswick, Nova Scotia, Prince Edward Island)	–	–	1969–72	1973–77	1978–82	1983–87	–
Canada, New Brunswick	1962–64	1965–66	–	–	1978–82	1983–86	1988–92
Canada, Newfoundland	1960–62	1963–66	1969–72	1973–77	1978–82	1983–87	1988–92
Canada, Northwest Territories & Yukon	–	–	–	1973–77	1978–82	1983–87	–
Canada, Northwest Territories	–	–	–	–	–	–	1983–92
Canada, Nova Scotia	–	–	–	–	1978–82	1983–87	1988–92
Canada, Ontario	–	–	–	1969–71	1978–82	1983–87	1988–92
Canada, Prince Edward Island	–	–	–	–	1978–82	1983–87	1988–92
Canada, Quebec	–	1963–66	1969–72	1973–77	1978–81	1983–87	1988–92
Canada, Saskatchewan	1960–62	1963–66	1969–72	1973–77	1978–82	1983–87	1988–92
Canada, Yukon	–	–	–	–	–	–	1983–92
USA, California, Alameda County:							
White	–	1960–64	1969–73	1973–77	1978–82	1983–87	–
Black	–	1960–64	1969–73	1973–77	1978–82	1983–87	–
USA, California, Central Valley:							
Non-Hispanic White	–	–	–	–	–	–	1988–92
Hispanic	–	–	–	–	–	–	1988–92
USA, California, Los Angeles County:							
Non-Hispanic White	–	–	–	–	–	–	1988–92
Hispanic White	–	–	–	–	–	–	1988–92
Other White	–	–	–	1972–77	1978–82	1983–87	–
Spanish-surnamed White	–	–	–	1972–77	1978–82	1983–87	–
Black	–	–	–	1972–77	1978–82	1983–87	1988–92
Japanese	–	–	–	1972–77	1978–82	1983–87	1988–92
Chinese	–	–	–	1972–77	1978–82	1983–87	1988–92
Filipino	–	–	–	–	1978–82	1983–87	1988–92
Korean	–	–	–	–	1978–82	1983–87	1988–92
USA, California, San Francisco Bay Area:							
Non-Hispanic White	–	–	–	–	–	–	1988–92
Hispanic White	–	–	–	–	–	–	1988–92
White	–	–	1969–73	1973–77	1978–82	1983–87	–
Black	–	–	1969–73	1973–77	1978–82	1983–87	1988–92
Chinese	–	–	1969–73	1973–77	1978–82	–	1988–92
	Vol. I	Vol. II	Vol. III	Vol. IV	Vol. V	Vol. VI	Vol. VII

Table 1.2. (Contd). Geographical coverage in the seven successive volumes of Cancer Incidence in Five Continents

	Vol. I	Vol. II	Vol. III	Vol. IV	Vol. V	Vol. VI	Vol. VII
Japanese	–	–	–	1973–77	1978–82	–	1988–92
Filipino	–	–	–	–	1978–82	–	1988–92
1960–62	1963–65	1968–72	1973–77	–	–	1988–92	
White	–	–	–	–	1978–82	1983–87	1988–92
USA, Connecticut:							
Black	–	–	–	–	1978–82	1983–87	1988–92
USA, Georgia, Atlanta:							
White	–	–	–	1975–77	1978–82	1983–87	1988–92
Black	–	–	–	1975–77	1978–82	1983–87	1988–92
USA, Iowa	–	–	1969–71	1973–77	1978–82	1983–87	1988–92
USA, Louisiana, Central Region:							
White	–	–	–	–	–	–	1988–92
Black	–	–	–	–	–	–	1988–92
USA, Louisiana, New Orleans:							
White	–	–	–	1974–77	1978–82	1983–87	1988–92
Black	–	–	–	1974–77	1978–82	1983–87	1988–92
USA, Michigan, Detroit:							
White	–	–	1969–71	1973–77	1978–82	1983–87	1988–92
Black	–	–	1969–71	1973–77	1978–82	1983–87	1988–92
USA, Nevada	–	1959–66	–	–	–	–	–
USA, New Mexico:	–	–	–	–	–	1983–87	–
Non-Hispanic White	–	–	–	–	–	–	1988–92
Hispanic White	–	–	–	–	–	–	1988–92
Hispanic	–	–	1969–72	1973–77	1978–82	–	–
Other White (Anglo)			1969–72	1973–77	1978–82	–	–
American Indian	–	–	1969–72	1973–77	1978–82	–	1988–92
USA, New York City	–	–	–	–	1978–82	1983–87	–
USA, New York State (less New York City)	1959–61	–	1969–71	1973–77	1978–82	1983–87	–
USA, Texas, El Paso:							
Latin	–	1960–66	1968–70	–	–	–	–
Other than Latin	–	1960–66	1968–70	–	–	–	–
USA, Utah	–	–	1966–70	1973–77	1978–82	1983–87	1988–92
USA, Washington, Seattle	–	–	–	1974–77	1978–82	1983–87	1988–92
USA, SEER:							
White	–	–	–	–	–	1983–87	1988–92
Black	–	–	–	–	–	1983–87	1988–92
ASIA							
China, Qidong County	–	–	–	–	–	1983–87	1988–92
China, Shanghai	–	–	–	1975	1978–82	1983–87	1988–92
China, Tianjin	–	–	–	–	1981–82	1983–87	1988–92
Hong Kong	–	–	–	1974–77	1978–82	1983–87	1988–92
India, Ahmedabad	–	–	–	–	–	1983–87	–
India, Bangalore	–	–	–	–	1982	1983–87	1988–92
India, Barshi, Paranda and Bhum	–	–	–	–	–	–	1988–92
India, Bombay	–	1964–66	1968–72	1973–75	1978–82	1983–87	1988–92
India, Karunagappally	–	–	–	–	–	–	1991–92
India, Madras	–	–	–	–	1982	1983–87	1988–92
India, Nagpur	–	–	–	–	1980–82	–	–
India, Poona	–	–	–	1973–77	1978–82	–	–

Table 1.2. (Contd). Geographical coverage in the seven successive volumes of Cancer Incidence in Five Continents

	Vol. I	Vol. II	Vol. III	Vol. IV	Vol. V	Vol. VI	Vol. VII
India, Trivandrum	–	–	–	–	–	–	1991–92
Israel:	1960–63	–	–	–	–	–	–
All Jews	–	1960–66	1967–71	1972–76	1977–81	1982–86	1988–92
Jews born in Israel	–	1960–66	1967–71	1972–76	1977–81	1982–86	1988–92
Israel:							
Jews born in Africa							
or Asia	–	1960–66	1967–71	1972–76	1977–81	1982–86	1988–92
Jews born in							
Europe or America	–	1960–66	1967–71	1972–76	1977–81	1982–86	1988–92
Non-Jews	–	1960–66	1967–71	1972–76	1977–81	1982–86	1988–92
Japan, Fukuoka	–	–	–	1974–75	–	–	–
Japan, Hiroshima	–	–	–	–	1978–80	1981–85	1986–90
Japan, Miyagi	1959–60	1962–64	1968–71	1973–77	1978–81	1983–87	1988–92
Japan, Nagasaki	–	–	–	1973–77	1978–82	1983–87	1988–92
Japan, Okayama	–	1966	1969	–	–	–	–
Japan, Osaka	–	–	1970–71	1973–77	1979–82	1983–87	1988–92
Japan, Saga	–	–	–	–	–	1984–86	1988–92
Japan, Yamagata	–	–	–	–	–	1983–86	1988–92
Korea, Kangwha County	–	–	–	–	–	–	1986–92
Kuwait:Non-Kuwaitis	–	–	–	–	1979–82	1983–87	1988–89
							1992–93
Kuwaitis	–	–	–	–	1979–82	1983–87	1988–89
							1992–93
Kyrgyzstan	–	–	–	–	–	1986–87	–
Philippines, Manila	–	–	–	–	–	1983–87	1988–92
Philippines, Rizal	–	–	–	–	1978–82	1983–87	–
Singapore:							
Chinese	1950–61	–	1968–72	1973–77	1978–82	1983–87	1988–92
Malay	–	–	1968–72	1973–77	1978–82	1983–87	1988–92
Indian	–	–	1968–72	1973–77	1978–82	1983–87	1988–92
Thailand, Chiang Mai	–	–	–	–	–	1983–87	1988–92
Thailand, Khon Kaen	–	–	–	–	–	1988–89	1990–93
Viet Nam, Hanoi	–	–	–	–	–	–	1991–93
EUROPE							
Austria, Tyrol	–	–	–	–	–	–	1988–92
Belarus	–	–	–	–	–	1983–87	1988–92
Croatia	–	–	–	–	–	–	1988–91
Czech Republic	–	–	–	–	–	1983–87	1988–92
Denmark	1953–57	1958–62	1963–67	1968–72	1978–82	1983–87	1988–92
				1973–76			
Estonia	–	–	–	–	–	1983–87	1988–92
Finland	1959–61	1962–65	1966–70	1971–76	1977–81	1982–86	1987–92
France, Bas-Rhin	–	–	–	1975–77	1978–81	1983–87	1988–92
France, Calvados	–	–	–	–	1978–82	1983–87	1988–92
France, Doubs	–	–	–	1977	1978–82	1983–87	1988–92
France, Haut-Rhin	–	–	–	–	–	–	1988–92
France, Hérault	–	–	–	–	–	–	1988–92
France, Isère	–	–	–	–	1979–82	1983–87	1988–92
France, Somme	–	–	–	–	–	1983–84	1988–92
France, Tarn	–	–	–	–	–	1983–87	1988–92
Germany, Eastern States							
(ex-GDR)	–	1964–66	1968–72	1973–77	1978–82	1983–87	1988–89
Germany, Hamburg	1960–62	1963–66	1969–72	1973–77	1978–79	–	–
Germany, Saarland	–	–	1968–72	1973–77	1978–82	1983–87	1988–92

Table 1.2. (Contd). Geographical coverage in the seven successive volumes of Cancer Incidence in Five Continents

	Vol. I	Vol. II	Vol. III	Vol. IV	Vol. V	Vol. VI	Vol. VII
Hungary, County Szabolcs-Szatmar	–	1962–66	1969–71	1973–77	1978–82	1983–87	–
Hungary, County Vas	–	1962–66	1968–72	1973–77	1978–82	1983–87	–
Hungary, Miskolc	–	1962–66	–	–	–	–	–
Iceland	1955–63	–	1964–72	–	1973–82	1983–87	1988–92
Ireland, Southern	–	–	–	–	1980–82	1983–86	1988–92
Italy, Ferrara Province	–	–	–	–	–	–	1991–92
Italy, Florence	–	–	–	–	–	1985–87	1988–91
Italy, Genoa	–	–	–	–	–	1986–87	1988–92
Italy, Latina	–	–	–	–	–	1983–85	1988–91
Italy, Macerata Province	–	–	–	–	–	–	1991–92
Italy, Modena	–	–	–	–	–	–	1988–92
Italy, Parma Province	–	–	–	–	1978–82	1983–87	1988–92
Italy, Ragusa	–	–	–	–	–	1986–87	1988–92
Italy, Romagna	–	–	–	–	–	1985–87	1989–92
Italy, Torino	–	–	–	–	–	1984–85	1988–91
Italy, Trieste	–	–	–	–	–	1983–87	1989–92
Italy, Varese Province	–	–	–	1976–77	1978–81	1983–87	1988–92
Italy, Venetian Region	–	–	–	–	–	–	1988–92
Latvia	–	–	–	–	–	1983–87	1988–92
Malta	–	–	1969–72	–	–	–	1992–93
Netherlands	–	–	–	–	–	–	1989–92
Netherlands, Three Provinces	1960–62	–	–	–	–	–	–
Netherlands, Eindhoven	–	–	–	–	1978–82	1983–87	1988–92
Netherlands, Maastricht	–	–	–	–	–	1986–88	1988–92
Norway	1959–61	1964–66	1968–72	1973–77	1978–82	1983–87	1988–92
Poland, Cieszyn Area	–	–	1968–72	1973–77	–	–	–
Poland, Cracow	–	1965–66	1968–72	1973–77	1978–81	1983–86	1988–92
Poland, Katowice District	–	1965–66	1970–72	1973–74	–	–	–
Poland, Kielce	–	–	–	–	–	–	1988–92
Poland, Lower Silesia	–	–	–	–	–	1984–87	1988–92
Poland, Nowy Sacz	–	–	1968–72	1973–77	1978–81	1983–86	–
Poland, Opole	–	–	–	–	–	1985–87	–
Poland, Warsaw City	–	1965–66	1968–72	1973–77	1980–82	1983–87	1989–92
Poland, Warsaw Rural Areas	–	1965–66	1968–72	1973–77	–	1983–87	–
Portugal, Vila Nova de Gaia	–	–	–	–	–	1983–87	–
Romania, Banat Region	–	1967	–	–	–	–	–
Romania, County Cluj	–	–	–	1974–78	1979–82	1983–87	–
Romania, County Timis	–	–	1970–72	–	–	–	–
Russian Federation, St Petersburg	–	–	–	–	–	1983–87	–
Slovakia	–	–	–	–	1978–82	1983–87	1988–92
Slovakia, Western	–	–	–	1973–77	–	–	–
Slovenia	1956–60	1961–65	1968–72	1973–76	1978–81	1982–87	1988–92
Spain, Albacete	–	–	–	–	–	–	1991–92
Spain, Asturias	–	–	–	–	–	–	1988–91
Spain, Basque Country	–	–	–	–	–	1986–87	1988–91
Spain, Granada	–	–	–	–	–	1985–87	1988–92
Spain, Mallorca	–	–	–	–	–	–	1988–92
Spain, Murcia	–	–	–	–	–	1984–87	1988–92
Spain, Navarra	–	–	–	1973–77	1978–82	1983–86	1987–91
Spain, Tarragona	–	–	–	–	1980–83	1984–87	1988–92
Spain, Zaragoza	–	–	1968–72	1973–77	1978–82	1983–85	1986–90

Table 1.2. (Contd). Geographical coverage in the seven successive volumes of Cancer Incidence in Five Continents

	Vol. I	Vol. II	Vol. III	Vol. IV	Vol. V	Vol. VI	Vol. VII
Sweden	1959–61	1962–65	1966–70	1971–75	1978–82	1983–87	1988–92
Switzerland, Basel	–	–	–	–	1981–82	1983–87	1988–92
Switzerland, Geneva	–	–	1970–72	1973–77	1979–82	1983–87	1988–92
Switzerland, Graubünden	–	–	–	–	–	–	1989–92
Switzerland, Neuchâtel	–	–	–	1974–76	1978–82	1983–87	1988–92
Switzerland, St Gall–Appenzell	–	–	–	–	–	1983–87	1988–92
Switzerland, Valais	–	–	–	–	–	–	1989–92
Switzerland, Vaud	–	–	–	1975–77	1978–82	1983–87	1988–92
Switzerland, Zürich	–	–	–	–	1980–82	1983–87	1988–92
UK, England & Wales	–	–	–	–	1979–82	1983–86	1988–90
UK, England, East Anglia	–	–	–	–	–	–	1988–92
UK, England, Merseyside and Cheshire	1959–63	1963–66	1968–72	1975–77	1978–82	1983–87	1988–92
UK, England, North Western	–	–	–	1973–77	1979–82	1983–87	1988–92
UK, England, Oxford Region	–	1963–66	1968–72	1974–77	1979–82	1983–87	1988–92
UK, England, South Thames (South Metropolitan)	1960–62	–	1963–66	1973–77 + 1967–71	1978–82	1983–87	1988–92
UK, England, South Western	1960–62	1962–65	1966–70	–	1979–82	1983–87	1988–92
UK, England, Trent	–	1963–66	1967–70	1974–76	1979–82	1983–87	–
UK, England, Wessex	–	–	–	–	–	–	1988–92
UK, England, West Midlands (Birmingham)	1960–62	1963–66	1968–72	1973–76	1979–82	1983–86	1988–92
UK, England, Yorkshire	–	–	–	–	–	1983–87	1988–92
UK, Scotland	–	1963–66	–	–	1978–82	1983–87	1988–92
UK, Scotland, Ayrshire	–	–	1970–72	–	–	–	–
UK, Scotland, East	–	–	–	1973–77	1978–82	1983–87	–
UK, Scotland, North	–	–	–	1973–77	1978–82	1983–87	–
UK, Scotland, North-East	–	–	–	1973–77	1978–82	1983–87	–
UK, Scotland, South-East	–	–	–	1973–77	1978–82	1983–87	–
UK, Scotland, West	–	–	–	1975–77	1978–82	1983–87	1988–92
Yugoslavia, Vojvodina	–	–	–	–	–	–	1988–92
OCEANIA							
Australian Capital Territory	–	–	–	–	1978–82	1983–87	1988–92
Australia, New South Wales	–	–	–	1973–77	1978–82	1983–87	1988–92
Australia, Queensland	–	–	–	–	1982	–	–
Australia, South	–	–	–	1977	1978–82	1983–87	1988–92
Australia, Tasmania	–	–	–	–	1978–82	1983–87	1988–92
Australia, Victoria	–	–	–	–	1982	1983–87	1988–92
Western Australia	–	–	–	–	1982	1983–87	1988–92
French Polynesia	–	–	–	–	–	–	1988–92
New Zealand	1960–62	–	–	–	–	–	1988–92
Maori	–	1962–66	1968–71	1972–76	1978–82	1983–87	1988–92
Non-Maori	–	1962–66	1968–71	1972–76	1978–82	1983–87	1988–92
Pacific Polynesian Islanders	–	–	–	–	1978–82	–	–
USA, Hawaii	1960–63	–	–	–	–	–	–
White	1960–63	1960–64	1968–72	1973–77	1978–82	1983–87	1988–92
Chinese	–	1960–64	1968–72	1973–77	1978–82	1983–87	1988–92
Japanese	1960–63	1960–64	1968–72	1973–77	1978–82	1983–87	1988–92
Filipino	–	1960–64	1968–72	1973–77	1978–82	1983–87	1988–92
Hawaiian	1960–63	1960–64	1968–72	1973–77	1978–82	1983–87	1988–92

Chapter 2. Techniques of registration

L. Raymond

In recent years, the objectives pursued by cancer registries have multiplied. For many registries, the initial aims were essentially to count numbers of cases in the population covered, in order to calculate incidence rates which could be compared with those from other countries or populations. The principal goal was to elaborate or to confirm etiological hypotheses. For other registries, it is true, the initial motivation was rather to assess public health needs in terms of resources for diagnosis and treatment. Today, many registries try to aim at both epidemiological and clinical objectives, in the context of a global system of cancer control, seeking to plan and develop prevention as well as future resources.

This expansion of the role of registries results for many in having to collect more data and more detailed information, while continuing to maintain completeness and validity. It is necessary to multiply the sources of data, to link them in an adequate manner to avoid duplication registrations and to ensure that the information collected is as complete and as precise as possible. The development of computer methodology has been of great help, not only in assisting registries to verify the validity of their data, but also in facilitating the identification of new cases and the registration of subsequent events, such as recurrence, complementary treatment and death. It must, however, be stated that the need to link computer files with identifying information is coming into conflict with the growing installation of legal dispositions limiting possibilities of linkage for reasons of confidentiality (Muir & Démaret, 1991).

The problems are evidently of another order for a number of new registries, in particular in those areas of the world where the health care system is less developed, and registration has to be active, with visits paid to each health care establishment and every institute where diagnosis could have been effected. In these conditions, the completeness of collection of diagnosed cases is the main preoccupation.

It is necessary to remember that there is a distinction between under-registration and under-diagnosis. The low level of incidence observed in certain registries may, of course, result from a lack of exploitation of certain data sources, but it also often reflects the existence of a significant proportion of non-diagnosed cases, for example because of lack of access to medical facilities. On the other hand, incidence may be artificially inflated, often temporarily, when a new diagnostic technique permits detection of tumours that would not otherwise have been diagnosed for a longer period, or perhaps ever. For evident reasons, this phenomenon of over-diagnosis complicates the interpretation not only of geographical comparisons, but also of trends over time.

1. The geographical distribution of the registries

Examination of the list of contributing registries grouped by continent (Table 2.1) shows clearly that the proportion of the population covered by cancer registration in this volume varies considerably from one continent to another. In Africa, where the total population is estimated at 645 million persons, the population living in areas covered by population based registries contributing to this volume amounts to only 4.5 million, i.e. a proportion of 0.7%. On the other hand, in Europe this proportion is 27%, and it is 14% in the United States. In addition, the average density of the population in areas covered by cancer registration is considerably higher than for the world as a whole. Even in Europe, where the average density is 75 inhabitants per square kilometre, that of most registries is around 200 (with the exception of the Nordic countries). In Asia, this phenomenon is even more accentuated, with an average density of 660. This illustrates what may also be seen from the maps – that many registries are confined to urban areas, rather than whole provinces, or countries. The predominance of registries situated in the northern hemisphere is overweighted in relation to the distribution of the world's population (Table 2.1).

In looking at Chapter 1, which includes the list of registries contributing to *Cancer Incidence in Five Continents* over time, with the periods for which data are available, the reader will note a considerable development of registration of cancer in the world. It is also evident from the maps at the beginning of the book that the majority of the new registries have set up at a local or regional rather than a national level, while those registries which have served as pioneers, particularly in Europe, cover the whole of a country. In part this is no doubt due to practical and financial problems (the cost of running a registry is high), but equally to the recognition that the methodology now exists to extrapolate from data established for limited areas to an entire country. In many countries, one therefore seeks to create a network of local registries which can, in certain conditions, constitute a representative data-set. The national and international associations of cancer registries, of which the number and the activities are on the increase, make this one of their principal objectives.

2. Legal reporting

Legislative or regulatory measures have been taken in nearly half of the registration areas to make notification of cancer diagnoses compulsory (Table 2.1). But it is far from sure whether a legal obligation is really important in inducing overworked medical practitioners to report cases, and hence it provides no assurance that reporting will be complete. Whatever the circumstances, it is more important to interest in a more or less permanent manner the doctors and the auxiliary medical personnel responsible for selecting the diagnoses which should be registered in the activities of the registry, for example, by sending detailed epidemiological data periodically. In many situations in which it is obligatory to declare cancer cases, the personnel has to verify that this has been properly achieved using an appropriate method of sampling on the database.

3. Data sources

The sources which the registries must use to identify new cases will obviously depend on the structure and the organization of the health care system. Registries generally try to achieve the most effective strategy, taking into account the sources which yield the most cases, and the frequency of actual visits required. The two sources without which it is impossible to achieve complete coverage are (1) pathology laboratories and (2) hospital diagnoses (public and private establishments). Table 2.2 shows that the large majority of registries have access to these sources. In countries where death certification is of sufficient quality, the certificate constitutes the third indispensable source of data. Specialized services of radiotherapy, polyclinics (out-patient clinics) and laboratories of haematology are, where they exist, a fruitful source of complementary information (note that in Table 2.2 radiotherapy services are included in hospital sources, as they are usually located in a hospital).

Table 2.2 concerns the sources of information used by the registries in case-finding. It was constructed on the basis of the replies to a very simple question, requiring yes/no answers to a list of 'sources of case-finding used by your registry'. No distinction was made between major primary sources, and those referred to more irregularly – for example to collect missing information, or to trace back death certificate notification (DCN) cases. Thus, one may wonder whether general practitioners do, in reality, provide such an important source of case-finding as seems to be implied in the table.

Certain sources are clearly used rather infrequently – for example, health insurance information and screening programmes. In the 'Other' category, several registries mentioned the importance of other local or specialized registries – for example, childhood cancer registries, mesothelioma registries, etc.

For general information on the different types of data sources and how best to use them, the reader should refer to Chapter 5 of *Cancer Registration: Principles and Methods* (Powell, 1991). Although multiple source reporting is employed to increase completeness of registration (and number of sources per case used as an index of completeness), it provides no absolute guarantee. The choice of sources depends of course upon a series of considerations, including their validity and the ease of access to them. In this general statement, the death certificate must be considered separately, not only because it is a means of finding cases, but also because death certificate notification provides an important method of evaluating completeness of registration (Parkin *et al.*, 1994).

4. Data collected

Certain variables are considered 'essential', and population-based registration should not be considered established unless they are all included in the database. Those which describe the case are:

– the name
– the sex
– the date of birth or age
– the usual place of residence

Determination of the usual place of residence is often difficult, largely because the information available in the medical record may relate to a temporary residence, for example staying with a relative. To the extent that the objective of registering the address is not only to better identify the individual, but also to permit the calculation of incidence rates for a geographical area, it is necessary to define place of residence according to the same criteria as those adopted for the census of the population from which the person-years at risk in the denominator are estimated.

The variables which are essential for full characterization of the tumour are:

– the date of incidence
– the most valid basis of diagnosis (distinguishing at least the cases confirmed histologically from cases diagnosed clinically)
– the primary site
– the morphological type
– the behaviour.

The problems posed by coding site and morphology are described in Chapter 3.

According to the responses supplied in the questionnaire, the vast majority of registries collect all of these essential data items (Table 2.3). In reality, several registries have not been able to provide data on morphology or on the behaviour of the tumour. The reader will also find more detail on this topic in Chapters 3, 5 and 6.

The decision as to which other variables will be collected and registered routinely by a registry depends in principle on its primary interests. Those registries which are mainly interested in etiological research and primary prevention will naturally aim to collect items describing the environmental factors which might be associated with variations in risk, such as ethnic group, civil status, religion and, of course, occupation.

Those registries which are more interested in early detection and in therapeutic needs, will emphasize the variables which characterize the tumour (date of symptoms, stage) and its treatment. Examination of Table 2.3 shows that, for whatever reason, there exists a great variety of data items. The most frequently collected information on the person relates to place of birth. As for occupation, the data relating to it are often judged insufficiently reliable to be of use in an epidemiological study. It is not indispensable to have data on the general population established according to the same definition (denominator) in order to interpret the information collected on the occupation of persons with cancer. In many cases, using a proportional rate, studies of a case–control type may prove effective.

For further detail on the problems posed by selection of the data items to collect, the reader should refer to *Cancer Registration: Principles and Methods* (Jensen *et al.*, 1991).

5. Follow-up

Nearly two thirds of the contributing registries reported that they carry out follow-up of cases. However, the questionnaire did not attempt to establish the completeness of such follow-up nor whether the purpose is to calculate survival rates, or simply to keep the files up to date for clinical type studies (Table 2.1). The fact that follow-up is only passive in many cases leads one to suppose that the second hypothesis is the more likely. The existence of active follow-up (to determine whether a person is alive or dead for each case registered at a date or interval which is fixed) suggests that the registry has a particular interest in studies of survival. In many cases, the date of death is a piece of information that is obtained automatically and in a routine fashion. When it concerns entire countries or large regions, which are little subject to migratory movement, follow-up of cases based exclusively on death registration permits the estimation of survival rates with satisfactory precision. It remains nonetheless preferable to verify actively that the persons with cancer presumed to be alive really are so, when it is a question of calculating such rates; if a substantial percentage of cases are 'lost' to follow-up, any estimate of survival is likely to be biased (Parkin & Hakulinen, 1991; Estève *et al.*, 1994).

As far as the maximum follow-up period is concerned, this was not given systematically in the questionnaire, but it appears that follow-up is nearly always carried out indefinitely.

References

Estève, J., Benhamou, E. & Raymond, L. (1994) Statistical Methods in Cancer Research, Volume IV, Descriptive Epidemiology (IARC Scientific Publications No. 128), Lyon, IARC

Jensen, O.M., Parkin, D.M., MacLennan, R., Muir, C.S. & Skeet, R.G., eds (1991) Cancer Registration: Principles and Methods (IARC Scientific Publications No. 95), Lyon IARC

Muir, C.S. & Démaret, E. (1991) Cancer registration: legal aspects and confidentiality. In: Jensen, O.M., Parkin, D.M., MacLennan, R., Muir, C.S. & Skeet, R.G., eds, Cancer Registration: Principles and Methods (IARC Scientific Publications No. 95), Lyon, IARC

Parkin, D.M., Chen, V.W., Ferlay, J., Galceran, J., Storm, H.H and Whelan, S.L. (1994) Comparability and Quality Control in Cancer Registration (IARC Technical Reports No. 19), Lyon, IARC

Parkin, D.M. & Hakulinen, T. (1991) Analysis of survival. In: Jensen, O.M., Parkin, D.M., MacLennan, R., Muir, C.S. & Skeet, R.G., eds, Cancer Registration: Principles and Methods (IARC Scientific Publications No. 95), Lyon, IARC

Powell, J. (1991) Data sources and reporting. In: Jensen, O.M., Parkin, D.M., MacLennan, R., Muir, C.S. & Skeet, R.G., eds, Cancer Registration: Principles and Methods (IARC Scientific Publications No. 95), Lyon, IARC

Table 2.1 Population, surface area, latitude, mandatory reporting and follow-up

	Population (thousands)	Surface area (km2)	Population density (per km2)	Latitude (°)	Reporting Voluntary/ Compulsary	Follow-up of registered cases		
						Active/ Passive	All/Selected cases	Maximum duration (years)
AFRICA								
Algeria, Sétif	1105	6504	169.8	35 N	V	A/P	A	10
France, La Réunion	598	2512	237.9	22 S	V	A	A	5
Mali, Bamako	708			13 N		A	A	3
Uganda, Kyadondo County	1035	75259	13.8	0	V			
Zimbabwe, Harare	1062	872	1218.4	19 S	V	P	S	
TOTAL AFRICA	**4508**							
CENTRAL AND SOUTH AMERICA								
Argentina, Concordia	139	3680	37.8	32 S	V			
Brazil, Belém	1333	1221	1091.6	1 S				
Brazil, Goiania	925	801	1154.8	17 S	V			
Brazil, Porto Alegre	1263	552	2288.8	30 S	V/C			
Colombia, Cali	1504	11938	126	4 N	V	P	A	
Costa Rica	3014	51200	58.9	10 N	C	P	A	
Ecuador, Quito	1191	19	62685.3	0	V	P	A	
Peru, Lima	6122			12 S		P	A	
Peru, Trujillo	456	314	1452.9	8 S	V/C	P	A	
USA, Puerto Rico	3481	8586	405.5	18 N	C	P	A	
Uruguay, Montevideo	1360			35 S	C			
TOTAL CENTRAL AND SOUTH AMERICA	**20790**							
NORTH AMERICA								
Canada	27745	9970610	2.8	45 N				
Canada, Alberta	2555	38233	66.8	53 N	C	P	A	
Canada, British Columbia	3299	947800	3.5	49 N	V/C	A/P	S	Indefinite
Canada, Manitoba	1110	547704	2	49 N	C	P	A	
Canada, New Brunswick	743	3437	216.2	47 N	V	P	S	
Canada, Newfoundland	579	370485	1.6	48 N	V	A	A	Indefinite.
Canada, Northwest Territories	55	3244608	0	63 N	C	P	S	
Canada, Nova Scotia	913	55491	16.4	44 N	C	P	A	
Canada, Ontario	10299	1068578	9.6	45 N	V	A/P	A	
Canada, Prince Edward Island	131	5660	23.1	47 N	V			
Canada, Quebec	7013	1667926	4.2	45 N	C	A	A	Indefinite.
Canada, Saskatchewan	1016	651900	1.6	51 N	C	A/P	S	25
Canada, Yukon	26	3244608	0	63 N	C	P	S	
USA, California, Central Valley	2111	64750	32.6	36 N	C			
USA, California, Los Angeles County	8558	10500	815	34 N	C	A/P	A	Indefinite
USA, California, San Francisco Bay Area	3585	6427	557.8	38 N	V/C	A/P	S	Indefinite
USA, Connecticut	3223	12973	248.4	41 N	C	A/P	A	Indefinite
USA, Georgia, Atlanta	2143	4378	489.4	34 N	V/C	A/P	A	Indefinite
USA, Iowa	2782	145800	19.1	42 N	C	A/P	A	Indefinite
USA, Louisiana, Central Region	312		16.9			P	A	

Table 2.1 (Contd). Population, surface area, latitude, mandatory reporting and follow-up

	Population (thousands)	Surface area (km2)	Population density (per km2)	Latitude (°)	Reporting Voluntary/ Compulsary	Follow-up of registered cases		
						Active/ Passive	All/Selected cases	Maximum duration (years)
USA, Louisiana, New Orleans	996	2672	36.9	30 N	C	P	A	
USA, Michigan, Detroit	3848	3259	1180.8	42 N	C	A/P	S	Indefinite
USA, New Mexico	1473	121600	12.1	35 N	C	A/P	A	Indefinite
USA, Utah	1741	84990	20.5	41 N	C	A/P	A	Indefinite
USA, Washington, Seattle	3375	45800	73.7	47 N	V/C	A/P	A	Indefinite
USA, SEER	21528					A	A	Indefinite
TOTAL NORTH AMERICA	**61885**							
ASIA								
China, Qidong County	1152	1157	996	32 N	V/C	A/P	A	
China, Shanghai	7110	792	8977.2	31 N	C	A/P	A	
China, Tianjin	3565	160	22279.8	39 N	C	A/P	A	
Hong Kong	5743	1075	5342	22 N	V	P	A	
India, Bangalore	4001	276	14495.1	13 N	V	P	S	7
India, Barshi, Paranda, Bhum	443	3713	119.2	18 N	V	A	A	Indefinite
India, Bombay	9706	603	16095.6	19 N		A/P	S	7
India, Karunagappally	385	192	2005.7	9 N				
India, Madras	3802	170	22363.8	13 N	V	A/P	A	Indefinite
India, Trivandrum	1065	336	3170.8	8 N				
Israel	4739	20700	228.9	32 N	C	P	A	
Japan, Hiroshima	1066	740	1440.5	34 N	V			
Japan, Miyagi Prefecture	2246	7291	308	38 N	V	P	A	
Japan, Nagasaki Prefecture	1565	4090	382.5	33 N	V	A/P	A	
Japan, Osaka Prefecture	8735	1882	4641.1	35 N	V	A/P	A	10
Japan, Saga Prefecture	878	2433	360.7	33 N	V	P	A	
Japan, Yamagata Prefecture	1258	9326	134.9	38 N	V	A/P	A	10
Korea, Kangwha County	74	408	181.3	38 N	V	A	A	Indefinite
Kuwait	1710	17818	95.9	29 N	C			
Philippines, Manila	4380	274	15984.2	15 N	C	P	A	
Singapore	2680	584	4589.5	1 N	V	P	A	
Thailand, Chiang Mai	1367	20107	68	16 N	C	A	A	10
Thailand, Khon Kaen	1621	13404	121	15 N	V/C	A/P	A	
Viet Nam, Hanoi	2116	921	2297.2	21 N	V			
TOTAL ASIA	**71404**							
EUROPE								
Austria, Tyrol	625	12648	49.4	46 N	C	A/P	S	Indefinite
Belarus	10187	207600	49.1	53 N	C	A	A	20
Croatia	4734	56538	83.7	45 N	C	A/P	A	
Czech Republic	10342	78864	131.1	50 N	C	A/P	A	Indefinite
Denmark	5145	43000	119.7	56 N	C	A/P	A	Indefinite
Estonia	1562	45215	34.6	58 N	C			
Finland	4981	337000	14.8	62 N	C			
France, Bas-Rhin	953	4800	198.6	48 N	V			
France, Calvados	626	5548	112.9	49 N	V	A	A	Indefinite
France, Doubs	490	5234	93.7	47 N	V	A/P	A	18
France, Haut-Rhin	679	3522	192.8	48 N	C			
France, Hérault	803	6101	131.6	44 N	V	A	S	5

Table 2.1 (Contd). Population, surface area, latitude, mandatory reporting and follow-up

	Population (thousands)	Surface area (km2)	Population density (per km2)	Latitude (°)	Reporting Voluntary/ Compulsary	Follow-up of registered cases		
						Active/ Passive	All/Selected cases	Maximum duration (years)
France, Isère	1015	7431	136.6	45 N	V	P	A	
France, Somme	554	6280	88.2	50 N	V	A/P	A	10
France, Tarn	346	5758	60.1	44 N	V	A/P	S	10
Germany, Eastern States	16648	108333	153.7	52 N	C	A/P	A	5
Germany, Saarland	1067	2567	415.7	50 N	V	A/P	A	Indefinite
Iceland	281	103000	2.7	65 N	V	P	A	
Ireland, Southern	532	12155	43.8	52 N	V	P	A	
Italy, Ferrara Province	361	2632	137.1	45 N	V	A/P	A	
Italy, Florence	1168	3814	306.2	44 N	C	A/P	A	Indefinite
Italy, Genoa	696	239.6	2904.8	44 N	C	A/P	A	
Italy, Latina	469	2250	208.4	41 N	C	A/P	A	
Italy, Macerata Province	282	2449	115	43 N	V	A/P	A	Indefinite
Italy, Modena	603	2689	224.1	45 N	V	A	A	Indefinite
Italy, Parma Province	391	3449	113.4	45 N	V	A	A	Indefinite
Italy, Ragusa	288	1614	178.3	37 N	V	A/P	A	Indefinite
Italy, Romagna	605	4769	126.8	45 N	V/C	P	A	
Italy, Torino	996	130	7665.1	45 N	V	A/P	A	Indefinite
Italy, Trieste	261	211.6	1234.3	46 N	V	P	A	
Italy, Varese Province	793	1199	661.7	45 N	V/C	A/P	A	Indefinite
Italy, Venetian Region	1150	3805	302.2	45 N	V/C	P	A	
Latvia	2654	64600	41.1	57 N	C	A/P	A	5
Malta	363	316	1148.7	36 N	V/C	P	A	
Netherlands	15014	41000	366.2	52 N		P	A	
Netherlands, Eindhoven	936	2500	374.3	53 N	V/C	A/P	A	Indefinite
Netherlands, Maastricht	847	1354	625.5	51 N	V	A/P	S	
Norway	4245	325000	13.1	61 N	C	P	A	
Poland, Cracow	748	5034	148.6	50 N	C	P	A	
Poland, Kielce	1141	9211	123.9	50 N	C	A	A	
Poland, Lower Silesia	2895	18870	153.4	52 N	C	A/P	A	5
Poland, Warsaw City	1625	495	3283.3	52 N	C	A	A	Indefinite
Slovakia	5298	49014	108.1	48 N	C			
Slovenia	1999	20255	98.7	46 N	C	A/P	A	Indefinite
Spain, Albacete	342	14862	23	39 N	V	P	A	Indefinite
Spain, Asturias	1097	10565	103.8	44 N	V	P	A	
Spain, Basque Country	2111	7261	290.7	43 N	V	A/P	A	
Spain, Granada	788	2531	311.3	37 N	V	A	S	
Spain, Mallorca	583	3626	160.7	40 N	V	A/P	A	Indefinite
Spain, Murcia	1037	11317	91.6	38 N	C/V			
Spain, Navarra	520	10491	49.6	43 N	V	A/P	A	
Spain, Tarragona	541	6283	86.2	41 N	V	P		
Spain, Zaragoza	831	17194	48.3	42 N	V	P	A	
Switzerland, Basel	429	465	922.8	47 N	V	A/P	A	Indefinite
Switzerland, Geneva	382	282	1352.8	46 N	V	A/P	A	Indefinite
Switzerland, Graubünden	173	7109	24.3	46 N	V			
Switzerland, Neuchâtel	159	796	199.6	47 N	V	P	A	
Switzerland, St Gall-Appenzell	484	2430	199.1	47 N	V	P	A	
Switzerland, Valais	253	5231	48.4	46 N	V	A/P	A	
Switzerland, Vaud	569	3211	177.2	46 N	V	A/P	A	
Switzerland, Zurich	1146	1729	663	47 N	V	A/P	S	
UK, England & Wales	50558	150800	335.3	52 N	V/C	P	A	

Table 2.1 (Contd). Population, surface area, latitude, mandatory reporting and follow-up

	Population (thousands)	Surface area (km2)	Population density (per km2)	Latitude (°)	Reporting Voluntary/ Compulsary	Follow-up of registered cases		
						Active/ Passive	All/Selected cases	Maximum duration (years)
UK, England, East Anglia	2062	500	4124.2	54 N	V/C	A	S	Indefinite
UK, England, Merseyside & Cheshire	2412	2980	809.4	45 N	V/C	P	A	
UK, England, North Western	4006	4500	890.2	54 N	V	P	A	
UK, England, Oxford Region	2545	8200	310.3	52 N	C	A/P	S	Indefinite
UK, England, South Thames	6651	17440	381.3	51 N	C/V	P	A	
UK, England, South Western	3285	17000	193.2	50 N	C	P	A	
UK, England, Wessex	2966	10000	296.6	51 N	C	P	A	
UK, England, West Midlands	5219	13014	401	52 N	V	P	A	
UK, England, Yorkshire	3658	13700	267	54 N	V	P	A	
UK, Scotland	5100	77179	66.1	56 N	V	P	A	
UK, Scotland, West	2725	22972	118.6	57 N				
Yugoslavia, Vojvodina	2019	21506	93.9	45 N	C	A/P	A	Indefinite
TOTAL EUROPE	**220602**							
OCEANIA								
Australian Capital Territory	283			35 S	C/V			
Australia, New South Wales	5835	801400	7.3	34 S	C	P	A	
South Australia	1435	984375	1.5	35 S	C	A/P	A	Indefinite
Australia, Tasmania	462	68300	6.8	42 S				
Australia, Victoria	4366	227600	19.2	38 S	C			
Western Australia	1604	2225500	0.7	32 S	C			
French Polynesia	197			19 S	C/V	P	A	
New Zealand	3349	270534	12.4	40 S	C			
USA, Hawaii	1007	16635.5	60.5	22 N	C/V	A/P	S	Indefinite
TOTAL OCEANIA	**18538**							

Table 2.2 Sources of data

	Public hospital records	Out patient clinics	Private clin./ hosp.	Path. lab.	Autop -sies	Haema tology	Death certificate	G.P.	Health insurance	Screening progr.	Others
AFRICA											
Algeria, Sétif	X	X	X	X	X	X	X	X			X
La Réunion	X		X	X		X	X	X		X	
Mali, Bamako	X	X	X	X	X	X	X	X	X		
Uganda, Kyadondo County	X	X	X	X	X			X			
Zimbabwe, Harare	X	X	X	X		X	X	X			X
CENTRAL AND SOUTH AMERICA											
Argentina, Concordia	X	X	X	X	X	X	X	X			X
Brazil, Belém	X	X	X	X	X	X	X			X	
Brazil, Goiania	X	X	X	X	X	X	X	X		X	
Brazil, Porto Alegre	X	X	X	X		X	X				
Colombia, Cali	X	X	X	X	X	X	X	X	X	X	
Costa Rica	X		X	X	X	X	X			X	
Ecuador, Quito	X		X	X	X	X	X	X			X
Peru, Lima											
Peru, Trujillo	X		X	X	X	X	X	X		X	
USA, Puerto Rico	X	X	X	X	X	X	X	X			
Uruguay, Montevideo	X	X	X	X		X	X	X		X	
NORTH AMERICA											
Canada											
Canada, Alberta	X	X	X	X	X	X	X	X			X
Canada, British Columbia	X		X	X			X	X		X	
Canada, Manitoba	X	X	X	X	X	X	X	X		X	
Canada, New Brunswick	X			X	X	X	X				
Canada, Newfoundland	X	X	X	X	X	X	X				
Canada, Northwest Territories	X	X	X	X	X	X	X	X			
Canada, Nova Scotia	X			X	X		X				
Canada, Ontario	X	X		X	X		X				
Canada, Prince Edward Island	X	X		X	X	X	X	X			
Canada, Quebec	X										X
Canada, Saskatchewan	X	X	X	X	X	X	X	X		X	X
Canada, Yukon	X		X	X	X	X	X		X		
USA, California, Central Valley	X	X	X	X	X	X	X				
USA, California, Los Angeles County											
USA, California, San Francisco Bay Area	X	X	X	X	X		X	X			X
USA, Connecticut	X	X	X	X	X	X	X				
USA, Georgia, Atlanta											
USA, Iowa	X	X	X	X	X	X	X	X			
USA, Louisiana, Central Region	X	X	X	X	X	X	X				X
USA, Louisiana, New Orleans	X	X	X	X	X	X	X			X	
USA, Michigan, Detroit	X	X	X	X	X	X	X				
USA, New Mexico	X	X	X	X	X	X	X	X			
USA, Utah	X	X	X	X	X		X	X			X
USA, Washington, Seattle	X	X	X	X	X		X				X
USA, SEER	X	X	X	X	X	X	X	X			

Table 2.2 (Contd). Sources of data

	Public hospital records	Out patient clinics	Private clin./ hosp.	Path. lab.	Autop -sies	Haema tology	Death certificate	G.P.	Health insurance	Screening progr.	Others
ASIA											
China, Qidong County	X	X		X			X	X		X	
China, Shanghai	X	X					X				
China, Tianjin	X	X	X				X				
Hong Kong	X	X	X	X		X	X	X			
India, Bangalore	X	X	X	X	X	X	X	X		X	
India, Barshi, Paranda, Bhum	X	X	X	X	X	X	X	X		X	
India, Bombay	X		X	X	X	X	X				
India, Karunagappaly	X		X	X		X	X	X	X		
India, Madras	X	X	X	X	X	X	X				
India, Trivandrum	X	X	X	X		X	X				
Israel	X	X	X	X	X	X	X				
Japan, Hiroshima	X	X	X	X	X	X	X	X			
Japan, Miyagi Prefecture	X	X	X	X	X	X		X		X	
Japan, Nagasaki Prefecture	X	X	X	X	X		X	X		X	
Japan, Osaka Prefecture	X	X	X	X	X	X	X	X		X	X
Japan, Saga Prefecture	X	X					X	X			
Japan, Yamagata Prefecture	X	X	X				X	X		X	
Korea, Kangwha County	X		X	X		X	X	X	X		
Kuwait	X	X		X	X	X	X				
Philippines, Manila	X	X	X	X	X	X	X				
Singapore	X		X	X	X	X	X	X			
Thailand, Chiang Mai	X	X	X	X	X	X	X	X			
Thailand, Khon Kaen	X	X	X	X	X	X	X			X	
Viet Nam, Hanoi	X	X		X	X	X	X				
EUROPE											
Austria, Tyrol	X	X	X	X	X	X	X			X	
Belarus	X	X		X	X	X	X				
Croatia	X		X	X	X		X	X			
Czech Republic	X	X	X	X	X	X	X				X
Denmark	X	X	X		X		X	X		X	X
Estonia	X	X	X	X	X	X	X	X			
Finland	X	X	X	X	X	X	X	X			
France, Bas-Rhin	X	X	X	X	X	X	X			X	
France, Calvados	X	X	X	X			X	X			
France, Doubs	X	X	X	X	X	X	X				
France, Haut-Rhin	X		X	X	X	X					
France, Hérault	X	X	X	X		X					X
France, Isère	X	X	X	X		X		X	X	X	
France, Somme	X	X	X	X	X		X			X	
France, Tarn	X	X	X	X			X	X	X		
Germany, Eastern States	X	X	X	X	X	X	X	X			
Germany, Saarland	X	X	X	X	X	X	X	X			
Iceland	X		X	X	X	X	X	X		X	
Ireland, Southern	X	X	X	X	X	X	X	X			
Italy, Ferrara Province	X	X	X	X	X		X	X			
Italy, Florence	X	X	X	X	X		X			X	
Italy, Genoa	X	X	X	X		X	X				
Italy, Latina	X	X	X	X	X	X	X				

Table 2.2 (Contd). Sources of data

	Public hospital records	Out patient clinics	Private clin./ hosp.	Path. lab.	Autop -sies	Haema tology	Death certificate	G.P.	Health insurance	Screening progr.	Others
Italy, Macerata Province	X	X	X	X		X	X	X			X
Italy, Modena	X	X	X	X	X	X	X	X			
Italy, Parma Province	X	X	X	X	X		X				
Italy, Ragusa	X	X	X	X			X		X		
Italy, Romagna	X	X	X	X	X	X	X	X		X	X
Italy, Torino	X		X	X	X		X				
Italy, Trieste	X	X	X	X	X	X	X	X	X		
Italy, Varese Province	X		X	X			X				X
Italy, Venetian Region	X			X	X	X	X				
Latvia	X	X	X		X		X	X		X	
Malta	X		X	X		X	X				X
Netherlands	X	X		X	X			X	X		
Netherlands, Eindhoven	X	X	X	X	X	X					
Netherlands, Maastricht	X	X		X	X	X				X	
Norway	X	X	X	X	X	X	X	X			
Poland, Cracow	X	X	X				X	X			
Poland, Kielce	X						X				
Poland, Lower Silesia	X	X	X	X	X	X	X	X	X		
Poland, Warsaw City	X	X	X				X	X		X	
Slovakia	X	X		X	X	X	X			X	X
Slovenia	X	X	X			X	X	X			
Spain, Albacete	X		X	X	X	X	X	X	X		
Spain, Asturias	X	X	X	X	X	X	X				
Spain, Basque Country	X	X	X	X	X	X	X				
Spain, Granada	X	X	X	X	X	X	X				X
Spain, Mallorca	X	X	X	X	X	X	X	X			X
Spain, Murcia	X	X	X	X	X	X	X		X	X	
Spain, Navarra	X	X	X	X	X	X	X	X		X	X
Spain, Tarragona	X	X	X	X	X	X	X	X		X	X
Spain, Zaragoza	X		X	X		X	X	X			
Sweden	X	X	X	X	X	X	X				X
Switzerland, Basel	X		X	X	X	X	X				
Switzerland, Geneva	X	X		X	X	X	X				X
Switzerland, Graubünden	X			X	X	X	X				
Switzerland, Neuchâtel	X			X	X		X				
Switzerland, St Gall-Appenzell	X	X		X	X	X	X				
Switzerland, Valais	X	X	X	X	X	X	X	X			
Switzerland, Vaud	X	X		X	X	X	X				
Switzerland, Zurich	X	X		X	X	X	X				
UK, England & Wales	X	X	X	X			X	X			X
UK, England, East Anglia	X	X	X	X	X	X	X	X		X	X
UK, England, Mersey	X	X	X	X	X	X	X	X		X	X
UK, England, North Western	X	X	X	X			X	X			
UK, England, Oxford Region	X	X	X	X	X	X	X	X			X
UK, England, South Thames	X	X	X	X	X	X	?			X	X
UK, England, South Western	X	X	X	X	X	X	X			X	
UK, England, Wessex	X	X	X	X	X	X	X	X		X	
UK, England, West Midlands	X			X	X	X	X			X	X
UK, England, Yorkshire	X	X	X	X		X	X	X		X	X
UK, Scotland	X	X	X	X	X	X	X			X	X

Table 2.2 (Contd). Sources of data

	Public hospital records	Out patient clinics	Private clin./ hosp.	Path. lab.	Autop -sies	Haema tology	Death certificate	G.P.	Health insurance	Screening progr.	Others
UK, Scotland, West Yugoslavia, Vojvodina	X	X		X			X	X		X	X
OCEANIA											
Australian Capital Territory	X		X	X			X				
Australia, New South Wales	X		X	X			X				
South Australia	X	X	X	X	X	X	X				
Australia, Tasmania	X		X	X	X	X	X	X		X	X
Australia, Victoria	X		X	X	X	X	X				
Western Australia			X	X	X	X					
French Polynesia	X	X		X		X	X	X			X
New Zealand	X		X	X	X	X	X	X			
USA, Hawaii	X	X	X	X	X		X	X			

Table 2.3 Information recorded

	Basic variables	Ethn. col./ nation.	Place of birth	Identity No.	Civil status	Religion	Occupation	Date of first symptom	Stage	First treatment	Subseq. treatment
AFRICA											
Algeria, Sétif	X		X								
France, La Réunion	X		X				X				
Mali, Bamako	X	X	X								
Uganda, Kyadondo County											
Zimbabwe, Harare											
CENTRAL AND SOUTH AMERICA											
Argentina, Concordia	X		X	X							
Brazil, Belém	X										
Brazil, Goiania											
Brazil, Porto Alegre											
Colombia, Cali	X		X						X	X	X
Costa Rica	X		X	X	X		X				
Ecuador, Quito	X		X	X			X		X		
Peru, Lima											
Peru, Trujillo	X										
USA, Puerto Rico	X		X	X	X		X	X	X	X	X
Uruguay, Montevideo	X	X	X	X	X		X		X	X	X
NORTH AMERICA											
Canada											
Canada, Alberta			X	X	X				X	X	
Canada, British Columbia	X	X	X	X	X	X	X		X	X	
Canada, Manitoba	X		X	X	X					X	X
Canada, New Brunswick	X			X	X				X	X	X
Canada, Newfoundland	X		X	X	X				X	X	X
Canada, Northwest Territories	X	X	X	X	X						
Canada, Nova Scotia	X			X	X					X	
Canada, Ontario	X									X	X
Canada, Prince Edward Island	X		X	X	X						
Canada, Quebec			X	X							
Canada, Saskatchewan	X	X	X	X	X				X	X	X
Canada, Yukon	X	X	X	X	X						
USA, California, Central Valley	X	X	X	X	X	X	X		X	X	
USA, California, Los Angeles County	X	X	X	X	X	X	X		X	X	
USA, California, San Francisco Bay Area	X	X	X	X	X	X	X		X	X	
USA, Connecticut	X	X	X	X	X				X	X	
USA, Georgia, Atlanta	X	X	X	X	X				X	X	
USA, Iowa	X	X	X	X	X		X		X	X	

Table 2.3 (Contd). Information recorded

	Basic variables	Ethn. col./ nation.	Place of birth	Identity No.	Civil status	Religion	Occupation	Date of first symptom	Stage	First treatment	Subseq. treatment
USA, Louisiana, Central Region	X	X	X	X	X	X	X			X	X
USA, Louisiana, New Orleans	X	X	X	X	X	X	X			X	X
USA, Michigan, Detroit	X	X	X	X	X		X			X	X
USA, New Mexico	X	X	X	X	X					X	X
USA, Utah	X	X	X	X	X					X	X
USA, Washington, Seattle	X	X	X	X	X		X			X	X
USA, SEER	X	X	X	X	X			X		X	X
ASIA											
China, Qidong County		X	X				X				
China, Shanghai	X						X				
China, Tianjin	X	X					X				
Hong Kong	X		X	X			X				
India, Bangalore	X	X	X		X	X		X		X	X
India, Barshi, Paranda, Bhum	X	X	X		X	X				X	X
India, Bombay	X	X	X		X	X	X			X	X
India, Karunagappally	X	X	X		X	X	X			X	
India, Madras	X		X		X	X				X	X
India, Trivandrum	X	X	X		X	X				X	X
Israel	X	X	X	X		X				X	X
Japan, Hiroshima	X							X		X	X
Japan, Miyagi Prefecture	X							X		X	X
Japan, Nagasaki Prefecture	X									X	X
Japan, Osaka Prefecture	X				X					X	X
Japan, Saga Prefecture	X						X			X	X
Japan, Yamagata Prefecture	X							X		X	
Korea, Kangwha County	X			X	X	X	X		X	X	X
Kuwait	X	X		X	X	X	X			X	X
Philippines, Manila	X	X	X		X					X	
Singapore	X	X	X	X	X			X	X		
Thailand, Chiang Mai	X								X	X	X
Thailand, Khon Kaen	X	X		X	X	X			X	X	X
Viet Nam, Hanoi	X										
EUROPE											
Austria, Tyrol	X								X	X	X
Belarus	X						X		X	X	X
Croatia	X		X	X			X		X	X	X
Czech Republic	X			X				X	X	X	X
Denmark	X			X	X		X		X	X	X

Table 2.3 (Contd). Information recorded

	Basic variables	Ethn. col./ nation.	Place of birth	Identity No.	Civil status	Religion	Occupation	Date of first symptom	Stage	First treatment	Subseq. treatment
Estonia	X	X	X		X				X	X	
Finland	X			X			X		X	X	X
France, Bas-Rhin	X		X								
France, Calvados	X		X				X		X	X	X
France, Doubs	X		X		X		X		X	X	X
France, Haut-Rhin	X										
France, Hérault	X		X								
France, Isère	X		X				X	X	X	X	
France, Somme	X		X		X		X	X	X	X	X
France, Tarn	X		X				X		X		
Germany, Eastern States	X			X					X	X	X
Germany, Saarland	X	X			X		X	X	X	X	X
Iceland	X		X	X	X		X				
Ireland, Southern	X				X		X			X	X
Italy, Ferrara Province	X		X								
Italy, Florence	X		X		X				X		
Italy, Genoa	X		X	X					X		
Italy, Latina	X		X		X		X		X	X	X
Italy, Macerata Province	X		X		X		X				
Italy, Modena	X		X		X				X		
Italy, Parma Province	X		X								
Italy, Ragusa	X										
Italy, Romagna	X	X	X		X						
Italy, Torino	X		X								
Italy, Trieste	X		X	X	X		X	X	X	X	X
Italy, Varese Province	X		X	X	X				X	X	X
Italy, Venetian Region	X		X							X	X
Latvia	X	X		X			X		X	X	X
Malta	X			X	X		X	X	X	X	
Netherlands	X		X						X		
Netherlands, Eindhoven	X		X						X	X	X
Netherlands, Maastricht	X		X						X	X	
Norway	X			X				X	X	X	X
Poland, Cracow	X								X	X	
Poland, Kielce	X			X					X	X	X
Poland, Lower Silesia	X						X	X	X	X	X
Poland, Warsaw City	X							X	X	X	X
Slovakia	X			X			X	X	X	X	
Slovenia	X	X	X	X					X	X	X
Spain, Albacete	X		X	X	X						
Spain, Asturias	X										
Spain, Basque Country	X			X							
Spain, Granada	X		X	X				X			
Spain, Mallorca	X		X	X							

Table 2.3 (Contd). Information recorded

	Basic variables	Ethn. col./ nation.	Place of birth	Identity No.	Civil status	Religion	Occupation	Date of first symptom	Stage	First treatment	Subseq. treatment
Spain, Murcia	X		X	X	X		X	X		X	
Spain, Navarra	X								X	X	
Spain, Tarragona	X		X	X							
Spain, Zaragoza	X		X	X	X		X	X	X	X	
Sweden				X							
Switzerland, Basel	X	X		X	X		X		X	X	
Switzerland, Geneva	X	X	X		X		X		X	X	
Switzerland, Graubünden	X	X			X		X		X	X	
Switzerland, Neuchâtel	X		X		X		X		X	X	
Switzerland, St Gall-Appenzell	X				X		X		X	X	
Switzerland, Valais	X	X	X				X		X	X	
Switzerland, Vaud	X	X			X		X		X		
Switzerland, Zurich	X	X			X		X		X	X	
UK, England & Wales		X		X	X		X				
UK, England, East Anglia	X		X	X	X		X			X	X
UK, England, Merseyside & Cheshire	X	X	X	X	X		X			X	X
UK, England, North Western	X		X	X	X		X			X	
UK, England, Oxford Region	X		X	X	X		X	X	X	X	X
UK, England, South Thames	X		X	X	X		X			X	
UK, England, South Western	X		X	X	X			X	X	X	X
UK, England, Wessex	X			X	X				X	X	X
UK, England, West Midlands	X	X	X	X	X		X		X	X	X
UK, England, Yorkshire	X		X	X	X	X	X	X	X	X	X
UK, Scotland				X	X						
UK, Scotland, West											
Yugoslavia, Vojvodina	X	X		X				X	X	X	X
OCEANIA											
Australian Capital Territory	X	X	X						X		
Australia, New South Wales	X	X	X						X		
South Australia			X				X				
Australia, Tasmania	X		X				X				
Australia, Victoria	X	X	X								
Western Australia	X	X	X				X				
French Polynesia	X	X	X				X			X	X
New Zealand	X	X	X	X			X		X		
USA, Hawaii	X	X	X	X	X			X	X	X	

Chapter 3. Classification and coding

S.L. Whelan and J. Young

1. Classification used to present data on incidence

The Cancer Incidence in Five Continents series has followed the evolution of the International Classification of Diseases through four revisions and the creation of a new coding scheme for oncology, the ICD-O, now in its second edition (ICD-O-2). Volumes I and II (Doll et al., 1966; 1970) presented the data on cancer incidence coded to the 7th Revision (ICD-7; WHO, 1957). Volume III (Waterhouse et al., 1976) published data using both the 7th and the 8th (ICD-8; WHO, 1967) Revisions with tables of equivalence, which left to the user the work of comparing data from registries coding to different revisions. ICD-8, which came into effect in 1968, was used in Volume IV (Waterhouse et al., 1982), presenting data for the years 1973–77.

The 9th Revision of the ICD (ICD-9; WHO, 1977) was used for Volumes V (Muir *et al.*, 1987), VI (Parkin *et al.*, 1992) and VII (Parkin *et al.*, 1997), three volumes spanning 15 years of data on cancer incidence, 1978–92, corresponding to a period of rapidly increasing conformity internationally to standard classification systems and coding rules. This was in large part due to the publication, in 1976, of the ICD-O (WHO, 1976) with clearly defined axes of anatomical location, histology and behaviour. For data published in Volume IV (1973–77), just over one-third of the registries used MOTNAC (ACS,1951; 1968), one-third had started to use ICD-O, 12% used SNOP (CAP,1951) and 10% did not record histology (Powell, 1982). 75% of contributors to Volume V used ICD-O to code histology, and this figure had risen to 90% for Volume VI (Powell, 1987; 1992). In the present volume 92% of contributors coded their histological data to ICD-O, either first or second edition.

2. Analysis of coding practices

The classification systems used by cancer registries over these years for topography (commonly so-called although 'topography' in the ICD includes both histological entities such as melanoma, and systemic disease, for example leukaemia), the successive revisions of the ICD, would in principle make the task of presenting data coded in a comparable manner a simple one. In practice, it has been a never-ending exercise in detection for the editors of *Cancer Incidence in Five Continents* to establish exactly how registries code cancer. A survey of coding practices was carried out among contributors to Volumes IV, V and VI in an attempt to ascertain how registries coded selected diagnostic terms, and to assess the effect this might have on comparability. 50-odd terms believed to present problems of inconsistency were selected, and the results were analysed and presented in the books as well as serving as the basis for the asterisks denoting variations in coding practices and the corresponding notes.

Data submitted for the first four volumes of *Cancer Incidence in Five Continents* were sent in tabular format, by sex, site and five-year age-group, on tape, diskette or, most frequently, the forms designed for the purpose. The only verification which could be made by the editors was to tally the columns and rows. For the fifth volume, registries were given the opportunity of sending the data in the form of a case-listing coded either to ICD-9 topography only or to ICD-9 or ICD-O topography plus ICD-O morphology. A very small minority of registries sent data coded to ICD-O. Contributors to Volume VI were encouraged to send data as a listing of cases, but 24% sent tabulated data.

Table 3.1. Coding practices							
Registry[1]	ICD-O-1 (T + M)	ICD-O-2 (T + M)	ICD-O-1+ ICD-O-2 (T + M)	ICD-O FT (T + M)	ICD-9(T)+ ICD-O-1/2 (M)	ICD-9 (T) No M	Other
Africa (5)	5	0	0	0	0	0	0
Central & S. America (11)	8	0	0	0	3	0	0
Canada (12)	0	0	10	0	2	0	0
USA (12)	0	12	0	0	0	0	0
Asia (24)	10	0	1	0	9	3	1
Europe (76)	35	1.5^2	1	4	26	3.5^2	3
Oceania (9)	2	1	0	0	5	1	0

1 Canada and SEER excluded from analysis
2 One registry changed from one classification to another in the middle of the period

For the present volume, registries were told that data had to be sent as a case listing. Of the 148 populations for which data are published in this volume (Canada and SEER are excluded from the analysis as they group registries for which data are also published individually), 91 (62%) sent a case listing coded to ICD-O topography and morphology, 45 (30%) a listing coded to ICD-9 topography and ICD-O morphology, 8 (5%) were not able to provide data on histology and coded topography to ICD-9 and four (3%) used different systems (Table 3.1). This made it possible in principle for the editors to see from the raw data what was being included in the different codes as well as to decide whether or not to include certain benign, uncertain or *in situ* diagnoses in the tables. Thus, for this volume the survey on coding practices was dropped. In practice, it was still necessary to ask registries some questions, notably in relation to non-melanoma skin and bladder cancer (see Table 3.2).

3. Comparability

3.1. Mesothelioma and pleura

In fairness, it has to be admitted that 'deviant' coding practices are frequently the result of a conscious effort on the part of individual registries to register the best possible information and to compensate for changing diagnostic criteria, imprecise terms or failure of the ICD to accommodate new concepts. For example, in ICD-8 mesothelioma of peritoneum and of pleura was considered malignant and mesothelioma of other or unspecified sites as benign. 10% of registries contributing to Volume IV excluded mesothelioma of peritoneum and pleura when this was not specified as malignant; the 'benign' mesotheliomas (as defined by the ICD-8 rules) were included in the malignant categories by 29%. The problem was recognized in the 9th Revision and mesothelioma NOS became a malignant neoplasm. The editors of the present volume have chosen to preempt the 10th Revision of the ICD, although the data are coded to the 9th Revision, by giving mesothelioma its own three-character category in the tables.

Mesothelioma has been separated from ICD-9 163, Pleura for all registries which provided data on histology in this volume. For these registries, the few remaining diagnoses in this site have been grouped with ICD-9 164, Malignant neoplasm of thymus, heart and mediastinum. The non-mesothelioma diagnoses in the peritoneum have been grouped with Other and Unspecified.

Diagnoses of mesothelioma were not available separately for registries which did not provide data on histology, and these remain in the Pleura. In this case both ICD-9 163-164 and mesothelioma are marked with dagger signs referring to notes on the 'population' pages. For these registries, the mesotheliomas (as well as the non-mesothelioma diagnoses) in the peritoneum have been grouped with Other and Unspecified.

3.2. Kaposi's sarcoma

Some registries did not provide data for ICD-9 173 Other skin. Given that, in SEER data for the period, 99% of Kaposi's sarcomas were coded to this site in ICD-9, the result is an under-enumeration of Kaposi's sarcoma. For example, the Canadian registries sent data coded to both ICD-O-1 and ICD-O-2, and did not provide data on non-melanoma skin cancer. Data for Kaposi's sarcoma are available only for the single year for which data were coded to ICD-O-2. A note on the tables for the registries concerned and a dagger against Kaposi's sarcoma draws attention to this fact.

3.3. Non-melanoma skin cancer

Registries were asked to apply the IARC/IACR rules for coding multiple primaries (IARC, 1994) to their data, or to describe their rules so that the IARC/IACR rules could be applied. This sometimes reduces the number of incident cases when compared with tabulations produced by the registries themselves, and an analysis of selected sites which would be most affected is presented in Chapter 5. The major numerical difference would concern skin cancer, for which many registries include two diagnoses within the epidermoid carcinomas, basal and squamous cell carcinomas. The first two columns of Table 3.2 analyse which skin cancers are registered and the multiple primary rules applied by individual contributors. For this volume, as described in Chapter 5, the data were, wherever possible, recoded using IARC/IACR rules, and this will have resulted in these being reduced to a single diagnosis. It should be noted that not all registries which collect data on non-melanoma skin cancer have provided those data for publication here.

3.4. Ovarian cancer

In ICD-9 borderline ovarian malignancies should be coded to 236.2, as a neoplasm of uncertain behaviour. Over half the registries in Volume IV of *Cancer Incidence in Five Continents* coded this borderline tumour as a malignant neoplasm (ICD-8 did not give guidelines about the coding of this diagnosis), as did nearly a quarter of the registries in Volume V (in opposition to ICD-9 guidelines). However, in Volume VI only 5% of registries counted the borderline ovarian cancers as malignant. The ICD-O Field Trial and Second editions categorize the borderline tumours as invasive, and registries using this rule for part of or the whole of their submission to this volume will have included such diagnoses in ICD-9 183. As registries were not asked about their coding of borderline ovarian cancer for this volume, it is not possible to know what proportion of registries using ICD-O-1 or ICD-9 continued to include them in the malignant category. Borderline ovarian tumours accounted for 13% of all ovarian cancers in the area served by the Fred Hutchinson Cancer Surveillance System in the US (Harlow & Weiss, 1989).

3.5. Bladder cancer

The problem of the coding of non-invasive tumours, taking into account recorded level of invasion and grade, and which to include in the tables as 'cancer of the bladder' has been the subject of debate. In Volume VI it was decided, for the sake of geographical comparability, to exclude tumours of benign, *in situ* and unspecified behaviour. Bladder was marked in the tables if such diagnoses were not excluded, and a note drew attention to the fact that ICD-9 188 included non-invasive tumours.

In principle, the availability of data on histological type and behaviour for this volume made it possible to publish only data on malignant cancer by excluding diagnoses with any behaviour code other than 3. Registries were, however, questioned about the behaviour codes used for the non-invasive and unspecified diagnoses of malignant bladder cancer (see Table 3.2) and 36 registries assigned the behaviour code 3 to both non-invasive and unspecified diagnoses, so making it impossible to distinguish such cases. The editors decided that the time had come to accept that non-invasive diagnoses of bladder cancer are considered malignant by pathologists in general and for Volume VII the bladder cancer category would include the in situ and unspecified categories wherever possible. For registries which sent a data-set including records with behaviour codes 1 and 2, the non-invasive bladder cancers have been included in the tables. A dagger draws attention, in this instance, to ICD-9 188 when non-malignant diagnoses are *not* included. It may well be that some contributors which register these non-invasive bladder cancers did not include them in the data which they provided.

3.6. Brain and central nervous system
Many registries choose to include benign and unspecified tumours of the brain and central nervous system in their data because the clinical course may be similar to that of a malignant tumour. In previous volumes these tumours were included with cancers of the brain and nervous system. However, the proportion of such cases varies widely between registries, so that for the present volume they are no longer included, and for registries which did include such diagnoses previously there will be an artefactual decline in incidence. Studies of trends in incidence should take into account the practice in previous volumes.

Table 3.2 Coding practices

Registry	Non-melanoma skin cancers		Behaviour codes used for bladder cancer		
	Non-melanoma skin cancer included in the data	Multiple primary rules used for skin cancers	Invasive malignant carcinoma	Non- invasive malignant carcinoma	Malignant carcinoma not otherwise specified
AFRICA					
Algeria, Sétif	All	IACR[1]	N	N	N
France, La Réunion	All	IACR	3	2	3
Mali, Bamako	BCC, SCC, small cell, fusiform cell	1BCC, 1SCC	N	N	N
Uganda, Kyadondo County	All	IACR	3	3	3
Zimbabwe, Harare	BCC, SCC	1BCC, 1SCC	3	3	3
CENTRAL AND SOUTH AMERICA					
Argentina, Concordia	All	BCC counted separately	3	3	3
Brazil, Belém	All	IACR	N	N	N
Brazil, Goiania	All	By site	3	3	3
Brazil, Porto Alegre	N	0	2	2	2
Colombia, Cali	All	NA	3	N	N
Costa Rica	BCC, SCC	Counted separately	3	2	3
Ecuador, Quito	BCC, SCC, dermatofibro- sarcoma	1BCC, 1SCC	3	3	3
Peru, Lima	BCC, SCC1	BCC, 1SCC	3	2	3
Peru, Trujillo	BCC, SCC, Merkel cell	1BCC, 1SCC	3	2	3
USA, Puerto Rico	SEER	SEER[2]	3	2	3
Uruguay, Montevideo	BCC, SCC, lymphomas sarcomas	IACR	3	2	3
NORTH AMERICA					
Canada, Alberta	BCC, SCC	1BCC, 1SCC	3	2	3
Canada, British Columbia	All	By site	3	2	2
Canada, Manitoba	All	1BCC, 1SCC	3	2	3
Canada, New Brunswick	BCC, SCC	1BCC, 1SCC	3	2	3
Canada, Newfoundland	BCC, SCC	1BCC, 1SCC	3	2	3
Canada, Northwest Territories	N	0	3	2	3
Canada, Nova Scotia	All	All counted	3	2	3
Canada, Ontario	N	0	3	2	3
Canada, Prince Edward Island	BCC, SCC	1BCC, 1SCC	3	2	3
Canada, Quebec	N	0	3	3	3

Table (Contd). 3.2 Coding practices

Registry	Non-melanoma skin cancers		Behaviour codes used forbladder cancer		
	Non-melanoma skin cancer included in the data	Multiple primary rules used for skin cancers	Invasive malignant carcinoma	Non- invasive malignant carcinoma	Malignant carcinoma not otherwise specified
Canada, Saskatchewan	All	HVBy digit, time, laterality	3	2	3
Canada, Yukon	All	By site	3	2	2
USA, California, Central Valley	All exc. BCC, SCC	SEER	3	2	3
USA, California, Los Angeles	All exc. BCC, SCC	By histology, laterality, time	3	2	3
USA, California, San Francisco Bay Area	All exc. BCC, SCC	SEER	3	2	3
USA, Connecticut	All exc. BCC, SCC	SEER	3	2	3
USA, Georgia, Atlanta	All exc. BCC, SCC	SEER	3	2	3
USA, Iowa	All exc. BCC, SCC	SEER	3	2	3
USA, Louisiana, Central Region	All exc. BCC, SCC	SEER	3	2	3
USA, Louisiana, New Orleans	All exc. BCC, SCC	SEER	3	2	3
USA, Michigan, Detroit	All exc. BCC, SCC	SEER	3	2	3
USA, New Mexico	All exc. BCC, SCC	SEER	3	2	3
USA, Utah	All exc. BCC, SCC	SEER	3	2	3
USA, Washington, Seattle	All exc. BCC, SCC	SEER	3	2	3
USA, SEER	All exc. BCC, SCC	SEER	3	2	3
ASIA					
China, Qidong County	All	None found	N	N	N
China, Shanghai	All	Counted separately	N	N	N
China, Tianjin	All	Counted separately	3	2	3
Hong Kong	BCC, SCC, sebaceous adenoca., dermatofibrosa.	1 tumour	3	3	3
India, Bangalore	All	1BCC. 1SCC	3	3	3
India, Barshi, Paranda, Bhum	All	Counted separately	3	3	3
India, Bombay	BCC, SCC	1BCC, 1SCC	3	N	3
India, Karunagappally	SCC, BCC, baso- squamous cell	By histological type	3	2	3
India, Madras	All	Counted separately	3	N	N
India, Trivandrum	All	By histological type	3	N	N
Israel	All	SEER	3	3	3
Japan, Hiroshima	All	SEER	3	3	3
Japan, Miyagi Prefecture	All	1 primary	3	2	3
Japan, Nagasaki Prefecture	BCC, SCC, Bowen's, adenoacanthoma, mycosis fungoides	IACR	3	2	3
Japan, Osaka Prefecture	All	IACR	3	2	3
Japan, Saga Prefecture	All	By histological type	N	N	N

Table (Contd). 3.2 Coding practices

Registry	Non-melanoma skin cancers		Behaviour codes used for bladder cancer		
	Non-melanoma skin cancer included in the data	Multiple primary rules used for skin cancers	Invasive malignant carcinoma	Non- invasive malignant carcinoma	Malignant carcinoma not otherwise specified
Japan, Yamagata Prefecture	All	1BCC, 1SCC	3	2	3
Korea, Kangwha County	All	Counted separately	3	2	3
Kuwait	All	IACR	3	3	3
Philippines, Manila	BCC, SCC, dermatofibrosarcoma	1BCC, 1SCC	3	2	3
Singapore	All	IACR	3	3	3
Thailand, Chiang Mai	BCC, SCC, carcinoma of skin appendage	IACR	3	3	3
Thailand, Khon Kaen	All	Separately by site	3	N	3
Viet Nam, Hanoi	All	IACR	3	2	3
EUROPE					
Austria, Tyrol	All	IACR	3	2	N
Belarus	All	1BCC, 1SCC	3	3	3
Croatia	N	0	3	2	3
Czech Republic	All	IACR	3	3	3
Denmark	BCC, SCC, epithelial ca. 8010-8011	By histology and 3-digit site	3	1+0+2	3
Estonia	All	1BCC, 1SCC	3	2	3
Finland	All	By histology	0	0	0
France, Bas-Rhin	SCC	SCC only	3	2	3
France, Calvados	All (BCC excl since 1990)	IACR	3	2	1
France, Doubs	All	By histology	3	2	3
France, Haut-Rhin	All (BCC excl. to 1990)	BCC counted separately	3	2	3
France, Hérault	SCC	SCC only	3	2	3
France, Isère	All exc. BCC	SCCs counted separately	3	1or2	3
France, Somme	All but BCC	By subsite	3	1	1
France, Tarn	SCC, others, not BCC	SCCs counted separately	3	2	1
Germany, Eastern States	All exc. BCC	1BCC, 1SCC	3	3	3
Germany, Saarland	BCC, SCC	1BCC, 1SCC	3	3	3
Iceland	All exc. BCC	By histology	3	1or0	3
Ireland, Southern	All	1BCC, 1SCC	3	3	3
Italy, Ferrara Province	All	IACR	3	2	1
Italy, Florence	All	1BCC, 1SCC	3	2	3
Italy, Genoa	All	IACR	3	3	3
Italy, Latina	All	IACR	3	3	3
Italy, Macerata Province	BCC, SCC, epithelioma	IACR	3	3	3
Italy, Modena	BCC, SCC	By 4th digit site	3	3	3
Italy, Parma Province	BCC, SCC	One cancer (worst)	3	3	3
Italy, Ragusa	All	1BCC, 1SCC	3	2	1
Italy, Romagna	All	IACR	3	2	3
Italy, Torino	All	IACR	3	2	3
Italy, Trieste	All	1BCC,1SCC	3	2	3
Italy, Varese Province	All	1BCC, 1SCC	3	2	3
Italy, Venetian Region	All	By histology			
Latvia	All	BCC counted separately			

Table (Contd). 3.2 Coding practices

Registry	Non-melanoma skin cancers		Behaviour codes used for bladder cancer		
	Non-melanoma skin cancer included in the data	Multiple primary rules used for skin cancers	Invasive malignant carcinoma	Non- invasive malignant carcinoma	Malignant carcinoma not otherwise specified
Malta	BCC, SCC	Separately			
Netherlands	All exc. BCC	IACR	3	2	3
Netherlands, Eindhoven	All (BCC in subset)	IACR	3	2	3
Netherlands, Maastricht	All exc. BCC	IACR	3	2	3
Norway	SCC, baso-squamous cell, skin adnexal ca.	IACR	3	3	3
Poland, Cracow	All	Counted separately	3	2	3
Poland, Kielce	All	Counted separately	3	2	1
Poland, Lower Silesia	All	1BCC, SCC subdivided	3	2	1
Poland, Warsaw City	All	By histology	3	3	3
Slovakia	All	1BCC, 1SCC	3	2	3
Slovenia	All	Counted separately	3	2	3
Spain, Albacete	All exc. BCC, SCC	IACR	3	2	3
Spain, Asturias	N	0	3	3	3
Spain, Basque Country	All exc. BCC, epidermoid ca.	IACR	3	2	3
Spain, Granada	All	1BCC, 1SCC	3	2	3
Spain, Mallorca	All	SCC and BCC = 1; others separate	3	2	2 or 3
Spain, Murcia	BCC, SCC	IACR	3	1	3
Spain, Navarra	All	Separately	3	3	3
Spain, Tarragona	All	1BCC, 1SCC	3	3	3
Spain, Zaragoza	All	IACR	3	2	3
Sweden	All exc. BCC	By histology	3	3	3
Switzerland, Basel	All	1BCC, every SCC, others by histology	3	4	N
Switzerland, Geneva	BCC, SCC	1BCC, 1SCC	3	2	2
Switzerland, Graubünden	All	By site and histology	3	2	2
Switzerland, Neuchâtel	All	1BCC, 1SCC	3	2	3
Switzerland, St Gall–Appenzell	All	IACR	3	8	3
Switzerland, Valais	SCC, BCC, adnexal ca., ca. of skin appendage	1BCC. 1SCC	3	2	3
Switzerland, Vaud	All	1BCC, 1SCC	3	2	3
Switzerland, Zurich	All exc. BCC	By histology	3	3	3
UK, England, East Anglia	All	1BCC, others counted separately	3	1	3
UK, England, Merseyside & Cheshire	All	1BCC, all others	3	2	3
UK, England, North Western	BCC, SCC	1BCC, 1SCC	3	1	3
UK, England, Oxford Region	All	1BCC, 1SCC	3	0	3
UK, England, South Thames	All	1BCC, 1SCC, others separate	3	2	3

Table (Contd). 3.2 Coding practices

Registry	Non-melanoma skin cancers		Behaviour codes used for bladder cancer		
	Non-melanoma skin cancer included in the data	Multiple primary rules used for skin cancers	Invasive malignant carcinoma	Non- invasive malignant carcinoma	Malignant carcinoma not otherwise specified
UK, England, South Western	BCC, SCC	1BCC,1SCC	3	2	3
UK, England, Wessex	BCC, SCC for 1988 only	1BCC, 1SCC	3	3	3
UK, England, West Midlands	BCC, SCC	1BCC,1SCC	3	3	3
UK, Yorkshire	All	1BCC, SCC counted separately	3	2	3
UK, Scotland	BCC, SCC	1BCC, up to 5 SCCs	3	3	3
UK, Scotland, West	BCC, SCC	1BCC, all SCC	3	3	3
Yugoslavia, Vojvodina	All	1BCC, 1SCC (1 tumour without HV)	3	3	3
OCEANIA					
Australian Capital Territory	N	0	3	2	3
Australia, New South Wales	N	0	3	2	3
South Australia	N	0			
Australia, Tasmania	N	0	3	2	3
Australia, Victoria	N	0	3	3	3
Western Australia	N	0	3	2	3
French Polynesia	N	0	2	1	9
New Zealand	All exc. BCC, SCC	By histology			
USA, Hawaii	N	0	3	2	3

N = not registered
1 IARC, 1994
2 SEER,1992

4. The effects of the Cancer Incidence in Five Continents data-processing

Data received at IARC were first verified using the IARC CHECK program (Parkin *et al.*, 1994). For the checking process, all data-sets coded to ICD-9 were converted to ICD-O-1. Once the data were checked, any not already so coded were converted to the 2nd edition of ICD-O. This permitted the creation of a database in which every case iscoded to the same classification, and all the data were converted from ICD-O-2 to ICD-9 in the same way.

In the process of converting from ICD-O-2 to ICD-9, some diagnoses disappeared from data sent coded to ICD-O-2. For example, following the conversion rules for ICD-O-2 to ICD-9, the diagnosis papillary mucinous cystadenoma, borderline malignancy (ICD-O-2 8473/3 – a malignant diagnosis) was converted to ICD-9 236.2, a neoplasm of uncertain behaviour and so excluded from the analysis. Similarly, Waldenstrom's macroglobulinaemia (ICD-O-29761/3),alpha heavy chain disease (ICD-O-2 9762/3) and gamma heavy chain disease, Franklin's disease (ICD-O-2 9763/3) convert to ICD-9 273, in the chapter on Endocrine, Nutritional and Metabolic Diseases and Immunity Disorders. So registries which submitted data coded to ICD-O-2 lost a few cases.

5. Classification used in this volume

A number of contributors sent at least part of their data coded to ICD-O-2. One of the first decisions the editors had to take was whether to present data in the present volume by ICD-9 or ICD-10. It was agreed that the ICD-9 classification would be retained as the second edition of ICD-O was not published until 1990, the mid-year of the average data period published in Volume VII, and ICD-10 was not widely used for coding of mortality data during the 1988–92 period. Nonetheless two ICD-10 three character rubrics are included in the tables, mesothelioma and Kaposi's sarcoma, because of their aetiological importance.

The data are presented by ICD-9 with certain modifications and groupings. An abbreviated title is given for each code. The data are published at the three-digit level in the individual registry tables except for one site, penis, for which the fourth digit sub-categories have been used (187.1–187.4 Penis and 187.5–187.9 Other male genital, again foreshadowing the ICD-10 categories C60 and C63). As in Volume VI, Malignant neoplasms of gum, floor of mouth and other and unspecified parts of mouth have been grouped (ICD-9 143-145). Lymphosarcoma (ICD-9 200) and Other reticuloses (ICD-9 202) have been combined under the title Non-Hodgkin lymphoma.

Site	Full title	Groupings used in tables	Short title used in tables
140	Malignant neoplasm of lip	–	Lip
141	Malignant neoplasm of tongue	–	Tongue
142	Malignant neoplasm of major salivary glands	–	Salivary gland
143	Malignant neoplasm of gum	143, 144 & 145 are grouped	Mouth
144	Malignant neoplasm of floor of mouth		
145	Malignant neoplasm of other and unspecified parts of mouth		
146	Malignant neoplasm of oropharynx	–	Oropharynx
147	Malignant neoplasm of nasopharynx		Nasopharynx
148	Malignant neoplasm of hypopharynx	–	Hypopharynx
149	Malignant neoplasm of other and ill-defined sites within the lip, oral cavity and pharynx	–	Pharynx unspecified
150	Malignant neoplasm of oesophagus	–	Oesophagus
151	Malignant neoplasm of stomach		Stomach
152	Malignant neoplasm of small intestine, including duodenum	–	Small intestine
153	Malignant neoplasm of colon	–	Colon
154	Malignant neoplasm of rectum, rectosigmoid junction and anus	–	Rectum
155	Malignant neoplasm of liver and intrahepatic bile ducts	–	Liver
156	Malignant neoplasm of gallbladder and extrahepatic bile ducts	–	Gallbladder etc.
157	Malignant neoplasm of pancreas	–	Pancreas
158	Malignant neoplasm of retroperitoneum and peritoneum	158 is included in Other and unspecified	
159	Malignant neoplasm of other and ill-defined sites within the digestive organs and peritoneum	159 is included in Other and unspecified	
160	Malignant neoplasm of nasal cavities, middle ear and accessory sinuses	–	Nose, sinuses, etc.
161	Malignant neoplasm of larynx	–	Larynx
162	Malignant neoplasm of trachea, bronchus and lung	–	Bronchus, lung
163–4	Malignant neoplasm of pleura, thymus, heart and mediastinum	–	Other thoracic organs
165	Malignant neoplasm of other and ill-defined sites within the respiratory system and intrathoracic organs	165 is included in Other and unspecified	
170	Malignant neoplasm of bone and articular cartilage	–	Bone
171	Malignant neoplasm of connective and other soft tissue	–	Connective tissue
MES	Mesothelioma	–	Mesothelioma
KAP	Kaposi's sarcoma	–	Kaposi's sarcoma
172	Malignant melanoma of skin	–	Melanoma of skin
173	Other malignant neoplasm of skin	–	Other skin
174	Malignant neoplasm of female breast	–	Breast
175	Malignant neoplasm of male breast	–	Breast
179	Malignant neoplasm of uterus, part unspecified	–	Uterus unspecified
180	Malignant neoplasm of cervix uteri	–	Cervix uteri
181	Malignant neoplasm of placenta	–	Placenta
182	Malignant neoplasm of body of uterus	–	Corpus uteri

Table 3.3. Classification used in incidence tables

Table 3.3. (Contd). Classification used in incidence tables

Site	Full title	Groupings used in tables	Short title used in tables
183	Malignant neoplasm of ovary and other uterine adnexa	–	Ovary etc.
184	Malignant neoplasm of other and unspecified female genital organs	–	Other female genital
185	Malignant neoplasm of prostate	–	Prostate
186	Malignant neoplasm of testis	–	Testis
187	Malignant neoplasm of penis and other male genital organs	Not used when data for 187.1–.9 are given	Penis etc.
187.1–.4	Malignant neoplasm of prepuce, glans penis, body of penis and penis, part unspecified	–	Penis
187.5–.9	Malignant neoplasm of epididymis, spermatic cord, scrotum, other and site unspecified	–	Other male genital
188	Malignant neoplasm of bladder	–	Bladder
189	Malignant neoplasm of kidney	–	Kidney etc.
190	Malignant neoplasm of eye	–	Eye
191	Malignant neoplasm of brain	191 & 192	Brain and
192	Malignant neoplasm of other and unspecified parts of nervous system	are grouped together	nervous system
193	Malignant neoplasm of throid gland	–	Thyroid
194	Malignant neoplasm of other endocrine glands and related structures	–	Other endocrine
195	Malignant neoplasm of other and ill-defined sites	195 is included in Other and unspecified	
196	Secondary and unspecified malignant neoplasm of lymph nodes	196 is included in Other and unspecified	
197	Secondary malignant neoplasm of respiratory and digestive system	197 is included in Other and unspecified	
198	Secondary malignant neoplasm of other specified sites	198 is included in Other and unspecified	
199	Malignant neoplasm with specification of site	199 is included in Other and unspecified	
200	Lymphosarcoma and reticulosarcoma	200 & 202 are grouped	Non-Hodgkin lymphoma
201	Hodgkin's disease	–	Hodgkin's disease
202	Other malignant neoplasm of lymphoid and histiocytic tissue	200 & 202 are grouped	Non-Hodgkin lymphoma
203	Multiple myeloma and immunoproliferative neoplasms	–	Multiple myeloma
204	Lymphoid leukaemia	–	Lymphoid leukaemia
205	Myeloid leukaemia	–	Myeloid leukaemia
206	Monocytic leukaemia	–	Monocytic leukaemia
207	Other specified leukaemia	–	Other leukaemia
208	Leukaemia of unspecified cell type	–	Leukaemia unspecified
O & U	Other and unspecified	Comprises 158 (excluding mesothelioma for registries with histological data), 159, 165, 195, 196, 197, 198 & 199	
ALL	All sites	–	All sites
ALLb	All sites but skin	–	All sites excluding Other skin cancer (ICD-9 173)

References

ACS (1951) Manual of tumor nomenclature and coding. New York, NY, American Cancer Society

ACS (1968) Manual of tumor nomenclature and coding. New York, NY, American Cancer Society

CAP (1965) Systematized nomenclature of pathology. Chicago, IL, College of American Pathologists

Doll, R., Payne, P. & Waterhouse, J. (eds) (1966) Cancer Incidence in Five Continents: A Technical Report. Berlin, Springer-Verlag (for UICC)

Doll, R., Muir, C. & Waterhouse, J. (eds) (1970) Cancer Incidence in Five Continents, Volume II. Berlin, Springer-Verlag (for UICC)

Harlow, B.L. & Weiss, N.S. (1989) A case-control study of borderline ovarian tumors: the influence of perineal exposure to talc. Am. J. Epidemiol.. 130, 390–394

IARC (1994) Multiple primaries. Internal Report No. 94/003, IARC, Lyon

Muir, C., Waterhouse, J., Mack, T., Powell, J. & Whelan, S. (eds) (1987) Cancer Incidence in Five Continents, Volume V (IARC Scientific Publications No. 88), Lyon, IARC

Parkin, D.M., Muir, C.S., Whelan, S.L., Gao, Y.-T., Ferlay, J. & Powell, J. (1992) Cancer Incidence in Five Continents, Volume VI. (IARC Scientific Publications No. 120), Lyon, IARC

Parkin, D.M., Chen, V.W., Ferlay, J., Galceran, J., Storm, H.H. & Whelan, S.L. (1994) Comparability and Quality Control in Cancer Registration (IARC Technical Reports No. 19), Lyon, IARC

Powell, J. (1982) Techniques of registration. In: Waterhouse, J., Muir, C., Shanmugaratnam, K. & Powell, J. (eds) Cancer Incidence in Five Continents, Volume IV (IARC Scientific Publications No. 42), Lyon, IARC

Powell, J. (1987) Techniques of registration. In: Muir, C., Waterhouse, J., Mack, T., Powell, J. & Whelan, S. (eds) Cancer Incidence in Five Continents, Volume V (IARC Scientific Publications No. 88), Lyon, IARC

Powell, J. (1992) Techniques of registration. In: Parkin, D.M., Muir, C.S., Whelan, S.L., Gao, Y.-T., Ferlay, J. & Powell, J. Cancer Incidence in Five Continents, Volume VI (IARC Scientific Publications No. 120), Lyon, IARC

SEER (1992) The SEER Program Code Manual, revised edition, Bethesda, MD, National Institutes of Health, National Cancer Institute

Waterhouse, J., Muir, C., Correa, P. & Powell, J. (eds) (1976) Cancer Incidence in Five Continents, Volume III (IARC Scientific Publications No. 15), Lyon, IARC

Waterhouse, J., Muir, C., Shanmugaratnam, K. & Powell, J. (eds) (1982) Cancer Incidence in Five Continents, Volume IV (IARC Scientific Publications No. 42), Lyon, IARC

WHO (1957) International Classification of Diseases, 1955 Revision, Geneva, World Health Organization

WHO (1967) International Classification of Diseases, 1965 Revision, Geneva, World Health Organization

WHO (1977) International Classification of Diseases, 1975 Revision, Geneva, World Health Organization

WHO (1976) International Classification of Diseases for Oncology, first edition, Geneva, World Health Organization

WHO (1990) International Classification of Diseases for Oncology, second edition, Geneva, World Health Organization

Chapter 4. Histological groups

D.M. Parkin, K. Shanmugaratnam, L. Sobin,

J. Ferlay and S.L. Whelan

In this volume, as in Volumes II (Doll et al., 1970) and IV (Waterhouse et al., 1982) of Cancer Incidence in Five Continents, data are presented according to the different histological groupings within certain cancers. The reasons now are as they were then, that the characteristics of certain cancers – particularly with respect to etiology, treatment and prognosis – are better defined by a combination of tumour site plus morphology, than by the largely site-based categories of the International Classification of Diseases (ICD).

Diagnostic subgroups are presented for just 14 cancers, as defined by the ICD-9 codes used in this volume (Table 4.1). These were selected based on several criteria:

- Tumours (ICD categories) that are relatively important numerically;
- Histological subgroups within the ICD categories that have clear etiological, therapeutic or prognostic significance;
- The histological subgroups could be constructed using the morphological terms of the International Classification of Diseases for Oncology (ICD-O). This generally excludes terminology based upon special staining techniques (e.g., glandular and diffuse neoplasms of the stomach (Lauren, 1965)) or immunological methods to detect surface antigens of various types;
- The morphological diagnosis should be relatively reproducible between pathologists, based upon light microscopy of tissue specimens stained with haematoxylin and eosin only.

Table 4.1. Cancers for which histological subtypes are defined in this volume

Site	ICD-9	ICD-10
1. Oesophagus	150	C15
2. Liver	155	C22
3. Lung	162	C34
4. Bone	170	C40 + 41
5. Cervix uteri	180	C53
6. Corpus uteri	182	C54
7. Ovary	183.0	C56
8. Testis	186	C62
9. Bladder	188	C67
10. Kidney etc.	189	C64
11. Eye	190	C69
12. Thyroid	193	C73
13. Hodgkin's disease	201	C81
14. Leukaemia	204–208	C91–95

Several criteria were followed in defining the histological groupings. First, they were specified in terms of the morphological terms (and their corresponding codes) from the ICD-O. Although these are presented below as codes from the second edition (ICD-O-2), the equivalent codes from the first edition (ICD-O-1) can be obtained from tables of conversion (Percy & Van Holten, 1992) or computer programs which perform these conversions (Ferlay, 1994).

Second, the general scheme adopted by Berg (1996) was adopted as the framework. This meant that a category for 'unspecified tumours' (ICD-O 8000–8004) was retained for each site. This category includes all cases that have unknown histology, either because no histological examination was performed or because the results were not interpretable.

Third, while bearing in mind previous publications proposing histological subgroupings within tumour site, an attempt was made to retain relatively broad groupings, at the expense of losing certain specific histological types within them. This principle was adopted in the spirit of trying to maintain maximum comparability between the data from different cancer registries. It also acknowledges that some of the data-sets are rather small, and too fine a categorization would result in very small numbers within some of them.

Only *malignant tumours* (behaviour code /3 in ICD-O) are considered.

The authors made reference to numerous publications by cancer registries during the decisions concerning allocations of terms/codes to different histological groups. The basic reference works were the *International Classification of Diseases for Oncology*, second edition (Percy et al., 1990), the *International Histological Classifications of Tumours* (IHCT; Sobin et al., 1978; Mostofi et al., 1981; Zimmerman, 1980 ; Kreyberg et al 1981; Hedinger et al 1988), and the *International Classification of Childhood Cancer* (Kramárová et al., 1996). Two publications in particular have proposed comprehensive groupings of morphologies within tumour site: the morphological groups of Berg (1996), which provided the basis of the categories employed in the analyses of the SEER population-based data for 1973–87 (Percy et al., 1995), and the EUROCIM database (EUROCIM User's Manual). Finally, articles examining the epidemiology of different histologically defined subgroups within the 15 cancers selected were also perused.

In reviewing the contents of each subgroup, reference was made to an enormous database of cancer registry records available at IARC. Primarily, this comprised the data-sets included in *Cancer Incidence in Five Continents* Volume VI (but excluding those for which histology was unverified), but it included in addition the data from the US SEER program from 1973–92, the EUROCIM database, and records from certain cancer registries, predominantly in Africa, Asia and Latin

America, in collaboration with IARC and for which validation and correction of the database had already been carried out. For the 14 sites under consideration, some three million records were included, of which some 79% were reported as histologically verified.

The tabulations in this volume comprise simply the frequency of different histological subtypes (including the category 'uncertain histology') within the total of morphologically verified cases for the particular ICD category. The total number of registrations at the site are also provided, to indicate the proportion of cases with morphological verification (the figure is reproduced in the tables of indicators of quality also). Restriction to morphologically verified cases loses some information on subtypes, particularly for those cancers for which a reasonably accurate diagnosis can be obtained without histological examination (e.g., melanoma, Kaposi's sarcoma, retinoblastoma). If one makes the assumption that cases without a diagnosis based on histology or cytology have the same profile of histological subtypes as those with a tissue diagnosis, the percentages shown can be applied to the total number of cases (and the crude incidence rate) for a given site.

We have not attempted in this volume to present the breakdown by age-group, nor to calculate incidence rates by histological subtype. This level of detail is available in the electronic publication IARC CancerBase No. 2 (Ferlay, 1997).

The subgroups used, and their content in terms of ICD-O-2 morphology codes, are reproduced below. The justification for the choice of subgroups, and of their constituent histolog-ical entities, is contained in an IARC Technical Report (Parkin *et al.*, in preparation), which also provides a comput-er soft-ware for creating the subgroups from case listings. A few notes on each cancer site and its subgroups are included here. In addition, the following general points are pertinent:

1. Within each cancer in Table 4.1, the ICD-O M codes within the histological subgrouping include virtually all of those observed within the huge IARC database referred to above. Some are extremely rare occurrences (and will normally have been 'flagged' as such by some verification procedure within the registry or at IARC). Only morphological entities which were deemed frankly impossible at a given site have been excluded, in order that cancer registries will not have difficulties in allocating rare tumours to the subgroups (the process can be performed by computer program, without the need for 'hand coding')

2. Within the first 12 tumour sites listed in Table 4.1, there are no cases of mesothelioma (ICD-O 9050–9055, Kaposi's sarcoma (9140), lymphoma (9590–9764) or leukaemia (9800–9941). These cancers have their own specific ICD codes within the 10th revision (and hence appear as separate lines in the tabulations by site in this volume).

3. ICD-O M code 8050 (papillary carcinoma NOS) is a term of variable meaning. When an organ contains an appreciable number of other epidermoid carcinomas, this term also is assumed to mean a papillary epidermoid carcinoma. Where the organ is the site of many adenocarcinomas and few epidermoid carcinomas, the term is assumed to refer to papillary adenocarcinomas. For organs where the majority of carcinomas are of transitional cell type (urinary tract), it is assumed to refer to papillary transitional cell carcinomas.

Table 4.2. Oesophagus

1	**Carcinoma**	**8010-8572**
	1.1 Squamous cell carcinoma	8050-8076
	1.2 Adenocarcinoma (include adenosquamous, mucinous, adenoid cystic, mucoepidermoid and Barrett carcinoma)	8140-8141, 8190-8231, 8260-8263, 8310, 8430, 8480-8490, 8560,
	1.3 Other specified carcinomas	8570-8572
	1.4 Unspecified carcinoma	8010-8034
2	**Sarcoma**	**8800-8811, 8830, 8840-8920, 8990-8991, 9040-9044, 9120-9133, 9150, 9540-9581**
3	**Other specified cancer (include melanoma, carcinosarcoma)**	
4	**Unspecified cancer**	**8000-8004**

Oesophagus

The Adenocarcinoma group excludes cancers which normally occur in gastric epithelium (linitis plastica (8142)), adenocarcinoma, intestinal type (8144), carcinoma, diffuse (8145)) . It includes mucoepidermoid carcinomas (8430), sometimes considered as distinct malignant tumours, but because of their rarity (1.4% of oesophageal tumours (7.4% of oesophageal adenocarcinomas)), the distinction appears hardly worthwhile. The principal cancers in the 'Other Specified Carcinomas' group are small cell carcinomas (8040–8045). In this category also is 'basaloid squamous cell carcinoma', a recently described high-grade tumour that does not yet have an ICD-O morphology code. Of the codes currently available, 8123 (basaloid carcinoma) is the most appropriate for this tumour.

Table 4.3. Liver

1	**Carcinoma**	**8010-8572**
	1.1 Hepatocellular carcinoma	8170-8171
	1.2[a] Cholangiocarcinoma (all intrahepatic biliary carcinomas, i.e. all adenocarcinomas and adenosquamous carcinoma)	8050, 8140-8141, 8160-8161, 8260, 8440, 8480-8500, 8550, 8560, 8570-8572
	1.3 Other specified carcinomas (include combined hepatocellular and cholangiocarcinoma, carcinoid)	
	1.4 Unspecified carcinoma	8010-8034
2	**Hepatoblastoma**	**8970**
3	**Sarcoma**	
	3.1 Haemangiosarcoma	9120-9133, 9161
	3.2 Other sarcomas	8800-8811, 8830, 8840-8920, 8990-8991, 9040-9044, 9150, 9170, 9540-9581
4	**Other specified cancer**	
5	**Unspecified cancer**	**8000-8004**

[a]The category Cholangiocarcinoma applies to all primary carcinomas of the liver of biliary epithelial type; i.e. all carcinomas other than hepatocellular carcinoma and combined hepatocellular and cholangiocarcinoma.

Liver

The groupings largely follow those of the IHCT (Gibson & Sobin, 1978). Combined hepatocellular and cholangiocarcinomas (8180), which comprised 0.12% of cancers of known histology in the IARC database, appear in the 'Other specified carcinomas' category.

<table>
<tr><td colspan="2">Table 4.4. Lung</td></tr>
<tr><td>1 Carcinoma</td><td>8010-8572</td></tr>
<tr><td>1.1 Squamous cell carcinoma</td><td>8050-8076</td></tr>
<tr><td>1.2 Adenocarcinoma</td><td>8140,
8211,
8230-8231,
8250-8260
8323,
8480-8490,
8550-8560,
8570-8572</td></tr>
<tr><td>1.3 Small-cell carcinoma</td><td>8040-8045</td></tr>
<tr><td>1.4 Large-cell carcinoma
(include giant cell, clear-cell
and large-cell undifferentiated
carcinoma)</td><td>8012-8031,
8310</td></tr>
<tr><td>1.5[a] Other specified carcinomas
(include adenoid cystic,
mucoepidermoid, and
large-cell neuroendocrine
carcinomas, and carcinoid tumour)</td><td></td></tr>
<tr><td>1.6 Unspecified carcinoma</td><td>8010-8011,
8032-8034</td></tr>
<tr><td>2 Sarcoma</td><td>8800-8811,
8830,
8840-8920,
8990-8991,
9040-9044,
9120-9133,
9150,
9540-9581</td></tr>
<tr><td>3 Other specified cancer
(include pulmonary blastoma)</td><td></td></tr>
<tr><td>4 Unspecified cancer</td><td>8000-8004</td></tr>
</table>

[a] The separation of bronchial gland carcinomas (adenoid cystic and mucoepidermoid carcinomas) from other adenocarcinomas, as in the WHO classification, is based on differences in etiology and prognosis.

Mesotheliomas are *not* included in any group, as they are tabulated separately in this volume. Mesothelioma in lung tissue, as opposed to pleura, must be very rare (1.5% and 81.5% of mesotheliomas, respectively, in the SEER database (Mack, 1995)).

Lung

In the scheme adopted here, there are six groups of carcinomas.

Squamous cell cancers correspond to group 1 of the IHCT (Kreyberg *et al.*, 1981) and include 'papillary carcinoma NOS' (8050). *Adenocarcinoma* excludes bronchial gland carcinomas (adenoid cystic (8200) and mucoepidermoid (8430)) which appear in 'other specified carcinomas'. *Small-cell carcinoma* corresponds to group 2 of the IHCT. *Large-cell carcinoma* corresponds to group 4 of the IHCT and includes cancers so described (8012) as well as undifferentiated carcinomas (8020-8022), giant cell carcinomas (8030, 8031), and clear cell adenocarcinoma (8310). *Other specified carcinoma* includes the carcinoid tumours, bronchiolar gland tumours and 'mixed' tumours and carcinosarcomas (categories 6, 7 and 8, respectively, in the IHCT).

Table 4.5. Bone cancer

1	**Sarcoma**	**8800-8920, 9040-9044, 9120-9133, 9150, 9180-9250, 9260, 9540-9581**
	1.1 Osteosarcoma	9180-9200
	1.2 Chondrosarcoma	9220-9240
	1.3 Ewing sarcoma	9260
	1.4 Fibrosarcoma and malignant fibrous histiocytoma	8810-8812, 8830
	1.5 Other specified sarcomas (include angiosarcoma, malignant giant cell tumour and PNET)	
	1.6 Unspecified sarcoma	8800-8804
2	**Other specified cancer** (include chordoma, adamantinoma of long bones)	
3	**Unspecified cancer**	**8000-8004**

Table 4.6. Cervix uteri

1	**Carcinoma**	**8010-8572**
	1.1 Squamous cell carcinoma	8051-8076
	1.2 Adenocarcinoma (include adenosquamous carcinoma, adenocarcinoma with squamous differentiation, mucoepidermoid and adenoid cystic carcinomas)	8050, 8140-8141, 8190-8211, 8230-8231, 8260-8263, 8310, 8380, 8430, 8440-8490, 8510, 8560, 8570-8572,
	1.3 Other specified carcinoma	
	1.4 Unspecified carcinoma	8010-8034
2	**Sarcoma**	**8800-8811, 8830, 8840-8920, 8990-8991, 9040-9044, 9120-9133, 9150, 9540-9581**
3	**Other specified cancer** (include mullerian mixed tumour, carcinosarcoma, melanoma)	
4	**Unspecified cancer**	**8000-8004**

Bone cancer

The groups proposed regroup the categories of the IHCT (Schajowicz *et al.*, 1972) with the exception of tumours of lymphoid tissue or bone marrow, which appear with the lymphomas.

The main categories are: Osteosarcomas (Group I); Chondrosarcomas (Group II), and Ewing's sarcoma (part of Group IV). These three groups contain the same ICD-O entities as groups a-c in the *International Incidence of Childhood Cancer* (Kramárová *et al.*, 1996). Fibrosarcoma (part of group VI), includes malignant fibrous histiocytoma arising in bone. The 'Other sarcomas' category includes principally malignant giant cell tumours (group III, 9250); angiosarcomas (group V, 9120-9133) and liposarcomas (part of group VI, 8850).

The other specified tumours include mesenchymomas, chordomas and adamantinomas.

Cervix uteri

The groupings divide the carcinomas into four categories: squamous, adenocarcinoma, other specified and unspecified. Certain carcinomas which do not occur in the cervical epithelium are omitted from the squamous cell and adenocarcinoma groups. Papillary carcinoma NOS (0.5% of cases in the IARC database) is included with the adenocarcinomas. No distinction is made between the various types of adenocarcinoma listed in the IHCT (Poulsen *et al.*, 1975). Adenosquamous carcinomas (8560–8570) are included with the adenocarcinmas – they comprise 7.6% of this group in the IARC database.

Table 4.7. Corpus uteri

1	**Carcinoma**	**8010-8572**
	1.1 Adenocarcinoma (include adenosquamous carcinoma and adenocarcinoma with squamous differentiation)	8050, 8140-8141, 8190-8211, 8230-8231, 8260-8263, 8310, 8380, 8430, 8440-8490, 8510, 8560, 8570-8572
	1.2 Other specified carcinoma (include squamous cell carcinoma, clear-cell carcinoma)	
	1.3 Unspecified carcinoma	8010-8034
2	**Sarcoma** (include leiomyosarcoma, endometrial stromal sarcoma)	**8800-8811, 8830, 8840-8920, 8990-8991, 9040-9044, 9120-9133, 9150, 9540-9581**
3	**Other specified cancer** (include mullerian mixed tumour, carcinosarcoma, adenosarcoma)	
4	**Unspecified cancer**	**8000-8004**

Table 4.8. Ovary

1	**Carcinoma**	**8010-8570, 9014-9015, 9110[1]**
	1.1 Serous carcinoma	8441-8462, 9014
	1.2 Mucinous carcinoma	8470-8490, 9015
	1.3 Endometrioid carcinoma	8380-8381, 8560, 8570
	1.4 Clear cell carcinoma	8310-8313, 9110
	1.5 Adenocarcinoma NOS	8140-8190, 8211-8231, 8260, 8440
	1.6 Other specified carcinomas	
	1.7 Unspecified carcinoma	8010-8034
2	**Sex cord-stromal tumours**	**8590-8671**
3	**Germ cell tumours**	**8240-8245, 9060-9102**
4	**Other specified cancers** (include malignant Brenner tumour, mullerian mixed tumour, carcinosarcoma)	
5	**Unspecified cancer**	**8000-8004**

1.1–1.2: Categories 1.1 and 1.2 include tumours of borderline malignancy (low malignant potential). Unlike other borderline tumours, ICD-O includes borderline tumours of serous and mucinous type with carcinomas. This approach remains to be fully validated.

1 Excludes 8240-8245

Corpus uteri

The groupings proposed are identical to those of cervix cancer, except that squamous cell carcinomas are grouped with 'other specified carcinomas' because of their rarity at this site (they comprise only 0.9% of carcinomas in the IARC database).

Ovary

The categories are based primarily upon those in the IHCT (Serov *et al.*, 1973). The first four 'epithelial' carcinomas correspond to malignant serous (IA), mucinous (IB), endometrioid (IC) and clear-cell (ID) tumours. Among the carcinomas not encompassed within these four groups, the majority in the IARC database were various adenocarcinomas which cannot be allocated to any of the above groups, and are hence included in a category labelled 'Adenocarcinoma, NOS'. Sex cord/stromal tumours (Group II of the IHCT) retain their own group. Germ cell tumours include dysgerminomas, embryonal carcinomas and teratomas, as well as the rare carcinoid tumours of the ovary (Group IV of the IHCT), and the very rare gonadoblastomas (Group V). Lipid-cell tumours (Group III), Brenner tumours (group IE) and sarcomas (group VI) are very rare (<1% of cases in the IARC database) and are consigned to the 'other specified' subgroup.

Table 4.9. Testis cancer

1	**Germ cell tumours**	**9060-9102**
	1.1 Seminoma	9060-9064
	1.2 Other germ cell tumours	
	1.2.1 Embryonal carcinoma (include yolk sac tumour)	9070-9073
	1.2.2 Malignant teratoma	9080-9085, 9102
	1.2.3 Choriocarcinoma	9100-9101
2	**Other specified cancers** (include sex cord-stromal tumour)	
3	**Unspecified cancer**	**8000-8004**

Testis cancer

The groupings proposed correspond to the IHCT (Mostofi & Sobin 1977). They separate germ cell tumours from other specified cancers, and recognize four specific types of germ cell tumours: seminomas (9060–9064), embryonal carcinomas (9070–9073), malignant teratomas (9080–9085, 9102), and (more rare) choriocarcinomas (9100–9101).

Table 4.10. Bladder

1	**Carcinoma**	**8010-8570**
	1.1 Squamous cell carcinoma	8051-8076
	1.2 Transitional cell carcinoma (include transitional cell	8050, 8120-8122, 8130
	carcinoma with squamous and/or glandular differentiation)	
	1.3 Adenocarcinoma	8140-8145, 8190-8231, 8260-8263, 8310, 8480-8490, 8560, 8570
	1.4 Other specified carcinoma	
	1.5 Unspecified carcinoma	8010-8034
2	**Sarcoma**	**8800-8811, 8830, 8840-8920, 8990-8991, 9040-9044, 9120-9133, 9150, 9540-9581**
3	**Other specified cancer** (phaeochromocytoma, malignant paraganglioma, melanoma, carcinosarcoma)	
4	**Unspecified cancer**	**8000-8004**

Bladder

Transitional cell carcinomas (groups ID and IE in the IHCT (Mostofi *et al.*, 1973)) comprise the majority of carcinomas. Tumours coded 8050 (papillary carcinoma NOS) are assumed to be papillary transitional cell carcinomas (8130). The adenocarcinoma group comprised only 2% of histologically verified cases in the IARC database.

Table 4.11. Kidney etc.

1	**Carcinoma**	**8010-8570**
	1.1 Squamous, transitional cell carcinomas (epithelial tumours of renal pelvis)	8050-8130
	1.2 Renal cell carcinoma	8140, 8260, 8270-8312
	1.3 Other specified carcinoma	
	1.4 Unspecified carcinoma	8010-8034
2	**Nephroblastoma** (Wilms tumour), (include rhabdoid tumour, clear cell sarcoma)	**8960-8964**
3	**Sarcoma**	**8800-8811, 8830, 8840-8920, 8990-8991, 9040-9044, 9120-9133, 9150, 9540-9581**
4	**Other specified cancer**	
5	**Unspecified cancer**	**8000-8004**

Table 4.12. Eye

1	**Retinoblastoma**	**9510-9512**
2	**Malignant melanoma**	**8720-8790**
3	**Carcinoma**	**8010-8572**
	3.1 Squamous cell carcinoma	8050-8082
	3.2 Other specified carcinomas	
	3.3 Unspecified carcinoma	8010-8034
4	**Sarcoma**	**8800-8811, 8830, 8840-8920, 8990-8991, 9040-9044, 9120-9133, 9150, 9540-9581**
5	**Other specified cancers** (include glial tumours)	
6	**Unspecified cancer**	**8000-8004**

Kidney etc.

The rubric 189 within the ICD-9 includes kidney (189.0), renal pelvis (189.1), ureter (189.2) and urethra (189.3) as well as 'Urinary system NOS' (189.9). Tumours labelled 'kidney' without further specification, are coded to the rubric 189.0. This means that certain tumours of the renal pelvis will be so recorded, and explains why tumours of the urinary epithelium (transitional cell carcinomas, papillary carcinomas, squamous cell carcinomas) are found within this rubric, although they are properly tumours of the renal pelvis, rather than the parenchyma of the kidney.

The groupings of carcinomas for tumours of the kidney thus provides for 'squamous, papillary and transitional cell carcinomas' (8050-8130) corresponding to group II (Epithelial tumours of the renal pelvis) in the International Histological Classification (Mostofi *et al.*, 1981).

Epithelial tumours of the renal parenchyma (Group I of the IHCT) are primarily renal cell carcinoma (8312). We include adenocarcinomas NOS (8140) with this group, as well as papillary adenocarcinoma NOS (8260), assuming that certain renal cell carcinomas may have been so specified, or coded, in cancer registry data.

Wilms' tumour (nephroblastoma) has its own subgroup, as do the sarcomas.

Eye

The ICD rubrics for 'eye' (190 in ICD-9, C69 in ICD-10) include adnexae such as the lacrimal gland and duct, as well as 'orbit'. Tumours of these structures are accommodated within the code groupings for 'eye' (Zimmermann and Sobin, 1980).

The principal eye cancers – retinoblastoma and malignant melanoma – form two groups. The carcinomas (11.4% of eye cancers in the IARC database) are divided into squamous cell carcinomas (70% of the carcinomas) – principally tumours of the conjunctiva and cornea, other carcinomas, which comprises almost entirely adenocarcinomas (14.6%), mainly originating in the lacrimal gland and duct, and unspecified carcinomas (14.3% of carcinomas) which could be either.

Table 4.13. Thyroid	
1 Carcinoma	**8010-8511**
1.1 Follicular carcinoma	8290, 8330-8334
1.2 Papillary carcinoma	8050, 8260, 8340, 8350, 8450
1.3 Medullary carcinoma	8510-8511
1.4 Anaplastic carcinoma (include undifferentiated carcinoma, giant cell carcinoma)	8020-8034
1.5 Other specified carcinoma	
1.6 Unspecified carcinoma	8010-8012
2 Sarcoma	**8800-8811, 8830, 8840-8920, 8990-8991, 9040-9044, 9120-9133, 9150, 9540-9581**
3 Other specified cancer	
4 Unspecified cancer	**8000-8004**

Table 4.14. Hodgkin's disease	
1 Lymphocytic predominance	**9657-9659, 9660**
2 Nodular sclerosis	**9663-9667**
3 Mixed cellularity	**9652**
4 Lymphocytic depletion	**9653-9655**
5 Unspecified Hodgkin's disease	**9650, 9661, 9662**

Hodgkin's disease
Subdivision of Hodgkin's disease is generally carried out according to the Rye classification (Lukes *et al.*, 1966), which delineates four subgroups: lymphocytic predominance, nodular sclerosis, mixed cellularity and lymphocytic depletion. Cases classified as 'paragranuloma' under the old Jackson–Parker (1944) classification can be regrouped with the lymphocytic predominance category, while cases described as 'Hodgkin's granuloma and sarcoma' are not readily reallocated, and so are left in a category termed 'other specified'.

Thyroid
The scheme proposed follows the most recent revision of the IHCT (Hedinger *et al.*, 1988). The follicular carcinomas and papillary carcinomas provide the majority of thyroid cancers, the latter includes follicular carcinomas with a papillary component (8340). The anaplastic carcinomas (undifferentiated, giant cell, spindle cell carcinomas) are separated from 'unspecified carcinomas'. Small cell carcinoma (8040–8045) is specifically excluded, since the great majority of tumours previously so diagnosed are in fact lymphomas (Hedinger *et al.*, 1989), and should thus appear with the lymphomas. Squamous carcinomas (0.6% of thyroid cancers) are no longer recognized as a major histological type in the IHCT and are included in 'Other specified carcinomas'.

Table 4.15. Leukaemias

LEUKAEMIA		**9800-9941**
1	**Lymphoid**	**9820-9827, 9940–1**[a]
	1.1 Acute	9821, 9826
	1.2 Chronic	9823
	1.3 Other specified leukemia	
	1.4 Unspecified	9820
2	**Myeloid**	**9860-9868, 9930**
	2.1 Acute	9861, 9866-9867
	2.2 Chronic	9863, 9868, 9870, 9880
	2.3 Other specified (include granulocytic sarcoma)	
	2.4 Unspecified	9860
3.	**Monocytic**	**9890-9894**
	3.1 Acute	9891
	3.2 Chronic	9893
	3.3 Other specified	
	3.4 Unspecified	9890
4	**Other specified leukaemia**[b]	**9801-9804, 9840-9850, 9870-9880, 9900-9910 9931-9932**
	4.1 Acute	9801, 9841, 9910, 9931, 9932
	4.2 Chronic	9803, 9842
	4.3 Other	
5	**Unspecified leukaemia**	**9800**

[a] Hairy cell leukaemia and Leukaemic reticuloendotheliosis included within lymphoid leukaemia in ICD-10.

[b] Plasma cell leukaemia (9830) is excluded (it is classified with myeloma in ICD-9 203.1 and ICD-10 C90.1). Hairy cell leukaemia (9940) and leukaemic reticuloendotheliosis (9941) are excluded (they are classified with the non-Hodgkin lymphomas in ICD-9 (202.4) and with lymphoid leukaemias in ICD-10 (C91.4).

Leukaemias

The groupings of codes proposed allow extraction of data to the main cellular types (lymphoid, myeloid and monocytic), or to examine all acute or chronic leukaemias as a group (by combining the --1 or --2 subgroups).

Subacute leukaemias have been left with the 'other specified' subgroups.

References

Berg, J.W. (1996) Morphologic classification of human cancer. In: Schottenfeld, D. & Fraumeni, J.F., Jr. Cancer Epidemiology and Prevention, 2nd edition, Chapter 3 of Section 1: Basic Concepts; Oxford, New York, Oxford University Press, pp. 28-44

Doll, R., Muir, C. & Waterhouse, J. eds. (1970) Cancer Incidence in Five Continents, Vol. II, International Union Against Cancer, Berlin, Heidelberg, New York, Springer-Verlag

European Cancer Incidence and Mortality Database (EUROCIM) User Manual (1995) 2nd edition

Ferlay, J. (1994) ICD Conversion Programs for Cancer (IARC Technical Report No. 21), Lyon, IARC

Ferlay, J. (1997) Cancer Incidence in Five Continents VII (IARC CancerBase No. 2), Lyon, IARC

Gibson, J.B. & Sobin, L.H. (1978) Histological Typing of Tumours of the Liver, Biliary Tract and Pancreas (IHCT No. 20), Geneva, World Health Organization

Hedinger, C., Williams, E.D. & Sobin, L.H. (1988) Histological Typing of Thyroid Cancers (IHCT No. 11, 2nd edition), Geneva, World Health Organization

Hedinger, C., Williams, E.D. & Sobin, L.H. (1989) The WHO histological classification of thyroid tumors: a commentary on the second edition. Cancer, 63, 908–911

Jackson, H. and Parker, F. (1944) Hodgkin's disease. II Pathology. New Engl. J. Med., 231, 35–44

Kramárová, E., Stiller, C.A., Ferlay, J., Parkin, D.M. Draper, G.J., Michaelis, J., Neglia, J. & Qureshi, S. (1996) The International Classifiction of Childhood Cancer (IARC Technical Report No. 29), Lyon, IARC

Kreyberg, L., Liebow, A.A. & Vehlinger, E.A. (1981) Histological Typing of Lung Tumours (IHCT No. 1, 2nd edition), Geneva, World Health Organization

Lauren, P. (1965) The two histological main types of gastric carcinoma: diffuse and so-called intestinal-type carcinoma. Acta Pathol. Microbiol. Scand., 64, 31–49

Lukes, R.J., Craver, L.F., Hall, T.C., Rappaport, H. & Ruben, P. (1966) Report of the nomenclature committee. Cancer Res., 26, 1311

Mack, T.M. (1995) Sarcomas and Other Malignancies of Soft Tissue, Retroperitoneum, Peritoneum, Pleura, Heart, Mediastinum, and Spleen. Histology of Cancer. Incidence and Prognosis: SEER Population-Based Data, 1973-1987. Supplement to Cancer, American Cancer Society, Philadelphia

Mostofi, F.K. & Sobin, L.H. (1977) Histological Typing of Testis Tumours (IHCT No 16) Geneva, World Health Organization

Mostofi, F.K., Sesterhenn, I.A. & Sobin, L.H. (1981) Histological Typing of Kidney Tumours (IHCT No 25) Geneva, World Health Organization

Mostofi, F.K., Sobin, L.H. & Torloni, H. (1973) Histological Typing of Urinary Bladder Tumours (IHCT No 10) Geneva, World Health Organization

Parkin, D.M., Sobin, L., Shanmugaratnam, K., Ferlay, J. & Whelan, S.L. (1997) Histological subtypes of common cancers: Diagnostic groups for comparative studies of incidence and survival (IARC Technical Reports), Lyon, IARC (in preparation)

Percy, C. & Van Holten, V. (1992) Conversion of Neoplasms by Topography and Morphology from the International Classification of Diseases for Oncology, 2nd edition (ICD-O-2) to International Classification of Diseases for Oncology (ICD-O), Bethesda, MD, National Cancer Institute

Percy, C., Van Holten, V. & Muir, C.S., eds (1990) International Classification of Diseases for Oncology, 2nd edition (ICD-O-2). Geneva, World Health Organization

Percy, C., Young, J.L. Jr., Muir, C., Ries, L., Hankey, B., Sobin, L.H. & Berg, J.W. (1995) Histology of Cancer. Incidence and Prognosis: SEER Population-Based Data, 1973-1987. Supplement to Cancer, American Cancer Society, Philadelphia

Poulsen, H.E., Taylor, C.W. & Sobin, L.H. (1975) Histological typing of female genetal tract tumours. (IHCT No. 13), Geneva, World Health Organization

Schajowicz, F., Ackerman, L.V. & Sissons, H.A. (1972) Histological Typing of Bone Tumours (IHCT No. 6), Geneva, World Health Organization

Serov, S.F. & Scully, R.E. (1973) Histological Typing of Ovarian Tumours. (IHCT No. 9) Geneva, World Health Organization

Sobin, L.H., Thomas, L.B., Percy, C. & Henson, D.E. (1978) A Coded Compendium of the International Histological Classification of Tumours, World Health Organization, Geneva

Waterhouse, J., Muir, C., Shanmugaratnam, K. & Powell, J. (1982) Cancer Incidence in Five Continents Vol IV (IARC Scientific Publications No. 42), Lyon, IARC

Zimmermann, L.E. & Sobin, L.H. (1980) Histological Typing of Tumours of the Eye and its Adnexa (IHCT No 24), Geneva, World Health Organization

Chapter 5. Comparability and quality of data

D.M. Parkin

The purpose of Cancer Incidence in Five Continents is to present comparable incidence rates of cancer from different populations world-wide. The process of selection of data to be included and the preparation of the data-sets by the editors therefore require careful attention to several aspects related to comparability. As far as the cases registered are concerned, these include :

(*a*)　The definition of an incident case of cancer,
(*b*)　The completeness of enumeration of cases in the population covered,
(*c*)　The accuracy of abstraction and coding of information.

In addition to these, the denominator, person-years at risk for the period under consideration, should be estimated as accurately as possible.

In this chapter we consider the evaluation of data quality undertaken by the editors for this volume, and introduce the traditional tables of 'Indices of Data Quality' with which the users themselves can make judgements on the completeness and validity of the different data-sets.

In contrast to recent volumes of *Cancer Incidence in Five Continents*, this chapter does not present a detailed description of the standard definitions used by cancer registries to define an incident cancer, or the indices of comparability or validity that are generally applied. This material is now to be found in the publication *Comparability and Quality Control in Cancer Registration* (Parkin *et al.*, 1994), to which reference will be made throughout the chapter.

The following chapter, on Processing of Data, makes it clear that a considerable amount of work is undertaken in verifying coding, identifying possible duplicate registrations, querying unlikely or impossible combinations of codes, and conversion to a standard format even before any tabulations are prepared for editorial evaluation. These steps in validation of the data are part of the routine to which the great majority of data-sets are subjected, and the fact that it has been completed more or less successfully forms part of the editorial evaluation. Eight data-sets, for which no morphological data were available, are marked with a special flag (+); see below.

At their formal meetings, the editors had available to them:

(*a*)　The questionnaire responses which relate to definitions used by the registry (Table 5.1),
(*b*)　The tables of age-, sex- and site-specific incidence rates which comprise the bulk of this volume (Age-Specific and Age-Standardized Incidence Rates),
(*c*)　A set of editorial tables (Table 5.3),
(*d*)　The estimated population at risk, with the method

of estimation used and, superposed upon it (for registries appearing in the previous volume), the estimated population five years previously (Figure 5.1)

1. Comparability
1.1. Definition of incidence
Particular attention is required in three broad areas:

(*a*)　The distinction between recurrence or extension of an existing cancer, and the development of a new primary,
(*b*)　The detection of cancers incidentally, in asymptomatic individuals,
(*c*)　The detection of cancers at autopsy.
The rules used to distinguish new primary cancers from extensions/recurrences are set out in the IARC/IACR definitions (IARC, 1994). All contributing registries were asked whether they had recorded new primary cancers according to these rules. If not, they were requested to either:

(*a*)　recode the data themselves according to these rules, or
(*b*)　state how their own rules differed, so that the dataset provided could be recoded according to the IARC/IACR rules (N.B., this required that all cancers in the same individual could be identified).

Because of more thorough efforts to achieve standardization for Volume VII, the majority of data-sets now conform with the standard definition, and are thus more comparable in this respect. (Exceptions are noted in Table 5.1.)

As a corollary, it should be noted that the results in *Cancer Incidence in Five Continents* may not be exactly the same as those published by the cancer registries themselves, using their own definition of multiple primaries (see also Chapter 3). Similarly, it is possible that there are minor divergences in the definitions used between Volumes VI and VII for certain registries (this can be verified by comparing Tables 6.1 in Volume VI and 5.1 in this volume).

The sites likely to be most affected by varying definitions of multiple primaries are shown in Table 5.2, together with the differences in incidence for the SEER registries of the United States, using their own rather generous definition of 'second primary' (SEER, 1992) and the IARC/IACR rules.

For those registries which record non-melanoma skin cancers, it should be noted that the IARC/IACR rules specify that only one epidermoid carcinoma be recorded as a primary tumour. Such registries will often have recorded separately squamous cell and basal cell carcinomas (Table 3.2). If their data have been recoded, they will find that the number of registered cases is considerably reduced in the tables in this volume.

Table 5.1. Registration practices

Registry	Multiple primary rules	Includes incidental prostate cancer	Cancer cases with necropsy (%)	Includes cases at necropsy only
AFRICA				
Algeria, Sétif	I	Y	NK	N
France, La Réunion	I	Y		N
Mali, Bamako	I (S)	Y	NK	N
Uganda, Kyadondo County	I	Y	1%	Y
Zimbabwe, Harare	I (S)	Y	NK	Y
CENTRAL AND SOUTH AMERICA				
Argentina, Concordia	I (S)	Y	NK	Y
Brazil, Belém	I	Y	NK	Y
Brazil, Goiania	I (S)	Y	NK	Y
Brazil, Porto Alegre	I	Y	NK	Y
Colombia, Cali	I	Y	NK	Y
Costa Rica	I (S)	Y	NK	Y
Ecuador, Quito	I (S)	Y	0.06%	Y
Peru, Lima	I (S)	Y		N
Peru, Trujillo	I (S)	Y	NK	Y
USA, Puerto Rico	I	Y	0.52%	Y
Uruguay, Montevideo	I	Y	NK	N
NORTH AMERICA				
Canada, Alberta	C1	Y	4.60%	Y
Canada, British Columbia	C2	Y	9%	Y
Canada, Manitoba	C3	Y	NK	Y
Canada, New Brunswick	I (S)	Y	NK	Y
Canada, Newfoundland	C4	Y	NK	Y
Canada, Northwest Territories	I	Y	NK	Y
Canada, Nova Scotia	C5	Y	NK	Y
Canada, Ontario	I	N	< 6%	Y
Canada, Prince Edward Island	C2	Y	~5%	Y
Canada, Quebec	I	N	3 to 5%	N
Canada, Saskatchewan	I	Y	3%	Y
Canada, Yukon				
USA, California, Central Valley	I*	Y	NK	Y
USA, California, Los Angeles County	I*	Y	NK	Y
USA, California, San Francisco Bay Area	I*	Y	NK	Y
USA, Connecticut	I*	Y	NK	Y
USA, Georgia, Atlanta	I*	Y	3.80%	Y
USA, Iowa	I*	Y	NK	Y
USA, Louisiana, Central Region	I*	Y	NK	Y
USA, Louisiana New Orleans	I*	Y	NK	Y
USA, Michigan, Detroit	I*	Y	NK	Y
USA, New Mexico	I*	Y	3-5%	Y
USA, Utah	I*			
USA, Washington, Seattle	I*	N	NK	Y
USA, SEER	I*	Y	NK	Y
ASIA				
China, Qidong County	I	N	< 0.1%	N
China, Shanghai	I (S)	Y	NK	Y
China, Tianjin	I (S)	Y	< 1%	Y
Hong Kong	I	Y	NK	N
Indian, Bangalore	I (S)	Y		Y

Table 5.1. (Contd). Registration practices

Registry	Multiple primary rules	Includes incidental prostate cancer	Cancer cases with necropsy (%)	Includes cases at necropsy only
India, Barshi, Paranda and Bhum	I (S)	Y	NK	Y
India, Bombay	I (S)	Y	NK	Y
India, Karunagappally	I (S)	Y		
India, Madras	M	Y	0%	NA
Indian, Trivandrum	I (S)	Y		
Israel	I	Y	NK	Y
Japan, Hiroshima	S	Y	5%	Y
Japan, Miyagi Prefecture	I	N	about 4%?	N
Japan, Nagasaki Prefecture	I	Y	NK	Y
Japan, Osaka Prefecture	I	N	8%(1990)	N
Japan, Saga Prefecture	I (S)	Y	2.6%	Y
Japan, Yamagata Prefecture	I (S)	Y	NK	N
Korea, Kangwha County	I (S)	N	0	NA
Kuwait	I	Y	NK	
Philippines, Manila	I (S)	Y	NK	Y
Singapore	I	Y	NK	Y
Thailand, Chiang Mai	I	Y		Y
Thailand, Khon Kaen	I (S)	N	NK	N
Viet Nam, Hanoi	I	Y	NK	Y
EUROPE				
Austria, Tyrol	I	Y	29,9%	Y
Belarus	I (S)	Y	NK	Y
Croatia	I	Y	7%	Y
Czech Republic	I	Y	31-37%	Y
Denmark	I (S)	Y	18%	Y
Estonia	I (S)	Y	21.30%	Y
Finland	I (S)	Y	NK	Y
France, Bas-Rhin	I (S)	Y	NK	Y
France, Calvados	I	N	0.50%	Y
France, Doubs	I (S)	Y	1%	Y
France, Haut-Rhin	I (S)	Y	9,9,%	Y
France, Hérault	I (S)	Y		N
France, Isère	I (S)	Y	0.04%	Y
France, Somme	F1	Y		Y
France, Tarn	F2	Y	0%	
Germany, Eastern States	I (S)	Y	45-50%	Y
Germany, Saarland	I (S)	Y	NK	Y
Iceland	Ic	Y	34%	Y
Ireland, Southern	I (S)	Y	NK	Y
Italy, Ferrara Province	I	Y	~2.6%	Y
Italy, Florence	I (S)	Y	1%	Y
Italy, Genoa	I	Y	NK	N
Italy, Latina	I	Y	<1%	Y
Italy, Macerata Province	I	Y	NK	N
Italy, Modena	I (S)	Y	1%	N
Italy, Parma Province	I	Y	NK	Y
Italy, Ragusa	I (S)	Y	NK	Y
Italy, Romagna	I	Y	NK	Y
Italy, Torino	I	Y		
Italy, Trieste	I (S)	Y	70%	Y
Italy, Varese Province	I (S)	Y	<10%	N

Table 5.1. (Contd). Registration practices

Registry	Multiple primary rules	Includes incidental prostate cancer	Cancer cases with necropsy (%)	Includes cases at necropsy only
Italy, Venetian Region	I	Y	2.70%	Y
Latvia	I (S)	Y	~25%(1992)	Y
Malta	I (S)	Y	NK	Y
Netherlands	I	Y	NK	Y
Netherlands, Eindhoven	I	Y	<10%	Y
Netherlands, Maastricht	I	Y		Y
Norway	I	Y	NK	Y
Poland, Cracow	I (S)	Y	NK	Y
Poland, Kielce	I (S)	Y	NK	Y
Poland, Lower Silesia	I (S)	Y	NK	Y
Poland, Warsaw City	I (S)	Y	0.1-0.2%	Y
Slovakia	I	Y	15%	Y
Slovenia	I	Y	6%	Y
Spain, Albacete	I (S)	Y	NK	N
Spain, Asturias	I		<0.25%	Y
Spain, Basque Contry	I	Y	NK	Y
Spain, Granada	I (S)	Y	1%	Y
Spain, Mallorca	I (S)	Y	0.002	N
Spain, Murcia	I	Y	0.2	Y
Spain,Navarra	I (S)	Y	NK	Y
Spain, Tarragona	I (S)	Y	4%	Y
Spain, Zaragoza	I	N	<1%	Y
Sweden	I (S)	Y	25-30%	Y
Switzerland, Basel	I (S)	Y	50%	Y
Switzerland, Geneva	I (S)	Y	30%(1990)	Y
Switzerland, Graubünden	I (S)	Y	~15%	Y
Switzerland, Neuchâtel	I (S)	N	< 5%	Y
Switzerland, St Gall-Appenzell	I	Y	25%(1990)	Y
Switzerland, Valais	I (S)	Y	3.20%	Y
Switzerland, Vaud	I (S)	Y	10-20%	Y
Switzerland, Zurich	I (S)	Y		Y
UK, England & Wales	E		NK	
UK, England, East Anglia	I (S)	Y	NK	Y
UK, England, Merseyside and Cheshire	I (S)			
UK, England, North Western	E	Y	NK	Y
UK, England, Oxford Region	I (S)	Y	NK	Y
UK, England, South Thames	E	Y	7%	Y
UK, England, South Western	I (S)			
UK, England, Wessex	I (S)	Y	NK	Y
UK, England, West Midlands	E	Y	NK	Y
UK, England, Yorkshire	I (S)	Y	NK	Y
UK, Scotland	Sc	Y	NK	Y
UK, Scotland, West	I (S)	Y	NK	Y
Yugoslavia, Vojvodina	I (S)	Y	NK	Y
OCEANIA				
Australian Capital Territory	A	Y		Y
Australia, New South Wales	A	Y		Y
South Australia	I	Y	NK	Y
Australia, Tasmania	I	Y	NK	Y
Australia, Victoria	I	Y	NK	Y
Western Australia	I	Y	4-9%	Y

Table 5.1. (Contd). Registration practices

Registry	Multiple primary rules	Includes incidental prostate cancer	Cancer cases with necropsy (%)	Includes cases at necropsy only
French Polynesia	I			
New Zealand	I	Y	NK	Y
USA, Hawaii	I	Y	NK	Y

I, IARC/IACR rules.

I(S), IARC/IACR rules, except for 'Other Skin' (ICD 173); see Table 3.2.

C1, Time-dependent (criteria not stated); see also 3.2.

C2, Canadian Cancer Registry rules since 1992; clinical opinion 1988–91; see also 3.2.

C3, L and R breast considered separately; see also 3.2.

C4, Only IACR/IARC rules 1 and 2 applied; see also 3.2.

C5, Canadian Cancer Registry rules; see also 3.2.

M, Bilateral tumours counted twice (except ovary, retinoblastoma); subsites considered separately for 153, 154, 170, 171, 173. No definition of 'different' for histological types.

F1, Except for breast, lung, colon - two tumours = two cases; see also table 3.2.

F2, Except for breast and colon'; see also table 3.2.

Ic, The pathologist decides (criteria unstated).

E, (1) Clinical statements take priority over rules.(2) Time: second primaries registered if interval >12 months (>5 years for breast, colon). (3) 91 categories of 'different' histologies. (4) Subsites considered separately for 140, 142, 143, 144, 145, 173 (melanoma), 187, 189, 190, 192, 194. S, SEER rules (SEER, 1992).

Sc, All subsequent primaries registered unless they were known or judged not to be independent primary tumours'.

A, One tumour per three-digit site (no account taken of 'different' histologies).

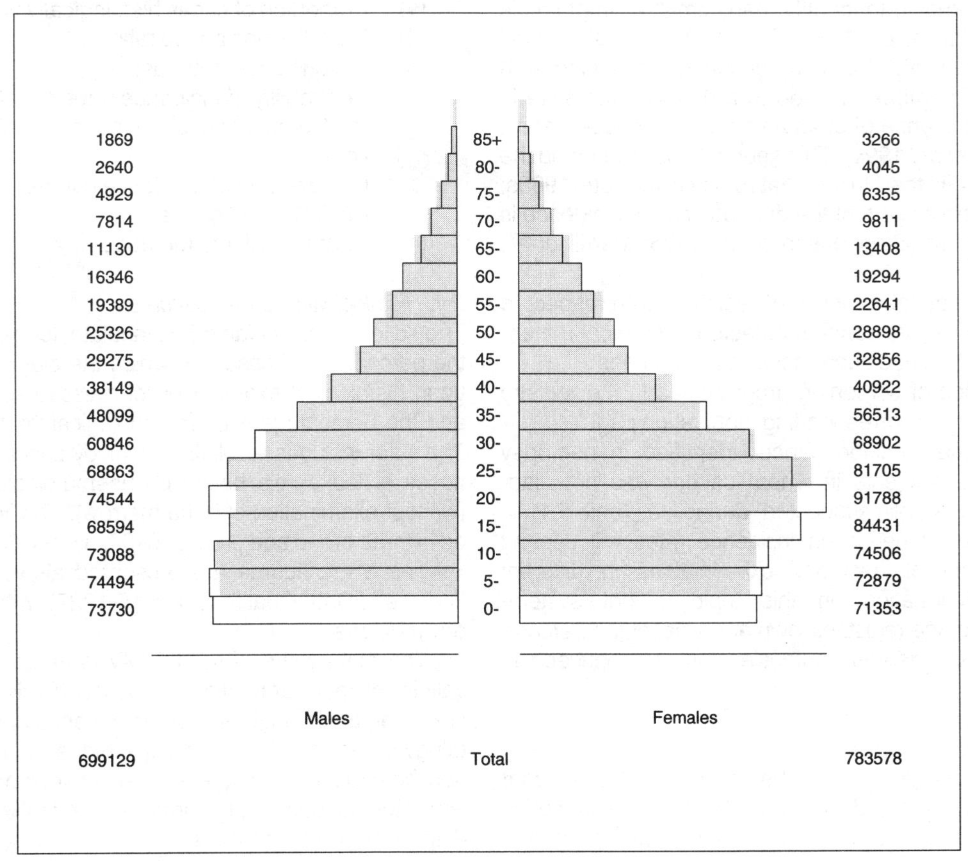

Figure 5.1. Population pyramid

Table 5.2. Percentage difference in incidence rates using multiple primary rules of SEER vs. IARC/IACR: SEER registries, 1988–92

Site	Difference (SEER/IACR) (%)			
	Male		Female	
	Crude	ASR	Crude	ASR
Breast	–	–	+ 5.8	+ 5.4
Colon	+ 5.0	+ 4.6	+ 4.7	+ 3.8
Melanoma	+ 3.3	+ 3.1	+ 2.0	+ 2.0
Kidney	+ 2.1	+ 1.9	+ 1.3	+ 1.8
Testis	+ 2.2	+ 1.9	–	–
Lung	+ 1.0	+ 1.0	+ 1.0	+ 1.2
All	+ 0.9	+ 0.8	+ 2.5	+ 2.3

1.1.2 Incidental diagnosis

Almost all registries include malignant tumours diagnosed during screening programmes, or histological specimens taken from individuals in whom there were no symptoms, or no clinical suspicion of cancer. These cases will increase incidence rates if the malignant cells so identified would never have resulted in a clinical cancer had they remained undetected.

The incidence of breast cancer appears to have been somewhat increased by the introduction of systematic mammographic screening for cancer. More striking, however, are the effects of such incidental diagnoses on the reported incidence of prostate cancer. The practice of careful histological examination of tissue removed by transurethral prostatectomy for benign prostatic hypotrophy has long been known to identify many small asymptomatic cancers (Sheldon *et al.*, 1980; Rohr 1987; Potosky *et al.*, 1990). More recently, the introduction of screening with prostate-specific antigen has led to a dramatic increase in the apparent incidence of prostate cancer (Jacobsen *et al.*, 1995; Potosky *et al.*, 1995). This seems to have affected the incidence rates in the United States since the late 1980s; there is some evidence that the dramatic rise in incidence is now slowing down (Stephenson *et al.*, 1995; Merrill *et al.*, 1996).

Table 5.1 notes the practice of registries with respect to registration of prostate cancers detected in surgical material; practically all include such 'incidental diagnoses'.

The presence of screening programmes in the registry area is noted on the corresponding 'population page'.

Most registries include cancer identified in necropsy examinations of subjects in whom cancer was not diagnosed (or perhaps even suspected) during life (Table 5.1).

The possible influence on incidence rates will depend upon the extent of necropsy examinations in different populations. Information on this topic is not systematically collected; the registries' own appraisal of the percentage of cancer deaths autopsied is reproduced in Table 5.1.

2. Completeness

Completeness of registration is the proportion of all incident cases in the registry population which have been included in the registry database. Completeness should be as close to 100% as possible, so that comparison of incidence rates between registries reflects true differences in cancer risk.

The Editors' main concern is with the possibility of incompleteness in the data submitted.

Duplicate registration of the same case should be avoided by careful attention to record linkage during the registration process. Because the case lists submitted do not contain personal identifying information, it is impossible for the Editors to check for possible duplicates. However, sometimes the existence of duplicate registration was suspected, e.g., by indices of completeness (see below) being higher than expected, and listings of possible duplicates (based on birthdate, sex, diagnosis and date of incidence) were returned to the registry for checking.

The following indices of completeness are routinely used during the editorial process:

(1) Proportion of cases histologically verified,
(2) Mortality : incidence ratio,
(3) Historic data methods:
  (*a*) Stability of incidence rates over time
  (*b*) Comparison of incidence in different populations
  (*c*) Age-specific incidence curves
  (*d*) Childhood cancer
(4) Death certificate methods

2.1. Histologically verified cancers

The editorial tables (Table 5.3) tabulate, for each site and sex, the percentage of cases for which the diagnosis was based upon histological examination of a tissue specimen (HV%), and the percentage with 'morphological verification' (MV%). The latter includes exfoliative cytology specimens, and diagnoses of leukaemia based on haematological examination (without examination of bone marrow). The MV% is presented in three broad age groups (0–34, 35–64, 65+).

The MV% figures are presented also in the tables of 'Indices of Data Quality' (pp. 1118-1227), without any breakdown by age.

The main value of the HV/MV is as an indicator of the validity of the diagnostic information (Parkin *et al.*, 1994). However, a very high proportion of cases diagnosed by histology or cytology/haematology – higher than might reasonably be expected – suggests over-reliance on the pathology laboratory as source of information, and failure to find cases diagnosed by other means.

In the editorial tables (Table 5.3), the column 'MV%' is accompanied by a flag (</>). '>' signifies that the number of cases so diagnosed is significantly greater than the value expected, based on the average percentage MV for the corresponding region (by sex and site) in *Cancer Incidence in Five Continents*, Volume VI. These means are reproduced in Table 5 of Parkin *et al.* (1994).

2.2. Mortality : incidence ratio

This is an important indicator of completeness, an example of the independent case ascertainment method (Parkin *et al.*, 1994). Registries are asked to provide the mortality data on cancer by sex, age group, and site, for the same period as the registered cases, from the local vital statistics office (municipal, provincial, national, etc.). Registry-generated mortality statistics (based on cases in the registry database who die during the period, or incorporating corrections to the certified cause of death) are *not* acceptable, since they do not constitute an independent data source.

When the quality of the mortality data are good, the M:I ratio is related to case fatality (1-survival). However, when mortality statistics are of poorer quality (incomplete certification, inaccurate cause of death statements) the relationship will be less close. Evaluation of the M:I ratio should take this into account. Since both survival and quality of mortality statistics are somewhat related to geographical region (both are poorer in developing countries) the regional location of the registry is important in evaluation of the statistic.

In the Editorial Tables (5.3), the M:I ratios for a given site are marked as being significantly greater (>) or less (<) than expected, based on the average regional values (13 of these) from *Cancer Incidence in Five Continents*, Volume VI (Table 7 of Parkin *et al.*, 1994).

The tables of indicators of quality (pp. 1118-1227) show the values of the M:I ratio for registries where official mortality statistics are available (and where their overall quality is not too hopeless to be used as an indicator of completeness). Thus, only for La Réunion among the African registries can an M:I ratio be calculated.

2.3. Stability of incidence rates over time

Changes in incidence rates over time which are greater than expected, and which cannot be ascribed to discrepancies in the estimation of person-years at risk, may well be related to changes in the completeness of case ascertainment. The change in incidence rates (as average percentage annual change) since Volume VI is presented in the column headed CH.V6 in the Editorial Tables (Table 5.3). Those changes which are statistically significant, based on a comparison of the age-standardized rate in Volume VI and Volume VII are marked in bold.

2.4. Comparison of incidence in different populations

The possibility of incomplete registration is also investigated by comparing the incidence rates observed with those in similar populations elsewhere. Formally, the Editorial Tables carried a flag (>/<) to the left of the 'site' name (Table 5.3) indicating whether the age-standardized rate was significantly different from the estimate for the corresponding world area in Table VI in Parkin *et al.* (1993). In addition, the editors frequently compared *ad hoc* tabulations from registries covering similar (geographically, ethnically) populations. The presence of lower than expected rates for several sites leads to under-registration being considered as an explanation.

2.5. Age-specific incidence curves

The draft tables, showing age-specific incidence rates by site and sex, are examined during the editorial process, in order to detect abnormal fluctuations in the anticipated patterns, including any fall-off in the rate of increase in incidence in older subjects (suggestive of under-ascertainment in the oldest age groups).

2.6. Childhood cancer

In general, the incidence of cancer (of all types) in the childhood age group shows much less variability than in adults, although there are well documented differences by geography or ethnicity for specific types of childhood cancer. The possibility of under-enumeration (or duplicate registrations) in this age range was investigated by comparing the observed age-specific rates in the childhood age range with the range of values observed in *Cancer Incidence in Five Continents* Volume VI. Values in the lowest and highest deciles, at ages 0–4, 5–9 and 10–14 were flagged by being reproduced in bold type in the Editorial Table (Table 5.3).

The limiting values for the lowest and highest deciles were as follows:

Age	Boys		Girls	
	Lowest	Highest	Lowest	Highest
0–4	<9.9	>24.1	<8.8	>21.2
5–9	<8.1	>14.6	<5.9	>12.4
10–14	<8.1	>14.8	<6.8	>12.9

2.7. Death certificate methods

Death certificates provide an important supplementary source of information for cancer registries. As far as incidence statistics are concerned, they function as a means of capturing information on cases which escaped the registration process during life. The means of using statistics on 'death certificate cases' to evaluate quality of cancer registry data was for many years a source of confusion. Recently, the concepts of death certificate notifications (DCN) and death certificate only (DCO) cases, as indices of completeness and validity, respectively, have been clearly defined (Parkin & Muir, 1992; Parkin *et al.*, 1994).

Completeness of registration may be evaluated on the basis of the proportion of incident cancers which first come to the registry's attention via a death certificate mentioning cancer (DCN cases). This information is not available to the editors of *Cancer Incidence in Five Continents,* who only know the numbers of DCO cases – that is, the residuum of cases remaining after various follow-back procedures have been carried out on DCN cases (see 3.2, below). For the most part, the proportion of DCO cases will be less – often considerably so – than the proportion of DCNs. Nevertheless, the DCN% will always be equal to, or greater than, the DCO%, so an elevated DCO% is suggestive of incompleteness. Even this must be interpreted in the light of local circumstances; in some developing countries, the quality of death certificates may be very poor, with a fair number of erroneous cancer deaths, which the registry may have difficulty tracing back to a hospital capable of confirming (or not) the death certificate statement. However, a low DCO% is thus no guarantee of completeness since, although it could indicate efficient case-finding, it could equally well result from the efficient traceback of DCN cases. Failure to use death certificates, when these are available and can be

Table 5.3 Editorial table

* EREWHON 1988-1992   FEMALE

S I T E	CASES	UNK%	R.F.	CR.R.	ST.R.	CH.V6	HV%	MV%	0-34	35-64	65+	DCO%	M/I	%.9	ICD-9
<Lip	10	0.0	0.1	0.1	0.2	3.6	80.0	80.0	0.0	75.0	100.0	20.0	10.0	40.0	140
Tongue	70	0.0	0.9	0.7	1.2	1.6	74.3	82.9	75.0	83.3	83.3	10.0	14.3<	58.6	141
Salivary gland	30	0.0	0.4	0.3	0.4	-4.1	90.0	96.7	100.0	100.0	80.0	3.3	10.0<	20.0	142
Mouth	534	0.2	7.0	5.6	8.9	-1.7	84.6	85.4	94.1	85.6	84.4	2.1	8.8<	16.9	143-5
Oropharynx	31	0.0	0.4	0.3	0.5	14.3	67.7	87.1	0.0	77.8	100.0	3.2	6.5<	16.1	146
Nasopharynx	19	0.0	0.2	0.2	0.2	7.0	57.9	73.7	100.0	62.5	33.3		15.8<		147
Hypopharynx	69	0.0	0.9	0.7	1.1	-2.7	66.7	76.8<	60.0	85.1	58.8	2.9	18.8<	10.1	148
Pharynx unspecified	22	0.0	0.3	0.2	0.4	2.6	72.7	72.7	50.0	66.7	100.0	18.2	22.7	0.0	149
Oesophagus	501	0.0	6.6	5.3	8.5	-0.8	70.9	74.3>	85.7	74.3	73.5	3.6	23.0<	38.3	150
>Stomach	321	0.0	4.2	3.4	5.1	-2.2	59.5	65.1<	82.1	69.7	50.5	14.0	31.5<	87.2	151
Small intestine	5	0.0	0.1	0.1	0.1	-21.6	80.0	80.0	50.0	100.0	100.0	20.0	20.0		152
>Colon	128	0.0	1.7	1.3	2.0	2.7	78.1	79.7	91.7	82.1	68.8	3.9	21.9<	42.2	153
Rectum	172	0.0	2.3	1.8	2.8	0.5	83.7	84.3	84.6	84.7	82.9	4.7	22.7<	3.5	154
<Liver	80	1.3	1.0	0.8	1.3	6.8	30.0	52.5>	50.0	58.9	33.3	32.5	55.0<		155
Gallbladder etc.	41	0.0	0.5	0.4	0.7	7.1	68.3	73.2>	0.0	77.8	64.3	12.2	29.3<	2.4	156
Pancreas	54	0.0	0.7	0.6	0.9	4.4	25.9	53.7>	60.0	62.5	35.3	16.7	46.3<	53.7	157
Nose, sinuses etc.	39	0.0	0.5	0.4	0.6	8.2	89.7	97.4>	100.0	96.3	100.0		10.3<	2.6	160
<Larynx	37	0.0	0.5	0.4	0.6	-4.3	64.9	78.4	75.0	84.0	62.5	10.8	16.2<	29.7	161
<Bronchus, lung	103	1.0	1.4	1.1	1.7	-2.4	52.4	75.7>	72.7	78.3	68.2	8.7	33.0<	93.2	162
Kaposi's sarcoma	0	0.0	0.0	0.0	0.0	0.0									KAP
Mesothelioma	2	0.0	0.0	0.0	0.0	-46.0	100.0	100.0	100.0	0.0	0.0				MES
Other thoracic organs	24	0.0	0.3	0.3	0.4	55.1	41.7	79.2	66.7	75.0	100.0	8.3		95.8	163(-MES),164
Bone	81	0.0	1.1	0.9	0.9	8.2	72.8	86.4>	91.7	80.0	75.0	7.4	12.3<	22.2	170
Connective tissue	66	0.0	0.9	0.7	0.9	1.4	84.8	97.0>	95.5	97.1	100.0	3.0	10.6<	18.2	171
Melanoma of Skin	14	0.0	0.2	0.1	0.2	-4.7	92.9	92.9	0.0	90.9	100.0		21.4<	7.1	172
Other Skin	90	0.0	1.2	0.9	1.4	-1.7	88.9	95.6>	100.0	96.7	90.5	2.2		16.7	173
Breast	1381	0.1	18.1	14.6	21.3	3.2	74.7	86.9<	90.6	86.9	84.5	2.4	30.1>	99.6	174
Uterus unspecified	24	0.0	0.3	0.3	0.3	-11.2	79.2	79.2>	77.8	80.0	80.0	12.5	16.7		179
Cervix uteri	1732	0.1	22.7	18.3	27.2	-2.6	87.2	88.2<	84.0	89.3	84.1	2.0	27.7>		180
Placenta	6	0.0	0.1	0.1	0.0	-23.7	66.7	66.7	66.7	0.0	0.0	16.7	33.3		181
Corpus uteri	118	0.8	1.5	1.2	1.9	3.4	95.8	96.6>	88.9	98.8	92.9	1.7	11.9<		182
<Ovary etc.	293	0.0	3.8	3.1	4.3	-2.5	75.4	85.3>	88.5	87.5	65.6	4.8	24.2<	0.7	183
Other female genital	85	0.0	1.1	0.9	1.4	2.3	94.1	94.1>	87.5	93.5	96.8		12.9<	1.2	184
Bladder	46	0.0	0.6	0.5	0.8	9.6	73.9	80.4	100.0	84.4	66.7	6.5	28.3<		188
Kidney, etc.	45	0.0	0.6	0.5	0.7	-2.9	82.2	93.3>	100.0	88.5	100.0		15.6<	0.0	189
Eye	21	0.0	0.3	0.2	0.3	15.3	85.7	85.7	85.7	100.0	80.0		9.5	9.5	190
Brain, nervous system	132	0.8	1.7	1.4	1.6	2.8	84.1	84.1>	84.8	84.7	66.7	9.1	25.0	28.8	191-2
Thyroid	233	0.0	3.1	2.5	3.2	2.5	75.5	90.1	96.2	87.8	84.4	0.4	6.4<		193
Other endocrine	4	0.0	0.1	0.0	0.1	-6.1	50.0	75.0	100.0	50.0	0.0	25.0	50.0	50.0	194
Non-Hodgkin's lymphoma	142	0.0	1.9	1.5	2.1	3.2	83.1	93.7>	87.9	96.2	93.5	3.5	38.7<	0.0	200,202
Hodgkin's Disease	52	0.0	0.7	0.5	0.6	4.3	90.4	98.1	100.0	100.0	83.3	1.9	17.3<	30.8	201
Multiple myeloma	36	0.0	0.5	0.4	0.6	0.1	19.4	86.1>	100.0	85.7	85.7	8.3	36.1<		203
>Lymphoid leukaemia	54	0.0	0.7	0.6	0.7	5.2	0.0	92.6>	92.5	100.0	90.0	7.4	44.4<	3.7	204
Myeloid leukaemia	127	0.0	1.7	1.3	1.6	6.0	1.6	94.5>	98.1	90.8	100.0	4.7	49.6<	0.8	205
Monocytic leukaemia	1	0.0	0.0	0.0	0.0	0.0	0.0	100.0	0.0	100.0	0.0		200.0	0.0	206
Other leukaemia	1	0.0	0.0	0.0	0.0	-25.6	0.0	100.0	0.0	100.0	0.0		200.0		207
Leukaemia,cell unspec.	36	0.0	0.5	0.4	0.5	10.3	2.8	55.6>	85.7	35.3	40.0	38.9	66.7	38.9	208
Other and unspecified	607	0.5	8.0#	6.4	9.5	5.3	13.3	17.1<	22.1	16.1	16.6	52.7			O&U
All Sites	7719	0.2	101.2	81.4	119.5	0.3	70.5	79.3>	83.3	80.5	72.6	8.1	29.1<		ALL
All Sites but 173	7629	0.2	100.0	80.4	118.1	0.3	70.3	79.1>	83.1	80.3	72.3	8.2	29.4<		

#R.F. for PSU is upper decile of CI5 VI (6.45)
%MV is significally <> from reference (chi2 > 3.84)
M/I is significally <> from reference (chi2 > 3.84)
Age specific rate (0-4):   8.8   7.1   21.2
Age specific rate (5-9):   5.9   4.7   12.4
Age specific rate (10-14): 6.8   5.8   12.9

Notes to Table 5.3

The title lists the registry, the period covered, and sex.

Site   The sites are those appearing in the main tables coded by ICD-9. The flags (<>) indicate when the age-standardized rate (STR) observed differs significantly (P<0.05) from the value estimated for the corresponding world area in Table VI of Parkin et al. (1993). The flag for 'lip' refers to the group 140–149, that for colon to 153–154 and that for lymphoid leukaemia to the group 204–208).

Cases   Number of cases registered during the period.

Unk%   Cases registered with unknown age. A flag (#) appears against the value for 'ALL sites but 173' if this lies in the top 10% of values of the data-sets published in Volume VI (see Table 6.3, p. 61 of Volume VI).

R.F.   Percentage of the total (All sites but 173). A flag (#) appears against the value for Other and Unspecified if this lies in the top 10% of values of the data-sets published in Volume VI (see Table 6.3, p61 of Volume VI).

CR.R.   The crude incidence rate, per 100 000.

ST.R.   The age-standardized rate (world standard) per 100 000. Values printed in bold are significantly different from those in Volume VI (test of Miettenen as described in Chapter 10, Volume VI).

CH.V6   The average annual change in the age-standardized rate since Volume VI. Values are printed in bold when the final rate is significantly different from that in Volume VI.

HV%   Percentage of cases with histological verification of diagnosis

MV%   Percentage of cases with morphological verification of diagnosis (i.e., including cytology and haematology). The flag (<,>) indicates when the number of cases so diagnosed is significantly less than, or greater than, expected based on the corresponding regional percentages in Table 5 of Parkin et al. (1994).

0–34;
35–64;
65+   MV% by age group

DCO%   Percentage of cases with diagnosis based on death certificate information only.

M/I   The ratio of deaths: cases registered, for the period indicated in the title. The flags (<,>) indicate whether the value is less than or greater than expected, based on the corresponding regional M/I percentages in Table 7 of Parkin et al. (1994).

%.9   The percentage of cases for which the fourth digit was .9 (or .8 for rectum, 154).

ICD-9   ICD-9 code

At the foot of the table

Three age-specific rates (0–4, 5–9, 10–14) are tested against the values observed in registries contributing data-sets to Volume VI. If they do not fall within the central 8 deciles, the observed value is printed in bold, together with the corresponding 'expected' range.

linked to the registry database (anonymous death certificates, as found in many Francophone countries, are useless in this respect), is generally taken to mean that some lack of completeness is likely to be present.

3. Validity
Validity is defined as the proportion of cases in a data-set with a given characteristic (e.g., site, age) which truly have the attribute.

Cancer Incidence in Five Continents uses five of the common indices of validity (Parkin *et al.*, 1994):

  Internal consistency
  Histological verification
  Death certificate only
  Primary site unknown
  Age unknown

The use of the IARC-CHECK program to perform consistency checks on the submitted data-sets is described in the chapter on data-processing (Chapter 6). Practically all data-sets were submitted to this process, and the cases queried checked by the registry before incorporation into the database. Very few registries provided data as case lists without histology, so precluding use of IARC-CHECK. These registries are identified by a flag (+) on the corresponding tables.

3.1. Histological verification
For most cases, the accuracy of the stated diagnosis is likely to be higher if it is based on histological examination by a pathologist. Previous surveys have shown that many cancer registries code diagnoses based on exfoliative cytology or on haematological examination of peripheral blood in the same category as histological examinations, so that it is impossible to distinguish between them. Partly for this reason, the tables of indices of data quality (pp..) concern the percentage of cases *morphologically verified*, and when this is not the case (i.e., excluding cytology/haematology), the percentage is shown in brackets [ ].

The Editorial Tables (5.3) include both histologically verified and morphologically verified percentages, the latter in three broad age groups. As noted above in Section 2.1, the flags (>/<) against the MV% column indicate whether the number of MV cases is greater than, or less than, that expected based on the regional average in *Cancer Incidence in Five Continents* Volume VI.

3.2. Death certificate only
In this volume, considerable effort has been made to ensure that what is reported as DCO cases in the Editorial Tables and Indices of Data Quality Tables does, indeed, refer to such cases. That is, they represent the residuum of cases – *after all trace-back manoeuvres have been completed* – for which no other information than a death certificate mentioning cancer could be obtained. Inasmuch as the diagnostic information on death certificates is well known to suffer from lack of accuracy, or lack of precision, a high proportion of DCO cases implies a lack of validity of the data. It would usually imply a lack of completeness also, as noted earlier (section 2.7).

Because of the many considerations involved in interpretation, and the sensitivity of the DCO% to local circumstances (availability of death certificates, quality of cause-of-death statements, facility to trace back cases), no objective criteria of acceptability of DCO% are applied. However, it will be noticed that no cancer registry has a DCO% (all

sites) in excess of 24%, and very few registries in North America, Western Europe, Australia/New Zealand with a DCO% (all sites) in excess of 12% have been included.

3.3. Other and unspecified
The content of this category is defined in detail in Chapter 3. A high proportion of cases assigned to these rubrics generally implies poor diagnostic precision (as evidenced by the low HV% observed for this rubric), or failure to specify the site of the primary cancer in cases diagnosed on the basis of tissue obtained from a metastasis.

Registries for whom the proportion of cases registered as 'Other and Unspecified' was in the upper decile of the contributions to the primary site uncertain category in *Cancer Incidence in Five Continents* Volume VI (6.67% for males, 6.45% for females) were marked with a flag (#) in the Editorial Tables (5.3).

The percentage of 'Other and Unspecified' cases, by registry, is given in Table 5.4

3.4. Age unknown
The proportion of cases for which age was unknown is reported, by registry, in Table 5.4.

In the Editorial Tables (5.3), a flag (#) was included if the value fell in the upper decile of that observed in *Cancer Incidence in Five Continents*, Volume VI (0.59% in males, 0.65% in females).

4. Population
Although it is easy to forget the fact, a 10% error in the estimation of population at risk produces just as much inaccuracy in the calculated incidence rate as a 10% error in enumeration of cases. However, cancer registries are generally not responsible for population estimates, and must rely upon various departments of central and local government to supply the required information. Registries should, however, inform themselves about the source of the population-at-risk figures which they use, and the methods used to produce estimates and projections. The Editors of this volume asked all contributing registries to provide this information, and it is summarized, along with the average annual population at risk for the period covered by the registrations, on the 'population page' of each entry.

The population data provided by a registry could rarely be subjected to verification by the Editors, although sometimes the appropriateness of the source of the information provided was queried. For registries which had provided data for Volume VI, a formal comparison was carried out between the population at risk in the two periods. Figure 1 shows the population pyramid for the current period with, in grey, that for the period five years earlier (as it appeared in volume VI), but moved upwards (aged) by five years, so that the general form of the two estimates can be compared.

Generally for Volume VII, which coincides with a period close to 1990, census data were available to registries, so that population estimates tended to be more accurate than those in Volume VI. Indeed, in some cases it was noted that the intercensal estimate used in Volume VI had been somewhat inaccurate.

Where it was considered that there may have been a problem in estimating population at risk, either for Volume VII or indeed for Volume VI, this is noted, together with other comments, on the population page. In some cases, likely inaccuracies in estimates of the population at risk contributed to the decision to add an asterisk to the registry's contribution.

5. Annotations to data-sets

5.1. Flagged data-sets (+)

As described above, several registries were unable to submit their data in the format requested (anonymous case listings with histology). For these data-sets, the internal consistency checks for data quality could not be performed. Another group of registries declined to verify the list of queries sent to them as part of the editorial process. These registries have been marked with a flag (+) as having undergone less rigorous quality control procedures than the majority.

5.2 The asterisk (*)

The presence of an asterisk implies that some care is required in interpretation of the numerical results for some or all cancer sites, and the reader should refer to the 'notes' section of the 'population page' for the registry for the precise reasons.

The principal use is to denote data-sets which were considered by the Editors to have characteristics suggesting questionable quality or completeness of information on cases or the population at risk. The criteria used in this judgement were not rigidly defined, the decision being based on examination of all of the indices described in this chapter and knowledge of the circumstances in which the registry operates. The intrinsic interest of the data-set in providing information on little known geographical and ethnic patterns, or continuity with earlier data from the same registry, were also taken into consideration.

For some data-sets, notes also warn readers to be cautious in the use of the results for the study of time trends. Thus, for certain registries, the material presented may be more accurate than that in earlier volumes of *Cancer Incidence in Five Continents* either because of more valid case data, or better information on the population at risk. The use of the asterisk for this purpose is explained on the relevant population page.

References

IARC, Lyon (1994). Multiple Primaries. Internal Report No. 94/003

Jacobsen, S.J., Katusic, S.K., Bergstrath, E.J., Oesterling, J.E., Ohst, D., Klee,. G.G., Chute, C.G. & Lieber, M.M. (1995) Incidence of prostate cancer diagnosis in the eras before and after serum prostate-specific antigen testing. J. Am. Med. Assoc., 247, 1445–1449

Merrill, R.M., Potosky, A.L. & Feuer, E.J. (1996) Changing trends in US Prostate Cancer Incidence Rates. J. Natl. Cancer Inst., 88, 1683–1685

Parkin, D.M. & Muir, C.S. (1992) Comparability and quality of data. In: Parkin, D.M., Muir, C.S., Whelan, S.L., Gao, Y.-T., Ferlay, J. & Powell, J. Cancer Incidence in Five Continents, Volume VI (IARC Scientific Publications No. 120), Lyon, IARC

Parkin, D.M., Pisani, P. & Ferlay, J. (1993) Estimates of the worldwide incidence of eighteen major cancers in 1985. Int. J. Cancer, 54, 594–606

Parkin, D.M., Chen, V.W., Ferlay, J., Galceran, J., Storm, H.H and Whelan, S.L. (1994) Comparability and Quality Control in Cancer Registration (IARC Technical Reports No. 19), Lyon, IARC

Potosky, A., Kessler, L., Gridley, G., Brown, C.C. & Horm, J.W. (1990) Rise in prostatic cancer incidence associated with increased use of transuretheral resection. J. Natl. Cancer Inst., 82, 1624–1628

Potosky, A.L., Miller, B.A., Albertsen, P.C. & Kramer, B.S. (1995) The role of increasing detection in the rising incidence of prostate cancer. J. Am. Med. Assoc., 273, 548–552

Rohr, L.R. (1987) Incidental adenocarcinoma in transuretheral resections of the prostate: partial versus complete microscopic examination. Am. J. Surg. Pathol., 11, 53–58

The SEER Program Code Manual, revised edition, 1992, Bethesda, MD, National Institutes of Health, National Cancer Institute

Sheldon, C.A., Williams, R.D. & Fraley, E.E. (1980) Incidental carcinoma of the prostate: a review of the literature and critical reappraisal of classification. J. Urol., 124, 626–631

Stephenson, R.A., Smart, C.R., Mineau, G.P., James, B.C., Janerich, D.T. & Dibble, R.L. (1995) The fall in incidence of prostate carcinoma. On the downside of prostate specific antigen included peak in incidence – data from the Utah Cancer Registry. Cancer, 77, 1342–1348

Table 5.4 PERCENTAGE OF OTHER AND UNSPECIFIED SITE (O&U) AND UNKNOWN AGE (UNK), ALL SITES

	MALE O&U	MALE UNK	FEMALE O&U	FEMALE UNK
AFRICA				
Algeria, Setif	5.2	-	3.6	-
France, La Reunion	3.8	-	3.2	-
Mali, Bamako	2.6	-	2.9	-
Uganda, Kyadondo	4.2	3.2	3.8	2.8
Zimbabwe, Harare: African	2.6	0.6	2.9	1.4
Zimbabwe, Harare: European	2.1	3.7	1.7	2.9
AMERICA, CENTRAL AND SOUTH				
Argentina, Concordia	11.1	-	8.2	-
Brazil, Belem	6.6	6.6	4.4	5.0
Brazil, Goiania	4.3	0.6	3.0	0.6
Brazil, Porto Alegre	4.1	6.1	4.6	6.0
Colombia, Cali	5.7	4.9	5.6	5.2
Costa Rica	4.2	0.7	4.0	0.8
Ecuador, Quito	4.3	1.6	4.8	1.0
Peru, Lima	4.9	2.2	4.1	1.1
Peru, Trujillo	4.4	1.8	3.9	2.0
US, Puerto Rico	4.1	0.8	4.4	0.6
Uruguay, Montevideo	7.7	-	7.1	-
AMERICA, NORTH				
Canada	3.8	0.1	4.0	-
Canada, Alberta	3.7	-	4.2	-
Canada, British Columbia	3.4	-	4.1	-
Canada, Manitoba	3.2	-	4.1	-
Canada, New Brunswick	3.3	0.1	4.5	0.2
Canada, Newfoundland	3.8	-	5.0	-
Canada, Northwest Territories	3.5	-	3.9	-
Canada, Nova Scotia	4.5	0.1	4.5	-
Canada, Ontario	4.5	0.1	3.9	0.1
Canada, Prince Edward Island	3.7	-	4.0	-
Canada, Quebec	3.2	-	3.8	-
Canada, Saskatchewan	2.9	-	3.6	-
Canada, Yukon	5.2	-	7.0	-
US, Cent. Calif.: Non-Hisp. White	3.3	-	3.4	-
US, Cent. Calif.: Hispanic	3.6	-	3.4	-
US, Los Angeles: Non-Hisp. White	3.0	-	3.6	-
US, Los Angeles: Hispanic White	3.4	-	3.6	-
US, Los Angeles: Black	3.4	-	3.9	-
US, Los Angeles: Chinese	4.2	-	4.2	-
US, Los Angeles: Filipino	3.7	-	2.6	0.1
US, Los Angeles: Korean	3.3	0.2	4.8	-
US, Los Angeles: Japanese	2.2	0.1	2.7	0.1
US, San Francisco: Non-Hisp. White	2.5	-	3.5	-
US, San Francisco: Hispanic White	2.4	0.1	3.2	-
US, San Francisco: Black	3.2	-	4.3	-
US, San Francisco: Chinese	3.6	-	3.9	-
US, San Francisco: Filipino	3.3	-	3.2	-
US, San Francisco: Japanese	2.0	-	2.7	-
US, Connecticut: White	3.0	-	3.5	-
US, Connecticut: Black	3.3	-	4.2	-
US, Atlanta: White	2.3	-	2.5	-
US, Atlanta: Black	4.1	-	4.2	-
US, Iowa	2.5	-	3.2	-

	MALE O&U	MALE UNK	FEMALE O&U	FEMALE UNK
US, Central Louisiana: White	3.9	0.1	4.1	0.1
US, Central Louisiana: Black	5.1	-	4.9	-
US, New Orleans: White	2.8	-	3.2	-
US, New Orleans: Black	3.9	-	4.4	-
US, Detroit: White	2.3	-	3.0	-
US, Detroit: Black	2.6	-	3.4	-
US, New Mexico: Non-Hisp. White	2.9	-	3.2	-
US, New Mexico: Hispanic White	3.6	-	3.6	-
US, New Mexico: American Indian	5.1	-	5.3	-
US, Utah	2.7	-	3.5	-
US, Seattle	2.1	-	2.7	-
US, SEER: White	2.5	-	3.2	-
US, SEER: Black	3.1	-	3.9	-
ASIA				
China, Qidong	0.4	-	0.7	-
China, Shanghai	2.8	-	3.3	-
China, Tianjin	2.5	-	3.0	-
Hong Kong	4.8	0.4	4.8	0.4
India, Bangalore	11.9	0.2	7.9	0.2
India, Barshi, Paranda and Bhum	12.6	-	7.6	-
India, Bombay	6.7	0.2	5.0	0.2
India, Karunagappally	13.7	2.4	9.1	2.7
India, Madras	7.9	-	5.3	-
India, Trivandrum	13.7	-	7.3	0.1
Israel: All Jews	5.9	0.2	5.7	0.3
Jews born in Israel	4.0	0.3	2.9	0.3
Jews born in America or Europe	5.9	0.2	6.5	0.3
Jews born in Africa or Asia	6.9	0.3	5.8	0.2
Non-Jews	7.4	0.2	6.6	0.2
Japan, Hiroshima	1.3	0.2	1.4	0.2
Japan, Miyagi	1.3	-	1.6	-
Japan, Nagasaki	1.3	0.1	1.6	0.2
Japan, Osaka	1.5	-	1.9	-
Japan, Saga	1.2	-	1.8	-
Japan, Yamagata	1.6	-	2.0	-
Korea, Kangwha	2.0	-	1.0	-
Kuwait: Non-Kuwaitis	3.6	0.3	3.1	0.2
Kuwait: Kuwaitis	5.9	0.3	4.6	0.3
Philippines, Manila	5.7	0.1	4.2	0.1
Singapore: Chinese	2.7	0.1	2.7	0.2
Singapore: Malay	4.0	-	3.2	-
Singapore: Indian	4.3	0.5	2.9	-
Thailand, Chiang Mai	11.9	-	10.7	-
Thailand, Khon Kaen	12.5	0.5	10.3	0.4
Viet Nam, Hanoi	4.0	1.9	3.9	2.4

PERCENTAGE OF OTHER AND UNSPECIFIED SITE (O&U) AND UNKNOWN AGE (UNK), ALL SITES

	MALE O&U	MALE UNK	FEMALE O&U	FEMALE UNK		MALE O&U	MALE UNK	FEMALE O&U	FEMALE UNK
EUROPE					Sweden	3.5	-	4.3	-
Austria, Tyrol	1.9	-	2.9	-	Switzerland, Basel	2.1	-	2.2	-
Belarus	2.0	-	1.7	-	Switzerland, Geneva	1.8	-	2.4	-
Croatia	5.2	1.1	6.7	1.7	Switzerland, Graubunden	2.1	-	2.9	-
Czech Republic	2.8	-	3.4	-	Switzerland, Neuchatel	1.7	-	2.8	-
Denmark	4.0	-	4.3	-	Switzerland, St Gall-Appenzell	1.9	-	2.4	-
Estonia	2.5	-	1.8	-	Switzerland, Valais	4.6	-	3.9	-
Finland	1.9	-	2.6	-	Switzerland, Vaud	2.3	-	2.8	-
France, Bas-Rhin	4.2	-	3.7	-	Switzerland, Zurich	2.6	-	3.6	-
France, Calvados	1.7	0.2	1.3	0.3	UK, England and Wales	5.3	-	5.6	0.1
France, Doubs	4.9	1.3	4.1	1.9	UK, East Anglia	4.6	-	5.1	-
France, Haut-Rhin	2.3	-	1.9	-	UK, Mersey	5.4	-	6.0	-
France, Herault	3.4	-	2.9	-	UK, North Western	5.8	-	6.1	-
France, Isere	4.5	-	4.0	-	UK, Oxford	4.4	0.2	5.3	0.2
France, Somme	2.9	-	3.1	-	UK, South Thames	4.8	-	5.5	-
France, Tarn	3.5	0.4	4.0	0.2	UK, South Western	0.5	-	0.7	-
Germany, Eastern States	1.0	-	1.3	-	UK, Wessex	4.7	-	5.5	-
Germany, Saarland	4.0	0.1	4.2	0.1	UK, West Midlands	5.4	-	5.7	-
Iceland	3.0	-	3.2	-	UK, Yorkshire	5.7	-	6.4	-
Ireland, Southern	4.1	-	5.1	-	UK, Scotland	4.9	-	5.3	-
Italy, Ferrara	2.6	-	2.5	-	UK, Scotland, West	5.2	-	5.6	-
Italy, Florence	2.6	-	3.6	-	Yugoslavia, Vojvodina	3.6	-	4.4	-
Italy, Genoa	3.0	-	3.4	-					
Italy, Latina	2.3	-	2.6	-	**OCEANIA**				
Italy, Macerata	2.3	-	3.4	-	Australian Capital Territory	4.0	-	3.7	-
Italy, Modena	2.8	-	3.3	-	Australia, New South Wales	4.8	-	5.3	-
Italy, Parma	2.6	-	2.7	-	South Australia	3.5	-	4.5	-
Italy, Ragusa	2.3	-	2.0	-	Australia, Tasmania	4.7	-	5.2	-
Italy, Romagna	2.1	-	2.8	-	Australia, Victoria	4.7	-	4.9	-
Italy, Torino	3.7	-	3.9	-	Western Australia	5.6	-	5.7	-
Italy, Trieste	-	-	-	-	French Polynesia	6.0	1.9	4.4	3.3
Italy, Varese	2.7	-	2.6	-	New Zealand: Non-Maori	5.3	-	5.8	-
Italy, Veneto	2.9	-	3.2	-	New Zealand: Maori	7.6	-	5.7	0.1
Latvia	1.0	-	1.0	-	US, Hawaii: White	2.2	-	3.2	-
Malta	3.9	2.2	3.4	1.5	US, Hawaii: Japanese	1.7	-	2.1	-
The Netherlands	4.6	-	4.3	-	US, Hawaii: Hawaiian	2.9	-	3.0	-
The Netherlands, Eindhoven	5.5	-	5.3	-	US, Hawaii: Filipino	2.7	-	1.7	-
The Netherlands, Maastricht	5.5	-	5.0	-	US, Hawaii: Chinese	2.4	-	3.1	-
Norway	3.6	-	4.5	-					
Poland, Cracow	5.4	-	5.8	-					
Poland, Kielce	2.3	-	3.2	-					
Poland, Lower Silesia	4.3	-	4.7	-					
Poland, Warsaw City	4.7	-	4.7	-					
Slovakia	1.9	-	2.7	-					
Slovenia	4.8	-	5.2	-					
Spain, Albacete	5.2	0.1	4.9	-					
Spain, Asturias	4.5	0.8	5.1	1.0					
Spain, Basque Country	5.9	0.1	6.4	0.1					
Spain, Granada	4.1	-	4.9	-					
Spain, Mallorca	4.1	1.1	4.4	1.4					
Spain, Murcia	3.8	0.9	4.6	1.0					
Spain, Navarra	3.3	0.3	3.8	0.2					
Spain, Tarragona	4.5	1.3	4.8	1.6					
Spain, Zaragoza	4.3	0.4	5.4	0.4					

Chapter 6. Processing of data

J. Ferlay

With the increasing numbers of cancer registries worldwide that are capable of supplying individual case data, it became clear that a regular procedure for data validation and storage had to be established and maintained in the unit of Descriptive Epidemiology (DEP) of IARC. A data-management process was therefore established, to provide accurate data for a growing number of projects managed in the unit. *Cancer Incidence in Five Continents* is obviously the largest such project and it was clear at an early stage that the preparation of the current volume would have to be integrated with the regular work, so that only the production of the tables remained specific. The data management process can be summarized by the following diagram:

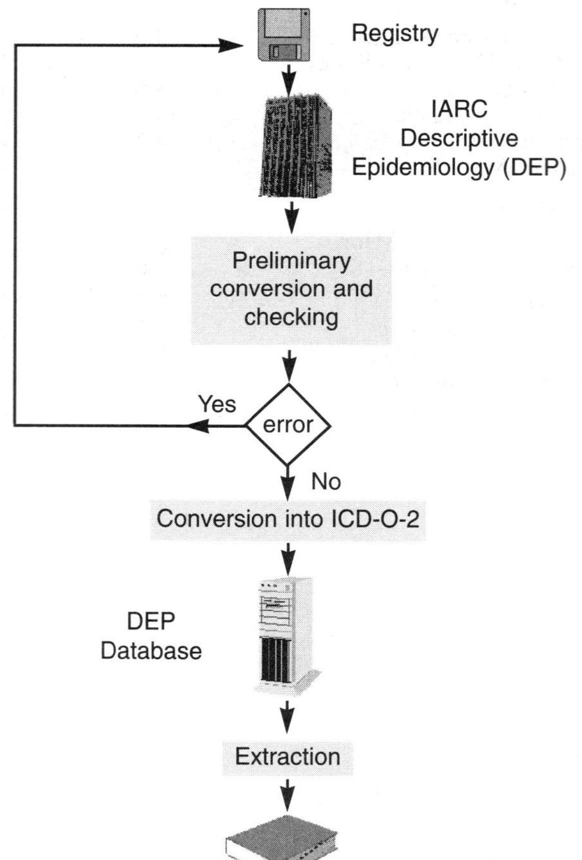

1. Data input processing

176 cancer registries replied to the invitation to participate by submitting data for volume VII. This resulted in the manipulation of around 8 500 000 individual records, and the production of around 250 preliminary data-sets to be examined carefully by the editors (including different ethnic groups or time periods). For each incident record, the minimum items required are:

1. a registration number which identifies the case
2. sex
3. ethnic group or race (optional)
4. age and/or birth date
5. date of incidence
6. site of the tumour
7. morphology of the tumour
8. behaviour of the tumour
9. basis of diagnosis

A description of all the codes used for these variables had to be provided with the data. However, it was not unusual that the code values did not match the description provided. In this case, the registry was asked for clarification and to provide the correct codes if necessary. This was particularly important when computing the percentage of histologically confirmed or death-certificate-only (DCO) cases used for the editorial process, because a misinterpretation of the basis of diagnosis codes could give a false picture of the data quality (see Chapter 5).

As usual, the data were accepted in any format and on any medium (paper forms, diskettes, tapes, electronic mail). Many different coding schemes were used for tumour site and morphology as summarized in Table 6.1.

2. Conversion into a full ICD-O coding schema

The checking process using the IARC-CHECK program (Parkin *et al.*, 1994) requires the data to be coded by ICD-O. As indicated in Table 6.1, around one third of the data-sets had to be converted into a full (topography and morphology) ICD-O coding schema before they could be handled by the program. For registries using a mixture of ICD-9 for topography and ICD-O for morphology, an ICD-9 (WHO, 1977) to ICD-O-1 (WHO, 1976) conversion program was prepared, and this proved to be particularly valuable in detecting incompatibilities between ICD-9 codes and ICD-O morphology and behaviour; these were transmitted back to the cancer registry for review and correction.

3. Behaviour code

Although the second edition of ICD-O (WHO, 1990) gives clear instructions that behaviour codes /6 and /9 should not be used by cancer registries (page xxv), these codes appeared in many data-sets, giving rise to problems with respect to the corresponding topography code. Usually, this was assumed to represent the site of the primary tumour. Where this was evidently not the case (carcinomas in lymph

Table 6.1. Coding of information about the tumour

Topography	Morphology	Number of data-sets(*)
ICD-9	No	13
ICD-7	MOTNAC (ACS, 1968)	1
ICD-9	MOTNAC (ACS, 1951)	1
ICD-9	WHO/HS/CANC/24.1(1956)	1
ICD-9	MOTNAC (1968)	1
ICD-9	User-defined system	2
ICD-9	ICD-O-1 (WHO, 1976)	53
ICD-O-1	ICD-O-1 (WHO, 1976)	82
ICD-O-1	ICD-O-Field Trial Edition (Percy & Van Holten, 1988)	5
ICD-O-2	ICD-O-2 (WHO, 1990)	34

* Total greater than 176: some registries used different classifications in the same data-set (see below).

nodes, bone etc.), a listing of such cases was sent back to the registries with a request for clarification. As a last resort, they were recoded to T199.9/C80.9 (primary site unknown).

Other difficulties that involved lengthy data-processing should also be mentioned:

• Some registries did not correct their original files at the same time as responding to the queries generated by the IARC-CHECK program. As a result, all the corrections had to be re-entered at IARC each time these registries re-submitted data.

• For registries submitting data coded to the main three-digit categories of ICD-9 only, a 'dummy' fourth digit had to be added to each ICD-9 code.

• For registries submitting records with ICD-9 codes without histology, a 'dummy' ICD-O-1 morphological code had to be assigned to each record to conform to the default data process. These registries are flagged using a '+' indicating that no check regarding the validity of the morphology or coherence between site, age and morphology could be performed (see chapter 5).

• Because ICD-O-2 was generally introduced into use in cancer registries around 1990, which corresponds to the middle of the period for this volume, some data-sets included both ICD-O-1 and 2 codes, depending on the year of incidence of the case. These data-sets had to be split into two (and for one which also used ICD-9 into three) data-sets before being checked.

• Some registries could not find an appropriate ICD-O (version 1 or 2) code and created their own codes. The corresponding cases had to be re-coded to the most appropriate and valid ICD-O-1 or 2 code.

4. Checking
The mortality data used for editorial purposes were generally provided as a tabulation of ICD-9 three-digit categories by sex and five-year age-group, so that no validity check (except the basic combination of sex and site) could be performed.

For the incidence data, once a data-set had been converted into ICD-O-1, or if it had been originally coded using ICD-O-1 or ICD-O-2 codes, it was submitted to the IARC CHECK program, which performed the following edits:

1. Code verification
    sex
    incidence and birth date (if provided)
    ICD-O version 1 or 2 topography and morphology

2. Consistency between items
    age versus birth/incidence dates
    sex versus site

Table 6.2. Examples of unlikely ICD-9 site/ICD-O morphology combinations

ICD-9		ICD-O first edition
202._	Non-Hodgkin lymphoma	Any ICD-O (M) code less than 9590.
201._	Hodgkin's disease	Any ICD-O (M) code less than 9650.
204-8	Leukaemia	Any ICD-O (M) code less than 9800.
204.0	ALL	9823/3 Chronic lymphocytic leukaemia
201.9	Hodgkin's disease, NOS	9590/3 Non-Hodgkin lymphoma, NOS
172.9	Melanoma of skin, NOS	8090/3 Basal cell carcinoma
162.9	Lung primary cancer	8140/6 Adenocarcinoma, metastatic
180.9	Cervical tumour, malignant	8070/2 In situ tumour

age versus site/histology
site versus histology
basis of diagnosis versus histology

3. Multiple primaries

When a data-set incorporated an identification number which was a *patient* identification number, it was possible to check for multiple primary tumours following the IACR rules (IARC, 1994). In that case, the data file was first sorted on the identification number, and within the identification number, by ascending incidence date. All the records concerning the patient were then passed through the following algorithm to detect multiple tumours or true duplicate registrations:

Suppose many records for the same patient

T(i)   being the topography (3 digits of ICD)
M(i)   being the morphology
TG(k) and MG(k) being the groups of topography and morphology considered to be different (Parkin *et al.*, 1994)

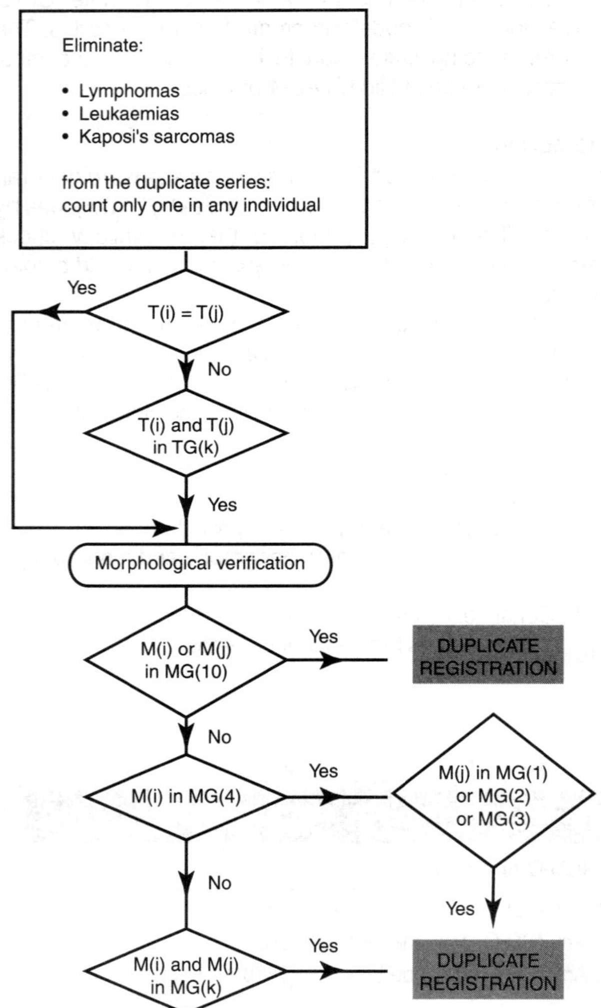

This program could detect all the duplicates which appeared during the period only if the cancer registry had submitted its complete data-set, including the years before the period for the current volume. Otherwise, some of the multiple tumours (generally those which occurred at the beginning of the current period) might not be detected because of lack of information on the prevalent cases.

All errors or unlikely or rare combinations of items were sent back to the cancer registry for verification. All amendments or new files resubmitted were then incorporated, converted (if necessary) and always checked again to ensure that no more errors were found. This long and tedious process for both cancer registry and IARC staff took several weeks or months; however, it ensured a maximum of data comparability and validity, although in some instances, the quality of the data was still not sufficient for inclusion in the present volume. This depended upon other considerations of comparability and quality, as described in Chapter 5.

When no more errors were detected, the incidence data were converted to both ICD-O-2 and ICD-9 codes, the mortality and population figures appropriately formatted, and all these were loaded into a central database.

5. Conversion into ICD-O-2

The data-sets which were not originally coded into ICD-O-2 were converted into this classification. This ensured that they were submitted to the same series of conversion programs, and that the final ICD-9 codes used in the publication followed a standard ICD-O-2 to ICD-9 conversion program (Percy *et al.*, 1992).

When a data-set was submitted coded to either ICD-9 or ICD-O-1, the series of conversion processes produced some unexpected results, for example new ICD-9 codes which were not originally recorded in the input file were created 'artificially'.

Suppose the following combination of ICD-9 (T) and ICD-O-1 (M) was found:

ICD-9	ICD-O (M)
199.0	8832/3
Unknown primary	

The first conversion into ICD-O-1 (T+M) will produce the following output codes:

ICD-O-1 (T+M)	
199.9	8832/3
Unknown primary	

The second conversion into ICD-O-2 (T+M) will produce the following output:

ICD-O-2 (T+M)	
C80.9	8832/3
Unknown primary	

Finally, the ICD-O-2 to ICD-9 conversion will produce the following ICD-9 code:

173.9	Skin, NOS

so that the final ICD-9 site does not correspond to that provided in the original record. Generally, such code changes will occur when the registry has not followed the rules in the ICD-O manuals; in the above example, a dermatofibrosarcoma (M8832/3) should have been coded to skin (T173._) if the site of the tumour was unspecified (rule 5 of ICD-O-1). But it also occurred with other specific morphological diagnoses such as basal cell carcinoma (M8090), osteosarcoma (M9180) which were converted to an ICD-9 topography code for skin or bone cancer. This explains why some cancer registries which submitted their data coded to ICD-9 found differences between their tabulations and those produced by the CI5 process.

All the conversion programs used in the data-entry process have been published as a PC DOS diskette (Ferlay, 1994). A Windows-based version of these programs which will include the ICD-9+ICD-O-1(M) into ICD-O-1 (T+M) conversion will become available during 1997.

6. Output data-processing

The DEP database contains all the incidence and mortality data-sets received in DEP, irrespective of the decision whether to include them in *Cancer Incidence in Five Continents* or not. The incidence data are stored as individual records and, as described above, checked and converted if necessary into ICD-O-2. These data can be easily converted to any other classification system. Using the DEP database, the production of the volume was quite fast. The data corresponding to the period of the registries accepted for publication were retrieved and converted into *Cancer Incidence in Five Continents* morphological groups (see Chapter 4). The tables presented in the book were then produced using specially designed programs running in batch mode. The production of the tables required around a week using the VAX™ computer, compared to the months necessary for checking the data.

7. CI5VII software

A diskette containing the incidence data together with a Windows PC-based software called *CI5VII* which manipulates these data will be published separately as an IARC electronic publication (Ferlay, 1997). This software was developed using object oriented programming (C++ language). It has graphic and basic statistical capabilities such as computation and comparison of incidence rates, and also permits aggregations of either registries or sites.

The data are stored in the traditional form of number of cases by sex and five-year age groups. A majority of the standard three-digit ICD-9 anatomical sites have been replaced by a set of 251 categories based on a combination of ICD-9 three- or four-digit sites and ICD-O-2 morphological groups. The four-digit categories were chosen to provide a correspondence between the three- or four-digit site codes used in ICD-9 and the three-digit site codes used in ICD-10, but some other sub-categories of epidemiological interest (such as the sub-divisions of the colon) have been used. For ICD-9 codes 150 (oesophagus), 162 (trachea, bronchus and lung), 170 (bone), 183 (ovary etc.) and 189 (kidney and other and unspecified urinary organs), this categorization permits access to the main site by either the morphological or the sub site level.

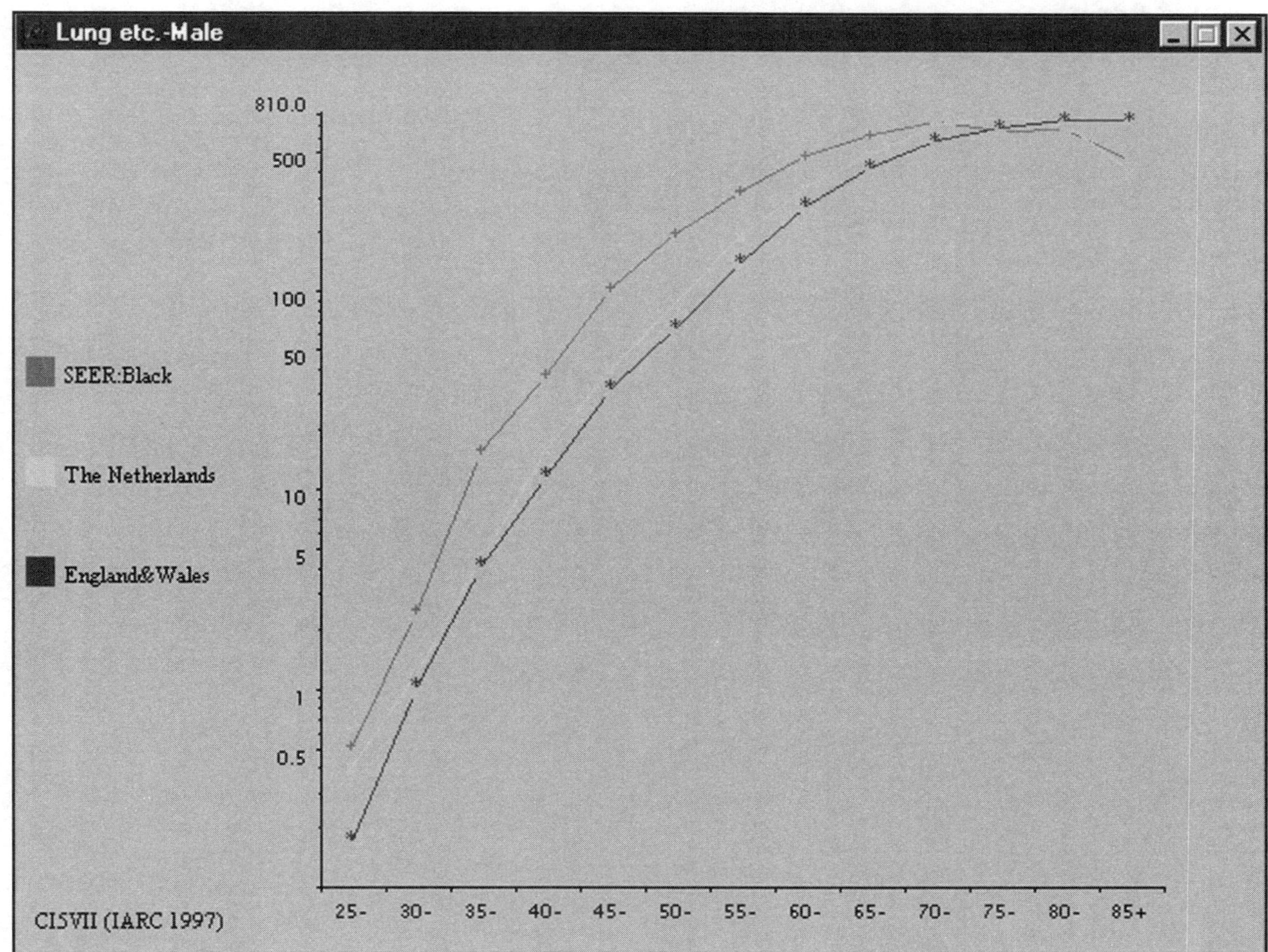

Figure 6.1. An example of the CI5VII graphical capabilities: the GraphIAge-specific option

Acknowledgement

The author would like to thank all the persons involved in the validation procedure for their patience and their unfailing help, and to particularly acknowledge the few contributors who checked their data using the IARC-CHECK program before submission. This was very helpful and much appreciated.

References

ACS (1951) Manual of Tumor Nomenclature and Coding, New York, NY, American Cancer Society

ACS (1968) Manual of Tumor Nomenclature and Coding New York, NY, American Cancer Society

Ferlay, J. (1994) ICD Conversion Programs for Cancer (IARC Technical Reports No. 21), Lyon, IARC

Ferlay, J. (1997) Cancer Incidence in Five Continents VII (IARC CancerBase No. 2), Lyon, IARC

Parkin, D.M., Chen, V.W., Ferlay, J., Galceran, J., Storm, H.H. & Whelan, S.L. (1994) Comparability and Quality Control in Cancer Registration (IARC Technical Reports No. 19), Lyon, IARC

Percy, C.L. & Van Holten, V. eds. (1988) ICD-O, International Classification of Diseases for Oncology, Field Trial Edition (developed by working party coordinated by IARC, Lyon).

Percy, C.L. ed. (1992) Conversion of Neoplasms by Topography and Morphology from the ICD-O-2 to ICD-9 and the ICD-9-CM. National Cancer Institute, Washington, USA.

WHO (World Health Organization) (1956) Histological classification of neoplasms, (WHO/HS/CANC/24.1), Geneva, World Health Organization

WHO (World Health Organization) (1976) International Classification of Diseases for Oncology (ICD-O), Geneva, World Health Organization

WHO (World Health Organization) (1990) International Classification of Diseases for Oncology, Second Edition (ICD-O), Geneva, World Health Organization

WHO (World Health Organization) (1957) Manual of the International Statistical Classification of Diseases, Injuries and Causes of Death (Based on the Recommendations of Seventh Revision Conference, 1955), Geneva, World Health Organization

WHO (World Health Organization) (1977) Manual of the International Statistical Classification of Diseases, Injuries and Causes of Death (Based on the Recommendations of Ninth Revision Conference, 1975), Geneva, World Health Organization

WHO (World Health Organization) (1992) Manual of the International Statistical Classification of Diseases, Injuries and Causes of Death (Based on the Recommendations of Tenth Revision Conference, 1990), Geneva, World Health Organization

Chapter 7. The tables

S.L. Whelan

1. The main tables

The largest set of tables in this book presents data on age-specific and age-standardized incidence for 183 populations. These tables follow Chapter 8 and are presented in sets of four pages:

(1)   An introductory text which describes the geographical area, the population covered, medical facilities and the registration practices.

(2)   The population page, which gives the population figures for the period by sex and five-year age-group in the form of an age-pyramid. For populations with persons of unknown age, the numbers are shown below the lowest age-group in the pyramid. This page also includes information on the source of the population data, the notes on the tables and a description of any screening programmes in the area.

(3)   The age-specific, standardized and cumulative rates, and the relative frequency, by ICD-9 site for males.

(4)   The age-specific, standardized and cumulative rates, and the relative frequency, by ICD-9 site for females.

1.1. Population-at-risk

Registries were asked to provide data on the population at risk each year, and most were able to do this. In general, the denominator is the average of the populations for the years for which data are presented. The year 1990, or around 1990, was a census year for many registries which resulted in a good level of accuracy. The intercensal estimates used in the previous volume were not always correct, and where this was known to have occurred, it has been pointed out in the notes on the population page. The user should also refer to Chapter 5 for a discussion of the denominator.

1.2. Age unknown

The numbers of persons of unknown age are included in the totals of the population figures by sex. The numbers of cases of unknown age are given in the incidence tables. They are included in the total numbers of cases and in the calculation of the all-ages crude rate, for each site and for all sites, but obviously do not appear in the age-specific rates. They are taken into account in the computation of the world standardized and cumulative incidence rates (see Chapter 8).

1.3. Tables of incidence by registry

The rates given in the body of these tables are the *average* annual incidence by sex, site and age-group per 100 000 population, i.e. they have been averaged over the number of years for which data are presented.

An example of the tables is given as Table 7.1. The column headings are defined below:

Site: A shortened version of the full ICD-9 title describes each site or site grouping (See Chapter 3 for details of the precise content of each 'site').

All ages: The total number of cases by site and for all sites.

Age unk: The numbers of cases of unknown age by site.

0-, 5-...:   The age-groups for which incidence data are presented. These usually end with the age-group 85+, but population data are not available above age 70 or 75 for some registries and in this case the incidence data finish at age 70+ or 75+.

Crude rate: The crude average annual incidence rate, based on the total number of registrations, of known and unknown ages, by site.

%:   The proportional frequency of each site to the total of all sites excluding ICD-9 173 (Other skin).

CR64 and
CR74:   The sum over each year of age of the age-specific incidence rates, taken from birth to age 64 and from birth to age 74 (see Chapter 8 and the Tables of Cumulative Incidence Rates).

ASR(W):   The world age-standardized incidence rate by site (see Chapter 8 and the Age-Standardized Rates Tables).

ICD(9th):   The ICD-9 code(s) corresponding to the site or group of sites given in the left-hand column.

Rate per case

At the foot of the table, on the left-hand side under 'All sites but 173' is the heading 'Rate from 1 case'. If the user wishes to calculate the numbers of cases for a particular age group, the age-specific rate should be divided by the rate from 1 case given at the bottom of the column concerned. For example, in Table 7.1, a rate of 2.0 in the age-group 0–4 for connective tissue is divided by 1.990, the rate from 1 case under the age 0–4 column, and the result is 1 case. There are 58 cases of lung cancer at age 80–84 (455.0/7.844).

TABLE 7.1

EREWHON 1988-1992

ANNUAL INCIDENCE PER 100,000 BY AGE GROUP (YEARS) - MALE

SITE	ALL AGES	AGE UNK	0-	5-	10-	15-	20-	25-	30-	35-	40-	45-	50-	55-	60-	65-	70-	75-	80-	85+	CRUDE RATE	%	CR 64	CR 74	ASR (W)	ICD (9th)
Lip	20	0	-	-	-	-	-	1.3	1.3	2.8	1.3	-	11.1	1.8	6.9	6.0	-	-	7.8	12.3	2.2	0.5	0.13	0.16	**1.6**	*140*
Tongue	51	0	-	-	-	-	1.5	-	-	5.5	6.6	1.4	22.2	9.0	16.1	9.0	22.0	22.1	7.8	12.3	5.6	1.2	0.31	0.47	**4.1**	*141*
Salivary gland	11	0	-	-	-	-	-	-	-	-	1.3	1.4	-	-	4.6	12.0	8.8	-	-	12.3	1.2	0.3	0.04	0.14	**0.9**	*142*
Mouth	59	0	-	-	-	-	-	-	-	1.4	11.9	6.8	14.2	16.3	18.4	15.1	4.4	22.1	23.5	61.7	6.5	1.3	0.34	0.44	**4.5**	*143-5*
Oropharynx	70	0	-	-	-	-	-	-	-	1.4	6.6	12.3	26.9	16.3	27.6	21.1	-	27.6	31.4	12.3	7.7	1.6	0.46	0.56	**5.4**	*146*
Nasopharynx	4	0	-	-	-	1.7	-	-	-	1.4	-	-	1.6	-	-	-	4.4	-	-	-	0.4	0.1	0.02	0.05	**0.4**	*147*
Hypopharynx	61	0	-	-	-	-	-	-	-	-	1.3	6.8	14.2	23.5	39.1	18.1	26.4	11.0	7.8	12.3	6.7	1.4	0.42	0.65	**5.0**	*148*
Pharynx unspecified	1	0	-	-	-	-	-	-	-	-	-	-	-	-	-	3.0	-	-	-	-	0.1	0.0	0.00	0.02	**0.1**	*149*
Oesophagus	95	0	-	-	-	-	-	-	-	-	5.3	2.7	14.2	27.1	43.7	39.2	39.5	44.1	94.1	49.4	10.5	2.2	0.47	0.86	**7.1**	*150*
Stomach	165	0	-	-	-	-	1.5	1.3	-	4.1	10.6	9.6	22.2	25.3	39.1	84.3	101.1	88.3	180.4	123.4	18.2	3.8	0.57	1.49	**12.3**	*151*
Small intestine	9	0	-	-	-	-	-	-	-	-	-	-	-	1.8	2.3	6.0	4.4	5.5	23.5	-	1.0	0.2	0.02	0.07	**0.6**	*152*
Colon	357	0	-	-	-	-	-	-	2.6	1.4	7.9	13.6	34.8	59.6	64.3	120.5	290.0	286.9	455.0	481.4	39.3	8.1	0.92	2.97	**25.2**	*153*
Rectum	166	0	-	-	-	-	-	-	3.8	4.1	5.3	6.8	12.7	23.5	62.0	84.3	79.1	137.9	133.4	185.1	18.3	3.8	0.59	1.41	**12.3**	*154*
Liver	149	0	-	-	-	-	-	-	1.3	-	2.6	4.1	14.2	27.1	48.3	78.3	101.1	154.5	86.3	123.4	16.4	3.4	0.49	1.38	**11.2**	*155*
Gallbladder etc.	27	0	-	-	-	-	-	-	-	-	1.4	-	-	1.8	2.3	3.0	17.6	38.6	70.6	37.0	3.0	0.6	0.03	0.13	**1.6**	*156*
Pancreas	125	0	-	-	-	-	-	-	1.3	-	4.0	5.5	12.7	23.5	32.2	60.2	92.3	110.3	125.5	61.7	13.8	2.8	0.40	1.16	**9.2**	*157*
Nose, sinuses etc.	10	0	-	-	-	-	-	-	1.3	-	-	1.4	4.7	1.8	2.3	-	-	11.0	-	12.3	1.1	0.2	0.06	0.06	**0.7**	*160*
Larynx	109	0	-	-	-	-	-	-	-	1.4	6.6	13.6	22.2	34.3	46.0	39.2	48.3	44.1	23.5	61.7	12.0	2.5	0.62	1.06	**8.6**	*161*
Bronchus, lung	696	0	-	-	-	-	-	-	2.6	9.7	22.5	34.1	83.9	146.3	291.8	361.5	408.6	391.7	455.0	518.4	76.6	15.9	2.95	6.80	**53.7**	*162*
Other thoracic organs	2	0	-	-	-	-	-	-	-	-	-	-	-	1.8	-	-	-	-	-	12.3	0.2	0.0	0.01	0.01	**0.1**	*163-4*
Bone	12	0	-	-	-	3.5	4.4	1.3	1.3	-	1.3	2.7	-	-	2.3	3.0	-	-	-	-	1.3	0.3	0.08	0.10	**1.3**	*170*
Connective tissue	20	0	2.0	-	-	1.7	-	1.3	1.3	-	-	2.7	1.6	1.8	6.9	3.0	13.2	16.6	7.8	12.3	2.2	0.5	0.10	0.18	**1.8**	*171*
Mesothelioma	9	0	-	-	-	-	-	-	-	-	-	-	-	7.2	2.3	6.0	4.4	5.5	-	-	1.0	0.2	0.05	0.10	**0.7**	*MES*
Kaposi's sarcoma	64	0	-	-	-	-	2.9	11.5	12.8	11.1	13.2	15.0	4.7	10.8	2.3	6.0	4.4	-	-	12.3	7.0	1.5	0.42	0.47	**5.4**	*KAP*
Melanoma of skin	130	0	-	-	4.0	1.7	1.5	6.4	9.0	9.7	11.9	10.9	23.7	25.3	41.4	30.1	52.7	60.7	62.8	24.7	14.3	3.0	0.73	1.14	**10.5**	*172*
Other skin	1468	0	-	-	-	3.5	5.9	6.4	20.5	29.0	64.7	96.9	201.1	263.7	438.9	608.5	799.6	1020.7	1161.0	1468.8	161.7		5.65	12.69	**109.7**	*173*
Breast	8	0	-	-	-	-	-	-	-	-	-	1.4	1.6	3.6	2.3	3.0	-	5.5	-	12.3	0.9	0.2	0.04	0.06	**0.6**	*175*
Prostate	708	0	-	-	-	-	-	-	-	-	2.6	2.7	15.8	45.2	135.6	349.4	553.6	789.0	941.3	1296.0	78.0	16.1	1.01	5.52	**49.0**	*185*
Testis	81	0	-	-	-	3.5	11.7	29.4	12.8	19.4	13.2	6.8	6.3	5.4	2.3	-	-	5.5	-	-	8.9	1.8	0.55	0.55	**7.4**	*186*
Penis	15	0	-	-	-	-	-	-	-	-	1.3	-	1.6	3.6	2.3	6.0	8.8	11.0	15.7	24.7	1.7	0.3	0.04	0.12	**1.1**	*187.1-.4*
Other male genital	7	0	-	-	-	-	-	-	-	-	-	1.4	-	-	2.3	6.0	4.4	5.5	-	12.3	0.8	0.2	0.02	0.07	**0.6**	*187.5-.9*
Bladder	443	0	-	-	-	-	1.5	-	-	2.8	7.9	19.1	47.5	88.5	131.0	213.9	259.2	397.2	423.6	345.6	48.8	10.1	1.49	3.86	**32.5**	*188*
Kidney etc.	133	0	-	-	-	-	-	-	-	1.4	5.3	10.9	3.2	19.9	25.3	114.5	83.5	88.3	133.4	74.1	14.6	3.0	0.33	1.32	**10.0**	*189*
Eye	9	0	-	-	-	-	-	-	-	-	1.3	1.4	-	3.6	4.6	3.0	-	5.5	7.8	-	1.0	0.2	0.05	0.07	**0.7**	*190*
Brain, nervous system	73	0	-	2.1	-	1.7	2.9	3.8	3.8	4.1	4.0	10.9	6.3	10.8	27.6	24.1	35.1	38.6	23.5	12.3	8.0	1.7	0.39	0.69	**6.1**	*191-2*
Thyroid	12	0	-	-	-	-	-	1.3	-	-	1.4	1.3	4.1	1.6	-	4.6	6.0	4.4	-	-	1.3	0.3	0.07	0.12	**1.0**	*193*
Other endocrine	5	0	2.0	-	-	-	-	-	-	-	-	-	-	1.8	-	4.4	-	15.7	-	-	0.6	0.1	0.02	0.04	**0.5**	*194*
Hodgkin's disease	31	0	-	-	-	3.5	1.5	5.1	2.6	2.8	2.6	1.4	4.7	3.6	11.5	6.0	4.4	11.0	-	24.7	3.4	0.7	0.20	0.25	**2.7**	*201*
Non-Hodgkin lymphoma	165	0	2.0	-	2.0	5.2	10.3	3.8	9.0	8.3	11.9	16.4	15.8	37.9	43.7	66.3	35.1	104.8	47.1	135.8	18.2	3.8	0.83	1.34	**13.5**	*200,202*
Multiple myeloma	47	0	-	-	-	-	-	-	-	-	1.3	5.5	1.6	9.0	11.5	6.0	48.3	44.1	15.7	98.7	5.2	1.1	0.14	0.42	**3.5**	*203*
Lymphoid leukaemia	63	0	10.0	-	4.0	5.2	1.5	-	-	-	-	1.4	7.9	7.2	9.2	18.1	57.1	33.1	54.9	74.1	6.9	1.4	0.23	0.61	**5.9**	*204*
Myeloid leukaemia	57	0	-	2.1	-	-	1.5	-	2.6	2.8	1.3	5.5	1.6	7.2	9.2	30.1	48.3	27.6	70.6	24.7	6.3	1.3	0.17	0.56	**4.4**	*205*
Monocytic leukaemia	0	0	-	-	-	-	-	-	-	-	-	-	-	-	-	-	-	-	-	-	0.0	0.0	0.00	0.00	**0.0**	*206*
Other leukaemia	0	0	-	-	-	-	-	-	-	-	-	-	-	-	-	-	-	-	-	-	0.0	0.0	0.00	0.00	**0.0**	*207*
Leukaemia unspecified	3	0	-	-	-	-	-	-	-	-	-	-	1.6	-	-	-	-	-	7.8	12.3	0.3	0.1	0.01	0.01	**0.2**	*208*
Other and unspecified	108	0	2.0	-	-	-	-	2.6	-	2.8	1.3	8.2	17.4	9.0	43.7	24.1	61.5	71.7	78.4	197.5	11.9	2.5	0.43	0.86	**8.2**	*O&U*
All sites	5858	0	17.9	4.2	9.9	31.5	48.4	75.5	89.8	130.0	240.4	345.3	677.7	1006.1	1707.3	2494.3	3330.4	4137.9	4792.9	5652.9	645.1		21.92	51.04	**442.0**	*ALL*
All sites but 173	4390	0	17.9	4.2	9.9	28.0	42.6	69.1	69.3	100.9	175.7	248.4	476.6	742.4	1268.4	1885.8	2530.8	3117.2	3631.9	4184.2	483.5	100.0	16.27	38.35	**332.3**	*ALLb*

| Rate from 1 case | | | 1.990 | 2.098 | 1.985 | 1.747 | 1.467 | 1.280 | 1.283 | 1.383 | 1.321 | 1.365 | 1.583 | 1.806 | 2.298 | 3.012 | 4.394 | 5.517 | 7.844 | 12.343 | | | | | | |

To overcome the problems posed by large populations (which result in zeroes after the decimal point), a scale factor is used, and the rate may be from 10 or from 100 cases instead of 1. In this instance, the calculation given above would be: 455.0/7.844×10, or 455.0/7.844×100.

Zero rate
A dash (–) means that there are no cases registered. 0.0 means an incidence rate less than 0.05.

1.4. Notes to the tables
An asterisk (*) beside the name of a registry indicates that there may be under-ascertainment of cases, possible lack of validity or potential inaccuracy in the denominator of the rates, for all sites or for some sites. The note on the population page explains the reason for the asterisk (see also Chapter 5).

A flag (+) denotes a registry for which it has not been possible to verify the data using the CHECK program designed to check for unlikely or impossible codes or combinations of codes (see Chapters 5 and 6).

A dagger (†) is used to denote variations in coding, for example for bladder, indicating that non-invasive diagnoses (normally included for this site – see Chapter 3) are *not* included, and for non-melanoma skin (Other skin). A note on the population page explains how the marked site differs from the standard contents defined in Chapter 3.

2. The age-standardized incidence rates tables
The tables which follow the main tables present the world age-standardized incidence rates and the cumulative rates for ages 0–74, with their standard errors (see Chapter 8). The first set of age-standardized rates and the cumulative rates are given by each of the sites in the main tables (see Chapter 3), with the addition of colon+rectum and all of the leukaemias. The Age-Standardized Incidence Rates (4-digit rubrics) present data for selected fourth-digit subdivisions of the three-digit ICD rubrics, for all registries providing fourth digits.

2.1. Key to conventions and symbols used in the tables

Small numbers
For rates based on less than 10 cases, the decimal is given by a comma and not a point, e.g. 3,4 rather than 3.4.

Unknown age
The letters 'm' (males) and/or 'f' (females) at the end of a row of figures signal rates based on data including more than 10% of cases of unknown age for males and/or females.

0.0/0,0
This figure shows that the rate or standard error is greater than 0 but less than 0.05.

0.00/0,00
The rate or standard error is greater than 0 but less than 0.005.

Previous volumes included truncated rates, and the cumulative rates for ages 0–64. These are no longer printed in this book.

3.Percentage distribution of microscopically verified cases by histological type
See Chapter 4.

4.Indices of data quality
4.1 Key to conventions and symbols used in the tables
For MV (% cases morphologically verified): a number in brackets signifies that cytological verification is excluded.

For MV and DCO (% cases based on a death certificate alone):

99	=	99% or more
Blank	=	MV/DCO not included for this site
0	=	cases registered but not morphologically verified/reported on the basis of a death certificate alone
–	=	no cases registered, although data for this site were submitted.

For M/I (ratio of mortality to incidence):

999	=	99% or more
Blank	=	M/I not included for this site
0	=	cases registered but no deaths
–	=	no cases and no deaths, although data on both cases and deaths collected for the site
NCR	=	no cases but one or more deaths.

See also Chapter 5.

Chapter 8. Age standardization

M. Plummer

The purpose of this chapter is to provide a brief introduction to the two summary measures of incidence used in this volume - the age-standardized rate and the cumulative rate. These statistics were discussed in more detail by Smith (1992) and Day (1992) in the previous volume in this series. Further discussion can be found in Jensen *et al.* (1991) and Estève *et al.* (1994).

The best way to analyse cancer incidence data is to use age-specific rates. However, it is often convenient to have a measure of overall incidence which can be used to compare different populations. The crude rate is not suitable for this purpose because it depends on the age structure of the population. Since the incidence of many types of cancer increases rapidly with age - in some cancers 500-fold over a 50-year span - the age structure of the population can be an important determinant of the crude rate. The aim of both the standardized rate and the cumulative rate is to provide a summary statistic which is independent of age and which is therefore more comparable between registries. There are other reasons why data may not be comparable, but they are not discussed in this chapter.

1. Standardized incidence rate

In order to calculate the standardized incidence rate, an external reference population with a given 'standard' age distribution is required. The standardized rate is the incidence rate that, theoretically, would have been observed if the population had the standard age distribution. The standardized rate is calculated first by estimating the age-specific rates and then applying these rates to the reference population. This process, called direct standardization, is illustrated in Table 8.1 using data on stomach cancer incidence among males in Denmark 1988–92 and the world population as a reference population. Age groups are indexed by the subscript i, d_i is the number of cases, y_i is the number of person-years at risk (given by multiplying the number of males in the Danish population by the observation period of five years) and w_i is the number of persons in age group i per 100 000 in the standard world population. The crude rate per 100 000 per annum is

$$10^5 \left(\sum_i d_i \right) \Big/ \left(\sum_i y_i \right) = 10^5 \times 1898/12678700$$
$$= 14.97$$

The age-standardized rate is given by

$$\sum_i d_i w_i / y_i = 9.03$$

In this example, the age-standardized rate is 40% lower than the crude rate because the standard world population has proportionally fewer males in the older age groups than the population of Denmark (14% over 70 years of age compared with 36%). Hence there would be fewer males at high risk of stomach cancer if the Danish population had the world standard age distribution.

The biggest problem with age-standardized rates is that the numbers used to make up the standard age distribution are arbitrary. The 'world', 'European' and 'African' populations have all been proposed as reference populations (Doll & Cook, 1967). In addition, truncated versions of these populations, which only include persons within a given age range, may be used to analyse cancers occurring in childhood or middle age. None of these reference populations is obviously correct, and they all give different results, both in terms of the absolute value of the standardized rates and the relative rankings of different registries. It is therefore very important, when reporting age-standardized rates, to report the population to which the rates have been standardized. The proliferation of different reference populations also interferes with the primary aim of age-standardization, which is comparability. For this reason, the only population used in this volume is the world population which is given in Table 8.1. It should be noted that, in this context the 'world' population has a very specific meaning. It is the population proposed by Doll for the first volume in this series (Doll et al., 1966) which simply rounded off the figures that Segi (1960) had derived from the pooled population of 46 countries. It is not meant to be identical to the current world population.

2. Cumulative rate

Before defining the cumulative rate, the concept of the cumulative risk will be introduced. The cumulative risk is the probability that an individual will develop the disease in question during a certain age period, in the absence of any competing cause of death. The age period over which the risk is accumulated must be specified. In this volume, the age range 0–74 is used, representing a lifetime risk of developing the disease. Other age ranges may be more appropriate for more specific needs, such as investigating childhood diseases.

If the cumulative risk from 0 to 74 is less than 10%, which is the case for most tumours, it can be approximated very well by the cumulative rate. The cumulative rate is, like the standardized rate, a weighted sum of age-specific incidence rates. However, the weights used to calculate the cumulative rate are not based on an external reference population, but are simply the widths of the age groups. In the example of males in Denmark, all the age groups are of five

Table 8.1. Computation of age-standardized incidence rates (stomach cancer, Denmark, males, 1988–92)

Age group i	No. of cases d_i	Person-years at risk y_i	Estimated incidence (per 10^5 years) $10^5(d_i/y_i)$	Standard world population w_i	Expected cases in standard population $d_i w_i/y_i$
0–	0	749 800	–	12 000	0.00
5–	0	695 500	–	10 000	0.00
10–	0	808 900	–	9 000	0.00
15–	1	931 100	0.1	9 000	0.01
20–	2	1 017 500	0.2	8 000	0.02
25–	6	1 032 700	0.6	8 000	0.05
30–	4	955 800	0.4	6 000	0.02
35–	16	946 500	1.7	6 000	0.10
40–	34	1 025 500	3.3	6 000	0.20
45–	76	926 900	8.2	6 000	0.49
50–	97	718 900	13.5	5 000	0.68
55–	150	626 800	23.9	4 000	0.96
60–	187	590 700	31.7	4 000	1.27
65–	302	553 100	54.6	3 000	1.64
70–	315	449 900	70.0	2 000	1.40
75–	309	337 200	91.6	1 000	0.92
80–	247	196 200	125.9	500	0.63
85+	152	115 700	131.4	500	0.66
Total	1898	12 678 700		100 000	9.03

years, so the cumulative rate from 0 to 74 is given by

$$5\sum_i d_i/y_i = 5 \times 208.2 \times 10^{-5}$$
$$= 0.0104$$

The cumulative rate is proportional to, but not identical to, an age-standardized rate which uses a uniform distribution between the two age limits as a standard age distribution. The cumulative rate is not, in fact, a rate but a dimensionless quantity. In other words, it is not expressed in units of 'per annum' but simply as a number. It is most conveniently expressed as a percentage, so the cumulative rate to age 74 in the above example would be given as 1.04.

The precise mathematical relationship between the cumulative rate and the cumulative risk is

$$\text{cumulative risk} = 1 - \exp(- \text{cumulative rate})$$

Table 8.2 shows the correction needed to convert the cumulative rate into the cumulative risk. For values under 10% the change is small.

The cumulative rate has two advantages over the age-standardized rate:

(a) as a form of direct standardization, it removes the problem of choosing an arbitrary reference population;

(b) as an approximation to the cumulative risk it has a greater intuitive appeal, and is more directly interpretable as a measurement of lifetime risk, ignoring mortality from other diseases.

3. Calculation of the standard error

Both the standardized and the cumulative rate can be expressed as a weighted sum of the age-specific rates, so the standard error can be derived in both cases from the same basic formula. If the age-specific rate in age-group i is estimated from d_i cases and y_i person-years, then the age-standardized rate (with w_i representing the standardization weights) given by

$$\sum_i w_i d_i/y_i$$

has an estimated variance (based on the Poisson distribution) of

$$\sum_i d_i\left(w_i/y_i\right)^2$$

and an estimated standard error of

$$\sqrt{\sum_i d_i\left(w_i/y_i\right)^2}$$

For the age-standardized rate, the weights are given by the number of persons in each age group per 100 000 in the standard population. For the cumulative rate, the weights are equal to the widths of the age-groups. When all the age-groups are five years across, the expression for the standard error of the cumulative rate (expressed as a percentage) reduces to

$$\text{S. E. (cumulative rate)} = 500 \sqrt{\sum_i d_i/y_i^2}$$

For the example of stomach cancer among males in Denmark, the estimates with standard errors are 9.03 (0.22) for the rate standardized to the world population and 1.04 (0.03) for the cumulative rate.

Table 8.2. Conversion of cumulative rates (100x) into the corresponding cumulative risk $100(1-e^{-x})$										
100x	0.1	0.5	1.0	5.0	7.0	10.0	15.0	20.0	30.0	40.0	50.0
$100(1-e^{-x})$	0.1	0.499	0.995	4.88	6.76	9.52	13.93	18.13	25.92	32.97	39.35

4. Cases of unknown age

In this volume, both summary measures of incidence have been adjusted to account for cases of unknown age. This was done simply by multiplying the standardized rate or cumulative rate, based on cases of known age, by T/K where T is the *total* number of cases of cancer of the same type in persons of the same sex, and K is the number occurring in persons of *known* age. The standard errors were also multiplied by the same correction factor (T/K).

The assumption underlying this correction is that the ages of cases are *missing at random*. In other words, the probability that the age of a case is unknown does not depend on the age of the case. Although this assumption is somewhat unrealistic - it is more likely that age is not recorded in older cases - it is important that *all* registered cases are used, so that the standardized or cumulative rate is not underestimated.

5. Comment

It should be stressed that neither the age-standardized rate nor the cumulative rate is a substitute for the age-specific incidence rates, which should always form the basis of a thorough analysis.

References

Day, N.E. (1992) Cumulative rate and cumulative risk. In: Parkin, D.M., Muir, C.S., Whelan, S.L., Gao, Y.-T., Ferlay, J. & Powell, J., eds, Cancer Incidence in Five Continents, Volume VI (IARC Scientific Publications No. 120), Lyon, IARC

Doll, R. & Cook, P. (1967) Summarizing indices for comparison of cancer incidence data. Int J Cancer, 2, 269-279

Doll, R., Payne, P. & Waterhouse, J., eds (1966) Cancer Incidence in Five Continents: A Technical Report, Berlin, Springer-Verlag (for UICC)

Estève, J., Benhamou, E. & Raymond, L (1994) Descriptive Epidemiology (IARC Scientific Publications No. 128), Lyon, IARC

Jensen, O.M., Parkin, D.M., MacLennan, R., Muir, C.S. & Skeet, R.G., eds (1991) Cancer registration principles and methods (IARC Scientific Publications No. 95), Lyon, IARC

Segi, M (1960) Cancer Mortality for Selected Sites in 24 Countries (1950–57), Sendai, Tohoku University School of Public Health

Smith, P. G. (1992) Comparison between registries: Age-standardized rates. In: Parkin, D.M., Muir, C.S., Whelan, S.L., Gao, Y.-T., Ferlay, J. & Powell, J., eds, Cancer Incidence in Five Continents, Volume VI (IARC Scientific Publications No. 120), Lyon, IARC

The Tables

Age-specific and age-standardized
incidence rates

Algeria, Sétif

The Cancer Registry of Sétif was established in January 1989, in collaboration with IARC, following a retrospective study on cancer incidence in Sétif between 1986 and 1988.

Cancer has become one of the major public health problems in Algeria, as diagnosis is often late and treatment is difficult and costly. Cancer accounts for 50% of the residents who seek treatment abroad. The registry is an indispensable tool in the fight against this serious illness and in making a precise evaluation of requirements for proper diagnosis, therapy and prevention.

The registry is attached to the department of public health information and biostatistics of the Service of Epidemiology and Preventive Medicine, situated in the mother and child hospital (Hôpital Mère Enfant) of the Centre Hospitalo-Universitaire (CHU) in Sétif.

The wilaya of Sétif covers an area of 6504 km², corresponding to 0.27% of the country. It is situated between Algiers to the west (the capital of the country), Constantine to the east, Boubie and Jijel (the coastal region) to the north and M'sila to the south. The wilaya of Sétif is called the capital of the highlands, having an altitude of 1200 m and a semi-arid continental climate with scorching summers and hard winters.

The population of the wilaya of Sétif was estimated at 1 225 688 on 31 December 1993, based on the last General Census of the National Population in 1987 (around 5% of the national population). The town is the second in importance in the country, after Algiers. The population density is 187 inhabitants per km², with 64% of the population living in rural areas. The birth rate is still high at 31.5 per 1000 and the mortality rate is declining slightly at 4.3 per 1000, giving an overall population growth rate of 2.7%. The number of persons per household is eight. The population is very young, 50% being in the age-group 0–15 years and 60% below the age of 19 years.

There are two main occupational sectors, agriculture and industry, with an active population numbering 271 414, of which 40% are without employment.

The wilaya of Sétif has eight hospitals, one a university hospital centre with 2025 hospital beds, providing 1.46 beds per 1000 inhabitants. There are 25 maternity hospitals, 15 polyclinics (one per 81 712 inhabitants), 49 health centres (one per 25 014 inhabitants) and 143 care units (one per 8 571 inhabitants). There are 108 medical specialists and 475 general practitioners (one doctor per 1691 inhabitants), 236 dentists (one per 5150 inhabitants), 90 pharmacists (one per 12 636 inhabitants) and 2081 paramedics (one for 438 inhabitants).

Cancer cases are diagnosed in Sétif, and radiotherapy treatment is carried out at the Pierre et Marie Curie Centre in Algiers or at the Anti-Cancer Centre in Constantine.

The registry uses the latest version of CANREG, NEWCRG, of IARC. Hospital data are obtained from the admissions department, the laboratories of pathology and biology, the haematology department, and all the medical departments in the CHU of Sétif as well as the Anti-Cancer Centre of Constantine and the Pierre et Marie Curie Centre in Algiers.

Data from non-hospital sources are collected from social security systems, from the municipal registry offices (death certificates) and from practitioners working in the private sector. These data are collected actively by a junior epidemiologist from the various sources.

Data entry and analysis are done in Sétif and verified using the IARC/IACR CHECK program. Duplicate entries are reduced to a minimum by careful inspection of the name, sex, dates of birth and of diagnosis.

The data are collected on a notification form for each new diagnosis of cancer. Data items comprise the personal identifying information (surname, first name, date of birth, place of residence), the date and basis of diagnosis, the diagnosis (site and morphology), and follow up (alive, dead, date and cause of death).

Certain items are coded directly at data collection, and others are coded centrally. The diagnosis is coded according to ICD-O.

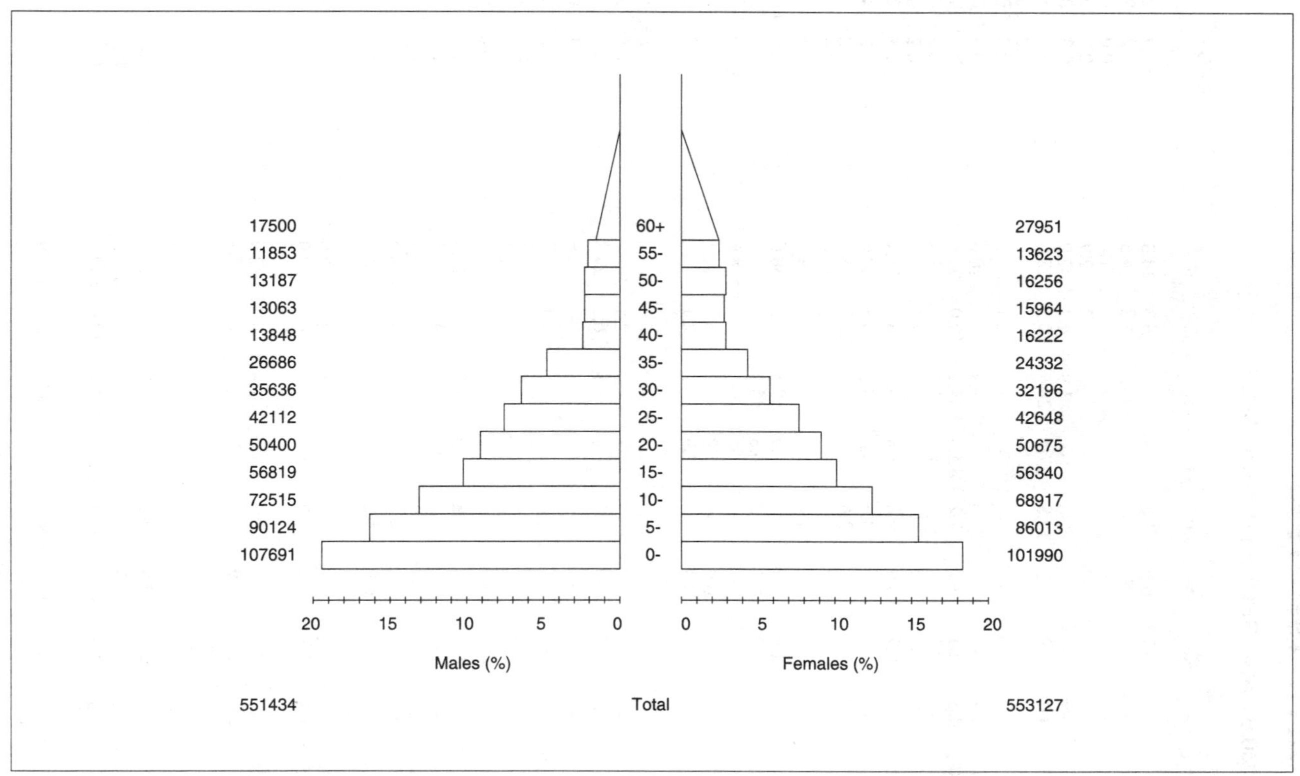

Algeria, Sétif

Source of population: 31 December 1991

Census: 31 December 1987. Recensement général de la population.

Estimate: On the basis of the 1987 census.

Notes to tables overleaf:

* There are very few cases registered on the basis of a death certificate alone, and the very high rate of histological verification for several sites, as well as low rates of incidence, indicate under-ascertainment of cases.

† 188 does not include non-invasive tumours.

Screening programmes in the area:

Since 1989 around 100 examinations have been carried out annually in the population aged over 15 for nasopharyngeal carcinoma.

* ALGERIA, SETIF 1990-1993

ANNUAL INCIDENCE PER 100,000 BY AGE GROUP (YEARS) - MALE

SITE	ALL AGES	AGE UNK	0-	5-	10-	15-	20-	25-	30-	35-	40-	45-	50-	55-	60+	CRUDE RATE	%	ASR (W)	ICD (9th)
Lip	20	0	-	0.3	-	0.4	-	-	0.7	0.9	1.8	1.9	1.9	6.3	14.3	0.9	2.1	**2.3**	140
Tongue	5	0	-	-	-	-	-	-	-	-	-	-	-	4.2	4.3	0.2	0.5	**0.6**	141
Salivary gland	1	0	-	-	-	-	-	-	-	-	-	-	-	-	1.4	0.0	0.1	**0.2**	142
Mouth	4	0	-	-	-	-	-	-	-	-	-	-	-	4.2	2.9	0.2	0.4	**0.5**	143-5
Oropharynx	6	0	-	-	0.3	-	-	-	-	-	-	-	1.9	4.2	2.9	0.3	0.6	**0.6**	146
Nasopharynx	85	0	-	-	0.7	2.2	3.5	3.0	4.9	3.7	10.8	17.2	28.4	10.5	28.6	3.9	8.8	**8.0**	147
Hypopharynx	0	0	-	-	-	-	-	-	-	-	-	-	-	-	-	0.0	0.0	**0.0**	148
Pharynx unspecified	1	0	-	-	-	-	-	-	-	-	-	-	-	2.1	-	0.0	0.1	**0.1**	149
Oesophagus	9	0	-	-	-	-	-	0.6	-	-	-	-	1.9	-	10.0	0.4	0.9	**1.2**	150
Stomach	113	0	-	-	-	-	1.0	0.6	2.1	3.7	7.2	13.4	34.1	19.0	92.9	5.1	11.7	**14.4**	151
Small intestine	4	0	-	-	-	-	-	-	0.7	-	-	1.9	1.9	-	1.4	0.2	0.4	**0.4**	152
Colon	4	0	-	-	-	-	-	0.6	-	-	-	-	-	2.1	2.9	0.2	0.4	**0.4**	153
Rectum	24	0	-	-	-	0.4	0.5	-	0.7	0.9	9.0	3.8	3.8	6.3	11.4	1.1	2.5	**2.6**	154
Liver	40	0	0.2	-	-	-	-	-	-	0.9	3.6	9.6	9.5	10.5	30.0	1.8	4.1	**5.1**	155
Gallbladder etc.	26	0	-	-	-	-	-	-	-	-	3.6	-	1.9	10.5	25.7	1.2	2.7	**3.6**	156
Pancreas	14	0	-	-	-	-	-	-	-	1.9	-	1.9	-	4.2	12.9	0.6	1.4	**1.8**	157
Nose, sinuses etc.	4	0	-	-	-	-	-	-	-	-	1.8	-	-	-	4.3	0.2	0.4	**0.6**	160
Larynx	44	0	-	-	-	-	-	-	1.4	0.9	1.8	1.9	9.5	14.8	38.6	2.0	4.6	**5.7**	161
Bronchus, lung	216	0	-	-	-	-	-	1.2	0.7	9.4	7.2	26.8	45.5	63.3	187.1	9.8	22.3	**28.1**	162
Other thoracic organs	7	0	-	-	-	-	-	0.6	-	-	-	-	-	-	8.6	0.3	0.7	**1.0**	163-4
Bone	23	0	-	0.6	0.7	1.8	1.0	-	-	0.9	-	1.9	-	6.3	11.4	1.0	2.4	**2.0**	170
Connective tissue	6	0	0.2	0.3	-	-	-	-	0.7	0.9	-	1.9	-	2.1	-	0.3	0.6	**0.4**	171
Mesothelioma	0	0	-	-	-	-	-	-	-	-	-	-	-	-	-	0.0	0.0	**0.0**	MES
Kaposi's sarcoma	0	0	-	-	-	-	-	-	-	-	-	-	-	-	-	0.0	0.0	**0.0**	KAP
Melanoma of skin	1	0	-	-	-	-	-	-	-	-	-	-	-	2.1	-	0.0	0.1	**0.1**	172
Other skin	33	0	0.5	0.3	-	0.4	-	0.6	0.7	-	5.4	3.8	3.8	6.3	24.3	1.5		**3.9**	173
Breast	2	0	-	-	-	-	-	-	-	-	-	-	-	-	2.9	0.1	0.2	**0.3**	175
Prostate	12	0	-	-	-	-	-	-	-	-	-	-	-	2.1	15.7	0.5	1.2	**1.8**	185
Testis	2	0	-	-	-	-	-	-	-	-	-	-	-	2.1	1.4	0.1	0.2	**0.2**	186
Penis	1	0	-	-	-	-	-	-	-	-	-	-	-	-	1.4	0.0	0.1	**0.2**	187.1-.4
Other male genital	0	0	-	-	-	-	-	-	-	-	-	-	-	-	-	0.0	0.0	**0.0**	187.5-.9
†Bladder	13	0	-	-	-	-	-	-	0.7	-	1.8	1.9	1.9	-	12.9	0.6	1.3	**1.8**	188
Kidney etc.	7	0	-	0.8	-	0.4	-	-	-	-	-	-	-	4.2	1.4	0.3	0.7	**0.4**	189
Eye	1	0	-	-	-	-	-	-	-	-	-	-	-	-	1.4	0.0	0.1	**0.2**	190
Brain, nervous system	14	0	-	0.3	-	0.4	-	0.6	-	-	3.6	-	1.9	2.1	10.0	0.6	1.4	**1.6**	191-2
Thyroid	3	0	-	-	-	-	-	-	-	0.9	1.8	-	-	-	1.4	0.1	0.3	**0.3**	193
Other endocrine	0	0	-	-	-	-	-	-	-	-	-	-	-	-	-	0.0	0.0	**0.0**	194
Hodgkin's disease	39	0	-	2.8	1.4	1.3	1.0	1.8	2.8	3.7	-	5.7	3.8	4.2	2.9	1.8	4.0	**2.2**	201
Non-Hodgkin lymphoma	70	0	1.6	1.1	1.4	0.9	2.5	1.8	2.8	3.7	7.2	5.7	7.6	6.3	32.9	3.2	7.2	**6.3**	200,202
Multiple myeloma	3	0	-	-	-	-	-	-	-	0.9	-	-	-	2.1	1.4	0.1	0.3	**0.3**	203
Lymphoid leukaemia	44	0	0.9	3.1	2.1	1.8	1.0	-	1.4	-	3.6	1.9	1.9	4.2	12.9	2.0	4.6	**2.9**	204
Myeloid leukaemia	28	0	0.5	0.3	1.0	2.2	-	2.4	2.1	0.9	1.8	3.8	-	2.1	7.1	1.3	2.9	**2.0**	205
Monocytic leukaemia	0	0	-	-	-	-	-	-	-	-	-	-	-	-	-	0.0	0.0	**0.0**	206
Other leukaemia	0	0	-	-	-	-	-	-	-	-	-	-	-	-	-	0.0	0.0	**0.0**	207
Leukaemia unspecified	19	0	0.5	0.3	1.0	0.9	-	0.6	2.8	-	1.8	-	1.9	-	5.7	0.9	2.0	**1.3**	208
Other and unspecified	52	0	0.5	0.6	0.7	-	-	2.4	2.1	2.8	3.6	3.8	1.9	10.5	37.1	2.4	5.4	**5.7**	O&U
All sites	1000	0	4.9	10.5	9.3	13.2	10.4	16.6	27.4	37.5	77.6	109.1	164.9	219.4	664.3	45.3		**111.0**	ALL
All sites but 173	967	0	4.4	10.3	9.3	12.8	10.4	16.0	26.7	37.5	72.2	105.3	161.1	213.0	640.0	43.8	100.0	**107.1**	ALLb

Rate from 1 case   0.232   0.277   0.345   0.440   0.496   0.594   0.702   0.937   1.805   1.914   1.896   2.109   1.429

†Important: see notes on population page

* ALGERIA, SETIF 1990-1993

ANNUAL INCIDENCE PER 100,000 BY AGE GROUP (YEARS) - FEMALE

SITE	ALL AGES	AGE UNK	0-	5-	10-	15-	20-	25-	30-	35-	40-	45-	50-	55-	60+	CRUDE RATE	%	ASR (W)	ICD (9th)
Lip	1	0	-	-	-	-	-	-	-	-	-	-	-	-	0.9	0.0	0.1	**0.1**	*140*
Tongue	1	0	-	-	-	-	-	-	-	-	-	-	-	1.8	-	0.0	0.1	**0.1**	*141*
Salivary gland	0	0	-	-	-	-	-	-	-	-	-	-	-	-	-	0.0	0.0	**0.0**	*142*
Mouth	2	0	-	-	-	-	-	-	-	-	3.1	-	-	-	-	0.1	0.2	**0.2**	*143-5*
Oropharynx	3	0	-	-	-	0.9	-	-	-	-	-	-	-	-	0.9	0.1	0.3	**0.2**	*146*
Nasopharynx	43	0	-	0.9	1.1	1.3	2.5	3.5	1.6	1.0	3.1	3.1	6.2	7.3	7.2	1.9	4.9	**2.7**	*147*
Hypopharynx	0	0	-	-	-	-	-	-	-	-	-	-	-	-	-	0.0	0.0	**0.0**	*148*
Pharynx unspecified	1	0	0.2	-	-	-	-	-	-	-	-	-	-	-	-	0.0	0.1	**0.0**	*149*
Oesophagus	4	0	-	-	-	-	-	-	-	-	1.5	-	-	5.5	-	0.2	0.5	**0.3**	*150*
Stomach	42	0	-	-	-	-	0.5	0.6	2.3	2.1	6.2	4.7	9.2	12.8	13.4	1.9	4.8	**3.5**	*151*
Small intestine	0	0	-	-	-	-	-	-	-	-	-	-	-	-	-	0.0	0.0	**0.0**	*152*
Colon	7	0	-	-	-	-	-	-	-	1.0	1.5	-	4.6	-	1.8	0.3	0.8	**0.6**	*153*
Rectum	27	0	-	-	-	-	0.5	0.6	-	2.1	4.6	4.7	6.2	1.8	10.7	1.2	3.1	**2.3**	*154*
Liver	25	0	-	-	-	-	0.5	-	0.8	1.0	3.1	3.1	1.5	1.8	14.3	1.1	2.9	**2.2**	*155*
Gallbladder etc.	118	0	-	-	-	-	-	1.2	-	3.1	18.5	14.1	35.4	42.2	41.1	5.3	13.5	**10.2**	*156*
Pancreas	8	0	-	-	-	-	-	-	-	-	3.1	1.6	3.1	-	2.7	0.4	0.9	**0.7**	*157*
Nose, sinuses etc.	5	0	-	-	-	-	-	0.6	-	-	-	-	1.5	1.8	1.8	0.2	0.6	**0.4**	*160*
Larynx	3	0	-	-	-	-	0.5	-	-	-	-	-	-	-	1.8	0.1	0.3	**0.2**	*161*
Bronchus, lung	33	0	-	-	-	-	0.5	0.6	0.8	-	1.5	3.1	4.6	9.2	17.0	1.5	3.8	**2.9**	*162*
Other thoracic organs	6	0	-	-	0.4	-	-	0.6	-	-	-	-	-	1.8	2.7	0.3	0.7	**0.4**	*163-4*
Bone	13	0	-	0.6	0.4	0.9	1.0	-	1.6	-	-	3.1	-	-	1.8	0.6	1.5	**0.7**	*170*
Connective tissue	7	0	-	0.3	0.4	0.4	0.5	-	-	2.1	-	-	-	-	0.9	0.3	0.8	**0.4**	*171*
Mesothelioma	0	0	-	-	-	-	-	-	-	-	-	-	-	-	-	0.0	0.0	**0.0**	*MES*
Kaposi's sarcoma	0	0	-	-	-	-	-	-	-	-	-	-	-	-	-	0.0	0.0	**0.0**	*KAP*
Melanoma of skin	1	0	-	-	-	-	-	-	-	-	-	-	-	1.8	-	0.0	0.1	**0.1**	*172*
Other skin	23	0	0.7	-	0.4	-	0.5	0.6	0.8	-	1.5	1.6	-	-	12.5	1.0		**1.8**	*173*
Breast	118	0	-	-	-	-	0.5	2.3	7.0	12.3	17.0	36.0	32.3	25.7	20.6	5.3	13.5	**9.5**	*174*
Uterus unspecified	1	0	-	-	-	-	-	-	-	-	1.6	-	-	-	-	0.0	0.1	**0.1**	*179*
Cervix uteri	166	0	-	-	-	-	-	1.8	5.4	16.4	50.9	39.2	33.8	36.7	35.8	7.5	19.0	**13.9**	*180*
Placenta	0	0	-	-	-	-	-	-	-	-	-	-	-	-	-	0.0	0.0	**0.0**	*181*
Corpus uteri	13	0	-	-	-	-	-	-	-	-	-	3.1	1.8	8.9		0.6	1.5	**1.2**	*182*
Ovary etc.	14	0	-	-	-	-	-	-	0.8	1.0	4.6	6.3	4.6	-	1.8	0.6	1.6	**1.2**	*183*
Other female genital	8	0	0.2	-	-	-	0.5	-	-	1.0	-	3.1	3.1	-	0.9	0.4	0.9	**0.6**	*184*
†Bladder	1	0	-	-	-	-	-	-	-	-	-	-	-	1.8	-	0.0	0.1	**0.1**	*188*
Kidney etc.	8	0	1.2	0.3	-	-	-	-	0.8	-	-	1.6	-	-	-	0.4	0.9	**0.3**	*189*
Eye	2	0	-	-	0.4	-	-	0.6	-	-	-	-	-	-	-	0.1	0.2	**0.1**	*190*
Brain, nervous system	11	0	0.5	0.3	0.4	0.4	0.5	-	0.8	-	1.5	3.1	-	1.8	-	0.5	1.3	**0.6**	*191-2*
Thyroid	9	0	-	-	-	-	-	-	2.3	-	-	-	3.1	1.8	2.7	0.4	1.0	**0.7**	*193*
Other endocrine	0	0	-	-	-	-	-	-	-	-	-	-	-	-	-	0.0	0.0	**0.0**	*194*
Hodgkin's disease	29	0	-	1.2	1.8	0.4	1.0	2.3	4.7	3.1	3.1	1.6	-	-	0.9	1.3	3.3	**1.4**	*201*
Non-Hodgkin lymphoma	37	0	0.5	0.3	0.4	-	1.5	1.8	1.6	2.1	7.7	4.7	1.5	3.7	10.7	1.7	4.2	**2.7**	*200,202*
Multiple myeloma	4	0	-	-	-	-	-	-	-	-	-	3.1	-	-	1.8	0.2	0.5	**0.4**	*203*
Lymphoid leukaemia	26	0	-	2.3	0.7	2.2	1.0	-	0.8	-	-	1.6	1.5	3.7	3.6	1.2	3.0	**1.3**	*204*
Myeloid leukaemia	29	0	0.2	1.5	0.4	1.8	1.0	1.2	0.8	3.1	6.2	-	1.5	-	4.5	1.3	3.3	**1.7**	*205*
Monocytic leukaemia	0	0	-	-	-	-	-	-	-	-	-	-	-	-	-	0.0	0.0	**0.0**	*206*
Other leukaemia	0	0	-	-	-	-	-	-	-	-	-	-	-	-	-	0.0	0.0	**0.0**	*207*
Leukaemia unspecified	14	0	0.5	1.2	-	0.9	-	-	1.0	-	-	4.6	-	1.8		0.6	1.6	**0.7**	*208*
Other and unspecified	32	0	0.2	0.3	-	-	-	0.6	0.8	7.2	3.1	11.0	3.1	1.8	8.0	1.4	3.7	**2.5**	*O&U*
All sites	895	0	4.4	9.0	6.5	9.3	12.8	18.8	33.4	59.6	141.8	151.9	164.6	167.0	233.4	40.5		**69.2**	*ALL*
All sites but 173	872	0	3.7	9.0	6.2	9.3	12.3	18.2	32.6	59.6	140.2	150.3	164.6	167.0	220.9	39.4	100.0	**67.4**	*ALLb*

Rate from 1 case 0.245 0.291 0.363 0.444 0.493 0.586 0.776 1.027 1.541 1.566 1.538 1.835 0.894

†Important: see notes on population page

France, La Réunion

Collection of data on cancer morbidity was initiated on the island of La Réunion in 1983. The population-based registry was established in 1988, with the aim of establishing the burden and patterns of cancer among residents of the island, whether diagnosed locally or elsewhere.

The island of La Réunion, one of the four overseas départements of France, is situated in the Indian Ocean, 9180 km away from Paris on longitude 55° 29′ E and latitude 21° 5′ S, between the equator and the Tropic of Capricorn. Like the islands of Mauritius and Rodriguez, it belongs to the Mascarene Archipelago, with Madagascar to the west and the Seychelles to the north. It is a volcanic and mountainous island, 2512 km^2 in area, dominated by the Piton des Neiges, the highest point in the Indian Ocean at 3069 m. The Piton de la Fournaise is still an active volcano, occupying the south-east third of the island.

The tropical climate is hot and humid; the high temperatures are moderated by the sea and the trade winds, which blow from the south-east. There are two seasons: summer or the hurricane period, hot and humid, from November to April, and winter which is dry and cool (May to October).

La Réunion was first inhabited in the 17th century, by European colonials and African and Malagasy slaves. After the abolition of slavery in 1848, the immigration of labourers from India and China added to this ethnic diversity. The population, at the 1990 census, amounted to 597 828 inhabitants (density 238 inhabitants per km^2). In 1990, the birth rate, although falling, remained high at 23 per 1000. With an annual increase of 1.9% (compared with 0.5% in metropolitan France), La Réunion is undergoing rapid demographic growth; in 1990, 40% of the inhabitants were under the age of 20 years. Only 9% of the population were born outside the département. There were 234 000 active members of the population, of whom 146 000 were employed.

On 1 January 1990, there were 933 doctors on the island, 521 of whom were general practitioners and 412 specialists (156 doctors per 100 000 inhabitants, compared with 262 on the mainland of France). There were 3237 hospital beds, of which 2286 were in the public sector and 951 private.

Registration is active. The first step involves collecting information from the principal sources, the public and private pathology and haematology laboratories. These data are then linked and supplemented with data from the treating physician. This step is fundamental since it permits the removal of cases diagnosed in previous years, recurrences or metastases from a cancer already registered, as well as cases among non-residents. The notification forms are kept for additional information to be added as received. The data are then coded and entered onto a personal computer. ICD-O-1 is used for coding topography and morphology. IARC/IACR rules are used for multiple tumours. Basal cell carcinomas of the skin are registered but excluded from analysis of the data.

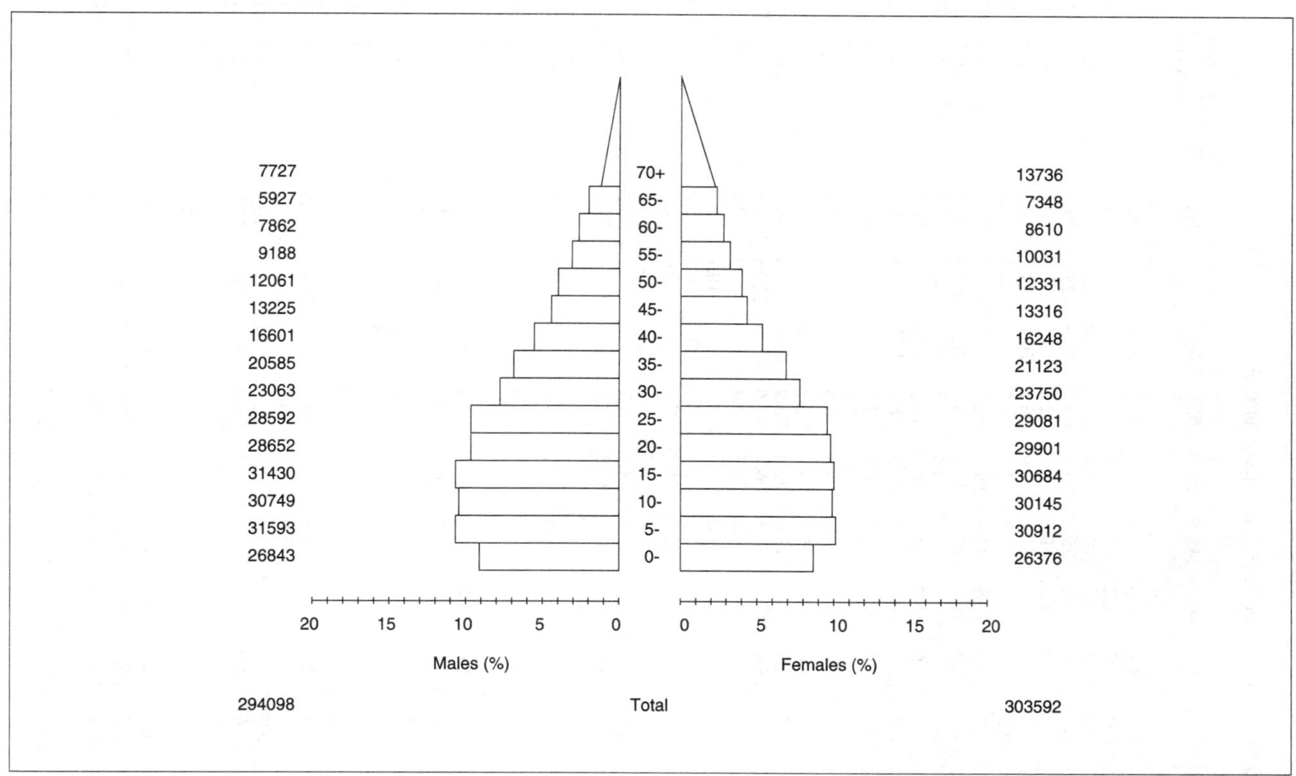

France, La Réunion
Source of population: 1990
Census: Recensement de la population 1990, Population de la France, Départements, arrondissements, cantons, communes. Direction Générale des Collectivités Locales, Institut National de la Statistique et des Etudes Economiques.

Notes to tables overleaf:
* The very high proportion of diagnoses based on histology and some rather high ratios of mortality to incidence suggest a degree of under-ascertainment.
† 173 does not include basal cell carcinoma
† 188 does not include non-invasive tumours

* FRANCE, LA REUNION 1988-1992

ANNUAL INCIDENCE PER 100,000 BY AGE GROUP (YEARS) - MALE

SITE	ALL AGES	AGE UNK	0-	5-	10-	15-	20-	25-	30-	35-	40-	45-	50-	55-	60-	65-	70+	CRUDE RATE	%	CR 64	ASR (W)	ICD (9th)
Lip	5	0	-	-	-	-	-	0.7	-	-	-	-	-	-	5.1	3.4	2.6	0.3	0.2	0.03	0.5	140
Tongue	63	0	-	-	-	-	-	0.7	1.7	5.8	6.0	9.1	23.2	21.8	20.4	10.1	20.7	4.3	2.8	0.44	5.4	141
Salivary gland	5	0	-	-	-	-	-	-	0.9	1.0	1.2	-	3.3	-	-	-	-	0.3	0.2	0.03	0.3	142
Mouth	69	0	-	-	-	-	-	-	0.9	2.9	6.0	19.7	13.3	34.8	28.0	16.9	18.1	4.7	3.1	0.53	6.2	143-5
Oropharynx	90	0	-	-	-	-	-	-	-	2.9	10.8	25.7	26.5	43.5	25.4	23.6	20.7	6.1	4.0	0.67	8.0	146
Nasopharynx	7	0	-	-	-	-	0.7	-	-	1.0	1.2	1.5	1.7	2.2	-	-	2.6	0.5	0.3	0.04	0.6	147
Hypopharynx	53	0	-	-	-	-	-	0.7	-	-	4.8	13.6	19.9	26.1	20.4	13.5	7.8	3.6	2.4	0.43	4.7	148
Pharynx unspecified	14	0	-	-	-	-	-	0.7	0.9	-	-	4.5	3.3	6.5	-	6.7	5.2	1.0	0.6	0.08	1.2	149
Oesophagus	240	0	-	-	-	-	-	-	1.7	6.8	10.8	37.8	68.0	102.3	119.6	101.2	82.8	16.3	10.7	1.74	22.1	150
Stomach	237	0	-	-	0.7	-	-	-	4.3	6.8	10.8	27.2	36.5	78.4	78.9	108.0	196.7	16.1	10.6	1.22	22.2	151
Small intestine	11	0	-	-	-	-	-	-	-	-	-	-	3.3	6.5	-	6.7	10.4	0.7	0.5	0.05	1.0	152
Colon	73	0	-	-	-	-	0.7	0.7	-	1.0	4.8	12.1	8.3	15.2	20.4	50.6	59.5	5.0	3.3	0.32	6.9	153
Rectum	63	0	-	-	-	-	0.7	1.4	0.9	1.9	6.0	3.0	13.3	8.7	17.8	30.4	56.9	4.3	2.8	0.27	5.8	154
Liver	29	0	-	-	-	-	-	0.7	-	1.0	2.4	-	9.9	2.2	17.8	20.2	12.9	2.0	1.3	0.17	2.7	155
Gallbladder etc.	13	0	-	-	-	-	-	-	-	-	-	-	-	6.5	-	10.1	18.1	0.9	0.6	0.03	1.3	156
Pancreas	30	0	-	-	-	-	-	-	-	1.0	1.2	1.5	8.3	10.9	17.8	13.5	15.5	2.0	1.3	0.20	2.8	157
Nose, sinuses etc.	11	0	0.7	-	-	-	-	-	-	1.0	-	3.3	2.2	7.6	-	-	5.2	0.7	0.5	0.08	1.0	160
Larynx	91	0	-	-	-	-	-	0.7	1.7	1.9	4.8	13.6	29.8	23.9	28.0	50.6	46.6	6.2	4.1	0.52	8.3	161
Bronchus, lung	360	0	-	-	-	-	-	2.1	-	3.9	13.3	34.8	66.3	93.6	160.3	229.5	271.8	24.5	16.1	1.87	34.5	162
Other thoracic organs	15	0	-	-	-	-	0.7	-	-	-	-	1.5	1.7	4.4	2.5	16.9	10.4	1.0	0.7	0.05	1.4	163-4
Bone	16	0	0.7	-	1.3	1.3	2.8	0.7	-	-	-	3.0	-	2.2	-	10.1	-	1.1	0.7	0.06	1.2	170
Connective tissue	15	0	-	-	0.7	0.6	0.7	-	0.9	1.0	2.4	1.5	1.7	2.2	2.5	6.7	5.2	1.0	0.7	0.07	1.2	171
Mesothelioma	6	0	-	-	-	-	-	-	-	-	1.2	1.5	1.7	2.2	-	3.4	2.6	0.4	0.3	0.03	0.5	MES
Kaposi's sarcoma	4	0	-	-	-	-	-	1.4	-	-	-	-	1.7	-	2.5	-	-	0.3	0.2	0.03	0.3	KAP
Melanoma of skin	17	0	-	-	-	-	-	0.7	0.9	-	2.4	4.5	3.3	8.7	5.1	-	5.2	1.2	0.8	0.13	1.4	172
†Other skin	108	0	0.7	-	-	-	-	1.4	1.7	1.0	4.8	10.6	13.3	32.7	45.8	57.4	85.4	7.3		0.56	10.2	173
Breast	5	0	-	-	-	-	-	-	-	-	-	-	-	6.5	-	-	5.2	0.3	0.2	0.03	0.5	175
Prostate	231	0	-	-	-	-	-	-	-	-	-	1.5	1.7	19.6	76.3	182.2	352.0	15.7	10.3	0.50	23.6	185
Testis	18	0	0.7	-	-	1.3	0.7	2.1	5.2	3.9	-	-	-	2.2	-	-	-	1.2	0.8	0.08	1.1	186
Penis	13	0	-	-	-	-	-	-	0.9	1.0	-	-	3.3	2.2	5.1	6.7	10.4	0.9	0.6	0.06	1.2	187.1-.4
Other male genital	2	0	-	-	-	-	-	0.7	-	-	-	-	-	-	-	-	2.6	0.1	0.1	0.00	0.2	187.5-.9
†Bladder	98	0	-	-	-	-	-	-	1.0	4.8	16.6	13.3	23.9	28.0	60.7	88.0	6.7	4.4	0.44	9.4	188
Kidney etc.	29	0	-	0.6	-	-	-	-	1.7	1.0	3.6	4.5	8.3	6.5	5.1	10.1	15.5	2.0	1.3	0.16	2.5	189
Eye	6	0	0.7	-	0.7	-	-	-	0.9	-	-	-	-	-	-	-	7.8	0.4	0.3	0.01	0.5	190
Brain, nervous system	26	0	2.2	0.6	0.7	-	-	2.1	2.6	-	2.4	4.5	3.3	6.5	7.6	-	5.2	1.8	1.2	0.16	2.1	191-2
Thyroid	10	0	-	-	-	-	-	0.7	1.7	-	-	4.5	-	2.2	2.5	3.4	2.6	0.7	0.4	0.06	0.8	193
Other endocrine	2	0	0.7	-	-	-	-	-	-	-	-	-	1.7	-	-	-	-	0.1	0.1	0.01	0.2	194
Hodgkin's disease	15	0	1.5	-	0.7	1.3	1.4	0.7	1.7	1.0	2.4	-	1.7	-	-	-	2.6	1.0	0.7	0.06	1.0	201
Non-Hodgkin lymphoma	57	0	1.5	1.9	2.6	1.3	-	0.7	1.7	2.9	8.4	4.5	6.6	10.9	20.4	10.1	25.9	3.9	2.6	0.32	4.8	200,202
Multiple myeloma	32	0	-	-	-	-	-	-	-	-	-	3.0	3.3	15.2	10.2	23.6	25.9	2.2	1.4	0.16	3.1	203
Lymphoid leukaemia	22	0	3.7	0.6	0.7	1.9	2.1	0.7	0.9	-	-	-	-	2.2	5.1	-	10.4	1.5	1.0	0.09	1.7	204
Myeloid leukaemia	38	0	0.7	-	-	1.9	1.4	0.7	2.6	1.0	2.4	1.5	5.0	4.4	12.7	10.1	28.5	2.6	1.7	0.17	3.3	205
Monocytic leukaemia	0	0	-	-	-	-	-	-	-	-	-	-	-	-	-	-	-	0.0	0.0	0.00	0.0	206
Other leukaemia	4	0	0.7	-	-	-	0.7	-	-	-	1.2	-	-	-	-	-	2.6	0.3	0.2	0.01	0.3	207
Leukaemia unspecified	2	0	0.7	-	-	-	-	-	-	-	-	-	-	-	-	-	2.6	0.1	0.1	0.00	0.2	208
Other and unspecified	88	0	1.5	0.6	-	1.3	-	0.7	1.7	2.9	3.6	15.1	11.6	26.1	33.1	47.2	46.6	6.0	3.9	0.49	8.0	O&U
All sites	2343	0	17.1	4.4	7.8	10.8	12.6	21.7	38.2	55.4	124.1	284.3	421.2	666.1	831.8	1143.9	1597.0	159.3		12.48	216.2	ALL
All sites but 173	2235	0	16.4	4.4	7.8	10.8	12.6	20.3	36.4	54.4	119.3	273.7	407.9	633.4	786.1	1086.6	1511.6	152.0	100.0	11.92	206.0	ALLb

Rate from 1 case   0.745 0.633 0.650 0.636 0.698 0.699 0.867 0.972 1.205 1.512 1.658 2.177 2.544 3.374 2.588

†Important: see notes on population page

* FRANCE, LA REUNION 1988-1992

ANNUAL INCIDENCE PER 100,000 BY AGE GROUP (YEARS) - FEMALE

SITE	ALL AGES	AGE UNK	0-	5-	10-	15-	20-	25-	30-	35-	40-	45-	50-	55-	60-	65-	70+	CRUDE RATE	%	CR 64	ASR (W)	ICD (9th)
Lip	2	0	-	-	-	-	-	-	-	-	-	-	-	2.0	2.3	2.7	-	0.1	0.1	0.01	**0.2**	*140*
Tongue	4	0	-	-	-	-	-	-	-	-	-	3.0	-	2.0	2.3	-	-	0.3	0.2	0.04	**0.4**	*141*
Salivary gland	3	0	-	-	-	-	-	0.8	-	-	-	-	-	4.0	-	-	-	0.2	0.2	0.02	**0.2**	*142*
Mouth	9	0	-	-	-	-	-	0.8	-	1.2	1.5	1.6	-	2.3	2.7	4.4	-	0.6	0.5	0.04	**0.6**	*143-5*
Oropharynx	5	0	-	-	-	-	-	0.8	-	-	1.5	-	2.0	2.3	-	1.5	-	0.3	0.3	0.03	**0.4**	*146*
Nasopharynx	3	0	-	-	-	0.7	-	-	-	-	-	1.6	-	-	-	1.5	-	0.2	0.2	0.01	**0.2**	*147*
Hypopharynx	4	0	-	-	-	-	-	-	-	-	1.5	1.6	4.0	-	-	-	-	0.3	0.2	0.04	**0.3**	*148*
Pharynx unspecified	2	0	-	-	-	-	-	0.7	-	-	-	-	1.6	-	-	-	-	0.1	0.1	0.01	**0.1**	*149*
Oesophagus	22	0	-	-	-	-	-	-	-	-	1.5	3.2	8.0	4.6	5.4	16.0		1.4	1.2	0.09	**1.6**	*150*
Stomach	117	0	0.8	-	-	-	-	0.7	2.5	3.8	4.9	10.5	6.5	27.9	25.6	49.0	72.8	7.7	6.6	0.42	**8.3**	*151*
Small intestine	13	0	-	-	-	-	-	-	-	-	1.2	1.5	1.6	-	7.0	8.2	5.8	0.9	0.7	0.06	**1.0**	*152*
Colon	76	0	-	0.6	-	2.0	-	-	1.7	2.8	4.9	10.5	9.7	8.0	18.6	35.4	36.4	5.0	4.3	0.29	**5.5**	*153*
Rectum	60	0	-	-	-	-	0.7	2.8	1.7	0.9	3.7	6.0	14.6	12.0	9.3	21.8	26.2	4.0	3.4	0.26	**4.3**	*154*
Liver	22	0	-	-	-	-	-	-	-	0.9	1.2	-	3.2	8.0	9.3	5.4	11.6	1.4	1.2	0.11	**1.6**	*155*
Gallbladder etc.	37	0	-	-	-	-	-	-	-	0.9	2.5	-	6.5	6.0	9.3	10.9	27.7	2.4	2.1	0.13	**2.6**	*156*
Pancreas	25	0	-	-	-	-	-	-	0.8	0.9	1.2	1.5	1.6	6.0	13.9	10.9	10.2	1.6	1.4	0.13	**1.9**	*157*
Nose, sinuses etc.	3	0	-	-	-	-	-	-	-	-	-	-	4.0	-	-	2.7	-	0.2	0.2	0.02	**0.2**	*160*
Larynx	4	0	-	-	-	-	-	0.8	-	-	-	-	-	-	2.3	-	2.9	0.3	0.2	0.02	**0.3**	*161*
Bronchus, lung	46	0	-	-	-	-	-	-	-	-	2.5	3.0	-	14.0	18.6	16.3	30.6	3.0	2.6	0.19	**3.3**	*162*
Other thoracic organs	10	0	0.8	-	-	-	-	-	-	-	1.2	3.0	1.6	-	2.3	-	5.8	0.7	0.6	0.04	**0.8**	*163-4*
Bone	13	0	-	0.6	0.7	0.7	-	0.7	-	1.9	2.5	-	-	4.0	-	-	4.4	0.9	0.7	0.05	**0.8**	*170*
Connective tissue	16	0	1.5	-	0.7	-	0.7	0.7	1.7	0.9	1.2	3.0	1.6	4.0	-	-	2.9	1.1	0.9	0.08	**1.1**	*171*
Mesothelioma	3	0	-	-	-	-	-	-	-	0.9	-	-	-	-	-	-	2.9	0.2	0.2	0.00	**0.2**	*MES*
Kaposi's sarcoma	0	0	-	-	-	-	-	-	-	-	-	-	-	-	-	-	-	0.0	0.0	0.00	**0.0**	*KAP*
Melanoma of skin	36	0	-	0.6	0.7	-	1.3	2.8	5.1	4.7	2.5	1.5	-	8.0	4.6	8.2	7.3	2.4	2.0	0.16	**2.3**	*172*
†Other skin	101	0	-	-	-	-	-	-	0.8	4.7	4.9	12.0	8.1	12.0	27.9	46.3	62.6	6.7		0.35	**7.2**	*173*
Breast	392	0	-	-	-	0.7	0.7	4.1	14.3	23.7	70.2	82.6	94.1	79.8	74.3	89.8	97.6	25.8	22.1	2.22	**29.4**	*174*
Uterus unspecified	18	0	-	-	-	-	-	0.7	-	0.9	1.2	-	6.5	4.0	2.3	10.9	5.8	1.2	1.0	0.08	**1.3**	*179*
Cervix uteri	338	0	-	-	-	-	2.0	10.3	24.4	35.0	41.9	69.1	64.9	71.8	65.0	84.4	56.8	22.3	19.1	1.92	**24.7**	*180*
Placenta	2	0	-	-	-	-	-	0.7	-	-	1.2	-	-	-	-	-	-	0.1	0.1	0.01	**0.1**	*181*
Corpus uteri	48	0	-	-	-	-	-	2.1	-	0.9	3.7	3.0	8.1	12.0	2.3	19.1	29.1	3.2	2.7	0.16	**3.3**	*182*
Ovary etc.	73	0	0.8	-	-	1.3	2.0	3.4	2.5	3.8	6.2	15.0	9.7	14.0	11.6	29.9	16.0	4.8	4.1	0.35	**5.3**	*183*
Other female genital	20	0	-	-	-	-	-	-	-	0.9	-	-	4.9	6.0	4.6	2.7	14.6	1.3	1.1	0.08	**1.4**	*184*
†Bladder	27	0	-	-	-	-	-	-	-	0.9	-	1.5	-	4.0	2.3	10.9	26.2	1.8	1.5	0.04	**1.8**	*188*
Kidney etc.	20	0	5.3	0.6	-	-	-	-	-	1.9	-	-	1.6	2.0	9.3	2.7	4.4	1.3	1.1	0.10	**1.6**	*189*
Eye	5	0	2.3	0.6	-	-	-	-	-	-	-	-	-	-	2.3	-	-	0.3	0.3	0.03	**0.4**	*190*
Brain, nervous system	30	0	0.8	0.6	2.7	3.9	0.7	2.1	1.7	1.9	-	-	1.6	2.0	9.3	5.4	2.9	2.0	1.7	0.14	**2.0**	*191-2*
Thyroid	24	0	-	-	-	0.7	1.3	1.4	1.7	0.9	4.9	3.0	1.6	8.0	2.3	5.4	2.9	1.6	1.4	0.13	**1.7**	*193*
Other endocrine	5	0	3.0	-	-	-	-	-	-	0.9	-	-	-	-	-	-	-	0.3	0.3	0.02	**0.4**	*194*
Hodgkin's disease	10	0	-	-	-	0.7	0.7	1.4	0.8	-	1.2	-	-	2.0	-	2.7	2.9	0.7	0.6	0.03	**0.6**	*201*
Non-Hodgkin lymphoma	55	0	1.5	1.3	0.7	-	0.7	1.4	4.2	1.9	2.5	3.0	1.6	6.0	4.6	27.2	29.1	3.6	3.1	0.15	**3.7**	*200,202*
Multiple myeloma	45	0	-	-	-	-	-	-	-	2.8	-	-	-	8.0	11.6	21.8	36.4	3.0	2.5	0.11	**3.1**	*203*
Lymphoid leukaemia	22	0	4.5	1.9	0.7	-	0.7	-	-	-	-	1.5	1.6	4.0	4.6	5.4	4.4	1.4	1.2	0.10	**1.7**	*204*
Myeloid leukaemia	39	0	-	0.6	0.7	1.3	1.3	1.4	0.8	1.9	-	3.0	6.5	8.0	4.6	13.6	16.0	2.6	2.2	0.15	**2.7**	*205*
Monocytic leukaemia	1	0	0.8	-	-	-	-	-	-	-	-	-	-	-	-	-	-	0.1	0.1	0.00	**0.1**	*206*
Other leukaemia	1	0	-	-	-	-	0.7	-	-	-	-	-	-	-	-	-	-	0.1	0.1	0.00	**0.1**	*207*
Leukaemia unspecified	2	0	-	-	-	-	-	-	0.8	-	-	-	-	-	-	-	1.5	0.1	0.1	0.00	**0.1**	*208*
Other and unspecified	59	0	0.8	-	-	-	1.3	1.4	0.8	1.9	1.2	3.0	11.4	8.0	23.2	35.4	20.4	3.9	3.3	0.26	**4.4**	*O&U*
All sites	1872	0	22.7	7.8	6.6	11.7	14.7	38.5	69.9	104.2	169.9	246.3	279.0	372.8	397.2	593.4	700.3	123.3		8.71	**135.4**	*ALL*
All sites but 173	1771	0	22.7	7.8	6.6	11.7	14.7	38.5	69.1	99.4	164.9	234.3	270.9	360.9	369.3	547.1	637.7	116.7	100.0	8.35	**128.2**	*ALLb*

Rate from 1 case   0.758 0.647 0.663 0.652 0.669 0.688 0.842 0.947 1.231 1.502 1.622 1.994 2.323 2.722 1.456

†Important: see notes on population page

Mali, Bamako

The Cancer Registry of Mali was created in January 1986 in the pathology service of the National Institute of Public Health Research (INSRP). This was the only pathology service in the country, and all cases of cancer diagnosed histologically are found there, so that this constitutes one of the main data sources for the registry.

From the beginning, the registry was conceived to cover the populations of the Bamako district (the capital) and its surrounding area.

Mali is situated in the centre of west Africa. It is a large country (1 240 000 km^2), consisting mostly of savannah and lateritic plains, merging into the sandy desert of the Sahara to the north; the west and south-west, however, have more highland and forested regions, and the two great rivers of western Africa, the Senegal and Niger, traverse the southern and western part of the country. The population in 1987 was 7 620 000, with 54% aged under 20 years, and an annual growth rate of 2.54%. The crude birth rate in 1987 was 43 per 1000, the crude mortality rate 18 per 1000 and the infant mortality rate 120 per 1000. Several ethnic groups are present, the principal ones being Mandinga, Bambara, Sarakolé, Seroulfo, Sourhai, Dogon and Peuhl. Most of the population are Moslem and 83% rural, engaged in agriculture growing principally millet, sorghum, rice, maize and tropical fruit for local consumption; cotton and groundnuts are the principal export crops. Stock-rearing, particularly of cattle, is the second most important rural activity, and fishing is carried out extensively in the major rivers.. There is very little industry.

In common with other developing countries, the health care infrastructure is far from adequate, and concentrated particularly in the capital of Bamako, where there are two major hospitals and two specialized institutes, one for dermatology and one for ophthalmology. The major health problems remain infectious diseases. Malaria is widespread at all ages, and gastroenteritis and respiratory infections are frequent. Bilharzia infection is common, particularly in the south.

Data collection for the registry is active. A technician is responsible for visiting regularly the principal health care structures used by the inhabitants of the area. These consist of three national hospitals, two institutes specializing in dermatology and in ophthalmology, and two maternal and child health centres run by gynaecologists.

In each service there is a correspondent of the registry, usually the head nurse who, under the supervision of the consulting physician, records the diagnosed cases on the registry forms. These are checked by the registry technician when he visits.

Another source of information is the death register of the town, in which all deaths and their causes are registered; this formality is required in order to obtain a burial certificate, without which no burial is possible, whether the death occurred in hospital or at home.

The notification form, designed in collaboration with the IARC, has a limited number of data items: the record number of the reporting service, the subject's first name and surname, sex, age, residence and ethnic group, the site of the primary cancer, basis of diagnosis, histology and date of death.

At the end of every three-month period, the data so collected are coded to the first edition of ICD-O.

The data are entered into a computer using the CAN-REG software which permits elimination of duplicate registrations.

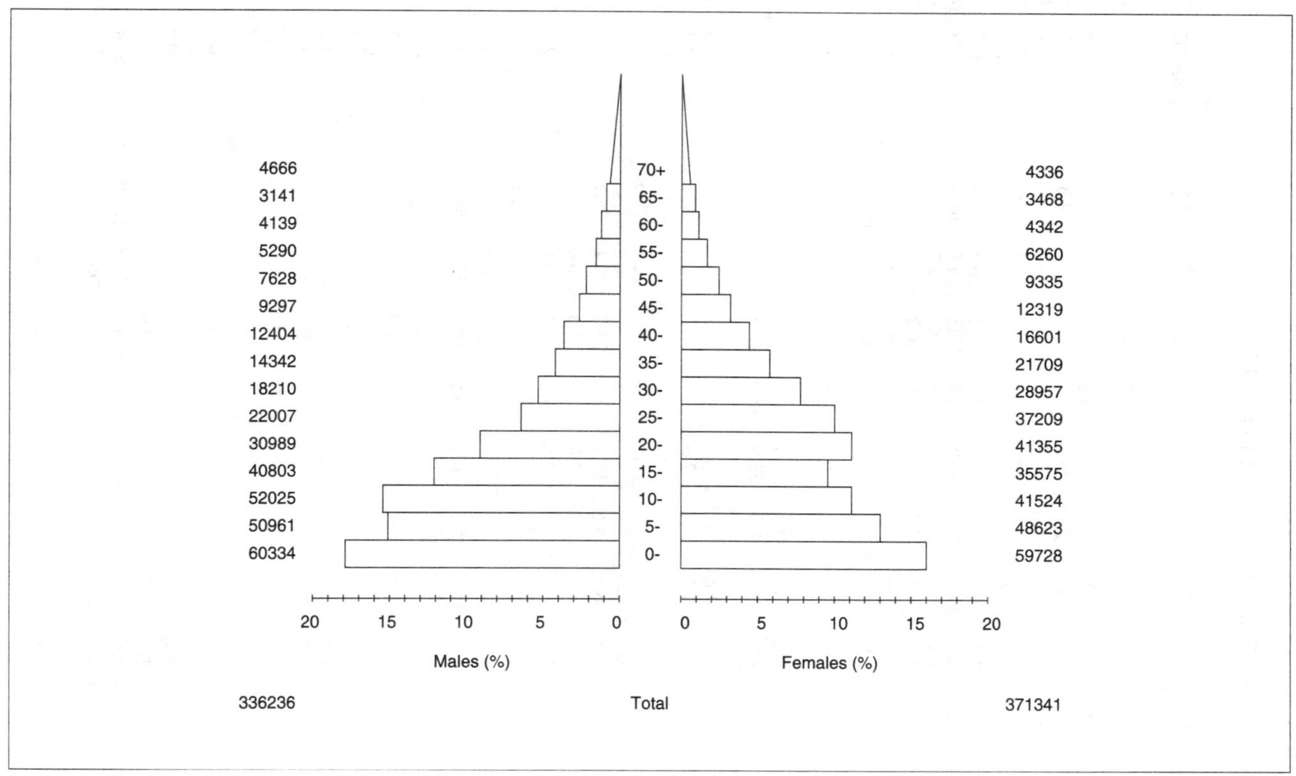

Mali, Bamako
Source of population: 1987–89
E*stimate*: An annual growth rate of 2.54% was applied to both sexes and all age-groups on the basis of the 1987 Census.
Census: Recensement Général de la Population et de l'Habitat 1987, Vol. 8.

Notes to tables overleaf:
* The time period largely overlaps that published in Volume VI and has been included for comparative purposes. The low incidence rates for several sites suggest under-ascertainment.
† 188 does not include non-invasive tumours.

* MALI, BAMAKO 1988-1992

ANNUAL INCIDENCE PER 100,000 BY AGE GROUP (YEARS) - MALE

SITE	ALL AGES	AGE UNK	0-	5-	10-	15-	20-	25-	30-	35-	40-	45-	50-	55-	60-	65-	70+	CRUDE RATE	%	CR 64	ASR (W)	ICD (9th)
Lip	2	0	-	-	-	-	-	-	-	-	1.6	-	-	3.8	-	-	-	0.1	0.2	0.03	**0.2**	140
Tongue	3	0	-	-	-	-	-	-	-	-	-	2.2	-	3.8	4.8	-	-	0.2	0.3	0.05	**0.5**	141
Salivary gland	0	0	-	-	-	-	-	-	-	-	-	-	-	-	-	-	-	0.0	0.0	0.00	**0.0**	142
Mouth	3	0	-	-	-	-	-	1.1	-	-	1.6	-	-	3.8	-	-	-	0.2	0.3	0.03	**0.3**	143-5
Oropharynx	2	0	-	-	-	-	-	-	-	-	-	2.2	-	-	-	-	4.3	0.1	0.2	0.01	**0.3**	146
Nasopharynx	1	0	-	-	-	-	-	-	-	-	-	-	2.6	-	-	-	-	0.1	0.1	0.01	**0.1**	147
Hypopharynx	0	0	-	-	-	-	-	-	-	-	-	-	-	-	-	-	-	0.0	0.0	0.00	**0.0**	148
Pharynx unspecified	4	0	-	-	-	-	-	-	-	2.8	1.6	2.2	-	-	-	-	-	0.2	0.4	0.03	**0.4**	149
Oesophagus	12	0	-	-	-	-	-	-	-	2.8	-	6.5	5.2	3.8	9.7	6.4	4.3	0.7	1.2	0.14	**1.7**	150
Stomach	143	0	-	0.8	-	0.5	1.3	2.7	7.7	16.7	12.9	32.3	83.9	52.9	77.3	95.5	68.6	8.5	14.3	1.45	**19.6**	151
Small intestine	4	0	-	-	-	-	-	-	-	1.4	-	-	-	3.8	-	12.7	-	0.2	0.4	0.03	**0.6**	152
Colon	22	0	-	-	-	-	0.6	-	-	2.8	4.8	2.2	10.5	7.6	24.2	-	17.1	1.3	2.2	0.26	**3.1**	153
Rectum	26	0	-	-	-	-	1.3	0.9	5.5	8.4	4.8	2.2	-	3.8	9.7	19.1	8.6	1.5	2.6	0.18	**2.9**	154
Liver	419	0	-	-	1.2	3.4	9.7	21.8	40.6	65.5	82.2	109.7	118.0	139.9	202.9	140.1	162.9	24.9	42.0	3.98	**51.1**	155
Gallbladder etc.	1	0	-	-	-	-	-	-	-	-	-	-	-	-	-	6.4	-	0.1	0.1	0.00	**0.2**	156
Pancreas	17	0	-	-	-	-	0.6	-	1.1	-	3.2	6.5	2.6	7.6	9.7	12.7	12.9	1.0	1.7	0.16	**2.4**	157
Nose, sinuses etc.	5	0	-	-	-	-	0.6	-	-	-	-	2.2	-	3.8	-	6.4	4.3	0.3	0.5	0.03	**0.7**	160
Larynx	15	0	-	-	-	-	0.6	-	-	1.4	-	2.2	7.9	3.8	19.3	12.7	8.6	0.9	1.5	0.18	**2.3**	161
Bronchus, lung	38	0	-	-	-	-	-	0.9	2.2	2.8	6.4	8.6	21.0	18.9	19.3	19.1	21.4	2.3	3.8	0.40	**5.3**	162
Other thoracic organs	0	0	-	-	-	-	-	-	-	-	-	-	-	-	-	-	-	0.0	0.0	0.00	**0.0**	163-4
Bone	9	0	0.3	-	0.4	1.0	0.6	-	-	-	1.6	-	-	3.8	4.8	-	4.3	0.5	0.9	0.06	**0.8**	170
Connective tissue	5	0	-	-	-	1.0	-	-	1.1	-	1.6	-	2.6	-	-	-	-	0.3	0.5	0.03	**0.4**	171
Mesothelioma	0	0	-	-	-	-	-	-	-	-	-	-	-	-	-	-	-	0.0	0.0	0.00	**0.0**	MES
Kaposi's sarcoma	19	0	-	-	-	-	0.6	1.8	5.5	-	1.6	4.3	10.5	3.8	-	6.4	8.6	1.1	1.9	0.14	**2.1**	KAP
Melanoma of skin	5	0	-	-	-	-	0.6	-	2.2	-	-	-	-	3.8	-	6.4	-	0.3	0.5	0.03	**0.5**	172
Other skin	36	0	-	0.4	-	-	0.6	-	1.1	4.2	6.4	8.6	13.1	11.3	24.2	19.1	25.7	2.1		0.35	**5.0**	173
Breast	3	0	-	-	-	-	-	-	-	-	-	2.6	-	4.8	6.4	-		0.2	0.3	0.04	**0.5**	175
Prostate	33	0	-	-	-	-	-	-	3.3	1.4	-	-	2.6	11.3	19.3	50.9	55.7	2.0	3.3	0.19	**5.4**	185
Testis	4	0	-	-	-	-	-	0.9	1.1	-	-	2.2	-	3.8	-	-	-	0.2	0.4	0.04	**0.4**	186
Penis	2	0	-	-	-	-	-	-	-	-	-	2.2	-	-	-	-	4.3	0.1	0.2	0.01	**0.3**	187.1-.4
Other male genital	1	0	-	-	-	-	-	-	-	-	-	-	-	-	-	6.4	-	0.1	0.1	0.00	**0.2**	187.5-.9
†Bladder	73	0	-	-	-	1.5	-	2.7	1.1	4.2	11.3	25.8	10.5	18.9	48.3	57.3	68.6	4.3	7.3	0.62	**10.6**	188
Kidney etc.	19	0	1.7	1.6	0.4	-	0.6	-	1.1	-	1.6	2.2	5.2	7.6	-	-	4.3	1.1	1.9	0.11	**1.5**	189
Eye	16	0	2.7	0.4	-	-	1.3	-	-	1.4	-	4.3	-	-	4.8	-	4.3	1.0	1.6	0.07	**1.2**	190
Brain, nervous system	4	0	-	-	-	-	0.6	-	-	-	1.6	-	-	-	4.8	-	4.3	0.2	0.4	0.04	**0.5**	191-2
Thyroid	3	0	-	-	0.4	-	-	0.9	-	1.4	-	-	-	-	-	-	-	0.2	0.3	0.01	**0.2**	193
Other endocrine	1	0	-	-	-	-	-	-	-	1.4	-	-	-	-	-	-	-	0.1	0.1	0.01	**0.1**	194
Hodgkin's disease	19	0	0.3	1.2	1.2	1.0	3.2	-	4.4	1.4	-	-	-	-	-	-	-	1.1	1.9	0.06	**1.0**	201
Non-Hodgkin lymphoma	25	0	-	0.8	0.4	0.5	1.3	1.8	4.4	4.2	1.6	-	2.6	3.8	9.7	12.7	12.9	1.5	2.5	0.16	**2.6**	200,202
Multiple myeloma	0	0	-	-	-	-	-	-	-	-	-	-	-	-	-	-	-	0.0	0.0	0.00	**0.0**	203
Lymphoid leukaemia	0	0	-	-	-	-	-	-	-	-	-	-	-	-	-	-	-	0.0	0.0	0.00	**0.0**	204
Myeloid leukaemia	2	0	-	-	-	-	0.6	-	-	1.4	-	-	-	-	-	-	-	0.1	0.2	0.01	**0.1**	205
Monocytic leukaemia	0	0	-	-	-	-	-	-	-	-	-	-	-	-	-	-	-	0.0	0.0	0.00	**0.0**	206
Other leukaemia	0	0	-	-	-	-	-	-	-	-	-	-	-	-	-	-	-	0.0	0.0	0.00	**0.0**	207
Leukaemia unspecified	10	0	0.3	-	-	-	1.3	0.9	-	2.8	3.2	4.3	-	-	-	-	-	0.6	1.0	0.06	**0.8**	208
Other and unspecified	27	0	-	0.8	-	1.0	1.3	0.9	-	4.2	3.2	-	5.2	-	29.0	19.1	17.1	1.6	2.7	0.23	**3.5**	O&U
All sites	1033	0	5.3	5.9	3.8	9.8	27.8	36.4	83.5	132.5	153.2	232.3	306.8	325.1	526.7	515.8	522.9	61.4		9.25	**129.5**	ALL
All sites but 173	997	0	5.3	5.5	3.8	9.8	27.1	36.4	82.4	128.3	146.7	223.7	293.7	313.8	502.5	496.7	497.2	59.3	100.0	8.90	**124.5**	ALLb

Rate from 1 case   0.331   0.392   0.384   0.490   0.645   0.909   1.098   1.395   1.612   2.151   2.622   3.781   4.832   6.367   4.286

†Important: see notes on population page

* MALI, BAMAKO 1988-1992

ANNUAL INCIDENCE PER 100,000 BY AGE GROUP (YEARS) - FEMALE

SITE	ALL AGES	AGE UNK	0-	5-	10-	15-	20-	25-	30-	35-	40-	45-	50-	55-	60-	65-	70+	CRUDE RATE	%	CR 64	ASR (W)	ICD (9th)
Lip	2	0	-	-	-	-	-	-	-	-	1.2	-	-	-	-	-	4.6	0.1	0.2	0.01	0.3	140
Tongue	3	0	-	-	-	-	-	-	0.7	0.9	-	-	-	-	-	5.8	-	0.2	0.3	0.01	0.3	141
Salivary gland	3	0	-	-	-	-	-	-	-	-	1.2	-	2.1	-	-	-	4.6	0.2	0.3	0.02	0.4	142
Mouth	3	0	-	-	-	-	0.5	0.5	-	-	-	-	-	-	-	5.8	-	0.2	0.3	0.01	0.3	143-5
Oropharynx	1	0	-	-	-	-	-	-	-	-	1.2	-	-	-	-	-	-	0.1	0.1	0.01	0.1	146
Nasopharynx	0	0	-	-	-	-	-	-	-	-	-	-	-	-	-	-	-	0.0	0.0	0.00	0.0	147
Hypopharynx	0	0	-	-	-	-	-	-	-	-	-	-	-	-	-	-	-	0.0	0.0	0.00	0.0	148
Pharynx unspecified	0	0	-	-	-	-	-	-	-	-	-	-	-	-	-	-	-	0.0	0.0	0.00	0.0	149
Oesophagus	7	0	-	-	-	-	-	-	1.4	2.8	-	-	-	-	-	11.5	-	0.4	0.8	0.02	0.6	150
Stomach	89	0	-	-	-	0.6	0.5	1.1	2.8	5.5	7.2	16.2	32.1	31.9	73.7	57.7	36.9	4.8	9.9	0.86	11.1	151
Small intestine	0	0	-	-	-	-	-	-	-	-	-	-	-	-	-	-	-	0.0	0.0	0.00	0.0	152
Colon	13	0	-	-	-	-	0.5	-	2.1	0.9	-	1.6	2.1	6.4	4.6	5.8	9.2	0.7	1.5	0.09	1.4	153
Rectum	8	0	-	-	-	-	0.5	0.5	0.7	-	1.2	1.6	4.3	-	-	-	4.6	0.4	0.9	0.04	0.7	154
Liver	164	0	0.3	-	0.5	2.8	2.4	5.4	8.3	15.7	20.5	26.0	34.3	54.3	73.7	98.0	64.6	8.8	18.3	1.22	17.5	155
Gallbladder etc.	0	0	-	-	-	-	-	-	-	-	-	-	-	-	-	-	-	0.0	0.0	0.00	0.0	156
Pancreas	6	0	-	-	-	-	-	-	-	-	-	1.6	4.3	-	4.6	11.5	-	0.3	0.7	0.05	0.8	157
Nose, sinuses etc.	3	0	-	-	-	-	-	-	-	-	1.2	-	2.1	-	-	-	4.6	0.2	0.3	0.02	0.4	160
Larynx	5	0	-	-	-	-	-	-	-	0.7	1.2	-	-	-	-	-	13.8	0.3	0.6	0.01	0.7	161
Bronchus, lung	13	0	-	-	-	-	-	1.1	-	-	1.2	1.6	4.3	12.8	9.2	-	4.6	0.7	1.5	0.15	1.5	162
Other thoracic organs	0	0	-	-	-	-	-	-	-	-	-	-	-	-	-	-	-	0.0	0.0	0.00	0.0	163-4
Bone	10	0	-	0.8	-	-	0.5	-	1.4	-	-	1.6	-	-	18.4	-	-	0.5	1.1	0.11	1.0	170
Connective tissue	3	0	-	-	-	-	-	0.5	-	-	-	-	-	-	9.2	-	-	0.2	0.3	0.05	0.4	171
Mesothelioma	0	0	-	-	-	-	-	-	-	-	-	-	-	-	-	-	-	0.0	0.0	0.00	0.0	MES
Kaposi's sarcoma	4	0	-	-	-	-	0.5	0.5	-	-	1.2	-	-	-	4.6	-	-	0.2	0.4	0.03	0.3	KAP
Melanoma of skin	8	0	0.3	-	-	-	-	-	-	-	-	3.2	-	3.2	18.4	-	-	0.4	0.9	0.13	1.1	172
Other skin	22	0	-	-	-	-	-	1.1	1.4	0.9	2.4	6.5	-	6.4	23.0	17.3	4.6	1.2		0.21	2.6	173
Breast	100	0	0.3	-	-	0.6	0.5	2.7	7.6	11.1	18.1	21.1	12.9	31.9	50.7	51.9	23.1	5.4	11.2	0.79	10.2	174
Uterus unspecified	25	0	-	-	0.5	-	1.0	0.5	1.4	4.6	1.2	1.6	15.0	3.2	4.6	11.5	4.6	1.3	2.8	0.17	2.3	179
Cervix uteri	248	0	-	0.4	-	-	-	9.7	20.0	30.4	53.0	50.3	62.1	63.9	82.9	69.2	60.0	13.4	27.7	1.86	23.5	180
Placenta	3	0	-	-	-	-	0.5	0.5	-	0.9	-	-	-	-	-	-	-	0.2	0.3	0.01	0.1	181
Corpus uteri	9	0	-	-	-	-	-	-	-	-	3.6	3.2	4.3	-	9.2	-	-	0.5	1.0	0.10	1.0	182
Ovary etc.	10	0	-	0.4	-	-	0.5	-	-	3.7	1.2	3.2	2.1	-	-	-	-	0.5	1.1	0.06	0.7	183
Other female genital	9	0	-	-	-	-	-	1.1	0.7	2.8	1.2	1.6	2.1	-	-	-	-	0.5	1.0	0.05	0.6	184
†Bladder	26	0	-	-	-	-	1.0	0.5	-	2.8	12.0	6.5	-	9.6	9.2	5.8	-	1.4	2.9	0.21	2.3	188
Kidney etc.	19	0	0.3	0.8	1.0	-	1.0	-	1.4	-	1.2	-	4.3	19.2	4.6	-	-	1.0	2.1	0.17	1.6	189
Eye	13	0	1.0	0.4	0.5	-	-	-	0.7	-	2.4	4.9	-	3.2	-	5.8	-	0.7	1.5	0.07	1.0	190
Brain, nervous system	4	0	-	0.4	-	-	0.5	0.5	-	0.9	-	-	-	-	-	-	-	0.2	0.4	0.01	0.2	191-2
Thyroid	17	0	-	-	-	-	0.5	-	0.7	1.8	7.2	-	6.4	-	-	5.8	13.8	0.9	1.9	0.08	1.7	193
Other endocrine	2	0	-	-	-	-	-	-	-	-	-	-	-	-	-	-	9.2	0.1	0.2	0.00	0.4	194
Hodgkin's disease	5	0	-	-	0.5	0.6	0.5	0.5	-	-	-	-	-	-	-	-	4.6	0.3	0.6	0.01	0.4	201
Non-Hodgkin lymphoma	10	0	-	-	-	0.6	1.0	1.1	0.7	0.9	-	-	-	3.2	-	-	9.2	0.5	1.1	0.04	0.8	200,202
Multiple myeloma	0	0	-	-	-	-	-	-	-	-	-	-	-	-	-	-	-	0.0	0.0	0.00	0.0	203
Lymphoid leukaemia	0	0	-	-	-	-	-	-	-	-	-	-	-	-	-	-	-	0.0	0.0	0.00	0.0	204
Myeloid leukaemia	11	0	-	-	-	-	1.0	0.5	0.7	-	-	-	6.4	6.4	-	5.8	4.6	0.6	1.2	0.08	1.1	205
Monocytic leukaemia	0	0	-	-	-	-	-	-	-	-	-	-	-	-	-	-	-	0.0	0.0	0.00	0.0	206
Other leukaemia	0	0	-	-	-	-	-	-	-	-	-	-	-	-	-	-	-	0.0	0.0	0.00	0.0	207
Leukaemia unspecified	12	0	0.3	0.8	1.0	-	0.5	-	0.7	0.9	-	4.9	-	-	-	5.8	-	0.6	1.3	0.05	0.8	208
Other and unspecified	27	0	-	-	3.4	-	-	1.1	1.4	0.9	2.4	1.6	6.4	3.2	9.2	5.8	23.1	1.5	3.0	0.15	2.7	O&U
All sites	917	0	2.7	4.1	7.2	5.1	13.5	29.6	55.3	88.4	143.4	159.1	207.8	258.8	409.9	380.6	304.4	49.4		6.92	92.8	ALL
All sites but 173	895	0	2.7	4.1	7.2	5.1	13.5	28.5	53.9	87.5	141.0	152.6	207.8	252.4	386.9	363.3	299.8	48.2	100.0	6.72	90.2	ALLb

Rate from 1 case

			0-	5-	10-	15-	20-	25-	30-	35-	40-	45-	50-	55-	60-	65-	70+
			0.335	0.411	0.482	0.562	0.484	0.538	0.691	0.921	1.205	1.624	2.142	3.195	4.606	5.767	4.613

†Important: see notes on population page

Uganda, Kyadondo County

The Kampala Cancer Registry was established in the Department of Pathology of Makerere Medical School in 1951 as a population-based cancer registry with the aim of determining cancer incidence in the population of Kyadondo county.

Kyadondo county comprises Kampala, the capital of Uganda, together with the peri-urban area. It lies on the equator at a longitude of approximately 34° E. The total registration area is 1914 km². The Ganda are the largest ethnic group in the county, constituting just over half of the population, but all other ethnic groups of Uganda are represented. There are also numerous ethnic groups from neighbouring countries. The total population has increased from 200 000 since the registry started to over 1 000 000 in the 1991 population census; 70% live in the Kampala conurbation. The principal occupations are administration, professional and para-professional, trade, clerical, sales, personal services, plant and machine operators. Subsistence farming is carried on in the outskirts of the city. The main foodstuffs consist of matooke (steamed green banana plant), posho (maize bread), beans and groundnuts. About half of the city dwellers receive a treated water supply from Lake Victoria. The religious affiliations of the population are Catholic (50%), Anglican (30%), Muslim (15%) and others (5%).

The county is served by one 900-bed hospital with an attached oncology institute and a radiotherapy unit, with national referral. Three missionary hospitals have 100 beds each. There are 150 doctors.

The two basic data sources used are (a) the records of the department of histopathology and those of private histopathology laboratory, and (b) hospital records from the four major hospitals in the county to which cancer cases may be admitted (Mulago, Mengo, Rubaga and Nsambya).

Data submission is voluntary and both active and passive registration are carried out. For hospital cases, the cancer registrar visits all hospital services at least once a month, and consults hospital records, personnel admission books, clinical registers and hospital records to identify patients diagnosed as having cancer. In the case of the histopathology laboratories, forms accompanying specimens for examination, which have all the information required for registration, are consulted by cancer registrars. For each case, data are collected on: source of information, inpatient or outpatient number, names, sex, age, usual residence, tribe, date of diagnosis, most valid basis, tumour site and histology.

The registration process itself is carried out both manually and with a microcomputer using the CANREG system. A search is made for duplicate records based on name, age, sex and tribe.

Henry Wabinga

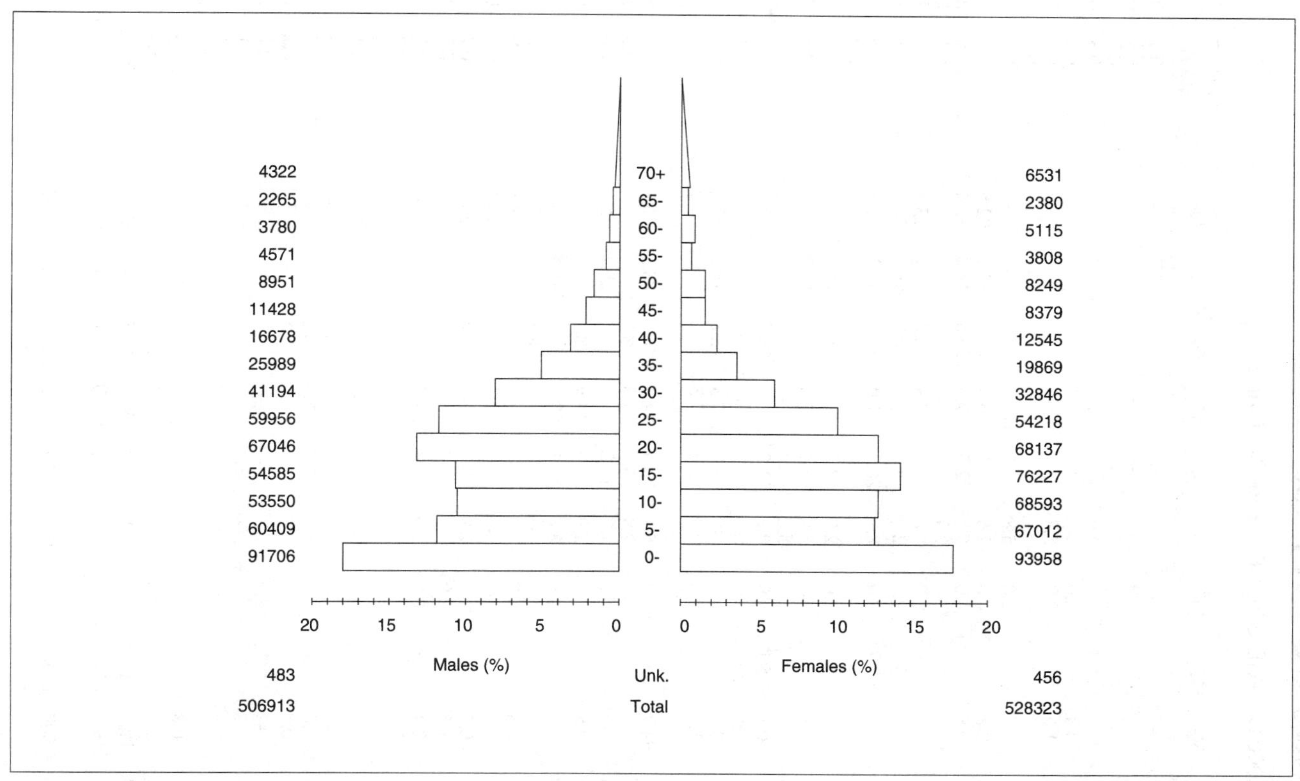

Uganda, Kyadondo County
Source of population: mid–95
Census: 1991
Estimate: Post-censal projected mid-year population based on the 1991 census.

Notes to the tables overleaf:
* The deficit of haematological cases indicates that the registry is failing to find these diagnoses.
† 188 does not include non-invasive tumours.

* UGANDA, KYADONDO COUNTY 1991-1993

ANNUAL INCIDENCE PER 100,000 BY AGE GROUP (YEARS) - MALE

SITE	ALL AGES	AGE UNK	0-	5-	10-	15-	20-	25-	30-	35-	40-	45-	50-	55-	60-	65-	70+	CRUDE RATE	%	CR 64	ASR (W)	ICD (9th)
Lip	1	0	-	-	-	-	-	-	-	-	-	-	-	-	-	14.7	-	0.1	0.1	0.00	**0.4**	*140*
Tongue	3	0	-	-	-	-	0.5	0.6	-	-	2.0	-	-	-	-	-	-	0.2	0.3	0.02	**0.2**	*141*
Salivary gland	3	0	-	-	-	-	-	0.6	-	-	2.0	2.9	-	-	-	-	-	0.2	0.3	0.03	**0.3**	*142*
Mouth	5	0	-	-	-	-	0.5	-	-	1.3	-	2.9	-	7.3	-	14.7	-	0.3	0.5	0.06	**1.0**	*143-5*
Oropharynx	5	0	-	-	-	-	-	0.6	0.8	-	2.0	-	3.7	7.3	-	-	-	0.3	0.5	0.07	**0.7**	*146*
Nasopharynx	9	0	-	0.6	-	-	-	0.6	1.6	1.3	2.0	5.8	3.7	-	-	-	-	0.6	0.8	0.08	**0.9**	*147*
Hypopharynx	1	0	-	-	-	-	-	-	-	-	-	-	-	-	8.8	-	-	0.1	0.1	0.04	**0.4**	*148*
Pharynx unspecified	3	0	-	-	-	-	-	-	-	-	2.0	5.8	-	-	-	-	-	0.2	0.3	0.04	**0.5**	*149*
Oesophagus	65	2	-	-	-	-	-	0.6	0.8	-	4.0	17.5	52.1	36.5	123.5	117.7	92.5	4.3	6.0	1.21	**18.2**	*150*
Stomach	25	1	-	-	-	0.6	1.0	0.6	0.8	-	4.0	5.8	22.3	7.3	26.5	44.2	15.4	1.6	2.3	0.36	**5.4**	*151*
Small intestine	1	0	-	-	-	-	-	-	-	-	-	2.9	-	-	-	-	-	0.1	0.1	0.01	**0.2**	*152*
Colon	16	1	-	-	-	-	-	-	2.4	2.6	2.0	8.8	-	7.3	8.8	14.7	23.1	1.1	1.5	0.17	**3.2**	*153*
Rectum	17	0	-	-	-	0.5	-	-	3.8	2.0	2.9	7.4	-	8.8	58.9	30.8		1.1	1.6	0.13	**4.3**	*154*
Liver	54	0	0.7	-	0.6	-	1.0	2.2	1.6	7.7	18.0	8.8	26.1	51.0	35.3	44.2	30.8	3.6	5.0	0.77	**9.9**	*155*
Gallbladder etc.	0	0	-	-	-	-	-	-	-	-	-	-	-	-	-	-	-	0.0	0.0	0.00	**0.0**	*156*
Pancreas	6	0	-	-	-	-	-	-	1.3	2.0	2.9	3.7	-	8.8	14.7	-		0.4	0.6	0.09	**1.4**	*157*
Nose, sinuses etc.	7	1	-	-	-	-	-	0.8	-	-	5.8	3.7	7.3	-	14.7	-		0.5	0.6	0.10	**1.5**	*160*
Larynx	6	0	-	-	-	-	0.6	0.8	-	-	5.8	7.4	-	-	-	-		0.4	0.6	0.07	**0.8**	*161*
Bronchus, lung	20	0	-	-	-	0.5	-	0.8	5.1	4.0	2.9	11.2	-	26.5	29.4	23.1		1.3	1.8	0.25	**4.2**	*162*
Other thoracic organs	1	0	-	-	-	-	-	-	-	-	-	-	7.3	-	-	-		0.1	0.1	0.04	**0.3**	*163-4*
Bone	14	0	-	1.1	0.6	1.8	0.5	-	0.8	-	-	3.7	7.3	8.8	14.7	15.4		0.9	1.3	0.12	**2.3**	*170*
Connective tissue	12	1	-	0.6	1.2	-	-	-	1.6	-	4.0	2.9	3.7	7.3	-	-	7.7	0.8	1.1	0.12	**1.6**	*171*
Mesothelioma	0	0	-	-	-	-	-	-	-	-	-	-	-	-	-	-	-	0.0	0.0	0.00	**0.0**	*MES*
Kaposi's sarcoma	524	16	10.2	9.9	5.0	3.1	24.9	56.7	94.7	85.9	91.9	55.4	74.5	94.8	26.5	88.3	46.3	34.5	48.2	3.27	**43.5**	*KAP*
Melanoma of skin	5	1	-	-	-	-	-	-	-	-	-	2.9	3.7	7.3	8.8	-	-	0.3	0.5	0.14	**1.3**	*172*
Other skin	15	1	0.4	-	0.6	-	-	0.6	-	-	-	11.7	11.2	-	-	29.4	15.4	1.0		0.13	**3.1**	*173*
Breast	6	1	-	-	-	-	-	-	0.8	-	-	2.9	-	14.6	8.8	-	-	0.4	0.6	0.16	**1.4**	*175*
Prostate	86	3	-	-	-	-	-	-	-	-	2.0	8.8	26.1	29.2	97.0	235.5	316.2	5.7	7.9	0.84	**27.7**	*185*
Testis	3	0	-	-	-	-	-	-	-	1.3	-	-	-	-	8.8	-	7.7	0.2	0.3	0.05	**0.7**	*186*
Penis	13	0	-	-	0.6	0.5	-	0.8	-	6.0	-	-	7.3	-	14.7	38.6		0.9	1.2	0.08	**2.8**	*187.1-.4*
Other male genital	4	0	-	-	-	0.6	-	-	-	-	-	-	7.3	-	-	15.4		0.3	0.4	0.04	**1.0**	*187.5-.9*
†Bladder	10	0	0.4	-	-	-	-	-	0.8	-	-	2.9	3.7	-	17.6	-	30.8	0.7	0.9	0.13	**2.4**	*188*
Kidney etc.	11	0	2.5	-	-	-	-	-	1.6	-	2.0	-	-	-	-	14.7	-	0.7	1.0	0.03	**1.0**	*189*
Eye	30	0	3.6	1.1	0.6	0.6	1.5	1.1	2.4	1.3	6.0	2.9	7.4	7.3	-	-	-	2.0	2.8	0.18	**2.3**	*190*
Brain, nervous system	3	0	0.4	0.6	-	-	-	-	-	-	-	-	-	-	8.8	-	-	0.2	0.3	0.05	**0.5**	*191-2*
Thyroid	5	0	-	-	-	0.6	-	1.1	-	-	-	2.9	-	-	8.8	-	-	0.3	0.5	0.07	**0.7**	*193*
Other endocrine	2	0	0.4	-	-	0.5	-	-	-	-	-	-	-	-	-	-	-	0.1	0.2	0.00	**0.1**	*194*
Hodgkin's disease	4	0	-	0.6	-	0.6	-	-	-	-	-	-	-	-	8.8	14.7	-	0.3	0.4	0.05	**0.9**	*201*
Non-Hodgkin lymphoma	48	1	3.6	6.1	3.7	1.8	2.0	1.7	1.6	2.6	2.0	5.8	3.7	7.3	8.8	-	-	3.2	4.4	0.26	**3.5**	*200,202*
Multiple myeloma	3	0	-	-	-	-	-	-	0.8	-	-	-	-	-	8.8	-	7.7	0.2	0.3	0.05	**0.7**	*203*
Lymphoid leukaemia	3	0	0.4	0.6	-	-	-	-	-	-	2.0	-	-	-	-	-	-	0.2	0.3	0.01	**0.2**	*204*
Myeloid leukaemia	1	0	-	-	-	-	-	-	-	-	-	-	3.7	-	-	-	-	0.1	0.1	0.02	**0.2**	*205*
Monocytic leukaemia	0	0	-	-	-	-	-	-	-	-	-	-	-	-	-	-	-	0.0	0.0	0.00	**0.0**	*206*
Other leukaemia	0	0	-	-	-	-	-	-	-	-	-	-	-	-	-	-	-	0.0	0.0	0.00	**0.0**	*207*
Leukaemia unspecified	6	0	-	-	1.2	0.6	0.5	-	0.8	1.3	-	-	-	-	-	-	-	0.4	0.6	0.02	**0.3**	*208*
Other and unspecified	46	6	1.5	1.1	1.2	0.6	1.0	1.1	2.4	6.4	10.0	2.9	11.2	29.2	26.5	14.7	15.4	3.0	4.2	0.55	**6.6**	*O&U*
All sites	1102	35	24.0	22.1	14.9	11.6	35.3	68.4	119.8	121.8	171.9	183.8	294.2	350.0	493.8	794.7	732.7	72.5		9.87	**158.2**	*ALL*
All sites but 173	1087	34	23.6	22.1	14.3	11.6	35.3	67.8	119.8	121.8	171.9	172.1	283.0	350.0	493.8	765.3	717.3	71.5	100.0	9.74	**155.2**	*ALLb*

| Rate from 1 case | | | 0.363 | 0.552 | 0.622 | 0.611 | 0.497 | 0.556 | 0.809 | 1.283 | 1.999 | 2.917 | 3.724 | 7.292 | 8.818 | 14.717 | 7.712 |

†Important: see notes on population page

* UGANDA, KYADONDO COUNTY 1991-1993

ANNUAL INCIDENCE PER 100,000 BY AGE GROUP (YEARS) - FEMALE

SITE	ALL AGES	AGE UNK	0-	5-	10-	15-	20-	25-	30-	35-	40-	45-	50-	55-	60-	65-	70+	CRUDE RATE	%	CR 64	ASR (W)	ICD (9th)
Lip	0	0	-	-	-	-	-	-	-	-	-	-	-	-	-	-	-	0.0	0.0	0.00	**0.0**	*140*
Tongue	1	0	-	-	-	-	-	-	-	-	-	-	-	-	-	-	5.1	0.1	0.1	0.00	**0.2**	*141*
Salivary gland	7	0	0.4	-	-	0.4	-	0.6	-	3.4	-	4.0	-	-	6.5	-	-	0.4	0.6	0.08	**0.8**	*142*
Mouth	7	1	-	-	-	-	-	-	-	1.7	-	8.0	-	-	6.5	14.0	5.1	0.4	0.6	0.09	**1.7**	*143-5*
Oropharynx	4	0	-	-	-	0.4	-	0.6	-	-	-	-	-	-	13.0	-	-	0.3	0.4	0.07	**0.6**	*146*
Nasopharynx	6	0	-	-	-	-	1.0	1.2	-	1.7	-	-	4.0	-	-	-	-	0.4	0.5	0.04	**0.5**	*147*
Hypopharynx	2	0	-	-	-	-	-	-	-	-	-	-	4.0	-	6.5	-	-	0.1	0.2	0.05	**0.5**	*148*
Pharynx unspecified	0	0	-	-	-	-	-	-	-	-	-	-	-	-	-	-	-	0.0	0.0	0.00	**0.0**	*149*
Oesophagus	37	1	-	-	-	-	-	-	1.0	-	10.6	15.9	24.2	26.3	45.6	28.0	45.9	2.3	3.4	0.64	**8.7**	*150*
Stomach	16	0	-	-	-	-	-	-	2.0	3.4	2.7	4.0	12.1	8.8	32.6	-	5.1	1.0	1.5	0.33	**3.2**	*151*
Small intestine	2	0	-	-	-	-	-	-	-	5.3	-	-	-	-	-	-	-	0.1	0.2	0.03	**0.3**	*152*
Colon	15	0	-	-	-	-	-	-	-	-	5.3	15.9	16.2	8.8	13.0	-	10.2	0.9	1.4	0.30	**3.4**	*153*
Rectum	11	0	-	-	-	-	0.5	0.6	1.0	1.7	2.7	-	8.1	8.8	-	-	15.3	0.7	1.0	0.12	**1.8**	*154*
Liver	30	1	-	-	-	0.4	1.0	1.8	6.1	1.7	18.6	-	8.1	8.8	6.5	42.0	10.2	1.9	2.7	0.27	**4.7**	*155*
Gallbladder etc.	0	0	-	-	-	-	-	-	-	-	-	-	-	-	-	-	-	0.0	0.0	0.00	**0.0**	*156*
Pancreas	4	0	-	-	-	-	-	-	-	-	1.7	2.7	-	4.0	-	6.5	-	0.3	0.4	0.07	**0.7**	*157*
Nose, sinuses etc.	6	0	-	-	1.0	0.4	0.5	-	1.0	1.7	-	-	-	-	-	-	-	0.4	0.5	0.02	**0.3**	*160*
Larynx	7	0	-	-	-	-	-	-	2.0	-	-	4.0	-	8.8	-	28.0	5.1	0.4	0.6	0.07	**1.8**	*161*
Bronchus, lung	4	1	-	-	-	0.5	-	1.0	-	-	-	-	-	-	-	-	5.1	0.3	0.4	0.01	**0.4**	*162*
Other thoracic organs	4	1	0.4	-	-	-	-	0.6	-	-	-	-	-	-	-	-	5.1	0.3	0.4	0.01	**0.4**	*163-4*
Bone	8	0	-	-	-	-	1.0	1.8	-	3.4	-	-	-	-	-	-	5.1	0.5	0.7	0.03	**0.6**	*170*
Connective tissue	16	0	0.4	0.5	1.0	0.9	1.5	0.6	2.0	3.4	-	8.0	-	-	-	-	-	1.0	1.5	0.09	**1.2**	*171*
Mesothelioma	0	0	-	-	-	-	-	-	-	-	-	-	-	-	-	-	-	0.0	0.0	0.00	**0.0**	*MES*
Kaposi's sarcoma	260	6	7.5	6.0	1.5	9.6	24.0	44.9	25.4	33.6	29.2	23.9	12.1	17.5	19.6	-	20.4	16.4	23.8	1.30	**18.0**	*KAP*
Melanoma of skin	5	0	-	-	-	-	-	0.6	-	-	-	-	4.0	8.8	6.5	-	5.1	0.3	0.5	0.10	**1.1**	*172*
Other skin	10	1	-	-	0.5	0.4	1.0	0.6	1.0	-	-	-	4.0	-	6.5	-	5.1	0.6		0.08	**1.0**	*173*
Breast	126	3	-	-	-	0.9	2.9	6.1	15.2	30.2	42.5	67.6	48.5	61.3	58.7	42.0	40.8	7.9	11.5	1.71	**20.7**	*174*
Uterus unspecified	3	0	-	-	-	-	-	-	-	-	-	8.0	-	-	14.0	-	-	0.2	0.3	0.04	**0.9**	*179*
Cervix uteri	248	6	-	-	-	-	3.9	14.8	30.4	63.8	101.0	135.3	84.9	113.8	117.3	84.0	61.2	15.6	22.7	3.41	**40.8**	*180*
Placenta	9	0	-	-	-	0.4	1.5	0.6	-	1.7	5.3	-	4.0	-	-	-	-	0.6	0.8	0.07	**0.8**	*181*
Corpus uteri	27	0	-	-	-	-	-	1.8	3.0	6.7	8.0	15.9	8.1	17.5	6.5	28.0	15.3	1.7	2.5	0.34	**5.0**	*182*
Ovary etc.	48	2	-	1.0	1.0	1.3	2.0	2.5	9.1	-	5.3	23.9	24.2	26.3	13.0	-	15.3	3.0	4.4	0.57	**6.6**	*183*
Other female genital	10	0	0.4	-	-	-	1.0	0.6	1.0	-	2.7	4.0	8.1	-	-	-	5.1	0.6	0.9	0.09	**1.2**	*184*
†Bladder	3	1	-	-	-	-	-	-	-	-	-	-	-	-	-	-	10.2	0.2	0.3	0.00	**0.6**	*188*
Kidney etc.	20	0	2.5	1.5	-	0.4	-	0.6	2.0	1.7	5.3	-	-	17.5	-	-	5.1	1.3	1.8	0.16	**2.0**	*189*
Eye	28	2	2.8	1.0	-	0.4	2.0	2.5	2.0	3.4	5.3	-	4.0	-	-	-	-	1.8	2.6	0.13	**1.8**	*190*
Brain, nervous system	3	0	-	-	0.5	-	-	-	1.0	-	-	4.0	-	-	-	-	-	0.2	0.3	0.03	**0.3**	*191-2*
Thyroid	19	2	-	-	0.5	-	1.0	0.6	2.0	1.7	2.7	4.0	-	17.5	13.0	14.0	15.3	1.2	1.7	0.24	**3.4**	*193*
Other endocrine	1	0	-	-	-	-	-	-	-	-	-	4.0	-	-	-	-	-	0.1	0.1	0.02	**0.2**	*194*
Hodgkin's disease	4	0	-	-	-	-	1.8	1.0	-	-	-	-	-	-	-	-	-	0.3	0.4	0.01	**0.2**	*201*
Non-Hodgkin lymphoma	36	1	2.1	4.0	1.9	1.7	1.5	2.5	2.0	-	5.3	4.0	-	-	-	-	5.1	2.3	3.3	0.13	**2.2**	*200,202*
Multiple myeloma	2	0	-	-	-	-	-	-	-	-	-	-	-	-	6.5	14.0	-	0.1	0.2	0.03	**0.7**	*203*
Lymphoid leukaemia	3	0	-	0.5	1.0	-	-	-	-	-	-	-	-	-	-	-	-	0.2	0.3	0.01	**0.1**	*204*
Myeloid leukaemia	3	0	-	0.5	-	-	-	-	-	-	-	-	-	-	13.0	-	-	0.2	0.3	0.07	**0.6**	*205*
Monocytic leukaemia	0	0	-	-	-	-	-	-	-	-	-	-	-	-	-	-	-	0.0	0.0	0.00	**0.0**	*206*
Other leukaemia	0	0	-	-	-	-	-	-	-	-	-	-	-	-	-	-	-	0.0	0.0	0.00	**0.0**	*207*
Leukaemia unspecified	7	0	0.4	0.5	0.5	0.4	0.5	-	-	1.7	-	-	-	-	-	-	5.1	0.4	0.6	0.02	**0.5**	*208*
Other and unspecified	42	2	1.1	-	0.5	0.9	2.0	1.2	8.1	6.7	8.0	4.0	16.2	35.0	6.5	28.0 ⋆	5.1	2.6	3.8	0.47	**5.9**	*O&U*
All sites	1104	31	17.7	15.4	9.7	19.2	48.9	89.8	119.8	174.5	268.4	358.0	299.0	385.2	404.0	336.1	331.8	69.7		11.37	**146.6**	*ALL*
All sites but 173	1094	30	17.7	15.4	9.2	18.8	47.9	89.1	118.7	174.5	268.4	358.0	295.0	385.2	397.5	336.1	326.6	69.0	100.0	11.29	**145.5**	*ALLb*

Rate from 1 case   0.355 0.497 0.486 0.437 0.489 0.615 1.015 1.678 2.657 3.978 4.041 8.754 6.517 14.006 5.104

†Important: see notes on population page

85

Zimbabwe, Harare

The National Cancer Registry (NCR) was established in 1985 in Harare as a result of an agreement between IARC and the Zimbabwean Ministry of Health. It was initially hospital-based, but adequate coverage for the population of the city of Harare was achieved in 1990. Although the registry records all cancer patients identified from its information sources, irrespective of residence, the present data for 1990–92 are confined to the Harare city population.

The activities of the registry are overseen by an advisory committee; the day-to-day administration is the responsibility of the registrar under the guidance of the medical director. The registry has four full-time staff comprising the registrar, secretary and two data collection clerks. It is located at Parirenyatwa Hospital, a large government referral centre and the location of the Medical School of the University of Zimbabwe. The project is supported by the Ministry of Health and Child Welfare, IARC and other organizations.

The first cancer registry in the country, then known as Rhodesia, was established in Bulawayo in 1963 and was one of the few on the African continent. It operated for 15 years until its operations were disrupted by the war of liberation, and is now being reactivated.

Harare is located in north-eastern Zimbabwe and is the country's largest city. According to the 1992 census, its population was almost 1 200 000, comprising 95% African (mainly Shona and Ndebele), 3% European and the remainder of Asian or mixed ethnicity.

Harare has a good health delivery system based on a network of primary health care facilities provided by the municipality with the government providing referral facilities. There is also a private sector that caters mainly for the middle- and higher-income groups.

Case-finding is mainly active, with registry staff visiting institutions within the health care system which are involved in the management of cancer patients. The registry's information sources include:

(1) Routine weekly visits to the inpatient wards of the two government central referral hospitals (Harare and Parirenyatwa).

(2) Medical records of discharged and deceased cancer patients from the two central hospitals and visits to oncology outpatient clinics.

(3) Histology reports from the public and private sectors.

(4) Completed notifications from the radiotherapy department.

(5) Death certificates of patients dying of cancer in greater Harare.

(6) Case series collected by interested clinicians, on, e.g., hepatoma, Kaposi's sarcoma and haematological malignancies.

Hospital inpatients are interviewed to verify the accuracy of reported age, residential status and other demographic data. Information recorded on each case includes sex, date of birth or age, residence, racial group, basis of diagnosis, tumour site and histology. Residence status is defined as the patient's place of residence during the last six months.

All notifications coming into the registry are thoroughly vetted to ensure that only incident cases are recorded. Incident cases are checked by doctors to confirm the diagnosis and completed forms are coded to the ICD-O system. The data are stored on a micro-computer using the CAN-REG system. Patient name lists are generated periodically to physically identify and eliminate duplicates. Data verification is done using the CHECK program and analysis is done using CANREG and EPIINFO.

When several lesions of the same histological type occur in a patient, only the first lesion is registered. Subsequent lesions are ignored. For example, the incidence of non-melanoma skin cancer is very high in the white community of Zimbabwe and many patients develop several lesions of the same histological type during their lifetime. However, if basal cell carcinoma and squamous cell carcinoma of the skin occur in the same patient affecting the same or different sites, they are recorded separately.

The registry observes the IARC/IACR rules regarding use of death certificates. All death certificates with a mention of cancer are abstracted on special forms and are matched with the registry's files. Follow-back is conducted for patients who do not have registry records but died in hospital, yielding death certificate notifications (DCN). If the death certificate is the only document available, registration has to be approved by the medical director.

Data from the registry are extensively utilized by both indigenous and foreign researchers, conference participants, lecturers, students, health educators and the Ministry of Health for management planning and national cancer control programmes.

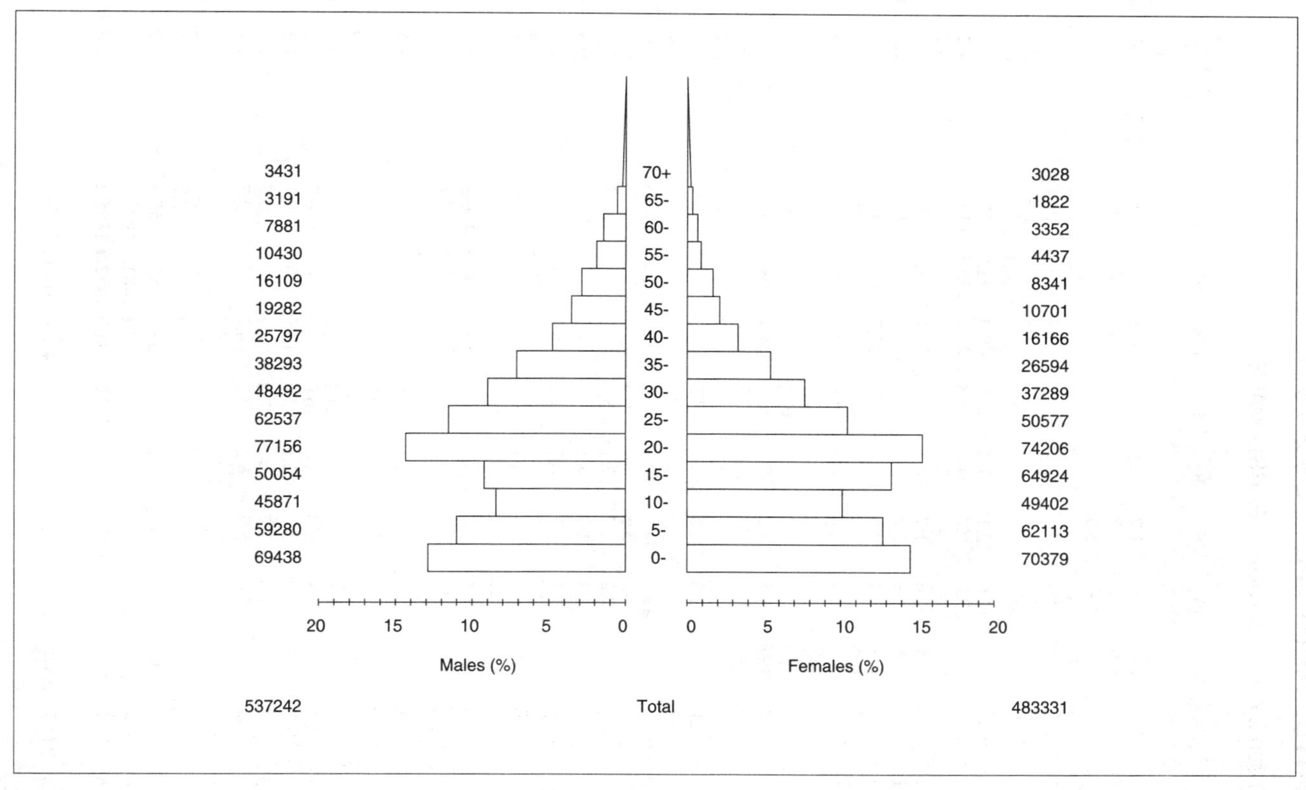

Zimbabwe, Harare City: African
Source of population: 1992
Census: 1992. Central Statistical Office 1993.
Notes to tables overleaf:
* The editors have doubts about the accuracy of enumeration of the older female population and the rates in this group should be interpreted with caution.
† 188 does not include non-invasive tumours.

* ZIMBABWE, HARARE: AFRICAN 1990-1992

ANNUAL INCIDENCE PER 100,000 BY AGE GROUP (YEARS) - MALE

SITE	ALL AGES	AGE UNK	0-	5-	10-	15-	20-	25-	30-	35-	40-	45-	50-	55-	60-	65-	70+	CRUDE RATE	%	CR 64	ASR (W)	ICD (9th)
Lip	0	0	-	-	-	-	-	-	-	-	-	-	-	-	-	-	-	0.0	0.0	0.00	0.0	140
Tongue	6	0	-	-	-	-	-	-	-	0.9	-	1.7	2.1	-	4.2	10.4	9.7	0.4	0.4	0.04	1.1	141
Salivary gland	5	0	-	-	-	-	-	0.5	-	0.9	-	1.7	-	-	-	10.4	9.7	0.3	0.3	0.02	0.9	142
Mouth	5	1	-	-	-	-	0.4	-	-	-	-	3.5	-	-	4.2	-	-	0.3	0.3	0.05	0.5	143-5
Oropharynx	0	0	-	-	-	-	-	-	-	-	-	-	-	-	-	-	-	0.0	0.0	0.00	0.0	146
Nasopharynx	13	0	-	-	-	0.7	-	0.5	2.7	-	1.3	-	2.1	-	4.2	20.9	19.4	0.8	0.8	0.06	2.0	147
Hypopharynx	2	0	-	-	-	0.4	-	-	-	-	-	-	-	-	4.2	-	-	0.1	0.1	0.02	0.2	148
Pharynx unspecified	2	0	-	-	-	-	-	-	-	-	-	-	-	3.2	-	10.4	-	0.1	0.1	0.02	0.4	149
Oesophagus	153	0	-	-	-	-	-	-	0.7	6.1	11.6	12.1	37.2	89.5	148.0	198.5	281.7	9.5	9.5	1.53	30.4	150
Stomach	68	0	-	-	-	-	-	-	1.4	2.6	9.0	5.2	24.8	28.8	21.1	135.8	136.0	4.2	4.2	0.46	13.8	151
Small intestine	1	0	-	-	-	-	-	-	-	-	-	-	2.1	-	-	-	-	0.1	0.1	0.01	0.1	152
Colon	39	0	-	-	-	0.7	1.7	1.1	-	3.5	2.6	1.7	10.3	12.8	21.1	41.8	68.0	2.4	2.4	0.28	6.6	153
Rectum	28	0	-	-	-	0.7	0.4	1.1	0.7	2.6	3.9	5.2	10.3	-	16.9	31.3	19.4	1.7	1.7	0.21	3.8	154
Liver	213	0	-	0.6	0.7	-	4.3	5.3	8.2	16.5	23.3	32.8	45.5	54.3	122.7	261.2	291.4	13.2	13.2	1.57	34.6	155
Gallbladder etc.	3	0	-	-	-	-	-	-	-	0.9	-	-	2.1	-	-	-	9.7	0.2	0.2	0.01	0.5	156
Pancreas	31	0	-	-	-	-	-	0.5	-	-	2.6	6.9	6.2	9.6	42.3	31.3	48.6	1.9	1.9	0.34	5.9	157
Nose, sinuses etc.	8	0	-	-	-	-	0.4	-	-	0.9	-	1.7	-	3.2	8.5	10.4	9.7	0.5	0.5	0.07	1.4	160
Larynx	23	1	-	-	-	-	-	-	-	-	-	3.5	4.1	19.2	25.4	31.3	29.1	1.4	1.4	0.27	4.5	161
Bronchus, lung	126	0	-	-	-	-	-	0.5	-	0.9	6.5	13.8	45.5	70.3	118.4	198.5	194.3	7.8	7.8	1.28	24.9	162
Other thoracic organs	2	0	-	-	-	0.7	-	-	-	-	-	-	-	3.2	-	-	-	0.1	0.1	0.02	0.2	163-4
Bone	12	0	-	0.6	0.7	2.0	0.9	-	-	-	-	-	2.1	-	12.7	-	9.7	0.7	0.7	0.09	1.4	170
Connective tissue	17	0	1.4	-	0.7	2.7	-	1.1	1.4	-	2.6	3.5	-	3.2	-	-	-	1.1	1.1	0.08	1.1	171
Mesothelioma	0	0	-	-	-	-	-	-	-	-	-	-	-	-	-	-	-	0.0	0.0	0.00	0.0	MES
Kaposi's sarcoma	380	2	2.9	0.6	-	-	12.1	41.0	64.6	51.4	49.1	34.6	49.7	47.9	50.8	20.9	19.4	23.6	23.6	2.03	24.6	KAP
Melanoma of skin	14	0	-	-	-	1.3	-	0.5	0.7	1.7	-	3.5	-	6.4	8.5	10.4	9.7	0.9	0.9	0.11	1.8	172
Other skin	22	2	-	-	-	-	0.4	1.1	-	2.6	2.6	1.7	2.1	3.2	8.5	31.3	38.9	1.4		0.12	4.0	173
Breast	5	0	-	-	-	-	-	-	-	-	1.3	1.7	4.1	-	4.2	-	-	0.3	0.3	0.06	0.6	175
Prostate	112	3	-	-	-	-	-	-	-	0.9	1.3	1.7	20.7	51.1	88.8	188.0	398.3	6.9	7.0	0.85	29.2	185
Testis	4	0	-	-	-	0.7	-	-	-	-	-	1.7	-	-	4.2	10.4	-	0.2	0.2	0.03	0.6	186
Penis	13	0	-	-	-	-	-	-	-	0.9	-	3.5	4.1	-	12.7	10.4	38.9	0.8	0.8	0.11	2.8	187.1-.4
Other male genital	0	0	-	-	-	-	-	-	-	-	-	-	-	-	-	-	-	0.0	0.0	0.00	0.0	187.5-.9
†Bladder	68	0	-	0.6	-	-	-	-	2.1	3.5	1.3	15.6	20.7	12.8	59.2	94.0	126.3	4.2	4.2	0.58	13.2	188
Kidney etc.	17	0	3.8	0.6	0.7	-	0.4	-	-	0.9	-	1.7	2.1	-	4.2	10.4	9.7	1.1	1.1	0.07	1.7	189
Eye	10	0	2.4	-	-	0.7	-	0.5	-	-	-	-	2.1	3.2	-	10.4	-	0.6	0.6	0.04	0.9	190
Brain, nervous system	29	0	1.4	0.6	2.2	2.7	0.9	1.6	0.7	2.6	2.6	-	4.1	9.6	4.2	-	9.7	1.8	1.8	0.17	2.4	191-2
Thyroid	9	0	-	-	-	-	0.4	0.5	-	0.9	-	1.7	-	6.4	8.5	-	9.7	0.6	0.6	0.09	1.2	193
Other endocrine	0	0	-	-	-	-	-	-	-	-	-	-	-	-	-	-	-	0.0	0.0	0.00	0.0	194
Hodgkin's disease	13	0	-	0.6	0.7	-	0.4	2.1	-	0.9	1.3	-	4.1	3.2	4.2	-	-	0.8	0.8	0.09	1.0	201
Non-Hodgkin lymphoma	58	0	1.0	5.1	0.7	2.0	0.4	4.8	2.7	4.4	7.8	6.9	12.4	16.0	4.2	10.4	9.7	3.6	3.6	0.34	4.7	200,202
Multiple myeloma	20	0	-	-	-	-	-	-	0.7	1.7	3.9	5.2	2.1	12.8	16.9	10.4	9.7	1.2	1.2	0.22	2.7	203
Lymphoid leukaemia	20	0	0.5	3.9	-	2.0	-	0.5	-	-	1.3	1.7	-	3.2	4.2	31.3	9.7	1.2	1.2	0.09	2.5	204
Myeloid leukaemia	34	0	1.0	0.6	3.6	3.3	0.4	2.1	1.4	2.6	2.6	5.2	6.2	3.2	4.2	-	9.7	2.1	2.1	0.18	2.7	205
Monocytic leukaemia	0	0	-	-	-	-	-	-	-	-	-	-	-	-	-	-	-	0.0	0.0	0.00	0.0	206
Other leukaemia	0	0	-	-	-	-	-	-	-	-	-	-	-	-	-	-	-	0.0	0.0	0.00	0.0	207
Leukaemia unspecified	2	0	-	-	-	-	-	-	-	-	-	-	-	-	4.2	-	9.7	0.1	0.1	0.02	0.6	208
Other and unspecified	43	1	-	-	0.7	1.3	0.4	1.1	1.4	4.4	2.6	-	6.2	16.0	33.8	52.2	58.3	2.7	2.7	0.35	7.2	O&U
All sites	1630	10	14.4	13.5	10.9	21.3	24.6	66.6	89.4	114.9	140.8	179.8	335.2	492.2	879.8	1483.3	1904.0	101.1		11.99	238.5	ALL
All sites but 173	1608	8	14.4	13.5	10.9	21.3	24.2	65.6	89.4	112.3	138.3	178.1	333.1	489.0	871.3	1452.0	1865.2	99.8	100.0	11.87	234.6	ALLb

Rate from 1 case: 0.480 0.562 0.727 0.666 0.432 0.533 0.687 0.870 1.292 1.729 2.069 3.196 4.230 10.446 9.714

†Important: see notes on population page

* ZIMBABWE, HARARE: AFRICAN 1990-1992

ANNUAL INCIDENCE PER 100,000 BY AGE GROUP (YEARS) - FEMALE

S I T E	ALL AGES	AGE UNK	0-	5-	10-	15-	20-	25-	30-	35-	40-	45-	50-	55-	60-	65-	70+	CRUDE RATE	%	CR 64	ASR (W)	ICD (9th)
Lip	0	0	-	-	-	-	-	-	-	-	-	-	-	-	-	-	-	0.0	0.0	0.00	0.0	140
Tongue	0	0	-	-	-	-	-	-	-	-	-	-	-	-	-	-	-	0.0	0.0	0.00	0.0	141
Salivary gland	1	0	-	-	-	-	-	-	-	-	-	-	-	-	-	-	11.0	0.1	0.1	0.00	0.4	142
Mouth	2	0	-	-	-	-	-	-	-	1.3	-	-	4.0	-	-	-	-	0.1	0.2	0.03	0.3	143-5
Oropharynx	0	0	-	-	-	-	-	-	-	-	-	-	-	-	-	-	-	0.0	0.0	0.00	0.0	146
Nasopharynx	3	0	-	-	-	-	-	-	-	-	-	3.1	-	7.5	-	-	11.0	0.2	0.3	0.05	0.9	147
Hypopharynx	1	0	-	-	-	-	-	-	-	-	-	-	-	-	-	-	11.0	0.1	0.1	0.00	0.4	148
Pharynx unspecified	2	0	-	-	-	-	-	-	-	-	-	3.1	-	-	9.9	-	-	0.1	0.2	0.07	0.6	149
Oesophagus	22	0	-	-	-	-	-	-	-	-	2.1	3.1	8.0	45.1	29.8	54.9	66.0	1.5	2.0	0.44	8.0	150
Stomach	54	0	-	-	-	-	-	2.0	-	2.5	2.1	6.2	55.9	22.5	49.7	219.5	132.1	3.7	5.0	0.70	18.4	151
Small intestine	1	0	-	-	-	-	-	-	-	-	-	-	-	-	-	18.3	-	0.1	0.1	0.00	0.5	152
Colon	11	0	-	-	-	-	-	0.7	-	-	2.1	6.2	4.0	15.0	19.9	-	22.0	0.8	1.0	0.24	3.0	153
Rectum	14	0	-	-	-	1.0	0.4	0.7	-	5.0	2.1	3.1	-	-	9.9	18.3	22.0	1.0	1.3	0.11	2.6	154
Liver	71	0	-	0.5	-	-	-	3.3	3.6	10.0	8.2	12.5	32.0	52.6	169.1	109.8	77.1	4.9	6.6	1.46	19.2	155
Gallbladder etc.	2	0	-	-	-	-	-	-	-	-	-	-	-	7.5	-	18.3	-	0.1	0.2	0.04	0.8	156
Pancreas	23	0	-	-	-	-	-	-	1.8	1.3	2.1	6.2	-	22.5	39.8	73.2	66.0	1.6	2.1	0.37	8.0	157
Nose, sinuses etc.	5	0	-	-	-	-	-	0.7	0.9	-	-	-	-	-	-	-	33.0	0.3	0.5	0.01	1.4	160
Larynx	2	0	-	-	-	-	-	-	-	-	-	-	-	-	-	18.3	11.0	0.1	0.2	0.00	1.0	161
Bronchus, lung	22	0	-	-	-	0.5	-	-	0.9	2.5	2.1	6.2	4.0	7.5	29.8	73.2	66.0	1.5	2.0	0.27	7.3	162
Other thoracic organs	2	0	-	-	-	-	-	-	-	-	-	3.1	4.0	-	-	-	-	0.1	0.2	0.04	0.4	163-4
Bone	9	0	-	-	-	0.5	1.3	-	-	5.0	-	-	-	-	9.9	-	-	0.6	0.8	0.08	0.9	170
Connective tissue	14	2	-	0.5	-	0.5	1.3	0.7	1.8	-	2.1	-	-	7.5	9.9	-	11.0	1.0	1.3	0.14	1.9	171
Mesothelioma	0	0	-	-	-	-	-	-	-	-	-	-	-	-	-	-	-	0.0	0.0	0.00	0.0	MES
Kaposi's sarcoma	108	1	0.9	1.1	-	2.6	5.8	21.7	17.9	21.3	8.2	18.7	12.0	15.0	-	-	-	7.4	10.1	0.63	7.9	KAP
Melanoma of skin	13	0	-	-	-	-	0.4	-	0.9	-	4.1	-	4.0	15.0	19.9	18.3	33.0	0.9	1.2	0.22	3.8	172
Other skin	12	0	-	-	-	-	-	-	0.9	-	4.1	3.1	-	-	9.9	54.9	44.0	0.8		0.09	4.3	173
Breast	117	3	-	-	-	-	0.4	6.6	9.8	33.8	28.9	37.4	55.9	67.6	69.6	73.2	55.0	8.1	10.9	1.59	20.4	174
Uterus unspecified	8	0	-	-	-	-	-	-	0.9	-	6.2	6.2	4.0	-	-	-	11.0	0.6	0.7	0.09	1.4	179
Cervix uteri	295	5	-	-	-	-	3.1	5.3	28.6	41.4	68.0	121.5	151.9	180.3	268.5	457.4	264.2	20.3	27.5	4.42	67.2	180
Placenta	15	0	-	-	-	0.5	2.2	2.6	3.6	-	-	3.1	-	-	-	-	-	1.0	1.4	0.06	0.8	181
Corpus uteri	17	0	-	-	-	-	0.4	-	0.9	1.3	2.1	-	24.0	15.0	19.9	18.3	22.0	1.2	1.6	0.32	4.3	182
Ovary etc.	36	0	-	-	0.7	0.5	0.9	2.0	2.7	2.5	4.1	21.8	4.0	30.1	59.7	36.6	22.0	2.5	3.4	0.64	8.0	183
Other female genital	4	1	-	0.5	-	-	-	-	-	-	-	3.1	-	-	-	18.3	-	0.3	0.4	0.02	1.1	184
†Bladder	43	0	-	0.5	-	-	-	0.7	1.8	2.5	12.4	6.2	24.0	15.0	79.6	54.9	110.1	3.0	4.0	0.71	12.5	188
Kidney etc.	9	0	3.3	0.5	-	-	-	-	-	-	-	-	4.0	-	-	-	-	0.6	0.8	0.04	0.7	189
Eye	8	2	1.9	1.1	-	-	-	-	-	-	-	-	-	-	-	-	-	0.6	0.7	0.02	0.4	190
Brain, nervous system	13	0	1.4	-	2.0	-	0.4	0.7	0.9	1.3	2.1	3.1	-	7.5	-	-	-	0.9	1.2	0.10	1.2	191-2
Thyroid	20	0	-	-	-	-	0.4	1.3	1.8	2.5	-	3.1	4.0	7.5	49.7	-	55.0	1.4	1.9	0.35	5.3	193
Other endocrine	2	0	0.5	-	-	-	-	-	-	1.3	-	-	-	-	-	-	-	0.1	0.2	0.01	0.1	194
Hodgkin's disease	6	0	-	-	0.7	0.5	-	1.3	-	-	-	-	8.0	-	-	-	-	0.4	0.6	0.05	0.6	201
Non-Hodgkin lymphoma	22	0	-	0.5	0.7	0.5	0.9	2.0	2.7	2.5	2.1	-	4.0	7.5	9.9	18.3	44.0	1.5	2.0	0.17	4.0	200,202
Multiple myeloma	12	0	-	-	-	-	-	-	-	-	2.1	6.2	8.0	-	29.8	36.6	22.0	0.8	1.1	0.23	4.1	203
Lymphoid leukaemia	14	0	0.9	1.6	1.3	0.5	-	-	0.9	-	-	-	4.0	7.5	19.9	-	11.0	1.0	1.3	0.18	2.2	204
Myeloid leukaemia	20	0	0.9	0.5	1.3	0.5	1.3	0.7	1.8	2.5	4.1	-	4.0	-	-	-	33.0	1.4	1.9	0.09	2.5	205
Monocytic leukaemia	0	0	-	-	-	-	-	-	-	-	-	-	-	-	-	-	-	0.0	0.0	0.00	0.0	206
Other leukaemia	0	0	-	-	-	-	-	-	-	-	-	-	-	-	-	-	-	0.0	0.0	0.00	0.0	207
Leukaemia unspecified	0	0	-	-	-	-	-	-	-	-	-	-	-	-	-	-	-	0.0	0.0	0.00	0.0	208
Other and unspecified	31	1	0.5	0.5	-	1.5	0.9	0.7	1.8	2.5	4.1	6.2	16.0	22.5	9.9	54.9	33.0	2.1	2.9	0.35	6.5	O&U
All sites	1086	15	10.4	8.0	6.7	9.8	20.7	53.4	86.7	142.9	175.3	292.8	443.6	578.5	1024.3	1445.3	1298.8	74.9		14.46	236.2	ALL
All sites but 173	1074	15	10.4	8.0	6.7	9.8	20.7	53.4	85.8	142.9	171.1	289.7	443.6	578.5	1014.3	1390.4	1254.8	74.1	100.0	14.38	231.9	ALLb

Rate from 1 case 0.474 0.537 0.675 0.513 0.449 0.659 0.894 1.253 2.062 3.115 3.996 7.513 9.944 18.295 11.007

†Important: see notes on population page

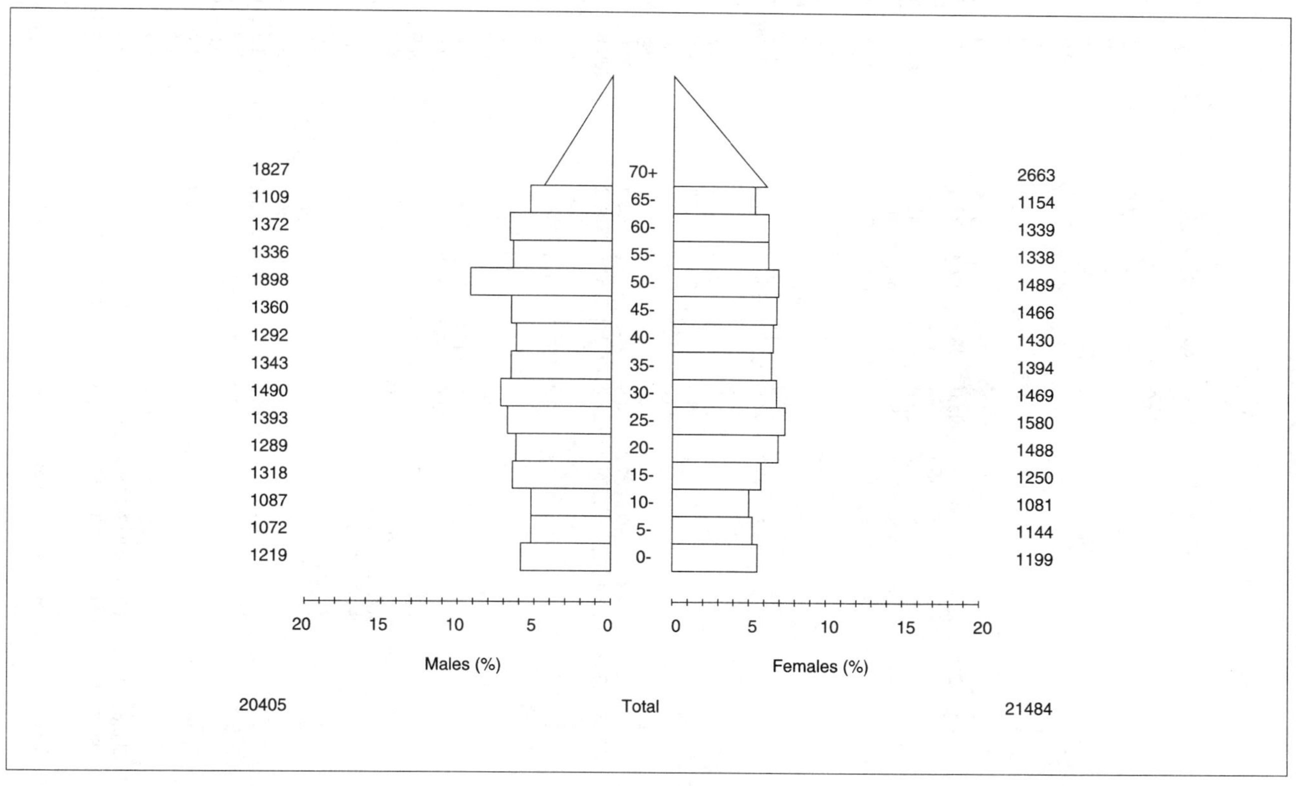

Zimbabwe, Harare City: European
Source of population: 1992
Census: 1992. Central Statistical Office, 1993.
Notes to tables overleaf:
* The rates are unstable due to small numbers, and the high proportion of DCO diagnoses indicates a degree of under-ascertainment.
† 188 does not include non-invasive tumours.

* ZIMBABWE, HARARE: EUROPEAN 1990-1992

ANNUAL INCIDENCE PER 100,000 BY AGE GROUP (YEARS) - MALE

SITE	ALL AGES	AGE UNK	0-	5-	10-	15-	20-	25-	30-	35-	40-	45-	50-	55-	60-	65-	70+	CRUDE RATE	%	CR 64	ASR (W)	ICD (9th)
Lip	1	0	-	-	-	-	-	-	-	-	-	-	-	25.0	-	-	-	1.6	0.3	0.12	1.0	140
Tongue	4	0	-	-	-	-	-	-	-	-	-	-	-	-	-	-	73.0	6.5	1.3	0.00	2.9	141
Salivary gland	0	0	-	-	-	-	-	-	-	-	-	-	-	-	-	-	-	0.0	0.0	0.00	0.0	142
Mouth	2	0	-	-	-	-	-	-	-	-	-	24.5	-	-	24.3	-	-	3.3	0.6	0.24	2.4	143-5
Oropharynx	0	0	-	-	-	-	-	-	-	-	-	-	-	-	-	-	-	0.0	0.0	0.00	0.0	146
Nasopharynx	0	0	-	-	-	-	-	-	-	-	-	-	-	-	-	-	-	0.0	0.0	0.00	0.0	147
Hypopharynx	0	0	-	-	-	-	-	-	-	-	-	-	-	-	-	-	-	0.0	0.0	0.00	0.0	148
Pharynx unspecified	0	0	-	-	-	-	-	-	-	-	-	-	-	-	-	-	-	0.0	0.0	0.00	0.0	149
Oesophagus	3	0	-	-	-	-	-	-	-	-	-	-	-	-	-	30.0	36.5	4.9	0.9	0.00	2.4	150
Stomach	9	0	-	-	-	-	-	-	-	24.8	-	-	-	25.0	48.6	30.0	73.0	14.7	2.8	0.49	8.3	151
Small intestine	2	0	-	-	-	-	-	-	-	-	-	-	35.1	-	-	-	-	3.3	0.6	0.18	1.8	152
Colon	20	0	-	-	-	-	-	-	-	-	25.8	24.5	17.6	25.0	72.9	90.1	182.4	32.7	6.3	0.83	17.8	153
Rectum	23	0	-	-	-	-	-	-	-	49.6	25.8	24.5	17.6	99.8	97.2	60.1	146.0	37.6	7.2	1.57	22.4	154
Liver	14	0	-	-	-	-	-	-	-	-	-	24.5	17.6	-	145.8	60.1	73.0	22.9	4.4	0.94	12.9	155
Gallbladder etc.	0	0	-	-	-	-	-	-	-	-	-	-	-	-	-	-	-	0.0	0.0	0.00	0.0	156
Pancreas	5	0	-	-	-	-	-	-	-	-	-	-	17.6	-	24.3	30.0	36.5	8.2	1.6	0.21	4.2	157
Nose, sinuses etc.	3	0	-	-	-	-	-	-	22.4	-	-	-	-	-	-	60.1	-	4.9	0.9	0.11	3.1	160
Larynx	11	0	-	-	-	-	-	-	-	-	-	-	-	25.0	145.8	30.0	54.7	18.0	3.5	0.85	9.9	161
Bronchus, lung	42	1	-	-	-	-	-	-	-	-	-	24.5	17.6	124.8	218.7	150.2	364.9	68.6	13.2	1.97	36.0	162
Other thoracic organs	0	0	-	-	-	-	-	-	-	-	-	-	-	-	-	-	-	0.0	0.0	0.00	0.0	163-4
Bone	1	0	-	-	-	-	-	-	-	-	-	-	-	-	-	30.0	-	1.6	0.3	0.00	0.9	170
Connective tissue	6	0	-	-	-	-	25.9	-	22.4	-	-	-	17.6	25.0	-	30.0	18.2	9.8	1.9	0.45	6.9	171
Mesothelioma	1	0	-	-	-	-	-	-	-	-	-	-	-	25.0	-	-	-	1.6	0.3	0.12	1.0	MES
Kaposi's sarcoma	2	0	-	-	-	-	-	-	-	24.8	25.8	-	-	-	-	-	-	3.3	0.6	0.25	3.0	KAP
Melanoma of skin	19	0	-	-	-	-	-	-	-	-	25.8	49.0	87.8	74.9	-	150.2	54.7	31.0	6.0	1.19	18.6	172
Other skin	551	28	-	31.1	-	50.6	51.7	95.7	201.3	273.0	464.4	735.1	1176.7	1921.2	1992.2	2162.8	2700.2	900.0		36.84	535.4	173
Breast	0	0	-	-	-	-	-	-	-	-	-	-	-	-	-	-	-	0.0	0.0	0.00	0.0	175
Prostate	67	2	-	-	-	-	-	-	-	-	-	49.0	17.6	99.8	267.2	210.3	729.8	109.4	21.1	2.23	55.7	185
Testis	0	0	-	-	-	-	-	-	-	-	-	-	-	-	-	-	-	0.0	0.0	0.00	0.0	186
Penis	1	0	-	-	-	-	-	-	-	-	-	-	-	-	-	30.0	-	1.6	0.3	0.00	0.9	187.1-.4
Other male genital	0	0	-	-	-	-	-	-	-	-	-	-	-	-	-	-	-	0.0	0.0	0.00	0.0	187.5-.9
†Bladder	31	0	-	-	-	-	-	-	22.4	-	-	24.5	-	74.9	145.8	210.3	237.2	50.6	9.7	1.34	27.4	188
Kidney etc.	3	0	-	-	-	-	-	-	-	-	-	-	-	25.0	24.3	30.0	-	4.9	0.9	0.25	2.9	189
Eye	3	0	-	-	-	25.3	-	-	-	-	-	-	17.6	-	24.3	-	-	4.9	0.9	0.34	4.1	190
Brain, nervous system	11	0	-	-	-	-	77.6	-	22.4	24.8	-	24.5	-	25.0	24.3	30.0	36.5	18.0	3.5	0.99	14.8	191-2
Thyroid	0	0	-	-	-	-	-	-	-	-	-	-	-	-	-	-	-	0.0	0.0	0.00	0.0	193
Other endocrine	0	0	-	-	-	-	-	-	-	-	-	-	-	-	-	-	-	0.0	0.0	0.00	0.0	194
Hodgkin's disease	0	0	-	-	-	-	-	-	-	-	-	-	-	-	-	-	-	0.0	0.0	0.00	0.0	201
Non-Hodgkin lymphoma	5	1	-	-	-	-	-	-	-	-	-	-	17.6	-	24.3	-	36.5	8.2	1.6	0.26	4.1	200,202
Multiple myeloma	2	0	-	-	-	-	-	-	-	-	-	-	-	-	-	-	36.5	3.3	0.6	0.00	1.5	203
Lymphoid leukaemia	2	0	-	-	-	-	-	-	-	-	-	-	-	25.0	-	-	18.2	3.3	0.6	0.12	1.7	204
Myeloid leukaemia	5	0	-	-	-	-	-	-	-	-	-	-	-	25.0	48.6	-	36.5	8.2	1.6	0.37	4.4	205
Monocytic leukaemia	0	0	-	-	-	-	-	-	-	-	-	-	-	-	-	-	-	0.0	0.0	0.00	0.0	206
Other leukaemia	1	0	-	-	-	-	-	-	-	-	-	-	-	-	-	-	18.2	1.6	0.3	0.00	0.7	207
Leukaemia unspecified	1	0	-	-	-	-	-	-	-	-	-	-	-	-	24.3	-	-	1.6	0.3	0.12	1.0	208
Other and unspecified	18	0	-	-	-	-	-	-	-	-	-	24.5	-	49.9	48.6	90.1	182.4	29.4	5.7	0.61	15.4	O&U
All sites	869	32	-	31.1	-	75.9	155.2	95.7	290.8	397.1	567.6	1029.2	1457.7	2694.6	3401.4	3514.6	5145.0	1419.4		52.93	825.4	ALL
All sites but 173	318	4	-	-	-	25.3	103.4	-	89.5	124.1	103.2	294.0	281.0	773.5	1409.1	1351.8	2444.8	519.4	100.0	16.22	290.6	ALLb
Rate from 1 case			27.345	31.095	30.656	25.284	25.860	23.929	22.366	24.820	25.800	24.504	17.562	24.950	24.295	30.039	18.245					

†Important: see notes on population page

* ZIMBABWE, HARARE: EUROPEAN 1990-1992

ANNUAL INCIDENCE PER 100,000 BY AGE GROUP (YEARS) - FEMALE

SITE	ALL AGES	AGE UNK	0-	5-	10-	15-	20-	25-	30-	35-	40-	45-	50-	55-	60-	65-	70+	CRUDE RATE	%	CR 64	ASR (W)	ICD (9th)
Lip	0	0	-	-	-	-	-	-	-	-	-	-	-	-	-	-	-	0.0	0.0	0.00	0.0	140
Tongue	6	1	-	-	-	-	-	-	-	-	-	-	-	-	74.7	57.8	-	9.3	1.8	0.45	5.7	141
Salivary gland	0	0	-	-	-	-	-	-	-	-	-	-	-	-	-	-	-	0.0	0.0	0.00	0.0	142
Mouth	1	0	-	-	-	-	-	-	-	-	-	-	-	-	-	28.9	-	1.6	0.3	0.00	0.9	143-5
Oropharynx	1	0	-	-	-	-	-	-	-	-	-	-	-	-	24.9	-	-	1.6	0.3	0.12	1.0	146
Nasopharynx	2	0	-	-	-	-	-	21.1	-	23.9	-	-	-	-	-	-	-	3.1	0.6	0.23	3.1	147
Hypopharynx	0	0	-	-	-	-	-	-	-	-	-	-	-	-	-	-	-	0.0	0.0	0.00	0.0	148
Pharynx unspecified	0	0	-	-	-	-	-	-	-	-	-	-	-	-	-	-	-	0.0	0.0	0.00	0.0	149
Oesophagus	3	0	-	-	-	-	-	-	-	-	-	-	-	-	-	-	37.6	4.7	0.9	0.00	1.5	150
Stomach	9	0	-	-	-	-	-	-	-	23.3	-	-	-	24.9	28.9	75.1	14.0	2.7	0.24	6.3	151
Small intestine	0	0	-	-	-	-	-	-	-	-	-	-	-	-	-	-	-	0.0	0.0	0.00	0.0	152
Colon	21	0	-	-	-	-	-	-	-	-	22.7	44.8	-	74.7	-	187.8	32.6	6.2	0.71	14.1	153
Rectum	10	0	-	-	-	-	-	-	23.9	-	-	24.9	49.8	-	75.1		15.5	2.9	0.49	7.4	154
Liver	8	0	-	-	-	-	-	-	-	-	-	-	-	57.8	75.1		12.4	2.4	0.00	4.7	155
Gallbladder etc.	0	0	-	-	-	-	-	-	-	-	-	-	-	-	-		0.0	0.0	0.00	0.0	156
Pancreas	8	0	-	-	-	-	-	-	-	-	44.8	-	24.9	28.9	50.1		12.4	2.4	0.35	6.1	157
Nose, sinuses etc.	2	0	-	-	-	-	-	-	-	-	-	-	-	-	25.0		3.1	0.6	0.00	1.0	160
Larynx	1	1	-	-	-	-	-	-	-	-	-	-	-	-	-		1.6	0.3	0.00	0.0	161
Bronchus, lung	24	0	-	-	-	-	-	-	-	22.7	22.4	49.8	124.5	86.7	150.2		37.2	7.1	1.10	18.1	162
Other thoracic organs	0	0	-	-	-	-	-	-	-	-	-	-	-	-	-		0.0	0.0	0.00	0.0	163-4
Bone	0	0	-	-	-	-	-	-	-	-	-	-	-	-	-		0.0	0.0	0.00	0.0	170
Connective tissue	1	0	-	-	-	22.4	-	-	-	-	-	-	-	-	-		1.6	0.3	0.11	1.8	171
Mesothelioma	0	0	-	-	-	-	-	-	-	-	-	-	-	-	-		0.0	0.0	0.00	0.0	MES
Kaposi's sarcoma	0	0	-	-	-	-	-	-	-	-	-	-	-	-	-		0.0	0.0	0.00	0.0	KAP
Melanoma of skin	17	0	-	-	-	-	-	47.8	23.3	45.5	-	74.7	24.9	-	100.1		26.4	5.0	1.08	15.0	172
Other skin	362	14	-	-	-	105.5	181.5	406.5	489.4	750.3	1046.3	1120.2	1646.4	1189.1		561.6		24.23	343.0	173
Breast	135	4	-	-	-	-	68.1	71.7	186.4	386.5	358.2	373.7	398.3	462.2	463.1		209.4	39.8	9.50	127.7	174
Uterus unspecified	2	0	-	-	-	-	-	23.3	-	-	-	-	12.5		3.1	0.6	0.12	1.9	179
Cervix uteri	10	0	-	-	-	-	45.4	-	46.6	22.7	22.4	-	-	28.9	37.6		15.5	2.9	0.69	10.4	180
Placenta	0	0	-	-	-	-	-	-	-	-	-	-	-		0.0	0.0	0.00	0.0	181
Corpus uteri	13	0	-	-	-	-	-	-	22.7	-	49.8	74.7	-	87.6		20.2	3.8	0.74	9.8	182
Ovary etc.	13	0	-	-	-	22.7	-	46.6	68.2	-	24.9	74.7	28.9	25.0		20.2	3.8	1.19	14.1	183
Other female genital	1	0	-	-	-	-	-	-	-	-	-	28.9	-		1.6	0.3	0.00	0.9	184
†Bladder	10	0	-	-	-	-	-	-	-	49.8	74.7	28.9	50.1		15.5	2.9	0.62	7.8	188
Kidney etc.	3	0	-	-	-	-	-	22.7	-	-	-	28.9	12.5		4.7	0.9	0.11	2.7	189
Eye	0	0	-	-	-	-	-	-	-	-	-	-	-		0.0	0.0	0.00	0.0	190
Brain, nervous system	11	0	-	-	30.8	-	-	-	23.3	22.7	-	49.8	24.9	28.9	50.1		17.1	3.2	0.76	11.4	191-2
Thyroid	2	0	-	-	-	-	-	-	22.7	-	-	28.9	-		3.1	0.6	0.11	2.2	193
Other endocrine	0	0	-	-	-	-	-	-	-	-	-	-	-		0.0	0.0	0.00	0.0	194
Hodgkin's disease	3	0	-	-	26.7	-	-	-	23.3	-	-	-	12.5		4.7	0.9	0.25	4.3	201
Non-Hodgkin lymphoma	4	0	-	-	-	-	-	23.9	-	-	49.8	-	12.5		6.2	1.2	0.37	3.9	200,202
Multiple myeloma	2	0	-	-	-	-	-	-	-	-	-	-	25.0		3.1	0.6	0.00	1.0	203
Lymphoid leukaemia	1	0	-	-	-	-	-	-	-	-	-	28.9	-		1.6	0.3	0.00	0.9	204
Myeloid leukaemia	3	0	-	-	-	-	-	-	-	22.4	-	28.9	12.5		4.7	0.9	0.11	2.5	205
Monocytic leukaemia	0	0	-	-	-	-	-	-	-	-	-	-	-		0.0	0.0	0.00	0.0	206
Other leukaemia	0	0	-	-	-	-	-	-	-	-	-	-	-		0.0	0.0	0.00	0.0	207
Leukaemia unspecified	0	0	-	-	-	-	-	-	-	-	-	-	-		0.0	0.0	0.00	0.0	208
Other and unspecified	12	0	-	-	-	-	-	-	-	-	-	24.9	74.7	57.8	75.1		18.6	3.5	0.50	8.7	O&U
All sites	701	20	-	-	30.8	26.7	22.4	126.6	317.6	597.8	885.6	1409.7	1074.5	1768.8	2315.2	2715.2	2841.4	1087.6		44.14	640.2	ALL
All sites but 173	339	6	-	-	30.8	26.7	22.4	21.1	136.1	191.3	396.2	659.4	514.9	722.5	1194.9	1068.7	1652.3	525.9	100.0	19.93	297.5	ALLb

Rate from 1 case

27.801 29.129 30.836 26.667 22.396 21.097 22.686 23.912 23.305 22.738 22.386 24.913 24.894 28.885 12.517

†Important: see notes on population page

Argentina, Concordia

The population-based Tumour Registry of Concordia, in the province of Entre Ríos, started operating in January 1990. It is located in the "Felipe Heras" Regional Hospital.

The registry covers the whole of the Department of Concordia, which is situated between latitudes 30°50´ and 31°47´ S and longitudes 57°56´and 58°36´ W.

Concordia had a population of 138 983 inhabitants (67 850 males and 71 133 females), according to the 1991 census. Distribution by age is similar to that of the world standard population. The population density is 37.8 inhabitants per km^2.

Immigration from Europe has formed the basis of the population of the area, which is therefore predominantly Caucasian white, with a low percentage of mixed race and no blacks.

It is a mainly rural area, where citrus fruits and rice are the most important crops. Poultry farming is also a major activity. The main industries are those related to food, drinks and wood.

The data sources for the registry are public and private hospitals, pathology and cytology laboratories, radiotherapy services, social work archives and death certificates provided by the local office of the National Registry Office.

Data collection is active and continuous. Information is collected on all invasive tumours occurring in residents of the Department of Concordia. Basal cell and squamous cell carcinomas are recorded as well as benign or uncertain-behaviour tumours of the central nervous system and bladder papillomas. Information about tumours *in situ* is also collected but these cases are not included.

Variables recorded are personal particulars, sources of information, basis and date of diagnosis, site, histological type and presence of multiple tumours. Site and morphology coding has so far been carried out by the registry pathologists, using ICD-O-1. Only primary tumours are included. Metastatic tumours with a non-defined primary site are coded as primary of unknown origin. The registry follows the IARC/IACR rules for multiple tumours. The CANREG software is used for data input and analysis, and the IARC CHECK program for checking for duplicates, mistakes and inconsistencies.

M.A. Prince
D. Loria
L. Herrera
E. Matos

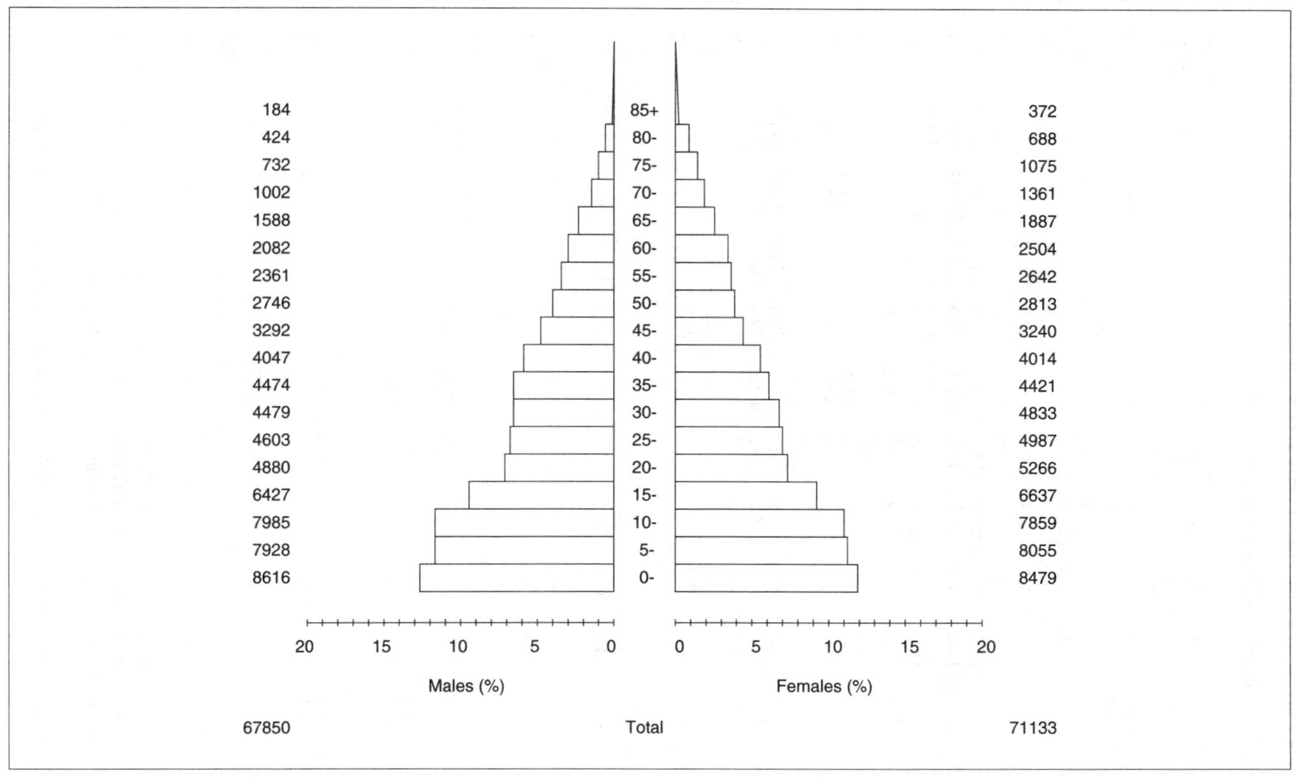

Argentina, Concordia
Source of population: 1991
Census: 1991. Instituto Nacional de Estadistica y Censos (INDEC). Censo Nacional de Poblacion y Vivienda 1991. Resultados definitivos total del Pais, Serie B, No. 25, 1993.
Notes to tables overleaf:
* The high proportion of diagnoses based on a death certificate alone indicates a degree of under-ascertainment. The childhood cancers are diagnosed outside the registry area and are under-registered.
† 188 does not include non-invasive tumours.

* ARGENTINA, CONCORDIA 1990-1994

ANNUAL INCIDENCE PER 100,000 BY AGE GROUP (YEARS) - MALE

SITE	ALL AGES	AGE UNK	0-	5-	10-	15-	20-	25-	30-	35-	40-	45-	50-	55-	60-	65-	70-	75-	80-	85+	CRUDE RATE	%	CR 64	CR 74	ASR (W)	ICD (9th)
Lip	5	0	-	-	-	-	-	-	-	-	-	14.6	-	-	12.6	20.0	27.3	-	-	1.5	0.7	0.07	0.24	**1.8**	*140*
Tongue	9	0	-	-	-	-	-	-	13.4	4.9	6.1	-	8.5	-	12.6	-	-	94.3	-	2.7	1.3	0.16	0.23	**2.7**	*141*
Salivary gland	3	0	-	-	-	-	-	-	-	4.9	-	8.5	-	-	-	20.0	-	-	-	0.9	0.4	0.07	0.17	**1.0**	*142*
Mouth	7	0	-	-	-	-	-	-	-	-	-	-	25.4	19.2	12.6	-	-	47.2	-	2.1	1.0	0.22	0.29	**2.4**	*143-5*
Oropharynx	6	0	-	-	-	-	-	4.5	-	-	6.1	7.3	25.4	-	-	-	-	-	-	1.8	0.9	0.22	0.22	**2.0**	*146*
Nasopharynx	0	0	-	-	-	-	-	-	-	-	-	-	-	-	-	-	-	-	-	0.0	0.0	0.00	0.00	**0.0**	*147*
Hypopharynx	7	0	-	-	-	-	-	-	-	-	-	7.3	8.5	19.2	-	39.9	27.3	-	-	2.1	1.0	0.17	0.37	**2.5**	*148*
Pharynx unspecified	3	0	-	-	-	-	-	-	-	4.5	-	-	9.6	12.6	-	-	-	-	-	0.9	0.4	0.07	0.13	**1.0**	*149*
Oesophagus	49	0	-	-	-	-	-	-	-	-	-	18.2	36.4	93.2	115.3	75.6	79.8	136.6	94.3	108.7	14.4	7.0	1.32	2.09	**17.5**	*150*
Stomach	70	0	-	-	-	-	-	-	8.9	4.5	29.7	12.2	51.0	76.2	76.8	113.4	179.6	218.6	283.0	326.1	20.6	9.9	1.30	2.76	**24.2**	*151*
Small intestine	2	0	-	-	-	-	-	-	-	-	-	-	-	-	-	20.0	-	-	108.7	0.6	0.3	0.00	0.10	**0.9**	*152*
Colon	49	0	-	-	-	-	-	4.5	4.5	4.9	12.2	29.1	42.4	19.2	63.0	139.7	191.3	377.4	652.2	14.4	7.0	0.58	1.60	**17.2**	*153*
Rectum	26	0	-	-	-	-	-	4.5	-	9.9	12.2	-	33.9	76.8	50.4	20.0	109.3	-	-	7.7	3.7	0.69	1.04	**9.0**	*154*
Liver	3	0	-	-	-	-	-	-	-	-	6.1	-	-	9.6	-	-	-	-	108.7	0.9	0.4	0.08	0.08	**1.3**	*155*
Gallbladder etc.	11	0	-	-	-	-	4.3	-	-	-	-	-	8.5	9.6	25.2	59.9	-	141.5	-	3.2	1.6	0.11	0.54	**3.7**	*156*
Pancreas	22	0	-	-	-	-	-	-	-	-	4.9	6.1	21.8	-	57.6	63.0	79.8	-	47.2	108.7	6.5	3.1	0.45	1.17	**8.3**	*157*
Nose, sinuses etc.	4	0	-	-	-	-	-	-	-	-	6.1	-	-	19.2	-	-	-	-	108.7	1.2	0.6	0.13	0.13	**1.7**	*160*
Larynx	24	0	-	-	-	-	4.3	-	-	4.9	24.3	29.1	16.9	57.6	-	39.9	27.3	94.3	108.7	7.1	3.4	0.69	0.89	**8.6**	*161*
Bronchus, lung	159	0	-	-	-	-	-	4.5	17.9	39.5	36.5	174.8	237.2	240.2	302.3	279.4	409.8	377.4	217.4	46.9	22.6	3.75	6.66	**55.5**	*162*
Other thoracic organs	6	0	-	-	-	-	4.3	-	-	9.9	6.1	-	-	19.2	-	-	-	-	-	1.8	0.9	0.20	0.20	**2.1**	*163-4*
Bone	6	0	-	2.5	-	9.3	8.2	-	-	-	-	-	-	-	-	-	-	-	-	1.8	0.9	0.10	0.10	**1.7**	*170*
Connective tissue	4	0	-	-	-	-	-	-	4.5	4.9	-	7.3	-	-	20.0	-	-	-	-	1.2	0.6	0.08	0.18	**1.3**	*171*
Mesothelioma	0	0	-	-	-	-	-	-	-	-	-	-	-	-	-	-	-	-	-	0.0	0.0	0.00	0.00	**0.0**	*MES*
Kaposi's sarcoma	1	0	-	-	-	-	-	-	-	4.9	-	-	-	-	-	-	-	-	-	0.3	0.1	0.02	0.02	**0.3**	*KAP*
Melanoma of skin	4	0	-	-	-	-	-	-	4.5	4.9	-	-	-	9.6	-	-	27.3	-	-	1.2	0.6	0.10	0.10	**1.2**	*172*
Other skin	133	0	-	-	-	-	-	4.3	8.9	17.9	9.9	60.8	94.7	135.5	182.5	214.1	379.2	355.2	283.0	1195.7	39.2		2.57	5.54	**48.6**	*173*
Breast	1	0	-	-	-	-	-	-	-	-	-	-	7.3	-	-	-	-	-	-	0.3	0.1	0.04	0.04	**0.4**	*175*
Prostate	48	0	-	-	-	-	-	-	-	-	-	-	7.3	8.5	48.0	125.9	179.6	273.2	471.7	217.4	14.1	6.8	0.32	1.85	**16.2**	*185*
Testis	9	0	-	-	-	4.1	8.7	4.5	8.9	-	6.1	-	16.9	-	-	-	-	-	-	2.7	1.3	0.25	0.25	**2.9**	*186*
Penis	2	0	-	-	-	-	-	-	-	4.9	-	-	-	-	-	27.3	-	-	-	0.6	0.3	0.02	0.02	**0.6**	*187.1-.4*
Other male genital	0	0	-	-	-	-	-	-	-	-	-	-	-	-	-	-	-	-	-	0.0	0.0	0.00	0.00	**0.0**	*187.5-.9*
†Bladder	26	0	-	-	-	-	-	-	-	-	6.1	-	33.9	48.0	25.2	99.8	191.3	47.2	108.7	7.7	3.7	0.44	1.06	**9.1**	*188*
Kidney etc.	8	0	-	-	-	-	-	-	-	-	-	-	16.9	9.6	25.2	39.9	-	-	108.7	2.4	1.1	0.13	0.46	**3.2**	*189*
Eye	3	0	-	-	-	-	-	-	-	-	4.9	-	-	8.5	9.6	-	-	-	-	0.9	0.4	0.12	0.12	**1.0**	*190*
Brain, nervous system	10	0	-	-	2.5	3.1	8.2	8.7	-	-	-	6.1	-	-	9.6	12.6	-	27.3	-	2.9	1.4	0.19	0.25	**3.3**	*191-2*
Thyroid	0	0	-	-	-	-	-	-	-	-	-	-	-	-	-	-	-	-	-	0.0	0.0	0.00	0.00	**0.0**	*193*
Other endocrine	0	0	-	-	-	-	-	-	-	-	-	-	-	-	-	-	-	-	-	0.0	0.0	0.00	0.00	**0.0**	*194*
Hodgkin's disease	4	0	-	5.0	-	-	-	-	-	-	4.9	-	-	-	9.6	-	-	-	-	1.2	0.6	0.10	0.10	**1.2**	*201*
Non-Hodgkin lymphoma	11	0	-	-	-	-	4.1	-	4.5	-	4.9	-	-	16.9	9.6	37.8	-	-	94.3	-	3.2	1.6	0.20	0.39	**3.6**	*200,202*
Multiple myeloma	0	0	-	-	-	-	-	-	-	-	-	-	-	-	-	-	-	-	-	0.0	0.0	0.00	0.00	**0.0**	*203*
Lymphoid leukaemia	5	0	-	-	-	-	-	-	-	-	-	-	-	-	19.2	25.2	-	-	47.2	-	1.5	0.7	0.10	0.22	**1.8**	*204*
Myeloid leukaemia	1	0	-	-	-	-	-	-	4.5	-	-	-	-	-	-	-	-	-	-	0.3	0.1	0.02	0.03	**0.3**	*205*
Monocytic leukaemia	0	0	-	-	-	-	-	-	-	-	-	-	-	-	-	-	-	-	-	0.0	0.0	0.00	0.00	**0.0**	*206*
Other leukaemia	0	0	-	-	-	-	-	-	-	-	-	-	-	-	-	-	-	-	-	0.0	0.0	0.00	0.00	**0.0**	*207*
Leukaemia unspecified	3	0	-	-	-	-	-	-	4.5	-	-	-	-	-	19.2	-	-	-	-	0.9	0.4	0.12	0.12	**1.0**	*208*
Other and unspecified	93	0	-	2.5	2.5	-	-	-	-	17.9	9.9	60.8	58.3	50.8	124.9	125.9	259.5	464.5	188.7	434.8	27.4	13.2	1.64	3.56	**32.5**	*O&U*
All sites	837	0	-	10.1	5.0	12.4	24.6	34.8	53.6	98.3	168.0	291.6	546.2	872.5	1248.8	1335.0	1956.1	2513.7	2688.7	3913.0	246.7		16.83	33.29	**293.5**	*ALL*
All sites but 173	704	0	-	10.1	5.0	12.4	24.6	30.4	44.7	80.5	158.1	230.9	451.6	737.0	1066.3	1120.9	1576.8	2158.5	2405.7	2717.4	207.5	100.0	14.26	27.75	**244.9**	*ALLb*

Rate from 1 case 2.321 2.523 2.505 3.112 4.098 4.345 4.465 4.470 4.942 6.075 7.283 8.471 9.606 12.594 19.960 27.322 47.170 108.696

†Important: see notes on population page

* ARGENTINA, CONCORDIA 1990-1994

ANNUAL INCIDENCE PER 100,000 BY AGE GROUP (YEARS) - FEMALE

SITE	ALL AGES	AGE UNK	0-	5-	10-	15-	20-	25-	30-	35-	40-	45-	50-	55-	60-	65-	70-	75-	80-	85+	CRUDE RATE	%	CR 64	CR 74	ASR (W)	ICD (9th)
Lip	1	0	-	-	-	-	-	-	-	-	-	-	-	-	-	-	-	-	-	53.8	0.3	0.1	0.00	0.00	**0.3**	*140*
Tongue	1	0	-	-	-	-	-	-	-	-	-	-	-	-	-	-	14.7	-	-	-	0.3	0.1	0.00	0.07	**0.3**	*141*
Salivary gland	3	0	-	-	2.5	-	-	-	-	-	5.0	-	-	-	-	-	14.7	-	-	-	0.8	0.4	0.04	0.11	**0.8**	*142*
Mouth	2	0	-	-	-	-	-	-	-	-	5.0	-	-	7.6	-	-	-	-	-	-	0.6	0.3	0.06	0.06	**0.6**	*143-5*
Oropharynx	1	0	-	-	-	-	-	-	-	-	-	-	-	-	8.0	-	-	-	-	-	0.3	0.1	0.04	0.04	**0.3**	*146*
Nasopharynx	2	0	-	-	-	-	-	-	-	-	-	-	-	15.1	-	-	-	-	-	-	0.6	0.3	0.08	0.08	**0.6**	*147*
Hypopharynx	1	0	-	-	-	-	-	-	-	-	-	-	-	-	-	-	-	-	-	53.8	0.3	0.1	0.00	0.00	**0.3**	*148*
Pharynx unspecified	0	0	-	-	-	-	-	-	-	-	-	-	-	-	-	-	-	-	-	-	0.0	0.0	0.00	0.00	**0.0**	*149*
Oesophagus	12	0	-	-	-	-	-	-	-	-	10.0	6.2	14.2	7.6	16.0	10.6	29.4	18.6	-	-	3.4	1.5	0.27	0.47	**3.7**	*150*
Stomach	36	0	-	-	-	-	-	-	4.5	-	10.0	-	35.5	30.3	16.0	42.4	73.5	93.0	87.2	268.8	10.1	4.6	0.48	1.06	**9.9**	*151*
Small intestine	4	0	-	-	-	-	-	-	-	-	5.0	-	-	-	10.6	-	-	18.6	-	53.8	1.1	0.5	0.02	0.08	**1.1**	*152*
Colon	56	0	-	-	-	-	-	8.0	-	13.6	-	12.3	35.5	22.7	39.9	95.4	88.2	223.3	116.3	268.8	15.7	7.2	0.66	1.58	**15.3**	*153*
Rectum	16	0	-	-	-	-	-	-	-	-	5.0	6.2	14.2	-	16.0	42.4	14.7	37.2	58.1	53.8	4.5	2.1	0.21	0.49	**4.5**	*154*
Liver	2	0	-	-	-	-	-	-	-	-	-	-	7.1	-	-	10.6	-	-	-	-	0.6	0.3	0.04	0.09	**0.7**	*155*
Gallbladder etc.	17	0	-	-	-	-	-	4.0	8.3	-	10.0	12.3	-	7.6	8.0	10.6	58.8	18.6	58.1	-	4.8	2.2	0.25	0.60	**4.7**	*156*
Pancreas	21	0	-	-	-	-	-	-	-	-	-	6.2	-	-	24.0	21.2	73.5	74.4	174.4	-	5.9	2.7	0.15	0.62	**5.1**	*157*
Nose, sinuses etc.	1	0	-	-	-	-	-	-	-	-	-	-	7.1	-	-	-	-	-	-	-	0.3	0.1	0.04	0.04	**0.4**	*160*
Larynx	6	0	-	-	-	-	-	-	4.5	-	-	6.2	-	7.6	8.0	10.6	-	18.6	-	-	1.7	0.8	0.13	0.18	**1.8**	*161*
Bronchus, lung	27	0	-	-	-	-	-	-	4.5	-	5.0	12.3	14.2	37.9	39.9	42.4	44.1	37.2	29.1	53.8	7.6	3.5	0.57	1.00	**8.1**	*162*
Other thoracic organs	10	0	-	-	-	-	-	-	-	-	-	6.2	7.1	-	8.0	31.8	14.7	37.2	-	53.8	2.8	1.3	0.11	0.34	**2.9**	*163-4*
Bone	5	0	-	-	-	-	-	-	-	-	5.0	-	-	7.6	-	31.8	-	-	-	-	1.4	0.6	0.06	0.22	**1.6**	*170*
Connective tissue	7	0	-	-	-	-	-	-	4.1	-	5.0	-	7.1	-	-	10.6	29.4	18.6	-	-	2.0	0.9	0.08	0.28	**2.0**	*171*
Mesothelioma	3	0	-	-	-	-	3.8	-	-	-	-	-	-	-	8.0	-	14.7	-	-	-	0.8	0.4	0.06	0.13	**0.9**	*MES*
Kaposi's sarcoma	0	0	-	-	-	-	-	-	-	-	-	-	-	-	-	-	-	-	-	-	0.0	0.0	0.00	0.00	**0.0**	*KAP*
Melanoma of skin	8	0	-	-	-	-	-	-	-	-	5.0	-	21.3	-	-	21.2	-	-	58.1	-	2.2	1.0	0.13	0.24	**2.3**	*172*
Other skin	124	0	-	-	-	-	-	4.0	12.4	13.6	14.9	49.4	49.8	75.7	63.9	95.4	264.5	427.9	581.4	591.4	34.9		1.42	3.22	**32.1**	*173*
Breast	207	0	-	-	-	-	-	12.0	20.7	31.7	69.8	80.2	113.8	166.5	207.7	328.6	426.2	353.5	319.8	591.4	58.2	26.6	3.51	7.29	**60.2**	*174*
Uterus unspecified	14	0	-	-	-	-	-	-	-	-	10.0	12.3	7.1	22.7	8.0	-	58.8	18.6	-	-	3.9	1.8	0.30	0.59	**4.3**	*179*
Cervix uteri	108	0	-	-	-	-	-	3.8	8.0	53.8	81.4	94.7	55.6	78.2	45.4	103.8	53.0	73.5	74.4	58.1	30.4	13.9	2.62	3.26	**32.0**	*180*
Placenta	0	0	-	-	-	-	-	-	-	-	-	-	-	-	-	-	-	-	-	-	0.0	0.0	0.00	0.00	**0.0**	*181*
Corpus uteri	28	0	-	-	-	-	-	4.0	-	-	10.0	6.2	21.3	30.3	31.9	74.2	44.1	37.2	29.1	-	7.9	3.6	0.52	1.11	**8.5**	*182*
Ovary etc.	26	0	-	-	-	-	11.4	-	4.1	-	-	12.3	21.3	22.7	24.0	31.8	44.1	55.8	29.1	53.8	7.3	3.3	0.48	0.86	**7.6**	*183*
Other female genital	13	0	-	-	-	-	-	4.0	4.1	4.5	-	-	-	-	8.0	63.6	-	18.6	29.1	53.8	3.7	1.7	0.10	0.42	**3.7**	*184*
†Bladder	14	0	-	-	-	-	-	-	-	-	5.0	-	14.2	15.1	24.0	-	14.7	18.6	58.1	107.5	3.9	1.8	0.29	0.36	**3.9**	*188*
Kidney etc.	11	0	-	-	-	-	-	4.0	-	-	-	-	7.1	-	16.0	21.2	44.1	18.6	-	53.8	3.1	1.4	0.14	0.46	**3.3**	*189*
Eye	3	0	-	-	-	-	-	-	-	-	-	-	14.2	-	-	-	-	-	-	53.8	0.8	0.4	0.07	0.07	**1.0**	*190*
Brain, nervous system	5	0	-	-	-	3.0	-	-	4.1	-	-	-	-	-	16.0	-	-	18.6	-	-	1.4	0.6	0.12	0.12	**1.3**	*191-2*
Thyroid	6	0	-	-	-	-	-	4.0	4.1	4.5	-	6.2	-	7.6	8.0	-	-	-	-	-	1.7	0.8	0.17	0.17	**1.8**	*193*
Other endocrine	0	0	-	-	-	-	-	-	-	-	-	-	-	-	-	-	-	-	-	-	0.0	0.0	0.00	0.00	**0.0**	*194*
Hodgkin's disease	2	0	-	-	-	-	3.8	-	-	-	-	-	7.1	-	-	-	-	-	-	-	0.6	0.3	0.05	0.05	**0.7**	*201*
Non-Hodgkin lymphoma	11	0	-	-	-	-	-	-	-	-	-	-	14.2	7.6	8.0	42.4	44.1	-	-	-	3.1	1.4	0.15	0.58	**3.5**	*200,202*
Multiple myeloma	1	0	-	-	-	-	-	-	-	-	-	-	-	-	-	-	-	14.7	-	-	0.3	0.1	0.00	0.07	**0.3**	*203*
Lymphoid leukaemia	6	0	-	2.5	-	3.0	-	-	-	-	-	-	-	15.1	8.0	10.6	-	-	-	-	1.7	0.8	0.14	0.20	**1.8**	*204*
Myeloid leukaemia	1	0	-	-	-	-	-	-	-	-	-	-	-	-	-	-	14.7	-	-	-	0.3	0.1	0.00	0.07	**0.3**	*205*
Monocytic leukaemia	0	0	-	-	-	-	-	-	-	-	-	-	-	-	-	-	-	-	-	-	0.0	0.0	0.00	0.00	**0.0**	*206*
Other leukaemia	0	0	-	-	-	-	-	-	-	-	-	-	-	-	-	-	-	-	-	-	0.0	0.0	0.00	0.00	**0.0**	*207*
Leukaemia unspecified	5	0	-	2.5	-	-	-	-	8.3	-	-	-	-	-	-	10.6	-	18.6	-	-	1.4	0.6	0.05	0.11	**1.2**	*208*
Other and unspecified	74	0	-	5.0	2.5	3.0	-	-	8.3	4.5	14.9	18.5	49.8	60.6	63.9	95.4	117.6	130.2	261.6	268.8	20.8	9.5	1.16	2.22	**20.4**	*O&U*
All sites	901	0	-	9.9	5.1	9.0	22.8	52.1	132.4	167.4	289.0	308.6	561.7	613.2	782.7	1218.9	1631.2	1786.0	1947.7	2634.4	253.3		14.77	29.02	**256.0**	*ALL*
All sites but 173	777	0	-	9.9	5.1	9.0	22.8	48.1	120.0	153.8	274.0	259.3	511.9	537.5	718.8	1123.5	1366.6	1358.1	1366.3	2043.0	218.5	100.0	13.35	25.80	**223.9**	*ALLb*
Rate from 1 case			2.359	2.483	2.545	3.013	3.798	4.010	4.138	4.524	4.983	6.173	7.110	7.570	7.987	10.599	14.695	18.605	29.070	53.763						

†Important: see notes on population page

Brazil, Belém

The Cancer Registry of Belém was set up in 1987, and is supported by the Secretary of State for Public Health of Para (Amazonia). It is located in the State Department of Public Health and is operated by the Research Sector of the Department. Cancer, which is the third greatest cause of death, has been increasing in importance as a public health problem due to uncontrolled industrialization and urbanization, as well as the control of infectious diseases. The objective was to study the burden and patterns of cancer in the population in order to formulate etiological hypotheses as a basis for analytical studies. At the same time it was recognized that a registry would help to identify groups at high risk of cancer, and provide the information necessary to set up and monitor the effect of screening programmes. The registry is also involved in public health education and contributes to planning of health services.

The metropolitan area of Belém is considered as the gateway to the Amazon, and includes the two municipalities of Belém and Ananindeua, both situated in the equatorial plain. It covers a total area of 1221 km^2, Belém having 736 km^2 and Ananindeua 485 km^2. The area is a prairie, with alternating dry and wet lands, lying no more than 14 m above sea level. The wetlands are constituted principally by the basins of the rivers Guamá, Acará and Moju, which form the bay of Guajará, bordering the city of Belém to the west and beyond which the rivers run directly into the Atlantic Ocean. The climate is humid and hot, with an average annual temperature of 32°C, reaching 37°C during the hottest months of the year. The average annual relative humidity is around 89%.

For 1990, the population was estimated to be 1 500 578 inhabitants. The median age was 17 years and 46% of the population was under the age of 20 years. The geometric annual growth rate during 1980–91 was 2.65%.

The sources of information used by the registry are covered by active registration. Data collection is from all hospitals in Belém, both public and private, via a planned programme of visits. Medical students act as data collectors. In addition, pathology reports and death certificates are used as primary sources of information. For the death certificates, home visits were undertaken for all deaths reported, since it was observed that certificates might contain erroneous diagnoses and sometimes addresses.

Following data collection, the data items on the notification form are checked for validity and consistency. The data are then entered onto a microcomputer using software prepared by the Department of Public Health. The data are coded to ICD-9 topography and ICD-O morphology.

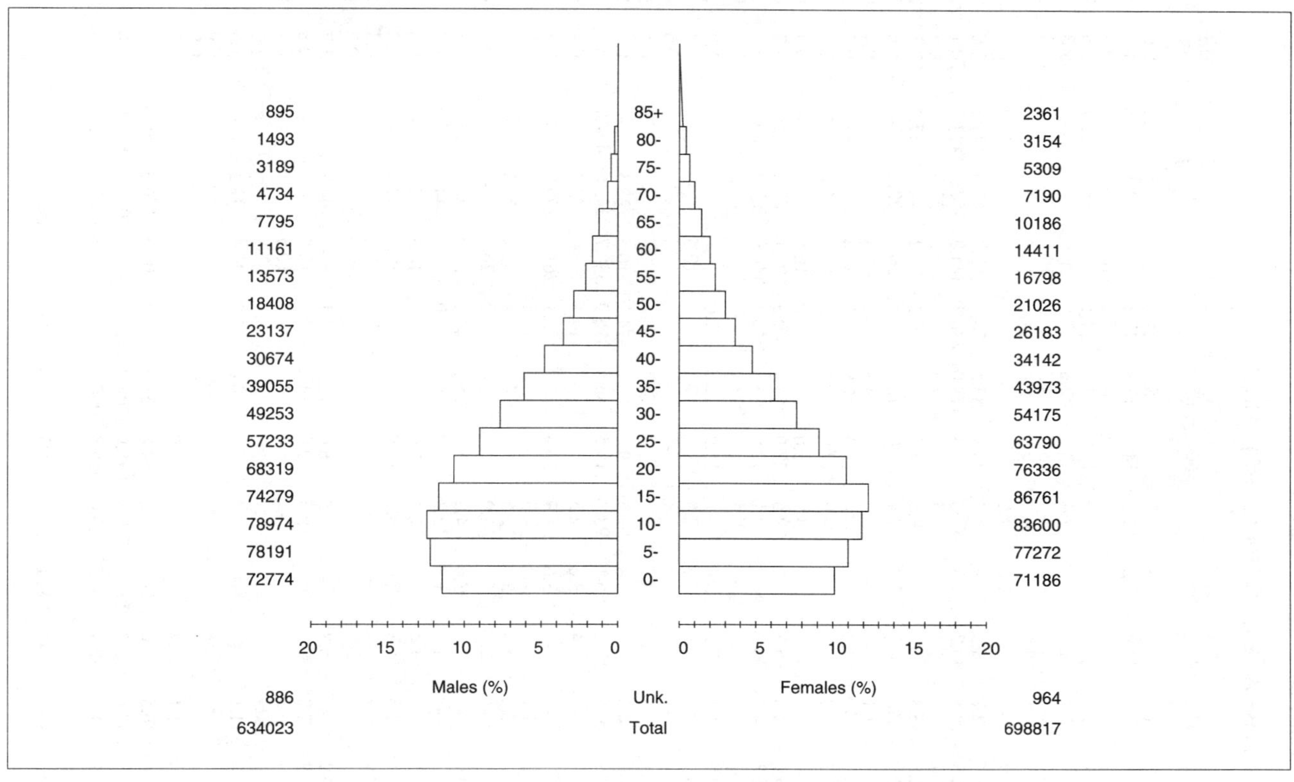

Brazil, Belém
Source of population: 1991
Census: 1991
Notes to tables overleaf:
* The high proportion of cases of unknown age, and of diagnoses ascribed to the Other and Unspecified category, as well as a large percentage of diagnoses based on a death certificate alone, suggest under-ascertainment of cases.
† 188 does not include non-invasive tumours

Screening programmes in the area:
60,000 cytological examinations are performed annually in the population between ages 20 and 60.

* BRAZIL, BELEM 1989-1991

ANNUAL INCIDENCE PER 100,000 BY AGE GROUP (YEARS) - MALE

SITE	ALL AGES	AGE UNK	0-	5-	10-	15-	20-	25-	30-	35-	40-	45-	50-	55-	60-	65-	70-	75-	80-	85+	CRUDE RATE	%	CR 64	CR 74	ASR (W)	ICD (9th)
Lip	12	0	-	-	-	-	-	-	1.4	-	1.1	-	1.8	2.5	-	8.6	21.1	-	22.3	37.2	0.6	0.7	0.03	0.18	**1.3**	140
Tongue	37	3	-	-	-	-	-	1.2	1.4	-	-	2.9	7.2	12.3	14.9	12.8	42.2	20.9	22.3	74.5	1.9	2.1	0.22	0.52	**4.0**	141
Salivary gland	9	0	-	-	-	-	0.5	-	-	-	-	-	3.6	2.5	6.0	4.3	7.0	10.5	-	-	0.5	0.5	0.06	0.12	**0.9**	142
Mouth	50	3	-	-	-	-	-	-	1.4	0.9	1.1	4.3	3.6	27.0	17.9	42.8	14.1	41.8	44.7	111.7	2.6	2.8	0.30	0.60	**5.5**	143-5
Oropharynx	19	0	-	-	-	-	-	-	-	0.9	1.1	1.4	-	7.4	3.0	42.8	-	20.9	-	-	1.0	1.1	0.07	0.28	**2.1**	146
Nasopharynx	6	0	-	0.9	-	-	-	-	-	-	-	-	1.8	-	3.0	4.3	-	10.5	-	-	0.3	0.3	0.03	0.05	**0.5**	147
Hypopharynx	19	2	-	-	-	-	-	-	-	0.9	1.1	2.9	3.6	9.8	3.0	8.6	14.1	10.5	22.3	-	1.0	1.1	0.12	0.25	**1.9**	148
Pharynx unspecified	5	0	-	-	-	-	0.5	-	-	0.9	-	-	1.8	2.5	-	-	-	-	-	37.2	0.3	0.3	0.03	0.03	**0.5**	149
Oesophagus	57	0	-	-	-	-	-	-	-	3.4	2.2	4.3	10.9	14.7	23.9	38.5	56.3	62.7	67.0	74.5	3.0	3.2	0.30	0.77	**6.3**	150
Stomach	383	32	-	-	-	-	0.5	0.6	3.4	12.8	18.5	43.2	59.8	86.0	137.4	278.0	288.7	344.9	357.2	484.2	20.1	21.6	1.98	5.07	**42.0**	151
Small intestine	8	0	-	-	-	-	-	0.6	-	1.7	-	1.4	-	2.5	-	4.3	-	10.5	22.3	-	0.4	0.5	0.03	0.05	**0.7**	152
Colon	43	3	-	-	-	0.4	0.5	-	0.7	2.6	3.3	-	1.8	9.8	14.9	12.8	56.3	73.2	44.7	37.2	2.3	2.4	0.18	0.55	**4.5**	153
Rectum	30	3	-	-	-	-	0.5	1.2	0.7	0.9	2.2	4.3	7.2	7.4	3.0	12.8	21.1	20.9	22.3	-	1.6	1.7	0.15	0.34	**2.8**	154
Liver	7	0	-	0.4	-	-	-	-	-	-	1.1	-	-	-	-	4.3	-	41.8	-	-	0.4	0.4	0.01	0.03	**0.7**	155
Gallbladder etc.	14	0	-	-	-	-	-	-	-	-	-	2.9	-	-	11.9	12.8	7.0	31.4	-	37.2	0.7	0.8	0.07	0.17	**1.7**	156
Pancreas	48	0	-	-	-	0.4	-	-	-	1.7	2.2	-	7.2	4.9	14.9	51.3	49.3	62.7	111.6	74.5	2.5	2.7	0.16	0.66	**5.5**	157
Nose, sinuses etc.	7	0	-	-	-	0.4	-	0.6	-	-	-	-	-	4.9	3.0	-	7.0	10.5	-	-	0.4	0.4	0.04	0.08	**0.6**	160
Larynx	79	8	-	-	-	0.4	-	-	1.4	0.9	4.3	5.8	10.9	19.6	23.9	64.1	49.3	94.1	67.0	111.7	4.2	4.5	0.37	1.00	**8.7**	161
Bronchus, lung	254	7	-	-	-	-	0.5	-	2.0	4.3	4.3	30.3	48.9	49.1	92.6	205.3	246.4	344.9	267.9	260.7	13.4	14.3	1.19	3.52	**28.6**	162
Other thoracic organs	10	2	-	-	-	-	-	1.2	-	-	-	1.4	-	7.4	-	8.6	-	-	-	-	0.5	0.6	0.06	0.12	**0.9**	163-4
Bone	36	1	0.5	1.3	0.8	1.3	1.0	1.7	2.0	0.9	1.1	7.2	5.4	-	11.9	12.8	7.0	-	-	-	1.9	2.0	0.18	0.28	**2.6**	170
Connective tissue	22	3	-	0.9	-	0.4	0.5	-	-	0.9	3.3	2.9	3.6	2.5	-	17.1	-	10.5	-	37.2	1.2	1.2	0.09	0.19	**1.9**	171
Mesothelioma	0	0	-	-	-	-	-	-	-	-	-	-	-	-	-	-	-	-	-	-	0.0	0.0	0.00	0.00	**0.0**	MES
Kaposi's sarcoma	1	0	-	-	-	-	-	-	-	-	-	-	-	-	-	4.3	-	-	-	-	0.1	0.1	0.00	0.02	**0.1**	KAP
Melanoma of skin	15	0	-	-	-	0.4	-	0.6	-	-	4.3	-	1.8	2.5	9.0	-	14.1	10.5	22.3	-	0.8	0.8	0.09	0.16	**1.4**	172
Other skin	318	21	-	-	-	-	0.5	2.3	2.0	7.7	20.6	17.3	56.1	93.3	119.5	145.4	316.9	386.7	245.6	484.2	16.7		1.71	4.18	**34.9**	173
Breast	7	0	-	-	-	-	-	-	-	-	-	1.4	3.6	2.5	-	-	14.1	-	22.3	-	0.4	0.4	0.04	0.11	**0.8**	175
Prostate	145	24	-	-	-	-	-	-	-	-	-	-	3.6	31.9	50.8	68.4	183.1	261.3	290.2	335.2	7.6	8.2	0.52	2.02	**17.9**	185
Testis	17	0	-	-	-	0.4	-	0.6	3.4	2.6	1.1	-	1.8	4.9	-	-	14.1	-	-	37.2	0.9	1.0	0.07	0.14	**1.3**	186
Penis	23	1	-	-	-	-	-	0.6	2.7	-	2.2	4.3	5.4	2.5	6.0	8.6	-	31.4	22.3	-	1.2	1.3	0.12	0.17	**2.0**	187.1-.4
Other male genital	7	0	-	-	-	-	-	-	-	-	-	2.9	-	4.9	-	-	7.0	20.9	-	-	0.4	0.4	0.04	0.07	**0.7**	187.5-.9
†Bladder	25	1	-	0.4	-	-	-	-	-	0.9	-	-	3.6	4.9	3.0	25.7	42.2	20.9	22.3	74.5	1.3	1.4	0.07	0.42	**3.0**	188
Kidney etc.	25	1	0.9	1.7	-	-	-	0.6	0.7	-	-	1.4	1.8	12.3	9.0	8.6	7.0	-	44.7	37.2	1.3	1.4	0.15	0.23	**2.3**	189
Eye	11	1	0.9	0.4	-	-	1.0	-	-	-	-	1.4	-	2.5	3.0	-	10.5	22.3	-	-	0.6	0.6	0.05	0.05	**0.8**	190
Brain, nervous system	41	1	1.4	3.0	0.4	0.4	1.5	0.6	-	-	3.3	5.8	3.6	4.9	14.9	17.1	-	10.5	22.3	74.5	2.2	2.3	0.20	0.29	**3.4**	191-2
Thyroid	5	1	-	-	-	0.4	-	-	0.7	0.9	-	-	-	-	-	-	7.0	-	-	-	0.3	0.3	0.01	0.06	**0.3**	193
Other endocrine	4	0	0.5	-	1.3	-	-	-	-	-	-	-	-	-	-	-	-	-	-	-	0.2	0.2	0.01	0.01	**0.2**	194
Hodgkin's disease	33	1	-	1.7	1.7	1.3	1.0	1.2	0.7	0.9	-	5.8	-	2.5	6.0	12.8	21.1	-	44.7	-	1.7	1.9	0.12	0.29	**2.5**	201
Non-Hodgkin lymphoma	54	1	-	4.3	2.1	1.3	0.5	0.6	2.0	0.9	2.2	-	9.1	19.6	9.0	34.2	14.1	10.5	-	-	2.8	3.0	0.26	0.51	**4.2**	200,202
Multiple myeloma	8	0	-	-	-	-	-	-	-	0.9	3.3	-	-	-	6.0	4.3	-	10.5	-	-	0.4	0.5	0.05	0.07	**0.7**	203
Lymphoid leukaemia	22	5	3.2	2.6	-	1.3	0.5	-	-	-	-	-	-	-	-	-	-	-	-	-	1.2	1.2	0.05	0.05	**1.0**	204
Myeloid leukaemia	25	1	-	0.9	1.3	0.4	0.5	1.2	1.4	-	1.1	-	-	7.4	6.0	8.6	7.0	31.4	22.3	-	1.3	1.4	0.10	0.19	**2.0**	205
Monocytic leukaemia	0	0	-	-	-	-	-	-	-	-	-	-	-	-	-	-	-	-	-	-	0.0	0.0	0.00	0.00	**0.0**	206
Other leukaemia	0	0	-	-	-	-	-	-	-	-	-	-	-	-	-	-	-	-	-	-	0.0	0.0	0.00	0.00	**0.0**	207
Leukaemia unspecified	13	0	0.9	0.4	0.4	0.4	0.5	0.6	-	2.6	1.1	1.4	-	-	3.0	-	-	-	-	-	0.7	0.7	0.06	0.06	**0.7**	208
Other and unspecified	139	13	1.4	-	0.4	0.4	1.5	2.9	2.0	3.4	6.5	8.6	27.2	44.2	44.8	51.3	91.5	104.5	156.3	149.0	7.3	7.8	0.79	1.58	**14.0**	O&U
All sites	2093	139	9.6	18.8	8.4	10.8	11.7	18.6	29.8	53.8	92.4	165.7	297.0	513.3	675.0	1235.8	1626.5	2132.3	2009.4	2569.8	110.0		10.20	25.53	**218.4**	ALL
All sites but 173	1775	118	9.6	18.8	8.4	10.8	11.2	16.3	27.7	46.1	71.7	148.4	240.8	420.0	555.5	1090.4	1309.7	1745.6	1763.8	2085.7	93.3	100.0	8.49	21.35	**183.5**	ALLb

Rate from 1 case   0.458 0.426 0.422 0.449 0.488 0.582 0.677 0.853 1.087 1.441 1.811 2.456 2.987 4.276 7.041 10.453 22.326 37.244

†Important: see notes on population page

* BRAZIL, BELEM 1989-1991

ANNUAL INCIDENCE PER 100,000 BY AGE GROUP (YEARS) - FEMALE

SITE	ALL AGES	AGE UNK	0-	5-	10-	15-	20-	25-	30-	35-	40-	45-	50-	55-	60-	65-	70-	75-	80-	85+	CRUDE RATE	%	CR 64	CR 74	ASR (W)	ICD (9th)
Lip	2	0	-	-	-	-	-	-	-	-	-	-	-	-	2.3	-	-	-	10.6	-	0.1	0.1	0.01	0.01	**0.1**	140
Tongue	22	0	-	-	-	-	-	0.5	-	0.8	1.0	2.5	1.6	2.0	-	22.9	13.9	18.8	10.6	14.1	1.0	0.9	0.04	0.23	**1.7**	141
Salivary gland	8	1	-	-	-	-	0.4	-	-	-	-	-	4.8	-	2.3	-	9.3	-	-	-	0.4	0.3	0.04	0.10	**0.6**	142
Mouth	27	1	-	-	-	-	-	-	-	0.8	-	1.3	1.6	4.0	2.3	13.1	13.9	50.2	42.3	14.1	1.3	1.1	0.05	0.19	**2.0**	143-5
Oropharynx	7	0	-	-	-	-	-	-	-	-	-	1.3	-	2.0	4.6	6.5	-	-	-	14.1	0.3	0.3	0.04	0.07	**0.6**	146
Nasopharynx	2	0	-	-	-	-	-	-	0.8	-	-	-	-	-	-	-	-	-	-	14.1	0.1	0.1	0.00	0.00	**0.1**	147
Hypopharynx	0	0	-	-	-	-	-	-	-	-	-	-	-	-	-	-	-	-	-	-	0.0	0.0	0.00	0.00	**0.0**	148
Pharynx unspecified	3	0	-	-	-	-	-	-	-	-	-	-	-	2.0	4.6	-	-	-	-	-	0.1	0.1	0.03	0.03	**0.3**	149
Oesophagus	20	1	-	-	-	-	-	-	0.6	-	2.9	2.5	3.2	2.0	4.6	3.3	18.5	6.3	10.6	14.1	1.0	0.8	0.08	0.20	**1.5**	150
Stomach	215	15	-	-	-	-	0.4	0.5	7.4	5.3	9.8	19.1	44.4	49.6	50.9	49.1	97.4	81.6	190.2	169.4	10.3	8.6	1.01	1.79	**16.0**	151
Small intestine	4	1	-	-	-	-	-	-	-	-	-	-	-	-	2.3	-	-	6.3	-	14.1	0.2	0.2	0.02	0.02	**0.3**	152
Colon	52	3	-	0.4	-	-	-	-	0.6	-	2.9	1.3	1.6	6.0	13.9	36.0	9.3	87.9	31.7	42.4	2.5	2.1	0.14	0.38	**3.9**	153
Rectum	60	2	-	-	-	-	-	0.5	2.5	1.5	3.9	6.4	7.9	11.9	23.1	19.6	46.4	12.6	10.6	28.2	2.9	2.4	0.30	0.64	**4.7**	154
Liver	6	1	-	-	-	-	-	-	-	-	1.0	-	1.6	-	2.3	-	9.3	-	-	-	0.3	0.2	0.03	0.08	**0.5**	155
Gallbladder etc.	38	3	-	-	-	-	-	-	-	-	1.0	3.8	3.2	9.9	16.2	16.4	18.5	25.1	21.1	28.2	1.8	1.5	0.19	0.37	**3.1**	156
Pancreas	31	1	-	-	0.4	-	-	-	1.2	-	2.0	3.8	4.8	4.0	-	6.5	27.8	25.1	31.7	28.2	1.5	1.2	0.08	0.26	**2.2**	157
Nose, sinuses etc.	3	0	-	-	-	-	0.4	-	-	-	-	1.3	-	2.0	-	-	-	-	-	-	0.1	0.1	0.02	0.02	**0.2**	160
Larynx	8	1	-	-	-	0.4	-	-	0.6	-	-	-	1.6	2.0	-	3.3	-	-	21.1	-	0.4	0.3	0.03	0.03	**0.5**	161
Bronchus, lung	90	4	-	-	0.4	0.8	0.4	-	-	-	1.0	6.4	11.1	25.8	30.1	49.1	37.1	44.0	42.3	127.1	4.3	3.6	0.40	0.85	**7.2**	162
Other thoracic organs	8	5	-	-	-	-	-	-	-	-	-	-	-	-	2.3	-	-	6.3	-	14.1	0.4	0.3	0.03	0.03	**0.6**	163-4
Bone	26	3	0.9	1.3	0.4	0.8	0.9	0.5	0.6	-	1.0	1.3	1.6	6.0	2.3	3.3	4.6	-	21.1	-	1.2	1.0	0.10	0.14	**1.5**	170
Connective tissue	32	0	-	0.4	0.4	0.4	0.9	0.5	1.2	2.3	2.9	1.3	1.6	4.0	4.6	6.5	9.3	44.0	-	14.1	1.5	1.3	0.10	0.18	**2.0**	171
Mesothelioma	1	0	-	-	-	-	-	-	-	-	-	-	-	-	-	-	-	-	10.6	-	0.0	0.0	0.00	0.00	**0.1**	MES
Kaposi's sarcoma	0	0	-	-	-	-	-	-	-	-	-	-	-	-	-	-	-	-	-	-	0.0	0.0	0.00	0.00	**0.0**	KAP
Melanoma of skin	14	1	-	-	-	-	0.4	-	1.8	1.5	-	1.3	1.6	4.0	4.6	3.3	-	-	-	-	0.7	0.6	0.08	0.10	**0.9**	172
Other skin	289	14	-	-	-	-	1.3	1.6	4.3	5.3	12.7	20.4	31.7	65.5	69.4	78.5	199.4	226.0	232.5	254.1	13.8		1.11	2.57	**21.9**	173
Breast	409	24	-	-	-	-	1.3	1.6	9.8	24.3	42.0	84.0	80.9	77.4	90.2	101.4	148.4	87.9	126.8	56.5	19.5	16.3	2.19	3.51	**30.2**	174
Uterus unspecified	27	0	-	-	-	-	0.9	0.5	-	0.8	2.0	6.4	6.3	6.0	4.6	3.3	13.9	12.6	-	14.1	1.3	1.1	0.14	0.22	**2.0**	179
Cervix uteri	931	23	-	-	-	0.4	3.9	13.1	35.7	78.8	116.2	170.6	187.1	200.4	194.3	193.1	153.0	175.8	306.5	84.7	44.4	37.2	5.13	6.90	**64.8**	180
Placenta	10	2	-	-	-	-	0.9	1.6	0.6	-	1.0	-	-	-	-	-	-	-	-	-	0.5	0.4	0.03	0.03	**0.4**	181
Corpus uteri	24	1	-	-	-	-	-	-	-	0.8	2.0	1.3	9.5	4.0	11.6	3.3	13.9	-	21.1	-	1.1	1.0	0.15	0.24	**1.9**	182
Ovary etc.	65	3	-	-	-	1.2	0.9	2.6	1.8	2.3	1.0	6.4	14.3	9.9	13.9	19.6	23.2	12.6	52.8	28.2	3.1	2.6	0.28	0.51	**4.5**	183
Other female genital	19	0	0.5	-	-	-	-	-	-	0.8	-	2.5	1.6	-	9.3	3.3	-	25.1	52.8	-	0.9	0.8	0.07	0.09	**1.3**	184
†Bladder	17	2	0.5	-	-	-	-	-	0.6	-	-	1.3	-	2.0	6.9	3.3	-	25.1	10.6	28.2	0.8	0.7	0.06	0.08	**1.2**	188
Kidney etc.	25	1	1.9	1.7	-	0.4	-	-	1.2	1.5	1.0	1.3	3.2	4.0	2.3	6.5	-	6.3	10.6	-	1.2	1.0	0.10	0.13	**1.5**	189
Eye	11	0	2.8	0.9	-	-	-	-	-	-	-	-	-	-	-	-	-	18.8	-	-	0.5	0.4	0.02	0.02	**0.6**	190
Brain, nervous system	35	2	1.4	2.2	1.2	0.4	1.7	1.0	1.8	2.3	2.0	1.3	3.2	4.0	-	-	4.6	6.3	-	-	1.7	1.4	0.12	0.14	**1.8**	191-2
Thyroid	23	4	-	-	-	-	1.3	1.0	3.1	1.5	1.0	1.3	3.2	-	4.6	-	-	-	-	14.1	1.1	0.9	0.10	0.10	**1.2**	193
Other endocrine	1	0	-	-	-	-	-	-	-	0.8	-	-	-	-	-	-	-	-	-	-	0.0	0.0	0.00	0.00	**0.0**	194
Hodgkin's disease	17	0	-	0.9	0.4	0.4	0.4	0.5	0.6	1.5	1.0	1.3	4.8	-	2.3	-	9.3	-	-	-	0.8	0.7	0.07	0.12	**1.0**	201
Non-Hodgkin lymphoma	31	1	0.9	1.7	0.4	0.4	0.4	1.0	1.2	-	1.0	2.5	4.8	4.0	6.9	16.4	4.6	-	-	-	1.5	1.2	0.13	0.24	**2.1**	200,202
Multiple myeloma	6	2	-	-	-	-	-	-	-	-	1.5	-	-	-	2.3	-	4.6	-	-	-	0.3	0.2	0.03	0.06	**0.4**	203
Lymphoid leukaemia	18	3	2.3	2.2	0.4	-	-	-	0.6	-	2.0	-	-	-	-	3.3	-	-	-	-	0.9	0.7	0.04	0.06	**0.9**	204
Myeloid leukaemia	19	1	0.5	0.4	0.4	1.5	0.4	-	0.6	-	-	3.9	2.5	1.6	2.0	-	-	6.3	-	-	0.9	0.8	0.07	0.07	**1.0**	205
Monocytic leukaemia	0	0	-	-	-	-	-	-	-	-	-	-	-	-	-	-	-	-	-	-	0.0	0.0	0.00	0.00	**0.0**	206
Other leukaemia	0	0	-	-	-	-	-	-	-	-	-	-	-	-	-	-	-	-	-	-	0.0	0.0	0.00	0.00	**0.0**	207
Leukaemia unspecified	14	0	0.9	-	0.8	-	-	2.6	0.6	-	1.0	-	-	-	-	-	2.3	6.5	-	-	0.7	0.6	0.04	0.07	**0.8**	208
Other and unspecified	124	15	1.4	0.4	0.8	-	0.4	0.5	-	3.8	4.9	7.6	20.6	29.8	27.8	39.3	32.5	56.5	126.8	70.6	5.9	5.0	0.56	0.97	**9.2**	O&U
All sites	2794	141	14.0	12.5	6.0	7.3	17.9	30.3	79.4	138.7	223.6	364.1	464.5	545.7	622.2	716.7	922.6	1067.4	1395.1	1087.1	133.3		13.30	21.93	**199.4**	ALL
All sites but 173	2505	127	14.0	12.5	6.0	7.3	16.6	28.7	75.1	133.4	210.9	343.7	432.8	480.2	552.8	638.1	723.2	841.3	1162.5	833.0	119.5	100.0	12.19	19.36	**177.5**	ALLb
Rate from 1 case			0.468	0.431	0.399	0.384	0.437	0.523	0.615	0.758	0.976	1.273	1.585	1.984	2.313	3.272	4.636	6.279	10.569	14.118						

†Important: see notes on population page

Brazil, Goiânia

The Population-Based Cancer Registry of Goiânia was instituted in September 1986 by the State Health Department under the supervision of the Federal Health Ministry. In November 1994, it was transferred to the Cancer Society of Goias (Associaçiao de Combate ao Cancer em Goiás).

Goiânia is the capital of the state of Goiás and was founded in 1933. The city, originally planned and designed to harbour 50 000 people, exhibits nowadays a high demographic expansion. Predominantly through the growth of the urban population, the city now has more than one million inhabitants.

Goiânia occupies an area of 801 km^2 and is located in the middle part of the Central Plateau of Brazil at an altitude of 800 m, at latitude 16°40′ S and longitude 49°15′ W. The climate is typically tropical, and the city is hot and sunny throughout almost the entire year. The average annual temperature ranges from 18 to 30°C. The humidity averages about 43% during the winter, but is much higher (74%) in the rainy season, from November to April. Two rivers split the city, and will provide the water for the city.

The city was planned and constructed to be the capital of the state of Goiás, replacing the old capital, many people from different states were attracted to Goiânia by job opportunities, during the time of its construction. Economic activities predominantly include commerce, and service assistance. A reasonable expansion has been demonstrated during the past few years for the construction, furniture, and textile industries. In contrast to the rest of the state of Goiás, agriculture is minimal in Goiânia, since only small rural properties are located in the city area.

The registry collects and processes data on all cancer cases who are residents in the Goiânia city area. All tumour cases classified as malignant, invasive or *in situ* are registered. The morphology and behaviour of the tumours are classified according to the ICD-O-1 M-code. Approximately 85% of the cancer cases collected by the registry are diagnosed based on microscopic procedures; 8% are detected by the analysis of death certificates, while the rest are diagnosed by surgery and other clinical procedures. The sources of information used by the registry include records from public and private hospitals, cancer hospital, private clinics, pathology and haematology laboratories, and also the death certificates provided by the official mortality registry of the state. Data obtained from these sources include the personal identification of the patient, comprising the name, sex, date of birth, residence address, and also the date of diagnosis. Data collection is made under strict control standards, considering the consistency of the information, checking of incomplete information and exclusion of duplicates.

Among the activities developed by the registry are the determination of incidence and distribution of all different malignant tumours in the population of the city of Goiânia, and the provision of reliable data necessary for the design of prevention and treatment programmes, as well as for the development of teaching and research programmes in schools and universities.

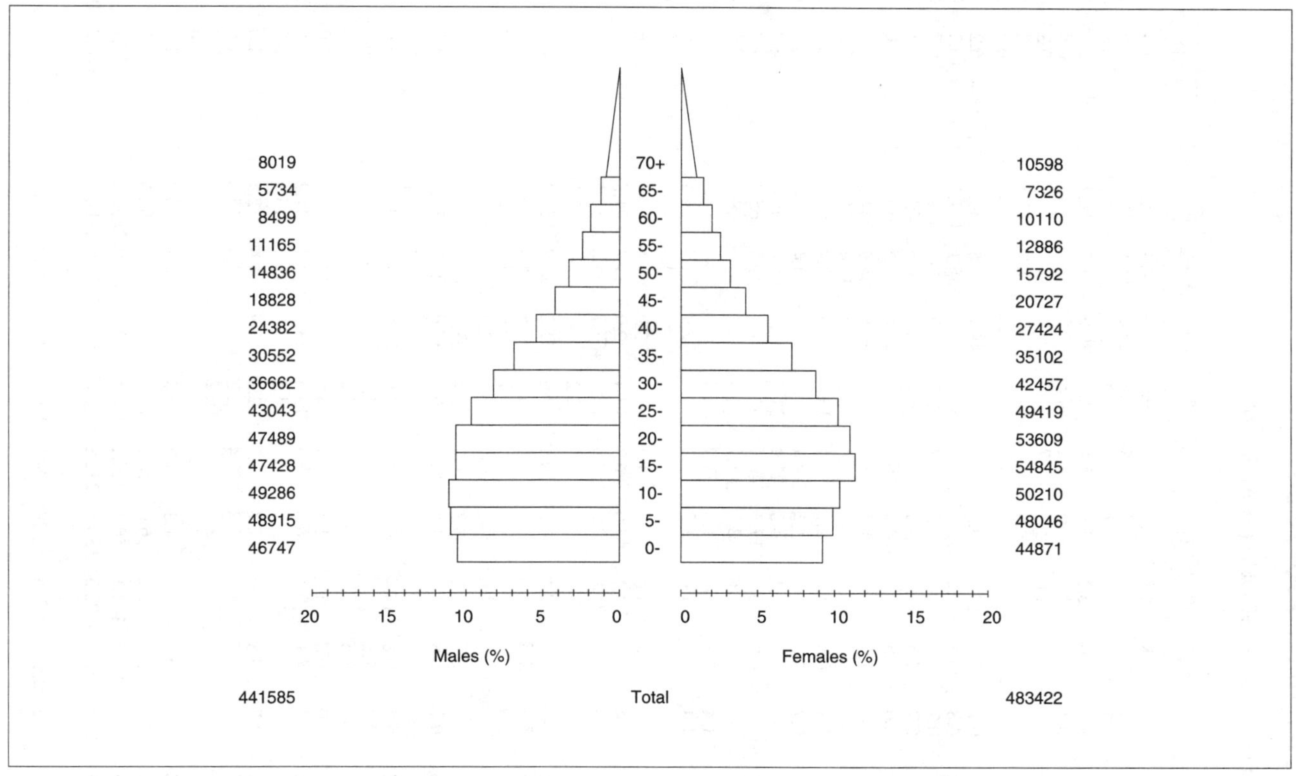

Brazil, Goiânia
Source of population: Average annual 1990–93
Census: 1991. Instituto Brasileiro de Geografia e Estatistica
Estimate: The populations for 1990, 1992 and 1993 were estimated by the Instituto Brasileiro de Geografia e Estastica on the basis of the 1991 census.
Notes to tables overleaf:
* The low rates and the ratios of mortality to incidence suggest under-ascertainment.

Note: The change in the rates since the previous period is probably due to a change in the population, which was estimated for data published in Volume VI and is based on a census for Volume VII.
† 188 does not include non-invasive tumours.

* BRAZIL, GOIANIA 1990-1993

ANNUAL INCIDENCE PER 100,000 BY AGE GROUP (YEARS) - MALE

SITE	ALL AGES	AGE UNK	0-	5-	10-	15-	20-	25-	30-	35-	40-	45-	50-	55-	60-	65-	70+	CRUDE RATE	%	CR 64	ASR (W)	ICD (9th)
Lip	24	0	-	-	-	-	0.5	0.6	0.7	0.8	4.1	1.3	1.7	9.0	-	4.4	28.1	1.4	1.3	0.09	2.2	140
Tongue	29	0	-	-	-	-	-	-	-	0.8	5.1	1.3	8.4	4.5	17.6	13.1	18.7	1.6	1.5	0.19	2.9	141
Salivary gland	11	0	-	-	-	-	-	-	0.7	-	1.0	1.3	3.4	2.2	8.8	4.4	3.1	0.6	0.6	0.09	1.0	142
Mouth	37	0	-	-	-	-	-	0.6	0.7	1.6	6.2	5.3	5.1	11.2	20.6	8.7	18.7	2.1	1.9	0.26	3.4	143-5
Oropharynx	15	0	-	-	-	0.5	-	-	0.7	-	1.0	4.0	8.4	4.5	5.9	-	-	0.8	0.8	0.13	1.2	146
Nasopharynx	6	0	-	-	0.5	-	0.5	0.6	-	-	1.0	1.3	1.7	-	-	-	-	0.3	0.3	0.03	0.4	147
Hypopharynx	15	0	-	-	-	-	-	-	-	-	-	4.0	6.7	4.5	-	8.7	12.5	0.8	0.8	0.08	1.5	148
Pharynx unspecified	3	0	-	-	-	-	-	-	-	-	-	1.3	1.7	2.2	-	-	-	0.2	0.2	0.03	0.3	149
Oesophagus	91	0	-	-	-	-	-	-	0.7	1.6	10.3	9.3	13.5	31.3	44.1	69.8	56.1	5.2	4.8	0.55	9.3	150
Stomach	182	0	-	-	-	-	1.1	1.2	4.8	3.3	9.2	11.9	18.5	53.7	76.5	135.1	177.7	10.3	9.5	0.90	19.2	151
Small intestine	6	0	-	-	-	-	-	-	0.7	-	-	1.3	1.7	2.2	2.9	-	3.1	0.3	0.3	0.04	0.5	152
Colon	54	0	-	-	-	-	-	-	0.7	2.5	1.0	9.3	5.1	6.7	38.2	30.5	49.9	3.1	2.8	0.32	5.8	153
Rectum	46	1	-	-	-	-	0.5	-	2.0	2.5	2.1	4.0	6.7	6.7	11.8	30.5	46.8	2.6	2.4	0.19	4.6	154
Liver	42	0	0.5	0.5	-	-	-	-	-	1.6	-	1.3	3.4	20.2	20.6	34.9	34.3	2.4	2.2	0.24	4.5	155
Gallbladder etc.	18	0	-	-	-	-	-	-	-	-	1.0	-	3.4	2.2	5.9	17.4	24.9	1.0	0.9	0.06	2.1	156
Pancreas	43	1	-	-	-	-	-	-	1.4	0.8	1.0	2.7	5.1	13.4	11.8	8.7	65.5	2.4	2.3	0.18	4.6	157
Nose, sinuses etc.	9	0	-	-	0.5	-	-	-	0.7	0.8	-	1.3	3.4	-	5.9	4.4	-	0.5	0.5	0.06	0.7	160
Larynx	75	0	0.5	-	-	-	0.5	-	-	3.3	2.1	4.0	21.9	31.3	20.6	65.4	46.8	4.2	3.9	0.42	7.7	161
Bronchus, lung	198	0	-	-	-	-	0.5	-	-	0.8	5.1	17.3	40.4	82.8	94.1	139.5	165.2	11.2	10.4	1.21	21.3	162
Other thoracic organs	11	0	-	-	-	-	0.5	0.6	-	-	1.0	2.7	1.7	4.5	-	-	9.4	0.6	0.6	0.05	0.9	163-4
Bone	20	0	1.1	-	1.0	3.2	1.1	0.6	1.4	0.8	-	1.3	1.7	4.5	-	-	-	1.1	1.0	0.08	1.1	170
Connective tissue	17	0	-	-	-	0.5	1.1	1.2	1.4	-	1.0	1.3	5.1	-	2.9	4.4	9.4	1.0	0.9	0.07	1.3	171
Mesothelioma	1	0	-	-	-	-	-	-	-	-	-	-	-	-	-	4.4	-	0.1	0.1	0.00	0.1	MES
Kaposi's sarcoma	11	0	-	-	-	-	0.5	1.7	1.4	0.8	1.0	-	1.7	-	2.9	4.4	-	0.6	0.6	0.05	0.7	KAP
Melanoma of skin	36	0	-	-	-	-	-	-	3.4	1.6	4.1	4.0	6.7	13.4	2.9	17.4	21.8	2.0	1.9	0.18	3.2	172
Other skin	1184	12	-	-	-	0.5	2.1	12.8	9.5	40.1	71.8	119.5	153.3	315.7	467.7	754.2	1116.1	67.0		6.03	123.2	173
Breast	2	0	-	-	-	-	-	-	-	-	-	-	-	2.2	-	-	3.1	0.1	0.1	0.01	0.2	175
Prostate	291	2	-	-	-	-	-	0.6	-	-	3.1	4.0	10.1	33.6	91.2	226.7	554.9	16.5	15.2	0.72	35.2	185
Testis	19	0	-	-	-	-	-	2.3	3.4	1.6	1.0	1.3	-	4.5	2.9	4.4	6.2	1.1	1.0	0.09	1.3	186
Penis	18	0	-	-	-	-	-	-	2.0	-	-	-	6.7	5.9	4.4	28.1		1.0	0.9	0.07	1.9	187.1-.4
Other male genital	2	0	-	-	-	-	-	-	-	-	1.0	-	-	-	2.9	-	-	0.1	0.1	0.02	0.2	187.5-.9
†Bladder	94	1	-	-	0.5	-	-	-	-	-	2.1	5.3	6.7	13.4	38.2	65.4	149.6	5.3	4.9	0.33	11.0	188
Kidney etc.	32	0	1.1	-	-	-	-	0.6	0.7	0.8	-	1.3	10.1	6.7	17.6	21.8	18.7	1.8	1.7	0.19	3.2	189
Eye	6	0	-	0.5	0.5	-	-	-	-	0.8	-	-	-	2.2	-	4.4	3.1	0.3	0.3	0.02	0.5	190
Brain, nervous system	99	0	1.6	2.0	1.5	1.6	3.7	1.2	6.8	9.8	14.4	10.6	11.8	9.0	17.6	17.4	37.4	5.6	5.2	0.46	7.2	191-2
Thyroid	13	0	-	-	-	-	-	1.7	0.7	1.6	-	-	3.4	4.5	2.9	-	6.2	0.7	0.7	0.07	1.0	193
Other endocrine	10	0	1.1	-	0.5	-	1.1	0.6	-	1.6	-	-	1.7	2.2	-	-	-	0.6	0.5	0.04	0.6	194
Hodgkin's disease	36	1	-	1.0	1.5	2.6	1.1	4.6	2.0	0.8	1.0	1.3	5.1	4.5	-	13.1	3.1	2.0	1.9	0.13	2.3	201
Non-Hodgkin lymphoma	62	1	2.1	1.0	1.5	1.6	1.6	1.2	1.4	4.1	3.1	6.6	3.4	13.4	23.5	13.1	31.2	3.5	3.2	0.33	5.1	200,202
Multiple myeloma	12	0	-	-	-	-	0.5	-	-	-	-	1.3	-	4.5	-	13.1	15.6	0.7	0.6	0.03	1.3	203
Lymphoid leukaemia	32	0	3.2	1.5	1.0	2.6	-	1.7	0.7	0.8	-	2.7	1.7	2.2	5.9	4.4	12.5	1.8	1.7	0.12	2.3	204
Myeloid leukaemia	29	0	0.5	-	1.0	1.1	1.6	1.2	2.7	2.5	1.0	2.7	3.4	2.2	-	4.4	15.6	1.6	1.5	0.10	2.0	205
Monocytic leukaemia	3	0	-	-	-	-	0.5	-	-	0.8	-	-	-	2.2	-	-	-	0.2	0.2	0.02	0.2	206
Other leukaemia	0	0	-	-	-	-	-	-	-	-	-	-	-	-	-	-	-	0.0	0.0	0.00	0.0	207
Leukaemia unspecified	17	0	1.1	-	0.5	0.5	0.5	0.6	-	0.8	2.1	1.3	1.7	4.5	-	8.7	6.2	1.0	0.9	0.07	1.3	208
Other and unspecified	134	0	1.1	0.5	0.5	1.1	1.6	2.3	2.7	5.7	6.2	6.6	16.9	26.9	61.8	109.0	96.6	7.6	7.0	0.67	13.4	O&U
All sites	3095	19	13.9	7.2	11.2	15.8	21.1	38.3	53.9	95.7	164.1	256.3	406.1	772.5	1132.4	1870.2	2896.2	175.2		15.03	314.1	ALL
All sites but 173	1911	7	13.9	7.2	11.2	15.3	19.0	25.6	44.3	55.6	92.3	136.8	252.8	456.8	664.7	1116.0	1780.1	108.2	100.0	9.01	190.9	ALLb

Rate from 1 case   0.535   0.511   0.507   0.527   0.526   0.581   0.682   0.818   1.025   1.328   1.685   2.239   2.941   4.359   3.117

†Important: see notes on population page

* BRAZIL, GOIANIA 1990-1993

ANNUAL INCIDENCE PER 100,000 BY AGE GROUP (YEARS) - FEMALE

SITE	ALL AGES	AGE UNK	0-	5-	10-	15-	20-	25-	30-	35-	40-	45-	50-	55-	60-	65-	70+	CRUDE RATE	%	CR 64	ASR (W)	ICD (9th)
Lip	7	1	-	-	-	-	-	-	0.6	-	0.9	1.2	1.6	-	2.5	3.4	-	0.4	0.3	0.04	**0.5**	*140*
Tongue	3	0	-	-	-	-	-	-	-	1.4	-	-	1.6	-	-	-	-	0.2	0.1	0.02	**0.2**	*141*
Salivary gland	7	0	-	-	-	-	0.5	0.5	-	-	-	-	-	1.9	2.5	6.8	2.4	0.4	0.3	0.03	**0.6**	*142*
Mouth	16	0	-	-	-	-	-	-	-	0.7	0.9	-	-	7.8	9.9	6.8	9.4	0.8	0.7	0.10	**1.4**	*143-5*
Oropharynx	7	0	-	-	-	-	-	-	0.6	-	-	-	1.6	-	2.5	3.4	7.1	0.4	0.3	0.02	**0.6**	*146*
Nasopharynx	2	0	-	-	-	-	-	-	-	-	-	1.2	1.6	-	-	-	-	0.1	0.1	0.01	**0.2**	*147*
Hypopharynx	1	0	-	-	-	-	-	-	-	-	0.9	-	-	-	-	-	-	0.1	0.0	0.00	**0.1**	*148*
Pharynx unspecified	0	0	-	-	-	-	-	-	-	-	-	-	-	-	-	-	-	0.0	0.0	0.00	**0.0**	*149*
Oesophagus	22	0	-	-	-	-	-	-	-	0.7	-	1.2	11.1	1.9	4.9	3.4	21.2	1.1	0.9	0.10	**1.9**	*150*
Stomach	128	0	-	-	-	-	-	1.5	1.2	5.0	8.2	16.9	22.2	19.4	37.1	75.1	75.5	6.6	5.2	0.56	**10.6**	*151*
Small intestine	12	0	-	-	-	-	-	-	0.6	-	1.8	1.2	1.6	3.9	2.5	10.2	2.4	0.6	0.5	0.06	**1.0**	*152*
Colon	107	2	-	-	-	-	-	2.0	1.8	2.8	4.6	4.8	19.0	15.5	29.7	40.9	96.7	5.5	4.3	0.41	**9.0**	*153*
Rectum	67	0	-	-	-	-	0.5	0.5	2.4	3.6	3.6	7.2	6.3	15.5	19.8	34.1	37.7	3.5	2.7	0.30	**5.3**	*154*
Liver	34	0	-	-	-	-	0.5	-	-	-	0.9	3.6	6.3	7.8	12.4	3.4	35.4	1.8	1.4	0.16	**2.9**	*155*
Gallbladder etc.	54	1	-	-	-	-	-	-	1.2	2.1	1.8	1.2	4.7	15.5	19.8	27.3	42.5	2.8	2.2	0.24	**4.6**	*156*
Pancreas	44	0	-	-	-	-	-	-	-	-	0.9	3.6	7.9	11.6	14.8	23.9	37.7	2.3	1.8	0.19	**4.0**	*157*
Nose, sinuses etc.	5	0	-	-	-	-	-	0.5	-	-	-	1.6	3.9	-	-	-	2.4	0.3	0.2	0.03	**0.4**	*160*
Larynx	14	0	-	-	-	-	-	0.5	-	-	1.8	2.4	3.2	1.9	2.5	6.8	7.1	0.7	0.6	0.06	**1.1**	*161*
Bronchus, lung	114	1	-	-	-	-	0.5	1.0	0.6	2.8	4.6	8.4	22.2	33.0	49.5	61.4	56.6	5.9	4.6	0.62	**9.7**	*162*
Other thoracic organs	5	0	-	-	-	-	0.5	-	-	-	-	-	-	3.9	2.5	-	2.4	0.3	0.2	0.03	**0.4**	*163-4*
Bone	23	0	-	0.5	3.0	2.7	1.9	0.5	0.6	0.7	0.9	-	-	-	-	3.4	2.4	1.2	0.9	0.05	**1.1**	*170*
Connective tissue	34	0	1.1	1.0	1.5	0.9	0.9	-	0.6	1.4	0.9	3.6	4.7	3.9	7.4	10.2	11.8	1.8	1.4	0.14	**2.4**	*171*
Mesothelioma	0	0	-	-	-	-	-	-	-	-	-	-	-	-	-	-	-	0.0	0.0	0.00	**0.0**	*MES*
Kaposi's sarcoma	0	0	-	-	-	-	-	-	-	-	-	-	-	-	-	-	-	0.0	0.0	0.00	**0.0**	*KAP*
Melanoma of skin	23	0	-	-	-	-	-	0.5	0.6	1.4	-	1.2	1.6	5.8	4.9	10.2	21.2	1.2	0.9	0.08	**1.9**	*172*
Other skin	1241	6	-	-	1.0	0.9	3.7	7.1	21.2	33.5	68.4	118.2	136.1	258.0	358.5	556.2	1004.9	64.2		5.06	**104.4**	*173*
Breast	548	2	-	-	-	0.5	1.4	4.0	13.5	32.8	69.3	115.8	126.6	114.5	106.3	105.8	188.7	28.3	22.3	2.93	**40.4**	*174*
Uterus unspecified	29	0	-	-	-	-	0.9	0.5	1.2	2.1	3.6	2.4	1.6	7.8	2.5	13.6	11.8	1.5	1.2	0.11	**2.0**	*179*
Cervix uteri	506	1	-	-	-	-	3.3	10.1	17.1	34.2	57.4	72.4	80.7	108.6	140.9	146.7	167.5	26.2	20.6	2.63	**37.1**	*180*
Placenta	0	0	-	-	-	-	-	-	-	-	-	-	-	-	-	-	-	0.0	0.0	0.00	**0.0**	*181*
Corpus uteri	48	0	-	-	-	-	-	0.5	-	-	1.8	2.4	4.7	17.5	27.2	30.7	25.9	2.5	2.0	0.27	**4.3**	*182*
Ovary etc.	75	1	-	-	0.5	-	1.4	1.5	1.8	3.6	4.6	8.4	15.8	19.4	19.8	23.9	28.3	3.9	3.0	0.39	**5.7**	*183*
Other female genital	27	0	-	-	-	-	-	0.5	-	1.4	1.8	2.4	1.6	3.9	7.4	20.5	18.9	1.4	1.1	0.10	**2.3**	*184*
†Bladder	30	0	-	-	-	-	-	-	0.6	-	1.8	-	7.9	5.8	4.9	17.1	28.3	1.6	1.2	0.11	**2.6**	*188*
Kidney etc.	37	0	2.2	0.5	0.5	0.5	0.5	-	1.8	1.4	1.8	3.6	7.9	7.8	9.9	-	14.2	1.9	1.5	0.19	**2.6**	*189*
Eye	12	0	1.1	-	-	0.5	-	0.5	-	0.7	1.8	-	-	3.9	2.5	-	4.7	0.6	0.5	0.05	**0.8**	*190*
Brain, nervous system	69	0	1.1	3.1	1.5	0.9	0.5	3.5	1.8	2.1	4.6	3.6	6.3	13.6	14.8	23.9	23.6	3.6	2.8	0.29	**4.8**	*191-2*
Thyroid	70	2	0.6	-	-	0.5	2.3	2.0	4.1	8.5	7.3	8.4	12.7	3.9	7.4	13.6	14.2	3.6	2.8	0.30	**4.3**	*193*
Other endocrine	13	0	1.7	-	-	1.4	-	-	0.6	1.4	0.9	-	-	-	2.5	-	4.7	0.7	0.5	0.04	**0.8**	*194*
Hodgkin's disease	30	0	1.1	-	1.0	0.5	0.5	1.0	1.2	3.6	3.6	3.6	-	1.9	4.9	3.4	9.4	1.6	1.2	0.11	**1.9**	*201*
Non-Hodgkin lymphoma	48	2	2.2	1.6	-	0.9	-	1.5	1.2	2.8	1.8	2.4	4.7	13.6	9.9	13.6	14.2	2.5	2.0	0.22	**3.4**	*200,202*
Multiple myeloma	16	0	-	-	-	-	-	-	-	-	-	1.2	1.6	1.9	7.4	23.9	7.1	0.8	0.7	0.06	**1.5**	*203*
Lymphoid leukaemia	20	0	5.0	1.0	-	1.4	-	-	-	-	-	-	1.6	1.9	-	3.4	7.1	1.0	0.8	0.05	**1.4**	*204*
Myeloid leukaemia	29	1	-	-	1.5	0.9	0.9	2.5	1.2	0.7	3.6	2.4	3.2	-	2.5	-	9.4	1.5	1.2	0.10	**1.7**	*205*
Monocytic leukaemia	1	0	-	-	-	-	-	-	-	-	0.9	-	-	-	-	-	-	0.1	0.0	0.00	**0.1**	*206*
Other leukaemia	0	0	-	-	-	-	-	-	-	-	-	-	-	-	-	-	-	0.0	0.0	0.00	**0.0**	*207*
Leukaemia unspecified	13	1	-	-	-	-	0.5	0.5	0.6	-	-	-	1.6	3.9	2.5	3.4	9.4	0.7	0.5	0.05	**1.0**	*208*
Other and unspecified	111	0	1.1	-	-	0.5	0.9	0.5	1.8	2.8	5.5	7.2	20.6	34.9	27.2	47.8	70.8	5.7	4.5	0.52	**9.1**	*O&U*
All sites	3702	21	17.3	7.8	10.5	12.8	21.9	44.0	80.1	154.5	273.5	412.5	554.1	776.0	984.1	1378.5	2134.8	191.4		16.84	**292.0**	*ALL*
All sites but 173	2461	15	17.3	7.8	9.5	11.9	18.2	36.9	58.9	121.1	205.1	294.3	417.9	518.0	625.6	822.3	1129.9	127.3	100.0	11.78	**187.6**	*ALLb*

Rate from 1 case   0.557   0.520   0.498   0.456   0.466   0.506   0.589   0.712   0.912   1.206   1.583   1.940   2.473   3.412   2.359

†Important: see notes on population page

Brazil, Porto Alegre

The population-based cancer registry of Porto Alegre was established in 1972, supported by the State Health Department of Rio Grande do Sul and by the Ministry of Health, becoming part of the Statistics Division of the State Health Department. Due to operational and financial difficulties, its activities were discontinued for a while, but in 1987 it was reactivated and data on malignant neoplasms for the years 1990-1992 are presented in this publication.

Porto Alegre is a city in the south of Brazil, and the capital of Rio Grande do Sul State. It is located on the east bank of the Guaiba River, near the confluence of the rivers Jacui, Cai, dos Sinos and Gravatai, and a lagoon, dos Patos. It lies on a series of hills up to 150 m above sea level. Separated from the Atlantic Ocean, the city experienced accelerated growth with the construction of railroads and roads, and became a major city of the extreme south of the country. With the opening of Mercosul, Porto Alegre has gained importance as a regional financial and tourist centre. Besides the administrative, political, cultural and commercial activities characteristic of all large urban centres, Porto Alegre also has important industrial activities, represented by textile, tannery and food manufacturers.

The climate is subtropical, influenced by polar air masses from the south of the continent and tropical ones from the Atlantic Ocean. Rainfall is well distributed throughout the year. The average annual temperature is 19°C.

The geographical area covered by the registry is 552 km^2 and the official population in 1991 was 1 263 403 inhabitants, of whom only 15 874 reside in rural areas.

The information sources for the cancer registry are general practice hospitals and oncology hospitals, pathology laboratories, radiotherapy centres and the death declaration. In 1991 the active collection of new cancer cases was responsible for 82.3% of registrations; the remaining 17.7% were sent by one pathology laboratory or were death-certificate-only registrations.

The present staff comprises three technicians and six trainers, all of them previously trained in specific courses of methodology in cancer registry. Besides, there are collaborators and members specialized in areas related to cancer.

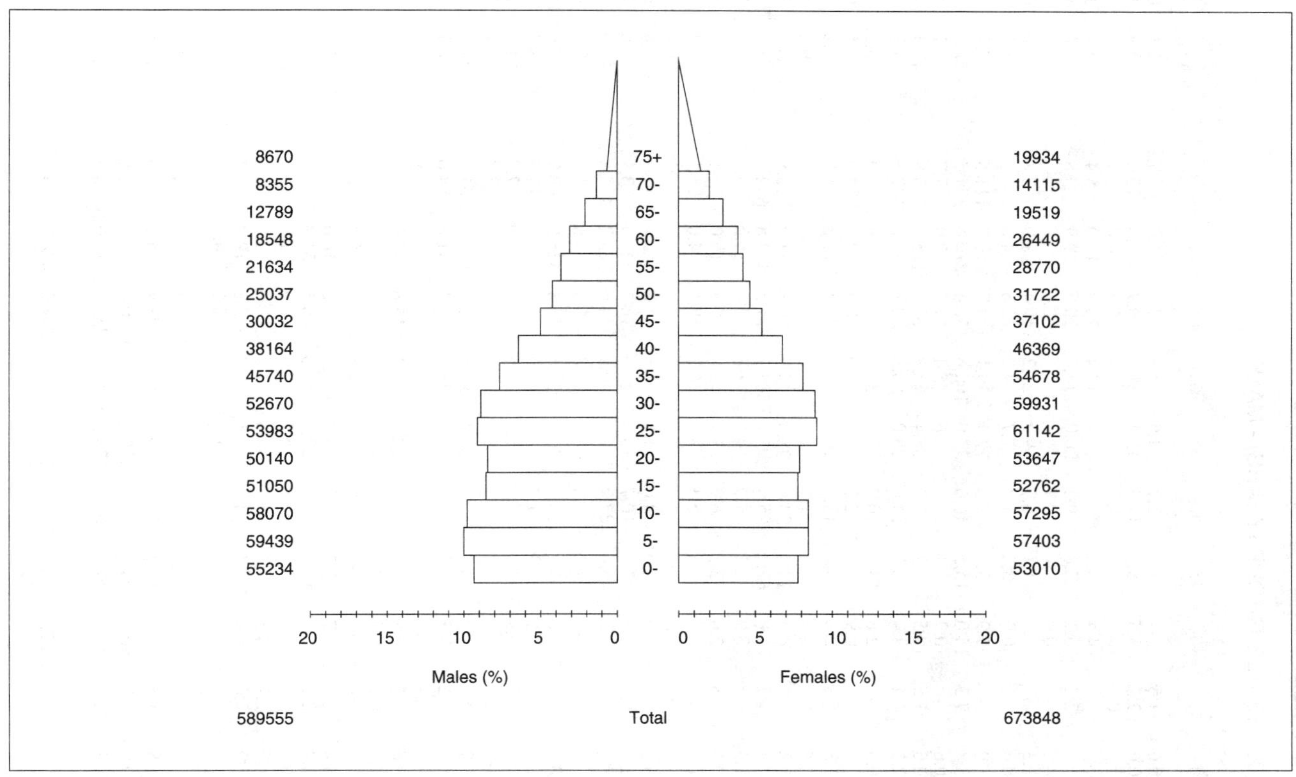

Brazil, Porto Alegre

Source of population: 1991

Census: 1991. Instituto Brasileiro de Geografia e Estatistica.

Notes to tables overleaf:

* Few cases have been registered from death certificates, implying under-ascertainment. The excessive number of unspecified morphological diagnoses and the high proportion of cases of unknown age indicate a lack of validity in the data.

Note: The change in the rates is probably due to a change in the population, which was estimated for Volume VI, and based on a more recent census for Volume VII.

† 188 does not include non-invasive tumours.

Screening programmes in the area:

300,000 cytological examinations were performed annually for cancer of the cervix in the population aged 18-65 between 1991 and 1995. 60,000 screening examinations for breast cancer were carried out annually in the population aged 25-80 from 1992.

* BRAZIL, PORTO ALEGRE 1990-1992

ANNUAL INCIDENCE PER 100,000 BY AGE GROUP (YEARS) - MALE

SITE	ALL AGES	AGE UNK	0-	5-	10-	15-	20-	25-	30-	35-	40-	45-	50-	55-	60-	65-	70-	75+	CRUDE RATE	%	CR 64	CR 74	ASR (W)	ICD (9th)
Lip	19	2	-	-	-	-	0.7	-	0.6	1.5	-	1.1	2.7	4.6	1.8	7.8	4.0	7.7	1.1	0.4	0.07	0.14	**1.2**	140
Tongue	69	3	-	-	-	-	-	0.6	0.6	2.2	3.5	8.9	17.3	15.4	21.6	20.9	8.0	15.4	3.9	1.5	0.37	0.52	**4.6**	141
Salivary gland	9	0	-	-	-	-	-	-	0.7	-	-	-	2.7	-	1.8	5.2	4.0	7.7	0.5	0.2	0.03	0.07	**0.6**	142
Mouth	54	1	-	-	-	-	-	-	-	-	4.4	5.5	13.3	13.9	14.4	20.9	16.0	15.4	3.1	1.2	0.26	0.45	**3.7**	143-5
Oropharynx	61	2	-	-	-	-	-	-	-	2.2	6.1	7.8	9.3	20.0	14.4	20.9	19.9	3.8	3.4	1.3	0.31	0.52	**4.0**	146
Nasopharynx	6	1	-	-	-	0.7	-	-	-	-	0.9	-	2.7	-	-	2.6	-	-	0.3	0.1	0.03	0.04	**0.4**	147
Hypopharynx	35	0	-	-	-	-	-	-	1.3	-	-	1.1	6.7	9.2	25.2	10.4	8.0	3.8	2.0	0.8	0.22	0.31	**2.4**	148
Pharynx unspecified	19	0	-	-	-	-	0.7	0.6	0.6	-	0.9	3.3	1.3	7.7	7.2	2.6	4.0	-	1.1	0.4	0.11	0.14	**1.2**	149
Oesophagus	269	10	-	-	-	-	0.7	1.9	1.9	-	7.9	13.3	49.3	72.4	79.1	114.7	119.7	111.5	15.2	5.8	1.18	2.39	**18.9**	150
Stomach	395	16	-	-	-	0.7	0.7	0.6	3.8	7.3	14.0	15.5	46.6	77.0	100.6	156.4	219.4	284.5	22.3	8.5	1.39	3.35	**27.9**	151
Small intestine	20	2	-	-	-	-	-	-	0.6	-	0.9	1.1	1.3	4.6	5.4	7.8	12.0	7.7	1.1	0.4	0.08	0.19	**1.4**	152
Colon	220	11	-	-	-	0.7	0.7	2.5	0.6	1.5	10.5	6.7	17.3	35.4	68.3	67.8	115.7	203.8	12.4	4.7	0.76	1.72	**15.7**	153
Rectum	175	3	-	-	-	0.7	1.3	-	2.5	4.4	4.4	6.7	24.0	20.0	50.3	80.8	83.8	142.3	9.9	3.8	0.58	1.42	**12.4**	154
Liver	117	3	-	-	-	0.7	-	-	0.6	-	2.6	13.3	10.7	27.7	39.5	57.3	55.9	50.0	6.6	2.5	0.49	1.07	**8.3**	155
Gallbladder etc.	27	1	-	-	-	-	-	-	-	-	0.9	-	2.7	3.1	9.0	10.4	12.0	34.6	1.5	0.6	0.08	0.20	**2.0**	156
Pancreas	128	1	-	-	-	-	-	0.6	1.3	5.8	2.6	4.4	13.3	26.2	34.1	41.7	71.8	111.5	7.2	2.7	0.45	1.02	**9.0**	157
Nose, sinuses etc.	5	0	-	-	-	-	-	-	0.6	0.7	0.9	-	1.3	-	1.8	-	-	-	0.3	0.1	0.03	0.03	**0.3**	160
Larynx	153	5	-	-	-	-	-	-	1.3	3.6	4.4	14.4	34.6	38.5	44.9	80.8	31.9	30.8	8.7	3.3	0.73	1.32	**10.5**	161
Bronchus, lung	946	12	-	-	-	0.7	0.7	3.7	4.4	11.7	21.0	62.2	95.9	203.4	303.7	427.5	474.8	642.1	53.5	20.3	3.58	8.15	**67.5**	162
Other thoracic organs	18	1	-	-	-	-	-	-	1.3	-	0.9	1.1	4.0	4.6	1.8	2.6	16.0	3.8	1.0	0.4	0.07	0.17	**1.2**	163-4
Bone	57	2	0.6	1.1	3.4	1.3	4.0	2.5	0.6	1.5	2.6	3.3	6.7	3.1	9.0	7.8	16.0	23.1	3.2	1.2	0.21	0.33	**3.6**	170
Connective tissue	42	3	1.2	0.6	1.1	-	0.7	1.2	0.6	0.7	-	3.3	5.3	3.1	16.2	10.4	4.0	23.1	2.4	0.9	0.18	0.26	**2.8**	171
Mesothelioma	0	0	-	-	-	-	-	-	-	-	-	-	-	-	-	-	-	-	0.0	0.0	0.00	0.00	**0.0**	MES
Kaposi's sarcoma	29	1	-	-	-	-	-	3.1	3.2	2.2	7.0	2.2	4.0	1.5	-	2.6	-	-	1.6	0.6	0.12	0.13	**1.5**	KAP
Melanoma of skin	82	4	-	-	1.1	-	0.7	1.2	1.9	5.1	7.9	5.5	10.7	13.9	21.6	18.2	27.9	23.1	4.6	1.8	0.37	0.61	**5.3**	172
Other skin	779	131	0.6	-	-	-	2.7	3.1	9.5	16.0	33.2	46.6	87.9	137.1	140.2	234.6	323.2	449.8	44.0		2.87	6.22	**53.9**	173
Breast	6	1	-	-	-	-	-	-	-	-	-	1.1	1.3	-	1.8	2.6	4.0	-	0.3	0.1	0.03	0.07	**0.4**	175
Prostate	566	32	-	-	-	-	-	0.6	0.6	-	2.6	1.1	20.0	40.1	127.6	216.3	426.9	868.9	32.0	12.2	1.02	4.43	**42.8**	185
Testis	61	5	-	-	-	1.3	2.7	8.0	8.2	2.9	7.9	3.3	1.3	3.1	3.6	-	-	11.5	3.4	1.3	0.23	0.23	**3.1**	186
Penis	17	3	-	-	-	-	-	-	0.6	0.7	0.9	2.2	1.3	1.5	3.6	2.6	8.0	7.7	1.0	0.4	0.07	0.13	**1.1**	187.1-.4
Other male genital	2	0	-	-	-	-	-	-	-	-	-	1.1	-	-	-	-	-	3.8	0.1	0.0	0.01	0.01	**0.1**	187.5-.9
†Bladder	251	17	-	-	-	-	-	1.2	1.9	2.2	-	3.3	10.7	32.4	57.5	132.9	171.6	261.4	14.2	5.4	0.59	2.22	**18.6**	188
Kidney etc.	143	4	1.8	-	-	-	-	0.6	1.3	2.2	1.7	6.7	18.6	21.6	57.5	44.3	91.8	84.6	8.1	3.1	0.58	1.28	**10.2**	189
Eye	10	3	-	-	-	-	-	-	-	-	-	1.1	2.7	4.6	-	-	-	3.8	0.6	0.2	0.06	0.06	**0.7**	190
Brain, nervous system	72	5	0.6	1.7	3.4	-	2.7	0.6	0.6	2.2	3.5	5.5	10.7	12.3	16.2	15.6	23.9	7.7	4.1	1.5	0.32	0.54	**4.6**	191-2
Thyroid	22	2	-	0.6	-	-	0.7	1.2	2.5	0.7	0.9	3.3	2.7	3.1	5.4	-	-	-	1.2	0.5	0.12	0.12	**1.2**	193
Other endocrine	9	1	0.6	-	-	-	-	-	-	-	-	-	4.0	1.5	1.8	-	4.0	3.8	0.5	0.2	0.04	0.07	**0.6**	194
Hodgkin's disease	42	5	-	-	1.1	-	1.3	1.2	4.4	2.9	1.7	2.2	2.7	3.1	1.8	7.8	16.0	15.4	2.4	0.9	0.13	0.26	**2.5**	201
Non-Hodgkin lymphoma	132	8	1.2	2.2	0.6	2.6	2.7	4.9	5.7	2.2	8.7	10.0	14.6	20.0	18.0	26.1	51.9	50.0	7.5	2.8	0.50	0.91	**8.4**	200,202
Multiple myeloma	35	0	-	0.6	-	0.7	-	-	0.6	-	-	3.3	5.3	6.2	7.2	13.0	31.9	15.4	2.0	0.8	0.12	0.34	**2.5**	203
Lymphoid leukaemia	47	11	2.4	1.7	1.1	0.7	1.3	-	-	2.2	3.5	-	1.3	4.6	1.8	-	12.0	34.6	2.7	1.0	0.13	0.21	**3.0**	204
Myeloid leukaemia	45	5	0.6	-	0.6	2.6	0.7	0.6	1.9	3.6	0.9	2.2	4.0	3.1	7.2	5.2	19.9	19.2	2.5	1.0	0.16	0.30	**2.8**	205
Monocytic leukaemia	3	0	-	-	-	-	-	-	-	-	-	-	-	1.5	-	2.6	4.0	-	0.2	0.1	0.01	0.04	**0.2**	206
Other leukaemia	0	0	-	-	-	-	-	-	-	-	-	-	-	-	-	-	-	-	0.0	0.0	0.00	0.00	**0.0**	207
Leukaemia unspecified	18	2	-	-	-	0.7	-	0.6	-	1.5	-	2.2	4.0	-	1.8	5.2	12.0	3.8	1.0	0.4	0.06	0.16	**1.2**	208
Other and unspecified	221	10	-	0.6	-	1.3	2.7	2.5	2.5	1.5	11.4	17.8	16.0	29.3	55.7	83.4	115.7	161.5	12.5	4.7	0.74	1.78	**15.5**	O&U
All sites	5436	329	9.7	9.0	12.6	15.0	27.9	43.8	69.0	91.8	180.8	294.1	592.5	930.6	1380.2	1970.4	2641.1	3748.6	307.4		19.46	44.01	**380.4**	ALL
All sites but 173	4657	198	9.1	9.0	12.6	15.0	25.3	40.8	59.5	75.8	147.6	247.5	504.6	793.5	1240.0	1735.9	2318.0	3298.7	263.3	100.0	16.61	37.78	**326.4**	ALLb

Rate from 1 case   0.603 0.561 0.574 0.653 0.665 0.617 0.633 0.729 0.873 1.110 1.331 1.541 1.797 2.606 3.990 3.845

†Important: see notes on population page

* BRAZIL, PORTO ALEGRE 1990-1992

ANNUAL INCIDENCE PER 100,000 BY AGE GROUP (YEARS) - FEMALE

SITE	ALL AGES	AGE UNK	0-	5-	10-	15-	20-	25-	30-	35-	40-	45-	50-	55-	60-	65-	70-	75+	CRUDE RATE	%	CR 64	CR 74	ASR (W)	ICD (9th)
Lip	2	0	-	-	-	-	-	-	0.6	-	-	-	-	-	-	-	-	1.7	0.1	0.0	0.00	0.00	**0.1**	*140*
Tongue	16	0	-	-	-	-	-	0.6	-	2.2	0.9	-	-	6.3	5.1	-	5.0	0.8	0.3	0.05	0.08	**0.7**	*141*
Salivary gland	13	0	-	-	-	-	1.2	-	-	0.6	1.4	0.9	-	-	2.5	-	2.4	6.7	0.6	0.3	0.03	0.05	**0.6**	*142*
Mouth	15	0	-	-	-	-	-	-	-	0.6	-	-	2.1	1.2	2.5	1.7	4.7	10.0	0.7	0.3	0.03	0.06	**0.6**	*143-5*
Oropharynx	7	0	-	-	-	-	-	-	-	-	0.7	0.9	-	-	2.5	1.7	-	3.3	0.3	0.1	0.02	0.03	**0.3**	*146*
Nasopharynx	1	0	-	-	-	-	-	-	-	-	-	-	-	-	1.3	-	-	-	0.0	0.0	0.01	0.01	**0.1**	*147*
Hypopharynx	3	0	-	-	-	-	-	-	-	0.7	-	-	-	-	-	3.4	-	-	0.1	0.1	0.00	0.02	**0.1**	*148*
Pharynx unspecified	2	0	-	-	-	-	-	-	-	-	-	-	-	-	1.3	-	-	1.7	0.1	0.0	0.01	0.01	**0.1**	*149*
Oesophagus	95	2	-	-	-	-	-	-	-	3.0	0.7	4.5	6.3	7.0	15.1	18.8	30.7	56.9	4.7	1.9	0.19	0.44	**4.1**	*150*
Stomach	200	9	-	-	0.6	-	1.2	1.6	1.1	3.7	5.0	8.1	10.5	26.6	29.0	39.3	73.2	85.3	9.9	3.9	0.46	1.05	**8.9**	*151*
Small intestine	14	0	-	-	-	-	-	-	-	1.2	-	1.8	1.1	1.2	2.5	3.4	7.1	1.7	0.7	0.3	0.04	0.09	**0.7**	*152*
Colon	315	10	-	-	-	0.6	1.2	2.7	1.7	4.9	7.2	18.9	18.9	37.1	37.8	61.5	89.7	168.9	15.6	6.1	0.68	1.46	**13.7**	*153*
Rectum	152	5	-	-	-	-	-	1.6	1.7	3.0	3.6	7.2	12.6	16.2	26.5	41.0	44.9	55.2	7.5	3.0	0.37	0.82	**6.9**	*154*
Liver	83	3	-	-	-	-	-	-	0.6	1.2	1.4	5.4	3.2	8.1	13.9	10.2	21.3	55.2	4.1	1.6	0.17	0.34	**3.5**	*155*
Gallbladder etc.	158	1	-	-	-	-	0.6	1.1	0.6	1.2	2.2	3.6	7.4	11.6	25.2	51.2	61.4	85.3	7.8	3.1	0.27	0.84	**6.9**	*156*
Pancreas	145	3	-	-	-	-	-	0.5	0.6	1.2	1.4	4.5	3.2	9.3	22.7	46.1	56.7	85.3	7.2	2.8	0.22	0.75	**6.3**	*157*
Nose, sinuses etc.	6	0	-	-	-	-	-	-	-	-	0.7	1.8	1.1	-	-	1.7	-	1.7	0.3	0.1	0.02	0.03	**0.3**	*160*
Larynx	28	1	-	-	-	-	-	-	1.1	-	0.7	-	6.3	7.0	6.3	3.4	4.7	5.0	1.4	0.5	0.11	0.15	**1.3**	*161*
Bronchus, lung	319	13	-	-	-	-	0.6	-	2.8	3.0	8.6	15.3	29.4	60.2	63.0	58.1	73.2	118.7	15.8	6.2	0.95	1.64	**14.4**	*162*
Other thoracic organs	18	1	-	-	-	-	-	-	-	0.6	0.7	1.8	1.1	5.8	1.3	1.7	2.4	6.7	0.9	0.4	0.06	0.08	**0.8**	*163-4*
Bone	42	3	0.6	-	1.2	1.3	1.2	0.5	-	1.8	1.4	1.8	2.1	5.8	2.5	3.4	7.1	16.7	2.1	0.8	0.11	0.17	**1.9**	*170*
Connective tissue	45	2	0.6	0.6	0.6	0.6	-	1.1	0.6	2.4	0.7	2.7	3.2	9.3	8.8	6.8	2.4	8.4	2.2	0.9	0.16	0.21	**2.1**	*171*
Mesothelioma	0	0	-	-	-	-	-	-	-	-	-	-	-	-	-	-	-	-	0.0	0.0	0.00	0.00	**0.0**	*MES*
Kaposi's sarcoma	2	0	-	-	-	-	-	-	0.6	-	-	-	-	-	-	-	-	1.7	0.1	0.0	0.00	0.00	**0.1**	*KAP*
Melanoma of skin	112	12	-	0.6	-	1.3	1.2	2.2	4.4	4.9	8.6	6.3	9.5	3.5	15.1	17.1	18.9	23.4	5.5	2.2	0.32	0.52	**5.0**	*172*
Other skin	731	118	-	-	0.6	1.3	1.2	7.1	15.0	21.3	15.8	48.5	47.3	75.3	89.5	123.0	141.7	240.8	36.2		1.93	3.50	**32.4**	*173*
Breast	1334	65	-	-	-	-	4.3	6.0	15.6	40.2	75.5	157.2	138.7	169.2	206.7	263.0	266.9	280.9	66.0	26.0	4.28	7.06	**62.0**	*174*
Uterus unspecified	202	17	-	-	-	1.3	0.6	1.1	5.0	6.7	13.7	9.9	21.0	22.0	21.4	32.4	49.6	56.9	10.0	3.9	0.56	1.01	**9.0**	*179*
Cervix uteri	497	16	-	-	-	-	4.3	15.8	32.3	40.8	30.2	48.5	54.6	55.6	44.1	58.1	56.7	51.8	24.6	9.7	1.69	2.28	**22.1**	*180*
Placenta	1	0	-	-	-	-	-	0.5	-	-	-	-	-	-	-	-	-	-	0.0	0.0	0.00	0.00	**0.0**	*181*
Corpus uteri	135	5	-	-	-	-	-	-	1.1	-	6.5	1.8	9.5	20.9	27.7	39.3	52.0	38.5	6.7	2.6	0.35	0.82	**6.2**	*182*
Ovary etc.	183	9	-	-	1.2	0.6	-	2.2	0.6	4.9	7.9	13.5	11.6	25.5	29.0	39.3	61.4	45.1	9.1	3.6	0.51	1.04	**8.4**	*183*
Other female genital	83	10	-	-	-	-	0.6	-	0.6	2.4	1.4	2.7	4.2	7.0	11.3	10.2	28.3	41.8	4.1	1.6	0.17	0.39	**3.6**	*184*
†Bladder	78	3	-	-	0.6	-	-	0.5	-	1.2	2.2	3.6	3.2	11.6	10.1	20.5	21.3	36.8	3.9	1.5	0.17	0.39	**3.4**	*188*
Kidney etc.	85	6	0.6	0.6	0.6	-	-	0.5	0.6	1.2	1.4	3.6	4.2	16.2	16.4	25.6	23.6	16.7	4.2	1.7	0.25	0.51	**4.0**	*189*
Eye	11	3	0.6	-	-	-	-	-	-	0.6	0.7	-	-	-	-	1.7	2.4	5.0	0.5	0.2	0.01	0.04	**0.5**	*190*
Brain, nervous system	57	3	-	0.6	0.6	1.3	1.2	1.6	2.8	2.4	2.9	4.5	3.2	7.0	5.0	5.1	16.5	6.7	2.8	1.1	0.17	0.29	**2.6**	*191-2*
Thyroid	64	4	-	-	-	1.9	1.2	0.5	2.2	3.7	3.6	2.7	6.3	7.0	6.3	8.5	18.9	10.0	3.2	1.2	0.19	0.34	**2.9**	*193*
Other endocrine	11	1	0.6	-	-	-	-	-	-	0.6	1.4	0.9	3.2	2.3	-	-	-	-	0.5	0.2	0.05	0.05	**0.6**	*194*
Hodgkin's disease	24	3	-	-	0.6	-	1.9	1.1	-	1.8	-	-	1.1	2.3	2.5	5.1	2.4	5.0	1.2	0.5	0.06	0.11	**1.1**	*201*
Non-Hodgkin lymphoma	142	6	-	0.6	1.2	1.3	1.9	2.7	3.3	0.6	2.9	7.2	8.4	12.7	30.2	23.9	42.5	48.5	7.0	2.8	0.38	0.73	**6.4**	*200,202*
Multiple myeloma	37	0	-	-	-	-	-	1.1	-	-	-	2.7	2.1	5.8	5.0	18.8	11.8	8.4	1.8	0.7	0.08	0.24	**1.8**	*203*
Lymphoid leukaemia	43	5	1.9	2.3	0.6	0.6	-	2.2	1.7	0.6	-	0.9	2.1	1.2	5.0	1.7	7.1	15.0	2.1	0.8	0.11	0.16	**2.0**	*204*
Myeloid leukaemia	62	7	-	0.6	1.7	0.6	0.6	-	2.8	1.2	1.4	3.6	4.2	3.5	5.0	12.0	9.4	23.4	3.1	1.2	0.14	0.26	**2.7**	*205*
Monocytic leukaemia	0	0	-	-	-	-	-	-	-	-	-	-	-	-	-	-	-	-	0.0	0.0	0.00	0.00	**0.0**	*206*
Other leukaemia	1	0	-	-	-	-	-	-	-	-	-	-	-	-	-	-	2.4	-	0.0	0.0	0.00	0.01	**0.0**	*207*
Leukaemia unspecified	22	2	0.6	1.2	0.6	0.6	-	-	0.6	0.6	0.7	0.9	2.1	2.3	1.3	3.4	4.7	3.3	1.1	0.4	0.06	0.11	**1.1**	*208*
Other and unspecified	269	6	-	-	-	0.6	0.6	2.2	2.2	4.9	7.2	12.6	15.8	22.0	35.3	59.8	94.5	140.5	13.3	5.2	0.53	1.32	**11.7**	*O&U*
All sites	5865	354	5.7	7.0	10.5	13.9	26.1	56.7	102.3	170.1	223.6	411.5	460.2	678.9	838.1	1127.1	1414.6	1879.5	290.1		15.99	29.51	**264.0**	*ALL*
All sites but 173	5134	236	5.7	7.0	9.9	12.6	24.9	49.6	87.3	148.7	207.8	363.0	413.0	603.6	748.6	1004.2	1272.9	1638.7	254.0	100.0	14.05	25.99	**231.5**	*ALLb*

Rate from 1 case   0.629 0.581 0.582 0.632 0.621 0.545 0.556 0.610 0.719 0.898 1.051 1.159 1.260 1.708 2.362 1.672

†Important: see notes on population page

Colombia, Cali

Cali Cancer Registry is a programme of the Department of Pathology at the University of Valle that has operated continuously since 1962. The staff includes a director, who is a professor of pathology, three assessing pathologists, a statistician coordinator, three record clerks and a secretary. Once a year, a group of specially trained medical students is selected to carry out a field survey of files of all private physicians who diagnose or treat cancer patients. An advisory committee was created in 1992, comprising a pathologist, an epidemiologist and three oncologists specializing in paediatric, clinical and surgical oncology. The registry staff and part of the operating costs are covered by the University of Valle. Most of the operating costs are obtained from foundations and specific grants for each activity.

The registry covers the population of the urban area of Cali city, which covers 119 km^2. The conurbation is divided into 20 communes for administrative purposes. Cali is the capital of the Department of Valle, one of the 32 departments into which the country is divided politically. The department is located in the south-west of Colombia on the Pacific Ocean. Cali is situated 1000 m above sea level between the Cauca river to the east and the chain of the Andes to the west, at latitude 3°27′ N and longitude 7°31′ W. The average temperature is 24°C.

In 1990, the Municipality of Cali had a total population of 1 637 501 inhabitants, 98.5% of whom were urban. The rate of urban population growth has fallen from 7.8% in 1951–64 to 3.4% in 1973–88 as a result of both lower fertility and decreased immigration. The proportion of the population under 15 years of age fell from 46.6% in 1973 to 31.6% in 1985, while those above 60 years rose from 4.9% to 6.2% during the same period.

Most of the population are mestizos (a mixture of Spanish and Indian), with a minority of pure negroes and whites. More than half of the resident population are migrants from other areas of Colombia and from other countries, notably Lebanon, Italy, Germany and central Europe. The majority of the inhabitants are Catholics. The official language is Spanish.

Roughly 80% of the working population is engaged in manufacturing industry, in trade, restaurants and hotels, or in municipal, social and personal services. The average unemployment rate has been 11.2% over the last ten years.

Public services are available to the major part of the population, and are becoming progressively more available in the suburbs. Air pollution has been serious due to a high density of nearby industrial plants.

A basic network of health substructures has been planned for the whole urban territory using health centres, and programmes of primary care and prevention have been promoted. Mortality rates have been falling for the last 30 years, especially for infant mortality. Life expectancy at birth is 74.9 years for women and 65.5 years for men.

A screening programme for cancer of cervix uteri was initiated in 1967. This has led to a substantial reduction in rates of invasive cervical cancer. Other educational campaigns for cancer prevention and early detection have been launched.

About 60% of the cancer patients diagnosed in Cali are treated at Valle University Hospital, a public general hospital with a total of 630 beds. A hospital-based cancer registry was established in 1986, a team for the management of childhood cancer began activities in 1989 and a formal oncology department is to be initiated. The hospital also maintains radio- and chemotherapy facilities. Other facilities for cancer diagnosis and treatment include three major non-university hospitals, cytopathology and haematology laboratories, and chemotherapy and radiotherapy centres.

Cancer notification is not compulsory in Cali. Cancer case reports are obtained actively by visiting all sources of information annually. These sources include hospitals and clinics, both public and private, pathology and haematology laboratories, radiotherapy centres, physicians and death certificates. It is estimated that registration is at least 95% complete. The data concerning each case are registered on a special form at the source site. They are classified and revised at the registry office and the information is entered into a computer database for checking for duplicates, errors and inconsistencies. Difficult cases are discussed by the staff and resolved either by the registry director or by revisiting the source, and sometimes, if appropriate, reviewing the microscopic slides.

Topography and morphology are coded according to ICD-O.

No active follow-up of cancer patients is carried out. Continuous review of all death certificates reveals which registered patients have died in the area of Cali.

The incidence data are available since 1962. They have been used to study time trends in risk for cancers in the area, to assess cancer screening programmes, to provide data for epidemiological studies and for use in teaching.

Edwin Carrascal

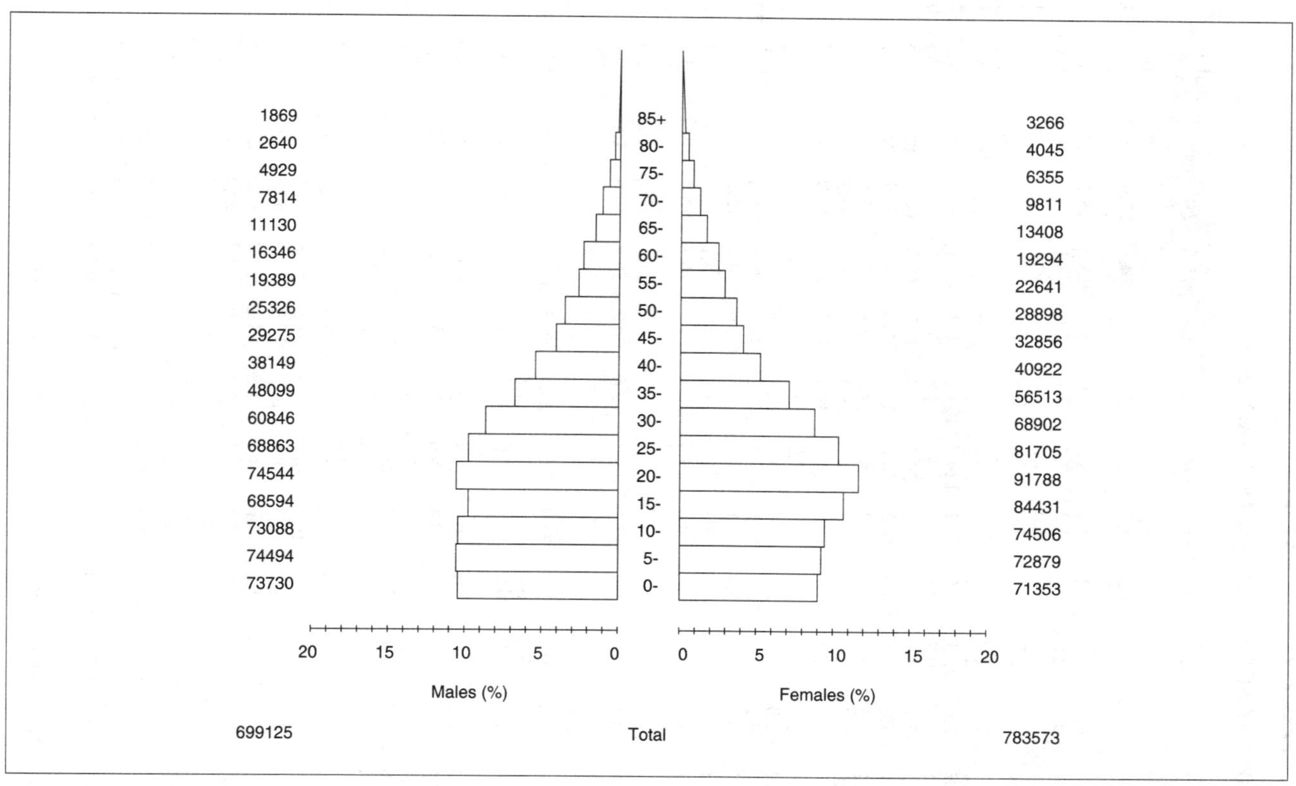

Colombia, Cali
Source of population: 1987–91
Census: The population-at-risk is the average of the 1985 and 1995 census populations.
Notes to tables overleaf:
† 188 does not include non-invasive tumours

Screening programmes in the area:
120,000 examinations have been performed annually for cervical cancer in the population over age 15 since 1967.

COLOMBIA, CALI 1987-1991

ANNUAL INCIDENCE PER 100,000 BY AGE GROUP (YEARS) - MALE

SITE	ALL AGES	AGE UNK	0-	5-	10-	15-	20-	25-	30-	35-	40-	45-	50-	55-	60-	65-	70-	75-	80-	85+	CRUDE RATE	%	CR 64	CR 74	ASR (W)	ICD (9th)
Lip	8	1	-	-	-	-	0.3	-	-	-	-	-	0.8	1.0	3.7	-	-	-	-	10.7	0.2	0.2	0.03	0.03	**0.3**	*140*
Tongue	27	0	-	-	-	-	-	-	-	-	1.0	-	1.6	4.1	4.9	10.8	5.1	4.1	37.9	10.7	0.8	0.6	0.06	0.14	**1.2**	*141*
Salivary gland	15	4	-	-	-	-	-	0.3	0.3	-	0.5	0.7	0.8	-	-	1.8	7.7	-	15.2	-	0.4	0.3	0.02	0.08	**0.6**	*142*
Mouth	52	6	-	0.3	-	-	-	0.3	1.0	0.4	0.5	0.7	3.2	4.1	8.6	18.0	15.4	16.2	15.2	10.7	1.5	1.2	0.11	0.30	**2.3**	*143-5*
Oropharynx	20	0	-	-	-	-	-	-	-	0.4	0.5	2.0	-	6.2	2.4	5.4	2.6	8.1	-	10.7	0.6	0.5	0.06	0.10	**0.9**	*146*
Nasopharynx	7	0	-	-	-	-	-	0.3	0.3	-	-	-	0.8	1.0	1.2	1.8	-	4.1	-	-	0.2	0.2	0.02	0.03	**0.3**	*147*
Hypopharynx	12	0	-	-	-	-	-	-	-	-	-	0.7	1.6	1.0	3.7	3.6	5.1	-	7.6	-	0.3	0.3	0.03	0.08	**0.6**	*148*
Pharynx unspecified	1	0	-	-	-	-	-	-	-	-	-	-	-	-	-	-	-	-	-	10.7	0.0	0.0	0.00	0.00	**0.1**	*149*
Oesophagus	86	4	-	-	-	-	-	-	-	0.4	1.6	2.0	7.1	4.1	17.1	21.6	30.7	52.7	30.3	74.9	2.5	2.0	0.17	0.44	**3.9**	*150*
Stomach	747	27	-	-	-	-	-	1.2	5.9	6.7	13.6	22.5	46.6	79.4	129.7	194.1	230.3	328.7	393.9	535.0	21.4	17.1	1.59	3.79	**33.3**	*151*
Small intestine	10	0	-	-	-	-	-	-	-	0.4	-	0.7	0.8	2.1	-	1.8	7.7	4.1	-	-	0.3	0.2	0.02	0.07	**0.4**	*152*
Colon	152	8	-	-	0.3	0.6	0.5	0.9	0.7	4.2	3.1	4.1	4.7	10.3	29.4	44.9	33.3	69.0	68.2	85.6	4.3	3.5	0.31	0.72	**6.6**	*153*
Rectum	124	5	-	-	-	0.6	0.5	0.3	1.0	2.1	1.0	4.8	9.5	16.5	23.2	27.0	35.8	44.6	37.9	53.5	3.5	2.8	0.31	0.64	**5.4**	*154*
Liver	61	4	-	-	-	-	-	0.3	0.3	1.2	1.6	1.4	5.5	7.2	6.1	18.0	12.8	24.3	45.5	10.7	1.7	1.4	0.13	0.29	**2.6**	*155*
Gallbladder etc.	85	1	-	-	-	-	-	-	0.3	0.8	0.5	6.1	3.9	10.3	14.7	25.2	28.2	28.4	37.9	74.9	2.4	1.9	0.19	0.46	**3.9**	*156*
Pancreas	119	2	-	-	-	-	-	0.3	0.7	-	2.1	1.4	7.1	15.5	20.8	39.5	48.6	52.7	53.0	64.2	3.4	2.7	0.24	0.69	**5.4**	*157*
Nose, sinuses etc.	26	1	-	-	-	-	-	0.3	0.7	-	1.0	1.4	2.4	3.1	1.2	9.0	7.7	4.1	7.6	10.7	0.7	0.6	0.05	0.14	**1.1**	*160*
Larynx	114	2	-	-	-	-	-	-	-	1.2	1.0	3.4	5.5	14.4	26.9	28.7	43.5	69.0	30.3	53.5	3.3	2.6	0.27	0.64	**5.2**	*161*
Bronchus, lung	536	20	-	-	0.3	-	-	0.6	0.3	1.7	4.2	13.0	30.8	57.8	110.1	140.2	199.6	308.4	325.8	224.7	15.3	12.3	1.14	2.90	**24.4**	*162*
Other thoracic organs	17	1	-	-	-	-	0.3	-	-	0.4	0.5	-	2.4	3.1	1.2	3.6	2.6	4.1	15.2	-	0.5	0.4	0.04	0.07	**0.7**	*163-4*
Bone	40	0	-	0.3	1.6	2.3	2.7	0.3	-	0.4	1.0	-	-	4.1	1.2	3.6	5.1	8.1	-	-	1.1	0.9	0.07	0.11	**1.2**	*170*
Connective tissue	64	8	-	0.3	0.3	0.9	0.5	1.2	1.0	2.1	2.1	1.4	-	8.3	8.6	10.8	7.7	16.2	15.2	10.7	1.8	1.5	0.15	0.26	**2.4**	*171*
Mesothelioma	1	0	-	-	-	-	-	-	-	-	-	-	-	-	1.2	-	-	-	-	-	0.0	0.0	0.01	0.01	**0.0**	*MES*
Kaposi's sarcoma	5	0	-	-	-	-	-	1.0	-	-	-	-	-	-	1.2	1.8	-	-	-	-	0.1	0.1	0.01	0.02	**0.2**	*KAP*
Melanoma of skin	69	8	-	-	0.3	-	0.5	0.6	2.0	0.8	3.1	6.1	2.4	3.1	8.6	12.6	10.2	28.4	7.6	10.7	2.0	1.6	0.16	0.28	**2.7**	*172*
Other skin	0	0	-	-	-	-	-	-	-	-	-	-	-	-	-	-	-	-	-	-	0.0		0.00	0.00	**0.0**	*173*
Breast	5	0	-	-	-	-	-	-	-	-	0.5	-	-	2.1	2.4	-	-	-	-	-	0.1	0.1	0.03	0.03	**0.2**	*175*
Prostate	693	47	-	-	-	-	-	-	-	-	1.0	0.7	5.5	34.0	71.0	226.4	386.5	539.7	613.6	577.8	19.8	15.9	0.60	3.89	**32.7**	*185*
Testis	64	2	1.4	-	-	1.2	1.6	1.7	6.2	2.9	3.7	2.0	0.8	-	-	1.8	-	8.1	7.6	-	1.8	1.5	0.11	0.12	**1.7**	*186*
Penis	28	2	-	-	-	-	-	0.3	-	0.4	1.6	2.0	0.8	3.1	4.9	5.4	2.6	12.2	15.2	10.7	0.8	0.6	0.07	0.11	**1.2**	*187.1-.4*
Other male genital	1	0	-	-	-	-	0.3	-	-	-	-	-	-	-	-	-	-	-	-	-	0.0	0.0	0.00	0.00	**0.0**	*187.5-.9*
†Bladder	164	10	-	-	-	-	-	0.3	0.3	1.7	3.1	1.4	2.4	9.3	24.5	53.9	71.7	89.3	174.2	53.5	4.7	3.8	0.23	0.90	**7.4**	*188*
Kidney etc.	62	1	1.4	0.8	-	-	0.3	0.3	0.3	0.4	3.1	2.7	7.1	8.3	8.6	12.6	5.1	16.2	-	21.4	1.8	1.4	0.17	0.26	**2.5**	*189*
Eye	18	2	1.6	-	-	-	-	-	0.3	0.4	1.0	1.4	-	-	1.2	1.8	-	8.1	-	-	0.5	0.4	0.03	0.04	**0.6**	*190*
Brain, nervous system	125	0	1.1	2.7	0.5	0.6	1.1	2.3	4.6	4.6	3.7	6.1	7.1	13.4	13.5	9.0	23.0	24.3	-	10.7	3.6	2.9	0.31	0.47	**4.4**	*191-2*
Thyroid	54	1	-	-	-	0.3	0.3	0.6	1.0	1.2	2.6	4.1	1.6	6.2	9.8	9.0	7.7	8.1	45.5	-	1.5	1.2	0.14	0.23	**2.1**	*193*
Other endocrine	7	0	0.8	-	-	0.6	-	-	-	-	0.5	-	-	-	1.2	-	-	-	-	-	0.2	0.2	0.02	0.02	**0.2**	*194*
Hodgkin's disease	61	3	1.1	2.1	1.1	1.2	1.1	1.7	1.6	0.8	1.0	2.7	3.9	4.1	2.4	-	7.7	-	-	10.7	1.7	1.4	0.13	0.17	**1.9**	*201*
Non-Hodgkin lymphoma	206	16	3.0	2.7	1.4	1.5	1.6	1.7	3.0	3.3	5.8	9.6	11.8	16.5	18.4	30.5	43.5	56.8	45.5	53.5	5.9	4.7	0.43	0.84	**7.9**	*200,202*
Multiple myeloma	51	3	-	-	-	-	-	-	-	-	0.5	1.4	3.2	8.3	8.6	10.8	17.9	12.2	60.6	21.4	1.5	1.2	0.12	0.27	**2.3**	*203*
Lymphoid leukaemia	66	3	3.3	3.2	0.8	2.3	1.1	0.6	0.7	-	-	3.4	1.6	1.0	1.2	1.8	5.1	16.2	15.2	21.4	1.9	1.5	0.10	0.14	**2.1**	*204*
Myeloid leukaemia	58	1	1.1	1.1	0.8	0.6	1.6	0.6	1.3	1.2	1.0	3.4	1.6	2.1	6.1	5.4	2.6	12.2	30.3	21.4	1.7	1.3	0.11	0.16	**2.0**	*205*
Monocytic leukaemia	2	0	-	-	-	-	-	-	-	-	-	-	-	1.0	-	-	-	-	7.6	-	0.1	0.0	0.01	0.01	**0.1**	*206*
Other leukaemia	1	0	-	-	-	-	-	-	-	-	-	-	-	-	-	1.8	-	-	-	-	0.0	0.0	0.00	0.01	**0.1**	*207*
Leukaemia unspecified	49	1	1.1	0.5	-	0.6	0.8	0.3	0.3	0.8	1.0	3.4	-	6.2	8.6	10.8	7.7	8.1	-	21.4	1.4	1.1	0.12	0.22	**2.0**	*208*
Other and unspecified	248	18	0.5	-	-	0.6	-	0.9	2.3	2.5	4.7	10.9	12.6	29.9	41.6	46.7	84.5	97.4	121.2	74.9	7.1	5.7	0.57	1.28	**10.7**	*O&U*
All sites	4361	212	16.3	14.0	7.4	13.7	15.0	18.0	37.5	43.7	74.4	127.8	197.4	402.3	649.7	1051.2	1405.1	1984.2	2280.3	2161.6	124.8		8.50	21.41	**187.6**	*ALL*
All sites but 173	4361	212	16.3	14.0	7.4	13.7	15.0	18.0	37.5	43.7	74.4	127.8	197.4	402.3	649.7	1051.2	1405.1	1984.2	2280.3	2161.6	124.8	100.0	8.50	21.41	**187.6**	*ALLb*

Rate from 1 case   0.271   0.268   0.274   0.292   0.268   0.290   0.329   0.416   0.524   0.683   0.790   1.032   1.224   1.797   2.559   4.058   7.576   10.701

†Important: see notes on population page

COLOMBIA, CALI 1987-1991

ANNUAL INCIDENCE PER 100,000 BY AGE GROUP (YEARS) - FEMALE

SITE	ALL AGES	AGE UNK	0-	5-	10-	15-	20-	25-	30-	35-	40-	45-	50-	55-	60-	65-	70-	75-	80-	85+	CRUDE RATE	%	CR 64	CR 74	ASR (W)	ICD (9th)
Lip	4	0	-	-	-	-	-	-	-	-	0.5	-	-	-	-	-	-	9.4	-	-	0.1	0.1	0.00	0.00	0.1	140
Tongue	27	0	-	-	-	-	-	-	-	0.4	0.5	0.6	3.5	0.9	5.2	4.5	8.2	6.3	14.8	6.1	0.7	0.5	0.05	0.12	1.0	141
Salivary gland	15	2	-	-	-	-	0.4	-	-	0.4	1.0	-	1.4	2.7	1.0	1.5	2.0	-	-	-	0.4	0.3	0.04	0.06	0.5	142
Mouth	37	3	-	-	-	-	-	-	-	-	1.8	2.1	2.7	5.2	8.9	10.2	9.4	14.8	18.4	-	0.9	0.6	0.06	0.17	1.4	143-5
Oropharynx	10	1	-	-	-	-	-	-	-	-	-	-	2.7	1.0	1.5	6.1	-	4.9	-	-	0.3	0.2	0.02	0.06	0.4	146
Nasopharynx	5	0	-	0.3	-	-	-	-	0.3	-	-	0.6	-	-	-	-	4.1	-	-	-	0.1	0.1	0.01	0.03	0.2	147
Hypopharynx	1	1	-	-	-	-	-	-	-	-	-	-	-	-	-	-	-	-	-	-	0.0	0.0	0.00	0.00	0.0	148
Pharynx unspecified	2	0	-	-	-	-	-	-	0.3	-	-	-	-	0.9	-	-	-	-	-	-	0.1	0.0	0.01	0.01	0.1	149
Oesophagus	65	3	-	-	-	-	-	-	0.6	-	-	0.6	4.2	1.8	6.2	23.9	12.2	31.5	29.7	42.9	1.7	1.1	0.07	0.26	2.3	150
Stomach	547	17	-	-	-	-	0.4	1.7	1.5	6.7	6.8	15.2	22.1	54.8	64.3	125.3	136.6	188.8	247.2	251.0	14.0	9.1	0.90	2.25	19.3	151
Small intestine	22	0	-	-	-	-	-	-	0.3	-	0.5	0.6	1.4	0.9	6.2	7.5	2.0	6.3	4.9	6.1	0.6	0.4	0.05	0.10	0.8	152
Colon	183	7	-	-	-	0.2	1.1	0.7	2.6	1.1	2.0	3.7	9.7	15.0	25.9	32.8	44.8	62.9	49.4	91.8	4.7	3.1	0.32	0.73	6.3	153
Rectum	130	8	-	-	-	0.2	0.4	-	2.0	0.7	1.0	5.5	9.0	9.7	18.7	19.4	34.7	50.3	34.6	24.5	3.3	2.2	0.25	0.54	4.5	154
Liver	63	1	-	0.3	-	0.2	-	-	0.3	-	1.0	1.8	3.5	2.7	9.3	10.4	22.4	34.6	24.7	18.4	1.6	1.1	0.10	0.26	2.2	155
Gallbladder etc.	228	3	-	-	-	-	0.2	0.2	0.6	1.4	1.5	3.7	14.5	27.4	33.2	55.2	69.3	78.7	84.0	67.3	5.8	3.8	0.42	1.05	8.3	156
Pancreas	107	2	-	-	-	-	-	-	0.3	0.7	1.5	2.4	4.8	8.8	18.7	14.9	26.5	50.3	44.5	73.5	2.7	1.8	0.19	0.40	3.8	157
Nose, sinuses etc.	24	1	-	-	-	0.2	-	0.5	-	-	1.0	2.4	0.7	3.5	3.1	4.5	2.0	3.1	4.9	-	0.6	0.4	0.06	0.09	0.8	160
Larynx	29	4	-	-	-	-	-	-	-	-	-	0.6	0.7	3.5	9.3	4.5	4.1	9.4	9.9	-	0.7	0.5	0.08	0.13	1.1	161
Bronchus, lung	261	15	-	-	-	-	-	0.7	0.3	0.4	3.4	6.1	9.7	31.8	44.6	52.2	59.1	122.7	84.0	67.3	6.7	4.4	0.51	1.10	9.5	162
Other thoracic organs	13	1	0.3	-	-	-	0.2	-	-	-	0.4	0.5	0.6	1.4	2.7	-	3.0	-	-	-	0.3	0.2	0.03	0.05	0.4	163-4
Bone	26	2	-	0.3	0.8	0.5	0.9	0.2	-	1.1	0.5	1.2	0.7	-	1.0	1.5	2.0	6.3	-	6.1	0.7	0.4	0.04	0.06	0.7	170
Connective tissue	82	4	0.6	0.3	0.3	1.4	1.5	-	2.6	1.8	1.5	4.9	5.5	4.4	2.1	7.5	12.2	9.4	4.9	36.7	2.1	1.4	0.14	0.24	2.4	171
Mesothelioma	1	0	-	-	-	-	-	-	-	-	-	0.6	-	-	-	-	-	-	-	-	0.0	0.0	0.00	0.00	0.0	MES
Kaposi's sarcoma	2	0	-	-	-	-	-	-	-	-	-	-	-	-	-	-	-	2.0	-	4.9	0.1	0.0	0.00	0.00	0.1	KAP
Melanoma of skin	102	8	-	-	0.3	-	0.9	1.2	2.0	3.9	5.9	4.3	5.5	7.1	10.4	7.5	14.3	12.6	14.8	12.2	2.6	1.7	0.22	0.34	3.1	172
Other skin	1	0	-	-	-	-	-	-	-	-	-	-	-	-	-	-	-	3.1	-	-	0.0		0.00	0.00	0.0	173
Breast	1151	77	-	-	-	-	0.7	3.9	17.4	27.6	64.5	81.0	90.7	98.9	123.4	144.7	169.2	173.1	138.4	165.3	29.4	19.2	2.72	4.40	38.8	174
Uterus unspecified	26	2	-	-	-	-	-	0.2	1.2	0.4	0.5	1.8	0.7	3.5	1.0	4.5	-	3.1	14.8	6.1	0.7	0.4	0.05	0.07	0.8	179
Cervix uteri	1061	58	-	-	-	-	1.3	9.3	20.0	38.2	52.8	64.5	85.1	106.0	121.3	117.8	89.7	125.9	138.4	104.1	27.1	17.7	2.64	3.73	34.4	180
Placenta	10	0	-	-	-	-	0.2	1.0	0.6	0.4	0.5	0.6	-	-	-	-	-	-	-	-	0.3	0.2	0.02	0.02	0.2	181
Corpus uteri	173	7	-	-	-	-	-	-	0.3	0.7	3.4	10.3	10.4	30.0	27.0	43.3	34.7	34.6	19.8	18.4	4.4	2.9	0.43	0.83	6.5	182
Ovary etc.	268	10	-	0.3	0.8	1.4	2.2	2.0	4.4	2.8	8.3	14.6	19.4	22.1	38.4	34.3	36.7	75.5	34.6	24.5	6.8	4.5	0.61	0.97	8.9	183
Other female genital	57	2	0.3	-	-	-	-	0.5	-	0.7	-	1.2	2.1	3.5	8.3	13.4	14.3	25.2	24.7	24.5	1.5	1.0	0.09	0.23	2.0	184
†Bladder	73	5	-	-	-	-	-	0.5	-	0.4	0.5	1.8	4.2	6.2	8.3	14.9	36.7	9.4	34.6	12.2	1.9	1.2	0.12	0.39	2.7	188
Kidney etc.	45	2	1.4	0.3	-	-	0.9	-	-	-	0.4	3.7	1.4	4.4	9.3	3.0	4.1	9.4	9.9	6.1	1.1	0.8	0.11	0.15	1.5	189
Eye	27	5	3.4	-	-	-	-	-	0.3	-	0.5	-	-	-	1.0	1.5	6.1	3.1	4.9	6.1	0.7	0.5	0.03	0.08	0.9	190
Brain, nervous system	110	2	1.7	1.4	0.8	0.7	0.4	1.0	3.5	2.1	3.9	2.4	6.2	11.5	12.4	13.4	14.3	6.3	9.9	6.1	2.8	1.8	0.24	0.39	3.5	191-2
Thyroid	237	14	-	-	0.3	0.7	2.4	6.9	8.7	9.2	7.8	12.2	11.1	15.0	15.5	10.4	22.4	44.1	29.7	12.2	6.0	4.0	0.48	0.65	6.7	193
Other endocrine	6	0	0.6	0.3	0.3	-	0.2	-	-	-	-	-	-	0.7	-	-	-	-	-	-	0.2	0.1	0.01	0.01	0.2	194
Hodgkin's disease	35	4	-	-	0.5	0.7	1.5	0.5	0.3	-	1.0	1.2	2.8	0.9	1.0	-	2.0	15.7	-	-	0.9	0.6	0.06	0.07	0.9	201
Non-Hodgkin lymphoma	175	11	1.1	0.8	1.1	-	0.7	0.5	2.9	1.8	4.9	4.3	8.3	17.7	22.8	34.3	34.7	44.1	19.8	24.5	4.5	2.9	0.36	0.72	6.0	200,202
Multiple myeloma	45	3	-	-	-	-	-	-	-	-	1.0	2.4	5.5	4.4	5.2	8.9	8.2	9.4	19.8	6.1	1.1	0.8	0.10	0.19	1.6	203
Lymphoid leukaemia	75	0	3.9	3.6	3.2	1.4	0.7	0.7	0.6	-	0.5	1.8	0.7	1.8	3.1	4.5	8.2	6.3	4.9	12.2	1.9	1.3	0.11	0.17	2.2	204
Myeloid leukaemia	61	1	0.8	0.3	0.8	0.7	0.2	0.7	1.2	2.1	1.5	0.6	3.5	7.1	6.2	4.5	4.1	15.7	9.9	6.1	1.6	1.0	0.13	0.17	1.9	205
Monocytic leukaemia	1	0	-	-	-	-	-	-	-	-	-	0.6	-	-	-	-	-	-	-	-	0.0	0.0	0.00	0.00	0.0	206
Other leukaemia	0	0	-	-	-	-	-	-	-	-	-	-	-	-	-	-	-	-	-	-	0.0	0.0	0.00	0.00	0.0	207
Leukaemia unspecified	42	0	0.8	0.3	-	0.9	0.2	0.2	0.9	1.1	1.0	0.6	2.1	3.5	2.1	3.0	6.1	15.7	9.9	12.2	1.1	0.7	0.07	0.11	1.3	208
Other and unspecified	335	23	0.6	0.3	0.3	0.2	0.2	1.0	1.2	1.8	5.4	6.7	19.4	27.4	51.8	65.6	81.5	97.6	128.5	128.6	8.6	5.6	0.62	1.41	12.0	O&U
All sites	6000	309	15.4	8.5	9.4	9.7	17.9	34.3	76.9	108.3	186.7	269.7	374.4	547.7	723.5	908.4	1047.7	1409.8	1329.8	1297.9	153.1		12.56	22.87	202.5	ALL
All sites but 173	5999	309	15.4	8.5	9.4	9.7	17.9	34.3	76.9	108.3	186.7	269.7	374.4	547.7	723.5	908.4	1047.7	1406.6	1329.8	1297.9	153.1	100.0	12.56	22.87	202.5	ALLb

| Rate from 1 case | | | 0.280 | 0.274 | 0.268 | 0.237 | 0.218 | 0.245 | 0.290 | 0.354 | 0.489 | 0.609 | 0.692 | 0.883 | 1.037 | 1.492 | 2.038 | 3.147 | 4.944 | 6.122 | | | | | | |

†Important: see notes on population page

Costa Rica

The Costa Rica National Tumour Registry was founded in December 1976, by Executive Decree, and started functioning in 1977, but nationwide coverage was achieved only in 1980. The aims were to collect data about cancer incidence and prevalence regarding age, sex, cancer site and geographical distribution within the country. The registry has moved from a manually operated system to a fully computerized one during the last four years.

The registry occupies a section of the Statistics Department of the Ministry of Health. A newly appointed medical director is in charge, and a medical registry technician and two statistical assistants are employed.

Costa Rica covers 51 200 km^2. At the 1984 national census, its population was 2 416 809 (1 208 216 male and 1 208 593 female), of whom 44.5% lived in cities and 55.5% in rural areas. The country has a national health care system and good quality vital statistics. It is estimated that the last census missed 5.7% of the population.

The official religion is Roman Catholic. The country's political constitution does not allow any differentiation between ethnic groups.

In 1992, the active population was employed in the following sectors: agriculture, hunting, forestry, fishing, 24.1%; mining and quarries, 0.1%; manufacturing industry, 18.9%; electricity, gas and water supply, 1.2%; building, 5.6%; sales (commerce), 16.6%; transport, communication, storage, 4.7%; finance, insurance and real estate, 3.6%; individual, social and city services, 24.1%.

It has been estimated that only 5% of the population seeks health care within private hospitals; special studies and treatments are offered mostly within the social security system.

The sources of information for the registry are the compulsory notification sheets on patients leaving hospitals, biopsy and autopsy reports with a diagnosis of cancer from all pathology services (public and private), and death certificates mentioning cancer, from the General Direction of Statistics and Census.

Except for death certificates, which have to be collected by the staff, data collection and case follow-up are passive. Death registration is complete, as it is compulsory to show this certificate before a burial. All cases notified are verified clinically or histologically, those that cannot be verified being discarded. Cases with a cytological diagnosis are accepted when localized in specific sites such as lung and cervix; however, the under-registration rate is still high with cytologies.

Each report sheet is checked against the Civil Registry database to verify the personal identification number, name and date of birth or death. Reports are then linked to the registry database, using software specially designed to find duplicates, to classify the case as incident or not. Each primary tumour case is given a unique identifying registry number and it is included in the registry database. Some consistency check edits are carried out during the inclusion of the case. Follow-up is passive. This whole process is being improved to reduce the probability of duplicates and inconsistencies. Multiple primaries are registered according to the IARC rules.

The registry has been used in various studies regarding occupational exposure cohorts and the risk of cancer during recent years and in descriptive and survival studies.

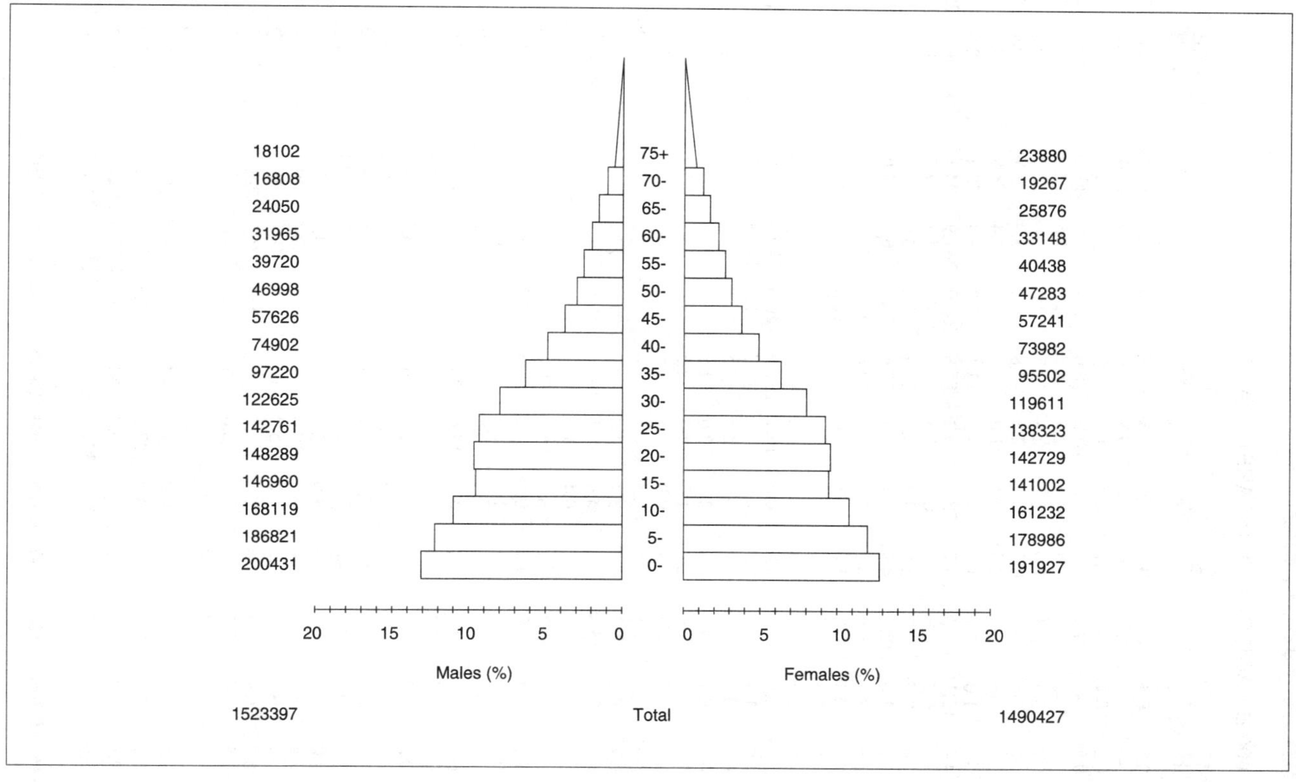

Costa Rica

Source of population: average annual 1988–92

Census: 1984. Ministerio de Planificación Nacional y Política Económica, Centro Latinoamericano de Demografía y Dirección General de Estadistica y Censos, Estimaciones y Proyecciones de Población por Sexo y Grupos de Edades, 1975-2000, Fascículo F/CR, San José, 1990.

Estimate: The population for each year was estimated on the basis of the 1984 Census, taking into account births and deaths, but not migration.

Notes to tables overleaf:

* The high percentage of death certificate only registrations with increases in incidence since Volume VI (e.g. for liver and brain cancers), and low level of morphological verification for some sites, suggest a lack of validity in the data.

† 188 does not include non-invasive tumours.

* COSTA RICA 1988-1992

ANNUAL INCIDENCE PER 100,000 BY AGE GROUP (YEARS) - MALE

SITE	ALL AGES	AGE UNK	0-	5-	10-	15-	20-	25-	30-	35-	40-	45-	50-	55-	60-	65-	70-	75+	CRUDE RATE	%	CR 64	CR 74	ASR (W)	ICD (9th)
Lip	63	1	-	-	-	-	0.1	0.3	0.5	0.4	0.3	0.7	2.1	3.5	3.8	5.0	10.7	19.9	0.8	0.7	0.06	0.14	1.3	140
Tongue	48	0	-	-	-	-	-	-	-	-	0.3	1.0	2.6	0.5	5.6	8.3	5.9	14.4	0.6	0.5	0.05	0.12	1.1	141
Salivary gland	19	0	-	-	-	0.1	-	0.1	0.2	0.4	-	0.7	0.9	1.0	2.5	1.7	-	2.2	0.2	0.2	0.03	0.04	0.4	142
Mouth	39	1	-	-	-	-	-	0.1	0.5	-	0.3	2.1	1.3	3.0	0.6	3.3	3.6	11.0	0.5	0.4	0.04	0.08	0.8	143-5
Oropharynx	37	0	-	-	-	-	-	-	-	-	-	1.4	0.9	2.5	4.4	4.2	3.6	12.2	0.5	0.4	0.05	0.08	0.8	146
Nasopharynx	40	0	-	0.3	0.2	0.4	0.7	0.4	0.2	0.6	0.3	1.0	1.7	2.5	1.3	2.5	-	2.2	0.5	0.4	0.05	0.06	0.7	147
Hypopharynx	32	0	-	-	-	-	-	-	-	-	-	0.3	1.3	2.5	3.8	4.2	5.9	7.7	0.4	0.4	0.04	0.09	0.7	148
Pharynx unspecified	18	0	-	-	0.1	0.1	-	-	-	-	-	0.3	0.4	1.0	-	1.7	2.4	8.8	0.2	0.2	0.01	0.03	0.4	149
Oesophagus	176	0	-	-	-	-	-	-	-	1.0	1.1	1.0	4.7	4.5	13.1	20.0	33.3	78.4	2.3	1.9	0.13	0.39	4.0	150
Stomach	2327	9	0.1	-	-	-	0.3	1.7	4.4	12.1	15.2	34.7	59.6	105.2	155.8	263.6	387.9	904.8	30.5	25.6	1.95	5.22	51.5	151
Small intestine	27	0	-	-	-	-	-	-	-	0.2	0.8	0.3	0.9	1.5	1.3	3.3	4.8	7.7	0.4	0.3	0.02	0.07	0.6	152
Colon	283	1	-	-	-	-	0.9	0.6	1.6	2.7	2.7	3.8	9.8	8.1	24.4	25.8	30.9	101.6	3.7	3.1	0.27	0.56	6.0	153
Rectum	221	0	-	-	-	0.1	0.3	0.7	1.0	1.0	2.1	4.9	5.1	11.6	15.6	26.6	36.9	63.0	2.9	2.4	0.21	0.53	4.8	154
Liver	317	0	0.1	-	0.2	0.1	0.8	1.4	1.6	3.1	5.6	4.2	8.1	9.1	24.4	29.1	50.0	95.0	4.2	3.5	0.29	0.69	6.6	155
Gallbladder etc.	119	0	-	-	-	-	0.1	0.3	0.2	0.4	0.8	1.0	3.8	5.0	8.1	12.5	22.6	45.3	1.6	1.3	0.10	0.27	2.6	156
Pancreas	270	2	-	-	-	-	-	0.1	0.5	0.8	1.9	1.7	6.8	10.1	24.4	25.8	52.4	108.3	3.5	3.0	0.23	0.63	6.1	157
Nose, sinuses etc.	23	0	-	0.1	0.1	-	0.1	-	-	0.2	-	0.3	0.9	0.5	1.9	5.0	1.2	5.5	0.3	0.3	0.02	0.05	0.5	160
Larynx	176	2	-	-	-	-	-	0.1	-	0.6	0.5	1.0	6.0	10.1	16.9	26.6	30.9	50.8	2.3	1.9	0.18	0.47	4.0	161
Bronchus, lung	686	3	-	-	-	0.1	0.4	-	1.0	1.4	2.4	5.2	14.9	24.2	71.3	91.5	146.4	234.2	9.0	7.5	0.61	1.80	15.6	162
Other thoracic organs	26	0	0.3	0.1	-	0.5	0.5	0.3	0.2	0.4	0.3	-	-	0.5	2.5	-	1.2	2.2	0.3	0.3	0.03	0.03	0.4	163-4
Bone	47	0	0.1	0.5	0.5	1.1	0.5	0.6	0.2	0.2	0.5	1.0	0.4	2.0	1.9	-	3.6	3.3	0.6	0.5	0.05	0.07	0.7	170
Connective tissue	97	1	1.0	0.1	0.5	0.8	0.7	0.4	1.6	1.2	1.9	2.4	1.3	4.5	2.5	5.8	3.6	12.2	1.3	1.1	0.10	0.14	1.6	171
Mesothelioma	6	0	-	-	-	-	-	-	0.2	-	0.3	-	0.9	0.5	0.6	-	-	-	0.1	0.1	0.01	0.01	0.1	MES
Kaposi's sarcoma	25	0	-	-	-	-	0.1	0.6	0.8	-	1.1	-	-	-	1.9	0.8	2.4	5.5	0.3	0.3	0.02	0.04	0.4	KAP
Melanoma of skin	99	0	0.1	0.1	-	-	0.4	-	0.7	0.6	1.3	1.7	3.4	4.0	6.3	7.5	14.3	33.1	1.3	1.1	0.09	0.20	2.1	172
Other skin	1907	38	0.3	0.1	0.1	0.4	1.5	3.2	6.2	12.3	23.0	35.4	53.6	79.1	141.4	210.4	277.2	603.2	25.0		1.82	4.31	41.3	173
Breast	12	0	-	-	-	-	-	-	-	-	-	-	0.4	1.0	1.9	-	2.4	4.4	0.2	0.1	0.02	0.03	0.3	175
Prostate	1179	8	0.1	-	-	-	-	-	-	0.2	0.8	1.7	6.8	25.7	70.1	132.2	255.8	671.7	15.5	13.0	0.53	2.48	27.0	185
Testis	161	0	0.9	-	0.1	1.6	2.6	4.6	5.1	4.7	2.9	1.7	0.9	1.5	2.5	1.7	3.6	3.3	2.1	1.8	0.15	0.17	2.1	186
Penis	61	0	-	-	-	-	-	-	0.2	1.0	0.8	1.7	1.7	2.5	3.1	5.8	10.7	18.8	0.8	0.7	0.06	0.14	1.3	187.1-.4
Other male genital	3	0	-	-	-	-	-	-	-	-	-	-	-	0.5	-	0.8	1.2	-	0.0	0.0	0.00	0.01	0.1	187.5-.9
†Bladder	298	1	0.3	-	-	-	0.1	0.4	0.3	0.8	2.4	2.1	4.7	14.6	26.9	37.4	50.0	109.4	3.9	3.3	0.26	0.70	6.6	188
Kidney etc.	155	0	0.6	0.4	-	-	0.1	-	0.2	0.4	2.4	2.8	5.5	12.1	12.5	22.5	19.0	26.5	2.0	1.7	0.19	0.39	3.3	189
Eye	44	0	1.6	0.1	-	0.1	-	-	0.2	0.2	0.5	0.7	1.3	1.5	0.6	0.8	3.6	9.9	0.6	0.5	0.03	0.06	0.8	190
Brain, nervous system	310	2	2.6	3.3	2.0	1.0	2.0	3.4	3.1	2.1	5.3	7.6	8.9	9.6	13.8	18.3	17.8	19.9	4.1	3.4	0.33	0.51	5.1	191-2
Thyroid	78	0	-	0.2	0.1	0.1	0.9	1.0	1.3	0.8	1.6	2.8	3.8	1.5	5.0	2.5	5.9	6.6	1.0	0.9	0.10	0.14	1.4	193
Other endocrine	19	0	0.3	0.1	0.1	0.1	0.1	-	-	0.2	-	0.3	0.4	1.5	0.6	-	1.2	4.4	0.2	0.2	0.02	0.03	0.3	194
Hodgkin's disease	172	1	1.0	2.1	1.9	1.8	0.8	1.5	2.0	4.3	1.1	3.8	3.0	2.0	7.5	7.5	4.8	12.2	2.3	1.9	0.17	0.23	2.6	201
Non-Hodgkin lymphoma	332	2	2.2	1.7	1.1	1.6	1.5	2.1	2.4	4.9	4.5	5.6	7.2	10.6	24.4	23.3	27.4	49.7	4.4	3.6	0.35	0.61	6.1	200,202
Multiple myeloma	112	0	-	-	-	-	-	0.1	-	0.4	0.5	0.3	3.8	5.0	10.0	15.8	19.0	39.8	1.5	1.2	0.10	0.28	2.5	203
Lymphoid leukaemia	270	0	6.9	4.3	3.1	2.9	2.0	1.5	0.7	0.4	0.8	1.4	5.1	2.5	6.3	8.3	16.7	26.5	3.5	3.0	0.19	0.31	4.0	204
Myeloid leukaemia	154	0	1.1	0.4	0.7	1.4	0.7	1.4	1.5	0.4	2.1	3.5	3.4	8.6	8.1	9.1	16.7	17.7	2.0	1.7	0.17	0.30	2.8	205
Monocytic leukaemia	6	0	0.1	-	-	-	-	-	-	0.4	0.3	0.3	-	-	-	-	-	1.1	0.1	0.1	0.01	0.01	0.1	206
Other leukaemia	0	0	-	-	-	-	-	-	-	-	-	-	-	-	-	-	-	-	0.0	0.0	0.00	0.00	0.0	207
Leukaemia unspecified	50	0	0.6	-	-	0.5	-	0.4	0.5	-	0.5	0.3	0.9	1.0	2.5	0.8	10.7	14.4	0.7	0.5	0.04	0.09	0.9	208
Other and unspecified	459	1	0.2	-	0.2	0.7	0.7	1.1	1.1	1.9	2.9	6.2	14.0	22.2	28.2	51.6	82.1	152.5	6.0	5.0	0.40	1.07	10.0	O&U
All sites	11003	73	20.5	14.1	11.2	15.8	19.2	28.6	39.8	63.2	92.1	149.6	263.0	420.9	760.2	1123.5	1680.1	3621.5	144.5		9.55	23.66	232.5	ALL
All sites but 173	9096	35	20.2	14.0	11.1	15.4	17.7	25.4	33.6	50.8	69.2	114.2	209.4	341.9	618.8	913.1	1402.8	3018.3	119.4	100.0	7.74	19.36	191.2	ALLb

Rate from 1 case   0.100   0.107   0.119   0.136   0.135   0.140   0.163   0.206   0.267   0.347   0.426   0.504   0.626   0.832   1.190   1.105

†Important: see notes on population page

* COSTA RICA 1988-1992

ANNUAL INCIDENCE PER 100,000 BY AGE GROUP (YEARS) - FEMALE

SITE	ALL AGES	AGE UNK	0-	5-	10-	15-	20-	25-	30-	35-	40-	45-	50-	55-	60-	65-	70-	75+	CRUDE RATE	%	CR 64	CR 74	ASR (W)	ICD (9th)
Lip	25	0	-	-	0.1	-	-	0.1	-	0.2	0.3	-	1.3	-	1.8	2.3	5.2	5.9	0.3	0.3	0.02	0.06	**0.5**	*140*
Tongue	29	0	-	-	-	-	-	-	0.2	0.2	0.3	0.3	0.8	1.5	3.0	3.1	2.1	7.5	0.4	0.3	0.03	0.06	**0.6**	*141*
Salivary gland	29	2	-	-	-	-	0.3	0.1	0.2	0.2	0.3	1.4	0.4	0.5	1.8	3.9	-	5.9	0.4	0.3	0.03	0.05	**0.5**	*142*
Mouth	31	0	0.1	-	-	0.1	-	-	-	-	0.8	1.0	0.8	0.5	1.8	0.8	4.2	10.1	0.4	0.3	0.03	0.05	**0.6**	*143-5*
Oropharynx	20	0	-	-	-	-	-	-	-	-	0.3	0.7	-	-	1.2	3.1	6.2	4.2	0.3	0.2	0.01	0.06	**0.4**	*146*
Nasopharynx	15	0	0.1	0.1	0.5	0.3	0.3	0.3	-	-	-	0.4	-	-	-	1.5	-	-	0.2	0.2	0.01	0.02	**0.2**	*147*
Hypopharynx	7	0	-	-	-	-	-	-	-	-	-	-	-	0.5	0.6	0.8	2.1	1.7	0.1	0.1	0.01	0.02	**0.1**	*148*
Pharynx unspecified	10	0	-	0.1	-	-	-	-	-	0.2	-	-	-	0.5	1.2	0.8	1.0	2.5	0.1	0.1	0.01	0.02	**0.2**	*149*
Oesophagus	72	0	-	-	-	-	-	-	-	0.2	0.5	0.3	1.3	3.5	7.2	6.2	16.6	18.4	1.0	0.8	0.07	0.18	**1.4**	*150*
Stomach	1199	6	0.2	-	-	0.3	0.8	1.4	3.5	7.7	11.1	18.2	29.2	37.6	60.9	109.0	155.7	406.2	16.1	13.4	0.86	2.19	**22.7**	*151*
Small intestine	25	0	-	-	-	0.1	-	-	0.2	0.2	-	-	1.7	2.5	1.2	3.1	3.1	3.4	0.3	0.3	0.03	0.06	**0.5**	*152*
Colon	343	2	-	-	-	0.3	0.6	1.2	1.3	2.1	3.8	6.6	9.3	13.4	27.2	22.4	36.3	98.8	4.6	3.8	0.33	0.63	**6.5**	*153*
Rectum	211	2	-	-	-	0.1	0.4	0.1	0.8	1.5	2.4	3.8	3.8	8.4	10.3	18.6	38.4	57.0	2.8	2.4	0.16	0.45	**4.0**	*154*
Liver	199	1	0.5	0.1	-	0.4	0.1	0.1	1.0	1.3	1.1	2.8	3.0	5.9	10.3	17.0	39.4	56.1	2.7	2.2	0.13	0.42	**3.7**	*155*
Gallbladder etc.	267	1	-	-	-	-	-	-	0.3	0.2	2.4	4.5	4.2	15.3	21.7	24.0	41.5	77.9	3.6	3.0	0.24	0.57	**5.3**	*156*
Pancreas	270	0	-	-	0.1	0.1	0.1	-	0.3	-	3.0	0.7	5.1	8.9	15.7	30.1	39.4	99.7	3.6	3.0	0.17	0.52	**5.2**	*157*
Nose, sinuses etc.	9	0	-	-	-	-	-	-	-	-	-	0.8	-	0.6	-	4.2	1.7	0.1	0.1	0.01	0.03	**0.2**	*160*
Larynx	31	0	-	-	-	-	-	-	0.2	-	-	1.3	1.0	2.4	5.4	4.2	8.4	0.4	0.3	0.02	0.07	**0.6**	*161*
Bronchus, lung	274	2	-	-	-	-	0.3	0.1	0.3	0.8	3.5	3.8	5.9	12.4	22.3	28.6	39.4	73.7	3.7	3.1	0.25	0.59	**5.4**	*162*
Other thoracic organs	9	0	0.2	-	-	0.3	-	-	0.2	-	-	-	-	-	-	0.8	2.1	0.8	0.1	0.1	0.00	0.02	**0.1**	*163-4*
Bone	43	0	0.2	0.4	1.1	0.7	0.8	-	-	-	0.3	0.7	-	1.5	1.8	0.8	3.1	3.4	0.6	0.5	0.04	0.06	**0.6**	*170*
Connective tissue	79	0	0.8	-	0.4	0.4	0.8	1.0	1.2	0.6	1.4	1.0	3.0	1.5	1.8	4.6	5.2	8.4	1.1	0.9	0.07	0.12	**1.3**	*171*
Mesothelioma	4	0	-	-	-	-	-	-	-	-	-	0.3	-	0.5	-	-	2.1	-	0.1	0.0	0.00	0.01	**0.1**	*MES*
Kaposi's sarcoma	5	0	-	-	-	-	-	-	0.2	0.2	-	-	-	-	-	0.8	-	1.7	0.1	0.1	0.00	0.01	**0.1**	*KAP*
Melanoma of skin	96	1	-	-	-	-	-	0.3	1.3	0.8	3.5	2.8	2.5	1.5	4.8	10.0	13.5	14.2	1.3	1.1	0.09	0.21	**1.8**	*172*
Other skin	2001	45	0.2	0.1	0.2	1.4	3.2	3.8	6.9	18.8	26.2	38.8	56.3	72.7	120.1	167.0	254.3	513.4	26.9		1.78	3.94	**37.9**	*173*
Breast	1513	6	-	-	-	-	0.7	3.0	10.0	23.5	46.2	70.2	67.3	91.0	95.9	100.5	115.2	162.5	20.3	17.0	2.05	3.13	**28.8**	*174*
Uterus unspecified	50	0	-	-	-	-	-	0.1	0.3	0.2	1.9	1.4	1.3	3.0	0.6	2.3	4.2	15.1	0.7	0.6	0.04	0.08	**0.9**	*179*
Cervix uteri	1381	6	-	-	-	-	2.2	11.0	21.7	31.0	41.1	48.2	61.8	59.8	70.6	81.2	84.1	121.4	18.5	15.5	1.74	2.57	**24.5**	*180*
Placenta	14	0	-	-	-	0.1	0.1	-	0.3	0.6	1.4	-	0.4	-	-	1.0	-	-	0.2	0.2	0.02	0.02	**0.2**	*181*
Corpus uteri	217	0	-	-	-	0.1	-	0.3	0.5	0.8	2.7	4.9	10.2	18.3	24.7	23.2	23.9	23.5	2.9	2.4	0.31	0.55	**4.4**	*182*
Ovary etc.	330	0	-	-	1.2	1.7	1.4	2.3	2.7	4.6	6.2	9.8	15.7	12.9	16.9	27.8	18.7	40.2	4.4	3.7	0.38	0.61	**5.9**	*183*
Other female genital	84	1	-	-	-	0.1	-	-	0.3	1.3	0.3	1.4	1.3	3.5	4.8	7.0	10.4	26.8	1.1	0.9	0.07	0.15	**1.6**	*184*
†Bladder	85	1	-	-	-	0.1	0.3	-	0.2	0.6	0.3	0.7	1.3	4.0	6.0	10.0	10.4	25.1	1.1	1.0	0.07	0.17	**1.6**	*188*
Kidney etc.	115	0	1.0	0.3	0.2	0.1	0.1	-	0.2	0.4	2.2	1.0	3.0	5.4	13.3	9.3	10.4	18.4	1.5	1.3	0.14	0.24	**2.2**	*189*
Eye	28	0	1.3	0.1	0.1	-	-	-	0.3	0.4	0.5	-	0.4	1.0	-	2.3	-	1.7	0.4	0.3	0.02	0.03	**0.4**	*190*
Brain, nervous system	245	0	2.8	1.6	1.6	1.4	0.8	2.2	3.2	4.2	5.4	3.8	6.3	7.4	7.2	17.8	10.4	12.6	3.3	2.7	0.24	0.38	**3.9**	*191-2*
Thyroid	315	1	-	-	-	0.7	2.9	4.6	6.0	7.5	8.1	10.8	12.7	11.9	10.9	12.4	21.8	11.7	4.2	3.5	0.38	0.55	**5.2**	*193*
Other endocrine	11	0	0.5	-	0.1	-	0.1	0.1	-	0.2	0.3	-	-	-	-	0.8	-	-	0.1	0.1	0.01	0.01	**0.1**	*194*
Hodgkin's disease	94	0	0.5	0.1	0.7	2.1	1.5	2.0	1.3	0.6	0.8	-	1.3	1.0	4.2	3.9	3.1	6.7	1.3	1.1	0.08	0.12	**1.4**	*201*
Non-Hodgkin lymphoma	204	1	0.3	1.0	0.7	1.3	0.6	1.3	1.8	0.8	1.6	4.2	5.9	7.9	10.3	17.8	21.8	32.7	2.7	2.3	0.19	0.39	**3.6**	*200,202*
Multiple myeloma	81	0	-	-	-	-	-	-	-	0.2	0.8	1.0	3.8	3.5	4.2	10.8	12.5	20.9	1.1	0.9	0.07	0.18	**1.6**	*203*
Lymphoid leukaemia	200	1	5.1	4.8	2.7	2.0	0.4	1.0	0.7	0.4	0.8	3.1	3.0	2.0	2.4	4.6	10.4	10.1	2.7	2.2	0.14	0.22	**2.8**	*204*
Myeloid leukaemia	162	2	1.0	0.8	0.6	1.0	1.8	2.7	1.3	2.1	2.7	1.0	4.7	3.5	7.2	5.4	6.2	20.9	2.2	1.8	0.15	0.21	**2.5**	*205*
Monocytic leukaemia	4	0	-	0.1	-	-	-	-	-	-	-	-	-	-	-	-	2.1	0.8	0.1	0.0	0.00	0.01	**0.1**	*206*
Other leukaemia	1	0	-	-	-	-	0.1	-	-	-	-	-	-	-	-	-	-	-	0.0	0.0	0.00	0.00	**0.0**	*207*
Leukaemia unspecified	47	0	0.2	-	0.1	0.3	0.1	0.3	0.2	0.6	-	2.4	0.8	1.0	0.6	3.9	3.1	12.6	0.6	0.5	0.03	0.07	**0.8**	*208*
Other and unspecified	435	2	0.6	0.3	0.4	0.1	0.6	0.7	2.2	1.7	3.5	7.3	14.0	18.8	29.0	41.7	50.9	112.2	5.8	4.9	0.40	0.86	**8.3**	*O&U*
All sites	10919	83	15.8	10.1	11.2	16.0	21.9	40.5	71.2	117.5	187.9	259.6	346.0	445.6	628.7	847.1	1139.7	2156.6	146.5		10.94	20.95	**201.7**	*ALL*
All sites but 173	8918	38	15.6	9.9	10.9	14.6	18.6	36.7	64.4	98.6	161.7	220.8	289.7	372.9	508.6	680.2	885.4	1643.2	119.7	100.0	9.16	17.02	**163.8**	*ALLb*

Rate from 1 case			0.104	0.112	0.124	0.142	0.140	0.145	0.167	0.209	0.270	0.349	0.423	0.495	0.603	0.773	1.038	0.838

†Important: see notes on population page

Ecuador, Quito

The National Cancer Registry of Ecuador was created in 1983 with the initial collaboration of PAHO/WHO. In 1984 the legal basis for the registry was established through a ministerial decree in which the Society for the Fight against Cancer, Quito section, was declared as the responsible institution, and the Society has also provided the financial support for the registry's activities so far. The registry depends on a Steering Committee and the President of the Society.

The registry's staff comprises a pathologist, who is the director of the registry, two epidemiologists, one in charge of the work of the registry and the other responsible for epidemiological research, who also acts as a consultant for the clinical research carried out by hospital physicians, and four registrars, one of them being a computer technician.

The registry has collected information on all cancer cases occurring in the City of Quito for 11 years, and has also promoted the creation of other registries in several towns in Ecuador. However, only one of these registries, covering the town of Portoviejo, has achieved an adequate degree of development. Another project supported by the Quito registry is the Hospital Cancer Registry in the Social Security Hospital, the largest hospital in the city.

The registry covers the town of Quito, the capital of Ecuador, with an area of 19 km^2, situated at 2810 m above sea level, in the Andes Cordillera. The town is surrounded by mountains and the average temperature is 17°C. The main industries in the city are textiles, food, plastics, drinks and metallurgy.

According to the 1990 census, Quito had a population of 1 187 000 inhabitants and a high annual rate of population growth (3.2%), mainly due to migration of farm workers. A high percentage of the population are of mixed race and the major religion is Catholic. Approximately 50% are under 20 years old.

The active population amounts to 46% of the total, and is distributed between economic sectors as follows: 59% in the tertiary sector, 24% in the secondary sector and 11% in the primary sector. There is a high percentage of self-employed workers (informal economy). As regards education, 4% of the population are illiterate, 38% have primary studies, 38% secondary studies and 17% higher studies.

The main hospitals rely on the Ministry of Public Health and the largest one, with 700 beds, belongs to the Institute of Social Security, attended by affiliated workers and, at the present time, a large group of farm workers.

There are many private clinics and surgeries as well as other autonomous or semi-autonomous services, such as the Society for the Fight against Cancer, the Municipality, the Childhood and Family Institute and religious organizations which own hospitals and surgeries.

The sources of information for the registry are the pathology and haematology laboratories, whether public or private, clinical records of public and private hospitals, as well as their statistics departments, radiotherapy services and medical surgeries. The registry has access to death certificates collected by the National Institute of Statistics and Censuses, and to the Hospital Discharge Survey from the same institution.

Cases are recorded on specially designed forms, and pathologists collaborate voluntarily writing down the morphological diagnosis, topographic site of the sample and the basis of diagnosis. This collaboration has always been very successful. All other data collection is active. Registrars review pathology archives and clinical records, and also interview private physicians. Collaboration at all levels is voluntary and an already high level of cooperation has increased as professionals have realized the importance of the registry.

No active follow-up is performed. Death registration is passive by review of death certificates.

The internal procedures for processing the information collected comprise several steps: quality control (internal consistency), coding (again controlling for quality), detection of duplicates (approximately 40% of collected forms are duplicates). Then electronic processing is carried out with software developed in the registry, which also runs quality and validation controls. Before publishing reports, a last quality control is performed, checking for consistency between morphology, site and age.

The majority of the scientific papers on cancer submitted to congresses or published in either national or international journals make use of the registry data.

A report, *Cáncer en Quito*, has been published annually since the registry began operating. The last two were prepared in both Spanish and English, and presented data coded to the second edition of ICD-O.

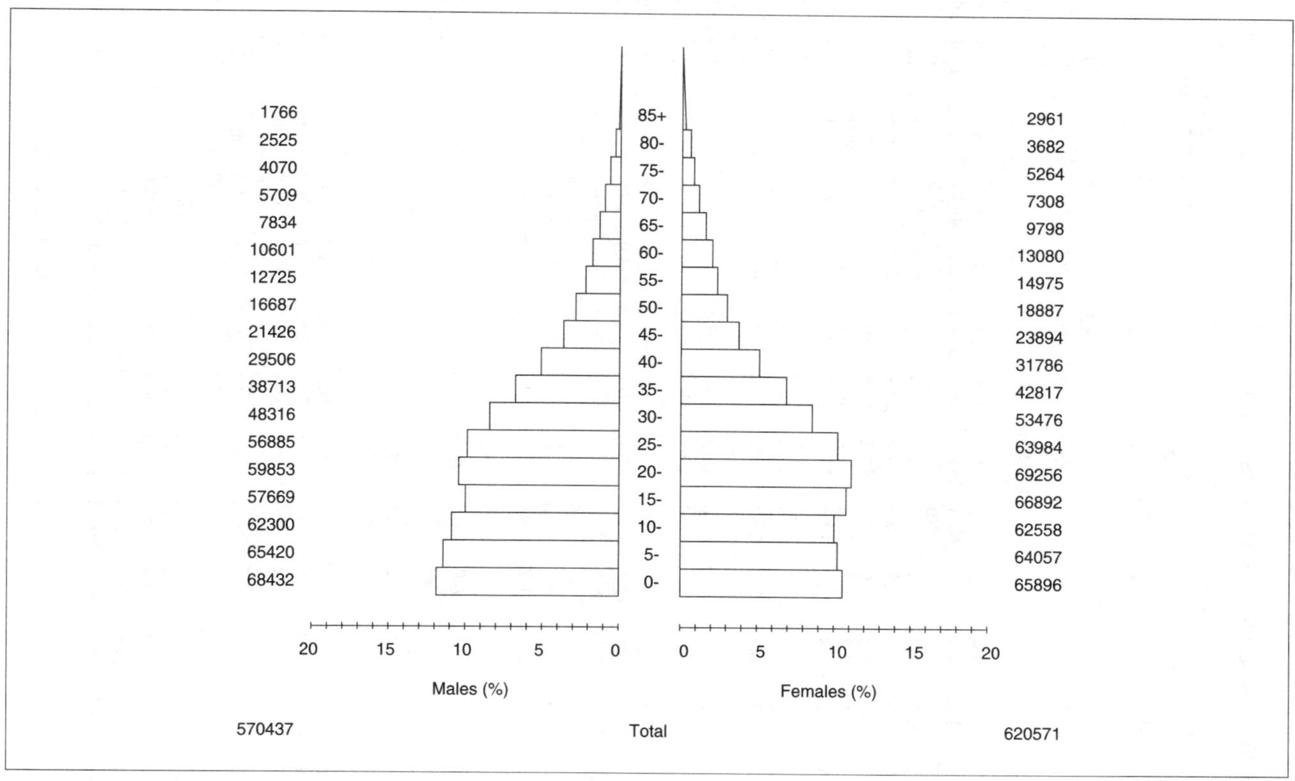

Ecuador, Quito

Source of population: average annual 1988–92
Census: 1990. Corrected for the non-response rate and for migration. Instituto Nacional de Estadística y Censos INEC. Censo de Población y IV de Vivienda 1990. Resultados Definitivos. Provincia de Pichincha. Ed. INEC. Quito, Ecuador, 1991.
Estimate: The populations for 1988 and 1989 were adjusted with the results of the 1982 and 1992 censuses. The populations for 1991 and 1992 were projected from the 1992 census, taking into account birth, deaths and migration.

Notes to tables overleaf:

* The high proportion of diagnoses based on a death certificate alone (DCO), in particular associated with the low level of lung cancer, suggests under-ascertainment.
Note: The change in the rates is probably due to a change in the population, estimated for Volume VI and based on a more recent Census for Volume VII.
† 188 does not include non-invasive tumours.

* ECUADOR, QUITO 1988-1992

ANNUAL INCIDENCE PER 100,000 BY AGE GROUP (YEARS) - MALE

SITE	ALL AGES	AGE UNK	0-	5-	10-	15-	20-	25-	30-	35-	40-	45-	50-	55-	60-	65-	70-	75-	80-	85+	CRUDE RATE	%	CR 64	CR 74	ASR (W)	ICD (9th)
Lip	3	0	-	-	-	-	-	-	-	-	0.7	-	-	1.6	-	2.6	-	-	-	-	0.1	0.1	0.01	0.02	0.2	140
Tongue	7	1	-	-	-	-	-	-	-	-	0.7	-	1.2	-	1.9	-	3.5	9.8	-	-	0.2	0.3	0.02	0.04	0.4	141
Salivary gland	9	0	-	-	-	-	-	-	-	0.5	0.7	-	-	3.1	-	5.1	-	14.7	-	-	0.3	0.3	0.02	0.05	0.5	142
Mouth	11	0	-	-	-	-	-	-	-	-	0.7	0.9	-	1.6	7.5	-	3.5	9.8	7.9	-	0.4	0.4	0.05	0.07	0.7	143-5
Oropharynx	3	0	-	-	-	-	-	-	-	-	-	-	-	-	-	2.6	-	9.8	-	-	0.1	0.1	0.00	0.01	0.2	146
Nasopharynx	2	1	-	-	0.3	-	-	-	-	-	-	-	-	-	-	-	-	-	-	-	0.1	0.1	0.00	0.00	0.1	147
Hypopharynx	0	0	-	-	-	-	-	-	-	-	-	-	-	-	-	-	-	-	-	-	0.0	0.0	0.00	0.00	0.0	148
Pharynx unspecified	3	0	-	-	-	-	-	-	-	-	-	-	-	-	1.6	-	2.6	-	-	11.3	0.1	0.1	0.01	0.02	0.2	149
Oesophagus	51	1	-	-	-	-	0.3	0.4	-	-	-	0.9	3.6	6.3	11.3	25.5	17.5	24.6	55.4	79.2	1.8	1.9	0.12	0.34	3.1	150
Stomach	543	21	-	-	-	-	0.7	1.4	5.8	9.3	14.9	23.3	52.7	64.4	145.3	196.6	224.2	235.9	483.1	283.0	19.0	20.5	1.65	3.84	32.2	151
Small intestine	12	0	-	-	-	-	-	-	0.4	0.5	-	-	-	1.6	7.5	5.1	3.5	4.9	7.9	-	0.4	0.5	0.05	0.09	0.7	152
Colon	64	1	-	-	-	-	0.3	-	0.4	1.0	0.7	2.8	2.4	6.3	15.1	17.9	52.5	54.1	23.8	56.6	2.2	2.4	0.15	0.51	3.9	153
Rectum	59	0	-	-	-	-	0.3	0.4	-	1.5	2.0	2.8	4.8	9.4	9.4	28.1	14.0	24.6	79.2	34.0	2.1	2.2	0.15	0.36	3.4	154
Liver	49	0	-	-	-	0.3	-	-	-	-	1.9	3.6	7.9	13.2	12.8	10.5	54.1	31.7	90.6	1.7	1.8	0.13	0.25	2.9	155
Gallbladder etc.	94	2	-	-	-	-	-	-	0.8	1.5	4.1	2.8	1.2	9.4	9.4	40.8	52.5	88.4	71.3	90.6	3.3	3.5	0.15	0.63	5.5	156
Pancreas	64	0	-	-	-	-	-	0.4	-	0.5	1.4	2.8	3.6	12.6	11.3	20.4	31.5	29.5	63.4	101.9	2.2	2.4	0.16	0.42	3.8	157
Nose, sinuses etc.	9	0	-	0.3	-	-	-	0.7	-	0.5	-	-	1.2	-	1.9	2.6	-	4.9	-	11.3	0.3	0.3	0.02	0.04	0.4	160
Larynx	24	0	-	-	-	-	-	-	-	0.5	1.4	-	-	6.3	5.7	5.1	17.5	14.7	7.9	34.0	0.8	0.9	0.07	0.18	1.5	161
Bronchus, lung	172	4	-	-	-	-	-	0.4	0.8	2.1	3.4	6.5	7.2	26.7	41.5	46.0	87.6	142.5	166.3	124.5	6.0	6.5	0.45	1.14	10.1	162
Other thoracic organs	0	0	-	-	-	-	-	-	-	-	-	-	-	-	-	-	-	-	-	-	0.0	0.0	0.00	0.00	0.0	163-4
Bone	27	0	0.3	-	1.3	2.4	1.0	1.8	1.2	-	0.7	-	-	1.6	1.9	-	3.5	-	-	-	0.9	1.0	0.06	0.08	0.9	170
Connective tissue	61	0	1.5	0.6	-	2.1	1.0	0.7	2.1	3.1	2.7	1.9	8.4	6.3	5.7	10.2	7.0	9.8	15.8	22.6	2.1	2.3	0.18	0.27	2.8	171
Mesothelioma	0	0	-	-	-	-	-	-	-	-	-	-	-	-	-	-	-	-	-	-	0.0	0.0	0.00	0.00	0.0	MES
Kaposi's sarcoma	2	0	-	-	-	-	-	-	-	-	0.7	-	1.2	-	-	-	-	-	-	-	0.1	0.1	0.01	0.01	0.1	KAP
Melanoma of skin	59	1	-	0.3	-	-	0.3	0.7	1.7	0.5	4.7	3.7	12.0	4.7	7.5	20.4	31.5	4.9	23.8	-	2.1	2.2	0.18	0.45	3.3	172
Other skin	380	1	-	-	-	-	-	1.8	6.6	10.3	12.9	16.8	39.6	51.9	107.5	89.4	161.1	201.5	261.4	260.4	13.3		1.24	2.50	21.9	173
Breast	6	1	-	-	-	-	-	0.4	-	-	-	-	-	1.6	-	-	3.5	-	7.9	11.3	0.2	0.2	0.01	0.03	0.3	175
Prostate	386	4	-	-	-	-	0.3	-	-	-	1.4	1.9	7.2	33.0	56.6	114.9	238.2	383.3	633.6	554.7	13.5	14.6	0.51	2.29	22.4	185
Testis	108	1	1.2	-	0.3	2.1	5.3	8.4	10.8	5.7	5.4	5.6	1.2	3.1	3.8	-	-	-	-	-	3.8	4.1	0.27	0.27	3.5	186
Penis	10	0	-	-	-	-	-	-	-	1.0	2.0	-	1.2	3.1	-	2.6	-	-	7.9	-	0.4	0.4	0.04	0.05	0.5	187.1-.4
Other male genital	2	0	-	-	-	-	-	-	-	-	-	-	-	-	3.8	-	-	-	-	-	0.1	0.1	0.02	0.02	0.2	187.5-.9
†Bladder	88	1	0.3	-	-	-	-	-	0.8	1.5	1.4	2.8	6.0	6.3	28.3	15.3	42.0	73.7	71.3	113.2	3.1	3.3	0.24	0.53	5.1	188
Kidney etc.	42	0	0.3	0.3	-	-	0.3	-	-	-	1.4	2.8	3.6	9.4	11.3	23.0	10.5	14.7	-	45.3	1.5	1.6	0.15	0.31	2.6	189
Eye	19	1	1.2	0.3	0.3	-	-	-	0.4	1.5	-	0.9	-	1.6	1.9	-	7.0	9.8	7.9	-	0.7	0.7	0.04	0.08	0.8	190
Brain, nervous system	60	0	1.2	2.4	1.0	1.7	0.7	1.4	0.8	1.5	2.7	4.7	2.4	4.7	7.5	12.8	14.0	9.8	-	-	2.1	2.3	0.16	0.30	2.8	191-2
Thyroid	51	0	-	0.6	0.6	1.0	1.3	1.4	1.2	3.1	2.0	1.9	2.4	4.7	13.2	10.2	7.0	9.8	7.9	11.3	1.8	1.9	0.17	0.25	2.4	193
Other endocrine	1	0	-	-	-	-	0.3	-	-	-	-	-	-	-	-	-	-	-	-	-	0.0	0.0	0.00	0.00	0.0	194
Hodgkin's disease	36	0	-	0.6	1.6	0.7	1.0	1.8	1.2	1.0	0.7	1.9	1.2	1.6	1.9	10.2	7.0	4.9	-	11.3	1.3	1.4	0.08	0.16	1.5	201
Non-Hodgkin lymphoma	170	1	0.9	3.1	1.6	1.4	3.0	2.5	4.6	4.1	12.2	15.9	10.8	18.9	24.5	25.5	35.0	44.2	71.3	56.6	6.0	6.4	0.52	0.82	8.2	200,202
Multiple myeloma	29	1	-	-	-	-	-	-	0.4	1.0	0.7	-	1.2	1.6	9.4	10.2	14.0	19.7	15.8	34.0	1.0	1.1	0.07	0.20	1.7	203
Lymphoid leukaemia	68	0	4.4	5.8	4.2	2.1	0.3	0.7	-	-	0.7	0.9	1.2	1.6	1.9	5.1	3.5	-	7.9	34.0	2.4	2.6	0.12	0.16	2.5	204
Myeloid leukaemia	81	2	1.5	0.3	1.0	1.7	1.3	1.8	1.7	2.6	5.4	4.7	8.4	7.9	3.8	7.7	24.5	24.6	7.9	45.3	2.8	3.1	0.21	0.38	3.8	205
Monocytic leukaemia	4	0	-	-	-	-	-	-	-	-	-	-	-	-	-	2.6	3.5	4.9	7.9	-	0.1	0.2	0.00	0.03	0.2	206
Other leukaemia	0	0	-	-	-	-	-	-	-	-	-	-	-	-	-	-	-	-	-	-	0.0	0.0	0.00	0.00	0.0	207
Leukaemia unspecified	34	0	0.3	0.6	-	1.0	0.7	-	-	2.1	0.7	-	4.8	4.7	5.7	2.6	7.0	9.8	23.8	34.0	1.2	1.3	0.10	0.15	1.7	208
Other and unspecified	129	3	-	0.6	0.3	0.7	0.3	1.4	1.2	2.6	4.7	8.4	13.2	15.7	17.0	30.6	59.6	78.6	103.0	45.3	4.5	4.9	0.34	0.80	7.1	O&U
All sites	3032	48	12.9	15.9	12.5	17.3	19.0	28.1	43.0	59.9	93.5	119.5	207.3	342.6	594.3	806.7	1198.1	1626.5	2273.1	2196.3	106.3		7.96	18.14	165.8	ALL
All sites but 173	2652	47	12.9	15.9	12.5	17.3	19.0	26.4	36.4	49.6	80.7	102.7	167.8	290.8	486.7	717.4	1036.9	1425.0	2011.7	1935.9	93.0	100.0	6.71	15.64	143.9	ALLb
Rate from 1 case			0.292	0.306	0.321	0.347	0.334	0.352	0.414	0.517	0.678	0.933	1.199	1.572	1.887	2.553	3.503	4.914	7.920	11.321						

†Important: see notes on population page

* ECUADOR, QUITO 1988-1992

ANNUAL INCIDENCE PER 100,000 BY AGE GROUP (YEARS) - FEMALE

SITE	ALL AGES	AGE UNK	0-	5-	10-	15-	20-	25-	30-	35-	40-	45-	50-	55-	60-	65-	70-	75-	80-	85+	CRUDE RATE	%	CR 64	CR 74	ASR (W)	ICD (9th)
Lip	0	0	-	-	-	-	-	-	-	-	-	-	-	-	-	-	-	-	-	-	0.0	0.0	0.00	0.00	0.0	140
Tongue	5	0	-	-	-	-	-	-	0.5	0.6	-	-	-	-	1.5	2.0	2.7	-	-	-	0.2	0.1	0.01	0.04	0.2	141
Salivary gland	9	0	-	-	-	0.3	0.3	-	0.4	-	-	-	-	-	-	-	8.2	3.8	-	13.5	0.3	0.2	0.00	0.05	0.3	142
Mouth	5	0	-	-	-	-	-	-	-	-	1.7	-	1.3	-	-	-	3.8	5.4	-	0.2	0.1	0.02	0.02	0.2	143-5
Oropharynx	2	0	-	-	-	-	0.3	-	-	-	1.1	-	-	-	-	-	-	-	-	-	0.1	0.1	0.01	0.01	0.1	146
Nasopharynx	0	0	-	-	-	-	-	-	-	-	-	-	-	-	-	-	-	-	-	-	0.0	0.0	0.00	0.00	0.0	147
Hypopharynx	0	0	-	-	-	-	-	-	-	-	-	-	-	-	-	-	-	-	-	-	0.0	0.0	0.00	0.00	0.0	148
Pharynx unspecified	1	1	-	-	-	-	-	-	-	-	-	-	-	-	-	-	-	-	-	-	0.0	0.0	0.00	0.00	0.0	149
Oesophagus	26	0	-	-	-	-	-	-	-	0.9	-	1.7	2.1	2.7	6.1	-	2.7	11.4	32.6	27.0	0.8	0.7	0.07	0.08	1.1	150
Stomach	435	7	-	-	-	-	0.6	0.9	4.9	8.4	12.0	17.6	34.9	28.0	52.0	114.3	153.2	231.7	271.5	276.9	14.0	11.5	0.81	2.17	19.5	151
Small intestine	18	1	-	-	-	-	-	0.3	-	0.5	1.3	-	1.1	1.3	3.1	6.1	2.7	3.8	-	27.0	0.6	0.5	0.04	0.09	0.8	152
Colon	121	2	-	-	-	0.6	-	0.6	1.5	1.9	3.1	4.2	11.6	6.7	21.4	32.7	54.7	45.6	48.9	67.5	3.9	3.2	0.26	0.71	5.7	153
Rectum	89	2	-	-	-	0.3	1.2	1.3	1.1	1.4	3.1	1.7	8.5	5.3	15.3	20.4	32.8	38.0	32.6	33.8	2.9	2.3	0.20	0.47	4.0	154
Liver	64	2	-	-	-	-	-	-	-	-	-	3.3	5.3	6.7	13.8	8.2	5.5	38.0	70.6	67.5	2.1	1.7	0.15	0.22	2.8	155
Gallbladder etc.	180	2	-	-	-	-	-	0.3	0.4	1.9	2.5	5.9	19.1	29.4	26.0	51.0	62.9	102.6	76.0	101.3	5.8	4.7	0.43	1.01	8.6	156
Pancreas	91	2	-	-	-	-	-	-	0.7	-	-	2.5	2.1	14.7	16.8	36.7	35.6	41.8	54.3	54.0	2.9	2.4	0.19	0.56	4.4	157
Nose, sinuses etc.	8	0	-	-	-	-	-	-	0.4	-	-	-	-	-	3.1	-	5.5	7.6	5.4	-	0.3	0.2	0.02	0.04	0.4	160
Larynx	6	0	-	-	-	-	-	-	-	0.5	-	-	-	1.3	-	-	2.7	3.8	5.4	6.8	0.2	0.2	0.01	0.02	0.2	161
Bronchus, lung	78	0	-	-	-	-	0.3	-	-	0.9	1.9	6.7	5.3	9.3	6.1	20.4	27.4	49.4	32.6	60.8	2.5	2.1	0.15	0.39	3.6	162
Other thoracic organs	0	0	-	-	-	-	-	-	-	-	-	-	-	-	-	-	-	-	-	-	0.0	0.0	0.00	0.00	0.0	163-4
Bone	27	1	0.3	0.3	1.0	1.2	2.0	-	1.5	0.5	-	-	1.1	-	-	-	5.5	3.8	5.4	-	0.9	0.7	0.04	0.07	0.8	170
Connective tissue	44	0	-	0.3	0.6	0.3	1.4	0.6	1.1	2.3	3.1	2.5	4.2	2.7	6.1	2.0	5.5	7.6	5.4	6.8	1.4	1.2	0.13	0.16	1.7	171
Mesothelioma	0	0	-	-	-	-	-	-	-	-	-	-	-	-	-	-	-	-	-	-	0.0	0.0	0.00	0.00	0.0	MES
Kaposi's sarcoma	2	0	-	-	-	-	-	-	-	-	-	-	-	-	1.5	-	2.7	-	-	-	0.1	0.1	0.01	0.02	0.1	KAP
Melanoma of skin	80	0	-	-	-	0.6	0.3	1.3	1.9	0.5	3.8	5.9	4.2	13.4	16.8	20.4	19.2	19.0	10.9	33.8	2.6	2.1	0.24	0.44	3.7	172
Other skin	494	6	-	0.3	1.0	0.3	0.6	1.3	4.5	12.6	17.0	19.3	29.7	53.4	87.2	136.8	131.4	205.1	271.5	297.2	15.9		1.15	2.51	22.5	173
Breast	580	1	-	-	-	-	0.3	1.6	7.9	27.6	46.6	50.2	82.6	93.5	94.8	91.8	109.5	87.4	124.9	121.6	18.7	15.3	2.03	3.04	26.8	174
Uterus unspecified	55	1	-	-	-	-	-	0.6	0.4	0.5	1.9	1.7	7.4	8.0	3.1	16.3	16.4	19.0	32.6	40.5	1.8	1.5	0.12	0.28	2.5	179
Cervix uteri	697	6	-	-	-	0.9	1.7	5.0	15.7	36.4	46.6	65.3	90.0	113.5	87.2	134.7	131.4	83.6	119.5	60.8	22.5	18.4	2.33	3.67	31.7	180
Placenta	10	0	-	-	-	0.3	0.3	0.9	0.7	0.5	0.6	0.8	-	-	-	-	-	-	-	-	0.3	0.3	0.02	0.02	0.3	181
Corpus uteri	106	0	-	-	-	-	0.3	0.6	0.4	0.9	5.7	5.0	14.8	17.4	27.5	32.7	21.9	19.0	38.0	27.0	3.4	2.8	0.36	0.64	5.3	182
Ovary etc.	146	2	-	0.3	1.9	1.8	1.4	0.6	4.1	6.1	8.8	12.6	14.8	26.7	19.9	14.3	21.9	19.0	5.4	20.3	4.7	3.8	0.50	0.69	6.3	183
Other female genital	15	0	-	-	-	-	-	-	-	0.5	-	0.8	-	1.3	1.5	6.1	10.9	11.4	5.4	-	0.5	0.4	0.02	0.11	0.7	184
†Bladder	33	0	-	-	-	-	0.3	-	-	-	-	1.7	2.1	-	4.6	10.2	13.7	22.8	27.2	27.0	1.1	0.9	0.04	0.16	1.5	188
Kidney etc.	29	0	0.3	0.6	-	-	-	0.3	0.7	0.5	-	0.8	6.4	5.3	4.6	6.1	2.7	7.6	-	13.5	0.9	0.8	0.10	0.14	1.3	189
Eye	21	0	2.1	0.3	-	-	-	-	0.4	-	1.3	1.7	-	2.7	3.1	-	2.7	7.6	-	6.8	0.7	0.6	0.06	0.07	0.9	190
Brain, nervous system	51	1	0.6	0.3	0.6	1.2	1.7	0.6	1.9	0.9	1.9	0.8	3.2	6.7	7.6	4.1	2.7	3.8	21.7	6.8	1.6	1.3	0.14	0.18	1.9	191-2
Thyroid	194	2	-	-	-	1.2	2.6	7.8	9.3	6.5	10.1	13.4	15.9	16.0	12.2	20.4	30.1	38.0	59.7	40.5	6.3	5.1	0.48	0.74	7.4	193
Other endocrine	2	0	-	-	-	-	-	-	-	-	0.6	-	-	-	1.5	-	-	-	-	-	0.1	0.1	0.01	0.01	0.1	194
Hodgkin's disease	34	0	0.3	0.9	0.6	-	0.9	1.3	1.1	0.9	2.5	0.8	4.2	1.3	3.1	2.0	5.5	3.8	-	-	1.1	0.9	0.09	0.13	1.3	201
Non-Hodgkin lymphoma	140	1	0.3	1.6	0.6	1.5	0.3	1.3	4.9	4.2	5.0	5.9	7.4	18.7	16.8	28.6	43.8	41.8	48.9	13.5	4.5	3.7	0.34	0.71	6.0	200,202
Multiple myeloma	20	0	-	-	-	-	-	-	-	-	1.3	0.8	3.2	-	4.6	4.1	10.9	11.4	10.9	-	0.6	0.5	0.05	0.12	1.0	203
Lymphoid leukaemia	69	0	3.3	2.8	2.2	3.3	1.7	1.3	1.1	-	1.9	-	1.1	1.3	4.6	8.2	8.2	11.4	-	-	2.2	1.8	0.12	0.21	2.4	204
Myeloid leukaemia	65	2	0.6	0.3	0.6	2.1	1.2	0.6	2.6	2.3	2.5	3.3	1.1	5.3	3.1	6.1	8.2	15.2	27.2	20.3	2.1	1.7	0.13	0.21	2.3	205
Monocytic leukaemia	4	0	0.3	-	0.3	0.3	-	-	-	-	-	-	-	-	-	-	-	3.8	-	-	0.1	0.1	0.00	0.00	0.1	206
Other leukaemia	0	0	-	-	-	-	-	-	-	-	-	-	-	-	-	-	-	-	-	-	0.0	0.0	0.00	0.00	0.0	207
Leukaemia unspecified	27	2	0.6	0.3	0.6	0.3	-	0.6	0.7	0.9	0.6	-	2.1	2.7	1.5	2.0	2.7	7.6	10.9	6.8	0.9	0.7	0.06	0.09	1.0	208
Other and unspecified	204	2	-	-	-	0.3	0.6	0.6	3.7	2.3	5.7	10.0	8.5	28.0	39.8	55.1	43.8	87.4	114.0	128.3	6.6	5.4	0.50	1.00	9.3	O&U
All sites	4287	45	8.8	8.4	10.2	16.7	19.9	30.6	74.1	123.8	191.9	248.6	395.0	524.8	617.7	894.0	1048.1	1318.2	1574.9	1607.6	138.2		11.47	21.29	191.0	ALL
All sites but 173	3793	39	8.8	8.1	9.3	16.4	19.3	29.4	69.6	111.2	174.9	229.3	365.3	471.4	530.6	757.2	916.8	1113.1	1303.4	1310.4	122.2	100.0	10.32	18.78	168.5	ALLb

Rate from 1 case			0.304	0.312	0.320	0.299	0.289	0.313	0.374	0.467	0.629	0.837	1.059	1.335	1.529	2.041	2.737	3.799	5.431	6.754

†Important: see notes on population page

121

Peru, Trujillo

The Trujillo Cancer Registry began as an histological registry in 1983 and became population-based in 1984. It was officially recognized by the Ministry of Health in 1990. The registry is located in the pathology department of the largest hospital in the city. Two other general hospitals are subcentres of the registry. It operates under a cooperative agreement between the National University of Trujillo and IARC.

The city of Trujillo, capital of the Departamento de La Libertad, is located on the coast of Peru, 560 km north of Lima, the nation's capital. The city lies 34 m above the sea level and is situated at 8° S and 79.1° W. The climate is semitropical with an average of 22.2°C maximum and 15°C minimum. The average annual rainfall is less than 20 mm. The registration area covers 314 km² and includes the district of Trujillo as well as four poor suburban communities containing 52% of the population of metropolitan Trujillo, largely immigrants from the Andean region. The majority of people are mestizos (a mixture of Spanish and Indian).

The population in 1989 was 456 077 (density 1452 inhabitants per km²). More than one third (38%) are younger than 15 years and only 6.6% are 60 years of age or older. The population is 98% urban. Almost 90% are Roman Catholics. The annual rate of population growth is 2%. Illiteracy is 6.3% among those older than 15 years of age.

In 1993, the overall mortality rate was 4.21 per 1000. Infant mortality was 27%. In 1994, 20% of all deaths were attributed to cardiovascular conditions and cancer ranked second with 19%. A nutritional survey performed in 1993 revealed that 27% of six-year old children suffered from chronic malnutrition.

Sanitation is inadequate. 70% of the population have provision of drinking water from the public supply and 64% are connected to public sewerage. Electricity is available in 81% of houses.

The economically active population in 1993 represented 38% of the total. The main economic activities were commerce and services, 64%; manufacturing and construction 25%; and agriculture and fishing, 11%.

Trujillo has a faculty of medical sciences with schools of medicine and of dentistry, and a faculty of nursing. There are three major general hospitals with a total of 770 beds and two major private clinics with 100 beds, as well as one radiotherapy department with a telecobalt unit. 14 qualified oncologists work in the area. The League for the Fight Against Cancer conducts a programme for prevention of cervix cancer, but in 1993 only 20% of the female population at risk for cervical cancer was screened.

Data for the registry are collected from the three major hospitals, from private clinics, and from oncologists, radiologists and pathologists. In the private sector, collection is carried out by medical students trained for the work. In general, the information is not easily available and the process of collection is slow. Cancer mortality data are obtained from the death certificates and Municipal Civil Registries. Death certificates mentioning cancer for cases not previously registered are traced back through the certifying doctor or by visiting the family of the deceased for additional information. Duplicates are avoided by using an alphabetical file for all registrations. Site and histology are coded according to ICD-O. The minimal identification details entered into the computer are: name, sex, date of birth, age and address of usual residence of the patient; the site and histology of the tumour, incidence date, most valid basis of diagnosis and source of information are registered. No follow-up of cases is attempted on grounds of cost. The second version of CANREG is used in the processing of data and for validation the IARC CHECK program.

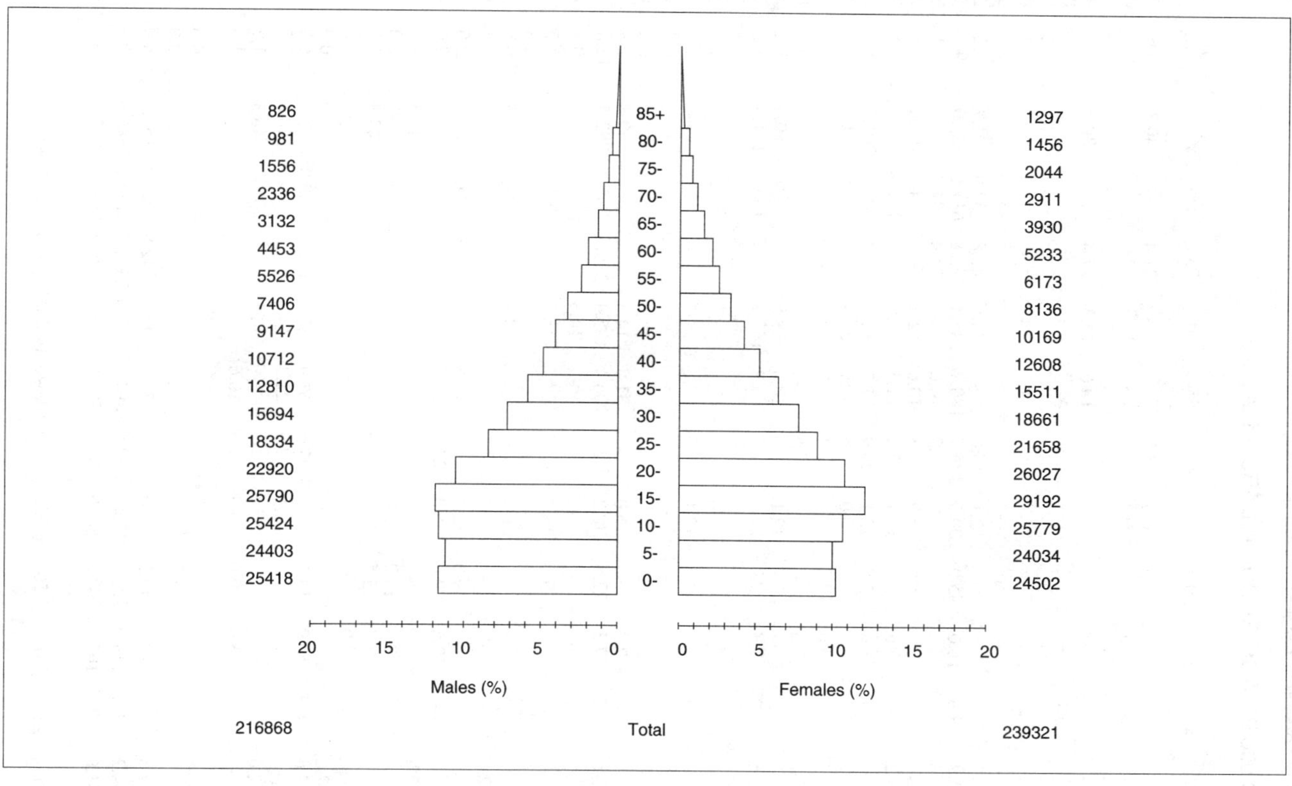

Peru, Trujillo
Source of population: average annual 1988–90
Census: Censos Nacionales: VIII de Poblacion y III de Vivienda (12 de Julio de 1981), Resultados Definitivos, Volumen A, Tomo 1, Departamento de la Libertad, Instituto Nacional de Estadistica, Lima, Peru, Enero 1984.
Censos Nacionales: IX de Poblacion y IV de Vivienda (11 de Julio de 1993), Resultados Definitivos a nivel Provincial y Distrital (Departamento de La Libertad, Provincia de Trujillo). Tomo 1. Direccion Nacional de Censos y Encuestas. Instituto Nacional de Estadistica e Informatica. Lima, Mayo de 1994.

Estimate: The population data were estimated by linear interpolation on the basis of the 1981 and 1993 National Censuses. The projection was made by sex and age-group.
Notes to tables overleaf:
† 188 does not include non-invasive tumours.

PERU, TRUJILLO 1988-1990

ANNUAL INCIDENCE PER 100,000 BY AGE GROUP (YEARS) - MALE

SITE	ALL AGES	AGE UNK	0-	5-	10-	15-	20-	25-	30-	35-	40-	45-	50-	55-	60-	65-	70-	75-	80-	85+	CRUDE RATE	%	CR 64	CR 74	ASR (W)	ICD (9th)
Lip	4	0	-	-	-	-	-	-	-	-	-	-	-	6.0	7.5	-	-	21.4	-	40.3	0.6	0.6	0.07	0.07	**1.0**	140
Tongue	3	0	-	-	-	-	-	-	-	-	-	3.6	-	6.0	-	-	14.3	-	-	-	0.5	0.5	0.05	0.12	**0.7**	141
Salivary gland	0	0	-	-	-	-	-	-	-	-	-	-	-	-	-	-	-	-	-	-	0.0	0.0	0.00	0.00	**0.0**	142
Mouth	6	0	-	-	-	-	1.5	-	-	-	-	-	-	-	-	10.6	14.3	21.4	-	80.7	0.9	0.9	0.01	0.13	**1.3**	143-5
Oropharynx	4	0	-	-	-	-	-	-	-	-	3.1	-	-	-	-	31.9	-	-	-	-	0.6	0.6	0.02	0.18	**1.1**	146
Nasopharynx	1	0	-	-	-	-	-	-	-	-	-	-	-	-	7.5	-	-	-	-	-	0.2	0.2	0.04	0.04	**0.3**	147
Hypopharynx	2	0	-	-	-	-	-	-	-	-	-	-	-	-	-	21.3	-	-	-	-	0.3	0.3	0.00	0.11	**0.6**	148
Pharynx unspecified	2	0	-	-	-	-	-	-	-	2.6	-	-	-	-	-	-	-	-	34.0	-	0.3	0.3	0.01	0.01	**0.3**	149
Oesophagus	14	0	-	-	-	-	-	-	-	-	-	-	-	-	12.1	15.0	-	28.5	42.8	34.0	201.7	2.2	2.1	0.14	0.28	**3.3**	150
Stomach	128	2	-	-	-	-	1.5	-	12.7	5.2	9.3	14.6	45.0	90.5	134.7	180.9	285.3	192.8	611.6	121.0	19.7	19.5	1.59	3.96	**31.1**	151
Small intestine	7	1	-	-	-	1.3	-	-	-	2.6	-	-	-	-	7.5	10.6	-	21.4	34.0	-	1.1	1.1	0.07	0.13	**1.5**	152
Colon	20	0	-	-	-	-	2.9	-	2.1	-	-	7.3	4.5	6.0	7.5	10.6	42.8	64.3	34.0	161.4	3.1	3.1	0.15	0.42	**4.4**	153
Rectum	16	0	-	-	-	-	-	-	2.1	5.2	-	3.6	-	12.1	22.5	21.3	28.5	-	101.9	-	2.5	2.4	0.23	0.48	**3.8**	154
Liver	33	0	-	1.4	1.3	-	1.5	1.8	-	-	3.1	3.6	22.5	12.1	29.9	21.3	14.3	107.1	101.9	201.7	5.1	5.0	0.39	0.56	**7.2**	155
Gallbladder etc.	16	0	-	-	-	-	-	-	-	-	3.1	-	-	6.0	7.5	31.9	28.5	42.8	68.0	161.4	2.5	2.4	0.08	0.39	**3.8**	156
Pancreas	21	0	-	-	-	-	-	-	-	-	-	3.6	13.5	-	52.4	42.6	28.5	64.3	34.0	-	3.2	3.2	0.35	0.70	**5.6**	157
Nose, sinuses etc.	2	0	-	-	-	-	-	-	-	-	-	3.6	-	-	7.5	-	-	-	-	-	0.3	0.3	0.06	0.06	**0.5**	160
Larynx	8	0	-	-	-	-	-	-	-	-	-	-	-	12.1	15.0	10.6	28.5	-	-	40.3	1.2	1.2	0.14	0.33	**2.2**	161
Bronchus, lung	47	0	-	-	-	-	-	-	2.1	2.6	3.1	7.3	9.0	24.1	67.4	63.9	142.7	85.7	135.9	121.0	7.2	7.2	0.58	1.61	**11.9**	162
Other thoracic organs	3	0	1.3	-	1.3	-	-	-	-	-	-	-	-	-	-	-	-	21.4	-	-	0.5	0.5	0.01	0.01	**0.5**	163-4
Bone	7	1	-	1.4	-	3.9	-	1.8	-	-	-	-	-	6.0	-	-	-	-	-	-	1.1	1.1	0.08	0.08	**1.0**	170
Connective tissue	7	0	-	-	-	-	-	3.6	-	-	3.1	-	4.5	12.1	7.5	-	-	-	-	-	1.1	1.1	0.15	0.15	**1.5**	171
Mesothelioma	0	0	-	-	-	-	-	-	-	-	-	-	-	-	-	-	-	-	-	-	0.0	0.0	0.00	0.00	**0.0**	MES
Kaposi's sarcoma	1	0	-	-	-	-	-	-	-	-	-	-	-	-	-	14.3	-	-	-	-	0.2	0.2	0.00	0.07	**0.3**	KAP
Melanoma of skin	12	2	-	-	-	-	-	-	-	-	-	7.3	9.0	6.0	-	31.9	14.3	-	-	40.3	1.8	1.8	0.13	0.41	**3.1**	172
Other skin	77	3	-	-	-	1.3	-	-	2.1	2.6	6.2	7.3	22.5	30.2	52.4	106.4	185.4	235.6	305.8	282.4	11.8		0.65	2.17	**18.6**	173
Breast	1	0	-	-	-	-	-	-	-	-	-	-	-	-	-	14.3	-	-	-	-	0.2	0.2	0.00	0.07	**0.3**	175
Prostate	89	1	-	-	-	-	-	-	-	-	-	-	9.0	18.1	67.4	127.7	256.8	406.9	441.7	484.1	13.7	13.6	0.48	2.42	**21.8**	185
Testis	17	0	1.3	-	-	3.9	1.5	9.1	10.6	2.6	3.1	-	-	-	-	-	-	-	-	-	2.6	2.6	0.16	0.16	**2.3**	186
Penis	5	0	-	-	-	-	-	-	-	-	3.1	-	-	6.0	-	-	14.3	-	34.0	40.3	0.8	0.8	0.05	0.12	**1.1**	187.1-.4
Other male genital	2	0	-	-	-	-	-	-	-	2.6	-	-	-	-	-	14.3	-	-	-	-	0.3	0.3	0.01	0.08	**0.4**	187.5-.9
†Bladder	13	1	-	-	-	-	-	1.8	-	-	3.1	-	9.0	12.1	-	10.6	-	42.8	34.0	80.7	2.0	2.0	0.14	0.20	**2.8**	188
Kidney etc.	13	0	3.9	-	-	-	-	-	-	-	-	3.6	9.0	6.0	22.5	21.3	14.3	-	-	-	2.0	2.0	0.23	0.40	**3.2**	189
Eye	9	0	5.2	-	1.3	-	-	-	2.1	2.6	-	-	-	-	7.5	-	-	-	-	40.3	1.4	1.4	0.09	0.09	**1.5**	190
Brain, nervous system	13	0	2.6	1.4	1.3	1.3	-	-	4.2	-	-	3.6	18.0	6.0	-	-	-	-	-	-	2.0	2.0	0.19	0.19	**2.3**	191-2
Thyroid	10	0	-	-	-	-	-	1.8	-	-	-	7.3	13.5	-	15.0	-	14.3	-	-	40.3	1.5	1.5	0.19	0.26	**2.3**	193
Other endocrine	1	0	-	-	-	-	-	-	-	-	-	3.6	-	-	-	-	-	-	-	-	0.2	0.2	0.02	0.02	**0.2**	194
Hodgkin's disease	6	0	2.6	2.7	1.3	-	-	-	-	2.6	-	-	-	-	-	-	-	-	-	-	0.9	0.9	0.05	0.05	**0.9**	201
Non-Hodgkin lymphoma	42	2	2.6	-	1.3	1.3	1.5	3.6	2.1	2.6	6.2	10.9	13.5	12.1	7.5	63.9	57.1	171.3	68.0	-	6.5	6.4	0.34	0.98	**9.3**	200,202
Multiple myeloma	10	0	-	-	-	-	-	-	-	-	-	7.3	-	12.1	7.5	21.3	14.3	21.4	-	40.3	1.5	1.5	0.13	0.31	**2.6**	203
Lymphoid leukaemia	11	0	-	4.1	1.3	2.6	1.5	-	2.1	2.6	-	-	-	-	-	14.3	-	-	40.3	-	1.7	1.7	0.07	0.14	**1.6**	204
Myeloid leukaemia	10	0	-	-	2.6	1.3	-	-	-	2.1	-	3.6	9.0	6.0	7.5	10.6	-	-	-	-	1.5	1.5	0.16	0.21	**2.0**	205
Monocytic leukaemia	1	0	-	1.4	-	-	-	-	-	-	-	-	-	-	-	-	-	-	-	-	0.2	0.2	0.01	0.01	**0.1**	206
Other leukaemia	0	0	-	-	-	-	-	-	-	-	-	-	-	-	-	-	-	-	-	-	0.0	0.0	0.00	0.00	**0.0**	207
Leukaemia unspecified	6	0	-	-	-	1.3	1.5	1.8	2.1	-	-	-	-	-	-	10.6	14.3	-	-	-	0.9	0.9	0.03	0.16	**1.1**	208
Other and unspecified	32	0	1.3	-	-	-	1.5	1.8	6.4	7.8	-	10.9	13.5	6.0	7.5	31.9	42.8	42.8	101.9	161.4	4.9	4.9	0.28	0.66	**6.7**	O&U
All sites	732	13	21.0	12.3	11.8	18.1	14.5	27.3	53.1	44.2	46.7	113.0	225.0	325.7	583.8	894.0	1340.9	1606.3	2174.7	2380.0	112.5		7.62	18.99	**168.3**	ALL
All sites but 173	655	10	21.0	12.3	11.8	16.8	14.5	27.3	51.0	41.6	40.5	105.7	202.5	295.6	531.4	787.6	1155.5	1370.7	1868.8	2097.6	100.7	100.0	6.97	16.83	**149.8**	ALLb
Rate from 1 case			1.311	1.366	1.311	1.292	1.454	1.818	2.124	2.602	3.112	3.644	4.501	6.032	7.485	10.643	14.265	21.418	33.979	40.339						

†Important: see notes on population page

PERU, TRUJILLO 1988-1990

ANNUAL INCIDENCE PER 100,000 BY AGE GROUP (YEARS) - FEMALE

SITE	ALL AGES	AGE UNK	0-	5-	10-	15-	20-	25-	30-	35-	40-	45-	50-	55-	60-	65-	70-	75-	80-	85+	CRUDE RATE	%	CR 64	CR 74	ASR (W)	ICD (9th)
Lip	2	0	-	-	-	-	-	-	-	-	-	-	4.1	-	-	-	-	-	22.9	-	0.3	0.2	0.02	0.02	**0.3**	*140*
Tongue	1	0	-	-	-	-	-	-	-	-	-	-	-	-	-	-	-	-	-	25.7	0.1	0.1	0.00	0.00	**0.1**	*141*
Salivary gland	3	0	-	-	-	-	-	-	-	-	2.6	-	4.1	-	-	-	-	16.3	-	-	0.4	0.3	0.03	0.03	**0.5**	*142*
Mouth	3	0	-	-	-	-	-	-	1.8	-	-	3.3	-	-	-	-	-	-	-	25.7	0.4	0.3	0.03	0.03	**0.4**	*143-5*
Oropharynx	0	0	-	-	-	-	-	-	-	-	-	-	-	-	-	-	-	-	-	-	0.0	0.0	0.00	0.00	**0.0**	*146*
Nasopharynx	0	0	-	-	-	-	-	-	-	-	-	-	-	-	-	-	-	-	-	-	0.0	0.0	0.00	0.00	**0.0**	*147*
Hypopharynx	0	0	-	-	-	-	-	-	-	-	-	-	-	-	-	-	-	-	-	-	0.0	0.0	0.00	0.00	**0.0**	*148*
Pharynx unspecified	1	0	-	-	-	-	-	-	-	-	-	-	4.1	-	-	-	-	-	-	-	0.1	0.1	0.02	0.02	**0.2**	*149*
Oesophagus	3	0	-	-	-	-	-	-	-	-	-	-	-	-	-	17.0	-	16.3	-	-	0.4	0.3	0.00	0.08	**0.7**	*150*
Stomach	112	2	-	-	-	-	2.6	-	5.4	4.3	10.6	13.1	8.2	21.6	101.9	84.8	125.9	309.7	320.4	488.3	15.6	10.9	0.85	1.93	**20.1**	*151*
Small intestine	4	0	-	-	-	-	-	-	-	-	-	-	4.1	-	-	-	22.9	16.3	-	-	0.6	0.4	0.02	0.13	**0.8**	*152*
Colon	24	1	-	-	-	-	-	-	-	-	2.6	-	4.1	16.2	38.2	42.4	-	32.6	22.9	102.8	3.3	2.3	0.32	0.54	**5.0**	*153*
Rectum	22	0	-	-	-	-	-	-	-	-	-	6.6	4.1	5.4	19.1	25.4	22.9	81.5	68.6	51.4	3.1	2.1	0.18	0.42	**4.2**	*154*
Liver	35	0	-	-	-	-	2.6	-	3.6	4.3	5.3	3.3	8.2	10.8	19.1	33.9	11.4	81.5	137.3	77.1	4.9	3.4	0.29	0.51	**5.9**	*155*
Gallbladder etc.	46	0	-	-	-	-	-	-	-	4.3	2.6	13.1	16.4	5.4	38.2	67.9	80.1	130.4	68.6	51.4	6.4	4.5	0.40	1.14	**9.3**	*156*
Pancreas	14	0	-	-	-	-	-	-	-	-	-	-	4.1	21.6	12.7	17.0	22.9	16.3	22.9	25.7	1.9	1.4	0.19	0.39	**3.0**	*157*
Nose, sinuses etc.	3	0	-	-	-	-	-	-	2.1	-	-	-	-	-	6.4	-	-	16.3	-	-	0.4	0.3	0.04	0.04	**0.5**	*160*
Larynx	2	0	-	-	-	-	-	-	4.3	-	-	-	-	-	-	-	-	-	-	-	0.3	0.2	0.02	0.02	**0.3**	*161*
Bronchus, lung	22	0	-	-	-	-	1.5	-	2.1	5.3	3.3	12.3	10.8	6.4	17.0	34.3	32.6	45.8	51.4	3.1	2.1	0.21	0.47	**4.1**	*162*
Other thoracic organs	2	0	-	-	-	-	1.5	-	-	-	-	-	-	-	-	-	11.4	-	-	-	0.3	0.2	0.01	0.06	**0.4**	*163-4*
Bone	5	0	-	-	2.6	2.3	-	1.5	-	-	-	-	-	-	-	-	-	-	-	-	0.7	0.5	0.03	0.03	**0.6**	*170*
Connective tissue	6	0	-	-	-	-	1.3	-	-	-	-	-	-	5.4	12.7	-	11.4	-	22.9	-	0.8	0.6	0.10	0.15	**1.2**	*171*
Mesothelioma	0	0	-	-	-	-	-	-	-	-	-	-	-	-	-	-	-	-	-	-	0.0	0.0	0.00	0.00	**0.0**	*MES*
Kaposi's sarcoma	2	1	-	-	-	-	-	-	-	-	-	-	-	-	-	-	16.3	-	-	-	0.3	0.2	0.00	0.00	**0.3**	*KAP*
Melanoma of skin	8	0	-	-	-	-	1.3	1.5	-	-	-	3.3	-	5.4	12.7	17.0	-	-	-	-	1.1	0.8	0.12	0.21	**1.7**	*172*
Other skin	85	2	-	-	-	-	-	3.1	3.6	6.4	5.3	9.8	28.7	32.4	63.7	50.9	160.3	130.4	228.8	257.0	11.8		0.78	1.86	**15.9**	*173*
Breast	160	5	-	-	-	-	-	1.5	12.5	40.8	50.2	95.1	106.5	97.2	44.6	84.8	80.1	65.2	137.3	51.4	22.3	15.6	2.31	3.17	**29.7**	*174*
Uterus unspecified	5	0	-	-	-	-	-	-	-	-	-	3.3	-	-	8.5	-	32.6	22.9	-	-	0.7	0.5	0.02	0.06	**0.9**	*179*
Cervix uteri	288	4	-	-	-	-	1.3	7.7	35.7	55.9	108.4	118.0	131.1	145.8	165.6	195.1	171.7	309.7	205.9	102.8	40.1	28.1	3.90	5.76	**53.5**	*180*
Placenta	1	0	-	-	-	1.1	-	-	-	-	-	-	-	-	-	-	-	-	-	-	0.1	0.1	0.01	0.01	**0.1**	*181*
Corpus uteri	14	0	-	-	-	-	-	-	1.8	-	-	6.6	16.4	5.4	6.4	17.0	22.9	-	22.9	-	1.9	1.4	0.18	0.38	**2.9**	*182*
Ovary etc.	41	0	1.4	-	-	-	1.3	4.6	5.4	6.4	10.6	6.6	20.5	21.6	19.1	59.4	11.4	48.9	22.9	-	5.7	4.0	0.49	0.84	**7.6**	*183*
Other female genital	18	1	-	-	-	-	-	-	-	-	-	6.6	4.1	5.4	6.4	17.0	34.3	16.3	45.8	102.8	2.5	1.8	0.12	0.39	**3.4**	*184*
†Bladder	3	0	-	-	-	-	-	-	-	-	-	-	-	-	12.7	-	11.4	-	-	-	0.4	0.3	0.06	0.12	**0.7**	*188*
Kidney etc.	18	1	2.7	-	-	-	-	1.5	-	2.1	-	6.6	16.4	10.8	6.4	8.5	-	-	22.9	51.4	2.5	1.8	0.25	0.29	**3.3**	*189*
Eye	5	1	-	1.4	-	-	-	-	-	-	-	-	-	-	-	-	22.9	16.3	-	-	0.7	0.5	0.01	0.15	**0.9**	*190*
Brain, nervous system	10	0	1.4	2.8	1.3	1.1	-	-	-	4.3	-	3.3	-	5.4	6.4	-	-	-	-	-	1.4	1.0	0.13	0.13	**1.6**	*191-2*
Thyroid	31	0	-	-	-	2.3	2.6	3.1	5.4	4.3	7.9	9.8	4.1	5.4	12.7	33.9	34.3	48.9	-	-	4.3	3.0	0.29	0.63	**5.4**	*193*
Other endocrine	0	0	-	-	-	-	-	-	-	-	-	-	-	-	-	-	-	-	-	-	0.0	0.0	0.00	0.00	**0.0**	*194*
Hodgkin's disease	1	0	-	-	-	-	1.3	-	-	-	-	-	-	-	-	-	-	-	-	-	0.1	0.1	0.01	0.01	**0.1**	*201*
Non-Hodgkin lymphoma	30	3	-	-	1.3	-	1.3	-	-	8.6	5.3	9.8	4.1	10.8	6.4	25.4	22.9	32.6	114.4	-	4.2	2.9	0.26	0.53	**5.2**	*200,202*
Multiple myeloma	7	0	-	-	-	-	-	-	-	-	-	3.3	4.1	5.4	6.4	-	22.9	16.3	-	-	1.0	0.7	0.10	0.21	**1.5**	*203*
Lymphoid leukaemia	11	0	2.7	5.5	-	1.1	-	3.1	-	-	-	4.1	-	6.4	-	-	-	-	-	-	1.5	1.1	0.11	0.11	**1.7**	*204*
Myeloid leukaemia	15	0	1.4	1.4	-	-	-	-	-	-	-	8.2	5.4	12.7	25.4	11.4	65.2	-	-	-	2.1	1.5	0.15	0.33	**3.1**	*205*
Monocytic leukaemia	1	0	-	-	-	-	-	-	-	2.6	-	-	-	-	-	-	-	-	-	-	0.1	0.1	0.01	0.01	**0.2**	*206*
Other leukaemia	0	0	-	-	-	-	-	-	-	-	-	-	-	-	-	-	-	-	-	-	0.0	0.0	0.00	0.00	**0.0**	*207*
Leukaemia unspecified	2	0	-	1.4	-	-	-	-	-	2.6	-	-	-	-	-	-	-	-	-	-	0.3	0.2	0.02	0.02	**0.3**	*208*
Other and unspecified	43	1	-	-	-	-	-	1.5	1.8	-	7.9	9.8	8.2	16.2	57.3	50.9	11.4	97.8	114.4	51.4	6.0	4.2	0.53	0.85	**8.4**	*O&U*
All sites	1109	22	9.5	12.5	5.2	8.0	15.4	32.3	76.8	150.4	230.0	334.3	430.2	469.8	700.6	899.1	961.8	1646.6	1670.5	1516.3	154.5		12.63	22.12	**205.9**	*ALL*
All sites but 173	1024	20	9.5	12.5	5.2	8.0	15.4	29.2	73.2	144.0	224.7	324.5	401.5	437.4	636.9	848.2	801.5	1516.1	1441.6	1259.3	142.6	100.0	11.84	20.25	**190.0**	*ALLb*

Rate from 1 case   1.360   1.387   1.293   1.142   1.281   1.539   1.786   2.149   2.644   3.278   4.097   5.400   6.369   8.482   11.450   16.303   22.883   25.700

†Important: see notes on population page

Peru, Lima

The Lima Metropolitan Cancer Registry was founded in 1968 as a function of the Institute of Neoplastic Diseases in the city of Lima. From the beginning it was conceived as population-based covering the population of metropolitan Lima. The registry operated until 1979 and has published reports in 1973, 1981 and 1982. Its activities were then discontinued until 1990,when it was re-established as a part of the "Maes-Heller" Cancer Research Centre. A report on cancer incidence and mortality for 1990–91 has been published.

The city of Lima is the capital of Peru, located in the central part of the western coast of South America, at latitude 12°5′ S and longitude 77°2′ W. The altitude ranges from sea level to 300 m.

The area covered by the registry is 2812 km^2. The population of metropolitan Lima according to the 1993 national census was 6 434 322 inhabitants (density 2288 per km^2), with a crude natality rate of 19.3 per 1000 and a crude mortality rate of 4.1 per 1000, resulting in population growth and an unbalanced structure: 4.7% of the population is over 65 years of age and 29.8% less than 15 years of age.

In the summer temperatures can reach 30°C and in winter 18°C, with the average monthly temperature 19.3°C. The relative humidity ranges between 70 and 90%, averaging 83%. The average monthly precipitation is 0.4 mm. Metropolitan Lima has a high level of environmental contamination due to the fact that 73% of the manufacturing industry and 66% of the automobiles in the country are located there.

The registry depends upon active data collection. Cases are collected by specially trained abstractors from the various private or public hospital services, pathology departments, private doctors and radiotherapy services. The proportion of deaths autopsied is very small. Death certificates are used as a source of information and, where cancer is a stated cause of death, are routinely reviewed from the Civil Registries of the District Municipalities.

Registration details include: name, marital status, sex, age, occupation, anatomical location of the tumour, histological type of the tumour and method of diagnosis.

At present, there is no active follow-up of registered patients.

The registry operates a computer system that permits identification of duplicate registrations and record linkage allowing automatic identification of patients with multiple primaries. After collection, the data are coded according to ICD-O-1. In Peru two family names are used and the first check for duplicates is done manually in alphabetic order. The information is then entered in a specially designed computer program which checks for consistency between: age vs date of birth and vs date of incidence; sex vs tumour site; tumour site vs histology and histology vs basis of diagnosis. Basal cell carcinoma of the skin and all carcinomas *in situ* are reported but analysed separately.

The registry regularly publishes statistical reports which are circulated within the country and internationally, promoting the use of the data for clinical and epidemiological research, planning purposes, medical, audit, education and general information.

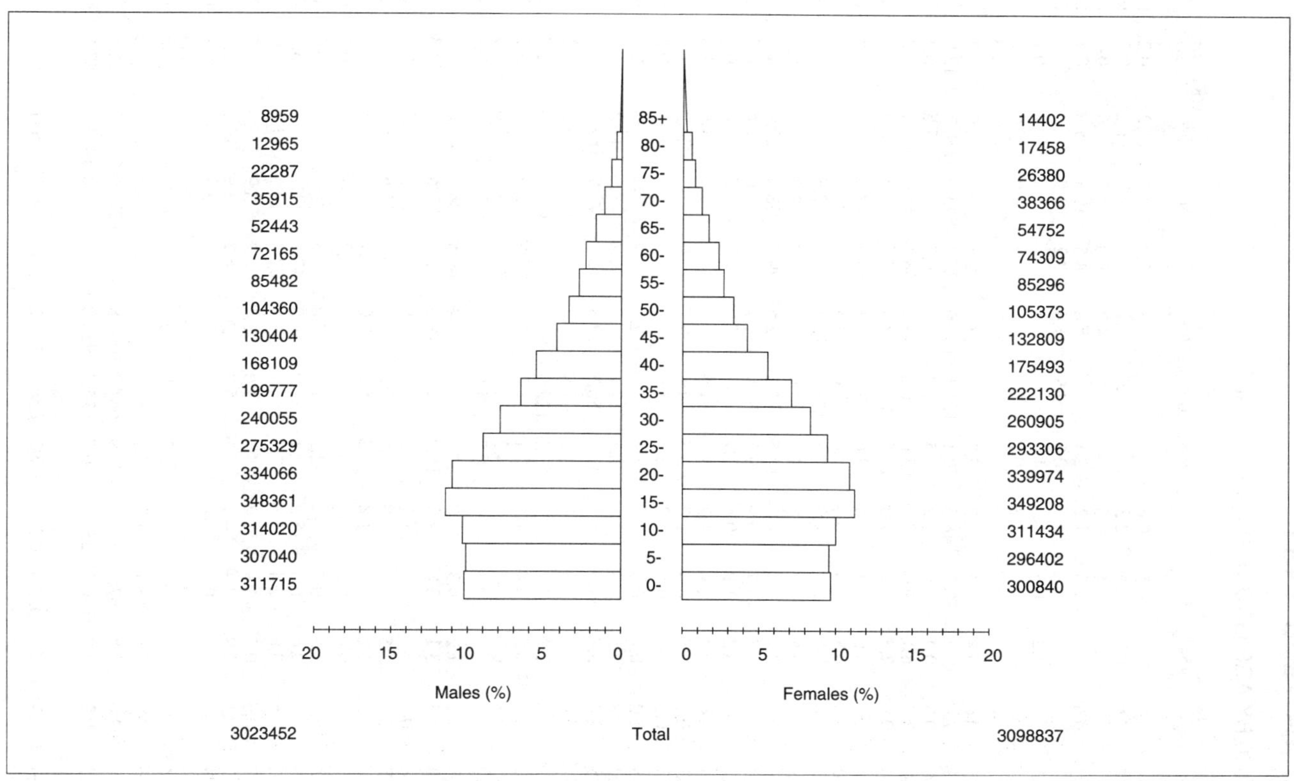

Peru, Lima
Source of population: 1990–91
Census: Censo Nacional de 1993. Instituto de Estadistica e Informatica (INEI). Lima, Peru
Estimate: The data for 1990–91 were estimated on the basis of the 1993 national census.

Notes to tables overleaf:
* Rates are low in comparison with earlier time periods suggesting incompleteness.
† 188 does not include non-invasive tumours.

* PERU, LIMA 1990-1991

ANNUAL INCIDENCE PER 100,000 BY AGE GROUP (YEARS) - MALE

SITE	ALL AGES	AGE UNK	0-	5-	10-	15-	20-	25-	30-	35-	40-	45-	50-	55-	60-	65-	70-	75-	80-	85+	CRUDE RATE	%	CR 64	CR 74	ASR (W)	ICD (9th)
Lip	12	0	-	-	-	-	-	-	-	-	-	-	0.5	0.6	2.8	-	2.8	2.2	3.9	11.2	0.2	0.2	0.02	0.03	**0.3**	140
Tongue	19	0	-	-	-	-	-	-	-	-	0.6	0.8	0.5	2.3	-	1.9	4.2	2.2	7.7	11.2	0.3	0.4	0.02	0.05	**0.5**	141
Salivary gland	26	1	-	-	-	-	-	-	0.2	-	-	1.5	2.4	0.6	-	3.8	4.2	9.0	7.7	5.6	0.4	0.5	0.02	0.07	**0.6**	142
Mouth	23	0	-	-	-	-	-	0.5	0.2	-	0.6	-	1.0	1.2	2.1	-	2.8	4.5	19.3	5.6	0.4	0.4	0.03	0.04	**0.5**	143-5
Oropharynx	8	0	-	-	-	-	-	-	0.2	-	-	-	-	0.7	2.9	1.4	2.2	3.9	-	-	0.1	0.2	0.00	0.03	**0.2**	146
Nasopharynx	8	0	-	-	-	-	-	-	-	0.3	-	1.2	0.5	-	1.4	-	1.4	-	-	-	0.1	0.2	0.02	Na.02	**0.2**	147
Hypopharynx	10	0	-	-	-	-	-	-	-	-	-	-	-	1.2	0.7	2.9	-	4.5	3.9	5.6	0.2	0.2	0.01	Hy.02	**0.3**	148
Pharynx unspecified	0	0	-	-	-	-	-	-	-	-	-	-	-	-	-	-	-	-	-	-	0.0	0.0	0.00	Ph.00	**0.0**	149
Oesophagus	73	1	-	-	-	-	-	-	0.5	0.6	0.8	1.4	7.0	6.2	7.6	13.9	22.4	30.9	33.5	1.2	1.4	0.08	0.19	**1.8**	150
Stomach	780	15	-	-	-	0.3	0.9	0.7	2.3	5.3	7.7	12.7	30.2	48.5	72.1	121.1	135.0	177.2	243.0	256.7	12.9	14.7	0.92	2.23	**19.1**	151
Small intestine	19	0	-	-	-	-	-	-	-	-	0.3	0.4	0.5	1.8	3.5	2.9	1.4	6.7	-	5.6	0.3	0.4	0.03	0.05	**0.5**	152
Colon	228	8	-	-	-	0.1	-	0.5	0.2	2.0	3.3	6.1	9.6	9.9	23.6	26.7	43.2	56.1	54.0	61.4	3.8	4.3	0.29	0.65	**5.6**	153
Rectum	135	3	-	-	-	-	0.1	-	0.8	2.0	0.9	2.7	3.4	7.0	12.5	25.7	22.3	33.7	38.6	22.3	2.2	2.6	0.15	0.40	**3.3**	154
Liver	153	5	0.2	0.2	0.6	0.1	0.7	1.5	1.2	2.8	2.7	3.5	3.8	3.5	7.6	17.2	22.3	35.9	42.4	39.1	2.5	2.9	0.15	0.35	**3.4**	155
Gallbladder etc.	81	0	-	-	-	-	-	-	-	-	1.0	0.3	0.8	3.4	6.4	9.0	7.6	19.5	24.7	27.0	16.7	1.3	1.5	0.10	0.24	**2.0**	156
Pancreas	120	1	-	-	-	-	0.1	0.2	0.6	0.8	1.8	2.7	2.9	9.9	17.3	14.3	22.3	24.7	7.7	33.5	2.0	2.3	0.18	0.37	**3.0**	157
Nose, sinuses etc.	37	0	0.2	-	-	-	-	0.4	0.4	0.8	-	0.8	1.9	2.9	2.1	2.9	11.1	6.7	3.9	-	0.6	0.7	0.05	0.12	**0.9**	160
Larynx	98	0	-	-	-	-	-	-	0.2	0.3	0.9	0.4	5.3	4.7	14.5	14.3	12.5	29.2	38.6	27.9	1.6	1.9	0.13	0.27	**2.4**	161
Bronchus, lung	635	2	-	-	-	0.1	0.4	1.5	2.3	1.5	11.5	18.7	50.9	79.7	82.9	126.7	197.4	162.0	167.4	10.5	12.0	0.83	1.89	**15.9**	162
Other thoracic organs	25	0	-	-	0.2	-	0.6	0.4	-	0.5	-	0.4	1.9	0.6	0.7	-	7.0	2.2	7.7	5.6	0.4	0.5	0.03	0.06	**0.5**	163-4
Bone	58	1	-	0.7	1.4	1.6	0.9	0.7	0.6	0.3	0.6	0.4	1.4	1.2	2.8	1.9	-	4.5	7.7	5.6	1.0	1.1	0.06	0.07	**1.0**	170
Connective tissue	85	4	1.0	0.3	-	0.9	0.9	1.1	1.7	1.3	0.3	1.5	3.4	2.3	3.5	4.8	9.7	9.0	-	27.9	1.4	1.6	0.09	0.17	**1.7**	171
Mesothelioma	11	0	-	-	0.2	-	-	-	-	0.3	0.3	-	0.5	1.2	2.1	1.0	1.4	-	-	-	0.2	0.2	0.02	0.03	**0.3**	MES
Kaposi's sarcoma	19	0	-	-	-	-	-	-	0.2	0.5	1.2	0.4	0.5	-	1.4	4.8	2.8	2.2	-	-	0.3	0.4	0.02	Ka.06	**0.4**	KAP
Melanoma of skin	71	2	-	-	-	0.3	-	0.2	0.4	1.0	1.8	1.5	4.8	3.5	6.9	7.6	13.9	6.7	3.9	11.2	1.2	1.3	0.11	0.22	**1.7**	172
Other skin	427	20	-	-	0.3	0.3	0.4	0.4	1.5	3.5	2.4	8.8	11.0	21.1	31.2	56.3	73.8	116.7	173.5	184.2	7.1		0.42	1.11	**10.3**	173
Breast	8	0	-	-	-	-	-	-	-	-	0.6	-	1.0	0.6	-	1.0	1.4	-	-	5.6	0.1	0.2	0.01	0.02	**0.2**	175
Prostate	767	18	-	0.2	-	0.1	-	-	0.2	-	0.6	2.3	3.4	22.8	62.4	122.0	196.3	287.2	474.4	457.6	12.7	14.5	0.47	2.10	**19.4**	185
Testis	187	4	1.4	0.2	0.5	2.2	5.5	7.3	5.8	3.0	4.2	1.5	3.4	1.8	2.1	1.0	1.4	4.5	3.9	11.2	3.1	3.5	0.20	0.21	**2.9**	186
Penis	31	0	-	-	-	-	-	0.4	0.4	-	0.3	0.8	-	1.2	4.2	3.8	5.6	11.2	7.7	5.6	0.5	0.6	0.04	0.08	**0.7**	187.1-.4
Other male genital	4	0	-	-	-	-	-	-	-	-	-	-	0.5	-	0.7	1.0	-	2.2	-	-	0.1	0.1	0.01	0.01	**0.1**	187.5-.9
†Bladder	220	7	-	-	0.2	-	-	0.2	0.4	0.8	1.2	1.2	4.3	7.0	21.5	31.5	72.4	69.5	88.7	44.6	3.6	4.2	0.19	0.73	**5.5**	188
Kidney etc.	140	7	0.8	0.2	-	-	0.1	-	0.2	1.0	1.5	3.1	3.8	9.9	15.2	22.9	19.5	33.7	27.0	5.6	2.3	2.6	0.19	0.41	**3.4**	189
Eye	31	1	1.6	0.8	-	-	-	0.2	0.2	0.8	0.3	-	-	1.2	0.7	1.0	2.8	2.2	-	11.2	0.5	0.6	0.03	0.05	**0.6**	190
Brain, nervous system	160	2	1.1	2.0	1.8	1.4	1.6	1.3	2.1	2.8	2.1	3.5	6.2	7.0	11.1	10.5	2.8	6.7	11.6	16.7	2.6	3.0	0.22	0.29	**3.1**	191-2
Thyroid	50	0	-	-	0.2	0.3	-	0.4	0.6	1.0	1.5	1.2	2.9	1.8	4.2	5.7	7.0	6.7	-	5.6	0.8	0.9	0.07	0.13	**1.1**	193
Other endocrine	7	0	-	0.2	0.2	-	0.1	-	-	-	-	0.4	0.5	-	0.7	-	-	2.2	-	-	0.1	0.1	0.01	0.01	**0.1**	194
Hodgkin's disease	53	1	0.3	1.8	1.0	0.1	0.9	0.5	0.8	0.3	0.3	1.5	0.5	-	2.1	1.0	7.0	4.5	-	5.6	0.9	1.0	0.05	Ho.09	**1.0**	201
Non-Hodgkin lymphoma	332	11	1.1	1.3	1.4	1.1	1.9	2.5	4.2	3.8	6.2	9.6	16.3	15.2	20.1	21.9	39.0	47.1	61.7	22.3	5.5	6.3	0.44	0.75	**7.1**	200,202
Multiple myeloma	63	0	-	-	-	-	-	0.4	-	-	0.6	0.8	2.4	5.3	7.6	6.7	11.1	22.4	19.3	11.2	1.0	1.2	0.09	0.17	**1.5**	203
Lymphoid leukaemia	108	2	3.7	2.0	2.7	1.9	1.0	0.5	0.6	0.3	0.6	0.8	1.9	1.2	4.8	1.0	8.4	2.2	3.9	5.6	1.8	2.0	0.11	0.16	**1.9**	204
Myeloid leukaemia	84	0	0.8	0.8	1.1	0.7	0.4	0.7	1.0	1.3	1.5	1.9	2.4	4.1	2.1	5.7	9.7	6.7	3.9	16.7	1.4	1.6	0.09	0.17	**1.7**	205
Monocytic leukaemia	5	0	-	-	-	-	-	-	0.3	-	-	-	0.5	-	-	1.0	1.4	-	3.9	-	0.1	0.1	0.00	0.02	**0.1**	206
Other leukaemia	1	0	-	-	-	-	-	-	-	-	-	-	0.5	-	-	-	-	-	-	-	0.0	0.0	0.00	0.00	**0.0**	207
Leukaemia unspecified	28	2	0.5	0.3	0.3	0.1	-	0.4	0.2	0.3	-	-	-	1.2	0.7	1.0	5.6	6.7	-	16.7	0.5	0.5	0.02	0.06	**0.6**	208
Other and unspecified	279	9	0.3	0.2	-	0.1	0.6	0.9	1.5	1.0	3.0	5.8	8.1	11.7	27.7	32.4	57.1	83.0	84.8	55.8	4.6	5.3	0.31	0.78	**6.7**	O&U
All sites	5719	127	13.0	10.9	11.9	11.8	17.4	22.5	30.6	41.3	52.0	92.8	167.7	280.2	491.9	681.7	1003.8	1379.7	1677.6	1635.2	94.6		6.36	14.98	**134.1**	ALL
All sites but 173	5292	107	13.0	10.9	11.6	11.5	16.9	22.2	29.2	37.8	49.7	84.0	156.7	259.1	460.7	625.4	930.0	1263.1	1504.0	1451.1	87.5	100.0	5.94	13.87	**123.8**	ALLb

Rate from 1 case   0.160   0.163   0.159   0.144   0.150   0.182   0.208   0.250   0.297   0.383   0.479   0.585   0.693   0.953   1.392   2.243   3.857   5.581

†Important: see notes on population page

* PERU, LIMA 1990-1991

ANNUAL INCIDENCE PER 100,000 BY AGE GROUP (YEARS) - FEMALE

SITE	ALL AGES	AGE UNK	0-	5-	10-	15-	20-	25-	30-	35-	40-	45-	50-	55-	60-	65-	70-	75-	80-	85+	CRUDE RATE	%	CR 64	CR 74	ASR (W)	ICD (9th)
Lip	8	0	-	0.2	-	-	-	-	-	-	-	-	-	-	-	0.9	1.3	1.9	2.9	10.4	0.1	0.1	0.00	0.01	**0.2**	*140*
Tongue	24	0	-	-	-	-	-	-	0.2	0.2	0.3	1.1	0.9	1.2	0.7	1.8	5.2	1.9	5.7	13.9	0.4	0.3	0.02	0.06	**0.5**	*141*
Salivary gland	22	1	-	-	-	-	-	-	0.2	0.2	0.6	0.4	-	1.2	3.4	3.7	1.3	1.9	2.9	6.9	0.4	0.3	0.03	0.06	**0.5**	*142*
Mouth	27	0	-	-	-	-	-	-	-	0.2	0.9	0.4	0.5	1.8	2.7	1.8	5.2	5.7	5.7	10.4	0.4	0.4	0.03	0.07	**0.6**	*143-5*
Oropharynx	8	0	-	-	-	-	-	-	-	-	-	-	-	-	-	-	2.6	7.6	2.9	3.5	0.1	0.1	0.00	0.01	**0.2**	*146*
Nasopharynx	5	0	-	-	-	-	-	-	-	-	-	-	0.5	0.6	-	0.9	1.3	-	-	3.5	0.1	0.1	0.01	0.02	**0.1**	*147*
Hypopharynx	4	0	-	-	-	-	-	-	-	-	0.3	-	-	0.6	0.7	0.9	-	-	-	-	0.1	0.1	0.01	0.01	**0.1**	*148*
Pharynx unspecified	1	0	-	-	-	-	-	-	-	-	-	-	-	-	-	-	-	-	-	3.5	0.0	0.0	0.00	0.00	**0.0**	*149*
Oesophagus	27	1	-	-	-	-	-	-	-	-	0.3	-	0.5	2.9	4.0	3.7	5.2	1.9	5.7	6.9	0.4	0.4	0.04	0.09	**0.6**	*150*
Stomach	626	12	-	-	0.2	0.3	0.3	1.0	3.1	5.6	9.1	16.2	20.9	29.9	47.1	67.6	113.4	147.8	117.4	145.8	10.1	8.8	0.68	1.60	**13.7**	*151*
Small intestine	19	0	-	-	-	-	-	-	-	-	0.3	-	0.5	2.3	2.0	1.8	2.6	-	2.9	17.4	0.3	0.3	0.03	0.05	**0.4**	*152*
Colon	242	5	-	-	0.2	0.1	-	0.5	0.8	1.8	2.0	5.3	5.7	15.8	16.1	26.5	46.9	64.4	54.4	62.5	3.9	3.4	0.25	0.62	**5.3**	*153*
Rectum	156	6	-	-	-	-	0.3	0.3	0.8	1.1	2.8	1.1	5.2	11.1	15.5	13.7	18.2	30.3	51.6	27.8	2.5	2.2	0.20	0.37	**3.3**	*154*
Liver	161	1	0.2	0.5	-	0.1	0.4	1.2	1.0	0.9	1.4	3.0	2.8	8.2	13.5	20.1	22.2	34.1	40.1	41.7	2.6	2.3	0.17	0.38	**3.4**	*155*
Gallbladder etc.	190	4	-	-	-	-	0.4	0.2	0.4	0.9	0.6	4.1	9.5	18.2	21.5	24.7	18.2	26.5	45.8	31.2	3.1	2.7	0.29	0.50	**4.3**	*156*
Pancreas	154	1	-	-	-	-	-	-	0.4	0.5	0.6	2.3	6.6	8.8	17.5	24.7	31.3	32.2	28.6	27.8	2.5	2.2	0.18	0.47	**3.6**	*157*
Nose, sinuses etc.	20	0	-	-	-	0.1	0.1	-	0.2	0.2	-	0.8	-	1.8	0.7	4.6	3.9	-	2.9	3.5	0.3	0.3	0.02	0.06	**0.4**	*160*
Larynx	19	0	-	-	-	-	0.1	0.2	0.2	0.2	-	-	0.5	1.8	2.0	3.7	2.6	3.8	-	-	0.3	0.3	0.02	0.06	**0.4**	*161*
Bronchus, lung	284	4	-	-	-	-	-	0.2	0.4	2.5	3.1	4.1	11.9	16.4	29.6	31.0	49.5	64.4	74.5	52.1	4.6	4.0	0.35	0.75	**6.3**	*162*
Other thoracic organs	12	1	-	-	-	-	-	-	-	0.2	0.3	-	-	0.6	0.7	0.9	2.6	1.9	8.6	-	0.2	0.2	0.01	0.03	**0.2**	*163-4*
Bone	50	1	-	0.5	0.8	0.7	0.4	0.3	0.2	0.2	-	2.6	2.4	2.3	2.7	1.8	1.3	3.8	5.7	6.9	0.8	0.7	0.07	0.08	**1.0**	*170*
Connective tissue	112	0	0.8	0.5	0.3	0.9	1.3	2.0	0.4	0.7	2.8	3.4	2.4	7.0	4.0	3.7	9.1	11.4	17.2	17.4	1.8	1.6	0.13	0.20	**2.1**	*171*
Mesothelioma	1	0	-	-	-	-	-	-	-	-	-	0.4	-	-	-	-	-	-	-	-	0.0	0.0	0.00	0.00	**0.0**	*MES*
Kaposi's sarcoma	4	0	-	-	-	-	-	0.2	-	-	-	0.4	-	0.6	0.7	-	-	-	-	-	0.1	0.1	0.01	0.01	**0.1**	*KAP*
Melanoma of skin	71	2	-	0.2	-	0.1	0.1	0.9	0.6	1.1	0.9	2.3	2.4	5.3	4.0	8.2	7.8	5.7	14.3	3.5	1.1	1.0	0.09	0.17	**1.5**	*172*
Other skin	391	13	-	-	0.2	-	0.6	0.7	1.0	2.0	5.7	7.2	10.0	24.0	30.3	39.3	67.8	87.2	97.4	118.0	6.3		0.42	0.98	**8.5**	*173*
Breast	1521	2	-	-	-	0.3	0.9	4.1	14.2	31.3	54.4	70.4	81.6	104.9	117.1	130.6	121.2	134.6	108.8	90.3	24.5	21.3	2.40	3.66	**32.3**	*174*
Uterus unspecified	34	1	-	-	-	-	-	-	0.2	-	0.2	1.1	0.4	1.9	1.8	3.4	3.7	3.9	-	11.5	10.4	0.5	0.5	0.05	0.09	**0.7**	*179*
Cervix uteri	1294	11	-	-	0.2	0.4	1.5	5.3	11.7	29.3	38.2	66.3	80.2	102.6	82.1	93.1	93.8	83.4	91.6	72.9	20.9	18.1	2.11	3.05	**27.3**	*180*
Placenta	40	1	-	-	-	0.1	1.5	1.7	1.5	0.9	0.6	0.4	0.5	-	-	1.8	-	-	-	-	0.6	0.6	0.04	0.05	**0.6**	*181*
Corpus uteri	184	3	-	-	-	0.1	-	-	0.4	0.9	2.8	8.7	12.8	18.8	18.2	17.4	23.5	13.3	28.6	3.5	3.0	2.6	0.32	0.53	**4.3**	*182*
Ovary etc.	296	2	-	0.5	0.8	0.4	1.3	2.0	3.4	4.5	11.7	9.4	19.0	18.2	20.2	16.4	20.9	28.4	14.3	10.4	4.8	4.1	0.46	0.65	**6.0**	*183*
Other female genital	62	1	0.2	-	-	-	0.1	0.3	-	0.2	0.6	0.8	1.9	2.3	4.7	5.5	14.3	22.7	14.3	10.4	1.0	0.9	0.06	0.16	**1.4**	*184*
†Bladder	76	0	0.2	-	-	-	0.3	-	0.4	-	0.6	1.1	3.8	2.9	3.4	14.6	14.3	15.2	20.0	20.8	1.2	1.1	0.06	0.21	**1.7**	*188*
Kidney etc.	89	1	0.8	0.8	-	-	-	0.2	0.4	0.5	1.7	2.6	2.8	8.8	6.7	8.2	13.0	11.4	8.6	3.5	1.4	1.2	0.13	0.24	**2.0**	*189*
Eye	24	0	1.5	0.3	-	-	-	-	0.4	-	0.3	-	-	-	-	3.7	1.3	3.8	-	10.4	0.4	0.3	0.01	0.04	**0.5**	*190*
Brain, nervous system	139	0	1.0	1.3	1.4	1.1	1.3	0.5	2.7	2.5	1.4	4.9	4.3	8.2	4.7	10.0	9.1	7.6	-	3.5	2.2	1.9	0.18	0.27	**2.6**	*191-2*
Thyroid	260	2	-	-	-	0.6	2.5	4.3	5.2	5.6	7.4	4.5	11.4	10.0	14.8	17.4	16.9	24.6	17.2	27.8	4.2	3.6	0.33	0.51	**4.9**	*193*
Other endocrine	6	0	0.2	-	0.3	-	-	-	0.2	-	-	-	-	0.7	0.9	-	-	-	-	-	0.1	0.1	0.01	0.01	**0.1**	*194*
Hodgkin's disease	43	0	0.3	0.2	0.5	0.1	0.3	0.5	0.4	0.9	1.4	0.4	2.4	3.5	1.3	2.7	2.6	1.9	-	-	0.7	0.6	0.06	0.09	**0.8**	*201*
Non-Hodgkin lymphoma	277	2	0.8	0.7	1.6	1.0	1.2	1.0	2.9	2.3	4.8	7.5	12.8	9.4	17.5	27.4	41.7	41.7	40.1	20.8	4.5	3.9	0.32	0.67	**5.8**	*200,202*
Multiple myeloma	41	0	-	-	-	-	-	-	0.2	0.2	-	0.6	1.1	2.8	4.1	2.0	6.4	3.9	11.4	2.9	3.5	0.7	0.6	0.06	0.11	**0.9**	*203*
Lymphoid leukaemia	91	0	2.5	2.0	2.4	2.1	0.3	1.0	0.4	0.9	0.6	1.5	1.4	-	1.3	-	5.2	1.9	8.6	3.5	1.5	1.3	0.08	0.11	**1.5**	*204*
Myeloid leukaemia	97	0	0.8	0.5	0.5	0.4	0.6	1.4	0.8	2.0	2.8	2.3	3.8	2.3	7.4	4.6	6.5	5.7	11.5	6.9	1.6	1.4	0.13	0.18	**1.9**	*205*
Monocytic leukaemia	1	0	-	-	-	-	-	-	0.2	-	-	-	-	-	-	-	-	-	-	-	0.0	0.0	0.00	0.00	**0.0**	*206*
Other leukaemia	0	0	-	-	-	-	-	-	-	-	-	-	-	-	-	-	-	-	-	-	0.0	0.0	0.00	0.00	**0.0**	*207*
Leukaemia unspecified	21	1	0.3	0.2	-	0.1	-	-	0.4	-	0.3	0.8	0.9	1.2	-	1.8	2.6	3.8	-	3.5	0.3	0.3	0.02	0.05	**0.4**	*208*
Other and unspecified	306	5	0.2	-	0.2	0.1	0.1	1.0	1.1	0.9	4.0	4.5	11.4	15.2	24.2	30.1	53.4	83.4	83.1	76.4	4.9	4.3	0.32	0.75	**6.6**	*O&U*
All sites	7540	84	9.8	8.4	9.5	9.6	16.2	31.4	56.2	101.7	167.2	242.5	338.8	476.6	549.1	682.2	868.0	1029.2	1048.2	992.9	121.7		10.20	18.04	**159.7**	*ALL*
All sites but 173	7149	71	9.8	8.4	9.3	9.6	15.6	30.7	55.2	99.7	161.5	235.3	328.8	452.5	518.8	642.9	800.2	942.0	950.9	874.9	115.3	100.0	9.77	17.06	**151.2**	*ALLb*
Rate from 1 case			0.166	0.169	0.161	0.143	0.147	0.170	0.192	0.225	0.285	0.376	0.475	0.586	0.673	0.913	1.303	1.895	2.864	3.472						

†Important: see notes on population page

USA, Puerto Rico

The Central Cancer Registry of Puerto Rico was was created at the end of 1950 as a result of a preliminary survey on cancer incidence in selected hospitals throughout the island. The following year the reporting of cancer cases to the registry was made compulsory. The registry is the only one that has monitored a homogeneous Latin-American population for more than 40 years.

Puerto Rico is a small island (8959 km^2) in the Caribbean, with a homogeneous population in terms of its demographic and cultural characteristics. The inhabitants of Puerto Rico are descendants of a mixture of the Indian natives and the African and Spanish migrants of the Conquest era. The cancer registry does not classify cases by race.

All cancer cases among residents in the island are processed in the registry. Sources of information are pathology laboratories, hospital records, private practitioners, radiotherapy centres and the death certificate archives of the Health Statistics Office of Puerto Rico.

The information gathered is checked to avoid duplicates and for completeness; it is then entered to a computer data storage system, tabulated, analysed and published. Additional information beyond that found in the annual reports is provided to hospitals and researchers upon request.

In 1972, the registry joined the National Cancer Institute's Surveillance, Epidemiology and End Results (SEER) programme, leading to improvements in the search of new cases, collection, editing and compilation of information and follow-up of cases. During the 1980s, the National Cancer Institute provided a minicomputer for the exclusive use of the registry. Functions were more precisely defined, skilled staff recruited and staff training intensified. However, in 1989, the association with the SEER programme was discontinued. Access to annual training and workshops was no longer available. Staff were lost and by 1994 half of the staff positions were vacant. Active follow-up of registered cases was discontinued and limited to review of death certificate archives. The minicomputer was becoming obsolete and was overwhelmed by the volume of the database (approximately 176 000 records accumulated since 1950).

Between 1992 and 1995, the Secretary of Health approved the re-organization of the cancer registry, giving priority to the collection, processing and publication of cancer incidence data. The Central Cancer Registry of Puerto Rico now consists of four working units: data collection; edition, analysis and classification; follow-up; and data-processing. In July 1994 a new director was appointed and a year later, a modern computer with 13 unit stations was installed, replacing the old minicomputer. In addition three portable personal computers were obtained for the data collection field unit.

Although cancer notification is compulsory by law, most hospitals limit their reporting to sending copies of pathology reports. Thus, abstractors from the registry have always completed the information on cases by reviewing medical records in hospitals where there are no tumour registries and at private physician's offices. Only 12 hospitals have a tumour registry and these usually send complete information to the registry.

The registry recently secured access to computerized death certificate records for Puerto Rico, in which all causes of death are coded and listed in the corresponding order based on the criteria used by the National Center for Health Statistics of the US Department of Health and Human Services (Multiple Cause Tapes). These files will be automatically matched with the registry files.

The first monograph published was *Cancer in Puerto Rico: 1950–1964*. Annual reports of *Cancer in Puerto Rico* have been published regularly since that time.

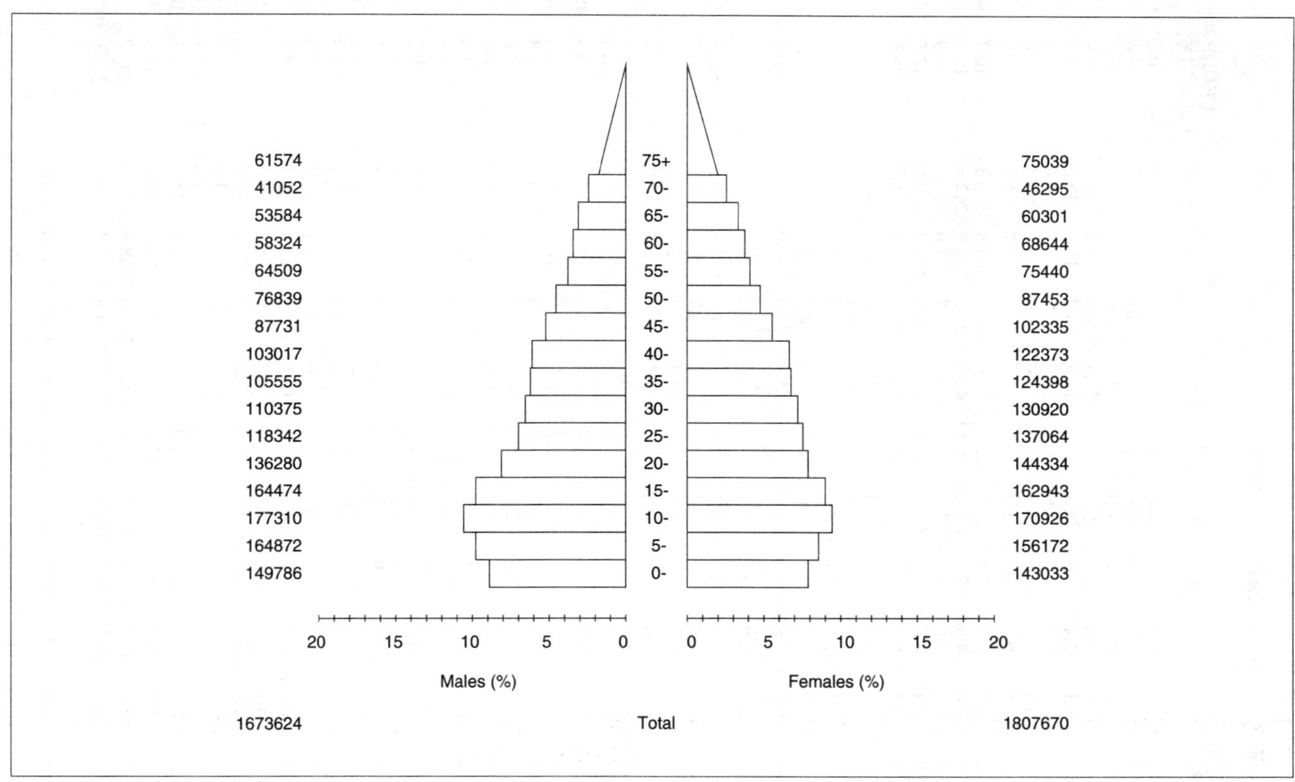

USA, Puerto Rico
Source of population: average annual 1988–91
Census: 1990
Notes to tables overleaf:
† 173 does not include basal cell or squamous cell carcinoma
† 188 does not include the uncertain or in situ category

USA, PUERTO RICO 1988-1991

ANNUAL INCIDENCE PER 100,000 BY AGE GROUP (YEARS) - MALE

SITE	ALL AGES	AGE UNK	0-	5-	10-	15-	20-	25-	30-	35-	40-	45-	50-	55-	60-	65-	70-	75+	CRUDE RATE	%	CR 64	CR 74	ASR (W)	ICD (9th)
Lip	52	0	-	-	-	-	-	-	0.2	-	0.2	-	1.0	1.9	1.7	3.7	7.9	6.9	0.8	0.3	0.03	0.08	**0.6**	*140*
Tongue	311	2	-	-	-	-	-	-	0.2	0.9	1.9	4.8	9.4	15.1	19.7	20.1	23.8	33.7	4.6	1.8	0.26	0.48	**4.1**	*141*
Salivary gland	36	0	-	-	0.1	-	0.2	0.2	0.2	0.2	0.2	1.1	1.0	0.4	0.9	1.9	1.2	5.7	0.5	0.2	0.02	0.04	**0.4**	*142*
Mouth	316	0	-	0.2	-	-	-	-	0.7	1.4	3.6	3.1	9.1	13.2	22.3	20.5	28.0	30.9	4.7	1.8	0.27	0.51	**4.2**	*143-5*
Oropharynx	228	1	-	-	-	-	0.2	-	0.2	1.4	2.4	6.8	8.5	11.6	14.6	18.2	11.6	15.0	3.4	1.3	0.23	0.38	**3.2**	*146*
Nasopharynx	41	0	-	-	0.1	0.2	0.2	0.2	-	0.2	0.5	0.9	1.6	0.4	3.9	4.2	1.8	1.6	0.6	0.2	0.04	0.07	**0.6**	*147*
Hypopharynx	238	0	-	-	-	-	-	-	-	0.2	1.2	3.7	6.5	10.5	12.9	15.9	20.1	30.5	3.6	1.4	0.17	0.35	**3.1**	*148*
Pharynx unspecified	45	0	-	-	-	-	-	0.2	-	0.5	0.2	-	1.0	1.9	2.1	3.7	3.7	5.7	0.7	0.3	0.03	0.07	**0.6**	*149*
Oesophagus	719	1	-	-	-	-	0.4	-	0.2	1.4	3.4	8.8	16.3	22.1	41.6	49.9	64.6	100.3	10.7	4.2	0.47	1.04	**9.0**	*150*
Stomach	1181	5	-	-	-	-	0.2	0.2	1.1	2.8	4.9	5.7	15.0	32.6	42.9	74.2	116.9	217.6	17.6	6.9	0.53	1.49	**13.6**	*151*
Small intestine	59	0	-	-	-	-	0.2	-	0.2	0.2	1.0	1.1	2.0	1.6	3.4	3.7	3.0	6.9	0.9	0.3	0.05	0.08	**0.8**	*152*
Colon	1170	5	-	-	-	-	0.4	2.5	2.3	3.3	7.8	12.5	22.1	34.5	62.2	91.9	112.7	149.0	17.5	6.8	0.74	1.77	**14.8**	*153*
Rectum	656	3	-	-	-	-	-	-	0.9	2.1	6.3	7.7	15.9	24.0	35.1	54.1	54.8	76.3	9.8	3.8	0.46	1.01	**8.5**	*154*
Liver	315	0	0.2	-	-	-	0.2	-	0.2	-	2.4	3.4	7.8	12.8	13.7	21.0	33.5	41.0	4.7	1.8	0.20	0.48	**4.0**	*155*
Gallbladder etc.	118	0	-	-	-	-	-	-	-	-	0.7	1.1	1.6	4.7	6.0	6.1	12.2	19.1	1.8	0.7	0.07	0.16	**1.4**	*156*
Pancreas	431	0	-	-	-	-	0.2	0.4	0.2	1.2	2.4	5.7	7.5	11.2	19.3	33.1	40.8	63.7	6.4	2.5	0.24	0.61	**5.3**	*157*
Nose, sinuses etc.	49	0	-	0.2	0.1	0.5	0.2	-	-	0.2	0.5	0.9	1.6	0.4	3.4	4.2	2.4	4.1	0.7	0.3	0.04	0.07	**0.7**	*160*
Larynx	441	1	-	-	-	-	-	-	0.2	0.2	2.4	6.8	11.4	17.8	28.3	37.3	42.0	43.8	6.6	2.6	0.34	0.73	**5.8**	*161*
Bronchus, lung	1505	1	-	-	-	-	0.2	0.8	0.7	1.7	8.0	15.1	23.4	55.4	90.9	113.4	158.9	191.6	22.5	8.8	0.98	2.34	**19.1**	*162*
Other thoracic organs	30	0	0.3	0.2	-	-	0.4	0.6	0.7	0.9	0.7	0.9	0.7	0.8	-	0.9	1.2	0.4	0.4	0.2	0.03	0.04	**0.5**	*163-4*
Bone	54	1	0.2	0.3	1.8	0.8	0.9	0.6	1.4	0.7	-	0.3	0.3	0.8	-	1.4	1.8	2.0	0.8	0.3	0.04	0.06	**0.7**	*170*
Connective tissue	112	3	0.7	0.5	0.3	0.6	0.7	0.4	0.5	1.9	1.0	2.0	2.3	3.5	4.7	4.7	6.1	8.9	1.7	0.7	0.10	0.15	**1.5**	*171*
Mesothelioma	22	0	-	-	-	-	-	-	-	0.2	0.2	-	1.0	1.2	0.4	1.4	2.4	2.4	0.3	0.1	0.02	0.03	**0.3**	*MES*
Kaposi's sarcoma	229	11	-	-	-	-	2.2	7.4	9.1	10.4	3.6	6.3	1.3	2.7	2.6	5.6	4.3	5.7	3.4	1.3	0.24	0.29	**3.3**	*KAP*
Melanoma of skin	108	3	-	-	-	0.2	0.2	0.8	0.7	1.2	1.2	1.4	2.3	2.3	5.6	6.5	7.9	11.4	1.6	0.6	0.08	0.16	**1.4**	*172*
†Other skin	25	0	-	-	-	0.2	0.2	-	0.5	0.2	0.5	-	0.7	0.8	-	-	2.4	4.1	0.4		0.01	0.03	**0.3**	*173*
Breast	23	0	-	-	-	-	-	-	-	-	0.2	0.3	0.7	1.6	0.9	1.4	3.0	2.0	0.3	0.1	0.02	0.04	**0.3**	*175*
Prostate	4831	59	-	-	-	0.2	-	-	-	-	1.7	6.3	21.8	83.7	180.0	396.6	610.2	888.0	72.2	28.1	1.49	6.58	**54.7**	*185*
Testis	85	0	0.8	0.3	0.1	0.9	2.2	5.3	3.9	1.4	0.5	0.9	0.7	-	-	0.5	0.6	0.8	1.3	0.5	0.08	0.09	**1.3**	*186*
Penis	176	1	-	-	-	-	-	0.2	0.2	1.2	1.5	2.6	2.9	4.3	10.7	11.7	15.8	23.1	2.6	1.0	0.12	0.26	**2.2**	*187.1-.4*
Other male genital	19	0	-	-	-	0.2	-	-	0.2	-	0.2	-	1.0	1.9	0.4	0.5	0.6	2.0	0.3	0.1	0.02	0.03	**0.3**	*187.5-.9*
†Bladder	737	3	-	-	-	-	0.2	-	0.2	0.7	2.9	7.4	6.5	18.2	25.3	50.4	76.1	134.8	11.0	4.3	0.31	0.94	**8.5**	*188*
Kidney etc.	296	0	1.0	0.5	-	-	0.2	-	0.2	1.2	2.2	3.7	9.8	12.8	17.1	20.1	26.8	27.6	4.4	1.7	0.24	0.48	**4.0**	*189*
Eye	47	2	0.5	-	-	-	0.2	0.2	0.7	0.9	0.5	1.1	0.3	1.2	2.1	2.3	1.2	4.5	0.7	0.3	0.04	0.06	**0.6**	*190*
Brain, nervous system	243	0	3.8	1.1	2.0	1.2	1.3	2.1	1.6	3.3	3.9	3.4	6.2	7.0	8.1	12.1	9.7	11.0	3.6	1.4	0.22	0.33	**3.5**	*191-2*
Thyroid	73	0	-	0.3	-	0.3	0.9	1.1	1.4	0.7	1.5	0.9	1.0	1.6	3.9	3.7	2.4	5.3	1.1	0.4	0.07	0.10	**1.0**	*193*
Other endocrine	10	0	0.3	0.3	-	-	-	-	-	-	-	-	0.3	-	0.4	-	0.6	1.2	0.1	0.1	0.01	0.01	**0.1**	*194*
Hodgkin's disease	158	2	-	1.2	1.6	1.5	3.3	4.0	3.2	1.7	3.2	1.1	2.0	5.0	2.6	3.7	2.4	6.1	2.4	0.9	0.15	0.18	**2.2**	*201*
Non-Hodgkin lymphoma	587	6	0.7	0.6	1.4	1.4	1.7	4.4	6.8	8.8	9.7	8.5	10.7	18.6	21.0	33.1	34.7	52.4	8.8	3.4	0.48	0.82	**7.8**	*200,202*
Multiple myeloma	245	2	-	-	-	-	0.2	-	0.2	0.2	0.2	3.1	4.2	8.5	14.1	14.0	25.0	36.1	3.7	1.4	0.16	0.35	**3.0**	*203*
Lymphoid leukaemia	180	12	5.0	3.2	0.8	2.3	0.7	0.8	-	0.7	-	0.6	2.0	1.6	4.7	4.7	6.7	16.6	2.7	1.0	0.12	0.18	**2.5**	*204*
Myeloid leukaemia	239	8	0.7	0.6	0.6	0.9	1.1	2.1	1.6	2.1	2.2	2.3	4.9	5.8	7.3	7.9	17.1	29.2	3.6	1.4	0.17	0.30	**3.1**	*205*
Monocytic leukaemia	6	0	0.2	-	-	-	-	-	-	-	-	-	-	-	-	0.5	-	1.6	0.1	0.0	0.00	0.00	**0.1**	*206*
Other leukaemia	6	0	-	-	-	-	-	-	-	-	-	0.6	-	-	-	-	-	1.6	0.1	0.0	0.00	0.00	**0.1**	*207*
Leukaemia unspecified	71	2	0.2	0.2	0.1	0.3	0.4	1.1	0.9	0.9	0.2	0.6	0.3	1.2	2.1	1.9	2.4	11.8	1.1	0.4	0.04	0.07	**0.9**	*208*
Other and unspecified	698	8	0.5	0.2	0.1	0.2	0.7	0.2	0.7	1.7	5.6	6.8	16.9	17.4	31.7	42.0	57.2	108.4	10.4	4.1	0.42	0.92	**8.5**	*O&U*
All sites	17221	142	15.0	9.6	9.3	11.6	20.0	36.1	42.1	59.4	93.7	150.5	263.2	474.4	770.7	1204.6	1658.9	2442.6	257.2		9.86	24.30	**212.8**	*ALL*
All sites but 173	17196	142	15.0	9.6	9.3	11.4	19.8	36.1	41.7	59.2	93.2	150.5	262.6	473.6	770.7	1204.6	1656.4	2438.5	256.9	100.0	9.84	24.27	**212.5**	*ALLb*

Rate from 10 cases   1.669   1.516   1.410   1.520   1.834   2.113   2.265   2.368   2.427   2.850   3.254   3.875   4.286   4.666   6.090   4.060

†Important: see notes on population page

USA, PUERTO RICO 1988-1991

ANNUAL INCIDENCE PER 100,000 BY AGE GROUP (YEARS) - FEMALE

SITE	ALL AGES	AGE UNK	0-	5-	10-	15-	20-	25-	30-	35-	40-	45-	50-	55-	60-	65-	70-	75+	CRUDE RATE	%	CR 64	CR 74	ASR (W)	ICD (9th)
Lip	22	0	-	-	-	-	-	0.2	-	-	-	-	-	0.3	1.8	0.4	1.6	3.7	0.3	0.2	0.01	0.02	**0.2**	*140*
Tongue	79	1	-	-	0.1	-	-	-	-	-	0.2	0.2	1.7	2.3	2.9	4.6	6.5	10.3	1.1	0.6	0.04	0.09	**0.8**	*141*
Salivary gland	34	1	-	-	0.1	0.2	0.2	0.2	0.2	0.2	0.8	0.2	0.3	0.7	1.5	1.2	1.1	3.3	0.5	0.3	0.02	0.04	**0.4**	*142*
Mouth	131	2	-	-	-	-	-	-	0.2	0.2	0.4	1.5	2.9	2.3	5.1	7.9	7.6	18.3	1.8	1.0	0.06	0.14	**1.4**	*143-5*
Oropharynx	43	0	-	-	-	-	-	-	-	-	0.4	0.2	-	1.7	2.9	2.5	2.7	5.3	0.6	0.3	0.03	0.05	**0.5**	*146*
Nasopharynx	10	0	-	-	-	-	0.2	-	0.4	-	-	0.2	0.6	-	0.7	-	1.1	-	0.1	0.1	0.01	0.02	**0.1**	*147*
Hypopharynx	25	0	-	-	-	-	-	-	-	0.2	0.2	0.2	-	0.3	1.5	1.7	1.6	3.3	0.3	0.2	0.01	0.03	**0.3**	*148*
Pharynx unspecified	11	0	-	-	-	-	-	-	-	-	-	-	-	0.3	0.7	0.4	-	2.3	0.2	0.1	0.01	0.01	**0.1**	*149*
Oesophagus	235	2	-	-	-	-	-	-	-	0.4	0.8	1.0	1.4	4.6	7.6	10.8	20.5	39.6	3.3	1.8	0.08	0.24	**2.2**	*150*
Stomach	617	6	-	-	-	0.2	0.2	0.4	0.6	1.0	3.7	3.4	8.3	12.9	18.9	25.3	58.9	92.3	8.5	4.6	0.25	0.67	**6.1**	*151*
Small intestine	47	0	-	-	-	-	-	-	-	0.4	0.6	0.2	1.7	1.7	3.6	2.1	3.2	3.0	0.7	0.4	0.04	0.07	**0.6**	*152*
Colon	1138	10	-	-	-	0.2	-	1.3	2.5	5.0	6.5	8.3	16.9	34.1	53.2	60.9	83.7	135.3	15.7	8.5	0.65	1.38	**12.1**	*153*
Rectum	554	5	-	-	-	0.2	-	0.7	1.5	1.4	3.7	7.6	9.1	14.9	24.8	35.7	40.5	58.0	7.7	4.1	0.32	0.71	**6.1**	*154*
Liver	159	1	-	-	-	-	0.2	-	0.2	-	0.6	1.0	1.7	3.0	6.9	9.5	9.7	24.7	2.2	1.2	0.07	0.17	**1.6**	*155*
Gallbladder etc.	221	0	-	-	-	-	-	0.2	-	0.4	1.0	1.2	4.3	3.6	9.1	15.8	20.5	27.0	3.1	1.6	0.10	0.28	**2.3**	*156*
Pancreas	312	0	-	-	-	-	-	0.3	0.5	-	0.2	0.8	2.2	4.6	8.4	15.8	30.8	50.0	4.3	2.3	0.10	0.33	**3.0**	*157*
Nose, sinuses etc.	30	0	-	-	-	-	-	-	0.2	-	0.2	-	0.3	0.7	0.7	2.1	1.1	5.3	0.4	0.2	0.01	0.03	**0.3**	*160*
Larynx	79	2	-	-	-	-	-	-	0.2	0.4	0.2	0.5	0.6	2.0	2.9	7.0	7.0	8.3	1.1	0.6	0.03	0.11	**0.8**	*161*
Bronchus, lung	625	0	-	-	0.1	0.2	0.2	0.2	0.4	1.6	1.8	3.9	8.3	19.9	25.1	41.9	61.6	71.0	8.6	4.7	0.31	0.83	**6.6**	*162*
Other thoracic organs	12	0	0.7	-	-	0.2	-	-	-	-	-	-	0.3	-	-	0.8	0.5	1.0	0.2	0.1	0.01	0.01	**0.2**	*163-4*
Bone	49	0	-	1.0	1.0	1.4	0.7	0.4	0.6	0.4	0.4	-	0.3	0.7	-	1.2	1.1	2.0	0.7	0.4	0.03	0.05	**0.6**	*170*
Connective tissue	81	1	0.7	0.3	0.1	0.3	0.2	0.7	1.1	1.0	0.4	1.0	0.9	2.3	2.2	3.3	2.7	6.7	1.1	0.6	0.06	0.09	**1.0**	*171*
Mesothelioma	10	0	-	-	-	-	-	-	-	-	0.2	-	-	-	0.4	0.4	2.7	0.7	0.1	0.1	0.00	0.02	**0.1**	*MES*
Kaposi's sarcoma	25	0	-	-	-	-	0.3	-	0.2	1.2	0.2	0.2	-	0.3	0.7	-	0.5	3.3	0.3	0.2	0.02	0.02	**0.3**	*KAP*
Melanoma of skin	92	0	-	-	0.1	0.2	0.2	0.2	0.4	1.6	1.6	1.0	2.9	2.7	3.3	3.3	4.3	7.7	1.3	0.7	0.07	0.11	**1.1**	*172*
†Other skin	33	0	-	-	-	0.3	0.2	0.2	1.0	0.8	-	0.5	0.3	0.3	0.7	0.8	2.2	2.7	0.5		0.02	0.04	**0.4**	*173*
Breast	3770	10	-	-	-	0.2	0.5	4.9	17.0	41.8	78.2	101.1	105.8	149.5	162.1	179.9	185.2	197.2	52.1	28.1	3.31	5.14	**45.7**	*174*
Uterus unspecified	47	0	-	-	-	-	-	0.4	-	0.2	0.6	0.2	0.6	1.3	1.1	2.1	2.7	7.0	0.7	0.4	0.02	0.05	**0.5**	*179*
Cervix uteri	813	2	-	-	-	0.2	0.5	5.1	9.2	11.9	21.2	21.0	20.6	20.5	29.5	31.5	35.1	42.0	11.2	6.1	0.70	1.03	**9.8**	*180*
Placenta	7	0	-	-	0.1	0.2	-	0.2	-	0.6	0.2	-	-	-	-	-	-	-	0.1	0.1	0.01	0.01	**0.1**	*181*
Corpus uteri	728	2	-	-	-	-	0.3	1.1	3.2	3.8	6.9	10.3	17.4	34.1	35.0	55.1	41.0	45.6	10.1	5.4	0.56	1.05	**8.6**	*182*
Ovary etc.	448	0	-	-	0.4	0.6	1.6	2.6	1.9	4.8	5.5	7.8	10.0	10.3	17.8	23.6	31.3	31.6	6.2	3.3	0.32	0.59	**5.2**	*183*
Other female genital	227	5	-	-	-	0.2	-	-	0.2	0.6	0.4	1.2	3.4	4.0	7.6	14.1	20.5	31.0	3.1	1.7	0.09	0.27	**2.3**	*184*
†Bladder	274	2	-	-	-	-	0.7	-	0.2	0.4	0.6	1.5	3.1	4.3	7.6	15.8	26.5	41.3	3.8	2.0	0.09	0.31	**2.7**	*188*
Kidney etc.	200	1	1.2	0.8	-	0.2	0.5	0.2	0.2	0.8	1.2	2.4	4.3	7.3	7.6	11.2	16.2	15.3	2.8	1.5	0.13	0.27	**2.4**	*189*
Eye	20	0	0.9	-	-	-	-	0.4	-	0.4	0.2	-	0.3	0.3	0.4	-	1.1	1.7	0.3	0.1	0.01	0.02	**0.3**	*190*
Brain, nervous system	198	1	1.9	2.2	2.3	0.8	1.0	0.7	1.5	1.2	2.5	2.2	3.4	3.3	6.6	9.5	8.1	9.3	2.7	1.5	0.15	0.24	**2.5**	*191-2*
Thyroid	271	0	-	-	0.1	0.9	4.3	6.2	5.3	6.2	4.3	4.2	5.1	7.6	5.5	5.8	8.1	7.7	3.7	2.0	0.25	0.32	**3.4**	*193*
Other endocrine	12	0	0.9	-	-	-	0.2	-	0.2	-	0.4	0.2	-	-	-	0.5	0.3	0.3	0.2	0.1	0.01	0.01	**0.2**	*194*
Hodgkin's disease	136	0	-	0.5	0.3	2.3	3.8	2.0	1.9	3.0	1.8	1.7	1.4	1.3	1.5	4.1	2.2	5.0	1.9	1.0	0.11	0.14	**1.7**	*201*
Non-Hodgkin lymphoma	456	2	0.2	1.1	0.3	1.1	0.9	1.6	1.7	2.4	3.7	5.1	9.4	13.3	14.2	21.6	32.4	46.3	6.3	3.4	0.28	0.55	**5.0**	*200,202*
Multiple myeloma	193	3	-	-	-	-	-	0.2	-	0.2	1.0	1.7	2.9	4.0	6.9	12.0	13.5	27.0	2.7	1.4	0.09	0.22	**2.0**	*203*
Lymphoid leukaemia	161	11	4.7	2.9	0.9	2.1	0.7	0.7	0.4	0.4	0.6	2.0	1.1	1.0	0.7	2.9	4.9	12.3	2.2	1.2	0.10	0.14	**2.1**	*204*
Myeloid leukaemia	182	8	0.7	0.3	0.6	0.5	1.0	1.8	1.7	1.2	2.5	2.4	2.3	7.0	2.9	6.6	7.6	13.7	2.5	1.4	0.13	0.20	**2.1**	*205*
Monocytic leukaemia	7	0	-	-	0.3	-	-	-	-	-	-	-	-	-	0.8	1.1	0.3	0.1	0.1	0.00	0.01	**0.1**	*206*
Other leukaemia	4	0	-	-	-	-	-	-	0.2	-	0.2	-	-	-	0.4	-	0.5	-	0.1	0.0	0.00	0.01	**0.0**	*207*
Leukaemia unspecified	44	1	-	0.2	0.1	0.3	0.2	0.2	0.4	-	-	0.2	0.6	0.3	1.1	1.7	1.6	7.0	0.6	0.3	0.02	0.04	**0.4**	*208*
Other and unspecified	587	7	0.3	-	-	0.3	0.2	1.1	0.8	1.0	2.9	4.2	8.0	12.6	18.2	32.3	43.7	84.6	8.1	4.4	0.25	0.64	**5.9**	*O&U*
All sites	13459	86	12.2	9.3	7.3	12.7	19.2	34.5	55.6	97.5	160.0	204.2	265.6	398.3	512.4	686.1	857.5	1211.4	186.1		9.00	16.77	**152.2**	*ALL*
All sites but 173	13426	86	12.2	9.3	7.3	12.4	19.1	34.3	54.6	96.7	160.0	203.7	265.3	398.0	511.7	685.3	855.4	1208.7	185.7	100.0	8.98	16.73	**151.8**	*ALLb*

Rate from 10 cases

	0-	5-	10-	15-	20-	25-	30-	35-	40-	45-	50-	55-	60-	65-	70-	75+
	1.748	1.601	1.463	1.534	1.732	1.824	1.910	2.010	2.043	2.443	2.859	3.314	3.642	4.146	5.400	3.332

†Important: see notes on population page

Uruguay, Montevideo

The Registro Nacional de Cáncer of Uruguay was created by law in 1984, but it began collecting data on cancer incidence and mortality in Montevideo only in August 1987. Since 1992 it has been located at the National Institute of Oncology, which belongs to the Ministry of Health. It is the first population-based cancer registry in the country.

The initial objectives of the registry were to develop and maintain a source of information on cancer incidence, mortality and prevalence in the country, mainly descriptive. In 1993 the registry expanded its fields of interest and began to undertake analytical and descriptive epidemiological studies on the Uruguayan population. These studies were mainly supported by funds coming from a national NGO, the Comisión Honoraria de Lucha Contra el Cáncer. Further financial support was provided by IARC.

The registry employs a medical director with training in pathology and epidemiology, an assistant epidemiologist, one clerk with coding expertise, a computer analyst, two consultant pathologists with special training in cancer, a medical doctor who supervises coding and staging, and ten data abstractors.

The county of Montevideo (530 km^2) is the area covered by the registry. It includes the capital city of Uruguay, Montevideo city, which contains almost half of the national population, and a small rural area which accounts for 4.6% of the population of the county. It is located at latitude 35° S and longitude 56° W, and represents 0.3% of the country's area. According to the last nation-wide census of 1985, the population of Montevideo was 1 309 100, including about 75 000 foreign immigrants, especially from Spain, Italy and Eastern Europe, who arrived during the first decades of this century. The population is mainly Caucasian, with no Indians; blacks constitute 3% of the total population. Internal migration from other counties used to be frequent in the past, but since 1965 has stabilized and is no longer a problem in calculating the true population at risk.

Though cancer cases are required by law to be reported, data collection is performed in an active way by a trained staff of abstractors. Data are obtained from state and private medical institutions, laboratories of pathology, oncology and radiotherapy clinics, outpatient clinics, and the Bureau of Vital Statistics of the Ministry of Health.

Though the cancer mortality data come from the death certificates of the whole country, the main area covered by the registry is Montevideo. Information is also obtained on incident cases of cancer residing outside Montevideo, but who are treated in hospitals in the city.

The registry is equipped with two personal computers that can process large databases and perform several kinds of data analysis. Each new case is registered, considering the date of diagnosis as date of incidence. Skin cancers and *in situ* cancers are registered, in all cases following the ICD-O. Consistency checks are performed periodically, and duplication checks are also carried out by hand, in all cases by the medical staff.

Due to shortage of personnel and to lack of funds, no trace-back of death certificate notifications was performed until 1993. Since 1995, active follow-up of incident cases is being performed, with the aim of obtaining survival rates.

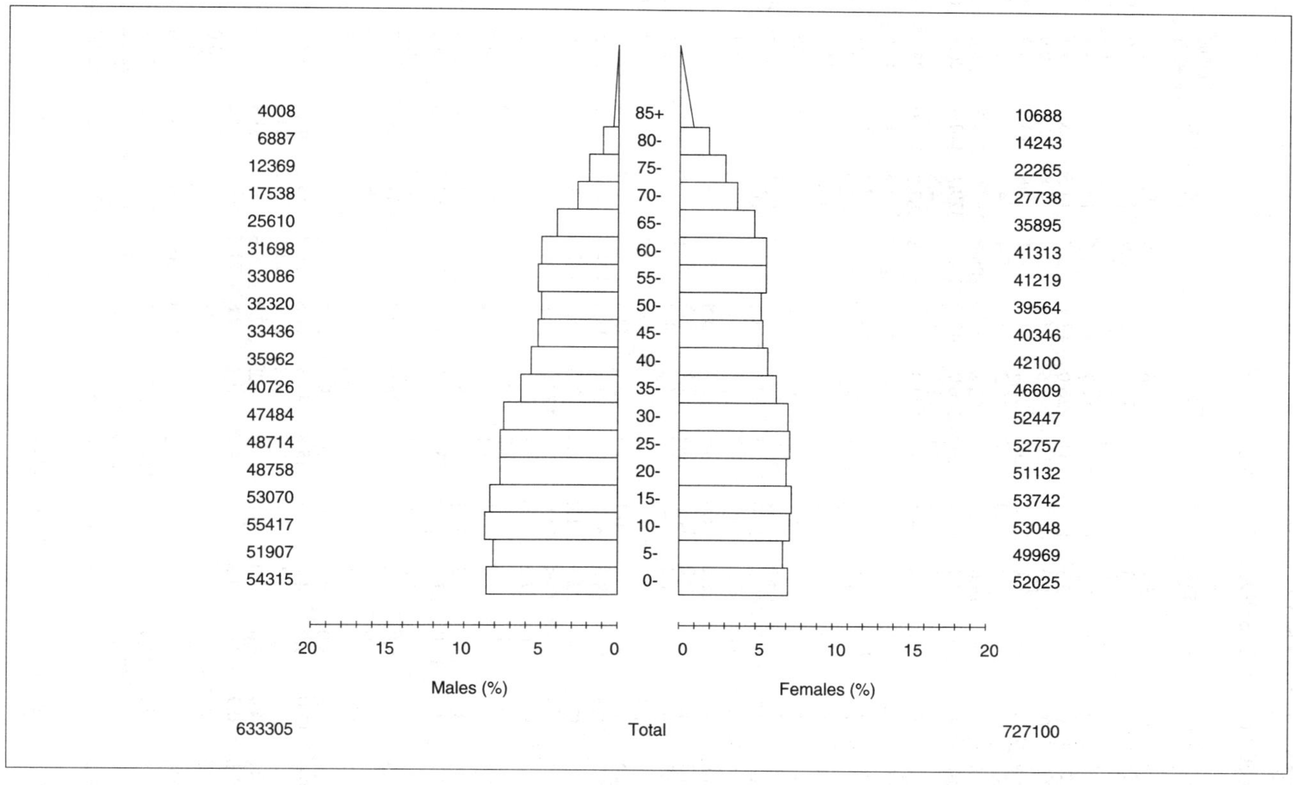

Uruguay, Montevideo

Source of population: average annual 1990–92

Census: 1975 and 1985. Dirección General de Estadísticas y Censos: Tercer Censo Nacional de Población y Vivienda. Montevideo, 1975. Dirección General de Estadísticas y Censos: Cuarto Censo Nacional de Población y Vivienda. Montevideo, 1985.

Estimate: The populations were estimated on the basis of the 1975 and 1985 censuses, taking into account births, deaths and migration and using a demographic/mathematical model for the cohorts. References: Dane-Celade, Seminario Internacional sobre Proyecciones Subnacionales de Población, Girardot, Colombia, 1988; Duchesne, Louis, Método de relación de cohortes, CELADE, Santiago, Chile, 1987; Rincón, M. y Hernández, H., Programe para elabor proyecciones de población de áreas pequeñas por sexo y grupos de edades, CELADE, San José, Costa Rica, 1988.

Notes to tables overleaf:

* The high level of diagnoses based on a death certificate alone (DCO) indicates a degree of under-ascertainment.

† 188 does not include non-invasive tumours.

Screening programmes in the area:

During the period some 10,000 examinations for breast cancer were carried out annually in the population aged 30-65.

* URUGUAY, MONTEVIDEO 1990-1992

ANNUAL INCIDENCE PER 100,000 BY AGE GROUP (YEARS) - MALE

SITE	ALL AGES	AGE UNK	0-	5-	10-	15-	20-	25-	30-	35-	40-	45-	50-	55-	60-	65-	70-	75-	80-	85+	CRUDE RATE	%	CR 64	CR 74	ASR (W)	ICD (9th)
Lip	24	0	-	-	-	-	-	-	-	-	0.9	1.0	3.1	2.0	4.2	2.6	7.6	13.5	9.7	-	1.3	0.3	0.06	0.11	**0.9**	140
Tongue	74	0	-	-	-	-	-	-	-	-	0.9	2.0	9.3	11.1	14.7	15.6	22.8	26.9	14.5	-	3.9	0.9	0.19	0.38	**2.9**	141
Salivary gland	26	0	-	-	-	-	-	0.7	2.1	-	1.9	3.0	1.0	1.0	1.1	2.6	5.7	13.5	14.5	8.3	1.4	0.3	0.05	0.10	**1.0**	142
Mouth	66	0	-	-	-	-	-	-	-	-	-	3.0	7.2	18.1	13.7	11.7	13.3	13.5	19.4	-	3.5	0.8	0.21	0.34	**2.7**	143-5
Oropharynx	78	0	-	-	-	-	-	-	-	-	1.9	4.0	9.3	12.1	16.8	26.0	17.1	2.7	14.5	16.6	4.1	1.0	0.22	0.44	**3.3**	146
Nasopharynx	17	0	-	-	0.6	0.6	-	-	-	0.8	0.9	-	1.0	1.0	1.1	2.6	7.6	2.7	4.8	16.6	0.9	0.2	0.03	0.08	**0.7**	147
Hypopharynx	79	0	-	-	-	-	-	-	-	-	0.9	4.0	3.1	16.1	23.1	23.4	13.3	8.1	4.8	33.3	4.2	1.0	0.24	0.42	**3.3**	148
Pharynx unspecified	24	0	-	-	-	-	-	-	-	-	-	-	5.2	2.0	5.3	5.2	7.6	5.4	4.8	8.3	1.3	0.3	0.06	0.13	**1.0**	149
Oesophagus	311	1	-	-	-	-	-	-	0.7	0.8	1.9	10.0	18.6	35.3	47.3	63.8	108.3	88.9	154.9	224.5	16.4	3.8	0.57	1.44	**11.9**	150
Stomach	510	0	-	-	-	0.6	-	-	0.7	3.3	4.6	22.9	30.9	37.3	73.6	106.7	142.5	196.7	329.1	340.9	26.8	6.3	0.87	2.12	**19.3**	151
Small intestine	15	0	-	-	-	-	-	-	-	-	-	-	3.1	2.0	2.1	3.9	1.9	5.4	4.8	8.3	0.8	0.2	0.04	0.07	**0.6**	152
Colon	637	0	-	-	-	-	0.7	-	0.7	5.7	4.6	12.0	24.8	48.4	89.4	122.3	224.3	266.8	387.2	523.9	33.5	7.8	0.93	2.66	**23.6**	153
Rectum	334	0	-	-	-	-	0.7	0.7	0.7	1.6	3.7	7.0	23.7	18.1	51.5	78.1	89.3	159.0	188.8	191.3	17.6	4.1	0.54	1.38	**12.5**	154
Liver	43	0	-	-	-	-	-	-	-	1.6	0.9	1.0	2.1	3.0	9.5	5.2	15.2	21.6	19.4	8.3	2.3	0.5	0.09	0.19	**1.6**	155
Gallbladder etc.	83	0	-	-	-	-	-	-	-	-	0.9	1.0	2.1	6.0	10.5	9.1	28.5	53.9	62.9	66.5	4.4	1.0	0.10	0.29	**2.9**	156
Pancreas	226	0	-	-	-	-	-	-	-	1.6	4.6	6.0	15.5	27.2	23.1	50.8	53.2	99.7	116.2	174.6	11.9	2.8	0.39	0.91	**8.6**	157
Nose, sinuses etc.	18	0	-	-	-	-	-	-	-	-	1.9	2.0	-	3.0	3.2	6.5	3.8	-	-	8.3	0.9	0.2	0.05	0.10	**0.8**	160
Larynx	308	0	-	-	-	-	-	-	-	1.6	3.7	12.0	24.8	47.4	58.9	75.5	91.2	83.5	87.1	66.5	16.2	3.8	0.74	1.58	**12.2**	161
Bronchus, lung	1778	1	-	-	-	-	0.7	0.7	4.2	16.4	48.2	64.8	140.3	215.6	316.5	403.5	543.6	517.4	566.3	632.0	93.6	21.9	4.04	8.78	**70.6**	162
Other thoracic organs	21	0	-	-	-	-	0.7	-	2.1	0.8	-	5.0	2.1	1.0	4.2	2.6	3.8	-	-	-	1.1	0.3	0.08	0.11	**1.0**	163-4
Bone	22	0	-	0.6	1.8	1.3	1.4	-	0.7	0.8	-	-	2.1	1.0	3.2	-	3.8	5.4	4.8	8.3	1.2	0.3	0.06	0.08	**1.0**	170
Connective tissue	68	0	0.6	-	-	1.3	0.7	-	1.4	3.3	3.7	3.0	7.2	13.1	8.4	7.8	9.5	16.2	9.7	33.3	3.6	0.8	0.21	0.30	**2.9**	171
Mesothelioma	11	0	-	-	-	-	-	-	-	0.8	1.9	1.0	1.0	-	5.3	1.3	1.9	2.7	-	-	0.6	0.1	0.04	0.06	**0.5**	MES
Kaposi's sarcoma	7	0	-	-	-	-	0.7	0.7	0.7	0.8	1.9	-	-	-	-	-	2.7	-	-	-	0.4	0.1	0.02	0.02	**0.3**	KAP
Melanoma of skin	89	0	-	-	-	0.6	1.4	-	4.2	4.9	3.7	8.0	5.2	10.1	9.5	13.0	32.3	5.4	38.7	8.3	4.7	1.1	0.24	0.46	**3.8**	172
Other skin	466	0	0.6	-	-	1.3	0.7	0.7	5.6	5.7	11.1	8.0	18.6	31.2	65.2	91.1	133.0	194.0	266.2	399.1	24.5		0.74	1.86	**17.6**	173
Breast	19	0	-	-	-	-	-	-	-	-	0.9	-	2.1	1.0	3.2	2.6	1.9	21.6	4.8	-	1.0	0.2	0.04	0.06	**0.7**	175
Prostate	939	0	-	-	-	-	-	-	-	-	0.9	2.0	15.5	21.2	83.1	177.0	366.8	509.3	798.6	1147.5	49.4	11.5	0.61	3.33	**32.6**	185
Testis	97	0	-	-	-	2.5	9.6	9.6	11.9	13.9	9.3	4.0	7.2	5.0	2.1	-	-	2.7	9.7	-	5.1	1.2	0.38	0.38	**4.8**	186
Penis	21	0	-	-	-	-	-	-	-	-	-	1.0	-	-	4.2	10.4	7.6	8.1	-	8.3	1.1	0.3	0.03	0.12	**0.8**	187.1-.4
Other male genital	3	0	-	-	-	-	0.7	-	-	-	-	-	-	-	1.1	-	1.9	-	-	-	0.2	0.0	0.01	0.02	**0.1**	187.5-.9
†Bladder	531	0	-	1.3	-	-	-	-	0.7	-	3.7	12.0	26.8	39.3	75.7	115.8	180.6	210.2	353.3	332.6	27.9	6.5	0.80	2.28	**19.7**	188
Kidney etc.	262	0	2.5	-	-	-	-	-	1.4	4.1	3.7	13.0	21.7	31.2	43.1	66.4	64.6	75.5	82.3	91.5	13.8	3.2	0.60	1.26	**10.6**	189
Eye	9	0	1.2	-	-	-	-	-	-	-	-	1.0	1.0	2.1	1.3	-	2.7	4.8	-	-	0.5	0.1	0.03	0.03	**0.4**	190
Brain, nervous system	146	0	1.8	3.2	3.6	1.9	1.4	2.1	2.8	2.5	10.2	15.0	7.2	15.1	11.6	26.0	30.4	26.9	38.7	33.3	7.7	1.8	0.39	0.67	**6.6**	191-2
Thyroid	27	0	-	-	0.6	-	-	1.4	0.7	-	-	2.0	5.2	7.1	2.1	3.9	1.9	2.7	9.7	-	1.4	0.3	0.09	0.12	**1.2**	193
Other endocrine	8	0	-	0.6	0.6	-	-	-	0.7	-	0.9	-	2.1	-	-	1.3	-	2.7	-	-	0.4	0.1	0.02	0.03	**0.4**	194
Hodgkin's disease	70	0	0.6	2.6	2.4	1.9	4.1	4.1	3.5	4.1	2.8	3.0	8.3	5.0	1.1	9.1	11.4	5.4	4.8	-	3.7	0.9	0.22	0.32	**3.4**	201
Non-Hodgkin lymphoma	239	0	1.2	3.2	1.2	1.9	2.1	3.4	6.3	10.6	12.0	15.0	14.4	20.1	35.8	44.3	41.8	59.3	53.2	99.8	12.6	2.9	0.64	1.07	**10.3**	200,202
Multiple myeloma	57	0	-	-	-	-	-	-	-	-	-	3.0	8.3	4.0	6.3	5.2	17.1	21.6	24.2	83.2	3.0	0.7	0.11	0.22	**2.3**	203
Lymphoid leukaemia	68	0	4.9	1.3	3.6	1.9	2.1	-	-	-	0.9	3.0	1.0	5.0	1.1	5.2	19.0	29.6	29.0	33.3	3.6	0.8	0.12	0.24	**3.1**	204
Myeloid leukaemia	69	0	-	1.9	1.8	-	0.7	0.7	2.1	4.1	0.9	2.0	9.3	8.1	4.2	5.2	22.8	21.6	14.5	16.6	3.6	0.8	0.18	0.32	**3.0**	205
Monocytic leukaemia	0	0	-	-	-	-	-	-	-	-	-	-	-	-	-	-	-	-	-	-	0.0	0.0	0.00	0.00	**0.0**	206
Other leukaemia	0	0	-	-	-	-	-	-	-	-	-	-	-	-	-	-	-	-	-	-	0.0	0.0	0.00	0.00	**0.0**	207
Leukaemia unspecified	37	0	0.6	-	0.6	-	1.4	-	0.7	1.6	-	-	1.0	2.0	4.2	11.7	13.3	10.8	9.7	8.3	1.9	0.5	0.06	0.19	**1.5**	208
Other and unspecified	660	0	-	-	-	-	-	2.1	2.1	3.3	13.9	22.9	37.1	67.5	111.5	125.0	205.3	245.2	329.1	332.6	34.7	8.1	1.30	2.95	**25.3**	O&U
All sites	8597	2	14.1	14.8	16.8	15.7	29.4	26.7	56.9	94.9	163.1	278.1	529.1	795.9	1253.5	1741.5	2567.7	3061.4	4089.6	4964.2	452.5		16.45	38.00	**334.2**	ALL
All sites but 173	8131	2	13.5	14.8	16.8	14.4	28.7	26.0	51.2	89.2	152.0	270.2	510.5	764.7	1188.3	1650.4	2434.7	2867.4	3823.4	4565.1	428.0	100.0	15.71	36.14	**316.6**	ALLb

| Rate from 1 case | | | 0.614 | 0.642 | 0.601 | 0.628 | 0.684 | 0.684 | 0.702 | 0.818 | 0.927 | 0.997 | 1.031 | 1.007 | 1.052 | 1.302 | 1.901 | 2.695 | 4.840 | 8.315 |

†Important: see notes on population page

* URUGUAY, MONTEVIDEO 1990-1992

ANNUAL INCIDENCE PER 100,000 BY AGE GROUP (YEARS) - FEMALE

SITE	ALL AGES	AGE UNK	0-	5-	10-	15-	20-	25-	30-	35-	40-	45-	50-	55-	60-	65-	70-	75-	80-	85+	CRUDE RATE	%	CR 64	CR 74	ASR (W)	ICD (9th)
Lip	3	0	-	-	-	-	-	-	0.6	-	-	0.8	-	-	-	-	-	-	-	3.1	0.1	0.0	0.01	0.01	**0.1**	*140*
Tongue	20	0	-	-	-	-	-	-	0.6	-	-	-	2.5	0.8	1.6	1.9	3.6	4.5	9.4	3.1	0.9	0.2	0.03	0.06	**0.5**	*141*
Salivary gland	15	0	-	-	-	-	0.7	-	-	-	-	-	-	0.8	3.2	-	3.6	4.5	4.7	-	0.7	0.2	0.03	0.05	**0.4**	*142*
Mouth	41	0	-	-	-	-	-	0.6	0.6	-	-	-	-	3.2	2.4	1.9	8.4	10.5	14.0	31.2	1.9	0.4	0.03	0.09	**0.9**	*143-5*
Oropharynx	10	0	-	-	-	-	-	-	-	-	-	-	-	0.8	0.8	1.9	3.6	1.5	2.3	3.1	0.5	0.1	0.01	0.04	**0.2**	*146*
Nasopharynx	8	0	-	-	0.6	-	0.7	-	-	0.7	0.8	0.8	-	-	-	-	2.4	1.5	-	-	0.4	0.1	0.02	0.03	**0.3**	*147*
Hypopharynx	6	0	-	-	-	-	-	-	-	-	-	1.7	-	-	0.8	-	-	3.0	2.3	-	0.3	0.1	0.01	0.01	**0.2**	*148*
Pharynx unspecified	3	0	-	-	-	-	-	-	-	-	-	-	-	-	-	-	-	-	4.7	3.1	0.1	0.0	0.00	0.00	**0.0**	*149*
Oesophagus	152	0	-	-	-	-	-	-	-	-	1.6	1.7	5.1	5.7	8.9	22.3	31.2	31.4	53.8	93.6	7.0	1.7	0.11	0.38	**3.4**	*150*
Stomach	399	0	-	-	-	-	-	1.3	3.2	1.4	4.8	4.1	8.4	19.4	25.8	53.9	78.1	107.8	147.4	171.5	18.3	4.4	0.34	1.00	**9.0**	*151*
Small intestine	14	0	-	-	-	-	-	-	-	-	-	0.8	0.8	2.4	0.8	-	6.0	9.4	-	-	0.6	0.2	0.02	0.02	**0.3**	*152*
Colon	793	0	-	-	-	-	3.3	0.6	1.3	6.4	7.1	15.7	21.1	38.0	50.8	81.7	168.2	182.6	287.8	436.6	36.4	8.7	0.72	1.97	**18.0**	*153*
Rectum	306	0	-	-	-	-	-	-	0.6	2.1	5.5	9.1	12.6	21.8	25.0	54.8	46.9	70.4	88.9	87.3	14.0	3.4	0.38	0.89	**7.7**	*154*
Liver	27	0	0.6	-	-	-	-	-	0.6	1.4	0.8	-	-	1.6	1.6	4.6	7.2	4.5	4.7	6.2	1.2	0.3	0.03	0.09	**0.8**	*155*
Gallbladder etc.	184	0	-	-	-	-	-	-	0.6	-	0.7	1.6	3.3	6.7	5.7	16.9	21.4	38.5	53.9	63.2	68.6	8.4	2.0	0.18	0.48	**4.2**	*156*
Pancreas	254	0	-	-	-	-	-	-	-	0.7	0.8	4.1	5.9	12.9	29.0	37.1	43.3	64.4	72.5	118.5	11.6	2.8	0.27	0.67	**5.9**	*157*
Nose, sinuses etc.	15	0	-	-	-	-	-	-	-	-	0.8	0.8	-	1.6	3.2	0.9	-	3.0	2.3	9.4	0.7	0.2	0.03	0.04	**0.4**	*160*
Larynx	32	0	-	-	-	-	-	-	-	-	2.4	1.7	4.2	2.4	8.1	0.9	2.4	4.5	2.3	6.2	1.5	0.4	0.09	0.11	**1.0**	*161*
Bronchus, lung	275	0	-	-	-	-	0.7	1.9	-	2.9	4.0	10.7	16.9	21.0	27.4	44.6	55.3	43.4	51.5	74.9	12.6	3.0	0.43	0.93	**7.5**	*162*
Other thoracic organs	11	0	-	-	-	-	-	-	-	0.7	-	0.8	-	0.8	0.8	0.9	1.2	3.0	2.3	6.2	0.5	0.1	0.02	0.03	**0.3**	*163-4*
Bone	22	0	-	-	1.2	1.3	0.6	0.6	1.4	1.6	0.8	1.7	0.8	-	0.9	1.2	1.5	9.4	3.1	-	1.0	0.2	0.05	0.06	**0.8**	*170*
Connective tissue	82	0	0.6	0.7	1.9	2.5	-	0.6	-	0.7	4.0	5.0	5.1	4.9	7.3	13.0	7.2	12.0	16.4	12.5	3.8	0.9	0.17	0.27	**2.7**	*171*
Mesothelioma	8	0	-	-	-	-	-	-	-	0.7	0.8	-	1.7	0.8	0.8	-	1.2	1.5	-	-	0.4	0.1	0.02	0.03	**0.3**	*MES*
Kaposi's sarcoma	1	0	-	-	-	-	-	-	-	-	-	-	-	0.8	-	-	-	-	-	-	0.0	0.0	0.00	0.00	**0.0**	*KAP*
Melanoma of skin	80	0	-	-	-	0.6	3.3	0.6	2.5	2.1	3.2	6.6	2.5	4.0	8.1	5.6	12.0	9.0	14.0	25.0	3.7	0.9	0.17	0.26	**2.5**	*172*
Other skin	379	0	-	-	0.6	-	-	3.2	2.5	2.1	9.5	9.9	16.9	17.8	33.1	46.4	63.7	86.8	121.7	143.5	17.4		0.48	1.03	**9.5**	*173*
Breast	3118	0	-	-	-	-	2.6	5.1	29.2	60.8	110.8	193.3	230.8	274.1	341.3	402.1	496.3	486.6	498.5	564.5	142.9	34.2	6.24	10.73	**92.6**	*174*
Uterus unspecified	41	0	-	-	-	-	-	-	0.6	-	2.4	3.3	4.2	1.6	0.8	6.5	7.2	12.0	7.0	3.1	1.9	0.4	0.06	0.13	**1.2**	*179*
Cervix uteri	528	0	-	-	-	-	3.9	10.7	26.7	42.2	48.3	55.4	38.8	42.1	34.7	32.5	49.3	40.4	32.8	56.1	24.2	5.8	1.51	1.92	**19.3**	*180*
Placenta	2	0	-	-	-	-	-	-	0.6	0.7	-	-	-	-	0.7	-	-	-	-	-	0.1	0.0	0.01	0.01	**0.1**	*181*
Corpus uteri	455	0	-	-	-	-	0.7	-	2.5	5.0	2.4	14.9	29.5	42.1	70.2	68.7	96.1	62.9	70.2	68.6	20.9	5.0	0.84	1.66	**12.8**	*182*
Ovary etc.	300	0	0.6	0.7	-	-	0.7	3.2	7.6	12.2	9.5	20.7	20.2	33.2	38.7	39.9	36.1	25.5	30.4	31.2	13.8	3.3	0.74	1.12	**9.8**	*183*
Other female genital	86	1	-	-	-	-	-	0.6	-	-	1.6	4.1	1.7	2.4	9.7	14.9	14.4	15.0	21.1	40.5	3.9	0.9	0.10	0.25	**2.2**	*184*
†Bladder	167	0	-	-	-	-	-	1.3	1.3	-	0.8	1.7	5.1	9.7	9.7	15.8	33.6	49.4	58.5	84.2	7.7	1.8	0.15	0.39	**3.7**	*188*
Kidney etc.	137	0	0.6	2.0	-	-	-	-	1.3	1.4	0.8	1.7	7.6	10.5	15.3	20.4	32.4	26.9	28.1	18.7	6.3	1.5	0.21	0.47	**3.8**	*189*
Eye	5	0	1.3	0.7	-	-	-	-	-	-	-	-	-	-	-	0.9	-	1.5	-	-	0.2	0.1	0.01	0.01	**0.3**	*190*
Brain, nervous system	155	0	3.2	2.0	1.9	1.2	2.6	1.9	2.5	2.1	9.5	4.1	11.0	10.5	21.8	13.0	15.6	21.0	32.8	9.4	7.1	1.7	0.37	0.52	**5.3**	*191-2*
Thyroid	115	0	-	-	0.6	4.3	3.9	3.8	11.4	6.4	6.3	4.1	6.7	9.7	10.5	8.4	2.4	3.0	9.4	15.6	5.3	1.3	0.34	0.39	**4.4**	*193*
Other endocrine	5	0	1.3	0.7	-	-	-	-	-	-	0.7	-	-	-	-	-	-	1.2	-	-	0.2	0.1	0.01	0.02	**0.3**	*194*
Hodgkin's disease	54	0	-	-	0.6	4.3	5.2	3.8	1.9	0.7	0.8	2.5	2.5	2.4	4.8	1.9	2.4	4.5	4.7	9.4	2.5	0.6	0.15	0.17	**2.2**	*201*
Non-Hodgkin lymphoma	261	0	1.3	1.3	0.6	3.1	2.0	1.3	4.4	4.3	4.0	6.6	13.5	13.7	31.5	29.7	50.5	61.4	37.4	53.0	12.0	2.9	0.44	0.84	**7.5**	*200,202*
Multiple myeloma	79	0	-	-	-	-	-	0.6	-	-	1.6	1.7	1.7	2.4	8.1	11.1	20.4	24.0	16.4	21.8	3.6	0.9	0.08	0.24	**1.9**	*203*
Lymphoid leukaemia	61	0	2.6	2.0	0.6	-	3.3	-	-	-	0.8	0.8	-	4.0	7.3	3.7	9.6	13.5	14.0	15.6	2.8	0.7	0.11	0.17	**2.0**	*204*
Myeloid leukaemia	71	0	0.6	-	1.3	-	1.3	-	0.6	2.1	1.6	1.7	3.4	6.5	0.8	7.4	18.0	19.5	16.4	6.2	3.3	0.8	0.10	0.23	**2.0**	*205*
Monocytic leukaemia	1	0	-	-	-	-	-	-	-	-	-	-	-	0.8	-	-	-	-	-	-	0.0	0.0	0.00	0.00	**0.0**	*206*
Other leukaemia	0	0	-	-	-	-	-	-	-	-	-	-	-	-	-	-	-	-	-	-	0.0	0.0	0.00	0.00	**0.0**	*207*
Leukaemia unspecified	41	0	0.6	0.7	-	0.6	0.7	-	-	0.7	1.6	1.7	0.8	2.4	1.6	2.8	6.0	12.0	11.7	15.6	1.9	0.4	0.06	0.10	**1.2**	*208*
Other and unspecified	670	0	0.6	1.3	0.6	-	-	1.3	1.9	2.9	5.5	11.6	16.0	30.7	46.0	89.1	120.2	178.2	248.1	315.0	30.7	7.4	0.59	1.64	**15.2**	*O&U*
All sites	9492	1	14.1	12.0	9.4	18.0	36.5	43.6	106.1	166.6	257.3	408.1	506.4	666.4	910.1	1163.6	1591.0	1768.1	2122.6	2635.4	435.1		15.78	29.55	**264.7**	*ALL*
All sites but 173	9113	1	14.1	12.0	8.8	18.0	36.5	40.4	103.6	164.5	247.8	398.2	489.5	648.6	877.0	1117.1	1527.4	1681.2	2000.9	2491.9	417.8	100.0	15.30	28.52	**255.2**	*ALLb*

Rate from 1 case   0.641 0.667 0.628 0.620 0.652 0.632 0.636 0.715 0.792 0.826 0.843 0.809 0.807 0.929 1.202 1.497 2.340 3.119

†Important: see notes on population page

137

Canada

Since 1969, Statistics Canada, Canada's central statistical agency, has collected population-based cancer incidence data. Starting with the 1992 data year, these data have been compiled by the Canadian Cancer Registry (CCR), replacing the event-oriented National Cancer Incidence Reporting System that functioned from 1969 to 1991. The goal of CCR is to provide incidence and survival information required for cancer control from a single national database. Reporting of cancer data from the ten provinces and two territories is coordinated by the Canadian Council of Cancer Registries, which includes representatives from each of the provincial or territorial registries (PTCRs), Statistics Canada, Health Canada, the National Cancer Institute of Canada, the Canadian Institute for Health Information and the Canadian Society for Epidemiology and Biostatistics.

Canada is the second largest country in the world, with an area of 9 970 610 km^2 extending from longitude 53° to 141° W and from latitude 42° to 83° N. It is bounded to the west by the Pacific Ocean and Alaska, to the north by the Arctic Ocean, to the east by the Atlantic Ocean and to the south by the USA.

The population numbered over 27 000 000 at the 1991 census, of whom 28% were under 20 years of age and 12% aged 65 or over. Most of this population lives in a corridor about 300 km wide along the southern border, and 32% is concentrated in the cities of Toronto, Montreal and Vancouver. A total of 77% live in urban areas.

Canada attracts about 200 000 or more immigrants annually (a higher proportion of its population than most other countries), with the majority going to Ontario (55%), British Columbia (17%), Quebec (14%) and Alberta (10%). Between 1986 and 1991, only Ontario, British Columbia and the Yukon gained population through inter-provincial migration, while Saskatchewan, Manitoba, Quebec, Alberta and Newfoundland lost more residents than they gained.

Canada's population is diverse with respect to ethnic origin, and almost 30% reported more than one ethnic background in 1991. For the 71% reporting single origins, major groups included British (28%), French (23%), German (3.4%), Italian (2.8%), Chinese (2.2%) and Ukrainian (1.5%). The aboriginal population of Canada, comprising native Indians, Métis, and Inuit, accounts for 3.7%. Languages spoken reflect these origins, the most frequently reported mother tongues being English (60%) and French (24%). The major religious denominations are Catholic (46%), Protestant (36%).

In 1991, the 7.8 million men in the labour force were distributed among the following major occupational groups: managerial and administrative (14%), construction (11%), service (10%), sales (9%) and product fabricating and assembling (9%). Major occupations among the 6.4 million women in the labour force included clerical and related (32%), service (16%), managerial and administrative (10%), sales (9%) and medicine and health (9%).

Health care delivery, including cancer registration, is a provincial/territorial responsibility. Centralized cancer care is provided in most provinces through provincial cancer agencies, which treat close to half of all registered cancer patients and which house population-based cancer registries for the province. Cancer registries for other provinces and both territories are generally organized through the departments of health. Each year, the registries of the ten provinces and of the Northwest Territories and Yukon report to Statistics Canada, by computer diskette, full information on incident cancer cases. Agreements have been signed between most provincial and territorial governments and Statistics Canada to provide a legal basis for transmission of data to the national level.

Information on each new patient and tumour is reported by the PTCRs using the standard record layouts and coding structures defined by the CCR. A set of validity and correlation checks is then applied, and any records failing to meet these (usually less than 1%) are rejected and returned for correction. The CCR operates in ICD-O-2, and defines multiple primaries based on a set of rules that involves four-digit ICD-O-T-2 codes, ICD-O-M-2 groupings, and laterality. By contrast, the event-oriented NCRS collected data from 1988-1991 in ICD-O-1; these procedures were described in Volume VI.

The CCR is organized as a patient-oriented SAS database on an IBM mainframe. Incoming patient and tumour records are checked for duplicates based on provincial registry numbers. An additional check for duplicate patients and tumours is conducted annually using all records in the database from 1992 onwards. In the first such run, based on 140 000 records, an internal duplication rate of 0.2% was found, about half the duplicates occurring between PTCRs and the remainder within PTCRs.

The Canadian Council of Cancer Registries has established a Data Quality Committee to make recommendations on matters relating to data quality and standardization for Canadian cancer registries. While reporting is considered to be greater than 95% complete, vigilance is always necessary to register cases from new sources, as medical care patterns change.

The annual publication, *Canadian Cancer Statistics*, developed in collaboration with the National Cancer Institute of Canada, Health Canada and PTCRs, is widely used. A historical monograph, *The Making of the Canadian Cancer Registry: Cancer Incidence in Canada and its Regions, 1969–1988* was published in 1993, and an atlas of cancer incidence is being prepared at Health Canada. Data from the National Cancer Incidence Reporting System and the CCR are being used for a variety of record-linkage studies. Epidemiological research includes an international study of cancer patterns among circumpolar Inuit, in collaboration with Denmark, Alaska and Russia, and an evaluation of screening for neuroblastoma, in collaboration with the University of Minnesota. Data for Canadian registries are published annually in *Cancer Incidence in North America*, a publication of the NAACCR.

Leslie Gaudette

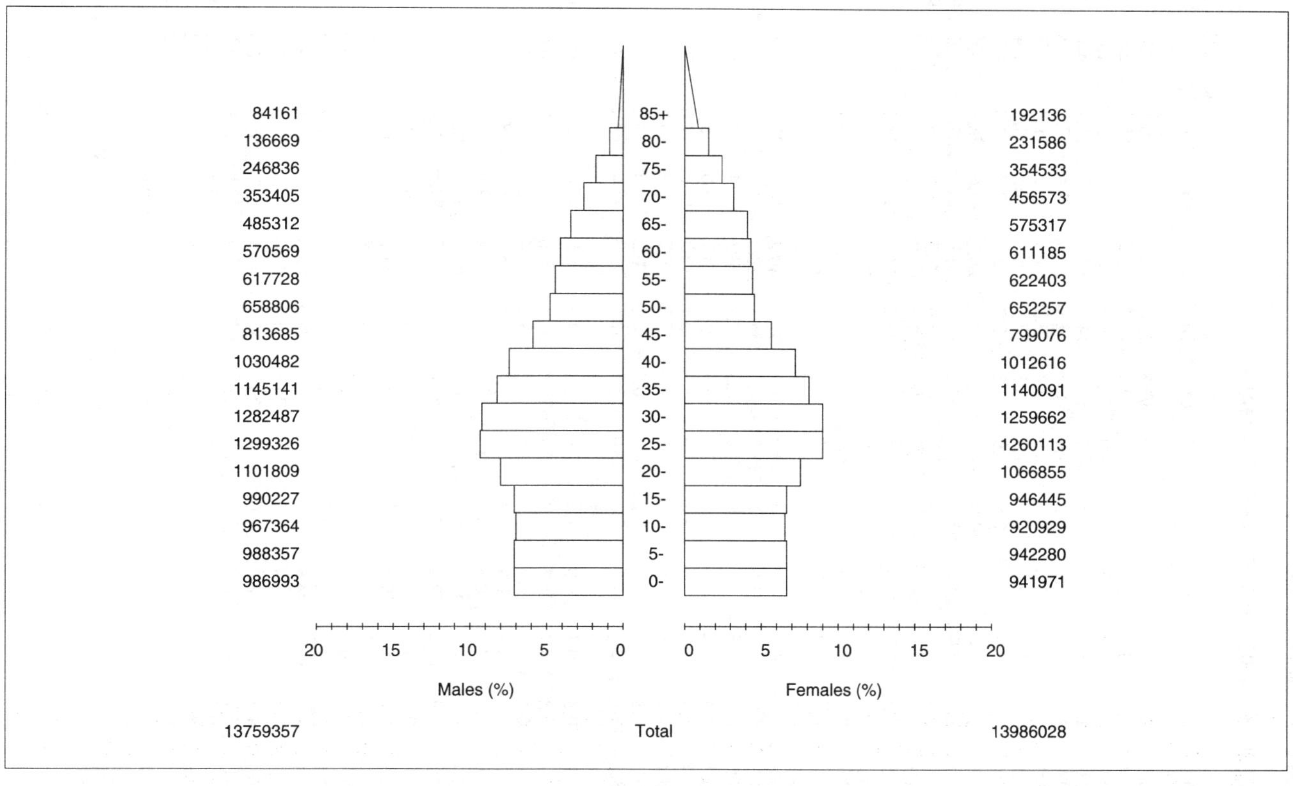

Canada

Source of population: average annual 1988-92
Census: Statistics Canada June 1991
Estimate: The populations were estimated at 1 July each year, based on revised intercensal estimates for 1988-91 and post-censal estimates for 1992. In 1993 revised estimates dating back to 1971 were implemented by Statistics Canada and population data from 1971 now include estimates of net census undercoverage, plus non-permanent residents defined as persons claiming refugee status, foreign students, work permit holders, or holders of Minister's permits, and non-Canadian-born dependants of such individuals. References: Statistics Canada, Catalogue 91-537, Revised intercensal population and family estimates, July 1, 1971–91, and Catalogue 91-213, Annual demographic statistics 1993 (for 1992 data).

Notes to tables overleaf:
† Kaposi's sarcoma is under-reported in this volume because cases of skin cancer (ICD-9 173) were not provided
† 173 not available
† 188 does not include non-invasive tumours for Newfoundland, the Northwest Territories and Ontario and registries differ across Canada as to how invasive tumours are defined.

Screening programmes in the area:
Organized breast screening programmes were set up between mid–88 and mid–91 in British Columbia, Alberta, Saskatchewan, Ontario, Noval Scotia and Yukon. A considerable amount of non-organized mammography screening has also been carried out since the mid–80s in all provinces.

CANADA 1988-1992

ANNUAL INCIDENCE PER 100,000 BY AGE GROUP (YEARS) - MALE

SITE	ALL AGES	AGE UNK	0-	5-	10-	15-	20-	25-	30-	35-	40-	45-	50-	55-	60-	65-	70-	75-	80-	85+	CRUDE RATE	%	CR 64	CR 74	ASR (W)	ICD (9th)
Lip	2842	2	-	-	-	0.0	0.1	0.3	0.6	0.7	1.6	3.5	5.4	8.2	12.0	17.2	25.6	32.2	40.5	46.3	4.1	1.0	0.16	0.38	**3.3**	*140*
Tongue	1774	1	0.0	0.0	-	0.1	0.1	0.2	0.5	0.9	1.5	3.3	5.4	8.8	10.4	10.5	11.4	10.5	11.3	11.6	2.6	0.6	0.16	0.27	**2.2**	*141*
Salivary gland	671	0	0.0	0.0	0.1	0.1	0.1	0.3	0.4	0.4	0.7	0.9	1.3	2.0	3.0	3.3	4.9	6.2	6.9	9.3	1.0	0.2	0.05	0.09	**0.8**	*142*
Mouth	2139	2	-	-	0.0	0.1	0.1	0.1	0.4	0.6	1.4	3.6	6.1	10.7	14.1	13.3	14.9	14.5	14.0	11.4	3.1	0.8	0.19	0.33	**2.7**	*143-5*
Oropharynx	1175	0	-	-	-	-	0.0	0.0	0.1	0.4	1.1	2.3	3.9	5.9	7.0	8.5	7.3	7.0	4.4	7.1	1.7	0.4	0.10	0.18	**1.5**	*146*
Nasopharynx	624	0	0.0	0.0	0.0	0.2	0.1	0.2	0.5	1.0	1.6	1.1	2.6	2.6	2.9	2.4	2.2	1.6	1.9	1.7	0.9	0.2	0.06	0.09	**0.8**	*147*
Hypopharynx	993	0	-	-	-	-	-	-	0.1	0.1	0.2	1.2	2.8	5.3	7.3	8.1	7.1	5.8	7.5	4.3	1.4	0.4	0.08	0.16	**1.2**	*148*
Pharynx unspecified	458	1	-	-	-	-	0.0	0.0	0.0	0.0	0.3	0.5	1.2	2.8	3.0	3.3	2.9	2.9	2.8	4.0	0.7	0.2	0.04	0.07	**0.6**	*149*
Oesophagus	3465	0	0.0	-	-	0.0	-	0.0	0.1	0.3	1.0	2.4	7.2	11.8	19.9	27.2	32.0	36.2	37.6	46.1	5.0	1.3	0.21	0.51	**4.1**	*150*
Stomach	9323	7	-	-	-	0.0	0.1	0.5	0.7	2.0	3.9	7.9	14.7	25.5	40.0	63.2	87.3	114.8	146.3	163.7	13.6	3.4	0.48	1.23	**10.6**	*151*
Small intestine	750	0	0.0	-	-	0.0	0.0	0.1	0.2	0.3	0.6	0.9	1.4	2.7	3.8	4.9	5.9	7.7	8.9	6.7	1.1	0.3	0.05	0.10	**0.9**	*152*
Colon	23539	10	-	-	-	0.2	0.3	0.8	1.7	4.0	8.9	18.1	35.7	64.2	110.6	162.1	229.4	289.7	359.1	377.6	34.2	8.5	1.22	3.18	**26.9**	*153*
Rectum	13732	6	-	-	-	0.0	0.1	0.5	0.8	2.6	6.0	12.8	26.6	47.9	71.3	100.9	127.2	148.0	163.3	149.5	20.0	5.0	0.84	1.98	**16.1**	*154*
Liver	2580	0	0.6	0.1	0.1	0.1	0.1	0.2	0.5	0.9	1.5	2.6	4.4	8.3	11.8	20.1	22.8	25.7	28.0	26.1	3.8	0.9	0.16	0.37	**3.1**	*155*
Gallbladder etc.	1626	0	-	0.0	-	-	-	0.1	0.0	0.3	0.5	1.3	2.4	3.9	6.0	11.5	15.8	23.3	26.6	30.7	2.4	0.6	0.07	0.21	**1.8**	*156*
Pancreas	6702	2	0.0	-	-	0.0	0.0	0.1	0.3	0.8	2.7	6.6	10.6	21.0	32.1	47.2	61.7	76.9	97.5	109.1	9.7	2.4	0.37	0.92	**7.7**	*157*
Nose, sinuses etc.	528	0	0.0	0.1	0.0	0.1	0.1	0.1	0.1	0.4	0.4	0.8	1.0	1.7	2.4	3.8	3.7	4.9	4.4	5.0	0.8	0.2	0.04	0.07	**0.6**	*160*
Larynx	5087	1	-	-	-	-	0.1	0.0	0.2	0.9	2.2	6.1	14.1	24.6	33.2	38.6	39.6	40.2	34.4	27.8	7.4	1.8	0.41	0.80	**6.3**	*161*
Bronchus, lung	55768	22	0.1	-	0.1	0.1	0.3	0.5	1.6	4.4	14.8	41.2	95.5	190.1	315.3	454.3	555.8	628.3	611.3	500.7	81.1	20.1	3.32	8.37	**65.4**	*162*
Other thoracic organs	508	0	0.4	0.1	0.1	0.3	0.3	0.5	0.3	0.6	0.5	0.6	1.1	1.1	1.4	2.3	3.4	3.3	4.4	3.3	0.7	0.2	0.04	0.07	**0.6**	*163-4*
Bone	832	0	0.1	0.7	1.2	1.9	1.1	0.7	0.7	0.7	0.9	1.0	0.9	1.8	2.0	2.6	3.1	3.7	5.6	5.7	1.2	0.3	0.07	0.10	**1.1**	*170*
Connective tissue	1703	3	1.1	0.5	0.6	0.9	1.1	1.0	1.2	1.4	1.8	2.8	2.9	3.4	5.5	8.3	9.1	12.3	13.6	21.6	2.5	0.6	0.12	0.21	**2.2**	*171*
Mesothelioma	935	0	-	-	0.0	-	0.0	0.0	0.1	0.2	0.5	1.1	2.8	3.6	5.6	6.5	7.5	9.7	6.9	4.5	1.4	0.3	0.07	0.14	**1.1**	*MES*
†Kaposi's sarcoma	236	0	-	-	-	-	0.0	0.5	0.8	0.9	0.8	0.6	0.2	0.1	0.1	0.2	0.1	0.2	0.6	0.2	0.3	0.1	0.02	0.02	**0.3**	*KAP*
Melanoma of skin	6286	13	0.0	0.0	0.2	0.8	1.8	3.4	5.4	8.3	11.1	12.7	17.1	20.4	25.0	27.4	32.4	35.3	35.0	39.2	9.1	2.3	0.53	0.83	**7.7**	*172*
†Other skin																										
Breast	510	1	-	-	-	-	0.0	0.0	0.1	0.1	0.3	0.4	0.9	1.5	2.6	3.3	4.2	5.8	7.6	8.1	0.7	0.2	0.03	0.07	**0.6**	*175*
Prostate	59546	22	0.0	0.0	-	0.0	0.1	0.1	0.1	0.2	0.8	5.7	25.5	92.0	238.4	470.8	731.5	956.6	1116.1	1178.0	86.6	21.5	1.82	7.83	**64.7**	*185*
Testis	3083	2	0.5	0.1	0.1	2.4	6.8	10.5	9.9	8.1	6.1	3.9	2.6	2.3	1.6	1.5	1.8	1.4	0.9	2.1	4.5	1.1	0.27	0.29	**3.8**	*186*
Penis	499	0	-	-	-	0.0	0.0	0.0	0.1	0.1	0.4	0.9	0.8	1.7	2.3	2.7	3.4	5.1	8.0	8.8	0.7	0.2	0.03	0.06	**0.6**	*187.1-.4*
Other male genital	177	1	0.0	0.1	-	0.0	0.1	0.0	0.1	0.1	0.1	0.3	0.3	0.5	0.6	0.9	1.3	1.4	2.5	3.3	0.3	0.1	0.01	0.02	**0.2**	*187.5-.9*
†Bladder	16385	2	0.1	0.0	0.0	0.1	0.3	0.7	1.4	3.0	5.9	11.8	23.0	43.1	76.9	116.4	155.7	204.3	246.9	284.5	23.8	5.9	0.83	2.19	**18.7**	*188*
Kidney etc.	9209	5	1.9	0.4	0.1	0.2	0.2	0.4	1.3	3.6	6.9	13.2	22.2	32.2	46.9	60.8	74.6	84.2	89.4	81.0	13.4	3.3	0.65	1.33	**11.1**	*189*
Eye	698	2	1.3	0.1	0.0	0.1	0.0	0.1	0.3	0.6	0.6	1.1	1.5	1.9	3.0	3.5	5.3	4.5	4.4	6.7	1.0	0.3	0.05	0.10	**0.9**	*190*
Brain, nervous system	5320	1	4.2	3.4	2.5	2.4	2.4	3.4	4.2	4.8	6.2	8.7	10.8	15.6	20.7	25.7	26.4	27.8	27.1	19.2	7.7	1.9	0.45	0.71	**7.0**	*191-2*
Thyroid	1419	0	-	0.1	0.2	0.5	0.7	1.6	1.8	2.4	2.9	3.4	3.3	3.9	4.2	6.0	5.5	4.4	5.6	5.0	2.1	0.5	0.12	0.18	**1.8**	*193*
Other endocrine	383	0	1.3	0.2	0.2	0.4	0.3	0.2	0.2	0.2	0.3	0.4	0.4	0.9	0.7	1.2	1.5	1.8	1.7	1.2	0.6	0.1	0.03	0.05	**0.6**	*194*
Hodgkin's disease	2191	0	0.1	0.5	1.7	3.7	5.0	4.4	3.8	3.4	3.3	3.2	3.1	3.8	3.3	4.4	4.5	3.6	4.2	4.8	3.2	0.8	0.20	0.24	**2.9**	*201*
Non-Hodgkin lymphoma	10763	7	1.3	1.6	1.5	2.3	2.6	3.8	6.2	9.4	12.1	18.2	24.5	31.0	42.2	57.0	76.0	84.9	87.4	92.9	15.6	3.9	0.78	1.45	**13.1**	*200,202*
Multiple myeloma	3517	1	-	-	0.0	-	0.1	0.1	0.3	0.4	1.5	2.6	5.4	9.9	14.4	24.7	35.3	45.5	51.1	60.1	5.1	1.3	0.17	0.47	**4.0**	*203*
Lymphoid leukaemia	4408	1	6.8	3.3	2.0	1.6	0.8	0.4	0.6	1.0	1.3	3.0	6.0	9.0	17.4	23.2	33.6	47.1	53.7	72.0	6.4	1.6	0.27	0.55	**5.7**	*204*
Myeloid leukaemia	3069	2	0.7	0.4	0.6	0.9	1.1	1.6	1.5	2.3	2.7	4.3	5.3	7.2	10.3	15.9	21.3	27.4	37.8	44.0	4.5	1.1	0.19	0.38	**3.7**	*205*
Monocytic leukaemia	147	0	0.1	0.0	-	0.1	0.0	0.0	0.0	0.1	0.2	0.1	0.1	0.3	0.4	0.6	1.0	1.5	3.1	3.1	0.2	0.1	0.01	0.02	**0.2**	*206*
Other leukaemia	126	0	0.2	0.0	0.1	0.0	0.1	0.1	0.1	0.1	0.1	0.1	0.2	0.2	0.5	0.5	0.8	0.8	1.9	1.0	0.2	0.0	0.01	0.02	**0.2**	*207*
Leukaemia unspecified	844	4	0.3	0.2	0.1	0.0	0.1	0.2	0.2	0.2	0.2	0.2	0.5	0.8	1.6	3.1	4.1	7.1	12.1	15.4	22.6	1.2	0.3	0.04	0.09	**1.0**	*208*
Other and unspecified	10543	23	0.7	0.0	0.0	0.2	0.3	0.8	1.4	2.4	3.7	7.9	15.6	27.2	44.5	66.8	94.5	127.8	169.6	242.2	15.3	3.8	0.52	1.33	**12.0**	*O&U*
All sites																										
All sites but 173	277113	144	22.2	12.0	11.7	20.0	27.3	38.7	50.7	75.6	122.0	225.4	419.8	764.0	1280.1	1937.8	2598.7	3188.7	3605.9	3753.7	402.8	100.0	15.35	38.05	**322.1**	*ALLb*

Rate from 10 cases   0.203   0.202   0.207   0.202   0.182   0.154   0.156   0.175   0.194   0.246   0.304   0.324   0.351   0.412   0.566   0.810   1.463   2.376

†Important: see notes on population page

CANADA 1988-1992

ANNUAL INCIDENCE PER 100,000 BY AGE GROUP (YEARS) - FEMALE

SITE	ALL AGES	AGE UNK	0-	5-	10-	15-	20-	25-	30-	35-	40-	45-	50-	55-	60-	65-	70-	75-	80-	85+	CRUDE RATE	%	CR 64	CR 74	ASR (W)	ICD (9th)
Lip	532	3	-	-	0.0	-	0.0	0.0	0.1	0.1	0.2	0.5	0.7	1.3	1.6	2.2	3.5	4.0	6.4	8.4	0.8	0.2	0.02	0.05	**0.5**	*140*
Tongue	781	2	-	0.0	-	0.0	0.1	0.1	0.2	0.5	0.5	1.0	1.3	2.5	3.0	3.7	4.9	5.0	7.4	5.9	1.1	0.3	0.05	0.09	**0.8**	*141*
Salivary gland	510	1	0.0	0.0	0.0	0.1	0.2	0.3	0.3	0.6	0.7	0.6	1.2	1.1	1.8	2.0	1.8	2.3	3.3	5.1	0.7	0.2	0.04	0.05	**0.5**	*142*
Mouth	1183	1	-	-	0.1	0.1	0.1	0.3	0.2	0.4	0.6	1.5	2.3	4.0	5.5	6.0	6.4	7.4	9.1	10.4	1.7	0.5	0.08	0.14	**1.2**	*143-5*
Oropharynx	434	0	-	-	-	0.0	0.0	0.0	0.0	0.2	0.4	0.7	1.1	1.9	2.4	2.7	2.3	2.3	1.9	1.4	0.6	0.2	0.03	0.06	**0.5**	*146*
Nasopharynx	271	0	0.1	0.0	0.0	0.0	0.1	0.2	0.3	0.4	0.4	0.6	1.0	0.7	1.0	1.0	1.0	1.0	0.3	0.6	0.4	0.1	0.02	0.03	**0.3**	*147*
Hypopharynx	221	0	-	-	-	-	-	-	-	0.0	0.1	0.3	0.6	0.9	1.4	1.1	1.5	1.5	0.9	0.7	0.3	0.1	0.02	0.03	**0.2**	*148*
Pharynx unspecified	154	0	0.0	-	-	-	0.0	0.0	0.0	0.0	0.1	0.2	0.4	0.6	0.9	0.6	1.2	1.2	0.5	0.9	0.2	0.1	0.01	0.02	**0.2**	*149*
Oesophagus	1492	1	-	-	-	-	0.0	-	0.1	0.1	0.2	0.9	1.3	3.3	5.3	8.1	10.6	12.6	18.7	21.8	2.1	0.6	0.06	0.15	**1.3**	*150*
Stomach	5322	1	-	-	0.0	0.0	0.1	0.3	0.7	1.7	2.4	3.6	6.8	9.3	15.6	24.1	33.4	49.8	67.0	81.4	7.6	2.1	0.20	0.49	**4.5**	*151*
Small intestine	700	0	-	-	-	0.0	0.0	0.1	0.2	0.3	0.5	0.7	1.1	1.8	2.4	3.8	5.2	5.6	6.0	4.6	1.0	0.3	0.04	0.08	**0.7**	*152*
Colon	24275	6	0.0	-	0.1	0.1	0.4	0.9	1.7	4.2	8.8	18.0	32.6	55.0	81.4	120.6	164.0	223.6	279.7	311.4	34.7	9.7	1.02	2.44	**21.3**	*153*
Rectum	9864	3	0.0	-	-	0.1	0.1	0.6	1.0	2.1	4.8	9.8	17.0	27.4	38.3	50.5	64.9	80.7	92.1	103.2	14.1	4.0	0.51	1.08	**9.2**	*154*
Liver	1345	1	0.3	0.1	0.1	0.0	0.1	0.2	0.3	0.3	0.6	0.9	1.8	2.8	4.5	6.5	7.9	11.4	13.7	18.9	1.9	0.5	0.06	0.13	**1.2**	*155*
Gallbladder etc.	2403	0	-	-	-	-	-	0.0	0.1	0.4	0.6	1.6	2.8	4.7	8.0	12.0	17.3	21.7	27.8	36.5	3.4	1.0	0.09	0.24	**2.1**	*156*
Pancreas	6408	3	0.0	0.0	0.0	0.0	0.1	0.2	0.3	0.6	1.8	3.7	7.0	12.2	20.7	33.3	48.1	58.7	76.9	90.1	9.2	2.6	0.23	0.64	**5.5**	*157*
Nose, sinuses etc.	344	0	0.1	0.0	0.1	0.1	0.1	0.1	0.1	0.2	0.3	0.5	0.8	1.0	1.2	1.6	1.8	2.5	1.6	2.9	0.5	0.1	0.02	0.04	**0.4**	*160*
Larynx	1070	1	-	-	-	-	0.0	0.0	0.1	0.3	0.8	1.7	2.8	5.4	6.4	6.1	6.4	4.9	4.1	2.8	1.5	0.4	0.09	0.15	**1.2**	*161*
Bronchus, lung	27377	10	0.1	-	0.0	0.1	0.3	0.6	2.3	5.4	14.7	33.3	60.4	92.9	136.7	173.7	193.7	192.3	154.5	117.3	39.1	11.0	1.73	3.57	**28.0**	*162*
Other thoracic organs	332	0	0.4	0.0	0.1	0.0	0.1	0.2	0.2	0.2	0.4	0.5	0.7	0.7	1.1	1.7	1.3	2.0	1.9	1.4	0.5	0.1	0.02	0.04	**0.4**	*163-4*
Bone	667	1	0.2	0.5	1.4	1.4	0.6	0.5	0.6	0.6	0.6	0.8	0.9	1.1	1.7	1.9	2.0	2.4	2.1	2.8	1.0	0.3	0.05	0.07	**0.9**	*170*
Connective tissue	1460	2	0.8	0.6	0.6	0.8	1.0	1.1	1.0	1.5	1.5	1.8	2.6	2.9	4.1	5.3	5.9	8.1	7.7	11.0	2.1	0.6	0.10	0.16	**1.6**	*171*
Mesothelioma	230	0	-	-	-	-	-	-	-	0.0	0.1	0.2	0.3	0.8	0.8	1.2	1.5	1.3	1.0	1.1	1.0	0.3	0.1	0.02	0.03	**0.2**	*MES*
†Kaposi's sarcoma	11	0	-	-	-	-	-	0.0	-	0.0	-	-	-	-	-	-	0.1	0.1	-	0.3	0.1	0.0	0.0	0.00	0.00	**0.0**	*KAP*
Melanoma of skin	6206	2	0.0	0.1	0.2	1.2	3.6	5.3	7.9	11.2	13.6	13.5	13.2	16.1	16.4	17.5	19.4	21.7	21.5	23.7	8.9	2.5	0.51	0.70	**6.9**	*172*
†Other skin																											
Breast	72027	21	-	-	-	0.1	0.8	6.1	21.1	51.8	107.6	162.9	199.4	229.0	285.5	332.6	372.8	393.9	381.5	364.6	103.0	28.8	5.32	8.85	**76.8**	*174*
Uterus unspecified	558	0	-	0.0	-	-	0.0	0.1	0.1	0.2	0.5	0.9	1.0	1.6	1.8	2.1	2.9	3.4	5.2	8.8	0.8	0.2	0.03	0.06	**0.5**	*179*
Cervix uteri	7020	6	0.0	-	-	0.0	1.9	7.7	13.4	16.7	16.0	15.7	13.5	15.2	16.1	19.7	19.4	22.1	20.0	16.3	10.0	2.8	0.58	0.78	**7.8**	*180*
Placenta	35	0	0.0	-	-	-	0.1	0.1	0.3	0.1	0.0	-	-	-	-	-	-	-	-	-	0.0	0.0	0.00	0.00	**0.0**	*181*
Corpus uteri	13582	5	-	-	-	0.0	0.1	0.5	1.5	4.1	9.2	15.3	35.5	53.7	67.7	85.7	91.0	81.6	67.8	47.6	19.4	5.4	0.94	1.82	**14.3**	*182*
Ovary etc.	9793	4	0.1	0.2	0.7	1.2	1.9	2.4	3.8	6.3	11.0	17.9	26.7	32.6	39.3	43.9	51.2	53.3	52.8	50.9	14.0	3.9	0.72	1.20	**10.5**	*183*
Other female genital	2005	1	0.1	0.0	-	0.1	0.2	0.4	1.0	1.5	1.5	2.6	3.4	3.6	6.1	8.3	11.6	14.8	17.2	26.9	2.9	0.8	0.10	0.20	**1.9**	*184*
†Bladder	5600	2	0.0	-	-	0.1	0.2	0.3	0.8	1.2	2.7	4.8	7.6	12.6	19.2	26.7	36.8	50.9	59.5	71.2	8.0	2.2	0.25	0.57	**5.0**	*188*
Kidney etc.	5712	2	2.1	0.7	0.1	0.1	0.2	0.6	1.2	2.6	4.2	6.8	12.1	17.3	22.9	29.3	33.7	37.6	45.6	38.8	8.2	2.3	0.35	0.67	**5.9**	*189*
Eye	601	0	1.1	0.1	0.2	0.1	0.1	0.2	0.3	0.5	0.7	0.7	1.2	1.3	2.1	2.3	3.1	2.8	3.9	3.9	0.9	0.2	0.04	0.07	**0.7**	*190*
Brain, nervous system	4178	0	3.5	3.0	2.2	1.9	1.6	2.1	3.3	3.3	4.0	4.6	8.3	10.1	14.4	16.2	20.5	20.5	19.6	12.8	6.0	1.7	0.31	0.50	**5.0**	*191-2*
Thyroid	4142	0	0.0	0.1	0.6	2.0	4.6	6.3	7.5	8.6	8.6	8.8	9.8	9.6	8.3	8.1	8.8	7.8	8.5	7.2	5.9	1.7	0.38	0.46	**4.9**	*193*
Other endocrine	378	0	1.5	0.4	0.2	0.1	0.1	0.2	0.2	0.4	0.3	0.5	0.8	1.0	0.9	1.1	1.6	1.1	0.9	0.6	0.5	0.2	0.03	0.05	**0.6**	*194*
Hodgkin's disease	1765	1	0.0	0.3	1.2	4.9	5.4	4.1	2.5	2.4	1.9	1.8	1.6	1.8	2.3	2.5	3.4	3.4	3.7	2.3	2.5	0.7	0.15	0.18	**2.3**	*201*
Non-Hodgkin lymphoma	9088	12	0.7	0.6	0.5	1.0	1.3	2.3	3.0	4.5	7.0	10.9	18.2	24.8	31.8	44.2	53.4	67.7	71.0	66.1	13.0	3.6	0.53	1.02	**9.0**	*200,202*
Multiple myeloma	3043	1	-	-	-	0.0	-	0.0	0.1	0.3	0.8	2.2	4.1	6.7	10.6	16.1	23.6	28.5	34.5	32.6	4.4	1.2	0.12	0.32	**2.7**	*203*
Lymphoid leukaemia	3046	2	6.6	2.8	1.5	0.8	0.6	0.4	0.4	0.5	0.9	1.6	2.9	4.2	8.3	11.2	15.3	23.0	29.4	39.2	4.4	1.2	0.16	0.29	**3.4**	*204*
Myeloid leukaemia	2488	2	0.6	0.2	0.6	0.9	0.9	1.1	1.4	2.2	2.5	3.4	3.9	4.3	6.9	9.8	13.4	15.3	19.1	24.7	3.6	1.0	0.14	0.26	**2.5**	*205*
Monocytic leukaemia	127	0	0.1	0.0	-	0.0	0.0	0.0	-	0.1	-	0.1	0.1	0.3	0.3	0.5	1.1	1.3	1.3	1.1	0.2	0.1	0.00	0.01	**0.1**	*206*
Other leukaemia	119	0	0.2	-	0.0	0.0	0.0	0.1	0.1	0.1	0.0	0.2	0.2	0.4	0.3	0.5	0.8	0.9	1.7	0.2	0.0	0.01	0.01	**0.1**	*207*
Leukaemia unspecified	832	0	0.3	0.1	0.0	0.1	0.1	0.1	0.2	0.2	0.3	0.5	0.6	1.2	1.6	2.9	4.7	6.9	12.0	18.2	1.2	0.3	0.03	0.07	**0.7**	*208*
Other and unspecified	9979	22	1.0	0.1	0.0	0.2	0.4	0.7	1.1	2.7	4.3	7.5	12.2	20.5	28.9	43.3	60.6	87.3	119.5	167.7	14.3	4.0	0.40	0.92	**8.6**	*O&U*
All sites																											
All sites but 173	249710	119	20.0	10.0	10.6	18.3	27.7	47.1	80.9	141.4	238.7	366.2	524.3	701.8	938.1	1194.4	1435.3	1647.7	1780.2	1867.8	357.1	100.0	15.63	28.79	**252.8**	*ALLb*

Rate from 10 cases   0.212 0.212 0.217 0.211 0.187 0.159 0.159 0.175 0.198 0.250 0.307 0.321 0.327 0.348 0.438 0.564 0.864 1.041

†Important: see notes on population page

Canada, Alberta

Alberta, with an area of 661 688 km^2, lies between latitudes 49° and 60° W. The population in 1991 consisted of 1 267 530 females and 1 274 425 males. Just over three quarters of the population is urban and over half lives in the two large cities (Edmonton and Calgary). About half of the population are of British extraction, the remainder including German, Ukrainian, French, Indian and Chinese. Although the main economic activity in the past has been related to agriculture and animal husbandry, and these are still very important, the petrochemical industry has become a dominant feature of Alberta's economy. The resulting job opportunities produced a great deal of migration from other parts of Canada in the past, although in recent years this trend has been lessened.

Records kept on cancer patients in Alberta since 1941 have been used for a population-based registry since 1951. All records since 1941 are now stored on computer tape. The registry is administered by the Department of Epidemiology, Prevention and Screening of the Alberta Cancer Board.

Since 1973 steps have been taken to improve the collection and recording of data to upgrade the registry to a true population-based system. Legislation was introduced to empower the Board to seek registration of all cancer cases diagnosed in the province. All pathology reports mentioning malignancy, whether from a hospital or a private laboratory, are sent to the cancer clinics. When a physician wishes to treat a person with cancer without the consulta-tion of the cancer clinic staff, he/she completes an information form supplying the cancer registry with basic identification and classification information on the patient. Vital statistics abstracts are received for cancer-related deaths.

An extensive system of case tracking has been established within the Cancer Clinic Appointments, Medical Records and Cancer Registry Departments to ensure that any information concerning a cancer case is followed up and the maximum amount of data gathered.

A patient index report is produced from the cancer registry system which contains identification information on all patients ever seen in any of the cancer clinics. As far as the registry is concerned, the primary use of this report is to determine whether or not a patient with cancer has ever attended a cancer clinic. Therefore it is the major system of case identification operational in the cancer clinic. It ensures that all reports relevant to a case of cancer are filled in an accessible patient record.

Pathology reports and vital statistics abstracts received are first extensively followed up to try to obtain complete registration information. When this information is not forthcoming (a small number of cases), the information is abstracted and coded in the cancer registry under a special prefix, therefore making the registry a complete count of all malignancies discovered.

Follow-up information stored in the registry consists of whether the patient is presumed alive or known to be dead.

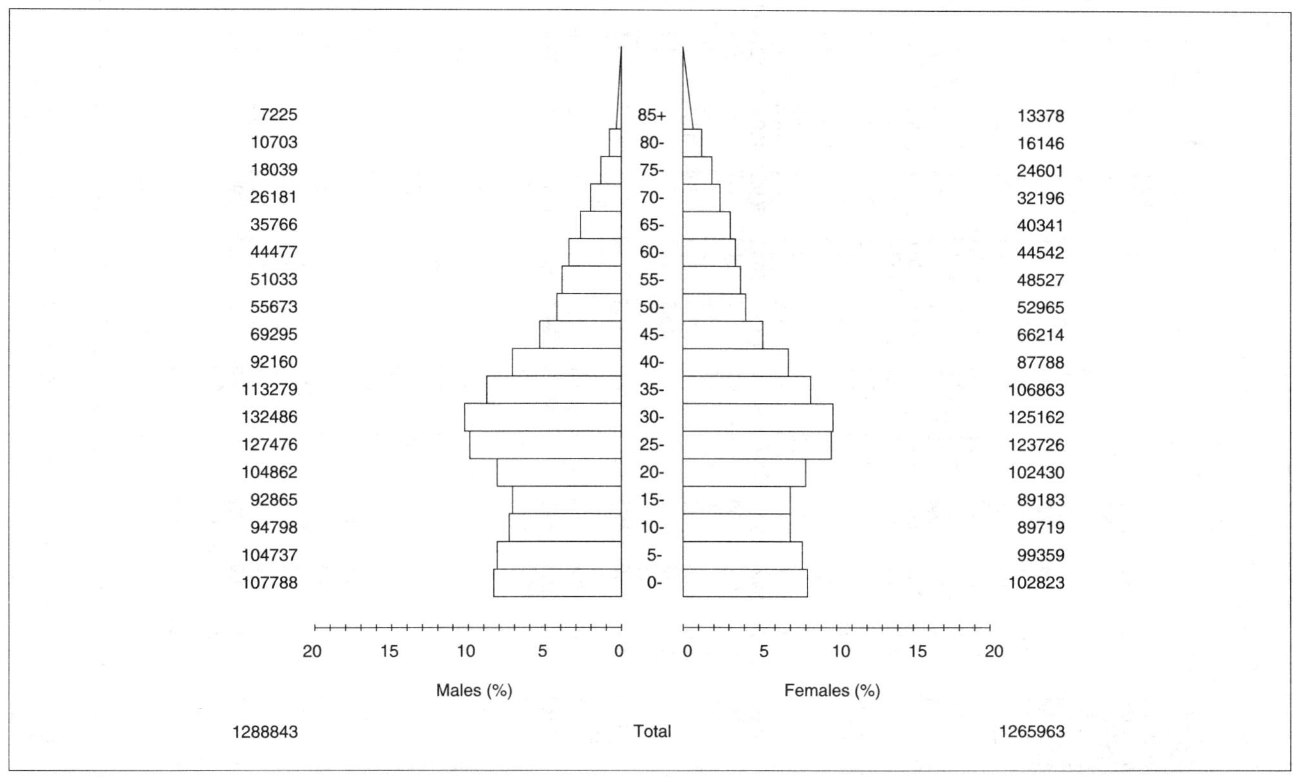

Canada, Alberta

Source of population: average annual 1988-92
Census: Statistics Canada June 1991
Estimate: The populations were estimated at 1 July each year, based on revised intercensal estimates for 1988-91 and post-censal estimates for 1992. In 1993 revised estimates dating back to 1971 were implemented by Statistics Canada and population data from 1971 now include estimates of net census undercoverage, plus non-permanent residents defined as persons claiming refugee status, foreign students, work permit holders, or holders of Minister's permits, and non-Canadian-born dependants of such individuals. References: Statistics Canada, Catalogue 91-537, Revised intercensal population and family estimates, July 1, 1971–91, and Catalogue 91-213, Annual demographic statistics 1993 (for 1992 data).

Notes to tables overleaf:
† Kaposi's sarcoma is under-reported in this volume because cases of skin cancer (ICD-9 173) were not provided
‡ 173 not available
Screening programmes in the area:
A breast screening programme in women aged 50-69 was started in 1990.

CANADA, ALBERTA 1988-1992

ANNUAL INCIDENCE PER 100,000 BY AGE GROUP (YEARS) - MALE

SITE	ALL AGES	AGE UNK	0-	5-	10-	15-	20-	25-	30-	35-	40-	45-	50-	55-	60-	65-	70-	75-	80-	85+	CRUDE RATE	%	CR 64	CR 74	ASR (W)	ICD (9th)
Lip	319	0	-	-	-	-	0.2	0.2	0.6	0.7	1.1	4.9	8.3	11.4	17.1	25.2	43.5	48.8	69.1	38.8	5.0	1.6	0.22	0.57	4.7	140
Tongue	95	0	-	-	-	-	-	0.2	0.6	0.9	0.9	1.2	4.0	3.1	9.4	9.5	8.4	5.5	5.6	2.8	1.5	0.5	0.10	0.19	1.5	141
Salivary gland	41	0	0.2	-	-	-	0.2	-	0.2	-	0.4	-	1.1	3.1	4.0	2.8	3.1	3.3	7.5	-	0.6	0.2	0.05	0.08	0.6	142
Mouth	130	0	-	-	-	-	0.4	0.2	0.6	0.2	2.0	2.3	5.4	8.6	8.5	8.4	13.8	4.4	9.3	19.4	2.0	0.7	0.14	0.25	2.0	143-5
Oropharynx	66	0	-	-	-	-	-	-	-	0.4	1.3	3.2	1.4	2.7	4.5	7.8	3.8	3.3	5.6	2.8	1.0	0.3	0.07	0.13	1.0	146
Nasopharynx	62	0	-	-	0.2	-	-	0.2	0.3	1.2	2.4	2.3	1.4	2.7	5.4	2.8	2.3	1.1	-	-	1.0	0.3	0.08	0.11	0.9	147
Hypopharynx	57	0	-	-	-	-	-	-	0.3	-	0.2	0.6	1.1	5.1	3.6	6.2	6.1	5.5	5.6	2.8	0.9	0.3	0.05	0.12	0.9	148
Pharynx unspecified	18	0	-	-	-	-	-	-	-	-	-	-	1.1	1.6	1.8	0.6	2.3	1.1	1.9	2.8	0.3	0.1	0.02	0.04	0.3	149
Oesophagus	166	0	-	-	-	-	-	-	0.2	0.7	0.6	7.9	6.3	12.1	16.8	19.9	21.1	7.5	44.3	2.6	0.8	0.14	0.32	2.6	150
Stomach	673	0	-	-	-	0.2	0.2	0.8	0.8	0.7	3.5	6.1	16.9	22.3	35.1	62.1	77.9	117.5	127.1	141.2	10.4	3.4	0.43	1.13	9.8	151
Small intestine	53	0	-	-	-	0.2	-	-	-	-	0.4	0.3	2.2	2.4	3.6	4.5	6.1	5.5	5.6	13.8	0.8	0.3	0.05	0.10	0.8	152
Colon	1508	0	-	-	-	-	0.2	0.5	1.2	3.0	6.7	17.3	27.3	55.6	95.3	125.8	194.8	220.6	306.4	318.3	23.4	7.7	1.04	2.64	22.2	153
Rectum	1049	0	-	-	-	-	0.2	0.3	0.8	1.9	5.9	16.5	25.1	48.2	74.2	77.7	123.8	157.4	171.9	146.7	16.3	5.3	0.87	1.87	15.7	154
Liver	192	0	0.7	0.6	-	0.2	-	0.8	0.7	0.7	2.3	4.7	8.2	10.3	17.9	22.2	25.5	26.2	24.9	3.0	1.0	0.15	0.35	2.9	155
Gallbladder etc.	106	0	-	-	-	-	-	0.2	0.2	0.2	0.2	1.2	1.4	5.5	4.9	7.8	12.2	17.7	20.6	33.2	1.6	0.5	0.07	0.17	1.5	156
Pancreas	591	0	-	-	-	-	-	-	0.2	0.9	2.2	6.1	7.5	25.1	36.9	54.2	65.7	85.4	127.1	163.3	9.2	3.0	0.39	0.99	8.7	157
Nose, sinuses etc.	43	0	-	0.2	0.2	-	0.2	0.3	0.2	0.9	1.3	1.2	-	0.8	2.2	3.9	1.5	2.2	5.6	2.8	0.7	0.2	0.04	0.06	0.6	160
Larynx	278	0	-	-	-	-	-	-	-	0.7	1.1	3.2	11.5	19.2	18.0	27.4	31.3	35.5	16.8	16.6	4.3	1.4	0.27	0.56	4.3	161
Bronchus, lung	3351	1	-	-	0.2	-	0.4	0.3	0.6	2.3	10.0	27.7	59.6	132.1	239.2	347.8	430.1	564.3	569.9	420.8	52.0	17.1	2.36	6.25	50.0	162
Other thoracic organs	27	0	0.2	-	-	0.9	0.2	-	0.2	0.7	0.9	0.9	0.7	0.4	0.4	0.6	0.8	1.1	3.7	-	0.4	0.1	0.03	0.03	0.4	163-4
Bone	64	0	-	0.8	1.5	1.9	1.0	0.3	0.6	1.1	0.7	0.6	-	1.6	2.7	1.7	3.1	3.3	3.7	-	1.0	0.3	0.06	0.09	1.0	170
Connective tissue	110	0	0.9	0.6	0.6	1.1	0.6	0.8	0.9	0.7	1.3	4.0	3.6	2.7	2.2	5.0	7.6	11.1	1.9	11.1	1.7	0.6	0.10	0.16	1.7	171
Mesothelioma	75	0	-	-	-	-	0.2	-	0.2	-	0.4	0.9	1.8	6.7	4.0	4.5	13.0	11.1	3.7	-	1.2	0.4	0.07	0.16	1.1	MES
†Kaposi's sarcoma	0	0	-	-	-	-	-	-	-	-	-	-	-	-	-	-	-	-	-	-	0.0	0.0	0.00	0.00	0.0	KAP
Melanoma of skin	520	0	-	-	-	0.9	1.1	3.9	6.2	7.8	11.5	14.4	12.6	25.5	22.9	28.0	31.3	23.3	35.5	41.5	8.1	2.6	0.53	0.83	7.5	172
†Other skin																										
Breast	36	0	-	-	-	-	-	0.2	0.2	-	0.2	0.6	0.4	1.6	3.6	3.4	3.8	2.2	5.6	5.5	0.6	0.2	0.03	0.07	0.5	175
Prostate	4470	0	-	-	-	-	0.2	-	-	-	0.2	4.6	23.4	86.2	231.1	456.8	729.5	965.7	1128.6	1123.9	69.4	22.8	1.73	7.66	63.4	185
Testis	324	0	0.7	0.2	0.2	3.2	5.3	11.6	12.4	9.2	5.4	4.6	3.2	2.4	1.3	1.1	3.8	-	1.9	-	5.0	1.7	0.30	0.32	4.1	186
Penis	33	0	-	-	-	-	-	-	-	-	0.4	0.6	0.7	2.0	1.8	1.1	2.3	5.5	3.7	16.6	0.5	0.2	0.03	0.04	0.5	187.1-.4
Other male genital	14	0	-	0.2	-	-	0.2	-	-	-	-	0.6	-	0.4	0.9	1.1	2.3	1.1	1.9	-	0.2	0.1	0.01	0.03	0.2	187.5-.9
Bladder	1199	0	0.2	-	-	-	-	0.3	1.1	4.6	4.8	12.1	20.1	48.2	76.4	101.8	151.3	174.1	252.3	215.9	18.6	6.1	0.84	2.10	17.6	188
Kidney etc.	754	0	1.5	1.0	-	0.2	0.2	0.6	1.2	4.1	4.8	13.3	25.5	32.5	39.6	68.2	81.0	87.6	100.9	91.3	11.7	3.8	0.62	1.37	11.4	189
Eye	54	0	0.7	0.4	-	0.4	-	-	0.3	-	0.7	1.2	1.4	1.2	3.6	3.9	3.8	5.5	5.6	5.5	0.8	0.3	0.05	0.09	0.9	190
Brain, nervous system	439	0	4.5	4.2	1.5	2.4	3.1	5.2	3.8	3.7	6.1	7.8	8.6	13.7	16.2	24.0	29.0	31.0	24.3	22.1	6.8	2.2	0.40	0.67	6.7	191-2
Thyroid	145	0	-	-	0.6	0.2	1.0	2.8	1.2	2.8	3.7	1.7	4.0	3.5	6.3	6.7	8.4	6.7	9.3	8.3	2.3	0.7	0.14	0.21	2.1	193
Other endocrine	18	0	-	0.2	0.2	1.1	-	0.2	0.2	-	-	-	0.4	0.4	0.9	0.6	0.8	1.1	1.9	2.8	0.3	0.1	0.02	0.02	0.3	194
Hodgkin's disease	190	0	-	0.2	0.8	3.7	4.0	5.0	3.9	3.0	2.6	1.7	4.3	5.9	1.8	6.2	4.6	3.3	3.7	2.8	2.9	1.0	0.18	0.24	2.7	201
Non-Hodgkin lymphoma	783	0	2.0	2.1	1.5	1.5	1.7	4.1	3.8	7.1	9.3	16.7	21.6	31.7	37.3	50.3	72.6	80.9	86.0	49.8	12.2	4.0	0.70	1.32	11.7	200,202
Multiple myeloma	268	0	-	-	-	-	-	-	-	0.5	2.2	2.3	5.7	9.0	15.3	23.5	29.0	44.3	59.8	60.9	4.2	1.4	0.18	0.44	3.9	203
Lymphoid leukaemia	326	0	6.1	2.9	1.7	1.7	0.6	0.2	1.1	1.2	1.1	1.7	6.8	9.0	18.0	17.9	24.4	39.9	50.5	66.4	5.1	1.7	0.26	0.47	5.1	204
Myeloid leukaemia	222	0	0.4	0.4	0.8	0.6	2.1	1.7	1.2	3.2	3.7	3.2	2.9	5.1	8.1	8.9	13.8	32.2	39.2	33.2	3.4	1.1	0.17	0.28	3.1	205
Monocytic leukaemia	12	0	0.7	-	-	-	-	-	0.2	-	-	0.3	-	0.4	-	0.6	-	2.2	3.7	-	0.2	0.1	0.01	0.01	0.2	206
Other leukaemia	1	0	-	-	-	-	-	-	-	-	-	-	-	-	-	-	0.8	-	-	-	0.0	0.0	0.00	0.00	0.0	207
Leukaemia unspecified	27	0	0.2	-	0.2	-	-	0.2	-	0.2	-	0.3	-	0.8	2.2	0.6	5.3	4.4	-	8.3	0.4	0.1	0.02	0.05	0.4	208
Other and unspecified	721	0	1.1	-	-	0.2	-	0.9	0.8	3.5	1.5	6.9	13.7	19.6	39.1	62.1	80.2	102.0	171.9	213.1	11.2	3.7	0.44	1.15	10.4	O&U
All sites																										
All sites but 173	19630	1	20.2	13.7	10.3	20.7	23.3	40.9	46.2	68.1	102.2	197.7	349.2	674.5	1122.4	1687.6	2371.2	2965.7	3488.6	3374.4	304.6	100.0	13.45	33.74	288.0	ALLb

Rate from 1 case   0.186   0.191   0.211   0.215   0.191   0.157   0.151   0.177   0.217   0.289   0.359   0.392   0.450   0.559   0.764   1.109   1.869   2.768

†Important: see notes on population page

CANADA, ALBERTA 1988-1992

ANNUAL INCIDENCE PER 100,000 BY AGE GROUP (YEARS) - FEMALE

SITE	ALL AGES	AGE UNK	0-	5-	10-	15-	20-	25-	30-	35-	40-	45-	50-	55-	60-	65-	70-	75-	80-	85+	CRUDE RATE	%	CR 64	CR 74	ASR (W)	ICD (9th)
Lip	69	0	-	-	-	-	-	-	-	-	0.7	-	1.9	1.6	4.5	5.5	7.5	5.7	7.4	16.4	1.1	0.4	0.04	0.11	0.9	140
Tongue	56	0	-	-	-	-	-	-	0.3	0.7	0.7	0.6	0.4	1.2	4.9	4.0	3.1	4.1	6.2	10.5	0.9	0.3	0.04	0.08	0.7	141
Salivary gland	31	0	-	-	0.2	-	-	0.2	0.3	0.6	1.4	0.3	2.3	1.2	1.3	0.5	0.6	1.6	-	1.5	0.5	0.2	0.04	0.04	0.5	142
Mouth	90	0	-	-	-	-	-	0.5	0.3	0.6	0.5	2.4	1.5	4.5	5.4	6.9	8.1	4.9	8.7	7.5	1.4	0.5	0.08	0.15	1.2	143-5
Oropharynx	20	0	-	-	-	-	-	-	-	0.2	0.2	0.9	0.8	0.4	0.9	2.5	1.2	1.6	1.2	-	0.3	0.1	0.02	0.04	0.3	146
Nasopharynx	16	0	0.2	0.2	-	-	0.2	0.2	0.2	0.2	0.5	0.3	0.4	0.4	0.9	1.0	-	0.8	-	-	0.3	0.1	0.02	0.02	0.2	147
Hypopharynx	11	0	-	-	-	-	-	-	-	-	-	0.3	0.8	-	1.8	1.0	-	0.8	1.2	-	0.2	0.1	0.01	0.02	0.2	148
Pharynx unspecified	8	0	-	-	-	-	-	-	-	-	0.2	0.3	0.4	0.4	0.9	-	-	-	1.2	1.5	0.1	0.0	0.01	0.01	0.1	149
Oesophagus	81	0	-	-	-	-	-	-	-	-	-	0.6	1.9	4.5	3.6	5.9	7.5	11.4	8.7	14.9	1.3	0.4	0.05	0.12	1.0	150
Stomach	343	0	-	-	-	-	0.2	0.3	1.1	0.9	0.7	3.3	7.6	9.5	13.0	18.8	27.3	42.3	55.7	94.2	5.4	1.9	0.18	0.41	4.0	151
Small intestine	69	0	-	-	-	-	-	0.3	0.3	0.9	1.4	0.9	1.1	1.6	2.2	5.9	6.8	6.5	7.4	3.0	1.1	0.4	0.04	0.11	0.9	152
Colon	1382	0	-	-	-	-	-	0.3	1.4	2.2	7.1	9.7	19.3	43.7	67.4	89.7	119.9	179.7	231.6	309.4	21.8	7.6	0.76	1.80	16.2	153
Rectum	686	0	-	-	-	-	0.2	0.3	0.6	1.5	5.0	9.1	17.4	20.2	41.8	44.1	63.4	79.7	85.5	109.1	10.8	3.8	0.48	1.02	8.7	154
Liver	80	0	0.2	0.2	0.4	-	-	0.2	0.2	0.4	0.9	0.6	1.1	1.6	2.2	5.5	6.2	8.1	14.9	16.4	1.3	0.4	0.04	0.10	1.0	155
Gallbladder etc.	160	0	-	-	-	-	-	-	-	0.4	0.5	0.6	2.6	4.5	7.2	8.9	21.1	26.0	17.3	32.9	2.5	0.9	0.08	0.23	1.9	156
Pancreas	483	0	-	-	-	-	-	-	0.3	0.2	0.9	3.0	8.3	14.0	22.9	34.7	47.2	54.5	83.0	118.1	7.6	2.7	0.25	0.66	5.7	157
Nose, sinuses etc.	26	0	-	-	-	-	-	-	-	0.6	0.7	0.6	0.4	1.6	0.9	3.0	0.6	3.3	-	-	0.4	0.1	0.02	0.04	0.4	160
Larynx	55	0	-	-	-	-	-	-	-	0.4	0.2	0.3	2.3	4.5	4.5	5.9	4.3	0.8	3.7	1.5	0.9	0.3	0.06	0.11	0.8	161
Bronchus, lung	1771	1	-	-	-	-	-	0.6	1.8	2.8	10.3	32.0	54.0	73.8	120.8	151.7	189.5	161.0	154.8	95.7	28.0	9.8	1.48	3.19	24.6	162
Other thoracic organs	15	0	0.4	-	-	-	-	0.2	-	-	-	-	0.8	0.8	-	2.0	-	1.6	1.2	1.5	0.2	0.1	0.01	0.02	0.2	163-4
Bone	48	0	0.2	0.4	1.3	0.9	1.0	0.3	0.3	0.9	0.5	0.9	1.1	-	0.4	2.0	1.2	2.4	2.5	1.5	0.8	0.3	0.04	0.06	0.7	170
Connective tissue	100	0	0.6	0.2	0.9	0.4	1.0	0.3	1.0	0.7	1.6	0.9	3.4	2.1	1.8	8.4	3.7	8.9	9.9	4.5	1.6	0.6	0.07	0.14	1.4	171
Mesothelioma	15	0	-	-	-	-	-	-	-	-	0.5	0.3	-	1.2	0.4	1.0	3.1	-	-	1.5	0.2	0.1	0.01	0.03	0.2	MES
†Kaposi's sarcoma	0	0	-	-	-	-	-	-	-	-	-	-	-	-	-	-	-	-	-	-	0.0	0.0	0.00	0.00	0.0	KAP
Melanoma of skin	552	0	-	-	-	2.5	2.9	7.3	8.3	10.7	15.5	16.3	18.5	12.8	17.5	10.9	18.0	29.3	28.5	31.4	8.7	3.1	0.56	0.71	7.5	172
†Other skin																										
Breast	5539	0	-	-	-	-	0.8	6.5	20.6	48.3	108.0	170.4	209.6	222.1	293.7	349.0	378.3	399.2	367.9	330.4	87.5	30.6	5.40	9.04	78.0	174
Uterus unspecified	33	0	-	-	-	-	-	0.2	-	-	0.9	0.6	1.9	-	1.8	2.0	1.2	2.4	3.7	7.5	0.5	0.2	0.03	0.04	0.4	179
Cervix uteri	634	0	-	-	-	1.8	7.9	12.1	19.7	21.6	19.3	8.7	18.5	13.9	23.3	25.5	13.0	23.5	20.9		10.0	3.5	0.62	0.86	8.4	180
Placenta	3	0	-	-	-	0.4	-	0.2	-	-	-	-	-	-	-	-	-	-	-	-	0.0	0.0	0.00	0.00	0.0	181
Corpus uteri	1065	0	-	-	-	-	-	0.5	1.4	4.1	9.6	17.8	35.1	55.2	83.1	91.2	87.6	86.2	69.4	46.3	16.8	5.9	1.03	1.93	15.2	182
Ovary etc.	743	0	0.2	-	0.7	2.5	2.9	3.2	3.8	7.1	9.8	17.8	28.7	29.3	41.8	37.7	52.2	47.2	54.5	40.4	11.7	4.1	0.74	1.19	10.5	183
Other female genital	143	0	0.2	-	-	-	-	0.2	0.5	1.5	1.8	2.7	3.4	3.3	9.9	5.5	9.9	11.4	13.6	32.9	2.3	0.8	0.12	0.19	1.8	184
Bladder	401	0	-	-	-	0.2	1.2	0.5	0.6	1.5	2.1	6.3	6.8	13.2	22.5	30.2	32.9	45.5	59.5	46.3	6.3	2.2	0.27	0.59	5.1	188
Kidney etc.	435	0	1.6	0.2	-	-	-	0.2	0.6	2.4	5.7	7.9	10.6	19.0	22.0	33.7	31.7	35.0	50.8	46.3	6.9	2.4	0.35	0.68	5.9	189
Eye	52	0	1.0	0.4	0.4	0.2	0.2	-	0.5	0.4	0.5	0.6	2.3	0.8	1.8	2.5	5.0	1.6	3.7	3.0	0.8	0.3	0.08	-	0.8	190
Brain, nervous system	312	0	2.7	3.4	2.0	1.1	1.8	1.0	3.2	4.1	3.4	3.9	6.0	11.1	17.1	15.9	14.9	16.3	19.8	13.5	4.9	1.7	0.30	0.46	4.6	191-2
Thyroid	384	0	-	-	0.2	2.7	4.3	6.5	8.6	9.2	10.7	10.3	14.7	7.0	9.0	7.4	9.9	5.7	5.0	10.5	6.1	2.1	0.42	0.50	5.4	193
Other endocrine	25	0	1.0	-	0.2	-	0.2	0.2	-	0.6	0.7	-	0.4	0.4	0.9	1.5	0.6	1.6	1.2	-	0.4	0.1	0.02	0.03	0.4	194
Hodgkin's disease	124	0	-	0.2	1.1	2.9	6.1	2.9	1.8	1.9	1.1	1.2	1.1	2.9	1.8	1.0	3.7	0.8	3.7	-	2.0	0.7	0.12	0.15	1.8	201
Non-Hodgkin lymphoma	620	0	0.8	-	0.4	0.7	1.2	1.8	3.0	4.9	4.6	10.0	19.6	25.6	33.2	42.1	42.2	57.7	53.3	61.3	9.8	3.4	0.53	0.95	8.4	200,202
Multiple myeloma	199	0	-	-	-	-	-	-	0.2	0.4	0.7	2.4	6.0	7.8	7.6	15.4	20.5	22.8	27.3	28.4	3.1	1.1	0.13	0.31	2.5	203
Lymphoid leukaemia	230	0	6.4	2.4	2.2	0.9	0.8	0.6	0.6	0.2	0.5	1.2	4.9	5.4	9.9	9.9	14.9	15.4	22.3	34.4	3.6	1.3	0.18	0.30	3.4	204
Myeloid leukaemia	170	0	0.2	-	0.2	1.1	0.2	0.5	1.3	2.1	2.3	1.8	4.5	3.7	7.2	7.9	9.3	13.8	21.1	32.9	2.7	0.9	0.13	0.21	2.1	205
Monocytic leukaemia	8	0	-	-	-	-	-	0.2	-	-	-	-	0.4	-	-	1.2	1.6	2.5	-		0.1	0.0	0.00	0.01	0.1	206
Other leukaemia	6	0	0.2	-	-	-	-	-	-	-	0.3	-	0.4	0.4	0.5	-	-	1.2	-		0.1	0.0	0.01	0.01	0.1	207
Leukaemia unspecified	30	0	-	-	-	-	0.2	0.2	-	0.4	0.5	-	-	0.4	0.4	2.0	3.1	1.6	3.7	12.0	0.5	0.2	0.01	0.04	0.3	208
Other and unspecified	761	0	0.6	-	0.2	0.2	0.4	0.5	1.0	2.1	4.3	5.7	12.5	23.1	26.9	46.6	66.5	95.1	164.7	143.5	12.0	4.2	0.39	0.95	8.8	O&U
All sites																										
All sites but 173	18084	1	16.3	7.6	10.7	16.4	27.7	44.3	76.5	135.5	238.3	364.6	524.9	656.1	932.1	1145.2	1351.7	1508.9	1703.2	1783.4	285.7	100.0	15.26	27.74	243.5	ALLb

| Rate from 1 case | | | 0.195 | 0.201 | 0.223 | 0.224 | 0.195 | 0.162 | 0.160 | 0.187 | 0.228 | 0.302 | 0.378 | 0.412 | 0.449 | 0.496 | 0.621 | 0.813 | 1.239 | 1.495 | | | | | | |

†Important: see notes on population page

Canada, British Columbia

The British Columbia Cancer Registry is part of a combined population-based registry and clinical database maintained by the British Columbia Cancer Agency (BCCA). The BCCA is a provincial government agency responsible for cancer care, control, and research in British Columbia.

Notification of cancer cases has been required since 1935. Legislation for the present registry was passed in 1987. In 1966, a register of all known deceased cancer cases was instituted within the provincial Division of Vital Statistics. A population-based register has been maintained since 1969. In 1980, responsibility for the registry was transferred to the BCCA, and a historical patient file (no diagnoses available) of cases referred to treatment clinics since 1932 was added to the database in 1985. There are now more than 450 000 cases recorded in the cancer registry.

The registry was originally set up to monitor cancer incidence and mortality in the province, but is now extensively used for health services planning and epidemiological research. The registry covers all of British Columbia (987 800 km^2), with a population of 3 131 700 (as of June 1990). British Columbia is the most westerly province of Canada, bordered by Alberta to the east and by the Pacific Ocean to the west.

The province lies between latitudes 49° and 60° N and longitudes 120° and 130° W. A considerable portion is mountainous. Most of the population lives within 100 m of sea level and is concentrated in the south-west corner of the province, where the climate is the mildest in Canada.

British Columbia is a major receiving area for internal migration within Canada and from abroad. Based on the 1981 census, the main ethnic groups are: British 51% of the population, other European groups 27%, and aboriginal 2%. Over the last two decades, immigration from Europe has declined, while migration from eastern and south-eastern Asia has increased, so that Asians are now the major immigrant group.

The major religions are United Church of Canada (Protestant) 20%, Roman Catholic 19%, and Anglican (Protestant) 14%. Approximately 80% of the population is urban. The largest components of the working population are employed in manufacturing industries (20%) and in independent business and service industries (20%). Approximately 16% of the working population is employed in trade, 12% in the construction industry, and 11.5% in transport and communications. Other important industries include: forestry, 4% of the labour force; agriculture, 2.5%, and fishing 1%.

Over 90% of cases are registered either by submission of pathology reports or following attendance at a BCCA treatment clinic. About 60% of cancer cases are treated at a BCCA clinic at some time, as the clinics operate all the radiotherapy treatment facilities and most of the chemotherapy services in the province. The registry receives listings of all deaths in the province from the Division of Vital Statistics. Death certificates account for about 7% of registrations. Other sources of registration, such as haematology laboratories and special treatment centres (e.g., the Children's Hospital) are exploited whenever possible. In addition to the registry's passive registration from multiple sources, active annual letter follow-up of all cases is carried out.

Registry data are used as a source of cases for surveys and case–control studies, and as outcome data for cohort studies of occupational groups. Registry statistics, and estimates of future incidence trends, have also been used in conjunction with clinic referral data for cancer services budgeting and facilities planning.

Mary McBride
Beth Tompkins

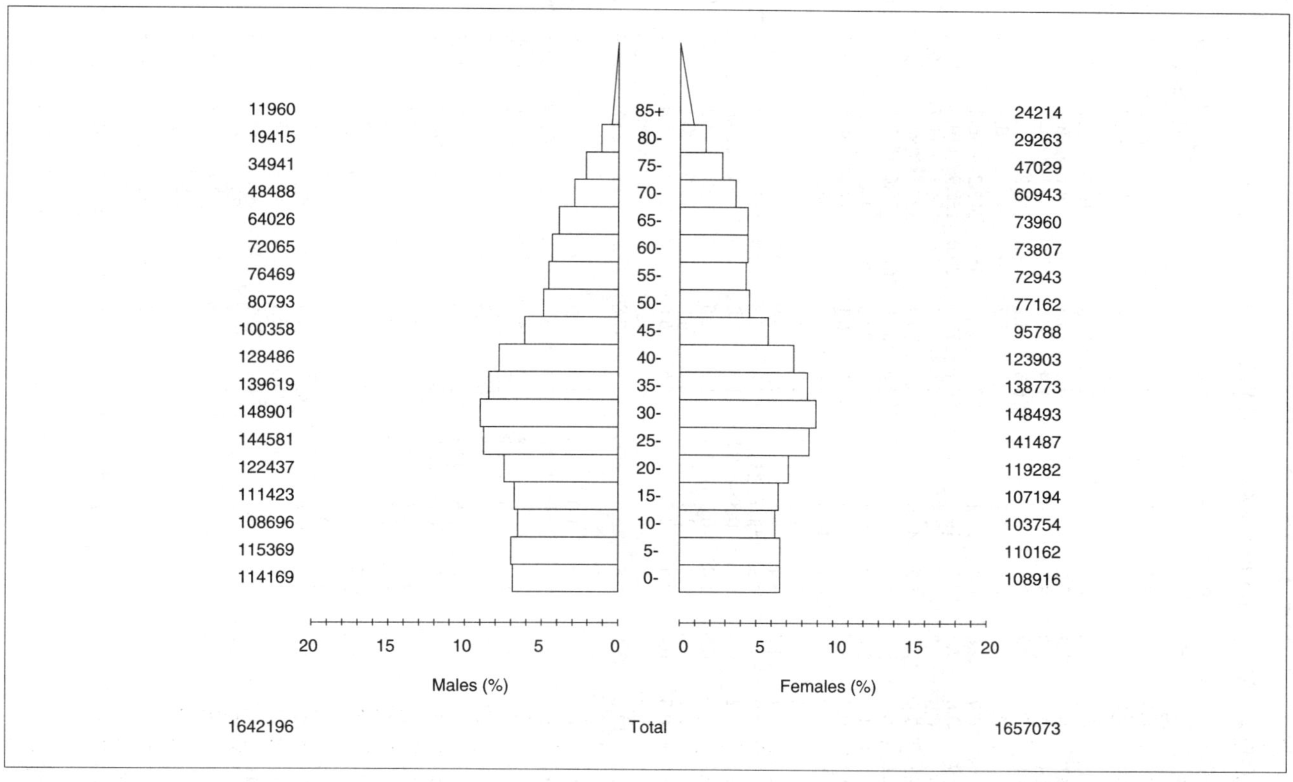

Canada, British Columbia
Source of population: average annual 1988-92
Census: Statistics Canada June 1991
Estimate: The populations were estimated at 1 July each year, based on revised intercensal estimates for 1988-91 and post-censal estimates for 1992. In 1993 revised estimates dating back to 1971 were implemented by Statistics Canada and population data from 1971 now include estimates of net census undercoverage, plus non-permanent residents defined as persons claiming refugee status, foreign students, work permit holders, or holders of Minister's permits, and non-Canadian-born dependants of such individuals. References: Statistics Canada, Catalogue 91-537, Revised intercensal population and family estimates, July 1, 1971–91, and Catalogue 91-213, Annual demographic statistics 1993 (for 1992 data).

Notes to tables overleaf:
† Kaposi's sarcoma is under-reported in this volume because cases of skin cancer (ICD-9 173) were not provided
‡ 173 not available
Screening programmes in the area:
640,000 examinations have been carried out annually for cervical cancer in females over 14 years of age since 1951. Breast cancer screening, comprising over 150,000 examinations a year, has been carried out in the population over age 40 (with active recruitment of 50-69 year olds) since 1988.

CANADA, BRITISH COLUMBIA 1988-1992

ANNUAL INCIDENCE PER 100,000 BY AGE GROUP (YEARS) - MALE

SITE	ALL AGES	AGE UNK	0-	5-	10-	15-	20-	25-	30-	35-	40-	45-	50-	55-	60-	65-	70-	75-	80-	85+	CRUDE RATE	%	CR 64	CR 74	ASR (W)	ICD (9th)
Lip	197	0	-	-	-	-	-	0.1	0.3	0.3	0.8	2.2	3.2	4.7	6.7	10.0	11.5	16.6	17.5	25.1	2.4	0.6	0.09	0.20	**1.7**	140
Tongue	232	0	-	-	-	-	0.2	0.1	1.2	1.6	1.6	2.8	6.7	8.9	8.3	7.8	14.0	10.9	11.3	10.0	2.8	0.7	0.16	0.27	**2.2**	141
Salivary gland	74	0	-	-	-	-	-	0.4	0.3	0.3	0.5	1.2	1.7	1.6	2.2	3.1	5.4	4.6	2.1	6.7	0.9	0.2	0.04	0.08	**0.7**	142
Mouth	305	0	-	-	-	0.4	0.2	-	0.1	0.4	1.2	4.6	6.9	13.1	15.8	14.1	14.8	15.5	16.5	13.4	3.7	0.9	0.21	0.36	**3.0**	143-5
Oropharynx	165	0	-	-	-	-	-	-	0.3	0.3	0.2	2.4	5.2	6.5	8.3	9.4	10.3	5.2	4.1	6.7	2.0	0.5	0.12	0.21	**1.6**	146
Nasopharynx	102	0	-	-	-	-	0.2	0.7	0.3	1.6	2.8	0.8	3.7	1.8	5.3	1.9	2.5	2.9	3.1	-	1.2	0.3	0.09	0.11	**1.0**	147
Hypopharynx	123	0	-	-	-	-	-	-	-	0.1	-	0.8	2.5	4.7	7.8	6.6	8.2	6.9	5.2	6.7	1.5	0.3	0.08	0.15	**1.2**	148
Pharynx unspecified	39	0	-	-	-	-	-	0.1	-	-	0.2	-	0.5	2.1	2.5	3.7	1.2	0.6	-	3.3	0.5	0.1	0.03	0.05	**0.4**	149
Oesophagus	489	0	-	-	-	0.2	-	-	-	0.4	0.9	2.6	6.4	11.8	22.2	27.2	35.1	45.8	42.2	36.8	6.0	1.4	0.22	0.53	**4.3**	150
Stomach	1078	0	-	-	-	-	0.5	0.3	0.5	1.9	3.6	7.2	12.1	19.9	37.7	58.1	75.5	99.0	131.9	110.4	13.1	3.1	0.42	1.09	**9.2**	151
Small intestine	72	0	-	-	-	-	-	-	0.1	-	0.6	1.0	0.5	2.6	3.1	3.1	4.5	4.0	4.1	11.7	0.9	0.2	0.04	0.08	**0.7**	152
Colon	2450	0	-	-	-	0.4	0.2	0.4	1.1	3.2	7.9	12.2	25.2	45.5	78.0	136.5	179.4	221.5	325.5	284.3	29.8	7.0	0.87	2.45	**20.7**	153
Rectum	1877	0	-	-	-	-	-	0.6	0.7	2.1	6.1	9.2	26.5	46.0	64.7	109.6	150.6	168.3	158.6	147.1	22.9	5.3	0.78	2.08	**16.4**	154
Liver	364	0	0.5	-	-	0.2	-	0.3	0.4	1.1	1.2	3.4	5.0	8.9	10.8	20.3	22.3	25.8	44.3	36.8	4.4	1.0	0.16	0.37	**3.2**	155
Gallbladder etc.	205	0	-	-	-	-	-	0.1	0.1	0.3	0.3	1.0	2.7	3.9	6.9	11.6	16.1	20.6	14.4	28.4	2.5	0.6	0.08	0.22	**1.8**	156
Pancreas	803	0	-	-	-	-	-	0.1	-	0.1	2.0	4.6	10.1	16.5	28.3	40.6	54.9	76.7	98.9	110.4	9.8	2.3	0.31	0.79	**6.8**	157
Nose, sinuses etc.	63	0	0.2	-	-	-	0.3	-	-	-	0.5	0.4	0.2	2.1	2.2	4.7	3.7	2.3	6.2	6.7	0.8	0.2	0.03	0.07	**0.6**	160
Larynx	518	0	-	-	-	-	-	-	0.4	0.3	1.4	4.8	8.4	14.6	28.9	29.1	30.5	40.6	29.9	31.8	6.3	1.5	0.29	0.59	**4.8**	161
Bronchus, lung	6262	0	-	-	-	-	-	0.1	0.7	4.2	10.9	34.3	74.3	153.0	255.3	394.8	465.3	563.8	541.8	463.2	76.3	17.8	2.66	6.96	**54.9**	162
Other thoracic organs	48	0	0.2	0.2	0.4	0.5	-	1.0	0.3	0.1	0.2	0.4	0.5	0.8	0.8	1.6	1.2	2.9	4.1	5.0	0.6	0.1	0.03	0.04	**0.5**	163-4
Bone	76	0	-	0.9	1.1	1.1	0.8	0.8	0.3	0.7	0.9	0.6	1.0	0.5	1.1	1.6	2.5	3.4	3.1	3.3	0.9	0.2	0.05	0.07	**0.8**	170
Connective tissue	192	0	1.2	0.5	0.2	0.4	0.8	1.1	1.6	1.1	2.2	1.8	3.2	2.4	4.2	8.1	4.9	12.0	15.5	20.1	2.3	0.5	0.10	0.17	**1.9**	171
Mesothelioma	137	0	-	-	-	-	-	0.1	-	0.1	0.5	0.4	2.5	3.7	8.9	5.6	6.6	13.7	13.4	5.0	1.7	0.4	0.08	0.14	**1.2**	MES
†Kaposi's sarcoma	2	0	-	-	-	-	-	-	-	0.1	0.2	-	-	-	-	-	-	-	-	-	0.0	0.0	0.00	0.00	**0.0**	KAP
Melanoma of skin	1021	0	-	-	0.6	1.3	4.7	4.8	6.3	12.6	12.6	15.9	20.5	25.6	33.3	33.7	47.8	42.9	29.9	36.8	12.4	2.9	0.69	1.10	**9.9**	172
†Other skin																										
Breast	52	0	-	-	-	-	-	0.2	-	-	0.1	0.3	-	1.0	1.0	1.4	1.9	3.3	4.6	8.2	8.4	0.6	0.1	0.02	0.05	**0.4**	175
Prostate	10473	0	-	-	-	-	-	0.1	-	0.1	0.8	9.4	39.4	128.9	332.8	655.4	948.3	1202.6	1329.8	1302.6	127.5	29.8	2.56	10.58	**84.9**	185
Testis	409	0	0.2	-	0.2	2.7	6.5	11.9	11.0	10.5	6.7	4.6	3.5	3.7	2.8	-	1.2	1.1	1.0	1.7	5.0	1.2	0.32	0.33	**4.2**	186
Penis	60	0	-	-	-	-	-	-	0.3	0.3	0.3	1.0	1.0	1.8	1.9	2.2	2.5	2.9	8.2	8.4	0.7	0.2	0.03	0.06	**0.5**	187.1-.4
Other male genital	21	0	-	-	-	-	-	0.1	0.1	0.3	0.2	0.2	0.2	-	0.6	0.9	0.4	1.7	4.1	1.7	0.3	0.1	0.01	0.02	**0.2**	187.5-.9
Bladder	1339	0	-	-	-	-	0.3	-	0.3	1.4	2.8	5.6	14.6	22.5	44.1	79.7	97.3	130.5	153.5	178.9	16.3	3.8	0.46	1.34	**11.3**	188
Kidney etc.	1016	0	2.8	0.3	0.2	0.2	0.3	0.7	1.5	3.3	5.0	13.4	18.6	26.2	38.9	48.1	70.5	65.3	61.8	70.2	12.4	2.9	0.56	1.15	**9.6**	189
Eye	84	0	1.2	-	-	-	-	-	0.5	1.0	0.5	1.2	1.7	2.1	3.1	2.5	2.1	5.2	4.1	8.4	1.0	0.2	0.06	0.08	**0.9**	190
Brain, nervous system	605	0	4.2	1.9	3.1	1.6	2.3	3.5	5.2	3.7	4.2	9.4	9.9	12.3	18.9	24.1	22.7	29.2	19.6	15.0	7.4	1.7	0.40	0.63	**6.3**	191-2
Thyroid	144	0	-	-	0.2	0.2	0.3	1.2	1.9	1.9	3.0	2.6	2.5	3.7	3.3	4.4	2.9	2.9	5.2	8.4	1.8	0.4	0.10	0.14	**1.4**	193
Other endocrine	20	0	0.5	0.2	0.4	0.4	-	0.1	-	-	-	0.4	0.2	0.5	0.3	0.6	-	1.1	1.0	-	0.2	0.1	0.02	0.02	**0.3**	194
Hodgkin's disease	206	0	-	-	2.0	3.8	2.6	3.0	3.1	2.1	2.5	3.0	1.2	3.1	3.1	4.7	4.1	4.6	3.1	5.0	2.5	0.6	0.15	0.19	**2.2**	201
Non-Hodgkin lymphoma	1399	0	1.4	2.1	0.7	1.1	2.0	4.6	6.7	10.0	12.1	19.5	23.5	26.9	40.5	57.5	77.1	97.3	87.6	97.0	17.0	4.0	0.76	1.43	**13.0**	200,202
Multiple myeloma	412	0	-	-	-	-	0.3	-	0.1	0.3	1.7	2.8	3.5	7.6	15.5	25.3	30.1	32.1	47.4	45.1	5.0	1.2	0.16	0.44	**3.6**	203
Lymphoid leukaemia	418	0	7.0	2.6	2.8	1.1	1.0	0.6	0.3	0.6	0.6	1.8	5.4	7.6	10.3	15.3	23.9	34.9	37.1	35.1	5.1	1.2	0.21	0.40	**4.4**	204
Myeloid leukaemia	308	0	1.2	0.2	0.4	0.5	0.7	1.1	1.7	2.3	2.2	4.0	5.7	6.0	7.5	13.4	15.7	12.6	23.7	35.1	3.8	0.9	0.17	0.31	**3.0**	205
Monocytic leukaemia	21	0	0.4	-	-	-	-	0.1	-	-	-	0.2	0.5	0.5	0.3	-	1.6	2.3	2.1	3.3	0.3	0.1	0.01	0.02	**0.2**	206
Other leukaemia	7	0	-	-	-	-	-	-	-	-	-	-	0.2	0.3	0.6	-	0.4	0.6	1.0	-	0.1	0.0	0.01	0.01	**0.1**	207
Leukaemia unspecified	92	0	-	-	0.2	-	-	0.3	-	-	-	0.4	0.2	1.3	2.2	3.7	2.9	8.0	22.7	30.1	1.1	0.3	0.02	0.06	**0.7**	208
Other and unspecified	1219	0	0.9	0.2	-	-	0.5	0.4	1.3	1.7	3.6	6.4	12.6	23.5	35.0	61.5	78.8	109.3	152.5	227.4	14.8	3.5	0.43	1.13	**10.4**	O&U
All sites																										
All sites but 173	35199	0	21.9	9.0	12.3	15.8	24.8	39.1	49.0	72.8	105.5	200.1	375.3	680.8	1206.1	1943.9	2554.8	3155.0	3497.2	3491.4	428.7	100.0	14.06	36.56	**307.0**	ALLb

Rate from 1 case   0.175 0.173 0.184 0.179 0.163 0.138 0.134 0.143 0.156 0.199 0.248 0.262 0.278 0.312 0.412 0.572 1.030 1.672

†Important: see notes on population page

CANADA, BRITISH COLUMBIA 1988-1992

ANNUAL INCIDENCE PER 100,000 BY AGE GROUP (YEARS) - FEMALE

SITE	ALL AGES	AGE UNK	0-	5-	10-	15-	20-	25-	30-	35-	40-	45-	50-	55-	60-	65-	70-	75-	80-	85+	CRUDE RATE	%	CR 64	CR 74	ASR (W)	ICD (9th)
Lip	39	0	-	-	-	-	-	-	-	-	0.5	0.4	-	1.4	0.5	1.1	2.0	2.6	4.8	3.3	0.5	0.1	0.01	0.03	0.3	140
Tongue	127	0	-	-	-	-	-	0.1	-	1.0	0.6	1.7	1.8	2.5	4.6	3.5	7.9	6.4	8.2	8.3	1.5	0.4	0.06	0.12	1.0	141
Salivary gland	64	0	-	-	-	0.4	0.2	0.1	0.3	0.4	0.8	0.2	1.6	0.8	2.4	1.9	2.0	2.1	2.7	7.4	0.8	0.2	0.04	0.06	0.5	142
Mouth	170	0	-	-	-	0.4	-	0.4	0.3	0.6	0.6	2.1	2.6	4.7	5.7	6.2	6.9	8.5	11.6	13.2	2.1	0.5	0.09	0.15	1.4	143-5
Oropharynx	63	0	-	-	-	-	-	-	0.1	0.3	0.5	0.2	0.8	2.2	3.3	1.9	4.3	3.4	2.1	1.7	0.8	0.2	0.04	0.07	0.5	146
Nasopharynx	51	0	-	-	-	-	0.3	0.3	0.5	0.6	0.5	1.0	3.1	0.5	0.8	0.8	1.6	1.3	1.4	0.8	0.6	0.2	0.04	0.05	0.5	147
Hypopharynx	29	0	-	-	-	-	-	-	-	-	0.2	0.2	-	1.4	0.8	0.8	3.3	1.7	0.7	0.8	0.4	0.1	0.01	0.03	0.2	148
Pharynx unspecified	10	0	-	-	-	-	-	-	-	-	0.2	-	-	-	0.5	0.5	1.0	0.4	-	0.8	0.1	0.0	0.00	0.01	0.1	149
Oesophagus	235	0	-	-	-	-	-	-	0.1	0.1	-	1.0	2.9	3.3	7.3	7.3	15.4	15.7	25.3	24.8	2.8	0.7	0.07	0.19	1.6	150
Stomach	580	0	-	-	-	-	0.2	0.6	0.7	1.6	2.3	2.5	4.7	8.8	14.9	21.1	26.9	47.6	64.2	51.2	7.0	1.8	0.18	0.42	3.9	151
Small intestine	64	0	-	-	-	-	-	-	-	-	0.2	0.4	1.3	1.1	1.1	3.0	3.6	6.4	4.8	3.3	0.8	0.2	0.02	0.05	0.5	152
Colon	2606	0	-	-	-	0.2	0.2	1.0	1.1	4.2	6.9	14.6	25.4	38.4	64.8	109.0	131.6	209.2	230.3	278.3	31.5	8.3	0.78	1.99	17.7	153
Rectum	1318	0	-	-	-	0.2	-	0.8	0.9	1.9	6.1	11.5	20.5	30.2	41.2	49.8	65.0	85.9	109.4	93.3	15.9	4.2	0.57	1.14	9.9	154
Liver	194	0	0.4	0.2	0.4	0.2	-	0.4	0.1	0.3	0.5	1.5	1.6	4.4	4.6	7.6	9.2	14.0	11.6	22.3	2.3	0.6	0.07	0.16	1.4	155
Gallbladder etc.	274	0	-	-	-	-	-	-	0.1	0.6	0.5	1.9	4.1	2.5	7.3	10.5	12.1	19.1	27.3	36.3	3.3	0.9	0.09	0.20	1.9	156
Pancreas	787	0	-	-	-	-	-	0.1	0.1	1.0	2.3	2.3	6.7	11.8	17.1	31.4	46.6	59.5	82.0	85.1	9.5	2.5	0.21	0.60	5.1	157
Nose, sinuses etc.	50	0	-	-	-	0.2	-	0.1	0.4	0.3	0.6	1.8	1.1	2.4	1.9	2.0	1.3	0.7	2.5	0.6	0.2	0.04	0.05	0.5	160	
Larynx	106	0	-	-	-	-	-	-	0.1	0.2	0.3	1.6	3.6	4.6	5.7	3.8	4.3	4.1	3.3	1.3	0.3	0.05	0.12	0.9	161	
Bronchus, lung	3922	0	0.4	-	-	0.4	0.5	0.8	2.2	5.2	13.2	36.5	60.9	94.9	140.6	211.7	233.7	230.5	201.6	138.8	47.3	12.5	1.78	4.01	31.1	162
Other thoracic organs	37	0	-	-	0.2	-	-	0.3	-	-	0.2	0.6	1.3	0.5	1.1	3.0	0.7	2.1	0.7	-	0.4	0.1	0.02	0.04	0.3	163-4
Bone	67	0	0.2	0.9	1.9	1.3	0.3	0.1	0.5	0.4	0.3	0.4	0.5	0.8	1.6	1.4	1.0	1.3	2.1	4.1	0.8	0.2	0.05	0.06	0.8	170
Connective tissue	165	0	1.8	0.4	0.8	0.7	0.7	0.8	0.7	1.7	0.6	1.0	2.6	1.9	3.3	4.6	5.9	8.1	6.8	13.2	2.0	0.5	0.09	0.14	1.5	171
Mesothelioma	26	0	-	-	-	-	-	-	-	-	-	0.2	0.5	1.6	1.4	1.1	1.3	0.9	0.7	0.8	0.3	0.1	0.02	0.03	0.2	MES
†Kaposi's sarcoma	0	0	-	-	-	-	-	-	-	-	-	-	-	-	-	-	-	-	-	-	0.0	0.0	0.00	0.00	0.0	KAP
Melanoma of skin †Other skin	1093	0	-	-	-	1.7	6.7	7.1	11.7	15.7	19.2	21.1	20.5	26.0	22.5	27.6	25.6	31.5	24.6	25.6	13.2	3.5	0.76	1.03	10.2	172
Breast	9903	0	-	-	-	0.2	1.0	7.5	21.1	52.2	121.9	183.3	200.1	249.0	308.1	376.4	435.5	443.6	417.6	413.8	119.5	31.5	5.72	9.78	84.3	174
Uterus unspecified	43	0	-	-	-	-	-	0.1	-	-	-	0.6	0.5	0.8	0.5	1.1	0.3	3.0	6.8	8.3	0.5	0.1	0.01	0.02	0.3	179
Cervix uteri	728	0	-	-	-	-	1.2	7.2	11.7	12.7	16.1	12.5	11.1	14.3	15.2	14.9	12.8	20.0	13.0	19.8	8.8	2.3	0.51	0.65	6.7	180
Placenta	2	0	0.2	-	-	-	-	-	0.1	-	-	-	-	-	-	-	-	-	-	-	0.0	0.0	0.00	0.00	0.0	181
Corpus uteri	1672	0	-	-	-	0.2	-	0.4	1.2	3.7	8.6	15.7	35.5	52.9	62.6	84.9	94.5	79.9	60.8	53.7	20.2	5.3	0.90	1.80	14.0	182
Ovary etc.	1244	0	-	0.2	1.0	0.7	1.3	1.3	3.0	4.0	10.2	17.7	27.2	32.6	35.8	53.0	56.8	57.4	62.2	56.2	15.0	4.0	0.68	1.22	10.5	183
Other female genital	231	0	-	-	-	0.2	-	0.9	0.6	1.6	2.1	3.6	3.6	4.6	6.2	11.8	12.8	19.1	31.4	2.8	0.7	0.09	0.18	1.6	184	
Bladder	462	0	-	-	-	-	-	0.1	0.8	0.1	1.1	1.9	4.4	6.6	8.7	18.1	26.6	34.4	39.6	64.4	5.6	1.5	0.12	0.34	3.0	188
Kidney etc.	565	0	2.0	0.7	-	-	-	0.7	0.8	1.6	3.1	4.6	9.8	12.1	17.1	27.3	26.3	31.5	32.1	33.0	6.8	1.8	0.26	0.53	4.6	189
Eye	74	0	1.5	-	0.4	0.4	-	0.1	0.3	0.4	0.6	0.6	1.3	2.2	2.2	1.6	2.6	1.7	4.8	2.5	0.9	0.2	0.05	0.07	0.8	190
Brain, nervous system	426	0	3.1	3.4	2.3	1.5	2.0	2.1	3.2	2.6	4.2	4.6	8.0	9.0	8.7	13.0	13.5	15.3	13.7	9.9	5.1	1.4	0.27	0.41	4.3	191-2
Thyroid	439	0	-	-	0.2	1.9	4.0	4.9	6.5	8.5	7.9	7.5	9.3	9.3	7.0	7.3	7.5	5.5	8.2	5.0	5.3	1.4	0.34	0.41	4.3	193
Other endocrine	28	0	1.1	0.5	-	0.2	-	0.1	-	0.1	0.3	0.4	-	0.8	0.3	0.8	0.7	0.9	-	0.8	0.3	0.1	0.02	0.03	0.4	194
Hodgkin's disease	179	0	0.2	0.5	0.8	5.0	5.2	3.1	2.0	2.2	1.9	1.7	1.6	0.3	2.2	3.0	2.0	1.7	2.1	1.7	2.2	0.6	0.13	0.16	2.1	201
Non-Hodgkin lymphoma	1084	0	0.9	1.1	0.8	1.3	2.2	2.5	2.7	4.6	4.8	8.8	16.6	19.5	29.0	44.9	52.2	57.8	74.5	78.5	13.1	3.4	0.47	0.96	8.5	200,202
Multiple myeloma	336	0	-	-	-	-	-	-	0.1	0.3	0.6	1.0	2.9	5.8	10.3	11.9	20.3	29.3	31.4	27.3	4.1	1.1	0.11	0.27	2.3	203
Lymphoid leukaemia	290	0	7.3	2.5	1.7	0.9	0.7	0.3	0.7	0.3	1.3	1.9	3.9	2.2	6.5	9.7	6.6	11.5	17.8	29.7	3.5	0.9	0.15	0.23	3.0	204
Myeloid leukaemia	259	0	0.4	0.2	1.0	0.6	1.5	1.7	1.2	2.5	2.4	2.7	2.1	4.7	5.1	9.5	8.9	12.8	10.9	17.3	3.1	0.8	0.13	0.22	2.2	205
Monocytic leukaemia	14	0	0.2	-	-	-	-	-	0.3	-	-	-	-	-	0.3	0.8	1.0	1.3	0.7	-	0.2	0.0	0.00	0.01	0.1	206
Other leukaemia	3	0	-	-	-	-	-	-	-	-	-	-	-	-	-	0.3	0.4	0.7	-	-	0.0	0.0	0.00	0.00	0.0	207
Leukaemia unspecified	82	0	-	-	-	-	-	0.4	0.3	-	0.3	0.2	0.3	0.3	0.5	2.7	4.6	6.0	10.3	14.0	1.0	0.3	0.01	0.05	0.5	208
Other and unspecified	1296	0	0.6	-	-	-	0.5	0.4	0.4	2.5	4.8	10.2	13.7	25.0	29.0	48.1	71.9	78.7	105.9	165.2	15.6	4.1	0.44	1.04	9.1	O&U
All sites																										
All sites but 173	31437	0	20.2	10.7	11.4	18.7	28.7	46.4	76.8	135.3	248.6	381.0	518.6	695.1	908.0	1248.5	1473.5	1669.2	1759.9	1851.8	379.4	100.0	15.50	29.11	254.4	ALLb

Rate from 1 case 0.184 0.182 0.193 0.187 0.168 0.141 0.135 0.144 0.161 0.209 0.259 0.274 0.271 0.270 0.328 0.425 0.683 0.826

†Important: see notes on population page

Canada, Manitoba

In 1937 the Province of Manitoba created a central registry to enumerate cancer cases. In 1950 this registry was reorganized on a population basis. Further changes took place in 1956, 1969, 1974 and 1982, that enabled the department to compile more detailed data for the purposes of (a) providing an accurate cancer incidence database for health-care planning and quality assurance; and (b) providing a research database for detailed study of malignant diseases including epidemiological studies, health-care analysis and natural history studies.

The registry is situated in and administered by the Manitoba Cancer Treatment and Research Foundation. Registry personnel comprise a director, a supervisor, and several health record technicians and clerical support staff, as well as computer staff.

The registry covers all of Manitoba, the most central province of Canada, bordered to the east by Ontario and Hudson Bay, to the west by Saskatchewan, to the north by the Northwest Territories and to the south by the USA, between latitudes 49° and 60° N and longitudes 90° and 102° W. The altitude varies from sea level to 823 m and the province covers an area of 649 950 km^2.

The average annual population during 1988–92 consisted of 550 886 males and 559 127 females. Nearly half of the population is of British extraction, with most of the rest being of European extraction. A small proportion of the population are Jewish, native Indian or Eskimo. Predominant occupations include clerical, service occupations, construction and production work, and farming.

Essentially all cancer cases are reported to the registry in accordance with the Public Health Act. Major information sources include pathology, cytology and autopsy reports; hospital admission/separation data; vital statistics death listings; and reports of malignant neoplasms from physicians. The health record technicians in the registry gather and compile data; the registry also has abstracting privileges in all of the active care hospitals in the City of Winnipeg.

Incidence of new primary cancers and mortality rates are published in the Manitoba Cancer Foundation Annual Report. Data are provided to the medical staff, the Epidemiology Department, and researchers, as well as to other registries.

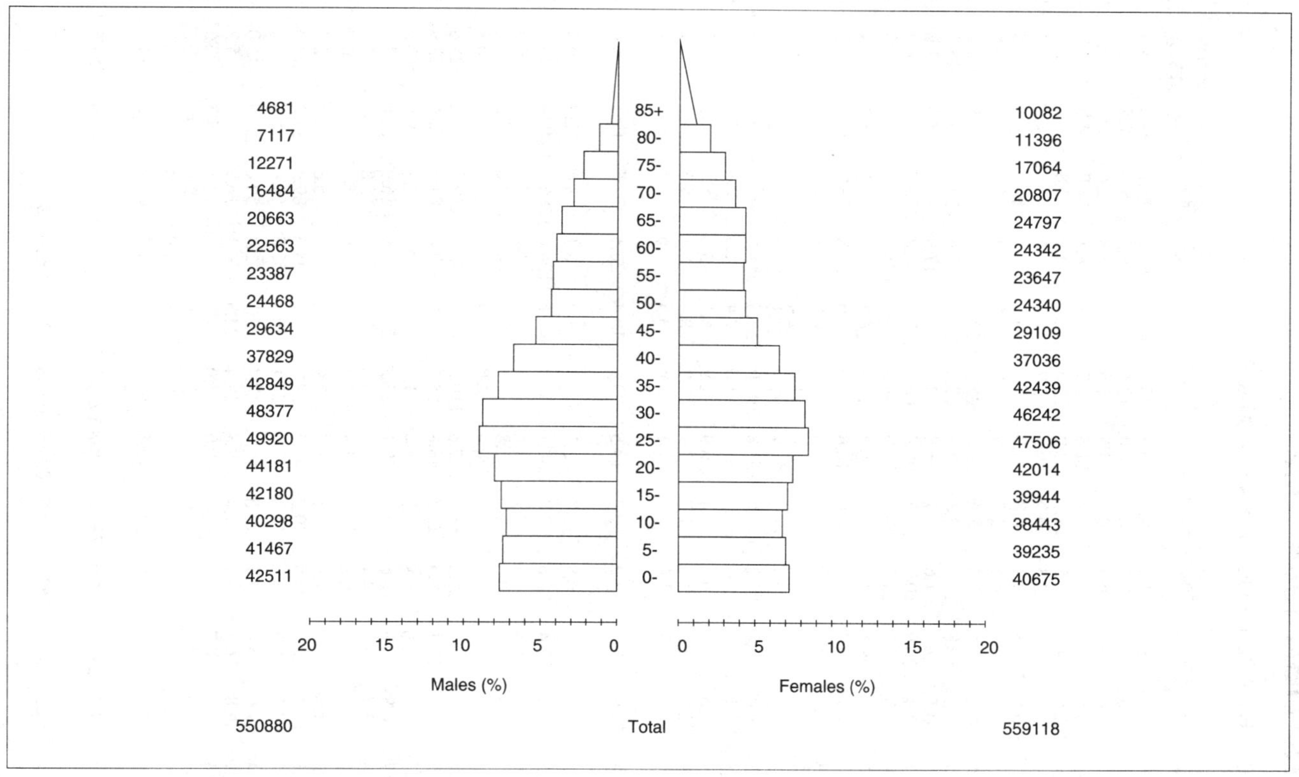

Canada, Manitoba

Source of population: average annual 1988-92

Census: Statistics Canada June 1991

Estimate: The populations were estimated at 1 July each year, based on revised intercensal estimates for 1988-91 and post-censal estimates for 1992. In 1993 revised estimates dating back to 1971 were implemented by Statistics Canada and population data from 1971 now include estimates of net census undercoverage, plus non-permanent residents defined as persons claiming refugee status, foreign students, work permit holders, or holders of Minister's permits, and non-Canadian-born dependants of such individuals. References: Statistics Canada, Catalogue 91-537, Revised intercensal population and family estimates, July 1, 1971–91, and Catalogue 91-213, Annual demographic statistics 1993 (for 1992 data).

Notes to tables overleaf:

† Kaposi's sarcoma is under-reported in this volume because cases of skin cancer (ICD-9 173) were not provided

† 173 not available

CANADA, MANITOBA 1988-1992

ANNUAL INCIDENCE PER 100,000 BY AGE GROUP (YEARS) - MALE

SITE	ALL AGES	AGE UNK	0-	5-	10-	15-	20-	25-	30-	35-	40-	45-	50-	55-	60-	65-	70-	75-	80-	85+	CRUDE RATE	%	CR 64	CR 74	ASR (W)	ICD (9th)
Lip	237	0	-	-	-	-	0.5	0.4	1.7	1.9	3.2	8.8	11.4	9.4	20.4	35.8	41.3	65.2	73.1	98.3	8.6	1.9	0.29	0.67	**6.2**	140
Tongue	67	0	-	0.5	-	-	-	0.4	0.4	0.5	2.6	2.7	3.3	8.6	8.0	12.6	9.7	6.5	8.4	12.8	2.4	0.5	0.13	0.25	**2.0**	141
Salivary gland	25	0	-	-	-	-	-	0.8	-	0.5	1.6	0.7	0.8	0.9	3.5	1.9	4.9	3.3	5.6	8.5	0.9	0.2	0.04	0.08	**0.7**	142
Mouth	79	0	-	-	-	-	-	-	0.4	-	0.5	4.7	8.2	15.4	11.5	7.7	12.1	8.1	14.0	4.3	2.9	0.6	0.20	0.30	**2.5**	143-5
Oropharynx	63	0	-	-	-	-	-	-	-	-	1.6	4.0	2.5	11.1	8.9	13.6	12.1	4.9	2.8	-	2.3	0.5	0.14	0.27	**2.0**	146
Nasopharynx	18	0	-	-	-	-	-	-	0.8	0.9	-	0.7	2.5	0.9	0.9	3.9	1.2	1.6	2.8	4.3	0.7	0.1	0.03	0.06	**0.5**	147
Hypopharynx	50	0	-	-	-	-	-	-	-	-	0.5	1.3	4.1	6.8	8.9	7.7	13.3	-	14.0	-	1.8	0.4	0.11	0.21	**1.5**	148
Pharynx unspecified	17	0	-	-	-	-	-	0.4	-	-	-	-	-	0.8	1.7	3.5	2.9	3.6	3.3	2.8	-	0.6	0.1	0.03	0.07	**0.5**	149
Oesophagus	140	0	-	-	-	-	-	-	-	0.5	0.5	3.4	2.5	8.6	26.6	22.3	29.1	31.0	28.1	59.8	5.1	1.1	0.21	0.47	**3.8**	150
Stomach	433	0	-	-	-	-	-	0.4	0.8	3.3	2.6	10.8	12.3	23.1	43.4	67.8	101.9	107.6	137.7	179.4	15.7	3.5	0.48	1.33	**11.1**	151
Small intestine	33	0	-	-	-	-	-	0.4	-	-	0.5	-	1.6	1.7	1.8	2.9	6.1	17.9	11.2	8.5	1.2	0.3	0.03	0.08	**0.8**	152
Colon	1071	0	-	-	-	-	1.4	0.8	2.1	3.7	7.4	20.9	40.1	66.7	95.7	166.5	207.5	304.8	370.9	474.3	38.9	8.6	1.19	3.06	**27.1**	153
Rectum	592	0	-	-	-	-	-	1.6	1.2	0.9	4.8	14.8	24.5	41.9	78.9	108.4	108.0	128.8	177.0	175.2	21.5	4.7	0.84	1.93	**16.0**	154
Liver	106	0	0.5	-	0.5	-	-	-	0.4	-	1.1	5.4	3.3	6.0	6.2	14.5	26.7	27.7	25.3	51.3	3.8	0.9	0.12	0.32	**2.8**	155
Gallbladder etc.	84	0	-	-	-	-	-	-	-	-	1.1	0.7	0.8	6.0	10.6	12.6	17.0	22.8	33.7	34.2	3.0	0.7	0.10	0.24	**2.1**	156
Pancreas	305	0	-	-	-	-	-	0.4	0.4	0.9	2.1	7.4	9.0	15.4	24.8	47.4	70.4	83.1	112.4	132.5	11.1	2.4	0.30	0.89	**7.6**	157
Nose, sinuses etc.	10	0	-	-	-	-	-	-	-	0.5	0.5	0.7	0.8	-	0.9	1.9	2.4	-	2.8	-	0.4	0.1	0.02	0.04	**0.3**	160
Larynx	149	0	-	-	-	-	0.5	-	-	0.5	1.1	6.1	12.3	11.1	21.3	27.1	29.1	27.7	33.7	12.8	5.4	1.2	0.26	0.54	**4.3**	161
Bronchus, lung	2217	0	-	-	-	-	0.5	0.4	2.1	4.7	9.0	33.7	84.2	171.0	258.8	394.9	553.3	555.8	606.9	499.9	80.5	17.8	2.82	7.56	**58.4**	162
Other thoracic organs	19	0	-	-	-	-	0.5	1.2	0.4	1.9	1.1	-	1.7	-	1.0	2.4	1.6	2.8	4.3	-	0.7	0.2	0.03	0.05	**0.5**	163-4
Bone	33	0	-	0.5	-	2.4	0.5	-	0.4	-	1.6	2.0	0.8	3.4	0.9	2.9	6.1	3.3	5.6	4.3	1.2	0.3	0.06	0.11	**1.0**	170
Connective tissue	58	0	0.9	0.5	1.0	0.5	0.9	0.4	1.7	0.9	2.6	1.3	1.6	1.7	7.1	3.9	8.5	8.1	5.6	25.6	2.1	0.5	0.11	0.17	**1.8**	171
Mesothelioma	47	0	-	-	-	-	-	0.4	-	0.9	-	2.7	1.6	4.3	7.1	13.6	8.5	1.6	8.4	-	-	1.7	0.4	0.09	0.20	**1.4**	MES
†Kaposi's sarcoma	1	0	-	-	-	-	-	-	0.4	-	-	-	-	-	-	-	-	-	-	-	0.0	0.0	0.00	0.00	**0.0**	KAP
Melanoma of skin	230	0	-	-	0.5	0.9	3.6	5.6	3.7	9.8	10.0	17.5	13.9	13.7	19.5	30.0	19.4	26.1	22.5	17.1	8.4	1.8	0.49	0.74	**7.1**	172
†Other skin																										
Breast	25	0	-	-	-	-	-	0.4	0.4	-	-	-	0.8	1.7	2.7	4.8	1.2	8.1	8.4	12.8	0.9	0.2	0.03	0.06	**0.6**	175
Prostate	3322	0	-	-	-	0.5	0.5	-	-	0.5	0.5	7.4	28.6	93.2	288.1	550.7	896.6	1194.6	1286.9	1448.4	120.6	26.7	2.10	9.33	**77.3**	185
Testis	127	0	-	-	-	1.4	9.5	8.4	8.3	9.8	8.5	6.1	4.1	4.3	1.8	-	2.4	1.6	2.8	-	4.6	1.0	0.31	0.32	**4.0**	186
Penis	19	0	-	-	-	-	-	-	-	0.5	0.5	1.3	0.8	1.7	1.8	2.9	2.4	4.9	2.8	4.3	0.7	0.2	0.03	0.06	**0.5**	187.1-.4
Other male genital	8	0	-	-	-	-	-	-	-	0.5	0.5	-	-	-	0.9	1.0	2.4	1.6	-	4.3	0.3	0.1	0.01	0.03	**0.2**	187.5-.9
Bladder	706	0	-	-	0.5	0.5	-	0.4	2.1	4.7	4.8	10.8	18.0	31.6	65.6	110.3	160.2	233.1	219.2	269.2	25.6	5.7	0.69	2.05	**17.5**	188
Kidney etc.	384	0	0.9	0.5	-	-	-	-	1.2	1.9	7.4	12.1	28.6	25.7	48.8	58.1	59.5	107.6	84.3	72.6	13.9	3.1	0.64	1.22	**10.7**	189
Eye	23	0	0.5	-	-	-	-	0.4	0.4	-	-	2.0	0.8	1.7	4.4	1.0	2.4	3.3	5.6	8.5	0.8	0.2	0.05	0.07	**0.7**	190
Brain, nervous system	211	0	5.2	4.3	3.0	1.4	1.4	4.4	5.4	4.7	4.8	8.8	10.6	12.8	30.1	22.3	21.8	17.9	16.9	12.8	7.7	1.7	0.48	0.70	**7.0**	191-2
Thyroid	62	0	-	-	-	0.5	0.5	1.6	2.1	1.9	3.7	3.4	4.1	7.7	4.4	5.8	8.5	3.3	2.8	-	2.3	0.5	0.15	0.22	**1.9**	193
Other endocrine	18	0	0.9	0.5	-	-	-	0.4	-	0.5	-	-	0.8	4.3	1.8	2.9	1.2	1.6	-	-	0.7	0.1	0.05	0.07	**0.6**	194
Hodgkin's disease	77	0	-	1.4	2.5	1.9	2.7	5.2	5.8	2.3	1.6	-	1.6	5.1	3.5	2.9	3.6	1.6	5.6	12.8	2.8	0.6	0.17	0.20	**2.5**	201
Non-Hodgkin lymphoma	496	0	0.5	1.9	3.0	3.3	2.3	4.8	6.2	6.1	13.7	20.9	27.8	40.2	43.4	69.7	78.9	94.5	89.9	81.2	18.0	4.0	0.87	1.61	**14.4**	200,202
Multiple myeloma	172	0	-	-	-	-	-	-	0.4	0.5	3.7	0.7	8.2	10.3	12.4	27.1	36.4	52.2	64.6	55.5	6.2	1.4	0.18	0.50	**4.3**	203
Lymphoid leukaemia	165	0	5.6	2.9	1.0	1.4	-	-	0.8	1.4	1.6	5.4	4.1	12.0	16.8	17.4	23.1	42.4	50.6	29.9	6.0	1.3	0.27	0.47	**4.9**	204
Myeloid leukaemia	142	0	1.4	-	0.5	2.4	1.4	1.6	2.1	1.9	4.8	6.1	5.7	9.4	9.8	18.4	24.3	24.4	16.9	42.7	5.2	1.1	0.23	0.45	**4.2**	205
Monocytic leukaemia	7	0	-	-	-	-	-	-	-	-	-	0.7	-	-	0.9	1.0	1.2	-	2.8	4.3	0.3	0.1	0.01	0.02	**0.2**	206
Other leukaemia	5	0	-	-	-	-	-	-	0.4	-	-	-	-	-	-	2.9	-	-	2.8	-	0.2	0.0	0.00	0.02	**0.1**	207
Leukaemia unspecified	18	0	-	-	-	-	-	-	0.4	-	-	-	-	-	2.7	2.9	3.6	4.9	8.4	8.5	0.7	0.1	0.02	0.05	**0.4**	208
Other and unspecified	394	0	1.4	-	0.5	0.5	-	0.4	1.2	1.4	2.6	9.4	6.5	20.5	49.6	52.3	97.1	104.3	106.8	166.6	14.3	3.2	0.47	1.22	**10.2**	O&U
All sites																										
All sites but 173	12465	0	17.9	13.0	12.9	17.5	26.3	41.7	54.2	70.9	114.7	245.7	394.0	713.2	1258.7	1958.1	2721.4	3342.7	3686.5	4041.9	452.5	100.0	14.90	38.30	**324.6**	ALLb
Rate from 1 case			0.470	0.482	0.496	0.474	0.453	0.401	0.413	0.467	0.529	0.675	0.817	0.855	0.886	0.968	1.213	1.630	2.810	4.273							

†Important: see notes on population page

CANADA, MANITOBA 1988-1992

ANNUAL INCIDENCE PER 100,000 BY AGE GROUP (YEARS) - FEMALE

SITE	ALL AGES	AGE UNK	0-	5-	10-	15-	20-	25-	30-	35-	40-	45-	50-	55-	60-	65-	70-	75-	80-	85+	CRUDE RATE	%	CR 64	CR 74	ASR (W)	ICD (9th)
Lip	42	0	-	-	-	-	-	0.4	-	0.5	-	0.7	1.6	4.2	3.3	3.2	6.7	7.0	7.0	13.9	1.5	0.4	0.05	0.10	**0.9**	*140*
Tongue	43	0	-	-	-	-	0.5	-	-	0.9	-	2.1	3.3	5.9	0.8	4.0	6.7	7.0	5.3	7.9	1.5	0.4	0.07	0.12	**1.0**	*141*
Salivary gland	19	0	-	-	-	-	-	-	0.9	-	1.1	0.7	-	0.8	4.9	4.0	-	2.3	-	-	0.7	0.2	0.04	0.06	**0.5**	*142*
Mouth	59	0	-	-	-	-	0.5	-	-	0.5	-	1.4	4.1	4.2	2.5	6.5	8.7	10.5	19.3	9.9	2.1	0.5	0.07	0.14	**1.2**	*143-5*
Oropharynx	18	0	-	-	-	-	-	-	-	-	0.5	-	0.8	1.7	0.8	5.6	1.9	1.2	1.8	4.0	0.6	0.2	0.02	0.06	**0.4**	*146*
Nasopharynx	15	0	-	-	-	-	-	0.4	0.4	-	0.5	-	0.8	0.8	1.6	2.4	1.9	2.3	-	2.0	0.5	0.1	0.02	0.05	**0.4**	*147*
Hypopharynx	10	0	-	-	-	-	-	-	-	-	-	0.7	-	1.6	4.0	1.0	1.2	-	-	-	0.4	0.1	0.01	0.04	**0.3**	*148*
Pharynx unspecified	5	0	-	-	-	-	-	-	-	-	-	-	0.8	-	0.8	-	1.9	-	-	2.0	0.2	0.0	0.01	0.02	**0.1**	*149*
Oesophagus	68	0	-	-	-	-	0.5	-	-	-	-	-	0.8	4.2	4.9	9.7	12.5	11.7	14.0	23.8	2.4	0.6	0.05	0.16	**1.3**	*150*
Stomach	237	0	-	-	-	-	-	-	0.9	2.4	1.6	3.4	13.1	6.8	14.0	23.4	23.1	50.4	80.7	77.4	8.5	2.2	0.21	0.44	**4.4**	*151*
Small intestine	28	0	-	-	-	-	-	-	0.4	-	-	-	-	1.7	4.9	0.8	2.9	7.0	8.8	7.9	1.0	0.3	0.04	0.05	**0.5**	*152*
Colon	1140	0	-	-	-	0.5	-	1.7	1.7	4.7	9.7	22.7	35.3	71.9	100.2	135.5	159.6	206.3	273.8	305.5	40.8	10.3	1.24	2.72	**23.4**	*153*
Rectum	426	0	-	-	-	-	-	0.4	2.2	2.4	2.7	8.9	17.3	27.9	38.6	54.0	69.2	76.2	77.2	95.2	15.2	3.9	0.50	1.12	**9.2**	*154*
Liver	57	0	0.5	-	-	-	-	-	0.4	-	-	0.7	5.8	-	1.6	7.3	9.6	4.7	17.5	23.8	2.0	0.5	0.05	0.13	**1.1**	*155*
Gallbladder etc.	111	0	-	-	-	-	-	0.4	-	-	0.5	1.4	-	5.1	7.4	13.7	17.3	32.8	28.1	25.8	4.0	1.0	0.07	0.23	**2.0**	*156*
Pancreas	292	0	-	-	-	0.5	-	-	-	0.9	1.6	8.9	7.4	14.4	18.1	35.5	43.3	58.6	72.0	89.3	10.4	2.7	0.26	0.65	**5.7**	*157*
Nose, sinuses etc.	10	0	-	-	-	-	-	-	0.4	-	-	0.7	-	0.8	0.8	2.4	-	-	3.5	2.0	0.4	0.1	0.01	0.03	**0.2**	*160*
Larynx	30	0	-	-	-	-	-	-	-	-	0.5	1.4	1.6	4.2	6.6	5.6	4.8	-	-	-	1.1	0.3	0.07	0.12	**0.9**	*161*
Bronchus, lung	1203	0	-	-	-	-	-	-	0.4	2.4	14.6	32.3	57.5	99.0	148.7	167.8	199.0	201.6	186.0	123.0	43.0	10.9	1.77	3.61	**28.3**	*162*
Other thoracic organs	15	0	1.5	-	-	-	-	-	0.9	0.5	0.5	-	-	0.8	0.8	-	1.9	1.2	3.5	2.0	0.5	0.1	0.03	0.03	**0.4**	*163-4*
Bone	22	0	-	1.0	1.0	1.5	-	0.8	-	0.5	2.2	0.7	-	-	1.6	1.6	-	1.2	1.8	2.0	0.8	0.2	0.05	0.05	**0.7**	*170*
Connective tissue	51	0	-	1.5	0.5	1.0	1.4	0.4	0.9	0.5	1.1	1.4	3.3	2.5	3.3	2.4	4.8	8.2	5.3	9.9	1.8	0.5	0.09	0.13	**1.4**	*171*
Mesothelioma	7	0	-	-	-	-	-	-	-	0.5	-	0.7	-	-	0.8	1.6	1.9	-	-	-	0.3	0.1	0.01	0.03	**0.2**	*MES*
†Kaposi's sarcoma	1	0	-	-	-	-	-	-	-	-	-	-	-	-	-	-	-	-	1.8	-	0.0	0.0	0.00	0.00	**0.0**	*KAP*
Melanoma of skin	253	0	-	-	0.5	2.5	2.9	3.8	9.1	10.8	14.6	11.0	13.1	16.1	18.9	16.9	25.0	18.8	21.1	23.8	9.0	2.3	0.52	0.73	**7.0**	*172*
†Other skin																										
Breast	3142	0	-	-	-	-	0.5	5.1	19.9	50.0	102.6	156.0	207.1	268.1	281.0	342.0	400.8	475.8	358.0	392.8	112.4	28.5	5.45	9.16	**79.3**	*174*
Uterus unspecified	32	0	-	-	-	-	-	-	-	-	-	-	2.5	1.7	1.6	2.4	7.7	7.0	3.5	11.9	1.1	0.3	0.03	0.08	**0.6**	*179*
Cervix uteri	290	0	-	-	-	-	2.4	10.5	19.0	15.1	17.8	14.4	8.2	16.9	15.6	19.4	17.3	24.6	22.8	9.9	10.4	2.6	0.60	0.78	**8.1**	*180*
Placenta	0	0	-	-	-	-	-	-	-	-	-	-	-	-	-	-	-	-	-	-	0.0	0.0	0.00	0.00	**0.0**	*181*
Corpus uteri	668	0	-	-	-	-	-	0.8	2.2	5.7	13.0	22.7	44.4	66.8	76.4	100.8	93.2	93.8	64.9	53.6	23.9	6.1	1.16	2.13	**17.0**	*182*
Ovary etc.	386	0	-	-	1.0	0.5	1.0	3.4	4.3	6.6	10.3	17.2	25.5	38.9	36.2	43.6	36.5	44.5	49.1	51.6	13.8	3.5	0.72	1.12	**10.0**	*183*
Other female genital	103	0	-	-	-	-	1.0	0.4	0.4	2.8	1.6	4.1	4.9	7.6	7.4	8.9	18.3	17.6	15.8	11.9	3.7	0.9	0.15	0.29	**2.4**	*184*
Bladder	261	0	-	-	-	-	-	-	0.9	0.9	1.6	7.6	10.7	14.4	17.3	28.2	45.2	55.1	57.9	59.5	9.3	2.4	0.27	0.63	**5.3**	*188*
Kidney etc.	250	0	2.5	0.5	-	1.0	0.5	1.7	1.7	1.4	4.9	10.3	9.0	18.6	18.9	23.4	41.3	34.0	64.9	23.8	8.9	2.3	0.35	0.68	**6.0**	*189*
Eye	37	0	2.0	-	-	0.5	-	-	-	-	-	1.4	3.3	0.8	4.1	5.6	4.8	2.3	5.3	6.0	1.3	0.3	0.06	0.11	**1.1**	*190*
Brain, nervous system	161	0	4.4	3.6	0.5	3.0	0.5	2.5	5.6	3.3	3.2	4.1	8.2	9.3	11.5	12.9	19.2	17.6	14.0	9.9	5.8	1.5	0.30	0.46	**4.7**	*191-2*
Thyroid	156	0	-	-	0.5	4.0	3.8	5.5	8.2	8.5	5.9	6.2	9.9	11.0	10.7	4.0	9.6	10.5	10.5	2.0	5.6	1.4	0.37	0.44	**4.7**	*193*
Other endocrine	12	0	1.0	0.5	-	-	-	-	0.4	0.5	1.1	0.7	-	1.7	-	-	1.0	1.2	-	-	0.4	0.1	0.03	0.03	**0.4**	*194*
Hodgkin's disease	50	0	-	0.5	1.0	2.0	3.3	2.9	1.7	1.4	2.7	0.7	2.5	2.5	1.6	-	1.9	3.5	5.3	-	1.8	0.5	0.12	0.12	**1.6**	*201*
Non-Hodgkin lymphoma	469	0	0.5	0.5	0.5	1.5	2.4	1.3	2.6	5.7	10.3	16.5	20.5	22.8	41.9	46.8	68.2	75.0	94.8	87.3	16.8	4.3	0.63	1.21	**10.7**	*200,202*
Multiple myeloma	147	0	-	-	-	-	-	-	-	0.5	1.1	3.4	-	11.0	5.8	21.0	20.2	38.7	35.1	37.7	5.3	1.3	0.11	0.31	**2.8**	*203*
Lymphoid leukaemia	112	0	7.4	4.1	0.5	0.5	-	0.8	-	0.5	0.5	2.7	3.3	2.5	4.9	6.5	7.7	23.4	26.3	29.8	4.0	1.0	0.14	0.21	**3.0**	*204*
Myeloid leukaemia	109	0	0.5	0.5	0.5	0.5	1.0	-	2.6	2.4	2.7	2.7	2.5	4.2	8.2	11.3	17.3	17.6	21.1	11.9	3.9	1.0	0.14	0.28	**2.5**	*205*
Monocytic leukaemia	5	0	-	-	-	-	-	-	-	0.5	-	-	-	-	-	0.8	1.0	-	1.8	2.0	0.2	0.0	0.00	0.01	**0.1**	*206*
Other leukaemia	2	0	-	-	-	-	-	-	-	-	-	-	-	-	-	0.8	1.0	-	-	-	0.1	0.0	0.00	0.01	**0.0**	*207*
Leukaemia unspecified	15	0	-	-	-	-	-	-	-	-	-	0.7	-	-	0.8	-	2.9	-	7.0	11.9	0.5	0.1	0.01	0.02	**0.2**	*208*
Other and unspecified	448	0	1.5	0.5	-	-	-	1.7	1.3	2.4	3.2	9.6	10.7	21.1	28.8	50.0	60.6	84.4	107.0	160.7	16.0	4.1	0.40	0.96	**8.8**	*O&U*
All sites																										
All sites but 173	11017	0	21.6	13.3	6.8	19.5	21.9	45.0	89.5	135.3	234.4	380.6	539.8	793.3	960.5	1236.4	1479.3	1736.9	1793.5	1825.0	394.1	100.0	16.31	29.89	**261.3**	*ALLb*

Rate from 1 case   0.492   0.510   0.520   0.501   0.476   0.421   0.433   0.471   0.540   0.687   0.822   0.846   0.822   0.807   0.961   1.172   1.755   1.984

†Important: see notes on population page

Canada, New Brunswick

The New Brunswick Provincial Cancer Registry was formed in 1955 to register all malignant diseases as well as selected benign cases in the province. The personnel consists of a director, three full-time employees and one casual employee. The registry came under the jurisdiction of the Department of Health in 1992.

The area covered by the registry is the entire Province of New Brunswick, an area of 73 437 km^2. There are seven cities, none of which has more than 100 000 inhabitants. The total population in the 1991 census was 723 900. 47.7% of the population is urban and 52.3% rural. New Brunswick is bordered by the provinces of Quebec and Nova Scotia, with the St Lawrence River to the north and the Bay of Fundy to the south.

The sources of data on patients with cancer include pathology laboratories, radiation oncology centres, cytology and haematology laboratories, death certificates and autopsies. The reporting of cancer incidence is voluntary. A programme for follow-up of all patients is being initiated. The registry receives death certificates with a mention of cancer. All data are recorded by computer and the hard copy is filed. The data from 1955 to 1971 were recorded on hand-punched cards and forwarded to Statistics Canada. From 1972 to 1984, data were forwarded on IBM punch cards. The 1985 to 1988 data were forwarded on tape by the Department of Health. The 1989 and later data are now registered by computer and converted to disk to be forwarded to the Canadian Cancer Registry. The completeness of the registry is ensured by checking pathologies, utilizing further follow-up information, including autopsies, radiation oncologists, surgeons, consultations with family doctors and edits in the reporting program. The registry maintains a patient record and a tumour record which permits the recording of multiple tumours for one person.

The data are used for analysis of trends, for surveys and studies and for reporting of incidence to the Canadian Cancer Registry, Statistics Canada.

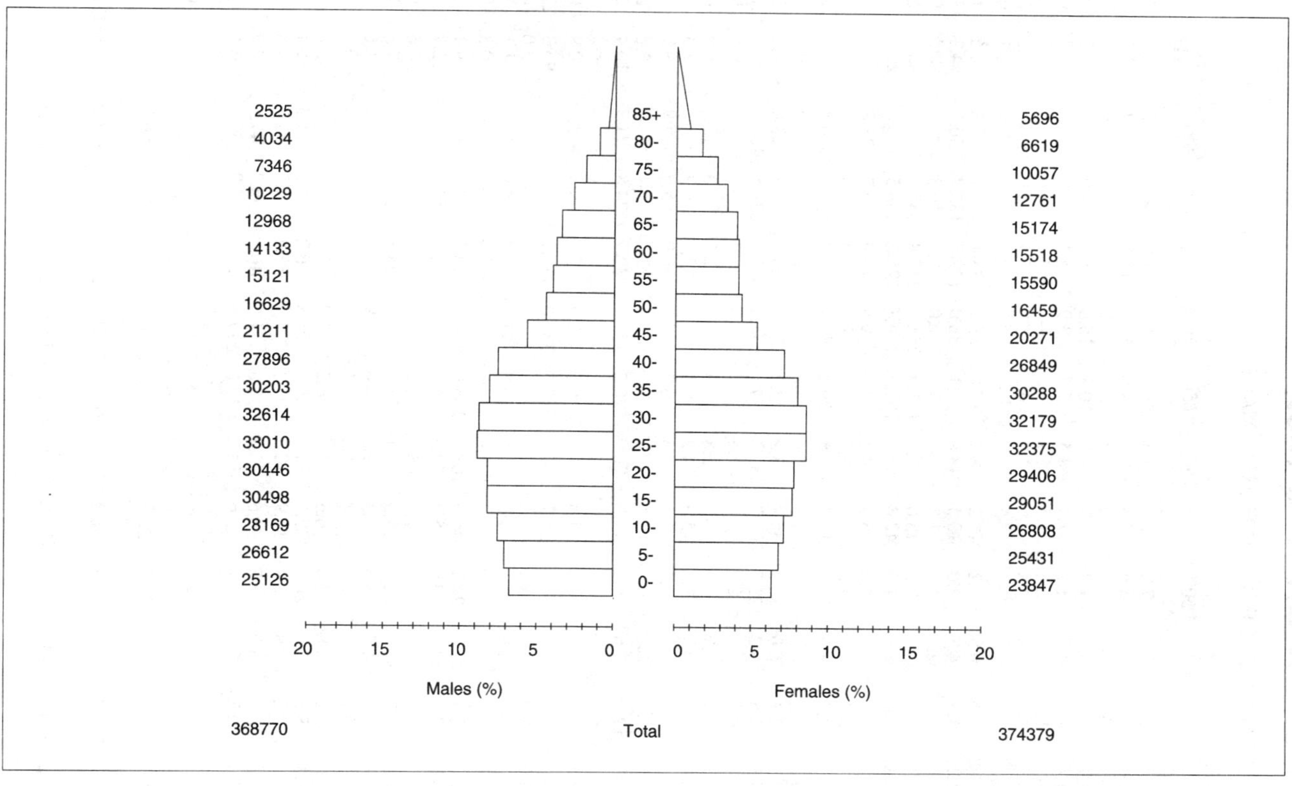

Canada, New Brunswick
Source of population: average annual 1988-92
Census: Statistics Canada June 1991
Estimate: The populations were estimated at 1 July each year, based on revised intercensal estimates for 1988-91 and post-censal estimates for 1992. In 1993 revised estimates dating back to 1971 were implemented by Statistics Canada and population data from 1971 now include estimates of net census undercoverage, plus non-permanent residents defined as persons claiming refugee status, foreign students, work permit holders, or holders of Minister's permits, and non-Canadian-born dependants of such individuals. References: Statistics Canada, Catalogue 91-537, Revised intercensal population and family estimates, July 1, 1971–91, and Catalogue 91-213, Annual demographic statistics 1993 (for 1992 data).

Notes to tables overleaf:
† Kaposi's sarcoma is under-reported in this volume because cases of skin cancer (ICD-9 173) were not provided
† 173 not available

CANADA, NEW BRUNSWICK 1988-1992

ANNUAL INCIDENCE PER 100,000 BY AGE GROUP (YEARS) - MALE

SITE	ALL AGES	AGE UNK	0-	5-	10-	15-	20-	25-	30-	35-	40-	45-	50-	55-	60-	65-	70-	75-	80-	85+	CRUDE RATE	%	CR 64	CR 74	ASR (W)	ICD (9th)
Lip	68	0	-	-	-	-	-	0.6	-	-	2.2	1.9	7.2	6.6	11.3	20.0	21.5	21.8	34.7	31.7	3.7	0.9	0.15	0.36	**3.0**	140
Tongue	43	0	-	-	-	0.7	-	-	-	2.0	-	5.7	3.6	9.3	9.9	4.6	13.7	13.6	-	7.9	2.3	0.6	0.16	0.25	**2.1**	141
Salivary gland	13	0	-	-	-	-	-	-	0.6	-	-	-	-	4.0	4.2	3.1	2.0	2.7	5.0	7.9	0.7	0.2	0.04	0.07	**0.6**	142
Mouth	50	1	-	-	-	-	-	-	-	1.3	-	4.7	7.2	5.3	11.3	10.8	15.6	5.4	14.9	31.7	2.7	0.6	0.15	0.29	**2.4**	143-5
Oropharynx	31	0	-	-	-	-	-	-	-	0.7	1.4	4.7	1.2	7.9	8.5	7.7	3.9	5.4	5.0	-	1.7	0.4	0.12	0.18	**1.5**	146
Nasopharynx	12	0	-	-	-	-	-	-	-	-	1.4	-	2.4	1.3	5.7	1.5	-	2.7	5.0	-	0.7	0.2	0.05	0.06	**0.6**	147
Hypopharynx	23	0	-	-	-	-	-	-	-	-	-	2.8	3.6	2.6	5.7	6.2	7.8	5.4	5.0	-	1.2	0.3	0.07	0.14	**1.1**	148
Pharynx unspecified	2	0	-	-	-	-	-	-	-	-	-	-	-	-	-	-	-	2.7	-	7.9	0.1	0.0	0.00	0.00	**0.1**	149
Oesophagus	84	0	-	-	-	-	-	-	-	-	1.4	0.9	7.2	13.2	18.4	17.0	33.2	38.1	39.7	15.8	4.6	1.1	0.21	0.46	**3.6**	150
Stomach	263	0	-	-	-	-	-	0.6	0.6	2.0	4.3	4.7	12.0	18.5	48.1	77.1	86.0	122.5	153.7	150.5	14.3	3.4	0.45	1.27	**10.8**	151
Small intestine	15	0	-	-	-	-	-	-	-	-	0.7	2.8	1.2	1.3	-	3.1	2.0	5.4	19.8	-	0.8	0.2	0.03	0.06	**0.6**	152
Colon	677	1	-	-	-	0.7	-	0.6	0.6	1.3	7.9	20.7	32.5	78.0	110.4	171.2	256.1	315.8	347.0	364.3	36.7	8.8	1.27	3.41	**28.1**	153
Rectum	371	1	-	-	-	0.7	-	-	0.6	1.3	8.6	12.3	31.3	42.3	87.7	100.2	119.3	125.2	168.5	118.8	20.1	4.8	0.93	2.03	**16.3**	154
Liver	45	0	-	-	-	-	-	-	0.6	-	-	0.9	6.0	5.3	4.2	17.0	9.8	10.9	39.7	23.8	2.4	0.6	0.09	0.22	**1.9**	155
Gallbladder etc.	29	0	-	-	-	-	-	-	-	-	0.7	-	1.2	-	2.8	10.8	9.8	21.8	14.9	15.8	1.6	0.4	0.02	0.13	**1.1**	156
Pancreas	175	1	-	-	-	-	-	-	-	-	0.7	8.5	12.0	13.2	36.8	29.3	56.7	89.8	104.1	126.7	9.5	2.3	0.36	0.79	**7.3**	157
Nose, sinuses etc.	15	0	-	0.8	-	-	-	-	-	-	0.7	0.7	-	-	1.3	1.4	-	7.8	8.2	9.9	7.9	0.8	0.2	0.02	0.06	**0.6**	160
Larynx	154	0	-	-	-	-	-	-	-	0.7	2.2	6.6	22.9	35.7	38.2	43.2	29.3	54.4	19.8	23.8	8.4	2.0	0.53	0.89	**7.3**	161
Bronchus, lung	1679	2	-	-	-	-	-	0.6	0.6	5.3	13.6	46.2	122.7	207.7	362.3	479.6	658.9	675.1	639.5	467.3	91.1	21.8	3.80	9.50	**72.9**	162
Other thoracic organs	7	0	-	-	-	-	-	0.6	-	-	0.7	-	2.4	-	2.8	-	2.0	-	-	-	0.4	0.1	0.03	0.04	**0.4**	163-4
Bone	17	0	-	-	2.8	2.0	-	-	-	1.3	1.4	0.9	-	-	2.8	1.5	-	2.7	5.0	-	0.9	0.2	0.06	0.06	**0.9**	170
Connective tissue	42	0	0.8	-	1.4	-	1.3	1.8	-	2.0	0.7	0.9	3.6	5.3	4.2	9.3	2.0	27.2	9.9	-	2.3	0.5	0.11	0.17	**1.9**	171
Mesothelioma	16	0	-	-	-	-	-	-	-	-	-	-	2.4	1.3	2.8	6.2	2.0	10.9	5.0	7.9	0.9	0.2	0.03	0.07	**0.7**	MES
†Kaposi's sarcoma	0	0	-	-	-	-	-	-	-	-	-	-	-	-	-	-	-	-	-	-	0.0	0.0	0.00	0.00	**0.0**	KAP
Melanoma of skin	192	0	-	-	0.7	-	2.6	4.2	5.5	11.3	17.2	17.0	19.2	17.2	26.9	26.2	41.1	32.7	24.8	71.3	10.4	2.5	0.61	0.95	**8.8**	172
†Other skin																										
Breast	16	0	-	-	-	-	-	-	-	0.7	-	-	1.2	1.3	-	6.2	3.9	5.4	9.9	23.8	0.9	0.2	0.02	0.07	**0.6**	175
Prostate	1775	0	0.8	-	-	-	-	-	-	-	1.4	7.5	16.8	121.7	267.5	510.5	739.0	971.9	1194.7	1283.0	96.3	23.0	2.08	8.33	**69.2**	185
Testis	56	0	0.8	-	-	3.9	2.6	7.3	5.5	4.6	5.0	4.7	4.8	-	-	-	2.0	-	-	-	3.0	0.7	0.20	0.21	**2.7**	186
Penis	20	0	-	-	-	-	-	-	0.6	-	-	1.9	-	1.3	2.8	1.5	11.7	5.4	14.9	15.8	1.1	0.3	0.03	0.10	**0.8**	187.1-.4
Other male genital	5	0	-	-	-	-	-	-	-	-	-	-	1.3	1.4	-	-	-	5.4	-	7.9	0.3	0.1	0.01	0.01	**0.2**	187.5-.9
Bladder	537	0	-	-	-	0.7	-	0.6	1.8	2.0	7.9	22.6	24.1	45.0	103.3	165.0	166.2	198.7	327.2	285.1	29.1	7.0	1.04	2.70	**22.6**	188
Kidney etc.	234	1	0.8	-	-	-	-	0.6	2.5	4.0	7.2	13.2	9.6	35.7	42.5	64.8	70.4	92.6	59.5	63.4	12.7	3.0	0.58	1.26	**10.3**	189
Eye	11	0	-	-	-	-	-	-	-	-	-	-	-	1.3	5.7	3.1	3.9	-	5.0	7.9	0.6	0.1	0.03	0.07	**0.5**	190
Brain, nervous system	135	0	2.4	3.0	2.1	1.3	2.6	0.6	4.3	6.0	5.7	11.3	13.2	18.5	24.1	21.6	19.6	24.5	24.8	15.8	7.3	1.8	0.48	0.68	**6.6**	191-2
Thyroid	29	0	-	-	0.7	-	-	-	-	1.3	3.6	4.7	3.6	1.3	2.8	4.6	5.9	2.7	5.0	15.8	1.6	0.4	0.09	0.14	**1.4**	193
Other endocrine	15	0	2.4	0.8	0.7	-	-	-	-	-	0.7	-	2.4	-	4.2	3.1	3.9	-	-	-	0.8	0.2	0.06	0.09	**0.9**	194
Hodgkin's disease	52	0	-	-	0.7	3.3	5.9	3.6	1.8	2.0	2.2	2.8	3.6	6.6	1.4	6.2	5.9	5.4	5.0	-	2.8	0.7	0.17	0.23	**2.5**	201
Non-Hodgkin lymphoma	279	0	-	1.5	0.7	2.6	2.0	2.4	6.7	9.3	8.6	20.7	26.5	29.1	31.1	66.3	95.8	76.2	54.5	71.3	15.1	3.6	0.71	1.52	**12.6**	200,202
Multiple myeloma	88	0	-	-	-	-	-	-	-	-	2.2	1.9	8.4	11.9	12.7	29.3	37.1	35.4	14.9	31.7	4.8	1.1	0.19	0.52	**3.9**	203
Lymphoid leukaemia	79	0	6.4	1.5	1.4	1.3	0.7	-	1.2	-	0.7	0.9	4.8	6.6	5.7	10.8	21.5	40.8	39.7	47.5	4.3	1.0	0.16	0.32	**3.7**	204
Myeloid leukaemia	67	0	-	-	-	-	2.0	3.0	1.8	2.6	0.7	2.8	1.2	2.6	14.2	17.0	17.6	27.2	5.0	31.7	3.6	0.9	0.16	0.33	**2.9**	205
Monocytic leukaemia	2	0	-	-	-	-	-	-	-	-	-	-	-	-	-	-	3.9	-	-	-	0.1	0.0	0.00	0.02	**0.1**	206
Other leukaemia	0	0	-	-	-	-	-	-	-	-	-	-	-	-	-	-	-	-	-	-	0.0	0.0	0.00	0.00	**0.0**	207
Leukaemia unspecified	34	0	0.8	1.5	-	-	0.7	0.6	0.6	0.7	0.7	-	-	2.6	4.2	6.2	5.9	21.8	19.8	15.8	1.8	0.4	0.06	0.12	**1.4**	208
Other and unspecified	255	1	-	-	-	-	-	1.2	1.2	1.3	2.2	7.5	21.6	23.8	38.2	60.1	70.4	98.0	208.2	166.3	13.8	3.3	0.49	1.14	**10.5**	O&U
All sites	7712	8																								
All sites but 173			15.1	9.0	11.4	17.0	20.4	29.1	37.4	64.2	114.7	245.1	443.8	788.3	1368.4	2021.8	2664.8	3212.3	3658.4	3563.8	418.2	100.0	15.84	39.29	**327.9**	ALLb
Rate from 1 case			0.796	0.752	0.710	0.656	0.657	0.606	0.613	0.662	0.717	0.943	1.203	1.323	1.415	1.542	1.955	2.722	4.957	7.920						

†Important: see notes on population page

CANADA, NEW BRUNSWICK 1988-1992

ANNUAL INCIDENCE PER 100,000 BY AGE GROUP (YEARS) - FEMALE

SITE	ALL AGES	AGE UNK	0-	5-	10-	15-	20-	25-	30-	35-	40-	45-	50-	55-	60-	65-	70-	75-	80-	85+	CRUDE RATE	%	CR 64	CR 74	ASR (W)	ICD (9th)
Lip	6	0	-	-	-	-	-	-	-	-	-	1.0	-	-	1.3	-	1.6	6.0	-	-	0.3	0.1	0.01	0.02	0.2	140
Tongue	14	0	-	-	-	-	-	0.6	-	0.7	-	-	-	1.3	2.6	-	3.1	9.9	3.0	3.5	0.7	0.2	0.03	0.04	0.4	141
Salivary gland	9	0	-	-	-	-	-	0.6	0.6	0.7	-	1.0	-	-	1.3	1.3	1.6	2.0	-	3.5	0.5	0.1	0.02	0.04	0.3	142
Mouth	26	0	-	-	-	-	-	-	-	-	-	2.0	3.6	5.1	2.6	5.3	7.8	2.0	9.1	7.0	1.4	0.4	0.07	0.13	1.0	143-5
Oropharynx	9	0	-	-	-	-	-	-	-	-	-	2.0	1.2	2.6	2.6	1.3	1.6	-	-	-	0.5	0.1	0.04	0.06	0.5	146
Nasopharynx	6	0	-	-	-	-	-	0.6	-	1.5	-	1.2	-	1.3	1.3	-	-	-	-	-	0.3	0.1	0.02	0.03	0.3	147
Hypopharynx	5	0	-	-	-	-	-	-	-	-	-	1.2	1.3	1.3	1.3	1.6	-	-	-	-	0.3	0.1	0.02	0.03	0.2	148
Pharynx unspecified	2	0	-	-	-	-	-	-	-	-	-	1.2	-	1.3	-	-	-	-	-	-	0.1	0.0	0.01	0.01	0.1	149
Oesophagus	29	0	-	-	-	-	-	-	-	-	-	1.2	1.3	5.2	5.3	11.0	8.0	9.1	17.6	1.5	0.5	0.04	0.12	0.9	150
Stomach	143	0	-	-	-	-	-	-	1.2	3.3	2.2	5.9	8.5	9.0	14.2	21.1	23.5	53.7	63.4	80.8	7.6	2.2	0.22	0.44	4.5	151
Small intestine	13	0	-	-	-	0.7	-	-	-	-	-	-	2.4	-	1.3	-	6.3	-	12.1	3.5	0.7	0.2	0.02	0.05	0.4	152
Colon	696	0	0.8	-	-	-	0.7	-	1.9	2.6	11.2	21.7	34.0	65.4	76.0	133.1	169.3	262.5	247.7	312.5	37.2	10.9	1.07	2.58	22.6	153
Rectum	279	1	-	-	-	-	-	1.2	0.6	1.3	8.2	9.9	10.9	39.8	30.9	55.4	72.1	85.5	90.6	94.8	14.9	4.4	0.52	1.16	9.6	154
Liver	26	1	-	-	-	-	0.7	0.6	-	0.7	0.7	-	-	2.6	5.2	2.6	3.1	13.9	3.0	10.5	1.4	0.4	0.05	0.08	0.9	155
Gallbladder etc.	45	0	-	-	-	-	-	-	-	0.7	2.2	1.0	3.6	7.7	7.7	5.3	3.1	15.9	15.1	21.1	2.4	0.7	0.11	0.16	1.6	156
Pancreas	143	1	-	-	-	-	-	-	-	1.3	-	4.9	6.1	6.4	20.6	26.4	34.5	37.8	78.6	77.2	7.6	2.2	0.20	0.50	4.4	157
Nose, sinuses etc.	10	0	-	-	-	-	-	0.6	-	-	-	2.0	2.4	-	1.3	3.1	2.0	-	3.5	0.5	0.2	0.03	0.05	0.4	160
Larynx	19	0	-	-	-	-	-	-	-	-	-	2.0	2.4	2.6	5.2	5.3	6.3	2.0	-	-	1.0	0.3	0.06	0.12	0.9	161
Bronchus, lung	687	3	-	-	-	-	-	0.6	1.2	5.3	16.4	38.5	60.8	101.3	146.9	152.9	177.1	147.2	120.8	91.3	36.7	10.7	1.86	3.52	27.5	162
Other thoracic organs	7	0	-	-	-	-	0.7	-	-	-	-	-	1.2	-	-	4.0	1.6	-	-	3.5	0.4	0.1	0.01	0.04	0.3	163-4
Bone	11	0	0.8	-	-	1.4	-	0.6	-	-	-	-	2.4	-	1.3	1.3	-	4.0	-	3.5	0.6	0.2	0.03	0.04	0.5	170
Connective tissue	44	0	-	-	0.7	1.4	0.7	1.9	-	1.3	1.5	-	4.9	2.6	6.4	7.9	7.8	6.0	15.1	10.5	2.4	0.7	0.11	0.19	1.7	171
Mesothelioma	2	0	-	-	-	-	-	-	-	-	-	-	-	-	-	1.3	1.6	-	-	-	0.1	0.0	0.00	0.01	0.1	MES
†Kaposi's sarcoma	0	0	-	-	-	-	-	-	-	-	-	-	-	-	-	-	-	-	-	-	0.0	0.0	0.00	0.00	0.0	KAP
Melanoma of skin	185	0	-	-	-	2.1	5.4	7.4	9.3	9.9	20.9	12.8	13.4	19.2	20.6	25.0	17.2	19.9	15.1	14.0	9.9	2.9	0.61	0.82	8.1	172
†Other skin																										
Breast	1835	1	-	-	-	-	-	6.2	21.8	42.9	113.2	131.2	187.1	221.9	287.4	328.2	374.6	344.0	368.6	372.2	98.0	28.7	5.06	8.58	73.3	174
Uterus unspecified	11	0	-	-	-	-	-	-	-	-	-	-	-	-	2.6	2.6	1.6	4.0	3.0	10.5	0.6	0.2	0.01	0.03	0.3	179
Cervix uteri	173	0	0.8	-	-	-	0.7	8.6	11.8	17.8	11.9	10.9	7.3	14.1	28.4	17.1	20.4	15.9	24.2	10.5	9.2	2.7	0.56	0.75	7.3	180
Placenta	1	0	-	-	-	-	0.7	-	-	-	-	-	-	-	-	-	-	-	-	-	0.1	0.0	0.00	0.00	0.1	181
Corpus uteri	315	0	-	-	-	-	-	1.2	0.6	5.3	6.0	10.9	30.4	41.0	47.7	77.8	90.9	85.5	48.3	52.7	16.8	4.9	0.72	1.56	12.0	182
Ovary etc.	227	1	-	-	0.7	-	1.4	-	3.7	8.6	6.7	15.8	25.5	28.2	24.5	36.9	43.9	51.7	69.5	42.1	12.1	3.6	0.58	0.98	8.7	183
Other female genital	56	0	-	-	-	-	-	-	0.6	2.0	-	5.9	1.2	3.8	10.3	4.0	18.8	13.9	18.1	17.6	3.0	0.9	0.12	0.24	2.0	184
Bladder	179	0	0.8	-	-	-	0.7	0.6	1.2	0.7	3.7	8.9	4.9	18.0	19.3	38.2	40.7	57.7	63.4	73.7	9.6	2.8	0.29	0.69	6.0	188
Kidney etc.	167	0	0.8	1.6	0.7	-	-	0.6	1.9	0.7	6.7	7.9	14.6	23.1	27.1	21.1	43.9	39.8	48.3	35.1	8.9	2.6	0.43	0.75	6.5	189
Eye	14	0	1.7	-	-	-	-	-	-	-	-	-	-	-	-	2.6	9.4	4.0	3.0	3.5	0.7	0.2	0.01	0.07	0.5	190
Brain, nervous system	112	0	4.2	1.6	4.5	3.4	0.7	1.9	1.9	5.3	5.2	3.0	6.1	5.1	15.5	19.8	15.7	27.8	18.1	10.5	6.0	1.8	0.29	0.47	5.0	191-2
Thyroid	90	0	-	-	0.7	3.4	1.4	2.5	5.6	4.0	6.0	15.8	13.4	6.4	11.6	4.0	7.8	6.0	6.0	3.5	4.8	1.4	0.35	0.41	4.3	193
Other endocrine	8	0	0.8	-	-	-	-	0.6	-	-	-	-	-	-	-	1.3	7.8	-	-	-	0.4	0.1	0.01	0.05	0.3	194
Hodgkin's disease	45	0	-	1.5	2.8	4.1	6.2	1.9	2.0	-	2.0	3.6	1.3	1.3	1.3	3.1	6.0	9.1	3.5	2.4	0.7	0.13	0.15	2.1	201
Non-Hodgkin lymphoma	236	2	-	0.7	0.7	2.0	1.2	3.7	2.0	1.5	15.8	18.2	20.5	21.9	39.5	48.6	89.5	96.7	49.2	12.6	3.7	0.45	0.89	8.2	200,202
Multiple myeloma	72	0	-	-	-	0.7	-	-	-	1.3	1.5	-	6.1	3.8	16.8	9.2	25.1	25.9	21.1	10.5	3.8	1.1	0.15	0.32	2.6	203
Lymphoid leukaemia	63	0	7.5	1.6	2.2	0.7	1.4	0.6	-	0.7	1.5	2.0	2.4	5.1	6.4	7.9	9.4	8.0	27.2	14.0	3.4	1.0	0.16	0.25	3.0	204
Myeloid leukaemia	50	0	-	-	-	-	0.7	1.9	-	0.7	0.7	3.0	2.4	2.6	9.0	10.5	14.1	8.0	12.1	17.6	2.7	0.8	0.10	0.23	1.9	205
Monocytic leukaemia	4	0	-	-	-	-	-	-	-	-	-	-	-	1.3	-	1.3	-	2.0	3.0	-	0.2	0.1	0.01	0.01	0.1	206
Other leukaemia	2	0	-	-	-	-	-	-	-	-	-	1.0	-	-	1.6	-	-	-	-	0.1	0.0	0.00	0.01	0.1	207
Leukaemia unspecified	29	0	-	0.8	0.7	-	-	-	-	-	0.7	1.0	-	1.3	1.3	2.6	4.7	2.0	24.2	31.6	1.5	0.5	0.03	0.07	0.8	208
Other and unspecified	286	0	0.8	-	-	-	1.4	1.2	0.6	1.3	3.7	6.9	12.2	21.8	32.2	35.6	78.4	103.4	120.8	158.0	15.3	4.5	0.41	0.98	8.9	O&U
All sites																										
All sites but 173	6391	10	19.3	5.5	12.7	17.2	23.1	47.6	70.9	122.8	234.6	346.3	498.2	687.6	918.9	1120.3	1415.2	1573.0	1667.7	1674.7	341.4	100.0	15.05	27.74	241.6	ALLb

Rate from 1 case   0.839   0.786   0.746   0.688   0.680   0.618   0.622   0.660   0.745   0.987   1.215   1.283   1.289   1.318   1.567   1.989   3.021   3.511

†Important: see notes on population page

Canada, Newfoundland

The Provincial Cancer Registry was started by the Department of Radiotherapy of the St John's General Hospital in 1954. In 1974, the registry came under the jurisdiction of the Newfoundland Cancer Treatment and Research Foundation (NCTRF), which was given a mandate by a legislative act to deliver a cancer control programme for the people of Newfoundland and Labrador.

The province of Newfoundland and Labrador is located on the east coast of Canada. The island of Newfoundland is surrounded by the Atlantic Ocean. Labrador is bounded by the Atlantic to the east and the province of Quebec to the west and south. The land mass of the province extends between latitudes 47 and 61° N and longitudes 52 and 76° W. The altitude varies from sea level to 1600 m in the interior of Labrador. The total area is 371 634 km^2.

The 1991 census showed a population of 568 475, which represents a growth of less than 1% over a ten-year period. The low population growth results from a large emigration of young people annually and correlates with a high rate of unemployment in the province. Fishing, pulp and paper industry and mining were the traditional occupations of Newfoundlanders and Labradorians. The fishing moratorium of the early 1990s resulted in a major exodus of people from the province and a shift to other industries such as tourism, offshore oil and information technology.

From 1954 to 1979, the Provincial Cancer Registry used many methods of classification including coding to regional site, ICD-8 and MOTNAC. In 1982, the registry was computerized and all records from 1969 were converted to ICD-O-1 and ICD-9. All leukaemia and lymphomas are coded to C42 (ICD-O-2) and also coded using ICD-9.

The NCTRF information network was enhanced during 1996 with the acquisition and implementation of an Oncology Patient Information System (OPIS). This system makes possible more efficient management and improved quality of patient information for the cancer treatment centre and community oncology programmes, cancer registration and screening registries.

In May 1996 all registry data back to 1969 were converted to the OPIS database. The introduction of OPIS allows linkage of cancer registry data with patient care information generated in clinical programmes. The next developmental phase will be the linkage of clinical data with financial information. Linkage of databases will permit evaluation of the various treatment modalities in terms of morbidity, survival rates, quality of cancer care and cost.

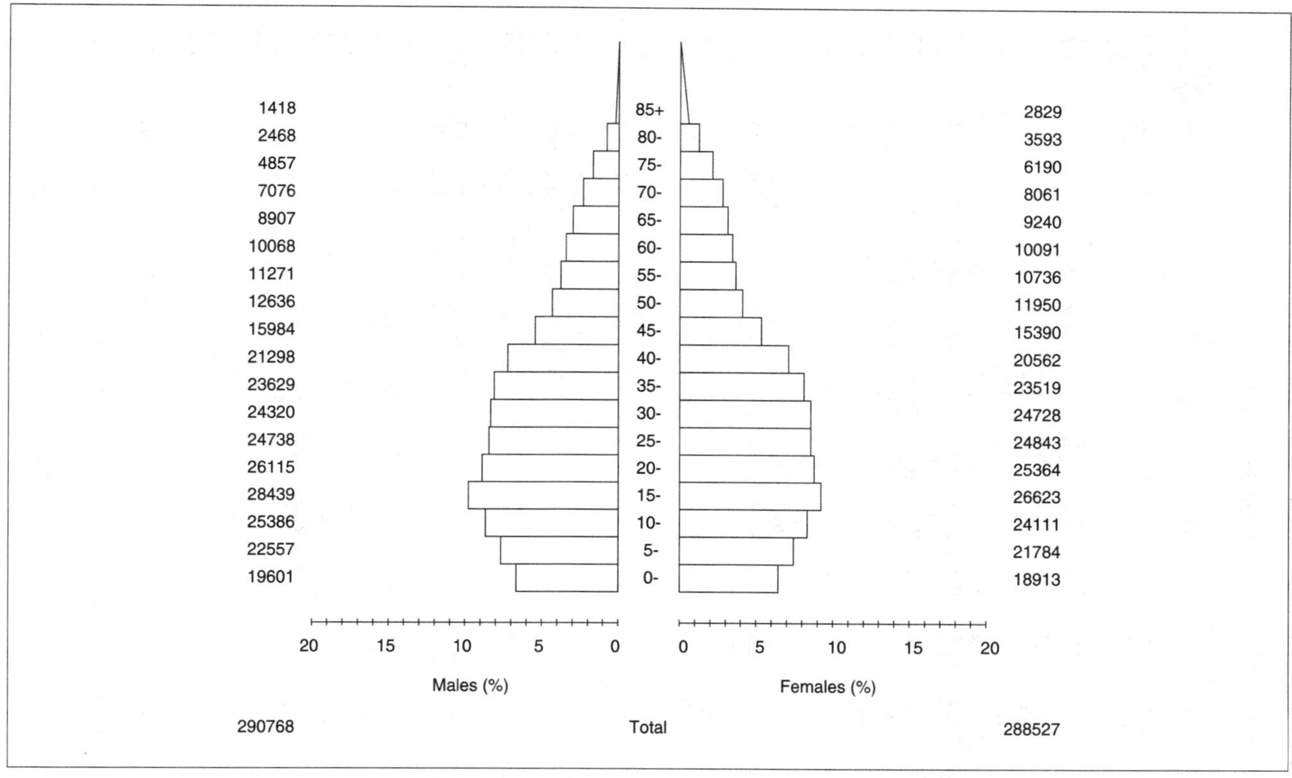

Canada, Newfoundland
Source of population: average annual 1988-92
Census: Statistics Canada June 1991
Estimate: The populations were estimated at 1 July each year, based on revised intercensal estimates for 1988-91 and post-censal estimates for 1992. In 1993 revised estimates dating back to 1971 were implemented by Statistics Canada and population data from 1971 now include estimates of net census undercoverage, plus non-permanent residents defined as persons claiming refugee status, foreign students, work permit holders, or holders of Minister's permits, and non-Canadian-born dependants of such individuals. References: Statistics Canada, Catalogue 91-537, Revised intercensal population and family estimates, July 1, 1971–91, and Catalogue 91-213, Annual demographic statistics 1993 (for 1992 data).

Notes to tables overleaf:
† Kaposi's sarcoma is under-reported in this volume because cases of skin cancer (ICD-9 173) were not provided
† 173 not available
† 188 does not include non-invasive tumours
Screening programmes in the area:
92,000 examinations for cervical cancer have been performed annually in the age-group 18-69 since 1969.

CANADA, NEWFOUNDLAND 1988-1992

ANNUAL INCIDENCE PER 100,000 BY AGE GROUP (YEARS) - MALE

SITE	ALL AGES	AGE UNK	0-	5-	10-	15-	20-	25-	30-	35-	40-	45-	50-	55-	60-	65-	70-	75-	80-	85+	CRUDE RATE	%	CR 64	CR 74	ASR (W)	ICD (9th)
Lip	203	0	-	-	-	-	-	-	4.1	2.5	12.2	17.5	14.2	35.5	43.7	74.1	101.7	86.5	105.3	197.3	14.0	4.5	0.65	1.53	12.7	140
Tongue	23	0	-	-	-	-	0.8	-	-	1.7	0.9	1.3	-	10.6	4.0	9.0	2.8	16.5	-	14.1	1.6	0.5	0.10	0.16	1.4	141
Salivary gland	11	0	-	-	-	-	-	-	-	0.8	-	1.3	3.2	3.5	2.0	-	2.8	4.1	8.1	14.1	0.8	0.2	0.05	0.07	0.7	142
Mouth	30	0	-	-	-	-	0.8	0.8	-	-	0.9	2.5	6.3	8.9	13.9	4.5	11.3	12.4	-	-	2.1	0.7	0.17	0.25	2.0	143-5
Oropharynx	20	0	-	-	-	-	-	-	1.6	-	-	2.5	6.3	3.5	7.9	6.7	5.7	-	8.1	-	1.4	0.4	0.11	0.17	1.4	146
Nasopharynx	14	0	-	-	-	-	-	-	-	-	0.9	1.3	1.6	5.3	6.0	4.5	8.5	-	-	-	1.0	0.3	0.08	0.14	1.0	147
Hypopharynx	15	0	-	-	-	-	-	-	-	-	0.9	1.3	3.2	7.1	4.0	6.7	-	8.2	-	-	1.0	0.3	0.08	0.12	1.0	148
Pharynx unspecified	10	0	-	-	-	-	-	-	-	-	0.9	1.3	4.7	1.8	-	6.7	-	-	-	14.1	0.7	0.2	0.04	0.08	0.7	149
Oesophagus	66	0	-	-	-	-	-	-	-	-	-	3.8	6.3	12.4	15.9	33.7	36.7	20.6	81.0	14.1	4.5	1.5	0.19	0.54	4.1	150
Stomach	301	0	-	-	-	-	0.8	0.8	0.8	4.2	4.7	13.8	17.4	37.3	83.4	89.8	175.2	168.8	243.1	422.9	20.7	6.6	0.82	2.14	18.5	151
Small intestine	11	0	-	-	-	-	-	-	-	-	-	1.3	-	-	6.0	4.5	-	16.5	8.1	-	0.8	0.2	0.04	0.06	0.7	152
Colon	504	0	-	-	-	-	-	1.6	4.1	9.3	16.0	15.0	60.1	79.8	166.9	181.9	234.6	312.9	283.6	211.4	34.7	11.1	1.76	3.85	31.4	153
Rectum	254	0	-	-	-	-	-	-	0.8	4.2	9.4	13.8	14.2	51.5	69.5	101.0	124.4	115.3	178.3	211.4	17.5	5.6	0.82	1.94	15.9	154
Liver	16	0	-	-	-	-	-	-	-	-	-	0.9	1.3	-	1.8	9.9	6.7	5.7	12.4	-	1.1	0.4	0.07	0.13	1.0	155
Gallbladder etc.	18	0	-	-	-	-	-	-	-	-	-	0.9	1.3	1.6	3.5	-	2.2	11.3	16.5	24.3	14.1	1.2	0.4	0.04	0.10	1.0	156
Pancreas	67	0	-	-	-	-	-	-	-	2.5	-	-	5.0	7.9	12.4	15.9	29.2	36.7	8.2	56.7	70.5	4.6	1.5	0.22	0.55	4.3	157
Nose, sinuses etc.	12	0	-	-	-	-	-	0.8	-	-	-	-	1.3	-	1.8	7.9	6.7	5.7	-	-	0.8	0.3	0.06	0.12	0.8	160
Larynx	89	0	-	-	-	-	-	-	-	-	1.7	1.9	2.5	12.7	30.2	37.7	24.7	36.7	41.2	40.5	-	6.1	2.0	0.43	0.74	5.8	161
Bronchus, lung	892	0	-	-	0.8	-	-	-	-	-	2.5	14.1	28.8	98.1	209.4	294.0	415.4	455.0	494.1	348.4	183.3	61.4	19.7	3.24	7.59	57.0	162
Other thoracic organs	3	0	-	-	-	-	-	-	-	-	0.8	-	-	-	-	-	2.2	2.8	-	-	0.2	0.1	0.00	0.03	0.2	163-4
Bone	12	0	-	-	0.8	2.1	-	-	1.6	-	0.9	2.5	1.6	-	-	-	-	16.2	-	-	0.8	0.3	0.05	0.05	0.7	170
Connective tissue	38	0	1.0	1.8	-	-	0.8	2.4	3.3	-	0.9	3.8	4.7	5.3	4.0	15.7	8.5	8.2	16.2	14.1	2.6	0.8	0.14	0.26	2.5	171
Mesothelioma	12	0	-	-	-	-	-	-	-	-	-	1.3	4.7	5.3	2.0	6.7	-	4.1	-	-	0.8	0.3	0.07	0.10	0.8	MES
†Kaposi's sarcoma	0	0	-	-	-	-	-	-	-	-	-	-	-	-	-	-	-	-	-	-	0.0	0.0	0.00	0.00	0.0	KAP
Melanoma of skin	59	0	-	-	-	-	1.4	1.5	1.6	1.6	1.7	4.7	8.8	11.1	10.6	13.9	18.0	8.5	12.4	8.1	28.2	4.1	1.3	0.28	0.42	3.9	172
†Other skin																										
Breast	10	0	-	-	-	-	-	-	-	-	-	-	1.3	-	3.5	-	-	11.3	-	16.2	14.1	0.7	0.2	0.02	0.08	0.6	175
Prostate	711	0	-	-	-	-	-	-	-	-	1.9	2.5	9.5	49.7	139.0	285.2	477.7	687.6	688.8	775.3	48.9	15.7	1.01	4.83	40.6	185
Testis	40	0	1.0	-	-	2.1	2.3	6.5	8.2	5.1	3.8	-	1.6	3.5	-	-	2.8	-	8.1	-	2.8	0.9	0.17	0.18	2.4	186
Penis	11	0	-	-	-	-	-	-	-	-	0.9	1.3	3.2	3.5	4.0	-	-	8.2	8.1	-	0.8	0.2	0.06	0.06	0.7	187.1-.4
Other male genital	2	0	-	-	-	-	0.8	-	-	-	-	1.6	-	-	-	-	-	-	-	-	0.1	0.0	0.01	0.01	0.1	187.5-.9
†Bladder	348	0	-	-	-	-	0.8	1.6	2.5	5.9	2.8	18.8	20.6	40.8	83.4	132.5	149.8	271.8	340.3	267.8	23.9	7.7	0.89	2.30	20.7	188
Kidney etc.	152	0	1.0	-	-	0.7	-	-	-	5.1	6.6	13.8	22.2	31.9	41.7	65.1	73.5	45.3	40.5	28.2	10.5	3.4	0.61	1.31	10.0	189
Eye	6	0	-	-	-	-	-	-	-	1.7	-	-	1.6	-	-	6.7	-	-	-	-	0.4	0.1	0.02	0.05	0.4	190
Brain, nervous system	74	0	5.1	1.8	3.9	-	1.5	1.6	1.6	5.1	0.9	5.0	19.0	14.2	7.9	15.7	22.6	16.5	16.2	-	5.1	1.6	0.34	0.53	5.2	191-2
Thyroid	24	0	-	-	-	0.7	0.8	1.6	0.8	0.8	0.9	3.8	-	-	6.0	15.7	5.7	4.1	-	14.1	1.7	0.5	0.08	0.18	1.6	193
Other endocrine	1	0	-	-	-	-	-	-	-	-	-	-	1.8	-	-	-	-	-	-	-	0.1	0.0	0.01	0.01	0.1	194
Hodgkin's disease	30	0	-	0.9	1.6	0.7	3.8	2.4	5.8	1.7	0.9	1.3	-	5.3	2.0	2.2	-	4.1	8.1	-	2.1	0.7	0.13	0.14	1.8	201
Non-Hodgkin lymphoma	126	0	2.0	1.8	0.8	2.1	3.8	2.4	4.1	4.2	4.7	15.0	12.7	21.3	31.8	42.7	39.6	32.9	24.3	42.3	8.7	2.8	0.53	0.94	8.4	200,202
Multiple myeloma	43	0	-	-	-	-	-	-	-	-	1.9	1.3	3.2	7.1	19.9	13.5	17.0	37.1	24.3	-	3.0	0.9	0.17	0.32	2.7	203
Lymphoid leukaemia	37	0	6.1	3.5	2.4	2.8	0.8	-	-	-	0.9	1.3	-	3.5	11.9	9.0	-	4.1	32.4	-	2.5	0.8	0.17	0.21	2.8	204
Myeloid leukaemia	49	0	1.0	-	-	1.4	1.5	3.2	1.6	2.5	5.6	3.8	4.7	3.5	-	18.0	22.6	4.1	16.2	28.2	3.4	1.1	0.15	0.35	3.1	205
Monocytic leukaemia	1	0	-	-	-	-	-	-	-	-	-	-	-	-	-	2.2	-	-	-	-	0.1	0.0	0.00	0.01	0.1	206
Other leukaemia	2	0	-	-	-	-	-	-	0.8	-	-	-	-	-	-	-	-	4.1	-	-	0.1	0.0	0.00	0.00	0.1	207
Leukaemia unspecified	7	0	-	1.8	-	-	-	-	-	-	-	-	1.6	1.8	-	4.5	2.8	-	-	-	0.5	0.2	0.03	0.06	0.5	208
Other and unspecified	173	0	-	-	-	-	0.8	-	1.6	-	3.8	6.3	19.0	39.0	31.8	65.1	93.3	123.5	72.9	141.0	11.9	3.8	0.51	1.30	10.7	O&U
All sites	4527	0																			311.4	100.0	14.41	34.03	282.0	ALLb
All sites but 173			17.3	11.5	10.2	14.1	21.4	27.5	45.2	64.3	107.0	207.7	400.4	768.3	1187.8	1729.0	2193.3	2602.2	2722.6	2720.6						
Rate from 1 case			1.020	0.887	0.788	0.703	0.766	0.808	0.822	0.846	0.939	1.251	1.583	1.774	1.986	2.245	2.826	4.117	8.103	14.096						

†Important: see notes on population page

CANADA, NEWFOUNDLAND 1988-1992

ANNUAL INCIDENCE PER 100,000 BY AGE GROUP (YEARS) - FEMALE

SITE	ALL AGES	AGE UNK	0-	5-	10-	15-	20-	25-	30-	35-	40-	45-	50-	55-	60-	65-	70-	75-	80-	85+	CRUDE RATE	%	CR 64	CR 74	ASR (W)	ICD (9th)
Lip	12	0	-	-	-	-	-	-	-	0.9	-	-	-	5.6	7.9	6.5	-	3.2	-	-	0.8	0.3	0.07	0.10	**0.8**	140
Tongue	11	0	-	-	-	-	-	-	-	1.7	1.0	-	-	1.9	2.0	2.2	5.0	3.2	5.6	7.1	0.8	0.3	0.03	0.07	**0.6**	141
Salivary gland	6	0	-	-	-	-	-	-	-	-	1.0	1.3	1.7	3.7	2.0	-	-	-	-	-	0.4	0.2	0.05	0.05	**0.4**	142
Mouth	13	0	-	-	-	-	-	-	-	0.9	-	-	1.7	-	4.0	-	7.4	6.5	16.7	7.1	0.9	0.3	0.03	0.07	**0.6**	143-5
Oropharynx	7	0	-	-	-	-	-	-	-	-	1.0	2.6	-	-	2.0	2.2	5.0	-	-	-	0.5	0.2	0.03	0.06	**0.5**	146
Nasopharynx	9	0	-	-	-	-	-	-	0.8	-	-	2.6	1.7	-	2.0	-	5.0	3.2	5.6	-	0.6	0.2	0.04	0.06	**0.5**	147
Hypopharynx	5	0	-	-	-	-	-	-	-	-	-	-	1.7	1.9	-	2.2	-	3.2	-	7.1	0.3	0.1	0.02	0.03	**0.3**	148
Pharynx unspecified	1	0	-	-	-	-	-	-	-	-	-	-	-	-	-	2.2	-	-	-	-	0.1	0.0	0.00	0.01	**0.1**	149
Oesophagus	23	0	-	-	-	-	-	-	-	-	1.0	1.3	1.7	1.9	2.0	4.3	7.4	12.9	44.5	7.1	1.6	0.6	0.04	0.10	**1.0**	150
Stomach	151	0	-	-	-	-	-	0.8	0.8	2.6	2.9	3.9	15.1	13.0	33.7	41.1	74.4	74.3	105.7	113.1	10.5	4.0	0.36	0.94	**7.9**	151
Small intestine	10	0	-	-	-	-	-	-	-	-	-	1.7	3.7	2.0	6.5	5.0	3.2	-	-	-	0.7	0.3	0.04	0.09	**0.6**	152
Colon	503	0	-	-	-	0.8	0.8	0.8	4.0	2.6	19.5	15.6	51.9	89.4	122.9	166.7	235.7	200.3	295.0	226.2	34.9	13.3	1.54	3.55	**28.1**	153
Rectum	175	0	1.1	-	-	0.8	-	0.8	1.6	3.4	6.8	18.2	20.1	31.7	35.7	58.4	62.0	87.2	55.7	63.6	12.1	4.6	0.60	1.20	**10.2**	154
Liver	10	0	-	-	-	-	-	-	-	0.9	-	1.3	-	-	4.0	2.2	7.4	3.2	-	7.1	0.7	0.3	0.03	0.08	**0.6**	155
Gallbladder etc.	42	0	-	-	-	-	-	-	0.8	1.7	-	2.6	8.4	3.7	9.9	15.2	19.8	16.2	27.8	-	2.9	1.1	0.14	0.31	**2.4**	156
Pancreas	54	0	-	0.9	-	-	-	-	-	0.9	1.0	2.6	3.3	3.7	15.9	26.0	22.3	19.4	33.4	28.3	3.7	1.4	0.14	0.38	**3.0**	157
Nose, sinuses etc.	7	0	-	-	-	-	-	-	-	-	-	1.7	-	2.0	4.3	-	-	-	5.6	14.1	0.5	0.2	0.02	0.04	**0.4**	160
Larynx	7	0	-	-	-	-	-	-	-	-	-	1.3	1.7	1.9	5.9	-	-	3.2	-	-	0.5	0.2	0.05	0.05	**0.5**	161
Bronchus, lung	225	0	-	-	-	-	-	-	0.8	1.7	8.8	19.5	28.4	61.5	63.4	97.4	91.8	64.6	44.5	42.4	15.6	5.9	0.92	1.87	**14.1**	162
Other thoracic organs	1	0	-	-	-	-	-	-	-	-	-	-	-	-	-	-	-	3.2	-	-	0.1	0.0	0.00	0.00	**0.0**	163-4
Bone	7	0	-	-	0.8	0.8	-	-	-	-	-	1.3	-	1.9	-	4.3	2.5	-	-	-	0.5	0.2	0.02	0.06	**0.5**	170
Connective tissue	21	0	-	-	-	-	1.6	-	-	1.7	-	2.6	1.7	1.9	5.9	10.8	-	12.9	5.6	-	1.5	0.6	0.08	0.13	**1.3**	171
Mesothelioma	3	0	-	-	-	-	-	-	-	-	-	-	-	-	-	-	2.5	6.5	-	-	0.2	0.1	0.00	0.01	**0.1**	MES
†Kaposi's sarcoma	0	0	-	-	-	-	-	-	-	-	-	-	-	-	-	-	-	-	-	-	0.0	0.0	0.00	0.00	**0.0**	KAP
Melanoma of skin	86	0	-	-	-	-	7.1	8.9	4.9	11.9	5.8	11.7	8.4	7.5	7.9	10.8	12.4	16.2	-	21.2	6.0	2.3	0.37	0.49	**5.2**	172
†Other skin																										
Breast	1044	0	-	-	-	-	-	5.6	23.5	52.7	88.5	137.7	180.7	167.7	204.1	246.7	297.7	368.3	361.8	247.4	72.4	27.6	4.30	7.03	**62.6**	174
Uterus unspecified	15	0	-	-	-	-	-	-	-	-	-	1.3	3.3	7.5	4.0	-	5.0	6.5	11.1	-	1.0	0.4	0.08	0.11	**0.9**	179
Cervix uteri	189	0	-	-	-	-	1.6	13.7	24.3	20.4	22.4	19.5	16.7	35.4	27.7	21.6	17.4	35.5	27.8	14.1	13.1	5.0	0.91	1.10	**11.3**	180
Placenta	0	0	-	-	-	-	-	-	-	-	-	-	-	-	-	-	-	-	-	-	0.0	0.0	0.00	0.00	**0.0**	181
Corpus uteri	206	0	-	-	-	-	0.8	-	3.2	8.5	9.7	22.1	31.8	54.0	57.5	80.1	59.5	54.9	22.3	35.3	14.3	5.4	0.94	1.64	**13.2**	182
Ovary etc.	154	0	-	-	0.8	-	-	2.4	5.7	5.1	11.7	22.1	40.2	20.5	37.7	28.1	52.1	35.5	27.8	28.3	10.7	4.1	0.73	1.13	**9.8**	183
Other female genital	37	0	-	-	-	0.8	-	0.8	0.8	0.9	3.9	2.6	3.3	5.6	4.0	13.0	5.0	3.2	27.8	42.4	2.6	1.0	0.11	0.20	**2.0**	184
†Bladder	94	0	-	-	-	-	-	-	0.8	2.6	2.9	3.9	8.4	7.5	21.8	28.1	54.6	25.8	50.1	84.8	6.5	2.5	0.24	0.65	**5.1**	188
Kidney etc.	105	0	2.1	-	-	-	0.8	2.4	2.4	2.6	4.9	5.2	16.7	16.8	25.8	45.5	34.7	32.3	33.4	7.1	7.3	2.8	0.40	0.80	**6.5**	189
Eye	4	0	-	-	-	-	-	-	0.8	-	-	-	-	3.7	-	2.2	-	-	-	-	0.3	0.1	0.02	0.03	**0.3**	190
Brain, nervous system	45	0	3.2	4.6	2.5	1.5	-	0.8	0.8	1.7	1.0	2.6	8.4	9.3	5.9	6.5	9.9	3.2	11.1	14.1	3.1	1.2	0.21	0.29	**3.2**	191-2
Thyroid	64	0	-	-	0.8	0.8	2.4	1.6	3.2	5.1	8.8	9.1	10.0	11.2	15.9	4.3	9.9	3.2	22.3	-	4.4	1.7	0.34	0.42	**4.1**	193
Other endocrine	3	0	-	-	0.8	0.8	-	0.8	-	-	-	-	-	-	-	-	-	-	-	-	0.2	0.1	0.01	0.01	**0.2**	194
Hodgkin's disease	33	0	-	0.9	0.8	7.5	3.9	1.6	3.2	2.6	-	1.3	-	-	4.0	4.3	2.5	-	-	7.1	2.3	0.9	0.13	0.16	**2.1**	201
Non-Hodgkin lymphoma	93	0	2.1	-	-	0.8	0.8	-	0.8	5.1	3.9	13.0	15.1	22.4	13.9	30.3	27.3	42.0	5.6	7.1	6.4	2.5	0.39	0.68	**5.9**	200,202
Multiple myeloma	39	0	-	-	-	-	-	-	-	0.9	1.0	2.6	3.3	5.6	13.9	15.2	12.4	22.6	16.7	7.1	2.7	1.0	0.14	0.27	**2.3**	203
Lymphoid leukaemia	29	0	10.6	1.8	0.8	-	-	-	-	-	-	2.6	-	1.9	-	8.7	12.4	3.2	11.1	7.1	2.0	0.8	0.09	0.19	**2.4**	204
Myeloid leukaemia	45	0	3.2	1.8	-	0.8	2.4	0.8	2.4	3.4	2.9	1.3	5.0	3.7	7.9	6.5	12.4	12.9	5.6	14.1	3.1	1.2	0.18	0.27	**2.9**	205
Monocytic leukaemia	0	0	-	-	-	-	-	-	-	-	-	-	-	-	-	-	-	-	-	-	0.0	0.0	0.00	0.00	**0.0**	206
Other leukaemia	1	0	-	-	-	-	-	-	-	-	-	-	-	-	-	-	-	-	5.6	-	0.1	0.0	0.00	0.00	**0.0**	207
Leukaemia unspecified	6	0	-	-	-	-	-	-	-	-	-	-	-	-	2.0	2.2	5.0	3.2	5.6	-	0.4	0.2	0.01	0.05	**0.3**	208
Other and unspecified	191	0	3.2	0.9	-	-	0.8	0.8	3.2	1.7	6.8	7.8	10.0	26.1	31.7	77.9	54.6	103.4	116.9	134.3	13.2	5.0	0.47	1.13	**10.3**	O&U
All sites																										
All sites but 173	3786	0	25.4	11.0	7.5	15.0	22.9	42.7	89.0	143.7	216.9	343.1	503.7	633.4	808.6	1084.4	1238.0	1298.8	1408.1	1194.6	262.4	100.0	14.31	25.93	**225.1**	ALLb

Rate from 1 case   1.057 0.918 0.829 0.751 0.788 0.805 0.809 0.850 0.973 1.299 1.674 1.863 1.982 2.164 2.481 3.231 5.566 7.069

†Important: see notes on population page

161

Canada, Northwest Territories

A formal system for collection of cancer incidence and mortality data operates under the direction of the Department of Health, Government of the Northwest Territories (NWT). Data back to 1969 are recorded on a mainframe computer.

All forms of malignancy have been reportable in the NWT since late 1990. However, the very extensive circumpolar geographic area which constitutes this jurisdiction (comprising one third of the land area of Canada) results in an additional reliance on diagnostic service and reporting from a number of contiguous provinces. This often means reduced timeliness and completeness of data reporting. Still, some cancer data have been collected since the 1950s.

The area which the registry covers is the largest in Canada, but it is the most sparsely populated. The NWT comprises the area north of the 60th parallel, lying between the Yukon Territory and the Beaufort Sea to the west and the Hudson Bay, Davis Strait and Greenland to the east. The Arctic Ocean forms the northern border, which reaches as far as the 83rd parallel.

The mid-1990 population of the NWT was about 58 000 persons living or based in some 64 communities, half of which had populations of under 500 residents. There is a population increase of almost 3% annually, and one third of the population is under 15 years of age. Health programmes and services are provided by seven regional health and/or hospital boards, reflecting eight official language groups in four ethnic categories (Dene, Inuit, Metis, and non-Aboriginal). Two thirds of the population are Aboriginal people

Most formal health services and programmes in the NWT are provided through community health centres, staffed by nurses, and visited by itinerant physicians. The patterns of illness observed are those of both first-world and third-world populations. Cancer-enhancing behaviours include smoking rates of about 70%. Cancer screening is comprehensive only for cervical cancer.

Data are supplied to the registry by a variety of sources. Due to the vast area which the registry covers and the wide dispersal of the population, health care delivery occurs primarily through nursing stations. Few centres within the NWT have the facilities to identify most cancers, so that health care facilities in southern Canada play an important role in diagnosing and treating NWT residents with cancer. Therefore the Alberta, Manitoba and Quebec cancer registries register a large majority of the cancer cases occurring among NWT residents who are treated or who die in their jurisdictions. Other Canadian provincial registries register cases to a lesser degree.

Collection of data is voluntary, but new legislation will make reporting mandatory. Follow-up of cases is passive; when new information is received, the files are updated.

The database is utilized for health-care planning and delivery and it will form a basis for future intervention studies.

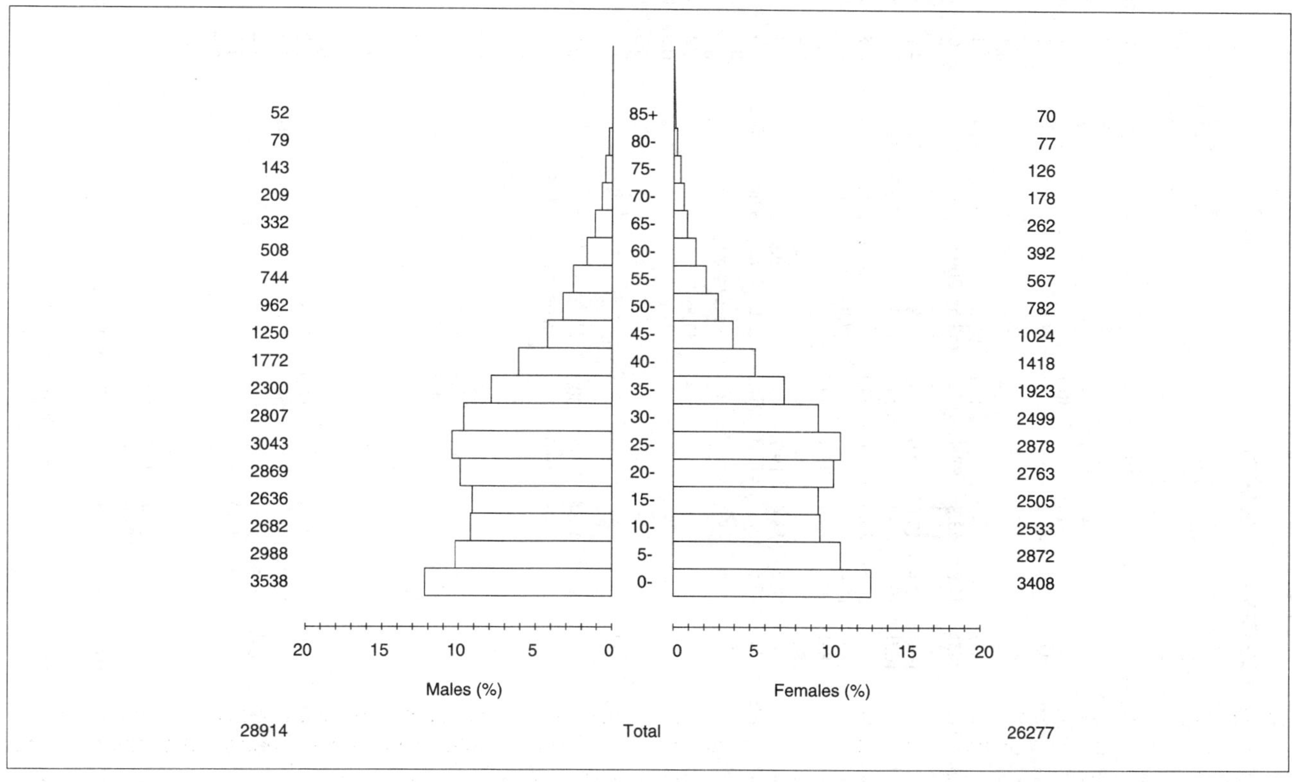

Canada, Northwest Territories

Source of population: average annual 1988-92
Census: Statistics Canada June 1991
Estimate: The populations were estimated at 1 July each year, based on revised intercensal estimates for 1988-91 and post-censal estimates for 1992. In 1993 revised estimates dating back to 1971 were implemented by Statistics Canada and population data from 1971 now include estimates of net census undercoverage, plus non-permanent residents defined as persons claiming refugee status, foreign students, work permit holders, or holders of Minister's permits, and non-Canadian-born dependants of such individuals. References: Statistics Canada, Catalogue 91-537, Revised intercensal population and family estimates, July 1, 1971–91, and Catalogue 91-213, Annual demographic statistics 1993 (for 1992 data).

Notes to tables overleaf:

† Kaposi's sarcoma is under-reported in this volume because cases of skin cancer (ICD-9 173) were not provided

† 173 not available

† 188 does not include non-invasive tumours

Screening programmes in the area:

2,821 cytological examinations a year were performed in women over age 15 for cervical cancer during 1988-92.

CANADA, NORTHWEST TERRITORIES 1983-1992

ANNUAL INCIDENCE PER 100,000 BY AGE GROUP (YEARS) - MALE

SITE	ALL AGES	AGE UNK	0-	5-	10-	15-	20-	25-	30-	35-	40-	45-	50-	55-	60-	65-	70-	75-	80-	85+	CRUDE RATE	%	CR 64	CR 74	ASR (W)	ICD (9th)
Lip	1	0	-	-	-	-	-	-	-	-	-	-	-	-	-	-	47.8	-	-	-	0.3	0.2	0.00	0.24	**1.0**	*140*
Tongue	2	0	-	-	-	-	-	3.3	-	-	-	-	-	-	19.7	-	-	-	-	-	0.7	0.5	0.11	0.11	**1.1**	*141*
Salivary gland	10	0	-	-	-	-	13.9	3.3	-	4.3	-	8.0	10.4	-	39.4	-	-	-	-	-	3.5	2.5	0.40	0.40	**4.2**	*142*
Mouth	1	0	-	-	-	-	-	-	-	-	-	-	-	-	19.7	-	-	-	-	-	0.3	0.2	0.10	0.10	**0.8**	*143-5*
Oropharynx	2	0	-	-	-	-	-	-	-	-	5.6	-	-	-	-	30.1	-	-	-	-	0.7	0.5	0.03	0.18	**1.2**	*146*
Nasopharynx	15	0	-	-	-	-	-	-	-	8.7	5.6	24.0	20.8	40.3	19.7	30.1	47.8	-	126.3	-	5.2	3.7	0.60	0.98	**8.2**	*147*
Hypopharynx	0	0	-	-	-	-	-	-	-	-	-	-	-	-	-	-	-	-	-	-	0.0	0.0	0.00	0.00	**0.0**	*148*
Pharynx unspecified	1	0	-	-	-	-	-	-	-	-	-	-	-	-	-	-	47.8	-	-	-	0.3	0.2	0.00	0.24	**1.0**	*149*
Oesophagus	4	0	-	-	-	-	-	-	-	-	-	8.0	-	-	-	30.1	95.6	-	-	-	1.4	1.0	0.04	0.67	**3.3**	*150*
Stomach	29	0	-	-	-	-	-	-	4.3	11.3	24.0	41.6	53.8	98.4	90.2	143.5	209.6	126.3	-	10.0	7.2	1.17	2.33	**18.8**	*151*
Small intestine	2	0	-	-	-	-	-	-	-	-	-	-	13.4	-	-	47.8	-	-	-	-	0.7	0.5	0.07	0.31	**1.5**	*152*
Colon	12	0	-	-	-	-	-	3.6	-	-	16.0	10.4	13.4	59.0	-	47.8	69.9	-	380.2	4.1	3.0	0.51	0.75	**8.1**	*153*
Rectum	22	0	-	-	-	-	3.3	-	4.3	-	16.0	10.4	-	137.8	120.2	191.3	-	126.3	190.1	7.6	5.5	0.86	2.42	**16.5**	*154*
Liver	8	0	-	-	-	3.5	-	-	-	5.6	-	20.8	13.4	-	30.1	-	69.9	126.3	-	2.8	2.0	0.22	0.37	**4.4**	*155*
Gallbladder etc.	5	0	-	-	-	-	-	-	-	5.6	8.0	10.4	-	-	-	47.8	-	126.3	-	1.7	1.2	0.12	0.36	**2.9**	*156*
Pancreas	10	0	-	-	-	-	-	-	-	-	8.0	10.4	13.4	39.4	30.1	95.6	-	252.5	-	3.5	2.5	0.36	0.98	**7.2**	*157*
Nose, sinuses etc.	1	0	-	-	-	-	-	-	-	-	8.0	-	-	-	-	-	-	-	-	0.3	0.2	0.04	0.04	**0.5**	*160*
Larynx	4	0	-	-	-	-	-	-	-	-	-	10.4	13.4	19.7	-	-	69.9	-	-	1.4	1.0	0.22	0.22	**2.5**	*161*
Bronchus, lung	126	0	-	-	-	-	-	-	-	-	28.2	32.0	145.5	322.5	472.3	661.3	813.0	768.7	378.8	380.2	43.6	31.4	5.00	12.37	**90.3**	*162*
Other thoracic organs	1	0	-	-	-	-	-	-	-	4.3	-	-	-	-	-	-	-	-	-	-	0.3	0.2	0.02	0.02	**0.3**	*163-4*
Bone	2	0	2.8	-	3.7	-	-	-	-	-	-	-	-	-	-	-	-	-	-	-	0.7	0.5	0.03	0.03	**0.7**	*170*
Connective tissue	4	0	2.8	-	-	-	-	-	-	8.7	-	-	-	-	-	-	47.8	-	-	-	1.4	1.0	0.06	0.30	**1.8**	*171*
Mesothelioma	0	0	-	-	-	-	-	-	-	-	-	-	-	-	-	-	-	-	-	-	0.0	0.0	0.00	0.00	**0.0**	*MES*
†Kaposi's sarcoma	0	0	-	-	-	-	-	-	-	-	-	-	-	-	-	-	-	-	-	-	0.0	0.0	0.00	0.00	**0.0**	*KAP*
Melanoma of skin	3	0	-	-	-	-	-	-	-	4.3	-	8.0	-	-	-	-	-	126.3	-	1.0	0.7	0.06	0.06	**1.4**	*172*
†Other skin																									
Breast	2	0	-	-	-	-	-	-	-	-	-	-	13.4	-	30.1	-	-	-	-	0.7	0.5	0.07	0.22	**1.4**	*175*
Prostate	25	0	-	-	-	-	-	3.6	-	-	-	-	40.3	59.0	180.3	286.9	209.6	378.8	-	8.6	6.2	0.51	2.85	**19.3**	*185*
Testis	16	0	-	-	-	3.5	9.9	24.9	4.3	16.9	8.0	-	-	-	-	-	-	-	-	5.5	4.0	0.34	0.34	**4.3**	*186*
Penis	1	0	-	-	-	-	-	-	-	-	-	-	13.4	-	-	-	-	-	-	0.3	0.2	0.07	0.07	**0.5**	*187.1-.4*
Other male genital	0	0	-	-	-	-	-	-	-	-	-	-	-	-	-	-	-	-	-	-	0.0	0.0	0.00	0.00	**0.0**	*187.5-.9*
†Bladder	11	0	-	-	-	-	-	-	-	-	-	10.4	26.9	78.7	30.1	47.8	69.9	126.3	-	3.8	2.7	0.58	0.97	**7.9**	*188*
Kidney etc.	16	0	-	-	-	-	-	-	-	-	-	52.0	26.9	118.1	60.1	47.8	-	-	-	5.5	4.0	0.98	1.52	**11.2**	*189*
Eye	1	0	-	-	-	-	-	-	-	-	10.4	-	-	-	-	-	-	-	-	0.3	0.2	0.05	0.05	**0.5**	*190*
Brain, nervous system	12	0	-	3.3	3.7	-	-	-	10.7	4.3	5.6	16.0	-	13.4	19.7	-	47.8	-	-	4.1	3.0	0.38	0.62	**5.2**	*191-2*
Thyroid	3	0	-	-	-	-	-	-	-	-	-	-	10.4	-	39.4	-	-	-	-	1.0	0.7	0.25	0.25	**2.1**	*193*
Other endocrine	2	0	5.7	-	-	-	-	-	-	-	-	-	-	-	-	-	-	-	-	0.7	0.5	0.03	0.03	**0.7**	*194*
Hodgkin's disease	1	0	-	-	-	-	-	-	3.6	-	-	-	-	-	-	-	-	-	-	0.3	0.2	0.02	0.02	**0.2**	*201*
Non-Hodgkin lymphoma	17	0	-	-	-	-	-	-	7.1	13.0	16.9	8.0	-	40.3	-	60.1	95.6	69.9	-	5.9	4.2	0.43	1.21	**8.7**	*200,202*
Multiple myeloma	4	0	-	-	-	-	-	-	-	-	-	-	10.4	-	19.7	30.1	-	-	190.1	1.4	1.0	0.15	0.30	**3.2**	*203*
Lymphoid leukaemia	4	0	2.8	-	-	-	-	-	-	-	-	16.0	10.4	-	-	-	-	-	-	1.4	1.0	0.15	0.15	**1.8**	*204*
Myeloid leukaemia	5	0	-	-	-	3.8	-	-	3.6	-	-	-	20.8	13.4	-	-	-	-	-	1.7	1.2	0.21	0.21	**2.1**	*205*
Monocytic leukaemia	0	0	-	-	-	-	-	-	-	-	-	-	-	-	-	-	-	-	-	0.0	0.0	0.00	0.00	**0.0**	*206*
Other leukaemia	1	0	-	-	-	3.8	-	-	-	-	-	-	-	-	-	-	-	-	-	0.3	0.2	0.02	0.02	**0.3**	*207*
Leukaemia unspecified	1	0	-	-	-	3.8	-	-	-	-	-	-	-	-	-	-	-	-	-	0.3	0.2	0.02	0.02	**0.3**	*208*
Other and unspecified	14	0	2.8	-	-	-	-	-	-	-	4.3	-	-	20.8	13.4	19.7	60.1	191.3	69.9	-	190.1	4.8	3.5	0.31	1.56	**10.2**	*O&U*
All sites																									
All sites but 173	401	0	17.0	3.3	7.5	11.4	20.9	19.7	57.0	65.2	101.5	207.9	436.5	685.4	1279.3	1472.8	2391.2	1607.3	1893.9	1330.8	138.7	100.0	14.56	33.88	**257.8**	*ALLb*

Rate from 1 case

		0-	5-	10-	15-	20-	25-	30-	35-	40-	45-	50-	55-	60-	65-	70-	75-	80-	85+
		2.826	3.346	3.727	3.793	3.485	3.285	3.562	4.347	5.640	7.996	10.394	13.439	19.681	30.057	47.824	69.881	126.263	190.114

†Important: see notes on population page

CANADA, NORTHWEST TERRITORIES 1983-1992

ANNUAL INCIDENCE PER 100,000 BY AGE GROUP (YEARS) - FEMALE

SITE	ALL AGES	AGE UNK	0-	5-	10-	15-	20-	25-	30-	35-	40-	45-	50-	55-	60-	65-	70-	75-	80-	85+	CRUDE RATE	%	CR 64	CR 74	ASR (W)	ICD (9th)
Lip	0	0	-	-	-	-	-	-	-	-	-	-	-	-	-	-	-	-	-	-	0.0	0.0	0.00	0.00	0.0	140
Tongue	2	0	-	-	-	4.0	-	-	-	-	-	-	-	17.6	-	-	-	-	-	-	0.8	0.5	0.11	0.11	1.1	141
Salivary gland	3	0	-	-	-	-	-	-	5.2	-	-	-	-	17.6	25.5	-	-	-	-	-	1.1	0.8	0.24	0.24	2.0	142
Mouth	0	0	-	-	-	-	-	-	-	-	-	-	-	-	-	-	-	-	-	-	0.0	0.0	0.00	0.00	0.0	143-5
Oropharynx	0	0	-	-	-	-	-	-	-	-	-	-	-	-	-	-	-	-	-	-	0.0	0.0	0.00	0.00	0.0	146
Nasopharynx	9	0	-	-	-	-	-	-	-	15.6	7.1	9.8	12.8	35.2	-	38.1	-	-	-	-	3.4	2.4	0.40	0.59	5.1	147
Hypopharynx	0	0	-	-	-	-	-	-	-	-	-	-	-	-	-	-	-	-	-	-	0.0	0.0	0.00	0.00	0.0	148
Pharynx unspecified	0	0	-	-	-	-	-	-	-	-	-	-	-	-	-	-	-	-	-	-	0.0	0.0	0.00	0.00	0.0	149
Oesophagus	6	0	-	-	-	-	-	-	4.0	-	-	-	-	-	-	76.3	111.8	-	-	141.8	2.3	1.6	0.02	0.96	5.5	150
Stomach	8	0	-	-	-	-	-	-	8.0	-	7.1	9.8	-	17.6	-	-	55.9	-	128.7	141.8	3.0	2.1	0.21	0.49	4.7	151
Small intestine	0	0	-	-	-	-	-	-	-	-	-	-	-	-	-	-	-	-	-	-	0.0	0.0	0.00	0.00	0.0	152
Colon	16	0	-	-	-	-	-	-	-	-	-	9.8	51.1	35.2	25.5	76.3	223.6	-	-	283.7	6.1	4.2	0.61	2.11	13.7	153
Rectum	13	0	-	-	-	-	-	-	-	-	14.1	19.5	25.6	17.6	25.5	-	55.9	158.6	128.7	141.8	4.9	3.4	0.51	0.79	9.1	154
Liver	0	0	-	-	-	-	-	-	-	-	-	-	-	-	-	-	-	-	-	-	0.0	0.0	0.00	0.00	0.0	155
Gallbladder etc.	5	0	-	-	-	-	-	-	-	-	7.1	9.8	-	17.6	-	38.1	55.9	-	-	-	1.9	1.3	0.17	0.64	4.0	156
Pancreas	8	0	-	-	-	-	-	-	4.0	5.2	-	9.8	25.6	35.2	-	-	55.9	-	-	-	3.0	2.1	0.40	0.68	4.9	157
Nose, sinuses etc.	0	0	-	-	-	-	-	-	-	-	-	-	-	-	-	-	-	-	-	-	0.0	0.0	0.00	0.00	0.0	160
Larynx	1	0	-	-	-	-	-	-	-	-	-	-	-	-	55.9	-	-	-	-	-	0.4	0.3	0.00	0.28	1.1	161
Bronchus, lung	80	0	-	-	-	-	-	3.5	-	5.2	14.1	78.1	153.3	229.0	408.2	419.5	279.5	475.8	386.1	283.7	30.4	21.0	4.46	7.95	65.6	162
Other thoracic organs	0	0	-	-	-	-	-	-	-	-	-	-	-	-	-	-	-	-	-	-	0.0	0.0	0.00	0.00	0.0	163-4
Bone	2	0	-	-	-	4.0	-	-	-	5.2	-	-	-	-	-	-	-	-	-	-	0.8	0.5	0.05	0.05	0.7	170
Connective tissue	1	0	-	-	-	-	-	-	4.0	-	-	-	-	-	-	-	-	-	-	-	0.4	0.3	0.02	0.02	0.2	171
Mesothelioma	0	0	-	-	-	-	-	-	-	-	-	-	-	-	-	-	-	-	-	-	0.0	0.0	0.00	0.00	0.0	MES
†Kaposi's sarcoma	0	0	-	-	-	-	-	-	-	-	-	-	-	-	-	-	-	-	-	-	0.0	0.0	0.00	0.00	0.0	KAP
Melanoma of skin	4	0	-	-	-	-	3.6	-	4.0	5.2	-	-	-	-	25.5	-	-	-	-	-	1.5	1.0	0.19	0.19	1.9	172
†Other skin																										
Breast	88	0	-	-	-	-	-	3.5	16.0	26.0	91.7	156.2	127.8	211.3	255.1	228.8	111.8	237.9	643.5	141.8	33.5	23.1	4.44	6.14	58.1	174
Uterus unspecified	2	0	-	-	-	-	-	-	-	5.2	-	-	-	-	-	-	-	79.3	-	-	0.8	0.5	0.03	0.03	1.1	179
Cervix uteri	32	0	-	-	-	-	18.1	13.9	8.0	41.6	35.3	19.5	-	70.4	-	38.1	55.9	-	-	-	12.2	8.4	1.03	1.50	13.9	180
Placenta	2	0	-	-	-	4.0	-	-	-	-	-	-	-	17.6	-	-	-	-	-	-	0.8	0.5	0.11	0.11	1.1	181
Corpus uteri	9	0	-	-	-	-	-	-	-	-	-	19.5	63.9	17.6	25.5	-	-	-	-	-	3.4	2.4	0.63	0.63	6.1	182
Ovary etc.	14	0	-	-	-	-	-	3.5	4.0	10.4	-	29.3	-	52.8	51.0	-	-	79.3	-	141.8	5.3	3.7	0.76	0.76	8.6	183
Other female genital	1	0	-	-	-	-	-	-	-	-	-	-	-	17.6	-	-	-	-	-	-	0.4	0.3	0.09	0.09	0.7	184
†Bladder	3	0	-	-	-	-	-	3.5	4.0	-	-	-	-	-	-	38.1	-	-	-	-	1.1	0.8	0.04	0.23	1.7	188
Kidney etc.	11	0	-	3.5	-	-	-	-	-	5.2	-	19.5	25.6	17.6	51.0	-	55.9	79.3	-	-	4.2	2.9	0.61	0.89	7.8	189
Eye	1	0	2.9	-	-	-	-	-	-	-	-	-	-	-	-	-	-	-	-	-	0.4	0.3	0.01	0.01	0.4	190
Brain, nervous system	7	0	2.9	-	-	-	10.9	-	4.0	-	-	-	-	17.6	-	-	55.9	-	-	-	2.7	1.8	0.18	0.46	3.3	191-2
Thyroid	7	0	-	-	-	4.0	-	3.5	4.0	5.2	14.1	-	-	-	-	-	-	79.3	-	-	2.7	1.8	0.15	0.15	2.8	193
Other endocrine	1	0	2.9	-	-	-	-	-	-	-	-	-	-	-	-	-	-	-	-	-	0.4	0.3	0.01	0.01	0.4	194
Hodgkin's disease	1	0	-	-	-	-	3.6	-	-	-	-	-	-	-	-	-	-	-	-	-	0.4	0.3	0.02	0.02	0.3	201
Non-Hodgkin lymphoma	17	0	-	-	-	-	-	-	8.0	15.6	-	29.3	12.8	35.2	25.5	76.3	-	-	386.1	-	6.5	4.5	0.63	1.01	10.5	200,202
Multiple myeloma	2	0	-	-	-	-	-	-	-	-	-	-	-	-	-	38.1	-	-	128.7	-	0.8	0.5	0.00	0.19	1.8	203
Lymphoid leukaemia	3	0	2.9	3.5	3.9	-	-	-	-	-	-	-	-	-	-	-	-	-	-	-	1.1	0.8	0.05	0.05	1.1	204
Myeloid leukaemia	4	0	5.9	-	-	4.0	-	-	-	-	5.2	-	-	-	-	-	-	-	-	-	1.5	1.0	0.08	0.08	1.4	205
Monocytic leukaemia	2	0	5.9	-	-	-	-	-	-	-	-	-	-	-	-	-	-	-	-	-	0.8	0.5	0.03	0.03	0.7	206
Other leukaemia	0	0	-	-	-	-	-	-	-	-	-	-	-	-	-	-	-	-	-	-	0.0	0.0	0.00	0.00	0.0	207
Leukaemia unspecified	1	0	-	-	-	-	-	-	-	-	-	-	12.8	-	-	-	-	-	-	-	0.4	0.3	0.06	0.06	0.6	208
Other and unspecified	15	0	-	-	-	-	-	-	4.0	-	21.2	9.8	25.6	17.6	-	38.1	167.7	158.6	-	141.8	5.7	3.9	0.39	1.42	10.9	O&U
All sites																										
All sites but 173	381	0	23.5	7.0	3.9	20.0	36.2	31.3	76.0	155.9	211.5	429.5	536.7	898.2	918.4	1106.0	1341.5	1348.1	1801.8	1418.4	144.9	100.0	16.74	28.98	252.5	ALLb

Rate from 1 case   2.933 3.482 3.948 3.992 3.618 3.474 4.001 5.198 7.051 9.762 12.778 17.612 25.510 38.139 55.897 79.302 128.700 141.844

†Important: see notes on population page

Canada, Nova Scotia

The Nova Scotia Cancer Registry dates back to 1964, at which time it was administered jointly by the Department of Health and the Medical Society of Nova Scotia. In 1981, responsibility for its operation was transferred to the newly formed Cancer Treatment and Research Foundation of Nova Scotia, which is in turn supported by the Nova Scotia Department of Health.

The registry covers the whole of the province of Nova Scotia, one of the three Maritime provinces of Canada, which lies to the south of the St Lawrence River, east of the Gulf of Maine and south of the provinces of New Brunswick and Prince Edward Island. Although joined to New Brunswick by a central peninsula to the north, it is separated from Prince Edward Island by the Northumberland Strait; to the south, west and east lies the Atlantic. Most of the province lies less than 200 m above sea level, the highest point being at 529 m in the Cape Breton peninsula. The province lies between longitudes 59 and 67° W and latitudes 43 and 47° N. It covers an area of 55 491 km^2.

At the 1991 census, the total population of Nova Scotia was 918 000, of which 44% were of British origin, 6% French and 5% other European. A further 5% were of other single ethnic origins, while the remaining 40% were of multiple ethnic origin. At that time, the active labour force (447 000) of Nova Scotia was employed in the following broad categories of industry: wholesale and retail trade, 18%; manufacturing, 11%; primary industry (agriculture, fishing, forestry, mining), 7%; construction 7%; transport 4%. The remainder were employed in occupations in the service, government, education or health-care sectors. Of the 1991 population, 54% lived in designated urban areas, 44% lived in rural non-farm residences and 2% on rural farms.

Throughout the registry's history, there has been a legal requirement to register all newly diagnosed cases of cancer. The sources of cancer registration have expanded over the years from completed Nova Scotia Cancer Registry Forms (1964 to present), to include pathology reports (since 1982) and the Nova Scotia Vital Statistics Department. Deaths that occurred between 1969 and 1989 were added through a record linkage contract with Statistics Canada, and include deaths of former Nova Scotia residents who died elsewhere in Canada. Since 1989 death certificate information for all provincial deaths has been added as part of an annual probabilistic record linkage process. A benefit of this record linkage step is a second and independent search for duplicate registrations.

All residents of the province are covered by a provincially-funded comprehensive health insurance scheme. The plan's unique identity number aids considerably in the maintenance of the unduplicated patient index.

The Nova Scotia Cancer Registry is active in the Canadian Council of Cancer Registries, and is a full member of the North American Association of Central Cancer Registries. Affiliation with the cancer registries in other Atlantic provinces (New Brunswick, Prince Edward Island and Newfoundland) has also proved fruitful. Active lines of communication within the region facilitate the rapid notification of registration information to ensure that residents of one province receiving treatment in another are correctly allocated to their home provinces. Reliability trials performed cooperatively with the other Atlantic registries have served to enhance the consistency of the application of coding rules. At the end of each calendar year, a series of edit checks ensures the quality of the data, which are then sent to Statistics Canada to become part of the Canadian Cancer Registry. The province's cancer statistics are published annually and given to users and to the providers of the information

Ron Dewar

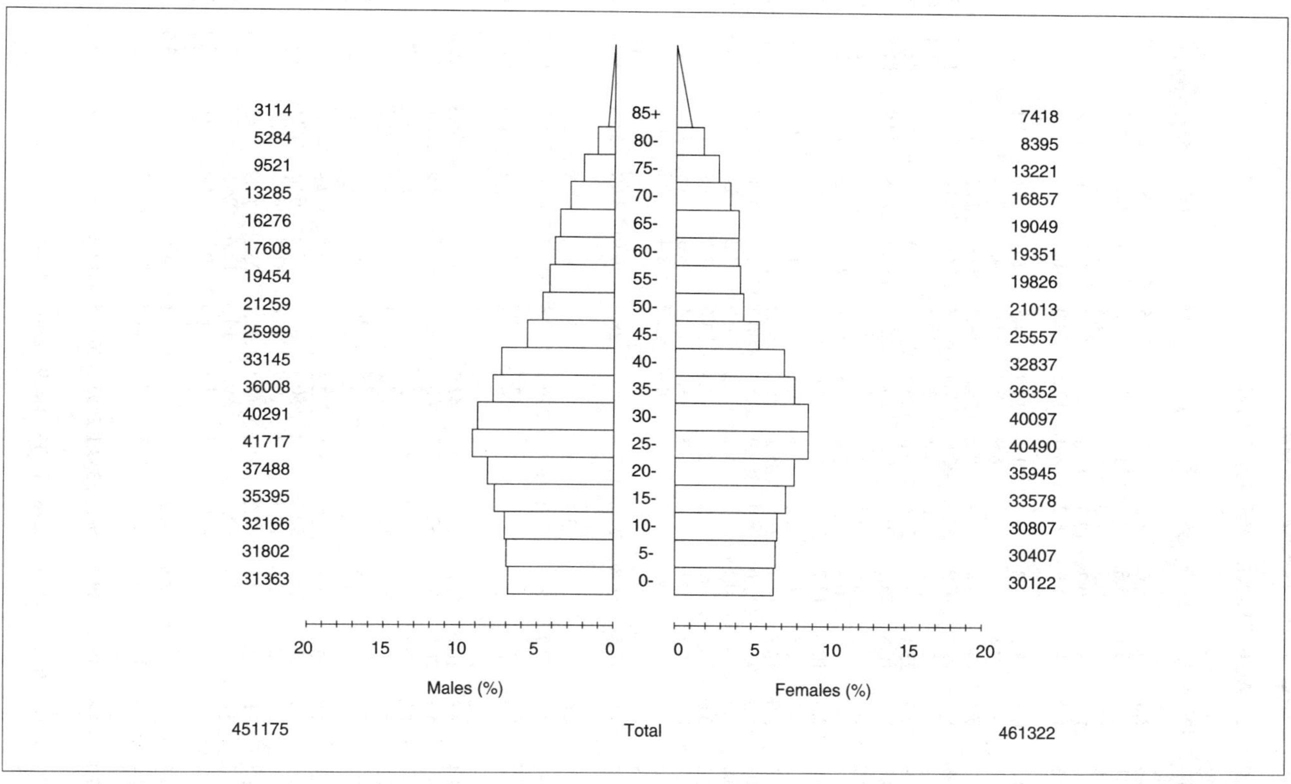

Canada, Nova Scotia
Source of population: average annual 1988-92
Census: Statistics Canada June 1991
Estimate: The populations were estimated at 1 July each year, based on revised intercensal estimates for 1988-91 and post-censal estimates for 1992. In 1993 revised estimates dating back to 1971 were implemented by Statistics Canada and population data from 1971 now include estimates of net census undercoverage, plus non-permanent residents defined as persons claiming refugee status, foreign students, work permit holders, or holders of Minister's permits, and non-Canadian-born dependants of such individuals. References: Statistics Canada, Catalogue 91-537, Revised intercensal population and family estimates, July 1, 1971–91, and Catalogue 91-213, Annual demographic statistics 1993 (for 1992 data).

Notes to tables overleaf:
† Kaposi's sarcoma is under-reported in this volume because cases of skin cancer (ICD-9 173) were not provided
‡ 173 not available

CANADA, NOVA SCOTIA 1988-1992

ANNUAL INCIDENCE PER 100,000 BY AGE GROUP (YEARS) - MALE

SITE	ALL AGES	AGE UNK	0-	5-	10-	15-	20-	25-	30-	35-	40-	45-	50-	55-	60-	65-	70-	75-	80-	85+	CRUDE RATE	%	CR 64	CR 74	ASR (W)	ICD (9th)
Lip	106	0	-	-	-	-	0.5	0.5	0.5	0.6	3.0	3.8	6.6	8.2	9.1	22.1	22.6	35.7	56.8	25.7	4.7	1.0	0.16	0.39	3.5	140
Tongue	58	0	0.6	-	-	-	-	-	-	1.1	-	3.1	5.6	8.2	11.4	12.3	13.5	8.4	11.4	6.4	2.6	0.6	0.15	0.28	2.2	141
Salivary gland	25	0	-	-	-	-	-	0.5	-	0.6	-	-	0.9	1.0	5.7	3.7	4.5	10.5	3.8	25.7	1.1	0.2	0.04	0.08	0.8	142
Mouth	87	0	-	-	-	-	-	1.0	-	-	1.8	6.2	10.3	17.0	16.0	12.0	16.8	18.9	12.8	-	3.9	0.9	0.24	0.38	3.3	143-5
Oropharynx	42	0	-	-	-	-	0.5	-	-	0.6	1.2	1.5	1.9	6.2	8.0	12.3	9.0	6.3	3.8	6.4	1.9	0.4	0.10	0.21	1.6	146
Nasopharynx	4	0	-	-	-	-	-	-	0.5	-	-	-	-	-	2.1	-	-	2.1	-	-	0.2	0.0	0.01	0.01	0.1	147
Hypopharynx	50	0	-	-	-	-	-	-	-	0.6	0.6	3.1	2.8	9.3	11.4	14.7	4.5	6.3	7.6	12.8	2.2	0.5	0.14	0.23	1.9	148
Pharynx unspecified	18	0	-	-	-	-	-	-	-	-	-	0.8	-	4.1	6.8	3.7	3.0	4.2	-	-	0.8	0.2	0.06	0.09	0.7	149
Oesophagus	121	0	0.6	-	-	-	-	-	-	-	1.2	3.1	2.8	11.3	18.2	24.6	43.7	33.6	49.2	38.5	5.4	1.2	0.19	0.53	4.0	150
Stomach	373	0	-	-	-	-	-	1.0	0.5	3.3	5.4	9.2	16.9	30.8	32.9	77.4	93.3	117.6	200.6	205.5	16.5	3.7	0.50	1.35	12.0	151
Small intestine	32	0	-	-	-	-	-	-	-	1.1	0.6	2.3	-	1.0	3.4	7.4	10.5	10.5	15.1	-	1.4	0.3	0.04	0.13	1.0	152
Colon	962	1	-	-	-	-	-	-	2.5	7.8	10.9	23.1	43.3	57.6	136.3	169.6	278.5	310.9	484.4	468.7	42.6	9.5	1.41	3.65	31.1	153
Rectum	489	1	-	-	-	-	0.5	-	0.5	3.9	6.0	10.8	26.3	49.3	77.2	113.0	123.4	123.9	177.9	199.0	21.7	4.8	0.87	2.06	16.7	154
Liver	51	0	0.6	-	-	-	-	-	0.5	0.6	-	-	0.9	3.1	6.8	8.6	22.6	25.2	15.1	-	2.3	0.5	0.06	0.22	1.6	155
Gallbladder etc.	42	0	-	-	-	-	-	-	-	-	-	-	0.9	1.0	3.4	9.8	15.1	21.0	26.5	12.8	1.9	0.4	0.03	0.15	1.2	156
Pancreas	258	0	0.6	-	-	-	-	-	0.5	1.1	3.6	10.0	13.2	21.6	40.9	66.4	63.2	75.6	75.7	77.1	11.4	2.5	0.46	1.11	8.9	157
Nose, sinuses etc.	19	0	-	-	-	-	-	-	-	-	-	1.5	1.9	2.1	1.1	6.1	4.5	4.2	3.8	6.4	0.8	0.2	0.03	0.09	0.7	160
Larynx	185	0	-	-	-	-	-	-	0.5	1.7	3.0	3.8	14.1	21.6	35.2	45.5	54.2	39.9	34.1	19.3	8.2	1.8	0.40	0.90	6.6	161
Bronchus, lung	2218	1	0.6	-	-	-	-	0.5	3.0	3.3	16.3	47.7	111.0	196.4	351.0	538.2	630.7	745.7	738.0	571.5	98.3	21.9	3.65	9.50	74.6	162
Other thoracic organs	20	0	-	-	-	-	1.1	1.0	1.5	0.6	1.2	-	0.9	-	1.1	1.2	6.0	4.2	3.8	-	0.9	0.2	0.04	0.07	0.7	163-4
Bone	25	0	-	0.6	0.6	0.6	1.6	1.0	1.0	2.2	0.6	-	-	2.3	2.5	3.0	2.1	3.8	12.8	-	1.1	0.2	0.05	0.08	0.9	170
Connective tissue	64	0	1.9	-	1.2	0.6	1.6	1.0	1.0	1.7	1.8	0.8	2.8	7.2	2.3	11.1	15.1	6.3	26.5	19.3	2.8	0.6	0.12	0.25	2.4	171
Mesothelioma	33	0	-	-	-	-	-	-	-	-	0.6	-	2.3	4.1	3.4	8.6	12.0	8.4	7.6	6.4	1.5	0.3	0.05	0.16	1.1	MES
†Kaposi's sarcoma	0	0	-	-	-	-	-	-	-	-	-	-	-	-	-	-	-	-	-	-	0.0	0.0	0.00	0.00	0.0	KAP
Melanoma of skin	258	0	-	-	1.2	1.1	1.6	3.8	6.0	9.4	14.5	16.9	19.8	23.6	37.5	41.8	28.6	39.9	37.8	57.8	11.4	2.5	0.68	1.03	9.6	172
†Other skin																										
Breast	11	0	-	-	-	-	-	-	-	-	0.6	-	3.1	1.1	-	3.0	4.2	3.8	6.4	-	0.5	0.1	0.02	0.04	0.4	175
Prostate	1971	1	-	-	-	-	1.1	-	-	-	0.6	3.1	26.3	81.2	213.5	390.7	639.8	953.7	1048.4	1245.7	87.4	19.4	1.63	6.79	59.0	185
Testis	110	0	0.6	-	-	2.8	6.9	9.1	12.4	10.0	9.1	0.8	1.9	2.1	1.1	4.9	3.0	2.1	-	6.4	4.9	1.1	0.28	0.32	4.0	186
Penis	27	0	-	-	-	-	0.5	-	0.6	1.2	0.8	-	-	-	5.7	6.1	7.5	6.3	11.4	3.8	1.2	0.3	0.04	0.11	0.9	187.1-.4
Other male genital	2	0	-	-	-	-	-	-	-	-	-	0.9	-	-	-	-	-	-	3.8	-	0.1	0.0	0.00	0.00	0.1	187.5-.9
Bladder	667	0	-	-	-	0.6	-	1.0	-	4.4	10.3	10.0	28.2	44.2	90.9	147.5	146.0	245.8	291.4	385.3	29.6	6.6	0.95	2.42	21.7	188
Kidney etc.	384	0	3.2	0.6	0.6	0.6	-	-	2.0	6.7	15.7	20.8	26.3	32.9	44.3	66.4	85.8	94.5	124.9	122.0	17.0	3.8	0.77	1.53	13.6	189
Eye	26	1	1.3	0.6	-	-	-	-	-	-	1.2	0.8	2.8	1.0	4.5	2.5	3.0	4.2	7.6	19.3	1.2	0.3	0.06	0.09	1.0	190
Brain, nervous system	159	0	3.2	1.9	1.2	1.7	2.1	4.3	5.0	2.2	6.6	6.9	13.2	13.4	18.2	17.2	27.1	25.2	30.3	25.7	7.0	1.6	0.40	0.62	6.1	191-2
Thyroid	31	0	-	-	-	0.6	0.5	1.0	-	1.1	0.6	5.4	3.8	3.1	1.1	7.4	3.0	2.1	-	-	1.4	0.3	0.09	0.14	1.3	193
Other endocrine	7	0	1.3	-	-	-	1.1	0.5	-	-	-	-	1.9	-	-	-	-	-	-	-	0.3	0.1	0.02	0.02	0.4	194
Hodgkin's disease	72	0	-	1.3	1.2	1.7	6.9	3.8	3.5	3.9	4.8	3.8	5.6	2.1	1.1	2.5	4.5	2.1	7.6	-	3.2	0.7	0.20	0.23	2.8	201
Non-Hodgkin lymphoma	338	0	-	1.9	1.2	2.3	0.5	2.9	5.0	10.6	9.7	20.0	22.6	30.8	52.2	50.4	63.2	67.2	64.3	122.0	15.0	3.3	0.80	1.37	12.3	200,202
Multiple myeloma	94	0	-	-	-	-	-	-	-	-	2.4	2.3	2.8	10.3	11.4	19.7	25.6	31.5	41.6	32.1	4.2	0.9	0.15	0.37	3.1	203
Lymphoid leukaemia	97	0	6.4	1.9	1.2	1.1	1.1	-	-	1.7	0.6	3.1	2.8	7.2	10.2	11.1	21.1	23.1	18.9	77.1	4.3	1.0	0.19	0.35	3.9	204
Myeloid leukaemia	65	0	-	-	-	0.6	0.5	1.4	-	0.6	3.0	3.8	4.7	7.2	5.7	9.8	10.5	12.6	26.5	25.7	2.9	0.6	0.14	0.24	2.3	205
Monocytic leukaemia	11	0	-	-	-	-	-	0.5	-	-	-	-	-	-	3.4	1.2	1.5	6.3	3.8	6.4	-	0.5	0.1	0.00	0.03	0.4	206
Other leukaemia	2	0	-	-	-	-	-	-	-	-	-	-	-	-	1.2	1.5	-	-	-	-	0.1	0.0	0.00	0.01	0.1	207
Leukaemia unspecified	67	1	0.6	1.3	-	-	-	-	1.5	0.6	1.2	2.3	2.8	4.1	4.5	7.4	24.1	31.5	3.8	32.1	-	3.0	0.7	0.10	0.26	2.3	208
Other and unspecified	453	0	1.3	-	-	-	-	-	1.0	2.2	5.4	15.4	28.2	29.8	47.7	90.9	114.4	172.3	189.2	211.9	20.1	4.5	0.66	1.68	14.9	O&U
All sites	10134	6																								
All sites but 173			23.0	10.1	8.7	14.1	27.7	35.5	49.6	85.0	144.8	249.2	458.1	754.6	1339.1	2053.3	2658.5	3344.2	3879.3	4109.4	449.2	100.0	16.01	39.58	337.6	ALLb
Rate from 1 case			0.638	0.629	0.622	0.565	0.534	0.479	0.496	0.555	0.603	0.769	0.941	1.028	1.136	1.229	1.505	2.101	3.785	6.421						

†Important: see notes on population page

CANADA, NOVA SCOTIA 1988-1992

ANNUAL INCIDENCE PER 100,000 BY AGE GROUP (YEARS) - FEMALE

SITE	ALL AGES	AGE UNK	0-	5-	10-	15-	20-	25-	30-	35-	40-	45-	50-	55-	60-	65-	70-	75-	80-	85+	CRUDE RATE	%	CR 64	CR 74	ASR (W)	ICD (9th)
Lip	8	0	-	-	-	-	-	-	-	-	-	0.8	1.0	-	2.1	-	1.2	-	4.8	2.7	0.3	0.1	0.02	0.02	0.2	140
Tongue	23	0	-	-	-	-	-	-	-	-	0.6	0.8	1.0	3.0	1.0	1.0	4.7	9.1	2.4	10.8	1.0	0.3	0.03	0.06	0.6	141
Salivary gland	14	0	-	-	-	-	-	1.0	-	0.6	-	-	-	3.0	-	-	3.6	3.0	2.4	5.4	0.6	0.2	0.02	0.04	0.4	142
Mouth	37	0	-	-	-	0.6	-	-	0.5	-	0.6	2.3	1.9	2.0	8.3	2.1	4.7	6.1	14.3	8.1	1.6	0.4	0.08	0.12	1.1	143-5
Oropharynx	15	0	-	-	-	-	-	-	-	-	0.6	-	1.0	4.0	1.0	6.3	1.2	1.5	-	-	0.7	0.2	0.03	0.07	0.5	146
Nasopharynx	4	0	-	-	-	0.6	-	-	-	-	-	-	-	-	-	3.1	-	-	-	-	0.2	0.0	0.00	0.02	0.1	147
Hypopharynx	9	0	-	-	-	-	-	-	-	-	-	1.6	1.0	-	1.0	-	3.6	1.5	-	2.7	0.4	0.1	0.02	0.04	0.3	148
Pharynx unspecified	11	0	0.7	-	-	-	-	-	-	0.6	-	-	1.0	2.0	1.0	2.1	-	-	-	8.1	0.5	0.1	0.03	0.04	0.4	149
Oesophagus	56	0	-	-	-	-	-	-	0.5	-	-	-	-	3.0	5.2	7.3	13.1	12.1	14.3	40.4	2.4	0.6	0.04	0.15	1.2	150
Stomach	218	0	-	-	-	-	-	1.5	1.0	4.4	3.0	1.6	7.6	10.1	16.5	22.0	38.0	56.0	57.2	134.8	9.5	2.4	0.23	0.53	5.1	151
Small intestine	31	0	-	-	-	-	-	1.0	-	-	1.8	1.6	2.9	2.0	5.2	3.1	3.6	4.5	7.1	5.4	1.3	0.3	0.07	0.11	1.0	152
Colon	1028	1	-	-	0.6	0.6	0.6	1.0	3.0	5.5	14.6	15.7	38.1	52.5	101.3	138.6	196.9	261.7	357.3	407.1	44.6	11.3	1.17	2.85	25.2	153
Rectum	372	0	-	-	-	-	-	1.5	1.0	2.2	6.7	8.6	7.6	29.3	51.7	47.2	79.5	87.7	102.4	110.5	16.1	4.1	0.54	1.18	9.8	154
Liver	42	0	0.7	-	-	-	-	0.5	-	-	0.6	0.8	-	3.0	3.1	9.4	5.9	1.5	26.2	16.2	1.8	0.5	0.04	0.12	1.1	155
Gallbladder etc.	72	0	-	-	-	-	-	-	-	-	-	0.8	2.9	3.0	8.3	10.5	14.2	15.1	19.1	45.8	3.1	0.8	0.07	0.20	1.7	156
Pancreas	246	1	0.7	-	-	-	-	-	-	-	0.6	3.9	4.8	9.1	30.0	27.3	48.6	65.0	81.0	137.5	10.7	2.7	0.25	0.63	5.7	157
Nose, sinuses etc.	15	0	-	-	-	-	1.1	-	-	-	-	0.8	1.0	1.0	-	3.1	2.4	7.6	-	-	0.7	0.2	0.02	0.05	0.4	160
Larynx	30	0	-	-	-	-	-	-	-	0.6	1.2	0.8	1.9	2.0	7.2	2.1	2.4	13.6	4.8	-	1.3	0.3	0.07	0.09	0.9	161
Bronchus, lung	1049	2	0.7	-	-	-	-	-	2.5	2.8	17.7	37.6	65.7	129.1	170.5	199.5	202.9	213.3	126.3	113.2	45.5	11.5	2.14	4.15	32.4	162
Other thoracic organs	5	0	0.7	-	-	-	-	-	0.5	-	-	-	-	-	1.0	2.4	-	-	-	-	0.2	0.1	0.01	0.02	0.2	163-4
Bone	25	0	-	0.7	1.3	0.6	1.1	-	1.0	0.6	1.2	0.8	1.0	3.0	4.1	1.0	1.2	-	2.4	5.4	1.1	0.3	0.08	0.09	1.0	170
Connective tissue	78	0	2.0	-	-	2.4	0.6	2.0	2.0	1.1	3.7	1.6	4.8	6.1	6.2	6.3	11.9	7.6	19.1	16.2	3.4	0.9	0.16	0.25	2.6	171
Mesothelioma	5	0	-	-	-	-	-	-	-	-	0.6	-	-	-	1.0	2.1	1.2	-	-	-	0.2	0.1	0.01	0.02	0.2	MES
†Kaposi's sarcoma	0	0	-	-	-	-	-	-	-	-	-	-	-	-	-	-	-	-	-	-	0.0	0.0	0.00	0.00	0.0	KAP
Melanoma of skin	280	0	-	-	-	1.2	5.0	4.9	11.0	19.3	17.7	15.7	24.7	15.1	21.7	21.0	28.5	24.2	38.1	40.4	12.1	3.1	0.68	0.93	9.3	172
†Other skin																										
Breast	2513	0	-	-	-	-	0.6	5.4	19.0	44.0	101.7	151.0	204.6	221.9	302.8	355.9	403.4	406.9	452.6	423.3	108.9	27.5	5.26	9.05	77.8	174
Uterus unspecified	10	0	-	-	-	-	-	-	-	-	0.6	0.8	1.0	2.0	1.0	-	1.2	1.5	-	5.4	0.4	0.1	0.03	0.03	0.3	179
Cervix uteri	322	0	-	-	-	-	3.3	9.9	20.9	22.0	18.9	18.0	17.1	18.2	27.9	27.3	36.8	27.2	28.6	27.0	14.0	3.5	0.78	1.10	10.7	180
Placenta	0	0	-	-	-	-	-	-	-	-	-	-	-	-	-	-	-	-	-	-	0.0	0.0	0.00	0.00	0.0	181
Corpus uteri	428	0	-	-	-	-	-	1.0	1.5	5.5	13.4	14.1	40.9	47.4	59.9	88.2	72.4	54.5	54.8	56.6	18.6	4.7	0.92	1.72	13.7	182
Ovary etc.	329	0	-	-	0.6	1.8	1.1	1.0	6.0	5.0	5.5	17.2	24.7	28.2	47.5	44.1	47.5	48.4	64.3	75.5	14.3	3.6	0.69	1.15	10.1	183
Other female genital	91	0	-	-	-	-	-	-	1.5	3.9	1.8	1.6	3.8	6.1	9.3	15.7	15.4	18.2	16.7	27.0	3.9	1.0	0.14	0.30	2.5	184
Bladder	230	0	-	-	-	1.2	0.6	0.5	1.0	3.3	3.0	9.4	13.3	14.1	22.7	30.4	35.6	60.5	57.2	75.5	10.0	2.5	0.35	0.68	6.2	188
Kidney etc.	236	0	1.3	1.3	-	-	0.6	-	2.5	3.9	3.0	5.5	10.5	19.2	28.9	38.8	34.4	56.0	61.9	51.2	10.2	2.6	0.39	0.75	6.7	189
Eye	24	0	0.7	-	-	-	-	-	-	-	0.6	0.8	1.9	4.0	2.1	6.3	4.7	1.5	4.8	-	1.0	0.3	0.05	0.11	0.8	190
Brain, nervous system	115	0	2.0	3.3	0.6	2.4	-	2.5	4.0	1.7	3.0	2.3	2.9	12.1	8.3	16.8	15.4	27.2	14.3	5.4	5.0	1.3	0.23	0.39	3.8	191-2
Thyroid	112	0	-	-	1.3	1.8	3.3	3.5	8.5	6.6	8.5	5.5	7.6	6.1	8.3	9.4	11.9	-	4.8	2.7	4.9	1.2	0.30	0.41	4.1	193
Other endocrine	4	0	-	0.7	-	-	-	0.5	-	-	-	-	-	-	-	-	1.2	-	2.4	-	0.2	0.0	0.01	0.01	0.1	194
Hodgkin's disease	61	0	-	0.7	0.6	4.8	4.5	5.9	2.0	2.8	1.2	3.1	1.0	-	2.1	4.2	2.4	4.5	2.4	8.1	2.6	0.7	0.14	0.18	2.3	201
Non-Hodgkin lymphoma	296	0	2.7	0.7	1.9	0.6	1.7	2.0	3.0	3.9	4.9	15.7	14.3	23.2	33.1	31.5	55.8	65.0	69.1	53.9	12.8	3.2	0.54	0.97	8.8	200,202
Multiple myeloma	93	0	-	-	-	-	-	-	-	-	-	4.7	3.8	11.1	12.4	11.5	21.4	22.7	26.2	13.5	4.0	1.0	0.16	0.32	2.6	203
Lymphoid leukaemia	67	0	6.6	3.9	1.3	1.2	-	0.5	-	1.1	-	1.6	1.0	2.0	6.2	6.3	10.7	13.6	11.9	10.8	2.9	0.7	0.13	0.21	2.6	204
Myeloid leukaemia	66	0	-	-	-	1.2	0.6	2.0	1.5	2.8	1.8	3.1	2.9	3.0	1.0	11.5	10.7	12.1	7.1	16.2	2.9	0.7	0.10	0.21	2.0	205
Monocytic leukaemia	9	0	-	-	-	-	-	-	-	-	-	-	2.0	1.0	2.1	3.6	1.5	-	-	-	0.4	0.1	0.02	0.04	0.3	206
Other leukaemia	1	0	-	-	-	-	-	-	-	-	-	-	-	1.0	-	-	-	-	-	-	0.0	0.0	0.01	0.01	0.0	207
Leukaemia unspecified	45	0	0.7	-	-	-	0.6	-	-	0.6	-	1.6	-	2.0	2.1	5.2	9.5	7.6	19.1	27.0	2.0	0.5	0.04	0.11	1.1	208
Other and unspecified	409	0	1.3	-	-	-	0.6	-	3.0	3.9	2.4	14.1	20.0	25.2	31.0	53.5	70.0	104.4	123.9	172.5	17.7	4.5	0.51	1.13	10.4	O&U
All sites																										
All sites but 173	9134	4	20.6	11.2	8.4	20.8	25.6	48.4	97.3	148.0	241.8	365.4	540.6	730.3	1055.2	1275.7	1535.2	1724.5	1901.0	2162.2	396.0	100.0	16.58	30.64	268.4	ALLb

	0-	5-	10-	15-	20-	25-	30-	35-	40-	45-	50-	55-	60-	65-	70-	75-	80-	85+
Rate from 1 case	0.664	0.658	0.649	0.596	0.556	0.494	0.499	0.550	0.609	0.783	0.952	1.009	1.034	1.050	1.186	1.513	2.382	2.696

†Important: see notes on population page

Canada, Ontario

The Ontario Cancer Registry is the largest patient-specific population-based cancer incidence registry in Canada. Operated by the Ontario Cancer Treatment and Research Foundation (OCTRF) since 1964, it covers the entire province of Ontario, registering all newly diagnosed cases of invasive neoplasia, except non-melanoma skin cancer. While cancer is not a legally reportable disease in Ontario, the Cancer Act provides a legal mandate for this undertaking, ensuring that the OCTRF provides for "the adequate reporting of cancer cases and the recording and compilation of data". In addition, the Cancer Act provides legal protection for physicians, dentists and health care agencies who report information on cases of cancer to the OCTRF.

Ontario, one of ten provinces of Canada, covers an area of 1 068 578 km^2 and lies between Quebec to the east and Manitoba to the west, located between latitudes 42 to 56° N. The altitude varies from 75 to 693 m above sea level. The population in 1991, according to the census of Canada, was 4 953 075 males and 5 131 805 females. Approximately 82% of the population live in urban areas and 74% were born in Canada. Of the people reporting single ethnic origins in the 1991 census, 37% are of British extraction and 8% of French descent. Approximately 70 000 North American Indians live in Ontario. The primary occupations for Ontario workers are: clerical (19%); management and administration (14%); service (12%); and sales (9%).

The process of cancer registration in Ontario is passive, relying almost completely on records collected for other purposes. Since 1977, the registry has relied on four major data sources: hospital discharge summaries which include a diagnosis of cancer; pathology reports with any mention of cancer; records of patients referred to the OCTRF's eight Regional Cancer Centres or the Princess Margaret Hospital; and death certificates with cancer as the underlying cause of death. All records except pathology reports are coded at the source and provided to the registry in machine-readable form. Paper copies of pathology reports are sent to the registry by all hospital and private pathology laboratories and are coded and key-entered by the registry staff into a computerized database. Since cancer is increasingly being diagnosed and managed on an outpatient basis, the registry has recently begun to receive hospital day surgery reports from all public hospitals in Ontario. Currently, over 400 000 records are received each year.

Reports pertaining to the same patient are identified through computerized probabilistic record linkage, in which identifying variables are compared across all records. The reported information is summarized on a case record, including details on such variables as primary site, morphology, earliest date of diagnosis, hospital of diagnosis, age at diagnosis and area of residence at diagnosis. The case resolution rules are designed to resolve all reports, including those with conflicting information. The net effect is to generate a small increase in the number of cancers resolved to non-specific sites (e.g., ICD-9 code 199), as well as to under-report multiple primaries. Another computer program (called COMPOSITE) summarizes important identifying and demographic variables from the linked source records and captures these values on the Patient Header record.

The primary site of cancer is coded according to ICD-9. Tumour morphology is coded according to ICD-O-1. ICD-O-2 was introduced in 1993. Under-registration resulting from cancer patients never coming into contact with the usual reporting sources appears to be very low. Where incompleteness exists, it is more likely to represent some defect in the reporting procedures. This is why the registry relies on multiple source reporting. Several statistical studies of the completeness of registration have been undertaken, following the technique of capture–recapture statistical estimation. These studies have estimated a completeness in excess of 95%, with highest rates for deep-seated organs and lowest rates (but still in excess of 90%) for melanomas.

Over the 1980s, the proportions of registered cases with microscopic verification were 84.4% for women and 82.3% for men. While these compare favourably with the overall Canadian rate of 85%, they are somewhat below a rate of approximately 95% reported by established active registries in North America. It is recognized that the registry does not receive all pathology reports for registered cases. Further, in a recent follow-up study of cases missing such reports (hospital-only cases), it was estimated that approximately 20% of such cases did not have invasive neoplasia.

The registry is used by a number of investigators as a source of subjects for case–control studies of cancer etiology and as the end-point for cohort studies involving occupational and environmental exposure. Increasingly, the registry is also used for health services research and supports cancer control planning efforts at provincial and regional levels. Three new monographs describing temporal trends, geographic patterns and cancer survival in Ontario have been published recently.

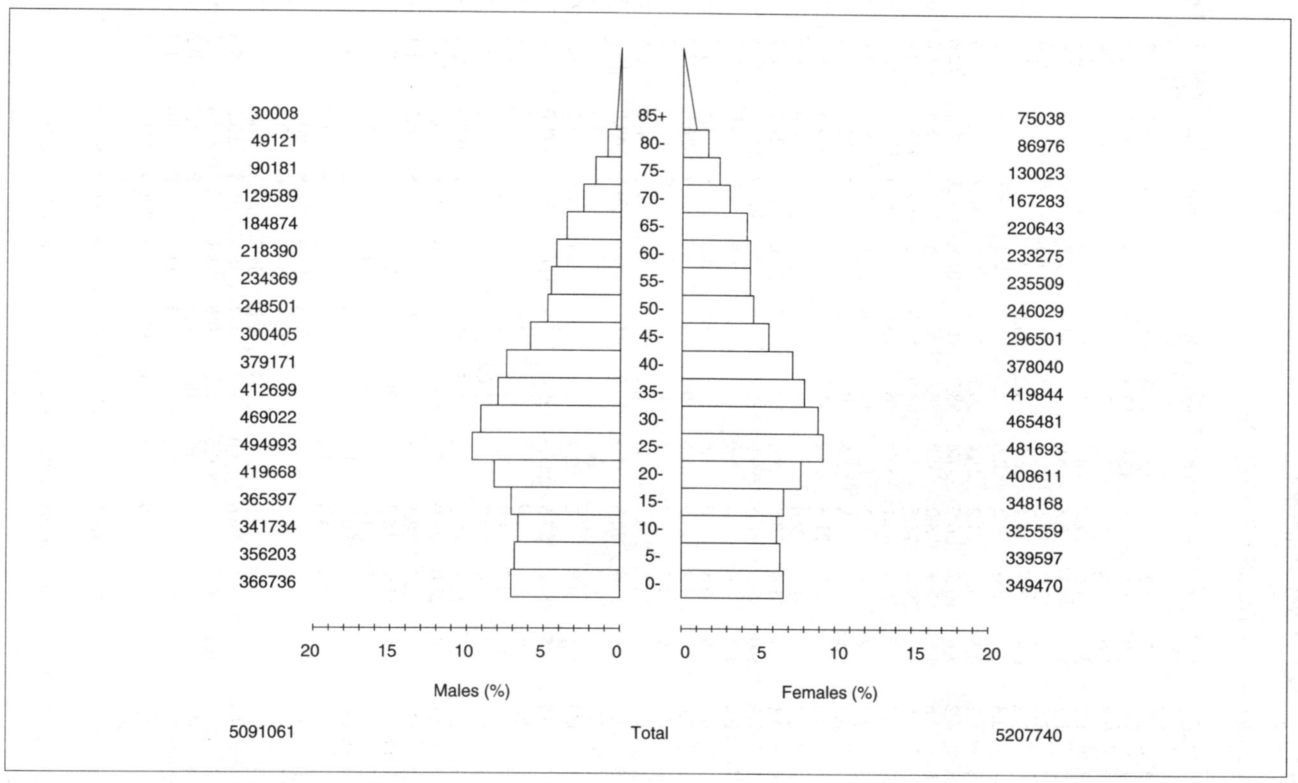

Canada, Ontario
Source of population: average annual 1988-92
Census: Statistics Canada June 1991
Estimate: The populations were estimated at 1 July each year, based on revised intercensal estimates for 1988-91 and postcensal estimates for 1992. In 1993 revised estimates dating back to 1971 were implemented by Statistics Canada and population data from 1971 now include estimates of net census undercoverage, plus non-permanent residents defined as persons claiming refugee status, foreign students, work permit holders, or holders of Minister's permits, and non-Canadian-born dependants of such individuals. References: Statistics Canada, Catalogue 91-537, Revised intercensal population and family estimates, July 1, 1971–91, and Catalogue 91-213, Annual demographic statistics 1993 (for 1992 data).
Notes to tables overleaf:
† Kaposi's sarcoma is under-reported in this volume because cases of skin cancer (ICD-9 173) were not provided
† 173 not available
† 188 does not include non-invasive tumours

Screening programmes in the area:
Opportunistic screening for breast cancer grew rapidly in the 1980s, and by 1992 there were approximately 0.5 million mammograms taken, largely for screening purposes. In 1990, the OCTRF implemented an organized screening programme for breast cancer, targeted at women 50-69 years of age. Growth has also been rapid in this programme, although it currently accounts only for the minority of women screened for breast cancer. Cervical cancer screening began in the 1960s. This programme is mostly opportunistic, focusing on women in their reproductive years. By 1992 there were approximately 1.7 million smears taken annually.

CANADA, ONTARIO 1988-1992

ANNUAL INCIDENCE PER 100,000 BY AGE GROUP (YEARS) - MALE

SITE	ALL AGES	AGE UNK	0-	5-	10-	15-	20-	25-	30-	35-	40-	45-	50-	55-	60-	65-	70-	75-	80-	85+	CRUDE RATE	%	CR 64	CR 74	ASR (W)	ICD (9th)
Lip	991	2	-	-	-	0.1	0.0	0.4	0.5	1.0	2.0	3.7	5.2	7.8	12.7	15.6	22.7	29.1	33.0	36.7	3.9	1.0	0.17	0.36	3.1	140
Tongue	732	1	-	-	-	0.1	0.0	0.2	0.4	0.7	1.8	4.0	5.6	9.8	12.0	12.3	10.5	12.6	13.8	10.7	2.9	0.7	0.17	0.29	2.4	141
Salivary gland	258	0	-	-	0.1	0.1	0.0	0.4	0.6	0.5	0.8	1.0	1.0	1.7	2.2	3.5	5.7	7.1	7.3	11.3	1.0	0.2	0.04	0.09	0.8	142
Mouth	821	0	-	-	0.1	0.1	0.2	0.2	0.5	0.7	1.1	3.1	5.6	9.5	16.6	14.0	15.6	16.9	13.4	10.0	3.2	0.8	0.19	0.34	2.7	143-5
Oropharynx	420	0	-	-	-	-	-	-	0.0	0.3	1.7	1.5	4.1	6.3	6.0	7.7	7.3	7.5	2.9	6.0	1.6	0.4	0.10	0.17	1.4	146
Nasopharynx	263	0	0.1	0.1	0.1	0.3	0.2	0.1	0.9	1.2	1.8	1.3	3.0	2.5	2.7	2.3	2.6	1.3	1.6	2.7	1.0	0.3	0.07	0.10	0.9	147
Hypopharynx	342	0	-	-	-	-	-	-	0.0	-	0.2	0.9	2.5	4.4	6.7	8.2	6.6	4.7	9.4	4.0	1.3	0.3	0.07	0.15	1.1	148
Pharynx unspecified	178	1	-	-	-	-	-	0.0	0.0	-	0.3	0.5	2.0	3.2	2.6	2.7	3.2	2.4	3.3	4.0	0.7	0.2	0.04	0.07	0.6	149
Oesophagus	1414	0	-	-	-	-	-	0.1	0.1	0.4	1.3	2.5	8.5	14.2	21.4	30.7	32.9	36.8	38.7	50.7	5.6	1.4	0.24	0.56	4.5	150
Stomach	3198	7	-	-	-	0.1	0.0	0.4	0.7	1.8	4.2	7.6	15.5	26.5	37.4	58.7	80.1	101.8	120.1	136.6	12.6	3.1	0.47	1.17	9.9	151
Small intestine	318	0	0.1	-	-	-	-	0.1	0.2	0.6	0.6	1.1	1.9	3.0	4.2	5.7	6.5	8.6	9.0	5.3	1.2	0.3	0.06	0.12	1.0	152
Colon	9781	8	-	-	-	0.1	0.4	0.9	1.9	4.3	9.5	19.7	39.4	71.5	124.8	183.9	255.0	333.1	384.4	428.6	38.4	9.4	1.36	3.56	30.1	153
Rectum	4749	4	-	-	-	-	0.1	0.4	0.8	2.7	5.4	11.5	25.4	46.1	69.2	96.5	113.7	131.5	149.0	122.6	18.7	4.6	0.81	1.86	15.0	154
Liver	973	0	0.6	0.1	0.1	0.1	-	0.3	0.6	1.3	2.2	2.8	5.6	8.3	12.7	19.5	23.6	23.1	22.8	18.7	3.8	0.9	0.17	0.39	3.1	155
Gallbladder etc.	584	0	-	-	-	-	-	0.0	0.0	0.2	0.4	1.5	2.7	3.8	5.8	10.5	16.2	22.8	25.7	25.3	2.3	0.6	0.07	0.21	1.8	156
Pancreas	2404	1	-	-	-	-	-	0.1	0.4	0.6	3.5	6.8	9.7	21.3	30.2	45.0	58.8	75.0	91.6	99.3	9.4	2.3	0.36	0.88	7.5	157
Nose, sinuses etc.	219	0	0.1	0.1	-	0.1	0.1	0.2	0.0	0.3	0.5	0.5	1.4	2.0	3.0	3.6	5.6	5.5	5.5	6.0	0.9	0.2	0.04	0.09	0.7	160
Larynx	1715	1	-	-	-	-	0.0	0.1	0.2	0.9	2.1	5.7	11.4	20.5	28.1	39.5	36.7	35.0	30.5	24.7	6.7	1.6	0.35	0.73	5.6	161
Bronchus, lung	19759	17	0.1	-	0.1	0.1	0.6	0.8	1.7	4.7	14.0	39.0	89.6	178.5	299.9	436.4	519.8	592.8	565.9	514.5	77.6	19.0	3.15	7.93	62.2	162
Other thoracic organs	186	0	0.5	0.1	0.1	0.2	0.3	0.5	0.2	0.4	0.5	1.1	1.4	1.2	1.0	2.7	3.5	1.8	2.9	4.0	0.7	0.2	0.04	0.07	0.7	163-4
Bone	310	0	0.1	0.8	1.1	2.2	1.3	1.0	0.8	0.5	0.7	0.9	0.6	2.0	1.6	1.8	3.9	3.3	6.1	3.3	1.2	0.3	0.07	0.10	1.1	170
Connective tissue	682	3	1.1	0.3	0.6	1.3	1.1	1.1	1.3	1.7	2.0	2.6	3.2	2.9	5.6	9.3	9.7	13.8	15.9	26.0	2.7	0.7	0.13	0.22	2.3	171
Mesothelioma	293	0	-	-	0.1	-	-	-	0.1	0.1	0.6	1.0	2.3	3.3	4.2	6.3	6.0	7.8	4.9	1.3	1.2	0.3	0.06	0.12	1.0	MES
†Kaposi's sarcoma	170	0	-	-	-	-	0.1	1.1	1.6	2.1	1.3	1.4	0.5	0.3	-	0.4	-	-	1.2	0.7	0.7	0.2	0.04	0.04	0.5	KAP
Melanoma of skin	2966	13	-	0.1	0.2	0.8	1.7	3.9	7.3	9.8	15.3	14.6	21.6	26.8	31.5	33.3	41.7	48.8	50.5	48.0	11.7	2.9	0.67	1.05	9.6	172
†Other skin																										
Breast	180	1	-	-	-	-	0.0	-	0.1	0.1	0.3	0.6	0.9	1.2	2.4	3.4	4.5	5.1	6.9	4.7	0.7	0.2	0.03	0.07	0.6	175
Prostate	21472	20	0.1	0.1	-	0.1	0.0	0.1	0.1	0.2	0.7	5.5	24.8	87.5	227.9	455.4	713.9	931.5	1110.3	1171.0	84.4	20.6	1.74	7.59	63.0	185
Testis	1238	2	0.4	0.1	0.3	2.5	7.7	11.8	10.3	8.6	6.9	4.4	2.3	2.0	1.6	1.7	1.5	0.9	0.4	3.3	4.9	1.2	0.30	0.31	4.1	186
Penis	185	0	-	-	-	0.1	-	0.0	0.1	0.0	0.5	0.9	0.7	1.5	2.7	3.1	2.6	4.7	9.4	8.0	0.7	0.2	0.03	0.06	0.6	187.1-.4
Other male genital	83	1	0.1	0.1	-	0.1	0.0	0.1	0.1	0.1	0.1	0.3	0.4	0.7	0.7	1.0	1.9	1.6	2.4	6.0	0.3	0.1	0.01	0.03	0.3	187.5-.9
†Bladder	5794	2	0.1	0.1	-	-	0.5	0.8	1.3	2.3	5.3	10.0	22.1	41.7	76.2	107.5	147.4	190.7	242.7	287.3	22.8	5.6	0.80	2.08	17.8	188
Kidney etc.	3438	4	2.0	0.3	0.1	0.2	0.3	0.4	1.1	3.2	7.8	12.4	23.0	33.0	50.8	60.8	71.0	81.6	90.8	70.0	13.5	3.3	0.67	1.33	11.2	189
Eye	276	1	1.6	0.1	0.1	-	0.0	0.1	0.2	0.7	0.7	1.1	1.5	2.1	2.8	3.7	5.9	4.7	4.5	6.7	1.1	0.3	0.06	0.10	1.0	190
Brain, nervous system	2085	1	4.1	4.0	2.6	2.6	2.3	3.0	4.2	4.7	7.4	8.9	11.1	18.3	21.7	27.3	27.2	28.8	29.3	20.0	8.2	2.0	0.48	0.75	7.4	191-2
Thyroid	594	0	-	0.2	0.2	0.5	0.8	1.9	2.5	3.2	3.0	4.0	3.1	4.0	4.8	6.6	5.4	4.2	5.3	4.7	2.3	0.6	0.14	0.20	2.0	193
Other endocrine	176	0	1.5	0.2	0.2	0.3	0.4	0.2	0.2	0.4	0.7	0.7	1.4	0.6	1.5	1.5	2.5	2.2	1.2	1.3	0.7	0.2	0.04	0.06	0.7	194
Hodgkin's disease	864	0	0.2	0.3	2.0	4.5	6.3	5.1	4.0	3.1	3.4	3.0	2.9	3.3	3.8	3.8	4.5	3.1	3.3	4.7	3.4	0.8	0.21	0.25	3.1	201
Non-Hodgkin lymphoma	4123	7	1.1	1.5	1.3	2.6	3.3	3.8	7.0	11.0	13.7	17.2	24.5	31.1	43.0	58.3	77.6	84.9	92.8	90.0	16.2	4.0	0.81	1.49	13.4	200,202
Multiple myeloma	1434	1	-	-	-	-	0.0	0.1	0.4	0.4	1.3	3.1	5.2	10.6	15.9	25.9	38.1	51.2	56.6	82.6	5.6	1.4	0.18	0.50	4.4	203
Lymphoid leukaemia	1837	1	6.8	3.4	2.5	1.8	0.7	0.4	0.5	1.3	1.8	4.0	7.0	9.9	18.8	25.9	42.4	51.5	53.3	90.0	7.2	1.8	0.29	0.64	6.4	204
Myeloid leukaemia	1431	2	0.8	0.4	0.6	1.0	1.5	1.9	1.6	2.5	3.1	5.1	6.7	9.6	13.0	19.9	26.7	36.1	55.4	55.3	5.6	1.4	0.24	0.47	4.6	205
Monocytic leukaemia	40	0	0.1	-	-	-	0.0	0.0	-	0.1	-	0.1	0.2	0.3	0.3	0.3	0.9	1.1	2.4	4.0	0.2	0.0	0.00	0.01	0.1	206
Other leukaemia	51	0	0.4	-	0.1	-	0.0	0.1	0.1	0.1	0.1	0.1	0.2	0.2	0.5	0.5	0.5	1.1	2.0	1.3	0.2	0.0	0.01	0.01	0.2	207
Leukaemia unspecified	326	3	0.3	0.1	0.1	-	0.1	0.1	0.2	0.1	0.1	0.5	0.9	1.5	2.5	3.6	8.5	13.5	17.9	32.0	1.3	0.3	0.03	0.09	1.0	208
Other and unspecified	4684	22	0.2	0.1	-	0.2	0.2	1.1	2.1	3.0	4.1	8.8	15.9	31.9	54.5	76.1	115.4	161.9	206.4	297.3	18.4	4.5	0.61	1.58	14.3	O&U
All sites																										
All sites but 173	104037	126	22.5	12.2	12.5	21.8	30.9	43.0	57.0	82.5	134.7	226.7	424.4	768.5	1287.9	1936.3	2586.3	3183.6	3600.5	3841.0	408.7	100.0	15.64	38.28	325.7	ALLb

Rate from 10 cases 0.545 0.561 0.585 0.547 0.477 0.404 0.426 0.485 0.527 0.666 0.805 0.853 0.916 1.082 1.543 2.218 4.072 6.665

†Important: see notes on population page

CANADA, ONTARIO 1988-1992

ANNUAL INCIDENCE PER 100,000 BY AGE GROUP (YEARS) - FEMALE

SITE	ALL AGES	AGE UNK	0-	5-	10-	15-	20-	25-	30-	35-	40-	45-	50-	55-	60-	65-	70-	75-	80-	85+	CRUDE RATE	%	CR 64	CR 74	ASR (W)	ICD (9th)
Lip	269	3	-	-	0.1	-	0.1	0.1	0.2	0.2	0.1	0.8	0.8	1.5	1.7	2.8	4.4	5.8	9.7	11.5	1.0	0.3	0.03	0.06	**0.6**	*140*
Tongue	318	2	-	0.1	-	-	0.0	0.2	0.3	0.4	0.6	1.0	1.8	2.0	3.1	4.4	5.6	4.6	9.7	5.3	1.2	0.3	0.05	0.10	**0.8**	*141*
Salivary gland	215	1	-	0.1	-	0.1	0.2	0.3	0.3	0.5	0.8	0.8	1.2	1.1	1.6	2.4	2.0	1.8	5.7	6.4	0.8	0.2	0.04	0.06	**0.6**	*142*
Mouth	522	1	-	-	-	0.1	0.1	0.4	0.3	0.5	0.8	1.7	2.8	4.6	6.4	7.7	7.4	8.6	9.7	10.9	2.0	0.5	0.09	0.16	**1.4**	*143-5*
Oropharynx	182	0	-	-	-	0.1	-	0.0	0.0	0.1	0.5	0.8	1.1	2.0	2.9	3.4	1.4	2.9	2.8	1.3	0.7	0.2	0.04	0.06	**0.5**	*146*
Nasopharynx	119	0	-	0.1	0.1	0.1	0.2	0.2	0.3	0.6	0.4	0.7	0.9	1.0	1.5	1.2	0.6	0.8	-	0.8	0.5	0.1	0.03	0.04	**0.4**	*147*
Hypopharynx	96	0	-	-	-	-	-	-	-	0.1	0.1	0.2	0.9	1.4	1.5	1.2	1.1	2.0	1.4	0.8	0.4	0.1	0.02	0.03	**0.3**	*148*
Pharynx unspecified	68	0	-	-	-	-	-	-	0.0	-	0.1	0.1	0.6	0.8	0.9	0.8	1.7	1.7	0.5	0.5	0.3	0.1	0.01	0.02	**0.2**	*149*
Oesophagus	633	1	-	-	-	-	-	0.1	0.1	0.3	1.4	1.4	4.0	5.5	9.7	11.0	14.5	21.2	23.7	2.4	0.7	0.06	0.17	**1.4**	*150*
Stomach	1855	1	-	-	0.1	0.1	0.1	0.3	0.6	1.5	2.4	3.5	5.6	9.9	15.1	24.2	30.1	41.8	55.0	81.8	7.1	1.9	0.20	0.47	**4.2**	*151*
Small intestine	277	0	-	-	-	-	-	0.1	0.2	0.4	0.4	0.7	0.7	2.6	2.8	4.4	4.8	6.8	5.7	4.0	1.1	0.3	0.04	0.09	**0.7**	*152*
Colon	9765	5	-	-	0.1	0.2	0.6	1.2	1.8	4.0	8.3	19.8	38.0	57.4	86.0	128.7	180.2	237.6	299.2	324.4	37.5	10.1	1.09	2.63	**22.8**	*153*
Rectum	3356	2	-	-	-	0.2	0.1	0.6	1.0	2.3	3.7	8.8	15.2	24.5	33.1	47.0	60.3	71.2	77.3	100.7	12.9	3.5	0.45	0.98	**8.3**	*154*
Liver	488	0	0.3	0.1	0.1	0.1	0.2	0.2	0.4	0.3	0.3	0.9	2.0	2.5	4.9	5.8	6.9	12.2	12.6	18.7	1.9	0.5	0.06	0.12	**1.2**	*155*
Gallbladder etc.	889	0	-	-	-	-	-	0.1	-	0.3	0.5	1.9	2.0	4.6	8.5	12.6	17.6	20.5	27.1	34.4	3.4	0.9	0.09	0.24	**2.0**	*156*
Pancreas	2430	1	-	-	0.1	-	0.1	0.2	0.5	0.6	2.1	4.1	6.6	11.8	19.5	35.2	49.3	57.8	75.9	91.4	9.3	2.5	0.23	0.65	**5.5**	*157*
Nose, sinuses etc.	136	0	0.1	-	0.1	-	0.1	0.1	0.1	0.1	0.3	0.5	0.9	1.1	0.9	1.6	2.4	2.0	2.3	4.5	0.5	0.1	0.02	0.04	**0.4**	*160*
Larynx	365	1	-	-	-	-	0.0	0.0	0.1	0.1	0.7	1.3	2.1	5.4	5.6	4.3	6.2	5.8	5.1	2.7	1.4	0.4	0.08	0.13	**1.0**	*161*
Bronchus, lung	10413	4	-	-	0.1	-	0.5	0.6	1.9	4.8	13.0	31.7	60.6	92.7	139.7	174.9	200.4	204.0	149.9	125.3	40.0	10.8	1.73	3.61	**28.2**	*162*
Other thoracic organs	128	0	0.5	-	-	0.1	0.1	0.3	0.3	0.4	0.4	0.6	0.6	0.8	1.2	1.4	0.8	1.7	1.8	0.8	0.5	0.1	0.03	0.04	**0.4**	*163-4*
Bone	244	1	0.2	0.5	1.2	1.7	0.6	0.6	0.5	0.6	0.4	0.6	0.7	1.4	1.7	1.5	2.2	2.3	2.3	2.4	0.9	0.3	0.05	0.07	**0.9**	*170*
Connective tissue	567	2	0.7	0.6	0.6	0.6	0.8	1.0	1.2	1.3	1.7	2.2	2.2	3.0	4.6	5.3	6.7	7.5	7.1	12.3	2.2	0.6	0.10	0.16	**1.7**	*171*
Mesothelioma	77	0	-	-	-	-	-	-	0.1	0.1	0.1	0.3	1.1	0.8	1.0	1.3	1.0	0.5	1.4	-	0.3	0.1	0.02	0.03	**0.2**	*MES*
†Kaposi's sarcoma	7	0	-	-	-	-	-	0.0	-	0.0	-	-	-	-	-	-	0.2	-	0.5	0.3	0.0	0.0	0.00	0.00	**0.0**	*KAP*
Melanoma of skin	2687	2	0.1	0.2	0.4	0.9	3.7	5.9	8.7	12.6	16.6	16.1	14.1	20.2	19.5	21.1	21.9	23.8	23.9	28.5	10.3	2.8	0.60	0.81	**8.0**	*172*
†Other skin																										
Breast	27349	20	-	-	-	0.3	1.2	5.4	20.2	52.7	108.7	168.6	210.7	234.6	290.0	335.7	366.9	385.0	377.8	369.7	105.0	28.3	5.47	8.98	**78.1**	*174*
Uterus unspecified	161	0	-	-	-	-	-	0.0	0.1	0.3	0.4	1.1	0.4	0.7	1.4	1.5	1.7	2.0	4.8	8.5	0.6	0.2	0.02	0.04	**0.4**	*179*
Cervix uteri	2780	6	-	-	-	-	2.1	7.5	13.9	18.5	16.5	18.4	16.1	15.7	17.3	20.8	20.1	23.2	16.1	13.6	10.7	2.9	0.63	0.84	**8.4**	*180*
Placenta	12	0	-	-	-	-	-	0.1	0.3	0.1	0.1	-	-	-	-	-	-	-	-	-	0.0	0.0	0.00	0.00	**0.0**	*181*
Corpus uteri	5300	5	-	-	-	0.1	0.2	0.7	1.5	4.1	9.1	15.2	35.2	59.7	72.1	89.3	97.0	79.8	66.7	46.1	20.4	5.5	0.99	1.92	**14.9**	*182*
Ovary etc.	3928	3	0.2	0.1	0.5	1.4	1.9	2.4	3.7	6.6	11.6	17.7	28.1	35.9	41.9	46.3	57.1	57.2	58.6	56.2	15.1	4.1	0.76	1.28	**11.1**	*183*
Other female genital	816	1	0.1	0.1	-	0.2	0.3	0.5	1.3	1.7	1.5	2.8	3.5	4.0	5.4	9.5	12.3	17.4	16.6	29.9	3.1	0.8	0.11	0.22	**2.0**	*184*
†Bladder	2041	1	0.1	-	0.1	0.1	0.1	0.3	0.6	1.2	2.1	4.0	8.0	11.2	18.9	26.0	33.1	52.0	61.6	71.2	7.8	2.1	0.23	0.53	**4.8**	*188*
Kidney etc.	2094	2	2.1	0.6	0.1	0.1	0.2	0.6	1.3	3.1	4.3	7.2	12.8	17.8	22.5	27.1	32.6	36.8	36.8	36.5	8.0	2.2	0.36	0.66	**5.8**	*189*
Eye	234	0	1.1	0.2	-	0.1	0.1	0.2	0.3	0.5	0.9	0.8	1.1	1.4	2.7	1.8	2.2	3.4	4.1	5.1	0.9	0.2	0.05	0.07	**0.7**	*190*
Brain, nervous system	1728	0	3.7	2.7	2.3	2.0	1.8	2.4	3.6	3.5	4.2	5.7	9.2	11.3	16.5	17.5	23.7	23.8	21.6	14.1	6.6	1.8	0.34	0.55	**5.4**	*191-2*
Thyroid	1870	0	-	0.1	0.6	2.0	6.3	8.9	9.2	11.7	10.4	10.9	11.5	10.7	8.7	9.2	8.1	8.2	10.6	6.7	7.2	1.9	0.46	0.54	**5.9**	*193*
Other endocrine	159	0	1.2	0.3	0.1	0.2	0.2	0.2	0.3	0.6	0.4	0.4	0.9	1.3	1.0	1.0	1.3	2.0	1.6	1.1	0.6	0.2	0.04	0.05	**0.6**	*194*
Hodgkin's disease	709	1	-	0.3	1.7	5.7	6.3	4.9	2.6	2.4	1.7	1.2	1.4	1.7	2.1	2.0	4.3	3.8	4.8	1.3	2.7	0.7	0.16	0.19	**2.5**	*201*
Non-Hodgkin lymphoma	3464	10	0.5	0.9	0.5	1.3	1.1	3.1	3.4	4.9	8.5	11.1	17.7	26.2	31.5	44.9	54.2	67.5	66.9	60.5	13.3	3.6	0.55	1.05	**9.3**	*200,202*
Multiple myeloma	1276	1	-	-	-	-	-	0.0	0.1	0.3	1.2	3.0	5.4	5.9	11.2	19.1	26.2	30.3	36.6	38.6	4.9	1.3	0.14	0.36	**3.0**	*203*
Lymphoid leukaemia	1295	2	6.0	2.5	1.4	1.0	0.7	0.4	0.3	0.7	1.1	1.7	2.8	4.8	10.9	12.2	18.7	28.8	30.6	49.3	5.0	1.3	0.17	0.33	**3.7**	*204*
Myeloid leukaemia	1168	2	0.5	0.2	0.6	1.1	0.9	1.4	1.4	2.7	3.1	4.5	5.0	4.8	8.2	11.1	19.0	19.1	27.8	31.2	4.5	1.2	0.17	0.32	**3.1**	*205*
Monocytic leukaemia	37	0	0.1	-	-	-	0.0	0.0	-	0.0	-	0.1	-	0.2	0.3	0.5	0.7	1.2	0.9	0.8	0.1	0.0	0.00	0.01	**0.1**	*206*
Other leukaemia	43	0	0.1	-	-	0.1	-	0.1	0.1	0.0	0.1	-	0.2	0.3	0.4	0.3	0.5	1.4	0.2	1.6	0.2	0.0	0.01	0.01	**0.1**	*207*
Leukaemia unspecified	359	0	0.2	0.1	-	0.2	-	0.1	0.3	0.1	0.3	0.4	0.7	1.4	2.1	3.1	3.8	8.6	15.2	24.0	1.4	0.4	0.03	0.06	**0.7**	*208*
Other and unspecified	3816	22	0.4	0.1	-	0.3	0.5	0.6	1.2	3.3	4.3	6.8	12.4	19.8	28.9	43.4	56.9	86.8	124.6	184.4	14.7	3.9	0.40	0.90	**8.6**	*O&U*
All sites																										
All sites but 173	96745	103	17.8	9.8	10.4	20.2	31.6	52.4	84.9	151.3	245.0	382.2	547.2	726.3	963.3	1224.9	1466.5	1676.6	1792.2	1943.8	371.5	100.0	16.23	29.70	**261.1**	*ALLb*

Rate from 10 cases   0.572 0.589 0.614 0.574 0.489 0.415 0.430 0.476 0.529 0.675 0.813 0.849 0.857 0.906 1.196 1.538 2.299 2.665

†Important: see notes on population page

Canada, Prince Edward Island

Formerly part of the Department of Health and Social Services, the Prince Edward Island Cancer Registry is now part of the Oncology Clinic at the Queen Elizabeth Hospital, the largest hospital on Prince Edward Island. Participation in the national cancer reporting system commenced in 1969. The personnel consists of the director of the clinic (a medical oncologist) and two health records technicians (one full-time and one part-time).

The registry covers all of Prince Edward Island, the smallest province of Canada, which is situated to the southwest of the Gulf of St Lawrence, lying between longitudes 62° and 65° W and latitudes 46° and 48°N. It covers an area of 5660 km^2, all lying at an altitude of less than 100 m above sea level.

The population according to the 1991 census consisted of 63 965 males and 65 800 females. Of these approximately 23% of the males and 22% of the females were under 15 years of age. Approximately 40% of the population live in urban areas while 60% live in rural areas. Most are of British, Irish or French origin, with small percentages of Lebanese or Dutch extraction. The predominant religions are Roman Catholic and Protestant Christian denominations. The major occupations are farming, fishing and tourism. There is no heavy industry.

The main source of data for the registry is pathology reports with a diagnosis of cancer, copies of which are sent to the registry from the two provincial laboratories and, on occasion, from other provinces in Canada. Additional data necessary for cancer registration may be obtained from either the oncology clinic, hospital records, or other physicians. Death certificates as the only source of information comprise a small number of the registrations and this proportion has fallen considerably over a 15-year period. The methods of collection are entirely voluntary. Legislation exists to cover active collection of data. The registry assesses completeness and quality of its data to be very high; this is due in part to the small size of the province, which makes follow-back information on registrations more accessible. With the future implementation of an island-wide health information system, it is expected that the completeness will be even further improved.

Cancer incidence registration data have been maintained and stored on computer since 1984 and have been used for some local studies as well as being forwarded to the National Registry. A new computer registration system on Prince Edward Island was installed to correlate with the national implementation of the Canadian Cancer Registry. This new system follows the Canadian Cancer Registry Data Dictionary rules and guidelines for reporting and has many edit checks to reduce the number of errors in data that have to be returned to the province for correction. Prince Edward Island has submitted two years of data to date and has had approximately 0.003% errors. In 1995 the registry upgraded the computer hardware.

Hospital organization and practice are based on a comprehensive government organized health insurance scheme. There are no private hospital facilities.

Dagny E. Dryer
Kim Vriends

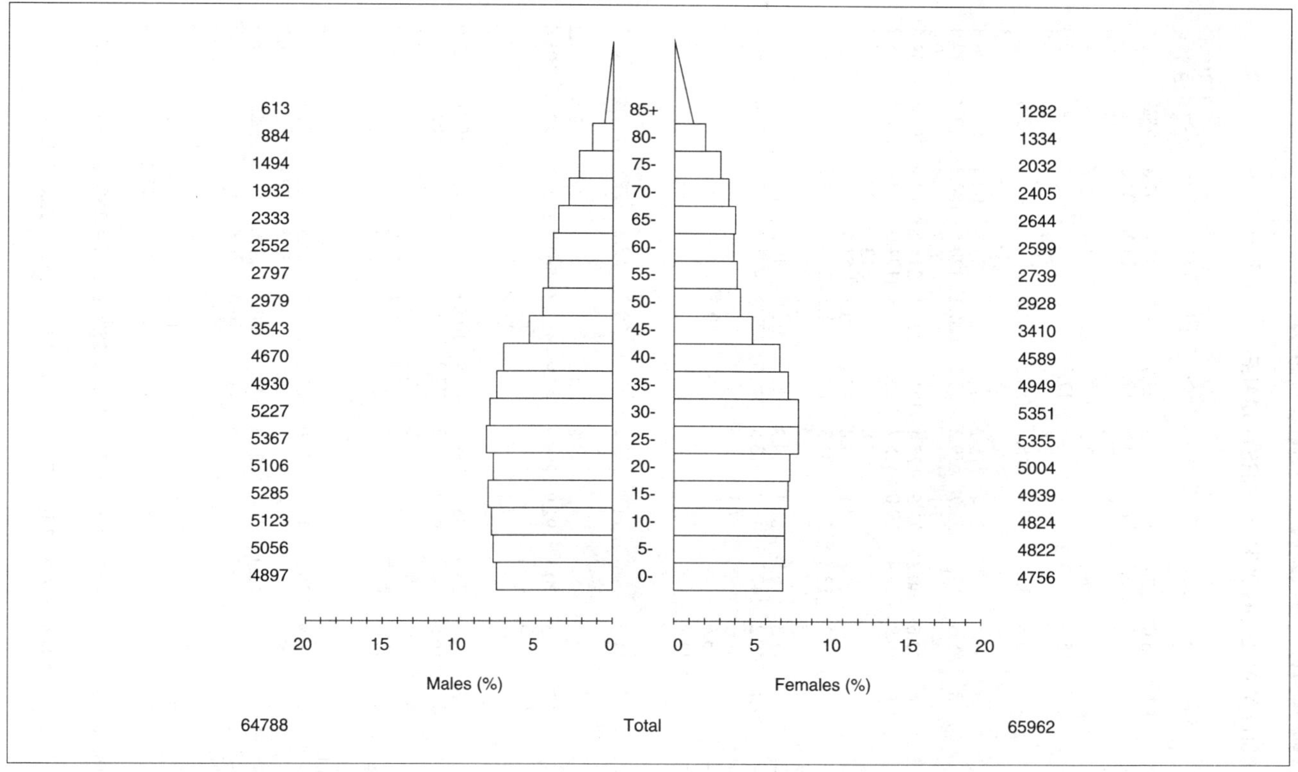

Canada, Prince Edward Island
Source of population: average annual 1988-92
Census: Statistics Canada June 1991
Estimate: The populations were estimated at 1 July each year, based on revised intercensal estimates for 1988-91 and post-censal estimates for 1992. In 1993 revised estimates dating back to 1971 were implemented by Statistics Canada and population data from 1971 now include estimates of net census undercoverage, plus non-permanent residents defined as persons claiming refugee status, foreign students, work permit holders, or holders of Minister's permits, and non-Canadian-born dependants of such individuals. References: Statistics Canada, Catalogue 91-537, Revised intercensal population and family estimates, July 1, 1971–91, and Catalogue 91-213, Annual demographic statistics 1993 (for 1992 data).

Notes to tables overleaf:
† Kaposi's sarcoma is under-reported in this volume because cases of skin cancer (ICD-9 173) were not provided
† 173 not available

CANADA, PRINCE EDWARD ISLAND 1988-1992

ANNUAL INCIDENCE PER 100,000 BY AGE GROUP (YEARS) - MALE

SITE	ALL AGES	AGE UNK	0-	5-	10-	15-	20-	25-	30-	35-	40-	45-	50-	55-	60-	65-	70-	75-	80-	85+	CRUDE RATE	%	CR 64	CR 74	ASR (W)	ICD (9th)
Lip	36	0	-	-	-	-	-	-	3.8	-	8.6	5.6	13.4	14.3	31.3	25.7	51.7	93.7	67.8	195.6	11.1	2.5	0.39	0.77	**7.6**	140
Tongue	12	0	-	-	-	-	-	-	-	-	-	5.6	6.7	21.4	23.5	17.1	-	13.4	22.6	-	3.7	0.8	0.29	0.37	**3.2**	141
Salivary gland	3	0	-	-	-	3.8	-	-	-	-	-	-	-	7.1	7.8	-	-	-	-	-	0.9	0.2	0.09	0.09	**0.9**	142
Mouth	12	0	-	-	-	-	-	-	-	-	-	-	6.7	35.7	7.8	-	31.0	13.4	22.6	-	3.7	0.8	0.25	0.41	**2.9**	143-5
Oropharynx	3	0	-	-	-	-	-	-	-	-	-	5.6	-	-	-	17.1	-	-	-	-	0.9	0.2	0.03	0.11	**0.9**	146
Nasopharynx	3	0	-	-	-	-	-	-	-	-	-	-	-	7.1	7.8	-	-	13.4	-	-	0.9	0.2	0.07	0.07	**0.7**	147
Hypopharynx	9	0	-	-	-	-	-	-	-	-	-	5.6	13.4	7.1	15.7	8.6	10.3	-	-	32.6	2.8	0.6	0.21	0.30	**2.6**	148
Pharynx unspecified	1	0	-	-	-	-	-	-	-	-	-	-	-	-	-	8.6	-	-	-	-	0.3	0.1	0.00	0.04	**0.3**	149
Oesophagus	22	0	-	-	-	-	-	-	-	4.1	-	-	-	21.4	15.7	34.3	20.7	53.5	90.4	65.2	6.8	1.5	0.21	0.48	**4.5**	150
Stomach	55	0	-	-	-	-	-	-	-	-	4.3	5.6	13.4	35.7	39.2	77.2	124.2	120.5	180.8	97.8	17.0	3.9	0.49	1.50	**11.7**	151
Small intestine	3	0	-	-	-	-	-	-	-	-	-	-	-	7.1	-	-	-	26.8	-	-	0.9	0.2	0.04	0.04	**0.6**	152
Colon	123	0	-	-	-	-	-	-	-	8.1	21.4	22.6	40.3	71.5	125.4	171.5	227.7	214.2	293.9	293.4	38.0	8.6	1.45	3.44	**27.8**	153
Rectum	59	0	-	-	-	-	-	-	-	-	8.6	16.9	13.4	50.0	15.7	85.7	113.8	174.0	113.0	130.4	18.2	4.1	0.52	1.52	**12.6**	154
Liver	4	0	-	-	-	-	-	-	-	-	-	-	-	-	7.8	-	-	13.4	22.6	32.6	1.2	0.3	0.04	0.04	**0.7**	155
Gallbladder etc.	10	0	-	-	-	-	-	-	-	-	-	-	-	7.1	7.8	17.1	20.7	53.5	-	-	3.1	0.7	0.07	0.26	**2.1**	156
Pancreas	50	0	-	-	-	-	-	-	-	-	-	11.3	13.4	28.6	31.3	102.9	51.7	133.9	158.2	130.4	15.4	3.5	0.42	1.20	**10.6**	157
Nose, sinuses etc.	3	0	-	-	-	3.8	-	-	-	-	-	11.3	-	-	-	-	-	-	-	-	0.9	0.2	0.08	0.08	**1.0**	160
Larynx	24	0	-	-	-	-	-	-	-	4.1	-	11.3	6.7	21.4	39.2	25.7	31.0	40.2	67.8	-	7.4	1.7	0.41	0.70	**5.8**	161
Bronchus, lung	259	0	-	-	-	-	-	-	-	-	17.1	45.2	147.7	143.0	313.5	342.9	527.8	495.3	632.9	293.4	79.9	18.1	3.33	7.69	**59.8**	162
Other thoracic organs	4	0	-	-	-	3.8	-	-	-	4.1	-	-	-	7.1	-	8.6	-	-	-	-	1.2	0.3	0.07	0.12	**1.1**	163-4
Bone	4	0	-	-	-	3.8	-	-	-	-	-	5.6	-	-	-	-	10.3	-	22.6	-	1.2	0.3	0.05	0.10	**1.0**	170
Connective tissue	11	0	-	-	-	-	7.8	3.7	3.8	-	-	11.3	-	14.3	7.8	8.6	-	-	22.6	-	3.4	0.8	0.24	0.29	**3.1**	171
Mesothelioma	2	0	-	-	-	-	-	-	-	-	-	-	-	7.1	-	8.6	-	-	-	-	0.6	0.1	0.04	0.08	**0.5**	MES
†Kaposi's sarcoma	0	0	-	-	-	-	-	-	-	-	-	-	-	-	-	-	-	-	-	-	0.0	0.0	0.00	0.00	**0.0**	KAP
Melanoma of skin	36	0	-	-	-	3.8	-	14.9	3.8	16.2	4.3	11.3	-	14.3	39.2	42.9	20.7	53.5	22.6	130.4	11.1	2.5	0.54	0.86	**8.8**	172
†Other skin																										
Breast	4	0	-	-	-	-	-	-	-	-	-	-	-	-	7.8	8.6	-	-	22.6	32.6	1.2	0.3	0.04	0.08	**0.8**	175
Prostate	342	0	-	-	-	-	-	-	-	-	4.3	11.3	20.1	92.9	289.9	642.9	921.0	562.2	1220.6	847.7	105.6	23.9	2.09	9.91	**70.9**	185
Testis	9	0	-	-	-	-	-	14.9	3.8	4.1	4.3	11.3	-	-	-	-	-	-	-	-	2.8	0.6	0.19	0.19	**2.6**	186
Penis	7	0	-	-	-	-	-	-	-	-	4.3	-	-	7.1	7.8	-	10.3	13.4	45.2	-	2.2	0.5	0.10	0.15	**1.4**	187.1-.4
Other male genital	0	0	-	-	-	-	-	-	-	-	-	-	-	-	-	-	-	-	-	-	0.0	0.0	0.00	0.00	**0.0**	187.5-.9
Bladder	71	0	-	-	-	-	-	-	-	-	4.3	-	26.9	35.7	39.2	102.9	103.5	187.4	316.5	195.6	21.9	5.0	0.53	1.56	**14.2**	188
Kidney etc.	51	0	-	-	-	-	-	-	-	8.1	8.6	16.9	6.7	64.3	86.2	77.2	31.0	66.9	90.4	65.2	15.7	3.6	0.95	1.50	**12.8**	189
Eye	5	0	4.1	-	-	-	-	-	-	-	4.3	-	6.7	-	7.8	8.6	-	-	-	-	1.5	0.4	0.11	0.16	**1.7**	190
Brain, nervous system	24	0	-	4.0	3.9	7.6	-	-	3.8	-	-	16.9	13.4	28.6	15.7	17.1	41.4	26.8	-	-	7.4	1.7	0.47	0.76	**6.7**	191-2
Thyroid	5	0	-	-	3.9	-	-	-	-	-	-	11.3	-	7.1	-	-	-	13.4	-	-	1.5	0.4	0.11	0.11	**1.4**	193
Other endocrine	1	0	-	-	-	-	-	-	-	4.1	-	-	-	-	-	-	-	-	-	-	0.3	0.1	0.02	0.02	**0.2**	194
Hodgkin's disease	9	0	-	-	-	-	11.8	-	7.7	8.1	4.3	-	-	7.1	-	-	-	-	-	-	2.8	0.6	0.19	0.19	**2.4**	201
Non-Hodgkin lymphoma	42	0	4.1	-	3.9	-	-	-	3.8	-	12.8	16.9	26.9	14.3	47.0	85.7	41.4	53.5	22.6	32.6	13.0	2.9	0.67	1.30	**11.2**	200,202
Multiple myeloma	20	0	-	-	-	-	-	-	-	-	-	-	-	21.4	7.8	60.0	41.4	53.5	22.6	-	6.2	1.4	0.15	0.65	**4.4**	203
Lymphoid leukaemia	21	0	8.2	-	-	-	-	-	-	-	-	-	13.4	-	23.5	42.9	20.7	26.8	67.8	65.2	6.5	1.5	0.23	0.54	**5.2**	204
Myeloid leukaemia	12	0	-	-	3.9	3.8	3.9	-	3.8	-	-	-	-	-	7.8	8.6	10.3	26.8	67.8	-	3.7	0.8	0.12	0.21	**2.6**	205
Monocytic leukaemia	1	0	-	-	-	3.8	-	-	-	-	-	-	-	-	-	-	-	-	-	-	0.3	0.1	0.02	0.02	**0.3**	206
Other leukaemia	1	0	-	-	-	-	-	-	-	-	4.3	-	-	-	-	-	-	-	-	-	0.3	0.1	0.02	0.02	**0.3**	207
Leukaemia unspecified	2	0	-	-	-	-	-	-	-	-	-	-	-	-	-	-	10.3	-	-	32.6	0.6	0.1	0.00	0.05	**0.4**	208
Other and unspecified	53	0	-	-	-	-	-	-	-	-	12.8	5.6	13.4	35.7	54.9	68.6	82.8	133.9	45.2	228.2	16.4	3.7	0.61	1.37	**11.8**	O&U
All sites																										
All sites but 173	1428	0	16.3	4.0	15.6	34.1	27.4	33.5	34.4	60.9	128.5	265.3	402.8	836.4	1332.2	2126.0	2556.1	2677.4	3661.8	2901.9	440.8	100.0	15.96	39.37	**322.4**	ALLb
Rate from 1 case			4.084	3.955	3.904	3.784	3.917	3.726	3.826	4.057	4.282	5.644	6.713	7.148	7.836	8.573	10.349	13.387	22.604	32.605						

†Important: see notes on population page

CANADA, PRINCE EDWARD ISLAND 1988-1992

ANNUAL INCIDENCE PER 100,000 BY AGE GROUP (YEARS) - FEMALE

SITE	ALL AGES	AGE UNK	0-	5-	10-	15-	20-	25-	30-	35-	40-	45-	50-	55-	60-	65-	70-	75-	80-	85+	CRUDE RATE	%	CR 64	CR 74	ASR (W)	ICD (9th)
Lip	1	0	-	-	-	-	-	-	-	-	-	-	-	-	-	-	8.3	-	-	-	0.3	0.1	0.00	0.04	0.2	140
Tongue	4	0	-	-	-	-	-	-	-	-	-	-	-	7.3	7.7	-	8.3	-	-	15.6	1.2	0.3	0.07	0.12	0.8	141
Salivary gland	1	0	-	-	-	-	-	-	-	-	-	-	-	-	7.7	-	-	-	-	-	0.3	0.1	0.04	0.04	0.3	142
Mouth	8	0	-	-	-	-	-	-	-	-	-	5.9	-	21.9	23.1	-	8.3	-	-	-	2.4	0.6	0.25	0.30	2.3	143-5
Oropharynx	1	0	-	-	-	-	-	-	-	-	-	-	-	-	-	7.6	-	-	-	-	0.3	0.1	0.00	0.04	0.2	146
Nasopharynx	1	0	-	-	-	-	-	-	-	-	-	-	-	-	-	-	-	9.8	-	-	0.3	0.1	0.00	0.00	0.1	147
Hypopharynx	1	0	-	-	-	-	-	-	-	-	-	-	-	-	-	-	-	9.8	-	-	0.3	0.1	0.00	0.00	0.1	148
Pharynx unspecified	0	0	-	-	-	-	-	-	-	-	-	-	-	-	-	-	-	-	-	-	0.0	0.0	0.00	0.00	0.0	149
Oesophagus	2	0	-	-	-	-	-	-	-	4.0	-	-	-	-	-	-	8.3	-	-	-	0.6	0.2	0.02	0.06	0.4	150
Stomach	35	0	-	-	-	-	4.0	-	3.7	-	4.4	-	13.7	7.3	15.4	22.7	41.6	19.7	74.9	187.1	10.6	2.7	0.24	0.56	5.4	151
Small intestine	3	0	-	-	-	-	-	-	-	-	-	-	-	7.3	7.7	-	-	-	15.0	-	0.9	0.2	0.07	0.07	0.7	152
Colon	152	0	-	-	-	-	-	-	-	12.1	13.1	23.5	41.0	43.8	69.3	105.9	182.9	403.4	389.7	280.7	46.1	11.7	1.01	2.46	23.7	153
Rectum	55	0	-	-	-	-	-	-	-	4.0	4.4	-	41.0	29.2	46.2	52.9	66.5	59.0	74.9	171.5	16.7	4.2	0.62	1.22	10.3	154
Liver	3	0	-	-	-	-	-	-	-	-	-	-	-	-	-	-	-	9.8	15.0	15.6	0.9	0.2	0.00	0.00	0.3	155
Gallbladder etc.	10	0	-	-	-	-	-	-	-	-	4.4	-	-	14.6	7.7	-	-	-	30.0	62.4	3.0	0.8	0.13	0.13	1.6	156
Pancreas	40	0	-	-	-	-	-	-	3.7	-	-	-	13.7	7.3	30.8	30.3	74.8	88.5	60.0	93.6	12.1	3.1	0.28	0.80	6.5	157
Nose, sinuses etc.	0	0	-	-	-	-	-	-	-	-	-	-	-	-	-	-	-	-	-	-	0.0	0.0	0.00	0.00	0.0	160
Larynx	3	0	-	-	-	-	-	-	-	-	-	-	-	7.3	-	-	-	19.7	-	-	0.9	0.2	0.04	0.04	0.5	161
Bronchus, lung	161	0	-	-	-	-	-	-	-	16.2	17.4	64.5	123.0	116.8	169.3	219.3	166.3	196.8	134.9	124.7	48.8	12.4	2.54	4.46	36.6	162
Other thoracic organs	2	0	-	-	-	-	-	-	-	-	-	-	-	-	7.7	7.6	-	-	-	-	0.6	0.2	0.04	0.08	0.5	163-4
Bone	2	0	-	-	-	4.0	-	-	-	-	-	-	-	-	-	-	8.3	-	-	-	0.6	0.2	0.02	0.06	0.5	170
Connective tissue	5	0	-	-	-	-	-	-	-	-	-	-	-	7.3	-	15.1	-	9.8	-	15.6	1.5	0.4	0.04	0.11	0.9	171
Mesothelioma	0	0	-	-	-	-	-	-	-	-	-	-	-	-	-	-	-	-	-	-	0.0	0.0	0.00	0.00	0.0	MES
†Kaposi's sarcoma	0	0	-	-	-	-	-	-	-	-	-	-	-	-	-	-	-	-	-	-	0.0	0.0	0.00	0.00	0.0	KAP
Melanoma of skin	38	0	-	-	-	4.0	4.0	7.5	7.5	12.1	21.8	17.6	20.5	36.5	15.4	15.1	24.9	19.7	30.0	31.2	11.5	2.9	0.73	0.93	9.4	172
†Other skin																										
Breast	363	0	-	-	-	-	-	3.7	18.7	44.4	95.9	187.7	170.8	306.6	292.4	257.1	473.9	462.4	404.7	343.1	110.1	28.0	5.60	9.26	79.2	174
Uterus unspecified	6	0	-	-	-	-	-	-	-	-	-	-	5.9	-	7.7	-	16.6	-	-	31.2	1.8	0.5	0.07	0.15	1.1	179
Cervix uteri	40	0	-	-	-	-	4.0	3.7	14.9	40.4	17.4	11.7	27.3	14.6	30.8	15.1	8.3	-	74.9	-	12.1	3.1	0.82	0.94	9.9	180
Placenta	1	0	-	-	-	-	-	3.7	-	-	-	-	-	-	-	-	-	-	-	-	0.3	0.1	0.02	0.02	0.3	181
Corpus uteri	56	0	-	-	-	-	-	-	-	-	-	5.9	13.7	29.2	46.2	128.6	83.1	59.0	89.9	62.4	17.0	4.3	0.47	1.53	10.9	182
Ovary etc.	35	0	-	-	-	4.0	-	-	3.7	4.0	17.4	23.5	13.7	36.5	23.1	30.3	24.9	29.5	15.0	46.8	10.6	2.7	0.63	0.91	8.4	183
Other female genital	15	0	-	-	-	-	-	-	-	-	8.7	-	6.8	7.3	23.1	7.6	24.9	-	15.0	46.8	4.5	1.2	0.23	0.39	3.1	184
Bladder	36	0	-	-	-	-	-	-	-	-	4.4	5.9	6.8	-	46.2	15.1	41.6	49.2	104.9	124.7	10.9	2.8	0.32	0.60	5.7	188
Kidney etc.	25	0	-	-	-	-	-	-	-	-	-	-	6.8	-	23.1	22.7	33.3	29.5	74.9	93.6	7.6	1.9	0.15	0.43	3.7	189
Eye	2	0	-	-	-	-	-	-	-	-	-	-	-	7.3	-	-	8.3	-	-	-	0.6	0.2	0.04	0.08	0.5	190
Brain, nervous system	22	0	-	4.1	4.1	4.0	-	-	3.7	8.1	8.7	-	6.8	7.3	7.7	30.3	33.3	-	30.0	15.6	6.7	1.7	0.27	0.59	5.1	191-2
Thyroid	14	0	-	-	-	-	4.0	11.2	11.2	8.1	4.4	-	6.8	-	-	7.6	8.3	9.8	-	-	4.2	1.1	0.23	0.31	3.5	193
Other endocrine	0	0	-	-	-	-	-	-	-	-	-	-	-	-	-	-	-	-	-	-	0.0	0.0	0.00	0.00	0.0	194
Hodgkin's disease	7	0	-	-	-	8.1	-	3.7	-	-	-	-	-	-	-	-	8.3	19.7	-	15.6	2.1	0.5	0.06	0.10	1.5	201
Non-Hodgkin lymphoma	53	0	-	-	-	4.0	4.0	-	3.7	8.1	13.1	35.2	13.7	14.6	30.8	30.3	99.8	78.7	45.0	62.4	16.1	4.1	0.64	1.29	11.0	200,202
Multiple myeloma	19	0	-	-	-	-	-	-	-	-	-	-	13.7	-	23.1	15.1	24.9	-	60.0	78.0	5.8	1.5	0.18	0.38	3.2	203
Lymphoid leukaemia	9	0	8.4	4.1	-	-	-	-	-	-	-	-	-	14.6	-	7.6	8.3	9.8	15.0	-	2.7	0.7	0.14	0.22	2.6	204
Myeloid leukaemia	13	0	-	-	-	-	-	-	-	-	4.4	11.7	-	-	15.4	7.6	8.3	29.5	-	46.8	3.9	1.0	0.16	0.24	2.5	205
Monocytic leukaemia	0	0	-	-	-	-	-	-	-	-	-	-	-	-	-	-	-	-	-	-	0.0	0.0	0.00	0.00	0.0	206
Other leukaemia	0	0	-	-	-	-	-	-	-	-	-	-	-	-	-	-	-	-	-	-	0.0	0.0	0.00	0.00	0.0	207
Leukaemia unspecified	1	0	-	-	-	-	-	-	-	-	-	-	-	-	-	-	-	-	-	15.6	0.3	0.1	0.00	0.00	0.1	208
Other and unspecified	52	0	-	-	-	-	-	-	-	-	-	5.9	-	7.3	15.4	37.8	74.8	88.5	209.8	171.5	15.8	4.0	0.14	0.71	6.7	O&U
All sites																										
All sites but 173	1297	0	8.4	8.3	4.1	28.3	20.0	33.6	71.0	161.6	239.7	404.6	539.6	751.9	992.7	1089.1	1579.6	1711.9	1963.4	2151.9	393.2	100.0	16.32	29.66	260.4	ALLb

Rate from 1 case   4.205   4.147   4.146   4.049   3.997   3.734   3.737   4.041   4.357   5.864   6.831   7.300   7.695   7.563   8.314   9.839   14.988   15.593

†Important: see notes on population page

Canada, Quebec

The Quebec Cancer Registry was created in 1961 at the suggestion of the National Cancer Institute of Canada, but it was only in April 1981 that notification of all cases hospitalized in Quebec with a diagnosis of cancer became obligatory. Non-hospitalized cases treated in surgical departments during the day were added to this source of notification in September 1983. The Ministry of Health and Social Services of Quebec is responsible for the functioning of the registry.

Quebec is the largest of the ten Canadian provinces, covering a surface area of 1 667 926 km^2, 11% of which is water and only 2.3% serves as urban or agricultural land. The rest is composed of forests, tundra and taiga.

Quebec contains nearly 7 000 000 inhabitants (49% men and 51% women), of whom nearly 80% live in an urban environment. Life expectancy at birth is 73.7 years for men and 80.9 for women. More than 11% of the population is over age 65, and the ageing of the population is becoming more accentuated.

In 1991, immigrants comprised nearly 10% of the population. These come mostly from Italy (13%), France (7%) and Haiti (6%), and establish themselves primarily in the metropolitan area of Montreal (88%). 80% of the population has French as mother tongue, and 12% English. There are 64 000 aboriginals in the Quebec population, of whom 89% are Amerindians and 11% Inuit. 86% of the population is Catholic and 6% Protestant.

In 1990, unemployment in Quebec accounted for about 14% of the active population. The working population is divided into three main sectors, 3% in agriculture, forestry, fishing and mining; 25% in manufacturing and construction industries and 72% in services.

The medical records clerks of each of some 150 hospital centres code the medical information (site and morphology of the cancer) according to rules provided by the registry. The primary sites of cancer (ICD-9 140–195 and 200–208) are collected by the cancer registry. Secondary malignant cancers (ICD-9 196–198) and unspecified sites (ICD-9 199) are kept only for cases for which there is no mention of a more specific diagnosis for the same individual. *In situ* diagnoses (ICD-9 230–234) are not collected.

The registry does not collect information on occupation, ethnic origin, religion or race for the cases. Extent of disease, stage at time of diagnosis and treatment are not recorded. Multiple primaries are recorded according to the IARC/IACR recommendations.

The methodology used in the registry assures a good level of quality, both in terms of completeness (more than 90% of new cancer cases are notified, with the exception of non-melanoma skin cancers) and in terms of the reliability of the information collected. Nonetheless, an effort must be made to diversify the sources of data on cancer in order to maintain the high level of quality in the cancer registry. Quebec is going through a period of cutbacks in health care costs and a reduction in hospital admissions. At the same time, medical personnel increasingly use diagnostic techniques and surgical procedures which are as little invasive as possible. Certain localized tumours at easily accessible sites or a very early stage, and even certain advanced cases, are increasingly diagnosed and treated entirely in out-patient departments or in a doctor's surgery without hospitalization or day-surgery. As a consequence, the use of a single source of notifications risks limiting the reliability of the registry in the medium term. The potential under-notification is more critical in that it would probably not be random but systematically concentrated in certain categories of cases.

The priorities of the Quebec Cancer Registry for the years to come are the following:

(*a*) to develop a more versatile computerized system to process the data;

(*b*) to diversify the sources of data to ensure completeness of cancer notification;

(*c*) to shorten the time taken to produce the data;

(*d*) to produce a databank centred on the person;

(*e*) to facilitate access to the data while protecting personal identifying information;

(*f*) to adapt to the specifications of the Canadian Cancer Registry;

(*g*) to reduce the amount of manual work required to identify new cases of primary cancer;

(*h*) to proceed to a linkage system with the death registry in order to obtain confirmation of death ('death clearance'), and to add the cases notified on the basis of death certificate only to the database.

The persons responsible for the registry have as their principal role, apart from monitoring the quality of the data, to support researchers using the registry. An annual report describes striking features of the data on incidence and mortality, how to obtain access to the registry data and the quality of the data. In April 1993, a study on survival related to cancer on the basis of the registry data was published.

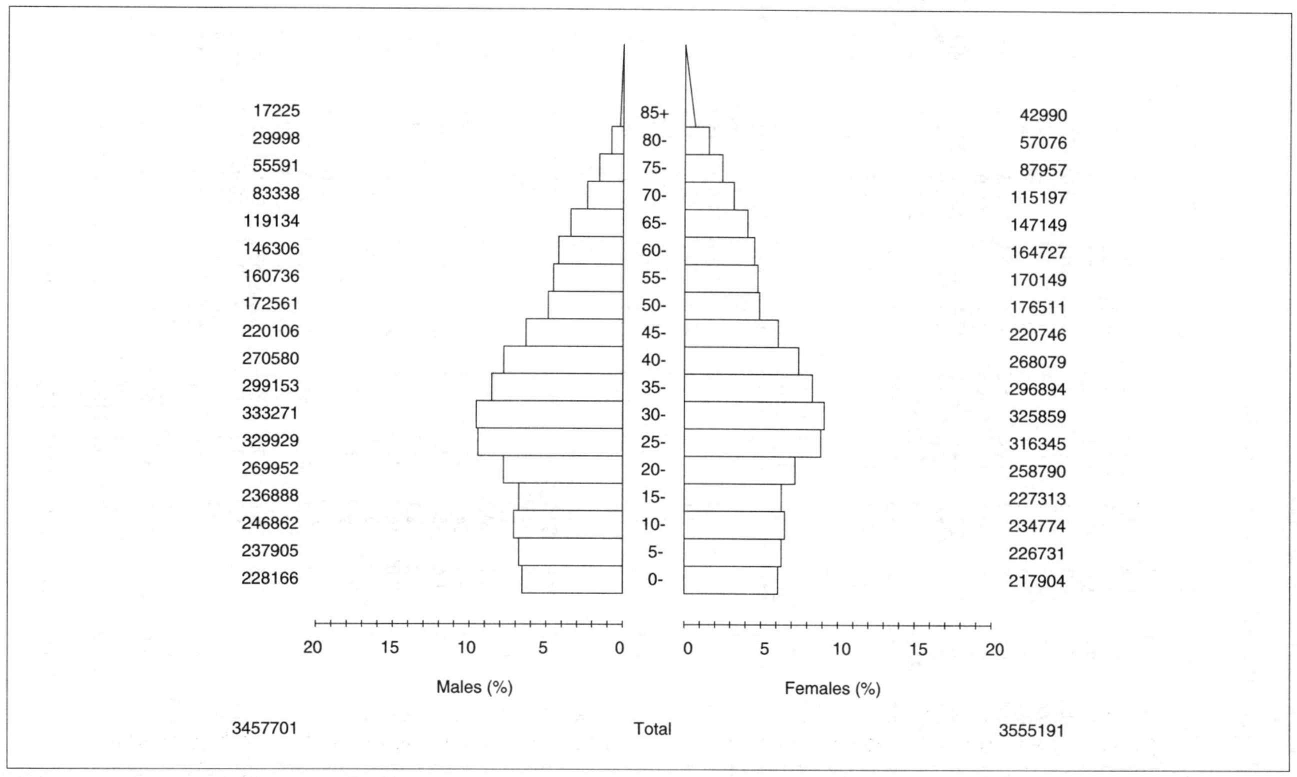

Canada, Quebec

Source of population: average annual 1988-92
Census: Statistics Canada June 1991
Estimate: The populations were estimated at 1 July each year, based on revised intercensal estimates for 1988-91 and post-censal estimates for 1992. In 1993 revised estimates dating back to 1971 were implemented by Statistics Canada and population data from 1971 now include estimates of net census undercoverage, plus non-permanent residents defined as persons claiming refugee status, foreign students, work permit holders, or holders of Minister's permits, and non-Canadian-born dependants of such individuals. References: Statistics Canada, Catalogue 91-537, Revised intercensal population and family estimates, July 1, 1971–91, and Catalogue 91-213, Annual demographic statistics 1993 (for 1992 data).

Notes to tables overleaf:
+ The editors were unable to verify these data
† Kaposi's sarcoma is under-reported in this volume because cases of skin cancer (ICD-9 173) were not provided
† 173 not available

+ CANADA, QUEBEC 1988-1992

ANNUAL INCIDENCE PER 100,000 BY AGE GROUP (YEARS) - MALE

SITE	ALL AGES	AGE UNK	0-	5-	10-	15-	20-	25-	30-	35-	40-	45-	50-	55-	60-	65-	70-	75-	80-	85+	CRUDE RATE	%	CR 64	CR 74	ASR (W)	ICD (9th)
Lip	400	0	-	-	-	-	0.1	0.2	0.3	0.2	0.4	1.4	2.0	5.0	7.1	8.2	13.9	21.6	38.0	40.6	2.3	0.6	0.08	0.19	1.9	140
Tongue	469	0	-	-	-	0.1	-	0.3	0.4	0.7	1.3	3.3	6.3	9.5	10.8	10.2	13.2	10.4	13.3	20.9	2.7	0.7	0.16	0.28	2.3	141
Salivary gland	193	0	-	0.1	0.2	0.1	0.1	0.3	0.4	0.5	0.7	1.1	1.4	2.5	3.7	4.0	5.0	8.3	8.0	10.4	1.1	0.3	0.05	0.10	0.9	142
Mouth	578	0	-	-	-	-	-	0.1	0.4	0.8	2.0	3.6	5.9	12.2	13.1	16.5	16.3	15.8	18.0	10.4	3.3	0.8	0.19	0.35	2.8	143-5
Oropharynx	340	0	-	-	-	-	-	0.1	0.2	0.6	0.6	2.9	4.9	5.5	8.2	9.2	7.7	10.8	6.0	16.3	2.0	0.5	0.11	0.20	1.7	146
Nasopharynx	122	0	-	-	-	0.2	0.1	0.2	0.2	0.5	0.8	0.9	2.3	2.9	1.6	2.4	1.7	1.4	1.3	2.3	0.7	0.2	0.05	0.07	0.6	147
Hypopharynx	291	0	-	-	-	-	-	-	0.1	0.1	0.1	1.5	3.6	6.2	9.3	8.6	8.2	9.0	5.3	4.6	1.7	0.4	0.10	0.19	1.5	148
Pharynx unspecified	163	0	-	-	-	-	0.1	-	0.1	0.1	0.4	0.8	0.8	3.2	4.6	5.0	4.3	5.8	5.3	7.0	0.9	0.2	0.05	0.10	0.8	149
Oesophagus	829	0	-	-	-	-	-	-	0.2	0.2	0.9	2.5	7.0	9.7	19.0	28.2	32.2	37.1	38.0	51.1	4.8	1.2	0.20	0.50	4.0	150
Stomach	2568	0	-	-	-	-	0.1	0.5	0.9	2.5	4.1	8.6	15.1	27.2	44.4	68.2	97.4	142.5	188.7	220.6	14.9	3.6	0.52	1.35	12.1	151
Small intestine	174	0	-	-	-	-	0.1	0.2	0.2	0.3	0.7	0.5	1.3	2.5	4.0	4.9	4.8	6.1	10.0	5.8	1.0	0.2	0.05	0.10	0.8	152
Colon	5558	0	-	-	-	0.3	0.1	0.8	1.7	3.7	8.5	18.0	34.8	66.3	109.1	155.6	231.1	280.6	354.0	361.1	32.1	7.9	1.22	3.15	26.4	153
Rectum	3734	0	-	-	-	-	0.1	0.5	1.0	3.1	6.6	14.6	30.3	53.5	78.5	108.8	142.3	173.8	180.0	177.6	21.6	5.3	0.94	2.20	18.0	154
Liver	756	0	0.7	0.1	0.2	0.2	0.3	0.3	0.4	0.8	1.3	2.5	3.5	10.3	14.9	26.9	27.1	34.9	34.7	30.2	4.4	1.1	0.18	0.45	3.7	155
Gallbladder etc.	472	0	-	0.1	-	-	-	0.1	-	0.5	0.9	1.5	2.5	4.2	7.0	14.6	16.6	29.1	35.3	41.8	2.7	0.7	0.08	0.24	2.2	156
Pancreas	1790	0	-	-	-	0.1	0.1	0.1	0.3	1.1	2.5	6.7	13.6	22.9	37.3	51.5	73.4	79.5	101.3	112.6	10.4	2.5	0.42	1.05	8.6	157
Nose, sinuses etc.	119	0	-	0.1	0.1	-	-	-	0.1	0.5	0.2	0.7	1.2	1.9	1.9	3.9	1.4	6.5	3.3	5.8	0.7	0.2	0.03	0.06	0.6	160
Larynx	1828	0	-	-	-	-	0.1	-	0.1	1.3	3.5	9.4	21.9	38.2	48.5	50.2	55.4	54.0	54.7	47.6	10.6	2.6	0.62	1.14	9.1	161
Bronchus, lung	17079	0	0.2	-	-	0.2	0.1	0.5	2.1	5.3	20.2	53.4	122.7	247.9	398.1	559.2	708.7	785.0	767.4	592.1	98.8	24.2	4.25	10.59	82.5	162
Other thoracic organs	182	0	0.7	0.1	0.2	0.4	0.7	0.2	0.4	0.7	0.4	0.2	1.3	1.5	3.0	3.4	5.8	7.9	9.3	4.6	1.1	0.3	0.05	0.09	0.9	163-4
Bone	265	0	0.3	0.7	1.4	1.8	1.2	0.7	1.0	0.9	1.0	1.1	1.6	2.4	3.1	5.0	2.4	5.0	6.0	15.1	1.5	0.4	0.09	0.12	1.4	170
Connective tissue	441	0	0.9	0.6	0.3	1.0	1.0	0.8	1.0	1.5	1.5	3.7	2.3	4.1	7.1	8.4	12.0	13.3	12.7	23.2	2.6	0.6	0.13	0.23	2.3	171
Mesothelioma	296	0	-	-	-	-	0.1	0.1	0.1	0.3	0.6	1.5	4.5	3.2	7.8	7.1	10.1	13.0	7.3	13.9	1.7	0.4	0.09	0.18	1.5	MES
†Kaposi's sarcoma	61	0	-	-	-	-	-	0.4	0.9	0.7	1.2	0.4	0.1	0.1	0.3	0.2	0.2	0.7	0.7	-	0.4	0.1	0.02	0.02	0.3	KAP
Melanoma of skin	749	0	0.2	0.1	0.1	0.7	0.7	1.5	2.5	4.1	4.3	6.8	10.8	7.7	12.0	12.4	14.2	16.5	18.0	20.9	4.3	1.1	0.26	0.39	3.7	172
†Other skin																										
Breast	150	0	-	-	-	-	-	0.1	-	0.4	0.4	1.0	1.9	3.6	3.9	5.0	9.4	7.3	10.4	0.9	0.2	0.04	0.08	0.7	175
Prostate	12117	0	-	-	-	-	-	0.1	0.3	0.8	4.7	22.8	82.7	208.1	397.4	632.4	803.7	982.7	1106.5	70.1	17.2	1.60	6.75	56.2	185
Testis	657	0	0.4	-	-	1.7	7.0	8.9	8.2	6.3	4.2	2.7	2.4	2.0	1.4	2.2	1.2	2.5	0.7	2.3	3.8	0.9	0.23	0.24	3.1	186
Penis	105	0	-	-	-	-	0.1	0.1	0.1	-	0.1	0.6	0.7	1.7	1.5	2.5	3.8	5.4	5.3	9.3	0.6	0.1	0.02	0.06	0.5	187.1-.4
Other male genital	33	0	-	0.1	-	0.1	0.1	-	0.1	0.1	0.1	0.4	0.1	0.5	0.3	0.7	0.5	1.1	2.7	2.3	0.2	0.0	0.01	0.01	0.2	187.5-.9
Bladder	4961	0	0.2	-	-	0.1	0.3	1.2	2.0	3.3	8.2	15.4	29.4	54.3	93.5	142.5	202.5	266.2	293.3	375.0	28.7	7.0	1.04	2.77	23.6	188
Kidney etc.	2372	0	1.9	0.5	-	0.1	0.1	0.5	1.4	3.5	6.6	13.6	21.6	35.1	47.2	62.1	81.4	88.1	104.0	108.0	13.7	3.4	0.66	1.38	11.7	189
Eye	167	0	1.4	0.1	-	0.2	0.1	0.1	0.2	0.7	0.4	1.3	1.2	2.1	2.2	3.0	6.7	5.0	4.0	4.6	1.0	0.2	0.05	0.10	0.9	190
Brain, nervous system	1403	0	4.2	3.3	2.3	3.5	2.8	3.6	4.1	5.9	6.1	8.6	10.0	14.2	21.3	28.5	30.2	31.7	36.0	24.4	8.1	2.0	0.45	0.74	7.3	191-2
Thyroid	307	0	-	0.1	-	0.8	0.9	1.1	1.3	1.8	2.4	2.5	3.4	3.4	3.6	5.2	4.8	5.0	6.7	2.3	1.8	0.4	0.11	0.16	1.5	193
Other endocrine	119	0	2.5	0.2	0.4	0.4	0.4	0.2	0.3	0.4	0.3	0.3	0.5	0.9	1.4	2.5	2.4	2.2	-	1.2	0.7	0.2	0.04	0.06	0.8	194
Hodgkin's disease	616	0	0.1	0.9	1.8	4.0	4.3	3.9	3.7	4.9	4.4	4.5	3.5	3.9	3.7	5.2	5.8	4.0	6.0	5.8	3.6	0.9	0.22	0.27	3.2	201
Non-Hodgkin lymphoma	2737	0	1.5	1.4	1.8	2.7	2.7	3.9	6.4	9.0	12.5	19.0	26.3	31.1	43.7	56.4	75.6	84.2	97.3	117.3	15.8	3.9	0.81	1.47	13.5	200,202
Multiple myeloma	827	0	-	-	0.1	-	-	-	0.5	0.6	1.3	2.5	5.8	9.3	12.2	21.8	39.1	48.6	51.3	52.2	4.8	1.2	0.16	0.47	3.9	203
Lymphoid leukaemia	1169	0	6.9	4.5	1.4	1.5	1.0	0.5	1.0	0.9	1.0	2.5	4.6	8.6	19.0	25.9	36.0	57.2	76.0	98.7	6.8	1.7	0.27	0.58	6.3	204
Myeloid leukaemia	646	0	0.8	0.7	0.6	1.1	0.4	1.1	1.1	1.9	1.9	4.0	3.6	5.7	8.7	12.3	22.3	28.1	30.0	45.3	3.7	0.9	0.16	0.33	3.2	205
Monocytic leukaemia	39	0	-	0.2	-	0.2	-	-	0.1	0.1	0.6	0.1	-	0.1	0.4	0.7	1.0	1.1	4.0	3.5	0.2	0.1	0.01	0.02	0.2	206
Other leukaemia	56	0	0.2	0.1	0.2	0.1	0.1	0.1	0.2	0.1	-	0.5	0.3	0.5	0.8	0.7	2.2	1.1	4.0	2.3	0.3	0.1	0.02	0.03	0.3	207
Leukaemia unspecified	248	0	0.5	0.2	0.1	0.1	0.4	0.3	0.4	0.3	0.3	0.6	1.0	2.0	4.8	5.9	7.4	14.0	16.7	17.4	1.4	0.4	0.06	0.12	1.2	208
Other and unspecified	2257	0	1.0	-	-	0.3	0.3	0.7	0.9	1.9	4.1	7.0	17.2	25.6	39.0	61.3	83.0	102.5	148.0	224.1	13.1	3.2	0.49	1.21	10.9	O&U
All sites																										
All sites but 173	70443	0	24.5	13.9	10.9	21.9	26.0	33.9	46.9	72.9	120.3	238.9	456.9	836.2	1370.7	2013.0	2748.8	3329.6	3792.8	4049.8	407.5	100.0	16.37	40.18	339.8	ALLb

Rate from 1 case	0.088	0.084	0.081	0.084	0.074	0.061	0.060	0.067	0.074	0.091	0.116	0.124	0.137	0.168	0.240	0.360	0.667	1.161

†Important: see notes on population page

+ CANADA, QUEBEC 1988-1992

ANNUAL INCIDENCE PER 100,000 BY AGE GROUP (YEARS) - FEMALE

SITE	ALL AGES	AGE UNK	0-	5-	10-	15-	20-	25-	30-	35-	40-	45-	50-	55-	60-	65-	70-	75-	80-	85+	CRUDE RATE	%	CR 64	CR 74	ASR (W)	ICD (9th)
Lip	55	0	-	-	-	-	-	-	-	0.1	-	0.4	0.3	0.4	0.8	0.7	1.2	1.8	2.1	5.1	0.3	0.1	0.01	0.02	**0.2**	*140*
Tongue	162	0	-	-	-	-	0.1	0.1	0.1	0.3	0.4	0.8	0.7	2.9	2.3	3.5	3.5	4.5	4.9	3.7	0.9	0.3	0.04	0.07	**0.6**	*141*
Salivary gland	128	0	0.2	-	0.1	-	0.2	0.3	0.3	0.9	0.4	0.6	1.0	0.8	1.7	2.0	1.9	3.0	2.5	5.1	0.7	0.2	0.03	0.05	**0.5**	*142*
Mouth	215	0	-	-	0.3	-	0.1	0.3	-	0.2	0.3	0.8	1.1	3.2	4.6	3.8	4.0	6.8	5.3	9.3	1.2	0.3	0.05	0.09	**0.8**	*143-5*
Oropharynx	108	0	-	-	-	-	0.1	-	0.1	0.2	0.3	0.7	1.5	1.8	2.3	1.2	3.0	2.0	1.8	1.9	0.6	0.2	0.03	0.06	**0.5**	*146*
Nasopharynx	40	0	0.2	-	-	-	-	0.1	0.1	0.2	0.1	0.4	0.3	0.5	0.6	0.4	1.0	0.9	-	0.5	0.2	0.1	0.01	0.02	**0.2**	*147*
Hypopharynx	48	0	-	-	-	-	-	-	-	-	0.1	0.2	0.5	0.6	1.3	1.0	1.9	0.7	1.1	0.5	0.3	0.1	0.01	0.03	**0.2**	*148*
Pharynx unspecified	46	0	-	-	-	-	0.1	0.1	-	-	-	0.3	0.2	0.8	1.1	0.4	1.2	2.0	1.1	0.5	0.3	0.1	0.01	0.02	**0.2**	*149*
Oesophagus	311	0	-	-	-	-	-	-	0.1	0.2	0.2	0.5	0.6	2.5	4.9	7.9	7.8	10.0	17.2	17.2	1.7	0.5	0.04	0.12	**1.0**	*150*
Stomach	1577	0	-	-	-	-	-	0.1	0.6	1.8	3.0	4.2	7.7	9.2	16.1	28.0	43.4	64.3	89.7	83.3	8.9	2.5	0.21	0.57	**5.2**	*151*
Small intestine	174	0	-	-	-	-	0.1	0.1	0.3	0.3	0.6	0.7	1.6	1.2	1.9	2.6	6.8	4.1	5.6	6.5	1.0	0.3	0.03	0.08	**0.6**	*152*
Colon	6105	0	-	-	0.1	-	0.2	0.8	1.7	5.2	9.1	19.0	29.5	57.6	80.6	114.6	164.9	223.3	285.6	301.5	34.3	9.8	1.02	2.42	**21.1**	*153*
Rectum	2817	0	-	-	-	-	0.1	0.4	0.8	2.1	5.5	10.3	18.7	31.4	42.5	56.3	71.4	93.2	112.5	111.2	15.8	4.5	0.56	1.20	**10.2**	*154*
Liver	404	0	0.5	0.1	-	-	0.2	0.3	0.2	0.2	1.0	1.1	2.3	3.4	5.3	8.2	9.9	13.4	16.5	20.5	2.3	0.6	0.07	0.16	**1.5**	*155*
Gallbladder etc.	678	0	-	-	-	-	-	-	0.1	0.3	0.7	1.4	3.2	5.2	8.5	13.6	19.1	24.3	31.5	44.7	3.8	1.1	0.10	0.26	**2.3**	*156*
Pancreas	1664	0	-	-	-	-	0.2	0.2	0.1	0.7	2.1	3.4	7.3	13.4	22.8	33.3	50.7	64.3	76.7	81.4	9.4	2.7	0.25	0.67	**5.7**	*157*
Nose, sinuses etc.	80	0	0.2	0.1	0.2	0.3	0.1	0.1	0.1	0.1	0.5	0.2	0.5	0.7	1.6	0.8	1.2	3.2	1.1	1.4	0.5	0.1	0.02	0.03	**0.4**	*160*
Larynx	432	0	-	-	-	-	-	-	0.1	0.6	1.3	3.4	5.0	7.6	9.6	10.5	8.9	5.5	4.9	5.6	2.4	0.7	0.14	0.23	**1.9**	*161*
Bronchus, lung	7023	0	-	-	0.1	0.1	0.2	0.6	3.6	7.9	18.8	35.0	62.9	94.6	132.7	163.4	181.4	184.9	155.2	110.7	39.5	11.3	1.78	3.51	**27.9**	*162*
Other thoracic organs	111	0	0.2	0.2	0.2	-	0.1	0.1	0.1	0.2	0.5	0.5	0.8	0.9	1.6	1.5	2.6	3.4	3.2	3.3	0.6	0.2	0.03	0.05	**0.5**	*163-4*
Bone	217	0	0.2	0.4	1.8	1.2	0.7	0.6	0.9	0.7	0.8	1.1	1.5	1.2	1.7	2.9	3.3	3.6	2.5	3.7	1.2	0.3	0.06	0.09	**1.1**	*170*
Connective tissue	379	0	0.6	0.7	0.5	1.1	1.2	1.6	0.7	2.0	1.3	1.9	2.6	2.9	4.0	4.5	5.2	9.3	6.3	10.2	2.1	0.6	0.11	0.15	**1.7**	*171*
Mesothelioma	88	0	-	-	-	-	-	-	0.1	0.1	0.4	0.4	0.9	0.8	1.9	2.3	1.2	2.3	1.8	3.3	0.5	0.1	0.02	0.04	**0.3**	*MES*
†Kaposi's sarcoma	2	0	-	-	-	-	-	-	-	-	-	-	-	-	-	0.1	0.2	-	-	-	0.0	0.0	0.00	0.00	**0.0**	*KAP*
Melanoma of skin	785	0	0.1	0.1	0.2	0.5	1.9	2.4	3.8	5.7	5.4	6.1	6.0	7.9	8.0	8.4	10.9	12.5	14.0	10.2	4.4	1.3	0.24	0.34	**3.3**	*172*
†Other skin																										
Breast	17503	0	-	-	-	-	0.5	7.1	22.7	53.4	103.3	152.7	182.1	212.2	266.9	298.1	338.9	368.4	372.5	331.2	98.5	28.0	5.00	8.19	**71.7**	*174*
Uterus unspecified	234	0	-	0.1	-	-	0.1	0.1	0.3	0.3	0.7	1.0	1.6	3.5	3.0	4.3	5.9	5.2	6.7	10.7	1.3	0.4	0.05	0.11	**0.9**	*179*
Cervix uteri	1602	0	-	-	-	0.1	1.8	6.7	11.7	13.3	12.2	12.1	13.3	12.2	13.0	18.5	19.8	21.6	25.6	19.5	9.0	2.6	0.48	0.67	**6.7**	*180*
Placenta	16	0	-	-	-	-	0.2	0.3	0.5	0.1	-	-	-	-	-	-	-	-	-	-	0.1	0.0	0.01	0.01	**0.1**	*181*
Corpus uteri	3369	0	-	-	-	-	0.1	0.2	1.6	3.2	8.6	13.7	34.6	46.2	64.1	78.8	89.6	88.9	77.1	42.8	19.0	5.4	0.86	1.70	**13.4**	*182*
Ovary etc.	2376	0	0.1	0.1	1.0	1.1	2.2	2.5	4.1	6.3	11.8	18.3	23.9	29.4	38.0	40.1	43.9	51.2	42.0	43.3	13.4	3.8	0.69	1.11	**9.9**	*183*
Other female genital	451	0	0.2	-	-	0.1	0.2	0.7	0.7	1.2	1.4	2.1	2.7	2.0	6.1	7.6	9.2	13.9	17.2	24.7	2.5	0.7	0.09	0.17	**1.6**	*184*
Bladder	1652	0	-	-	-	-	0.1	0.4	1.0	1.2	4.4	5.2	7.9	16.3	22.5	28.4	45.3	59.8	67.3	81.9	9.3	2.6	0.29	0.66	**5.8**	*188*
Kidney etc.	1588	0	2.3	0.8	0.2	0.2	0.2	0.6	1.0	2.6	4.0	6.8	12.7	18.1	25.9	31.4	35.1	40.0	58.2	46.5	8.9	2.5	0.38	0.71	**6.3**	*189*
Eye	137	0	1.0	0.1	0.3	-	-	0.2	0.3	0.7	0.6	0.6	0.9	0.9	1.6	2.0	3.5	3.0	1.8	2.8	0.8	0.2	0.04	0.06	**0.6**	*190*
Brain, nervous system	1140	0	4.1	2.7	2.3	1.7	1.9	2.3	2.9	3.4	4.4	4.4	8.8	9.4	15.4	17.1	24.3	22.3	23.8	15.8	6.4	1.8	0.32	0.53	**5.2**	*191-2*
Thyroid	888	0	0.1	0.2	0.9	1.6	3.6	4.2	5.8	5.7	6.6	6.4	6.3	9.5	7.2	8.3	9.5	9.6	8.1	11.6	5.0	1.4	0.29	0.38	**4.0**	*193*
Other endocrine	126	0	3.3	0.5	0.2	0.2	-	0.1	0.3	0.3	0.1	0.7	1.2	1.1	1.2	1.8	2.3	0.5	0.4	0.5	0.7	0.2	0.05	0.07	**0.8**	*194*
Hodgkin's disease	507	0	0.1	0.2	1.0	5.2	5.2	4.2	3.1	2.8	2.7	2.7	2.2	2.5	3.0	3.3	3.3	3.6	2.8	4.2	2.9	0.8	0.17	0.21	**2.6**	*201*
Non-Hodgkin lymphoma	2385	0	0.8	0.5	0.4	0.7	1.0	2.0	2.8	4.0	7.0	9.9	19.5	25.3	32.2	45.4	54.9	72.8	75.0	78.2	13.4	3.8	0.53	1.03	**9.1**	*200,202*
Multiple myeloma	761	0	-	-	-	-	-	-	0.1	0.2	0.7	1.4	2.6	6.7	10.9	15.6	24.1	29.8	36.1	34.4	4.3	1.2	0.11	0.31	**2.6**	*203*
Lymphoid leukaemia	776	0	6.3	3.5	1.4	0.6	0.5	0.3	0.3	0.3	0.7	1.3	2.2	3.4	5.2	11.4	18.4	24.8	39.2	45.1	4.4	1.2	0.13	0.28	**3.3**	*204*
Myeloid leukaemia	522	0	1.0	0.3	0.7	0.7	0.7	0.5	1.4	1.5	2.0	3.3	3.4	4.2	6.3	8.3	8.2	11.6	14.4	22.8	2.9	0.8	0.13	0.21	**2.2**	*205*
Monocytic leukaemia	43	0	0.2	-	-	0.1	0.1	-	-	0.1	-	0.1	0.2	0.2	0.2	0.3	1.6	1.6	2.1	2.8	0.2	0.1	0.01	0.02	**0.2**	*206*
Other leukaemia	59	0	0.4	-	0.2	0.1	0.1	0.2	0.2	0.1	-	0.6	0.5	0.1	0.4	0.4	0.7	0.9	2.5	4.7	0.3	0.1	0.01	0.02	**0.3**	*207*
Leukaemia unspecified	249	0	0.8	-	0.1	0.4	0.2	0.2	0.1	0.3	0.4	0.8	1.2	2.0	1.9	3.3	6.9	9.6	10.9	13.0	1.4	0.4	0.04	0.09	**0.9**	*208*
Other and unspecified	2382	0	2.1	0.2	-	0.2	0.2	0.8	1.0	2.6	4.4	7.2	11.0	18.6	28.4	37.0	57.3	87.1	113.2	162.4	13.4	3.8	0.38	0.85	**8.2**	*O&U*
All sites																										
All sites but 173	62415	0	24.9	10.7	12.0	16.1	24.1	41.9	75.9	133.8	229.2	344.6	495.3	675.3	912.1	1133.1	1409.2	1669.4	1839.3	1839.9	351.1	100.0	14.98	27.69	**244.4**	*ALLb*

Rate from 1 case   0.092   0.088   0.085   0.088   0.077   0.063   0.061   0.067   0.075   0.091   0.113   0.117   0.121   0.136   0.174   0.227   0.350   0.465

†Important: see notes on population page

Canada, Saskatchewan

The Saskatchewan Cancer Commission Act of 1930 authorized a commission to establish a cancer control programme in Saskatchewan. In 1932, comprehensive diagnostic and treatment services for cancer for all residents of the province were established. Registration dates from this time. In 1944, the costs of these services and of hospitalization were transferred from the patient to the Provincial Department of Health. In 1979, the Saskatchewan Cancer Foundation Act was passed establishing a Foundation to replace the Cancer Commission. The Foundation conducts a programme for the diagnosis, prevention and treatment of cancer. The Foundation maintains two service outlets—the Allan Blair Memorial Clinic in Regina and the Saskatoon Cancer Clinic. The clinics provide diagnosis, radiotherapy, chemotherapy and follow-up services. Registry services are an integral part of each clinic. The provincial screening programme for breast cancer was established in 1990.

The registry covers all of Saskatchewan, which lies between Alberta to the west, Manitoba to the east, the Northwest Territories to the north and the USA to the south, between latitudes 49° and 60° N and longitudes 102° and 110° W. Most of the province lies at altitudes of 300 m or above, and the majority of the population live in the southern half of the province. The total registration area covers 651 903 km^2.

At the 1989 census, the population consisted of 504 365 males and 505 250 females, some 32% of whom were under 20 years of age.

English is the main language of 91% of the population, while French is used by 1% and native Indian languages by approximately 2%.

In 1991, approximately 67% of the population resided in urban areas, with 35% living in the two largest cities (Regina and Saskatoon); 27% of the total population resides in rural areas while 6% live on reservations.

Agriculture is a primary occupation with approximately 24% of the male work force involved; sales, service and construction account for a further 27% of the workforce. 57% of women are employed in clerical and sales and service occupations.

The province is covered by a universal comprehensive health insurance plan. To be eligible for cancer payments under this plan, physicians are required to report all new cancer diagnoses to the registry. To complement this, copies of all malignant pathology reports are sent to the appropriate cancer clinic. These two notifications cover approximately 98% of all new cases diagnosed within the province. Further cases (1–2%) are discovered through death certificates which are received on a biweekly basis from the Vital Statistics branch of Saskatchewan Health.

The registry is patient-oriented. Data are coded according to ICD-O. Complete computerized information is available on all cancers diagnosed since 1967. For some major cancer sites (breast), conversion has been done back to 1950. In total there are currently about 158 500 patients on the database and about 203 000 case records. The growth rate of the file is about 7000 cases per year including all non-melanoma skin cancer.

Follow-up is active. Each case diagnosed (excluding non-melanoma skin cancers) is reviewed at least once a year either through a clinical examination or by letter to the referring/family physician. In situ cancers are followed for a disease-free period of three years and are then discontinued from the follow-up programme. Information on deaths within Saskatchewan is received directly from the vital statistics office every two weeks and matched against the active file. The rate of follow-up (excluding non-melanoma skin cancers) is currently 98.5% of all active cases.

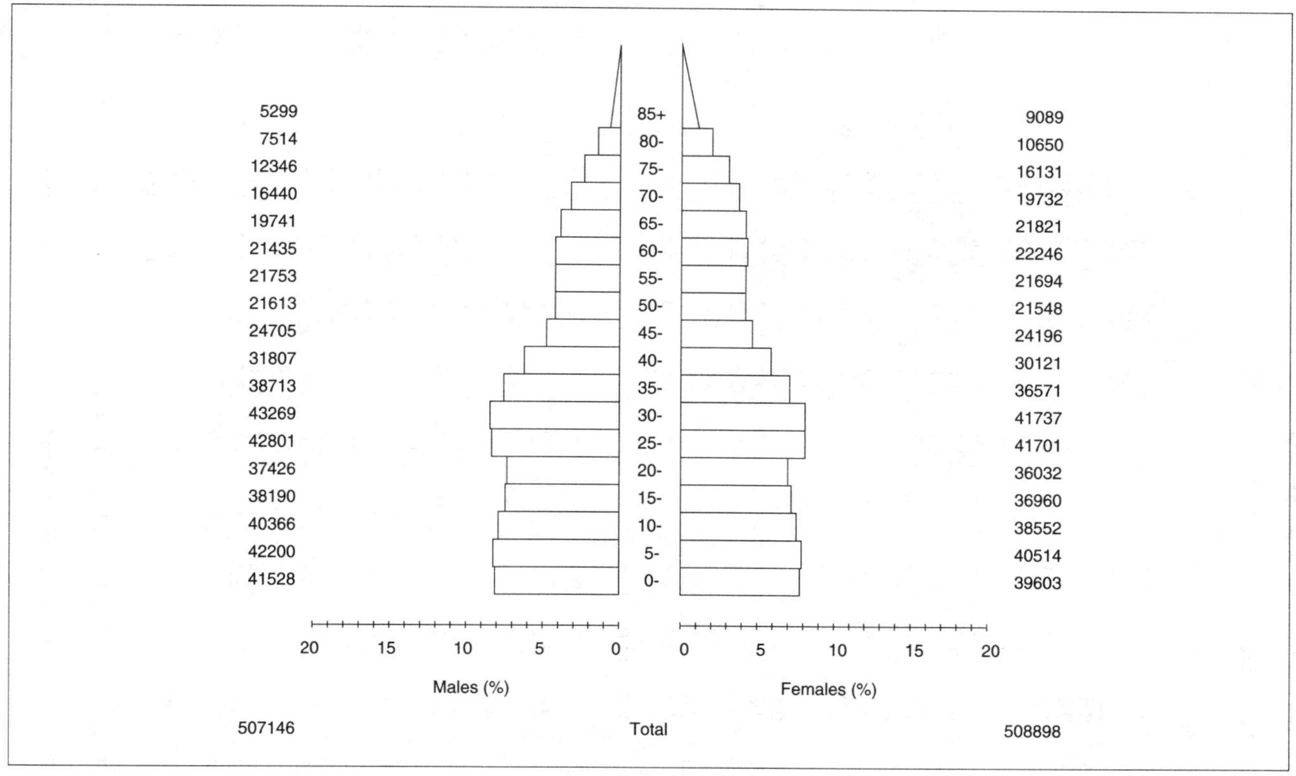

Canada, Saskatchewan
Source of population: average annual 1988-92
Census: Statistics Canada June 1991
Estimate: The populations were estimated at 1 July each year, based on revised intercensal estimates for 1988-91 and post-censal estimates for 1992. In 1993 revised estimates dating back to 1971 were implemented by Statistics Canada and population data from 1971 now include estimates of net census undercoverage, plus non-permanent residents defined as persons claiming refugee status, foreign students, work permit holders, or holders of Minister's permits, and non-Canadian-born dependants of such individuals. References: Statistics Canada, Catalogue 91-537, Revised intercensal population and family estimates, July 1, 1971–91, and Catalogue 91-213, Annual demographic statistics 1993 (for 1992 data).

Notes to tables overleaf:
† Kaposi's sarcoma is under-reported in this volume because cases of skin cancer (ICD-9 173) were not provided
† 173 not available
Screening programmes in the area:
Screening for breast cancer started in the 50-69 year old age-group in 1990.

CANADA, SASKATCHEWAN 1988-1992

ANNUAL INCIDENCE PER 100,000 BY AGE GROUP (YEARS) - MALE

SITE	ALL AGES	AGE UNK	0-	5-	10-	15-	20-	25-	30-	35-	40-	45-	50-	55-	60-	65-	70-	75-	80-	85+	CRUDE RATE	%	CR 64	CR 74	ASR (W)	ICD (9th)
Lip	283	0	-	-	-	-	-	-	1.8	1.0	2.5	6.5	21.3	25.7	22.4	44.6	73.0	64.8	55.9	94.3	11.2	2.5	0.41	0.99	**7.9**	140
Tongue	43	0	-	-	-	-	-	-	-	0.5	1.9	4.9	2.8	5.5	3.7	5.1	10.9	3.2	5.3	7.5	1.7	0.4	0.10	0.18	**1.4**	141
Salivary gland	21	0	-	-	-	0.5	-	-	-	-	1.3	-	1.9	0.9	1.9	3.0	2.4	1.6	16.0	3.8	0.8	0.2	0.03	0.06	**0.6**	142
Mouth	46	1	-	-	-	-	-	-	-	0.5	0.6	4.9	3.7	3.7	4.7	5.1	8.5	14.6	2.7	7.5	1.8	0.4	0.09	0.16	**1.4**	143-5
Oropharynx	24	0	-	-	-	-	-	-	-	-	0.6	0.8	-	4.6	6.5	3.0	-	4.9	8.0	3.8	0.9	0.2	0.06	0.08	**0.7**	146
Nasopharynx	18	0	-	-	-	0.5	-	-	-	1.0	1.3	-	1.9	3.7	-	4.1	2.4	-	2.7	-	0.7	0.2	0.04	0.07	**0.6**	147
Hypopharynx	33	0	-	-	-	-	-	-	-	-	1.9	0.8	2.8	6.4	1.9	9.1	2.4	3.2	10.6	-	1.3	0.3	0.07	0.13	**1.0**	148
Pharynx unspecified	11	0	-	-	-	-	-	-	-	-	-	0.8	-	2.8	1.9	1.0	1.2	3.2	2.7	-	0.4	0.1	0.03	0.04	**0.3**	149
Oesophagus	128	0	-	-	-	-	-	-	-	-	0.8	7.4	15.6	15.9	18.2	25.5	32.4	39.9	41.5	5.0	1.1	0.20	0.42	**3.5**	150
Stomach	360	0	-	-	-	-	-	-	0.5	0.6	5.7	6.5	22.1	28.9	54.7	80.3	102.1	143.7	192.5	14.2	3.2	0.32	1.00	**8.7**	151
Small intestine	37	0	-	-	-	-	-	-	0.5	0.5	-	-	0.9	4.6	5.6	6.1	10.9	4.9	10.6	3.8	1.5	0.3	0.06	0.15	**1.0**	152
Colon	890	0	-	-	-	-	-	2.3	0.9	4.1	11.3	17.0	37.0	43.2	87.7	123.6	187.3	265.7	319.4	358.5	35.1	8.0	1.02	2.57	**22.8**	153
Rectum	534	0	-	-	-	-	-	0.5	0.5	2.6	5.0	16.2	23.1	43.2	43.9	89.2	121.6	139.3	167.7	162.3	21.1	4.8	0.67	1.73	**14.3**	154
Liver	68	0	-	0.5	-	-	1.1	0.5	0.5	0.5	0.6	0.8	1.9	5.5	5.6	14.2	12.2	16.2	8.0	34.0	2.7	0.6	0.09	0.22	**1.9**	155
Gallbladder etc.	73	0	-	-	-	-	-	-	-	-	0.6	0.8	2.8	-	2.8	12.2	17.0	19.4	37.3	49.1	2.9	0.7	0.04	0.18	**1.7**	156
Pancreas	248	0	-	-	-	-	-	-	-	0.5	2.5	6.5	6.5	22.1	23.3	48.6	42.6	76.1	77.2	75.5	9.8	2.2	0.31	0.76	**6.5**	157
Nose, sinuses etc.	24	0	-	-	-	0.5	-	-	0.5	-	-	1.6	-	1.8	1.9	4.1	2.4	9.7	10.6	-	0.9	0.2	0.03	0.06	**0.6**	160
Larynx	143	0	-	-	-	-	-	-	-	-	0.6	0.8	6.5	23.0	32.7	23.3	29.2	24.3	18.6	18.9	5.6	1.3	0.32	0.58	**4.3**	161
Bronchus, lung	1936	1	-	-	-	-	-	0.5	1.4	2.1	13.8	25.9	77.7	146.2	267.8	379.9	455.0	479.5	508.3	403.8	76.3	17.3	2.68	6.85	**53.0**	162
Other thoracic organs	12	0	0.5	-	-	-	0.5	-	0.5	-	-	-	0.9	0.9	0.9	2.0	1.2	3.2	2.7	-	0.5	0.1	0.02	0.04	**0.4**	163-4
Bone	24	0	0.5	-	0.5	2.1	0.5	-	0.5	-	-	0.8	1.9	1.8	-	1.0	2.4	6.5	5.3	3.8	0.9	0.2	0.05	0.06	**0.8**	170
Connective tissue	65	0	1.9	0.5	2.0	1.0	2.1	0.9	0.5	2.6	3.8	1.6	2.8	2.8	7.5	3.0	4.9	3.2	13.3	22.6	2.6	0.6	0.15	0.19	**2.3**	171
Mesothelioma	24	0	-	-	-	-	-	-	0.5	-	1.3	0.8	1.9	1.8	2.8	2.0	3.6	8.1	8.0	-	0.9	0.2	0.05	0.07	**0.7**	MES
†Kaposi's sarcoma	2	0	-	-	-	-	-	0.5	-	-	-	-	-	-	-	-	1.2	-	-	-	0.1	0.0	0.00	0.01	**0.1**	KAP
Melanoma of skin	251	0	-	-	-	0.5	2.7	1.4	6.5	9.3	9.4	14.6	19.4	29.4	21.5	31.4	31.6	32.4	37.3	37.7	9.9	2.2	0.57	0.89	**8.0**	172
†Other skin																										175
Breast	23	0	-	-	-	-	-	-	1.0	-	1.6	0.9	0.9	2.8	3.0	2.4	4.9	10.6	7.5	-	0.9	0.2	0.04	0.06	**0.6**	175
Prostate	2857	1	-	-	-	-	-	-	-	-	0.6	4.9	24.1	105.7	242.6	509.6	733.5	1041.6	1099.2	1079.3	112.7	25.6	1.89	8.11	**66.8**	185
Testis	98	0	1.4	-	-	2.6	4.3	8.9	8.8	6.7	8.2	5.7	-	2.8	1.9	1.0	3.6	3.2	-	-	3.9	0.9	0.26	0.28	**3.5**	186
Penis	30	0	-	-	-	-	-	-	0.9	-	-	1.6	1.9	2.8	1.9	3.0	4.9	9.7	10.6	7.5	1.2	0.3	0.05	0.08	**0.8**	187.1-.4
Other male genital	9	0	-	-	-	-	0.5	-	-	-	0.6	-	0.9	-	-	2.0	3.6	-	2.7	-	0.4	0.1	0.01	0.04	**0.3**	187.5-.9
Bladder	748	0	-	0.5	-	-	0.5	0.9	0.5	5.7	6.3	17.0	20.4	48.7	68.1	131.7	167.9	196.0	239.5	279.3	29.5	6.7	0.84	2.34	**19.5**	188
Kidney etc.	415	0	2.4	0.9	-	-	0.5	-	1.8	5.2	4.4	12.1	24.1	23.0	46.7	72.9	87.6	116.6	90.5	75.5	16.4	3.7	0.61	1.41	**11.8**	189
Eye	45	0	0.5	0.5	-	-	-	0.5	0.9	1.0	1.9	-	2.8	1.8	5.6	8.1	14.6	3.2	2.7	3.8	1.8	0.4	0.08	0.19	**1.4**	190
Brain, nervous system	171	0	5.8	1.9	4.0	0.5	1.1	3.3	2.3	5.2	5.7	6.5	14.8	15.6	17.7	22.3	15.8	13.0	16.0	15.1	6.7	1.5	0.42	0.61	**6.2**	191-2
Thyroid	76	0	-	-	-	0.5	0.5	0.5	2.8	2.1	5.7	6.5	5.6	10.1	4.7	6.1	12.2	6.5	8.0	3.8	3.0	0.7	0.19	0.29	**2.6**	193
Other endocrine	8	0	-	-	-	1.0	-	-	0.5	-	-	0.8	-	-	0.9	-	1.2	1.6	-	3.8	0.3	0.1	0.02	0.02	**0.3**	194
Hodgkin's disease	73	0	-	-	1.0	1.6	6.9	5.6	1.8	2.6	1.9	4.9	7.4	2.8	2.8	4.1	2.4	4.9	2.7	3.8	2.9	0.7	0.20	0.23	**2.7**	201
Non-Hodgkin lymphoma	431	0	1.0	0.5	2.5	1.6	2.1	2.8	4.6	8.3	7.5	16.2	26.8	42.3	42.0	50.7	83.9	92.3	74.5	105.7	17.0	3.9	0.79	1.46	**12.9**	200,202
Multiple myeloma	155	0	-	-	-	-	-	0.5	0.5	-	0.6	4.0	9.3	13.8	12.1	30.4	31.6	42.1	37.3	49.1	6.1	1.4	0.20	0.51	**4.2**	203
Lymphoid leukaemia	253	0	10.1	1.9	2.5	2.6	-	-	-	0.5	3.8	5.7	13.0	10.1	30.8	45.6	37.7	61.6	55.9	41.5	10.0	2.3	0.40	0.82	**8.0**	204
Myeloid leukaemia	122	0	-	-	0.5	-	0.5	2.3	2.3	2.1	3.1	3.2	11.1	3.7	13.1	22.3	10.9	19.4	37.3	37.7	4.8	1.1	0.21	0.38	**3.6**	205
Monocytic leukaemia	13	0	-	-	-	-	0.5	-	-	0.5	-	0.8	-	0.9	0.9	3.0	-	3.2	8.0	-	0.5	0.1	0.02	0.03	**0.4**	206
Other leukaemia	1	0	0.5	-	-	-	-	-	-	-	-	-	-	-	-	-	-	-	-	-	0.0	0.0	0.00	0.00	**0.1**	207
Leukaemia unspecified	23	0	-	-	-	-	-	-	-	-	0.6	-	0.9	-	2.8	4.1	2.4	8.1	16.0	3.8	0.9	0.2	0.02	0.05	**0.5**	208
Other and unspecified	322	0	0.5	-	-	0.5	1.1	0.5	1.4	2.6	1.9	5.7	5.6	19.3	25.2	39.5	54.7	90.7	130.4	211.3	12.7	2.9	0.32	0.79	**7.9**	O&U
All sites																										
All sites but 173	11171	3	25.0	7.1	12.9	16.2	25.1	33.2	43.4	69.7	112.6	209.7	400.7	721.7	1114.1	1847.9	2401.3	3037.2	3353.5	3449.2	440.5	100.0	13.96	35.21	**298.5**	ALLb
Rate from 1 case			0.482	0.474	0.495	0.524	0.534	0.467	0.462	0.517	0.629	0.810	0.925	0.919	0.933	1.013	1.216	1.620	2.661	3.774						

†Important: see notes on population page

CANADA, SASKATCHEWAN 1988-1992

ANNUAL INCIDENCE PER 100,000 BY AGE GROUP (YEARS) - FEMALE

SITE	ALL AGES	AGE UNK	0-	5-	10-	15-	20-	25-	30-	35-	40-	45-	50-	55-	60-	65-	70-	75-	80-	85+	CRUDE RATE	%	CR 64	CR 74	ASR (W)	ICD (9th)
Lip	30	0	-	-	-	-	-	-	0.5	-	-	-	0.9	1.8	-	4.6	8.1	2.5	13.1	8.8	1.2	0.3	0.02	0.08	0.6	140
Tongue	21	0	-	-	-	-	-	0.5	-	-	-	0.8	0.9	3.7	1.8	1.8	1.0	1.2	13.1	2.2	0.8	0.2	0.04	0.05	0.5	141
Salivary gland	22	0	-	-	-	-	1.1	0.5	0.5	0.5	0.7	0.8	0.9	1.8	0.9	2.7	3.0	3.7	1.9	2.2	0.9	0.2	0.04	0.07	0.6	142
Mouth	42	0	-	-	-	-	-	0.5	1.0	0.5	0.7	0.8	3.7	1.8	3.6	7.3	6.1	5.0	1.9	15.4	1.7	0.5	0.06	0.13	1.1	143-5
Oropharynx	9	0	-	-	-	-	-	-	-	-	-	-	-	3.7	-	2.7	2.0	-	-	-	0.4	0.1	0.02	0.04	0.3	146
Nasopharynx	4	0	-	-	-	-	-	-	-	-	-	-	0.9	-	-	-	2.0	-	1.9	-	0.2	0.0	0.00	0.01	0.1	147
Hypopharynx	6	0	-	-	-	-	-	-	-	-	-	-	0.9	-	2.7	0.9	-	1.2	-	-	0.2	0.1	0.02	0.02	0.2	148
Pharynx unspecified	3	0	-	-	-	-	-	-	0.5	-	-	-	-	-	0.9	-	1.0	-	-	-	0.1	0.0	0.01	0.01	0.1	149
Oesophagus	53	0	-	-	-	-	0.6	-	-	-	0.7	0.8	0.9	0.9	6.3	3.7	11.1	11.2	13.1	22.0	2.1	0.6	0.05	0.13	1.1	150
Stomach	178	0	-	-	-	-	-	1.0	0.5	1.6	2.0	3.3	4.6	5.5	19.8	14.7	27.4	38.4	50.7	68.2	7.0	2.0	0.19	0.40	3.7	151
Small intestine	31	0	-	-	-	-	-	-	0.5	-	0.7	1.7	-	0.9	1.8	10.1	5.1	5.0	3.8	4.4	1.2	0.3	0.03	0.10	0.8	152
Colon	885	0	-	-	-	-	-	-	1.0	4.4	8.0	16.5	33.4	51.6	71.9	117.3	136.8	172.3	247.9	301.4	34.8	9.7	0.93	2.20	19.1	153
Rectum	363	0	-	-	-	-	-	0.5	1.0	0.5	2.7	9.1	15.8	20.3	39.6	55.0	47.6	69.4	86.4	114.4	14.3	4.0	0.45	0.96	8.3	154
Liver	40	0	-	-	-	-	-	-	0.5	-	0.7	-	-	3.7	3.6	3.7	7.1	8.7	9.4	15.4	1.6	0.4	0.04	0.10	0.8	155
Gallbladder etc.	116	0	-	-	-	-	-	-	-	0.5	1.3	0.8	3.7	6.5	4.5	10.1	25.3	21.1	43.2	44.0	4.6	1.3	0.09	0.26	2.2	156
Pancreas	262	0	-	-	-	-	-	-	-	-	1.3	0.8	8.4	14.8	21.6	29.3	50.7	57.0	82.6	83.6	10.3	2.9	0.23	0.63	5.3	157
Nose, sinuses etc.	10	0	-	-	-	-	-	-	-	-	-	-	-	0.9	-	0.9	2.0	5.0	1.9	2.2	0.4	0.1	0.00	0.02	0.2	160
Larynx	22	0	-	-	-	-	-	0.5	-	-	1.3	-	2.8	3.7	3.6	5.5	2.0	-	-	-	0.9	0.2	0.06	0.10	0.8	161
Bronchus, lung	866	0	-	-	-	-	-	-	2.4	6.0	16.6	27.3	54.8	80.2	127.7	161.3	133.8	121.5	105.2	92.4	34.0	9.5	1.57	3.05	23.9	162
Other thoracic organs	11	0	0.5	-	-	-	-	-	0.5	0.5	0.7	1.7	-	0.9	-	1.8	1.0	-	1.9	-	0.4	0.1	0.02	0.04	0.4	163-4
Bone	22	0	-	0.5	1.0	2.2	1.1	1.0	0.5	0.5	-	0.8	-	-	2.7	0.9	1.0	3.7	-	-	0.9	0.2	0.05	0.06	0.8	170
Connective tissue	49	0	1.5	0.5	-	0.5	1.1	0.5	1.4	1.1	1.3	2.5	0.9	3.7	2.7	5.5	4.1	5.0	9.4	8.8	1.9	0.5	0.09	0.14	1.5	171
Mesothelioma	7	0	-	-	-	-	-	-	-	-	-	-	0.9	-	1.8	0.9	-	1.2	1.9	2.2	0.3	0.1	0.01	0.02	0.2	MES
†Kaposi's sarcoma	1	0	-	-	-	-	-	-	-	-	-	-	-	-	-	0.9	-	-	-	-	0.0	0.0	0.00	0.00	0.0	KAP
Melanoma of skin	242	0	-	-	-	1.1	2.8	7.2	11.5	18.0	14.6	14.9	14.9	11.1	16.2	16.5	21.3	19.8	20.7	24.2	9.5	2.7	0.56	0.75	7.6	172
†Other skin																										
Breast	2757	0	-	-	-	-	-	3.8	24.0	53.6	95.6	144.7	201.4	236.9	312.9	376.7	384.1	389.3	364.3	356.4	108.4	30.3	5.36	9.17	77.9	174
Uterus unspecified	11	0	-	-	-	-	-	-	-	-	-	-	0.9	1.8	-	-	2.0	2.5	3.8	4.4	0.4	0.1	0.01	0.02	0.2	179
Cervix uteri	240	0	-	-	-	-	2.8	9.6	10.5	18.6	21.2	18.2	10.2	11.1	8.1	22.0	10.1	31.0	15.0	13.2	9.4	2.6	0.55	0.71	7.7	180
Placenta	0	0	-	-	-	-	-	-	-	-	-	-	-	-	-	-	-	-	-	-	0.0	0.0	0.00	0.00	0.0	181
Corpus uteri	494	0	-	-	-	-	-	1.4	1.0	4.9	11.3	18.2	40.8	51.6	54.8	73.3	72.0	75.6	82.6	52.8	19.4	5.4	0.92	1.65	13.6	182
Ovary etc.	359	0	-	2.0	-	1.1	2.8	3.8	2.9	8.2	12.0	16.5	26.0	35.0	38.7	40.3	49.7	55.8	31.9	37.4	14.1	4.0	0.74	1.19	10.6	183
Other female genital	60	0	-	-	-	-	-	0.5	0.5	0.5	-	3.3	5.6	2.8	3.6	8.2	7.1	12.4	20.7	6.6	2.4	0.7	0.08	0.16	1.5	184
Bladder	243	1	-	-	-	-	-	0.5	1.9	0.5	3.3	7.4	8.4	13.8	23.4	33.9	38.5	43.4	54.5	72.6	9.5	2.7	0.30	0.66	5.6	188
Kidney etc.	237	0	3.0	0.5	-	-	1.1	0.5	1.0	3.3	2.7	5.0	12.1	14.8	21.6	33.9	44.6	42.2	45.1	37.4	9.3	2.6	0.33	0.72	6.1	189
Eye	22	0	1.0	-	-	-	-	-	-	0.5	1.3	0.8	-	-	1.8	3.7	1.0	3.7	5.6	6.6	0.9	0.2	0.03	0.05	0.6	190
Brain, nervous system	113	0	3.0	3.5	2.6	2.2	0.6	1.9	3.8	1.6	2.7	2.5	8.4	6.5	10.8	11.9	14.2	7.4	9.4	4.4	4.4	1.2	0.25	0.38	3.9	191-2
Thyroid	120	0	-	-	-	2.2	3.3	6.2	4.3	4.4	7.3	8.3	8.4	10.1	8.1	8.2	9.1	11.2	-	6.6	4.7	1.3	0.31	0.40	4.1	193
Other endocrine	12	0	-	0.5	0.5	-	0.6	-	-	1.1	-	0.8	1.9	-	0.9	0.9	2.0	-	-	-	0.5	0.1	0.03	0.05	0.5	194
Hodgkin's disease	47	0	-	-	1.0	2.7	3.3	1.9	2.4	1.6	1.3	2.5	-	1.8	1.8	4.6	3.0	5.0	1.9	-	1.8	0.5	0.10	0.14	1.6	201
Non-Hodgkin lymphoma	375	0	0.5	0.5	0.5	-	1.7	0.5	2.9	3.8	10.0	6.6	17.6	32.3	42.3	47.7	52.7	75.6	84.5	46.2	14.7	4.1	0.60	1.10	9.5	200,202
Multiple myeloma	98	0	-	-	-	-	-	-	0.5	-	-	0.8	1.9	8.3	6.3	9.2	23.3	16.1	43.2	19.8	3.9	1.1	0.09	0.25	2.0	203
Lymphoid leukaemia	172	0	7.6	3.0	1.6	1.6	-	-	1.0	0.5	0.7	1.7	6.5	11.1	18.9	19.2	15.2	38.4	37.6	26.4	6.8	1.9	0.27	0.44	4.8	204
Myeloid leukaemia	82	0	1.0	-	0.5	0.5	1.7	2.4	1.4	0.5	2.7	-	2.8	1.8	4.5	9.2	15.2	18.6	11.3	13.2	3.2	0.9	0.10	0.22	2.1	205
Monocytic leukaemia	7	0	-	0.5	-	-	-	-	-	-	-	-	0.9	-	0.9	0.9	1.0	1.2	-	2.2	0.3	0.1	0.01	0.02	0.2	206
Other leukaemia	2	0	0.5	-	-	-	-	-	-	-	-	-	0.9	-	-	-	-	-	-	-	0.1	0.0	0.01	0.01	0.1	207
Leukaemia unspecified	16	0	-	-	-	-	-	-	-	-	0.7	0.8	-	-	-	2.7	-	2.5	5.6	13.2	0.6	0.2	0.01	0.02	0.3	208
Other and unspecified	324	0	-	-	-	-	-	0.5	1.4	1.1	4.6	3.3	8.4	16.6	34.2	35.7	45.6	76.9	80.7	116.6	12.7	3.6	0.35	0.76	6.9	O&U
All sites																										
All sites but 173	9086	1	18.7	11.4	7.8	14.1	24.4	45.6	81.5	139.5	230.4	324.0	511.4	673.9	927.8	1200.7	1290.3	1461.7	1607.5	1648.0	357.1	100.0	15.05	27.51	239.8	ALLb

Rate from 1 case: 0.505   0.494   0.519   0.541   0.555   0.480   0.479   0.547   0.664   0.827   0.928   0.922   0.899   0.917   1.014   1.240   1.878   2.200

†Important: see notes on population page

Canada, Yukon

Formed in 1994, the Yukon Cancer Registry includes historical data back to the mid-1980s. The British Columbia Cancer Agency maintains the Yukon Registry along with its own provincial data.

Located in the north-western corner of Canada, the Yukon Territory borders Canada's Northwest Territories to the east and the province of British Columbia to the south. The Yukon represents 5% of Canada's total land area (483 450 km^2), making it the eighth largest of Canada's ten provinces and two territories.

With a population of 31 395 in 1992, the Yukon is Canada's least populated province or territory. Whitehorse, the territorial capital, is home to over 70% of the population. Eleven of Yukon's 16 communities have a population of under 500 people. In the last ten years, the annual rate of population increase in the Yukon was 2.4%. The Yukon has a relatively young population, with 24% under the age of 15 years and an overall average age of 32 years. Only 4% of the population is over 65 years old. Despite the small population and high number of small communities, all communities but one are accessible by road. One quarter of the population is of aboriginal origin (mainly Athapaskan and Tlinkit).

Health programmes and services in the Yukon are provided through 11 health centres, 4 nursing stations and 2 hospitals. Many Yukon residents are sent outside the territory for diagnosis and treatment of cancer due to a lack of resident specialized services. As a result, diagnosis and reporting of cancer incidence and mortality in Yukon residents occur in other provinces (primarily in British Columbia) as well as in the Yukon.

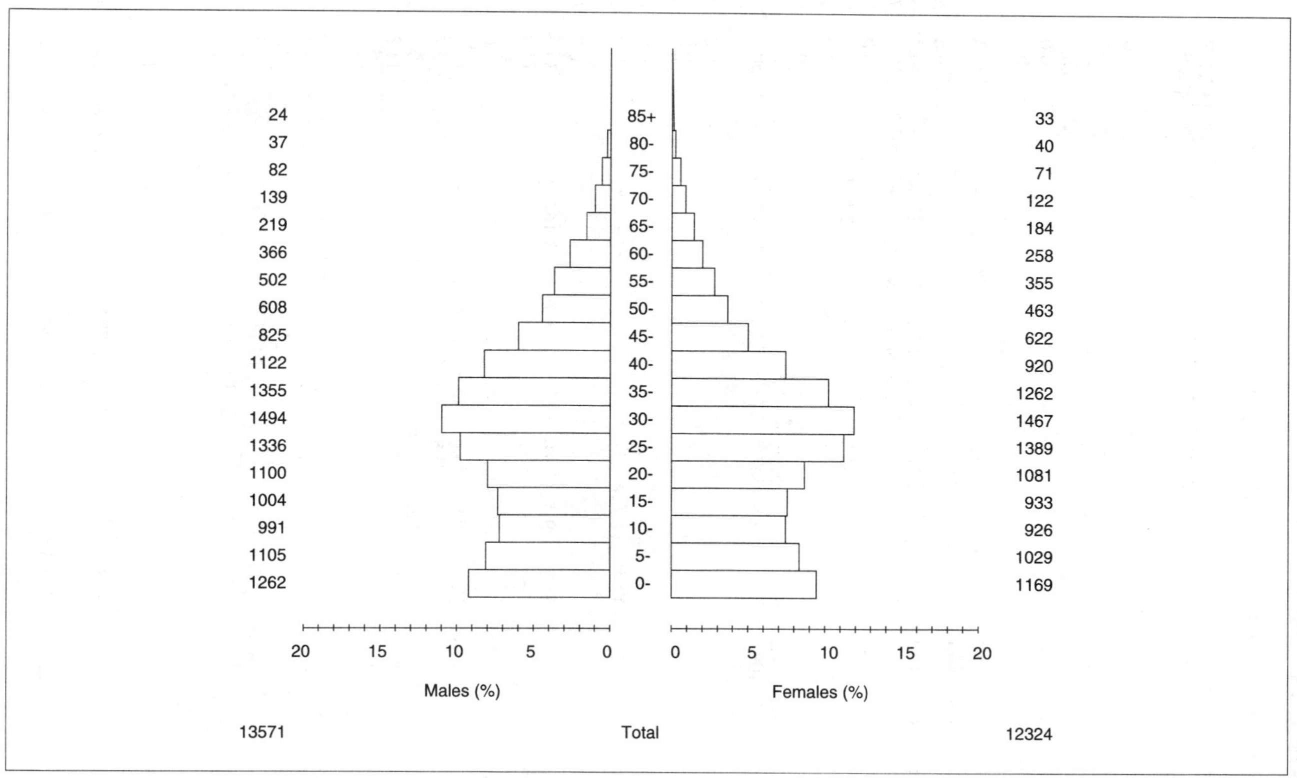

Canada, Yukon
Source of population: average annual 1988-92
Census: Statistics Canada June 1991
Estimate: The populations were estimated at 1 July each year, based on revised intercensal estimates for 1988-91 and post-censal estimates for 1992. In 1993 revised estimates dating back to 1971 were implemented by Statistics Canada and population data from 1971 now include estimates of net census undercoverage, plus non-permanent residents defined as persons claiming refugee status, foreign students, work permit holders, or holders of Minister's permits, and non-Canadian-born dependants of such individuals. References: Statistics Canada, Catalogue 91-537, Revised intercensal population and family estimates, July 1, 1971–91, and Catalogue 91-213, Annual demographic statistics 1993 (for 1992 data).

Notes to tables overleaf:
† Kaposi's sarcoma is under-reported in this volume because cases of skin cancer (ICD-9 173) were not provided
† 173 not available

CANADA, YUKON 1983-1992

ANNUAL INCIDENCE PER 100,000 BY AGE GROUP (YEARS) - MALE

SITE	ALL AGES	AGE UNK	0-	5-	10-	15-	20-	25-	30-	35-	40-	45-	50-	55-	60-	65-	70-	75-	80-	85+	CRUDE RATE	%	CR 64	CR 74	ASR (W)	ICD (9th)
Lip	3	0	-	-	-	-	-	-	-	14.8	-	-	-	-	27.3	-	-	-	-	-	2.2	0.9	0.21	0.21	**2.0**	140
Tongue	0	0	-	-	-	-	-	-	-	-	-	-	-	-	-	-	-	-	-	-	0.0	0.0	0.00	0.00	**0.0**	141
Salivary gland	1	0	-	-	-	-	-	-	-	-	-	-	16.4	-	-	-	-	-	-	-	0.7	0.3	0.08	0.08	**0.8**	142
Mouth	9	0	-	-	-	-	-	-	-	-	-	24.2	32.9	19.9	54.6	-	143.9	-	-	-	6.6	2.8	0.66	1.38	**9.0**	143-5
Oropharynx	1	0	-	-	-	-	-	-	-	-	-	-	16.4	-	-	-	-	-	-	-	0.7	0.3	0.08	0.08	**0.8**	146
Nasopharynx	0	0	-	-	-	-	-	-	-	-	-	-	-	-	-	-	-	-	-	-	0.0	0.0	0.00	0.00	**0.0**	147
Hypopharynx	0	0	-	-	-	-	-	-	-	-	-	-	-	-	-	-	-	-	-	-	0.0	0.0	0.00	0.00	**0.0**	148
Pharynx unspecified	2	0	-	-	-	-	-	-	-	-	-	-	-	-	-	-	143.9	-	-	-	1.5	0.6	0.00	0.72	**2.9**	149
Oesophagus	6	0	-	-	-	-	-	-	-	-	-	12.1	-	-	109.2	-	-	121.1	-	-	4.4	1.8	0.61	0.61	**6.3**	150
Stomach	7	0	-	-	-	-	-	-	-	-	17.8	24.2	16.4	-	27.3	45.6	-	-	-	-	5.2	2.2	0.43	0.66	**5.8**	151
Small intestine	0	0	-	-	-	-	-	-	-	-	-	-	-	-	-	-	-	-	-	-	0.0	0.0	0.00	0.00	**0.0**	152
Colon	14	0	-	-	-	-	-	-	-	7.4	8.9	12.1	-	39.8	27.3	91.2	143.9	121.1	810.8	-	10.3	4.3	0.48	1.65	**15.3**	153
Rectum	25	0	-	-	-	-	-	-	-	-	-	-	32.9	-	-	365.0	431.7	847.5	-	803.2	18.4	7.7	0.16	4.15	**33.7**	154
Liver	0	0	-	-	-	-	-	-	-	-	-	-	-	-	-	-	-	-	-	-	0.0	0.0	0.00	0.00	**0.0**	155
Gallbladder etc.	3	0	-	-	-	-	-	-	-	-	-	-	54.6	-	-	-	-	270.3	-	-	2.2	0.9	0.27	0.27	**3.5**	156
Pancreas	4	0	-	-	-	-	-	-	-	-	-	-	39.8	27.3	-	71.9	-	-	-	-	2.9	1.2	0.34	0.70	**4.1**	157
Nose, sinuses etc.	0	0	-	-	-	-	-	-	-	-	-	-	-	-	-	-	-	-	-	-	0.0	0.0	0.00	0.00	**0.0**	160
Larynx	4	0	-	-	-	-	-	-	-	-	-	24.2	-	-	-	91.2	-	-	-	-	2.9	1.2	0.12	0.58	**4.2**	161
Bronchus, lung	69	0	7.9	-	-	-	-	-	-	-	8.9	109.0	296.0	198.8	382.2	273.7	503.6	242.1	270.3	-	50.8	21.2	5.01	8.90	**68.1**	162
Other thoracic organs	0	0	-	-	-	-	-	-	-	-	-	-	-	-	-	-	-	-	-	-	0.0	0.0	0.00	0.00	**0.0**	163-4
Bone	0	0	-	-	-	-	-	-	-	-	-	-	-	-	-	-	-	-	-	-	0.0	0.0	0.00	0.00	**0.0**	170
Connective tissue	0	0	-	-	-	-	-	-	-	-	-	-	-	-	-	-	-	-	-	-	0.0	0.0	0.00	0.00	**0.0**	171
Mesothelioma	0	0	-	-	-	-	-	-	-	-	-	-	-	-	-	-	-	-	-	-	0.0	0.0	0.00	0.00	**0.0**	MES
†Kaposi's sarcoma	0	0	-	-	-	-	-	-	-	-	-	-	-	-	-	-	-	-	-	-	0.0	0.0	0.00	0.00	**0.0**	KAP
Melanoma of skin	9	0	-	-	-	-	-	-	-	44.3	-	-	49.3	-	-	-	-	-	-	-	6.6	2.8	0.47	0.47	**5.1**	172
†Other skin																										175
Breast	1	0	-	-	-	-	-	-	-	-	-	-	-	-	-	-	-	121.1	-	-	0.7	0.3	0.00	0.00	**1.2**	175
Prostate	53	0	-	-	-	-	-	-	-	-	-	-	65.8	99.4	273.0	638.7	719.4	484.3	1621.6	-	39.0	16.3	2.19	8.98	**64.7**	185
Testis	19	0	-	-	-	-	27.3	-	53.5	36.9	26.7	-	-	-	-	-	-	-	-	-	14.0	5.8	0.72	0.72	**9.2**	186
Penis	1	0	-	-	-	-	-	-	-	-	-	-	16.4	-	-	-	-	-	-	-	0.7	0.3	0.08	0.08	**0.8**	187.1-.4
Other male genital	0	0	-	-	-	-	-	-	-	-	-	-	-	-	-	-	-	-	-	-	0.0	0.0	0.00	0.00	**0.0**	187.5-.9
Bladder	15	0	-	-	-	-	-	-	-	-	-	12.1	16.4	19.9	54.6	45.6	503.6	242.1	-	-	11.0	4.6	0.52	3.26	**18.4**	188
Kidney etc.	7	0	-	-	-	-	-	-	-	-	17.8	-	-	-	81.9	-	-	242.1	-	-	5.2	2.2	0.50	0.50	**6.8**	189
Eye	1	0	-	-	-	-	-	-	-	-	-	-	-	19.9	-	-	-	-	-	-	0.7	0.3	0.10	0.10	**0.8**	190
Brain, nervous system	16	0	-	-	-	-	18.2	29.9	6.7	-	-	36.3	82.2	-	27.3	-	-	-	-	-	11.8	4.9	1.00	1.00	**11.6**	191-2
Thyroid	1	0	-	-	-	-	-	-	-	-	-	12.1	-	-	-	-	-	-	-	-	0.7	0.3	0.06	0.06	**0.7**	193
Other endocrine	0	0	-	-	-	-	-	-	-	-	-	-	-	-	-	-	-	-	-	-	0.0	0.0	0.00	0.00	**0.0**	194
Hodgkin's disease	8	0	-	-	-	-	18.2	-	-	7.4	-	-	-	-	-	-	-	605.3	-	-	5.9	2.5	0.13	0.13	**7.9**	201
Non-Hodgkin lymphoma	8	0	-	-	-	-	-	20.1	-	-	-	24.2	-	-	81.9	-	-	-	-	-	5.9	2.5	0.63	0.63	**5.9**	200,202
Multiple myeloma	6	0	-	-	-	-	-	7.5	-	14.8	-	-	-	19.9	-	-	143.9	-	-	-	4.4	1.8	0.21	0.93	**5.2**	203
Lymphoid leukaemia	11	0	7.9	-	-	19.9	-	-	-	-	-	24.2	16.4	79.5	-	-	71.9	-	-	-	8.1	3.4	0.74	1.10	**9.6**	204
Myeloid leukaemia	2	0	-	-	-	-	-	-	-	-	-	12.1	-	-	27.3	-	-	-	-	-	1.5	0.6	0.20	0.20	**1.8**	205
Monocytic leukaemia	2	0	-	-	-	-	-	-	-	-	17.8	-	-	-	-	-	-	-	-	-	1.5	0.6	0.09	0.09	**1.1**	206
Other leukaemia	0	0	-	-	-	-	-	-	-	-	-	-	-	-	-	-	-	-	-	-	0.0	0.0	0.00	0.00	**0.0**	207
Leukaemia unspecified	0	0	-	-	-	-	-	-	-	-	-	-	-	-	-	-	-	-	-	-	0.0	0.0	0.00	0.00	**0.0**	208
Other and unspecified	17	0	-	-	-	-	-	-	-	-	8.9	24.2	-	59.7	81.9	273.7	-	242.1	-	-	12.5	5.2	0.87	2.24	**18.3**	O&U
All sites	325	0	15.8	-	-	19.9	63.6	37.4	80.3	125.4	106.9	351.1	657.8	596.5	1337.7	1824.8	2877.7	3268.8	2973.0	803.2	239.3	100.0	16.96	40.48	**325.7**	ALLb
All sites but 173																										

Rate from 1 case 7.919 9.042 10.084 9.955 9.083 7.483 6.692 7.375 8.909 12.108 16.445 19.885 27.300 45.620 71.942 121.07 270.27 401.61

†Important: see notes on population page

CANADA, YUKON 1983-1992

ANNUAL INCIDENCE PER 100,000 BY AGE GROUP (YEARS) - FEMALE

SITE	ALL AGES	UNK	0-	5-	10-	15-	20-	25-	30-	35-	40-	45-	50-	55-	60-	65-	70-	75-	80-	85+	CRUDE RATE	%	CR 64	CR 74	ASR (W)	ICD (9th)
Lip	1	0	-	-	-	-	-	-	-	-	-	-	-	-	-	54.1	-	-	-	-	0.8	0.4	0.00	0.27	**1.6**	140
Tongue	2	0	-	-	-	-	-	-	-	-	-	-	-	-	77.4	-	-	-	-	-	1.6	0.7	0.39	0.39	**3.1**	141
Salivary gland	0	0	-	-	-	-	-	-	-	-	-	-	-	-	-	-	-	-	-	-	0.0	0.0	0.00	0.00	**0.0**	142
Mouth	1	0	-	-	-	-	-	-	-	-	-	-	-	-	-	54.1	-	-	-	-	0.8	0.4	0.00	0.27	**1.6**	143-5
Oropharynx	2	0	-	-	-	-	-	-	-	-	-	16.1	21.6	-	-	-	-	-	-	-	1.6	0.7	0.19	0.19	**2.0**	146
Nasopharynx	0	0	-	-	-	-	-	-	-	-	-	-	-	-	-	-	-	-	-	-	0.0	0.0	0.00	0.00	**0.0**	147
Hypopharynx	1	0	-	-	-	-	-	-	-	-	-	-	-	-	-	-	-	139.3	-	-	0.8	0.4	0.00	0.00	**1.4**	148
Pharynx unspecified	2	0	-	-	-	-	-	-	-	-	21.7	-	-	-	-	-	-	-	-	-	1.6	0.7	0.11	0.11	**1.3**	149
Oesophagus	0	0	-	-	-	-	-	-	-	-	-	-	-	-	-	-	-	-	-	-	0.0	0.0	0.00	0.00	**0.0**	150
Stomach	4	0	-	-	-	-	-	-	-	-	21.7	-	-	-	-	-	163.3	-	-	-	3.2	1.5	0.11	0.93	**4.6**	151
Small intestine	0	0	-	-	-	-	-	-	-	-	-	-	-	-	-	-	-	-	-	-	0.0	0.0	0.00	0.00	**0.0**	152
Colon	7	0	-	-	-	-	-	-	-	-	-	16.1	21.6	84.5	-	-	163.3	-	-	-	5.7	2.6	0.61	1.43	**8.7**	153
Rectum	12	0	-	-	-	-	-	-	-	-	-	-	107.9	84.5	-	-	-	139.3	248.1	595.2	9.7	4.4	0.96	0.96	**14.4**	154
Liver	1	0	8.6	-	-	-	-	-	-	-	-	-	-	-	-	-	-	-	-	-	0.8	0.4	0.04	0.04	**1.0**	155
Gallbladder etc.	2	0	-	-	-	-	-	-	-	-	-	-	-	28.2	-	-	-	-	248.1	-	1.6	0.7	0.14	0.14	**2.4**	156
Pancreas	3	0	-	-	-	-	-	-	-	-	-	-	-	-	-	108.3	-	139.3	-	-	2.4	1.1	0.00	0.54	**4.6**	157
Nose, sinuses etc.	0	0	-	-	-	-	-	-	-	-	-	-	-	-	-	-	-	-	-	-	0.0	0.0	0.00	0.00	**0.0**	160
Larynx	0	0	-	-	-	-	-	-	-	-	-	-	-	-	-	-	-	-	-	-	0.0	0.0	0.00	0.00	**0.0**	161
Bronchus, lung	39	0	-	-	-	-	-	-	-	7.9	43.5	32.1	107.9	337.8	232.1	270.7	244.9	139.3	-	-	31.6	14.3	3.81	6.38	**47.6**	162
Other thoracic organs	0	0	-	-	-	-	-	-	-	-	-	-	-	-	-	-	-	-	-	-	0.0	0.0	0.00	0.00	**0.0**	163-4
Bone	0	0	-	-	-	-	-	-	-	-	-	-	-	-	-	-	-	-	-	-	0.0	0.0	0.00	0.00	**0.0**	170
Connective tissue	3	0	-	-	-	-	-	-	23.8	-	-	-	-	-	-	-	-	-	-	-	2.4	1.1	0.12	0.12	**1.4**	171
Mesothelioma	0	0	-	-	-	-	-	-	-	-	-	-	-	-	-	-	-	-	-	-	0.0	0.0	0.00	0.00	**0.0**	MES
†Kaposi's sarcoma	0	0	-	-	-	-	-	-	-	-	-	-	-	-	-	-	-	-	-	-	0.0	0.0	0.00	0.00	**0.0**	KAP
Melanoma of skin	11	0	-	-	-	-	-	-	13.6	31.7	21.7	48.2	-	-	-	-	-	-	-	-	8.9	4.0	0.58	0.58	**6.9**	172
†Other skin																										
Breast	77	0	-	-	-	-	-	-	68.1	55.4	87.0	273.0	237.4	225.2	-	270.7	571.4	-	744.4	297.6	62.4	28.2	4.73	8.94	**74.7**	174
Uterus unspecified	0	0	-	-	-	-	-	-	-	-	-	-	-	-	-	-	-	-	-	-	0.0	0.0	0.00	0.00	**0.0**	179
Cervix uteri	15	0	-	-	-	-	37.0	-	20.4	7.9	-	32.1	21.6	-	-	108.3	-	-	496.3	-	12.2	5.5	0.60	1.14	**13.4**	180
Placenta	0	0	-	-	-	-	-	-	-	-	-	-	-	-	-	-	-	-	-	-	0.0	0.0	0.00	0.00	**0.0**	181
Corpus uteri	15	0	-	-	-	-	-	-	-	-	10.9	-	43.2	84.5	232.1	162.4	-	-	-	-	12.2	5.5	1.85	2.67	**20.3**	182
Ovary etc.	17	0	-	-	-	-	-	7.2	6.8	7.9	-	64.2	21.6	56.3	38.7	270.7	81.6	-	-	-	13.8	6.2	1.01	2.78	**19.9**	183
Other female genital	1	0	-	-	-	-	-	-	6.8	-	-	-	-	-	-	-	-	-	-	-	0.8	0.4	0.03	0.03	**0.4**	184
Bladder	0	0	-	-	-	-	-	-	-	-	-	-	-	-	-	-	-	-	-	-	0.0	0.0	0.00	0.00	**0.0**	188
Kidney etc.	5	0	17.1	-	-	-	-	-	-	-	10.9	-	-	-	77.4	-	-	-	-	-	4.1	1.8	0.53	0.53	**5.8**	189
Eye	0	0	-	-	-	-	-	-	-	-	-	-	-	-	-	-	-	-	-	-	0.0	0.0	0.00	0.00	**0.0**	190
Brain, nervous system	1	0	-	-	-	-	-	-	-	-	-	-	-	28.2	-	-	-	-	-	-	0.8	0.4	0.14	0.14	**1.1**	191-2
Thyroid	6	0	-	-	-	-	-	14.4	-	-	21.7	32.1	-	-	-	-	-	-	-	-	4.9	2.2	0.34	0.34	**4.4**	193
Other endocrine	0	0	-	-	-	-	-	-	-	-	-	-	-	-	-	-	-	-	-	-	0.0	0.0	0.00	0.00	**0.0**	194
Hodgkin's disease	6	0	-	-	-	10.7	18.5	14.4	-	7.9	-	-	-	-	-	-	-	-	-	-	4.9	2.2	0.26	0.26	**4.1**	201
Non-Hodgkin lymphoma	5	0	-	-	-	-	-	-	-	7.9	-	16.1	-	-	-	77.4	54.1	-	-	-	4.1	1.8	0.51	0.78	**6.2**	200,202
Multiple myeloma	4	0	-	-	-	-	-	-	-	-	-	-	21.6	84.5	-	-	-	-	-	-	3.2	1.5	0.53	0.53	**4.5**	203
Lymphoid leukaemia	10	0	34.2	-	-	-	-	-	-	-	-	64.2	-	-	-	77.4	-	-	-	-	8.1	3.7	0.88	0.88	**11.1**	204
Myeloid leukaemia	1	0	-	-	-	-	-	-	-	-	10.9	-	-	-	-	-	-	-	-	-	0.8	0.4	0.05	0.05	**0.7**	205
Monocytic leukaemia	0	0	-	-	-	-	-	-	-	-	-	-	-	-	-	-	-	-	-	-	0.0	0.0	0.00	0.00	**0.0**	206
Other leukaemia	0	0	-	-	-	-	-	-	-	-	-	-	-	-	-	-	-	-	-	-	0.0	0.0	0.00	0.00	**0.0**	207
Leukaemia unspecified	0	0	-	-	-	-	-	-	-	-	-	-	-	-	-	-	-	-	-	-	0.0	0.0	0.00	0.00	**0.0**	208
Other and unspecified	19	0	17.1	-	-	-	-	-	-	-	10.9	-	43.2	-	-	216.6	81.6	1114.2	-	297.6	15.4	7.0	0.36	1.85	**25.6**	O&U
All sites																										
All sites but 173	273	0	77.0	-	-	10.7	55.5	36.0	115.8	150.5	260.9	594.2	647.5	1013.5	812.4	1570.1	1306.1	1671.3	1737.0	1190.5	221.4	100.0	18.87	33.25	**294.8**	ALLb

Rate from 1 case   8.551   9.716   10.799   10.715   9.243   7.199   6.814   7.921   10.870   16.059   21.584   28.153   38.685   54.142   81.633   139.28   248.14   297.62

†Important: see notes on population page

USA, California, Central Valley

The Cancer Registry of Central California is the population-based cancer registry that monitors all newly diagnosed cancers and cancer deaths in the Central Valley of California. It began operations in 1987 and was population-based beginning in 1988 and data are now available through 1993. It is one of ten regional registries which provide data to the California Cancer Registry (CCR), the state-wide central registry in Sacramento.

The area covered by the registry includes nine counties extending from Kern County in the south (latitude 35° N) to Stanislaus County in the north (latitude 37° N). It is bounded to the east by the Sierra Nevada mountains and to the west by the coastal range. In 1993 the population of the Central Valley was approximately 2 500 000, the majority living in Fresno (670 000), Kern (544 000), Stanislaus (370 000) and Tulare (311 000) counties. Two counties lying on the western slopes of the Sierra Nevada are sparsely populated (Mariposa County with a population of 14 000 and Tuolumne County with a population of 48 000).

The population of the region is ethnically diverse: 32% are Hispanic, 57% are non-Hispanic whites, 4% blacks and 7% Asian or other. The age-distribution in the Central Valley is younger than in the rest of California. For example, 27% of all Californians are less than 17 years of age, compared with more than 30% of Central Valley residents. More residents of the Central Valley live below the poverty level than elsewhere in the state and the median family income in this area is less than $30 000 per year compared to more than $40 000 per year throughout the state. Both the birth rate and the fertility rate among females in the Central Valley are much higher than in the rest of the state. These rates are germane to risk of breast cancer and cervical cancer in the region.

Cigarette smoking is more common among males in the Central Valley than elsewhere: while 20.3% of males throughout California are current smokers, for the Central Valley the figure is 24%. The percentage of former smokers is higher as well.

Agriculture is the dominant industry in the Central Valley. Fresno County alone is the leading producer of agricultural commodities in the United States. For this reason there is a distinct population of seasonal and migrant farm workers. Half of the state's approximately 800 000 live and work in the Central Valley and pose a special data-collection challenge in that many of them are migrant and undocumented.

The sources of cancer diagnoses in the region are the hospital record and the pathology report. There are 52 hospitals in the region, of which 11 are approved by the American College of Surgeons (ACoS). These ACoS hospitals have in-house registries and report all new diagnoses directly to the registry electronically. It is estimated that 65% of all diagnoses occur in the ACoS-approved hospitals. The rest of the hospitals are visited by state-approved subcontractors who periodically review records and complete cancer abstract forms or by regional registry staff who do the same. All abstracts are completed using the same computer program wherever the information is originally collected.

The cancer abstract form itself includes information on the patient, diagnostic procedures, physician(s), tumour data, and treatment data. Follow-up information is available only on patients seen at the ACoS hospitals.

The primary function of the registry is to provide numerator data allowing the calculation of accurate incidence rates. Since the Central Valley of California has been the location of several reported cancer clusters, accurate incidence rates are very valuable. Also, the registry serves an analytical purpose in that population-based case–control studies can be conducted utilizing its resources. Also, the registry provides qualified researchers with non-confidential information on such variables as stage at diagnosis, grade and histology for selected cancer sites of interest. The first annual report from the registry (*Cancer Incidence in the Central Valley, 1988-1993*) includes information on more than 50 000 incident cancers.

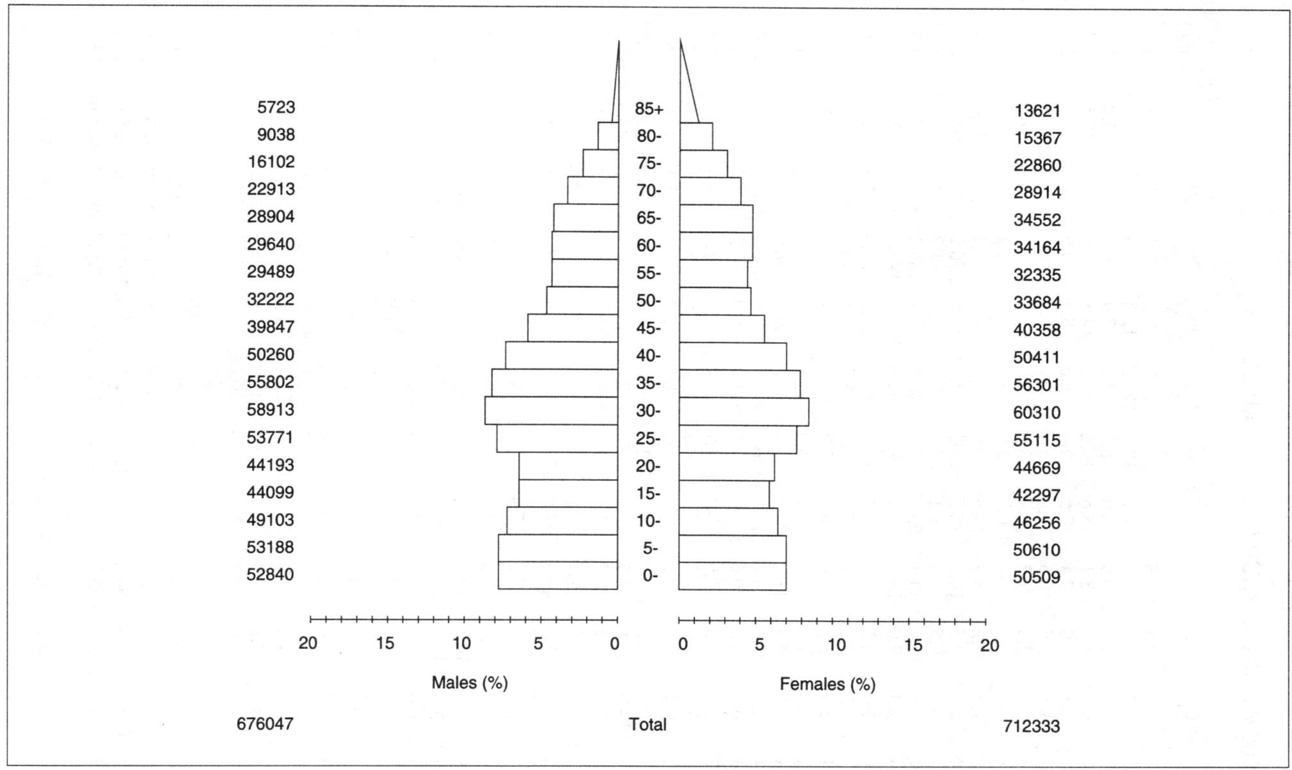

USA, California, Central Valley: Non-Hispanic White

Source of population: average annual 1988–92

Estimate: Annual mid-year population estimates by age, race/ethnicity and sex to the county level for non-Hispanic whites, non-Hispanic blacks, Hispanics and non-Hispanic Asian/Others were obtained from the California Department of Finance (DOF) Demographic Research Unit. Estimates for 1988, 1989 and 1990 are from a special population summary for 1970–90 with gender, age and race-ethnic detail released by DOF in April 1993, benchmarked to the 1990 Census.

Estimates for 1991 and 1992 are from current estimates of the California population with gender, age and race/ethnic detail consistent with Report 93 E-2. Reference: California Department of Finance. Population Estimates for California State and Counties: Report 93 E-2. Sacramento, CA: California Department of Finance, Demographic Research Unit, February 1994.

Notes to tables overleaf:

+ The editors were unable to verify these data

† 173 does not include basal cell or squamous cell carcinoma

+ USA, CALIFORNIA, CENTRAL VALLEY: NON-HISPANIC WHITE 1988-1992

ANNUAL INCIDENCE PER 100,000 BY AGE GROUP (YEARS) - MALE

SITE	ALL AGES	AGE UNK	0-	5-	10-	15-	20-	25-	30-	35-	40-	45-	50-	55-	60-	65-	70-	75-	80-	85+	CRUDE RATE	%	CR 64	CR 74	ASR (W)	ICD (9th)
Lip	141	0	-	-	-	-	-	0.4	1.0	-	0.8	3.5	5.6	11.5	12.1	18.7	17.5	22.4	19.9	34.9	4.2	0.8	0.17	0.36	3.0	140
Tongue	106	0	-	-	-	-	-	0.7	-	1.1	1.2	2.5	5.0	14.2	13.5	15.2	12.2	2.5	11.1	3.5	3.1	0.6	0.19	0.33	2.5	141
Salivary gland	47	0	-	-	-	0.5	-	-	-	0.7	-	3.0	0.6	2.0	6.1	4.2	7.9	6.2	6.6	7.0	1.4	0.3	0.06	0.12	1.0	142
Mouth	125	0	-	-	-	-	0.5	0.4	-	1.1	0.8	4.0	8.1	13.6	14.2	13.1	14.8	14.9	11.1	10.5	3.7	0.7	0.21	0.35	2.9	143-5
Oropharynx	72	0	-	-	-	-	-	-	-	-	1.6	2.0	7.4	7.5	9.4	9.0	5.2	9.9	-	-	2.1	0.4	0.14	0.21	1.7	146
Nasopharynx	29	0	-	-	-	0.5	-	0.4	-	0.4	1.6	1.5	0.6	1.4	5.4	0.7	1.7	1.2	6.6	3.5	0.9	0.2	0.06	0.07	0.7	147
Hypopharynx	48	0	-	-	-	-	-	-	-	-	-	2.0	1.2	6.1	3.4	5.5	7.9	6.2	8.9	7.0	1.4	0.3	0.06	0.13	1.0	148
Pharynx unspecified	15	0	-	-	-	-	-	-	-	-	-	-	0.7	2.0	2.8	5.2	1.2	-	-	-	0.4	0.1	0.01	0.05	0.3	149
Oesophagus	183	0	-	-	-	-	0.5	-	0.7	0.4	1.2	5.0	8.7	13.6	20.9	23.5	31.4	12.4	37.6	14.0	5.4	1.0	0.25	0.53	4.0	150
Stomach	358	0	-	-	-	-	0.5	-	0.3	1.4	2.4	4.5	10.6	18.3	24.3	38.1	58.5	78.2	99.6	94.3	10.6	2.0	0.31	0.79	6.9	151
Small intestine	59	0	-	-	-	-	-	-	-	1.1	-	0.5	3.1	6.1	3.4	9.0	6.1	11.2	13.3	3.5	1.7	0.3	0.07	0.15	1.2	152
Colon	1295	0	-	0.4	-	-	-	1.1	0.7	3.9	11.1	13.6	34.1	53.6	85.7	144.6	218.2	288.1	360.7	377.4	38.3	7.4	1.02	2.84	24.4	153
Rectum	742	0	-	-	-	-	-	0.4	1.0	3.6	8.0	9.0	24.8	33.2	68.8	92.0	128.3	144.1	137.2	143.3	22.0	4.2	0.74	1.85	14.8	154
Liver	127	0	0.8	-	0.4	-	0.5	-	-	1.1	2.4	3.5	2.5	6.8	11.5	13.1	20.1	23.6	13.3	31.4	3.8	0.7	0.15	0.31	2.7	155
Gallbladder etc.	79	0	-	-	-	-	-	-	-	-	1.2	1.0	1.9	2.0	6.7	8.3	13.1	19.9	13.3	31.4	2.3	0.4	0.06	0.17	1.5	156
Pancreas	387	0	-	-	-	0.5	-	0.4	0.3	0.4	2.4	5.5	9.9	18.3	31.7	51.2	72.4	79.5	77.4	69.9	11.4	2.2	0.35	0.97	7.6	157
Nose, sinuses etc.	37	0	-	-	-	-	-	-	-	0.4	-	1.5	1.9	4.7	2.0	2.8	6.1	5.0	6.6	7.0	1.1	0.2	0.05	0.10	0.8	160
Larynx	277	0	-	-	-	-	-	0.4	-	0.4	2.0	6.5	11.2	20.3	33.1	36.0	40.2	46.0	39.8	24.5	8.2	1.6	0.37	0.75	5.9	161
Bronchus, lung	3487	1	-	-	-	0.5	-	0.4	0.3	5.4	12.7	45.7	118.6	217.7	356.3	496.1	572.6	675.7	564.3	464.8	103.2	19.9	3.79	9.13	71.1	162
Other thoracic organs	13	0	-	-	-	-	0.5	0.4	-	0.4	0.8	0.5	0.6	-	1.4	0.9	2.5	2.2	-	-	0.4	0.1	0.02	0.03	0.3	163-4
Bone	43	0	-	0.4	2.4	1.8	1.4	0.4	-	0.7	2.0	0.5	1.9	0.7	2.7	1.4	4.4	3.7	4.4	-	1.3	0.2	0.07	0.10	1.2	170
Connective tissue	95	0	1.9	-	0.8	0.9	0.9	0.4	1.0	1.8	2.0	-	4.3	5.4	4.7	13.8	7.0	8.7	24.3	7.0	2.8	0.5	0.12	0.23	2.2	171
Mesothelioma	66	0	-	-	-	-	-	-	0.3	-	0.4	1.0	2.5	3.4	5.4	8.3	12.2	12.4	11.1	14.0	2.0	0.4	0.07	0.17	1.3	MES
Kaposi's sarcoma	66	0	-	-	-	-	1.8	5.6	5.4	3.6	2.4	1.5	-	4.1	1.3	-	-	3.7	-	3.5	2.0	0.4	0.13	0.13	1.6	KAP
Melanoma of skin	537	0	-	-	-	0.9	2.3	6.3	9.2	10.8	14.3	23.6	21.7	27.1	43.9	57.4	56.7	58.4	55.3	45.4	15.9	3.1	0.80	1.37	12.1	172
†Other skin	48	0	-	-	-	-	0.5	-	0.3	0.7	0.4	0.5	1.2	1.4	4.7	4.2	8.7	8.7	8.9	14.0	1.4		0.05	0.11	1.0	173
Breast	18	0	-	-	-	-	-	-	-	-	-	0.5	1.2	2.0	1.3	2.1	1.7	5.0	2.2	-	0.5	0.1	0.03	0.04	0.4	175
Prostate	5078	2	-	-	-	-	-	-	0.3	-	2.0	15.6	42.8	154.0	350.9	735.5	1057.9	1227.1	1332.1	1251.0	150.2	28.9	2.83	11.80	91.9	185
Testis	191	0	-	0.4	-	2.3	8.1	13.8	13.9	14.0	7.6	6.5	3.7	2.0	2.0	2.1	1.7	-	2.2	-	5.7	1.1	0.37	0.39	5.0	186
Penis	31	0	-	-	-	-	-	-	-	-	0.4	0.5	0.6	2.7	3.4	2.8	6.1	2.5	11.1	3.5	0.9	0.2	0.04	0.08	0.6	187.1-.4
Other male genital	11	0	-	-	-	-	-	0.4	-	-	-	1.0	0.6	-	2.0	-	0.9	3.7	-	-	0.3	0.1	0.02	0.02	0.3	187.5-.9
Bladder	926	0	-	-	-	-	-	0.4	0.7	1.8	8.0	10.5	18.6	48.2	76.9	102.4	139.7	190.0	267.8	279.6	27.4	5.3	0.83	2.04	17.7	188
Kidney etc.	470	0	1.1	0.8	-	-	-	-	-	2.5	4.4	12.5	23.0	35.9	41.2	63.0	58.5	83.2	68.6	52.4	13.9	2.7	0.61	1.21	10.1	189
Eye	46	0	1.1	-	-	-	-	0.4	0.7	-	0.8	1.5	1.2	4.7	7.4	2.1	4.4	3.7	4.4	7.0	1.4	0.3	0.09	0.12	1.1	190
Brain, nervous system	291	0	3.4	2.6	2.0	2.3	2.3	3.7	3.1	4.7	7.6	8.5	16.1	23.1	16.9	22.8	34.0	22.4	28.8	14.0	8.6	1.7	0.48	0.77	7.2	191-2
Thyroid	98	0	-	0.4	0.8	0.5	1.8	2.2	2.4	3.2	3.2	3.5	6.2	4.7	4.0	6.9	7.0	9.9	8.9	-	2.9	0.6	0.16	0.23	2.4	193
Other endocrine	24	0	0.8	-	0.4	0.9	1.4	0.4	-	-	0.4	1.0	0.6	0.7	2.7	-	3.5	1.2	2.2	-	0.7	0.1	0.05	0.06	0.7	194
Hodgkin's disease	104	0	-	-	0.8	3.6	5.0	3.0	4.8	3.9	1.2	3.0	2.5	5.4	3.4	4.8	7.0	7.5	4.4	3.5	3.1	0.6	0.18	0.24	2.7	201
Non-Hodgkin lymphoma	635	0	1.1	1.5	2.0	0.9	1.8	1.9	7.8	3.6	13.5	17.1	20.5	36.6	41.2	51.9	91.6	111.8	141.6	101.3	18.8	3.6	0.75	1.47	13.2	200,202
Multiple myeloma	175	0	-	-	-	-	-	-	0.3	1.1	2.0	4.0	5.6	10.2	17.5	22.1	21.8	23.6	37.6	52.4	5.2	1.0	0.20	0.42	3.6	203
Lymphoid leukaemia	205	0	3.8	3.4	2.0	0.5	1.4	-	1.0	1.1	0.4	3.5	3.1	4.7	15.5	15.2	31.4	32.3	57.5	62.9	6.1	1.2	0.20	0.44	4.5	204
Myeloid leukaemia	198	0	0.8	0.8	0.4	3.2	0.5	1.9	3.4	3.9	3.6	4.0	4.3	8.8	12.8	20.8	24.4	26.1	26.6	41.9	5.9	1.1	0.24	0.47	4.4	205
Monocytic leukaemia	10	0	-	-	-	0.5	-	-	-	-	-	-	-	-	-	2.1	1.7	5.0	-	-	0.3	0.1	0.00	0.02	0.2	206
Other leukaemia	2	0	-	-	-	-	-	-	-	-	-	0.5	-	-	-	0.9	-	-	-	-	0.1	0.0	0.00	0.01	0.0	207
Leukaemia unspecified	36	0	-	-	-	-	-	-	-	0.4	0.4	0.5	1.2	-	2.0	5.5	4.4	6.2	17.7	7.0	1.1	0.2	0.02	0.07	0.7	208
Other and unspecified	575	0	0.4	-	0.4	-	0.5	1.5	1.0	5.0	4.4	9.5	16.1	35.9	48.6	59.5	78.6	101.8	154.9	146.8	17.0	3.3	0.62	1.31	11.5	O&U
All sites	17606	3	15.1	10.5	12.6	19.5	32.1	46.9	60.1	84.2	131.3	246.4	456.2	873.5	1423.1	2192.0	2906.6	3409.3	3702.1	3435.0	520.8		17.06	42.56	351.8	ALL
All sites but 173	17558	3	15.1	10.5	12.6	19.5	31.7	46.9	59.7	83.5	130.9	245.9	455.0	872.2	1418.3	2187.9	2897.9	3400.7	3693.2	3421.0	519.4	100.0	17.01	42.45	350.9	ALLb

| Rate from 1 case | | | 0.378 | 0.376 | 0.407 | 0.454 | 0.453 | 0.372 | 0.339 | 0.358 | 0.398 | 0.502 | 0.621 | 0.678 | 0.675 | 0.692 | 0.873 | 1.242 | 2.213 | 3.494 |

†Important: see notes on population page

+ USA, CALIFORNIA, CENTRAL VALLEY: NON-HISPANIC WHITE 1988-1992

ANNUAL INCIDENCE PER 100,000 BY AGE GROUP (YEARS) - FEMALE

SITE	ALL AGES	AGE UNK	0-	5-	10-	15-	20-	25-	30-	35-	40-	45-	50-	55-	60-	65-	70-	75-	80-	85+	CRUDE RATE	%	CR 64	CR 74	ASR (W)	ICD (9th)
Lip	24	0	-	-	-	-	-	-	-	-	0.4	-	1.2	-	0.6	4.1	0.7	5.2	3.9	4.4	0.7	0.2	0.01	0.03	**0.3**	140
Tongue	67	0	-	-	-	-	0.4	-	-	1.1	1.2	3.0	3.0	3.1	5.9	2.9	11.8	5.2	3.9	4.4	1.9	0.4	0.09	0.16	**1.3**	141
Salivary gland	30	0	-	-	-	-	-	-	0.3	-	0.4	-	0.6	0.6	2.9	2.3	4.2	4.4	3.9	4.4	0.8	0.2	0.02	0.06	**0.5**	142
Mouth	93	0	-	-	-	-	-	-	-	0.4	-	0.5	4.2	4.3	7.6	8.1	12.5	13.1	13.0	10.3	2.6	0.6	0.08	0.19	**1.5**	143-5
Oropharynx	31	0	-	-	-	-	-	-	-	-	0.8	1.0	0.6	2.5	4.1	2.3	4.8	1.7	2.6	-	0.9	0.2	0.04	0.08	**0.6**	146
Nasopharynx	14	0	-	0.4	0.4	0.5	-	-	-	-	0.4	-	-	1.2	1.8	1.2	-	2.6	-	-	0.4	0.1	0.02	0.03	**0.3**	147
Hypopharynx	16	0	-	-	-	-	-	-	-	-	0.4	-	1.2	-	1.8	2.3	2.8	1.7	-	-	0.4	0.1	0.02	0.04	**0.3**	148
Pharynx unspecified	5	0	-	-	-	-	-	-	-	-	-	-	-	0.6	-	0.6	0.7	0.9	-	1.5	0.1	0.0	0.00	0.01	**0.1**	149
Oesophagus	74	0	-	-	-	-	-	-	-	-	-	1.0	0.6	1.2	4.7	11.0	6.9	14.0	13.0	8.8	2.1	0.5	0.04	0.13	**1.0**	150
Stomach	210	0	-	-	-	-	-	-	-	0.7	1.6	3.5	1.8	9.3	10.5	17.9	20.1	28.0	42.9	52.9	5.9	1.4	0.14	0.33	**2.9**	151
Small intestine	48	0	-	-	-	-	0.4	-	0.3	0.4	0.4	1.0	2.4	1.9	0.6	1.2	6.9	5.2	13.0	8.8	1.3	0.3	0.04	0.08	**0.7**	152
Colon	1432	0	-	-	-	-	0.4	1.5	-	3.6	9.1	12.9	26.7	37.7	74.3	112.9	163.9	222.2	283.7	339.2	40.2	9.2	0.83	2.22	**19.5**	153
Rectum	544	0	-	-	-	-	0.4	-	1.0	1.8	6.7	7.4	13.7	18.6	34.0	48.6	62.9	73.5	93.7	89.6	15.3	3.5	0.42	0.98	**8.2**	154
Liver	77	0	-	-	-	-	-	-	-	1.1	0.8	1.5	1.8	3.7	5.3	9.8	6.2	7.0	11.7	11.7	2.2	0.5	0.07	0.15	**1.3**	155
Gallbladder etc.	91	0	-	-	-	-	-	-	-	0.4	-	1.0	-	6.2	2.9	5.8	9.7	14.9	20.8	23.5	2.6	0.6	0.05	0.13	**1.2**	156
Pancreas	399	0	-	-	-	-	0.4	-	0.7	1.1	1.6	2.0	6.5	16.7	18.7	34.7	49.8	65.6	74.2	74.9	11.2	2.6	0.24	0.66	**5.5**	157
Nose, sinuses etc.	24	0	-	-	-	-	-	-	0.3	0.4	-	0.5	-	0.6	2.3	2.9	2.8	1.7	2.6	4.4	0.7	0.2	0.02	0.05	**0.4**	160
Larynx	72	0	-	-	-	-	-	-	-	-	1.6	2.0	3.0	5.6	7.0	11.6	5.5	2.6	3.9	5.9	2.0	0.5	0.10	0.18	**1.4**	161
Bronchus, lung	2267	1	-	-	-	-	0.4	0.4	2.0	4.3	13.9	43.6	86.7	131.1	196.1	258.2	309.2	258.1	206.9	121.9	63.6	14.6	2.39	5.23	**39.5**	162
Other thoracic organs	10	0	-	-	-	-	-	-	-	-	0.4	1.0	-	0.6	1.2	-	0.7	1.7	1.3	-	0.3	0.1	0.02	0.02	**0.2**	163-4
Bone	36	0	-	2.4	2.6	0.5	-	-	0.7	0.4	1.6	1.0	1.2	1.2	1.8	1.2	0.7	1.7	-	2.9	1.0	0.2	0.07	0.08	**1.0**	170
Connective tissue	99	0	1.6	1.2	0.4	1.4	0.9	0.7	2.0	1.4	0.8	3.5	3.6	1.9	4.1	5.8	5.5	7.9	13.0	17.6	2.8	0.6	0.12	0.17	**2.0**	171
Mesothelioma	22	0	-	-	-	-	-	-	0.3	-	-	0.5	-	0.6	2.9	2.9	2.1	2.6	1.3	2.9	0.6	0.1	0.02	0.05	**0.4**	MES
Kaposi's sarcoma	4	0	-	-	-	-	0.4	-	-	-	-	-	-	-	-	-	-	0.9	1.3	1.5	0.1	0.0	0.00	0.00	**0.1**	KAP
Melanoma of skin	417	0	-	-	0.9	2.8	4.9	10.2	10.3	16.0	15.1	15.4	13.1	19.8	13.5	21.4	23.5	21.9	39.0	32.3	11.7	2.7	0.61	0.83	**8.6**	172
†Other skin	29	0	-	-	0.4	0.5	-	-	-	1.1	0.8	1.5	0.6	0.6	1.8	1.2	2.8	4.4	2.6	1.5	0.8		0.04	0.06	**0.6**	173
Breast	4665	1	-	-	-	0.5	0.4	6.2	23.5	51.5	106.7	187.8	210.8	256.1	329.6	387.8	453.8	496.1	429.5	331.8	131.0	30.0	5.87	10.08	**86.2**	174
Uterus unspecified	17	0	-	-	-	-	-	-	-	-	-	0.5	-	-	0.6	0.6	0.7	3.5	1.3	11.7	0.5	0.1	0.01	0.01	**0.2**	179
Cervix uteri	356	0	-	-	-	-	4.9	7.3	13.3	17.8	13.1	16.4	14.8	14.8	18.7	16.8	13.1	13.1	18.2	16.2	10.0	2.3	0.61	0.76	**7.8**	180
Placenta	2	0	-	-	0.5	-	-	-	-	0.4	-	-	-	-	-	-	-	-	-	-	0.1	0.0	0.00	0.00	**0.1**	181
Corpus uteri	925	1	-	-	-	-	0.4	-	2.0	4.6	10.3	18.8	41.6	61.2	79.6	104.8	103.1	99.7	76.8	47.0	26.0	6.0	1.09	2.13	**16.7**	182
Ovary etc.	598	0	-	0.4	0.9	0.9	2.7	2.2	6.3	3.9	10.7	18.8	28.5	26.6	48.6	48.0	60.9	51.6	53.4	60.2	16.8	3.9	0.75	1.30	**11.2**	183
Other female genital	114	0	-	-	-	-	-	0.7	0.7	-	2.4	2.0	4.2	2.5	7.0	11.6	8.3	16.6	15.6	20.6	3.2	0.7	0.10	0.20	**1.8**	184
Bladder	255	0	-	-	-	-	-	0.4	0.3	0.4	1.2	3.5	6.5	10.5	19.3	23.2	27.0	28.9	46.9	48.5	7.2	1.6	0.21	0.46	**3.9**	188
Kidney etc.	330	0	2.0	0.8	-	-	-	0.4	1.0	2.8	2.8	6.9	11.9	16.1	26.3	27.2	38.0	35.0	46.9	30.8	9.3	2.1	0.35	0.68	**5.8**	189
Eye	27	0	-	-	-	-	0.4	0.4	-	0.7	-	2.0	1.2	2.5	1.2	1.2	0.7	3.5	2.6	2.9	0.8	0.2	0.04	0.05	**0.5**	190
Brain, nervous system	247	0	3.6	3.2	3.0	3.3	2.7	1.8	4.6	3.6	4.4	4.0	9.5	12.4	10.5	14.5	24.2	21.0	22.1	10.3	6.9	1.6	0.33	0.53	**5.3**	191-2
Thyroid	201	0	-	0.4	0.9	1.4	4.0	5.8	6.3	9.2	7.9	7.4	8.3	9.3	8.8	9.3	6.2	10.5	10.4	1.5	5.6	1.3	0.35	0.43	**4.6**	193
Other endocrine	12	0	0.8	-	0.4	-	-	0.4	0.7	-	-	-	-	1.2	-	0.6	0.7	0.9	-	1.5	0.3	0.1	0.02	0.02	**0.3**	194
Hodgkin's disease	96	0	-	-	0.4	4.7	5.8	5.4	4.0	3.2	2.4	-	1.8	1.9	2.3	2.9	3.5	4.4	3.9	2.9	2.7	0.6	0.16	0.19	**2.4**	201
Non-Hodgkin lymphoma	519	0	0.4	0.8	0.9	1.4	1.8	0.4	3.0	4.6	6.0	12.9	17.8	24.1	34.0	37.6	57.4	67.4	66.4	58.7	14.6	3.3	0.54	1.01	**8.9**	200,202
Multiple myeloma	176	1	-	-	-	-	-	-	-	0.7	1.2	4.0	4.2	6.8	7.6	15.6	18.7	28.9	37.7	22.0	4.9	1.1	0.12	0.30	**2.6**	203
Lymphoid leukaemia	167	0	5.9	2.0	0.9	0.5	0.9	0.4	0.3	0.7	0.4	2.5	3.0	1.9	9.4	11.6	15.2	18.4	29.9	32.3	4.7	1.1	0.14	0.28	**3.1**	204
Myeloid leukaemia	160	0	1.2	0.4	1.3	2.4	1.3	0.7	2.7	2.1	2.8	1.5	3.0	5.6	4.1	9.3	18.0	22.7	13.0	29.4	4.5	1.0	0.14	0.28	**2.8**	205
Monocytic leukaemia	8	0	-	-	-	-	-	-	-	-	-	-	-	1.9	0.6	0.6	0.7	0.9	-	1.5	0.2	0.1	0.01	0.02	**0.1**	206
Other leukaemia	4	0	0.4	-	-	-	-	-	-	-	-	-	0.6	-	-	-	-	1.7	-	-	0.1	0.0	0.00	0.00	**0.1**	207
Leukaemia unspecified	22	0	-	-	-	0.5	-	-	-	-	-	-	-	-	0.6	2.3	2.8	4.4	5.2	4.4	0.6	0.1	0.01	0.03	**0.3**	208
Other and unspecified	525	0	0.4	-	-	-	0.4	0.4	0.7	2.8	4.4	3.0	9.5	16.7	30.4	40.5	58.1	62.1	109.3	133.6	14.7	3.4	0.34	0.84	**7.3**	O&U
All sites	15561	4	16.2	11.9	13.4	21.8	34.5	45.7	87.2	142.8	234.5	395.5	549.2	741.6	1045.5	1336.5	1627.6	1760.2	1841.6	1692.9	436.9		16.70	31.53	**271.2**	ALL
All sites but 173	15532	4	16.2	11.9	13.0	21.3	34.5	45.7	87.2	141.7	233.7	394.0	548.6	741.0	1043.8	1335.4	1624.8	1755.9	1839.0	1691.4	436.1	100.0	16.67	31.47	**270.7**	ALLb

| Rate from 1 case | | | 0.396 | 0.395 | 0.432 | 0.473 | 0.448 | 0.363 | 0.332 | 0.355 | 0.397 | 0.496 | 0.594 | 0.619 | 0.585 | 0.579 | 0.692 | 0.875 | 1.301 | 1.468 | |

†Important: see notes on population page

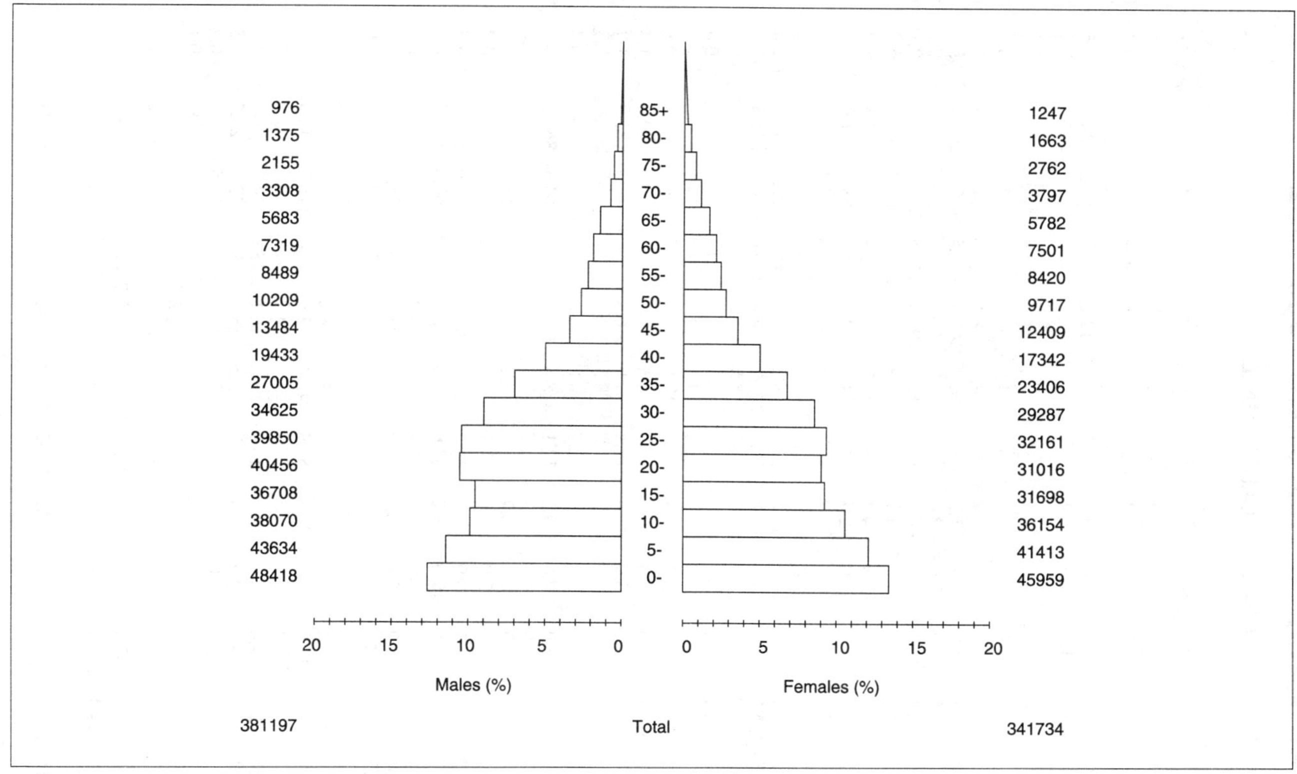

USA, California, Central Valley: Hispanic

Source of population: average annual 1988–92

Estimate: Annual mid-year population estimates by age, race/ethnicity and sex to the county level for non-Hispanic whites, non-Hispanic blacks, Hispanics and non-Hispanic Asian/Others were obtained from the California Department of Finance (DOF) Demographic Research Unit. Estimates for 1988, 1989 and 1990 are from a special population summary for 1970–90 with gender, age and race-ethnic detail released by DOF in April 1993, benchmarked to the 1990 Census. Estimates for 1991 and 1992 are from current estimates of the California population with gender, age and race/ethnic detail consistent with Report 93 E-2. Reference: California Department of Finance. Population Estimates for California State and Counties: Report 93 E-2. Sacramento, CA: California Department of Finance, Demographic Research Unit, February 1994.

Notes to tables overleaf:

+ The editors were unable to verify these data

† 173 does not include basal cell or squamous cell carcinoma

+ USA, CALIFORNIA, CENTRAL VALLEY: HISPANIC 1988-1992

ANNUAL INCIDENCE PER 100,000 BY AGE GROUP (YEARS) - MALE

SITE	ALL AGES	AGE UNK	0-	5-	10-	15-	20-	25-	30-	35-	40-	45-	50-	55-	60-	65-	70-	75-	80-	85+	CRUDE RATE	%	CR 64	CR 74	ASR (W)	ICD (9th)
Lip	14	0	-	-	-	-	-	-	-	-	1.0	3.0	-	9.4	8.2	3.5	18.1	-	-	-	0.7	0.5	0.11	0.22	**1.4**	140
Tongue	17	0	-	-	-	-	0.5	-	-	-	-	1.5	-	2.4	2.7	14.1	24.2	46.4	-	-	0.9	0.6	0.04	0.23	**1.7**	141
Salivary gland	6	0	-	-	-	-	-	-	1.7	0.7	-	-	-	-	-	-	-	-	-	41.0	0.3	0.2	0.01	0.01	**0.4**	142
Mouth	12	0	-	-	-	-	-	-	-	0.7	-	-	5.9	2.4	8.2	-	12.1	-	14.5	20.5	0.6	0.5	0.09	0.15	**1.2**	143-5
Oropharynx	7	0	-	-	-	0.5	-	-	-	-	2.1	1.5	2.0	2.4	2.7	-	-	-	-	-	0.4	0.3	0.06	0.06	**0.6**	146
Nasopharynx	5	0	-	-	-	-	-	-	0.6	0.7	1.0	-	-	-	2.7	-	6.0	-	-	-	0.3	0.2	0.03	0.06	**0.4**	147
Hypopharynx	7	0	-	-	-	-	-	-	-	-	1.0	-	-	4.7	2.7	7.0	-	9.3	-	-	0.4	0.3	0.04	0.08	**0.7**	148
Pharynx unspecified	4	0	-	-	-	-	-	0.5	-	-	-	1.5	-	2.4	-	3.5	-	-	-	-	0.2	0.2	0.02	0.04	**0.3**	149
Oesophagus	24	0	-	-	-	-	-	-	-	0.7	-	5.9	-	2.4	8.2	28.2	18.1	18.6	14.5	20.5	1.3	0.9	0.09	0.32	**2.4**	150
Stomach	105	0	-	-	-	-	-	0.5	1.7	4.4	3.1	5.9	11.8	21.2	43.7	56.3	66.5	111.4	116.3	204.8	5.5	3.9	0.46	1.08	**9.9**	151
Small intestine	5	0	-	-	-	-	-	-	-	-	1.0	-	3.9	2.4	2.7	-	-	-	-	-	0.3	0.2	0.05	0.05	**0.5**	152
Colon	173	0	-	-	-	-	1.0	0.5	0.6	4.4	2.1	11.9	11.8	44.8	46.4	112.6	193.5	148.5	218.1	327.7	9.1	6.5	0.62	2.15	**17.0**	153
Rectum	129	0	-	-	-	-	-	0.5	0.6	0.7	6.2	5.9	23.5	37.7	46.4	80.9	96.7	157.8	160.0	81.9	6.8	4.8	0.61	1.50	**12.5**	154
Liver	58	0	0.8	0.5	-	-	0.5	0.5	-	-	2.1	8.9	9.8	9.4	27.3	31.7	18.1	102.1	29.1	20.5	3.0	2.2	0.30	0.55	**5.4**	155
Gallbladder etc.	30	0	-	-	-	-	-	-	-	0.7	-	1.5	2.0	2.4	13.7	14.1	24.2	46.4	58.2	81.9	1.6	1.1	0.10	0.29	**2.9**	156
Pancreas	71	0	-	-	-	-	-	-	0.6	-	3.1	3.0	3.9	25.9	41.0	45.7	66.5	37.1	87.2	61.5	3.7	2.7	0.39	0.95	**7.1**	157
Nose, sinuses etc.	4	0	-	-	-	-	-	-	-	0.7	1.0	-	2.0	-	-	-	9.3	-	-	-	0.2	0.2	0.02	0.02	**0.3**	160
Larynx	39	0	-	-	-	-	0.5	-	-	-	2.1	-	3.9	11.8	16.4	28.2	36.3	46.4	29.1	41.0	2.0	1.5	0.17	0.50	**3.9**	161
Bronchus, lung	347	0	-	-	-	-	0.5	-	2.3	1.5	4.1	14.8	35.3	84.8	158.5	225.2	314.4	529.0	436.2	225.3	18.2	13.0	1.51	4.21	**34.5**	162
Other thoracic organs	4	0	-	-	-	-	0.5	0.5	-	-	1.0	-	-	-	-	3.5	-	-	-	-	0.2	0.2	0.01	0.03	**0.2**	163-4
Bone	11	0	-	0.5	0.5	-	1.0	1.0	-	-	2.1	3.0	-	-	-	-	9.3	-	-	0.6	0.4	0.04	0.04	**0.6**	170
Connective tissue	27	0	1.7	-	-	-	1.0	1.5	1.2	0.7	1.0	1.5	-	16.4	3.5	12.1	27.8	14.5	-	1.4	1.0	0.12	0.20	**2.0**	171
Mesothelioma	16	0	-	-	-	-	-	-	0.6	-	-	1.5	3.9	7.1	-	17.6	6.0	9.3	29.1	-	0.8	0.6	0.07	0.18	**1.5**	MES
Kaposi's sarcoma	26	0	-	-	-	-	1.0	1.5	4.0	3.7	4.1	3.0	2.0	-	3.5	-	-	-	-	20.5	1.4	1.0	0.10	0.11	**1.4**	KAP
Melanoma of skin	37	1	0.4	-	1.1	-	1.0	1.0	1.2	0.7	1.0	1.5	5.9	11.8	16.4	7.0	6.0	-	43.6	81.9	1.9	1.4	0.22	0.28	**3.0**	172
†Other skin	6	0	-	-	-	1.1	0.5	0.5	0.6	-	-	-	-	-	3.5	-	-	-	-	-	0.3		0.01	0.03	**0.3**	173
Breast	6	0	-	-	-	-	-	-	-	0.7	-	-	-	-	2.7	10.6	6.0	-	-	-	0.3	0.2	0.02	0.10	**0.6**	175
Prostate	659	0	-	-	-	-	-	-	-	-	-	5.9	17.6	89.5	213.1	478.6	925.0	1104.4	1163.3	860.3	34.6	24.7	1.63	8.65	**67.4**	185
Testis	58	0	0.8	-	-	0.5	4.0	9.5	7.5	5.2	3.1	3.0	-	4.7	2.7	-	-	-	-	-	3.0	2.2	0.21	0.21	**2.6**	186
Penis	11	0	-	-	-	-	-	0.5	1.2	-	-	1.5	-	4.7	-	3.5	18.1	-	14.5	-	0.6	0.4	0.04	0.15	**0.9**	187.1-.4
Other male genital	4	0	-	-	-	-	-	-	-	-	1.0	-	2.0	-	2.7	-	-	9.3	-	-	0.2	0.2	0.03	0.03	**0.4**	187.5-.9
Bladder	84	0	-	-	-	-	-	0.5	0.6	0.7	1.0	1.5	3.9	18.8	46.4	31.7	96.7	120.6	130.9	102.4	4.4	3.2	0.37	1.01	**8.3**	188
Kidney etc.	123	0	1.7	0.5	-	0.5	-	-	0.6	3.7	2.1	14.8	19.6	18.8	54.6	88.0	72.6	74.2	160.0	102.4	6.5	4.6	0.58	1.39	**11.6**	189
Eye	10	0	1.7	-	-	0.5	-	-	0.6	0.7	1.0	-	-	-	2.7	-	6.0	-	-	-	0.5	0.4	0.04	0.07	**0.6**	190
Brain, nervous system	79	0	4.1	2.8	2.6	0.5	1.5	2.0	1.7	4.4	4.1	5.9	9.8	18.8	10.9	21.1	24.2	18.6	58.2	-	4.1	3.0	0.35	0.57	**5.6**	191-2
Thyroid	20	0	-	-	-	0.5	1.0	0.5	1.2	1.5	2.1	-	-	4.7	8.2	-	-	37.1	14.5	-	1.0	0.8	0.10	0.10	**1.4**	193
Other endocrine	8	0	0.4	0.5	1.1	0.5	1.0	0.5	-	-	-	-	-	-	-	-	-	-	-	-	0.4	0.3	0.02	0.02	**0.4**	194
Hodgkin's disease	31	0	0.4	0.5	2.1	3.3	0.5	2.5	1.7	-	3.1	4.4	2.0	-	-	3.5	6.0	9.3	-	-	1.6	1.2	0.10	0.15	**1.8**	201
Non-Hodgkin lymphoma	124	0	0.4	1.8	-	1.1	2.0	1.5	3.5	8.1	6.2	11.9	19.6	25.9	51.9	42.2	72.6	-	116.3	143.4	6.5	4.7	0.67	1.24	**10.5**	200,202
Multiple myeloma	35	0	-	-	-	-	-	-	-	0.7	2.1	1.5	5.9	7.1	27.3	17.6	24.2	46.4	14.5	-	1.8	1.3	0.22	0.43	**3.5**	203
Lymphoid leukaemia	78	0	6.2	6.0	3.7	4.4	-	1.0	2.3	0.7	2.1	3.0	5.9	11.8	13.7	17.6	18.1	18.6	14.5	-	4.1	2.9	0.30	0.48	**5.1**	204
Myeloid leukaemia	47	0	0.4	0.5	1.6	1.6	1.5	2.0	2.3	2.2	3.1	4.4	3.9	7.1	13.7	3.5	18.1	9.3	43.6	20.5	2.5	1.8	0.22	0.33	**3.3**	205
Monocytic leukaemia	4	0	-	0.5	-	-	-	-	-	-	-	-	2.0	-	-	3.5	-	-	14.5	-	0.2	0.2	0.01	0.03	**0.3**	206
Other leukaemia	2	0	-	0.5	-	-	0.5	-	-	-	-	-	-	-	-	-	-	-	-	-	0.1	0.1	0.00	0.00	**0.1**	207
Leukaemia unspecified	6	0	-	-	-	0.5	-	-	-	1.5	-	-	-	-	-	-	-	6.0	-	41.0	0.3	0.2	0.01	0.04	**0.5**	208
Other and unspecified	97	0	-	-	-	-	-	0.5	1.2	-	4.1	8.9	17.6	28.3	30.1	31.7	60.5	129.9	101.8	245.8	5.1	3.6	0.45	0.91	**9.3**	O&U
All sites	2670	1	19.0	14.2	12.6	15.8	19.8	29.6	39.9	51.1	74.1	142.4	237.0	525.3	945.4	1442.7	2273.3	2886.3	3097.3	2744.8	140.1		10.63	29.22	**246.2**	ALL
All sites but 173	2664	1	19.0	14.2	12.6	14.7	19.3	29.1	39.3	51.1	74.1	142.4	237.0	525.3	945.4	1439.2	2273.3	2886.3	3097.3	2744.8	139.8	100.0	10.62	29.19	**245.9**	ALLb

Rate from 1 case   0.413 0.458 0.525 0.545 0.494 0.502 0.578 0.741 1.029 1.483 1.959 2.356 2.732 3.519 6.046 9.281 14.541 20.483

†Important: see notes on population page

+ USA, CALIFORNIA, CENTRAL VALLEY: HISPANIC 1988-1992

ANNUAL INCIDENCE PER 100,000 BY AGE GROUP (YEARS) - FEMALE

SITE	ALL AGES	AGE UNK	0-	5-	10-	15-	20-	25-	30-	35-	40-	45-	50-	55-	60-	65-	70-	75-	80-	85+	CRUDE RATE	%	CR 64	CR 74	ASR (W)	ICD (9th)
Lip	1	0	-	-	-	-	-	-	-	-	-	-	2.1	-	-	-	-	-	-	-	0.1	0.0	0.01	0.01	0.1	140
Tongue	8	0	-	-	-	-	-	-	-	0.9	1.2	-	-	2.4	2.7	10.4	-	7.2	-	-	0.5	0.3	0.04	0.09	0.7	141
Salivary gland	10	0	-	-	-	-	-	0.6	1.4	1.7	-	-	-	2.4	2.7	-	5.3	-	12.0	16.0	0.6	0.4	0.04	0.07	0.7	142
Mouth	6	0	-	-	-	-	-	0.6	-	-	-	1.6	-	2.4	-	-	15.8	-	-	-	0.4	0.2	0.02	0.10	0.6	143-5
Oropharynx	2	0	-	-	-	-	-	-	-	-	-	-	-	2.4	-	-	-	7.2	-	-	0.1	0.1	0.01	0.01	0.2	146
Nasopharynx	2	0	0.4	-	-	-	-	-	-	-	-	1.6	-	-	-	-	-	-	-	-	0.1	0.1	0.01	0.01	0.1	147
Hypopharynx	1	0	-	-	-	-	-	-	-	-	-	-	-	-	-	3.5	-	-	-	-	0.1	0.0	0.00	0.02	0.1	148
Pharynx unspecified	0	0	-	-	-	-	-	-	-	-	-	-	-	-	-	-	-	-	-	-	0.0	0.0	0.00	0.00	0.0	149
Oesophagus	6	0	-	-	-	-	-	-	-	0.9	-	-	-	-	-	6.9	5.3	-	12.0	16.0	0.4	0.2	0.00	0.07	0.5	150
Stomach	74	0	-	-	-	-	0.6	0.6	1.4	3.4	-	4.8	2.1	19.0	29.3	31.1	63.2	72.4	60.1	112.2	4.3	3.0	0.31	0.78	6.5	151
Small intestine	10	0	-	-	-	-	-	-	-	-	-	-	4.1	-	-	3.5	5.3	7.2	48.1	16.0	0.6	0.4	0.02	0.06	0.8	152
Colon	118	0	-	-	-	-	0.6	0.6	0.7	2.6	5.8	12.9	20.6	16.6	37.3	51.9	84.3	130.3	156.3	96.2	6.9	4.8	0.49	1.17	10.4	153
Rectum	73	0	-	-	-	-	-	0.6	-	1.7	4.6	11.3	22.6	16.6	42.7	34.6	26.3	21.7	60.1	32.1	4.3	3.0	0.50	0.81	6.9	154
Liver	40	0	0.9	-	-	-	-	0.6	-	2.6	2.3	1.6	10.3	7.1	2.7	27.7	26.3	29.0	48.1	16.0	2.3	1.6	0.14	0.41	3.4	155
Gallbladder etc.	53	0	-	-	-	-	-	-	-	-	1.2	4.8	8.2	23.8	2.7	31.1	42.1	50.7	72.1	64.1	3.1	2.2	0.20	0.57	4.8	156
Pancreas	64	0	-	-	-	-	-	0.6	-	0.9	1.2	1.6	10.3	14.3	10.7	41.5	47.4	72.4	84.2	112.2	3.7	2.6	0.20	0.64	5.7	157
Nose, sinuses etc.	0	0	-	-	-	-	-	-	-	-	-	-	-	-	-	-	-	-	-	-	0.0	0.0	0.00	0.00	0.0	160
Larynx	2	0	-	-	-	-	-	-	-	-	-	-	-	-	2.7	-	-	7.2	-	-	0.1	0.1	0.01	0.01	0.2	161
Bronchus, lung	166	0	-	-	-	-	-	-	0.7	2.6	5.8	12.9	24.7	57.0	82.6	89.9	100.1	130.3	180.3	64.1	9.7	6.8	0.93	1.88	15.4	162
Other thoracic organs	3	0	0.4	-	-	-	-	-	-	-	-	-	-	-	2.7	-	5.3	-	-	-	0.2	0.1	0.02	0.04	0.3	163-4
Bone	11	0	-	0.5	1.7	1.9	-	0.6	0.7	-	-	-	2.1	-	2.7	-	-	-	-	-	0.6	0.5	0.05	0.05	0.7	170
Connective tissue	22	0	1.3	0.5	0.6	1.3	0.6	0.6	-	0.9	4.6	-	2.1	-	2.7	6.9	10.5	-	-	32.1	1.3	0.9	0.08	0.16	1.6	171
Mesothelioma	5	0	-	-	-	-	-	0.6	0.7	-	-	-	-	2.4	2.7	3.5	-	-	-	-	0.3	0.2	0.03	0.05	0.4	MES
Kaposi's sarcoma	1	0	-	-	-	-	0.6	-	-	-	-	-	-	-	-	-	-	-	-	-	0.1	0.0	0.00	0.00	0.1	KAP
Melanoma of skin	40	0	-	0.6	-	1.3	1.9	4.1	3.4	4.6	4.8	6.2	2.4	10.7	10.4	10.5	21.7	12.0	-	-	2.3	1.6	0.20	0.30	2.9	172
†Other skin	8	0	-	-	1.3	1.3	1.2	-	-	1.2	-	-	-	-	-	-	12.0	-	-	-	0.5		0.02	0.02	0.4	173
Breast	629	0	-	-	-	-	1.3	7.5	24.6	50.4	75.0	122.5	150.3	144.9	152.0	238.7	258.1	195.5	324.6	256.5	36.8	25.8	3.64	6.13	53.6	174
Uterus unspecified	1	0	-	-	-	-	-	-	-	-	-	-	-	-	-	-	-	-	-	16.0	0.1	0.0	0.00	0.00	0.1	179
Cervix uteri	232	0	-	-	-	-	4.5	13.1	16.4	40.2	25.4	48.4	30.9	33.3	50.7	38.0	52.7	43.4	60.1	16.0	13.6	9.5	1.31	1.77	17.1	180
Placenta	2	0	-	-	-	-	-	1.2	-	-	-	-	-	-	-	-	-	-	-	-	0.1	0.1	0.01	0.01	0.1	181
Corpus uteri	143	0	-	-	-	-	0.6	2.5	4.8	6.8	10.4	25.8	20.6	47.5	42.7	62.3	94.8	79.6	24.0	48.1	8.4	5.9	0.81	1.59	12.7	182
Ovary etc.	112	0	0.4	0.5	1.7	3.8	3.2	3.1	2.0	5.1	3.5	14.5	14.4	35.6	29.3	34.6	68.5	57.9	60.1	16.0	6.6	4.6	0.59	1.10	9.3	183
Other female genital	26	0	-	-	0.6	-	-	-	0.7	0.9	1.2	6.4	2.1	2.4	8.0	10.4	26.3	-	36.1	32.1	1.5	1.1	0.11	0.29	2.3	184
Bladder	31	1	-	-	-	-	-	-	-	-	1.2	-	4.1	2.4	13.3	20.8	21.1	29.0	36.1	64.1	1.8	1.3	0.11	0.32	2.8	188
Kidney etc.	68	0	2.2	0.5	-	-	-	-	2.7	1.7	3.5	3.2	8.2	9.5	21.3	41.5	47.4	43.4	72.1	32.1	4.0	2.8	0.26	0.71	5.8	189
Eye	7	0	1.7	-	-	-	-	-	-	-	-	1.6	-	-	3.5	-	7.2	-	-	-	0.4	0.3	0.02	0.03	0.5	190
Brain, nervous system	51	0	3.5	2.4	1.7	1.3	3.2	-	0.7	4.3	-	3.2	4.1	9.5	10.7	17.3	-	29.0	-	16.0	3.0	2.1	0.22	0.31	3.6	191-2
Thyroid	92	0	-	-	1.1	1.3	3.2	9.3	10.9	12.0	12.7	6.4	4.1	9.5	16.0	13.8	-	14.5	24.0	48.1	5.4	3.8	0.43	0.50	5.9	193
Other endocrine	3	0	1.3	-	-	-	-	-	-	-	-	-	-	-	-	-	-	-	-	-	0.2	0.1	0.01	0.01	0.2	194
Hodgkin's disease	21	0	-	0.5	0.6	1.9	-	2.5	-	1.7	1.2	1.6	2.1	2.4	2.7	6.9	5.3	7.2	12.0	-	1.2	0.9	0.08	0.15	1.5	201
Non-Hodgkin lymphoma	101	0	-	1.4	-	1.3	0.6	0.6	2.0	3.4	6.9	16.1	10.3	21.4	21.3	51.9	52.7	86.9	60.1	112.2	5.9	4.1	0.43	0.95	8.6	200,202
Multiple myeloma	31	0	-	-	-	-	-	-	-	-	1.7	3.2	6.2	4.8	16.0	20.8	15.8	29.0	24.0	16.0	1.8	1.3	0.16	0.34	2.9	203
Lymphoid leukaemia	51	0	7.0	2.4	4.4	1.9	1.3	1.2	0.7	-	-	3.2	2.1	4.8	5.3	10.4	5.3	14.5	12.0	-	3.0	2.1	0.17	0.25	3.2	204
Myeloid leukaemia	25	0	0.9	1.0	1.1	-	-	1.2	1.4	-	1.7	2.3	3.2	2.1	2.4	2.7	6.9	-	21.7	-	16.0	1.5	1.0	0.10	0.13	1.7	205
Monocytic leukaemia	2	0	-	-	-	-	-	-	0.7	-	-	-	-	-	-	-	5.3	-	-	-	0.1	0.1	0.00	0.03	0.1	206
Other leukaemia	4	0	-	-	1.1	-	-	-	-	-	-	-	-	2.4	-	3.5	-	-	-	-	0.2	0.2	0.02	0.03	0.3	207
Leukaemia unspecified	5	0	-	-	0.6	0.6	-	-	-	-	-	-	-	2.4	-	3.5	-	-	-	16.0	0.3	0.2	0.02	0.04	0.4	208
Other and unspecified	84	0	0.9	-	-	-	1.9	0.6	1.4	1.7	3.5	8.1	10.3	14.3	29.3	45.0	42.1	57.9	60.1	160.3	4.9	3.4	0.36	0.79	7.3	O&U
All sites	2447	1	20.9	9.7	15.5	16.4	25.1	52.2	78.5	153.0	178.8	325.6	387.0	517.8	658.5	982.3	1142.8	1274.3	1562.9	1443.0	143.2		12.20	22.83	203.3	ALL
All sites but 173	2439	1	20.9	9.7	15.5	15.1	23.9	51.0	78.5	153.0	177.6	325.6	387.0	517.8	658.5	982.3	1142.8	1274.3	1550.9	1443.0	142.7	100.0	12.17	22.80	202.8	ALLb

| Rate from 1 case | | | 0.435 | 0.483 | 0.553 | 0.631 | 0.645 | 0.622 | 0.683 | 0.854 | 1.153 | 1.612 | 2.058 | 2.375 | 2.666 | 3.459 | 5.266 | 7.240 | 12.022 | 16.033 | | | | | | |

†Important: see notes on population page

197

USA, California, Los Angeles County

The Cancer Surveillance Program (CSP) of Los Angeles County was started at the University of Southern California in 1970 as part of an epidemiology and biostatistics programme. It was designed explicitly for purposes of etiological research. Complete ascertainment began in 1972. In June 1987, the CSP became one of the ten regional registries of the California Cancer Registry, a population-based cancer registry for the State of California. This registry was established by California law in 1985 and places the obligation for identifying and abstracting cancer cases on those facilities where cancer is diagnosed and treated.

Los Angeles County is an urban area covering more than 10 000 km^2 and has the largest population of any county in the United States, with nearly nine million residents in 1990. Among these residents are more than two million self-declared Latinos including more than 1 500 000 Mexicans, 40 000 Puerto Ricans, 50 000 Cubans and sizeable populations representing various Central and South American countries. There are more than one million blacks in the county and between 100 000 and 300 000 each of Japanese, Chinese, Koreans and Filipinos. Other major south-east Asian groups include Vietnamese, Cambodians and Thais. The principal religious groups include Catholics, Protestants, Jews, Mormons, Buddhists and Seventh-day Adventists. There is wide variation in socioeconomic as well as sociocultural characteristics in the county.

The CSP combines elements of an active and a passive surveillance system. Under the active surveillance component, the CSP personnel systematically screen pathology and other relevant files at all facilities to obtain pathology reports for each cancer case diagnosed or treated at hospitals, some treatment facilities and free-standing pathology laboratories, although full medical charts are reviewed only for patients who may be eligible for analytical (such as case–control) studies and for a sample of other patients. For passive surveillance, each hospital or other reporting facility completes a full abstract, including stage and treatment information, on every cancer case diagnosed and/or treated in that facility. For each cancer case, 134 data items including disease or medical variables, demographics and administrative descriptors are coded and computerized. Occupation and industry of employment are available for most cases of working age. Data regarding race, nationality, birthplace, religion, social security number, surname and first name are collected to allow classification of the cases with regard to ethnicity, religion and migrant status.

The responsibility for completing reporting at some hospitals is contracted back to the CSP; currently about 15% of all hospital reports in Los Angeles County are so reported. All of the completed abstracts are record-linked by the CSP to the pathology reports obtained under active surveillance to assure that one abstract is completed on each histologically verified cancer case.

Before 1992, linkage with the State of California death tapes was the only means of passive follow-up. However, beginning with 1992 diagnoses, the CSP instituted complete follow-up as a function of its new affiliation with the National Cancer Institute's Surveillance, Epidemiology and End Results (SEER) Program. Follow-up data are collected by record linkages with multiple sources as well as incorporating active follow-up information provided by hospitals. In addition, the CSP manually screens all death certificates of Los Angeles County residents to identify any cancer cases with clinical evidence of cancer, but in whom a pathological confirmation was deemed unnecessary or impossible. This review also provides feedback on the efficiency of case ascertainment procedures.

Manual and computerized record linkages are performed separately with a variety of external data sources, using a sophisticated probabilistic methodology. Multiple primaries are noted by a tumour sequence number. Each data item is checked as an allowable code, and selected inter-field checks are performed.

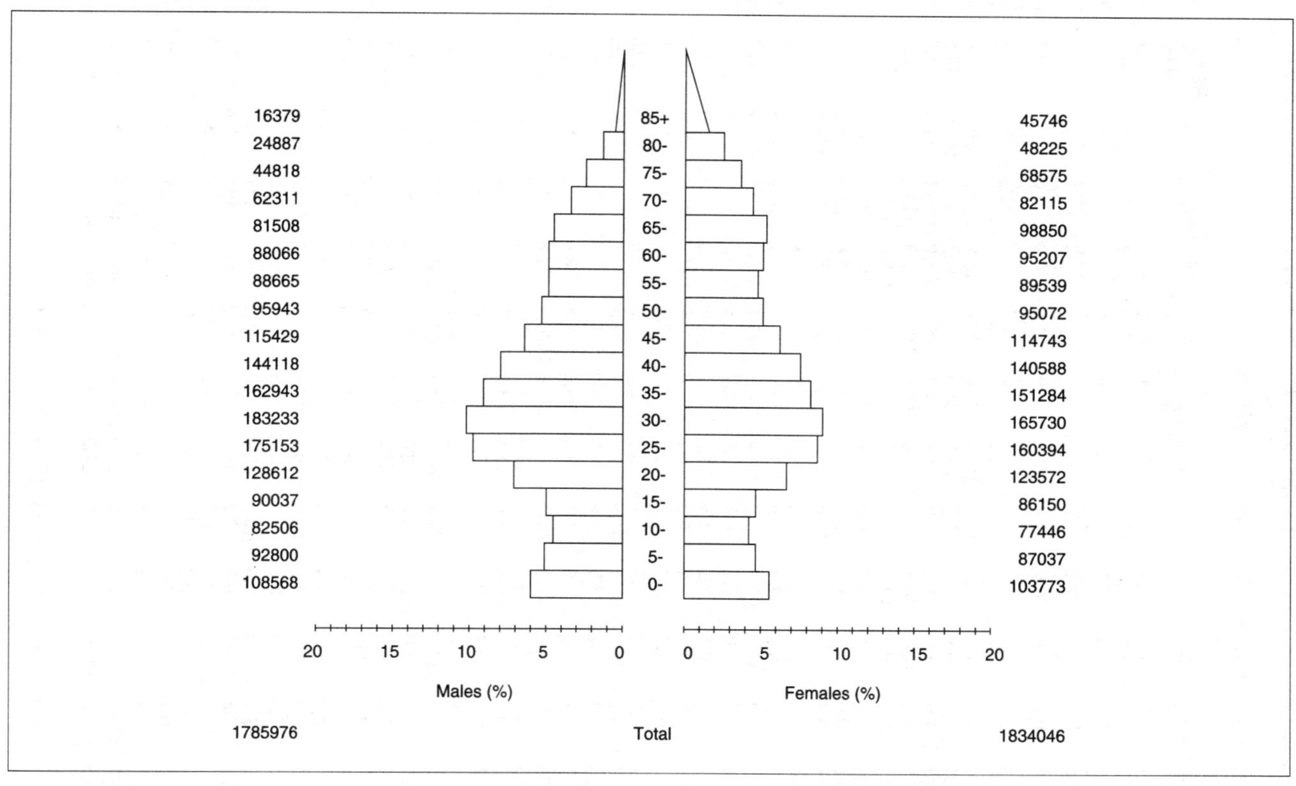

USA, California, Los Angeles County: Non-Hispanic White
Source of population: 1990
Census: 1990 Census.
Notes to tables overleaf:
† 173 does not include basal cell or squamous cell carcinoma
The denominators are not the same populations as those published in Volume VI and the data for this ethnic group are not comparable.

USA, CALIFORNIA, LOS ANGELES COUNTY: NON-HISPANIC WHITE 1988-1992

ANNUAL INCIDENCE PER 100,000 BY AGE GROUP (YEARS) - MALE

SITE	ALL AGES	AGE UNK	0-	5-	10-	15-	20-	25-	30-	35-	40-	45-	50-	55-	60-	65-	70-	75-	80-	85+	CRUDE RATE	%	CR 64	CR 74	ASR (W)	ICD (9th)
Lip	239	0	-	-	-	-	-	0.3	0.5	0.6	1.9	1.7	2.3	4.1	6.8	9.1	12.8	14.3	13.7	20.8	2.7	0.5	0.09	0.20	1.7	140
Tongue	383	0	-	-	-	-	-	0.3	0.1	1.0	1.7	4.7	5.8	12.2	13.6	16.2	17.0	19.2	12.9	14.7	4.3	0.7	0.20	0.36	3.0	141
Salivary gland	142	0	-	-	-	-	0.2	0.2	0.2	0.6	1.2	1.2	1.7	2.0	3.4	6.4	5.5	7.1	11.3	13.4	1.6	0.3	0.05	0.11	1.0	142
Mouth	391	0	-	-	-	-	-	0.2	0.1	0.7	0.4	4.2	8.8	11.3	14.8	14.5	22.1	15.6	19.3	13.4	4.4	0.7	0.20	0.39	3.0	143-5
Oropharynx	216	0	-	-	-	-	-	-	0.1	0.2	1.0	4.0	4.4	8.1	7.9	9.3	8.3	6.2	8.0	3.7	2.4	0.4	0.13	0.22	1.7	146
Nasopharynx	62	0	-	-	-	0.4	-	-	-	0.2	0.1	0.9	0.8	2.9	1.8	2.9	2.6	0.9	4.0	-	0.7	0.1	0.04	0.06	0.5	147
Hypopharynx	168	0	-	-	-	-	-	-	-	0.4	1.4	2.5	4.3	9.1	7.1	9.0	7.6	5.6	6.1	1.9	0.3	0.09	0.17	1.3	148
Pharynx unspecified	50	0	-	-	-	-	-	0.1	0.2	0.3	0.5	-	2.0	1.8	3.2	2.2	1.3	1.6	-	0.6	0.1	0.02	0.05	0.4	149
Oesophagus	502	0	-	-	-	-	-	0.1	0.1	0.4	1.2	1.9	7.9	11.5	18.6	22.1	29.9	21.9	40.2	29.3	5.6	1.0	0.21	0.47	3.7	150
Stomach	1115	0	-	-	-	-	-	0.6	0.7	1.5	2.5	6.8	11.9	19.2	29.5	41.0	57.1	80.3	98.0	141.6	12.5	2.1	0.36	0.85	7.6	151
Small intestine	172	0	-	-	-	-	0.2	-	0.3	0.6	1.0	1.2	3.5	2.9	5.5	7.4	5.8	8.0	16.1	11.0	1.9	0.3	0.08	0.14	1.3	152
Colon	4331	0	-	-	-	-	0.5	0.9	2.4	5.5	6.8	14.9	36.5	67.4	113.8	165.6	250.7	346.3	415.5	481.1	48.5	8.2	1.24	3.33	28.9	153
Rectum	1947	0	-	-	-	-	0.5	0.9	1.3	2.2	5.7	9.5	19.8	38.3	59.3	85.9	104.0	129.9	161.5	144.1	21.8	3.7	0.69	1.64	13.6	154
Liver	402	0	0.7	-	-	-	-	0.1	0.3	0.9	0.7	3.1	4.2	9.0	11.6	20.6	17.3	27.7	26.5	24.4	4.5	0.8	0.15	0.34	2.9	155
Gallbladder etc.	223	0	-	-	-	-	-	-	-	0.1	0.6	0.5	1.7	2.9	5.2	8.6	13.8	15.6	24.9	33.0	2.5	0.4	0.06	0.17	1.5	156
Pancreas	1161	0	-	-	-	-	-	0.3	0.3	0.5	3.3	5.4	12.7	18.0	35.7	52.8	61.3	75.4	97.2	124.5	13.0	2.2	0.38	0.95	8.1	157
Nose, sinuses etc.	89	0	-	-	-	0.2	-	0.1	-	0.4	0.6	0.5	1.5	1.8	3.0	3.9	3.9	3.6	4.8	8.5	1.0	0.2	0.04	0.08	0.7	160
Larynx	802	0	-	-	-	-	0.2	-	0.3	1.2	2.8	5.9	12.7	21.9	33.4	37.8	43.7	31.2	42.6	19.5	9.0	1.5	0.39	0.80	6.1	161
Bronchus, lung	8425	0	0.2	-	-	-	0.8	1.4	1.4	5.9	11.9	38.3	95.1	187.2	293.4	386.2	475.4	558.7	619.6	467.7	94.3	16.0	3.18	7.49	59.7	162
Other thoracic organs	57	0	0.4	-	-	-	0.3	0.7	0.7	0.6	0.7	1.0	0.2	0.7	1.6	1.2	1.3	1.3	-	2.4	0.6	0.1	0.03	0.05	0.5	163-4
Bone	102	0	-	0.9	1.9	1.6	1.1	0.7	0.3	1.1	0.8	0.7	2.1	1.4	1.1	2.2	2.6	1.3	2.4	4.9	1.1	0.2	0.07	0.09	1.1	170
Connective tissue	338	0	1.5	0.2	0.7	0.7	0.9	1.6	1.6	1.8	2.8	4.3	4.6	6.5	5.7	9.6	13.5	14.7	16.9	20.8	3.8	0.6	0.17	0.28	2.8	171
Mesothelioma	166	0	-	-	-	-	-	-	-	0.1	0.1	1.0	1.9	3.2	6.1	8.1	7.1	14.7	14.7	9.6	9.8	1.9	0.3	0.06	0.14	1.2	MES
Kaposi's sarcoma	1789	0	-	-	-	-	3.4	23.8	45.3	52.7	39.8	32.9	21.3	13.1	5.5	2.2	4.2	4.9	6.4	15.9	20.0	3.4	1.19	1.22	14.5	KAP
Melanoma of skin	2020	2	-	-	0.2	2.0	5.6	8.2	9.9	14.9	21.5	29.6	36.7	41.5	51.3	57.7	64.5	72.7	88.4	81.8	22.6	3.8	1.11	1.72	16.0	172
†Other skin	155	0	-	-	-	0.4	-	0.3	1.4	0.6	1.4	1.7	2.5	1.8	2.0	5.9	5.8	10.3	8.8	8.5	1.7		0.06	0.12	1.1	173
Breast	131	0	-	-	-	-	-	-	0.2	0.7	1.0	1.5	2.3	3.4	6.6	6.4	8.9	9.6	8.5	1.5	0.2	0.05	0.11	0.9	175
Prostate	14961	2	0.2	0.2	-	-	-	-	0.1	0.4	1.2	11.8	40.6	161.1	382.0	749.6	1170.9	1321.8	1337.2	1167.3	167.5	28.4	2.99	12.59	96.3	185
Testis	658	0	0.6	-	0.2	3.8	10.4	14.7	18.9	13.5	8.7	6.1	3.8	3.2	1.6	1.5	1.9	2.7	2.4	-	7.4	1.2	0.43	0.44	5.8	186
Penis	64	0	-	-	-	-	-	-	0.1	-	0.1	0.5	0.6	1.6	1.1	1.7	4.2	3.1	9.6	6.1	0.7	0.1	0.02	0.05	0.4	187.1-.4
Other male genital	36	0	0.2	-	-	-	0.2	-	0.1	0.3	0.2	0.4	1.1	1.1	0.7	1.6	1.3	4.0	2.4	0.4	0.1	0.02	0.03	0.3	187.5-.9
Bladder	2526	0	0.2	-	-	-	0.2	0.6	1.2	1.5	2.8	10.6	18.6	38.6	72.2	112.4	149.9	192.8	215.4	258.9	28.3	4.8	0.73	2.04	17.1	188
Kidney etc.	1365	0	1.3	0.9	-	0.2	0.6	0.9	1.4	3.8	4.6	12.3	16.3	31.1	42.9	53.7	69.0	81.2	82.8	84.3	15.3	2.6	0.58	1.20	10.1	189
Eye	111	0	0.9	0.2	-	0.2	-	0.1	0.3	0.6	1.1	1.9	2.3	1.8	2.0	3.2	3.5	6.7	5.6	2.4	1.2	0.2	0.06	0.09	0.9	190
Brain, nervous system	886	0	5.2	4.3	1.7	3.3	2.8	3.8	5.1	5.2	6.5	8.3	12.5	18.7	22.5	27.2	28.2	34.8	29.7	30.5	9.9	1.7	0.50	0.78	7.8	191-2
Thyroid	335	0	-	-	-	-	1.7	1.6	3.4	2.8	5.7	6.6	7.1	6.3	7.0	6.9	7.4	8.5	6.4	7.3	3.8	0.6	0.21	0.28	2.8	193
Other endocrine	53	0	2.6	0.6	0.2	0.4	-	0.2	0.5	0.1	-	-	0.6	1.1	0.9	1.5	0.6	1.3	1.6	-	0.6	0.1	0.04	0.05	0.7	194
Hodgkin's disease	353	0	0.2	0.4	0.7	3.6	5.8	6.5	5.0	4.1	4.4	4.0	3.5	4.5	3.9	3.7	5.1	4.0	2.4	7.3	4.0	0.7	0.23	0.28	3.3	201
Non-Hodgkin lymphoma	2396	1	1.5	1.5	1.9	2.0	3.0	7.9	17.7	24.2	23.7	31.4	34.2	39.2	49.3	64.0	83.5	106.7	122.2	118.4	26.8	4.5	1.19	1.93	18.5	200,202
Multiple myeloma	512	1	-	-	-	-	-	0.1	0.7	0.5	0.6	2.4	5.8	6.8	12.9	21.1	32.4	41.9	40.2	44.0	5.7	1.0	0.15	0.42	3.5	203
Lymphoid leukaemia	642	0	6.6	3.4	2.9	2.4	0.5	0.6	0.7	1.2	1.1	2.6	6.5	10.6	16.4	21.3	28.2	37.0	49.0	62.3	7.2	1.2	0.28	0.53	5.6	204
Myeloid leukaemia	643	1	1.5	0.4	1.0	1.3	1.6	1.1	2.0	2.3	2.6	4.5	6.7	9.2	14.1	22.6	27.0	43.7	44.2	68.4	7.2	1.2	0.24	0.49	4.8	205
Monocytic leukaemia	29	0	0.2	-	-	-	-	-	0.1	-	-	0.2	0.2	0.2	0.7	1.2	1.3	2.7	2.4	3.7	0.3	0.1	0.01	0.02	0.2	206
Other leukaemia	14	0	-	-	-	-	-	-	0.1	-	-	-	0.2	0.2	-	1.0	1.0	1.3	0.8	-	0.2	0.0	0.00	0.01	0.1	207
Leukaemia unspecified	84	0	0.4	-	-	0.2	-	0.2	0.2	0.1	0.4	0.3	-	0.5	1.1	3.2	4.5	6.7	8.0	14.7	0.9	0.2	0.02	0.06	0.6	208
Other and unspecified	1577	0	0.6	-	0.5	-	0.2	0.7	1.0	2.8	6.4	11.1	13.8	29.5	46.6	51.0	79.0	104.9	142.2	189.3	17.7	3.0	0.57	1.22	11.0	O&U
All sites	52823	7	24.7	13.1	12.1	22.9	40.3	79.9	126.2	158.1	182.4	293.7	478.0	863.0	1423.3	2141.6	2946.8	3503.1	3871.9	3776.8	591.5		18.59	44.04	374.5	ALL
All sites but 173	52668	7	24.7	13.1	12.1	22.4	40.3	79.6	124.8	157.5	181.0	292.0	475.5	861.2	1421.2	2135.7	2941.1	3492.8	3863.1	3768.2	589.8	100.0	18.53	43.92	373.4	ALLb

| Rate from 1 case | | | 0.184 | 0.216 | 0.242 | 0.222 | 0.156 | 0.114 | 0.109 | 0.123 | 0.139 | 0.173 | 0.208 | 0.226 | 0.227 | 0.245 | 0.321 | 0.446 | 0.804 | 1.221 | | | | | | |

†Important: see notes on population page

USA, CALIFORNIA, LOS ANGELES COUNTY: NON-HISPANIC WHITE 1988-1992

ANNUAL INCIDENCE PER 100,000 BY AGE GROUP (YEARS) - FEMALE

SITE	ALL AGES	AGE UNK	0-	5-	10-	15-	20-	25-	30-	35-	40-	45-	50-	55-	60-	65-	70-	75-	80-	85+	CRUDE RATE	%	CR 64	CR 74	ASR (W)	ICD (9th)
Lip	54	0	-	-	-	-	0.2	0.1	0.2	0.1	0.3	-	0.4	0.7	1.3	1.4	2.7	1.2	2.5	3.5	0.6	0.1	0.02	0.04	0.3	140
Tongue	212	0	-	-	-	-	0.2	-	0.1	0.7	0.9	1.6	2.9	3.1	6.5	8.3	7.3	7.0	8.7	6.6	2.3	0.4	0.08	0.16	1.3	141
Salivary gland	113	1	-	-	-	0.2	-	0.2	0.5	0.7	0.9	1.4	1.3	1.3	2.7	2.8	4.6	2.6	5.0	3.1	1.2	0.2	0.05	0.08	0.7	142
Mouth	322	1	-	-	-	-	0.2	0.4	0.1	-	1.3	1.2	3.8	7.1	9.9	10.9	13.4	15.5	8.3	9.2	3.5	0.6	0.12	0.24	1.9	143-5
Oropharynx	148	0	-	0.2	-	-	-	-	0.1	0.3	0.4	1.0	1.5	3.8	4.4	5.9	5.4	6.1	5.4	2.2	1.6	0.3	0.06	0.11	0.9	146
Nasopharynx	34	0	0.2	-	-	-	-	-	0.1	-	-	0.7	0.8	0.9	0.4	1.6	1.0	0.9	0.8	0.4	0.4	0.1	0.02	0.03	0.2	147
Hypopharynx	59	0	-	-	-	-	-	0.1	-	-	0.3	0.2	0.6	2.2	2.5	3.2	1.2	2.0	0.8	-	0.6	0.1	0.03	0.05	0.4	148
Pharynx unspecified	32	0	0.2	-	-	-	-	-	-	0.1	0.1	0.2	1.3	0.2	0.6	1.7	1.2	1.2	1.3	0.3	0.1	0.01	0.02	0.2	149
Oesophagus	316	1	-	-	-	-	-	-	-	-	0.1	1.0	2.1	6.3	6.5	11.5	12.7	10.8	15.8	24.0	3.4	0.6	0.08	0.20	1.6	150
Stomach	682	0	-	-	-	-	-	0.4	0.5	0.9	0.9	3.0	7.8	8.0	10.9	13.6	23.1	29.7	44.8	64.7	7.4	1.4	0.16	0.35	3.2	151
Small intestine	151	0	-	-	-	-	-	0.1	0.2	0.3	1.0	1.7	1.7	2.2	4.2	3.8	5.6	5.8	6.6	5.7	1.6	0.3	0.06	0.10	0.9	152
Colon	4566	2	-	-	-	0.5	-	0.5	1.6	3.2	6.8	13.2	31.8	48.7	70.2	113.3	175.1	241.2	323.5	353.3	49.8	9.1	0.88	2.33	20.6	153
Rectum	1747	0	-	-	-	0.2	-	0.6	0.6	2.4	5.1	7.7	17.9	28.6	33.6	57.1	63.6	73.8	101.6	97.9	19.1	3.5	0.48	1.09	9.1	154
Liver	208	0	0.2	-	-	-	0.3	0.2	0.4	0.1	0.3	1.4	1.9	2.5	3.6	4.2	7.1	10.8	13.3	14.4	2.3	0.4	0.05	0.11	1.1	155
Gallbladder etc.	301	0	-	-	-	-	-	-	0.1	0.1	0.1	1.0	2.9	3.1	3.2	8.1	8.3	17.2	21.6	28.0	3.3	0.6	0.05	0.14	1.3	156
Pancreas	1206	0	-	-	-	-	0.2	-	0.4	1.3	1.6	4.5	7.8	9.6	21.4	35.6	50.9	66.5	73.4	80.0	13.2	2.4	0.23	0.67	5.6	157
Nose, sinuses etc.	59	0	-	-	-	0.2	-	-	-	0.1	0.4	0.2	0.6	1.1	0.8	2.0	2.2	2.6	2.1	3.5	0.6	0.1	0.02	0.04	0.3	160
Larynx	194	0	-	-	-	-	-	0.1	-	0.3	0.7	1.2	2.1	4.0	8.0	9.3	8.5	4.7	3.3	3.5	2.1	0.4	0.08	0.17	1.3	161
Bronchus, lung	6674	0	-	-	-	0.2	-	0.4	1.6	5.0	14.8	39.6	76.6	126.4	178.3	260.8	298.1	307.4	250.5	147.8	72.8	13.3	2.21	5.01	38.6	162
Other thoracic organs	21	0	0.2	-	0.3	-	-	-	-	0.4	0.1	0.2	-	0.7	0.4	0.8	0.5	-	0.8	0.4	0.2	0.0	0.01	0.02	0.2	163-4
Bone	89	0	0.2	0.7	2.1	1.9	0.3	0.5	1.0	0.7	0.7	0.2	0.8	1.8	1.1	1.4	1.5	1.5	2.1	1.7	1.0	0.2	0.06	0.07	0.9	170
Connective tissue	276	0	1.3	0.9	0.3	0.2	1.9	0.7	1.8	2.2	1.3	2.1	4.4	3.8	6.1	4.0	6.8	8.2	10.0	10.9	3.0	0.5	0.14	0.19	2.0	171
Mesothelioma	51	0	-	-	-	-	-	-	-	0.1	0.1	0.2	0.6	0.9	1.1	2.8	1.9	0.9	1.2	3.5	0.6	0.1	0.02	0.04	0.3	MES
Kaposi's sarcoma	31	1	-	-	-	-	-	0.2	0.5	0.1	-	-	-	0.2	0.2	0.4	-	2.0	2.9	2.2	0.3	0.1	0.01	0.01	0.1	KAP
Melanoma of skin	1489	0	-	-	0.5	2.3	6.8	13.2	16.1	16.1	18.2	22.5	23.4	18.1	30.5	28.7	30.0	28.9	21.6	28.0	16.2	3.0	0.84	1.13	11.3	172
†Other skin	132	1	-	-	-	-	0.2	0.9	0.8	0.8	1.3	0.9	1.7	2.2	1.5	3.4	2.4	4.4	5.0	7.4	1.4		0.05	0.08	0.8	173
Breast	15823	3	-	-	-	-	0.8	6.7	26.2	63.9	128.9	225.5	274.7	329.0	407.3	451.0	508.6	507.8	481.9	403.5	172.5	31.5	7.32	12.12	103.7	174
Uterus unspecified	32	0	-	-	-	-	-	-	-	-	0.1	0.5	0.2	0.4	0.6	0.2	1.5	1.2	1.7	3.1	0.3	0.1	0.01	0.02	0.2	179
Cervix uteri	935	0	-	-	-	0.2	1.0	5.6	12.4	15.6	13.5	17.6	13.0	20.3	14.5	16.8	13.4	14.6	13.3	10.5	10.2	1.9	0.57	0.72	7.2	180
Placenta	4	0	-	-	-	-	-	0.1	0.2	0.1	-	-	-	-	-	-	-	-	-	-	0.0	0.0	0.00	0.00	0.0	181
Corpus uteri	3294	1	-	-	-	-	-	0.4	2.9	5.6	10.1	24.1	41.9	71.5	94.1	130.7	145.6	128.3	93.7	60.3	35.9	6.6	1.25	2.63	20.2	182
Ovary etc.	2012	0	-	0.7	0.3	2.1	1.3	1.6	4.1	8.3	11.1	24.2	29.5	43.3	52.3	61.3	69.2	67.7	65.5	45.5	21.9	4.0	0.89	1.55	13.1	183
Other female genital	363	0	0.6	-	-	-	0.2	0.2	0.6	1.1	1.6	3.0	2.9	4.2	7.8	6.9	9.7	17.2	24.9	23.2	4.0	0.7	0.11	0.19	1.9	184
Bladder	886	0	-	-	-	-	-	0.1	0.6	0.3	1.1	3.0	5.7	11.2	16.4	24.5	37.3	40.5	61.0	60.3	9.7	1.8	0.19	0.50	4.2	188
Kidney etc.	813	0	2.1	0.5	-	-	-	0.4	0.5	1.7	2.3	8.2	9.9	13.4	17.0	24.3	34.3	35.9	32.3	29.3	8.9	1.6	0.28	0.57	4.9	189
Eye	94	0	1.9	-	-	-	-	0.5	0.6	0.3	0.1	1.9	0.8	1.6	3.2	1.8	1.7	2.0	2.9	2.2	1.0	0.2	0.05	0.07	0.8	190
Brain, nervous system	670	0	2.5	4.6	1.5	1.9	2.9	3.5	3.9	4.4	4.1	5.4	7.6	8.9	10.7	16.0	18.8	23.9	27.8	8.7	7.3	1.3	0.31	0.48	5.1	191-2
Thyroid	779	0	-	0.2	1.8	3.5	6.5	8.4	11.3	13.1	9.0	10.8	13.7	10.5	9.9	10.9	11.2	7.0	13.3	7.0	8.5	1.6	0.49	0.60	6.6	193
Other endocrine	38	0	1.9	0.2	-	-	-	-	0.1	-	0.1	0.2	0.6	-	0.8	1.0	0.7	1.5	1.2	0.4	0.4	0.1	0.02	0.03	0.4	194
Hodgkin's disease	279	0	-	0.2	0.3	3.7	5.3	5.9	4.7	4.6	1.6	1.9	1.5	1.8	2.5	2.2	3.4	5.2	4.6	1.7	3.0	0.6	0.17	0.20	2.5	201
Non-Hodgkin lymphoma	1725	0	0.6	0.5	0.5	1.6	1.3	2.1	3.1	5.0	6.7	11.0	16.8	25.2	34.9	52.2	66.2	69.4	84.2	79.6	18.8	3.4	0.55	1.14	9.8	200,202
Multiple myeloma	469	0	-	-	-	-	-	-	0.1	0.5	0.7	1.4	4.0	6.5	12.2	12.5	18.3	23.3	29.9	24.5	5.1	0.9	0.13	0.28	2.4	203
Lymphoid leukaemia	523	0	5.4	2.3	1.0	0.5	0.2	0.6	0.4	0.1	0.6	2.1	2.7	6.0	9.5	11.9	19.5	21.9	26.5	39.3	5.7	1.0	0.16	0.31	3.3	204
Myeloid leukaemia	502	0	1.3	0.9	0.3	1.4	1.0	1.1	2.2	2.5	2.7	4.5	4.2	6.7	6.9	12.5	16.3	16.6	23.2	27.1	5.5	1.0	0.18	0.32	3.2	205
Monocytic leukaemia	16	0	-	-	-	-	-	-	0.1	-	0.1	-	0.4	0.2	0.8	-	0.2	0.3	0.8	1.3	0.2	0.0	0.01	0.01	0.1	206
Other leukaemia	22	0	0.4	-	-	-	0.2	-	-	-	-	-	-	-	0.6	0.8	0.2	1.5	1.7	0.9	0.2	0.0	0.01	0.01	0.1	207
Leukaemia unspecified	90	0	-	0.2	0.3	0.2	0.2	-	-	0.1	-	0.9	0.2	0.4	1.3	2.0	1.9	4.4	7.9	8.3	1.0	0.2	0.02	0.04	0.4	208
Other and unspecified	1837	0	-	0.2	-	-	0.3	0.4	1.1	1.9	5.0	9.4	12.0	23.0	36.8	45.7	73.8	90.1	106.2	126.8	20.0	3.7	0.45	1.05	9.0	O&U
All sites	50373	11	19.1	12.4	9.0	20.9	31.2	56.5	101.9	165.1	257.2	462.4	638.0	873.1	1149.5	1481.2	1787.5	1933.1	2037.1	1866.8	549.3		18.99	35.33	304.3	ALL
All sites but 173	50241	10	19.1	12.4	9.0	20.9	31.1	55.6	101.0	164.3	255.9	461.6	636.4	870.9	1148.0	1477.8	1785.1	1928.7	2032.1	1859.4	547.9	100.0	18.93	35.25	303.5	ALLb

Rate from 1 case   0.193   0.223   0.258   0.232   0.162   0.125   0.121   0.132   0.142   0.174   0.210   0.223   0.210   0.202   0.244   0.292   0.415   0.437

†Important: see notes on population page

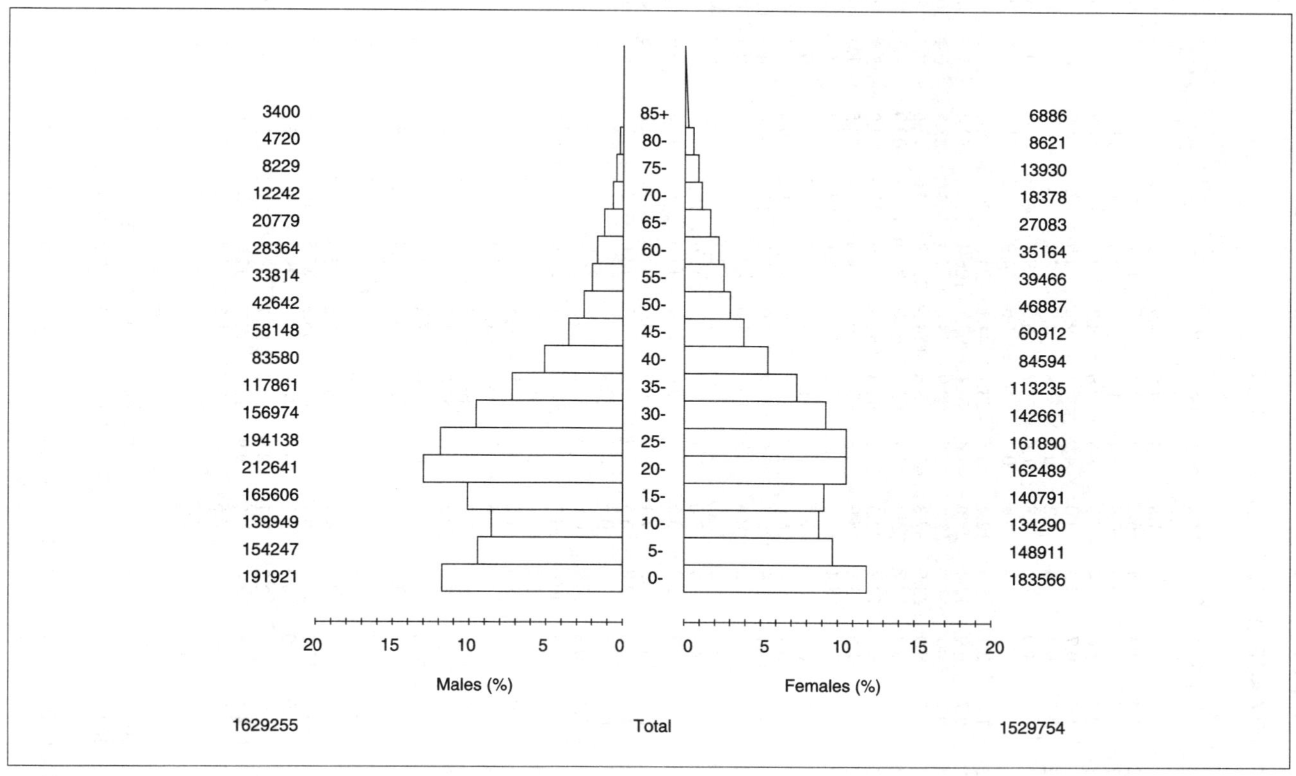

USA, California, Los Angeles County: Hispanic White
Source of population: 1990
Census: 1990 Census.
Notes to tables overleaf:
† 173 does not include basal cell or squamous cell carcinoma
The denominators are not the same populations as those published in Volume VI and the data for this ethnic group are not comparable.

USA, CALIFORNIA, LOS ANGELES COUNTY: HISPANIC WHITE 1988-1992

ANNUAL INCIDENCE PER 100,000 BY AGE GROUP (YEARS) - MALE

SITE	ALL AGES	AGE UNK	0-	5-	10-	15-	20-	25-	30-	35-	40-	45-	50-	55-	60-	65-	70-	75-	80-	85+	CRUDE RATE	%	CR 64	CR 74	ASR (W)	ICD (9th)
Lip	23	0	-	-	-	-	-	-	-	-	1.0	-	1.8	1.4	4.8	4.9	7.3	4.2	17.6		0.3	0.2	0.02	0.07	0.6	140
Tongue	59	0	-	-	-	-	-	0.1	-	0.2	1.0	2.4	3.8	6.5	5.6	7.7	6.5	12.2	8.5	-	0.7	0.6	0.10	0.17	1.4	141
Salivary gland	23	0	-	-	-	0.1	0.2	0.2	0.1	0.7	0.5	-	0.9	0.6	1.4	1.9	-	2.4	4.2	11.8	0.3	0.2	0.02	0.03	0.4	142
Mouth	54	0	-	-	-	-	-	0.1	-	0.3	0.5	1.0	1.4	5.9	8.5	9.6	8.2	2.4	12.7	11.8	0.7	0.5	0.09	0.18	1.4	143-5
Oropharynx	43	0	-	-	-	-	-	-	0.1	-	1.0	0.7	2.3	3.0	4.9	6.7	9.8	4.9	12.7	5.9	0.5	0.4	0.06	0.14	1.1	146
Nasopharynx	20	0	-	0.1	-	0.1	-	-	-	0.2	0.7	0.7	0.5	1.2	0.7	4.8	3.3	2.4	-	-	0.2	0.2	0.02	0.06	0.5	147
Hypopharynx	25	0	-	-	-	-	-	-	-	-	-	1.0	1.9	1.8	1.4	1.9	6.5	9.7	12.7	-	0.3	0.2	0.03	0.07	0.6	148
Pharynx unspecified	8	0	-	-	-	-	-	-	-	-	-	-	-	0.6	0.7	-	1.6	4.9	4.2	11.8	0.1	0.1	0.01	0.01	0.2	149
Oesophagus	140	0	-	-	-	-	0.1	0.1	-	0.3	1.0	2.1	5.6	12.4	13.4	23.1	44.1	24.3	29.7	35.3	1.7	1.3	0.18	0.51	3.7	150
Stomach	481	0	-	-	-	-	0.2	0.4	2.2	2.9	5.7	6.9	17.4	26.6	44.4	74.1	93.1	126.4	148.3	182.4	5.9	4.6	0.53	1.37	11.8	151
Small intestine	29	0	-	-	-	-	-	-	0.3	-	0.7	-	-	2.4	2.8	2.9	8.2	7.3	4.2	23.5	0.4	0.3	0.03	0.09	0.7	152
Colon	668	0	-	-	-	-	0.2	0.4	1.5	1.7	5.7	8.9	23.5	37.3	62.1	113.6	158.5	213.9	207.6	217.6	8.2	6.3	0.71	2.07	17.1	153
Rectum	384	0	-	-	-	0.2	0.2	0.5	1.0	2.2	2.9	6.2	12.7	23.7	44.4	65.5	67.0	92.4	127.1	100.0	4.7	3.6	0.47	1.13	9.5	154
Liver	264	0	0.8	0.1	0.1	0.1	0.1	0.3	0.8	1.2	2.6	4.1	12.2	22.5	26.1	41.4	58.8	38.9	33.9	52.9	3.2	2.5	0.36	0.86	6.5	155
Gallbladder etc.	83	0	0.1	-	-	-	-	-	0.1	0.2	1.0	1.0	3.8	5.9	6.3	13.5	19.6	14.6	42.4	23.5	1.0	0.8	0.09	0.26	2.1	156
Pancreas	275	0	-	-	-	-	0.1	0.2	0.4	0.7	1.7	5.2	8.4	16.6	34.6	42.4	65.3	68.1	59.3	129.4	3.4	2.6	0.34	0.88	7.2	157
Nose, sinuses etc.	25	0	-	-	-	-	0.1	0.2	0.1	0.2	1.4	0.7	0.5	1.2	1.4	1.0	3.3	2.4	8.5	5.9	0.3	0.2	0.03	0.05	0.5	160
Larynx	157	0	-	-	-	-	-	-	0.3	1.4	3.1	7.0	16.6	21.9	21.2	40.8	21.9	21.2	29.4	1.9	1.5	0.25	0.56	4.1	161
Bronchus, lung	1183	0	-	-	0.1	0.4	0.2	0.2	1.7	2.0	4.8	14.1	36.6	70.4	117.0	199.2	285.9	413.2	377.1	500.0	14.5	11.2	1.24	3.66	31.0	162
Other thoracic organs	31	0	0.4	-	0.3	0.6	0.6	0.5	0.3	0.2	-	-	0.5	0.6	0.7	-	1.6	2.4	-	5.9	0.4	0.3	0.02	0.03	0.4	163-4
Bone	77	0	0.1	0.4	1.9	2.4	1.3	0.8	0.6	0.2	1.2	0.7	0.5	-	1.4	-	-	2.4	4.2	-	0.9	0.7	0.06	0.06	0.9	170
Connective tissue	118	0	1.8	0.3	0.9	1.2	0.6	0.4	1.0	1.0	2.2	3.8	1.9	3.0	7.1	6.7	1.6	17.0	12.7	11.8	1.4	1.1	0.12	0.17	2.0	171
Mesothelioma	45	0	-	-	-	-	-	-	-	0.2	0.2	0.3	1.9	3.5	3.5	9.6	11.4	14.6	8.5	11.8	0.6	0.4	0.05	0.15	1.2	MES
Kaposi's sarcoma	718	0	0.1	-	-	0.1	2.7	13.6	25.1	28.5	22.3	15.1	11.3	7.1	1.4	6.7	3.3	7.3	4.2	11.8	8.8	6.8	0.64	0.69	8.1	KAP
Melanoma of skin	102	0	-	-	0.1	-	0.7	0.3	1.5	1.5	1.7	2.8	2.8	6.5	9.2	9.6	8.2	14.6	8.5	11.8	1.3	1.0	0.14	0.22	2.0	172
†Other skin	25	0	0.1	0.1	0.1	-	-	0.2	0.8	0.3	0.7	0.9	0.7	0.6	0.7	2.9	-	-	4.2	-	0.3		0.03	0.04	0.4	173
Breast	13	0	-	-	-	-	-	-	-	-	0.2	0.3	0.9	0.6	1.4	1.0	3.3	2.4	4.2	5.9	0.2	0.1	0.02	0.04	0.3	175
Prostate	2192	1	-	-	-	-	-	-	-	1.2	6.5	30.0	76.9	220.0	444.7	753.1	840.9	940.7	1000.0		26.9	20.8	1.67	7.67	60.4	185
Testis	303	0	1.1	-	-	2.2	4.9	8.7	7.8	6.4	5.0	1.7	1.4	3.0	2.1	1.9	-	-	-	-	3.7	2.9	0.22	0.23	3.0	186
Penis	37	0	-	-	-	-	-	0.1	0.3	0.3	1.0	0.7	2.3	1.2	2.1	5.8	6.5	4.9	8.5	11.8	0.5	0.4	0.04	0.10	0.8	187.1-.4
Other male genital	9	0	0.2	-	-	-	-	0.1	-	0.2	-	-	-	0.6	0.7	-	1.6	2.4	-	5.9	0.1	0.1	0.01	0.02	0.2	187.5-.9
Bladder	317	0	-	-	-	-	0.2	0.3	0.6	-	2.9	2.1	5.2	17.2	31.7	49.1	91.5	114.2	122.9	123.5	3.9	3.0	0.30	1.00	8.3	188
Kidney etc.	377	1	1.6	0.4	-	0.2	-	0.3	0.6	1.0	3.8	11.4	17.4	30.8	30.3	51.0	71.9	75.3	76.3	88.2	4.6	3.6	0.49	1.11	9.2	189
Eye	30	0	1.6	-	-	0.1	0.2	-	-	0.2	0.5	0.3	-	1.2	0.7	1.0	3.3	2.4	-	5.9	0.4	0.3	0.02	0.04	0.5	190
Brain, nervous system	286	0	4.1	2.5	1.6	1.7	1.9	1.9	3.6	3.1	3.8	3.8	7.5	4.7	12.7	22.1	16.3	19.4	16.9	29.4	3.5	2.7	0.26	0.46	4.7	191-2
Thyroid	100	0	-	0.1	-	0.2	0.5	1.4	1.0	2.5	1.9	3.8	1.4	7.1	3.5	1.0	11.4	12.2	8.5	5.9	1.2	0.9	0.12	0.18	1.7	193
Other endocrine	33	0	2.0	0.6	0.3	0.1	0.1	-	-	0.2	0.2	-	0.5	0.6	-	1.0	-	-	-	-	0.4	0.3	0.02	0.03	0.4	194
Hodgkin's disease	149	0	0.4	0.6	1.1	1.6	1.9	1.8	1.8	2.7	2.2	2.1	2.3	4.7	6.3	5.8	1.6	7.3	12.7	11.8	1.8	1.4	0.15	0.18	2.1	201
Non-Hodgkin lymphoma	633	0	1.7	1.2	2.0	1.7	1.7	4.0	7.8	12.9	10.1	17.2	22.0	36.1	31.7	43.3	55.5	87.5	76.3	47.1	7.8	6.0	0.75	1.24	11.7	200,202
Multiple myeloma	145	0	-	-	-	-	0.2	-	0.5	0.5	1.0	1.0	6.6	14.2	13.4	28.9	26.1	29.2	33.9	35.3	1.8	1.4	0.19	0.46	3.7	203
Lymphoid leukaemia	272	0	8.0	4.5	3.0	1.9	1.5	0.9	1.4	1.5	1.7	1.4	2.3	7.1	8.5	11.6	14.7	19.4	21.2	23.5	3.3	2.6	0.22	0.35	4.2	204
Myeloid leukaemia	193	0	1.4	0.6	1.1	1.4	1.4	1.5	1.9	2.0	4.1	2.8	3.8	6.5	9.9	10.6	14.7	12.2	25.4	52.9	2.4	1.8	0.19	0.32	3.3	205
Monocytic leukaemia	10	0	0.1	-	-	-	0.2	0.1	-	0.2	0.2	-	0.6	-	1.0	1.6	2.4	-	-	-	0.1	0.1	0.01	0.02	0.2	206
Other leukaemia	4	0	0.2	-	-	-	-	-	-	-	-	-	-	-	-	-	2.4	4.2	-	-	0.0	0.0	0.00	0.00	0.1	207
Leukaemia unspecified	39	0	0.1	0.3	-	0.1	0.4	0.3	0.3	0.5	-	1.0	0.5	2.4	1.4	2.9	3.3	14.6	-	11.8	0.5	0.4	0.04	0.07	0.7	208
Other and unspecified	364	0	0.4	-	-	0.5	0.2	0.8	1.4	1.7	3.1	7.2	12.2	16.0	33.8	51.0	81.7	85.1	105.9	158.8	4.5	3.5	0.39	1.05	8.9	O&U
All sites	10566	2	26.3	11.9	12.7	17.1	22.3	40.9	66.5	80.9	103.4	145.8	274.4	509.3	833.5	1404.3	2069.9	2462.0	2618.6	3029.4	129.7		10.73	28.10	239.7	ALL
All sites but 173	10541	2	26.2	11.8	12.6	17.1	22.3	40.7	65.7	80.6	102.9	145.1	273.4	508.7	832.7	1401.4	2069.9	2462.0	2614.4	3029.4	129.4	100.0	10.70	28.06	239.4	ALLb

Rate from 1 case   0.104   0.130   0.143   0.121   0.094   0.103   0.127   0.170   0.239   0.344   0.469   0.591   0.705   0.963   1.634   2.430   4.237   5.882

†Important: see notes on population page

USA, CALIFORNIA, LOS ANGELES COUNTY: HISPANIC WHITE 1988-1992

ANNUAL INCIDENCE PER 100,000 BY AGE GROUP (YEARS) - FEMALE

SITE	ALL AGES	AGE UNK	0-	5-	10-	15-	20-	25-	30-	35-	40-	45-	50-	55-	60-	65-	70-	75-	80-	85+	CRUDE RATE	%	CR 64	CR 74	ASR (W)	ICD (9th)
Lip	8	0	-	-	-	0.1	-	-	-	-	-	-	-	-	0.6	-	2.2	1.4	4.6	2.9	0.1	0.1	0.00	0.01	0.1	140
Tongue	32	0	-	-	-	-	-	-	0.6	0.4	0.7	0.3	3.4	1.5	2.3	3.0	1.1	-	-	5.8	0.4	0.3	0.05	0.07	0.6	141
Salivary gland	27	0	-	-	0.1	-	-	0.2	0.6	0.2	0.5	1.6	-	1.5	1.7	1.5	-	2.9	4.6	-	0.4	0.2	0.03	0.04	0.4	142
Mouth	33	0	-	-	0.1	-	0.1	0.1	0.3	0.2	0.7	0.3	1.3	1.5	-	0.7	4.4	7.2	11.6	5.8	0.4	0.3	0.02	0.05	0.5	143-5
Oropharynx	10	0	-	-	-	-	-	-	-	-	0.2	-	0.9	0.5	-	0.7	2.2	2.9	2.3	-	0.1	0.1	0.01	0.02	0.2	146
Nasopharynx	12	0	-	-	-	0.4	-	-	0.1	-	-	-	0.4	0.5	0.6	2.2	-	-	4.6	-	0.2	0.1	0.01	0.02	0.2	147
Hypopharynx	2	0	-	-	-	-	-	-	-	-	-	-	-	-	-	-	-	2.9	-	-	0.0	0.0	0.00	0.00	0.0	148
Pharynx unspecified	5	0	-	-	-	-	-	0.1	-	-	-	-	-	-	0.6	-	1.1	1.4	-	2.9	0.1	0.0	0.00	0.01	0.1	149
Oesophagus	31	0	-	-	-	-	-	0.1	-	-	-	0.3	0.4	2.0	3.4	2.2	5.4	5.7	9.3	5.8	0.4	0.3	0.03	0.07	0.6	150
Stomach	403	0	-	-	0.1	0.1	0.2	0.6	3.1	2.8	5.4	5.6	9.8	18.8	21.0	36.2	42.4	54.6	97.4	148.1	5.3	3.5	0.34	0.73	6.9	151
Small intestine	28	0	-	-	-	-	-	-	-	0.4	-	0.3	0.4	2.0	2.8	4.4	2.2	4.3	4.6	5.8	0.4	0.2	0.03	0.06	0.5	152
Colon	660	0	-	-	-	-	0.1	0.5	1.1	2.5	5.9	9.9	17.1	31.4	36.4	59.1	104.5	127.8	178.6	203.3	8.6	5.7	0.52	1.34	11.8	153
Rectum	342	0	-	-	-	-	0.1	0.6	1.3	2.3	3.5	7.9	10.2	14.7	21.6	42.8	51.1	45.9	34.8	92.9	4.5	3.0	0.31	0.78	6.3	154
Liver	123	0	0.5	0.1	0.1	0.1	0.2	0.4	0.1	0.4	0.2	0.7	3.0	5.6	9.1	9.6	20.7	17.2	27.8	40.7	1.6	1.1	0.10	0.25	2.2	155
Gallbladder etc.	228	0	-	-	-	-	-	-	0.6	0.4	1.7	1.6	7.3	10.6	15.9	28.1	32.6	35.9	71.9	58.1	3.0	2.0	0.19	0.49	4.2	156
Pancreas	288	0	-	-	-	0.1	-	0.1	0.1	0.4	2.1	3.9	6.4	8.6	21.6	30.3	44.6	73.2	71.9	81.3	3.8	2.5	0.22	0.59	5.2	157
Nose, sinuses etc.	27	0	-	-	-	-	0.1	0.1	0.3	0.5	-	0.7	2.1	0.5	1.7	3.7	1.1	1.4	2.3	2.9	0.4	0.2	0.03	0.05	0.5	160
Larynx	22	0	-	-	-	-	-	0.1	0.1	0.2	-	-	0.9	0.5	3.4	1.5	4.4	4.3	2.3	-	0.3	0.2	0.03	0.06	0.4	161
Bronchus, lung	762	0	0.1	-	0.1	-	-	0.1	0.3	2.6	4.3	13.1	18.8	35.5	62.0	88.6	144.7	143.6	132.2	148.1	10.0	6.6	0.68	1.85	14.5	162
Other thoracic organs	10	0	0.3	-	-	0.1	-	-	-	-	-	0.3	0.9	-	0.6	0.7	1.1	-	-	-	0.1	0.1	0.01	0.02	0.2	163-4
Bone	64	0	-	0.9	1.9	2.6	0.2	0.5	0.1	0.4	0.7	0.7	1.3	1.5	2.8	-	-	-	2.3	-	0.8	0.6	0.07	0.07	0.9	170
Connective tissue	103	0	1.0	0.5	0.6	0.9	0.7	0.5	0.7	2.3	2.1	2.3	3.4	1.5	2.8	5.2	3.3	7.2	11.6	-	1.3	0.9	0.10	0.14	1.5	171
Mesothelioma	16	0	-	-	-	0.1	-	0.1	0.3	0.2	-	0.3	-	-	1.1	-	2.2	5.7	2.3	2.9	0.2	0.1	0.01	0.02	0.2	MES
Kaposi's sarcoma	18	0	-	-	-	-	-	0.5	0.6	0.2	0.7	0.7	-	-	-	-	1.1	-	4.6	2.9	0.2	0.2	0.01	0.02	0.2	KAP
Melanoma of skin	139	1	-	-	0.1	0.4	0.2	1.4	1.3	2.5	3.1	2.6	4.7	4.6	4.0	11.1	7.6	20.1	13.9	23.2	1.8	1.2	0.13	0.22	2.2	172
†Other skin	41	0	-	-	0.3	0.4	0.5	0.2	1.1	0.2	1.2	0.7	1.7	-	1.1	1.5	2.2	2.9	2.3	2.9	0.5		0.04	0.06	0.6	173
Breast	3186	1	-	-	-	-	1.0	4.9	18.9	47.0	75.4	133.3	141.6	184.5	193.4	245.2	285.1	268.5	290.0	200.4	41.7	27.7	4.00	6.65	57.4	174
Uterus unspecified	9	0	-	-	-	-	-	-	0.1	-	-	0.3	-	-	0.6	-	1.1	-	4.6	8.7	0.1	0.1	0.01	0.01	0.1	179
Cervix uteri	1172	0	-	-	0.1	0.3	2.8	10.1	25.0	29.3	40.9	40.7	45.6	47.1	40.4	48.0	32.6	35.9	48.7	31.9	15.3	10.2	1.41	1.82	17.9	180
Placenta	13	0	-	-	-	0.1	0.2	0.5	0.3	0.5	0.2	-	-	-	-	-	-	-	-	-	0.2	0.1	0.01	0.01	0.1	181
Corpus uteri	608	0	-	-	-	0.1	0.4	1.5	2.2	5.3	9.0	21.3	35.0	32.4	52.3	62.0	54.4	44.5	58.0	43.6	7.9	5.3	0.80	1.38	11.5	182
Ovary etc.	514	0	0.1	0.4	1.3	2.3	1.7	2.2	2.8	4.6	9.5	12.8	20.0	25.3	32.4	44.3	47.9	50.3	46.4	43.6	6.7	4.5	0.58	1.04	9.0	183
Other female genital	84	0	0.1	-	-	-	-	0.1	0.1	0.2	0.5	1.0	2.1	6.1	3.4	5.9	13.1	21.5	27.8	14.5	1.1	0.7	0.07	0.16	1.5	184
Bladder	135	0	-	-	-	-	0.1	-	0.1	-	1.2	2.0	4.7	2.0	6.8	17.0	28.3	24.4	41.8	31.9	1.8	1.2	0.08	0.31	2.5	188
Kidney etc.	266	0	1.7	0.4	0.4	-	0.1	0.5	1.1	1.1	4.0	4.9	9.0	13.7	17.6	29.5	23.9	37.3	32.5	34.9	3.5	2.3	0.27	0.54	4.8	189
Eye	24	0	1.1	-	-	-	-	0.1	0.1	0.5	0.2	0.7	0.9	-	-	0.7	1.1	1.4	-	2.9	0.3	0.2	0.02	0.03	0.3	190
Brain, nervous system	233	0	3.5	2.0	1.9	1.0	1.2	2.0	2.4	1.9	3.5	3.9	9.0	5.6	7.4	8.9	16.3	8.6	4.6	14.5	3.0	2.0	0.23	0.35	3.6	191-2
Thyroid	384	0	-	0.1	0.3	2.6	3.2	7.4	7.9	7.1	11.1	9.5	11.5	11.1	11.9	5.9	10.9	4.3	20.9	14.5	5.0	3.3	0.42	0.50	5.4	193
Other endocrine	22	0	1.1	-	-	-	0.1	0.1	0.3	-	0.2	-	0.9	1.0	0.6	1.5	-	-	-	-	0.3	0.2	0.02	0.03	0.3	194
Hodgkin's disease	105	0	0.1	0.1	1.8	2.0	2.0	1.5	1.1	0.9	1.2	1.6	0.4	2.0	3.4	3.0	6.5	4.3	-	5.8	1.4	0.9	0.09	0.14	1.5	201
Non-Hodgkin lymphoma	405	0	1.1	0.3	0.3	1.6	1.4	1.1	2.8	1.9	3.8	6.6	16.6	19.8	22.8	36.2	45.7	51.7	71.9	49.4	5.3	3.5	0.40	0.81	7.1	200,202
Multiple myeloma	134	0	-	-	-	-	-	0.1	0.1	-	1.7	1.3	3.0	6.1	9.7	17.0	25.0	27.3	32.5	17.4	1.8	1.2	0.11	0.32	2.5	203
Lymphoid leukaemia	205	0	6.6	4.6	2.7	1.3	1.4	0.6	0.6	0.4	0.9	1.6	2.1	4.6	5.7	5.2	7.6	7.2	7.0	17.4	2.7	1.8	0.17	0.23	3.0	204
Myeloid leukaemia	180	0	1.2	0.7	0.4	0.9	1.2	1.7	2.2	2.6	4.0	1.3	4.3	8.1	6.8	6.6	13.1	11.5	18.6	11.6	2.4	1.6	0.18	0.28	2.7	205
Monocytic leukaemia	3	0	-	-	-	-	-	-	-	-	0.2	-	-	-	-	0.7	1.1	-	-	-	0.0	0.0	0.00	0.01	0.1	206
Other leukaemia	3	0	0.1	0.1	-	-	-	-	-	-	-	-	-	-	0.6	-	-	-	-	-	0.0	0.0	0.00	0.00	0.0	207
Leukaemia unspecified	18	0	0.4	-	0.1	-	-	0.1	-	0.4	-	-	0.9	-	-	2.2	-	2.9	2.3	5.8	0.2	0.2	0.01	0.02	0.3	208
Other and unspecified	413	1	0.2	0.1	-	0.4	0.1	0.2	1.1	1.9	3.8	4.3	8.5	20.3	29.0	33.2	52.2	71.8	118.3	145.2	5.4	3.6	0.35	0.78	7.3	O&U
All sites	11550	3	19.4	10.5	13.3	18.0	19.7	41.4	82.0	124.3	204.5	301.1	410.3	533.1	662.0	906.1	1148.1	1241.9	1524.2	1530.6	151.0		12.20	22.48	200.0	ALL
All sites but 173	11509	3	19.4	10.5	13.0	17.6	19.2	41.1	80.9	124.2	203.3	300.4	408.6	533.1	660.9	904.6	1145.9	1239.1	1521.9	1527.7	150.5	100.0	12.16	22.42	199.4	ALLb

Rate from 1 case   0.109   0.134   0.149   0.142   0.123   0.124   0.140   0.177   0.236   0.328   0.427   0.507   0.569   0.738   1.088   1.436   2.320   2.904

†Important: see notes on population page

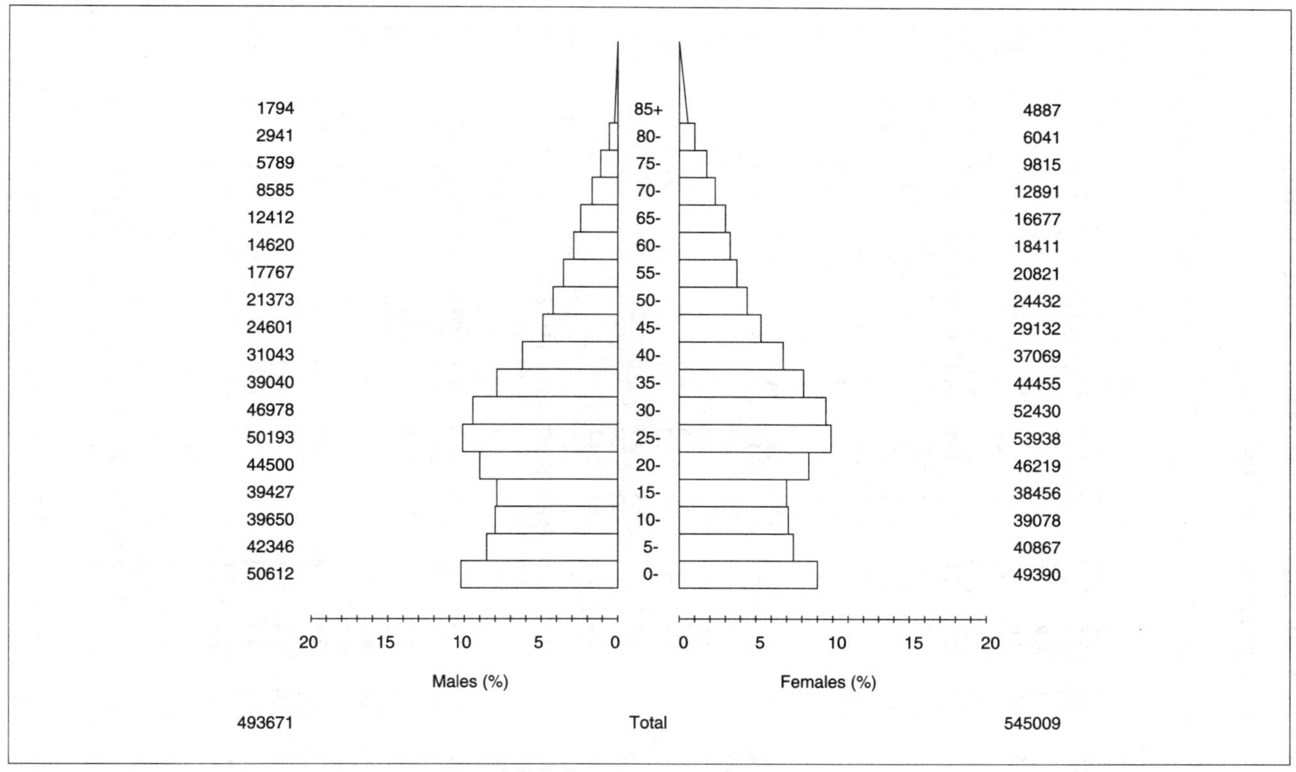

USA, California, Los Angeles County: Black
Source of population: 1990
Census: 1990 Census.
Notes to tables overleaf:
† 173 does not include basal cell or squamous cell carcinoma
The denominators are not the same populations as those published in Volume VI and the data for this ethnic group are not comparable.

USA, CALIFORNIA, LOS ANGELES COUNTY: BLACK 1988-1992

ANNUAL INCIDENCE PER 100,000 BY AGE GROUP (YEARS) - MALE

SITE	ALL AGES	AGE UNK	0-	5-	10-	15-	20-	25-	30-	35-	40-	45-	50-	55-	60-	65-	70-	75-	80-	85+	CRUDE RATE	%	CR 64	CR 74	ASR (W)	ICD (9th)
Lip	0	0	-	-	-	-	-	-	-	-	-	-	-	-	-	-	-	-	-	-	0.0	0.0	0.00	0.00	0.0	140
Tongue	86	0	-	-	-	-	0.4	0.8	0.4	2.0	3.9	4.9	10.3	20.3	12.3	25.8	11.6	10.4	13.6	22.3	3.5	0.9	0.28	0.46	3.9	141
Salivary gland	19	0	-	-	0.5	0.5	-	-	-	1.0	0.6	1.6	0.9	3.4	4.1	3.2	4.7	-	-	11.1	0.8	0.2	0.06	0.10	0.9	142
Mouth	93	0	-	-	-	0.5	-	-	0.4	0.5	1.9	13.8	12.2	14.6	28.7	14.5	14.0	20.7	13.6	-	3.8	1.0	0.36	0.51	4.4	143-5
Oropharynx	57	0	-	-	-	0.5	-	-	0.4	0.5	1.3	3.3	7.5	13.5	17.8	16.1	7.0	3.5	6.8	-	2.3	0.6	0.22	0.34	2.7	146
Nasopharynx	22	0	-	0.5	0.5	1.5	-	-	0.4	-	1.3	0.8	1.9	2.3	2.7	3.2	4.7	3.5	13.6	-	0.9	0.2	0.06	0.10	1.0	147
Hypopharynx	36	0	-	-	-	-	-	-	-	0.5	0.6	1.6	6.6	4.5	6.8	16.1	7.0	3.5	13.6	-	1.5	0.4	0.10	0.22	1.7	148
Pharynx unspecified	20	0	-	-	-	-	-	0.4	0.5	-	-	2.8	3.4	5.5	8.1	7.0	-	-	-	-	0.8	0.2	0.06	0.14	0.9	149
Oesophagus	198	0	-	-	-	-	0.4	0.4	1.5	1.9	7.3	25.3	34.9	47.9	58.0	60.6	51.8	40.8	55.7		8.0	2.1	0.60	1.19	9.2	150
Stomach	304	0	-	-	-	-	0.4	0.9	4.1	7.7	12.2	17.8	41.7	38.3	96.7	123.5	114.0	149.6	156.1		12.3	3.2	0.62	1.72	13.6	151
Small intestine	36	0	-	-	-	-	-	-	-	2.6	3.3	2.8	9.0	8.2	6.4	7.0	6.9	-	22.3		1.5	0.4	0.13	0.20	1.7	152
Colon	771	0	-	-	-	-	-	1.2	1.7	4.6	21.9	29.3	55.2	81.0	145.0	217.5	244.6	373.1	401.2	457.1	31.2	8.1	1.70	4.01	34.8	153
Rectum	290	0	-	-	-	0.5	-	0.4	1.7	4.1	8.4	11.4	27.1	39.4	65.7	83.8	58.2	110.6	129.2	100.3	11.7	3.1	0.79	1.50	13.1	154
Liver	111	0	0.8	-	-	-	-	-	1.3	-	2.6	5.7	7.5	15.8	34.2	17.7	44.3	38.0	40.8	11.1	4.5	1.2	0.34	0.65	5.1	155
Gallbladder etc.	33	0	-	-	-	-	-	0.4	-	0.5	0.6	0.8	3.7	1.1	6.8	1.6	21.0	3.5	20.4	55.7	1.3	0.3	0.07	0.18	1.5	156
Pancreas	233	1	-	-	-	-	-	-	-	1.0	3.9	7.3	18.7	16.9	36.9	70.9	102.5	103.6	170.0	111.5	9.4	2.5	0.43	1.30	10.5	157
Nose, sinuses etc.	23	0	-	-	-	-	-	-	0.9	1.0	-	-	1.9	4.5	5.5	3.2	9.3	6.9	6.8	-	0.9	0.2	0.07	0.13	1.0	160
Larynx	213	0	-	-	-	-	-	-	-	-	1.0	8.4	6.5	17.8	43.9	52.0	69.3	55.9	51.8	47.6	55.7	8.6	2.3	0.65	1.27	9.9	161
Bronchus, lung	1925	0	-	-	-	-	1.3	-	1.3	11.8	43.2	91.9	177.8	311.8	429.5	544.6	663.9	649.5	571.2	445.9	78.0	20.3	5.34	11.39	88.7	162
Other thoracic organs	12	0	0.8	0.5	-	-	-	0.4	-	0.5	0.6	0.8	2.8	1.1	1.4	-	-	-	-	-	0.5	0.1	0.04	0.04	0.5	163-4
Bone	21	0	-	0.5	0.5	1.5	0.9	0.4	0.9	0.5	0.6	1.6	0.9	1.1	2.7	3.2	2.3	-	-	-	0.9	0.2	0.06	0.09	0.9	170
Connective tissue	52	0	2.0	-	2.0	1.0	1.8	0.4	1.3	1.5	2.6	3.3	3.7	2.3	5.5	4.8	2.3	20.7	6.8	11.1	2.1	0.5	0.14	0.17	2.2	171
Mesothelioma	15	0	-	-	-	-	-	-	-	-	1.6	0.9	2.3	2.7	1.6	4.7	10.4	6.8	11.1	0.6	0.2	0.04	0.07	0.7	MES
Kaposi's sarcoma	273	0	-	-	-	0.5	1.8	19.5	37.5	29.2	19.3	17.1	9.4	6.8	2.7	-	2.3	10.4	-	11.1	11.1	2.9	0.72	0.73	9.0	KAP
Melanoma of skin	20	0	0.4	-	-	-	-	0.9	0.4	-	0.5	-	-	-	2.3	2.7	-	7.0	10.4	27.2	11.1	0.8	0.2	0.04	0.07	0.8	172
†Other skin	21	0	-	-	-	-	-	-	0.9	2.0	4.5	0.8	2.8	1.1	4.1	-	-	-	-	-	0.9		0.08	0.08	0.8	173
Breast	12	0	-	-	-	-	-	-	0.5	-	-	0.9	1.1	2.7	1.6	4.7	6.9	6.8	11.1	0.5	0.1	0.03	0.06	0.5	175
Prostate	2865	2	-	-	-	-	-	-	-	-	4.5	15.4	73.9	247.7	593.7	1010.3	1418.8	1551.2	1740.9	1817.2	116.1	30.3	4.68	16.83	130.6	185
Testis	35	0	0.4	-	0.5	0.5	2.7	2.0	5.5	3.1	-	-	0.9	-	-	-	3.5	-	-		1.4	0.4	0.08	0.08	1.1	186
Penis	24	0	-	-	-	-	-	-	0.5	1.3	0.8	1.9	1.1	1.4	3.2	9.3	17.3	20.4	22.3		1.0	0.3	0.03	0.10	1.0	187.1-.4
Other male genital	2	0	0.4	-	-	-	-	-	-	-	-	-	-	1.6	-	-	-	-	-		0.1	0.0	0.00	0.01	0.1	187.5-.9
Bladder	206	0	-	-	-	-	-	0.4	0.9	3.1	5.2	4.9	7.5	15.8	32.8	41.9	100.2	110.6	142.8	167.2	8.3	2.2	0.35	1.06	9.1	188
Kidney etc.	237	0	2.8	1.4	-	0.5	-	0.8	1.3	2.0	3.2	7.3	30.9	29.3	45.1	70.9	72.2	69.1	61.2	78.0	9.6	2.5	0.62	1.34	10.9	189
Eye	6	0	0.4	-	-	-	-	-	-	-	1.6	-	1.1	1.4	-	-	-	6.8	-		0.2	0.1	0.02	0.02	0.3	190
Brain, nervous system	105	0	3.2	2.8	1.0	1.0	1.3	2.8	4.7	1.5	3.9	3.3	8.4	10.1	15.0	14.5	18.6	13.8	20.4	-	4.3	1.1	0.30	0.46	4.5	191-2
Thyroid	25	0	-	0.5	-	-	0.4	1.2	0.9	1.5	0.6	4.1	1.9	2.3	-	3.2	-	6.9	-	11.1	1.0	0.3	0.07	0.08	1.0	193
Other endocrine	10	0	0.8	0.5	0.5	-	0.4	0.4	-	0.5	-	0.8	-	-	-	-	2.3	-	6.8	-	0.4	0.1	0.02	0.03	0.4	194
Hodgkin's disease	53	0	-	-	0.5	1.5	4.5	2.8	1.3	5.1	1.9	2.4	2.8	4.5	2.7	1.6	-	3.5	6.8	11.1	2.1	0.6	0.15	0.16	2.0	201
Non-Hodgkin lymphoma	255	0	1.2	0.5	1.5	0.5	2.2	4.0	8.5	14.3	14.8	22.0	19.7	24.8	23.3	38.7	48.9	41.5	68.0	78.0	10.3	2.7	0.69	1.12	10.6	200,202
Multiple myeloma	212	0	-	-	-	-	-	0.4	0.4	1.5	3.9	3.3	21.5	30.4	38.3	53.2	51.3	100.2	156.4	133.8	8.6	2.2	0.50	1.02	9.5	203
Lymphoid leukaemia	101	0	1.6	0.9	1.0	-	0.4	0.8	1.7	1.5	1.9	4.9	13.1	7.9	24.6	14.5	30.3	20.7	20.4	44.6	4.1	1.1	0.30	0.53	4.6	204
Myeloid leukaemia	108	0	1.2	0.5	0.5	-	0.9	2.4	2.6	2.6	5.8	8.1	5.6	11.3	8.2	11.3	18.6	44.9	81.6	33.4	4.4	1.1	0.25	0.40	4.4	205
Monocytic leukaemia	6	0	-	-	-	-	-	-	-	-	-	0.8	0.9	-	1.6	-	6.9	6.8	-		0.2	0.1	0.01	0.02	0.2	206
Other leukaemia	1	0	-	-	-	-	-	-	-	-	-	-	-	1.4	-	-	-	-	-		0.0	0.0	0.01	0.01	0.1	207
Leukaemia unspecified	12	0	-	-	-	-	-	-	-	0.6	0.8	1.9	1.1	-	3.2	4.7	3.5	6.8	11.1	0.5	0.1	0.02	0.06	0.5	208
Other and unspecified	325	0	1.2	-	-	0.5	0.4	-	0.9	3.6	7.1	21.1	25.3	50.7	57.5	74.1	97.8	120.9	176.8	122.6	13.2	3.4	0.84	1.70	14.7	O&U
All sites	9484	3	17.0	8.5	9.1	11.2	20.7	42.6	79.2	110.7	193.3	328.4	635.4	1117.8	1818.1	2612.0	3343.0	3724.3	4209.5	4091.4	384.2		21.97	51.75	425.8	ALL
All sites but 173	9463	3	17.0	8.5	9.1	11.2	20.7	42.6	78.3	108.6	188.8	327.6	632.6	1116.7	1814.0	2612.0	3343.0	3724.3	4209.5	4091.4	383.4	100.0	21.88	51.67	424.9	ALLb

Rate from 1 case   0.395   0.472   0.504   0.507   0.449   0.398   0.426   0.512   0.644   0.813   0.936   1.126   1.368   1.611   2.330   3.455   6.800   11.148

†Important: see notes on population page

USA, CALIFORNIA, LOS ANGELES COUNTY: BLACK 1988-1992

ANNUAL INCIDENCE PER 100,000 BY AGE GROUP (YEARS) - FEMALE

SITE	ALL AGES	AGE UNK	0-	5-	10-	15-	20-	25-	30-	35-	40-	45-	50-	55-	60-	65-	70-	75-	80-	85+	CRUDE RATE	%	CR 64	CR 74	ASR (W)	ICD (9th)
Lip	1	0	-	-	-	-	-	-	-	-	-	-	-	-	-	1.2	-	-	-	-	0.0	0.0	0.00	0.01	0.0	140
Tongue	21	0	-	-	-	-	-	-	0.8	1.3	-	0.7	-	4.8	1.1	6.0	4.7	2.0	-	-	0.8	0.3	0.04	0.10	0.7	141
Salivary gland	13	0	-	-	-	-	0.4	0.4	0.8	-	1.1	0.7	0.8	2.9	1.1	-	-	-	-	4.1	0.5	0.2	0.04	0.04	0.4	142
Mouth	45	0	-	-	-	0.5	0.4	-	0.4	1.3	1.6	2.1	3.3	4.8	5.4	8.4	7.8	8.2	6.6	4.1	1.7	0.6	0.10	0.18	1.5	143-5
Oropharynx	26	0	-	-	-	-	-	-	-	0.5	3.4	3.3	4.8	3.3	3.6	6.2	-	-	4.1	1.0	0.3	0.08	0.13	1.0	146
Nasopharynx	5	0	-	-	-	-	-	0.4	0.4	-	-	-	0.8	1.0	1.1	-	-	-	-	0.2	0.1	0.02	0.02	0.2	147
Hypopharynx	6	0	-	-	-	-	-	-	-	-	-	0.7	-	2.9	-	1.2	1.6	-	-	-	0.2	0.1	0.02	0.03	0.2	148
Pharynx unspecified	5	0	-	-	-	-	-	-	-	-	-	-	0.8	1.0	2.2	-	-	2.0	-	-	0.2	0.1	0.02	0.02	0.2	149
Oesophagus	95	0	-	-	-	-	-	-	-	0.9	1.1	4.1	7.4	12.5	25.0	10.8	23.3	12.2	13.2	24.6	3.5	1.2	0.25	0.43	3.3	150
Stomach	206	0	-	-	-	-	-	0.4	1.5	0.4	3.2	3.4	8.2	16.3	14.1	26.4	62.1	77.4	89.4	90.0	7.6	2.6	0.24	0.68	5.9	151
Small intestine	36	0	-	-	-	-	-	-	0.4	0.4	0.5	2.1	3.3	4.8	5.4	7.2	9.3	4.1	3.3	4.1	1.3	0.5	0.08	0.17	1.3	152
Colon	860	0	-	-	-	-	0.4	0.4	0.8	5.8	14.0	22.7	54.8	53.8	114.1	152.3	198.6	254.7	291.3	360.1	31.6	10.8	1.33	3.09	26.5	153
Rectum	322	0	-	-	-	-	-	-	0.4	2.7	8.6	8.9	18.8	28.8	39.1	52.8	85.3	106.0	89.4	77.8	11.8	4.0	0.54	1.23	10.1	154
Liver	68	0	-	-	0.5	0.5	-	-	0.8	0.9	1.6	3.4	0.8	5.8	6.5	19.2	14.0	22.4	9.9	8.2	2.5	0.9	0.10	0.27	2.2	155
Gallbladder etc.	51	0	-	-	-	-	-	-	0.8	-	-	2.1	1.6	4.8	4.3	4.8	7.8	10.2	39.7	36.8	1.9	0.6	0.07	0.13	1.4	156
Pancreas	280	0	-	-	-	-	0.4	-	0.4	0.9	2.7	6.2	9.0	19.2	32.6	39.6	83.8	93.7	129.1	118.7	10.3	3.5	0.36	0.97	8.2	157
Nose, sinuses etc.	10	0	-	-	-	0.5	-	-	-	0.4	-	-	0.8	1.0	2.2	-	3.1	2.0	-	4.1	0.4	0.1	0.02	0.04	0.3	160
Larynx	55	0	-	-	-	-	-	0.4	-	-	0.5	2.1	3.3	6.7	6.5	16.8	12.4	12.2	6.6	12.3	2.0	0.7	0.10	0.24	1.8	161
Bronchus, lung	1035	0	-	-	-	0.5	0.9	0.7	1.5	8.5	17.8	42.6	76.1	138.3	165.1	245.8	198.6	207.8	162.2	159.6	38.0	13.0	2.26	4.48	35.4	162
Other thoracic organs	6	0	-	-	0.5	-	-	-	0.4	-	-	0.7	-	1.0	1.1	1.2	-	-	-	-	0.2	0.1	0.02	0.02	0.2	163-4
Bone	6	0	-	-	-	1.0	-	-	-	0.4	-	-	-	-	-	1.1	-	1.6	-	3.3	0.2	0.1	0.01	0.02	0.2	170
Connective tissue	56	0	1.2	0.5	-	1.0	1.3	1.1	1.9	0.9	1.6	2.7	2.5	3.8	5.4	12.0	1.6	2.0	13.2	8.2	2.1	0.7	0.12	0.19	1.9	171
Mesothelioma	6	0	-	-	-	-	-	-	-	-	-	1.4	-	-	-	2.4	-	-	3.3	4.1	0.2	0.1	0.01	0.02	0.2	MES
Kaposi's sarcoma	7	0	-	-	0.5	-	0.4	0.7	-	0.4	-	-	-	-	-	-	-	-	3.3	4.1	0.3	0.1	0.01	0.01	0.2	KAP
Melanoma of skin	20	0	-	-	-	-	0.4	0.4	-	0.4	0.5	-	1.6	1.9	2.2	1.2	4.7	4.1	9.9	4.1	0.7	0.3	0.04	0.07	0.6	172
†Other skin	26	0	-	-	0.5	1.0	0.4	1.1	1.1	-	1.1	2.1	-	-	1.1	3.6	4.7	2.0	6.6	4.1	1.0		0.04	0.08	0.8	173
Breast	2389	1	-	-	-	-	1.3	13.3	27.5	67.9	130.6	195.0	207.9	244.0	277.0	335.8	327.4	319.9	374.1	311.0	87.7	29.9	5.82	9.14	80.9	174
Uterus unspecified	10	0	-	-	-	-	0.4	-	-	-	-	-	-	3.3	3.6	-	4.1	3.3	-	-	0.4	0.1	0.02	0.04	0.3	179
Cervix uteri	361	0	-	-	-	0.5	4.3	7.4	13.4	18.0	21.0	23.3	24.6	26.9	23.9	39.6	43.4	46.9	39.7	24.6	13.2	4.5	0.82	1.23	11.6	180
Placenta	2	0	-	-	-	-	0.4	-	0.4	-	-	-	-	-	-	-	-	-	-	-	0.1	0.0	0.00	0.00	0.1	181
Corpus uteri	325	0	-	-	-	-	0.4	0.4	1.9	4.0	2.7	11.7	18.0	36.5	55.4	61.2	76.0	87.6	79.5	36.8	11.9	4.1	0.66	1.34	10.7	182
Ovary etc.	246	0	0.4	0.5	0.5	-	3.5	1.9	3.1	1.8	9.7	9.6	18.8	18.3	25.0	43.2	57.4	50.9	36.4	49.1	9.0	3.1	0.46	0.97	8.1	183
Other female genital	47	0	0.4	-	-	-	-	0.4	0.4	0.9	1.6	2.7	3.3	1.0	9.8	9.6	3.1	8.2	16.6	8.2	1.7	0.6	0.10	0.17	1.6	184
Bladder	122	0	-	-	-	-	0.4	-	-	0.4	0.5	1.4	3.3	10.6	15.2	16.8	27.9	32.6	66.2	81.8	4.5	1.5	0.16	0.38	3.5	188
Kidney etc.	172	0	1.6	0.5	-	0.5	0.4	1.5	1.5	1.3	3.8	8.9	12.3	19.2	30.4	24.0	26.4	30.6	33.1	36.8	6.3	2.2	0.41	0.66	5.9	189
Eye	6	0	1.2	-	-	-	-	-	-	-	-	1.4	-	-	-	1.2	-	-	-	-	0.2	0.1	0.01	0.02	0.3	190
Brain, nervous system	90	0	2.8	3.4	2.6	2.6	0.9	1.1	0.8	2.7	2.7	3.4	2.5	4.8	8.7	8.4	7.8	20.4	6.6	12.3	3.3	1.1	0.19	0.28	3.2	191-2
Thyroid	91	0	-	-	-	0.5	1.7	2.2	4.6	2.7	5.9	8.2	8.2	3.8	9.8	2.4	6.2	10.2	9.9	8.2	3.3	1.1	0.24	0.28	3.0	193
Other endocrine	8	0	0.8	0.5	0.5	-	-	-	-	-	-	0.7	1.6	1.0	-	-	-	-	-	-	0.3	0.1	0.03	0.03	0.4	194
Hodgkin's disease	53	0	-	1.0	0.5	1.0	2.2	3.3	3.1	3.1	1.6	0.7	2.5	1.9	2.2	2.4	3.1	2.0	6.6	4.1	1.9	0.7	0.12	0.14	1.7	201
Non-Hodgkin lymphoma	187	0	0.4	1.0	-	1.6	0.4	1.1	4.6	5.8	5.9	8.9	12.3	11.5	18.5	28.8	31.0	30.6	26.5	69.6	6.9	2.3	0.36	0.66	6.0	200,202
Multiple myeloma	162	0	-	-	-	-	-	-	0.4	0.4	2.7	6.9	10.6	13.4	15.2	28.8	40.3	55.0	56.3	40.9	5.9	2.0	0.25	0.59	5.0	203
Lymphoid leukaemia	53	0	2.0	0.5	-	-	-	0.4	1.1	-	1.1	2.1	3.3	4.8	6.5	9.6	6.2	12.2	3.3	16.4	1.9	0.7	0.11	0.19	1.8	204
Myeloid leukaemia	94	0	0.8	1.0	1.0	0.5	1.3	1.5	1.1	2.7	3.2	4.8	5.7	1.9	6.5	12.0	14.0	14.3	33.1	28.6	3.4	1.2	0.16	0.29	3.0	205
Monocytic leukaemia	1	0	-	-	-	0.5	-	-	-	-	-	-	-	-	-	-	-	-	-	-	0.0	0.0	0.00	0.00	0.0	206
Other leukaemia	0	0	-	-	-	-	-	-	-	-	-	-	-	-	-	-	-	-	-	-	0.0	0.0	0.00	0.00	0.0	207
Leukaemia unspecified	17	0	0.4	-	-	-	-	0.4	-	-	1.1	-	0.8	-	3.3	3.6	1.6	-	6.6	12.3	0.6	0.2	0.03	0.06	0.5	208
Other and unspecified	310	0	-	0.5	-	-	0.9	0.4	1.5	1.3	4.3	15.1	9.8	30.7	50.0	50.4	71.4	61.1	82.8	147.3	11.4	3.9	0.57	1.18	9.9	O&U
All sites	8013	1	12.1	9.3	7.2	13.0	23.8	41.2	77.4	139.5	255.2	416.7	542.7	751.2	1000.5	1297.6	1473.9	1609.8	1761.3	1821.2	294.1		16.45	30.31	262.4	ALL
All sites but 173	7987	1	12.1	9.3	6.7	12.0	23.4	40.0	76.3	139.5	254.1	414.7	542.7	751.2	999.4	1294.0	1469.2	1607.7	1754.7	1817.1	293.1	100.0	16.41	30.23	261.5	ALLb

Rate from 1 case: 0.405 0.489 0.512 0.520 0.433 0.371 0.381 0.450 0.540 0.687 0.819 0.961 1.086 1.199 1.551 2.038 3.311 4.092

†Important: see notes on population page

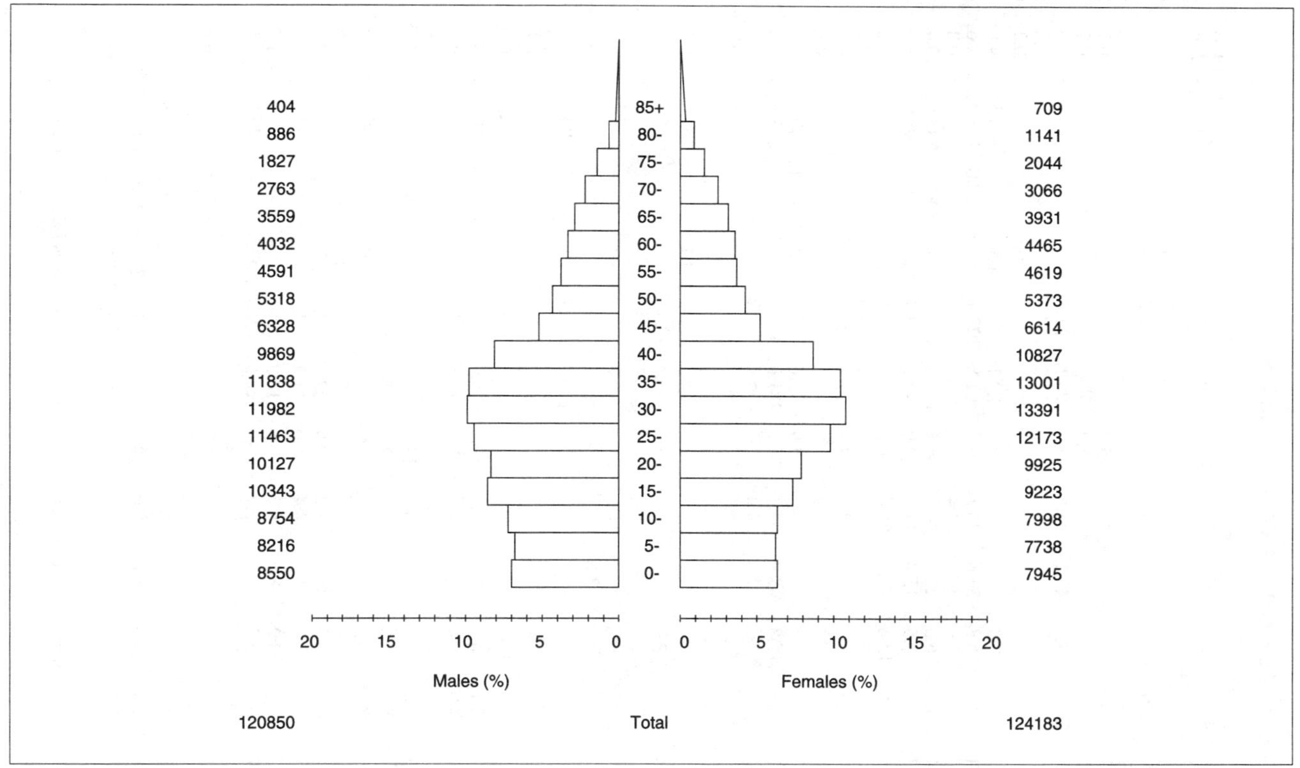

USA, California, Los Angeles County: Chinese
Source of population: 1990
Census: 1990 Census.
Notes to tables overleaf:
† 173 does not include basal cell or squamous cell carcinoma
The denominators are not the same populations as those published in Volume VI and the data for this ethnic group are not comparable.

USA, CALIFORNIA, LOS ANGELES COUNTY: CHINESE 1988-1992

ANNUAL INCIDENCE PER 100,000 BY AGE GROUP (YEARS) - MALE

SITE	ALL AGES	AGE UNK	0-	5-	10-	15-	20-	25-	30-	35-	40-	45-	50-	55-	60-	65-	70-	75-	80-	85+	CRUDE RATE	%	CR 64	CR 74	ASR (W)	ICD (9th)
Lip	1	0	-	-	-	-	-	-	-	-	-	-	-	-	-	-	-	10.9	-	-	0.2	0.1	0.00	0.00	0.1	140
Tongue	5	0	-	-	-	-	2.0	-	-	1.7	2.0	-	-	-	5.0	-	7.2	-	-	-	0.8	0.4	0.05	0.09	0.7	141
Salivary gland	5	0	-	-	-	-	-	-	-	1.7	-	-	3.8	8.7	-	-	7.2	-	-	-	0.8	0.4	0.07	0.11	0.8	142
Mouth	4	0	2.3	-	-	-	-	-	1.7	-	-	-	-	-	5.0	-	7.2	-	-	-	0.7	0.3	0.04	0.08	0.7	143-5
Oropharynx	1	0	-	-	-	-	-	-	-	-	-	-	-	-	5.0	-	-	-	-	-	0.2	0.1	0.02	0.02	0.2	146
Nasopharynx	62	0	-	-	-	-	-	3.5	1.7	13.5	20.3	19.0	45.1	43.6	24.8	28.1	21.7	-	-	-	10.3	5.3	0.86	1.11	9.8	147
Hypopharynx	6	0	-	-	-	-	-	-	-	-	-	-	-	-	-	11.2	14.5	-	45.1	-	1.0	0.5	0.00	0.13	0.9	148
Pharynx unspecified	1	0	-	-	-	-	-	-	-	-	-	-	-	-	-	-	-	10.9	-	-	0.2	0.1	0.00	0.00	0.1	149
Oesophagus	24	0	-	-	-	-	-	-	-	-	-	3.2	7.5	8.7	9.9	28.1	21.7	65.7	-	148.5	4.0	2.0	0.15	0.40	4.0	150
Stomach	76	0	-	-	-	-	-	-	1.7	3.4	4.1	6.3	37.6	26.1	9.9	61.8	123.1	131.4	158.0	198.0	12.6	6.5	0.45	1.37	11.7	151
Small intestine	2	0	-	-	-	-	-	-	-	1.7	-	-	-	4.4	-	-	-	-	-	-	0.3	0.2	0.03	0.03	0.3	152
Colon	117	0	-	-	-	-	-	1.7	3.3	3.4	8.1	6.3	22.6	34.9	64.5	134.9	144.8	218.9	180.6	346.5	19.4	9.9	0.72	2.12	18.3	153
Rectum	56	0	-	-	-	-	-	-	1.7	1.7	12.2	9.5	15.0	17.4	9.9	45.0	72.4	120.4	90.3	99.0	9.3	4.8	0.34	0.92	8.3	154
Liver	103	0	-	-	-	1.9	-	-	6.7	13.5	4.1	12.6	26.3	56.6	84.3	39.3	123.1	131.4	158.0	198.0	17.0	8.8	1.03	1.84	16.1	155
Gallbladder etc.	13	0	-	-	-	-	-	-	-	-	2.0	-	-	-	-	28.1	29.0	10.9	45.1	-	2.2	1.1	0.01	0.30	1.9	156
Pancreas	26	0	-	-	-	-	-	-	-	1.7	2.0	-	11.3	13.1	9.9	22.5	21.7	54.7	67.7	49.5	4.3	2.2	0.19	0.41	3.9	157
Nose, sinuses etc.	3	0	-	-	-	-	-	1.7	-	-	-	-	-	4.4	-	-	-	10.9	-	-	0.5	0.3	0.03	0.03	0.4	160
Larynx	9	0	-	-	-	-	-	-	-	-	-	-	-	-	14.9	5.6	7.2	10.9	45.1	49.5	1.5	0.8	0.07	0.14	1.5	161
Bronchus, lung	232	0	-	-	-	-	-	1.7	-	5.1	4.1	15.8	48.9	65.3	114.1	281.0	361.9	383.1	496.6	643.6	38.4	19.7	1.27	4.49	36.5	162
Other thoracic organs	4	0	-	-	-	-	-	-	-	-	-	-	3.8	4.4	-	5.6	7.2	-	-	-	0.7	0.3	0.04	0.10	0.7	163-4
Bone	2	0	-	-	-	-	-	1.7	1.7	-	-	-	-	-	-	-	-	-	-	-	0.3	0.2	0.02	0.02	0.2	170
Connective tissue	9	0	4.7	-	-	-	-	-	-	-	-	-	-	-	14.9	11.2	14.5	-	-	-	1.5	0.8	0.10	0.23	1.8	171
Mesothelioma	1	0	-	-	-	-	-	-	-	-	-	-	-	-	-	-	-	10.9	-	-	0.2	0.1	0.00	0.00	0.1	MES
Kaposi's sarcoma	6	0	-	-	-	-	-	3.3	3.4	-	3.2	-	-	5.0	-	-	-	-	-	-	1.0	0.5	0.07	0.07	0.8	KAP
Melanoma of skin	0	0	-	-	-	-	-	-	-	-	-	-	-	-	-	-	-	-	-	-	0.0	0.0	0.00	0.00	0.0	172
†Other skin	2	0	-	-	-	-	-	-	-	-	-	-	-	-	-	-	-	10.9	-	49.5	0.3		0.00	0.00	0.4	173
Breast	1	0	-	-	-	-	-	-	-	-	-	-	3.8	-	-	-	-	-	-	-	0.2	0.1	0.02	0.02	0.2	175
Prostate	137	0	-	-	-	-	-	-	-	-	-	3.2	-	-	49.6	106.8	275.1	328.4	609.5	594.1	22.7	11.6	0.26	2.17	20.2	185
Testis	7	0	4.7	-	-	-	-	3.5	3.3	1.7	-	-	-	-	-	-	-	-	-	-	1.2	0.6	0.07	0.07	1.1	186
Penis	3	0	-	-	-	-	-	-	-	-	-	3.2	-	-	-	-	7.2	10.9	-	-	0.5	0.3	0.02	0.05	0.4	187.1-.4
Other male genital	0	0	-	-	-	-	-	-	-	-	-	-	-	-	-	-	-	-	-	-	0.0	0.0	0.00	0.00	0.0	187.5-.9
Bladder	49	0	-	-	-	-	-	-	-	-	6.1	6.3	7.5	8.7	19.8	45.0	79.6	87.6	158.0	99.0	8.1	4.2	0.24	0.87	7.4	188
Kidney etc.	29	0	-	-	-	-	-	-	1.7	-	2.0	6.3	7.5	8.7	9.9	16.9	79.6	21.9	67.7	-	4.8	2.5	0.18	0.66	4.4	189
Eye	0	0	-	-	-	-	-	-	-	-	-	-	-	-	-	-	-	-	-	-	0.0	0.0	0.00	0.00	0.0	190
Brain, nervous system	15	0	-	2.4	-	-	-	3.5	1.7	3.4	2.0	-	-	4.4	14.9	5.6	7.2	-	45.1	-	2.5	1.3	0.16	0.23	2.3	191-2
Thyroid	11	0	-	-	-	1.9	-	-	1.7	1.7	8.1	3.2	-	-	5.0	5.6	-	10.9	-	-	1.8	0.9	0.11	0.14	1.5	193
Other endocrine	2	0	-	-	-	-	-	-	-	-	-	-	-	-	-	-	-	10.9	-	49.5	0.3	0.2	0.00	0.00	0.4	194
Hodgkin's disease	3	0	-	-	-	-	-	-	-	-	-	-	3.8	-	-	5.6	-	10.9	-	-	0.5	0.3	0.02	0.05	0.5	201
Non-Hodgkin lymphoma	51	0	-	2.4	-	3.9	3.9	-	5.0	3.4	10.1	6.3	15.0	21.8	9.9	22.5	57.9	87.6	45.1	49.5	8.4	4.3	0.41	0.81	7.6	200,202
Multiple myeloma	11	0	-	-	-	-	-	-	-	-	-	-	-	4.4	5.0	11.2	7.2	21.9	45.1	99.0	1.8	0.9	0.05	0.14	1.8	203
Lymphoid leukaemia	9	0	2.3	-	-	1.9	2.0	-	-	-	-	3.2	3.8	8.7	-	11.2	-	-	-	-	1.5	0.8	0.11	0.17	1.7	204
Myeloid leukaemia	27	0	-	-	-	1.9	-	3.5	3.3	1.7	6.1	3.2	7.5	8.7	-	22.5	29.0	43.8	-	49.5	4.5	2.3	0.18	0.44	4.0	205
Monocytic leukaemia	1	0	-	-	-	-	-	-	-	-	-	3.2	-	-	-	-	-	-	-	-	0.2	0.1	0.02	0.02	0.2	206
Other leukaemia	2	0	-	-	-	-	-	-	-	-	-	-	-	-	5.0	-	-	-	22.6	-	0.3	0.2	0.02	0.02	0.3	207
Leukaemia unspecified	0	0	-	-	-	-	-	-	-	-	-	-	-	-	-	-	-	-	-	-	0.0	0.0	0.00	0.00	0.0	208
Other and unspecified	50	0	-	-	-	-	-	-	-	-	8.1	9.5	15.0	26.1	24.8	33.7	36.2	65.7	90.3	346.5	8.3	4.3	0.42	0.77	8.4	O&U
All sites	1178	0	14.0	4.9	-	11.6	7.9	20.9	38.4	62.5	101.3	123.3	285.8	379.0	520.8	989.0	1563.5	1882.9	2370.2	3069.3	195.0		7.85	20.62	182.3	ALL
All sites but 173	1176	0	14.0	4.9	-	11.6	7.9	20.9	38.4	62.5	101.3	123.3	285.8	379.0	520.8	989.0	1563.5	1871.9	2370.2	3019.8	194.6	100.0	7.85	20.62	181.9	ALLb

Rate from 1 case 2.339 2.434 2.285 1.934 1.975 1.745 1.669 1.689 2.027 3.161 3.761 4.356 4.960 5.620 7.239 10.947 22.573 49.505

†Important: see notes on population page

USA, CALIFORNIA, LOS ANGELES COUNTY: CHINESE 1988-1992

ANNUAL INCIDENCE PER 100,000 BY AGE GROUP (YEARS) - FEMALE

SITE	ALL AGES	AGE UNK	0-	5-	10-	15-	20-	25-	30-	35-	40-	45-	50-	55-	60-	65-	70-	75-	80-	85+	CRUDE RATE	%	CR 64	CR 74	ASR (W)	ICD (9th)
Lip	1	0	-	-	-	-	-	-	-	-	-	-	-	-	-	-	-	-	17.5	-	0.2	0.1	0.00	0.00	**0.1**	*140*
Tongue	4	0	-	-	-	-	-	-	-	-	-	3.0	-	4.3	-	-	-	9.8	-	28.2	0.6	0.4	0.04	0.04	**0.6**	*141*
Salivary gland	3	0	-	-	-	-	-	1.6	-	1.5	-	-	3.7	-	-	-	-	-	-	-	0.5	0.3	0.03	0.03	**0.4**	*142*
Mouth	1	0	-	-	-	-	-	-	-	-	-	-	-	-	-	-	-	-	17.5	-	0.2	0.1	0.00	0.00	**0.1**	*143-5*
Oropharynx	2	0	-	-	-	-	-	-	-	-	-	-	-	-	-	-	5.1	9.8	-	-	0.3	0.2	0.00	0.03	**0.3**	*146*
Nasopharynx	22	0	-	-	-	-	-	-	1.5	4.6	5.5	6.0	3.7	4.3	-	15.3	32.6	9.8	35.1	-	3.5	2.1	0.13	0.37	**2.8**	*147*
Hypopharynx	0	0	-	-	-	-	-	-	-	-	-	-	-	-	-	-	-	-	-	-	0.0	0.0	0.00	0.00	**0.0**	*148*
Pharynx unspecified	1	0	-	-	-	-	-	-	-	-	-	-	-	-	-	-	-	-	-	28.2	0.2	0.1	0.00	0.00	**0.1**	*149*
Oesophagus	9	0	-	-	-	-	-	-	-	-	-	-	-	-	-	13.0	29.4	52.6	28.2	1.4	0.9	0.00	0.07	**1.0**	*150*
Stomach	57	0	-	-	-	-	-	-	3.0	6.2	1.8	6.0	11.2	8.7	17.9	40.7	52.2	97.8	52.6	282.1	9.2	5.4	0.27	0.74	**7.6**	*151*
Small intestine	1	0	-	-	-	-	-	-	-	-	-	-	-	-	-	-	-	-	-	28.2	0.2	0.1	0.00	0.00	**0.1**	*152*
Colon	94	0	-	-	-	-	-	-	1.5	4.6	3.7	9.1	11.2	34.6	31.4	45.8	130.5	156.6	210.3	282.1	15.1	8.9	0.48	1.36	**12.3**	*153*
Rectum	53	0	-	-	-	-	-	-	3.0	6.2	11.1	6.0	-	26.0	31.4	35.6	58.7	58.7	52.6	28.2	8.5	5.0	0.42	0.89	**7.1**	*154*
Liver	31	0	-	-	-	-	-	-	-	-	-	6.0	-	8.7	35.8	15.3	32.6	48.9	52.6	84.6	5.0	2.9	0.25	0.49	**4.4**	*155*
Gallbladder etc.	18	0	-	-	-	-	-	-	-	-	-	3.0	-	-	4.5	5.1	19.6	58.7	70.1	56.4	2.9	1.7	0.04	0.16	**2.1**	*156*
Pancreas	19	0	-	-	-	-	-	-	1.5	-	1.8	3.0	3.7	-	4.5	20.4	26.1	19.6	52.6	28.2	3.1	1.8	0.07	0.31	**2.5**	*157*
Nose, sinuses etc.	1	0	-	-	-	-	-	-	-	-	-	-	-	-	-	5.1	-	-	-	-	0.2	0.1	0.00	0.03	**0.2**	*160*
Larynx	1	0	-	-	-	-	-	-	-	-	-	-	-	-	-	-	6.5	-	-	-	0.2	0.1	0.00	0.03	**0.1**	*161*
Bronchus, lung	126	0	-	-	-	-	-	-	-	1.5	7.4	9.1	11.2	21.6	49.3	96.7	195.7	244.6	298.0	225.7	20.3	11.9	0.50	1.96	**16.4**	*162*
Other thoracic organs	0	0	-	-	-	-	-	-	-	-	-	-	-	-	-	-	-	-	-	-	0.0	0.0	0.00	0.00	**0.0**	*163-4*
Bone	2	0	-	-	-	2.2	-	-	1.5	-	-	-	-	-	-	-	-	-	-	-	0.3	0.2	0.02	0.02	**0.3**	*170*
Connective tissue	9	0	-	-	2.5	-	2.0	-	1.5	1.5	1.8	-	-	-	-	-	5.1	6.5	9.8	17.5	1.4	0.9	0.05	0.11	**1.1**	*171*
Mesothelioma	0	0	-	-	-	-	-	-	-	-	-	-	-	-	-	-	-	-	-	-	0.0	0.0	0.00	0.00	**0.0**	*MES*
Kaposi's sarcoma	0	0	-	-	-	-	-	-	-	-	-	-	-	-	-	-	-	-	-	-	0.0	0.0	0.00	0.00	**0.0**	*KAP*
Melanoma of skin	4	0	-	-	-	-	-	-	1.5	-	-	3.0	-	-	4.5	-	-	-	-	28.2	0.6	0.4	0.04	0.04	**0.6**	*172*
†Other skin	2	0	-	-	-	-	-	-	-	-	1.8	-	3.7	-	-	-	-	-	-	-	0.3		0.03	0.03	**0.3**	*173*
Breast	266	0	-	-	-	-	-	1.6	16.4	52.3	77.6	99.8	100.5	86.6	107.5	81.4	156.6	205.5	105.2	197.5	42.8	25.1	2.71	3.90	**36.8**	*174*
Uterus unspecified	2	0	-	-	-	-	-	-	-	1.5	-	3.0	-	-	-	-	-	-	-	-	0.3	0.2	0.02	0.02	**0.3**	*179*
Cervix uteri	53	0	-	-	-	-	-	-	-	9.2	9.2	21.2	11.2	26.0	31.4	40.7	32.6	39.1	17.5	28.2	8.5	5.0	0.54	0.91	**7.7**	*180*
Placenta	0	0	-	-	-	-	-	-	-	-	-	-	-	-	-	-	-	-	-	-	0.0	0.0	0.00	0.00	**0.0**	*181*
Corpus uteri	46	0	-	-	-	-	-	-	3.0	4.6	3.7	3.0	18.6	34.6	49.3	30.5	19.6	39.1	-	28.2	7.4	4.3	0.58	0.83	**7.0**	*182*
Ovary etc.	47	0	-	-	-	-	4.0	-	4.5	4.6	12.9	12.1	11.2	26.0	17.9	35.6	13.0	19.6	52.6	28.2	7.6	4.4	0.47	0.71	**6.6**	*183*
Other female genital	4	0	-	-	-	-	-	-	-	-	1.5	-	-	-	-	6.5	9.8	17.5	-	-	0.6	0.4	0.01	0.04	**0.4**	*184*
Bladder	15	0	2.5	-	-	-	-	-	-	-	-	3.0	-	-	4.5	5.1	26.1	29.4	35.1	56.4	2.4	1.4	0.05	0.21	**2.1**	*188*
Kidney etc.	13	0	-	-	-	-	-	-	-	-	-	-	-	-	17.9	10.2	26.1	29.4	-	-	2.1	1.2	0.09	0.27	**1.8**	*189*
Eye	1	0	-	-	-	-	-	-	-	-	-	1.8	-	-	-	-	-	-	-	-	0.2	0.1	0.01	0.01	**0.1**	*190*
Brain, nervous system	7	0	-	-	-	-	-	1.6	-	1.5	-	-	7.4	4.3	-	5.1	6.5	-	-	-	1.1	0.7	0.07	0.13	**1.1**	*191-2*
Thyroid	26	0	-	-	-	-	2.0	3.3	6.0	6.2	3.7	9.1	11.2	4.3	9.0	5.1	6.5	19.6	-	-	4.2	2.5	0.27	0.33	**3.5**	*193*
Other endocrine	0	0	-	-	-	-	-	-	-	-	-	-	-	-	-	-	-	-	-	-	0.0	0.0	0.00	0.00	**0.0**	*194*
Hodgkin's disease	4	0	-	-	-	-	-	-	1.5	3.1	-	-	-	-	-	4.5	-	-	-	-	0.6	0.4	0.05	0.05	**0.5**	*201*
Non-Hodgkin lymphoma	36	0	2.5	-	-	-	2.0	4.9	4.5	3.1	3.7	9.1	3.7	17.3	9.0	20.4	13.0	19.6	70.1	56.4	5.8	3.4	0.30	0.47	**5.0**	*200,202*
Multiple myeloma	7	0	-	-	-	-	-	-	-	-	1.8	-	-	4.3	-	10.2	-	-	17.5	56.4	1.1	0.7	0.03	0.08	**1.0**	*203*
Lymphoid leukaemia	10	0	5.0	-	-	-	-	-	-	-	-	3.0	11.2	-	-	15.3	-	9.8	-	-	1.6	0.9	0.10	0.17	**1.9**	*204*
Myeloid leukaemia	13	0	-	-	-	-	-	1.6	1.5	-	1.8	3.0	11.2	4.3	9.0	10.2	-	9.8	-	-	2.1	1.2	0.16	0.21	**2.0**	*205*
Monocytic leukaemia	1	0	-	-	2.5	-	-	-	-	-	-	-	-	-	-	-	-	-	-	-	0.2	0.1	0.01	0.01	**0.2**	*206*
Other leukaemia	0	0	-	-	-	-	-	-	-	-	-	-	-	-	-	-	-	-	-	-	0.0	0.0	0.00	0.00	**0.0**	*207*
Leukaemia unspecified	3	0	-	-	-	-	-	-	-	-	-	-	-	-	-	-	5.1	6.5	-	17.5	0.5	0.3	0.00	0.06	**0.4**	*208*
Other and unspecified	45	0	-	-	-	-	-	1.6	3.0	4.6	3.7	3.0	-	17.3	13.4	15.3	45.7	48.9	17.5	366.7	7.2	4.3	0.23	0.54	**6.0**	*O&U*
All sites	1060	0	10.1	-	5.0	2.2	10.1	16.4	55.3	118.5	155.2	223.8	234.5	333.4	452.4	580.0	932.8	1232.9	1279.6	1946.4	170.7		8.08	15.65	**144.8**	*ALL*
All sites but 173	1058	0	10.1	-	5.0	2.2	10.1	16.4	55.3	118.5	153.3	223.8	230.8	333.4	452.4	580.0	932.8	1232.9	1279.6	1946.4	170.4	100.0	8.06	15.62	**144.5**	*ALLb*

Rate from 1 case 2.517 2.585 2.501 2.168 2.015 1.643 1.494 1.538 1.847 3.024 3.722 4.330 4.479 5.088 6.523 9.785 17.528 28.209

†Important: see notes on population page

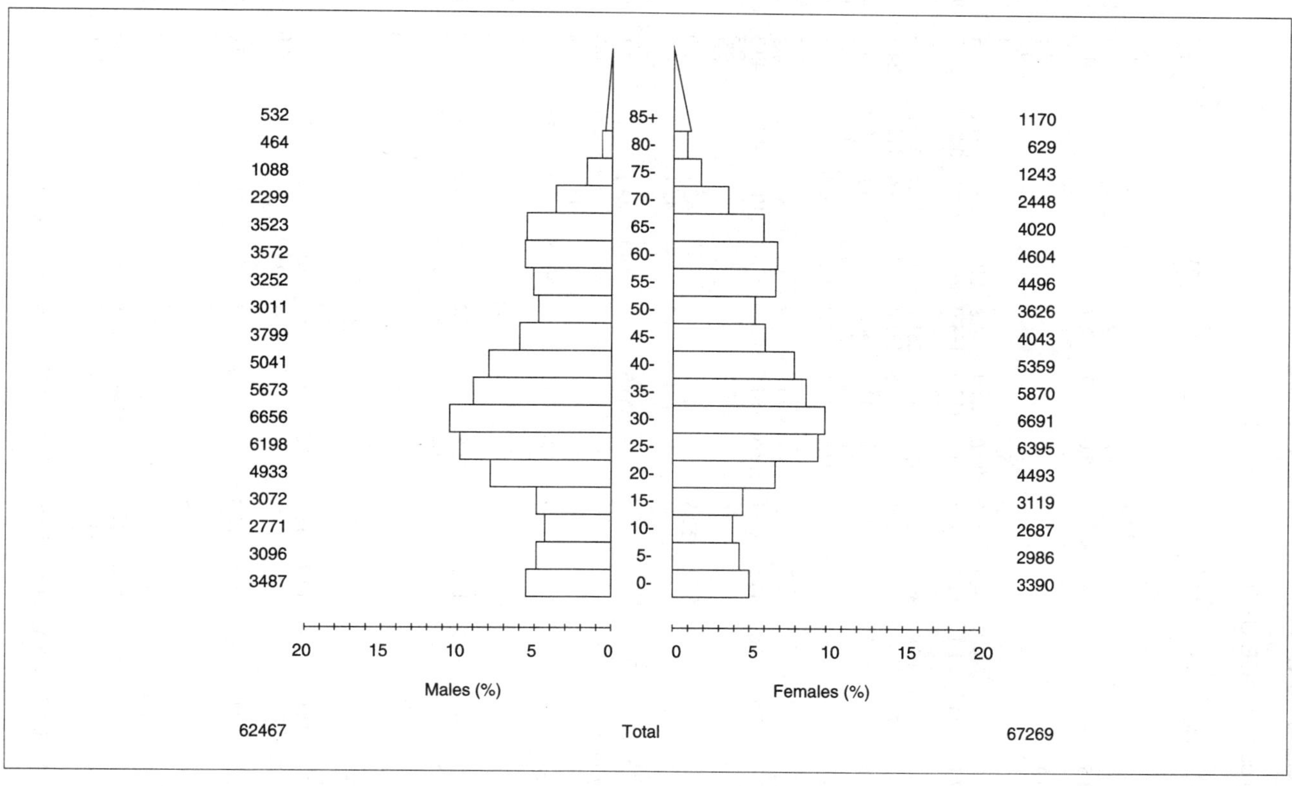

USA, California, Los Angeles County: Japanese
Source of population: 1990
Census: 1990 Census.
Notes to tables overleaf:
† 173 does not include basal cell or squamous cell carcinoma
The denominators are not the same populations as those published in Volume VI and the data for this ethnic group are not comparable.

USA, CALIFORNIA, LOS ANGELES COUNTY: JAPANESE 1988-1992

ANNUAL INCIDENCE PER 100,000 BY AGE GROUP (YEARS) - MALE

SITE	ALL AGES	AGE UNK	0-	5-	10-	15-	20-	25-	30-	35-	40-	45-	50-	55-	60-	65-	70-	75-	80-	85+	CRUDE RATE	%	CR 64	CR 74	ASR (W)	ICD (9th)
Lip	0	0	-	-	-	-	-	-	-	-	-	-	-	-	-	-	-	-	-	-	0.0	0.0	0.00	0.00	0.0	140
Tongue	6	0	-	-	-	-	-	-	-	-	-	-	-	12.3	-	11.4	8.7	18.4	-	-	1.9	0.6	0.06	0.16	1.2	141
Salivary gland	2	0	-	-	-	-	-	-	-	-	-	-	-	-	5.6	-	8.7	-	-	-	0.6	0.2	0.03	0.07	0.4	142
Mouth	4	0	-	-	-	-	-	-	-	3.5	-	-	-	-	5.6	5.7	8.7	-	-	-	1.3	0.4	0.05	0.12	0.8	143-5
Oropharynx	2	0	-	-	-	-	-	-	-	-	-	-	-	-	-	-	-	-	-	75.2	0.6	0.2	0.00	0.00	0.4	146
Nasopharynx	1	0	-	-	-	-	-	-	-	3.5	-	-	-	-	-	-	-	-	-	-	0.3	0.1	0.02	0.02	0.2	147
Hypopharynx	2	0	-	-	-	-	-	-	-	-	-	-	-	-	11.2	-	-	-	-	-	0.6	0.2	0.06	0.06	0.4	148
Pharynx unspecified	1	0	-	-	-	-	-	-	-	-	-	-	-	-	5.6	-	-	-	-	-	0.3	0.1	0.03	0.03	0.2	149
Oesophagus	27	0	-	-	-	-	-	-	-	-	-	-	19.9	18.5	28.0	11.4	34.8	110.3	129.3	37.6	8.6	2.5	0.33	0.56	5.8	150
Stomach	102	0	-	6.5	-	-	4.1	-	3.0	7.1	4.0	21.1	13.3	80.0	44.8	113.5	174.0	257.4	258.6	338.3	32.7	9.6	0.92	2.36	21.2	151
Small intestine	2	0	-	-	-	-	-	3.2	-	-	-	-	-	-	-	5.7	-	-	-	-	0.6	0.2	0.02	0.04	0.4	152
Colon	131	0	-	-	-	-	-	-	-	-	-	15.8	39.9	92.3	95.2	119.2	261.0	349.3	387.9	413.5	41.9	12.3	1.22	3.12	26.7	153
Rectum	77	0	-	-	-	-	-	-	-	-	7.9	-	13.3	30.8	78.4	113.5	121.8	202.2	258.6	112.8	24.7	7.3	0.65	1.83	15.2	154
Liver	27	0	-	-	-	-	-	-	-	3.5	-	10.5	-	12.3	61.6	11.4	34.8	-	43.1	150.4	8.6	2.5	0.44	0.67	5.8	155
Gallbladder etc.	13	0	-	-	-	-	-	-	-	-	-	5.3	-	18.5	5.6	5.7	26.1	36.8	-	75.2	4.2	1.2	0.15	0.31	2.7	156
Pancreas	38	0	-	-	-	-	-	-	-	3.5	-	-	-	30.8	28.0	34.1	34.8	165.4	86.2	225.6	12.2	3.6	0.31	0.66	7.5	157
Nose, sinuses etc.	1	0	-	-	-	-	-	-	-	-	-	-	6.6	-	-	-	-	-	-	-	0.3	0.1	0.03	0.03	0.3	160
Larynx	6	0	-	-	-	-	-	-	-	-	-	-	-	-	5.6	17.0	8.7	18.4	-	-	1.9	0.6	0.03	0.16	1.1	161
Bronchus, lung	154	0	-	-	-	-	-	-	-	7.1	7.9	15.8	46.5	61.5	156.8	164.6	313.2	330.9	301.7	451.1	49.3	14.5	1.48	3.87	31.2	162
Other thoracic organs	1	0	-	-	-	-	-	3.2	-	-	-	-	-	-	-	-	-	-	-	-	0.3	0.1	0.02	0.02	0.3	163-4
Bone	1	0	-	-	-	-	4.1	-	-	-	-	-	-	-	-	-	-	-	-	-	0.3	0.1	0.02	0.02	0.3	170
Connective tissue	6	0	-	-	-	-	-	-	-	-	-	-	-	12.3	5.6	11.4	-	-	43.1	-	1.9	0.6	0.09	0.15	1.3	171
Mesothelioma	2	0	-	-	-	-	-	-	-	-	-	-	-	-	-	-	8.7	-	43.1	-	0.6	0.2	0.00	0.04	0.4	MES
Kaposi's sarcoma	13	0	-	-	-	-	-	3.2	9.0	3.5	15.9	21.1	-	-	-	-	-	-	-	-	4.2	1.2	0.26	0.26	3.2	KAP
Melanoma of skin	5	0	-	-	-	-	-	-	3.0	-	-	-	-	-	-	11.4	-	18.4	43.1	-	1.6	0.5	0.02	0.07	0.9	172
†Other skin	2	0	-	-	-	-	-	-	3.0	3.5	-	-	-	-	-	-	-	-	-	-	0.6		0.03	0.03	0.4	173
Breast	3	0	-	-	-	-	-	-	-	-	-	-	-	-	-	-	17.4	-	43.1	-	1.0	0.3	0.00	0.09	0.6	175
Prostate	252	1	-	-	-	-	-	-	-	-	-	-	-	36.9	156.8	334.9	574.2	808.8	991.4	939.8	80.7	23.7	0.97	5.54	47.2	185
Testis	4	0	-	-	-	-	-	3.2	3.0	3.5	-	-	-	-	5.6	-	-	-	-	-	1.3	0.4	0.08	0.08	0.9	186
Penis	0	0	-	-	-	-	-	-	-	-	-	-	-	-	-	-	-	-	-	-	0.0	0.0	0.00	0.00	0.0	187.1-.4
Other male genital	1	0	-	-	-	-	-	-	-	-	-	-	-	-	-	-	-	18.4	-	-	0.3	0.1	0.00	0.00	0.2	187.5-.9
Bladder	32	0	-	-	-	-	-	-	-	-	4.0	5.3	13.3	12.3	16.8	34.1	52.2	91.9	86.2	150.4	10.2	3.0	0.26	0.69	6.5	188
Kidney etc.	21	0	-	-	-	-	-	-	3.0	3.5	4.0	5.3	13.3	12.3	11.2	28.4	26.1	18.4	43.1	37.6	6.7	2.0	0.26	0.54	4.5	189
Eye	0	0	-	-	-	-	-	-	-	-	-	-	-	-	-	-	-	-	-	-	0.0	0.0	0.00	0.00	0.0	190
Brain, nervous system	6	0	-	-	-	-	4.1	-	3.0	3.5	-	-	-	12.3	-	5.7	-	-	-	-	1.9	0.6	0.11	0.14	1.4	191-2
Thyroid	4	0	-	-	-	-	-	6.5	-	-	-	-	6.6	6.2	-	-	-	-	-	-	1.3	0.4	0.10	0.10	1.1	193
Other endocrine	1	0	-	-	-	-	-	-	-	-	-	-	-	-	-	-	8.7	-	-	-	0.3	0.1	0.00	0.04	0.2	194
Hodgkin's disease	2	0	-	-	-	-	-	-	-	-	-	-	-	-	-	-	17.4	-	-	-	0.6	0.2	0.00	0.09	0.3	201
Non-Hodgkin lymphoma	58	0	5.7	-	-	-	4.1	6.5	3.0	7.1	15.9	5.3	19.9	18.5	39.2	34.1	95.7	165.4	43.1	225.6	18.6	5.5	0.63	1.27	12.6	200,202
Multiple myeloma	3	0	-	-	-	-	-	-	-	-	-	-	-	-	-	5.7	8.7	18.4	-	-	1.0	0.3	0.00	0.07	0.5	203
Lymphoid leukaemia	2	0	5.7	6.5	-	-	-	-	-	-	-	-	-	-	-	-	-	-	-	-	0.6	0.2	0.06	0.06	1.3	204
Myeloid leukaemia	22	0	-	6.5	-	-	-	-	-	-	4.0	-	6.6	12.3	-	28.4	43.5	73.5	43.1	75.2	7.0	2.1	0.15	0.51	4.8	205
Monocytic leukaemia	1	0	-	-	-	-	-	-	-	-	-	-	6.6	-	-	-	-	-	-	-	0.3	0.1	0.03	0.03	0.3	206
Other leukaemia	2	0	-	-	-	-	-	-	-	-	-	-	6.6	6.2	-	-	-	-	-	-	0.6	0.2	0.06	0.06	0.6	207
Leukaemia unspecified	1	0	-	-	-	-	-	-	-	-	-	-	-	-	-	-	8.7	-	-	-	0.3	0.1	0.00	0.04	0.2	208
Other and unspecified	23	0	-	-	-	-	-	-	-	-	4.0	15.8	6.6	-	16.8	17.0	26.1	36.8	215.5	75.2	7.4	2.2	0.22	0.43	5.0	O&U
All sites	1064	1	11.5	19.4	-	-	16.2	25.8	30.0	52.9	67.4	121.1	219.2	485.9	783.9	1124.0	1922.6	2739.0	3060.3	3383.5	340.7		9.17	24.42	216.7	ALL
All sites but 173	1062	1	11.5	19.4	-	-	16.2	25.8	27.0	49.4	67.4	121.1	219.2	485.9	783.9	1124.0	1922.6	2739.0	3060.3	3383.5	340.0	100.0	9.14	24.39	216.3	ALLb
Rate from 1 case			5.736	6.460	7.218	6.510	4.054	3.227	3.005	3.525	3.967	5.265	6.642	6.150	5.599	5.677	8.699	18.382	43.103	37.594						

†Important: see notes on population page

USA, CALIFORNIA, LOS ANGELES COUNTY: JAPANESE 1988-1992

ANNUAL INCIDENCE PER 100,000 BY AGE GROUP (YEARS) - FEMALE

SITE	ALL AGES	AGE UNK	0-	5-	10-	15-	20-	25-	30-	35-	40-	45-	50-	55-	60-	65-	70-	75-	80-	85+	CRUDE RATE	%	CR 64	CR 74	ASR (W)	ICD (9th)
Lip	0	0	-	-	-	-	-	-	-	-	-	-	-	-	-	-	-	-	-	-	0.0	0.0	0.00	0.00	0.0	140
Tongue	7	0	-	-	-	-	-	-	3.0	-	-	-	5.5	-	8.7	-	8.2	16.1	-	17.1	2.1	0.7	0.09	0.13	1.2	141
Salivary gland	0	0	-	-	-	-	-	-	-	-	-	-	-	-	-	-	-	-	-	-	0.0	0.0	0.00	0.00	0.0	142
Mouth	7	0	-	-	-	-	-	-	-	-	-	4.9	5.5	8.9	-	-	-	16.1	31.8	17.1	2.1	0.7	0.10	0.10	1.3	143-5
Oropharynx	1	0	-	-	-	-	-	-	-	-	-	-	-	-	-	5.0	-	-	-	-	0.3	0.1	0.00	0.02	0.1	146
Nasopharynx	2	0	-	-	-	-	-	-	-	-	-	-	-	4.4	-	5.0	-	-	-	-	0.6	0.2	0.02	0.05	0.3	147
Hypopharynx	0	0	-	-	-	-	-	-	-	-	-	-	-	-	-	-	-	-	-	-	0.0	0.0	0.00	0.00	0.0	148
Pharynx unspecified	1	0	-	-	-	-	-	-	-	-	-	-	-	-	-	-	8.2	-	-	-	0.3	0.1	0.00	0.04	0.2	149
Oesophagus	6	0	-	-	-	-	-	-	-	-	-	-	5.5	-	8.7	-	8.2	-	31.8	17.1	1.8	0.6	0.07	0.11	1.0	150
Stomach	76	0	-	-	-	-	-	6.3	3.0	10.2	3.7	-	27.6	53.4	21.7	29.9	73.5	128.7	190.8	307.7	22.6	7.5	0.63	1.15	12.0	151
Small intestine	1	0	-	-	-	-	-	-	-	-	-	-	-	-	-	-	-	-	-	17.1	0.3	0.1	0.00	0.00	0.1	152
Colon	133	0	-	-	-	-	-	-	6.0	-	3.7	9.9	22.1	57.8	65.2	124.4	228.8	209.2	190.8	410.3	39.5	13.1	0.82	2.59	20.6	153
Rectum	64	0	-	-	-	-	-	-	3.0	6.8	3.7	19.8	11.0	17.8	43.4	64.7	81.7	80.5	95.4	153.8	19.0	6.3	0.53	1.26	10.6	154
Liver	20	0	-	-	-	-	-	-	-	-	-	-	11.0	17.8	13.0	19.9	16.3	-	63.6	51.3	5.9	2.0	0.21	0.39	3.3	155
Gallbladder etc.	10	0	-	-	-	-	-	-	-	-	-	4.9	5.5	4.4	4.3	5.0	16.3	16.1	31.8	17.1	3.0	1.0	0.10	0.20	1.8	156
Pancreas	40	0	-	-	-	-	-	-	3.0	-	3.7	4.9	5.5	17.8	13.0	39.8	40.8	96.5	159.0	85.5	11.9	3.9	0.24	0.64	6.4	157
Nose, sinuses etc.	0	0	-	-	-	-	-	-	-	-	-	-	-	-	-	-	-	-	-	-	0.0	0.0	0.00	0.00	0.0	160
Larynx	1	0	-	-	-	-	-	-	-	-	-	-	-	4.3	-	-	-	-	-	-	0.3	0.1	0.02	0.02	0.2	161
Bronchus, lung	71	0	-	-	-	-	-	-	-	3.4	3.7	9.9	44.1	48.9	47.8	49.8	89.9	112.6	127.2	85.5	21.1	7.0	0.79	1.49	12.6	162
Other thoracic organs	0	0	-	-	-	-	-	-	-	-	-	-	-	-	-	-	-	-	-	-	0.0	0.0	0.00	0.00	0.0	163-4
Bone	0	0	-	-	-	-	-	-	-	-	-	-	-	-	-	-	-	-	-	-	0.0	0.0	0.00	0.00	0.0	170
Connective tissue	6	0	5.9	-	-	-	-	-	-	-	-	4.9	5.5	-	-	10.0	-	-	31.8	-	1.8	0.6	0.08	0.13	1.7	171
Mesothelioma	1	0	-	-	-	-	-	-	-	-	-	-	-	-	-	4.3	-	-	-	-	0.3	0.1	0.02	0.02	0.2	MES
Kaposi's sarcoma	0	0	-	-	-	-	-	-	-	-	-	-	-	-	-	-	-	-	-	-	0.0	0.0	0.00	0.00	0.0	KAP
Melanoma of skin	4	0	-	-	-	-	-	3.0	-	3.4	-	4.9	-	-	-	-	-	-	31.8	-	1.2	0.4	0.06	0.06	0.8	172
†Other skin	4	0	-	-	-	-	-	-	-	-	-	-	-	-	-	5.0	8.2	16.1	-	17.1	1.2		0.00	0.07	0.6	173
Breast	319	0	-	-	-	-	4.5	12.5	12.0	34.1	115.7	163.2	198.6	177.9	173.8	288.6	220.6	289.6	318.0	119.7	94.8	31.4	4.46	7.01	63.0	174
Uterus unspecified	0	0	-	-	-	-	-	-	-	-	-	-	-	-	-	-	-	-	-	-	0.0	0.0	0.00	0.00	0.0	179
Cervix uteri	20	0	-	-	-	-	-	-	3.0	6.8	18.7	4.9	16.5	17.8	4.3	-	8.2	-	-	34.2	5.9	2.0	0.36	0.40	4.1	180
Placenta	0	0	-	-	-	-	-	-	-	-	-	-	-	-	-	-	-	-	-	-	0.0	0.0	0.00	0.00	0.0	181
Corpus uteri	44	0	-	-	-	-	-	-	6.0	6.8	18.7	9.9	5.5	40.0	17.4	29.9	81.7	32.2	31.8	-	13.1	4.3	0.52	1.08	8.1	182
Ovary etc.	44	0	-	-	-	-	-	6.3	3.0	10.2	-	14.8	44.1	22.2	34.8	34.8	16.3	48.3	-	34.2	13.1	4.3	0.68	0.93	8.7	183
Other female genital	5	1	-	-	-	-	-	-	-	-	-	-	-	-	8.7	-	16.1	31.8	-	-	1.5	0.5	0.05	0.05	0.8	184
Bladder	10	0	-	-	-	-	-	-	-	-	-	-	-	8.9	8.7	-	16.3	16.1	63.6	17.1	3.0	1.0	0.09	0.17	1.6	188
Kidney etc.	13	0	-	-	-	-	-	-	3.0	-	-	-	5.5	13.3	4.3	5.0	24.5	16.1	31.8	17.1	3.9	1.3	0.13	0.28	2.2	189
Eye	1	0	-	-	-	-	-	-	-	-	3.7	-	-	-	-	-	-	-	-	-	0.3	0.1	0.02	0.02	0.2	190
Brain, nervous system	6	0	-	-	-	-	-	-	3.0	-	3.7	-	-	4.4	-	5.0	8.2	-	31.8	-	1.8	0.6	0.06	0.12	1.1	191-2
Thyroid	18	0	-	-	-	-	-	15.6	6.0	-	7.5	-	11.0	17.8	4.3	5.0	8.2	-	-	-	5.4	1.8	0.31	0.38	3.8	193
Other endocrine	1	0	5.9	-	-	-	-	-	-	-	-	-	-	-	-	-	-	-	-	-	0.3	0.1	0.03	0.03	0.7	194
Hodgkin's disease	2	0	-	-	-	-	-	-	-	-	-	-	-	-	-	10.0	-	-	-	-	0.6	0.2	0.00	0.05	0.3	201
Non-Hodgkin lymphoma	32	0	-	-	-	-	4.5	-	-	-	-	-	19.8	22.2	13.0	19.9	57.2	80.5	31.8	34.2	9.5	3.1	0.30	0.68	5.8	200,202
Multiple myeloma	3	0	-	-	-	-	-	-	-	-	-	-	-	4.4	-	-	8.2	16.1	-	-	0.9	0.3	0.02	0.06	0.5	203
Lymphoid leukaemia	7	0	17.7	6.7	7.4	-	-	-	-	-	-	-	-	-	-	5.0	8.2	-	-	-	2.1	0.7	0.16	0.22	3.8	204
Myeloid leukaemia	13	0	5.9	-	-	6.4	-	3.1	3.0	3.4	-	-	5.5	-	8.7	5.0	16.3	16.1	-	17.1	3.9	1.3	0.18	0.29	3.3	205
Monocytic leukaemia	0	0	-	-	-	-	-	-	-	-	-	-	-	-	-	-	-	-	-	-	0.0	0.0	0.00	0.00	0.0	206
Other leukaemia	0	0	-	-	-	-	-	-	-	-	-	-	-	-	-	-	-	-	-	-	0.0	0.0	0.00	0.00	0.0	207
Leukaemia unspecified	0	0	-	-	-	-	-	-	-	-	-	-	-	-	-	-	-	-	-	-	0.0	0.0	0.00	0.00	0.0	208
Other and unspecified	28	0	-	-	-	-	-	-	-	-	-	3.7	-	22.1	8.9	13.0	29.9	24.5	32.2	31.8	102.6	8.3	2.8	0.24	0.51	4.6	O&U
All sites	1021	1	35.4	6.7	7.4	6.4	8.9	43.8	59.8	85.2	190.3	277.0	457.8	569.4	525.6	796.0	1078.4	1255.0	1558.0	1572.6	303.6		11.38	20.76	187.6	ALL
All sites but 173	1017	1	35.4	6.7	7.4	6.4	8.9	43.8	59.8	85.2	190.3	277.0	457.8	569.4	525.6	791.0	1070.3	1238.9	1558.0	1555.6	302.4	100.0	11.38	20.70	187.1	ALLb

Rate from 1 case   5.900 6.698 7.443 6.412 4.451 3.127 2.989 3.407 3.732 4.947 5.516 4.448 4.344 4.975 8.170 16.090 31.797 17.094

†Important: see notes on population page

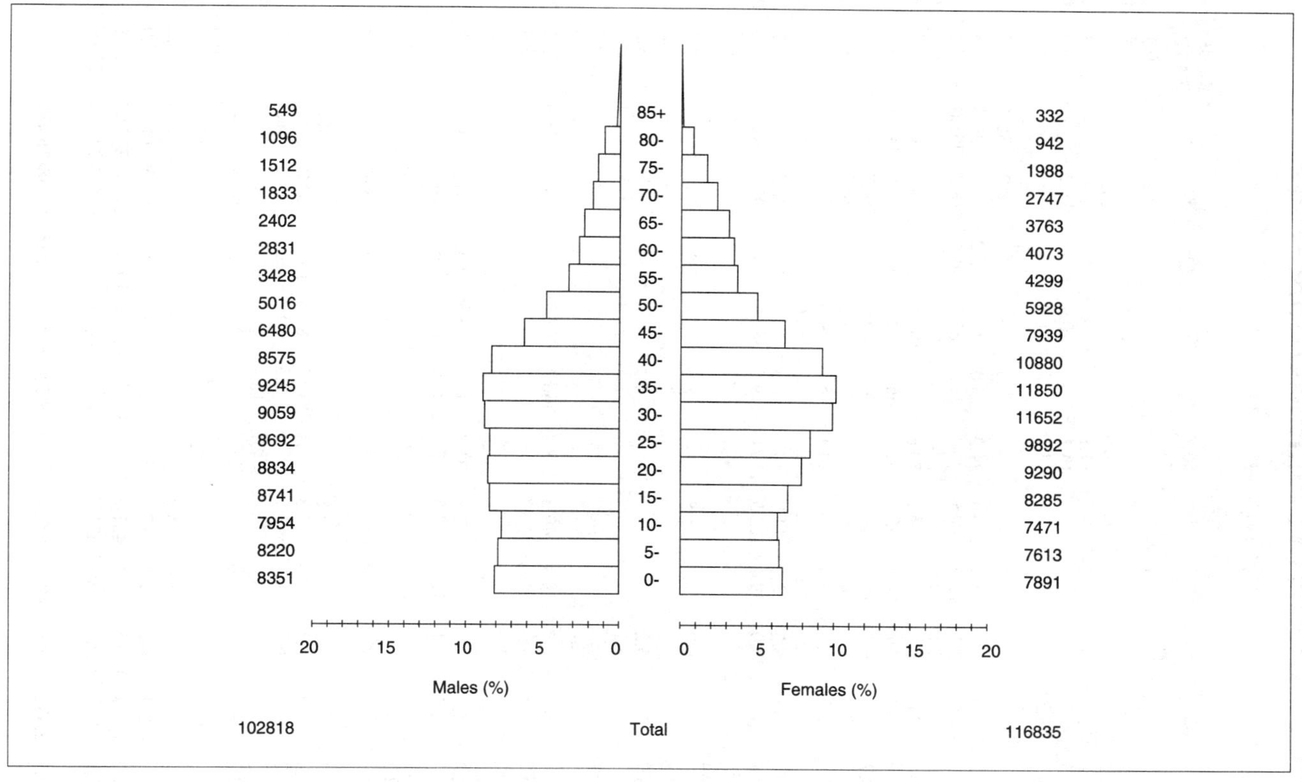

USA, California, Los Angeles County: Filipino
Source of population: 1990
Census: 1990 Census.
Notes to tables overleaf:
† 173 does not include basal cell or squamous cell carcinoma
The denominators are not the same populations as those published in Volume VI and the data for this ethnic group are not comparable.

USA, CALIFORNIA, LOS ANGELES COUNTY: FILIPINO 1988-1992

ANNUAL INCIDENCE PER 100,000 BY AGE GROUP (YEARS) - MALE

SITE	ALL AGES	AGE UNK	0-	5-	10-	15-	20-	25-	30-	35-	40-	45-	50-	55-	60-	65-	70-	75-	80-	85+	CRUDE RATE	%	CR 64	CR 74	ASR (W)	ICD (9th)
Lip	2	0	-	-	-	-	-	-	2.2	-	-	-	4.0	-	-	-	-	-	-	-	0.4	0.2	0.03	0.03	**0.3**	*140*
Tongue	2	0	-	-	-	-	-	-	-	-	-	-	-	-	-	-	21.8	-	-	-	0.4	0.2	0.00	0.11	**0.4**	*141*
Salivary gland	3	0	-	-	-	2.3	-	-	-	2.2	-	-	-	-	-	-	-	-	18.2	-	0.6	0.3	0.02	0.02	**0.4**	*142*
Mouth	4	0	-	-	-	-	-	-	-	-	-	-	-	-	14.1	-	-	26.5	-	-	0.8	0.4	0.07	0.07	**0.8**	*143-5*
Oropharynx	5	0	-	-	-	-	-	-	-	-	3.1	-	-	-	14.1	-	10.9	-	18.2	-	1.0	0.4	0.09	0.14	**1.1**	*146*
Nasopharynx	21	0	-	-	-	-	-	2.3	8.8	4.3	9.3	9.3	-	11.7	14.1	8.3	21.8	-	-	-	4.1	1.9	0.30	0.45	**3.8**	*147*
Hypopharynx	1	0	-	-	-	-	-	-	-	-	-	-	-	-	-	-	-	13.2	-	-	0.2	0.1	0.00	0.00	**0.1**	*148*
Pharynx unspecified	3	0	-	-	-	-	-	-	-	-	-	-	-	-	-	8.3	-	-	18.2	36.4	0.6	0.3	0.00	0.04	**0.5**	*149*
Oesophagus	9	0	-	-	-	-	-	-	-	-	-	-	4.0	-	21.2	25.0	-	13.2	-	36.4	1.8	0.8	0.13	0.25	**2.1**	*150*
Stomach	37	0	-	-	-	-	-	-	-	2.2	4.7	3.1	19.9	17.5	-	25.0	65.5	105.8	18.2	255.0	7.2	3.3	0.24	0.69	**6.8**	*151*
Small intestine	3	0	-	-	-	2.3	-	-	-	-	-	3.1	4.0	-	-	-	-	-	-	-	0.6	0.3	0.05	0.05	**0.6**	*152*
Colon	73	0	-	-	-	-	-	-	-	-	7.0	6.2	31.9	29.2	70.6	91.6	109.1	66.1	200.7	291.4	14.2	6.5	0.72	1.73	**14.4**	*153*
Rectum	46	0	-	-	-	-	-	-	-	-	7.0	3.1	12.0	35.0	35.3	66.6	32.7	119.0	73.0	145.7	8.9	4.1	0.46	0.96	**9.0**	*154*
Liver	49	0	2.4	-	2.5	-	-	-	6.6	8.7	7.0	6.2	15.9	40.8	21.2	50.0	43.6	39.7	54.7	182.1	9.5	4.4	0.56	1.02	**9.5**	*155*
Gallbladder etc.	9	0	-	-	-	-	-	-	-	-	-	2.3	-	4.0	5.8	-	8.3	21.8	13.2	36.5	-	1.8	0.8	0.06	0.21	**1.6**	*156*
Pancreas	25	0	-	-	-	-	-	-	-	2.2	2.3	-	8.0	-	14.1	16.7	54.6	105.8	73.0	-	4.9	2.2	0.13	0.49	**4.2**	*157*
Nose, sinuses etc.	2	0	-	-	-	-	-	-	-	-	-	-	-	-	-	10.9	-	-	36.4	0.4	0.2	0.00	0.05	**0.4**	*160*
Larynx	14	0	-	-	-	-	-	-	-	2.2	-	-	6.2	8.0	11.7	14.1	8.3	-	26.5	36.5	-	2.7	1.3	0.21	0.25	**2.6**	*161*
Bronchus, lung	222	0	-	-	-	-	-	2.3	2.2	10.8	21.0	37.0	79.7	122.5	219.0	299.8	381.9	304.2	401.5	218.6	43.2	19.9	2.47	5.88	**44.9**	*162*
Other thoracic organs	1	0	-	-	-	2.3	-	-	-	-	-	-	-	-	-	-	-	-	-	-	0.2	0.1	0.01	0.01	**0.2**	*163-4*
Bone	3	0	-	-	2.5	-	-	2.3	-	2.2	-	-	-	-	-	-	-	-	-	-	0.6	0.3	0.03	0.03	**0.5**	*170*
Connective tissue	12	0	2.4	2.4	-	-	-	-	2.2	-	-	6.2	4.0	5.8	-	8.3	10.9	13.2	36.5	-	2.3	1.1	0.12	0.21	**2.2**	*171*
Mesothelioma	1	0	-	-	-	-	-	-	-	2.2	-	-	-	-	-	-	-	-	-	-	0.2	0.1	0.01	0.01	**0.1**	*MES*
Kaposi's sarcoma	17	0	-	-	-	-	2.3	-	11.0	8.7	11.7	6.2	-	-	-	-	-	-	-	-	3.3	1.5	0.20	0.20	**2.4**	*KAP*
Melanoma of skin	4	0	-	-	-	-	-	-	-	-	-	3.1	-	-	-	-	21.8	-	-	36.4	0.8	0.4	0.02	0.12	**0.8**	*172*
†Other skin	2	0	-	-	-	-	2.3	-	2.2	-	-	-	-	-	-	-	-	-	-	-	0.4	0.2	0.02	0.02	**0.3**	*173*
Breast	0	0	-	-	-	-	-	-	-	-	-	-	-	-	-	-	-	-	-	-	0.0	0.0	0.00	0.00	**0.0**	*175*
Prostate	258	0	-	-	-	-	-	-	-	-	-	-	19.9	40.8	148.4	366.4	501.9	701.1	1094.9	801.5	50.2	23.1	1.05	5.39	**46.1**	*185*
Testis	7	0	2.4	-	-	-	2.3	-	4.4	6.5	-	-	-	-	-	-	-	-	-	-	1.4	0.6	0.08	0.08	**1.1**	*186*
Penis	0	0	-	-	-	-	-	-	-	-	-	-	-	-	-	-	-	-	-	-	0.0	0.0	0.00	0.00	**0.0**	*187.1-.4*
Other male genital	0	0	-	-	-	-	-	-	-	-	-	-	-	-	-	-	-	-	-	-	0.0	0.0	0.00	0.00	**0.0**	*187.5-.9*
Bladder	27	0	-	-	-	-	-	-	-	-	2.2	4.7	-	5.8	35.3	41.6	65.5	52.9	36.5	36.4	5.3	2.4	0.24	0.78	**5.5**	*188*
Kidney etc.	29	0	4.8	-	-	-	-	2.3	-	-	2.3	3.1	12.0	17.5	42.4	41.6	43.6	26.5	18.2	-	5.6	2.6	0.42	0.85	**6.6**	*189*
Eye	0	0	-	-	-	-	-	-	-	-	-	-	-	-	-	-	-	-	-	-	0.0	0.0	0.00	0.00	**0.0**	*190*
Brain, nervous system	19	0	4.8	2.4	5.0	2.3	2.3	2.3	-	2.2	4.7	-	4.0	5.8	7.1	-	54.6	-	-	-	3.7	1.7	0.21	0.49	**4.1**	*191-2*
Thyroid	22	0	-	-	-	-	-	-	2.2	8.7	11.7	3.1	8.0	17.5	21.2	8.3	-	13.2	18.2	-	4.3	2.0	0.36	0.40	**4.0**	*193*
Other endocrine	1	0	-	-	2.5	-	-	-	-	-	-	-	-	-	-	-	-	-	-	-	0.2	0.1	0.01	0.01	**0.2**	*194*
Hodgkin's disease	9	0	-	2.4	-	2.3	2.3	-	-	4.3	2.3	-	-	5.8	-	-	-	-	18.2	36.4	1.8	0.8	0.10	0.10	**1.5**	*201*
Non-Hodgkin lymphoma	59	0	7.2	-	-	6.9	-	2.3	4.4	4.3	7.0	3.1	12.0	23.3	14.1	33.3	87.3	132.3	164.2	145.7	11.5	5.3	0.42	1.03	**10.5**	*200,202*
Multiple myeloma	16	0	-	-	-	-	-	-	-	-	2.2	-	6.2	4.0	11.7	7.1	8.3	10.9	26.5	73.0	36.4	3.1	1.4	0.16	0.25	**2.7**	*203*
Lymphoid leukaemia	16	0	4.8	7.3	2.5	-	-	-	2.2	2.2	2.3	-	8.0	-	7.1	16.7	10.9	-	18.2	-	3.1	1.4	0.18	0.32	**3.4**	*204*
Myeloid leukaemia	37	0	4.8	2.4	2.5	2.3	-	-	4.4	2.2	9.3	12.3	8.0	-	21.2	33.3	21.8	52.9	109.5	-	7.2	3.3	0.35	0.62	**6.7**	*205*
Monocytic leukaemia	0	0	-	-	-	-	-	-	-	-	-	-	-	-	-	-	-	-	-	-	0.0	0.0	0.00	0.00	**0.0**	*206*
Other leukaemia	0	0	-	-	-	-	-	-	-	-	-	-	-	-	-	-	-	-	-	-	0.0	0.0	0.00	0.00	**0.0**	*207*
Leukaemia unspecified	6	0	2.4	-	-	-	-	2.3	-	-	-	2.3	-	4.0	5.8	-	-	-	-	36.4	1.2	0.5	0.08	0.08	**1.2**	*208*
Other and unspecified	41	0	-	-	-	-	-	-	2.2	-	2.3	6.2	8.0	17.5	35.3	16.7	43.6	145.5	109.5	145.7	8.0	3.7	0.36	0.66	**7.3**	*O&U*
All sites	1117	0	35.9	17.0	17.6	18.3	13.6	16.1	57.4	77.9	121.3	126.5	283.1	431.7	777.1	1182.3	1647.6	1997.4	2646.0	2477.2	217.3		9.97	24.12	**211.1**	*ALL*
All sites but 173	1115	0	35.9	17.0	17.6	18.3	11.3	16.1	55.2	77.9	121.3	126.5	283.1	431.7	777.1	1182.3	1647.6	1997.4	2646.0	2477.2	216.9	100.0	9.95	24.10	**210.8**	*ALLb*

Rate from 1 case   2.395   2.433   2.514   2.288   2.264   2.301   2.208   2.163   2.332   3.086   3.987   5.834   7.065   8.326   10.911   13.228   18.248   36.430

†Important: see notes on population page

USA, CALIFORNIA, LOS ANGELES COUNTY: FILIPINO 1988-1992

ANNUAL INCIDENCE PER 100,000 BY AGE GROUP (YEARS) - FEMALE

SITE	ALL AGES	AGE UNK	0-	5-	10-	15-	20-	25-	30-	35-	40-	45-	50-	55-	60-	65-	70-	75-	80-	85+	CRUDE RATE	%	CR 64	CR 74	ASR (W)	ICD (9th)
Lip	0	0	-	-	-	-	-	-	-	-	-	-	-	-	-	-	-	-	-	-	0.0	0.0	0.00	0.00	0.0	140
Tongue	6	0	-	-	-	-	-	-	-	-	-	2.5	-	-	4.9	10.6	-	-	42.5	-	1.0	0.5	0.04	0.09	0.9	141
Salivary gland	6	0	-	-	-	-	-	-	-	-	1.8	2.5	3.4	-	9.8	5.3	-	-	-	-	1.0	0.5	0.09	0.11	1.0	142
Mouth	4	0	-	-	-	-	-	-	1.7	-	-	-	-	-	-	-	7.3	20.1	-	-	0.7	0.3	0.01	0.04	0.4	143-5
Oropharynx	1	0	-	-	-	-	-	-	-	-	-	-	-	-	-	-	-	10.1	-	-	0.2	0.1	0.00	0.00	0.1	146
Nasopharynx	2	0	-	-	-	-	-	2.0	-	-	-	2.5	-	-	-	-	-	-	-	-	0.3	0.2	0.02	0.02	0.3	147
Hypopharynx	0	0	-	-	-	-	-	-	-	-	-	-	-	-	-	-	-	-	-	-	0.0	0.0	0.00	0.00	0.0	148
Pharynx unspecified	0	0	-	-	-	-	-	-	-	-	-	-	-	-	-	-	-	-	-	-	0.0	0.0	0.00	0.00	0.0	149
Oesophagus	0	0	-	-	-	-	-	-	-	-	-	-	-	-	-	-	-	-	-	-	0.0	0.0	0.00	0.00	0.0	150
Stomach	26	0	-	-	-	-	-	-	1.7	1.7	3.7	2.5	-	4.7	14.7	26.6	36.4	30.2	42.5	120.5	4.5	2.1	0.14	0.46	4.0	151
Small intestine	2	0	-	-	-	-	-	-	-	1.7	-	-	-	-	-	-	-	10.1	-	-	0.3	0.2	0.01	0.01	0.2	152
Colon	55	0	-	-	-	-	2.2	2.0	-	1.7	3.7	5.0	10.1	14.0	24.6	42.5	109.2	50.3	169.9	60.2	9.4	4.4	0.32	1.07	8.1	153
Rectum	44	0	-	-	-	-	-	-	-	5.1	5.5	12.6	13.5	23.3	14.7	42.5	29.1	80.5	21.2	-	7.5	3.5	0.37	0.73	6.4	154
Liver	20	0	-	-	-	-	-	-	1.7	-	-	3.4	14.0	9.8	10.6	36.4	10.1	42.5	180.7	3.4	1.6	0.14	0.38	3.5	155
Gallbladder etc.	13	0	-	-	-	-	-	-	-	-	1.8	-	-	4.7	4.9	-	36.4	20.1	42.5	60.2	2.2	1.0	0.06	0.24	1.9	156
Pancreas	34	0	-	-	-	-	-	-	-	-	-	-	6.7	9.3	-	31.9	80.1	50.3	84.9	241.0	5.8	2.7	0.08	0.64	5.4	157
Nose, sinuses etc.	4	0	-	-	-	2.4	-	-	-	-	-	-	4.7	-	10.6	-	-	-	-	-	0.7	0.3	0.04	0.09	0.7	160
Larynx	5	0	-	-	-	-	-	-	-	-	-	-	-	-	4.9	10.6	7.3	10.1	-	-	0.9	0.4	0.02	0.11	0.8	161
Bronchus, lung	83	0	-	-	-	-	-	-	1.7	3.4	7.4	12.6	27.0	23.3	44.2	74.4	123.8	140.8	63.7	60.2	14.2	6.6	0.60	1.59	12.3	162
Other thoracic organs	0	0	-	-	-	-	-	-	-	-	-	-	-	-	-	-	-	-	-	-	0.0	0.0	0.00	0.00	0.0	163-4
Bone	4	0	-	-	-	-	4.0	1.7	-	-	-	3.4	-	-	-	-	-	-	-	-	0.7	0.3	0.05	0.05	0.6	170
Connective tissue	14	0	2.5	-	5.4	-	2.0	1.7	-	1.8	2.5	3.4	14.0	-	10.6	-	-	21.2	-	2.4	1.1	0.17	0.22	2.5	171
Mesothelioma	1	0	-	-	-	-	-	-	-	-	-	-	-	-	5.3	-	-	-	-	-	0.2	0.1	0.00	0.03	0.2	MES
Kaposi's sarcoma	0	0	-	-	-	-	-	-	-	-	-	-	-	-	-	-	-	-	-	-	0.0	0.0	0.00	0.00	0.0	KAP
Melanoma of skin	1	0	-	-	-	-	-	-	-	-	1.8	-	-	-	-	-	-	-	-	-	0.2	0.1	0.01	0.01	0.1	172
†Other skin	3	0	-	-	-	-	-	-	-	3.4	-	-	-	-	-	-	7.3	-	-	-	0.5		0.02	0.05	0.3	173
Breast	480	0	-	-	-	-	-	8.1	37.8	55.7	154.4	188.9	236.2	176.8	171.9	271.1	203.9	261.6	254.8	120.5	82.2	38.2	5.15	7.52	69.3	174
Uterus unspecified	0	0	-	-	-	-	-	-	-	-	-	-	-	-	-	-	-	-	-	-	0.0	0.0	0.00	0.00	0.0	179
Cervix uteri	59	0	-	-	-	-	-	6.1	3.4	11.8	12.9	5.0	16.9	41.9	14.7	53.1	58.2	20.1	21.2	-	10.1	4.7	0.56	1.12	8.6	180
Placenta	0	0	-	-	-	-	-	-	-	-	-	-	-	-	-	-	-	-	-	-	0.0	0.0	0.00	0.00	0.0	181
Corpus uteri	74	0	-	-	-	-	-	2.0	3.4	10.1	12.9	15.1	47.2	65.1	24.6	31.9	51.0	30.2	42.5	60.2	12.7	5.9	0.90	1.32	11.4	182
Ovary etc.	62	0	-	5.3	-	2.4	-	10.1	1.7	8.4	7.4	25.2	16.9	46.5	24.6	26.6	36.4	20.1	21.2	60.2	10.6	4.9	0.74	1.06	9.9	183
Other female genital	5	0	-	-	-	-	-	-	-	1.8	-	-	4.7	-	5.3	-	-	-	120.5	0.9	0.4	0.03	0.06	1.1	184
Bladder	6	0	-	-	-	-	-	-	-	-	-	-	-	-	14.7	5.3	7.3	10.1	-	-	1.0	0.5	0.07	0.14	1.0	188
Kidney etc.	18	0	-	-	-	-	-	-	-	-	1.8	-	3.4	-	19.6	10.6	14.6	70.4	-	60.2	3.1	1.4	0.12	0.25	2.7	189
Eye	0	0	-	-	-	-	-	-	-	-	-	-	-	-	-	-	-	-	-	-	0.0	0.0	0.00	0.00	0.0	190
Brain, nervous system	14	0	2.5	-	-	-	2.2	-	3.4	3.4	-	5.0	-	14.0	-	15.9	-	-	-	-	2.4	1.1	0.15	0.23	2.2	191-2
Thyroid	78	0	2.5	-	-	-	10.8	10.1	10.3	21.9	23.9	17.6	20.2	37.2	34.4	15.9	7.3	20.1	21.2	-	13.4	6.2	0.95	1.06	11.2	193
Other endocrine	0	0	-	-	-	-	-	-	-	-	-	-	-	-	-	-	-	-	-	-	0.0	0.0	0.00	0.00	0.0	194
Hodgkin's disease	5	0	-	-	2.7	2.4	-	2.0	-	-	-	-	3.4	-	-	5.3	-	-	-	-	0.9	0.4	0.05	0.08	0.9	201
Non-Hodgkin lymphoma	49	0	-	-	-	2.4	4.3	-	5.1	1.7	5.5	2.5	3.4	14.0	14.7	31.9	51.0	90.5	148.6	120.5	8.4	3.9	0.27	0.68	7.0	200,202
Multiple myeloma	12	0	-	-	-	-	-	-	-	-	-	2.5	-	4.7	-	10.6	29.1	40.2	-	-	2.1	1.0	0.04	0.23	1.6	203
Lymphoid leukaemia	11	0	17.7	-	-	-	-	-	-	-	-	-	-	-	9.8	5.3	-	-	-	60.2	1.9	0.9	0.14	0.16	3.0	204
Myeloid leukaemia	19	0	-	-	8.0	-	2.2	4.0	-	-	-	5.5	5.0	-	4.7	4.9	10.6	-	40.2	-	3.3	1.5	0.17	0.22	3.0	205
Monocytic leukaemia	1	0	2.5	-	-	-	-	-	-	-	-	-	-	-	-	-	-	-	-	-	0.2	0.1	0.01	0.01	0.3	206
Other leukaemia	1	0	-	-	-	2.4	-	-	-	-	-	-	-	-	-	-	-	-	-	-	0.2	0.1	0.01	0.01	0.2	207
Leukaemia unspecified	3	0	-	-	-	-	-	-	-	-	-	1.8	-	-	-	4.9	-	-	10.1	-	0.5	0.2	0.03	0.03	0.4	208
Other and unspecified	33	1	2.5	2.6	-	-	-	2.0	-	1.7	1.8	7.6	6.7	14.0	9.8	26.6	36.4	20.1	42.5	180.7	5.6	2.6	0.25	0.58	5.7	O&U
All sites	1258	1	30.4	7.9	16.1	12.1	21.5	54.6	73.8	133.3	257.4	317.4	425.1	535.0	481.2	807.9	968.3	1066.4	1082.8	1506.0	215.3		11.84	20.73	189.2	ALL
All sites but 173	1255	1	30.4	7.9	16.1	12.1	21.5	54.6	73.8	130.0	257.4	317.4	425.1	535.0	481.2	807.9	961.0	1066.4	1082.8	1506.0	214.8	100.0	11.82	20.67	188.9	ALLb

Rate from 1 case: 2.535 2.627 2.677 2.414 2.153 2.022 1.716 1.688 1.838 2.519 3.374 4.652 4.910 5.315 7.281 10.060 21.231 60.241

†Important: see notes on population page

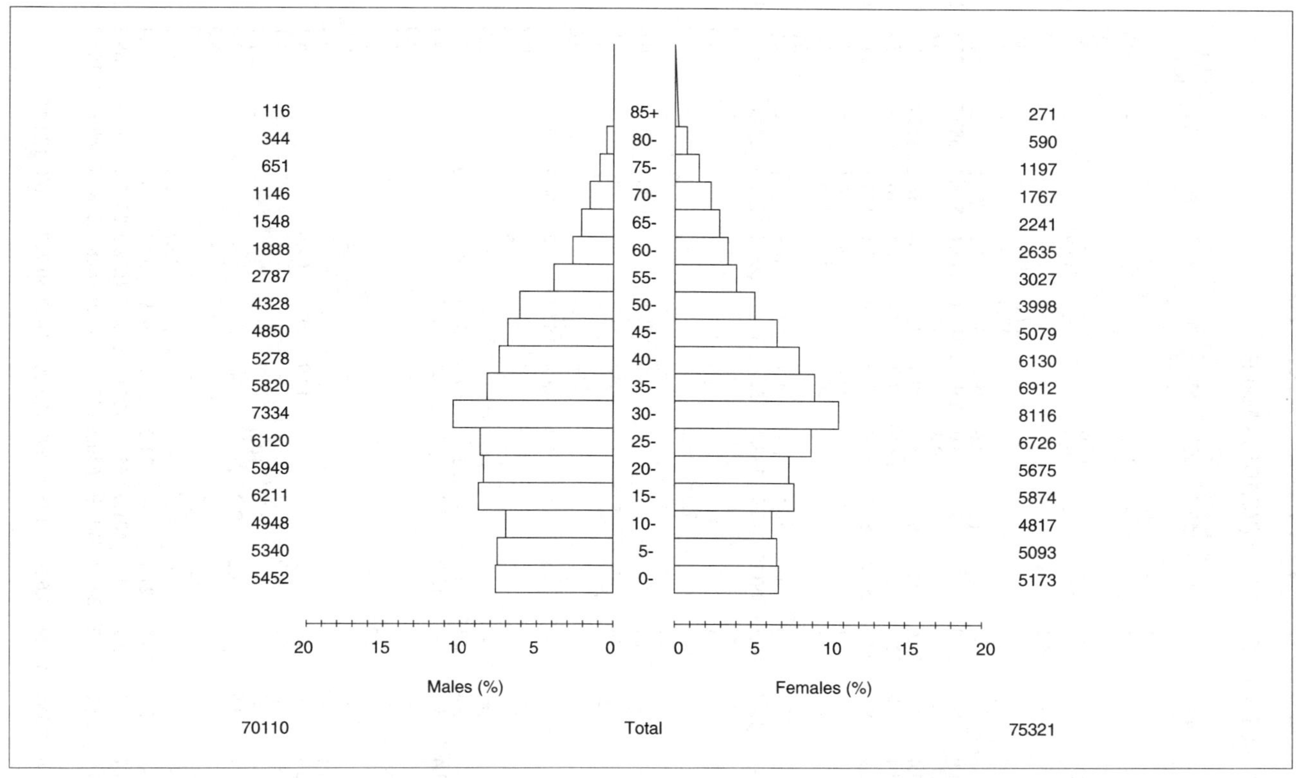

USA, California, Los Angeles County: Korean
Source of population: 1990
Census: 1990 Census.
Notes to tables overleaf:
† 173 does not include basal cell or squamous cell carcinoma
The denominators are not the same populations as those published in Volume VI and the data for this ethnic group are not comparable.

USA, CALIFORNIA, LOS ANGELES COUNTY: KOREAN 1988-1992

ANNUAL INCIDENCE PER 100,000 BY AGE GROUP (YEARS) - MALE

SITE	ALL AGES	AGE UNK	0-	5-	10-	15-	20-	25-	30-	35-	40-	45-	50-	55-	60-	65-	70-	75-	80-	85+	CRUDE RATE	%	CR 64	CR 74	ASR (W)	ICD (9th)
Lip	1	0	-	-	-	-	-	-	-	-	-	4.1	-	-	-	-	-	-	-	-	0.3	0.2	0.02	0.02	0.2	140
Tongue	3	0	-	-	-	-	-	-	-	-	-	4.1	-	-	21.2	-	-	-	-	-	0.9	0.5	0.13	0.13	1.1	141
Salivary gland	0	0	-	-	-	-	-	-	-	-	-	-	-	-	-	-	-	-	-	-	0.0	0.0	0.00	0.00	0.0	142
Mouth	1	0	-	-	-	-	-	-	-	-	-	-	-	-	10.6	-	-	-	-	-	0.3	0.2	0.05	0.05	0.4	143-5
Oropharynx	3	0	-	-	-	-	-	-	3.4	-	-	-	-	-	10.6	-	-	30.7	-	-	0.9	0.5	0.07	0.07	0.9	146
Nasopharynx	1	0	-	-	-	-	-	-	-	-	-	4.1	-	-	-	-	-	-	-	-	0.3	0.2	0.02	0.02	0.2	147
Hypopharynx	3	0	-	-	-	-	-	-	-	-	-	-	-	-	-	-	17.5	61.4	-	-	0.9	0.5	0.00	0.09	1.0	148
Pharynx unspecified	1	0	-	-	-	-	-	-	-	-	-	-	-	-	-	-	17.5	-	-	-	0.3	0.2	0.00	0.09	0.3	149
Oesophagus	15	0	-	-	-	-	-	-	-	-	-	4.6	14.4	10.6	38.8	34.9	92.2	58.1	344.8	-	4.3	2.6	0.15	0.52	6.0	150
Stomach	109	0	-	-	-	-	-	3.3	13.6	6.9	15.2	28.9	64.7	93.3	53.0	258.4	314.1	215.1	523.3	689.7	31.1	18.8	1.39	4.26	35.5	151
Small intestine	2	0	-	-	-	-	-	-	-	-	-	-	-	-	10.6	-	17.5	-	-	-	0.6	0.3	0.05	0.14	0.8	152
Colon	42	0	-	-	-	-	-	-	2.7	3.4	3.8	20.6	9.2	50.2	63.6	90.4	139.6	61.4	58.1	172.4	12.0	7.3	0.77	1.92	14.1	153
Rectum	26	0	-	-	-	-	-	-	2.7	3.4	3.8	12.4	13.9	-	31.8	51.7	104.7	61.4	116.3	-	7.4	4.5	0.34	1.12	8.1	154
Liver	75	1	-	-	-	-	-	-	-	6.9	18.9	20.6	50.8	86.1	158.9	155.0	52.4	215.1	116.3	-	21.4	13.0	1.73	2.79	23.9	155
Gallbladder etc.	8	0	-	-	-	-	-	-	-	-	-	4.1	-	-	-	38.8	34.9	30.7	58.1	-	2.3	1.4	0.02	0.39	2.7	156
Pancreas	14	0	-	-	-	-	-	-	-	-	7.6	4.1	-	-	31.8	64.6	-	30.7	116.3	-	4.0	2.4	0.22	0.54	4.8	157
Nose, sinuses etc.	0	0	-	-	-	-	-	-	-	-	-	-	-	-	-	-	-	-	-	-	0.0	0.0	0.00	0.00	0.0	160
Larynx	17	0	-	-	-	-	-	-	-	-	-	8.2	4.6	28.7	10.6	51.7	34.9	61.4	58.1	-	4.8	2.9	0.26	0.69	5.5	161
Bronchus, lung	110	0	-	-	-	-	-	-	2.7	-	15.2	16.5	60.1	78.9	148.3	232.6	331.6	399.4	639.5	344.8	31.4	19.0	1.61	4.43	36.7	162
Other thoracic organs	0	0	-	-	-	-	-	-	-	-	-	-	-	-	-	-	-	-	-	-	0.0	0.0	0.00	0.00	0.0	163-4
Bone	3	0	-	-	4.0	-	-	-	-	-	-	4.1	-	-	12.9	-	-	-	-	-	0.9	0.5	0.04	0.11	1.0	170
Connective tissue	7	0	3.7	-	-	3.2	-	-	5.5	-	-	-	-	7.2	21.2	-	-	-	-	-	2.0	1.2	0.20	0.20	2.2	171
Mesothelioma	0	0	-	-	-	-	-	-	-	-	-	-	-	-	-	-	-	-	-	-	0.0	0.0	0.00	0.00	0.0	MES
Kaposi's sarcoma	2	0	-	-	-	-	-	-	-	-	-	4.1	-	-	-	17.5	-	-	-	-	0.6	0.3	0.02	0.11	0.6	KAP
Melanoma of skin	0	0	-	-	-	-	-	-	-	-	-	-	-	-	-	-	-	-	-	-	0.0	0.0	0.00	0.00	0.0	172
†Other skin	0	0	-	-	-	-	-	-	-	-	-	-	-	-	-	-	-	-	-	-	0.0	0.0	0.00	0.00	0.0	173
Breast	0	0	-	-	-	-	-	-	-	-	-	-	-	-	-	-	-	-	-	-	0.0	0.0	0.00	0.00	0.0	175
Prostate	29	0	-	-	-	-	-	-	-	-	-	4.6	14.4	31.8	38.8	157.1	153.6	290.7	172.4	-	8.3	5.0	0.25	1.23	10.2	185
Testis	3	0	-	-	-	-	3.4	-	2.7	-	-	-	-	-	12.9	-	-	-	-	-	0.9	0.5	0.03	0.10	0.8	186
Penis	1	0	-	-	-	-	-	-	-	-	-	-	-	-	-	-	30.7	-	-	-	0.3	0.2	0.00	0.00	0.3	187.1-.4
Other male genital	0	0	-	-	-	-	-	-	-	-	-	-	-	-	-	-	-	-	-	-	0.0	0.0	0.00	0.00	0.0	187.5-.9
Bladder	16	0	3.7	-	-	-	-	-	-	-	3.8	4.1	4.6	-	10.6	64.6	52.4	30.7	116.3	-	4.6	2.8	0.13	0.72	5.4	188
Kidney etc.	19	0	-	-	-	-	-	-	3.4	3.8	-	13.9	7.2	-	103.4	52.4	-	116.3	-	-	5.4	3.3	0.14	0.92	6.1	189
Eye	0	0	-	-	-	-	-	-	-	-	-	-	-	-	-	-	-	-	-	-	0.0	0.0	0.00	0.00	0.0	190
Brain, nervous system	5	0	-	-	-	3.2	-	3.3	-	3.4	-	-	-	-	-	-	17.5	30.7	-	-	1.4	0.9	0.05	0.14	1.4	191-2
Thyroid	6	0	-	-	-	-	-	3.3	5.5	-	-	8.2	-	7.2	-	-	-	-	-	-	1.7	1.0	0.12	0.12	1.4	193
Other endocrine	0	0	-	-	-	-	-	-	-	-	-	-	-	-	-	-	-	-	-	-	0.0	0.0	0.00	0.00	0.0	194
Hodgkin's disease	1	0	-	-	-	-	-	-	-	3.4	-	-	-	-	-	-	-	-	-	-	0.3	0.2	0.02	0.02	0.2	201
Non-Hodgkin lymphoma	18	0	-	-	4.0	-	-	3.3	2.7	6.9	7.6	4.1	13.9	-	-	12.9	69.8	61.4	-	-	5.1	3.1	0.21	0.63	5.0	200,202
Multiple myeloma	4	0	-	-	-	-	-	-	-	-	-	4.1	4.6	7.2	-	-	-	-	-	172.4	1.1	0.7	0.08	0.08	1.6	203
Lymphoid leukaemia	4	0	7.3	3.7	-	-	-	-	-	-	-	-	-	-	10.6	-	-	-	-	-	1.1	0.7	0.11	0.11	1.7	204
Myeloid leukaemia	7	0	-	-	4.0	-	-	-	2.7	3.4	3.8	-	9.2	7.2	-	-	-	-	-	-	2.0	1.2	0.15	0.15	1.7	205
Monocytic leukaemia	0	0	-	-	-	-	-	-	-	-	-	-	-	-	-	-	-	-	-	-	0.0	0.0	0.00	0.00	0.0	206
Other leukaemia	0	0	-	-	-	-	-	-	-	-	-	-	-	-	-	-	-	-	-	-	0.0	0.0	0.00	0.00	0.0	207
Leukaemia unspecified	4	0	-	-	4.0	-	-	-	-	-	-	-	4.6	-	-	-	-	30.7	58.1	-	1.1	0.7	0.04	0.04	1.2	208
Other and unspecified	19	0	-	-	-	-	-	-	-	-	3.8	16.5	27.7	-	21.2	25.8	34.9	30.7	58.1	-	5.4	3.3	0.35	0.65	5.5	O&U
All sites	579	1	14.7	3.7	16.2	6.4	3.4	13.1	40.9	44.7	87.2	173.2	291.1	401.9	656.8	1253.2	1500.9	1628.3	2383.7	1896.6	165.2		8.78	22.58	188.8	ALL
All sites but 173	579	1	14.7	3.7	16.2	6.4	3.4	13.1	40.9	44.7	87.2	173.2	291.1	401.9	656.8	1253.2	1500.9	1628.3	2383.7	1896.6	165.2	100.0	8.78	22.58	188.8	ALLb

Rate from 1 case   3.668 3.745 4.042 3.220 3.362 3.268 2.727 3.436 3.789 4.124 4.621 7.176 10.593 12.920 17.452 30.722 58.140 172.41

†Important: see notes on population page

USA, CALIFORNIA, LOS ANGELES COUNTY: KOREAN 1988-1992

ANNUAL INCIDENCE PER 100,000 BY AGE GROUP (YEARS) - FEMALE

SITE	ALL AGES	AGE UNK	0-	5-	10-	15-	20-	25-	30-	35-	40-	45-	50-	55-	60-	65-	70-	75-	80-	85+	CRUDE RATE	%	CR 64	CR 74	ASR (W)	ICD (9th)
Lip	0	0	-	-	-	-	-	-	-	-	-	-	-	-	-	-	-	-	-	-	0.0	0.0	0.00	0.00	0.0	140
Tongue	1	0	-	-	-	-	-	-	2.5	-	-	-	-	-	-	-	-	-	-	-	0.3	0.2	0.01	0.01	0.1	141
Salivary gland	0	0	-	-	-	-	-	-	-	-	-	-	-	-	-	-	-	-	-	-	0.0	0.0	0.00	0.00	0.0	142
Mouth	1	0	-	-	-	-	-	-	-	-	-	-	-	-	-	-	-	16.7	-	-	0.3	0.2	0.00	0.00	0.2	143-5
Oropharynx	0	0	-	-	-	-	-	-	-	-	-	-	-	-	-	-	-	-	-	-	0.0	0.0	0.00	0.00	0.0	146
Nasopharynx	1	0	-	-	-	-	-	-	-	-	-	3.9	-	-	-	-	-	-	-	-	0.3	0.2	0.02	0.02	0.2	147
Hypopharynx	0	0	-	-	-	-	-	-	-	-	-	-	-	-	-	-	-	-	-	-	0.0	0.0	0.00	0.00	0.0	148
Pharynx unspecified	0	0	-	-	-	-	-	-	-	-	-	-	-	-	-	-	-	-	-	-	0.0	0.0	0.00	0.00	0.0	149
Oesophagus	1	0	-	-	-	-	-	-	-	-	-	-	-	-	7.6	-	-	-	-	-	0.3	0.2	0.04	0.04	0.3	150
Stomach	70	0	-	-	-	-	-	5.9	9.9	8.7	16.3	19.7	15.0	39.6	30.4	71.4	169.8	117.0	135.6	295.2	18.6	12.0	0.73	1.93	16.2	151
Small intestine	4	0	-	-	-	-	-	-	-	-	-	3.9	10.0	-	-	-	-	16.7	-	-	1.1	0.7	0.07	0.07	0.9	152
Colon	35	0	-	-	-	-	-	-	-	8.7	6.5	11.8	10.0	13.2	15.2	71.4	34.0	50.1	169.5	147.6	9.3	6.0	0.33	0.85	8.2	153
Rectum	28	0	-	-	-	-	3.0	-	-	-	16.3	3.9	15.0	6.6	30.4	17.8	45.3	50.1	33.9	221.4	7.4	4.8	0.38	0.69	6.9	154
Liver	24	0	-	-	-	-	-	-	-	-	3.3	7.9	20.0	13.2	22.8	8.9	56.6	50.1	101.7	-	6.4	4.1	0.34	0.66	5.5	155
Gallbladder etc.	24	0	-	-	-	-	-	-	-	-	-	-	10.0	19.8	30.4	17.8	56.6	33.4	67.8	295.2	6.4	4.1	0.30	0.67	6.3	156
Pancreas	21	0	-	-	-	-	-	3.0	-	-	3.3	3.9	20.0	6.6	22.8	17.8	45.3	-	67.8	147.6	5.6	3.6	0.30	0.61	5.4	157
Nose, sinuses etc.	1	0	-	-	-	-	-	-	-	-	3.9	-	-	-	-	-	-	-	-	-	0.3	0.2	0.02	0.02	0.2	160
Larynx	4	0	-	-	-	-	-	-	-	-	-	-	-	-	7.6	8.9	22.6	-	-	-	1.1	0.7	0.04	0.20	1.0	161
Bronchus, lung	52	0	-	-	-	-	-	-	-	-	9.8	11.8	15.0	19.8	53.1	71.4	113.2	167.1	101.7	147.6	13.8	9.0	0.55	1.47	12.3	162
Other thoracic organs	1	0	-	-	-	-	-	-	-	-	-	-	-	-	-	-	-	33.9	-	-	0.3	0.2	0.00	0.00	0.2	163-4
Bone	1	0	-	-	-	-	3.0	-	-	-	-	-	-	-	-	-	-	-	-	-	0.3	0.2	0.01	0.01	0.2	170
Connective tissue	5	0	3.9	-	-	-	-	-	-	-	-	3.9	-	-	7.6	8.9	-	16.7	-	-	1.3	0.9	0.08	0.12	1.4	171
Mesothelioma	0	0	-	-	-	-	-	-	-	-	-	-	-	-	-	-	-	-	-	-	0.0	0.0	0.00	0.00	0.0	MES
Kaposi's sarcoma	0	0	-	-	-	-	-	-	-	-	-	-	-	-	-	-	-	-	-	-	0.0	0.0	0.00	0.00	0.0	KAP
Melanoma of skin	2	0	-	-	-	-	-	-	-	-	-	-	5.0	-	-	-	-	-	33.9	-	0.5	0.3	0.03	0.03	0.4	172
†Other skin	1	0	-	-	-	-	-	2.5	-	-	-	-	-	-	-	-	-	-	-	-	0.3		0.01	0.01	0.1	173
Breast	97	0	-	-	-	-	10.6	-	7.4	43.4	58.7	78.8	70.0	52.9	7.6	17.8	90.5	50.1	33.9	73.8	25.8	16.7	1.65	2.19	21.4	174
Uterus unspecified	1	0	-	-	-	-	-	-	-	-	-	-	-	-	-	-	-	16.7	-	-	0.3	0.2	0.00	0.00	0.2	179
Cervix uteri	59	0	-	-	-	-	-	-	9.9	23.1	19.6	11.8	25.0	39.6	60.7	71.4	56.6	83.5	33.9	-	15.7	10.2	0.95	1.59	13.4	180
Placenta	0	0	-	-	-	-	-	-	-	-	-	-	-	-	-	-	-	-	-	-	0.0	0.0	0.00	0.00	0.0	181
Corpus uteri	10	0	-	-	-	-	-	-	-	-	3.3	-	10.0	13.2	15.2	17.8	11.3	-	-	-	2.7	1.7	0.21	0.35	2.6	182
Ovary etc.	19	0	-	-	-	-	7.0	-	-	2.9	6.5	7.9	25.0	13.2	30.4	8.9	-	-	-	-	5.0	3.3	0.46	0.51	4.9	183
Other female genital	2	0	3.9	-	-	-	-	-	-	-	-	3.9	-	-	-	-	-	-	-	-	0.5	0.3	0.04	0.04	0.7	184
Bladder	8	0	-	-	-	-	-	-	-	-	-	-	-	6.6	15.2	8.9	34.0	16.7	-	-	2.1	1.4	0.11	0.32	2.0	188
Kidney etc.	15	0	3.9	-	-	-	-	-	-	-	-	3.9	-	19.8	-	44.6	34.0	-	-	147.6	4.0	2.6	0.14	0.53	4.2	189
Eye	0	0	-	-	-	-	-	-	-	-	-	-	-	-	-	-	-	-	-	-	0.0	0.0	0.00	0.00	0.0	190
Brain, nervous system	7	0	-	3.9	4.2	-	-	-	-	2.9	3.3	-	-	-	7.6	8.9	-	-	33.9	-	1.9	1.2	0.11	0.15	1.9	191-2
Thyroid	21	0	-	-	3.4	3.5	3.0	2.5	11.6	3.3	-	10.0	13.2	-	53.5	-	16.7	33.9	-	-	5.6	3.6	0.25	0.52	4.8	193
Other endocrine	0	0	-	-	-	-	-	-	-	-	-	-	-	-	-	-	-	-	-	-	0.0	0.0	0.00	0.00	0.0	194
Hodgkin's disease	1	0	-	-	-	-	-	3.0	-	-	-	-	-	-	-	-	-	-	-	-	0.3	0.2	0.01	0.01	0.2	201
Non-Hodgkin lymphoma	18	0	-	-	-	-	-	-	2.5	-	3.3	3.9	15.0	33.0	-	-	45.3	16.7	33.9	73.8	4.8	3.1	0.29	0.51	4.3	200,202
Multiple myeloma	4	0	-	-	-	-	-	-	-	-	-	-	-	-	7.6	-	-	33.4	33.9	-	1.1	0.7	0.04	0.04	0.8	203
Lymphoid leukaemia	5	0	3.9	3.9	-	3.4	-	-	-	-	-	-	13.2	-	-	-	-	-	-	-	1.3	0.9	0.12	0.12	1.7	204
Myeloid leukaemia	9	0	-	-	-	3.4	3.5	-	4.9	5.8	-	3.9	-	-	7.6	-	-	-	33.9	-	2.4	1.5	0.15	0.15	1.9	205
Monocytic leukaemia	0	0	-	-	-	-	-	-	-	-	-	-	-	-	-	-	-	-	-	-	0.0	0.0	0.00	0.00	0.0	206
Other leukaemia	0	0	-	-	-	-	-	-	-	-	-	-	-	-	-	-	-	-	-	-	0.0	0.0	0.00	0.00	0.0	207
Leukaemia unspecified	1	0	-	-	-	-	-	-	-	-	-	-	-	-	7.6	-	-	-	-	-	0.3	0.2	0.04	0.04	0.3	208
Other and unspecified	28	0	-	-	-	-	-	-	-	5.8	-	3.9	5.0	19.8	30.4	35.7	56.6	66.8	101.7	73.8	7.4	4.8	0.32	0.79	6.6	O&U
All sites	582	0	15.5	7.9	4.2	10.2	24.7	20.8	41.9	112.8	153.3	193.0	280.1	343.6	417.5	562.2	871.5	818.7	1084.7	1623.6	154.5		8.13	15.30	138.1	ALL
All sites but 173	581	0	15.5	7.9	4.2	10.2	24.7	20.8	39.4	112.8	153.3	193.0	280.1	343.6	417.5	562.2	871.5	818.7	1084.7	1623.6	154.3	100.0	8.11	15.28	138.0	ALLb

Rate from 1 case	0-	5-	10-	15-	20-	25-	30-	35-	40-	45-	50-	55-	60-	65-	70-	75-	80-	85+
	3.866	3.927	4.152	3.405	3.524	2.974	2.464	2.894	3.263	3.938	5.003	6.607	7.590	8.925	11.319	16.708	33.898	73.801

†Important: see notes on population page

USA, California, San Francisco Bay Area

A population-based cancer registration system began in May 1972, in five San Francisco Bay Area counties: Alameda, Contra Costa, Marin, San Francisco and San Mateo. In 1973 the registry became part of the Surveillance, Epidemiology, and End Results (SEER) Program of the National Cancer Institute. Since 1988, the registry has been one of the ten regional registries contributing data to the California Cancer Registry.

The registry is operated by the Northern California Cancer Center (NCCC). Since 1988, the NCCC has operated an additional population-based registry covering four adjacent counties immediately to the south of the San Francisco Bay Area.

The San Francisco-Oakland area is located along the coast of northern California between longitudes 122° and 123° W and latitudes 38° and 39° N, covering 6427 km². The population at the 1990 census was 3 699 901, made up of 59% non-Hispanic white, 14% white Hispanic, 11% black, 6.9% Chinese, 4.5% Filipino, 1.2% Japanese 0.8% Vietnamese, 0.8% Asian Indian, 0.7% Korean, and 1.1% other Asian. The Hispanic and Asian populations are increasing most rapidly, mainly through migration to the Bay Area. Thus, the area is multi-cultural and many languages are spoken. Approximately 98% of the population lives in urban areas.

From 1969 to 1986 cancer registration was voluntary, although there was complete participation by hospitals in the area. Registry staff visited large hospitals in neighboring counties to identify cases who lived in the five-county Bay Area. Staff identified additional cases by visiting pathology laboratories, radiation centres, surgery centres and nursing homes. These records were supplemented by information from residents' death certificates on which cancer was listed as the underlying cause of death or mentioned on the death certificate.

In 1987 a California State law created the California Cancer Registry and made reporting from hospitals mandatory, as well as requiring physicians to report cases who are not seen at a hospital. Registry staff continue to visit radiation and surgery centres. In addition, there is an increasing tendency for cancer cases to be diagnosed and treated as outpatients. Therefore, the registry staff now visits all pathology laboratories in the area to identify cases independently to assure completeness. Staff also continue to review death certificates. The California Cancer Registry provides for the sharing of cases between reporting regions and for the ascertainment of cases from some neighbouring states, so that Bay Area residents who are diagnosed or treated elsewhere are reported to the Bay Area Registry. Twice a year the database is linked to the State of California death tapes to identify any cases not already reported. It is estimated that over 95% of cases are identified and reported to the registry.

Currently in the area there are 58 hospitals and more than 2000 physicians who treat cancer patients. In addition, there are eight free-standing radiation centres, 30 surgery centres and 69 pathology laboratories involved in cancer diagnosis and treatment.

The registry collects data not only on cancer incidence but also on diagnostic procedures, cancer characteristics (including stage and grade), treatment and survival. To monitor survival, the registry has been engaging in annual lifetime follow-up of all patients to determine vital status, beginning with patients diagnosed in 1973. Both active and passive follow-up methods are used. Active follow-up includes letters to physicians and telephone calls to patients. Most follow-up is passive, and involves methods such as computer linkages to vital statistics, drivers' license, medicare, voter and credit records. These provide follow-up information for over 95% of patients.

The registry supports a hospital-based computer software program that allows institutions to collect, edit and store data in electronic files for submission to the registry. At the registry, data are visually edited for completeness and accuracy and then checked again by computer edit for allowable codes and compatibility between different data fields. The data are then linked to the database using a "soundex" code, birth date, and social security number. New cases are added, and new information on existing cases is merged. Multiple primaries are noted with a multiple sequence number. Each case is given a unique identification number.

The demographic diversity of the San Francisco Bay Area makes the registry data, representing over 20 years of information on over 400 000 cancer cases, especially useful for descriptive and analytic epidemiology research, cancer control studies and health care planning. In addition, studies of costs of care, treatment patterns, survival factors, and accuracy in classification of racial and ethnic groups have been completed. The registry is a resource for researchers, public health workers, the news media and hospitals. Confidential data on patients are released only to qualified investigators after a request for data is approved for scientific merit, human subject concerns (including protection of confidentiality), and for compatibility with the State cancer reporting law. Data for such studies are released only for the specific study, and names are never used in reports.

Dee W. West
Sally L. Glaser
Lilia C. O'Connor

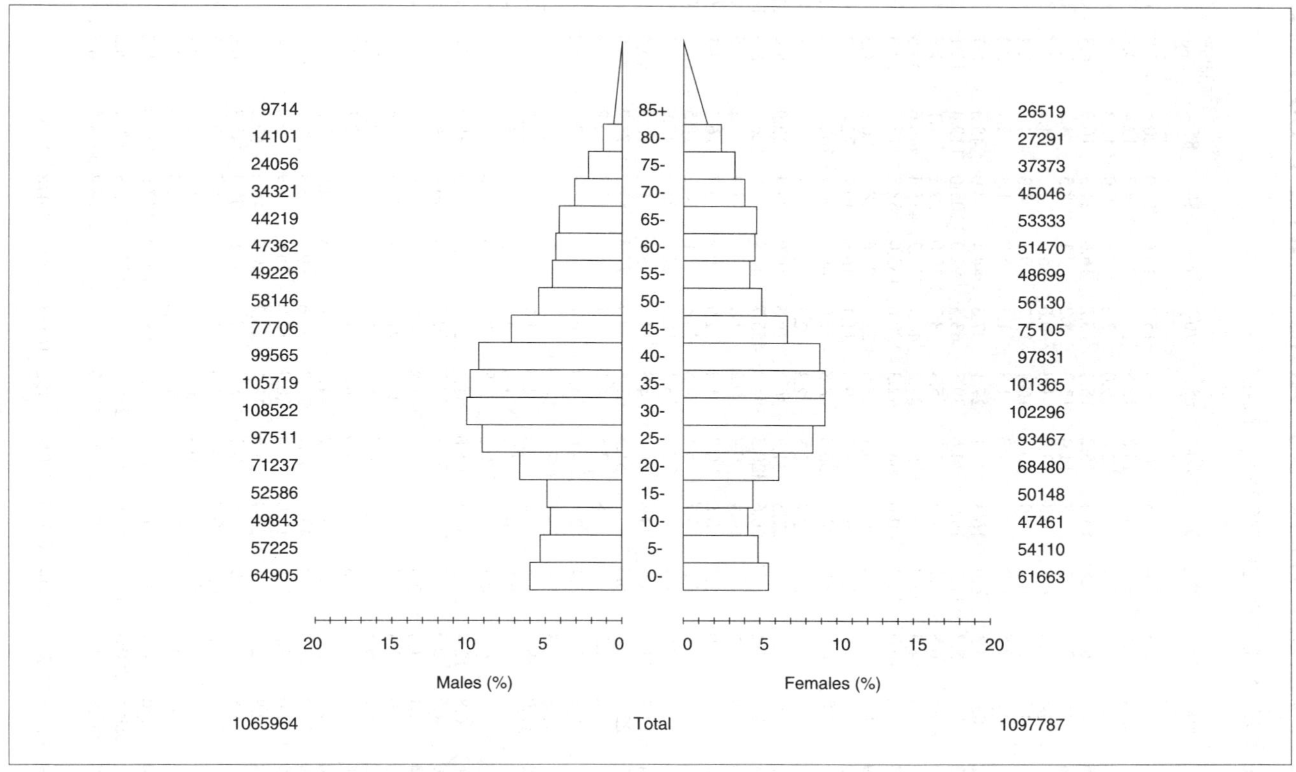

USA, California, San Francisco Bay Area: Non-Hispanic White
Source of population: average annual 1988-92
Estimate: NCI estimates based on U.S. Bureau of Census population estimates by county for the years 1988–92.

Notes to tables overleaf:
† 173 does not include basal cell or squamous cell carcinoma

USA, CALIFORNIA, SAN FRANCISCO BAY AREA: NON-HISPANIC WHITE 1988-1992

ANNUAL INCIDENCE PER 100,000 BY AGE GROUP (YEARS) - MALE

SITE	ALL AGES	AGE UNK	0-	5-	10-	15-	20-	25-	30-	35-	40-	45-	50-	55-	60-	65-	70-	75-	80-	85+	CRUDE RATE	%	CR 64	CR 74	ASR (W)	ICD (9th)
Lip	149	0	-	-	-	-	-	0.2	1.1	0.4	2.6	0.3	3.8	4.5	6.3	9.0	15.7	16.6	17.0	20.6	2.8	0.5	0.10	0.22	1.8	140
Tongue	230	0	-	-	-	-	-	0.4	0.7	0.4	1.4	4.4	6.2	13.4	14.8	18.5	18.1	20.0	14.2	12.4	4.3	0.7	0.21	0.39	3.1	141
Salivary gland	96	0	-	-	-	-	0.3	0.4	-	0.4	1.4	2.1	2.4	1.6	3.8	9.0	7.6	9.1	9.9	10.3	1.8	0.3	0.06	0.14	1.2	142
Mouth	231	0	-	-	-	-	-	0.2	0.7	0.6	2.0	6.4	4.8	15.4	15.2	15.4	15.2	16.6	21.3	10.3	4.3	0.7	0.23	0.38	3.2	143-5
Oropharynx	144	0	-	-	-	-	-	0.2	0.2	0.9	1.0	2.8	4.1	9.8	11.4	11.3	8.2	9.1	8.5	4.1	2.7	0.4	0.15	0.25	2.0	146
Nasopharynx	38	0	-	-	0.8	0.8	0.6	0.4	0.2	-	0.4	1.0	0.3	0.8	3.0	1.8	0.6	5.0	-	4.1	0.7	0.1	0.04	0.05	0.6	147
Hypopharynx	126	0	-	-	-	-	-	-	-	-	0.2	1.3	4.1	6.9	10.6	10.4	15.7	9.1	4.3	4.1	2.4	0.4	0.12	0.25	1.8	148
Pharynx unspecified	22	0	-	-	-	-	-	-	-	-	0.2	0.5	0.3	-	1.3	1.8	1.7	5.0	1.4	2.1	0.4	0.1	0.01	0.03	0.3	149
Oesophagus	358	0	-	-	-	-	-	-	0.2	0.2	0.6	3.3	6.9	16.3	21.1	27.1	37.3	44.1	44.0	45.3	6.7	1.1	0.24	0.56	4.5	150
Stomach	647	0	-	-	-	-	-	0.2	0.6	1.3	1.8	5.7	11.7	19.9	34.6	39.8	63.5	92.3	105.0	119.4	12.1	2.0	0.38	0.90	7.9	151
Small intestine	83	0	-	-	-	-	-	0.2	0.6	0.4	0.6	0.8	2.1	1.6	6.3	5.4	8.7	10.0	7.1	4.1	1.6	0.3	0.06	0.13	1.1	152
Colon	2374	0	-	-	-	-	0.3	1.0	3.1	2.8	6.8	14.9	32.0	66.6	116.1	173.2	240.1	329.2	435.4	440.6	44.5	7.3	1.22	3.29	28.3	153
Rectum	1187	0	-	-	-	-	-	1.2	2.8	3.4	6.2	16.0	18.9	40.6	68.0	92.3	120.6	133.0	158.8	115.3	22.3	3.7	0.79	1.85	15.0	154
Liver	230	0	0.3	-	-	0.8	-	-	0.2	0.9	1.6	1.5	4.8	9.3	13.1	18.5	22.7	21.6	28.4	26.8	4.3	0.7	0.16	0.37	3.0	155
Gallbladder etc.	117	0	-	-	-	-	-	-	-	0.2	0.4	-	2.1	6.1	3.8	9.0	11.1	16.6	19.9	22.6	2.2	0.4	0.06	0.16	1.4	156
Pancreas	655	0	-	-	-	-	-	-	0.7	0.6	2.8	6.9	7.9	20.3	36.3	48.8	67.0	86.5	100.7	102.9	12.3	2.0	0.38	0.96	8.0	157
Nose, sinuses etc.	42	0	-	0.3	-	-	0.3	-	0.2	0.2	0.2	0.3	2.1	2.4	2.5	2.3	2.3	3.3	7.1	-	0.8	0.1	0.04	0.07	0.6	160
Larynx	449	0	-	-	-	-	-	-	0.6	3.2	3.6	15.1	21.5	31.7	36.2	39.6	49.9	28.4	32.9	8.4	1.4	0.38	0.76	6.0	161
Bronchus, lung	4559	0	0.3	-	-	0.4	0.3	-	1.5	6.1	16.3	41.2	88.7	166.6	320.5	386.3	455.7	517.9	541.8	426.2	85.5	14.1	3.21	7.42	58.6	162
Other thoracic organs	26	0	0.3	-	-	0.4	0.6	1.2	-	0.4	0.4	0.5	-	0.4	0.4	0.5	1.2	2.5	1.4	2.1	0.5	0.1	0.02	0.03	0.4	163-4
Bone	57	0	0.3	0.7	1.2	1.1	-	0.4	0.6	1.1	1.6	1.0	1.7	0.8	0.8	1.4	2.9	0.8	5.7	6.2	1.1	0.2	0.06	0.08	0.9	170
Connective tissue	163	0	1.8	0.7	0.4	0.4	2.8	1.4	2.0	1.3	3.0	2.3	2.8	3.7	5.1	4.5	13.4	10.8	14.2	18.5	3.1	0.5	0.14	0.23	2.4	171
Mesothelioma	163	0	-	-	-	-	0.3	-	-	-	-	0.5	1.4	4.9	8.0	13.1	18.6	24.9	25.5	32.9	3.1	0.5	0.08	0.23	1.9	MES
Kaposi's sarcoma	2609	0	-	-	-	-	5.6	42.7	105.0	138.1	111.3	71.8	42.0	23.6	16.0	4.5	4.7	5.0	1.4	10.3	49.0	8.1	2.78	2.83	33.5	KAP
Melanoma of skin	1221	0	-	0.4	2.7	5.1	7.6	13.3	19.3	22.7	30.9	28.5	36.2	51.5	67.8	69.9	72.3	87.9	78.2	22.9	3.8	1.09	1.78	16.4	172
†Other skin	77	0	-	-	0.4	0.6	0.4	0.6	0.4	1.6	1.5	1.4	2.8	2.5	4.1	4.7	6.7	11.3	6.2	1.4		0.06	0.10	1.0	173
Breast	65	0	-	-	-	-	-	-	-	-	0.4	1.3	1.4	2.4	4.6	5.9	6.4	3.3	11.3	2.1	1.2	0.2	0.05	0.11	0.9	175
Prostate	8194	0	-	-	-	-	-	-	0.2	-	2.8	10.3	51.9	136.1	397.8	758.5	1138.6	1274.5	1354.5	1218.8	153.7	25.3	3.00	12.48	95.9	185
Testis	462	0	-	-	0.4	4.6	10.7	17.6	20.5	17.2	11.0	8.5	4.5	2.4	2.5	1.8	1.7	1.7	-	2.1	8.7	1.4	0.50	0.52	6.7	186
Penis	29	0	-	-	-	-	-	-	-	-	-	-	0.7	0.8	1.7	1.8	4.1	2.5	5.7	6.2	0.5	0.1	0.02	0.05	0.4	187.1-.4
Other male genital	20	0	-	-	0.4	-	-	-	0.2	0.2	-	0.3	0.7	0.4	0.8	1.8	0.6	3.3	2.8	-	0.4	0.1	0.01	0.03	0.3	187.5-.9
Bladder	2002	0	-	-	0.4	0.4	0.8	0.8	1.8	3.6	6.8	12.4	34.1	57.3	105.6	151.1	222.0	271.0	299.3	288.2	37.6	6.2	1.12	2.99	24.5	188
Kidney etc.	767	0	2.2	1.0	-	-	-	1.2	0.4	3.0	4.6	10.6	17.2	28.8	34.2	59.7	73.4	87.3	96.4	74.1	14.4	2.4	0.52	1.18	9.9	189
Eye	54	0	0.9	-	0.4	-	-	0.2	0.4	0.4	0.4	1.3	2.4	1.6	3.4	1.8	4.7	5.0	1.4	-	1.0	0.2	0.06	0.09	0.8	190
Brain, nervous system	499	0	3.7	2.1	3.2	1.9	4.5	4.9	4.4	7.0	8.0	11.8	13.4	16.3	19.8	23.5	21.6	29.1	28.4	22.6	9.4	1.5	0.51	0.73	7.5	191-2
Thyroid	175	0	-	-	-	0.8	0.8	2.3	4.2	4.2	3.2	3.6	4.8	3.7	9.7	8.6	5.8	4.2	4.3	2.1	3.3	0.5	0.19	0.26	2.5	193
Other endocrine	30	0	2.2	0.3	-	0.8	0.6	-	0.2	0.8	0.4	0.5	0.3	-	1.3	0.9	1.2	-	-	2.1	0.6	0.1	0.04	0.05	0.6	194
Hodgkin's disease	262	0	-	0.7	4.4	4.6	8.4	8.6	5.0	7.0	4.0	3.9	3.4	4.5	4.2	4.1	5.8	8.3	2.8	8.2	4.9	0.8	0.29	0.34	4.3	201
Non-Hodgkin lymphoma	1906	0	0.3	1.7	0.4	1.9	5.9	11.9	29.3	46.9	45.0	47.9	44.7	43.1	61.7	73.3	99.6	99.8	133.3	142.1	35.8	5.9	1.70	2.57	25.0	200,202
Multiple myeloma	320	0	-	-	-	-	0.3	-	0.4	0.9	2.0	2.3	7.2	10.6	17.3	20.4	32.6	46.6	36.9	45.3	6.0	1.0	0.21	0.47	4.0	203
Lymphoid leukaemia	349	0	8.0	4.2	1.6	1.9	1.4	0.4	0.4	0.8	2.8	2.3	5.8	8.9	11.8	18.1	26.2	39.9	46.8	67.9	6.5	1.1	0.25	0.47	5.4	204
Myeloid leukaemia	352	0	0.9	0.3	0.4	1.9	1.1	1.8	3.1	2.3	3.8	4.1	6.9	8.5	9.7	15.8	32.0	41.6	55.3	45.3	6.6	1.1	0.23	0.46	4.5	205
Monocytic leukaemia	24	0	-	-	-	0.4	-	0.2	-	-	-	1.0	0.3	0.8	-	1.8	1.7	2.5	5.7	2.1	0.5	0.1	0.01	0.03	0.3	206
Other leukaemia	5	0	-	-	-	-	-	-	-	-	-	-	0.3	-	0.4	0.5	-	-	1.4	2.1	0.1	0.0	0.00	0.01	0.1	207
Leukaemia unspecified	42	0	0.3	0.3	-	-	0.3	-	0.4	-	-	0.3	-	1.6	0.4	1.4	5.2	4.2	11.3	12.4	0.8	0.1	0.02	0.05	0.5	208
Other and unspecified	808	0	0.6	-	0.4	0.4	-	0.2	0.7	3.0	3.6	6.4	14.4	27.6	38.8	53.8	68.8	107.2	127.6	168.8	15.2	2.5	0.48	1.09	9.9	O&U
All sites	32418	0	22.2	12.6	14.8	26.2	51.4	108.5	205.7	277.1	289.5	350.3	510.8	851.6	1530.7	2216.7	3019.1	3550.0	3925.8	3670.7	608.2		21.26	47.44	409.0	ALL
All sites but 173	32341	0	22.2	12.6	14.8	25.9	50.8	108.1	205.1	276.8	287.9	348.7	509.4	848.7	1528.2	2212.6	3014.4	3543.3	3914.4	3664.5	606.8	100.0	21.20	47.33	407.9	ALLb

| Rate from 1 case | | | 0.308 | 0.349 | 0.401 | 0.380 | 0.281 | 0.205 | 0.184 | 0.189 | 0.201 | 0.257 | 0.344 | 0.406 | 0.422 | 0.452 | 0.583 | 0.831 | 1.418 | 2.059 |

†Important: see notes on population page

USA, CALIFORNIA, SAN FRANCISCO BAY AREA: NON-HISPANIC WHITE 1988-1992

ANNUAL INCIDENCE PER 100,000 BY AGE GROUP (YEARS) - FEMALE

SITE	ALL AGES	AGE UNK	0-	5-	10-	15-	20-	25-	30-	35-	40-	45-	50-	55-	60-	65-	70-	75-	80-	85+	CRUDE RATE	%	CR 64	CR 74	ASR (W)	ICD (9th)
Lip	36	0	-	-	-	-	-	-	-	-	-	0.5	-	0.8	0.8	3.7	2.7	1.1	5.9	3.0	0.7	0.1	0.01	0.04	**0.3**	140
Tongue	154	0	-	-	-	-	0.6	0.2	0.2	0.6	0.8	1.3	3.2	8.2	6.2	9.4	12.0	9.6	5.1	12.1	2.8	0.5	0.11	0.21	**1.7**	141
Salivary gland	59	0	-	-	0.4	-	-	0.2	0.8	0.6	0.8	1.1	0.7	1.2	1.6	3.4	3.6	4.8	4.4	0.8	1.1	0.2	0.04	0.07	**0.6**	142
Mouth	210	0	-	-	-	0.4	0.3	-	0.2	0.6	0.6	2.4	4.6	6.2	8.2	12.4	17.8	17.7	15.4	12.1	3.8	0.7	0.12	0.27	**2.1**	143-5
Oropharynx	85	0	-	-	-	-	-	-	0.2	0.2	0.2	0.5	2.9	2.9	5.1	5.6	8.9	5.4	3.7	1.5	1.5	0.3	0.06	0.13	**1.0**	146
Nasopharynx	17	0	-	-	-	-	-	-	-	0.2	-	0.5	1.4	0.4	0.8	0.4	0.9	1.1	-	1.5	0.3	0.1	0.02	0.02	**0.2**	147
Hypopharynx	48	0	-	-	-	-	-	-	-	-	-	0.3	0.7	3.7	1.9	3.0	4.4	3.7	3.7	0.8	0.9	0.2	0.03	0.07	**0.5**	148
Pharynx unspecified	19	0	-	-	-	-	-	-	-	-	-	0.5	-	1.2	0.4	1.5	2.2	1.1	1.5	-	0.3	0.1	0.01	0.03	**0.2**	149
Oesophagus	169	0	-	-	-	-	-	-	-	-	0.2	0.5	2.9	4.5	5.1	10.9	13.8	18.2	11.7	18.1	3.1	0.6	0.07	0.19	**1.5**	150
Stomach	372	0	-	-	-	-	-	-	0.2	0.4	1.8	2.1	4.3	7.4	8.5	17.6	25.8	30.5	45.4	57.3	6.8	1.3	0.12	0.34	**3.0**	151
Small intestine	61	0	-	-	-	-	-	-	-	0.2	0.2	0.3	1.8	2.1	1.6	4.5	5.8	3.2	5.1	4.5	1.1	0.2	0.03	0.08	**0.6**	152
Colon	2576	0	-	-	-	-	0.3	0.2	1.2	3.0	5.9	11.2	26.7	45.6	82.0	110.6	186.0	252.6	326.8	341.6	46.9	8.9	0.88	2.36	**20.7**	153
Rectum	999	0	-	-	-	0.4	-	0.4	1.2	1.6	5.1	8.5	13.2	26.3	35.7	48.0	65.7	104.9	98.2	95.0	18.2	3.4	0.46	1.03	**9.0**	154
Liver	122	0	0.6	0.4	-	-	-	0.4	-	0.6	0.8	0.8	2.1	2.9	4.3	5.6	8.9	7.0	15.4	10.6	2.2	0.4	0.06	0.14	**1.2**	155
Gallbladder etc.	162	0	-	-	-	-	-	-	-	0.4	0.4	1.6	1.1	4.1	3.5	3.7	15.1	16.1	18.3	23.4	3.0	0.6	0.06	0.15	**1.3**	156
Pancreas	730	0	-	-	-	-	-	-	0.4	0.2	1.8	4.8	6.8	18.5	25.6	34.1	49.7	76.0	79.9	87.5	13.3	2.5	0.29	0.71	**6.2**	157
Nose, sinuses etc.	28	0	-	-	-	-	-	-	-	0.6	-	-	0.4	0.4	0.8	1.9	1.3	2.7	1.5	4.5	0.5	0.1	0.01	0.03	**0.2**	160
Larynx	127	0	-	-	-	-	-	-	-	0.2	0.6	1.3	1.8	7.4	8.2	8.2	10.7	6.4	7.3	4.5	2.3	0.4	0.10	0.19	**1.4**	161
Bronchus, lung	3906	0	-	-	-	0.4	-	0.2	2.3	5.5	12.1	33.0	79.8	131.8	203.6	262.5	323.2	344.1	243.3	157.6	71.2	13.5	2.34	5.27	**40.4**	162
Other thoracic organs	8	0	-	-	-	-	-	-	-	0.4	-	-	-	-	0.4	0.4	0.4	-	1.5	0.8	0.1	0.0	0.00	0.01	**0.1**	163-4
Bone	41	0	0.3	0.4	0.8	1.2	0.9	0.4	0.4	0.8	0.4	0.3	0.7	0.4	1.6	0.4	2.7	2.1	0.7	0.8	0.7	0.1	0.04	0.06	**0.7**	170
Connective tissue	132	0	1.3	-	-	0.4	1.8	1.1	0.8	1.2	1.6	1.3	2.1	3.7	5.4	4.1	6.7	7.0	6.6	12.1	2.4	0.5	0.10	0.16	**1.6**	171
Mesothelioma	27	0	-	-	-	-	-	-	0.2	-	0.4	-	1.1	0.4	1.6	1.9	0.4	2.1	2.2	2.3	0.5	0.1	0.02	0.03	**0.3**	MES
Kaposi's sarcoma	18	0	-	-	-	-	-	0.2	-	0.4	0.2	-	-	0.4	-	-	0.4	1.1	5.1	2.3	0.3	0.1	0.01	0.01	**0.1**	KAP
Melanoma of skin	940	0	-	-	-	2.0	5.5	12.8	16.6	15.0	23.3	24.5	23.2	22.6	32.6	28.9	28.4	32.1	34.4	27.9	17.1	3.2	0.89	1.18	**11.9**	172
†Other skin	77	0	-	-	-	0.4	0.9	1.3	0.8	0.8	0.8	1.1	1.1	1.2	2.3	1.1	4.0	8.0	2.9	6.0	1.4		0.05	0.08	**0.9**	173
Breast	9080	0	-	-	0.4	-	1.5	5.3	21.1	68.9	137.4	222.4	268.7	330.2	393.6	477.7	470.2	494.5	503.5	429.9	165.4	31.3	7.25	11.99	**103.3**	174
Uterus unspecified	23	0	-	-	-	-	-	-	-	-	0.4	0.3	-	-	-	0.4	1.3	1.6	2.9	6.8	0.4	0.1	0.00	0.01	**0.1**	179
Cervix uteri	502	0	-	-	-	-	0.6	5.8	11.1	10.3	14.1	12.5	11.8	9.4	20.2	20.2	9.8	13.4	12.5	16.6	9.1	1.7	0.48	0.63	**6.2**	180
Placenta	8	0	-	-	0.4	0.8	-	0.6	0.2	0.2	-	-	-	-	-	-	-	-	-	-	0.1	0.0	0.01	0.01	**0.2**	181
Corpus uteri	1760	0	-	-	-	-	-	0.6	0.8	3.9	8.4	18.4	41.0	64.1	97.5	121.5	126.5	128.4	120.9	65.6	32.1	6.1	1.17	2.41	**18.8**	182
Ovary etc.	1164	0	-	-	-	2.8	1.2	3.6	2.9	7.7	10.6	19.7	29.9	48.0	55.2	56.6	69.3	70.6	71.1	58.1	21.2	4.0	0.91	1.54	**13.2**	183
Other female genital	188	0	0.3	-	-	-	0.6	0.2	0.4	1.0	3.1	2.9	1.8	3.3	6.6	9.7	11.1	14.4	15.4	16.6	3.4	0.6	0.10	0.21	**1.8**	184
Bladder	748	0	-	-	-	0.4	0.3	0.2	0.8	1.8	2.2	4.8	7.5	20.5	25.3	39.7	45.3	71.2	77.7	90.5	13.6	2.6	0.32	0.74	**6.5**	188
Kidney etc.	457	0	1.3	0.4	0.4	-	0.3	0.2	0.6	1.4	4.1	5.9	7.8	13.6	16.7	22.9	31.5	41.7	34.4	31.7	8.3	1.6	0.26	0.54	**4.7**	189
Eye	58	0	1.3	-	-	-	-	0.9	0.2	0.4	0.2	1.1	0.7	1.6	2.7	1.9	3.6	5.4	2.2	2.3	1.1	0.2	0.05	0.07	**0.7**	190
Brain, nervous system	400	0	3.2	2.6	2.9	1.2	4.7	4.1	3.1	4.7	5.5	5.3	7.8	12.3	13.6	18.7	20.0	17.7	18.3	8.3	7.3	1.4	0.36	0.55	**5.5**	191-2
Thyroid	470	0	-	-	1.7	4.0	12.3	9.4	9.2	15.2	13.9	10.7	8.6	6.6	11.3	6.4	10.2	8.0	6.6	3.8	8.6	1.6	0.51	0.60	**6.8**	193
Other endocrine	25	0	1.3	0.4	-	-	-	0.4	0.2	-	-	0.3	0.7	1.6	0.4	0.7	0.9	1.6	0.7	0.8	0.5	0.1	0.03	0.03	**0.4**	194
Hodgkin's disease	184	0	-	-	0.8	4.8	13.4	5.8	4.3	2.8	2.2	1.9	1.1	2.1	2.3	3.4	2.2	2.1	3.7	4.5	3.4	0.6	0.21	0.24	**3.2**	201
Non-Hodgkin lymphoma	1005	0	1.0	0.4	0.4	1.6	3.2	3.0	2.5	6.5	6.5	10.1	18.5	22.2	35.7	49.5	61.3	86.2	90.9	76.9	18.3	3.5	0.56	1.11	**10.0**	200,202
Multiple myeloma	269	0	-	-	-	-	-	-	-	0.2	0.8	2.9	3.9	4.5	10.1	16.1	15.5	25.7	33.0	25.6	4.9	0.9	0.11	0.27	**2.4**	203
Lymphoid leukaemia	228	0	6.2	3.0	0.4	0.8	0.3	0.2	-	0.4	1.2	1.3	2.9	4.5	4.3	8.6	13.3	16.1	23.5	28.7	4.2	0.8	0.13	0.24	**2.8**	204
Myeloid leukaemia	265	0	1.6	0.4	-	1.2	0.6	1.1	2.0	1.8	2.0	3.5	5.7	2.5	5.4	10.5	10.2	25.2	30.0	24.1	4.8	0.9	0.14	0.24	**2.7**	205
Monocytic leukaemia	11	0	-	0.4	-	-	-	-	0.3	-	-	-	0.4	-	-	0.4	1.6	1.5	0.8	-	0.2	0.0	0.01	0.01	**0.1**	206
Other leukaemia	9	0	0.3	-	-	-	-	-	-	0.2	-	0.4	0.4	0.4	-	0.4	0.5	-	1.5	-	0.2	0.0	0.01	0.01	**0.1**	207
Leukaemia unspecified	42	0	-	-	-	-	0.2	0.4	-	0.4	-	-	0.4	0.4	1.6	1.1	2.2	3.7	5.1	6.8	0.8	0.1	0.02	0.03	**0.3**	208
Other and unspecified	1026	0	1.0	-	-	-	0.3	0.2	0.8	1.2	3.3	5.9	11.0	23.0	36.5	45.7	65.7	84.6	123.8	147.1	18.7	3.5	0.42	0.97	**8.6**	O&U
All sites	29045	0	19.8	8.1	8.8	22.7	49.6	59.5	86.0	161.6	275.0	428.5	612.5	875.6	1187.1	1495.5	1772.4	2072.6	2123.7	1935.2	529.2		18.97	35.31	**306.3**	ALL
All sites but 173	28968	0	19.8	8.1	8.8	22.3	48.8	58.2	85.2	160.8	274.1	427.4	611.4	874.3	1184.8	1494.4	1768.4	2064.6	2120.8	1929.2	527.7	100.0	18.92	35.23	**305.4**	ALLb
Rate from 1 case			0.324	0.370	0.421	0.399	0.292	0.214	0.196	0.197	0.204	0.266	0.356	0.411	0.389	0.375	0.444	0.535	0.733	0.754						

†Important: see notes on population page

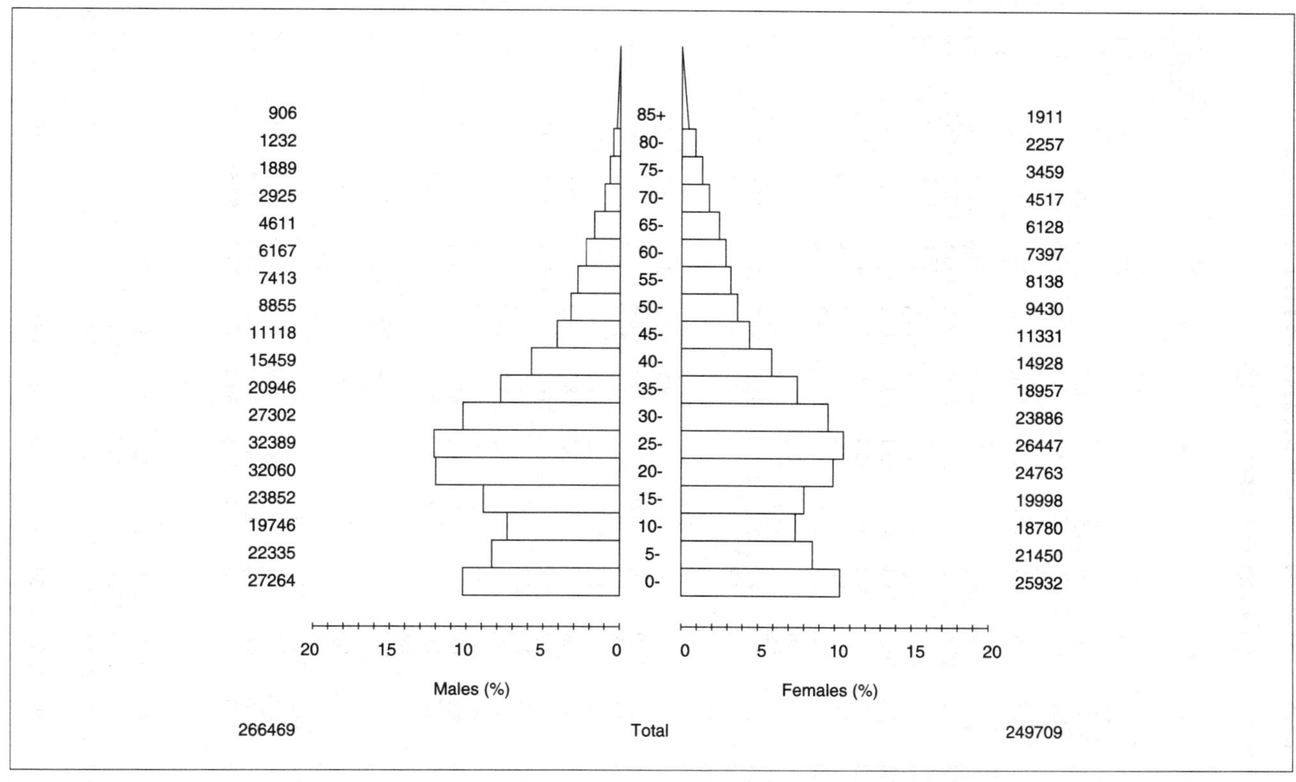

USA, California, San Francisco Bay Area: Hispanic White
Source of population: average annual 1988–92
Estimate: The years 1988-89 and 1991-92 are bench-marked to the 1990 census, making allowance for births, deaths, and migration into and out of the registration area. Sex-specific totals were apportioned to specific Asian populations based on a 5% sample of the census. The resulting race- and sex-specific population estimates were then apportioned to 5-year age categories based on the race- and sex-specific age distribution in the 100% census counts.

Notes to tables overleaf:
† 173 does not include basal cell or squamous cell carcinoma

USA, CALIFORNIA, SAN FRANCISCO BAY AREA: HISPANIC WHITE 1988-1992

ANNUAL INCIDENCE PER 100,000 BY AGE GROUP (YEARS) - MALE

SITE	ALL AGES	AGE UNK	0-	5-	10-	15-	20-	25-	30-	35-	40-	45-	50-	55-	60-	65-	70-	75-	80-	85+	CRUDE RATE	%	CR 64	CR 74	ASR (W)	ICD (9th)
Lip	4	0	-	-	-	-	-	-	-	-	-	1.8	2.3	-	-	4.3	-	10.6	-	-	0.3	0.1	0.02	0.04	**0.5**	140
Tongue	18	0	-	-	-	-	-	-	0.7	-	-	5.4	4.5	8.1	9.7	8.7	13.7	21.2	-	-	1.4	0.6	0.14	0.25	**2.1**	141
Salivary gland	8	0	-	-	-	-	-	-	-	-	1.3	-	2.7	9.7	-	13.7	-	-	-	22.1	0.6	0.3	0.07	0.14	**1.0**	142
Mouth	15	0	-	-	-	-	-	-	-	-	-	3.6	4.5	5.4	-	8.7	6.8	31.8	16.2	44.2	1.1	0.5	0.07	0.15	**1.7**	143-5
Oropharynx	15	0	-	-	-	-	-	-	-	-	2.6	3.6	4.5	2.7	13.0	4.3	-	31.8	-	-	1.1	0.5	0.13	0.15	**1.7**	146
Nasopharynx	4	0	-	-	-	-	0.6	-	-	-	-	-	2.3	-	-	4.3	-	-	-	22.1	0.3	0.1	0.01	0.04	**0.4**	147
Hypopharynx	16	0	-	-	-	-	-	-	-	-	1.3	1.8	4.5	10.8	6.5	13.0	-	31.8	-	-	1.2	0.6	0.12	0.19	**1.8**	148
Pharynx unspecified	2	0	-	-	-	-	-	-	-	-	-	-	-	-	3.2	-	-	10.6	-	-	0.2	0.1	0.02	0.02	**0.2**	149
Oesophagus	30	0	-	-	-	-	-	-	0.7	-	1.3	3.6	4.5	2.7	9.7	21.7	54.7	10.6	48.7	66.2	2.3	1.1	0.11	0.49	**3.5**	150
Stomach	114	0	-	-	-	-	1.2	-	1.5	3.8	5.2	14.4	20.3	27.0	32.4	82.4	116.2	158.8	178.5	66.2	8.6	4.0	0.53	1.52	**12.6**	151
Small intestine	7	0	-	-	-	-	-	-	-	-	-	-	-	8.1	6.5	-	-	10.6	16.2	-	0.5	0.2	0.07	0.07	**0.8**	152
Colon	189	0	-	-	-	0.8	-	-	0.7	3.8	3.9	14.4	22.6	67.4	38.9	134.5	239.3	243.5	340.8	331.1	14.2	6.6	0.76	2.63	**21.4**	153
Rectum	123	0	-	-	-	-	-	-	0.7	4.8	7.8	10.8	15.8	48.6	55.1	82.4	75.2	211.7	178.5	44.2	9.2	4.3	0.72	1.51	**13.6**	154
Liver	60	0	0.7	-	-	-	0.6	-	-	1.0	7.8	5.4	9.0	29.7	45.4	26.0	20.5	42.3	32.5	88.3	4.5	2.1	0.50	0.73	**6.7**	155
Gallbladder etc.	18	0	-	-	-	-	-	-	-	-	-	2.6	-	4.5	5.4	3.2	4.3	13.7	31.8	64.9	22.1	1.4	0.6	0.08	0.17	**1.9**	156
Pancreas	57	0	-	-	-	-	-	-	-	-	1.0	-	7.2	11.3	13.5	16.2	21.7	34.2	201.1	97.4	44.2	4.3	2.0	0.25	0.53	**6.3**	157
Nose, sinuses etc.	5	0	-	-	-	-	-	-	-	-	-	3.6	-	-	6.5	-	-	-	16.2	-	0.4	0.2	0.05	0.05	**0.6**	160
Larynx	30	0	-	-	-	-	0.6	-	-	-	-	7.2	4.5	13.5	22.7	17.3	27.3	10.6	32.5	-	2.3	1.1	0.24	0.47	**3.5**	161
Bronchus, lung	323	1	-	-	-	-	-	1.2	0.7	4.8	7.8	27.0	49.7	75.5	152.4	225.5	389.7	434.0	535.5	287.0	24.2	11.3	1.60	4.69	**37.2**	162
Other thoracic organs	5	0	-	-	2.0	0.8	-	0.6	-	-	-	-	2.3	-	-	-	-	-	-	-	0.4	0.2	0.03	0.03	**0.4**	163-4
Bone	12	0	-	0.9	2.0	0.8	1.2	1.2	-	1.0	1.3	-	-	-	6.5	-	-	-	-	-	0.9	0.4	0.07	0.07	**0.9**	170
Connective tissue	26	0	1.5	-	1.0	-	1.9	-	1.5	2.9	-	3.6	11.3	2.7	9.7	4.3	6.8	21.2	-	-	2.0	0.9	0.18	0.24	**2.4**	171
Mesothelioma	18	0	-	-	-	-	-	-	0.7	1.0	-	-	-	5.4	3.2	8.7	41.0	31.8	16.2	22.1	1.4	0.6	0.05	0.30	**2.0**	MES
Kaposi's sarcoma	314	0	-	-	-	1.7	5.0	22.2	60.1	92.6	56.9	54.0	13.6	10.8	6.5	-	6.8	-	-	44.2	23.6	11.0	1.62	1.65	**19.9**	KAP
Melanoma of skin	30	0	-	-	-	0.8	-	-	0.7	2.9	7.8	1.8	11.3	5.4	9.7	21.7	13.7	10.6	-	-	2.3	1.1	0.20	0.38	**3.1**	172
†Other skin	5	0	-	-	-	-	1.2	-	1.0	-	-	-	2.3	-	3.2	-	-	-	-	-	0.4		0.04	0.04	**0.4**	173
Breast	7	0	-	-	-	-	-	-	-	-	-	1.8	-	-	3.2	8.7	6.8	-	32.5	-	0.5	0.2	0.03	0.10	**0.8**	175
Prostate	578	2	-	-	-	-	-	-	-	-	1.3	7.2	24.8	91.7	246.4	516.2	861.4	1058.6	1038.6	905.1	43.4	20.3	1.86	8.78	**68.5**	185
Testis	62	0	0.7	-	-	2.5	9.4	6.8	13.2	5.7	3.9	3.6	2.3	2.7	-	-	6.8	-	-	-	4.7	2.2	0.25	0.29	**3.5**	186
Penis	8	0	-	-	-	-	-	-	0.7	1.0	-	-	-	-	3.2	4.3	13.7	-	16.2	22.1	0.6	0.3	0.02	0.11	**0.8**	187.1-.4
Other male genital	2	0	-	-	-	-	-	-	-	-	-	-	-	-	-	6.8	10.6	-	-	-	0.2	0.1	0.00	0.03	**0.2**	187.5-.9
Bladder	92	0	-	-	-	-	-	0.6	-	1.0	3.9	1.8	9.0	13.5	48.6	65.1	88.9	158.8	194.7	154.5	6.9	3.2	0.39	1.16	**10.4**	188
Kidney etc.	91	0	2.2	-	-	-	-	-	-	1.9	6.5	12.6	18.1	32.4	51.9	69.4	61.5	74.1	32.5	88.3	6.8	3.2	0.63	1.28	**10.5**	189
Eye	5	0	1.5	-	-	0.8	-	-	-	-	-	1.8	-	-	3.2	-	-	-	-	-	0.4	0.2	0.04	0.04	**0.5**	190
Brain, nervous system	74	0	2.2	4.5	3.0	2.5	1.2	1.9	5.9	2.9	3.9	9.0	13.6	13.5	16.2	17.3	68.4	21.2	32.5	44.2	5.6	2.6	0.40	0.83	**7.1**	191-2
Thyroid	32	0	-	-	-	1.7	1.9	2.5	1.5	2.9	2.6	5.4	2.3	10.8	3.2	8.7	6.8	31.8	-	22.1	2.4	1.1	0.17	0.25	**2.7**	193
Other endocrine	7	0	0.7	-	1.0	-	1.2	0.6	-	-	-	1.8	-	2.7	-	-	-	-	-	-	0.5	0.2	0.04	0.04	**0.5**	194
Hodgkin's disease	30	0	-	1.8	1.0	3.4	3.1	4.3	2.9	1.9	-	1.8	-	-	3.2	4.3	6.8	10.6	-	-	2.3	1.1	0.12	0.17	**2.1**	201
Non-Hodgkin lymphoma	232	0	1.5	1.8	2.0	2.5	3.1	10.5	13.2	34.4	37.5	25.2	29.4	48.6	45.4	86.7	95.7	127.0	64.9	198.7	17.4	8.1	1.27	2.19	**20.8**	200,202
Multiple myeloma	37	0	-	-	-	-	-	0.6	-	1.0	1.3	1.8	2.3	8.1	32.4	26.0	27.3	42.3	32.5	66.2	2.8	1.3	0.24	0.50	**4.3**	203
Lymphoid leukaemia	39	0	7.3	3.6	4.1	2.5	1.2	0.6	0.7	-	2.6	3.6	2.3	2.7	6.5	4.3	13.7	21.2	16.2	-	2.9	1.4	0.19	0.28	**3.6**	204
Myeloid leukaemia	40	0	-	0.9	1.0	0.8	2.5	-	1.5	1.9	1.3	3.6	9.0	5.4	19.5	30.4	13.7	21.2	32.5	22.1	3.0	1.4	0.24	0.46	**4.1**	205
Monocytic leukaemia	0	0	-	-	-	-	-	-	-	-	-	-	-	-	-	-	-	-	-	-	0.0	0.0	0.00	0.00	**0.0**	206
Other leukaemia	0	0	-	-	-	-	-	-	-	-	-	-	-	-	-	-	-	-	-	-	0.0	0.0	0.00	0.00	**0.0**	207
Leukaemia unspecified	5	0	-	-	-	-	-	-	-	-	-	-	-	2.7	-	-	6.8	-	48.7	-	0.4	0.2	0.01	0.05	**0.5**	208
Other and unspecified	70	0	-	-	-	-	1.2	-	2.2	1.9	3.9	10.8	13.6	10.8	42.2	34.7	47.9	74.1	64.9	110.4	5.3	2.5	0.43	0.85	**7.6**	O&U
All sites	2859	3	18.3	13.4	17.2	21.8	36.2	55.0	109.9	176.6	175.9	260.8	332.0	590.8	995.5	1570.2	2406.5	3207.7	3180.8	2737.3	214.6		14.03	33.94	**295.0**	ALL
All sites but 173	2854	3	18.3	13.4	17.2	21.8	36.2	53.7	109.9	175.7	175.9	260.8	329.7	590.8	992.3	1570.2	2406.5	3207.7	3180.8	2737.3	214.2	100.0	13.99	33.90	**294.6**	ALLb

Rate from 1 case   0.734   0.895   1.013   0.838   0.624   0.617   0.733   0.955   1.294   1.799   2.259   2.698   3.243   4.337   6.837   10.586   16.228   22.075

†Important: see notes on population page

USA, CALIFORNIA, SAN FRANCISCO BAY AREA: HISPANIC WHITE 1988-1992

ANNUAL INCIDENCE PER 100,000 BY AGE GROUP (YEARS) - FEMALE

SITE	ALL AGES	AGE UNK	0-	5-	10-	15-	20-	25-	30-	35-	40-	45-	50-	55-	60-	65-	70-	75-	80-	85+	CRUDE RATE	%	CR 64	CR 74	ASR (W)	ICD (9th)
Lip	1	0	-	-	-	-	-	-	-	-	-	-	-	2.5	-	-	-	-	-	-	0.1	0.0	0.01	0.01	**0.1**	140
Tongue	6	0	-	-	-	-	-	-	-	-	-	1.8	4.2	4.9	-	3.3	-	-	-	-	0.5	0.2	0.05	0.07	**0.6**	141
Salivary gland	8	0	-	-	-	-	0.8	0.8	0.8	-	1.3	-	-	4.9	-	-	-	5.8	-	10.5	0.6	0.3	0.04	0.04	**0.6**	142
Mouth	13	0	-	-	-	-	-	0.8	0.8	1.1	-	-	2.1	-	8.1	3.3	8.9	11.6	8.9	-	1.0	0.5	0.06	0.12	**1.0**	143-5
Oropharynx	5	0	-	-	-	-	-	-	-	-	-	-	4.2	2.5	5.4	-	-	-	-	-	0.4	0.2	0.06	0.06	**0.5**	146
Nasopharynx	2	0	-	-	-	-	-	-	-	-	-	-	-	-	-	-	-	5.8	8.9	-	0.2	0.1	0.00	0.00	**0.1**	147
Hypopharynx	1	0	-	-	-	-	-	-	-	-	-	-	-	-	-	-	4.4	-	-	-	0.1	0.0	0.00	0.02	**0.1**	148
Pharynx unspecified	0	0	-	-	-	-	-	-	-	-	-	-	-	-	-	-	-	-	-	-	0.0	0.0	0.00	0.00	**0.0**	149
Oesophagus	6	0	-	-	-	-	-	-	-	-	-	-	-	-	5.4	-	8.9	-	17.7	-	0.5	0.2	0.03	0.07	**0.5**	150
Stomach	64	0	-	-	-	-	-	0.8	0.8	3.2	4.0	8.8	10.6	4.9	13.5	16.3	26.6	57.8	44.3	136.0	5.1	2.3	0.23	0.45	**4.8**	151
Small intestine	7	0	-	-	-	-	-	-	-	-	-	-	2.1	-	2.7	-	4.4	5.8	8.9	20.9	0.6	0.3	0.02	0.05	**0.5**	152
Colon	201	0	-	-	-	-	0.8	-	-	1.1	6.7	17.6	25.4	24.6	56.8	81.6	124.0	179.2	327.8	209.3	16.1	7.3	0.67	1.69	**15.5**	153
Rectum	85	0	-	-	-	-	-	0.8	-	2.1	1.3	3.5	14.8	17.2	37.9	35.9	66.4	40.5	106.3	62.8	6.8	3.1	0.39	0.90	**7.1**	154
Liver	31	0	-	1.9	-	-	-	-	-	-	1.3	8.8	2.1	4.9	5.4	3.3	17.7	46.3	17.7	31.4	2.5	1.1	0.12	0.23	**2.5**	155
Gallbladder etc.	22	0	-	-	-	-	-	-	-	2.1	-	-	-	4.9	8.1	9.8	8.9	34.7	26.6	10.5	1.8	0.8	0.08	0.17	**1.7**	156
Pancreas	69	0	-	-	-	-	-	-	-	1.1	2.7	5.3	6.4	7.4	16.2	49.0	26.6	52.0	88.6	115.1	5.5	2.5	0.19	0.57	**5.3**	157
Nose, sinuses etc.	7	0	-	-	-	-	-	-	-	1.1	1.3	-	-	2.7	9.8	-	-	-	8.9	-	0.6	0.3	0.03	0.07	**0.6**	160
Larynx	7	0	-	-	-	-	-	-	-	-	-	2.1	4.9	5.4	-	4.4	5.8	-	-	-	0.6	0.3	0.06	0.08	**0.7**	161
Bronchus, lung	268	0	-	-	-	-	-	-	-	4.2	6.7	19.4	38.2	66.4	94.6	163.2	203.7	185.0	239.2	136.0	21.5	9.7	1.15	2.98	**22.9**	162
Other thoracic organs	2	0	-	-	-	-	-	-	0.8	-	-	-	-	-	-	3.3	-	-	-	-	0.2	0.1	0.00	0.02	**0.1**	163-4
Bone	6	0	-	-	1.1	1.0	-	-	1.7	1.1	-	-	-	-	2.7	-	-	-	-	-	0.5	0.2	0.04	0.04	**0.5**	170
Connective tissue	18	0	2.3	-	-	1.0	-	0.8	0.8	2.1	-	1.8	2.1	4.9	5.4	3.3	-	11.6	-	10.5	1.4	0.7	0.11	0.12	**1.5**	171
Mesothelioma	5	0	-	-	-	-	-	-	-	-	-	1.8	-	2.5	2.7	6.5	-	-	-	-	0.4	0.2	0.03	0.07	**0.5**	MES
Kaposi's sarcoma	2	0	-	-	-	-	0.8	-	-	-	-	-	-	-	-	-	-	8.9	-	-	0.2	0.1	0.00	0.00	**0.1**	KAP
Melanoma of skin	60	0	-	-	2.1	1.0	4.8	4.5	5.9	3.2	12.1	5.3	6.4	12.3	5.4	19.6	17.7	11.6	-	10.5	4.8	2.2	0.31	0.50	**4.8**	172
†Other skin	7	0	-	-	-	2.0	0.8	0.8	-	-	-	-	-	-	-	3.3	-	-	-	20.9	0.6		0.02	0.03	**0.5**	173
Breast	815	0	-	-	-	-	-	10.6	27.6	42.2	87.1	153.6	195.1	216.3	256.8	290.5	349.8	370.0	380.9	272.1	65.3	29.5	4.95	8.15	**70.8**	174
Uterus unspecified	2	0	-	-	-	-	-	-	-	-	-	-	2.1	-	-	-	4.4	-	-	-	0.2	0.1	0.01	0.03	**0.2**	179
Cervix uteri	157	0	-	-	-	-	-	6.8	12.6	28.5	25.5	30.0	19.1	41.8	48.7	26.1	31.0	23.1	26.6	41.9	12.6	5.7	1.06	1.35	**12.9**	180
Placenta	2	0	-	-	-	-	-	0.8	0.8	-	-	-	-	-	-	-	-	-	-	-	0.2	0.1	0.01	0.01	**0.1**	181
Corpus uteri	153	0	-	-	-	1.0	-	1.5	4.2	6.3	12.1	19.4	25.4	46.7	48.7	91.4	93.0	63.6	53.2	41.9	12.3	5.5	0.83	1.75	**13.5**	182
Ovary etc.	109	0	-	-	1.1	2.0	1.6	0.8	2.5	2.1	10.7	24.7	17.0	31.9	46.0	45.7	53.1	52.0	8.9	20.9	8.7	3.9	0.70	1.20	**9.9**	183
Other female genital	17	0	-	-	-	-	-	-	-	1.1	-	1.8	-	4.9	8.1	3.3	4.4	11.6	26.6	31.4	1.4	0.6	0.08	0.12	**1.3**	184
Bladder	28	0	-	-	-	-	-	-	-	-	1.3	1.8	-	-	-	10.8	9.8	17.7	23.1	44.3	62.8	2.2	1.0	0.07	0.21	**2.0**	188
Kidney etc.	64	0	2.3	1.9	-	-	-	0.8	0.8	1.1	5.4	12.4	6.4	9.8	16.2	42.4	35.4	40.5	17.7	20.9	5.1	2.3	0.28	0.67	**5.6**	189
Eye	7	0	3.1	0.9	-	-	-	-	-	-	-	-	-	2.5	-	3.3	-	-	-	-	0.6	0.3	0.03	0.05	**0.7**	190
Brain, nervous system	51	0	0.8	3.7	1.1	-	4.8	2.3	5.0	2.1	2.7	-	2.1	9.8	16.2	13.1	22.1	23.1	8.9	10.5	4.1	1.8	0.25	0.43	**4.0**	191-2
Thyroid	105	0	-	-	1.1	2.0	7.3	10.6	20.9	9.5	12.1	14.1	8.5	9.8	13.5	16.3	8.9	28.9	26.6	-	8.4	3.8	0.55	0.67	**7.5**	193
Other endocrine	3	0	1.5	-	-	1.0	-	-	-	-	-	-	-	-	-	-	-	-	-	-	0.2	0.1	0.01	0.03	**0.3**	194
Hodgkin's disease	24	0	-	-	1.1	3.0	2.4	0.8	1.7	2.1	4.0	3.5	-	4.9	-	-	8.9	-	17.7	10.5	1.9	0.9	0.12	0.16	**1.8**	201
Non-Hodgkin lymphoma	126	0	1.5	-	1.1	-	0.8	-	3.3	1.1	10.7	17.6	25.4	41.8	48.7	42.4	53.1	75.2	70.9	62.8	10.1	4.6	0.76	1.24	**11.0**	200,202
Multiple myeloma	27	0	-	-	-	-	-	-	-	-	-	3.5	6.4	4.9	8.1	13.1	17.7	28.9	17.7	20.9	2.2	1.0	0.11	0.27	**2.3**	203
Lymphoid leukaemia	39	0	5.4	3.7	4.3	1.0	2.4	1.5	-	-	1.3	-	2.1	7.4	5.4	9.8	17.7	5.8	17.7	10.5	3.1	1.4	0.17	0.31	**3.4**	204
Myeloid leukaemia	46	0	0.8	0.9	-	1.0	-	2.3	1.7	1.1	2.7	7.1	6.4	9.8	24.3	16.3	17.7	11.6	17.7	20.9	3.7	1.7	0.29	0.46	**4.0**	205
Monocytic leukaemia	0	0	-	-	-	-	-	-	-	-	-	-	-	-	-	-	-	-	-	-	0.0	0.0	0.00	0.00	**0.0**	206
Other leukaemia	1	0	-	-	-	-	-	-	-	-	-	-	-	-	-	-	-	3.3	-	-	0.1	0.0	0.00	0.02	**0.1**	207
Leukaemia unspecified	3	0	-	-	-	-	0.8	-	-	-	-	-	-	-	2.7	-	4.4	-	-	-	0.2	0.1	0.02	0.04	**0.3**	208
Other and unspecified	88	0	2.3	-	-	1.0	-	-	-	4.2	1.3	10.6	2.1	17.2	29.7	26.1	48.7	69.4	106.3	115.1	7.0	3.2	0.34	0.72	**6.9**	O&U
All sites	2770	0	20.1	13.1	12.8	17.0	27.5	48.4	92.9	123.4	214.4	374.2	439.0	629.1	862.4	1063.9	1310.6	1480.0	1754.1	1517.4	221.9		14.37	26.24	**231.7**	ALL
All sites but 173	2763	0	20.1	13.1	12.8	15.0	26.7	47.6	92.9	123.4	214.4	374.2	439.0	629.1	862.4	1060.6	1310.6	1480.0	1754.1	1496.4	221.3	100.0	14.35	26.21	**231.1**	ALLb

Rate from 1 case   0.771   0.932   1.065   1.000   0.808   0.756   0.837   1.055   1.340   1.765   2.121   2.458   2.704   3.263   4.428   5.781   8.859   10.465

†Important: see notes on population page

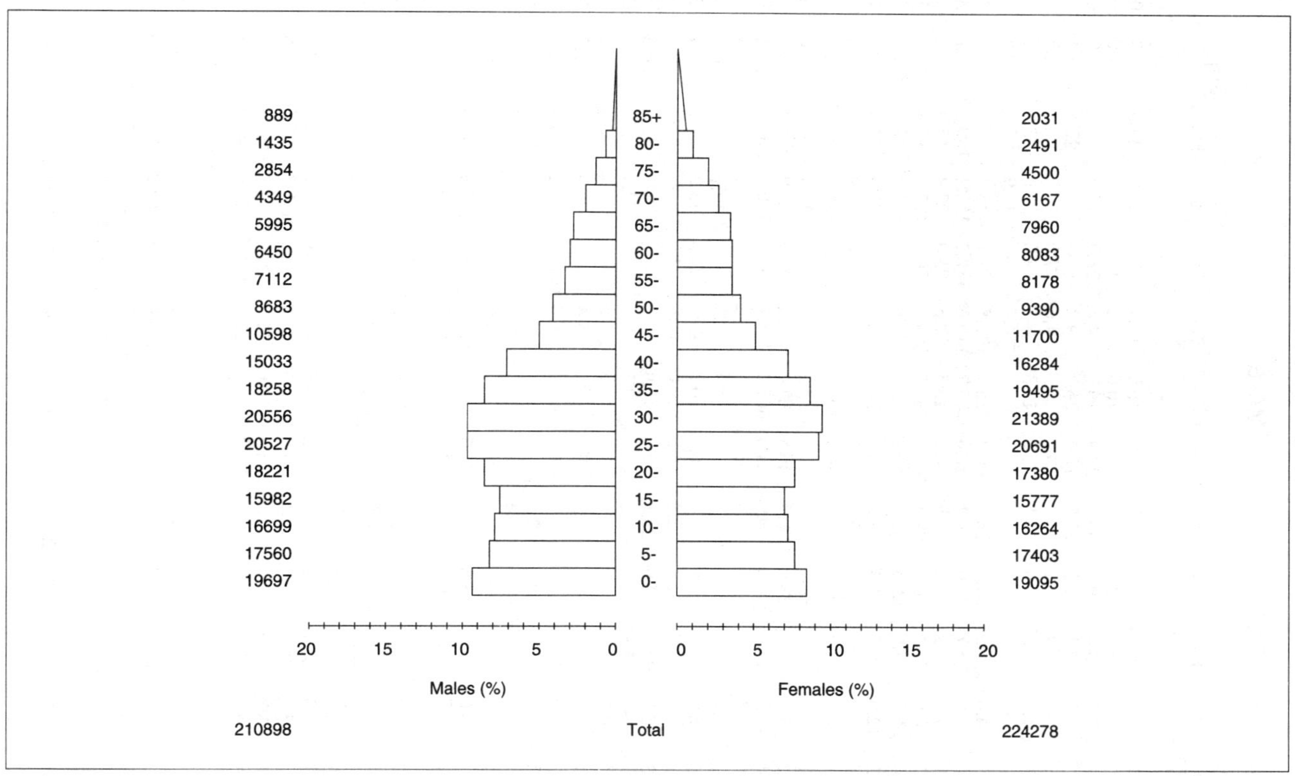

USA, California, San Francisco Bay Area: Black
Source of population: average annual 1988–92
Estimate: NCI estimates based on U.S. Bureau of Census population estimates by county for the years 1988–92.

Notes to tables overleaf:
† 173 does not include basal cell or squamous cell carcinoma

USA, CALIFORNIA, SAN FRANCISCO BAY AREA: BLACK 1988-1992

ANNUAL INCIDENCE PER 100,000 BY AGE GROUP (YEARS) - MALE

SITE	ALL AGES	AGE UNK	0-	5-	10-	15-	20-	25-	30-	35-	40-	45-	50-	55-	60-	65-	70-	75-	80-	85+	CRUDE RATE	%	CR 64	CR 74	ASR (W)	ICD (9th)
Lip	2	0	-	-	-	-	-	-	-	-	-	1.9	-	-	-	3.3	-	-	-	-	0.2	0.0	0.01	0.03	**0.2**	140
Tongue	41	0	-	-	-	-	-	-	-	1.1	4.0	5.7	16.1	11.2	34.1	10.0	18.4	7.0	27.9	45.0	3.9	0.8	0.36	0.50	**4.4**	141
Salivary gland	11	0	-	-	-	-	-	-	-	-	-	1.9	2.3	5.6	-	10.0	4.6	14.0	13.9	-	1.0	0.2	0.05	0.12	**1.1**	142
Mouth	42	0	-	-	-	-	-	-	-	1.1	2.7	3.8	9.2	36.6	27.9	16.7	4.6	28.0	13.9	-	4.0	0.9	0.41	0.51	**4.4**	143-5
Oropharynx	36	0	-	-	-	-	-	-	1.0	-	2.7	9.4	11.5	22.5	12.4	26.7	9.2	-	-	22.5	3.4	0.7	0.30	0.48	**3.9**	146
Nasopharynx	7	0	-	-	-	-	1.1	-	-	-	-	1.9	4.6	-	3.1	-	4.6	7.0	-	-	0.7	0.1	0.05	0.08	**0.7**	147
Hypopharynx	27	0	-	-	-	-	-	-	-	1.1	1.3	3.8	4.6	14.1	21.7	13.3	-	14.0	27.9	22.5	2.6	0.6	0.23	0.30	**2.8**	148
Pharynx unspecified	6	0	-	-	-	-	-	-	-	-	-	1.9	-	-	9.3	-	4.6	-	13.9	-	0.6	0.1	0.06	0.08	**0.6**	149
Oesophagus	116	0	-	-	-	-	-	-	1.0	-	4.0	7.5	34.5	36.6	40.3	86.7	105.8	98.1	55.7	-	11.0	2.4	0.62	1.58	**11.5**	150
Stomach	159	0	-	-	-	-	1.1	-	1.0	4.4	8.0	5.7	23.0	39.4	80.6	76.7	119.6	182.2	153.2	180.0	15.1	3.3	0.82	1.80	**15.4**	151
Small intestine	23	0	-	-	-	-	-	-	-	1.1	1.3	1.9	-	2.8	6.2	13.3	27.6	21.0	27.9	45.0	2.2	0.5	0.07	0.27	**2.1**	152
Colon	353	0	-	-	-	-	-	-	2.9	3.3	10.6	28.3	36.9	98.4	102.3	233.5	289.7	350.3	473.7	517.4	33.5	7.3	1.41	4.03	**33.8**	153
Rectum	135	0	-	-	-	-	-	1.9	2.9	4.4	5.3	17.0	25.3	28.1	52.7	83.4	105.8	105.1	153.2	22.5	12.8	2.8	0.69	1.63	**13.0**	154
Liver	81	0	2.0	-	-	-	-	-	1.0	2.2	12.0	5.7	11.5	11.2	62.0	30.0	78.2	42.0	27.9	22.5	7.7	1.7	0.54	1.08	**8.1**	155
Gallbladder etc.	11	0	-	-	-	-	-	-	-	-	1.1	-	-	5.6	6.2	3.3	9.2	7.0	27.9	-	1.0	0.2	0.06	0.13	**1.0**	156
Pancreas	132	0	-	-	-	-	-	-	1.0	1.1	4.0	17.0	25.3	36.6	46.5	106.8	73.6	112.1	125.4	135.0	12.5	2.7	0.66	1.56	**13.1**	157
Nose, sinuses etc.	6	0	-	-	1.2	-	-	1.0	-	1.1	-	1.9	-	-	-	3.3	-	-	13.9	-	0.6	0.1	0.03	0.04	**0.5**	160
Larynx	91	0	-	-	-	-	-	-	-	-	2.2	4.0	13.2	23.0	30.9	46.5	63.4	59.8	49.0	27.9	45.0	8.6	1.9	0.60	1.22	**9.4**
Bronchus, lung	1003	0	-	-	-	-	1.1	1.0	3.9	16.4	45.2	115.1	230.3	314.9	524.0	607.2	726.5	630.6	710.5	562.4	95.1	20.7	6.26	12.93	**101.5**	162
Other thoracic organs	4	0	-	-	-	-	-	-	1.0	-	1.3	-	-	2.8	3.1	-	-	-	-	-	0.4	0.1	0.04	0.04	**0.4**	163-4
Bone	7	0	-	-	1.2	2.5	-	-	1.0	1.1	-	-	-	-	-	3.3	-	-	13.9	-	0.7	0.1	0.03	0.05	**0.6**	170
Connective tissue	36	0	1.0	-	1.2	-	-	4.9	1.0	1.1	6.7	5.7	6.9	8.4	6.2	10.0	13.8	21.0	13.9	22.5	3.4	0.7	0.22	0.33	**3.4**	171
Mesothelioma	14	0	-	-	-	-	-	-	1.0	-	-	3.8	2.3	2.8	-	10.0	13.8	21.0	-	-	1.3	0.3	0.05	0.17	**1.3**	MES
Kaposi's sarcoma	281	0	-	-	-	-	8.8	28.3	62.3	84.3	75.8	34.0	23.0	28.1	9.3	10.0	-	-	-	45.0	26.6	5.8	1.77	1.82	**21.5**	KAP
Melanoma of skin	8	0	-	-	-	-	-	1.0	-	-	-	1.9	-	5.6	-	3.3	-	7.0	27.9	-	0.8	0.2	0.04	0.06	**0.7**	172
†Other skin	11	0	-	-	-	-	-	1.9	1.0	3.3	4.0	-	-	-	-	3.3	4.6	-	-	-	1.0		0.05	0.09	**0.8**	173
Breast	13	0	-	-	-	-	-	-	-	1.1	1.3	-	-	11.2	3.1	-	18.4	-	27.9	-	1.2	0.3	0.08	0.18	**1.2**	175
Prostate	1345	0	-	-	-	-	-	-	-	-	4.0	18.9	69.1	227.8	524.0	924.1	1526.6	1632.5	1783.2	1844.8	127.5	27.8	4.22	16.47	**127.6**	185
Testis	12	0	-	-	-	-	2.2	3.9	1.0	2.2	2.7	-	2.8	-	-	-	-	-	-	-	1.1	0.2	0.07	0.07	**0.9**	186
Penis	5	0	-	-	-	-	-	-	-	-	-	-	2.8	3.1	-	9.2	7.0	-	-	-	0.5	0.1	0.03	0.08	**0.5**	187.1-.4
Other male genital	2	0	-	-	-	-	-	-	-	-	-	-	-	-	-	4.6	7.0	-	-	-	0.2	0.0	0.00	0.02	**0.2**	187.5-.9
Bladder	112	0	-	-	-	-	-	1.0	1.0	-	4.0	3.8	13.8	22.5	46.5	86.7	110.4	98.1	139.3	45.0	10.6	2.3	0.46	1.45	**10.8**	188
Kidney etc.	102	0	1.0	-	-	-	1.1	-	2.9	2.2	6.7	9.4	20.7	33.7	34.1	53.4	87.4	42.0	125.4	67.5	9.7	2.1	0.56	1.26	**10.0**	189
Eye	5	0	1.0	-	-	-	-	-	1.0	-	-	-	-	-	3.1	-	4.6	7.0	-	-	0.5	0.1	0.03	0.05	**0.5**	190
Brain, nervous system	53	0	10.2	5.7	7.2	2.5	-	5.8	1.9	1.1	1.3	9.4	6.9	2.8	9.3	10.0	23.0	-	-	-	5.0	1.1	0.32	0.49	**5.5**	191-2
Thyroid	11	0	-	-	1.2	-	-	-	1.0	1.1	-	3.8	-	2.8	3.1	3.3	4.6	7.0	-	22.5	1.0	0.2	0.06	0.10	**1.1**	193
Other endocrine	4	0	1.0	-	-	-	-	-	-	1.1	-	-	-	-	-	3.3	4.6	-	-	-	0.4	0.1	0.01	0.05	**0.4**	194
Hodgkin's disease	35	0	-	-	2.4	3.8	1.1	7.8	4.9	3.3	5.3	1.9	4.6	2.8	3.1	6.7	9.2	-	-	-	3.3	0.7	0.20	0.28	**3.0**	201
Non-Hodgkin lymphoma	157	0	-	-	2.4	1.3	2.2	8.8	14.6	30.7	20.0	26.4	29.9	25.3	37.2	30.0	46.0	56.0	83.6	90.0	14.9	3.2	0.99	1.37	**14.0**	200,202
Multiple myeloma	100	0	-	-	-	-	-	1.0	2.9	1.1	4.0	5.7	23.0	28.1	27.9	53.4	82.8	91.1	139.3	67.5	9.5	2.1	0.47	1.15	**9.5**	203
Lymphoid leukaemia	45	0	3.0	3.4	3.6	1.3	1.1	1.0	1.0	-	1.3	1.9	4.6	8.4	15.5	10.0	41.4	21.0	27.9	67.5	4.3	0.9	0.23	0.49	**4.6**	204
Myeloid leukaemia	39	0	-	1.1	-	2.5	1.1	1.0	2.9	4.4	5.3	5.7	4.6	5.6	6.2	16.7	13.8	14.0	27.9	45.0	3.7	0.8	0.20	0.35	**3.6**	205
Monocytic leukaemia	3	0	-	1.1	-	-	-	-	-	-	1.3	-	-	-	-	-	-	7.0	-	-	0.3	0.1	0.01	0.01	**0.3**	206
Other leukaemia	1	0	-	-	-	-	-	-	-	-	-	-	-	-	-	-	4.6	-	-	-	0.1	0.0	0.00	0.02	**0.1**	207
Leukaemia unspecified	7	0	-	-	-	-	-	1.0	-	-	-	-	-	2.8	-	3.3	9.2	-	27.9	-	0.7	0.1	0.02	0.08	**0.6**	208
Other and unspecified	154	0	1.0	-	-	-	-	-	1.9	4.4	2.7	20.8	39.2	42.2	86.8	63.4	115.0	70.1	167.2	180.0	14.6	3.2	0.99	1.89	**15.7**	O&U
All sites	4848	0	20.3	11.4	20.4	13.8	20.9	71.1	118.7	182.9	252.8	396.3	707.1	1164.1	1897.4	2692.2	3788.9	3776.4	4499.9	4117.0	459.7		24.39	56.79	**466.3**	ALL
All sites but 173	4837	0	20.3	11.4	20.4	13.8	20.9	69.2	117.7	179.6	248.8	396.3	707.1	1164.1	1897.4	2688.9	3784.3	3776.4	4499.9	4117.0	458.7	100.0	24.33	56.70	**465.4**	ALLb

| Rate from 1 case | | | 1.015 | 1.139 | 1.198 | 1.251 | 1.098 | 0.974 | 0.973 | 1.095 | 1.330 | 1.887 | 2.303 | 2.812 | 3.100 | 3.336 | 4.598 | 7.006 | 13.931 | 22.497 |

†Important: see notes on population page

USA, CALIFORNIA, SAN FRANCISCO BAY AREA: BLACK 1988-1992

ANNUAL INCIDENCE PER 100,000 BY AGE GROUP (YEARS) - FEMALE

SITE	ALL AGES	AGE UNK	0-	5-	10-	15-	20-	25-	30-	35-	40-	45-	50-	55-	60-	65-	70-	75-	80-	85+	CRUDE RATE	%	CR 64	CR 74	ASR (W)	ICD (9th)
Lip	0	0	-	-	-	-	-	-	-	-	-	-	-	-	-	-	-	-	-	-	0.0	0.0	0.00	0.00	**0.0**	*140*
Tongue	9	0	-	-	-	-	-	-	-	-	-	3.4	2.1	4.9	-	2.5	3.2	4.4	8.0	-	0.8	0.2	0.05	0.08	**0.7**	*141*
Salivary gland	6	0	1.0	-	-	1.3	-	-	-	-	-	-	-	2.4	-	2.5	3.2	4.4	-	-	0.5	0.2	0.02	0.05	**0.5**	*142*
Mouth	20	0	-	-	-	-	-	1.0	-	-	3.4	4.3	12.2	12.4	5.0	-	4.4	-	-	19.7	1.8	0.5	0.17	0.19	**1.8**	*143-5*
Oropharynx	10	0	-	-	-	-	-	-	-	-	1.2	1.7	-	2.4	9.9	5.0	3.2	-	-	-	0.9	0.3	0.08	0.12	**0.9**	*146*
Nasopharynx	2	0	-	1.1	-	-	-	-	-	-	-	-	-	-	2.5	-	-	-	-	-	0.2	0.1	0.02	0.02	**0.2**	*147*
Hypopharynx	8	0	-	-	-	-	-	-	-	-	1.2	1.7	4.3	4.9	2.5	-	3.2	-	-	-	0.7	0.2	0.07	0.09	**0.7**	*148*
Pharynx unspecified	4	0	-	-	-	-	-	-	0.9	-	-	1.7	-	2.4	-	2.5	-	-	-	-	0.4	0.1	0.03	0.04	**0.3**	*149*
Oesophagus	46	0	-	-	-	-	-	-	-	-	2.5	6.8	10.6	17.1	14.8	25.1	22.7	17.8	8.0	-	4.1	1.2	0.26	0.50	**3.8**	*150*
Stomach	112	0	-	-	-	-	1.2	1.0	1.9	3.1	6.1	1.7	23.4	22.0	14.8	37.7	32.4	66.7	88.3	216.6	10.0	3.0	0.38	0.73	**7.6**	*151*
Small intestine	14	0	-	-	-	-	-	-	-	1.0	1.2	1.7	2.1	2.4	4.9	2.5	9.7	4.4	8.0	9.8	1.2	0.4	0.07	0.13	**1.0**	*152*
Colon	408	0	-	-	-	-	-	-	4.7	8.2	11.1	23.9	61.8	68.5	91.6	158.3	207.5	297.7	385.3	354.4	36.4	10.9	1.35	3.18	**27.9**	*153*
Rectum	119	0	-	-	-	-	1.2	1.9	-	6.2	7.4	12.0	21.3	19.6	29.7	25.1	64.9	71.1	112.4	68.9	10.6	3.2	0.50	0.95	**8.5**	*154*
Liver	27	0	-	-	-	-	-	-	-	-	1.2	1.7	2.1	12.2	14.8	5.0	6.5	13.3	8.0	49.2	2.4	0.7	0.16	0.22	**2.1**	*155*
Gallbladder etc.	14	0	-	-	-	-	-	-	-	-	1.2	-	-	4.9	2.5	5.0	13.0	4.4	8.0	19.7	1.2	0.4	0.04	0.13	**1.0**	*156*
Pancreas	159	0	-	-	-	-	-	-	1.9	3.1	4.9	-	10.6	46.5	56.9	55.3	87.6	115.5	136.4	108.3	14.2	4.2	0.62	1.33	**11.0**	*157*
Nose, sinuses etc.	4	0	-	-	-	-	-	-	-	1.0	1.2	-	-	2.4	-	2.5	-	-	-	-	0.4	0.1	0.02	0.04	**0.3**	*160*
Larynx	25	0	-	-	-	-	-	-	-	1.0	-	5.1	8.5	2.4	12.4	15.1	6.5	-	8.0	19.7	2.2	0.7	0.15	0.26	**2.1**	*161*
Bronchus, lung	562	0	-	-	-	-	-	1.0	-	8.2	28.2	53.0	112.9	156.5	235.1	248.7	295.1	248.8	256.8	88.6	50.1	15.0	2.97	5.69	**44.3**	*162*
Other thoracic organs	4	0	-	-	-	-	-	1.0	-	1.0	-	-	-	-	2.5	2.5	-	-	-	-	0.4	0.1	0.02	0.03	**0.3**	*163-4*
Bone	6	0	-	-	1.2	-	-	-	1.9	-	-	1.7	-	-	-	2.5	-	-	-	9.8	0.5	0.2	0.02	0.04	**0.5**	*170*
Connective tissue	21	0	-	1.1	1.2	-	2.3	-	1.9	2.1	1.2	3.4	4.3	-	7.4	7.5	3.2	4.4	-	-	1.9	0.6	0.12	0.18	**1.8**	*171*
Mesothelioma	4	0	-	-	-	-	-	-	-	-	-	-	-	-	-	2.5	3.2	-	-	19.7	0.4	0.1	0.00	0.03	**0.2**	*MES*
Kaposi's sarcoma	2	0	-	-	-	-	-	-	0.9	-	-	-	-	-	-	-	4.4	-	-	-	0.2	0.1	0.00	0.00	**0.1**	*KAP*
Melanoma of skin	8	0	-	-	-	-	1.2	-	0.9	-	2.5	-	2.1	-	2.5	-	4.4	-	-	9.8	0.7	0.2	0.05	0.05	**0.6**	*172*
†Other skin	14	0	-	-	1.2	-	-	3.9	0.9	3.1	-	3.4	2.1	2.4	-	2.5	-	-	-	-	1.2		0.09	0.10	**1.1**	*173*
Breast	1056	0	-	-	-	-	1.2	7.7	32.7	74.9	132.6	193.2	240.7	266.6	282.1	321.6	321.1	373.3	272.9	364.2	94.2	28.1	6.16	9.37	**83.7**	*174*
Uterus unspecified	13	0	-	-	-	-	-	-	-	2.5	3.4	2.1	-	-	10.0	3.2	4.4	-	-	19.7	1.2	0.3	0.04	0.11	**1.0**	*179*
Cervix uteri	139	0	-	-	-	-	2.3	5.8	10.3	16.4	33.2	30.8	17.0	19.6	17.3	27.6	22.7	35.5	24.1	68.9	12.4	3.7	0.76	1.01	**10.5**	*180*
Placenta	1	0	-	-	-	-	-	-	-	-	1.2	-	-	-	-	-	-	-	-	-	0.1	0.0	0.01	0.01	**0.1**	*181*
Corpus uteri	147	0	-	-	-	-	-	-	0.9	3.1	6.1	6.8	17.0	51.4	74.2	60.3	68.1	66.7	72.2	59.1	13.1	3.9	0.80	1.44	**11.4**	*182*
Ovary etc.	125	0	-	-	1.2	2.5	2.3	2.9	1.9	4.1	4.9	12.0	21.3	14.7	42.1	57.8	58.4	48.9	56.2	78.7	11.1	3.3	0.55	1.13	**9.5**	*183*
Other female genital	21	0	-	-	-	-	-	1.9	0.9	1.0	1.2	3.4	6.4	2.4	2.5	7.5	9.7	4.4	-	19.7	1.9	0.6	0.10	0.19	**1.6**	*184*
Bladder	61	0	-	-	-	-	-	-	-	-	-	5.1	8.5	12.2	14.8	22.6	38.9	31.1	40.1	98.4	5.4	1.6	0.20	0.51	**4.3**	*188*
Kidney etc.	78	0	4.2	-	-	1.3	1.2	-	2.8	2.1	6.1	10.3	8.5	19.6	27.2	37.7	22.7	40.0	16.1	-	7.0	2.1	0.42	0.72	**6.3**	*189*
Eye	2	0	2.1	-	-	-	-	-	-	-	-	-	-	-	-	-	-	-	-	-	0.2	0.1	0.01	0.01	**0.3**	*190*
Brain, nervous system	34	0	6.3	-	1.2	5.1	-	1.9	0.9	2.1	1.2	6.8	4.3	2.4	-	5.0	13.0	13.3	8.0	-	3.0	0.9	0.16	0.25	**3.0**	*191-2*
Thyroid	37	0	-	-	-	-	4.6	1.0	2.8	7.2	3.7	6.8	4.3	9.8	4.9	2.5	13.0	4.4	-	9.8	3.3	1.0	0.23	0.30	**2.9**	*193*
Other endocrine	4	0	-	2.3	-	-	-	-	-	-	-	-	-	2.4	2.5	-	-	-	-	-	0.4	0.1	0.04	0.04	**0.4**	*194*
Hodgkin's disease	25	0	-	1.1	-	2.5	4.6	1.9	1.9	2.1	2.5	3.4	-	2.4	4.9	5.0	6.5	4.4	-	-	2.2	0.7	0.14	0.19	**2.1**	*201*
Non-Hodgkin lymphoma	100	0	-	-	-	-	1.2	3.9	0.9	7.2	7.4	6.8	14.9	19.6	24.7	32.7	45.4	44.4	64.2	68.9	8.9	2.7	0.43	0.82	**7.3**	*200,202*
Multiple myeloma	86	0	-	-	-	1.3	-	-	-	-	6.1	3.4	10.6	14.7	39.6	35.2	51.9	40.0	64.2	39.4	7.7	2.3	0.38	0.81	**6.4**	*203*
Lymphoid leukaemia	40	0	2.1	5.7	1.2	1.3	1.2	-	-	-	-	5.1	2.1	7.3	9.9	10.0	6.5	13.3	48.2	39.4	3.6	1.1	0.18	0.26	**3.2**	*204*
Myeloid leukaemia	24	0	1.0	3.4	-	1.3	-	-	1.9	1.9	1.0	2.5	1.7	2.1	2.4	-	2.5	22.2	8.0	19.7	2.1	0.6	0.10	0.11	**1.8**	*205*
Monocytic leukaemia	3	0	1.0	-	-	-	-	-	-	-	-	-	-	2.4	-	2.5	-	-	-	-	0.3	0.1	0.02	0.03	**0.3**	*206*
Other leukaemia	1	0	-	-	-	-	-	-	-	-	-	-	-	-	-	-	-	-	8.0	-	0.1	0.0	0.00	0.00	**0.0**	*207*
Leukaemia unspecified	4	0	-	-	-	-	-	-	1.0	-	-	-	-	-	-	2.5	-	4.4	8.0	-	0.4	0.1	0.02	0.02	**0.3**	*208*
Other and unspecified	164	0	1.0	-	-	-	1.2	1.9	2.8	3.1	3.7	18.8	8.5	26.9	42.1	52.8	81.1	142.2	104.3	167.3	14.6	4.4	0.55	1.22	**11.2**	*O&U*
All sites	3773	0	18.9	14.9	7.4	16.5	25.3	41.6	76.7	162.1	286.2	444.4	641.1	863.3	1108.5	1309.0	1527.4	1759.7	1822.0	2047.4	336.4		18.53	32.72	**287.1**	*ALL*
All sites but 173	3759	0	18.9	14.9	6.1	16.5	25.3	37.7	75.7	159.0	286.2	441.0	638.9	860.8	1108.5	1306.5	1527.4	1759.7	1822.0	2047.4	335.2	100.0	18.45	32.62	**286.0**	*ALLb*
Rate from 1 case			1.047	1.149	1.230	1.268	1.151	0.967	0.935	1.026	1.228	1.709	2.130	2.446	2.474	2.512	3.243	4.444	8.026	9.843						

†Important: see notes on population page

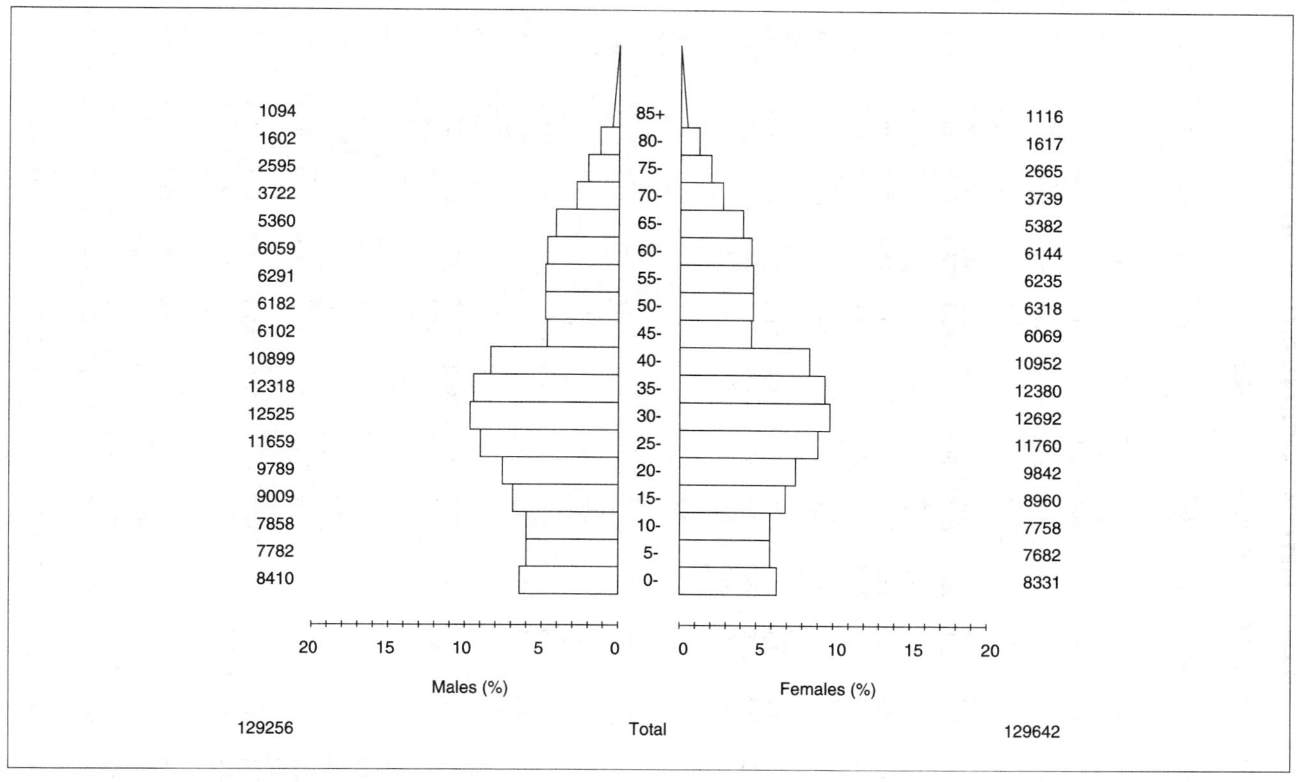

USA, California, San Francisco Bay Area: Chinese
Source of population: average annual 1988-92
Estimate: The years 1988-89 and 1991-92 are bench-marked to the 1990 census, making allowance for births, deaths, and migration into and out of the registration area. Sex-specific totals were apportioned to specific Asian populations based on a 5% sample of the census. The resulting race- and sex-specific population estimates were then apportioned to 5-year age categories based on the race- and sex-specific age distribution in the 100% census counts.

Notes to tables overleaf:
† 173 does not include basal cell or squamous cell carcinoma

USA, CALIFORNIA, SAN FRANCISCO BAY AREA: CHINESE 1988-1992

ANNUAL INCIDENCE PER 100,000 BY AGE GROUP (YEARS) - MALE

SITE	ALL AGES	AGE UNK	0-	5-	10-	15-	20-	25-	30-	35-	40-	45-	50-	55-	60-	65-	70-	75-	80-	85+	CRUDE RATE	%	CR 64	CR 74	ASR (W)	ICD (9th)
Lip	0	0	-	-	-	-	-	-	-	-	-	-	-	-	-	-	-	-	-	-	0.0	0.0	0.00	0.00	0.0	140
Tongue	9	0	-	-	-	-	-	-	3.2	-	1.8	-	-	-	3.3	3.7	-	30.8	-	-	1.4	0.5	0.04	0.06	0.9	141
Salivary gland	6	0	-	-	-	-	-	-	-	-	-	3.3	3.2	3.2	3.3	3.7	-	7.7	-	-	0.9	0.3	0.06	0.08	0.8	142
Mouth	14	0	-	-	-	-	-	-	-	-	1.8	-	-	6.4	9.9	3.7	10.7	23.1	25.0	-	2.2	0.7	0.09	0.16	1.4	143-5
Oropharynx	3	0	-	-	-	-	-	-	-	1.6	-	3.3	-	-	-	-	-	-	-	18.3	0.5	0.2	0.02	0.02	0.4	146
Nasopharynx	'92	0	-	-	-	-	-	6.9	9.6	16.2	16.5	16.4	45.3	44.5	49.5	29.8	16.1	23.1	12.5	-	14.2	4.7	1.02	1.25	11.6	147
Hypopharynx	4	0	-	-	-	-	-	-	-	1.6	-	-	-	3.2	-	3.7	5.4	-	-	-	0.6	0.2	0.02	0.07	0.4	148
Pharynx unspecified	2	0	-	-	-	-	-	-	-	-	-	-	-	-	-	-	-	-	12.5	18.3	0.3	0.1	0.00	0.00	0.2	149
Oesophagus	34	0	-	-	-	-	-	-	-	-	3.7	6.6	-	19.1	9.9	14.9	32.2	46.2	37.4	36.6	5.3	1.7	0.20	0.43	3.7	150
Stomach	99	0	-	-	-	-	2.0	-	3.2	1.6	3.7	13.1	16.2	25.4	39.6	63.4	91.3	123.3	74.9	146.2	15.3	5.1	0.52	1.30	10.9	151
Small intestine	7	0	-	-	-	-	-	-	-	1.6	-	-	-	6.4	-	3.7	-	-	37.4	-	1.1	0.4	0.04	0.06	0.7	152
Colon	189	0	-	-	-	-	-	1.7	-	9.7	5.5	19.7	25.9	54.0	62.7	97.0	188.1	185.0	324.5	329.0	29.2	9.6	0.90	2.32	20.0	153
Rectum	113	0	-	-	-	-	-	3.4	1.6	3.2	3.7	3.3	25.9	25.4	59.4	97.0	96.7	115.6	49.9	146.2	17.5	5.8	0.63	1.60	12.7	154
Liver	172	0	-	-	-	-	-	-	6.4	9.7	14.7	19.7	74.4	73.1	79.2	104.5	102.1	131.0	62.4	164.5	26.6	8.8	1.39	2.42	20.5	155
Gallbladder etc.	23	0	-	-	-	-	-	-	-	-	1.8	-	3.2	6.4	9.9	14.9	26.9	30.8	25.0	18.3	3.6	1.2	0.11	0.32	2.4	156
Pancreas	58	0	-	-	-	-	-	-	-	-	-	-	9.7	9.5	36.3	29.8	59.1	77.1	62.4	127.9	9.0	3.0	0.28	0.72	6.1	157
Nose, sinuses etc.	7	0	-	-	-	-	-	-	-	-	3.3	3.2	3.2	3.3	7.5	-	7.7	-	-	-	1.1	0.4	0.06	0.10	0.9	160
Larynx	26	0	-	-	-	-	-	-	-	-	1.8	3.3	-	3.2	13.2	29.8	21.5	38.5	12.5	18.3	4.0	1.3	0.11	0.36	2.8	161
Bronchus, lung	366	0	-	-	-	-	-	-	1.6	3.2	5.5	22.9	55.0	114.4	181.5	246.3	354.6	470.1	461.8	274.2	56.6	18.7	1.92	4.93	39.4	162
Other thoracic organs	7	0	-	-	-	-	-	1.7	-	-	-	-	6.5	6.4	-	3.7	-	7.7	-	-	1.1	0.4	0.07	0.09	0.9	163-4
Bone	4	0	-	2.6	5.1	-	-	-	-	-	-	-	3.2	-	-	-	-	-	-	-	0.6	0.2	0.05	0.05	0.9	170
Connective tissue	12	0	2.4	-	-	2.2	-	-	-	-	-	3.3	-	3.2	3.3	14.9	10.7	7.7	-	-	1.9	0.6	0.07	0.20	1.7	171
Mesothelioma	5	0	-	-	-	-	-	-	-	-	-	-	-	-	-	7.5	10.7	-	12.5	-	0.8	0.3	0.00	0.09	0.5	MES
Kaposi's sarcoma	14	0	-	-	-	-	-	3.4	3.2	1.6	9.2	6.6	-	3.2	3.3	-	-	-	-	-	2.2	0.7	0.15	0.15	1.8	KAP
Melanoma of skin	1	0	-	-	-	-	-	-	-	-	-	-	-	-	-	3.7	-	-	-	-	0.2	0.1	0.00	0.02	0.1	172
†Other skin	2	0	-	-	-	-	-	-	-	-	-	-	-	3.2	-	-	5.4	-	-	-	0.3		0.02	0.04	0.2	173
Breast	3	0	-	-	-	-	-	-	-	1.6	-	-	-	-	-	-	10.7	-	-	-	0.5	0.2	0.01	0.06	0.3	175
Prostate	268	0	-	-	-	-	-	-	-	-	-	3.3	-	38.1	46.2	223.9	349.2	408.5	486.8	438.7	41.5	13.7	0.44	3.30	26.0	185
Testis	16	0	-	-	-	-	2.0	8.6	1.6	6.5	3.7	3.3	3.2	3.2	-	-	-	-	-	-	2.5	0.8	0.16	0.16	2.0	186
Penis	1	0	-	-	-	-	-	-	-	-	-	-	-	-	-	3.7	-	-	-	-	0.2	0.1	0.00	0.02	0.1	187.1-.4
Other male genital	4	0	-	-	-	-	-	-	-	-	1.8	-	-	3.2	-	3.7	-	7.7	-	-	0.6	0.2	0.03	0.04	0.4	187.5-.9
Bladder	85	0	-	-	-	-	-	-	-	-	-	6.6	9.7	19.1	29.7	89.5	80.6	92.5	87.4	127.9	13.2	4.3	0.33	1.18	9.1	188
Kidney etc.	29	0	-	-	-	-	-	-	-	-	1.8	3.3	3.2	12.7	16.5	37.3	10.7	23.1	12.5	18.3	4.5	1.5	0.19	0.43	3.4	189
Eye	0	0	-	-	-	-	-	-	-	-	-	-	-	-	-	-	-	-	-	-	0.0	0.0	0.00	0.00	0.0	190
Brain, nervous system	23	0	-	2.6	7.6	2.2	4.1	-	4.8	1.6	3.7	-	16.2	3.2	3.3	3.7	5.4	7.7	-	-	3.6	1.2	0.25	0.29	3.4	191-2
Thyroid	20	0	-	-	-	-	-	-	1.6	4.9	1.8	-	9.7	-	9.9	14.9	16.1	15.4	-	-	3.1	1.0	0.14	0.29	2.3	193
Other endocrine	6	0	-	5.1	-	-	1.7	1.6	-	-	-	-	3.2	3.3	-	-	-	-	-	-	0.9	0.3	0.07	0.07	1.0	194
Hodgkin's disease	7	0	-	-	-	2.2	2.0	-	-	-	-	3.3	6.5	-	3.3	-	5.4	-	-	-	1.1	0.4	0.09	0.11	1.1	201
Non-Hodgkin lymphoma	96	0	2.4	2.6	-	-	4.1	6.9	9.6	6.5	7.3	6.6	9.7	47.7	23.1	48.5	37.6	107.9	99.9	91.4	14.9	4.9	0.63	1.06	10.8	200,202
Multiple myeloma	12	0	-	-	-	-	-	-	-	-	-	-	3.2	-	6.6	11.2	21.5	-	12.5	18.3	1.9	0.6	0.05	0.21	1.3	203
Lymphoid leukaemia	26	0	9.5	10.3	2.5	4.4	-	-	-	1.6	1.8	-	-	12.7	-	18.7	5.4	7.7	12.5	18.3	4.0	1.3	0.21	0.33	4.4	204
Myeloid leukaemia	22	0	4.8	-	-	2.2	4.1	1.7	-	3.2	1.8	3.3	-	3.2	-	7.5	26.9	15.4	12.5	18.3	3.4	1.1	0.12	0.29	2.9	205
Monocytic leukaemia	0	0	-	-	-	-	-	-	-	-	-	-	-	-	-	-	-	-	-	-	0.0	0.0	0.00	0.00	0.0	206
Other leukaemia	0	0	-	-	-	-	-	-	-	-	-	-	-	-	-	-	-	-	-	-	0.0	0.0	0.00	0.00	0.0	207
Leukaemia unspecified	4	0	-	-	-	-	-	-	-	1.6	-	-	-	-	-	-	-	5.4	7.7	12.5	0.6	0.2	0.01	0.03	0.3	208
Other and unspecified	70	0	-	-	-	-	-	-	4.8	-	1.8	3.3	19.4	19.1	16.5	33.6	75.2	84.8	124.8	73.1	10.8	3.6	0.32	0.87	7.3	O&U
All sites	1961	0	19.0	23.1	15.3	13.3	18.4	36.0	52.7	77.9	95.4	157.3	352.6	578.6	726.1	1279.8	1681.7	2104.0	2071.9	2102.0	303.4		10.83	25.64	218.3	ALL
All sites but 173	1959	0	19.0	23.1	15.3	13.3	18.4	36.0	52.7	77.9	95.4	157.3	352.6	575.4	726.1	1279.8	1676.3	2104.0	2071.9	2102.0	303.1	100.0	10.81	25.59	218.0	ALLb

Rate from 1 case   2.378   2.570   2.545   2.220   2.043   1.715   1.597   1.624   1.835   3.278   3.235   3.179   3.301   3.731   5.373   7.707   12.481   18.278

†Important: see notes on population page

USA, CALIFORNIA, SAN FRANCISCO BAY AREA: CHINESE 1988-1992

ANNUAL INCIDENCE PER 100,000 BY AGE GROUP (YEARS) - FEMALE

SITE	ALL AGES	AGE UNK	0-	5-	10-	15-	20-	25-	30-	35-	40-	45-	50-	55-	60-	65-	70-	75-	80-	85+	CRUDE RATE	%	CR 64	CR 74	ASR (W)	ICD (9th)
Lip	1	0	-	-	-	-	-	-	-	-	-	-	-	-	-	-	-	7.5	-	-	0.2	0.1	0.00	0.00	0.1	140
Tongue	7	0	-	-	-	-	-	-	4.7	-	-	-	-	-	3.3	3.7	5.3	-	12.4	-	1.1	0.4	0.04	0.09	0.7	141
Salivary gland	3	0	-	-	-	-	-	-	1.6	-	-	-	-	-	3.3	-	-	7.5	-	-	0.5	0.2	0.02	0.02	0.3	142
Mouth	4	0	-	-	-	-	-	-	-	-	-	3.3	3.2	-	-	3.7	5.3	-	-	-	0.6	0.2	0.03	0.08	0.6	143-5
Oropharynx	2	0	-	-	-	-	-	-	-	-	-	-	-	-	-	-	-	-	24.7	-	0.3	0.1	0.00	0.00	0.1	146
Nasopharynx	33	0	-	-	-	-	-	5.1	4.7	3.2	12.8	3.3	3.2	9.6	9.8	18.6	10.7	7.5	-	35.8	5.1	1.8	0.26	0.40	3.8	147
Hypopharynx	0	0	-	-	-	-	-	-	-	-	-	-	-	-	-	-	-	-	-	-	0.0	0.0	0.00	0.00	0.0	148
Pharynx unspecified	0	0	-	-	-	-	-	-	-	-	-	-	-	-	-	-	-	-	-	-	0.0	0.0	0.00	0.00	0.0	149
Oesophagus	9	0	-	-	-	-	-	-	-	-	-	-	-	6.5	-	3.7	5.3	7.5	37.1	17.9	1.4	0.5	0.03	0.08	0.8	150
Stomach	68	0	-	-	-	-	-	1.7	4.7	1.6	1.8	3.3	12.7	9.6	22.8	22.3	42.8	82.6	86.6	268.8	10.5	3.8	0.29	0.62	6.9	151
Small intestine	4	0	-	-	-	-	-	-	-	-	1.8	3.3	-	-	3.3	-	5.3	-	-	-	0.6	0.2	0.04	0.07	0.5	152
Colon	198	0	-	-	-	-	-	1.7	4.7	6.5	11.0	19.8	47.5	67.4	52.1	96.6	133.7	232.6	235.0	447.9	30.5	11.0	1.05	2.20	21.1	153
Rectum	97	0	-	-	-	-	-	1.7	-	1.6	5.5	-	19.0	19.2	42.3	74.3	64.2	112.6	173.1	107.5	15.0	5.4	0.45	1.14	10.0	154
Liver	56	0	-	-	-	-	-	-	-	1.6	5.5	9.9	19.0	9.6	13.0	29.7	42.8	67.5	111.3	35.8	8.6	3.1	0.29	0.66	6.0	155
Gallbladder etc.	23	0	-	-	-	-	-	-	-	-	-	3.3	-	-	3.3	11.1	26.7	45.0	61.8	35.8	3.5	1.3	0.03	0.22	2.1	156
Pancreas	49	0	-	-	-	-	-	-	-	1.6	1.8	-	6.3	22.5	13.0	7.4	53.5	52.5	111.3	107.5	7.6	2.7	0.23	0.53	4.9	157
Nose, sinuses etc.	3	0	-	-	-	-	-	-	-	-	-	-	3.2	3.2	-	-	5.3	-	-	-	0.5	0.2	0.03	0.06	0.4	160
Larynx	3	0	-	-	-	-	-	-	-	-	-	-	-	3.2	-	3.7	-	7.5	-	-	0.5	0.2	0.02	0.03	0.3	161
Bronchus, lung	227	0	-	-	-	-	-	-	-	6.5	14.6	13.2	47.5	57.7	65.1	144.9	181.8	322.7	160.8	519.6	35.0	12.6	1.02	2.66	24.0	162
Other thoracic organs	1	0	-	-	-	-	-	-	-	-	-	-	-	-	-	3.7	-	-	-	-	0.2	0.1	0.00	0.02	0.1	163-4
Bone	2	0	-	-	-	2.2	-	-	-	-	-	-	-	-	3.2	-	-	-	-	-	0.3	0.1	0.03	0.03	0.3	170
Connective tissue	9	0	-	-	2.6	-	-	3.4	-	-	-	-	3.3	3.2	-	6.5	3.7	-	12.4	-	1.4	0.5	0.09	0.11	1.3	171
Mesothelioma	0	0	-	-	-	-	-	-	-	-	-	-	-	-	-	-	-	-	-	-	0.0	0.0	0.00	0.00	0.0	MES
Kaposi's sarcoma	0	0	-	-	-	-	-	-	-	-	-	-	-	-	-	-	-	-	-	-	0.0	0.0	0.00	0.00	0.0	KAP
Melanoma of skin	3	0	-	-	-	-	-	-	-	-	-	-	3.2	3.2	3.3	-	-	-	-	-	0.5	0.2	0.05	0.05	0.4	172
†Other skin	1	0	-	-	-	-	-	-	-	1.6	-	-	-	-	-	-	-	-	-	-	0.2		0.01	0.01	0.1	173
Breast	459	0	-	-	-	-	2.0	10.2	26.8	53.3	69.4	158.2	129.8	134.7	162.7	204.4	251.4	292.7	210.2	447.9	70.8	25.4	3.74	6.01	55.2	174
Uterus unspecified	5	0	-	-	-	-	-	-	-	-	-	-	3.2	3.2	3.3	-	5.3	7.5	-	-	0.8	0.3	0.05	0.07	0.6	179
Cervix uteri	53	0	-	-	-	-	-	-	-	9.7	7.3	3.3	25.3	12.8	19.5	33.4	21.4	52.5	37.1	17.9	8.2	2.9	0.39	0.66	6.0	180
Placenta	0	0	-	-	-	-	-	-	-	-	-	-	-	-	-	-	-	-	-	-	0.0	0.0	0.00	0.00	0.0	181
Corpus uteri	91	0	-	-	-	-	-	-	1.6	6.5	11.0	26.4	31.7	35.3	42.3	48.3	85.6	37.5	12.4	53.8	14.0	5.0	0.77	1.44	11.3	182
Ovary etc.	66	0	-	-	2.6	-	-	-	4.7	12.9	7.3	9.9	31.7	38.5	13.0	18.6	26.7	15.0	74.2	53.8	10.2	3.7	0.60	0.83	7.8	183
Other female genital	6	0	-	-	-	-	-	-	-	-	1.6	-	-	6.4	-	-	10.7	-	12.4	-	0.9	0.3	0.04	0.09	0.6	184
Bladder	32	0	-	-	-	-	-	-	1.6	-	1.8	-	-	9.6	-	14.9	37.4	22.5	98.9	89.6	4.9	1.8	0.07	0.33	3.0	188
Kidney etc.	25	0	-	-	-	-	-	-	-	1.6	5.5	-	3.2	19.2	6.5	7.4	10.7	37.5	12.4	35.8	3.9	1.4	0.18	0.27	2.7	189
Eye	2	0	-	-	-	-	-	-	-	-	-	1.8	-	-	3.3	-	-	-	-	-	0.3	0.1	0.03	0.03	0.2	190
Brain, nervous system	23	0	2.4	2.6	-	2.2	-	3.4	1.6	-	1.8	9.9	3.2	6.4	3.3	7.4	5.3	30.0	12.4	17.9	3.5	1.3	0.18	0.25	3.1	191-2
Thyroid	53	0	-	-	2.6	8.9	16.3	3.4	4.7	12.9	9.1	13.2	6.3	3.2	16.3	18.6	16.0	7.5	12.4	-	8.2	2.9	0.48	0.66	7.1	193
Other endocrine	2	0	-	-	-	-	-	-	-	3.2	-	-	-	-	-	-	-	-	-	-	0.3	0.1	0.02	0.02	0.2	194
Hodgkin's disease	4	0	-	-	-	4.5	-	3.4	-	-	-	-	-	-	-	-	-	-	-	-	0.6	0.2	0.04	0.04	0.7	201
Non-Hodgkin lymphoma	56	0	2.4	-	-	6.7	2.0	5.1	1.6	6.5	-	13.2	12.7	16.0	13.0	33.4	16.0	67.5	37.1	35.8	8.6	3.1	0.40	0.64	6.9	200,202
Multiple myeloma	20	0	-	-	-	-	-	-	-	-	1.8	3.3	-	6.4	3.3	7.4	26.7	22.5	49.5	17.9	3.1	1.1	0.07	0.24	2.0	203
Lymphoid leukaemia	9	0	2.4	2.6	-	-	-	-	-	-	-	3.7	-	-	-	-	5.3	7.5	-	53.8	1.4	0.5	0.04	0.07	1.2	204
Myeloid leukaemia	23	0	2.4	-	-	2.2	-	5.1	-	-	1.6	-	13.2	-	9.8	7.4	21.4	7.5	24.7	17.9	3.5	1.3	0.17	0.32	3.1	205
Monocytic leukaemia	0	0	-	-	-	-	-	-	-	-	-	-	-	-	-	-	-	-	-	-	0.0	0.0	0.00	0.00	0.0	206
Other leukaemia	0	0	-	-	-	-	-	-	-	-	-	-	-	-	-	-	-	-	-	-	0.0	0.0	0.00	0.00	0.0	207
Leukaemia unspecified	4	0	-	-	-	-	-	-	-	-	-	-	-	-	-	-	-	7.4	-	35.8	0.6	0.2	0.00	0.04	0.4	208
Other and unspecified	71	0	-	-	-	-	-	1.7	3.2	3.2	7.3	9.9	6.3	22.5	19.5	14.9	37.4	82.6	160.8	161.3	11.0	3.9	0.37	0.63	7.2	O&U
All sites	1807	0	9.6	5.2	7.7	26.8	20.3	45.9	66.2	137.3	182.6	322.9	421.0	522.9	563.1	851.0	1160.6	1643.5	1780.9	2616.0	278.8		11.66	21.72	204.3	ALL
All sites but 173	1806	0	9.6	5.2	7.7	26.8	20.3	45.9	66.2	135.7	182.6	322.9	421.0	522.9	563.1	851.0	1160.6	1643.5	1780.9	2616.0	278.6	100.0	11.65	21.71	204.2	ALLb
Rate from 1 case			2.400	2.603	2.578	2.232	2.032	1.701	1.576	1.615	1.826	3.295	3.165	3.208	3.255	3.716	5.348	7.505	12.367	17.918						

†Important: see notes on population page

241

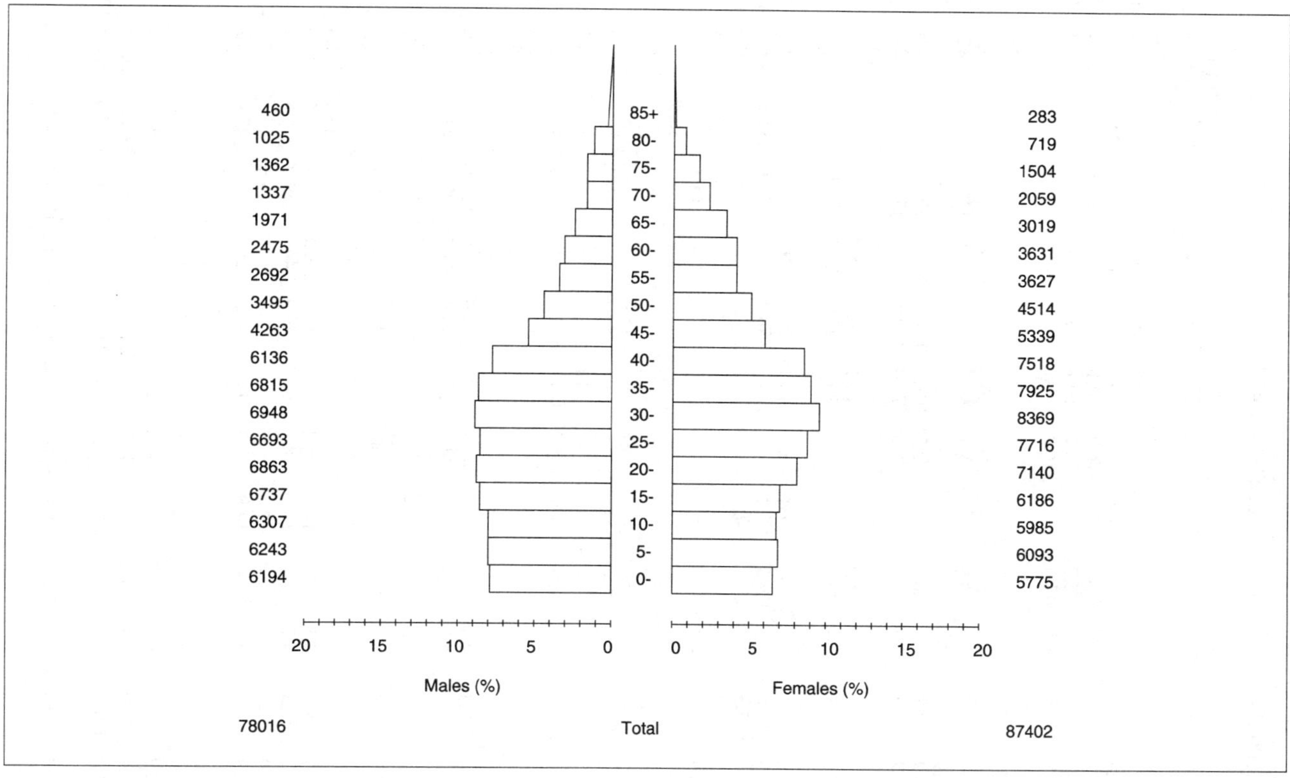

USA, California, San Francisco Bay Area: Filipino
Source of population: average annual 1988–92
Estimate: The years 1988-89 and 1991-92 are bench-marked to the 1990 census, making allowance for births, deaths, and migration into and out of the registration area. Sex-specific totals were apportioned to specific Asian populations based on a 5% sample of the census. The resulting race- and sex-specific population estimates were then apportioned to 5-year age categories based on the race- and sex-specific age distribution in the 100% census counts.
Notes to tables overleaf:
† 173 does not include basal cell or squamous cell carcinoma

USA, CALIFORNIA, SAN FRANCISCO BAY AREA: FILIPINO 1988-1992

ANNUAL INCIDENCE PER 100,000 BY AGE GROUP (YEARS) - MALE

SITE	ALL AGES	AGE UNK	0-	5-	10-	15-	20-	25-	30-	35-	40-	45-	50-	55-	60-	65-	70-	75-	80-	85+	CRUDE RATE	%	CR 64	CR 74	ASR (W)	ICD (9th)
Lip	0	0	-	-	-	-	-	-	-	-	-	-	-	-	-	-	-	-	-	-	0.0	0.0	0.00	0.00	0.0	140
Tongue	5	0	-	-	-	-	-	3.0	-	-	-	-	-	-	-	20.3	15.0	-	-	43.4	1.3	0.5	0.01	0.19	1.4	141
Salivary gland	5	0	-	-	-	-	-	-	-	2.9	-	-	-	7.4	-	-	-	14.7	19.5	43.4	1.3	0.5	0.05	0.05	0.9	142
Mouth	4	0	-	-	-	-	-	-	-	-	-	-	-	-	16.2	10.1	-	-	19.5	-	1.0	0.4	0.08	0.13	1.0	143-5
Oropharynx	4	0	-	-	-	-	-	-	-	-	-	-	5.7	-	8.1	10.1	15.0	-	-	-	1.0	0.4	0.07	0.19	1.2	146
Nasopharynx	18	0	-	-	-	-	-	6.0	5.8	8.8	9.8	9.4	11.4	-	16.2	-	15.0	14.7	-	-	4.6	1.8	0.34	0.41	4.2	147
Hypopharynx	0	0	-	-	-	-	-	-	-	-	-	-	-	-	-	-	-	-	-	-	0.0	0.0	0.00	0.00	0.0	148
Pharynx unspecified	0	0	-	-	-	-	-	-	-	-	-	-	-	-	-	-	-	-	-	-	0.0	0.0	0.00	0.00	0.0	149
Oesophagus	12	0	-	-	-	-	-	-	-	-	-	9.4	5.7	-	-	30.4	-	-	58.5	130.3	3.1	1.2	0.08	0.23	2.7	150
Stomach	32	0	-	-	-	-	-	-	2.9	-	-	-	5.7	-	8.1	50.7	89.7	161.5	117.1	43.4	8.2	3.1	0.08	0.79	6.5	151
Small intestine	2	0	-	-	-	-	-	-	-	-	2.9	-	-	7.4	-	-	-	-	-	-	0.5	0.2	0.05	0.05	0.5	152
Colon	82	0	-	-	-	3.0	2.9	-	2.9	5.9	9.8	14.1	40.1	37.1	72.7	101.4	164.5	161.5	273.1	173.7	21.0	8.0	0.94	2.27	19.0	153
Rectum	50	0	-	-	-	-	-	3.0	2.9	5.9	3.3	4.7	11.4	37.1	48.5	71.0	119.6	73.4	175.6	86.8	12.8	4.9	0.58	1.54	11.8	154
Liver	42	0	3.2	-	-	-	-	-	2.9	-	-	14.1	-	59.4	48.5	30.4	134.6	58.7	78.0	130.3	10.8	4.1	0.64	1.47	11.0	155
Gallbladder etc.	10	0	-	-	-	-	-	-	-	-	-	-	5.7	-	10.1	29.9	58.7	19.5	43.4	2.6	1.0	0.03	0.23	2.1	156
Pancreas	27	0	-	-	-	-	-	-	-	2.9	3.3	9.4	17.2	14.9	16.2	10.1	29.9	88.1	78.0	130.3	6.9	2.6	0.32	0.52	5.9	157
Nose, sinuses etc.	4	0	-	-	-	-	-	3.0	-	-	-	-	5.7	-	-	10.1	-	-	19.5	-	1.0	0.4	0.04	0.09	0.9	160
Larynx	6	0	-	-	-	-	-	-	-	-	-	-	-	7.4	8.1	10.1	15.0	29.4	-	-	1.5	0.6	0.08	0.20	1.5	161
Bronchus, lung	182	0	-	-	-	-	-	-	-	5.9	13.0	28.1	108.7	156.0	234.3	284.0	358.9	367.1	273.1	434.2	46.7	17.8	2.73	5.95	46.8	162
Other thoracic organs	3	0	-	-	-	3.0	-	-	-	-	3.3	-	-	7.4	-	-	-	-	-	-	0.8	0.3	0.07	0.07	0.8	163-4
Bone	2	0	-	-	-	-	-	3.0	-	-	3.3	-	-	-	-	-	-	-	-	-	0.5	0.2	0.03	0.03	0.4	170
Connective tissue	5	0	-	-	-	-	-	-	-	5.9	3.3	4.7	-	-	-	-	-	-	19.5	-	1.3	0.5	0.07	0.07	0.9	171
Mesothelioma	4	0	-	-	-	-	-	-	-	-	-	-	-	-	8.1	-	-	14.7	-	86.8	1.0	0.4	0.04	0.04	0.9	MES
Kaposi's sarcoma	22	0	-	-	-	-	-	9.0	8.6	14.7	16.3	28.1	-	-	-	-	-	-	-	-	5.6	2.1	0.38	0.38	4.8	KAP
Melanoma of skin	4	0	-	-	-	3.0	-	-	-	-	-	-	-	-	8.1	-	15.0	-	-	43.4	1.0	0.4	0.06	0.13	1.1	172
†Other skin	0	0	-	-	-	-	-	-	-	-	-	-	-	-	-	-	-	-	-	-	0.0	0.0	0.00	0.00	0.0	173
Breast	2	0	-	-	-	-	-	-	-	-	-	-	-	-	-	10.1	-	-	-	43.4	0.5	0.2	0.00	0.05	0.5	175
Prostate	243	0	-	-	-	-	-	-	-	-	-	4.7	28.6	14.9	145.5	314.5	822.4	734.1	975.4	1346.1	62.3	23.7	0.97	6.65	53.0	185
Testis	7	0	-	-	-	-	-	6.0	5.8	-	6.5	-	-	-	-	15.0	-	-	-	-	1.8	0.7	0.09	0.17	1.5	186
Penis	1	0	-	-	-	-	-	-	-	-	-	-	-	-	-	-	-	14.7	-	-	0.3	0.1	0.00	0.00	0.1	187.1-.4
Other male genital	1	0	-	-	-	-	-	-	-	-	-	-	-	-	-	-	-	14.7	-	-	0.3	0.1	0.00	0.00	0.1	187.5-.9
Bladder	35	0	-	-	-	-	-	-	2.9	-	3.3	9.4	17.2	14.9	40.4	-	134.6	88.1	117.1	-	9.0	3.4	0.44	1.11	8.2	188
Kidney etc.	27	0	-	-	-	3.0	-	-	-	-	-	14.1	22.9	7.4	24.2	30.4	44.9	58.7	78.0	43.4	6.9	2.6	0.36	0.73	6.5	189
Eye	0	0	-	-	-	-	-	-	-	-	-	-	-	-	-	-	-	-	-	-	0.0	0.0	0.00	0.00	0.0	190
Brain, nervous system	20	0	3.2	-	-	-	-	-	8.6	5.9	3.3	4.7	-	29.7	8.1	20.3	74.8	-	-	-	5.1	2.0	0.32	0.79	5.4	191-2
Thyroid	15	0	-	-	-	-	-	-	5.8	5.9	3.3	-	11.4	-	16.2	-	44.9	14.7	39.0	-	3.8	1.5	0.21	0.44	3.4	193
Other endocrine	2	0	3.2	-	-	-	-	-	2.9	-	-	-	-	-	-	-	-	-	-	-	0.5	0.2	0.03	0.03	0.6	194
Hodgkin's disease	5	0	-	-	6.3	3.0	-	-	2.9	-	-	-	-	-	-	-	-	-	-	43.4	1.2	0.5	0.06	0.06	1.2	201
Non-Hodgkin lymphoma	48	0	-	-	-	-	-	-	5.8	14.7	9.8	23.5	5.7	14.9	24.2	60.9	119.6	102.8	97.5	43.4	12.3	4.7	0.49	1.39	11.0	200,202
Multiple myeloma	20	0	-	-	-	-	-	-	-	-	3.3	4.7	-	14.9	8.1	60.9	29.9	44.0	39.0	86.8	5.1	2.0	0.15	0.61	4.9	203
Lymphoid leukaemia	13	0	9.7	-	-	-	5.8	-	5.8	2.9	-	-	11.4	7.4	-	-	-	14.7	19.5	-	3.3	1.3	0.22	0.22	3.3	204
Myeloid leukaemia	19	0	-	3.2	3.2	-	2.9	-	2.9	2.9	3.3	9.4	-	14.9	32.3	10.1	15.0	29.4	-	43.4	4.9	1.9	0.37	0.50	4.9	205
Monocytic leukaemia	2	0	-	-	-	-	-	-	-	-	-	-	-	-	-	10.1	-	-	19.5	-	0.5	0.2	0.00	0.05	0.4	206
Other leukaemia	2	0	-	-	-	-	-	-	-	-	-	-	-	7.4	-	-	-	14.7	-	-	0.5	0.2	0.04	0.04	0.4	207
Leukaemia unspecified	3	0	-	-	-	-	-	-	-	-	-	4.7	-	-	-	-	15.0	14.7	-	-	0.8	0.3	0.02	0.10	0.7	208
Other and unspecified	34	0	-	-	-	-	2.9	-	-	2.9	3.3	9.4	22.9	29.7	56.6	20.3	15.0	102.8	58.5	43.4	8.7	3.3	0.64	0.81	8.2	O&U
All sites	1024	0	19.4	3.2	9.5	14.8	14.6	32.9	69.1	91.0	101.0	206.4	337.6	490.3	848.5	1186.9	2332.5	2290.4	2594.6	3082.9	262.5		11.19	28.79	240.7	ALL
All sites but 173	1024	0	19.4	3.2	9.5	14.8	14.6	32.9	69.1	91.0	101.0	206.4	337.6	490.3	848.5	1186.9	2332.5	2290.4	2594.6	3082.9	262.5	100.0	11.19	28.79	240.7	ALLb

Rate from 1 case: 3.229 3.203 3.171 2.969 2.914 2.988 2.878 2.935 3.259 4.691 5.722 7.429 8.081 10.144 14.952 14.682 19.508 43.422

†Important: see notes on population page

USA, CALIFORNIA, SAN FRANCISCO BAY AREA: FILIPINO 1988-1992

ANNUAL INCIDENCE PER 100,000 BY AGE GROUP (YEARS) - FEMALE

SITE	ALL AGES	AGE UNK	0-	5-	10-	15-	20-	25-	30-	35-	40-	45-	50-	55-	60-	65-	70-	75-	80-	85+	CRUDE RATE	%	CR 64	CR 74	ASR (W)	ICD (9th)
Lip	3	0	-	-	-	-	-	-	-	-	2.7	-	-	-	-	-	19.4	-	-	-	0.7	0.3	0.01	0.11	**0.5**	*140*
Tongue	3	0	-	-	-	-	-	-	-	-	2.7	-	-	-	5.5	-	-	-	-	70.6	0.7	0.3	0.04	0.04	**0.7**	*141*
Salivary gland	8	0	-	-	-	-	-	-	5.0	-	2.7	-	8.9	-	11.0	6.6	-	-	-	-	1.8	0.8	0.14	0.17	**1.5**	*142*
Mouth	9	0	-	-	-	-	-	2.6	-	2.5	-	-	-	5.5	-	19.9	19.4	13.3	-	-	2.1	0.9	0.05	0.25	**1.7**	*143-5*
Oropharynx	3	0	-	-	-	-	-	-	-	-	-	-	-	-	-	6.6	-	13.3	27.8	-	0.7	0.3	0.00	0.03	**0.5**	*146*
Nasopharynx	5	0	-	-	-	-	-	-	-	-	2.7	3.7	4.4	5.5	-	-	9.7	-	-	-	1.1	0.5	0.08	0.13	**1.0**	*147*
Hypopharynx	2	0	-	-	-	-	-	-	-	-	-	-	4.4	-	5.5	-	-	-	-	-	0.5	0.2	0.05	0.05	**0.4**	*148*
Pharynx unspecified	0	0	-	-	-	-	-	-	-	-	-	-	-	-	-	-	-	-	-	-	0.0	0.0	0.00	0.00	**0.0**	*149*
Oesophagus	1	0	-	-	-	-	-	-	-	-	-	-	-	-	-	6.6	-	-	-	-	0.2	0.1	0.00	0.03	**0.2**	*150*
Stomach	21	0	-	-	-	-	-	-	-	-	2.7	3.7	-	-	11.0	53.0	19.4	39.9	55.6	141.2	4.8	2.1	0.09	0.45	**4.2**	*151*
Small intestine	0	0	-	-	-	-	-	-	-	-	-	-	-	-	-	-	-	-	-	-	0.0	0.0	0.00	0.00	**0.0**	*152*
Colon	45	0	-	-	-	-	-	2.6	-	-	8.0	18.7	17.7	27.6	33.0	46.4	38.8	53.2	139.0	70.6	10.3	4.5	0.54	0.96	**8.9**	*153*
Rectum	46	0	-	-	-	-	-	-	7.2	5.0	8.0	7.5	17.7	33.1	22.0	46.4	77.7	66.5	55.6	-	10.5	4.6	0.50	1.12	**8.6**	*154*
Liver	22	0	-	-	-	-	-	-	-	2.5	2.7	-	4.4	5.5	11.0	19.9	38.8	93.1	-	141.2	5.0	2.2	0.13	0.42	**4.2**	*155*
Gallbladder etc.	13	0	-	-	-	-	-	-	-	-	2.7	-	4.4	-	5.5	26.5	9.7	26.6	55.6	70.6	3.0	1.3	0.06	0.24	**2.5**	*156*
Pancreas	27	0	-	-	3.3	-	-	-	-	-	2.7	3.7	4.4	-	16.5	39.7	58.3	66.5	55.6	70.6	6.2	2.7	0.15	0.64	**5.2**	*157*
Nose, sinuses etc.	3	0	-	-	-	-	-	-	2.4	-	2.7	-	-	-	-	-	-	13.3	-	-	0.7	0.3	0.03	0.03	**0.4**	*160*
Larynx	3	0	-	-	-	-	-	-	-	-	-	-	8.9	-	5.5	-	-	-	-	-	0.7	0.3	0.07	0.07	**0.7**	*161*
Bronchus, lung	82	0	-	-	-	-	-	2.6	4.8	7.6	5.3	22.5	53.2	44.1	33.0	72.9	165.1	132.9	83.4	70.6	18.8	8.1	0.87	2.05	**15.9**	*162*
Other thoracic organs	1	0	-	-	-	-	-	-	-	-	-	-	-	-	-	-	-	13.3	-	-	0.2	0.1	0.00	0.00	**0.1**	*163-4*
Bone	4	0	-	-	-	3.2	2.8	-	-	-	2.7	-	4.4	-	-	-	-	-	-	-	0.9	0.4	0.07	0.07	**0.9**	*170*
Connective tissue	5	0	-	-	-	-	-	-	2.4	-	-	3.7	4.4	5.5	-	-	9.7	-	-	-	1.1	0.5	0.08	0.13	**1.0**	*171*
Mesothelioma	1	0	-	-	-	-	-	-	-	-	-	-	-	-	-	-	9.7	-	-	-	0.2	0.1	0.00	0.00	**0.2**	*MES*
Kaposi's sarcoma	0	0	-	-	-	-	-	-	-	-	-	-	-	-	-	-	-	-	-	-	0.0	0.0	0.00	0.00	**0.0**	*KAP*
Melanoma of skin	5	0	-	-	-	-	-	-	-	-	-	3.7	-	5.5	-	6.6	-	26.6	-	-	1.1	0.5	0.05	0.08	**0.9**	*172*
†Other skin	2	0	-	-	-	-	2.8	-	-	-	-	-	4.4	-	-	-	-	-	-	-	0.5		0.04	0.04	**0.4**	*173*
Breast	333	0	-	-	-	-	-	7.8	26.3	73.2	103.7	191.0	168.4	193.0	214.8	238.5	242.7	226.0	194.7	211.9	76.2	33.1	4.89	7.30	**65.3**	*174*
Uterus unspecified	1	0	-	-	-	-	-	-	-	-	-	-	4.4	-	-	-	-	-	-	-	0.2	0.1	0.02	0.02	**0.2**	*179*
Cervix uteri	49	0	-	-	-	-	-	2.6	9.6	17.7	10.6	37.5	22.2	16.5	27.5	39.7	19.4	13.3	-	70.6	11.2	4.9	0.72	1.02	**9.7**	*180*
Placenta	1	0	-	-	-	-	2.8	-	-	-	-	-	-	-	-	-	-	-	-	-	0.2	0.1	0.01	0.01	**0.2**	*181*
Corpus uteri	48	0	-	-	-	-	-	-	-	10.1	16.0	22.5	39.9	22.1	38.6	53.0	9.7	39.9	-	-	11.0	4.8	0.75	1.06	**9.5**	*182*
Ovary etc.	36	0	-	-	6.7	3.2	2.8	2.6	2.4	5.0	5.3	3.7	22.2	33.1	27.5	26.5	19.4	26.6	27.8	-	8.2	3.6	0.57	0.80	**7.4**	*183*
Other female genital	7	0	-	-	-	-	-	2.6	-	2.5	-	-	-	5.5	11.0	6.6	9.7	-	-	-	1.6	0.7	0.11	0.19	**1.4**	*184*
Bladder	11	0	-	-	-	-	-	2.6	-	-	-	-	4.4	-	16.5	13.2	9.7	13.3	27.8	70.6	2.5	1.1	0.12	0.23	**2.3**	*188*
Kidney etc.	14	0	-	-	-	-	-	2.6	-	2.5	-	3.7	8.9	-	11.0	6.6	19.4	26.6	55.6	-	3.2	1.4	0.14	0.27	**2.6**	*189*
Eye	0	0	-	-	-	-	-	-	-	-	-	-	-	-	-	-	-	-	-	-	0.0	0.0	0.00	0.00	**0.0**	*190*
Brain, nervous system	13	0	-	-	3.3	3.2	-	5.2	-	-	5.3	3.7	4.4	11.0	5.5	-	9.7	-	-	70.6	3.0	1.3	0.21	0.26	**3.0**	*191-2*
Thyroid	56	0	-	-	-	-	8.4	13.0	11.9	27.8	8.0	7.5	22.2	33.1	27.5	13.2	38.8	53.2	-	70.6	12.8	5.6	0.80	1.06	**10.6**	*193*
Other endocrine	1	0	-	-	-	-	-	-	-	-	-	-	4.4	-	-	-	-	-	-	-	0.2	0.1	0.02	0.02	**0.2**	*194*
Hodgkin's disease	4	0	-	-	-	-	2.8	-	4.8	-	-	-	-	-	-	6.6	-	-	-	-	0.9	0.4	0.04	0.07	**0.7**	*201*
Non-Hodgkin lymphoma	42	0	-	-	-	-	-	-	2.4	2.5	2.7	11.2	4.4	16.5	22.0	39.7	106.8	79.8	55.6	211.9	9.6	4.2	0.31	1.04	**8.4**	*200,202*
Multiple myeloma	12	0	-	-	-	-	-	-	-	-	-	3.7	4.4	11.0	-	-	19.4	66.5	-	70.6	2.7	1.2	0.10	0.19	**2.3**	*203*
Lymphoid leukaemia	12	0	6.9	13.1	-	-	-	2.6	2.4	-	-	-	4.4	-	5.5	-	-	26.6	-	-	2.7	1.2	0.17	0.17	**3.2**	*204*
Myeloid leukaemia	17	0	-	6.6	-	-	-	2.6	-	2.5	-	7.5	8.9	16.5	-	13.2	9.7	26.6	27.8	-	3.9	1.7	0.22	0.34	**3.6**	*205*
Monocytic leukaemia	1	0	-	-	-	-	-	-	-	-	-	3.7	-	-	-	-	-	-	-	-	0.2	0.1	0.02	0.02	**0.2**	*206*
Other leukaemia	1	0	-	-	-	-	-	-	-	-	-	-	-	-	-	-	-	-	27.8	-	0.2	0.1	0.00	0.00	**0.1**	*207*
Leukaemia unspecified	4	0	6.9	-	-	-	-	-	-	-	-	-	-	-	5.5	6.6	-	-	-	-	0.9	0.4	0.06	0.10	**1.3**	*208*
Other and unspecified	32	0	3.5	-	-	-	2.8	-	-	5.0	2.7	22.5	4.4	-	11.0	46.4	9.7	26.6	222.5	-	7.3	3.2	0.26	0.54	**6.1**	*O&U*
All sites	1009	0	17.3	19.7	13.4	9.7	25.2	51.8	76.5	171.6	202.2	385.8	469.7	490.8	583.8	861.1	1000.1	1183.2	1112.3	1412.4	230.9		12.59	21.89	**199.2**	*ALL*
All sites but 173	1007	0	17.3	19.7	13.4	9.7	22.4	51.8	76.5	171.6	202.2	385.8	465.2	490.8	583.8	861.1	1000.1	1183.2	1112.3	1412.4	230.4	100.0	12.55	21.86	**198.8**	*ALLb*

Rate from 1 case   3.463 3.282 3.342 3.233 2.801 2.592 2.390 2.523 2.660 3.745 4.431 5.514 5.508 6.624 9.710 13.294 27.809 70.621

†Important: see notes on population page

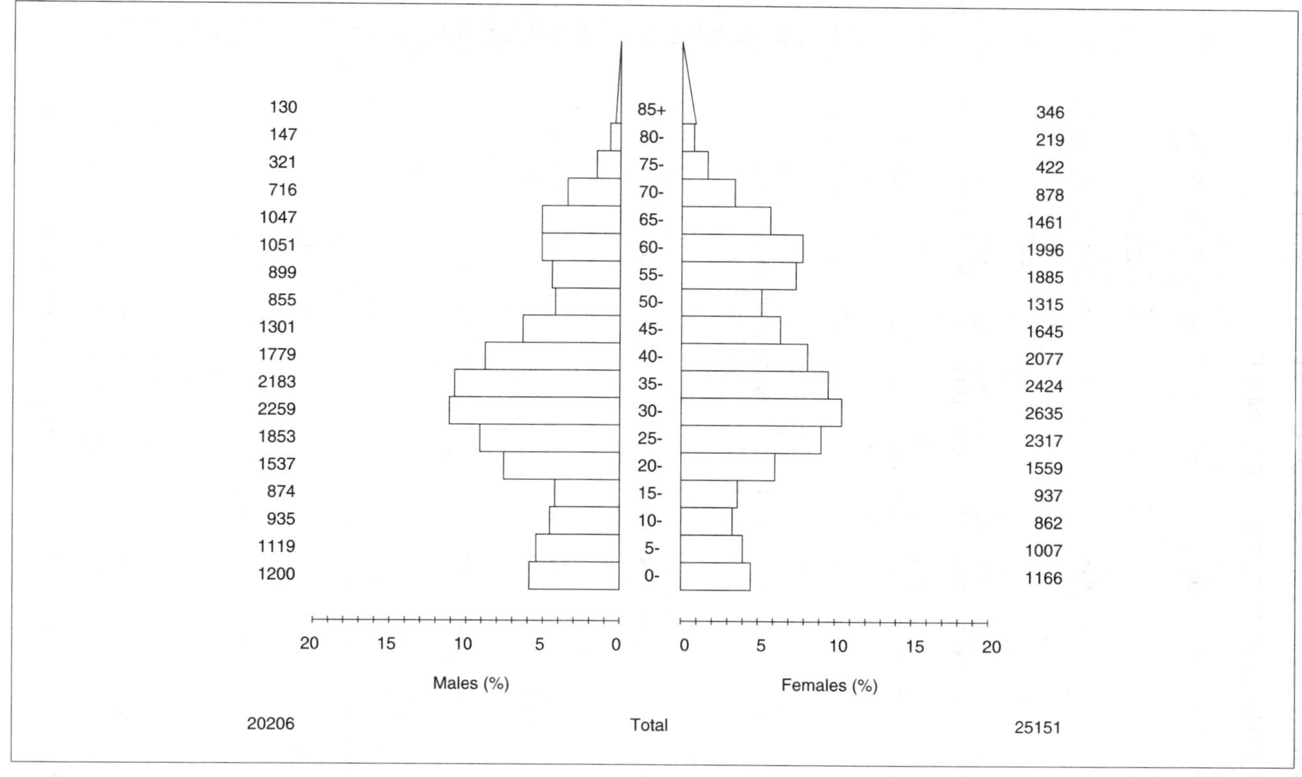

USA, California, San Francisco Bay Area: Japanese
Source of population: average annual 1988–92
Estimate: The years 1988-89 and 1991-92 are bench-marked to the 1990 census, making allowance for births, deaths, and migration into and out of the registration area. Sex-specific totals were apportioned to specific Asian populations based on a 5% sample of the census. The resulting race- and sex-specific population estimates were then apportioned to 5-year age categories based on the race- and sex-specific age distribution in the 100% census counts.

Notes to tables overleaf:
† 173 does not include basal cell or squamous cell carcinoma

USA, CALIFORNIA, SAN FRANCISCO BAY AREA: JAPANESE 1988-1992

ANNUAL INCIDENCE PER 100,000 BY AGE GROUP (YEARS) - MALE

SITE	ALL AGES	UNK	0-	5-	10-	15-	20-	25-	30-	35-	40-	45-	50-	55-	60-	65-	70-	75-	80-	85+	CRUDE RATE	%	CR 64	CR 74	ASR (W)	ICD (9th)
Lip	0	0	-	-	-	-	-	-	-	-	-	-	-	-	-	-	-	-	-	-	0.0	0.0	0.00	0.00	0.0	140
Tongue	1	0	-	-	-	-	-	-	-	-	-	-	-	-	-	-	-	62.2	-	-	1.0	0.3	0.00	0.00	0.6	141
Salivary gland	0	0	-	-	-	-	-	-	-	-	-	-	-	-	-	-	-	-	-	-	0.0	0.0	0.00	0.00	0.0	142
Mouth	2	0	-	-	-	-	-	-	-	-	-	-	46.8	-	-	-	-	-	-	-	2.0	0.6	0.23	0.23	2.3	143-5
Oropharynx	0	0	-	-	-	-	-	-	-	-	-	-	-	-	-	-	-	-	-	-	0.0	0.0	0.00	0.00	0.0	146
Nasopharynx	0	0	-	-	-	-	-	-	-	-	-	-	-	-	-	-	-	-	-	-	0.0	0.0	0.00	0.00	0.0	147
Hypopharynx	1	0	-	-	-	-	-	-	-	-	-	-	-	-	-	-	-	62.2	-	-	1.0	0.3	0.00	0.00	0.6	148
Pharynx unspecified	0	0	-	-	-	-	-	-	-	-	-	-	-	-	-	-	-	-	-	-	0.0	0.0	0.00	0.00	0.0	149
Oesophagus	14	0	-	-	-	-	-	-	-	9.2	-	-	23.4	44.5	38.0	95.5	55.9	62.2	-	-	13.9	3.9	0.58	1.33	9.6	150
Stomach	36	0	-	-	-	22.9	-	-	-	-	-	30.7	23.4	22.2	95.1	114.6	195.5	124.3	680.3	921.7	35.6	10.1	0.97	2.52	26.4	151
Small intestine	0	0	-	-	-	-	-	-	-	-	-	-	-	-	-	-	-	-	-	-	0.0	0.0	0.00	0.00	0.0	152
Colon	39	0	-	-	-	-	-	-	-	-	-	15.4	23.4	111.2	38.0	171.9	335.2	248.6	272.1	460.8	38.6	10.9	0.94	3.48	26.1	153
Rectum	28	0	-	-	-	-	-	-	-	9.2	11.2	15.4	-	44.5	171.2	76.4	139.7	62.2	408.2	153.6	27.7	7.8	1.26	2.34	19.3	154
Liver	8	0	-	-	-	-	-	-	-	-	-	-	-	44.5	38.0	-	55.9	124.3	-	-	7.9	2.2	0.41	0.69	5.7	155
Gallbladder etc.	4	0	-	-	-	-	-	-	-	-	-	15.4	-	-	-	-	55.9	-	-	153.6	4.0	1.1	0.08	0.36	2.8	156
Pancreas	11	0	-	-	-	-	-	-	-	-	-	-	23.4	-	-	19.1	27.9	248.6	272.1	307.2	10.9	3.1	0.12	0.35	7.7	157
Nose, sinuses etc.	1	0	-	-	-	-	-	-	-	-	-	-	-	-	19.0	-	-	-	-	-	1.0	0.3	0.10	0.10	0.8	160
Larynx	4	0	-	-	-	-	-	-	-	-	11.2	-	-	-	38.0	-	-	-	136.1	-	4.0	1.1	0.25	0.25	2.9	161
Bronchus, lung	54	0	-	-	-	-	-	-	8.9	-	11.2	30.7	23.4	88.9	133.1	191.0	363.1	683.7	408.2	153.6	53.4	15.1	1.48	4.25	35.7	162
Other thoracic organs	0	0	-	-	-	-	-	-	-	-	-	-	-	-	-	-	-	-	-	-	0.0	0.0	0.00	0.00	0.0	163-4
Bone	1	0	-	-	-	-	-	-	-	-	-	-	-	-	-	19.1	-	-	-	-	1.0	0.3	0.00	0.10	0.6	170
Connective tissue	3	0	-	-	-	22.9	-	-	-	9.2	-	15.4	-	-	-	-	-	-	-	-	3.0	0.8	0.24	0.24	3.5	171
Mesothelioma	1	0	-	-	-	-	-	-	-	-	-	-	-	-	-	-	-	62.2	-	-	1.0	0.3	0.00	0.00	0.6	MES
Kaposi's sarcoma	8	0	-	-	-	-	-	-	8.9	18.3	22.5	15.4	23.4	-	-	-	-	62.2	-	-	7.9	2.2	0.44	0.44	5.7	KAP
Melanoma of skin	1	0	-	-	-	-	-	-	-	-	-	-	-	-	-	-	27.9	-	-	-	1.0	0.3	0.00	0.14	0.6	172
†Other skin	0	0	-	-	-	-	-	-	-	-	-	-	-	-	-	-	-	-	-	-	0.0	0.0	0.00	0.00	0.0	173
Breast	0	0	-	-	-	-	-	-	-	-	-	-	-	-	-	-	-	-	-	-	0.0	0.0	0.00	0.00	0.0	175
Prostate	66	0	-	-	-	-	-	-	-	-	-	-	46.8	88.9	19.0	229.2	446.9	994.4	1224.5	921.7	65.3	18.4	0.77	4.15	43.1	185
Testis	8	0	-	-	-	-	-	54.0	-	18.3	11.2	-	-	-	-	-	-	-	-	-	7.9	2.2	0.42	0.42	6.1	186
Penis	1	0	-	-	-	-	-	-	-	-	-	-	-	-	-	-	19.1	-	-	-	1.0	0.3	0.00	0.10	0.6	187.1-.4
Other male genital	0	0	-	-	-	-	-	-	-	-	-	-	-	-	-	-	-	-	-	-	0.0	0.0	0.00	0.00	0.0	187.5-.9
Bladder	17	0	-	-	-	-	-	-	8.9	-	-	15.4	23.4	-	19.0	95.5	55.9	124.3	-	614.4	16.8	4.7	0.33	1.09	11.7	188
Kidney etc.	8	0	16.7	-	-	-	-	-	-	-	-	-	-	76.1	38.2	-	62.2	-	-	-	7.9	2.2	0.46	0.65	6.8	189
Eye	0	0	-	-	-	-	-	-	-	-	-	-	-	-	-	-	-	-	-	-	0.0	0.0	0.00	0.00	0.0	190
Brain, nervous system	4	0	-	-	-	-	-	-	-	-	11.2	15.4	-	-	-	19.1	-	62.2	-	-	4.0	1.1	0.13	0.23	2.8	191-2
Thyroid	3	0	-	-	-	-	-	10.8	-	-	-	-	23.4	-	-	-	-	27.9	-	-	3.0	0.8	0.17	0.31	2.6	193
Other endocrine	1	0	-	-	-	-	-	-	8.9	-	-	-	-	-	-	-	-	-	-	-	1.0	0.3	0.04	0.04	0.5	194
Hodgkin's disease	3	0	-	-	-	-	-	10.8	-	-	-	-	-	-	-	19.1	-	62.2	-	-	3.0	0.8	0.05	0.15	2.1	201
Non-Hodgkin lymphoma	14	0	-	-	-	-	-	-	-	9.2	11.2	30.7	23.4	-	19.0	38.2	55.9	124.3	136.1	153.6	13.9	3.9	0.47	0.94	10.0	200,202
Multiple myeloma	3	0	-	-	-	-	-	-	-	-	-	-	23.4	-	-	19.1	-	62.2	-	-	3.0	0.8	0.12	0.21	2.4	203
Lymphoid leukaemia	1	0	-	17.9	-	-	-	-	-	-	-	-	-	-	-	-	-	-	-	-	1.0	0.3	0.09	0.09	1.8	204
Myeloid leukaemia	5	0	-	-	-	-	-	-	-	-	11.2	15.4	-	22.2	-	-	-	-	62.2	-	153.6	4.9	1.4	0.24	0.24	3.9	205
Monocytic leukaemia	0	0	-	-	-	-	-	-	-	-	-	-	-	-	-	-	-	-	-	-	0.0	0.0	0.00	0.00	0.0	206
Other leukaemia	0	0	-	-	-	-	-	-	-	-	-	-	-	-	-	-	-	-	-	-	0.0	0.0	0.00	0.00	0.0	207
Leukaemia unspecified	0	0	-	-	-	-	-	-	-	-	-	-	-	-	-	-	-	-	-	-	0.0	0.0	0.00	0.00	0.0	208
Other and unspecified	7	0	-	-	-	-	-	-	-	-	-	-	-	-	19.0	38.2	55.9	-	-	307.2	6.9	2.0	0.10	0.57	4.6	O&U
All sites	358	0	16.7	17.9	-	45.7	-	75.6	35.4	73.3	101.2	-	327.5	466.9	722.7	1203.4	1899.4	3356.1	3537.4	4301.1	354.3		10.49	26.00	250.3	ALL
All sites but 173	358	0	16.7	17.9	-	45.7	-	75.6	35.4	73.3	101.2	-	327.5	466.9	722.7	1203.4	1899.4	3356.1	3537.4	4301.1	354.3	100.0	10.49	26.00	250.3	ALLb

Rate from 1 case   16.664 17.867 21.390 22.873 13.006 10.793 8.852 9.160 11.240 15.370 23.392 22.232 19.019 19.102 27.933 62.150 136.05 153.61

†Important: see notes on population page

USA, CALIFORNIA, SAN FRANCISCO BAY AREA: JAPANESE 1988-1992

ANNUAL INCIDENCE PER 100,000 BY AGE GROUP (YEARS) - FEMALE

SITE	ALL AGES	AGE UNK	0-	5-	10-	15-	20-	25-	30-	35-	40-	45-	50-	55-	60-	65-	70-	75-	80-	85+	CRUDE RATE	%	CR 64	CR 74	ASR (W)	ICD (9th)
Lip	1	0	-	-	-	-	-	-	-	-	-	-	15.2	-	-	-	-	-	-	-	0.8	0.2	0.08	0.08	**0.8**	140
Tongue	4	0	-	-	-	-	-	-	-	-	-	-	-	10.6	10.0	13.7	22.8	-	-	-	3.2	0.9	0.10	0.29	**1.7**	141
Salivary gland	3	0	-	-	-	-	-	-	8.2	-	-	-	-	-	-	-	45.6	-	-	-	2.4	0.7	0.04	0.27	**1.4**	142
Mouth	2	0	-	-	-	-	-	-	-	-	12.2	-	-	-	-	-	-	-	-	57.7	1.6	0.5	0.06	0.06	**1.0**	143-5
Oropharynx	0	0	-	-	-	-	-	-	-	-	-	-	-	-	-	-	-	-	-	-	0.0	0.0	0.00	0.00	**0.0**	146
Nasopharynx	0	0	-	-	-	-	-	-	-	-	-	-	-	-	-	-	-	-	-	-	0.0	0.0	0.00	0.00	**0.0**	147
Hypopharynx	0	0	-	-	-	-	-	-	-	-	-	-	-	-	-	-	-	-	-	-	0.0	0.0	0.00	0.00	**0.0**	148
Pharynx unspecified	0	0	-	-	-	-	-	-	-	-	-	-	-	-	-	-	-	-	-	-	0.0	0.0	0.00	0.00	**0.0**	149
Oesophagus	1	0	-	-	-	-	-	-	-	-	-	-	-	-	10.0	-	-	-	-	-	0.8	0.2	0.05	0.05	**0.4**	150
Stomach	25	0	-	-	-	-	-	-	7.6	-	9.6	24.3	45.6	31.8	30.1	27.4	91.1	-	91.2	288.7	19.9	5.7	0.75	1.34	**11.8**	151
Small intestine	0	0	-	-	-	-	-	-	-	-	-	-	-	-	-	-	-	-	-	-	0.0	0.0	0.00	0.00	**0.0**	152
Colon	57	0	-	-	-	-	-	8.6	7.6	8.2	-	12.2	106.4	53.1	80.1	95.8	250.6	283.8	365.0	288.7	45.3	13.0	1.38	3.11	**27.0**	153
Rectum	19	0	-	-	-	-	-	-	-	-	28.9	-	-	10.6	30.1	41.1	91.1	94.6	91.2	115.5	15.1	4.3	0.35	1.01	**8.4**	154
Liver	5	0	-	-	-	-	-	-	-	-	-	-	-	21.2	10.0	13.7	-	-	91.2	-	4.0	1.1	0.16	0.22	**2.1**	155
Gallbladder etc.	8	0	-	-	-	-	-	-	-	-	-	-	-	10.6	10.0	-	68.3	-	91.2	115.5	6.4	1.8	0.10	0.44	**3.2**	156
Pancreas	9	0	-	-	-	-	-	-	-	-	-	12.2	-	-	20.0	13.7	-	47.3	-	230.9	7.2	2.1	0.16	0.23	**3.6**	157
Nose, sinuses etc.	0	0	-	-	-	-	-	-	-	-	-	-	-	-	-	-	-	-	-	-	0.0	0.0	0.00	0.00	**0.0**	160
Larynx	1	0	-	-	-	-	-	-	-	-	-	-	-	10.6	-	-	-	-	-	-	0.8	0.2	0.05	0.05	**0.4**	161
Bronchus, lung	32	0	-	-	-	-	-	-	-	-	9.6	12.2	60.8	53.1	70.1	82.1	68.3	141.9	-	115.5	25.4	7.3	1.03	1.78	**15.1**	162
Other thoracic organs	0	0	-	-	-	-	-	-	-	-	-	-	-	-	-	-	-	-	-	-	0.0	0.0	0.00	0.00	**0.0**	163-4
Bone	0	0	-	-	-	-	-	-	-	-	-	-	-	-	-	-	-	-	-	-	0.0	0.0	0.00	0.00	**0.0**	170
Connective tissue	2	0	17.1	-	-	-	-	-	-	-	-	-	-	-	-	13.7	-	-	-	-	1.6	0.5	0.09	0.15	**2.5**	171
Mesothelioma	0	0	-	-	-	-	-	-	-	-	-	-	-	-	-	-	-	-	-	-	0.0	0.0	0.00	0.00	**0.0**	MES
Kaposi's sarcoma	0	0	-	-	-	-	-	-	-	-	-	-	-	-	-	-	-	-	-	-	0.0	0.0	0.00	0.00	**0.0**	KAP
Melanoma of skin	1	0	-	-	-	-	-	8.6	-	-	-	-	-	-	-	-	-	-	-	-	0.8	0.2	0.04	0.04	**0.7**	172
†Other skin	0	0	-	-	-	-	-	-	-	-	-	-	-	-	-	-	-	-	-	-	0.0	0.0	0.00	0.00	**0.0**	173
Breast	138	0	-	-	-	-	-	17.3	37.9	41.2	134.8	145.9	152.0	212.2	180.3	314.8	341.7	378.4	182.5	230.9	109.7	31.6	4.61	7.89	**68.4**	174
Uterus unspecified	0	0	-	-	-	-	-	-	-	-	-	-	-	-	-	-	-	-	-	-	0.0	0.0	0.00	0.00	**0.0**	179
Cervix uteri	11	0	-	-	-	-	-	8.6	7.6	-	19.3	24.3	-	10.6	20.0	13.7	-	-	91.2	-	8.7	2.5	0.45	0.52	**5.9**	180
Placenta	0	0	-	-	-	-	-	-	-	-	-	-	-	-	-	-	-	-	-	-	0.0	0.0	0.00	0.00	**0.0**	181
Corpus uteri	33	0	-	-	-	-	-	-	-	8.2	19.3	36.5	45.6	31.8	40.1	95.8	136.7	189.2	-	-	26.2	7.6	0.91	2.07	**16.5**	182
Ovary etc.	16	0	-	-	-	-	-	-	-	8.2	-	12.2	15.2	53.1	10.0	41.1	22.8	94.6	-	57.7	12.7	3.7	0.49	0.81	**7.4**	183
Other female genital	0	0	-	-	-	-	-	-	-	-	-	-	-	-	-	-	-	-	-	-	0.0	0.0	0.00	0.00	**0.0**	184
Bladder	8	0	-	-	-	-	-	-	-	-	-	-	-	21.2	20.0	13.7	45.6	47.3	-	-	6.4	1.8	0.21	0.50	**3.4**	188
Kidney etc.	3	0	-	-	-	-	-	-	-	-	-	-	-	-	-	-	22.8	-	91.2	57.7	2.4	0.7	0.00	0.11	**1.2**	189
Eye	1	0	-	-	-	-	-	-	-	-	-	-	-	-	-	-	-	47.3	-	-	0.8	0.2	0.00	0.00	**0.5**	190
Brain, nervous system	3	0	-	-	-	-	12.8	-	-	-	-	-	-	10.6	-	13.7	-	-	-	-	2.4	0.7	0.12	0.19	**1.9**	191-2
Thyroid	13	0	-	-	-	-	12.8	-	7.6	24.7	28.9	12.2	15.2	10.6	-	27.4	-	-	-	-	10.3	3.0	0.56	0.70	**7.4**	193
Other endocrine	0	0	-	-	-	-	-	-	-	-	-	-	-	-	-	-	-	-	-	-	0.0	0.0	0.00	0.00	**0.0**	194
Hodgkin's disease	1	0	-	-	-	-	-	-	-	-	-	-	-	10.0	-	-	-	-	-	-	0.8	0.2	0.05	0.05	**0.4**	201
Non-Hodgkin lymphoma	23	0	-	-	-	-	-	-	-	-	9.6	12.2	15.2	21.2	60.1	95.8	-	47.3	273.7	57.7	18.3	5.3	0.59	1.07	**10.3**	200,202
Multiple myeloma	1	0	-	-	-	-	-	-	-	-	9.6	-	-	-	-	-	-	-	-	-	0.8	0.2	0.05	0.05	**0.6**	203
Lymphoid leukaemia	1	0	-	-	-	-	-	-	-	-	-	-	-	-	-	-	22.8	-	-	-	0.8	0.2	0.00	0.11	**0.5**	204
Myeloid leukaemia	3	0	-	-	-	-	-	-	-	-	9.6	-	-	-	10.0	-	22.8	-	-	-	2.4	0.7	0.10	0.21	**1.4**	205
Monocytic leukaemia	0	0	-	-	-	-	-	-	-	-	-	-	-	-	-	-	-	-	-	-	0.0	0.0	0.00	0.00	**0.0**	206
Other leukaemia	0	0	-	-	-	-	-	-	-	-	-	-	-	-	-	-	-	-	-	-	0.0	0.0	0.00	0.00	**0.0**	207
Leukaemia unspecified	0	0	-	-	-	-	-	-	-	-	-	-	-	-	-	-	-	-	-	-	0.0	0.0	0.00	0.00	**0.0**	208
Other and unspecified	12	0	-	-	-	-	-	-	-	-	9.6	-	-	10.6	10.0	27.4	22.8	141.9	182.5	57.7	9.5	2.7	0.15	0.40	**5.3**	O&U
All sites	437	0	17.1	-	-	-	25.7	43.2	68.3	99.0	288.8	316.1	471.3	583.6	631.1	944.3	1275.6	1513.7	1551.1	1674.4	347.4		12.72	23.82	**211.2**	ALL
All sites but 173	437	0	17.1	-	-	-	25.7	43.2	68.3	99.0	288.8	316.1	471.3	583.6	631.1	944.3	1275.6	1513.7	1551.1	1674.4	347.4	100.0	12.72	23.82	**211.2**	ALLb

Rate from 1 case

17.147 19.857 23.196 21.331 12.825 8.631 7.588 8.248 9.627 12.158 15.205 10.610 10.018 13.686 22.779 47.304 91.241 57.737

†Important: see notes on population page

249

USA, Connecticut

The Connecticut Tumor Registry, which is located in the Connecticut Department of Health in Hartford, Connecticut, contains reports on all malignant, *in situ* and certain benign tumours diagnosed in residents of Connecticut since 1935. The reporting of cancer by hospitals was voluntary until 1971 when reporting became mandatory by law. This law was amended in 1983 to include private pathology laboratories. The registry is funded by the State of Connecticut and the federal government. Since 1973 it has been participating in the Surveillance, Epidemiology and End Results (SEER) Program sponsored by the National Cancer Institute.

The registry covers the entire State of Connecticut, which is bounded by Massachusetts to the north, Rhode Island to the east, Long Island Sound to the south and New York to the west. It lies between latitudes 41°15′ and 42°00′ N and longitudes 71°45′ and 73°30′ W. The total registration area is 12 973 km². At the 1990 census, the population of the state was 3 287 116 (87% white and 9.3% black). Approximately 6.5% of the population is Hispanic, mostly of Puerto Rican origin.

Reports are prepared by tumour registrars located in all general and state hospitals and submitted to the registry. Registry field staff abstract cancer reports from state mental institutions, federal hospitals and selected out-of-state hospitals where Connecticut residents traditionally go for diagnosis and/or treatment. The registry is also notified of Connecticut residents who are hospitalized in the states of New York, Massachusetts, Rhode Island, New Hampshire and Florida through reciprocal cancer reporting agreements with these states.

All death certificates with a mention of cancer are reviewed and checked against the registry files for prior registration. Follow-back is initiated on all death certificates which do not match to a patient in the registry in order to verify whether the patient was diagnosed with cancer when alive.

Stringent controls prevent duplication of case reporting. Quality control of information is maintained through the use of data-processing editing techniques, case-finding audits and reviews of coded and abstracted data.

From its inception, the registry has maintained lifetime follow-up on all malignant and *in situ* tumours. The registry now contains over 550 000 cases, with approximately 110 000 under active follow-up.

The formation of a state-wide tumour registry was largely due to the physicians of the Connecticut State Medical Society, who established a Cancer Coordinating Committee which has been actively involved in guiding and evaluating registry procedures for over forty years. The committee utilizes registry data in programmes aimed at early detection, successful therapy and annual follow-up of cancer patients.

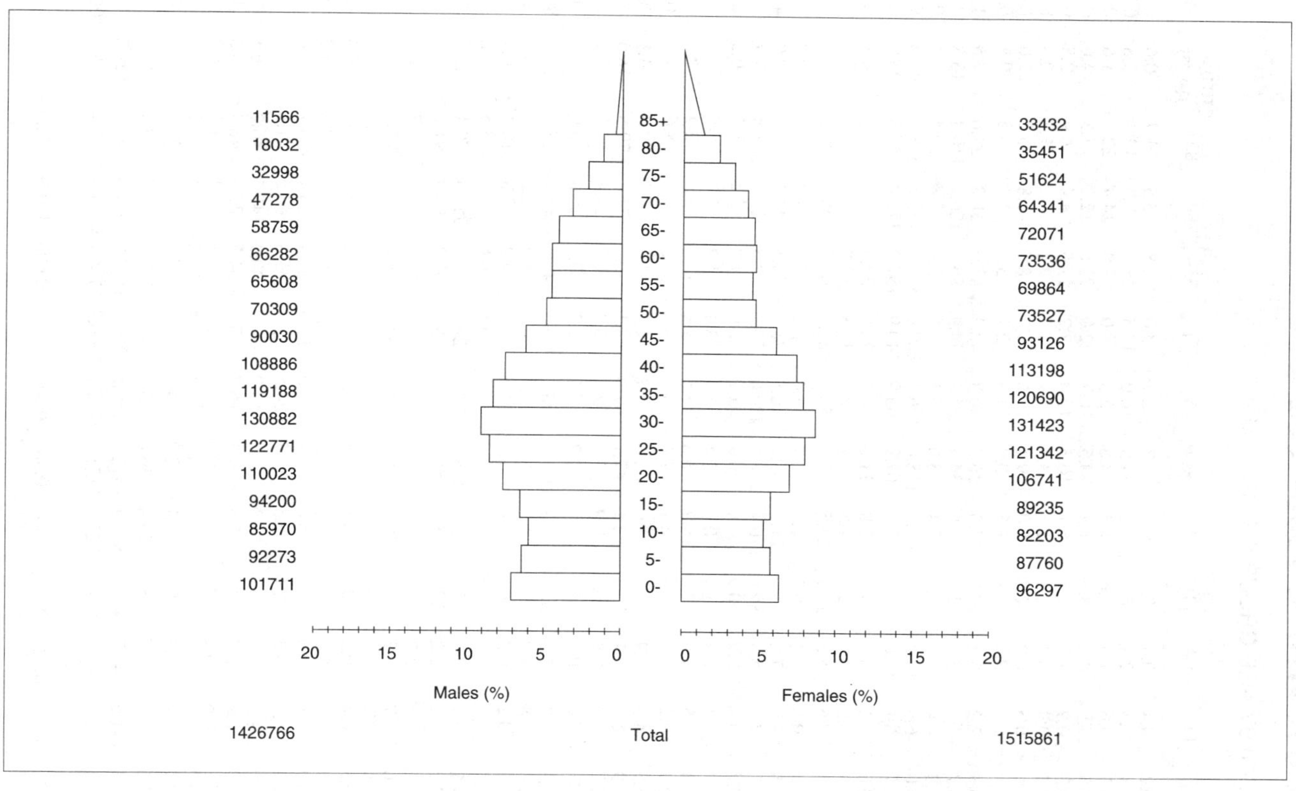

USA, Connecticut: White
Source of population: average annual 1988-92
Estimate: NCI estimates based on U.S. Bureau of Census population estimates by county for the years 1988–92.

Notes to tables overleaf:
† 173 does not include basal cell or squamous cell carcinoma

USA, CONNECTICUT: WHITE 1988-1992

ANNUAL INCIDENCE PER 100,000 BY AGE GROUP (YEARS) - MALE

SITE	ALL AGES	AGE UNK	0-	5-	10-	15-	20-	25-	30-	35-	40-	45-	50-	55-	60-	65-	70-	75-	80-	85+	CRUDE RATE	%	CR 64	CR 74	ASR (W)	ICD (9th)
Lip	42	0	-	-	-	-	-	-	-	0.2	0.4	0.4	0.3	0.9	1.2	2.7	3.0	4.8	5.5	1.7	0.6	0.1	0.02	0.05	0.4	140
Tongue	269	0	-	-	-	-	0.2	-	0.2	1.8	1.5	2.4	6.5	12.8	14.5	16.0	13.5	15.8	13.3	12.1	3.8	0.7	0.20	0.35	2.8	141
Salivary gland	112	0	-	-	-	-	-	-	-	0.5	0.6	1.3	2.6	1.2	3.6	5.8	8.0	7.9	14.4	22.5	1.6	0.3	0.05	0.12	1.1	142
Mouth	329	0	-	-	-	-	0.2	-	-	0.5	1.8	4.2	8.5	11.3	20.5	16.7	22.0	23.6	12.2	17.3	4.6	0.9	0.24	0.43	3.4	143-5
Oropharynx	180	0	-	-	-	-	-	-	0.2	0.2	0.9	2.2	5.4	6.7	10.3	15.0	7.2	11.5	4.4	6.9	2.5	0.5	0.13	0.24	1.9	146
Nasopharynx	60	0	-	-	-	0.2	-	-	0.2	0.3	0.9	0.7	2.3	1.5	3.3	5.1	1.7	2.4	-	1.7	0.8	0.2	0.05	0.08	0.7	147
Hypopharynx	141	0	-	-	-	-	-	-	-	-	0.6	0.9	2.8	4.0	9.1	11.6	9.7	8.5	7.8	5.2	2.0	0.4	0.09	0.19	1.4	148
Pharynx unspecified	31	0	-	-	-	-	-	-	-	-	-	0.4	0.9	1.5	0.9	1.4	2.1	3.6	1.1	3.5	0.4	0.1	0.02	0.04	0.3	149
Oesophagus	537	0	-	-	-	0.2	-	-	0.2	0.3	2.2	3.8	10.2	14.3	26.3	36.8	42.3	43.0	38.8	34.6	7.5	1.4	0.29	0.68	5.3	150
Stomach	986	0	-	-	-	-	-	0.3	0.8	0.7	3.7	8.0	14.8	21.6	34.4	55.1	74.9	86.1	126.4	150.4	13.8	2.6	0.42	1.07	9.2	151
Small intestine	98	0	-	0.2	-	-	-	0.2	0.3	1.0	0.4	1.3	1.1	3.4	3.0	6.1	7.6	3.6	7.8	10.4	1.4	0.3	0.05	0.12	1.0	152
Colon	3395	0	-	-	-	-	-	0.5	0.8	1.8	4.0	6.6	14.2	31.0	63.7	118.0	196.4	269.9	358.2	483.6	518.8	47.6	9.0	1.20	3.54	30.4	153
Rectum	1706	0	-	-	-	-	-	-	0.7	0.9	2.7	6.1	11.6	21.3	46.0	67.9	105.9	140.9	157.6	173.0	145.3	23.9	4.5	0.79	2.02	16.1	154
Liver	343	0	0.4	-	-	-	0.2	0.2	0.6	0.8	1.5	3.8	4.8	9.8	11.8	20.4	22.8	30.9	34.4	36.3	4.8	0.9	0.17	0.39	3.3	155
Gallbladder etc.	166	0	-	-	-	-	-	-	-	0.2	0.9	0.4	2.3	1.5	5.1	8.2	14.8	17.0	20.0	39.8	2.3	0.4	0.05	0.17	1.5	156
Pancreas	836	0	-	-	-	-	-	0.2	0.2	0.5	2.6	5.8	11.7	23.5	30.5	55.1	68.1	67.9	95.4	88.2	11.7	2.2	0.37	0.99	7.9	157
Nose, sinuses etc.	55	0	-	-	-	-	0.2	0.2	-	-	0.6	0.4	0.3	1.2	2.1	3.4	2.5	5.5	8.9	5.2	0.8	0.1	0.02	0.05	0.5	160
Larynx	641	0	-	-	-	-	-	-	-	1.5	2.9	7.8	13.9	21.9	31.7	40.5	38.1	54.5	44.4	27.7	9.0	1.7	0.40	0.79	6.5	161
Bronchus, lung	6541	0	-	-	-	0.2	0.5	0.3	2.0	5.7	14.3	45.8	89.6	170.4	288.5	420.0	523.7	632.8	623.3	511.8	91.7	17.4	3.09	7.81	62.1	162
Other thoracic organs	46	0	0.4	0.2	-	0.2	0.4	0.5	0.5	0.7	0.4	0.9	0.9	-	0.9	1.7	3.0	1.2	2.2	3.5	0.6	0.1	0.03	0.05	0.5	163-4
Bone	68	0	-	-	0.9	1.7	1.3	1.3	0.3	0.7	0.4	0.4	1.1	0.9	2.4	1.4	3.4	1.2	2.2	-	1.0	0.2	0.06	0.08	0.9	170
Connective tissue	209	0	2.4	0.2	0.2	0.6	1.3	0.5	0.9	1.3	3.5	1.6	2.8	5.2	6.0	6.5	11.8	14.5	5.5	32.9	2.9	0.6	0.13	0.22	2.3	171
Mesothelioma	108	0	-	-	-	-	-	-	-	0.3	0.2	0.7	1.4	2.1	2.4	9.5	8.0	8.5	17.7	8.6	1.5	0.3	0.04	0.12	1.0	MES
Kaposi's sarcoma	222	0	-	-	-	-	1.1	4.6	7.2	5.5	4.8	4.9	2.8	3.0	2.1	2.7	2.5	1.8	5.5	19.0	3.1	0.6	0.18	0.21	2.4	KAP
Melanoma of skin	1323	0	-	-	0.2	0.6	2.9	4.6	12.1	11.9	16.7	21.1	32.1	42.1	47.1	47.0	68.1	70.9	77.6	79.5	18.5	3.5	0.96	1.53	13.8	172
†Other skin	86	0	-	-	-	-	0.5	0.7	0.8	0.7	1.7	0.9	0.6	0.9	1.8	2.4	3.4	6.7	14.4	12.1	1.2		0.04	0.07	0.8	173
Breast	89	0	-	-	-	-	-	-	-	-	0.4	1.4	2.1	2.7	6.1	7.2	10.9	10.0	6.9		1.2	0.2	0.03	0.10	0.8	175
Prostate	9189	0	-	-	0.2	-	-	-	-	0.2	1.8	7.8	38.4	113.7	295.4	595.3	929.8	1140.7	1244.4	1217.3	128.8	24.4	2.29	9.91	79.1	185
Testis	442	0	1.2	0.2	-	4.2	7.3	17.1	15.0	12.4	8.8	4.2	4.3	1.5	0.3	1.4	0.8	1.2	2.2	-	6.2	1.2	0.38	0.39	5.3	186
Penis	51	0	-	-	-	-	-	-	-	0.2	0.2	0.2	0.6	2.4	1.8	1.7	4.7	4.2	3.3	10.4	0.7	0.1	0.03	0.06	0.5	187.1-.4
Other male genital	11	0	-	-	-	0.2	0.2	-	-	-	-	-	0.3	0.3	0.6	-	0.8	0.6	-	3.5	0.2	0.0	0.01	0.01	0.1	187.5-.9
Bladder	3053	0	0.2	-	-	0.4	1.1	0.7	2.1	4.2	9.4	23.1	37.0	73.2	114.4	177.7	224.2	300.6	359.3	389.1	42.8	8.1	1.33	3.34	28.4	188
Kidney etc.	1177	0	2.0	0.2	-	-	0.2	0.5	1.4	3.2	6.1	12.2	20.2	35.4	56.7	69.1	75.7	93.3	90.9	91.6	16.5	3.1	0.69	1.41	11.8	189
Eye	45	0	0.4	0.7	-	-	-	0.2	-	0.3	0.7	0.7	1.1	1.2	0.9	1.4	2.1	1.8	4.4	5.2	0.6	0.1	0.03	0.05	0.5	190
Brain, nervous system	643	0	4.1	4.1	2.1	2.8	2.9	3.6	5.2	4.0	5.7	8.2	13.9	20.1	16.9	24.8	34.3	29.1	33.3	24.2	9.0	1.7	0.47	0.76	7.4	191-2
Thyroid	212	0	-	0.2	1.2	0.2	0.7	1.6	2.9	2.9	2.8	4.4	5.1	5.5	6.9	8.5	5.5	9.7	6.7	1.7	3.0	0.6	0.17	0.24	2.4	193
Other endocrine	28	0	1.2	0.2	-	0.2	0.2	-	-	0.3	0.4	0.2	0.3	0.6	0.3	0.7	1.3	1.2	3.3	-	0.4	0.1	0.02	0.03	0.4	194
Hodgkin's disease	333	0	0.4	0.2	0.9	4.9	10.0	8.1	5.5	5.9	3.5	3.1	4.6	4.0	4.2	6.1	5.1	6.1	6.7	8.6	4.7	0.9	0.28	0.33	4.1	201
Non-Hodgkin lymphoma	1473	0	0.4	2.2	0.9	2.3	3.5	6.2	8.4	8.7	15.1	20.0	26.2	36.6	45.9	63.0	82.9	107.3	123.1	133.1	20.6	3.9	0.88	1.61	15.0	200,202
Multiple myeloma	381	0	-	-	-	-	-	-	0.3	0.2	1.3	3.3	2.8	9.5	15.7	24.5	28.3	35.8	45.5	41.5	5.3	1.0	0.17	0.43	3.5	203
Lymphoid leukaemia	436	0	5.9	2.4	1.9	1.5	1.5	-	0.9	1.0	1.5	1.8	5.4	11.9	15.4	19.7	24.5	30.9	45.5	46.7	6.1	1.2	0.25	0.48	4.9	204
Myeloid leukaemia	379	0	0.2	0.9	0.9	0.6	0.9	1.6	2.3	3.0	2.9	3.8	4.3	5.8	9.1	16.7	23.7	34.5	35.5	48.4	5.3	1.0	0.18	0.38	3.7	205
Monocytic leukaemia	24	0	0.4	-	-	-	-	0.2	0.2	0.2	0.6	0.2	0.6	0.3	0.6	0.7	1.3	1.8	1.1	1.7	0.3	0.1	0.02	0.03	0.3	206
Other leukaemia	10	0	-	-	-	-	-	0.2	-	0.2	-	-	0.3	-	0.3	0.7	0.4	0.6	1.1	1.7	0.1	0.0	0.00	0.01	0.1	207
Leukaemia unspecified	110	0	0.2	-	0.2	0.4	-	-	0.5	0.7	0.4	1.3	0.6	2.1	2.7	4.8	7.6	7.3	18.9	20.8	1.5	0.3	0.05	0.11	1.0	208
Other and unspecified	1145	0	0.8	0.2	0.2	-	0.2	1.3	1.8	1.5	4.8	8.7	13.9	28.4	36.8	53.4	76.1	103.0	176.3	197.1	16.1	3.0	0.49	1.14	10.6	O&U
All sites	37761	0	20.4	12.1	10.0	21.7	37.6	56.2	75.3	91.1	141.6	249.7	453.4	826.1	1372.9	2169.5	2909.5	3560.8	4051.6	4044.5	529.3		16.84	42.24	357.5	ALL
All sites but 173	37675	0	20.4	12.1	10.0	21.7	37.1	55.6	74.6	90.4	140.0	248.8	452.9	825.2	1371.1	2167.1	2906.2	3554.1	4037.1	4032.4	528.1	100.0	16.80	42.17	356.7	ALLb
Rate from 1 case			0.197	0.217	0.233	0.212	0.182	0.163	0.153	0.168	0.184	0.222	0.284	0.305	0.302	0.340	0.423	0.606	1.109	1.729						

†Important: see notes on population page

USA, CONNECTICUT: WHITE 1988-1992

ANNUAL INCIDENCE PER 100,000 BY AGE GROUP (YEARS) - FEMALE

SITE	ALL AGES	AGE UNK	0-	5-	10-	15-	20-	25-	30-	35-	40-	45-	50-	55-	60-	65-	70-	75-	80-	85+	CRUDE RATE	%	CR 64	CR 74	ASR (W)	ICD (9th)
Lip	16	0	-	-	-	-	-	-	-	0.2	-	0.2	-	-	0.8	0.6	0.6	-	2.3	1.8	0.2	0.0	0.01	0.01	**0.1**	*140*
Tongue	143	0	-	-	-	-	0.2	0.2	0.8	0.3	0.7	0.4	2.4	2.3	6.8	6.9	5.3	6.6	7.9	7.8	1.9	0.4	0.07	0.13	**1.1**	*141*
Salivary gland	94	0	-	0.5	-	0.4	0.2	0.3	0.5	1.0	0.7	0.9	1.9	1.1	2.4	4.7	2.8	3.9	3.4	4.8	1.2	0.3	0.05	0.09	**0.8**	*142*
Mouth	196	0	-	-	-	-	0.4	0.2	0.2	-	0.9	1.5	2.7	4.9	7.9	8.3	11.2	7.4	11.3	11.4	2.6	0.5	0.09	0.19	**1.5**	*143-5*
Oropharynx	86	0	0.2	-	-	-	-	-	-	0.2	0.2	0.9	2.2	4.0	4.1	3.1	4.7	4.6	1.7	0.6	1.1	0.2	0.06	0.10	**0.8**	*146*
Nasopharynx	20	0	-	-	-	-	-	-	0.2	0.2	0.2	0.6	-	0.6	0.8	1.4	0.6	1.2	-	-	0.3	0.1	0.01	0.02	**0.2**	*147*
Hypopharynx	59	0	-	-	-	-	-	-	-	-	0.2	0.2	1.6	2.3	1.6	4.2	3.4	2.7	0.6	1.8	0.8	0.2	0.03	0.07	**0.5**	*148*
Pharynx unspecified	24	0	-	-	-	-	-	-	-	-	-	0.6	0.8	0.3	0.8	1.1	1.9	0.4	1.1	0.6	0.3	0.1	0.01	0.03	**0.2**	*149*
Oesophagus	209	0	-	-	-	-	-	-	-	-	0.2	0.9	1.6	4.9	8.2	8.3	12.7	9.7	13.0	19.1	2.8	0.6	0.08	0.18	**1.4**	*150*
Stomach	632	0	-	-	-	-	-	-	0.9	1.3	1.6	1.3	8.2	7.4	13.3	18.6	28.3	44.9	61.5	68.8	8.3	1.7	0.17	0.40	**3.8**	*151*
Small intestine	123	0	-	-	-	-	-	0.3	-	0.3	0.9	0.9	1.4	2.9	2.7	6.7	4.4	5.4	9.0	10.2	1.6	0.3	0.05	0.10	**0.9**	*152*
Colon	3612	0	-	-	0.2	-	0.2	0.8	1.5	4.3	7.2	17.8	25.6	45.2	78.1	128.5	176.2	246.4	335.7	385.8	47.7	9.7	0.91	2.43	**21.6**	*153*
Rectum	1404	0	-	-	-	0.2	-	0.5	1.7	2.0	4.8	7.7	15.0	22.0	41.3	53.8	79.6	88.3	99.9	104.7	18.5	3.8	0.48	1.14	**9.4**	*154*
Liver	169	0	0.6	-	-	-	0.2	0.3	-	-	0.5	1.5	1.1	3.4	2.7	5.6	8.1	12.0	16.9	12.0	2.2	0.5	0.05	0.12	**1.1**	*155*
Gallbladder etc.	278	0	-	-	-	-	-	0.2	-	0.5	0.4	0.9	2.2	4.6	5.7	6.7	17.1	18.6	27.1	28.7	3.7	0.7	0.07	0.19	**1.6**	*156*
Pancreas	955	0	-	-	-	-	0.2	0.2	0.2	1.0	1.6	3.2	7.3	15.5	22.3	37.7	47.9	69.3	77.3	91.5	12.6	2.6	0.26	0.69	**5.9**	*157*
Nose, sinuses etc.	47	0	-	0.2	-	-	-	-	0.2	0.3	0.2	0.2	0.5	1.7	1.6	1.9	1.2	3.1	1.1	3.6	0.6	0.1	0.02	0.04	**0.4**	*160*
Larynx	191	0	-	-	-	-	-	-	0.2	-	0.5	1.7	4.1	7.4	10.3	8.6	11.2	7.4	4.5	3.6	2.5	0.5	0.12	0.22	**1.7**	*161*
Bronchus, lung	4540	0	-	-	-	0.7	0.2	0.7	1.1	3.8	15.9	34.1	76.7	123.4	165.1	229.2	263.3	263.1	212.1	122.6	59.9	12.2	2.11	4.57	**35.2**	*162*
Other thoracic organs	31	0	0.6	0.2	0.2	-	-	0.2	0.2	0.3	0.2	-	-	0.9	1.1	0.6	0.9	1.9	1.1	1.2	0.4	0.1	0.02	0.03	**0.3**	*163-4*
Bone	68	0	-	-	1.2	1.1	0.9	0.8	0.6	0.5	0.4	0.6	1.1	0.9	1.1	1.4	1.9	3.1	2.8	0.6	0.9	0.2	0.05	0.06	**0.7**	*170*
Connective tissue	163	0	0.6	0.2	0.2	1.3	0.6	1.3	0.9	1.3	1.9	1.3	1.9	1.7	4.6	4.2	5.9	6.2	4.5	13.2	2.2	0.4	0.09	0.14	**1.5**	*171*
Mesothelioma	44	0	-	-	-	-	-	0.2	-	-	0.5	0.2	0.5	1.4	1.6	1.4	2.2	2.7	2.3	1.8	0.6	0.1	0.02	0.04	**0.3**	*MES*
Kaposi's sarcoma	22	0	-	-	-	-	-	0.2	0.5	0.2	-	-	-	-	-	0.3	0.3	-	1.2	2.8	4.2	0.3	0.1	0.01	0.01	**0.1**	*KAP*
Melanoma of skin	1188	0	-	-	0.2	1.6	4.7	7.9	13.2	17.7	20.0	25.6	23.1	29.5	24.2	27.8	31.1	31.4	31.0	40.7	15.7	3.2	0.84	1.13	**11.2**	*172*
†Other skin	72	0	-	-	-	-	0.2	0.7	0.3	0.3	1.4	0.9	1.4	1.4	2.2	1.1	2.2	2.7	4.5	4.2	0.9		0.04	0.06	**0.6**	*173*
Breast	11135	0	-	-	-	-	1.1	8.1	21.9	65.3	124.4	200.6	230.9	283.7	360.9	402.9	443.0	485.8	503.2	427.1	146.9	30.0	6.48	10.71	**93.3**	*174*
Uterus unspecified	73	0	0.2	-	-	-	-	-	-	0.3	0.9	0.9	0.5	0.9	1.6	3.1	1.6	3.5	6.2	8.4	1.0	0.2	0.03	0.05	**0.5**	*179*
Cervix uteri	714	0	-	-	-	-	1.5	8.9	11.9	15.1	14.3	18.5	12.8	10.9	15.0	13.9	10.9	13.6	18.1	14.4	9.4	1.9	0.54	0.67	**7.0**	*180*
Placenta	3	0	-	-	-	-	-	-	0.2	0.2	-	-	-	-	0.3	-	-	-	-	-	0.0	0.0	0.00	0.00	**0.0**	*181*
Corpus uteri	2222	0	-	-	-	-	-	1.3	2.0	5.3	12.5	25.6	53.6	67.3	78.6	100.7	114.7	100.7	93.7	59.8	29.3	6.0	1.23	2.31	**18.4**	*182*
Ovary etc.	1383	0	-	0.9	-	1.6	1.7	3.0	3.3	6.8	12.0	19.1	29.1	33.8	46.8	51.1	55.6	62.4	63.7	54.4	18.2	3.7	0.79	1.32	**11.6**	*183*
Other female genital	292	0	-	-	-	-	-	0.3	0.5	0.7	1.2	2.6	1.6	5.4	5.2	7.8	14.0	19.0	22.6	34.7	3.9	0.8	0.09	0.20	**1.8**	*184*
Bladder	1104	0	-	-	-	-	-	0.2	0.5	1.3	3.0	7.1	13.6	24.6	29.6	46.3	54.4	65.9	77.9	87.3	14.6	3.0	0.40	0.90	**7.6**	*188*
Kidney etc.	751	0	2.7	0.7	0.5	0.4	-	0.2	1.1	1.7	5.1	4.7	9.8	18.6	23.9	30.5	39.2	39.9	43.4	34.1	9.9	2.0	0.35	0.70	**5.9**	*189*
Eye	47	0	0.8	0.5	-	-	0.2	-	0.2	0.3	0.4	0.2	0.5	0.9	0.5	1.9	2.5	1.2	1.7	3.6	0.6	0.1	0.02	0.04	**0.5**	*190*
Brain, nervous system	475	0	4.4	2.7	2.7	2.2	2.2	1.6	3.3	2.8	3.0	5.2	5.4	7.2	12.2	15.0	23.0	18.2	16.4	15.0	6.3	1.3	0.28	0.47	**4.7**	*191-2*
Thyroid	464	0	-	-	0.5	2.9	4.5	5.1	5.6	10.8	8.0	9.0	10.6	6.6	7.6	10.3	9.0	8.1	7.9	8.4	6.1	1.3	0.36	0.45	**4.8**	*193*
Other endocrine	14	0	0.6	-	0.2	0.2	0.2	-	-	-	-	0.3	-	-	0.6	0.3	0.4	0.6	-	0.2	0.2	0.0	0.01	0.01	**0.2**	*194*
Hodgkin's disease	307	0	-	0.5	0.7	6.1	9.7	8.6	5.5	4.6	4.4	1.9	1.6	2.9	2.7	2.2	3.1	5.0	6.8	2.4	4.1	0.8	0.25	0.27	**3.6**	*201*
Non-Hodgkin lymphoma	1389	0	0.2	0.2	0.5	2.0	2.2	3.8	3.3	5.1	8.5	10.7	20.4	26.3	42.4	53.3	64.7	72.1	82.4	80.8	18.3	3.7	0.63	1.22	**10.6**	*200,202*
Multiple myeloma	359	0	-	-	-	-	-	-	-	-	0.9	1.5	2.7	5.2	13.6	12.8	22.7	18.6	31.6	27.5	4.7	1.0	0.12	0.30	**2.3**	*203*
Lymphoid leukaemia	326	0	5.4	2.3	1.9	0.7	0.6	0.2	0.6	0.5	0.5	0.6	1.1	6.3	7.6	8.6	16.5	13.9	19.2	32.3	4.3	0.9	0.14	0.27	**2.9**	*204*
Myeloid leukaemia	303	0	0.8	0.2	0.5	0.9	0.7	1.6	0.8	2.3	1.9	3.2	4.6	5.4	5.2	9.4	14.6	13.9	15.8	19.7	4.0	0.8	0.14	0.26	**2.5**	*205*
Monocytic leukaemia	17	0	0.2	0.5	-	-	-	-	0.2	-	-	0.4	-	0.6	0.3	-	0.9	1.2	-	1.2	0.2	0.0	0.01	0.02	**0.2**	*206*
Other leukaemia	17	0	-	-	-	-	-	-	-	-	0.2	-	-	-	0.3	0.6	0.9	1.5	2.8	0.6	0.2	0.0	0.00	0.01	**0.1**	*207*
Leukaemia unspecified	101	0	-	0.2	-	-	-	0.2	-	0.5	0.2	0.6	0.8	1.1	2.4	2.5	4.0	6.2	10.2	12.0	1.3	0.3	0.03	0.06	**0.6**	*208*
Other and unspecified	1303	0	0.6	0.5	-	0.2	0.4	0.3	0.9	1.7	3.0	6.0	9.5	15.5	29.9	36.6	60.3	84.5	116.2	169.3	17.2	3.5	0.34	0.83	**7.8**	*O&U*
All sites	37185	0	18.1	10.3	9.7	22.9	33.0	58.3	84.5	161.1	265.4	422.7	593.0	812.7	1098.5	1382.5	1680.4	1879.7	2075.5	2038.1	490.6		17.95	33.26	**290.0**	*ALL*
All sites but 173	37113	0	18.1	10.3	9.7	22.9	32.8	57.7	84.2	160.7	264.0	421.8	591.6	811.3	1096.3	1381.4	1678.2	1877.0	2071.0	2033.9	489.7	100.0	17.91	33.20	**289.4**	*ALLb*
Rate from 1 case			0.208	0.228	0.243	0.224	0.187	0.165	0.152	0.166	0.177	0.215	0.272	0.286	0.272	0.277	0.311	0.387	0.564	0.598						

†Important: see notes on population page

253

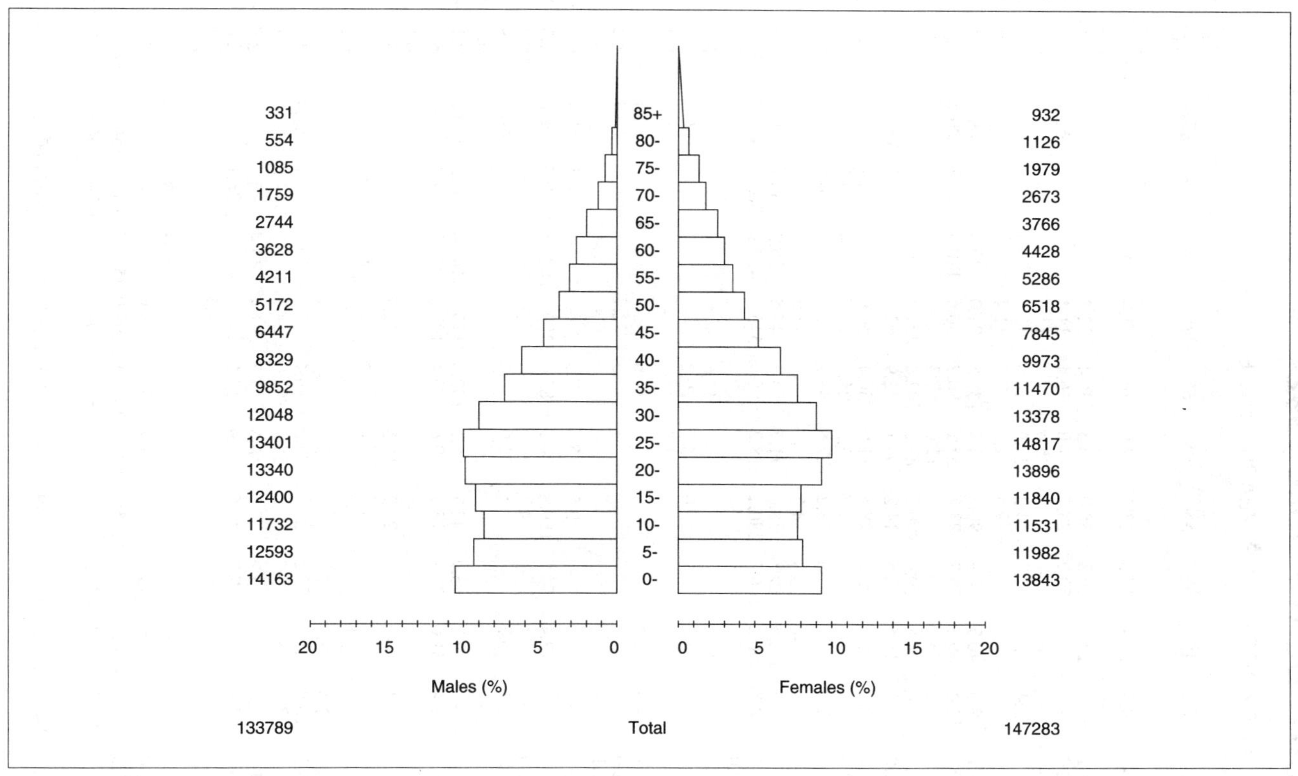

USA, Connecticut: Black
Source of population: average annual 1988-92
Estimate: NCI estimates based on U.S. Bureau of Census population estimates by county for the years 1988–92.
Notes to tables overleaf:
† 173 does not include basal cell or squamous cell carcinoma
Note: There was an error in the population data for Blacks in Volume VI and this results in artificial large increases in the incidence data published in this volume.

USA, CONNECTICUT: BLACK 1988-1992

ANNUAL INCIDENCE PER 100,000 BY AGE GROUP (YEARS) - MALE

SITE	ALL AGES	AGE UNK	0-	5-	10-	15-	20-	25-	30-	35-	40-	45-	50-	55-	60-	65-	70-	75-	80-	85+	CRUDE RATE	%	CR 64	CR 74	ASR (W)	ICD (9th)
Lip	0	0	-	-	-	-	-	-	-	-	-	-	-	-	-	-	-	-	-	-	0.0	0.0	0.00	0.00	**0.0**	*140*
Tongue	31	0	-	-	-	-	-	-	-	-	9.6	21.7	15.5	23.7	22.0	36.4	11.4	18.4	-	-	4.6	1.5	0.46	0.70	**6.0**	*141*
Salivary gland	3	0	-	1.6	-	-	-	-	-	-	-	-	-	-	11.0	-	-	-	-	-	0.4	0.1	0.06	0.06	**0.6**	*142*
Mouth	35	0	-	-	-	-	-	-	-	4.1	-	27.9	19.3	38.0	16.5	36.4	22.7	-	36.1	-	5.2	1.6	0.53	0.83	**6.8**	*143-5*
Oropharynx	29	0	-	-	-	-	-	-	-	2.0	4.8	12.4	30.9	23.7	11.0	36.4	11.4	-	-	60.4	4.3	1.4	0.42	0.66	**5.7**	*146*
Nasopharynx	6	0	-	-	-	1.6	-	-	1.7	-	-	6.2	-	-	5.5	-	11.4	-	-	-	0.9	0.3	0.07	0.13	**1.1**	*147*
Hypopharynx	17	0	-	-	-	-	-	-	-	-	2.4	3.1	7.7	14.2	27.6	14.6	11.4	36.9	-	-	2.5	0.8	0.28	0.40	**3.4**	*148*
Pharynx unspecified	6	0	-	-	-	-	-	-	-	-	-	-	-	9.5	11.0	7.3	11.4	-	-	-	0.9	0.3	0.10	0.20	**1.3**	*149*
Oesophagus	100	0	-	-	-	-	-	-	-	4.1	9.6	40.3	30.9	90.2	93.7	138.5	91.0	129.0	72.2	60.4	14.9	4.7	1.34	2.49	**20.1**	*150*
Stomach	65	0	-	-	-	-	1.5	-	1.7	-	14.4	9.3	23.2	23.7	55.1	80.2	136.4	110.6	72.2	120.7	9.7	3.1	0.64	1.73	**13.2**	*151*
Small intestine	7	0	-	-	-	-	-	-	-	-	4.8	3.1	-	4.7	11.0	7.3	-	-	-	-	1.0	0.3	0.12	0.15	**1.3**	*152*
Colon	153	0	-	-	-	-	1.5	1.5	-	4.1	9.6	24.8	69.6	90.2	88.2	182.2	227.4	276.4	685.4	301.8	22.9	7.2	1.45	3.50	**30.9**	*153*
Rectum	59	0	-	-	-	1.6	-	-	-	2.0	7.2	15.5	42.5	14.2	33.1	72.9	102.3	73.7	108.2	181.1	8.8	2.8	0.58	1.46	**12.1**	*154*
Liver	36	0	1.4	-	-	-	-	-	1.7	2.0	7.2	9.3	23.2	28.5	11.0	36.4	56.9	18.4	72.2	-	5.4	1.7	0.42	0.89	**6.9**	*155*
Gallbladder etc.	13	0	-	-	-	-	-	-	1.7	2.0	-	3.1	-	4.7	5.5	21.9	22.7	18.4	36.1	60.4	1.9	0.6	0.09	0.31	**2.6**	*156*
Pancreas	42	0	-	-	-	-	-	-	-	2.0	12.0	6.2	11.6	33.2	27.6	43.7	79.6	73.7	36.1	60.4	6.3	2.0	0.46	1.08	**8.3**	*157*
Nose, sinuses etc.	3	0	-	-	-	-	-	-	-	-	-	-	3.9	4.7	-	-	11.4	-	-	-	0.4	0.1	0.04	0.10	**0.6**	*160*
Larynx	51	0	-	-	-	-	-	-	-	-	9.6	12.4	19.3	38.0	71.7	58.3	45.5	55.3	36.1	60.4	7.6	2.4	0.75	1.27	**10.4**	*161*
Bronchus, lung	422	0	-	-	-	-	-	-	1.7	24.4	28.8	96.2	166.3	280.2	518.2	568.5	545.8	423.9	505.1	422.5	63.1	19.9	5.58	11.15	**86.2**	*162*
Other thoracic organs	5	0	2.8	-	-	-	-	3.0	-	2.0	-	-	-	-	-	-	-	-	-	-	0.7	0.2	0.04	0.04	**0.7**	*163-4*
Bone	5	0	-	-	1.7	-	-	1.5	1.7	-	-	-	-	-	-	14.6	-	-	-	-	0.7	0.2	0.02	0.10	**0.8**	*170*
Connective tissue	21	0	1.4	-	-	3.2	1.5	4.5	-	-	-	6.2	7.7	19.0	5.5	29.2	-	-	-	60.4	3.1	1.0	0.25	0.39	**3.9**	*171*
Mesothelioma	3	0	-	-	-	-	-	-	-	-	-	3.1	-	-	11.0	-	-	-	-	-	0.4	0.1	0.07	0.07	**0.6**	*MES*
Kaposi's sarcoma	29	0	-	-	-	-	-	3.0	16.6	16.2	4.8	12.4	-	-	-	14.6	-	-	-	60.4	4.3	1.4	0.27	0.34	**4.0**	*KAP*
Melanoma of skin	8	0	-	-	-	-	-	-	1.7	2.0	-	-	7.7	-	-	7.3	22.7	-	-	60.4	1.2	0.4	0.06	0.21	**1.6**	*172*
†Other skin	6	0	-	-	-	-	-	-	1.7	6.1	2.4	3.1	-	-	-	-	-	-	-	-	0.9	0.3	0.07	0.07	**0.8**	*173*
Breast	6	0	-	-	-	-	-	-	-	-	-	-	-	9.5	5.5	7.3	-	-	36.1	60.4	0.9	0.3	0.08	0.11	**1.3**	*175*
Prostate	564	0	-	-	-	-	-	-	-	-	-	-	12.4	54.1	189.9	424.5	1085.9	1250.7	1824.5	1659.5	1508.8	84.3	26.6	3.40	15.09	**119.7**	*185*
Testis	5	0	-	-	-	-	1.5	-	1.7	2.0	-	3.1	-	4.7	-	-	-	-	-	-	0.7	0.2	0.07	0.07	**0.7**	*186*
Penis	6	0	-	-	-	-	1.5	-	-	-	-	2.4	6.2	-	-	11.0	-	-	-	-	60.4	0.9	0.3	0.10	0.10	**1.3**	*187.1-.4*
Other male genital	1	0	-	-	-	-	1.5	-	-	-	-	-	-	-	-	-	-	-	-	-	-	0.1	0.0	0.01	0.01	**0.1**	*187.5-.9*
Bladder	61	0	-	-	-	-	-	1.5	-	-	-	9.3	3.9	42.7	55.1	102.0	113.7	147.4	108.2	120.7	9.1	2.9	0.56	1.64	**12.7**	*188*
Kidney etc.	57	0	-	-	-	-	-	-	3.3	2.0	2.4	31.0	27.1	23.7	49.6	36.4	102.3	73.7	144.3	-	8.5	2.7	0.70	1.39	**11.2**	*189*
Eye	1	0	1.4	-	-	-	-	-	-	-	-	-	-	-	-	-	-	-	-	-	0.1	0.0	0.01	0.01	**0.2**	*190*
Brain, nervous system	21	0	2.8	1.6	-	3.2	-	-	3.0	1.7	4.1	2.4	-	23.7	16.5	-	22.7	-	-	-	3.1	1.0	0.30	0.41	**3.6**	*191-2*
Thyroid	7	0	-	-	-	-	1.5	-	-	-	4.1	-	-	4.7	5.5	7.3	-	18.4	-	-	1.0	0.3	0.08	0.12	**1.2**	*193*
Other endocrine	2	0	1.4	-	-	-	-	-	-	-	-	3.1	-	-	-	-	-	-	-	-	0.3	0.1	0.02	0.02	**0.4**	*194*
Hodgkin's disease	13	0	-	1.6	1.7	1.6	1.5	1.5	-	6.1	2.4	3.1	7.7	-	5.5	-	-	-	-	-	1.9	0.6	0.16	0.16	**2.0**	*201*
Non-Hodgkin lymphoma	81	0	1.4	6.4	5.1	1.6	4.5	7.5	16.6	18.3	16.8	21.7	23.2	23.7	27.6	36.4	45.5	73.7	36.1	60.4	12.1	3.8	0.87	1.28	**13.2**	*200,202*
Multiple myeloma	34	0	-	-	-	-	-	-	-	-	7.2	3.1	7.7	9.5	55.1	51.0	34.1	18.4	144.3	60.4	5.1	1.6	0.41	0.84	**7.0**	*203*
Lymphoid leukaemia	19	0	4.2	-	-	-	-	1.5	-	4.1	2.4	3.1	3.9	9.5	16.5	7.3	11.4	18.4	72.2	-	2.8	0.9	0.23	0.32	**3.4**	*204*
Myeloid leukaemia	19	0	-	-	-	-	1.5	-	1.7	6.1	4.8	-	7.7	9.5	22.0	14.6	11.4	-	36.1	-	2.8	0.9	0.27	0.40	**3.4**	*205*
Monocytic leukaemia	1	0	-	-	-	-	-	-	-	-	-	-	-	-	-	-	11.4	-	-	-	0.1	0.0	0.00	0.06	**0.2**	*206*
Other leukaemia	0	0	-	-	-	-	-	-	-	-	-	-	-	-	-	-	-	-	-	-	0.0	0.0	0.00	0.00	**0.0**	*207*
Leukaemia unspecified	4	0	-	1.6	-	-	-	-	-	-	-	-	-	4.7	-	-	-	18.4	36.1	-	0.6	0.2	0.03	0.03	**0.7**	*208*
Other and unspecified	71	0	-	-	-	-	1.5	1.5	5.0	2.0	12.0	27.9	19.3	19.0	71.7	80.2	79.6	73.7	144.3	181.1	10.6	3.3	0.80	1.60	**14.0**	*O&U*
All sites	2128	0	16.9	12.7	8.5	12.9	16.5	31.3	59.8	121.8	180.1	440.5	634.2	1115.9	1802.5	2835.1	3104.0	3501.7	4076.5	3560.7	318.1		22.27	51.96	**426.0**	*ALL*
All sites but 173	2122	0	16.9	12.7	8.5	12.9	16.5	31.3	58.1	115.7	177.7	437.4	634.2	1115.9	1802.5	2835.1	3104.0	3501.7	4076.5	3560.7	317.2	100.0	22.20	51.90	**425.2**	*ALLb*
Rate from 1 case			1.412	1.588	1.705	1.613	1.499	1.492	1.660	2.030	2.401	3.102	3.867	4.749	5.512	7.288	11.370	18.430	36.075	60.350						

†Important: see notes on population page

USA, CONNECTICUT: BLACK 1988-1992

ANNUAL INCIDENCE PER 100,000 BY AGE GROUP (YEARS) - FEMALE

SITE	ALL AGES	AGE UNK	0-	5-	10-	15-	20-	25-	30-	35-	40-	45-	50-	55-	60-	65-	70-	75-	80-	85+	CRUDE RATE	%	CR 64	CR 74	ASR (W)	ICD (9th)
Lip	0	0	-	-	-	-	-	-	-	-	-	-	-	-	-	-	-	-	-	-	0.0	0.0	0.00	0.00	0.0	140
Tongue	11	0	-	-	-	-	-	-	-	1.7	6.0	5.1	3.1	-	9.0	5.3	7.5	-	-	-	1.5	0.6	0.12	0.19	1.6	141
Salivary gland	8	0	-	-	-	-	-	1.5	-	-	2.0	2.5	6.1	3.8	-	-	-	-	17.8	21.4	1.1	0.4	0.08	0.08	1.0	142
Mouth	12	0	-	-	-	-	-	-	-	1.7	-	7.6	-	3.8	9.0	5.3	15.0	10.1	17.8	-	1.6	0.6	0.11	0.21	1.7	143-5
Oropharynx	8	0	-	-	-	-	-	-	-	-	2.0	-	6.1	3.8	4.5	10.6	7.5	-	-	-	1.1	0.4	0.08	0.17	1.2	146
Nasopharynx	3	0	-	-	-	1.7	-	-	1.5	-	2.0	-	-	-	-	-	-	-	-	-	0.4	0.2	0.03	0.03	0.4	147
Hypopharynx	5	0	-	-	-	-	-	-	-	1.7	-	-	6.1	-	-	5.3	-	10.1	-	-	0.7	0.3	0.04	0.07	0.7	148
Pharynx unspecified	3	0	-	-	-	-	-	-	-	-	2.0	2.5	-	-	4.5	-	-	-	-	-	0.4	0.2	0.05	0.05	0.5	149
Oesophagus	26	0	-	-	-	-	-	-	-	-	2.0	-	6.1	18.9	22.6	37.2	15.0	10.1	17.8	42.9	3.5	1.3	0.25	0.51	3.9	150
Stomach	49	0	-	-	-	-	-	1.3	1.5	1.7	2.0	5.1	6.1	18.9	27.1	37.2	67.3	30.3	106.5	107.2	6.7	2.5	0.32	0.84	6.7	151
Small intestine	11	0	-	-	-	-	-	-	-	1.7	2.0	2.5	-	3.8	9.0	10.6	-	10.1	35.5	-	1.5	0.6	0.10	0.15	1.5	152
Colon	188	0	-	-	-	-	-	-	6.0	7.0	14.0	15.3	61.4	75.7	76.8	122.1	164.6	252.7	301.8	493.2	25.5	9.6	1.28	2.71	25.2	153
Rectum	63	0	-	-	-	-	-	-	-	5.2	2.0	7.6	18.4	26.5	40.6	58.4	67.3	60.6	106.5	42.9	8.6	3.2	0.50	1.13	9.0	154
Liver	10	0	-	-	-	-	-	-	-	-	-	2.5	6.1	-	4.5	10.6	15.0	-	35.5	-	1.4	0.5	0.07	0.19	1.4	155
Gallbladder etc.	11	0	-	-	-	-	-	1.3	-	-	-	-	3.1	3.8	9.0	10.6	7.5	20.2	-	21.4	1.5	0.6	0.09	0.18	1.6	156
Pancreas	60	0	-	-	-	-	-	1.3	-	1.7	2.0	2.5	6.1	26.5	27.1	47.8	74.8	131.4	106.5	64.3	8.1	3.1	0.34	0.95	8.0	157
Nose, sinuses etc.	5	0	-	-	-	-	-	1.3	-	1.7	2.0	-	3.8	-	-	-	-	10.1	-	-	0.7	0.3	0.04	0.04	0.6	160
Larynx	12	0	-	-	-	-	-	-	-	-	2.0	-	12.3	-	4.5	21.2	15.0	-	-	-	1.6	0.6	0.09	0.28	1.9	161
Bronchus, lung	227	0	-	-	-	-	-	1.3	3.0	12.2	20.1	28.0	70.6	98.4	158.1	270.8	209.5	161.7	266.3	42.9	30.8	11.6	1.96	4.36	33.2	162
Other thoracic organs	3	0	-	-	-	-	-	-	-	-	-	-	5.1	-	4.5	-	-	-	-	-	0.4	0.2	0.05	0.05	0.5	163-4
Bone	2	0	-	-	-	-	1.4	-	1.5	-	-	-	-	-	-	-	-	-	-	-	0.3	0.1	0.01	0.01	0.2	170
Connective tissue	18	0	-	1.7	1.7	-	-	4.0	1.5	-	2.0	7.6	3.1	7.6	-	15.9	7.5	10.1	-	-	2.4	0.9	0.15	0.26	2.5	171
Mesothelioma	0	0	-	-	-	-	-	-	-	-	-	-	-	-	-	-	-	-	-	-	0.0	0.0	0.00	0.00	0.0	MES
Kaposi's sarcoma	2	0	-	-	-	-	-	-	-	1.7	-	-	-	4.5	-	-	-	-	-	-	0.3	0.1	0.03	0.03	0.3	KAP
Melanoma of skin	7	0	-	-	-	-	-	1.3	-	-	-	-	3.1	3.8	4.5	-	7.5	10.1	-	21.4	1.0	0.4	0.06	0.10	1.0	172
†Other skin	7	0	-	-	-	-	1.4	1.3	1.5	1.7	4.0	-	-	3.8	-	-	-	-	-	-	1.0		0.07	0.07	0.8	173
Breast	604	0	-	-	-	-	1.4	9.4	32.9	64.5	126.3	186.1	224.0	268.6	298.1	355.8	321.7	343.6	372.9	557.6	82.0	30.9	6.06	9.44	84.5	174
Uterus unspecified	9	0	-	-	-	-	-	-	-	-	1.7	4.0	-	-	-	9.0	5.3	7.5	20.2	-	1.2	0.5	0.07	0.14	1.2	179
Cervix uteri	97	0	-	-	-	1.7	1.4	10.8	6.0	15.7	22.1	20.4	43.0	30.3	45.2	42.5	37.4	30.3	53.3	85.8	13.2	5.0	0.98	1.38	13.2	180
Placenta	1	0	-	-	-	-	-	-	-	-	1.7	-	-	-	-	-	-	-	-	-	0.1	0.1	0.01	0.01	0.1	181
Corpus uteri	86	0	-	-	-	-	-	-	1.5	5.2	6.0	2.5	27.6	34.0	54.2	95.6	119.7	70.7	71.0	64.3	11.7	4.4	0.66	1.73	12.5	182
Ovary etc.	47	0	-	-	1.7	5.1	2.9	1.3	3.0	1.7	-	2.5	27.6	15.1	31.6	42.5	37.4	30.3	-	-	6.4	2.4	0.46	0.86	7.0	183
Other female genital	11	0	-	-	-	-	-	-	-	3.5	2.0	-	3.8	9.0	5.3	7.5	20.2	-	21.4	-	1.5	0.6	0.09	0.16	1.5	184
Bladder	33	0	-	-	-	-	-	-	-	1.7	-	-	3.1	7.6	9.0	26.6	74.8	40.4	88.8	64.3	4.5	1.7	0.11	0.61	4.4	188
Kidney etc.	39	0	1.4	-	-	1.7	-	2.7	1.5	3.5	-	7.6	3.1	26.5	22.6	5.3	15.0	60.6	71.0	-	64.3	5.3	2.0	0.35	0.45	5.2	189
Eye	1	0	1.4	-	-	-	-	-	-	-	-	-	-	-	-	-	-	-	-	-	0.1	0.1	0.01	0.01	0.2	190
Brain, nervous system	15	0	-	5.0	-	1.7	-	-	1.5	-	-	2.5	3.1	11.3	-	15.9	-	10.1	17.8	-	2.0	0.8	0.13	0.21	2.2	191-2
Thyroid	30	0	-	-	-	-	-	1.3	4.5	5.2	10.0	7.6	12.3	3.8	9.0	15.9	22.4	10.1	17.8	-	4.1	1.5	0.27	0.46	4.0	193
Other endocrine	2	0	2.9	-	-	-	-	-	-	-	-	-	-	-	-	-	-	-	-	-	0.3	0.1	0.01	0.01	0.3	194
Hodgkin's disease	14	0	-	-	-	5.1	2.9	-	3.0	3.5	-	2.5	-	7.6	9.0	-	-	-	-	-	1.9	0.7	0.17	0.17	1.9	201
Non-Hodgkin lymphoma	67	0	-	-	5.2	-	2.9	4.0	7.5	5.2	8.0	20.4	18.4	18.9	27.1	47.8	37.4	40.4	35.5	42.9	9.1	3.4	0.59	1.01	9.2	200,202
Multiple myeloma	29	0	-	-	-	-	-	-	-	3.5	-	2.5	18.4	7.6	27.1	31.9	15.0	-	53.3	21.4	3.9	1.5	0.30	0.53	4.3	203
Lymphoid leukaemia	20	0	1.4	5.0	-	-	-	-	-	-	1.7	-	2.5	-	11.3	4.5	26.6	-	40.4	17.8	2.7	1.0	0.13	0.27	2.9	204
Myeloid leukaemia	19	0	-	1.7	-	-	-	1.3	1.5	3.5	4.0	7.6	3.1	7.6	13.5	5.3	7.5	-	-	21.4	2.6	1.0	0.22	0.28	2.7	205
Monocytic leukaemia	0	0	-	-	-	-	-	-	-	-	-	-	-	-	-	-	-	-	-	-	0.0	0.0	0.00	0.00	0.0	206
Other leukaemia	1	0	-	-	-	-	-	-	-	-	-	-	-	-	-	-	-	-	17.8	-	0.1	0.1	0.00	0.00	0.1	207
Leukaemia unspecified	4	0	-	-	-	-	-	-	-	-	-	-	-	-	-	4.5	10.6	7.5	-	-	0.5	0.2	0.02	0.11	0.6	208
Other and unspecified	82	0	-	-	1.7	-	1.4	-	-	3.5	4.0	10.2	15.3	7.6	45.2	58.4	97.3	91.0	159.8	278.8	11.1	4.2	0.44	1.22	11.0	O&U
All sites	1962	0	7.2	13.4	10.4	16.9	15.8	44.5	80.7	165.6	254.7	369.6	616.7	764.2	1038.7	1460.4	1489.0	1536.1	1988.6	2080.2	266.4		16.99	31.74	274.0	ALL
All sites but 173	1955	0	7.2	13.4	10.4	16.9	14.4	43.2	79.2	163.9	250.7	369.6	616.7	760.4	1038.7	1460.4	1489.0	1536.1	1988.6	2080.2	265.5	100.0	16.92	31.67	273.2	ALLb
Rate from 1 case			1.445	1.669	1.734	1.689	1.439	1.350	1.495	1.744	2.005	2.549	3.068	3.783	4.516	5.311	7.482	10.106	17.756	21.445						

†Important: see notes on population page

USA, Georgia, Atlanta

The Georgia Center for Cancer Statistics (GCCS), a division of the Department of Epidemiology in the Rollins School of Public Health at Emory University, was founded in 1976 to provide population-based incidence data for a five-county region in the south-eastern United States. Metropolitan Atlanta was a logical choice, as it was included in the First, Second, and Third National Cancer Surveys. Since its inception, the population covered by the Metropolitan Atlanta SEER Registry has increased dramatically, but the geographical boundaries have not changed.

The GCCS also operates the Rural Georgia SEER Registry (since 1978), the Georgia portion of the Savannah River Region Health Information System (since 1991), and the Georgia Cancer Registry (since 1995). It collaborates with the the Surveillance, Epidemiology and End Results (SEER) Program of the National Cancer Institute, the Cancer Control Program of the State of Georgia, the National Program of Cancer Registries at the Centers for Disease Control and the US Department of Energy on these various cancer registry projects.

The Metropolitan Atlanta area covered by the data presented here amounts to 4500 km^2, and is situated at latitude 33°45′ N and longitude 84°23′ W. The total population is 2 142 502, of which about 30% is black, while less than 3.3% comprises other 'non-white' races. The area has one of the fastest growing populations in the United States, with an increase of more than 489 000 (29%) between 1980 and 1990. Occupations are diverse, with an emphasis on office employment rather than manufacturing industry. Atlanta lies at an altitude of over 320 metres, enjoying a mild climate. Air pollution has become a problem in recent years.

Cancer is a reportable disease in Georgia; however, for the 1988–92 data, the Metropolitan Atlanta SEER Registry did not rely on passive reporting. Data are collected by specially trained abstractors from hospital inpatient and outpatient services, free-standing pathology laboratories, offices of private physicians, autopsies and death certificates.

Follow-up is accomplished through hospital tumour registries and treating physicians and by matching the registry file against death certificates for residents of Georgia, the records of the US Health Care Financing Administration and the county voter registration files. Through these sources, vital status is known to within one year of the current date for 95% of all registrants. Data are collected on a laptop computer system and stored and processed using central registry software developed at the GCCS. Automated and visual screening are performed to avoid duplicate records. Fifty employees are involved in data collection, coding, editing, data-processing and analytical research at the GCCS, although not all are directly involved with the Atlanta Registry.

All hospitals in the area allow access to their data. The GCCS exchanges information with individual hospital tumour registries to their mutual benefit. Time has proved that the Center maintains the confidentiality it promises, and comfortable working relationships generally have been established with hospitals and physicians.

A number of population-based analytical epidemiological investigations have been conducted using the registry for case-finding. Several investigations have focused on factors which may relate to observed high incidence and low survival rates from cancer among blacks. Such studies have included cancers of the prostate, pancreas, oesophagus, breast, ovary and colo-rectum, and multiple myeloma. The Center also has been involved in collaborative case–control studies of passive exposure to cigarette smoking and lung cancer in non-smoking women, breast cancer in young women, Agent Orange exposure in Vietnam, lymphomas and soft tissue sarcomas in young men, breast cancer survival, and risk factors for oral and ovarian cancer, among others.

Jonathan M. Liff
J. William Eley

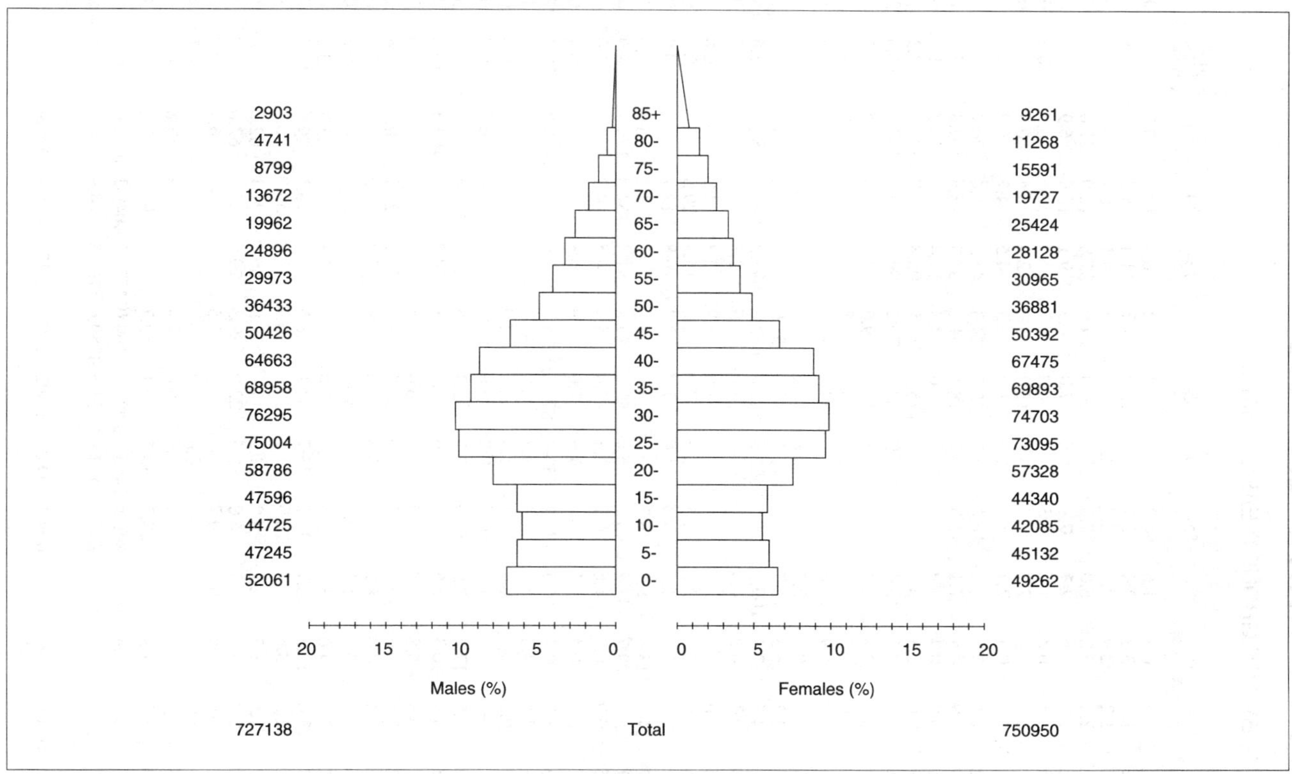

USA, Georgia, Atlanta: White
Source of population: average annual 1988-92
Estimate: NCI estimates based on U.S. Bureau of Census population estimates by county for the years 1988–92.

Notes to tables overleaf:
† 173 does not include basal cell or squamous cell carcinoma

USA, GEORGIA, ATLANTA: WHITE 1988-1992

ANNUAL INCIDENCE PER 100,000 BY AGE GROUP (YEARS) - MALE

SITE	ALL AGES	AGE UNK	0-	5-	10-	15-	20-	25-	30-	35-	40-	45-	50-	55-	60-	65-	70-	75-	80-	85+	CRUDE RATE	%	CR 64	CR 74	ASR (W)	ICD (9th)
Lip	45	0	-	-	-	-	-	0.3	0.3	-	0.6	0.4	1.6	4.7	4.0	9.0	10.2	6.8	12.7	20.7	1.2	0.3	0.06	0.16	1.2	140
Tongue	66	0	-	-	-	-	0.3	0.3	0.5	1.2	1.2	3.2	4.4	2.7	5.6	13.0	11.7	11.4	4.2	-	1.8	0.5	0.10	0.22	1.7	141
Salivary gland	35	0	-	-	0.4	0.4	-	-	0.3	1.2	1.2	2.0	0.5	2.7	2.4	2.0	4.4	9.1	8.4	-	1.0	0.2	0.06	0.09	0.9	142
Mouth	129	0	-	-	-	-	-	-	0.3	1.2	2.2	5.2	6.0	7.3	15.3	24.0	24.9	31.8	16.9	27.6	3.5	0.9	0.19	0.43	3.5	143-5
Oropharynx	61	0	-	-	-	-	-	-	-	0.6	1.9	3.6	2.7	7.3	5.6	7.0	7.3	9.1	16.9	6.9	1.7	0.4	0.11	0.18	1.6	146
Nasopharynx	18	0	-	-	-	0.4	-	-	0.3	0.3	0.3	0.8	1.6	1.3	1.6	4.0	-	-	-	6.9	0.5	0.1	0.03	0.05	0.5	147
Hypopharynx	48	0	-	-	-	-	-	-	-	-	0.6	0.4	2.7	5.3	4.8	13.0	13.2	2.3	8.4	6.9	1.3	0.3	0.07	0.20	1.4	148
Pharynx unspecified	17	0	-	-	-	-	-	-	-	-	0.3	0.4	2.7	1.3	1.6	1.0	1.5	4.5	4.2	6.9	0.5	0.1	0.03	0.04	0.5	149
Oesophagus	154	0	-	-	-	-	-	0.5	-	1.2	1.5	3.6	6.6	14.0	17.7	25.0	29.3	45.5	46.4	20.7	4.2	1.1	0.23	0.50	4.1	150
Stomach	192	0	-	-	-	-	0.3	-	0.8	0.9	1.9	4.4	7.1	13.3	13.7	28.1	51.2	65.9	46.4	103.3	5.3	1.3	0.21	0.61	5.2	151
Small intestine	49	0	-	-	-	-	-	-	0.5	0.6	0.9	0.4	4.9	5.3	6.4	2.0	7.3	11.4	8.4	13.8	1.3	0.3	0.10	0.14	1.3	152
Colon	992	0	-	-	-	-	-	0.5	1.8	4.9	8.0	16.3	36.2	52.0	103.6	176.3	216.5	306.8	438.7	434.0	27.3	7.0	1.12	3.08	27.0	153
Rectum	421	0	-	-	-	-	-	0.8	1.0	4.1	5.3	9.1	15.4	38.7	57.0	69.1	70.2	90.9	109.7	137.8	11.6	3.0	0.66	1.35	11.5	154
Liver	107	0	0.4	-	0.4	0.8	-	0.3	-	-	0.9	2.4	2.2	4.7	15.3	28.1	19.0	27.3	29.5	20.7	2.9	0.7	0.14	0.37	3.0	155
Gallbladder etc.	60	0	-	-	-	-	-	-	-	-	0.6	-	2.7	4.7	8.0	6.0	20.5	18.2	25.3	13.8	1.7	0.4	0.08	0.21	1.6	156
Pancreas	271	0	-	-	-	0.4	-	0.3	0.8	1.5	1.9	5.9	12.6	17.3	25.7	52.1	70.2	63.6	84.4	75.8	7.5	1.9	0.33	0.94	7.4	157
Nose, sinuses etc.	26	0	-	-	-	-	-	-	0.5	0.9	0.3	0.8	2.2	2.0	0.8	6.0	2.9	4.5	-	-	0.7	0.2	0.04	0.08	0.7	160
Larynx	263	0	-	-	-	-	-	0.3	0.3	-	0.3	2.2	6.3	13.7	20.7	41.0	49.1	57.0	52.3	38.0	68.9	7.2	1.8	0.42	0.95	7.4	161
Bronchus, lung	2603	0	0.4	-	-	-	-	0.3	1.0	4.6	14.5	42.4	109.8	209.5	332.6	532.0	637.8	693.2	662.2	482.2	71.6	18.2	3.58	9.42	72.4	162
Other thoracic organs	18	0	-	0.4	-	0.4	1.0	0.5	0.3	0.9	0.3	0.8	0.5	-	-	1.0	1.5	2.3	-	-	0.5	0.1	0.03	0.04	0.4	163-4
Bone	28	0	-	0.4	0.4	1.3	0.3	1.1	1.6	1.5	0.6	-	-	-	1.0	2.9	2.3	4.2	-	0.8	0.2	0.04	0.06	0.7	170
Connective tissue	89	0	2.7	-	1.8	1.3	0.3	1.1	0.8	1.5	0.6	2.8	2.2	5.3	5.6	9.0	13.2	15.9	29.5	13.8	2.4	0.6	0.13	0.24	2.5	171
Mesothelioma	33	0	-	-	-	-	-	-	-	-	0.6	1.2	1.6	3.3	1.6	7.0	7.3	6.8	12.7	-	0.9	0.2	0.04	0.11	0.9	MES
Kaposi's sarcoma	494	0	-	-	-	-	1.7	17.9	33.8	43.2	24.4	13.5	8.2	6.7	0.8	3.0	-	4.2	6.9	-	13.6	3.5	0.75	0.77	9.3	KAP
Melanoma of skin	688	0	0.4	-	-	-	2.7	9.1	12.1	17.1	25.4	29.7	41.2	40.7	55.4	52.1	87.8	61.4	54.8	179.1	18.9	4.8	1.17	1.87	17.1	172
†Other skin	37	0	-	-	-	-	0.3	-	0.5	1.5	0.9	0.8	1.6	0.7	2.4	7.0	4.4	4.5	4.2	27.6	1.0	-	0.04	0.10	1.0	173
Breast	15	0	-	-	-	-	-	-	0.3	0.3	0.3	0.4	1.1	-	1.6	2.0	2.9	6.8	-	-	0.4	0.1	0.02	0.04	0.4	175
Prostate	3972	0	-	-	-	-	-	-	-	0.3	1.9	13.1	63.7	176.2	457.9	876.6	1274.1	1522.9	1505.8	1439.8	109.2	27.8	3.56	14.32	111.2	185
Testis	221	0	0.4	-	-	3.8	8.2	12.3	13.9	9.9	7.4	4.8	3.8	3.3	3.2	2.0	-	-	-	-	6.1	1.5	0.35	0.36	4.7	186
Penis	13	0	-	-	-	-	-	-	0.3	0.3	-	0.5	1.3	1.6	2.0	2.9	4.5	-	-	-	0.4	0.1	0.02	0.05	0.3	187.1-.4
Other male genital	8	0	-	-	-	-	-	-	-	-	-	1.1	0.7	0.8	3.0	-	-	-	-	6.9	0.2	0.1	0.01	0.03	0.2	187.5-.9
Bladder	836	0	-	-	-	-	-	0.5	0.8	4.4	6.5	17.8	17.0	54.0	89.2	143.3	191.6	261.4	375.4	337.6	23.0	5.9	0.95	2.63	22.7	188
Kidney etc.	387	0	1.5	1.3	0.4	0.4	-	-	0.8	2.3	4.9	10.3	16.5	30.0	38.6	61.1	73.1	118.2	101.2	103.3	10.6	2.7	0.54	1.21	10.6	189
Eye	35	0	0.4	-	-	-	-	0.5	0.5	0.3	0.3	0.8	2.2	4.0	4.8	6.0	4.4	2.3	-	-	1.0	0.2	0.07	0.12	1.0	190
Brain, nervous system	268	0	3.5	3.4	2.7	4.2	3.1	4.3	3.9	5.2	5.3	10.3	13.7	9.3	28.9	21.0	29.3	22.7	21.1	20.7	7.4	1.9	0.49	0.74	7.3	191-2
Thyroid	97	0	-	-	0.4	0.4	0.7	1.6	2.4	4.6	3.4	4.0	8.2	4.7	8.8	1.0	5.9	2.3	4.2	6.9	2.7	0.7	0.20	0.23	2.3	193
Other endocrine	11	0	0.8	0.4	-	-	0.3	-	-	0.3	-	0.8	1.1	0.7	-	-	1.5	-	-	-	0.3	0.1	0.02	0.03	0.3	194
Hodgkin's disease	116	0	-	0.4	0.9	1.7	4.8	5.9	4.5	1.7	3.1	4.0	5.5	1.3	3.2	5.0	7.3	2.3	4.2	13.8	3.2	0.8	0.18	0.25	2.8	201
Non-Hodgkin lymphoma	589	0	1.2	0.8	1.3	5.5	2.4	8.0	13.1	17.4	13.0	17.8	30.7	34.7	33.7	64.1	58.5	88.6	118.1	89.6	16.2	4.1	0.90	1.51	14.6	200,202
Multiple myeloma	149	0	-	-	-	-	-	0.3	0.3	0.9	2.5	3.6	5.5	10.0	14.5	19.0	30.7	40.9	59.0	82.7	4.1	1.0	0.19	0.44	4.0	203
Lymphoid leukaemia	144	0	4.6	3.0	2.7	2.5	1.0	0.5	1.0	1.2	1.5	1.2	2.2	8.0	11.2	17.0	21.9	36.4	21.1	62.0	4.0	1.0	0.20	0.40	4.3	204
Myeloid leukaemia	143	0	-	-	0.4	1.0	0.8	0.8	2.0	2.2	4.0	7.1	6.0	5.6	22.0	29.3	29.5	67.5	62.0	3.9	1.0	0.15	0.41	3.7	205
Monocytic leukaemia	7	0	-	-	-	-	-	0.3	-	-	0.8	0.5	0.7	-	1.5	-	-	6.9	0.1	0.0	0.01	0.02	0.2	206
Other leukaemia	3	0	-	-	-	-	0.3	-	-	-	-	-	0.8	1.0	-	-	-	0.1	0.0	0.01	0.01	0.1	207
Leukaemia unspecified	18	0	-	-	-	-	-	0.3	-	0.3	-	-	1.3	1.6	5.0	4.4	-	8.4	13.8	0.5	0.1	0.02	0.06	0.5	208
Other and unspecified	329	0	0.8	-	-	-	1.0	0.8	0.5	2.0	3.1	7.9	11.0	28.7	30.5	60.1	52.7	86.4	92.8	172.2	9.0	2.3	0.43	1.00	9.0	O&U
All sites	14305	0	16.9	10.2	11.6	24.0	30.3	68.8	100.1	142.1	155.0	257.8	483.1	846.8	1465.2	2438.5	3164.0	3773.1	4049.1	4092.0	393.5		18.06	46.07	385.0	ALL
All sites but 173	14268	0	16.9	10.2	11.6	24.0	29.9	68.8	99.6	140.7	154.0	257.0	481.4	846.1	1462.8	2431.5	3159.6	3768.5	4044.9	4064.5	392.4	100.0	18.02	45.97	384.0	ALLb

Rate from 1 case   0.384   0.423   0.447   0.420   0.340   0.267   0.262   0.290   0.309   0.397   0.549   0.667   0.803   1.002   1.463   2.273   4.218   6.889

†Important: see notes on population page

USA, GEORGIA, ATLANTA: WHITE 1988-1992

ANNUAL INCIDENCE PER 100,000 BY AGE GROUP (YEARS) - FEMALE

SITE	ALL AGES	AGE UNK	0-	5-	10-	15-	20-	25-	30-	35-	40-	45-	50-	55-	60-	65-	70-	75-	80-	85+	CRUDE RATE	%	CR 64	CR 74	ASR (W)	ICD (9th)
Lip	8	0	-	-	-	-	-	-	0.3	-	-	-	-	-	1.4	-	1.0	2.6	1.8	2.2	0.2	0.1	0.01	0.01	**0.1**	*140*
Tongue	45	0	-	-	-	-	-	-	0.3	0.6	0.6	1.2	0.5	3.2	3.6	6.3	11.2	2.6	8.9	-	1.2	0.3	0.05	0.14	**0.9**	*141*
Salivary gland	23	0	-	-	-	-	0.3	0.5	0.3	0.3	1.2	0.4	1.1	0.6	-	0.8	4.1	3.8	1.8	2.2	0.6	0.2	0.02	0.05	**0.4**	*142*
Mouth	94	0	-	-	-	-	0.3	-	0.3	0.6	1.2	3.6	2.2	8.4	8.5	5.5	15.2	10.3	10.6	25.9	2.5	0.7	0.13	0.23	**1.9**	*143-5*
Oropharynx	30	0	-	-	-	-	-	-	-	-	-	1.2	1.6	2.6	5.7	1.6	6.1	3.8	1.8	-	0.8	0.2	0.06	0.09	**0.7**	*146*
Nasopharynx	16	0	-	-	-	-	-	-	0.3	0.3	0.4	0.5	1.9	-	0.8	3.0	3.8	3.5	-	0.4	0.1	0.02	0.04	**0.3**	*147*
Hypopharynx	14	0	-	-	-	-	-	-	-	-	0.4	-	1.9	0.7	1.6	3.0	1.3	1.8	4.3	0.4	0.1	0.02	0.04	**0.3**	*148*
Pharynx unspecified	16	0	-	-	-	-	-	-	-	-	-	1.1	0.6	3.6	1.6	3.0	1.3	1.8	2.2	0.4	0.1	0.03	0.05	**0.4**	*149*
Oesophagus	60	0	-	-	-	-	0.3	-	0.3	-	1.2	2.2	5.2	7.1	3.9	12.2	5.1	16.0	6.5	1.6	0.5	0.08	0.16	**1.2**	*150*
Stomach	128	0	-	-	-	-	0.5	0.5	0.6	0.6	1.2	3.8	5.2	7.8	14.2	16.2	25.7	37.3	34.6	3.4	1.0	0.10	0.25	**2.3**	*151*
Small intestine	43	0	-	-	-	-	-	-	0.9	1.2	0.4	3.8	0.6	1.4	5.5	6.1	3.8	8.9	8.6	1.1	0.3	0.04	0.10	**0.8**	*152*
Colon	1113	0	-	-	-	-	1.4	1.6	2.3	6.8	13.1	25.5	45.9	82.5	123.5	140.9	233.5	300.0	339.1	29.6	8.4	0.90	2.22	**20.0**	*153*
Rectum	401	0	-	-	-	-	0.3	1.1	4.9	5.0	6.0	17.4	16.8	32.7	46.4	60.8	61.6	63.9	86.4	10.7	3.0	0.42	0.96	**7.9**	*154*
Liver	51	0	0.4	-	0.5	-	-	-	-	0.3	0.3	-	1.6	1.3	6.4	6.3	6.1	14.1	8.9	6.5	1.4	0.4	0.05	0.12	**1.0**	*155*
Gallbladder etc.	64	0	-	-	-	-	-	-	-	-	-	0.9	-	1.1	3.9	4.3	8.7	8.1	14.1	12.4	21.6	1.7	0.5	0.05	0.13	**1.2**	*156*
Pancreas	259	0	-	-	-	-	0.3	-	0.3	0.6	0.9	2.4	4.9	12.3	16.4	30.7	35.5	51.3	69.2	90.7	6.9	2.0	0.19	0.52	**4.6**	*157*
Nose, sinuses etc.	15	0	-	0.4	-	-	-	-	0.3	0.3	-	-	-	1.3	2.8	1.6	2.0	1.3	-	2.2	0.4	0.1	0.03	0.04	**0.4**	*160*
Larynx	74	0	-	-	-	-	-	-	0.5	0.9	0.6	1.2	3.8	5.8	9.2	16.5	6.1	5.1	5.3	2.2	2.0	0.6	0.11	0.22	**1.7**	*161*
Bronchus, lung	1663	0	-	-	-	0.5	1.4	0.8	1.3	5.2	9.8	30.6	61.8	123.4	191.3	225.0	292.0	241.2	220.1	133.9	44.3	12.6	2.13	4.71	**35.5**	*162*
Other thoracic organs	14	0	0.8	-	0.5	-	-	-	0.5	0.9	0.6	0.4	-	-	-	0.8	1.0	1.3	-	-	0.4	0.1	0.02	0.03	**0.3**	*163-4*
Bone	24	0	-	0.4	1.4	0.9	0.3	0.3	0.5	0.6	0.3	-	1.1	0.6	0.7	1.6	2.0	-	1.8	4.3	0.6	0.2	0.04	0.05	**0.6**	*170*
Connective tissue	69	0	2.8	0.4	-	-	1.0	1.4	0.8	1.7	2.4	2.8	1.6	1.9	1.4	1.6	4.1	5.1	8.9	13.0	1.8	0.5	0.09	0.12	**1.5**	*171*
Mesothelioma	11	0	-	-	-	-	-	-	0.3	-	0.3	-	0.5	-	2.8	-	-	6.4	-	-	0.3	0.1	0.02	0.02	**0.2**	*MES*
Kaposi's sarcoma	6	0	-	-	-	-	0.3	-	-	-	0.4	-	0.6	-	-	-	1.3	-	-	4.3	0.2	0.0	0.01	0.01	**0.1**	*KAP*
Melanoma of skin	570	0	-	-	-	5.4	7.0	10.1	17.9	21.7	22.2	25.8	21.1	23.9	30.6	22.8	25.3	28.2	26.6	17.3	15.2	4.3	0.93	1.17	**12.0**	*172*
†Other skin	21	0	-	0.4	0.5	-	0.3	-	0.3	0.6	0.3	1.2	-	0.6	0.7	-	1.0	3.8	3.5	6.5	0.6		0.02	0.03	**0.4**	*173*
Breast	4253	0	-	-	-	-	1.0	9.9	21.7	73.0	125.4	196.1	244.6	279.0	328.5	380.7	402.5	405.3	456.1	349.9	113.3	32.2	6.40	10.31	**89.9**	*174*
Uterus unspecified	3	0	-	-	-	-	-	-	-	-	-	-	-	1.3	-	-	-	1.3	-	-	0.1	0.0	0.01	0.01	**0.1**	*179*
Cervix uteri	348	0	-	-	-	-	2.4	8.2	14.2	12.9	13.6	11.9	15.2	13.6	14.9	14.2	17.2	23.1	16.0	10.8	9.3	2.6	0.53	0.69	**7.0**	*180*
Placenta	4	0	-	-	-	-	-	0.8	-	0.3	-	-	-	-	-	-	-	-	-	-	0.1	0.0	0.01	0.01	**0.1**	*181*
Corpus uteri	710	0	-	-	-	-	0.3	1.4	1.1	6.3	11.0	18.7	35.8	53.0	76.1	90.5	90.2	89.8	67.4	58.3	18.9	5.4	1.02	1.92	**15.4**	*182*
Ovary etc.	547	0	-	-	1.0	2.3	2.4	3.3	3.5	6.0	12.7	17.9	22.2	33.6	45.5	48.0	61.8	75.7	63.9	54.0	14.6	4.1	0.75	1.30	**11.5**	*183*
Other female genital	109	0	-	-	-	-	0.3	0.5	1.1	1.7	1.8	5.2	2.7	7.8	3.6	11.0	11.2	10.3	12.4	32.4	2.9	0.8	0.12	0.23	**2.1**	*184*
Bladder	284	0	-	-	-	-	0.3	1.4	-	0.3	3.6	5.2	7.6	14.9	22.0	26.7	45.6	44.9	65.7	71.3	7.6	2.1	0.28	0.64	**5.4**	*188*
Kidney etc.	229	0	3.2	0.4	-	0.5	-	0.5	0.5	0.3	2.1	5.6	9.2	12.9	16.4	22.8	38.5	38.5	30.2	41.0	6.1	1.7	0.26	0.56	**4.9**	*189*
Eye	25	0	1.2	-	-	-	-	-	0.3	0.3	0.3	-	1.1	0.6	2.1	2.4	4.3	3.8	3.5	2.2	0.7	0.2	0.03	0.06	**0.6**	*190*
Brain, nervous system	239	0	5.7	4.4	4.3	1.8	1.7	2.7	2.1	5.4	6.8	5.6	7.6	9.0	9.2	22.8	25.3	16.7	21.3	6.5	6.4	1.8	0.33	0.57	**5.8**	*191-2*
Thyroid	302	0	-	-	1.0	2.7	7.7	7.9	9.6	10.6	12.2	13.9	13.0	9.0	11.4	10.2	11.2	11.5	5.3	8.6	8.0	2.3	0.49	0.60	**6.5**	*193*
Other endocrine	13	0	1.6	-	-	-	0.3	0.3	0.3	0.3	0.3	0.4	-	0.6	-	1.6	-	-	-	-	0.3	0.1	0.02	0.03	**0.4**	*194*
Hodgkin's disease	107	0	-	0.9	0.5	5.0	4.9	4.4	5.6	2.3	2.1	1.2	1.6	0.6	0.7	1.6	7.1	5.1	10.6	-	2.8	0.8	0.15	0.19	**2.4**	*201*
Non-Hodgkin lymphoma	505	0	0.4	-	1.0	0.5	1.0	4.1	4.0	4.9	5.3	11.1	20.6	29.1	41.2	59.0	54.7	59.0	97.6	73.4	13.4	3.8	0.62	1.18	**10.3**	*200,202*
Multiple myeloma	116	0	-	-	-	-	-	-	0.3	0.3	1.2	2.8	3.8	5.8	9.2	11.8	16.2	21.8	24.8	25.9	3.1	0.9	0.12	0.26	**2.2**	*203*
Lymphoid leukaemia	113	0	6.1	1.8	1.0	0.5	0.7	0.5	0.3	-	1.5	0.8	2.7	3.9	4.3	9.4	13.2	15.4	24.8	23.8	3.0	0.9	0.12	0.23	**2.7**	*204*
Myeloid leukaemia	134	0	0.4	0.9	-	0.5	0.7	1.4	0.5	1.1	0.9	2.4	3.3	5.8	7.8	11.8	13.2	23.1	28.4	43.2	3.6	1.0	0.13	0.25	**2.6**	*205*
Monocytic leukaemia	14	0	-	-	-	-	0.3	-	0.3	-	0.3	-	0.5	-	-	0.8	2.0	1.3	3.5	8.6	0.4	0.1	0.01	0.02	**0.2**	*206*
Other leukaemia	3	0	0.4	-	0.5	-	-	-	-	-	-	-	-	-	-	-	-	1.3	-	-	0.1	0.0	0.00	0.00	**0.1**	*207*
Leukaemia unspecified	9	0	-	-	-	-	-	-	-	-	-	0.4	-	0.6	-	0.8	1.0	2.6	3.5	2.2	0.2	0.1	0.01	0.01	**0.1**	*208*
Other and unspecified	337	0	0.8	-	-	-	0.3	-	0.8	0.9	3.0	5.2	8.7	16.8	29.2	40.9	43.6	47.5	72.8	105.8	9.0	2.6	0.33	0.75	**6.5**	*O&U*
All sites	13236	0	24.0	10.2	11.9	20.3	35.9	63.2	92.9	170.0	259.4	397.7	557.5	766.7	1043.8	1294.1	1524.8	1630.3	1822.8	1732.0	352.5		17.27	31.36	**273.6**	*ALL*
All sites but 173	13215	0	24.0	9.7	11.4	20.3	35.6	63.2	92.6	169.4	259.1	396.5	557.5	766.0	1043.1	1294.1	1523.8	1626.5	1819.2	1725.5	352.0	100.0	17.24	31.33	**273.2**	*ALLb*

Rate from 1 case   0.406   0.443   0.475   0.451   0.349   0.274   0.268   0.286   0.296   0.397   0.542   0.646   0.711   0.787   1.014   1.283   1.775   2.160

†Important: see notes on population page

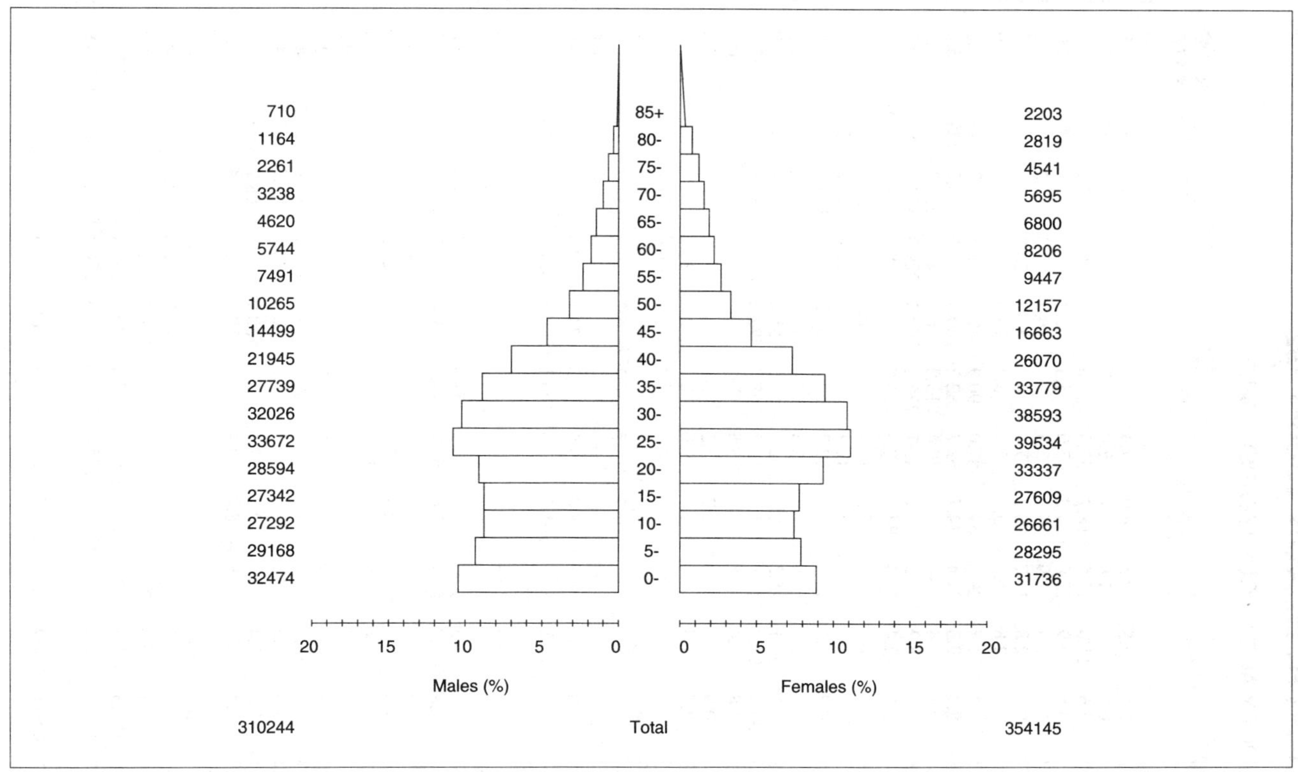

USA, Georgia, Atlanta: Black
Source of population: average annual 1988-92
Estimate: NCI estimates based on U.S. Bureau of Census population estimates by county for the years 1988–92.
Notes to tables overleaf:
† 173 does not include basal cell or squamous cell carcinoma

Note: There was an error in the population data for Blacks in Volume VI and this results in artificial large increases in the incidence data published in this volume.

USA, GEORGIA, ATLANTA: BLACK 1988-1992

ANNUAL INCIDENCE PER 100,000 BY AGE GROUP (YEARS) - MALE

SITE	ALL AGES	AGE UNK	0-	5-	10-	15-	20-	25-	30-	35-	40-	45-	50-	55-	60-	65-	70-	75-	80-	85+	CRUDE RATE	%	CR 64	CR 74	ASR (W)	ICD (9th)
Lip	0	0	-	-	-	-	-	-	-	-	-	-	-	-	-	-	-	-	-	-	0.0	0.0	0.00	0.00	0.0	140
Tongue	43	0	-	-	-	-	-	-	-	-	0.7	6.4	5.5	17.5	24.0	17.4	8.7	24.7	-	34.4	-	2.8	1.0	0.36	0.52	4.2	141
Salivary gland	10	0	-	-	-	-	-	-	-	-	-	0.9	1.4	1.9	2.7	7.0	8.7	6.2	-	-	28.1	0.6	0.2	0.07	0.14	1.1	142
Mouth	48	0	-	-	-	-	0.7	-	-	0.7	3.6	11.0	17.5	18.7	31.3	26.0	6.2	8.8	17.2	-	3.1	1.1	0.42	0.58	4.9	143-5
Oropharynx	31	0	-	-	-	-	-	-	0.6	-	3.6	6.9	15.6	24.0	7.0	4.3	6.2	-	-	-	2.0	0.7	0.29	0.34	2.9	146
Nasopharynx	17	0	-	0.7	-	0.7	-	1.2	0.6	0.7	1.8	2.8	1.9	5.3	3.5	-	6.2	8.8	17.2	-	1.1	0.4	0.10	0.13	1.3	147
Hypopharynx	24	0	-	-	-	-	-	-	-	0.7	0.9	2.8	11.7	10.7	17.4	8.7	-	26.5	-	-	1.5	0.6	0.22	0.26	2.5	148
Pharynx unspecified	14	0	-	-	-	-	-	-	-	-	-	2.8	5.8	5.3	3.5	8.7	18.5	8.8	-	-	0.9	0.3	0.09	0.22	1.5	149
Oesophagus	137	0	-	-	-	-	-	-	0.6	0.7	6.4	31.7	29.2	69.4	87.0	90.9	49.4	70.8	17.2	28.1	8.8	3.2	1.13	1.83	14.7	150
Stomach	129	0	-	-	-	-	0.7	-	2.5	4.3	8.2	19.3	21.4	34.7	62.7	82.2	80.3	79.6	68.7	225.2	8.3	3.0	0.77	1.58	13.4	151
Small intestine	20	0	-	-	-	-	-	-	0.6	1.4	0.9	1.4	-	5.3	10.4	13.0	6.2	44.2	17.2	-	1.3	0.5	0.10	0.20	1.9	152
Colon	300	0	-	-	-	0.7	1.4	0.6	1.9	5.8	16.4	26.2	31.2	88.1	142.7	225.1	290.3	229.9	343.5	365.9	19.3	7.0	1.57	4.15	32.4	153
Rectum	109	0	-	-	-	-	-	0.6	2.5	5.0	3.6	12.4	23.4	34.7	38.3	64.9	80.3	88.4	51.5	197.0	7.0	2.5	0.60	1.33	11.2	154
Liver	38	0	-	-	-	-	0.7	0.6	1.2	5.8	3.6	-	7.8	5.3	17.4	-	30.9	17.7	51.5	28.1	2.4	0.9	0.21	0.37	3.2	155
Gallbladder etc.	16	0	-	-	-	-	-	-	-	0.7	-	-	1.9	2.7	10.4	-	24.7	35.4	17.2	28.1	1.0	0.4	0.08	0.20	1.7	156
Pancreas	95	0	-	-	-	-	-	0.6	1.2	1.4	0.9	4.1	13.6	34.7	52.2	64.9	86.5	70.8	154.6	140.7	6.1	2.2	0.54	1.30	10.5	157
Nose, sinuses etc.	8	0	-	-	-	-	-	-	0.6	-	-	-	3.9	-	3.5	-	18.5	-	17.2	-	0.5	0.2	0.04	0.13	0.8	160
Larynx	107	0	-	-	-	-	-	-	0.6	0.7	9.1	22.1	25.3	40.0	62.7	60.6	55.6	53.1	34.4	56.3	6.9	2.5	0.80	1.38	11.2	161
Bronchus, lung	892	0	-	-	-	-	-	1.2	1.9	10.8	35.5	93.8	214.3	331.0	515.2	558.4	772.0	689.8	687.0	309.6	57.5	20.8	6.02	12.67	97.3	162
Other thoracic organs	11	0	0.6	-	0.7	0.7	-	-	0.6	-	1.8	1.4	5.8	-	3.5	-	-	-	-	-	0.7	0.3	0.08	0.08	0.9	163-4
Bone	9	0	-	-	0.7	2.2	0.7	-	0.6	-	0.9	-	-	2.7	3.5	-	-	-	-	-	0.6	0.2	0.06	0.06	0.7	170
Connective tissue	22	0	1.2	-	1.5	0.7	-	0.6	-	0.7	2.7	1.4	1.9	5.3	7.0	8.7	12.4	17.7	-	-	1.4	0.5	0.12	0.22	2.0	171
Mesothelioma	8	0	-	-	-	-	-	-	-	1.4	-	2.8	-	-	3.5	4.3	-	8.8	17.2	-	0.5	0.2	0.04	0.06	0.7	MES
Kaposi's sarcoma	92	0	-	-	-	-	2.8	14.8	15.6	17.3	4.6	8.3	1.9	2.7	-	-	-	-	17.2	-	5.9	2.1	0.34	0.34	4.4	KAP
Melanoma of skin	8	0	-	-	-	-	-	-	-	-	-	-	-	2.7	3.5	8.7	6.2	17.7	17.2	-	0.5	0.2	0.03	0.10	0.9	172
†Other skin	9	0	-	-	0.7	-	0.7	1.2	0.6	2.2	-	1.4	-	-	-	-	-	-	-	-	0.6		0.03	0.03	0.5	173
Breast	14	0	-	-	-	-	-	-	-	-	0.9	-	5.8	8.0	3.5	4.3	24.7	8.8	-	-	0.9	0.3	0.09	0.24	1.5	175
Prostate	1235	0	-	-	-	-	-	-	-	-	1.8	24.8	113.0	301.7	640.6	1160.1	1278.5	1821.9	2009.6	1745.0	79.6	28.7	5.41	17.60	142.3	185
Testis	10	0	-	0.7	0.7	-	0.7	-	-	1.4	3.6	1.4	-	-	-	-	-	-	-	-	0.6	0.2	0.04	0.04	0.6	186
Penis	12	0	-	-	-	-	-	-	-	-	-	2.8	3.9	-	10.4	8.7	6.2	8.8	17.2	-	0.8	0.3	0.09	0.16	1.3	187.1-.4
Other male genital	3	0	-	-	-	-	-	-	-	-	0.9	-	-	-	3.5	-	-	-	17.2	-	0.2	0.1	0.02	0.02	0.3	187.5-.9
Bladder	93	0	0.6	0.7	-	-	-	-	0.6	1.4	3.6	5.5	17.5	32.0	34.8	51.9	67.9	70.8	274.8	56.3	6.0	2.2	0.48	1.08	9.6	188
Kidney etc.	144	0	4.3	-	0.7	-	-	1.8	1.2	4.3	12.8	24.8	50.7	32.0	62.7	43.3	49.4	115.0	103.1	-	9.3	3.4	0.98	1.44	13.6	189
Eye	8	0	1.8	0.7	-	-	-	-	-	-	0.9	-	-	7.0	-	-	8.8	-	-	-	0.5	0.2	0.05	0.05	0.7	190
Brain, nervous system	46	0	2.5	0.7	4.4	1.5	-	1.2	1.9	2.2	4.6	6.9	3.9	2.7	7.0	4.3	30.9	26.5	17.2	-	3.0	1.1	0.20	0.37	3.6	191-2
Thyroid	21	0	-	-	0.7	-	-	0.6	0.6	2.2	0.9	1.4	3.9	5.3	17.4	4.3	12.4	-	-	28.1	1.4	0.5	0.17	0.25	2.0	193
Other endocrine	4	0	-	0.7	-	1.5	-	-	-	-	-	1.4	-	-	-	-	-	-	-	-	0.3	0.1	0.02	0.02	0.3	194
Hodgkin's disease	33	0	-	1.4	-	1.5	2.1	1.8	1.2	5.8	4.6	4.1	1.9	2.7	3.5	8.7	-	-	-	-	2.1	0.8	0.15	0.20	2.1	201
Non-Hodgkin lymphoma	137	0	0.6	-	0.7	0.7	1.4	8.3	11.9	12.3	18.2	13.8	23.4	24.0	20.9	30.3	61.8	17.7	85.9	28.1	8.8	3.2	0.68	1.14	10.2	200,202
Multiple myeloma	76	0	-	-	-	-	-	-	1.9	2.2	4.6	5.5	7.8	13.3	48.7	47.6	80.3	44.2	85.9	112.6	4.9	1.8	0.42	1.06	8.2	203
Lymphoid leukaemia	44	0	3.1	3.4	-	0.7	1.4	0.6	-	-	1.8	1.4	3.9	10.7	17.4	17.3	30.9	17.7	68.7	28.1	2.8	1.0	0.22	0.46	4.2	204
Myeloid leukaemia	39	0	0.6	2.1	0.7	0.7	1.4	1.2	1.9	2.9	2.7	2.8	1.9	8.0	10.4	17.3	18.5	8.8	34.4	-	2.5	0.9	0.19	0.37	3.2	205
Monocytic leukaemia	0	0	-	-	-	-	-	-	-	-	-	-	-	-	-	-	-	-	-	-	0.0	0.0	0.00	0.00	0.0	206
Other leukaemia	1	0	-	-	-	-	-	-	-	-	0.9	-	-	-	-	-	-	-	-	-	0.1	0.0	0.00	0.00	0.1	207
Leukaemia unspecified	11	0	-	-	-	-	-	-	0.6	-	-	1.4	3.9	-	7.0	-	18.5	8.8	17.2	-	0.7	0.3	0.06	0.16	1.1	208
Other and unspecified	177	0	-	-	-	1.5	0.7	1.2	1.9	9.4	7.3	16.6	21.4	72.1	90.5	82.2	129.7	141.5	120.2	253.3	11.4	4.1	1.11	2.17	18.3	O&U
All sites	4305	0	15.4	11.0	11.7	13.2	15.4	38.0	56.2	105.3	182.3	373.8	717.0	1262.7	2095.8	2727.0	3390.8	3776.4	4431.5	3658.9	277.5		24.49	55.08	450.5	ALL
All sites but 173	4296	0	15.4	11.0	11.0	13.2	14.7	36.8	55.6	103.1	182.3	372.4	717.0	1262.7	2095.8	2727.0	3390.8	3776.4	4431.5	3658.9	276.9	100.0	24.45	55.04	450.1	ALLb

Rate from 1 case   0.616   0.686   0.733   0.731   0.699   0.594   0.624   0.721   0.911   1.379   1.948   2.670   3.481   4.329   6.176   8.844   17.176   28.145

†Important: see notes on population page

USA, GEORGIA, ATLANTA: BLACK 1988-1992

ANNUAL INCIDENCE PER 100,000 BY AGE GROUP (YEARS) - FEMALE

SITE	ALL AGES	AGE UNK	0-	5-	10-	15-	20-	25-	30-	35-	40-	45-	50-	55-	60-	65-	70-	75-	80-	85+	CRUDE RATE	%	CR 64	CR 74	ASR (W)	ICD (9th)
Lip	1	0	-	-	-	-	-	-	-	-	-	-	-	-	-	-	3.5	-	-	-	0.1	0.0	0.00	0.02	**0.1**	*140*
Tongue	12	0	-	-	-	-	-	0.5	-	0.8	-	6.6	4.2	4.9	2.9	-	-	-	9.1	0.7	0.3	0.08	0.10	**0.9**	*141*
Salivary gland	13	0	-	-	0.8	-	-	1.0	0.5	0.6	0.8	-	1.6	2.1	7.3	2.9	3.5	-	-	-	0.7	0.3	0.07	0.11	**0.9**	*142*
Mouth	29	0	-	-	-	0.7	-	-	0.5	1.8	0.8	4.8	8.2	8.5	4.9	5.9	10.5	4.4	7.1	9.1	1.6	0.7	0.15	0.23	**2.0**	*143-5*
Oropharynx	14	0	-	-	-	-	-	-	-	0.6	0.8	3.6	6.6	2.1	2.4	5.9	-	-	7.1	-	0.8	0.4	0.08	0.11	**1.0**	*146*
Nasopharynx	4	0	-	-	-	-	-	0.5	0.5	-	-	-	-	-	2.9	3.5	-	-	-	-	0.2	0.1	0.01	0.04	**0.2**	*147*
Hypopharynx	10	0	-	-	-	-	-	-	-	-	0.8	1.2	3.3	2.1	2.4	5.9	3.5	4.4	-	-	0.6	0.3	0.05	0.10	**0.8**	*148*
Pharynx unspecified	9	0	-	-	-	-	-	-	-	-	-	-	-	-	2.4	11.8	-	8.8	7.1	9.1	0.5	0.2	0.01	0.07	**0.6**	*149*
Oesophagus	63	0	-	-	-	-	-	-	-	1.2	1.5	7.2	19.7	19.1	19.5	38.2	14.0	26.4	-	9.1	3.6	1.6	0.34	0.60	**4.9**	*150*
Stomach	81	0	-	-	-	-	0.6	1.5	1.6	1.2	2.3	-	4.9	29.6	19.5	11.8	38.6	48.4	63.8	81.7	4.6	2.1	0.31	0.56	**5.0**	*151*
Small intestine	19	0	-	-	-	-	0.6	-	-	0.6	-	1.2	3.3	4.2	2.4	14.7	14.0	-	7.1	9.1	1.1	0.5	0.06	0.21	**1.4**	*152*
Colon	400	0	-	-	-	-	-	1.0	2.6	8.3	13.0	14.4	41.1	80.4	95.0	182.4	182.6	229.0	312.1	344.9	22.6	10.3	1.28	3.10	**26.2**	*153*
Rectum	129	0	-	-	-	-	-	1.0	1.6	4.7	3.8	12.0	11.5	29.6	36.6	61.8	59.7	52.9	49.6	72.6	7.3	3.3	0.50	1.11	**8.8**	*154*
Liver	25	0	0.6	-	-	-	-	-	0.5	0.6	2.3	1.2	-	2.1	4.9	20.6	-	-	35.5	27.2	1.4	0.6	0.06	0.16	**1.6**	*155*
Gallbladder etc.	23	0	-	-	-	-	-	-	-	0.6	-	2.4	-	12.7	2.4	5.9	10.5	13.2	28.4	9.1	1.3	0.6	0.09	0.17	**1.5**	*156*
Pancreas	135	0	-	-	-	-	1.2	-	-	1.2	3.8	9.6	6.6	27.5	36.6	58.8	63.2	96.9	99.3	108.9	7.6	3.5	0.43	1.04	**8.9**	*157*
Nose, sinuses etc.	4	0	-	-	-	0.7	-	-	-	-	0.8	1.2	1.6	-	-	-	-	-	-	-	0.2	0.1	0.02	0.02	**0.3**	*160*
Larynx	31	0	-	-	-	-	-	-	-	1.2	2.3	2.4	11.5	10.6	7.3	11.8	7.0	4.4	-	18.2	1.8	0.8	0.18	0.27	**2.3**	*161*
Bronchus, lung	402	0	-	-	-	-	-	1.0	4.1	5.9	16.1	38.4	72.4	91.0	165.7	205.9	179.1	123.3	92.2	108.9	22.7	10.4	1.97	3.90	**29.8**	*162*
Other thoracic organs	7	0	0.6	-	-	-	0.6	-	0.5	-	1.5	-	-	-	2.4	2.9	-	-	-	-	0.4	0.2	0.03	0.04	**0.4**	*163-4*
Bone	13	0	-	1.4	1.5	0.7	1.2	-	-	1.2	-	1.2	1.6	4.2	-	-	-	-	-	-	0.7	0.3	0.07	0.07	**0.8**	*170*
Connective tissue	32	0	1.9	-	-	1.4	1.2	0.5	1.0	1.8	1.5	2.4	-	4.2	4.9	5.9	10.5	13.2	7.1	18.2	1.8	0.8	0.10	0.19	**1.9**	*171*
Mesothelioma	2	0	-	-	-	-	-	-	-	-	0.8	1.2	-	-	-	-	-	-	-	-	0.1	0.1	0.01	0.01	**0.1**	*MES*
Kaposi's sarcoma	4	0	-	-	-	-	-	0.5	0.6	-	-	-	-	-	-	-	-	7.1	9.1	-	0.2	0.1	0.01	0.01	**0.1**	*KAP*
Melanoma of skin	8	0	-	-	-	-	-	-	-	-	1.5	-	-	2.1	-	-	3.5	4.4	14.2	9.1	0.5	0.2	0.02	0.04	**0.4**	*172*
†Other skin	17	0	-	-	0.8	-	-	1.0	1.0	2.4	3.1	1.2	-	2.1	2.4	-	3.5	-	-	-	1.0		0.07	0.09	**0.9**	*173*
Breast	1158	0	-	-	0.8	-	3.0	12.1	34.2	56.8	127.3	157.2	182.6	207.5	229.1	273.5	291.5	400.8	453.9	317.7	65.4	29.9	5.05	7.88	**72.3**	*174*
Uterus unspecified	8	0	-	-	-	-	0.6	-	-	-	-	-	1.6	-	2.4	2.9	10.5	4.4	-	-	0.5	0.2	0.02	0.09	**0.6**	*179*
Cervix uteri	205	0	-	-	-	0.7	1.8	8.1	9.8	14.2	23.0	26.4	26.3	27.5	36.6	44.1	31.6	39.6	49.6	54.5	11.6	5.3	0.87	1.25	**12.0**	*180*
Placenta	2	0	-	-	-	-	1.2	-	-	-	-	-	-	-	-	-	-	-	-	-	0.1	0.1	0.01	0.01	**0.1**	*181*
Corpus uteri	155	0	-	-	-	-	-	1.0	2.6	3.6	1.5	10.8	6.6	29.6	53.6	73.5	94.8	70.5	92.2	90.8	8.8	4.0	0.55	1.39	**10.6**	*182*
Ovary etc.	118	0	-	-	-	1.4	1.2	1.5	2.6	4.1	3.8	13.2	28.0	27.5	24.4	44.1	10.5	48.4	42.6	72.6	6.7	3.0	0.54	0.81	**7.8**	*183*
Other female genital	35	0	-	-	-	-	-	0.5	1.0	-	-	6.0	3.3	6.4	4.9	14.7	14.0	22.0	28.4	18.2	2.0	0.9	0.11	0.25	**2.3**	*184*
Bladder	57	0	-	-	-	-	-	-	-	1.2	0.8	3.6	4.9	4.2	2.4	32.4	35.1	52.9	42.6	54.5	3.2	1.5	0.09	0.42	**3.5**	*188*
Kidney etc.	77	0	-	0.7	0.8	-	-	0.5	1.0	3.0	3.8	8.4	4.9	16.9	24.4	44.1	17.6	22.0	35.5	36.3	4.3	2.0	0.32	0.63	**5.3**	*189*
Eye	2	0	1.3	-	-	-	-	-	-	-	-	-	-	-	-	-	-	-	-	-	0.1	0.1	0.01	0.01	**0.2**	*190*
Brain, nervous system	56	0	2.5	2.1	3.8	-	1.2	1.0	2.6	2.4	2.3	3.6	3.3	4.2	19.5	8.8	10.5	22.0	14.2	-	3.2	1.4	0.24	0.34	**3.6**	*191-2*
Thyroid	59	0	-	0.7	-	0.7	3.0	3.0	2.6	2.4	5.4	3.6	9.9	4.2	14.6	5.9	3.5	13.2	28.4	27.2	3.3	1.5	0.25	0.30	**3.4**	*193*
Other endocrine	3	0	-	-	-	-	-	-	-	-	-	-	-	-	5.9	3.5	-	-	-	-	0.2	0.1	0.00	0.05	**0.2**	*194*
Hodgkin's disease	34	0	-	-	0.8	0.7	3.6	4.6	4.1	1.8	-	2.4	3.3	-	2.4	-	3.5	-	-	-	1.9	0.9	0.12	0.14	**1.6**	*201*
Non-Hodgkin lymphoma	98	0	0.6	-	0.8	0.7	0.6	3.5	1.0	2.4	4.6	7.2	13.2	6.4	39.0	38.2	56.2	30.8	28.4	18.2	5.5	2.5	0.40	0.87	**6.7**	*200,202*
Multiple myeloma	93	0	-	-	-	-	-	-	-	1.8	1.5	3.6	6.6	23.3	19.5	44.1	38.6	70.5	78.0	81.7	5.3	2.4	0.28	0.70	**6.1**	*203*
Lymphoid leukaemia	35	0	3.2	1.4	0.8	1.4	1.2	-	-	-	0.8	1.2	-	4.2	9.7	5.9	10.5	22.0	21.3	18.2	2.0	0.9	0.12	0.20	**2.3**	*204*
Myeloid leukaemia	45	0	-	2.8	2.3	1.4	-	2.0	2.1	1.2	2.3	-	-	4.2	21.9	5.9	3.5	30.8	-	18.2	2.5	1.2	0.20	0.25	**2.8**	*205*
Monocytic leukaemia	0	0	-	-	-	-	-	-	-	-	-	-	-	-	-	-	-	-	-	-	0.0	0.0	0.00	0.00	**0.0**	*206*
Other leukaemia	0	0	-	-	-	-	-	-	-	-	-	-	-	-	-	-	-	-	-	-	0.0	0.0	0.00	0.00	**0.0**	*207*
Leukaemia unspecified	4	0	-	-	-	-	-	-	-	0.6	-	-	-	-	-	2.9	3.5	-	7.1	-	0.2	0.1	0.00	0.04	**0.2**	*208*
Other and unspecified	165	0	1.3	-	0.8	-	0.6	1.0	2.1	2.4	6.9	7.2	11.5	27.5	29.2	52.9	101.8	88.1	113.5	190.6	9.3	4.3	0.45	1.23	**10.3**	*O&U*
All sites	3896	0	12.0	9.2	13.5	10.9	23.4	46.5	81.4	132.0	242.4	360.1	506.7	732.5	957.7	1358.8	1352.0	1567.9	1773.2	1851.7	220.0		15.64	29.20	**253.7**	*ALL*
All sites but 173	3879	0	12.0	9.2	12.8	10.9	23.4	45.5	80.3	129.7	239.4	358.9	506.7	730.4	955.3	1358.8	1348.5	1567.9	1773.2	1851.7	219.1	100.0	15.57	29.11	**252.8**	*ALLb*
Rate from 1 case			0.630	0.707	0.750	0.724	0.600	0.506	0.518	0.592	0.767	1.200	1.645	2.117	2.437	2.941	3.512	4.404	7.093	9.077						

†Important: see notes on population page

USA, Iowa

Cancer data collection for the entire state of Iowa began in 1969 with the Third National Cancer Survey sponsored by the National Cancer Institute (NCI). With the completion of the survey in 1971, no further funding for cancer registration was available, therefore 1972 data are incomplete. In 1973, the State Health Registry of Iowa, frequently referred to as the Iowa Cancer Registry, became part of the NCI Surveillance, Epidemiology and End Results (SEER) Program and state-wide incidence recording was reinstated. Thus, population-based incidence data are available for the years 1969–71 and 1973 to the present.

The registry is administratively within the Department of Preventive Medicine and Environmental Health of the University of Iowa College of Medicine and functions as a collaborative programme with the Iowa Department of Public Health.

The state of Iowa is located near the geographical middle of the United States and is part of the American agricultural heartland. Bordered to the north by Minnesota, the south by Missouri, the east by Illinois, and the west by Nebraska, it lies between 40°30′ and 43°30′ N, and 91°30′ and 93°30′ W. The total area is about 145 800 km², with elevations ranging between 146 and 505 m above sea level. The climate is humid continental, with an average annual temperature of 9.5°C and average annual precipitation of approximately 80 cm.

The state had a population of 2 780 000 in 1990, of whom about 40% lived in rural locations including places with less than 2500 inhabitants. Only two towns had populations exceeding 100 000, although 11 of the 99 counties are currently designated as metropolitan areas. The principal ethnic group is Caucasian, with Germans, Danes and Swedes accounting for a large segment of the population. Over 80% of Iowa residents are native-born. The 1990 population was 96.6% white, 1.7% black and 1.7% other races. The population is primarily Christian, the most prevalent denominations being Roman Catholic, Lutheran and Methodist.

Iowa is a predominantly agricultural state, the main crops being corn and soybeans. Meat production is also important, the state being responsible for 25% of US production of pork. Food-processing and farm-equipment manufacture are the major industrial activities.

Cancer became a reportable disease in Iowa in 1982. The Iowa Department of Public Health has designated responsibility for cancer data collection to the registry. Cancer data for Iowa residents are obtained from 150 hospitals, clinics and private pathology laboratories located both within the state and in places bordering the state where Iowans may go for cancer care. Three neighbouring states exchange cancer data with the registry. Data are collected by hospital cancer registrars and by nineteen field staff employed by the registry, who visit assigned hospitals and free-standing pathology laboratories. The field staff abstract cancer data using laptop computers and transmit the data via modem to the registry. The data are then extensively edited at the registry.

Although some Iowans who leave the state for care are missed, ascertainment is thought to be about 99% complete. Sources of ascertainment within hospitals include medical records, radiation oncology and pathology departments. Cancer cases are also ascertained by registry staff from pathology laboratories that are not associated with a hospital. Death certificates that mention cancer and were not previously ascertained are followed back to determine if the cases are reportable. The registry applies a number of passive follow-up mechanisms to obtain survival data. These include computerized linkage of SEER incidence data with (1) death certificate data, (2) driver's license files from the Iowa Department of Transportation, and (3) medicare files provided by the Health Care Financing Administration. Active patient follow-up is conducted on an annual basis using a combination of methodologies, including patient and/or physician postal follow-up, hospital registries through both manual review and computer data linkage, and hospital readmission reviews.

The unit of registration within the registry is the tumour rather than the patient. Careful checking is carried out to avoid duplicate registration both of the patients and of the same tumour within a patient. Quality control activities in the areas of abstracting, coding and data management involve a significant portion of the registry's operation.

Registry data have been extensively used in a number of national and international epidemiological studies.

Charles F. Lynch
Charles E. Platz
Kathleen M. McKeen

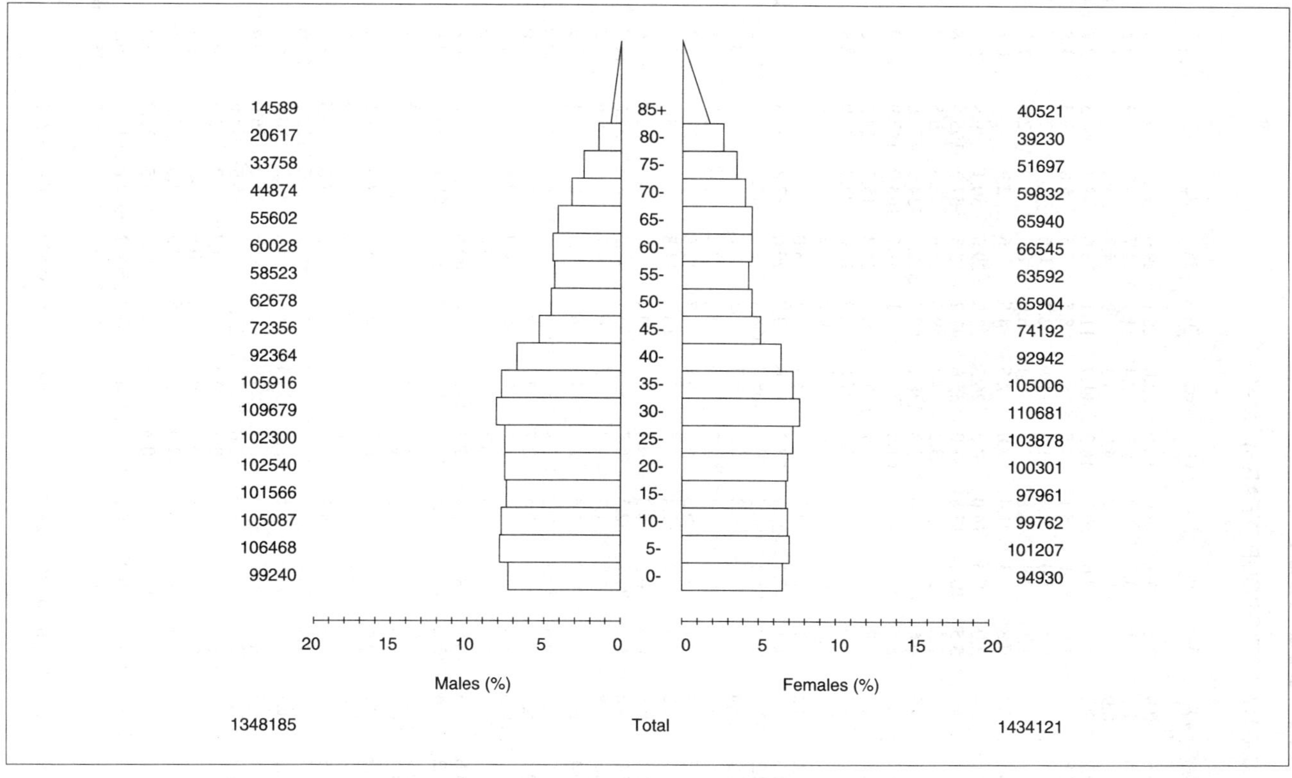

USA, Iowa
Source of population: average annual 1988-92
Estimate: NCI estimates based on U.S. Bureau of Census population estimates by county for the years 1988–92.

Notes to tables overleaf:
† 173 does not include basal cell or squamous cell carcinoma

USA, IOWA 1988-1992

ANNUAL INCIDENCE PER 100,000 BY AGE GROUP (YEARS) - MALE

SITE	ALL AGES	AGE UNK	0-	5-	10-	15-	20-	25-	30-	35-	40-	45-	50-	55-	60-	65-	70-	75-	80-	85+	CRUDE RATE	%	CR 64	CR 74	ASR (W)	ICD (9th)
Lip	358	0	-	-	-	0.2	0.2	-	0.7	0.6	0.9	2.2	7.7	8.9	16.0	23.0	28.1	29.6	35.9	34.3	5.3	1.0	0.19	0.44	**3.6**	*140*
Tongue	148	0	-	-	-	0.2	-	0.2	0.4	0.8	1.1	1.1	3.5	6.2	9.7	9.4	11.1	4.7	8.7	6.9	2.2	0.4	0.12	0.22	**1.7**	*141*
Salivary gland	75	0	-	-	-	0.2	-	0.4	0.4	-	0.9	0.3	1.9	1.7	4.0	4.3	4.9	4.7	5.8	6.9	1.1	0.2	0.05	0.09	**0.8**	*142*
Mouth	249	0	-	-	-	0.2	-	0.2	0.4	0.2	3.2	5.8	8.6	10.3	16.3	11.9	11.1	13.6	8.7	16.5	3.7	0.7	0.23	0.34	**2.9**	*143-5*
Oropharynx	120	0	-	-	-	-	-	-	-	0.8	0.9	1.9	5.1	5.1	4.7	8.3	8.5	6.5	5.8	1.4	1.8	0.3	0.09	0.18	**1.4**	*146*
Nasopharynx	31	0	-	-	-	-	-	0.2	0.4	-	-	0.6	1.0	2.4	1.0	1.8	2.2	0.6	-	2.7	0.5	0.1	0.03	0.05	**0.4**	*147*
Hypopharynx	123	0	-	-	-	-	-	-	-	-	-	1.1	3.8	4.8	7.7	10.4	8.9	8.9	3.9	2.7	1.8	0.3	0.09	0.18	**1.4**	*148*
Pharynx unspecified	48	0	-	-	-	-	-	-	0.2	0.2	0.8	1.3	1.4	3.0	2.5	4.5	3.6	2.9	-	0.7	0.1	0.03	0.07	**0.5**	*149*
Oesophagus	401	0	-	-	-	-	-	0.2	0.9	0.4	3.0	8.0	14.0	20.0	26.3	33.0	29.0	30.1	39.8	5.9	1.1	0.23	0.53	**4.1**	*150*
Stomach	661	0	-	-	-	-	-	0.2	0.4	1.5	4.1	5.5	10.2	18.8	31.0	35.6	47.2	53.3	57.2	105.6	9.8	1.8	0.36	0.77	**6.6**	*151*
Small intestine	114	0	-	-	-	-	-	0.2	-	-	0.9	2.2	2.6	3.1	3.3	4.7	9.4	13.6	12.6	5.5	1.7	0.3	0.06	0.13	**1.1**	*152*
Colon	3321	0	-	-	-	-	0.6	0.6	2.4	4.5	6.9	16.6	42.4	77.6	122.3	178.1	268.8	337.1	434.6	471.6	49.3	9.2	1.37	3.60	**30.7**	*153*
Rectum	1474	0	-	-	-	-	0.2	1.0	0.7	2.1	5.0	8.6	20.7	42.7	61.6	78.1	139.1	131.5	163.0	143.9	21.9	4.1	0.71	1.80	**14.3**	*154*
Liver	244	0	0.6	-	-	-	0.2	-	0.4	0.6	0.9	0.8	2.9	6.8	9.7	18.3	20.1	24.3	15.5	23.3	3.6	0.7	0.11	0.31	**2.4**	*155*
Gallbladder etc.	159	0	0.2	-	-	-	-	0.2	0.2	0.6	0.2	0.6	1.9	2.7	6.3	7.6	12.9	16.6	22.3	21.9	2.4	0.4	0.06	0.17	**1.5**	*156*
Pancreas	787	0	-	-	-	-	-	-	0.7	1.3	1.7	4.4	10.8	22.6	32.3	41.7	60.2	81.2	89.2	102.8	11.7	2.2	0.37	0.88	**7.5**	*157*
Nose, sinuses etc.	55	0	0.2	-	-	-	-	0.2	0.2	0.4	0.2	1.1	1.0	2.1	2.3	1.4	3.6	3.0	8.7	4.1	0.8	0.2	0.04	0.06	**0.6**	*160*
Larynx	599	0	-	-	-	-	-	-	-	1.3	1.7	4.1	12.4	22.9	37.3	53.6	39.7	29.0	37.8	34.3	8.9	1.7	0.40	0.87	**6.5**	*161*
Bronchus, lung	6688	0	-	-	0.4	-	0.2	0.2	1.6	4.3	12.6	39.8	95.4	188.3	320.8	468.7	568.3	631.0	644.1	452.4	99.2	18.5	3.32	8.50	**65.9**	*162*
Other thoracic organs	23	0	0.8	-	-	0.2	-	0.2	0.4	0.2	0.6	-	-	0.3	0.3	0.7	1.3	0.6	-	4.1	0.3	0.1	0.02	0.03	**0.3**	*163-4*
Bone	73	0	0.2	0.2	2.1	1.8	0.8	0.6	1.1	0.6	0.4	1.7	0.6	1.4	1.7	1.4	2.2	2.4	1.0	2.7	1.1	0.2	0.07	0.08	**1.0**	*170*
Connective tissue	217	0	0.6	0.9	0.6	0.2	1.8	1.2	1.6	1.5	2.8	2.8	4.8	5.5	5.0	6.8	14.7	13.6	11.6	23.3	3.2	0.6	0.15	0.25	**2.5**	*171*
Mesothelioma	102	0	-	-	-	-	-	-	-	0.2	0.2	1.4	1.9	2.4	2.7	5.8	10.7	11.8	9.7	5.5	1.5	0.3	0.04	0.13	**1.0**	*MES*
Kaposi's sarcoma	41	0	-	-	-	-	-	1.8	2.7	1.1	0.6	0.8	0.3	0.3	0.3	-	0.4	-	-	1.4	0.6	0.1	0.04	0.04	**0.5**	*KAP*
Melanoma of skin	862	0	0.2	0.2	-	0.8	1.4	4.9	6.6	14.0	15.8	16.3	21.7	32.5	26.7	33.8	35.7	43.2	48.5	57.6	12.8	2.4	0.70	1.05	**9.9**	*172*
†Other skin	83	0	-	-	0.6	-	0.2	0.4	0.2	0.9	0.9	1.1	1.9	1.7	2.3	2.5	6.2	4.1	9.7	9.6	1.2	-	0.05	0.09	**0.9**	*173*
Breast	58	0	-	-	-	-	-	-	-	0.4	0.4	-	0.3	1.4	2.0	4.7	6.2	3.6	6.8	4.1	0.9	0.2	0.02	0.08	**0.6**	*175*
Prostate	10112	0	0.2	0.2	-	-	-	-	0.2	0.2	1.1	6.6	39.9	122.3	322.8	639.9	1030.9	1256.6	1388.2	1347.5	150.0	28.0	2.47	10.82	**86.4**	*185*
Testis	334	0	-	-	-	3.3	9.9	10.9	14.4	9.4	6.3	4.1	4.1	2.4	2.7	2.2	0.9	-	1.0	-	5.0	0.9	0.34	0.35	**4.5**	*186*
Penis	71	0	-	-	-	-	-	0.4	-	0.6	1.4	0.6	1.0	1.7	5.4	6.7	4.7	7.8	6.9	1.1	0.2	0.03	0.09	**0.7**	*187.1-.4*
Other male genital	19	0	0.4	-	-	0.2	-	0.2	-	-	-	-	-	1.4	0.3	0.7	2.2	0.6	1.0	1.4	0.3	0.1	0.01	0.03	**0.2**	*187.5-.9*
Bladder	2478	0	-	0.2	0.2	0.2	0.2	1.2	2.9	3.6	7.6	16.0	28.1	42.4	92.3	141.7	198.8	269.6	307.5	327.6	36.8	6.9	0.97	2.68	**22.9**	*188*
Kidney etc.	1006	0	1.4	0.9	-	0.2	0.6	0.4	1.6	4.2	5.4	15.2	18.8	35.5	40.3	57.9	70.9	82.4	95.1	49.4	14.9	2.8	0.62	1.27	**10.6**	*189*
Eye	77	0	1.0	0.2	-	-	0.2	-	0.4	0.9	0.4	0.3	3.5	2.4	1.3	2.9	4.0	7.1	4.9	5.5	1.1	0.2	0.05	0.09	**0.9**	*190*
Brain, nervous system	565	0	3.2	4.3	2.9	3.3	3.1	3.5	3.6	5.5	6.7	8.6	12.1	14.0	18.3	23.4	24.1	26.7	30.1	27.4	8.4	1.6	0.45	0.68	**7.0**	*191-2*
Thyroid	210	0	-	-	0.2	0.2	1.6	2.9	3.3	4.5	4.1	3.0	6.4	5.8	6.3	7.6	6.2	8.3	4.9	4.1	3.1	0.6	0.19	0.26	**2.6**	*193*
Other endocrine	28	0	1.6	0.2	-	0.6	0.4	0.4	-	0.2	0.2	-	0.3	-	0.7	0.7	-	2.4	-	1.4	0.4	0.1	0.02	0.03	**0.4**	*194*
Hodgkin's disease	235	0	0.2	0.2	1.5	3.3	4.5	5.1	4.2	4.5	3.0	2.5	4.5	4.1	2.3	8.3	6.7	3.6	7.8	5.5	3.5	0.7	0.20	0.27	**3.1**	*201*
Non-Hodgkin lymphoma	1390	0	0.2	1.3	1.7	1.8	2.5	2.7	5.8	9.3	11.5	17.4	26.8	35.5	47.6	71.2	94.9	94.2	124.2	152.2	20.6	3.9	0.82	1.65	**14.6**	*200,202*
Multiple myeloma	458	0	-	-	-	-	-	-	0.4	1.1	1.7	2.8	4.8	9.6	15.0	28.4	41.0	46.8	49.5	58.9	6.8	1.3	0.18	0.52	**4.3**	*203*
Lymphoid leukaemia	635	0	6.0	3.6	1.5	1.4	1.2	0.2	0.9	1.1	1.5	4.1	10.2	14.7	22.3	25.9	41.4	51.5	65.0	96.0	9.4	1.8	0.34	0.68	**6.8**	*204*
Myeloid leukaemia	404	0	1.0	0.4	0.4	1.2	1.4	1.0	2.0	1.9	2.6	2.8	6.4	8.9	12.0	18.3	29.4	37.3	35.9	48.0	6.0	1.1	0.21	0.45	**4.1**	*205*
Monocytic leukaemia	26	0	-	-	-	0.2	-	-	-	0.2	-	0.3	-	0.7	0.4	2.7	4.7	3.9	2.7	-	0.4	0.1	0.01	0.02	**0.2**	*206*
Other leukaemia	8	0	-	-	0.2	-	-	-	-	-	-	0.3	-	0.3	0.7	0.4	0.4	0.6	-	-	0.1	0.0	0.01	0.01	**0.1**	*207*
Leukaemia unspecified	93	0	0.6	-	0.2	-	-	0.2	0.4	0.4	0.6	0.3	0.3	1.0	2.0	3.6	5.8	9.5	13.6	23.3	1.4	0.3	0.03	0.08	**0.8**	*208*
Other and unspecified	905	0	0.8	-	-	0.2	0.2	1.0	0.9	1.7	3.0	8.3	11.2	17.1	30.3	46.8	58.4	92.4	113.5	172.7	13.4	2.5	0.37	0.90	**8.4**	*O&U*
All sites	36168	0	19.5	12.8	12.4	19.9	31.2	42.2	62.9	87.6	120.2	218.6	450.9	806.2	1370.0	2126.9	2984.3	3500.2	3927.8	3915.1	536.5		16.27	41.83	**349.1**	*ALL*
All sites but 173	36085	0	19.5	12.8	11.8	19.9	31.0	41.8	62.7	86.7	119.3	217.5	449.0	804.5	1367.7	2124.4	2978.1	3496.1	3918.1	3905.5	535.3	100.0	16.22	41.73	**348.2**	*ALLb*

Rate from 1 case | | | 0.202 | 0.188 | 0.190 | 0.197 | 0.195 | 0.196 | 0.182 | 0.189 | 0.217 | 0.276 | 0.319 | 0.342 | 0.333 | 0.360 | 0.446 | 0.592 | 0.970 | 1.371 |

†Important: see notes on population page

USA, IOWA 1988-1992

ANNUAL INCIDENCE PER 100,000 BY AGE GROUP (YEARS) - FEMALE

SITE	ALL AGES	AGE UNK	0-	5-	10-	15-	20-	25-	30-	35-	40-	45-	50-	55-	60-	65-	70-	75-	80-	85+	CRUDE RATE	%	CR 64	CR 74	ASR (W)	ICD (9th)
Lip	51	0	-	-	-	-	-	-	0.2	0.2	0.4	0.5	0.6	1.6	1.2	1.5	2.3	4.3	3.1	2.5	0.7	0.2	0.02	0.04	**0.4**	140
Tongue	100	0	-	-	-	-	-	0.4	0.4	0.4	0.9	1.1	1.8	3.1	4.2	3.6	5.3	3.5	3.6	5.9	1.4	0.3	0.06	0.11	**0.9**	141
Salivary gland	62	0	-	0.2	-	0.4	-	0.8	0.5	0.2	0.6	1.1	0.6	1.3	0.9	2.1	2.7	1.5	4.6	3.5	0.9	0.2	0.03	0.06	**0.6**	142
Mouth	160	0	-	-	0.4	0.4	0.2	-	0.2	0.6	0.4	0.5	3.0	4.4	6.0	6.4	7.7	5.0	10.7	12.3	2.2	0.5	0.08	0.15	**1.3**	143-5
Oropharynx	55	0	-	-	-	-	-	-	-	-	0.2	1.6	0.9	1.6	3.3	4.5	2.0	1.2	2.0	0.5	0.8	0.2	0.04	0.07	**0.6**	146
Nasopharynx	19	0	-	-	0.4	0.2	-	-	0.2	0.2	-	0.5	-	1.3	0.6	0.3	0.7	0.4	0.5	0.5	0.3	0.1	0.02	0.02	**0.2**	147
Hypopharynx	25	0	-	-	-	-	-	-	-	-	0.2	0.3	0.3	1.9	1.2	1.2	1.3	-	1.5	0.5	0.3	0.1	0.02	0.03	**0.2**	148
Pharynx unspecified	12	0	-	-	-	-	-	-	-	-	-	0.3	-	0.3	0.3	0.6	-	1.2	0.5	1.5	0.2	0.0	0.00	0.01	**0.1**	149
Oesophagus	126	0	-	-	-	-	-	0.2	-	-	-	-	0.9	2.5	3.9	6.7	5.7	8.9	9.7	9.9	1.8	0.4	0.04	0.10	**0.8**	150
Stomach	379	0	-	-	-	-	-	-	0.2	1.0	0.6	2.7	2.4	3.8	6.9	12.1	17.7	29.4	31.1	42.9	5.3	1.1	0.09	0.24	**2.2**	151
Small intestine	112	0	-	-	-	-	-	0.2	-	0.4	0.6	1.6	1.5	2.2	3.9	5.8	5.3	5.0	6.6	6.9	1.6	0.3	0.05	0.11	**0.9**	152
Colon	3999	0	-	-	-	0.2	-	1.9	2.0	3.8	8.0	19.7	29.1	70.1	103.7	148.6	186.5	268.9	336.5	385.0	55.8	12.0	1.19	2.87	**25.1**	153
Rectum	1254	0	-	-	-	-	0.4	0.4	1.3	2.9	2.8	7.3	15.8	22.6	36.7	52.2	66.2	75.4	86.2	102.7	17.5	3.8	0.45	1.04	**8.7**	154
Liver	140	0	0.2	0.2	-	-	-	0.4	0.2	0.4	-	1.9	1.5	1.3	3.6	4.5	7.4	8.9	13.8	8.9	2.0	0.4	0.05	0.11	**1.0**	155
Gallbladder etc.	291	0	-	-	-	-	-	-	-	0.8	0.4	1.1	1.8	5.0	6.3	11.2	13.7	22.1	21.9	29.6	4.1	0.9	0.08	0.20	**1.8**	156
Pancreas	841	0	-	-	-	0.2	0.2	-	0.2	0.4	1.9	3.8	7.9	11.0	18.3	28.5	49.5	61.9	60.7	83.9	11.7	2.5	0.22	0.61	**5.2**	157
Nose, sinuses etc.	46	0	-	-	-	-	0.2	0.2	0.2	0.2	0.4	0.3	0.9	0.9	1.8	1.5	1.7	1.9	4.6	1.5	0.6	0.1	0.03	0.04	**0.4**	160
Larynx	127	0	-	-	-	-	-	-	0.2	-	-	1.3	4.2	7.2	6.6	9.7	4.7	1.9	2.5	3.0	1.8	0.4	0.10	0.17	**1.3**	161
Bronchus, lung	3437	0	-	-	-	-	0.2	0.8	1.8	3.0	8.8	28.6	61.9	101.9	144.6	194.7	203.9	185.7	160.6	100.2	47.9	10.3	1.76	3.75	**28.6**	162
Other thoracic organs	15	0	0.4	-	-	-	-	-	0.2	-	-	0.5	0.6	0.6	-	0.3	0.3	0.8	0.5	0.5	0.2	0.0	0.01	0.02	**0.2**	163-4
Bone	77	0	-	0.6	2.4	1.8	0.6	0.2	0.2	1.1	0.6	0.3	0.3	0.9	1.5	2.1	1.7	2.7	4.1	1.0	1.1	0.2	0.05	0.07	**0.9**	170
Connective tissue	200	0	1.1	0.6	0.6	1.0	0.2	1.5	0.9	2.1	2.4	1.6	2.4	3.8	4.2	7.3	7.7	7.4	8.7	12.3	2.8	0.6	0.11	0.19	**1.9**	171
Mesothelioma	29	0	-	-	-	-	-	-	0.2	-	-	0.3	0.6	0.3	0.6	1.5	1.0	2.3	1.0	3.0	0.4	0.1	0.01	0.02	**0.2**	MES
Kaposi's sarcoma	4	0	-	-	-	-	-	-	-	-	-	-	-	-	-	-	-	0.8	0.5	0.5	0.1	0.0	0.00	0.00	**0.0**	KAP
Melanoma of skin	833	0	-	-	0.4	1.2	5.0	8.9	11.7	15.6	14.0	14.8	17.6	15.7	16.2	19.1	22.1	24.4	24.5	42.0	11.6	2.5	0.61	0.81	**8.4**	172
†Other skin	57	0	0.2	0.2	-	0.2	-	0.4	0.4	0.8	0.9	-	1.2	0.6	1.5	1.2	1.7	1.5	5.1	3.9	0.8		0.03	0.05	**0.5**	173
Breast	9716	0	-	-	-	-	1.6	5.4	25.7	64.2	116.6	178.7	226.1	233.4	302.7	374.9	419.2	474.7	451.7	443.7	135.5	29.2	5.77	9.74	**85.3**	174
Uterus unspecified	23	0	-	-	-	-	-	-	-	0.2	-	0.8	0.9	0.6	-	-	0.7	-	0.5	5.4	0.3	0.1	0.01	0.02	**0.2**	179
Cervix uteri	727	0	-	-	-	0.2	2.0	10.8	15.0	17.0	17.2	16.4	17.3	12.6	17.4	17.3	16.4	13.2	13.8	12.3	10.1	2.2	0.63	0.80	**8.2**	180
Placenta	5	0	-	-	-	-	0.2	0.2	0.2	0.4	-	-	-	-	-	-	-	-	-	-	0.1	0.0	0.00	0.00	**0.1**	181
Corpus uteri	2025	0	-	-	-	-	-	0.6	2.2	7.6	12.9	21.8	41.9	68.9	81.1	106.2	99.6	102.1	75.5	70.1	28.2	6.1	1.19	2.21	**17.7**	182
Ovary etc.	1359	0	0.2	-	0.2	3.1	2.6	3.3	4.7	7.4	11.0	22.6	24.9	34.0	39.7	57.0	62.2	68.5	61.2	58.7	19.0	4.1	0.77	1.36	**12.0**	183
Other female genital	295	0	0.2	-	-	-	-	0.2	1.3	0.6	1.3	1.6	3.3	7.9	8.7	7.9	15.0	14.3	19.4	29.6	4.1	0.9	0.13	0.24	**2.1**	184
Bladder	862	0	-	-	-	-	0.4	0.6	0.4	1.0	2.4	3.5	8.2	15.7	24.9	36.1	42.5	57.6	58.6	77.0	12.0	2.6	0.29	0.68	**5.7**	188
Kidney etc.	748	0	2.1	0.6	-	-	0.4	0.6	0.7	2.1	4.9	8.1	11.2	16.7	24.3	30.9	37.1	42.9	47.4	36.5	10.4	2.2	0.36	0.70	**6.1**	189
Eye	77	0	1.5	0.2	-	0.4	0.2	0.2	-	0.2	-	0.3	1.2	2.5	2.1	3.6	2.7	4.6	2.5	3.5	1.1	0.2	0.04	0.08	**0.8**	190
Brain, nervous system	478	0	2.5	3.0	2.0	1.2	2.0	3.9	2.2	3.6	4.1	4.9	11.2	9.1	11.1	18.5	17.0	28.6	15.8	8.4	6.7	1.4	0.30	0.48	**4.9**	191-2
Thyroid	530	0	-	-	1.2	2.2	7.0	10.0	11.0	10.3	11.0	12.9	12.1	12.3	9.6	9.7	8.7	7.4	7.1	4.9	7.4	1.6	0.50	0.59	**6.5**	193
Other endocrine	36	0	1.3	0.6	-	-	0.2	-	0.2	-	0.2	0.8	0.6	0.9	2.1	0.3	1.0	1.2	-	1.0	0.5	0.1	0.03	0.04	**0.5**	194
Hodgkin's disease	205	0	-	-	1.2	5.1	6.8	6.9	4.3	2.5	1.7	1.9	0.9	1.6	0.6	3.3	0.7	4.6	5.1	3.5	2.9	0.6	0.17	0.19	**2.6**	201
Non-Hodgkin lymphoma	1371	0	0.4	0.4	0.4	1.6	1.2	2.1	3.1	4.0	5.6	15.9	18.5	28.6	36.7	44.9	79.6	77.4	92.8	86.4	19.1	4.1	0.59	1.21	**10.4**	200,202
Multiple myeloma	417	0	-	-	-	-	0.2	-	-	0.4	0.6	2.4	3.9	7.2	12.6	16.4	21.4	34.4	35.7	23.2	5.8	1.3	0.14	0.33	**2.8**	203
Lymphoid leukaemia	461	0	5.3	2.2	1.6	1.2	0.2	0.2	-	1.0	1.5	1.6	2.7	4.7	8.1	16.1	22.7	24.4	33.6	44.4	6.4	1.4	0.15	0.35	**3.6**	204
Myeloid leukaemia	361	0	1.1	0.4	0.6	0.6	0.8	1.0	2.0	1.3	3.4	3.2	4.9	3.8	9.3	11.8	13.7	20.9	20.4	29.6	5.0	1.1	0.16	0.29	**2.9**	205
Monocytic leukaemia	29	0	0.2	-	-	0.2	-	0.2	-	-	0.2	0.3	-	0.3	0.9	1.2	1.7	0.8	0.5	3.9	0.4	0.1	0.01	0.03	**0.2**	206
Other leukaemia	9	0	0.2	-	-	-	-	-	-	0.2	-	-	0.3	0.3	-	0.3	0.7	-	0.5	0.5	0.1	0.0	0.01	0.01	**0.1**	207
Leukaemia unspecified	71	0	0.2	-	-	-	-	0.4	-	0.4	-	-	-	-	0.6	3.3	2.0	3.9	7.1	11.4	1.0	0.2	0.01	0.03	**0.4**	208
Other and unspecified	1064	0	-	-	0.2	-	0.2	0.6	0.7	1.5	3.0	6.2	7.0	15.4	22.8	30.3	43.8	63.8	102.5	130.8	14.8	3.2	0.29	0.66	**6.2**	O&U
All sites	33320	0	17.1	9.1	11.6	21.6	32.9	63.2	94.5	159.6	242.1	395.7	555.4	742.5	993.6	1317.6	1526.9	1772.2	1856.7	1949.6	464.7		16.69	30.92	**271.2**	ALL
All sites but 173	33263	0	16.9	8.9	11.6	21.4	32.9	62.8	94.1	158.8	241.2	395.7	554.1	741.9	992.1	1316.3	1525.3	1770.7	1851.6	1945.6	463.9	100.0	16.66	30.87	**270.7**	ALLb

| Rate from 1 case | | | 0.211 | 0.198 | 0.201 | 0.204 | 0.199 | 0.193 | 0.181 | 0.191 | 0.215 | 0.270 | 0.303 | 0.314 | 0.300 | 0.303 | 0.334 | 0.387 | 0.510 | 0.494 | | | | | | |

†Important: see notes on population page

USA, Louisiana, Central Region

The Louisiana Tumor Registry was established in 1974 to carry out cancer registration in the three counties of the metropolitan New Orleans area. Its coverage was expanded in 1983 to include South Louisiana, and in 1988 to the north, completing the statewide population-based registry. The registry consists of a central office and eight regional offices. Data from two of the eight regions, the rural Central Louisiana and the urban new Orleans area, are presented in this volume.

The registry functioned within the Office of Public Health of the Louisiana Department of Health and Hospitals until 1995, when it was transferred to the Louisiana State University Medical Center in New Orleans (LSUMC-NO). Funding for the registry came from the state's general funds before the transfer and now comes from LSUMC-NO. Since 1994, the Centers for Disease Control and Prevention have provided additional funds. The operations of the cancer registry are mandated by Louisiana law. An amendment to the law passed in 1995 requires all hospitals, pathology laboratories, radiation centres and clinicians who diagnose or treat cancer patients to report them to the registry, and allows for interstate exchange of cases. The same law mandates strict confidentiality of the data. The registry follows the rules and procedures of the Surveillance, Epidemiology and End Results (SEER) Program and uses the standards established by the North American Association of Central Cancer Registries (NAACCR).

Central Louisiana is the most rural and sparsely populated area and experiences the lowest cancer incidence in the state. The region stretches across the state from the Sabine River to the Mississippi River, encompassing a large national forest and two military bases. Alexandria is its largest city (population in 1990: 49 188). The population in 1990 was 311 982, of whom 25% were blacks and 73% whites (density 16.9 people per km^2 versus 36.9 in Louisiana as a whole). Median household incomes and the percentage of high-school graduates in Central Louisiana are significantly lower than in the state as a whole.

The principal economic activities are farming, mining, and lumber production. In addition, Alexandria derives many jobs from the military bases and as the commercial, cultural, and medical centre. Manufacturing, principally of wood products, and oil and gas extraction are also important. The leading agricultural crops are cotton and soybeans, as well as smaller amounts of rice, sugar, corn, and farm-raised fish. Pine trees, used mainly for paper pulp, are also harvested.

Air quality was not monitored in Central Louisiana. In 1987–94, industrial releases of toxic substances in the two most industrialized counties ranked in the highest quartile in the state. Other parts of the region reported no toxic industrial releases. The region derives its water mainly from wells. Water from all sources is monitored for compliance with federal water safety standards.

This presentation of cancer incidence data is restricted to patients who were residents of the registration area at the time of diagnosis. About half of the cases came from hospitals with cancer programmes accredited by the American College of Surgeons. These cases are abstracted by specially trained hospital registrars and submitted to the registry. The central registry staff screen and abstract cases from the remaining hospitals and from pathology laboratories and radiation centres that are not affiliated with hospitals. They also investigate death certificates mentioning cancer as a cause of death if the deceased was not included in the registry system. In 1988–92, death-certificate-only cases accounted for 2.8–3.5% in the Central Region.

Each patient in the registry is assigned a unique identification number. This allows identification of patients with multiple primaries. In defining multiple primaries, the registry follows the SEER rules, which vary slightly from the rules of IACR. The registry does not have an active follow-up programme, but hospitals with registries accredited by the American College of Surgeons obtain survival data on their patients annually, and death information is recorded at the registry as received.

Quality assurance in the registry is the responsibility of both the regional offices and the central registry. Rescreening and reabstracting are performed annually. An assessment of case completeness and data quality by the NAACCR on 1992 cases for the entire state showed a completeness rate of 97.6% and an overall data quality error rate of 5.9%. The 1988–92 data have been subjected to a wide range of computerized tests for invalid codes, inconsistencies and duplications using programs developed by the registry as well as by SEER and IARC.

The registry publishes periodic reports in the form of monographs. The *Cancer in Louisiana* series has provided information on cancer incidence and mortality rates, time trends and childhood cancers in New Orleans and South Louisiana, as well as comparisons among regions and with the national rates. Articles on cancer incidence are published in the *Journal of the Louisiana State Medical Society*. Other registry-based research has focused on stage at diagnosis and socioeconomic determinants as explanations for the discrepancies between incidence and mortality rates.

Vivien W. Chen
Catherine N. Correa
Patricia A. Andrews
Xiao Cheng Wu
Pelayo Correa

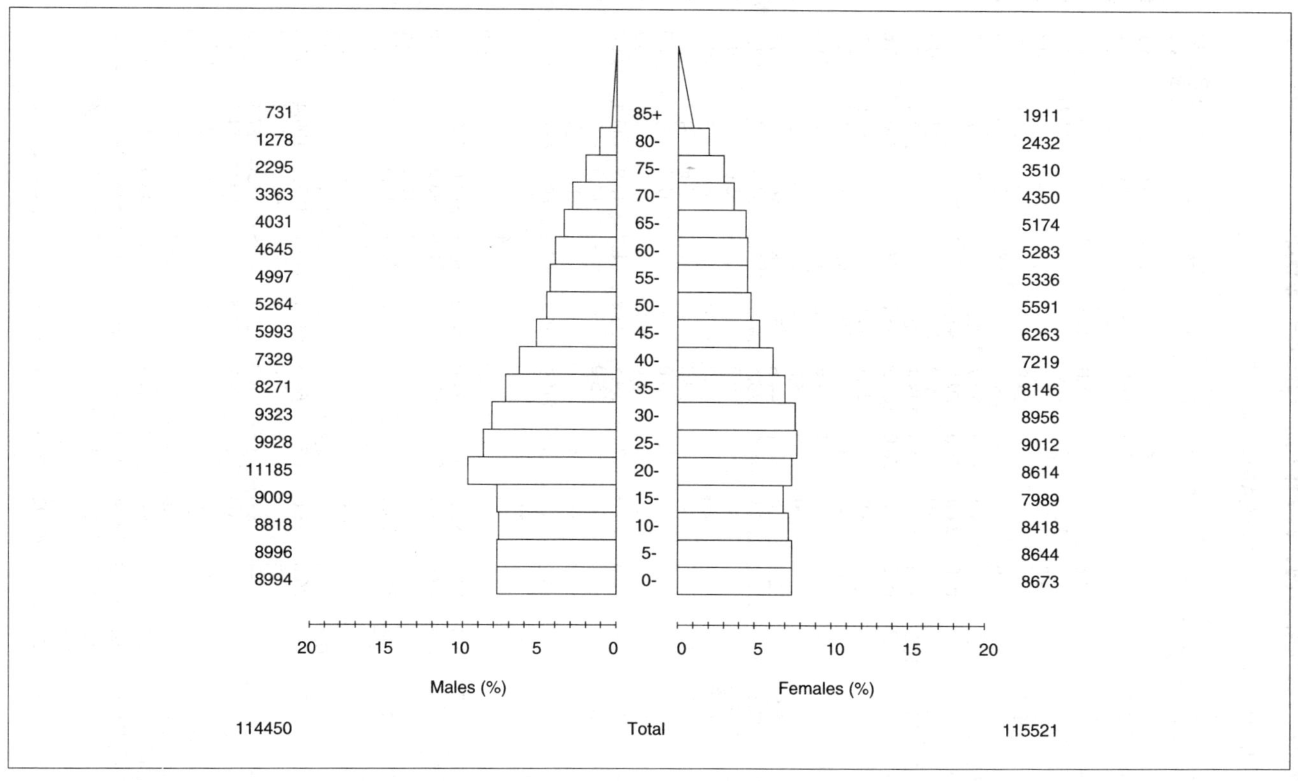

USA, Louisiana, Central Region: White
Source of population: average annual 1988–92
Census: 1990
Estimate: Population estimates from the U.S. Bureau of the Census, obtained from the National Cancer Institute.

Notes to tables overleaf:
† 173 does not include basal cell or squamous cell carcinoma

USA, LOUISIANA, CENTRAL REGION: WHITE 1988-1992

ANNUAL INCIDENCE PER 100,000 BY AGE GROUP (YEARS) - MALE

SITE	ALL AGES	AGE UNK	0-	5-	10-	15-	20-	25-	30-	35-	40-	45-	50-	55-	60-	65-	70-	75-	80-	85+	CRUDE RATE	%	CR 64	CR 74	ASR (W)	ICD (9th)
Lip	18	1	-	-	-	-	-	-	-	-	2.7	-	-	8.0	17.2	19.8	5.9	17.4	15.6	54.7	3.1	0.8	0.15	0.28	2.6	140
Tongue	18	0	-	-	-	-	-	2.0	-	-	2.7	-	3.8	12.0	21.5	19.8	-	-	15.6	54.7	3.1	0.8	0.21	0.31	2.8	141
Salivary gland	5	0	-	-	-	-	-	-	-	-	2.7	-	-	-	-	-	5.9	17.4	-	27.4	0.9	0.2	0.01	0.04	0.6	142
Mouth	7	0	-	-	-	-	1.8	-	-	-	-	3.3	3.8	-	-	5.0	11.9	8.7	-	-	1.2	0.3	0.04	0.13	1.0	143-5
Oropharynx	5	0	-	-	-	-	-	-	-	-	2.7	-	-	12.0	-	-	-	-	-	27.4	0.9	0.2	0.07	0.07	0.8	146
Nasopharynx	2	0	-	-	-	-	-	-	-	-	-	-	3.8	-	-	5.0	-	-	-	-	0.3	0.1	0.02	0.04	0.3	147
Hypopharynx	6	0	-	-	-	-	-	-	-	-	2.7	-	-	-	-	14.9	5.9	-	-	27.4	1.0	0.3	0.01	0.12	0.9	148
Pharynx unspecified	8	0	-	-	-	-	-	-	-	-	2.7	-	7.6	4.0	-	9.9	-	8.7	15.6	-	1.4	0.3	0.07	0.12	1.2	149
Oesophagus	26	0	-	-	-	-	-	-	-	4.8	-	6.7	3.8	8.0	12.9	39.7	23.8	8.7	31.3	27.4	4.5	1.1	0.18	0.50	3.8	150
Stomach	42	0	-	-	-	-	-	2.0	-	-	-	10.0	19.0	24.0	21.5	29.8	41.6	52.3	46.9	-	7.3	1.8	0.38	0.74	6.0	151
Small intestine	4	0	-	-	-	-	-	-	-	-	-	-	-	4.0	-	9.9	-	-	-	27.4	0.7	0.2	0.02	0.07	0.6	152
Colon	217	0	-	-	-	-	1.8	-	2.1	7.3	13.6	16.7	30.4	64.0	124.9	148.8	285.4	374.7	328.6	191.5	37.9	9.1	1.30	3.48	28.1	153
Rectum	89	0	-	-	-	-	-	2.0	2.1	-	2.7	3.3	15.2	32.0	56.0	104.2	83.2	87.1	93.9	246.2	15.6	3.7	0.57	1.50	12.3	154
Liver	15	0	-	-	-	-	-	-	2.1	-	-	-	-	4.0	8.6	24.8	11.9	8.7	-	82.1	2.6	0.6	0.07	0.26	2.1	155
Gallbladder etc.	15	0	-	-	-	-	-	-	-	-	-	-	-	-	4.3	-	29.7	43.6	31.3	54.7	2.6	0.6	0.02	0.17	1.6	156
Pancreas	63	0	-	-	-	-	-	-	4.3	2.4	2.7	10.0	7.6	8.0	30.1	44.6	77.3	113.3	109.5	82.1	11.0	2.6	0.33	0.94	8.0	157
Nose, sinuses etc.	2	0	-	-	-	-	-	-	-	-	-	-	-	4.0	-	5.0	-	-	-	-	0.3	0.1	0.02	0.04	0.3	160
Larynx	60	0	-	-	-	-	-	-	-	-	-	5.5	3.3	22.8	20.0	51.7	44.6	77.3	78.4	46.9	-	10.5	2.5	0.52	1.13	8.4	161
Bronchus, lung	562	0	-	-	-	-	-	-	4.3	2.4	27.3	50.1	110.2	260.1	374.6	585.4	564.8	723.2	657.3	410.3	98.2	23.6	4.14	9.90	77.4	162
Other thoracic organs	5	0	-	-	-	-	-	-	-	2.4	-	-	-	-	-	9.9	-	8.7	15.6	-	0.9	0.2	0.01	0.06	0.6	163-4
Bone	4	0	-	-	-	2.2	-	2.0	-	-	-	3.3	-	4.0	-	-	-	-	-	-	0.7	0.2	0.06	0.06	0.7	170
Connective tissue	16	1	-	-	-	-	1.8	-	-	4.8	5.5	3.3	-	-	4.3	19.8	-	8.7	15.6	54.7	2.8	0.7	0.11	0.21	2.3	171
Mesothelioma	6	0	-	-	-	-	-	-	-	-	-	-	-	-	12.9	5.0	-	-	31.3	-	1.0	0.3	0.06	0.09	0.8	MES
Kaposi's sarcoma	4	0	-	-	-	-	-	-	2.1	-	-	-	-	-	14.9	-	-	-	-	-	0.7	0.2	0.01	0.09	0.6	KAP
Melanoma of skin	63	0	-	-	-	-	-	-	8.6	9.7	5.5	33.4	30.4	28.0	17.2	59.5	23.8	8.7	46.9	109.4	11.0	2.6	0.66	1.08	9.9	172
†Other skin	4	0	-	-	-	-	-	-	-	2.4	2.7	-	-	-	-	5.0	-	-	15.6	-	0.7		0.03	0.05	0.5	173
Breast	4	0	-	-	-	-	-	-	-	-	-	-	3.8	4.0	4.3	-	-	-	-	27.4	0.7	0.2	0.06	0.06	0.7	175
Prostate	537	0	-	-	-	-	-	-	-	-	-	-	15.2	88.0	245.4	391.9	749.2	993.3	1189.4	1613.8	93.8	22.6	1.74	7.45	64.8	185
Testis	19	0	-	-	-	2.2	5.4	6.0	8.6	9.7	5.5	-	-	4.0	4.3	-	-	-	-	-	3.3	0.8	0.23	0.23	2.9	186
Penis	2	0	-	-	-	-	-	-	-	-	-	-	-	-	-	-	-	17.4	-	-	0.3	0.1	0.00	0.00	0.2	187.1-.4
Other male genital	0	0	-	-	-	-	-	-	-	-	-	-	-	-	-	-	-	-	-	-	0.0	0.0	0.00	0.00	0.0	187.5-.9
Bladder	160	0	-	-	-	-	-	2.0	-	-	2.7	13.3	53.2	52.0	77.5	124.0	202.2	165.5	313.0	300.9	28.0	6.7	1.00	2.63	21.5	188
Kidney etc.	63	0	-	-	-	-	1.8	-	2.1	2.4	-	3.3	19.0	24.0	21.5	49.6	83.2	78.4	93.9	109.4	11.0	2.6	0.37	1.04	8.3	189
Eye	5	0	2.2	-	-	-	-	-	-	-	-	-	-	-	-	-	5.9	17.4	15.6	-	0.9	0.2	0.01	0.04	0.6	190
Brain, nervous system	40	0	4.4	-	-	-	1.8	4.0	8.6	9.7	5.5	3.3	11.4	20.0	8.6	39.7	17.8	17.4	15.6	-	7.0	1.7	0.39	0.67	6.1	191-2
Thyroid	7	0	-	-	-	-	1.8	4.0	-	2.4	2.7	3.3	-	4.0	-	-	-	-	-	-	1.2	0.3	0.09	0.09	1.1	193
Other endocrine	2	0	2.2	-	-	-	-	-	-	-	-	-	-	4.0	-	-	-	-	-	-	0.3	0.1	0.03	0.03	0.4	194
Hodgkin's disease	10	0	-	-	2.3	-	-	-	-	2.4	-	10.0	7.6	-	4.3	-	-	-	31.3	-	1.7	0.4	0.13	0.13	1.7	201
Non-Hodgkin lymphoma	102	0	-	2.2	-	2.2	5.4	4.0	6.4	4.8	5.5	-	26.6	28.0	47.4	64.5	101.1	148.1	187.8	109.4	17.8	4.3	0.66	1.49	13.4	200,202
Multiple myeloma	19	0	-	-	-	-	-	-	-	-	5.5	-	7.6	8.0	8.6	5.0	11.9	34.9	46.9	27.4	3.3	0.8	0.15	0.23	2.5	203
Lymphoid leukaemia	22	0	2.2	2.2	2.3	-	-	-	-	-	-	-	-	8.0	8.6	14.9	29.7	43.6	15.6	27.4	3.8	0.9	0.12	0.34	3.0	204
Myeloid leukaemia	26	0	-	-	-	-	1.8	2.0	4.3	-	2.7	3.3	3.8	8.0	4.3	9.9	23.8	8.7	109.5	54.7	4.5	1.1	0.15	0.32	3.3	205
Monocytic leukaemia	0	0	-	-	-	-	-	-	-	-	-	-	-	-	-	-	-	-	-	-	0.0	0.0	0.00	0.00	0.0	206
Other leukaemia	0	0	-	-	-	-	-	-	-	-	-	-	-	-	-	-	-	-	-	-	0.0	0.0	0.00	0.00	0.0	207
Leukaemia unspecified	6	0	-	-	2.3	2.2	-	-	-	-	-	-	-	4.0	-	-	5.9	8.7	15.6	-	1.0	0.3	0.04	0.07	0.8	208
Other and unspecified	94	0	-	-	-	-	-	-	4.3	2.4	8.2	10.0	11.4	44.0	51.7	64.5	101.1	148.1	46.9	246.2	16.4	3.9	0.66	1.49	12.8	O&U
All sites	2384	2	11.1	4.4	6.8	8.9	23.2	30.2	60.1	70.1	120.1	190.2	417.9	796.4	1244.2	1989.3	2580.4	3250.0	3599.4	3993.4	416.6		14.93	37.80	318.4	ALL
All sites but 173	2380	2	11.1	4.4	6.8	8.9	23.2	30.2	60.1	67.7	117.3	190.2	417.9	796.4	1244.2	1984.3	2580.4	3250.0	3583.7	3993.4	415.9	100.0	14.90	37.75	317.9	ALLb

Rate from 1 case   2.224   2.223   2.268   2.220   1.788   2.014   2.145   2.418   2.729   3.337   3.799   4.002   4.305   4.961   5.946   8.713   15.649   27.352

†Important: see notes on population page

USA, LOUISIANA, CENTRAL REGION: WHITE 1988-1992

ANNUAL INCIDENCE PER 100,000 BY AGE GROUP (YEARS) - FEMALE

SITE	ALL AGES	AGE UNK	0-	5-	10-	15-	20-	25-	30-	35-	40-	45-	50-	55-	60-	65-	70-	75-	80-	85+	CRUDE RATE	%	CR 64	CR 74	ASR (W)	ICD (9th)
Lip	1	0	-	-	-	-	-	-	-	-	-	-	-	-	-	3.9	-	-	-	-	0.2	0.1	0.00	0.02	**0.1**	140
Tongue	9	0	-	-	-	-	-	-	-	-	-	-	-	3.7	7.6	11.6	9.2	5.7	-	-	1.6	0.5	0.06	0.16	**1.0**	141
Salivary gland	2	0	-	-	-	-	-	-	-	-	-	-	-	3.7	-	-	-	-	-	10.5	0.3	0.1	0.02	0.02	**0.2**	142
Mouth	10	0	-	2.3	-	-	-	-	-	-	-	-	-	-	-	11.6	9.2	-	24.7	10.5	1.7	0.5	0.01	0.12	**0.9**	143-5
Oropharynx	5	0	-	-	-	-	-	-	-	-	-	-	7.5	7.6	-	4.6	-	-	-	0.9	0.3	0.08	0.10	**0.7**	146
Nasopharynx	2	0	-	-	-	-	-	-	-	-	-	-	3.7	-	-	4.6	-	-	-	0.3	0.1	0.02	0.04	**0.2**	147
Hypopharynx	0	0	-	-	-	-	-	-	-	-	-	-	-	-	-	-	-	-	-	0.0	0.0	0.00	0.00	**0.0**	148
Pharynx unspecified	2	0	-	-	-	-	-	-	-	-	-	3.2	-	-	-	-	-	-	8.2	-	0.3	0.1	0.02	0.02	**0.2**	149
Oesophagus	7	0	-	-	-	-	-	-	-	-	-	3.2	-	3.7	-	7.7	-	5.7	8.2	10.5	1.2	0.4	0.03	0.07	**0.7**	150
Stomach	26	0	-	-	-	-	-	-	-	-	2.8	-	-	-	7.6	19.3	32.2	22.8	41.1	20.9	4.5	1.3	0.05	0.31	**2.2**	151
Small intestine	5	0	-	-	-	-	-	-	-	-	-	-	-	3.7	3.8	-	4.6	-	-	20.9	0.9	0.3	0.04	0.06	**0.5**	152
Colon	209	0	-	-	-	-	2.3	2.2	2.2	4.9	13.9	22.4	28.6	26.2	45.4	108.2	179.3	182.3	287.8	324.3	36.2	10.8	0.74	2.18	**19.0**	153
Rectum	66	0	-	-	-	-	-	-	-	2.5	-	3.2	14.3	26.2	15.1	34.8	69.0	57.0	57.6	83.7	11.4	3.4	0.31	0.83	**6.4**	154
Liver	12	0	2.3	-	-	-	-	-	-	-	-	3.2	-	-	7.6	3.9	4.6	-	24.7	31.4	2.1	0.6	0.07	0.11	**1.3**	155
Gallbladder etc.	19	0	-	-	-	-	-	-	-	-	-	-	3.6	-	7.6	11.6	23.0	45.6	-	-	3.3	1.0	0.06	0.23	**1.7**	156
Pancreas	68	0	-	-	-	-	-	-	2.2	2.5	-	16.0	10.7	15.0	26.5	11.6	64.4	51.3	82.2	115.1	11.8	3.5	0.36	0.74	**6.6**	157
Nose, sinuses etc.	4	0	-	-	-	-	-	-	-	-	-	-	-	3.7	-	3.9	-	-	16.4	-	0.7	0.2	0.02	0.04	**0.3**	160
Larynx	17	0	-	-	-	-	-	2.2	-	-	-	6.4	-	15.0	11.4	7.7	4.6	11.4	16.4	-	2.9	0.9	0.17	0.24	**2.1**	161
Bronchus, lung	246	0	-	-	-	-	-	-	-	-	8.3	25.5	53.6	82.5	174.1	189.4	156.3	182.3	156.2	188.3	42.6	12.7	1.72	3.45	**27.3**	162
Other thoracic organs	4	0	-	-	-	-	-	-	-	-	2.5	-	-	-	-	3.9	4.6	-	8.2	-	0.7	0.2	0.01	0.05	**0.4**	163-4
Bone	7	0	-	-	2.4	2.5	-	-	-	-	2.8	-	3.6	-	-	3.9	-	-	-	20.9	1.2	0.4	0.06	0.08	**1.0**	170
Connective tissue	10	0	-	2.3	2.4	2.5	2.3	2.2	-	2.5	2.8	3.2	-	-	7.7	-	-	-	-	-	1.7	0.5	0.10	0.14	**1.8**	171
Mesothelioma	0	0	-	-	-	-	-	-	-	-	-	-	-	-	-	-	-	-	-	-	0.0	0.0	0.00	0.00	**0.0**	MES
Kaposi's sarcoma	1	0	-	-	-	-	-	-	-	-	-	-	-	-	-	-	-	5.7	-	-	0.2	0.1	0.00	0.00	**0.1**	KAP
Melanoma of skin	63	0	-	-	-	-	7.0	8.9	-	7.4	19.4	12.8	-	22.5	18.9	23.2	23.0	57.0	32.9	62.8	10.9	3.3	0.48	0.71	**7.5**	172
†Other skin	6	0	-	-	-	-	-	4.4	-	2.5	-	-	3.6	-	-	-	4.6	-	8.2	-	1.0		0.05	0.08	**0.8**	173
Breast	521	0	-	-	-	-	-	4.4	20.1	46.6	83.1	121.3	157.4	183.7	246.1	274.4	285.0	319.0	386.4	303.4	90.2	26.9	4.31	7.11	**62.3**	174
Uterus unspecified	3	0	-	-	-	-	-	-	-	-	-	-	-	-	-	-	-	5.7	-	20.9	0.5	0.2	0.00	0.00	**0.2**	179
Cervix uteri	49	0	-	-	-	-	-	8.9	20.1	14.7	16.6	6.4	21.5	18.7	7.6	15.5	13.8	5.7	-	10.5	8.5	2.5	0.57	0.72	**7.2**	180
Placenta	0	0	-	-	-	-	-	-	-	-	-	-	-	-	-	-	-	-	-	-	0.0	0.0	0.00	0.00	**0.0**	181
Corpus uteri	75	0	-	-	-	-	-	-	2.2	2.5	8.3	9.6	7.2	22.5	53.0	61.8	46.0	45.6	32.9	73.2	13.0	3.9	0.53	1.07	**8.5**	182
Ovary etc.	77	0	-	-	-	2.5	-	4.4	2.2	2.5	13.9	3.2	28.6	33.7	26.5	61.8	41.4	45.6	32.9	52.3	13.3	4.0	0.59	1.10	**9.3**	183
Other female genital	14	0	-	-	-	-	2.3	-	-	-	2.8	6.4	-	7.5	3.8	7.7	-	11.4	16.4	10.5	2.4	0.7	0.11	0.15	**1.7**	184
Bladder	43	0	-	-	-	-	-	2.2	2.2	-	-	3.2	-	7.5	15.1	7.7	32.2	45.6	74.0	83.7	7.4	2.2	0.15	0.35	**3.5**	188
Kidney etc.	37	0	4.6	-	-	-	-	-	-	7.4	-	3.2	14.3	3.7	15.1	15.5	32.2	22.8	49.3	10.5	6.4	1.9	0.24	0.48	**4.3**	189
Eye	5	0	-	-	-	-	-	-	-	-	-	-	-	3.7	-	11.6	-	-	8.2	-	0.9	0.3	0.02	0.08	**0.5**	190
Brain, nervous system	38	0	2.3	-	4.8	2.5	2.3	4.4	2.2	2.5	2.8	6.4	7.2	7.5	11.4	27.1	23.0	22.8	8.2	20.9	6.6	2.0	0.28	0.53	**5.1**	191-2
Thyroid	29	0	-	-	2.4	2.5	4.6	6.7	6.7	7.4	-	9.6	3.6	3.7	3.8	11.6	9.2	22.8	-	10.5	5.0	1.5	0.25	0.36	**4.1**	193
Other endocrine	4	0	2.3	-	-	-	-	-	-	-	-	-	3.8	-	-	-	11.4	-	-	-	0.7	0.2	0.03	0.03	**0.5**	194
Hodgkin's disease	13	0	-	-	-	7.5	-	4.4	6.7	4.9	-	-	-	-	3.8	3.9	-	5.7	-	-	2.3	0.7	0.14	0.16	**2.1**	201
Non-Hodgkin lymphoma	77	1	-	-	-	5.0	-	2.2	-	-	5.5	12.8	14.3	22.5	34.1	46.4	55.2	45.6	65.8	83.7	13.3	4.0	0.49	1.00	**8.5**	200,202
Multiple myeloma	26	0	-	-	-	-	-	-	-	-	-	3.2	3.6	3.7	11.4	15.5	36.8	22.8	24.7	10.5	4.5	1.3	0.11	0.37	**2.6**	203
Lymphoid leukaemia	19	0	-	2.3	-	-	-	-	-	-	-	3.2	3.6	-	15.1	3.9	4.6	39.9	8.2	20.9	3.3	1.0	0.12	0.16	**2.0**	204
Myeloid leukaemia	25	0	-	-	-	-	-	-	-	-	-	3.2	-	3.7	3.8	15.5	23.0	22.8	32.9	52.3	4.3	1.3	0.05	0.25	**2.1**	205
Monocytic leukaemia	1	0	-	-	-	-	-	-	-	-	-	-	-	-	-	-	4.6	-	-	-	0.2	0.1	0.00	0.02	**0.1**	206
Other leukaemia	1	0	-	-	-	-	-	-	-	-	-	-	-	-	-	-	-	-	8.2	-	0.2	0.1	0.00	0.00	**0.0**	207
Leukaemia unspecified	2	0	-	-	-	-	-	-	-	-	-	-	-	-	-	-	-	5.7	-	10.5	0.3	0.1	0.00	0.00	**0.1**	208
Other and unspecified	80	0	-	-	-	-	-	-	-	2.5	8.3	9.6	14.3	11.2	26.5	38.7	59.8	39.9	115.1	156.9	13.8	4.1	0.36	0.85	**7.6**	O&U
All sites	1940	1	11.5	6.9	11.9	25.0	20.9	57.7	67.0	115.4	191.1	300.2	393.4	551.0	813.9	1082.3	1264.1	1367.2	1636.2	1830.9	335.8		12.84	24.57	**215.2**	ALL
All sites but 173	1934	1	11.5	6.9	11.9	25.0	20.9	53.3	67.0	112.9	191.1	300.2	389.9	551.0	813.9	1082.3	1259.5	1367.2	1628.0	1830.9	334.8	100.0	12.78	24.50	**214.4**	ALLb

Rate from 1 case   2.306 2.314 2.376 2.503 2.322 2.219 2.233 2.455 2.770 3.193 3.577 3.748 3.786 3.865 4.597 5.697 8.222 10.462

†Important: see notes on population page

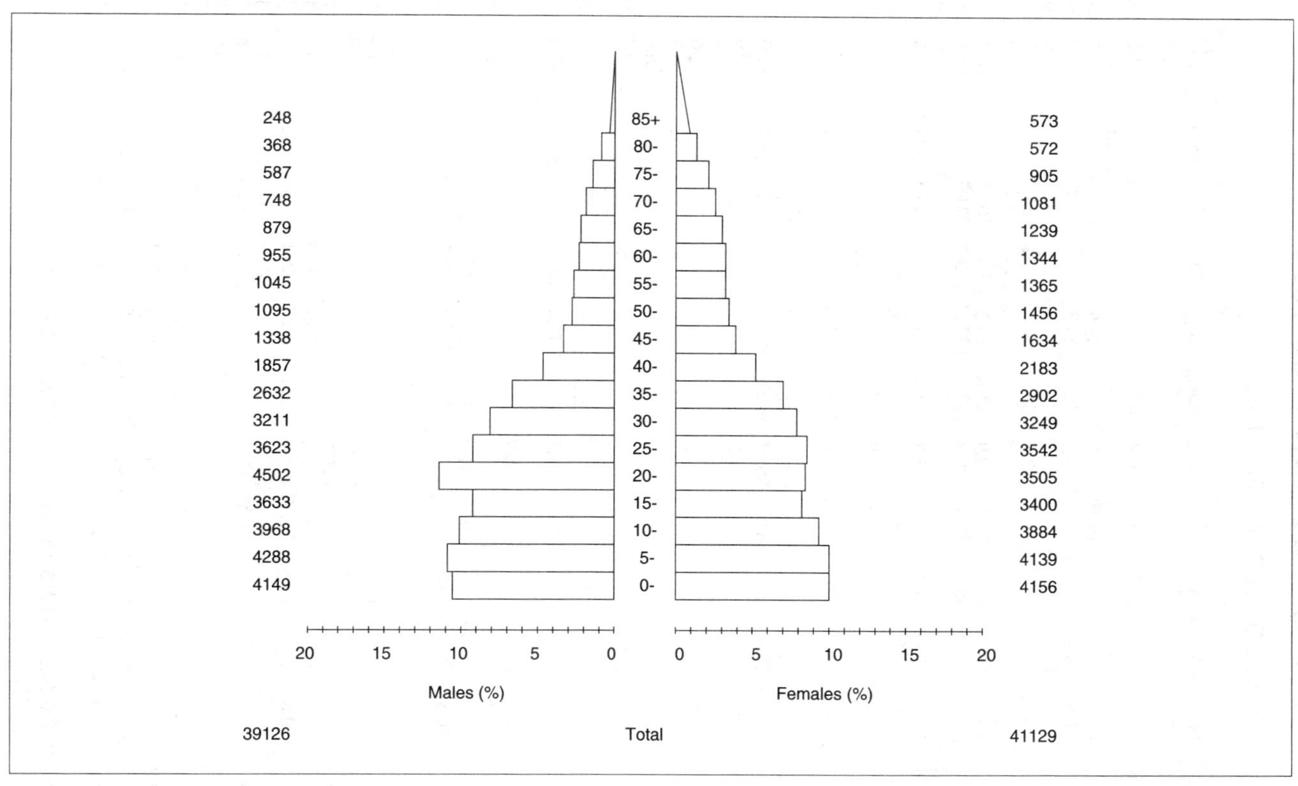

USA, Louisiana, Central Region: Black
Source of population: average annual 1988–92
Census: 1990
Estimate: Population estimates from the U.S. Bureau of the Census, obtained from the National Cancer Institute.

Notes to tables overleaf:
† 173 does not include basal cell or squamous cell carcinoma

USA, LOUISIANA, CENTRAL REGION: BLACK 1988-1992

ANNUAL INCIDENCE PER 100,000 BY AGE GROUP (YEARS) - MALE

SITE	ALL AGES	AGE UNK	0-	5-	10-	15-	20-	25-	30-	35-	40-	45-	50-	55-	60-	65-	70-	75-	80-	85+	CRUDE RATE	%	CR 64	CR 74	ASR (W)	ICD (9th)
Lip	0	0	-	-	-	-	-	-	-	-	-	-	-	-	-	-	-	-	-	-	0.0	0.0	0.00	0.00	**0.0**	140
Tongue	6	0	-	-	-	-	-	-	-	7.6	-	-	18.3	19.1	20.9	45.5	-	-	-	-	3.1	0.9	0.33	0.56	**4.3**	141
Salivary gland	1	0	-	-	-	-	-	-	-	-	-	-	-	-	-	-	-	-	-	80.6	0.5	0.1	0.00	0.00	**0.4**	142
Mouth	3	0	-	-	-	-	-	-	-	-	-	-	-	19.1	-	-	53.5	-	-	-	1.5	0.4	0.10	0.36	**1.8**	143-5
Oropharynx	6	0	-	-	-	-	-	-	-	-	21.5	29.9	-	-	22.8	26.7	-	-	-	-	3.1	0.9	0.26	0.50	**4.3**	146
Nasopharynx	2	0	-	-	-	5.5	-	-	-	-	-	14.9	-	-	-	-	-	-	-	-	1.0	0.3	0.10	0.10	**1.4**	147
Hypopharynx	8	0	-	-	-	-	-	-	-	-	-	-	-	-	62.8	45.5	-	68.1	54.3	-	4.1	1.2	0.31	0.54	**4.8**	148
Pharynx unspecified	0	0	-	-	-	-	-	-	-	-	-	-	-	-	-	-	-	-	-	-	0.0	0.0	0.00	0.00	**0.0**	149
Oesophagus	21	0	-	-	-	-	-	-	-	10.8	-	-	91.3	57.4	20.9	91.0	80.2	34.0	108.7	80.6	10.7	3.1	0.90	1.76	**14.0**	150
Stomach	27	0	-	-	-	-	-	-	-	-	-	-	36.5	38.3	20.9	113.8	187.2	170.1	271.7	-	13.8	3.9	0.48	1.98	**14.4**	151
Small intestine	2	0	-	-	-	-	-	-	-	-	7.6	-	19.1	-	-	-	-	-	-	-	1.0	0.3	0.13	0.13	**1.2**	152
Colon	50	0	-	-	-	-	4.4	5.5	-	7.6	21.5	29.9	91.3	95.7	83.8	91.0	133.7	170.1	543.5	403.2	25.6	7.3	1.70	2.82	**27.9**	153
Rectum	16	0	-	-	-	-	-	-	-	7.6	10.8	14.9	54.8	19.1	41.9	45.5	26.7	68.1	-	161.3	8.2	2.3	0.75	1.11	**10.6**	154
Liver	8	0	-	-	5.0	-	-	-	6.2	-	-	-	-	38.3	41.9	22.8	-	-	54.3	-	4.1	1.2	0.46	0.57	**5.0**	155
Gallbladder etc.	3	0	-	-	-	-	-	-	-	-	-	14.9	-	-	-	-	26.7	34.0	-	-	1.5	0.4	0.07	0.21	**1.8**	156
Pancreas	38	0	-	-	-	-	-	-	-	-	-	14.9	36.5	95.7	62.8	113.8	160.4	272.2	326.1	161.3	19.4	5.6	1.05	2.42	**20.8**	157
Nose, sinuses etc.	1	0	-	-	-	-	-	-	-	-	-	-	-	-	-	-	-	54.3	-	-	0.5	0.1	0.00	0.00	**0.3**	160
Larynx	11	0	-	-	-	-	-	-	-	7.6	-	14.9	18.3	19.1	20.9	68.3	26.7	-	108.7	-	5.6	1.6	0.40	0.88	**7.0**	161
Bronchus, lung	172	0	-	-	-	-	-	-	-	7.6	32.3	29.9	127.8	382.7	565.4	910.1	802.1	714.5	760.9	564.5	87.9	25.1	5.73	14.29	**105.6**	162
Other thoracic organs	0	0	-	-	-	-	-	-	-	-	-	-	-	-	-	-	-	-	-	-	0.0	0.0	0.00	0.00	**0.0**	163-4
Bone	0	0	-	-	-	-	-	-	-	-	-	-	-	-	-	-	-	-	-	-	0.0	0.0	0.00	0.00	**0.0**	170
Connective tissue	4	0	-	-	-	-	-	-	-	-	10.8	14.9	-	-	-	-	-	53.5	-	-	2.0	0.6	0.13	0.40	**2.6**	171
Mesothelioma	0	0	-	-	-	-	-	-	-	-	-	-	-	-	-	-	-	-	-	-	0.0	0.0	0.00	0.00	**0.0**	MES
Kaposi's sarcoma	1	0	-	-	-	-	4.4	-	-	-	-	-	-	-	-	-	-	-	-	-	0.5	0.1	0.02	0.02	**0.4**	KAP
Melanoma of skin	0	0	-	-	-	-	-	-	-	-	-	-	-	-	-	-	-	-	-	-	0.0	0.0	0.00	0.00	**0.0**	172
†Other skin	0	0	-	-	-	-	-	-	-	-	-	-	-	-	-	-	-	-	-	-	0.0	0.0	0.00	0.00	**0.0**	173
Breast	2	0	-	-	-	-	-	-	7.6	-	-	-	-	-	22.8	-	-	-	-	-	1.0	0.3	0.04	0.15	**1.1**	175
Prostate	163	0	-	-	-	-	-	-	-	-	-	-	54.8	172.2	251.3	546.1	775.4	986.7	1739.1	2016.1	83.3	23.8	2.39	9.00	**80.2**	185
Testis	1	0	-	-	-	-	-	-	-	-	-	-	18.3	-	-	-	-	-	-	-	0.5	0.1	0.09	0.09	**0.9**	186
Penis	5	0	-	-	-	-	-	-	-	-	-	14.9	-	-	20.9	-	-	34.0	-	161.3	2.6	0.7	0.18	0.18	**2.9**	187.1-.4
Other male genital	1	0	-	-	-	-	-	-	-	-	10.8	-	-	-	-	-	-	-	-	-	0.5	0.1	0.05	0.05	**0.6**	187.5-.9
Bladder	25	0	-	-	-	-	-	-	-	-	-	-	36.5	19.1	41.9	159.3	133.7	68.1	217.4	161.3	12.8	3.7	0.49	1.95	**14.3**	188
Kidney etc.	24	0	-	-	-	-	-	-	6.2	-	10.8	29.9	54.8	76.5	-	45.5	107.0	136.1	163.0	-	12.3	3.5	0.89	1.65	**14.3**	189
Eye	1	0	4.8	-	-	-	-	-	-	-	-	-	-	-	-	-	-	-	-	-	0.5	0.1	0.02	0.02	**0.6**	190
Brain, nervous system	3	0	4.8	4.7	5.0	-	-	-	-	-	-	-	-	-	-	-	-	-	-	-	1.5	0.4	0.07	0.07	**1.5**	191-2
Thyroid	2	0	-	-	-	-	-	-	-	-	-	-	18.3	19.1	-	-	-	-	-	-	1.0	0.3	0.19	0.19	**1.7**	193
Other endocrine	0	0	-	-	-	-	-	-	-	-	-	-	-	-	-	-	-	-	-	-	0.0	0.0	0.00	0.00	**0.0**	194
Hodgkin's disease	4	0	4.8	-	-	-	4.4	-	-	7.6	-	-	-	-	20.9	-	-	-	-	-	2.0	0.6	0.19	0.19	**2.2**	201
Non-Hodgkin lymphoma	13	0	-	4.7	-	-	-	-	6.2	7.6	-	14.9	18.3	19.1	83.8	22.8	26.7	34.0	-	-	6.6	1.9	0.77	1.02	**8.8**	200,202
Multiple myeloma	10	0	-	-	-	-	-	-	-	-	10.8	-	18.3	57.4	-	22.8	26.7	68.1	-	80.6	5.1	1.5	0.43	0.68	**6.2**	203
Lymphoid leukaemia	8	0	4.8	9.3	5.0	-	-	-	-	-	-	-	-	19.1	-	-	-	102.1	-	-	4.1	1.2	0.19	0.19	**3.8**	204
Myeloid leukaemia	5	0	-	-	-	-	-	-	-	7.6	-	-	18.3	38.3	-	-	-	-	54.3	-	2.6	0.7	0.32	0.32	**3.2**	205
Monocytic leukaemia	0	0	-	-	-	-	-	-	-	-	-	-	-	-	-	-	-	-	-	-	0.0	0.0	0.00	0.00	**0.0**	206
Other leukaemia	0	0	-	-	-	-	-	-	-	-	-	-	-	-	-	-	-	-	-	-	0.0	0.0	0.00	0.00	**0.0**	207
Leukaemia unspecified	2	0	-	-	-	-	-	-	-	-	-	-	-	19.1	-	22.8	-	-	-	-	1.0	0.3	0.10	0.21	**1.4**	208
Other and unspecified	35	0	-	-	-	-	-	-	-	22.8	-	44.8	-	57.4	41.9	136.5	160.4	170.1	108.7	403.2	17.9	5.1	0.83	2.32	**19.6**	O&U
All sites	684	0	19.3	18.7	15.1	5.5	13.3	5.5	18.7	98.8	140.0	283.9	711.9	1301.2	1403.1	2548.4	2807.5	3130.3	4565.2	4274.2	349.6		20.18	46.95	**391.9**	ALL
All sites but 173	684	0	19.3	18.7	15.1	5.5	13.3	5.5	18.7	98.8	140.0	283.9	711.9	1301.2	1403.1	2548.4	2807.5	3130.3	4565.2	4274.2	349.6	100.0	20.18	46.95	**391.9**	ALLb

Rate from 1 case   4.820 4.663 5.039 5.504 4.442 5.520 6.228 7.598 10.770 14.941 18.255 19.135 20.942 22.753 26.738 34.025 54.348 80.645

†Important: see notes on population page

USA, LOUISIANA, CENTRAL REGION: BLACK 1988-1992

ANNUAL INCIDENCE PER 100,000 BY AGE GROUP (YEARS) - FEMALE

SITE	ALL AGES	AGE UNK	0-	5-	10-	15-	20-	25-	30-	35-	40-	45-	50-	55-	60-	65-	70-	75-	80-	85+	CRUDE RATE	%	CR 64	CR 74	ASR (W)	ICD (9th)
Lip	0	0	-	-	-	-	-	-	-	-	-	-	-	-	-	-	-	-	-	-	0.0	0.0	0.00	0.00	0.0	140
Tongue	0	0	-	-	-	-	-	-	-	-	-	-	-	-	-	-	-	-	-	-	0.0	0.0	0.00	0.00	0.0	141
Salivary gland	1	0	-	-	-	-	-	-	-	-	-	-	13.7	-	-	-	-	-	-	-	0.5	0.2	0.07	0.07	0.7	142
Mouth	3	0	-	-	-	-	-	-	-	-	-	-	13.7	14.6	-	-	-	22.1	-	-	1.5	0.6	0.14	0.14	1.5	143-5
Oropharynx	0	0	-	-	-	-	-	-	-	-	-	-	-	-	-	-	-	-	-	-	0.0	0.0	0.00	0.00	0.0	146
Nasopharynx	0	0	-	-	-	-	-	-	-	-	-	-	-	-	-	-	-	-	-	-	0.0	0.0	0.00	0.00	0.0	147
Hypopharynx	1	0	-	-	-	-	-	-	6.9	-	-	-	-	-	-	-	-	-	-	-	0.5	0.2	0.03	0.03	0.4	148
Pharynx unspecified	1	0	-	-	-	-	-	-	-	-	-	12.2	-	-	-	-	-	-	-	-	0.5	0.2	0.06	0.06	0.7	149
Oesophagus	5	0	-	-	-	-	-	-	-	-	-	-	13.7	14.6	-	16.1	18.5	22.1	-	-	2.4	1.0	0.14	0.32	2.3	150
Stomach	13	0	-	-	-	-	-	-	-	-	-	-	27.5	14.6	29.8	32.3	18.5	66.3	34.9	34.9	6.3	2.7	0.36	0.61	5.5	151
Small intestine	0	0	-	-	-	-	-	-	-	-	-	-	-	-	-	-	-	-	-	-	0.0	0.0	0.00	0.00	0.0	152
Colon	60	0	-	-	-	-	5.7	-	-	-	18.3	24.5	68.7	73.2	59.5	177.6	222.0	132.5	279.4	139.6	29.2	12.3	1.25	3.25	25.0	153
Rectum	12	0	-	-	-	-	-	-	-	6.9	-	-	-	-	44.6	32.3	37.0	-	104.8	34.9	5.8	2.5	0.26	0.60	4.6	154
Liver	2	0	4.8	-	-	-	-	-	-	-	-	-	-	-	-	-	-	34.9	-	-	1.0	0.4	0.02	0.02	0.8	155
Gallbladder etc.	3	0	-	-	-	-	-	-	-	-	-	-	-	29.8	-	-	-	-	-	34.9	1.5	0.6	0.15	0.15	1.4	156
Pancreas	22	0	-	-	-	-	-	-	-	6.9	-	-	-	43.9	14.9	80.7	55.5	66.3	69.9	139.6	10.7	4.5	0.33	1.01	8.0	157
Nose, sinuses etc.	1	0	-	-	-	-	-	-	-	-	-	-	-	-	-	-	18.5	-	-	-	0.5	0.2	0.00	0.09	0.4	160
Larynx	3	0	-	-	-	-	-	-	-	-	-	-	13.7	-	14.9	-	18.5	-	-	-	1.5	0.6	0.14	0.24	1.7	161
Bronchus, lung	64	0	-	-	-	-	-	6.2	6.9	-	-	-	68.7	102.5	133.9	161.4	259.0	220.8	104.8	139.6	31.1	13.1	1.59	3.69	27.1	162
Other thoracic organs	1	0	-	-	-	-	-	-	-	-	-	-	-	-	-	-	18.5	-	-	-	0.5	0.2	0.00	0.09	0.4	163-4
Bone	1	0	-	-	5.1	-	-	-	-	-	-	-	-	-	-	-	-	-	-	-	0.5	0.2	0.03	0.03	0.5	170
Connective tissue	8	0	-	-	5.1	-	5.7	-	-	-	-	-	-	14.6	-	16.1	37.0	22.1	34.9	-	3.9	1.6	0.13	0.39	3.1	171
Mesothelioma	0	0	-	-	-	-	-	-	-	-	-	-	-	-	-	-	-	-	-	-	0.0	0.0	0.00	0.00	0.0	MES
Kaposi's sarcoma	2	0	-	-	-	-	-	-	-	-	-	-	-	-	14.9	-	-	22.1	-	-	1.0	0.4	0.07	0.07	0.8	KAP
Melanoma of skin	2	0	-	-	-	-	-	-	-	-	9.2	-	-	14.6	-	-	-	-	-	-	1.0	0.4	0.12	0.12	1.1	172
†Other skin	2	0	-	-	-	-	-	-	-	-	-	-	13.7	-	-	-	-	-	-	34.9	1.0		0.07	0.07	0.9	173
Breast	123	0	-	-	-	-	5.7	28.2	24.6	68.9	73.3	110.1	109.9	205.1	238.1	226.0	222.0	242.9	174.6	209.4	59.8	25.3	4.32	6.56	58.1	174
Uterus unspecified	6	0	-	-	-	-	-	-	-	-	-	-	-	14.6	-	48.4	-	22.1	-	34.9	2.9	1.2	0.07	0.32	2.4	179
Cervix uteri	25	0	-	-	-	-	5.7	5.6	18.5	34.5	27.5	12.2	-	29.3	29.8	16.1	55.5	44.2	34.9	-	12.2	5.1	0.82	1.17	11.0	180
Placenta	0	0	-	-	-	-	-	-	-	-	-	-	-	-	-	-	-	-	-	-	0.0	0.0	0.00	0.00	0.0	181
Corpus uteri	22	0	-	-	-	-	-	-	-	-	-	12.2	13.7	29.3	59.5	64.6	55.5	-	69.9	174.5	10.7	4.5	0.57	1.17	9.2	182
Ovary etc.	17	0	-	-	5.1	-	-	-	-	-	-	-	27.5	29.3	44.6	80.7	18.5	22.1	34.9	34.9	8.3	3.5	0.53	1.03	8.2	183
Other female genital	5	0	-	-	-	-	-	-	-	-	-	-	-	14.9	16.1	37.0	-	-	-	34.9	2.4	1.0	0.07	0.34	2.0	184
Bladder	11	0	-	-	-	-	-	-	-	-	-	12.2	-	-	14.9	-	55.5	22.1	69.9	104.7	5.3	2.3	0.14	0.41	3.5	188
Kidney etc.	10	0	9.6	-	-	-	-	-	-	-	-	-	13.7	14.6	29.8	16.1	-	22.1	34.9	34.9	4.9	2.1	0.34	0.42	4.7	189
Eye	0	0	-	-	-	-	-	-	-	-	-	-	-	-	-	-	-	-	-	-	0.0	0.0	0.00	0.00	0.0	190
Brain, nervous system	5	0	4.8	-	-	-	-	-	-	-	-	-	-	14.6	-	16.1	-	22.1	34.9	-	2.4	1.0	0.10	0.18	2.0	191-2
Thyroid	5	0	-	-	-	-	-	-	-	13.8	-	12.2	-	-	-	-	-	22.1	34.9	-	2.4	1.0	0.13	0.13	2.0	193
Other endocrine	1	0	-	-	-	-	-	-	-	-	-	-	-	-	-	-	-	22.1	-	-	0.5	0.2	0.00	0.00	0.2	194
Hodgkin's disease	1	0	-	-	-	-	-	-	-	-	-	-	-	14.9	-	-	-	-	-	-	0.5	0.2	0.07	0.07	0.6	201
Non-Hodgkin lymphoma	12	0	-	-	-	-	5.7	-	6.2	-	-	-	13.7	-	44.6	16.1	18.5	44.2	34.9	34.9	5.8	2.5	0.35	0.52	4.9	200,202
Multiple myeloma	9	0	-	-	-	-	-	-	-	-	-	-	13.7	14.6	14.9	-	37.0	44.2	34.9	34.9	4.4	1.8	0.22	0.40	3.4	203
Lymphoid leukaemia	2	0	-	-	-	-	-	-	-	-	-	-	-	-	-	16.1	-	22.1	-	-	1.0	0.4	0.00	0.08	0.7	204
Myeloid leukaemia	3	0	-	-	-	-	-	-	-	-	-	-	-	-	-	-	-	22.1	34.9	34.9	1.5	0.6	0.00	0.00	0.6	205
Monocytic leukaemia	0	0	-	-	-	-	-	-	-	-	-	-	-	-	-	-	-	-	-	-	0.0	0.0	0.00	0.00	0.0	206
Other leukaemia	1	0	-	-	-	-	-	-	-	-	-	-	-	-	-	-	18.5	-	-	-	0.5	0.2	0.00	0.09	0.4	207
Leukaemia unspecified	0	0	-	-	-	-	-	-	-	-	-	-	-	-	-	-	-	-	-	-	0.0	0.0	0.00	0.00	0.0	208
Other and unspecified	24	0	-	-	-	-	-	-	-	-	-	12.2	41.2	-	89.3	16.1	37.0	66.3	139.7	139.6	11.7	4.9	0.71	0.98	9.6	O&U
All sites	489	0	19.2	-	15.4	-	28.5	33.9	55.4	144.7	128.3	208.1	466.9	644.5	937.5	1049.2	1257.9	1214.7	1397.1	1431.1	237.8		13.41	24.95	210.4	ALL
All sites but 173	487	0	19.2	-	15.4	-	28.5	33.9	55.4	144.7	128.3	208.1	453.2	644.5	937.5	1049.2	1257.9	1214.7	1397.1	1396.2	236.8	100.0	13.34	24.88	209.6	ALLb

| Rate from 1 case | | | 4.811 | 4.831 | 5.149 | 5.881 | 5.705 | 5.646 | 6.155 | 6.892 | 9.161 | 12.238 | 13.732 | 14.648 | 14.881 | 16.142 | 18.498 | 22.085 | 34.928 | 34.904 | | | | | | |

†Important: see notes on population page

USA, Louisiana, New Orleans

The Louisiana Tumor Registry was established in 1974 to carry out cancer registration in the three counties (Orleans, Jefferson and St Bernard) of the metropolitan New Orleans area. Its coverage was expanded in 1983 to include South Louisiana, and in 1988 to the north, and statewide population-based registration was achieved. The structure and operation of the registry as a whole are described above in the section on Louisiana Central Region.

New Orleans is located in the southeastern United States, on the delta of the Mississippi River. Land elevations rarely reach 15 feet (5 metres), and over half of the land is uninhabitable wetlands. The climate is subtropical and humid. Although the Mississippi River drains a large agricultural and industrial region, levels of herbicides and pesticides, volatile organic compounds and trihalomethanes in drinking water are in compliance with US Environmental Protection Agency standards. Since 1981, the Air Pollutant Standards Index, a composite indicator of levels of ambient particulate matter, oxides and ozone, has classified over 80% of days each year in New Orleans in its most salubrious range, and on only two days did air quality fall to the "unhealthful" level.

The metropolitan New Orleans area has a population of 1 010 067. About 99% live in urban areas. Whites constitute 58.0%, blacks 38.6% and Asians 2.0%. Immigrants amount to 4.8%, the largest groups coming from Europe, Viet Nam and Central America.

The economy of the region is oriented to service industries; only 9.4% of employed persons are engaged in manufacturing. Tourism, retail and wholesale trade, health services, restaurants and business services are the leading non-manufacturing industries. Since it has two medical schools and several large referral hospital complexes, the New Orleans region draws cancer patients from a wide area for diagnosis and treatment.

The cancer incidence data presented here are restricted to patients who were residents of the New Orleans area at the time of diagnosis. Over half of the cases came from hospitals with cancer programmes accredited by the American College of Surgeons. These cases were abstracted by specially trained hospital registrars and submitted to the Louisiana Tumor Registry. The central registry staff screen and abstract cases from the remaining hospitals and from pathology laboratories and radiation centres that are not affiliated with hospitals. They also investigate death certificates that mention cancer as a cause of death if the deceased was not included in the registry system. In 1988–92, death-certificate-only cases accounted for 2.2% of the total.

Each patient in the registry is assigned a unique identification number. This allows identification of patients with multiple primaries. In defining multiple primaries, the registry follows the SEER rules, which vary slightly from the rules of IACR. The registry does not have an active follow-up programme, but hospitals with registries accredited by the American College of Surgeons obtain survival data on their patients annually, and death information is recorded at the registry as received.

Quality assurance in the registry is the responsibility of both the regional offices and the central registry. Rescreening and reabstracting are performed annually. An assessment of case completeness and data quality by the NAACCR on 1992 cases for the entire state showed a completeness rate of 97.6% and an overall data quality error rate of 5.9%. The 1988–92 data have been subjected to a wide range of computerized tests for invalid codes, inconsistencies and duplications using programs developed by the registry as well as by SEER and IARC.

The registry publishes periodic reports in the form of monographs. The *Cancer in Louisiana* series has provided information on cancer incidence and mortality rates, time trends and childhood cancers in New Orleans and South Louisiana, as well as comparisons among regions and with the national rates. Articles on cancer incidence are published in the *Journal of the Louisiana State Medical Society.* Other registry-based research has focused on stage at diagnosis and socioeconomic determinants as explanations for the discrepancies between incidence and mortality rates

Vivien W. Chen
Patricia A. Andrews
Catherine N. Correa
Xian Cheng Wu
Pelayo Correa

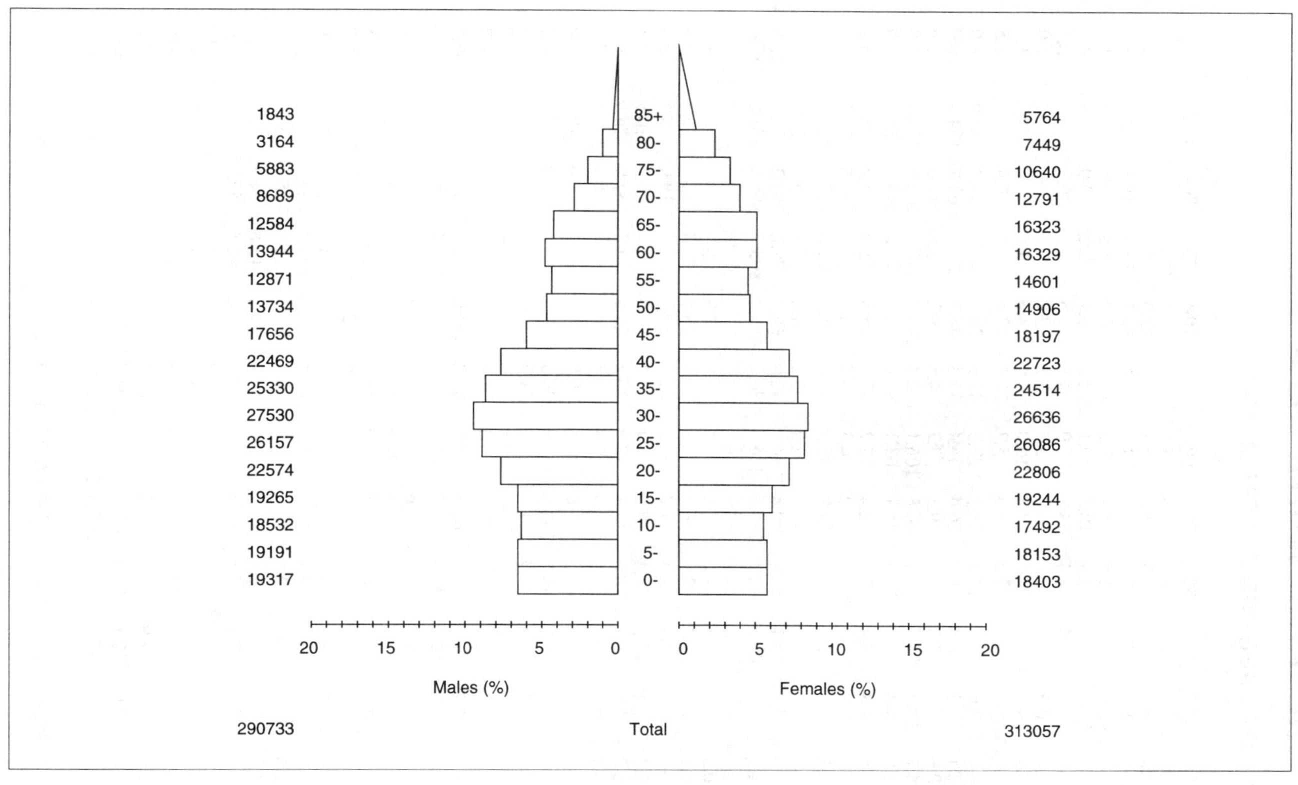

USA, Louisiana, New Orleans: White
Source of population: average annual 1988–92
Census: 1990
Estimate: Population estimates from the U.S. Bureau of the Census, obtained from the National Cancer Institute.

Notes to tables overleaf:
† 173 does not include basal cell or squamous cell carcinoma

USA, LOUISIANA, NEW ORLEANS: WHITE 1988-1992

ANNUAL INCIDENCE PER 100,000 BY AGE GROUP (YEARS) - MALE

SITE	ALL AGES	AGE UNK	0-	5-	10-	15-	20-	25-	30-	35-	40-	45-	50-	55-	60-	65-	70-	75-	80-	85+	CRUDE RATE	%	CR 64	CR 74	ASR (W)	ICD (9th)
Lip	26	0	-	-	-	-	-	-	-	0.8	0.9	-	1.5	1.6	5.7	6.4	13.8	17.0	19.0	-	1.8	0.3	0.05	0.15	1.2	140
Tongue	48	0	-	-	-	-	-	-	-	0.8	1.8	7.9	5.8	7.8	4.3	11.1	16.1	17.0	25.3	32.5	3.3	0.6	0.14	0.28	2.5	141
Salivary gland	24	0	-	-	-	-	0.9	0.8	-	-	0.9	-	1.5	3.1	7.2	7.9	6.9	6.8	6.3	21.7	1.7	0.3	0.07	0.15	1.3	142
Mouth	68	0	-	-	-	-	-	-	-	-	-	7.9	7.3	18.6	20.1	22.2	16.1	10.2	19.0	32.5	4.7	0.9	0.27	0.46	3.7	143-5
Oropharynx	30	0	-	-	-	-	-	-	-	-	-	3.4	4.4	14.0	12.9	4.8	4.6	-	6.3	-	2.1	0.4	0.17	0.22	1.8	146
Nasopharynx	15	0	-	-	-	-	-	-	-	0.8	0.9	-	-	4.7	5.7	3.2	9.2	-	-	-	1.0	0.2	0.06	0.12	0.8	147
Hypopharynx	24	0	-	-	-	-	-	-	-	0.8	0.9	1.1	-	7.8	10.0	9.5	4.6	3.4	-	-	1.7	0.3	0.10	0.17	1.3	148
Pharynx unspecified	22	0	-	-	-	-	-	-	-	-	-	-	2.9	1.6	5.7	11.1	13.8	3.4	6.3	-	1.5	0.3	0.05	0.18	1.1	149
Oesophagus	116	0	-	-	-	-	-	-	0.7	-	3.6	3.4	13.1	17.1	27.3	42.9	36.8	40.8	44.2	75.9	8.0	1.5	0.33	0.72	5.9	150
Stomach	145	0	-	-	-	-	-	-	0.7	2.4	1.8	6.8	8.7	26.4	34.4	33.4	48.3	57.8	63.2	184.4	10.0	1.8	0.41	0.81	7.4	151
Small intestine	27	0	-	-	-	-	-	0.8	-	0.8	-	2.3	2.9	9.3	5.7	4.8	9.2	6.8	12.6	-	1.9	0.3	0.11	0.18	1.5	152
Colon	609	0	-	-	-	-	-	-	2.9	4.7	12.5	21.5	26.2	66.8	106.1	190.7	269.3	295.7	404.5	466.5	41.9	7.7	1.20	3.50	29.1	153
Rectum	291	0	-	-	-	-	-	0.8	2.2	1.6	5.3	9.1	20.4	45.1	63.1	85.8	140.4	129.2	145.4	86.8	20.0	3.7	0.74	1.87	14.3	154
Liver	74	0	-	-	-	-	-	0.8	0.7	-	1.8	3.4	2.9	12.4	17.2	17.5	25.3	51.0	37.9	21.7	5.1	0.9	0.20	0.41	3.6	155
Gallbladder etc.	37	0	-	-	-	-	-	-	-	-	0.9	-	2.9	6.2	4.3	9.5	13.8	23.8	31.6	32.5	2.5	0.5	0.07	0.19	1.7	156
Pancreas	187	0	-	-	-	-	-	-	0.7	1.6	2.7	6.8	13.1	24.9	37.3	52.4	71.4	102.0	120.1	119.3	12.9	2.4	0.44	1.05	9.1	157
Nose, sinuses etc.	12	0	-	-	-	2.1	-	-	0.7	-	-	-	-	-	2.9	3.2	4.6	3.4	6.3	10.8	0.8	0.2	0.03	0.07	0.7	160
Larynx	181	0	-	-	-	-	-	-	0.7	1.6	2.7	9.1	26.2	40.4	44.5	42.9	66.7	78.2	63.2	32.5	12.5	2.3	0.63	1.17	9.4	161
Bronchus, lung	1707	0	-	-	-	-	-	-	3.6	4.7	17.8	45.3	112.1	253.3	436.0	586.4	662.9	805.7	865.8	661.8	117.4	21.6	4.36	10.61	84.0	162
Other thoracic organs	12	0	-	-	-	1.0	1.8	-	-	-	2.7	-	-	3.1	2.9	3.2	-	-	-	-	0.8	0.2	0.06	0.07	0.7	163-4
Bone	16	0	1.0	-	-	1.0	2.7	0.8	1.5	0.8	-	1.1	1.5	1.6	1.4	-	2.3	6.8	-	-	1.1	0.2	0.07	0.08	1.0	170
Connective tissue	46	0	1.0	2.1	1.1	2.1	1.8	1.5	2.2	3.2	1.8	3.4	2.9	4.7	4.3	7.9	13.8	6.8	12.6	10.8	3.2	0.6	0.16	0.27	2.7	171
Mesothelioma	49	0	-	-	-	-	-	-	-	-	-	1.1	1.5	7.8	11.5	20.7	20.7	17.0	19.0	43.4	3.4	0.6	0.11	0.32	2.4	MES
Kaposi's sarcoma	190	0	-	-	-	1.0	1.8	26.8	34.1	40.3	23.1	15.9	4.4	7.8	1.4	3.2	-	3.4	6.3	10.8	13.1	2.4	0.78	0.80	10.0	KAP
Melanoma of skin	132	0	-	-	-	-	3.5	3.8	4.4	8.7	8.0	18.1	14.6	17.1	17.2	22.2	29.9	27.2	37.9	75.9	9.1	1.7	0.48	0.74	7.1	172
†Other skin	10	0	-	-	-	-	-	-	0.7	0.8	0.9	-	-	1.6	2.9	4.8	-	-	-	-	0.7		0.03	0.06	0.5	173
Breast	15	0	-	-	-	-	-	-	-	-	-	-	1.5	1.6	1.4	9.5	4.6	3.4	12.6	10.8	1.0	0.2	0.02	0.09	0.7	175
Prostate	1835	0	-	-	-	1.0	-	-	1.5	-	0.9	7.9	49.5	133.6	334.2	646.8	902.2	1132.0	1282.9	1475.5	126.2	23.3	2.64	10.39	84.5	185
Testis	89	0	-	-	-	4.2	5.3	15.3	16.7	9.5	13.4	5.7	2.9	1.6	-	1.6	-	-	-	-	6.1	1.1	0.37	0.38	5.0	186
Penis	10	0	-	-	-	-	-	0.8	-	-	-	1.1	-	-	4.3	-	4.6	6.8	6.3	-	0.7	0.1	0.03	0.05	0.5	187.1-.4
Other male genital	3	0	-	-	-	-	-	-	-	-	-	-	-	1.4	1.6	-	3.4	-	-	-	0.2	0.0	0.01	0.02	0.1	187.5-.9
Bladder	575	0	-	-	-	-	-	-	2.9	7.1	6.2	11.3	24.8	66.8	111.9	173.2	191.0	356.9	391.8	520.8	39.6	7.3	1.16	2.98	27.2	188
Kidney etc.	288	0	4.1	-	-	2.1	0.9	0.8	2.2	3.9	8.9	12.5	30.6	37.3	61.7	65.2	103.6	122.4	158.0	173.6	19.8	3.7	0.82	1.67	14.9	189
Eye	17	0	1.0	-	-	1.0	-	-	0.7	-	-	1.1	-	1.6	4.3	3.2	2.3	13.6	6.3	10.8	1.2	0.2	0.05	0.08	0.9	190
Brain, nervous system	101	0	5.2	-	1.1	1.0	2.7	3.1	2.9	4.7	8.9	5.7	5.8	15.5	21.5	19.1	16.1	13.6	25.3	65.1	6.9	1.3	0.39	0.57	5.9	191-2
Thyroid	40	0	-	-	-	1.0	-	-	1.5	3.2	3.6	2.3	8.7	4.7	12.9	11.1	-	-	6.3	10.8	2.8	0.5	0.19	0.24	2.3	193
Other endocrine	4	0	-	-	-	-	-	-	-	-	-	-	1.5	-	1.4	1.6	2.3	-	-	-	0.3	0.1	0.01	0.03	0.2	194
Hodgkin's disease	58	0	-	-	1.1	3.1	9.7	7.6	4.4	3.2	5.3	3.4	2.9	4.7	2.9	-	6.9	3.4	12.6	10.8	4.0	0.7	0.24	0.28	3.5	201
Non-Hodgkin lymphoma	302	0	-	3.1	2.2	2.1	0.9	6.9	10.9	18.9	16.9	26.1	23.3	31.1	43.0	60.4	103.6	102.0	107.4	86.8	20.8	3.8	0.93	1.75	15.7	200,202
Multiple myeloma	65	0	-	-	-	-	-	-	0.7	2.4	-	-	2.9	9.3	14.3	19.1	34.5	23.8	25.3	54.2	4.5	0.8	0.15	0.42	3.2	203
Lymphoid leukaemia	77	0	9.3	2.1	2.2	1.0	1.8	1.5	0.7	2.4	-	1.1	4.4	6.2	12.9	17.5	23.0	13.6	44.2	65.1	5.3	1.0	0.23	0.43	4.8	204
Myeloid leukaemia	72	0	-	1.0	-	-	2.7	1.5	1.5	0.8	2.7	3.4	5.8	12.4	8.6	12.7	18.4	40.8	56.9	21.7	5.0	0.9	0.20	0.36	3.6	205
Monocytic leukaemia	8	0	-	-	-	1.0	-	-	1.5	-	-	-	-	-	1.4	1.6	2.3	3.4	-	10.8	0.6	0.1	0.02	0.04	0.4	206
Other leukaemia	3	0	-	-	-	-	-	-	-	-	-	-	-	-	1.6	2.3	3.4	-	-		0.2	0.0	0.00	0.02	0.1	207
Leukaemia unspecified	13	0	-	-	-	1.0	0.9	0.8	-	-	-	-	-	-	1.4	1.6	2.3	13.6	6.3	21.7	0.9	0.2	0.02	0.04	0.7	208
Other and unspecified	222	0	-	-	-	-	-	-	0.7	2.4	4.5	7.9	13.1	34.2	43.0	68.3	78.3	88.4	132.7	227.8	15.3	2.8	0.53	1.26	11.0	O&U
All sites	7895	0	21.7	8.3	7.6	26.0	37.2	74.2	104.6	132.6	162.0	257.1	454.3	965.0	1574.8	2323.5	2999.1	3657.7	4234.3	4687.0	543.1		19.13	45.74	389.9	ALL
All sites but 173	7885	0	21.7	8.3	7.6	26.0	37.2	74.2	103.9	131.9	161.1	257.1	454.3	963.4	1572.0	2318.7	2999.1	3657.7	4228.0	4687.0	542.4	100.0	19.09	45.68	389.4	ALLb
Rate from 1 case			1.035	1.042	1.079	1.038	0.886	0.765	0.726	0.790	0.890	1.133	1.456	1.554	1.434	1.589	2.302	3.399	6.320	10.850						

†Important: see notes on population page

USA, LOUISIANA, NEW ORLEANS: WHITE 1988-1992

ANNUAL INCIDENCE PER 100,000 BY AGE GROUP (YEARS) - FEMALE

SITE	ALL AGES	AGE UNK	0-	5-	10-	15-	20-	25-	30-	35-	40-	45-	50-	55-	60-	65-	70-	75-	80-	85+	CRUDE RATE	%	CR 64	CR 74	ASR (W)	ICD (9th)
Lip	4	0	-	-	-	-	-	-	-	-	-	-	-	-	-	2.5	-	-	2.7	3.5	0.3	0.1	0.00	0.01	**0.1**	*140*
Tongue	27	0	-	-	-	-	-	-	-	-	3.3	-	-	7.3	7.4	6.3	7.5	2.7	10.4	1.7	0.4	0.05	0.12	**1.0**	*141*
Salivary gland	16	0	-	-	-	1.0	-	0.8	1.5	-	0.9	-	-	1.4	1.2	3.7	7.8	1.9	-	-	1.0	0.2	0.03	0.09	**0.7**	*142*
Mouth	45	0	-	-	-	1.0	-	-	-	-	-	-	2.7	8.2	2.4	9.8	20.3	7.5	21.5	3.5	2.9	0.6	0.07	0.22	**1.6**	*143-5*
Oropharynx	10	0	-	-	-	-	-	-	-	-	0.9	-	-	2.7	1.2	6.1	-	1.9	-	-	0.6	0.1	0.02	0.05	**0.4**	*146*
Nasopharynx	13	0	-	-	-	-	-	-	0.8	1.8	1.1	1.3	2.7	1.2	3.7	1.6	-	-	3.5	0.8	0.2	0.04	0.07	**0.6**	*147*
Hypopharynx	5	0	-	-	-	-	-	-	-	-	-	-	-	3.7	1.2	-	-	2.7	-	0.3	0.1	0.02	0.02	**0.2**	*148*
Pharynx unspecified	7	0	-	-	-	-	-	-	-	-	0.9	-	1.3	-	2.4	-	1.6	1.9	2.7	-	0.4	0.1	0.02	P.03	**0.3**	*149*
Oesophagus	44	0	-	-	-	-	-	-	-	-	-	-	-	6.8	7.3	11.0	9.4	13.2	16.1	17.3	2.8	0.6	0.07	0.17	**1.4**	*150*
Stomach	93	0	-	-	-	-	-	-	-	-	1.8	6.6	6.7	9.6	4.9	12.3	15.6	30.1	40.3	62.5	5.9	1.3	0.15	0.29	**2.9**	*151*
Small intestine	19	0	-	-	-	-	-	-	0.8	-	2.7	4.1	-	1.2	-	5.6	10.7	17.3	1.2	0.3	0.04	0.04	**0.6**	*152*
Colon	789	0	-	-	-	-	-	0.8	3.3	7.0	12.1	29.5	69.9	84.5	116.4	204.8	283.8	346.3	405.9	50.4	10.9	1.04	2.64	**23.2**	*153*
Rectum	239	0	-	-	-	-	-	-	-	2.4	3.5	2.2	20.1	21.9	29.4	44.1	57.8	77.1	77.9	111.0	15.3	3.3	0.40	0.91	**7.7**	*154*
Liver	33	0	-	-	-	-	-	-	-	-	0.9	1.1	-	2.7	6.1	3.7	4.7	15.0	18.8	10.4	2.1	0.5	0.05	0.10	**1.0**	*155*
Gallbladder etc.	45	0	-	-	-	-	-	-	-	-	-	1.1	4.0	1.4	7.3	3.7	6.3	16.9	16.1	41.6	2.9	0.6	0.07	0.12	**1.3**	*156*
Pancreas	217	0	-	-	-	-	-	-	0.8	-	0.9	3.3	8.1	11.0	23.3	34.3	64.1	84.6	75.2	128.4	13.9	3.0	0.24	0.73	**6.2**	*157*
Nose, sinuses etc.	4	0	-	-	-	-	-	-	-	-	-	1.1	-	-	-	3.1	-	-	-	0.3	0.1	0.01	0.03	**0.2**	*160*
Larynx	71	0	-	-	-	-	-	-	-	-	1.8	1.1	5.4	15.1	17.1	18.4	14.1	18.8	8.1	6.9	4.5	1.0	0.20	0.36	**2.8**	*161*
Bronchus, lung	1115	0	-	-	-	-	-	2.3	0.8	7.3	12.3	40.7	80.5	142.4	203.3	263.4	325.2	300.7	217.5	197.8	71.2	15.4	2.45	5.39	**41.2**	*162*
Other thoracic organs	10	0	-	-	-	-	0.9	-	-	0.8	0.9	2.2	-	2.7	2.4	-	-	1.9	-	-	0.6	0.1	0.05	0.05	**0.5**	*163-4*
Bone	8	0	-	-	1.1	-	-	0.8	1.5	-	0.9	-	-	-	1.2	1.2	-	1.9	-	-	0.5	0.1	0.03	0.03	**0.4**	*170*
Connective tissue	48	0	-	1.1	-	1.0	-	0.8	0.8	0.8	2.6	3.3	6.7	5.5	3.7	7.4	12.5	3.8	18.8	6.9	3.1	0.7	0.13	0.23	**2.1**	*171*
Mesothelioma	17	0	-	-	-	-	0.9	0.8	-	0.8	1.8	-	1.3	4.1	-	3.7	1.6	5.6	2.7	-	1.1	0.2	0.05	0.07	**0.7**	*MES*
Kaposi's sarcoma	4	0	-	-	-	-	0.9	0.8	0.8	-	-	-	-	-	-	-	1.9	-	-	0.3	0.1	0.01	Kap.01	**0.2**	*KAP*
Melanoma of skin	89	0	1.1	-	-	1.0	0.9	3.1	6.8	1.6	6.2	3.3	12.1	8.2	11.0	14.7	15.6	7.5	16.1	17.3	5.7	1.2	0.28	0.43	**4.0**	*172*
†Other skin	14	0	-	-	-	-	-	0.8	-	0.9	1.1	2.7	-	2.4	2.5	1.6	5.6	-	3.5	0.9		0.04	0.06	**0.6**	*173*
Breast	2160	0	-	-	-	1.8	6.1	20.3	65.3	120.6	164.9	216.0	249.3	347.8	410.5	411.2	453.0	434.9	444.1	138.0	29.8	5.96	10.07	**87.0**	*174*
Uterus unspecified	19	0	-	-	-	-	-	-	-	-	1.1	2.7	2.7	-	3.7	6.3	1.9	5.4	13.9	1.2	0.3	0.03	0.08	**0.7**	*179*
Cervix uteri	139	0	-	-	-	3.5	7.7	12.8	13.9	16.7	16.5	10.7	11.0	6.1	19.6	9.4	9.4	16.1	10.4	8.9	1.9	0.49	0.64	**6.7**	*180*
Placenta	2	0	-	-	-	0.9	-	-	-	-	0.9	-	-	-	-	-	-	-	-	0.1	0.0	0.01	0.01	**0.1**	*181*
Corpus uteri	235	0	-	-	-	0.9	-	1.5	4.9	7.0	20.9	24.2	27.4	29.4	55.1	57.8	39.5	48.3	55.5	15.0	3.2	0.58	1.15	**9.3**	*182*
Ovary etc.	274	0	-	-	2.1	-	3.1	6.0	13.1	9.7	24.2	25.5	39.7	34.3	44.1	40.7	58.3	88.6	31.2	17.5	3.8	0.79	1.21	**11.2**	*183*
Other female genital	51	0	-	-	-	-	0.8	0.8	0.8	2.6	4.4	2.7	2.7	7.3	11.0	6.3	15.0	18.8	10.4	3.3	0.7	0.11	0.20	**1.9**	*184*
Bladder	222	0	-	-	-	-	0.8	0.8	0.8	6.2	5.5	10.7	21.9	31.8	39.2	61.0	50.7	75.2	107.6	14.2	3.1	0.39	0.89	**7.4**	*188*
Kidney etc.	193	0	3.3	-	-	-	-	0.8	0.8	2.6	6.6	18.8	20.5	25.7	47.8	42.2	58.3	56.4	38.2	12.3	2.7	0.40	0.85	**7.2**	*189*
Eye	20	0	1.1	-	-	-	2.3	0.8	-	-	-	2.7	2.7	-	2.5	3.1	5.6	2.7	10.4	1.3	0.3	0.05	0.08	**0.9**	*190*
Brain, nervous system	74	0	5.4	5.5	1.1	1.0	3.5	1.5	3.8	2.4	2.6	5.5	1.3	5.5	9.8	11.0	12.5	7.5	8.1	10.4	4.7	1.0	0.25	0.36	**4.1**	*191-2*
Thyroid	125	0	-	-	-	3.1	3.5	8.4	9.8	10.6	11.4	16.5	14.8	8.2	6.1	9.8	14.1	20.7	5.4	3.5	8.0	1.7	0.46	0.58	**6.3**	*193*
Other endocrine	12	0	1.1	-	-	-	-	0.8	-	0.9	-	2.7	4.1	-	1.2	1.6	-	5.4	-	0.8	0.2	0.05	0.06	**0.6**	*194*
Hodgkin's disease	44	0	-	-	6.9	3.1	4.4	6.1	3.8	0.8	4.4	4.4	-	2.7	1.2	1.2	-	3.8	2.7	-	2.8	0.6	0.19	0.20	**2.8**	*201*
Non-Hodgkin lymphoma	253	0	-	-	-	-	1.8	1.5	3.0	5.7	7.9	12.1	22.8	27.4	30.6	41.7	53.2	60.1	83.2	86.7	16.2	3.5	0.56	1.04	**9.2**	*200,202*
Multiple myeloma	56	0	-	-	-	-	-	-	-	-	1.8	1.1	-	2.7	6.1	13.5	18.8	22.6	13.4	20.8	3.6	0.8	0.06	0.22	**1.7**	*203*
Lymphoid leukaemia	71	0	9.8	1.1	-	1.0	-	-	-	-	1.8	1.1	4.0	2.7	4.9	7.4	18.8	30.1	21.5	20.8	4.5	1.0	0.13	0.26	**3.2**	*204*
Myeloid leukaemia	77	0	1.1	1.1	1.1	1.0	0.9	-	1.5	0.8	1.8	1.1	9.4	5.5	11.0	8.6	26.6	11.3	34.9	10.4	4.9	1.1	0.18	0.36	**3.1**	*205*
Monocytic leukaemia	4	0	-	1.1	1.1	-	-	-	-	-	-	-	-	-	1.2	1.2	-	-	-	0.3	0.1	0.02	0.02	**0.3**	*206*
Other leukaemia	1	0	-	-	-	-	-	-	-	-	1.1	-	-	-	-	-	-	-	-	0.1	0.0	0.01	0.01	**0.1**	*207*
Leukaemia unspecified	16	0	-	2.2	-	-	-	0.8	0.8	-	-	-	-	1.4	1.2	-	-	3.8	8.1	17.3	1.0	0.2	0.03	0.03	**0.6**	*208*
Other and unspecified	236	0	-	-	-	-	-	-	2.3	1.6	0.9	11.0	8.1	11.0	31.8	39.2	54.7	62.0	102.0	145.7	15.1	3.3	0.33	0.80	**7.2**	*O&U*
All sites	7270	0	22.8	12.1	11.4	15.6	24.6	48.3	83.3	140.3	245.6	381.4	562.2	769.8	1010.4	1341.6	1612.0	1808.1	1927.6	2085.1	464.4		16.64	31.41	**273.2**	*ALL*
All sites but 173	7256	0	22.8	12.1	11.4	15.6	24.6	48.3	82.6	140.3	244.7	380.3	559.5	769.8	1008.0	1339.2	1610.4	1802.5	1927.6	2081.7	463.5	100.0	16.60	31.35	**272.6**	*ALLb*

Rate from 1 case	1.087	1.102	1.143	1.039	0.877	0.767	0.751	0.816	0.880	1.099	1.342	1.370	1.225	1.225	1.564	1.880	2.685	3.469

†Important: see notes on population page

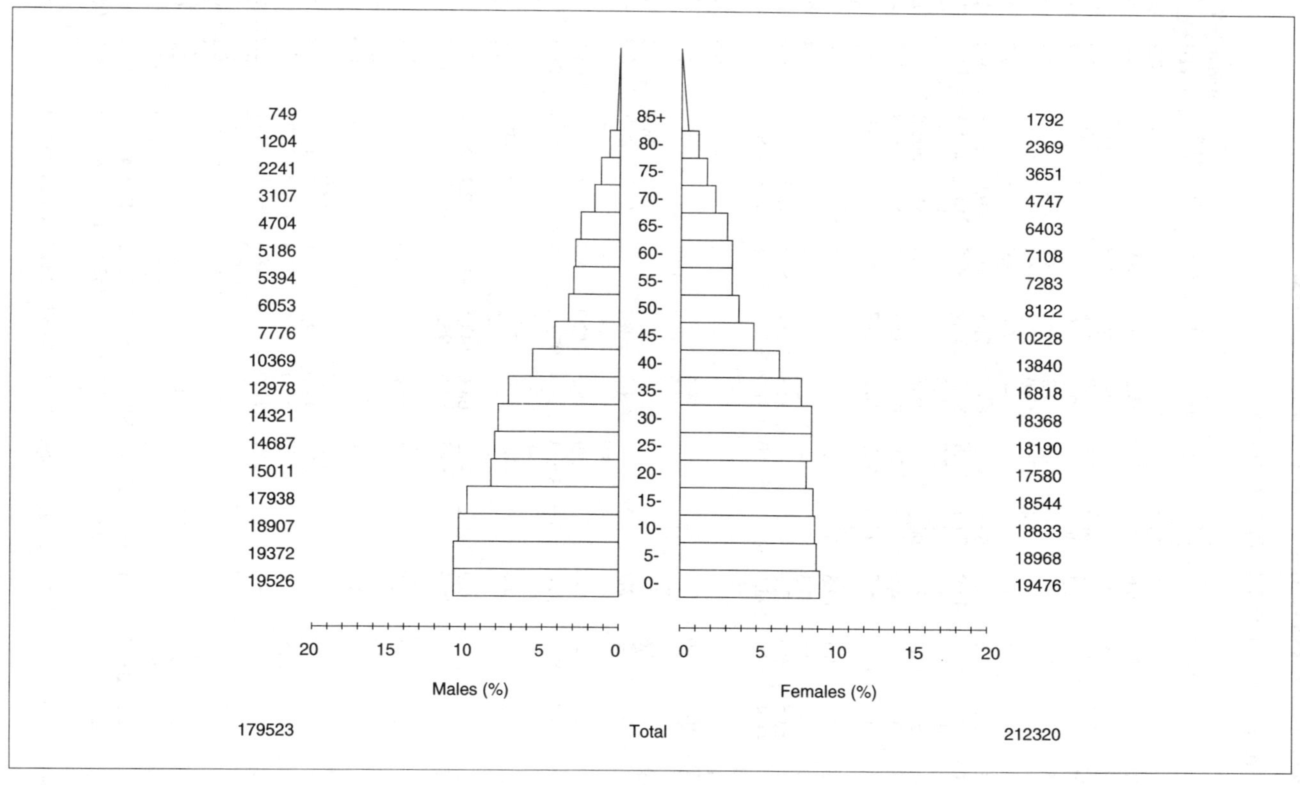

USA, Louisiana, New Orleans: Black
Source of population: average annual 1988–92
Census: 1990
Estimate: Population estimates from the U.S. Bureau of the Census, obtained from the National Cancer Institute.

Notes to tables overleaf:
† 173 does not include basal cell or squamous cell carcinoma

USA, LOUISIANA, NEW ORLEANS: BLACK 1988-1992

ANNUAL INCIDENCE PER 100,000 BY AGE GROUP (YEARS) - MALE

SITE	ALL AGES	AGE UNK	0-	5-	10-	15-	20-	25-	30-	35-	40-	45-	50-	55-	60-	65-	70-	75-	80-	85+	CRUDE RATE	%	CR 64	CR 74	ASR (W)	ICD (9th)
Lip	2	0	-	-	-	-	-	-	-	-	-	-	3.3	3.7	-	-	-	-	-		0.2	0.1	0.04	0.04	**0.3**	140
Tongue	20	0	-	-	-	-	-	-	-	3.1	-	12.9	6.6	11.1	15.4	8.5	6.4	8.9	-	-	2.2	0.6	0.25	0.32	**2.8**	141
Salivary gland	10	0	-	-	-	2.2	-	-	-	1.5	-	2.6	-	-	3.9	8.5	6.4	8.9	-	26.7	1.1	0.3	0.05	0.13	**1.2**	142
Mouth	35	0	-	-	-	-	1.3	-	-	1.5	5.8	20.6	23.1	14.8	15.4	17.0	6.4	-	-	53.3	3.9	1.1	0.41	0.53	**5.1**	143-5
Oropharynx	24	0	-	-	-	-	-	-	-	4.6	3.9	2.6	13.2	26.0	7.7	12.8	12.9	-	-	-	2.7	0.7	0.29	0.42	**3.3**	146
Nasopharynx	10	0	-	-	-	1.1	2.7	-	1.4	1.5	-	5.1	-	-	3.9	4.3	-	8.9	-	-	1.1	0.3	0.08	0.10	**1.2**	147
Hypopharynx	17	0	-	-	-	-	-	-	-	-	-	7.7	6.6	7.4	7.7	17.0	19.3	8.9	-	-	1.9	0.5	0.15	0.33	**2.4**	148
Pharynx unspecified	6	0	-	-	-	-	-	-	-	-	-	5.1	3.3	-	-	6.4	8.9	16.6	-		0.7	0.2	0.04	0.07	**0.8**	149
Oesophagus	83	0	-	-	-	-	-	1.4	1.5	5.8	7.7	36.3	55.6	46.3	63.8	51.5	80.3	49.8	53.3		9.2	2.5	0.77	1.35	**11.1**	150
Stomach	134	0	1.0	-	-	-	-	1.4	2.8	4.6	7.7	10.3	43.0	37.1	57.8	85.0	135.2	169.5	215.9	213.4	14.9	4.1	0.83	1.93	**16.8**	151
Small intestine	9	0	-	-	-	-	-	-	-	-	1.9	2.6	3.3	3.7	7.7	8.5	-	-	16.6	-	1.0	0.3	0.10	0.14	**1.2**	152
Colon	247	0	-	-	-	-	-	5.6	-	15.4	15.4	72.7	100.1	115.7	178.5	206.0	303.4	381.9	506.8		27.5	7.5	1.62	3.55	**31.4**	153
Rectum	86	0	-	1.0	-	-	-	-	-	6.2	15.4	12.9	6.6	26.0	54.0	89.3	83.7	53.5	33.2	80.0	9.6	2.6	0.61	1.47	**11.2**	154
Liver	58	0	-	-	1.1	-	-	-	-	-	3.9	12.9	16.5	44.5	34.7	42.5	25.7	35.7	49.8	80.0	6.5	1.8	0.57	0.91	**7.9**	155
Gallbladder etc.	10	0	-	-	-	-	-	-	-	-	1.9	-	3.3	3.7	-	4.3	6.4	17.8	33.2	26.7	1.1	0.3	0.04	0.10	**1.2**	156
Pancreas	75	0	-	-	-	-	-	-	1.4	4.6	7.7	5.1	19.8	33.4	19.3	63.8	57.9	89.2	149.5	53.3	8.4	2.3	0.46	1.07	**9.2**	157
Nose, sinuses etc.	12	0	-	1.0	-	-	2.7	-	-	3.1	-	2.6	3.3	-	12.8	-	17.8	-	-		1.3	0.4	0.06	0.13	**1.4**	160
Larynx	84	0	-	-	-	-	-	-	-	-	13.5	10.3	23.1	48.2	54.0	38.3	109.4	53.5	116.2	-	9.4	2.6	0.75	1.48	**11.1**	161
Bronchus, lung	842	0	-	1.0	-	-	1.3	-	5.6	15.4	44.4	113.2	198.2	355.9	590.0	641.9	888.3	713.8	929.9	666.8	93.8	25.6	6.62	14.28	**110.8**	162
Other thoracic organs	4	0	1.0	-	-	-	2.7	-	-	1.5	-	-	-	-	-	-	-	-	-		0.4	0.1	0.03	0.03	**0.4**	163-4
Bone	8	0	-	2.1	1.1	-	-	-	-	3.1	-	-	-	-	-	4.3	6.4	8.9	-	-	0.9	0.2	0.03	0.08	**0.8**	170
Connective tissue	22	0	1.0	-	-	-	-	2.7	-	9.2	1.9	2.6	-	11.1	3.9	12.8	19.3	-	-	26.7	2.5	0.7	0.16	0.32	**2.7**	171
Mesothelioma	16	0	-	-	-	-	-	-	1.4	1.5	3.9	-	6.6	11.1	3.9	8.5	12.9	17.8	-	-	1.8	0.5	0.14	0.25	**2.0**	MES
Kaposi's sarcoma	30	0	-	-	-	-	4.0	5.4	7.0	13.9	11.6	2.6	-	-	3.9	-	-	-	-	26.7	3.3	0.9	0.24	0.24	**3.1**	KAP
Melanoma of skin	7	0	-	1.1	-	-	-	-	-	-	-	-	3.3	3.7	-	4.3	6.4	-	16.6	26.7	0.8	0.2	0.04	0.09	**0.9**	172
†Other skin	3	0	-	-	1.1	-	1.4	-	-	-	-	-	-	-	3.9	-	-	-	-		0.3		0.03	0.03	**0.4**	173
Breast	9	0	-	-	-	-	-	-	-	-	1.9	-	-	-	3.9	8.5	12.9	8.9	33.2	-	1.0	0.3	0.03	0.14	**1.0**	175
Prostate	794	0	-	-	-	-	-	-	-	-	-	5.8	23.1	49.6	215.0	339.3	701.4	972.0	1311.6	1527.7	1760.5	88.5	24.1	3.16	11.53	**96.4**	185
Testis	13	0	-	-	-	3.3	-	4.1	2.8	4.6	1.9	-	3.7	-	-	-	-	-	-	-	1.4	0.4	0.10	0.10	**1.3**	186
Penis	11	0	-	-	-	-	-	-	-	-	1.9	5.1	3.3	7.4	11.6	-	-	-	16.6	26.7	1.2	0.3	0.15	0.15	**1.6**	187.1-.4
Other male genital	1	0	-	-	-	-	-	-	-	1.5	-	-	-	-	-	-	-	-	-		0.1	0.0	0.01	0.01	**0.1**	187.5-.9
Bladder	111	0	-	-	-	-	-	-	-	1.5	-	12.9	9.9	22.2	46.3	68.0	148.1	205.2	182.7	293.4	12.4	3.4	0.46	1.54	**13.5**	188
Kidney etc.	94	0	1.0	-	-	-	-	1.4	-	1.5	1.9	20.6	36.3	11.1	34.7	80.8	90.1	89.2	182.7	133.4	10.5	2.9	0.54	1.40	**12.0**	189
Eye	1	0	-	-	-	-	-	-	-	-	2.6	-	-	-	-	-	-	-	-		0.1	0.0	0.01	0.01	**0.2**	190
Brain, nervous system	37	0	5.1	2.1	2.1	-	1.3	1.4	2.8	-	1.9	2.6	3.3	18.5	19.3	29.8	6.4	26.8	-	-	4.1	1.1	0.30	0.48	**4.6**	191-2
Thyroid	5	0	-	-	-	-	1.3	-	1.4	-	-	2.6	3.3	-	-	6.4	-	-	-		0.6	0.2	0.04	0.08	**0.6**	193
Other endocrine	3	0	-	-	-	-	-	-	1.4	-	-	-	3.3	-	3.9	-	-	-	-		0.3	0.1	0.04	0.04	**0.4**	194
Hodgkin's disease	16	0	-	-	2.1	-	-	5.4	1.4	3.1	1.9	5.1	-	3.9	4.3	-	8.9	16.6	-		1.8	0.5	0.11	0.14	**1.8**	201
Non-Hodgkin lymphoma	76	0	-	1.0	1.1	1.1	2.7	4.1	12.6	7.7	13.5	18.0	29.7	14.8	23.1	17.0	32.2	44.6	33.2	133.4	8.5	2.3	0.65	0.89	**9.4**	200,202
Multiple myeloma	68	0	-	-	-	-	-	-	-	-	3.9	12.9	16.5	29.7	27.0	51.0	57.9	71.4	116.2	133.4	7.6	2.1	0.45	0.99	**8.7**	203
Lymphoid leukaemia	29	0	2.0	3.1	1.1	2.2	-	1.4	1.4	1.5	-	5.1	6.6	7.4	23.1	17.0	-	8.9	-	26.7	3.2	0.9	0.28	0.36	**3.7**	204
Myeloid leukaemia	30	0	1.0	-	1.1	4.5	1.3	2.7	4.2	1.5	-	-	9.9	7.4	11.6	12.8	-	8.9	33.2	106.7	3.3	0.9	0.22	0.28	**3.6**	205
Monocytic leukaemia	2	0	-	-	-	-	-	1.4	1.4	-	-	-	-	-	-	-	-	-	-		0.2	0.1	0.01	0.01	**0.2**	206
Other leukaemia	1	0	-	-	-	-	-	-	-	-	1.9	-	-	-	-	-	-	-	-		0.1	0.0	0.01	0.01	**0.1**	207
Leukaemia unspecified	14	0	-	-	-	-	-	-	2.8	-	1.9	2.6	-	3.7	11.6	4.3	19.3	8.9	-	26.7	1.6	0.4	0.11	0.23	**1.8**	208
Other and unspecified	127	0	1.0	-	-	-	-	-	-	3.1	19.3	20.6	43.0	44.5	50.1	80.8	83.7	133.8	166.1	293.4	14.1	3.9	0.91	1.73	**16.4**	O&U
All sites	3296	0	13.3	11.4	8.5	16.7	21.3	32.7	58.7	103.2	202.5	388.3	707.1	1182.6	1658.1	2401.8	3096.2	3533.2	4317.5	4774.6	367.2		22.02	49.51	**418.2**	ALL
All sites but 173	3293	0	13.3	11.4	8.5	15.6	21.3	31.3	58.7	103.2	202.5	388.3	707.1	1182.6	1654.2	2401.8	3096.2	3533.2	4317.5	4774.6	366.8	100.0	21.99	49.48	**417.9**	ALLb

Rate from 1 case   1.024 1.032 1.058 1.115 1.332 1.362 1.397 1.541 1.929 2.572 3.304 3.707 3.856 4.251 6.437 8.922 16.606 26.674

†Important: see notes on population page

USA, LOUISIANA, NEW ORLEANS: BLACK 1988-1992

ANNUAL INCIDENCE PER 100,000 BY AGE GROUP (YEARS) - FEMALE

SITE	ALL AGES	AGE UNK	0-	5-	10-	15-	20-	25-	30-	35-	40-	45-	50-	55-	60-	65-	70-	75-	80-	85+	CRUDE RATE	%	CR 64	CR 74	ASR (W)	ICD (9th)
Lip	0	0	-	-	-	-	-	-	-	-	-	-	-	-	-	-	-	-	-	-	0.0	0.0	0.00	0.00	0.0	140
Tongue	7	0	-	-	-	-	-	-	-	-	-	3.9	2.5	2.7	-	6.2	4.2	-	-	-	0.7	0.2	0.05	0.10	0.7	141
Salivary gland	7	0	-	-	-	-	-	1.1	2.2	-	-	3.9	2.5	-	-	-	4.2	-	-	-	0.7	0.2	0.05	0.07	0.7	142
Mouth	11	0	-	-	-	-	-	-	2.2	1.2	-	2.0	2.5	8.2	-	-	4.2	5.5	8.4	-	1.0	0.4	0.08	0.10	1.0	143-5
Oropharynx	5	0	-	-	-	-	-	-	-	-	-	-	-	5.6	-	-	5.5	16.9	-	-	0.5	0.2	0.03	0.03	0.4	146
Nasopharynx	5	0	-	-	-	1.1	-	-	1.1	1.2	-	2.5	-	-	-	5.5	-	-	-	-	0.5	0.2	0.03	0.03	0.4	147
Hypopharynx	2	0	-	-	-	-	-	-	-	-	-	-	-	2.8	-	-	5.5	-	-	-	0.2	0.1	0.01	0.01	0.2	148
Pharynx unspecified	4	0	-	-	-	-	-	-	-	-	1.4	2.0	2.5	-	-	-	-	-	-	11.2	0.4	0.1	0.03	0.03	0.4	149
Oesophagus	27	0	-	-	-	-	-	-	-	-	-	2.0	9.8	13.7	14.1	9.4	12.6	27.4	8.4	-	2.5	0.9	0.20	0.31	2.6	150
Stomach	86	0	-	-	-	-	-	1.1	2.4	1.4	2.0	12.3	13.7	28.1	25.0	29.5	98.6	126.6	145.1	8.1	2.8	0.31	0.58	6.4	151
Small intestine	18	0	-	-	-	-	-	1.1	2.4	-	4.9	11.0	2.8	3.1	12.6	16.4	8.4	-	1.7	0.6	0.11	0.19	1.6	152
Colon	314	0	-	-	-	-	2.2	2.2	3.6	11.6	19.6	44.3	74.1	95.7	134.3	219.1	241.0	244.7	468.8	29.6	10.1	1.27	3.03	25.8	153
Rectum	85	0	-	-	-	-	2.2	-	2.4	2.9	9.8	2.5	27.5	22.5	59.3	42.1	71.2	42.2	89.3	8.0	2.7	0.35	0.86	7.2	154
Liver	24	0	1.0	-	-	-	2.3	-	-	-	-	7.4	5.5	8.4	21.9	8.4	5.5	25.3	-	2.3	0.8	0.12	0.27	2.2	155
Gallbladder etc.	28	0	-	-	-	-	1.1	-	-	-	-	2.5	13.7	11.3	21.9	8.4	16.4	50.6	-	2.6	0.9	0.14	0.29	2.4	156
Pancreas	117	0	-	-	-	-	-	-	-	-	9.8	2.5	24.7	42.2	65.6	71.6	131.5	118.2	111.6	11.0	3.8	0.40	1.09	9.3	157
Nose, sinuses etc.	9	0	-	-	-	-	-	1.1	-	-	-	-	2.7	11.3	-	8.4	-	-	11.2	0.8	0.3	0.08	0.12	0.8	160
Larynx	22	0	-	-	-	-	-	-	1.2	1.4	-	9.8	-	11.3	25.0	4.2	5.5	16.9	-	2.1	0.7	0.12	0.26	2.1	161
Bronchus, lung	415	0	-	-	-	-	-	-	5.4	10.7	21.7	41.1	78.8	98.9	168.8	281.1	198.0	306.7	244.7	167.4	39.1	13.4	2.13	4.52	36.9	162
Other thoracic organs	2	0	-	-	-	-	-	-	-	-	-	-	-	-	2.8	-	4.2	-	-	0.2	0.1	0.01	0.04	0.2	163-4
Bone	5	0	-	-	2.1	-	1.1	-	-	-	-	-	2.7	-	-	-	-	11.2	0.5	0.2	0.03	0.03	0.4	170
Connective tissue	14	0	-	-	-	1.1	1.1	1.1	-	3.6	1.4	2.0	-	8.2	2.8	6.2	-	-	-	1.3	0.5	0.11	0.14	1.3	171
Mesothelioma	3	0	-	-	-	-	-	-	-	-	-	-	2.5	-	3.1	4.2	-	-	-	0.3	0.1	0.01	0.05	0.3	MES
Kaposi's sarcoma	3	0	-	-	-	-	-	-	-	-	1.4	-	-	-	-	-	5.5	-	11.2	0.3	0.1	0.01	0.01	0.2	KAP
Melanoma of skin	1	0	-	-	-	-	-	-	-	-	-	-	-	-	-	-	-	-	11.2	0.1	0.0	0.00	0.00	0.1	172
†Other skin	8	0	-	-	-	1.1	-	-	1.1	1.2	-	-	2.5	2.7	2.8	3.1	4.2	-	-	0.8	0.06	0.09	0.8	173
Breast	931	0	-	-	-	-	3.4	19.8	38.1	86.8	153.2	201.4	231.5	219.7	247.6	309.2	362.3	367.0	337.6	435.3	87.7	30.0	6.01	9.36	84.9	174
Uterus unspecified	11	0	-	-	-	1.1	-	-	-	-	-	2.0	2.5	2.7	-	6.2	-	11.0	-	33.5	1.0	0.4	0.04	0.07	0.9	179
Cervix uteri	170	0	-	-	-	1.1	3.4	11.0	18.5	34.5	43.4	25.4	22.2	49.4	25.3	15.6	46.3	27.4	42.2	55.8	16.0	5.5	1.17	1.48	14.8	180
Placenta	2	0	-	-	-	-	1.1	1.1	-	-	-	-	-	-	-	-	-	-	-	-	0.2	0.1	0.01	0.01	0.2	181
Corpus uteri	101	0	-	-	-	-	1.1	1.1	2.2	5.9	2.9	3.9	9.8	19.2	56.3	62.5	80.0	49.3	33.8	55.8	9.5	3.3	0.51	1.23	9.0	182
Ovary etc.	84	0	-	1.1	-	3.2	1.1	6.6	1.1	3.6	4.3	19.6	7.4	22.0	28.1	31.2	33.7	21.9	50.6	78.1	7.9	2.7	0.49	0.81	7.6	183
Other female genital	29	0	-	-	-	-	-	1.1	-	-	-	9.8	4.9	8.2	16.9	3.1	16.9	21.9	8.4	22.3	2.7	0.9	0.20	0.30	2.7	184
Bladder	51	0	-	-	-	-	-	-	-	-	4.3	2.0	4.9	2.7	22.5	21.9	25.3	32.9	101.3	55.8	4.8	1.6	0.18	0.42	3.9	188
Kidney etc.	83	0	4.1	-	-	-	-	-	1.1	5.9	15.9	9.8	4.9	19.2	19.7	40.6	25.3	38.3	59.1	89.3	7.8	2.7	0.40	0.73	7.1	189
Eye	0	0	-	-	-	-	-	-	-	-	-	-	-	-	-	-	-	-	-	-	0.0	0.0	0.00	0.00	0.0	190
Brain, nervous system	30	0	4.1	3.2	2.1	1.1	-	3.3	1.1	-	2.9	-	7.4	2.7	2.8	6.2	12.6	16.4	8.4	-	2.8	1.0	0.15	0.25	2.8	191-2
Thyroid	49	0	-	-	-	2.2	1.1	6.6	7.6	9.5	8.7	7.8	7.4	11.0	5.6	3.1	8.4	16.4	-	-	4.6	1.6	0.34	0.40	4.3	193
Other endocrine	6	0	1.0	-	2.1	-	-	-	-	-	1.4	-	-	2.7	-	-	-	-	8.4	-	0.6	0.2	0.04	0.04	0.6	194
Hodgkin's disease	16	0	-	-	-	2.2	3.4	4.4	1.1	2.4	-	2.0	-	2.7	2.8	3.1	-	-	-	-	1.5	0.5	0.10	0.12	1.5	201
Non-Hodgkin lymphoma	64	0	-	1.1	-	-	-	-	2.2	3.6	10.1	7.8	7.4	8.2	30.9	28.1	12.6	21.9	50.6	89.3	6.0	2.1	0.36	0.56	5.5	200,202
Multiple myeloma	68	0	-	-	-	-	-	-	-	1.2	4.3	3.9	12.3	16.5	19.7	15.6	54.8	49.3	67.5	100.4	6.4	2.2	0.29	0.64	5.5	203
Lymphoid leukaemia	20	0	5.1	-	2.1	-	1.1	1.1	-	-	-	-	2.5	2.7	5.6	6.2	8.4	-	8.4	22.3	1.9	0.6	0.10	0.18	2.0	204
Myeloid leukaemia	26	0	-	3.2	-	-	-	1.1	1.1	2.4	-	3.9	2.5	2.7	14.1	6.2	8.4	16.4	16.9	11.2	2.4	0.8	0.15	0.23	2.3	205
Monocytic leukaemia	2	0	-	-	-	-	-	-	-	-	-	-	-	-	2.8	-	-	-	11.2	0.2	0.1	0.01	0.01	0.2	206
Other leukaemia	1	0	-	-	-	-	-	-	-	-	-	-	-	-	-	-	5.5	-	-	0.1	0.0	0.00	0.00	0.1	207
Leukaemia unspecified	5	0	-	1.1	-	-	-	1.1	-	1.2	-	-	-	-	-	-	4.2	-	8.4	-	0.5	0.2	0.02	0.04	0.4	208
Other and unspecified	137	0	1.0	1.1	-	-	-	1.1	2.2	3.6	8.7	17.6	22.2	16.5	30.9	56.2	101.1	109.5	92.8	167.4	12.9	4.4	0.52	1.31	11.3	O&U
All sites	3108	0	16.4	10.5	8.5	14.0	20.5	67.1	93.6	190.3	303.5	414.5	541.7	719.5	965.1	1280.6	1440.8	1752.8	1806.1	2265.6	292.8		16.83	30.43	271.8	ALL
All sites but 173	3100	0	16.4	10.5	8.5	12.9	20.5	67.1	92.5	189.1	303.5	414.5	539.3	716.7	962.2	1277.5	1436.6	1752.8	1806.1	2265.6	292.0	100.0	16.77	30.34	271.0	ALLb

Rate from 1 case   1.027 1.054 1.062 1.078 1.138 1.099 1.089 1.189 1.445 1.955 2.462 2.746 2.814 3.123 4.213 5.477 8.440 11.161

†Important: see notes on population page

285

USA, Michigan, Detroit

The Metropolitan Detroit Cancer Surveillance Section (MDCSS) is a unit in the Epidemiology Section of the Karmanos Cancer Institute. It began in 1949 as a pathology registry for 25 collaborating hospitals and in 1960 became a central statistical resource for these hospitals.

The MDCSS was organized in its current form to participate in the Third National Cancer Survey for the years 1969–71. In 1973, the MDCSS became one of the founding participants in the National Cancer Institute's SEER (Surveillance, Epidemiology, and End Results) Program. In Michigan, cancer is a reportable disease, with the MDCSS functioning as the official designate of the Michigan Department of Community Health for collecting this information in the Detroit Metropolitan area. Effective from January 1985, the Public Health Statutes of Michigan authorized the establishment of a state-wide cancer incidence reporting system. Data for the tri-county Detroit area are being provided to the new state-wide system by the MDCSS.

Metropolitan Detroit is on the eastern border of Michigan, facing Canada, between longitudes 82 and 83° W and latitudes 42 and 43° N. The total registration area is 3259 km^2. The population covered by the MDCSS was 3 912 679 in the 1990 census. Of these, 73.5% were white, 24.0% black and 2% of Spanish origin. Foreign-born persons residing in the Metropolitan area are primarily of Arabic, Greek, Polish, Italian, German, English, Irish or Scottish origin. The area is predominantly urban and is heavily industrialized, as the centre of the United States automobile manufacturing industry.

The MDCSS provides both incidence and survival reporting for the Metropolitan Detroit area. Data are collected by the MDCSS abstracting staff from 50 hospitals as well as from private pathology laboratories, radiation therapy facilities and selected clinics and physicians' offices. These facilities include all those located in Metropolitan Detroit as well as facilities outside the tri-county area which routinely provide care for cancer patients resident in the MDCSS registration area. Active follow-up is maintained for all cases, with requests for information sent to physicians on a bi-monthly basis. Readmissions to hospitals are also abstracted for follow-up data; additionally, telephone contacts are made with physicians' offices and with patients as routine elements of active follow-up. Death certificates for the State of Michigan, and for other states which are retirement areas for local residents, are linked by computer tape each quarter to provide up-to-date information about death and causes of death.

Epidemiological research based upon MDCSS data is conducted by the Epidemiology Section of the Karmanos Cancer Institute. Primary areas of interest are studies of racial and ethnic diversity and occupational etiologies of cancer. Particular emphasis is placed upon studies of risk determination; delineating occupational cancer risk among blacks and women as well as white men, understanding differences in cancer incidence among blacks and whites, and identifying genetic and familial patterns of cancer occurrence.

In addition to providing a research base, MDCSS data are utilized extensively by local health departments, by the Michigan Department of Community Health, and by area health professionals for planning, evaluation, and educational purposes. Community concerns about cancer risk are also addressed through utilization of the MDCSS data.

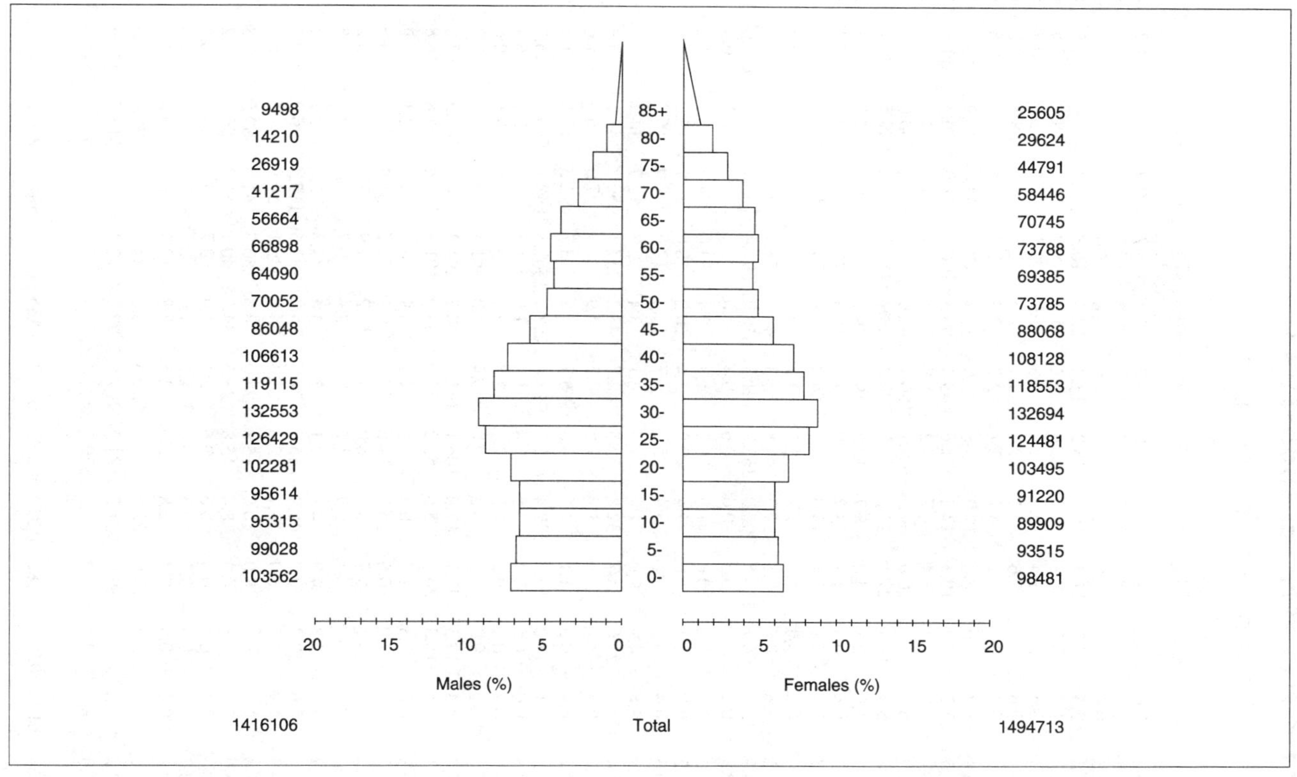

USA, Michigan, Detroit: White
Source of population: average annual 1988-92
Estimate: NCI estimates based on U.S. Bureau of Census population estimates by county for the years 1988–92.

Notes to tables overleaf:
† 173 does not include basal cell or squamous cell carcinoma

USA, MICHIGAN, DETROIT: WHITE 1988-1992

ANNUAL INCIDENCE PER 100,000 BY AGE GROUP (YEARS) - MALE

SITE	ALL AGES	AGE UNK	0-	5-	10-	15-	20-	25-	30-	35-	40-	45-	50-	55-	60-	65-	70-	75-	80-	85+	CRUDE RATE	%	CR 64	CR 74	ASR (W)	ICD (9th)
Lip	83	0	-	-	-	-	-	0.2	0.3	0.2	0.6	0.2	1.1	2.8	4.8	4.9	4.4	6.7	9.9	14.7	1.2	0.2	0.05	0.10	0.9	140
Tongue	284	0	0.2	-	-	0.2	-	0.3	0.6	1.3	1.3	4.4	9.1	13.1	14.4	15.9	19.4	17.1	9.9	10.5	4.0	0.7	0.22	0.40	3.2	141
Salivary gland	86	0	-	-	-	0.2	0.2	0.5	0.2	0.8	0.9	-	2.6	2.2	3.3	4.6	5.8	5.9	2.8	16.8	1.2	0.2	0.05	0.11	0.9	142
Mouth	320	0	-	0.2	-	0.2	-	0.2	0.8	0.5	2.3	4.2	11.4	14.7	18.2	13.4	22.3	16.3	16.9	27.4	4.5	0.8	0.26	0.44	3.6	143-5
Oropharynx	178	0	-	-	-	-	-	0.2	0.7	1.9	2.6	8.3	6.9	8.4	9.2	11.2	8.9	11.3	8.4	2.5	0.5	0.14	0.25	2.0	146
Nasopharynx	48	0	-	-	0.2	-	0.2	0.2	0.2	0.3	0.6	0.7	1.4	2.2	2.1	2.8	1.9	2.2	1.4	2.1	0.7	0.1	0.04	0.06	0.6	147
Hypopharynx	143	0	-	-	-	-	-	-	-	-	0.6	1.4	2.6	4.1	9.6	12.4	12.6	8.2	5.6	8.4	2.0	0.4	0.09	0.22	1.6	148
Pharynx unspecified	45	0	-	-	-	-	-	-	-	-	0.2	0.2	-	4.1	2.1	2.8	2.9	3.7	1.4	6.3	0.6	0.1	0.03	0.06	0.5	149
Oesophagus	461	0	-	-	-	-	-	0.2	0.5	0.3	1.3	4.0	8.0	17.2	23.6	27.9	38.8	47.5	39.4	37.9	6.5	1.2	0.27	0.61	4.9	150
Stomach	841	0	-	-	-	-	0.2	0.2	0.6	1.5	3.2	7.2	10.3	17.2	32.6	43.4	80.5	106.2	121.0	126.3	11.9	2.2	0.36	0.98	8.5	151
Small intestine	135	0	-	-	-	-	-	-	0.3	-	0.8	1.2	3.4	4.7	4.2	8.8	13.6	11.1	11.3	14.7	1.9	0.4	0.07	0.18	1.4	152
Colon	3048	0	-	-	-	-	0.4	1.9	2.6	2.9	6.0	20.5	36.0	64.0	109.1	186.7	242.6	397.5	499.6	558.0	43.0	7.9	1.22	3.36	30.5	153
Rectum	1534	0	-	-	-	-	0.6	0.5	1.4	1.8	3.9	14.4	21.1	44.6	71.5	100.2	123.7	164.2	194.2	149.5	21.7	4.0	0.80	1.92	15.9	154
Liver	294	0	1.0	-	-	-	-	-	-	0.5	1.9	2.8	4.0	8.7	10.2	19.1	29.1	27.5	28.1	35.8	4.2	0.8	0.15	0.39	3.1	155
Gallbladder etc.	162	0	-	-	-	-	-	-	0.2	0.3	0.4	0.5	1.1	3.7	7.2	7.4	15.5	22.3	25.3	29.5	2.3	0.4	0.07	0.18	1.6	156
Pancreas	828	0	-	-	-	-	-	-	0.3	1.7	3.4	5.1	12.6	19.0	33.8	54.0	67.9	94.4	115.4	117.9	11.7	2.1	0.38	0.99	8.5	157
Nose, sinuses etc.	59	0	-	-	-	0.4	-	0.3	0.2	-	0.8	0.9	1.4	2.8	2.7	2.1	2.4	5.2	4.2	4.2	0.8	0.2	0.05	0.07	0.7	160
Larynx	748	0	-	-	-	-	-	0.3	0.8	1.2	3.6	9.5	19.1	29.3	42.8	53.3	48.5	55.7	39.4	33.7	10.6	1.9	0.53	1.04	8.3	161
Bronchus, lung	7125	0	-	-	-	0.2	0.2	0.2	2.1	6.5	15.2	46.7	118.5	206.9	367.7	491.3	640.0	692.4	757.2	627.5	100.6	18.5	3.82	9.48	74.6	162
Other thoracic organs	21	0	-	0.2	0.2	-	0.4	0.2	0.3	0.2	0.2	-	0.6	0.6	0.6	0.4	1.0	-	2.8	2.1	0.3	0.1	0.02	0.02	0.3	163-4
Bone	85	0	-	0.6	2.1	2.5	0.6	1.1	0.8	1.2	0.4	1.6	0.6	1.6	1.2	1.8	2.4	3.0	4.2	2.1	1.2	0.2	0.07	0.09	1.1	170
Connective tissue	201	0	1.2	0.4	-	2.5	0.8	1.1	1.2	1.2	0.8	2.1	4.0	4.4	7.2	7.4	10.2	18.6	19.7	19.0	2.8	0.5	0.13	0.22	2.3	171
Mesothelioma	113	0	-	-	-	-	-	-	-	0.3	0.4	0.9	-	3.4	5.7	6.7	11.6	12.6	9.9	16.8	1.6	0.3	0.05	0.15	1.2	MES
Kaposi's sarcoma	188	0	-	-	-	-	0.4	3.5	4.5	5.7	5.6	4.9	2.0	1.6	1.5	2.1	3.4	2.2	12.7	14.7	2.7	0.5	0.15	0.18	2.1	KAP
Melanoma of skin	984	0	-	-	0.8	1.7	2.9	3.6	7.5	11.4	13.5	21.6	25.7	32.8	39.5	42.7	43.2	37.1	50.7	59.0	13.9	2.6	0.81	1.23	11.2	172
†Other skin	70	0	-	-	-	-	0.4	0.6	1.4	0.7	0.4	1.2	-	1.2	1.5	3.2	4.9	5.9	7.0	6.3	1.0	0.2	0.04	0.08	0.7	173
Breast	80	0	-	-	-	-	-	-	-	0.2	0.4	0.5	1.1	1.6	3.3	6.7	8.2	3.7	11.3	12.6	1.1	0.2	0.03	0.11	0.8	175
Prostate	11059	0	-	-	-	-	-	0.3	0.5	0.3	2.1	13.0	56.0	179.4	432.3	793.1	1258.7	1507.5	1648.1	1530.8	156.2	28.7	3.42	13.68	108.2	185
Testis	455	0	0.2	0.2	0.2	2.7	9.6	14.7	16.4	12.3	9.0	6.5	3.4	2.5	2.4	1.8	1.0	1.5	1.4	2.1	6.4	1.2	0.40	0.41	5.4	186
Penis	46	0	-	-	-	-	-	-	-	-	0.2	0.7	0.3	1.2	2.1	2.8	2.9	5.2	7.0	8.4	0.6	0.1	0.02	0.05	0.5	187.1-.4
Other male genital	14	0	0.2	-	-	-	-	-	-	-	-	0.2	0.6	0.3	0.6	0.4	1.0	1.5	2.8	-	0.2	0.0	0.01	0.02	0.2	187.5-.9
Bladder	2661	0	-	-	-	-	-	0.6	1.4	4.2	8.4	19.3	43.7	69.0	106.1	161.3	240.7	294.2	330.7	383.2	37.6	6.9	1.26	3.27	27.4	188
Kidney etc.	1189	0	1.9	0.4	0.2	-	0.2	0.5	0.5	2.7	7.5	16.3	26.6	35.6	53.2	72.0	99.0	101.8	108.4	75.8	16.8	3.1	0.73	1.58	12.9	189
Eye	62	0	1.4	0.2	-	-	-	-	0.2	0.3	0.8	0.5	1.7	0.3	1.8	4.2	3.9	4.5	7.0	2.1	0.9	0.2	0.04	0.08	0.7	190
Brain, nervous system	606	0	5.6	4.6	4.0	3.3	2.5	4.0	5.0	6.5	6.2	7.0	10.6	15.0	14.6	22.6	30.1	34.2	39.4	25.3	8.6	1.6	0.44	0.71	7.5	191-2
Thyroid	228	0	-	-	0.2	0.6	0.8	1.9	2.4	3.2	3.9	5.1	5.7	3.7	6.0	9.9	11.2	11.9	7.0	12.6	3.2	0.6	0.17	0.27	2.6	193
Other endocrine	35	0	1.7	0.2	0.4	0.2	0.2	0.3	0.3	-	0.4	-	-	0.9	1.2	0.7	2.4	0.7	-	-	0.5	0.1	0.03	0.05	0.5	194
Hodgkin's disease	297	0	0.4	0.4	1.9	4.4	6.8	5.9	6.9	4.7	4.9	3.3	4.9	4.1	2.1	5.6	4.4	7.4	5.6	2.1	4.2	0.8	0.25	0.30	3.7	201
Non-Hodgkin lymphoma	1392	0	0.6	1.0	1.5	2.3	2.3	5.7	5.1	9.9	15.6	20.9	27.7	45.9	45.7	72.7	75.7	122.6	115.4	96.9	19.7	3.6	0.92	1.66	15.3	200,202
Multiple myeloma	412	0	-	-	-	-	-	-	0.2	0.3	1.9	2.6	8.0	13.7	12.0	25.4	34.0	46.1	54.9	69.5	5.8	1.1	0.19	0.49	4.2	203
Lymphoid leukaemia	515	0	7.9	4.2	2.1	2.5	1.2	0.5	0.8	1.3	1.3	4.0	8.0	10.0	15.8	24.0	28.6	50.5	61.9	69.5	7.3	1.3	0.30	0.56	6.3	204
Myeloid leukaemia	442	0	1.2	0.2	0.6	0.4	1.4	1.6	1.7	3.0	2.6	3.3	4.9	8.4	15.8	23.6	34.5	40.1	56.3	56.9	6.2	1.1	0.23	0.52	4.7	205
Monocytic leukaemia	34	0	0.2	0.2	0.2	-	0.2	0.3	-	-	0.2	0.5	0.5	0.6	0.6	2.1	1.9	3.7	4.2	4.2	0.5	0.1	0.02	0.04	0.4	206
Other leukaemia	19	0	0.2	-	-	-	-	-	-	0.2	-	0.5	0.3	0.3	0.6	1.1	1.0	2.2	2.8	2.1	0.3	0.0	0.01	0.02	0.2	207
Leukaemia unspecified	105	0	0.6	0.6	-	-	0.2	0.2	0.8	0.2	0.2	0.5	0.9	2.8	3.9	2.5	7.8	13.4	19.7	16.8	1.5	0.3	0.05	0.10	1.1	208
Other and unspecified	894	0	1.0	-	0.2	-	-	1.3	1.5	2.0	3.9	5.3	10.6	22.5	35.9	50.5	70.8	86.9	121.0	195.8	12.6	2.3	0.42	1.03	9.3	O&U
All sites	38629	0	25.3	13.7	14.9	24.5	32.7	52.5	70.0	92.7	139.2	268.5	519.9	931.5	1581.2	2407.5	3377.7	4112.3	4606.5	4516.6	545.6		18.83	47.76	402.0	ALL
All sites but 173	38559	0	25.3	13.7	14.9	24.5	32.3	51.9	68.7	92.0	138.8	267.3	519.9	930.2	1579.7	2404.3	3372.9	4106.3	4599.5	4510.3	544.6	100.0	18.80	47.68	401.3	ALLb

Rate from 1 case   0.193 0.202 0.210 0.209 0.196 0.158 0.151 0.168 0.188 0.232 0.285 0.312 0.299 0.353 0.485 0.743 1.407 2.106

†Important: see notes on population page

USA, MICHIGAN, DETROIT: WHITE 1988-1992

ANNUAL INCIDENCE PER 100,000 BY AGE GROUP (YEARS) - FEMALE

SITE	ALL AGES	AGE UNK	0-	5-	10-	15-	20-	25-	30-	35-	40-	45-	50-	55-	60-	65-	70-	75-	80-	85+	CRUDE RATE	%	CR 64	CR 74	ASR (W)	ICD (9th)
Lip	18	0	-	-	-	-	-	-	-	-	0.2	-	0.3	0.3	-	0.8	0.3	2.2	2.0	2.3	0.2	0.1	0.00	0.01	**0.1**	*140*
Tongue	119	0	0.2	-	-	0.2	-	0.3	0.2	0.7	0.4	0.9	3.3	4.0	4.1	5.7	6.8	3.6	5.4	5.5	1.6	0.3	0.07	0.13	**1.1**	*141*
Salivary gland	87	0	-	-	-	0.2	0.2	0.5	0.2	0.5	0.7	1.1	3.0	2.0	2.2	2.5	4.1	2.2	2.7	10.2	1.2	0.3	0.05	0.09	**0.8**	*142*
Mouth	203	0	-	-	-	-	0.4	-	0.5	0.5	1.5	0.9	3.0	5.8	8.9	8.5	9.2	11.2	16.2	10.2	2.7	0.6	0.11	0.20	**1.7**	*143-5*
Oropharynx	77	0	-	-	-	-	-	-	-	0.2	0.2	1.4	1.4	2.9	3.3	4.5	5.5	3.1	0.7	1.6	1.0	0.2	0.05	0.10	**0.7**	*146*
Nasopharynx	19	0	-	-	-	-	-	0.2	-	-	0.4	-	0.5	-	0.5	0.6	1.7	0.4	0.7	2.3	0.3	0.1	0.01	0.02	**0.2**	*147*
Hypopharynx	38	0	-	-	-	-	-	-	-	-	-	-	0.3	2.0	2.4	2.3	2.1	2.7	0.7	-	0.5	0.1	0.02	0.05	**0.3**	*148*
Pharynx unspecified	16	0	-	-	-	-	-	-	-	-	-	-	0.3	0.6	0.8	0.8	0.7	0.4	1.4	1.6	0.2	0.0	0.01	0.02	**0.1**	*149*
Oesophagus	179	0	-	-	-	-	-	-	0.2	-	0.2	0.2	2.4	5.5	5.7	6.8	13.0	9.8	14.9	16.4	2.4	0.5	0.07	0.17	**1.3**	*150*
Stomach	521	0	-	-	-	0.2	-	-	0.5	0.2	0.9	1.6	3.3	6.6	13.3	22.9	31.1	44.7	52.0	55.5	7.0	1.5	0.13	0.40	**3.5**	*151*
Small intestine	101	0	-	-	-	-	-	0.3	0.2	0.2	0.6	1.4	0.8	3.2	1.4	5.4	6.5	5.8	4.7	8.6	1.4	0.3	0.04	0.10	**0.8**	*152*
Colon	3037	0	-	-	-	0.4	-	0.6	2.9	3.4	8.3	17.7	27.6	44.7	69.9	104.0	175.9	248.7	305.2	361.6	40.6	8.7	0.88	2.28	**20.5**	*153*
Rectum	1254	0	-	-	-	0.2	-	0.2	0.9	2.0	3.0	8.2	22.5	28.0	41.5	58.0	68.4	82.6	93.2	94.5	16.8	3.6	0.53	1.16	**9.7**	*154*
Liver	176	0	-	-	-	0.2	0.8	-	0.5	0.2	-	1.6	1.9	3.2	5.7	6.5	10.3	10.7	16.9	14.8	2.4	0.5	0.07	0.15	**1.3**	*155*
Gallbladder etc.	304	0	-	-	-	-	-	-	-	0.3	0.7	1.4	2.2	5.2	8.1	11.9	16.8	23.2	30.4	37.5	4.1	0.9	0.09	0.23	**2.1**	*156*
Pancreas	851	0	-	-	-	0.2	-	0.2	0.3	1.0	0.6	2.7	7.9	12.7	24.7	33.6	58.5	66.1	79.0	83.6	11.4	2.4	0.25	0.71	**5.8**	*157*
Nose, sinuses etc.	46	0	-	-	-	-	0.2	0.3	-	0.5	0.2	0.5	1.1	0.6	0.8	1.7	1.7	3.6	2.7	3.9	0.6	0.1	0.02	0.04	**0.4**	*160*
Larynx	173	0	-	-	-	-	-	0.3	0.2	0.3	0.2	2.7	4.3	7.5	8.9	6.5	9.9	8.5	2.7	3.9	2.3	0.5	0.12	0.20	**1.6**	*161*
Bronchus, lung	4772	0	-	-	-	0.2	0.4	1.0	0.6	4.7	13.9	44.1	90.5	151.9	196.0	249.6	275.8	275.1	243.7	165.6	63.9	13.7	2.52	5.14	**40.2**	*162*
Other thoracic organs	19	0	0.4	-	-	0.2	-	-	0.3	-	-	0.2	0.5	0.6	0.8	0.3	0.7	0.4	1.4	-	0.3	0.1	0.02	0.02	**0.2**	*163-4*
Bone	57	0	0.4	1.3	0.7	0.4	1.0	0.2	0.5	0.5	0.6	0.9	0.3	0.6	1.1	0.8	0.3	3.1	2.0	3.1	0.8	0.2	0.04	0.05	**0.7**	*170*
Connective tissue	173	0	2.0	0.2	0.4	0.9	0.8	1.3	1.2	0.8	1.3	1.4	1.9	3.2	4.9	4.5	5.5	10.7	12.8	5.5	2.3	0.5	0.10	0.15	**1.7**	*171*
Mesothelioma	30	0	-	-	-	0.2	-	-	0.3	0.2	-	0.5	-	0.6	1.4	1.1	1.7	0.4	4.1	0.8	0.4	0.1	0.02	0.03	**0.2**	*MES*
Kaposi's sarcoma	17	0	-	-	-	-	-	-	-	0.5	-	0.2	-	-	-	-	1.0	0.9	0.7	5.5	0.2	0.0	0.00	0.01	**0.1**	*KAP*
Melanoma of skin	727	0	-	0.2	0.4	1.1	3.5	6.1	11.3	11.3	11.3	15.7	13.6	19.0	19.5	17.5	16.1	19.2	15.5	21.9	9.7	2.1	0.56	0.73	**7.3**	*172*
†Other skin	76	0	-	-	0.2	-	-	1.4	1.4	0.8	0.7	0.7	0.8	2.0	1.4	1.1	1.7	2.2	4.1	7.8	1.0		0.05	0.06	**0.7**	*173*
Breast	10265	0	-	-	-	-	0.8	6.7	27.3	57.9	125.8	192.6	222.3	277.6	354.0	408.5	463.3	481.8	449.6	417.1	137.4	29.5	6.32	10.68	**91.9**	*174*
Uterus unspecified	29	0	-	-	-	-	-	-	0.2	0.2	0.7	0.8	0.3	0.3	1.1	1.4	1.8	1.4	3.9	0.4	0.1	0.01	0.02	**0.2**	*179*
Cervix uteri	781	0	-	-	-	0.9	2.5	8.2	11.9	14.8	16.1	17.7	17.3	13.8	17.9	15.5	18.1	20.5	14.2	21.9	10.5	2.2	0.61	0.77	**7.9**	*180*
Placenta	5	0	-	-	-	-	-	0.2	0.6	-	-	-	-	-	-	-	-	-	-	-	0.1	0.0	0.00	0.00	**0.0**	*181*
Corpus uteri	2217	0	-	-	-	0.2	-	1.0	2.7	6.9	16.8	25.0	49.3	61.1	95.7	113.4	121.1	102.7	89.8	66.4	29.7	6.4	1.29	2.47	**19.6**	*182*
Ovary etc.	1392	0	-	-	0.2	1.3	1.7	3.4	3.8	9.6	12.9	21.1	29.0	35.7	46.3	60.5	63.0	61.6	60.8	64.0	18.6	4.0	0.83	1.44	**12.4**	*183*
Other female genital	288	0	0.2	-	-	0.2	0.2	0.8	0.8	0.8	1.9	1.8	2.3	3.8	5.5	7.0	9.3	15.7	17.4	21.6	27.3	3.9	0.8	0.12	0.25	**2.2**	*184*
Bladder	967	0	-	-	-	-	0.8	0.3	1.2	0.8	2.2	5.2	11.7	17.3	29.5	44.7	60.9	56.7	79.0	94.5	12.9	2.8	0.35	0.87	**7.1**	*188*
Kidney etc.	736	0	2.2	0.9	0.4	-	0.2	0.3	0.8	1.7	3.3	7.3	13.6	20.5	30.6	26.6	38.7	46.0	37.8	39.8	9.8	2.1	0.41	0.73	**6.4**	*189*
Eye	46	0	1.0	-	-	-	-	0.2	0.3	0.2	0.7	0.2	0.5	1.7	1.4	1.1	2.1	1.8	1.4	2.3	0.6	0.1	0.03	0.05	**0.5**	*190*
Brain, nervous system	488	0	4.3	2.8	2.0	3.1	1.9	2.4	2.9	2.0	4.3	4.8	7.6	8.9	11.7	16.4	21.6	24.6	23.6	14.1	6.5	1.4	0.29	0.48	**5.0**	*191-2*
Thyroid	634	0	-	-	0.9	2.9	6.2	8.2	12.2	11.0	11.3	12.9	8.7	14.7	11.9	14.7	13.3	9.4	12.8	9.4	8.5	1.8	0.50	0.64	**6.7**	*193*
Other endocrine	35	0	1.0	0.2	0.2	-	-	-	-	0.2	0.2	0.9	-	0.3	1.9	1.7	1.7	0.9	0.7	-	0.5	0.1	0.02	0.04	**0.4**	*194*
Hodgkin's disease	227	0	-	0.2	1.6	7.0	6.4	6.4	3.6	5.4	1.8	1.6	1.4	1.2	1.9	2.8	2.4	1.3	2.0	1.6	3.0	0.7	0.19	0.22	**2.9**	*201*
Non-Hodgkin lymphoma	1275	0	0.4	0.2	1.1	0.9	1.5	2.4	3.9	4.2	8.3	13.4	18.4	28.0	38.2	50.3	65.4	87.5	72.9	82.8	17.1	3.7	0.61	1.18	**10.4**	*200,202*
Multiple myeloma	391	0	-	-	-	-	-	-	-	0.5	0.9	1.8	4.9	5.8	10.3	15.8	22.9	29.0	43.2	36.7	5.2	1.1	0.12	0.31	**2.7**	*203*
Lymphoid leukaemia	380	0	5.5	1.9	1.1	0.7	0.6	0.3	0.3	0.3	1.8	1.6	3.3	5.2	9.8	15.0	16.4	24.6	29.7	34.4	5.1	1.1	0.16	0.32	**3.4**	*204*
Myeloid leukaemia	398	0	0.8	0.4	0.2	2.2	0.6	1.1	1.4	2.4	3.3	3.0	4.6	7.8	8.7	13.0	19.8	21.4	31.1	33.6	5.3	1.1	0.18	0.35	**3.3**	*205*
Monocytic leukaemia	17	0	-	-	-	-	-	-	0.2	-	-	0.5	0.8	0.3	0.3	1.4	0.3	0.4	0.7	0.8	0.2	0.0	0.01	0.02	**0.2**	*206*
Other leukaemia	13	0	-	-	-	-	-	-	-	-	-	0.2	-	0.3	0.8	1.1	-	0.4	2.0	-	0.2	0.0	0.01	0.01	**0.1**	*207*
Leukaemia unspecified	95	0	0.4	-	-	0.2	-	-	0.2	0.2	1.1	0.2	1.4	1.2	0.8	4.0	6.5	4.0	8.8	12.5	1.3	0.3	0.03	0.08	**0.7**	*208*
Other and unspecified	1056	0	0.8	-	-	-	0.4	0.3	1.2	1.5	3.7	5.5	8.7	15.3	26.6	33.1	56.8	75.5	113.4	143.7	14.1	3.0	0.32	0.77	**7.1**	*O&U*
All sites	34825	0	19.7	8.3	9.6	24.3	30.9	55.1	96.8	150.5	262.5	424.2	601.5	834.8	1132.7	1408.1	1737.0	1911.1	2011.8	2030.9	466.0		18.25	33.98	**294.2**	*ALL*
All sites but 173	34749	0	19.7	8.3	9.3	24.3	30.9	53.7	95.4	149.6	261.7	423.5	600.7	832.7	1131.3	1407.0	1735.3	1908.8	2007.8	2023.0	465.0	100.0	18.21	33.92	**293.6**	*ALLb*

Rate from 1 case   0.203 0.214 0.222 0.219 0.193 0.161 0.151 0.169 0.185 0.227 0.271 0.288 0.271 0.283 0.342 0.447 0.675 0.781

†Important: see notes on population page

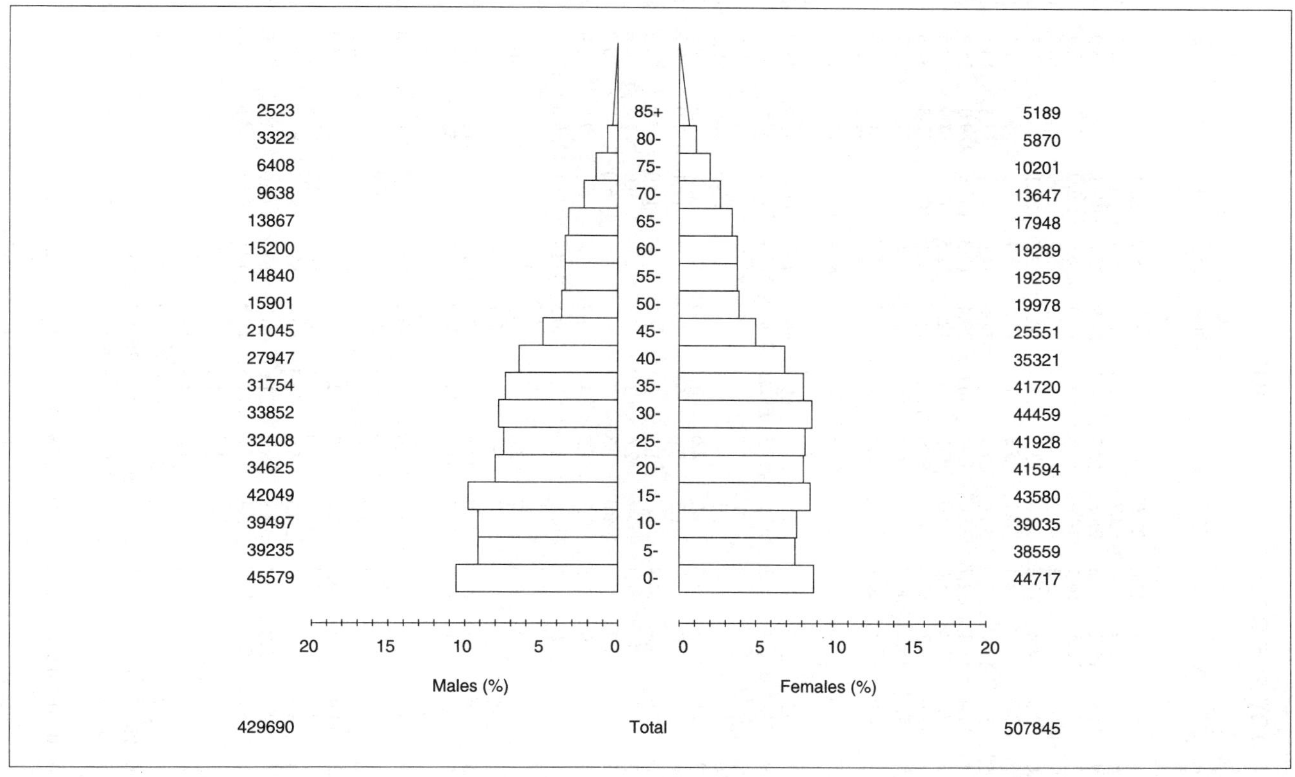

USA, Michigan, Detroit: Black
Source of population: average annual 1988-92
Estimate: NCI estimates based on U.S. Bureau of Census population estimates by county for the years 1988–92.
Notes to tables overleaf:
† 173 does not include basal cell or squamous cell carcinoma

Note: There was an error in the population data for Blacks in Volume VI and this results in artificial large increases in the incidence data published in this volume.

USA, MICHIGAN, DETROIT: BLACK 1988-1992

ANNUAL INCIDENCE PER 100,000 BY AGE GROUP (YEARS) - MALE

SITE	ALL AGES	AGE UNK	0-	5-	10-	15-	20-	25-	30-	35-	40-	45-	50-	55-	60-	65-	70-	75-	80-	85+	CRUDE RATE	%	CR 64	CR 74	ASR (W)	ICD (9th)
Lip	0	0	-	-	-	-	-	-	-	-	-	-	-	-	-	-	-	-	-	-	0.0	0.0	0.00	0.00	**0.0**	140
Tongue	100	0	-	-	-	-	-	-	1.3	8.6	9.5	22.6	27.0	9.2	14.4	18.7	18.7	30.1	7.9	4.7	1.0	0.39	0.56	**4.9**	141
Salivary gland	16	0	-	-	0.5	0.5	-	0.6	-	0.6	1.4	1.0	-	2.7	2.6	1.4	2.1	9.4	-	-	0.7	0.2	0.05	0.07	**0.7**	142
Mouth	126	0	-	-	-	-	-	-	0.6	1.9	11.4	16.2	22.6	25.6	19.7	20.2	24.9	25.0	18.1	-	5.9	1.2	0.49	0.72	**6.2**	143-5
Oropharynx	72	0	-	-	-	-	-	-	-	1.3	7.2	10.5	16.4	14.8	11.8	10.1	10.4	6.2	6.0	7.9	3.4	0.7	0.31	0.41	**3.7**	146
Nasopharynx	11	0	-	-	-	-	-	-	1.2	-	-	1.0	2.5	1.3	-	1.4	4.2	6.2	-	-	0.5	0.1	0.03	0.06	**0.5**	147
Hypopharynx	70	0	-	-	-	-	-	-	0.6	0.6	2.9	4.8	17.6	14.8	13.2	15.9	10.4	12.5	24.1	-	3.3	0.7	0.27	0.40	**3.5**	148
Pharynx unspecified	23	0	-	-	-	-	-	-	0.6	0.7	1.0	2.5	8.1	5.3	1.4	12.5	3.1	-	-	-	1.1	0.2	0.09	0.16	**1.1**	149
Oesophagus	288	0	-	-	-	-	-	0.6	2.5	5.0	18.1	39.0	56.6	67.1	77.9	72.6	74.9	78.2	55.5	13.4	2.7	0.94	1.70	**13.7**	150
Stomach	338	0	-	-	-	-	0.6	-	3.0	4.4	11.4	11.4	32.7	35.0	43.4	96.6	120.4	112.3	132.4	229.8	15.7	3.2	0.71	1.79	**14.9**	151
Small intestine	54	0	-	-	-	-	-	-	0.6	1.3	2.1	3.8	5.0	4.0	10.5	21.6	12.5	12.5	18.1	7.9	2.5	0.5	0.14	0.31	**2.5**	152
Colon	806	0	-	-	0.5	-	-	0.6	1.8	10.7	18.6	25.7	52.8	88.9	156.6	191.8	273.9	358.9	463.5	372.5	37.5	7.7	1.78	4.11	**35.0**	153
Rectum	294	0	-	-	-	-	-	1.2	1.8	5.0	7.2	15.2	30.2	40.4	56.6	88.0	78.9	99.9	102.3	79.3	13.7	2.8	0.79	1.62	**13.4**	154
Liver	147	0	0.9	-	-	0.5	-	-	0.6	1.3	3.6	15.2	16.4	22.9	31.6	37.5	35.3	31.2	54.2	31.7	6.8	1.4	0.46	0.83	**7.0**	155
Gallbladder etc.	31	0	-	-	-	-	-	-	-	-	2.9	-	-	-	5.3	10.1	4.2	15.6	36.1	23.8	1.4	0.3	0.04	0.11	**1.2**	156
Pancreas	287	0	-	-	-	-	-	-	1.8	2.5	5.0	12.4	23.9	43.1	55.3	90.9	87.2	87.4	120.4	111.0	13.4	2.7	0.72	1.61	**12.9**	157
Nose, sinuses etc.	8	0	-	-	-	-	-	-	0.6	-	-	-	1.3	-	2.6	2.9	-	6.2	-	-	0.4	0.1	0.02	0.04	**0.4**	160
Larynx	256	0	-	-	-	-	-	-	-	1.3	9.3	23.8	30.2	45.8	65.8	69.2	60.2	49.9	66.2	31.7	11.9	2.4	0.88	1.53	**12.3**	161
Bronchus, lung	2263	0	-	-	-	-	-	-	1.8	18.9	44.4	116.9	186.1	362.5	467.1	692.3	794.8	727.1	710.2	467.6	105.3	21.5	5.99	13.42	**103.2**	162
Other thoracic organs	8	0	-	-	0.5	-	0.6	-	1.2	-	0.7	-	2.5	-	1.3	-	-	-	-	-	0.4	0.1	0.03	0.03	**0.4**	163-4
Bone	12	0	-	0.5	0.5	1.9	0.6	-	-	0.6	1.4	-	-	1.3	-	1.4	-	-	-	-	0.6	0.1	0.03	0.04	**0.5**	170
Connective tissue	47	0	0.4	1.0	1.5	2.9	1.2	0.6	1.8	1.9	2.9	1.9	2.5	4.0	2.6	4.3	8.3	15.6	-	7.9	2.2	0.4	0.13	0.19	**2.1**	171
Mesothelioma	14	0	-	-	-	-	-	-	-	0.6	-	1.0	-	1.3	2.6	5.8	2.1	-	18.1	7.9	0.7	0.1	0.03	0.07	**0.6**	MES
Kaposi's sarcoma	77	0	-	-	-	-	1.2	11.1	14.8	5.0	7.9	3.8	3.8	-	1.3	1.4	2.1	-	12.0	7.9	3.6	0.7	0.24	0.26	**3.3**	KAP
Melanoma of skin	13	0	-	-	-	-	-	0.6	0.6	1.3	0.7	-	1.3	-	2.6	2.9	4.2	-	6.0	-	0.6	0.1	0.04	0.07	**0.6**	172
†Other skin	19	0	-	-	0.5	-	-	1.2	3.1	-	2.9	1.3	4.0	1.3	2.9	-	-	6.0	-	-	0.9	-	0.07	0.09	**0.9**	173
Breast	19	0	-	-	-	-	-	-	-	2.1	1.9	2.5	2.7	1.3	4.3	4.2	9.4	-	7.9	-	0.9	0.2	0.05	0.10	**0.9**	175
Prostate	3397	0	-	-	-	-	1.2	-	-	5.0	8.6	93.1	270.9	598.7	1104.7	1560.5	1838.2	1944.1	1735.6	158.1	32.3	4.89	18.21	**141.5**	185
Testis	15	0	0.4	-	-	0.5	1.2	1.2	2.4	1.3	-	-	1.3	-	1.4	2.1	-	-	-	-	0.7	0.1	0.04	0.06	**0.7**	186
Penis	13	0	-	-	-	-	-	-	-	-	-	1.0	1.3	2.7	2.6	4.3	-	3.1	18.1	-	0.6	0.1	0.04	0.06	**0.6**	187.1-.4
Other male genital	3	0	-	0.5	-	-	-	-	-	-	-	-	-	-	1.3	-	-	2.1	-	-	0.1	0.0	0.01	0.02	**0.1**	187.5-.9
Bladder	273	0	-	0.5	-	-	-	0.6	3.0	2.5	3.6	9.5	20.1	29.6	47.4	67.8	62.3	171.6	162.5	111.0	12.7	2.6	0.58	1.23	**11.7**	188
Kidney etc.	263	0	1.8	-	-	-	0.6	-	2.4	1.9	7.9	17.1	34.0	37.7	51.3	59.1	74.7	96.7	78.2	55.5	12.2	2.5	0.77	1.44	**12.2**	189
Eye	5	0	1.3	-	-	-	-	-	-	-	0.7	-	-	-	1.4	-	-	-	-	-	0.2	0.0	0.01	0.02	**0.2**	190
Brain, nervous system	85	0	3.5	2.5	2.0	1.9	0.6	1.9	3.0	1.9	5.7	7.6	3.8	5.4	7.9	7.2	10.4	28.1	24.1	-	4.0	0.8	0.24	0.33	**3.9**	191-2
Thyroid	36	0	-	-	-	-	2.3	0.6	2.4	1.9	0.7	1.9	3.8	5.4	6.6	4.3	4.2	6.2	12.0	-	1.7	0.3	0.13	0.17	**1.6**	193
Other endocrine	6	0	0.9	-	-	-	-	0.6	-	0.6	-	-	-	-	2.7	-	-	-	-	-	0.3	0.1	0.02	0.02	**0.3**	194
Hodgkin's disease	65	0	-	1.5	1.0	3.8	1.7	6.8	7.1	6.3	1.4	2.9	3.8	2.7	5.3	2.9	-	-	-	-	3.0	0.6	0.22	0.24	**2.9**	201
Non-Hodgkin lymphoma	286	0	-	0.5	1.0	1.4	3.5	8.0	11.2	21.4	13.6	24.7	21.4	41.8	31.6	36.1	56.0	59.3	72.2	63.4	13.3	2.7	0.90	1.36	**12.9**	200,202
Multiple myeloma	195	0	-	-	-	-	-	-	-	4.4	3.6	8.6	15.1	24.3	36.8	50.5	80.9	53.1	84.3	87.2	9.1	1.9	0.46	1.12	**8.7**	203
Lymphoid leukaemia	82	0	0.9	2.5	2.5	1.4	-	0.6	0.6	1.3	0.7	3.8	6.3	14.8	9.2	21.6	18.7	15.6	12.0	31.7	3.8	0.8	0.22	0.43	**3.8**	204
Myeloid leukaemia	100	0	0.9	1.5	-	-	0.6	1.9	0.6	0.6	3.6	5.7	11.3	5.4	15.8	17.3	35.3	40.6	48.2	23.8	4.7	1.0	0.24	0.50	**4.5**	205
Monocytic leukaemia	6	0	-	0.5	-	-	-	-	-	-	-	-	-	1.3	1.3	1.4	-	6.2	-	-	0.3	0.1	0.02	0.02	**0.3**	206
Other leukaemia	10	0	-	0.5	-	-	-	-	0.6	-	-	-	-	-	5.3	1.4	-	6.2	-	7.9	0.5	0.1	0.03	0.04	**0.4**	207
Leukaemia unspecified	15	0	-	-	-	-	-	0.6	-	0.6	-	-	-	-	1.3	4.3	16.6	3.1	-	-	0.7	0.1	0.01	0.12	**0.6**	208
Other and unspecified	271	0	1.3	-	-	-	-	1.2	1.8	3.1	5.7	14.3	16.4	31.0	53.9	60.6	87.2	103.0	102.3	190.2	12.6	2.6	0.64	1.38	**12.0**	O&U
All sites	10525	0	12.3	12.2	10.1	15.2	14.4	40.1	69.1	114.6	209.7	402.9	747.1	1284.4	1911.8	2913.2	3654.2	4113.2	4460.1	3764.5	489.9		24.22	57.06	**465.1**	ALL
All sites but 173	10506	0	12.3	12.2	9.6	15.2	14.4	40.1	67.9	111.5	209.7	400.1	745.8	1280.3	1910.5	2910.3	3654.2	4113.2	4454.1	3764.5	489.0	100.0	24.15	56.97	**464.2**	ALLb

Rate from 1 case   0.439   0.510   0.506   0.476   0.578   0.617   0.591   0.630   0.716   0.950   1.258   1.348   1.316   1.442   2.075   3.121   6.019   7.925

†Important: see notes on population page

USA, MICHIGAN, DETROIT: BLACK 1988-1992

ANNUAL INCIDENCE PER 100,000 BY AGE GROUP (YEARS) - FEMALE

SITE	ALL AGES	AGE UNK	0-	5-	10-	15-	20-	25-	30-	35-	40-	45-	50-	55-	60-	65-	70-	75-	80-	85+	CRUDE RATE	%	CR 64	CR 74	ASR (W)	ICD (9th)
Lip	2	0	-	-	-	-	-	-	0.4	-	-	-	-	-	-	1.1	-	-	-	-	0.1	0.0	0.00	0.01	**0.1**	*140*
Tongue	30	0	0.4	-	-	-	-	-	0.4	0.5	0.6	3.9	5.0	4.2	4.1	6.7	-	3.9	-	-	1.2	0.4	0.10	0.13	**1.2**	*141*
Salivary gland	14	0	-	-	-	-	-	-	0.4	-	2.3	-	1.0	1.0	1.0	1.1	2.9	-	10.2	-	0.6	0.2	0.03	0.05	**0.4**	*142*
Mouth	61	0	-	-	-	-	0.5	0.5	0.4	1.0	1.7	5.5	6.0	7.3	8.3	13.4	7.3	7.8	3.4	11.6	2.4	0.7	0.16	0.26	**2.2**	*143-5*
Oropharynx	27	0	-	-	-	-	-	-	-	-	1.7	0.8	2.0	7.3	2.1	6.7	5.9	2.0	-	3.9	1.1	0.3	0.07	0.13	**1.0**	*146*
Nasopharynx	5	0	-	-	-	-	-	-	0.4	0.5	0.6	-	-	1.0	1.0	-	-	-	-	-	0.2	0.1	0.02	0.02	**0.2**	*147*
Hypopharynx	8	0	-	-	-	-	-	-	-	-	0.8	1.0	2.1	2.1	1.1	1.5	-	-	-	-	0.3	0.1	0.03	0.04	**0.3**	*148*
Pharynx unspecified	6	0	-	-	-	-	-	-	-	-	0.8	2.0	-	1.0	1.1	1.5	-	-	-	-	0.2	0.1	0.02	0.03	**0.3**	*149*
Oesophagus	102	0	-	-	-	-	-	-	-	-	1.1	5.5	7.0	19.7	14.5	18.9	23.4	21.6	13.6	19.3	4.0	1.2	0.24	0.45	**3.5**	*150*
Stomach	195	0	-	-	-	0.9	-	0.5	0.4	2.9	2.3	3.9	10.0	6.2	22.8	23.4	49.8	70.6	92.0	77.1	7.7	2.3	0.25	0.62	**5.6**	*151*
Small intestine	41	0	-	-	-	-	-	-	-	-	1.1	-	3.0	4.2	4.1	6.7	10.3	9.8	20.4	15.4	1.6	0.5	0.06	0.15	**1.2**	*152*
Colon	899	0	-	-	-	-	0.5	1.4	4.5	7.2	13.6	18.8	42.0	73.7	131.7	171.6	221.3	245.1	282.8	265.9	35.4	10.8	1.47	3.43	**27.9**	*153*
Rectum	273	0	-	-	-	-	-	-	0.9	2.4	2.3	9.4	16.0	32.2	34.2	50.1	71.8	62.7	78.4	80.9	10.8	3.3	0.49	1.10	**8.7**	*154*
Liver	74	0	0.9	-	-	-	-	-	-	-	1.7	3.9	5.0	5.2	10.4	11.1	13.2	19.6	30.7	23.1	2.9	0.9	0.14	0.26	**2.4**	*155*
Gallbladder etc.	57	0	-	-	-	-	-	-	0.4	-	0.6	-	4.0	3.1	8.3	11.1	17.6	9.8	23.8	23.1	2.2	0.7	0.08	0.23	**1.7**	*156*
Pancreas	303	0	-	0.5	-	-	-	-	0.9	2.4	2.8	10.2	6.0	26.0	40.4	61.3	71.8	84.3	112.4	104.1	11.9	3.6	0.45	1.11	**9.2**	*157*
Nose, sinuses etc.	21	0	0.4	-	0.5	0.5	0.5	-	-	-	0.8	2.1	2.1	1.1	1.5	1.5	9.8	3.4	-	-	0.8	0.3	0.05	0.07	**0.8**	*160*
Larynx	75	0	-	-	-	-	-	-	-	1.0	2.3	3.1	15.0	11.4	12.4	14.5	11.7	2.0	10.2	7.7	3.0	0.9	0.23	0.36	**2.9**	*161*
Bronchus, lung	1213	0	-	-	-	0.5	-	1.0	4.5	7.2	15.9	48.5	109.1	146.4	212.6	263.0	282.8	229.4	197.6	138.7	47.8	14.6	2.73	5.46	**42.0**	*162*
Other thoracic organs	4	0	-	-	-	-	-	-	0.4	-	-	0.8	1.0	-	-	-	1.5	-	-	-	0.2	0.0	0.01	0.02	**0.2**	*163-4*
Bone	17	0	-	0.5	1.0	0.5	1.0	0.5	-	0.5	0.6	2.3	-	1.0	2.1	-	2.9	-	-	-	0.7	0.2	0.05	0.06	**0.7**	*170*
Connective tissue	44	0	1.3	-	-	0.9	1.9	1.4	0.4	1.0	2.3	3.1	-	3.1	1.0	2.2	5.9	3.9	20.4	11.6	1.7	0.5	0.08	0.12	**1.5**	*171*
Mesothelioma	6	0	-	-	-	-	-	-	-	-	1.6	1.0	1.0	-	2.2	-	-	-	-	-	0.2	0.1	0.02	0.03	**0.3**	*MES*
Kaposi's sarcoma	10	0	-	-	-	-	-	1.0	0.9	1.0	-	0.8	-	-	2.2	-	-	3.4	-	-	0.4	0.1	0.02	0.03	**0.3**	*KAP*
Melanoma of skin	11	0	-	-	-	-	0.5	-	-	-	-	-	1.0	1.0	1.0	-	1.5	3.9	10.2	3.9	0.4	0.1	0.02	0.03	**0.3**	*172*
†Other skin	26	0	0.4	-	0.5	0.5	0.5	0.5	0.4	2.4	2.8	3.1	-	1.0	1.0	1.1	2.9	2.0	-	-	1.0		0.07	0.09	**0.9**	*173*
Breast	2328	0	-	-	-	0.5	1.4	10.0	30.6	63.3	134.8	183.2	199.2	253.4	265.4	328.7	366.4	352.9	402.0	343.0	91.7	27.9	5.71	9.18	**80.8**	*174*
Uterus unspecified	12	0	-	-	-	-	-	-	-	-	1.1	-	-	-	4.1	1.1	-	2.0	6.8	7.7	0.5	0.1	0.03	0.03	**0.4**	*179*
Cervix uteri	369	0	-	-	-	1.4	2.9	6.2	13.5	21.6	19.3	25.8	26.0	37.4	39.4	37.9	23.4	52.9	54.5	46.2	14.5	4.4	0.97	1.27	**12.7**	*180*
Placenta	3	0	-	-	-	-	-	1.0	0.4	-	-	-	-	-	-	-	-	-	-	-	0.1	0.0	0.01	0.01	**0.1**	*181*
Corpus uteri	350	0	-	-	-	0.5	-	0.5	3.1	6.7	6.2	11.0	16.0	31.2	76.7	64.6	71.8	76.5	54.5	77.1	13.8	4.2	0.76	1.44	**11.6**	*182*
Ovary etc.	243	0	-	-	2.6	1.8	-	2.9	2.7	5.8	7.4	11.7	15.0	18.7	18.7	53.5	38.1	45.1	68.1	54.0	9.6	2.9	0.44	0.89	**8.0**	*183*
Other female genital	64	0	0.4	-	-	-	0.5	1.4	0.4	1.4	2.8	3.9	5.0	2.1	4.1	7.8	8.8	15.7	27.3	19.3	2.5	0.8	0.11	0.19	**2.0**	*184*
Bladder	150	0	-	-	-	-	0.5	-	0.4	0.5	1.7	3.9	4.0	10.4	13.5	26.7	26.4	56.9	71.5	77.1	5.9	1.8	0.17	0.44	**4.2**	*188*
Kidney etc.	180	0	2.7	0.5	-	-	-	0.5	1.3	1.4	9.6	7.8	15.0	20.8	18.7	25.6	39.6	39.2	37.5	19.3	7.1	2.2	0.39	0.72	**6.2**	*189*
Eye	5	0	1.3	0.5	-	-	0.5	-	-	-	-	-	-	-	-	1.0	-	-	-	-	0.2	0.1	0.01	0.01	**0.3**	*190*
Brain, nervous system	93	0	5.8	5.2	1.5	1.4	1.9	2.4	0.9	2.4	4.0	4.7	2.0	6.2	7.3	5.6	10.3	13.7	-	3.9	3.7	1.1	0.23	0.31	**3.7**	*191-2*
Thyroid	96	0	-	-	-	0.9	2.4	1.0	4.5	4.8	6.2	9.4	3.0	2.1	10.4	14.5	10.3	7.8	3.4	15.4	3.8	1.2	0.22	0.35	**3.3**	*193*
Other endocrine	11	0	1.3	-	-	-	0.5	-	0.9	0.5	-	0.8	-	-	1.0	1.1	-	2.0	-	-	0.4	0.1	0.03	0.03	**0.4**	*194*
Hodgkin's disease	51	0	-	-	1.5	3.2	2.4	2.9	1.8	1.4	3.4	3.9	2.0	1.0	5.2	1.1	2.9	2.0	-	-	2.0	0.6	0.14	0.16	**1.9**	*201*
Non-Hodgkin lymphoma	195	0	0.9	-	-	-	4.3	1.4	2.2	6.2	7.9	7.0	13.0	13.5	31.1	25.6	46.9	31.4	23.8	23.1	7.7	2.3	0.44	0.80	**6.7**	*200,202*
Multiple myeloma	208	0	-	-	-	-	-	0.5	0.4	0.5	2.3	5.5	8.0	21.8	30.1	35.7	55.7	41.2	85.2	77.1	8.2	2.5	0.35	0.80	**6.4**	*203*
Lymphoid leukaemia	82	0	3.6	2.1	1.0	0.9	0.5	0.5	-	-	1.1	0.8	1.0	6.2	5.2	13.4	14.7	19.6	27.3	34.7	3.2	1.0	0.11	0.25	**2.7**	*204*
Myeloid leukaemia	87	0	0.9	-	-	0.5	1.0	0.5	0.4	1.9	4.0	5.5	9.0	2.1	3.1	17.8	11.7	17.6	23.8	30.8	3.4	1.0	0.14	0.29	**2.8**	*205*
Monocytic leukaemia	4	0	-	-	-	-	-	-	0.4	-	-	-	-	-	-	1.1	-	-	6.8	-	0.2	0.0	0.00	0.01	**0.1**	*206*
Other leukaemia	2	0	-	-	-	-	-	0.5	-	-	-	-	-	-	-	-	-	-	-	3.9	0.1	0.0	0.00	0.00	**0.1**	*207*
Leukaemia unspecified	18	0	-	-	-	-	-	0.5	-	1.0	1.1	-	1.0	2.1	1.0	-	2.9	3.9	3.4	15.4	0.7	0.2	0.03	0.05	**0.5**	*208*
Other and unspecified	287	0	0.4	-	0.5	0.5	1.4	0.5	0.9	3.8	7.4	11.0	14.0	26.0	28.0	45.7	39.6	84.3	115.8	123.3	11.3	3.4	0.47	0.90	**8.7**	*O&U*
All sites	8362	0	21.0	9.3	9.2	15.1	25.5	39.6	81.4	152.9	276.3	423.5	574.6	815.2	1081.4	1379.5	1578.3	1652.7	1924.8	1757.4	329.3		17.63	32.42	**279.4**	*ALL*
All sites but 173	8336	0	20.6	9.3	8.7	14.7	25.0	39.1	81.0	150.5	273.5	420.3	574.6	814.1	1080.4	1378.4	1575.4	1650.7	1924.8	1757.4	328.3	100.0	17.56	32.33	**278.4**	*ALLb*

Rate from 1 case   0.447   0.519   0.512   0.459   0.481   0.477   0.450   0.479   0.566   0.783   1.001   1.038   1.037   1.114   1.466   1.960   3.407   3.854

†Important: see notes on population page

USA, New Mexico

The New Mexico Tumour registry, located at the University of New Mexico Cancer Research and Treatment Center in Albuquerque, began its operation in 1967 and expanded state-wide in 1969. Cancer reporting has been required (but not enforced) by a State Health Agency regulation since 1922. The registry became the official repository for cancer data for the State Health Agency in 1975. Funding for the registry initially came from the New Mexico Regional Medical Program and since 1973 primarily from the National Cancer Institute's Surveillance, Epidemiology and End results (SEER) Program.

In area, New Mexico is the fifth largest state in the USA. Its population is about 1.5 million, of whom approximately one third live in the Albuquerque metropolitan area; the remainder live in cities with fewer than 100 000 inhabitants or in villages. Located in the south-west of the country (latitude 30°10′ to 37° N), it has extensive high desert and mountain terrain, the altitude ranging from 859 to 4010 m above sea level. Rainfall and humidity are low.

The people of New Mexico come from diverse ethnic backgrounds: 38% have Spanish and/or Mexican-American heritage (Hispanics); 9% are American Indians (Navajo, Pueblo, Apache); 2% are Black, less than 1% are Asian; the remaining 50% are non-Hispanic white, of European descent. A sizeable subgroup of New Mexico's Hispanic population lives in small mountain communities in the northern part of the state and traces its ancestry to Spanish soldiers and colonists who settled in New Mexico during the 17th and 18th centuries. Their genetic make-up, habits, diet, etc. differ greatly from those of the Hispanic persons in southern New Mexico, who are of recent Mexican descent.

Median levels of education and per capita income are in the lowest decile of the 50 states.

The registry abstracts and follows all cases of known malignancy. Multiple primary tumours are counted separately, by assigning cancer sequence numbers within the records of individual patients. Patients entered into the registry system are followed for life. Direct contact with patients is permitted only with the physician's consent.

Some of the larger hospitals employ tumour registrars, and abstractors from the central registry travel to the other hospitals and clinics throughout the state to review and abstract cancer patient records. The majority of the registry's cases are registered from hospital admission and out-patient records. Regular visits to all New Mexico non-hospital diagnostic or treatment centres provide additional cases. Within hospitals, pathology reports and all available billing and diagnostic indices are reviewed to assure complete coverage. Other methods of case-finding are used to obtain information on cancer cases not seen in reporting hospitals. Radiation therapy records and death certificates are reviewed regularly.

Data from the medical chart are entered directly onto diskettes via portable laptop computers using a software package assembled locally. This allows collection of supplemental data items of special interest to individual hospitals and physicians. It also allows each hospital to analyse its own 25+-year complete data-set and to compare it with a state-wide analytical data-set of individual records that have been stripped of personal identifiers.

The data from the abstractors' diskettes are edited, linked and merged into the master file that is maintained on a mini-computer in the central office.

Abstracted cases are reviewed for thoroughness and accuracy in the registry. The medical director of the registry, a pathologist, is consulted on problem cases. Diagnoses are coded to ICD-O (2nd edition). The file is ordered by computer-generated accession numbers, but can be sorted by any item of data. Numerous routine cross-checks are made to ensure that the file does not contain duplicate cases. Periodically, reports are sent to participating hospitals and individual physicians. Over 100 special requests for cancer data are also handled by the registry annually.

Descriptive epidemiological analyses have shown that the Hispanics and American Indians have lower rates than the non-Hispanic white population for skin, breast, endometrium, lung and colorectal cancers and higher rates for stomach, uterine cervix and gallbladder cancers.

The registry has been a case-finding source for a variety of population-based case–control studies relating to cancer etiology. It has also been used to monitor patterns of cancer care and survival in relation to factors such as ethnicity, age and marital status.

The development of new laboratory techniques for investigating molecular and cellular changes in preserved tissue specimens has created requests for the registry to help select cases from the file that have documentation of different clinical courses and outcomes.

The registry is conducting a large cohort study of underground uranium miners.

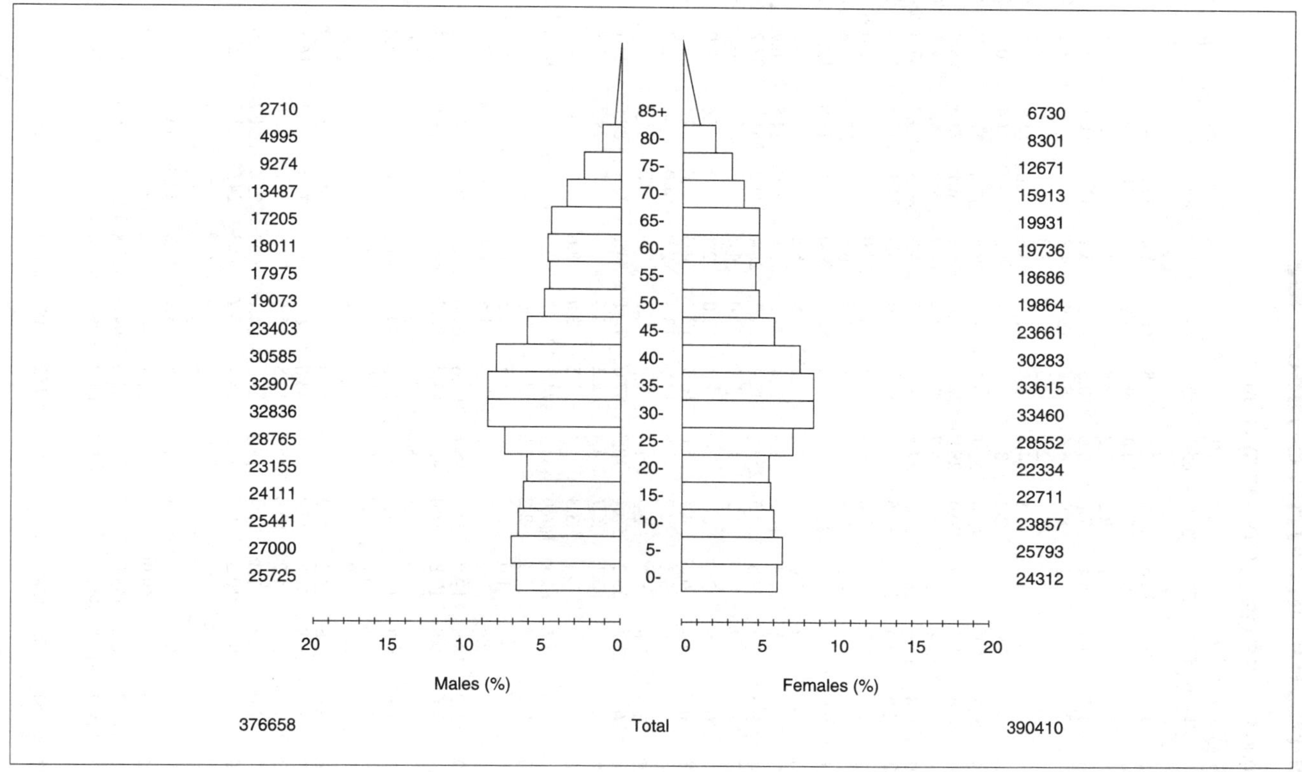

USA, New Mexico: Non-Hispanic White
Source of population: average annual 1988-92
Estimate: NCI estimates based on U.S. Bureau of Census population estimates by county for the years 1988–92.

Notes to tables overleaf:
† 173 does not include basal cell or squamous cell carcinoma

USA, NEW MEXICO: NON-HISPANIC WHITE 1988-1992

ANNUAL INCIDENCE PER 100,000 BY AGE GROUP (YEARS) - MALE

SITE	ALL AGES	AGE UNK	0-	5-	10-	15-	20-	25-	30-	35-	40-	45-	50-	55-	60-	65-	70-	75-	80-	85+	CRUDE RATE	%	CR 64	CR 74	ASR (W)	ICD (9th)
Lip	123	0	-	-	-	-	-	-	1.8	1.2	1.3	6.8	12.6	10.0	17.8	19.8	31.1	41.0	36.0	36.9	6.5	1.2	0.26	0.51	4.4	140
Tongue	60	0	-	-	-	-	0.9	0.7	-	2.4	3.9	6.0	9.4	7.8	4.4	9.3	8.9	6.5	12.0	7.4	3.2	0.6	0.18	0.27	2.4	141
Salivary gland	29	0	-	-	-	-	-	0.6	-	0.7	0.9	2.1	2.2	2.2	5.8	7.4	12.9	4.0	22.1		1.5	0.3	0.04	0.11	1.0	142
Mouth	63	0	-	-	-	-	-	-	0.6	1.3	0.9	8.4	7.8	10.0	10.5	13.3	15.1	32.0	14.8		3.3	0.6	0.14	0.26	2.3	143-5
Oropharynx	35	0	-	-	-	-	-	-	-	2.0	3.4	3.1	8.9	4.4	5.8	8.9	4.3	-	-		1.9	0.3	0.11	0.18	1.4	146
Nasopharynx	6	0	-	-	-	-	0.7	-	-	-	-	-	-	2.2	2.3	-	2.2	-	-		0.3	0.1	0.01	0.03	0.2	147
Hypopharynx	22	0	-	-	-	-	-	-	-	-	-	1.0	1.1	4.4	5.8	1.5	8.6	16.0	14.8		1.2	0.2	0.03	0.07	0.7	148
Pharynx unspecified	14	0	-	-	-	-	-	0.6	-	-	0.9	-	2.2	3.3	2.3	3.0	4.3	-	7.4		0.7	0.1	0.04	0.06	0.5	149
Oesophagus	108	0	-	-	-	-	-	-	0.6	0.7	2.6	10.5	13.4	21.1	15.1	28.2	38.8	32.0	29.5		5.7	1.0	0.24	0.46	3.8	150
Stomach	157	0	-	-	-	-	-	-	0.6	2.6	4.3	4.2	20.0	28.9	32.5	32.6	43.1	76.1	73.8		8.3	1.5	0.30	0.63	5.4	151
Small intestine	39	0	-	-	-	0.8	-	-	-	0.7	3.4	3.1	3.3	6.7	7.0	7.4	12.9	8.0	14.8		2.1	0.4	0.09	0.16	1.5	152
Colon	696	0	-	-	-	-	-	0.7	2.4	3.0	9.8	12.0	28.3	64.5	84.4	139.5	185.4	265.3	284.3	420.7	37.0	6.7	1.03	2.65	23.1	153
Rectum	325	0	-	-	-	-	-	0.6	1.2	4.6	6.0	22.0	35.6	52.2	61.6	83.0	103.5	124.1	147.6		17.3	3.1	0.61	1.33	11.3	154
Liver	68	0	-	-	-	-	-	-	0.6	-	1.3	1.7	1.0	7.8	6.7	13.9	16.3	28.0	24.0	51.7	3.6	0.7	0.10	0.25	2.3	155
Gallbladder etc.	31	0	-	-	-	-	-	-	-	-	-	-	4.2	3.3	1.1	9.3	4.4	6.5	24.0	22.1	1.6	0.3	0.04	0.11	1.1	156
Pancreas	240	0	-	-	-	-	-	-	-	1.8	2.0	4.3	9.4	28.9	41.1	52.3	68.2	69.0	96.1	73.8	12.7	2.3	0.44	1.04	8.2	157
Nose, sinuses etc.	15	0	-	-	-	-	-	-	0.6	-	0.9	1.0	2.2	1.1	2.3	5.9	6.5	-	-		0.8	0.1	0.03	0.07	0.5	160
Larynx	127	0	-	-	-	-	0.9	-	-	0.7	5.1	11.5	17.8	18.9	31.4	28.2	47.4	20.0	14.8		6.7	1.2	0.27	0.57	4.6	161
Bronchus, lung	1548	0	-	-	-	-	-	-	1.8	9.8	26.5	78.6	133.5	253.2	392.9	464.2	528.4	524.5	361.6		82.2	15.0	2.52	6.80	52.5	162
Other thoracic organs	13	0	-	-	-	0.8	0.9	-	0.6	1.2	-	0.9	-	1.1	1.1	1.2	3.0	4.3	-	-	0.7	0.1	0.03	0.05	0.5	163-4
Bone	18	0	-	0.7	0.8	0.8	3.5	0.7	-	-	0.7	0.9	2.1	-	-	2.3	3.0	2.2	-	7.4	1.0	0.2	0.05	0.08	0.9	170
Connective tissue	69	0	0.8	1.5	-	0.8	0.9	2.1	1.2	1.8	0.7	3.4	6.3	4.5	5.6	16.3	19.3	4.3	12.0	29.5	3.7	0.7	0.15	0.32	2.8	171
Mesothelioma	41	0	-	-	-	-	-	-	0.6	0.6	-	0.9	3.1	2.2	5.6	13.9	13.3	12.9	4.0	-	2.2	0.4	0.06	0.20	1.4	MES
Kaposi's sarcoma	67	0	-	-	-	-	-	9.0	9.1	11.5	3.9	2.6	5.2	2.2	1.1	1.2	-	-	4.0	7.4	3.6	0.6	0.22	0.23	2.8	KAP
Melanoma of skin	435	0	-	-	0.8	2.5	3.5	13.9	14.6	20.7	26.2	22.2	25.2	50.1	48.9	57.0	77.1	84.1	72.1	88.6	23.1	4.2	1.14	1.81	16.8	172
†Other skin	36	0	-	-	-	-	-	0.7	1.2	0.6	2.6	-	3.1	6.7	4.4	2.3	4.4	6.5	12.0	29.5	1.9		0.10	0.13	1.4	173
Breast	14	0	-	-	-	-	-	-	-	0.6	-	-	-	3.3	1.1	3.5	3.0	8.6	-	-	0.7	0.1	0.03	0.06	0.5	175
Prostate	3593	0	-	-	-	-	-	-	-	-	2.0	14.5	60.8	166.9	451.9	874.2	1370.2	1492.3	1593.6	1417.0	190.8	34.7	3.48	14.70	112.4	185
Testis	119	0	-	-	-	5.8	12.1	16.0	12.2	14.0	9.2	3.4	6.3	2.2	2.2	2.3	3.0	-	-	-	6.3	1.2	0.42	0.44	5.7	186
Penis	17	0	-	-	-	-	-	-	0.6	-	-	1.0	2.2	4.4	3.5	1.5	8.6	4.0	-		0.9	0.2	0.04	0.07	0.6	187.1-.4
Other male genital	6	0	-	-	-	-	-	-	-	-	0.9	-	-	-	-	1.5	6.5	-	-	7.4	0.3	0.1	0.00	0.01	0.2	187.5-.9
Bladder	705	0	-	-	-	-	-	-	2.4	4.9	5.2	18.8	19.9	54.5	84.4	168.6	204.6	243.7	316.3	324.7	37.4	6.8	0.95	2.82	23.2	188
Kidney etc.	234	0	2.3	-	-	-	-	-	-	2.4	2.6	6.8	17.8	23.4	43.3	44.2	68.2	64.7	64.1	59.0	12.4	2.3	0.49	1.06	8.5	189
Eye	19	0	1.6	-	-	-	-	-	0.6	-	-	-	-	1.1	5.6	2.3	5.9	8.6	-	-	1.0	0.2	0.04	0.09	0.8	190
Brain, nervous system	146	0	4.7	2.2	2.4	2.5	2.6	2.8	2.4	6.7	4.6	10.3	11.5	11.1	11.1	18.6	34.1	15.1	32.0	36.9	7.8	1.4	0.37	0.64	6.3	191-2
Thyroid	68	0	-	-	-	1.7	0.9	2.1	3.0	3.6	1.3	5.1	5.2	7.8	8.9	11.6	10.4	10.8	-	7.4	3.6	0.7	0.20	0.31	2.8	193
Other endocrine	7	0	-	-	-	1.7	0.9	-	-	-	0.7	-	1.0	-	-	1.2	-	2.2	-	-	0.4	0.1	0.02	0.03	0.4	194
Hodgkin's disease	61	0	-	-	0.8	4.1	8.6	4.2	3.7	3.6	2.6	2.6	4.2	2.2	3.3	2.3	5.9	6.5	4.0	7.4	3.2	0.6	0.20	0.24	3.0	201
Non-Hodgkin lymphoma	316	0	0.8	2.2	0.8	0.8	3.5	5.6	7.3	7.9	8.5	18.8	27.3	27.8	35.5	43.0	66.7	79.8	76.1	125.5	16.8	3.1	0.73	1.28	12.1	200,202
Multiple myeloma	98	0	-	-	-	-	-	-	-	1.2	1.3	3.4	4.2	10.0	15.5	12.8	35.6	32.3	32.0	36.9	5.2	0.9	0.18	0.42	3.4	203
Lymphoid leukaemia	143	0	7.8	5.2	0.8	1.7	-	0.7	1.2	-	2.0	3.4	7.3	12.2	18.9	23.2	34.1	32.3	52.1	51.7	7.6	1.4	0.31	0.59	6.0	204
Myeloid leukaemia	112	0	-	-	2.4	1.7	1.7	0.7	2.4	1.8	2.6	0.9	10.5	6.7	11.1	24.4	25.2	32.3	24.0	51.7	5.9	1.1	0.21	0.46	4.2	205
Monocytic leukaemia	7	0	-	-	-	-	-	-	0.6	-	-	-	2.2	-	-	1.5	4.3	-	-	7.4	0.4	0.1	0.01	0.02	0.2	206
Other leukaemia	2	0	-	-	-	-	-	-	-	-	-	-	-	-	1.2	1.5	-	-	-		0.1	0.0	0.00	0.01	0.1	207
Leukaemia unspecified	27	0	-	-	-	-	0.9	-	-	-	-	0.9	-	1.1	1.1	2.3	8.9	17.3	20.0	14.8	1.4	0.3	0.02	0.08	0.8	208
Other and unspecified	301	0	-	-	-	-	0.9	1.4	0.6	1.2	4.6	12.8	19.9	24.5	34.4	51.1	94.9	99.2	104.1	155.0	16.0	2.9	0.50	1.23	10.4	O&U
All sites	10380	0	17.9	11.9	8.6	25.7	42.3	61.9	70.7	99.1	122.3	218.8	453.0	796.7	1363.6	2204.0	3094.8	3523.8	3739.7	3778.6	551.2		16.46	42.96	355.3	ALL
All sites but 173	10344	0	17.9	11.9	8.6	25.7	42.3	61.2	69.4	98.5	119.7	218.8	449.9	790.0	1359.2	2201.7	3090.4	3517.4	3727.7	3749.1	549.3	100.0	16.36	42.83	354.0	ALLb
Rate from 1 case			0.777	0.741	0.786	0.829	0.864	0.695	0.609	0.608	0.654	0.855	1.049	1.113	1.110	1.162	1.483	2.157	4.004	7.380						

†Important: see notes on population page

USA, NEW MEXICO: NON-HISPANIC WHITE 1988-1992

ANNUAL INCIDENCE PER 100,000 BY AGE GROUP (YEARS) - FEMALE

SITE	ALL AGES	AGE UNK	0-	5-	10-	15-	20-	25-	30-	35-	40-	45-	50-	55-	60-	65-	70-	75-	80-	85+	CRUDE RATE	%	CR 64	CR 74	ASR (W)	ICD (9th)
Lip	25	0	-	-	-	-	-	-	0.6	1.2	-	-	-	2.1	2.0	3.0	6.3	6.3	9.6	5.9	1.3	0.3	0.03	0.08	0.6	140
Tongue	30	0	-	-	-	-	-	-	-	-	1.3	1.7	1.0	2.1	5.1	10.0	1.3	1.6	7.2	8.9	1.5	0.4	0.06	0.11	0.9	141
Salivary gland	18	0	-	-	-	-	-	1.4	-	-	1.3	-	-	-	1.0	4.0	3.8	3.2	7.2	3.0	0.9	0.2	0.02	0.06	0.5	142
Mouth	43	0	-	-	-	0.9	-	-	-	-	1.3	3.4	3.0	4.3	5.1	6.0	10.1	9.5	9.6	-	2.2	0.5	0.09	0.17	1.4	143-5
Oropharynx	11	0	-	-	-	-	-	-	0.6	-	-	-	1.0	3.2	1.0	2.0	1.3	-	2.4	3.0	0.6	0.1	0.03	0.05	0.4	146
Nasopharynx	4	0	-	-	-	-	-	-	-	-	-	0.8	1.0	-	1.0	-	1.3	-	-	-	0.2	0.0	0.01	0.02	0.2	147
Hypopharynx	5	0	-	-	-	-	-	-	-	-	-	-	1.1	2.0	-	1.3	1.6	-	-	-	0.3	0.1	0.02	0.02	0.2	148
Pharynx unspecified	4	0	-	-	-	-	-	-	-	-	-	-	-	-	-	2.5	1.6	-	3.0		0.2	0.0	0.00	0.01	0.1	149
Oesophagus	45	0	-	-	-	-	-	-	-	-	0.7	-	2.0	-	8.1	8.0	10.1	14.2	16.9	5.9	2.3	0.5	0.05	0.14	1.2	150
Stomach	91	0	-	-	-	-	-	0.7	-	0.6	2.0	0.8	7.0	7.5	8.1	9.0	21.4	25.3	31.3	23.8	4.7	1.1	0.13	0.29	2.5	151
Small intestine	26	0	-	-	-	-	-	0.7	-	1.8	0.7	0.8	2.0	-	3.0	2.0	3.8	6.3	7.2	8.9	1.3	0.3	0.05	0.07	0.8	152
Colon	699	0	-	-	-	-	0.9	-	0.6	3.6	11.9	14.4	25.2	34.3	64.9	96.3	140.8	213.1	236.1	279.3	35.8	8.4	0.78	1.96	17.5	153
Rectum	248	0	-	-	-	-	0.9	-	-	1.8	5.9	5.9	15.1	26.8	24.3	33.1	57.8	52.1	69.9	68.4	12.7	3.0	0.40	0.86	7.1	154
Liver	39	0	0.8	-	-	-	-	0.7	0.6	0.6	1.3	0.8	-	1.1	6.1	2.0	10.1	6.3	19.3	8.9	2.0	0.5	0.06	0.12	1.1	155
Gallbladder etc.	54	0	-	-	-	-	-	-	-	-	0.7	-	2.0	1.1	2.0	6.0	8.8	18.9	21.7	41.6	2.8	0.6	0.03	0.10	1.1	156
Pancreas	208	0	-	-	-	-	0.9	-	1.2	-	0.7	1.7	3.0	19.3	15.2	37.1	51.5	56.8	69.9	68.4	10.7	2.5	0.21	0.65	5.2	157
Nose, sinuses etc.	19	0	-	-	-	-	-	-	-	-	1.3	1.7	2.0	2.1	2.0	4.0	2.5	3.2	-	3.0	1.0	0.2	0.05	0.08	0.7	160
Larynx	38	0	-	-	-	-	-	-	-	-	-	-	2.0	7.5	8.1	10.0	7.5	7.9	-	-	1.9	0.5	0.09	0.18	1.3	161
Bronchus, lung	955	0	-	-	-	-	0.9	-	1.2	3.6	5.9	22.8	49.3	112.4	152.0	192.7	228.7	183.1	185.5	115.9	48.9	11.5	1.74	3.85	28.8	162
Other thoracic organs	7	0	0.8	-	-	-	-	-	-	-	-	-	1.0	1.1	1.0	2.0	-	-	2.4	-	0.4	0.1	0.02	0.03	0.3	163-4
Bone	15	0	-	0.8	4.2	0.9	-	0.7	-	0.6	-	0.8	-	1.1	-	1.0	2.5	-	-	3.0	0.8	0.2	0.05	0.06	0.8	170
Connective tissue	56	0	1.6	-	-	-	1.8	0.7	1.2	2.4	2.0	4.2	5.0	2.1	6.1	2.0	11.3	6.3	14.5	8.9	2.9	0.7	0.14	0.20	2.0	171
Mesothelioma	14	0	-	-	-	-	-	-	-	-	-	-	2.0	1.1	-	2.0	2.5	9.5	2.4	-	0.7	0.2	0.02	0.04	0.4	MES
Kaposi's sarcoma	2	0	-	-	-	-	-	-	-	-	-	-	-	-	-	-	1.6	-	-	3.0	0.1	0.0	0.00	0.00	0.0	KAP
Melanoma of skin	329	0	-	-	1.7	4.4	11.6	9.1	21.5	16.7	18.5	24.5	26.2	25.7	29.4	20.1	28.9	31.6	48.2	38.6	16.9	4.0	0.95	1.19	12.5	172
†Other skin	33	0	-	-	-	-	1.8	0.7	2.4	2.4	2.6	2.5	1.0	1.1	-	1.0	3.8	3.2	9.6	8.9	1.7		0.07	0.10	1.1	173
Breast	2625	0	-	-	-	-	-	11.2	23.9	55.9	121.5	189.3	227.5	243.0	313.1	368.3	438.6	446.7	445.7	359.6	134.5	31.6	5.93	9.96	86.3	174
Uterus unspecified	11	0	-	-	-	-	-	-	-	0.6	-	0.8	1.0	-	-	2.0	1.3	1.6	2.4	8.9	0.6	0.1	0.01	0.03	0.3	179
Cervix uteri	235	0	-	0.8	-	-	2.7	11.2	15.5	19.0	14.5	22.0	13.1	24.6	19.3	22.1	11.3	14.2	12.0	26.7	12.0	2.8	0.71	0.88	9.1	180
Placenta	0	0	-	-	-	-	-	-	-	-	-	-	-	-	-	-	-	-	-	-	0.0	0.0	0.00	0.00	0.0	181
Corpus uteri	486	0	-	-	-	-	-	0.7	4.8	4.8	11.2	31.3	34.2	50.3	78.0	70.2	110.6	97.9	67.5	26.7	24.9	5.8	1.08	1.98	15.8	182
Ovary etc.	330	0	-	0.8	-	0.9	1.8	4.2	4.2	7.7	10.6	17.8	26.2	35.3	41.5	40.1	64.1	53.7	38.5	65.4	16.9	4.0	0.75	1.28	11.0	183
Other female genital	71	0	-	-	-	-	-	0.7	1.2	3.0	2.0	2.5	3.0	7.5	8.1	9.0	6.3	17.4	19.3	17.8	3.6	0.9	0.14	0.22	2.1	184
Bladder	211	0	-	-	-	-	-	-	2.4	0.6	0.7	5.1	8.1	17.1	21.3	24.1	40.2	67.9	67.5	80.2	10.8	2.5	0.28	0.60	5.4	188
Kidney etc.	140	0	4.1	0.8	-	-	-	1.4	1.2	1.8	4.0	2.5	14.1	9.6	18.2	25.1	26.4	26.8	12.0	26.7	7.2	1.7	0.29	0.55	4.8	189
Eye	15	0	0.8	0.8	-	-	-	-	-	0.6	-	-	-	1.1	2.0	5.0	2.5	1.6	2.4	-	0.8	0.2	0.03	0.06	0.6	190
Brain, nervous system	115	0	1.6	1.6	1.7	1.8	3.6	2.8	3.0	4.2	8.6	3.4	7.0	5.4	15.2	13.0	15.1	4.7	21.7	17.8	5.9	1.4	0.30	0.44	4.4	191-2
Thyroid	161	0	-	-	-	5.3	6.3	9.1	13.2	10.1	14.5	10.1	11.1	11.8	9.1	6.0	8.8	17.4	12.0	5.9	8.2	1.9	0.50	0.58	6.6	193
Other endocrine	5	0	1.6	0.8	-	-	-	-	-	-	-	1.7	-	-	-	-	-	-	-	-	0.3	0.1	0.02	0.02	0.4	194
Hodgkin's disease	48	0	-	-	0.8	4.4	7.2	2.8	1.2	1.8	2.6	1.7	-	1.1	2.0	2.0	7.5	4.7	4.8	8.9	2.5	0.6	0.13	0.18	2.2	201
Non-Hodgkin lymphoma	289	0	-	-	0.8	1.8	1.8	1.4	2.4	4.8	8.6	10.1	14.1	21.4	22.3	34.1	66.6	60.0	94.0	74.3	14.8	3.5	0.45	0.95	8.3	200,202
Multiple myeloma	92	0	-	-	-	-	0.9	-	0.6	-	0.7	2.5	2.0	3.2	11.1	15.1	18.9	23.7	38.5	26.7	4.7	1.1	0.11	0.27	2.4	203
Lymphoid leukaemia	91	0	4.9	2.3	2.5	0.9	-	1.4	2.4	1.2	0.7	1.7	3.0	6.4	5.1	9.0	16.3	26.8	19.3	17.8	4.7	1.1	0.16	0.29	3.3	204
Myeloid leukaemia	94	0	-	-	1.7	1.8	0.9	-	1.8	1.8	5.9	3.4	6.0	5.4	7.1	10.0	8.8	12.6	33.7	38.6	4.8	1.1	0.18	0.27	2.9	205
Monocytic leukaemia	5	0	0.8	-	-	-	-	-	-	-	-	-	-	1.1	-	1.0	1.3	1.6	-	-	0.3	0.1	0.01	0.02	0.2	206
Other leukaemia	0	0	-	-	-	-	-	-	-	-	-	-	-	-	-	-	-	-	-	-	0.0	0.0	0.00	0.00	0.0	207
Leukaemia unspecified	33	0	-	0.8	-	-	-	-	-	-	-	0.8	1.0	-	3.0	6.0	5.0	4.7	7.2	32.7	1.7	0.4	0.03	0.08	0.8	208
Other and unspecified	271	0	0.8	-	-	-	0.9	-	0.6	-	1.3	3.4	10.1	15.0	25.3	43.1	45.2	72.6	91.6	148.6	13.9	3.3	0.29	0.73	6.7	O&U
All sites	8346	0	18.1	9.3	13.4	22.9	44.8	61.6	107.6	153.5	265.5	397.3	532.6	716.0	949.5	1159.0	1514.5	1619.4	1761.2	1693.9	427.6		16.46	29.83	262.1	ALL
All sites but 173	8313	0	18.1	9.3	13.4	22.9	43.0	60.9	105.2	151.1	262.9	394.7	531.6	715.0	949.5	1158.0	1510.7	1616.3	1751.6	1685.0	425.9	100.0	16.39	29.73	261.0	ALLb

Rate from 1 case   0.823 0.775 0.838 0.881 0.895 0.700 0.598 0.595 0.660 0.845 1.007 1.070 1.013 1.003 1.257 1.578 2.409 2.972

†Important: see notes on population page

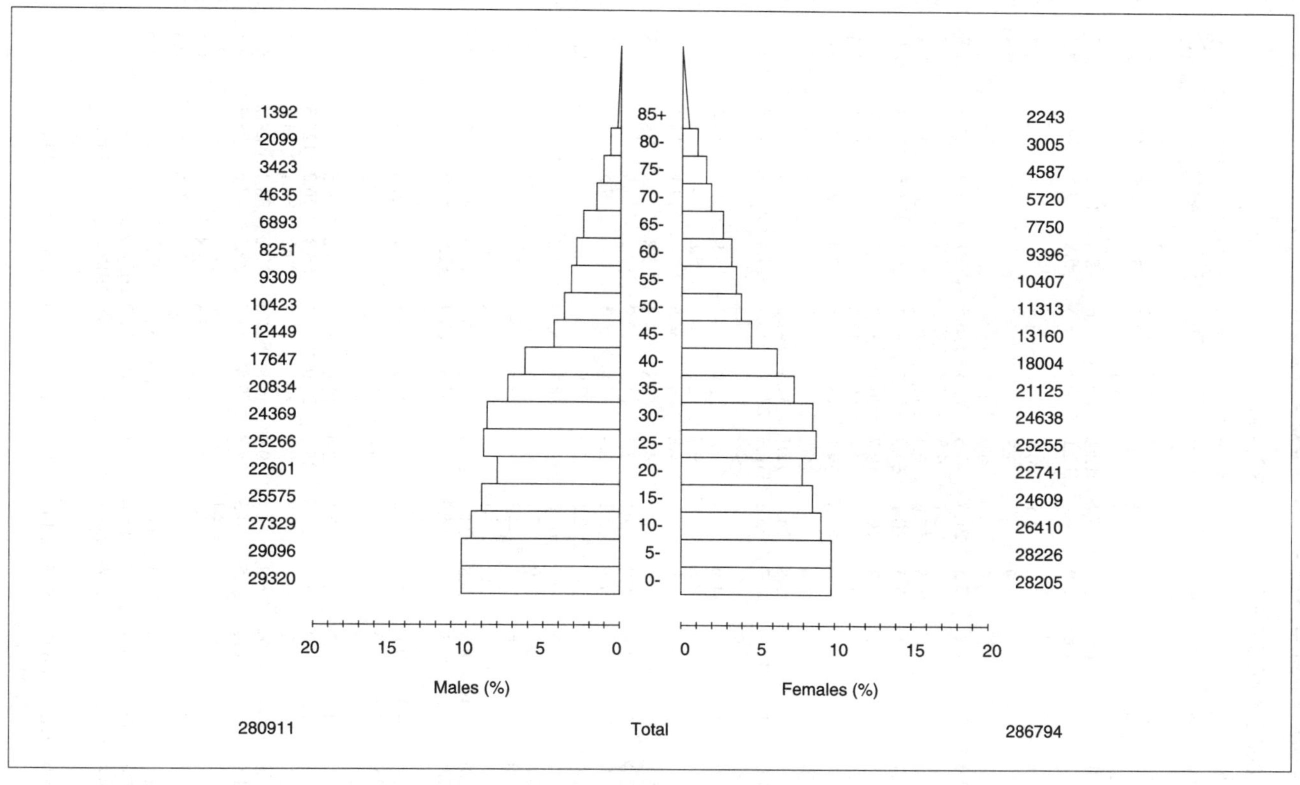

USA, New Mexico: Hispanic White
Source of population: average annual 1988-92
Estimate: *NCI estimates based on U.S. Bureau of* Census
population estimates by county for the years 1988–92.

Notes to tables overleaf:
† 173 does not include basal cell or squamous cell carcinoma

USA, NEW MEXICO: HISPANIC WHITE 1988-1992

ANNUAL INCIDENCE PER 100,000 BY AGE GROUP (YEARS) - MALE

SITE	ALL AGES	AGE UNK	0-	5-	10-	15-	20-	25-	30-	35-	40-	45-	50-	55-	60-	65-	70-	75-	80-	85+	CRUDE RATE	%	CR 64	CR 74	ASR (W)	ICD (9th)
Lip	22	0	-	-	-	-	-	-	-	-	1.1	-	3.8	-	7.3	11.6	12.9	11.7	19.1	71.8	1.6	0.7	0.06	0.18	**1.7**	140
Tongue	23	0	-	-	-	-	-	-	-	-	2.3	3.2	5.8	4.3	7.3	8.7	12.9	5.8	9.5	43.1	1.6	0.7	0.11	0.22	**1.9**	141
Salivary gland	2	0	-	-	0.7	-	-	-	-	-	-	-	-	-	2.9	-	-	-	-	-	0.1	0.1	0.00	0.02	**0.2**	142
Mouth	24	0	-	-	-	-	1.6	1.0	-	1.6	5.8	6.4	12.1	11.6	8.6	5.8	19.1	-	1.7	0.7	0.14	0.24	**2.0**	143-5
Oropharynx	13	0	-	-	-	-	-	-	-	-	1.6	1.9	-	12.1	2.9	8.6	5.8	9.5	14.4	0.9	0.4	0.08	0.14	**1.1**	146
Nasopharynx	2	0	-	-	-	-	-	-	-	-	1.6	-	-	-	-	4.3	-	-	-	0.1	0.1	0.01	0.03	**0.2**	147
Hypopharynx	8	0	-	-	-	-	-	-	-	-	-	-	-	2.1	9.7	5.8	4.3	-	-	-	0.6	0.2	0.06	0.11	**0.7**	148
Pharynx unspecified	4	0	-	-	-	-	-	-	-	-	-	1.9	-	7.3	-	-	-	-	-	0.3	0.1	0.05	0.05	**0.4**	149
Oesophagus	29	0	-	-	-	-	-	-	-	-	1.6	3.8	-	9.7	20.3	17.3	46.7	9.5	28.7	2.1	0.9	0.08	0.26	**2.3**	150
Stomach	166	0	-	-	-	0.8	-	0.8	-	2.9	6.8	4.8	17.3	21.5	43.6	72.5	116.5	181.1	142.9	244.3	11.8	5.1	0.49	1.44	**12.7**	151
Small intestine	10	0	-	-	-	-	-	-	0.8	-	-	-	-	2.1	4.8	2.9	12.9	11.7	-	-	0.7	0.3	0.04	0.12	**0.8**	152
Colon	250	0	-	-	-	-	0.9	-	1.6	3.8	3.4	8.0	34.5	55.9	99.4	133.5	138.1	204.5	200.1	229.9	17.8	7.6	1.04	2.40	**20.0**	153
Rectum	169	0	-	-	-	-	0.9	-	1.6	2.9	3.4	14.5	17.3	30.1	67.9	110.3	73.4	128.5	171.5	71.8	12.0	5.2	0.69	1.61	**13.5**	154
Liver	59	0	-	0.7	-	-	-	-	-	-	5.7	3.2	7.7	19.3	9.7	26.1	30.2	35.1	85.8	43.1	4.2	1.8	0.23	0.51	**4.5**	155
Gallbladder etc.	23	0	-	-	-	-	-	-	-	-	-	-	1.9	-	4.8	11.6	17.3	29.2	57.2	14.4	1.6	0.7	0.03	0.18	**1.6**	156
Pancreas	98	0	-	-	-	-	-	-	1.6	1.0	6.8	3.2	13.4	23.6	29.1	46.4	47.5	58.4	76.2	172.4	7.0	3.0	0.39	0.86	**7.7**	157
Nose, sinuses etc.	9	0	-	-	-	-	-	-	-	1.0	-	3.2	1.9	-	-	-	11.7	9.5	28.7	0.6	0.3	0.03	0.03	**0.7**	160
Larynx	47	0	-	-	-	-	-	-	0.8	-	-	3.2	3.8	15.0	12.1	34.8	47.5	35.1	9.5	-	3.3	1.4	0.18	0.59	**3.9**	161
Bronchus, lung	344	0	-	-	-	0.8	-	-	-	1.0	3.4	12.9	30.7	75.2	116.3	223.4	215.7	321.4	247.7	344.8	24.5	10.5	1.20	3.40	**27.5**	162
Other thoracic organs	10	0	-	-	0.7	-	1.8	0.8	-	-	-	1.6	-	4.3	2.4	2.9	4.3	-	-	-	0.7	0.3	0.06	0.09	**0.8**	163-4
Bone	15	0	-	-	0.7	-	1.8	2.4	-	1.0	2.3	-	1.9	4.3	-	2.9	-	5.8	-	14.4	1.1	0.5	0.07	0.09	**1.1**	170
Connective tissue	23	0	1.4	0.7	1.5	1.6	-	0.8	1.6	-	-	1.6	3.8	-	9.7	2.9	8.6	5.8	-	28.7	1.6	0.7	0.11	0.17	**1.8**	171
Mesothelioma	18	0	-	-	-	-	-	-	0.8	-	-	-	1.9	-	4.8	8.7	34.5	-	19.1	14.4	1.3	0.5	0.04	0.25	**1.5**	MES
Kaposi's sarcoma	40	0	-	-	-	-	1.8	5.5	8.2	10.6	1.1	1.6	-	-	4.8	5.8	4.3	5.8	-	28.7	2.8	1.2	0.17	0.22	**2.5**	KAP
Melanoma of skin	36	0	-	-	-	-	1.8	3.2	2.5	3.8	3.4	1.6	5.8	2.1	7.3	14.5	12.9	17.5	9.5	-	2.6	1.1	0.16	0.29	**2.7**	172
†Other skin	14	0	-	0.7	0.7	-	0.9	0.8	-	1.0	2.3	-	1.9	2.1	2.4	5.8	4.3	-	9.5	-	1.0		0.06	0.11	**1.0**	173
Breast	3	0	-	-	-	-	-	-	-	-	-	-	-	2.1	2.4	2.9	-	-	-	-	0.2	0.1	0.02	0.04	**0.3**	175
Prostate	967	0	-	-	-	-	-	-	-	-	1.1	3.2	30.7	101.0	283.6	568.7	863.0	1034.2	1152.9	1293.1	68.8	29.5	2.10	9.26	**74.1**	185
Testis	68	0	1.4	-	-	2.3	10.6	13.5	13.1	5.8	5.7	4.8	1.9	2.1	4.8	-	-	-	-	-	4.8	2.1	0.33	0.33	**4.4**	186
Penis	16	0	-	-	-	-	-	-	-	1.0	1.1	1.6	-	4.3	-	11.6	-	5.8	28.6	43.1	1.1	0.5	0.04	0.10	**1.2**	187.1-.4
Other male genital	1	0	-	-	-	-	-	-	-	-	-	-	-	2.1	-	-	-	-	-	-	0.1	0.0	0.01	0.01	**0.1**	187.5-.9
Bladder	135	0	-	-	-	-	-	-	-	1.0	3.4	8.0	5.8	23.6	50.9	78.3	86.3	116.9	95.3	201.1	9.6	4.1	0.46	1.29	**10.7**	188
Kidney etc.	122	0	2.0	-	-	-	-	-	2.5	1.9	10.2	24.1	19.2	15.0	46.1	63.8	60.4	52.6	57.2	43.1	8.7	3.7	0.61	1.23	**10.1**	189
Eye	7	0	2.0	-	0.7	-	-	-	-	-	-	-	-	2.1	-	2.9	4.3	-	-	-	0.5	0.2	0.02	0.06	**0.6**	190
Brain, nervous system	51	0	2.0	2.1	1.5	0.8	-	2.4	1.6	1.9	6.8	4.8	7.7	6.4	14.5	23.2	4.3	11.7	9.5	14.4	3.6	1.6	0.26	0.40	**4.0**	191-2
Thyroid	24	0	-	-	-	0.8	-	1.6	0.8	2.9	2.3	1.6	5.8	4.3	4.8	5.8	21.6	-	-	-	1.7	0.7	0.12	0.26	**1.9**	193
Other endocrine	7	0	1.4	-	0.7	-	-	-	-	1.0	-	1.6	-	2.1	-	-	-	9.5	-	0.5	0.2	0.03	0.03	**0.5**	194
Hodgkin's disease	34	0	-	1.4	1.5	0.8	1.8	0.8	4.9	1.9	4.5	3.2	1.9	2.1	2.4	11.6	12.9	5.8	9.5	-	2.4	1.0	0.14	0.26	**2.4**	201
Non-Hodgkin lymphoma	118	0	0.7	0.7	0.7	-	3.5	2.4	8.2	4.8	4.5	8.0	21.1	23.6	33.9	29.0	43.1	64.3	76.2	129.3	8.4	3.6	0.56	0.92	**9.0**	200,202
Multiple myeloma	36	0	-	-	-	-	0.9	-	-	1.0	1.1	3.2	3.8	4.3	7.3	20.3	12.9	29.2	38.1	71.8	2.6	1.1	0.11	0.27	**2.8**	203
Lymphoid leukaemia	68	0	12.3	4.8	1.5	1.6	0.9	3.2	0.8	1.9	-	1.6	5.8	2.1	19.4	5.8	21.6	29.2	38.1	28.7	4.8	2.1	0.28	0.42	**5.2**	204
Myeloid leukaemia	47	0	0.7	1.4	-	1.6	2.7	0.8	0.8	1.9	3.4	6.4	11.5	4.3	4.8	5.8	17.3	29.2	47.6	28.7	3.3	1.4	0.20	0.32	**3.5**	205
Monocytic leukaemia	2	0	-	-	-	-	-	-	-	-	-	1.9	2.1	-	-	-	-	-	-	-	0.1	0.1	0.02	0.02	**0.2**	206
Other leukaemia	2	0	-	-	-	-	-	-	-	-	-	-	-	-	-	-	4.3	5.8	-	-	0.1	0.1	0.00	0.02	**0.1**	207
Leukaemia unspecified	4	0	-	-	-	-	-	-	-	-	1.1	1.6	-	-	-	-	2.9	-	-	9.5	0.3	0.1	0.01	0.03	**0.3**	208
Other and unspecified	117	0	-	-	-	-	-	0.8	0.8	1.0	3.4	4.8	15.4	12.9	24.2	46.4	82.0	105.2	133.4	244.3	8.3	3.6	0.32	0.96	**8.9**	O&U
All sites	3287	0	23.9	12.4	11.0	10.9	30.1	39.6	55.0	57.6	90.7	147.8	299.3	485.6	984.1	1648.0	2071.2	2617.6	2810.9	3491.4	234.0		11.24	29.84	**255.0**	ALL
All sites but 173	3273	0	23.9	11.7	10.2	10.9	29.2	38.8	55.0	56.6	88.4	147.8	297.4	483.4	981.7	1642.2	2066.9	2617.6	2801.3	3491.4	233.0	100.0	11.18	29.72	**254.0**	ALLb

Rate from 1 case			0.682	0.687	0.732	0.782	0.885	0.792	0.821	0.960	1.133	1.607	1.919	2.148	2.424	2.901	4.315	5.843	9.528	14.368

†Important: see notes on population page

USA, NEW MEXICO: HISPANIC WHITE 1988-1992

ANNUAL INCIDENCE PER 100,000 BY AGE GROUP (YEARS) - FEMALE

SITE	ALL AGES	AGE UNK	0-	5-	10-	15-	20-	25-	30-	35-	40-	45-	50-	55-	60-	65-	70-	75-	80-	85+	CRUDE RATE	%	CR 64	CR 74	ASR (W)	ICD (9th)
Lip	3	0	-	-	-	-	-	-	0.8	-	-	-	-	1.9	-	-	-	-	-	8.9	0.2	0.1	0.01	0.01	0.2	140
Tongue	2	0	-	-	-	-	-	-	-	-	-	-	1.8	-	-	-	-	-	-	8.9	0.1	0.1	0.01	0.01	0.1	141
Salivary gland	6	0	-	-	-	-	-	-	1.9	-	-	-	-	-	4.3	-	-	-	6.7	8.9	0.4	0.2	0.03	0.03	0.4	142
Mouth	4	0	-	-	-	-	-	-	-	-	-	-	3.5	1.9	-	-	-	-	6.7	-	0.3	0.1	0.03	0.03	0.3	143-5
Oropharynx	3	0	-	-	-	-	-	-	0.9	-	-	-	-	-	2.1	2.6	-	-	-	-	0.2	0.1	0.02	0.03	0.2	146
Nasopharynx	4	0	-	-	-	-	0.9	-	-	-	-	-	1.8	-	2.1	-	-	4.4	-	-	0.3	0.1	0.02	0.02	0.3	147
Hypopharynx	0	0	-	-	-	-	-	-	-	-	-	-	-	-	-	-	-	-	-	-	0.0	0.0	0.00	0.00	0.0	148
Pharynx unspecified	0	0	-	-	-	-	-	-	-	-	-	-	-	-	-	-	-	-	-	-	0.0	0.0	0.00	0.00	0.0	149
Oesophagus	9	0	-	-	-	-	-	-	-	-	-	-	-	-	-	2.6	3.5	4.4	6.7	44.6	0.6	0.3	0.00	0.03	0.4	150
Stomach	98	0	-	-	-	-	-	-	-	3.8	1.1	13.7	7.1	9.6	36.2	18.1	49.0	65.4	86.5	80.2	6.8	3.4	0.36	0.69	6.3	151
Small intestine	9	0	-	-	-	-	-	-	0.8	-	-	1.5	1.8	1.9	2.1	-	3.5	8.7	-	8.9	0.6	0.3	0.04	0.06	0.6	152
Colon	229	0	-	-	-	-	-	0.8	4.1	1.9	11.1	12.2	28.3	40.4	40.4	56.8	115.4	152.6	219.6	214.0	16.0	7.9	0.70	1.56	14.2	153
Rectum	94	0	-	-	-	-	-	-	-	0.9	6.7	10.6	15.9	9.6	21.3	43.9	28.0	48.0	66.6	89.2	6.6	3.3	0.33	0.68	6.3	154
Liver	34	0	2.1	-	-	-	-	-	1.6	-	-	-	3.5	5.8	4.3	12.9	14.0	21.8	26.6	35.7	2.4	1.2	0.09	0.22	2.1	155
Gallbladder etc.	72	0	-	-	-	-	-	-	-	0.9	2.2	3.0	14.1	13.5	17.0	28.4	42.0	21.8	59.9	62.4	5.0	2.5	0.25	0.61	4.8	156
Pancreas	87	0	-	-	-	-	0.9	0.8	0.8	1.9	-	4.6	8.8	9.6	8.5	31.0	49.0	56.7	106.5	89.2	6.1	3.0	0.18	0.58	5.2	157
Nose, sinuses etc.	4	0	-	-	-	-	-	-	0.8	-	-	-	-	1.9	2.1	-	-	-	6.7	-	0.3	0.1	0.02	0.02	0.2	160
Larynx	11	0	-	-	-	-	-	-	0.8	-	1.1	-	-	3.8	-	10.3	3.5	-	13.3	-	0.8	0.4	0.03	0.10	0.7	161
Bronchus, lung	207	0	-	-	-	-	-	-	0.8	-	7.8	13.7	21.2	34.6	78.8	69.7	101.4	109.0	146.4	178.3	14.4	7.2	0.78	1.64	13.8	162
Other thoracic organs	5	0	0.7	-	-	-	-	-	-	-	-	-	-	-	1.9	2.1	2.6	-	4.4	-	0.3	0.2	0.02	0.04	0.4	163-4
Bone	13	0	1.4	-	1.5	0.8	0.9	0.8	-	-	1.1	1.5	-	1.9	-	-	-	8.7	6.7	-	0.9	0.5	0.05	0.05	0.9	170
Connective tissue	25	0	-	1.4	0.8	-	0.9	0.8	0.8	0.9	2.2	-	5.3	1.9	4.3	10.3	3.5	8.7	6.7	17.8	1.7	0.9	0.10	0.17	1.7	171
Mesothelioma	3	0	-	-	-	-	-	-	-	-	-	-	-	-	-	5.2	-	-	6.7	-	0.2	0.1	0.00	0.03	0.2	MES
Kaposi's sarcoma	3	0	-	-	-	-	-	-	-	-	-	-	-	-	-	-	3.5	4.4	-	8.9	0.2	0.1	0.00	0.02	0.2	KAP
Melanoma of skin	48	0	-	-	-	3.3	-	0.8	6.5	5.7	1.1	10.6	3.5	7.7	6.4	5.2	21.0	4.4	6.7	17.8	3.3	1.7	0.23	0.36	3.3	172
†Other skin	13	0	-	-	-	-	0.9	2.4	1.6	1.9	-	1.5	1.8	-	2.1	-	3.5	-	6.7	-	0.9		0.06	0.08	0.8	173
Breast	856	0	-	-	-	-	0.9	4.8	30.0	46.4	93.3	152.0	160.9	174.9	206.5	252.9	279.7	322.7	159.7	214.0	59.7	29.7	4.35	7.01	61.3	174
Uterus unspecified	5	0	-	-	-	-	-	-	-	0.9	-	-	1.8	-	-	3.5	-	-	17.8		0.3	0.2	0.01	0.03	0.3	179
Cervix uteri	144	0	-	-	-	-	1.8	11.1	13.0	18.9	16.7	18.2	24.8	9.6	27.7	33.5	7.0	43.6	26.6	35.7	10.0	5.0	0.71	0.91	9.7	180
Placenta	2	0	-	-	-	-	-	-	1.6	-	-	-	-	-	-	-	-	-	-	-	0.1	0.1	0.01	0.01	0.1	181
Corpus uteri	134	0	-	-	-	-	-	2.4	4.9	4.7	15.6	15.2	24.8	26.9	27.7	56.8	31.5	61.0	39.9	35.7	9.3	4.6	0.61	1.05	9.4	182
Ovary etc.	121	0	-	0.7	2.3	0.8	-	2.4	0.8	5.7	7.8	18.2	19.4	28.8	31.9	33.5	42.0	48.0	39.9	35.7	8.4	4.2	0.59	0.97	8.6	183
Other female genital	22	0	-	-	-	-	-	-	0.8	1.9	1.1	-	3.5	-	4.3	5.2	7.0	8.7	39.9	17.8	1.5	0.8	0.06	0.12	1.2	184
Bladder	49	0	-	-	-	-	-	-	-	0.9	-	3.0	3.5	1.9	21.3	7.7	35.0	34.9	46.6	44.6	3.4	1.7	0.15	0.37	3.1	188
Kidney etc.	76	0	2.1	-	-	-	-	-	1.6	1.9	1.1	7.6	12.4	19.2	23.4	25.8	35.0	39.2	13.3	35.7	5.3	2.6	0.35	0.65	5.4	189
Eye	2	0	1.4	-	-	-	-	-	-	-	-	-	-	-	-	-	-	-	-	-	0.1	0.1	0.01	0.01	0.2	190
Brain, nervous system	50	0	4.3	1.4	3.0	1.6	1.8	-	1.6	3.8	2.2	3.0	7.1	3.8	6.4	7.7	17.5	26.2	6.7	-	3.5	1.7	0.20	0.33	3.5	191-2
Thyroid	120	0	-	-	-	0.8	7.9	10.3	13.8	12.3	12.2	15.2	17.7	13.5	21.3	18.1	14.0	21.8	6.7	17.8	8.4	4.2	0.62	0.79	8.2	193
Other endocrine	3	0	-	0.7	-	-	-	-	0.8	-	-	-	-	-	-	-	-	4.4	-	-	0.2	0.1	0.01	0.01	0.2	194
Hodgkin's disease	21	0	-	-	1.5	0.8	4.4	-	2.4	0.9	-	-	7.1	-	-	2.6	3.5	4.4	13.3	-	1.5	0.7	0.09	0.12	1.4	201
Non-Hodgkin lymphoma	84	0	0.7	1.4	-	-	-	1.6	1.6	3.8	5.6	3.0	10.6	11.5	27.7	23.2	35.0	26.2	59.9	62.4	5.9	2.9	0.34	0.63	5.6	200,202
Multiple myeloma	38	0	-	-	-	-	-	-	-	-	-	3.0	7.1	5.8	14.9	10.3	31.5	17.4	20.0	17.8	2.6	1.3	0.15	0.36	2.7	203
Lymphoid leukaemia	27	0	3.5	2.1	0.8	0.8	-	2.4	-	-	-	-	1.8	-	8.5	7.7	3.5	8.7	13.3	8.9	1.9	0.9	0.10	0.16	1.9	204
Myeloid leukaemia	35	0	1.4	1.4	1.5	0.8	-	2.4	1.6	3.8	1.1	4.6	-	3.8	8.5	5.2	7.0	8.7	13.3	8.9	2.4	1.2	0.15	0.22	2.4	205
Monocytic leukaemia	4	0	-	-	-	-	1.8	-	-	-	1.1	-	-	-	2.6	-	-	-	-	-	0.3	0.1	0.01	0.03	0.3	206
Other leukaemia	1	0	-	-	-	-	-	-	-	-	-	-	-	-	-	-	3.5	-	-	-	0.1	0.0	0.00	0.02	0.1	207
Leukaemia unspecified	12	0	0.7	-	-	-	-	-	0.8	-	-	0.9	-	1.5	1.8	1.9	-	5.2	3.5	20.0	0.8	0.4	0.04	0.08	0.8	208
Other and unspecified	104	0	1.4	-	-	-	-	1.6	-	-	1.1	7.6	3.5	9.6	19.2	33.5	38.5	69.8	119.8	178.3	7.3	3.6	0.22	0.58	6.1	O&U
All sites	2896	0	19.9	9.2	11.4	9.8	22.9	48.3	91.7	127.8	193.3	325.2	426.1	459.3	683.3	831.0	1038.5	1268.8	1424.3	1605.0	202.0		12.14	21.49	195.7	ALL
All sites but 173	2883	0	19.9	9.2	11.4	9.8	22.0	45.9	90.1	125.9	193.3	323.7	424.3	459.3	681.1	831.0	1035.0	1268.8	1417.6	1605.0	201.1	100.0	12.08	21.41	194.9	ALLb

Rate from 1 case			0.709	0.709	0.757	0.813	0.879	0.792	0.812	0.947	1.111	1.520	1.768	1.922	2.129	2.581	3.497	4.360	6.656	8.917

†Important: see notes on population page

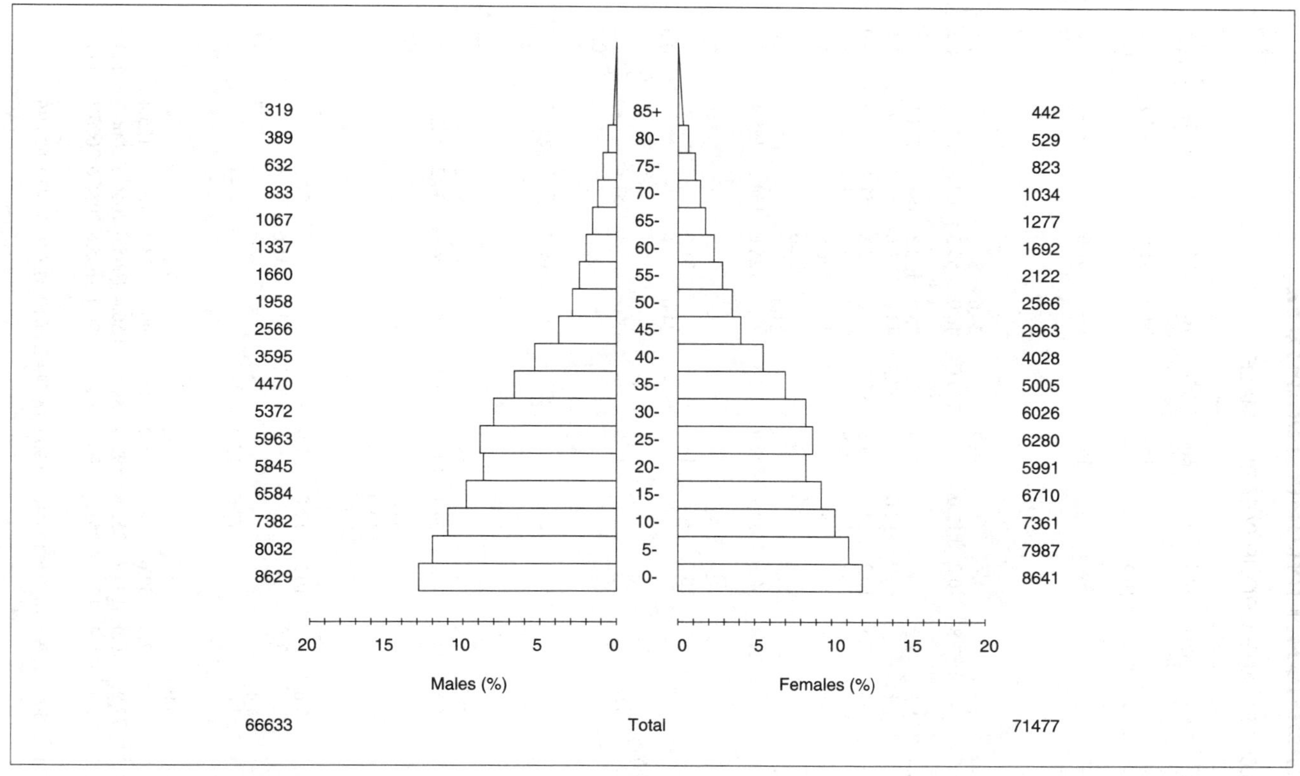

USA, New Mexico: American Indian
Source of population: average annual 1988-92
Estimate: NCI estimates based on U.S. Bureau of Census population estimates by county for the years 1988–92.

Notes to tables overleaf:
† 173 does not include basal cell or squamous cell carcinoma

USA, NEW MEXICO: AMERICAN INDIAN 1988-1992

ANNUAL INCIDENCE PER 100,000 BY AGE GROUP (YEARS) - MALE

SITE	ALL AGES	AGE UNK	0-	5-	10-	15-	20-	25-	30-	35-	40-	45-	50-	55-	60-	65-	70-	75-	80-	85+	CRUDE RATE	%	CR 64	CR 74	ASR (W)	ICD (9th)
Lip	4	0	-	-	-	-	-	-	-	-	-	-	-	-	15.0	-	24.0	31.6	-	62.7	1.2	1.1	0.07	0.19	**1.7**	140
Tongue	1	0	-	-	-	-	-	-	-	-	-	-	10.2	-	-	-	-	-	-	-	0.3	0.3	0.05	0.05	**0.5**	141
Salivary gland	0	0	-	-	-	-	-	-	-	-	-	-	-	-	-	-	-	-	-	-	0.0	0.0	0.00	0.00	**0.0**	142
Mouth	2	0	-	-	-	-	-	-	-	-	-	-	-	-	15.0	-	-	31.6	-	-	0.6	0.5	0.07	0.07	**0.9**	143-5
Oropharynx	0	0	-	-	-	-	-	-	-	-	-	-	-	-	-	-	-	-	-	-	0.0	0.0	0.00	0.00	**0.0**	146
Nasopharynx	0	0	-	-	-	-	-	-	-	-	-	-	-	-	-	-	-	-	-	-	0.0	0.0	0.00	0.00	**0.0**	147
Hypopharynx	0	0	-	-	-	-	-	-	-	-	-	-	-	-	-	-	-	-	-	-	0.0	0.0	0.00	0.00	**0.0**	148
Pharynx unspecified	0	0	-	-	-	-	-	-	-	-	-	-	-	-	-	-	-	-	-	-	0.0	0.0	0.00	0.00	**0.0**	149
Oesophagus	5	0	-	-	-	-	-	-	-	-	5.6	-	-	-	29.9	-	24.0	31.6	-	-	1.5	1.3	0.18	0.30	**2.3**	150
Stomach	21	0	-	-	-	-	-	3.4	3.7	-	-	7.8	10.2	12.0	-	150.0	48.0	63.3	102.8	125.4	6.3	5.7	0.19	1.18	**9.2**	151
Small intestine	1	0	-	-	-	-	-	-	-	-	-	-	-	-	-	18.7	-	-	-	-	0.3	0.3	0.00	0.09	**0.6**	152
Colon	26	0	-	-	-	-	-	-	3.7	13.4	11.1	7.8	-	-	44.9	18.7	96.0	158.2	154.2	188.1	7.8	7.0	0.40	0.98	**9.7**	153
Rectum	12	0	-	-	-	-	-	-	7.4	-	11.1	-	10.2	12.0	-	37.5	48.0	31.6	51.4	-	3.6	3.2	0.20	0.63	**4.8**	154
Liver	23	0	-	-	-	-	-	-	-	-	-	7.8	10.2	24.1	59.8	93.7	48.0	158.2	51.4	125.4	6.9	6.2	0.51	1.22	**10.6**	155
Gallbladder etc.	11	0	-	-	-	-	-	-	-	-	-	-	-	12.0	29.9	18.7	72.0	63.3	51.4	62.7	3.3	3.0	0.21	0.66	**4.9**	156
Pancreas	16	0	-	-	-	-	-	-	-	-	-	7.8	-	24.1	-	75.0	48.0	126.6	154.2	-	4.8	4.3	0.16	0.77	**6.7**	157
Nose, sinuses etc.	1	0	-	-	-	-	-	-	-	-	-	-	-	-	-	-	-	31.6	-	-	0.3	0.3	0.00	0.00	**0.3**	160
Larynx	2	0	-	-	-	-	-	-	-	-	-	-	-	-	-	-	24.0	-	-	62.7	0.6	0.5	0.00	0.12	**0.8**	161
Bronchus, lung	24	0	-	-	-	-	-	-	-	-	-	-	23.4	30.6	24.1	29.9	37.5	72.0	126.6	154.2	125.4	7.2	6.5	0.54	1.09	**10.3**	162
Other thoracic organs	0	0	-	-	-	-	-	-	-	-	-	-	-	-	-	-	-	-	-	-	0.0	0.0	0.00	0.00	**0.0**	163-4
Bone	1	0	-	-	-	3.0	-	-	-	-	-	-	-	-	-	-	-	-	-	-	0.3	0.3	0.02	0.02	**0.3**	170
Connective tissue	5	0	-	-	5.4	-	-	-	-	-	-	-	10.2	-	15.0	-	-	31.6	-	-	1.5	1.3	0.15	0.15	**1.9**	171
Mesothelioma	2	0	-	-	-	-	-	-	-	-	-	-	-	-	-	-	24.0	31.6	-	-	0.6	0.5	0.00	0.12	**0.8**	MES
Kaposi's sarcoma	2	0	-	-	-	-	-	-	3.7	4.5	-	-	-	-	-	-	-	-	-	-	0.6	0.5	0.04	0.04	**0.5**	KAP
Melanoma of skin	4	0	-	2.5	-	-	-	-	-	-	5.6	-	-	-	15.0	-	-	-	51.4	-	1.2	1.1	0.12	0.12	**1.4**	172
†Other skin	0	0	-	-	-	-	-	-	-	-	-	-	-	-	-	-	-	-	-	-	0.0	0.0	0.00	0.00	**0.0**	173
Breast	1	0	-	-	-	-	-	-	-	-	-	-	-	-	15.0	-	-	-	-	-	0.3	0.3	0.07	0.07	**0.6**	175
Prostate	89	0	-	-	-	-	-	-	-	-	-	7.8	30.6	24.1	119.7	299.9	336.1	506.3	771.2	877.7	26.7	24.0	0.91	4.09	**36.8**	185
Testis	10	0	-	-	-	3.0	6.8	10.1	7.4	4.5	-	7.8	-	-	-	-	-	-	-	-	3.0	2.7	0.20	0.20	**2.8**	186
Penis	1	0	-	-	-	-	-	-	-	-	-	-	-	12.0	-	-	-	-	-	-	0.3	0.3	0.06	0.06	**0.5**	187.1-.4
Other male genital	0	0	-	-	-	-	-	-	-	-	-	-	-	-	-	-	-	-	-	-	0.0	0.0	0.00	0.00	**0.0**	187.5-.9
Bladder	7	0	2.3	-	-	-	-	-	-	-	5.6	7.8	-	-	15.0	-	-	31.6	51.4	62.7	2.1	1.9	0.15	0.15	**2.6**	188
Kidney etc.	29	0	-	-	-	-	-	-	-	-	5.6	23.4	40.9	24.1	104.7	56.2	48.0	94.9	154.2	62.7	8.7	7.8	0.99	1.51	**13.6**	189
Eye	2	0	-	5.0	-	-	-	-	-	-	-	-	-	-	-	-	-	-	-	-	0.6	0.5	0.02	0.02	**0.5**	190
Brain, nervous system	9	0	2.3	2.5	-	-	3.4	-	-	-	11.1	-	-	24.1	15.0	-	24.0	-	-	-	2.7	2.4	0.29	0.41	**3.5**	191-2
Thyroid	3	0	-	-	-	-	3.4	-	-	-	-	-	12.0	15.0	-	-	-	-	-	-	0.9	0.8	0.15	0.15	**1.3**	193
Other endocrine	0	0	-	-	-	-	-	-	-	-	-	-	-	-	-	-	-	-	-	-	0.0	0.0	0.00	0.00	**0.0**	194
Hodgkin's disease	1	0	-	-	-	-	3.4	-	-	-	-	-	-	-	-	-	-	-	-	-	0.3	0.3	0.02	0.02	**0.3**	201
Non-Hodgkin lymphoma	10	0	-	-	-	3.0	-	-	3.7	4.5	5.6	-	10.2	12.0	29.9	-	-	-	102.8	-	3.0	2.7	0.34	0.34	**3.8**	200,202
Multiple myeloma	7	0	-	-	-	-	-	-	-	-	-	7.8	-	-	-	18.7	24.0	31.6	102.8	62.7	2.1	1.9	0.04	0.25	**2.7**	203
Lymphoid leukaemia	10	0	2.3	5.0	5.4	6.1	-	3.4	-	-	5.6	-	-	-	-	-	-	-	-	62.7	3.0	2.7	0.14	0.14	**2.7**	204
Myeloid leukaemia	8	0	2.3	-	-	3.0	3.4	-	3.7	4.5	5.6	-	-	12.0	15.0	-	-	-	-	-	2.4	2.2	0.25	0.25	**2.7**	205
Monocytic leukaemia	0	0	-	-	-	-	-	-	-	-	-	-	-	-	-	-	-	-	-	-	0.0	0.0	0.00	0.00	**0.0**	206
Other leukaemia	0	0	-	-	-	-	-	-	-	-	-	-	-	-	-	-	-	-	-	-	0.0	0.0	0.00	0.00	**0.0**	207
Leukaemia unspecified	2	0	-	-	-	-	3.4	-	-	-	5.6	-	-	-	-	-	-	-	-	-	0.6	0.5	0.04	0.04	**0.6**	208
Other and unspecified	19	0	-	2.5	-	-	-	-	-	-	-	7.8	30.6	24.1	15.0	18.7	96.0	63.3	102.8	125.4	5.7	5.1	0.40	0.97	**8.1**	O&U
All sites	371	0	9.3	17.4	10.8	18.2	17.1	23.5	33.5	31.3	77.9	116.9	194.1	253.0	598.4	843.5	1056.4	1645.6	2056.6	2006.3	111.4		7.01	16.51	**151.3**	ALL
All sites but 173	371	0	9.3	17.4	10.8	18.2	17.1	23.5	33.5	31.3	77.9	116.9	194.1	253.0	598.4	843.5	1056.4	1645.6	2056.6	2006.3	111.4	100.0	7.01	16.51	**151.3**	ALLb

Rate from 1 case   2.318   2.490   2.709   3.038   3.422   3.354   3.723   4.474   5.563   7.794   10.215   12.048   14.959   18.744   24.010   31.646   51.414   62.696

†Important: see notes on population page

USA, NEW MEXICO: AMERICAN INDIAN 1988-1992

ANNUAL INCIDENCE PER 100,000 BY AGE GROUP (YEARS) - FEMALE

SITE	ALL AGES	AGE UNK	0-	5-	10-	15-	20-	25-	30-	35-	40-	45-	50-	55-	60-	65-	70-	75-	80-	85+	CRUDE RATE	%	CR 64	CR 74	ASR (W)	ICD (9th)
Lip	1	0	-	-	-	-	-	-	-	-	5.0	-	-	-	-	-	-	-	-	-	0.3	0.2	0.02	0.02	**0.3**	*140*
Tongue	1	0	-	-	-	-	-	-	-	-	-	-	-	-	-	15.7	-	-	-	-	0.3	0.2	0.00	0.08	**0.5**	*141*
Salivary gland	1	0	-	-	-	-	-	3.2	-	-	-	-	-	-	-	-	-	-	-	-	0.3	0.2	0.02	0.02	**0.3**	*142*
Mouth	1	0	-	-	-	-	-	-	-	-	-	-	-	-	-	-	19.3	-	-	-	0.3	0.2	0.00	0.10	**0.4**	*143-5*
Oropharynx	0	0	-	-	-	-	-	-	-	-	-	-	-	-	-	-	-	-	-	-	0.0	0.0	0.00	0.00	**0.0**	*146*
Nasopharynx	2	0	-	-	-	-	-	-	-	-	-	-	-	-	11.8	15.7	-	-	-	-	0.6	0.5	0.06	0.14	**0.9**	*147*
Hypopharynx	0	0	-	-	-	-	-	-	-	-	-	-	-	-	-	-	-	-	-	-	0.0	0.0	0.00	0.00	**0.0**	*148*
Pharynx unspecified	0	0	-	-	-	-	-	-	-	-	-	-	-	-	-	-	-	-	-	-	0.0	0.0	0.00	0.00	**0.0**	*149*
Oesophagus	1	0	-	-	-	-	-	-	-	-	-	-	-	-	-	-	-	-	37.8	-	0.3	0.2	0.00	0.00	**0.2**	*150*
Stomach	24	0	-	-	-	-	3.3	-	-	-	9.9	6.7	-	37.7	35.5	31.3	19.3	97.2	75.6	181.0	6.7	5.5	0.47	0.72	**7.8**	*151*
Small intestine	0	0	-	-	-	-	-	-	-	-	-	-	-	-	-	-	-	-	-	-	0.0	0.0	0.00	0.00	**0.0**	*152*
Colon	21	0	-	-	-	-	-	-	-	4.0	5.0	-	23.4	18.9	11.8	15.7	116.1	121.5	37.8	-	5.9	4.8	0.32	0.97	**7.1**	*153*
Rectum	14	0	-	-	-	-	-	-	-	4.0	9.9	13.5	-	28.3	-	47.0	-	24.3	-	90.5	3.9	3.2	0.28	0.51	**4.9**	*154*
Liver	7	0	-	-	-	-	-	-	-	-	-	-	7.8	18.9	-	-	19.3	24.3	-	90.5	2.0	1.6	0.13	0.23	**2.2**	*155*
Gallbladder etc.	35	0	-	-	-	-	-	-	-	-	-	13.5	15.6	37.7	70.9	78.3	77.4	121.5	151.2	135.7	9.8	8.1	0.69	1.47	**12.5**	*156*
Pancreas	18	0	-	-	-	-	-	-	-	-	-	6.7	-	9.4	11.8	62.6	58.0	121.5	-	135.7	5.0	4.2	0.14	0.74	**6.2**	*157*
Nose, sinuses etc.	5	0	-	-	-	-	-	-	-	4.0	5.0	-	-	-	-	38.7	-	-	-	45.2	1.4	1.2	0.04	0.24	**1.5**	*160*
Larynx	0	0	-	-	-	-	-	-	-	-	-	-	-	-	-	-	-	-	-	-	0.0	0.0	0.00	0.00	**0.0**	*161*
Bronchus, lung	12	0	-	-	-	-	-	-	-	-	-	-	7.8	18.9	23.6	15.7	19.3	24.3	75.6	90.5	3.4	2.8	0.25	0.43	**4.0**	*162*
Other thoracic organs	0	0	-	-	-	-	-	-	-	-	-	-	-	-	-	-	-	-	-	-	0.0	0.0	0.00	0.00	**0.0**	*163-4*
Bone	2	0	-	2.5	-	-	-	-	-	-	-	-	-	-	-	15.7	-	-	-	-	0.6	0.5	0.01	0.09	**0.7**	*170*
Connective tissue	7	0	2.3	-	-	-	3.3	3.2	-	4.0	5.0	-	-	9.4	-	-	19.3	-	-	-	2.0	1.6	0.14	0.23	**2.1**	*171*
Mesothelioma	1	0	-	-	-	-	-	-	-	-	-	-	-	-	-	15.7	-	-	-	-	0.3	0.2	0.00	0.08	**0.5**	*MES*
Kaposi's sarcoma	0	0	-	-	-	-	-	-	-	-	-	-	-	-	-	-	-	-	-	-	0.0	0.0	0.00	0.00	**0.0**	*KAP*
Melanoma of skin	3	0	-	-	-	-	-	-	-	8.0	-	-	-	-	-	-	-	-	-	45.2	0.8	0.7	0.04	0.04	**0.7**	*172*
†Other skin	1	0	-	-	-	-	-	3.3	-	-	-	-	-	-	-	-	-	-	-	-	0.3		0.02	0.02	**0.2**	*173*
Breast	80	0	-	-	-	-	-	6.4	6.6	28.0	64.5	94.5	77.9	66.0	70.9	141.0	38.7	121.5	75.6	45.2	22.4	18.5	2.07	2.97	**28.3**	*174*
Uterus unspecified	1	0	-	-	-	-	-	-	-	-	5.0	-	-	-	-	-	-	-	-	-	0.3	0.2	0.02	0.02	**0.3**	*179*
Cervix uteri	28	0	-	-	-	-	-	-	10.0	16.0	9.9	13.5	15.6	47.1	23.6	15.7	19.3	24.3	37.8	181.0	7.8	6.5	0.68	0.85	**8.8**	*180*
Placenta	0	0	-	-	-	-	-	-	-	-	-	-	-	-	-	-	-	-	-	-	0.0	0.0	0.00	0.00	**0.0**	*181*
Corpus uteri	24	0	-	-	-	-	-	-	-	8.0	9.9	27.0	23.4	37.7	35.5	62.6	19.3	24.3	-	-	6.7	5.5	0.71	1.12	**9.3**	*182*
Ovary etc.	36	0	-	-	-	8.9	3.3	3.2	6.6	8.0	19.9	20.2	23.4	28.3	82.7	62.6	19.3	24.3	37.8	-	10.1	8.3	1.02	1.43	**12.9**	*183*
Other female genital	4	0	-	-	-	-	-	-	-	-	-	-	-	-	-	-	19.3	24.3	37.8	45.2	1.1	0.9	0.00	0.10	**1.0**	*184*
Bladder	2	0	-	-	-	-	-	-	-	-	-	-	-	9.4	-	-	-	-	-	45.2	0.6	0.5	0.05	0.05	**0.6**	*188*
Kidney etc.	21	0	-	2.5	-	-	-	-	12.0	-	-	6.7	31.2	9.4	35.5	31.3	58.0	72.9	-	-	5.9	4.8	0.49	0.93	**7.6**	*189*
Eye	1	0	2.3	-	-	-	-	-	-	-	-	-	-	-	-	-	-	-	-	-	0.3	0.2	0.01	0.01	**0.3**	*190*
Brain, nervous system	7	0	2.3	-	5.4	3.0	6.7	-	-	-	4.0	-	-	-	-	-	-	-	-	-	2.0	1.6	0.11	0.11	**1.8**	*191-2*
Thyroid	12	0	-	-	-	-	3.3	3.2	3.3	8.0	-	6.7	23.4	9.4	-	15.7	19.3	-	-	-	3.4	2.8	0.29	0.46	**4.0**	*193*
Other endocrine	2	0	-	-	-	-	-	-	-	-	-	-	-	9.4	-	15.7	-	-	-	-	0.6	0.5	0.05	0.13	**0.8**	*194*
Hodgkin's disease	1	0	-	-	-	-	-	-	-	-	-	-	-	-	-	-	-	24.3	-	-	0.3	0.2	0.00	0.00	**0.2**	*201*
Non-Hodgkin lymphoma	12	0	-	-	-	-	-	-	-	-	14.9	6.7	-	18.9	11.8	31.3	-	24.3	37.8	45.2	3.4	2.8	0.26	0.42	**4.1**	*200,202*
Multiple myeloma	10	0	-	-	-	-	-	-	-	-	-	-	7.8	28.3	11.8	15.7	19.3	24.3	37.8	45.2	2.8	2.3	0.24	0.41	**3.5**	*203*
Lymphoid leukaemia	8	0	4.6	5.0	-	3.0	3.3	-	-	-	5.0	-	-	9.4	-	-	-	-	-	-	2.2	1.8	0.15	0.15	**2.3**	*204*
Myeloid leukaemia	5	0	-	-	2.7	-	-	-	3.3	4.0	-	-	-	7.8	-	-	-	-	37.8	-	1.4	1.2	0.09	0.09	**1.3**	*205*
Monocytic leukaemia	0	0	-	-	-	-	-	-	-	-	-	-	-	-	-	-	-	-	-	-	0.0	0.0	0.00	0.00	**0.0**	*206*
Other leukaemia	0	0	-	-	-	-	-	-	-	-	-	-	-	-	-	-	-	-	-	-	0.0	0.0	0.00	0.00	**0.0**	*207*
Leukaemia unspecified	0	0	-	-	-	-	-	-	-	-	-	-	-	-	-	-	-	-	-	-	0.0	0.0	0.00	0.00	**0.0**	*208*
Other and unspecified	23	0	-	-	-	-	-	-	-	4.0	-	-	-	18.9	47.3	31.3	77.4	121.5	37.8	181.0	6.4	5.3	0.35	0.89	**7.7**	*O&U*
All sites	434	0	11.6	10.0	8.2	14.9	23.4	19.1	33.2	115.9	168.8	216.0	265.0	471.3	484.6	736.1	677.0	1020.7	718.3	1402.7	121.4		9.21	16.27	**147.8**	*ALL*
All sites but 173	433	0	11.6	10.0	8.2	14.9	23.4	19.1	29.9	115.9	168.8	216.0	265.0	471.3	484.6	736.1	677.0	1020.7	718.3	1402.7	121.2	100.0	9.19	16.26	**147.6**	*ALLb*
Rate from 1 case			2.315	2.504	2.717	2.981	3.338	3.185	3.319	3.996	4.965	6.750	7.794	9.425	11.820	15.662	19.342	24.301	37.807	45.249						

†Important: see notes on population page

USA, Utah

The Utah Cancer Registry was established in 1966 as a state-wide, population-based registry under the Regional Medical Program. In 1973 the registry expanded its interests, began a number of epidemiological studies, and joined the National Cancer Institute's Surveillance, Epidemiology and End Results (SEER) Program, then being implemented. The registry is part of the University of Utah School of Medicine, and is a core resource of the Utah Regional Cancer Center.

The State of Utah contains approximately 1.9 million people, predominantly of northern European ancestry. The population is growing at the rate of about 3% per year, due primarily to a high birth rate. Approximately 78% of the population lives in an urban four-county area; the remaining population resides primarily in scattered small communities where the major activity is farming, although coal-mining is important in at least three rural counties. The racial distribution (1990) is 96% white (4.7% Hispanic), 0.7% black, 1.4% native American, and 1.9% Asian and Pacific islanders. About 70% of the population are members of the Church of Jesus Christ of Later-Day Saints (Mormon), which is noted for its emphasis on health practices. Active members abstain from alcohol, tobacco, coffee and tea. This is largely responsible for Utah having the lowest overall cancer incidence rate in the SEER Program. Data indicate a substantial difference in cancer risk between the Mormon and non-Mormon segments of the population, especially for sites related to alcohol and tobacco use. The level of medical service in Utah is high, and all deaths are medically certified.

Cancer cases are identified and followed using information obtained from hospitals, nursing homes, pathology laboratories, radiation treatment centres, physician offices, the Utah Department of Vital Statistics and central registries located in seven surrounding states, and by direct patient contact. Reporting of cancer data in Utah is legislatively mandated.

Thirteen hospitals in Utah have computerized hospital cancer registries. Case abstracts from these hospitals are submitted monthly on diskette by hospital registrars. This system covers approximately 80% of the cancer cases in the state. Six radiation therapy facilities also submit monthly abstracts. Central registry personnel travel to outlying counties to identify and abstract cases in the remaining 30 smaller rural hospitals on an annual basis. All hospital and private pathology laboratories are visited monthly to identify non-hospitalized cases and as a quality control measure for hospitalized cases. Physicians may also report cases directly to the registry.

The State of Utah provides computer tapes of all deaths in Utah on a quarterly basis. The Utah Bureau of Vital Statistics also provides annually a tape including death certificate data on Utah residents dying in surrounding states. These are matched with the registry's files by computer, supplemented by manual comparisons when needed. Besides providing death certificate data on cases already on file, this process reveals cases which may have been missed. These are accepted as incident cases if no other record can be found after search of inpatient, outpatient and pathology laboratory records.

Follow-up letters are sent annually, serving as a physician reminder and providing data to the registry on treatment and patient status. Active follow-up is pursued by both hospital registrars and central registry personnel. Intermittent additional matches are performed with other data-bases such as the US Health Care Financing Administration, the Utah Drivers License Bureau, and Voters Registration.

Data are coded by hospital registrars and by central registry personnel, depending on field. Hospitals submit abstracts and copies of pathology reports to facilitate central coding, which includes SEER Program extent of disease and site-specific surgery.

Quality control of hospital registrars and central registry personnel is conducted by specific programmes within SEER and separately by procedures within the registry. These include computer on-line editing of data entry, numerous edit checks of previously entered data, sample reabstracting and recoding of cases, and repeat searches for cases at hospitals and laboratories.

In addition to being used by SEER, Utah data have been used in numerous studies of various cancer sites, which have evaluated environmental exposures and differences in risk by religion. The large families, good genealogical records and health consciousness of the Mormon population have fostered studies on the genetics of cancer and predisposing lesions. In addition, the registry publishes and provides to all Utah physicians an overall review of cancer in Utah every five years and a review of particular topics on a regular basis.

J.L. Stanford
R. Dibble

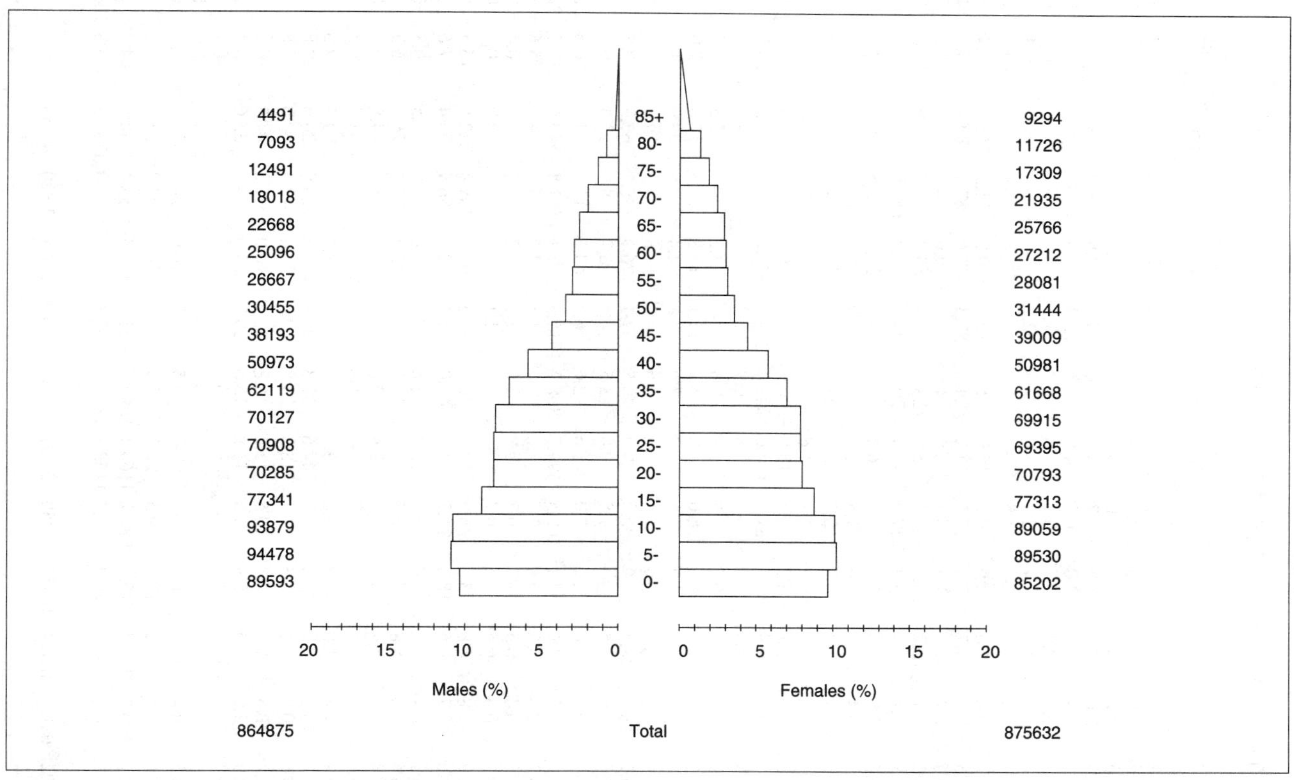

USA, Utah
Source of population: average annual 1988-92
Estimate: NCI estimates based on U.S. Bureau of Census population estimates by county for the years 1988–92.

Notes to tables overleaf:
† 173 does not include basal cell or squamous cell carcinoma

USA, UTAH 1988-1992

ANNUAL INCIDENCE PER 100,000 BY AGE GROUP (YEARS) - MALE

SITE	ALL AGES	AGE UNK	0-	5-	10-	15-	20-	25-	30-	35-	40-	45-	50-	55-	60-	65-	70-	75-	80-	85+	CRUDE RATE	%	CR 64	CR 74	ASR (W)	ICD (9th)
Lip	168	0	-	-	-	-	-	0.8	0.9	1.9	0.8	4.7	6.6	12.7	11.2	30.9	30.0	22.4	59.2	31.2	3.9	1.3	0.20	0.50	4.1	140
Tongue	63	0	0.2	-	-	-	0.3	-	0.3	0.6	2.0	2.1	2.0	9.7	6.4	14.1	3.3	8.0	2.8	-	1.5	0.5	0.12	0.21	1.7	141
Salivary gland	41	0	-	-	-	0.3	-	-	-	1.0	1.2	0.5	1.3	3.0	4.8	6.2	6.7	6.4	2.8	13.4	0.9	0.3	0.06	0.12	1.0	142
Mouth	70	0	-	-	-	-	0.3	0.3	0.3	0.6	2.0	2.6	5.3	6.7	4.8	14.1	5.5	9.6	8.5	8.9	1.6	0.5	0.11	0.21	1.8	143-5
Oropharynx	26	0	-	-	-	-	-	-	-	-	0.4	2.1	2.0	0.7	4.8	3.5	2.2	4.8	-	8.9	0.6	0.2	0.05	0.08	0.7	146
Nasopharynx	9	0	-	0.2	-	-	0.3	-	-	-	0.4	0.5	0.7	0.7	1.6	-	1.1	-	-	-	0.2	0.1	0.02	0.03	0.2	147
Hypopharynx	18	0	-	-	-	-	-	-	-	-	-	1.6	0.7	2.2	4.0	2.6	2.2	-	-	4.5	0.4	0.1	0.04	0.07	0.5	148
Pharynx unspecified	5	0	-	-	-	-	-	-	-	-	0.4	-	-	1.5	-	1.8	-	-	-	-	0.1	0.0	0.01	0.02	0.1	149
Oesophagus	102	0	-	-	-	-	-	-	0.3	0.3	0.8	2.6	3.9	9.0	15.9	21.2	12.2	20.8	11.3	13.4	2.4	0.8	0.16	0.33	2.6	150
Stomach	239	0	-	-	-	-	0.6	0.3	0.6	0.6	3.1	4.7	7.9	13.5	23.1	24.7	53.3	57.6	67.7	89.1	5.5	1.8	0.27	0.66	5.6	151
Small intestine	38	0	-	-	-	-	-	0.6	-	0.6	0.4	1.6	1.3	3.7	2.4	4.4	4.4	9.6	14.1	-	0.9	0.3	0.05	0.10	0.9	152
Colon	943	0	-	-	-	0.3	0.3	0.6	2.6	3.5	7.1	16.2	26.3	56.2	66.9	128.8	192.0	265.8	307.3	342.9	21.8	7.2	0.90	2.50	21.7	153
Rectum	472	0	-	-	-	-	-	0.3	0.8	0.6	1.9	3.1	8.9	14.4	39.0	45.4	70.6	94.3	108.9	112.8	138.0	10.9	3.6	0.57	1.40	11.4	154
Liver	85	0	0.9	-	0.2	0.5	-	-	-	0.6	0.8	1.0	2.6	4.5	6.4	13.2	10.0	22.4	22.6	35.6	2.0	0.6	0.09	0.20	2.0	155
Gallbladder etc.	34	0	-	-	-	-	-	-	-	-	0.4	1.0	2.6	1.5	1.6	3.5	8.9	9.6	14.1	-	0.8	0.3	0.04	0.10	0.8	156
Pancreas	251	0	-	-	-	-	-	-	0.6	1.0	2.7	5.2	10.5	12.7	28.7	27.4	49.9	70.5	84.6	44.5	5.8	1.9	0.31	0.69	5.9	157
Nose, sinuses etc.	15	0	-	-	-	-	0.3	-	-	-	1.2	-	0.7	0.7	1.6	2.6	-	3.2	5.6	-	0.3	0.1	0.02	0.04	0.4	160
Larynx	129	0	-	-	-	-	-	-	0.6	0.3	0.4	3.1	5.9	17.2	15.9	26.5	18.9	16.0	22.6	8.9	3.0	1.0	0.22	0.44	3.4	161
Bronchus, lung	1215	0	-	-	-	0.3	-	1.1	0.9	1.6	5.9	19.9	38.7	81.0	150.6	203.8	273.1	288.2	251.0	209.3	28.1	9.3	1.50	3.88	29.8	162
Other thoracic organs	22	0	1.1	-	-	-	-	0.8	0.9	0.3	1.2	1.0	-	-	0.8	0.9	2.2	-	-	4.5	0.5	0.2	0.03	0.05	0.5	163-4
Bone	59	0	-	0.8	1.1	4.4	1.7	2.0	0.3	1.9	0.4	1.0	0.7	1.5	0.8	2.6	2.2	-	3.2	-	4.5	1.4	0.4	0.08	0.10	1.3	170
Connective tissue	88	0	0.7	0.4	0.6	0.5	0.3	1.1	1.7	2.6	2.7	2.6	1.3	6.0	4.0	5.3	11.1	12.8	11.3	17.8	2.0	0.7	0.12	0.21	2.0	171
Mesothelioma	42	0	-	-	-	-	-	-	-	-	0.8	1.0	1.3	1.5	3.2	7.9	7.8	14.4	8.5	8.9	1.0	0.3	0.04	0.12	1.0	MES
Kaposi's sarcoma	49	0	-	-	-	-	0.3	1.7	4.0	3.5	3.5	0.5	0.7	1.5	-	0.9	-	1.6	-	-	8.9	1.1	0.4	0.08	0.08	1.0	KAP
Melanoma of skin	539	0	-	-	0.6	1.8	4.0	4.2	8.8	16.7	18.4	28.8	28.9	30.0	39.0	48.5	57.7	76.9	36.7	62.3	12.5	4.1	0.91	1.44	13.3	172
†Other skin	38	0	0.2	0.2	0.2	0.5	-	0.6	1.4	1.0	0.4	1.6	-	1.5	0.8	3.5	4.4	3.2	8.5	13.4	0.9	-	0.04	0.08	0.8	173
Breast	28	0	-	-	-	-	-	-	-	-	0.4	1.0	2.0	3.0	1.6	2.6	6.7	3.2	11.3	4.5	0.6	0.2	0.04	0.09	0.7	175
Prostate	5087	0	-	-	-	-	-	-	-	-	2.7	13.1	57.1	208.5	499.7	868.2	1315.3	1577.1	1581.8	1549.6	117.6	38.8	3.91	14.82	115.9	185
Testis	244	0	0.7	-	-	4.4	8.8	16.4	13.7	10.3	9.8	5.8	3.9	3.7	1.6	-	1.1	3.2	5.6	4.5	5.6	1.9	0.40	0.40	5.4	186
Penis	17	0	-	-	-	-	-	-	-	0.3	0.4	0.5	-	0.7	0.8	3.5	1.1	3.2	11.3	4.5	0.4	0.1	0.01	0.04	0.4	187.1-.4
Other male genital	6	0	-	-	-	-	-	-	-	-	0.4	0.5	-	0.7	-	-	1.1	-	-	8.9	0.1	0.0	0.01	0.01	0.2	187.5-.9
Bladder	712	0	-	0.4	-	0.3	-	0.3	1.4	2.9	7.8	6.8	23.0	36.0	53.4	96.2	144.3	193.7	284.8	222.6	16.5	5.4	0.66	1.86	16.2	188
Kidney etc.	327	0	2.7	0.8	-	-	0.6	-	2.3	0.6	2.7	12.6	18.4	21.7	34.3	45.0	51.1	62.4	56.4	53.4	7.6	2.5	0.48	0.96	8.3	189
Eye	34	0	0.9	-	-	0.5	0.3	-	-	0.3	0.4	-	2.0	2.2	4.8	2.6	7.8	1.6	2.8	4.5	0.8	0.3	0.06	0.11	0.9	190
Brain, nervous system	272	0	4.0	2.8	4.3	3.4	2.6	4.5	3.1	6.4	5.5	5.8	15.1	10.5	7.2	26.5	24.4	22.4	25.4	26.7	6.3	2.1	0.38	0.63	6.5	191-2
Thyroid	121	0	-	-	0.2	0.5	1.1	2.0	3.4	5.8	7.8	8.4	3.9	4.5	2.4	10.6	5.5	8.0	8.5	4.5	2.8	0.9	0.20	0.28	2.9	193
Other endocrine	15	0	0.9	0.4	0.2	0.5	0.3	-	0.3	0.6	-	-	-	-	-	1.8	-	-	-	-	0.3	0.1	0.02	0.03	0.3	194
Hodgkin's disease	86	0	0.2	0.6	1.3	2.6	2.8	4.5	2.3	2.3	1.6	1.0	3.3	2.2	3.2	2.6	1.1	3.2	-	4.5	2.0	0.7	0.14	0.16	2.0	201
Non-Hodgkin lymphoma	554	0	0.9	0.8	1.5	2.8	2.0	2.8	4.0	5.5	13.3	18.9	25.6	26.2	44.6	57.3	97.7	110.5	110.0	84.6	12.8	4.2	0.75	1.52	13.3	200,202
Multiple myeloma	163	0	-	-	-	-	0.3	-	-	0.6	0.8	3.1	5.3	12.7	18.3	23.8	30.0	38.4	42.3	49.0	3.8	1.2	0.21	0.47	4.0	203
Lymphoid leukaemia	186	0	4.5	2.5	2.1	1.3	0.9	1.1	1.4	0.3	0.8	1.6	5.3	10.5	11.2	16.8	22.2	40.0	31.0	44.5	4.3	1.4	0.22	0.41	4.4	204
Myeloid leukaemia	145	0	0.7	0.2	0.2	0.3	1.1	0.3	2.3	2.9	2.0	2.6	5.9	4.5	12.8	15.0	30.0	24.0	25.4	35.6	3.4	1.1	0.18	0.40	3.4	205
Monocytic leukaemia	5	0	-	-	-	-	-	0.3	-	-	-	-	1.3	-	-	0.9	1.1	-	-	-	0.1	0.0	0.01	0.02	0.1	206
Other leukaemia	1	0	-	-	-	-	-	-	-	-	-	-	-	-	-	-	-	-	-	4.5	0.0	0.0	0.00	0.00	0.0	207
Leukaemia unspecified	41	0	-	-	-	0.3	0.3	-	-	0.3	0.4	1.6	0.7	-	-	3.5	6.7	16.0	14.1	35.6	0.9	0.3	0.02	0.07	0.9	208
Other and unspecified	349	0	0.7	0.6	-	0.3	0.3	0.6	0.3	1.6	3.5	5.2	10.5	19.5	28.7	45.9	73.3	86.5	93.0	138.0	8.1	2.7	0.36	0.95	8.2	O&U
All sites	13153	0	19.2	11.0	12.6	25.6	29.6	47.7	59.0	82.1	120.8	203.7	349.4	686.2	1169.1	1892.5	2671.7	3229.5	3355.4	3348.6	304.2		14.08	36.90	308.7	ALL
All sites but 173	13115	0	19.0	10.8	12.4	25.1	29.6	47.1	57.6	81.1	120.5	202.1	349.4	684.7	1168.3	1888.9	2667.3	3226.3	3347.0	3335.3	303.3	100.0	14.04	36.82	307.8	ALLb

Rate from 1 case: 0.223 0.212 0.213 0.259 0.285 0.282 0.285 0.322 0.392 0.524 0.657 0.750 0.797 0.882 1.110 1.601 2.820 4.453

†Important: see notes on population page

USA, UTAH 1988-1992

ANNUAL INCIDENCE PER 100,000 BY AGE GROUP (YEARS) - FEMALE

SITE	ALL AGES	AGE UNK	0-	5-	10-	15-	20-	25-	30-	35-	40-	45-	50-	55-	60-	65-	70-	75-	80-	85+	CRUDE RATE	%	CR 64	CR 74	ASR (W)	ICD (9th)
Lip	36	0	-	-	-	-	0.3	0.6	0.9	-	0.4	0.5	1.9	1.4	0.7	3.9	2.7	2.3	10.2	12.9	0.8	0.3	0.03	0.07	**0.7**	140
Tongue	44	0	-	-	-	-	-	0.9	-	0.3	0.4	3.1	1.9	2.8	2.2	7.0	2.7	5.8	5.1	6.5	1.0	0.4	0.06	0.11	**1.0**	141
Salivary gland	21	0	-	0.2	0.2	0.3	-	0.6	-	-	0.4	2.1	1.3	1.4	-	0.8	0.9	4.6	1.7	-	0.5	0.2	0.03	0.04	**0.5**	142
Mouth	42	0	-	-	-	-	0.3	0.6	-	0.3	0.4	2.1	2.5	2.1	2.2	2.3	5.5	3.5	11.9	8.6	1.0	0.4	0.05	0.09	**0.9**	143-5
Oropharynx	7	0	-	-	-	-	-	0.3	-	-	-	-	-	0.7	2.2	-	0.9	1.2	-	-	0.2	0.1	0.02	0.02	**0.2**	146
Nasopharynx	6	0	0.2	0.2	-	-	-	-	-	-	-	-	0.6	-	-	0.8	-	2.3	-	-	0.1	0.1	0.01	0.01	**0.1**	147
Hypopharynx	7	0	-	-	-	-	-	-	-	-	-	-	0.6	-	-	1.6	1.8	-	3.4	-	0.2	0.1	0.00	0.02	**0.1**	148
Pharynx unspecified	6	0	-	-	-	-	-	-	-	-	-	-	-	0.7	0.7	1.6	-	1.2	-	2.2	0.1	0.1	0.01	0.01	**0.1**	149
Oesophagus	23	0	-	-	-	-	-	-	-	-	-	-	0.6	-	2.9	7.8	2.7	3.5	1.7	2.2	0.5	0.2	0.02	0.07	**0.5**	150
Stomach	152	0	-	-	-	-	-	-	0.3	2.0	1.5	9.5	8.5	8.8	16.3	14.6	24.3	32.4	58.1	3.5	1.4	0.15	0.31	**2.9**	151
Small intestine	40	0	-	-	-	-	-	-	0.3	1.2	1.5	2.5	1.4	2.2	4.7	5.5	5.8	6.8	6.5	0.9	0.4	0.05	0.10	**0.8**	152
Colon	873	0	-	-	-	-	0.6	2.0	4.2	7.8	13.8	17.8	44.9	61.7	86.2	119.4	164.1	235.4	230.3	19.9	8.1	0.76	1.79	**15.8**	153
Rectum	339	0	-	-	-	-	0.6	-	2.6	3.9	7.7	11.4	22.1	23.5	41.9	45.6	64.7	56.3	64.6	7.7	3.1	0.36	0.80	**6.7**	154
Liver	62	0	0.7	-	-	-	-	-	0.3	0.6	0.4	2.1	0.6	2.8	5.1	3.1	7.3	11.6	17.1	15.1	1.4	0.6	0.06	0.12	**1.2**	155
Gallbladder etc.	94	0	-	-	-	-	-	-	0.6	1.0	2.0	0.5	2.5	2.8	7.3	9.3	15.5	12.7	32.4	12.9	2.1	0.9	0.08	0.21	**1.7**	156
Pancreas	254	0	-	0.2	-	-	-	-	0.3	-	0.4	3.6	3.8	17.1	8.1	33.4	34.6	55.5	73.3	66.7	5.8	2.4	0.17	0.51	**4.4**	157
Nose, sinuses etc.	19	0	-	-	0.4	-	-	-	-	0.6	0.8	0.5	1.9	0.7	0.7	-	2.7	-	5.1	2.2	0.4	0.2	0.03	0.04	**0.4**	160
Larynx	21	0	-	-	-	-	-	0.3	-	-	0.8	-	0.6	0.7	2.9	3.1	1.8	2.3	5.1	2.2	0.5	0.2	0.03	0.05	**0.4**	161
Bronchus, lung	603	0	-	-	-	-	0.3	0.6	0.3	1.6	4.7	13.8	27.4	44.2	65.4	90.0	93.9	83.2	66.5	66.7	13.8	5.6	0.79	1.71	**13.1**	162
Other thoracic organs	13	0	-	0.2	-	-	0.3	-	-	0.3	0.4	0.5	1.3	-	-	1.6	1.8	2.3	-	-	0.3	0.1	0.02	0.03	**0.3**	163-4
Bone	33	0	0.2	0.7	2.0	0.3	0.8	1.2	0.6	0.3	-	-	1.3	-	1.5	0.8	1.8	-	1.7	2.2	0.8	0.3	0.04	0.06	**0.7**	170
Connective tissue	80	0	0.9	-	0.7	0.3	0.8	1.7	1.7	1.3	2.0	1.5	1.3	4.3	2.2	10.1	3.6	4.6	13.6	10.8	1.8	0.7	0.09	0.16	**1.7**	171
Mesothelioma	11	0	-	-	-	-	-	-	-	0.6	-	-	1.3	-	1.5	0.8	2.7	1.2	-	-	0.3	0.1	0.02	0.03	**0.3**	MES
Kaposi's sarcoma	2	0	-	-	-	-	-	-	-	-	-	-	-	-	-	0.9	-	-	-	2.2	0.0	0.0	0.00	0.00	**0.0**	KAP
Melanoma of skin	502	0	-	0.4	1.1	2.3	8.5	10.4	15.7	15.6	23.1	16.9	20.4	23.5	27.9	17.9	29.2	22.0	37.5	55.9	11.5	4.7	0.83	1.06	**11.0**	172
†Other skin	41	0	-	0.2	0.4	-	0.8	1.2	0.3	1.3	-	0.5	4.5	1.4	3.7	2.3	-	4.6	5.1	2.2	0.9	-	0.07	0.08	**0.9**	173
Breast	3394	0	-	-	-	-	0.6	5.5	17.4	49.9	93.0	158.4	197.2	232.2	285.2	350.8	382.9	376.7	400.8	333.5	77.5	31.5	5.20	8.87	**75.8**	174
Uterus unspecified	12	0	-	-	-	-	-	-	-	-	-	-	0.7	1.5	-	0.9	3.5	5.1	4.3	-	0.3	0.1	0.01	0.02	**0.2**	179
Cervix uteri	342	0	-	-	-	0.3	2.5	9.5	10.6	15.2	22.0	13.3	14.6	19.9	13.2	16.3	12.8	11.6	25.6	8.6	7.8	3.2	0.61	0.75	**7.7**	180
Placenta	7	0	-	-	-	0.3	0.3	0.6	0.3	-	-	0.5	-	-	0.8	-	-	-	-	-	0.2	0.1	0.01	0.01	**0.2**	181
Corpus uteri	833	0	-	-	-	-	0.3	1.4	2.0	5.5	11.8	22.6	38.8	78.3	97.0	108.7	128.6	93.6	78.5	38.7	19.0	7.7	1.29	2.47	**19.0**	182
Ovary etc.	468	0	-	-	0.7	1.0	0.3	1.4	3.7	8.4	8.2	17.9	23.5	39.9	39.7	47.3	45.6	52.0	56.3	51.6	10.7	4.3	0.72	1.19	**10.3**	183
Other female genital	83	0	-	-	-	-	0.8	-	0.3	1.3	1.2	2.6	2.5	3.6	8.1	6.2	5.5	12.7	22.2	19.4	1.9	0.8	0.10	0.16	**1.6**	184
Bladder	187	0	0.2	-	-	0.3	-	0.9	0.6	1.0	0.8	4.1	5.1	8.5	11.8	14.7	19.1	34.7	47.8	71.0	4.3	1.7	0.17	0.34	**3.3**	188
Kidney etc.	184	0	0.9	0.7	-	0.3	0.3	0.6	0.6	1.9	3.5	5.1	9.5	13.5	16.9	17.1	22.8	20.8	13.6	34.4	4.2	1.7	0.27	0.47	**4.1**	189
Eye	17	0	0.5	-	0.2	-	-	-	-	0.3	0.4	-	-	2.1	1.5	1.6	2.7	1.2	1.7	-	0.4	0.2	0.03	0.05	**0.4**	190
Brain, nervous system	245	0	4.2	1.8	3.8	2.1	1.4	3.7	2.3	3.6	6.3	8.7	10.8	10.7	10.3	16.3	14.6	24.3	22.2	15.1	5.6	2.3	0.35	0.50	**5.5**	191-2
Thyroid	347	0	-	-	0.4	1.8	5.9	13.0	12.0	14.6	18.4	15.9	21.0	16.4	11.0	7.0	10.0	5.8	11.9	8.6	7.9	3.2	0.65	0.74	**8.1**	193
Other endocrine	17	0	2.1	-	-	0.3	-	-	0.3	0.3	0.4	0.5	-	0.7	0.8	-	1.2	-	-	-	0.4	0.2	0.02	0.03	**0.4**	194
Hodgkin's disease	93	0	-	0.9	1.8	2.8	2.5	4.3	2.9	2.6	1.6	1.0	1.9	2.8	0.7	3.1	2.7	4.6	5.1	-	2.1	0.9	0.13	0.16	**2.0**	201
Non-Hodgkin lymphoma	469	0	-	0.4	1.1	1.3	1.7	2.0	2.9	4.5	8.2	10.3	14.6	29.2	29.4	35.7	78.4	71.6	78.5	75.3	10.7	4.3	0.53	1.10	**9.3**	200,202
Multiple myeloma	124	0	-	-	-	-	-	-	-	-	0.4	1.5	4.5	3.6	6.6	16.3	19.1	35.8	20.5	30.1	2.8	1.1	0.08	0.26	**2.2**	203
Lymphoid leukaemia	138	0	6.8	2.9	2.9	1.3	1.1	0.9	0.6	0.6	2.0	1.0	0.6	2.1	3.7	7.8	10.9	12.7	10.2	25.8	3.2	1.3	0.13	0.23	**2.9**	204
Myeloid leukaemia	131	0	0.7	0.4	0.7	0.3	0.8	0.9	2.9	2.9	2.4	1.0	3.2	2.8	9.6	5.4	11.9	27.7	22.2	21.5	3.0	1.2	0.14	0.23	**2.5**	205
Monocytic leukaemia	5	0	0.2	-	-	-	-	-	-	-	0.4	-	-	-	-	-	0.9	1.2	1.7	-	0.1	0.0	0.00	0.01	**0.1**	206
Other leukaemia	3	0	0.2	-	-	-	-	-	-	-	0.4	-	-	-	0.8	-	-	-	-	-	0.1	0.0	0.00	0.01	**0.1**	207
Leukaemia unspecified	20	0	-	-	0.2	-	-	-	-	-	-	0.5	-	0.7	2.2	1.6	-	3.5	8.5	8.6	0.5	0.2	0.02	0.03	**0.3**	208
Other and unspecified	378	0	2.1	-	-	0.3	-	0.6	0.6	1.6	4.7	3.6	7.6	18.5	22.8	39.6	43.8	67.0	83.6	139.9	8.6	3.5	0.31	0.73	**6.8**	O&U
All sites	10828	0	20.2	9.4	16.8	15.3	30.8	64.6	82.4	145.9	237.0	340.9	473.2	669.5	805.5	1044.8	1211.8	1344.9	1538.4	1517.1	247.3		14.56	25.84	**229.2**	ALL
All sites but 173	10787	0	20.2	9.2	16.4	15.3	29.9	63.4	82.1	144.6	237.0	340.4	468.8	668.1	801.8	1042.4	1211.8	1340.3	1533.3	1514.9	246.4	100.0	14.49	25.76	**228.3**	ALLb
Rate from 1 case			0.235	0.223	0.225	0.259	0.283	0.288	0.286	0.324	0.392	0.513	0.636	0.712	0.735	0.776	0.912	1.155	1.706	2.152						

†Important: see notes on population page

USA, Washington, Seattle

The Cancer Surveillance System (CSS) of the Fred Hutchinson Cancer Research Center has participated in the Surveillance, Epidemiology, and End Results (SEER) Program of the US National Cancer Institute since 1974. Its purposes are: (*a*) to provide data on the incidence of all neoplasms in the area covered by the registry, (*b*) to provide data on survival on all cancer cases, and (*c*) to serve as a resource for epidemiological studies of cancer etiology and patterns of care.

The CSS covers thirteen contiguous counties in the north-west portion of Washington State. According to the 1990 census, the population covered was 3 366 824, approximately 70% of the state population. About 76% of these reside in two main conurbations. According to the census, 88% of the population is white, 4% black, 1.5% native American, 5.5% Asian and 1% other races. Approximately 3% were of Spanish origin, of whom two thirds were white Hispanic and one third other Hispanic. The major industries in the area are logging and wood products, fishing, shipping, aerospace, biotechnology and software development.

Medical care is largely obtained from private physicians and hospitals. There is one major prepaid health maintenance organization in the Seattle area and additional smaller plans have been established in recent years. There are also military, veteran and other federal hospitals that provide service to select groups.

The primary sources of data are the medical records in the 49 area hospitals. Cases are also identified from the records in independent pathology laboratories, radiotherapy offices, surgical centres and selected physician offices. In 1990, cancer became a reportable disease in Washington State, but most health-care providers have participated voluntarily in the registry since 1974.

CSS performs computerized linkages between electronic versions of case-finding sources and its own database. Most recently, complete electronic versions of pathology reports have been incorporated into the database, eliminating the need to abstract the data from the medical record. From the electronic pathology reports, the results of all laboratory tests become part of the patient's electronic file in the database. Although it is not feasible to code all of the data for potential future analysis, it is possible to maintain the text information in a central database and if necessary the entire database can be searched by key words.

Incidence, treatment and survival data are collected and coded by CSS personnel using standardized definitions from the SEER Program. In addition to the SEER edit package, CSS uses its own package with over 450 edits, including range, inter-field, inter-record and inter-database edits.

Routinely performed validity checks include: sex versus site, histology versus organ, laterality versus site, histology behaviour code versus extent of disease, and consistency of dates. Duplicates are identified and eliminated via routine searches for similar first and last name, birthdate, social security number and address.

Current follow-up information is available for approximately 95% of all cases, through both active and passive collection. Computerized matching of registry files is performed quarterly with Washington State death certificates, and annually with data from several state and federal agencies including the Department of Motor Vehicles, Health Care Financing Administration and the Bureau of Vital Statistics. The State of Washington maintains a Comprehensive Hospital Abstract Reporting System (CHARS), and linkages with this database provide a means of assessing case-finding from area hospitals. Non-cancer as well as cancer-related hospital admissions are also used to update follow-up information for cancer patients already registered.

Almost 80% of the cases are actively followed by registry staff at area hospitals. CSS personnel perform active follow-up for all other cases. Centralized follow-up letters are generated to request the physician's last date of contact with a patient, and to enquire about missing race, stage and treatment information.

In 1974, less than 1% of all incident cases were diagnosed and treated solely in an outpatient setting. In 1992, this percentage had increased to 35%, necessitating major changes in data collection methods, particularly regarding collection of treatment information. CSS developed the Treatment Query System, which is incorporated into the follow-up letter generation program. CSS utilized the NCI Physician Data Query (PDQ) State-of-the-Art Treatment Information guidelines to generate treatment queries that are appropriate for each combination of site, stage, tumour histology, age, and other factors that may affect treatment decisions.

CSS serves as a resource for numerous descriptive, correlational, and population-based case–control and cohort studies of cancer etiology as well as for studies of survival and cancer care. CSS routinely responds to requests for cancer-related information from physicians, hospitals, local and regional health authorities, as well as media representatives and members of the public.

D.B. Thomas
J.L Standford
M. Potts

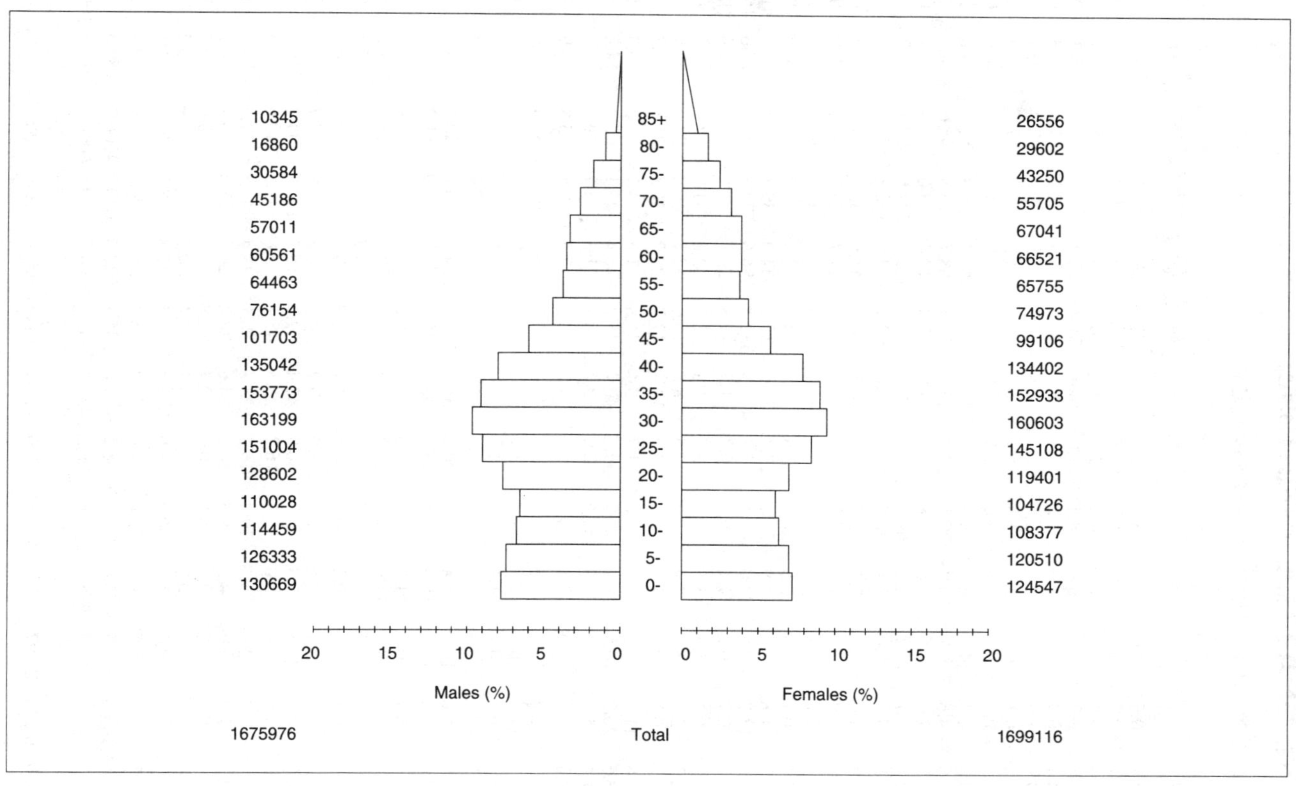

USA, Washington, Seattle

Source of population: average annual 1988-92

Estimate: NCI estimates based on U.S. Bureau of Census population estimates by county for the years 1988–92.

Notes to tables overleaf:

† 173 does not include basal cell or squamous cell carcinoma

Screening programmes in the area:

Hospitals in the area periodically offer screening programmes. These, however, are conducted separately from registry activities.

USA, WASHINGTON, SEATTLE 1988-1992

ANNUAL INCIDENCE PER 100,000 BY AGE GROUP (YEARS) - MALE

SITE	ALL AGES	AGE UNK	0-	5-	10-	15-	20-	25-	30-	35-	40-	45-	50-	55-	60-	65-	70-	75-	80-	85+	CRUDE RATE	%	CR 64	CR 74	ASR (W)	ICD (9th)
Lip	195	0	-	-	-	-	0.2	0.1	0.2	0.4	0.6	2.0	1.8	4.3	8.3	13.3	12.8	20.9	15.4	30.9	2.3	0.5	0.09	0.22	**1.9**	*140*
Tongue	252	0	-	-	-	-	0.2	0.1	0.1	1.2	0.9	4.7	6.6	6.2	13.9	14.7	16.4	13.1	20.2	13.5	3.0	0.6	0.17	0.32	**2.6**	*141*
Salivary gland	89	0	-	-	0.2	0.2	-	0.3	0.2	0.4	0.4	1.4	1.1	4.0	2.3	3.9	6.2	6.5	9.5	5.8	1.1	0.2	0.05	0.10	**0.9**	*142*
Mouth	260	0	0.2	-	-	0.2	0.3	0.1	-	0.5	0.9	3.9	6.8	8.4	11.6	14.4	21.2	22.2	9.5	11.6	3.1	0.6	0.16	0.34	**2.7**	*143-5*
Oropharynx	111	0	-	-	-	-	-	-	0.4	0.5	0.9	0.6	2.9	5.6	5.3	8.1	6.2	3.9	7.1	1.9	1.3	0.3	0.08	0.15	**1.2**	*146*
Nasopharynx	56	0	-	-	0.2	-	0.3	0.4	0.2	0.9	1.0	0.6	0.8	1.6	1.3	1.8	4.0	1.3	1.2	3.9	0.7	0.1	0.04	0.07	**0.6**	*147*
Hypopharynx	109	0	-	-	-	-	-	-	-	-	0.1	0.6	3.2	4.3	5.9	8.1	8.4	5.9	7.1	7.7	1.3	0.3	0.07	0.15	**1.2**	*148*
Pharynx unspecified	48	0	-	-	-	-	-	-	-	0.3	-	0.5	4.0	2.6	2.5	4.0	3.9	1.2	-	0.6	0.1	0.04	0.07	**0.5**	*149*
Oesophagus	483	0	-	-	-	-	-	-	0.8	1.3	4.7	6.0	14.9	23.1	35.1	38.5	41.2	30.8	52.2	5.8	1.2	0.25	0.62	**4.9**	*150*
Stomach	762	0	-	0.2	-	-	-	-	0.9	2.6	4.6	6.9	10.2	20.5	32.0	43.1	55.3	68.7	73.5	98.6	9.1	1.9	0.39	0.88	**7.5**	*151*
Small intestine	119	0	-	-	-	-	0.5	-	0.2	0.5	1.0	1.6	2.6	2.8	5.3	4.9	5.8	12.4	13.0	5.8	1.4	0.3	0.07	0.13	**1.2**	*152*
Colon	2778	0	-	-	-	0.4	0.2	0.7	1.6	2.5	6.7	13.2	32.3	69.5	111.3	159.3	221.3	315.8	347.6	409.9	33.2	6.9	1.19	3.09	**26.5**	*153*
Rectum	1378	0	-	-	-	-	0.2	0.4	0.7	2.1	4.4	9.6	22.1	38.2	64.7	80.0	102.7	143.9	138.8	141.1	16.4	3.4	0.71	1.63	**13.6**	*154*
Liver	351	0	0.5	-	0.2	0.2	0.2	0.1	0.4	0.9	1.6	3.7	8.4	5.3	13.2	20.7	20.4	41.9	33.2	34.8	4.2	0.9	0.17	0.38	**3.5**	*155*
Gallbladder etc.	168	0	-	-	-	0.2	-	-	0.1	0.3	0.9	0.4	1.6	4.3	5.9	6.0	12.4	17.7	29.7	40.6	2.0	0.4	0.07	0.16	**1.6**	*156*
Pancreas	760	0	-	-	-	-	0.2	-	0.1	1.3	2.5	5.7	10.5	18.3	29.4	47.0	64.6	77.2	86.6	83.1	9.1	1.9	0.34	0.90	**7.3**	*157*
Nose, sinuses etc.	65	0	-	-	-	0.2	0.5	0.3	0.1	0.4	0.1	1.8	0.5	0.6	3.6	3.9	4.0	3.3	1.2	7.7	0.8	0.2	0.04	0.08	**0.7**	*160*
Larynx	528	0	-	-	-	-	-	0.1	0.1	0.5	1.8	3.9	11.8	21.1	29.7	38.6	38.1	34.0	39.1	11.6	6.3	1.3	0.35	0.73	**5.5**	*161*
Bronchus, lung	6332	0	-	-	-	0.2	0.2	0.5	1.1	4.6	13.8	42.5	93.0	182.1	314.7	431.8	537.3	586.6	577.7	483.3	75.6	15.6	3.26	8.11	**63.2**	*162*
Other thoracic organs	36	0	0.3	0.2	-	0.4	0.3	0.4	0.6	0.1	0.7	0.2	1.1	0.3	0.7	1.4	1.3	-	-	-	0.4	0.1	0.03	0.04	**0.4**	*163-4*
Bone	88	0	0.2	0.2	1.6	1.6	0.9	0.7	0.5	0.7	0.4	1.8	1.6	1.2	2.6	1.8	2.2	2.0	1.2	7.7	1.1	0.2	0.07	0.09	**1.0**	*170*
Connective tissue	244	0	1.4	0.3	1.4	0.4	0.9	0.7	1.6	2.2	2.7	3.1	2.9	5.0	7.6	8.8	10.6	13.7	19.0	23.2	2.9	0.6	0.15	0.25	**2.5**	*171*
Mesothelioma	225	0	-	-	-	-	-	0.1	-	-	0.1	0.8	1.6	5.0	9.9	14.4	17.7	22.2	46.3	25.1	2.7	0.6	0.09	0.25	**2.1**	*MES*
Kaposi's sarcoma	530	0	-	-	-	-	1.2	8.6	17.3	19.8	11.7	8.5	5.5	1.6	1.7	0.4	1.8	1.3	4.7	-	6.3	1.3	0.38	0.39	**4.7**	*KAP*
Melanoma of skin	1191	0	-	0.2	0.2	1.8	2.6	6.1	8.9	12.6	20.3	20.5	29.4	32.3	39.6	40.7	48.2	46.4	45.1	67.7	14.2	2.9	0.87	1.32	**12.2**	*172*
†Other skin	100	0	0.2	-	-	0.4	0.5	0.7	0.4	1.4	1.2	1.6	1.6	1.6	2.0	3.2	3.1	11.1	4.7	9.7	1.2		0.06	0.09	**1.0**	*173*
Breast	75	0	-	-	-	-	-	-	-	0.3	-	1.0	2.1	4.3	2.0	4.2	3.5	7.2	7.1	5.8	0.9	0.2	0.05	0.09	**0.8**	*175*
Prostate	14042	0	0.2	-	-	-	-	-	0.1	2.8	12.8	89.0	230.5	562.7	1045.1	1465.1	1705.5	1691.6	1637.5	167.6	34.7	4.49	17.04	**131.5**	*185*
Testis	529	0	0.3	-	0.2	2.2	9.3	12.2	16.5	11.8	11.0	6.5	2.4	1.9	1.7	1.1	0.9	2.0	1.2	-	6.3	1.3	0.38	0.39	**5.1**	*186*
Penis	36	0	-	-	-	-	-	0.1	-	-	0.3	0.4	1.1	0.9	1.7	0.7	2.7	2.6	4.7	5.8	0.4	0.1	0.02	0.04	**0.4**	*187.1-.4*
Other male genital	26	0	-	0.2	-	0.2	-	-	0.1	0.1	0.4	-	0.9	0.9	1.0	1.1	0.9	0.3	0.1	1.0	0.3	0.1	0.01	0.02	**0.3**	*187.5-.9*
Bladder	2423	0	0.2	-	0.2	0.4	0.8	0.9	1.5	5.1	5.6	10.2	28.4	63.3	90.8	134.7	211.1	254.4	306.0	330.6	28.9	6.0	1.04	2.77	**23.1**	*188*
Kidney etc.	1002	0	2.0	1.4	0.2	-	0.2	0.4	0.7	2.7	5.3	13.0	18.9	33.8	43.6	48.4	75.7	73.9	81.9	81.2	12.0	2.5	0.61	1.23	**10.3**	*189*
Eye	74	0	1.7	0.2	0.2	-	-	0.1	0.1	0.4	0.7	0.8	1.6	2.8	3.3	1.4	5.8	1.3	2.4	1.9	0.9	0.2	0.06	0.10	**0.9**	*190*
Brain, nervous system	683	0	5.4	4.9	2.8	2.7	2.5	3.7	3.7	5.6	7.8	8.3	11.0	20.2	19.2	22.5	31.4	32.0	20.2	15.5	8.2	1.7	0.49	0.76	**7.6**	*191-2*
Thyroid	209	0	-	-	-	-	1.7	1.9	2.5	4.4	2.7	4.9	2.6	4.0	5.3	4.9	6.2	5.9	8.3	7.7	2.5	0.5	0.15	0.21	**2.1**	*193*
Other endocrine	31	0	1.7	0.2	0.3	0.4	0.3	-	0.1	-	0.1	-	0.3	0.6	0.7	1.1	0.9	0.7	-	-	0.4	0.1	0.02	0.03	**0.4**	*194*
Hodgkin's disease	292	0	-	0.8	1.0	4.7	5.0	7.0	4.3	3.5	3.7	4.1	2.6	2.5	3.0	3.2	4.4	4.6	5.9	7.7	3.5	0.7	0.21	0.25	**3.1**	*201*
Non-Hodgkin lymphoma	1599	0	1.5	1.1	2.3	2.4	2.3	6.8	9.7	15.0	13.2	20.6	31.3	43.7	46.9	62.4	89.4	115.1	112.7	94.7	19.1	3.9	0.98	1.74	**16.0**	*200,202*
Multiple myeloma	442	0	-	-	-	-	-	0.1	-	0.1	1.5	2.9	5.0	11.2	16.2	25.3	48.2	43.8	49.8	40.6	5.3	1.1	0.19	0.55	**4.2**	*203*
Lymphoid leukaemia	509	0	6.6	3.3	1.9	1.8	0.8	0.3	0.2	1.3	1.3	2.6	8.1	12.4	16.2	25.3	30.1	33.4	41.5	71.5	6.1	1.3	0.28	0.56	**5.7**	*204*
Myeloid leukaemia	394	0	0.5	0.2	-	0.5	1.1	2.5	0.9	2.5	2.2	4.7	4.5	9.3	10.6	24.6	28.3	26.2	28.5	36.7	4.7	1.0	0.20	0.46	**3.9**	*205*
Monocytic leukaemia	19	0	0.2	0.2	0.2	-	-	0.1	0.1	0.1	0.1	0.2	0.3	0.6	0.3	0.4	1.8	-	-	3.9	0.2	0.0	0.01	0.02	**0.2**	*206*
Other leukaemia	17	0	0.5	-	-	-	-	-	-	-	-	-	0.3	0.6	1.0	0.7	0.4	0.7	3.6	1.9	0.2	0.0	0.01	0.02	**0.2**	*207*
Leukaemia unspecified	89	0	0.5	0.5	-	0.4	0.3	0.1	0.1	-	0.4	0.4	1.3	0.9	3.0	3.2	5.3	11.8	8.3	17.4	1.1	0.2	0.04	0.08	**0.9**	*208*
Other and unspecified	833	0	0.6	0.2	-	0.2	0.3	0.3	0.5	2.5	4.3	5.5	9.7	18.6	31.0	44.2	58.4	79.1	104.4	164.3	9.9	2.1	0.37	0.88	**8.0**	*O&U*
All sites	40582	0	24.2	13.9	12.9	21.8	33.7	57.0	76.8	112.6	144.5	243.5	486.6	926.1	1608.3	2461.6	3335.1	3920.3	4043.9	4106.3	484.3		18.81	47.79	**395.5**	*ALL*
All sites but 173	40482	0	24.0	13.9	12.9	21.4	33.3	56.3	76.5	111.2	143.4	241.9	485.1	924.6	1606.3	2458.4	3332.0	3909.2	4039.1	4096.6	483.1	100.0	18.75	47.71	**394.6**	*ALLb*

| Rate from 1 case | | | 0.153 | 0.158 | 0.175 | 0.182 | 0.156 | 0.132 | 0.123 | 0.130 | 0.148 | 0.197 | 0.263 | 0.310 | 0.330 | 0.351 | 0.443 | 0.654 | 1.186 | 1.933 |

†Important: see notes on population page

USA, WASHINGTON, SEATTLE 1988-1992

ANNUAL INCIDENCE PER 100,000 BY AGE GROUP (YEARS) - FEMALE

SITE	ALL AGES	AGE UNK	0-	5-	10-	15-	20-	25-	30-	35-	40-	45-	50-	55-	60-	65-	70-	75-	80-	85+	CRUDE RATE	%	CR 64	CR 74	ASR (W)	ICD (9th)
Lip	35	0	-	-	-	-	-	-	0.1	0.1	0.3	0.6	0.5	0.6	0.6	2.1	2.2	1.4	2.7	1.5	0.4	0.1	0.01	0.04	0.3	140
Tongue	134	0	-	-	-	-	0.2	-	0.1	0.7	0.4	0.8	2.1	5.8	6.9	4.8	6.1	8.8	7.4	5.3	1.6	0.4	0.09	0.14	1.2	141
Salivary gland	80	0	-	-	-	-	0.3	0.4	0.4	1.2	0.9	1.6	0.8	0.9	2.4	4.5	2.9	1.4	2.0	4.5	0.9	0.2	0.04	0.08	0.7	142
Mouth	215	0	-	-	-	-	-	0.3	0.5	0.5	1.2	1.2	4.8	6.1	10.5	12.2	12.6	11.6	5.4	6.8	2.5	0.6	0.13	0.25	1.9	143-5
Oropharynx	73	0	-	-	-	-	-	-	0.1	0.1	0.4	1.6	2.1	4.5	3.3	5.0	4.6	2.7	1.5		0.9	0.2	0.04	0.09	0.7	146
Nasopharynx	38	0	-	0.2	0.2	-	0.5	-	0.2	-	1.0	0.6	0.3	0.9	0.6	2.7	1.1	1.4	-	-	0.4	0.1	0.02	0.04	0.4	147
Hypopharynx	41	0	-	-	-	-	-	-	-	-	0.2	0.3	2.1	3.6	1.5	2.5	2.3	-	2.3	0.5	0.1	0.03	0.05	0.4	148
Pharynx unspecified	35	0	-	-	-	-	-	-	-	-	-	0.5	1.8	1.5	1.2	2.2	2.8	1.4	3.0	0.4	0.1	0.02	0.04	0.3	149
Oesophagus	219	0	-	-	-	-	-	-	0.1	0.1	0.4	1.9	4.9	7.8	12.8	14.0	20.3	19.6	8.3	2.6	0.6	0.08	0.21	1.6	150
Stomach	426	0	-	-	-	-	0.8	0.4	1.7	2.2	2.4	4.0	7.0	12.9	13.1	20.1	31.9	38.5	52.7	5.0	1.3	0.16	0.32	3.0	151
Small intestine	100	0	-	-	-	-	0.1	0.1	0.3	0.7	1.4	1.6	2.1	5.1	3.3	5.0	4.6	8.1	1.2	0.3	0.06	0.10	0.8	152
Colon	2903	0	-	-	-	0.4	0.2	1.1	1.5	3.5	8.0	12.5	28.8	49.0	77.6	106.5	168.4	236.8	294.6	328.4	34.2	8.5	0.91	2.29	20.2	153
Rectum	1127	0	-	-	-	-	0.3	0.6	1.0	1.4	5.5	8.9	16.3	26.5	38.2	50.7	62.5	68.4	95.3	85.1	13.3	3.3	0.49	1.06	8.8	154
Liver	178	0	0.5	-	-	-	-	0.1	0.1	0.4	0.6	0.4	2.9	3.0	7.5	7.8	9.3	15.7	12.2	10.5	2.1	0.5	0.08	0.16	1.4	155
Gallbladder etc.	220	0	-	-	-	-	0.3	-	0.2	0.5	0.7	0.6	1.3	4.3	6.3	7.8	11.5	15.7	25.0	26.4	2.6	0.6	0.07	0.17	1.5	156
Pancreas	937	0	0.2	-	0.2	-	-	0.3	0.4	1.2	1.3	3.8	10.4	15.2	24.7	39.7	57.1	71.2	93.2	103.9	11.0	2.8	0.29	0.77	6.6	157
Nose, sinuses etc.	36	0	-	0.2	-	-	-	0.3	-	0.3	0.4	-	0.8	0.6	1.2	0.3	2.2	1.8	2.7	3.0	0.4	0.1	0.02	0.03	0.3	160
Larynx	130	0	-	-	-	-	-	0.1	0.2	0.4	0.4	1.2	4.0	3.6	6.9	6.9	7.9	5.5	4.1	1.5	1.5	0.4	0.09	0.16	1.2	161
Bronchus, lung	4413	0	-	-	-	0.2	0.5	1.0	1.0	2.1	10.4	29.1	73.9	136.0	197.2	242.2	293.0	298.3	220.9	138.6	51.9	13.0	2.26	4.93	37.6	162
Other thoracic organs	24	0	0.5	-	0.2	-	-	-	0.2	0.5	0.3	-	0.3	-	0.6	-	2.5	0.5	0.7	-	0.3	0.1	0.01	0.03	0.2	163-4
Bone	79	0	0.3	1.2	1.3	1.5	1.3	0.3	0.7	0.5	1.3	0.8	1.1	0.6	1.5	0.6	1.1	1.4	1.4	0.8	0.9	0.2	0.06	0.07	0.9	170
Connective tissue	202	0	2.1	0.8	0.7	0.8	0.8	1.0	1.0	2.0	1.3	2.8	2.7	3.3	4.5	5.7	6.5	9.2	6.1	12.0	2.4	0.6	0.12	0.18	2.0	171
Mesothelioma	48	0	-	-	-	-	-	-	0.1	0.3	0.6	0.4	0.5	0.3	1.8	2.1	2.2	4.6	3.4	1.5	0.6	0.1	0.02	0.04	0.4	MES
Kaposi's sarcoma	5	0	-	-	-	0.2	-	0.1	-	-	-	-	-	-	-	-	-	1.4	-	-	0.1	0.0	0.00	0.00	0.0	KAP
Melanoma of skin	1127	0	0.2	-	-	2.1	7.2	11.0	13.4	16.6	19.6	20.2	24.3	21.9	25.0	26.8	25.5	25.4	27.0	17.3	13.3	3.3	0.81	1.07	10.7	172
†Other skin	104	0	-	-	0.6	0.6	0.5	1.0	0.5	1.3	1.8	0.8	1.6	2.1	2.1	2.1	3.9	1.8	7.4	3.8	1.2		0.06	0.09	0.9	173
Breast	10380	0	-	-	-	-	0.2	7.0	25.5	56.4	119.9	195.1	234.8	285.9	358.1	415.0	457.0	467.0	445.2	433.0	122.2	30.5	6.41	10.77	92.5	174
Uterus unspecified	8	0	-	-	-	-	-	-	0.1	-	-	-	-	0.3	0.3	1.1	-	-	1.5	0.1	0.0	0.00	0.01	0.1	179
Cervix uteri	791	0	-	-	-	0.2	2.5	8.8	12.5	14.9	15.3	14.9	20.3	13.4	15.6	19.7	10.8	8.8	10.1	13.6	9.3	2.3	0.59	0.74	7.6	180
Placenta	13	0	-	-	-	0.2	0.8	0.1	0.4	0.1	-	0.4	-	-	-	-	-	-	-		0.2	0.0	0.01	0.01	0.1	181
Corpus uteri	2225	0	-	-	-	-	-	0.6	2.2	4.3	9.2	21.8	42.7	67.2	103.4	119.9	135.7	127.6	85.1	70.0	26.2	6.5	1.26	2.54	19.6	182
Ovary etc.	1359	0	0.2	0.3	-	0.2	1.5	2.9	3.4	7.2	9.1	17.2	22.9	46.2	48.7	57.3	65.0	62.9	69.6	64.0	16.0	4.0	0.80	1.41	11.9	183
Other female genital	279	0	0.2	-	-	0.2	0.2	0.4	0.6	1.8	1.0	3.6	3.7	6.4	6.3	7.5	15.1	15.7	23.0	28.6	3.3	0.8	0.12	0.24	2.1	184
Bladder	786	0	-	-	-	-	0.5	0.6	0.7	1.6	1.6	2.8	12.0	19.2	26.2	39.1	40.9	50.4	56.1	78.3	9.3	2.3	0.33	0.73	6.1	188
Kidney etc.	641	0	1.8	0.3	-	0.4	-	1.0	0.7	0.9	2.7	7.1	15.5	13.1	21.0	31.3	27.6	38.8	50.0	31.6	7.5	1.9	0.32	0.62	5.5	189
Eye	66	0	1.1	-	-	-	0.2	0.1	0.6	0.5	0.1	0.2	1.3	1.5	0.9	3.6	2.5	2.3	4.7	1.5	0.8	0.2	0.03	0.06	0.6	190
Brain, nervous system	504	0	3.1	4.5	1.8	2.3	1.5	2.1	2.6	3.4	4.8	8.1	6.9	12.2	9.6	14.6	21.9	22.7	16.2	9.0	5.9	1.5	0.31	0.50	5.1	191-2
Thyroid	628	0	-	0.2	0.4	2.5	5.9	9.5	9.5	12.7	12.1	13.5	9.6	10.6	8.1	7.5	9.0	7.9	8.1	7.5	7.4	1.8	0.47	0.55	6.2	193
Other endocrine	26	0	0.8	0.2	0.2	-	0.2	-	0.1	0.3	0.3	0.3	-	0.9	1.2	-	-	1.4	-	-	0.3	0.1	0.02	0.03	0.3	194
Hodgkin's disease	226	0	0.2	-	2.0	3.4	5.5	4.7	2.9	2.4	1.9	2.0	0.8	2.4	3.0	3.3	4.7	5.5	3.4	2.3	2.7	0.7	0.16	0.20	2.4	201
Non-Hodgkin lymphoma	1227	0	0.8	0.5	-	1.5	1.3	2.9	3.4	3.9	10.1	10.5	18.1	24.6	35.8	52.5	62.1	78.6	83.1	71.5	14.4	3.6	0.57	1.14	10.0	200,202
Multiple myeloma	385	0	-	-	-	-	-	0.3	-	0.7	0.9	3.6	4.5	7.9	12.9	19.4	23.0	28.7	34.5	19.6	4.5	1.1	0.15	0.37	3.0	203
Lymphoid leukaemia	340	0	5.9	2.3	1.1	0.8	0.5	0.4	1.0	0.3	1.2	2.2	2.4	5.8	5.1	11.0	17.2	19.9	30.4	19.6	4.0	1.0	0.15	0.29	3.1	204
Myeloid leukaemia	320	0	1.1	-	0.7	1.3	1.0	1.0	1.1	1.2	2.2	3.6	3.5	6.4	5.1	11.6	17.2	13.4	25.0	25.6	3.8	0.9	0.14	0.29	2.7	205
Monocytic leukaemia	16	0	-	-	-	-	0.2	0.1	0.1	-	-	-	-	0.3	0.9	0.6	0.7	0.9	1.4	0.8	0.2	0.0	0.01	0.01	0.1	206
Other leukaemia	9	0	0.3	-	-	-	-	-	-	-	-	-	-	-	0.6	-	0.4	0.9	1.4	-	0.1	0.0	0.00	0.01	0.1	207
Leukaemia unspecified	70	0	0.3	0.2	-	-	0.2	0.3	0.1	0.1	0.3	0.8	0.3	0.6	2.1	1.2	4.3	3.2	7.4	9.0	0.8	0.2	0.03	0.05	0.5	208
Other and unspecified	931	0	0.6	-	-	0.4	0.5	0.3	1.2	1.6	1.2	4.4	7.5	19.8	24.4	36.1	55.3	56.4	81.1	133.3	11.0	2.7	0.31	0.77	6.6	O&U
All sites	34159	0	20.1	10.8	9.4	19.1	34.8	61.5	91.3	149.9	253.7	403.4	594.9	844.3	1140.7	1413.2	1698.6	1860.8	1918.8	1844.4	402.1		18.17	33.73	290.6	ALL
All sites but 173	34055	0	20.1	10.8	8.9	18.5	34.3	60.5	90.8	148.6	251.9	402.6	593.3	842.2	1138.6	1411.1	1694.6	1858.9	1911.3	1840.6	400.9	100.0	18.11	33.63	289.6	ALLb

Rate from 1 case   0.161 0.166 0.185 0.191 0.168 0.138 0.125 0.131 0.149 0.202 0.267 0.304 0.301 0.298 0.359 0.462 0.676 0.753

†Important: see notes on population page

USA, The 'SEER' Program

The Surveillance, Epidemiology and End Results (SEER) Program is a continuing project of the Surveillance Program of the National Cancer Institute (NCI). The Program was initiated in 1973 as an outgrowth of two earlier NCI programmes: the End Results Program and the three National Cancer Surveys. Data are classified according to sex, race, age and residence of the patient; anatomical site and histological type of cancer as well as first course of treatment.

The aims of the programme can be summarized as follows: (1) to determine the incidence of cancer in selected geographical areas of the USA in relation to demographic and social characteristics of the population; (2) to estimate cancer incidence for the USA on an annual basis; (3) to monitor trends in the incidence of individual primary sites and histological types of cancer in relation to geographical area and the demographic and social characteristics of the population; (4) to determine periodically the survival experience of cancer patients in selected geographical areas; (5) to monitor trends in cancer patient survival in relation to site of cancer, extent of disease, type of therapy and to identify demographic, socioeconomic, and other parameters of prognostic importance; (6) to identify possible etiological factors by conducting studies which can reveal groups of the population at high or low cancer risk, which may be defined by social, occupational, environmental, dietary or other characteristics, and by drug history; (7) to promote specialist training in epidemiology and biostatistics, and in the methodology, operation and management of cancer registries.

Participants in the SEER Program were selected on the basis of their ability to operate and maintain a population-based cancer reporting system and for their population sub-groups which were of special epidemiological interest rather than the degree to which the SEER areas are representative of the demographic characteristics of the US population. Seven participants began collecting data for cases diagnosed in 1973, one began with 1974 and one began in 1975. (The nine participants include the five states of Connecticut, Iowa, New Mexico, Utah and Hawaii and four metropolitan areas: the San Francisco Bay area in California, the Detroit metropolitan area in Michigan, the Atlanta, Georgia metropolitan area and the Seattle, Washington area.) This represents about 10% of the total population of the US and is fairly representative with respect to selected demographic variables. With regard to race, blacks are under-represented whereas other minority populations (Chinese, Japanese, Hawaiians and American Indians) are over-represented. Rural populations, especially rural blacks, are also under-represented. In addition to contributing to SEER, each of these nine SEER Programs reports data from their own registry in this volume.

Each participant is required to maintain a cancer information reporting system in its geographical area of coverage; to utilize abstracts of records of all cancer patients resident in the area who are seen in any hospital in or outside the coverage area; to abstract all death certificates on which cancer is mentioned for residents dying within the area, as well as those for any case listed in the reporting system; to utilize the records of private laboratories, radiotherapy units and nursing homes to ensure complete coverage of cases, and to maintain a reporting system so as to produce valid incidence rates within 13 months after the end of each calendar year.

All participants are required to report all malignant and *in situ* neoplasms as defined in ICD-O, excepting papillary, squamous, basal cell and carcinomas NOS of skin. They must collect complete information about the extent of disease, and the first course of cancer-directed therapy on all patients diagnosed and residing in the area and should, by every possible means, obtain active follow-up on all cases.

The data collected must include sufficient detail for each cancer to be classified according to the variables described in the Code Manual of the SEER Program and hence provide to the NCI computer tapes which contain data on the incidence of cancer, extent of disease at time of diagnosis, cancer site and type, tumour-directed therapy, and patient survival information. Neither the patient's name nor the name of the hospital is provided to NCI. Each participant is responsible for consolidating all data concerning an individual cancer case into one record. The total file for each area is then submitted to the NCI. Data are computer-edited for legitimate codes and for internal consistency by both the participant and the NCI.

Participants are asked to cooperate with the NCI field staff to re-abstract samples of hospital medical records, and by providing a review of various sources of case identification, such as pathology logs, diagnostic indices, radiotherapy schedules, and autopsy reports, to ensure that all cancer cases are being reported.

Staff members attend various workshops and meetings of the SEER Program to ensure that all staff implement new codes and procedures in the same manner and to allow the exchange of ideas and problems among the various participants. For example, when the ICD-O was being field-tested and it included a new lymphoma section, special workshops were given in the different registries to ensure understanding and comparability.

The registries are encouraged to maintain core staff of professional and technical people available for: (a) conducting and reporting detailed analyses of the data in the registry, together with presentation of the data on which they are based; (b) responding to NCI requests to participate in collaborative epidemiological studies within the SEER Program; (c) developing etiological hypotheses, based on analyses of the registry data and on research opportunities in the local area, and formulating study plans to test these hypotheses; (d) conducting the administrative activities necessary to maintain the cooperation of physicians and hospitals in special studies.

Mortality tapes containing data on all deaths occurring within the USA are obtained annually from the National Center for Health Statistics (NCHS). From these tapes, a file of all cancer deaths classifiable by age, sex, race and cancer site is extracted so that cancer mortality for the entire USA and each SEER area can be determined.

Each year since 1985 the NCI has published an 'Annual Cancer Statistics Review', which comprises principally SEER data (incidence), and survival and mortality from NCHS. These publications are available free on request. The most recent available Annual Cancer Statistics Review is for the years 1973–93 on the SEER WEB page www-seer.ims.nci.nih.gov.

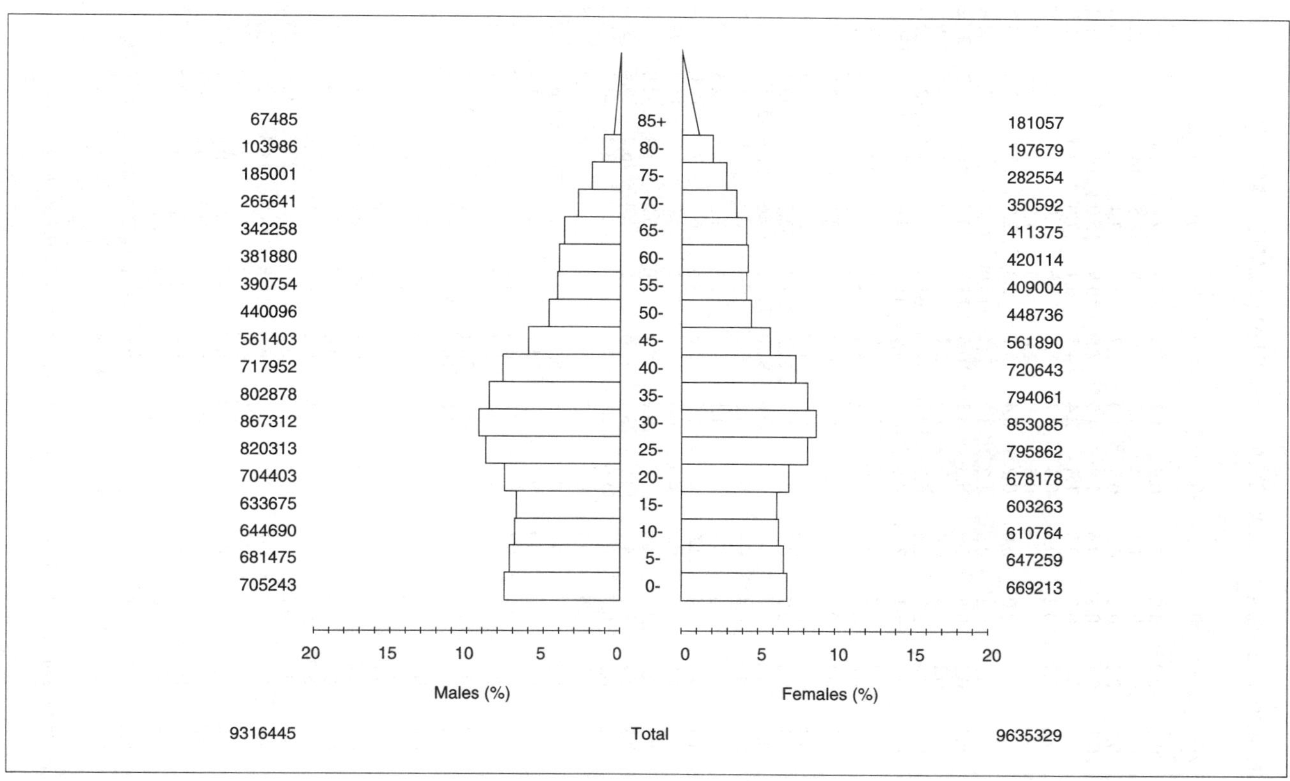

USA, SEER: White
Source of population: average annual 1988-92
Estimate: NCI estimates based on U.S. Bureau of Census population estimates by county for the years 1988–92.

Notes to tables overleaf:
† 173 does not include basal cell or squamous cell carcinoma

USA, SEER: WHITE 1988-1992

ANNUAL INCIDENCE PER 100,000 BY AGE GROUP (YEARS) - MALE

SITE	ALL AGES	AGE UNK	0-	5-	10-	15-	20-	25-	30-	35-	40-	45-	50-	55-	60-	65-	70-	75-	80-	85+	CRUDE RATE	%	CR 64	CR 74	ASR (W)	ICD (9th)
Lip	1155	0	-	-	-	-	0.1	0.2	0.5	0.4	0.9	1.3	3.3	4.8	7.1	12.1	14.2	16.6	20.8	23.7	2.5	0.5	0.09	0.22	**1.9**	140
Tongue	1415	0	0.0	-	-	0.1	0.1	0.2	0.4	1.1	1.4	3.5	6.0	9.5	11.8	14.6	14.2	12.5	11.7	10.1	3.0	0.6	0.17	0.31	**2.5**	141
Salivary gland	567	0	-	-	0.1	0.2	0.1	0.2	0.2	0.5	0.9	1.0	1.7	2.1	3.4	5.1	6.5	6.8	7.5	12.2	1.2	0.2	0.05	0.11	**1.0**	142
Mouth	1685	0	0.0	0.0	-	0.1	0.1	0.1	0.3	0.6	1.9	4.5	7.5	10.9	15.0	14.7	17.1	18.2	14.2	16.6	3.6	0.7	0.21	0.36	**3.0**	143-5
Oropharynx	903	0	-	-	-	-	-	0.0	0.1	0.5	1.3	2.4	4.5	6.4	7.8	9.5	7.8	8.0	6.7	4.7	1.9	0.4	0.12	0.20	**1.6**	146
Nasopharynx	259	0	-	0.0	0.1	0.1	0.2	0.1	0.2	0.2	0.4	0.7	1.1	1.6	2.0	2.6	1.7	1.9	0.2	3.0	0.6	0.1	0.03	0.06	**0.5**	147
Hypopharynx	758	0	-	-	-	-	-	-	-	-	0.3	1.0	2.8	4.5	7.9	9.9	9.8	7.5	5.8	5.6	1.6	0.3	0.08	0.18	**1.3**	148
Pharynx unspecified	242	0	-	-	-	0.0	-	-	0.0	0.0	0.2	0.4	0.7	2.3	2.2	2.1	2.6	3.7	1.5	2.4	0.5	0.1	0.03	0.05	**0.4**	149
Oesophagus	2657	0	-	-	-	0.0	-	0.1	0.2	0.5	1.2	3.7	7.4	14.0	21.4	29.0	35.0	39.6	33.9	38.5	5.7	1.2	0.24	0.56	**4.5**	150
Stomach	4669	0	-	0.0	-	0.0	0.2	0.2	0.6	1.3	3.3	6.2	10.5	18.2	30.7	41.4	61.7	77.2	91.2	117.4	10.0	2.0	0.36	0.87	**7.5**	151
Small intestine	692	0	-	0.0	-	0.0	0.1	0.1	0.3	0.4	0.7	1.3	2.4	3.5	4.6	5.8	8.5	9.7	10.6	7.7	1.5	0.3	0.07	0.14	**1.2**	152
Colon	17985	0	-	-	-	0.1	0.3	0.8	2.3	3.4	6.7	15.7	34.5	65.4	108.5	173.4	238.6	329.6	416.6	462.6	38.6	7.9	1.19	3.25	**28.1**	153
Rectum	8756	0	-	-	-	-	0.2	0.7	1.1	2.5	4.9	10.8	19.9	41.4	64.0	87.2	116.6	139.1	158.1	140.8	18.8	3.8	0.73	1.75	**14.3**	154
Liver	1786	0	0.6	0.0	0.1	0.2	0.1	0.1	0.2	0.6	1.5	2.4	4.0	7.7	11.3	19.1	21.3	29.1	28.7	33.5	3.8	0.8	0.14	0.35	**3.0**	155
Gallbladder etc.	931	0	-	-	-	-	-	0.0	0.1	0.2	0.5	0.3	2.1	3.4	5.3	7.3	13.2	16.8	23.5	29.0	2.0	0.4	0.06	0.16	**1.4**	156
Pancreas	4791	0	-	-	-	0.0	0.0	0.1	0.4	1.1	2.6	5.6	10.9	20.1	32.1	48.2	64.6	79.4	95.0	94.2	10.3	2.1	0.36	0.93	**7.7**	157
Nose, sinuses etc.	340	0	0.0	0.0	-	0.1	0.1	0.2	0.1	0.2	0.4	0.9	1.0	1.7	2.4	2.6	2.9	4.2	6.0	3.9	0.7	0.1	0.04	0.06	**0.6**	160
Larynx	3589	0	-	-	-	-	0.1	0.1	0.2	0.8	2.3	5.7	13.3	22.7	32.7	43.0	40.1	42.5	36.0	27.3	7.7	1.6	0.39	0.80	**6.3**	161
Bronchus, lung	37191	0	0.1	-	0.1	0.2	0.2	0.4	1.4	4.6	13.3	39.6	91.0	171.9	301.6	422.8	521.5	583.5	590.1	467.7	79.8	16.3	3.12	7.84	**61.3**	162
Other thoracic organs	214	0	0.4	0.1	0.1	0.2	0.4	0.5	0.4	0.4	0.4	0.5	0.5	0.4	0.7	1.0	1.7	1.0	1.0	2.4	0.5	0.1	0.02	0.04	**0.4**	163-4
Bone	502	0	0.1	0.4	1.4	2.0	0.9	1.0	0.6	0.9	0.7	1.1	1.0	1.1	1.5	1.6	2.5	2.2	2.3	3.9	1.1	0.2	0.06	0.09	**1.0**	170
Connective tissue	1306	0	1.4	0.4	0.7	0.9	1.1	1.0	1.4	1.6	2.1	2.5	3.6	4.5	6.2	7.2	12.0	13.4	13.3	22.5	2.8	0.6	0.14	0.23	**2.4**	171
Mesothelioma	872	0	-	-	-	-	0.0	0.0	0.1	0.2	0.3	0.9	1.4	3.5	5.3	9.7	13.0	14.8	19.2	15.1	1.9	0.4	0.06	0.17	**1.4**	MES
Kaposi's sarcoma	4582	0	-	-	-	0.1	1.5	11.3	24.3	31.0	23.5	15.9	8.7	5.0	3.2	1.9	2.0	1.9	4.0	9.2	9.8	2.0	0.62	0.64	**7.6**	KAP
Melanoma of skin	7457	0	0.1	0.1	0.3	1.4	2.9	5.8	9.7	14.3	18.9	23.1	28.6	35.5	41.4	46.9	55.6	57.0	59.2	72.0	16.0	3.3	0.91	1.42	**13.1**	172
†Other skin	526	0	0.1	0.1	0.2	0.2	0.3	0.5	0.7	0.8	1.0	1.0	1.1	1.7	2.0	3.2	4.4	6.2	9.4	11.0	1.1		0.05	0.09	**0.9**	173
Breast	432	0	-	-	-	-	-	0.0	0.2	0.2	0.7	1.1	2.1	2.6	4.9	5.9	5.8	8.5	5.6	0.9	0.2	0.04	0.09	**0.7**	175
Prostate	66227	0	0.1	0.0	0.0	-	0.0	0.1	0.1	2.1	10.5	55.3	159.5	405.5	775.8	1176.0	1372.1	1448.8	1376.6	142.2	29.0	3.17	12.93	**100.8**	185
Testis	2970	0	0.5	0.1	0.1	3.6	9.7	14.4	15.9	12.3	9.1	5.8	3.9	2.4	2.1	1.5	1.1	1.1	1.3	0.9	6.4	1.3	0.40	0.41	**5.4**	186
Penis	298	0	-	-	-	-	-	0.0	0.1	0.1	0.3	0.5	0.6	1.3	1.8	2.9	3.6	4.1	6.2	7.1	0.6	0.1	0.02	0.06	**0.5**	187.1-.4
Other male genital	105	0	0.1	0.0	0.0	0.1	0.0	0.0	0.0	0.0	0.0	0.2	0.3	0.5	0.5	0.8	1.1	1.7	1.3	2.7	0.2	0.0	0.01	0.02	**0.2**	187.5-.9
Bladder	15168	0	0.1	0.1	0.1	0.2	0.4	0.7	1.7	4.1	7.1	15.5	30.1	57.5	96.0	149.0	209.5	265.9	317.3	332.8	32.6	6.6	1.07	2.86	**24.0**	188
Kidney etc.	6315	0	2.1	0.7	0.1	0.1	0.2	0.4	1.0	2.8	5.7	13.0	19.8	32.0	45.4	59.8	75.8	85.2	89.8	73.8	13.6	2.8	0.62	1.29	**10.8**	189
Eye	408	0	1.1	0.2	0.1	0.1	0.1	0.1	0.2	0.4	0.6	0.6	1.9	1.8	2.5	2.6	4.3	3.7	3.5	3.0	0.9	0.2	0.05	0.08	**0.8**	190
Brain, nervous system	3810	0	4.3	3.8	3.1	3.0	2.9	3.9	4.2	5.6	6.5	8.7	12.3	15.6	17.8	23.2	28.9	28.3	29.4	23.7	8.2	1.7	0.46	0.72	**7.3**	191-2
Thyroid	1384	0	-	0.0	0.3	0.5	1.2	2.0	2.9	4.0	3.5	4.6	5.2	4.9	6.8	7.8	7.2	8.1	5.8	5.6	3.0	0.6	0.18	0.25	**2.5**	193
Other endocrine	197	0	1.3	0.3	0.2	0.4	0.4	0.1	0.1	0.2	0.3	0.2	0.3	0.5	0.6	0.8	1.0	1.1	0.8	0.6	0.4	0.1	0.03	0.03	**0.5**	194
Hodgkin's disease	1754	0	0.2	0.6	1.6	3.8	6.2	6.3	4.9	4.4	3.5	3.2	4.0	3.4	3.1	5.3	5.3	5.4	5.4	6.5	3.8	0.8	0.23	0.28	**3.4**	201
Non-Hodgkin lymphoma	9548	0	0.7	1.4	1.5	2.3	3.0	6.2	10.7	16.1	18.1	23.6	30.2	39.1	46.8	65.6	85.9	104.4	116.9	123.9	20.5	4.2	1.00	1.75	**16.3**	200,202
Multiple myeloma	2455	0	-	-	-	-	0.1	0.1	0.2	0.6	1.6	2.9	5.2	10.7	15.1	23.7	34.6	41.5	46.4	52.5	5.3	1.1	0.18	0.47	**3.9**	203
Lymphoid leukaemia	2997	0	6.7	3.6	2.0	1.9	1.1	0.6	0.8	0.9	1.6	2.7	6.6	10.8	15.8	21.3	29.1	39.1	48.7	67.9	6.4	1.3	0.27	0.53	**5.6**	204
Myeloid leukaemia	2455	0	0.6	0.4	0.5	0.8	1.4	1.4	1.8	2.5	2.6	3.6	6.0	7.3	11.1	19.9	28.8	34.4	40.8	47.7	5.3	1.1	0.20	0.44	**4.1**	205
Monocytic leukaemia	144	0	0.1	0.1	0.0	0.1	0.0	0.1	0.1	0.1	0.1	0.4	0.4	0.6	0.3	0.9	1.7	2.3	2.3	3.0	0.3	0.1	0.01	0.02	**0.2**	206
Other leukaemia	68	0	0.1	-	0.0	-	0.0	0.0	-	0.0	-	0.1	0.2	0.2	0.5	0.6	0.7	0.8	1.3	1.5	0.1	0.0	0.01	0.01	**0.1**	207
Leukaemia unspecified	535	0	0.3	0.2	0.1	0.2	0.2	0.1	0.3	0.2	0.3	0.6	0.5	1.5	2.2	3.3	6.5	9.3	14.6	18.7	1.1	0.2	0.03	0.08	**0.8**	208
Other and unspecified	5734	0	0.7	0.1	0.1	0.1	0.3	0.8	0.9	2.0	3.8	7.0	12.1	22.5	33.5	50.0	68.0	92.3	123.9	177.5	12.3	2.5	0.42	1.01	**9.2**	O&U
All sites	228834	0	21.5	12.8	12.7	22.7	36.2	61.0	91.6	125.1	158.4	256.3	465.6	838.1	1442.2	2241.4	3063.9	3629.0	3979.4	3968.2	491.2		17.72	44.25	**371.7**	ALL
All sites but 173	228308	0	21.5	12.7	12.6	22.5	35.9	60.6	90.9	124.3	157.4	255.3	464.4	836.3	1440.2	2238.2	3059.5	3622.8	3969.9	3957.3	490.1	100.0	17.67	44.16	**370.9**	ALLb

| Rate from 10 cases | | | 0.284 | 0.293 | 0.310 | 0.316 | 0.284 | 0.244 | 0.231 | 0.249 | 0.279 | 0.356 | 0.454 | 0.512 | 0.524 | 0.584 | 0.753 | 1.081 | 1.923 | 2.964 | | | | | | |

†Important: see notes on population page

USA, SEER: WHITE 1988-1992

ANNUAL INCIDENCE PER 100,000 BY AGE GROUP (YEARS) - FEMALE

SITE	ALL AGES	AGE UNK	0-	5-	10-	15-	20-	25-	30-	35-	40-	45-	50-	55-	60-	65-	70-	75-	80-	85+	CRUDE RATE	%	CR 64	CR 74	ASR (W)	ICD (9th)
Lip	216	0	-	-	-	-	0.0	0.1	0.2	0.1	0.1	0.3	0.3	0.7	0.8	1.7	1.8	1.9	3.5	3.0	0.4	0.1	0.01	0.03	**0.3**	*140*
Tongue	776	0	0.0	-	-	0.0	0.1	0.2	0.3	0.5	0.6	1.1	2.3	4.0	5.0	6.1	6.4	5.7	5.9	6.8	1.6	0.4	0.07	0.13	**1.1**	*141*
Salivary gland	450	0	0.0	0.1	0.1	0.2	0.2	0.5	0.3	0.6	0.8	1.1	1.2	1.2	1.6	3.1	3.1	2.9	3.4	4.2	0.9	0.2	0.04	0.07	**0.7**	*142*
Mouth	1180	0	-	-	0.1	0.1	0.2	0.2	0.2	0.5	0.9	1.7	3.3	5.1	7.6	8.2	11.1	9.9	11.6	10.6	2.4	0.6	0.10	0.20	**1.6**	*143-5*
Oropharynx	430	0	0.0	-	-	-	-	-	0.0	0.2	0.1	0.9	1.6	2.4	3.8	3.5	4.5	3.3	1.9	1.0	0.9	0.2	0.05	0.09	**0.6**	*146*
Nasopharynx	132	0	0.0	0.1	0.1	0.0	0.0	0.0	0.0	0.1	0.2	0.4	0.4	0.6	0.6	0.9	1.1	1.1	0.5	0.7	0.3	0.1	0.01	0.02	**0.2**	*147*
Hypopharynx	243	0	-	-	-	-	-	-	-	-	0.1	0.2	0.5	2.1	1.8	2.2	2.8	1.9	1.3	1.1	0.5	0.1	0.02	0.05	**0.3**	*148*
Pharynx unspecified	134	0	-	-	-	-	-	-	-	-	-	0.2	0.4	0.7	0.9	1.1	1.4	1.2	1.0	1.4	0.3	0.1	0.01	0.02	**0.2**	*149*
Oesophagus	1044	0	-	-	-	-	-	0.1	0.0	0.1	0.2	0.4	1.7	3.8	6.2	8.2	11.1	11.6	13.0	13.1	2.2	0.5	0.06	0.16	**1.2**	*150*
Stomach	2822	0	-	-	-	0.0	-	0.2	0.4	0.9	1.3	2.1	5.0	6.5	10.9	16.1	23.7	35.5	44.5	54.2	5.9	1.4	0.14	0.34	**3.1**	*151*
Small intestine	616	0	-	-	-	-	-	0.2	0.1	0.4	0.7	1.0	1.6	2.1	2.8	4.9	5.4	5.0	6.8	7.5	1.3	0.3	0.04	0.10	**0.8**	*152*
Colon	19227	0	-	-	0.0	0.1	0.1	0.8	1.7	3.5	7.7	15.3	26.5	48.9	78.8	115.6	169.2	240.4	312.2	351.9	39.9	9.4	0.92	2.34	**20.8**	*153*
Rectum	7176	0	-	-	-	0.1	0.1	0.4	1.0	2.1	4.4	8.0	16.4	23.6	36.2	50.5	65.7	78.4	89.2	94.0	14.9	3.5	0.46	1.04	**8.7**	*154*
Liver	969	0	0.5	0.1	0.0	0.0	0.1	0.2	0.2	0.3	0.4	1.2	1.5	2.6	5.0	5.3	8.7	11.3	14.8	11.7	2.0	0.5	0.06	0.13	**1.2**	*155*
Gallbladder etc.	1552	0	-	-	-	-	0.0	0.0	0.1	0.5	0.7	0.9	2.1	4.4	6.3	8.8	14.6	18.8	24.8	28.6	3.2	0.8	0.08	0.19	**1.7**	*156*
Pancreas	5166	0	0.0	0.0	0.0	0.1	0.1	0.1	0.1	0.3	0.7	1.2	3.4	7.4	14.2	20.9	35.2	49.9	65.3	76.6	88.5	10.7	2.5	0.24	0.67	**5.7**	*157*
Nose, sinuses etc.	268	0	-	0.1	0.1	-	0.1	0.1	0.1	0.1	0.4	0.3	0.2	0.8	1.0	1.4	1.6	1.7	2.5	2.6	3.0	0.6	0.1	0.02	0.04	**0.4**	*160*
Larynx	901	0	-	-	-	-	-	0.1	0.2	0.2	0.4	1.4	3.2	6.2	7.8	8.4	8.1	5.9	4.2	3.0	1.9	0.4	0.10	0.18	**1.4**	*161*
Bronchus, lung	24781	0	-	-	-	0.2	0.4	0.7	1.1	3.6	11.2	31.3	69.4	118.9	169.8	220.4	255.2	248.7	203.4	129.6	51.4	12.1	2.03	4.41	**33.8**	*162*
Other thoracic organs	136	0	0.4	0.1	0.1	0.0	0.0	0.0	0.2	0.3	0.1	0.2	0.4	0.5	0.6	0.5	1.0	0.9	0.9	0.4	0.3	0.1	0.01	0.02	**0.2**	*163-4*
Bone	399	0	0.2	0.6	1.5	1.0	0.8	0.5	0.5	0.6	0.6	0.5	0.7	0.7	1.2	1.1	1.5	2.2	2.2	1.4	0.8	0.2	0.05	0.06	**0.8**	*170*
Connective tissue	1105	0	1.4	0.4	0.5	0.7	0.8	1.2	1.1	1.6	1.8	1.9	2.4	3.0	4.4	5.1	6.0	7.6	8.4	11.3	2.3	0.5	0.11	0.16	**1.7**	*171*
Mesothelioma	219	0	-	-	-	-	0.0	0.0	0.1	0.1	0.3	0.2	0.6	0.6	1.4	1.6	1.4	2.8	2.2	1.5	0.5	0.1	0.02	0.03	**0.3**	*MES*
Kaposi's sarcoma	80	0	-	-	-	-	-	0.1	0.1	0.2	0.0	0.1	-	0.1	0.0	0.0	0.3	1.1	1.5	2.5	0.2	0.0	0.00	0.00	**0.1**	*KAP*
Melanoma of skin	6383	0	0.0	0.1	0.5	2.0	5.7	9.3	13.9	16.0	18.5	20.8	20.3	22.2	23.8	22.9	25.2	26.2	27.6	32.3	13.2	3.1	0.77	1.01	**10.2**	*172*
†Other skin	472	0	0.0	0.1	0.2	0.2	0.4	0.9	0.6	0.8	0.9	0.9	1.4	1.4	1.8	1.3	2.3	3.0	4.7	5.1	1.0		0.05	0.06	**0.7**	*173*
Breast	62413	0	-	-	0.0	-	0.9	7.0	23.8	61.0	121.2	194.5	231.5	273.2	340.5	403.6	439.4	466.3	459.4	415.8	129.6	30.4	6.27	10.48	**90.7**	*174*
Uterus unspecified	188	0	0.0	-	-	-	-	-	0.0	0.2	0.2	0.4	0.4	0.4	0.5	0.9	1.2	1.5	2.2	5.3	0.4	0.1	0.01	0.02	**0.2**	*179*
Cervix uteri	4650	0	-	0.0	-	0.2	2.0	8.8	12.4	15.1	15.7	16.0	15.7	13.5	17.3	17.3	13.1	15.0	15.3	15.7	9.7	2.3	0.58	0.74	**7.5**	*180*
Placenta	48	0	-	-	0.0	0.1	0.2	0.3	0.3	0.2	-	0.1	-	-	0.0	0.0	-	-	-	-	0.1	0.0	0.01	0.01	**0.1**	*181*
Corpus uteri	12727	0	-	-	-	0.1	0.1	1.0	2.1	5.6	12.1	22.7	43.2	63.2	87.8	107.6	116.1	107.0	87.2	63.1	26.4	6.2	1.19	2.31	**18.2**	*182*
Ovary etc.	8259	0	0.1	0.2	0.4	1.6	1.5	3.1	3.6	7.6	11.0	20.0	26.6	38.4	46.3	54.2	61.3	63.9	62.7	58.8	17.1	4.0	0.80	1.38	**11.9**	*183*
Other female genital	1628	0	0.1	-	-	0.1	0.3	0.4	0.7	1.4	1.7	2.7	2.8	5.6	6.6	8.4	12.7	15.7	20.4	27.0	3.4	0.8	0.11	0.22	**2.0**	*184*
Bladder	5225	0	0.0	-	-	0.1	0.3	0.5	0.7	1.1	2.2	4.8	9.5	17.7	25.4	36.9	46.6	57.0	67.5	83.0	10.8	2.5	0.31	0.73	**6.2**	*188*
Kidney etc.	3994	0	2.2	0.6	0.2	0.2	0.1	0.5	0.8	1.4	3.7	6.3	11.4	15.6	22.6	27.6	34.2	39.8	38.2	34.7	8.3	1.9	0.33	0.64	**5.5**	*189*
Eye	357	0	1.1	0.2	0.0	0.1	0.1	0.2	0.2	0.3	0.3	0.3	0.8	1.6	1.5	2.4	2.6	2.7	2.4	2.5	0.7	0.2	0.03	0.06	**0.6**	*190*
Brain, nervous system	3047	0	3.7	3.0	2.6	2.1	2.4	2.7	2.8	3.6	4.9	5.8	7.8	9.5	11.7	16.6	20.3	21.7	18.4	11.2	6.3	1.5	0.31	0.50	**5.1**	*191-2*
Thyroid	3719	0	-	0.0	0.8	2.7	7.0	9.1	10.2	11.8	11.8	12.3	11.1	10.7	10.2	9.9	10.0	9.1	8.7	7.1	7.7	1.8	0.49	0.59	**6.4**	*193*
Other endocrine	176	0	1.2	0.2	0.1	0.1	0.1	0.1	0.2	0.2	0.1	0.2	0.4	0.4	0.9	0.8	0.6	0.8	0.5	0.3	0.4	0.1	0.02	0.03	**0.4**	*194*
Hodgkin's disease	1441	0	0.0	0.3	1.4	4.7	6.8	5.8	3.9	3.2	2.4	1.7	1.3	1.9	2.0	2.8	3.3	3.8	5.0	3.0	3.0	0.7	0.18	0.21	**2.7**	*201*
Non-Hodgkin lymphoma	7693	0	0.4	0.4	0.6	1.3	1.7	2.7	3.1	4.6	7.8	11.7	18.4	26.2	36.9	48.9	65.8	76.0	85.4	79.8	16.0	3.7	0.58	1.15	**10.1**	*200,202*
Multiple myeloma	2177	0	-	-	-	-	0.1	0.1	0.0	0.3	0.8	2.4	4.0	5.6	11.2	15.3	20.8	26.9	33.0	26.5	4.5	1.1	0.12	0.30	**2.5**	*203*
Lymphoid leukaemia	2123	0	5.8	2.4	1.6	0.8	0.5	0.5	0.5	0.5	1.3	1.2	2.3	4.9	6.6	11.1	16.5	19.3	25.5	31.7	4.4	1.0	0.14	0.28	**3.2**	*204*
Myeloid leukaemia	2054	0	0.9	0.3	0.6	1.1	0.6	1.2	1.4	1.8	2.5	3.1	4.3	5.2	7.4	10.9	14.3	18.8	24.4	27.2	4.3	1.0	0.15	0.28	**2.7**	*205*
Monocytic leukaemia	118	0	0.1	0.1	-	-	0.1	0.1	0.1	-	0.1	0.2	0.2	0.3	0.4	0.6	0.9	1.1	0.9	1.9	0.2	0.1	0.01	0.02	**0.2**	*206*
Other leukaemia	65	0	0.2	-	0.0	-	-	-	-	0.0	0.1	0.1	0.0	0.1	0.1	0.3	0.4	0.5	0.6	1.1	0.4	0.1	0.00	0.01	**0.1**	*207*
Leukaemia unspecified	449	0	0.1	0.1	0.0	0.0	0.1	0.2	0.1	0.2	0.2	0.4	0.5	0.7	1.4	2.5	3.7	4.0	7.7	10.6	0.9	0.2	0.02	0.05	**0.5**	*208*
Other and unspecified	6535	0	0.9	0.1	0.0	0.2	0.3	0.3	0.9	1.4	2.8	5.3	8.4	16.9	27.5	36.9	54.0	70.6	103.4	143.3	13.6	3.2	0.32	0.78	**7.1**	*O&U*
All sites	205963	0	19.7	9.5	11.5	20.3	34.6	60.1	90.6	155.1	256.6	408.1	572.1	789.2	1066.4	1350.0	1620.9	1816.4	1938.3	1917.2	427.5		17.47	32.32	**281.6**	*ALL*
All sites but 173	205491	0	19.7	9.5	11.3	20.1	34.2	59.3	90.0	154.3	255.7	407.3	570.8	787.9	1064.6	1348.7	1618.6	1813.3	1933.6	1912.1	426.5	100.0	17.42	32.26	**280.9**	*ALLb*

| Rate from 10 cases | | | 0.299 | 0.309 | 0.327 | 0.332 | 0.295 | 0.251 | 0.234 | 0.252 | 0.278 | 0.356 | 0.446 | 0.489 | 0.476 | 0.486 | 0.570 | 0.708 | 1.012 | 1.105 |

†Important: see notes on population page

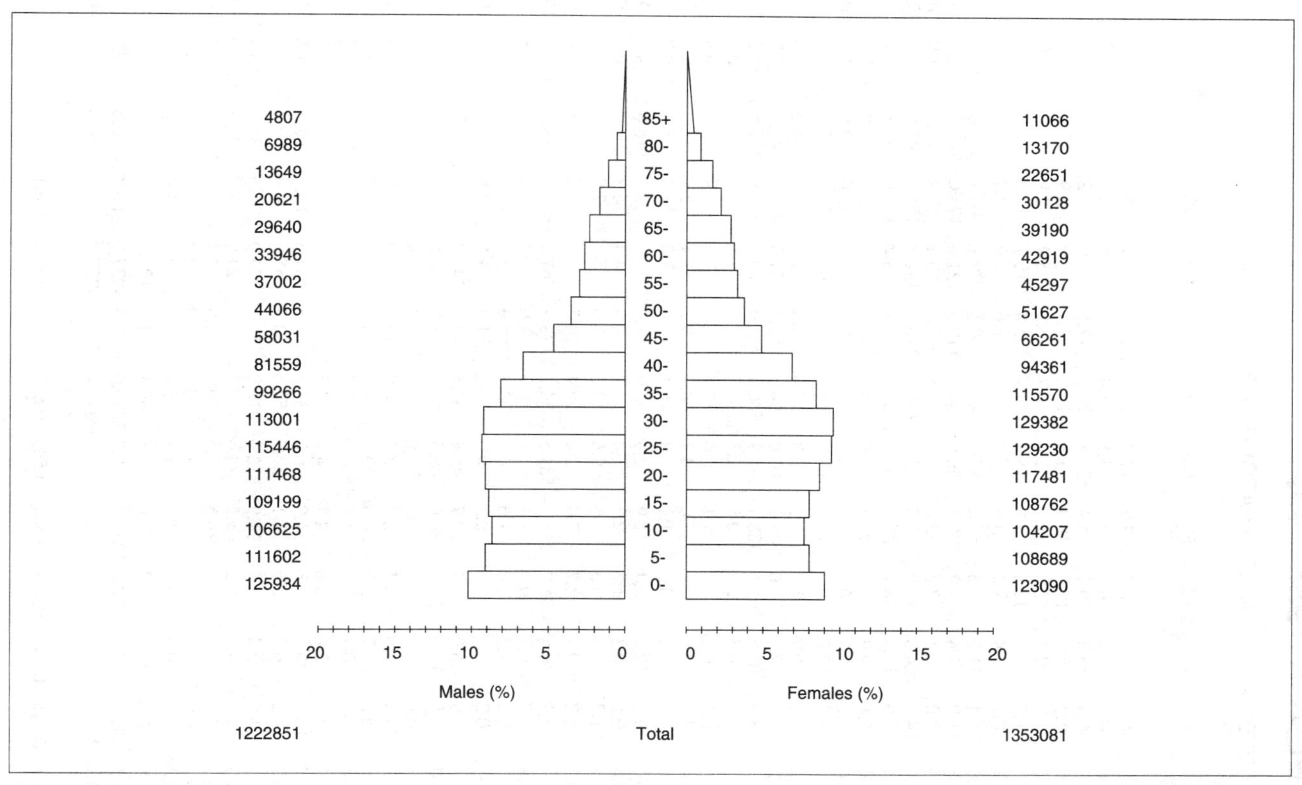

USA, SEER: Black
Source of population: average annual 1988-92
Estimate: NCI estimates based on U.S. Bureau of Census population estimates by county for the years 1988–92.
Notes to tables overleaf:
† 173 does not include basal cell or squamous cell carcinoma

Note: There was an error in the population data for Blacks in Volume VI for Connecticut, Atlanta and Detroit. This results in artificial large increases in incidence in Blacks in the SEER data.

USA, SEER: BLACK 1988-1992

ANNUAL INCIDENCE PER 100,000 BY AGE GROUP (YEARS) - MALE

SITE	ALL AGES	AGE UNK	0-	5-	10-	15-	20-	25-	30-	35-	40-	45-	50-	55-	60-	65-	70-	75-	80-	85+	CRUDE RATE	%	CR 64	CR 74	ASR (W)	ICD (9th)
Lip	2	0	-	-	-	-	-	-	-	-	-	0.3	-	-	-	0.7	-	-	-	-	0.0	0.0	0.00	0.01	**0.0**	*140*
Tongue	226	0	-	-	-	0.2	-	-	-	0.8	6.4	8.3	18.2	22.2	17.7	13.5	19.4	11.7	25.8	12.5	3.7	1.0	0.37	0.53	**4.5**	*141*
Salivary gland	45	0	-	0.2	0.2	0.2	-	0.2	-	0.6	0.7	1.0	0.9	3.2	4.1	4.0	2.9	8.8	2.9	4.2	0.7	0.2	0.06	0.09	**0.9**	*142*
Mouth	270	0	-	-	-	-	0.2	-	0.4	1.4	6.4	13.4	19.1	25.4	22.4	20.9	17.5	19.0	17.2	-	4.4	1.1	0.44	0.63	**5.4**	*143-5*
Oropharynx	178	0	-	-	-	-	-	-	0.5	0.6	4.7	8.6	15.9	18.4	11.8	15.5	9.7	2.9	2.9	12.5	2.9	0.8	0.30	0.43	**3.6**	*146*
Nasopharynx	48	0	-	0.2	-	0.4	0.4	0.3	0.7	0.4	1.0	2.1	2.3	2.7	2.4	0.7	4.8	5.9	2.9	-	0.8	0.2	0.06	0.09	**0.9**	*147*
Hypopharynx	149	0	-	-	-	-	-	-	0.2	0.6	1.7	3.4	12.3	13.5	18.3	14.2	5.8	16.1	17.2	4.2	2.4	0.6	0.25	0.35	**3.0**	*148*
Pharynx unspecified	52	0	-	-	-	-	-	-	-	0.2	0.2	1.4	2.3	5.4	5.9	2.7	13.6	2.9	2.9	-	0.9	0.2	0.08	0.16	**1.1**	*149*
Oesophagus	679	0	-	-	-	-	-	-	0.5	1.6	5.4	21.0	34.5	56.8	67.2	82.3	80.5	79.1	60.1	41.6	11.1	2.9	0.93	1.75	**13.8**	*150*
Stomach	756	0	-	-	-	-	0.7	-	2.3	3.6	11.0	11.4	27.2	35.7	56.0	84.3	118.3	121.6	123.0	203.8	12.4	3.2	0.74	1.75	**14.5**	*151*
Small intestine	114	0	-	-	-	-	-	-	0.5	1.0	2.0	3.1	2.3	3.8	8.8	15.5	13.6	23.4	17.2	12.5	1.9	0.5	0.11	0.25	**2.1**	*152*
Colon	1752	0	-	-	0.2	0.2	0.7	0.7	1.6	6.9	14.7	24.5	44.9	93.0	133.1	206.5	276.4	332.6	454.9	391.0	28.7	7.4	1.60	4.02	**33.6**	*153*
Rectum	662	0	-	-	-	0.2	-	0.9	2.1	4.4	5.6	15.9	28.1	35.1	50.1	81.0	92.1	98.2	103.0	95.7	10.8	2.8	0.71	1.58	**12.8**	*154*
Liver	334	0	0.8	-	-	0.2	0.2	0.2	0.9	2.6	5.6	9.3	13.6	15.7	33.0	33.7	45.6	33.7	48.6	25.0	5.5	1.4	0.41	0.81	**6.5**	*155*
Gallbladder etc.	78	0	-	-	-	-	-	-	-	0.2	0.6	1.2	0.7	0.5	2.7	5.9	8.1	10.7	19.0	28.6	20.8	1.3	0.3	0.06	0.15	**1.4**	*156*
Pancreas	605	0	-	-	-	-	-	0.2	1.1	2.0	3.9	10.0	20.0	40.5	47.1	85.0	79.5	93.8	123.0	120.6	9.9	2.6	0.62	1.45	**11.8**	*157*
Nose, sinuses etc.	29	0	-	-	0.2	-	-	0.2	0.4	0.2	-	0.7	1.8	1.1	1.8	2.0	4.8	2.9	5.7	4.2	0.5	0.1	0.03	0.07	**0.5**	*160*
Larynx	541	0	-	-	-	-	-	-	0.2	1.2	7.4	17.9	25.0	41.1	63.0	64.8	55.3	51.3	45.8	41.6	8.8	2.3	0.78	1.38	**11.0**	*161*
Bronchus, lung	4964	0	-	-	-	-	0.4	0.5	2.5	15.7	38.3	105.5	201.5	328.1	494.9	636.3	741.9	669.6	683.9	457.6	81.2	21.0	5.94	12.83	**99.1**	*162*
Other thoracic organs	28	0	0.5	-	0.2	0.4	-	0.5	0.7	0.2	1.0	0.3	2.3	0.5	1.8	-	-	-	-	-	0.5	0.1	0.04	0.04	**0.5**	*163-4*
Bone	37	0	-	0.2	0.8	1.6	0.7	0.2	0.5	0.6	0.7	0.3	-	1.1	0.6	2.7	-	-	2.9	-	0.6	0.2	0.04	0.05	**0.6**	*170*
Connective tissue	143	0	1.1	0.5	1.3	1.6	0.5	1.7	1.2	1.4	3.7	2.8	3.6	7.0	4.7	8.1	9.7	16.1	5.7	12.5	2.3	0.6	0.16	0.25	**2.5**	*171*
Mesothelioma	43	0	-	-	-	-	-	-	0.2	0.6	-	2.1	0.5	1.1	2.9	6.1	4.8	7.3	11.4	8.3	0.7	0.2	0.04	0.09	**0.8**	*MES*
Kaposi's sarcoma	506	0	-	-	-	-	2.5	13.3	23.7	24.6	19.1	12.4	6.4	5.9	2.9	4.0	1.9	-	8.6	16.6	8.3	2.1	0.55	0.58	**7.0**	*KAP*
Melanoma of skin	42	0	-	-	-	-	0.3	0.5	0.6	0.5	0.3	1.8	2.2	1.8	4.0	4.8	4.4	14.3	4.2	-	0.7	0.2	0.04	0.08	**0.7**	*172*
†Other skin	48	0	-	-	0.4	-	0.2	0.7	0.9	3.0	1.2	2.1	0.5	1.6	0.6	2.0	1.0	-	2.9	-	0.8		0.06	0.07	**0.7**	*173*
Breast	59	0	-	-	-	-	-	-	-	0.2	1.2	0.7	2.7	7.0	2.4	5.4	10.7	5.9	8.6	8.3	1.0	0.2	0.07	0.15	**1.2**	*175*
Prostate	7129	0	-	-	-	-	-	0.3	-	-	3.7	14.5	86.7	266.5	581.5	1076.2	1473.2	1767.1	1879.9	1755.6	116.6	30.1	4.77	17.51	**137.0**	*185*
Testis	49	0	0.2	0.2	0.2	0.2	1.1	1.2	1.4	1.8	1.7	0.7	0.9	1.1	-	0.7	1.0	-	-	-	0.8	0.2	0.05	0.06	**0.7**	*186*
Penis	38	0	-	0.2	-	-	-	-	-	-	0.2	1.7	1.4	1.6	4.7	3.4	2.9	5.9	14.3	4.2	0.6	0.2	0.05	0.08	**0.7**	*187.1-.4*
Other male genital	9	0	-	0.2	-	-	0.2	-	-	-	0.2	-	-	0.5	0.6	-	1.9	1.5	2.9	-	0.1	0.0	0.01	0.02	**0.2**	*187.5-.9*
Bladder	584	0	0.2	0.4	-	-	-	0.5	1.2	1.2	3.9	6.9	16.8	29.7	45.4	67.5	83.4	131.9	174.5	95.7	9.6	2.5	0.53	1.29	**11.1**	*188*
Kidney etc.	609	0	2.1	0.4	0.2	-	0.4	0.5	2.1	3.0	7.8	17.9	32.2	34.6	49.5	54.0	71.8	86.5	97.3	45.8	10.0	2.6	0.75	1.38	**11.8**	*189*
Eye	20	0	1.4	0.2	-	-	-	-	0.2	-	0.5	-	-	1.8	0.7	1.0	2.9	-	-	-	0.3	0.1	0.02	0.03	**0.4**	*190*
Brain, nervous system	233	0	4.0	2.7	3.0	2.4	0.2	2.4	2.1	2.2	4.4	7.6	5.4	6.5	8.2	8.8	16.5	19.0	14.3	-	3.8	1.0	0.26	0.38	**4.1**	*191-2*
Thyroid	80	0	-	-	0.4	-	0.7	0.5	1.1	2.4	0.5	1.7	2.7	4.3	7.7	4.0	4.8	5.9	5.7	8.3	1.3	0.3	0.11	0.15	**1.4**	*193*
Other endocrine	18	0	1.0	0.2	-	0.4	0.2	-	-	0.4	-	0.7	-	1.1	-	0.7	1.0	-	-	-	0.3	0.1	0.02	0.03	**0.3**	*194*
Hodgkin's disease	159	0	-	1.1	0.9	3.1	1.8	4.3	3.5	5.2	3.2	2.8	3.6	2.7	4.1	4.7	1.9	-	-	-	2.6	0.7	0.18	0.22	**2.5**	*201*
Non-Hodgkin lymphoma	719	0	0.3	0.9	1.5	1.5	3.2	8.3	11.9	19.7	15.7	20.7	23.6	31.9	30.0	33.7	53.3	51.3	68.7	62.4	11.8	3.0	0.85	1.28	**12.3**	*200,202*
Multiple myeloma	444	0	-	-	-	-	-	0.2	1.1	2.2	4.2	6.2	13.6	21.1	37.7	52.6	84.4	58.6	94.4	83.2	7.3	1.9	0.43	1.12	**8.6**	*203*
Lymphoid leukaemia	210	0	2.5	2.3	1.5	0.9	0.7	0.7	0.4	1.2	1.2	2.4	5.4	11.9	12.4	16.9	24.2	24.9	28.6	33.3	3.4	0.9	0.22	0.42	**4.0**	*204*
Myeloid leukaemia	218	0	0.6	1.3	0.2	0.7	0.9	1.4	1.6	3.0	4.2	4.5	6.8	6.5	13.6	17.5	23.3	24.9	37.2	20.8	3.6	0.9	0.23	0.43	**3.9**	*205*
Monocytic leukaemia	12	0	0.2	0.4	-	-	-	-	-	0.2	-	-	0.5	0.6	0.7	1.9	4.4	-	-	-	0.2	0.1	0.01	0.02	**0.2**	*206*
Other leukaemia	12	0	-	0.2	-	-	-	-	0.2	-	0.2	-	-	-	2.4	0.7	1.0	2.9	-	4.2	0.2	0.1	0.01	0.02	**0.2**	*207*
Leukaemia unspecified	42	0	0.2	0.4	-	-	-	0.3	0.2	0.2	-	0.3	0.9	1.1	1.8	3.4	12.6	7.3	11.4	-	0.7	0.2	0.03	0.11	**0.8**	*208*
Other and unspecified	728	0	0.6	-	-	0.4	0.5	0.9	2.1	4.8	6.4	16.9	22.7	40.0	67.8	66.1	101.8	105.5	117.3	199.7	11.9	3.1	0.82	1.66	**14.1**	*O&U*
All sites	23703	0	15.6	11.6	11.1	14.5	16.3	41.6	70.8	123.3	202.1	385.0	710.8	1232.4	1930.7	2816.5	3587.5	3927.0	4366.4	3810.6	387.7		23.83	55.85	**455.3**	*ALL*
All sites but 173	23655	0	15.6	11.6	10.7	14.5	16.1	40.9	69.9	120.3	200.8	382.9	710.3	1230.7	1930.1	2814.4	3586.5	3927.0	4363.5	3810.6	386.9	100.0	23.77	55.78	**454.5**	*ALLb*

| Rate from 1 case | | | 0.159 | 0.179 | 0.188 | 0.183 | 0.179 | 0.173 | 0.177 | 0.201 | 0.245 | 0.345 | 0.454 | 0.541 | 0.589 | 0.675 | 0.970 | 1.465 | 2.861 | 4.160 |

†Important: see notes on population page

USA, SEER: BLACK 1988-1992

ANNUAL INCIDENCE PER 100,000 BY AGE GROUP (YEARS) - FEMALE

SITE	ALL AGES	AGE UNK	0-	5-	10-	15-	20-	25-	30-	35-	40-	45-	50-	55-	60-	65-	70-	75-	80-	85+	CRUDE RATE	%	CR 64	CR 74	ASR (W)	ICD (9th)
Lip	3	0	-	-	-	-	-	-	0.2	-	-	-	-	-	-	0.5	0.7	-	-	-	0.0	0.0	0.00	0.01	**0.0**	140
Tongue	66	0	0.2	-	-	-	-	-	0.3	0.3	1.1	2.7	4.3	4.0	4.2	5.1	2.0	2.6	1.5	1.8	1.0	0.3	0.09	0.12	**1.1**	141
Salivary gland	47	0	0.2	-	0.2	0.2	-	0.6	0.6	0.2	1.3	0.6	1.5	2.2	1.9	2.0	2.7	0.9	6.1	1.8	0.7	0.2	0.05	0.07	**0.7**	142
Mouth	126	0	-	-	-	0.2	0.2	0.3	0.6	1.0	0.8	4.8	5.0	7.9	8.4	8.7	6.6	6.2	4.6	10.8	1.9	0.7	0.15	0.22	**1.9**	143-5
Oropharynx	62	0	-	-	-	-	-	0.2	-	0.2	1.3	1.5	3.1	4.4	4.2	6.1	4.0	0.9	1.5	3.6	0.9	0.3	0.07	0.12	**1.0**	146
Nasopharynx	17	0	-	0.2	-	0.2	0.3	0.2	0.5	0.2	0.4	-	-	0.9	0.9	0.5	0.7	-	-	-	0.3	0.1	0.02	0.02	**0.2**	147
Hypopharynx	32	0	-	-	-	-	-	-	-	0.2	0.4	0.9	2.7	2.2	2.3	2.0	2.0	1.8	-	-	0.5	0.2	0.04	0.06	**0.5**	148
Pharynx unspecified	23	0	-	-	-	-	-	-	0.2	-	0.2	0.9	0.8	0.4	1.9	3.1	0.7	1.8	1.5	1.8	0.3	0.1	0.02	0.04	**0.3**	149
Oesophagus	253	0	-	-	-	-	-	-	-	0.3	1.5	5.1	11.6	19.0	16.8	26.5	19.3	20.3	9.1	14.5	3.7	1.3	0.27	0.50	**3.9**	150
Stomach	460	0	-	-	-	0.4	0.3	0.9	1.1	2.2	2.8	2.4	10.1	16.3	21.0	26.0	45.1	60.0	83.5	106.6	6.8	2.4	0.29	0.64	**5.9**	151
Small intestine	91	0	-	-	-	-	0.2	-	-	0.5	1.1	1.2	2.3	3.5	4.7	7.7	9.3	7.1	16.7	10.8	1.3	0.5	0.07	0.15	**1.2**	152
Colon	2005	0	-	-	-	0.2	0.2	0.8	3.7	7.4	13.1	17.8	48.4	73.3	108.1	161.8	201.8	249.9	311.3	321.7	29.6	10.5	1.37	3.18	**26.8**	153
Rectum	611	0	-	-	-	-	0.2	0.6	0.8	4.3	3.4	9.7	15.9	28.7	33.6	45.9	65.1	61.8	79.0	72.3	9.0	3.2	0.49	1.04	**8.5**	154
Liver	144	0	0.5	-	-	-	-	-	-	0.2	0.5	1.5	2.4	3.1	5.3	9.3	11.2	9.3	12.4	25.8	27.1	2.1	0.8	0.11	0.22	**2.0**	155
Gallbladder etc.	113	0	-	-	-	-	-	-	0.2	0.2	0.2	0.6	0.9	2.3	5.3	6.1	8.2	13.3	10.6	19.7	21.7	1.7	0.6	0.08	0.19	**1.5**	156
Pancreas	700	0	-	0.2	-	-	-	0.3	0.2	0.9	2.2	3.4	6.9	7.0	28.7	41.0	58.7	71.0	101.5	112.4	101.2	10.3	3.7	0.45	1.10	**9.3**	157
Nose, sinuses etc.	36	0	0.2	-	0.2	0.4	0.2	0.2	-	0.3	0.6	0.6	1.9	1.8	0.9	1.5	1.3	5.3	1.5	-	0.5	0.2	0.04	0.05	**0.5**	160
Larynx	147	0	-	-	-	-	-	-	-	0.9	1.7	2.7	12.8	7.5	9.8	13.8	10.0	1.8	6.1	10.8	2.2	0.8	0.18	0.30	**2.4**	161
Bronchus, lung	2558	0	-	-	-	0.2	-	1.1	3.1	7.6	18.7	42.3	91.8	132.0	200.8	252.6	252.3	198.7	194.4	113.9	37.8	13.4	2.49	5.01	**38.5**	162
Other thoracic organs	20	0	0.3	-	-	-	0.2	0.2	0.3	0.2	0.6	0.9	0.4	-	1.4	1.0	0.7	-	-	-	0.3	0.1	0.02	0.03	**0.3**	163-4
Bone	46	0	-	0.7	1.3	0.6	0.9	0.2	0.6	0.7	0.2	1.8	0.4	1.3	1.4	0.5	1.3	-	-	1.8	0.7	0.2	0.05	0.06	**0.7**	170
Connective tissue	129	0	1.3	0.4	0.4	0.7	1.4	1.2	0.9	1.2	1.9	3.3	1.5	3.1	3.7	6.6	8.0	6.2	10.6	10.8	1.9	0.7	0.11	0.18	**1.8**	171
Mesothelioma	14	0	-	-	-	-	-	-	-	-	0.2	0.9	0.4	0.4	-	1.5	1.3	-	-	5.4	0.2	0.1	0.01	0.02	**0.2**	MES
Kaposi's sarcoma	19	0	-	-	-	0.2	-	0.3	0.6	0.7	-	0.3	-	-	0.5	1.0	-	0.9	3.0	1.8	0.3	0.1	0.01	0.02	**0.2**	KAP
Melanoma of skin	38	0	-	-	-	-	0.3	0.3	0.2	-	0.8	-	1.2	1.8	1.4	0.5	2.7	4.4	7.6	7.2	0.6	0.2	0.03	0.05	**0.5**	172
†Other skin	73	0	0.2	-	0.6	0.4	0.3	1.4	1.1	2.6	2.5	2.1	0.4	1.8	0.9	1.0	2.0	1.8	-	1.8	1.1		0.07	0.09	**1.0**	173
Breast	5488	0	-	-	0.2	0.2	1.9	10.4	31.2	64.0	132.3	175.7	203.4	244.6	267.9	319.0	334.6	357.6	375.1	352.4	81.1	28.7	5.66	8.93	**79.3**	174
Uterus unspecified	43	0	-	-	-	-	0.2	-	-	0.2	1.3	0.6	0.8	-	3.3	3.6	3.3	5.3	3.0	7.2	0.6	0.2	0.03	0.07	**0.6**	179
Cervix uteri	865	0	-	-	-	0.9	2.0	7.6	11.7	17.3	22.7	26.0	26.0	30.9	34.5	35.7	27.9	41.5	45.6	54.2	12.8	4.5	0.90	1.22	**12.0**	180
Placenta	7	0	-	-	-	-	0.3	0.3	0.2	0.2	0.2	-	-	-	-	-	-	-	-	-	0.1	0.0	0.01	0.01	**0.1**	181
Corpus uteri	794	0	-	-	-	0.2	-	0.5	2.3	5.4	4.7	9.1	14.7	35.8	71.8	67.9	77.7	72.4	71.4	72.3	11.7	4.1	0.72	1.45	**11.4**	182
Ovary etc.	567	0	-	-	1.3	2.0	1.4	2.3	2.5	4.3	4.7	10.9	21.3	19.4	26.6	51.5	36.5	45.0	50.1	56.0	8.4	3.0	0.48	0.92	**8.1**	183
Other female genital	148	0	0.3	-	-	-	0.2	0.9	0.6	1.0	1.5	4.2	4.3	4.9	5.1	8.7	13.3	14.1	18.2	18.1	2.2	0.8	0.12	0.22	**2.0**	184
Bladder	335	0	-	-	-	-	0.2	-	0.2	0.9	0.8	3.6	6.6	8.8	12.6	27.6	35.8	53.0	57.7	75.9	5.0	1.7	0.17	0.49	**4.3**	188
Kidney etc.	410	0	1.8	0.4	0.2	0.4	0.3	1.4	1.5	2.2	6.4	8.5	10.5	20.8	21.9	28.6	29.2	37.1	38.0	25.3	6.1	2.1	0.38	0.67	**5.9**	189
Eye	14	0	1.6	0.2	0.2	-	0.2	-	-	-	-	-	-	-	-	0.5	-	-	-	-	0.2	0.1	0.01	0.01	**0.3**	190
Brain, nervous system	208	0	4.2	3.3	1.9	1.5	1.2	1.4	1.5	1.9	2.3	4.2	2.7	5.3	7.0	7.1	10.0	14.1	6.1	1.8	3.1	1.1	0.19	0.28	**3.2**	191-2
Thyroid	243	0	-	0.2	-	0.7	2.6	1.5	4.3	4.7	5.9	6.6	7.4	4.9	9.3	9.7	10.6	7.9	9.1	14.5	3.6	1.3	0.24	0.34	**3.3**	193
Other endocrine	22	0	0.8	0.6	-	-	0.2	-	0.3	0.2	-	0.3	-	0.4	0.9	2.0	0.7	0.9	-	-	0.3	0.1	0.02	0.03	**0.4**	194
Hodgkin's disease	141	0	-	0.2	1.2	2.9	3.7	3.1	2.5	1.9	1.7	3.0	1.9	1.8	5.1	1.5	3.3	2.6	-	-	2.1	0.7	0.15	0.17	**2.0**	201
Non-Hodgkin lymphoma	494	0	0.5	-	0.8	0.4	2.4	2.8	2.5	5.0	7.2	8.1	14.3	15.5	30.3	31.1	47.8	33.6	31.9	32.5	7.3	2.6	0.45	0.84	**7.0**	200,202
Multiple myeloma	448	0	-	-	-	0.2	-	0.2	0.2	1.2	2.8	4.2	8.9	19.0	29.4	37.8	47.1	44.1	77.4	65.1	6.6	2.3	0.33	0.75	**6.1**	203
Lymphoid leukaemia	186	0	2.6	2.6	1.0	1.1	0.9	0.2	-	0.2	0.6	1.8	0.8	6.2	7.9	12.2	10.0	20.3	27.3	28.9	2.7	1.0	0.13	0.24	**2.6**	204
Myeloid leukaemia	192	0	0.6	1.5	0.6	0.7	0.5	1.4	1.5	1.6	3.2	3.9	4.6	4.9	7.5	10.7	8.0	18.5	12.1	23.5	2.8	1.0	0.16	0.26	**2.7**	205
Monocytic leukaemia	8	0	0.2	-	-	-	-	0.2	-	0.2	-	-	-	0.4	-	1.5	-	-	3.0	-	0.1	0.0	0.00	0.01	**0.1**	206
Other leukaemia	4	0	-	-	-	-	-	0.2	-	-	-	-	-	-	-	-	-	-	3.0	1.8	0.1	0.0	0.00	0.00	**0.0**	207
Leukaemia unspecified	33	0	-	-	-	-	-	0.3	-	0.7	0.6	0.3	0.4	0.9	1.4	1.5	2.7	2.6	4.6	7.2	0.5	0.2	0.02	0.04	**0.4**	208
Other and unspecified	743	0	0.6	-	0.6	0.2	1.0	0.8	1.4	3.1	5.7	11.2	12.4	26.5	32.6	48.5	67.7	98.0	113.9	159.0	11.0	3.9	0.48	1.06	**9.7**	O&U
All sites	19226	0	16.1	10.3	10.6	14.9	24.0	43.8	80.5	150.0	264.7	395.1	569.9	802.7	1060.1	1361.0	1498.9	1625.5	1843.6	1845.2	284.2		17.21	31.51	**272.6**	ALL
All sites but 173	19153	0	15.9	10.3	10.0	14.5	23.7	42.4	79.5	147.4	262.2	393.0	569.5	800.9	1059.2	1360.0	1496.9	1623.8	1843.6	1843.4	283.1	100.0	17.14	31.43	**271.6**	ALLb

Rate from 1 case			0.162	0.184	0.192	0.184	0.170	0.155	0.155	0.173	0.212	0.302	0.387	0.442	0.466	0.510	0.664	0.883	1.519	1.807

†Important: see notes on population page

China, Qidong

A population-based cancer registry covering the whole region and all its residents has operated since 1972 when the Qidong Liver Cancer Institute (QLCI) was founded. The main aim of the registry, run by the Department of Epidemiology, as part of the Institute's cancer control initiatives, was initially to conduct epidemiological and etiological research on liver cancer.

Qidong City, in Jiangsu Province, is situated at the mouth of the Yangtze River (*Chang Jiang*), by the Yellow Sea (*Huang Hai*), to the north of Shanghai. It lies at latitude 31°50′ N and longitude 121°39′ E, covering an area of about 1600 km² and has a population of 1 180 000 (density: 750 per km²). The climate is generally warm and humid in spring and summer, cool in autumn and slightly cold in winter with almost no snow.

Qidong is situated in Shanghai Economic Zone. Farming used to be the major occupation but industrialization has been increasing in recent years. It is famous for production of beans, grain and cotton. The Lushi fishing ground is one of the four biggest fishing areas in China.

Qidong Cancer Registry depends for data collection upon small registries at district level and township level, with usually one full-time physician or health care person. These together form the Qidong Anti-cancer Network, which in addition to cancer and death registration is responsible for prevention and treatment of cancers in this area.

In 1974, a system for certification of deaths from all causes was established under the supervision of the Health Ministry of PR China. The data from this system together with the cancer incidence and mortality data from the cancer registration system are widely used not only for liver cancer epidemiological research, but also in monitoring cancer incidence for all sites, for evaluation of cancer control programmes, and for disease control activities.

Both active and passive methods are used for case-finding. District and township hospitals are responsible for the registration of incident cases and deaths from cancers in the outpatient departments, hospitalization (including those back home hospitalized out of Qidong), follow-up, autopsies, and biopsies. For any patient with cancer in the registration area, after a first check to see whether it is a new case, the registry personnel request information such as name, gender, age, address, marriage, occupation, and medical items such as date and basis of diagnosis, treatment (if any), and hospital name. These data are recorded and are reported by monthly lists to the next higher level registry.

When an incident case dies at home after a period in hospital, the registration personnel add the date of death to the record that already exists. A death certificate is issued by the registration personnel if there is none from the physician who was in charge of the case. If information on death is received without any prior notification, a disease record review or a home visit will be made to obtain full information.

All data files received from the lower registries are checked with cancer report lists and death certificate notification cards in order to reduce omissions and exclude duplicate registrations. Because of the follow-back efforts, the proportion of death-certificate-only registrations is very low. After finishing annual analysis and a data-set report (to provincial and national health authorities), all records are kept in paper form classified by year and by township and also as a computer database.

There are three general hospitals in Qidong, each with some 200–500 doctors, nurses and other staff. In addition, there are 100 beds for liver cancer patients in QLCI. The registration personnel in the record departments of these hospitals keep in touch with those at the cancer registry for monthly linkage with the discharge record of the cancer patients.

Each township hospital usually contains 20–50 beds and outpatient departments for various kinds of diseases. Under the hospital there are 15 village clinics on average with one to three health workers, whose main tasks are vaccinations, injections and treatment of various disorders. At least one of the village health workers is responsible for collecting information from patients with cancer who go to see doctors at a higher-level hospital and/or from those who have been discharged from any hospital.

Facilities for treating patients with cancer are also available in 'tumour wards' of hospitals as well as at QLCI where both internal medicine treatment and surgical operations are performed. Most cancer patients visit a hospital at least once for diagnosis and treatment. Almost all liver cancer patients go to QLCI for serum alpha-fetoprotein assay; more than half have diagnostic examinations as an outpatient, and nearly a quarter are hospitalized in the QLCI.

Several other city hospitals have their own pathology or histology departments; pathology records of all patients, including those diagnosed and treated in local hospitals, are reviewed by pathologists at the QLCI or other city hospitals, or directly abstracted from disease records made by the big city hospitals such as those of Nanjing, Shanghai and Beijing.

Jian-Guo Chen
Wen-Guang Li

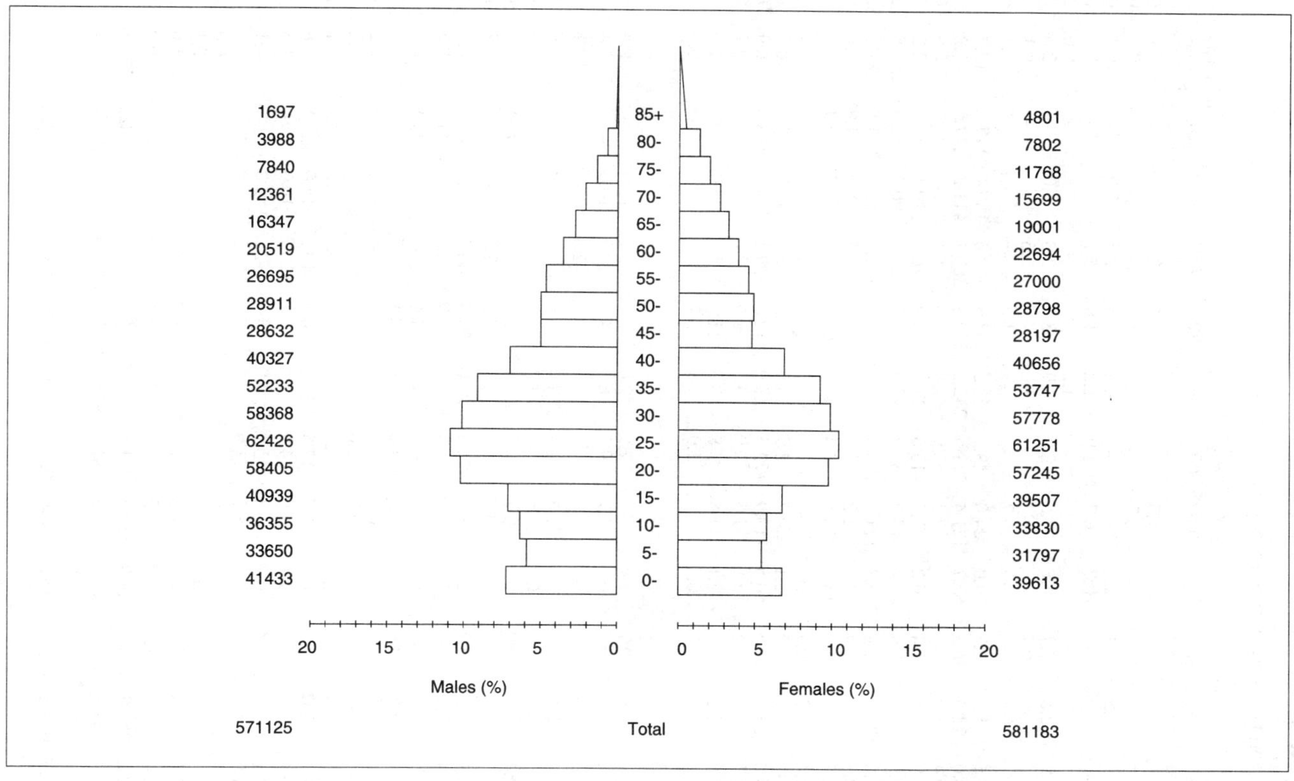

China, Qidong
Source of population: 1988–92
Notes to data overleaf:
* The low rates of childhood cancer, rather high ratios of mortality to incidence and the fall in incidence in the oldest age-groups indicate a degree of under-ascertainment.
+ The editors were unable to verify these data
† 163-164 includes mesothelioma of the pleura
† Mesothelioma not available separately
† Kaposi's sarcoma not available separately
† 188 does not include non-invasive tumours
Note: Data in Volume VI covered the city of Qidong; the registry has extended its coverage to the County in Volume VII.

Screening programmes in the area:
Some 10,000 examinations for cervical cancer are carried out annually in the population aged 25-70. 7,000 annual examinations for liver cancer are performed in the age-group 30-59.

+* CHINA, QIDONG COUNTY 1988-1992

ANNUAL INCIDENCE PER 100,000 BY AGE GROUP (YEARS) - MALE

SITE	ALL AGES	AGE UNK	0-	5-	10-	15-	20-	25-	30-	35-	40-	45-	50-	55-	60-	65-	70-	75-	80-	85+	CRUDE RATE	%	CR 64	CR 74	ASR (W)	ICD (9th)
Lip	4	0	-	-	-	-	-	-	-	-	-	-	-	1.5	-	-	1.6	2.6	-	-	0.1	0.1	0.01	0.02	**0.1**	140
Tongue	4	0	-	-	-	-	-	0.3	-	-	-	-	-	0.7	-	-	3.2	-	-	-	0.1	0.1	0.01	0.02	**0.1**	141
Salivary gland	11	0	-	-	-	-	-	-	-	-	0.5	1.4	2.1	-	-	2.4	1.6	2.6	5.0	-	0.4	0.2	0.02	0.04	**0.4**	142
Mouth	8	0	-	-	-	-	-	-	-	-	-	-	0.7	0.7	1.9	1.2	1.6	5.1	-	-	0.3	0.1	0.02	0.03	**0.3**	143-5
Oropharynx	1	0	-	-	-	-	-	-	-	-	-	-	-	-	-	1.2	-	-	-	-	0.0	0.0	0.00	0.01	**0.0**	146
Nasopharynx	58	0	-	-	-	-	0.7	-	1.4	1.9	2.5	7.7	4.8	7.5	2.9	4.9	8.1	2.6	5.0	-	2.0	0.9	0.15	0.21	**1.9**	147
Hypopharynx	3	0	-	-	-	-	-	-	-	-	-	-	0.7	-	-	1.2	-	2.6	-	-	0.1	0.0	0.00	0.01	**0.1**	148
Pharynx unspecified	2	0	-	-	-	-	-	-	-	-	-	-	-	0.7	-	-	1.6	-	-	-	0.1	0.0	0.00	0.01	**0.1**	149
Oesophagus	347	0	-	-	-	-	-	0.6	0.3	1.1	1.5	7.7	9.0	24.0	49.7	68.5	134.3	132.6	150.4	117.8	12.2	5.5	0.47	1.48	**11.5**	150
Stomach	1292	0	-	-	-	1.0	1.0	3.8	6.2	10.0	22.3	36.3	65.7	121.4	211.5	242.2	339.8	380.1	411.2	247.5	45.2	20.3	2.40	5.31	**42.7**	151
Small intestine	15	0	-	-	-	-	-	-	-	0.4	1.0	-	-	2.2	3.9	2.4	1.6	5.1	-	-	0.5	0.2	0.04	0.06	**0.5**	152
Colon	64	0	-	-	-	-	-	0.3	-	1.9	1.5	1.4	6.2	7.5	13.6	11.0	4.9	10.2	20.1	-	2.2	1.0	0.16	0.24	**2.1**	153
Rectum	224	0	-	-	0.5	0.7	0.6	1.7	-	4.6	3.5	8.4	10.4	14.2	32.2	40.4	61.5	51.0	90.3	82.5	7.8	3.5	0.38	0.89	**7.4**	154
Liver	2336	0	-	-	2.2	2.4	4.5	22.4	71.3	147.8	194.9	192.1	206.8	171.6	173.5	154.1	135.9	122.4	85.3	11.8	81.8	36.7	5.95	7.40	**72.1**	155
Gallbladder etc.	41	0	-	-	-	-	-	0.3	-	2.3	-	1.4	2.8	2.2	3.9	12.2	9.7	7.7	5.0	11.8	1.4	0.6	0.06	0.17	**1.4**	156
Pancreas	212	0	-	-	-	0.5	0.3	0.6	1.4	2.7	3.0	4.2	18.0	13.5	27.3	41.6	66.3	48.5	75.2	47.1	7.4	3.3	0.36	0.90	**7.0**	157
Nose, sinuses etc.	10	0	-	-	-	-	-	-	-	0.4	0.5	0.7	-	-	1.2	-	12.8	5.0	-	-	0.4	0.2	0.01	0.01	**0.3**	160
Larynx	19	0	-	-	-	-	-	-	-	-	-	0.7	2.1	0.7	3.9	4.9	1.6	5.1	-	11.8	0.7	0.3	0.04	0.07	**0.7**	161
Bronchus, lung	1053	0	-	-	-	1.0	0.7	0.3	0.3	5.0	11.9	19.6	50.5	110.9	172.5	223.9	312.3	329.1	315.9	188.5	36.9	16.6	1.86	4.54	**35.0**	162
†Other thoracic organs	20	0	-	-	-	-	-	-	-	1.1	-	1.4	2.8	1.5	2.9	3.7	1.6	2.6	5.0	-	0.7	0.3	0.05	0.08	**0.7**	163-4
Bone	46	0	-	-	0.6	1.5	0.3	0.3	1.0	0.8	1.5	2.8	2.1	1.5	5.8	8.6	11.3	5.1	5.0	-	1.6	0.7	0.09	0.19	**1.6**	170
Connective tissue	9	0	-	-	-	-	-	0.6	-	-	0.5	0.7	0.7	-	1.9	-	3.2	-	-	-	0.3	0.1	0.02	0.04	**0.3**	171
†Mesothelioma																										
†Kaposi's sarcoma																										
Melanoma of skin	12	0	-	-	-	-	0.3	-	-	-	-	0.7	1.4	-	2.9	2.4	-	2.6	10.0	-	0.4	0.2	0.03	0.04	**0.4**	172
Other skin	40	0	-	-	-	0.5	-	-	-	0.8	0.5	0.7	0.7	3.7	9.7	6.1	4.9	12.8	10.0	47.1	1.4		0.08	0.14	**1.4**	173
Breast	3	0	-	-	-	-	-	-	-	-	1.0	-	-	-	-	-	-	2.6	-	-	0.1	0.0	0.00	0.00	**0.1**	175
Prostate	15	0	-	-	-	-	-	-	-	-	0.5	-	-	1.5	1.9	4.9	6.5	-	10.0	-	0.5	0.2	0.02	0.08	**0.5**	185
Testis	8	0	-	-	-	-	0.3	0.6	-	-	-	-	0.7	1.5	-	1.2	-	2.6	-	-	0.3	0.1	0.02	0.02	**0.2**	186
Penis	12	0	-	-	-	-	-	-	-	0.4	-	0.7	2.1	0.7	-	-	3.2	5.1	5.0	11.8	0.4	0.2	0.02	0.04	**0.4**	187.1-.4
Other male genital	5	0	-	-	-	-	-	0.3	-	-	-	-	0.7	-	-	3.2	2.6	-	-	-	0.2	0.1	0.01	0.02	**0.1**	187.5-.9
†Bladder	118	0	-	-	-	-	-	-	-	1.1	0.5	4.2	5.5	8.2	22.4	22.0	24.3	48.5	50.1	47.1	4.1	1.9	0.21	0.44	**4.0**	188
Kidney etc.	15	0	-	-	-	-	0.7	-	-	0.4	1.0	-	1.4	0.7	1.9	-	4.9	2.6	-	11.8	0.5	0.2	0.03	0.05	**0.5**	189
Eye	3	0	-	-	-	-	-	-	-	-	-	-	-	-	-	1.2	1.6	-	-	11.8	0.1	0.0	0.00	0.01	**0.1**	190
Brain, nervous system	97	0	-	1.2	1.7	1.0	1.4	2.2	1.7	3.4	2.5	4.9	6.2	10.5	14.6	8.6	8.1	7.7	-	-	3.4	1.5	0.26	0.34	**3.2**	191-2
Thyroid	5	0	-	-	-	-	-	0.3	0.3	-	0.5	-	-	0.7	-	1.2	-	-	-	-	0.2	0.1	0.01	0.02	**0.1**	193
Other endocrine	3	0	-	-	0.6	-	-	-	-	-	-	-	-	0.7	1.0	-	-	-	-	-	0.1	0.0	0.01	0.01	**0.1**	194
Hodgkin's disease	2	0	-	-	-	-	-	-	0.3	-	-	-	0.7	-	-	-	-	-	-	-	0.1	0.0	0.01	0.01	**0.1**	201
Non-Hodgkin lymphoma	104	0	-	0.6	1.7	1.5	-	1.0	1.4	1.1	2.0	7.7	6.2	6.7	17.5	23.2	14.6	10.2	15.0	11.8	3.6	1.6	0.24	0.43	**3.7**	200,202
Multiple myeloma	37	0	-	-	0.6	1.0	-	0.3	0.3	0.4	-	2.1	1.4	3.0	4.9	7.3	8.1	10.2	10.0	-	1.3	0.6	0.07	0.15	**1.3**	203
Lymphoid leukaemia	31	0	1.0	1.2	-	0.5	0.3	1.0	0.3	1.1	1.0	1.4	0.7	1.5	1.9	4.9	4.9	2.6	5.0	-	1.1	0.5	0.06	0.11	**1.1**	204
Myeloid leukaemia	53	0	1.0	1.2	2.2	0.5	1.0	0.6	1.4	1.9	1.5	2.1	2.1	3.7	1.9	7.3	3.2	12.8	5.0	-	1.9	0.8	0.11	0.16	**1.8**	205
Monocytic leukaemia	0	0	-	-	-	-	-	-	-	-	-	-	-	-	-	-	-	-	-	-	0.0	0.0	0.00	0.00	**0.0**	206
Other leukaemia	2	0	-	-	-	-	0.3	-	-	-	-	-	0.7	-	-	-	-	-	-	-	0.1	0.0	0.01	0.01	**0.1**	207
Leukaemia unspecified	29	0	0.5	-	0.6	-	0.3	0.3	1.7	1.1	0.5	1.4	0.7	1.5	2.9	1.2	9.7	2.6	-	-	1.0	0.5	0.06	0.11	**0.9**	208
Other and unspecified	27	0	-	-	-	0.5	0.3	-	-	0.4	1.5	1.4	2.8	2.2	-	7.3	6.5	2.6	5.0	-	0.9	0.4	0.05	0.11	**0.9**	O&U
All sites	6400	0	2.4	4.2	9.9	12.2	13.4	36.8	91.5	192.2	257.9	314.3	417.8	530.4	791.5	924.9	1205.3	1255.1	1313.9	860.2	224.1		13.37	24.02	**207.1**	ALL
All sites but 173	6360	0	2.4	4.2	9.9	11.7	13.4	36.8	91.5	191.4	257.4	313.6	417.1	526.7	781.7	918.8	1200.5	1242.3	1303.8	813.1	222.7	100.0	13.29	23.89	**205.7**	ALLb

Rate from 1 case: 0.483 0.594 0.550 0.489 0.342 0.320 0.343 0.383 0.496 0.699 0.692 0.749 0.975 1.223 1.618 2.551 5.015 11.784

†Important: see notes on population page

324

+* CHINA, QIDONG COUNTY 1988-1992

ANNUAL INCIDENCE PER 100,000 BY AGE GROUP (YEARS) - FEMALE

SITE	ALL AGES	AGE UNK	0-	5-	10-	15-	20-	25-	30-	35-	40-	45-	50-	55-	60-	65-	70-	75-	80-	85+	CRUDE RATE	%	CR 64	CR 74	ASR (W)	ICD (9th)
Lip	2	0	-	-	-	-	-	-	-	-	-	-	0.7	-	0.9	-	-	-	-	-	0.1	0.1	0.01	0.01	0.1	140
Tongue	6	0	-	-	-	-	-	-	-	-	-	-	-	1.5	-	-	3.8	1.7	-	-	0.2	0.2	0.01	0.03	0.2	141
Salivary gland	3	0	-	-	-	-	-	-	-	0.7	-	-	-	-	-	-	-	-	-	4.2	0.1	0.1	0.00	0.00	0.1	142
Mouth	8	0	-	-	-	-	-	-	-	0.4	-	-	1.4	0.7	0.9	2.1	1.3	-	-	-	0.3	0.2	0.02	0.03	0.2	143-5
Oropharynx	5	0	-	-	-	-	-	-	0.3	-	0.5	-	-	0.7	-	-	1.3	-	2.6	-	0.2	0.1	0.01	0.01	0.1	146
Nasopharynx	40	0	-	-	-	-	-	0.3	-	1.5	2.0	1.4	2.1	2.2	6.2	3.2	1.3	10.2	10.3	8.3	1.4	1.1	0.08	0.10	1.1	147
Hypopharynx	0	0	-	-	-	-	-	-	-	-	-	-	-	-	-	-	-	-	-	-	0.0	0.0	0.00	0.00	0.0	148
Pharynx unspecified	0	0	-	-	-	-	-	-	-	-	-	-	-	-	-	-	-	-	-	-	0.0	0.0	0.00	0.00	0.0	149
Oesophagus	181	0	-	-	-	-	-	0.3	-	0.7	2.0	4.3	5.6	13.3	15.0	25.3	42.0	59.5	53.8	50.0	6.2	5.0	0.21	0.54	4.6	150
Stomach	780	0	-	-	-	-	1.4	1.3	6.2	8.9	19.7	21.3	34.7	48.1	91.7	100.0	172.0	166.6	210.2	129.1	26.8	21.4	1.17	2.53	20.7	151
Small intestine	17	0	-	-	-	-	-	-	-	0.4	0.5	-	-	1.5	0.9	2.1	1.3	5.1	15.4	-	0.6	0.5	0.02	0.03	0.4	152
Colon	79	0	-	-	-	0.5	-	0.3	1.0	0.7	1.0	2.1	3.5	5.9	5.3	6.3	16.6	22.1	20.5	33.3	2.7	2.2	0.10	0.22	2.0	153
Rectum	262	0	-	-	-	-	0.7	1.0	2.1	3.7	4.4	5.0	13.2	17.0	33.5	25.3	67.5	71.4	38.5	45.8	9.0	7.2	0.40	0.87	7.0	154
Liver	648	0	0.5	-	-	0.5	1.4	4.2	18.7	30.9	47.2	50.4	44.4	57.8	58.2	44.2	49.7	42.5	25.6	4.2	22.3	17.8	1.57	2.04	19.1	155
Gallbladder etc.	37	0	-	-	-	-	-	0.3	-	-	0.5	0.7	2.8	2.2	6.2	9.5	5.1	8.5	5.1	-	1.3	1.0	0.06	0.14	1.1	156
Pancreas	180	0	-	-	-	-	0.3	0.3	0.3	1.5	1.5	4.3	3.5	9.6	24.7	33.7	45.9	49.3	33.3	33.3	6.2	4.9	0.23	0.63	4.8	157
Nose, sinuses etc.	7	0	-	-	-	-	-	-	-	-	-	1.4	-	-	0.9	1.1	1.3	1.7	2.6	-	0.2	0.2	0.01	0.02	0.2	160
Larynx	2	0	-	-	-	-	-	-	-	-	-	-	-	-	0.9	-	-	1.7	-	-	0.1	0.1	0.00	0.00	0.1	161
Bronchus, lung	405	0	-	-	-	-	0.3	1.0	1.7	3.7	7.4	10.6	16.7	38.5	39.7	72.6	94.3	78.2	89.7	45.8	13.9	11.1	0.60	1.43	11.0	162
†Other thoracic organs	11	0	-	-	-	-	-	0.3	-	-	-	0.7	0.7	3.0	1.8	1.1	1.3	-	-	-	0.4	0.3	0.03	0.04	0.3	163-4
Bone	37	0	0.5	-	0.6	0.5	0.7	0.7	0.3	0.7	0.5	2.1	0.7	3.0	1.8	8.4	3.8	1.7	5.1	8.3	1.3	1.0	0.06	0.12	1.1	170
Connective tissue	6	0	-	-	-	-	0.3	-	0.3	-	0.5	-	-	0.7	0.9	-	-	-	2.6	-	0.2	0.2	0.01	0.01	0.2	171
†Mesothelioma																										
†Kaposi's sarcoma																										
Melanoma of skin	11	0	-	-	-	-	-	0.3	0.3	0.7	0.5	-	-	0.7	-	2.1	-	-	2.6	8.3	0.4	0.3	0.01	0.02	0.3	172
Other skin	48	0	-	-	-	-	-	-	0.3	0.4	1.5	1.4	1.4	1.5	0.9	2.1	10.2	11.9	28.2	33.3	1.7		0.04	0.10	1.1	173
Breast	371	0	-	-	-	-	-	2.3	6.2	18.2	26.1	36.9	32.6	25.9	35.3	22.1	30.6	18.7	23.1	20.8	12.8	10.2	0.92	1.18	11.2	174
Uterus unspecified	33	0	-	-	-	0.5	-	0.3	0.7	0.7	1.5	1.4	4.2	5.2	0.9	4.2	1.3	5.1	-	-	1.1	0.9	0.08	0.10	1.0	179
Cervix uteri	97	0	-	-	-	-	0.3	0.3	0.3	0.4	3.4	1.4	9.7	6.7	13.2	7.4	16.6	15.3	28.2	25.0	3.3	2.7	0.18	0.30	2.6	180
Placenta	17	0	-	-	-	-	0.7	1.6	1.7	1.1	0.5	0.7	-	-	-	-	-	-	-	-	0.6	0.5	0.03	0.03	0.4	181
Corpus uteri	19	0	-	-	-	-	-	0.3	0.7	-	0.5	1.4	2.1	1.5	1.8	2.1	2.5	1.7	2.6	-	0.7	0.5	0.04	0.06	0.6	182
Ovary etc.	37	0	-	-	-	-	0.3	0.3	0.7	-	1.5	1.4	6.9	1.5	5.3	7.4	-	3.4	2.6	-	1.3	1.0	0.09	0.13	1.2	183
Other female genital	1	0	-	-	-	-	-	-	-	-	-	-	-	-	-	1.1	-	-	-	-	0.0	0.0	0.00	0.01	0.0	184
†Bladder	30	0	-	-	-	-	-	-	0.3	-	-	-	1.4	1.5	2.6	3.2	10.2	5.1	15.4	8.3	1.0	0.8	0.03	0.10	0.7	188
Kidney etc.	15	0	-	-	0.6	-	0.3	-	-	0.4	0.5	0.7	-	1.5	2.6	3.2	2.5	-	-	-	0.5	0.4	0.03	0.06	0.5	189
Eye	2	0	0.5	-	-	-	-	-	-	-	-	-	-	-	-	-	1.7	-	-	-	0.1	0.1	0.00	0.00	0.1	190
Brain, nervous system	62	0	1.5	1.3	1.2	1.0	0.3	0.7	1.7	2.6	1.0	2.8	6.3	6.7	2.6	4.2	5.1	5.1	-	-	2.1	1.7	0.15	0.19	2.0	191-2
Thyroid	17	0	-	-	-	-	0.7	-	0.3	0.7	1.5	1.4	1.4	0.7	-	2.1	1.3	-	2.6	-	0.6	0.5	0.03	0.05	0.5	193
Other endocrine	2	0	-	-	-	0.5	-	-	-	0.4	-	-	-	-	-	-	-	-	-	-	0.1	0.1	0.00	0.00	0.1	194
Hodgkin's disease	1	0	-	-	-	-	-	-	-	-	-	-	-	-	-	-	-	1.7	-	-	0.0	0.0	0.00	0.00	0.0	201
Non-Hodgkin lymphoma	64	0	-	-	-	-	0.3	1.3	1.0	2.2	1.0	4.3	3.5	3.7	6.2	7.4	6.4	11.9	12.8	4.2	2.2	1.8	0.12	0.19	1.8	200,202
Multiple myeloma	20	0	-	-	-	-	-	-	0.3	-	0.5	0.7	-	0.7	3.5	3.2	1.3	3.4	10.3	8.3	0.7	0.5	0.03	0.05	0.5	203
Lymphoid leukaemia	20	0	0.5	0.6	-	1.0	0.3	0.7	0.7	0.4	0.5	1.4	-	0.7	1.8	3.2	-	1.7	-	-	0.7	0.5	0.04	0.06	0.7	204
Myeloid leukaemia	57	0	1.5	1.3	1.2	-	2.1	0.3	1.0	2.6	1.0	2.8	2.1	2.2	2.6	7.4	10.2	1.7	2.6	4.2	2.0	1.6	0.10	0.19	1.8	205
Monocytic leukaemia	1	0	-	-	-	-	-	-	-	-	-	-	-	-	-	-	-	-	-	-	0.0	0.0	0.00	0.00	0.0	206
Other leukaemia	3	0	-	-	0.6	-	-	-	-	0.4	-	-	-	0.7	-	-	-	-	-	-	0.1	0.1	0.01	0.01	0.1	207
Leukaemia unspecified	21	0	-	1.3	1.2	-	1.0	0.3	-	0.4	-	1.5	-	0.7	-	5.3	1.1	-	2.6	-	0.7	0.6	0.06	0.06	0.7	208
Other and unspecified	26	0	0.5	-	-	-	-	-	0.7	0.7	0.4	0.5	0.7	1.4	1.5	4.4	4.2	2.5	3.4	4.2	0.9	0.7	0.05	0.09	0.8	O&U
All sites	3691	0	5.6	4.4	5.3	4.6	11.9	19.9	48.1	86.0	130.9	163.8	202.8	269.6	378.1	422.1	608.9	613.5	648.5	479.0	127.0		6.65	11.81	102.9	ALL
All sites but 173	3643	0	5.6	4.4	5.3	4.6	11.9	19.9	47.8	85.6	129.4	162.4	201.4	268.1	377.2	420.0	598.7	601.6	620.3	445.7	125.4	100.0	6.62	11.71	101.9	ALLb

Rate from 1 case			0.505	0.629	0.591	0.506	0.349	0.327	0.346	0.372	0.492	0.709	0.694	0.741	0.881	1.053	1.274	1.700	2.563	4.165

†Important: see notes on population page

325

China, Shanghai

The population-based Shanghai Cancer Registry, the oldest in China, was established and started operating in 1963. According to a regulation issued by the Shanghai Municipal Bureau of Public Health, all medical facilities (more than 150 units) in Shanghai are responsible for notifying all newly diagnosed cancer cases and benign tumours of the central nervous system to the registry.

Shanghai is situated on the east coast of China at the outlet of Yangtzi River, with an altitude above sea level of about 4 m, at latitude 31°14′ N and longitude 121°29′ E. The area is 6340 km^2 (urban area about 792 km^2). The average annual temperature is about 15°C.

Shanghai is the largest industrial city in China. There are about 13 million inhabitants in the municipality. The urban area has expanded in recent years. In 1990, the inhabitants in the urban area numbered 7.2 million. In 1990, cancer caused 27% of all deaths in the Shanghai urban area.

A well organized administrative system for recording households in urban Shanghai has existed for several decades. All permanent residents in Shanghai must be registered in the local resident offices. The Municipal Bureau of Public Security can thus provide quite accurate total numbers of males and females at the end of each year. Complete city censuses were taken in 1973, 1979, 1982, 1985, 1990 and 1992, so the population by sex and age-group in urban Shanghai for each year can be estimated.

A standardized notification card, which includes information on names, date of birth, sex, address, occupation, cancer site, date and basis of cancer diagnosis, is used for reporting cancer cases. The notifications completed by physicians or medical clerks are sent to the cancer registry and filed according to the name of the patient and administrative district of residence. Using this file, the registry staff can determine if a patient has already been reported to the registry, so as to avoid duplication.

Death certificates for all cancer patients are obtained monthly from the Vital Statistics Section of the Shanghai Hygiene and Anti-epidemic Centre and compared with the file of new cases kept in the registry. If the deceased was not registered before death, the registry staff interview relatives to obtain information on the hospital where the case was diagnosed and treated, and the date and basis of cancer diagnosis. Such information is also collected from the hospital if there is any doubt about the accuracy of the information provided by the relatives. Since the late 1980s, the registry has obtained information on the vital status of cancer patients by both active and passive follow-up.

Data from all cancer notification cards are computerized, using specially designed software in which Chinese characters are read directly. Records with similar contents in terms of name, sex, date of birth, address and cancer site are printed out and examined to detect and then delete any duplications.

All cancer cases registered before 1983 were classified according to the three-digit rubrics of ICD-9 and later according to the four-digit rubrics of ICD-9.

Cancer incidence and mortality rates are calculated by sex, age and site of cancer. Age-adjusted rates are calculated by use of the direct method of standardization with the world population as the standard. The accumulated data of the registry are used for cancer control activities and cancer epidemiological studies in Shanghai.

Gao Yu Tang
Jin Fan

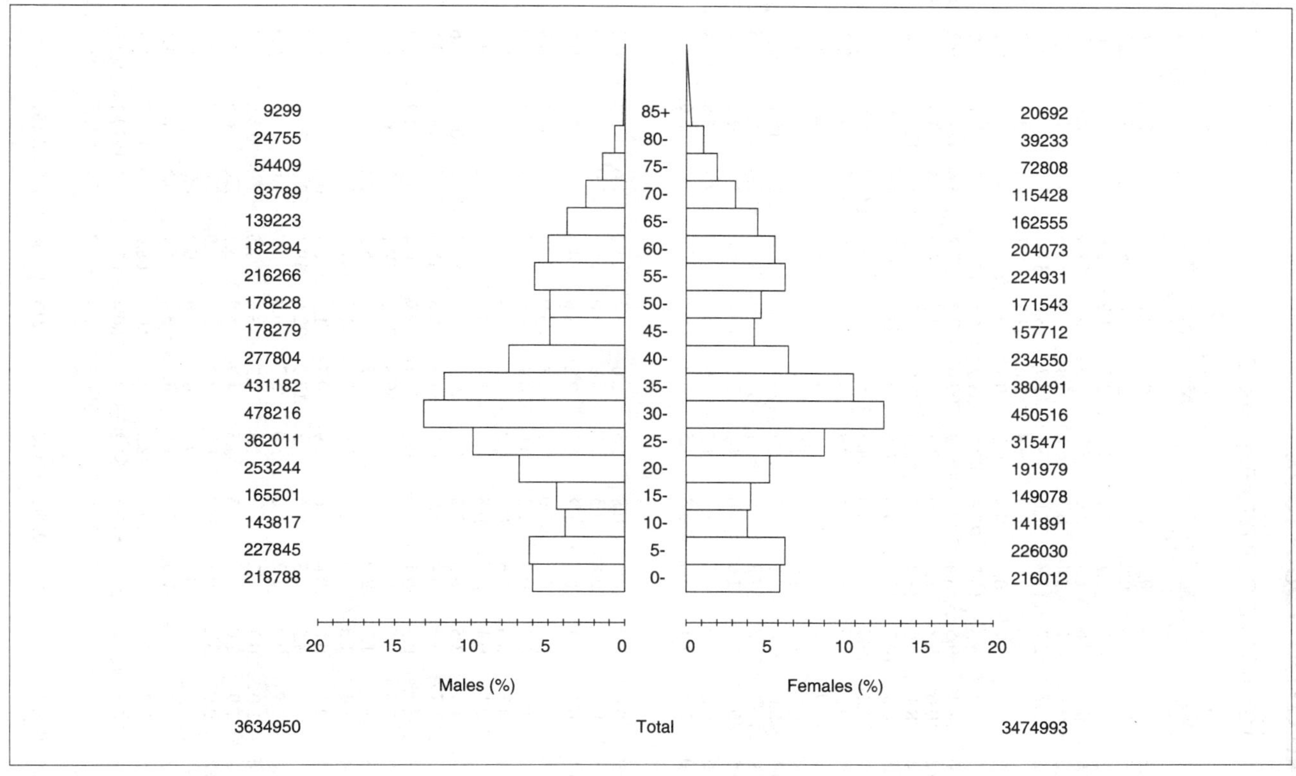

China, Shanghai
Source of population: average annual 1988–92
Census: 1990
Estimate: The sex and age distribution of the 1988 and 1989 populations were estimated by interpolation of the sex and age distributions of the 1985 and 1990 censuses. The 1991 and 1992 populations were based on the 1990 census data.

Notes to tables overleaf:
+ The editors were unable to verify these data
† 163-164 includes mesothelioma of the pleura
† Mesothelioma not available separately
† Kaposi's sarcoma not available separately
† 188 does not include non-invasive tumours
† 191-2 includes non-invasive tumours (number unknown)

+ CHINA, SHANGHAI 1988-1992

ANNUAL INCIDENCE PER 100,000 BY AGE GROUP (YEARS) - MALE

SITE	ALL AGES	AGE UNK	0-	5-	10-	15-	20-	25-	30-	35-	40-	45-	50-	55-	60-	65-	70-	75-	80-	85+	CRUDE RATE	%	CR 64	CR 74	ASR (W)	ICD (9th)
Lip	26	0	-	-	-	-	0.1	-	-	0.1	-	0.3	0.3	0.1	0.1	0.7	0.2	2.2	1.6	2.2	0.1	0.0	0.01	0.01	**0.1**	140
Tongue	152	0	-	-	-	-	-	0.2	0.1	0.5	0.6	1.6	0.8	2.7	2.4	3.2	2.6	5.5	1.6	8.6	0.8	0.3	0.04	0.07	**0.7**	141
Salivary gland	111	0	-	0.1	0.1	-	0.1	0.2	0.2	0.2	0.6	0.7	0.7	2.1	1.6	2.2	1.9	1.8	4.8	4.3	0.6	0.2	0.03	0.05	**0.5**	142
Mouth	223	0	-	-	0.1	-	0.3	0.1	0.6	0.5	0.6	1.5	2.6	3.7	5.3	8.1	7.4	11.3	10.8	1.2	0.4	0.05	0.12	**1.0**	143-5
Oropharynx	61	0	-	-	-	-	-	-	0.2	0.0	0.1	0.1	0.4	0.6	0.8	1.4	3.4	2.6	0.8	4.3	0.3	0.1	0.01	0.04	**0.3**	146
Nasopharynx	999	0	-	-	0.8	0.8	0.4	1.0	2.8	4.2	7.7	12.2	11.8	12.0	15.1	15.7	13.6	11.8	7.3	-	5.5	1.9	0.35	0.49	**4.5**	147
Hypopharynx	30	0	-	-	-	-	0.1	-	-	-	-	-	0.3	0.8	1.0	1.3	0.7	2.4	2.2	0.2	0.1	0.01	Hy.02	**0.1**	148
Pharynx unspecified	11	0	-	-	-	-	0.1	-	0.0	-	0.1	0.1	0.1	0.2	0.1	0.1	0.6	-	-	-	0.1	0.0	0.00	0.01	**0.1**	149
Oesophagus	2855	0	-	-	-	-	-	0.1	0.5	0.9	1.7	3.5	10.8	27.6	49.0	83.2	135.4	156.2	163.2	187.1	15.7	5.5	0.47	1.56	**12.5**	150
Stomach	10761	0	-	-	-	0.2	0.5	2.6	8.2	14.0	18.4	30.5	58.4	109.7	193.9	309.6	407.7	499.2	473.4	421.6	59.2	20.7	2.18	5.77	**46.5**	151
Small intestine	151	0	-	-	-	-	-	0.1	0.1	0.2	0.6	0.8	1.5	2.6	2.3	4.0	4.3	4.0	2.4	4.3	0.8	0.3	0.04	0.08	**0.7**	152
Colon	2797	0	-	-	0.1	0.1	0.3	1.0	3.3	4.4	8.1	13.0	16.4	30.1	48.4	73.0	97.2	113.2	104.2	122.6	15.4	5.4	0.63	1.48	**12.2**	153
Rectum	2129	0	-	-	-	0.1	0.1	1.4	2.6	4.3	6.2	10.7	15.3	24.0	36.6	49.3	69.7	80.1	84.8	92.5	11.7	4.1	0.51	1.10	**9.3**	154
Liver	6459	0	0.7	0.4	0.1	0.5	1.0	3.6	8.0	15.7	24.3	39.3	66.5	98.6	114.5	138.9	157.6	169.1	172.9	135.5	35.5	12.4	1.87	3.35	**28.2**	155
Gallbladder etc.	577	0	-	-	-	-	-	-	0.2	0.5	0.8	1.5	3.7	5.5	9.9	15.1	26.9	24.6	37.2	23.7	3.2	1.1	0.11	0.32	**2.5**	156
Pancreas	1445	0	-	-	-	-	-	0.4	0.5	1.2	3.0	6.3	7.4	14.8	27.8	39.2	54.8	67.3	70.3	49.5	8.0	2.8	0.31	0.78	**6.3**	157
Nose, sinuses etc.	163	0	-	-	0.1	0.1	0.2	0.2	0.4	0.4	0.7	1.1	1.2	1.3	2.5	3.0	5.8	4.0	8.1	-	0.9	0.3	0.04	0.09	**0.7**	160
Larynx	767	1	-	-	-	0.1	-	-	0.3	0.3	0.6	2.4	3.7	10.5	16.3	24.3	28.4	28.3	32.3	15.1	4.2	1.5	0.17	0.44	**3.3**	161
Bronchus, lung	13000	0	-	-	-	0.4	0.4	0.9	2.7	5.9	11.3	21.8	57.8	138.6	264.1	407.1	568.5	596.6	555.0	436.6	71.5	25.0	2.52	7.40	**56.1**	162
†Other thoracic organs	260	0	0.2	0.1	-	0.2	0.6	0.4	0.3	0.5	0.9	1.3	1.9	1.8	4.6	5.2	10.4	7.0	12.1	2.2	1.4	0.5	0.06	0.14	**1.2**	163-4
Bone	353	0	0.3	0.4	0.3	1.9	0.3	0.6	0.8	1.0	0.6	0.9	2.5	3.1	4.5	6.8	14.7	9.6	12.9	6.5	1.9	0.7	0.09	0.19	**1.6**	170
Connective tissue	354	0	0.9	0.5	0.6	0.8	1.1	0.8	1.3	1.0	1.4	2.1	3.3	3.8	4.5	6.0	6.2	5.5	4.8	8.6	1.9	0.7	0.11	0.17	**1.7**	171
†Mesothelioma																										
†Kaposi's sarcoma																										
Melanoma of skin	77	0	-	-	-	-	-	-	0.0	0.0	0.4	0.4	0.4	0.8	1.5	2.0	3.4	2.2	1.6	2.2	0.4	0.1	0.02	0.05	**0.3**	172
Other skin	362	0	-	-	-	-	0.2	0.2	0.1	0.3	0.3	0.8	2.1	2.8	3.5	5.8	7.8	13.0	15.1	21.0	34.4	2.0		0.08	0.18	**1.7**	173
Breast	86	0	-	-	-	-	-	-	0.1	0.1	0.1	1.1	0.6	1.2	1.2	2.2	2.6	4.4	-	2.2	0.5	0.2	0.02	0.05	**0.4**	175
Prostate	530	0	-	-	-	-	-	-	0.1	0.1	-	0.3	1.1	3.0	6.7	12.8	26.0	47.8	50.1	34.4	2.9	1.0	0.06	0.25	**2.3**	185
Testis	172	0	0.9	0.1	-	0.2	0.6	0.4	1.7	1.5	1.4	0.6	0.4	1.2	0.9	0.9	0.9	1.5	3.2	4.3	0.9	0.3	0.05	0.06	**0.7**	186
Penis	66	0	-	-	-	-	-	-	0.1	0.1	0.3	0.3	0.6	0.7	0.8	1.0	2.8	3.7	2.4	4.3	0.4	0.1	0.01	0.03	**0.3**	187.1-.4
Other male genital	38	0	-	-	0.1	-	-	-	0.0	-	0.1	0.1	-	0.3	1.0	1.4	0.6	1.8	3.2	-	0.2	0.1	0.01	0.02	**0.2**	187.5-.9
†Bladder	1562	0	-	-	-	0.2	0.2	0.3	0.6	1.8	1.9	3.5	6.6	13.9	28.3	40.1	63.3	82.7	100.2	105.4	8.6	3.0	0.29	0.80	**6.9**	188
Kidney etc.	631	0	0.9	0.1	0.1	0.5	0.2	0.3	0.5	1.0	1.7	3.3	6.4	8.9	10.8	14.9	18.8	15.8	20.2	19.4	3.5	1.2	0.17	0.34	**2.9**	189
Eye	33	0	0.6	-	-	-	-	-	0.1	0.1	-	0.3	0.1	0.4	0.2	0.4	0.9	0.4	0.8	4.3	0.2	0.1	0.01	0.02	**0.2**	190
†Brain, nervous system	1180	0	2.0	2.7	2.5	2.4	2.3	1.9	3.6	4.8	5.5	5.5	10.8	11.4	16.6	19.8	27.1	19.1	17.8	6.5	6.5	2.3	0.36	0.59	**5.6**	191-2
Thyroid	241	0	-	0.2	-	0.4	0.5	0.8	1.0	1.3	1.6	1.7	2.0	2.3	3.3	2.7	3.6	5.5	2.4	-	1.3	0.5	0.07	0.11	**1.0**	193
Other endocrine	207	0	0.1	0.8	0.8	0.7	0.2	0.3	0.8	1.4	1.4	1.6	1.9	2.5	3.0	1.7	1.1	1.5	0.8	-	1.1	0.4	0.08	0.09	**1.0**	194
Hodgkin's disease	88	0	0.2	0.4	0.3	0.2	0.6	0.4	0.5	0.5	0.1	0.6	0.4	0.6	0.9	0.7	1.5	0.7	0.8	-	0.5	0.2	0.03	0.04	**0.4**	201
Non-Hodgkin lymphoma	926	0	2.2	1.2	0.4	1.2	1.3	1.5	2.4	2.5	4.0	3.5	6.3	9.6	15.3	17.7	22.6	19.1	32.3	28.0	5.1	1.8	0.26	0.46	**4.3**	200,202
Multiple myeloma	162	0	-	0.1	-	-	-	0.1	0.1	0.0	0.3	0.9	1.2	2.0	3.0	5.7	6.8	3.7	1.6	-	0.9	0.3	0.04	0.10	**0.7**	203
Lymphoid leukaemia	235	0	2.4	2.6	2.5	1.1	0.4	0.3	0.9	0.6	1.0	0.7	1.2	1.4	1.4	2.2	3.6	1.5	7.3	8.6	1.3	0.5	0.08	0.11	**1.5**	204
Myeloid leukaemia	374	0	0.5	1.0	0.6	1.1	0.9	1.7	2.2	1.9	1.9	2.0	3.4	2.5	3.5	4.9	5.8	3.7	2.4	6.5	2.1	0.7	0.12	0.17	**1.7**	205
Monocytic leukaemia	114	0	0.3	0.4	0.3	0.2	0.2	0.2	0.3	0.2	0.6	0.7	0.7	0.9	1.8	2.6	2.6	2.9	2.4	2.2	0.6	0.2	0.03	0.06	**0.6**	206
Other leukaemia	22	0	0.1	-	-	-	0.1	0.1	0.0	-	-	-	0.1	0.2	0.8	0.6	0.4	0.4	0.8	-	0.1	0.0	0.01	0.01	**0.1**	207
Leukaemia unspecified	197	0	0.8	0.3	0.3	0.6	0.7	0.6	0.4	0.7	0.9	1.1	0.9	2.0	1.6	3.2	3.4	5.1	6.5	12.9	1.1	0.4	0.05	0.09	**1.0**	208
Other and unspecified	1479	0	0.2	0.1	0.1	0.5	0.2	0.6	1.3	2.5	2.7	4.9	8.2	15.2	22.3	37.6	50.3	68.0	94.5	114.0	8.1	2.8	0.29	0.73	**6.6**	O&U
All sites	52466	1	13.3	11.4	10.4	15.1	13.8	23.0	49.7	77.4	114.8	185.4	322.1	577.1	934.2	1377.1	1880.4	2103.3	2136.1	1927.1	288.7		11.74	28.03	**230.5**	ALL
All sites but 173	52104	1	13.3	11.4	10.4	14.9	13.7	22.9	49.5	77.1	114.0	183.3	319.3	573.6	928.4	1369.3	1867.4	2088.2	2115.1	1892.7	286.7	100.0	11.66	27.84	**228.8**	ALLb

Rate from 1 case   0.091   0.088   0.139   0.121   0.079   0.055   0.042   0.046   0.072   0.112   0.112   0.092   0.110   0.144   0.213   0.368   0.808   2.151

†Important: see notes on population page

+ CHINA, SHANGHAI 1988-1992

ANNUAL INCIDENCE PER 100,000 BY AGE GROUP (YEARS) - FEMALE

SITE	ALL AGES	AGE UNK	0-	5-	10-	15-	20-	25-	30-	35-	40-	45-	50-	55-	60-	65-	70-	75-	80-	85+	CRUDE RATE	%	CR 64	CR 74	ASR (W)	ICD (9th)
Lip	12	0	-	-	-	-	-	-	-	-	-	-	-	0.1	0.4	0.2	0.7	0.3	-	-	0.1	0.0	0.00	0.01	0.0	140
Tongue	128	0	-	-	-	-	-	-	0.4	0.4	0.3	1.1	1.3	1.7	1.2	2.7	2.1	2.7	6.1	1.0	0.7	0.3	0.03	0.06	0.5	141
Salivary gland	98	0	-	-	0.1	-	0.1	0.1	0.4	0.7	0.9	0.5	1.0	0.8	1.0	1.1	1.4	1.6	3.6	1.0	0.6	0.3	0.03	0.04	0.4	142
Mouth	200	0	-	0.1	-	-	0.3	0.1	0.4	0.4	0.8	1.0	0.9	1.8	3.9	4.7	4.7	4.9	2.0	4.8	1.2	0.5	0.05	0.10	0.8	143-5
Oropharynx	35	0	-	-	-	-	-	-	-	0.2	-	0.1	0.1	0.4	0.7	0.7	0.5	1.6	1.5	-	0.2	0.1	0.01	0.01	0.1	146
Nasopharynx	389	0	-	-	0.1	0.5	0.7	1.1	1.0	2.5	2.7	6.0	3.7	4.4	4.3	4.2	4.5	4.1	2.5	3.9	2.2	1.0	0.14	0.18	1.8	147
Hypopharynx	11	0	-	-	-	-	-	-	-	-	0.1	-	-	0.2	0.2	0.5	-	-	1.0	-	0.1	0.0	0.00	0.00	0.0	148
Pharynx unspecified	4	0	-	-	-	-	-	-	-	-	-	-	-	-	-	0.1	-	0.3	0.5	1.0	0.0	0.0	0.00	0.00	0.0	149
Oesophagus	1338	0	-	-	-	-	-	-	0.1	0.3	0.5	1.5	6.4	12.1	21.0	32.7	44.9	52.2	63.2	65.7	7.7	3.5	0.21	0.60	4.8	150
Stomach	5584	0	-	-	0.3	0.1	1.1	3.9	10.4	14.0	16.1	23.8	30.8	51.8	71.2	115.8	156.1	179.4	193.7	176.9	32.1	14.6	1.12	2.48	21.0	151
Small intestine	109	0	-	-	-	0.1	0.1	0.1	0.0	0.2	0.3	0.6	0.9	1.2	1.9	2.3	2.1	2.7	4.6	1.9	0.6	0.3	0.03	0.05	0.4	152
Colon	2762	0	0.1	-	0.1	0.1	0.5	1.6	3.1	4.8	9.6	13.8	20.5	35.6	44.9	58.2	71.4	75.0	48.4	57.0	15.9	7.2	0.67	1.32	10.8	153
Rectum	1890	0	-	-	-	-	0.5	1.8	3.5	5.5	7.8	9.4	14.8	21.5	30.2	36.4	39.7	47.8	50.0	30.9	10.9	4.9	0.48	0.86	7.3	154
Liver	2579	0	0.6	-	0.1	0.5	0.1	1.5	1.7	3.5	4.3	10.3	19.8	27.0	37.8	54.0	72.1	90.9	94.8	72.5	14.8	6.7	0.54	1.17	9.8	155
Gallbladder etc.	971	0	-	-	0.1	-	0.1	0.3	0.4	1.1	2.5	5.0	10.3	17.2	23.1	32.9	36.8	28.5	19.3	5.6	2.5	0.19	0.47	3.6	156
Pancreas	1118	0	-	-	-	-	-	0.2	0.4	0.4	1.2	3.3	6.2	10.8	17.7	25.7	39.3	42.0	42.8	30.0	6.4	2.9	0.20	0.53	4.1	157
Nose, sinuses etc.	100	0	0.1	-	-	0.1	-	0.2	0.2	0.2	0.3	0.5	0.9	1.4	1.4	1.2	2.4	1.9	3.6	2.9	0.6	0.3	0.03	0.05	0.4	160
Larynx	98	0	-	-	-	-	-	-	-	0.1	-	0.1	0.9	0.6	1.4	3.0	2.4	4.4	4.1	3.9	0.6	0.3	0.02	0.04	0.4	161
Bronchus, lung	4898	0	-	-	-	0.1	0.3	0.8	2.1	4.8	7.7	15.5	27.7	44.7	75.1	122.5	168.8	178.0	148.9	108.3	28.2	12.8	0.89	2.35	18.2	162
†Other thoracic organs	157	0	0.1	-	0.1	0.3	0.7	0.4	0.4	0.6	0.3	1.1	0.8	1.2	1.6	3.2	2.8	4.4	3.6	3.9	0.9	0.4	0.04	0.07	0.7	163-4
Bone	286	0	-	0.6	1.1	0.8	0.5	0.5	0.8	0.4	0.5	1.1	1.3	2.0	3.2	5.9	8.0	8.2	7.1	6.8	1.6	0.7	0.06	0.13	1.3	170
Connective tissue	273	0	1.2	0.2	0.1	0.5	0.5	1.1	1.2	1.2	1.5	2.4	2.0	2.4	2.4	3.7	3.3	3.8	2.5	7.7	1.6	0.7	0.08	0.12	1.3	171
†Mesothelioma																										
†Kaposi's sarcoma																										
Melanoma of skin	68	1	0.1	-	-	-	-	0.2	0.1	0.2	0.1	0.3	0.3	0.6	1.4	0.6	1.9	1.9	2.0	1.9	0.4	0.2	0.02	0.03	0.3	172
Other skin	276	0	-	-	-	-	0.2	0.1	0.1	0.5	0.6	1.1	1.6	2.1	4.7	4.3	6.1	9.6	16.3	21.3	1.6		0.06	0.11	1.1	173
Breast	6084	0	-	-	-	0.3	1.0	4.2	15.1	32.8	63.8	83.3	70.1	72.2	69.5	74.3	74.3	73.1	75.4	65.7	35.0	15.9	2.06	2.80	26.5	174
Uterus unspecified	166	0	-	-	-	-	-	-	0.2	0.3	1.2	0.5	0.9	1.3	1.5	3.1	3.1	9.3	8.2	7.7	1.0	0.4	0.03	0.06	0.6	179
Cervix uteri	860	0	-	-	-	-	0.1	0.1	0.4	0.7	1.8	3.3	5.0	8.5	16.8	19.3	28.9	24.7	22.9	16.4	4.9	2.2	0.18	0.43	3.3	180
Placenta	18	0	-	-	-	-	0.2	0.1	0.2	0.3	0.1	-	0.1	-	-	0.1	-	-	-	-	0.1	0.0	0.01	0.01	0.1	181
Corpus uteri	856	0	-	-	-	0.1	0.1	0.4	1.2	1.1	4.3	7.5	15.2	19.7	13.8	13.3	8.0	9.6	2.5	4.8	4.9	2.2	0.32	0.42	3.7	182
Ovary etc.	1321	0	-	0.1	0.6	1.9	1.7	2.3	4.0	5.9	9.0	13.6	15.9	16.7	16.2	17.5	18.9	15.4	14.8	9.7	7.6	3.5	0.44	0.62	5.8	183
Other female genital	129	0	-	-	-	-	-	0.1	0.3	-	0.4	0.9	1.5	1.8	3.0	3.6	3.8	6.1	3.9	0.7	0.3	0.02	0.06	0.5	184
†Bladder	486	0	-	-	-	-	-	0.3	0.2	0.4	0.6	1.5	2.1	3.2	5.4	11.4	16.8	20.1	28.0	21.3	2.8	1.3	0.07	0.21	1.8	188
Kidney etc.	371	0	1.2	0.4	0.1	-	0.4	0.4	0.5	0.6	1.2	2.7	3.1	4.3	6.9	6.2	7.1	8.0	5.1	8.7	2.1	1.0	0.11	0.18	1.6	189
Eye	30	0	0.5	-	0.1	-	-	0.1	0.0	0.1	0.3	0.5	0.3	0.1	0.3	0.2	0.3	0.3	0.5	-	0.2	0.1	0.01	0.01	0.2	190
†Brain, nervous system	1019	0	2.6	2.0	1.7	1.3	2.0	2.3	2.8	4.4	6.6	6.6	8.4	13.4	13.7	15.5	11.4	11.8	7.6	2.9	5.9	2.7	0.34	0.47	4.7	191-2
Thyroid	670	0	-	-	0.1	1.1	1.0	2.0	4.4	5.6	7.2	8.5	6.6	4.4	5.7	5.3	5.4	4.1	3.6	1.0	3.9	1.8	0.23	0.29	3.0	193
Other endocrine	382	0	-	0.4	0.7	1.1	2.1	3.2	4.5	3.1	3.2	2.5	1.9	1.8	1.9	1.5	0.7	0.8	-	1.0	2.2	1.0	0.13	0.14	1.7	194
Hodgkin's disease	60	0	-	0.3	-	0.4	0.5	0.1	0.2	0.2	0.3	0.1	0.2	0.3	0.9	1.1	1.2	-	1.5	1.0	0.3	0.2	0.02	0.03	0.3	201
Non-Hodgkin lymphoma	579	0	0.4	1.2	0.7	1.1	1.0	1.2	1.2	1.5	2.7	3.3	4.4	5.9	7.4	9.1	12.1	11.8	14.8	9.7	3.3	1.5	0.16	0.27	2.5	200,202
Multiple myeloma	117	0	-	-	-	-	-	-	0.0	-	0.4	0.8	0.3	2.0	2.1	2.8	3.6	2.5	1.5	1.9	0.7	0.3	0.03	0.06	0.5	203
Lymphoid leukaemia	180	0	2.4	1.6	0.6	0.8	0.5	0.6	0.6	0.4	0.9	0.5	1.0	1.7	1.7	1.4	1.6	1.9	2.0	1.0	1.0	0.5	0.07	0.08	1.1	204
Myeloid leukaemia	273	0	0.6	0.4	0.8	0.9	0.6	1.0	1.2	1.3	1.3	1.9	2.6	2.3	3.1	3.6	2.8	2.7	4.6	1.0	1.6	0.7	0.09	0.12	1.3	205
Monocytic leukaemia	83	0	0.2	0.2	0.1	-	0.3	0.1	0.2	0.3	0.4	0.3	0.7	1.1	1.1	1.5	1.9	0.8	0.5	1.0	0.5	0.2	0.02	0.04	0.4	206
Other leukaemia	17	0	0.1	-	-	-	-	-	0.0	0.1	0.1	-	0.1	0.1	0.3	0.5	0.5	-	0.5	-	0.1	0.0	0.00	0.01	0.1	207
Leukaemia unspecified	185	0	0.6	0.4	0.6	0.3	0.4	0.3	0.4	0.5	0.5	0.5	0.9	1.2	1.5	3.7	4.0	6.0	4.1	8.7	1.1	0.5	0.04	0.08	0.8	208
Other and unspecified	1254	0	0.7	0.4	0.3	0.1	0.2	1.0	1.6	1.6	3.9	4.1	8.2	10.1	15.9	23.1	33.4	47.5	56.1	65.7	7.2	3.3	0.24	0.52	4.8	O&U
All sites	38524	1	11.5	8.3	8.7	12.9	18.1	33.7	65.9	102.6	166.4	238.5	296.4	406.6	531.8	724.4	907.8	1009.2	992.0	855.4	221.7		9.51	17.67	154.3	ALL
All sites but 173	38248	1	11.5	8.3	8.7	12.9	17.9	33.5	65.8	102.1	165.8	237.4	294.7	404.5	527.1	720.1	901.7	999.6	975.7	834.1	220.1	100.0	9.45	17.56	153.2	ALLb
Rate from 1 case			0.093	0.088	0.141	0.134	0.104	0.063	0.044	0.053	0.085	0.127	0.117	0.089	0.098	0.123	0.173	0.275	0.510	0.966						

†Important: see notes on population page

329

China, Tianjin

The Tianjin Cancer Registry was established at the section of Cancer Epidemiology, Tianjin Cancer Institute and Hospital in 1978 to perform descriptive epidemiology and etiological research. Since 1984, the cancer incidence and mortality data provided by the registry have been used to monitor the effectiveness of the Tianjin non-communicable disease control project.

Tianjin is the third largest city in China and has a population of nine million, 98% of Han nationality. Tianjin is an industrial and commercial city. The registry covers the central urban area of 160 km^2, with a population of over three million. The city is situated at latitude 39°8′ N and longitude 117°12′ E and lies at an altitude of one to three metres above sea level.

All physicians and medical clerks in the registry area are responsible for filling out a report form for each new case diagnosed as a malignant tumour.

Death certificates for malignant tumours have to be registered as such at the local police station and the residential file is checked against this source. All cancer deaths without a previous record in the registry are traced to his/her family, clinic and employer. Only permanent residents who are filed at the local police station are registered, so death-certificate-only registrations are rare. The registry conducts an active re-checking programme periodically to review all patient records of every medical unit located in the registry area to complete the incidence and mortality data. A total of 15 data items previously recorded (serial number, name, sex code, age, occupation code, working unit code, address code, cancer site code, code of diagnostic basis, year of diagnosis, month of diagnosis, medical unit code, year of death, month of death and reporting source code) have been supplemented with the morphology code according to ICD-O and the fourth digit of ICD-9 topography code for the present data-set.

For the purpose of data management and processing, a Chinese software package is used, which was developed at the registry and is revised periodically. Each data item is checked as being an allowable code, and certain selected combinations of items are also checked. Possible duplicate records from different sources are identified by computer as well as by hand.

In 1994, an occupational cancer study based on the data of the Tianjin Cancer Registry was carried out and published as IARC Technical Report No. 22. A survival analysis and study of cancer trends is in progress. With the support of a grant, the registry data will be used for follow-up in the cohort study of 140 000 women that started in 1984.

Qing-sheng Wang
Ke-xin Chen

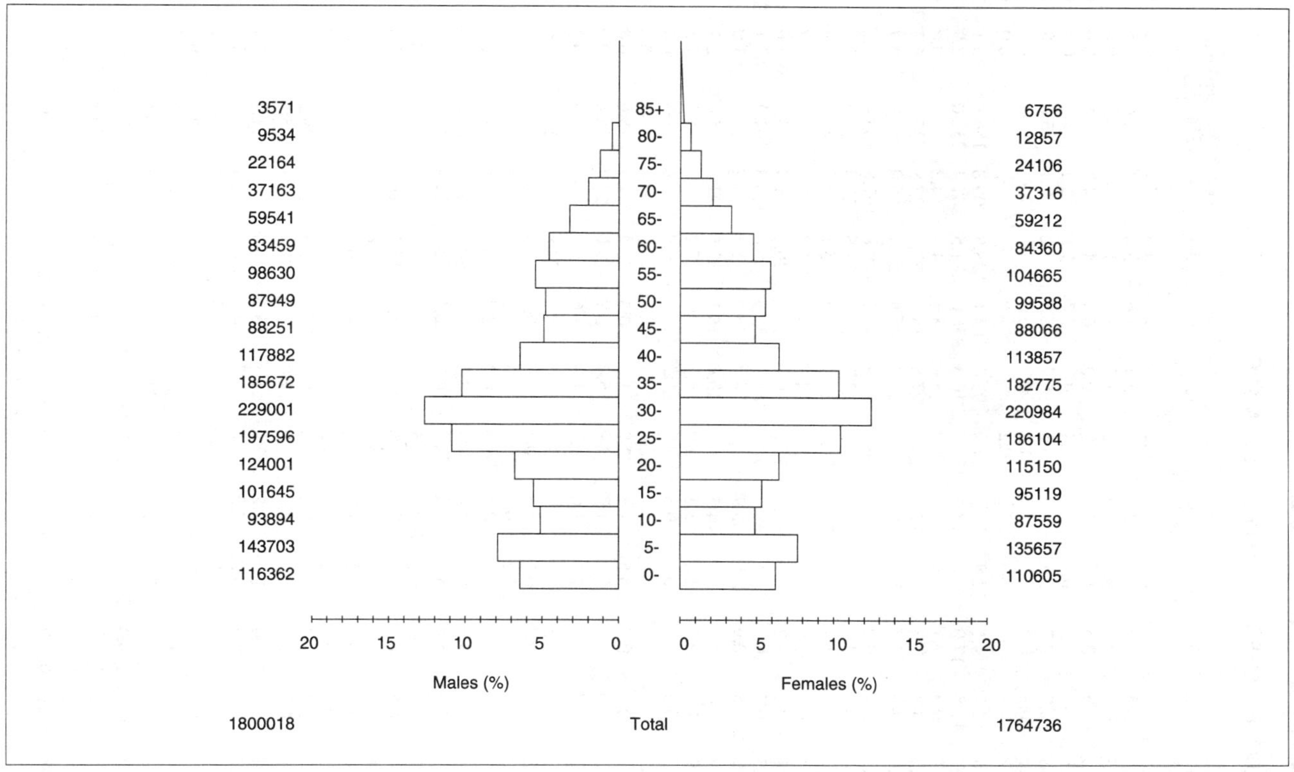

China, Tianjin

Source of population: average annual 1988–92

Census: A file of permanent residents is maintained at the police station. At the beginning of each year data at 31 December of the preceding year are obtained from the police station.

Estimate: The population for each year is estimated by taking the population at 31 December of that year plus the population at 31 December of the preceding year and dividing by 2.

Notes to tables overleaf:

† 188 does not include non-invasive tumours

Screening programmes in the area:

20,000 examinations for cervical cancer and 40,000 for breast cancer were carried out annually in the age group over 35 during the period 1988-90.

CHINA, TIANJIN 1988-1992

ANNUAL INCIDENCE PER 100,000 BY AGE GROUP (YEARS) - MALE

SITE	ALL AGES	AGE UNK	0-	5-	10-	15-	20-	25-	30-	35-	40-	45-	50-	55-	60-	65-	70-	75-	80-	85+	CRUDE RATE	%	CR 64	CR 74	ASR (W)	ICD (9th)
Lip	14	0	-	-	-	-	-	-	-	-	-	-	0.2	0.4	0.2	1.0	1.1	3.6	2.1	-	0.2	0.1	0.00	0.01	**0.1**	140
Tongue	47	0	-	-	-	-	-	-	0.1	-	0.5	0.2	1.1	2.0	1.7	3.4	1.6	3.6	4.2	5.6	0.5	0.3	0.03	0.05	**0.5**	141
Salivary gland	37	0	-	-	-	0.4	-	0.1	0.3	0.3	0.3	0.5	0.5	0.6	2.2	1.7	1.1	1.8	-	-	0.4	0.2	0.03	0.04	**0.4**	142
Mouth	78	0	0.2	-	-	-	0.2	0.1	0.3	0.2	0.3	0.5	1.8	2.4	1.9	6.0	6.5	4.5	4.2	5.6	0.9	0.4	0.04	0.10	**0.8**	143-5
Oropharynx	28	0	-	0.1	-	-	0.2	-	-	0.1	-	-	0.5	0.6	2.4	0.7	2.7	1.8	2.1	-	0.3	0.1	0.02	0.04	**0.3**	146
Nasopharynx	161	0	-	-	0.2	0.2	0.3	0.5	0.4	0.8	2.0	2.7	5.7	5.9	5.5	5.7	6.5	7.2	2.1	5.6	1.8	0.9	0.12	0.18	**1.6**	147
Hypopharynx	19	0	-	-	-	-	-	-	-	0.1	0.3	0.2	-	0.2	1.2	1.7	2.2	-	-	-	0.2	0.1	0.01	0.03	**0.2**	148
Pharynx unspecified	3	0	-	-	-	-	-	-	-	0.1	-	-	0.2	0.2	-	-	-	-	-	-	0.0	0.0	0.00	0.00	**0.0**	149
Oesophagus	1359	0	-	-	-	-	0.2	0.1	0.2	0.6	1.7	4.5	11.8	25.3	51.0	93.4	163.1	198.5	209.8	156.8	15.1	7.2	0.48	1.76	**14.0**	150
Stomach	2959	0	-	-	-	-	0.6	1.7	3.8	4.7	11.5	17.0	35.5	77.1	128.9	210.3	276.6	281.5	287.4	252.0	32.9	15.8	1.40	3.84	**29.8**	151
Small intestine	54	0	-	-	-	-	-	-	0.1	0.1	0.2	0.7	0.9	1.4	1.9	4.0	5.4	4.5	4.2	-	0.6	0.3	0.03	0.07	**0.5**	152
Colon	566	0	-	-	-	-	0.5	1.4	1.9	2.5	4.8	7.3	9.3	17.0	20.1	27.5	38.2	52.3	37.8	33.6	6.3	3.0	0.32	0.65	**5.6**	153
Rectum	622	0	-	-	-	0.2	0.3	0.1	2.8	2.6	4.4	5.7	8.6	16.2	29.5	27.9	46.8	51.4	65.0	67.2	6.9	3.3	0.35	0.73	**6.2**	154
Liver	2266	0	0.5	-	0.4	0.2	0.6	0.9	2.3	6.5	13.7	29.0	44.1	84.2	106.2	118.9	148.5	149.8	167.8	134.4	25.2	12.1	1.44	2.78	**22.7**	155
Gallbladder etc.	236	0	-	-	-	-	0.2	-	0.3	0.4	0.8	2.3	2.3	5.3	6.9	13.1	31.8	31.6	29.4	5.6	2.6	1.3	0.09	0.32	**2.4**	156
Pancreas	528	0	-	0.1	-	-	-	0.4	0.1	1.7	2.4	5.7	6.8	12.4	26.1	33.9	45.2	45.1	50.3	44.8	5.9	2.8	0.28	0.67	**5.4**	157
Nose, sinuses etc.	63	0	0.2	0.1	-	-	-	0.2	0.3	0.4	0.2	0.9	0.9	1.6	1.9	4.7	4.3	2.7	2.1	-	0.7	0.3	0.03	0.08	**0.6**	160
Larynx	323	0	-	-	-	-	-	-	-	0.1	0.8	3.2	4.3	14.4	15.8	20.5	19.9	26.2	29.4	33.6	3.6	1.7	0.19	0.40	**3.3**	161
Bronchus, lung	5589	0	-	-	-	0.2	0.3	1.7	3.6	7.3	20.5	46.2	79.4	169.9	278.2	384.3	472.0	465.6	415.3	291.2	62.1	29.8	3.04	7.32	**55.9**	162
Other thoracic organs	89	0	-	0.1	0.4	-	0.2	0.1	0.5	0.2	0.5	0.9	2.0	3.9	1.9	4.0	5.9	5.4	4.2	11.2	1.0	0.5	0.05	0.10	**0.9**	163-4
Bone	200	0	-	0.3	0.6	1.0	-	0.6	1.0	0.9	1.4	1.6	2.5	4.5	6.9	10.4	16.1	13.5	21.0	5.6	2.2	1.1	0.11	0.24	**2.0**	170
Connective tissue	116	0	0.5	-	0.2	0.2	0.5	0.4	0.7	0.9	1.0	2.5	1.8	3.7	1.0	4.7	9.7	7.2	-	5.6	1.3	0.6	0.07	0.14	**1.2**	171
Mesothelioma	18	0	-	-	-	-	-	0.1	0.1	-	0.3	-	0.2	0.8	0.7	1.7	-	0.9	-	-	0.2	0.1	0.01	0.02	**0.2**	MES
Kaposi's sarcoma	0	0	-	-	-	-	-	-	-	-	-	-	-	-	-	-	-	-	-	-	0.0	0.0	0.00	0.00	**0.0**	KAP
Melanoma of skin	37	0	-	-	-	-	-	-	-	0.5	0.5	0.5	1.4	2.2	1.7	0.5	5.4	2.1	5.6	-	0.4	0.2	0.02	0.04	**0.4**	172
Other skin	79	0	-	-	-	-	-	-	0.3	1.0	-	1.4	1.2	2.9	5.0	5.9	9.0	14.7	16.8	-	0.9		0.03	0.09	**0.8**	173
Breast	34	0	-	-	-	-	-	-	0.2	0.2	0.7	0.9	1.1	1.0	1.0	1.3	1.6	0.9	-	-	0.4	0.2	0.03	0.04	**0.3**	175
Prostate	177	0	-	-	-	-	-	-	0.3	0.2	0.3	0.5	0.2	3.4	3.1	13.4	18.3	29.8	35.7	67.2	2.0	0.9	0.04	0.20	**1.9**	185
Testis	50	0	0.9	0.1	-	0.2	-	0.6	0.7	0.8	0.7	0.7	0.7	0.6	0.5	1.0	0.5	1.8	2.1	-	0.6	0.3	0.03	0.04	**0.5**	186
Penis	23	0	-	-	-	-	-	0.2	0.2	0.2	0.3	-	0.2	0.2	0.2	1.0	1.6	1.8	8.4	-	0.2	0.1	0.01	0.02	**0.2**	187.1-.4
Other male genital	17	0	-	-	-	-	-	-	0.2	-	0.2	-	-	0.2	1.0	0.7	2.7	0.9	2.1	-	0.2	0.1	0.01	0.02	**0.2**	187.5-.9
†Bladder	608	0	-	0.1	0.2	-	0.2	0.2	0.5	1.4	3.1	3.9	5.5	13.6	24.4	37.3	57.6	69.5	96.5	84.0	6.8	3.2	0.27	0.74	**6.3**	188
Kidney etc.	335	0	1.4	0.3	0.4	0.2	0.3	-	0.9	1.1	1.5	5.4	5.9	8.3	15.1	14.8	22.1	32.5	29.4	11.2	3.7	1.8	0.20	0.39	**3.5**	189
Eye	13	0	0.3	0.1	-	-	0.2	-	-	0.2	-	0.2	0.2	0.2	0.5	-	-	0.9	2.1	-	0.1	0.1	0.01	0.01	**0.2**	190
Brain, nervous system	494	0	1.9	2.2	1.9	1.4	1.6	2.1	3.0	4.6	6.8	8.6	8.9	7.3	14.6	20.2	24.2	13.5	18.9	-	5.5	2.6	0.32	0.55	**5.1**	191-2
Thyroid	82	0	-	0.1	-	0.4	0.5	0.2	0.4	1.1	1.0	1.8	1.6	1.0	3.4	2.7	3.2	1.8	6.3	-	0.9	0.4	0.06	0.09	**0.8**	193
Other endocrine	72	0	-	0.1	-	0.2	0.2	0.3	0.8	0.8	2.5	0.5	1.1	1.2	1.9	3.4	1.6	0.9	-	-	0.8	0.4	0.05	0.07	**0.7**	194
Hodgkin's disease	34	0	0.2	-	0.2	-	0.2	0.3	0.5	0.5	0.2	0.2	1.1	1.2	1.0	-	-	-	-	-	0.4	0.2	0.03	0.03	**0.3**	201
Non-Hodgkin lymphoma	424	0	1.0	1.7	1.5	0.8	1.5	1.2	1.6	1.7	3.7	5.2	8.6	9.5	15.3	19.5	23.7	20.8	29.4	39.2	4.7	2.3	0.27	0.48	**4.5**	200,202
Multiple myeloma	49	0	-	-	-	-	-	0.1	0.1	0.1	0.5	0.2	0.2	2.6	1.9	2.0	3.2	5.4	2.1	5.6	0.5	0.3	0.03	0.06	**0.5**	203
Lymphoid leukaemia	103	0	2.4	1.0	1.3	0.6	0.3	0.5	0.8	0.4	0.8	1.4	0.2	2.2	2.9	1.3	3.2	5.4	-	11.2	1.1	0.5	0.07	0.10	**1.3**	204
Myeloid leukaemia	166	0	1.2	0.6	1.1	1.4	1.3	1.3	0.8	2.3	1.7	2.5	3.2	2.2	4.6	3.7	4.3	6.3	2.1	-	1.8	0.9	0.12	0.16	**1.8**	205
Monocytic leukaemia	19	0	-	-	-	-	0.2	0.3	-	0.2	0.3	0.5	0.5	-	1.0	-	0.5	1.8	-	-	0.2	0.1	0.01	0.02	**0.2**	206
Other leukaemia	10	0	-	-	-	-	-	-	0.1	0.1	0.2	-	0.9	-	0.2	-	0.5	-	-	5.6	0.1	0.1	0.01	0.01	**0.1**	207
Leukaemia unspecified	155	0	1.0	1.0	1.1	0.6	0.6	1.0	1.1	1.5	0.7	1.8	1.8	2.8	1.9	6.0	7.5	11.7	10.5	5.6	1.7	0.8	0.09	0.15	**1.6**	208
Other and unspecified	469	0	0.9	0.4	0.2	0.2	1.0	0.5	0.9	1.8	4.6	4.3	7.7	12.6	21.8	23.5	33.9	34.3	27.3	22.4	5.2	2.5	0.28	0.57	**4.7**	O&U
All sites	18825	0	12.5	8.6	9.8	8.3	11.9	17.4	31.8	50.2	99.3	170.4	272.0	523.0	813.8	1138.0	1521.9	1613.4	1627.7	1332.7	209.2		10.14	23.44	**190.0**	ALL
All sites but 173	18746	0	12.5	8.6	9.8	8.3	11.9	17.4	31.8	49.9	98.2	170.4	270.6	521.7	810.9	1133.0	1516.0	1604.4	1613.0	1315.9	208.3	100.0	10.11	23.36	**189.2**	ALLb

Rate from 1 case   0.172 0.139 0.213 0.197 0.161 0.101 0.087 0.108 0.170 0.227 0.227 0.203 0.240 0.336 0.538 0.902 2.098 5.600

†Important: see notes on population page

CHINA, TIANJIN 1988-1992

ANNUAL INCIDENCE PER 100,000 BY AGE GROUP (YEARS) - FEMALE

SITE	ALL AGES	AGE UNK	0-	5-	10-	15-	20-	25-	30-	35-	40-	45-	50-	55-	60-	65-	70-	75-	80-	85+	CRUDE RATE	%	CR 64	CR 74	ASR (W)	ICD (9th)
Lip	6	0	-	-	-	-	-	-	-	-	-	-	0.2	-	-	1.0	0.5	-	-	3.0	0.1	0.0	0.00	0.01	**0.1**	140
Tongue	51	0	-	-	-	-	-	0.1	0.1	0.2	-	0.2	0.6	1.9	2.1	3.0	3.8	3.3	3.1	5.9	0.6	0.3	0.03	0.06	**0.5**	141
Salivary gland	27	0	-	-	-	0.2	-	0.3	0.3	-	0.2	1.6	1.2	0.2	-	0.3	0.5	1.7	1.6	-	0.3	0.2	0.02	0.02	**0.3**	142
Mouth	44	0	-	-	0.2	-	0.2	0.2	0.3	0.2	-	0.7	0.6	0.8	0.7	3.0	4.8	0.8	4.7	-	0.5	0.3	0.02	0.06	**0.4**	143-5
Oropharynx	22	0	-	-	-	-	-	-	0.1	-	0.2	0.2	0.8	1.0	0.2	2.4	0.5	-	-	3.0	0.2	0.1	0.01	0.03	**0.2**	146
Nasopharynx	68	0	-	-	-	-	-	0.4	0.4	0.3	0.9	0.9	1.6	1.5	4.3	1.7	2.7	0.8	3.1	3.0	0.8	0.4	0.05	0.07	**0.6**	147
Hypopharynx	4	0	-	-	-	-	-	-	-	-	-	-	0.2	-	0.2	0.3	0.5	-	-	-	0.0	0.0	0.00	0.01	**0.0**	148
Pharynx unspecified	0	0	-	-	-	-	-	-	-	-	-	-	-	-	-	-	-	-	-	-	0.0	0.0	0.00	0.00	**0.0**	149
Oesophagus	654	0	-	-	-	-	-	-	0.2	0.8	0.7	1.8	5.6	14.7	27.7	49.0	55.2	73.8	82.4	62.2	7.4	4.2	0.26	0.78	**6.2**	150
Stomach	1193	0	-	-	0.2	-	1.6	1.3	3.5	4.8	6.9	10.9	26.5	25.2	42.7	57.4	101.8	95.4	91.8	68.1	13.5	7.7	0.62	1.41	**11.4**	151
Small intestine	41	0	-	-	-	-	-	-	0.2	0.1	0.2	0.9	1.2	0.8	1.7	3.0	2.1	1.7	1.6	-	0.5	0.3	0.03	0.05	**0.4**	152
Colon	521	0	-	-	-	-	0.2	0.8	1.4	2.0	3.0	6.6	9.4	15.3	21.1	27.0	28.4	48.1	37.3	5.9	5.9	3.3	0.30	0.58	**4.9**	153
Rectum	609	0	0.2	-	-	-	0.3	0.3	3.9	3.5	5.4	5.7	10.4	15.1	23.2	25.7	34.8	54.8	43.6	23.7	6.9	3.9	0.34	0.64	**5.6**	154
Liver	934	0	0.4	-	-	0.2	0.3	0.6	0.9	2.4	3.0	7.5	13.1	24.1	43.9	58.1	69.1	86.3	70.0	44.4	10.6	6.0	0.48	1.12	**8.9**	155
Gallbladder etc.	196	0	-	-	-	-	0.2	0.2	0.1	0.8	0.9	1.6	2.0	2.7	9.7	17.2	15.0	14.9	12.4	8.9	2.2	1.3	0.09	0.25	**1.9**	156
Pancreas	358	0	-	0.1	-	-	0.3	-	0.4	1.4	1.4	2.3	5.0	9.9	16.6	22.6	22.5	32.4	31.1	14.8	4.1	2.3	0.19	0.41	**3.4**	157
Nose, sinuses etc.	36	0	0.2	0.1	-	-	0.2	0.1	0.2	0.1	0.4	0.5	0.8	1.0	0.9	2.0	2.1	0.8	1.6	-	0.4	0.2	0.02	0.04	**0.4**	160
Larynx	170	0	0.2	-	-	-	-	-	0.1	-	0.7	1.1	3.2	4.6	10.2	11.1	10.2	13.3	6.2	11.8	1.9	1.1	0.10	0.21	**1.7**	161
Bronchus, lung	3870	0	-	0.1	-	-	0.3	0.9	2.1	5.6	10.9	27.7	63.5	113.5	194.9	262.8	299.1	277.1	216.2	177.6	43.9	24.9	2.10	4.91	**37.0**	162
Other thoracic organs	47	0	0.2	0.1	0.2	-	0.2	0.2	0.4	0.2	-	0.2	0.8	1.1	2.4	3.7	1.6	-	-	-	0.5	0.3	0.03	0.06	**0.5**	163-4
Bone	182	0	-	0.3	1.8	1.1	0.9	0.3	0.8	1.8	0.5	1.6	2.0	3.6	7.3	6.4	12.9	12.4	6.2	5.9	2.1	1.2	0.11	0.21	**1.8**	170
Connective tissue	91	0	0.4	0.1	0.5	0.2	0.3	0.3	0.6	1.0	0.9	1.8	1.4	2.3	3.1	2.0	2.7	6.6	-	-	1.0	0.6	0.06	0.09	**0.9**	171
Mesothelioma	20	0	-	-	-	-	-	0.1	0.2	0.3	0.4	0.5	0.6	-	0.9	0.7	0.5	-	-	-	0.2	0.1	0.01	0.02	**0.2**	MES
Kaposi's sarcoma	0	0	-	-	-	-	-	-	-	-	-	-	-	-	-	-	-	-	-	-	0.0	0.0	0.00	0.00	**0.0**	KAP
Melanoma of skin	27	0	-	0.1	-	-	-	0.1	0.2	0.1	0.4	0.7	0.4	0.8	0.5	-	1.6	1.7	3.1	5.9	0.3	0.2	0.02	0.02	**0.3**	172
Other skin	76	0	0.2	-	-	0.2	-	0.2	0.1	0.1	0.5	0.9	0.8	1.0	3.3	3.7	4.8	4.1	12.4	20.7	0.9		0.04	0.08	**0.8**	173
Breast	2586	0	-	-	-	0.2	1.9	4.4	16.2	30.3	61.0	77.7	66.3	60.2	62.4	71.9	67.0	70.5	76.2	23.7	29.3	16.6	1.90	2.60	**24.6**	174
Uterus unspecified	91	0	-	-	-	-	-	0.1	0.1	0.2	1.1	1.4	2.2	1.3	3.6	4.1	6.4	9.1	9.3	3.0	1.0	0.6	0.05	0.10	**0.9**	179
Cervix uteri	454	0	-	-	-	-	0.2	0.3	0.8	4.8	4.2	8.8	20.6	38.2	42.9	42.3	23.3	8.9	-	-	5.1	2.9	0.20	0.61	**4.4**	180
Placenta	54	0	0.2	-	-	-	1.2	1.7	1.4	0.2	0.7	0.9	0.2	-	-	1.0	-	0.8	-	-	0.6	0.3	0.03	0.04	**0.5**	181
Corpus uteri	280	0	-	-	-	-	0.2	0.5	0.4	1.3	2.6	6.6	9.6	12.0	13.5	7.4	6.4	7.5	4.7	-	3.2	1.8	0.23	0.30	**2.7**	182
Ovary etc.	535	0	0.4	0.6	0.9	0.6	0.7	1.9	2.8	3.9	9.5	13.2	14.1	11.1	18.7	18.9	17.7	16.6	3.1	8.9	6.1	3.4	0.39	0.57	**5.3**	183
Other female genital	57	0	-	-	-	-	-	-	0.3	0.4	0.5	0.4	1.0	4.0	3.0	4.8	3.3	4.7	3.0	-	0.6	0.4	0.03	0.07	**0.5**	184
†Bladder	214	0	-	-	-	-	0.2	0.2	0.2	0.4	0.5	1.4	1.6	3.4	7.1	12.2	19.8	25.7	42.0	26.6	2.4	1.4	0.08	0.24	**2.0**	188
Kidney etc.	174	0	0.5	0.4	-	-	-	-	0.2	0.8	0.7	0.9	3.6	6.3	10.2	7.4	7.5	10.0	6.2	8.9	2.0	1.1	0.12	0.19	**1.7**	189
Eye	11	0	0.2	-	-	-	-	0.1	0.2	0.2	0.2	-	0.2	0.2	-	0.3	-	-	-	3.0	0.1	0.1	0.01	0.01	**0.1**	190
Brain, nervous system	501	0	1.4	0.6	0.9	0.8	1.4	2.8	2.6	4.4	4.9	5.5	10.2	13.8	21.1	19.3	17.7	14.9	9.3	-	5.7	3.2	0.35	0.54	**4.8**	191-2
Thyroid	216	0	-	-	-	0.2	1.0	1.4	2.1	3.9	3.3	3.9	5.6	2.7	4.7	6.8	5.9	4.1	3.1	3.0	2.4	1.4	0.14	0.21	**2.0**	193
Other endocrine	64	0	-	0.1	-	-	-	0.9	0.7	0.9	1.2	1.1	1.4	1.3	1.7	1.7	0.5	-	-	-	0.7	0.4	0.05	0.06	**0.6**	194
Hodgkin's disease	32	0	-	-	-	0.2	0.2	0.3	0.3	0.9	0.4	1.1	0.6	-	0.5	0.7	-	1.7	-	-	0.4	0.2	0.02	0.03	**0.3**	201
Non-Hodgkin lymphoma	279	0	0.2	-	0.7	0.2	1.4	1.1	1.5	1.2	2.3	1.8	4.6	8.4	10.2	14.2	13.4	15.8	10.9	11.8	3.2	1.8	0.17	0.31	**2.6**	200,202
Multiple myeloma	36	0	-	-	-	-	-	-	-	-	0.2	-	0.6	0.6	2.6	3.0	2.1	2.5	1.6	3.0	0.4	0.2	0.02	0.05	**0.3**	203
Lymphoid leukaemia	53	0	1.8	1.2	1.1	-	0.2	0.1	0.3	0.3	0.4	0.5	1.0	1.1	0.7	1.0	0.5	-	-	-	0.6	0.3	0.04	0.05	**0.7**	204
Myeloid leukaemia	128	0	1.1	1.2	0.9	0.8	1.0	1.4	1.4	1.5	2.5	1.8	0.8	2.5	1.2	2.4	1.1	4.1	-	-	1.5	0.8	0.09	0.11	**1.4**	205
Monocytic leukaemia	14	0	0.4	0.1	-	-	0.2	-	-	0.3	-	0.5	0.4	0.4	0.2	-	-	-	-	-	0.2	0.1	0.01	0.01	**0.2**	206
Other leukaemia	7	0	0.4	-	-	-	-	-	0.1	-	-	-	0.2	-	-	1.0	-	-	-	-	0.1	0.0	0.00	0.01	**0.1**	207
Leukaemia unspecified	141	0	1.3	1.0	0.9	1.1	0.5	0.6	0.4	1.2	1.1	2.5	2.6	1.9	4.5	2.4	5.9	9.1	7.8	3.0	1.6	0.9	0.10	0.14	**1.6**	208
Other and unspecified	475	0	1.1	0.1	0.2	0.4	0.3	0.8	1.1	2.1	4.2	6.1	11.8	14.7	15.4	19.9	33.8	28.2	20.2	11.8	5.4	3.1	0.29	0.56	**4.6**	O&U
All sites	15649	0	10.5	6.6	8.7	6.5	15.5	25.1	48.5	81.0	135.1	207.8	294.4	392.7	620.7	801.2	931.5	996.4	850.9	583.2	177.4		9.27	17.93	**149.9**	ALL
All sites but 173	15573	0	10.3	6.6	8.7	6.3	15.5	24.9	48.4	80.9	134.6	206.9	293.6	391.7	617.4	797.5	926.7	992.3	838.5	562.5	176.5	100.0	9.23	17.85	**149.2**	ALLb
Rate from 1 case			0.181	0.147	0.228	0.210	0.174	0.107	0.091	0.109	0.176	0.227	0.201	0.191	0.237	0.338	0.536	0.830	1.556	2.960						

†Important: see notes on population page

Hong Kong

The Hong Kong Cancer Registry is a population-based cancer registry that was established within the Medical and Health Department Institute of Radiology and Oncology in 1963. With the splitting of this institute and later taking over of all public hospitals by the Hospital Authority in 1991, the registry is now affiliated to the Hospital Authority of Hong Kong.

The total land area of Hong Kong is 1075 km^2. The population at the 1991 census was about 5 800 000. The current population is around 98% Chinese, of whom 90% have come from, or are descended from, people in the Guangdong Province of southern China. Hong Kong is one of the most densely populated places in the world, with an overall population density of 5353 persons per km^2 at the end of 1991.

Hong Kong had a workforce of 2.8 million in 1991, of whom 63% were male and 37% were female. Of this workforce, 26.5% were engaged in wholesale and retail trades, restaurants and hotels, 9.7% in transport, storage and communications, 8.3% in construction, 8.4% in finance, insurance, real estate and business services, and 26.4% in manufacturing.

Information on cancer site (topography) and histology (morphology) in relation to incidence and mortality is continuously collected. Basic demographic data are also collected for epidemiological studies.

Cancer notification is on a voluntary basis. However, the registry staff have access to most hospital and laboratory tumour registries, whether they are privately run or publicly funded, allowing data on clinical and histopathological diagnoses to be extracted from their registers of cancer cases. There are a number of channels through which data are collected: (1) voluntary notification from medical practitioners; (2) all five departments of radiotherapy and oncology in Hospital Authority hospitals; (3) all pathology departments of Hospital Authority hospitals and the Department of Health; (4) discharge summaries from all Hospital Authority regional hospitals; (5) case summaries from two radiotherapy departments in the private sector; (6) most pathology departments/institutes in the private sector; (7) cancer deaths from the Births, Deaths & Marriages Registry of the government.

Notifications from the above sources amount to about 65 000 separate entries per annum. All extracted data are coded and checked for eligibility by a series of comprehensive cross-checking programs with on a microcomputer network before they are registered. Multiple neoplasms for the same person are counted separately. Valid data are then entered and updated in the database. Over 16 000 new cases and 9000 cancer deaths are reported each year.

The demographic information is the key to checking and eliminating duplicate registrations of the same patient. The unique identity card number for each individual helps greatly in the process of cross-checking. There are a number of procedures used to check the accuracy and validity of data. These are performed by a series of computer programs, which look for compatibility between sex and site and consistency between site and morphology. However, for childhood cancers, there are difficulties in cross-checking multiple entries, since children have no identity card. In addition, Chinese parents may change a child's name after a diagnosis of cancer, believing that this may bring better luck to the child. The new name would appear as a new entry.

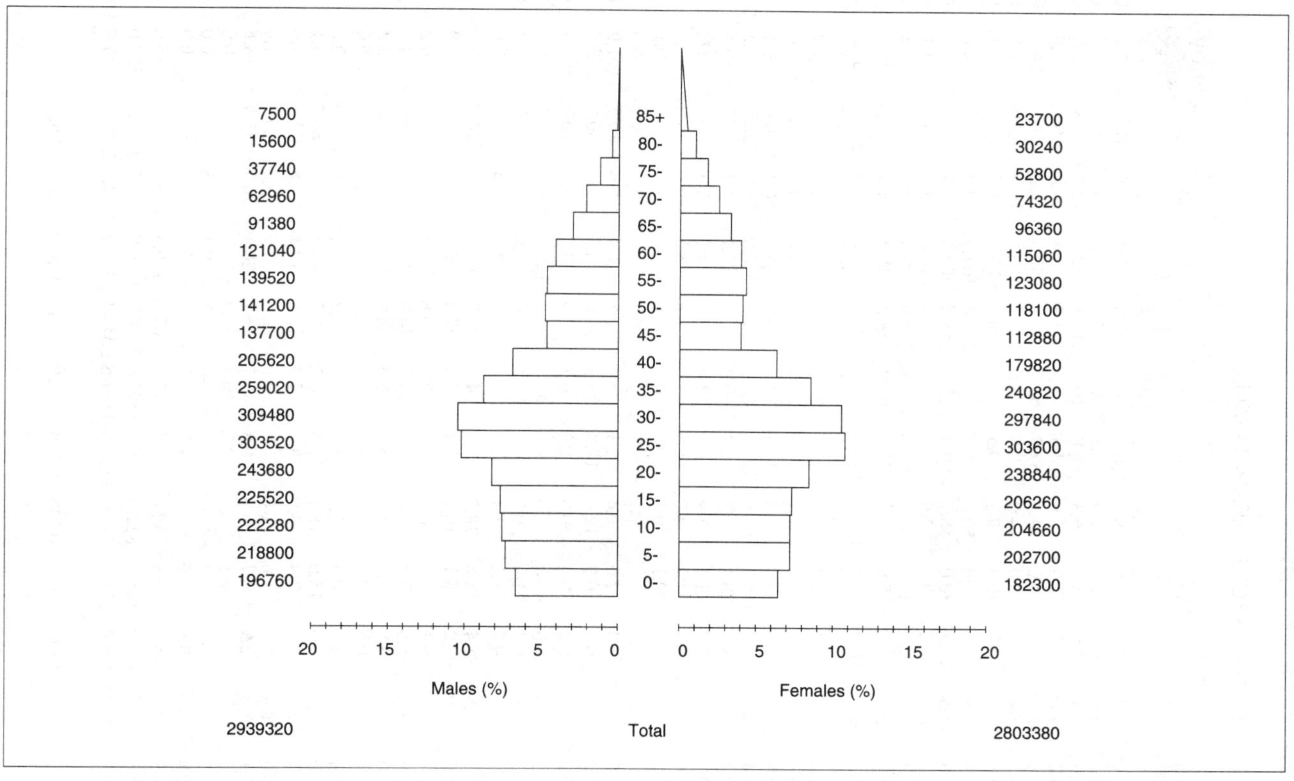

Hong Kong

Source of population: average annual 1988-92

Census: 1991. Census and Statistics Department of Government.

Estimate: Mid-year estimates of the populations for 1988, 1989 and 1990 were produced by the Census and Statistics Department on the basis of the 1986 By-Census, making allowance for births, deaths and migration. The 1992 estimate was based on the 1991 Census, making allowance for births, deaths and migration.

Note: 4th digit data are not available

HONG KONG 1988-1992

ANNUAL INCIDENCE PER 100,000 BY AGE GROUP (YEARS) - MALE

SITE	ALL AGES	AGE UNK	0-	5-	10-	15-	20-	25-	30-	35-	40-	45-	50-	55-	60-	65-	70-	75-	80-	85+	CRUDE RATE	%	CR 64	CR 74	ASR (W)	ICD (9th)
Lip	13	1	-	-	-	-	-	-	-	0.1	-	-	0.1	0.4	0.3	0.2	0.6	0.5	1.3	-	0.1	0.0	0.01	0.01	**0.1**	140
Tongue	327	2	-	-	-	-	0.2	0.5	0.8	0.9	1.8	2.9	4.8	8.6	10.4	9.2	7.6	9.0	11.5	10.7	2.2	0.7	0.16	0.24	**2.1**	141
Salivary gland	115	1	-	-	-	-	0.2	0.3	0.3	0.2	1.0	0.9	1.4	2.9	2.3	2.8	3.5	4.2	5.1	10.7	0.8	0.2	0.05	0.08	**0.7**	142
Mouth	292	1	-	-	-	0.3	0.2	0.1	0.1	0.6	1.4	2.5	3.4	6.3	8.8	10.3	13.3	12.2	12.8	5.3	2.0	0.6	0.12	0.24	**1.9**	143-5
Oropharynx	145	0	-	-	-	-	0.1	-	0.3	0.2	1.0	1.5	2.0	3.6	4.3	5.5	3.8	5.3	3.8	5.3	1.0	0.3	0.06	0.11	**0.9**	146
Nasopharynx	3935	3	-	-	0.1	1.4	1.9	9.3	19.1	36.8	52.1	67.7	70.0	74.8	67.9	62.2	51.1	40.3	28.2	21.3	26.8	8.4	2.01	2.57	**24.3**	147
Hypopharynx	236	0	-	-	-	-	0.1	-	-	-	1.4	3.3	4.0	4.0	8.6	8.8	6.7	9.5	10.3	8.0	1.6	0.5	0.11	0.18	**1.6**	148
Pharynx unspecified	17	0	-	-	-	-	-	-	0.1	0.1	-	0.1	0.3	0.3	0.5	0.9	0.3	0.5	1.3	-	0.1	0.0	0.01	0.01	**0.1**	149
Oesophagus	2179	4	-	-	-	-	0.3	0.1	0.6	1.3	4.5	12.8	27.9	50.6	71.2	85.6	102.6	104.9	100.0	101.3	14.8	4.7	0.85	1.79	**14.2**	150
Stomach	3008	13	-	-	-	0.4	0.7	1.1	2.6	5.6	11.5	15.3	30.0	48.7	69.9	115.3	158.2	200.3	215.4	221.3	20.5	6.5	0.93	2.31	**19.4**	151
Small intestine	163	0	-	-	-	-	0.1	0.3	0.3	0.5	0.6	2.2	0.8	2.6	3.5	5.3	7.6	10.6	12.8	5.3	1.1	0.3	0.05	0.12	**1.0**	152
Colon	3472	9	-	-	0.1	0.9	0.7	2.2	4.2	6.9	12.1	19.9	30.9	54.9	85.9	124.3	176.0	227.9	264.1	304.0	23.6	7.4	1.10	2.60	**22.5**	153
Rectum	1954	8	-	-	0.2	0.3	0.2	0.9	2.3	5.9	5.8	11.2	25.9	33.1	51.7	63.0	84.5	119.2	151.3	133.3	13.3	4.2	0.69	1.43	**12.6**	154
Liver	5628	10	0.4	0.5	0.6	1.2	1.2	4.3	10.0	21.1	36.6	56.9	88.7	115.7	146.9	170.1	197.3	189.2	197.4	213.3	38.3	12.1	2.43	4.27	**36.2**	155
Gallbladder etc.	551	0	-	-	-	0.1	0.2	0.1	0.4	0.2	1.5	2.2	3.0	8.0	11.6	23.4	29.5	48.8	61.5	56.0	3.7	1.2	0.14	0.40	**3.6**	156
Pancreas	615	0	0.1	-	0.1	-	0.1	0.2	0.5	0.5	2.5	2.9	7.2	11.2	15.9	22.1	29.9	39.7	51.3	34.7	4.2	1.3	0.21	0.47	**4.0**	157
Nose, sinuses etc.	144	1	-	0.1	-	-	-	0.1	0.4	0.5	0.9	1.6	2.7	2.4	3.0	5.3	3.8	6.4	7.7	-	1.0	0.3	0.06	0.10	**0.9**	160
Larynx	1193	1	-	-	-	0.1	0.1	0.1	0.4	0.7	2.5	5.5	13.5	21.8	37.5	54.3	64.8	65.7	56.4	40.0	8.1	2.6	0.41	1.01	**7.7**	161
Bronchus, lung	11531	32	-	-	0.5	1.5	1.8	4.8	10.4	24.2	54.6	114.2	202.6	327.5	480.2	627.7	706.9	826.9	698.7	78.5	24.7	3.72	9.28	**74.7**	162
Other thoracic organs	57	0	0.1	-	0.1	0.1	0.2	0.3	0.3	0.2	0.7	1.0	0.4	0.7	1.2	0.9	0.3	2.1	1.3	2.7	0.4	0.1	0.03	0.03	**0.4**	163-4
Bone	170	1	-	0.3	1.4	1.8	1.1	0.3	0.8	0.5	1.5	0.7	1.1	1.9	2.3	2.4	4.1	4.2	7.7	-	1.2	0.4	0.07	0.10	**1.1**	170
Connective tissue	339	0	0.8	0.7	0.1	0.8	0.8	1.2	1.3	2.0	3.0	3.3	4.4	4.7	5.3	8.1	8.3	8.5	9.0	8.0	2.3	0.7	0.14	0.22	**2.2**	171
Mesothelioma	9	0	-	0.1	-	-	-	-	-	-	0.1	0.1	0.1	-	0.7	0.6	-	-	-	-	0.1	0.0	0.00	0.01	**0.1**	MES
Kaposi's sarcoma	2	0	-	-	-	-	-	-	-	-	-	-	-	-	-	0.3	-	-	-	-	0.0	0.0	0.00	0.00	**0.0**	KAP
Melanoma of skin	150	2	-	-	-	-	0.2	0.3	0.3	0.3	0.8	1.3	1.9	2.0	2.4	2.8	3.9	2.5	6.4	6.4	10.7	1.0	0.3	0.06	0.10	**1.0**	172
Other skin	846	41	-	-	-	0.3	0.9	1.1	1.1	2.2	3.5	6.4	10.9	12.6	17.8	24.3	35.6	38.7	64.1	80.0	5.8		0.30	0.61	**5.6**	173
Breast	49	0	-	-	-	-	0.1	-	0.1	0.2	-	0.3	0.4	0.9	1.3	0.7	2.9	3.7	3.8	10.7	0.3	0.1	0.02	0.03	**0.3**	175
Prostate	1185	7	-	-	-	-	-	0.1	-	0.2	0.6	1.0	2.4	7.0	18.0	45.7	81.6	142.0	219.2	213.3	8.1	2.5	0.15	0.79	**7.9**	185
Testis	203	2	1.7	0.3	0.3	0.4	1.1	2.6	2.6	1.5	2.1	0.7	1.0	0.7	0.8	1.1	1.0	2.6	1.3	5.3	1.4	0.4	0.08	0.09	**1.3**	186
Penis, other male genital	92	0	0.1	-	-	0.2	-	0.1	0.1	-	0.1	0.7	1.1	1.1	2.5	3.5	4.1	4.8	11.5	2.7	0.6	0.2	0.03	0.07	**0.6**	187
Bladder	2215	17	-	-	-	0.4	0.5	0.7	1.0	2.7	3.8	8.4	18.8	28.2	58.5	84.9	129.9	161.6	203.8	224.0	15.1	4.8	0.62	1.70	**14.5**	188
Kidney etc.	567	5	1.3	0.5	0.1	0.1	0.4	0.3	1.0	1.0	2.9	3.2	5.1	10.2	15.4	19.0	22.2	29.1	29.5	42.7	3.9	1.2	0.21	0.42	**3.8**	189
Eye	31	2	1.5	0.1	-	-	0.1	0.1	0.1	-	-	0.1	-	0.1	0.2	0.9	0.6	0.5	-	-	0.2	0.1	0.01	0.02	**0.3**	190
Brain, nervous system	655	1	2.4	2.8	2.0	1.5	1.9	2.0	2.8	3.9	3.2	5.5	7.4	9.6	10.1	14.7	14.9	11.7	26.9	13.3	4.5	1.4	0.28	0.42	**4.3**	191-2
Thyroid	331	2	0.1	0.1	0.1	0.4	1.8	1.4	2.1	2.0	2.2	3.8	4.4	4.4	6.3	5.3	6.0	8.5	10.3	8.0	2.3	0.7	0.15	0.20	**2.0**	193
Other endocrine	95	0	2.0	0.6	0.4	0.6	0.3	0.1	0.3	0.4	-	0.9	0.6	0.6	1.2	1.8	2.2	1.6	1.3	-	0.6	0.2	0.04	0.06	**0.8**	194
Hodgkin's disease	94	0	-	0.7	0.6	0.6	0.6	0.4	0.2	0.4	0.5	1.0	1.0	1.1	1.8	1.5	1.3	1.1	2.6	5.3	0.6	0.2	0.04	0.06	**0.6**	201
Non-Hodgkin lymphoma	1342	4	1.6	1.7	2.2	2.8	3.2	3.6	4.5	6.0	8.2	9.0	15.0	18.1	27.3	32.2	49.2	44.5	66.7	66.7	9.1	2.9	0.52	0.93	**8.7**	200,202
Multiple myeloma	270	3	-	-	-	0.1	0.2	0.3	0.3	0.8	0.6	1.3	2.4	4.9	8.1	7.7	10.8	19.1	21.8	21.3	1.8	0.6	0.10	0.19	**1.7**	203
Lymphoid leukaemia	286	4	6.2	5.9	3.0	1.1	1.4	0.5	0.9	0.5	0.4	0.9	1.0	1.6	1.8	2.6	2.5	1.1	3.8	5.3	1.9	0.6	0.13	0.15	**2.4**	204
Myeloid leukaemia	528	2	1.7	0.6	1.0	1.6	2.0	2.1	3.0	3.1	3.3	2.9	6.7	6.3	6.8	7.7	16.2	20.1	16.7	18.7	3.6	1.1	0.21	0.33	**3.4**	205
Monocytic leukaemia	7	0	-	-	-	-	-	0.1	0.1	-	-	-	0.1	-	0.2	0.4	0.3	-	-	-	0.0	0.0	0.00	0.01	**0.0**	206
Other leukaemia	6	0	0.1	-	-	-	-	-	-	-	-	-	0.3	-	-	0.3	0.5	1.3	-	-	0.0	0.0	0.00	0.00	**0.0**	207
Leukaemia unspecified	138	3	0.5	0.3	0.9	0.2	0.5	0.6	0.4	0.8	0.6	0.9	2.0	1.9	1.5	1.5	4.1	6.4	3.8	-	0.9	0.3	0.06	0.09	**0.9**	208
Other and unspecified	2292	11	0.2	0.3	0.4	1.4	1.7	1.5	2.4	4.9	9.1	15.0	26.8	40.6	57.5	75.7	109.6	119.8	156.4	146.7	15.6	4.9	0.81	1.74	**14.9**	O&U
All sites	47477	193	21.0	15.6	13.8	19.8	27.1	41.2	72.8	126.6	208.7	333.0	545.6	812.4	1176.1	1595.8	2080.7	2439.9	2888.5	2757.3	323.0		17.14	35.60	**307.2**	ALL
All sites but 173	46631	152	21.0	15.6	13.8	19.5	26.2	40.1	71.7	124.5	205.2	326.7	534.7	799.7	1158.3	1571.5	2045.1	2401.2	2824.4	2677.3	317.3	100.0	16.84	34.98	**301.7**	ALLb

Rate from 1 case   0.102   0.091   0.090   0.089   0.082   0.066   0.065   0.077   0.097   0.145   0.142   0.143   0.165   0.219   0.318   0.530   1.282   2.667

HONG KONG 1988-1992

ANNUAL INCIDENCE PER 100,000 BY AGE GROUP (YEARS) - FEMALE

SITE	ALL AGES	AGE UNK	0-	5-	10-	15-	20-	25-	30-	35-	40-	45-	50-	55-	60-	65-	70-	75-	80-	85+	CRUDE RATE	%	CR 64	CR 74	ASR (W)	ICD (9th)
Lip	6	0	-	-	-	-	-	-	-	-	-	-	0.2	-	-	0.2	0.3	0.4	1.3	-	0.0	0.0	0.00	0.00	0.0	140
Tongue	194	1	-	-	-	-	0.3	0.4	0.5	1.1	1.4	1.4	3.4	4.1	3.3	5.8	5.7	4.9	4.6	6.8	1.4	0.5	0.08	0.14	1.2	141
Salivary gland	106	0	-	-	-	0.4	0.5	0.3	0.7	0.4	1.6	1.2	1.2	1.1	2.1	0.8	1.6	2.7	5.3	3.4	0.8	0.3	0.05	0.06	0.6	142
Mouth	133	0	0.1	-	-	0.3	-	0.1	0.2	0.3	0.1	1.4	1.7	1.8	2.8	4.2	5.7	6.4	5.3	6.8	0.9	0.4	0.04	0.09	0.8	143-5
Oropharynx	33	0	-	-	-	-	-	0.1	-	0.3	0.3	0.2	0.3	1.0	0.7	0.6	0.5	0.4	1.3	2.5	0.2	0.1	0.01	0.02	0.2	146
Nasopharynx	1462	2	-	-	-	0.4	2.3	3.6	8.5	15.4	21.5	22.3	29.1	26.8	26.2	23.7	18.0	17.0	12.6	7.6	10.4	4.1	0.78	0.99	9.5	147
Hypopharynx	25	1	-	-	-	-	0.1	0.1	-	-	0.1	-	0.3	0.2	1.0	0.4	0.8	1.9	-	1.7	0.2	0.1	0.01	0.02	0.1	148
Pharynx unspecified	3	0	-	-	-	-	-	-	-	-	-	-	0.2	-	0.2	-	0.3	0.4	-	-	0.0	0.0	0.00	0.00	0.0	149
Oesophagus	565	3	-	-	-	0.1	0.3	0.1	0.1	0.6	2.1	2.3	4.4	6.5	11.0	24.3	22.6	30.7	36.4	40.5	4.0	1.6	0.14	0.37	3.2	150
Stomach	1752	6	0.1	-	-	0.2	0.8	1.4	4.0	5.7	7.2	9.0	12.5	18.0	32.7	45.0	69.2	98.5	129.0	140.1	12.5	4.9	0.46	1.03	9.5	151
Small intestine	116	0	-	-	-	-	-	0.1	-	0.1	0.6	1.1	1.9	1.6	3.8	2.9	2.7	5.7	7.9	7.6	0.8	0.3	0.05	0.07	0.7	152
Colon	3288	10	-	-	-	0.1	1.3	1.9	4.3	6.9	8.7	20.0	31.2	56.1	74.2	102.7	132.7	164.8	193.8	188.2	23.5	9.3	1.03	2.21	18.8	153
Rectum	1602	8	-	-	-	-	0.6	1.3	2.6	3.7	4.7	11.3	16.8	26.5	34.9	48.4	61.4	77.7	91.3	92.8	11.4	4.5	0.51	1.07	9.2	154
Liver	1665	3	0.7	0.1	0.2	0.7	0.4	1.1	2.4	3.6	6.9	8.9	15.1	28.6	35.8	46.7	70.5	84.1	97.9	89.5	11.9	4.7	0.52	1.11	9.5	155
Gallbladder etc.	514	1	-	-	-	-	-	0.1	0.3	0.3	1.0	1.4	2.5	7.1	8.9	14.7	24.0	34.8	41.7	52.3	3.7	1.4	0.11	0.30	2.7	156
Pancreas	522	2	-	-	0.1	-	0.3	0.3	0.5	0.2	1.2	2.1	3.0	8.0	11.1	17.4	23.7	23.9	45.6	38.0	3.7	1.5	0.13	0.34	2.9	157
Nose, sinuses etc.	68	1	-	-	-	-	-	0.1	0.4	0.2	0.4	0.5	0.7	1.1	1.7	1.5	1.6	2.3	6.0	0.8	0.5	0.2	0.03	0.04	0.4	160
Larynx	126	0	-	-	-	-	-	0.1	-	0.2	0.2	0.9	1.4	2.1	3.1	5.6	8.1	4.2	3.3	2.5	0.9	0.4	0.04	0.11	0.8	161
Bronchus, lung	5655	21	-	-	0.1	0.3	0.9	1.5	3.0	8.1	13.6	20.7	41.2	70.4	108.1	176.8	274.0	358.0	426.6	384.8	40.3	15.9	1.34	3.61	30.7	162
Other thoracic organs	32	0	-	-	-	-	0.1	0.1	0.1	0.2	0.2	0.2	0.2	0.3	0.9	1.0	0.8	1.1	-	1.7	0.2	0.1	0.01	0.02	0.2	163-4
Bone	131	1	0.3	0.5	1.3	1.2	0.4	0.5	0.6	0.8	0.6	0.9	1.2	1.6	1.2	1.5	1.9	3.0	5.3	1.7	0.9	0.4	0.06	0.07	0.9	170
Connective tissue	314	1	0.8	0.8	0.9	1.7	1.2	1.3	1.3	1.6	2.0	3.4	2.5	3.7	4.9	6.6	7.3	8.3	6.0	5.1	2.2	0.9	0.13	0.20	2.1	171
Mesothelioma	10	0	-	-	-	-	0.2	-	-	-	-	-	0.2	0.2	-	-	0.8	-	1.3	-	0.1	0.0	0.00	0.01	0.1	MES
Kaposi's sarcoma	0	0	-	-	-	-	-	-	-	-	-	-	-	-	-	-	-	-	-	-	0.0	0.0	0.00	0.00	0.0	KAP
Melanoma of skin	132	0	-	-	0.1	-	0.2	0.3	0.8	0.6	0.6	0.9	1.4	2.1	1.7	4.4	2.7	6.4	5.3	7.6	0.9	0.4	0.04	0.08	0.7	172
Other skin	803	19	-	0.1	-	0.1	0.8	1.4	1.4	1.6	2.7	5.8	5.9	8.3	14.8	19.9	27.4	39.8	56.9	80.2	5.7		0.22	0.46	4.4	173
Breast	5392	20	-	-	-	0.4	1.8	6.4	19.3	43.8	74.7	84.9	80.9	79.6	93.2	116.0	125.9	136.7	141.5	150.2	38.5	15.2	2.43	3.65	34.0	174
Uterus unspecified	41	0	-	-	-	-	-	0.3	-	0.4	0.3	0.5	0.5	0.6	0.2	1.2	0.5	0.8	2.6	3.4	0.3	0.1	0.01	0.02	0.2	179
Cervix uteri	2389	11	-	-	-	-	0.8	2.5	8.3	16.0	27.5	34.5	38.1	49.1	54.1	55.8	59.7	47.3	47.6	38.8	17.0	6.7	1.16	1.74	15.3	180
Placenta	7	0	-	-	0.1	-	0.1	-	0.3	-	-	-	-	-	-	-	-	-	-	-	0.0	0.0	0.00	0.00	0.0	181
Corpus uteri	1040	3	-	-	-	-	0.1	0.8	2.6	4.7	9.9	20.6	23.9	25.7	25.0	21.8	21.0	20.1	19.8	11.8	7.4	2.9	0.57	0.78	7.0	182
Ovary etc.	1164	0	0.2	-	0.7	2.5	3.5	3.4	5.0	8.3	10.6	15.9	16.6	16.9	24.2	25.1	25.0	25.0	19.8	21.1	8.3	3.3	0.54	0.79	7.4	183
Other female genital	195	1	-	-	-	0.1	-	0.1	0.5	0.7	0.6	1.1	1.7	4.1	3.3	8.3	7.5	5.7	11.9	7.6	1.4	0.5	0.06	0.14	1.1	184
Bladder	821	2	-	0.1	-	0.3	0.3	0.4	0.5	0.9	1.2	3.2	5.4	5.5	12.7	24.9	43.9	61.4	67.5	61.6	5.9	2.3	0.15	0.50	4.3	188
Kidney etc.	378	1	0.7	0.4	0.1	0.2	0.8	0.5	0.6	1.2	1.1	2.3	4.6	6.5	8.9	11.0	12.6	14.0	17.2	16.9	2.7	1.1	0.14	0.26	2.3	189
Eye	37	1	2.2	0.1	0.1	-	-	-	0.1	0.1	0.2	0.2	0.2	-	-	0.4	0.8	0.4	1.3	-	0.3	0.1	0.02	0.02	0.4	190
Brain, nervous system	502	0	1.6	3.2	2.1	1.7	1.7	1.5	2.2	2.5	2.2	4.1	5.8	5.0	8.0	12.2	11.0	13.6	8.6	5.9	3.6	1.4	0.21	0.32	3.4	191-2
Thyroid	1146	2	-	0.1	0.7	2.7	5.2	5.9	8.6	11.0	13.6	12.4	14.2	16.4	18.6	17.0	12.6	16.7	13.9	15.2	8.2	3.2	0.55	0.70	7.1	193
Other endocrine	101	2	1.9	0.9	0.2	0.1	0.4	0.4	0.5	0.8	0.6	0.5	0.2	1.0	1.0	1.7	1.1	1.9	0.7	1.7	0.7	0.3	0.04	0.06	0.8	194
Hodgkin's disease	42	0	-	-	0.1	0.5	0.3	0.3	0.4	0.2	0.1	0.4	-	0.6	0.3	1.2	0.3	0.4	0.7	0.8	0.3	0.1	0.02	0.02	0.3	201
Non-Hodgkin lymphoma	1036	3	1.2	0.9	0.8	2.0	2.1	2.6	4.3	4.2	4.9	9.2	9.3	14.3	19.6	23.5	33.9	33.7	41.7	52.3	7.4	2.9	0.38	0.67	6.2	200,202
Multiple myeloma	287	0	-	-	0.1	0.1	0.3	0.1	0.1	0.6	0.6	1.8	2.7	4.4	5.4	9.3	11.6	14.8	19.8	22.8	2.0	0.8	0.08	0.18	1.6	203
Lymphoid leukaemia	194	0	4.3	2.8	2.2	1.5	0.3	0.4	0.7	0.5	0.8	0.4	0.7	1.1	1.2	1.7	3.2	1.9	4.6	3.4	1.4	0.5	0.08	0.11	1.6	204
Myeloid leukaemia	392	5	0.9	1.5	1.2	1.3	1.2	1.1	2.5	2.2	4.3	2.3	3.6	2.8	5.6	6.6	10.8	9.1	9.9	10.1	2.8	1.1	0.15	0.24	2.5	205
Monocytic leukaemia	8	0	0.2	-	0.1	-	-	-	-	-	-	-	-	0.3	-	-	0.8	0.7	-	-	0.1	0.0	0.00	0.00	0.1	206
Other leukaemia	3	0	-	-	-	-	-	-	-	-	-	-	-	-	0.2	-	0.4	-	0.8	-	0.0	0.0	0.00	0.00	0.0	207
Leukaemia unspecified	108	2	0.8	0.2	0.3	0.2	0.3	0.5	0.1	0.4	0.3	0.7	0.7	1.6	1.2	2.5	3.2	5.3	2.6	4.2	0.8	0.3	0.04	0.07	0.7	208
Other and unspecified	1751	15	0.2	0.4	0.7	0.5	0.8	1.8	3.0	4.2	6.8	9.2	16.9	23.4	33.4	51.1	71.3	90.2	103.8	108.9	12.5	4.9	0.51	1.13	9.9	O&U
All sites	36291	148	16.1	11.9	11.9	19.6	30.2	45.4	90.9	155.3	237.9	320.2	404.1	536.2	701.2	946.7	1220.1	1477.3	1720.9	1699.6	258.9		12.96	23.84	215.5	ALL
All sites but 173	35488	129	16.1	11.8	11.9	19.5	29.5	44.0	89.5	153.7	235.2	314.3	398.1	527.9	686.4	926.7	1192.7	1437.5	1664.0	1619.4	253.2	100.0	12.74	23.37	211.1	ALLb
Rate from 1 case			0.101	0.099	0.098	0.097	0.084	0.066	0.067	0.083	0.111	0.177	0.169	0.162	0.174	0.208	0.269	0.379	0.661	0.844						

India, Bangalore

The population-based cancer registry at Bangalore was established at Kidwai Memorial Institute of Oncology (KIMIO) in 1981 as part of the National Cancer Registry Programme of the Indian Council of Medical Research. Data collection started from 1 January 1982. The KIMIO is a referral hospital for cancer patients and is a comprehensive cancer centre with all modern facilities for cancer diagnosis and treatment. The registry staff comprises a medical officer, statisticians and social investigators and the basic working of the registry has been computerized.

The registry covers the area of Bangalore Urban Agglomeration (that includes Bangalore city and certain peripheral urban areas) with a total area of 212 km^2. Bangalore is one of the fastest growing cities (38.87% growth between 1981 and 1991) in Asia and is the home of most of the computer software and electronic industries of India. It is located at an altitude of 914 m above sea level and has pleasant cool temperatures throughout most of the year. The population according to the 1991 census was 4 090 000, with a male:female ratio of 1.1. The proportion of literates was 54.5% among males and 62.9% among females. The proportion of total workers was 52% among males and 12.5% among females.

With the growing population, medical facilities have rapidly improved both in number and quality and particularly in oncology services. In the past six years, four additional private cancer care centres with facilities for radiotherapy have opened, taking the total number of radiotherapy machines in the city to nine.

The KIMIO is the main source of data for the registry, accounting for over 60% of cancers registered during the period 1988–92. Data collection is active and is carried out by social investigators visiting the principal sources of information according to a regular weekly schedule. Information on deaths is collected from 14 units of the Bangalore Municipal Corporation. Follow-up of cases is done only when special studies on selected sites of cancer are conducted.

Computerized data entry, range and consistency checks, tabulations etc. are all carried out with programs developed in-house. Duplicate checks are carried out by a combination of computer programming and manual verification.

Active follow-up through visits to homes of patients has been done for selected sites of cancer and results of survival have been published. The registry is now in the process of undertaking specific exercises to determine completeness of coverage as well as look into the quality of data collection.

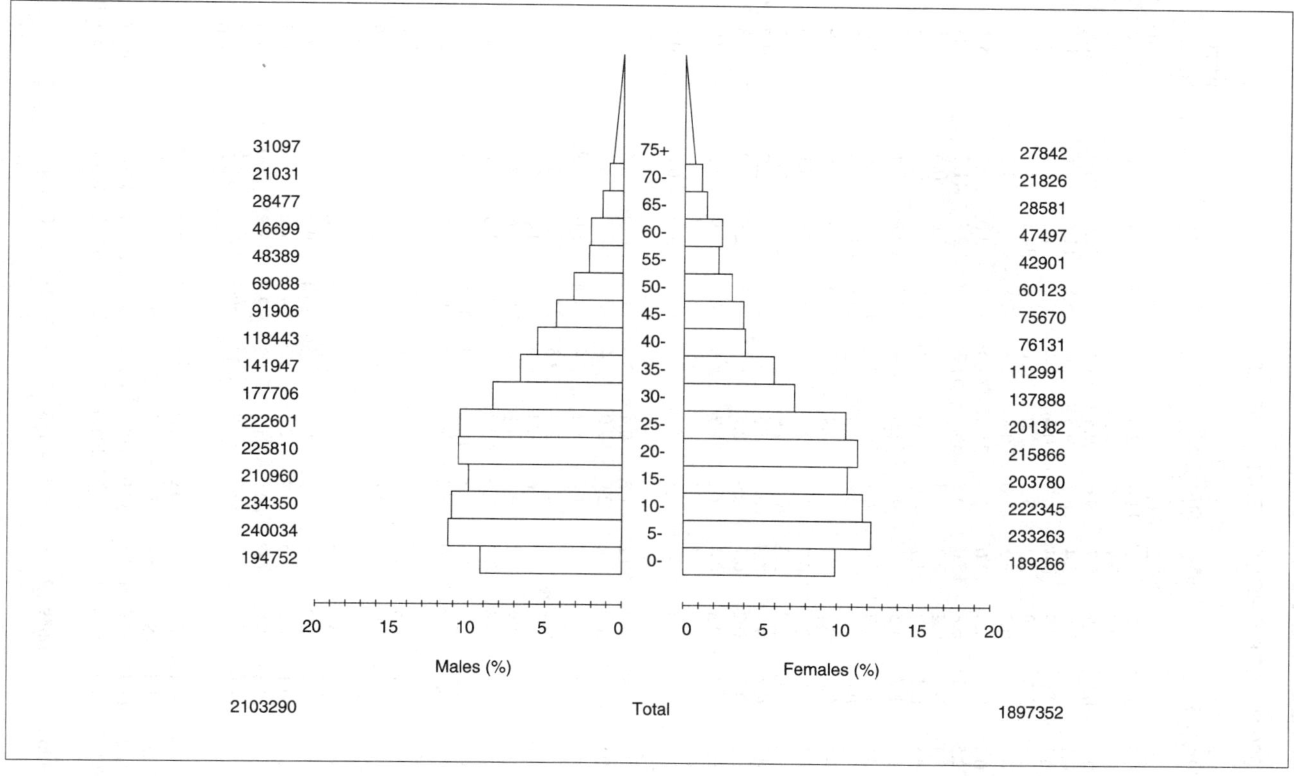

India, Bangalore
Source of population: average annual 1988-92
Census: 1991
Estimate: The population data for 1988, 1989 and 1990 were intercensal estimates; the 1992 population was a postcensal estimate.

Notes to tables overleaf:
*   The 1991 census figures were only available for all ages, and the incidence patterns indicate that the increase in the total population may have been wrongly allocated within the different age-groups. The childhood rates show evidence of under-ascertainment.

* INDIA, BANGALORE 1988-1992

ANNUAL INCIDENCE PER 100,000 BY AGE GROUP (YEARS) - MALE

SITE	ALL AGES	AGE UNK	0-	5-	10-	15-	20-	25-	30-	35-	40-	45-	50-	55-	60-	65-	70-	75+	CRUDE RATE	%	CR 64	CR 74	ASR (W)	ICD (9th)
Lip	11	0	-	-	-	-	-	-	0.1	-	-	0.2	0.3	-	1.3	0.7	-	2.6	0.1	0.2	0.01	0.01	**0.2**	140
Tongue	228	1	-	-	-	-	-	0.4	0.3	1.3	1.7	5.7	11.6	12.0	15.8	18.3	17.1	16.1	2.2	3.4	0.24	0.42	**3.5**	141
Salivary gland	42	0	-	0.1	0.1	0.1	-	0.3	0.1	-	0.2	0.9	2.6	1.2	1.7	2.8	4.8	3.2	0.4	0.6	0.04	0.07	**0.6**	142
Mouth	188	0	0.1	-	0.1	0.1	0.3	0.2	0.2	0.8	1.9	5.7	9.6	9.5	13.3	7.0	20.0	10.9	1.8	2.8	0.21	0.34	**2.8**	143-5
Oropharynx	136	0	-	-	-	-	0.1	0.3	0.1	-	2.0	2.4	6.7	9.5	8.6	15.5	11.4	5.1	1.3	2.0	0.15	0.28	**2.2**	146
Nasopharynx	30	0	-	-	0.3	0.3	0.2	0.1	0.1	0.6	0.5	0.4	1.2	0.4	0.4	0.7	1.9	1.3	0.3	0.4	0.02	0.04	**0.3**	147
Hypopharynx	366	0	-	-	-	-	-	0.2	0.2	0.5	2.0	2.9	5.2	15.3	19.0	29.1	41.4	37.1	24.4	3.5	5.5	0.37	0.76	**5.8**	148
Pharynx unspecified	32	0	-	-	-	-	-	0.1	-	0.1	-	0.2	1.1	2.0	0.8	2.6	2.8	-	3.2	0.3	0.5	0.03	0.05	**0.5**	149
Oesophagus	557	0	-	-	-	-	-	0.2	0.2	0.7	2.1	4.4	12.0	26.9	31.0	33.0	58.3	58.0	39.9	5.3	8.3	0.55	1.13	**8.8**	150
Stomach	666	0	-	-	-	0.1	0.2	0.3	2.5	3.4	6.8	15.0	20.8	36.0	52.2	59.0	72.3	41.2	6.3	9.9	0.69	1.34	**10.3**	151
Small intestine	6	0	-	-	-	-	-	-	0.1	-	0.2	0.2	0.3	-	-	1.0	0.6	0.1	0.1	0.00	0.01	**0.1**	152
Colon	162	1	-	-	-	-	0.4	0.8	0.5	0.4	2.2	4.1	4.6	7.0	7.7	19.7	14.3	9.6	1.5	2.4	0.14	0.31	**2.4**	153
Rectum	212	0	-	-	-	-	0.5	0.4	1.5	1.7	1.5	6.3	4.6	11.6	8.1	19.7	22.8	15.4	2.0	3.2	0.18	0.39	**3.1**	154
Liver	185	0	0.6	0.1	0.3	-	0.1	0.2	0.8	1.7	1.7	3.0	6.7	10.7	9.0	14.7	19.0	11.6	1.8	2.8	0.17	0.34	**2.7**	155
Gallbladder etc.	36	0	-	-	-	-	-	-	0.2	0.6	-	1.3	0.6	2.5	1.3	3.5	1.9	3.9	0.3	0.5	0.03	0.06	**0.5**	156
Pancreas	95	0	-	-	-	-	-	0.2	0.1	0.6	0.8	1.3	2.6	5.4	8.1	10.5	5.7	9.6	0.9	1.4	0.10	0.18	**1.5**	157
Nose, sinuses etc.	49	0	-	0.2	-	0.2	-	0.1	0.3	0.3	0.3	0.7	1.4	2.5	2.6	3.5	2.9	5.1	0.5	0.7	0.04	0.08	**0.7**	160
Larynx	267	1	-	-	-	-	0.3	0.2	0.1	1.8	1.2	3.3	10.4	17.4	21.8	30.9	24.7	16.7	2.5	4.0	0.28	0.56	**4.3**	161
Bronchus, lung	495	0	-	-	-	-	-	0.5	0.8	4.1	8.3	20.8	28.5	36.8	55.5	63.7	32.2	4.7	7.4	0.50	1.10	**8.1**	162
Other thoracic organs	35	0	-	-	-	0.1	-	0.1	0.1	0.3	0.2	0.7	0.9	2.5	1.7	2.8	2.9	3.9	0.3	0.5	0.03	0.06	**0.5**	163-4
Bone	97	0	0.2	0.3	0.8	2.4	1.3	0.7	0.1	0.7	0.5	0.4	1.2	1.7	2.6	0.7	2.9	3.2	0.9	1.4	0.06	0.08	**1.0**	170
Connective tissue	74	0	0.1	0.2	0.4	0.4	1.1	0.4	0.5	0.8	1.0	0.4	1.7	-	3.9	5.6	4.8	-	0.7	1.1	0.05	0.11	**0.9**	171
Mesothelioma	9	0	-	-	-	-	-	-	-	-	0.3	-	0.3	-	-	2.8	1.0	0.6	0.1	0.1	0.00	0.02	**0.2**	MES
Kaposi's sarcoma	0	0	-	-	-	-	-	-	-	-	-	-	-	-	-	-	-	-	0.0	0.0	0.00	0.00	**0.0**	KAP
Melanoma of skin	21	0	-	-	-	-	-	0.1	0.1	0.3	0.2	0.2	1.2	0.4	3.0	1.4	-	0.6	0.2	0.3	0.03	0.03	**0.3**	172
Other skin	104	0	-	-	-	-	-	0.3	0.5	1.5	1.0	2.6	2.9	7.0	3.4	10.5	4.8	8.4	1.0		0.10	0.17	**1.5**	173
Breast	18	0	-	-	-	-	-	0.1	-	0.3	-	0.2	1.2	1.2	0.4	1.4	1.0	1.9	0.2	0.3	0.02	0.03	**0.3**	175
Prostate	289	1	-	-	-	-	-	-	-	-	0.2	1.1	4.3	5.8	19.3	31.6	58.0	65.6	2.7	4.3	0.15	0.60	**4.7**	185
Testis	50	0	0.3	0.1	-	0.3	0.4	0.6	1.0	1.1	1.0	-	0.6	0.4	0.9	0.7	1.0	0.6	0.5	0.7	0.03	0.04	**0.5**	186
Penis	98	1	-	-	-	-	-	0.3	0.1	1.1	1.9	2.4	2.3	4.1	6.4	6.3	7.6	8.4	0.9	1.5	0.09	0.16	**1.4**	187.1-.4
Other male genital	15	0	-	-	-	-	-	-	0.2	0.1	0.3	0.2	0.6	0.4	-	0.7	1.0	2.6	0.1	0.2	0.01	0.02	**0.2**	187.5-.9
Bladder	217	1	-	0.1	-	-	0.1	0.2	0.6	1.5	2.0	2.6	6.1	12.4	13.3	17.6	24.7	25.1	2.1	3.2	0.20	0.41	**3.3**	188
Kidney etc.	78	0	0.9	0.2	0.2	0.1	0.1	0.1	-	0.3	1.0	2.0	3.2	2.9	3.4	9.8	2.9	1.3	0.7	1.2	0.07	0.13	**1.2**	189
Eye	12	0	0.2	0.2	-	-	-	-	0.1	-	-	-	0.6	0.4	0.4	-	1.0	0.6	0.1	0.2	0.01	0.01	**0.2**	190
Brain, nervous system	262	0	1.3	0.9	1.0	0.8	1.2	1.3	2.7	2.8	4.2	4.6	8.1	9.5	7.3	9.1	7.6	7.1	2.5	3.9	0.23	0.31	**3.1**	191-2
Thyroid	92	2	-	-	0.3	0.3	0.4	0.8	0.8	0.8	0.7	1.4	1.7	3.8	1.7	2.1	3.5	6.7	5.1	0.9	1.4	0.07	0.12	**1.1**	193
Other endocrine	4	0	-	-	-	-	0.2	0.1	-	0.1	-	-	-	-	-	0.1	-	-	0.0	0.1	0.00	0.00	**0.0**	194
Hodgkin's disease	122	1	0.2	0.8	1.0	1.0	0.6	0.7	0.8	1.7	2.0	1.5	2.3	2.1	4.3	2.8	2.9	1.9	1.2	1.8	0.10	0.13	**1.3**	201
Non-Hodgkin lymphoma	281	1	0.4	0.9	0.5	1.8	1.7	0.7	1.7	2.7	2.9	4.6	7.2	9.1	11.6	20.4	19.0	11.6	2.7	4.2	0.23	0.43	**3.7**	200,202
Multiple myeloma	43	0	-	-	-	-	-	-	-	0.1	0.3	1.5	1.4	2.1	2.6	4.2	7.6	1.9	0.4	0.6	0.04	0.10	**0.7**	203
Lymphoid leukaemia	103	0	2.1	1.4	1.5	0.9	0.4	0.3	0.1	0.4	0.8	0.7	0.9	1.2	1.3	2.8	3.8	1.9	1.0	1.5	0.06	0.09	**1.1**	204
Myeloid leukaemia	161	0	0.9	0.4	0.8	1.0	1.3	0.5	1.0	2.7	2.0	2.6	4.9	5.4	1.3	6.3	4.8	4.5	1.5	2.4	0.12	0.18	**1.9**	205
Monocytic leukaemia	3	0	-	-	-	-	-	0.1	-	-	0.2	-	-	-	-	-	-	-	0.0	0.0	0.00	0.00	**0.0**	206
Other leukaemia	1	0	-	-	-	-	-	0.1	-	-	-	-	-	-	-	-	-	0.6	0.0	0.0	0.00	0.00	**0.0**	207
Leukaemia unspecified	43	0	0.4	0.3	0.2	0.3	0.4	0.3	-	0.4	0.2	0.7	0.9	1.2	0.4	1.4	1.9	2.6	0.4	0.6	0.03	0.04	**0.5**	208
Other and unspecified	813	2	1.4	0.6	0.5	0.9	1.2	2.1	2.0	3.5	8.9	15.9	28.4	35.5	57.8	56.2	76.1	58.5	7.7	12.1	0.80	1.46	**12.0**	O&U
All sites	6808	12	9.2	6.9	7.8	11.2	12.7	13.3	21.2	41.4	65.0	123.6	233.9	312.0	400.9	563.3	621.9	471.4	64.7		6.31	12.24	**99.8**	ALL
All sites but 173	6704	12	9.2	6.9	7.8	11.2	12.7	13.0	20.7	39.9	64.0	121.0	231.0	305.0	397.4	552.7	617.2	463.1	63.7	100.0	6.21	12.07	**98.3**	ALLb

Rate from 10 cases   1.027   0.833   0.853   0.948   0.886   0.898   1.125   1.409   1.689   2.176   2.895   4.133   4.283   7.023   9.510   6.431

* INDIA, BANGALORE 1988-1992

ANNUAL INCIDENCE PER 100,000 BY AGE GROUP (YEARS) - FEMALE

SITE	ALL AGES	AGE UNK	0-	5-	10-	15-	20-	25-	30-	35-	40-	45-	50-	55-	60-	65-	70-	75+	CRUDE RATE	%	CR 64	CR 74	ASR (W)	ICD (9th)
Lip	10	0	-	-	-	-	-	-	-	-	0.3	0.5	-	1.9	0.4	-	-	1.4	0.1	0.1	0.02	0.02	0.2	140
Tongue	70	0	-	-	-	-	-	0.2	0.3	0.5	0.5	1.3	2.3	3.3	5.1	7.7	9.2	6.5	0.7	0.9	0.07	0.15	1.2	141
Salivary gland	30	0	-	0.3	-	-	0.4	0.1	0.1	0.4	0.8	0.8	2.0	-	0.8	0.7	-	2.9	0.3	0.4	0.03	0.03	0.4	142
Mouth	534	1	-	-	-	0.1	0.1	0.4	1.6	4.6	14.4	14.5	26.9	32.2	34.9	41.3	34.8	35.9	5.6	7.0	0.65	1.03	8.9	143-5
Oropharynx	31	0	-	-	-	-	-	-	-	0.2	0.8	1.1	1.0	1.4	1.7	4.2	1.8	3.6	0.3	0.4	0.03	0.06	0.5	146
Nasopharynx	19	0	-	-	0.2	0.2	0.3	-	0.1	0.4	-	0.3	0.3	0.5	1.3	1.4	-	0.7	0.2	0.2	0.02	0.02	0.2	147
Hypopharynx	69	0	-	-	-	-	-	0.2	0.4	1.1	2.1	2.4	2.0	2.8	5.1	3.5	4.6	5.0	0.7	0.9	0.08	0.12	1.1	148
Pharynx unspecified	22	0	-	-	-	-	0.1	-	0.1	-	0.8	0.3	1.0	1.4	2.1	2.1	1.8	-	0.2	0.3	0.03	0.05	0.4	149
Oesophagus	501	0	-	-	-	-	0.3	0.1	0.4	3.4	7.4	17.7	25.3	32.6	33.3	39.9	48.6	32.3	5.3	6.6	0.60	1.04	8.5	150
Stomach	321	0	-	-	-	0.3	0.3	0.8	2.0	4.4	7.4	8.5	9.3	18.6	18.9	27.3	22.0	23.0	3.4	4.2	0.35	0.60	5.1	151
Small intestine	5	0	-	-	-	-	0.1	0.1	-	-	0.3	-	0.3	-	-	0.7	-	-	0.1	0.1	0.00	0.01	0.1	152
Colon	128	0	-	-	-	0.1	0.2	0.4	0.7	1.6	2.4	3.7	7.3	5.1	8.0	6.3	11.9	7.2	1.3	1.7	0.15	0.24	2.0	153
Rectum	172	0	-	-	-	0.1	0.4	0.3	0.7	1.6	2.9	5.8	8.6	13.1	9.3	9.1	9.2	12.9	1.8	2.3	0.21	0.31	2.8	154
Liver	80	1	0.1	-	0.1	0.1	0.1	0.2	0.3	0.7	1.3	2.4	4.7	4.7	5.9	4.9	3.7	2.9	0.8	1.0	0.10	0.15	1.3	155
Gallbladder etc.	41	0	-	-	-	-	-	-	-	-	0.4	1.3	1.1	1.0	3.3	2.5	0.7	7.3	3.6	0.4	0.5	0.05	0.09	0.7	156
Pancreas	54	0	-	-	-	-	-	0.1	-	0.6	0.5	1.8	1.9	1.3	1.4	3.4	3.5	5.5	4.3	0.6	0.7	0.05	0.10	0.9	157
Nose, sinuses etc.	39	0	-	-	-	0.1	-	-	0.4	0.2	0.5	0.8	1.7	2.8	4.2	2.1	1.8	2.2	0.4	0.5	0.05	0.07	0.6	160
Larynx	37	0	-	-	-	0.2	-	-	0.3	0.9	1.1	1.3	0.7	2.8	1.3	2.8	0.9	2.2	0.4	0.5	0.04	0.06	0.6	161
Bronchus, lung	103	1	-	-	-	0.1	0.1	0.5	0.6	0.5	1.6	2.6	6.7	6.5	6.7	8.4	5.5	2.9	1.1	1.4	0.13	0.20	1.7	162
Other thoracic organs	24	0	-	0.1	0.2	-	-	-	-	0.4	0.3	0.3	1.7	0.9	2.1	1.4	0.9	1.4	0.3	0.3	0.03	0.04	0.4	163-4
Bone	81	0	0.2	0.7	0.8	1.6	0.7	0.3	0.3	0.4	1.3	2.6	1.7	-	1.3	2.8	0.9	2.2	0.9	1.1	0.06	0.08	0.9	170
Connective tissue	66	0	-	0.2	-	0.4	0.5	0.5	0.9	1.1	1.8	1.6	2.7	1.4	1.7	2.8	1.8	2.9	0.7	0.9	0.06	0.09	0.9	171
Mesothelioma	2	0	-	-	-	-	-	-	0.3	-	-	-	-	-	-	-	-	-	0.0	0.0	0.00	0.00	0.0	MES
Kaposi's sarcoma	0	0	-	-	-	-	-	-	-	-	-	-	-	-	-	-	-	-	0.0	0.0	0.00	0.00	0.0	KAP
Melanoma of skin	14	0	-	-	-	-	-	-	-	0.4	0.5	0.5	0.3	0.9	0.8	-	2.7	-	0.1	0.2	0.02	0.03	0.2	172
Other skin	90	0	0.1	-	-	0.1	0.4	0.2	0.1	1.2	3.2	2.1	3.0	5.6	5.1	3.5	10.1	3.6	0.9		0.11	0.17	1.4	173
Breast	1381	2	-	-	-	0.5	1.0	3.6	12.6	25.3	49.4	50.7	62.2	68.5	68.6	64.4	51.3	51.7	14.6	18.1	1.72	2.29	21.3	174
Uterus unspecified	24	0	-	-	-	-	0.2	0.2	0.7	0.2	-	0.5	1.3	-	1.3	2.1	-	1.4	0.3	0.3	0.02	0.03	0.3	179
Cervix uteri	1732	2	-	-	-	0.3	0.8	4.0	11.5	32.0	56.7	69.5	83.5	96.0	96.8	85.4	60.5	46.0	18.3	22.7	2.26	2.99	27.2	180
Placenta	6	0	-	-	-	-	0.2	0.2	0.3	-	-	-	-	-	-	-	-	-	0.1	0.1	0.00	0.00	0.0	181
Corpus uteri	118	1	-	-	0.1	0.1	0.1	-	0.9	1.1	2.9	2.6	6.0	8.9	6.7	7.0	11.0	4.3	1.2	1.5	0.15	0.24	1.9	182
Ovary etc.	293	0	-	0.2	0.2	1.1	1.1	1.8	2.3	4.8	8.7	10.0	12.6	16.8	11.8	12.6	6.4	5.0	3.1	3.8	0.36	0.45	4.3	183
Other female genital	85	0	0.1	-	-	-	0.1	0.3	0.4	0.7	1.6	2.1	1.3	6.1	4.6	6.3	15.6	3.6	0.9	1.1	0.09	0.20	1.4	184
Bladder	46	0	0.1	-	-	-	-	-	0.1	0.2	-	2.4	0.7	3.7	5.1	2.1	2.7	4.3	0.5	0.6	0.06	0.09	0.8	188
Kidney etc.	45	0	0.5	0.1	0.1	-	0.3	0.2	0.3	0.2	1.3	1.1	1.0	2.8	2.9	0.7	2.7	0.7	0.5	0.6	0.05	0.07	0.7	189
Eye	21	0	1.0	0.3	-	-	-	-	0.1	-	0.3	-	0.3	-	-	1.4	0.9	1.4	0.2	0.3	0.01	0.02	0.3	190
Brain, nervous system	132	1	0.8	1.0	1.0	0.7	0.6	1.3	1.2	2.5	2.6	2.9	2.7	3.7	3.4	1.4	3.7	-	1.4	1.7	0.12	0.15	1.6	191-2
Thyroid	233	0	-	-	0.4	0.9	1.1	2.4	4.1	3.2	6.0	6.3	6.0	9.3	8.4	9.1	6.4	8.6	2.5	3.1	0.24	0.32	3.2	193
Other endocrine	4	0	0.1	-	-	-	-	0.1	-	-	-	0.3	0.3	-	-	-	-	-	0.0	0.1	0.00	0.00	0.1	194
Hodgkin's disease	52	0	-	0.1	0.3	0.5	0.4	0.5	1.0	0.7	1.6	0.5	0.3	2.3	1.3	1.4	2.7	0.7	0.5	0.7	0.05	0.07	0.6	201
Non-Hodgkin lymphoma	142	0	0.5	0.3	0.2	0.3	0.8	0.4	1.0	2.3	2.1	4.8	4.3	5.6	5.9	9.1	8.2	6.5	1.5	1.9	0.14	0.23	2.1	200,202
Multiple myeloma	36	0	0.1	-	-	-	-	-	-	0.2	1.6	1.1	1.3	3.3	2.5	2.8	1.8	0.7	0.4	0.5	0.05	0.07	0.6	203
Lymphoid leukaemia	54	0	2.2	0.7	0.4	0.4	0.1	-	0.1	0.4	0.3	-	-	0.5	-	2.8	4.6	0.7	0.6	0.7	0.03	0.06	0.7	204
Myeloid leukaemia	127	0	0.1	0.3	0.8	0.4	1.5	1.0	1.5	1.6	1.6	3.2	4.7	7.9	2.9	2.1	3.7	0.7	1.3	1.7	0.14	0.17	1.6	205
Monocytic leukaemia	1	0	-	-	-	-	-	-	-	0.2	-	-	-	-	-	-	-	-	0.0	0.0	0.00	0.00	0.0	206
Other leukaemia	1	0	-	-	-	-	-	-	-	-	-	-	0.3	-	-	-	-	-	0.0	0.0	0.00	0.00	0.0	207
Leukaemia unspecified	36	0	0.3	-	0.3	0.3	0.2	0.2	0.1	0.7	0.3	0.8	1.0	1.4	1.3	2.1	0.9	0.7	0.4	0.5	0.03	0.05	0.5	208
Other and unspecified	607	3	0.7	0.5	0.7	1.2	0.8	1.8	3.8	6.9	9.7	19.3	20.3	37.8	32.0	40.6	36.7	38.1	6.4	8.0	0.68	1.07	9.5	O&U
All sites	7719	12	7.1	4.7	5.8	9.9	13.2	22.1	52.5	107.6	201.2	252.1	322.0	417.7	411.4	430.4	405.0	334.7	81.4		9.15	13.33	119.5	ALL
All sites but 173	7629	12	7.0	4.7	5.8	9.8	12.9	21.9	52.4	106.4	198.1	250.0	319.0	412.1	406.3	426.9	394.9	331.2	80.4	100.0	9.05	13.16	118.1	ALLb

Rate from 10 cases   1.057   0.857   0.899   0.981   0.926   0.993   1.450   1.770   2.627   2.643   3.326   4.662   4.211   6.998   9.163   7.183

India, Barshi, Paranda and Bhum

Since all existing cancer registeries in India served urban populations and 76% of the population still resides in rural areas, the Indian Council of Medical Research decided about 10 years ago to set up rural cancer registries under its National Cancer Registry Programme. The usual methods of registration were modified to overcome deficiencies in diagnostic services in the rural setting and the first rural cancer registry was set up in 1987 at Barshi, in the state of Maharashtra, in western India.

The registry area comprises rural areas of three sub-districts, viz., Barshi in Solapur district and Paranda and Bhum in Osmanabad district, situated in the vicinity of Nargis Dutt Memorial Cancer Hospital (located on the outskirts of Barshi Town), with a total population of about 400 000 in 346 villages spread over 3713 km^2. The registry area is situated between latitudes 17.1° and 18.4° N and longitudes 76° and 76.4° E.

A village is the basic administrative unit in rural areas and is defined as having greater than 25% of the male working population engaged in agricultural activities, a population of less than 400 persons per km^2, and a total population of generally less than 5000.

As the age–sex distribution from the 1991 decennial census is not yet published, the age–sex distribution of the extrapolated population for 1991 (based on 1971–81 growth rates) was applied to the 1991 reported population, to derive the exponential growth rates required for estimating the requisite population estimates.

Trained field-investigators visit the villages regularly and interact with the rural community to identify and motivate likely cancer cases to visit a hospital for early diagnosis and treatment. To screen symptomatic cases, Cancer Detection Camps are periodically arranged for groups of villages. Data on cancer cases from the registry area are also collected from various hospitals and diagnostic laboratories in urban centres which serve the population.

Information on deaths is collected from village death records and also directly from the local community. As deaths are generally not medically certified, relatives of all deceased are visited to collect relevant information to assist in a 'follow-back' to the medical records in the treating hospital or physician.

All cancer patients are followed up every six months to ascertain their vital status.

The data are evaluated for completeness by conducting annual house-to-house surveys in a sample of villages. The evaluation has indicated that a diagnosed case has not been missed by the registry. Under-registration due to probable cancer cases dying before confirmation of diagnosis is about 1%, while under-registration due to patients not reaching even a general practitioner or patients under the care of local medical personnel not reaching diagnostic centres before death seems to be in the range of 6 to 16%. However, there are indications that the registry has reached near complete registration for cancers of the breast and cervix uteri.

Smoking-related cancers have a low incidence since smoking is not common in the population, as indicated by a tobacco survey in this area.

The data on cervical cancer cases showed that the innovative methodology adopted at the registry has resulted in improved stages at diagnosis of cervical cancer as well as improved survival three years after the inception of the registry, owing to enhanced awareness of cancer symptoms in the population. Motivation of symptomatic women to seek medical care through repeated home visits by the registry personnel is also likely to be a contributing factor.

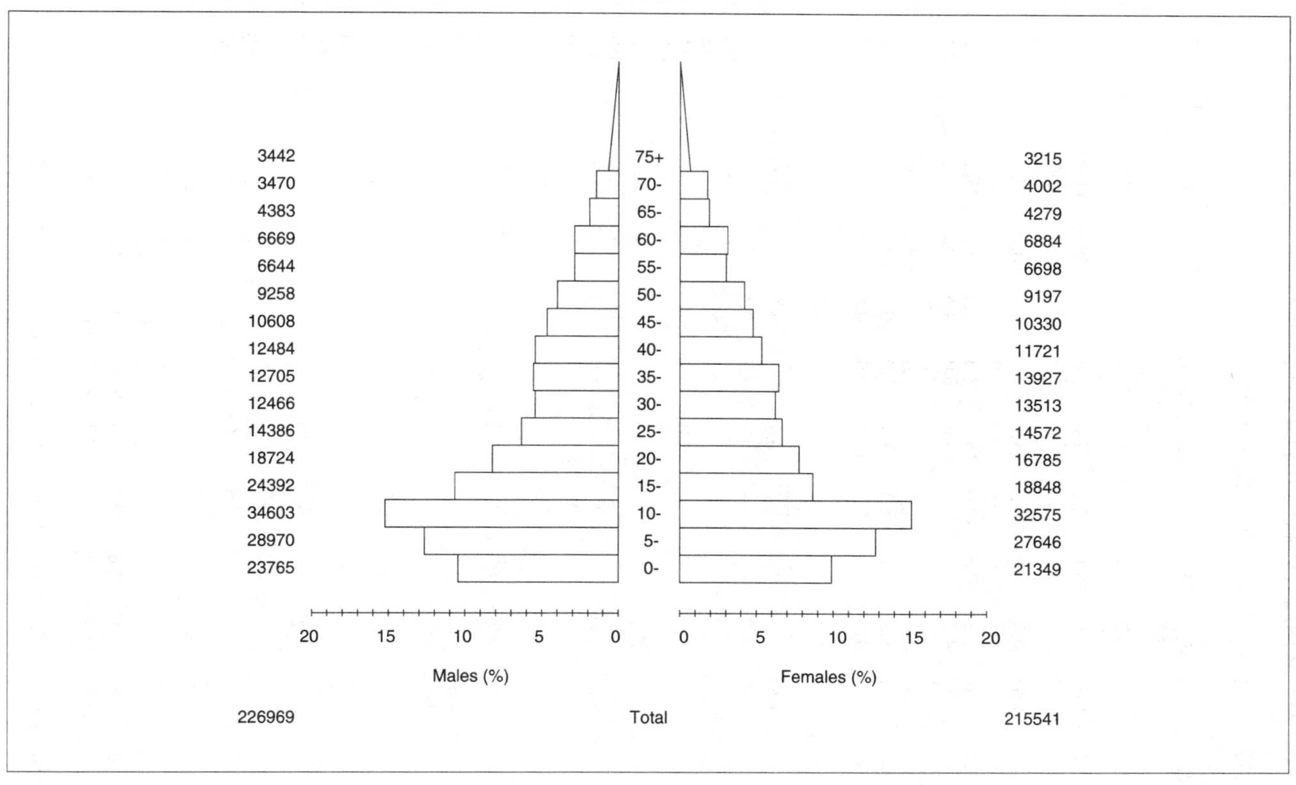

India, Barshi, Paranda and Bhum

Source of population: average annual 1988–92

Census: Census of India 1991. Banthia, J.K. Series 14, Maharashtra. Provincial population totals. Government photozinco press, Pune 1991. Census of India 1981, District Census Handbooks, Solapur and Osmanabad. Maharashtra Census Directorate, Government Printing Stationary and Publications, Maharashtra State, Bombay, 1986. Census of India 1971, District Census Handbooks, Osmanabad and Solapur. Maharashtra Census Directorate, Government Printing Stationary and Publications, Maharashtra State, 1976. Mahana, P.P. Census of India 1981, Series 12, Part IV-A, Social and Cultural tables, Central Government Publications, New Delhi, 1986.

Estimate: Population data for each village in the area are available by sex in the decennial census reports of Maharashtra. The age distribution is not available for the rural population of each tahsil. It is available only for the rural population of the whole district obtained by extrapolating from the distributions observed in the 20% area sample surveys conducted during the decennial census (Chari 1976; Mahana 1986). The 1991 Census has published figures for the entire population, but data are not yet available by age. For each tahsil, by sex, exponential growth rates were determined from the reported age distributions for 1971 and 1981. Based on these growth rates the age-specific population for 1991 was extrapolated, and the age distribution of this extrapolated population was applied to the provisional total population of 1991. The exponential growth rates in the age-groups during 1981–91 were then estimated, to produce population data for 1 July in each of the years 1988-92.

Notes to the tables overleaf:

* The rates show evidence of under-diagnosis.

Screening programmes in the area:

Cancer detection camps are held twice a year throughout the registration area. All patients visiting the camps are examined, however only symptomatic cases are actively encouraged to visit the camps.

* INDIA, BARSHI, PARANDA AND BHUM 1988-1992

ANNUAL INCIDENCE PER 100,000 BY AGE GROUP (YEARS) - MALE

SITE	ALL AGES	AGE UNK	0-	5-	10-	15-	20-	25-	30-	35-	40-	45-	50-	55-	60-	65-	70-	75+	CRUDE RATE	%	CR 64	CR 74	ASR (W)	ICD (9th)
Lip	3	0	-	-	-	-	-	-	-	-	-	1.9	-	3.0	-	-	5.8	-	0.3	0.7	0.02	0.05	**0.3**	140
Tongue	19	0	-	-	-	-	-	-	1.6	1.6	3.2	-	-	6.0	21.0	22.8	-	5.8	1.7	4.3	0.17	0.28	**2.3**	141
Salivary gland	4	0	-	-	-	-	-	-	-	-	1.6	-	-	-	-	4.6	11.5	-	0.4	0.9	0.01	0.09	**0.5**	142
Mouth	33	0	-	-	-	-	-	1.4	3.2	1.6	1.6	15.1	2.2	15.1	6.0	22.8	28.8	11.6	2.9	7.5	0.23	0.49	**3.8**	143-5
Oropharynx	6	0	-	-	-	-	-	-	-	-	-	-	-	3.0	3.0	13.7	-	5.8	0.5	1.4	0.03	0.10	**0.8**	146
Nasopharynx	0	0	-	-	-	-	-	-	-	-	-	-	-	-	-	-	-	-	0.0	0.0	0.00	0.00	**0.0**	147
Hypopharynx	56	0	-	-	-	-	1.1	1.4	-	1.6	4.8	9.4	6.5	15.1	33.0	73.0	40.3	17.4	4.9	12.7	0.36	0.93	**6.7**	148
Pharynx unspecified	6	0	-	-	-	0.8	-	1.4	-	-	1.6	-	-	6.0	-	-	-	5.8	0.5	1.4	0.05	0.05	**0.6**	149
Oesophagus	49	0	-	-	-	-	-	-	1.6	-	3.2	7.5	13.0	15.1	33.0	36.5	46.1	23.2	4.3	11.1	0.37	0.78	**5.8**	150
Stomach	7	0	-	-	-	-	-	-	-	-	4.8	-	-	3.0	3.0	4.6	5.8	-	0.6	1.6	0.05	0.11	**0.8**	151
Small intestine	1	0	-	-	-	-	-	-	-	-	-	-	-	-	3.0	-	-	-	0.1	0.2	0.01	0.01	**0.1**	152
Colon	6	0	-	-	-	-	-	-	-	1.6	-	-	2.2	-	3.0	4.6	5.8	5.8	0.5	1.4	0.03	0.09	**0.7**	153
Rectum	23	0	-	-	-	-	-	5.6	1.6	-	3.2	1.9	6.5	9.0	6.0	9.1	23.1	5.8	2.0	5.2	0.17	0.33	**2.6**	154
Liver	15	0	-	-	-	-	-	-	-	-	1.6	1.9	2.2	12.0	15.0	4.6	5.8	5.8	1.3	3.4	0.16	0.22	**1.8**	155
Gallbladder etc.	1	0	-	-	-	-	-	-	-	-	-	-	-	-	-	-	5.8	-	0.1	0.2	0.00	0.03	**0.1**	156
Pancreas	4	0	-	-	-	-	-	-	-	-	-	1.9	-	-	-	4.6	11.5	-	0.4	0.9	0.01	0.09	**0.5**	157
Nose, sinuses etc.	3	0	-	-	-	-	-	1.4	-	-	-	-	2.2	-	-	-	-	5.8	0.3	0.7	0.02	0.02	**0.3**	160
Larynx	21	0	-	-	-	-	-	-	-	1.6	1.6	3.8	2.2	6.0	3.0	31.9	23.1	11.6	1.9	4.8	0.09	0.37	**2.5**	161
Bronchus, lung	11	0	-	-	-	-	-	-	-	-	4.8	1.9	2.2	6.0	3.0	9.1	5.8	-	1.0	2.5	0.09	0.16	**1.3**	162
Other thoracic organs	0	0	-	-	-	-	-	-	-	-	-	-	-	-	-	-	-	-	0.0	0.0	0.00	0.00	**0.0**	163-4
Bone	4	0	-	-	0.6	-	1.1	-	1.6	-	-	1.9	-	-	-	-	-	-	0.4	0.9	0.03	0.03	**0.3**	170
Connective tissue	6	0	0.8	0.7	0.6	0.8	-	-	-	-	-	1.9	-	3.0	-	-	-	-	0.5	1.4	0.04	0.04	**0.5**	171
Mesothelioma	0	0	-	-	-	-	-	-	-	-	-	-	-	-	-	-	-	-	0.0	0.0	0.00	0.00	**0.0**	MES
Kaposi's sarcoma	0	0	-	-	-	-	-	-	-	-	-	-	-	-	-	-	-	-	0.0	0.0	0.00	0.00	**0.0**	KAP
Melanoma of skin	0	0	-	-	-	-	-	-	-	-	-	-	-	-	-	-	-	-	0.0	0.0	0.00	0.00	**0.0**	172
Other skin	12	0	-	-	-	-	-	-	-	1.6	1.6	-	2.2	-	6.0	9.1	17.3	11.6	1.1	-	0.06	0.19	**1.4**	173
Breast	0	0	-	-	-	-	-	-	-	-	-	-	-	-	-	-	-	-	0.0	0.0	0.00	0.00	**0.0**	175
Prostate	12	0	-	-	-	-	-	-	-	-	-	-	6.5	-	12.0	13.7	5.8	5.8	1.1	2.7	0.09	0.19	**1.4**	185
Testis	3	0	-	-	-	-	1.1	-	-	-	-	-	2.2	-	-	4.6	-	-	0.3	0.7	0.02	0.04	**0.3**	186
Penis	29	0	-	-	-	-	-	-	3.2	3.1	1.6	3.8	8.6	12.0	15.0	13.7	28.8	5.8	2.6	6.6	0.24	0.45	**3.3**	187.1-.4
Other male genital	5	0	-	-	-	-	-	-	1.6	-	1.6	-	2.2	-	3.0	-	-	5.8	0.4	1.1	0.04	0.04	**0.5**	187.5-.9
Bladder	9	0	-	-	-	-	-	-	-	1.6	-	-	4.3	-	-	9.1	5.8	17.4	0.8	2.0	0.03	0.10	**1.0**	188
Kidney etc.	4	0	-	0.7	-	-	-	-	-	1.6	-	-	-	-	-	-	11.5	-	0.4	0.9	0.01	0.07	**0.4**	189
Eye	0	0	-	-	-	-	-	-	-	-	-	-	-	-	-	-	-	-	0.0	0.0	0.00	0.00	**0.0**	190
Brain, nervous system	4	0	-	0.7	-	0.8	-	-	-	-	-	1.9	2.2	-	-	-	-	-	0.4	0.9	0.03	0.03	**0.4**	191-2
Thyroid	5	0	-	-	-	1.1	1.4	-	-	-	3.2	-	-	-	-	-	-	5.8	0.4	1.1	0.03	0.03	**0.5**	193
Other endocrine	0	0	-	-	-	-	-	-	-	-	-	-	-	-	-	-	-	-	0.0	0.0	0.00	0.00	**0.0**	194
Hodgkin's disease	5	0	-	-	0.6	0.8	1.1	-	1.6	-	-	-	-	-	-	-	5.8	-	0.4	1.1	0.02	0.05	**0.4**	201
Non-Hodgkin lymphoma	9	0	0.8	0.7	-	-	-	2.8	-	-	3.2	-	-	6.0	-	4.6	-	-	0.8	2.0	0.07	0.09	**1.0**	200,202
Multiple myeloma	1	0	-	-	-	-	-	-	-	-	-	-	2.2	-	-	-	-	-	0.1	0.2	0.01	0.01	**0.1**	203
Lymphoid leukaemia	9	0	-	2.8	1.2	0.8	-	1.4	-	-	-	-	-	-	-	-	-	5.8	0.8	2.0	0.03	0.03	**0.7**	204
Myeloid leukaemia	10	0	-	-	0.6	-	-	2.8	1.6	-	-	-	6.5	3.0	3.0	-	-	5.8	0.9	2.3	0.09	0.09	**1.1**	205
Monocytic leukaemia	0	0	-	-	-	-	-	-	-	-	-	-	-	-	-	-	-	-	0.0	0.0	0.00	0.00	**0.0**	206
Other leukaemia	0	0	-	-	-	-	-	-	-	-	-	-	-	-	-	-	-	-	0.0	0.0	0.00	0.00	**0.0**	207
Leukaemia unspecified	1	0	-	0.7	-	-	-	-	-	-	-	-	-	-	-	-	-	-	0.1	0.2	0.00	0.00	**0.1**	208
Other and unspecified	57	0	-	0.7	-	0.8	1.1	2.8	1.6	-	3.2	1.9	6.5	21.1	30.0	54.8	40.3	52.3	5.0	12.9	0.35	0.82	**6.7**	O&U
All sites	453	0	1.7	6.9	3.5	4.9	6.4	22.2	19.3	15.7	46.5	56.6	82.1	138.5	206.9	351.4	334.3	220.8	39.9		3.06	6.48	**51.8**	ALL
All sites but 173	441	0	1.7	6.9	3.5	4.9	6.4	22.2	19.3	14.2	44.9	56.6	79.9	138.5	200.9	342.2	317.0	209.1	38.9	100.0	3.00	6.29	**50.4**	ALLb

Rate from 1 case   0.842   0.690   0.578   0.820   1.068   1.390   1.604   1.574   1.602   1.885   2.160   3.010   2.999   4.563   5.763   5.810

* INDIA, BARSHI, PARANDA AND BHUM 1988-1992

ANNUAL INCIDENCE PER 100,000 BY AGE GROUP (YEARS) - FEMALE

SITE	ALL AGES	AGE UNK	0-	5-	10-	15-	20-	25-	30-	35-	40-	45-	50-	55-	60-	65-	70-	75+	CRUDE RATE	%	CR 64	CR 74	ASR (W)	ICD (9th)
Lip	0	0	-	-	-	-	-	-	-	-	-	-	-	-	-	-	-	-	0.0	0.0	0.00	0.00	0.0	140
Tongue	3	0	-	-	-	-	-	-	-	-	-	1.9	-	-	2.9	-	5.0	-	0.3	0.6	0.02	0.05	0.3	141
Salivary gland	1	0	-	-	0.6	-	-	-	-	-	-	-	-	-	-	-	-	-	0.1	0.2	0.00	0.00	0.1	142
Mouth	7	0	-	-	-	-	-	-	-	-	-	-	6.5	-	5.8	4.7	-	6.2	0.6	1.4	0.06	0.09	0.8	143-5
Oropharynx	1	0	-	-	-	-	-	-	-	-	-	-	2.2	-	-	-	-	-	0.1	0.2	0.01	0.01	0.1	146
Nasopharynx	0	0	-	-	-	-	-	-	-	-	-	-	-	-	-	-	-	-	0.0	0.0	0.00	0.00	0.0	147
Hypopharynx	5	0	-	-	-	-	-	-	1.5	1.4	-	1.9	-	-	-	4.7	5.0	-	0.5	1.0	0.02	0.07	0.5	148
Pharynx unspecified	0	0	-	-	-	-	-	-	-	-	-	-	-	-	-	-	-	-	0.0	0.0	0.00	0.00	0.0	149
Oesophagus	16	0	-	-	-	-	-	-	-	-	1.7	5.8	2.2	6.0	14.5	14.0	-	6.2	1.5	3.3	0.15	0.22	1.9	150
Stomach	8	0	-	-	-	-	-	-	1.5	-	-	1.9	2.2	9.0	2.9	-	-	6.2	0.7	1.6	0.09	0.09	0.9	151
Small intestine	0	0	-	-	-	-	-	-	-	-	-	-	-	-	-	-	-	-	0.0	0.0	0.00	0.00	0.0	152
Colon	4	0	-	-	-	-	-	-	-	1.4	-	1.9	-	6.0	-	-	-	-	0.4	0.8	0.05	0.05	0.4	153
Rectum	10	0	-	-	-	-	-	2.7	1.5	-	5.1	1.9	2.2	-	-	-	5.0	6.2	0.9	2.0	0.07	0.09	1.1	154
Liver	6	0	-	-	-	-	-	1.4	-	1.4	-	3.9	2.2	3.0	-	-	-	-	0.6	1.2	0.06	0.06	0.7	155
Gallbladder etc.	2	0	-	-	-	-	-	-	-	-	1.7	-	-	-	2.9	-	-	-	0.2	0.4	0.02	0.02	0.2	156
Pancreas	2	0	-	-	-	-	-	-	-	-	-	1.9	2.2	-	-	-	-	-	0.2	0.4	0.02	0.02	0.2	157
Nose, sinuses etc.	2	0	-	-	-	-	-	-	-	1.4	-	-	-	-	-	4.7	-	-	0.2	0.4	0.01	0.03	0.2	160
Larynx	0	0	-	-	-	-	-	-	-	-	-	-	-	-	-	-	-	-	0.0	0.0	0.00	0.00	0.0	161
Bronchus, lung	3	0	-	-	-	-	-	-	-	-	1.7	1.9	-	-	2.9	-	-	-	0.3	0.6	0.03	0.03	0.3	162
Other thoracic organs	0	0	-	-	-	-	-	-	-	-	-	-	-	-	-	-	-	-	0.0	0.0	0.00	0.00	0.0	163-4
Bone	5	0	-	-	-	-	1.2	-	-	1.4	-	1.9	-	-	-	4.7	5.0	-	0.5	1.0	0.02	0.07	0.5	170
Connective tissue	2	0	-	-	-	-	-	-	-	-	-	3.9	-	-	-	-	-	-	0.2	0.4	0.02	0.02	0.2	171
Mesothelioma	0	0	-	-	-	-	-	-	-	-	-	-	-	-	-	-	-	-	0.0	0.0	0.00	0.00	0.0	MES
Kaposi's sarcoma	0	0	-	-	-	-	-	-	-	-	-	-	-	-	-	-	-	-	0.0	0.0	0.00	0.00	0.0	KAP
Melanoma of skin	1	0	-	-	-	-	-	-	-	-	-	-	-	3.0	-	-	-	-	0.1	0.2	0.01	0.01	0.1	172
Other skin	10	0	-	-	-	-	-	-	1.5	-	3.4	-	-	3.0	5.8	-	15.0	6.2	0.9		0.07	0.14	1.1	173
Breast	78	0	-	-	-	-	-	-	5.9	10.1	18.8	19.4	19.6	23.9	40.7	46.7	25.0	-	7.2	15.9	0.69	1.05	8.7	174
Uterus unspecified	0	0	-	-	-	-	-	-	-	-	-	-	-	-	-	-	-	-	0.0	0.0	0.00	0.00	0.0	179
Cervix uteri	252	0	-	-	-	-	-	2.7	20.7	46.0	63.1	71.6	71.8	89.6	130.7	51.4	35.0	24.9	23.4	51.2	2.48	2.91	27.4	180
Placenta	0	0	-	-	-	-	-	-	-	-	-	-	-	-	-	-	-	-	0.0	0.0	0.00	0.00	0.0	181
Corpus uteri	3	0	-	-	-	-	-	-	-	-	1.7	-	2.2	3.0	-	-	-	-	0.3	0.6	0.03	0.03	0.3	182
Ovary etc.	12	0	-	-	-	1.1	1.2	-	-	5.7	3.4	1.9	-	3.0	2.9	4.7	-	-	1.1	2.4	0.10	0.12	1.2	183
Other female genital	8	0	-	-	-	-	-	-	-	1.4	-	-	2.2	3.0	2.9	4.7	-	18.7	0.7	1.6	0.05	0.07	0.9	184
Bladder	0	0	-	-	-	-	-	-	-	-	-	-	-	-	-	-	-	-	0.0	0.0	0.00	0.00	0.0	188
Kidney etc.	1	0	-	-	-	-	-	-	-	-	1.4	-	-	-	-	-	-	-	0.1	0.2	0.01	0.01	0.1	189
Eye	1	0	0.9	-	-	-	-	-	-	-	-	-	-	-	-	-	-	-	0.1	0.2	0.00	0.00	0.1	190
Brain, nervous system	2	0	-	-	-	-	-	-	1.5	-	1.7	-	-	-	-	-	-	-	0.2	0.4	0.02	0.02	0.2	191-2
Thyroid	2	0	-	-	-	-	-	-	-	-	1.7	-	-	-	-	-	-	6.2	0.2	0.4	0.01	0.01	0.2	193
Other endocrine	0	0	-	-	-	-	-	-	-	-	-	-	-	-	-	-	-	-	0.0	0.0	0.00	0.00	0.0	194
Hodgkin's disease	0	0	-	-	-	-	-	-	-	-	-	-	-	-	-	-	-	-	0.0	0.0	0.00	0.00	0.0	201
Non-Hodgkin lymphoma	5	0	0.9	-	-	-	-	-	-	-	-	1.9	-	3.0	2.9	4.7	-	-	0.5	1.0	0.04	0.07	0.6	200,202
Multiple myeloma	1	0	-	-	-	-	-	-	-	-	-	1.9	-	-	-	-	-	-	0.1	0.2	0.01	0.01	0.1	203
Lymphoid leukaemia	6	0	0.9	0.7	1.8	-	-	1.4	-	-	-	-	-	-	-	-	-	-	0.6	1.2	0.02	0.02	0.5	204
Myeloid leukaemia	5	0	-	0.7	0.6	1.1	-	-	-	1.4	-	-	-	-	2.9	-	-	-	0.5	1.0	0.03	0.03	0.4	205
Monocytic leukaemia	0	0	-	-	-	-	-	-	-	-	-	-	-	-	-	-	-	-	0.0	0.0	0.00	0.00	0.0	206
Other leukaemia	0	0	-	-	-	-	-	-	-	-	-	-	-	-	-	-	-	-	0.0	0.0	0.00	0.00	0.0	207
Leukaemia unspecified	0	0	-	-	-	-	-	-	-	-	-	-	-	-	-	-	-	-	0.0	0.0	0.00	0.00	0.0	208
Other and unspecified	38	0	0.9	-	-	-	-	1.4	1.5	2.9	6.8	5.8	8.7	17.9	20.3	4.7	15.0	31.1	3.5	7.7	0.33	0.43	4.3	O&U
All sites	502	0	3.7	1.4	3.1	2.1	2.4	9.6	35.5	76.1	110.9	131.6	124.0	173.2	241.1	149.6	109.9	112.0	46.6		4.57	5.87	55.0	ALL
All sites but 173	492	0	3.7	1.4	3.1	2.1	2.4	9.6	34.0	76.1	107.5	131.6	124.0	170.2	235.3	149.6	95.0	105.7	45.7	100.0	4.51	5.73	53.9	ALLb

Rate from 1 case	0-	5-	10-	15-	20-	25-	30-	35-	40-	45-	50-	55-	60-	65-	70-	75+
	0.937	0.723	0.614	1.061	1.192	1.372	1.480	1.436	1.706	1.936	2.175	2.986	2.905	4.674	4.998	6.220

India, Bombay

The Bombay Cancer Registry was established in June 1963 as a unit of the Indian Cancer Society at Bombay, with the aim of obtaining reliable morbidity and mortality data on cancer from a precisely defined urban population (Greater Bombay). The actual compilation of data began in 1964. Until then, no continuing activity on registration of cancer cases in a population had been undertaken anywhere in India. The project started in collaboration with and received financial support up to 1975 from the Biometry Branch of the US National Cancer Institute. During 1976–80 the project received financial support from the Department of Science and Technology, Government of India at New Delhi and the Indian Cancer Society. Since 1981–82, the registry has been funded in part by the Indian Council of Medical Resarch.

The registry covers the resident population of Greater Bombay, a densely populated metropolis on the west coast of India, occupying an area of 603 km^2, situated between latitudes 18°54′ and 19°16′ N, and longitudes 70°47′ and 73° E. Greater Bombay is, in fact, an island, joined to the mainland by bridges, and has a warm, humid climate.

The estimated population of Greater Bombay as of 1 July 1990 was 9 700 000. The city is the industrial heart of India. As a result of continuing immigration, it has a multireligious and multi-lingual population, representing every state in the Union, approximately 68.8% being Hindus, 14.1% Muslims, 6.3% Christians (mostly Hindu converts), 4.8% Neo-Buddhists and 4.1% Jains (an ultra-conservative Hindu sect), 1.1% Parsis (Zoroastrians) and 0.1% Sikhs.

A total of about 22 500 hospital beds are available in the registration area.

Information is obtained on all cancer patients registered in 150 government hospitals/institutions and private hospitals or nursing homes in Bombay which are under the care of specialists (surgeons, physicians, pathologists, radiologists and gynaecologists). The majority of hospitals in Bombay are maintained by the Municipal Corporation and State Government, which are responsible for the organization of public health care and medical services in the city. The major source of data is the Tata Memorial Centre, which is a postgraduate university teaching centre for cancer research. The city has five medical colleges. The diagnosis and treatment of cancer is centralized in certain hospitals. Major cancer surgery is undertaken in all the major hospitals and well equipped private nursing homes in the city. Facilities for cobalt-60 therapy are available in five hospitals, while ortho-voltage deep X-ray therapy is available in 15 hospitals in the city.

General medical practitioners are not contacted individually as, according to local practice, only specialists assume charge of cancer patients in private hospitals and nursing homes, and even the few patients who are not admitted for hospital care are at one stage or another referred to specialists by a general practitioner.

Staff members of the registry visit the wards of all cooperating hospitals at least once a week, to personally interview each cancer patient as well as those suspected of having cancer. All files maintained by the various departments of these hospitals are also cross-checked individually. Care is taken to prevent duplication of an entry relating to a patient already registered.

With the exception of the Tata Memorial Hospital for cancer, hospital outpatient records are not included in the registry files, because of a paucity of clinical details and lack of specific information on the residential status of patients attending these clinics.

Supplementary information is gleaned from the death records maintained by the Municipal Corporation. This makes it possible to check on a number of missed cases. Every cancer death not traceable to an entry in the files is labelled as an unmatched death and is so registered for the corresponding year.

The reliability of the data and the quality of the registration have considerably improved. At present the percentage of microscopically confirmed cases is 76% and the percentage of cases diagnosed through death certificates alone is 7%. The ratio of deaths to incident cases is 52%.

The registry collects information on multiple cancer cases. For determining the presence of multiple primary cancers, the IACR rules are used.

The registry records follow-up information for selected primary sites.

The registry publishes yearly reports, and has published numerous journal articles and monographs. The data are also used by public health workers for etiological and cancer control studies. As the oldest registry in the country, the registry is a rich source of data for studying time trends in cancer incidence and mortality.

D.J. Jussawalla
B.B. Yeole

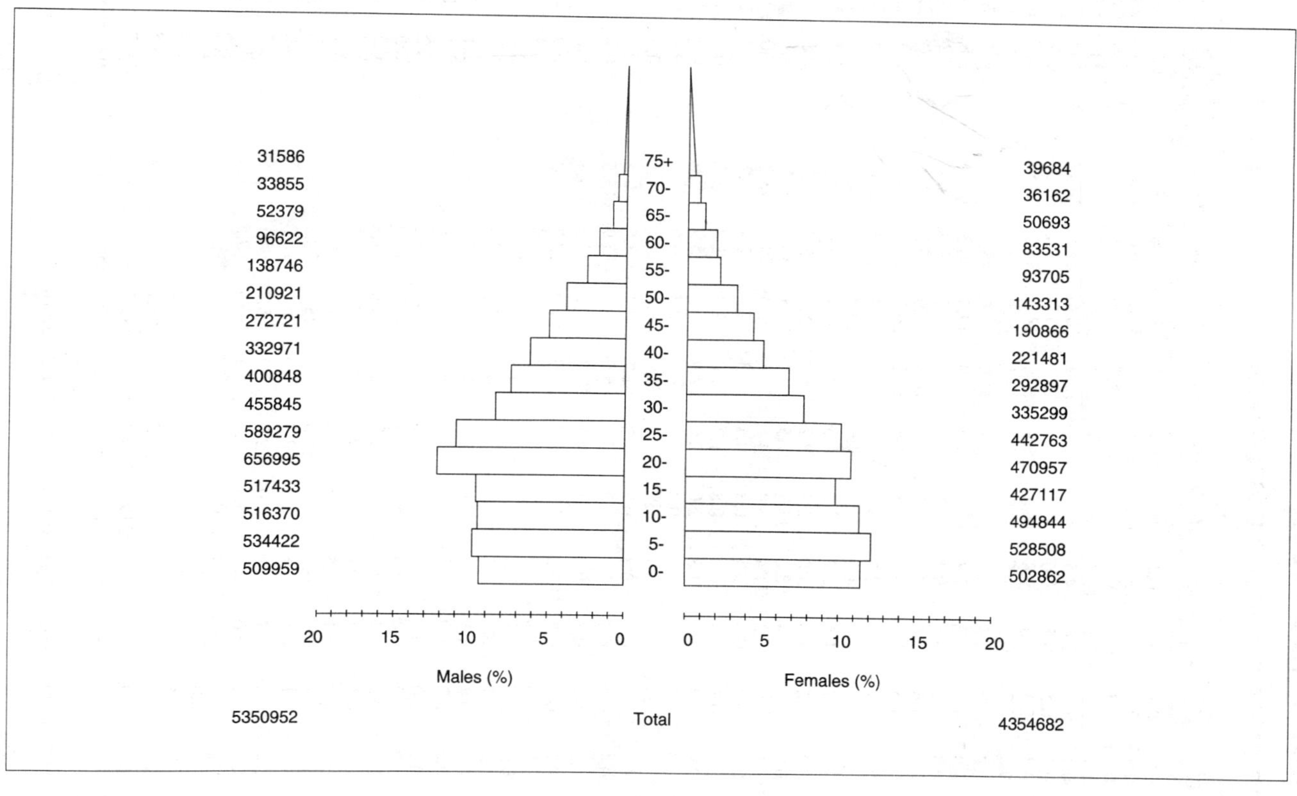

India, Bombay
Source of population: average annual 1988–92
Census: Census of India 1991: Series 1, India, Paper 2 of 1991, Provisional Population Totals: Rural-Urban Distribution. Census of India 1991, Maharashtra, Part IV(B)ii, Religion Tables. Census of India 1981, Series 12, Maharashtra, Part IIA, General Population Tables. Census of India 1981, Series 12, Maharashtra, Part V, A&B, Migration Tables, pp 594-595. Zakariah, K.C., Migrants in Greater Bombay.

Estimate: The population on 1 July of each year between 1988 and 1992 was estimated from the 1981 and 1991 Census Reports, assuming a geometric rate of growth for each sex. The age-distribution was assumed to be that of the 1981 Census. The estimates were corrected by eliminating all migrants whose duration of residence in Bombay was less than one year.

Notes to tables overleaf:
† 188 does not include non-invasive tumours

INDIA, BOMBAY 1988-1992

ANNUAL INCIDENCE PER 100,000 BY AGE GROUP (YEARS) - MALE

SITE	ALL AGES	AGE UNK	0-	5-	10-	15-	20-	25-	30-	35-	40-	45-	50-	55-	60-	65-	70-	75+	CRUDE RATE	%	CR 64	CR 74	ASR (W)	ICD (9th)
Lip	54	0	-	0.0	-	-	-	-	0.1	0.1	0.1	0.7	0.7	1.4	1.4	1.1	2.4	3.2	0.2	0.3	0.02	0.04	**0.4**	140
Tongue	950	3	-	-	-	-	0.1	0.3	0.9	2.4	4.8	9.6	13.3	21.5	27.5	38.2	36.6	45.0	3.6	5.1	0.40	0.78	**6.5**	141
Salivary gland	97	0	0.0	-	0.0	-	0.0	0.3	0.2	0.3	0.7	0.6	1.1	0.9	2.7	5.7	4.1	1.9	0.4	0.5	0.03	0.08	**0.6**	142
Mouth	1023	3	-	0.0	-	0.1	0.3	0.4	1.4	3.9	6.1	12.3	16.7	22.3	23.2	32.5	23.0	30.4	3.8	5.5	0.44	0.71	**6.2**	143-5
Oropharynx	482	0	-	-	-	0.0	-	0.1	0.4	1.5	1.6	4.5	7.3	10.1	13.9	20.6	27.2	24.1	1.8	2.6	0.20	0.44	**3.5**	146
Nasopharynx	120	0	0.1	0.1	0.2	0.3	0.2	0.2	0.2	0.5	0.7	0.6	0.8	2.0	2.3	5.0	2.4	1.9	0.4	0.6	0.04	0.08	**0.7**	147
Hypopharynx	1167	1	0.0	-	-	-	0.1	0.3	0.7	2.3	5.3	9.8	16.6	26.5	41.6	48.9	54.3	54.5	4.4	6.3	0.52	1.03	**8.3**	148
Pharynx unspecified	226	0	-	-	0.0	-	-	0.1	0.0	0.3	0.9	1.5	2.9	4.3	9.1	11.1	12.4	16.5	0.8	1.2	0.10	0.21	**1.8**	149
Oesophagus	1383	1	-	-	-	0.0	0.2	0.3	0.7	1.7	4.6	8.5	18.3	33.3	46.0	62.6	85.7	108.3	5.2	7.4	0.57	1.31	**10.8**	150
Stomach	1010	1	0.0	0.0	0.1	0.2	0.2	0.5	1.0	1.8	3.3	7.3	12.5	19.9	32.9	49.3	60.3	67.1	3.8	5.4	0.40	0.95	**7.7**	151
Small intestine	49	0	-	-	0.0	-	-	-	0.0	0.2	0.3	0.4	0.4	0.9	1.4	2.3	3.0	3.2	0.2	0.3	0.02	0.04	**0.4**	152
Colon	522	0	-	-	0.0	0.1	0.4	0.4	1.0	1.6	2.1	3.7	5.1	9.4	16.8	16.0	26.0	41.2	2.0	2.8	0.20	0.41	**3.7**	153
Rectum	537	0	-	-	-	0.0	0.3	0.4	0.7	1.5	1.9	3.9	6.5	11.4	13.2	26.3	24.2	38.0	2.0	2.9	0.20	0.45	**3.9**	154
Liver	506	2	0.4	0.1	0.2	0.1	0.1	0.1	0.4	1.1	1.6	2.7	6.1	9.1	15.9	29.4	34.9	26.6	1.9	2.7	0.19	0.51	**3.9**	155
Gallbladder etc.	249	0	-	-	-	0.1	0.1	0.1	0.5	0.2	1.3	1.9	3.2	4.6	7.9	10.7	10.0	16.5	0.9	1.3	0.10	0.20	**1.8**	156
Pancreas	302	1	-	-	-	-	-	0.1	0.2	0.7	1.4	2.2	3.5	5.6	9.5	17.9	14.8	19.0	1.1	1.6	0.12	0.28	**2.3**	157
Nose, sinuses etc.	157	1	0.0	0.0	-	0.1	0.1	0.1	0.2	0.6	1.0	1.0	2.7	2.2	5.0	5.3	5.9	5.1	0.6	0.8	0.07	0.12	**1.0**	160
Larynx	1093	2	-	0.0	-	0.0	0.2	0.1	0.9	1.4	3.4	8.2	13.7	27.5	40.6	56.1	57.3	55.7	4.1	5.9	0.48	1.05	**8.2**	161
Bronchus, lung	1867	2	-	0.0	0.0	0.0	0.2	0.4	1.1	2.0	5.2	11.4	23.9	44.1	77.6	102.3	108.1	96.2	7.0	10.0	0.83	1.88	**14.5**	162
Other thoracic organs	54	0	0.1	0.0	0.1	0.0	0.1	0.1	0.1	0.2	0.3	0.1	0.3	0.4	2.3	1.5	2.4	3.2	0.2	0.3	0.02	0.04	**0.4**	163-4
Bone	200	0	0.1	0.4	1.2	1.7	1.0	0.3	0.7	0.3	0.4	0.3	0.8	1.3	1.0	2.3	1.2	3.2	0.7	1.1	0.05	0.07	**0.8**	170
Connective tissue	239	0	0.5	0.3	0.4	0.4	0.4	0.5	0.9	0.9	1.2	1.8	2.0	2.0	2.9	6.1	5.9	7.6	0.9	1.3	0.07	0.13	**1.3**	171
Mesothelioma	15	0	-	-	0.0	0.0	-	-	0.0	0.0	0.2	-	0.3	0.4	-	0.4	0.6	-	0.1	0.1	0.01	0.01	**0.1**	MES
Kaposi's sarcoma	0	0	-	-	-	-	-	-	-	-	-	-	-	-	-	-	-	-	0.0	0.0	0.00	0.00	**0.0**	KAP
Melanoma of skin	53	0	-	-	-	-	0.1	0.1	-	-	0.1	0.3	0.7	1.2	1.7	3.4	3.5	2.5	0.2	0.3	0.02	0.06	**0.4**	172
Other skin	244	2	0.0	0.0	-	0.1	0.1	0.2	0.4	0.8	0.8	1.8	2.7	5.6	5.0	6.9	15.9	15.8	0.9		0.09	0.20	**1.7**	173
Breast	75	0	-	-	-	-	-	-	0.0	-	0.3	0.7	1.1	1.6	2.3	3.8	5.3	4.4	0.3	0.4	0.03	0.08	**0.6**	175
Prostate	764	1	-	0.0	-	-	-	0.1	-	0.1	0.1	0.3	1.2	3.2	8.8	21.9	51.9	98.7	145.0	2.9	4.1	0.18	0.93	**7.9**	185
Testis	229	0	0.4	0.1	0.0	0.5	0.7	1.4	1.8	1.4	1.2	1.2	0.9	0.4	1.2	1.5	3.5	1.9	0.9	1.2	0.06	0.08	**0.9**	186
Penis	219	0	-	-	-	-	0.1	0.2	0.4	1.0	1.1	2.1	2.7	2.5	4.8	8.0	11.2	17.1	0.8	1.2	0.07	0.17	**1.5**	187.1-.4
Other male genital	11	1	-	-	-	-	-	0.1	-	-	0.1	0.1	-	-	0.2	-	2.4	-	0.0	0.1	0.00	0.02	**0.1**	187.5-.9
†Bladder	554	3	-	0.0	0.0	-	0.1	0.1	0.4	0.8	1.1	2.3	5.6	8.5	17.0	37.8	44.9	59.5	2.1	3.0	0.18	0.60	**4.8**	188
Kidney etc.	301	1	0.9	0.3	0.0	0.1	0.1	0.0	0.2	0.9	1.0	2.3	4.3	5.3	9.1	12.2	10.6	10.1	1.1	1.6	0.12	0.24	**2.0**	189
Eye	48	0	1.1	0.2	-	0.0	-	-	0.1	0.0	0.1	-	0.4	0.1	0.2	-	1.2	1.3	0.2	0.3	0.01	0.02	**0.2**	190
Brain, nervous system	660	1	1.1	2.1	1.3	1.2	0.9	1.2	1.9	3.0	3.4	3.4	5.5	9.7	8.1	13.7	13.0	12.7	2.5	3.5	0.21	0.35	**3.3**	191-2
Thyroid	133	2	-	0.0	0.1	0.1	0.2	0.3	0.5	0.2	0.4	1.0	1.7	2.7	2.5	4.6	1.8	5.7	0.5	0.7	0.05	0.08	**0.8**	193
Other endocrine	54	0	0.9	0.3	0.1	0.2	0.1	0.1	-	0.1	0.1	0.2	0.1	0.3	0.2	-	-	-	0.2	0.3	0.01	0.01	**0.2**	194
Hodgkin's disease	283	0	0.4	1.2	0.9	0.9	0.7	0.8	0.6	1.0	1.1	1.5	1.8	2.5	3.3	1.9	6.5	3.2	1.1	1.5	0.08	0.13	**1.3**	201
Non-Hodgkin lymphoma	696	0	0.5	0.8	0.8	1.0	1.3	1.5	1.8	2.3	3.5	3.2	5.9	11.0	12.4	25.6	18.3	25.3	2.6	3.7	0.23	0.45	**4.1**	200,202
Multiple myeloma	158	0	-	-	-	0.0	-	0.0	-	0.1	0.5	1.6	2.3	2.7	6.6	6.1	10.0	9.5	0.6	0.8	0.07	0.15	**1.2**	203
Lymphoid leukaemia	324	0	2.6	1.5	1.5	1.2	0.7	0.4	0.4	0.3	0.7	0.9	1.0	2.0	3.3	5.7	4.1	7.6	1.2	1.7	0.08	0.13	**1.6**	204
Myeloid leukaemia	416	1	0.4	0.8	0.8	0.7	0.7	1.3	2.0	2.0	2.6	2.1	3.3	4.0	4.1	6.9	9.5	7.0	1.6	2.2	0.12	0.21	**2.0**	205
Monocytic leukaemia	7	0	0.1	-	-	-	-	-	0.0	-	-	0.1	0.1	-	0.2	-	-	-	0.0	0.0	0.00	0.00	**0.0**	206
Other leukaemia	14	0	0.0	0.1	-	0.2	-	0.0	-	0.0	0.1	0.1	-	-	0.2	-	-	-	0.1	0.1	0.00	0.00	**0.1**	207
Leukaemia unspecified	84	0	0.2	0.3	0.3	0.5	0.1	0.2	0.0	0.2	0.4	0.2	0.7	1.2	0.6	1.5	1.2	1.3	0.3	0.5	0.02	0.04	**0.4**	208
Other and unspecified	1275	1	0.2	0.1	0.1	0.4	0.3	0.7	0.9	2.3	4.9	8.5	16.8	28.5	39.7	68.7	59.7	68.4	4.8	6.8	0.52	1.16	**9.4**	O&U
All sites	18904	30	10.2	9.2	8.2	10.2	10.4	13.8	23.9	42.9	72.1	128.0	219.4	359.8	539.4	812.1	923.9	1066.3	70.7		7.25	15.94	**133.1**	ALL
All sites but 173	18660	28	10.2	9.2	8.2	10.2	10.3	13.6	23.4	42.0	71.3	126.1	216.7	354.2	534.5	805.3	908.0	1050.5	69.7	100.0	7.16	15.74	**131.4**	ALLb

Rate from 10 cases: 0.392 0.374 0.387 0.387 0.304 0.339 0.439 0.499 0.601 0.733 0.948 1.441 2.070 3.818 5.907 6.332

†Important: see notes on population page

INDIA, BOMBAY 1988-1992

ANNUAL INCIDENCE PER 100,000 BY AGE GROUP (YEARS) - FEMALE

SITE	ALL AGES	AGE UNK	0-	5-	10-	15-	20-	25-	30-	35-	40-	45-	50-	55-	60-	65-	70-	75+	CRUDE RATE	%	CR 64	CR 74	ASR (W)	ICD (9th)
Lip	37	0	0.0	-	-	-	-	-	0.1	-	0.1	0.7	0.4	1.5	1.7	2.0	-	2.0	0.2	0.2	0.02	0.03	**0.3**	140
Tongue	287	0	0.0	-	-	-	0.1	0.4	0.5	1.2	2.2	2.9	5.2	10.9	9.6	8.3	11.6	13.6	1.3	1.7	0.16	0.26	**2.3**	141
Salivary gland	48	0	-	-	0.1	-	0.0	0.1	0.2	0.7	0.4	0.4	0.8	-	1.4	1.2	0.6	2.5	0.2	0.3	0.02	0.03	**0.3**	142
Mouth	584	1	0.0	-	-	0.0	0.2	0.4	0.8	2.6	5.1	6.6	13.1	14.9	21.3	18.9	23.8	26.2	2.7	3.5	0.33	0.54	**4.6**	143-5
Oropharynx	57	0	-	-	-	-	0.0	-	0.1	0.2	0.4	0.5	0.7	1.3	1.4	3.6	2.8	6.0	0.3	0.3	0.02	0.05	**0.5**	146
Nasopharynx	39	0	-	-	-	0.1	0.3	0.2	0.1	-	0.4	0.5	0.4	1.1	-	1.2	0.6	2.0	0.2	0.2	0.02	0.02	**0.3**	147
Hypopharynx	262	1	-	-	-	0.0	0.2	0.3	0.7	1.6	1.5	2.6	6.4	6.0	10.8	7.9	10.0	8.1	1.2	1.6	0.15	0.24	**2.0**	148
Pharynx unspecified	78	0	-	-	-	-	-	0.1	0.1	0.2	0.3	0.8	0.6	2.1	3.4	3.2	5.0	8.1	0.4	0.5	0.04	0.08	**0.7**	149
Oesophagus	962	1	-	-	-	-	0.1	0.4	1.0	2.3	4.8	11.5	18.7	25.6	36.4	45.0	47.6	66.0	4.4	5.8	0.50	0.97	**8.3**	150
Stomach	462	1	-	-	-	0.0	0.2	0.2	1.4	1.7	2.0	5.7	7.3	14.1	15.6	16.6	25.4	27.7	2.1	2.8	0.24	0.45	**3.8**	151
Small intestine	30	0	-	-	-	-	0.1	0.0	0.1	0.1	-	0.1	0.7	0.6	1.4	0.8	1.7	1.0	0.1	0.2	0.02	0.03	**0.2**	152
Colon	354	0	0.0	-	-	0.1	0.1	0.2	0.9	1.2	2.3	3.2	4.3	8.1	12.0	13.0	23.2	30.2	1.6	2.1	0.16	0.34	**3.0**	153
Rectum	330	0	-	-	0.1	0.1	0.3	0.7	0.5	0.7	2.6	4.5	5.2	5.3	8.6	14.2	19.4	21.7	1.5	2.0	0.14	0.31	**2.7**	154
Liver	226	2	0.6	0.1	-	0.0	0.1	0.2	0.3	0.5	1.3	2.3	2.7	3.8	5.3	10.3	17.7	17.1	1.0	1.4	0.09	0.23	**1.9**	155
Gallbladder etc.	324	0	-	-	-	-	-	0.2	0.4	1.5	2.2	3.6	7.1	9.2	10.3	14.2	15.5	16.1	1.5	1.9	0.17	0.32	**2.7**	156
Pancreas	214	0	-	-	-	-	0.0	0.0	0.6	0.6	1.4	1.9	3.8	7.7	5.0	10.7	12.2	13.6	1.0	1.3	0.11	0.22	**1.8**	157
Nose, sinuses etc.	96	0	0.0	-	-	0.1	0.1	0.2	0.2	0.3	0.6	0.5	3.1	1.7	3.4	2.8	5.0	3.0	0.4	0.6	0.05	0.09	**0.7**	160
Larynx	163	1	-	-	-	-	0.0	-	0.3	0.5	1.2	1.7	2.1	4.5	5.5	7.9	7.7	13.6	0.7	1.0	0.08	0.16	**1.4**	161
Bronchus, lung	432	1	-	0.0	0.1	0.0	0.1	0.2	0.5	1.1	3.1	4.4	7.1	9.6	13.2	24.9	26.5	28.7	2.0	2.6	0.20	0.46	**3.7**	162
Other thoracic organs	39	0	-	0.0	0.0	0.0	-	0.0	0.1	0.3	0.3	0.3	0.1	0.4	1.2	1.6	2.8	3.0	0.2	0.2	0.01	0.04	**0.3**	163-4
Bone	105	0	0.2	0.3	0.7	0.6	0.3	0.4	0.2	0.2	0.5	0.5	1.0	0.9	0.7	2.0	2.8	3.5	0.5	0.6	0.03	0.06	**0.6**	170
Connective tissue	156	0	0.5	0.1	0.3	0.3	0.3	0.5	0.5	0.8	1.4	1.5	2.2	2.1	1.9	4.3	5.0	1.5	0.7	0.9	0.06	0.11	**1.0**	171
Mesothelioma	8	0	-	-	-	-	-	0.1	0.1	0.1	0.1	-	0.1	-	-	0.4	-	-	0.0	0.0	0.00	0.00	**0.0**	MES
Kaposi's sarcoma	2	0	-	-	-	-	-	-	-	0.1	-	-	0.1	-	-	-	-	-	0.0	0.0	0.00	0.00	**0.0**	KAP
Melanoma of skin	43	0	0.0	-	-	0.0	0.0	0.1	0.1	0.2	-	0.4	0.6	0.6	1.9	1.6	2.8	2.5	0.2	0.3	0.02	0.04	**0.3**	172
Other skin	159	1	-	0.1	-	0.1	0.2	0.1	0.4	0.8	0.9	2.2	2.2	2.8	5.5	3.6	8.3	11.1	0.7		0.08	0.14	**1.2**	173
Breast	3864	3	-	-	0.0	0.3	0.7	3.6	13.3	26.6	44.2	55.9	79.7	93.7	94.6	112.4	107.8	119.4	17.7	23.2	2.06	3.17	**28.2**	174
Uterus unspecified	152	0	-	-	-	0.0	0.1	0.2	0.7	1.0	1.2	2.4	3.4	5.3	4.3	10.5	14.6		0.7	0.9	0.07	0.15	**1.3**	179
Cervix uteri	2818	6	-	-	0.0	-	0.6	3.2	7.9	21.1	33.4	44.3	60.0	77.5	73.3	76.5	61.4	44.9	12.9	16.9	1.61	2.30	**20.2**	180
Placenta	45	1	-	-	0.0	0.0	0.6	0.5	0.2	0.5	0.2	0.2	-	-	0.4	0.6	0.5		0.2	0.3	0.01	0.02	**0.2**	181
Corpus uteri	296	1	-	-	-	0.0	-	0.1	0.3	0.5	1.9	3.8	6.3	10.2	12.0	15.0	8.8	12.6	1.4	1.8	0.18	0.30	**2.5**	182
Ovary etc.	989	3	0.1	0.3	0.4	1.0	0.9	1.1	2.5	4.2	10.5	14.6	18.3	25.8	28.0	31.2	24.3	23.7	4.5	5.9	0.54	0.82	**7.2**	183
Other female genital	181	1	0.0	-	-	-	0.1	0.1	0.5	0.7	1.1	1.8	2.9	2.8	6.9	5.9	12.7	12.6	0.8	1.1	0.09	0.18	**1.5**	184
†Bladder	132	0	0.1	-	-	0.0	0.0	-	0.1	0.3	0.5	0.9	2.0	3.0	3.8	7.5	12.7	11.6	0.6	0.8	0.05	0.15	**1.2**	188
Kidney etc.	130	1	0.9	0.2	0.0	0.0	0.2	0.1	0.4	0.5	0.8	1.5	0.4	2.8	4.1	5.1	2.8	3.0	0.6	0.8	0.06	0.10	**0.9**	189
Eye	35	0	0.8	0.2	0.1	-	0.0	-	-	-	0.1	-	0.1	-	0.2	0.4	0.6	1.0	0.2	0.2	0.01	0.01	**0.2**	190
Brain, nervous system	357	0	0.7	1.0	1.3	1.1	0.8	0.9	0.8	1.6	2.3	2.4	4.6	5.8	5.7	7.9	6.1	9.1	1.6	2.1	0.15	0.22	**2.2**	191-2
Thyroid	326	0	-	0.0	-	0.4	0.9	1.3	2.2	2.3	2.8	2.9	4.3	4.7	7.4	5.9	7.7	11.6	1.5	2.0	0.15	0.22	**2.1**	193
Other endocrine	26	0	0.6	0.1	0.1	0.0	0.0	0.1	-	-	-	-	-	-	-	-	-	-	0.1	0.2	0.01	0.01	**0.1**	194
Hodgkin's disease	107	1	0.1	0.3	0.2	0.5	0.3	0.4	0.3	0.3	0.7	0.9	1.3	1.7	1.4	2.0	3.3	1.5	0.5	0.6	0.04	0.07	**0.6**	201
Non-Hodgkin lymphoma	377	0	0.3	0.6	0.6	0.7	0.6	0.6	0.8	1.6	2.1	3.5	4.5	8.1	12.2	12.6	12.7	13.6	1.7	2.3	0.18	0.31	**2.7**	200,202
Multiple myeloma	103	0	-	-	-	-	-	-	-	0.2	0.5	0.6	2.0	4.5	3.8	7.1	5.0	5.5	0.5	0.6	0.06	0.12	**0.9**	203
Lymphoid leukaemia	194	0	1.6	1.3	0.5	1.0	0.3	0.5	0.2	0.6	0.4	0.4	0.7	1.7	1.4	3.9	5.0	5.5	0.9	1.2	0.05	0.10	**1.1**	204
Myeloid leukaemia	254	0	0.6	0.6	0.7	0.8	0.5	0.8	1.1	1.8	1.6	1.6	3.2	3.0	3.4	3.6	7.2	5.0	1.2	1.5	0.10	0.15	**1.5**	205
Monocytic leukaemia	3	0	-	-	-	-	-	-	0.1	-	-	-	0.1	-	-	-	-	-	0.0	0.0	0.00	0.00	**0.0**	206
Other leukaemia	5	0	0.1	-	0.0	-	-	-	-	-	-	0.1	-	-	-	-	-	0.5	0.0	0.0	0.00	0.00	**0.0**	207
Leukaemia unspecified	59	0	0.4	0.3	0.4	0.1	0.1	0.0	0.3	-	-	0.2	-	0.4	0.7	2.0	2.2	3.5	0.3	0.4	0.01	0.04	**0.4**	208
Other and unspecified	835	1	0.4	0.1	0.2	0.4	0.5	0.8	1.4	2.7	4.6	9.7	15.4	20.7	24.2	37.5	41.5	47.4	3.8	5.0	0.41	0.80	**6.8**	O&U
All sites	16785	27	8.1	5.5	6.0	8.5	10.2	19.1	42.8	85.6	143.4	206.0	304.1	404.7	465.9	561.0	610.6	676.3	77.1		8.56	14.43	**126.6**	ALL
All sites but 173	16626	26	8.1	5.4	6.0	8.4	10.0	19.0	42.4	84.9	142.5	203.8	301.9	401.9	460.4	557.5	602.3	665.3	76.4	100.0	8.49	14.29	**125.4**	ALLb

Rate from 10 cases   0.398   0.378   0.404   0.468   0.425   0.452   0.596   0.683   0.903   1.048   1.396   2.134   2.394   3.945   5.531   5.040

†Important: see notes on population page

India, Karunagappally

The Rural Cancer Registry of Karunagappally, in Kerala, India, was initiated in 1990 by the Regional Cancer Centre in Trivandrum, with funding from the Department of Atomic Energy, Bombay, to study cancer occurrence in relation to the high natural background radiation present in a coastal area of Kerala. Kerala is a small south-western coastal state, unique in flora and fauna, and the vital indices of the people differ greatly from those in other parts of the country. The state language is Malayalam and English education has been in vogue for the past two centuries.

Karunagappally taluk (a taluk is a governmental local administration unit) in Quilon district is about 105 km north of Trivandrum, the capital city of the state of Kerala. The coastal areas have monazite-rich sands which emit radiation. The area and population of the taluk are divided into panchayats with populations of 25 000–30 000. Each panchayat is further divided into panchayat wards, usually 12 in number.

The census of 1991 indicated an annual exponential growth rate of 1.09% in the area. The total census population by sex has been published by the government, but the five-year age distribution is yet to be published. To obtain the age distribution, we have taken a 10% sample of the 1991 population from six panchayats and the age structure of this sample was used for estimating the age distribution of the total population of the taluk.

The population-based cancer registry was established to cover the total 383 514 population (189 647 males, 193 867 females at the 1991 census) spread over an area of 212 km^2, of which around 20 km^2 are lagoons and canals. The density of population was thus almost 2000 persons per km^2. About 100 000 people live in the areas of high background radiation. The largely rural population (99%) is engaged in agriculture, coir-making, fishing and cashew production. As in other parts of Kerala, the expectation of life at birth is above 65 years for males and 70 years for females. The literacy rate is more than 85% and the male to female ratio is 0.98:1. Immigration and emigration are believed to be negligible or minimal.

There are no dedicated cancer hospitals in the area, the nearest cancer centre being the Regional Cancer Centre at Trivandrum. Cancer case-finding is done through record scrutiny of 47 general hospitals situated within the taluk (34) and also in the adjoining Quilon town (9), the Medical College Cancer Registry Trivandrum, the Regional Cancer Centre, Trivandrum and two major pathology laboratories, one in Trivandrum and one in Kottayam, 90 km away.

The case records of cancer patients (inpatients only) are abstracted from these sources and brought to the field office at Vavvakkavu in the taluk and processed with the assistance of a statistician and sociologist. The trained enumerators visit all households and enumerate every individual in the household, collect information on residence, occupation, lifestyle habits (especially of tobacco and alcohol consumption), marital and pregnancy status etc., as well as other socio-demographic information. The purpose of this exercise was to develop a cohort with sufficient person-years of observation to increase the analytical power of the study with regard to radiation exposure. Gamma radiation levels outside and inside each house are recorded by using micro g-scintillometers provided by the Bhabha Atomic Research Centre, Bombay. Attempts are being made to record total dosimetry.

Birth and death registration in the area has a high coverage, reflecting the high literacy rate and intense governmental propaganda for registration of births and deaths. Although registration of deaths appears to be almost complete, the quality of registration of cause of death is not optimal. Even when the record indicates the presence of 'cancer', often no information regarding the primary site or type of cancer is available. Hence the proportion of cases in ICD 199 'unknown primary' is somewhat high. Almost 7% of all deaths were found to be from cancer.

The current incidence rates obtained are for the first reporting years of the registry. Death-certificate-only registrations amount to 13%, a rate expected to decrease with time. The current report covers the years 1991–92. Microscopic verification of cases was 80%.

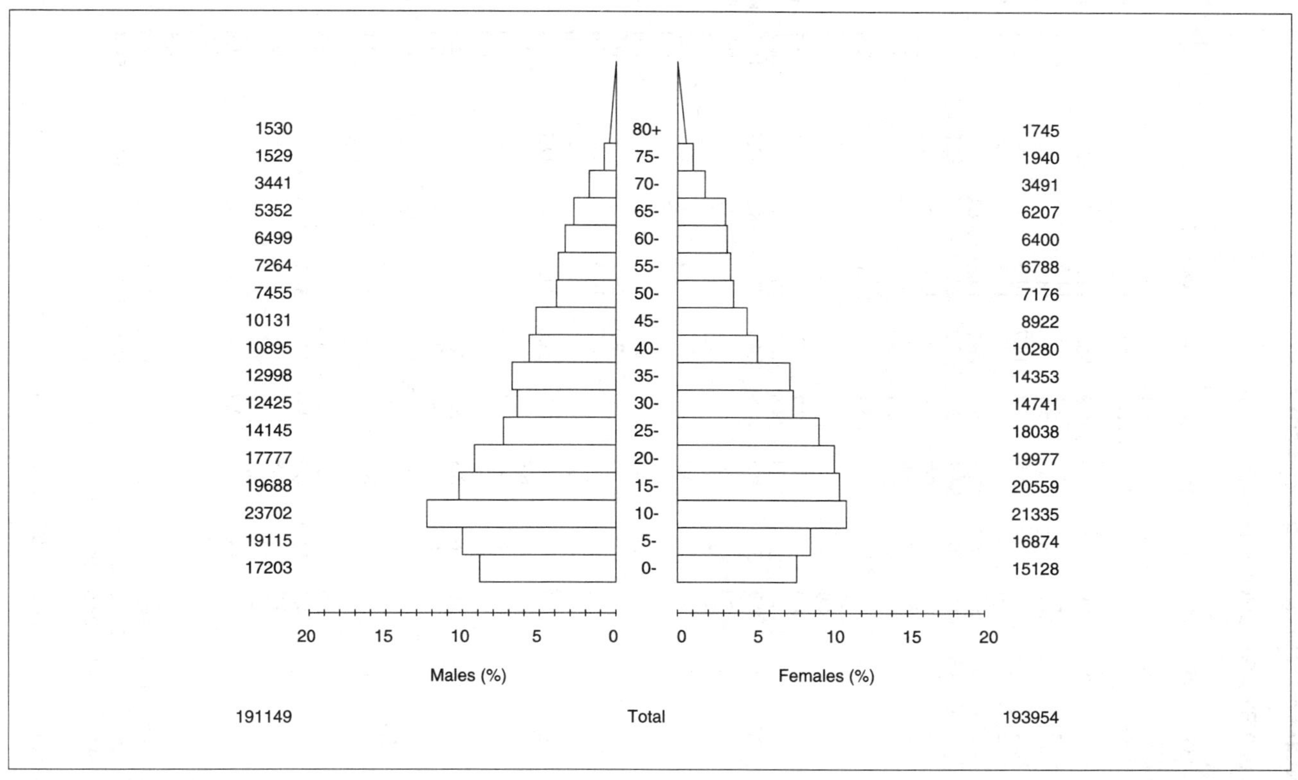

India, Karunagappally
Source of population: 1991
Census: Census of India 1991. Final Population Totals: p.54.
Series 12, Kerala: Paper 3 of 1991. N.M. Samuel, MA. LLB,
Director of Census Operations, Kerala.
Estimate: The age-distribution was estimated from a 10% ran-
dom sample of households obtained from house-to-house sur-
vey returns of 10 Panchayats. The age distribution of persons
in these households was used to estimate the age distribution
of the total taluks population.

Notes to tables overleaf:
* There is some evidence of under-registration and childhood
  cancer is certainly under-ascertained in the area
† 188 does not include non-invasive tumours

* INDIA, KARUNAGAPPALLY 1991-1992

ANNUAL INCIDENCE PER 100,000 BY AGE GROUP (YEARS) - MALE

SITE	ALL AGES	AGE UNK	0-	5-	10-	15-	20-	25-	30-	35-	40-	45-	50-	55-	60-	65-	70-	75-	80+	CRUDE RATE	%	CR 64	CR 74	ASR (W)	ICD (9th)
Lip	2	0	-	-	-	-	-	-	-	-	-	-	-	-	15.4	-	-	-	-	0.5	0.5	0.08	0.08	**0.6**	140
Tongue	18	0	-	-	-	-	-	-	3.8	-	-	-	33.5	27.5	23.1	28.0	-	32.7	32.7	4.7	4.9	0.44	0.58	**5.4**	141
Salivary gland	2	0	-	-	-	-	-	-	-	-	-	-	-	6.9	-	-	-	32.7	-	0.5	0.5	0.03	0.03	**0.6**	142
Mouth	24	1	-	-	-	2.5	-	-	-	-	9.2	4.9	13.4	20.6	30.8	56.1	14.5	32.7	65.4	6.3	6.5	0.43	0.79	**7.0**	143-5
Oropharynx	9	0	-	-	-	-	-	4.0	-	-	-	4.9	-	6.9	23.1	-	14.5	65.4	-	2.4	2.4	0.19	0.27	**2.7**	146
Nasopharynx	6	0	-	-	-	-	-	4.0	-	-	-	4.9	6.7	-	7.7	9.3	14.5	-	-	1.6	1.6	0.12	0.24	**1.8**	147
Hypopharynx	10	0	-	-	-	-	-	3.5	4.0	-	4.6	-	6.7	13.8	7.7	18.7	14.5	-	-	2.6	2.7	0.20	0.37	**2.8**	148
Pharynx unspecified	2	0	-	-	-	-	-	-	-	-	-	4.9	-	-	-	-	14.5	-	-	0.5	0.5	0.02	0.10	**0.6**	149
Oesophagus	23	0	-	-	-	-	-	-	-	-	-	4.9	6.7	27.5	76.9	46.7	14.5	32.7	-	6.0	6.2	0.58	0.89	**6.8**	150
Stomach	21	0	-	-	-	-	-	3.5	4.0	-	4.6	14.8	20.1	34.4	23.1	9.3	29.1	-	32.7	5.5	5.7	0.52	0.71	**6.2**	151
Small intestine	2	0	-	-	-	-	-	-	-	-	-	-	-	6.9	-	-	14.5	-	-	0.5	0.5	0.03	0.11	**0.6**	152
Colon	5	1	-	-	-	-	-	-	-	-	-	-	6.7	20.6	-	-	-	-	-	1.3	1.3	0.17	0.17	**1.5**	153
Rectum	6	0	-	-	-	-	2.8	-	4.0	-	-	4.9	-	6.9	7.7	9.3	-	-	-	1.6	1.6	0.13	0.18	**1.6**	154
Liver	9	0	-	-	-	-	-	-	-	-	9.2	-	13.4	-	23.1	-	29.1	-	-	2.4	2.4	0.23	0.37	**2.7**	155
Gallbladder etc.	0	0	-	-	-	-	-	-	-	-	-	-	-	-	-	-	-	-	-	0.0	0.0	0.00	0.00	**0.0**	156
Pancreas	7	2	-	-	-	-	-	-	-	-	-	4.9	6.7	-	15.4	9.3	-	-	-	1.8	1.9	0.19	0.25	**2.1**	157
Nose, sinuses etc.	2	0	-	-	-	-	-	-	-	-	-	4.9	-	-	7.7	-	-	-	-	0.5	0.5	0.06	0.06	**0.6**	160
Larynx	17	0	-	-	-	-	-	-	-	-	-	-	20.1	13.8	38.5	46.7	29.1	-	-	4.4	4.6	0.36	0.74	**5.1**	161
Bronchus, lung	58	2	-	-	-	2.5	-	-	-	7.7	9.2	9.9	53.7	89.5	76.9	84.1	72.7	98.1	32.7	15.2	15.6	1.29	2.10	**17.0**	162
Other thoracic organs	0	0	-	-	-	-	-	-	-	-	-	-	-	-	-	-	-	-	-	0.0	0.0	0.00	0.00	**0.0**	163-4
Bone	2	0	-	-	-	-	-	-	-	-	-	-	6.7	-	-	-	14.5	-	-	0.5	0.5	0.03	0.11	**0.6**	170
Connective tissue	5	0	-	2.6	-	-	-	-	4.0	-	-	-	-	6.9	-	-	14.5	-	32.7	1.3	1.3	0.07	0.14	**1.4**	171
Mesothelioma	0	0	-	-	-	-	-	-	-	-	-	-	-	-	-	-	-	-	-	0.0	0.0	0.00	0.00	**0.0**	MES
Kaposi's sarcoma	0	0	-	-	-	-	-	-	-	-	-	-	-	-	-	-	-	-	-	0.0	0.0	0.00	0.00	**0.0**	KAP
Melanoma of skin	3	0	-	-	-	-	-	-	-	-	-	-	-	-	-	-	9.3	29.1	-	0.8	0.8	0.00	0.19	**0.9**	172
Other skin	9	0	-	-	-	2.5	-	-	-	3.8	4.6	-	-	-	-	46.7	14.5	-	-	2.4		0.05	0.36	**2.4**	173
Breast	0	0	-	-	-	-	-	-	-	-	-	-	-	-	-	-	-	-	-	0.0	0.0	0.00	0.00	**0.0**	175
Prostate	13	0	-	-	-	-	-	-	-	3.8	-	4.9	-	-	7.7	28.0	43.6	98.1	32.7	3.4	3.5	0.08	0.44	**3.9**	185
Testis	2	0	-	-	-	2.5	-	-	-	-	-	-	-	6.9	-	-	-	-	-	0.5	0.5	0.05	0.05	**0.5**	186
Penis	4	0	-	-	-	-	-	-	-	-	-	4.9	6.7	-	7.7	9.3	-	-	-	1.0	1.1	0.10	0.14	**1.2**	187.1-.4
Other male genital	0	0	-	-	-	-	-	-	-	-	-	-	-	-	-	-	-	-	-	0.0	0.0	0.00	0.00	**0.0**	187.5-.9
†Bladder	9	0	-	-	-	-	-	-	-	-	-	4.9	6.7	13.8	15.4	28.0	-	-	-	2.4	2.4	0.20	0.34	**2.6**	188
Kidney etc.	3	0	-	-	-	-	-	-	-	-	-	-	6.7	-	-	9.3	14.5	-	-	0.8	0.8	0.03	0.15	**0.9**	189
Eye	0	0	-	-	-	-	-	-	-	-	-	-	-	-	-	-	-	-	-	0.0	0.0	0.00	0.00	**0.0**	190
Brain, nervous system	9	0	-	2.6	-	-	-	-	8.0	15.4	-	-	6.7	-	-	-	14.5	-	-	2.4	2.4	0.16	0.24	**2.3**	191-2
Thyroid	8	1	-	-	-	-	2.8	-	4.0	-	4.6	-	-	6.9	-	-	29.1	32.7	-	2.1	2.2	0.10	0.27	**2.2**	193
Other endocrine	1	0	-	-	-	-	-	-	-	-	-	-	-	-	7.7	-	-	-	-	0.3	0.3	0.04	0.04	**0.3**	194
Hodgkin's disease	3	0	-	-	-	-	2.8	-	-	-	-	4.9	-	-	-	9.3	-	-	-	0.8	0.8	0.04	0.09	**0.8**	201
Non-Hodgkin lymphoma	18	0	-	-	-	10.2	-	-	-	-	-	4.9	13.4	6.9	15.4	18.7	58.1	65.4	-	4.7	4.9	0.25	0.64	**5.1**	200,202
Multiple myeloma	2	0	-	-	-	-	-	-	-	-	-	4.9	-	6.9	-	-	-	-	-	0.5	0.5	0.06	0.06	**0.6**	203
Lymphoid leukaemia	5	0	-	5.2	-	5.1	-	-	-	-	-	-	-	6.9	-	-	-	-	-	1.3	1.3	0.09	0.09	**1.3**	204
Myeloid leukaemia	7	0	-	-	-	2.5	-	3.5	4.0	3.8	-	-	13.4	-	7.7	-	-	-	-	1.8	1.9	0.18	0.18	**2.0**	205
Monocytic leukaemia	0	0	-	-	-	-	-	-	-	-	-	-	-	-	-	-	-	-	-	0.0	0.0	0.00	0.00	**0.0**	206
Other leukaemia	0	0	-	-	-	-	-	-	-	-	-	-	-	-	-	-	-	-	-	0.0	0.0	0.00	0.00	**0.0**	207
Leukaemia unspecified	2	0	-	-	2.1	-	-	-	4.0	-	-	-	-	-	-	-	-	-	-	0.5	0.5	0.03	0.03	**0.4**	208
Other and unspecified	52	2	-	-	-	-	2.8	7.1	4.0	7.7	13.8	14.8	40.2	48.2	38.5	93.4	58.1	163.5	32.7	13.6	14.0	0.92	1.71	**15.2**	O&U
All sites	380	9	-	10.5	2.1	27.9	11.3	17.7	48.3	46.2	59.7	108.6	288.4	378.6	477.0	569.9	552.2	654.0	261.4	99.4		7.56	13.31	**110.4**	ALL
All sites but 173	371	9	-	10.5	2.1	25.4	11.3	17.7	48.3	42.3	55.1	108.6	288.4	378.6	477.0	523.2	537.6	654.0	261.4	97.0	100.0	7.51	12.94	**108.0**	ALLb

Rate from 1 case   2.906   2.616   2.110   2.540   2.813   3.535   4.024   3.847   4.589   4.935   6.707   6.883   7.693   9.342   14.531   32.701   32.680

†Important: see notes on population page

* INDIA, KARUNAGAPPALLY 1991-1992

ANNUAL INCIDENCE PER 100,000 BY AGE GROUP (YEARS) - FEMALE

SITE	ALL AGES	AGE UNK	0-	5-	10-	15-	20-	25-	30-	35-	40-	45-	50-	55-	60-	65-	70-	75-	80+	CRUDE RATE	%	CR 64	CR 74	ASR (W)	ICD (9th)
Lip	3	0	-	-	-	-	-	-	-	-	-	-	13.9	-	-	-	14.3	-	-	0.8	1.0	0.07	0.14	**1.0**	*140*
Tongue	14	0	-	-	-	-	-	-	3.4	-	-	5.6	-	-	7.8	48.3	28.6	51.5	28.7	3.6	4.9	0.08	0.47	**3.7**	*141*
Salivary gland	0	0	-	-	-	-	-	-	-	-	-	-	-	-	-	-	-	-	-	0.0	0.0	0.00	0.00	**0.0**	*142*
Mouth	22	2	-	-	-	-	-	-	-	3.5	4.9	11.2	13.9	7.4	39.1	40.3	14.3	51.5	-	5.7	7.7	0.44	0.74	**6.3**	*143-5*
Oropharynx	0	0	-	-	-	-	-	-	-	-	-	-	-	-	-	-	-	-	-	0.0	0.0	0.00	0.00	**0.0**	*146*
Nasopharynx	3	0	-	-	-	-	-	-	-	-	-	-	-	7.4	7.8	-	-	25.8	-	0.8	1.0	0.08	0.08	**0.9**	*147*
Hypopharynx	2	0	-	-	-	-	-	-	-	-	-	-	-	7.4	7.8	-	-	-	-	0.5	0.7	0.08	0.08	**0.6**	*148*
Pharynx unspecified	0	0	-	-	-	-	-	-	-	-	-	-	-	-	-	-	-	-	-	0.0	0.0	0.00	0.00	**0.0**	*149*
Oesophagus	11	0	-	-	-	-	-	-	-	-	-	11.2	7.0	14.7	23.4	16.1	-	25.8	-	2.8	3.8	0.28	0.36	**3.3**	*150*
Stomach	11	1	-	-	-	-	2.5	-	-	-	-	-	-	14.7	23.4	8.1	28.6	-	28.7	2.8	3.8	0.22	0.43	**3.1**	*151*
Small intestine	0	0	-	-	-	-	-	-	-	-	-	-	-	-	-	-	-	-	-	0.0	0.0	0.00	0.00	**0.0**	*152*
Colon	5	0	-	-	-	-	-	-	-	3.5	-	5.6	-	7.4	-	8.1	-	25.8	-	1.3	1.7	0.08	0.12	**1.3**	*153*
Rectum	1	0	-	-	-	-	-	-	-	-	-	-	-	-	7.8	-	-	-	-	0.3	0.3	0.04	0.04	**0.3**	*154*
Liver	6	0	-	-	-	-	-	-	3.4	3.5	-	5.6	13.9	-	-	-	14.3	-	-	1.5	2.1	0.13	0.20	**1.7**	*155*
Gallbladder etc.	0	0	-	-	-	-	-	-	-	-	-	-	-	-	-	-	-	-	-	0.0	0.0	0.00	0.00	**0.0**	*156*
Pancreas	1	0	-	-	-	-	-	-	3.4	-	-	-	-	-	-	-	-	-	-	0.3	0.3	0.02	0.02	**0.2**	*157*
Nose, sinuses etc.	1	0	-	-	-	-	-	-	-	3.5	-	-	-	-	-	-	-	-	-	0.3	0.3	0.02	0.02	**0.2**	*160*
Larynx	0	0	-	-	-	-	-	-	-	-	-	-	-	-	-	-	-	-	-	0.0	0.0	0.00	0.00	**0.0**	*161*
Bronchus, lung	10	0	-	-	-	-	-	-	-	-	-	-	-	7.4	7.8	56.4	-	-	28.7	2.6	3.5	0.08	0.36	**2.6**	*162*
Other thoracic organs	0	0	-	-	-	-	-	-	-	-	-	-	-	-	-	-	-	-	-	0.0	0.0	0.00	0.00	**0.0**	*163-4*
Bone	1	0	-	-	2.3	-	-	-	-	-	-	-	-	-	-	-	-	-	-	0.3	0.3	0.01	0.01	**0.2**	*170*
Connective tissue	2	0	-	-	-	-	-	-	-	3.5	-	5.6	-	-	-	-	-	-	-	0.5	0.7	0.05	0.05	**0.5**	*171*
Mesothelioma	0	0	-	-	-	-	-	-	-	-	-	-	-	-	-	-	-	-	-	0.0	0.0	0.00	0.00	**0.0**	*MES*
Kaposi's sarcoma	0	0	-	-	-	-	-	-	-	-	-	-	-	-	-	-	-	-	-	0.0	0.0	0.00	0.00	**0.0**	*KAP*
Melanoma of skin	0	0	-	-	-	-	-	-	-	-	-	-	-	-	-	-	-	-	-	0.0	0.0	0.00	0.00	**0.0**	*172*
Other skin	10	0	-	-	-	-	-	2.8	-	3.5	-	-	7.0	14.7	7.8	24.2	14.3	-	-	2.6		0.18	0.37	**2.7**	*173*
Breast	56	2	-	-	-	-	-	2.8	23.7	41.8	14.6	16.8	55.7	66.3	46.9	24.2	-	51.5	-	14.4	19.6	1.39	1.52	**15.1**	*174*
Uterus unspecified	0	0	-	-	-	-	-	-	-	-	-	-	-	-	-	-	-	-	-	0.0	0.0	0.00	0.00	**0.0**	*179*
Cervix uteri	54	2	-	-	-	-	-	-	6.8	13.9	14.6	50.4	34.8	36.8	70.3	56.4	71.6	25.8	57.3	13.9	18.9	1.18	1.85	**15.7**	*180*
Placenta	0	0	-	-	-	-	-	-	-	-	-	-	-	-	-	-	-	-	-	0.0	0.0	0.00	0.00	**0.0**	*181*
Corpus uteri	4	0	-	-	-	-	-	-	3.4	-	-	11.2	7.0	-	-	-	-	-	-	1.0	1.4	0.11	0.11	**1.2**	*182*
Ovary etc.	7	0	-	-	2.4	-	-	-	-	-	-	5.6	7.0	14.7	-	16.1	-	-	-	1.8	2.4	0.15	0.23	**2.0**	*183*
Other female genital	2	0	-	-	-	-	-	-	-	-	-	5.6	-	7.4	-	-	-	-	-	0.5	0.7	0.06	0.06	**0.6**	*184*
†Bladder	2	0	-	-	-	-	-	-	3.5	-	-	-	-	-	-	8.1	-	-	-	0.5	0.7	0.02	0.06	**0.5**	*188*
Kidney etc.	0	0	-	-	-	-	-	-	-	-	-	-	-	-	-	-	-	-	-	0.0	0.0	0.00	0.00	**0.0**	*189*
Eye	0	0	-	-	-	-	-	-	-	-	-	-	-	-	-	-	-	-	-	0.0	0.0	0.00	0.00	**0.0**	*190*
Brain, nervous system	9	1	-	-	-	2.4	-	2.8	3.4	3.5	-	5.6	7.0	7.4	7.8	-	-	-	-	2.3	3.1	0.22	0.22	**2.4**	*191-2*
Thyroid	15	0	-	-	2.3	-	-	8.3	6.8	3.5	-	16.8	7.0	14.7	-	8.1	-	25.8	-	3.9	5.2	0.30	0.34	**3.9**	*193*
Other endocrine	0	0	-	-	-	-	-	-	-	-	-	-	-	-	-	-	-	-	-	0.0	0.0	0.00	0.00	**0.0**	*194*
Hodgkin's disease	1	0	-	-	-	-	-	-	-	-	-	-	7.0	-	-	-	-	-	-	0.3	0.3	0.03	0.03	**0.3**	*201*
Non-Hodgkin lymphoma	4	0	-	-	-	2.4	-	-	-	-	-	-	-	7.4	7.8	-	14.3	-	-	1.0	1.4	0.09	0.16	**1.1**	*200,202*
Multiple myeloma	5	0	-	-	-	-	-	-	-	-	4.9	-	-	-	-	-	14.3	77.3	-	1.3	1.7	0.02	0.10	**1.4**	*203*
Lymphoid leukaemia	4	0	-	3.0	-	2.4	-	2.8	-	-	4.9	-	-	-	-	-	-	-	-	1.0	1.4	0.07	0.07	**1.0**	*204*
Myeloid leukaemia	2	0	-	-	-	-	-	-	-	-	4.9	-	-	-	7.8	-	-	-	-	0.5	0.7	0.06	0.06	**0.6**	*205*
Monocytic leukaemia	0	0	-	-	-	-	-	-	-	-	-	-	-	-	-	-	-	-	-	0.0	0.0	0.00	0.00	**0.0**	*206*
Other leukaemia	0	0	-	-	-	-	-	-	-	-	-	-	-	-	-	-	-	-	-	0.0	0.0	0.00	0.00	**0.0**	*207*
Leukaemia unspecified	1	0	-	-	-	-	-	2.8	-	-	-	-	-	-	-	-	-	-	-	0.3	0.3	0.01	0.01	**0.2**	*208*
Other and unspecified	27	0	-	-	-	-	5.0	-	-	-	9.7	5.6	20.9	29.5	23.4	32.2	71.6	25.8	57.3	7.0	9.4	0.47	0.99	**7.7**	*O&U*
All sites	296	8	-	3.0	4.7	9.7	7.5	22.2	54.3	87.1	58.4	162.5	202.1	265.2	296.9	346.4	286.5	386.6	200.6	76.3		6.03	9.28	**82.5**	*ALL*
All sites but 173	286	8	-	3.0	4.7	9.7	7.5	19.4	54.3	83.6	58.4	162.5	195.1	250.4	289.1	322.2	272.1	386.6	200.6	73.7	100.0	5.85	8.91	**79.8**	*ALLb*

Rate from 1 case   3.305   2.963   2.344   2.432   2.503   2.772   3.392   3.484   4.864   5.604   6.968   7.366   7.813   8.055   14.323   25.773   28.653

†Important: see notes on population page

India, Madras

The Madras Metropolitan Tumour Registry, a population-based cancer registry, was established in 1981 at the Cancer Institute, Madras, as part of the National Cancer Registry Programme (NCRP) of the Indian Council of Medical Research. It is the only population-based registry in Tamilnadu.

Madras, the capital of the state of Tamilnadu, is located on the eastern coast of India at latitude 13.04° N and longitude 80.17° E. It lies at sea level and has average temperatures varying between 15° and 47°C. The registration area corresponds to the metropolitan boundaries encompassing an area of 170 km².

The registry covers a population of 3 800 000 (males, 52.6%; females, 47.4), an increase in ten years of 17%. The total population of the state is 55 858 946 (urban: 19 077 592; rural: 36 781 354). Literacy in the Madras population is 72%. Tamil is the predominant spoken language. The majority are Hindus (84%), followed by Muslims (8%), Christians (7%) and other religious groups (1%). The census figures on occupation of the residents of Madras, classified according to National Industrial Classification (1970), reveal that 31% are categorized as 'main workers' while the rest are either 'marginal workers' or 'nonworkers'. The break-down of main workers is as follows: trade and commerce 26%, industry 24%, transport/communication 11%, construction workers 6%, livestock/mining 1% and other services 32%.

Cancer is not a notifiable disease in India. Registration of cases is entirely active. The more than 200 sources of data are government and private hospitals, nursing homes, clinics, consultants, radiotherapy centres, pathology laboratories and imaging centres. Mortality information is collected from the Vital Statistics Division of the Corporation of Madras. Investigators from the registry visit all these sources on a fixed schedule, to collect data by interviewing the case wherever possible and/or from medical records using a standard form. The criteria for inclusion of cases in the registry is that the cases should have been residing in Madras for at least a year at the time of first diagnosis of cancer. This helps to avoid registering cases from a floating population. The base institution accounts for 17% of the total cancer cases registered, government hospitals for 63% and private institutions 14%. Death-certificate-only registrations were 6%. Systematic trace-back of cancer cases first identified through a death certificate, in the form of visits to relevant houses and hospitals, is carried out for cases registered since 1983. Periodic as well as annual checks for completeness of coverage are performed independently at all sources of intake by re-screening of cases. Registry operations are constantly monitored with emphasis on the quality of data collected and the number of cases registered from different sources.

Until 1991, data on mortality were collected from the Vital Statistics Department from death certificates which mentioned 'tumour' or 'cancer' as the cause of death. Since 1992, information on all deaths that occur in the city of Madras, irrespective of the stated cause in death certificate, has been abstracted and computerized in the registry. This mortality database is matched against the morbidity database. This has resulted in an increase in the mortality to incidence ratio from 41% during 1982–91 to 60% in 1992–93. Active follow-up of cases registered during 1982–91 was the other source of mortality information in the registry until 1991. Madras was the first registry in the NCRP network to start active follow-up of cases and is the only one to follow the modified method of mortality data collection.

Data-processing has been progressively computerized to minimize the manual work and improve the quality and efficiency. Special programmes to identify duplicate cases and for matching and linking of mortality data with the morbidity database and data entry with in-built checks for consistency have been developed to enhance the quality of data.

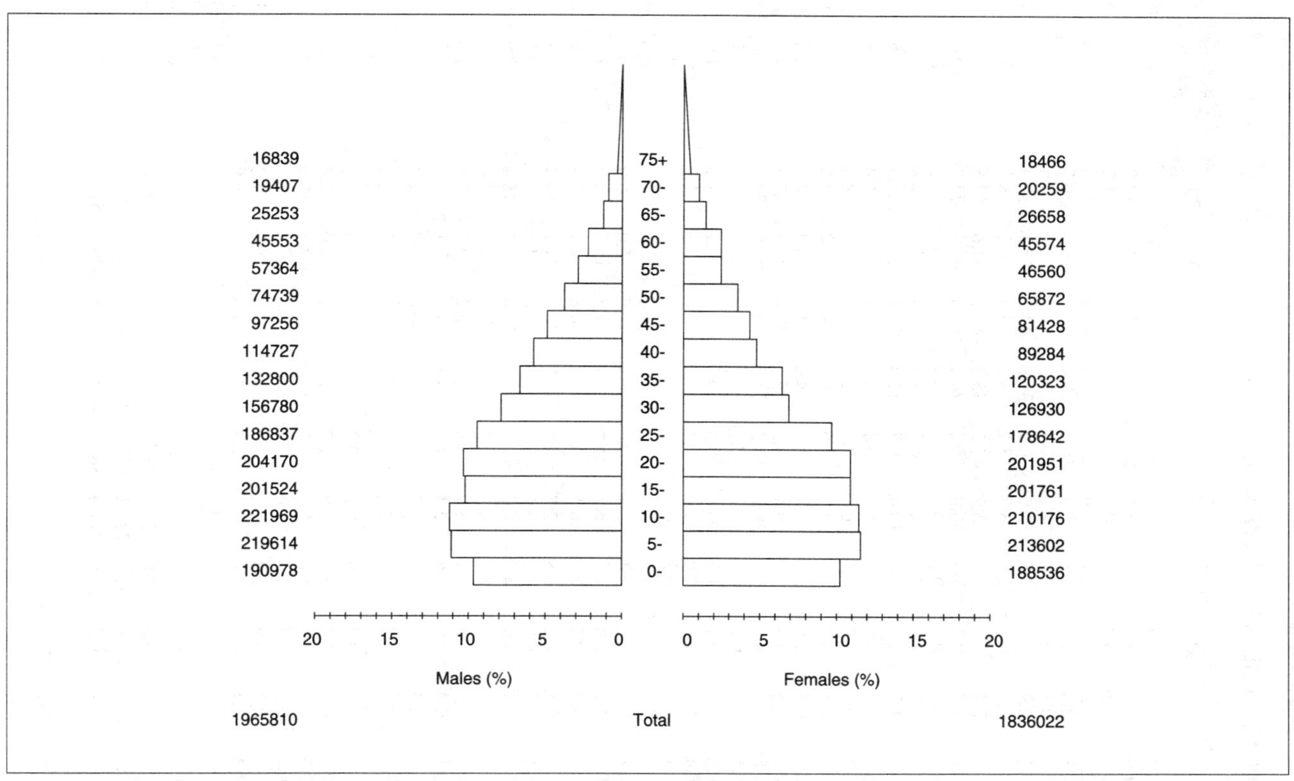

India, Madras

Source of population: average annual 1988–92

Census: Census of India 1981, Series 20, Tamil Nadu, Social and Cultural Tables Part IVA, Table C6, p. 329. Census of India 1991, Series 1, India, Paper 2 of 1991, Provisional Population Totals: Rural-Urban Distribution

Estimate: The 1991 Census figures were not available by age. The population at 1 July was estimated for each year applying the exponential growth rate method to the 1981 and 1991 Census figures, using the 1981 figures to estimate the age distribution.

Notes to tables overleaf:

† 188 does not include non-invasive tumours

INDIA, MADRAS 1988-1992

ANNUAL INCIDENCE PER 100,000 BY AGE GROUP (YEARS) - MALE

SITE	ALL AGES	AGE UNK	0-	5-	10-	15-	20-	25-	30-	35-	40-	45-	50-	55-	60-	65-	70-	75+	CRUDE RATE	%	CR 64	CR 74	ASR (W)	ICD (9th)
Lip	28	0	-	-	-	-	-	-	0.3	-	0.5	1.4	1.1	0.7	2.6	2.4	1.0	-	0.3	0.4	0.03	0.05	**0.4**	140
Tongue	371	0	0.1	-	-	0.1	0.1	0.3	1.0	2.7	5.1	9.0	15.3	23.0	25.9	35.6	23.7	19.0	3.8	4.9	0.41	0.71	**5.8**	141
Salivary gland	34	0	-	-	-	-	0.1	0.2	0.3	0.5	0.7	0.2	0.5	1.4	1.3	7.1	2.1	1.2	0.3	0.4	0.03	0.07	**0.5**	142
Mouth	465	0	-	-	-	-	0.3	0.2	0.4	3.2	4.0	11.7	20.9	29.3	34.2	47.5	22.7	40.4	4.7	6.1	0.52	0.87	**7.5**	143-5
Oropharynx	162	0	-	-	-	-	0.1	0.1	0.1	0.8	1.4	4.3	5.9	10.8	9.7	18.2	18.5	10.7	1.6	2.1	0.17	0.35	**2.7**	146
Nasopharynx	67	0	-	-	0.3	0.3	0.9	0.6	0.5	0.3	0.5	1.0	2.1	1.4	3.5	3.2	5.2	3.6	0.7	0.9	0.06	0.10	**0.9**	147
Hypopharynx	403	0	-	-	0.1	0.3	0.4	0.3	0.8	2.9	3.0	8.6	17.9	20.9	31.6	42.8	27.8	33.3	4.1	5.3	0.43	0.79	**6.5**	148
Pharynx unspecified	69	0	-	-	-	-	-	-	0.3	0.8	0.5	2.3	3.7	3.1	3.1	5.5	4.1	8.3	0.7	0.9	0.07	0.12	**1.1**	149
Oesophagus	641	0	-	-	-	0.1	0.2	0.2	1.3	2.4	5.4	13.6	26.2	45.3	45.2	65.7	54.6	54.6	6.5	8.4	0.70	1.30	**10.5**	150
Stomach	979	0	-	-	-	-	0.6	1.2	3.1	6.3	9.2	17.9	40.9	55.8	74.2	114.0	67.0	77.2	10.0	12.9	1.05	1.95	**15.9**	151
Small intestine	10	0	-	-	-	-	0.1	-	0.1	-	0.5	0.2	0.3	-	0.9	-	-	1.2	0.1	0.1	0.01	0.01	**0.1**	152
Colon	122	0	-	-	-	-	0.1	0.2	0.5	1.2	2.1	3.7	4.8	4.9	8.3	7.9	12.4	4.8	1.2	1.6	0.13	0.23	**1.8**	153
Rectum	245	0	-	-	-	0.2	0.5	0.9	1.3	1.2	3.7	6.4	10.4	9.8	11.4	22.2	16.5	27.3	2.5	3.2	0.23	0.42	**3.8**	154
Liver	161	0	0.5	-	-	-	-	0.2	0.3	1.5	1.7	3.1	8.0	9.4	10.5	13.5	9.3	11.9	1.6	2.1	0.18	0.29	**2.5**	155
Gallbladder etc.	35	0	-	-	-	-	-	-	0.4	0.5	0.9	0.2	0.8	2.4	2.6	1.6	3.1	2.4	0.4	0.5	0.04	0.06	**0.5**	156
Pancreas	92	0	-	-	-	-	0.1	0.6	0.5	0.5	0.9	1.2	4.5	5.6	6.6	7.9	5.2	4.8	0.9	1.2	0.10	0.17	**1.4**	157
Nose, sinuses etc.	58	0	-	0.1	-	-	0.1	0.2	0.3	0.5	1.0	0.8	2.7	0.7	4.0	4.8	8.2	4.8	0.6	0.8	0.05	0.12	**0.9**	160
Larynx	309	0	-	-	-	-	0.1	0.1	0.6	0.8	4.4	7.4	9.4	19.5	25.0	30.1	27.8	27.3	3.1	4.1	0.34	0.63	**5.1**	161
Bronchus, lung	789	0	-	-	0.1	0.1	0.2	0.5	1.5	2.9	9.8	19.9	29.2	51.3	64.5	86.3	52.6	39.2	8.0	10.4	0.90	1.59	**12.6**	162
Other thoracic organs	14	0	-	-	0.1	0.2	0.3	0.1	0.1	-	0.2	0.4	0.3	0.7	-	-	-	-	0.1	0.2	0.01	0.01	**0.1**	163-4
Bone	101	0	-	0.5	1.2	3.0	1.3	0.9	0.6	1.4	0.7	1.0	0.8	0.3	0.9	-	2.1	1.2	1.0	1.3	0.06	0.07	**1.0**	170
Connective tissue	87	0	0.7	0.3	0.3	0.5	1.3	1.2	0.4	1.5	0.7	1.0	1.9	1.4	1.3	4.0	3.1	1.2	0.9	1.1	0.06	0.10	**1.0**	171
Mesothelioma	5	0	-	-	-	-	0.1	-	0.1	-	-	0.2	0.5	-	-	-	-	-	0.1	0.1	0.00	0.00	**0.1**	MES
Kaposi's sarcoma	0	0	-	-	-	-	-	-	-	-	-	-	-	-	-	-	-	-	0.0	0.0	0.00	0.00	**0.0**	KAP
Melanoma of skin	27	0	-	0.1	0.1	-	-	0.1	0.3	0.2	0.4	2.1	0.3	0.9	1.6	1.0	5.9	0.3	0.4	0.02	0.04	**0.4**	172
Other skin	107	0	-	-	-	0.1	-	0.2	0.3	1.2	1.6	1.9	3.5	5.6	6.1	11.9	13.4	5.9	1.1		0.10	0.23	**1.7**	173
Breast	17	0	-	-	-	-	0.1	-	0.2	0.2	0.4	0.5	0.7	0.4	0.8	2.1	4.8		0.2	0.2	0.01	0.03	**0.3**	175
Prostate	179	0	0.1	-	-	-	-	-	0.1	0.5	0.2	0.8	2.7	4.5	11.9	26.1	37.1	59.4	1.8	2.4	0.10	0.42	**3.6**	185
Testis	60	0	0.3	-	-	0.5	0.5	0.6	1.3	1.2	0.2	1.0	2.1	1.0	0.4	0.8	4.1	-	0.6	0.8	0.05	0.07	**0.7**	186
Penis	196	0	-	-	-	0.1	0.5	1.1	1.4	1.9	4.1	8.0	12.2	12.3	19.0	11.3	15.4	2.0	2.6	0.21	0.36	**3.0**	187.1-.4
Other male genital	5	0	-	-	-	-	-	-	-	-	-	-	0.3	0.4	-	2.1	1.2	0.1	0.1	0.00	0.01	**0.1**	187.5-.9
†Bladder	162	0	-	0.1	-	0.2	0.2	0.1	0.1	0.3	1.6	2.1	5.9	5.9	12.7	22.2	22.7	19.0	1.6	2.1	0.15	0.37	**2.8**	188
Kidney etc.	67	0	0.8	-	-	-	0.1	0.1	0.1	0.3	0.9	1.6	2.4	4.2	4.8	4.8	3.1	-	0.7	0.9	0.08	0.12	**1.0**	189
Eye	35	0	2.2	0.5	0.2	-	0.1	-	-	0.2	-	-	0.5	-	-	0.8	1.0	1.2	0.4	0.5	0.02	0.03	**0.4**	190
Brain, nervous system	188	0	1.2	1.5	0.8	0.7	0.9	1.5	2.2	3.2	3.3	2.7	3.2	4.2	6.1	7.1	2.1	3.6	1.9	2.5	0.16	0.20	**2.2**	191-2
Thyroid	53	0	-	-	-	0.1	-	0.2	0.1	-	0.7	0.8	2.9	3.8	3.1	0.8	6.2	5.9	0.5	0.7	0.06	0.09	**0.8**	193
Other endocrine	16	0	0.4	0.2	-	0.1	0.1	0.2	-	-	0.2	0.6	0.3	0.3	-	-	-	-	0.2	0.2	0.01	0.01	**0.2**	194
Hodgkin's disease	123	0	0.5	1.7	1.4	1.2	0.8	0.7	0.8	0.9	2.3	2.1	1.9	1.7	1.3	3.2	1.0	2.4	1.3	1.6	0.09	0.11	**1.3**	201
Non-Hodgkin lymphoma	287	0	0.6	1.5	1.6	2.2	1.6	1.6	2.3	2.3	2.8	5.6	6.4	8.4	14.9	11.1	7.2	16.6	2.9	3.8	0.26	0.35	**3.7**	200,202
Multiple myeloma	52	0	-	-	-	-	0.2	0.2	0.3	0.2	0.3	1.2	1.6	3.1	2.6	6.3	7.2	1.2	0.5	0.7	0.05	0.12	**0.8**	203
Lymphoid leukaemia	134	0	3.5	2.9	1.4	0.8	1.0	1.2	1.0	0.3	0.9	0.2	-	-	0.4	1.6	5.2	1.2	1.4	1.8	0.07	0.10	**1.4**	204
Myeloid leukaemia	109	0	0.5	0.5	0.3	0.4	1.1	0.9	1.8	1.4	0.9	1.4	2.1	2.4	2.6	4.8	5.2	5.9	1.1	1.4	0.08	0.13	**1.3**	205
Monocytic leukaemia	5	0	-	0.1	-	-	0.1	0.1	-	-	-	-	0.3	-	0.4	-	-	-	0.1	0.1	0.01	0.01	**0.1**	206
Other leukaemia	0	0	-	-	-	-	-	-	-	-	-	-	-	-	-	-	-	-	0.0	0.0	0.00	0.00	**0.0**	207
Leukaemia unspecified	17	0	0.1	-	0.1	0.4	0.3	0.3	0.3	0.2	0.2	-	-	0.3	-	-	-	-	0.2	0.2	0.01	0.01	**0.2**	208
Other and unspecified	609	0	0.6	-	0.3	0.4	1.1	0.5	2.6	5.1	6.8	13.8	20.3	31.7	40.8	52.3	44.3	60.6	6.2	8.0	0.62	1.10	**9.5**	O&U
All sites	7695	0	12.3	9.9	8.0	11.8	14.8	17.3	29.1	50.3	81.8	156.5	275.1	388.7	490.0	695.3	543.1	584.3	78.3		7.73	13.92	**118.2**	ALL
All sites but 173	7588	0	12.3	9.9	8.0	11.7	14.8	17.1	28.8	49.1	80.2	154.6	271.6	383.2	483.8	683.5	529.7	578.4	77.2	100.0	7.63	13.69	**116.5**	ALLb

Rate from 1 case   0.105   0.091   0.090   0.099   0.098   0.107   0.128   0.151   0.174   0.206   0.268   0.349   0.439   0.792   1.031   1.188

†Important: see notes on population page

INDIA, MADRAS 1988-1992

ANNUAL INCIDENCE PER 100,000 BY AGE GROUP (YEARS) - FEMALE

SITE	ALL AGES	AGE UNK	0-	5-	10-	15-	20-	25-	30-	35-	40-	45-	50-	55-	60-	65-	70-	75+	CRUDE RATE	%	CR 64	CR 74	ASR (W)	ICD (9th)
Lip	25	0	-	-	-	-	-	-	-	-	-	0.5	0.9	1.3	2.6	3.0	3.9	3.2	0.3	0.3	0.03	0.06	0.5	140
Tongue	117	0	-	-	-	-	0.2	0.3	0.2	0.8	1.3	3.2	7.6	7.3	8.3	8.3	8.9	6.5	1.3	1.4	0.15	0.23	1.9	141
Salivary gland	29	0	0.1	-	-	0.2	0.1	0.3	0.5	-	0.2	1.0	1.8	1.3	-	0.8	3.0	1.1	0.3	0.3	0.03	0.05	0.4	142
Mouth	495	0	0.1	0.1	-	0.2	0.1	0.4	2.2	2.8	9.2	10.3	30.1	29.2	43.0	37.5	29.6	29.2	5.4	5.9	0.64	0.97	8.2	143-5
Oropharynx	32	0	-	-	0.1	-	0.1	-	0.2	-	0.7	1.2	1.2	3.0	1.8	2.3	2.0	1.1	0.3	0.4	0.04	0.06	0.5	146
Nasopharynx	27	0	-	-	0.2	-	0.6	0.3	0.2	0.3	0.2	0.7	1.2	0.4	0.4	2.3	-	-	0.3	0.3	0.02	0.03	0.3	147
Hypopharynx	164	0	-	-	-	0.1	0.1	0.9	1.3	3.5	3.1	5.9	9.4	11.2	6.1	4.5	5.9	4.3	1.8	2.0	0.21	0.26	2.4	148
Pharynx unspecified	15	0	-	-	-	-	-	0.1	-	-	0.2	-	-	1.3	2.2	3.0	-	1.1	0.2	0.2	0.02	0.03	0.3	149
Oesophagus	423	0	-	-	-	0.2	-	0.3	2.0	3.2	7.2	13.0	23.1	27.5	26.3	31.5	40.5	19.5	4.6	5.0	0.51	0.87	7.0	150
Stomach	433	0	-	-	-	0.1	0.3	1.5	2.2	4.5	8.1	14.0	21.3	30.9	22.8	31.5	16.8	31.4	4.7	5.1	0.53	0.77	7.0	151
Small intestine	5	0	-	-	-	-	-	0.1	-	-	-	0.2	-	0.4	-	0.8	1.0	-	0.1	0.1	0.00	0.01	0.1	152
Colon	84	0	-	-	0.1	-	-	0.1	0.5	0.8	1.3	2.5	5.2	7.3	5.7	4.5	3.0	2.2	0.9	1.0	0.12	0.15	1.3	153
Rectum	174	0	-	0.1	0.2	0.2	0.3	1.6	1.1	0.8	1.3	2.0	7.6	10.3	16.2	12.0	10.9	14.1	1.9	2.1	0.21	0.32	2.8	154
Liver	32	0	0.1	0.1	-	-	0.1	0.1	0.6	0.2	0.4	0.2	1.8	2.6	0.9	1.5	2.0	2.2	0.3	0.4	0.04	0.05	0.5	155
Gallbladder etc.	26	0	-	-	-	-	-	-	-	0.2	-	0.2	1.8	2.1	1.8	4.5	2.0	1.1	0.3	0.3	0.03	0.06	0.5	156
Pancreas	43	0	-	-	-	0.1	-	0.2	-	1.2	0.9	1.0	0.9	1.7	2.2	3.8	5.9	2.2	0.5	0.5	0.04	0.09	0.7	157
Nose, sinuses etc.	45	0	-	-	-	0.1	0.3	0.2	0.2	0.2	0.9	0.5	0.6	4.7	3.5	3.0	2.0	4.3	0.5	0.5	0.06	0.08	0.7	160
Larynx	38	0	-	-	-	0.1	-	-	0.5	0.2	0.9	0.5	0.6	3.4	4.4	3.0	1.0	2.2	0.4	0.5	0.05	0.07	0.6	161
Bronchus, lung	142	0	-	-	-	-	0.1	0.1	0.5	0.8	3.1	3.9	7.3	10.7	11.0	15.0	3.9	4.3	1.5	1.7	0.19	0.28	2.4	162
Other thoracic organs	4	0	-	0.1	-	0.1	-	-	-	-	-	-	0.3	-	-	0.8	-	-	0.0	0.0	0.00	0.01	0.1	163-4
Bone	34	0	-	0.2	0.6	0.9	0.3	0.3	0.5	0.3	0.2	-	-	0.9	0.9	-	1.0	-	0.4	0.4	0.03	0.03	0.4	170
Connective tissue	83	0	0.5	0.3	0.3	1.0	0.9	0.7	0.9	1.0	1.1	2.5	0.9	2.1	1.8	3.8	2.0	1.1	0.9	1.0	0.07	0.10	1.0	171
Mesothelioma	3	0	-	-	-	-	-	0.1	-	-	-	-	-	-	0.4	-	1.0	-	0.0	0.0	0.00	0.01	0.0	MES
Kaposi's sarcoma	0	0	-	-	-	-	-	-	-	-	-	-	-	-	-	-	-	-	0.0	0.0	0.00	0.00	0.0	KAP
Melanoma of skin	16	0	-	-	0.1	-	-	-	-	-	0.4	0.2	0.6	1.3	1.3	-	3.0	1.1	0.2	0.2	0.02	0.03	0.3	172
Other skin	71	0	-	-	-	0.2	0.2	0.3	0.6	0.8	0.7	2.9	2.7	3.0	3.1	3.8	3.0	9.7	0.8		0.07	0.11	1.1	173
Breast	1525	0	-	-	-	-	0.9	4.9	7.7	28.4	46.1	59.4	62.2	83.8	68.0	75.8	71.1	82.3	16.6	18.1	1.81	2.54	23.5	174
Uterus unspecified	25	0	-	-	-	-	-	0.2	-	0.7	1.5	1.5	0.9	0.9	1.5	1.0	2.2		0.3	0.3	0.03	0.04	0.4	179
Cervix uteri	2540	0	-	-	-	0.9	3.8	17.6	40.6	72.1	99.0	133.9	164.9	133.0	105.8	98.7	50.9		27.7	30.2	3.33	4.35	38.9	180
Placenta	22	0	-	-	0.1	0.9	0.7	0.3	0.5	0.2	-	-	-	-	-	-	-		0.2	0.3	0.01	0.01	0.2	181
Corpus uteri	127	0	-	-	-	-	-	0.2	0.5	0.8	1.8	3.7	5.8	10.7	8.3	14.3	3.9	8.7	1.4	1.5	0.16	0.25	2.2	182
Ovary etc.	390	0	0.1	0.3	1.1	0.7	1.3	1.8	2.5	6.3	8.7	14.0	14.9	19.3	16.2	21.8	20.7	7.6	4.2	4.6	0.44	0.65	5.7	183
Other female genital	116	0	-	0.1	-	-	0.2	0.3	0.5	0.7	3.1	3.7	3.3	3.0	9.2	5.3	19.7	8.7	1.3	1.4	0.12	0.25	1.9	184
†Bladder	53	0	-	-	-	-	-	-	-	0.5	-	1.2	2.1	3.0	3.5	7.5	8.9	4.3	0.6	0.6	0.05	0.13	1.0	188
Kidney etc.	44	0	0.5	-	-	-	0.2	-	0.2	0.3	0.7	1.0	2.1	1.3	2.6	5.3	2.0	2.2	0.5	0.5	0.04	0.08	0.7	189
Eye	30	0	1.7	0.6	0.1	-	-	0.1	-	-	0.2	0.2	-	0.9	0.9	-	-	-	0.3	0.4	0.02	0.02	0.4	190
Brain, nervous system	84	0	0.8	0.6	0.3	0.2	0.2	0.8	1.1	1.8	0.7	2.0	2.1	4.7	1.3	3.0	1.0	1.1	0.9	1.0	0.08	0.10	1.1	191-2
Thyroid	112	0	-	-	-	0.1	0.8	0.9	0.8	1.3	2.5	4.4	4.9	3.9	4.4	3.0	9.9	4.3	1.2	1.3	0.12	0.18	1.6	193
Other endocrine	8	0	0.1	-	-	0.1	-	0.1	0.2	-	0.2	0.2	-	0.4	-	-	-	1.1	0.1	0.1	0.01	0.01	0.1	194
Hodgkin's disease	55	0	0.3	0.6	0.4	0.3	1.2	0.6	0.5	0.5	0.7	1.0	1.2	0.4	0.9	0.8	-	1.1	0.6	0.7	0.04	0.05	0.6	201
Non-Hodgkin lymphoma	149	0	0.1	1.0	0.4	0.8	1.7	1.3	1.1	1.2	2.9	4.4	1.8	5.6	5.3	9.8	5.9	1.1	1.6	1.8	0.14	0.22	2.0	200,202
Multiple myeloma	24	0	-	-	-	-	-	-	-	-	0.4	1.0	1.5	2.6	1.3	-	3.0	1.1	0.3	0.3	0.03	0.05	0.4	203
Lymphoid leukaemia	70	0	1.5	1.3	1.1	0.3	0.5	0.1	0.3	-	1.3	0.5	-	1.3	1.3	1.5	2.0	1.1	0.8	0.8	0.05	0.07	0.8	204
Myeloid leukaemia	74	0	-	0.5	0.5	0.6	0.8	0.2	1.3	0.3	0.7	1.2	2.1	3.9	2.6	3.8	1.0	2.2	0.8	0.9	0.07	0.10	1.0	205
Monocytic leukaemia	3	0	-	-	-	-	-	0.1	-	0.2	-	-	-	-	-	0.8	-	-	0.0	0.0	0.00	0.01	0.0	206
Other leukaemia	1	0	-	-	0.1	-	-	-	-	-	-	-	-	-	-	-	-	-	0.0	0.0	0.00	0.00	0.0	207
Leukaemia unspecified	16	0	0.1	-	0.2	0.3	0.3	-	0.2	-	0.2	0.2	0.3	0.4	-	0.8	1.0	-	0.2	0.2	0.01	0.02	0.2	208
Other and unspecified	452	0	0.3	0.2	0.4	0.9	1.2	1.2	2.7	4.2	9.6	16.0	18.8	27.5	21.1	27.8	26.7	24.9	4.9	5.4	0.52	0.79	7.1	O&U
All sites	8480	0	6.5	5.9	6.1	7.8	14.7	25.6	51.4	109.2	194.7	281.2	385.6	502.6	447.6	468.9	428.4	346.6	92.4		10.19	14.68	130.9	ALL
All sites but 173	8409	0	6.5	5.9	6.1	7.6	14.5	25.3	50.7	108.4	194.0	278.3	382.9	499.6	444.6	465.1	425.5	336.8	91.6	100.0	10.12	14.57	129.8	ALLb
Rate from 1 case			0.106	0.094	0.095	0.099	0.099	0.112	0.158	0.166	0.224	0.246	0.304	0.430	0.439	0.750	0.987	1.083						

†Important: see notes on population page

India, Trivandrum

The population-based Trivandrum Cancer Registry was initiated in 1994 by the Regional Cancer Centre, Trivandrum, Kerala in collaboration with IARC. Kerala, the most southwesterly state of India, has different socio-demographic features compared with other parts of the country. It has a very high density of population (749 persons/km^2) with easily accessible health care facilities. The infant mortality rate has been consistently low (17 per 1000 live births), which has pushed up the average life expectancy to 65 years for men and 71 years for women. The state has the lowest birth and death rates, 18.1 and 6.0 per 1000 persons, respectively.

The Kerala Government has implemented a Cancer Control Programme that includes health education, early detection, community-based intervention trials and augmentation of diagnostic and therapeutic facilities.

Trivandrum is situated at latitude 8° 29´ N and longitude 76° 57´ E, at an altitude of 64 m above sea level.

The registry covers both urban and rural populations in Trivandrum Corporation limits and the three Community Development blocks in Trivandrum District. The estimated population of this area at the 1991 census was 1 066 322 (524 130 males and 542 192 females). Trivandrum city corporation area covers 75 km^2 and has a population of 524 006. The rural Kazhakkuttam and Chirayinkil community development blocks comprise an area of 261 km^2 with 542 316 population. The major part of the population is of Hindu religion (57%), followed by Muslims (23%) and Christians (19%).

The estimates of the population at risk were obtained from the decennial census figures. The census data for the year 1981 is available by sex and five-year age groups and for the year 1991, census data is available by sex, but not by five-year age group. The population at risk for the year 1991 in each age group has been estimated by extrapolating the percentage distribution of five-year age-groups of the 1981 census to the total population of the 1991 census. The 1992 population is estimated using an exponential growth rate and based on the 1991 population.

Data on cancer are generated by visiting the major hospitals which cater to the area. Trivandrum city has a large number of hospitals including private and government sectors. There is a Medical College and a Regional Cancer Centre, both of which have histopathology services. The registry covers 70 hospitals and five pathology laboratories. The major source of cancer cases for the registry is the Hospital Cancer Registry, which has been functioning at the Regional Cancer Centre in Trivandrum since 1982. This centre has excellent diagnostic and treatment facilities. Patients come from all parts of Kerala and also from adjoining areas of Tamil Nadu. 80% of all registrations have been obtained from the Medical College Hospital and the Regional Cancer Centre.

Other data sources include government and private hospitals, pathology laboratories and radiological diagnostic centres. Every case with a diagnosis of malignancy from these sources is recorded. Death records of Trivandrum corporation and Kazhakuttam and Chirayinkil panchayat offices provide additional information about cancer patients and deaths. Death certification by a registered medical practitioner is not mandatory. The deaths in the area specified as 'cancer deaths' reported to these offices are believed to be under-registered. Autopsy is not regularly practised in the area except for medico-legal purposes.

All deaths identified by the registry are matched with the Hospital Cancer Registry database consisting of all cases from 1982. Cases where the death certificate is the only source of information are also included, with the date of death taken as the date of first diagnosis.

For government and private hospitals, nursing homes, pathologists and radiologists, an introductory letter was sent describing the basic purpose of the registry and requesting their cooperation in the collection of data on cancer patients. The principal investigator of the registry conducts classes in the regular meetings of medical officers from various hospitals in the registry area, to make them aware of the purpose of the registry and to get their cooperation.

A dedicated computer program was developed in-house for checking consistency of data and generating tables. Initially the data are checked for inconsistencies in data entry. Inconsistency checks on the variables sex, site (ICD-9), age, basis of diagnosis and date of death are performed. Thereafter checks for duplicate entries are carried out and duplicates eliminated.

The registry collects follow-up information of all cancer patients from time to time. All the patients attending the Regional Cancer Centre, Trivandrum are instructed to attend for follow-up every 6–12 months. Reply-paid postcards written in local language were sent to the lost to follow-up cases and the patients reported from other hospitals to enquire about the status of the patient.

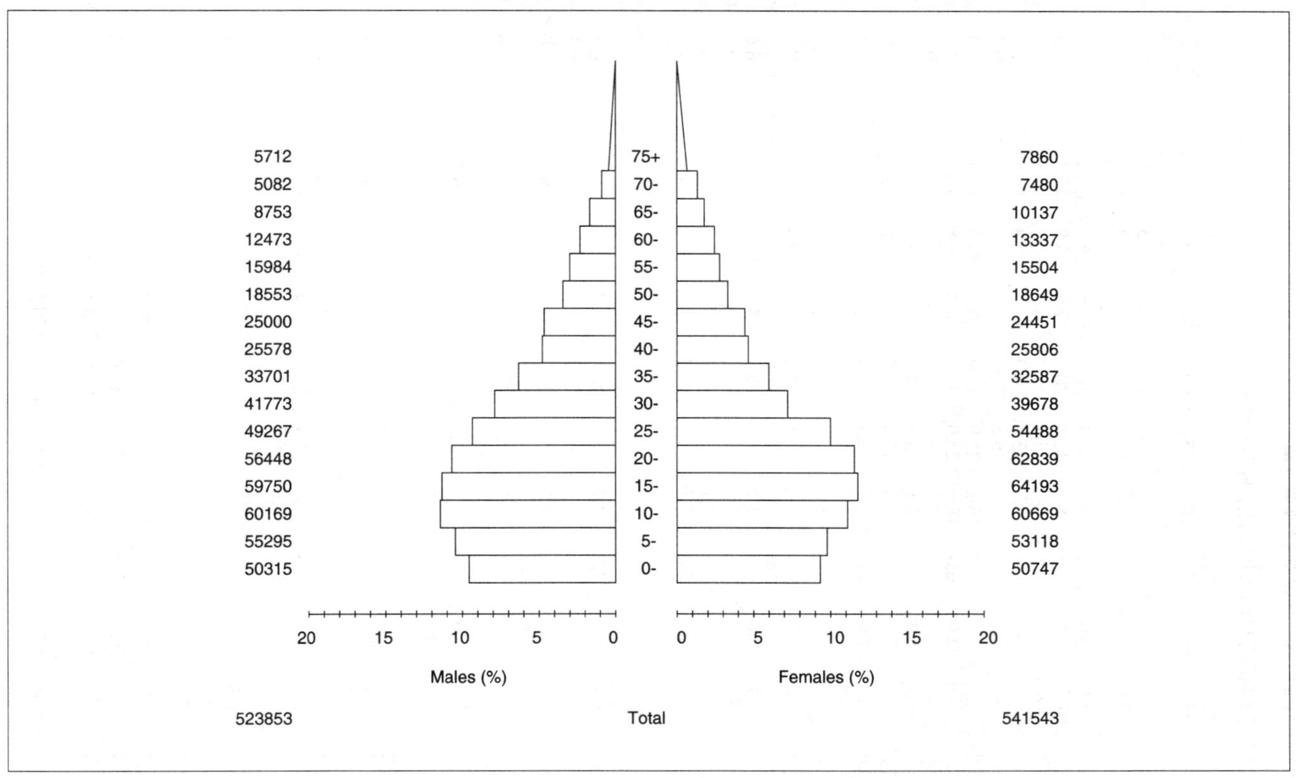

India, Trivandrum

Source of population: average annual 1991–92
Census: Census of India 1991. Final Population Totals: p.54. Series 12, Kerala: Paper 3 of 1991. N.M. Samuel, MA. LLB, Director of Census Operations, Kerala.
Estimate: The 1992 population is estimated on the basis of the 1991 Census, taking into account births and deaths but not migration.

Notes to tables overleaf:

* There is evidence of under-registration and childhood cancer is certainly under-ascertained in the area
† 188 does not include non-invasive tumours

* INDIA, TRIVANDRUM 1991-1992

ANNUAL INCIDENCE PER 100,000 BY AGE GROUP (YEARS) - MALE

SITE	ALL AGES	AGE UNK	0-	5-	10-	15-	20-	25-	30-	35-	40-	45-	50-	55-	60-	65-	70-	75+	CRUDE RATE	%	CR 64	CR 74	ASR (W)	ICD (9th)
Lip	6	0	-	-	-	-	-	-	-	-	-	-	-	-	4.0	5.7	29.5	8.8	0.6	0.8	0.02	0.20	1.1	140
Tongue	31	0	-	-	-	-	-	2.0	-	3.0	2.0	2.0	16.2	15.6	20.0	22.8	29.5	17.5	3.0	4.2	0.30	0.57	4.4	141
Salivary gland	0	0	-	-	-	-	-	-	-	-	-	-	-	-	-	-	-	-	0.0	0.0	0.00	0.00	0.0	142
Mouth	72	0	-	-	-	-	-	-	-	4.5	5.9	12.0	26.9	31.3	60.1	51.4	39.4	105.0	6.9	9.8	0.70	1.16	10.8	143-5
Oropharynx	21	0	-	-	-	-	-	-	-	1.5	-	2.0	5.4	12.5	20.0	17.1	9.8	35.0	2.0	2.8	0.21	0.34	3.2	146
Nasopharynx	3	0	-	-	-	-	-	-	-	-	-	-	-	3.1	-	5.7	-	8.8	0.3	0.4	0.02	0.04	0.5	147
Hypopharynx	12	0	-	-	-	-	-	-	-	-	-	-	2.7	3.1	4.0	34.3	9.8	17.5	1.1	1.6	0.05	0.27	2.0	148
Pharynx unspecified	2	0	-	-	-	-	-	-	-	-	-	-	-	6.3	-	-	-	-	0.2	0.3	0.03	0.03	0.3	149
Oesophagus	31	0	-	-	-	-	-	-	1.2	-	-	6.0	16.2	21.9	16.0	28.6	29.5	17.5	3.0	4.2	0.31	0.60	4.6	150
Stomach	45	0	-	-	-	-	-	-	-	-	2.0	6.0	18.9	25.0	32.1	74.3	9.8	35.0	4.3	6.1	0.42	0.84	6.8	151
Small intestine	1	0	-	-	-	-	-	-	-	-	-	-	2.7	-	-	-	-	-	0.1	0.1	0.01	0.01	0.1	152
Colon	17	0	-	-	-	0.8	0.9	-	-	1.5	5.9	-	8.1	3.1	4.0	22.8	19.7	-	1.6	2.3	0.12	0.33	2.4	153
Rectum	21	0	-	-	-	-	-	-	1.2	-	3.9	-	13.5	12.5	4.0	22.8	9.8	26.3	2.0	2.8	0.18	0.34	3.0	154
Liver	23	0	-	-	-	-	-	1.0	2.4	1.5	5.9	6.0	2.7	6.3	4.0	28.6	-	35.0	2.2	3.1	0.15	0.29	3.1	155
Gallbladder etc.	2	0	-	-	-	-	0.9	-	-	-	-	-	2.7	-	-	-	-	-	0.2	0.3	0.02	0.02	0.2	156
Pancreas	17	0	-	-	-	-	0.9	-	2.4	-	-	10.0	5.4	-	4.0	11.4	29.5	8.8	1.6	2.3	0.11	0.32	2.4	157
Nose, sinuses etc.	6	0	-	-	-	-	-	-	-	-	2.0	-	-	3.1	8.0	-	9.8	8.8	0.6	0.8	0.07	0.11	0.9	160
Larynx	34	0	-	-	-	-	-	-	-	-	3.9	4.0	2.7	12.5	12.0	74.3	29.5	52.5	3.2	4.6	0.18	0.69	5.5	161
Bronchus, lung	69	0	-	-	-	-	-	-	-	3.0	7.8	10.0	8.1	37.5	76.2	45.7	118.1	35.0	6.6	9.3	0.71	1.53	10.6	162
Other thoracic organs	2	0	-	-	-	0.8	0.9	-	-	-	-	-	-	-	-	-	-	-	0.2	0.3	0.01	0.01	0.1	163-4
Bone	4	0	-	-	-	1.7	-	-	-	-	-	-	2.7	-	-	5.7	-	-	0.4	0.5	0.02	0.05	0.5	170
Connective tissue	11	0	-	-	0.8	-	-	-	2.4	-	2.0	2.0	2.7	3.1	8.0	5.7	-	8.8	1.0	1.5	0.11	0.13	1.4	171
Mesothelioma	0	0	-	-	-	-	-	-	-	-	-	-	-	-	-	-	-	-	0.0	0.0	0.00	0.00	0.0	MES
Kaposi's sarcoma	0	0	-	-	-	-	-	-	-	-	-	-	-	-	-	-	-	-	0.0	0.0	0.00	0.00	0.0	KAP
Melanoma of skin	2	0	1.0	-	-	-	-	-	-	-	-	-	-	-	-	-	9.8	-	0.2	0.3	0.00	0.05	0.3	172
Other skin	8	0	-	-	-	-	-	-	-	1.5	-	2.0	2.7	6.3	8.0	5.7	-	-	0.8		0.10	0.13	1.1	173
Breast	3	0	-	-	-	-	-	-	-	1.5	-	-	-	-	-	5.7	9.8	-	0.3	0.4	0.01	0.09	0.5	175
Prostate	42	0	-	-	-	-	-	-	-	-	-	-	2.7	3.1	20.0	62.8	68.9	148.8	4.0	5.7	0.13	0.79	7.3	185
Testis	4	0	-	-	-	0.8	0.9	-	-	-	3.9	-	-	-	-	-	-	-	0.4	0.5	0.03	0.03	0.4	186
Penis	8	0	-	-	-	-	-	-	-	1.5	-	-	-	3.1	8.0	-	19.7	17.5	0.8	1.1	0.06	0.16	1.3	187.1-.4
Other male genital	0	0	-	-	-	-	-	-	-	-	-	-	-	-	-	-	-	-	0.0	0.0	0.00	0.00	0.0	187.5-.9
†Bladder	15	0	-	-	-	-	-	-	-	-	2.0	2.0	-	3.1	4.0	11.4	59.0	26.3	1.4	2.0	0.06	0.41	2.6	188
Kidney etc.	4	0	2.0	-	-	-	-	-	-	-	-	-	2.7	3.1	-	-	-	-	0.4	0.5	0.04	0.04	0.5	189
Eye	1	0	1.0	-	-	-	-	-	-	-	-	-	-	-	-	-	-	-	0.1	0.1	0.00	0.00	0.1	190
Brain, nervous system	19	0	1.0	-	-	0.8	-	1.0	1.2	-	3.9	6.0	2.7	3.1	4.0	17.1	9.8	26.3	1.8	2.6	0.12	0.25	2.6	191-2
Thyroid	19	0	-	-	-	0.8	2.7	1.0	2.4	4.5	2.0	2.0	13.5	-	-	5.7	-	8.8	1.8	2.6	0.14	0.17	2.0	193
Other endocrine	1	0	-	-	-	-	-	-	-	-	-	2.0	-	-	-	-	-	-	0.1	0.1	0.01	0.01	0.1	194
Hodgkin's disease	7	0	-	1.8	-	-	-	2.0	1.2	-	-	-	-	-	4.0	5.7	-	-	0.7	0.9	0.05	0.07	0.7	201
Non-Hodgkin lymphoma	33	0	1.0	1.8	-	0.8	0.9	1.0	1.2	1.5	9.8	6.0	5.4	3.1	24.1	11.4	39.4	17.5	3.1	4.5	0.28	0.54	4.5	200,202
Multiple myeloma	18	0	-	-	-	-	-	-	-	-	2.0	6.0	10.8	6.3	-	34.3	-	17.5	1.7	2.4	0.12	0.30	2.6	203
Lymphoid leukaemia	18	0	3.0	1.8	1.7	0.8	2.7	-	-	-	-	-	5.4	-	12.0	11.4	-	-	1.7	2.4	0.14	0.19	2.1	204
Myeloid leukaemia	9	0	1.0	-	0.8	0.8	1.8	1.0	-	1.5	-	2.0	-	-	-	5.7	-	-	0.9	1.2	0.04	0.07	0.9	205
Monocytic leukaemia	0	0	-	-	-	-	-	-	-	-	-	-	-	-	-	-	-	-	0.0	0.0	0.00	0.00	0.0	206
Other leukaemia	1	0	-	-	-	-	-	-	1.2	-	-	-	-	-	-	-	-	-	0.1	0.1	0.01	0.01	0.1	207
Leukaemia unspecified	2	0	1.0	-	-	-	0.9	-	-	-	-	-	-	-	-	-	-	-	0.2	0.3	0.01	0.01	0.2	208
Other and unspecified	102	0	-	-	-	0.8	-	-	1.2	4.5	11.7	14.0	24.3	46.9	56.1	120.0	98.4	131.3	9.7	13.8	0.80	1.89	15.5	O&U
All sites	746	0	10.9	5.4	3.3	9.2	13.3	9.1	18.0	31.2	76.2	102.0	207.5	275.3	416.9	754.0	688.7	814.1	71.2		5.89	13.11	109.2	ALL
All sites but 173	738	0	10.9	5.4	3.3	9.2	13.3	9.1	18.0	29.7	76.2	100.0	204.8	269.0	408.9	748.3	688.7	814.1	70.4	100.0	5.79	12.97	108.1	ALLb

Rate from 1 case 0.994 0.904 0.831 0.837 0.886 1.015 1.197 1.484 1.955 2.000 2.695 3.128 4.009 5.712 9.839 8.754

†Important: see notes on population page

* INDIA, TRIVANDRUM 1991-1992

ANNUAL INCIDENCE PER 100,000 BY AGE GROUP (YEARS) - FEMALE

SITE	ALL AGES	AGE UNK	0-	5-	10-	15-	20-	25-	30-	35-	40-	45-	50-	55-	60-	65-	70-	75+	CRUDE RATE	%	CR 64	CR 74	ASR (W)	ICD (9th)
Lip	0	0	-	-	-	-	-	-	-	-	-	-	-	-	-	-	-	-	0.0	0.0	0.00	0.00	0.0	140
Tongue	14	0	-	-	-	-	-	0.9	-	1.5	1.9	-	2.7	9.7	7.5	4.9	13.4	12.7	1.3	2.0	0.12	0.21	1.8	141
Salivary gland	6	0	-	-	-	-	-	0.9	1.3	-	-	-	2.7	3.2	3.7	-	-	6.4	0.6	0.9	0.06	0.06	0.7	142
Mouth	43	0	-	-	-	-	-	-	-	1.5	-	4.1	2.7	25.8	45.0	39.5	26.7	44.5	4.0	6.1	0.40	0.73	5.9	143-5
Oropharynx	3	0	-	-	-	-	-	-	-	-	-	2.0	2.7	-	-	-	-	6.4	0.3	0.4	0.02	0.02	0.4	146
Nasopharynx	4	0	-	-	-	-	-	-	1.3	-	-	2.0	2.7	-	3.7	-	-	-	0.4	0.6	0.05	0.05	0.5	147
Hypopharynx	6	0	-	-	-	-	-	0.9	-	-	-	2.0	2.7	3.2	-	4.9	6.7	-	0.6	0.9	0.04	0.10	0.7	148
Pharynx unspecified	0	0	-	-	-	-	-	-	-	-	-	-	-	-	-	-	-	-	0.0	0.0	0.00	0.00	0.0	149
Oesophagus	10	0	-	-	-	-	-	-	-	-	-	-	-	12.9	3.7	4.9	13.4	12.7	0.9	1.4	0.08	0.17	1.3	150
Stomach	18	0	-	-	-	-	-	-	-	-	-	4.1	5.4	9.7	15.0	19.7	6.7	12.7	1.7	2.6	0.17	0.30	2.5	151
Small intestine	1	0	-	-	-	-	-	-	-	-	-	2.0	-	-	-	-	-	-	0.1	0.1	0.01	0.01	0.1	152
Colon	8	0	-	-	-	-	-	-	-	3.1	3.9	-	-	3.2	7.5	4.9	-	-	0.7	1.1	0.09	0.11	1.0	153
Rectum	18	0	-	-	-	0.8	0.8	-	1.3	-	-	-	-	3.2	11.2	14.8	26.7	25.4	1.7	2.6	0.09	0.29	2.3	154
Liver	9	0	-	-	-	-	0.8	-	1.3	-	-	2.0	2.7	3.2	11.2	-	6.7	-	0.8	1.3	0.11	0.14	1.1	155
Gallbladder etc.	5	0	-	-	-	-	-	-	-	-	-	-	2.7	9.7	-	-	-	6.4	0.5	0.7	0.06	0.06	0.6	156
Pancreas	8	0	-	-	-	-	-	-	-	-	-	6.1	2.7	-	-	9.9	13.4	-	0.7	1.1	0.04	0.16	1.1	157
Nose, sinuses etc.	5	0	-	-	-	-	-	-	-	-	-	4.1	2.7	-	3.7	-	6.7	-	0.5	0.7	0.05	0.09	0.7	160
Larynx	3	0	-	-	-	-	-	-	-	-	-	-	-	-	-	4.9	6.7	6.4	0.3	0.4	0.06	0.06	0.4	161
Bronchus, lung	14	0	-	-	-	-	-	0.9	-	-	-	-	2.7	3.2	18.7	4.9	20.1	12.7	1.3	2.0	0.13	0.25	1.9	162
Other thoracic organs	1	0	-	-	-	-	-	-	-	1.5	-	-	-	-	-	-	-	-	0.1	0.1	0.01	0.01	0.1	163-4
Bone	4	0	-	-	0.8	0.8	-	-	1.3	-	-	-	-	-	-	4.9	-	-	0.4	0.6	0.01	0.04	0.4	170
Connective tissue	7	0	-	-	-	1.6	0.8	-	-	-	-	-	5.4	3.2	-	4.9	-	-	0.6	1.0	0.05	0.08	0.7	171
Mesothelioma	1	0	-	-	-	0.8	-	-	-	-	-	-	-	-	-	-	-	-	0.1	0.1	0.00	0.00	0.1	MES
Kaposi's sarcoma	0	0	-	-	-	-	-	-	-	-	-	-	-	-	-	-	-	-	0.0	0.0	0.00	0.00	0.0	KAP
Melanoma of skin	1	0	-	-	-	-	-	-	-	-	-	-	-	3.2	-	-	-	-	0.1	0.1	0.02	0.02	0.1	172
Other skin	8	0	-	-	-	-	0.8	-	-	-	-	-	2.7	-	15.0	4.9	-	6.4	0.7		0.09	0.12	1.1	173
Breast	156	0	-	-	-	-	3.2	2.8	12.6	24.5	42.6	40.9	56.3	67.7	56.2	54.3	53.5	31.8	14.4	22.2	1.53	2.07	18.8	174
Uterus unspecified	4	0	-	-	-	-	0.8	-	-	-	1.9	2.0	-	-	-	6.7	-	-	0.4	0.6	0.02	0.06	0.4	179
Cervix uteri	125	0	-	-	-	-	-	-	6.3	13.8	25.2	42.9	34.9	54.8	56.2	64.1	66.8	57.3	11.5	17.8	1.17	1.83	15.9	180
Placenta	0	0	-	-	-	-	-	-	-	-	-	-	-	-	-	-	-	-	0.0	0.0	0.00	0.00	0.0	181
Corpus uteri	17	0	-	-	-	-	-	-	1.3	3.1	1.9	-	5.4	12.9	3.7	14.8	13.4	6.4	1.6	2.4	0.14	0.28	2.1	182
Ovary etc.	34	0	-	-	-	1.6	-	0.9	2.5	1.5	7.8	10.2	16.1	3.2	3.7	39.5	20.1	-	3.1	4.8	0.24	0.54	4.2	183
Other female genital	6	0	1.0	-	-	-	-	-	-	-	-	-	2.7	3.2	3.7	4.9	-	6.4	0.6	0.9	0.05	0.08	0.8	184
†Bladder	2	0	-	-	-	-	-	-	-	-	-	-	-	-	-	9.9	-	-	0.2	0.3	0.00	0.05	0.3	188
Kidney etc.	3	0	-	-	-	-	-	1.8	-	1.9	-	-	-	-	-	-	-	-	0.3	0.4	0.02	0.02	0.3	189
Eye	2	0	2.0	-	-	-	-	-	-	-	-	-	-	-	-	-	-	-	0.2	0.3	0.01	0.01	0.2	190
Brain, nervous system	16	0	-	-	0.8	0.8	-	1.8	2.5	1.5	-	-	8.0	3.2	7.5	9.9	6.7	-	1.5	2.3	0.13	0.21	1.8	191-2
Thyroid	41	0	-	-	-	0.8	3.2	8.3	7.6	9.2	5.8	4.1	5.4	3.2	3.7	9.9	6.7	19.1	3.8	5.8	0.26	0.34	3.9	193
Other endocrine	0	0	-	-	-	-	-	-	-	-	-	-	-	-	-	-	-	-	0.0	0.0	0.00	0.00	0.0	194
Hodgkin's disease	4	0	-	-	-	0.8	-	-	1.3	-	1.9	-	2.7	-	-	-	-	-	0.4	0.6	0.03	0.03	0.4	201
Non-Hodgkin lymphoma	17	0	-	-	-	0.8	0.8	0.9	1.3	-	1.9	4.1	2.7	3.2	15.0	14.8	6.7	-	1.6	2.4	0.15	0.26	2.1	200,202
Multiple myeloma	3	0	-	-	-	-	-	-	-	-	-	2.0	-	6.4	-	-	-	-	0.3	0.4	0.04	0.04	0.4	203
Lymphoid leukaemia	12	0	1.0	0.9	2.5	0.8	0.8	0.9	1.3	-	-	2.0	5.4	-	-	-	-	-	1.1	1.7	0.08	0.08	1.1	204
Myeloid leukaemia	15	0	-	-	-	-	-	1.8	2.5	1.5	3.9	4.1	5.4	3.2	3.7	4.9	6.7	-	1.4	2.1	0.13	0.19	1.7	205
Monocytic leukaemia	0	0	-	-	-	-	-	-	-	-	-	-	-	-	-	-	-	-	0.0	0.0	0.00	0.00	0.0	206
Other leukaemia	0	0	-	-	-	-	-	-	-	-	-	-	-	-	-	-	-	-	0.0	0.0	0.00	0.00	0.0	207
Leukaemia unspecified	4	1	-	-	-	-	-	-	1.3	-	-	-	-	-	-	4.9	-	6.4	0.4	0.6	0.01	0.04	0.5	208
Other and unspecified	52	0	-	-	0.8	-	-	1.8	-	6.1	-	16.4	24.1	22.6	18.7	39.5	26.7	25.4	4.8	7.4	0.45	0.78	6.7	O&U
All sites	710	1	3.9	0.9	4.9	9.3	11.9	24.8	46.6	69.0	100.8	157.5	211.8	277.3	318.7	399.5	361.0	305.3	65.6		6.20	10.00	87.1	ALL
All sites but 173	702	1	3.9	0.9	4.9	9.3	11.1	24.8	46.6	69.0	100.8	157.5	209.1	277.3	303.7	394.6	361.0	299.0	64.8	100.0	6.10	9.89	86.0	ALLb

| Rate from 1 case | | | 0.985 | 0.941 | 0.824 | 0.779 | 0.796 | 0.918 | 1.260 | 1.534 | 1.938 | 2.045 | 2.681 | 3.225 | 3.749 | 4.932 | 6.684 | 6.361 |

†Important: see notes on population page

Israel

The Israel Cancer Registry, founded in 1960, is a national population/tumour-based registry. Its mission is to keep a dynamic national database for cancer incidence and mortality, to provide information regarding incidence and mortality, trends and survival to support health policy determination and to participate in the evaluation of technologies and treatments. It also functions as part of the Israel Centre for Disease Control. The legal basis for reporting to the registry was established by Public Health Ordinance Amendment in 1982, which made notification of cancer cases mandatory.

The registry's staff consists of a medical and administrative director, a registration medical director (chief abstractor), a chief statistician, three medical record librarians, four medical secretaries, one part-time archivist, part-time medical students in statistics and medical registration, and an abstractor for quality control.

Population data by sex and five-year age group are available from censuses in 1961, 1972 and 1983, and as yearly intercensus estimates. The data of the last census in 1996 are being analysed. In 1995, the population of Israel was 5 339 300 (2 675 800 males and 2 723 500 females). The Jewish population constitutes the large majority (80%); the non-Jewish population comprises Moslems, Christians and Druze. Among the Jewish population, 60% are Israel-born, and the rest born in the USA or Europe (25%) or in Asia or Africa (15%). In the period 1990–93 approximately 700 000 people migrated from the former Soviet Union to Israel. Cultural and possible genetic differences between the various population groups are reflected in wide differences in cancer incidence.

The population is relatively young compared with those of other European countries, with marked differences in age structure between the Jewish and non-Jewish populations. However, the proportion of children under 15 years declined during the last 25 years, while the proportion of people aged 65 and over nearly doubled.

An identity number assigned to each person in Israel upon birth or immigration is used on medical documents, facilitating identification of registered patients and linkage with other information, such as occupational rosters.

The registry relies mainly on passive registration, using existing records, such as copies of hospital case summaries, pathological, cytological and haematological reports, death certificates, oncology reports, etc. Computer files from oncological departments are also available from 1994 and are being used to complete the database. Passive follow-up is possible through the population register, by updated linkage to the mortality and immigration files. Efforts are being made to increase active registration and medical abstractors visited all the private pathological laboratories throughout the country to retrieve cases that had not been reported. The completeness of the data in the registry is estimated to be over 90%.

Demographic data recorded include: family, given and father's names, family soundex, personal identity number, gender, date of birth, residence status; for immigrants, country of birth and year of immigration, or, for younger Israel-born (0–29 years old), parent's country of origin, and country and hospital of tumour diagnosis. Medical data recorded are: date and place of diagnosis, basis of diagnosis, tumour site and morphology (including behaviour code), clinical stage of disease at diagnosis, laterality of tumour, treatment (radiological, surgical and chemotherapy), date, place and cause of death. Medical information is coded according to ICD-9 and ICD-O for morphology. The whole file is SEER-compatible.

Quality control is made primarily by a basic set of logical computerized checks, systematic search for duplicates, and routine follow-up and updating. Data are processed by an on-line system with the master file, allowing for continual checking of new cases, recurrence of former cases, multiple primary tumours and passive follow-up. A multi-purpose retrieval program is used for printing out part of the file, and for counts of cases and tabulations.

The percentage of registered cases based on death certificates only is 3.4%. This source of information provides information mainly on pancreatic and lung cancer, as survival time in these cases is rather short.

Outputting data from public or medical databases which includes personal information or identifiers is forbidden by law. In studies using the registry's data, researchers cannot have personal information on patients. In case there is a need to verify some of the information, this is done by the registry's director or staff. Contacting patients or their families is possible only through the patient's physician who must obtain the patient's consent.

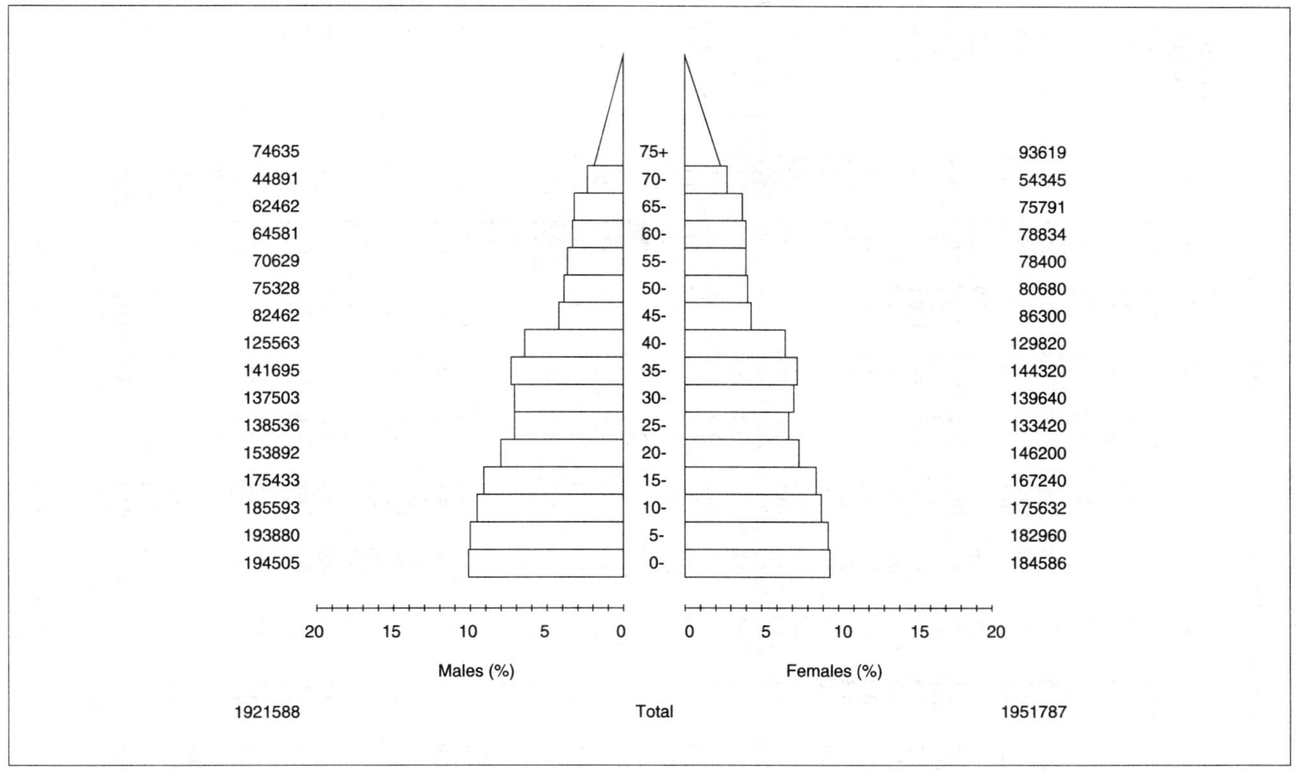

Israel: All Jews
Source of population: average annual 1988–92
Estimate: The Population Register has recorded details of each Israeli citizen (born in Israel or immigrant), with their personal identity number. It is continuously updated for births and deaths, immigration and emigration, and changes of address, civil status or names. Annual population estimates from the Population Register are published by the Central Bureau of Statistics.

ISRAEL: ALL JEWS 1988-1992

ANNUAL INCIDENCE PER 100,000 BY AGE GROUP (YEARS) - MALE

SITE	ALL AGES	AGE UNK	0-	5-	10-	15-	20-	25-	30-	35-	40-	45-	50-	55-	60-	65-	70-	75+	CRUDE RATE	%	CR 64	CR 74	ASR (W)	ICD (9th)
Lip	359	0	0.1	-	-	-	0.3	0.7	1.2	3.1	4.8	5.3	4.5	7.1	9.3	15.4	21.4	27.1	3.7	1.3	0.18	0.37	3.3	140
Tongue	79	0	-	-	-	-	-	-	-	0.4	0.8	1.0	1.6	3.1	2.5	4.2	4.9	4.8	0.8	0.3	0.05	0.09	0.8	141
Salivary gland	81	0	0.1	0.3	-	0.1	-	-	-	1.3	0.6	0.5	2.1	0.8	1.9	3.8	4.9	5.6	0.8	0.3	0.04	0.08	0.7	142
Mouth	82	0	-	0.1	-	0.1	0.1	-	0.1	0.1	0.8	1.0	1.3	3.1	3.1	2.6	4.9	6.2	0.9	0.3	0.05	0.09	0.8	143-5
Oropharynx	26	0	-	-	-	-	-	-	-	-	-	0.5	0.3	0.6	2.2	1.0	1.3	2.1	0.3	0.1	0.02	0.03	0.3	146
Nasopharynx	102	3	0.1	-	0.2	0.6	0.1	0.3	0.6	1.0	2.4	1.5	3.5	3.1	2.8	3.5	2.2	1.9	1.1	0.4	0.08	0.11	1.1	147
Hypopharynx	25	0	-	-	-	-	-	0.1	-	0.1	0.2	0.2	0.5	0.6	-	1.0	1.8	2.7	0.3	0.1	0.01	0.02	0.2	148
Pharynx unspecified	7	0	-	-	-	-	-	-	-	0.1	-	-	0.5	-	0.3	-	0.9	0.3	0.1	0.0	0.00	0.01	0.1	149
Oesophagus	215	0	-	-	-	-	-	0.1	-	0.3	0.6	1.0	1.1	2.3	4.6	9.9	15.6	29.7	2.2	0.8	0.05	0.18	1.7	150
Stomach	1563	6	-	0.2	-	-	-	0.4	1.2	2.1	4.8	9.5	16.2	25.2	51.1	72.0	106.0	182.8	16.3	5.8	0.56	1.45	13.0	151
Small intestine	73	1	-	-	-	-	-	0.1	0.1	0.1	0.8	1.2	1.3	2.0	3.4	2.2	4.5	5.1	0.8	0.3	0.05	0.08	0.7	152
Colon	3039	5	-	-	0.1	-	0.5	0.9	1.5	3.2	6.8	13.6	22.8	49.6	88.9	159.1	233.9	354.0	31.6	11.3	0.94	2.91	24.9	153
Rectum	1675	7	-	-	-	-	0.1	0.3	0.3	1.7	6.5	10.9	17.8	35.7	58.2	89.0	117.2	172.3	17.4	6.2	0.66	1.70	14.4	154
Liver	365	0	0.2	-	-	-	-	0.1	0.3	0.7	1.0	0.7	3.2	6.2	15.2	25.6	34.3	28.4	3.8	1.4	0.14	0.44	3.2	155
Gallbladder etc.	190	0	-	-	-	-	-	0.1	-	0.3	0.3	0.5	2.7	5.1	4.3	8.3	12.0	23.6	2.0	0.7	0.07	0.17	1.5	156
Pancreas	865	5	-	-	-	-	-	0.3	0.9	1.0	1.0	5.6	9.6	19.5	20.4	47.4	62.8	95.4	9.0	3.2	0.29	0.85	7.2	157
Nose, sinuses etc.	39	0	-	0.1	-	0.2	0.3	-	-	-	0.3	0.5	0.3	0.8	1.9	1.9	2.2	2.4	0.4	0.1	0.02	0.04	0.4	160
Larynx	489	0	-	-	-	0.1	-	-	-	0.4	2.1	3.4	10.1	17.6	27.9	29.5	29.4	29.5	5.1	1.8	0.31	0.60	4.7	161
Bronchus, lung	2925	13	-	0.1	-	0.1	-	0.6	0.9	3.5	9.1	24.0	42.7	86.9	133.8	173.5	195.6	224.6	30.4	10.9	1.52	3.37	27.0	162
Other thoracic organs	48	0	0.5	-	-	0.2	-	0.4	0.1	0.4	0.2	1.0	1.9	0.3	0.3	2.2	1.8	2.4	0.5	0.2	0.03	0.05	0.5	163-4
Bone	144	0	0.2	0.4	1.8	2.4	1.8	1.0	1.3	1.1	1.4	2.2	0.8	2.0	0.9	3.2	4.0	3.2	1.5	0.5	0.09	0.12	1.4	170
Connective tissue	288	0	1.4	0.2	0.8	1.3	0.9	0.9	1.3	3.0	3.0	5.3	4.2	5.1	7.4	9.3	10.2	16.1	3.0	1.1	0.17	0.27	2.8	171
Mesothelioma	47	0	-	-	-	-	-	-	0.3	-	0.5	0.2	0.5	2.3	2.5	1.6	3.1	2.9	0.5	0.2	0.03	0.06	0.4	MES
Kaposi's sarcoma	320	0	-	-	0.1	0.3	0.6	1.7	1.7	1.0	2.4	2.7	5.9	8.7	11.8	19.6	35.6	3.3	1.2	0.13	0.28	2.7	KAP	
Melanoma of skin	946	1	-	0.2	1.1	1.7	4.0	6.7	12.1	16.4	22.3	20.2	23.2	29.1	35.5	30.7	35.6	9.8	3.5	0.69	1.02	9.5	172	
Other skin	324	1	-	0.1	0.1	0.1	0.9	0.7	1.2	1.4	3.3	4.9	4.5	5.1	8.7	15.4	14.3	28.4	3.4		0.16	0.30	2.9	173
Breast	130	0	-	-	-	-	-	0.1	0.3	0.4	1.1	1.7	1.3	2.5	5.9	5.8	7.6	11.3	1.4	0.5	0.07	0.13	1.2	175
Prostate	3147	3	0.1	-	-	0.1	-	-	0.3	-	0.3	1.9	9.0	28.3	71.8	169.4	279.3	430.9	32.8	11.7	0.56	2.81	23.9	185
Testis	294	0	0.1	-	0.2	1.3	6.2	5.5	8.3	5.2	6.5	4.4	2.1	2.3	2.8	1.6	2.2	1.6	3.1	1.1	0.22	0.24	3.0	186
Penis	6	0	-	-	-	-	-	-	-	0.1	-	-	-	0.3	-	0.3	0.9	0.3	0.1	0.0	0.00	0.01	0.1	187.1-.4
Other male genital	17	0	0.1	0.1	-	0.1	-	-	-	-	-	0.2	-	0.6	0.9	-	0.4	1.9	0.2	0.1	0.01	0.01	0.2	187.5-.9
Bladder	2897	4	0.1	-	-	0.6	0.1	0.4	2.3	4.0	7.8	14.6	30.3	60.3	115.2	171.6	199.6	280.6	30.2	10.8	1.18	3.04	25.1	188
Kidney etc.	1143	2	1.0	0.1	-	-	-	0.6	0.9	2.8	5.9	7.8	13.5	30.0	44.0	67.6	89.1	86.0	11.9	4.3	0.53	1.32	10.4	189
Eye	83	0	1.0	0.1	0.1	-	-	-	-	0.6	0.8	1.2	0.5	2.0	2.5	3.8	2.7	5.9	0.9	0.3	0.04	0.08	0.8	190
Brain, nervous system	569	3	2.7	3.1	1.9	2.2	2.9	2.5	3.2	4.5	4.1	7.3	11.4	15.3	15.5	20.5	23.2	16.3	5.9	2.1	0.38	0.60	5.8	191-2
Thyroid	268	0	0.1	0.2	0.4	0.3	1.2	1.9	2.8	2.4	4.0	7.0	5.8	4.2	8.1	9.6	8.9	8.8	2.8	1.0	0.19	0.28	2.7	193
Other endocrine	45	0	1.4	0.4	0.2	-	-	0.3	-	-	0.6	0.7	0.3	0.6	0.6	1.9	1.3	0.5	0.5	0.2	0.03	0.04	0.5	194
Hodgkin's disease	284	0	0.3	0.8	1.2	3.6	5.2	4.3	3.3	4.7	4.3	4.9	4.0	1.4	3.4	3.2	1.8	3.2	3.0	1.1	0.21	0.23	2.9	201
Non-Hodgkin lymphoma	1336	2	1.5	3.0	1.7	2.4	2.1	3.3	4.4	7.9	12.3	14.3	21.2	33.1	47.1	56.7	61.0	88.2	13.9	5.0	0.77	1.36	12.6	200,202
Multiple myeloma	287	1	-	-	-	-	-	-	0.3	1.6	0.2	1.0	2.7	5.4	10.5	11.5	25.4	30.0	3.0	1.1	0.11	0.29	2.4	203
Lymphoid leukaemia	382	2	2.3	2.5	1.4	2.2	1.3	0.4	0.7	0.7	1.9	1.5	4.8	5.7	12.1	10.9	20.9	27.6	4.0	1.4	0.19	0.35	3.5	204
Myeloid leukaemia	289	2	0.7	0.4	1.0	1.0	0.6	1.0	2.0	2.0	2.1	3.6	3.5	5.4	7.7	10.6	12.5	19.3	3.0	1.1	0.16	0.27	2.7	205
Monocytic leukaemia	29	1	-	-	0.1	0.1	0.1	-	0.1	-	0.5	0.5	-	0.8	0.6	0.3	1.3	2.7	0.3	0.1	0.02	0.02	0.3	206
Other leukaemia	19	0	-	-	-	-	-	-	0.1	-	0.2	-	-	0.8	0.3	0.6	0.9	2.4	0.2	0.1	0.01	0.01	0.1	207
Leukaemia unspecified	86	0	0.2	0.2	0.2	-	0.1	-	0.3	0.1	1.1	0.2	1.9	0.6	2.5	2.2	2.7	10.2	0.9	0.3	0.04	0.06	0.7	208
Other and unspecified	1589	5	0.8	0.2	0.1	0.2	0.1	1.0	1.5	1.4	5.4	11.4	20.2	37.7	48.9	64.7	108.7	173.9	16.5	5.9	0.65	1.52	13.5	O&U
All sites	27216	67	15.2	12.7	11.9	20.6	27.0	33.2	50.5	77.8	127.7	203.2	309.3	550.5	889.7	1341.9	1790.1	2524.3	283.3		11.68	27.37	238.6	ALL
All sites but 173	26892	66	15.2	12.6	11.7	20.5	26.1	32.5	49.3	76.4	124.4	198.4	304.8	545.4	881.1	1326.6	1775.8	2495.9	279.9	100.0	11.52	27.07	235.7	ALLb

Rate from 10 cases   1.028 1.032 1.078 1.140 1.300 1.444 1.455 1.411 1.593 2.425 2.655 2.832 3.097 3.202 4.455 2.680

ISRAEL: ALL JEWS 1988-1992

ANNUAL INCIDENCE PER 100,000 BY AGE GROUP (YEARS) - FEMALE

SITE	ALL AGES	AGE UNK	0-	5-	10-	15-	20-	25-	30-	35-	40-	45-	50-	55-	60-	65-	70-	75+	CRUDE RATE	%	CR 64	CR 74	ASR (W)	ICD (9th)
Lip	122	0	-	-	-	-	0.1	-	0.3	0.8	0.9	1.4	1.0	1.5	3.0	4.0	6.3	10.0	1.3	0.4	0.05	0.10	0.9	140
Tongue	78	0	-	-	-	-	-	-	0.1	0.3	0.3	0.9	1.2	1.0	1.8	2.4	6.6	5.6	0.8	0.3	0.03	0.07	0.6	141
Salivary gland	67	0	-	-	0.1	0.1	0.1	0.4	0.4	-	0.9	0.7	1.0	1.3	1.5	0.8	2.6	5.1	0.7	0.2	0.03	0.05	0.5	142
Mouth	77	0	-	-	0.1	-	0.3	-	0.1	0.3	0.6	0.2	1.2	1.3	2.0	2.4	2.2	7.0	0.8	0.3	0.03	0.05	0.6	143-5
Oropharynx	10	0	-	-	-	0.1	-	-	-	-	0.2	-	0.2	-	0.3	0.3	1.1	0.4	0.1	0.0	0.00	0.01	0.1	146
Nasopharynx	45	0	-	0.1	0.3	0.1	0.1	-	-	0.8	0.5	1.2	0.5	1.0	1.0	2.1	0.4	1.3	0.5	0.2	0.03	0.04	0.4	147
Hypopharynx	5	0	-	-	-	-	-	-	-	-	-	-	-	-	-	0.5	0.4	0.4	0.1	0.0	0.00	0.00	0.0	148
Pharynx unspecified	0	0	-	-	-	-	-	-	-	-	-	-	-	-	-	-	-	-	0.0	0.0	0.00	0.00	0.0	149
Oesophagus	158	1	-	-	-	-	-	-	0.3	0.3	0.5	0.7	2.0	3.8	5.3	12.9	15.0	1.6	0.5	0.04	0.13	1.1	150	
Stomach	884	5	-	0.1	-	-	0.1	0.4	1.1	1.2	3.2	5.3	9.2	12.0	22.6	38.5	42.3	81.0	9.1	3.0	0.28	0.69	6.2	151
Small intestine	59	0	-	-	-	-	-	-	0.1	0.1	0.3	0.9	0.5	2.0	1.8	2.4	4.0	3.0	0.6	0.2	0.03	0.06	0.5	152
Colon	2778	10	-	-	-	0.5	0.4	1.0	2.4	3.2	8.3	13.0	31.0	50.3	79.2	116.4	159.7	233.9	28.5	9.5	0.95	2.34	19.9	153
Rectum	1532	6	-	-	-	0.1	0.1	0.7	1.4	2.4	6.6	10.2	21.3	26.8	45.7	60.2	94.2	117.5	15.7	5.3	0.58	1.35	11.4	154
Liver	224	1	0.3	-	-	0.2	-	-	0.1	0.1	0.6	0.7	1.7	1.8	8.1	9.5	15.1	18.4	2.3	0.8	0.07	0.19	1.6	155
Gallbladder etc.	354	1	-	-	-	-	-	-	-	-	0.6	0.9	3.0	5.4	7.6	17.7	23.9	32.0	3.6	1.2	0.09	0.30	2.4	156
Pancreas	816	2	-	0.1	-	-	-	0.1	-	0.3	0.4	1.4	4.6	7.2	12.2	20.3	33.5	51.9	75.4	8.4	2.8	0.23	0.66	5.7	157
Nose, sinuses etc.	44	0	0.1	-	-	-	-	-	-	0.3	-	0.7	0.2	1.8	0.8	1.1	3.3	3.0	0.5	0.2	0.02	0.04	0.3	160
Larynx	91	0	-	-	-	-	-	-	-	0.3	0.9	0.9	1.0	3.3	3.3	4.5	3.7	4.7	0.9	0.3	0.05	0.09	0.7	161
Bronchus, lung	1210	3	0.2	-	-	0.1	0.3	0.4	0.4	1.4	4.5	9.7	11.9	29.6	41.4	55.9	67.0	84.2	12.4	4.2	0.50	1.12	9.2	162
Other thoracic organs	39	0	0.3	-	0.1	0.1	0.1	0.3	0.3	0.6	0.5	0.5	0.2	0.5	1.0	1.3	1.1	1.1	0.4	0.1	0.02	0.03	0.4	163-4
Bone	106	0	-	0.4	1.1	1.6	0.7	1.3	0.6	0.4	0.6	1.6	1.5	1.5	0.8	1.8	2.6	3.8	1.1	0.4	0.06	0.08	1.0	170
Connective tissue	258	0	1.3	0.5	0.5	1.4	0.8	0.6	2.0	1.2	2.9	2.5	4.7	4.1	3.3	7.9	8.1	13.2	2.6	0.9	0.13	0.21	2.2	171
Mesothelioma	21	0	-	-	-	-	-	-	-	-	0.2	0.2	-	0.8	0.8	1.3	1.1	1.1	0.2	0.1	0.01	0.02	0.2	MES
Kaposi's sarcoma	128	0	-	-	-	0.1	0.1	0.3	-	-	0.5	0.2	0.5	1.8	1.3	5.3	5.9	15.0	1.3	0.4	0.02	0.08	0.8	KAP
Melanoma of skin	1075	1	-	-	0.7	1.4	3.3	6.4	9.2	15.7	19.4	21.6	20.6	20.9	25.9	24.3	32.8	31.0	11.0	3.7	0.73	1.01	9.8	172
Other skin	349	0	-	-	0.2	0.5	0.5	0.4	1.1	2.2	3.9	4.9	5.5	5.6	8.4	13.2	12.1	22.6	3.6		0.17	0.29	2.8	173
Breast	8628	16	-	-	-	-	1.1	4.9	28.2	62.4	130.0	201.4	207.2	225.3	257.8	307.2	316.9	310.0	88.4	29.6	5.60	8.73	77.4	174
Uterus unspecified	75	0	-	-	-	-	-	0.1	0.1	0.8	0.3	1.2	1.7	2.0	2.0	3.4	1.1	4.5	0.8	0.3	0.04	0.06	0.6	179
Cervix uteri	554	4	-	-	-	0.4	0.8	2.5	6.6	8.6	9.9	16.2	12.1	11.7	12.7	12.9	13.6	10.9	5.7	1.9	0.41	0.54	5.3	180
Placenta	6	0	-	-	-	-	-	0.1	-	0.1	0.2	0.2	0.5	-	-	-	-	-	0.1	0.0	0.01	0.01	0.1	181
Corpus uteri	1246	4	-	-	-	-	0.1	0.6	1.3	1.7	7.5	13.2	32.7	45.7	49.7	60.4	54.1	48.5	12.8	4.3	0.77	1.34	10.8	182
Ovary etc.	1299	8	0.1	0.2	0.3	0.8	2.1	2.2	2.0	5.4	14.3	25.7	25.5	41.1	49.2	47.8	46.7	48.1	13.3	4.5	0.85	1.33	11.6	183
Other female genital	220	1	0.1	-	0.1	0.2	0.1	0.4	0.3	0.3	0.8	1.2	2.2	1.8	5.1	10.0	13.6	18.4	2.3	0.8	0.06	0.18	1.6	184
Bladder	723	2	0.1	-	0.1	0.4	-	0.6	1.1	1.2	1.4	4.4	8.4	13.3	18.5	32.7	39.7	59.0	7.4	2.5	0.25	0.61	5.3	188
Kidney etc.	672	1	1.1	0.7	0.1	-	0.1	0.3	0.7	1.0	2.2	6.3	9.7	13.3	23.6	35.9	35.7	38.7	6.9	2.3	0.30	0.65	5.4	189
Eye	80	0	1.3	0.2	0.1	-	0.1	0.1	0.1	0.6	0.3	0.2	0.5	2.3	1.8	1.8	3.7	4.3	0.8	0.3	0.04	0.07	0.7	190
Brain, nervous system	463	0	2.7	3.4	1.3	1.6	1.5	2.2	2.7	3.3	4.6	4.4	4.7	9.9	9.9	19.0	12.5	13.2	4.7	1.6	0.26	0.42	4.2	191-2
Thyroid	804	0	-	0.1	0.8	3.0	5.7	6.6	8.5	12.3	14.9	14.1	15.4	19.9	18.8	17.4	13.2	13.5	8.2	2.8	0.60	0.75	7.7	193
Other endocrine	45	0	1.3	0.3	0.1	0.1	0.1	0.4	0.1	0.3	0.6	0.2	0.7	1.0	0.8	0.5	0.4	0.6	0.5	0.2	0.03	0.04	0.5	194
Hodgkin's disease	284	0	-	0.2	1.6	3.3	8.1	5.5	5.6	3.3	2.8	2.3	1.5	1.8	2.0	2.1	2.9	3.4	2.9	1.0	0.19	0.22	2.8	201
Non-Hodgkin lymphoma	1273	6	1.4	1.3	1.1	1.1	2.6	2.7	4.2	4.9	10.8	12.7	20.3	26.0	34.0	47.5	57.0	73.5	13.0	4.4	0.62	1.14	10.4	200,202
Multiple myeloma	258	2	-	-	-	-	-	-	0.1	0.4	0.9	3.5	3.5	5.4	5.8	11.6	13.6	19.7	2.6	0.9	0.10	0.23	1.9	203
Lymphoid leukaemia	268	0	1.6	2.2	1.3	1.1	0.7	0.1	0.3	0.4	-	0.9	1.7	2.6	4.6	6.6	8.5	24.6	2.7	0.9	0.09	0.16	2.0	204
Myeloid leukaemia	250	1	0.3	0.5	0.2	0.6	0.7	1.6	1.7	1.5	1.7	3.2	5.0	5.1	5.6	4.0	11.0	13.5	2.6	0.9	0.14	0.22	2.1	205
Monocytic leukaemia	25	0	0.2	0.1	-	0.1	-	0.4	-	0.1	0.2	-	-	0.5	0.8	0.8	1.1	1.1	0.3	0.1	0.01	0.02	0.2	206
Other leukaemia	5	0	-	-	-	-	-	-	-	0.1	-	-	-	-	0.3	0.5	-	0.2	0.1	0.0	0.00	0.00	0.0	207
Leukaemia unspecified	73	1	0.1	-	-	0.1	-	0.1	-	0.1	0.3	0.5	0.2	1.8	1.0	2.9	2.9	7.0	0.7	0.3	0.02	0.05	0.5	208
Other and unspecified	1675	7	0.9	0.4	0.1	0.4	0.3	1.6	1.9	2.5	5.5	10.4	16.1	20.7	36.5	68.3	85.4	159.4	17.2	5.8	0.49	1.26	11.7	O&U
All sites	29456	83	13.5	11.0	10.5	19.6	31.6	46.3	85.8	143.4	267.3	405.8	495.8	639.5	825.8	1105.9	1295.1	1657.6	301.8		15.02	27.06	242.1	ALL
All sites but 173	29107	83	13.5	11.0	10.2	19.1	31.1	45.9	84.6	141.2	263.4	400.9	490.3	633.9	817.4	1092.7	1282.9	1634.9	298.3	100.0	14.86	26.77	239.3	ALLb

Rate from 10 cases: 1.084 1.093 1.139 1.196 1.368 1.499 1.432 1.386 1.541 2.317 2.479 2.551 2.537 2.639 3.680 2.136

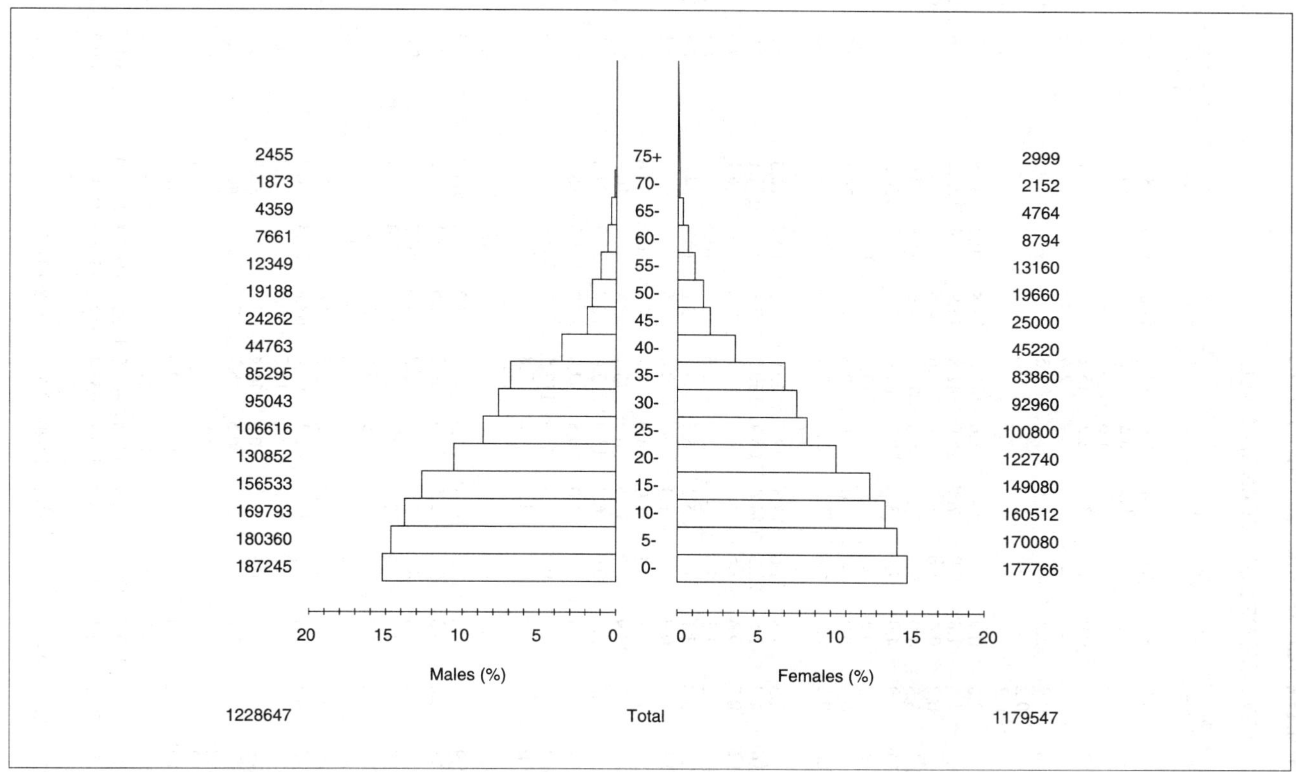

Israel: Jews Born in Israel
Source of population: average annual 1988–92
Estimate: The Population Register has recorded details of each Israeli citizen (born in Israel or immigrant), with their personal identity number. It is continuously updated for births and deaths, immigration and emigration, and changes of address, civil status or names. Annual population estimates from the Population Register are published by the Central Bureau of Statistics.

ISRAEL: JEWS BORN IN ISRAEL 1988-1992

ANNUAL INCIDENCE PER 100,000 BY AGE GROUP (YEARS) - MALE

SITE	ALL AGES	AGE UNK	0-	5-	10-	15-	20-	25-	30-	35-	40-	45-	50-	55-	60-	65-	70-	75+	CRUDE RATE	%	CR 64	CR 74	ASR (W)	ICD (9th)
Lip	88	0	0.1	-	-	-	0.3	0.6	1.1	3.5	8.5	6.6	9.4	13.0	13.1	41.3	32.0	8.1	1.4	2.4	0.28	0.65	**4.8**	*140*
Tongue	13	0	-	-	-	-	-	-	-	-	1.3	-	1.0	6.5	5.2	-	10.7	16.3	0.2	0.3	0.07	0.12	**1.1**	*141*
Salivary gland	12	0	0.1	0.3	-	0.1	-	-	-	0.9	-	-	2.1	1.6	-	-	-	-	0.2	0.3	0.03	0.03	**0.3**	*142*
Mouth	15	0	-	0.1	-	0.1	-	-	0.2	-	0.9	-	3.1	3.2	5.2	-	-	24.4	0.2	0.4	0.06	0.06	**1.1**	*143-5*
Oropharynx	1	0	-	-	-	-	-	-	-	-	-	-	-	-	2.6	-	-	-	0.0	0.0	0.01	0.01	**0.1**	*146*
Nasopharynx	27	0	0.1	-	0.1	0.6	0.2	0.4	0.8	0.9	2.2	-	3.1	-	2.6	-	-	-	0.4	0.7	0.06	0.06	**0.6**	*147*
Hypopharynx	3	0	-	-	-	-	-	0.2	-	0.2	-	-	1.0	-	-	-	-	-	0.0	0.1	0.01	0.01	**0.1**	*148*
Pharynx unspecified	1	0	-	-	-	-	-	-	-	0.2	-	-	-	-	-	-	-	-	0.0	0.0	0.00	0.00	**0.0**	*149*
Oesophagus	17	0	-	-	-	-	-	0.2	-	0.5	0.9	-	-	1.6	7.8	13.8	10.7	32.6	0.3	0.5	0.06	0.18	**1.8**	*150*
Stomach	101	1	-	0.2	-	-	-	0.2	1.1	1.6	1.8	9.9	7.3	25.9	41.8	45.9	53.4	122.2	1.6	2.7	0.45	0.95	**8.9**	*151*
Small intestine	7	0	-	-	-	-	-	-	-	0.2	0.4	1.6	1.0	-	2.6	4.6	-	-	0.1	0.2	0.03	0.05	**0.4**	*152*
Colon	230	1	-	-	0.1	-	0.5	0.9	1.3	3.5	4.0	9.9	27.1	45.3	73.1	137.6	341.6	277.0	3.7	6.2	0.83	3.24	**23.9**	*153*
Rectum	119	1	-	-	-	-	0.2	0.2	0.4	1.9	4.0	4.9	13.5	29.2	67.9	64.2	42.7	130.3	1.9	3.2	0.62	1.16	**10.7**	*154*
Liver	18	0	0.2	-	-	-	-	0.2	0.4	0.5	0.4	-	-	3.2	13.1	4.6	10.7	8.1	0.3	0.5	0.09	0.17	**1.3**	*155*
Gallbladder etc.	14	0	-	-	-	-	-	0.2	-	0.5	0.9	-	1.0	4.9	2.6	4.6	-	24.4	0.2	0.4	0.05	0.07	**1.1**	*156*
Pancreas	74	1	-	-	-	-	-	0.4	0.6	0.5	0.9	5.8	7.3	22.7	26.1	50.5	32.0	97.8	1.2	2.0	0.33	0.74	**7.0**	*157*
Nose, sinuses etc.	6	0	-	0.1	-	0.1	0.3	-	-	-	-	-	-	1.6	-	-	10.7	-	0.1	0.2	0.01	0.06	**0.3**	*160*
Larynx	46	0	-	-	-	0.1	-	-	-	0.5	1.8	1.6	7.3	22.7	20.9	22.9	10.7	16.3	0.7	1.2	0.27	0.44	**3.6**	*161*
Bronchus, lung	279	4	-	0.1	-	0.1	-	0.6	0.6	4.2	12.5	22.3	44.8	66.4	130.5	123.9	128.1	171.1	4.5	7.5	1.43	2.71	**22.6**	*162*
Other thoracic organs	20	0	0.5	-	-	0.3	-	0.4	0.2	0.7	0.4	1.6	1.0	-	-	9.2	-	8.1	0.3	0.5	0.03	0.07	**0.8**	*163-4*
Bone	79	0	0.2	0.4	1.8	2.6	2.0	1.1	1.3	1.2	1.3	2.5	-	-	2.6	-	10.7	-	1.3	2.1	0.08	0.14	**1.4**	*170*
Connective tissue	97	0	1.5	0.2	0.7	1.3	1.1	0.9	1.5	3.0	3.1	7.4	5.2	6.5	5.2	9.2	10.7	24.4	1.6	2.6	0.19	0.29	**3.2**	*171*
Mesothelioma	6	0	-	-	-	-	-	-	0.2	-	0.9	-	1.0	-	2.6	4.6	-	-	0.1	0.2	0.02	0.05	**0.4**	*MES*
Kaposi's sarcoma	45	0	-	-	-	0.1	0.3	0.6	2.3	1.4	1.3	4.1	1.0	4.9	7.8	9.2	10.7	32.6	0.7	1.2	0.12	0.22	**2.3**	*KAP*
Melanoma of skin	375	0	-	-	0.2	1.1	1.7	4.1	7.4	14.1	25.9	43.7	52.1	56.7	73.1	63.3	-	16.3	6.1	10.0	1.40	1.63	**15.6**	*172*
Other skin	68	0	-	0.1	0.1	-	0.8	0.6	1.3	1.6	3.6	9.9	6.3	11.3	7.8	18.4	21.3	24.4	1.1	-	0.22	0.42	**3.7**	*173*
Breast	22	0	-	-	-	-	-	0.2	0.2	0.2	0.4	3.3	1.0	6.5	7.8	9.2	21.3	16.3	0.4	0.6	0.10	0.25	**1.9**	*175*
Prostate	237	0	0.1	-	-	0.1	-	-	0.2	-	-	0.8	6.3	35.6	117.5	252.3	362.9	578.4	3.9	6.4	0.80	3.88	**32.9**	*185*
Testis	178	0	0.1	-	0.2	1.3	6.1	5.6	8.0	5.6	8.0	4.9	4.2	3.2	7.8	-	-	-	2.9	4.8	0.28	0.28	**3.3**	*186*
Penis	0	0	-	-	-	-	-	-	-	-	-	-	-	-	-	-	-	-	0.0	0.0	0.00	0.00	**0.0**	*187.1-.4*
Other male genital	4	0	0.1	0.1	-	0.1	-	-	-	-	-	0.8	-	-	-	-	-	-	0.1	0.1	0.01	0.01	**0.1**	*187.5-.9*
Bladder	255	0	0.1	-	-	0.4	0.2	0.6	1.9	3.0	7.6	17.3	35.4	61.5	99.2	165.2	170.8	203.7	4.2	6.8	1.14	2.82	**22.5**	*188*
Kidney etc.	129	0	1.1	0.1	-	-	-	0.6	0.8	3.0	6.3	9.1	12.5	24.3	39.2	82.6	53.4	65.2	2.1	3.5	0.48	1.16	**9.3**	*189*
Eye	26	0	1.0	0.1	0.1	-	-	-	-	0.2	1.3	4.1	2.1	-	5.2	4.6	10.7	-	0.4	0.7	0.07	0.15	**1.1**	*190*
Brain, nervous system	208	0	2.7	3.1	1.9	2.2	3.1	2.3	2.5	4.7	4.0	8.2	12.5	17.8	23.5	13.8	32.0	8.1	3.4	5.6	0.44	0.67	**6.1**	*191-2*
Thyroid	85	0	0.1	0.2	0.5	0.4	1.1	2.1	2.7	1.6	4.9	7.4	6.3	4.9	7.8	22.9	-	-	1.4	2.3	0.20	0.31	**2.9**	*193*
Other endocrine	23	0	1.5	0.4	0.1	-	-	0.2	-	-	0.4	-	-	-	2.6	-	10.7	-	0.4	0.6	0.03	0.08	**0.6**	*194*
Hodgkin's disease	169	0	0.3	0.9	1.1	3.6	5.0	5.3	4.0	4.5	1.8	7.4	5.2	1.6	2.6	4.6	-	8.1	2.8	4.5	0.22	0.24	**3.2**	*201*
Non-Hodgkin lymphoma	312	1	1.5	3.0	1.6	2.7	1.8	4.1	4.2	6.8	13.4	19.8	25.0	42.1	60.0	68.8	85.4	16.3	5.1	8.4	0.93	1.71	**13.5**	*200,202*
Multiple myeloma	32	0	-	-	-	-	-	-	0.4	1.2	-	0.8	4.2	3.2	15.7	36.7	21.3	16.3	0.5	0.9	0.13	0.42	**3.0**	*203*
Lymphoid leukaemia	111	1	2.0	2.4	1.4	2.2	1.1	0.6	0.8	0.9	1.8	0.8	4.2	6.5	10.4	13.8	-	16.3	1.8	3.0	0.18	0.25	**2.9**	*204*
Myeloid leukaemia	77	2	0.6	0.3	0.8	0.9	0.6	0.6	1.7	1.6	3.1	3.3	4.2	6.5	5.2	9.2	21.3	40.7	1.3	2.1	0.15	0.31	**3.2**	*205*
Monocytic leukaemia	4	0	-	-	-	-	0.2	-	0.2	-	-	0.8	-	1.6	-	-	-	-	0.1	0.1	0.01	0.01	**0.1**	*206*
Other leukaemia	3	0	-	-	-	-	-	-	0.2	-	-	-	-	-	-	4.6	-	8.1	0.0	0.1	0.00	0.02	**0.3**	*207*
Leukaemia unspecified	14	0	0.2	0.2	0.2	-	0.2	-	0.2	0.2	0.4	-	1.0	-	2.6	-	-	16.3	0.2	0.4	0.03	0.03	**0.6**	*208*
Other and unspecified	150	0	0.9	0.2	0.1	0.1	0.2	0.8	1.5	1.4	5.8	9.9	22.9	38.9	41.8	32.1	21.3	195.5	2.4	4.0	0.62	0.89	**11.0**	*O&U*
All sites	3800	12	15.1	12.9	11.2	20.6	26.6	34.3	50.3	76.9	136.7	230.8	342.9	581.4	963.2	1330.4	1547.7	2224.0	61.9		12.55	26.99	**235.5**	*ALL*
All sites but 173	3732	12	15.1	12.8	11.1	20.6	25.8	33.8	49.0	75.3	133.1	220.9	336.7	570.1	955.4	1312.0	1526.3	2199.6	60.7	100.0	12.34	26.58	**231.9**	*ALLb*

Rate from 1 case 0.107 0.111 0.118 0.128 0.153 0.188 0.210 0.234 0.447 0.824 1.042 1.620 2.610 4.588 10.673 8.147

ISRAEL: JEWS BORN IN ISRAEL 1988-1992

ANNUAL INCIDENCE PER 100,000 BY AGE GROUP (YEARS) - FEMALE

SITE	ALL AGES	AGE UNK	0-	5-	10-	15-	20-	25-	30-	35-	40-	45-	50-	55-	60-	65-	70-	75+	CRUDE RATE	%	CR 64	CR 74	ASR (W)	ICD (9th)
Lip	24	0	-	-	-	-	0.2	-	0.2	0.7	1.3	2.4	3.1	3.0	2.3	16.8	-	20.0	0.4	0.5	0.07	0.15	**1.6**	*140*
Tongue	9	0	-	-	-	-	-	-	0.2	0.5	-	0.8	1.0	3.0	-	8.4	-	-	0.2	0.2	0.03	0.07	**0.5**	*141*
Salivary gland	20	0	-	-	0.1	0.1	0.2	0.4	0.4	-	1.8	1.6	2.0	3.0	-	-	-	20.0	0.3	0.4	0.05	0.05	**0.9**	*142*
Mouth	14	0	-	-	0.1	-	0.2	-	0.2	0.5	0.4	-	2.0	-	2.3	-	9.3	26.7	0.2	0.3	0.03	0.08	**1.0**	*143-5*
Oropharynx	1	0	-	-	-	0.1	-	-	-	-	-	-	-	-	-	-	-	-	0.0	0.0	0.00	0.00	**0.0**	*146*
Nasopharynx	15	0	-	0.1	0.4	0.1	0.2	-	-	0.5	0.9	1.6	-	1.5	-	4.2	-	6.7	0.3	0.3	0.03	0.05	**0.6**	*147*
Hypopharynx	0	0	-	-	-	-	-	-	-	-	-	-	-	-	-	-	-	-	0.0	0.0	0.00	0.00	**0.0**	*148*
Pharynx unspecified	0	0	-	-	-	-	-	-	-	-	-	-	-	-	-	-	-	-	0.0	0.0	0.00	0.00	**0.0**	*149*
Oesophagus	12	1	-	-	-	-	-	-	-	-	0.4	-	1.0	3.0	4.5	-	-	33.3	0.2	0.2	0.05	0.05	**1.1**	*150*
Stomach	72	0	-	0.1	-	-	-	0.6	0.9	1.2	3.1	3.2	6.1	6.1	25.0	42.0	65.0	66.7	1.2	1.4	0.23	0.77	**6.0**	*151*
Small intestine	5	0	-	-	-	-	-	-	-	0.2	0.4	-	1.0	1.5	-	-	9.3	-	0.1	0.1	0.02	0.06	**0.3**	*152*
Colon	253	0	-	-	-	0.4	0.5	1.0	2.2	3.3	8.8	12.0	27.5	63.8	59.1	121.7	111.5	313.4	4.3	4.8	0.89	2.06	**20.2**	*153*
Rectum	147	2	-	-	-	-	0.2	0.2	1.3	2.4	8.0	12.8	13.2	35.0	43.2	58.8	83.6	100.0	2.5	2.8	0.59	1.31	**10.9**	*154*
Liver	15	0	0.3	-	-	0.1	-	-	-	0.2	-	-	1.0	-	4.5	12.6	27.9	6.7	0.3	0.3	0.03	0.23	**1.4**	*155*
Gallbladder etc.	11	0	-	-	-	-	-	-	-	-	0.4	1.6	1.0	4.6	2.3	-	9.3	13.3	0.2	0.2	0.05	0.10	**0.9**	*156*
Pancreas	65	0	-	0.1	-	-	-	0.2	-	0.2	0.7	1.3	5.6	11.2	16.7	15.9	25.2	55.8	53.3	1.1	1.2	0.26	0.66	**5.3**	*157*
Nose, sinuses etc.	6	0	0.1	-	-	-	-	-	-	-	-	-	6.1	-	4.2	-	-	-	0.1	0.1	0.03	0.05	**0.4**	*160*
Larynx	15	0	-	-	-	-	-	-	-	0.5	1.3	0.8	1.0	7.6	6.8	-	-	-	0.3	0.3	0.09	0.09	**0.8**	*161*
Bronchus, lung	141	0	0.2	-	-	0.1	0.2	0.4	0.4	1.4	4.4	12.8	17.3	42.6	40.9	63.0	55.8	113.3	2.4	2.7	0.60	1.20	**10.7**	*162*
Other thoracic organs	15	0	0.3	-	0.1	0.1	0.2	0.4	0.4	0.2	0.9	-	-	1.5	2.3	-	-	-	0.3	0.3	0.03	0.03	**0.4**	*163-4*
Bone	52	0	-	0.5	1.1	1.7	0.7	1.8	0.9	-	0.4	1.6	3.1	-	2.3	-	-	13.3	0.9	1.0	0.07	0.07	**1.2**	*170*
Connective tissue	62	0	1.4	0.5	0.4	1.1	0.8	0.6	2.2	1.4	1.3	1.6	1.0	3.0	-	4.2	18.6	-	1.1	1.2	0.08	0.19	**1.5**	*171*
Mesothelioma	0	0	-	-	-	-	-	-	-	-	-	-	-	-	-	-	-	-	0.0	0.0	0.00	0.00	**0.0**	*MES*
Kaposi's sarcoma	5	0	-	-	-	-	-	-	-	-	0.4	-	-	-	-	-	-	26.7	0.1	0.1	0.00	0.00	**0.6**	*KAP*
Melanoma of skin	425	0	-	-	0.5	1.3	3.4	6.5	10.5	20.5	30.1	43.2	46.8	27.4	36.4	42.0	27.9	46.7	7.2	8.1	1.13	1.48	**14.9**	*172*
Other skin	87	0	-	-	0.2	0.4	0.7	0.6	1.5	3.1	6.2	6.4	9.2	7.6	20.5	12.6	18.6	33.3	1.5		0.28	0.44	**4.2**	*173*
Breast	1802	7	-	-	-	-	1.1	5.4	27.5	58.2	150.8	247.2	231.9	300.9	311.6	377.8	297.4	360.0	30.6	34.4	6.70	10.09	**90.5**	*174*
Uterus unspecified	9	0	-	-	-	-	-	0.2	0.2	0.7	-	-	4.1	-	-	-	-	-	0.2	0.2	0.03	0.03	**0.3**	*179*
Cervix uteri	183	1	-	-	-	0.3	0.8	2.4	6.9	9.5	11.5	19.2	12.2	22.8	15.9	12.6	9.3	20.0	3.1	3.5	0.51	0.62	**6.3**	*180*
Placenta	2	0	-	-	-	-	-	0.2	-	-	-	0.8	-	-	-	-	-	-	0.0	0.0	0.00	0.00	**0.1**	*181*
Corpus uteri	202	1	-	-	-	-	0.2	0.6	1.3	1.4	8.0	16.0	43.7	36.5	63.7	92.3	74.3	146.7	3.4	3.9	0.86	1.70	**15.1**	*182*
Ovary etc.	255	2	0.1	0.2	0.4	0.9	1.8	2.6	2.4	6.2	13.3	35.2	31.5	50.2	52.3	25.2	65.0	33.3	4.3	4.9	0.99	1.45	**12.4**	*183*
Other female genital	21	0	0.1	-	0.1	0.3	0.2	0.2	0.4	0.2	-	-	1.0	1.5	6.8	8.4	46.5	-	0.4	0.4	0.05	0.33	**1.7**	*184*
Bladder	69	0	0.1	-	0.1	0.4	-	0.6	1.3	1.2	2.2	2.4	6.1	15.2	18.2	21.0	27.9	66.7	1.2	1.3	0.24	0.48	**4.7**	*188*
Kidney etc.	74	0	0.8	0.7	0.1	-	0.2	0.2	0.9	0.5	2.2	6.4	4.1	7.6	25.0	25.2	65.0	40.0	1.3	1.4	0.24	0.69	**5.2**	*189*
Eye	21	0	1.4	0.1	0.1	-	-	0.2	-	0.7	-	-	-	1.5	-	-	-	13.3	0.4	0.4	0.02	0.02	**0.6**	*190*
Brain, nervous system	161	0	2.6	3.5	1.4	1.5	1.6	2.4	2.8	2.6	4.9	3.2	7.1	10.6	6.8	12.6	9.3	26.7	2.7	3.1	0.26	0.36	**4.2**	*191-2*
Thyroid	278	0	-	0.1	0.7	3.0	5.9	5.4	8.2	13.4	15.0	10.4	15.3	22.8	20.5	4.2	9.3	26.7	4.7	5.3	0.60	0.67	**7.4**	*193*
Other endocrine	26	0	1.4	0.4	0.1	-	0.2	0.4	0.2	0.5	1.3	0.8	-	-	-	-	-	-	0.4	0.5	0.03	0.03	**0.4**	*194*
Hodgkin's disease	175	0	-	0.2	1.7	3.6	8.1	5.6	5.2	2.9	2.7	4.0	4.1	1.5	4.5	-	-	-	3.0	3.3	0.22	0.22	**2.9**	*201*
Non-Hodgkin lymphoma	253	1	1.5	1.4	1.2	1.2	2.4	3.2	5.4	5.5	12.8	9.6	23.4	24.3	40.9	67.2	55.8	60.0	4.3	4.8	0.67	1.28	**11.1**	*200,202*
Multiple myeloma	24	1	-	-	-	-	-	-	0.2	0.5	0.4	3.2	1.0	9.1	9.1	-	27.9	6.7	0.4	0.5	0.12	0.27	**1.8**	*203*
Lymphoid leukaemia	71	0	1.4	2.0	1.4	1.2	0.8	-	0.2	0.5	-	0.8	2.0	4.6	2.3	4.2	27.9	20.0	1.2	1.4	0.09	0.25	**2.2**	*204*
Myeloid leukaemia	65	1	0.2	0.6	0.2	0.4	0.7	1.8	1.3	1.2	1.3	4.0	3.1	7.6	9.1	16.8	9.3	20.0	1.1	1.2	0.16	0.29	**2.8**	*205*
Monocytic leukaemia	8	0	0.2	0.1	-	0.1	-	0.6	-	-	0.4	-	-	-	-	-	-	-	0.1	0.2	0.01	0.01	**0.1**	*206*
Other leukaemia	1	0	-	-	-	-	-	-	-	-	-	-	-	-	2.3	-	-	-	0.0	0.0	0.01	0.01	**0.1**	*207*
Leukaemia unspecified	6	0	0.1	-	-	0.1	-	0.2	-	0.2	-	-	1.0	-	-	4.2	-	-	0.1	0.1	0.01	0.03	**0.2**	*208*
Other and unspecified	152	0	0.9	0.4	0.1	0.4	0.3	1.8	1.9	1.2	5.7	10.4	17.3	22.8	15.9	54.6	65.0	180.0	2.6	2.9	0.40	0.99	**10.5**	*O&U*
All sites	5329	17	13.1	11.1	10.8	19.2	31.6	46.2	87.8	144.5	304.7	481.6	557.5	776.6	873.3	1141.8	1282.4	1913.6	90.4		16.84	29.00	**265.6**	*ALL*
All sites but 173	5242	17	13.1	11.1	10.6	18.8	31.0	45.6	86.3	141.4	298.5	475.2	548.3	769.0	852.8	1129.2	1263.8	1880.3	88.9	100.0	16.56	28.57	**261.4**	*ALLb*

| Rate from 1 case | | | 0.113 | 0.118 | 0.125 | 0.134 | 0.163 | 0.198 | 0.215 | 0.238 | 0.442 | 0.800 | 1.017 | 1.520 | 2.274 | 4.198 | 9.293 | 6.668 | | | | | | |

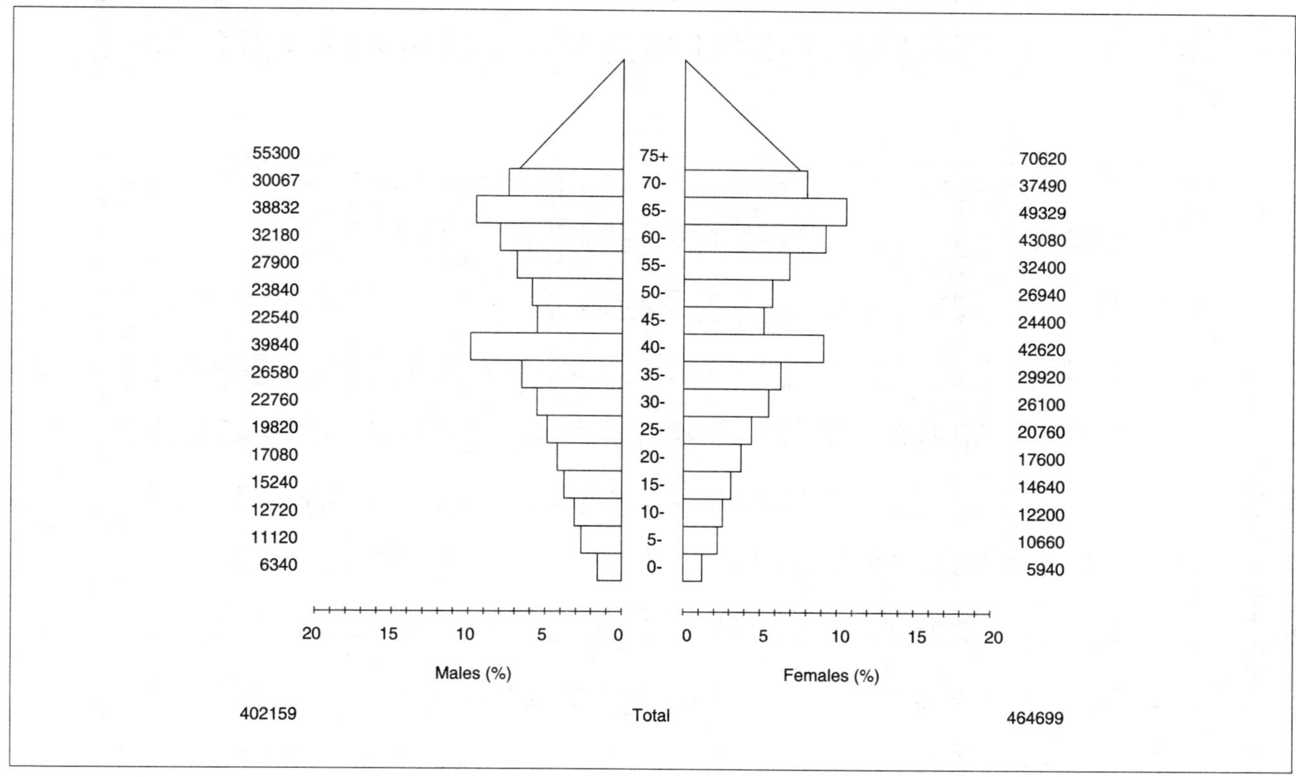

Israel: Jews Born in Europe or America

Source of population: average annual 1988–92

Estimate: The Population Register has recorded details of each Israeli citizen (born in Israel or immigrant), with their personal identity number. It is continuously updated for births and deaths, immigration and emigration, and changes of address, civil status or names. Annual population estimates from the Population Register are published by the Central Bureau of Statistics.

ISRAEL: JEWS BORN IN EUROPE OR AMERICA 1988-1992

ANNUAL INCIDENCE PER 100,000 BY AGE GROUP (YEARS) - MALE

SITE	ALL AGES	AGE UNK	0-	5-	10-	15-	20-	25-	30-	35-	40-	45-	50-	55-	60-	65-	70-	75+	CRUDE RATE	%	CR 64	CR 74	ASR (W)	ICD (9th)
Lip	227	0	-	-	-	-	-	1.0	0.9	1.5	4.0	7.1	5.9	7.9	13.7	17.0	26.6	34.0	11.3	1.4	0.21	0.43	**3.8**	140
Tongue	39	0	-	-	-	-	-	-	-	1.5	1.0	1.8	3.4	2.9	1.9	3.6	2.7	4.0	1.9	0.2	0.06	0.09	**0.9**	141
Salivary gland	49	0	-	-	-	-	-	-	-	0.8	1.5	0.9	3.4	0.7	3.1	3.6	6.7	6.1	2.4	0.3	0.05	0.10	**0.9**	142
Mouth	37	0	-	-	-	-	1.2	-	-	0.8	0.5	1.8	1.7	2.2	1.2	2.1	4.7	5.1	1.8	0.2	0.05	0.08	**0.8**	143-5
Oropharynx	14	0	-	-	-	-	-	-	-	-	-	-	-	1.4	1.9	1.0	1.3	1.8	0.7	0.1	0.02	0.03	**0.2**	146
Nasopharynx	26	0	-	-	-	-	-	-	-	-	2.0	0.9	1.7	2.9	1.2	3.6	0.7	1.8	1.3	0.2	0.04	0.06	**0.6**	147
Hypopharynx	13	0	-	-	-	-	-	-	-	-	-	-	-	-	-	1.0	2.7	2.5	0.6	0.1	0.00	0.02	**0.1**	148
Pharynx unspecified	4	0	-	-	-	-	-	-	-	-	-	0.8	-	-	-	-	1.3	0.4	0.2	0.0	0.00	0.01	**0.1**	149
Oesophagus	146	0	-	-	-	-	-	-	-	-	1.8	2.5	0.7	3.7	10.3	16.6	32.2	7.3	0.9	0.04	0.18	**1.7**	150	
Stomach	1103	4	-	-	-	-	-	2.0	1.8	3.8	7.0	11.5	22.7	27.2	58.4	89.1	114.4	202.2	54.9	6.7	0.67	1.70	**15.2**	151
Small intestine	40	1	-	-	-	-	-	1.0	0.9	-	0.5	0.9	-	2.2	3.7	2.6	5.3	4.7	2.0	0.2	0.05	0.09	**0.7**	152
Colon	2265	2	-	-	-	-	-	1.0	0.9	3.8	9.0	19.5	33.6	65.2	111.2	196.7	270.1	404.3	112.6	13.7	1.22	3.56	**30.2**	153
Rectum	1153	6	-	-	-	-	-	1.0	-	0.8	8.5	11.5	29.4	43.7	62.8	96.8	135.7	190.2	57.3	7.0	0.79	1.96	**16.6**	154
Liver	233	0	-	-	-	-	-	-	-	1.5	0.5	0.9	5.9	7.2	16.8	26.8	33.3	30.0	11.6	1.4	0.16	0.46	**3.5**	155
Gallbladder etc.	114	0	-	-	-	-	-	-	-	-	-	-	2.5	4.3	3.7	7.7	11.3	24.2	5.7	0.7	0.05	0.15	**1.4**	156
Pancreas	588	2	-	-	-	-	-	-	1.8	3.0	1.5	4.4	12.6	18.6	22.4	52.5	72.5	102.7	29.2	3.5	0.32	0.95	**8.0**	157
Nose, sinuses etc.	16	0	-	-	-	-	-	-	-	-	1.0	0.9	0.8	-	-	2.7	2.9	0.8	0.1	0.01	0.03	**0.3**	160	
Larynx	262	0	-	-	-	-	-	-	-	-	3.5	2.7	8.4	16.5	22.4	30.4	29.9	28.6	13.0	1.6	0.27	0.57	**4.4**	161
Bronchus, lung	1692	6	-	-	-	-	-	1.0	0.9	1.5	7.0	22.2	38.6	91.8	129.9	166.4	199.6	230.4	84.1	10.2	1.47	3.31	**26.5**	162
Other thoracic organs	21	0	-	-	-	-	-	1.0	-	-	-	0.9	1.7	0.7	0.6	2.1	2.7	2.5	1.0	0.1	0.02	0.05	**0.4**	163-4
Bone	40	0	-	-	3.1	1.3	1.2	1.0	0.9	0.8	0.5	3.5	1.7	2.9	0.6	3.1	4.0	3.3	2.0	0.2	0.09	0.12	**1.4**	170
Connective tissue	130	0	-	-	1.6	1.3	-	-	0.9	3.0	3.0	6.2	3.4	3.6	8.7	10.3	12.0	17.7	6.5	0.8	0.16	0.27	**2.6**	171
Mesothelioma	32	0	-	-	-	-	-	-	0.9	-	-	0.9	0.8	3.6	4.4	1.0	3.3	3.6	1.6	0.2	0.05	0.07	**0.6**	MES
Kaposi's sarcoma	147	0	-	-	-	-	-	1.0	0.9	2.3	3.6	1.7	3.6	5.0	6.7	14.6	32.5	7.3	0.9	0.08	0.19	**1.9**	KAP	
Melanoma of skin	489	0	-	-	-	1.3	2.3	5.0	7.9	16.6	16.1	29.3	16.8	28.0	33.6	46.4	40.6	43.8	24.3	3.0	0.78	1.22	**11.3**	172
Other skin	207	0	-	-	-	1.3	2.3	1.0	1.8	1.5	3.5	4.4	6.7	5.0	11.2	16.0	17.3	35.1	10.3		0.19	0.36	**3.6**	173
Breast	78	0	-	-	-	-	-	-	0.9	0.8	-	0.9	2.5	2.9	6.8	5.7	8.6	11.9	3.9	0.5	0.07	0.15	**1.2**	175
Prostate	2067	1	-	-	-	-	-	-	-	-	0.5	1.8	13.4	28.7	64.6	164.8	271.4	425.0	102.8	12.5	0.55	2.73	**23.4**	185
Testis	92	0	-	-	-	1.3	8.2	6.1	15.8	6.0	8.5	7.1	2.5	2.2	3.7	2.6	2.7	2.2	4.6	0.6	0.31	0.33	**4.0**	186
Penis	3	0	-	-	-	-	-	-	-	-	0.8	-	-	-	-	-	0.7	0.4	0.1	0.0	0.00	0.01	**0.1**	187.1-.4
Other male genital	8	0	-	-	-	-	-	-	-	-	-	-	-	0.7	1.2	-	0.7	1.4	0.4	0.0	0.01	0.01	**0.1**	187.5-.9
Bladder	1898	2	-	-	-	2.6	-	-	3.5	6.0	9.5	16.0	37.8	64.5	126.2	176.1	208.9	307.8	94.4	11.5	1.33	3.26	**27.5**	188
Kidney etc.	803	2	-	-	-	-	-	1.0	1.8	3.0	7.5	15.1	15.1	42.3	54.7	83.4	110.4	97.3	39.9	4.8	0.70	1.68	**13.0**	189
Eye	42	0	-	-	-	-	-	-	-	1.5	0.5	-	-	3.6	2.5	3.6	2.7	6.9	2.1	0.3	0.04	0.07	**0.7**	190
Brain, nervous system	247	1	3.2	3.6	3.1	1.3	2.3	5.0	4.4	3.8	3.5	8.0	13.4	15.1	17.4	25.2	25.9	19.5	12.3	1.5	0.42	0.68	**6.6**	191-2
Thyroid	109	0	-	-	-	-	-	2.0	2.6	2.3	2.5	5.3	6.7	4.3	9.9	9.3	9.3	10.1	5.4	0.7	0.18	0.27	**2.5**	193
Other endocrine	14	0	-	-	1.6	-	-	-	-	-	1.0	0.9	-	-	0.6	2.6	1.3	0.7	0.7	0.1	0.02	0.04	**0.4**	194
Hodgkin's disease	65	0	-	-	3.1	3.9	7.0	2.0	3.5	6.0	5.5	4.4	2.5	0.7	3.1	3.1	0.7	2.9	3.2	0.4	0.21	0.23	**3.0**	201
Non-Hodgkin lymphoma	705	1	3.2	3.6	1.6	-	2.3	-	1.8	13.5	10.0	9.8	18.5	35.1	52.2	62.3	66.5	98.0	35.1	4.3	0.76	1.40	**12.8**	200,202
Multiple myeloma	173	0	-	-	-	-	-	-	-	1.5	-	-	-	6.5	9.3	8.8	25.9	32.9	8.6	1.0	0.09	0.26	**2.2**	203
Lymphoid leukaemia	186	0	9.5	1.8	1.6	2.6	3.5	-	0.9	0.8	1.0	1.8	7.6	8.6	14.3	8.2	22.0	27.8	9.3	1.1	0.27	0.42	**4.8**	204
Myeloid leukaemia	139	0	3.2	1.8	3.1	1.3	1.2	3.0	3.5	2.3	2.0	6.2	3.4	5.7	9.3	10.3	12.0	17.0	6.9	0.8	0.23	0.34	**3.8**	205
Monocytic leukaemia	16	1	-	-	1.6	1.3	-	-	-	-	0.5	-	-	1.4	0.6	-	0.7	2.9	0.8	0.1	0.03	0.03	**0.5**	206
Other leukaemia	13	0	-	-	-	-	-	-	-	-	-	-	-	0.7	0.6	0.5	1.3	2.9	0.6	0.1	0.01	0.02	**0.2**	207
Leukaemia unspecified	49	0	-	-	-	-	-	-	0.9	-	1.0	-	2.5	0.7	3.7	2.6	3.3	9.4	2.4	0.3	0.04	0.07	**0.7**	208
Other and unspecified	981	4	-	-	-	1.3	-	3.0	2.6	0.8	5.5	13.3	21.8	35.8	49.1	74.2	105.1	175.8	48.8	5.9	0.67	1.57	**14.1**	O&U
All sites	16775	33	18.9	10.8	20.4	21.0	31.6	38.3	62.4	91.8	130.5	225.4	354.0	602.2	952.1	1440.0	1912.4	2699.5	834.2		12.82	29.62	**259.1**	ALL
All sites but 173	16568	33	18.9	10.8	20.4	19.7	29.3	37.3	60.6	90.3	127.0	220.9	347.3	597.1	941.0	1424.1	1895.1	2664.4	824.0	100.0	12.63	29.26	**255.5**	ALLb

| Rate from 1 case | | | 3.155 | 1.799 | 1.572 | 1.312 | 1.171 | 1.009 | 0.879 | 0.752 | 0.502 | 0.887 | 0.839 | 0.717 | 0.622 | 0.515 | 0.665 | 0.362 | | | | | | |

ISRAEL: JEWS BORN IN EUROPE OR AMERICA 1988-1992

ANNUAL INCIDENCE PER 100,000 BY AGE GROUP (YEARS) - FEMALE

SITE	ALL AGES	AGE UNK	0-	5-	10-	15-	20-	25-	30-	35-	40-	45-	50-	55-	60-	65-	70-	75+	CRUDE RATE	%	CR 64	CR 74	ASR (W)	ICD (9th)
Lip	79	0	-	-	-	-	-	-	-	0.7	0.5	1.6	0.7	0.6	4.6	4.1	8.5	10.5	3.4	0.5	0.04	0.11	**0.9**	140
Tongue	49	0	-	-	-	-	-	-	-	-	0.5	-	0.7	0.6	2.3	2.8	7.5	5.7	2.1	0.3	0.02	0.07	**0.5**	141
Salivary gland	32	0	-	-	-	-	-	-	-	-	-	0.8	-	0.6	1.9	0.8	3.2	5.1	1.4	0.2	0.02	0.04	**0.3**	142
Mouth	44	0	-	-	-	-	-	-	-	-	0.5	0.8	0.7	1.9	1.4	3.2	2.7	6.2	1.9	0.3	0.03	0.06	**0.5**	143-5
Oropharynx	5	0	-	-	-	-	-	-	-	-	-	-	0.7	-	0.5	-	1.6	-	0.2	0.0	0.01	0.01	**0.1**	146
Nasopharynx	11	0	-	-	-	-	-	-	-	1.3	-	-	-	-	0.5	2.0	-	0.8	0.5	0.1	0.01	0.02	**0.2**	147
Hypopharynx	4	0	-	-	-	-	-	-	-	-	-	-	-	-	-	0.4	0.5	0.6	0.2	0.0	0.00	0.00	**0.0**	148
Pharynx unspecified	0	0	-	-	-	-	-	-	-	-	-	-	-	-	-	-	-	-	0.0	0.0	0.00	0.00	**0.0**	149
Oesophagus	93	0	-	-	-	-	-	-	-	-	-	0.8	0.7	-	4.2	4.5	14.4	12.5	4.0	0.5	0.03	0.12	**0.9**	150
Stomach	603	4	-	-	-	-	-	-	1.5	1.3	3.8	8.2	12.6	14.8	25.1	35.7	45.9	87.2	26.0	3.5	0.34	0.75	**6.9**	151
Small intestine	43	0	-	-	-	-	-	-	0.8	-	0.5	2.5	0.7	3.1	2.3	3.2	4.8	2.8	1.9	0.2	0.05	0.09	**0.7**	152
Colon	1982	8	-	-	-	1.4	-	1.0	0.8	2.0	9.9	18.0	41.6	58.0	91.9	134.6	186.2	253.8	85.3	11.3	1.13	2.74	**23.0**	153
Rectum	1052	3	-	-	-	1.4	-	1.9	1.5	2.7	6.6	9.8	22.3	30.9	54.8	65.7	105.1	129.4	45.3	6.0	0.66	1.52	**12.8**	154
Liver	129	1	-	-	-	1.4	-	-	-	-	-	0.8	3.0	1.9	7.4	7.3	14.4	16.4	5.6	0.7	0.07	0.18	**1.5**	155
Gallbladder etc.	249	1	-	-	-	-	-	-	-	-	1.4	0.8	3.7	5.6	7.4	19.5	25.1	33.7	10.7	1.4	0.09	0.32	**2.6**	156
Pancreas	561	2	-	-	-	-	-	-	0.8	-	0.9	4.1	7.4	13.6	21.8	37.7	51.7	79.9	24.1	3.2	0.24	0.69	**5.9**	157
Nose, sinuses etc.	30	0	-	-	-	-	-	-	-	0.7	-	-	-	1.2	1.4	1.2	4.8	3.4	1.3	0.2	0.02	0.05	**0.3**	160
Larynx	54	0	-	-	-	-	-	-	-	-	0.9	1.6	0.7	3.1	3.2	5.3	3.7	4.8	2.3	0.3	0.05	0.09	**0.8**	161
Bronchus, lung	860	2	-	-	-	-	1.1	-	0.8	2.0	5.2	7.4	13.4	35.2	52.9	66.9	80.6	92.9	37.0	4.9	0.59	1.33	**10.7**	162
Other thoracic organs	16	0	-	-	-	-	-	-	-	0.7	0.5	0.8	0.7	0.6	0.5	1.6	1.1	1.1	0.7	0.1	0.02	0.03	**0.3**	163-4
Bone	31	0	-	-	-	-	1.1	-	-	0.7	0.9	0.8	0.7	1.2	0.5	2.0	3.2	3.1	1.3	0.2	0.03	0.06	**0.5**	170
Connective tissue	139	0	-	1.9	-	4.1	1.1	1.0	1.5	2.0	4.7	3.3	7.4	3.7	3.7	9.3	8.5	14.4	6.0	0.8	0.17	0.26	**2.8**	171
Mesothelioma	16	0	-	-	-	-	-	-	-	-	0.5	0.8	-	1.2	0.5	2.0	1.1	1.1	0.7	0.1	0.01	0.03	**0.3**	MES
Kaposi's sarcoma	81	0	-	-	-	1.4	1.1	1.9	-	-	0.5	0.8	1.5	1.9	1.4	3.6	5.9	13.3	3.5	0.5	0.05	0.10	**1.1**	KAP
Melanoma of skin	566	1	-	-	3.3	2.7	3.4	7.7	11.5	15.4	23.0	23.0	21.5	30.2	33.4	31.2	40.5	37.4	24.4	3.2	0.88	1.24	**11.9**	172
Other skin	220	0	-	-	-	1.4	-	-	-	2.0	4.2	7.4	7.4	8.0	8.4	16.2	14.9	25.2	9.5		0.19	0.35	**3.3**	173
Breast	4838	5	-	-	-	-	1.1	3.9	29.1	69.5	133.3	236.1	261.3	251.9	297.1	348.3	355.8	336.4	208.2	27.7	6.42	9.95	**87.9**	174
Uterus unspecified	51	0	-	-	-	-	-	-	-	1.3	-	3.3	2.2	3.7	3.2	2.8	1.6	5.4	2.2	0.3	0.07	0.09	**0.9**	179
Cervix uteri	187	2	-	-	-	1.4	1.1	1.0	4.6	4.7	8.4	10.7	11.1	7.4	7.9	12.2	14.4	10.5	8.0	1.1	0.29	0.43	**4.1**	180
Placenta	1	0	-	-	-	-	-	-	-	-	0.5	-	-	-	-	-	-	-	0.0	0.0	0.00	0.00	**0.0**	181
Corpus uteri	764	1	-	-	-	-	-	-	1.5	4.0	8.9	17.2	40.1	60.5	54.8	66.1	57.1	49.6	32.9	4.4	0.94	1.55	**12.6**	182
Ovary etc.	778	4	-	-	-	-	4.5	1.9	1.5	5.3	22.5	23.8	31.2	50.0	59.4	53.9	52.8	56.1	33.5	4.5	1.01	1.54	**13.5**	183
Other female genital	140	1	-	-	-	-	-	1.9	-	0.7	1.9	1.6	3.0	-	6.0	9.3	12.3	19.0	6.0	0.8	0.08	0.18	**1.7**	184
Bladder	491	2	-	-	-	-	-	1.0	0.8	2.7	1.4	8.2	10.4	17.3	24.6	35.7	45.3	57.2	21.1	2.8	0.33	0.74	**6.2**	188
Kidney etc.	473	1	10.1	-	-	-	-	-	-	2.0	2.3	9.0	18.6	21.6	28.3	40.5	39.5	43.9	20.4	2.7	0.46	0.86	**7.8**	189
Eye	47	0	-	1.9	-	-	1.1	-	-	0.7	0.5	-	0.7	4.9	1.9	2.4	4.8	4.2	2.0	0.3	0.06	0.09	**0.9**	190
Brain, nervous system	217	0	6.7	-	-	2.7	1.1	1.9	3.1	4.7	4.7	6.6	3.0	13.6	13.5	21.9	14.4	12.7	9.3	1.2	0.31	0.49	**4.9**	191-2
Thyroid	297	0	-	-	-	2.7	4.5	8.7	10.0	11.4	11.3	7.4	19.3	22.8	20.0	18.2	13.9	11.9	12.8	1.7	0.59	0.75	**7.4**	193
Other endocrine	18	0	-	-	-	1.4	-	1.0	-	-	0.5	-	1.5	2.5	1.4	0.8	0.5	0.8	0.8	0.1	0.04	0.05	**0.5**	194
Hodgkin's disease	82	0	-	-	-	1.4	10.2	7.7	7.7	4.7	2.8	2.5	0.7	1.9	2.3	2.8	4.3	4.0	3.5	0.5	0.21	0.24	**3.1**	201
Non-Hodgkin lymphoma	718	2	-	-	-	-	2.3	-	2.3	3.3	10.8	14.8	23.8	27.2	33.9	46.6	60.3	81.6	30.9	4.1	0.59	1.13	**9.9**	200,202
Multiple myeloma	144	1	-	-	-	-	-	-	-	0.7	0.9	3.3	4.5	5.6	4.6	9.3	11.7	18.7	6.2	0.8	0.10	0.20	**1.8**	203
Lymphoid leukaemia	145	0	6.7	3.8	-	-	-	1.0	-	0.7	-	1.6	0.7	3.1	4.2	7.3	9.1	24.6	6.2	0.8	0.11	0.19	**2.6**	204
Myeloid leukaemia	129	0	3.4	-	-	2.7	-	-	2.3	2.0	2.8	4.9	5.2	5.6	5.6	4.1	12.3	13.3	5.6	0.7	0.17	0.25	**2.7**	205
Monocytic leukaemia	14	0	-	-	-	-	-	-	-	0.7	-	-	-	0.6	1.4	1.2	0.5	1.4	0.6	0.1	0.01	0.02	**0.2**	206
Other leukaemia	3	0	-	-	-	-	-	-	-	0.7	-	-	-	-	-	0.4	-	0.3	0.1	0.0	0.00	0.01	**0.1**	207
Leukaemia unspecified	50	0	-	-	-	-	-	-	-	-	-	0.5	-	-	2.5	1.9	2.0	4.3	7.9	2.2	0.3	0.02	0.06	**0.5**	208
Other and unspecified	1148	4	-	1.9	-	-	-	1.9	2.3	3.3	6.6	16.4	17.1	19.1	43.6	75.0	93.4	167.4	49.4	6.6	0.56	1.41	**12.9**	O&U
All sites	17684	45	26.9	9.4	3.3	26.0	34.1	45.3	84.3	154.4	285.3	461.5	602.8	739.5	947.5	1222.0	1444.1	1768.3	761.1		17.15	30.51	**271.5**	ALL
All sites but 173	17464	45	26.9	9.4	3.3	24.6	34.1	45.3	84.3	152.4	281.1	454.1	595.4	731.5	939.2	1205.8	1429.2	1743.1	751.6	100.0	16.95	30.16	**268.2**	ALLb
Rate from 1 case			3.367	1.876	1.639	1.366	1.136	0.963	0.766	0.668	0.469	0.820	0.742	0.617	0.464	0.405	0.533	0.283						

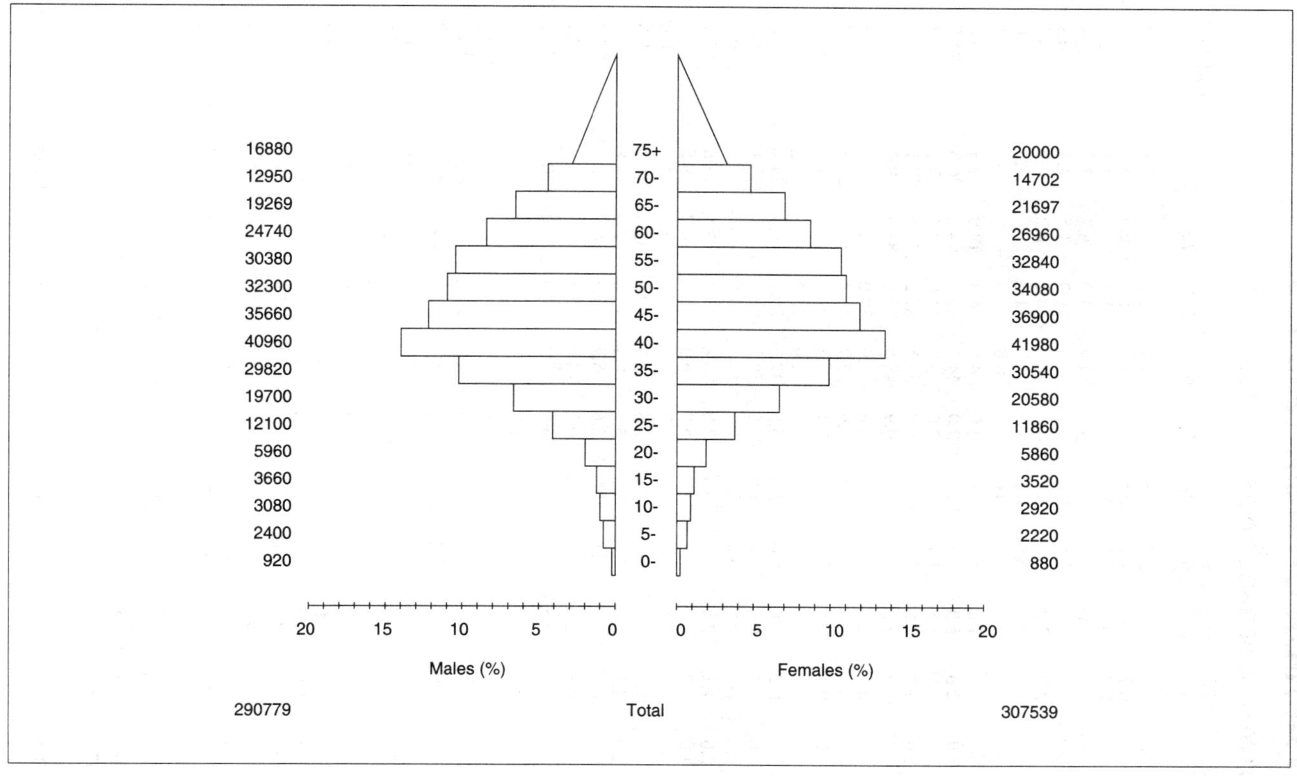

Israel: Jews Born in Africa or Asia
Source of population: average annual 1988–92
Estimate: The Population Register has recorded details of each Israeli citizen (born in Israel or immigrant), with their personal identity number. It is continuously updated for births and deaths, immigration and emigration, and changes of address, civil status or names. Annual population estimates from the Population Register are published by the Central Bureau of Statistics.

ISRAEL: JEWS BORN IN AFRICA OR ASIA 1988-1992

ANNUAL INCIDENCE PER 100,000 BY AGE GROUP (YEARS) - MALE

SITE	ALL AGES	AGE UNK	0-	5-	10-	15-	20-	25-	30-	35-	40-	45-	50-	55-	60-	65-	70-	75+	CRUDE RATE	%	CR 64	CR 74	ASR (W)	ICD (9th)
Lip	44	0	-	-	-	-	-	1.7	2.0	3.4	1.5	3.4	0.6	3.9	2.4	6.2	7.7	7.1	3.0	0.7	0.09	0.16	**1.5**	*140*
Tongue	26	0	-	-	-	-	-	-	-	0.7	-	1.1	0.6	2.0	2.4	6.2	9.3	4.7	1.8	0.4	0.03	0.11	**0.8**	*141*
Salivary gland	19	0	-	-	-	-	-	-	-	2.7	0.5	0.6	1.2	0.7	0.8	5.2	-	4.7	1.3	0.3	0.03	0.06	**0.6**	*142*
Mouth	30	0	-	-	-	-	-	-	-	-	1.0	1.1	-	3.9	4.9	4.2	6.2	7.1	2.1	0.5	0.05	0.11	**0.9**	*143-5*
Oropharynx	11	0	-	-	-	-	-	-	-	-	-	1.1	0.6	-	2.4	1.0	1.5	3.6	0.8	0.2	0.02	0.03	**0.3**	*146*
Nasopharynx	49	3	-	-	6.5	-	-	-	-	2.0	2.9	2.8	5.0	4.6	4.9	4.2	6.2	2.4	3.4	0.8	0.15	0.21	**2.1**	*147*
Hypopharynx	9	0	-	-	-	-	-	-	-	-	0.5	0.6	0.6	1.3	-	1.0	-	3.6	0.6	0.1	0.01	0.02	**0.2**	*148*
Pharynx unspecified	2	0	-	-	-	-	-	-	-	-	-	-	0.6	-	0.8	-	-	-	0.1	0.0	0.01	0.01	**0.1**	*149*
Oesophagus	52	0	-	-	-	-	-	-	-	-	1.0	1.1	0.6	3.9	4.9	8.3	13.9	21.3	3.6	0.8	0.06	0.17	**1.5**	*150*
Stomach	356	0	-	-	-	-	-	-	1.0	2.0	5.9	7.3	16.7	23.0	44.5	43.6	94.2	126.8	24.5	5.5	0.50	1.19	**10.2**	*151*
Small intestine	26	0	-	-	-	-	-	-	-	-	1.5	1.1	2.5	2.6	3.2	1.0	3.1	7.1	1.8	0.4	0.05	0.08	**0.7**	*152*
Colon	540	2	-	-	-	-	3.4	-	3.0	2.0	7.8	12.3	12.4	36.9	63.1	87.2	134.4	199.1	37.1	8.3	0.71	1.82	**15.7**	*153*
Rectum	400	0	-	-	-	-	-	-	-	2.0	7.3	14.6	11.8	30.9	48.5	77.8	83.4	119.7	27.5	6.1	0.58	1.38	**11.6**	*154*
Liver	113	0	-	-	-	-	-	-	-	0.7	2.0	1.1	3.1	6.6	12.9	28.0	40.2	26.1	7.8	1.7	0.13	0.47	**3.3**	*155*
Gallbladder etc.	62	0	-	-	-	-	-	-	-	-	-	1.1	3.7	5.9	5.7	10.4	15.4	21.3	4.3	0.9	0.08	0.21	**1.8**	*156*
Pancreas	203	2	-	-	-	-	-	-	1.0	0.7	0.5	6.2	8.7	19.1	16.2	36.3	44.8	71.1	14.0	3.1	0.26	0.67	**5.8**	*157*
Nose, sinuses etc.	17	0	-	-	-	5.5	-	-	-	-	-	0.6	-	1.3	4.9	6.2	-	1.2	1.2	0.3	0.06	0.09	**1.0**	*160*
Larynx	180	0	-	-	-	-	-	-	-	0.7	1.0	5.0	12.4	16.5	37.2	29.1	30.9	34.4	12.4	2.8	0.36	0.66	**5.3**	*161*
Bronchus, lung	945	3	-	-	-	-	-	-	2.0	3.4	6.8	26.4	44.6	89.5	138.2	196.2	196.1	212.1	65.0	14.5	1.56	3.53	**27.8**	*162*
Other thoracic organs	7	0	-	-	-	-	-	-	-	-	-	0.6	2.5	-	-	1.0	-	1.2	0.5	0.1	0.02	0.02	**0.2**	*163-4*
Bone	25	0	-	-	-	-	-	-	2.0	1.3	2.4	1.1	0.6	2.0	0.8	4.2	3.1	3.6	1.7	0.4	0.05	0.09	**0.8**	*170*
Connective tissue	59	0	-	-	-	-	-	1.7	1.0	2.7	2.4	3.4	4.3	5.9	6.5	6.2	6.2	9.5	4.1	0.9	0.14	0.20	**1.9**	*171*
Mesothelioma	9	0	-	-	-	-	-	-	-	-	0.5	-	-	2.0	-	2.1	3.1	1.2	0.6	0.1	0.01	0.04	**0.3**	*MES*
Kaposi's sarcoma	128	0	-	-	-	-	-	-	-	2.0	1.0	2.2	4.3	8.6	13.7	22.8	32.4	46.2	8.8	2.0	0.16	0.44	**3.7**	*KAP*
Melanoma of skin	81	0	-	-	-	-	-	1.7	2.0	2.7	6.3	3.4	3.7	5.3	9.7	11.4	12.4	11.8	5.6	1.2	0.17	0.29	**2.6**	*172*
Other skin	47	0	-	-	-	-	-	1.7	-	0.7	2.9	1.7	1.9	2.6	5.7	13.5	6.2	5.9	3.2		0.09	0.18	**1.5**	*173*
Breast	30	0	-	-	-	-	-	-	-	0.7	2.9	1.1	0.6	0.7	4.0	5.2	3.1	8.3	2.1	0.5	0.05	0.09	**0.9**	*175*
Prostate	832	1	-	-	-	-	-	-	1.0	-	0.5	2.8	7.4	25.0	66.3	159.8	282.6	420.6	57.2	12.7	0.52	2.73	**23.2**	*185*
Testis	23	0	-	-	-	-	3.4	3.3	1.0	2.7	2.9	2.2	0.6	2.0	-	1.5	-	-	1.6	0.4	0.09	0.10	**1.2**	*186*
Penis	3	0	-	-	-	-	-	-	-	-	-	-	-	0.7	-	1.0	1.5	-	0.2	0.0	0.00	0.02	**0.1**	*187.1-.4*
Other male genital	5	0	-	-	-	-	-	-	-	-	-	-	-	-	0.7	-	-	3.6	0.3	0.1	0.01	0.01	**0.1**	*187.5-.9*
Bladder	735	1	-	-	-	-	-	-	3.0	4.7	6.3	11.8	21.7	56.0	105.9	160.9	180.7	197.9	50.6	11.3	1.05	2.76	**21.5**	*188*
Kidney etc.	208	0	-	-	-	-	-	-	-	2.0	3.9	2.2	13.0	21.1	31.5	32.2	44.8	48.6	14.3	3.2	0.37	0.75	**6.1**	*189*
Eye	15	0	21.7	-	-	-	-	-	-	0.7	0.5	-	-	1.3	1.6	4.2	1.5	3.6	1.0	0.2	0.13	0.16	**3.0**	*190*
Brain, nervous system	111	2	-	-	-	-	-	-	5.1	4.7	4.9	6.2	8.7	14.5	10.5	12.5	15.4	5.9	7.6	1.7	0.28	0.42	**3.5**	*191-2*
Thyroid	74	0	-	-	-	-	6.7	-	3.0	4.7	4.4	7.9	5.0	3.9	5.7	7.3	9.3	5.9	5.1	1.1	0.21	0.29	**2.9**	*193*
Other endocrine	8	0	-	-	-	-	1.7	-	-	-	0.5	1.1	0.6	1.3	-	1.0	-	-	0.6	0.1	0.03	0.03	**0.3**	*194*
Hodgkin's disease	49	0	-	-	-	3.4	-	-	4.0	5.9	3.4	4.3	2.0	4.0	3.1	4.6	3.6		3.4	0.8	0.13	0.17	**1.8**	*201*
Non-Hodgkin lymphoma	314	0	-	-	6.5	-	3.4	1.7	8.1	6.0	12.7	12.9	21.1	27.0	36.4	42.6	44.8	65.2	21.6	4.8	0.68	1.12	**10.4**	*200,202*
Multiple myeloma	81	1	-	-	-	-	-	-	-	2.7	0.5	1.7	3.7	5.3	10.5	11.4	24.7	21.3	5.6	1.2	0.12	0.31	**2.4**	*203*
Lymphoid leukaemia	85	1	-	8.3	-	-	-	-	-	-	2.9	1.7	3.1	2.6	9.7	15.6	21.6	28.4	5.8	1.3	0.14	0.33	**3.3**	*204*
Myeloid leukaemia	73	0	-	-	-	5.5	-	1.7	2.0	2.7	1.0	2.2	3.1	4.6	6.5	11.4	12.4	23.7	5.0	1.1	0.15	0.26	**2.8**	*205*
Monocytic leukaemia	9	0	-	-	-	-	-	-	-	-	1.0	0.6	-	-	0.8	1.0	3.1	2.4	0.6	0.1	0.01	0.03	**0.3**	*206*
Other leukaemia	3	0	-	-	-	-	-	-	-	-	0.5	-	-	1.3	-	-	-	-	0.2	0.0	0.01	0.01	**0.1**	*207*
Leukaemia unspecified	22	0	-	-	-	-	-	-	-	-	2.0	0.6	1.9	0.7	0.8	2.1	-	11.8	1.5	0.3	0.03	0.04	**0.6**	*208*
Other and unspecified	455	1	-	-	-	-	-	-	-	2.0	4.9	11.2	17.3	38.8	50.9	52.9	129.7	161.1	31.3	7.0	0.63	1.54	**13.0**	*O&U*
All sites	6575	17	21.7	8.3	13.0	10.9	20.1	14.9	37.6	67.1	113.8	169.4	255.1	488.5	780.1	1137.5	1532.0	1964.5	452.2		10.03	23.41	**199.7**	*ALL*
All sites but 173	6528	17	21.7	8.3	13.0	10.9	20.1	13.2	37.6	66.4	110.8	167.7	253.3	485.8	774.5	1124.0	1525.8	1958.5	449.0	100.0	9.94	23.23	**198.2**	*ALLb*

Rate from 1 case   21.739   8.333   6.494   5.464   3.356   1.653   1.015   0.671   0.488   0.561   0.619   0.658   0.808   1.038   1.544   1.185

ISRAEL: JEWS BORN IN AFRICA OR ASIA 1988-1992

ANNUAL INCIDENCE PER 100,000 BY AGE GROUP (YEARS) - FEMALE

SITE	ALL AGES	AGE UNK	0-	5-	10-	15-	20-	25-	30-	35-	40-	45-	50-	55-	60-	65-	70-	75+	CRUDE RATE	%	CR 64	CR 74	ASR (W)	ICD (9th)
Lip	17	0	-	-	-	-	-	-	1.0	1.3	1.0	0.5	-	1.2	0.7	0.9	1.4	6.0	1.1	0.3	0.03	0.04	**0.5**	140
Tongue	18	0	-	-	-	-	-	-	-	-	0.5	1.1	1.8	0.6	1.5	-	5.4	5.0	1.2	0.3	0.03	0.05	**0.5**	141
Salivary gland	15	0	-	-	-	-	-	1.7	1.0	-	1.0	-	1.2	1.2	1.5	0.9	1.4	3.0	1.0	0.2	0.04	0.05	**0.5**	142
Mouth	19	0	-	-	-	-	3.4	-	-	-	1.0	-	1.2	1.2	3.0	0.9	-	7.0	1.2	0.3	0.05	0.05	**0.7**	143-5
Oropharynx	4	0	-	-	-	-	-	-	-	-	0.5	-	-	-	-	0.9	-	2.0	0.3	0.1	0.00	0.01	**0.1**	146
Nasopharynx	19	0	-	-	-	-	-	-	-	1.3	0.5	1.6	1.2	1.8	2.2	1.8	1.4	2.0	1.2	0.3	0.04	0.06	**0.5**	147
Hypopharynx	1	0	-	-	-	-	-	-	-	-	-	-	-	-	-	0.9	-	-	0.1	0.0	0.00	0.00	**0.0**	148
Pharynx unspecified	0	0	-	-	-	-	-	-	-	-	-	-	-	-	-	-	-	-	0.0	0.0	0.00	0.00	**0.0**	149
Oesophagus	52	0	-	-	-	-	-	-	-	1.3	0.5	0.5	0.6	3.7	3.0	8.3	10.9	20.0	3.4	0.8	0.05	0.14	**1.3**	150
Stomach	206	1	-	-	-	-	3.4	-	1.9	1.3	2.9	4.9	7.6	11.6	17.1	44.2	29.9	60.0	13.4	3.3	0.25	0.63	**5.6**	151
Small intestine	11	0	-	-	-	-	-	-	-	-	-	0.5	-	1.2	1.5	0.9	1.4	4.0	0.7	0.2	0.02	0.03	**0.3**	152
Colon	535	1	-	-	-	-	-	1.7	5.8	3.3	6.2	9.8	24.6	36.5	64.5	73.7	97.9	150.0	34.8	8.5	0.76	1.62	**14.1**	153
Rectum	329	1	-	-	-	-	-	3.4	1.9	2.0	4.8	8.7	25.2	19.5	31.9	46.1	68.0	77.0	21.4	5.2	0.49	1.06	**8.9**	154
Liver	80	0	-	-	-	-	-	-	1.0	-	1.9	1.1	1.2	2.4	10.4	13.8	15.0	27.0	5.2	1.3	0.09	0.23	**2.1**	155
Gallbladder etc.	92	0	-	-	-	-	-	-	-	-	-	0.5	3.5	4.9	9.6	17.5	23.1	28.0	6.0	1.5	0.09	0.30	**2.3**	156
Pancreas	189	0	-	-	-	-	-	-	-	-	1.9	4.3	4.7	9.1	19.3	24.9	51.7	63.0	12.3	3.0	0.20	0.58	**4.8**	157
Nose, sinuses etc.	8	0	-	-	-	-	-	-	-	0.7	-	1.6	0.6	0.6	-	-	-	2.0	0.5	0.1	0.02	0.02	**0.2**	160
Larynx	22	0	-	-	-	-	-	-	-	-	0.5	0.5	1.2	1.8	2.2	3.7	4.1	5.0	1.4	0.3	0.03	0.07	**0.6**	161
Bronchus, lung	203	1	-	-	-	-	-	1.7	-	0.7	3.8	9.2	7.6	18.9	20.8	28.6	34.0	47.0	13.2	3.2	0.31	0.63	**5.4**	162
Other thoracic organs	8	0	-	-	-	-	-	-	-	1.3	-	0.5	-	-	1.5	0.9	1.4	1.0	0.5	0.1	0.02	0.03	**0.2**	163-4
Bone	23	0	-	-	6.8	-	-	-	-	1.3	0.5	2.2	1.2	2.4	0.7	1.8	1.4	5.0	1.5	0.4	0.08	0.09	**1.2**	170
Connective tissue	56	0	-	-	6.8	5.7	-	-	-	1.9	-	2.9	2.7	4.7	4.3	3.7	5.5	5.4	11.0	3.6	0.9	0.16	0.22	**2.6**	171
Mesothelioma	5	0	-	-	-	-	-	-	-	-	-	-	-	0.6	1.5	-	1.4	1.0	0.3	0.1	0.01	0.02	**0.1**	MES
Kaposi's sarcoma	40	0	-	-	-	-	-	-	-	-	0.5	-	-	2.4	1.5	10.1	6.8	17.0	2.6	0.6	0.02	0.11	**1.0**	KAP
Melanoma of skin	80	0	-	-	-	-	-	3.4	-	2.6	4.3	5.4	4.7	8.5	10.4	4.6	12.2	5.0	5.2	1.3	0.20	0.28	**2.5**	172
Other skin	42	0	-	-	-	-	-	-	1.0	-	1.0	2.2	1.8	2.4	4.5	6.5	4.1	12.0	2.7		0.06	0.12	**1.1**	173
Breast	1963	2	-	-	-	-	-	3.4	29.2	66.1	103.4	146.3	147.9	168.1	174.3	195.4	216.3	207.0	127.7	31.1	4.20	6.26	**56.4**	174
Uterus unspecified	14	0	-	-	-	-	-	-	-	0.7	1.0	0.5	-	1.2	0.7	4.6	-	2.0	0.9	0.2	0.02	0.04	**0.4**	179
Cervix uteri	184	1	-	-	-	-	-	6.7	7.8	9.8	9.5	17.9	12.9	11.6	19.3	14.7	12.2	11.0	12.0	2.9	0.48	0.62	**6.1**	180
Placenta	3	0	-	-	-	-	-	-	-	0.7	-	-	1.2	-	-	-	-	-	0.2	0.0	0.01	0.01	**0.1**	181
Corpus uteri	279	2	-	-	-	-	-	1.7	1.0	-	5.7	8.7	20.5	34.7	37.1	39.6	43.5	30.0	18.1	4.4	0.55	0.97	**7.7**	182
Ovary etc.	261	0	-	-	-	-	-	-	-	3.3	7.1	20.6	17.0	28.6	31.2	38.7	28.6	22.0	17.0	4.1	0.54	0.88	**7.3**	183
Other female genital	59	0	-	-	-	-	-	-	-	-	0.5	1.6	2.3	3.7	3.0	12.0	12.2	19.0	3.8	0.9	0.06	0.18	**1.5**	184
Bladder	161	0	-	-	-	-	-	-	1.0	-	0.5	3.3	8.2	8.5	8.9	28.6	27.2	62.0	10.5	2.6	0.15	0.43	**4.0**	188
Kidney etc.	123	0	-	-	-	-	-	1.7	1.0	1.3	1.9	4.3	5.9	7.3	15.6	25.8	21.8	20.0	8.0	1.9	0.19	0.43	**3.5**	189
Eye	11	0	-	-	-	-	-	-	1.0	-	0.5	0.5	0.6	-	1.5	0.9	1.4	3.0	0.7	0.2	0.02	0.03	**0.3**	190
Brain, nervous system	84	0	-	9.0	-	-	-	1.7	1.9	3.9	3.8	3.8	4.7	6.1	5.2	13.8	8.2	13.0	5.5	1.3	0.20	0.31	**3.4**	191-2
Thyroid	228	0	-	-	6.8	5.7	6.8	13.5	7.8	10.5	18.6	21.1	12.3	15.8	15.6	18.4	12.2	17.0	14.8	3.6	0.67	0.83	**9.2**	193
Other endocrine	1	0	-	-	-	-	-	-	-	-	-	-	0.6	-	-	-	-	-	0.1	0.0	0.00	0.00	**0.0**	194
Hodgkin's disease	27	0	-	-	-	-	-	1.7	4.9	3.3	2.9	1.1	0.6	1.8	0.7	0.9	-	2.0	1.8	0.4	0.08	0.09	**1.1**	201
Non-Hodgkin lymphoma	299	2	-	-	-	-	6.8	3.4	1.0	4.6	8.6	13.6	15.8	25.0	31.9	45.2	47.6	47.0	19.4	4.7	0.56	1.02	**8.9**	200,202
Multiple myeloma	90	0	-	-	-	-	-	-	-	-	1.4	3.8	4.1	3.7	6.7	19.4	16.3	25.0	5.9	1.4	0.10	0.28	**2.3**	203
Lymphoid leukaemia	52	0	22.7	9.0	-	-	-	-	-	1.0	-	-	0.5	2.3	1.2	5.9	5.5	4.1	25.0	3.4	0.8	0.21	0.26	**4.9**	204
Myeloid leukaemia	56	0	-	-	-	-	-	3.4	3.4	2.9	2.0	1.0	1.6	5.9	3.7	4.5	0.9	8.2	13.0	3.6	0.9	0.14	0.19	**2.1**	205
Monocytic leukaemia	2	0	-	-	-	-	-	-	-	-	-	-	-	-	-	-	2.7	-	0.1	0.0	0.00	0.01	**0.1**	206
Other leukaemia	1	0	-	-	-	-	-	-	-	-	-	-	-	-	-	0.9	-	-	0.1	0.0	0.00	0.00	**0.0**	207
Leukaemia unspecified	16	1	-	-	-	-	-	-	-	-	-	0.5	1.1	-	1.8	-	4.6	-	4.0	1.0	0.3	0.02	0.04	**0.4**	208
Other and unspecified	367	2	-	-	-	-	-	-	1.0	5.2	3.8	6.0	13.5	21.3	31.9	55.3	66.7	127.0	23.9	5.8	0.42	1.03	**9.3**	O&U
All sites	6355	14	22.7	18.0	20.5	11.4	23.9	48.9	76.8	128.4	206.3	314.4	370.9	481.1	606.8	823.1	907.3	1209.0	413.3		11.68	20.35	**186.3**	ALL
All sites but 173	6313	14	22.7	18.0	20.5	11.4	23.9	48.9	75.8	128.4	205.3	312.2	369.1	478.7	602.4	816.7	903.3	1197.0	410.5	100.0	11.61	20.23	**185.1**	ALLb

Rate from 1 case   22.727   9.009   6.849   5.682   3.413   1.686   0.972   0.655   0.476   0.542   0.587   0.609   0.742   0.922   1.360   1.000

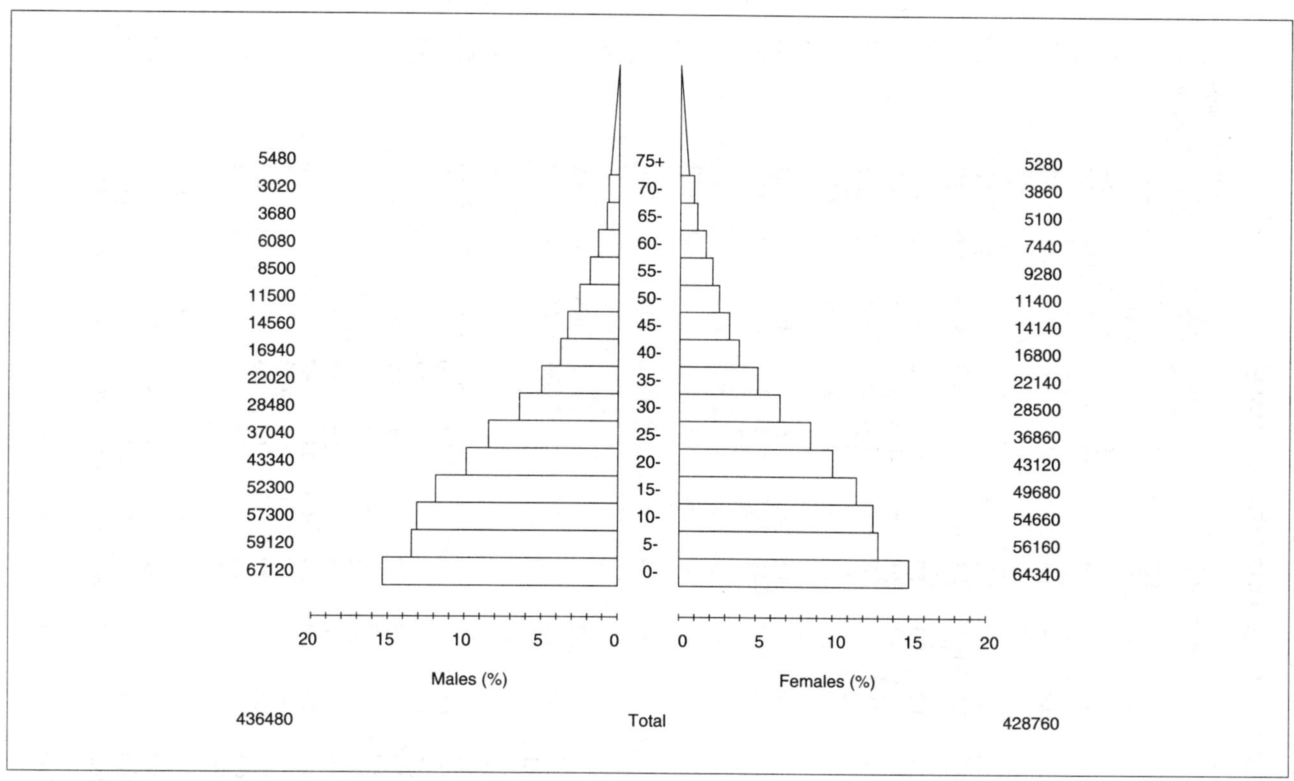

Israel: Non-Jews
Source of population: average annual 1988–92
Estimate: The Population Register has recorded details of each Israeli citizen (born in Israel or immigrant), with their personal identity number. It is continuously updated for births and deaths, immigration and emigration, and changes of address, civil status or names. Annual population estimates from the Population Register are published by the Central Bureau of Statistics.

ISRAEL: NON-JEWS 1988-1992

ANNUAL INCIDENCE PER 100,000 BY AGE GROUP (YEARS) - MALE

SITE	ALL AGES	AGE UNK	0-	5-	10-	15-	20-	25-	30-	35-	40-	45-	50-	55-	60-	65-	70-	75+	CRUDE RATE	%	CR 64	CR 74	ASR (W)	ICD (9th)
Lip	16	0	-	-	-	-	-	-	-	-	-	2.7	7.0	9.4	3.3	5.4	-	14.6	0.7	1.1	0.11	0.14	**1.5**	140
Tongue	1	0	-	-	-	-	-	-	-	-	-	-	-	-	-	5.4	-	-	0.0	0.1	0.00	0.03	**0.2**	141
Salivary gland	2	0	-	-	-	-	-	-	-	-	-	-	-	2.4	-	-	-	3.6	0.1	0.1	0.01	0.01	**0.2**	142
Mouth	5	0	-	-	-	-	-	-	-	-	-	1.4	-	2.4	-	-	13.2	3.6	0.2	0.3	0.02	0.08	**0.5**	143-5
Oropharynx	1	0	-	-	-	-	-	-	-	-	-	-	-	-	-	-	6.6	-	0.0	0.1	0.00	0.03	**0.1**	146
Nasopharynx	12	0	-	-	-	0.4	0.5	-	-	0.9	2.4	1.4	3.5	2.4	-	5.4	-	7.3	0.5	0.8	0.06	0.08	**0.9**	147
Hypopharynx	1	0	-	-	-	-	-	-	-	-	-	-	-	-	-	-	-	3.6	0.0	0.1	0.00	0.00	**0.1**	148
Pharynx unspecified	0	0	-	-	-	-	-	-	-	-	-	-	-	-	-	-	-	-	0.0	0.0	0.00	0.00	**0.0**	149
Oesophagus	5	0	-	-	-	0.4	-	-	-	-	-	-	1.7	-	-	-	13.2	3.6	0.2	0.3	0.01	0.08	**0.5**	150
Stomach	71	0	-	-	-	-	0.5	0.5	0.7	1.8	10.6	1.4	13.9	25.9	9.9	43.5	59.6	62.0	3.3	4.9	0.33	0.84	**6.8**	151
Small intestine	4	0	0.3	-	-	-	-	-	-	-	1.2	-	-	-	-	5.4	-	3.6	0.2	0.3	0.01	0.03	**0.3**	152
Colon	66	0	-	-	-	-	-	2.1	1.8	8.3	2.7	8.7	23.5	6.6	38.0	53.0	73.0	3.0	4.6	0.27	0.72	**6.2**	153
Rectum	31	0	-	-	-	-	0.5	-	-	2.4	4.1	10.4	7.1	13.2	27.2	-	25.5	1.4	2.2	0.19	0.32	**3.1**	154
Liver	31	0	0.9	-	-	-	-	1.4	0.9	-	2.7	1.7	9.4	9.9	5.4	13.2	43.8	1.4	2.2	0.13	0.23	**2.6**	155
Gallbladder etc.	15	0	-	-	-	0.5	-	-	0.9	-	-	1.7	4.7	3.3	16.3	6.6	18.2	0.7	1.0	0.06	0.17	**1.5**	156
Pancreas	39	0	-	-	-	-	-	-	0.9	1.2	4.1	7.0	7.1	13.2	27.2	33.1	47.4	1.8	2.7	0.17	0.47	**4.0**	157
Nose, sinuses etc.	5	0	0.3	-	-	-	-	0.5	-	-	-	-	2.4	-	-	-	7.3	0.2	0.3	0.02	0.02	**0.3**	160
Larynx	39	0	-	-	-	-	-	-	-	0.9	1.2	4.1	10.4	23.5	19.7	10.9	6.6	32.8	1.8	2.7	0.30	0.39	**3.7**	161
Bronchus, lung	284	1	-	-	-	-	1.1	1.4	3.6	11.8	22.0	64.3	108.2	134.9	184.8	165.6	240.9	13.0	19.7	1.74	3.50	**29.1**	162
Other thoracic organs	7	0	0.6	-	-	0.8	-	0.5	-	-	-	-	2.4	-	-	5.4	-	0.3	0.5	0.02	0.05	**0.4**	163-4
Bone	16	0	-	0.7	0.7	0.8	0.9	1.1	-	-	3.5	-	1.7	-	-	5.4	-	3.6	0.7	1.1	0.05	0.07	**0.9**	170
Connective tissue	20	0	0.3	-	0.7	-	1.4	0.5	2.1	-	2.4	1.4	3.5	2.4	-	-	6.6	10.9	0.9	1.4	0.07	0.11	**1.2**	171
Mesothelioma	1	0	-	-	-	-	-	-	-	-	-	-	-	-	-	6.6	-	-	0.0	0.1	0.00	0.03	**0.1**	MES
Kaposi's sarcoma	8	0	-	-	-	-	0.5	0.5	-	-	-	1.4	1.7	2.4	-	10.9	-	3.6	0.4	0.6	0.03	0.09	**0.7**	KAP
Melanoma of skin	10	0	-	-	-	-	0.5	1.6	-	-	-	1.4	3.5	2.4	-	-	-	7.3	0.5	0.7	0.05	0.05	**0.7**	172
Other skin	8	0	-	-	-	-	0.5	0.5	-	0.9	2.4	1.4	-	4.7	-	-	-	-	0.4		0.05	0.05	**0.5**	173
Breast	5	0	-	-	-	-	-	-	-	-	1.2	-	-	-	-	10.9	6.6	3.6	0.2	0.3	0.01	0.09	**0.6**	175
Prostate	98	1	0.3	-	-	-	-	-	-	-	1.2	-	7.0	9.4	16.4	119.6	92.7	167.9	4.5	6.8	0.17	1.25	**10.4**	185
Testis	14	0	0.3	-	-	0.4	1.8	1.1	2.1	-	1.2	1.4	-	2.4	-	-	-	-	0.6	1.0	0.05	0.05	**0.7**	186
Penis	0	0	-	-	-	-	-	-	-	-	-	-	-	-	-	-	-	-	0.0	0.0	0.00	0.00	**0.0**	187.1-.4
Other male genital	0	0	-	-	-	-	-	-	-	-	-	-	-	-	-	-	-	-	0.0	0.0	0.00	0.00	**0.0**	187.5-.9
Bladder	128	1	-	-	-	-	-	1.1	0.7	1.8	1.2	13.7	15.7	44.7	36.2	114.1	72.8	146.0	5.9	8.9	0.58	1.52	**13.1**	188
Kidney etc.	36	0	0.9	0.3	-	-	0.5	0.5	-	0.9	-	4.1	5.2	9.4	23.0	5.4	33.1	21.9	1.6	2.5	0.22	0.42	**3.3**	189
Eye	13	0	2.1	0.3	-	-	-	-	0.7	0.9	1.2	-	-	-	3.3	-	6.6	-	0.6	0.9	0.04	0.08	**0.7**	190
Brain, nervous system	43	0	1.5	3.0	1.7	1.1	-	0.5	1.4	2.7	4.7	2.7	-	7.1	6.6	16.3	6.6	-	2.0	3.0	0.17	0.28	**2.6**	191-2
Thyroid	19	0	-	-	-	-	0.9	1.1	1.4	1.8	3.5	2.7	1.7	9.4	-	-	6.6	-	0.9	1.3	0.11	0.15	**1.3**	193
Other endocrine	9	0	1.2	0.3	-	0.4	-	-	-	0.9	1.2	1.4	-	-	-	-	-	-	0.4	0.6	0.03	0.03	**0.4**	194
Hodgkin's disease	50	0	-	3.4	1.0	2.7	2.3	2.7	4.9	2.7	2.4	5.5	1.7	4.7	3.3	-	-	-	2.3	3.5	0.19	0.19	**2.4**	201
Non-Hodgkin lymphoma	116	0	2.1	3.7	3.1	0.8	1.8	3.8	4.9	4.5	9.4	12.4	10.4	28.2	19.7	32.6	33.1	43.8	5.3	8.1	0.53	0.85	**8.3**	200,202
Multiple myeloma	20	0	-	-	-	-	-	-	-	-	-	1.4	7.0	9.4	13.2	5.4	13.2	14.6	0.9	1.4	0.15	0.25	**2.1**	203
Lymphoid leukaemia	49	0	2.1	1.7	2.4	2.3	-	1.1	0.7	1.8	-	2.7	1.7	7.1	3.3	-	13.2	36.5	2.2	3.4	0.13	0.20	**2.7**	204
Myeloid leukaemia	28	0	0.6	1.7	0.3	-	1.4	1.6	0.7	0.9	-	1.4	1.7	4.7	6.6	10.9	13.2	7.3	1.3	1.9	0.11	0.23	**2.0**	205
Monocytic leukaemia	0	0	-	-	-	-	-	-	-	-	-	-	-	-	-	-	-	-	0.0	0.0	0.00	0.00	**0.0**	206
Other leukaemia	2	0	0.3	-	-	-	-	-	-	-	-	-	-	-	3.3	-	-	-	0.1	0.1	0.02	0.02	**0.2**	207
Leukaemia unspecified	14	0	-	-	0.3	0.8	0.9	-	-	1.2	-	-	1.7	-	6.6	10.9	-	10.9	0.6	1.0	0.06	0.11	**1.1**	208
Other and unspecified	106	0	1.5	0.3	-	0.4	0.5	-	0.7	1.8	3.5	9.6	10.4	30.6	49.3	65.2	53.0	113.1	4.9	7.4	0.54	1.13	**10.2**	O&U
All sites	1448	3	15.2	15.6	10.5	11.1	15.7	20.5	26.0	33.6	79.1	111.3	205.2	409.4	404.6	788.0	735.1	1182.5	66.3		6.80	14.43	**128.3**	ALL
All sites but 173	1440	3	15.2	15.6	10.5	11.1	15.2	20.0	26.0	32.7	76.7	109.9	205.2	404.7	404.6	788.0	735.1	1182.5	66.0	100.0	6.75	14.38	**127.7**	ALLb

| Rate from 1 case | | | 0.298 | 0.338 | 0.349 | 0.382 | 0.461 | 0.540 | 0.702 | 0.908 | 1.181 | 1.374 | 1.739 | 2.353 | 3.289 | 5.435 | 6.623 | 3.650 |

ISRAEL: NON-JEWS 1988-1992

ANNUAL INCIDENCE PER 100,000 BY AGE GROUP (YEARS) - FEMALE

SITE	ALL AGES	AGE UNK	0-	5-	10-	15-	20-	25-	30-	35-	40-	45-	50-	55-	60-	65-	70-	75+	CRUDE RATE	%	CR 64	CR 74	ASR (W)	ICD (9th)
Lip	10	0	-	-	-	-	-	-	-	0.9	1.2	-	1.8	2.2	5.4	7.8	5.2	3.8	0.5	0.8	0.06	0.12	**0.9**	140
Tongue	5	0	-	-	-	-	-	-	-	-	1.2	-	-	2.2	-	-	10.4	3.8	0.2	0.4	0.02	0.07	**0.4**	141
Salivary gland	2	0	-	-	-	-	-	0.5	-	-	-	-	-	-	-	-	-	3.8	0.1	0.2	0.00	0.00	**0.1**	142
Mouth	5	0	-	-	-	-	-	-	0.7	-	1.2	-	-	-	2.7	3.9	-	3.8	0.2	0.4	0.02	0.04	**0.4**	143-5
Oropharynx	0	0	-	-	-	-	-	-	-	-	-	-	-	-	-	-	-	-	0.0	0.0	0.00	0.00	**0.0**	146
Nasopharynx	2	0	-	-	0.4	-	-	-	0.7	-	-	-	-	-	-	-	-	-	0.1	0.2	0.01	0.01	**0.1**	147
Hypopharynx	2	0	-	-	-	-	-	-	-	-	-	-	1.8	-	-	3.9	-	-	0.1	0.2	0.01	0.03	**0.2**	148
Pharynx unspecified	0	0	-	-	-	-	-	-	-	-	-	-	-	-	-	-	-	-	0.0	0.0	0.00	0.00	**0.0**	149
Oesophagus	3	0	-	-	-	-	-	-	0.7	-	-	-	-	-	-	-	-	7.6	0.1	0.3	0.00	0.00	**0.2**	150
Stomach	40	1	-	-	-	-	-	0.5	1.4	4.5	1.2	5.7	5.3	4.3	5.4	7.8	31.1	41.7	1.9	3.3	0.14	0.34	**3.2**	151
Small intestine	5	0	-	0.4	-	-	-	-	-	-	-	2.8	-	2.2	2.7	-	-	-	0.2	0.4	0.04	0.04	**0.4**	152
Colon	70	0	-	-	-	-	-	1.1	-	-	4.8	11.3	5.3	19.4	21.5	27.5	31.1	87.1	3.3	5.8	0.32	0.61	**6.1**	153
Rectum	36	0	-	-	-	-	-	0.5	-	-	4.8	9.9	5.3	6.5	10.8	19.6	15.5	22.7	1.7	3.0	0.19	0.36	**3.2**	154
Liver	18	0	0.3	-	0.4	-	0.5	-	-	0.9	1.2	1.4	3.5	-	5.4	7.8	5.2	18.9	0.8	1.5	0.07	0.13	**1.4**	155
Gallbladder etc.	34	0	-	-	-	-	-	-	-	1.8	1.2	1.4	8.8	8.6	16.1	31.4	10.4	18.9	1.6	2.8	0.19	0.40	**3.2**	156
Pancreas	31	0	-	-	-	-	-	-	-	-	-	2.8	3.5	8.6	13.4	23.5	15.5	34.1	1.4	2.6	0.14	0.34	**2.9**	157
Nose, sinuses etc.	2	0	-	-	-	-	-	-	-	-	1.4	-	-	2.7	-	-	-	-	0.1	0.2	0.02	0.02	**0.2**	160
Larynx	0	0	-	-	-	-	-	-	-	-	-	-	-	-	-	-	-	-	0.0	0.0	0.00	0.00	**0.0**	161
Bronchus, lung	41	0	-	-	0.4	-	-	-	1.4	-	-	1.4	14.0	8.6	21.5	23.5	15.5	30.3	1.9	3.4	0.24	0.43	**3.7**	162
Other thoracic organs	3	0	-	-	-	-	0.9	-	-	0.9	-	-	-	-	-	-	-	-	0.1	0.3	0.01	0.01	**0.1**	163-4
Bone	9	0	0.3	0.4	1.8	0.4	-	0.5	-	-	-	-	-	-	-	-	-	-	0.4	0.8	0.02	0.02	**0.3**	170
Connective tissue	16	0	0.3	0.4	-	1.2	0.5	0.5	0.7	-	1.2	1.4	3.5	2.2	2.7	-	-	7.6	0.7	1.3	0.07	0.07	**1.0**	171
Mesothelioma	5	0	-	-	-	-	-	0.5	-	-	-	-	1.8	2.2	-	-	-	7.6	0.2	0.4	0.02	0.02	**0.4**	MES
Kaposi's sarcoma	4	0	-	0.4	-	-	-	-	-	-	1.2	-	-	-	-	-	10.4	-	0.2	0.3	0.01	0.06	**0.3**	KAP
Melanoma of skin	8	0	-	-	-	-	-	-	-	-	2.4	1.4	1.8	2.2	2.7	-	-	7.6	0.4	0.7	0.05	0.05	**0.7**	172
Other skin	9	0	-	-	-	-	0.5	1.1	-	1.8	-	-	-	-	2.7	-	5.2	7.6	0.4		0.03	0.06	**0.6**	173
Breast	262	0	-	-	-	-	-	0.9	1.6	11.2	28.0	36.9	59.4	52.6	84.1	80.6	54.9	51.8	53.0	12.2	21.9	1.78	2.31	**21.3**	174
Uterus unspecified	1	0	-	-	-	-	-	-	-	-	1.2	-	-	-	-	-	-	-	0.0	0.1	0.01	0.01	**0.1**	179
Cervix uteri	40	1	-	-	-	-	-	0.5	0.7	10.8	4.8	9.9	10.5	6.5	8.1	3.9	-	3.8	1.9	3.3	0.27	0.29	**3.0**	180
Placenta	0	0	-	-	-	-	-	-	-	-	-	-	-	-	-	-	-	-	0.0	0.0	0.00	0.00	**0.0**	181
Corpus uteri	55	0	-	-	-	-	-	-	0.7	3.6	4.8	12.7	8.8	21.6	21.5	27.5	20.7	11.4	2.6	4.6	0.37	0.61	**4.9**	182
Ovary etc.	37	0	-	-	-	0.8	0.5	0.5	0.7	3.6	3.6	4.2	7.0	6.5	18.8	11.8	5.2	15.2	1.7	3.1	0.23	0.32	**3.0**	183
Other female genital	8	0	-	-	-	-	-	-	0.7	-	1.2	-	-	4.3	5.4	-	10.4	-	0.4	0.7	0.06	0.11	**0.7**	184
Bladder	16	0	-	-	-	-	0.5	-	-	-	1.2	-	3.5	-	-	11.8	10.4	26.5	0.7	1.3	0.03	0.14	**1.4**	188
Kidney etc.	24	0	0.6	1.1	-	0.4	-	-	-	-	1.2	1.4	5.3	6.5	10.8	3.9	5.2	15.2	1.1	2.0	0.14	0.18	**1.9**	189
Eye	10	0	2.2	-	-	-	-	-	-	-	1.2	-	-	-	-	3.9	-	3.8	0.5	0.8	0.02	0.04	**0.5**	190
Brain, nervous system	42	0	1.6	1.8	1.1	2.4	0.5	1.1	1.4	2.7	-	5.7	-	4.3	13.4	3.9	5.2	7.6	2.0	3.5	0.18	0.23	**2.5**	191-2
Thyroid	61	0	-	-	0.4	2.0	1.9	3.8	3.5	6.3	6.0	8.5	12.3	8.6	13.4	3.9	10.4	7.6	2.8	5.1	0.33	0.40	**4.1**	193
Other endocrine	8	0	0.6	0.4	0.4	-	-	-	-	-	1.2	2.8	-	2.2	-	-	-	-	0.4	0.7	0.04	0.04	**0.5**	194
Hodgkin's disease	28	0	-	1.1	0.7	3.2	1.4	1.1	-	2.7	-	-	1.8	-	8.1	7.8	5.2	-	1.3	2.3	0.10	0.17	**1.6**	201
Non-Hodgkin lymphoma	86	0	0.6	2.1	0.4	1.6	0.9	2.2	3.5	4.5	6.0	7.1	8.8	17.2	10.8	39.2	46.6	41.7	4.0	7.2	0.33	0.76	**6.5**	200,202
Multiple myeloma	17	0	-	-	-	-	-	-	-	-	-	4.2	5.3	4.3	8.1	7.8	10.4	7.6	0.8	1.4	0.11	0.20	**1.6**	203
Lymphoid leukaemia	24	1	1.6	1.4	1.1	0.4	-	-	-	1.8	1.2	-	1.8	-	2.7	-	10.4	11.4	1.1	2.0	0.06	0.12	**1.3**	204
Myeloid leukaemia	33	0	0.9	-	0.4	2.0	0.9	1.6	1.4	4.5	2.4	-	-	-	2.7	3.9	20.7	15.2	1.5	2.8	0.08	0.21	**2.0**	205
Monocytic leukaemia	0	0	-	-	-	-	-	-	-	-	-	-	-	-	-	-	-	-	0.0	0.0	0.00	0.00	**0.0**	206
Other leukaemia	1	0	0.3	-	-	-	-	-	-	-	-	-	-	-	-	-	-	-	0.0	0.1	0.00	0.00	**0.0**	207
Leukaemia unspecified	14	0	0.3	-	-	-	-	1.1	-	-	-	2.4	-	-	-	10.8	-	5.2	15.2	0.7	1.2	0.07	0.10	**1.1**	208
Other and unspecified	79	0	0.3	1.1	-	-	-	0.5	1.4	0.9	2.4	7.1	7.0	23.7	34.9	35.3	36.3	75.8	3.7	6.6	0.40	0.75	**6.9**	O&U
All sites	1206	3	9.9	10.3	7.3	14.5	9.7	19.5	30.9	80.4	98.8	164.1	180.7	258.6	365.6	376.5	409.3	617.4	56.3		6.27	10.21	**95.0**	ALL
All sites but 173	1197	3	9.9	10.3	7.3	14.5	9.3	18.4	30.9	78.6	98.8	164.1	180.7	258.6	362.9	376.5	404.1	609.8	55.8	100.0	6.24	10.15	**94.5**	ALLb

| Rate from 1 case | | | 0.311 | 0.356 | 0.366 | 0.403 | 0.464 | 0.543 | 0.702 | 0.903 | 1.190 | 1.414 | 1.754 | 2.155 | 2.688 | 3.922 | 5.181 | 3.788 | | | | | | |

Japan, Hiroshima

The Hiroshima Tumour Registry was established in 1957 under the auspices of the Hiroshima City Medical Association and with technical support from the Atomic Bomb Casualty Commission, the predecessor of the Radiation Effects Research Foundation (RERF). The objectives were to develop and maintain a source of information on tumours diagnosed in the community and to provide cancer incidence data for studies on the effects of exposure to radiation from the atomic bombing in 1945.

Hiroshima City, the capital of Hiroshima Prefecture, is located in the western part of Japan. It covers an area of 740 km² (latitude 34° N, longitude 132° E, altitude from sea level to 890 m). Hiroshima City is an administratively defined area which does not completely correspond with Hiroshima metropolitan area. The latter includes the city itself and its surrounding suburban areas. After its destruction in the atomic bombing of 1945, Hiroshima City developed as an administrative centre in the Chugoku and Shikoku areas. Its major industries include shipbuilding, automobile, metalworking, machinery and other manufacturing. The population in 1990 was 1 090 000 (density 1467 per km²), of whom 99% were Japanese. The proportion 65 years and over was 10% in 1990, compared with 7% in 1980. The population is primarily urban; 69% of employees are in sales, trade and service industries, 29% in construction and manufacturing industries and only 2% in agriculture and related work. The number of hospital beds per 100 000 population was 1310 in 1993; the number of physicians per 100 000 population was 246 in 1992.

The case-finding and data-collection procedures combine both active and passive approaches. All physicians and hospitals in the city are requested by the Medical Association to report tumour cases to the registry. Reportable tumours include all malignant neoplasms, neoplasms of uncertain nature and benign neoplasms of the central nervous system. However, a great majority (about 80%) of cases are accessed by means of hospital visits. RERF field personnel visit most of the large hospitals in the area and review all the hospital records, including clinical records, surgical reports, radiology reports, and cytology, pathology and autopsy reports. Causes of death are also ascertained.

The Hiroshima Tissue Registry, a prefecture-wide registry started in 1973 under the auspices of the Hiroshima Prefectural Medical Association, serves as an additional source of information. This registry is designed to collect and examine surgically removed tumour tissues; tumours are classified and tissue slides are stored. Malignant cases residing in the city and identified through the Tissue Registry are added to the Tumour Registry file.

Information obtained for the Tumour Registry includes name, address, sex, date of birth, tumour site and morphology, methods of diagnosis and date of diagnosis. Cases identified from various hospitals and sources are collated, and data are stored in computerized files. Checking for duplicate entries is performed manually with the assistance of a computer. All cases with possible multiple primary tumours are reviewed; pathology slides from the Tissue Registry are also reviewed, if necessary. Two or more tumours in one person are recorded separately under the same personal identity. Edit checks are performed including: sex versus site; age versus site; site versus morphology; and year of birth and year of death versus year of diagnosis. The completeness of registration is assessed by conventional indices as well as data from independent *ad hoc* surveys. The current rate of death-certificate-only registrations is about 7%. Since a majority of cases are ascertained by visits to large hospitals, cases missed by not including all area hospitals present a source of concern. However, a recent survey of three medium-sized hospitals that are not included in the regular data abstraction schedule indicated that missed cases from such hospitals represent less than 1% of all cancers.

Long-term epidemiological studies of the atomic bombing survivors have shown excess leukaemia risk, which was seen mostly in the early years after the bombing, and excess solid cancer risk which still persists. However, excess cancer cases due to atomic bomb radiation constitute a very small proportion of the overall population cancer incidence rate for Hiroshima. Excess incident cancer cases that occurred in the atomic bomb survivors residing in Hiroshima are estimated, very roughly, to be fewer than 200 for the period 1986–90 covered in this report. This is about 1% of a total of over 17 000 incident cases reported for the entire population of Hiroshima for the same period.

K. Mabuchi
Y. Fujita

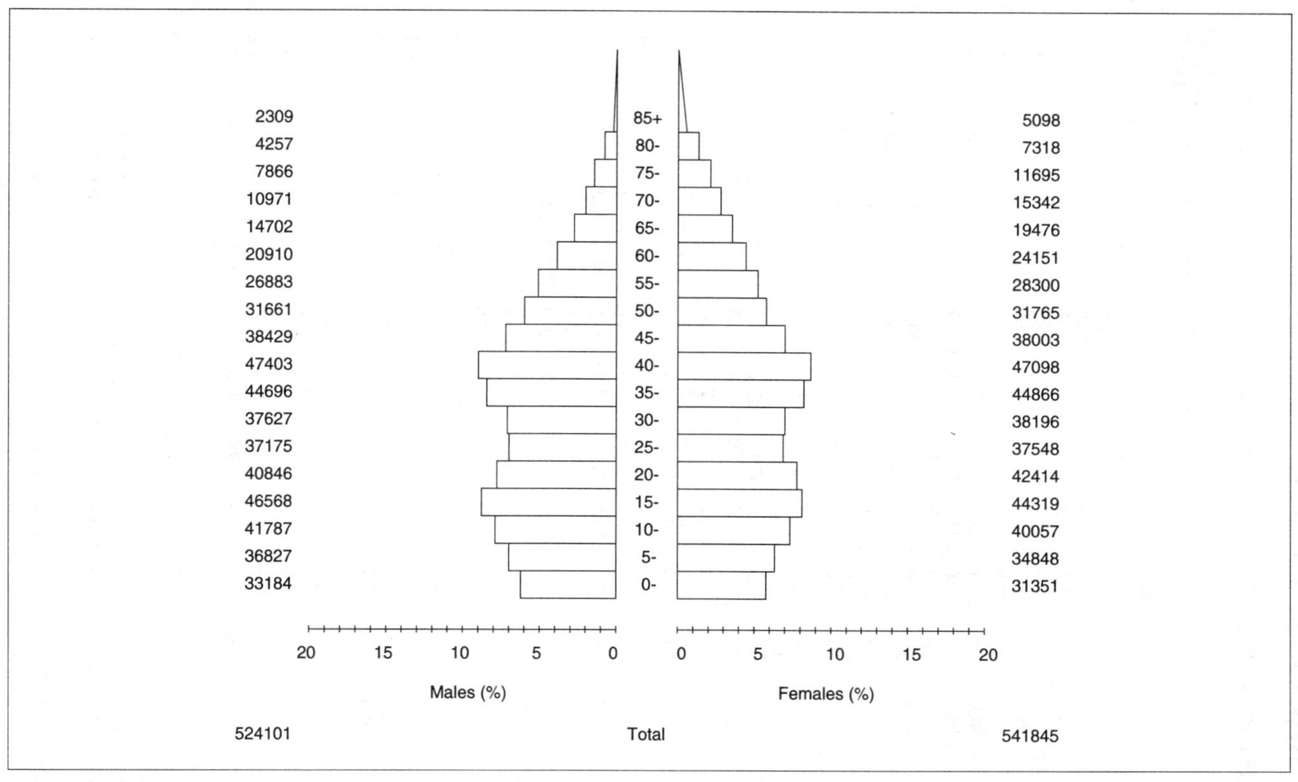

Japan, Hiroshima

Source of population: average annual 1986–90

Census: 1990 Population Census of Japan, Statistics Bureau, Management and Coordination Agency, 1991. 1985 Population Census of Japan, Statistics Bureau, Management and Coordination Agency, 1986.

Estimate: The data for each year are estimated by linear interpolation of the 1985 and 1990 Census data.

Screening programmes in the area:

There has been a screening programme for women over age 30 for cervical cancer since 1983 and for breast cancer since 1987 (20,000 examinations for each site in 1993). The population over age 40 has been screened for stomach cancer since 1983 (20,000 examinations in 1993) and lung cancer since 1987 (2,000 examinations in 1993).

JAPAN, HIROSHIMA 1986-1990

ANNUAL INCIDENCE PER 100,000 BY AGE GROUP (YEARS) - MALE

SITE	ALL AGES	AGE UNK	0-	5-	10-	15-	20-	25-	30-	35-	40-	45-	50-	55-	60-	65-	70-	75-	80-	85+	CRUDE RATE	%	CR 64	CR 74	ASR (W)	ICD (9th)
Lip	1	0	-	-	-	-	-	-	-	-	-	-	0.6	-	-	-	-	-	-	-	0.0	0.0	0.00	0.00	0.0	140
Tongue	60	0	-	-	-	-	0.5	0.5	1.1	0.9	2.1	3.1	5.1	5.2	8.6	9.5	7.3	15.3	4.7	8.7	2.3	0.6	0.14	0.22	2.0	141
Salivary gland	24	0	-	0.5	-	-	0.5	-	-	0.4	0.4	1.0	1.9	3.7	1.9	1.4	1.8	7.6	14.1	-	0.9	0.2	0.05	0.07	0.8	142
Mouth	47	0	-	-	-	-	-	-	-	0.9	-	2.1	5.1	6.0	5.7	10.9	10.9	7.6	4.7	8.7	1.8	0.5	0.10	0.21	1.6	143-5
Oropharynx	21	0	-	-	-	-	-	-	-	-	-	0.5	2.5	4.5	3.8	5.4	3.6	-	-	-	0.8	0.2	0.06	0.10	0.7	146
Nasopharynx	17	0	-	-	-	-	0.5	-	-	0.4	1.3	2.6	0.6	2.2	1.0	-	3.6	-	-	-	0.6	0.2	0.04	0.06	0.5	147
Hypopharynx	35	0	-	-	-	-	-	-	-	-	0.4	-	1.3	6.0	4.8	10.9	5.5	10.2	9.4	17.3	1.3	0.4	0.06	0.14	1.2	148
Pharynx unspecified	8	0	-	-	-	-	-	-	-	-	-	-	0.6	0.7	2.9	-	1.8	5.1	-	-	0.3	0.1	0.02	0.03	0.3	149
Oesophagus	317	0	-	-	-	-	0.5	0.5	-	-	0.8	8.8	16.4	38.7	60.3	62.6	87.5	81.4	98.7	69.3	12.1	3.3	0.63	1.38	10.7	150
Stomach	2508	7	-	-	-	-	1.0	2.7	10.6	26.0	40.1	85.4	142.8	234.3	327.1	508.8	630.7	747.5	789.2	796.8	95.7	26.1	4.36	10.08	83.1	151
Small intestine	15	0	-	-	-	-	-	-	-	-	-	1.6	0.6	0.7	3.8	-	1.8	5.1	9.4	8.7	0.6	0.2	0.03	0.04	0.5	152
Colon	939	0	-	-	-	-	-	-	4.3	5.8	13.5	23.4	55.0	88.5	149.2	212.2	220.6	269.5	272.5	329.1	35.8	9.8	1.70	3.86	31.6	153
Rectum	576	4	-	-	-	-	-	1.1	1.6	5.8	8.9	17.2	35.4	60.3	89.0	112.9	156.8	106.8	159.7	216.5	22.0	6.0	1.10	2.46	19.4	154
Liver	1352	1	-	-	-	-	-	1.1	2.1	4.0	18.1	27.1	92.9	219.5	272.6	273.4	242.4	259.3	239.6	233.8	51.6	14.1	3.19	5.77	45.5	155
Gallbladder etc.	185	1	-	-	-	-	-	-	-	-	2.5	2.6	5.1	15.6	15.3	53.1	45.6	78.8	108.0	86.6	7.1	1.9	0.21	0.70	6.1	156
Pancreas	264	1	-	-	-	-	-	-	-	0.9	2.5	5.2	10.7	23.1	42.1	69.4	62.0	89.0	89.3	121.3	10.1	2.7	0.42	1.08	9.0	157
Nose, sinuses etc.	32	0	-	-	-	-	-	0.5	0.5	-	1.3	1.6	3.2	5.2	4.8	5.4	3.6	2.5	-	-	1.2	0.3	0.09	0.13	1.1	160
Larynx	117	0	-	-	-	-	-	-	-	-	-	4.2	2.5	19.3	19.1	24.5	38.3	28.0	32.9	17.3	4.5	1.2	0.23	0.54	3.9	161
Bronchus, lung	1193	2	-	-	-	-	0.5	0.5	1.1	3.6	7.6	10.9	27.2	93.0	179.8	238.1	368.2	511.0	653.0	580.3	45.5	12.4	1.62	4.66	39.6	162
Other thoracic organs	34	0	3.6	-	-	0.9	-	-	1.6	0.9	1.7	0.5	1.9	2.2	1.9	1.4	1.8	5.1	14.1	8.7	1.3	0.4	0.08	0.09	1.3	163-4
Bone	18	0	-	-	1.0	1.7	0.5	-	0.5	-	-	1.0	-	2.2	-	2.7	-	2.5	9.4	-	0.7	0.2	0.03	0.05	0.6	170
Connective tissue	33	0	0.6	-	-	0.4	1.0	1.6	0.5	0.9	1.7	0.5	0.6	2.2	2.9	5.4	3.6	7.6	4.7	8.7	1.3	0.3	0.06	0.11	1.2	171
Mesothelioma	13	0	-	-	-	-	-	-	-	0.4	-	1.0	1.3	0.7	1.0	2.7	3.6	5.1	-	-	0.5	0.1	0.02	0.05	0.4	MES
Kaposi's sarcoma	0	0	-	-	-	-	-	-	-	-	-	-	-	-	-	-	-	-	-	-	0.0	0.0	0.00	0.00	0.0	KAP
Melanoma of skin	13	0	-	0.5	-	-	-	-	-	-	0.4	0.5	1.9	-	1.9	2.7	3.6	-	4.7	-	0.5	0.1	0.03	0.06	0.5	172
Other skin	164	3	-	0.5	0.5	-	-	-	0.5	3.1	1.3	3.6	5.7	14.9	19.1	21.8	36.5	68.6	112.7	43.3	6.3		0.25	0.55	5.2	173
Breast	7	0	-	-	-	-	-	-	-	-	-	-	-	1.9	2.7	3.6	2.5	-	-	-	0.3	0.1	0.01	0.04	0.3	175
Prostate	329	1	-	-	-	-	-	-	-	-	-	-	2.5	6.0	30.6	61.2	129.4	193.2	249.0	337.8	12.6	3.4	0.20	1.15	10.9	185
Testis	49	0	1.2	-	-	0.9	2.4	5.9	3.2	3.1	3.0	1.0	2.5	1.5	-	-	1.8	-	-	-	1.9	0.5	0.12	0.13	1.7	186
Penis	11	0	-	-	-	-	-	-	-	-	0.4	0.5	-	2.2	1.9	-	3.6	5.1	-	-	0.4	0.1	0.03	0.04	0.3	187.1-.4
Other male genital	8	0	-	-	-	-	-	-	-	0.5	-	-	1.0	-	1.5	-	3.6	2.5	-	-	0.3	0.1	0.02	0.03	0.3	187.5-.9
Bladder	388	1	-	-	-	-	-	-	-	2.7	6.3	11.4	13.3	30.5	42.1	88.4	113.0	134.8	173.8	181.9	14.8	4.0	0.53	1.54	12.9	188
Kidney etc.	231	0	-	-	-	-	-	1.1	0.5	2.7	3.4	4.7	12.0	15.6	36.3	57.1	58.3	63.6	79.9	95.3	8.8	2.4	0.38	0.96	7.8	189
Eye	6	0	2.4	0.5	-	-	-	-	-	-	-	-	0.5	-	-	-	-	-	-	-	0.2	0.1	0.02	0.02	0.4	190
Brain, nervous system	65	0	0.6	1.1	1.4	0.9	0.5	1.1	3.7	2.2	2.5	3.1	1.3	5.2	6.7	6.8	9.1	10.2	-	-	2.5	0.7	0.15	0.23	2.2	191-2
Thyroid	90	0	-	-	-	-	1.5	1.6	0.5	3.1	4.6	6.2	5.1	8.2	7.7	9.5	10.9	25.4	4.7	17.3	3.4	0.9	0.19	0.29	2.9	193
Other endocrine	10	0	1.8	-	1.0	0.9	-	-	-	-	-	-	-	-	1.9	-	1.8	-	-	-	0.4	0.1	0.03	0.04	0.5	194
Hodgkin's disease	8	0	-	-	-	0.4	-	-	-	0.4	-	-	0.6	1.5	1.0	1.4	1.8	-	-	-	0.3	0.1	0.02	0.04	0.3	201
Non-Hodgkin lymphoma	248	1	3.6	2.7	2.4	0.9	1.0	3.2	2.7	4.5	4.6	8.3	10.1	20.1	29.7	32.6	52.9	66.1	75.2	86.6	9.5	2.6	0.47	0.90	8.6	200,202
Multiple myeloma	53	1	-	-	-	-	-	-	0.5	-	0.4	1.6	1.3	3.0	5.7	6.8	27.3	20.3	9.4	43.3	2.0	0.6	0.06	0.24	1.8	203
Lymphoid leukaemia	46	0	2.4	0.5	2.4	2.1	-	0.5	0.5	1.3	0.8	1.0	2.5	2.2	1.9	5.4	9.1	7.6	-	8.7	1.8	0.5	0.09	0.17	1.8	204
Myeloid leukaemia	105	0	-	1.1	1.9	1.3	1.5	-	1.1	3.6	2.5	3.6	5.7	10.4	9.6	9.5	21.9	35.6	4.7	26.0	4.0	1.1	0.21	0.37	3.5	205
Monocytic leukaemia	3	0	0.6	-	-	-	-	-	-	-	-	-	-	-	-	-	-	5.1	-	-	0.1	0.0	0.00	0.00	0.1	206
Other leukaemia	0	0	-	-	-	-	-	-	-	-	-	-	-	-	-	-	-	-	-	-	0.0	0.0	0.00	0.00	0.0	207
Leukaemia unspecified	12	0	0.6	-	-	0.4	-	0.5	-	0.9	0.4	-	-	-	1.0	2.7	3.6	2.5	-	-	0.5	0.1	0.02	0.05	0.5	208
Other and unspecified	123	1	0.6	0.5	-	-	-	-	1.6	0.4	1.7	3.1	5.7	11.2	17.2	15.0	29.2	43.2	56.4	69.3	4.7	1.3	0.21	0.43	4.1	O&U
All sites	9778	24	18.1	8.1	10.5	10.7	11.8	22.6	39.3	79.2	135.4	250.9	483.2	967.9	1413.7	1934.4	2422.6	2931.5	3283.7	3421.1	373.1		17.30	39.14	327.5	ALL
All sites but 173	9614	21	18.1	7.6	10.1	10.7	11.8	22.6	38.8	76.1	134.2	247.2	477.6	953.0	1394.5	1912.6	2386.1	2862.9	3170.9	3377.8	366.9	100.0	17.05	38.59	322.3	ALLb
Rate from 1 case			0.603	0.543	0.479	0.429	0.490	0.538	0.532	0.447	0.422	0.520	0.632	0.744	0.956	1.360	1.823	2.543	4.698	8.661						

JAPAN, HIROSHIMA 1986-1990

ANNUAL INCIDENCE PER 100,000 BY AGE GROUP (YEARS) - FEMALE

SITE	ALL AGES	AGE UNK	0-	5-	10-	15-	20-	25-	30-	35-	40-	45-	50-	55-	60-	65-	70-	75-	80-	85+	CRUDE RATE	%	CR 64	CR 74	ASR (W)	ICD (9th)
Lip	1	0	-	-	-	-	-	-	-	-	-	-	-	-	-	1.0	-	-	-	-	0.0	0.0	0.00	0.01	**0.0**	*140*
Tongue	27	0	-	-	-	-	0.9	-	-	-	-	1.1	4.4	1.4	3.3	2.1	1.3	3.4	8.2	7.8	1.0	0.4	0.06	0.07	**0.8**	*141*
Salivary gland	8	0	-	-	-	-	-	0.5	-	-	-	-	0.6	-	3.3	-	1.3	1.7	-	-	0.3	0.1	0.02	0.03	**0.2**	*142*
Mouth	27	1	-	-	-	-	-	-	0.5	-	-	0.5	1.3	1.4	0.8	3.1	7.8	8.6	8.2	7.8	1.0	0.4	0.02	0.08	**0.7**	*143-5*
Oropharynx	3	0	-	-	-	-	-	-	-	0.4	-	0.5	-	-	-	-	1.3	-	-	-	0.1	0.0	0.00	0.01	**0.1**	*146*
Nasopharynx	9	0	-	-	-	-	-	0.5	0.5	-	-	1.6	-	0.7	0.8	1.0	-	1.7	-	-	0.3	0.1	0.02	0.03	**0.3**	*147*
Hypopharynx	4	0	-	-	-	-	-	-	-	-	-	-	0.6	0.7	-	1.0	1.3	-	-	-	0.1	0.1	0.01	0.02	**0.1**	*148*
Pharynx unspecified	2	0	-	-	-	-	-	-	-	-	-	-	-	-	-	-	2.6	-	-	-	0.1	0.0	0.00	0.01	**0.1**	*149*
Oesophagus	69	0	-	-	-	-	-	-	-	-	0.4	0.5	6.3	3.5	6.6	7.2	9.1	32.5	21.9	11.8	2.5	1.0	0.09	0.17	**1.7**	*150*
Stomach	1384	0	-	-	-	0.9	0.9	5.9	9.9	29.4	35.2	43.7	61.1	80.6	123.4	187.9	242.5	318.1	300.6	364.8	51.1	19.1	1.96	4.11	**35.9**	*151*
Small intestine	11	0	-	-	-	-	-	-	-	-	-	1.1	0.6	-	2.5	1.0	2.6	1.7	2.7	-	0.4	0.2	0.02	0.04	**0.3**	*152*
Colon	717	1	-	-	-	0.5	0.5	1.1	1.0	5.3	15.3	17.4	30.2	54.4	75.4	89.3	122.5	179.6	194.0	219.7	26.5	9.9	1.01	2.07	**18.2**	*153*
Rectum	360	1	-	-	-	-	0.9	-	2.1	3.1	6.8	13.2	19.5	29.7	39.7	61.6	57.4	71.8	60.1	62.8	13.3	5.0	0.58	1.17	**9.7**	*154*
Liver	440	0	-	-	-	0.5	0.5	-	-	0.9	1.3	3.7	10.7	33.2	54.7	88.3	110.8	90.6	128.4	98.1	16.2	6.1	0.53	1.52	**11.4**	*155*
Gallbladder etc.	246	1	-	-	-	-	-	0.5	1.0	0.9	1.7	3.2	5.7	12.0	24.8	20.5	69.1	68.4	98.4	98.1	9.1	3.4	0.25	0.70	**5.9**	*156*
Pancreas	235	0	-	-	-	-	-	-	-	1.3	1.7	3.2	7.6	12.7	14.1	30.8	67.8	54.7	82.0	121.6	8.7	3.2	0.20	0.70	**5.7**	*157*
Nose, sinuses etc.	14	0	-	-	-	-	0.5	0.5	-	0.8	-	0.6	2.1	0.8	2.1	-	3.4	2.7	-	0.5	0.2	0.03	0.04	**0.4**	*160*
Larynx	10	0	-	-	-	-	0.5	0.5	-	-	-	-	1.4	-	3.1	-	5.1	-	-	-	0.4	0.1	0.01	0.03	**0.3**	*161*
Bronchus, lung	469	0	-	-	0.5	-	-	-	1.0	2.7	7.2	11.1	16.4	30.4	39.7	66.7	101.7	123.1	155.8	129.4	17.3	6.5	0.55	1.39	**11.7**	*162*
Other thoracic organs	19	0	0.6	-	-	-	0.5	0.5	-	0.4	0.8	0.5	1.9	0.7	1.7	3.1	1.3	3.4	-	-	0.7	0.3	0.04	0.06	**0.6**	*163-4*
Bone	16	0	-	-	0.5	0.5	0.9	0.5	-	1.3	0.8	1.1	-	-	2.5	1.0	-	-	-	-	0.6	0.2	0.04	0.05	**0.5**	*170*
Connective tissue	32	0	3.2	-	0.5	-	-	0.5	1.0	1.3	0.4	1.1	1.9	2.8	0.8	4.1	1.3	1.7	5.5	3.9	1.2	0.4	0.07	0.10	**1.2**	*171*
Mesothelioma	5	0	-	-	-	-	0.5	-	0.5	-	-	-	-	-	0.8	-	-	3.4	-	-	0.2	0.1	0.01	0.01	**0.1**	*MES*
Kaposi's sarcoma	0	0	-	-	-	-	-	-	-	-	-	-	-	-	-	-	-	-	-	-	0.0	0.0	0.00	0.00	**0.0**	*KAP*
Melanoma of skin	16	0	-	-	-	0.5	-	0.5	0.5	0.9	0.4	1.1	1.3	-	0.8	-	2.6	-	2.7	7.8	0.6	0.2	0.03	0.04	**0.5**	*172*
Other skin	155	1	-	0.6	-	0.9	-	2.7	0.5	1.3	3.0	1.6	4.4	10.6	11.6	11.3	30.0	29.1	43.7	113.8	5.7		0.19	0.39	**3.9**	*173*
Breast	1172	4	-	-	-	0.5	0.5	0.5	16.2	38.8	75.2	106.3	89.4	89.0	111.0	107.8	87.3	77.0	82.0	74.5	43.3	16.2	2.65	3.62	**33.4**	*174*
Uterus unspecified	29	0	-	-	-	-	-	-	-	1.3	0.8	0.5	2.5	0.7	1.7	1.0	1.3	5.1	8.2	31.4	1.1	0.4	0.04	0.05	**0.7**	*179*
Cervix uteri	456	1	-	-	-	-	0.9	3.7	10.5	22.3	23.8	17.9	29.0	28.3	47.2	43.1	43.0	56.4	62.9	47.1	16.8	6.3	0.92	1.35	**12.6**	*180*
Placenta	1	0	-	-	-	-	-	-	-	0.4	-	-	-	-	-	-	-	-	-	-	0.0	0.0	0.00	0.00	**0.0**	*181*
Corpus uteri	171	0	-	-	-	-	0.9	1.6	1.6	2.2	6.4	6.8	16.4	19.8	23.2	17.5	20.9	17.1	5.5	11.8	6.3	2.4	0.39	0.59	**5.0**	*182*
Ovary etc.	224	1	0.6	1.1	0.5	0.9	2.4	4.3	4.2	8.5	9.3	14.7	12.6	19.8	19.9	18.5	14.3	20.5	16.4	31.4	8.3	3.1	0.50	0.66	**6.6**	*183*
Other female genital	32	0	-	-	-	-	-	-	-	0.4	0.4	1.1	1.3	2.8	4.1	5.1	6.5	6.8	2.7	7.8	1.2	0.4	0.05	0.11	**0.9**	*184*
Bladder	114	1	-	-	-	-	-	-	-	0.4	0.8	1.1	6.3	5.7	5.0	21.6	28.7	22.2	46.5	43.1	4.2	1.6	0.10	0.35	**2.8**	*188*
Kidney etc.	115	0	1.9	-	-	-	0.5	-	1.6	0.4	1.3	2.1	4.4	10.6	14.9	13.3	24.8	23.9	30.1	11.8	4.2	1.6	0.19	0.38	**3.2**	*189*
Eye	2	0	0.6	-	-	-	-	-	0.5	-	-	-	-	-	-	-	-	-	-	-	0.1	0.0	0.01	0.01	**0.1**	*190*
Brain, nervous system	54	0	1.9	2.3	2.0	3.2	0.9	0.5	1.0	0.9	0.8	2.6	3.1	2.8	2.5	4.1	5.2	1.7	2.7	-	2.0	0.7	0.12	0.17	**2.0**	*191-2*
Thyroid	321	0	-	-	0.5	0.5	3.3	5.9	7.9	11.1	18.3	21.1	23.9	21.2	29.8	24.6	31.3	20.5	19.1	27.5	11.8	4.4	0.72	1.00	**9.4**	*193*
Other endocrine	9	0	3.2	-	-	-	-	-	-	-	0.4	0.5	0.6	-	-	1.0	-	-	-	-	0.3	0.1	0.02	0.03	**0.5**	*194*
Hodgkin's disease	11	0	-	-	-	0.9	-	1.1	-	-	-	1.1	-	0.7	1.7	2.1	-	-	-	-	0.4	0.2	0.03	0.04	**0.4**	*201*
Non-Hodgkin lymphoma	164	2	-	0.6	0.5	0.5	-	2.1	1.6	2.2	2.1	8.4	6.3	8.5	9.9	21.6	36.5	39.3	35.5	27.5	6.1	2.3	0.22	0.51	**4.4**	*200,202*
Multiple myeloma	43	0	-	-	-	-	-	-	-	-	0.8	2.6	1.9	1.4	5.0	9.2	3.9	1.7	30.1	3.9	1.6	0.6	0.06	0.12	**1.1**	*203*
Lymphoid leukaemia	25	0	1.9	1.7	-	0.5	0.9	-	1.0	0.9	0.8	0.5	0.6	0.7	0.8	2.1	1.3	1.7	5.5	-	0.9	0.3	0.05	0.07	**0.9**	*204*
Myeloid leukaemia	71	0	1.3	0.6	-	1.4	-	2.1	1.6	1.3	0.8	2.1	4.4	2.8	2.5	8.2	14.3	8.6	19.1	15.7	2.6	1.0	0.10	0.22	**2.1**	*205*
Monocytic leukaemia	2	0	-	-	-	-	-	-	-	-	-	-	-	-	0.8	-	-	1.7	-	-	0.1	0.0	0.00	0.01	**0.1**	*206*
Other leukaemia	1	0	-	-	-	-	-	-	-	-	-	-	-	-	-	1.0	-	-	-	-	0.0	0.0	0.00	0.01	**0.0**	*207*
Leukaemia unspecified	8	0	-	-	-	-	-	-	-	-	-	-	-	-	0.8	-	2.6	5.1	-	7.8	0.3	0.1	0.00	0.02	**0.2**	*208*
Other and unspecified	104	1	-	-	-	0.5	-	-	1.0	1.8	0.4	1.1	5.0	7.8	6.6	11.3	20.9	22.2	38.3	47.1	3.8	1.4	0.12	0.28	**2.6**	*O&U*
All sites	7408	15	15.3	6.9	5.0	12.2	16.0	36.2	68.6	142.6	218.7	296.3	382.8	501.1	695.6	899.5	1177.1	1333.9	1519.4	1635.7	273.4		12.01	22.42	**198.9**	*ALL*
All sites but 173	7253	14	15.3	6.3	5.0	11.3	16.0	33.6	68.1	141.3	215.7	294.7	378.4	490.5	684.0	888.2	1147.1	1304.8	1475.7	1522.0	267.7	100.0	11.82	22.02	**195.0**	*ALLb*

Rate from 1 case			0.638	0.574	0.499	0.451	0.472	0.533	0.524	0.446	0.425	0.526	0.630	0.707	0.828	1.027	1.304	1.710	2.733	3.923

Japan, Miyagi Prefecture

The Miyagi Prefectural Cancer Registry (formerly Miyagi Cancer Registry, initiated in 1951 by the late Professor Mitsuo Segi at the Department of Public Health at Tohoku University School of Medicine in Sendai) marked its 36th year since registration was restarted in 1959. The registry has covered the entire prefecture from the beginning. The office has been located in the Miyagi Cancer Society since 1976. Miyagi Prefecture makes grants for registration, and the Miyagi Cancer Society also supports it financially. All the work of the registry is the responsibility of the Registry Committee which comprises representatives of the Miyagi Medical Association, Tohoku University School of Medicine, public and private medical institutions, Miyagi Prefecture and the Miyagi Cancer Society.

Miyagi Prefecture is situated in the northern part of Japan, between latitudes 37°46′ and 39°00′ N and longitudes 140°17′ and 140°41′ E, and is flanked on the east by the Pacific Ocean. Sendai, the prefectural seat of Miyagi Prefecture, is situated about 350 km north of Tokyo. The annual mean temperature in Sendai is 12.3°C, and the annual rainfall is about 1200 mm. The altitude ranges from sea level to 1841 m. The total registration area is 7291 km², and the population is 2 248 558 (1 105 103 males and 1 143 455 females) including 2730 male and 2694 female foreigners.

Japanese citizens are with very few exceptions of a single religion, race and language, and there are very few immigrants in Japan.

No data are available on labour force status, industry or employment status in the 1990 census because of privacy protection.

Cancer cases are registered from clinics and hospitals (inpatients and outpatients), radiology and pathology departments, autopsy records, mass-screening records and death certificates. Since reporting by clinics and hospitals is voluntary, information collection has always been largely active. Except for the cases reported from clinics and a few hospitals, all the rest are collected by abstracting the relevant cases from medical records of hospitals, pathology and autopsy records, etc. More than 90% of the incidence reports are collected by this active method. Despite the resulting delay, this active form of information collection ensures satisfactory completeness of registration.

All death certificates of Miyagi Prefecture are collated with the registered cases. Cases which have not been registered are given an estimated year of incidence by counting half of the stated 'duration of illness'. The recent percentage of cases registered from death certificates has been around 10% of the total.

Since the inception of the registry, the population of the prefecture has risen from 1 743 195 (1960 census) to 2 248 558 (1990 census), while the number of incident cases rose from about 2400 to 7400 per year and the number of cancer deaths from about 2000 to 4000.

Many patients come to Miyagi Prefecture from other prefectures for treatment, but relatively few have gone from Miyagi to other prefectures for treatment. However, the latter are slightly increasing each year. Therefore, regular visits to hospitals in other prefectures are becoming indispensable for case-finding and data-collection. This development, combined with some increase in the numbers of elderly patients dying outside medical institutions, is making it difficult to improve the completeness of coverage.

Until 1985, follow-up was passive, with only perusal of all death certificates. It is now possible to follow patients by referring back to hospitals when there is no information on death. Patients are followed both actively and passively, but not regularly at present.

Data are stored both manually and on computer disks since 1978. The computer has been used since 1972, but it was only in 1981 that a system was developed which enabled effective information retrieval. Data are entered and updated directly. Multiple neoplasms for the same person are counted separately, and up to two primaries can be retrieved.

Akira Takano
Yoshi Okuno

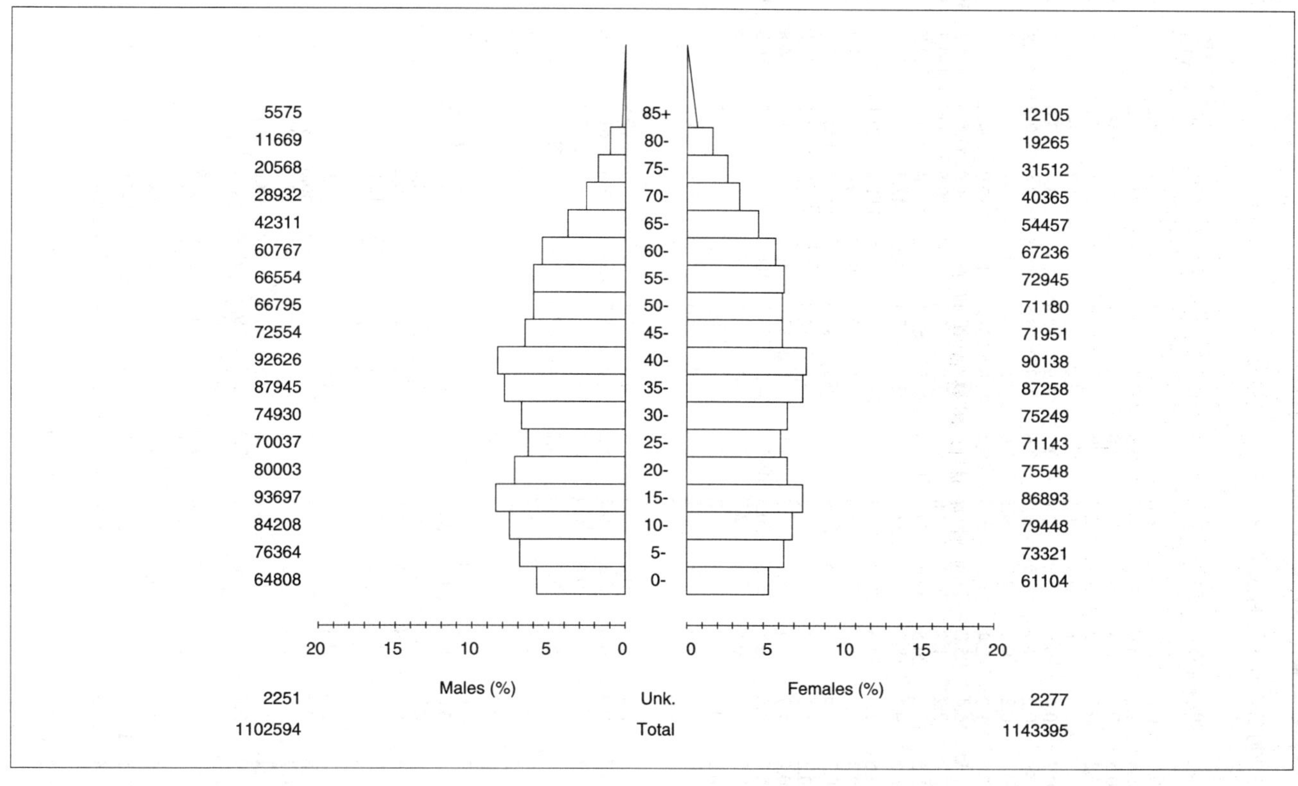

Japan, Miyagi Prefecture

Source of population: average annual 1988–92
Census: 1990 Population Census of Japan, Vol. 2, Results of the First Basic Complete Tabulation, Part 2, 04 Miyagi-ken. 1985 Population Census of Japan, Vol. 2, Results of the First Basic Complete Tabulation, Part 2, 04 Miyagi-ken.
Estimate: The population data for 1988, 1989, 1991 and 1992 were estimated from the Census results of 1985 and 1990.
Notes to tables overleaf:
† 188 does not include the uncertain category

Screening programmes in the area:

196,500 annual examinations have been carried out annually in women over age 30 since 1961, and 49,500 examinations in women over age 35 for breast cancer since 1977. The population over age 40 has been screened for stomach cancer since 1960 (201 800 examinations a year), and for large bowel cancer since 1981 (20 000 annual examinations). The population over age 50 has been screened for lung cancer since 1982 (388 600 X-ray and 15 500 cytological examinations annually).

JAPAN, MIYAGI PREFECTURE 1988-1992

ANNUAL INCIDENCE PER 100,000 BY AGE GROUP (YEARS) - MALE

SITE	ALL AGES	AGE UNK	0-	5-	10-	15-	20-	25-	30-	35-	40-	45-	50-	55-	60-	65-	70-	75-	80-	85+	CRUDE RATE	%	CR 64	CR 74	ASR (W)	ICD (9th)
Lip	17	0	-	-	-	-	-	-	-	0.2	0.2	-	-	0.6	1.0	-	3.5	2.9	1.7	3.6	0.3	0.1	0.01	0.03	**0.2**	140
Tongue	117	0	-	-	-	-	0.2	-	0.8	1.4	1.9	3.6	4.2	6.3	4.6	7.1	5.5	5.8	10.3	3.6	2.1	0.6	0.12	0.18	**1.6**	141
Salivary gland	39	0	-	-	-	-	-	0.5	0.5	0.6	0.3	0.6	2.1	2.0	3.3	3.5	1.0	5.1	-	0.7	0.2	0.03	0.07	**0.5**	142
Mouth	69	0	-	-	-	-	0.3	0.3	0.2	0.2	1.9	3.3	3.3	3.9	3.8	3.5	5.8	5.1	7.2	1.3	0.3	0.07	0.10	**0.9**	143-5
Oropharynx	29	0	-	-	-	-	-	-	-	-	1.1	0.3	1.5	2.6	2.4	2.8	1.0	1.7	-	0.5	0.1	0.03	0.05	**0.4**	146
Nasopharynx	40	0	-	-	-	0.2	0.7	0.3	-	0.2	0.4	0.8	1.2	2.4	0.7	1.9	2.8	3.9	3.4	3.6	0.7	0.2	0.03	0.06	**0.6**	147
Hypopharynx	66	0	-	-	-	-	0.2	-	-	-	0.2	1.7	1.5	4.2	3.6	5.7	3.5	6.8	3.4	7.2	1.2	0.3	0.06	0.10	**0.9**	148
Pharynx unspecified	12	0	-	-	-	-	-	-	-	-	0.2	0.3	0.6	0.3	1.6	0.5	-	1.0	-	-	0.2	0.1	0.02	0.02	**0.2**	149
Oesophagus	1075	0	-	-	-	-	-	-	0.5	1.1	1.9	12.4	24.6	46.6	69.4	90.8	105.1	112.8	132.0	104.0	19.5	5.1	0.78	1.76	**14.0**	150
Stomach	6323	0	0.3	-	-	-	0.7	1.7	10.7	27.1	46.4	85.2	147.9	251.2	342.3	494.4	630.4	709.8	671.9	645.7	114.7	30.2	4.57	10.19	**82.7**	151
Small intestine	40	0	-	-	-	-	-	-	-	-	0.2	1.1	1.2	0.6	1.6	3.8	1.4	6.8	8.6	7.2	0.7	0.2	0.02	0.05	**0.5**	152
Colon	1902	0	-	-	0.2	-	0.5	1.4	4.3	5.5	11.2	26.5	49.4	79.0	112.6	139.9	163.1	203.2	231.4	215.2	34.5	9.1	1.45	2.97	**24.9**	153
Rectum	1274	0	-	-	-	-	0.6	1.9	3.6	9.1	18.2	36.8	57.1	72.4	98.3	105.1	126.4	147.4	114.8	23.1	6.1	1.00	2.02	**16.7**	154
Liver	1175	0	-	-	-	-	-	0.3	1.9	3.6	7.3	14.6	29.9	73.3	69.1	86.0	94.0	88.5	111.4	129.1	21.3	5.6	1.00	1.90	**15.4**	155
Gallbladder etc.	616	0	-	-	-	-	0.2	-	0.5	0.9	1.7	4.1	7.2	15.0	26.3	50.6	82.3	96.3	120.0	132.7	11.2	2.9	0.28	0.94	**7.9**	156
Pancreas	850	0	-	-	-	-	-	-	0.5	0.7	4.5	6.6	12.6	27.9	47.7	67.1	96.1	122.5	133.7	125.6	15.4	4.1	0.50	1.32	**10.9**	157
Nose, sinuses etc.	108	0	0.3	-	0.2	-	0.2	0.3	-	0.2	1.3	2.2	2.4	7.2	5.6	5.7	6.9	8.8	12.0	7.2	2.0	0.5	0.10	0.16	**1.4**	160
Larynx	266	0	-	-	-	-	-	-	0.3	0.2	1.7	1.4	5.1	11.4	14.5	26.0	32.5	30.1	20.6	21.5	4.8	1.3	0.17	0.47	**3.5**	161
Bronchus, lung	3106	0	-	-	-	-	0.6	1.9	5.7	8.6	18.5	38.6	80.5	165.2	290.7	365.7	486.2	500.5	466.4	56.3	14.8	1.60	4.88	**39.6**	162
Other thoracic organs	45	0	-	0.3	-	-	0.2	0.6	0.3	0.2	0.4	0.8	1.8	2.7	0.3	2.4	4.8	4.9	1.7	-	0.8	0.2	0.04	0.07	**0.6**	163-4
Bone	43	0	-	0.5	1.0	2.1	0.5	0.3	0.5	0.2	0.6	1.1	0.3	1.2	1.3	-	0.7	1.9	-	7.2	0.8	0.2	0.05	0.05	**0.7**	170
Connective tissue	100	0	2.5	0.8	0.7	0.2	1.2	0.3	0.5	2.0	1.3	1.4	1.2	2.1	4.3	2.4	4.1	11.7	8.6	17.9	1.8	0.5	0.09	0.13	**1.6**	171
Mesothelioma	15	0	-	-	-	-	-	-	-	-	0.4	0.3	0.6	0.3	0.3	1.4	1.4	1.9	1.7	-	0.3	0.1	0.01	0.02	**0.2**	MES
Kaposi's sarcoma	0	0	-	-	-	-	-	-	-	-	-	-	-	-	-	-	-	-	-	-	0.0	0.0	0.00	0.00	**0.0**	KAP
Melanoma of skin	42	0	-	-	-	-	-	0.5	-	0.4	1.1	0.6	0.6	1.3	4.3	2.1	9.7	1.7	10.8	0.8	0.2	0.02	0.05	**0.6**	172
Other skin	197	0	0.3	0.3	0.2	-	0.2	-	0.3	0.7	0.9	0.6	3.3	5.7	8.2	15.6	18.7	27.2	39.4	61.0	3.6		0.10	0.27	**2.6**	173
Breast	22	0	-	-	-	-	-	-	-	0.2	-	-	0.6	0.9	0.7	1.4	3.5	-	6.9	7.2	0.4	0.1	0.01	0.04	**0.3**	175
Prostate	737	0	-	-	-	-	0.3	0.5	-	0.6	0.3	2.7	7.8	25.7	53.4	97.5	173.1	214.2	215.2	13.4	3.5	0.19	0.94	**9.0**	185	
Testis	91	0	0.9	0.3	-	0.4	3.0	4.9	5.3	3.2	0.9	1.4	1.2	1.2	0.3	0.5	-	-	1.7	7.2	1.7	0.4	0.11	0.12	**1.6**	186
Penis	19	0	-	-	-	-	-	-	0.3	0.2	-	-	0.6	0.6	1.0	1.9	2.1	1.9	1.7	-	0.3	0.1	0.01	0.03	**0.2**	187.1-.4
Other male genital	15	0	0.3	-	-	-	-	-	-	-	0.2	-	-	1.0	-	2.8	3.9	1.7	3.6	0.3	0.1	0.01	0.02	**0.2**	187.5-.9
†Bladder	696	0	-	-	-	0.2	-	0.9	1.6	3.2	3.9	5.2	12.0	22.2	30.6	54.8	77.4	101.1	99.4	136.3	12.6	3.3	0.40	1.06	**9.0**	188
Kidney etc.	486	0	1.2	-	-	-	0.2	0.3	1.1	1.8	5.0	9.6	11.1	23.1	28.3	26.5	47.0	42.8	53.1	39.5	8.8	2.3	0.41	0.78	**6.5**	189
Eye	11	0	0.9	-	-	-	-	-	-	-	0.2	-	-	0.3	1.0	0.5	-	-	3.4	-	0.2	0.1	0.01	0.01	**0.2**	190
Brain, nervous system	150	0	1.5	2.1	1.0	1.5	1.0	1.1	2.7	3.0	2.2	2.5	4.2	4.5	6.6	4.3	9.0	2.9	3.4	-	2.7	0.7	0.17	0.24	**2.4**	191-2
Thyroid	110	0	-	-	-	0.2	-	1.1	1.1	2.0	1.9	2.5	4.5	3.3	4.9	6.1	2.8	7.8	12.0	3.6	2.0	0.5	0.11	0.15	**1.5**	193
Other endocrine	21	0	2.5	-	0.5	0.6	0.2	-	-	0.2	-	-	-	0.3	0.3	0.9	0.7	1.0	-	-	0.4	0.1	0.02	0.03	**0.5**	194
Hodgkin's disease	31	0	-	-	-	-	1.0	0.3	0.5	-	0.6	0.3	0.6	0.3	1.3	1.9	3.5	-	6.9	-	0.6	0.1	0.02	0.05	**0.4**	201
Non-Hodgkin lymphoma	463	0	1.9	2.4	1.9	1.7	1.0	2.0	2.4	3.6	3.5	6.6	11.7	18.6	21.1	25.5	31.8	39.9	66.8	39.5	8.4	2.2	0.39	0.68	**6.5**	200,202
Multiple myeloma	118	0	-	-	-	-	-	-	-	0.2	-	0.8	1.2	3.3	4.3	11.3	19.4	14.6	22.3	21.5	2.1	0.6	0.05	0.20	**1.5**	203
Lymphoid leukaemia	113	0	6.8	2.4	2.4	0.9	0.2	1.1	0.5	1.4	1.1	2.2	0.9	3.6	1.6	3.3	2.1	3.9	8.6	10.8	2.0	0.5	0.13	0.15	**2.3**	204
Myeloid leukaemia	197	0	1.2	0.3	0.5	1.7	0.5	0.9	1.9	3.0	3.0	3.0	4.8	5.7	7.9	12.8	9.0	20.4	5.1	32.3	3.6	0.9	0.17	0.28	**2.9**	205
Monocytic leukaemia	5	0	-	-	-	0.2	-	-	-	0.2	-	-	-	-	0.9	0.7	-	-	-	-	0.1	0.0	0.00	0.01	**0.1**	206
Other leukaemia	13	0	0.3	-	-	-	-	-	0.3	-	-	-	-	0.3	1.0	0.5	1.4	2.9	1.7	-	0.2	0.1	0.01	0.02	**0.2**	207
Leukaemia unspecified	38	0	0.9	0.3	0.2	-	-	-	-	-	0.2	0.3	0.3	0.9	1.6	3.3	2.1	6.8	3.4	10.8	0.7	0.2	0.02	0.05	**0.6**	208
Other and unspecified	265	0	2.8	0.3	0.5	0.2	0.5	0.3	0.3	0.5	1.9	1.7	3.3	6.0	8.6	15.1	28.3	44.7	58.3	75.3	4.8	1.3	0.13	0.35	**3.6**	O&U
All sites	21167	0	24.7	9.7	9.3	10.2	13.0	19.7	44.6	77.1	127.4	242.0	434.8	786.7	1110.5	1628.9	2080.1	2544.7	2744.0	2694.2	383.9		14.55	33.09	**278.5**	ALL
All sites but 173	20970	0	24.4	9.4	9.0	10.2	12.7	19.7	44.3	76.4	126.5	241.5	431.5	781.0	1102.2	1613.3	2061.4	2517.5	2704.6	2633.2	380.4	100.0	14.44	32.82	**275.9**	ALLb

Rate from 1 case   0.309   0.262   0.238   0.213   0.250   0.286   0.267   0.227   0.216   0.276   0.299   0.301   0.329   0.473   0.691   0.972   1.714   3.587

†Important: see notes on population page

JAPAN, MIYAGI PREFECTURE 1988-1992

ANNUAL INCIDENCE PER 100,000 BY AGE GROUP (YEARS) - FEMALE

SITE	ALL AGES	AGE UNK	0-	5-	10-	15-	20-	25-	30-	35-	40-	45-	50-	55-	60-	65-	70-	75-	80-	85+	CRUDE RATE	%	CR 64	CR 74	ASR (W)	ICD (9th)
Lip	8	0	-	-	-	-	-	-	-	-	0.2	0.3	0.3	0.3	0.3	-	-	1.3	-	1.7	0.1	0.1	0.01	0.01	0.1	140
Tongue	64	0	-	-	-	-	-	-	0.3	0.5	0.9	1.7	0.8	1.4	3.6	1.5	4.5	4.4	7.3	6.6	1.1	0.4	0.05	0.07	0.7	141
Salivary gland	25	0	-	-	-	-	-	0.6	0.5	-	0.4	0.6	1.4	0.5	0.9	0.4	1.0	1.3	2.1	-	0.4	0.2	0.02	0.03	0.3	142
Mouth	51	0	-	-	-	0.2	-	-	-	-	-	-	1.4	1.6	1.8	4.0	4.5	3.2	6.2	3.3	0.9	0.3	0.03	0.07	0.5	143-5
Oropharynx	2	0	-	-	-	-	-	-	-	-	-	-	-	0.3	-	0.4	-	-	-	-	0.0	0.0	0.00	0.00	0.0	146
Nasopharynx	11	0	-	-	-	-	-	-	-	-	0.2	0.3	0.3	0.3	0.3	1.1	0.5	1.3	-	-	0.2	0.1	0.01	0.01	0.1	147
Hypopharynx	20	0	-	-	-	-	-	-	-	0.2	-	-	0.6	0.5	1.8	0.7	1.0	3.2	-	-	0.3	0.1	0.02	0.02	0.2	148
Pharynx unspecified	4	0	-	-	-	-	-	-	-	-	-	-	0.3	-	-	-	0.5	0.6	-	1.7	0.1	0.0	0.00	0.00	0.0	149
Oesophagus	240	0	-	-	-	-	-	-	0.3	-	0.7	0.8	2.5	4.1	8.3	16.2	19.3	24.1	42.6	31.4	4.2	1.6	0.08	0.26	2.2	150
Stomach	3120	0	-	-	0.3	0.2	1.3	5.9	8.2	23.6	30.4	48.4	56.5	79.0	113.3	161.6	236.8	267.2	280.3	277.6	54.6	20.3	1.84	3.83	32.8	151
Small intestine	30	0	-	-	-	-	-	-	-	0.2	0.2	0.8	1.1	0.5	1.2	1.5	1.5	1.9	1.0	6.6	0.5	0.2	0.02	0.04	0.3	152
Colon	1571	0	-	-	-	-	0.8	1.1	2.1	6.0	8.2	17.8	28.7	37.8	64.5	82.3	109.5	158.7	179.6	171.8	27.5	10.2	0.84	1.79	15.7	153
Rectum	861	0	-	-	-	-	0.5	-	1.1	3.7	5.5	12.2	21.9	29.3	29.7	50.7	62.9	71.7	64.4	74.3	15.1	5.6	0.52	1.09	9.0	154
Liver	546	0	0.3	-	-	0.2	0.3	0.8	0.3	0.5	2.9	3.6	6.2	12.9	25.0	30.5	45.6	57.1	48.8	76.0	9.6	3.5	0.26	0.65	5.4	155
Gallbladder etc.	747	0	-	-	-	-	0.3	-	0.3	0.9	1.3	2.8	7.0	11.8	24.1	38.9	62.9	87.0	118.3	152.0	13.1	4.9	0.24	0.75	6.8	156
Pancreas	581	0	-	-	-	-	-	0.3	0.3	0.5	1.3	4.7	7.3	12.6	22.0	27.5	51.5	64.7	73.7	92.5	10.2	3.8	0.24	0.64	5.5	157
Nose, sinuses etc.	70	0	-	-	-	-	-	0.3	-	0.5	0.4	1.1	1.1	0.5	2.1	3.7	5.5	9.5	6.2	9.9	1.2	0.5	0.03	0.08	0.7	160
Larynx	15	0	-	-	-	-	-	0.3	-	-	-	-	0.6	0.3	0.6	0.7	1.5	1.9	1.0	-	0.3	0.1	0.01	0.02	0.2	161
Bronchus, lung	1041	0	-	-	-	-	-	0.8	1.3	2.5	5.3	11.4	15.7	28.2	39.0	54.0	90.7	107.9	114.2	94.2	18.2	6.8	0.52	1.25	10.3	162
Other thoracic organs	26	0	-	-	-	-	-	-	0.5	0.2	0.2	0.3	-	1.9	0.6	1.1	2.5	1.9	-	1.7	0.5	0.2	0.02	0.04	0.3	163-4
Bone	33	0	0.3	0.3	0.5	1.2	0.8	0.8	0.3	0.9	0.4	0.6	-	1.4	0.3	0.4	-	-	1.0	1.7	0.6	0.2	0.04	0.04	0.6	170
Connective tissue	69	0	1.6	-	0.5	0.5	-	0.3	2.1	1.1	0.7	1.7	2.8	1.1	1.5	1.5	1.5	0.6	4.2	9.9	1.2	0.4	0.07	0.08	1.0	171
Mesothelioma	3	0	-	-	-	-	-	-	-	-	0.3	-	0.3	-	0.4	-	-	-	-	-	0.1	0.0	0.00	0.00	0.0	MES
Kaposi's sarcoma	0	0	-	-	-	-	-	-	-	-	-	-	-	-	-	-	-	-	-	-	0.0	0.0	0.00	0.00	0.0	KAP
Melanoma of skin	24	0	-	-	0.3	-	-	-	0.3	-	-	-	0.6	0.5	0.3	1.8	2.5	1.3	4.2	1.7	0.4	0.2	0.01	0.03	0.2	172
Other skin	177	0	-	-	0.5	0.2	0.3	-	-	0.7	0.9	1.9	2.8	3.0	4.2	8.1	10.9	20.9	24.9	38.0	3.1		0.07	0.17	1.7	173
Breast	2440	0	-	-	-	-	0.5	5.1	17.8	44.7	77.9	110.4	81.2	77.3	77.9	84.5	84.2	72.4	50.9	23.1	42.7	15.8	2.46	3.31	31.1	174
Uterus unspecified	56	0	-	-	-	-	-	-	0.3	0.2	0.2	0.3	0.6	1.1	1.2	1.1	4.0	3.8	16.6	14.9	1.0	0.4	0.02	0.04	0.5	179
Cervix uteri	525	0	-	-	-	-	0.3	4.8	6.6	8.3	15.3	12.2	11.5	12.3	17.6	20.9	26.3	25.4	27.0	19.8	9.2	3.4	0.44	0.68	6.4	180
Placenta	8	0	-	-	-	0.2	-	0.8	0.5	-	0.2	-	-	-	-	-	0.5	-	-	-	0.1	0.1	0.01	0.01	0.1	181
Corpus uteri	339	0	-	-	-	-	-	1.1	0.8	3.7	6.2	8.9	12.6	16.7	17.3	12.5	13.4	8.9	9.3	13.2	5.9	2.2	0.34	0.47	4.1	182
Ovary etc.	494	0	-	-	0.3	1.8	1.6	2.5	2.4	6.2	10.4	15.0	20.5	17.0	17.0	15.1	14.4	20.9	26.0	21.5	8.6	3.2	0.47	0.62	6.1	183
Other female genital	36	0	-	-	-	-	-	-	-	0.2	0.2	0.8	-	0.3	2.1	1.1	4.5	3.2	3.1	5.0	0.6	0.2	0.02	0.05	0.4	184
†Bladder	269	0	-	-	-	0.2	0.3	-	0.3	0.5	1.6	1.7	2.5	6.6	7.1	12.1	21.8	33.6	35.3	49.6	4.7	1.7	0.10	0.27	2.5	188
Kidney etc.	216	0	1.6	-	-	-	0.5	0.3	0.5	0.9	1.8	3.6	3.4	6.9	8.0	14.0	15.9	18.4	16.6	3.3	3.8	1.4	0.14	0.29	2.5	189
Eye	6	0	0.3	0.3	-	-	-	-	-	-	0.2	-	-	0.3	-	0.7	-	-	-	-	0.1	0.0	0.01	0.01	0.1	190
Brain, nervous system	110	0	2.3	1.4	2.0	0.7	0.5	1.4	1.3	0.7	2.0	2.5	2.5	3.6	2.4	4.4	3.5	1.9	2.1	-	1.9	0.7	0.12	0.16	1.8	191-2
Thyroid	688	0	0.3	0.3	0.8	0.7	2.6	3.4	7.7	12.6	18.4	24.5	24.2	27.7	22.9	18.0	20.3	17.1	15.6	11.6	12.0	4.5	0.73	0.92	9.0	193
Other endocrine	25	0	4.3	-	-	-	-	0.3	-	-	-	1.4	-	0.3	0.3	-	-	2.5	-	-	0.4	0.2	0.03	0.03	0.7	194
Hodgkin's disease	15	0	-	-	-	0.5	0.5	0.3	-	0.2	0.2	-	0.3	0.5	-	0.4	1.0	1.0	0.6	-	1.7	0.3	0.1	0.01	0.02	0.2	201
Non-Hodgkin lymphoma	380	0	0.3	0.5	0.8	0.7	1.1	1.7	1.6	3.4	2.4	5.8	7.9	7.4	14.6	19.1	23.3	34.3	38.4	23.1	6.6	2.5	0.24	0.45	4.2	200,202
Multiple myeloma	147	0	-	-	-	-	-	-	-	-	0.4	0.6	2.8	2.2	7.1	8.4	8.9	19.0	17.6	21.5	2.6	1.0	0.07	0.15	1.4	203
Lymphoid leukaemia	72	0	2.6	1.4	1.5	0.2	0.8	0.3	0.5	0.7	2.2	0.6	0.8	1.6	2.4	0.7	2.0	3.2	1.0	3.3	1.3	0.5	0.08	0.09	1.3	204
Myeloid leukaemia	126	0	0.7	0.3	0.3	0.2	0.8	0.6	1.6	1.6	1.6	1.4	2.0	3.8	5.9	5.1	4.0	8.3	9.3	9.9	2.2	0.8	0.10	0.15	1.5	205
Monocytic leukaemia	10	0	0.3	-	-	-	-	-	-	0.5	0.2	-	0.3	-	0.3	0.7	-	1.3	-	-	0.2	0.1	0.01	0.01	0.1	206
Other leukaemia	9	0	0.3	-	-	-	-	0.5	-	-	-	-	0.3	-	1.0	-	1.0	1.7	0.2	0.1	0.01	0.01	0.1	207
Leukaemia unspecified	22	0	-	-	-	-	0.3	-	-	0.2	-	-	1.4	0.3	0.3	0.4	2.0	2.5	2.1	3.3	0.4	0.1	0.01	0.02	0.2	208
Other and unspecified	247	0	1.0	-	-	0.5	-	0.6	0.3	0.2	0.7	1.4	2.5	4.9	6.8	12.1	17.8	28.6	40.5	44.6	4.3	1.6	0.09	0.24	2.4	O&U
All sites	15579	0	16.4	4.4	7.6	8.3	14.0	34.3	60.6	126.8	202.6	302.2	337.2	421.1	556.8	720.2	985.5	1197.6	1292.5	1323.4	272.5		10.46	18.99	171.6	ALL
All sites but 173	15402	0	16.4	4.4	7.0	8.1	13.8	34.3	60.6	126.1	201.7	300.2	334.4	418.1	552.7	712.1	974.6	1176.7	1267.6	1285.4	269.4	100.0	10.39	18.82	169.9	ALLb

| Rate from 1 case | | | 0.327 | 0.273 | 0.252 | 0.230 | 0.265 | 0.281 | 0.266 | 0.229 | 0.222 | 0.278 | 0.281 | 0.274 | 0.297 | 0.367 | 0.495 | 0.635 | 1.038 | 1.652 |

†Important: see notes on population page

Japan, Nagasaki Prefecture

Since 1958, the Radiation Effects Research Foundation (RERF; formerly called the Atomic Bomb Casualty Commission) has run a population-based tumour registry among the inhabitants of Nagasaki City under the supervision of the Nagasaki City Medical Association Tumor Statistics Committee. Nagasaki is home to many survivors of the 1945 atomic bombing of the city. The Nagasaki City Cancer Registry was launched in order to accurately determine the cancer incidence among these people, and its coverage was extended to the greater Nagasaki Prefecture area as of 1985.

The registry collects information on all malignant tumours and benign tumours of the brain. The actual registry work is carried out by RERF and conducted in cooperation with Nagasaki University and local medical associations.

Nagasaki Prefecture is located on the western edge of the Japanese archipelago and is characterized by its large number of remote islands (71 inhabited islands) and beautiful scenery. The total area is 4090 km^2, and the population is about 1 563 000 (737 000 males and 826 000 females). Non-Japanese persons account for only 2.7% of the population and therefore are not included in the cancer registry. Approximately half of the prefecture population lives in either Nagasaki City or Sasebo City. Shipbuilding is the main industry in both of these cities.

Although cancer information (diagnosis, treatment, staging, etc.) depends partly on reports from physicians, this source is insufficient because physicians are under no obligation to provide information. From the very beginning, an aggressive approach was adopted in order to obtain complete information, staff members going to medical institutions and collecting data from patients' charts. Information on pathological diagnoses has been obtained for almost all cases in Nagasaki Prefecture. Information on most of these cases is collected through the Tissue Registry. This registry has covered all of Nagasaki Prefecture except the northern part since 1973, and collects not only pathological information but also tissue specimens to facilitate the review of diagnoses. The pathological information collected is sent to the cancer registry. All death information for prefecture residents collected by local administrative bodies is also sent to the registry office.

The registry produces an annual report on cancer incidence and mortality in Nagasaki Prefecture.

Midori Soda
Takayoshi Ikeda

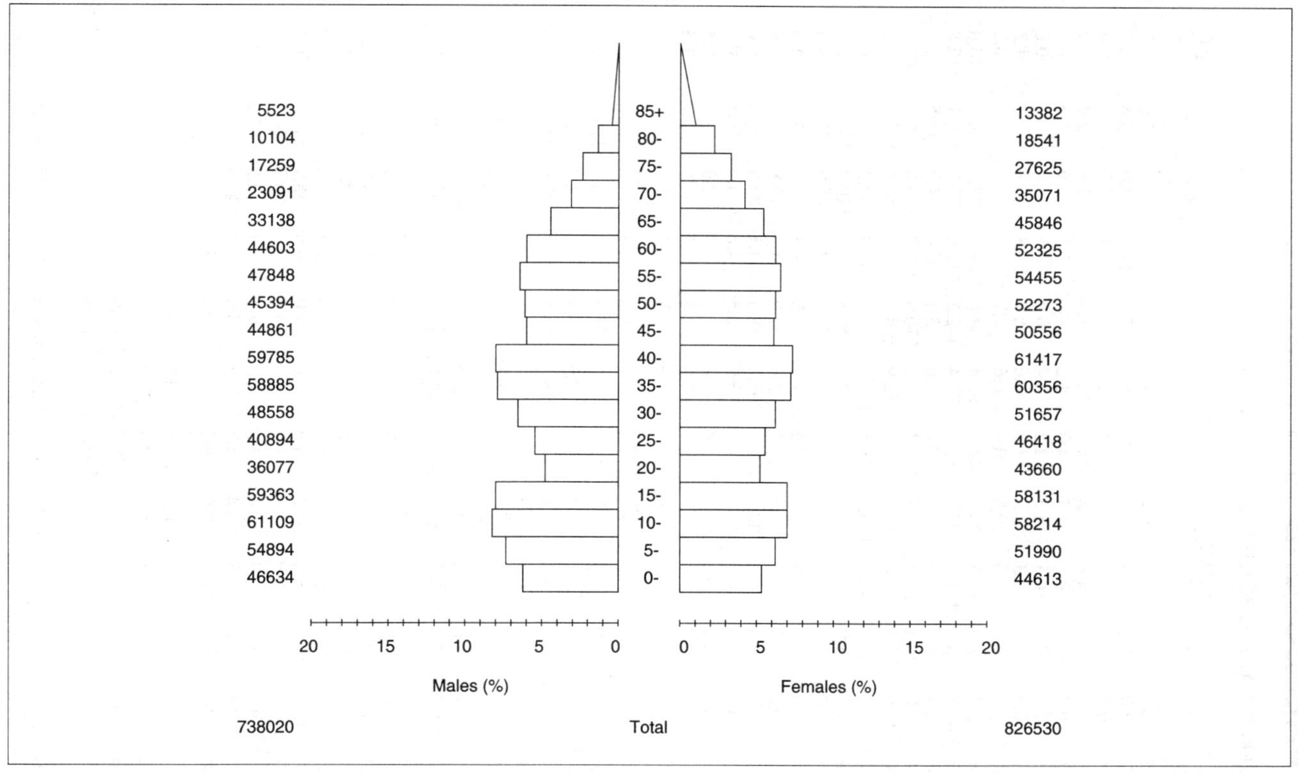

Japan, Nagasaki Prefecture

Source of population: average annual 1988–92

Census: 1990 Population Census of Japan, Statistics Bureau, Management and Coordination Agency, 1991. 1985 Population Census of Japan, Statistics Bureau, Management and Coordination Agency, 1986.

Estimate: The population data for 1988, 1989, 1991 and 1992 were estimated from the Census results of 1985 and 1990.

Note: the registration area has been expanded to cover the Prefecture as well as the City since the period published in Volume VI and the data are not comparable.

Notes to tables overleaf:

† 188 does not include the uncertain category

Screening programmes in the area:

Women over age 30 have been screened for cervical cancer since 1983 (46 461 examinations annually) and for breast cancer since 1987 (38 568 examinations annually). The population over age 40 has been screened for stomach cancer since 1983 (50 213 annual examinations), lung cancer since 1987 (55 273 annual examinations) and large bowel since 1992 (20 414 annual examinations).

JAPAN, NAGASAKI PREFECTURE 1988-1992

ANNUAL INCIDENCE PER 100,000 BY AGE GROUP (YEARS) - MALE

SITE	ALL AGES	AGE UNK	0-	5-	10-	15-	20-	25-	30-	35-	40-	45-	50-	55-	60-	65-	70-	75-	80-	85+	CRUDE RATE	%	CR 64	CR 74	ASR (W)	ICD (9th)
Lip	6	0	-	-	-	-	-	-	-	0.3	-	-	-	0.4	-	1.8	-	-	-	3.6	0.2	0.0	0.00	0.01	0.1	140
Tongue	81	0	-	-	-	-	0.6	-	-	0.7	2.0	1.8	2.6	6.7	7.2	6.6	5.2	11.6	4.0	3.6	2.2	0.5	0.11	0.17	1.5	141
Salivary gland	21	0	-	-	-	0.3	-	-	0.4	0.3	0.3	0.4	1.8	-	2.2	1.8	0.9	1.2	4.0	-	0.6	0.1	0.03	0.04	0.4	142
Mouth	108	0	-	-	-	-	-	0.5	-	-	1.7	1.8	4.8	3.8	13.5	10.3	11.3	11.6	11.9	7.2	2.9	0.6	0.13	0.24	1.9	143-5
Oropharynx	27	0	0.4	-	-	-	-	-	-	0.3	0.7	-	0.4	1.7	4.0	1.2	-	3.5	5.9	3.6	0.7	0.2	0.04	0.04	0.5	146
Nasopharynx	29	0	-	-	-	-	0.6	-	-	-	1.7	0.4	0.4	3.3	2.2	2.4	0.9	3.5	-	-	0.8	0.2	0.04	0.06	0.5	147
Hypopharynx	46	0	-	-	-	-	-	-	-	-	0.3	0.4	1.3	2.5	3.6	6.6	6.9	5.8	5.9	-	1.2	0.3	0.04	0.11	0.8	148
Pharynx unspecified	8	0	-	-	-	-	-	-	-	-	-	0.4	-	0.8	0.9	0.6	1.7	-	-	-	0.2	0.0	0.01	0.02	0.1	149
Oesophagus	516	1	-	-	-	-	-	-	-	2.4	3.7	8.0	15.4	25.5	44.4	60.4	54.6	84.6	73.2	39.8	14.0	3.1	0.50	1.07	8.7	150
Stomach	4164	4	-	-	-	0.3	0.6	2.9	13.2	20.7	45.2	65.5	119.4	207.7	315.2	372.4	542.2	611.9	673.0	706.1	112.8	24.8	3.96	8.53	71.0	151
Small intestine	40	0	-	-	-	-	-	-	-	-	0.7	0.9	1.3	1.3	3.1	3.6	5.2	5.8	4.0	14.5	1.1	0.2	0.04	0.08	0.7	152
Colon	1509	3	-	-	-	0.3	-	0.5	2.1	6.1	10.0	22.3	52.4	85.7	126.4	134.6	170.6	219.0	233.6	246.2	40.9	9.0	1.53	3.06	25.7	153
Rectum	1040	1	-	-	0.3	0.3	1.1	1.0	1.2	2.0	11.0	18.3	30.0	56.0	76.2	112.9	129.9	133.3	150.4	181.1	28.2	6.2	0.99	2.20	18.0	154
Liver	1871	0	1.3	-	-	-	-	0.5	2.5	4.8	15.7	40.1	73.6	156.3	178.5	166.0	200.9	144.9	162.3	206.4	50.7	11.1	2.37	4.20	33.3	155
Gallbladder etc.	475	0	-	-	-	0.3	-	-	-	1.4	1.7	4.0	6.6	18.8	31.4	53.1	59.8	86.9	110.8	137.6	12.9	2.8	0.32	0.89	7.7	156
Pancreas	545	0	-	-	-	-	-	0.5	-	2.4	5.4	7.1	12.8	16.3	43.9	50.7	77.9	98.5	108.9	90.5	14.8	3.2	0.44	1.09	9.0	157
Nose, sinuses etc.	67	0	-	-	-	-	-	-	-	1.4	2.0	0.4	1.8	1.3	4.9	9.1	7.8	9.3	7.9	7.2	1.8	0.4	0.06	0.14	1.2	160
Larynx	208	1	-	-	-	-	-	-	-	-	0.7	0.9	3.5	10.9	24.2	25.3	32.0	24.3	17.8	21.7	5.6	1.2	0.20	0.49	3.5	161
Bronchus, lung	2584	1	-	-	-	-	-	1.6	5.1	9.4	22.3	37.9	80.7	172.6	298.1	418.3	498.3	583.9	434.5	70.0	15.4	1.65	5.23	41.7	162
Other thoracic organs	34	0	0.4	-	-	-	-	-	-	0.3	0.7	1.3	0.9	1.3	1.8	3.0	2.6	4.6	4.0	14.5	0.9	0.2	0.03	0.06	0.6	163-4
Bone	20	0	0.4	1.1	0.3	1.7	1.1	-	-	-	0.3	0.4	0.4	-	0.9	0.6	-	1.2	2.0	-	0.5	0.1	0.03	0.04	0.6	170
Connective tissue	57	0	1.7	1.1	-	1.3	0.6	1.0	1.2	-	1.0	0.9	-	1.7	2.7	1.8	4.3	9.3	5.9	21.7	1.5	0.3	0.07	0.10	1.3	171
Mesothelioma	25	0	-	-	-	-	-	-	-	0.3	-	1.3	0.4	0.8	1.3	2.4	2.6	4.6	4.0	7.2	0.7	0.1	0.02	0.05	0.4	MES
Kaposi's sarcoma	0	0	-	-	-	-	-	-	-	-	-	-	-	-	-	-	-	-	-	-	0.0	0.0	0.00	0.00	0.0	KAP
Melanoma of skin	25	0	-	-	0.3	-	0.6	0.5	-	0.3	0.3	1.3	0.9	1.7	1.3	1.8	1.7	1.2	2.0	3.6	0.7	0.1	0.04	0.05	0.5	172
Other skin	314	1	-	-	1.0	-	0.5	0.4	1.4	3.0	4.0	7.0	11.7	19.3	26.6	35.5	42.9	85.1	123.1	8.5		0.24	0.55	5.2	173
Breast	8	0	-	-	-	-	-	-	-	-	-	-	0.4	0.4	0.6	0.9	1.2	4.0	3.6	0.2	0.0	0.00	0.01	0.1	175
Prostate	619	0	-	-	-	-	-	-	-	-	0.4	3.5	9.6	26.9	45.3	93.5	185.4	227.6	249.9	16.8	3.7	0.20	0.90	9.1	185
Testis	28	0	0.9	-	-	0.3	2.8	3.4	1.2	1.4	1.0	-	0.4	0.4	-	0.9	-	-	-	0.8	0.2	0.06	0.06	0.9	186
Penis	25	0	-	-	-	-	-	-	-	-	-	-	0.8	3.1	1.8	3.5	4.6	4.0	10.9	0.7	0.1	0.02	0.05	0.4	187.1-.4
Other male genital	16	0	-	-	-	-	-	-	-	-	0.4	-	3.0	2.6	2.3	5.9	7.2	0.4	0.1	0.00	0.03	0.2	187.5-.9
†Bladder	681	0	-	-	-	-	-	-	1.2	1.7	6.7	11.6	7.9	24.7	48.9	68.2	85.7	110.1	166.3	181.1	18.5	4.1	0.51	1.28	11.2	188
Kidney etc.	340	0	0.9	0.4	-	-	-	-	1.2	1.4	5.0	7.6	11.9	15.9	27.8	36.8	39.8	45.2	33.7	29.0	9.2	2.0	0.36	0.74	6.1	189
Eye	13	0	2.1	-	-	-	0.6	-	0.4	0.3	0.3	-	0.8	-	-	0.9	1.2	-	-	0.4	0.1	0.02	0.03	0.4	190
Brain, nervous system	129	0	1.3	1.8	2.3	1.7	2.2	1.5	1.6	1.7	3.0	4.0	4.4	4.6	5.8	6.0	13.0	9.3	11.9	7.2	3.5	0.8	0.18	0.27	2.9	191-2
Thyroid	76	0	-	-	0.7	-	-	0.5	0.4	0.3	2.7	2.7	2.2	5.0	4.5	6.0	8.7	1.2	9.9	14.5	2.1	0.5	0.09	0.17	1.4	193
Other endocrine	17	0	2.6	0.4	-	0.7	1.1	-	-	-	0.3	0.4	0.4	-	0.9	-	-	-	2.0	-	0.5	0.1	0.03	0.03	0.6	194
Hodgkin's disease	13	0	-	0.4	0.3	0.3	-	-	-	-	-	0.4	0.9	-	0.4	-	2.6	2.3	2.0	-	0.4	0.1	0.01	0.03	0.3	201
Non-Hodgkin lymphoma	745	0	1.7	0.7	1.6	0.7	4.4	2.0	2.9	5.8	10.4	12.5	26.4	37.2	54.7	70.0	71.0	108.9	85.1	112.3	20.2	4.4	0.80	1.51	13.5	200,202
Multiple myeloma	101	0	-	-	-	-	-	-	-	0.7	1.3	1.3	0.9	5.0	9.0	4.8	15.6	17.4	25.7	14.5	2.7	0.6	0.09	0.19	1.6	203
Lymphoid leukaemia	64	0	6.0	2.2	1.3	3.0	0.6	1.0	0.4	1.0	0.7	1.3	0.9	0.4	1.8	1.8	4.3	1.2	2.0	7.2	1.7	0.4	0.10	0.13	2.0	204
Myeloid leukaemia	133	0	-	-	1.0	1.7	1.7	1.5	1.6	2.0	2.3	4.0	1.8	8.4	5.8	7.8	15.6	16.2	17.8	7.2	3.6	0.8	0.16	0.28	2.6	205
Monocytic leukaemia	6	0	0.4	-	-	-	-	-	-	0.3	0.3	-	0.4	0.4	0.4	-	-	1.2	-	-	0.2	0.0	0.01	0.01	0.1	206
Other leukaemia	5	0	-	-	-	-	-	-	-	-	-	-	-	0.9	-	-	2.3	-	3.6	0.1	0.0	0.00	0.00	0.1	207
Leukaemia unspecified	48	0	1.3	-	-	0.3	0.6	-	0.4	0.3	1.0	0.9	0.4	0.4	1.8	4.2	5.2	7.0	9.9	21.7	1.3	0.3	0.04	0.08	1.0	208
Other and unspecified	214	0	0.4	-	-	-	-	-	0.8	1.4	2.7	2.2	3.5	5.9	13.5	19.3	24.3	33.6	67.3	68.8	5.8	1.3	0.15	0.37	3.5	O&U
All sites	17101	12	21.9	8.0	8.2	14.5	18.8	17.6	35.0	68.6	155.2	254.1	441.5	817.2	1288.7	1629.5	2160.9	2567.9	2935.5	3012.7	463.4		15.76	34.72	293.2	ALL
All sites but 173	16787	11	21.9	8.0	8.2	13.5	18.8	17.1	34.6	67.2	152.2	250.1	434.4	805.5	1269.4	1603.0	2125.4	2525.1	2850.4	2889.6	454.9	100.0	15.51	34.17	288.0	ALLb

Rate from 1 case   0.429   0.364   0.327   0.337   0.554   0.489   0.412   0.340   0.335   0.446   0.441   0.418   0.448   0.604   0.866   1.159   1.979   3.621

†Important: see notes on population page

JAPAN, NAGASAKI PREFECTURE 1988-1992

ANNUAL INCIDENCE PER 100,000 BY AGE GROUP (YEARS) - FEMALE

SITE	ALL AGES	AGE UNK	0-	5-	10-	15-	20-	25-	30-	35-	40-	45-	50-	55-	60-	65-	70-	75-	80-	85+	CRUDE RATE	%	CR 64	CR 74	ASR (W)	ICD (9th)
Lip	0	0	-	-	-	-	-	-	-	-	-	-	-	-	-	-	-	-	-	-	0.0	0.0	0.00	0.00	0.0	140
Tongue	52	1	-	-	-	0.3	-	-	0.8	1.3	0.7	0.4	2.3	1.8	1.9	3.9	2.9	0.7	7.6	4.5	1.3	0.4	0.05	0.08	0.7	141
Salivary gland	22	0	-	-	0.3	-	-	0.9	-	-	1.0	0.8	0.8	0.4	0.8	1.7	1.1	0.7	-	3.0	0.5	0.2	0.02	0.04	0.4	142
Mouth	44	0	-	-	-	-	-	0.4	0.4	0.3	0.3	0.4	0.4	1.5	3.8	2.6	3.4	5.1	2.2	4.5	1.1	0.3	0.04	0.07	0.6	143-5
Oropharynx	9	0	-	-	-	-	-	-	-	-	0.3	-	-	0.7	-	0.4	-	0.7	3.2	1.5	0.2	0.1	0.01	0.01	0.1	146
Nasopharynx	15	0	-	-	-	-	-	-	0.3	-	-	0.4	1.5	-	0.8	0.4	2.3	-	2.2	-	0.4	0.1	0.02	0.03	0.2	147
Hypopharynx	9	0	-	-	-	-	-	-	-	-	-	0.4	-	1.1	0.4	0.4	-	0.7	2.2	-	0.2	0.1	0.01	0.01	0.1	148
Pharynx unspecified	4	0	-	-	0.3	-	-	-	-	-	0.3	-	-	-	-	0.4	-	-	1.1	-	0.1	0.0	0.00	0.01	0.1	149
Oesophagus	113	0	-	-	-	-	-	-	-	-	-	2.0	1.1	1.5	1.9	6.5	9.7	13.8	22.7	35.9	2.7	0.9	0.03	0.11	1.1	150
Stomach	2503	2	-	-	-	1.4	0.5	4.3	15.5	28.5	29.0	41.5	52.4	75.7	111.2	143.5	180.2	259.2	325.8	339.3	60.6	19.5	1.80	3.42	31.3	151
Small intestine	24	0	-	-	-	-	-	-	-	-	0.3	-	-	0.4	1.5	1.7	1.7	3.6	3.2	4.5	0.6	0.2	0.01	0.03	0.3	152
Colon	1295	1	-	-	0.3	0.3	0.9	-	3.1	6.6	11.7	20.2	31.0	40.8	60.8	80.7	90.1	141.9	157.5	207.7	31.3	10.1	0.88	1.73	15.7	153
Rectum	730	2	-	-	-	-	0.5	-	2.3	6.0	7.5	12.7	22.2	25.0	35.2	48.9	66.7	60.1	58.2	95.6	17.7	5.7	0.56	1.14	9.5	154
Liver	662	0	0.9	-	-	-	0.5	-	1.5	0.7	1.3	8.7	10.7	26.4	36.7	52.8	59.3	57.9	86.3	68.7	16.0	5.1	0.44	1.00	8.1	155
Gallbladder etc.	675	0	-	-	-	-	-	-	0.8	1.3	3.3	5.1	10.7	13.2	24.5	36.2	58.2	86.9	129.4	139.0	16.3	5.2	0.29	0.77	7.1	156
Pancreas	441	0	-	-	-	-	-	-	-	1.0	1.6	2.8	3.4	11.8	17.6	31.8	46.8	52.9	68.0	71.7	10.7	3.4	0.19	0.58	4.8	157
Nose, sinuses etc.	34	0	-	-	-	-	-	-	0.4	0.3	0.3	1.2	1.5	-	2.3	3.5	1.7	3.6	2.2	-	0.8	0.3	0.03	0.06	0.5	160
Larynx	15	0	-	-	-	-	-	-	-	-	-	0.4	-	-	0.4	0.9	2.3	1.4	-	7.5	0.4	0.1	0.00	0.02	0.2	161
Bronchus, lung	1070	2	-	-	-	0.3	0.9	1.3	1.2	3.6	6.2	9.9	19.5	22.8	38.6	70.7	97.5	133.9	153.2	194.3	25.9	8.3	0.52	1.37	12.1	162
Other thoracic organs	21	0	0.4	-	-	-	-	-	0.4	-	0.7	0.8	-	1.5	0.8	1.3	-	0.7	2.2	4.5	0.5	0.2	0.02	0.03	0.3	163-4
Bone	23	0	-	0.8	1.4	0.3	0.5	-	0.4	0.7	-	0.4	-	0.4	1.1	-	1.1	1.4	1.1	3.0	0.6	0.2	0.03	0.04	0.5	170
Connective tissue	44	0	1.3	0.4	0.7	0.7	0.9	0.4	0.4	0.3	-	0.4	0.8	1.8	1.5	2.6	1.7	0.7	3.2	9.0	1.1	0.3	0.05	0.07	0.9	171
Mesothelioma	4	0	-	-	-	-	-	-	-	-	0.3	0.4	0.4	0.4	-	-	-	-	-	-	0.1	0.0	0.01	0.01	0.1	MES
Kaposi's sarcoma	0	0	-	-	-	-	-	-	-	-	-	-	-	-	-	-	-	-	-	-	0.0	0.0	0.00	0.00	0.0	KAP
Melanoma of skin	31	0	-	0.4	-	-	-	-	0.8	0.3	-	0.4	0.8	0.4	0.8	0.9	1.7	2.9	5.4	10.5	0.8	0.2	0.02	0.03	0.4	172
Other skin	350	1	-	-	-	0.3	0.5	0.4	2.3	0.3	2.3	2.8	5.7	7.0	8.4	17.0	24.5	31.1	72.3	115.1	8.5		0.15	0.36	3.7	173
Breast	1612	5	-	-	-	-	-	7.8	15.5	40.1	65.5	90.6	68.9	69.4	80.3	68.1	60.4	55.0	55.0	44.8	39.0	12.5	2.20	2.84	27.1	174
Uterus unspecified	67	0	-	-	-	-	-	0.4	-	0.3	-	1.2	1.5	1.1	1.9	1.7	4.6	8.7	10.8	23.9	1.6	0.5	0.03	0.06	0.7	179
Cervix uteri	702	2	-	-	-	0.3	1.8	5.2	14.7	24.5	20.8	21.4	20.3	27.9	29.8	37.1	33.6	37.6	31.3	31.4	17.0	5.5	0.84	1.19	11.3	180
Placenta	4	0	-	-	-	-	-	0.4	-	0.3	-	0.4	0.4	-	-	-	-	-	-	-	0.1	0.0	0.01	0.01	0.1	181
Corpus uteri	257	4	-	-	-	-	0.5	0.9	1.2	1.7	3.6	13.1	15.7	20.2	15.7	9.2	10.8	7.2	6.5	7.5	6.2	2.0	0.37	0.47	4.2	182
Ovary etc.	387	2	-	0.8	1.7	2.4	4.1	5.6	3.9	5.6	10.4	15.8	17.2	15.4	13.0	17.9	17.7	22.4	20.5	10.5	9.4	3.0	0.48	0.66	6.7	183
Other female genital	48	0	-	-	-	-	-	-	-	-	-	0.4	1.1	0.7	2.3	2.2	6.3	6.5	8.6	4.5	1.2	0.4	0.02	0.07	0.5	184
†Bladder	215	1	-	-	-	-	-	-	0.4	0.7	1.3	2.8	0.8	2.9	8.8	13.5	16.0	26.8	38.8	52.3	5.2	1.7	0.09	0.24	2.3	188
Kidney etc.	172	0	1.3	0.8	-	-	-	0.4	0.4	1.3	-	2.0	2.7	4.4	10.3	10.5	17.7	15.2	20.5	22.4	4.2	1.3	0.12	0.26	2.3	189
Eye	5	0	1.3	-	-	-	-	-	-	-	-	0.4	-	-	-	-	-	-	1.1	-	0.1	0.0	0.01	0.01	0.2	190
Brain, nervous system	109	0	4.5	1.2	1.4	1.0	1.8	0.9	1.9	0.7	1.6	2.4	2.3	2.9	2.7	2.6	7.4	5.8	14.0	6.0	2.6	0.8	0.13	0.18	2.2	191-2
Thyroid	389	1	-	-	0.3	0.7	4.1	3.4	8.9	9.6	12.7	15.8	18.0	12.5	12.2	14.4	21.7	21.7	15.1	13.5	9.4	3.0	0.49	0.67	6.7	193
Other endocrine	9	0	-	1.2	-	-	-	-	-	-	-	0.4	0.4	-	1.1	-	-	-	-	1.5	0.2	0.1	0.02	0.02	0.2	194
Hodgkin's disease	5	0	-	-	-	0.3	0.5	-	-	0.3	-	-	-	-	-	-	-	0.7	-	1.5	0.1	0.0	0.01	0.01	0.1	201
Non-Hodgkin lymphoma	521	0	0.9	0.4	1.4	0.7	-	2.2	2.7	4.0	8.1	11.5	12.6	18.7	24.8	31.0	33.1	48.5	64.7	43.3	12.6	4.1	0.44	0.76	7.1	200,202
Multiple myeloma	109	0	-	-	-	-	-	-	-	0.7	-	0.8	0.8	2.6	5.4	11.3	10.8	10.1	17.3	10.5	2.6	0.8	0.05	0.16	1.2	203
Lymphoid leukaemia	42	0	5.8	1.9	1.4	1.0	1.4	0.4	0.4	-	0.3	1.2	0.4	0.4	-	0.9	1.1	0.7	1.1	-	1.0	0.3	0.07	0.08	1.5	204
Myeloid leukaemia	130	0	0.9	1.2	0.7	1.7	2.3	0.9	1.2	2.3	1.6	2.4	4.2	3.3	3.1	6.1	10.3	8.0	10.8	13.5	3.1	1.0	0.13	0.21	2.2	205
Monocytic leukaemia	3	0	-	-	-	-	-	-	-	-	0.3	0.4	-	-	-	-	-	-	-	1.5	0.1	0.0	0.00	0.00	0.1	206
Other leukaemia	5	0	1.3	-	-	-	-	-	-	-	-	-	-	-	-	-	-	-	1.1	1.5	0.1	0.0	0.01	0.01	0.2	207
Leukaemia unspecified	25	0	-	0.4	-	-	-	-	0.4	0.3	-	0.4	0.4	0.4	0.4	-	2.9	2.9	5.4	6.0	0.6	0.2	0.01	0.03	0.3	208
Other and unspecified	205	1	0.4	-	-	-	-	-	0.8	0.3	2.0	2.0	1.1	5.1	5.0	9.2	13.1	26.1	34.5	70.2	5.0	1.6	0.08	0.20	2.1	O&U
All sites	13211	25	19.3	9.2	10.0	12.0	21.5	36.2	82.5	144.5	195.4	296.3	334.0	422.7	568.0	744.7	920.4	1164.2	1465.9	1685.8	319.7		10.78	19.12	177.8	ALL
All sites but 173	12861	24	19.3	9.2	10.0	11.7	21.1	35.8	80.1	144.1	193.1	293.5	328.3	415.8	559.6	727.6	895.9	1133.0	1393.6	1570.7	311.2	100.0	10.63	18.76	174.0	ALLb
Rate from 1 case			0.448	0.385	0.344	0.344	0.458	0.431	0.387	0.331	0.326	0.396	0.383	0.367	0.382	0.436	0.570	0.724	1.079	1.495						

†Important: see notes on population page

393

Japan, Osaka Prefecture

In 1962 the Osaka Prefectural Government, the Osaka Medical Association, and the Osaka Medical Centre for Cancer and Cardiovascular Diseases (OMCCCD) started prefecture-wide cancer registration on a voluntary basis in order to obtain information about the nature and extent of the cancer problem in Osaka and to assist planning and evaluation of cancer control programmes. The Osaka Cancer Registry is based in the Department of Cancer Control and Statistics of the OMCCCD. The Prefectural Department of Environment and Public Health is responsible for the budgetary support for registration.

Osaka prefecture is located in the central part of Japan. In area it is the second smallest, but its population density is the highest among all prefectures in Japan. During the past 30 years the population has increased from 6.0 to 8.7 million, as of the 1990 census. 98% of the population is Japanese, 1.8% Korean and 0.2% Chinese and others.

Within the prefecture, Osaka city is surrounded by 31 satellite cities, 12 towns and one village. Of all workers, 36% are engaged in industry, 41% in commerce, 21% in personal services and 0.6% in agriculture.

The Osaka Medical Association requests physicians and hospitals to mail cancer reports to it. Monthly cancer reports are transferred from the Association to the registry and cancer death certificates from the health centres. Data entries are conducted on a yearly basis. Record linkage is carried out by computer and uncertainties are resolved manually referring to the original cards. All items in a report are checked for consistency before and after computer entry. Between any two reports belonging to one patient, items are cross-checked for consistency after every collation and also at the final stage of the registration procedures.

Multiple primary cancers are counted separately in computing incidence. It has been estimated that the present number of registered cases corresponds to 85–94% of all actual cancer cases occurring in Osaka.

Since 1975, in order to assess patients' prognosis, all non-deceased registered cases have been collated every year with death certificates of all causes of death for Osaka residents. Living cases are surveyed to confirm their prognosis by health centre staff five years after the first diagnosis of cancer. The staff matches the file of living patients with the citizen registry file at the city office of the patient's address to confirm whether they are alive or dead. Patients occasionally move outside the prefecture. These are traced by sending a questionnaire to the city office of the patient's new address. The proportion of lost cases was less than 5%. Expected survival rates calculated from mortality in Japan are used in computing relative survival rates.

The registry started a cancer information service programme in 1975. Prognosis of reported patients as well as cancer statistics of each hospital are provided free at the request of participating hospitals or hospital doctors. The registry has held a conference annually to report cancer registration activities in Osaka, inviting representatives from all large and medium-sized general hospitals and clinical departments of medical university hospitals.

Since the registry was founded, it has prepared an annual report, published by the Department of Environment and Public Health for distribution to all participating hospitals and the authorities concerned.

The major trends observed by the registry are: (1) cancers of the stomach and cervix have been decreasing, and cancers of the colon, liver, lung, gallbladder, pancreas, breast, corpus, ovary, prostate and other sites increasing; (2) medical care for cancer patients has been improving; (3) five-year relative survival rates have substantially improved for cancers of the stomach, colon, rectum and breast, and to a limited extent in cancers of the oesophagus, liver, gallbladder, lung, ovary, lymphoma and leukaemia. However, no improvement has been made for cancers of the pancreas, uterus and bladder, although the latter two showed high rates from the start.

Cancer has been the leading cause of death in Osaka Prefecture since 1972. The rank order of Osaka was first among all 49 prefectures in Japan in mortality for all sites of cancer among males as well as among females in 1990.

Aya Hanai
Wakiko Ajiki
Hideaki Tsukuma
Akira Oshima
Isaburo Fujimoto

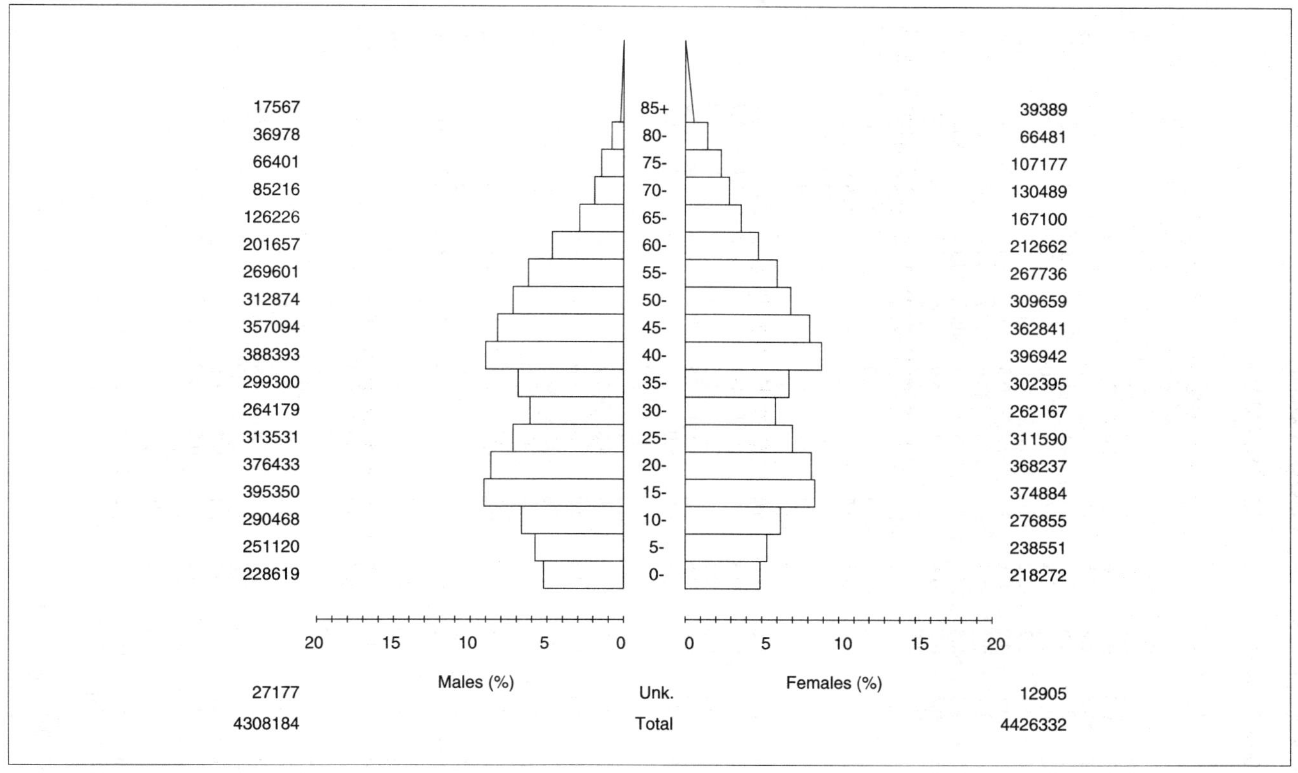

Japan, Osaka Prefecture

Source of population: average annual 1988–92

Census: 1990. Statistics Bureau, Management and Coordination Agency, Government of Japan, 1990 Population Census of Japan, Vol. 2-2-27 Osaka-Fu, Tokyo, 1991. 1985. Statistics Bureau, Management and Coordination Agency, Government of Japan, 1985 Population Census of Japan, Vol. 2-2-27 Osaka-Fu, Tokyo, 1986.

Estimate: The data for 1988, 1989, 1991 and 1992 were estimated by linear extrapolation from the 1985 and 1990 Census data.

Notes to tables overleaf:

† 188 does not include non-invasive tumours

Screening programmes in the area:

Data on screening were not available for Osaka City. For the rest of the Prefecture, data are provided for the screening offered by the municipal governments. An unknown number of workers will also have benefitted from screening offered by their employers. Women over age 30 have been screened for cervical cancer since 1958 (average 178 826 annual examinations during this period), and for breast cancer since 1987 (average 99 816 annual examinations). The population over age 40 has been screened for stomach cancer since 1961 (100 237 average annual examinations), lung cancer since 1987 (96 123 average annual examinations) and large bowel since 1992 (53 893 examinations in that year).

JAPAN, OSAKA PREFECTURE 1988-1992

ANNUAL INCIDENCE PER 100,000 BY AGE GROUP (YEARS) - MALE

SITE	ALL AGES	AGE UNK	0-	5-	10-	15-	20-	25-	30-	35-	40-	45-	50-	55-	60-	65-	70-	75-	80-	85+	CRUDE RATE	%	CR 64	CR 74	ASR (W)	ICD (9th)
Lip	12	0	-	-	-	-	-	-	-	-	0.1	-	0.3	0.2	-	0.2	0.6	0.5	-	0.1	0.0	0.00	0.00	**0.0**	140
Tongue	427	0	-	-	-	0.1	-	0.4	0.6	0.9	1.2	2.7	3.7	5.3	6.5	8.4	6.3	7.8	9.7	8.0	2.0	0.6	0.11	0.18	**1.6**	141
Salivary gland	118	0	-	-	-	0.1	-	0.3	0.3	0.1	0.3	0.4	0.6	1.4	1.4	2.7	2.8	3.0	4.3	3.4	0.5	0.2	0.02	0.05	**0.4**	142
Mouth	378	0	-	-	0.1	0.1	-	-	-	0.2	0.8	1.8	2.5	5.5	5.1	7.3	10.8	10.5	11.9	12.5	1.8	0.5	0.08	0.17	**1.4**	143-5
Oropharynx	177	0	-	-	-	-	-	-	0.1	0.1	0.5	0.5	1.9	2.1	4.1	4.1	3.5	3.0	2.7	1.1	0.8	0.2	0.05	0.08	**0.7**	146
Nasopharynx	155	0	-	0.1	0.1	0.3	0.4	-	-	0.4	0.7	1.2	1.4	1.6	1.5	3.0	2.6	2.1	2.2	-	0.7	0.2	0.04	0.07	**0.6**	147
Hypopharynx	319	0	-	-	-	-	-	-	-	0.1	0.4	1.2	2.2	3.6	5.0	7.8	10.3	8.1	11.9	15.9	1.5	0.4	0.06	0.15	**1.2**	148
Pharynx unspecified	29	0	-	-	-	-	-	-	-	-	0.1	0.2	0.1	0.2	0.2	0.5	1.6	0.6	2.7	1.1	0.1	0.0	0.00	0.01	**0.1**	149
Oesophagus	2424	0	-	0.1	-	-	-	0.6	1.4	7.3	17.1	26.8	44.3	59.9	69.7	79.8	89.8	85.4	11.3	3.4	0.49	1.14	**9.1**	150
Stomach	17241	1	-	-	-	0.1	0.4	2.2	5.5	17.0	29.5	56.5	100.2	162.5	268.8	386.4	505.1	619.6	770.7	850.5	80.0	24.1	3.21	7.67	**65.0**	151
Small intestine	167	0	-	-	-	-	-	0.1	0.2	0.3	0.8	0.8	0.8	1.4	3.1	3.0	3.8	5.1	4.9	6.8	0.8	0.2	0.04	0.07	**0.6**	152
Colon	5505	0	-	-	0.1	0.1	0.4	1.0	1.6	4.5	9.5	15.9	32.1	57.0	84.6	121.2	155.8	211.4	221.8	293.7	25.6	7.7	1.03	2.42	**20.7**	153
Rectum	3594	1	-	-	0.1	0.1	0.2	0.4	1.1	3.1	7.6	14.1	25.1	41.1	60.5	74.3	93.4	94.6	125.5	173.1	16.7	5.0	0.77	1.61	**13.5**	154
Liver	12445	1	1.1	0.1	0.3	-	0.2	0.3	1.4	5.5	12.1	28.5	71.6	195.9	288.3	302.3	286.3	288.2	307.8	286.9	57.8	17.4	3.03	5.97	**46.7**	155
Gallbladder etc.	1621	0	-	-	-	-	0.1	0.3	0.1	1.1	0.9	2.4	5.5	10.5	23.2	35.5	58.0	80.1	116.8	142.3	7.5	2.3	0.22	0.69	**6.2**	156
Pancreas	2531	0	0.2	-	-	-	0.1	0.1	0.3	1.4	3.8	6.4	12.1	23.3	37.4	59.3	79.1	102.4	126.0	168.5	11.7	3.5	0.43	1.12	**9.6**	157
Nose, sinuses etc.	233	0	-	0.1	0.1	0.1	0.1	0.1	0.2	0.5	0.6	1.0	1.4	2.2	2.9	5.7	6.1	7.5	9.2	4.6	1.1	0.3	0.05	0.10	**0.9**	160
Larynx	897	0	-	-	-	-	-	-	-	0.1	0.7	1.9	4.5	10.5	15.7	24.1	28.9	29.8	42.2	30.7	4.2	1.3	0.17	0.43	**3.4**	161
Bronchus, lung	11305	0	-	-	-	0.1	0.2	0.5	1.6	5.0	10.0	18.6	32.4	76.0	151.5	278.4	437.2	584.6	733.4	790.1	52.5	15.8	1.48	5.06	**43.5**	162
Other thoracic organs	144	0	0.6	-	0.1	0.2	0.3	0.4	0.2	0.6	0.2	0.4	0.8	1.0	1.4	2.7	4.5	4.5	1.1	5.7	0.7	0.2	0.03	0.07	**0.6**	163-4
Bone	136	0	0.2	0.3	1.0	1.2	0.5	0.4	0.5	0.6	0.4	0.5	0.3	0.3	0.5	1.6	1.6	3.0	1.1	2.3	0.6	0.2	0.03	0.05	**0.6**	170
Connective tissue	212	0	2.9	0.6	0.2	0.4	0.4	0.4	0.3	0.3	0.9	0.6	0.6	1.6	1.5	2.5	4.5	4.5	4.9	5.7	1.0	0.3	0.05	0.09	**1.1**	171
Mesothelioma	96	0	-	-	-	-	-	-	-	0.2	0.1	0.2	0.5	1.0	1.0	3.6	2.3	3.6	3.2	5.7	0.4	0.1	0.02	0.05	**0.4**	MES
Kaposi's sarcoma	2	0	-	-	-	-	-	0.1	-	-	-	-	-	-	0.2	-	-	-	-	-	0.0	0.0	0.00	0.00	**0.0**	KAP
Melanoma of skin	58	0	-	-	-	0.1	-	0.1	0.1	0.3	0.2	0.3	0.3	0.4	1.1	1.1	1.4	0.9	2.7	1.1	0.3	0.1	0.01	0.03	**0.2**	172
Other skin	320	0	-	-	0.1	0.1	0.1	0.1	0.4	0.3	0.7	0.7	1.5	1.9	4.8	5.4	7.5	13.6	22.7	35.3	1.5		0.05	0.12	**1.2**	173
Breast	38	0	-	-	-	0.1	-	-	-	-	0.1	0.1	0.3	0.2	1.3	1.0	0.5	1.5	-	2.3	0.2	0.1	0.01	0.02	**0.1**	175
Prostate	1758	0	0.1	-	-	-	-	-	-	0.2	0.6	1.5	5.6	14.7	34.5	69.2	129.2	179.6	252.7	8.2	2.5	0.11	0.63	**6.8**	185
Testis	317	0	1.7	0.1	0.1	0.5	1.2	3.2	3.8	2.5	2.7	1.1	1.5	0.7	0.8	0.6	0.7	1.5	0.5	-	1.5	0.4	0.10	0.11	**1.4**	186
Penis	58	0	-	-	-	-	-	-	-	0.1	0.2	0.2	0.4	0.7	0.8	0.8	1.6	1.8	2.2	4.6	0.3	0.1	0.01	0.02	**0.2**	187.1-.4
Other male genital	26	0	-	-	-	-	0.1	-	-	-	0.1	0.1	0.2	0.6	0.6	0.2	1.2	0.5	3.4	0.1	0.0	0.01	0.01	**0.1**	187.5-.9
†Bladder	1926	0	-	-	-	0.1	0.1	0.1	0.5	1.1	2.6	4.0	7.7	14.5	24.8	42.9	66.0	84.9	122.8	167.4	8.9	2.7	0.28	0.82	**7.4**	188
Kidney etc.	1423	0	1.5	0.3	0.2	-	0.1	0.1	0.4	0.9	3.0	3.8	7.5	14.5	22.0	31.8	41.1	53.6	62.7	54.6	6.6	2.0	0.27	0.64	**5.5**	189
Eye	28	0	1.0	0.1	0.1	-	-	-	-	-	0.1	0.1	0.1	0.4	0.2	0.5	0.6	0.5	-	0.1	0.0	0.01	0.01	**0.2**	190
Brain, nervous system	667	0	2.4	2.5	2.4	1.1	0.7	1.3	1.7	1.6	1.9	2.7	3.5	4.2	6.9	10.9	12.2	15.7	10.3	13.7	3.1	0.9	0.17	0.28	**3.0**	191-2
Thyroid	295	0	-	-	0.1	0.2	0.3	0.4	0.4	1.3	1.1	0.8	1.6	3.0	3.9	4.6	7.7	7.8	5.4	14.8	1.4	0.4	0.07	0.13	**1.1**	193
Other endocrine	119	0	2.9	0.4	0.3	0.4	0.4	0.2	0.2	0.1	0.1	0.2	0.4	0.7	1.0	0.3	1.2	3.3	1.1	2.3	0.6	0.2	0.04	0.04	**0.7**	194
Hodgkin's disease	123	0	0.1	-	0.2	0.3	0.2	0.4	0.2	0.3	0.6	0.6	0.5	0.7	1.8	2.5	2.6	1.5	2.2	4.6	0.6	0.2	0.03	0.05	**0.5**	201
Non-Hodgkin lymphoma	1565	1	0.8	1.5	1.7	1.4	0.9	1.4	2.3	2.1	3.2	5.9	8.8	13.2	20.3	33.4	38.3	48.5	60.0	53.5	7.3	2.2	0.32	0.68	**6.1**	200,202
Multiple myeloma	406	0	-	-	-	-	-	-	-	0.3	0.6	0.8	1.2	2.4	6.7	9.3	13.6	19.3	26.5	31.9	1.9	0.6	0.06	0.17	**1.6**	203
Lymphoid leukaemia	407	0	3.4	3.3	1.6	1.2	0.5	0.6	0.5	0.7	1.3	2.0	1.7	2.7	3.8	4.9	5.2	3.0	6.5	8.0	1.9	0.6	0.12	0.17	**2.0**	204
Myeloid leukaemia	678	0	0.5	0.9	0.6	1.3	1.2	1.5	2.3	1.7	3.5	3.5	3.6	5.6	6.3	7.9	13.4	15.1	15.1	17.1	3.1	0.9	0.16	0.27	**2.7**	205
Monocytic leukaemia	59	0	0.4	0.1	0.1	0.2	0.2	0.1	-	0.1	0.4	0.1	0.3	0.1	0.7	1.0	0.7	1.5	1.6	2.3	0.3	0.1	0.01	0.01	**0.3**	206
Other leukaemia	32	0	-	-	0.1	-	0.1	-	0.1	-	0.2	0.1	0.3	0.5	0.8	0.7	0.6	0.5	1.1	0.1	0.0	0.01	0.01	**0.1**	207
Leukaemia unspecified	159	0	0.4	0.1	0.4	0.2	0.2	0.3	0.2	0.3	0.3	0.2	0.7	1.0	1.6	2.4	3.3	7.8	7.6	11.4	0.7	0.2	0.03	0.06	**0.7**	208
Other and unspecified	1084	0	0.9	0.3	0.2	0.3	0.2	0.3	0.5	1.1	0.7	2.4	4.8	9.3	14.9	22.2	29.1	51.2	61.7	85.4	5.0	1.5	0.18	0.44	**4.2**	O&U
All sites	71714	4	21.2	10.8	10.1	9.5	9.5	16.9	27.6	57.6	105.7	193.5	365.2	713.2	1148.2	1613.8	2091.2	2618.9	3197.0	3661.4	332.9		13.45	31.97	**274.0**	ALL
All sites but 173	71394	4	21.2	10.8	10.1	9.5	9.5	16.8	27.2	57.3	105.0	192.8	363.7	711.3	1143.4	1608.4	2083.6	2605.4	3174.3	3626.1	331.4	100.0	13.39	31.85	**272.8**	ALLb

Rate from 1 case			0.087	0.080	0.069	0.051	0.053	0.064	0.076	0.067	0.051	0.056	0.064	0.074	0.099	0.158	0.235	0.301	0.541	1.138

†Important: see notes on population page

JAPAN, OSAKA PREFECTURE 1988-1992

ANNUAL INCIDENCE PER 100,000 BY AGE GROUP (YEARS) - FEMALE

SITE	ALL AGES	AGE UNK	0-	5-	10-	15-	20-	25-	30-	35-	40-	45-	50-	55-	60-	65-	70-	75-	80-	85+	CRUDE RATE	%	CR 64	CR 74	ASR (W)	ICD (9th)
Lip	12	0	-	-	-	-	-	-	-	-	-	-	0.1	0.1	0.3	-	-	0.4	0.3	1.5	0.1	0.0	0.00	0.00	**0.0**	140
Tongue	223	1	-	-	-	-	0.1	0.5	0.4	0.7	1.0	0.7	1.8	2.2	1.8	1.8	4.6	3.0	4.8	6.6	1.0	0.4	0.05	0.08	**0.7**	141
Salivary gland	70	0	-	-	-	-	0.1	0.1	0.2	0.1	0.2	0.2	0.6	0.4	0.5	0.8	0.6	1.3	2.7	4.1	0.3	0.1	0.01	0.02	**0.2**	142
Mouth	204	0	-	0.1	-	0.1	-	0.1	0.1	0.3	0.2	0.8	0.8	1.5	3.3	3.1	4.8	3.9	5.7	5.6	0.9	0.4	0.04	0.08	**0.6**	143-5
Oropharynx	45	0	-	-	-	-	-	-	-	0.1	0.2	0.1	0.4	0.6	0.7	0.6	1.1	0.4	0.6	0.5	0.2	0.1	0.01	0.02	**0.1**	146
Nasopharynx	69	0	-	-	-	-	0.2	-	0.1	0.3	0.2	0.4	0.5	0.8	0.8	1.2	0.5	0.9	0.9	1.0	0.3	0.1	0.02	0.02	**0.2**	147
Hypopharynx	55	0	-	-	-	-	-	-	-	-	0.1	0.2	0.4	0.3	0.6	1.1	0.9	1.7	2.1	1.0	0.2	0.1	0.01	0.02	**0.2**	148
Pharynx unspecified	14	0	-	-	-	-	-	-	-	-	0.1	-	0.1	-	0.1	0.5	0.5	-	0.3	1.0	0.1	0.0	0.00	0.01	**0.0**	149
Oesophagus	582	0	-	-	-	-	-	-	-	0.2	0.7	1.0	2.1	4.0	5.8	7.9	13.8	16.2	28.0	32.5	2.6	1.1	0.07	0.18	**1.6**	150
Stomach	9509	4	-	-	-	0.2	0.6	2.8	7.6	16.3	28.9	31.8	48.8	63.5	84.2	133.6	169.8	243.3	330.6	418.4	43.0	18.5	1.42	2.94	**27.3**	151
Small intestine	106	0	-	-	-	-	-	0.1	0.1	-	0.3	0.2	0.7	0.8	1.0	1.7	2.1	3.0	2.7	3.6	0.5	0.2	0.02	0.04	**0.3**	152
Colon	4535	3	-	-	-	-	0.3	0.8	1.5	4.1	7.7	12.6	23.6	33.9	53.6	72.9	90.9	117.2	152.2	166.0	20.5	8.8	0.69	1.51	**13.1**	153
Rectum	2298	0	-	-	-	0.1	0.1	0.7	1.4	2.7	5.3	10.1	14.9	21.7	26.0	34.2	37.7	51.5	52.9	78.2	10.4	4.5	0.41	0.77	**6.8**	154
Liver	3905	0	0.9	0.1	0.1	0.1	0.1	-	0.3	1.0	2.6	4.5	10.3	29.2	58.2	85.9	95.9	107.7	115.5	134.0	17.6	7.6	0.54	1.45	**11.5**	155
Gallbladder etc.	2227	0	-	-	-	0.1	0.1	0.1	0.2	0.3	1.6	2.7	7.0	11.2	18.4	36.5	54.7	86.0	102.3	111.7	10.1	4.3	0.21	0.66	**6.0**	156
Pancreas	1981	0	0.1	0.1	-	0.1	0.1	0.1	0.7	0.5	1.4	3.1	6.5	10.5	15.1	33.3	45.2	70.7	89.6	113.2	9.0	3.9	0.19	0.58	**5.4**	157
Nose, sinuses etc.	161	0	0.1	-	0.1	0.1	0.1	0.1	-	0.3	0.1	0.7	0.6	1.0	1.5	2.4	2.8	5.0	4.2	7.6	0.7	0.3	0.02	0.05	**0.5**	160
Larynx	107	0	-	-	0.1	-	-	-	-	0.1	0.1	0.1	0.4	1.1	2.3	3.1	2.8	4.2	3.6	0.5	0.2	0.01	0.04	**0.3**	161
Bronchus, lung	4526	0	0.1	-	-	0.1	0.1	0.5	0.9	3.4	4.5	7.6	14.5	25.5	37.8	73.8	115.1	154.3	199.2	202.1	20.5	8.8	0.48	1.42	**12.4**	162
Other thoracic organs	109	0	0.5	0.3	0.1	0.1	0.1	0.1	0.2	0.1	0.1	0.6	0.7	0.8	1.2	1.7	1.5	1.3	1.8	2.5	0.5	0.2	0.02	0.04	**0.4**	163-4
Bone	107	0	0.3	0.4	0.9	0.5	0.2	0.4	0.4	0.1	0.3	0.2	0.5	0.2	0.8	0.8	2.0	1.5	0.9	0.5	0.5	0.2	0.03	0.04	**0.5**	170
Connective tissue	200	0	2.7	0.8	0.2	0.4	0.4	0.3	0.4	0.1	0.7	0.4	0.8	1.0	1.7	1.6	2.9	3.2	4.5	2.5	0.9	0.4	0.05	0.07	**0.9**	171
Mesothelioma	63	0	-	-	-	-	-	-	0.1	0.1	0.3	0.3	0.1	0.4	0.9	0.8	1.4	1.9	1.8	1.0	0.3	0.1	0.01	0.02	**0.2**	MES
Kaposi's sarcoma	0	0	-	-	-	-	-	-	-	-	-	-	-	-	-	-	-	-	-	-	0.0	0.0	0.00	0.00	**0.0**	KAP
Melanoma of skin	67	0	0.1	-	0.1	0.1	0.1	0.1	0.1	0.1	0.4	0.5	0.3	0.4	0.8	0.2	1.4	0.9	1.2	0.5	0.3	0.1	0.02	0.02	**0.2**	172
Other skin	266	0	-	-	0.1	0.1	0.1	0.1	0.2	0.3	0.6	0.4	0.9	1.6	2.4	3.6	5.2	5.4	9.0	26.4	1.2		0.03	0.08	**0.8**	173
Breast	7544	2	-	-	-	0.2	0.4	2.5	12.8	29.3	53.8	74.0	70.1	64.5	69.2	74.6	74.9	63.4	62.6	64.5	34.1	14.7	1.88	2.63	**24.3**	174
Uterus unspecified	440	0	-	-	-	-	-	-	0.3	0.3	0.3	1.1	1.8	2.5	3.5	4.8	6.9	12.5	25.9	35.0	2.0	0.9	0.05	0.11	**1.2**	179
Cervix uteri	2839	0	-	-	-	0.2	0.7	3.5	8.1	12.7	17.5	18.4	20.4	21.0	28.8	35.1	34.6	36.6	35.2	27.4	12.8	5.5	0.66	1.00	**9.2**	180
Placenta	14	0	-	-	-	0.1	0.1	0.2	0.2	0.1	0.1	0.1	0.1	-	-	-	0.2	-	-	-	0.1	0.0	0.00	0.00	**0.1**	181
Corpus uteri	932	1	-	-	-	0.1	0.1	0.3	0.8	1.0	3.1	6.1	11.8	13.5	13.4	11.5	7.5	7.1	6.3	8.1	4.2	1.8	0.25	0.35	**3.0**	182
Ovary etc.	1722	0	0.2	0.4	0.7	0.6	1.5	2.6	2.6	4.8	7.3	11.3	15.5	16.1	17.0	21.1	17.2	21.1	20.8	32.5	7.8	3.4	0.40	0.59	**5.6**	183
Other female genital	151	0	0.1	0.1	-	-	-	0.1	-	0.1	0.2	0.3	0.6	1.0	1.7	2.5	2.6	4.3	7.8	5.6	0.7	0.3	0.02	0.05	**0.4**	184
†Bladder	654	0	-	0.1	-	0.1	0.1	0.1	0.3	0.2	0.5	0.9	1.7	3.4	6.0	9.1	15.2	19.4	32.2	47.7	3.0	1.3	0.07	0.19	**1.8**	188
Kidney etc.	629	0	1.0	0.1	0.1	0.2	-	0.1	0.3	0.3	1.2	1.5	2.8	4.4	7.3	10.9	12.1	16.2	20.8	22.8	2.8	1.2	0.10	0.21	**1.9**	189
Eye	19	0	0.7	0.1	0.1	0.1	0.1	-	0.1	-	0.1	-	0.1	-	0.1	-	0.1	-	0.4	0.3	0.1	0.0	0.01	0.01	**0.1**	190
Brain, nervous system	541	0	2.8	1.7	2.5	1.0	1.1	1.3	0.8	1.6	1.2	2.3	2.4	2.5	5.1	5.6	6.4	6.3	10.2	8.6	2.4	1.1	0.13	0.19	**2.2**	191-2
Thyroid	1083	0	-	0.1	0.2	0.7	1.3	1.5	2.8	3.8	5.5	7.5	7.6	8.7	10.3	8.1	12.7	18.3	16.2	17.3	4.9	2.1	0.25	0.35	**3.5**	193
Other endocrine	76	0	2.5	0.3	0.1	0.1	0.2	0.2	0.1	0.1	-	0.2	0.2	0.2	0.7	0.2	1.4	0.4	1.2	-	0.3	0.1	0.02	0.03	**0.5**	194
Hodgkin's disease	62	0	0.2	0.1	-	0.4	0.5	0.3	0.2	0.1	-	-	0.3	0.6	0.9	0.2	0.6	0.7	0.6	-	0.3	0.1	0.02	0.02	**0.2**	201
Non-Hodgkin lymphoma	1103	0	1.5	0.8	0.7	0.8	0.8	1.2	1.8	1.5	2.5	3.7	5.7	7.3	12.0	14.6	23.0	23.5	28.0	25.9	5.0	2.1	0.20	0.39	**3.6**	200,202
Multiple myeloma	367	0	-	-	-	-	0.1	0.1	-	0.3	0.3	0.7	1.4	2.5	4.6	6.0	7.4	12.9	11.1	18.3	1.7	0.7	0.05	0.12	**1.0**	203
Lymphoid leukaemia	341	0	4.2	1.7	1.1	1.0	0.8	0.6	0.5	1.1	1.1	1.5	1.4	1.6	2.4	2.5	2.8	3.4	4.8	3.6	1.5	0.7	0.09	0.12	**1.6**	204
Myeloid leukaemia	468	0	0.5	0.8	1.1	1.0	0.5	0.8	1.2	1.8	1.9	2.3	2.3	3.5	2.5	4.1	5.2	7.7	10.5	11.2	2.1	0.9	0.10	0.15	**1.6**	205
Monocytic leukaemia	37	0	-	-	-	0.1	0.1	0.1	0.2	-	0.2	0.2	0.1	0.5	0.3	0.5	0.8	0.6	0.3	-	0.2	0.1	0.01	0.01	**0.1**	206
Other leukaemia	21	0	0.1	0.1	-	0.1	-	0.1	-	-	0.3	-	0.2	0.3	-	0.4	0.2	0.7	0.3	0.5	0.1	0.0	0.00	0.01	**0.1**	207
Leukaemia unspecified	98	0	0.5	0.4	0.1	0.1	0.2	0.1	0.1	0.1	0.1	0.3	0.4	0.4	0.5	0.5	1.5	2.8	3.9	5.1	0.4	0.2	0.02	0.03	**0.4**	208
Other and unspecified	997	1	1.5	0.3	0.1	0.1	0.2	0.3	0.7	0.6	1.2	2.4	2.4	4.6	9.4	14.0	18.7	27.2	48.4	70.1	4.5	1.9	0.12	0.28	**2.9**	O&U
All sites	51579	12	20.4	8.7	8.5	8.4	11.1	22.8	48.4	90.8	154.9	213.8	286.4	371.4	514.1	728.7	910.1	1169.3	1465.7	1729.9	233.1		8.80	17.00	**155.5**	ALL
All sites but 173	51313	12	20.4	8.7	8.5	8.3	11.0	22.7	48.2	90.5	154.3	213.4	285.5	369.8	511.8	725.1	904.9	1163.9	1456.7	1703.5	231.9	100.0	8.77	16.92	**154.8**	ALLb

| Rate from 1 case | | | 0.092 | 0.084 | 0.072 | 0.053 | 0.054 | 0.064 | 0.076 | 0.066 | 0.050 | 0.055 | 0.065 | 0.075 | 0.094 | 0.120 | 0.153 | 0.187 | 0.301 | 0.508 |

†Important: see notes on population page

Japan, Saga Prefecture

The Saga Cancer Survey was run by the Prefectural Health Department in cooperation with the Saga Medical Association, from 1973 until it was re-designed as the Population-based Saga Cancer Registry in 1984. This registry aims to obtain information on the nature and extent of cancer problems, and to assist in planning and evaluation of cancer control programmes in Saga Prefecture. The Prefectural Department of Health Promotion and Environment is responsible for budgetary support for registration.

Saga is located in the north of Kyushu, in the southwestern part of Japan, and its surface area is 2433 km^2, between latitudes 32°57′ and 33°37′ N and longitudes 129°44′ and 130°33′ E. The population covered by the registry was approximately 880 000 at the 1990 census, of whom more than 99% were of Japanese nationality. There are 7 cities, 37 towns, and 5 villages in the prefecture. Saga is not a highly industrialized prefecture and its major industries are agriculture and fishery. Saga is famous for its pottery works named Imari, Arita and Karatsu.

Case-finding and data-collection are carried out both actively and passively. Two of the staff, including a medical doctor, abstract cancer cases from medical records of major hospitals in Saga and neighbouring prefectures. All physicians and medical institutions are requested to report cancer cases to the registry on a voluntary basis. Since cancer registries have been organized in the adjacent prefectures (Nagasaki and Fukuoka), relevant case reports are exchanged between registries. Reportable tumours include all malignant neoplasms, carcinoma *in situ*, and neoplasms of uncertain nature. Official death certificates are routinely obtained to be used for cancer registration. They are mainly employed to follow up incident cancer cases, to track down deceased cases without case reports, and to register death-certificate-only cases.

An unique personal computer system has been developed to process registration data since 1992. Information recorded includes name, sex, date of birth, age, usual residence, principal occupation, date of first diagnosis, diagnosis (site and morphology), clinical stage, methods of diagnosis, histological diagnosis, nature of treatment, date of death, cause of death, and so on. Cancer cases abstracted and/or reported are collated and coded; they are then stored not only on the hard disk of the computer but also on floppy disk. Duplicate entries are identified by linking items of date of birth, name, sex, cancer (site and morphology) and address by the computer as well as manually. Reports of possible multiple primary tumours are carefully reviewed in terms of cancer site, histological type and time at diagnosis. Then, if they are not regarded as either metastasis or recurrence, they are evaluated as multiple primary tumours and are counted separately in computing incidence.

Partly due to limitations of finance and staffing, follow-up of cancer patients has not been undertaken routinely, and effective utilization of the cancer registry data has been rather limited. However, an annual report of cancer statistics in the prefecture is published in Japanese for physicians and health professionals. These data have been utilized for several epidemiological studies on primary, secondary, and tertiary prevention of cancer.

Mitsuru Mori
Junichi Naramoto,
Masatoshi Ishizuka
Eisuke Nakazato
Ayako Maeda

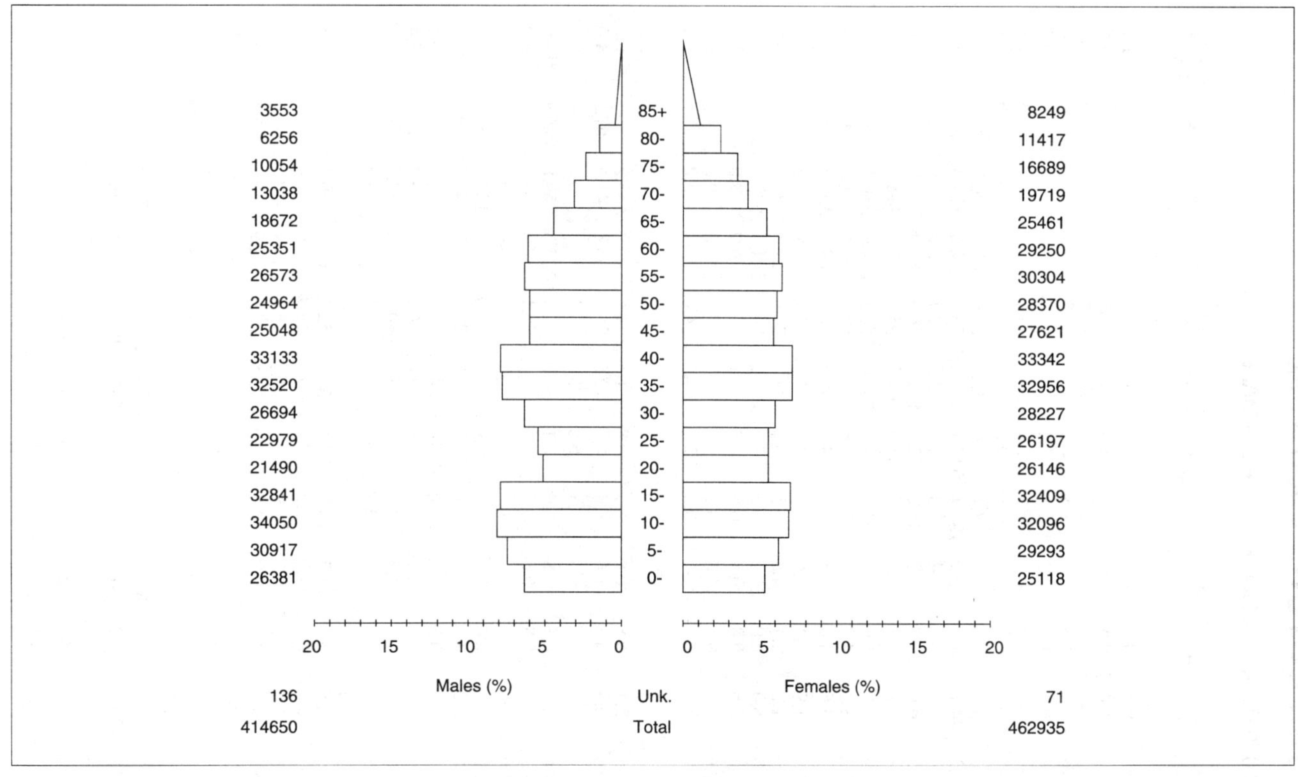

Japan, Saga Prefecture
Source of population: average annual 1988–92
Census: 1990 Population Census of Japan, Statistics Bureau, Management and Coordination Agency, 1991. 1985 Population Census of Japan, Statistics Bureau, Management and Coordination Agency, 1986.
Estimate: Figures for 1988 and 1989 were estimated on the basis of the 1985 Census, adding births and immigrants and subtracting deaths and emigrants. The methodology for 1991 and 1992 was the same, based on the 1990 Census.
Notes to the tables overleaf:
* The high proportion of diagnoses based on a death certificate alone indicate under-ascertainment.
+ The editors were unable to verify these data
† 163-164 includes mesothelioma of the pleura

† Mesothelioma not available separately
† Kaposi's sarcoma not available separately
† 188 does not include non-invasive tumours
Screening programmes in the area:
Women over age 30 have been screened annually for cervical cancer since 1983. The population over age 40 has been screened annually for stomach cancer since 1983, lung cancer since 1988 and large bowel cancer since 1992.

+* JAPAN, SAGA PREFECTURE 1988-1992

ANNUAL INCIDENCE PER 100,000 BY AGE GROUP (YEARS) - MALE

SITE	ALL AGES	AGE UNK	0-	5-	10-	15-	20-	25-	30-	35-	40-	45-	50-	55-	60-	65-	70-	75-	80-	85+	CRUDE RATE	%	CR 64	CR 74	ASR (W)	ICD (9th)
Lip	3	0	-	-	-	-	-	-	-	-	-	-	-	-	-	-	1.5	2.0	3.2	-	0.1	0.0	0.00	0.01	**0.1**	140
Tongue	39	0	-	-	-	-	-	-	-	0.6	0.6	0.8	4.0	1.5	4.7	11.8	10.7	4.0	9.6	-	1.9	0.4	0.06	0.17	**1.2**	141
Salivary gland	17	0	-	-	-	-	-	-	0.7	-	1.2	0.8	-	1.5	1.6	1.1	4.6	2.0	3.2	16.9	0.8	0.2	0.03	0.06	**0.5**	142
Mouth	49	0	-	-	-	-	0.9	-	-	-	-	-	2.4	4.5	6.3	10.7	13.8	13.9	12.8	5.6	2.4	0.5	0.07	0.19	**1.5**	143-5
Oropharynx	20	0	-	-	-	-	-	-	-	0.6	-	1.6	-	1.5	4.7	-	7.7	6.0	3.2	-	1.0	0.2	0.04	0.08	**0.6**	146
Nasopharynx	14	0	-	-	-	-	-	-	-	-	0.6	1.6	3.2	1.5	2.4	-	1.5	2.0	-	-	0.7	0.2	0.05	0.05	**0.5**	147
Hypopharynx	22	0	-	-	-	-	-	-	-	-	-	1.6	0.8	3.0	3.9	4.3	4.6	2.0	-	11.3	1.1	0.2	0.05	0.09	**0.7**	148
Pharynx unspecified	2	0	-	-	-	-	-	-	-	-	-	-	-	-	0.8	-	-	-	-	5.6	0.1	0.0	0.00	0.00	**0.1**	149
Oesophagus	243	0	-	-	-	-	-	-	-	-	3.0	4.8	6.4	18.1	41.0	42.8	66.0	65.6	76.7	45.0	11.7	2.7	0.37	0.91	**7.0**	150
Stomach	2420	0	-	-	-	-	2.8	1.7	6.0	17.2	44.1	51.1	100.9	182.1	317.1	407.0	573.7	622.6	824.8	827.3	116.7	26.6	3.62	8.52	**70.7**	151
Small intestine	18	0	-	-	-	-	-	-	-	-	-	-	2.4	0.8	1.6	3.2	3.1	2.0	6.4	22.5	0.9	0.2	0.02	0.06	**0.5**	152
Colon	664	0	-	-	-	-	0.9	0.7	5.5	6.0	20.0	31.2	48.2	72.6	106.0	156.5	183.0	239.8	309.5	32.0	7.3	0.93	2.24	**19.3**	153
Rectum	387	0	-	-	-	-	1.7	-	1.8	7.2	10.4	22.4	44.4	45.0	64.3	95.1	81.6	118.3	73.2	18.7	4.3	0.67	1.46	**11.6**	154
Liver	1352	0	-	-	0.6	0.6	-	-	4.5	4.9	16.3	35.9	77.7	164.8	229.6	241.0	253.1	254.6	310.1	236.4	65.2	14.9	2.67	5.15	**41.0**	155
Gallbladder etc.	277	0	-	-	-	-	0.9	-	-	1.2	3.0	4.0	9.6	15.1	27.6	31.1	69.0	93.5	111.9	230.8	13.4	3.0	0.31	0.81	**7.7**	156
Pancreas	344	0	-	-	-	-	-	-	-	-	3.6	4.0	8.8	18.1	39.4	82.5	58.3	109.4	153.5	168.8	16.6	3.8	0.37	1.07	**9.5**	157
Nose, sinuses etc.	43	0	-	-	-	-	-	-	-	1.2	1.8	3.2	1.6	3.0	3.9	6.4	9.2	11.9	3.2	22.5	2.1	0.5	0.07	0.15	**1.4**	160
Larynx	131	0	-	-	-	-	-	-	-	-	1.2	2.4	4.8	13.5	16.6	32.1	27.6	31.8	35.2	33.8	6.3	1.4	0.19	0.49	**3.8**	161
Bronchus, lung	1429	0	-	-	-	-	0.9	-	5.5	6.0	16.0	26.4	59.5	177.5	259.2	394.2	521.1	623.4	540.3	68.9	15.7	1.46	4.73	**39.2**	162
†Other thoracic organs	24	0	1.5	0.6	-	-	0.9	-	-	-	0.6	0.8	0.8	0.8	3.2	2.1	-	6.0	9.6	22.5	1.2	0.3	0.05	0.06	**0.9**	163-4
Bone	15	0	-	-	-	1.2	-	1.7	-	0.6	-	0.8	1.6	0.8	-	-	-	2.0	9.6	11.3	0.7	0.2	0.03	0.03	**0.6**	170
Connective tissue	17	0	0.8	-	0.6	-	-	-	-	-	-	-	-	0.8	3.9	4.3	4.6	-	3.2	5.6	0.8	0.2	0.03	0.07	**0.6**	171
†Mesothelioma																										
†Kaposi's sarcoma																										
Melanoma of skin	18	0	0.8	-	-	-	-	-	-	-	2.4	0.8	0.8	1.5	0.8	1.1	1.5	9.9	3.2	-	0.9	0.2	0.04	0.05	**0.6**	172
Other skin	95	0	-	-	-	-	-	0.9	-	0.6	0.6	0.8	1.6	6.8	8.7	9.6	26.1	35.8	41.6	67.5	4.6		0.10	0.28	**2.6**	173
Breast	8	0	-	-	-	-	-	-	-	-	-	-	0.8	1.5	0.8	1.1	3.1	-	3.2	-	0.4	0.1	0.02	0.04	**0.2**	175
Prostate	267	0	-	-	-	-	-	-	-	0.6	-	0.8	0.8	3.0	18.1	30.0	76.7	133.3	159.8	236.4	12.9	2.9	0.12	0.65	**6.7**	185
Testis	19	0	-	-	-	0.6	0.9	3.5	3.0	1.2	-	0.8	0.8	1.5	-	-	3.1	2.0	-	-	0.9	0.2	0.06	0.08	**0.9**	186
Penis, other male genital	5	0	-	-	-	-	-	-	-	0.6	-	-	-	1.5	-	-	-	2.0	3.2	-	0.2	0.1	0.01	0.01	**0.1**	187
†Bladder	273	0	-	0.6	-	-	0.9	-	0.7	1.2	1.8	6.4	7.2	14.3	22.9	51.4	66.0	79.6	134.3	152.0	13.2	3.0	0.28	0.87	**7.7**	188
Kidney etc.	160	0	-	-	-	-	-	0.9	-	2.5	3.0	4.8	10.4	15.1	19.7	31.1	27.6	35.8	44.8	39.4	7.7	1.8	0.28	0.58	**4.9**	189
Eye	3	0	1.5	-	-	-	-	-	-	-	0.8	-	-	-	-	-	-	-	-	-	0.1	0.0	0.01	0.01	**0.2**	190
Brain, nervous system	70	0	1.5	1.9	0.6	0.6	0.9	0.9	1.5	1.2	4.2	0.8	3.2	7.5	7.9	9.6	6.1	9.9	6.4	28.1	3.4	0.8	0.16	0.24	**2.6**	191-2
Thyroid	32	0	-	-	-	-	-	-	-	1.2	-	1.6	1.6	2.3	2.4	5.4	10.7	6.0	9.6	11.3	1.5	0.4	0.05	0.13	**1.0**	193
Other endocrine	7	0	0.8	-	-	0.6	-	0.9	-	-	-	-	0.8	-	-	-	-	-	9.6	-	0.3	0.1	0.01	0.01	**0.3**	194
Hodgkin's disease	3	0	-	0.6	-	-	-	-	-	-	0.6	-	-	-	-	-	-	-	-	5.6	0.1	0.0	0.01	0.01	**0.1**	201
Non-Hodgkin lymphoma	275	0	1.5	1.3	0.6	3.0	5.6	0.9	3.7	5.5	4.8	6.4	11.2	15.8	28.4	50.3	52.2	65.6	99.1	67.5	13.3	3.0	0.44	0.96	**8.8**	200,202
Multiple myeloma	66	0	-	-	-	-	-	-	-	-	0.6	0.8	4.0	6.0	7.1	10.7	19.9	21.9	22.4	5.6	3.2	0.7	0.09	0.25	**1.9**	203
Lymphoid leukaemia	117	0	3.8	4.5	1.8	3.0	0.9	2.6	3.0	1.8	3.0	4.8	8.0	9.8	10.3	11.8	13.8	17.9	19.2	22.5	5.6	1.3	0.29	0.41	**4.6**	204
Myeloid leukaemia	105	0	1.5	0.6	1.2	1.2	0.9	-	2.2	5.5	3.0	3.2	7.2	4.5	7.9	11.8	23.0	17.9	35.2	28.1	5.1	1.2	0.20	0.37	**3.5**	205
Monocytic leukaemia	1	0	-	-	-	-	-	-	-	-	0.6	-	-	-	-	-	-	-	-	-	0.0	0.0	0.00	0.00	**0.0**	206
Other leukaemia	4	0	-	-	0.6	-	-	-	-	-	-	0.8	-	0.8	-	-	-	-	3.2	-	0.2	0.0	0.01	0.01	**0.1**	207
Leukaemia unspecified	15	0	0.8	-	1.2	-	-	-	-	-	-	-	-	1.6	2.1	1.5	4.0	12.8	5.6	0.7	0.2	0.02	0.04	**0.5**	208
Other and unspecified	110	0	0.8	0.6	-	-	-	1.5	-	1.2	0.8	1.6	3.0	12.6	17.1	21.5	43.8	57.5	61.9	5.3	1.2	0.11	0.30	**3.0**	O&U
All sites	9183	0	15.2	11.0	7.0	11.0	15.8	17.4	27.7	61.5	121.3	194.0	364.5	678.1	1153.4	1553.1	2107.6	2502.3	3222.5	3320.6	442.9		13.39	31.69	**269.4**	ALL
All sites but 173	9088	0	15.2	11.0	7.0	11.0	15.8	16.5	27.7	60.9	120.7	193.2	362.9	671.4	1144.7	1543.4	2081.5	2466.5	3180.9	3253.0	438.3	100.0	13.29	31.42	**266.8**	ALLb

| Rate from 1 case | | | 0.758 | 0.647 | 0.587 | 0.609 | 0.931 | 0.870 | 0.749 | 0.615 | 0.604 | 0.798 | 0.801 | 0.753 | 0.789 | 1.071 | 1.534 | 1.989 | 3.197 | 5.628 | | | | | | |

†Important: see notes on population page

+* JAPAN, SAGA PREFECTURE 1988-1992

ANNUAL INCIDENCE PER 100,000 BY AGE GROUP (YEARS) - FEMALE

SITE	ALL AGES	AGE UNK	0-	5-	10-	15-	20-	25-	30-	35-	40-	45-	50-	55-	60-	65-	70-	75-	80-	85+	CRUDE RATE	%	CR 64	CR 74	ASR (W)	ICD (9th)
Lip	1	0	-	-	-	-	-	-	-	-	-	-	-	-	-	-	-	-	-	2.4	0.0	0.0	0.00	0.00	**0.0**	*140*
Tongue	23	0	0.8	-	-	-	-	0.8	-	-	-	0.7	2.1	-	1.4	1.6	3.0	2.4	10.5	4.8	1.0	0.4	0.03	0.05	**0.6**	*141*
Salivary gland	9	0	-	-	-	-	0.8	-	-	0.6	-	0.7	0.7	1.3	-	0.8	-	1.2	1.8	-	0.4	0.1	0.02	0.02	**0.3**	*142*
Mouth	29	0	-	-	-	-	-	-	-	-	0.6	0.7	2.1	2.6	1.4	3.1	6.1	2.4	5.3	7.3	1.3	0.4	0.04	0.08	**0.6**	*143-5*
Oropharynx	3	0	-	-	-	-	-	0.8	-	-	-	-	-	-	0.7	-	1.0	-	-	-	0.1	0.0	0.01	0.01	**0.1**	*146*
Nasopharynx	6	0	-	-	-	-	-	-	0.6	-	-	-	-	-	0.7	0.8	2.0	-	1.8	-	0.3	0.1	0.01	Nas.02	**0.1**	*147*
Hypopharynx	6	0	-	-	-	-	-	-	-	-	-	0.7	0.7	1.4	-	1.0	-	1.8	-		0.3	0.1	0.01	Hyp.02	**0.1**	*148*
Pharynx unspecified	1	0	-	-	-	-	-	-	-	-	-	-	-	-	-	-	-	-	-	2.4	0.0	0.0	0.00	Pha.nx	**0.0**	*149*
Oesophagus	49	0	-	-	-	-	-	-	-	-	-	1.4	2.0	1.4	4.7	10.1	8.4	17.5	21.8		2.1	0.8	0.02	0.10	**0.8**	*150*
Stomach	1331	0	-	-	-	-	-	5.3	10.6	16.4	29.4	37.7	39.5	71.3	97.1	122.5	192.7	256.5	325.8	312.8	57.5	20.5	1.54	3.11	**28.1**	*151*
Small intestine	16	0	-	-	-	-	-	-	-	-	0.6	1.4	0.7	-	1.4	0.8	2.0	3.6	5.3	2.4	0.7	0.2	0.02	0.03	**0.4**	*152*
Colon	630	0	-	-	-	-	-	1.4	0.6	10.8	15.9	21.1	37.0	47.9	60.5	105.5	107.9	141.9	191.5		27.2	9.7	0.67	1.50	**12.8**	*153*
Rectum	312	0	-	-	-	-	0.8	0.8	0.7	0.6	4.2	7.2	11.3	23.1	29.4	34.6	46.7	45.5	70.1	70.3	13.5	4.8	0.39	0.80	**6.7**	*154*
Liver	603	0	0.8	-	-	-	0.8	-	0.7	-	4.2	2.2	10.6	28.4	41.7	71.5	119.7	153.4	141.9	128.5	26.1	9.3	0.45	1.40	**11.3**	*155*
Gallbladder etc.	417	0	-	-	-	-	-	-	-	3.0	1.2	6.5	9.2	16.5	28.7	51.1	58.8	74.3	122.6	160.0	18.0	6.4	0.33	0.88	**7.8**	*156*
Pancreas	313	0	-	-	-	-	-	-	1.4	0.6	1.2	2.2	5.6	11.2	16.4	31.4	48.7	85.1	94.6	104.3	13.5	4.8	0.19	0.59	**5.5**	*157*
Nose, sinuses etc.	21	0	-	-	-	0.6	-	0.7	-	0.6	-	-	0.7	2.7	0.8	2.0	7.2	1.8	7.3		0.9	0.3	0.03	0.04	**0.5**	*160*
Larynx	7	0	-	-	-	-	-	-	-	-	-	0.7	-	-	2.1	1.6	-	-	2.4		0.3	0.1	0.01	0.02	**0.2**	*161*
Bronchus, lung	502	0	-	-	-	-	-	0.8	2.1	1.8	6.6	8.7	14.8	17.8	34.2	56.6	90.3	93.5	136.6	138.2	21.7	7.7	0.43	1.17	**9.8**	*162*
†Other thoracic organs	19	0	-	-	-	-	-	-	-	-	-	1.4	0.7	2.6	2.1	3.1	1.0	2.4	3.5	-	0.8	0.3	0.03	0.06	**0.5**	*163-4*
Bone	13	0	-	0.7	1.2	0.6	0.8	-	-	0.6	0.6	-	-	1.3	0.7	0.8	-	-	-	4.8	0.6	0.2	0.03	0.04	**0.5**	*170*
Connective tissue	12	0	-	-	-	0.6	-	-	-	-	0.6	-	1.4	3.3	0.7	-	-	1.2	1.8	-	0.5	0.2	0.03	0.03	**0.3**	*171*
†Mesothelioma																										
†Kaposi's sarcoma																										
Melanoma of skin	21	0	-	-	-	-	-	-	0.6	1.2	0.7	-	1.3	-	3.1	3.0	3.6	1.8	9.7		0.9	0.3	0.02	0.05	**0.5**	*172*
Other skin	64	0	-	-	-	-	-	0.7	-	0.6	-	0.7	0.7	2.7	2.4	7.1	14.4	21.0	53.3		2.8		0.03	0.07	**1.0**	*173*
Breast	657	0	-	-	-	-	0.8	2.3	15.6	17.6	45.6	55.0	49.3	65.3	58.8	52.6	46.7	56.3	33.3	38.8	28.4	10.1	1.55	2.05	**19.1**	*174*
Uterus unspecified	59	0	-	-	-	-	-	0.8	-	-	1.2	2.2	3.5	3.3	4.1	1.6	9.1	6.0	14.0	31.5	2.5	0.9	0.08	0.13	**1.3**	*179*
Cervix uteri	263	0	-	-	0.6	0.8	3.1	8.5	14.6	11.4	13.0	16.2	16.5	23.2	14.9	24.3	38.3	31.5	21.8		11.4	4.1	0.54	0.74	**7.2**	*180*
Placenta	2	0	-	-	-	-	-	-	-	-	0.6	-	0.7	-	-	-	-	-	-	-	0.1	0.0	0.01	0.01	**0.1**	*181*
Corpus uteri	90	0	-	-	-	-	-	1.4	1.2	3.0	2.9	8.5	11.9	10.3	5.5	5.1	16.8	8.8	2.4		3.9	1.4	0.20	0.25	**2.3**	*182*
Ovary etc.	186	0	-	-	0.6	2.3	2.3	4.3	0.6	10.2	13.0	13.4	15.2	15.0	13.4	18.3	25.2	17.5	17.0		8.0	2.9	0.38	0.54	**5.2**	*183*
Other female genital	22	0	-	-	-	-	-	-	-	0.6	2.2	-	1.3	2.1	1.6	2.0	6.0	5.3	2.4		1.0	0.3	0.03	0.05	**0.5**	*184*
†Bladder	99	0	-	-	-	-	-	-	-	0.6	0.7	2.1	2.6	3.4	4.7	9.1	20.4	47.3	63.0		4.3	1.5	0.05	0.12	**1.5**	*188*
Kidney etc.	89	0	-	-	-	-	0.7	0.6	-	3.6	4.2	2.0	2.9	9.6	12.6	7.1	16.8	21.0	24.2		3.8	1.4	0.10	0.20	**1.9**	*189*
Eye	1	0	-	-	-	-	-	-	-	-	-	0.7	-	-	-	-	-	-	-		0.0	0.0	0.00	0.00	**0.0**	*190*
Brain, nervous system	64	0	4.0	2.0	-	2.5	0.8	2.3	-	1.8	-	2.2	3.5	3.3	6.2	6.3	3.0	6.0	5.3	9.7	2.8	1.0	0.14	0.19	**2.3**	*191-2*
Thyroid	103	0	-	-	-	-	0.8	1.5	1.4	2.4	4.2	6.5	4.9	4.0	8.2	8.6	15.2	9.6	17.5	21.8	4.4	1.6	0.17	0.29	**2.6**	*193*
Other endocrine	3	0	-	-	-	-	-	-	-	0.6	-	0.7	-	-	-	-	-	1.2	-		0.1	0.0	0.01	0.01	**0.1**	*194*
Hodgkin's disease	5	0	-	-	-	0.6	-	-	-	0.6	-	0.7	-	-	-	2.0	-	-	-		0.2	0.1	0.01	Hod.02	**0.2**	*201*
Non-Hodgkin lymphoma	145	0	-	0.7	0.6	-	-	2.3	-	1.2	3.6	3.6	4.9	6.6	13.0	17.3	24.3	18.0	35.0	24.2	6.3	2.2	0.18	0.39	**3.3**	*200,202*
Multiple myeloma	58	0	-	-	-	-	-	-	-	0.6	0.6	-	0.7	3.3	4.8	11.0	7.1	14.4	10.5	9.7	2.5	0.9	0.05	0.14	**1.1**	*203*
Lymphoid leukaemia	87	0	4.0	1.4	-	1.2	-	-	2.1	1.8	3.0	5.1	4.2	4.0	8.2	5.5	8.1	12.0	10.5	12.1	3.8	1.3	0.17	0.24	**2.7**	*204*
Myeloid leukaemia	70	0	-	-	0.6	2.5	-	1.5	3.5	0.6	4.2	0.7	2.1	4.0	3.4	7.9	7.1	7.2	8.8	17.0	3.0	1.1	0.12	0.19	**1.9**	*205*
Monocytic leukaemia	0	0	-	-	-	-	-	-	-	-	-	-	-	-	-	-	-	-	-	-	0.0	0.0	0.00	0.00	**0.0**	*206*
Other leukaemia	2	0	0.8	-	-	-	-	-	-	-	-	-	-	-	0.7	-	-	-	-	-	0.1	0.0	0.01	0.01	**0.1**	*207*
Leukaemia unspecified	18	0	0.8	-	-	-	-	0.8	-	1.2	-	0.7	0.7	-	-	-	2.0	4.8	8.8	2.4	0.8	0.3	0.02	0.03	**0.5**	*208*
Other and unspecified	118	0	1.6	0.7	-	-	2.3	-	-	1.2	0.6	1.4	2.8	3.3	12.3	7.9	9.1	16.8	42.0	55.8	5.1	1.8	0.13	0.22	**2.5**	*O&U*
All sites	6549	0	12.7	5.5	2.5	9.9	10.7	25.2	56.0	72.2	151.8	201.3	244.6	368.9	497.8	622.9	900.6	1138.4	1424.1	1578.3	282.9		8.30	15.91	**144.9**	*ALL*
All sites but 173	6485	0	12.7	5.5	2.5	9.9	10.7	25.2	55.3	72.2	151.2	201.3	243.9	368.3	495.0	620.6	893.5	1124.1	1403.1	1525.0	280.2	100.0	8.27	15.84	**144.0**	*ALLb*
Rate from 1 case			0.796	0.683	0.623	0.617	0.765	0.763	0.709	0.607	0.600	0.724	0.705	0.660	0.684	0.786	1.014	1.198	1.752	2.424							

†Important: see notes on population page

Japan, Yamagata Prefecture

In 1974 the Yamagata Prefectural Cancer Registry was established by the Yamagata Prefectural Government, cooperating with the Yamagata Medical Association and the Yamagata Prefectural Medical Centre for Adults. The Yamagata Prefectural Health Department is responsible for the financial support of this registry.

Yamagata prefecture is located in the northern part of Japan, between latitudes 37°43′ and 39°12′ N and longitudes 139°31′ and 140°39′ E), and is bordered to the west by the Sea of Japan. It covers an area of 9323 km². Yamagata city, the capital of Yamagata Prefecture, is situated about 290 km north of Tokyo. The annual mean temperature of Yamagata city is 11.2°C and the annual rainfall is about 1100 mm. The maximum altitude in Yamagata prefecture is 2236 m above sea level. The population of the prefecture is about 1 250 000, 99.8% of whom are Japanese. The population density is among the lowest in Japan, because the country is mountainous and cold. There are 13 cities, 27 towns and 4 villages. About 657 000 people are employed: 35.7% in industry, 15.4% in agriculture, 21.2% in commerce and 18.9% in personal services.

Hospital provision consists of some 14 000 beds in 70 hospitals. This gives an overall provision of approximately 11.4 beds per 1000 residents. The Yamagata Medical Association requests physicians and hospital doctors to report voluntarily on cancer patients newly diagnosed or treated. The central registry, which is located in the Yamagata Prefectural Medical Centre for Adults, collects cancer reports transferred from the Yamagata Medical Association and copies of all death certificates from eight health centres in the prefecture.

Collection of data on cancer cases depends upon voluntary case reports, lists of mass screening and death certificates. The rate of death-certificate-only registrations is 16.3% (1974–92) of all incident cases. Unfortunately, cancer registration from all hospitals is not yet complete in Yamagata prefecture. Members of the Yamagata Prefectural Medical Centre for Adults visit several large hospitals to search for cancer patients in the pathological and surgical lists, and the physicians then record the clinical stage, diagnostic procedures, etc. The case cards are sent to the Cancer Registration Centre through the Yamagata Medical Association. Case cards from this system constitute about 20% of all registrations. It is not difficult to follow up registered patients because only a few move out of the prefecture. Those who died outside the prefecture make up about 0.1% of incident cases.

Cancer registration is essential for evaluation of mass screening. The survival rate of gastric cancer in Yamagata prefecture is improving as a result of the increasing percentage of gastric cancer diagnosed by mass screening. The participation rate in such screening in the prefecture is about 26% among people over 40 years old. The relative ten-year survival rates of patients participating in mass screening for gastric cancer were 83% (male) and 84% (female), and in those without screening 36% and 37%. The corresponding figures for mass screening for lung cancer were 20% (male) and 38% (female), and 7% and 8% without screening. Patients with mass screening for uterine cancer had a relative ten-year survival rate of 97%, and those without screening 62%. These results show that mass screening, especially for gastric and uterine cancer, is of great medical value.

The results of cancer registration are published as annual reports, giving the standard statistics on cancer incidence and the five-year survival rates.

Yukio Sato
Toru Matsuda

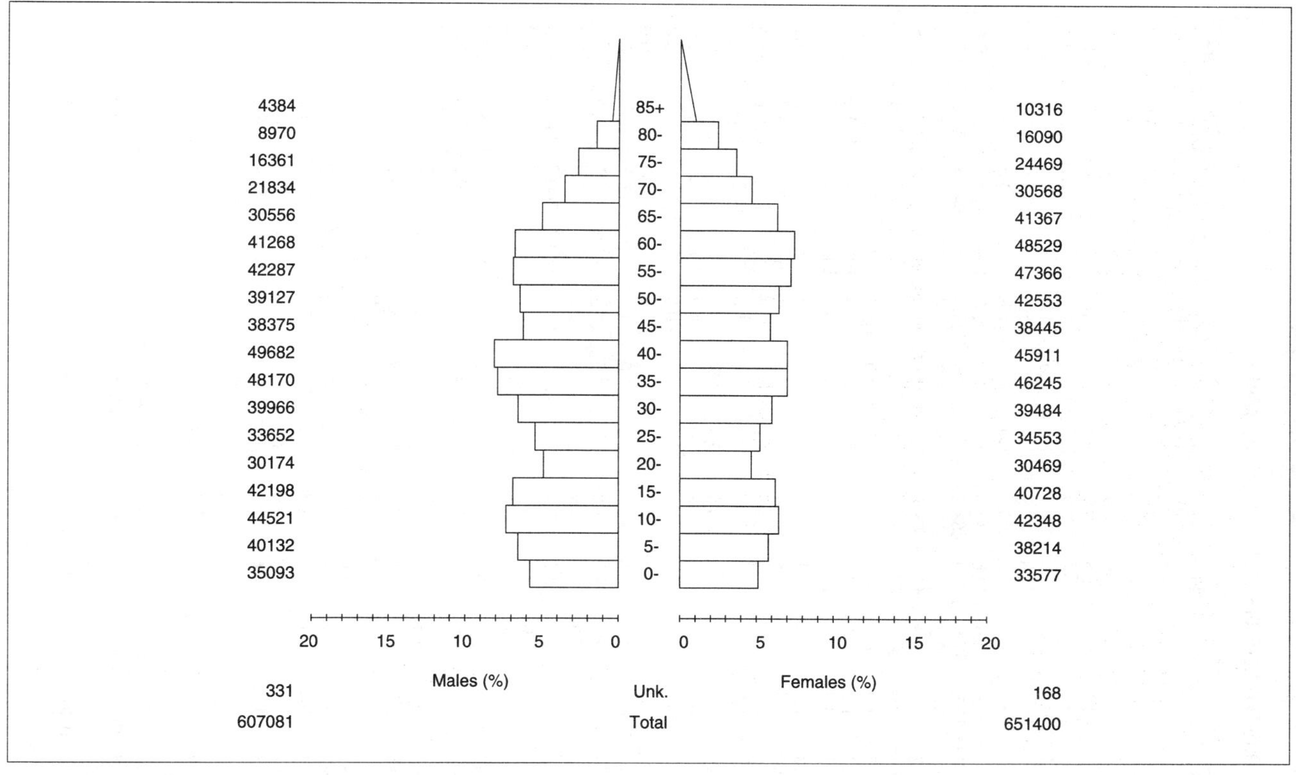

Japan, Yamagata Prefecture

Source of population: average annual 1988–92

Census: 1990 Population Census of Japan, Vol. 2, Part 2: 06 Yamagata-ken. 1985 Population Census of Japan, Statistics Bureau.

Estimate: The 1988 and 1989 population figures are postcensal estimates based on the 1985 Census, and those for 1991 and 1992 are postcensal estimates based on the 1990 Census.

Notes to tables overleaf:

† 188 does not include non-invasive tumours

Note: The high proportion of cases coded to carcinoma NOS (in the absence of histological confirmation) rendered the histological data non-comparable with those from other registries and the data on histology have not been published.

Screening programmes in the area:

The female population over age 30 has been screened for cervical cancer since 1964 (65 000 examinations annually) and for breast cancer since 1985 (46 000 examinations annually). The population over age 40 has been screened for stomach cancer since 1964 (110 000 examinations a year), lung cancer since 1984 (36 000 examinations a year) and large bowel cancer since 1989 (51 000 examinations a year).

JAPAN, YAMAGATA PREFECTURE 1988-1992

ANNUAL INCIDENCE PER 100,000 BY AGE GROUP (YEARS) - MALE

SITE	ALL AGES	AGE UNK	0-	5-	10-	15-	20-	25-	30-	35-	40-	45-	50-	55-	60-	65-	70-	75-	80-	85+	CRUDE RATE	%	CR 64	CR 74	ASR (W)	ICD (9th)
Lip	4	0	-	-	-	-	-	-	-	-	-	-	-	0.5	-	-	-	1.2	2.2	4.6	0.1	0.0	0.00	0.00	**0.1**	*140*
Tongue	24	0	-	-	-	-	-	-	-	0.4	-	1.0	1.0	-	1.5	3.3	1.8	4.9	11.1	-	0.8	0.2	0.02	0.05	**0.4**	*141*
Salivary gland	22	0	-	-	-	-	0.7	0.6	-	0.4	-	0.5	1.0	0.9	0.5	3.9	-	3.7	8.9	-	0.7	0.2	0.02	0.04	**0.5**	*142*
Mouth	41	0	-	-	-	-	-	-	-	-	0.4	0.5	1.5	0.9	5.3	2.6	6.4	2.4	15.6	13.7	1.4	0.3	0.04	0.09	**0.8**	*143-5*
Oropharynx	8	0	-	-	-	-	-	-	-	-	-	-	-	0.9	0.5	0.7	1.8	1.2	2.2	-	0.3	0.1	0.01	0.02	**0.1**	*146*
Nasopharynx	20	0	-	-	-	0.5	-	-	-	0.4	0.4	-	2.0	0.9	1.5	2.0	1.8	3.7	-	-	0.7	0.1	0.03	0.05	**0.4**	*147*
Hypopharynx	37	0	-	-	-	-	-	-	-	-	-	0.5	2.0	1.9	3.4	3.3	5.5	3.7	15.6	-	1.2	0.3	0.04	0.08	**0.7**	*148*
Pharynx unspecified	9	0	-	-	-	-	-	-	-	-	-	0.5	-	-	1.0	1.3	1.8	-	4.5	-	0.3	0.1	0.01	0.02	**0.2**	*149*
Oesophagus	596	0	-	-	-	-	-	-	-	-	1.6	3.6	22.0	37.8	62.0	71.3	81.5	106.3	69.1	82.1	19.6	4.3	0.64	1.40	**11.0**	*150*
Stomach	5071	0	1.1	-	-	0.5	0.7	4.2	11.0	34.0	56.8	87.0	177.4	268.2	415.3	523.6	723.6	825.1	947.5	853.0	167.1	36.3	5.28	11.52	**95.5**	*151*
Small intestine	23	0	-	-	-	-	0.7	0.6	-	0.8	0.4	0.5	-	1.4	1.5	3.3	0.9	3.7	2.2	4.6	0.8	0.2	0.03	0.05	**0.5**	*152*
Colon	1138	0	-	-	0.9	-	-	0.6	2.0	4.2	10.5	20.3	42.9	58.2	88.7	112.6	169.5	202.9	211.8	218.9	37.5	8.1	1.14	2.55	**21.3**	*153*
Rectum	862	0	-	-	-	-	-	1.5	5.4	9.3	20.3	27.6	47.8	68.8	81.8	129.2	132.0	182.8	141.4	28.4	6.2	0.90	1.96	**16.2**	*154*	
Liver	794	0	-	-	-	-	-	-	1.0	1.7	3.2	6.8	21.5	53.9	77.5	108.0	105.3	111.2	113.7	132.3	26.2	5.7	0.83	1.89	**14.8**	*155*
Gallbladder etc.	391	0	-	-	-	-	-	-	0.5	1.7	1.2	3.1	8.2	10.9	17.0	36.0	62.3	105.1	136.0	150.5	12.9	2.8	0.21	0.70	**6.7**	*156*
Pancreas	522	0	-	-	-	-	-	-	-	0.8	3.2	8.3	13.8	24.6	35.4	56.9	79.7	100.2	124.8	146.0	17.2	3.7	0.43	1.11	**9.5**	*157*
Nose, sinuses etc.	64	0	-	-	-	-	-	-	-	0.8	1.6	1.6	3.1	2.8	5.8	7.2	6.4	6.1	-	36.5	2.1	0.5	0.08	0.15	**1.3**	*160*
Larynx	137	0	-	-	-	-	-	-	-	0.4	0.4	2.1	4.6	11.4	12.6	16.4	21.1	18.3	13.4	13.7	4.5	1.0	0.16	0.34	**2.6**	*161*
Bronchus, lung	2022	0	-	-	-	-	-	-	1.5	4.6	6.8	20.3	32.7	81.3	154.1	231.0	345.3	425.4	490.5	456.1	66.6	14.5	1.51	4.39	**35.9**	*162*
Other thoracic organs	28	0	-	-	-	-	1.3	-	-	-	1.2	-	-	0.9	3.9	4.6	1.8	3.7	2.2	-	0.9	0.2	0.04	0.07	**0.6**	*163-4*
Bone	10	0	-	-	-	1.9	-	0.6	-	-	-	-	0.5	0.5	0.5	0.7	-	-	2.2	-	0.3	0.1	0.02	0.02	**0.3**	*170*
Connective tissue	29	0	0.6	-	-	-	0.7	-	-	0.4	0.4	1.6	1.5	1.4	1.9	1.3	1.8	6.1	-	13.7	1.0	0.2	0.04	0.06	**0.7**	*171*
Mesothelioma	1	0	-	-	-	-	-	-	-	-	-	-	-	-	-	-	0.9	-	-	-	0.0	0.0	0.00	0.00	**0.0**	*MES*
Kaposi's sarcoma	0	0	-	-	-	-	-	-	-	-	-	-	-	-	-	-	-	-	-	-	0.0	0.0	0.00	0.00	**0.0**	*KAP*
Melanoma of skin	21	0	-	-	-	-	-	-	-	-	0.8	2.1	0.5	-	1.0	2.0	1.8	4.9	6.7	-	0.7	0.2	0.02	0.04	**0.4**	*172*
Other skin	60	0	-	-	-	-	-	-	-	0.8	1.6	0.5	1.5	1.9	3.9	2.6	9.2	13.4	17.8	22.8	2.0		0.05	0.11	**1.1**	*173*
Breast	9	0	-	-	-	-	-	0.6	-	-	-	0.5	-	0.9	-	-	1.8	2.4	2.2	-	0.3	0.1	0.01	0.02	**0.2**	*175*
Prostate	496	0	-	-	-	-	-	-	-	-	0.4	0.5	1.5	7.1	17.4	36.7	85.2	180.9	200.7	241.8	16.3	3.5	0.13	0.74	**7.9**	*185*
Testis	40	0	0.6	-	-	0.9	1.3	5.3	4.0	2.1	1.6	1.6	1.0	0.5	-	-	2.4	2.2	-	1.3	0.3	0.09	0.09	**1.3**	*186*
Penis, other male genital	13	0	-	-	-	-	-	-	-	-	0.5	-	0.5	0.5	0.7	2.7	3.7	2.2	9.1	0.4	0.1	0.01	0.02	**0.2**	*187*
†Bladder	416	0	-	-	-	-	-	-	2.0	0.8	1.6	1.0	8.2	22.2	29.6	38.0	59.5	85.6	118.2	155.1	13.7	3.0	0.33	0.81	**7.4**	*188*
Kidney etc.	248	0	-	-	-	-	1.3	-	-	2.1	2.4	3.6	10.2	11.4	17.9	28.1	43.1	41.6	40.1	22.8	8.2	1.8	0.24	0.60	**4.7**	*189*
Eye	0	0	-	-	-	-	-	-	-	-	-	-	-	-	-	-	-	-	-	-	0.0	0.0	0.00	0.00	**0.0**	*190*
Brain, nervous system	70	0	1.7	1.5	0.9	0.5	-	-	1.5	2.1	0.8	3.1	4.6	3.8	5.3	3.3	3.7	6.1	6.7	-	2.3	0.5	0.13	0.16	**1.8**	*191-2*
Thyroid	46	0	-	-	-	-	0.7	-	0.5	0.8	2.8	1.0	2.6	0.9	4.4	5.9	3.7	1.2	4.5	4.6	1.5	0.3	0.07	0.12	**1.0**	*193*
Other endocrine	8	0	-	-	-	0.5	-	0.6	-	-	-	-	1.0	0.5	1.0	-	0.9	-	-	-	0.3	0.1	0.02	0.02	**0.2**	*194*
Hodgkin's disease	5	0	-	0.5	-	-	-	-	-	-	-	-	1.0	-	-	0.7	0.9	-	-	-	0.2	0.0	0.01	0.02	**0.1**	*201*
Non-Hodgkin lymphoma	237	0	0.6	1.0	0.4	1.4	0.7	1.8	2.5	3.3	2.0	5.2	6.6	8.5	14.5	25.5	33.0	36.7	55.7	31.9	7.8	1.7	0.24	0.54	**4.8**	*200,202*
Multiple myeloma	101	0	-	-	-	-	-	-	-	0.4	0.4	2.1	1.0	4.3	4.4	13.1	17.4	14.7	26.8	54.7	3.3	0.7	0.06	0.22	**1.9**	*203*
Lymphoid leukaemia	39	0	2.3	1.5	1.8	0.9	0.7	1.2	0.5	0.4	0.4	1.0	2.0	0.9	2.4	1.3	0.9	2.4	2.2	4.6	1.3	0.3	0.08	0.09	**1.3**	*204*
Myeloid leukaemia	111	0	-	0.5	1.3	0.5	1.3	-	2.0	3.3	1.2	2.1	3.6	7.6	5.8	5.9	16.5	17.1	11.1	18.2	3.7	0.8	0.15	0.26	**2.4**	*205*
Monocytic leukaemia	6	0	-	-	-	-	-	-	-	-	-	0.4	-	-	0.5	0.7	1.8	1.2	-	-	0.2	0.0	0.00	0.02	**0.1**	*206*
Other leukaemia	6	0	-	-	-	-	-	-	-	-	-	-	-	0.9	1.5	-	-	1.2	-	-	0.2	0.0	0.01	0.01	**0.1**	*207*
Leukaemia unspecified	26	0	-	-	-	-	-	-	-	0.8	0.8	-	2.4	2.9	2.0	3.7	3.7	-	4.6	0.9	0.2	0.03	0.06	**0.5**	*208*
Other and unspecified	224	0	0.6	-	-	-	-	0.6	1.0	1.7	0.8	1.6	7.2	5.2	11.1	17.7	38.5	51.3	75.8	82.1	7.4	1.6	0.15	0.43	**4.0**	*O&U*
All sites	14035	0	7.4	5.0	5.4	7.6	9.9	16.6	31.5	74.7	115.5	205.3	416.1	686.7	1082.7	1455.7	2072.9	2537.7	2929.5	2919.3	462.4		13.32	30.97	**261.6**	*ALL*
All sites but 173	13975	0	7.4	5.0	5.4	7.6	9.9	16.6	31.5	73.9	113.9	204.8	414.5	684.8	1078.8	1453.0	2063.7	2524.2	2911.7	2896.5	460.4	100.0	13.27	30.86	**260.6**	*ALLb*

| Rate from 1 case | | | 0.570 | 0.498 | 0.449 | 0.474 | 0.663 | 0.594 | 0.500 | 0.415 | 0.403 | 0.521 | 0.511 | 0.473 | 0.485 | 0.655 | 0.916 | 1.222 | 2.229 | 4.561 |

†Important: see notes on population page

JAPAN, YAMAGATA PREFECTURE 1988-1992

ANNUAL INCIDENCE PER 100,000 BY AGE GROUP (YEARS) - FEMALE

SITE	ALL AGES	AGE UNK	0-	5-	10-	15-	20-	25-	30-	35-	40-	45-	50-	55-	60-	65-	70-	75-	80-	85+	CRUDE RATE	%	CR 64	CR 74	ASR (W)	ICD (9th)
Lip	5	0	-	-	-	-	-	-	-	-	-	-	0.5	-	-	-	2.0	-	1.2	-	0.2	0.0	0.00	0.01	**0.1**	*140*
Tongue	24	0	-	-	-	-	-	-	0.5	0.4	0.4	0.5	0.9	1.3	0.4	1.0	1.3	2.5	5.0	5.8	0.7	0.2	0.02	0.03	**0.4**	*141*
Salivary gland	17	0	-	-	-	-	-	-	-	-	-	-	-	0.8	1.2	1.5	2.0	0.8	5.0	1.9	0.5	0.2	0.01	0.03	**0.2**	*142*
Mouth	22	0	-	-	-	-	-	-	-	-	0.4	-	0.5	0.4	0.4	1.0	3.3	2.5	6.2	5.8	0.7	0.2	0.01	0.03	**0.3**	*143-5*
Oropharynx	5	0	-	-	-	-	-	-	-	-	-	-	-	-	-	-	1.6	2.5	1.9	-	0.2	0.0	0.00	0.00	**0.0**	*146*
Nasopharynx	5	0	-	-	-	-	-	-	-	-	-	1.0	0.5	-	-	0.5	-	-	1.2	-	0.2	0.0	0.01	0.01	**0.1**	*147*
Hypopharynx	7	0	-	-	-	-	-	-	-	0.4	-	-	0.5	-	0.4	1.0	0.7	-	1.2	-	0.2	0.1	0.01	0.01	**0.1**	*148*
Pharynx unspecified	5	0	-	-	-	-	-	-	-	-	-	-	-	0.4	-	0.5	0.7	-	-	3.9	0.2	0.0	0.00	0.01	**0.1**	*149*
Oesophagus	133	0	-	-	-	-	-	-	-	0.9	0.4	1.6	1.4	2.1	4.5	11.6	9.8	20.4	27.3	42.7	4.1	1.3	0.05	0.16	**1.6**	*150*
Stomach	2813	0	-	-	-	0.5	2.6	4.1	11.7	25.5	39.2	44.7	68.2	92.5	143.8	202.1	285.9	385.0	390.3	368.4	86.4	28.0	2.16	4.60	**40.1**	*151*
Small intestine	14	0	-	-	-	-	-	-	-	-	-	-	0.9	0.4	0.4	-	2.6	2.5	2.5	1.9	0.4	0.1	0.01	0.02	**0.2**	*152*
Colon	1171	0	-	-	-	0.5	0.7	1.2	2.0	6.1	9.1	20.8	28.7	41.4	57.3	79.8	125.6	147.9	205.1	168.7	36.0	11.6	0.84	1.87	**16.1**	*153*
Rectum	620	0	-	-	0.5	-	-	-	1.5	5.2	10.5	15.1	16.0	29.1	35.9	43.5	64.1	60.5	77.1	71.7	19.0	6.2	0.57	1.11	**9.3**	*154*
Liver	384	0	0.6	-	-	-	-	-	-	2.2	0.9	2.6	3.8	7.2	22.3	35.8	47.8	45.8	59.7	79.5	11.8	3.8	0.20	0.61	**5.0**	*155*
Gallbladder etc.	587	0	-	-	-	-	-	-	-	0.9	1.7	5.2	6.1	12.2	21.8	37.7	58.9	92.4	129.3	176.4	18.0	5.8	0.24	0.72	**6.9**	*156*
Pancreas	382	0	-	-	-	-	-	-	-	1.3	1.3	1.6	5.6	8.0	16.5	31.9	45.8	60.5	79.6	54.3	11.7	3.8	0.17	0.56	**4.7**	*157*
Nose, sinuses etc.	18	0	-	-	-	-	-	-	-	-	-	-	-	0.8	0.4	1.9	2.6	2.5	3.7	1.9	0.6	0.2	0.01	0.03	**0.2**	*160*
Larynx	4	0	-	-	-	-	-	-	-	-	-	-	0.5	-	-	0.5	0.7	0.8	-	-	0.1	0.0	0.00	0.01	**0.1**	*161*
Bronchus, lung	649	0	-	-	-	-	-	1.7	1.0	0.9	5.7	4.7	13.6	14.8	30.5	41.1	73.9	106.3	103.2	137.7	19.9	6.5	0.36	0.94	**8.3**	*162*
Other thoracic organs	6	0	-	-	-	-	-	-	-	-	-	-	-	0.4	1.2	-	-	-	2.5	-	0.2	0.1	0.01	0.01	**0.1**	*163-4*
Bone	17	0	-	0.5	0.5	1.0	-	0.6	-	-	1.7	-	0.5	-	0.8	1.0	0.7	0.8	1.2	-	0.5	0.2	0.03	0.04	**0.4**	*170*
Connective tissue	22	0	-	-	-	0.5	0.7	0.6	-	-	0.4	0.5	1.4	1.7	-	-	1.3	-	5.0	7.8	0.7	0.2	0.03	0.04	**0.4**	*171*
Mesothelioma	2	0	-	-	-	-	-	-	-	-	0.4	-	-	-	-	0.5	-	-	-	-	0.1	0.0	0.00	0.00	**0.0**	*MES*
Kaposi's sarcoma	0	0	-	-	-	-	-	-	-	-	-	-	-	-	-	-	-	-	-	-	0.0	0.0	0.00	0.00	**0.0**	*KAP*
Melanoma of skin	22	0	-	-	-	-	-	-	-	0.9	-	-	0.5	-	2.1	1.5	-	2.5	7.5	3.9	0.7	0.2	0.02	0.02	**0.3**	*172*
Other skin	82	0	-	-	-	0.5	-	-	-	-	-	2.6	2.4	2.1	2.1	3.9	3.3	18.0	13.7	29.1	2.5		0.05	0.08	**1.1**	*173*
Breast	1111	0	-	-	-	-	-	4.1	11.7	42.0	66.2	74.4	53.6	53.2	58.9	51.2	58.9	40.9	48.5	40.7	34.1	11.1	1.82	2.37	**22.7**	*174*
Uterus unspecified	45	0	-	-	-	-	-	-	-	-	1.0	0.9	0.8	1.6	2.9	3.3	4.9	11.2	17.4	-	1.4	0.4	0.02	0.05	**0.6**	*179*
Cervix uteri	292	0	-	-	-	-	-	2.9	3.0	13.4	12.6	12.0	12.2	12.2	11.1	16.0	18.3	25.3	18.6	17.4	9.0	2.9	0.40	0.57	**5.5**	*180*
Placenta	3	0	-	-	-	-	-	-	0.5	-	-	0.5	-	0.4	-	-	-	-	-	-	0.1	0.0	0.01	0.01	**0.1**	*181*
Corpus uteri	168	0	-	-	-	-	-	0.6	1.0	1.3	3.5	6.2	17.4	11.4	12.4	10.2	8.5	7.4	3.7	3.9	5.2	1.7	0.27	0.36	**3.2**	*182*
Ovary etc.	256	0	-	-	0.5	1.0	1.3	2.9	2.0	4.3	9.1	12.0	12.2	11.8	14.0	13.1	19.0	14.7	18.6	21.3	7.9	2.5	0.36	0.52	**4.9**	*183*
Other female genital	19	0	-	-	-	-	-	-	-	-	1.3	-	-	2.5	0.5	0.7	4.9	1.2	1.2	1.9	0.6	0.2	0.02	0.02	**0.3**	*184*
†Bladder	143	0	-	-	-	-	0.7	-	-	-	0.9	1.6	0.9	3.0	3.7	6.3	19.0	23.7	29.8	46.5	4.4	1.4	0.05	0.18	**1.7**	*188*
Kidney etc.	134	0	-	-	-	-	-	-	0.5	-	1.7	1.0	3.8	5.1	7.4	8.7	9.2	14.7	28.6	31.0	4.1	1.3	0.10	0.19	**1.8**	*189*
Eye	1	0	-	-	-	-	-	-	-	-	-	-	-	-	-	-	-	1.2	-	-	0.0	0.0	0.00	0.00	**0.0**	*190*
Brain, nervous system	75	0	2.4	0.5	1.9	-	0.7	-	2.0	0.9	1.7	1.0	2.4	3.4	4.5	6.3	5.9	4.9	-	1.9	2.3	0.7	0.11	0.17	**1.7**	*191-2*
Thyroid	269	0	-	-	-	1.5	2.6	2.9	4.1	10.8	14.8	12.5	13.6	11.8	15.2	12.1	11.8	9.0	11.2	17.4	8.3	2.7	0.45	0.57	**5.7**	*193*
Other endocrine	7	0	1.2	0.5	-	-	-	-	-	-	-	-	-	-	0.4	0.5	-	-	1.2	-	0.2	0.1	0.01	0.02	**0.2**	*194*
Hodgkin's disease	2	0	-	-	-	-	-	-	0.4	-	-	-	-	0.4	-	-	-	-	-	-	0.1	0.0	0.00	0.00	**0.1**	*201*
Non-Hodgkin lymphoma	155	0	1.8	0.5	0.9	1.0	-	0.6	1.0	1.7	2.6	3.6	4.2	3.0	8.2	9.2	11.1	20.4	24.9	19.4	4.8	1.5	0.15	0.25	**2.6**	*200,202*
Multiple myeloma	81	0	-	-	-	-	-	-	-	-	-	-	-	0.9	1.7	3.3	7.3	6.5	15.5	23.6	2.5	0.8	0.03	0.10	**0.9**	*203*
Lymphoid leukaemia	38	0	3.0	-	0.5	-	1.3	0.6	0.5	0.9	0.9	1.6	-	2.1	0.8	1.9	1.3	5.7	-	1.9	1.2	0.4	0.06	0.08	**1.0**	*204*
Myeloid leukaemia	78	0	0.6	0.5	1.4	1.5	-	0.6	0.5	3.0	2.2	2.6	1.9	2.5	3.3	3.4	7.2	7.4	5.0	3.9	2.4	0.8	0.10	0.16	**1.6**	*205*
Monocytic leukaemia	8	0	-	-	-	-	-	-	0.5	0.4	0.4	-	-	0.4	-	1.0	0.7	-	-	1.9	0.2	0.1	0.01	0.02	**0.2**	*206*
Other leukaemia	5	0	-	-	-	-	-	-	-	-	-	-	0.5	0.4	-	0.5	-	-	2.5	-	0.2	0.0	0.00	0.01	**0.1**	*207*
Leukaemia unspecified	23	0	-	-	-	-	0.7	1.2	-	-	-	0.4	0.5	2.4	0.8	0.4	0.5	2.6	3.3	1.2	0.7	0.2	0.03	0.05	**0.5**	*208*
Other and unspecified	206	0	-	-	-	-	0.7	0.6	0.5	0.9	0.9	1.0	5.6	4.6	5.8	15.5	15.0	29.4	48.5	58.2	6.3	2.0	0.10	0.26	**2.6**	*O&U*
All sites	10135	0	9.5	2.6	6.1	7.9	11.8	24.9	44.6	124.6	191.7	232.5	284.8	345.0	496.2	664.8	931.7	1185.2	1409.5	1456.0	311.2		8.91	16.89	**153.8**	*ALL*
All sites but 173	10053	0	9.5	2.6	6.1	7.4	11.8	24.9	44.6	124.6	191.7	229.9	282.5	342.9	494.1	660.9	928.4	1167.2	1395.9	1426.9	308.7	100.0	8.86	16.81	**152.8**	*ALLb*
Rate from 1 case			0.596	0.523	0.472	0.491	0.656	0.579	0.507	0.432	0.436	0.520	0.470	0.422	0.412	0.483	0.654	0.817	1.243	1.939						

†Important: see notes on population page

Korea, Kangwha County

The Kangwha County Cancer Registry was started in 1983 when nationwide medical insurance was implemented in the area. Teaching faculty and house staff of the Department of Preventive Medicine and Public Health at the College of Medicine of Yonsei University were involved in launching the cancer registry in the county, where a health research programme had started in 1975. The registry is the only community-based cancer registry in Korea.

Kangwha county—a rural area, actually an island connected by a bridge to the mainland—is about 50 km from Seoul, the capital of Korea. Nearly half of the employed population are farmers. There are a limited number of small factories that may pollute the environment. Air pollution is minimal and water is less polluted than in Seoul. Consumption of petroleum products is low due to the small number and size of factories and the limited number of cars.

Among the population of Kangwha county, some 56% have no religion, 23% are Christians and 15% Buddhists. All are ethnically Korean and nearly all were born in Korea.

About 40% of cancer patients in the county are treated in the Kangwha hospital which is the only hospital in the area; the remainder make use of more than 50 hospitals in the Seoul metropolitan area.

A registered nurse takes care of data collection under the supervision of the director of the registry. Data were stored on magnetic tape at the beginning of the registry but were subsequently transferred to a personal computer.

Cancer registration is not popular in Korea. Many medium-sized hospitals are not willing to show their medical records and in many cases their medical records are incomplete, missing pathological reports, or even unable to be found.

A major difficulty is the low proportion of known cause of mortality. Korean people, particularly the elderly in rural areas, wish to die in their homes rather than in hospital. It is not against the law to bury the dead without a medical doctor's death certificate. A document prepared by ten neighbours gives the right to bury the dead. For this reason the proportion of known cause of mortality is very low in Korea. Although the National Statistical Office is expected to provide the number of cancer deaths in Kangwha, the mortality/incidence ratio is liable to be as low as 20–30%.

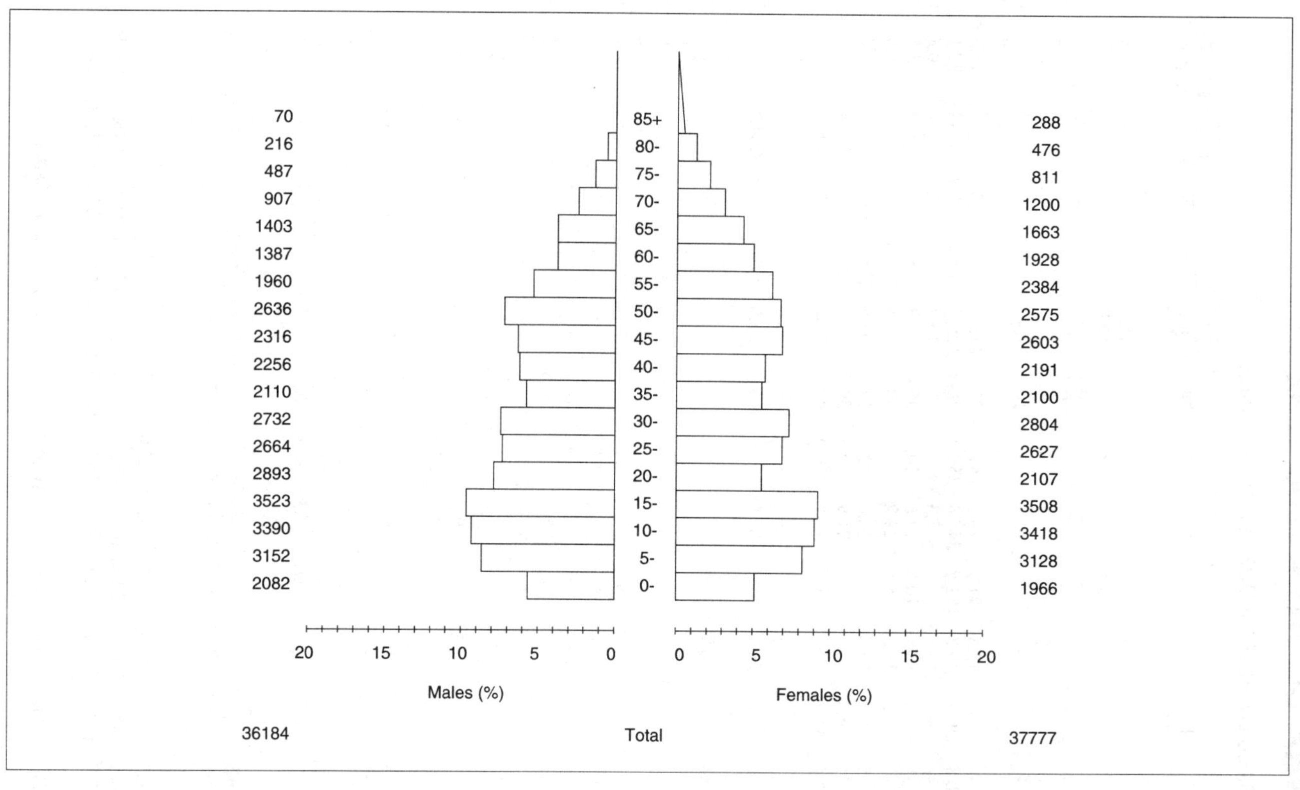

Korea, Kangwha County

Source of population: average annual 1988–90 and 1992 (+1993)

Census: 1990. National Census Data. R.O.K. De facto population, 1990.

Estimate: The estimated populations for 1988, 1989 and 1992 were obtained from the Statistics Year Books, Kangwha County, Citizenship register data published in 1989, 1990 and 1993.

Notes to tables overleaf:

* The rates are based on small numbers, and suggest some under-ascertainment in childhood and the oldest age-groups.

† 188 does not include non-invasive tumours

Note: 9 male cases and 13 female cases of unknown primary site were erroneously omitted from these data.

* KOREA, KANGWHA COUNTY 1986-1992

ANNUAL INCIDENCE PER 100,000 BY AGE GROUP (YEARS) - MALE

SITE	ALL AGES	AGE UNK	0-	5-	10-	15-	20-	25-	30-	35-	40-	45-	50-	55-	60-	65-	70-	75-	80-	85+	CRUDE RATE	%	CR 64	CR 74	ASR (W)	ICD (9th)
Lip	0	0	-	-	-	-	-	-	-	-	-	-	-	-	-	-	-	-	-	-	0.0	0.0	0.00	0.00	0.0	140
Tongue	2	0	-	-	-	-	-	-	-	-	-	6.2	-	-	-	-	15.8	-	-	-	0.8	0.3	0.03	0.11	0.7	141
Salivary gland	5	0	-	-	-	-	-	-	-	-	-	-	10.8	7.3	10.3	-	15.8	-	-	-	2.0	0.8	0.14	0.22	1.6	142
Mouth	2	0	-	-	-	-	-	-	-	-	-	-	-	-	-	20.4	-	-	-	-	0.8	0.3	0.00	0.10	0.6	143-5
Oropharynx	3	0	-	-	-	-	-	5.4	-	-	-	-	-	-	-	20.4	-	-	-	-	1.2	0.5	0.03	0.13	1.0	146
Nasopharynx	2	0	-	-	-	-	-	-	-	-	-	6.2	-	7.3	-	-	-	-	-	-	0.8	0.3	0.07	0.07	0.7	147
Hypopharynx	1	0	-	-	-	-	-	-	-	-	-	-	-	-	10.2	-	-	-	-	-	0.4	0.2	0.00	0.05	0.3	148
Pharynx unspecified	0	0	-	-	-	-	-	-	-	-	-	-	-	-	-	-	-	-	-	-	0.0	0.0	0.00	0.00	0.0	149
Oesophagus	32	0	-	-	-	-	-	-	-	-	-	12.3	21.7	29.2	41.2	71.3	110.3	88.0	66.1	-	12.6	5.4	0.52	1.43	10.2	150
Stomach	203	0	-	-	-	-	4.9	10.7	10.5	6.8	50.7	49.3	151.7	247.8	350.2	336.0	425.3	586.7	330.7	-	80.1	33.9	4.41	8.22	65.9	151
Small intestine	2	0	-	-	-	-	-	-	-	-	-	-	-	7.3	-	-	15.8	-	-	-	0.8	0.3	0.04	0.12	0.6	152
Colon	14	0	-	-	-	-	-	-	-	-	6.3	-	10.8	14.6	20.6	20.4	47.3	58.7	-	-	5.5	2.3	0.26	0.60	4.5	153
Rectum	25	0	-	-	-	-	-	-	-	-	6.3	18.5	5.4	29.2	51.5	50.9	31.5	117.3	-	-	9.9	4.2	0.55	0.97	8.3	154
Liver	85	0	-	-	-	-	-	10.7	5.2	13.5	25.3	55.5	75.9	116.6	92.7	112.0	94.5	176.0	330.7	-	33.6	14.2	1.98	3.01	27.7	155
Gallbladder etc.	13	0	-	-	-	-	-	-	-	-	6.3	-	10.8	21.9	10.3	30.5	-	29.3	66.1	204.1	5.1	2.2	0.25	0.40	4.8	156
Pancreas	20	0	-	-	-	-	-	-	-	6.8	12.7	-	21.7	14.6	20.6	40.7	47.3	-	66.1	204.1	7.9	3.3	0.38	0.82	7.2	157
Nose, sinuses etc.	0	0	-	-	-	-	-	-	-	-	-	-	-	-	-	-	-	-	-	-	0.0	0.0	0.00	0.00	0.0	160
Larynx	4	0	-	-	-	-	-	-	-	-	-	6.2	-	7.3	10.3	10.2	-	-	-	-	1.6	0.7	0.12	0.17	1.4	161
Bronchus, lung	104	0	-	-	-	-	-	-	-	13.5	19.0	24.7	81.3	87.5	123.6	285.1	252.0	293.3	66.1	204.1	41.1	17.4	1.75	4.43	33.8	162
Other thoracic organs	0	0	-	-	-	-	-	-	-	-	-	-	-	-	-	-	-	-	-	-	0.0	0.0	0.00	0.00	0.0	163-4
Bone	7	0	-	-	4.2	4.1	4.9	5.4	-	6.8	-	6.2	-	-	-	-	15.8	-	-	-	2.8	1.2	0.16	0.24	2.7	170
Connective tissue	0	0	-	-	-	-	-	-	-	-	-	-	-	-	-	-	-	-	-	-	0.0	0.0	0.00	0.00	0.0	171
Mesothelioma	0	0	-	-	-	-	-	-	-	-	-	-	-	-	-	-	-	-	-	-	0.0	0.0	0.00	0.00	0.0	MES
Kaposi's sarcoma	1	0	-	-	-	-	-	-	-	-	6.3	-	-	-	-	-	-	-	-	-	0.4	0.2	0.03	0.03	0.4	KAP
Melanoma of skin	1	0	-	-	-	-	-	-	-	-	-	-	5.4	-	-	-	-	-	-	-	0.4	0.2	0.03	0.03	0.3	172
Other skin	7	0	-	-	-	-	-	-	-	13.5	6.3	-	5.4	-	10.3	-	-	58.7	-	-	2.8		0.18	0.18	2.5	173
Breast	1	0	-	-	-	-	-	-	-	-	-	-	-	-	-	10.2	-	-	-	-	0.4	0.2	0.00	0.05	0.3	175
Prostate	3	0	-	-	-	-	-	-	-	-	-	-	-	7.3	-	20.4	-	-	-	-	1.2	0.5	0.04	0.14	0.9	185
Testis	1	0	-	-	-	-	-	-	5.2	-	-	-	-	-	-	-	-	-	-	-	0.4	0.2	0.03	0.03	0.3	186
Penis	2	0	-	-	-	-	-	-	-	-	-	-	-	-	-	10.2	-	29.3	-	-	0.8	0.3	0.00	0.05	0.6	187.1-.4
Other male genital	0	0	-	-	-	-	-	-	-	-	-	-	-	-	-	-	-	-	-	-	0.0	0.0	0.00	0.00	0.0	187.5-.9
†Bladder	10	0	-	-	-	-	-	-	-	-	-	6.2	-	29.2	-	20.4	31.5	-	66.1	-	3.9	1.7	0.18	0.44	3.1	188
Kidney etc.	5	0	-	-	-	4.1	-	-	5.2	-	-	-	-	7.3	20.6	-	-	-	-	-	2.0	0.8	0.19	0.19	1.8	189
Eye	0	0	-	-	-	-	-	-	-	-	-	-	-	-	-	-	-	-	-	-	0.0	0.0	0.00	0.00	0.0	190
Brain, nervous system	9	0	-	-	-	4.1	-	5.4	5.2	6.8	-	6.2	-	14.6	-	-	15.8	-	-	204.1	3.6	1.5	0.21	0.29	3.8	191-2
Thyroid	2	0	-	-	-	-	-	-	10.5	-	-	-	-	-	-	-	-	-	-	-	0.8	0.3	0.05	0.05	0.6	193
Other endocrine	0	0	-	-	-	-	-	-	-	-	-	-	-	-	-	-	-	-	-	-	0.0	0.0	0.00	0.00	0.0	194
Hodgkin's disease	1	0	-	-	-	-	4.9	-	-	-	-	-	-	-	-	-	-	-	-	-	0.4	0.2	0.02	0.02	0.4	201
Non-Hodgkin lymphoma	9	0	-	-	-	-	-	-	5.2	-	6.3	-	10.8	7.3	10.3	20.4	15.8	-	-	-	3.6	1.5	0.20	0.38	2.9	200,202
Multiple myeloma	2	0	-	-	-	-	-	-	-	-	-	-	-	7.3	-	-	15.8	-	-	-	0.8	0.3	0.04	0.12	0.6	203
Lymphoid leukaemia	4	0	13.7	-	-	4.1	-	5.4	-	-	-	-	-	-	-	-	-	-	-	-	1.6	0.7	0.12	0.12	2.4	204
Myeloid leukaemia	7	0	-	-	4.2	4.1	-	10.7	-	6.8	-	-	5.4	7.3	-	-	-	-	-	-	2.8	1.2	0.19	0.19	2.6	205
Monocytic leukaemia	0	0	-	-	-	-	-	-	-	-	-	-	-	-	-	-	-	-	-	-	0.0	0.0	0.00	0.00	0.0	206
Other leukaemia	1	0	-	-	-	4.1	-	-	-	-	-	-	-	-	-	-	-	-	-	-	0.4	0.2	0.02	0.02	0.4	207
Leukaemia unspecified	3	0	13.7	-	4.2	-	-	-	-	-	-	-	-	-	-	-	-	-	-	-	1.2	0.5	0.09	0.09	2.0	208
Other and unspecified	12	0	-	-	-	-	-	-	-	6.8	-	12.3	5.4	14.6	20.6	10.2	-	58.7	66.1	-	4.7	2.0	0.30	0.35	4.0	O&U
All sites	605	0	27.4	-	12.6	24.3	14.8	53.6	47.1	81.2	145.6	209.7	422.7	685.1	793.1	1099.7	1149.8	1496.0	1058.2	816.3	238.9		12.59	23.83	201.7	ALL
All sites but 173	598	0	27.4	-	12.6	24.3	14.8	53.6	47.1	67.7	139.3	209.7	417.3	685.1	782.8	1099.7	1149.8	1437.4	1058.2	816.3	236.1	100.0	12.41	23.66	199.2	ALLb

Rate from 1 case   6.862   4.532   4.214   4.055   4.938   5.363   5.229   6.770   6.332   6.168   5.419   7.289   10.300   10.182   15.751   29.334   66.138   204.082

†Important: see notes on population page

* KOREA, KANGWHA COUNTY 1986-1992

ANNUAL INCIDENCE PER 100,000 BY AGE GROUP (YEARS) - FEMALE

SITE	ALL AGES	AGE UNK	0-	5-	10-	15-	20-	25-	30-	35-	40-	45-	50-	55-	60-	65-	70-	75-	80-	85+	CRUDE RATE	%	CR 64	CR 74	ASR (W)	ICD (9th)
Lip	1	0	-	-	-	-	-	-	-	-	-	-	-	-	-	-	-	17.6	-	-	0.4	0.3	0.00	0.00	**0.2**	140
Tongue	1	0	-	-	-	-	-	-	-	-	-	-	-	-	-	8.6	-	-	-	-	0.4	0.3	0.00	0.04	**0.3**	141
Salivary gland	0	0	-	-	-	-	-	-	-	-	-	-	-	-	-	-	-	-	-	-	0.0	0.0	0.00	0.00	**0.0**	142
Mouth	3	0	-	-	-	-	-	-	5.1	-	-	-	-	-	-	-	11.9	17.6	-	-	1.1	0.8	0.03	0.08	**0.7**	143-5
Oropharynx	0	0	-	-	-	-	-	-	-	-	-	-	-	-	-	-	-	-	-	-	0.0	0.0	0.00	0.00	**0.0**	146
Nasopharynx	1	0	-	-	-	-	-	-	-	-	-	-	-	-	7.4	-	-	-	-	-	0.4	0.3	0.04	0.00	**0.3**	147
Hypopharynx	0	0	-	-	-	-	-	-	-	-	-	-	-	-	-	-	-	-	-	-	0.0	0.0	0.00	0.00	**0.0**	148
Pharynx unspecified	1	0	-	-	-	-	-	-	-	-	-	-	-	6.0	-	-	-	-	-	-	0.4	0.3	0.03	0.03	**0.2**	149
Oesophagus	2	0	-	-	-	-	-	-	-	-	-	-	-	-	-	8.6	-	-	-	49.6	0.8	0.5	0.00	0.04	**0.5**	150
Stomach	91	0	-	-	-	4.1	13.6	16.3	5.1	27.2	13.0	27.4	44.4	65.9	96.3	128.9	154.8	193.8	60.0	-	34.4	23.6	1.57	2.98	**25.0**	151
Small intestine	3	0	-	-	-	-	-	-	-	-	-	5.5	-	-	14.8	-	-	-	-	-	1.1	0.8	0.10	0.10	**0.9**	152
Colon	7	0	-	-	-	-	-	-	-	6.8	13.0	-	5.5	-	14.8	-	11.9	-	-	-	2.6	1.8	0.20	0.26	**2.3**	153
Rectum	20	0	-	-	-	-	-	-	10.2	6.8	-	16.5	5.5	6.0	22.2	34.4	11.9	35.2	60.0	-	7.6	5.2	0.34	0.57	**5.3**	154
Liver	29	0	-	-	-	-	-	-	5.1	6.8	-	16.5	33.3	18.0	29.6	25.8	47.6	70.5	-	-	11.0	7.5	0.55	0.91	**7.7**	155
Gallbladder etc.	16	0	-	-	-	-	-	-	-	-	-	-	5.5	18.0	14.8	34.4	11.9	70.5	-	49.6	6.1	4.2	0.19	0.42	**3.8**	156
Pancreas	11	0	-	-	-	-	-	-	-	-	-	-	-	18.0	-	34.4	47.6	-	-	-	4.2	2.9	0.09	0.50	**2.7**	157
Nose, sinuses etc.	1	0	-	-	-	-	-	-	-	-	-	-	5.5	-	-	-	-	-	-	-	0.4	0.3	0.03	0.03	**0.3**	160
Larynx	1	0	-	-	-	-	-	-	-	-	-	-	-	-	-	8.6	-	-	-	-	0.4	0.3	0.00	0.04	**0.3**	161
Bronchus, lung	32	0	-	-	-	-	-	-	-	-	26.1	-	11.1	30.0	29.6	60.1	59.5	35.2	60.0	49.6	12.1	8.3	0.48	1.08	**8.4**	162
Other thoracic organs	3	0	-	-	-	-	-	-	-	-	-	5.5	-	-	17.2	-	-	-	-	-	1.1	0.8	0.03	0.11	**0.8**	163-4
Bone	2	0	-	-	-	4.1	-	-	-	6.8	-	-	-	-	-	-	-	-	-	-	0.8	0.5	0.05	0.05	**0.8**	170
Connective tissue	0	0	-	-	-	-	-	-	-	-	-	-	-	-	-	-	-	-	-	-	0.0	0.0	0.00	0.00	**0.0**	171
Mesothelioma	0	0	-	-	-	-	-	-	-	-	-	-	-	-	-	-	-	-	-	-	0.0	0.0	0.00	0.00	**0.0**	MES
Kaposi's sarcoma	0	0	-	-	-	-	-	-	-	-	-	-	-	-	-	-	-	-	-	-	0.0	0.0	0.00	0.00	**0.0**	KAP
Melanoma of skin	1	0	-	-	-	-	-	-	-	-	-	-	-	-	-	-	-	17.6	-	-	0.4	0.3	0.00	0.00	**0.2**	172
Other skin	2	0	-	-	-	-	-	-	-	-	-	-	-	6.0	7.4	-	-	-	-	-	0.8		0.07	0.07	**0.5**	173
Breast	23	0	-	-	-	-	-	-	-	-	52.2	5.5	16.6	36.0	22.2	8.6	11.9	-	-	-	8.7	6.0	0.66	0.76	**7.1**	174
Uterus unspecified	1	0	-	-	-	-	-	-	-	-	-	-	-	-	7.4	-	-	-	-	-	0.4	0.3	0.04	0.04	**0.3**	179
Cervix uteri	71	0	-	-	-	-	16.3	20.4	47.6	58.7	22.0	61.0	71.9	96.3	34.4	11.9	17.6	30.0	49.6	26.8	18.4	1.97	2.20	**21.8**	180
Placenta	0	0	-	-	-	-	-	-	-	-	-	-	-	-	-	-	-	-	-	-	0.0	0.0	0.00	0.00	**0.0**	181
Corpus uteri	1	0	-	-	-	-	-	-	-	-	-	5.5	-	-	-	-	-	-	-	0.4	0.3	0.03	0.03	**0.3**	182
Ovary etc.	8	0	-	-	-	6.8	5.4	5.1	-	-	11.0	5.5	6.0	7.4	-	-	-	-	-	3.0	2.1	0.24	0.24	**2.8**	183
Other female genital	1	0	-	-	-	-	-	-	-	-	-	-	-	8.6	-	-	-	-	-	0.4	0.3	0.00	0.04	**0.3**	184
†Bladder	5	0	-	-	-	-	5.4	-	-	-	-	-	6.0	-	8.6	11.9	17.6	-	-	1.9	1.3	0.06	0.16	**1.3**	188
Kidney etc.	4	0	-	4.2	-	-	-	-	6.8	-	-	-	-	-	-	11.9	17.6	-	-	1.5	1.0	0.05	0.11	**1.2**	189
Eye	0	0	-	-	-	-	-	-	-	-	-	-	-	-	-	-	-	-	-	-	0.0	0.0	0.00	0.00	**0.0**	190
Brain, nervous system	6	0	-	4.6	-	-	-	-	-	-	-	-	5.5	6.0	14.8	8.6	-	-	-	-	2.3	1.6	0.15	0.20	**1.8**	191-2
Thyroid	17	0	-	-	-	6.8	5.4	5.1	20.4	19.6	22.0	-	6.0	14.8	-	-	-	30.0	-	6.4	4.4	0.50	0.50	**6.0**	193
Other endocrine	0	0	-	-	-	-	-	-	-	-	-	-	-	-	-	-	-	-	-	-	0.0	0.0	0.00	0.00	**0.0**	194
Hodgkin's disease	0	0	-	-	-	-	-	-	-	-	-	-	-	-	-	-	-	-	-	-	0.0	0.0	0.00	0.00	**0.0**	201
Non-Hodgkin lymphoma	6	0	-	-	-	-	6.8	-	-	-	-	11.0	-	-	7.4	-	11.9	17.6	-	-	2.3	1.6	0.13	0.19	**1.9**	200,202
Multiple myeloma	4	0	-	-	-	-	-	-	-	-	6.8	-	5.5	12.0	-	-	-	-	-	-	1.5	1.0	0.12	0.12	**1.2**	203
Lymphoid leukaemia	2	0	-	-	-	4.1	-	-	-	-	-	-	-	-	7.4	-	-	-	-	-	0.8	0.5	0.06	0.06	**0.7**	204
Myeloid leukaemia	4	0	-	-	4.2	4.1	-	-	-	-	-	-	5.5	-	-	8.6	-	-	-	-	1.5	1.0	0.07	0.11	**1.3**	205
Monocytic leukaemia	0	0	-	-	-	-	-	-	-	-	-	-	-	-	-	-	-	-	-	-	0.0	0.0	0.00	0.00	**0.0**	206
Other leukaemia	0	0	-	-	-	-	-	-	-	-	-	-	-	-	-	-	-	-	-	-	0.0	0.0	0.00	0.00	**0.0**	207
Leukaemia unspecified	2	0	-	-	-	-	-	-	-	-	-	-	5.5	-	-	-	-	17.6	-	-	0.8	0.5	0.03	0.03	**0.5**	208
Other and unspecified	4	0	-	-	-	-	-	-	-	-	6.5	-	5.5	6.0	-	-	-	17.6	-	-	1.5	1.0	0.09	0.09	**1.1**	O&U
All sites	387	0	-	4.6	8.4	16.3	33.9	48.9	56.0	136.1	189.1	142.7	227.5	317.6	414.9	438.1	416.7	563.7	240.1	198.4	146.3		7.98	12.25	**110.7**	ALL
All sites but 173	385	0	-	4.6	8.4	16.3	33.9	48.9	56.0	136.1	189.1	142.7	227.5	311.6	407.5	438.1	416.7	563.7	240.1	198.4	145.6	100.0	7.91	12.19	**110.2**	ALLb

Rate from 1 case: 7.266 4.567 4.180 4.072 6.780 5.438 5.095 6.803 6.520 5.488 5.548 5.992 7.410 8.590 11.905 17.615 30.012 49.603

†Important: see notes on population page

Kuwait

The Kuwait Cancer Registry was established in 1971 in the Radiotherapy Department at the Al-Sabah hospital. The initial purpose of the registry was to study the incidence and morphology of cancers in the Kuwaiti population and to use this information as the basis for establishing a comprehensive service for diagnosis, treatment, follow-up and care of cancer patients. After the establishment of the Kuwait Cancer Control Centre in 1982, the registry became a separate department of the hospital.

The state of Kuwait is situated in the north-western corner of the Arabian Gulf. It is an oil-producing country with an area of 17 818 km^2. The mainland is a generally flat sandy desert with a scattering of oases. There are a few rocky hills of heights ranging from 180 to 300 m above sea level. Kuwait experiences wide variations in temperature, ranging from an average of 45°C in July to an average of 8°C in January. There is also wide variation in annual rainfall, ranging from as little as 22 mm to 352 mm, which falls almost entirely between November and April.

According to the 1985 census, the total population was 1 697 301, of whom 37% were children aged below 15 years. Kuwaiti nationals constituted about 40% and expatriates 60% of the population. Expatriates from more than 50 different countries live in Kuwait, of whom the majority are Arabs and south and south-east Asians.

For administrative purposes, the country is divided into five health regions: Capital, Hawali, AlFarwania, Al-Ahmadi, and Al-Jahra. The medical services in each health region comprise a number of primary health care clinics which provide general, maternal, child, and dental health care services, and a general public hospital. Besides these clinics and hospitals, there are also specialized centres, including the Kuwait Cancer Control Centre. The latter, established in 1982, is the only specialized cancer treatment hospital in the country, and offers modern facilities in various modalities of cancer diagnosis, treatment and follow-up.

Notification of cancer is compulsory through a Ministerial Decree. Cancer registrations are reasonably comprehensive as almost all cases not initially diagnosed or treated at the Kuwait Cancer Control Centre (including those who receive initial treatment abroad) are referred to this centre for further treatment or follow-up. The registry maintains a separate alphabetical and numeric index which includes information such as case note number, nationality, name, sex, age, year of diagnosis and site. Pathology reports and death certificates are filed numerically by year. All new registrations are checked against these indices to avoid duplication.

The registry collects information on malignant neoplasms according to the recommendations of the IARC. The sources of information are: case notes from the Cancer Control Centre and other hospitals; reports from the pathology departments of the Cancer Control Centre and of other hospitals; and mortality data from the Vital and Health Statistics Division of the Ministry of Health.

The registry includes data on all neoplasms classified as malignant. For the period 1979–92, the data have been coded according to ICD-O-1 and ICD-9. From 1 January 1993, the registry has adopted ICD-O-2 and ICD-10.

In this volume, data are presented for the periods 1988–89 and 1992–93. Reliable incidence and population data for the years 1990–91 are not available due to the disruption brought about by the occupation of the country in 1990.

Anjum Memon
Ali N. Al-Muhanna

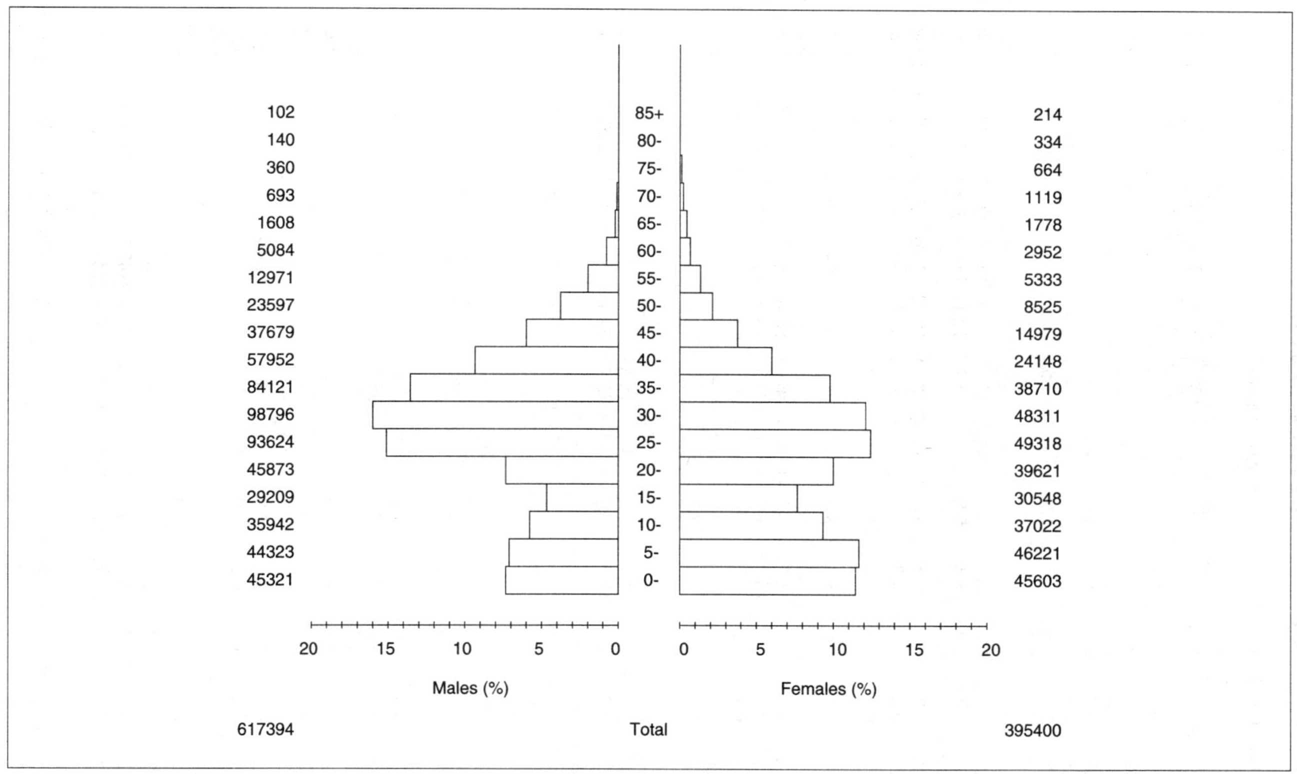

Kuwait: Non-Kuwaitis

Source of population: average annual 1988-89 and 1992-93
Census: 1985
Estimate: The populations for inter-censal years are estimated by the Central Statistical Office and the Vital & Health Statistics Division using the second degree polynomial (parabola) method.

Notes to tables overleaf:
* Comparisons with the data published in previous volumes may be misleading (or may not be possible) due to the heterogeneous and transitory nature of the non-Kuwaiti population.

* KUWAIT: NON-KUWAITIS 1988-1989,1992-1993

ANNUAL INCIDENCE PER 100,000 BY AGE GROUP (YEARS) - MALE

SITE	ALL AGES	AGE UNK	0-	5-	10-	15-	20-	25-	30-	35-	40-	45-	50-	55-	60-	65-	70-	75-	80-	85+	CRUDE RATE	%	CR 64	CR 74	ASR (W)	ICD (9th)
Lip	8	0	-	-	-	-	-	-	0.3	-	1.3	1.3	1.1	-	-	15.5	-	-	-	-	0.3	0.7	0.02	0.10	**0.7**	*140*
Tongue	10	0	-	-	-	-	-	-	0.5	0.6	1.3	0.7	1.1	-	-	15.5	-	-	-	-	0.4	0.8	0.02	0.10	**0.7**	*141*
Salivary gland	7	0	-	-	-	-	-	-	0.3	-	0.4	1.3	2.1	-	-	15.5	-	-	-	-	0.3	0.6	0.02	0.10	**0.7**	*142*
Mouth	10	0	-	-	0.7	-	-	-	0.3	0.6	0.9	0.7	1.1	1.9	4.9	-	-	-	-	-	0.4	0.8	0.05	0.05	**0.5**	*143-5*
Oropharynx	4	0	-	-	-	-	0.5	-	-	0.3	0.4	-	-	-	-	-	-	-	-	243.3	0.2	0.3	0.01	0.01	**1.3**	*146*
Nasopharynx	23	0	-	-	0.7	-	-	0.3	0.5	1.5	1.3	4.6	2.1	1.9	-	15.5	-	-	-	-	0.9	1.9	0.06	0.14	**1.2**	*147*
Hypopharynx	4	0	-	-	-	-	-	-	0.5	-	0.4	0.7	-	-	-	-	-	-	-	-	0.2	0.3	0.01	0.01	**0.1**	*148*
Pharynx unspecified	1	0	-	-	-	-	-	-	0.3	-	-	-	-	-	-	-	-	-	-	-	0.0	0.1	0.00	0.00	**0.0**	*149*
Oesophagus	10	0	-	-	-	-	-	-	-	0.6	-	2.7	-	-	9.8	-	-	138.6	-	-	0.4	0.8	0.07	0.07	**2.0**	*150*
Stomach	52	1	-	-	-	-	0.5	0.8	0.8	1.5	0.4	8.0	5.3	5.8	34.4	77.7	72.1	138.6	178.6	243.3	2.1	4.4	0.29	1.06	**10.1**	*151*
Small intestine	0	0	-	-	-	-	-	-	-	-	-	-	-	-	-	-	-	-	-	-	0.0	0.0	0.00	0.00	**0.0**	*152*
Colon	56	0	-	-	-	-	-	0.5	1.3	1.8	2.2	6.6	7.4	13.5	24.6	46.6	-	138.6	535.7	243.3	2.3	4.7	0.29	0.52	**9.3**	*153*
Rectum	33	0	-	-	-	0.9	0.5	0.3	0.5	1.5	0.4	6.6	4.2	1.9	19.7	15.5	36.1	69.3	-	-	1.3	2.8	0.18	0.44	**3.6**	*154*
Liver	48	0	0.6	-	-	-	-	0.3	0.8	0.6	0.9	2.0	8.5	21.2	54.1	46.6	72.1	69.3	-	-	1.9	4.0	0.44	1.04	**7.3**	*155*
Gallbladder etc.	11	0	-	-	-	-	-	-	0.3	-	-	1.3	2.1	3.9	14.7	-	-	69.3	-	-	0.4	0.9	0.11	0.11	**1.6**	*156*
Pancreas	35	0	-	-	-	-	-	-	-	0.3	1.3	4.0	5.3	13.5	19.7	77.7	36.1	69.3	357.1	-	1.4	2.9	0.22	0.79	**7.5**	*157*
Nose, sinuses etc.	3	0	-	-	-	-	-	-	-	-	-	-	-	1.9	-	-	36.1	69.3	-	-	0.1	0.3	0.01	0.19	**1.5**	*160*
Larynx	34	0	-	-	-	-	-	-	-	0.3	1.7	4.6	3.2	15.4	19.7	46.6	36.1	69.3	178.6	243.3	1.4	2.9	0.22	0.64	**6.9**	*161*
Bronchus, lung	141	0	-	-	-	-	-	0.3	1.3	1.5	4.3	11.3	18.0	34.7	137.7	264.3	324.6	415.8	1071.4	486.6	5.7	11.9	1.04	3.99	**35.3**	*162*
Other thoracic organs	7	0	-	-	-	-	1.1	-	-	-	0.9	0.7	1.1	-	-	-	-	-	-	-	0.3	0.6	0.02	0.02	**0.3**	*163-4*
Bone	17	0	-	0.6	0.7	3.4	1.1	0.5	0.3	0.3	-	1.3	-	3.9	4.9	-	-	-	-	-	0.7	1.4	0.08	0.08	**1.0**	*170*
Connective tissue	31	0	0.6	-	1.4	1.7	1.6	0.3	1.0	1.2	1.3	2.7	1.1	7.7	9.8	-	-	-	-	-	1.3	2.6	0.15	0.15	**1.6**	*171*
Mesothelioma	4	0	-	-	-	-	-	-	-	0.3	-	0.7	1.1	1.9	-	-	-	-	-	-	0.2	0.3	0.02	0.02	**0.2**	*MES*
Kaposi's sarcoma	2	0	-	-	-	-	-	-	-	-	0.4	-	-	1.9	-	-	-	-	-	-	0.1	0.2	0.01	0.01	**0.1**	*KAP*
Melanoma of skin	11	0	-	-	-	-	-	-	0.8	0.9	-	-	1.1	3.9	4.9	15.5	-	-	-	-	0.4	0.9	0.06	0.14	**1.0**	*172*
Other skin	43	0	-	-	-	-	-	-	0.5	0.3	4.7	4.0	5.3	17.3	19.7	31.1	72.1	-	-	243.3	1.7		0.26	0.78	**5.9**	*173*
Breast	5	0	-	-	-	-	-	-	-	0.9	-	-	2.1	-	-	-	-	-	-	-	0.2	0.4	0.02	0.02	**0.2**	*175*
Prostate	32	0	-	-	-	-	-	-	-	-	-	-	2.1	1.9	19.7	124.4	180.3	485.1	535.7	486.6	1.3	2.7	0.12	1.64	**18.3**	*185*
Testis	35	0	-	-	0.7	0.9	1.6	2.4	1.5	0.9	0.9	3.3	4.2	-	-	15.5	-	-	-	-	1.4	2.9	0.08	0.16	**1.5**	*186*
Penis	3	0	-	-	-	-	-	-	-	-	0.3	0.4	-	-	1.9	-	-	-	-	-	0.1	0.3	0.01	0.01	**0.1**	*187.1-.4*
Other male genital	2	0	0.6	-	-	-	-	-	0.3	-	-	-	-	-	-	-	-	-	-	-	0.1	0.2	0.00	0.00	**0.1**	*187.5-.9*
Bladder	79	0	-	-	-	-	-	0.5	1.0	2.4	2.2	6.0	15.9	15.4	39.3	108.8	288.5	138.6	178.6	486.6	3.2	6.6	0.41	2.40	**17.5**	*188*
Kidney etc.	32	0	-	0.6	-	-	-	-	0.8	0.9	1.3	5.3	1.1	5.8	19.7	62.2	36.1	69.3	-	-	1.3	2.7	0.18	0.67	**4.9**	*189*
Eye	0	0	-	-	-	-	-	-	-	-	-	-	-	-	-	-	-	-	-	-	0.0	0.0	0.00	0.00	**0.0**	*190*
Brain, nervous system	57	0	3.3	2.3	0.7	0.9	1.6	1.3	1.5	2.1	3.5	4.0	3.2	5.8	19.7	-	-	-	-	-	2.3	4.8	0.25	0.25	**2.8**	*191-2*
Thyroid	40	0	-	-	-	-	-	1.1	1.5	0.9	4.7	3.3	2.1	7.7	-	15.5	36.1	69.3	357.1	-	1.6	3.4	0.11	0.36	**4.8**	*193*
Other endocrine	3	0	1.1	-	-	-	-	-	-	-	-	0.7	-	-	-	-	-	-	-	-	0.1	0.3	0.01	0.01	**0.2**	*194*
Hodgkin's disease	48	0	1.1	2.8	1.4	3.4	2.2	0.8	2.0	2.1	1.3	0.7	8.5	1.9	-	-	-	-	-	-	1.9	4.0	0.14	0.14	**2.0**	*201*
Non-Hodgkin lymphoma	121	0	2.8	4.5	2.1	0.9	2.7	3.2	2.5	3.3	7.3	8.6	17.0	19.3	19.7	31.1	72.1	-	357.1	-	4.9	10.2	0.47	0.99	**9.4**	*200,202*
Multiple myeloma	20	0	-	-	-	-	-	-	-	0.9	0.9	2.0	3.2	3.9	9.8	46.6	36.1	-	178.6	-	0.8	1.7	0.10	0.52	**3.9**	*203*
Lymphoid leukaemia	52	0	8.3	4.5	2.1	0.9	1.1	1.1	0.5	1.2	0.4	1.3	3.2	5.8	4.9	15.5	36.1	69.3	-	-	2.1	4.4	0.18	0.43	**4.6**	*204*
Myeloid leukaemia	46	0	-	-	0.7	0.9	-	2.7	1.5	2.4	2.2	4.0	4.2	3.9	14.7	-	-	-	-	-	1.9	3.9	0.19	0.19	**1.9**	*205*
Monocytic leukaemia	1	0	-	-	-	-	-	-	-	-	-	-	1.1	-	-	-	-	-	-	-	0.0	0.1	0.01	0.01	**0.1**	*206*
Other leukaemia	0	0	-	-	-	-	-	-	-	-	-	-	-	-	-	-	-	-	-	-	0.0	0.0	0.00	0.00	**0.0**	*207*
Leukaemia unspecified	6	0	-	-	-	-	0.5	0.3	-	-	0.4	0.7	1.1	1.9	-	-	-	-	-	-	0.2	0.5	0.02	0.02	**0.3**	*208*
Other and unspecified	44	3	1.1	0.6	0.7	0.9	0.5	0.8	0.3	0.9	1.7	3.3	5.3	7.7	24.6	31.1	72.1	69.3	-	-	1.8	3.7	0.26	0.81	**5.8**	*O&U*
All sites	1231	4	19.3	15.8	11.8	14.6	15.8	17.6	23.3	33.0	51.8	108.8	145.1	235.1	550.7	1135.0	1442.5	2148.3	3928.6	2676.4	49.8		6.23	19.16	**178.6**	*ALL*
All sites but 173	1188	4	19.3	15.8	11.8	14.6	15.8	17.6	22.8	32.7	47.0	104.8	139.8	217.8	531.0	1103.9	1370.4	2148.3	3928.6	2433.1	48.1	100.0	5.97	18.39	**172.7**	*ALLb*

Rate from 1 case   0.552   0.564   0.696   0.856   0.545   0.267   0.253   0.297   0.431   0.663   1.059   1.927   4.917   15.547   36.062   69.300   178.571   243.309

* KUWAIT: NON-KUWAITIS 1988-1989,1992-1993

ANNUAL INCIDENCE PER 100,000 BY AGE GROUP (YEARS) - FEMALE

SITE	ALL AGES	AGE UNK	0-	5-	10-	15-	20-	25-	30-	35-	40-	45-	50-	55-	60-	65-	70-	75-	80-	85+	CRUDE RATE	%	CR 64	CR 74	ASR (W)	ICD (9th)
Lip	1	0	-	-	-	-	-	-	-	-	1.0	-	-	-	-	-	-	-	-	-	0.1	0.1	0.01	0.01	0.1	140
Tongue	3	0	-	-	-	-	0.6	-	-	-	1.0	-	-	-	8.5	-	-	-	-	-	0.2	0.3	0.05	0.05	0.5	141
Salivary gland	4	0	-	0.5	-	-	-	1.5	-	-	-	-	-	-	-	-	-	-	-	-	0.3	0.4	0.01	0.01	0.2	142
Mouth	3	0	-	-	-	0.8	-	-	-	-	-	-	-	-	16.9	-	-	-	-	-	0.2	0.3	0.09	0.09	0.8	143-5
Oropharynx	0	0	-	-	-	-	-	-	-	-	-	-	-	-	-	-	-	-	-	-	0.0	0.0	0.00	0.00	0.0	146
Nasopharynx	2	0	-	-	-	-	-	0.5	-	-	-	1.7	-	-	-	-	-	-	-	-	0.1	0.2	0.01	0.01	0.1	147
Hypopharynx	0	0	-	-	-	-	-	-	-	-	-	-	-	-	-	-	-	-	-	-	0.0	0.0	0.00	0.00	0.0	148
Pharynx unspecified	0	0	-	-	-	-	-	-	-	-	-	-	-	-	-	-	-	-	-	-	0.0	0.0	0.00	0.00	0.0	149
Oesophagus	4	0	-	-	-	-	-	0.5	-	0.6	-	-	-	4.7	8.5	-	-	-	-	-	0.3	0.4	0.07	0.07	0.6	150
Stomach	16	0	-	-	-	-	0.6	0.5	0.5	0.6	1.0	6.7	8.8	9.4	-	-	22.3	-	74.8	-	1.0	1.8	0.14	0.25	2.3	151
Small intestine	1	0	-	-	-	-	-	-	-	-	-	1.7	-	-	-	-	-	-	-	-	0.1	0.1	0.01	0.01	0.1	152
Colon	13	0	-	-	-	-	0.6	-	0.5	0.6	-	3.3	8.8	9.4	16.9	14.1	-	-	-	-	0.8	1.5	0.20	0.27	2.2	153
Rectum	13	0	-	-	-	0.8	-	-	0.5	2.6	-	1.7	2.9	4.7	16.9	-	44.7	-	-	-	0.8	1.5	0.15	0.37	2.3	154
Liver	8	0	-	-	-	-	-	-	-	-	-	-	2.9	-	16.9	28.1	22.3	37.6	-	116.4	0.5	0.9	0.10	0.35	3.1	155
Gallbladder etc.	11	0	-	-	-	-	-	-	-	-	-	1.7	2.9	14.1	-	42.2	22.3	37.6	74.8	-	0.7	1.2	0.09	0.42	3.3	156
Pancreas	12	0	-	-	-	-	-	-	-	-	-	5.0	5.9	14.1	8.5	-	44.7	-	-	116.4	0.8	1.3	0.17	0.39	3.0	157
Nose, sinuses etc.	1	0	-	-	-	-	-	-	-	-	1.0	-	-	-	-	-	-	-	-	-	0.1	0.1	0.01	0.01	0.1	160
Larynx	1	0	-	-	-	-	-	-	-	-	-	1.7	-	-	-	-	-	-	-	-	0.1	0.1	0.01	0.01	0.1	161
Bronchus, lung	37	0	-	-	-	-	-	-	0.5	1.3	-	6.7	11.7	32.8	16.9	126.5	134.0	37.6	74.8	-	2.3	4.1	0.35	1.65	10.3	162
Other thoracic organs	5	0	0.5	-	-	0.8	-	-	-	-	1.0	1.7	-	-	-	14.1	-	-	-	-	0.3	0.6	0.02	0.09	0.7	163-4
Bone	5	0	-	0.5	0.7	1.6	-	0.5	-	-	-	-	-	-	-	-	-	-	-	-	0.3	0.6	0.02	0.02	0.3	170
Connective tissue	9	0	-	0.5	0.7	-	0.6	0.5	1.0	0.6	-	-	-	4.7	-	-	-	37.6	-	-	0.6	1.0	0.04	0.04	0.9	171
Mesothelioma	2	0	-	-	-	-	-	-	1.0	-	-	-	-	-	-	-	-	-	-	-	0.1	0.2	0.01	0.01	0.1	MES
Kaposi's sarcoma	1	0	-	-	-	-	-	-	-	-	-	-	2.9	-	-	-	-	-	-	-	0.1	0.1	0.01	0.01	0.1	KAP
Melanoma of skin	4	0	-	-	-	-	-	-	-	-	-	-	-	-	-	-	22.3	75.3	-	116.4	0.3	0.4	0.00	0.11	1.8	172
Other skin	19	0	-	-	-	-	-	0.5	1.9	3.1	1.7	17.6	-	8.5	14.1	22.3	75.3	-	-	-	1.2		0.17	0.35	3.3	173
Breast	309	0	-	-	-	-	-	4.1	12.4	34.2	71.4	108.5	120.2	103.1	110.1	112.4	22.3	75.3	-	349.2	19.5	34.5	2.82	3.49	34.8	174
Uterus unspecified	1	0	-	-	-	-	-	-	-	-	-	-	-	8.5	-	-	-	-	-	-	0.1	0.1	0.04	0.04	0.3	179
Cervix uteri	56	0	-	-	-	-	-	2.0	2.1	8.4	14.5	15.0	14.7	14.1	16.9	-	22.3	-	74.8	-	3.5	6.2	0.44	0.55	5.4	180
Placenta	5	0	-	-	-	-	-	0.5	1.0	0.6	-	1.7	-	-	-	-	-	-	-	-	0.3	0.6	0.02	0.02	0.2	181
Corpus uteri	17	0	-	-	-	-	-	-	-	0.6	2.1	-	2.9	18.8	33.9	56.2	-	37.6	-	-	1.1	1.9	0.29	0.57	4.5	182
Ovary etc.	45	0	-	-	0.7	0.8	-	1.5	1.6	1.3	9.3	10.0	20.5	4.7	33.9	56.2	67.0	-	-	116.4	2.8	5.0	0.42	1.04	7.8	183
Other female genital	4	0	-	-	-	-	0.6	-	-	-	1.0	1.7	-	-	-	-	-	-	-	116.4	0.3	0.4	0.02	0.02	0.8	184
Bladder	15	0	0.5	-	-	-	-	-	-	0.6	1.0	3.3	2.9	-	8.5	14.1	89.3	75.3	74.8	-	0.9	1.7	0.08	0.60	4.2	188
Kidney etc.	14	0	1.1	0.5	-	0.8	0.6	0.5	-	-	-	-	2.9	-	16.9	28.1	44.7	37.6	-	-	0.9	1.6	0.12	0.48	3.3	189
Eye	0	0	-	-	-	-	-	-	-	-	-	-	-	-	-	-	-	-	-	-	0.0	0.0	0.00	0.00	0.0	190
Brain, nervous system	32	0	0.5	2.7	2.0	1.6	0.6	3.0	1.6	2.6	1.0	3.3	2.9	-	8.5	28.1	-	-	-	-	2.0	3.6	0.15	0.29	2.8	191-2
Thyroid	78	0	-	-	-	2.5	3.8	7.1	8.3	6.5	9.3	11.7	11.7	14.1	16.9	14.1	-	75.3	74.8	-	4.9	8.7	0.46	0.53	6.6	193
Other endocrine	6	0	1.6	1.1	-	-	-	-	-	-	1.0	-	-	-	-	-	-	-	-	-	0.4	0.7	0.02	0.02	0.4	194
Hodgkin's disease	24	0	-	1.6	0.7	2.5	2.5	0.5	2.1	0.6	1.0	5.0	2.9	-	8.5	-	22.3	-	-	-	1.5	2.7	0.14	0.25	2.1	201
Non-Hodgkin lymphoma	44	0	1.6	1.1	2.0	0.8	0.6	1.5	1.0	1.3	4.1	13.4	11.7	4.7	33.9	28.1	44.7	37.6	-	116.4	2.8	4.9	0.39	0.75	6.7	200,202
Multiple myeloma	7	0	-	-	-	-	-	-	-	-	-	-	2.9	9.4	16.9	-	-	75.3	-	-	0.4	0.8	0.15	0.15	2.0	203
Lymphoid leukaemia	32	0	6.0	1.6	0.7	1.6	2.5	1.5	0.5	1.3	-	-	-	-	8.5	14.1	-	75.3	-	116.4	2.0	3.6	0.12	0.19	3.6	204
Myeloid leukaemia	19	0	-	-	-	1.9	0.5	3.1	1.9	3.1	-	-	5.9	-	8.5	-	-	-	-	-	1.2	2.1	0.12	0.12	1.3	205
Monocytic leukaemia	0	0	-	-	-	-	-	-	-	-	-	-	-	-	-	-	-	-	-	-	0.0	0.0	0.00	0.00	0.0	206
Other leukaemia	0	0	-	-	-	-	-	-	-	-	-	-	-	-	-	-	-	-	-	-	0.0	0.0	0.00	0.00	0.0	207
Leukaemia unspecified	4	0	-	-	-	-	-	-	-	-	1.0	-	-	-	-	14.1	44.7	-	-	-	0.3	0.4	0.01	0.30	1.4	208
Other and unspecified	28	2	0.5	-	0.7	0.8	0.6	0.5	1.0	0.6	4.1	3.3	8.8	4.7	16.9	28.1	44.7	37.6	74.8	-	1.8	3.1	0.23	0.62	5.0	O&U
All sites	915	2	12.6	10.3	8.1	15.5	16.4	27.4	39.3	69.1	132.5	210.3	275.6	267.2	465.7	632.5	736.9	828.0	523.6	1164.1	57.9		7.77	14.63	129.1	ALL
All sites but 173	896	2	12.6	10.3	8.1	15.5	16.4	27.4	38.8	67.2	129.4	208.6	258.0	267.2	457.2	618.4	714.6	752.7	523.6	1164.1	56.7	100.0	7.60	14.28	125.8	ALLb
Rate from 1 case			0.548	0.541	0.675	0.818	0.631	0.507	0.517	0.646	1.035	1.669	2.932	4.688	8.467	14.055	22.331	37.636	74.794	116.414						

413

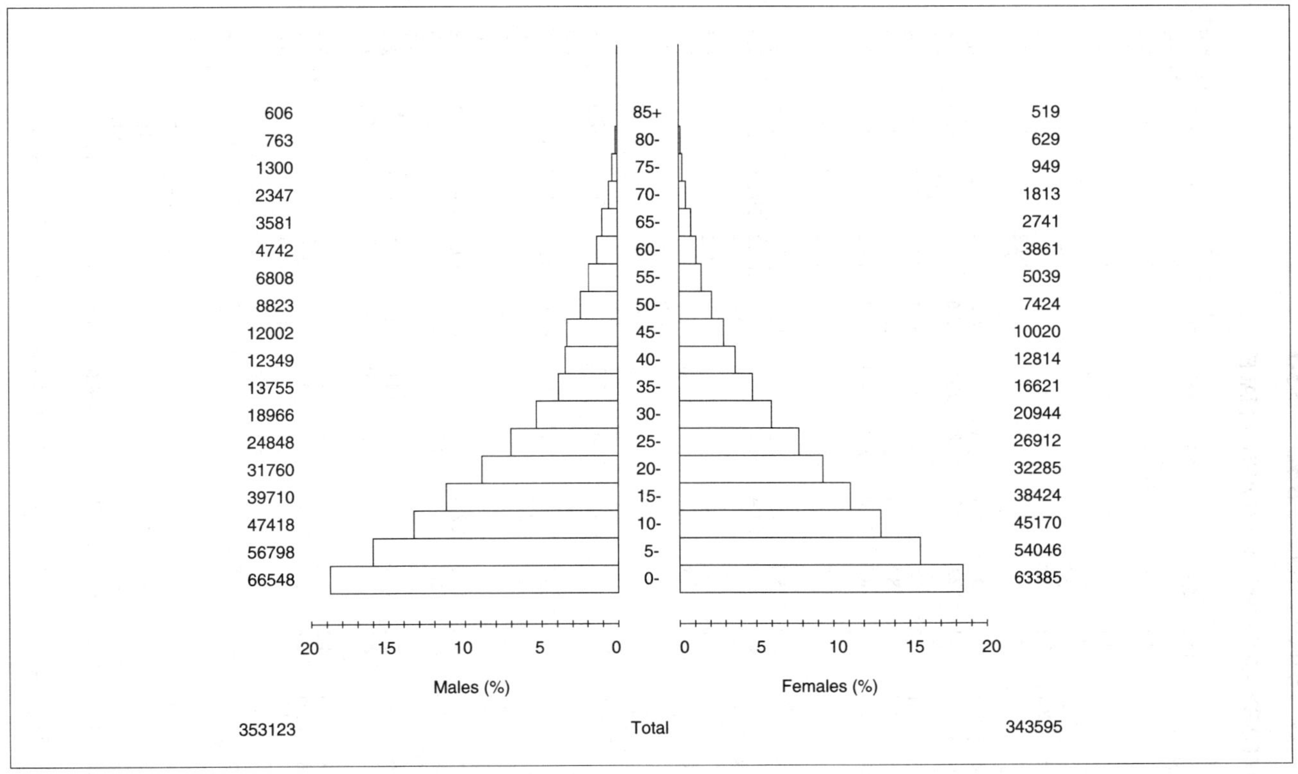

Kuwait: Kuwaitis
Source of population: average annual 1988-89 and 1992-93
Census: 1985
Estimate: The populations for inter-censal years are estimated by the Central Statistical Office and the Vital & Health Statistics Division using the second degree polynomial (parabola) method.

Notes to tables overleaf:
* The high proportion of diagnoses based on a death certificate alone indicates under-ascertainment.

* KUWAIT: KUWAITIS 1988-1989,1992-1993

ANNUAL INCIDENCE PER 100,000 BY AGE GROUP (YEARS) - MALE

SITE	ALL AGES	AGE UNK	0-	5-	10-	15-	20-	25-	30-	35-	40-	45-	50-	55-	60-	65-	70-	75-	80-	85+	CRUDE RATE	%	CR 64	CR 74	ASR (W)	ICD (9th)
Lip	3	0	-	-	-	-	-	-	-	-	-	2.1	-	-	-	-	-	19.2	-	41.2	0.2	0.4	0.01	0.01	**0.5**	*140*
Tongue	1	0	-	-	-	-	-	-	-	-	-	-	-	-	5.3	-	-	-	-	-	0.1	0.1	0.03	0.03	**0.2**	*141*
Salivary gland	4	0	-	0.4	-	-	-	-	1.3	-	-	2.1	-	-	-	-	-	19.2	-	-	0.3	0.6	0.02	0.02	**0.4**	*142*
Mouth	3	0	-	-	-	-	-	-	-	-	-	-	-	-	5.3	7.0	-	-	-	41.2	0.2	0.4	0.03	0.06	**0.6**	*143-5*
Oropharynx	2	0	-	-	-	-	-	-	-	-	-	-	5.7	-	-	-	-	-	-	-	0.1	0.3	0.03	0.03	**0.3**	*146*
Nasopharynx	16	0	-	-	-	-	-	-	-	5.5	8.1	2.1	8.5	7.3	-	20.9	-	-	-	-	1.1	2.3	0.16	0.26	**2.3**	*147*
Hypopharynx	5	0	-	-	-	-	-	-	-	-	-	-	-	7.3	5.3	-	-	19.2	-	41.2	0.4	0.7	0.06	0.06	**0.9**	*148*
Pharynx unspecified	0	0	-	-	-	-	-	-	-	-	-	-	-	-	-	-	-	-	-	-	0.0	0.0	0.00	0.00	**0.0**	*149*
Oesophagus	9	0	-	-	-	-	-	-	-	-	-	-	2.8	3.7	5.3	14.0	10.6	38.5	-	41.2	0.6	1.3	0.06	0.18	**1.7**	*150*
Stomach	25	0	-	-	0.5	-	0.8	1.0	2.6	-	-	2.1	2.8	14.7	15.8	20.9	42.6	38.5	-	82.4	1.8	3.7	0.20	0.52	**4.1**	*151*
Small intestine	2	0	-	-	-	-	-	-	-	-	-	-	-	-	-	-	-	-	32.7	41.2	0.1	0.3	0.00	0.00	**0.4**	*152*
Colon	22	0	-	-	-	0.6	-	1.0	1.3	1.8	6.1	4.2	-	3.7	-	20.9	21.3	57.7	65.5	82.4	1.6	3.2	0.09	0.30	**3.5**	*153*
Rectum	22	0	-	-	-	-	-	-	1.3	-	4.0	-	8.5	7.3	10.5	27.9	10.6	19.2	32.7	206.1	1.6	3.2	0.16	0.35	**3.9**	*154*
Liver	41	0	-	-	0.5	0.6	-	-	-	3.6	2.0	6.2	8.5	11.0	58.0	14.0	85.2	19.2	-	206.1	2.9	6.0	0.45	0.95	**7.3**	*155*
Gallbladder etc.	10	0	-	-	-	-	-	-	-	-	-	2.1	-	-	5.3	-	21.3	19.2	32.7	164.9	0.7	1.5	0.04	0.14	**1.9**	*156*
Pancreas	26	0	-	-	-	-	-	-	2.6	-	-	2.1	11.3	-	21.1	41.9	63.9	19.2	32.7	41.2	1.8	3.8	0.19	0.71	**4.8**	*157*
Nose, sinuses etc.	0	0	-	-	-	-	-	-	-	-	-	-	-	-	-	-	-	-	-	-	0.0	0.0	0.00	0.00	**0.0**	*160*
Larynx	15	0	-	-	-	-	-	-	-	1.8	-	4.2	5.7	11.0	5.3	7.0	10.6	57.7	-	41.2	1.1	2.2	0.14	0.23	**2.5**	*161*
Bronchus, lung	111	0	-	-	-	0.6	-	-	-	3.6	-	8.3	34.0	51.4	84.3	118.7	149.1	269.2	294.6	329.8	7.9	16.3	0.91	2.25	**20.3**	*162*
Other thoracic organs	5	0	0.8	-	-	-	-	-	1.3	1.8	-	-	-	-	-	-	10.6	-	-	-	0.4	0.7	0.02	0.07	**0.5**	*163-4*
Bone	7	0	-	-	-	1.3	0.8	1.0	1.3	-	-	2.1	-	-	-	-	-	19.2	-	-	0.5	1.0	0.03	0.03	**0.7**	*170*
Connective tissue	9	0	0.8	0.4	0.5	-	0.8	1.0	-	1.8	-	-	2.8	-	-	7.0	-	-	-	-	0.6	1.3	0.04	0.08	**0.8**	*171*
Mesothelioma	3	0	-	-	-	-	-	-	-	-	-	-	-	3.7	5.3	-	10.6	-	-	-	0.2	0.4	0.04	0.10	**0.6**	*MES*
Kaposi's sarcoma	3	0	-	-	-	-	-	-	-	-	-	-	7.3	-	-	-	-	-	-	41.2	0.2	0.4	0.04	0.04	**0.5**	*KAP*
Melanoma of skin	3	0	-	-	-	-	0.8	-	-	-	-	-	-	-	-	-	10.6	-	32.7	-	0.2	0.4	0.00	0.06	**0.4**	*172*
Other skin	16	0	-	-	-	-	-	-	-	-	6.1	-	-	14.7	10.5	7.0	-	57.7	32.7	82.4	1.1		0.16	0.19	**2.7**	*173*
Breast	0	0	-	-	-	-	-	-	-	-	-	-	-	-	-	-	-	-	-	-	0.0	0.0	0.00	0.00	**0.0**	*175*
Prostate	33	0	-	-	-	-	-	-	-	-	-	-	5.7	11.0	36.9	20.9	63.9	38.5	65.5	329.8	2.3	4.8	0.27	0.69	**6.5**	*185*
Testis	8	0	0.4	-	-	-	-	2.0	1.3	3.6	2.0	-	-	3.7	-	-	-	-	-	-	0.6	1.2	0.07	0.07	**0.8**	*186*
Penis	0	0	-	-	-	-	-	-	-	-	-	-	-	-	-	-	-	-	-	-	0.0	0.0	0.00	0.00	**0.0**	*187.1-.4*
Other male genital	0	0	-	-	-	-	-	-	-	-	-	-	-	-	-	-	-	-	-	-	0.0	0.0	0.00	0.00	**0.0**	*187.5-.9*
Bladder	40	0	-	-	-	-	-	-	-	5.5	-	4.2	11.3	22.0	42.2	27.9	42.6	19.2	196.4	82.4	2.8	5.9	0.43	0.78	**7.0**	*188*
Kidney etc.	14	0	0.8	-	-	-	-	-	-	1.8	2.0	4.2	5.7	-	10.5	-	42.6	-	-	-	1.0	2.1	0.12	0.34	**2.1**	*189*
Eye	2	0	0.4	-	-	-	-	-	-	-	-	-	-	-	-	-	-	-	32.7	-	0.1	0.3	0.00	0.00	**0.2**	*190*
Brain, nervous system	33	0	0.8	0.9	2.1	2.5	0.8	2.0	1.3	3.6	-	6.2	11.3	-	-	14.0	42.6	19.2	32.7	-	2.3	4.8	0.16	0.44	**3.7**	*191-2*
Thyroid	14	0	-	-	-	-	1.6	1.0	-	5.5	2.0	2.1	-	-	5.3	14.0	-	19.2	32.7	41.2	1.0	2.1	0.09	0.16	**2.0**	*193*
Other endocrine	3	0	-	0.4	0.5	-	-	-	-	-	-	-	-	-	-	7.0	-	-	-	-	0.2	0.4	0.00	0.04	**0.3**	*194*
Hodgkin's disease	41	0	-	4.0	2.6	1.9	1.6	4.0	2.6	1.8	4.0	4.2	11.3	-	5.3	27.9	10.6	19.2	-	-	2.9	6.0	0.22	0.41	**4.0**	*201*
Non-Hodgkin lymphoma	47	0	0.4	1.3	1.6	1.3	1.6	7.0	1.3	1.8	2.0	16.7	2.8	29.4	5.3	20.9	10.6	38.5	65.5	-	3.3	6.9	0.36	0.52	**5.5**	*200,202*
Multiple myeloma	7	0	-	-	-	-	-	-	-	-	4.0	-	-	-	5.3	-	21.3	19.2	32.7	-	0.5	1.0	0.05	0.15	**1.2**	*203*
Lymphoid leukaemia	18	0	1.5	2.2	1.6	0.6	1.6	1.0	-	-	-	-	-	-	5.3	7.0	-	-	-	-	1.3	2.6	0.07	0.10	**1.2**	*204*
Myeloid leukaemia	20	0	0.4	-	0.5	1.9	-	1.0	2.6	5.5	-	4.2	2.8	11.0	-	-	21.3	-	32.7	-	1.4	2.9	0.15	0.26	**2.3**	*205*
Monocytic leukaemia	1	0	-	-	-	0.6	-	-	-	-	-	-	-	-	-	-	-	-	-	-	0.1	0.1	0.00	0.00	**0.1**	*206*
Other leukaemia	0	0	-	-	-	-	-	-	-	-	-	-	-	-	-	-	-	-	-	-	0.0	0.0	0.00	0.00	**0.0**	*207*
Leukaemia unspecified	13	0	-	0.9	1.1	0.6	-	-	-	-	4.0	-	2.8	-	-	5.3	-	-	65.5	82.4	0.9	1.9	0.07	0.07	**1.6**	*208*
Other and unspecified	41	2	0.4	0.4	0.5	-	-	1.0	2.6	1.8	2.0	4.2	11.3	22.0	21.1	48.9	31.9	-	130.9	41.2	2.9	6.0	0.35	0.78	**6.4**	*O&U*
All sites	698	2	6.4	11.0	12.1	12.6	10.2	23.1	23.7	50.9	48.6	83.3	155.8	242.4	379.6	495.6	734.8	846.2	1243.9	2061.0	49.4		5.31	11.48	**106.7**	*ALL*
All sites but 173	682	2	6.4	11.0	12.1	12.6	10.2	23.1	23.7	50.9	42.5	83.3	155.8	227.7	369.0	488.6	734.8	788.5	1211.1	1978.6	48.3	100.0	5.16	11.29	**103.9**	*ALLb*
Rate from 1 case			0.376	0.440	0.527	0.630	0.787	1.006	1.318	1.817	2.024	2.083	2.834	3.672	5.272	6.980	10.650	19.231	32.733	41.220						

* KUWAIT: KUWAITIS 1988-1989,1992-1993

ANNUAL INCIDENCE PER 100,000 BY AGE GROUP (YEARS) - FEMALE

SITE	ALL AGES	AGE UNK	0-	5-	10-	15-	20-	25-	30-	35-	40-	45-	50-	55-	60-	65-	70-	75-	80-	85+	CRUDE RATE	%	CR 64	CR 74	ASR (W)	ICD (9th)
Lip	0	0	-	-	-	-	-	-	-	-	-	-	-	-	-	-	-	-	-	-	0.0	0.0	0.00	0.00	**0.0**	140
Tongue	2	0	-	-	-	0.7	-	-	-	-	-	-	-	5.0	-	-	-	-	-	-	0.1	0.3	0.03	0.03	**0.3**	141
Salivary gland	5	0	-	-	-	-	-	-	2.4	-	-	2.5	-	5.0	-	9.1	-	-	-	-	0.4	0.7	0.05	0.09	**0.8**	142
Mouth	4	0	-	-	-	-	-	-	-	-	2.0	2.5	3.4	-	6.5	-	-	-	-	-	0.3	0.5	0.07	0.07	**0.7**	143-5
Oropharynx	3	0	-	-	-	-	-	-	-	-	-	-	-	6.5	9.1	-	26.3	-	-	-	0.2	0.4	0.03	0.08	**0.8**	146
Nasopharynx	6	0	-	-	-	-	1.5	-	-	3.0	2.0	2.5	-	-	-	-	-	-	-	-	0.4	0.8	0.05	0.05	**0.6**	147
Hypopharynx	7	0	-	-	-	-	-	-	-	-	2.0	-	10.1	-	6.5	18.2	-	-	-	-	0.5	0.9	0.09	0.18	**1.4**	148
Pharynx unspecified	0	0	-	-	-	-	-	-	-	-	-	-	-	-	-	-	-	-	-	-	0.0	0.0	0.00	0.00	**0.0**	149
Oesophagus	10	0	-	-	-	-	-	-	-	-	-	2.5	-	5.0	-	27.4	27.6	52.7	-	48.1	0.7	1.3	0.04	0.31	**2.5**	150
Stomach	23	0	-	-	-	-	-	0.9	-	3.0	-	-	10.1	19.8	32.4	18.2	13.8	26.3	79.4	96.2	1.7	3.1	0.33	0.49	**4.8**	151
Small intestine	2	0	-	-	-	-	-	-	-	-	-	-	3.4	-	-	-	-	-	39.7	-	0.1	0.3	0.02	0.02	**0.4**	152
Colon	25	0	-	-	-	-	0.8	0.9	1.2	3.0	3.9	2.5	10.1	14.9	13.0	18.2	55.1	26.3	-	96.2	1.8	3.3	0.25	0.62	**4.8**	153
Rectum	11	0	-	-	-	-	-	0.9	-	1.5	2.0	-	13.5	5.0	-	18.2	-	-	39.7	-	0.8	1.5	0.11	0.21	**1.9**	154
Liver	16	0	0.4	-	-	-	-	-	-	-	-	2.5	10.1	5.0	25.9	9.1	41.4	26.3	39.7	-	1.2	2.1	0.22	0.47	**3.5**	155
Gallbladder etc.	7	0	-	-	-	-	-	-	-	-	-	2.5	3.4	9.9	6.5	-	-	-	39.7	48.1	0.5	0.9	0.11	0.11	**1.4**	156
Pancreas	15	0	-	-	-	-	-	-	1.2	-	-	2.5	3.4	5.0	13.0	-	68.9	79.0	-	48.1	1.1	2.0	0.12	0.47	**3.5**	157
Nose, sinuses etc.	4	0	-	-	0.6	-	-	-	-	-	-	5.0	-	5.0	-	-	-	-	-	-	0.3	0.5	0.05	0.05	**0.5**	160
Larynx	5	0	-	0.5	-	-	-	-	-	-	-	5.0	-	-	-	9.1	-	26.3	-	-	0.4	0.7	0.03	0.07	**0.9**	161
Bronchus, lung	40	0	0.4	-	-	-	-	-	1.2	-	2.0	5.0	10.1	9.9	25.9	63.8	110.3	131.7	158.9	96.2	2.9	5.3	0.27	1.14	**9.2**	162
Other thoracic organs	1	0	-	-	-	-	-	-	-	-	-	-	-	-	6.5	-	-	-	-	-	0.1	0.1	0.03	0.03	**0.3**	163-4
Bone	10	0	-	0.9	1.7	-	1.5	0.9	1.2	-	-	-	-	-	-	-	-	26.3	-	-	0.7	1.3	0.03	0.03	**0.8**	170
Connective tissue	8	0	0.8	-	-	-	1.5	-	-	-	-	7.5	-	5.0	-	-	-	-	-	-	0.6	1.1	0.07	0.07	**0.9**	171
Mesothelioma	0	0	-	-	-	-	-	-	-	-	-	-	-	-	-	-	-	-	-	-	0.0	0.0	0.00	0.00	**0.0**	MES
Kaposi's sarcoma	1	0	-	-	-	-	-	-	1.2	-	-	-	-	-	-	-	-	-	-	-	0.1	0.1	0.01	0.01	**0.1**	KAP
Melanoma of skin	1	0	-	-	-	-	-	-	-	-	-	-	-	-	-	-	-	26.3	-	-	0.1	0.1	0.00	0.00	**0.3**	172
Other skin	8	0	-	-	-	-	-	-	-	1.5	-	5.0	3.4	5.0	6.5	9.1	13.8	-	-	-	0.6		0.11	0.22	**1.6**	173
Breast	208	0	-	-	-	-	2.3	9.3	16.7	49.6	56.6	82.3	80.8	69.5	90.7	218.8	68.9	79.0	79.4	-	15.1	27.6	2.29	3.73	**32.8**	174
Uterus unspecified	1	0	-	-	-	-	-	-	-	-	-	2.5	-	-	-	-	-	-	-	-	0.1	0.1	0.01	0.01	**0.1**	179
Cervix uteri	42	0	-	-	-	-	-	-	2.4	3.0	15.6	10.0	23.6	29.8	13.0	-	55.1	79.0	39.7	144.3	3.1	5.6	0.49	0.76	**7.6**	180
Placenta	6	0	-	-	-	-	-	0.9	-	1.5	3.9	5.0	-	-	-	-	-	-	-	-	0.4	0.8	0.06	0.06	**0.7**	181
Corpus uteri	14	0	-	-	-	-	-	-	2.4	3.0	2.0	5.0	3.4	5.0	13.0	9.1	13.8	-	39.7	-	1.0	1.9	0.17	0.28	**2.4**	182
Ovary etc.	25	0	0.4	-	0.6	-	0.8	-	1.2	-	3.9	2.5	16.8	14.9	19.4	27.4	41.4	-	-	48.1	1.8	3.3	0.30	0.65	**4.7**	183
Other female genital	3	0	-	-	-	-	-	-	-	-	-	-	-	-	-	9.1	-	26.3	39.7	-	0.2	0.4	0.00	0.05	**0.7**	184
Bladder	10	0	-	-	-	-	-	-	-	-	-	-	-	5.0	32.4	-	27.6	26.3	-	48.1	0.7	1.3	0.19	0.32	**2.5**	188
Kidney etc.	11	0	-	-	-	-	0.8	-	-	1.5	3.9	-	6.7	5.0	-	9.1	27.6	-	39.7	-	0.8	1.5	0.09	0.27	**1.9**	189
Eye	2	0	-	0.5	0.6	-	-	-	-	-	-	-	-	-	-	-	-	-	-	-	0.1	0.3	0.01	0.01	**0.1**	190
Brain, nervous system	27	0	2.0	0.9	2.2	-	2.3	2.8	1.2	1.5	-	2.5	-	9.9	6.5	-	27.6	26.3	39.7	-	2.0	3.6	0.16	0.30	**2.9**	191-2
Thyroid	48	0	-	-	-	0.7	3.9	5.6	6.0	18.0	7.8	7.5	6.7	-	19.4	18.2	-	26.3	-	192.4	3.5	6.4	0.38	0.47	**6.1**	193
Other endocrine	7	0	2.0	-	0.6	-	-	-	-	-	-	-	3.4	-	-	-	-	-	-	-	0.5	0.9	0.03	0.03	**0.5**	194
Hodgkin's disease	16	0	0.8	-	0.6	2.0	1.5	0.9	-	1.5	-	-	-	9.9	13.0	-	13.8	-	39.7	-	1.2	2.1	0.15	0.22	**2.0**	201
Non-Hodgkin lymphoma	43	0	2.4	-	1.7	2.0	-	0.9	1.2	-	3.9	5.0	6.7	49.6	25.9	45.6	27.6	26.3	-	48.1	3.1	5.7	0.50	0.86	**7.1**	200,202
Multiple myeloma	7	0	-	-	-	-	-	-	-	-	-	2.5	6.7	9.9	-	-	13.8	-	-	48.1	0.5	0.9	0.10	0.16	**1.4**	203
Lymphoid leukaemia	20	1	3.2	2.3	0.6	0.7	0.8	0.9	-	-	-	-	3.4	5.0	-	-	-	-	-	-	1.5	2.7	0.09	0.09	**1.3**	204
Myeloid leukaemia	18	1	0.8	-	-	1.3	-	0.9	1.2	3.0	2.0	5.0	-	-	25.9	9.1	-	26.3	-	-	1.3	2.4	0.21	0.26	**2.7**	205
Monocytic leukaemia	0	0	-	-	-	-	-	-	-	-	-	-	-	-	-	-	-	-	-	-	0.0	0.0	0.00	0.00	**0.0**	206
Other leukaemia	1	0	-	0.5	-	-	-	-	-	-	-	-	-	-	-	-	-	-	-	-	0.1	0.1	0.00	0.00	**0.0**	207
Leukaemia unspecified	3	0	-	-	-	-	0.8	-	-	-	-	-	-	-	-	-	-	13.8	-	48.1	0.2	0.4	0.00	0.07	**0.6**	208
Other and unspecified	35	0	0.8	0.5	-	-	-	0.9	-	-	3.9	5.0	6.7	9.9	25.9	36.5	82.7	79.0	119.1	144.3	2.5	4.6	0.27	0.86	**7.4**	O&U
All sites	761	2	13.8	6.0	8.9	7.2	18.6	26.9	40.6	94.8	117.1	182.1	245.8	322.5	433.8	592.7	744.5	843.0	834.0	1154.4	55.4		7.61	14.31	**127.3**	ALL
All sites but 173	753	2	13.8	6.0	8.9	7.2	18.6	26.9	40.6	93.3	117.1	177.1	242.4	317.5	427.4	583.6	730.7	843.0	834.0	1154.4	54.8	100.0	7.50	14.09	**125.8**	ALLb

| Rate from 1 case | | | 0.394 | 0.463 | 0.553 | 0.651 | 0.774 | 0.929 | 1.194 | 1.504 | 1.951 | 2.495 | 3.367 | 4.961 | 6.475 | 9.118 | 13.787 | 26.344 | 39.714 | 48.100 | | | | | | |

Philippines, Manila

The Philippine Cancer Society began cancer registration activity in 1959, with an attempt to organize a national cancer registry. Although this was not successful, it served as a pilot study. In 1968, the Society started the first formal registration activity in the Philippines when the Central Tumor Registry of the Philippines began collecting data from 25 hospitals in Metro Manila and one provincial hospital (Cebu), relying solely on passive notification of cases. This continued to function as a central registry for 26 hospitals until 1983, when it was converted to a population-based cancer registry covering the population of the four cities of Metropolitan Manila, namely Manila, Pasay, Caloocan and Quezon City. It was renamed as the Philippine Cancer Society–Manila Cancer Registry. Its first activity was retrospective collection of data on cancer occurring in the catchment area for the period 1980–82. Cancer registry clerks were trained to abstract pertinent cancer information from hospital records and death certificates.

The catchment area encompasses a land area of 274 km^2, located in the south-west portion of Luzon, and borders Manila Bay to the west, Bulacan to the north and Rizal province to the south-east. The city of Manila is the capital of the Philippines and is the country's main port, the hub of commerce and trade, and the seat of cultural and intellectual activites. It has the heaviest concentration of population in the Philippines, with a population density of 42 572 persons per km^2 in 1980–85.

The population of the four cities of Metropolitan Manila, based on the 1990 Census on Population and Housing conducted by the National Statistics Office, is 4 379 679, representing an increase of 19.8% as compared to that of the 1980 census. As a whole, the population is young.

Health services in the National Capital Region and the adjacent province of Rizal include 143 secondary and tertiary care hospitals, 43 primary care hospitals and 32 clinics of the Department of Health for outpatient consultations. Eight hospitals have radiotherapy facilities.

Since 1984, the registry has cooperated with the Department of Health – Rizal Cancer Registry to cover 94 hospitals within the National Capital Region and the Province of Rizal. Both registries use the same methods of data collection and the same forms.

Hospital data sources include medical records, radiotherapy records, pathology and haematology records and logs, radiology, ultrasound, nuclear medicine, CT scan and MRI reports and logs, and the hospital tumour registry (where available). Death certificates obtained from the office of the Local Civil Registrar are also reviewed.

Data are stored manually and on computer hard disk, with back-up diskettes. Checking for duplicate registrations is accomplished both manually and with the aid of the computer. Checks for consistency and validity of codes are performed with the CANREG program. Multiple primaries in a patient are coded according to the IARC/IACR rules and recorded separately under the same personal identity. Follow-up is not done except for a review of death certificates.

Problems encountered in the registry include: (a) the use of different names, particularly among the Chinese; (b) poor record-keeping in a number of hospitals; (c) absence of reports of private pathological examinations from the records of hospitals; (d) lack of manpower for data collection and other registry procedures; and (e) delay in data collection due to concern about confidentiality in some hospitals.

Data generated through the Manila and Rizal registries have served as a basis for planning most of the cancer control activities of the Philippine Cancer Control Programme of the Department of Health.

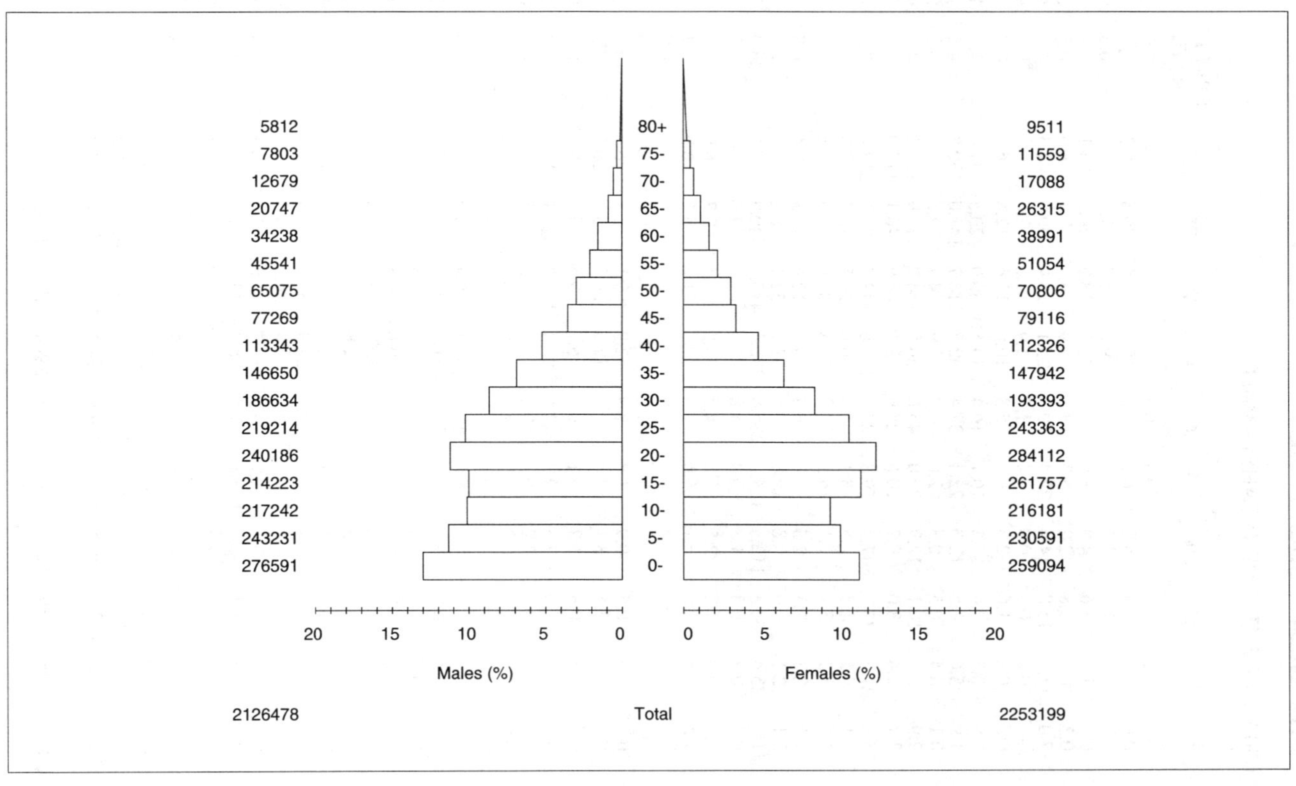

Philippines, Manila
Source of population: 1990
Census: 1990 Census on Population and Housing, Republic of the Philippines. National Statistics Office. Manila, June 1992.

Notes to tables overleaf:
* The high proportion of diagnoses based on a death certificate alone (DCO) indicate under-ascertainment.
† 188 does not include non-invasive tumours

* PHILIPPINES, MANILA 1988-1992

ANNUAL INCIDENCE PER 100,000 BY AGE GROUP (YEARS) - MALE

SITE	ALL AGES	AGE UNK	0-	5-	10-	15-	20-	25-	30-	35-	40-	45-	50-	55-	60-	65-	70-	75-	80+	CRUDE RATE	%	CR 64	CR 74	ASR (W)	ICD (9th)
Lip	5	0	-	-	-	-	-	0.1	-	-	0.2	-	-	0.9	0.6	-	-	-	-	0.0	0.0	0.01	0.01	**0.1**	*140*
Tongue	129	0	-	0.1	-	-	0.1	-	0.4	0.8	1.6	3.4	5.2	6.1	14.6	19.3	12.6	20.5	10.3	1.2	1.2	0.16	0.32	**2.6**	*141*
Salivary gland	68	0	0.1	0.1	0.1	0.4	0.1	0.3	0.2	0.7	0.4	1.8	3.7	1.3	5.3	9.6	6.3	7.7	-	0.6	0.6	0.07	0.15	**1.2**	*142*
Mouth	145	0	-	-	-	0.1	0.2	0.5	0.4	0.3	1.1	3.6	4.9	7.0	17.5	21.2	18.9	20.5	24.1	1.4	1.3	0.18	0.38	**3.1**	*143-5*
Oropharynx	52	2	-	-	-	-	-	0.2	0.1	0.3	0.9	0.8	2.2	5.3	4.1	2.9	4.7	7.7	6.9	0.5	0.5	0.07	0.11	**1.0**	*146*
Nasopharynx	490	1	-	0.2	0.6	0.8	1.1	2.8	3.8	7.0	11.3	15.8	14.4	22.4	29.2	25.1	28.4	30.8	41.3	4.6	4.5	0.55	0.82	**7.6**	*147*
Hypopharynx	12	0	-	-	-	-	-	-	0.1	-	0.2	0.3	0.3	0.4	1.8	1.9	1.6	2.6	-	0.1	0.1	0.02	0.03	**0.3**	*148*
Pharynx unspecified	71	0	0.1	-	0.1	0.2	-	0.1	0.1	0.5	0.2	1.6	2.5	4.4	5.8	10.6	12.6	12.8	6.9	0.7	0.7	0.08	0.19	**1.5**	*149*
Oesophagus	140	0	-	-	-	-	0.1	0.1	0.1	0.5	0.7	2.6	5.5	10.1	16.4	13.5	30.0	20.5	31.0	1.3	1.3	0.18	0.40	**3.1**	*150*
Stomach	494	1	-	0.1	-	0.1	0.2	0.6	2.1	1.9	5.6	7.5	12.0	22.4	37.4	62.7	116.7	141.0	130.8	4.6	4.6	0.45	1.35	**11.1**	*151*
Small intestine	23	0	-	-	-	-	-	-	0.1	0.1	0.4	0.5	0.3	2.6	1.8	2.9	4.7	2.6	-	0.2	0.2	0.03	0.07	**0.5**	*152*
Colon	512	0	-	-	-	0.5	0.3	1.3	1.5	2.9	5.1	10.1	12.9	29.0	45.6	66.5	64.7	117.9	151.4	4.8	4.7	0.55	1.20	**11.0**	*153*
Rectum	371	0	-	-	0.1	0.2	0.5	1.1	2.1	2.7	2.8	8.0	9.2	20.6	28.6	52.1	48.9	46.1	117.0	3.5	3.4	0.38	0.89	**7.7**	*154*
Liver	1307	1	0.4	0.1	0.7	0.3	1.0	2.9	9.8	15.8	21.4	35.7	47.3	59.3	87.6	111.8	149.9	171.7	213.4	12.3	12.1	1.41	2.72	**23.9**	*155*
Gallbladder etc.	65	0	-	-	-	-	-	0.1	0.2	0.3	0.1	0.5	1.3	2.5	3.1	1.8	10.6	20.5	10.3	13.8	0.6	0.6	0.05	0.20	**1.4**	*156*
Pancreas	211	0	-	-	-	-	-	0.1	0.2	0.2	1.5	1.2	3.1	7.1	14.5	22.8	30.8	37.9	33.3	41.3	2.0	2.0	0.25	0.60	**4.7**	*157*
Nose, sinuses etc.	88	0	-	-	0.1	0.1	0.2	0.2	0.4	1.1	2.3	2.3	2.5	4.0	6.4	5.8	12.6	10.3	3.4	0.8	0.8	0.10	0.19	**1.5**	*160*
Larynx	256	0	-	-	-	-	-	0.1	0.2	0.1	2.1	6.0	9.8	19.8	31.5	33.7	52.1	28.2	24.1	2.4	2.4	0.35	0.78	**5.6**	*161*
Bronchus, lung	2764	4	0.1	0.1	0.2	0.6	1.5	2.6	4.8	11.2	25.4	60.3	112.5	174.3	285.6	398.1	413.3	440.9	347.6	26.0	25.6	3.40	7.46	**58.7**	*162*
Other thoracic organs	31	0	-	-	-	0.3	0.3	0.5	0.1	0.3	0.2	0.3	1.8	0.9	1.8	1.0	1.6	2.6	-	0.3	0.3	0.03	0.04	**0.4**	*163-4*
Bone	107	0	0.1	0.1	1.0	1.6	1.4	0.5	0.6	0.4	0.9	1.3	2.5	1.8	4.7	4.8	9.5	7.7	6.9	1.0	1.0	0.08	0.16	**1.5**	*170*
Connective tissue	178	0	0.9	0.6	0.3	0.5	0.6	1.4	1.8	1.5	1.8	2.6	6.1	6.6	9.9	9.6	11.0	25.6	6.9	1.7	1.6	0.17	0.28	**2.6**	*171*
Mesothelioma	3	0	-	-	-	-	-	-	-	0.1	-	-	0.3	-	0.6	-	-	-	-	0.0	0.0	0.01	0.01	**0.0**	*MES*
Kaposi's sarcoma	4	0	-	-	-	-	-	0.1	0.1	-	-	-	-	-	1.2	-	-	-	-	0.0	0.0	0.01	0.01	**0.1**	*KAP*
Melanoma of skin	35	0	-	-	-	-	0.1	0.1	0.2	0.1	0.5	0.5	0.9	1.8	2.9	2.9	9.5	5.1	6.9	0.3	0.3	0.04	0.10	**0.7**	*172*
Other skin	135	0	-	-	0.1	0.2	0.3	0.3	1.0	0.8	2.1	2.6	3.1	7.0	12.3	12.5	20.5	23.1	20.6	1.3		0.15	0.31	**2.6**	*173*
Breast	41	0	-	0.1	0.1	-	-	-	-	0.5	0.4	0.8	1.2	3.1	0.6	6.7	9.5	5.1	10.3	0.4	0.4	0.03	0.11	**0.9**	*175*
Prostate	632	0	-	-	-	-	-	0.2	0.1	0.4	0.7	1.0	4.6	19.3	42.6	95.4	190.9	328.1	474.9	5.9	5.9	0.35	1.78	**17.6**	*185*
Testis	77	0	0.6	-	-	-	0.8	0.8	1.7	2.0	0.9	0.5	2.2	0.4	0.6	-	3.2	2.6	-	0.7	0.7	0.05	0.07	**0.7**	*186*
Penis	37	0	-	-	-	-	-	0.1	0.2	0.5	1.2	1.6	0.9	0.9	1.2	4.8	6.3	-	3.4	0.3	0.3	0.03	0.09	**0.7**	*187.1-.4*
Other male genital	4	0	-	-	-	-	0.1	0.1	-	-	-	-	-	0.4	-	-	-	2.6	-	0.0	0.0	0.00	0.00	**0.1**	*187.5-.9*
†Bladder	213	0	-	-	-	0.1	0.2	0.1	0.5	0.8	2.3	3.4	4.9	6.6	19.3	39.5	39.4	59.0	61.9	2.0	2.0	0.19	0.59	**4.9**	*188*
Kidney etc.	216	0	1.1	0.2	0.2	0.1	0.2	0.3	0.5	1.6	2.5	6.0	8.9	7.9	18.1	21.2	25.2	28.2	27.5	2.0	2.0	0.24	0.47	**4.0**	*189*
Eye	56	0	2.5	0.5	-	-	-	-	-	0.3	0.2	0.5	1.5	0.9	-	1.9	1.6	2.6	-	0.5	0.5	0.03	0.05	**0.6**	*190*
Brain, nervous system	183	0	0.7	1.5	1.3	1.0	0.5	1.2	0.8	1.1	2.1	3.9	5.2	7.5	8.2	10.6	6.3	7.7	13.8	1.7	1.7	0.17	0.26	**2.6**	*191-2*
Thyroid	175	0	-	0.2	0.2	0.2	0.7	1.4	1.8	1.8	2.5	1.6	4.6	8.3	13.4	18.3	17.4	12.8	10.3	1.6	1.6	0.18	0.36	**2.9**	*193*
Other endocrine	16	0	0.2	-	0.3	0.4	0.1	-	-	-	0.4	-	0.3	-	0.6	1.0	-	-	-	0.2	0.1	0.01	0.02	**0.2**	*194*
Hodgkin's disease	62	0	0.1	0.1	0.1	0.1	0.5	0.5	0.9	0.4	0.4	1.3	1.5	4.4	2.3	2.9	-	10.3	10.3	0.6	0.6	0.06	0.08	**0.9**	*201*
Non-Hodgkin lymphoma	353	0	0.8	0.5	0.7	2.1	1.7	1.6	2.8	3.1	3.7	5.7	7.7	17.1	20.4	28.9	33.1	35.9	34.4	3.3	3.3	0.34	0.65	**5.7**	*200,202*
Multiple myeloma	47	0	-	-	-	0.1	-	-	0.2	0.4	0.2	1.3	2.5	1.3	4.7	3.9	6.3	10.3	13.8	0.4	0.4	0.05	0.10	**1.0**	*203*
Lymphoid leukaemia	188	0	3.5	4.2	1.8	1.6	1.2	0.6	0.4	-	-	0.3	0.9	0.9	3.5	8.7	1.6	5.1	10.3	1.8	1.7	0.09	0.15	**2.0**	*204*
Myeloid leukaemia	169	0	1.1	1.5	1.4	1.4	1.7	0.7	0.6	1.9	1.9	1.3	2.5	3.1	1.8	8.7	14.2	7.7	6.9	1.6	1.6	0.10	0.22	**2.1**	*205*
Monocytic leukaemia	5	0	-	-	0.1	-	-	-	0.1	-	-	-	0.3	-	-	-	1.6	-	3.4	0.0	0.0	0.00	0.01	**0.1**	*206*
Other leukaemia	1	0	0.1	-	-	-	-	-	-	-	-	-	-	-	-	-	-	-	-	0.0	0.0	0.00	0.00	**0.0**	*207*
Leukaemia unspecified	139	0	0.8	1.4	2.1	0.8	1.2	0.9	0.4	1.9	0.7	1.6	0.6	1.8	3.5	3.9	12.6	5.1	3.4	1.3	1.3	0.09	0.17	**1.6**	*208*
Other and unspecified	626	2	0.7	0.8	0.6	1.3	1.2	0.7	2.8	3.5	6.9	13.7	23.7	30.7	47.9	67.5	82.0	102.5	96.4	5.9	5.8	0.67	1.42	**12.1**	*O&U*
All sites	10936	11	13.4	12.2	12.2	15.0	18.4	25.1	44.7	71.3	115.6	216.1	343.6	540.2	866.3	1233.9	1539.6	1814.7	1985.5	102.9		11.48	25.36	**215.1**	*ALL*
All sites but 173	10801	11	13.4	12.2	12.1	14.8	18.1	24.8	43.7	70.5	113.5	213.5	340.5	533.1	854.0	1221.4	1519.0	1791.6	1964.9	101.6	100.0	11.33	25.05	**212.5**	*ALLb*

Rate from 1 case   0.072 0.082 0.092 0.093 0.083 0.091 0.107 0.136 0.176 0.259 0.307 0.439 0.584 0.964 1.577 2.563 3.441

†Important: see notes on population page

* PHILIPPINES, MANILA 1988-1992

ANNUAL INCIDENCE PER 100,000 BY AGE GROUP (YEARS) - FEMALE

SITE	ALL AGES	AGE UNK	0-	5-	10-	15-	20-	25-	30-	35-	40-	45-	50-	55-	60-	65-	70-	75-	80+	CRUDE RATE	%	CR 64	CR 74	ASR (W)	ICD (9th)
Lip	6	0	-	-	-	-	-	0.2	-	-	-	-	0.3	0.8	0.5	0.8	-	1.7	-	0.1	0.0	0.01	0.01	**0.1**	*140*
Tongue	118	1	-	-	-	-	-	0.2	0.6	0.5	0.7	1.5	3.1	3.9	6.2	16.7	16.4	22.5	27.3	1.0	0.9	0.08	0.25	**2.1**	*141*
Salivary gland	63	0	-	-	-	0.1	0.1	0.1	0.3	0.5	1.6	1.0	0.8	3.9	1.5	8.4	7.0	6.9	6.3	0.6	0.5	0.05	0.13	**1.0**	*142*
Mouth	167	0	-	-	-	0.1	-	0.1	0.4	0.4	0.5	1.8	4.5	4.3	17.4	25.1	23.4	31.1	33.6	1.5	1.3	0.15	0.39	**3.2**	*143-5*
Oropharynx	40	0	-	-	-	-	0.1	0.2	-	0.4	0.2	0.5	1.1	1.6	3.6	6.1	1.2	10.4	2.1	0.4	0.3	0.04	0.07	**0.7**	*146*
Nasopharynx	259	0	-	0.1	-	0.3	0.6	0.7	1.8	3.5	3.7	7.8	9.6	15.3	11.8	11.4	15.2	19.0	14.7	2.3	2.0	0.28	0.41	**3.7**	*147*
Hypopharynx	7	0	-	-	-	-	-	-	0.1	-	-	0.5	0.8	-	-	0.8	-	-	-	0.1	0.1	0.01	0.01	**0.1**	*148*
Pharynx unspecified	52	0	-	-	-	-	0.1	0.2	-	-	0.2	0.5	1.4	1.6	2.6	8.4	8.2	10.4	14.7	0.5	0.4	0.03	0.12	**1.0**	*149*
Oesophagus	84	0	-	-	-	0.1	-	-	0.2	0.4	0.4	0.8	1.1	3.5	4.6	11.4	18.7	24.2	12.6	0.7	0.7	0.06	0.21	**1.6**	*150*
Stomach	366	1	-	-	-	-	0.4	0.8	1.1	1.9	4.5	5.3	9.3	13.3	26.7	37.2	51.5	57.1	71.5	3.2	2.8	0.32	0.76	**6.4**	*151*
Small intestine	17	0	-	0.1	-	-	-	0.1	-	-	0.9	0.3	0.6	0.4	1.0	1.5	1.2	-	2.1	0.2	0.1	0.02	0.03	**0.3**	*152*
Colon	506	1	-	-	0.1	0.2	0.4	1.1	1.4	2.0	3.4	8.3	12.7	21.2	34.9	55.5	63.2	100.4	105.1	4.5	3.9	0.43	1.02	**8.9**	*153*
Rectum	345	0	-	0.1	-	0.2	0.4	0.3	1.0	2.7	4.3	5.3	9.0	17.6	23.6	30.4	43.3	46.7	63.1	3.1	2.7	0.32	0.69	**5.9**	*154*
Liver	468	0	0.6	-	0.1	0.4	0.4	1.0	1.7	2.6	6.4	8.6	9.3	15.7	29.8	47.9	69.1	74.4	73.6	4.2	3.6	0.38	0.97	**8.0**	*155*
Gallbladder etc.	86	0	-	-	-	-	0.1	-	0.1	-	0.2	2.3	2.5	3.9	5.6	9.1	10.5	13.8	31.5	0.8	0.7	0.07	0.17	**1.6**	*156*
Pancreas	182	1	0.1	-	-	0.2	-	0.1	-	0.4	1.6	2.0	7.1	8.6	12.3	19.8	35.1	27.7	29.4	1.6	1.4	0.16	0.44	**3.3**	*157*
Nose, sinuses etc.	65	0	0.1	-	-	0.2	0.3	0.2	0.4	0.5	1.4	1.8	1.1	3.9	2.1	4.6	3.5	6.9	4.2	0.6	0.5	0.06	0.10	**0.9**	*160*
Larynx	52	0	-	-	-	-	0.1	-	0.3	-	0.4	0.8	0.6	2.7	5.6	5.3	4.7	12.1	10.5	0.5	0.4	0.05	0.10	**0.9**	*161*
Bronchus, lung	959	1	-	-	0.1	0.1	0.4	0.9	2.0	5.3	7.5	19.0	31.1	54.8	69.2	85.9	127.6	155.7	143.0	8.5	7.5	0.95	2.02	**16.8**	*162*
Other thoracic organs	18	0	-	-	-	0.2	-	0.2	0.3	-	0.4	0.5	0.3	0.8	1.0	-	-	1.7	-	0.2	0.1	0.02	0.02	**0.2**	*163-4*
Bone	91	0	-	0.3	1.2	1.3	0.4	0.1	0.2	0.5	1.4	1.0	0.8	4.3	2.6	3.0	5.9	5.2	6.3	0.8	0.7	0.07	0.11	**1.1**	*170*
Connective tissue	161	0	0.5	0.3	0.4	0.6	0.6	0.9	1.3	1.5	1.4	3.0	3.7	5.5	5.1	9.9	7.0	17.3	18.9	1.4	1.3	0.12	0.21	**2.1**	*171*
Mesothelioma	3	0	-	-	-	-	-	0.1	-	-	-	-	-	0.5	-	1.2	-	-	-	0.0	0.0	0.00	0.00	**0.1**	*MES*
Kaposi's sarcoma	0	0	-	-	-	-	-	-	-	-	-	-	-	-	-	-	-	-	-	0.0	0.0	0.00	0.00	**0.0**	*KAP*
Melanoma of skin	38	0	-	-	-	-	0.1	0.3	0.2	0.1	0.4	2.3	0.8	0.8	1.0	2.3	4.7	1.7	6.3	0.3	0.3	0.03	0.07	**0.6**	*172*
Other skin	115	1	-	-	-	-	0.4	0.2	1.2	0.5	2.1	1.8	3.1	4.3	5.1	11.4	8.2	8.7	23.1	1.0		0.10	0.19	**1.8**	*173*
Breast	3274	0	-	0.1	0.2	0.6	1.3	5.3	19.9	43.9	87.6	118.8	121.7	153.6	169.3	155.8	196.6	174.8	155.6	29.1	25.5	3.61	5.37	**47.7**	*174*
Uterus unspecified	242	0	-	-	-	0.1	0.3	1.1	1.4	3.1	3.7	9.4	9.0	11.0	8.7	12.9	19.9	10.4	25.2	2.1	1.9	0.24	0.40	**3.6**	*179*
Cervix uteri	1532	1	-	0.1	0.1	0.1	0.7	3.6	11.2	27.7	38.5	59.2	52.5	61.1	70.3	73.0	94.8	50.2	54.7	13.6	11.9	1.63	2.47	**21.6**	*180*
Placenta	55	0	-	-	-	0.2	1.1	0.9	0.7	1.1	0.9	1.0	0.3	0.4	-	-	-	-	-	0.5	0.4	0.03	0.03	**0.4**	*181*
Corpus uteri	362	0	-	-	-	0.1	0.2	0.6	0.9	3.0	6.1	8.8	20.9	26.2	23.1	29.6	17.6	10.4	10.5	3.2	2.8	0.45	0.69	**5.7**	*182*
Ovary etc.	692	2	0.5	0.5	0.6	1.2	2.0	3.9	3.5	8.9	12.8	22.0	24.9	23.9	35.4	25.8	36.3	39.8	29.4	6.1	5.4	0.70	1.01	**9.4**	*183*
Other female genital	64	0	-	-	-	-	-	-	0.2	0.4	0.9	2.3	2.3	2.4	4.6	3.8	7.0	8.7	12.6	0.6	0.5	0.07	0.12	**1.1**	*184*
†Bladder	82	0	-	-	-	-	0.1	-	0.3	0.1	0.4	1.5	1.4	3.5	4.6	11.4	15.2	15.6	18.9	0.7	0.6	0.06	0.19	**1.5**	*188*
Kidney etc.	161	0	0.9	0.2	-	0.2	0.1	0.2	0.6	1.4	2.5	2.5	4.2	5.5	12.8	16.0	18.7	10.4	6.3	1.4	1.3	0.16	0.33	**2.6**	*189*
Eye	38	0	1.5	0.2	0.1	0.2	0.1	0.2	-	0.3	0.4	-	-	0.5	-	1.2	1.7	6.3	-	0.3	0.3	0.02	0.02	**0.4**	*190*
Brain, nervous system	163	0	0.9	1.1	0.9	0.4	1.1	1.3	0.8	1.2	0.7	3.5	1.7	4.7	6.7	6.8	10.5	12.1	2.1	1.4	1.3	0.13	0.21	**2.0**	*191-2*
Thyroid	709	0	-	0.1	0.6	1.4	4.2	5.5	9.0	9.6	11.4	12.6	19.5	26.2	28.2	29.6	29.3	26.0	29.4	6.3	5.5	0.64	0.94	**8.7**	*193*
Other endocrine	12	0	-	0.1	-	0.1	0.1	0.2	0.2	0.3	-	-	0.6	-	0.5	-	-	-	-	0.1	0.1	0.01	0.01	**0.1**	*194*
Hodgkin's disease	34	0	0.1	0.1	-	0.2	0.3	0.4	0.3	0.3	0.2	0.8	0.8	0.8	0.5	0.8	1.2	3.5	2.1	0.3	0.3	0.02	0.03	**0.4**	*201*
Non-Hodgkin lymphoma	246	0	0.2	0.7	0.6	0.5	0.6	1.2	1.4	1.5	2.5	3.3	7.1	10.2	12.8	16.7	18.7	24.2	37.9	2.2	1.9	0.21	0.39	**3.6**	*200,202*
Multiple myeloma	34	0	-	-	-	0.1	-	-	-	0.3	0.2	0.5	1.4	2.7	1.0	2.3	3.5	8.7	6.3	0.3	0.3	0.03	0.06	**0.6**	*203*
Lymphoid leukaemia	142	0	3.2	2.3	1.5	0.8	0.8	0.4	0.5	0.8	0.2	0.8	1.1	0.4	1.0	2.3	3.5	1.7	4.2	1.3	1.1	0.07	0.10	**1.4**	*204*
Myeloid leukaemia	147	0	1.8	0.5	1.0	0.4	0.7	0.3	1.0	1.6	1.6	3.3	2.0	3.9	3.1	3.0	1.2	12.1	18.9	1.3	1.1	0.11	0.13	**1.7**	*205*
Monocytic leukaemia	8	0	-	-	-	-	0.1	-	0.3	-	-	0.5	-	-	-	0.8	-	-	-	0.1	0.1	0.00	0.01	**0.1**	*206*
Other leukaemia	1	0	-	-	-	-	-	-	-	-	-	-	-	-	-	0.8	-	-	-	0.0	0.0	0.00	0.00	**0.0**	*207*
Leukaemia unspecified	171	0	1.2	0.6	2.1	1.4	1.2	1.0	0.6	0.7	1.8	1.3	2.3	3.5	5.6	3.8	4.7	19.0	8.4	1.5	1.3	0.12	0.16	**1.9**	*208*
Other and unspecified	540	0	0.3	0.6	0.7	0.7	0.5	0.9	2.2	3.7	6.4	12.6	14.4	25.9	31.3	49.4	58.5	53.6	75.7	4.8	4.2	0.50	1.04	**8.8**	*O&U*
All sites	12977	9	12.0	8.0	10.5	12.4	20.1	34.7	70.0	133.7	222.0	341.3	403.1	558.6	694.5	857.3	1065.1	1138.5	1204.9	115.2		12.61	22.23	**195.6**	*ALL*
All sites but 173	12862	8	12.0	8.0	10.5	12.4	19.6	34.4	68.8	133.2	219.9	339.5	400.0	554.3	689.4	845.9	1056.9	1129.9	1181.8	114.2	100.0	12.52	22.04	**193.8**	*ALLb*

Rate from 1 case   0.077 0.087 0.093 0.076 0.070 0.082 0.103 0.135 0.178 0.253 0.282 0.392 0.513 0.760 1.170 1.730 2.103

†Important: see notes on population page

Singapore

Comprehensive population-based cancer registration began in January 1968. The registry was founded primarily to obtain information on cancer patterns in Singapore. It is staffed by one pathologist, three epidemiologists (all working part-time), two secretaries and one record-searcher (full-time). There is an Advisory Committee comprising representatives of the Ministry of Health, the Singapore Cancer Society and various hospital departments.

Registration covers the whole of the Republic of Singapore, situated in the centre of the Malayan archipelago at latitude 1°17′ N and longtitude 103°15′ E, comprising the main island of Singapore and several offshore islands which jointly cover an area of 641 km². The island lies at the southern tip of the Malayan peninsula, with which it is connected by a road and rail causeway. The highest point is 166 m above sea level. The maximum temperature is around 31°C and the minimum 24°C. The mean relative humidity is around 71%. The island generally has rainfall throughout the year (total annual rainfall approximately 2000 mm), but is particularly wet during the monsoon season from November to January.

The population (2 705 115 at the 1990 census) comprises several ethnic groups, the largest of which are Chinese (77.7%), Malays (14.1%) and Indians (7.1%). Overall, the population density is 4705 persons per km².

The Chinese in Singapore are for the most part derived from the south-eastern Chinese provinces of Fukien and Kwangtung. The major linguistic or dialect groups (1990 census) are Hokkiens, 42.2%; Teochew, 21.9%; Cantonese, 15.2%; Hakka, 7.3%; Hainanese, 7.0% and others, 6.4%. The Malays are derived from Malaysia and Indonesia. This racial group consists of Malays, 68.3%; Javanese,17.2%; Boyanese, 11.3%, and others 3.3%. The term "Indian" was used in the census to denote all persons derived from indigenous populations of the Indian sub-continent and includes Indians, Pakistanis and Sri Lankans. This population consists of Tamils, 63.9%; Malayalis, 8.6%; Sikhs, 6.7%, Hindustanis, 2.0% and others, 18.8%.

Sources of data for the cancer registry are: (a) cancer notifications from all sections of the medical profession, (b) pathology records, (c) hospital records, and (d) death certificates. Cancer notification is voluntary. All doctors in Singapore are provided with notification forms with prepaid postage. The registry ensures that notifications are as complete as possible by checking all pathology reports and death certificates issued in Singapore as well as records of all government hospitals. Cancer cases picked up from these sources are checked against registered cases and reminders are sent to doctors in charge of cases that have not been notified to the registry. Cancer cases not notified by doctors (approximately 10%) are registered by the registry staff on the basis of information derived from the sources mentioned above. Cancer registrations are reasonably comprehensive since all cases diagnosed histologically and all cases with a mention of cancer in hospital discharge forms and death certificates are included.

There is no personal contact with cases nor any patient follow-up by the registry. Information on diagnosis and survival is obtained through hospital pathology and death records.

The cancer notification forms and a register of cases are maintained on a current chronological basis. All relevant information is coded and the registry maintains a computerized file of all cases. Duplication of cases is avoided by checking all new cases against the master index.

The data have been used mainly to determine incidence levels and relative risks of cancers in Singapore by sex, ethnic groups and migrant status. Such information has formed the basis of epidemiological and clinical studies on specific cancers.

In 1990, there were 3423 registered medical practitioners (one for every 757 of the population), of whom 1593 were in private practice and 1831 in the full-time service of the Ministry of Health and National University of Singapore. A total of 9749 hospital beds (3.6 hospital beds per 1000 population) were available, 7922 in 11 government and institutional hospitals and 1827 in 10 private hospitals. The government also provides 18 maternal and child health clinics and 21 outpatient clinics offering an essentially general practitioner type of service, in addition to several hundred private clinics. Certification of death is virtually complete. In 1990, 96.4% of all deaths were certifed by qualified medical practitioners or the coroner and 3.6% by inspecting officers. The latter would certify a case as cancer only on the basis of a previous hospital diagnosis.

H.P. Lee
K.S. Chia
Adeline L.H. Seow
K. Shanmugaratnam

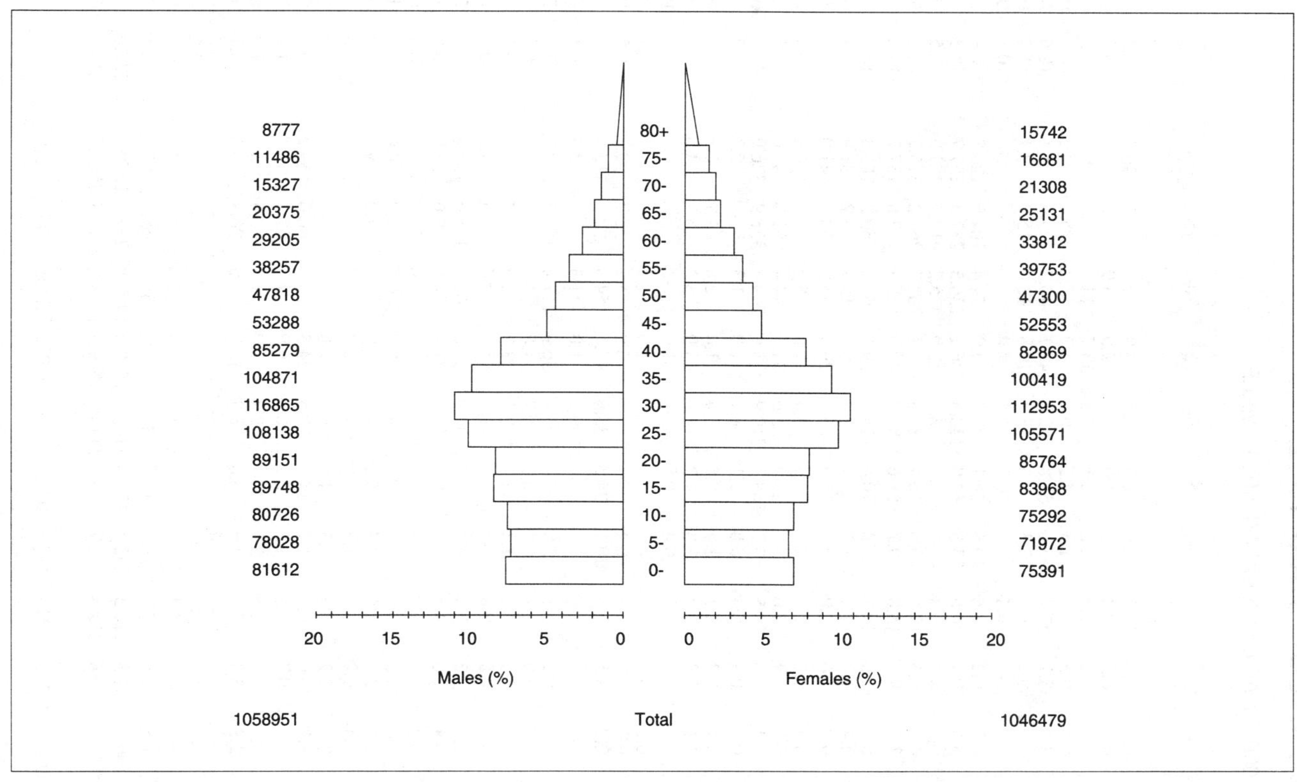

Singapore: Chinese
Source of population: 1990
Census: Census of Population 1990, Department of Statistics, Singapore

Notes to tables overleaf:
† 188 does not include non-invasive tumours

SINGAPORE: CHINESE 1988-1992

ANNUAL INCIDENCE PER 100,000 BY AGE GROUP (YEARS) - MALE

SITE	ALL AGES	AGE UNK	0-	5-	10-	15-	20-	25-	30-	35-	40-	45-	50-	55-	60-	65-	70-	75-	80+	CRUDE RATE	%	CR 64	CR 74	ASR (W)	ICD (9th)
Lip	1	0	-	-	-	-	-	-	-	-	-	0.4	-	-	-	-	-	-	-	0.0	0.0	0.00	0.00	0.0	140
Tongue	63	0	-	-	-	-	0.2	-	0.3	0.8	2.1	0.8	2.9	0.5	7.5	4.9	9.1	8.7	20.5	1.2	0.6	0.08	0.15	1.3	141
Salivary gland	34	0	-	-	0.2	0.2	0.4	1.1	0.2	0.6	0.5	0.4	2.9	1.0	-	2.0	3.9	5.2	-	0.6	0.3	0.04	0.07	0.6	142
Mouth	67	0	-	-	-	-	0.2	-	0.2	-	0.2	1.9	3.8	3.1	6.8	13.7	14.4	8.7	9.1	1.3	0.6	0.08	0.22	1.6	143-5
Oropharynx	39	0	-	-	-	-	-	-	-	0.2	0.5	-	1.3	4.2	6.8	3.9	5.2	5.2	9.1	0.7	0.3	0.06	0.11	0.9	146
Nasopharynx	985	2	-	-	0.2	1.3	1.6	5.9	14.0	23.3	38.7	57.4	55.6	51.8	52.0	47.1	40.5	29.6	25.1	18.6	8.7	1.51	1.95	18.5	147
Hypopharynx	70	0	-	-	0.2	-	-	-	-	-	0.2	-	3.3	7.3	8.2	10.8	13.0	15.7	9.1	1.3	0.6	0.10	0.22	1.7	148
Pharynx unspecified	6	0	-	-	-	-	-	-	-	-	-	0.4	-	0.5	1.4	2.0	-	-	-	0.1	0.1	0.01	0.02	0.2	149
Oesophagus	365	0	-	-	-	-	-	-	-	0.2	0.2	3.4	10.5	26.7	37.0	53.0	74.4	104.5	120.8	6.9	3.2	0.39	1.03	8.6	150
Stomach	1245	1	-	-	-	-	0.2	1.1	1.5	3.6	9.4	14.6	33.5	64.8	138.3	206.1	250.5	287.3	357.7	23.5	11.0	1.34	3.62	29.3	151
Small intestine	25	0	-	-	-	-	-	-	0.2	-	0.7	0.8	-	1.6	2.1	2.0	5.2	10.4	2.3	0.5	0.2	0.03	0.06	0.5	152
Colon	1063	2	-	-	0.2	0.2	1.1	1.5	2.4	4.2	10.6	17.6	40.6	60.1	84.9	153.1	202.3	261.2	275.7	20.1	9.4	1.12	2.90	24.2	153
Rectum	784	0	-	-	-	-	0.4	0.4	2.4	3.1	9.4	15.0	29.7	58.6	84.9	109.0	135.7	137.6	157.2	14.8	6.9	1.02	2.24	18.0	154
Liver	961	0	0.5	0.5	0.2	-	0.2	0.9	2.7	6.1	10.8	19.1	31.8	70.6	115.7	129.6	167.0	160.2	166.3	18.1	8.5	1.30	2.78	22.1	155
Gallbladder etc.	75	0	-	-	-	-	-	-	-	0.4	1.2	1.1	1.7	4.7	6.2	5.9	15.7	19.2	31.9	1.4	0.7	0.08	0.18	1.7	156
Pancreas	215	0	-	-	-	-	-	-	0.9	0.8	1.6	3.0	9.2	14.6	25.3	29.4	35.2	50.5	41.0	4.1	1.9	0.28	0.60	4.9	157
Nose, sinuses etc.	42	0	-	-	-	0.4	-	0.2	0.3	0.4	1.2	2.3	3.3	2.6	3.4	1.0	5.2	-	2.3	0.8	0.4	0.07	0.10	0.9	160
Larynx	236	0	-	-	-	-	-	-	0.3	0.6	1.9	3.0	5.0	20.9	31.4	44.4	52.2	41.0	-	4.5	2.1	0.33	0.71	5.5	161
Bronchus, lung	2620	2	-	-	0.2	0.2	-	0.4	1.5	3.4	11.0	34.5	70.7	168.3	310.9	433.9	549.4	558.9	726.9	49.5	23.1	3.01	7.93	62.7	162
Other thoracic organs	37	0	-	-	-	0.7	0.9	0.4	0.7	0.8	0.9	0.4	0.8	2.1	4.1	1.0	1.3	-	2.3	0.7	0.3	0.06	0.07	0.7	163-4
Bone	43	0	-	-	0.2	1.3	0.9	1.1	1.0	0.4	0.7	1.1	1.7	0.5	1.4	1.0	2.6	1.7	2.3	0.8	0.4	0.05	0.07	0.8	170
Connective tissue	86	0	0.2	0.5	0.2	1.1	1.1	1.5	0.9	1.1	2.3	2.3	3.3	4.7	4.8	3.9	5.2	5.2	4.6	1.6	0.8	0.12	0.17	1.7	171
Mesothelioma	3	0	-	-	-	-	-	-	-	-	-	-	0.4	0.5	-	1.0	-	-	-	0.1	0.0	0.00	0.01	0.1	MES
Kaposi's sarcoma	5	0	-	-	-	-	0.2	-	0.2	0.2	-	-	-	-	-	1.0	1.3	-	-	0.1	0.0	0.00	0.01	0.1	KAP
Melanoma of skin	27	0	-	-	-	0.2	-	-	-	0.2	0.2	1.1	0.4	-	-	6.9	5.2	8.7	9.1	0.5	0.2	0.01	0.07	0.6	172
Other skin	405	6	-	-	-	0.2	0.4	0.4	0.5	2.7	3.5	7.5	20.1	24.6	35.6	49.1	54.8	92.3	113.9	7.6		0.48	1.01	9.1	173
Breast	4	0	-	-	-	-	-	-	-	-	-	-	-	-	0.7	1.0	1.3	-	2.3	0.1	0.0	0.00	0.01	0.1	175
Prostate	415	2	-	-	-	-	-	-	-	-	0.2	-	2.9	8.9	27.4	56.9	121.4	160.2	239.3	7.8	3.7	0.20	1.09	9.8	185
Testis	49	0	2.5	0.3	0.2	0.7	0.4	1.3	0.7	1.7	0.9	1.1	0.8	0.5	0.7	1.0	-	-	-	0.9	0.4	0.06	0.06	0.9	186
Penis	30	0	-	0.3	-	-	-	0.4	-	-	0.5	-	1.3	3.7	2.7	3.9	3.9	1.7	6.8	0.6	0.3	0.04	0.08	0.7	187.1-.4
Other male genital	16	0	-	-	-	-	-	0.2	-	0.2	0.5	0.8	-	0.5	2.1	-	2.6	3.5	4.6	0.3	0.1	0.02	0.03	0.3	187.5-.9
†Bladder	331	0	-	-	-	-	0.2	0.4	1.0	1.0	1.2	3.4	9.2	11.5	34.9	54.0	61.3	101.0	109.4	6.3	2.9	0.31	0.89	7.7	188
Kidney etc.	184	0	0.5	0.5	0.2	0.2	0.4	0.4	0.5	0.4	2.6	4.5	5.4	9.9	17.8	31.4	32.6	29.6	31.9	3.5	1.6	0.22	0.54	4.3	189
Eye	16	0	2.9	-	-	-	-	-	-	0.2	-	-	0.4	-	-	-	2.6	-	-	0.3	0.1	0.02	0.03	0.4	190
Brain, nervous system	114	0	2.0	2.3	2.2	0.9	1.1	2.0	1.5	1.0	2.3	3.0	2.1	4.2	4.1	5.9	6.5	7.0	4.6	2.2	1.0	0.14	0.21	2.3	191-2
Thyroid	100	0	-	-	-	0.7	1.3	1.3	0.5	1.7	2.3	4.5	3.3	5.2	8.9	7.9	3.9	7.0	9.1	1.9	0.9	0.15	0.21	2.0	193
Other endocrine	30	0	1.0	0.5	0.5	0.4	0.9	-	0.3	0.4	0.2	-	1.3	1.6	1.4	2.0	1.3	-	-	0.6	0.3	0.04	0.06	0.6	194
Hodgkin's disease	22	0	-	-	1.0	1.1	0.2	-	0.2	0.2	0.2	0.4	1.3	1.0	0.7	2.0	-	-	-	0.4	0.2	0.03	0.04	0.5	201
Non-Hodgkin lymphoma	290	0	1.5	1.0	1.2	0.7	1.8	1.8	2.6	3.2	5.6	6.4	11.7	14.1	20.5	24.5	28.7	40.0	59.2	5.5	2.6	0.36	0.63	6.1	200,202
Multiple myeloma	53	0	-	-	-	-	-	0.2	0.2	-	0.7	1.5	1.7	2.1	6.8	6.9	7.8	12.2	13.7	1.0	0.5	0.07	0.14	1.2	203
Lymphoid leukaemia	99	0	6.1	3.8	2.7	3.1	0.9	0.7	0.7	0.4	-	1.5	2.1	-	2.7	2.9	1.3	3.5	2.3	1.9	0.9	0.12	0.15	2.3	204
Myeloid leukaemia	165	0	2.0	0.8	0.7	1.8	0.7	1.5	2.7	2.3	3.3	3.8	4.6	6.8	8.9	12.8	19.6	20.9	6.8	3.1	1.5	0.20	0.36	3.3	205
Monocytic leukaemia	1	0	-	-	-	-	-	-	-	-	-	-	0.4	-	-	-	-	-	-	0.0	0.0	0.00	0.00	0.0	206
Other leukaemia	0	0	-	-	-	-	-	-	-	-	-	-	-	-	-	-	-	-	-	0.0	0.0	0.00	0.00	0.0	207
Leukaemia unspecified	13	0	0.5	-	-	0.2	0.2	-	-	-	-	0.4	-	-	1.4	1.0	2.6	1.7	4.6	0.2	0.1	0.01	0.03	0.3	208
Other and unspecified	323	0	-	0.3	0.5	-	0.4	0.4	0.7	1.5	2.8	7.1	11.7	13.6	37.0	61.8	58.7	55.7	57.0	6.1	2.8	0.38	0.98	7.6	O&U
All sites	11757	15	19.6	10.8	11.1	16.0	16.8	25.3	41.9	66.9	131.3	226.3	392.7	678.0	1149.8	1578.4	1997.8	2267.1	2679.7	222.0		13.95	31.86	267.1	ALL
All sites but 173	11352	9	19.6	10.8	11.1	15.8	16.4	25.0	41.4	64.3	127.8	218.8	372.7	653.5	1114.2	1529.3	1943.0	2174.8	2565.7	214.4	100.0	13.47	30.84	258.0	ALLb

Rate from 1 case 0.245 0.256 0.248 0.223 0.224 0.185 0.171 0.191 0.235 0.375 0.418 0.523 0.685 0.982 1.305 1.741 2.279

†Important: see notes on population page

SINGAPORE: CHINESE 1988-1992

ANNUAL INCIDENCE PER 100,000 BY AGE GROUP (YEARS) - FEMALE

SITE	ALL AGES	AGE UNK	0-	5-	10-	15-	20-	25-	30-	35-	40-	45-	50-	55-	60-	65-	70-	75-	80+	CRUDE RATE	%	CR 64	CR 74	ASR (W)	ICD (9th)
Lip	0	0	-	-	-	-	-	-	-	-	-	-	-	-	-	-	-	-	-	0.0	0.0	0.00	0.00	0.0	140
Tongue	38	0	-	-	-	-	-	0.2	0.2	0.8	1.2	1.1	0.8	2.5	1.8	3.2	2.8	4.8	3.8	0.7	0.4	0.04	0.07	0.7	141
Salivary gland	32	1	-	-	0.5	0.2	0.2	0.2	0.4	0.8	0.7	0.8	0.8	0.5	1.2	2.4	3.8	2.4	1.3	0.6	0.3	0.03	0.06	0.6	142
Mouth	33	0	-	-	-	-	-	-	0.2	0.2	0.5	0.4	0.8	3.0	1.8	3.2	5.6	1.2	7.6	0.6	0.3	0.03	0.08	0.6	143-5
Oropharynx	13	0	-	-	-	-	-	-	-	0.2	0.5	0.4	-	1.0	0.6	0.8	0.9	2.4	2.5	0.2	0.1	0.01	0.02	0.2	146
Nasopharynx	421	2	-	-	0.3	-	1.2	2.8	8.3	12.5	14.5	18.6	24.5	17.6	20.1	16.7	13.1	14.4	6.4	8.0	3.9	0.61	0.76	7.3	147
Hypopharynx	5	0	-	-	-	-	-	-	-	-	-	-	-	-	0.6	1.6	-	2.4	-	0.1	0.0	0.00	0.01	0.1	148
Pharynx unspecified	1	0	-	-	-	-	-	-	-	-	-	-	-	-	-	-	-	1.2	-	0.0	0.0	0.00	Ph.00	0.0	149
Oesophagus	134	0	-	-	-	-	-	-	-	0.2	0.2	0.8	1.3	3.5	6.5	10.3	22.5	38.4	50.8	2.6	1.3	0.06	0.23	2.2	150
Stomach	769	1	-	-	-	0.2	-	0.6	2.5	6.2	6.5	11.0	17.8	38.2	44.4	81.2	113.6	125.9	180.4	14.7	7.2	0.64	1.61	13.6	151
Small intestine	24	0	-	-	-	-	-	-	-	-	0.5	0.4	0.8	2.5	1.8	1.6	0.9	3.6	6.4	0.5	0.2	0.03	0.04	0.4	152
Colon	1160	3	-	-	0.5	0.7	0.7	1.5	2.7	7.4	8.0	18.3	35.5	57.4	80.4	120.2	157.7	205.0	233.8	22.2	10.8	1.07	2.46	21.0	153
Rectum	561	0	-	-	0.3	-	-	0.6	1.8	2.4	4.6	10.7	20.3	23.6	36.1	64.5	87.3	87.5	108.0	10.7	5.2	0.50	1.26	10.3	154
Liver	320	0	1.3	0.6	-	0.5	-	0.4	-	0.8	2.7	4.6	6.8	11.6	19.5	42.2	36.6	67.1	78.8	6.1	3.0	0.24	0.64	5.8	155
Gallbladder etc.	104	0	-	-	-	-	-	0.2	-	0.8	-	2.7	3.4	4.5	8.3	8.8	19.7	10.8	25.4	2.0	1.0	0.10	0.24	1.9	156
Pancreas	181	0	-	-	0.5	-	0.2	-	0.2	1.4	1.0	3.8	5.5	7.5	11.2	19.1	31.0	30.0	34.3	3.5	1.7	0.16	0.41	3.3	157
Nose, sinuses etc.	21	0	-	-	-	0.2	0.2	-	0.2	0.2	0.5	-	1.7	0.5	3.5	0.8	0.9	1.2	1.3	0.4	0.2	0.04	0.04	0.4	160
Larynx	34	1	-	-	-	-	-	-	-	-	-	0.8	0.4	1.0	3.5	8.0	5.6	4.8	2.5	0.6	0.3	0.03	0.10	0.7	161
Bronchus, lung	1092	0	-	-	-	-	-	0.2	1.1	1.8	4.0	5.8	12.2	28.8	38.2	75.7	131.3	170.8	217.0	252.8	20.9	10.2	0.84	2.35	19.6	162
Other thoracic organs	27	1	-	-	-	-	-	-	0.4	0.4	0.4	0.5	1.5	2.1	1.5	1.2	0.8	-	2.4	1.3	0.5	0.3	0.04	0.05	0.5	163-4
Bone	50	0	0.5	0.3	0.8	1.4	0.5	1.5	1.6	0.4	1.2	0.4	0.8	0.5	0.6	1.6	3.8	-	1.3	1.0	0.5	0.05	0.08	0.9	170
Connective tissue	63	0	0.3	0.6	1.6	0.2	1.2	0.6	-	1.0	1.2	1.5	3.0	1.5	1.8	1.6	10.3	3.6	2.5	1.2	0.6	0.07	0.13	1.2	171
Mesothelioma	2	0	-	-	-	-	-	-	-	-	-	-	0.4	0.5	-	-	-	-	-	0.0	0.0	0.00	0.00	0.0	MES
Kaposi's sarcoma	0	0	-	-	-	-	-	-	-	-	-	-	-	-	-	-	-	-	-	0.0	0.0	0.00	0.00	0.0	KAP
Melanoma of skin	34	0	-	-	-	-	0.5	0.4	0.2	0.6	0.2	0.8	1.3	0.5	2.4	1.6	1.9	3.6	10.2	0.6	0.3	0.03	0.05	0.6	172
Other skin	471	3	-	-	-	-	0.5	0.8	2.3	2.8	4.3	8.8	9.7	13.1	24.3	35.0	65.7	76.7	160.1	9.0		0.33	0.84	8.0	173
Breast	2187	3	-	-	-	-	0.7	5.5	18.1	47.2	91.2	125.2	110.8	100.6	105.9	124.9	105.1	117.5	124.5	41.8	20.4	3.03	4.18	39.5	174
Uterus unspecified	0	0	-	-	-	-	-	-	-	-	-	-	-	-	-	-	-	-	-	0.0	0.0	0.00	0.00	0.0	179
Cervix uteri	879	1	-	-	-	0.5	0.2	1.3	5.1	17.1	32.1	45.7	50.3	51.8	45.0	60.5	46.0	58.7	35.6	16.8	8.2	1.25	1.78	16.3	180
Placenta	7	0	-	-	-	-	0.2	0.2	0.7	0.2	-	-	-	-	-	-	-	-	-	0.1	0.1	0.01	0.01	0.1	181
Corpus uteri	366	0	-	-	-	-	0.2	-	1.6	6.4	9.7	18.3	17.8	36.7	27.2	27.9	15.0	16.8	12.7	7.0	3.4	0.59	0.80	7.0	182
Ovary etc.	585	0	0.3	1.1	0.8	1.7	5.8	6.4	8.9	8.6	13.0	27.8	34.2	26.2	27.8	34.2	21.6	40.8	14.0	11.2	5.5	0.81	1.09	10.7	183
Other female genital	57	0	-	-	-	-	0.2	0.2	0.2	0.4	0.5	1.9	0.8	2.0	3.0	6.4	7.5	10.8	11.4	1.1	0.5	0.05	0.12	1.0	184
†Bladder	112	0	-	-	-	-	0.2	-	-	-	0.5	1.1	3.4	4.5	6.5	12.7	17.8	28.8	24.1	2.1	1.0	0.08	0.23	2.0	188
Kidney etc.	116	0	1.6	-	-	0.2	-	0.4	0.7	-	1.0	3.8	3.4	4.5	8.9	12.7	10.3	18.0	19.1	2.2	1.1	0.12	0.24	2.2	189
Eye	11	1	1.9	-	-	-	-	-	0.4	-	-	-	-	-	0.6	-	-	-	-	0.2	0.1	0.02	0.02	0.3	190
Brain, nervous system	93	0	1.1	1.7	1.9	1.0	0.9	1.1	1.4	1.8	0.5	1.1	1.7	1.0	4.7	8.0	5.6	4.8	7.6	1.8	0.9	0.10	0.17	1.8	191-2
Thyroid	353	2	-	-	0.8	1.9	5.8	5.5	8.1	7.6	8.4	13.3	10.1	12.6	11.8	13.5	16.9	18.0	16.5	6.7	3.3	0.43	0.59	6.0	193
Other endocrine	17	0	1.1	0.6	0.8	-	-	-	0.4	0.2	-	-	0.4	0.5	-	-	2.8	-	-	0.3	0.2	0.02	0.03	0.4	194
Hodgkin's disease	20	0	-	-	0.8	-	0.5	0.4	0.2	0.8	0.5	-	-	-	0.6	0.8	-	1.2	3.8	0.4	0.2	0.02	0.02	0.3	201
Non-Hodgkin lymphoma	232	0	1.1	0.3	0.8	0.7	1.2	1.1	1.2	2.6	2.7	8.0	3.4	9.1	22.5	24.7	28.2	21.6	19.1	4.4	2.2	0.27	0.54	4.5	200,202
Multiple myeloma	47	0	-	-	-	-	-	-	0.2	0.2	1.0	1.1	0.8	1.5	1.8	4.8	4.7	13.2	10.2	0.9	0.4	0.03	0.08	0.8	203
Lymphoid leukaemia	74	0	5.3	4.4	1.6	1.0	0.7	0.6	0.5	-	0.2	1.1	0.4	0.5	3.0	0.8	0.9	3.6	3.8	1.4	0.7	0.10	0.11	1.8	204
Myeloid leukaemia	115	0	0.8	0.6	-	1.9	2.1	2.1	1.2	1.2	2.7	2.7	0.8	6.0	4.1	1.6	10.3	13.2	7.6	2.2	1.1	0.13	0.19	2.0	205
Monocytic leukaemia	0	0	-	-	-	-	-	-	-	-	-	-	-	-	-	-	-	-	-	0.0	0.0	0.00	0.00	0.0	206
Other leukaemia	1	0	-	0.3	-	-	-	-	-	-	-	-	-	-	`	-	-	-	-	0.0	0.0	0.00	0.00	0.0	207
Leukaemia unspecified	14	0	1.1	-	-	0.5	-	0.2	-	-	-	0.4	-	0.5	-	-	-	4.8	1.3	0.3	0.1	0.01	0.01	0.3	208
Other and unspecified	306	0	1.1	-	-	-	0.2	0.8	-	3.0	3.1	4.9	8.9	19.1	14.8	32.6	44.1	48.0	55.9	5.8	2.9	0.28	0.66	5.6	O&U
All sites	11182	19	17.2	10.3	12.0	12.9	24.5	36.9	71.4	140.2	221.6	355.8	414.0	508.1	635.3	922.4	1091.6	1326.0	1538.5	213.7		12.32	22.41	202.5	ALL
All sites but 173	10711	16	17.2	10.3	12.0	12.9	24.0	36.2	69.1	137.4	217.2	347.1	404.2	495.1	611.0	887.4	1025.9	1249.3	1378.4	204.7	100.0	11.99	21.57	194.6	ALLb

Rate from 1 case			0.265	0.278	0.266	0.238	0.233	0.189	0.177	0.199	0.241	0.381	0.423	0.503	0.591	0.796	0.939	1.199	1.270

†Important: see notes on population page

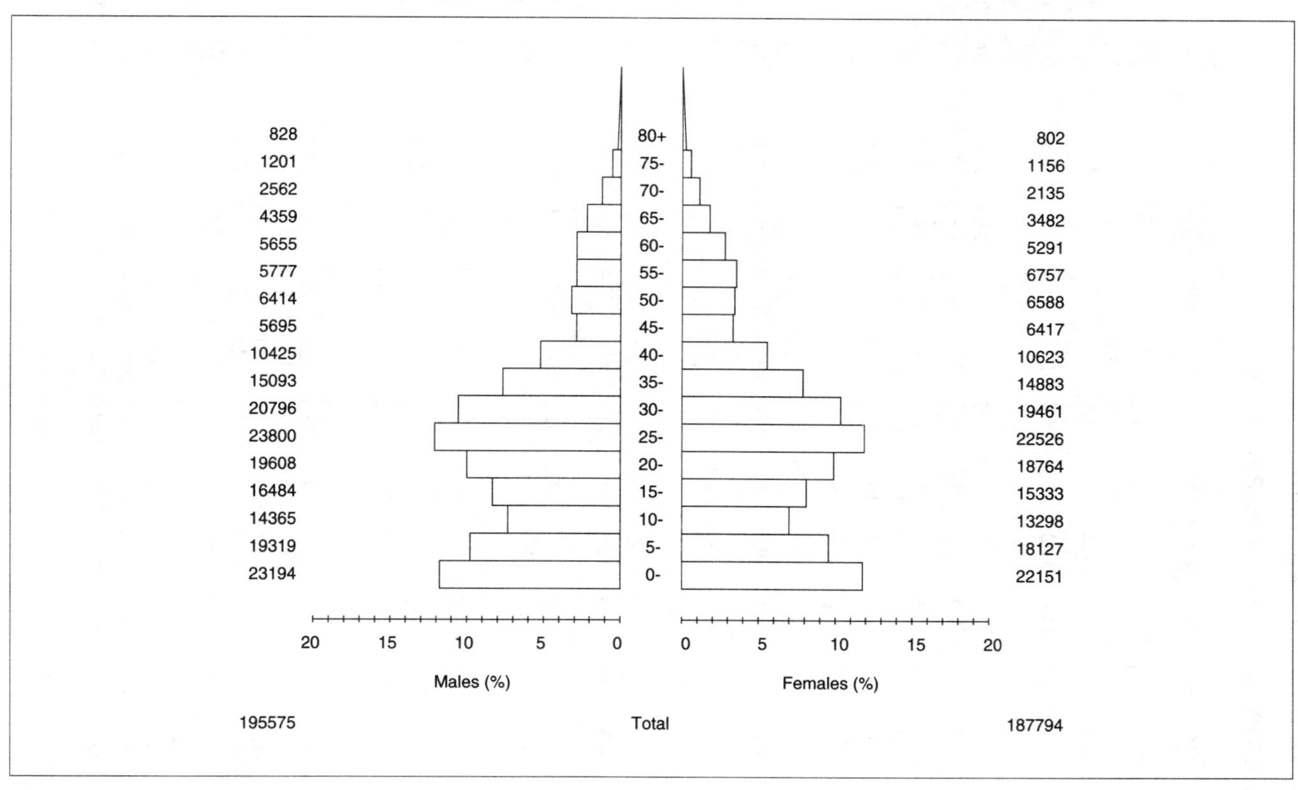

Singapore: Malay
Source of population: 1990
Census: Census of Population 1990, Department of Statistics, Singapore

Notes to tables overleaf:
† 188 does not include non-invasive tumours

SINGAPORE: MALAY 1988-1992

ANNUAL INCIDENCE PER 100,000 BY AGE GROUP (YEARS) - MALE

SITE	ALL AGES	AGE UNK	0-	5-	10-	15-	20-	25-	30-	35-	40-	45-	50-	55-	60-	65-	70-	75-	80+	CRUDE RATE	%	CR 64	CR 74	ASR (W)	ICD (9th)
Lip	0	0	-	-	-	-	-	-	-	-	-	-	-	-	-	-	-	-	-	0.0	0.0	0.00	0.00	0.0	140
Tongue	4	0	-	-	-	-	1.0	-	1.0	-	1.9	-	-	-	3.5	-	-	-	-	0.4	0.4	0.04	0.04	0.4	141
Salivary gland	4	0	-	-	-	-	-	-	-	-	-	-	-	3.5	13.8	-	-	-	-	0.4	0.4	0.02	0.09	0.6	142
Mouth	7	0	-	-	-	-	-	-	1.3	-	-	6.2	-	3.5	-	7.8	16.7	24.1		0.7	0.7	0.06	0.09	1.1	143-5
Oropharynx	6	0	-	-	-	-	-	-	-	-	-	3.1	-	7.1	-	7.8	33.3	-		0.6	0.6	0.05	0.09	0.9	146
Nasopharynx	50	0	-	-	-	2.4	1.0	-	7.7	1.3	7.7	14.0	31.2	24.2	24.8	18.4	15.6	-	-	5.1	5.0	0.57	0.74	6.5	147
Hypopharynx	1	0	-	-	-	-	-	-	-	-	-	-	-	-	-	7.8	-	-		0.1	0.1	0.00	0.04	0.2	148
Pharynx unspecified	0	0	-	-	-	-	-	-	-	-	-	-	-	-	-	-	-	-		0.0	0.0	0.00	0.00	0.0	149
Oesophagus	6	0	-	-	-	-	-	-	-	-	-	3.5	3.1	-	3.5	-	-	33.3	24.1	0.6	0.6	0.05	0e.05	1.1	150
Stomach	59	0	-	-	-	-	-	-	1.0	1.3	5.8	10.5	15.6	24.2	42.4	59.6	62.4	66.6	48.3	6.0	5.9	0.50	1.11	8.7	151
Small intestine	2	0	-	-	-	-	-	-	-	-	-	-	3.1	-	-	-	-	16.7	-	0.2	0.2	0.02	0.02	0.3	152
Colon	76	0	-	-	-	1.2	-	2.5	1.0	-	1.9	17.6	9.4	31.2	56.6	68.8	109.3	99.9	48.3	7.8	7.6	0.61	1.50	11.2	153
Rectum	52	0	-	-	-	-	-	-	-	2.7	3.8	14.0	24.9	17.3	31.8	45.9	46.8	99.9	-	5.3	5.2	0.47	0.94	7.8	154
Liver	83	0	-	-	-	-	1.0	0.8	4.8	8.0	13.4	14.0	12.5	10.4	42.4	91.8	62.4	133.2	96.5	8.5	8.3	0.54	1.31	11.6	155
Gallbladder etc.	12	0	-	-	-	-	-	-	1.0	-	3.8	-	3.1	-	3.5	13.8	15.6	16.7	24.1	1.2	1.2	0.06	0.20	1.7	156
Pancreas	13	0	0.9	-	-	-	-	-	-	-	-	7.0	3.1	3.5	7.1	13.8	15.6	16.7	-	1.3	1.3	0.11	0.25	2.0	157
Nose, sinuses etc.	4	0	-	-	-	-	1.0	-	-	-	-	-	3.1	3.5	-	4.6	-	-	-	0.4	0.4	0.04	0.06	0.5	160
Larynx	15	0	-	-	-	-	-	-	-	-	-	7.0	-	6.9	-	13.8	46.8	16.7	24.1	1.5	1.5	0.07	0.37	2.5	161
Bronchus, lung	240	0	-	-	-	1.2	-	1.7	1.0	4.0	19.2	35.1	49.9	86.5	145.0	197.3	351.2	366.4	506.8	24.5	23.9	1.72	4.46	37.2	162
Other thoracic organs	5	0	-	-	-	1.2	-	0.8	-	-	-	-	-	6.9	-	4.6	-	-	-	0.5	0.5	0.04	0.07	0.6	163-4
Bone	6	0	-	-	1.4	1.2	2.0	-	-	-	-	-	-	3.5	-	4.6	-	-	-	0.6	0.6	0.04	0.06	0.7	170
Connective tissue	13	0	0.9	-	-	-	-	1.7	-	-	1.9	7.0	3.1	-	-	18.4	15.6	-	-	1.3	1.3	0.07	0.24	1.8	171
Mesothelioma	0	0	-	-	-	-	-	-	-	-	-	-	-	-	-	-	-	-	-	0.0	0.0	0.00	Mes.00	0.0	MES
Kaposi's sarcoma	0	0	-	-	-	-	-	-	-	-	-	-	-	-	-	-	-	-	-	0.0	0.0	0.00	0.00	0.0	KAP
Melanoma of skin	1	0	-	-	-	-	-	0.8	-	-	-	-	-	-	-	-	-	-	-	0.1	0.1	0.00	0.00	0.1	172
Other skin	30	0	-	-	-	-	-	0.8	-	1.3	3.8	3.5	12.5	6.9	21.2	41.3	23.4	16.7	-	3.1		0.25	0.57	4.2	173
Breast	3	0	-	-	-	-	-	-	-	-	-	-	3.5	-	4.6	-	16.7	-		0.3	0.3	0.02	0.04	0.4	175
Prostate	55	0	-	-	-	-	-	-	-	-	-	3.5	-	13.8	31.8	50.5	117.1	99.9	217.2	5.6	5.5	0.25	1.08	9.1	185
Testis	9	0	2.6	-	-	1.2	1.0	-	-	1.3	-	-	6.2	-	-	4.6	-	-	-	0.9	0.9	0.06	0.08	1.0	186
Penis	0	0	-	-	-	-	-	-	-	-	-	-	-	-	-	-	-	-	-	0.0	0.0	0.00	0.00	0.0	187.1-.4
Other male genital	0	0	-	-	-	-	-	-	-	-	-	-	-	-	-	-	-	-	-	0.0	0.0	0.00	0.00	0.0	187.5-.9
†Bladder	46	0	-	-	-	-	2.0	-	1.0	-	1.9	3.5	3.1	17.3	17.7	50.5	39.0	149.9	120.7	4.7	4.6	0.23	0.68	7.1	188
Kidney etc.	18	0	0.9	-	-	-	-	-	-	2.7	1.9	-	6.2	17.3	17.7	-	7.8	16.7	-	1.8	1.8	0.23	0.27	2.4	189
Eye	2	0	0.9	-	-	-	-	-	-	-	-	-	-	-	-	-	-	-	24.1	0.2	0.2	0.00	0.00	0.3	190
Brain, nervous system	17	0	1.7	1.0	-	1.2	-	0.8	6.7	1.3	-	-	6.2	3.5	3.5	-	-	-	-	1.7	1.7	0.13	0.13	1.6	191-2
Thyroid	11	0	-	-	-	-	3.1	-	1.0	1.3	-	-	6.2	6.9	3.5	-	7.8	-	-	1.1	1.1	0.11	0.15	1.3	193
Other endocrine	5	0	1.7	1.0	-	1.2	1.0	-	-	-	-	-	-	-	-	-	-	-	-	0.5	0.5	0.02	0.02	0.5	194
Hodgkin's disease	12	0	-	1.0	-	1.2	1.0	-	-	5.3	1.9	3.5	3.1	-	3.5	-	7.8	-	-	1.2	1.2	0.10	0.14	1.4	201
Non-Hodgkin lymphoma	52	0	-	1.0	4.2	-	4.1	1.7	1.0	2.7	7.7	3.5	18.7	27.7	28.3	13.8	46.8	33.3	24.1	5.3	5.2	0.50	0.81	6.9	200,202
Multiple myeloma	19	0	-	-	-	-	-	-	-	1.3	-	3.5	6.2	10.4	10.6	18.4	23.4	33.3	-	1.9	1.9	0.16	0.37	2.8	203
Lymphoid leukaemia	17	0	5.2	4.1	-	2.4	-	-	-	1.3	-	-	3.1	3.5	-	4.6	-	16.7	-	1.7	1.7	0.10	0.12	1.9	204
Myeloid leukaemia	30	0	0.9	1.0	-	1.2	1.0	5.0	1.0	4.0	3.8	3.5	15.6	-	10.6	4.6	7.8	33.3	24.1	3.1	3.0	0.24	0.30	3.6	205
Monocytic leukaemia	1	0	-	-	-	-	-	-	-	-	-	-	-	-	-	-	-	16.7	-	0.1	0.1	0.00	0.00	0.2	206
Other leukaemia	1	0	0.9	-	-	-	-	-	-	-	-	-	-	-	-	-	-	-	-	0.1	0.1	0.00	0.00	0.1	207
Leukaemia unspecified	5	0	-	1.0	-	1.2	-	-	-	-	1.9	-	-	-	3.5	-	-	16.7	-	0.5	0.5	0.04	0.04	0.6	208
Other and unspecified	41	0	-	-	-	-	1.0	0.8	1.0	4.0	-	3.5	15.6	13.8	24.8	32.1	46.8	50.0	48.3	4.2	4.1	0.32	0.72	5.9	O&U
All sites	1033	0	16.4	10.4	5.6	17.0	20.4	17.6	28.9	45.1	82.5	158.0	274.4	342.7	551.7	793.8	1092.6	1415.5	1254.8	105.6		7.85	17.28	148.8	ALL
All sites but 173	1003	0	16.4	10.4	5.6	17.0	20.4	16.8	28.9	43.7	78.7	154.5	261.9	335.8	530.4	752.5	1069.1	1398.8	1254.8	102.6	100.0	7.60	16.71	144.6	ALLb

Rate from 1 case   0.862   1.035   1.392   1.213   1.020   0.840   0.962   1.325   1.918   3.512   3.118   3.462   3.536   4.588   7.804   16.653   24.131

†Important: see notes on population page

SINGAPORE: MALAY 1988-1992

ANNUAL INCIDENCE PER 100,000 BY AGE GROUP (YEARS) - FEMALE

SITE	ALL AGES	AGE UNK	0-	5-	10-	15-	20-	25-	30-	35-	40-	45-	50-	55-	60-	65-	70-	75-	80+	CRUDE RATE	%	CR 64	CR 74	ASR (W)	ICD (9th)
Lip	0	0	-	-	-	-	-	-	-	-	-	-	-	-	-	-	-	-	-	0.0	0.0	0.00	0.00	**0.0**	*140*
Tongue	2	0	-	-	-	-	-	-	-	1.3	-	-	3.0	-	-	-	-	-	-	0.2	0.2	0.02	0.02	**0.2**	*141*
Salivary gland	2	0	-	-	-	-	1.1	-	-	-	-	-	-	-	3.8	-	-	-	-	0.2	0.2	0.02	0.02	**0.2**	*142*
Mouth	3	0	-	-	-	-	-	-	-	-	-	-	-	3.0	3.8	-	-	17.3	-	0.3	0.3	0.03	0.03	**0.4**	*143-5*
Oropharynx	1	0	-	-	-	-	-	-	-	-	-	-	-	-	-	-	9.4	-	-	0.1	0.1	0.00	0.05	**0.2**	*146*
Nasopharynx	19	0	-	-	-	-	2.1	-	3.1	4.0	11.3	-	6.1	3.0	-	11.5	-	-	-	2.0	1.9	0.15	0.21	**2.0**	*147*
Hypopharynx	2	0	-	-	-	-	-	-	-	-	-	-	-	-	-	11.5	-	-	-	0.2	0.2	0.00	0.06	**0.3**	*148*
Pharynx unspecified	0	0	-	-	-	-	-	-	-	-	-	-	-	-	-	-	-	-	-	0.0	0.0	0.00	0.00	**0.0**	*149*
Oesophagus	4	0	-	-	-	-	-	-	-	-	-	-	3.0	3.8	5.7	-	-	24.9		0.4	0.4	0.03	0.06	**0.7**	*150*
Stomach	36	0	-	-	-	1.3	-	1.8	-	-	3.8	3.1	9.1	17.8	18.9	51.7	18.7	51.9	49.8	3.8	3.7	0.28	0.63	**5.5**	*151*
Small intestine	2	0	-	-	-	-	-	-	-	-	-	3.1	-	3.8	-	-	-	-	-	0.2	0.2	0.03	0.03	**0.3**	*152*
Colon	47	0	-	-	-	-	0.9	2.1	4.0	16.9	3.1	24.3	8.9	30.2	34.5	9.4	69.2	24.9	5.0	4.8	0.45	0.67	**6.6**	*153*
Rectum	49	0	-	-	-	-	0.9	-	2.7	5.6	3.1	30.4	11.8	45.4	23.0	46.8	51.9	99.7	5.2	5.0	0.50	0.85	**7.7**	*154*
Liver	25	0	-	-	-	-	-	2.1	-	1.9	6.2	12.1	3.0	15.1	34.5	18.7	51.9	-	2.7	2.5	0.20	0.47	**3.9**	*155*
Gallbladder etc.	13	0	-	-	-	-	-	-	-	1.3	5.6	12.5	3.0	-	3.8	5.7	18.7	-	-	1.4	1.3	0.13	0.25	**2.0**	*156*
Pancreas	8	0	-	-	-	-	-	-	-	1.9	-	6.1	3.0	7.6	5.7	9.4	-	-	0.9	0.8	0.09	0.17	**1.2**	*157*
Nose, sinuses etc.	7	0	-	-	-	-	-	0.9	-	-	1.9	-	3.0	-	11.5	18.7	-	-	0.7	0.7	0.03	0.18	**1.0**	*160*
Larynx	5	0	-	-	-	-	-	-	-	-	-	3.0	-	3.8	-	9.4	17.3	24.9	0.5	0.5	0.03	0.08	**0.9**	*161*
Bronchus, lung	61	0	-	-	-	-	-	-	3.1	1.3	3.8	6.2	24.3	14.8	30.2	68.9	84.3	173.0	24.9	6.5	6.2	0.42	1.18	**9.6**	*162*
Other thoracic organs	5	0	-	-	-	-	1.1	-	1.0	1.3	-	3.1	-	3.0	-	-	-	-	0.5	0.5	0.05	0.05	**0.5**	*163-4*
Bone	5	0	0.9	-	1.5	1.3	1.1	-	-	-	-	-	-	-	5.7	-	-	-	0.5	0.5	0.02	0.05	**0.6**	*170*
Connective tissue	11	0	-	-	-	-	3.2	2.7	1.0	2.7	-	3.1	-	-	5.7	-	-	-	1.2	1.1	0.06	0.09	**1.1**	*171*
Mesothelioma	0	0	-	-	-	-	-	-	-	-	-	-	-	-	-	-	-	-	-	0.0	0.0	0.00	0.00	**0.0**	*MES*
Kaposi's sarcoma	0	0	-	-	-	-	-	-	-	-	-	-	-	-	-	-	-	-	-	0.0	0.0	0.00	0.00	**0.0**	*KAP*
Melanoma of skin	2	0	0.9	-	-	-	-	-	-	-	1.9	-	-	-	-	-	-	-	-	0.2	0.2	0.01	0.01	**0.2**	*172*
Other skin	23	0	-	-	-	-	-	0.9	-	-	3.8	3.1	6.1	11.8	18.9	11.5	18.7	51.9	24.9	2.4		0.22	0.37	**3.5**	*173*
Breast	261	0	-	-	-	-	-	1.8	26.7	48.4	96.0	77.9	85.0	82.9	79.4	149.3	74.9	86.5	124.6	27.8	26.5	2.49	3.61	**33.9**	*174*
Uterus unspecified	0	0	-	-	-	-	-	-	-	-	-	-	-	-	-	-	-	-	-	0.0	0.0	0.00	0.00	**0.0**	*179*
Cervix uteri	79	0	-	-	-	-	-	0.9	1.0	10.8	11.3	37.4	42.5	44.4	49.1	28.7	18.7	34.6	-	8.4	8.0	0.99	1.22	**11.1**	*180*
Placenta	2	0	-	-	-	-	1.1	-	1.0	-	-	-	-	-	-	-	-	-	-	0.2	0.2	0.01	0.01	**0.1**	*181*
Corpus uteri	38	0	-	-	-	-	-	0.9	-	9.4	9.4	9.3	15.2	17.8	11.3	17.2	46.8	-	-	4.0	3.9	0.37	0.69	**5.1**	*182*
Ovary etc.	80	0	-	-	1.5	7.8	8.5	7.1	5.1	5.4	16.9	24.9	24.3	29.6	22.7	11.5	18.7	34.6	24.9	8.5	8.1	0.77	0.92	**9.9**	*183*
Other female genital	4	0	-	-	-	-	-	-	-	-	1.9	-	-	-	7.6	-	-	17.3	-	0.4	0.4	0.05	0.05	**0.6**	*184*
†Bladder	5	0	-	-	-	-	-	-	-	-	-	3.1	-	3.0	-	17.2	-	-	-	0.5	0.5	0.03	0.12	**0.8**	*188*
Kidney etc.	7	0	-	-	-	-	-	0.9	-	-	1.9	-	3.0	3.0	11.3	-	-	-	-	0.7	0.7	0.10	0.10	**0.9**	*189*
Eye	3	0	1.8	1.1	-	-	-	-	-	-	-	-	-	-	-	-	-	-	-	0.3	0.3	0.01	0.01	**0.3**	*190*
Brain, nervous system	9	0	-	2.2	1.5	-	2.1	-	1.0	-	-	-	-	3.0	-	-	9.4	17.3	-	1.0	0.9	0.05	0.10	**1.1**	*191-2*
Thyroid	60	0	0.9	-	1.5	3.9	11.7	8.9	5.1	6.7	13.2	15.6	15.2	5.9	3.8	11.5	18.7	-	-	6.4	6.1	0.46	0.61	**6.5**	*193*
Other endocrine	2	0	-	-	-	-	-	-	-	-	-	3.1	-	-	-	5.7	-	-	-	0.2	0.2	0.02	0.04	**0.4**	*194*
Hodgkin's disease	3	0	-	-	-	-	-	-	-	2.1	-	3.1	-	-	-	-	-	-	-	0.3	0.3	0.03	0.03	**0.3**	*201*
Non-Hodgkin lymphoma	43	0	-	2.2	1.5	-	1.1	1.8	1.0	9.4	9.4	6.2	12.1	11.8	18.9	34.5	28.1	-	-	4.6	4.4	0.38	0.69	**5.6**	*200,202*
Multiple myeloma	13	0	-	-	-	-	-	-	-	-	-	3.1	3.0	17.8	3.8	5.7	28.1	-	-	1.4	1.3	0.14	0.31	**1.9**	*203*
Lymphoid leukaemia	10	0	2.7	3.3	-	3.9	-	-	1.0	-	-	-	-	-	-	-	-	-	-	1.1	1.0	0.05	0.05	**1.1**	*204*
Myeloid leukaemia	24	0	0.9	1.1	-	2.6	1.1	3.6	-	4.0	-	6.2	6.1	3.0	15.1	5.7	9.4	-	24.9	2.6	2.4	0.22	0.29	**3.1**	*205*
Monocytic leukaemia	0	0	-	-	-	-	-	-	-	-	-	-	-	-	-	-	-	-	-	0.0	0.0	0.00	0.00	**0.0**	*206*
Other leukaemia	0	0	-	-	-	-	-	-	-	-	-	-	-	-	-	-	-	-	-	0.0	0.0	0.00	0.00	**0.0**	*207*
Leukaemia unspecified	1	0	-	1.1	-	-	-	-	-	-	-	-	-	-	-	-	-	-	-	0.1	0.1	0.01	0.01	**0.1**	*208*
Other and unspecified	32	0	0.9	-	-	-	-	-	3.1	2.7	-	9.3	9.1	11.8	18.9	11.5	46.8	51.9	24.9	3.4	3.2	0.28	0.57	**4.7**	*O&U*
All sites	1008	0	9.0	11.0	7.5	20.9	34.1	33.7	59.6	115.6	218.4	246.2	343.0	319.7	430.9	585.8	561.9	726.4	473.3	107.3		9.25	14.99	**136.5**	*ALL*
All sites but 173	985	0	9.0	11.0	7.5	20.9	34.1	32.9	59.6	115.6	214.6	243.1	337.0	307.8	412.0	574.3	543.1	674.5	448.4	104.9	100.0	9.03	14.61	**133.0**	*ALLb*

Rate from 1 case			0.903	1.103	1.504	1.304	1.066	0.888	1.028	1.344	1.883	3.117	3.036	2.960	3.780	5.743	9.364	17.295	24.913

†Important: see notes on population page

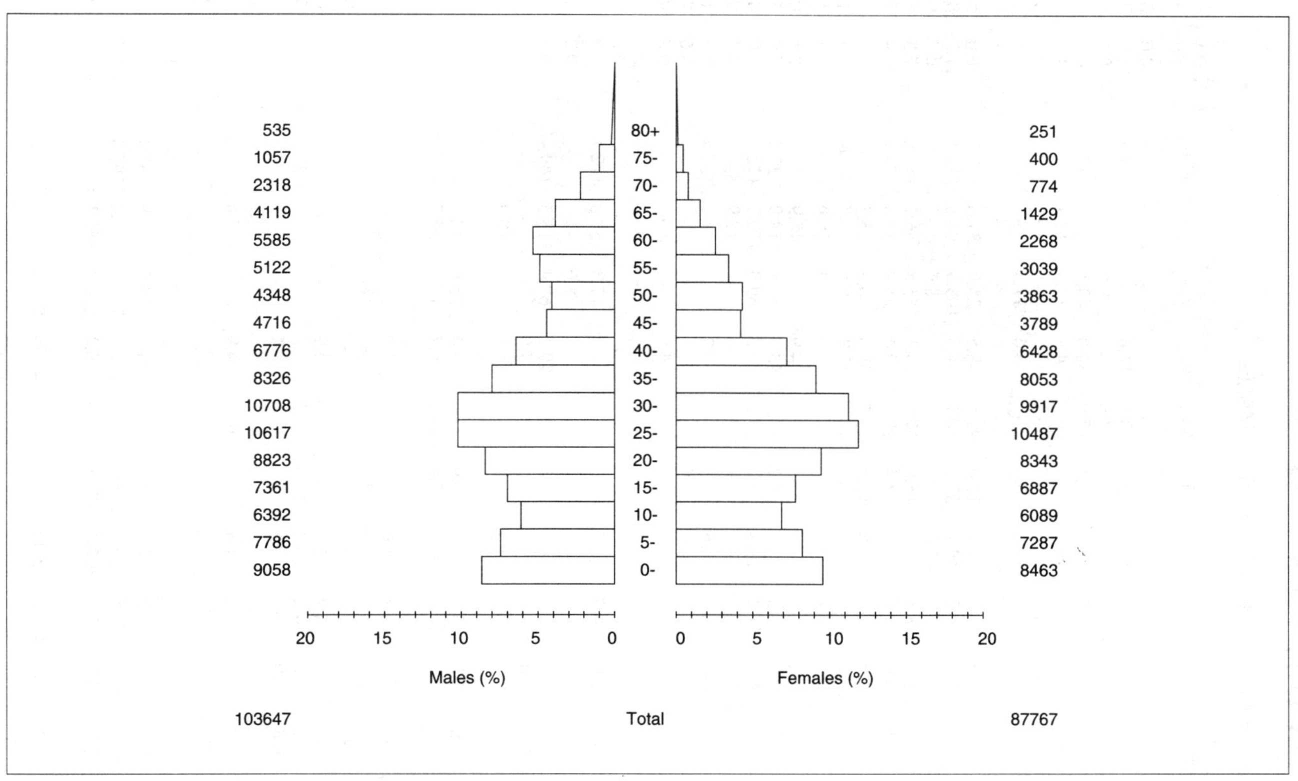

Singapore: Indian
Source of population: 1990
Census: Census of Population 1990, Department of Statistics, Singapore

Notes to tables overleaf:
† 188 does not include non-invasive tumours

SINGAPORE: INDIAN 1988-1992

ANNUAL INCIDENCE PER 100,000 BY AGE GROUP (YEARS) - MALE

SITE	ALL AGES	AGE UNK	0-	5-	10-	15-	20-	25-	30-	35-	40-	45-	50-	55-	60-	65-	70-	75-	80+	CRUDE RATE	%	CR 64	CR 74	ASR (W)	ICD (9th)
Lip	0	0	-	-	-	-	-	-	-	-	-	-	-	-	-	-	-	-	-	0.0	0.0	0.00	0.00	0.0	140
Tongue	15	0	-	-	-	-	-	-	-	-	-	-	18.4	23.4	3.6	14.6	-	-	37.4	2.9	2.5	0.23	0.30	2.8	141
Salivary gland	2	0	-	-	-	-	-	-	-	-	-	-	-	-	3.6	-	8.6	-	-	0.4	0.3	0.02	0.06	0.3	142
Mouth	22	0	-	-	-	-	-	-	-	-	-	4.2	-	11.7	17.9	34.0	43.1	-	37.4	4.2	3.7	0.17	0.55	3.7	143-5
Oropharynx	7	0	-	-	-	-	-	-	-	-	3.0	-	9.2	-	-	4.9	17.3	18.9	-	1.4	1.2	0.06	0.17	1.3	146
Nasopharynx	2	0	-	-	-	-	-	-	-	-	-	4.2	4.6	-	-	-	-	-	-	0.4	0.3	0.04	0.04	0.5	147
Hypopharynx	8	0	-	-	-	2.7	-	-	-	-	-	-	4.6	3.9	-	14.6	17.3	-	-	1.5	1.4	0.06	0.22	1.4	148
Pharynx unspecified	1	0	-	-	-	-	-	1.9	-	-	-	-	-	-	-	-	-	-	-	0.2	0.2	0.01	0.01	0.2	149
Oesophagus	31	0	-	-	-	-	-	-	-	-	3.0	-	9.2	15.6	21.5	48.5	25.9	37.8	112.1	6.0	5.3	0.25	0.62	5.6	150
Stomach	58	2	-	-	-	-	-	3.8	-	-	5.9	4.2	18.4	31.2	50.1	24.3	103.5	94.6	112.1	11.2	9.8	0.59	1.25	10.3	151
Small intestine	2	0	-	-	-	-	-	-	-	-	-	-	4.6	-	-	-	8.6	-	-	0.4	0.3	0.02	0.07	0.4	152
Colon	39	0	-	-	-	-	-	-	3.7	2.4	5.9	8.5	13.8	15.6	17.9	29.1	51.8	56.7	186.8	7.5	6.6	0.34	0.74	7.6	153
Rectum	33	0	-	-	-	-	-	-	-	2.4	5.9	4.2	18.4	23.4	28.6	19.4	25.9	37.8	74.7	6.4	5.6	0.42	0.64	6.0	154
Liver	39	0	-	-	-	-	-	-	-	-	3.0	-	4.6	19.5	21.5	58.3	86.3	75.7	-	7.5	6.6	0.24	0.97	6.3	155
Gallbladder etc.	8	0	-	-	-	-	-	-	-	-	-	-	-	-	10.7	19.4	8.6	-	-	1.5	1.4	0.05	0.19	1.2	156
Pancreas	9	0	-	-	-	-	-	-	-	-	-	4.2	9.2	-	7.2	4.9	17.3	18.9	-	1.7	1.5	0.10	0.21	1.7	157
Nose, sinuses etc.	4	0	-	-	-	2.7	-	-	-	-	3.0	-	-	-	-	4.9	-	18.9	-	0.8	0.7	0.03	0.05	0.8	160
Larynx	26	0	-	-	-	-	-	-	-	2.4	-	4.2	-	11.7	14.3	43.7	51.8	18.9	37.4	5.0	4.4	0.16	0.64	4.3	161
Bronchus, lung	83	0	-	-	-	-	-	-	1.9	2.4	5.9	21.2	18.4	31.2	57.3	126.2	69.0	170.2	112.1	16.0	14.1	0.69	1.67	14.3	162
Other thoracic organs	1	0	-	-	-	-	-	-	-	-	-	-	-	-	-	-	-	18.9	-	0.2	0.2	0.00	0.00	0.2	163-4
Bone	8	0	-	-	3.1	2.7	2.3	1.9	-	-	-	-	4.6	-	-	9.7	-	-	37.4	1.5	1.4	0.07	0.12	1.8	170
Connective tissue	3	0	2.2	-	-	-	-	-	-	-	-	-	4.6	3.9	-	-	-	-	-	0.6	0.5	0.05	0.05	0.7	171
Mesothelioma	1	0	-	-	-	-	-	-	-	-	-	-	-	-	-	4.9	-	-	-	0.2	0.2	0.00	0.02	0.1	MES
Kaposi's sarcoma	2	0	-	-	-	-	2.3	-	1.9	-	-	-	-	-	-	-	-	-	-	0.4	0.3	0.02	0.02	0.3	KAP
Melanoma of skin	0	0	-	-	-	-	-	-	-	-	-	-	-	-	-	-	-	-	-	0.0	0.0	0.00	0.00	0.0	172
Other skin	15	0	-	-	-	-	-	-	-	-	3.0	4.2	13.8	-	7.2	4.9	17.3	37.8	112.1	2.9		0.14	0.25	3.4	173
Breast	1	0	-	-	-	-	-	-	-	-	-	-	-	-	-	-	8.6	-	-	0.2	0.2	0.00	0.04	0.2	175
Prostate	35	0	-	-	-	-	-	-	-	-	-	-	-	19.5	25.1	29.1	60.4	113.5	149.4	6.8	5.9	0.22	0.67	6.5	185
Testis	12	0	-	-	-	-	9.1	1.9	1.9	7.2	3.0	4.2	-	-	-	4.9	-	-	-	2.3	2.0	0.14	0.16	2.0	186
Penis	5	0	-	-	-	-	-	-	-	-	-	-	4.6	-	-	14.6	-	18.9	-	1.0	0.8	0.02	0.10	0.9	187.1-.4
Other male genital	1	0	-	-	-	-	-	-	-	-	-	-	-	-	-	4.9	-	-	-	0.2	0.2	0.00	0.02	0.1	187.5-.9
†Bladder	21	0	-	-	-	-	2.3	-	1.9	4.8	3.0	4.2	9.2	3.9	3.6	19.4	25.9	18.9	112.1	4.1	3.6	0.16	0.39	4.2	188
Kidney etc.	17	0	-	-	-	-	-	-	-	-	-	12.7	4.6	7.8	14.3	9.7	17.3	56.7	-	3.3	2.9	0.20	0.33	3.1	189
Eye	0	0	-	-	-	-	-	-	-	-	-	-	-	-	-	-	-	-	-	0.0	0.0	0.00	0.00	0.0	190
Brain, nervous system	9	0	-	7.7	-	-	-	-	-	-	3.0	4.2	4.6	3.9	3.6	4.9	-	-	-	1.7	1.5	0.13	0.16	1.9	191-2
Thyroid	5	0	-	-	-	-	-	-	-	-	3.0	-	4.6	3.9	3.6	-	8.6	-	-	1.0	0.8	0.08	0.12	0.9	193
Other endocrine	0	0	-	-	-	-	-	-	-	-	-	-	-	-	-	-	-	-	-	0.0	0.0	0.00	0.00	0.0	194
Hodgkin's disease	5	0	-	-	3.1	2.7	-	-	-	-	-	4.2	4.6	-	-	4.9	-	-	-	1.0	0.8	0.07	0.10	1.2	201
Non-Hodgkin lymphoma	21	0	-	-	-	5.4	-	-	-	7.2	3.0	4.2	13.8	19.5	7.2	14.6	-	-	37.4	4.1	3.6	0.30	0.37	3.9	200,202
Multiple myeloma	10	0	-	-	-	-	-	-	-	4.8	3.0	-	4.6	3.9	3.6	19.4	-	-	-	1.9	1.7	0.10	0.20	1.6	203
Lymphoid leukaemia	7	0	2.2	-	3.1	2.7	2.3	3.8	-	-	-	-	-	3.9	-	-	-	-	-	1.4	1.2	0.09	0.09	1.4	204
Myeloid leukaemia	9	0	-	-	-	-	-	-	1.9	-	3.0	-	4.6	-	10.7	4.9	-	37.8	-	1.7	1.5	0.10	0.13	1.5	205
Monocytic leukaemia	0	0	-	-	-	-	-	-	-	-	-	-	-	-	-	-	-	-	-	0.0	0.0	0.00	0.00	0.0	206
Other leukaemia	0	0	-	-	-	-	-	-	-	-	-	-	-	-	-	-	-	-	-	0.0	0.0	0.00	0.00	0.0	207
Leukaemia unspecified	1	0	-	-	-	-	-	-	-	-	-	-	-	-	-	3.6	-	-	-	0.2	0.2	0.02	0.02	0.1	208
Other and unspecified	26	1	-	-	-	-	-	-	3.7	2.4	-	4.2	4.6	15.6	7.2	34.0	34.5	37.8	37.4	5.0	4.4	0.20	0.55	4.4	O&U
All sites	604	3	4.4	7.7	9.4	19.0	18.1	13.2	16.8	36.0	59.0	97.5	216.2	273.3	343.8	631.1	707.5	889.0	1195.4	116.5		5.60	12.33	108.9	ALL
All sites but 173	589	3	4.4	7.7	9.4	19.0	18.1	13.2	16.8	36.0	56.1	93.3	202.4	273.3	336.6	626.2	690.3	851.1	1083.3	113.6	100.0	5.46	12.08	105.5	ALLb

Rate from 1 case: 2.208 2.569 3.129 2.717 2.267 1.884 1.868 2.402 2.952 4.241 4.600 3.904 3.581 4.855 8.628 18.914 37.355

†Important: see notes on population page

SINGAPORE: INDIAN 1988-1992

ANNUAL INCIDENCE PER 100,000 BY AGE GROUP (YEARS) - FEMALE

SITE	ALL AGES	AGE UNK	0-	5-	10-	15-	20-	25-	30-	35-	40-	45-	50-	55-	60-	65-	70-	75-	80+	CRUDE RATE	%	CR 64	CR 74	ASR (W)	ICD (9th)
Lip	2	0	-	-	-	-	-	-	-	-	-	-	-	-	-	14.0	25.8	-	-	0.5	0.5	0.00	0.20	**0.9**	*140*
Tongue	2	0	-	-	-	-	-	-	-	-	-	5.3	5.2	-	-	-	-	-	-	0.5	0.5	0.05	0.05	**0.6**	*141*
Salivary gland	3	0	-	-	-	-	-	-	2.0	-	-	-	-	-	8.8	-	-	-	79.7	0.7	0.8	0.05	0.05	**1.3**	*142*
Mouth	11	0	-	-	-	-	2.4	1.9	-	-	-	5.3	10.4	-	17.6	42.0	-	50.0	-	2.5	2.8	0.19	0.40	**3.6**	*143-5*
Oropharynx	3	0	-	-	-	-	-	-	-	-	-	-	-	6.6	8.8	-	-	50.0	-	0.7	0.8	0.08	0.08	**1.1**	*146*
Nasopharynx	1	0	-	-	-	-	-	-	-	-	-	-	-	-	-	-	25.8	-	-	0.2	0.3	0.00	0.13	**0.5**	*147*
Hypopharynx	3	0	-	-	-	-	-	-	-	-	-	-	-	13.2	-	14.0	-	-	-	0.7	0.8	0.07	0.14	**0.9**	*148*
Pharynx unspecified	0	0	-	-	-	-	-	-	-	-	-	-	-	-	-	-	-	-	-	0.0	0.0	0.00	0.00	**0.0**	*149*
Oesophagus	12	0	-	-	-	-	-	-	-	-	3.1	-	5.2	26.3	26.4	28.0	25.8	-	-	2.7	3.0	0.31	0.57	**3.9**	*150*
Stomach	22	0	-	-	-	-	-	-	-	7.5	6.2	10.6	10.4	19.7	8.8	56.0	25.8	100.0	159.4	5.0	5.6	0.32	0.72	**7.9**	*151*
Small intestine	1	0	-	-	-	-	-	-	-	2.5	-	-	-	-	-	-	-	-	-	0.2	0.3	0.01	0.01	**0.1**	*152*
Colon	15	0	-	-	-	-	-	-	2.0	2.5	3.1	15.8	15.5	6.6	8.8	28.0	51.7	-	-	3.4	3.8	0.27	0.67	**4.7**	*153*
Rectum	16	0	-	-	-	-	-	1.9	-	2.5	-	5.3	-	6.6	8.8	42.0	180.8	50.0	-	3.6	4.0	0.13	1.24	**6.6**	*154*
Liver	6	0	-	-	-	-	-	-	-	-	-	-	-	6.6	8.8	14.0	-	100.0	79.7	1.4	1.5	0.08	0.15	**2.8**	*155*
Gallbladder etc.	5	0	-	-	-	-	-	-	-	-	3.1	5.3	10.4	-	8.8	-	-	-	-	1.1	1.3	0.14	0.14	**1.4**	*156*
Pancreas	4	0	-	-	-	-	-	-	-	-	-	-	5.2	-	8.8	14.0	-	50.0	-	0.9	1.0	0.07	0.14	**1.5**	*157*
Nose, sinuses etc.	2	0	-	-	-	-	2.4	-	-	-	-	-	-	-	8.8	-	-	-	-	0.5	0.5	0.06	0.06	**0.5**	*160*
Larynx	3	0	-	-	-	-	-	-	-	-	-	-	-	-	8.8	14.0	-	50.0	-	0.7	0.8	0.04	0.11	**1.3**	*161*
Bronchus, lung	10	0	-	-	-	-	-	-	-	-	6.2	-	5.2	13.2	8.8	14.0	77.5	-	-	2.3	2.5	0.17	0.62	**3.5**	*162*
Other thoracic organs	1	0	-	-	-	-	-	-	2.0	-	-	-	-	-	-	-	-	-	-	0.2	0.3	0.01	0.01	**0.1**	*163-4*
Bone	3	0	-	2.7	-	-	-	1.9	2.0	-	-	-	-	-	-	-	-	-	-	0.7	0.8	0.03	0.03	**0.5**	*170*
Connective tissue	2	0	-	-	-	-	-	-	-	2.5	-	-	-	6.6	-	-	-	-	-	0.5	0.5	0.05	0.05	**0.4**	*171*
Mesothelioma	0	0	-	-	-	-	-	-	-	-	-	-	-	-	-	-	-	-	-	0.0	0.0	0.00	0.00	**0.0**	*MES*
Kaposi's sarcoma	0	0	-	-	-	-	-	-	-	-	-	-	-	-	-	-	-	-	-	0.0	0.0	0.00	0.00	**0.0**	*KAP*
Melanoma of skin	0	0	-	-	-	-	-	-	-	-	-	-	-	-	-	-	-	-	-	0.0	0.0	0.00	0.00	**0.0**	*172*
Other skin	12	0	-	-	-	-	-	-	-	2.5	-	5.3	-	6.6	44.1	14.0	51.7	50.0	-	2.7		0.29	0.62	**4.4**	*173*
Breast	111	0	-	-	-	-	-	1.9	8.1	27.3	65.3	79.2	72.5	92.1	114.6	112.0	180.8	50.0	159.4	25.3	28.0	2.31	3.77	**31.9**	*174*
Uterus unspecified	0	0	-	-	-	-	-	-	-	-	-	-	-	-	-	-	-	-	-	0.0	0.0	0.00	0.00	**0.0**	*179*
Cervix uteri	32	0	-	-	-	-	-	-	2.0	9.9	21.8	21.1	31.1	32.9	-	14.0	51.7	100.0	-	7.3	8.1	0.59	0.92	**8.6**	*180*
Placenta	0	0	-	-	-	-	-	-	-	-	-	-	-	-	-	-	-	-	-	0.0	0.0	0.00	0.00	**0.0**	*181*
Corpus uteri	20	0	-	-	-	-	-	-	2.0	7.5	3.1	5.3	10.4	26.3	44.1	-	51.7	-	79.7	4.6	5.1	0.49	0.75	**6.2**	*182*
Ovary etc.	28	0	-	-	-	-	2.4	1.9	4.0	7.5	6.2	10.6	25.9	39.5	17.6	28.0	51.7	-	-	6.4	7.1	0.58	0.98	**7.5**	*183*
Other female genital	2	0	-	-	-	2.9	-	-	-	-	-	-	6.6	-	-	-	-	-	-	0.5	0.5	0.05	0.05	**0.5**	*184*
†Bladder	2	0	-	-	-	-	-	-	-	-	-	-	-	-	8.8	-	-	50.0	-	0.5	0.5	0.04	0.04	**0.9**	*188*
Kidney etc.	9	0	2.4	-	-	-	-	1.9	-	-	3.1	5.3	-	6.6	8.8	14.0	25.8	50.0	-	2.1	2.3	0.14	0.34	**3.0**	*189*
Eye	1	0	-	-	-	-	-	-	-	-	-	-	-	-	-	-	-	50.0	-	0.2	0.3	0.00	0.00	**0.5**	*190*
Brain, nervous system	7	0	2.4	-	-	-	-	-	-	-	-	5.3	10.4	-	8.8	14.0	25.8	-	-	1.6	1.8	0.13	0.33	**2.4**	*191-2*
Thyroid	13	0	-	3.3	-	-	-	1.9	2.0	5.0	9.3	5.3	5.2	13.2	8.8	-	-	-	-	3.0	3.3	0.27	0.27	**2.9**	*193*
Other endocrine	0	0	-	-	-	-	-	-	-	-	-	-	-	-	-	-	-	-	-	0.0	0.0	0.00	0.00	**0.0**	*194*
Hodgkin's disease	2	0	-	-	-	-	-	1.9	-	-	-	-	-	-	-	14.0	-	-	-	0.5	0.5	0.01	0.08	**0.6**	*201*
Non-Hodgkin lymphoma	10	0	-	2.7	-	-	-	-	2.0	5.0	3.1	-	5.2	6.6	-	14.0	51.7	-	-	2.3	2.5	0.12	0.45	**2.9**	*200,202*
Multiple myeloma	3	0	-	-	-	-	-	-	-	-	-	-	-	13.2	-	-	25.8	-	-	0.7	0.8	0.07	0.19	**1.0**	*203*
Lymphoid leukaemia	5	0	2.4	-	-	-	-	-	-	-	-	5.3	-	6.6	8.8	-	-	-	79.7	1.1	1.3	0.12	0.12	**2.0**	*204*
Myeloid leukaemia	10	0	-	2.7	-	2.9	-	-	-	-	3.1	5.3	10.4	6.6	17.6	14.0	-	-	-	2.3	2.5	0.24	0.31	**2.9**	*205*
Monocytic leukaemia	0	0	-	-	-	-	-	-	-	-	-	-	-	-	-	-	-	-	-	0.0	0.0	0.00	0.00	**0.0**	*206*
Other leukaemia	1	0	-	-	-	-	2.4	-	-	-	-	-	-	-	-	-	-	-	-	0.2	0.3	0.01	0.01	**0.2**	*207*
Leukaemia unspecified	1	0	2.4	-	-	-	-	-	-	-	-	-	-	-	-	-	-	-	-	0.2	0.3	0.01	0.01	**0.3**	*208*
Other and unspecified	12	0	-	-	-	-	-	-	4.0	2.5	-	5.3	5.2	13.2	8.8	28.0	25.8	-	79.7	2.7	3.0	0.19	0.46	**4.0**	*O&U*
All sites	408	0	9.5	8.2	3.3	5.8	9.6	15.3	32.3	84.4	136.9	200.5	243.3	375.1	432.0	545.8	955.6	799.6	717.1	93.0		7.78	15.29	**127.1**	*ALL*
All sites but 173	396	0	9.5	8.2	3.3	5.8	9.6	15.3	32.3	82.0	136.9	195.3	243.3	368.5	387.9	531.8	903.9	749.6	717.1	90.2	100.0	7.49	14.67	**122.7**	*ALLb*

Rate from 1 case | | | 2.363 | 2.745 | 3.284 | 2.904 | 2.397 | 1.907 | 2.017 | 2.484 | 3.111 | 5.278 | 5.177 | 6.581 | 8.816 | 13.996 | 25.826 | 49.975 | 79.681 |

†Important: see notes on population page

433

Thailand, Chiang Mai

The cancer unit of Chiang Mai University was established in 1963 as a hospital-based tumour registry. The population-based tumour registry was started in 1986 to study cancer incidence in Chiang Mai province during the years 1983–87.

Chiang Mai is one of the seventeen provinces of the northern part of Thailand, located about 697 km north of Bangkok, at latitude 16° N and longitude 99° E. It borders the Union of Myanmar to the north, the provinces of Lumpang and Lumpoon to the east, Tak to the south and Mae Hong Son to the west. Its total area is 20 107 km².

About 66% of the area is forests and mountains. These mountains are the branches of the Thong Chai and Laso Ranges. Another 21% is plains along both banks of the Ping River, that are are suitable for growing many kinds of plants.

The highest temperature is about 40°C during April, the lowest temperature 8°C during January. The average annual number of rainy days is around 115, while the average annual rainfall is 1217 mm. The rainy season runs from May to October.

As of 30 November 1990, Chiang Mai was administratively divided into 19 amphoes, 4 king amphure, 179 tambons and 1450 mubans. Local administration consists of "Changwat Administrative Organization", 1 municipality and 22 health districts.

The total population of the province according to the 1990 census was 1 367 183 persons (694 173 males and 673 010 females). Only 12.21% of the total population were living in the municipal area.

Data on patients diagnosed with cancer are collected actively from one university hospital (1800 beds), 10 private hospitals (1560 beds), one provincial hospital (256 beds), five government hospitals (290 beds) and 20 community hospitals (420 beds), under the care of 683 specialists. All patient identifications are compared and matched to exclude multiple registration.

For every cancer patient, the following information is recorded: name, tumour number, hospital, address, age, sex, race, date of first diagnosis, method of diagnosis, primary site of cancer, clinical staging, type of treatment, morphology, histological grading, multifocality, laterality, date last seen, date of death, and cause of death.

Mortality data are taken from death certificates obtained from the Public Health Service. All death certificates which mention cancer as the cause of death are matched against the file of registered cases. Every cancer death not traceable to an existing entry is labelled as a death-certificate-only; the date of death is taken as the date of diagnosis, and is also registered in the data files. In addition, copies of all death certificates found to mention cancer as a cause of death are individually scrutinized to confirm the statement on the certificate.

The details for each patient are cross-checked with the information collected from different hospitals, to ensure completeness of records. Additional information is obtained every time a cancer patient is re-admitted or re-examined. The same patient may be notified from two or more hospitals. Care is taken to see that multiple entries are not made in such cases; the medical information for each patient is combined.

The morphology code numbers consist of six digits; the first four identify the histological type of neoplasm, the fifth indicates its behaviour and the sixth indicates grading of morphology.

A second or third primary in a patient is registered only when all primary sites are confirmed histologically. A new registration number is given for each new site as indicated by the three-digit ICD code, thus no new registration is made for a second primary cancer occurring in the same site (first three digits), but a different sub-site (fourth digit), or occurring in the other of paired organs.

Follow-up is both active and passive. Information collected routinely is the date last seen, status of the patients (living with cancer, living with no evidence of cancer, living with unknown status or dead), and cause of death. This information is collected from a special clinic in the hospitals in Chiang Mai, by sending letters to the patients, by visiting the patients at home, and from casual sources.

The percentage of cases registered with histological verification of diagnosis was 68.7%. Only 8.2% of cases were registered on the basis of information from a death certificate only. The average mortality to incidence ratio for all cancer was 76.4%.

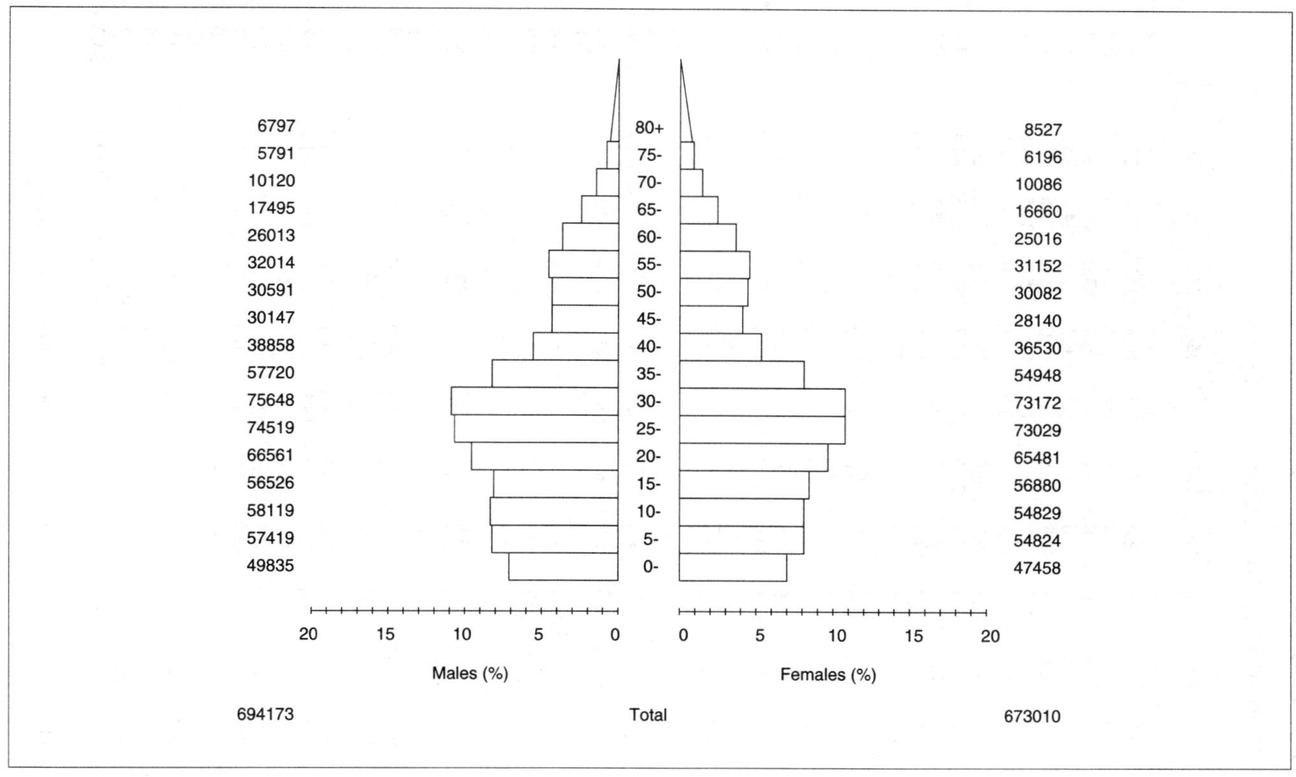

Thailand, Chiang Mai
Source of population: 1990
Census: 1990 Census of Population and Housing (1 April)

Notes to tables overleaf:
† 188 does not include non-invasive tumours

THAILAND, CHIANG MAI 1988-1992

ANNUAL INCIDENCE PER 100,000 BY AGE GROUP (YEARS) - MALE

SITE	ALL AGES	AGE UNK	0-	5-	10-	15-	20-	25-	30-	35-	40-	45-	50-	55-	60-	65-	70-	75-	80+	CRUDE RATE	%	CR 64	CR 74	ASR (W)	ICD (9th)
Lip	7	0	-	-	-	-	-	-	0.3	-	-	0.7	-	-	1.5	1.1	-	-	5.9	0.2	0.2	0.01	0.02	0.2	140
Tongue	59	0	-	-	-	-	-	-	-	0.3	1.5	2.7	2.0	2.5	8.5	10.3	21.7	20.7	20.6	1.7	1.3	0.09	0.25	2.0	141
Salivary gland	12	0	-	-	-	-	-	0.3	0.3	-	0.7	1.3	0.6	0.8	2.3	2.0	3.5	2.9	0.3	0.3	0.02	0.04	0.4	142
Mouth	77	0	-	-	-	-	-	-	-	0.7	1.5	2.0	2.0	3.7	9.2	6.9	33.6	41.4	38.3	2.2	1.7	0.10	0.30	2.5	143-5
Oropharynx	50	0	-	-	-	-	-	0.5	0.8	0.7	0.5	-	2.0	1.9	3.8	6.9	17.8	24.2	26.5	1.4	1.1	0.05	0.17	1.6	146
Nasopharynx	88	0	-	0.3	-	0.4	1.5	0.8	1.6	2.8	2.6	3.3	9.8	7.5	8.5	8.0	11.9	3.5	5.9	2.5	1.9	0.20	0.29	2.6	147
Hypopharynx	74	0	-	-	-	-	-	-	-	-	0.5	0.7	0.7	2.5	10.0	12.6	25.7	34.5	58.8	2.1	1.6	0.07	0.26	2.4	148
Pharynx unspecified	9	0	-	-	-	-	-	-	0.3	-	-	-	1.3	-	2.3	1.1	2.0	-	2.9	0.3	0.2	0.02	0.03	0.3	149
Oesophagus	70	0	-	-	-	-	-	-	-	0.3	0.5	1.3	5.2	6.9	8.5	13.7	19.8	24.2	20.6	2.0	1.5	0.11	0.28	2.3	150
Stomach	245	0	-	-	-	-	-	0.3	0.5	2.9	3.8	5.1	8.6	12.4	25.6	36.1	37.7	51.4	55.3	44.1	7.1	5.3	0.48	0.92	7.5	151
Small intestine	13	0	-	-	-	-	-	-	-	0.3	0.3	0.5	0.7	0.7	0.6	3.1	1.1	2.0	3.5	-	0.4	0.3	0.03	0.05	0.4	152
Colon	139	0	-	-	-	-	-	-	1.6	1.6	4.5	5.1	3.3	12.4	12.5	10.8	17.1	25.7	27.6	29.4	4.0	3.0	0.26	0.47	4.2	153
Rectum	101	0	-	-	-	-	0.9	0.3	2.1	1.7	2.6	1.3	4.6	6.2	10.0	27.4	17.8	27.6	17.7	2.9	2.2	0.15	0.37	3.1	154
Liver	659	0	-	0.3	0.3	0.7	1.2	2.7	9.0	15.9	23.2	31.8	42.5	61.8	76.9	102.9	124.5	96.7	67.7	19.0	14.1	1.33	2.47	20.1	155
Gallbladder etc.	104	0	-	-	-	-	-	-	0.5	2.8	0.5	6.6	7.2	9.4	13.1	13.7	29.6	20.7	20.6	3.0	2.2	0.20	0.42	3.3	156
Pancreas	85	0	-	-	-	-	-	0.3	0.3	0.5	1.4	3.6	3.3	6.5	8.1	7.7	14.9	19.8	17.3	11.8	2.4	1.8	0.16	0.33	2.7	157
Nose, sinuses etc.	32	0	-	-	-	-	-	0.5	-	1.0	0.5	1.3	1.3	3.7	3.1	3.4	9.9	10.4	2.9	0.9	0.7	0.06	0.12	1.0	160
Larynx	158	0	-	-	-	-	-	0.3	-	-	1.0	4.6	6.5	10.0	22.3	32.0	69.2	51.8	44.1	4.6	3.4	0.22	0.73	5.3	161
Bronchus, lung	1140	0	-	0.3	-	0.4	0.9	1.9	2.9	10.7	21.1	45.1	99.4	136.2	164.5	217.2	227.3	186.5	100.0	32.8	24.5	2.42	4.64	36.0	162
Other thoracic organs	2	0	-	-	-	-	-	-	0.3	-	-	-	-	-	-	1.1	-	-	-	0.1	0.0	0.00	0.01	0.1	163-4
Bone	23	0	0.4	-	1.7	1.8	0.6	0.5	1.1	0.3	-	-	0.7	-	-	1.1	-	-	2.9	0.7	0.5	0.04	0.04	0.6	170
Connective tissue	17	0	-	-	-	-	0.3	0.8	0.3	1.0	1.0	0.7	0.7	1.2	-	3.4	-	-	-	0.5	0.4	0.03	0.05	0.5	171
Mesothelioma	1	0	-	-	-	-	-	-	-	-	-	-	-	0.6	-	-	-	-	-	0.0	0.0	0.00	0.00	0.0	MES
Kaposi's sarcoma	1	0	-	-	-	-	-	0.3	-	-	-	-	-	-	-	-	-	-	-	0.0	0.0	0.00	0.00	0.0	KAP
Melanoma of skin	21	0	-	-	-	-	-	-	0.3	0.3	-	0.7	1.3	1.9	2.3	3.4	-	10.4	11.8	0.6	0.5	0.03	0.05	0.6	172
Other skin	132	0	-	-	-	-	0.9	0.3	0.8	0.7	2.6	5.3	5.9	8.1	13.1	29.7	29.6	44.9	50.0	3.8		0.19	0.48	4.2	173
Breast	2	0	-	-	-	-	-	-	-	-	-	-	-	-	1.5	-	-	-	-	0.1	0.0	0.01	0.01	0.1	175
Prostate	122	0	-	-	-	-	-	-	0.3	-	-	1.3	1.3	3.1	9.2	33.2	41.5	76.0	82.4	3.5	2.6	0.08	0.45	4.1	185
Testis	22	0	-	-	-	0.4	0.6	0.8	1.9	0.7	0.5	0.7	0.7	0.6	-	2.3	-	-	2.9	0.6	0.5	0.03	0.05	0.5	186
Penis	78	0	-	-	-	-	-	0.5	1.3	1.0	1.0	2.0	7.2	8.7	12.3	8.0	13.8	20.7	5.9	2.2	1.7	0.17	0.28	2.4	187.1-.4
Other male genital	0	0	-	-	-	-	-	-	-	-	-	-	-	-	-	-	-	-	-	0.0	0.0	0.00	0.00	0.0	187.5-.9
†Bladder	168	0	-	-	-	-	-	-	1.3	0.7	2.6	3.3	5.9	14.4	19.2	35.4	45.5	48.4	76.5	4.8	3.6	0.24	0.64	5.3	188
Kidney etc.	50	0	0.4	-	0.3	-	-	-	0.3	0.3	1.5	1.3	6.5	3.7	9.2	8.0	2.0	6.9	8.8	1.4	1.1	0.12	0.17	1.6	189
Eye	5	0	0.8	-	-	-	-	-	0.3	-	-	-	0.7	-	-	-	2.0	-	-	0.1	0.1	0.01	0.02	0.2	190
Brain, nervous system	66	0	1.6	1.0	1.4	1.1	2.1	1.1	1.3	1.4	3.1	2.0	3.9	1.9	5.4	4.6	2.0	6.9	-	1.9	1.4	0.14	0.17	2.0	191-2
Thyroid	37	0	-	-	-	-	0.3	1.1	0.5	0.7	0.5	2.7	3.3	1.2	5.4	5.7	2.0	-	8.8	1.1	0.8	0.08	0.12	1.1	193
Other endocrine	5	0	-	-	-	-	-	0.3	0.8	-	-	-	-	0.6	-	-	-	-	-	0.1	0.1	0.01	0.01	0.1	194
Hodgkin's disease	43	0	-	0.3	0.7	1.1	0.3	2.1	0.5	1.0	2.1	0.7	2.6	3.7	3.8	1.1	2.0	-	2.9	1.2	0.9	0.10	0.11	1.2	201
Non-Hodgkin lymphoma	131	0	0.4	0.3	1.4	2.1	1.8	3.2	2.9	3.1	2.1	4.6	7.8	7.5	13.8	11.4	19.8	13.8	11.8	3.8	2.8	0.26	0.41	3.8	200,202
Multiple myeloma	14	0	-	-	-	-	-	-	-	0.3	-	-	0.7	4.4	-	1.1	5.9	-	2.9	0.4	0.3	0.03	0.06	0.4	203
Lymphoid leukaemia	34	0	4.0	3.1	1.0	0.4	0.3	-	0.3	-	1.0	-	0.7	0.6	2.3	-	-	3.5	2.9	1.0	0.7	0.07	0.07	1.2	204
Myeloid leukaemia	93	0	-	0.3	1.7	2.5	1.8	2.1	2.6	2.8	2.6	0.7	5.9	5.0	6.9	6.9	7.9	6.9	11.8	2.7	2.0	0.17	0.25	2.6	205
Monocytic leukaemia	0	0	-	-	-	-	-	-	-	-	-	-	-	-	-	-	-	-	-	0.0	0.0	0.00	0.00	0.0	206
Other leukaemia	0	0	-	-	-	-	-	-	-	-	-	-	-	-	-	-	-	-	-	0.0	0.0	0.00	0.00	0.0	207
Leukaemia unspecified	30	0	-	1.0	0.3	1.1	1.2	0.3	0.3	1.0	1.0	-	0.7	3.1	3.1	-	4.0	-	-	0.9	0.6	0.07	0.09	0.8	208
Other and unspecified	572	0	-	-	-	0.4	1.8	5.6	7.7	9.0	15.4	25.2	45.8	55.6	73.8	93.7	88.9	65.6	58.8	16.5	12.3	1.20	2.11	17.4	O&U
All sites	4791	0	7.6	7.3	8.9	12.0	17.1	28.4	47.9	72.1	107.6	169.2	319.7	426.1	582.0	780.8	978.3	953.2	862.1	138.0		9.03	17.82	148.4	ALL
All sites but 173	4659	0	7.6	7.3	8.9	12.0	16.2	28.2	47.1	71.4	105.0	163.9	313.8	417.9	568.9	751.1	948.6	908.3	812.1	134.2	100.0	8.84	17.34	144.2	ALLb
Rate from 1 case			0.401	0.348	0.344	0.354	0.300	0.268	0.264	0.347	0.515	0.663	0.654	0.625	0.769	1.143	1.976	3.454	2.942						

†Important: see notes on population page

THAILAND, CHIANG MAI 1988-1992

ANNUAL INCIDENCE PER 100,000 BY AGE GROUP (YEARS) - FEMALE

SITE	ALL AGES	AGE UNK	0-	5-	10-	15-	20-	25-	30-	35-	40-	45-	50-	55-	60-	65-	70-	75-	80+	CRUDE RATE	%	CR 64	CR 74	ASR (W)	ICD (9th)
Lip	15	0	-	-	-	-	-	-	0.3	0.4	-	-	-	0.6	1.6	3.6	-	16.1	4.7	0.4	0.3	0.01	0.03	**0.4**	*140*
Tongue	37	0	-	-	-	-	-	-	-	0.4	0.5	1.4	2.0	3.2	4.8	6.0	15.9	6.5	9.4	1.1	0.8	0.06	0.17	**1.2**	*141*
Salivary gland	16	0	-	-	-	-	-	-	0.3	0.7	1.1	0.7	2.0	0.6	0.8	1.2	2.0	6.5	2.3	0.5	0.3	0.03	0.05	**0.5**	*142*
Mouth	66	0	-	-	0.4	-	0.3	-	0.3	0.7	0.5	0.7	4.7	5.8	7.2	13.2	13.9	6.5	32.8	2.0	1.3	0.10	0.24	**2.0**	*143-5*
Oropharynx	29	0	-	-	-	-	-	-	-	-	0.5	0.7	0.7	2.6	1.6	7.2	5.9	19.4	11.7	0.9	0.6	0.03	0.10	**0.9**	*146*
Nasopharynx	48	0	-	-	-	-	-	0.8	1.1	1.1	2.2	4.3	5.3	1.3	8.8	3.6	4.0	6.5	-	1.4	1.0	0.12	0.16	**1.5**	*147*
Hypopharynx	18	0	-	-	-	-	-	0.3	-	-	-	-	0.7	0.6	2.4	3.6	7.9	6.5	7.0	0.5	0.4	0.02	0.08	**0.6**	*148*
Pharynx unspecified	3	0	-	-	-	-	-	-	-	-	-	-	-	0.6	0.8	-	-	3.2	-	0.1	0.1	0.01	0.01	**0.1**	*149*
Oesophagus	46	0	-	-	-	-	-	-	-	0.4	0.5	1.4	1.3	4.5	5.6	7.2	21.8	12.9	11.7	1.4	0.9	0.07	0.21	**1.5**	*150*
Stomach	154	0	-	-	-	0.4	-	-	1.6	2.9	5.5	5.7	13.3	16.7	20.8	27.6	31.7	16.1	11.7	4.6	3.1	0.33	0.63	**4.9**	*151*
Small intestine	4	0	-	-	-	-	-	-	-	-	-	-	0.7	1.3	1.3	-	-	-	-	0.1	0.1	0.01	0.01	**0.1**	*152*
Colon	122	0	-	-	-	-	0.3	1.1	1.4	3.3	2.7	4.3	8.6	12.2	20.8	13.2	13.9	32.3	14.1	3.6	2.5	0.27	0.41	**3.7**	*153*
Rectum	92	0	-	-	-	-	-	0.8	2.7	1.5	2.7	4.3	7.3	5.1	12.8	15.6	13.9	16.1	9.4	2.7	1.9	0.19	0.33	**2.8**	*154*
Liver	303	0	0.4	-	-	1.1	0.6	1.1	2.5	4.4	5.5	17.8	23.9	27.6	42.4	51.6	63.5	42.0	39.9	9.0	6.2	0.64	1.21	**9.7**	*155*
Gallbladder etc.	92	0	-	-	-	-	-	-	0.3	-	1.6	5.7	4.7	6.4	15.2	24.0	13.9	19.4	25.8	2.7	1.9	0.17	0.36	**3.0**	*156*
Pancreas	74	0	-	-	-	-	-	0.8	-	1.1	-	1.4	6.0	6.4	12.0	15.6	19.8	16.1	9.4	2.2	1.5	0.14	0.32	**2.4**	*157*
Nose, sinuses etc.	20	0	0.4	-	-	-	-	-	0.8	0.4	1.1	-	0.7	2.6	3.2	-	4.0	3.2	2.3	0.6	0.4	0.05	0.07	**0.6**	*160*
Larynx	55	0	-	-	-	-	-	-	-	0.7	1.1	0.7	4.7	3.9	8.0	16.8	13.9	9.7	7.0	1.6	1.1	0.10	0.25	**1.8**	*161*
Bronchus, lung	941	0	-	-	-	-	0.9	2.2	1.9	5.1	18.6	36.2	74.5	124.6	163.1	158.5	214.2	135.6	75.1	28.0	19.2	2.14	4.00	**30.3**	*162*
Other thoracic organs	3	0	-	-	0.4	-	0.3	-	-	-	-	-	0.7	-	-	-	-	-	-	0.1	0.1	0.01	0.01	**0.1**	*163-4*
Bone	18	0	-	-	-	1.1	0.6	0.3	0.5	-	-	1.4	2.7	-	-	-	2.0	9.7	-	0.5	0.4	0.03	0.04	**0.6**	*170*
Connective tissue	20	0	1.3	-	-	0.4	0.3	0.3	0.3	0.7	0.5	2.1	0.7	1.9	0.8	-	4.0	-	-	0.6	0.4	0.05	0.07	**0.7**	*171*
Mesothelioma	0	0	-	-	-	-	-	-	-	-	-	-	-	-	-	-	-	-	-	0.0	0.0	0.00	0.00	**0.0**	*MES*
Kaposi's sarcoma	0	0	-	-	-	-	-	-	-	-	-	-	-	-	-	-	-	-	-	0.0	0.0	0.00	0.00	**0.0**	*KAP*
Melanoma of skin	15	0	-	-	-	0.4	-	0.3	-	-	0.5	-	1.3	2.6	1.6	1.2	2.0	3.2	2.3	0.4	0.3	0.03	0.05	**0.5**	*172*
Other skin	98	0	-	-	-	-	0.6	0.5	1.1	1.8	0.5	2.1	6.0	5.8	9.6	14.4	19.8	45.2	35.2	2.9		0.14	0.31	**3.0**	*173*
Breast	477	0	-	-	-	-	0.6	3.8	10.1	20.4	45.4	41.2	43.2	34.7	34.4	42.0	35.7	19.4	14.1	14.2	9.7	1.17	1.56	**14.6**	*174*
Uterus unspecified	0	0	-	-	-	-	-	-	-	-	-	-	-	-	-	-	-	-	-	0.0	0.0	0.00	0.00	**0.0**	*179*
Cervix uteri	864	0	-	-	-	-	3.7	7.7	20.0	51.0	67.3	70.4	65.2	75.1	57.6	67.2	57.5	29.1	18.8	25.7	17.6	2.09	2.71	**25.6**	*180*
Placenta	9	0	-	-	-	-	0.3	0.8	0.5	-	0.7	-	1.3	-	-	-	-	-	-	0.3	0.2	0.02	0.02	**0.2**	*181*
Corpus uteri	110	0	-	-	-	-	0.3	0.5	1.4	1.5	4.9	10.0	12.6	12.2	13.6	12.0	9.9	9.7	4.7	3.3	2.2	0.28	0.39	**3.5**	*182*
Ovary etc.	152	0	0.8	0.4	-	0.7	3.1	4.4	3.3	4.7	5.5	7.1	13.3	14.1	12.0	8.4	13.9	12.9	2.3	4.5	3.1	0.35	0.46	**4.4**	*183*
Other female genital	41	0	-	-	-	0.4	-	0.5	0.8	1.5	1.6	2.1	2.7	3.9	1.6	4.8	4.0	9.7	9.4	1.2	0.8	0.08	0.12	**1.2**	*184*
†Bladder	78	0	-	-	-	-	-	-	0.3	0.4	1.6	2.8	2.7	7.7	13.6	15.6	15.9	29.1	14.1	2.3	1.6	0.15	0.30	**2.5**	*188*
Kidney etc.	48	0	-	-	-	-	-	-	0.8	0.7	0.5	1.4	2.7	4.5	8.8	10.8	11.9	6.5	2.3	1.4	1.0	0.10	0.21	**1.5**	*189*
Eye	5	0	0.4	-	-	-	-	-	0.3	-	-	0.7	-	0.6	-	-	2.0	-	-	0.1	0.1	0.01	0.02	**0.2**	*190*
Brain, nervous system	55	0	2.1	1.5	1.5	0.4	0.9	1.4	0.8	1.1	2.2	2.1	1.3	1.9	7.2	4.8	2.0	-	2.3	1.6	1.1	0.12	0.16	**1.8**	*191-2*
Thyroid	88	0	-	-	-	-	0.6	1.9	1.6	5.5	5.5	1.4	6.6	6.4	6.4	12.0	11.9	3.2	2.3	2.6	1.8	0.18	0.30	**2.5**	*193*
Other endocrine	4	0	-	-	-	-	0.3	0.3	-	-	-	-	1.3	-	-	-	-	-	-	0.1	0.1	0.01	0.01	**0.1**	*194*
Hodgkin's disease	15	0	-	-	-	-	-	0.3	0.3	1.5	-	0.7	-	0.6	2.4	1.2	-	6.5	2.3	0.4	0.3	0.03	0.03	**0.4**	*201*
Non-Hodgkin lymphoma	84	0	0.8	1.5	0.7	1.8	1.2	0.8	1.1	2.2	2.7	2.8	4.0	5.1	6.4	12.0	7.9	16.1	9.4	2.5	1.7	0.16	0.26	**2.6**	*200,202*
Multiple myeloma	10	0	-	-	-	-	-	-	-	-	0.5	-	1.3	1.3	0.8	2.4	2.0	-	2.3	0.3	0.2	0.02	0.04	**0.3**	*203*
Lymphoid leukaemia	22	0	1.7	0.7	1.8	0.7	0.3	-	0.8	0.4	0.5	-	-	-	0.8	2.4	-	-	-	0.7	0.4	0.04	0.05	**0.7**	*204*
Myeloid leukaemia	88	0	2.9	0.4	1.5	1.1	1.8	1.6	2.7	2.5	2.7	4.3	3.3	2.6	7.2	7.2	13.9	3.2	2.3	2.6	1.8	0.17	0.28	**2.7**	*205*
Monocytic leukaemia	1	0	-	-	-	-	-	-	-	-	-	-	-	-	-	-	2.0	-	-	0.0	0.0	0.00	0.01	**0.0**	*206*
Other leukaemia	1	0	-	-	-	0.4	-	-	-	-	-	-	-	-	-	-	-	-	-	0.0	0.0	0.00	0.00	**0.0**	*207*
Leukaemia unspecified	28	0	0.8	-	-	1.1	0.3	-	0.5	0.4	1.1	2.1	2.0	1.9	1.6	4.8	4.0	-	-	0.8	0.6	0.06	0.10	**0.9**	*208*
Other and unspecified	537	0	1.7	0.4	-	2.5	2.7	3.0	7.1	10.2	19.7	24.9	35.2	50.7	82.3	79.2	73.4	64.6	51.6	16.0	10.9	1.20	1.97	**16.7**	*O&U*
All sites	5006	0	13.5	4.7	6.2	12.0	20.2	35.6	67.5	129.2	208.0	265.8	369.7	461.6	601.2	671.1	755.5	642.3	450.3	148.8		10.98	18.11	**155.6**	*ALL*
All sites but 173	4908	0	13.5	4.7	6.2	12.0	19.5	35.1	66.4	127.4	207.5	263.7	363.7	455.8	591.6	656.7	735.7	597.2	415.2	145.9	100.0	10.84	17.80	**152.6**	*ALLb*
Rate from 1 case			0.421	0.365	0.365	0.352	0.305	0.274	0.273	0.364	0.547	0.711	0.665	0.642	0.799	1.200	1.983	3.228	2.345						

†Important: see notes on population page

Thailand, Khon Kaen

Khon Kaen Cancer Registry was established in 1984 at the Faculty of Medicine and Srinagarind Hospital, Khon Kaen University. It started as the Hospital Cancer Registry to collect all cancer cases in Srinagarind University Hospital. The population-based cancer registry started officially in January 1988, after a preparatory period of some five months.

Khon Kaen Cancer Registry is under the management of the cancer unit and a cancer committee composed of 20 members. Two registered nurses, two practical nurses, one computer statistician and two clerks form the registration team of the Unit. Verification of the collected cases is performed by the team under the supervision of physicians who are chairman and secretariat of the cancer committee. The cancer committee as a whole plays a major advisory role.

The area covered by the registry comprises 25 districts of Khon Kaen province. Khon Kaen city is the capital of the north-eastern region of Thailand, and is situated between latitudes 10 and 19° N and longitudes 103 and 102° E, about 450 km north-east of Bangkok. The province is a high plateau about 200 m above sea level, covering an area of 13 404 km^2. The climate is generally hot and dry. The mean temperature is around 28°C and the average annual rainfall approximately 1188 mm.

The population of Khon Kaen is homogeneous. Most people are farmers working in rice and cassava fields. Their habit of eating raw fish is a major public health problem, causing about 50% of the population to be infected with liver flukes (*Opisthorchis viverrini*), which leads to quite a high incidence of cholangiocarcinoma in the area.

Most of the public hospitals in Khon Kaen belong to the Ministry of Public Health; the university hospital and another small army hospital are the only other government hospitals. In the last two years, three new hospitals have been established. Attempts to improve the referral system have gained some support but many patients still refer themselves according to their preference. Death certificates in remote villages are filled in by the headman of the village, and are sent to the office of the Khon Kaen Medical Officer.

The data sources for the registry are:

(1) Srinagarind Hospital (800-bed university hospital). The data from the active hospital cancer registry are selected for patients who resided in Khon Kaen during the time of collection. These data come from outpatient, inpatient, operating theatre, radiotherapy and pathology department records.

(2) Khon Kaen Provincial Hospital (580 beds). The data are collected from the outpatient records and the pathology department, and filed by the nurse in charge, supervised by the registry's registered nurses.

(3) Other hospitals in Khon Kaen. The outpatient records are used by the nurses in charge to complete the data forms.

Death certificates with a mention of cancer are collected from the office of the Chief Medical Officer. These data are reviewed and checked with existing registry files before data entry.

The Chief Medical Officer and all the directors of hospitals in Khon Kaen have agreed to make collection of data for the cancer registry compulsory. Registration is done both actively and passively.

Any follow-up data on cancer patients are updated on file. At the end of each year, a return-paid postcard is sent to each patient thought to be still alive, to ascertain their present status, whether alive or dead. If no answer is received, a second postcard is sent to the headman of the village for him to report on the patient's status.

Each completed data form is checked manually and entered into the database files in the registry microcomputer.

The name, age, sex, address and site of cancer are checked for any duplication. Any questionable case is traced to the original sources of information for clarification.

All multiple primary cases are clarified by physicians with their original records and with any other physicians concerned, if needed.

The rising trends of all cancer cases are being analysed. A cohort study of the population of areas with endemic liver fluke infestation is being conducted to monitor the high liver cancer incidence in relation to this risk factor.

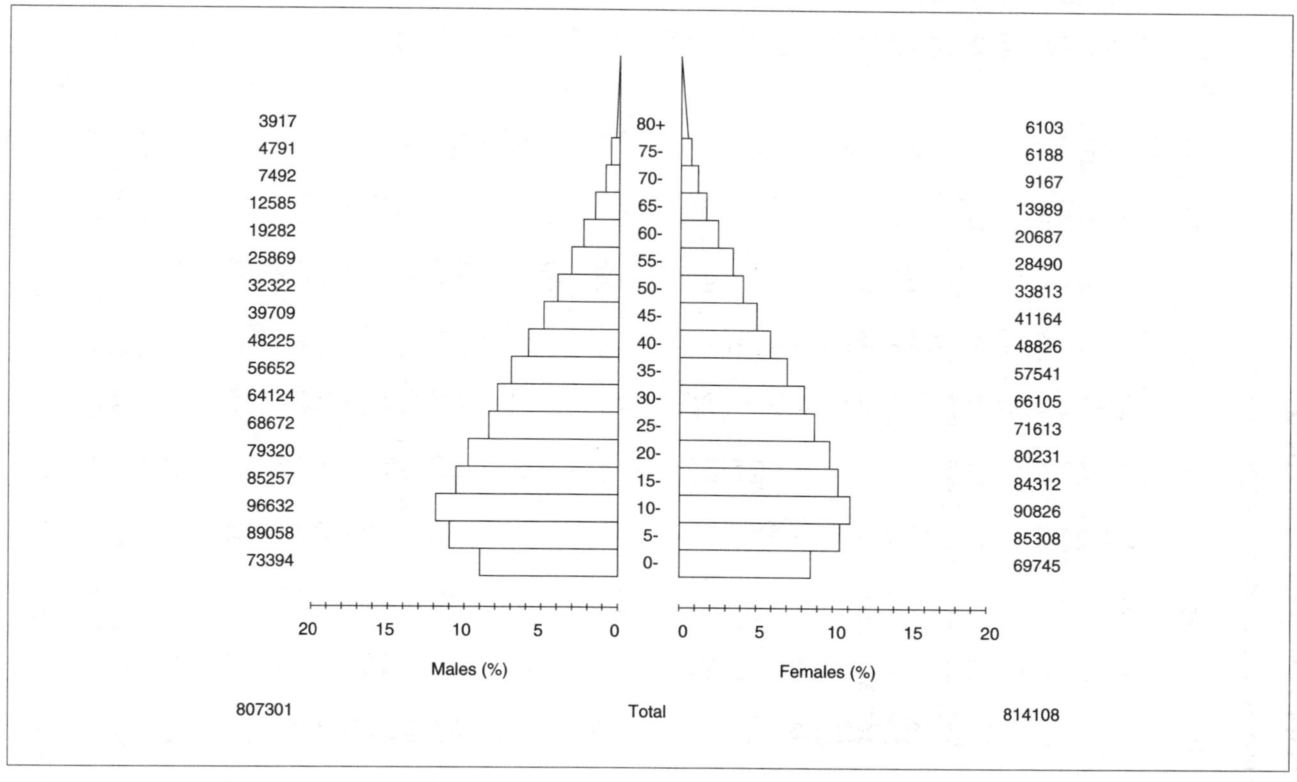

Thailand, Khon Kaen

Source of population: 1990

Census: 1990 Census of Population and Housing (1 April)

Notes to tables overleaf:

* The high proportion of diagnoses based on a death certificate alone, low rates of childhood cancer, and a high proportion of cases in the Other and unspecified category suggest problems in ascertainment and, possibly, data validity.

† 188 does not include non-invasive tumours

Screening programmes in the area

Since 1990 1 000 examinations were carried out annually in the population over age 35 for cervical and 1 000 for breast cancer. Some 2 000 annual screening examinations have been performed for liver cancer and for cancer of the oral cavity in the population over age 40 since 1990.

* THAILAND, KHON KAEN 1990-1993

ANNUAL INCIDENCE PER 100,000 BY AGE GROUP (YEARS) - MALE

SITE	ALL AGES	AGE UNK	0-	5-	10-	15-	20-	25-	30-	35-	40-	45-	50-	55-	60-	65-	70-	75-	80+	CRUDE RATE	%	CR 64	CR 74	ASR (W)	ICD (9th)
Lip	7	0	-	-	-	-	-	-	0.4	-	-	-	-	1.9	-	2.0	3.3	5.2	6.4	0.2	0.2	0.01	0.04	**0.3**	140
Tongue	22	0	-	-	-	-	-	1.1	-	-	0.5	0.6	1.5	3.9	3.9	6.0	13.3	5.2	-	0.7	0.5	0.06	0.15	**1.0**	141
Salivary gland	6	0	-	-	-	-	-	-	-	-	0.5	0.6	0.8	-	2.6	-	3.3	-	-	0.2	0.1	0.02	0.04	**0.3**	142
Mouth	33	0	-	-	0.3	-	-	-	0.4	-	0.5	1.3	3.1	2.9	6.5	7.9	16.7	15.7	25.5	1.0	0.8	0.07	0.20	**1.7**	143-5
Oropharynx	14	0	-	-	-	-	-	-	-	-	1.6	0.6	0.8	1.9	2.6	-	6.7	10.4	6.4	0.4	0.3	0.04	0.07	**0.7**	146
Nasopharynx	65	1	-	-	-	0.3	1.6	0.4	2.3	0.9	2.6	5.0	7.0	6.8	10.4	15.9	6.7	10.4	-	2.0	1.6	0.19	0.30	**2.6**	147
Hypopharynx	11	0	-	-	-	-	0.3	-	0.4	-	0.5	-	-	1.0	1.3	-	-	20.9	12.8	0.3	0.3	0.02	0.02	**0.5**	148
Pharynx unspecified	1	0	-	-	-	-	-	-	-	-	-	-	-	-	-	2.0	-	-	-	0.0	0.0	0.00	0.01	**0.1**	149
Oesophagus	34	1	-	-	-	-	0.3	-	0.4	-	2.1	1.3	2.3	7.7	5.2	9.9	6.7	15.7	-	1.1	0.8	0.10	0.18	**1.5**	150
Stomach	84	1	-	-	-	-	0.6	-	-	0.4	1.0	4.4	10.1	10.6	19.4	21.9	50.1	31.3	-	2.6	2.0	0.24	0.60	**4.1**	151
Small intestine	3	0	-	-	-	-	-	-	0.4	-	-	-	0.8	-	-	2.0	-	-	-	0.1	0.1	0.01	0.02	**0.1**	152
Colon	107	0	-	-	-	0.6	0.6	0.7	1.2	2.2	5.7	3.1	8.5	13.5	27.2	15.9	50.1	26.1	19.1	3.3	2.6	0.32	0.65	**4.9**	153
Rectum	63	0	-	-	-	-	-	-	2.6	0.5	4.4	6.2	8.7	10.4	9.9	40.0	36.5	-	-	2.0	1.5	0.16	0.41	**3.0**	154
Liver	2119	9	1.4	-	-	0.9	2.5	1.8	12.1	33.5	68.4	120.9	225.9	374.0	534.2	524.4	543.9	433.1	370.2	65.6	51.3	6.91	12.27	**97.4**	155
Gallbladder etc.	41	1	-	-	-	-	-	-	-	1.3	0.5	3.1	6.2	8.7	3.9	9.9	10.0	10.4	6.4	1.3	1.0	0.12	0.22	**1.8**	156
Pancreas	21	0	-	-	-	-	-	-	0.4	0.9	1.0	-	2.3	2.9	3.9	6.0	6.7	10.4	-	0.7	0.5	0.06	0.12	**0.9**	157
Nose, sinuses etc.	11	0	-	-	-	-	-	0.4	0.8	0.4	0.5	-	-	1.9	2.6	4.0	-	-	-	0.3	0.3	0.03	0.05	**0.4**	160
Larynx	22	0	-	-	-	-	-	-	-	-	-	-	0.8	1.9	5.2	7.9	13.3	31.3	6.4	0.7	0.5	0.04	0.15	**1.2**	161
Bronchus, lung	355	2	-	-	-	0.3	-	1.8	1.6	5.3	11.9	15.7	28.6	46.4	85.6	109.3	93.4	135.7	146.8	11.0	8.6	0.99	2.01	**17.0**	162
Other thoracic organs	8	0	-	-	-	-	0.3	0.4	0.4	0.4	-	-	-	2.9	-	2.0	-	-	-	0.2	0.2	0.02	0.03	**0.3**	163-4
Bone	29	0	-	-	0.5	0.9	-	0.7	-	0.4	0.5	1.9	3.1	3.9	3.9	-	16.7	5.2	-	0.9	0.7	0.08	0.16	**1.2**	170
Connective tissue	26	0	1.4	-	1.0	0.6	0.3	-	1.2	0.4	1.6	1.3	1.5	1.0	1.3	2.0	-	5.2	-	0.8	0.6	0.06	0.07	**0.9**	171
Mesothelioma	1	0	-	-	0.3	-	-	-	0.3	-	-	-	-	-	-	-	-	-	-	0.0	0.0	0.00	0.00	**0.0**	MES
Kaposi's sarcoma	0	0	-	-	-	-	-	-	-	-	-	-	-	-	-	-	-	-	-	0.0	0.0	0.00	0.00	**0.0**	KAP
Melanoma of skin	7	0	-	-	-	-	-	-	-	-	-	-	0.6	-	-	2.6	2.0	-	10.4	6.4	0.2	0.2	0.02	0.03	**0.4**	172
Other skin	77	0	-	-	0.3	-	-	0.7	0.4	0.9	2.6	1.9	5.4	9.7	15.6	19.9	40.0	-	76.6	2.4		0.19	0.49	**3.9**	173
Breast	0	0	-	-	-	-	-	-	-	-	-	-	-	-	-	-	-	-	-	0.0	0.0	0.00	0.00	**0.0**	175
Prostate	48	0	-	-	-	-	-	-	-	-	-	-	2.3	1.0	9.1	19.9	36.7	36.5	57.4	1.5	1.2	0.06	0.34	**2.8**	185
Testis	18	0	-	-	-	-	0.6	1.1	1.9	-	0.5	2.5	0.8	1.0	-	2.0	-	-	-	0.6	0.4	0.04	0.05	**0.6**	186
Penis	45	0	-	-	-	-	-	-	0.4	1.8	4.1	3.1	7.0	5.8	5.2	6.0	6.7	5.2	12.8	1.4	1.1	0.14	0.20	**1.8**	187.1-.4
Other male genital	0	0	-	-	-	-	-	-	-	-	-	-	-	-	-	-	-	-	-	0.0	0.0	0.00	0.00	**0.0**	187.5-.9
†Bladder	65	0	-	-	-	0.3	-	-	0.4	0.9	1.0	1.3	6.2	11.6	10.4	13.9	36.7	36.5	25.5	2.0	1.6	0.16	0.41	**3.2**	188
Kidney etc.	31	0	1.0	0.3	-	-	0.3	-	0.8	0.9	2.1	3.8	3.9	1.0	2.6	2.0	10.0	-	-	1.0	0.8	0.08	0.14	**1.2**	189
Eye	9	0	0.7	-	-	-	0.3	0.4	-	0.4	-	-	-	-	2.6	-	3.3	-	6.4	0.3	0.2	0.02	0.04	**0.4**	190
Brain, nervous system	72	0	2.4	1.1	1.6	0.9	1.3	2.2	2.7	1.3	1.6	3.8	0.8	5.8	6.5	13.9	6.7	5.2	6.4	2.2	1.7	0.16	0.26	**2.7**	191-2
Thyroid	23	0	-	-	-	0.3	0.3	-	0.4	0.4	1.6	1.3	1.5	1.9	5.2	2.0	10.0	10.4	-	0.7	0.6	0.06	0.12	**1.0**	193
Other endocrine	7	0	0.3	-	0.3	0.3	0.3	-	0.4	0.9	0.9	-	-	-	-	-	-	-	-	0.2	0.2	0.01	0.01	**0.2**	194
Hodgkin's disease	12	0	-	0.3	-	0.6	-	-	0.8	0.4	-	0.6	0.8	1.9	2.6	-	-	-	-	0.4	0.3	0.04	0.04	**0.4**	201
Non-Hodgkin lymphoma	69	0	0.7	0.6	0.5	1.5	1.6	1.1	1.6	1.8	3.1	3.1	7.0	1.9	5.2	9.9	16.7	15.7	19.1	2.1	1.7	0.15	0.28	**2.7**	200,202
Multiple myeloma	4	0	-	-	-	-	-	-	-	-	-	0.6	-	1.0	-	-	6.7	-	-	0.1	0.1	0.01	0.04	**0.2**	203
Lymphoid leukaemia	38	0	3.4	2.0	0.5	1.2	1.9	1.1	1.2	-	0.5	-	-	-	-	2.0	3.3	-	-	1.2	0.9	0.06	0.09	**1.2**	204
Myeloid leukaemia	41	0	0.7	-	1.6	0.9	0.9	1.5	0.8	1.3	1.6	1.3	0.8	3.9	3.9	7.9	3.3	-	-	1.3	1.0	0.09	0.15	**1.4**	205
Monocytic leukaemia	1	0	-	-	-	0.3	-	-	-	-	-	-	-	-	-	-	-	-	-	0.0	0.0	0.00	0.00	**0.0**	206
Other leukaemia	0	0	-	-	-	-	-	-	-	-	-	-	-	-	-	-	-	-	-	0.0	0.0	0.00	0.00	**0.0**	207
Leukaemia unspecified	33	1	0.7	-	0.3	1.8	-	2.5	0.8	0.4	2.1	-	0.8	1.9	1.3	4.0	6.7	5.2	-	1.0	0.8	0.06	0.12	**1.2**	208
Other and unspecified	524	6	2.0	1.1	0.3	0.9	1.9	3.6	3.5	10.1	16.1	27.7	60.3	83.1	118.0	123.2	113.5	93.9	76.6	16.2	12.7	1.66	2.86	**23.3**	O&U
All sites	4207	22	14.6	5.3	7.2	12.3	16.1	21.5	37.8	70.6	136.9	215.9	406.8	634.0	920.5	987.3	1181.3	1028.0	887.2	130.3		12.56	23.46	**190.6**	ALL
All sites but 173	4130	22	14.6	5.3	7.0	12.3	16.1	20.8	37.4	69.7	134.3	214.1	401.4	624.3	905.0	967.4	1141.2	1028.0	810.6	127.9	100.0	12.38	22.98	**186.8**	ALLb

Rate from 1 case			0.341	0.281	0.259	0.293	0.315	0.364	0.390	0.441	0.518	0.630	0.773	0.966	1.297	1.986	3.337	5.218	6.382

†Important: see notes on population page

* THAILAND, KHON KAEN 1990-1993

ANNUAL INCIDENCE PER 100,000 BY AGE GROUP (YEARS) - FEMALE

SITE	ALL AGES	AGE UNK	0-	5-	10-	15-	20-	25-	30-	35-	40-	45-	50-	55-	60-	65-	70-	75-	80+	CRUDE RATE	%	CR 64	CR 74	ASR (W)	ICD (9th)
Lip	59	2	-	-	-	-	-	-	-	0.4	-	1.8	0.7	6.1	10.9	23.2	27.3	12.1	41.0	1.8	1.8	0.10	0.36	2.7	140
Tongue	21	0	-	-	-	0.3	-	-	0.8	-	-	1.8	0.7	4.4	1.2	3.6	5.5	8.1	8.2	0.6	0.6	0.05	0.09	0.8	141
Salivary gland	8	0	-	-	-	-	0.6	0.3	0.4	0.4	-	-	-	0.9	1.2	-	2.7	-	-	0.2	0.2	0.02	0.03	0.3	142
Mouth	68	0	-	-	-	0.3	-	0.3	0.4	1.3	-	0.6	3.0	7.9	13.3	19.7	32.7	40.4	16.4	2.1	2.1	0.14	0.40	3.0	143-5
Oropharynx	6	0	-	-	-	-	-	-	-	-	-	-	0.7	0.9	-	-	-	8.1	8.2	0.2	0.2	0.01	0.01	0.2	146
Nasopharynx	23	0	-	-	-	-	-	0.3	0.4	1.3	2.0	1.8	1.5	1.8	3.6	3.6	5.5	-	-	0.7	0.7	0.06	0.11	0.9	147
Hypopharynx	1	0	-	-	-	-	-	-	-	0.4	-	-	-	-	-	-	-	-	-	0.0	0.0	0.00	0.00	0.0	148
Pharynx unspecified	1	0	-	-	-	-	-	-	-	0.4	-	-	-	-	-	-	-	-	-	0.0	0.0	0.00	0.00	0.0	149
Oesophagus	12	0	-	-	-	-	-	-	-	-	0.5	1.2	-	1.8	3.6	1.8	2.7	4.0	4.1	0.4	0.4	0.04	0.06	0.5	150
Stomach	52	0	-	-	-	-	0.3	0.7	1.5	1.3	0.5	2.4	5.2	4.4	12.1	10.7	10.9	12.1	8.2	1.6	1.6	0.14	0.25	2.1	151
Small intestine	3	0	-	-	-	-	-	-	-	-	0.7	-	0.7	-	1.2	-	4.0	-	-	0.1	0.1	0.01	0.01	0.1	152
Colon	81	0	-	-	-	0.3	-	0.3	1.1	1.7	2.0	3.6	12.6	10.5	9.7	17.9	24.5	16.2	8.2	2.5	2.5	0.21	0.42	3.3	153
Rectum	48	0	-	-	-	-	-	0.3	2.3	0.9	1.0	2.4	4.4	1.8	13.3	12.5	5.5	12.1	8.2	1.5	1.5	0.13	0.22	1.9	154
Liver	927	3	0.4	-	-	0.3	-	-	4.2	13.9	22.5	53.4	88.0	143.9	219.9	212.7	242.7	185.8	114.7	28.5	28.1	2.74	5.03	39.0	155
Gallbladder etc.	47	0	-	-	-	-	-	-	-	0.9	-	2.4	3.0	3.5	10.9	26.8	10.9	16.2	4.1	1.4	1.4	0.10	0.29	2.1	156
Pancreas	16	0	-	-	-	-	-	-	-	0.4	1.0	0.6	0.7	2.6	6.0	1.8	5.5	-	-	0.5	0.5	0.06	0.09	0.7	157
Nose, sinuses etc.	9	0	-	-	-	-	-	-	-	-	0.5	0.6	-	2.6	1.2	-	2.7	-	-	0.3	0.3	0.02	0.04	0.4	160
Larynx	5	0	-	-	-	-	-	-	-	-	0.5	0.6	-	0.9	-	1.8	2.7	-	8.2	0.2	0.2	0.01	0.03	0.2	161
Bronchus, lung	132	0	-	-	-	0.3	0.6	0.3	0.4	2.6	4.6	10.9	15.5	16.7	20.5	19.7	35.5	40.4	12.3	4.1	4.0	0.36	0.64	5.3	162
Other thoracic organs	2	0	-	-	-	-	-	-	-	-	-	-	0.7	-	1.2	-	-	-	-	0.1	0.1	0.01	0.01	0.1	163-4
Bone	40	0	-	-	0.3	0.6	0.6	0.3	-	0.4	1.0	1.8	3.0	3.5	8.5	5.4	24.5	4.0	-	1.2	1.2	0.10	0.25	1.7	170
Connective tissue	19	0	1.1	0.3	-	0.3	0.6	-	0.4	0.4	0.5	0.6	0.7	2.6	3.6	-	-	4.0	-	0.6	0.6	0.06	0.06	0.7	171
Mesothelioma	0	0	-	-	-	-	-	-	-	-	-	-	-	-	-	-	-	-	-	0.0	0.0	0.00	0.00	0.0	MES
Kaposi's sarcoma	0	0	-	-	-	-	-	-	-	-	-	-	-	-	-	-	-	-	-	0.0	0.0	0.00	0.00	0.0	KAP
Melanoma of skin	14	0	-	-	-	-	-	-	-	-	0.4	0.5	1.2	1.5	0.9	1.2	5.4	2.7	4.1	0.4	0.4	0.03	0.07	0.6	172
Other skin	81	0	-	-	0.3	0.6	0.3	0.3	0.4	0.4	1.0	1.8	4.4	7.0	19.3	17.9	10.9	48.5	53.3	2.5		0.18	0.32	3.4	173
Breast	236	0	-	-	-	-	-	1.0	7.2	11.7	22.5	26.7	22.9	21.1	25.4	21.4	16.4	12.1	8.2	7.2	7.1	0.69	0.88	8.4	174
Uterus unspecified	4	0	-	-	-	-	-	-	-	-	0.5	-	0.7	-	2.4	-	-	-	-	0.1	0.1	0.02	0.02	0.2	179
Cervix uteri	517	0	-	-	-	-	2.8	3.8	12.1	21.7	33.3	53.4	59.9	61.4	58.0	60.8	54.5	24.2	12.3	15.9	15.7	1.53	2.11	18.8	180
Placenta	13	0	-	-	-	-	1.2	1.7	1.1	-	-	0.6	-	-	-	-	-	-	-	0.4	0.4	0.02	0.02	0.3	181
Corpus uteri	54	0	-	-	-	-	-	-	0.4	0.9	2.6	7.9	11.8	6.1	4.8	5.4	2.7	8.1	-	1.7	1.6	0.17	0.21	2.0	182
Ovary etc.	126	0	-	-	0.3	0.9	1.6	2.1	3.8	5.6	4.6	11.5	12.6	14.9	16.9	8.9	8.2	-	16.4	3.9	3.8	0.37	0.46	4.4	183
Other female genital	19	0	-	-	-	-	-	-	0.4	1.7	0.5	-	0.7	2.6	4.8	5.4	5.5	-	-	0.6	0.6	0.05	0.11	0.8	184
†Bladder	14	0	-	-	-	-	-	-	0.4	0.9	-	1.8	0.7	0.9	2.4	1.8	2.7	-	8.2	0.4	0.4	0.04	0.06	0.5	188
Kidney etc.	19	1	1.1	0.3	-	0.3	-	-	0.4	-	2.0	1.2	2.2	0.9	2.4	-	-	-	-	0.6	0.6	0.06	0.06	0.7	189
Eye	11	0	1.4	-	0.6	-	0.3	0.3	0.4	-	-	0.6	-	-	-	-	-	-	4.1	0.3	0.3	0.02	0.02	0.4	190
Brain, nervous system	67	0	0.7	1.2	1.7	1.2	0.9	2.1	0.8	1.3	2.0	4.9	5.2	6.1	7.3	5.4	2.7	4.0	-	2.1	2.0	0.18	0.22	2.3	191-2
Thyroid	106	0	-	-	-	0.3	1.6	3.5	6.1	3.9	8.2	8.5	6.7	5.3	6.0	12.5	5.5	8.1	16.4	3.3	3.2	0.25	0.34	3.5	193
Other endocrine	6	0	-	0.3	-	-	-	-	0.8	-	-	-	0.7	1.8	-	-	-	-	-	0.2	0.2	0.02	0.02	0.2	194
Hodgkin's disease	12	0	-	-	-	-	0.9	-	0.4	0.4	-	0.7	0.9	2.4	3.6	2.7	-	-	-	0.4	0.4	0.03	0.06	0.5	201
Non-Hodgkin lymphoma	50	0	1.1	0.3	-	0.3	-	1.4	1.1	1.7	3.1	2.4	4.4	3.5	4.8	-	13.6	4.0	16.4	1.5	1.5	0.12	0.19	1.8	200,202
Multiple myeloma	3	0	-	-	-	-	-	-	-	-	-	-	0.6	-	1.8	-	-	-	-	0.1	0.1	0.01	0.01	0.1	203
Lymphoid leukaemia	27	1	1.4	0.9	1.1	0.9	1.2	0.3	0.4	0.4	1.0	0.6	0.7	0.9	-	-	-	-	-	0.8	0.8	0.05	0.05	0.8	204
Myeloid leukaemia	43	0	1.1	-	0.3	0.6	0.6	0.7	0.4	2.6	2.6	1.8	5.9	2.6	-	10.7	-	-	4.1	1.3	1.3	0.10	0.15	1.5	205
Monocytic leukaemia	1	0	-	-	-	-	-	-	-	-	-	-	-	-	-	-	2.7	-	-	0.0	0.0	0.00	0.01	0.1	206
Other leukaemia	0	0	-	-	-	-	-	-	-	-	-	-	-	-	-	-	-	-	-	0.0	0.0	0.00	0.00	0.0	207
Leukaemia unspecified	34	0	0.7	0.6	0.3	0.6	1.6	0.7	0.8	0.9	1.0	1.8	3.0	4.4	2.4	-	-	-	-	1.0	1.0	0.09	0.09	1.1	208
Other and unspecified	347	5	0.4	-	-	1.8	1.2	2.4	6.1	6.1	8.2	15.8	36.2	50.0	71.3	78.6	70.9	48.5	20.5	10.7	10.5	1.01	1.77	14.0	O&U
All sites	3384	12	9.3	3.8	4.7	9.8	17.1	23.7	54.8	87.8	130.6	230.2	322.4	409.8	574.0	598.7	643.6	529.3	405.5	103.9		9.42	15.66	132.4	ALL
All sites but 173	3303	12	9.3	3.8	4.4	9.2	16.8	23.4	54.5	87.3	129.5	228.4	317.9	402.8	554.7	580.8	632.7	480.8	352.3	101.4	100.0	9.24	15.33	129.0	ALLb

Rate from 1 case			0.358	0.293	0.275	0.297	0.312	0.349	0.378	0.434	0.512	0.607	0.739	0.878	1.208	1.787	2.727	4.040	4.096

†Important: see notes on population page

441

Viet Nam, Hanoi

Hanoi Cancer Registry was established in October 1987 at Hanoi Cancer Hospital; regular data collection started in January 1988. Its aim is to collect systematically information on newly diagnosed cancer cases in residents of Hanoi, so as to estimate as precisely as possible cancer incidence in the population for epidemiological and public health purposes.

Hanoi is the capital of Viet Nam and one of the most important economic and industrial centres. It is located in the Red River delta in northern Viet Nam, between latitude 20°53′ and 21°23′ N and longitude 105°44′ and 106°2′ E. The area covered is 921 km² and the population density is 2383 persons per km². 60% of the inhabitants of Hanoi live in rural areas. The crude death rate is 6.2 per thousand and the infant mortality rate is 32.0 per thousand. Life expectancy at birth is 69.7 years.

A comprehensive health service system has operated since 1955 in the north and 1975 in the south. A large network of medical centres and hospitals enables the entire population to obtain free medical service. Since 1990, some medical service expenditures have been charged to patients, but most is still subsidized by the government. Under the Ministry of Health, the health system in each province is the responsibility of the Provincial Health Department; each district has a district health department. In each province there exists a network of clinical and preventive establishments. The basic unit is the communal or sub-district health centre, which exists in more than 90% of communes and sub-districts.

Although the whole country shares the same structure of health services, Hanoi is privileged compared with other provinces in its large number of relatively modern medical research institutes, specialized hospitals and teaching-based hospitals. The four inner-city district general hospitals differ from other hospitals of the same administrative level by the quality of medical service (staff, equipment).

All 22 establishments, which are medical research institutes, specialized, teaching-based and general hospitals, military and professional hospitals, contribute to the registry. The private health care system, which consists of private consultations (there are no private hospitals), has no facilities for specific diagnosis of cancers and does not contribute to the registry. The death registry has functioned for a long time but in the absence of notification of medical cause of death cannot serve as a source of data.

In each hospital, a list of all possible sources of information (medical records of in- and out-patients, hospital check-in, departmental, consultation and laboratory logs including autopsy log) has been established and is periodically reviewed and updated by registry staff. An active mechanism of data collection is applied. The registry staff periodically visit hospitals at a frequency depending on the number of cases in each hospital, but no less than once every six months.

The items collected and data-processing procedures follow the recommendation of MacLennan in *Cancer Registration: Principles and Methods*. All available information on newly diagnosed cancer cases (including carcinoma *in situ*) having a permanent resident address mentioning Hanoi is collected on a registry card. The card then is verified for missing information, followed by duplicate checking based on an index file with the name, age, sex, address, date of diagnosis and localization. New cases are then coded and entered, and information on already registered cases is updated using CANREG software. The ICD-O was originally used for coding site and morphology. Checking for completeness is carried out once per year by the independent case ascertainment method. Data validity checking is carried out during data entry (CANREG) and periodically using the CHECK program of IARC/IACR for unlikely combinations of sex/site, age/site and site/histology.

Several problems confront the registry:

(1) The population is mobile due to informal emigration and changing of territory, but the national census is carried out only every tenth year and a formal population estimate is made only at five-year intervals.

(2) The absence of a post-code system and the rapid growth and changes in the city area cause some difficulties in ascertaining the permanent address of cases.

(3) The lack of medical causes in the death registry affects data completeness to some extent.

The cancer incidence estimates based on the data of the Hanoi Cancer Registry are periodically submitted to the Department of Planning and Department of Treatment of the Ministry of Health and are commonly used by students and researchers for theses and other studies. They are also used by the media for scientific and educational programmes.

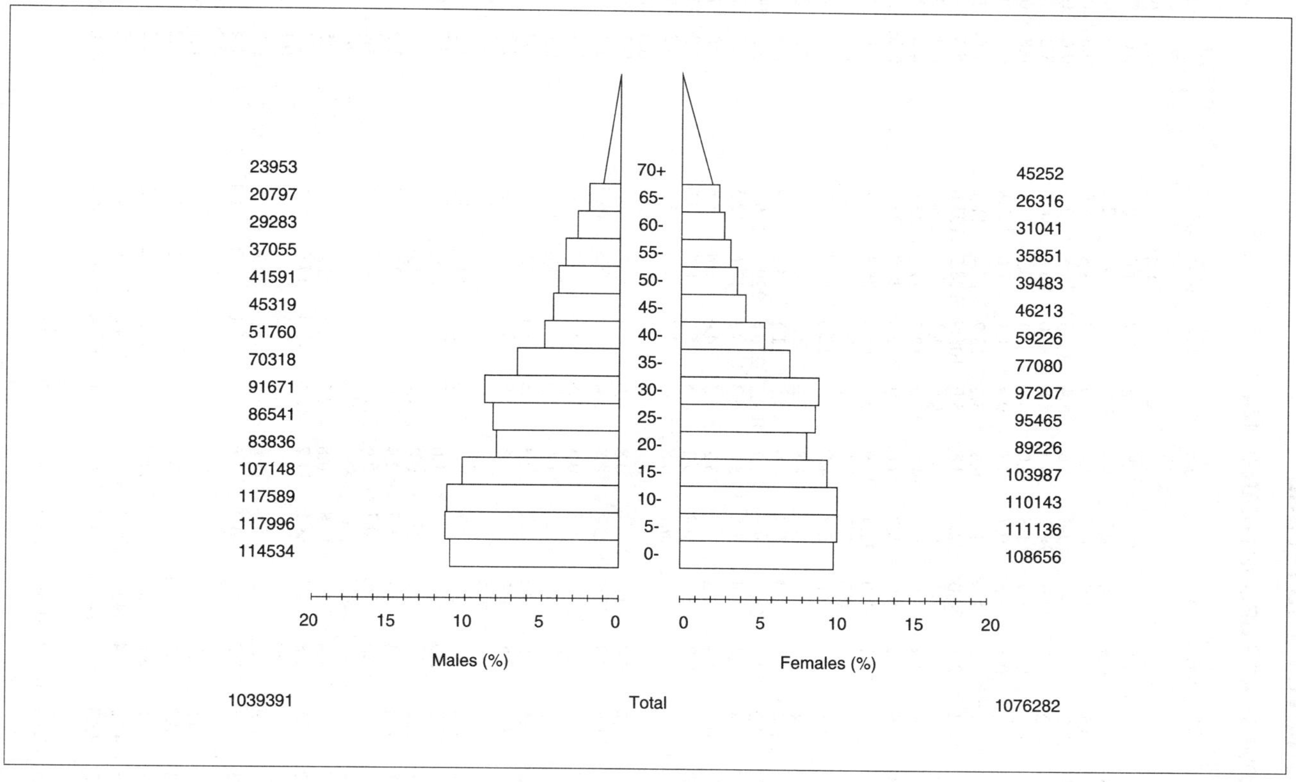

Viet Nam, Hanoi
Source of population: 1990,1995
Census: 1989
Estimate: 1990: estimate based on 1989 Census. P(1/7/1990) = P(1/4/1989) x Exp (1.25.r). r: annual growth rate between 1979 and 1989. 1995: component method, taking into account births, deaths and migration. Source: Projection of population, school enrolment and labour force, Vietnam, 1990-2005, Stat. Pub. House, 1994.

Notes to tables overleaf:
* Given the local circumstances, lack of death certification and low level of histological verification there is probably under-registration.
† 188 does not include non-invasive tumours

* VIET NAM, HANOI 1991-1993

ANNUAL INCIDENCE PER 100,000 BY AGE GROUP (YEARS) - MALE

SITE	ALL AGES	AGE UNK	0-	5-	10-	15-	20-	25-	30-	35-	40-	45-	50-	55-	60-	65-	70+	CRUDE RATE	%	CR 64	ASR (W)	ICD (9th)
Lip	2	0	-	-	-	-	-	-	-	-	-	-	-	-	-	1.6	1.4	0.1	0.1	0.00	0.1	140
Tongue	18	2	-	-	-	-	-	-	-	0.5	-	-	0.8	1.8	5.7	1.6	8.3	0.6	0.5	0.05	0.8	141
Salivary gland	19	1	-	0.3	-	0.3	-	0.8	-	0.5	0.6	0.7	4.8	0.9	2.3	-	2.8	0.6	0.6	0.06	0.7	142
Mouth	26	1	-	-	-	-	-	-	0.4	1.9	1.9	0.7	2.4	3.6	2.3	4.8	5.6	0.8	0.8	0.07	1.1	143-5
Oropharynx	20	0	-	-	-	-	-	0.4	0.4	-	-	2.2	1.6	5.4	2.3	4.8	2.8	0.6	0.6	0.06	0.8	146
Nasopharynx	255	5	-	0.3	1.1	2.2	2.4	1.9	2.2	8.5	21.9	28.7	24.8	28.8	33.0	25.6	30.6	8.2	7.4	0.79	10.3	147
Hypopharynx	26	0	-	-	-	-	-	-	-	0.5	1.9	1.5	4.0	0.9	3.4	3.2	12.5	0.8	0.8	0.06	1.2	148
Pharynx unspecified	11	0	-	-	-	0.3	-	-	-	0.5	1.3	0.7	0.8	0.9	1.1	1.6	2.8	0.4	0.3	0.03	0.5	149
Oesophagus	50	0	-	-	-	-	-	-	-	-	1.3	1.5	6.4	8.1	13.7	14.4	11.1	1.6	1.5	0.15	2.2	150
Stomach	482	7	-	0.3	-	0.6	1.6	1.5	6.2	12.3	20.0	32.4	39.3	45.0	105.9	128.2	103.0	15.5	14.0	1.34	20.9	151
Small intestine	3	0	-	-	-	-	-	-	-	-	-	0.7	-	0.9	1.1	-	-	0.1	0.1	0.01	0.1	152
Colon	126	2	-	-	1.1	0.3	0.4	0.4	1.8	4.3	5.8	8.1	19.2	11.7	12.5	27.2	25.0	4.0	3.7	0.33	5.2	153
Rectum	99	2	-	-	-	0.3	-	0.8	1.5	1.9	5.2	5.9	9.6	5.4	19.4	24.0	27.8	3.2	2.9	0.25	4.3	154
Liver	496	9	0.6	0.6	1.1	1.6	2.8	3.5	6.2	20.4	27.0	32.4	44.9	67.5	85.4	75.3	82.1	15.9	14.5	1.50	20.3	155
Gallbladder etc.	8	1	-	-	-	-	-	-	-	-	0.6	0.7	1.6	1.8	2.3	-	-	0.3	0.2	0.04	0.3	156
Pancreas	47	1	-	-	-	-	0.4	-	1.1	-	2.6	2.2	4.0	6.3	12.5	11.2	7.0	1.5	1.4	0.15	2.0	157
Nose, sinuses etc.	28	1	-	0.6	0.6	-	-	0.4	0.4	1.4	-	3.7	4.8	1.8	1.1	4.8	1.4	0.9	0.8	0.08	1.1	160
Larynx	20	0	-	-	-	-	-	-	0.4	-	1.3	0.7	4.0	4.5	1.1	3.2	4.2	0.6	0.6	0.06	0.8	161
Bronchus, lung	788	4	0.3	0.3	0.3	0.3	1.6	1.9	2.2	12.8	18.0	29.4	69.7	109.7	210.6	229.2	185.1	25.3	23.0	2.30	34.9	162
Other thoracic organs	48	0	-	-	-	-	-	-	0.4	1.4	1.9	1.5	3.2	6.3	9.1	17.6	12.5	1.5	1.4	0.12	2.1	163-4
Bone	57	2	0.3	-	0.3	2.8	3.2	-	0.7	1.4	3.2	3.7	3.2	4.5	4.6	6.4	5.6	1.8	1.7	0.14	2.1	170
Connective tissue	58	2	1.5	0.3	0.9	0.9	0.8	0.8	0.4	2.8	1.9	0.7	3.2	4.5	5.7	8.0	13.9	1.9	1.7	0.13	2.3	171
Mesothelioma	5	0	-	-	-	-	-	-	-	-	-	0.7	0.8	-	1.1	1.6	1.4	0.2	0.1	0.01	0.2	MES
Kaposi's sarcoma	1	0	-	-	-	-	-	-	-	-	-	-	0.8	-	-	-	-	0.0	0.0	0.00	0.0	KAP
Melanoma of skin	10	0	-	0.3	-	0.3	-	-	0.4	0.9	1.3	-	0.8	0.9	1.1	-	-	0.3	0.3	0.03	0.3	172
Other skin	67	6	-	-	0.3	-	-	-	1.5	0.9	2.6	2.9	4.8	5.4	15.9	9.6	19.5	2.1		0.19	2.9	173
Breast	12	0	-	-	-	-	0.4	-	-	-	-	1.5	0.8	1.8	4.6	3.2	-	0.4	0.3	0.05	0.5	175
Prostate	24	0	-	-	-	-	-	-	-	-	-	-	1.6	0.9	10.2	1.6	15.3	0.8	0.7	0.06	1.2	185
Testis	21	0	0.9	-	-	0.3	0.4	1.2	1.1	0.5	0.6	2.2	0.8	1.8	1.1	1.6	-	0.7	0.6	0.05	0.7	186
Penis	52	0	-	-	-	0.3	0.4	-	1.1	2.8	0.6	2.2	2.4	3.6	13.7	12.8	13.9	1.7	1.5	0.14	2.2	187.1-.4
Other male genital	2	0	-	-	-	-	-	-	-	-	0.6	-	-	-	-	-	1.4	0.1	0.1	0.00	0.1	187.5-.9
†Bladder	39	0	-	-	-	-	0.8	0.4	0.4	-	2.6	2.2	-	4.5	5.7	14.4	12.5	1.3	1.1	0.08	1.7	188
Kidney etc.	16	0	0.9	-	-	-	-	-	0.7	0.5	-	-	1.6	2.7	2.3	-	4.2	0.5	0.5	0.04	0.6	189
Eye	23	1	3.8	0.3	-	-	-	0.4	0.4	-	0.6	0.7	0.8	1.8	-	1.6	-	0.7	0.7	0.05	0.8	190
Brain, nervous system	37	0	0.3	0.8	0.6	0.6	1.6	0.8	0.4	2.4	1.9	1.5	2.4	-	4.6	3.2	4.2	1.2	1.1	0.09	1.3	191-2
Thyroid	30	0	-	-	-	-	0.4	0.8	1.5	0.5	0.6	0.7	5.6	1.8	5.7	6.4	2.8	1.0	0.9	0.09	1.2	193
Other endocrine	4	0	-	-	-	-	0.4	0.4	-	-	0.6	-	-	0.9	-	-	-	0.1	0.1	0.01	0.1	194
Hodgkin's disease	48	2	0.3	1.1	0.9	0.6	1.2	1.5	2.2	1.9	1.3	1.5	0.8	2.7	2.3	6.4	7.0	1.5	1.4	0.10	1.7	201
Non-Hodgkin lymphoma	167	11	3.5	0.6	2.0	1.6	1.2	4.2	5.1	3.8	7.1	8.1	11.2	13.5	19.4	17.6	20.9	5.4	4.9	0.43	6.3	200,202
Multiple myeloma	3	0	-	-	-	-	-	-	-	-	0.6	-	-	-	2.3	-	-	0.1	0.1	0.01	0.1	203
Lymphoid leukaemia	21	0	1.5	0.8	0.9	0.9	-	-	0.4	-	-	0.7	1.6	1.8	-	1.6	-	0.7	0.6	0.04	0.7	204
Myeloid leukaemia	45	0	0.6	1.1	0.6	3.7	-	1.2	1.5	2.8	1.3	0.7	1.6	2.7	1.1	3.2	1.4	1.4	1.3	0.09	1.4	205
Monocytic leukaemia	5	0	0.3	0.3	0.6	0.3	-	-	-	-	-	-	-	-	-	-	-	0.2	0.1	0.01	0.1	206
Other leukaemia	2	0	-	-	0.6	-	-	-	-	-	-	-	-	-	-	-	-	0.1	0.1	0.00	0.1	207
Leukaemia unspecified	38	1	2.6	1.1	1.1	0.3	1.2	0.8	0.7	0.5	0.6	1.5	3.2	-	1.1	3.2	1.4	1.2	1.1	0.08	1.3	208
Other and unspecified	139	7	0.9	0.8	1.1	1.2	2.8	3.5	3.6	3.8	3.9	7.4	11.2	9.0	17.1	19.2	23.7	4.5	4.1	0.35	5.4	O&U
All sites	3498	67	18.0	9.9	13.9	19.9	23.9	27.3	44.7	92.4	143.6	192.7	305.4	376.0	644.3	700.4	674.9	112.2		9.75	145.6	ALL
All sites but 173	3431	61	18.0	9.9	13.6	19.9	23.9	27.3	43.3	91.5	141.0	189.8	300.5	370.6	628.4	690.8	655.4	110.0	100.0	9.56	142.7	ALLb
Rate from 1 case			0.291	0.282	0.283	0.311	0.398	0.385	0.364	0.474	0.644	0.736	0.801	0.900	1.138	1.603	1.392					

†Important: see notes on population page

* VIET NAM, HANOI 1991-1993

ANNUAL INCIDENCE PER 100,000 BY AGE GROUP (YEARS) - FEMALE

SITE	ALL AGES	AGE UNK	0-	5-	10-	15-	20-	25-	30-	35-	40-	45-	50-	55-	60-	65-	70+	CRUDE RATE	%	CR 64	ASR (W)	ICD (9th)
Lip	7	0	-	-	-	-	-	-	-	-	-	-	0.8	-	1.1	1.3	2.9	0.2	0.3	0.01	0.2	140
Tongue	28	3	-	-	-	-	-	0.3	-	1.1	2.2	2.5	0.9	5.4	3.8	5.2	0.9	1.1	0.07	1.0	141
Salivary gland	17	2	-	-	-	0.3	0.4	0.7	0.7	0.4	-	-	0.8	1.9	1.1	1.3	2.2	0.5	0.7	0.04	0.5	142
Mouth	33	1	-	-	0.3	-	-	1.4	0.7	0.4	0.6	1.4	0.8	2.8	2.1	6.3	7.4	1.0	1.3	0.05	1.1	143-5
Oropharynx	7	1	-	-	-	-	-	-	0.3	0.9	-	-	0.8	1.9	-	-	-	0.2	0.3	0.02	0.2	146
Nasopharynx	137	14	-	-	0.3	1.3	2.2	4.2	3.4	2.2	7.9	13.0	10.1	9.3	15.0	12.7	5.2	4.2	5.4	0.38	4.8	147
Hypopharynx	12	0	-	-	-	-	-	-	0.3	-	1.4	-	-	3.2	1.3	3.7	0.4	0.5	0.03	0.4	148
Pharynx unspecified	2	0	-	-	-	-	-	-	-	-	-	-	-	-	2.5	-	0.1	0.1	0.00	0.1	149
Oesophagus	17	1	-	-	-	-	-	0.3	-	-	-	0.8	1.9	2.1	3.8	5.2	0.5	0.7	0.03	0.6	150
Stomach	297	3	-	-	-	-	2.6	1.7	8.6	10.4	12.9	16.6	18.6	27.0	52.6	54.5	32.4	9.2	11.6	0.76	10.4	151
Small intestine	0	0	-	-	-	-	-	-	-	-	-	-	-	-	-	-	-	0.0	0.0	0.00	0.0	152
Colon	81	1	-	-	-	-	0.4	0.7	1.4	2.2	3.4	7.9	10.1	6.5	10.7	7.6	11.8	2.5	3.2	0.22	2.9	153
Rectum	70	0	-	-	-	1.0	0.4	0.3	1.4	3.0	5.1	5.8	4.2	6.5	10.7	7.6	6.6	2.2	2.7	0.19	2.5	154
Liver	137	1	-	-	0.9	1.0	0.7	0.7	2.1	3.5	5.6	10.1	14.4	13.9	22.6	19.0	14.7	4.2	5.4	0.38	4.9	155
Gallbladder etc.	3	0	-	-	-	-	-	-	-	-	-	1.4	-	-	-	1.3	-	0.1	0.1	0.01	0.1	156
Pancreas	20	1	-	-	-	-	-	0.3	-	0.4	0.6	-	4.6	8.6	3.8	-	0.6	0.8	0.08	0.8	157
Nose, sinuses etc.	27	2	-	0.3	-	0.3	-	-	0.3	0.4	1.7	2.2	1.7	2.8	2.1	5.1	2.9	0.8	1.1	0.06	1.0	160
Larynx	2	0	-	-	-	-	-	-	-	-	1.1	-	-	-	-	-	0.1	0.1	0.01	0.1	161
Bronchus, lung	175	2	-	-	-	0.6	1.1	1.4	2.7	3.0	3.4	18.8	16.0	17.7	24.7	29.1	24.3	5.4	6.8	0.45	6.3	162
Other thoracic organs	24	1	-	-	-	0.3	-	-	1.0	0.9	0.6	-	2.5	3.7	4.3	5.1	0.7	0.7	0.9	0.07	0.8	163-4
Bone	28	0	0.3	-	-	1.0	0.7	1.0	0.7	1.7	1.1	1.4	1.7	1.9	2.1	2.5	0.7	0.9	1.1	0.07	0.9	170
Connective tissue	40	1	0.3	0.9	0.6	0.6	1.1	1.0	0.7	1.7	1.7	-	1.7	0.9	4.3	8.9	1.5	1.2	1.6	0.08	1.3	171
Mesothelioma	4	0	-	-	-	-	-	-	-	-	-	-	-	-	3.2	-	0.7	0.1	0.2	0.02	0.2	MES
Kaposi's sarcoma	0	0	-	-	-	-	-	-	-	-	-	-	-	-	-	-	-	0.0	0.0	0.00	0.0	KAP
Melanoma of skin	7	1	-	-	-	0.3	-	-	-	-	-	-	0.8	-	3.2	-	0.7	0.2	0.3	0.03	0.3	172
Other skin	70	4	-	-	-	0.3	-	0.3	0.7	1.3	0.6	1.4	7.6	4.6	11.8	8.9	17.7	2.2		0.15	2.4	173
Breast	504	4	-	-	0.3	0.3	1.1	5.2	9.6	23.8	52.3	80.1	57.4	41.8	43.0	17.7	19.2	15.6	19.7	1.59	18.2	174
Uterus unspecified	6	0	-	-	-	-	-	0.3	-	-	0.6	1.4	1.7	-	-	-	-	0.2	0.2	0.02	0.2	179
Cervix uteri	171	2	-	-	-	-	0.4	0.3	3.8	9.5	13.5	19.5	19.4	12.1	16.1	20.3	11.8	5.3	6.7	0.48	6.1	180
Placenta	63	1	-	-	0.3	7.5	5.2	3.1	2.2	3.4	2.2	2.5	-	-	-	-	2.0	2.5	0.13	1.8	181
Corpus uteri	41	0	0.3	-	-	-	-	-	0.3	3.0	2.3	5.8	4.2	3.7	4.3	6.3	1.5	1.3	1.6	0.12	1.5	182
Ovary etc.	82	0	-	-	0.3	1.0	0.7	3.5	0.7	2.6	9.0	5.8	4.2	2.8	16.1	3.8	5.9	2.5	3.2	0.23	2.9	183
Other female genital	46	1	-	-	-	-	-	0.3	1.0	0.4	0.6	2.9	1.7	8.4	5.4	8.9	8.8	1.4	1.8	0.11	1.6	184
†Bladder	6	0	-	-	-	-	-	0.3	-	-	-	0.7	-	-	1.1	1.3	1.5	0.2	0.2	0.01	0.2	188
Kidney etc.	10	0	0.9	0.3	-	-	-	-	-	0.4	-	0.7	-	1.9	-	1.3	0.7	0.3	0.4	0.02	0.4	189
Eye	17	0	0.9	0.9	0.3	-	-	0.7	0.7	-	-	0.7	1.7	-	-	1.3	1.5	0.5	0.7	0.03	0.5	190
Brain, nervous system	27	0	0.3	0.9	1.2	0.6	0.7	0.7	0.7	0.4	1.1	0.7	1.7	0.9	2.1	1.3	0.7	0.8	1.1	0.06	0.9	191-2
Thyroid	90	3	-	-	-	0.6	3.7	1.7	2.4	1.7	7.3	4.3	8.4	13.9	4.3	6.3	4.4	2.8	3.5	0.25	3.1	193
Other endocrine	2	0	-	-	0.3	-	0.4	-	-	-	-	-	-	-	-	-	-	0.1	0.1	0.00	0.1	194
Hodgkin's disease	28	1	0.3	-	0.3	-	1.1	1.4	0.7	1.3	2.8	0.7	3.4	-	1.1	1.3	0.7	0.9	1.1	0.07	0.9	201
Non-Hodgkin lymphoma	85	2	0.9	1.2	0.6	1.0	1.9	0.3	2.4	1.7	5.1	1.4	6.8	8.4	7.5	8.9	8.8	2.6	3.3	0.20	2.8	200,202
Multiple myeloma	0	0	-	-	-	-	-	-	-	-	-	-	-	-	-	-	-	0.0	0.0	0.00	0.0	203
Lymphoid leukaemia	14	0	0.3	1.2	1.2	-	-	-	-	0.4	-	0.7	-	0.9	1.1	1.3	-	0.4	0.5	0.03	0.5	204
Myeloid leukaemia	40	0	0.9	0.6	0.9	0.6	1.1	0.7	0.3	1.7	1.1	3.6	3.4	1.9	1.1	1.3	3.7	1.2	1.6	0.09	1.3	205
Monocytic leukaemia	1	0	-	-	0.3	-	-	-	-	-	-	-	-	-	-	-	-	0.0	0.0	0.00	0.0	206
Other leukaemia	1	0	-	-	-	-	-	-	-	-	-	-	0.9	-	-	-	-	0.0	0.0	0.00	0.0	207
Leukaemia unspecified	44	1	1.8	0.9	1.2	2.2	1.1	1.4	0.7	1.7	0.6	-	3.4	-	3.2	1.3	0.7	1.4	1.7	0.09	1.4	208
Other and unspecified	102	10	1.5	-	-	0.3	1.9	1.4	3.1	3.0	4.5	5.0	6.8	7.4	9.7	12.7	8.1	3.2	4.0	0.25	3.5	O&U
All sites	2625	64	8.9	7.2	8.8	14.4	31.4	37.7	55.2	86.5	151.4	220.0	222.9	213.8	307.1	281.2	224.7	81.3		7.00	91.8	ALL
All sites but 173	2555	60	8.9	7.2	8.8	14.1	31.4	37.4	54.5	85.2	150.8	218.6	215.3	209.2	295.3	272.3	207.0	79.1	100.0	6.84	89.4	ALLb

Rate from 1 case   0.307 0.300 0.303 0.321 0.374 0.349 0.343 0.432 0.563 0.721 0.844 0.930 1.074 1.267 0.737

†Important: see notes on population page

Austria, Tyrol

The Cancer Registry of Tyrol was founded at the end of 1986, and since 1988 cases have been collected on a population basis.

In Austria, a law passed in 1968 obliges hospitals to report every cancer case to the Austrian Federal Bureau of Statistics. In addition to this Austrian Cancer Registry, in some provinces a local cancer registry is responsible for cancer registration in the region.

The Cancer Registry of Tyrol is legally based on a contract between hospitals and the cancer registry. It is an independent institution, but clearly works in close connection with the Austrian Cancer Registry.

Tyrol is one of nine provinces of Austria, lying in the western part of Austria and bordered to the east and west by the provinces of Salzburg and Vorarlberg, to the north by Germany (Bavaria) and to the south by Italy (South Tyrol). The province covers 12 648 km^2, of which only some 12.5% is habitable. It lies between latitudes 46°46′ and 47°45′ N and longitudes 10°06′ and 12°58′ E. The average altitude of habitable regions is 738 m.

The population is 631 410 (1991 census), with about 20% living in the capital Innsbruck, which has more than 100 000 inhabitants, and the rest in smaller towns of less than 13 000 and in some 260 villages. 9% of the people are from foreign countries, mainly former Yugoslavia and Turkey. 90% are Roman Catholics, 2.4% Protestants, 2.3% Muslims, 5.3% others. The main occupational groups are personal services (32%), commerce and transport (22.2%), industry and trade (21.6%) and tourism (10.4%); about 7% are unemployed.

Medical facilities are offered by the University Hospital in Innsbruck (which offers both basic facilities for Innsbruck and surrounding areas and special facilities for the whole province), nine local hospitals in the rural districts and two semi-private hospitals in Innsbruck. Most pathology diagnoses are performed by one institute in Innsbruck, while two pathologists in Innsbruck perform diagnoses of melanomas and female cancers.

All hospitals are obliged to report cancer cases to the Austrian Federal Bureau of Statistics. These reports are sent initially to the local cancer registry and are then forwarded to the Federal Bureau of Statistics. The basic information consists of personal data including address, incidence date, most valid basis of diagnosis, topography, his-tology, behaviour, staging and summary of first treatment. Besides this basic reporting, some departments of the university hospital in Innsbruck use special report schemes, for example the surgical departments, urological departments and for melanomas. Further, all pathology diagnoses concerning cancer in the pathology departments mentioned above and all death certificates are sent to the registry. This leads in general to multiple notifications being received for each cancer case. Persons are identified by name, birth date, sex and address. Data linkage is carried out with a sophisticated program developed within the registry which computes a probability of identity based on name, birth date, sex, address and topography. The program also considers such information as phonetic similarities, frequent typographic errors, etc. The generated lists are manually checked; if necessary, registry staff contact the communities to clarify questions.

Multiple cancers in an individual are recorded separately on demand by physicians, but for reporting purposes, the IARC definition of multiple cancers is followed strictly.

Reporting of follow-up information depends on agreements with hospitals. Some hospitals send regular information on check-ups, others only on demand by the registry. For all cases, the date of next check-up is stored and the hospital contacted if no notification is received.

Topography and histology are classified according to ICD-O-DA (German edition), the classification is done by one trained documentalist in cooperation with a pathologist.

Programs for checking personal data (for example rare ages, sex and first name combination, ordering of date-values) were developed within the registry; for checking cancer data we use the IARC program for quality control in cancer registries.

Besides annual reports beginning with 1988, data are widely used by physicians (especially from the University Hospital in Innsbruck) for various purposes. For those departments sending regular follow-up information, we generate a report to the general practitioner. Two studies on etiology of renal cell cancers and on indoor radon in relation to lung cancer are in progress (in collaboration with research institutes in Germany).

W. Oberaigner

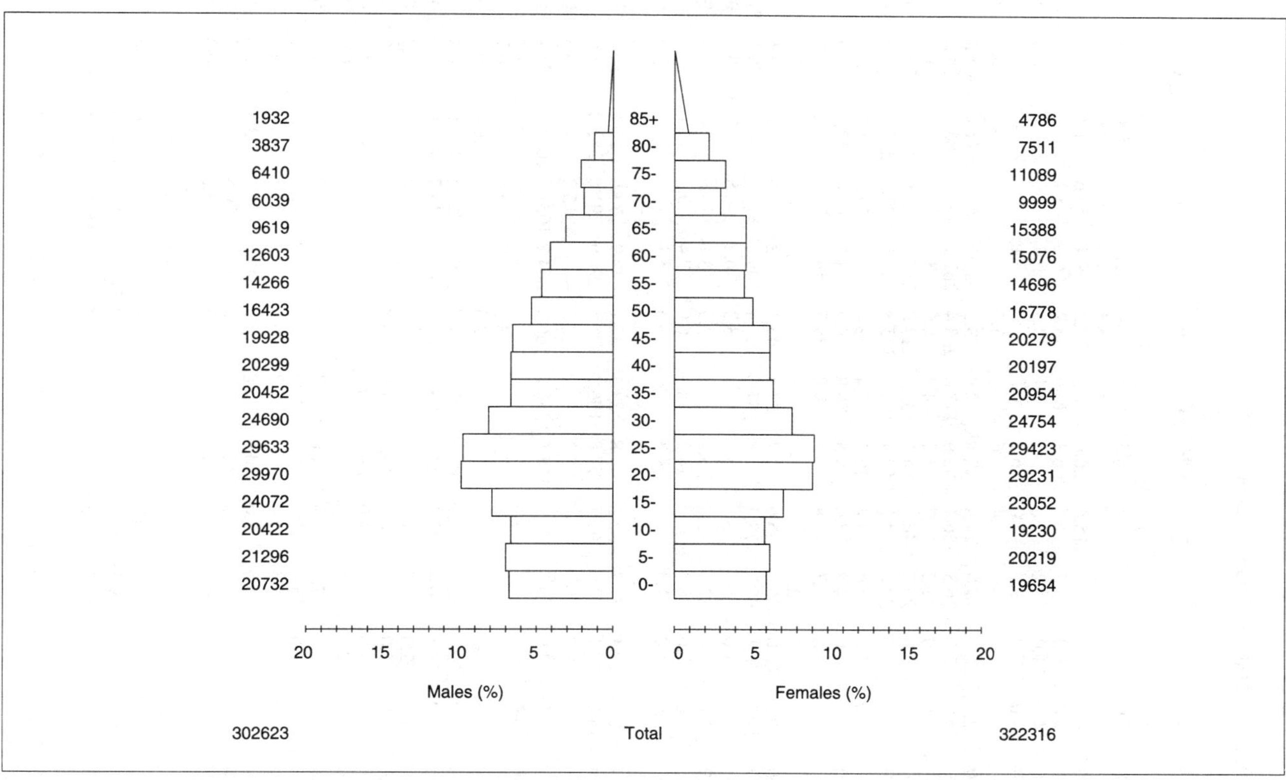

Austria, Tyrol
Source of population: average annual 1988–92
Census: 1991.
Estimate: The populations for 1988, 1989 and 1990 are estimates provided by the Federal Bureau of Statistics. The 1992 estimated population is an extrapolation from the 1991 census assuming linear growth in every age and sex group.

Screening programmes in the area:
10 000 screening examinations for prostate cancer have been carried out annually in the population over age 50 since 1992.

AUSTRIA, TYROL 1988-1992

ANNUAL INCIDENCE PER 100,000 BY AGE GROUP (YEARS) - MALE

SITE	ALL AGES	AGE UNK	0-	5-	10-	15-	20-	25-	30-	35-	40-	45-	50-	55-	60-	65-	70-	75-	80-	85+	CRUDE RATE	%	CR 64	CR 74	ASR (W)	ICD (9th)
Lip	6	0	-	-	-	-	-	-	-	-	1.0	1.0	-	1.4	-	4.2	-	-	-	10.4	0.4	0.1	0.02	0.04	**0.4**	*140*
Tongue	28	0	-	-	-	-	-	-	-	1.0	2.0	4.0	2.4	4.2	6.3	12.5	6.6	3.1	10.4	10.4	1.9	0.5	0.10	0.20	**1.6**	*141*
Salivary gland	11	0	-	-	-	-	0.7	-	-	-	-	-	1.2	1.4	-	2.1	3.3	9.4	10.4	10.4	0.7	0.2	0.02	0.04	**0.5**	*142*
Mouth	67	0	-	-	-	-	-	0.7	-	1.0	6.9	5.0	11.0	15.4	20.6	8.3	23.2	9.4	15.6	31.1	4.4	1.1	0.30	0.46	**3.9**	*143-5*
Oropharynx	37	0	-	-	-	-	-	0.7	-	-	2.0	6.0	9.7	1.4	6.3	16.6	13.2	6.2	5.2	-	2.4	0.6	0.13	0.28	**2.2**	*146*
Nasopharynx	12	0	-	0.9	-	-	-	-	-	1.0	1.0	1.0	1.2	2.8	-	2.1	3.3	9.4	-	-	0.8	0.2	0.04	0.07	**0.7**	*147*
Hypopharynx	26	0	-	-	-	-	-	-	-	1.0	1.0	3.0	9.7	7.0	6.3	6.2	-	3.1	-	-	1.7	0.4	0.14	0.17	**1.5**	*148*
Pharynx unspecified	3	0	-	-	-	-	-	-	-	-	-	-	1.4	1.6	-	3.3	-	-	-	-	0.2	0.1	0.01	0.03	**0.2**	*149*
Oesophagus	78	0	-	-	-	-	-	-	-	1.0	2.0	6.0	11.0	14.0	17.5	22.9	23.2	28.1	41.7	41.4	5.2	1.3	0.26	0.49	**4.2**	*150*
Stomach	517	0	-	-	-	-	-	1.3	1.6	5.9	9.9	12.0	26.8	56.1	93.6	178.8	238.4	262.1	390.9	486.5	34.2	8.7	1.04	3.12	**26.3**	*151*
Small intestine	15	0	-	-	-	-	-	-	-	-	-	1.0	1.2	4.2	3.2	4.2	6.6	3.1	15.6	-	1.0	0.3	0.05	0.10	**0.8**	*152*
Colon	397	0	-	-	-	-	0.7	2.0	2.4	4.9	5.9	6.0	20.7	46.3	84.1	133.1	218.6	212.2	265.8	217.4	26.2	6.7	0.87	2.62	**20.5**	*153*
Rectum	273	0	-	-	-	-	-	-	0.8	3.9	4.9	13.0	29.2	32.2	52.4	101.9	135.8	106.1	125.1	227.7	18.0	4.6	0.68	1.87	**14.8**	*154*
Liver	83	0	-	-	-	0.8	0.7	0.7	-	-	2.0	1.0	3.7	8.4	12.7	37.4	33.1	59.3	52.1	31.1	5.5	1.4	0.15	0.50	**4.2**	*155*
Gallbladder etc.	60	0	-	-	-	-	-	-	-	1.0	-	3.0	4.9	7.0	9.5	20.8	19.9	18.7	67.8	62.1	4.0	1.0	0.13	0.33	**3.0**	*156*
Pancreas	134	0	-	-	-	-	-	0.7	-	-	2.0	7.0	9.7	16.8	31.7	49.9	39.7	56.2	93.8	124.2	8.9	2.2	0.34	0.79	**7.0**	*157*
Nose, sinuses etc.	5	0	-	-	-	-	-	-	-	-	-	2.4	-	-	-	-	3.1	10.4	-	0.3	0.1	0.01	0.01	**0.2**	*160*
Larynx	137	0	-	-	-	-	-	-	-	2.0	6.9	12.0	26.8	26.6	31.7	37.4	43.1	31.2	46.9	51.8	9.1	2.3	0.53	0.93	**7.7**	*161*
Bronchus, lung	1031	0	-	-	-	-	1.3	-	3.2	2.9	17.7	36.1	93.8	179.4	261.8	357.6	397.4	505.4	515.9	465.8	68.1	17.3	2.98	6.76	**54.7**	*162*
Other thoracic organs	13	0	1.0	-	-	-	-	0.7	0.8	-	-	1.0	-	-	3.2	-	3.3	6.2	20.8	-	0.9	0.2	0.03	0.05	**0.6**	*163-4*
Bone	24	0	-	-	2.0	0.8	2.0	1.3	-	2.9	1.0	-	2.4	2.8	3.2	2.1	3.3	3.1	15.6	-	1.6	0.4	0.09	0.12	**1.4**	*170*
Connective tissue	44	0	4.8	0.9	1.0	1.7	-	0.7	0.8	-	1.0	2.0	8.5	-	14.3	8.3	6.6	9.4	5.2	41.4	2.9	0.7	0.18	0.25	**2.9**	*171*
Mesothelioma	8	0	-	-	-	-	-	-	-	-	1.0	1.0	1.2	-	4.8	-	3.3	3.1	-	-	0.5	0.1	0.04	0.06	**0.5**	*MES*
Kaposi's sarcoma	0	0	-	-	-	-	-	-	-	-	-	-	-	-	-	-	-	-	-	-	0.0	0.0	0.00	0.00	**0.0**	*KAP*
Melanoma of skin	224	0	-	-	4.2	4.7	16.9	4.9	14.7	8.9	19.1	31.7	32.2	42.8	33.3	33.1	49.9	73.0	62.1	14.8	3.8	0.90	1.23	**12.4**	*172*
Other skin	433	0	-	-	1.7	2.0	3.4	1.6	5.9	14.8	20.1	32.9	61.7	77.8	106.0	175.5	196.6	291.8	383.0	28.6	-	1.11	2.52	**22.4**	*173*
Breast	5	0	-	-	-	-	-	-	-	-	-	1.0	-	-	3.2	-	3.3	-	5.2	-	0.3	0.1	0.02	0.04	**0.3**	*175*
Prostate	1091	0	-	-	-	-	-	-	-	-	1.0	2.0	9.7	65.9	166.6	382.6	566.3	864.2	1031.9	1014.5	72.1	18.3	1.23	5.97	**51.6**	*185*
Testis	111	0	1.0	-	1.0	3.3	9.3	20.2	13.8	15.6	10.8	8.0	3.7	5.6	-	2.1	-	-	-	10.4	7.3	1.9	0.46	0.47	**6.3**	*186*
Penis	11	0	-	-	-	-	0.7	-	-	-	-	-	-	-	3.2	-	3.3	6.2	15.6	20.7	0.7	0.2	0.02	0.04	**0.5**	*187.1-.4*
Other male genital	2	0	-	-	-	-	-	-	-	-	-	-	-	-	-	-	3.3	-	-	10.4	0.1	0.0	0.00	0.02	**0.1**	*187.5-.9*
Bladder	551	0	-	-	-	2.5	-	1.3	3.2	7.8	8.9	10.0	30.4	51.9	106.3	207.9	251.7	330.7	323.1	434.8	36.4	9.2	1.11	3.41	**28.3**	*188*
Kidney etc.	268	0	-	-	-	0.8	-	0.7	0.8	6.8	9.9	19.1	30.4	29.4	58.7	93.6	109.3	109.2	114.7	113.9	17.7	4.5	0.78	1.80	**14.6**	*189*
Eye	18	0	1.9	0.9	-	-	-	-	-	2.0	1.0	2.0	3.7	1.4	3.2	-	-	6.2	10.4	-	1.2	0.3	0.08	0.08	**1.1**	*190*
Brain, nervous system	84	0	2.9	2.8	1.0	4.2	0.7	2.7	4.1	2.0	3.9	7.0	4.9	18.2	14.3	22.9	29.8	6.2	-	10.4	5.6	1.4	0.34	0.61	**5.3**	*191-2*
Thyroid	45	0	-	-	-	-	0.7	-	2.4	5.9	3.0	4.0	7.3	5.6	4.8	10.4	9.9	12.5	10.4	10.4	3.0	0.8	0.17	0.27	**2.5**	*193*
Other endocrine	13	0	1.0	0.9	-	-	-	-	-	1.0	1.0	2.0	2.4	-	1.6	6.2	-	3.1	-	-	0.9	0.2	0.05	0.08	**0.9**	*194*
Hodgkin's disease	44	0	-	1.9	2.0	0.8	3.3	3.4	2.4	2.9	3.9	1.0	7.3	5.6	1.6	4.2	6.6	6.2	5.2	-	2.9	0.7	0.18	0.23	**2.6**	*201*
Non-Hodgkin lymphoma	140	0	-	-	-	2.5	0.7	-	2.4	2.0	10.8	7.0	13.4	14.0	41.3	39.5	39.7	53.0	62.5	62.1	9.3	2.3	0.47	0.87	**7.6**	*200,202*
Multiple myeloma	61	0	-	-	-	-	-	-	0.8	-	1.0	4.0	7.3	5.6	19.0	31.2	26.5	18.7	15.6	10.4	4.0	1.0	0.19	0.48	**3.5**	*203*
Lymphoid leukaemia	100	0	5.8	3.8	2.9	4.2	0.7	1.3	1.6	1.0	1.0	3.0	8.5	7.0	20.6	20.8	16.6	40.6	52.1	93.2	6.6	1.7	0.31	0.49	**5.9**	*204*
Myeloid leukaemia	56	0	-	-	-	1.7	1.3	4.7	0.8	1.0	-	5.0	11.0	4.2	12.7	10.4	16.6	12.5	20.8	-	3.7	0.9	0.21	0.35	**3.1**	*205*
Monocytic leukaemia	4	0	-	-	-	-	-	-	-	-	-	-	-	-	1.6	-	3.3	3.1	5.2	-	0.3	0.1	0.01	0.02	**0.2**	*206*
Other leukaemia	0	0	-	-	-	-	-	-	-	-	-	-	-	-	-	-	-	-	-	-	0.0	0.0	0.00	0.00	**0.0**	*207*
Leukaemia unspecified	8	0	-	-	-	-	-	-	-	-	1.0	-	-	-	-	-	6.6	3.1	10.4	20.7	0.5	0.1	0.00	0.04	**0.4**	*208*
Other and unspecified	124	0	-	-	-	0.8	-	0.7	-	-	1.0	4.0	7.3	16.8	19.0	39.5	43.1	59.3	99.0	176.0	8.2	2.1	0.25	0.66	**6.2**	*O&U*
All sites	6402	0	18.3	12.2	9.8	29.9	28.7	64.8	48.6	96.8	149.8	239.9	489.5	754.2	1263.2	2016.8	2569.9	3129.3	3856.6	4244.3	423.1		16.03	38.96	**335.4**	*ALL*
All sites but 173	5969	0	18.3	12.2	9.8	28.2	26.7	61.4	47.0	90.9	135.0	219.8	456.7	692.5	1185.4	1910.8	2394.4	2932.7	3564.7	3861.3	394.5	100.0	14.92	36.45	**313.1**	*ALLb*

| Rate from 1 case | | | 0.965 | 0.939 | 0.979 | 0.831 | 0.667 | 0.675 | 0.810 | 0.978 | 0.985 | 1.004 | 1.218 | 1.402 | 1.587 | 2.079 | 3.312 | 3.120 | 5.212 | 10.352 | | | | | | |

AUSTRIA, TYROL 1988-1992

ANNUAL INCIDENCE PER 100,000 BY AGE GROUP (YEARS) - FEMALE

SITE	ALL AGES	AGE UNK	0-	5-	10-	15-	20-	25-	30-	35-	40-	45-	50-	55-	60-	65-	70-	75-	80-	85+	CRUDE RATE	%	CR 64	CR 74	ASR (W)	ICD (9th)
Lip	0	0	-	-	-	-	-	-	-	-	-	-	-	-	-	-	-	-	-	-	0.0	0.0	0.00	0.00	0.0	140
Tongue	5	0	-	-	-	-	-	-	-	-	1.0	-	-	1.4	-	1.3	2.0	-	2.7	-	0.3	0.1	0.01	0.03	0.2	141
Salivary gland	9	0	-	-	-	-	-	0.7	0.8	-	1.0	-	-	2.7	1.3	1.3	2.0	-	2.7	-	0.6	0.1	0.03	0.05	0.4	142
Mouth	25	0	-	-	-	-	-	-	0.8	-	2.0	1.0	9.5	1.4	4.0	7.8	-	3.6	2.7	-	1.6	0.4	0.09	0.13	1.2	143-5
Oropharynx	14	0	-	-	-	-	-	-	-	-	3.0	1.0	2.4	1.4	5.3	-	-	3.6	-	4.2	0.9	0.2	0.07	0.07	0.7	146
Nasopharynx	4	0	-	-	-	-	-	0.8	-	-	-	-	1.2	-	-	-	-	3.6	-	-	0.2	0.1	0.01	0.01	0.1	147
Hypopharynx	6	0	-	-	-	-	-	-	-	-	2.0	-	-	-	1.3	1.3	2.0	-	2.7	-	0.4	0.1	0.02	0.03	0.3	148
Pharynx unspecified	2	0	-	-	-	-	-	-	-	-	-	-	-	1.4	-	1.3	-	-	-	-	0.1	0.0	0.01	0.01	0.1	149
Oesophagus	14	0	-	-	-	-	-	-	-	-	-	1.0	1.2	1.4	2.7	2.6	2.0	3.6	8.0	4.2	0.9	0.2	0.03	0.05	0.5	150
Stomach	510	0	-	-	-	-	-	0.7	4.8	2.9	6.9	17.8	15.5	23.1	51.7	83.2	130.0	162.3	258.3	376.0	31.6	7.9	0.62	1.68	15.7	151
Small intestine	7	0	-	-	-	-	-	-	-	-	-	-	1.2	2.7	-	1.3	-	3.6	2.7	-	0.4	0.1	0.02	0.03	0.3	152
Colon	512	0	-	-	-	-	1.4	0.7	5.7	6.7	12.9	9.9	19.1	35.4	47.8	91.0	158.0	162.3	226.3	292.5	31.8	7.9	0.70	1.94	16.7	153
Rectum	268	0	-	-	-	-	-	-	-	1.0	4.0	7.9	19.1	24.5	25.2	45.5	84.0	106.4	93.2	129.5	16.6	4.1	0.41	1.06	8.9	154
Liver	64	0	1.0	-	-	-	-	-	-	-	-	3.0	2.4	-	6.6	11.7	12.0	25.2	24.0	62.7	4.0	1.0	0.06	0.18	2.0	155
Gallbladder etc.	96	0	-	-	-	-	-	0.7	-	-	-	1.0	1.2	2.7	10.6	15.6	22.0	43.3	53.3	66.9	6.0	1.5	0.08	0.27	2.6	156
Pancreas	204	0	-	-	-	-	-	-	0.8	1.0	1.0	2.0	3.6	13.6	13.3	33.8	52.0	95.6	133.1	87.7	12.7	3.2	0.18	0.60	5.7	157
Nose, sinuses etc.	9	0	-	-	-	-	-	-	1.0	-	-	2.0	1.2	-	-	-	2.0	3.6	5.3	-	0.6	0.1	0.02	0.03	0.3	160
Larynx	6	0	-	-	-	-	-	-	-	-	-	1.0	4.8	-	-	-	2.0	-	-	-	0.4	0.1	0.03	0.04	0.3	161
Bronchus, lung	302	0	-	-	-	-	-	0.7	0.8	3.8	13.9	16.8	29.8	19.1	39.8	53.3	98.0	83.0	109.2	79.4	18.7	4.7	0.62	1.38	11.3	162
Other thoracic organs	15	0	-	-	-	-	-	-	-	-	-	1.0	-	1.4	1.3	3.9	4.0	1.8	10.7	8.4	0.9	0.2	0.02	0.06	0.5	163-4
Bone	18	0	-	1.0	1.0	1.7	1.4	0.7	-	-	1.0	-	1.2	1.4	2.7	1.3	2.0	5.4	2.7	-	1.1	0.3	0.06	0.08	0.9	170
Connective tissue	48	0	2.0	1.0	-	-	1.4	4.1	-	1.9	2.0	2.0	1.2	5.4	1.3	10.4	10.0	12.6	13.3	-	3.0	0.7	0.11	0.21	2.2	171
Mesothelioma	6	0	-	-	-	-	-	-	-	-	-	2.0	-	-	-	1.3	4.0	-	2.7	-	0.4	0.1	0.01	0.04	0.3	MES
Kaposi's sarcoma	0	0	-	-	-	-	-	-	-	-	-	-	-	-	-	-	-	-	-	-	0.0	0.0	0.00	0.00	0.0	KAP
Melanoma of skin	324	0	-	-	-	6.9	10.3	12.2	19.4	15.3	31.7	26.6	32.2	38.1	41.1	37.7	42.0	36.1	39.9	54.3	20.1	5.0	1.17	1.57	15.6	172
Other skin	469	0	-	-	-	0.9	-	2.0	3.2	5.7	12.9	13.8	25.0	27.2	41.1	79.3	98.0	156.9	234.3	296.7	29.1		0.66	1.55	14.9	173
Breast	1541	0	-	-	-	-	-	2.7	11.3	39.1	103.0	148.9	190.7	172.8	218.9	243.0	342.0	322.8	359.5	430.4	95.6	23.8	4.44	7.36	64.9	174
Uterus unspecified	33	0	-	-	-	-	-	-	-	-	-	2.4	2.7	2.7	5.2	2.0	9.0	32.0	20.9	2.0	0.5	0.04	0.07	0.9	179		
Cervix uteri	367	0	-	-	-	-	2.7	10.9	23.4	33.4	42.6	37.5	41.7	49.0	31.8	45.5	44.0	39.7	42.6	50.1	22.8	5.7	1.37	1.81	17.7	180
Placenta	0	0	-	-	-	-	-	-	-	-	-	-	-	-	-	-	-	-	-	-	0.0	0.0	0.00	0.00	0.0	181
Corpus uteri	312	0	-	-	-	-	0.7	0.7	0.8	1.0	8.9	14.8	29.8	58.5	59.7	79.3	82.0	63.1	63.9	41.8	19.4	4.8	0.87	1.68	13.0	182
Ovary etc.	366	0	-	-	1.0	1.7	4.1	4.8	3.2	12.4	10.9	25.6	28.6	55.8	43.8	68.9	96.0	73.9	93.2	87.7	22.7	5.7	0.96	1.78	15.1	183
Other female genital	73	0	-	-	-	-	1.4	-	-	2.9	3.0	1.0	4.8	2.7	14.6	11.7	12.0	25.2	24.0	37.6	4.5	1.1	0.15	0.27	2.6	184
Bladder	196	0	-	-	-	-	0.7	-	0.8	3.8	3.0	7.9	3.6	1.7	23.9	37.7	58.0	72.1	77.2	75.2	12.2	3.0	0.31	0.79	6.6	188
Kidney etc.	199	0	3.1	1.0	-	0.9	-	-	-	3.8	-	9.9	9.5	17.7	19.9	42.9	62.0	90.2	47.9	50.1	12.3	3.1	0.33	0.85	7.3	189
Eye	16	0	-	-	-	-	-	-	0.8	1.9	-	3.0	1.2	-	4.0	1.3	4.0	-	5.3	4.2	1.0	0.2	0.05	0.08	0.7	190
Brain, nervous system	91	0	4.1	3.0	3.1	0.9	1.4	2.0	1.6	3.8	5.9	7.9	13.1	6.8	18.6	14.3	10.0	7.2	8.0	8.4	5.6	1.4	0.36	0.48	5.0	191-2
Thyroid	169	0	-	-	-	0.9	0.7	3.4	8.9	11.5	20.8	12.8	14.3	17.7	22.6	24.7	30.0	27.1	24.0	20.9	10.5	2.6	0.57	0.84	7.8	193
Other endocrine	10	0	-	-	1.0	0.9	-	-	-	-	-	1.0	-	1.4	1.3	2.6	4.0	1.8	-	-	0.6	0.2	0.03	0.06	0.5	194
Hodgkin's disease	35	0	-	1.0	-	1.7	4.8	2.0	4.0	1.0	2.0	3.0	2.4	1.4	2.7	2.6	2.0	1.8	-	8.4	2.2	0.5	0.13	0.15	1.9	201
Non-Hodgkin lymphoma	196	0	-	1.0	-	0.9	3.4	0.7	4.0	2.9	6.9	11.8	9.5	13.6	22.6	36.4	66.0	57.7	50.6	58.5	12.2	3.0	0.39	0.90	7.5	200,202
Multiple myeloma	72	0	-	-	-	-	-	-	-	-	1.0	3.0	6.0	2.7	14.6	13.0	18.0	27.1	21.3	33.4	4.5	1.1	0.14	0.29	2.5	203
Lymphoid leukaemia	66	0	5.1	2.0	-	3.5	-	0.7	0.8	1.0	1.0	3.0	2.4	6.8	5.3	10.4	6.0	16.2	24.0	33.4	4.1	1.0	0.16	0.24	3.0	204
Myeloid leukaemia	55	0	-	-	-	-	-	0.7	0.8	2.9	4.0	3.9	7.2	8.2	9.3	9.1	12.0	3.6	18.6	4.2	3.4	0.8	0.18	0.29	2.5	205
Monocytic leukaemia	2	0	-	-	-	-	-	-	-	-	-	1.4	-	-	-	2.7	-	-	0.1	0.0	0.01	0.01	0.1	206		
Other leukaemia	1	0	-	-	-	-	-	-	-	-	-	-	-	-	2.0	-	-	-	0.1	0.0	0.00	0.01	0.0	207		
Leukaemia unspecified	6	0	-	-	-	-	-	-	-	-	-	-	-	1.3	-	2.0	3.6	2.7	4.2	0.4	0.1	0.01	0.02	0.2	208	
Other and unspecified	202	0	1.0	1.0	-	-	-	-	0.8	1.9	4.0	7.9	4.8	6.8	13.3	41.6	20.0	61.3	109.2	204.7	12.5	3.1	0.21	0.52	6.0	O&U
All sites	6945	0	16.3	10.9	6.2	20.8	34.2	51.0	98.6	162.3	312.9	411.3	543.5	647.8	827.8	1174.9	1602.1	1816.1	2233.9	2636.5	430.9		15.72	29.60	267.4	ALL
All sites but 173	6476	0	16.3	10.9	6.2	20.0	34.2	48.9	95.3	156.5	300.0	397.4	518.5	620.6	786.6	1095.7	1504.1	1659.2	1999.6	2339.9	401.8	100.0	15.06	28.06	252.5	ALLb

| Rate from 1 case | | | 1.018 | 0.989 | 1.040 | 0.868 | 0.684 | 0.680 | 0.808 | 0.954 | 0.990 | 0.986 | 1.192 | 1.361 | 1.327 | 1.300 | 2.000 | 1.803 | 2.663 | 4.178 | | | | | | |

Belarus

Cancer registration in Belarus has been carried out since 1953. However, because of the small number of oncological hospitals, it was incomplete during the 1950s and 1960s. Efforts to improve cancer registration were undertaken in the late 60s and early 70s and the first satisfactory statistical data were obtained in this period.

In 1973 the central computerized cancer registry began to function in Belarus (at that time the Byelorussian SSR). The Belarusian Cancer Registry possesses such files since 1978, which contain information on new cancer cases, on living cancer patients, registered in the preceding years, and on cancer patients who died within the incidence year.

Until 1985 the information stored in the computer files had no names or addresses of persons with cancer diagnoses, leading to some difficulties in data correction and specification. In 1985 a computer system was set up in the oncological dispensaries which allowed long-term continuous data collection for each patient and easier follow-up. Since 1991 this system has functioned on personal computers in all the Belarusian oncological dispensaries.

The registry collects information about the cancer situation in the whole Republic of Belarus, which occupies 207 600 km^2. The capital is Minsk (population 1 613 000 according to the 1989 census). There are six regions in the republic (Brest, Grodno, Gomel, Minsk, Mogilev and Vitebsk). There are 14 cities with a population of more than 100 000, and 84 towns with more than 10 000. The main branches of industry are machine-building and metal-processing, including automobile and tractor manufacture (Minsk, Zhodino, Mogilev), radioelectronics, oil refinery and chemical industries (Svetlogorsk, Mogilev and Novopolotsk).

The population is 10 179 000 (males, 46.8%; females, 53.2%; 65.5% urban). Among these there are 77.9% Belarusians, 13.2% Russians, 4.1% Polish, 2.9% Ukrainians, 1.1% Jews and 0.8% others.

In 1986 the Chernobyl accident led to the exposure of one fifth of the Belarusian population to radiation. About 4 tonnes of nuclear fuel was emitted into the environment (more than 10^{18} Bq of iodine, caesium, cerium, barium, strontium, plutonium and other radionuclides).

In every rayon (an administrative subdivision of a region) of Belarus (also in every city outpatient clinic), there is an oncologist who is responsible for all cancer patients of his or her area. In every case where cancer is suspected, he or she should direct the patient to the regional specialized oncological hospital (oncological dispensary) for complete examination. Any medical institution where a cancer case is diagnosed must fill in a special notification form and send it to the oncological dispensary. Pathologists must also send a notification if they incidentally diagnose cancer as a result of an autopsy.

The fact that more than 85% of treated cancer patients have their treatment in oncological dispensaries makes data collection significantly easier. Every dispensary has a special department that collects data on all cancer cases in the region, including those diagnosed after death, and maintains the computerized database. Most of the required information is entered into a computer directly from patient's medical records kept in the dispensary. Each month the staff of this department checks the records of the regional population bureau, which keeps all death certificates, in order to find additional information on cancer cases. During this check they can also find information about death of known patients. Each cancer case so identified that was not previously known is checked by sending a letter to the treating hospital, requesting more detailed information.

The Belarusian Cancer Registry registers all cases of malignant neoplasms including diseases of the lymphatic and haematopoietic tissues, and carcinoma *in situ*.

The information collected by the registry is classified by person. There is one record in a computer file for each person, but it contains separate information on all diagnosed tumours and the treatment applied to each tumour.

Each person included in the registry file is identified by the region code, the dispensary code, the date of registration and registration card number

Tumours are coded according to ICD-9. For coding histology, a local classification is used.

Each tumour of a patient is recorded separately within the personal record, allowing the correct counting of all cancer cases. Independent primaries are defined as tumours of different organs or different parts of organs, according to four-digit ICD-9 classification. Multiple tumours of skin are always counted separately, independently of site and morphological characteristics.

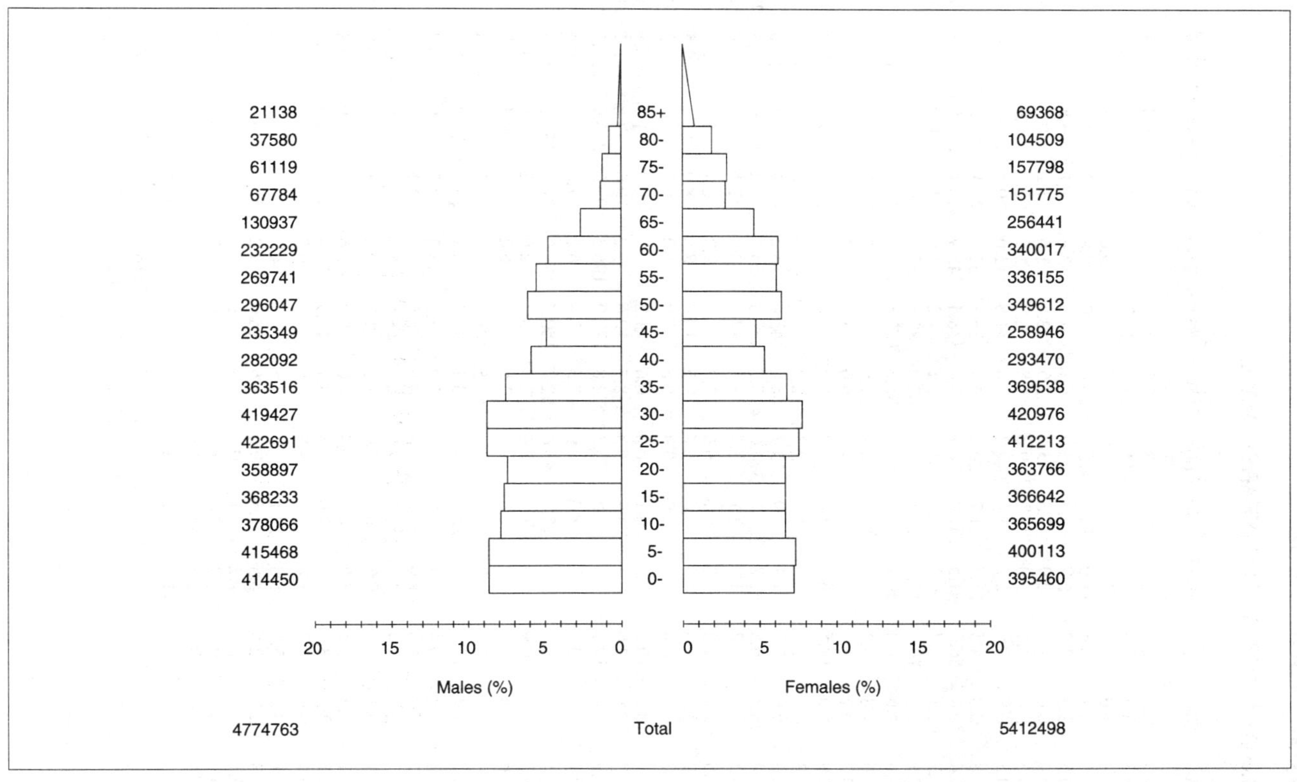

Belarus

Source of population: average annual 1988–92

Census: Statistical Collection (Number and Age Structure of Population of the Byelorussian SSR), 1989 All-Union Census, Minsk, 1994.

Estimate: The populations for 1988, 1990, 1991 and 1992 are estimates based on the 1989 census, taking into account births and deaths but not migration.

Notes to tables overleaf:

* The absence of official mortality data and use of non-standard classification made it difficult to assess the quality of the data, and there is evidence of under-registration in the older age-groups.

+ The editors were unable to verify these data.

Screening programmes in the area

The population over age 18 has been examined annually for cancer of the cervix and breast since 1972. Since 1986, all children and the adult population exposed to radiation as a result of the Chernobyl accident have been screened annually for thyroid cancer.

*+ BELARUS 1988-1992

ANNUAL INCIDENCE PER 100,000 BY AGE GROUP (YEARS) - MALE

SITE	ALL AGES	AGE UNK	0-	5-	10-	15-	20-	25-	30-	35-	40-	45-	50-	55-	60-	65-	70-	75-	80-	85+	CRUDE RATE	%	CR 64	CR 74	ASR (W)	ICD (9th)
Lip	1527	0	-	-	0.1	-	0.1	0.1	0.6	1.0	2.3	6.0	12.1	20.0	23.9	35.1	38.4	43.2	63.9	46.4	6.4	2.3	0.33	0.70	**5.8**	140
Tongue	676	0	-	-	-	-	-	0.0	0.5	1.3	3.5	5.9	9.3	9.1	11.1	11.2	11.2	4.3	4.3	2.8	2.8	1.0	0.20	0.31	**2.6**	141
Salivary gland	212	0	-	-	-	0.1	0.1	0.2	0.3	0.4	1.0	1.7	2.2	1.8	2.9	4.4	4.4	3.6	4.8	4.7	0.9	0.3	0.05	0.10	**0.8**	142
Mouth	944	0	-	-	-	-	0.1	0.1	0.3	1.3	5.7	8.6	11.0	14.6	15.7	15.4	13.0	8.8	4.3	4.7	4.0	1.4	0.29	0.43	**3.6**	143-5
Oropharynx	420	0	-	-	-	0.1	0.1	0.0	0.1	0.5	2.3	3.7	6.7	5.9	5.9	6.1	7.4	3.6	1.1	3.8	1.8	0.6	0.13	0.19	**1.6**	146
Nasopharynx	170	0	0.0	0.3	0.1	0.2	0.2	0.1	0.2	0.4	0.6	1.1	0.9	2.3	3.0	3.5	2.4	1.6	1.1	0.9	0.7	0.3	0.05	0.08	**0.7**	147
Hypopharynx	523	0	-	0.0	-	-	-	-	0.1	0.6	2.8	4.1	7.0	8.2	9.6	7.8	6.2	5.9	3.2	0.9	2.2	0.8	0.16	0.23	**2.0**	148
Pharynx unspecified	148	0	-	-	0.1	-	-	-	0.1	0.3	0.9	0.9	2.2	1.6	2.2	3.8	1.8	1.0	0.5	-	0.6	0.2	0.04	0.07	**0.6**	149
Oesophagus	1513	0	-	-	-	-	0.1	0.0	0.1	0.8	2.8	8.5	15.7	21.7	26.6	34.4	36.3	32.1	27.1	21.8	6.3	2.3	0.38	0.74	**5.8**	150
Stomach	12140	0	-	-	0.1	0.4	0.9	1.3	5.6	13.4	30.4	56.0	91.5	139.0	216.7	285.0	338.4	345.9	316.1	214.8	50.9	18.4	2.78	5.89	**46.8**	151
Small intestine	81	0	-	0.1	-	-	0.1	-	0.1	0.3	0.1	0.3	0.7	0.5	1.8	2.1	1.2	1.6	1.1	0.9	0.3	0.1	0.02	0.04	**0.3**	152
Colon	2507	0	-	0.1	0.2	0.1	0.4	0.4	1.5	2.1	5.7	10.7	18.2	26.1	41.9	62.9	82.3	87.4	60.7	28.4	10.5	3.8	0.54	1.26	**9.8**	153
Rectum	3163	0	0.0	-	-	0.1	0.2	0.7	1.0	1.8	4.6	8.8	20.2	33.4	54.9	86.6	106.8	104.1	113.4	71.0	13.2	4.8	0.63	1.60	**12.3**	154
Liver	1064	0	0.4	0.0	0.2	-	0.3	0.2	0.6	0.6	1.8	3.4	7.4	11.5	20.2	27.6	32.2	31.7	23.9	19.9	4.5	1.6	0.23	0.53	**4.1**	155
Gallbladder etc.	267	0	-	-	0.1	-	-	-	0.2	0.2	0.2	1.1	2.2	2.8	4.3	6.0	8.3	8.2	12.8	4.7	1.1	0.4	0.06	0.13	**1.0**	156
Pancreas	2194	1	-	-	-	0.1	0.1	0.2	0.5	1.9	5.0	10.5	16.2	24.8	37.0	58.2	67.6	63.8	51.6	39.7	9.2	3.3	0.48	1.11	**8.6**	157
Nose, sinuses etc.	142	0	-	0.0	0.1	-	-	-	0.1	0.3	0.7	0.8	1.5	1.5	2.3	2.9	3.5	2.6	1.6	1.9	0.6	0.2	0.04	0.07	**0.6**	160
Larynx	2769	0	-	-	0.2	-	0.1	0.1	0.5	2.6	9.6	19.7	31.7	43.9	53.7	55.6	43.4	26.8	23.4	13.2	11.6	4.2	0.81	1.31	**10.5**	161
Bronchus, lung	17510	4	-	0.0	0.1	0.2	0.1	0.9	2.1	8.2	28.1	70.8	147.8	252.1	374.0	445.7	439.3	365.2	243.2	141.0	73.3	26.5	4.42	8.85	**66.8**	162
Other thoracic organs	215	3	0.1	0.1	-	0.2	0.3	0.3	0.4	0.2	0.5	0.8	1.9	3.1	3.7	3.1	4.4	3.9	2.1	1.9	0.9	0.3	0.06	0.10	**0.8**	163-4
Bone	572	0	0.4	0.7	1.5	2.0	1.2	0.8	0.8	1.5	1.8	1.6	3.8	5.1	6.6	11.2	11.2	9.2	6.4	4.7	2.4	0.9	0.14	0.25	**2.3**	170
Connective tissue	595	0	0.4	0.3	0.6	1.1	0.9	1.4	1.1	1.9	3.3	3.6	4.3	4.6	6.7	9.5	10.0	8.5	8.0	12.3	2.5	0.9	0.15	0.25	**2.4**	171
Mesothelioma	57	0	-	-	0.1	-	-	0.0	-	0.2	0.1	0.4	0.8	0.9	0.9	0.8	0.9	1.0	0.5	-	0.2	0.1	0.02	0.02	**0.2**	MES
Kaposi's sarcoma	24	0	-	-	-	0.1	0.1	0.0	-	-	0.1	0.1	0.2	0.1	0.3	0.6	1.2	-	0.5	1.9	0.1	0.0	0.00	0.01	**0.1**	KAP
Melanoma of skin	496	0	-	0.0	0.2	0.2	0.4	0.6	1.4	1.8	3.8	2.0	4.7	4.2	5.3	8.7	10.6	7.2	10.6	7.6	2.1	0.8	0.12	0.22	**1.9**	172
Other skin	5177	2	0.0	0.0	0.1	0.3	0.3	0.6	2.5	4.9	12.8	19.8	31.3	47.5	73.3	124.8	172.9	196.3	198.5	246.9	21.7		0.97	2.46	**20.3**	173
Breast	83	0	-	-	-	-	-	-	-	0.1	-	0.3	0.7	1.0	0.9	2.3	2.4	6.2	1.1	-	0.3	0.1	0.01	0.04	**0.3**	175
Prostate	3049	1	-	-	0.1	0.1	-	0.0	0.0	0.1	0.6	2.1	6.2	18.2	46.4	92.7	150.5	179.0	172.4	136.2	12.8	4.6	0.37	1.59	**12.2**	185
Testis	338	5	0.1	0.1	-	0.7	2.7	3.3	1.9	1.5	1.5	0.9	0.9	1.2	2.4	2.3	3.2	2.0	3.2	3.8	1.4	0.5	0.09	0.12	**1.3**	186
Penis, other male genital	179	0	-	-	-	-	-	-	0.2	0.6	0.6	0.9	0.9	1.6	2.3	4.0	3.0	6.2	9.0	10.4	0.7	0.3	0.04	0.07	**0.7**	187
Bladder	3207	4	0.1	-	0.1	0.1	0.2	0.2	0.8	1.9	4.0	7.7	17.7	32.2	59.3	84.5	106.2	116.5	121.9	102.2	13.4	4.9	0.62	1.58	**12.4**	188
Kidney etc.	1964	0	1.5	0.7	0.3	0.1	0.4	0.4	1.0	2.9	7.7	12.2	17.6	25.1	34.5	43.1	44.3	23.9	27.7	13.2	8.2	3.0	0.52	0.96	**7.7**	189
Eye	183	0	0.8	0.0	0.1	0.1	0.1	0.2	0.3	0.3	0.4	0.4	1.4	2.0	3.0	2.9	4.1	3.3	3.2	2.8	0.8	0.3	0.05	0.08	**0.7**	190
Brain, nervous system	1003	0	2.3	2.2	2.0	1.3	1.4	1.9	2.8	3.7	5.8	6.0	8.9	11.4	9.6	9.6	6.5	3.9	2.1	3.8	4.2	1.5	0.30	0.38	**3.9**	191-2
Thyroid	357	0	0.0	1.7	1.7	0.9	0.5	0.5	0.9	1.3	2.1	1.4	2.2	2.3	2.4	4.7	5.6	5.2	1.1	3.8	1.5	0.5	0.09	0.14	**1.5**	193
Other endocrine	51	0	0.1	-	0.1	0.3	0.1	0.0	0.1	0.1	0.1	0.2	0.3	0.4	0.5	1.2	1.2	0.3	1.1	-	0.2	0.1	0.01	0.02	**0.2**	194
Hodgkin's disease	813	0	0.8	2.0	1.7	5.1	4.8	4.0	3.2	2.1	3.4	3.1	3.9	4.0	5.8	7.0	5.9	3.6	4.8	1.9	3.4	1.2	0.22	0.28	**3.3**	201
Non-Hodgkin lymphoma	809	0	1.2	1.8	1.0	1.5	0.9	0.9	1.3	2.1	2.3	3.4	5.3	7.0	10.5	14.7	15.9	15.4	14.4	11.4	3.4	1.2	0.19	0.35	**3.2**	200,202
Multiple myeloma	269	0	-	-	-	0.1	0.1	0.0	0.2	0.4	0.6	1.2	1.8	3.1	5.8	6.9	7.4	5.2	4.3	0.9	1.1	0.4	0.07	0.14	**1.0**	203
Lymphoid leukaemia	1480	0	2.9	2.3	1.2	1.7	1.2	1.3	1.2	1.1	3.3	5.1	8.8	12.5	24.8	34.8	38.7	34.0	26.1	17.0	6.2	2.2	0.34	0.70	**6.0**	204
Myeloid leukaemia	615	0	0.1	0.3	0.4	0.7	0.9	0.8	1.1	1.2	2.3	2.5	4.5	5.5	9.8	11.6	15.0	9.2	16.0	9.5	2.6	0.9	0.15	0.28	**2.4**	205
Monocytic leukaemia	25	0	0.0	-	-	0.1	0.1	-	0.0	0.1	-	0.1	0.2	0.1	0.2	0.8	0.6	0.3	1.1	-	0.1	0.0	0.00	0.01	**0.1**	206
Other leukaemia	56	0	0.0	-	0.1	0.1	-	0.0	-	0.2	0.2	0.3	0.7	0.4	1.1	1.1	0.9	0.3	1.1	0.9	0.2	0.1	0.02	0.03	**0.2**	207
Leukaemia unspecified	289	0	0.7	0.4	0.5	0.6	0.6	0.5	0.5	0.4	0.6	0.9	2.4	3.8	1.6	5.5	6.5	4.3	4.3	2.8	1.2	0.4	0.07	0.13	**1.2**	208
Other and unspecified	1416	1	0.6	0.4	0.4	0.7	0.5	1.1	1.0	1.5	3.3	5.2	11.7	16.7	23.2	34.4	38.4	32.1	25.5	14.2	5.9	2.1	0.33	0.70	**5.5**	O&U
All sites	71292	21	12.7	14.0	13.3	18.8	20.2	23.5	37.2	70.2	169.2	304.9	547.5	834.7	1248.8	1677.0	1911.4	1818.4	1624.8	1231.9	298.6		16.58	34.53	**276.0**	ALL
All sites but 173	66115	19	12.7	13.9	13.2	18.5	19.8	22.9	34.7	65.3	156.5	285.1	516.2	787.2	1175.5	1552.2	1738.5	1622.1	1426.3	984.9	276.9	100.0	15.61	32.07	**255.7**	ALLb
Rate from 10 cases			0.483	0.481	0.529	0.543	0.557	0.473	0.477	0.550	0.709	0.850	0.676	0.741	0.861	1.527	2.951	3.272	5.322	9.461						

*+ BELARUS 1988-1992

ANNUAL INCIDENCE PER 100,000 BY AGE GROUP (YEARS) - FEMALE

SITE	ALL AGES	AGE UNK	0-	5-	10-	15-	20-	25-	30-	35-	40-	45-	50-	55-	60-	65-	70-	75-	80-	85+	CRUDE RATE	%	CR 64	CR 74	ASR (W)	ICD (9th)
Lip	425	1	-	-	-	-	-	0.0	-	0.2	0.1	0.3	0.3	1.7	2.9	5.1	9.2	9.8	14.7	12.1	1.6	0.7	0.03	0.10	**0.8**	*140*
Tongue	99	0	-	-	-	-	0.1	0.0	0.1	0.1	0.3	0.2	0.6	0.7	1.2	1.2	1.7	0.9	1.1	0.9	0.4	0.2	0.02	0.03	**0.2**	*141*
Salivary gland	142	0	-	0.0	-	-	0.1	0.1	0.4	0.3	0.3	0.3	0.9	0.5	1.4	1.9	1.4	1.3	1.9	2.6	0.5	0.2	0.02	0.04	**0.3**	*142*
Mouth	176	0	-	-	-	-	0.1	0.3	0.1	0.3	0.4	0.4	0.6	1.4	1.1	1.7	3.2	2.3	3.3	4.6	0.7	0.3	0.02	0.05	**0.4**	*143-5*
Oropharynx	62	0	-	-	-	-	0.1	0.0	0.0	0.1	0.3	0.2	0.2	0.5	0.5	0.9	0.5	0.9	1.3	0.3	0.2	0.1	0.01	0.02	**0.1**	*146*
Nasopharynx	86	0	-	-	-	-	0.1	0.0	0.1	0.2	0.1	0.2	0.6	0.7	0.9	0.8	1.2	1.3	0.8	0.6	0.3	0.1	0.01	0.02	**0.2**	*147*
Hypopharynx	15	0	-	-	-	-	0.1	-	-	-	0.1	0.1	0.1	0.1	0.1	0.2	0.5	-	0.2	-	0.1	0.0	0.00	0.01	**0.0**	*148*
Pharynx unspecified	26	0	0.1	-	-	-	0.1	0.0	-	-	-	-	0.2	0.2	0.4	0.2	0.1	0.6	0.4	0.3	0.1	0.0	0.00	0.01	**0.1**	*149*
Oesophagus	298	0	-	-	-	-	-	-	-	0.2	0.3	0.5	0.3	1.0	2.5	4.3	6.1	7.2	7.5	6.3	1.1	0.5	0.02	0.08	**0.6**	*150*
Stomach	8879	2	0.1	0.1	0.1	0.4	1.0	1.6	3.7	9.1	15.1	21.2	33.9	51.6	81.2	128.0	162.6	162.7	148.1	85.9	32.8	15.3	1.10	2.55	**20.1**	*151*
Small intestine	83	1	0.1	-	-	0.1	-	-	0.1	0.1	0.1	0.5	0.6	0.9	0.8	0.9	0.9	0.6	1.0	0.3	0.3	0.1	0.02	0.03	**0.2**	*152*
Colon	3267	0	-	-	0.2	0.1	0.5	0.7	1.9	3.7	6.7	9.3	16.5	19.0	30.6	42.0	57.5	56.1	46.7	33.7	12.1	5.6	0.45	0.94	**7.6**	*153*
Rectum	3630	1	0.1	-	0.1	0.1	0.2	0.5	1.3	2.7	5.4	9.3	14.9	25.0	37.6	49.1	63.4	59.6	57.0	39.8	13.4	6.3	0.48	1.05	**8.3**	*154*
Liver	835	0	0.2	-	0.1	0.1	0.2	0.2	0.5	0.6	1.6	2.2	3.4	4.3	8.2	11.7	14.4	16.0	12.1	8.1	3.1	1.4	0.11	0.24	**1.9**	*155*
Gallbladder etc.	549	0	-	-	-	0.1	-	-	0.0	0.1	1.0	0.8	2.2	3.8	5.5	7.7	12.4	8.4	6.7	8.9	2.0	0.9	0.07	0.17	**1.2**	*156*
Pancreas	1684	2	-	-	-	0.1	0.1	0.1	0.2	0.9	1.7	3.0	6.5	9.9	15.3	22.5	30.0	35.6	33.3	22.8	6.2	2.9	0.19	0.45	**3.6**	*157*
Nose, sinuses etc.	105	0	0.1	-	-	0.1	-	0.1	0.0	0.2	0.3	0.2	0.5	1.0	0.9	1.0	1.4	1.3	1.7	0.9	0.4	0.2	0.02	0.03	**0.3**	*160*
Larynx	95	0	-	-	-	0.2	-	0.1	0.1	0.3	0.6	0.5	0.3	0.5	0.8	1.2	1.2	0.9	0.4	1.2	0.4	0.2	0.02	0.03	**0.3**	*161*
Bronchus, lung	2709	0	-	0.0	-	-	0.1	0.1	0.9	1.4	3.0	5.3	10.1	15.8	24.5	36.0	61.3	52.2	47.5	30.0	10.0	4.7	0.31	0.79	**6.0**	*162*
Other thoracic organs	122	0	0.1	0.0	0.1	-	0.2	0.0	0.3	0.2	0.7	0.3	0.5	0.5	0.9	1.7	1.4	1.3	2.1	0.6	0.5	0.2	0.02	0.04	**0.3**	*163-4*
Bone	440	0	0.2	0.6	1.6	1.1	1.0	0.5	0.6	1.2	1.1	1.7	1.5	2.7	3.2	3.0	5.5	4.6	4.4	2.3	1.6	0.8	0.09	0.13	**1.3**	*170*
Connective tissue	626	0	1.0	0.2	0.5	0.4	0.9	1.2	1.4	1.7	3.0	2.2	3.3	3.8	4.4	4.9	7.5	6.5	5.7	3.7	2.3	1.1	0.12	0.18	**1.8**	*171*
Mesothelioma	70	0	-	-	-	-	-	0.1	0.2	0.6	0.2	0.5	0.5	0.5	1.0	0.9	0.6	-	0.6	0.3	0.1	0.01	0.02	**0.2**	*MES*	
Kaposi's sarcoma	14	0	-	-	0.1	0.1	-	-	-	-	-	0.1	0.1	0.1	0.1	0.5	0.3	-	-	0.1	0.0	0.00	0.01	**0.0**	*KAP*	
Melanoma of skin	830	0	-	0.0	-	0.2	0.5	1.4	1.7	3.4	5.0	4.7	5.8	5.6	5.5	8.0	7.2	6.5	7.3	5.2	3.1	1.4	0.17	0.25	**2.3**	*172*
Other skin	7336	2	0.1	-	0.2	0.1	0.3	0.6	3.4	6.1	13.6	19.0	30.3	36.5	61.6	96.2	129.3	131.9	152.5	125.7	27.1		0.86	1.99	**16.3**	*173*
Breast	10424	0	-	-	-	0.3	0.5	4.8	16.4	36.9	68.2	82.1	86.3	78.5	93.9	99.3	87.0	60.8	46.5	39.8	38.5	18.0	2.34	3.27	**29.6**	*174*
Uterus unspecified	41	0	-	-	-	-	0.1	0.0	0.1	-	0.2	0.2	0.2	0.2	0.3	0.6	0.7	0.5	0.2	0.3	0.2	0.1	0.01	0.01	**0.1**	*179*
Cervix uteri	4029	1	-	-	0.1	0.3	1.4	4.5	10.7	16.3	22.6	23.6	24.7	26.0	34.8	43.4	42.8	30.5	21.2	13.0	14.9	6.9	0.83	1.26	**11.2**	*180*
Placenta	39	0	-	-	0.2	0.5	0.4	0.1	0.1	0.1	0.2	0.2	0.1	0.2	-	-	0.1	0.1	0.2	-	0.1	0.1	0.01	0.01	**0.1**	*181*
Corpus uteri	4096	0	-	-	0.2	0.4	0.6	1.9	3.7	9.8	18.6	37.5	45.9	51.7	51.6	39.9	22.2	19.7	9.5	15.1	7.1	0.85	1.31	**10.6**	*182*	
Ovary etc.	3970	0	-	0.0	0.7	1.3	1.5	2.2	5.5	7.7	15.3	21.5	30.7	32.8	40.9	46.3	42.7	31.6	22.6	8.9	14.7	6.8	0.80	1.25	**10.7**	*183*
Other female genital	813	0	-	-	-	-	0.1	0.2	0.2	0.5	0.7	1.2	2.5	3.7	7.3	13.4	17.0	14.8	15.3	11.2	3.0	1.4	0.08	0.23	**1.8**	*184*
Bladder	655	3	-	-	-	-	-	-	-	0.4	0.7	1.0	2.1	2.6	4.8	8.7	15.5	16.0	13.6	9.8	2.4	1.1	0.06	0.18	**1.4**	*188*
Kidney etc.	1454	0	1.8	0.7	0.3	0.2	0.4	0.4	1.1	2.1	3.2	5.3	9.6	13.6	16.8	18.6	19.5	10.1	7.7	3.7	5.4	2.5	0.28	0.47	**3.9**	*189*
Eye	204	0	0.7	0.1	0.1	-	0.2	0.2	0.1	0.4	0.5	1.1	1.1	1.3	1.4	2.3	1.8	3.0	1.7	1.4	0.8	0.4	0.04	0.06	**0.6**	*190*
Brain, nervous system	858	0	1.4	1.9	1.9	1.9	1.0	2.0	2.8	2.4	4.2	4.1	6.0	7.7	6.0	5.5	2.6	1.1	0.8	1.4	3.2	1.5	0.22	0.26	**2.8**	*191-2*
Thyroid	1166	0	0.3	2.1	1.9	1.1	2.0	2.4	4.5	5.4	8.0	6.5	6.2	6.9	7.9	6.7	7.4	4.9	5.9	4.0	4.3	2.0	0.28	0.35	**3.7**	*193*
Other endocrine	32	0	0.1	-	0.1	0.1	0.1	0.0	-	0.2	0.3	0.1	0.2	0.1	0.3	0.5	0.1	0.1	-	-	0.1	0.1	0.01	0.01	**0.1**	*194*
Hodgkin's disease	699	0	0.2	0.5	1.4	4.5	5.6	4.3	3.3	2.6	2.2	1.5	2.1	2.7	2.0	3.9	2.8	2.4	0.8	2.0	2.6	1.2	0.16	0.20	**2.5**	*201*
Non-Hodgkin lymphoma	654	0	0.6	0.5	0.5	0.8	0.5	0.9	0.9	1.2	1.6	1.7	3.1	3.9	6.6	6.6	8.4	7.5	6.3	5.8	2.4	1.1	0.11	0.19	**1.8**	*200,202*
Multiple myeloma	337	0	-	-	0.1	0.1	0.1	0.0	0.2	0.2	0.7	1.1	1.7	2.9	4.5	5.4	5.4	3.4	1.3	0.9	1.2	0.6	0.06	0.11	**0.8**	*203*
Lymphoid leukaemia	1119	0	1.6	2.0	1.8	0.7	0.5	0.6	1.0	1.3	2.4	1.9	4.7	6.8	10.1	15.2	18.2	13.6	8.2	6.3	4.1	1.9	0.18	0.34	**3.0**	*204*
Myeloid leukaemia	627	0	0.4	0.1	0.4	0.5	0.8	1.2	1.0	1.4	2.1	2.4	3.0	4.3	6.3	8.0	7.4	5.1	3.6	1.2	2.3	1.1	0.12	0.20	**1.7**	*205*
Monocytic leukaemia	25	0	0.1	-	-	-	-	0.0	0.1	0.1	-	0.1	0.1	0.4	0.2	0.4	0.4	0.4	-	0.1	0.0	0.00	0.01	**0.1**	*206*	
Other leukaemia	72	0	0.1	-	0.1	-	0.1	0.1	0.0	0.2	0.3	0.3	0.3	0.7	0.5	1.0	1.3	0.5	0.4	-	0.1	0.1	0.01	0.02	**0.2**	*207*
Leukaemia unspecified	298	0	0.5	0.6	0.4	0.4	0.2	0.3	0.4	0.6	0.7	1.2	1.8	1.9	2.7	2.7	4.0	2.4	1.9	1.2	1.1	0.5	0.06	0.09	**0.9**	*208*
Other and unspecified	1103	3	0.7	0.2	0.2	0.3	0.4	0.4	0.5	1.1	1.8	3.2	4.5	7.7	11.4	15.1	19.0	13.6	13.4	11.8	4.1	1.9	0.16	0.33	**2.7**	*O&U*
All sites	65318	16	9.7	10.2	12.6	15.9	22.0	33.5	67.7	117.8	207.1	261.4	363.5	438.9	603.2	786.3	925.6	813.9	749.4	529.6	241.4		10.82	19.38	**165.0**	*ALL*
All sites but 173	57982	14	9.7	10.2	12.4	15.8	21.7	32.9	64.3	111.7	193.5	242.4	333.2	402.4	541.6	690.1	796.3	682.0	596.9	403.9	214.3	100.0	9.96	17.40	**148.7**	*ALLb*
Rate from 10 cases			0.506	0.500	0.547	0.545	0.550	0.485	0.475	0.541	0.681	0.772	0.572	0.595	0.588	0.780	1.318	1.267	1.914	2.883							

Croatia

The Croatian National Cancer Registry was established in 1959. Initially it collected cancer mortality statistics, and started to record cancer case notifications in 1962. The registry was intended to supply basic data on cancer incidence and characteristics for the planning and evaluation of individual preventive measures and oncological services, for patient care planning. Underfinancing has led to occasional disruptions in the registry's operation. The registry's present full-time staff consists of a medical hygienic specialist as director, a senior statistician and two statisticians. The registry is part of the Epidemiology Service at the Croatian National Institute of Public Health.

The registration area is the whole of Croatia, which until 1991 formed part of the Yugoslav republic. Croatia borders on Slovenia to the north-west, Hungary to the north, Voiuodina (part of Serbia) to the east, and Bosnia-Herzegovina and Montenegro to the south. In the south-west, it opens onto the Adriatic Sea. Lying between latitudes 42°23′ and 46°33′ N, and longitudes 13°30′ and 19°27′ E, it covers an area of 56 538 km^2 and has 5790 km of coastline. While the north of the country has a continental climate, the coastal area has a Mediterranean climate.

The population according to the 1991 census was 4 784 265 (48.5% males; 51.5% females). Ethnically, Croats made up 78.1%. Roman Catholics accounted for 76.5% of the population. There was an economically active population of 2 039 833, working in mining and industry (32.5%), trade (10.1%), transport and communications (7.5%), central and local government bodies, funds, associations, health, welfare and social services (6.8%), construction (6.2%), catering and tourist trade (4.8%), agriculture and fisheries (4.1%) and 3.8% in invisible trade (financial, technical and other services). 285 216 inhabitants were working abroad.

In 1990, the health service had a workforce of 10 152 physicians (1 per 469 population). The health service entry points were general practitioners, industrial physicians, gynaecologists, paediatricians, school health specialists and medical stomatologists, affiliated to health centres with which, in principle, each commune was provided. When necessary, the primary health service referred patients to a polyclinic-consultant service or to a hospital. There were 104 hospitals with about 35 000 beds (7.4 per 1000 population). While 32 were general hospitals and the rest specialized, only one was dedicated to oncology. Most health institutions admitted oncology cases; special oncology units (with a full range of services) operated in bigger centres.

For the registry, the basic notification is the one completed for a patient at hospital discharge. Systems for outpatient notification and anatomical pathology reporting are still being set up. Mortality information is derived from death certificates with a mention of cancer. Notifications include the name of the health care provider (hospital or physician), so that these can be contacted for further information. Because the unique population identification number is not entered on every form, data-merging is time-consuming. Active follow-up is not undertaken. The registry still has a large percentage of death-certificate-only entries. This was particularly related, until 1990, to the fact that a significant part of the population received medical care at military hospitals or foreign hospitals, neither of which were obliged to send notifications. Registry involvement in under- and postgraduate education has made a significant contribution to improvement of data quality and completeness. A very close collaboration has been established with the Croatian Pathological Society.

The classifications used are ICD-9 and SNOP. Data are collected on all patients assigned any of the diagnostic codes 140–208, as well as benign and unspecified brain neoplasms, carcinomas *in situ*, polycythaemia and myelofibrosis.

The registry was first computerized in 1968, but a new system installed in 1992 has greatly improved its operation. At data entry, checks are first made for permissible values in each data field. Next, logical checks are performed for items such as discharge date vs date of admission and site/sex and site/age compatibility. Finally, the data on a new notification form are checked against possible earlier database items. Each primary cancer in the same individual is entered after checking, and is noted in the personal record by showing the number of incident diagnoses. This is checked with the clinicians who cared for the patient. Data are stored on a magnetic disk and on a tape (streamer). The paper notification cards have been kept since 1968.

Cancer incidence data appear each year in a special bulletin and in the institute's joint annual report. Analyses and observed trends are published in medical journals. The registry provides a database for various types of research and serves to assess the status of cancer and trends in individual cancer sites.

Marija Strnad

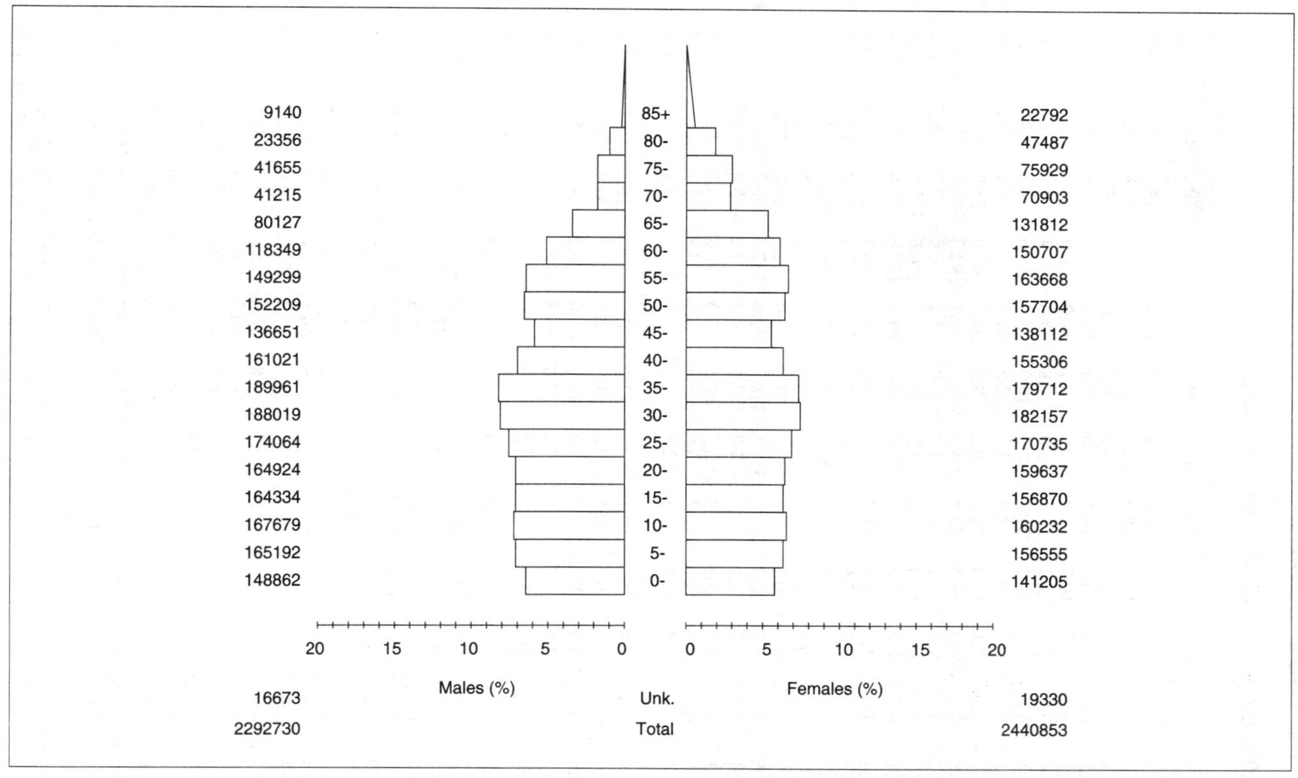

Croatia

Source of population: average of 1988, 1989 and 1991
Census: 1991 Census of population, 31 March 1991, Documentation 882, Republic of Croatia, Central Bureau of Statistics, Zagreb, 1994 (Popis stanovnistva 1991, Dokumentacija 882, Republika Hrvatska, Drzavni zavod za statistiku, Zagreb, 1994). 1981 Population Census, 31 March 1981, Document 501, Republic of Croatia, National Bureau of Statistics, Zagreb, 1982 (Popis stanovnistva 1981, Dokumentacija 501, Republika Hrvatska, Republicki zavod za statistiku, Zagreb, 1982)
Estimate: The population estimates for 1988 and 1989 are based on the 1981 census, taking into account births and deaths. References: Demogr. statistics 1988, Federal Bureau of Statistics, Beograd, 1990. Demograf. statistics 1989, Federal Bureau of Statistics, Beograd, 1991.

Notes to tables overleaf:
* Some of the indices of quality, for example unexpected ratios of mortality to incidence, indicate under-ascertainment
† 188 does not include non-invasive tumours

* CROATIA 1988-1991

ANNUAL INCIDENCE PER 100,000 BY AGE GROUP (YEARS) - MALE

SITE	ALL AGES	AGE UNK	0-	5-	10-	15-	20-	25-	30-	35-	40-	45-	50-	55-	60-	65-	70-	75-	80-	85+	CRUDE RATE	%	CR 64	CR 74	ASR (W)	ICD (9th)
Lip	358	8	-	-	-	-	-	-	0.5	0.3	1.7	2.7	5.6	9.0	11.4	19.7	19.4	21.0	35.3	35.6	3.9	1.1	0.16	0.36	**3.0**	*140*
Tongue	432	12	-	-	-	-	-	0.1	-	2.1	3.1	9.1	11.2	15.6	16.7	12.5	12.7	12.0	11.8	2.7	4.7	1.4	0.30	0.43	**3.6**	*141*
Salivary gland	161	2	-	0.2	-	-	0.2	0.3	0.7	0.5	1.1	2.9	2.8	4.7	4.2	6.2	3.0	11.4	9.6	13.7	1.8	0.5	0.09	0.14	**1.4**	*142*
Mouth	375	4	-	-	-	-	-	-	0.1	0.5	4.0	6.0	10.2	13.1	15.0	13.4	10.3	12.6	12.8	8.2	4.1	1.2	0.25	0.37	**3.1**	*143-5*
Oropharynx	342	2	-	-	-	-	-	-	-	0.8	2.9	7.7	10.7	13.9	12.5	9.7	10.9	6.0	5.4	5.5	3.7	1.1	0.24	0.35	**2.9**	*146*
Nasopharynx	82	1	-	-	0.1	-	0.2	0.1	0.1	0.4	0.9	1.3	2.1	2.3	3.0	2.8	3.0	2.4	1.1	2.7	0.9	0.3	0.05	0.08	**0.7**	*147*
Hypopharynx	524	5	-	-	-	0.2	-	-	0.1	1.2	4.3	9.7	15.1	21.3	20.7	19.0	15.2	9.0	8.6	2.7	5.7	1.6	0.37	0.54	**4.4**	*148*
Pharynx unspecified	55	0	-	-	-	-	-	-	0.1	0.3	0.7	0.7	2.8	1.9	2.5	1.2	3.0	2.1	2.1	2.7	0.6	0.2	0.03	0.05	**0.4**	*149*
Oesophagus	746	7	-	-	-	-	-	-	0.3	1.1	3.7	9.1	16.3	24.9	29.2	29.3	24.3	60.0	28.9	21.9	8.1	2.3	0.43	0.70	**6.1**	*150*
Stomach	3364	28	-	-	-	0.2	-	1.4	2.8	5.8	10.2	24.0	44.3	83.6	108.2	179.4	214.7	292.3	298.6	238.0	36.7	10.6	1.41	3.40	**28.1**	*151*
Small intestine	47	1	-	-	-	-	-	0.1	0.1	0.1	0.3	1.1	1.1	1.3	1.9	0.9	1.2	0.6	3.2	5.5	0.5	0.1	0.03	0.04	**0.4**	*152*
Colon	1513	24	-	-	0.1	0.5	0.6	1.1	1.3	5.1	8.5	10.6	19.4	30.6	47.3	72.1	103.7	126.6	135.9	125.8	16.5	4.8	0.64	1.53	**12.8**	*153*
Rectum	1597	29	-	-	-	-	0.5	0.3	0.9	2.4	4.3	10.4	23.5	35.7	52.6	81.4	104.9	127.8	167.0	123.1	17.4	5.0	0.66	1.61	**13.4**	*154*
Liver	555	2	0.3	0.2	0.1	-	0.2	0.4	0.3	1.4	1.4	4.2	8.7	13.7	20.1	28.4	38.2	40.2	43.9	21.9	6.1	1.7	0.26	0.59	**4.7**	*155*
Gallbladder etc.	255	1	-	-	-	-	-	-	0.4	0.3	0.2	2.0	1.6	5.7	7.6	14.7	14.0	32.4	27.8	19.1	2.8	0.8	0.09	0.23	**2.1**	*156*
Pancreas	1070	8	-	-	-	-	-	0.5	0.6	1.1	4.2	4.5	8.4	14.8	27.1	38.0	56.5	64.3	79.2	76.0	49.2	11.7	3.4	0.50	1.11	**9.0**	*157*
Nose, sinuses etc.	62	0	-	-	-	-	-	-	0.1	-	-	0.5	2.0	1.7	1.5	2.5	3.6	5.4	3.2	8.2	0.7	0.2	0.03	0.06	**0.5**	*160*
Larynx	1556	22	-	-	-	-	-	0.4	1.1	4.7	11.8	25.2	40.2	57.6	58.5	55.5	57.0	52.2	38.5	32.8	17.0	4.9	1.01	1.58	**13.1**	*161*
Bronchus, lung	8624	88	-	-	-	0.2	0.3	1.9	3.2	14.6	31.5	82.3	156.7	295.0	371.1	428.7	439.8	437.5	350.0	284.5	94.0	27.1	4.83	9.22	**72.5**	*162*
Other thoracic organs	82	0	0.7	0.2	-	0.3	0.3	0.6	0.3	0.4	0.3	0.5	1.8	1.7	1.3	3.4	4.2	4.2	5.4	5.5	0.9	0.3	0.04	0.08	**0.8**	*163-4*
Bone	167	2	0.7	1.1	1.5	1.8	2.4	0.6	0.7	1.3	1.2	1.5	2.3	1.8	3.2	2.5	3.0	10.8	4.3	16.4	1.8	0.5	0.10	0.13	**1.7**	*170*
Connective tissue	138	1	0.8	0.5	0.4	0.8	0.8	0.6	0.9	1.6	0.6	0.7	2.6	2.2	3.6	5.9	4.9	4.8	1.1	8.2	1.5	0.4	0.08	0.14	**1.3**	*171*
Mesothelioma	65	1	0.2	-	-	0.2	-	-	-	0.9	1.8	1.6	2.3	2.5	1.2	1.2	1.2	2.1	-		0.7	0.2	0.05	0.06	**0.6**	*MES*
Kaposi's sarcoma	1	0	-	-	-	-	-	0.1	-	-	-	-	-	-	-	-	-	-	-	-	0.0	0.0	0.00	0.00	**0.0**	*KAP*
Melanoma of skin	350	10	-	-	0.1	0.8	0.2	1.6	2.4	3.6	3.9	3.8	6.6	7.4	7.8	11.2	20.6	12.0	16.1	13.7	3.8	1.1	0.20	0.36	**3.1**	*172*
Other skin	117	0	-	-	-	-	-	-	-	-	-	-	0.5	0.5	0.6	1.9	6.7	13.8	36.4	93.0	1.3		0.01	0.05	**1.0**	*173*
Breast	66	0	-	-	-	-	-	-	-	0.3	0.5	0.5	0.3	1.8	3.2	2.2	3.0	4.2	9.6	5.5	0.7	0.2	0.03	0.06	**0.5**	*175*
Prostate	2096	27	-	-	-	-	0.2	-	0.4	0.1	0.5	2.4	7.2	17.9	40.6	92.0	198.3	315.1	410.0	478.7	22.9	6.6	0.35	1.82	**17.5**	*185*
Testis	238	3	0.3	0.3	0.1	2.0	5.5	8.9	4.9	2.9	3.6	2.0	0.7	1.2	0.8	0.6	3.0	1.8	1.1	-	2.6	0.7	0.17	0.19	**2.5**	*186*
Penis	47	1	-	-	-	-	-	-	0.1	0.3	0.2	0.4	0.3	0.7	1.7	2.8	1.8	1.2	7.5	13.7	0.5	0.1	0.02	0.04	**0.4**	*187.1-.4*
Other male genital	22	0	-	-	-	-	0.2	0.1	0.3	-	-	-	0.3	0.2	0.8	0.3	1.8	1.2	1.2	2.1	0.2	0.1	0.01	0.02	**0.2**	*187.5-.9*
†Bladder	1400	20	-	0.2	-	-	0.3	0.3	1.6	1.7	2.6	7.9	13.5	26.3	44.8	67.7	98.3	145.2	164.8	175.1	15.3	4.4	0.50	1.34	**11.7**	*188*
Kidney etc.	754	10	2.9	1.2	0.4	0.5	0.2	0.6	1.6	2.2	4.2	8.6	12.2	21.8	25.3	34.6	44.9	37.2	25.7	27.4	8.2	2.4	0.41	0.82	**6.8**	*189*
Eye	62	2	1.2	0.5	0.1	-	0.3	0.4	-	0.3	0.2	-	1.1	1.3	1.5	2.2	5.5	1.2	1.1	-	0.7	0.2	0.04	0.08	**0.7**	*190*
Brain, nervous system	905	5	5.2	3.6	2.7	1.4	3.0	3.7	4.7	7.9	8.8	11.5	17.7	24.6	27.5	32.8	18.2	12.6	12.8	10.9	9.9	2.8	0.62	0.87	**8.5**	*191-2*
Thyroid	130	2	-	-	-	0.3	0.8	0.4	0.7	2.0	1.4	2.0	2.8	2.2	4.0	2.5	3.0	3.6	7.5	8.2	1.4	0.4	0.08	0.11	**1.1**	*193*
Other endocrine	58	0	0.5	0.3	0.7	-	0.2	-	0.5	0.5	0.6	0.2	1.0	1.2	1.7	2.2	2.4	-	2.1	-	0.6	0.2	0.04	0.06	**0.6**	*194*
Hodgkin's disease	175	0	0.8	0.8	1.2	1.2	1.4	1.4	2.1	1.6	1.6	2.2	2.6	2.5	4.4	3.4	2.4	4.2	5.4	2.7	1.9	0.6	0.12	0.15	**1.7**	*201*
Non-Hodgkin lymphoma	564	5	1.5	3.0	2.2	1.2	1.5	2.0	3.3	4.5	3.6	6.4	7.9	10.2	14.8	21.5	29.1	24.0	25.7	16.4	6.1	1.8	0.31	0.57	**5.3**	*200,202*
Multiple myeloma	217	0	-	-	-	-	0.2	0.1	-	0.3	0.9	2.4	2.3	5.9	7.6	8.7	15.2	24.6	15.0	2.7	2.4	0.7	0.10	0.22	**1.8**	*203*
Lymphoid leukaemia	490	9	6.0	2.6	1.8	1.8	1.8	0.3	0.5	0.9	1.6	3.1	5.1	10.0	16.3	17.8	20.6	26.4	39.6	32.8	5.3	1.5	0.26	0.46	**4.8**	*204*
Myeloid leukaemia	333	4	1.7	0.9	0.9	0.5	0.9	1.0	1.2	2.0	1.9	3.8	4.4	6.5	7.8	16.8	10.3	18.6	25.7	13.7	3.6	1.0	0.17	0.31	**3.0**	*205*
Monocytic leukaemia	2	0	-	-	-	-	-	-	-	-	-	-	-	-	0.3	-	0.6	-	-	-	0.0	0.0	0.00	0.00	**0.0**	*206*
Other leukaemia	5	0	-	-	-	-	-	-	-	-	-	-	0.2	-	0.4	-	-	-	1.1	2.7	0.1	0.0	0.00	0.00	**0.0**	*207*
Leukaemia unspecified	76	1	0.2	-	-	0.2	-	-	0.1	0.3	0.3	0.2	1.3	1.2	1.5	4.1	4.2	6.0	9.6	16.4	0.8	0.2	0.03	0.07	**0.7**	*208*
Other and unspecified	1645	8	1.2	0.3	0.4	0.5	0.8	1.3	1.6	2.1	7.3	11.0	23.0	38.2	58.1	76.4	94.0	126.0	158.4	196.9	17.9	5.2	0.73	1.59	**14.0**	*O&U*
All sites	31923	355	24.2	15.6	13.3	14.1	22.9	31.0	41.1	82.3	141.6	291.3	506.4	849.3	1103.1	1450.5	1738.4	2132.4	2249.9	2152.6	348.1		15.86	31.98	**272.7**	*ALL*
All sites but 173	31806	355	24.2	15.6	13.3	14.1	22.9	31.0	41.1	82.3	141.6	291.3	505.9	848.8	1102.5	1448.6	1731.7	2118.6	2213.5	2059.6	346.8	100.0	15.85	31.93	**271.6**	*ALLb*

Rate from 1 case   0.168   0.151   0.149   0.152   0.152   0.144   0.133   0.132   0.155   0.183   0.164   0.167   0.211   0.312   0.607   0.600   1.070   2.735

†Important: see notes on population page

* CROATIA 1988-1991

ANNUAL INCIDENCE PER 100,000 BY AGE GROUP (YEARS) - FEMALE

SITE	ALL AGES	AGE UNK	0-	5-	10-	15-	20-	25-	30-	35-	40-	45-	50-	55-	60-	65-	70-	75-	80-	85+	CRUDE RATE	%	CR 64	CR 74	ASR (W)	ICD (9th)
Lip	114	2	-	-	-	-	-	-	-	0.1	-	0.7	0.8	1.4	1.8	3.2	5.3	5.9	11.1	12.1	1.2	0.4	0.02	0.07	0.6	140
Tongue	56	3	-	-	0.3	-	0.2	-	0.1	0.1	0.8	0.5	1.3	0.3	0.7	1.9	1.1	1.6	3.2	2.2	0.6	0.2	0.02	0.04	0.4	141
Salivary gland	79	1	-	-	0.2	0.2	0.3	0.1	0.1	0.7	0.8	0.4	1.0	0.8	0.7	2.5	2.1	3.6	3.7	8.8	0.8	0.3	0.03	0.05	0.5	142
Mouth	74	1	-	-	-	-	-	0.1	-	-	-	0.5	0.8	1.2	1.5	1.9	3.2	3.3	5.8	7.7	0.8	0.3	0.02	0.05	0.4	143-5
Oropharynx	39	0	-	-	-	-	-	-	-	-	0.3	0.9	0.6	0.9	1.3	0.8	1.4	1.3	-	2.2	0.4	0.1	0.02	0.03	0.3	146
Nasopharynx	25	0	-	-	-	-	-	0.1	0.3	-	0.6	0.4	0.3	0.2	1.3	0.4	0.4	0.3	-	1.1	0.3	0.1	0.02	0.02	0.2	147
Hypopharynx	48	1	-	-	-	-	0.2	0.1	0.4	-	0.5	0.7	0.3	0.8	2.0	0.9	0.4	2.3	1.1	1.1	0.5	0.2	0.03	0.03	0.3	148
Pharynx unspecified	6	0	-	-	-	-	-	-	-	-	-	0.2	-	-	-	0.2	-	-	0.5	3.3	0.1	0.0	0.00	0.00	0.0	149
Oesophagus	150	1	-	-	-	-	-	-	-	0.4	0.6	0.7	1.0	2.1	3.2	4.2	5.3	8.6	13.7	11.0	1.5	0.6	0.04	0.09	0.8	150
Stomach	2122	21	-	-	0.2	-	-	0.9	2.2	4.0	5.3	9.4	16.3	22.8	39.6	63.7	97.3	140.9	164.3	132.7	21.7	7.9	0.51	1.32	11.5	151
Small intestine	47	4	-	-	-	-	-	-	0.3	0.3	0.1	0.2	0.4	0.3	0.3	1.7	0.4	3.0	2.1	4.4	0.5	0.2	0.01	0.02	0.3	152
Colon	1557	36	-	-	0.2	-	0.2	0.7	1.0	3.8	2.7	11.4	17.8	20.2	31.2	48.6	59.2	85.6	103.7	95.4	15.9	5.8	0.46	1.01	8.9	153
Rectum	1450	24	-	-	-	-	0.2	0.7	0.5	2.5	5.0	9.4	15.1	20.0	31.4	44.0	60.6	82.3	89.5	83.4	14.9	5.4	0.43	0.96	8.3	154
Liver	447	6	0.2	-	-	-	-	0.4	0.5	1.0	1.4	2.9	3.3	7.5	7.8	12.7	18.7	25.7	31.1	29.6	4.6	1.7	0.13	0.29	2.5	155
Gallbladder etc.	577	12	-	-	-	-	-	-	0.1	0.4	0.5	2.0	3.8	6.6	12.6	18.0	27.1	38.2	41.1	41.7	5.9	2.2	0.13	0.36	3.1	156
Pancreas	896	15	-	-	-	-	-	0.4	0.5	1.4	2.1	3.1	6.8	11.6	19.7	28.3	45.8	48.1	58.4	65.8	9.2	3.4	0.23	0.61	5.0	157
Nose, sinuses etc.	59	0	-	-	-	-	-	-	-	-	0.2	0.6	0.9	1.7	1.7	1.8	2.3	6.8	4.4	4.4	0.6	0.2	0.02	0.03	0.3	160
Larynx	98	5	0.2	-	-	-	-	0.1	0.3	-	0.8	1.6	0.8	1.4	3.0	2.7	1.8	4.3	3.7	4.4	1.0	0.4	0.04	0.07	0.6	161
Bronchus, lung	1579	28	-	-	-	-	0.2	1.2	1.2	4.5	7.1	15.0	22.2	23.4	41.5	52.7	59.6	66.2	67.4	60.3	16.2	5.9	0.59	1.16	9.7	162
Other thoracic organs	54	0	0.4	0.2	0.2	0.5	0.3	-	0.1	0.1	0.2	0.9	0.5	0.5	1.3	1.5	0.7	1.6	2.1	4.4	0.6	0.2	0.03	0.04	0.4	163-4
Bone	139	1	0.2	1.1	1.1	1.9	0.9	1.0	0.7	1.4	1.0	0.5	0.5	1.7	2.0	2.7	3.9	3.3	3.2	7.7	1.4	0.5	0.07	0.10	1.2	170
Connective tissue	150	5	0.7	0.3	0.5	0.3	0.8	0.4	1.1	1.0	1.0	1.6	2.9	2.0	1.7	3.4	4.6	4.0	3.2	6.6	1.5	0.6	0.07	0.11	1.2	171
Mesothelioma	16	0	-	-	-	-	-	-	-	-	0.2	-	0.5	-	1.0	0.2	1.1	0.3	0.5	-	0.2	0.1	0.01	0.01	0.1	MES
Kaposi's sarcoma	0	0	-	-	-	-	-	-	-	-	-	-	-	-	-	-	-	-	-	-	0.0	0.0	0.00	0.00	0.0	KAP
Melanoma of skin	410	9	0.2	-	-	0.5	0.6	1.8	2.1	3.5	5.8	4.9	6.8	7.0	6.5	11.2	7.8	9.5	15.3	12.1	4.2	1.5	0.20	0.30	2.9	172
Other skin	187	2	-	-	-	-	-	-	-	-	-	0.2	0.5	-	0.3	2.3	2.8	12.5	30.0	70.2	1.9		0.00	0.03	0.8	173
Breast	5385	91	-	-	0.2	1.0	0.9	4.2	14.4	35.6	65.8	94.7	90.0	102.2	125.1	130.9	144.2	150.5	134.8	171.1	55.2	20.1	2.72	4.12	37.2	174
Uterus unspecified	288	0	-	-	-	-	-	-	0.4	0.6	1.4	3.4	3.2	2.6	4.3	6.3	11.6	16.5	25.8	27.4	2.9	1.1	0.08	0.17	1.6	179
Cervix uteri	1567	23	-	-	-	-	0.2	1.6	10.4	17.3	20.6	20.9	20.6	20.8	24.6	35.5	37.0	31.0	28.6	19.7	16.0	5.9	0.87	1.22	11.6	180
Placenta	7	0	-	-	-	-	0.2	0.2	0.1	-	0.1	0.2	0.4	-	-	-	-	-	-	-	0.1	0.0	0.01	0.01	0.1	181
Corpus uteri	1536	32	-	-	-	-	-	0.3	1.1	1.5	7.4	15.2	29.0	44.0	47.4	54.4	44.8	36.2	30.5	15.4	15.7	5.7	0.75	1.25	10.0	182
Ovary etc.	1484	22	-	0.3	0.9	1.8	2.2	2.3	4.5	8.1	11.4	21.0	26.9	31.5	36.2	40.2	43.7	42.1	33.7	14.3	15.2	5.5	0.75	1.17	10.3	183
Other female genital	282	10	-	-	-	-	0.2	-	0.3	1.4	0.6	1.4	2.4	4.4	5.6	8.7	10.6	13.5	16.8	21.9	2.9	1.1	0.08	0.18	1.6	184
†Bladder	454	13	-	-	-	-	0.3	0.1	0.4	0.3	1.1	2.4	2.4	6.3	9.0	12.9	18.3	26.7	37.9	32.9	4.6	1.7	0.11	0.28	2.5	188
Kidney etc.	556	6	3.2	0.6	0.2	-	0.2	0.6	0.4	1.9	2.6	6.5	6.8	10.5	15.3	15.7	21.2	19.8	18.4	12.1	5.7	2.1	0.25	0.43	3.9	189
Eye	86	0	0.9	-	0.2	-	0.3	0.1	-	0.3	0.2	0.2	1.3	0.8	2.3	2.1	3.2	2.3	6.3	7.7	0.9	0.3	0.03	0.06	0.6	190
Brain, nervous system	769	9	2.8	3.8	2.5	1.9	2.5	3.4	4.5	6.8	5.5	11.6	10.5	16.6	16.9	19.7	14.5	10.9	7.9	3.3	7.9	2.9	0.45	0.63	6.3	191-2
Thyroid	514	12	-	-	0.3	0.6	3.0	3.2	4.4	9.0	9.8	11.2	5.7	6.1	9.8	6.6	7.1	8.6	6.3	7.7	5.3	1.9	0.32	0.39	4.2	193
Other endocrine	64	2	1.6	0.6	0.5	0.5	0.2	0.1	0.4	0.4	0.4	0.2	1.1	0.9	1.8	0.6	0.4	0.7	-	-	0.7	0.2	0.05	0.05	0.7	194
Hodgkin's disease	141	2	0.2	-	0.6	3.0	3.4	1.2	1.4	1.3	1.9	0.7	0.8	1.4	1.7	1.3	1.4	3.0	2.6	1.1	1.4	0.5	0.09	0.10	1.3	201
Non-Hodgkin lymphoma	538	9	1.1	1.0	1.4	0.5	2.5	2.3	2.5	2.2	2.7	4.0	5.7	7.9	11.1	15.4	18.7	20.4	19.5	13.2	5.5	2.0	0.23	0.40	3.8	200,202
Multiple myeloma	275	9	0.2	-	-	-	0.2	-	0.1	0.3	1.1	0.7	4.0	5.3	6.3	11.8	10.9	10.9	8.9	9.9	2.8	1.0	0.09	0.21	1.7	203
Lymphoid leukaemia	363	8	3.2	2.7	1.1	0.8	0.8	0.6	0.7	0.1	1.1	1.8	2.9	4.9	6.8	10.2	12.0	19.4	14.7	11.0	3.7	1.4	0.14	0.25	2.7	204
Myeloid leukaemia	352	14	0.4	1.4	0.6	0.3	0.6	1.2	1.5	1.7	2.3	4.2	4.0	4.9	8.3	8.0	8.1	15.1	11.1	9.9	3.6	1.3	0.16	0.25	2.5	205
Monocytic leukaemia	2	0	-	-	-	-	-	-	-	-	-	-	-	-	0.2	0.4	-	-	-	-	0.0	0.0	0.00	0.00	0.0	206
Other leukaemia	3	0	-	-	-	-	-	0.1	-	-	-	-	-	-	-	-	-	0.3	0.5	-	0.0	0.0	0.00	0.00	0.0	207
Leukaemia unspecified	74	0	0.2	-	-	-	0.2	-	0.3	0.1	0.3	-	0.6	0.8	1.7	1.3	3.9	4.9	4.7	6.6	0.8	0.3	0.02	0.05	0.4	208
Other and unspecified	1808	14	1.8	0.5	0.2	0.6	0.3	0.4	1.6	3.1	4.2	6.0	8.4	20.2	29.0	46.3	72.6	112.9	165.8	230.3	18.5	6.8	0.38	0.98	9.7	O&U
All sites	26927	453	17.2	12.6	11.1	14.7	23.3	39.5	67.9	120.5	178.2	274.8	331.0	429.5	588.1	740.8	890.7	1098.1	1234.0	1287.7	275.8		10.72	19.02	172.9	ALL
All sites but 173	26740	451	17.2	12.6	11.1	14.7	23.3	39.5	67.9	120.5	178.2	274.6	330.5	429.5	587.7	738.6	887.8	1085.5	1204.0	1217.5	273.9	100.0	10.72	18.99	172.1	ALLb
Rate from 1 case			0.177	0.160	0.156	0.159	0.157	0.146	0.137	0.139	0.161	0.181	0.159	0.153	0.166	0.190	0.353	0.329	0.526	1.097						

†Important: see notes on population page

457

Czech Republic

The National Oncologic Registry of the Czech Republic (NOR) was founded in 1976 as a continuation of nationwide recording of newly notified malignant neoplasms which had been operating since 1956. In the 1980s the data quality and the functioning of the registry greatly improved. Since 1984, reporting of histology, if known, has been compulsory.

The Czech Republic covers an area of 78 864 km^2, and had a population of 10 302 215 in March 1991 (48.5% male, 51.5% female). The birth rate was 12.6 per thousand and the mortality rate 12.5 per thousand.

Transformation of the health services and privatization of health establishments have necessitated changes in registry practice in order to retain its quality. Since 1991, District Registries equipped with computers have been gradually established. In 1993 the National Oncologic Registry Board was established and started to manage the registry's performance as well as resolving conceptual and methodological problems. Eight Regional Administrators have been nominated who are responsible for the performance of the registry in the districts of their region (there are 85 districts in the Czech Republic); they are also members of the Board, which concentrates on improving the quality of controls and their unification in the framework of the registry.

Notification of neoplasms is mandatory by law for every physician who diagnoses a malignant neoplasm, a neoplasm *in situ* or a neoplasm of unknown character or morphology. The notification is sent to a specialized district health establishment where details are supplemented within three months with the morphology, date of diagnosis (i.e., of its verification), proposed plan of therapy, TNM, etc. Since 1994, all data for the national registry pass controls in regional workplaces.

During 1988–92 there were two routes of data entry into the national registry:

(*a*) The physician sent filled notifications to the specialized district oncological establishment, where they were supplemented by specialized data and, after checking, sent, directly or via regional workplaces, four times a year to the Institute of Health Information and Statistics (IHIS), where the data were entered, processed, checked and included in the national registry.

(*b*) The physician filled in the notification which was supplemented with specialized data in a district oncological establishment and entered, processed and checked at a district or regional oncological registry and sent to IHIS once a year for final checking and inclusion in the national registry.

The Institute of Health Information and Statistics receives data annually on population and deaths from the Czech Statistical Office. The data on deaths are compared with the registry data, which results in two files for manual checking, search and complementary notification. One file contains information on deaths from the Czech Statistical Office concerning persons already registered but not reported dead; it is checked whether they indeed have died and the cause of death is notified. The second file contains the cancer deaths in the Statistical Office data concerning persons not previously registered; a search is performed to find whether they were treated, and a positive result leads to complementary notification of the neoplasm; if they were not treated, complementary notifications are made as death-certificate-only cases with code 99.

The diagnosis of malignant tumours, cause of death, morphology and TNM were coded using ICD-9, ICD-O-1 and TNM classification (1978). Since January 1994, coding according to ICD-10 and ICD-O-2 has been mandatory. The registry created its own conversion between ICD-9 and ICD-10. Since 1995 the 4th edition of the 2nd revision of the TNM classification (1992) has been used.

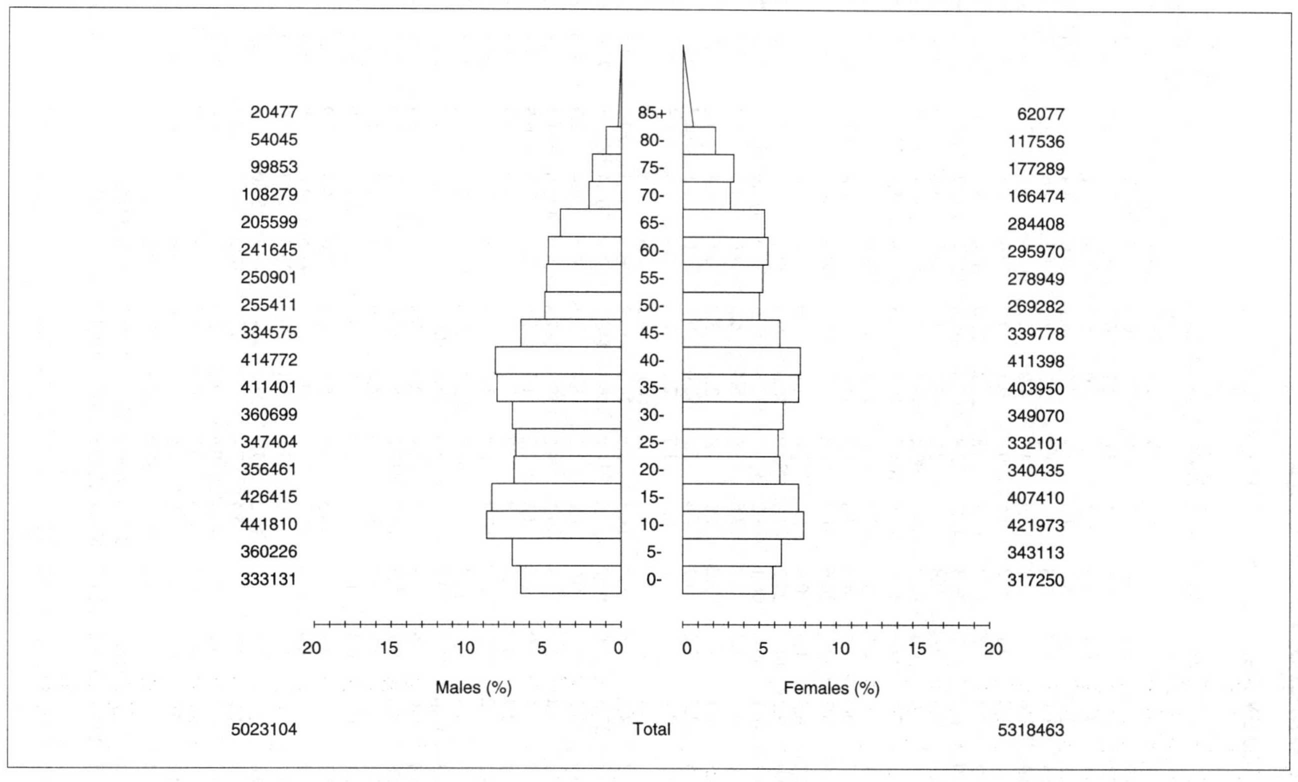

Czech Republic
Source of population:
Census: 1980 Census of population (CSO, Prague, 1982).
1991 Census of population (CSO, Prague, 1994)
Estimate: The Czech Statistical Office (CSO) carries out a population census every 10 years. In the meantime, CSO produces annual balance computations based on registered births, deaths and migration. The population estimates for 1988, 1989 and 1990 are based on the 1 November 1980 Census, and for 1991 and 1992 on the 3 March 1991 Census.

Notes to tables overleaf:
+ The editors were unable to verify these data
† 188 does not include non-invasive tumours

+ CZECH REPUBLIC 1988-1992

ANNUAL INCIDENCE PER 100,000 BY AGE GROUP (YEARS) - MALE

SITE	ALL AGES	AGE UNK	0-	5-	10-	15-	20-	25-	30-	35-	40-	45-	50-	55-	60-	65-	70-	75-	80-	85+	CRUDE RATE	%	CR 64	CR 74	ASR (W)	ICD (9th)
Lip	536	0	-	-	-	-	-	-	0.1	0.1	0.3	1.3	3.0	4.4	7.4	9.3	11.8	17.8	18.9	22.5	2.1	0.5	0.08	0.19	**1.6**	140
Tongue	649	0	-	-	-	0.0	0.1	0.1	0.6	0.9	2.9	6.0	9.4	7.7	6.9	7.5	6.3	5.8	5.2	3.9	2.6	0.7	0.17	0.24	**2.1**	141
Salivary gland	278	0	-	-	0.1	0.0	0.1	0.2	0.2	0.3	0.8	1.1	1.6	2.1	3.6	3.2	6.5	6.6	7.4	11.7	1.1	0.3	0.05	0.10	**0.9**	142
Mouth	669	0	-	-	-	-	-	0.1	0.2	1.5	3.8	6.1	7.5	9.4	7.8	7.0	5.7	5.4	4.1	3.9	2.7	0.7	0.18	0.25	**2.2**	143-5
Oropharynx	647	0	-	-	-	0.0	0.1	-	0.2	1.0	3.8	6.9	8.2	7.5	5.9	7.5	8.5	4.0	4.4	2.9	2.6	0.7	0.17	0.25	**2.1**	146
Nasopharynx	184	0	-	0.1	-	0.2	0.1	0.2	0.1	0.5	1.1	1.4	1.6	1.8	1.7	2.2	2.2	1.2	2.6	2.0	0.7	0.2	0.04	0.07	**0.6**	147
Hypopharynx	326	0	-	-	-	-	-	-	0.1	0.4	1.6	3.6	3.8	3.9	4.1	4.2	2.2	2.4	2.2	2.9	1.3	0.3	0.09	0.12	**1.1**	148
Pharynx unspecified	30	0	-	-	-	-	0.1	-	-	-	0.0	0.1	0.2	0.6	0.4	0.1	0.9	0.4	1.1	1.0	0.1	0.0	0.01	0.01	**0.1**	149
Oesophagus	1324	0	-	-	-	-	0.1	0.1	0.2	0.9	3.3	7.8	11.7	14.7	16.8	20.2	19.0	26.4	28.9	41.0	5.3	1.3	0.28	0.47	**4.2**	150
Stomach	6505	0	-	-	-	-	0.2	1.0	1.7	4.0	6.7	13.7	26.3	44.2	72.8	117.0	165.5	226.7	262.7	286.2	25.9	6.6	0.85	2.27	**19.5**	151
Small intestine	167	0	0.1	-	-	-	-	-	0.1	0.2	0.3	0.6	0.8	1.6	2.5	3.2	3.7	3.8	3.0	1.0	0.7	0.2	0.03	0.07	**0.5**	152
Colon	7936	0	-	0.1	0.0	0.2	0.7	0.8	2.1	3.6	7.9	18.4	31.9	63.7	99.4	153.7	213.2	245.8	263.1	236.4	31.6	8.1	1.14	2.98	**24.0**	153
Rectum	7970	0	-	-	-	0.1	0.3	0.9	1.1	4.1	7.8	22.5	41.6	76.8	101.9	145.5	184.3	234.9	255.7	214.9	31.7	8.1	1.29	2.93	**24.2**	154
Liver	2161	0	0.7	0.2	0.0	0.0	0.1	0.2	0.2	1.3	2.3	4.5	9.3	18.7	32.0	47.4	49.9	58.9	57.4	38.1	8.6	2.2	0.35	0.83	**6.6**	155
Gallbladder etc.	1570	0	-	-	-	-	0.1	0.1	0.1	0.5	0.9	2.3	4.5	9.8	16.7	33.9	41.6	57.9	71.8	59.6	6.3	1.6	0.17	0.55	**4.6**	156
Pancreas	3735	0	-	-	-	0.1	0.1	0.3	0.6	2.6	6.3	12.0	20.6	31.9	51.2	66.9	88.5	100.3	109.5	85.0	14.9	3.8	0.63	1.40	**11.4**	157
Nose, sinuses etc.	156	0	-	-	-	0.0	0.1	0.2	0.1	0.3	0.5	1.0	0.9	1.4	2.0	1.9	2.6	2.6	5.6	2.0	0.6	0.2	0.03	0.05	**0.5**	160
Larynx	2305	0	-	-	-	-	-	0.1	0.4	3.0	9.2	14.2	23.2	29.3	32.9	36.3	29.9	27.8	19.2	18.6	7.4	2.3	0.56	0.89	**7.4**	161
Bronchus, lung	24827	0	0.1	-	0.0	0.1	0.1	0.3	1.6	9.7	31.1	86.8	166.1	288.2	396.9	492.3	511.5	481.9	475.9	426.8	98.9	25.3	4.90	9.92	**77.8**	162
Other thoracic organs	299	0	0.4	-	0.0	0.2	0.3	0.1	0.3	0.2	0.7	1.2	2.2	2.6	3.6	5.4	6.6	4.6	4.8	3.9	1.2	0.3	0.06	0.12	**1.0**	163-4
Bone	291	0	0.3	0.5	1.1	2.0	1.1	0.3	0.3	0.5	1.1	1.1	2.0	1.1	1.4	2.3	3.0	2.6	4.4	6.8	1.2	0.3	0.06	0.09	**1.1**	170
Connective tissue	638	0	1.5	0.3	0.5	0.8	0.8	1.0	1.3	1.5	2.5	2.2	4.1	4.4	5.3	8.6	9.4	12.0	8.1	10.7	2.5	0.7	0.13	0.22	**2.2**	171
Mesothelioma	126	0	-	-	-	0.0	-	0.1	0.1	0.3	0.1	0.8	1.0	0.8	1.7	2.1	2.4	2.8	1.9	4.9	0.5	0.1	0.02	0.05	**0.4**	MES
Kaposi's sarcoma	28	0	-	-	-	-	-	0.1	0.1	0.1	-	0.1	-	0.4	0.2	0.6	0.2	1.0	0.4	2.0	0.1	0.0	0.00	0.01	**0.1**	KAP
Melanoma of skin	2057	0	0.1	0.1	0.2	0.6	1.4	1.6	3.7	4.7	8.1	11.4	14.3	18.3	22.8	29.2	30.8	36.7	37.4	20.5	8.2	2.1	0.44	0.74	**6.5**	172
Other skin	18476	0	-	-	0.2	0.3	0.7	2.4	5.3	11.9	23.3	48.5	80.2	136.5	211.0	316.1	448.3	613.1	706.4	825.3	73.6		2.60	6.42	**55.8**	173
Breast	157	0	-	-	-	0.0	0.1	-	-	0.1	0.2	0.4	0.9	1.4	1.7	3.4	3.1	4.6	4.4	2.9	0.6	0.2	0.02	0.06	**0.5**	175
Prostate	8481	0	0.1	-	-	-	0.1	0.1	-	0.1	0.4	2.7	8.5	30.7	76.8	158.3	287.8	425.0	472.6	404.4	33.8	8.6	0.60	2.83	**24.1**	185
Testis	1420	0	0.4	0.2	0.2	3.2	9.0	16.9	14.9	12.7	8.4	3.9	1.6	2.1	1.3	1.7	1.5	2.2	3.3	6.8	5.7	1.4	0.37	0.39	**5.2**	186
Penis	229	0	-	-	0.0	-	-	-	0.1	0.4	0.4	0.5	1.4	1.3	2.7	3.9	4.1	8.4	8.9	4.9	0.9	0.2	0.03	0.07	**0.7**	187.1-.4
Other male genital	71	0	0.1	0.1	-	-	0.1	0.1	0.1	0.2	0.2	0.2	0.3	0.8	0.4	1.0	1.8	1.8	1.9	-	0.3	0.1	0.01	0.03	**0.2**	187.5-.9
†Bladder	5093	0	0.1	-	-	-	0.1	0.3	0.5	2.4	3.8	9.1	22.2	41.0	68.5	102.4	133.5	154.0	172.1	158.2	20.3	5.2	0.74	1.92	**15.4**	188
Kidney etc.	5310	0	2.5	0.2	0.1	0.4	0.2	0.5	1.2	4.3	10.6	21.5	39.7	57.2	73.3	97.6	109.0	98.3	104.0	73.3	21.1	5.4	1.06	2.09	**16.9**	189
Eye	218	0	0.6	0.1	-	-	0.2	0.2	0.1	0.4	0.6	0.6	1.6	2.1	2.9	3.5	3.9	3.2	3.7	2.9	0.9	0.2	0.05	0.08	**0.7**	190
Brain, nervous system	1396	0	2.7	2.6	1.9	2.2	2.0	2.9	3.3	3.8	5.6	8.7	9.3	14.6	12.8	15.3	12.0	8.4	3.7	1.0	5.6	1.4	0.36	0.50	**5.0**	191-2
Thyroid	389	0	-	-	0.2	0.4	0.7	0.4	0.7	0.7	2.3	2.5	2.7	3.1	4.0	4.0	3.9	6.4	7.4	4.9	1.5	0.4	0.09	0.13	**1.3**	193
Other endocrine	137	0	0.8	0.1	0.0	0.2	0.2	0.2	0.1	0.1	0.1	0.3	1.2	1.0	1.4	2.0	3.1	2.0	1.5	1.0	0.5	0.1	0.03	0.05	**0.5**	194
Hodgkin's disease	835	0	0.8	0.8	1.2	4.1	4.8	3.1	3.1	3.1	2.6	3.1	4.4	4.3	6.0	5.5	6.8	6.4	6.3	2.9	3.3	0.9	0.21	0.27	**3.0**	201
Non-Hodgkin lymphoma	2122	0	1.6	1.8	2.2	1.9	2.2	1.7	2.4	3.8	5.4	8.4	10.6	16.7	23.3	30.5	38.4	41.5	44.0	51.8	8.4	2.2	0.41	0.76	**7.0**	200,202
Multiple myeloma	845	0	-	-	-	0.0	-	0.1	0.1	0.4	1.4	1.8	4.6	8.0	11.5	16.1	20.1	25.4	20.7	18.6	3.4	0.9	0.14	0.32	**2.6**	203
Lymphoid leukaemia	1587	0	5.5	2.6	2.0	1.3	0.6	0.6	0.5	0.8	1.5	3.5	5.6	10.2	17.3	23.2	34.9	43.7	50.0	50.8	6.3	1.6	0.26	0.55	**5.4**	204
Myeloid leukaemia	920	0	0.6	0.7	0.7	0.9	1.7	1.6	2.2	2.2	1.9	3.5	3.8	6.4	7.4	14.7	15.9	18.6	19.2	20.5	3.7	0.9	0.17	0.32	**3.0**	205
Monocytic leukaemia	55	0	0.1	0.1	0.1	-	0.1	-	-	0.0	0.1	0.1	0.1	0.4	0.4	0.5	2.0	1.4	3.0	1.0	0.2	0.1	0.01	0.02	**0.2**	206
Other leukaemia	57	0	0.1	-	-	0.0	0.1	-	-	0.1	0.0	0.2	0.4	0.3	0.7	0.6	1.7	1.8	1.5	2.0	0.2	0.1	0.01	0.02	**0.2**	207
Leukaemia unspecified	161	0	0.2	0.3	0.1	0.2	0.2	0.2	0.2	0.2	0.2	0.2	0.2	0.9	1.0	1.5	2.2	2.0	5.6	4.8	6.8	0.6	0.2	0.03	0.05	**0.5**	208
Other and unspecified	3215	0	1.1	0.2	0.1	0.4	0.3	0.7	1.1	2.4	5.3	9.8	16.0	26.5	37.8	53.3	67.2	90.5	120.3	134.8	12.8	3.3	0.51	1.11	**9.9**	O&U
All sites	116588	0	20.4	10.9	11.2	20.3	29.0	39.3	50.8	92.8	177.7	356.7	611.6	1010.6	1460.7	2063.3	2607.3	3133.0	3415.3	3283.7	464.2		19.46	42.81	**360.8**	ALL
All sites but 173	98112	0	20.4	10.9	11.0	20.0	28.3	36.8	45.5	80.8	154.4	308.2	531.5	874.1	1249.8	1747.3	2159.1	2519.9	2708.9	2458.4	390.6	100.0	16.86	36.39	**305.0**	ALLb

Rate from 10 cases   0.600   0.555   0.453   0.469   0.561   0.576   0.554   0.486   0.482   0.598   0.783   0.797   0.828   0.973   1.847   2.003   3.701   9.767

†Important: see notes on population page

+ CZECH REPUBLIC 1988-1992

ANNUAL INCIDENCE PER 100,000 BY AGE GROUP (YEARS) - FEMALE

SITE	ALL AGES	AGE UNK	0-	5-	10-	15-	20-	25-	30-	35-	40-	45-	50-	55-	60-	65-	70-	75-	80-	85+	CRUDE RATE	%	CR 64	CR 74	ASR (W)	ICD (9th)
Lip	189	0	-	-	-	-	-	-	-	-	0.1	0.3	0.5	0.6	0.7	1.9	2.0	5.1	6.6	9.0	0.7	0.2	0.01	0.03	**0.3**	*140*
Tongue	156	0	-	-	-	-	-	-	0.1	0.3	0.4	0.8	1.0	0.9	1.5	1.4	1.3	2.1	3.4	2.6	0.6	0.2	0.02	0.04	**0.4**	*141*
Salivary gland	225	0	0.1	0.1	-	0.1	0.4	0.1	0.5	0.2	0.4	0.6	1.0	1.0	1.2	2.0	2.6	4.5	3.4	7.7	0.8	0.2	0.03	0.05	**0.5**	*142*
Mouth	167	0	-	-	-	-	-	0.1	0.1	0.1	0.4	0.9	0.9	0.9	1.4	1.4	2.3	2.9	2.7	3.5	0.6	0.2	0.02	0.04	**0.4**	*143-5*
Oropharynx	113	0	-	-	-	-	0.1	-	0.1	0.1	0.3	0.2	0.7	1.1	1.2	1.0	1.6	1.8	1.7	0.6	0.4	0.1	0.02	0.03	**0.3**	*146*
Nasopharynx	79	0	-	0.1	0.1	0.0	0.1	0.1	0.3	0.2	0.1	0.5	0.9	0.6	0.5	0.2	0.8	0.8	0.3	1.3	0.3	0.1	0.02	0.02	**0.2**	*147*
Hypopharynx	36	0	-	-	-	-	-	-	-	0.0	0.1	0.5	0.4	0.4	0.4	0.7	-	0.3	0.3	0.1	0.0	0.01	0.01	**0.1**	*148*
Pharynx unspecified	8	0	-	-	-	-	-	-	-	-	0.1	-	-	-	-	-	0.1	0.2	-	-	0.6	0.0	0.0	0.00	0.00	**0.0**	*149*
Oesophagus	271	0	-	-	-	-	-	-	-	0.0	0.2	0.6	0.9	0.9	1.9	2.5	4.6	5.9	8.5	8.7	1.0	0.3	0.02	0.06	**0.5**	*150*
Stomach	4890	0	-	-	-	0.0	0.2	0.5	1.4	3.2	5.1	7.7	11.1	16.1	29.9	48.5	76.9	113.5	154.0	160.1	18.4	5.4	0.38	1.00	**9.2**	*151*
Small intestine	134	0	-	-	0.0	0.1	0.1	-	0.1	0.2	0.2	0.4	0.4	0.5	0.8	0.8	3.6	2.5	2.6	2.6	0.5	0.1	0.01	0.04	**0.3**	*152*
Colon	7685	0	-	0.1	0.2	0.5	0.6	0.9	1.8	4.1	8.5	15.1	23.4	41.0	61.0	85.4	127.1	161.5	180.2	176.2	28.9	8.5	0.79	1.85	**15.7**	*153*
Rectum	5602	0	-	-	-	0.1	0.2	0.5	1.4	3.2	6.3	11.8	18.3	34.4	45.9	65.4	84.0	113.3	131.9	114.1	21.1	6.2	0.61	1.36	**11.6**	*154*
Liver	1317	0	0.6	-	-	0.2	0.2	0.3	0.2	0.7	1.0	1.8	3.6	6.7	9.3	17.6	22.2	27.0	30.3	30.3	5.0	1.5	0.12	0.32	**2.7**	*155*
Gallbladder etc.	3691	0	-	-	-	-	-	0.1	0.2	0.5	1.4	4.4	8.5	16.7	29.1	46.8	57.2	81.6	103.8	103.4	13.9	4.1	0.30	0.82	**7.1**	*156*
Pancreas	3257	0	0.1	-	-	0.0	0.2	0.3	0.5	1.0	2.5	5.0	10.2	16.2	24.8	41.0	48.3	69.3	84.6	82.2	12.2	3.6	0.30	0.75	**6.5**	*157*
Nose, sinuses etc.	114	0	-	0.1	0.0	-	0.1	-	0.1	0.1	0.3	0.2	0.4	0.8	0.9	1.1	1.1	1.1	3.2	3.9	0.4	0.1	0.02	0.03	**0.3**	*160*
Larynx	168	0	-	-	-	-	-	-	0.2	0.1	0.5	0.8	0.7	1.5	1.4	2.0	2.8	1.6	2.2	2.6	0.6	0.2	0.03	0.05	**0.4**	*161*
Bronchus, lung	4469	0	-	-	-	-	0.1	0.2	0.5	2.6	6.9	13.8	22.1	33.3	47.6	54.8	65.0	69.0	73.2	63.5	16.8	4.9	0.64	1.23	**10.1**	*162*
Other thoracic organs	196	0	0.2	0.1	0.2	0.2	0.1	0.1	0.2	0.1	0.3	0.6	1.2	1.5	1.5	1.4	3.1	2.7	3.4	3.2	0.7	0.2	0.03	0.05	**0.5**	*163-4*
Bone	233	0	0.2	0.6	1.1	1.3	0.6	0.4	0.3	0.3	0.8	0.5	0.4	1.2	1.0	1.4	1.7	2.0	3.1	2.3	0.9	0.3	0.04	0.06	**0.7**	*170*
Connective tissue	611	0	0.9	0.5	0.8	0.3	1.0	0.9	0.9	1.2	1.8	2.1	3.3	3.4	4.1	4.9	7.6	7.3	7.1	9.7	2.3	0.7	0.11	0.17	**1.7**	*171*
Mesothelioma	109	0	-	-	-	-	0.1	0.1	0.1	0.0	0.3	0.5	0.8	0.9	0.8	1.2	1.3	0.8	1.4	2.6	0.4	0.1	0.02	0.03	**0.3**	*MES*
Kaposi's sarcoma	15	0	-	-	-	-	-	-	-	-	-	0.1	-	0.1	-	0.4	0.1	0.1	0.3	0.3	0.1	0.0	0.00	0.00	**0.0**	*KAP*
Melanoma of skin	2284	0	0.1	0.2	0.4	1.2	1.8	3.1	4.9	8.3	10.8	11.6	15.2	14.2	16.8	20.6	19.6	21.0	21.3	23.8	8.6	2.5	0.44	0.64	**6.1**	*172*
Other skin	17660	0	0.1	0.1	0.2	0.7	1.3	3.0	7.4	14.7	26.3	43.1	62.6	87.5	123.9	190.6	271.8	352.9	408.9	473.0	66.4		1.85	4.17	**36.6**	*173*
Breast	18156	0	-	-	-	0.1	0.4	3.4	15.6	32.9	65.2	108.5	115.2	137.8	163.1	179.4	194.3	212.3	224.6	229.1	68.3	20.1	3.21	5.08	**45.1**	*174*
Uterus unspecified	65	0	-	-	-	-	-	-	0.1	0.0	-	0.2	0.2	0.3	0.3	0.7	0.5	1.5	2.7	1.6	0.2	0.1	0.01	0.01	**0.1**	*179*
Cervix uteri	5705	0	0.1	-	-	0.1	2.6	14.0	26.9	35.5	39.4	39.1	29.3	30.5	37.3	37.9	33.8	34.9	30.6	25.8	21.5	6.3	1.27	1.63	**16.4**	*180*
Placenta	33	0	-	-	-	0.1	0.7	0.4	0.2	0.0	0.1	0.1	0.1	0.1	-	0.1	-	-	-	-	0.1	0.0	0.01	0.01	**0.1**	*181*
Corpus uteri	7096	0	-	-	-	-	0.3	0.4	1.3	4.6	10.9	29.7	53.0	69.3	87.0	91.1	92.6	74.7	66.2	50.6	26.7	7.8	1.28	2.20	**17.7**	*182*
Ovary etc.	5082	0	0.1	0.3	0.9	1.3	1.4	3.2	5.3	9.7	17.6	30.0	35.8	42.3	47.5	51.6	53.5	49.3	47.1	40.3	19.1	5.6	0.98	1.50	**13.3**	*183*
Other female genital	1103	0	-	-	-	-	0.1	-	0.6	0.8	1.6	2.4	2.7	4.4	8.3	10.9	14.9	23.6	31.0	35.8	4.1	1.2	0.10	0.23	**2.2**	*184*
†Bladder	1565	0	0.1	-	0.0	-	0.1	0.2	0.2	0.6	1.4	2.9	4.9	8.9	13.2	17.4	25.7	29.7	39.1	40.6	5.9	1.7	0.16	0.38	**3.2**	*188*
Kidney etc.	3516	0	2.3	0.7	0.1	0.0	0.2	0.4	0.9	2.2	4.3	12.9	19.2	28.5	37.8	46.1	47.2	51.8	41.5	38.3	13.2	3.9	0.55	1.01	**8.5**	*189*
Eye	210	0	0.7	0.1	0.0	0.0	-	0.1	0.3	0.3	0.7	0.8	1.4	1.4	1.9	1.8	2.3	2.6	2.6	1.9	0.8	0.2	0.04	0.06	**0.6**	*190*
Brain, nervous system	1220	0	2.2	2.2	1.9	1.5	1.5	2.2	2.6	3.0	4.3	6.2	7.5	8.7	12.7	10.1	8.5	6.8	4.3	1.9	4.6	1.3	0.28	0.38	**3.8**	*191-2*
Thyroid	1115	0	-	0.1	0.4	1.0	1.6	3.0	3.4	3.8	4.7	5.9	6.1	6.0	6.1	8.2	8.0	12.7	13.4	13.5	4.2	1.2	0.21	0.29	**3.0**	*193*
Other endocrine	121	0	0.8	-	0.1	0.0	0.1	0.1	0.1	0.4	0.6	0.3	0.9	0.5	0.8	1.0	1.8	0.5	1.5	1.0	0.5	0.1	0.02	0.04	**0.4**	*194*
Hodgkin's disease	726	0	0.1	0.3	1.4	5.1	6.0	2.9	2.5	2.4	1.8	1.7	1.9	1.7	2.7	3.7	4.3	6.1	5.6	4.2	2.7	0.8	0.15	0.19	**2.4**	*201*
Non-Hodgkin lymphoma	1887	0	0.9	0.5	0.6	0.9	0.8	1.2	1.8	1.9	4.1	5.8	7.6	9.7	15.1	20.8	25.9	31.2	32.8	34.2	7.1	2.1	0.25	0.49	**4.4**	*200,202*
Multiple myeloma	926	0	-	-	-	0.0	-	0.1	-	0.4	0.8	1.5	3.9	5.5	8.9	12.6	15.3	18.2	16.8	15.5	3.5	1.0	0.11	0.24	**2.0**	*203*
Lymphoid leukaemia	1093	0	4.6	2.1	1.6	0.7	0.6	0.4	0.2	0.9	0.6	1.2	2.0	4.4	6.8	10.5	13.0	20.8	24.2	29.6	4.1	1.2	0.13	0.25	**2.8**	*204*
Myeloid leukaemia	928	0	0.6	0.6	0.9	0.7	0.8	1.0	1.3	2.0	2.6	3.1	4.0	5.4	7.7	8.9	10.3	13.2	11.4	11.9	3.5	1.0	0.15	0.25	**2.4**	*205*
Monocytic leukaemia	42	0	0.1	-	0.1	-	0.1	-	0.1	0.1	0.1	0.1	0.2	-	0.2	0.4	0.2	0.6	1.4	1.3	0.2	0.0	0.01	0.01	**0.1**	*206*
Other leukaemia	44	0	0.1	0.1	0.0	-	0.1	-	0.1	0.0	-	0.3	0.4	0.3	0.3	0.2	1.0	0.3	1.9	0.2	0.0	0.01	0.01	**0.1**	*207*
Leukaemia unspecified	134	0	0.2	0.1	0.0	0.2	0.2	0.1	0.1	-	0.3	0.4	0.4	0.5	0.3	1.3	1.8	3.0	2.9	3.5	0.5	0.1	0.01	0.03	**0.3**	*208*
Other and unspecified	3665	0	0.8	0.2	0.0	0.0	0.5	0.7	1.1	1.6	3.6	7.6	8.5	16.0	24.9	36.4	51.2	78.5	104.5	132.1	13.8	4.1	0.33	0.77	**7.2**	*O&U*
All sites	108111	0	15.6	8.7	11.3	16.9	24.8	44.3	85.9	144.9	239.9	384.2	494.2	664.7	890.4	1146.2	1414.9	1723.1	1943.1	2002.7	406.5		15.13	27.93	**248.7**	*ALL*
All sites but 173	90451	0	15.5	8.7	11.1	16.2	23.5	41.3	78.6	130.2	213.6	341.0	431.6	577.2	766.6	955.5	1143.1	1370.2	1534.2	1529.7	340.1	100.0	13.28	23.77	**212.0**	*ALLb*
Rate from 10 cases			0.630	0.583	0.474	0.491	0.587	0.602	0.573	0.495	0.486	0.589	0.743	0.717	0.676	0.703	1.201	1.128	1.702	3.222						

†Important: see notes on population page

461

Denmark

The Danish Cancer Registry was founded in May 1942 as a nationwide programme to register all cancer cases in the population, excluding that of the Faroe Islands. Incidence figures are available from 1 January 1943. Data from Greenland with its Inuit population are not included in the present tabulations. The registry was, until January 1997, administratively part of the Danish Cancer Society, which received financial support for the registry from the National Board of Health. From January 1997, the registry has been the responsibility of the National Board of Health. The registry operates under the "Law on Public Authorities, Registers" with instructions established by the Minister of Health, and supervised by the National Data Protection Board.

The Kingdom of Denmark (excluding Greenland and the Faroe Islands) covers 43 080 km² between latitudes 55 and 58° N, and longitudes 8 and 12°30′ E. The population on 1 January 1986 was 5 100 000; it is of Caucasian stock and fairly homogeneous. Approximately 27% of the population live in the Greater Copenhagen area, 38% live in provincial towns of 10 000 to about 200 000 inhabitants, and 35% live in rural areas.

The medical care system is organized into a private sector of general practitioners and specialists under contract with the National Health Insurance, and a public sector operating hospitals under the authority of the counties and communities or the Danish States. Health care is provided free to all inhabitants. In 1990 there were approximately six hospital beds and two physicians per 1000 inhabitants.

Cancer surgery is carried out both at general hospitals and at oncological centres. The hospital departments are serviced by 28 institutes of pathology. Non-surgical cancer treatment is partially centralized at five regional radiotherapy and oncological centres. Almost the entire population is capable of reaching a regional cancer centre within a few hours by ground transport.

Medical certification of death by medical doctors is compulsory. Computerized medical information systems on hospital discharges have been operating nationally since 1977; registration of histopathological diagnoses covers, for the period of this volume, only part of the population.

Reporting of cancer is mandatory by administrative order from the National Board of Health. Legally, the responsibility for reporting to the registry lies with the head of clinical hospital departments, the head of pathology departments performing autopsies and a practising physician undertaking treatment or follow-up without referring the patient to hospital.

The registry is tumour-based, and with the exception of multiple cancers of the skin and cancer in paired organs with similar morphological characteristics, tumours are the units counted. All malignant neoplasms including carcinomas, sarcomas, leukaemias and lymphomas as well as all brain and central nervous system tumours and all bladder tumours irrespective of behaviour must be reported. Precancerous lesions of the cervix uteri are reportable but not included in tabulations.

The entire registry database is cross-checked annually by computerized record linkage with all deaths that occur in the country. Follow-back is accomplished by mailed enquiries to the certifying physician or hospital concerning cancer cases from death certificates not known to the registry. Less than 2% remain as death-certificate-only cases. Since 1987, cases are also captured from the patient discharge registry but only included if confirmed.

Assessments by linkage to patient discharge registers, pathology registers and patient series registry have shown that the completeness of the registry is 95–97%.

Since 1968 all inhabitants have been identified by a unique personal identifying number, used in most registration systems, including the cancer registry. A central computerized population register keeps a continuously updated file of personal information on all inhabitants. Reported cases of cancer are linked to the Central Population Registry using the personal identification number, the identity is checked and information corresponding to the date of diagnosis is transferred to the registry file.

Upon receipt at the registry, notifications are checked and coded. Medical coding is carried out by physicians and trained medical coding staff. Duplicate registrations are readily picked up with the help of the personal ID number. The entire coding process is supported by computer checks of consistency between variables (sex, codes, procedures, etc.), warning programmes and manual check procedures. New tumour cases are then included in the registry's computerized database and additions or corrections are made to previously notified cases. If the information received is incomplete or contradictory, an inquiry is made to the notifying clinician.

All data up to 1977 were classified according to a modified version of ICD-7 expanded to include certain information on histology and tumour behaviour. All cases diagnosed since 1978 have been classified according to the ICD-O as well as the modified ICD-7.

The registry produces morbidity statistics in relation to variation over time, geographical location, occupation and other factors. Since 1978, incidence data have been published for each year separately. These annually published data include non-invasive brain tumours, which is not the case in this volume.

The registry is used extensively as an end-point in cohort studies of environmental factors and medical procedures in relation to cancer risk. It conducts epidemiological research especially with a view to causes of cancer, and preventive measures taken.

Hans H. Storm

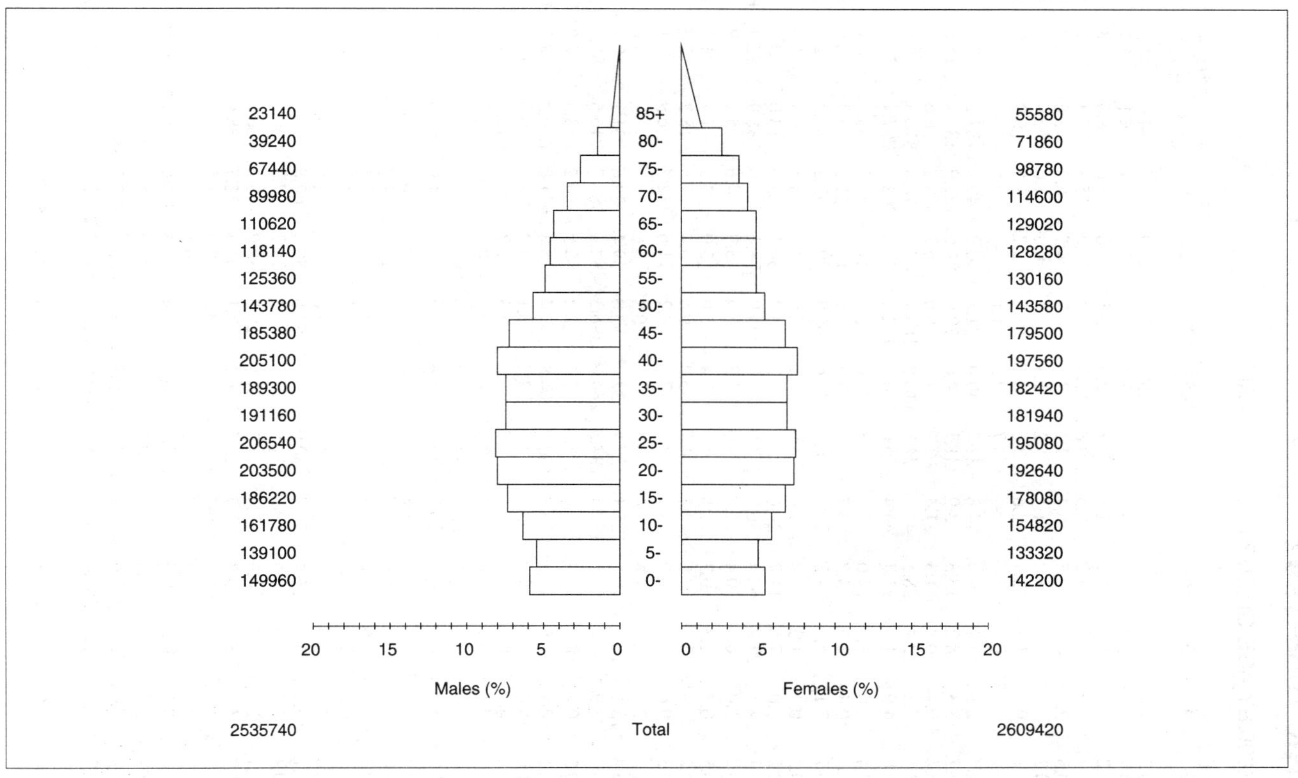

Denmark
Source of population: average annual 1988–92
Census: The population is monitored constantly by the Central Population Registry. For each year, the mean between the population on 1 January and on 31 December has been used.
Screening programmes in the area:
The population between ages 23 and 59 is screened every three years for cervical cancer. Women aged 50-69 in two areas of the country have been screened for breast cancer every other year since 1992. A trial of screening for large bowel cancer was conducted in Funen in 1990.

DENMARK 1988-1992

ANNUAL INCIDENCE PER 100,000 BY AGE GROUP (YEARS) - MALE

SITE	ALL AGES	AGE UNK	0-	5-	10-	15-	20-	25-	30-	35-	40-	45-	50-	55-	60-	65-	70-	75-	80-	85+	CRUDE RATE	%	CR 64	CR 74	ASR (W)	ICD (9th)
Lip	551	0	-	-	-	-	-	-	0.1	0.2	1.0	3.1	4.6	7.5	13.5	15.9	18.2	24.0	29.6	34.6	4.3	1.0	0.15	0.32	2.7	140
Tongue	217	0	-	-	-	-	-	0.1	0.2	0.7	1.2	2.2	2.6	5.4	4.2	7.1	5.8	5.0	4.1	6.1	1.7	0.4	0.08	0.15	1.2	141
Salivary gland	105	0	-	-	0.1	0.1	-	0.1	0.2	0.2	0.6	1.2	1.1	1.3	1.7	2.5	3.1	3.0	3.6	8.6	0.8	0.2	0.03	0.06	0.6	142
Mouth	467	0	-	-	0.1	0.1	0.1	-	0.1	0.7	2.9	4.7	8.2	8.3	9.8	12.1	11.3	13.0	15.8	17.3	3.7	0.8	0.18	0.29	2.6	143-5
Oropharynx	294	0	-	-	-	-	-	-	-	0.5	2.1	4.0	6.5	6.4	7.1	7.1	6.7	4.7	6.6	2.6	2.3	0.5	0.13	0.20	1.7	146
Nasopharynx	57	0	-	-	-	0.1	0.2	0.1	-	0.2	-	0.8	1.0	1.1	1.2	1.4	2.4	0.3	1.0	0.9	0.4	0.1	0.02	0.04	0.3	147
Hypopharynx	122	0	-	-	-	-	-	-	-	-	0.5	1.8	2.4	2.6	3.6	3.4	3.1	2.7	1.5	0.9	1.0	0.2	0.05	0.09	0.7	148
Pharynx unspecified	14	0	-	-	-	-	-	-	-	-	-	0.1	-	-	0.7	0.5	1.1	-	0.5	-	0.1	0.0	0.00	0.01	0.1	149
Oesophagus	955	0	-	-	-	-	-	-	0.1	0.4	2.3	5.1	9.5	14.8	22.7	30.0	31.1	40.9	49.4	37.2	7.5	1.7	0.27	0.58	4.8	150
Stomach	1898	0	-	-	-	0.1	0.2	0.6	0.4	1.7	3.3	8.2	13.5	23.9	31.7	54.6	70.0	91.6	125.9	131.4	15.0	3.5	0.42	1.04	9.0	151
Small intestine	149	0	-	-	-	-	-	-	-	0.4	0.4	0.8	1.3	1.4	2.7	4.7	6.0	6.2	8.2	8.6	1.2	0.3	0.03	0.09	0.7	152
Colon	4439	0	-	-	0.1	0.1	0.1	0.8	2.4	3.1	7.2	12.4	28.1	47.7	74.3	116.8	188.7	248.8	278.8	316.3	35.0	8.1	0.88	2.41	20.6	153
Rectum	3550	0	-	-	-	-	-	0.3	1.2	1.9	4.9	11.1	21.7	44.4	76.0	110.3	142.5	176.2	202.3	207.4	28.0	6.5	0.81	2.07	17.0	154
Liver	769	0	0.4	0.1	-	0.1	0.1	0.1	0.3	0.4	1.0	1.8	4.0	7.8	19.3	24.0	30.0	41.8	44.9	33.7	6.1	1.4	0.18	0.45	3.7	155
Gallbladder etc.	379	0	-	-	-	-	-	-	0.3	-	0.4	1.5	3.2	3.7	7.1	9.6	14.9	17.2	31.6	25.9	3.0	0.7	0.08	0.20	1.8	156
Pancreas	1625	0	-	0.1	-	-	0.1	0.3	0.5	0.7	3.1	5.3	9.3	20.1	36.2	48.6	66.9	80.7	92.3	83.8	12.8	3.0	0.38	0.96	7.8	157
Nose, sinuses etc.	160	0	-	-	-	-	-	0.1	0.1	0.3	0.4	1.3	1.8	2.6	3.0	6.1	6.0	4.4	4.1	6.9	1.3	0.3	0.05	0.11	0.9	160
Larynx	1024	0	-	-	-	0.1	-	-	0.2	0.5	3.0	7.6	11.7	20.6	28.8	34.2	33.8	37.1	26.0	13.0	8.1	1.9	0.36	0.70	5.5	161
Bronchus, lung	10445	0	-	-	-	0.2	0.2	0.6	1.0	3.7	14.1	27.8	68.4	156.8	247.8	387.3	473.9	478.1	423.0	286.9	82.4	19.0	2.60	6.91	51.9	162
Other thoracic organs	117	0	0.1	-	0.1	-	0.1	0.5	0.2	0.2	1.0	0.4	0.4	1.8	3.6	2.7	2.9	3.9	4.6	5.2	0.9	0.2	0.04	0.07	0.6	163-4
Bone	138	0	0.1	0.9	0.6	1.9	1.3	0.8	0.5	0.5	0.8	1.3	0.7	1.8	1.0	1.4	2.0	3.0	3.1	1.7	1.1	0.3	0.06	0.08	1.0	170
Connective tissue	341	0	0.9	0.7	0.7	1.2	1.0	1.1	1.3	2.2	1.9	2.2	3.1	4.1	4.7	5.2	9.6	10.4	7.6	18.2	2.7	0.6	0.13	0.20	2.1	171
Mesothelioma	267	0	-	-	0.1	-	0.1	-	0.1	0.3	0.6	1.1	3.9	4.1	7.1	7.2	8.2	11.6	12.7	6.9	2.1	0.5	0.09	0.16	1.4	MES
Kaposi's sarcoma	126	0	-	-	-	-	0.1	1.9	2.4	1.3	2.4	2.4	1.8	1.0	0.2	-	0.2	0.6	-	-	1.0	0.2	0.07	0.07	0.8	KAP
Melanoma of skin	1537	0	-	-	0.4	1.1	2.0	4.9	5.3	9.4	15.1	18.7	19.3	21.1	26.4	32.4	32.0	39.4	33.6	31.1	12.1	2.8	0.62	0.94	8.8	172
Other skin	10805	0	-	0.1	0.2	0.3	1.6	4.4	9.3	16.1	32.9	59.0	93.6	132.1	194.3	284.0	396.3	482.8	587.7	716.5	85.2		2.72	6.12	53.1	173
Breast	100	0	-	-	-	-	-	-	0.1	0.2	0.2	0.3	1.4	1.9	2.0	2.4	2.2	3.9	9.2	3.5	0.8	0.2	0.03	0.05	0.5	175
Prostate	7392	0	-	-	-	-	-	0.1	-	0.1	0.1	1.8	12.1	35.3	100.4	204.8	357.4	516.3	631.0	649.1	58.3	13.5	0.75	3.56	31.0	185
Testis	1338	0	1.1	-	0.1	5.4	14.5	25.4	27.1	21.6	15.0	9.3	9.0	5.4	2.5	2.2	3.1	3.0	4.1	6.9	10.6	2.4	0.68	0.71	9.2	186
Penis	177	0	-	-	-	-	-	0.2	-	0.2	0.6	0.9	1.7	2.1	3.7	5.2	5.3	7.7	10.7	10.4	1.4	0.3	0.05	0.10	0.9	187.1-.4
Other male genital	12	0	-	-	-	-	-	-	-	-	0.1	0.1	0.1	0.2	0.3	-	0.2	0.9	-	1.7	0.1	0.0	0.00	0.01	0.1	187.5-.9
Bladder	5822	0	0.1	-	-	0.1	0.4	0.8	1.3	3.5	9.0	15.3	32.7	68.6	123.8	195.8	242.9	298.9	311.4	292.1	45.9	10.6	1.28	3.47	27.9	188
Kidney etc.	1761	0	1.1	0.1	-	-	0.2	0.3	1.6	1.8	5.7	10.4	13.6	26.0	35.9	52.4	65.6	80.1	81.0	64.0	13.9	3.2	0.48	1.07	8.9	189
Eye	161	0	2.3	0.1	0.1	-	0.3	-	0.1	0.3	1.2	1.0	1.9	1.8	2.7	3.3	4.4	5.3	6.1	4.3	1.3	0.3	0.06	0.10	1.0	190
Brain, nervous system	1037	0	3.2	4.2	2.5	2.0	2.4	4.3	5.4	6.0	7.5	10.2	11.0	14.7	20.8	24.8	17.3	17.8	11.7	3.5	8.2	1.9	0.47	0.68	6.8	191-2
Thyroid	142	0	-	-	0.2	0.3	0.4	0.8	0.3	0.4	1.1	1.6	1.0	1.4	3.6	2.7	2.4	3.9	4.1	6.9	1.1	0.3	0.06	0.08	0.8	193
Other endocrine	45	0	0.8	0.4	0.4	0.4	0.1	0.1	0.2	-	0.2	0.1	0.4	0.5	0.8	0.4	1.1	0.3	1.0	0.9	0.4	0.1	0.02	0.03	0.4	194
Hodgkin's disease	429	0	0.4	0.3	1.0	3.1	3.7	4.7	4.7	3.4	4.5	3.0	3.2	3.8	4.6	4.2	3.6	6.8	4.6	3.5	3.4	0.8	0.20	0.24	2.9	201
Non-Hodgkin lymphoma	1806	0	0.4	1.6	1.5	2.1	2.2	2.9	5.1	7.1	10.4	15.0	16.4	21.7	30.0	42.8	57.6	59.6	67.8	73.5	14.2	3.3	0.58	1.08	9.8	200,202
Multiple myeloma	655	0	-	-	-	-	-	-	0.5	0.7	1.2	2.0	6.5	9.7	11.0	17.7	27.1	29.7	37.2	39.8	5.2	1.2	0.16	0.38	3.2	203
Lymphoid leukaemia	877	0	7.3	4.0	1.4	0.9	0.9	0.2	0.6	0.7	1.1	2.8	4.9	9.4	11.7	24.6	28.5	38.0	45.4	60.5	6.9	1.6	0.23	0.49	5.2	204
Myeloid leukaemia	768	0	1.2	0.4	0.6	1.1	1.3	1.1	1.7	1.9	3.0	3.1	5.3	9.7	13.5	18.1	27.1	31.4	36.7	38.0	6.1	1.4	0.22	0.45	4.1	205
Monocytic leukaemia	13	0	0.1	-	-	-	0.1	-	-	-	-	-	-	0.2	-	0.4	0.2	0.9	1.5	0.9	0.1	0.0	0.00	0.01	0.1	206
Other leukaemia	8	0	-	-	-	-	-	-	0.1	-	-	-	-	0.2	0.3	0.4	0.2	0.3	-	-	0.1	0.0	0.00	0.01	0.0	207
Leukaemia unspecified	54	0	-	-	0.1	0.1	-	-	0.1	-	0.1	0.2	0.4	0.2	0.8	0.5	2.4	2.4	5.6	5.2	0.4	0.1	0.01	0.03	0.2	208
Other and unspecified	2601	0	0.9	0.3	-	0.2	0.9	1.2	1.6	2.4	4.7	8.6	15.6	27.3	50.4	77.9	93.6	121.6	165.1	204.0	20.5	4.7	0.57	1.43	12.5	O&U
All sites	65749	0	20.5	13.5	10.5	21.3	34.4	58.5	76.9	96.2	168.6	271.7	459.0	782.2	1247.8	1889.9	2509.2	3056.1	3432.7	3470.2	518.6		16.31	38.30	327.0	ALL
All sites but 173	54944	0	20.5	13.4	10.3	20.9	32.8	54.1	67.6	80.2	135.7	212.6	365.4	650.1	1053.5	1605.9	2112.9	2573.3	2845.1	2753.7	433.4	100.0	13.59	32.18	273.9	ALLb

| Rate from 10 cases | | | 1.334 | 1.438 | 1.236 | 1.074 | 0.983 | 0.968 | 1.046 | 1.057 | 0.975 | 1.079 | 1.391 | 1.595 | 1.693 | 1.808 | 2.223 | 2.966 | 5.097 | 8.643 | | | | | | |

DENMARK 1988-1992

ANNUAL INCIDENCE PER 100,000 BY AGE GROUP (YEARS) - FEMALE

SITE	ALL AGES	AGE UNK	0-	5-	10-	15-	20-	25-	30-	35-	40-	45-	50-	55-	60-	65-	70-	75-	80-	85+	CRUDE RATE	%	CR 64	CR 74	ASR (W)	ICD (9th)
Lip	92	0	-	-	-	-	-	0.1	0.2	0.1	-	0.6	0.3	0.8	0.9	2.0	4.0	3.2	2.8	2.9	0.7	0.2	0.01	0.05	**0.3**	*140*
Tongue	120	0	-	-	-	-	-	0.1	-	0.1	0.3	0.9	1.4	1.2	3.3	2.3	2.3	2.6	4.2	4.3	0.9	0.2	0.04	0.06	**0.5**	*141*
Salivary gland	85	0	-	-	0.1	-	0.5	0.2	0.3	0.3	0.2	0.6	1.0	1.1	0.8	1.7	1.9	1.6	1.4	3.6	0.7	0.1	0.03	0.04	**0.4**	*142*
Mouth	304	0	-	0.2	0.1	0.2	0.1	0.2	0.2	0.4	1.1	2.0	2.4	4.1	5.9	6.5	6.5	7.7	11.1	8.3	2.3	0.5	0.09	0.15	**1.3**	*143-5*
Oropharynx	125	0	-	-	-	0.1	-	-	-	0.3	0.3	0.9	2.1	2.6	3.6	2.5	2.4	2.8	0.8	2.9	1.0	0.2	0.05	0.07	**0.6**	*146*
Nasopharynx	34	0	-	-	0.1	0.1	-	0.2	-	-	0.5	0.3	0.6	0.3	0.6	0.5	0.9	0.6	0.3	-	0.3	0.1	0.01	0.02	**0.2**	*147*
Hypopharynx	35	0	-	-	-	-	-	-	-	-	-	0.1	0.3	0.5	1.1	1.6	0.7	0.4	1.4	0.4	0.3	0.1	0.01	0.02	**0.2**	*148*
Pharynx unspecified	9	0	-	-	-	-	-	-	-	-	-	0.1	0.1	0.1	0.5	-	-	0.2	0.4	-	-	0.1	0.0	0.00	0.00	**0.0**	*149*
Oesophagus	387	0	-	-	-	-	-	-	-	-	0.1	1.2	2.1	4.1	5.6	7.9	12.4	14.0	13.6	20.5	3.0	0.7	0.07	0.17	**1.4**	*150*
Stomach	1348	0	-	-	-	-	0.1	0.5	1.0	1.5	2.5	5.3	6.8	14.0	16.2	23.4	31.9	43.1	66.2	78.1	10.3	2.3	0.24	0.52	**4.7**	*151*
Small intestine	128	0	-	-	-	-	-	0.1	0.2	0.1	0.3	0.7	0.6	1.7	2.2	3.3	3.5	2.2	4.7	6.1	1.0	0.2	0.03	0.06	**0.5**	*152*
Colon	5665	0	-	-	0.1	0.2	0.3	1.0	2.0	3.3	7.8	15.8	32.9	50.7	76.4	111.9	160.4	208.7	255.8	264.5	43.4	9.6	0.95	2.31	**19.9**	*153*
Rectum	2789	0	-	-	-	-	0.1	0.3	0.9	2.2	5.5	11.0	17.0	32.1	46.0	53.5	75.7	98.4	108.3	116.6	21.4	4.7	0.58	1.22	**10.4**	*154*
Liver	558	0	0.4	0.2	0.1	0.1	0.3	0.3	0.3	0.9	0.9	1.3	2.9	4.0	6.5	11.3	17.6	18.8	24.5	25.2	4.3	0.9	0.09	0.24	**2.0**	*155*
Gallbladder etc.	675	0	-	-	-	-	-	-	0.1	0.2	0.4	1.7	2.4	6.0	9.4	12.6	20.4	26.7	33.4	31.3	5.2	1.1	0.10	0.27	**2.3**	*156*
Pancreas	1825	0	-	-	-	0.1	0.1	-	0.2	0.8	2.8	4.7	8.1	17.1	26.7	34.7	60.4	65.0	83.8	76.3	14.0	3.1	0.30	0.78	**6.4**	*157*
Nose, sinuses etc.	116	0	0.1	-	-	0.1	0.1	-	0.2	0.1	0.3	0.6	0.4	1.8	1.9	2.5	3.5	3.0	4.2	3.2	0.9	0.2	0.03	0.06	**0.5**	*160*
Larynx	235	0	-	-	-	-	-	-	0.1	0.2	0.8	1.1	2.2	6.8	6.4	5.0	7.2	4.3	2.8	3.2	1.8	0.4	0.09	0.15	**1.1**	*161*
Bronchus, lung	5536	0	-	-	-	-	0.2	0.3	1.4	4.6	11.2	29.5	57.7	102.8	134.1	166.5	149.4	131.4	99.1	79.9	42.4	9.4	1.71	3.29	**25.4**	*162*
Other thoracic organs	64	0	0.3	-	-	0.1	-	0.1	0.2	0.1	0.3	0.3	0.7	0.9	0.8	1.4	1.0	1.2	3.1	1.1	0.5	0.1	0.02	0.03	**0.3**	*163-4*
Bone	94	0	0.1	0.8	0.9	0.9	0.3	0.2	0.1	0.4	0.5	0.9	0.3	0.9	1.1	1.2	1.4	1.4	1.4	2.5	0.7	0.2	0.04	0.05	**0.6**	*170*
Connective tissue	305	0	1.4	0.2	0.5	1.1	1.3	0.7	1.2	1.8	1.3	2.6	2.9	2.2	2.8	3.7	5.2	6.9	8.3	9.4	2.3	0.5	0.10	0.14	**1.6**	*171*
Mesothelioma	73	0	-	-	-	-	0.2	-	-	0.3	0.1	0.2	0.3	1.1	0.8	1.9	2.4	1.8	3.3	1.4	0.6	0.1	0.01	0.04	**0.3**	*MES*
Kaposi's sarcoma	2	0	-	-	-	-	-	-	-	-	-	-	-	-	-	0.2	-	-	-	0.4	0.0	0.0	0.00	0.00	**0.0**	*KAP*
Melanoma of skin	2142	0	-	0.2	0.6	1.9	6.9	9.2	11.8	16.2	21.0	27.7	24.2	23.7	27.1	32.2	37.5	30.4	28.4	27.0	16.4	3.6	0.85	1.20	**11.7**	*172*
Other skin	10468	0	-	-	0.5	0.6	3.0	5.6	12.9	26.1	46.8	70.3	103.4	110.5	148.0	199.0	250.6	282.2	348.2	414.5	80.2		2.64	4.89	**43.3**	*173*
Breast	15036	0	-	-	-	-	0.6	5.7	21.2	57.8	119.9	185.1	208.1	239.2	253.5	266.9	278.2	294.6	308.4	306.9	115.2	25.6	5.46	8.18	**73.3**	*174*
Uterus unspecified	126	0	-	0.2	-	-	-	0.1	-	-	0.2	1.1	1.3	2.5	1.9	1.9	3.1	3.8	4.7	3.2	1.0	0.2	0.04	0.06	**0.5**	*179*
Cervix uteri	2767	0	-	-	-	0.1	3.7	12.9	24.0	28.6	31.0	30.3	28.0	35.5	36.5	45.1	39.8	34.4	34.8	24.1	21.2	4.7	1.15	1.58	**15.2**	*180*
Placenta	9	0	-	-	-	-	0.2	0.2	0.2	0.2	0.1	-	-	-	-	-	-	-	-	-	0.1	0.0	0.00	0.00	**0.1**	*181*
Corpus uteri	3165	0	-	-	-	-	0.1	0.2	0.4	2.6	4.9	14.2	35.1	49.5	88.6	101.8	93.9	64.6	54.3	38.9	24.3	5.4	0.98	1.96	**14.7**	*182*
Ovary etc.	2874	0	-	0.3	0.1	1.5	2.9	2.8	5.1	7.8	13.0	26.3	35.5	42.4	56.6	68.7	67.2	56.7	57.3	41.0	22.0	4.9	0.97	1.65	**14.0**	*183*
Other female genital	585	0	0.1	-	-	0.1	0.2	0.3	0.9	1.3	1.5	2.5	2.6	4.1	8.3	10.5	13.1	20.0	24.8	32.7	4.5	1.0	0.11	0.23	**2.1**	*184*
Bladder	1979	0	0.1	-	0.1	0.1	0.2	0.5	0.4	1.6	2.7	6.2	13.7	24.6	34.9	47.4	56.9	64.2	69.0	67.7	15.2	3.4	0.43	0.95	**7.7**	*188*
Kidney etc.	1413	0	1.4	0.8	0.1	0.1	0.1	0.1	0.3	1.5	2.3	6.0	9.6	16.3	22.0	33.6	45.2	45.4	49.5	38.1	10.8	2.4	0.30	0.70	**5.7**	*189*
Eye	149	0	1.5	0.2	0.1	0.2	0.2	0.1	-	0.7	1.0	1.2	0.8	3.1	1.7	2.2	2.8	3.4	3.9	2.2	1.1	0.3	0.05	0.08	**0.9**	*190*
Brain, nervous system	816	0	4.6	3.3	2.3	1.5	1.5	2.4	2.3	3.2	4.0	6.6	7.9	12.9	12.6	19.4	14.1	13.4	10.6	4.3	6.3	1.4	0.33	0.49	**5.0**	*191-2*
Thyroid	400	0	-	-	0.1	0.3	1.6	2.1	4.6	3.6	3.6	3.0	4.3	2.8	3.7	4.2	5.4	7.7	7.8	9.4	3.1	0.7	0.15	0.20	**2.1**	*193*
Other endocrine	46	0	0.6	0.3	-	0.1	0.3	-	-	0.3	0.5	0.6	0.1	0.8	0.6	0.8	1.0	0.4	-	-	0.4	0.1	0.02	0.03	**0.3**	*194*
Hodgkin's disease	252	0	-	0.3	0.4	1.5	3.7	3.4	3.2	1.2	1.7	1.3	1.0	1.8	1.9	2.6	2.6	3.4	2.8	2.2	1.9	0.4	0.11	0.13	**1.6**	*201*
Non-Hodgkin lymphoma	1550	0	0.1	0.3	0.4	1.0	0.7	1.8	2.9	4.1	7.2	8.5	11.6	16.9	21.8	32.6	38.2	48.4	49.8	43.2	11.9	2.6	0.39	0.74	**6.5**	*200,202*
Multiple myeloma	584	0	-	-	-	-	-	-	-	0.2	0.9	2.0	2.8	6.9	10.6	15.5	18.7	18.2	21.2	17.6	4.5	1.0	0.12	0.29	**2.2**	*203*
Lymphoid leukaemia	618	0	5.8	2.9	0.8	0.4	0.3	0.2	0.5	0.4	1.0	1.0	1.3	3.5	6.9	9.8	15.0	20.9	27.0	32.4	4.7	1.1	0.13	0.25	**2.9**	*204*
Myeloid leukaemia	638	0	1.4	0.6	0.5	1.3	0.8	0.9	1.2	2.3	3.5	2.7	4.3	4.8	6.5	12.4	16.4	17.4	20.6	22.3	4.9	1.1	0.15	0.30	**2.9**	*205*
Monocytic leukaemia	6	0	-	-	-	-	-	-	-	-	0.1	-	-	0.2	0.3	-	-	0.6	-	-	0.0	0.0	0.00	0.00	**0.0**	*206*
Other leukaemia	10	0	-	-	-	-	-	-	-	-	0.1	-	-	0.2	0.2	0.2	0.3	0.2	0.3	0.7	0.1	0.0	0.00	0.00	**0.0**	*207*
Leukaemia unspecified	61	0	0.1	-	-	-	-	0.1	0.1	0.3	0.1	0.1	0.8	0.2	-	0.3	1.7	1.4	2.8	6.1	0.5	0.1	0.01	0.02	**0.2**	*208*
Other and unspecified	3004	0	0.8	0.2	-	0.3	-	0.7	0.9	3.1	5.4	10.4	18.4	28.0	47.2	55.7	75.7	112.4	119.4	147.9	23.0	5.1	0.58	1.23	**11.0**	*O&U*
All sites	69302	0	19.1	10.5	8.3	14.3	30.8	53.8	101.7	181.1	310.0	489.5	660.1	887.4	1144.4	1420.6	1649.2	1790.0	1980.5	2024.5	531.2		19.55	34.90	**304.9**	*ALL*
All sites but 173	58834	0	19.1	10.5	7.8	13.7	27.8	48.2	88.8	155.0	263.2	419.2	556.8	776.9	996.4	1221.5	1398.6	1507.8	1632.3	1609.9	450.9	100.0	16.92	30.02	**261.6**	*ALLb*

| Rate from 10 cases | | | 1.406 | 1.500 | 1.292 | 1.123 | 1.038 | 1.025 | 1.099 | 1.096 | 1.012 | 1.114 | 1.393 | 1.537 | 1.559 | 1.550 | 1.745 | 2.025 | 2.783 | 3.598 |

Estonia

Cancer registration in Estonia began in 1953, when compulsory registration of incident cases of cancer was introduced in the former USSR. During 1953–67, short and incomplete annual reports were produced; since 1961, cases detected on the basis of a death certificate have been added to the database. In 1968–70 cancer registration in Estonia was centralized, and thus core documentation and satisfactory incidence data are available since 1968. The Estonian Cancer Registry (ECR; Eesti Vähiregister) was founded on 16 January 1978.

Until the end of 1991, the registry consisted of two subdivisions. One of these—the Department of Cancer Statistics—belonged to the Estonian Cancer Centre (formerly Tallinn Cancer Dispensary), and its task was data collection. The other subdivision—now the Department of Epidemiology and Biostatistics, located in the Institute of Experimental and Clinical Medicine—was responsible for statistical and epidemiological analysis and interpretation of the data. Each year both subdivisions made a business contract with the former Public Health Information and Data Processing Centre, for data processing. In December 1991, the Department of Cancer Statistics was renamed the Estonian Cancer Registry, while, formally, the Department of Epidemiology and Biostatistics found itself excluded. In the period 1991–93 the registry was on the verge of extinction because of such external administrative manipulations as well as outdated hardware and software, but in 1994, major reorganization led to renewal of normal activities.

The registry covers the whole of Estonia, which is situated by the Baltic Sea, between latitudes 57°30′ and 59°49′ N and longitudes 21°45′ and 28°15′ E. The area is 45 215 km^2. The highest point is 318 m above sea level, and only 10% of the territory lies above 100 m. The average annual temperature is 4–6° C and the average annual precipitation 550–750 mm.

At the 1989 (12 January) census, the population was 731 392 males and 834 270 females. The largest towns were Tallinn (479 000 inhabitants), Tartu (113 400), Narva (81 200) and Kohtla-Järve (77 300). 28.5% of population lives in rural areas.

The 1989 census revealed great ethnic diversity, with 61.5% Estonians, 30.3% Russians, 3.1% Ukrainians and 1.5% Belorusians.

In 1989, 43% of the working population was employed in industry and trade, 17% in the health services, physical recreation and social security, education, science, culture and arts, 13% in agriculture, 10% in transport and communications, and 9% in public catering, state purchases, supply and sales.

Life expectancy at birth in 1986–91 was 65.7 years for males and 75.0 for females. The birth rate was 14.1 and the death rate 12.3 per thousand. The infant mortality rate was 12.4 per thousand live births.

In Estonia, during the years 1988–92 covered by this volume, every health-care institution where cancer was diagnosed was obliged to send a notification form to one of the 17 local cancer registries. Data recorded included name, sex, date of birth, place of birth, nationality, marital status, principal occupation, usual residence, duration of residence in Estonia, reason for presentation of the patient, date of first consultation, date of diagnosis, site of tumour, histological diagnosis, clinical stage and basis of diagnosis. The names of the notifying health-care institution and of that to which the patient was sent for treatment were also recorded.

Later, for each case of cancer registered, details including treatment, status of the patient at annual follow-ups, date and cause of death, etc. were abstracted from notifications, inpatient records, outpatient records and death certificates onto a follow-up card. A patient is followed until death, and follow-up data are collected routinely.

As one section of the ECR was located in a cancer institution where half of all cancer patients in Estonia were treated, the ECR often received more information than the local cancer registries. Therefore staff from the local registries visited the ECR quarterly to check the follow-up cards for completeness and to update them.

Follow-up cards stored in the ECR were checked and each patient was assigned a unique registration number. Multiple primaries were noted by a tumour sequence number. After coding, the data were entered into the database through an on-line data entry system. At the time of entry a limited amount of editing was performed. Additional intra- and inter-field edits were done after input. Manual and computer files were updated as new information was received and checked. If the information received was incomplete, the ECR made an inquiry to the health-care institution or population registry. The process of filing follow-up cards by names and different computerized lists of cancer cases allowed elimination of duplicate registrations.

At monthly intervals, all death certificates kept in the Estonian State Department of Statistics (now the Statistical Office of Estonia) were checked manually by an abstractor of the ECR. From each certificate where cancer was mentioned, the relevant information was sent to local cancer registries to be matched against other lists, made by registries' abstractors using regional civil registration office documentation.

There were no death-certificate-only cases. If a death certificate was the first notification of a cancer case, the certifying physician/hospital was contacted to obtain additional information. If the evidence for cancer was sufficiently strong, a notification and a follow-up card were filled in and the case was entered into the computer. For all other cases, the follow-up cards were filled in, but the information was not coded or computerized.

Up to 1991, annual incidence, mortality, prevalence and treatment data were routinely provided as a part of the Soviet Union public health statistics system. Related annual official statistical reports that had to be completed some weeks after the end of each calendar year were of questionable quality. Other, more informative and reliable tabulations concerning mainly absolute numbers, crude, age-specific and age-standardized incidence and prevalence rates, calculated and analysed at the Department of Epidemiology and Biostatistics, have been used for the purposes of descriptive epidemiology. In 1996, a statistical compendium *Cancer in Estonia 1968-1992: Incidence, Mortality, Prevalence, Survival* (in English) was published.

Mati Rahu

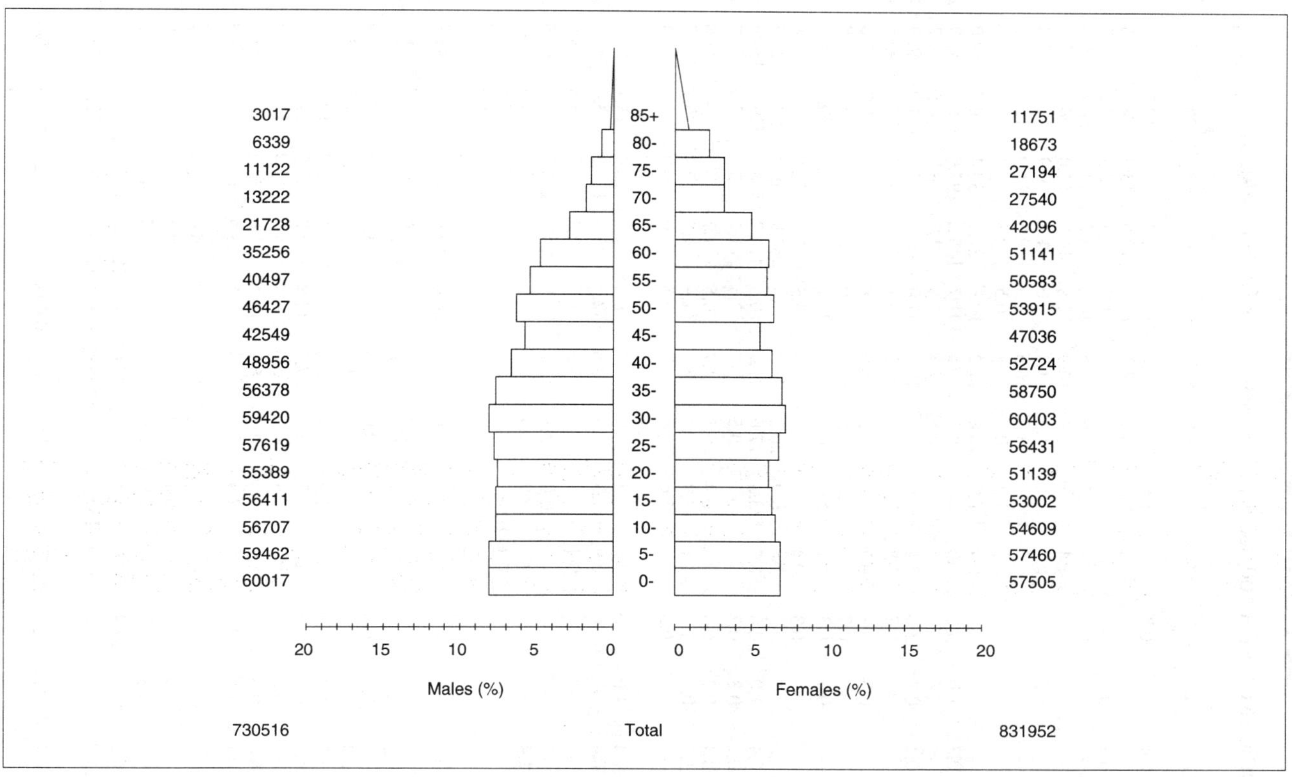

Estonia
Source of population: average annual 1988–92
Census: 12 January 1989. Eesti Vabariigi Riiklik Statistikaamet. Eesti Vabariigi maakondade, linnade ja alevite rahvistik. II osa. Rahvastiku sooline ja anuseline koosseis. 1989. a. rahvaloenduse andmed. Tallinn, 1991.
Estimate: Estonian Interuniversity Population Research Centre. The annual population estimates are based on the 1989 census, taking into account births and deaths, and migration.

Notes to tables overleaf:
† 188 does not include non-invasive tumours

ESTONIA 1988-1992

ANNUAL INCIDENCE PER 100,000 BY AGE GROUP (YEARS) - MALE

SITE	ALL AGES	AGE UNK	0-	5-	10-	15-	20-	25-	30-	35-	40-	45-	50-	55-	60-	65-	70-	75-	80-	85+	CRUDE RATE	%	CR 64	CR 74	ASR (W)	ICD (9th)
Lip	100	0	-	-	-	-	0.4	-	0.7	-	1.6	5.2	2.6	5.4	11.3	9.2	19.7	16.2	34.7	13.3	2.7	0.9	0.14	0.28	**2.3**	140
Tongue	107	0	-	-	-	-	-	-	-	1.4	0.4	6.1	8.6	11.9	13.0	13.8	4.5	3.6	3.2	6.6	2.9	0.9	0.21	0.30	**2.5**	141
Salivary gland	20	0	-	-	-	-	0.4	0.3	-	-	-	0.9	-	1.0	1.7	2.8	3.0	7.2	3.2	6.6	0.5	0.2	0.02	0.05	**0.5**	142
Mouth	178	0	-	-	-	-	-	-	0.3	1.4	7.4	8.9	15.5	20.2	18.2	14.7	6.1	10.8	3.2	-	4.9	1.6	0.36	0.46	**4.1**	143-5
Oropharynx	133	0	-	-	-	-	-	-	-	1.4	6.5	6.1	12.9	12.8	11.9	11.0	4.5	9.0	6.3	6.6	3.6	1.2	0.26	0.34	**3.1**	146
Nasopharynx	21	0	-	-	-	0.4	-	0.3	-	0.7	1.6	1.9	1.3	1.0	1.1	0.9	-	1.8	-	-	0.6	0.2	0.04	0.05	**0.5**	147
Hypopharynx	83	0	-	-	-	-	-	-	-	0.4	-	3.3	6.5	8.9	9.6	11.0	12.1	9.0	-	-	2.3	0.7	0.14	0.26	**1.9**	148
Pharynx unspecified	9	0	-	-	-	-	-	-	-	-	1.2	0.5	-	0.5	2.3	-	-	-	-	-	0.2	0.1	0.02	0.02	**0.2**	149
Oesophagus	237	0	-	-	-	-	-	-	-	0.4	2.9	10.8	17.2	19.3	27.2	30.4	30.3	18.0	34.7	33.1	6.5	2.1	0.39	0.69	**5.6**	150
Stomach	1450	0	-	-	0.4	0.7	1.0	4.0	11.0	22.1	38.1	71.5	101.7	145.2	197.9	246.6	258.9	258.7	225.3	39.7	12.7	1.98	4.20	**34.0**	151
Small intestine	22	0	-	-	-	-	-	-	-	-	0.5	1.3	1.5	1.7	3.7	4.5	7.2	3.2	-	0.6	0.2	0.02	0.07	**0.5**	152
Colon	602	0	-	-	-	-	0.4	0.3	3.0	3.2	8.6	10.3	19.4	37.0	60.7	87.4	121.0	140.3	132.5	112.7	16.5	5.3	0.71	1.76	**14.1**	153
Rectum	495	0	-	-	-	-	-	-	0.3	0.7	2.9	9.9	22.0	35.1	51.1	84.7	77.1	93.5	132.5	99.4	13.6	4.3	0.61	1.42	**11.5**	154
Liver	177	0	-	-	0.4	-	-	0.3	0.3	0.7	0.8	5.2	6.0	15.8	24.4	24.9	30.3	27.0	15.8	19.9	4.8	1.5	0.27	0.55	**4.2**	155
Gallbladder etc.	55	0	-	-	-	-	-	-	-	0.7	-	1.6	0.5	2.6	3.0	5.7	8.3	6.1	19.8	3.2	6.6	1.5	0.5	0.07	0.14	**1.3**	156
Pancreas	444	0	-	-	-	-	-	0.3	0.3	1.1	5.3	14.6	22.0	26.7	41.4	77.3	80.2	86.3	56.8	92.8	12.2	3.9	0.56	1.35	**10.7**	157
Nose, sinuses etc.	30	0	-	-	-	-	-	0.3	0.4	1.2	0.5	0.4	3.5	2.8	2.8	6.1	3.6	3.2	6.6	0.8	0.3	0.05	0.09	**0.7**	160
Larynx	389	0	-	-	-	-	-	-	-	2.8	6.9	20.2	23.3	37.5	53.9	49.7	33.3	23.4	18.9	6.6	10.6	3.4	0.72	1.14	**9.1**	161
Bronchus, lung	3221	0	0.3	-	-	0.4	0.4	1.0	2.0	8.2	23.3	77.6	141.7	310.6	414.7	506.2	529.4	436.9	315.5	212.1	88.2	28.2	4.90	10.08	**75.7**	162
Other thoracic organs	23	0	0.3	-	-	0.7	0.7	0.3	0.7	-	-	0.5	-	2.5	1.1	3.7	3.0	1.8	-	-	0.6	0.2	0.03	0.07	**0.6**	163-4
Bone	27	0	-	-	0.7	1.1	0.4	0.7	0.3	0.4	0.4	0.5	1.7	0.5	1.7	4.6	-	1.8	3.2	-	0.7	0.2	0.04	0.06	**0.7**	170
Connective tissue	89	0	3.0	0.7	0.7	2.1	1.1	0.3	1.3	1.1	2.9	0.9	3.4	4.9	4.5	7.4	6.1	9.0	15.8	13.3	2.4	0.8	0.14	0.20	**2.3**	171
Mesothelioma	21	0	-	-	-	-	-	-	0.3	-	1.6	-	1.7	0.5	4.0	0.9	-	5.4	-	-	0.6	0.2	0.04	0.05	**0.5**	MES
Kaposi's sarcoma	1	0	-	-	-	-	-	-	-	-	-	-	-	-	-	0.9	-	-	-	-	0.0	0.0	0.00	0.00	**0.0**	KAP
Melanoma of skin	147	0	-	-	0.4	3.5	1.4	1.0	1.0	2.5	3.3	4.7	7.3	8.4	14.7	16.6	15.1	16.2	6.3	13.3	4.0	1.3	0.24	0.40	**3.6**	172
Other skin	839	0	-	-	0.4	0.7	0.4	-	2.0	6.0	11.8	11.8	33.6	52.3	75.4	119.7	163.4	208.6	189.3	178.9	23.0		0.97	2.39	**19.6**	173
Breast	20	0	-	-	-	-	-	-	-	0.4	-	-	1.3	1.5	2.3	2.8	4.5	3.6	3.2	-	0.5	0.2	0.03	0.06	**0.5**	175
Prostate	931	0	-	-	-	-	-	-	-	-	2.0	3.3	11.2	36.5	74.9	153.7	249.6	368.6	366.0	225.3	25.5	8.1	0.64	2.66	**21.6**	185
Testis	66	0	-	-	-	0.7	1.4	4.2	4.4	4.3	2.9	2.4	0.4	-	1.1	1.8	4.5	-	6.3	6.6	1.8	0.6	0.11	0.14	**1.6**	186
Penis	34	0	-	-	-	-	-	-	0.7	0.4	0.8	0.5	2.2	1.5	2.8	2.8	7.6	5.4	6.3	13.3	0.9	0.3	0.04	0.10	**0.8**	187.1-.4
Other male genital	7	0	-	-	-	-	-	-	-	-	-	-	-	-	1.7	0.9	1.5	1.8	3.2	-	0.2	0.1	0.01	0.02	**0.2**	187.5-.9
†Bladder	475	0	0.3	-	-	-	-	0.3	0.3	0.7	2.9	8.5	13.4	29.1	56.2	69.0	95.3	127.7	97.8	106.0	13.0	4.2	0.56	1.38	**11.2**	188
Kidney etc.	484	0	1.7	0.7	-	0.4	0.4	-	0.7	1.1	7.8	16.0	27.1	46.9	50.5	73.6	51.4	57.5	50.5	53.0	13.3	4.2	0.77	1.39	**11.4**	189
Eye	36	0	0.7	0.3	-	-	-	0.7	-	-	-	0.5	3.0	4.4	2.8	4.6	3.0	1.8	3.2	-	1.0	0.3	0.06	0.10	**0.9**	190
Brain, nervous system	214	0	3.0	2.7	1.8	3.2	2.2	3.1	4.0	2.8	6.1	8.9	14.6	14.8	11.9	17.5	4.5	12.6	-	-	5.9	1.9	0.40	0.51	**5.4**	191-2
Thyroid	31	0	-	-	-	-	-	0.7	0.3	-	1.6	0.9	1.3	2.5	3.4	0.9	3.0	1.8	9.5	6.6	0.8	0.3	0.05	0.07	**0.7**	193
Other endocrine	16	0	-	-	-	0.4	0.4	-	-	-	-	-	1.3	1.5	1.1	2.8	1.5	3.6	-	-	0.4	0.1	0.02	0.04	**0.4**	194
Hodgkin's disease	106	0	-	1.3	2.1	1.8	3.6	4.2	4.7	2.1	1.2	3.8	2.6	4.0	5.1	2.8	10.6	7.2	3.2	-	2.9	0.9	0.18	0.25	**2.7**	201
Non-Hodgkin lymphoma	188	0	1.3	0.7	1.8	1.1	1.1	0.7	2.0	2.1	3.7	3.3	7.8	12.8	17.0	23.0	22.7	36.0	18.9	6.6	5.1	1.6	0.28	0.51	**4.5**	200,202
Multiple myeloma	72	0	-	-	-	-	-	0.3	-	0.7	0.4	1.9	5.6	4.9	8.5	11.0	13.6	5.4	6.3	-	2.0	0.6	0.11	0.24	**1.7**	203
Lymphoid leukaemia	218	0	3.7	2.0	2.5	-	0.4	0.3	1.3	1.1	-	4.7	6.9	11.4	21.6	32.2	24.2	53.9	34.7	39.8	6.0	1.9	0.28	0.56	**5.4**	204
Myeloid leukaemia	107	0	0.7	-	0.4	0.4	0.7	1.4	0.3	1.4	2.5	2.8	4.3	8.4	8.5	13.8	9.1	19.8	12.6	13.3	2.9	0.9	0.16	0.27	**2.5**	205
Monocytic leukaemia	4	0	-	-	-	0.4	-	-	-	-	-	0.5	-	-	1.5	1.8	-	-	-	-	0.1	0.0	0.00	0.01	**0.1**	206
Other leukaemia	13	0	-	-	-	-	-	-	-	0.4	-	0.5	-	-	0.6	1.8	9.1	1.8	3.2	-	0.4	0.1	0.01	0.06	**0.3**	207
Leukaemia unspecified	18	0	-	0.7	0.4	0.4	-	1.0	-	-	0.4	0.9	-	0.5	0.6	0.9	3.0	3.6	3.2	-	0.5	0.2	0.02	0.04	**0.5**	208
Other and unspecified	304	0	0.3	-	1.1	-	-	0.3	0.7	-	2.9	8.9	12.1	23.2	29.5	46.0	63.5	57.5	53.6	19.9	8.3	2.7	0.39	0.94	**7.2**	O&U
All sites	12264	0	15.3	9.1	12.3	17.7	16.2	23.6	37.4	61.0	149.5	307.4	537.6	926.5	1299.6	1752.5	1986.1	2186.5	1921.3	1544.2	335.8		17.07	35.76	**289.4**	ALL
All sites but 173	11425	0	15.3	9.1	12.0	17.0	15.9	23.6	35.3	55.0	137.7	295.7	504.0	874.1	1224.2	1632.9	1822.7	1978.0	1732.0	1365.2	312.8	100.0	16.09	33.37	**269.8**	ALLb

Rate from 1 case   0.333   0.336   0.353   0.355   0.361   0.347   0.337   0.355   0.409   0.470   0.431   0.494   0.567   0.920   1.513   1.798   3.155   6.627

†Important: see notes on population page

ESTONIA 1988-1992

ANNUAL INCIDENCE PER 100,000 BY AGE GROUP (YEARS) - FEMALE

SITE	ALL AGES	AGE UNK	0-	5-	10-	15-	20-	25-	30-	35-	40-	45-	50-	55-	60-	65-	70-	75-	80-	85+	CRUDE RATE	%	CR 64	CR 74	ASR (W)	ICD (9th)
Lip	24	0	-	-	-	-	-	-	-	-	-	-	-	0.4	0.8	2.9	1.5	6.6	2.1	3.4	0.6	0.2	0.01	0.03	**0.3**	140
Tongue	26	0	-	-	-	-	-	-	-	-	0.4	-	0.7	2.0	2.3	1.9	0.7	2.9	2.1	1.7	0.6	0.2	0.03	0.04	**0.4**	141
Salivary gland	30	0	-	-	-	-	-	-	0.3	0.3	0.8	0.9	1.5	0.8	1.2	1.0	4.4	2.2	1.1	5.1	0.7	0.3	0.03	0.06	**0.5**	142
Mouth	32	0	-	-	-	-	-	-	-	0.3	0.4	0.4	1.5	2.4	1.6	2.9	4.4	1.5	1.1	-	0.8	0.3	0.03	0.07	**0.5**	143-5
Oropharynx	10	0	-	-	-	-	0.4	-	-	-	-	-	1.5	0.4	1.2	-	-	0.7	-	-	0.2	0.1	0.02	0.02	**0.2**	146
Nasopharynx	14	0	-	-	-	-	-	-	-	0.3	0.4	0.4	-	0.4	0.8	0.5	1.5	2.9	1.1	-	0.3	0.1	0.01	0.02	**0.2**	147
Hypopharynx	5	0	-	-	-	-	-	-	-	-	0.4	-	-	-	0.8	0.5	0.7	-	-	-	0.1	0.0	0.01	0.01	**0.1**	148
Pharynx unspecified	1	0	-	-	-	-	-	-	-	-	0.4	-	-	-	-	-	-	-	-	-	0.0	0.0	0.00	0.00	**0.0**	149
Oesophagus	58	0	-	-	-	-	-	-	0.3	-	-	0.9	0.4	1.2	3.9	3.8	4.4	7.4	12.9	8.5	1.4	0.5	0.03	0.07	**0.7**	150
Stomach	1231	0	-	-	-	0.4	2.3	1.4	4.3	8.9	14.4	20.0	28.2	43.1	66.1	80.8	122.7	152.2	134.9	119.1	29.6	10.8	0.95	1.96	**16.6**	151
Small intestine	14	0	-	-	-	-	-	-	-	-	0.4	-	0.8	1.2	1.4	1.5	0.7	-	3.4	-	0.3	0.1	0.01	0.03	**0.2**	152
Colon	878	0	-	-	-	0.8	0.4	0.7	2.3	2.7	7.6	8.5	21.5	35.2	43.0	67.9	84.2	123.6	107.1	57.9	21.1	7.7	0.61	1.37	**11.4**	153
Rectum	578	0	-	-	-	0.4	-	0.4	1.0	1.7	2.7	6.0	14.1	25.7	30.1	45.1	53.7	69.9	77.1	52.8	13.9	5.1	0.41	0.90	**7.5**	154
Liver	141	0	-	-	-	0.4	-	-	0.3	0.3	0.8	2.1	1.9	5.9	10.2	13.3	11.6	14.0	20.3	5.1	3.4	1.2	0.11	0.23	**1.9**	155
Gallbladder etc.	137	0	-	-	-	-	-	-	0.3	-	0.8	1.7	3.3	5.5	7.8	10.0	13.1	16.9	17.1	15.3	3.3	1.2	0.10	0.21	**1.8**	156
Pancreas	457	0	-	-	-	-	-	-	0.3	1.0	2.7	4.7	4.8	12.7	28.2	37.1	53.7	67.7	52.5	42.5	11.0	4.0	0.27	0.73	**5.7**	157
Nose, sinuses etc.	28	0	-	-	-	0.4	-	-	0.7	0.3	0.4	0.4	1.5	0.4	1.2	2.4	1.5	2.2	1.1	5.1	0.7	0.2	0.03	0.05	**0.4**	160
Larynx	24	0	-	-	-	-	-	0.4	-	-	1.5	-	0.7	1.6	2.7	1.9	0.7	0.7	-	-	0.6	0.2	0.03	0.05	**0.4**	161
Bronchus, lung	606	0	-	-	-	-	-	0.7	1.0	2.0	3.4	8.5	12.2	22.5	37.9	62.2	71.2	57.4	47.1	47.7	14.6	5.3	0.44	1.11	**8.3**	162
Other thoracic organs	21	0	-	-	-	0.4	0.4	-	0.3	0.7	0.4	0.4	0.4	1.2	0.8	1.4	1.5	1.5	1.1	-	0.5	0.2	0.02	0.04	**0.4**	163-4
Bone	38	0	0.3	0.7	0.7	0.8	1.2	-	0.7	0.3	1.1	-	0.7	0.4	2.0	2.9	1.5	2.9	1.1	1.7	0.9	0.3	0.04	0.07	**0.8**	170
Connective tissue	118	0	1.7	0.7	1.5	0.4	-	0.7	2.0	-	1.9	2.6	4.8	5.9	3.5	7.1	9.4	5.1	10.7	8.5	2.8	1.0	0.13	0.21	**2.1**	171
Mesothelioma	11	0	-	-	-	-	-	-	-	-	1.7	0.7	0.4	0.4	-	2.2	-	-	-	-	0.3	0.1	0.02	0.03	**0.2**	MES
Kaposi's sarcoma	2	0	-	-	-	-	-	-	0.3	-	-	-	-	-	-	0.5	-	-	-	-	0.0	0.0	0.00	0.00	**0.0**	KAP
Melanoma of skin	239	0	-	-	-	1.1	0.4	3.5	4.3	4.8	7.6	8.1	10.8	8.7	8.2	16.6	10.2	14.0	10.7	15.3	5.7	2.1	0.29	0.42	**4.1**	172
Other skin	1291	0	-	-	-	-	0.4	0.4	3.3	3.4	10.6	27.6	29.3	44.7	62.2	94.5	114.7	166.2	147.8	177.0	31.0		0.91	1.96	**16.9**	173
Breast	2200	0	-	-	-	-	-	5.7	17.9	33.0	67.1	108.4	107.2	102.8	111.1	117.8	136.5	132.4	114.6	76.6	52.9	19.4	2.77	4.04	**36.5**	174
Uterus unspecified	0	0	-	-	-	-	-	-	-	-	-	-	-	-	-	-	-	-	-	-	0.0	0.0	0.00	0.00	**0.0**	179
Cervix uteri	817	0	-	-	-	-	1.2	7.1	12.3	21.4	33.8	30.2	30.8	29.3	39.1	58.0	50.1	36.0	30.0	15.3	19.6	7.2	1.03	1.57	**14.1**	180
Placenta	13	0	-	-	-	0.4	0.4	0.7	1.0	-	0.4	1.7	0.4	-	-	-	-	-	-	-	0.3	0.1	0.02	0.02	**0.3**	181
Corpus uteri	835	0	-	-	-	-	-	0.4	1.0	6.1	11.0	23.8	39.0	49.8	61.0	65.6	55.9	55.9	40.7	20.4	20.1	7.4	0.96	1.57	**12.9**	182
Ovary etc.	789	0	-	-	0.7	1.5	1.6	2.8	3.6	6.1	15.6	23.0	37.5	36.0	54.0	52.7	57.4	53.7	35.3	35.7	19.0	7.0	0.91	1.46	**12.5**	183
Other female genital	147	0	-	-	-	-	-	0.7	-	0.7	1.1	-	4.5	6.7	4.7	10.0	16.0	13.2	22.5	28.9	3.5	1.3	0.09	0.22	**1.9**	184
†Bladder	179	0	-	-	-	-	-	-	-	-	-	1.3	2.2	4.3	8.2	12.4	20.3	33.8	28.9	18.7	4.3	1.6	0.08	0.24	**2.0**	188
Kidney etc.	386	0	4.2	1.4	-	-	-	0.4	1.0	1.4	2.3	6.4	13.0	20.2	30.5	27.1	34.9	27.2	27.8	15.3	9.3	3.4	0.40	0.71	**6.0**	189
Eye	33	0	1.0	-	-	-	-	0.4	0.7	-	0.4	0.9	0.7	2.0	2.0	1.4	3.6	-	3.2	1.7	0.8	0.3	0.04	0.07	**0.6**	190
Brain, nervous system	200	0	4.2	3.8	2.6	2.3	1.2	2.5	2.6	2.4	3.8	6.0	12.2	10.3	10.6	8.1	3.6	4.4	1.1	-	4.8	1.8	0.32	0.38	**4.3**	191-2
Thyroid	157	0	-	-	-	0.4	-	1.1	3.0	4.1	4.2	5.5	6.3	2.0	8.6	9.0	10.2	10.3	12.9	8.5	3.8	1.4	0.18	0.27	**2.5**	193
Other endocrine	7	0	-	-	-	-	-	0.4	0.3	-	-	0.4	0.7	-	0.4	0.5	-	-	-	-	0.2	0.1	0.01	0.01	**0.1**	194
Hodgkin's disease	69	0	0.3	-	1.1	3.0	4.3	2.5	3.0	1.7	2.7	-	1.9	0.4	0.8	1.4	2.2	2.2	1.1	-	1.7	0.6	0.11	0.13	**1.6**	201
Non-Hodgkin lymphoma	153	0	0.3	1.0	0.7	1.1	0.8	0.7	0.7	1.4	1.9	3.0	4.8	5.5	7.4	13.3	12.3	13.2	9.6	6.8	3.7	1.3	0.15	0.28	**2.5**	200,202
Multiple myeloma	85	0	-	-	-	-	-	-	0.3	0.3	0.4	1.7	3.3	3.6	5.5	8.6	8.0	6.6	6.4	3.4	2.0	0.7	0.08	0.16	**1.2**	203
Lymphoid leukaemia	177	0	4.5	2.4	1.1	0.4	-	-	0.3	-	1.9	2.6	3.7	5.1	8.6	10.9	21.1	18.4	16.1	6.8	4.3	1.6	0.15	0.31	**3.0**	204
Myeloid leukaemia	104	0	1.0	0.3	-	-	0.4	1.4	1.3	1.7	2.7	2.1	1.5	4.7	3.5	5.7	14.5	8.1	4.3	3.4	2.5	0.9	0.10	0.20	**1.8**	205
Monocytic leukaemia	2	0	-	-	0.4	-	-	-	-	-	-	-	-	-	0.4	-	-	-	-	-	0.0	0.0	0.00	0.00	**0.0**	206
Other leukaemia	14	0	-	-	-	-	-	-	-	-	-	0.4	0.7	-	-	2.4	1.5	0.7	3.2	-	0.3	0.1	0.01	0.02	**0.2**	207
Leukaemia unspecified	36	0	0.7	0.3	-	1.1	-	-	0.3	-	-	0.9	1.9	0.8	-	2.3	1.9	5.8	-	2.1	0.9	0.3	0.04	0.08	**0.7**	208
Other and unspecified	224	0	0.3	-	-	-	0.4	-	-	1.0	2.7	3.0	5.6	6.3	15.3	13.8	21.1	30.2	26.8	18.7	5.4	2.0	0.17	0.35	**3.0**	O&U
All sites	12641	0	18.8	10.8	8.8	15.1	15.3	35.1	71.2	108.6	210.1	316.4	418.4	512.0	691.8	878.9	1045.7	1165.7	1035.7	830.6	303.9		12.16	21.79	**189.2**	ALL
All sites but 173	11350	0	18.8	10.8	8.8	15.1	14.9	34.7	67.9	105.2	199.5	288.7	389.1	467.4	629.6	784.4	931.0	999.5	887.9	653.6	272.9	100.0	11.25	19.83	**172.3**	ALLb
Rate from 1 case			0.348	0.348	0.366	0.377	0.391	0.354	0.331	0.340	0.379	0.425	0.371	0.395	0.391	0.475	0.726	0.735	1.071	1.702						

†Important: see notes on population page

Finland

The Finnish Cancer Registry (Institute for Statistical and Epidemiological Cancer Research) was established in 1952 on the initiative of the Cancer Society of Finland. Data on newly diagnosed cases of cancer have been collected since 1953.

The registry covers the whole of Finland (area 338 000 km²), which is bordered to the north by Norway, to the east by Russia, to the west by Sweden and the Gulf of Bothnia and to the south by the Gulf of Finland. The average altitude is 150 m. Finland has 31 570 km² of inland water and belongs to the coniferous forest zone. The population is 5 070 000 (1993). Ethnically, the Finns are Caucasians, and of mixed origin, including Baltic, Scandinavian and probably eastern elements; 86% are Lutherans. The official languages of the country are Finnish and Swedish; 6% of the population speak Swedish as their mother tongue (1993). The main occupational groups are: manufacturing and construction 25.4%, trade and transport 17.5%, health and welfare 12.3%, agriculture and forestry 8.6%, and education and research 6.7% (1991). Some 64% of the population live in urban municipalities. The population of Helsinki with its suburbs accounts for 17% of the total.

In 1993, Finland had 13 340 physicians (2.6 per 1000 inhabitants) and 53 900 hospital beds (excluding psychiatric hospitals). The country is divided into 22 health care districts, five of which (Helsinki, Turku, Oulu, Kuopio, Tampere) have a university teaching hospital. Diagnosis and treatment of cancer are only partly centralized; cancer surgery is practised in all major hospitals and also in many smaller units. Radiotherapy is available in nine hospitals. There are facilities for specialized paediatric oncology in the five university hospitals.

Reporting of cancer cases has been compulsory since 1961. Cases are notified from hospital in- and outpatient and radiotherapy departments, from pathological, cytological and haematological laboratories, from death certificates mentioning cancer, and from practising physicians. If the notification originates from a laboratory or from a death certificate alone, further information is requested. Follow-up for death is done by checking all death certificates issued in Finland annually against the Cancer Registry files. Patients are never contacted. Case identification is based on the personal identification number used in Finland since 1967. If multiple primary tumours are diagnosed in the same person, each is recorded separately, except for skin tumours of the same histology occurring within one year. Coding of the information takes place some two years after diagnosis and is supervised by a physician (pathologist).

Apart from providing routine statistics (annual incidence rates by sex, age, primary site, place of residence and health care district) and data for planning purposes, the registry is engaged in active research on cancer epidemiology and biometrics, and provides material for clinical and pathological studies and follow-up data on cancer patients. The registry also acts as a consultant body in Finland on cancer epidemiology problems.

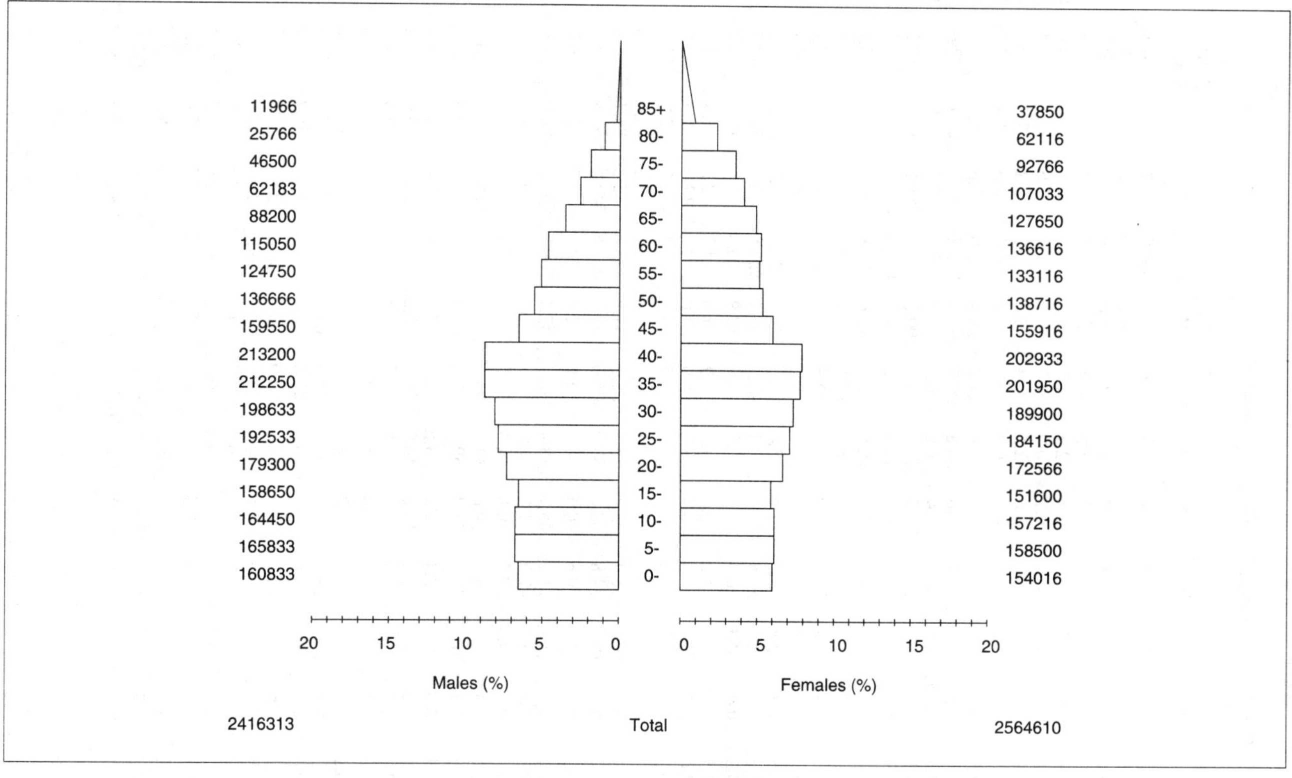

Finland
Source of population: average annual 1987–92
Census: Continuous census. Source: Statistics Finland FIN-REGION database.
Screening programmes in the area:
Women aged between ages 25/30 and 55/60 (depending on the municipality) have been screened for cervical cancer since 1963. Breast cancer screening has been carried out in the population aged 50-59/64 since 1987.

FINLAND 1987-1992

ANNUAL INCIDENCE PER 100,000 BY AGE GROUP (YEARS) - MALE

SITE	ALL AGES	AGE UNK	0-	5-	10-	15-	20-	25-	30-	35-	40-	45-	50-	55-	60-	65-	70-	75-	80-	85+	CRUDE RATE	%	CR 64	CR 74	ASR (W)	ICD (9th)
Lip	691	0	-	-	-	-	-	0.1	0.2	0.2	0.7	1.0	3.9	9.1	17.7	23.6	26.8	40.5	42.7	55.7	4.8	1.4	0.16	0.42	**3.5**	*140*
Tongue	180	0	-	-	-	0.1	0.2	0.3	0.3	0.5	0.7	2.0	2.7	3.3	3.3	4.9	4.6	5.0	3.2	7.0	1.2	0.4	0.07	0.11	**1.0**	*141*
Salivary gland	120	0	-	-	-	-	0.2	0.2	0.5	0.5	0.3	0.7	1.8	0.9	1.6	4.2	4.0	2.9	5.2	8.4	0.8	0.2	0.03	0.07	**0.6**	*142*
Mouth	188	0	-	0.1	-	0.1	-	0.1	0.2	0.6	0.8	1.3	2.6	3.6	3.5	4.3	5.6	6.8	5.2	13.9	1.3	0.4	0.06	0.11	**1.0**	*143-5*
Oropharynx	81	0	-	-	-	-	-	-	-	0.1	0.5	0.5	1.1	2.4	2.3	2.1	1.3	3.2	-	1.4	0.6	0.2	0.03	0.05	**0.4**	*146*
Nasopharynx	47	0	-	-	-	0.1	0.2	-	0.2	0.2	0.3	0.5	0.4	0.7	0.9	1.3	1.1	1.4	0.6	-	0.3	0.1	0.02	0.03	**0.3**	*147*
Hypopharynx	96	0	-	-	-	-	-	-	-	0.1	0.3	0.1	1.5	1.6	2.5	3.4	3.2	2.2	5.2	7.0	0.7	0.2	0.03	0.06	**0.5**	*148*
Pharynx unspecified	19	0	-	-	-	0.1	-	0.1	-	-	-	0.2	-	0.1	0.4	0.8	1.1	0.4	0.6	1.4	0.1	0.0	0.00	0.01	**0.1**	*149*
Oesophagus	670	0	-	-	-	-	-	0.1	0.5	0.7	2.2	5.2	9.2	13.9	21.2	28.4	38.0	33.6	66.9	4.6	1.4	0.16	0.41	**3.5**	*150*
Stomach	3279	0	-	-	-	-	0.1	0.2	1.6	2.7	6.6	12.0	19.8	41.0	60.8	96.4	135.6	196.4	237.4	284.1	22.6	6.8	0.72	1.88	**16.6**	*151*
Small intestine	190	0	-	-	-	-	0.2	-	0.2	0.1	0.8	1.6	2.0	2.4	4.8	4.7	6.2	9.7	8.4	7.0	1.3	0.4	0.06	0.11	**1.0**	*152*
Colon	2486	0	-	0.3	0.3	1.2	0.7	1.0	1.8	3.1	6.0	10.4	14.6	31.7	44.3	69.3	100.5	144.1	161.1	215.9	17.1	5.1	0.58	1.43	**12.8**	*153*
Rectum	2063	0	-	-	-	-	0.1	0.2	0.7	1.7	3.0	6.8	13.2	26.5	40.4	65.2	91.7	114.3	152.7	139.3	14.2	4.3	0.46	1.25	**10.5**	*154*
Liver	931	0	0.5	0.2	0.1	0.2	-	0.3	-	0.4	1.3	2.7	4.3	7.6	18.8	27.6	46.6	58.8	69.2	79.4	6.4	1.9	0.18	0.55	**4.8**	*155*
Gallbladder etc.	416	0	-	-	-	-	-	-	-	0.3	0.9	1.4	2.3	3.2	8.8	12.5	17.7	25.1	30.4	48.7	2.9	0.9	0.08	0.24	**2.1**	*156*
Pancreas	1848	0	-	-	-	-	0.1	0.1	0.1	1.4	3.8	7.3	12.4	22.0	38.4	55.4	81.7	105.7	119.0	139.3	12.7	3.8	0.43	1.11	**9.5**	*157*
Nose, sinuses etc.	107	0	-	-	0.2	-	-	-	0.2	0.2	0.5	0.7	1.0	1.2	2.8	3.0	3.2	4.3	6.5	1.4	0.7	0.2	0.03	0.06	**0.6**	*160*
Larynx	627	0	0.1	-	-	-	0.1	-	0.1	0.5	1.8	2.8	5.1	12.0	15.4	22.1	24.7	24.4	21.3	26.5	4.3	1.3	0.19	0.42	**3.3**	*161*
Bronchus, lung	10455	0	-	-	0.1	-	-	0.2	0.7	2.5	9.8	26.7	58.8	134.4	273.1	417.2	505.2	525.8	500.0	451.3	72.1	21.6	2.53	7.14	**54.3**	*162*
Other thoracic organs	98	0	-	-	-	-	0.1	0.2	0.1	0.2	0.4	0.3	0.5	1.3	1.6	1.9	2.9	6.8	5.8	13.9	0.7	0.2	0.02	0.05	**0.5**	*163-4*
Bone	139	0	0.1	0.2	1.1	1.6	0.5	1.0	1.0	0.5	0.5	1.3	1.2	0.9	1.3	1.9	1.6	3.2	3.2	1.4	1.0	0.3	0.06	0.07	**0.9**	*170*
Connective tissue	436	0	0.4	0.5	1.2	0.3	1.0	1.6	1.6	2.6	2.7	2.6	4.4	4.5	8.1	6.0	11.0	12.2	17.5	15.3	3.0	0.9	0.16	0.24	**2.4**	*171*
Mesothelioma	197	0	-	-	-	-	-	-	-	0.3	1.1	1.5	2.0	3.5	5.6	4.5	8.3	6.1	6.5	2.8	1.4	0.4	0.07	0.13	**1.0**	*MES*
Kaposi's sarcoma	75	0	-	-	-	-	-	0.3	0.8	0.5	0.1	-	0.1	0.5	0.3	1.7	2.4	3.2	7.1	12.5	0.5	0.2	0.01	0.03	**0.4**	*KAP*
Melanoma of skin	1438	0	0.1	-	0.1	0.6	2.1	2.6	4.5	8.1	9.7	14.6	18.4	23.8	23.8	25.3	31.9	35.8	45.3	55.7	9.9	3.0	0.54	0.83	**7.8**	*172*
Other skin	10688	0	-	0.1	-	0.9	1.4	2.9	7.9	13.2	26.3	48.1	74.8	109.0	189.0	302.0	452.7	611.8	744.5	963.8	73.7		2.37	6.14	**54.6**	*173*
Breast	59	0	-	-	-	-	-	-	0.3	0.1	0.1	0.4	0.6	0.5	0.9	2.5	2.4	2.2	3.2	2.8	0.4	0.1	0.01	0.04	**0.3**	*175*
Prostate	8559	0	-	-	0.1	-	-	-	-	0.1	0.3	3.2	11.1	48.1	118.4	248.3	482.4	709.3	938.6	988.9	59.0	17.7	0.91	4.56	**41.3**	*185*
Testis	395	0	1.3	-	0.1	2.3	5.0	5.0	4.6	4.8	2.8	2.8	2.7	1.9	0.9	1.7	2.1	1.1	3.2	1.4	2.7	0.8	0.17	0.19	**2.5**	*186*
Penis, other male genital	100	0	-	0.1	-	0.1	0.1	0.2	0.3	0.3	0.7	0.9	0.7	0.8	1.6	2.5	1.6	4.7	6.5	7.0	0.7	0.2	0.03	0.05	**0.5**	*187*
Bladder	3002	0	0.2	-	-	-	0.4	0.5	1.1	2.0	4.5	8.8	15.4	29.0	58.4	96.7	142.6	183.9	223.8	224.2	20.7	6.2	0.60	1.80	**15.2**	*188*
Kidney etc.	2245	0	2.8	0.7	-	0.1	0.3	0.3	1.3	2.5	6.7	11.7	23.0	35.4	50.8	70.9	87.4	92.1	79.6	100.3	15.5	4.6	0.68	1.47	**12.1**	*189*
Eye	162	0	1.7	0.1	-	0.2	-	0.3	0.2	0.4	0.9	0.8	2.4	1.5	3.6	2.6	3.8	5.0	7.8	4.2	1.1	0.3	0.06	0.09	**1.0**	*190*
Brain, nervous system	1179	0	8.9	4.1	3.6	2.6	3.3	5.4	6.2	5.6	6.6	8.6	13.4	10.0	16.7	20.8	18.2	23.3	21.3	8.4	8.1	2.4	0.48	0.67	**7.5**	*191-2*
Thyroid	323	0	0.1	-	-	0.4	0.8	1.0	1.3	2.0	2.4	3.4	3.4	4.5	4.8	6.0	5.1	6.5	11.0	15.3	2.2	0.7	0.12	0.18	**1.8**	*193*
Other endocrine	79	0	-	0.2	0.3	0.2	0.5	0.3	0.3	0.2	0.4	0.4	0.4	0.4	1.3	2.6	1.3	3.6	3.9	-	0.5	0.2	0.02	0.04	**0.4**	*194*
Hodgkin's disease	402	0	-	0.5	0.9	2.3	3.2	3.5	3.8	3.2	3.4	2.6	2.3	3.2	4.6	3.4	4.0	5.7	5.2	7.0	2.8	0.8	0.17	0.20	**2.4**	*201*
Non-Hodgkin lymphoma	1932	0	1.9	1.0	0.8	2.1	1.9	2.4	3.5	6.7	8.1	13.1	19.8	28.2	33.9	45.5	61.1	69.9	85.4	97.5	13.3	4.0	0.62	1.15	**10.5**	*200,202*
Multiple myeloma	679	0	-	-	-	-	0.1	0.1	0.2	0.6	1.2	2.4	4.6	8.1	13.5	20.4	31.1	33.3	51.7	55.7	4.7	1.4	0.15	0.41	**3.5**	*203*
Lymphoid leukaemia	626	0	5.9	3.3	2.2	2.1	0.8	0.5	0.6	1.1	2.0	1.3	3.4	3.3	7.7	15.9	19.3	24.0	35.6	51.5	4.3	1.3	0.17	0.35	**4.0**	*204*
Myeloid leukaemia	494	0	1.0	0.2	0.2	1.4	1.1	1.2	1.6	1.8	2.1	2.5	3.4	4.8	6.4	8.9	18.5	19.7	26.5	39.0	3.4	1.0	0.14	0.28	**2.7**	*205*
Monocytic leukaemia	24	0	-	-	-	-	0.1	0.1	-	-	-	-	-	0.4	0.4	1.1	2.5	0.6	7.0	0.2	0.0	0.00	0.01	**0.1**	*206*
Other leukaemia	12	0	-	-	-	-	-	-	-	-	-	0.1	0.1	-	0.3	0.4	0.3	0.4	1.9	1.4	0.1	0.0	0.00	0.01	**0.1**	*207*
Leukaemia unspecified	46	0	-	-	-	0.1	0.1	0.1	-	0.1	-	-	0.4	0.5	0.9	0.6	1.1	2.9	5.2	8.4	0.3	0.1	0.01	0.02	**0.2**	*208*
Other and unspecified	1115	0	0.1	-	0.1	0.1	0.1	0.3	0.4	0.9	1.5	3.0	6.6	13.5	20.7	32.9	42.3	63.1	93.1	129.5	7.7	2.3	0.24	0.61	**5.7**	*O&U*
All sites	58998	0	25.2	11.7	11.6	19.3	24.6	32.6	48.2	73.3	122.9	215.5	367.7	650.5	1129.1	1765.5	2525.9	3241.2	3836.4	4369.1	406.9		13.66	35.12	**305.6**	*ALL*
All sites but 173	48310	0	25.2	11.6	11.6	18.4	23.2	29.7	40.3	60.1	96.6	167.5	292.9	541.5	940.0	1463.5	2073.2	2629.4	3091.8	3405.3	333.2	100.0	11.29	28.98	**251.0**	*ALLb*

| Rate from 1 case | | | 0.104 | 0.101 | 0.101 | 0.105 | 0.093 | 0.087 | 0.084 | 0.079 | 0.078 | 0.104 | 0.122 | 0.134 | 0.145 | 0.189 | 0.268 | 0.358 | 0.647 | 1.393 | | | | | | |

FINLAND 1987-1992

ANNUAL INCIDENCE PER 100,000 BY AGE GROUP (YEARS) - FEMALE

SITE	ALL AGES	AGE UNK	0-	5-	10-	15-	20-	25-	30-	35-	40-	45-	50-	55-	60-	65-	70-	75-	80-	85+	CRUDE RATE	%	CR 64	CR 74	ASR (W)	ICD (9th)
Lip	225	0	-	-	-	-	-	-	0.1	0.1	0.2	-	0.1	1.6	1.6	4.4	7.9	6.5	12.1	12.3	1.5	0.4	0.02	0.08	**0.6**	*140*
Tongue	165	0	-	-	-	-	-	0.2	0.4	0.4	0.2	1.0	1.1	0.9	2.0	3.0	4.5	3.8	3.8	10.1	1.1	0.3	0.03	0.07	**0.6**	*141*
Salivary gland	139	0	-	-	0.1	0.1	0.3	0.2	0.4	0.7	0.3	1.2	0.6	1.1	1.5	2.6	2.2	2.3	4.8	5.3	0.9	0.3	0.03	0.06	**0.5**	*142*
Mouth	197	0	-	-	0.3	0.1	0.1	0.1	0.4	0.5	0.2	0.5	1.1	1.5	2.2	2.2	4.7	6.8	8.9	7.5	1.3	0.4	0.03	0.07	**0.7**	*143-5*
Oropharynx	30	0	-	-	-	-	-	0.1	-	0.1	-	0.4	0.4	-	0.4	0.4	0.5	1.4	0.8	0.4	0.2	0.1	0.01	0.01	**0.1**	*146*
Nasopharynx	31	0	-	0.1	-	-	0.2	-	0.1	0.1	0.2	-	-	0.4	0.4	0.3	1.1	0.5	0.8	1.3	0.2	0.1	0.01	0.01	**0.1**	*147*
Hypopharynx	35	0	-	-	-	-	-	-	-	0.1	0.1	0.3	0.1	0.1	0.1	0.5	1.2	1.8	0.8	0.9	0.2	0.1	0.00	0.01	**0.1**	*148*
Pharynx unspecified	7	0	-	-	-	-	-	-	-	-	-	-	0.1	-	0.1	0.1	0.2	0.4	-	0.4	0.0	0.0	0.00	0.00	**0.0**	*149*
Oesophagus	594	0	-	-	0.1	-	-	0.1	-	0.1	0.2	1.2	1.6	2.5	5.5	8.9	15.1	23.0	30.3	41.0	3.9	1.1	0.06	0.18	**1.7**	*150*
Stomach	2970	0	-	-	-	0.1	0.5	0.7	1.8	2.5	6.1	10.3	12.5	20.5	31.7	40.2	71.2	94.1	136.3	180.5	19.3	5.5	0.43	0.99	**9.2**	*151*
Small intestine	190	0	-	-	0.1	-	0.2	-	0.1	0.3	0.6	1.0	1.6	1.9	2.1	4.0	4.2	3.4	5.9	9.7	1.2	0.4	0.04	0.08	**0.7**	*152*
Colon	3654	0	-	0.4	0.7	1.4	1.5	2.4	1.8	3.5	6.7	9.4	18.1	21.7	41.7	55.9	84.2	132.4	155.6	177.9	23.7	6.8	0.55	1.25	**11.6**	*153*
Rectum	2051	0	-	-	-	-	0.1	0.5	0.7	1.7	3.1	6.9	10.8	18.3	21.6	35.8	50.6	69.7	80.5	94.2	13.3	3.8	0.32	0.75	**6.6**	*154*
Liver	896	0	0.4	-	0.1	0.2	0.2	0.2	0.2	0.9	1.1	2.8	2.4	4.9	8.3	12.3	25.5	29.6	39.7	59.4	5.8	1.7	0.11	0.30	**2.7**	*155*
Gallbladder etc.	1143	0	-	-	-	-	-	0.2	0.2	0.3	0.2	1.8	3.6	8.0	15.0	18.8	29.9	38.1	56.6	61.2	7.4	2.1	0.15	0.39	**3.4**	*156*
Pancreas	2368	0	-	-	-	-	0.1	0.2	0.7	0.7	2.5	4.3	7.6	14.0	23.9	41.4	65.2	82.6	111.9	129.9	15.4	4.4	0.27	0.80	**7.0**	*157*
Nose, sinuses etc.	75	0	-	-	-	-	-	0.1	-	-	0.2	0.2	0.4	0.5	1.1	1.0	1.9	2.5	3.0	4.0	0.5	0.1	0.01	0.03	**0.2**	*160*
Larynx	75	0	-	-	-	-	-	-	-	-	0.2	0.3	0.7	1.1	2.0	1.0	1.7	2.0	1.1	2.2	0.5	0.1	0.02	0.04	**0.3**	*161*
Bronchus, lung	2341	0	-	-	0.1	0.2	0.4	0.4	0.9	1.7	5.2	8.2	14.3	21.8	36.5	53.4	60.4	64.9	72.4	61.6	15.2	4.4	0.45	1.02	**8.2**	*162*
Other thoracic organs	63	0	-	-	-	-	-	-	-	0.2	0.1	0.1	0.2	0.1	0.9	0.8	1.7	2.0	3.2	4.0	0.4	0.1	0.01	0.02	**0.2**	*163-4*
Bone	135	0	0.1	0.2	0.6	0.9	1.3	0.7	0.4	1.1	0.3	0.7	1.0	1.4	0.6	1.0	2.0	1.8	1.3	3.5	0.9	0.3	0.05	0.06	**0.7**	*170*
Connective tissue	446	0	1.1	0.5	0.7	1.1	1.4	1.5	2.0	1.5	2.2	2.4	2.0	3.9	4.8	5.9	6.9	8.1	9.1	16.7	2.9	0.8	0.13	0.19	**2.0**	*171*
Mesothelioma	107	0	-	-	-	-	-	0.2	0.1	0.1	0.2	0.6	0.6	1.0	1.5	3.0	2.8	2.2	2.7	2.6	0.7	0.2	0.02	0.05	**0.4**	*MES*
Kaposi's sarcoma	34	0	-	-	-	-	-	-	-	-	0.1	-	-	-	0.1	0.1	0.6	1.3	3.8	2.6	0.2	0.1	0.00	0.00	**0.1**	*KAP*
Melanoma of skin	1513	0	-	-	0.2	1.2	4.1	4.8	6.8	7.7	10.5	12.9	15.4	15.3	15.9	17.1	21.5	27.7	28.7	33.5	9.8	2.8	0.47	0.67	**6.7**	*172*
Other skin	14884	0	-	-	0.6	0.8	2.7	5.3	10.0	18.2	34.6	56.2	79.7	108.4	161.2	230.6	353.0	489.9	611.2	711.1	96.7		2.39	5.31	**48.2**	*173*
Breast	15115	0	-	-	-	0.1	0.5	4.7	18.6	48.4	98.6	173.5	222.4	225.5	198.1	210.5	224.1	262.8	272.3	277.9	98.2	28.2	4.95	7.12	**65.0**	*174*
Uterus unspecified	66	0	-	-	-	-	-	-	-	0.1	0.1	0.2	-	0.9	0.9	0.7	0.5	1.6	3.5	7.9	0.4	0.1	0.01	0.02	**0.2**	*179*
Cervix uteri	893	0	-	-	-	0.2	1.2	2.6	3.3	5.0	5.9	5.8	5.5	7.9	8.9	14.2	16.2	17.1	24.1	19.8	5.8	1.7	0.23	0.38	**3.6**	*180*
Placenta	12	0	-	-	0.1	-	0.5	0.1	0.2	0.2	0.1	-	-	-	-	-	-	-	-	-	0.1	0.0	0.01	0.01	**0.1**	*181*
Corpus uteri	3283	0	-	-	-	-	0.3	0.5	1.0	2.6	7.0	16.7	32.4	52.0	62.7	70.9	75.2	68.6	64.4	63.4	21.3	6.1	0.88	1.61	**12.9**	*182*
Ovary etc.	2656	0	0.1	0.1	0.5	0.8	1.4	2.7	3.2	6.1	11.9	18.7	26.2	34.8	45.1	47.0	49.8	53.9	53.9	52.8	17.3	5.0	0.76	1.24	**10.9**	*183*
Other female genital	525	0	-	-	-	0.4	0.9	0.8	0.6	0.6	1.1	2.4	3.1	2.6	5.6	6.1	11.1	18.3	18.5	31.3	3.4	1.0	0.09	0.18	**1.8**	*184*
Bladder	1001	0	0.1	-	-	-	0.1	-	0.4	0.8	1.4	2.0	3.6	6.9	13.4	15.9	21.3	37.9	45.9	49.3	6.5	1.9	0.14	0.33	**3.1**	*188*
Kidney etc.	1805	0	3.0	0.3	0.2	0.2	0.2	0.5	0.9	1.7	3.6	5.8	11.2	16.0	27.7	44.1	46.4	46.9	47.5	49.8	11.7	3.4	0.36	0.81	**6.7**	*189*
Eye	179	0	1.0	-	-	0.1	0.2	-	-	0.8	0.6	1.6	2.5	2.3	2.3	3.7	3.0	2.3	2.7	3.1	1.2	0.3	0.06	0.09	**0.9**	*190*
Brain, nervous system	1084	0	5.4	5.2	3.0	2.6	3.3	3.0	4.5	5.0	5.5	6.3	7.0	10.6	13.2	14.5	14.6	18.3	14.0	7.9	7.0	2.0	0.37	0.52	**5.8**	*191-2*
Thyroid	1298	0	-	0.1	0.5	2.3	4.1	6.9	8.4	10.2	12.6	12.7	14.4	10.3	12.4	12.7	11.8	16.3	13.7	18.1	8.4	2.4	0.48	0.60	**6.4**	*193*
Other endocrine	62	0	0.1	-	0.1	0.1	0.2	0.2	0.2	-	0.6	1.0	0.7	1.0	0.2	0.5	0.9	1.1	0.5	1.3	0.4	0.1	0.02	0.03	**0.3**	*194*
Hodgkin's disease	321	0	-	0.3	1.4	3.5	1.9	2.5	2.9	2.2	1.2	1.5	1.8	2.0	1.7	2.2	2.2	5.4	5.1	4.8	2.1	0.6	0.12	0.14	**1.8**	*201*
Non-Hodgkin lymphoma	2106	0	0.8	0.6	0.8	0.4	1.5	2.2	2.2	5.4	8.5	9.0	13.2	18.3	28.4	36.3	48.1	55.5	66.8	57.2	13.7	3.9	0.46	0.88	**7.8**	*200,202*
Multiple myeloma	795	0	-	-	-	0.1	-	0.1	-	0.6	1.1	1.6	2.8	5.6	9.5	16.7	21.5	27.3	27.6	39.6	5.2	1.5	0.11	0.30	**2.5**	*203*
Lymphoid leukaemia	523	0	7.0	3.7	1.6	1.1	0.4	0.4	0.5	0.4	0.6	1.8	2.4	3.0	4.4	4.8	9.2	12.4	18.8	17.6	3.4	1.0	0.14	0.21	**2.8**	*204*
Myeloid leukaemia	490	0	1.0	0.2	1.0	0.5	1.4	0.9	1.1	0.7	1.6	2.7	2.6	3.5	6.8	8.0	10.3	12.0	13.4	11.4	3.2	0.9	0.12	0.21	**2.1**	*205*
Monocytic leukaemia	16	0	-	-	-	-	0.1	0.1	-	-	0.1	-	-	-	0.1	0.3	-	1.1	2.6	0.1	0.0	0.00	0.00	**0.1**	*206*	
Other leukaemia	13	0	-	-	-	-	-	-	-	0.2	0.2	0.1	-	0.3	0.4	0.7	0.9	1.4	4.8	6.2	0.1	0.0	0.00	0.00	**0.0**	*207*
Leukaemia unspecified	64	0	0.1	0.1	-	-	-	-	-	-	-	-	-	0.1	0.2	0.7	1.1	0.9	0.4	0.1	0.01	0.01	**0.2**	*208*	
Other and unspecified	1779	0	0.1	0.2	-	0.2	0.1	0.4	0.4	0.9	1.9	3.7	4.9	10.5	15.2	22.8	36.0	56.4	97.4	159.4	11.6	3.3	0.19	0.49	**5.0**	*O&U*
All sites	68454	0	20.3	12.1	12.9	19.1	30.6	46.5	75.3	134.1	239.3	390.1	532.7	664.8	839.6	1077.4	1424.3	1815.3	2182.5	2516.5	444.9		15.09	27.60	**252.3**	*ALL*
All sites but 173	53570	0	20.3	12.1	12.3	18.4	27.9	41.2	65.3	116.0	204.7	333.8	453.1	556.4	678.4	846.8	1071.3	1325.4	1571.2	1805.4	348.1	100.0	12.70	22.29	**204.1**	*ALLb*

Rate from 1 case   0.108   0.105   0.106   0.110   0.097   0.090   0.088   0.083   0.082   0.107   0.120   0.125   0.122   0.131   0.156   0.180   0.268   0.440

France, Bas-Rhin

The activity of the Cancer Registry of Bas-Rhin began in 1974. The registration of cases covers the resident population of the département of the Bas-Rhin.

This département constitutes the northern half of the Alsace region, occupying the east side of the plain drained by the Rhine, and reaching the massif of the Vosges on the west, with a total area of 4758 km². The town of Strasbourg is its regional centre. Forest covers 30% of the land area. The maximum altitude (1100 m) is reached in the Vosges, and the minimum (32 m) on the Rhine plain. The climate is temperate to semi-continental.

The population consisted of 953 219 inhabitants in 1982 (density 194 inhabitants per km²). 54.4% of the population live in an urban environment in agglomerations with over 5000 inhabitants, 27.6% in villages with less than 2000 inhabitants, and 40.8% in the urban agglomeration of Strasbourg. The population is slightly younger than the general French population.

The active population amounts to 46.0% of the total population: 51.7% of this population works in the services sector, 43.2% in industry, and 5.1% in agriculture.

The département is without mineral resources and does not produce any raw materials, but has a major energy-production industry (petrol refineries and hydroelectric stations). The mechanical and electrical construction industry and the food industry (including breweries and wine production) are the most important. Agriculture plays an important role in spite of the low percentage of the population employed in this sector.

Bas-Rhin is a relatively rich département: incomes are high, and the level of consumption is also high, notably for food. Life expectancy in 1990 was 71.6 years for males, and 79.7 years for females.

Bas-Rhin has a high level of medico-social equipment, with 9479 hospital beds in 1990 (1 bed per 80 inhabitants), 1359 general practitioners and 1638 specialists. Hospitals employ 37.4% of all doctors. A number of scattered rural small hospitals permits hospitalization close to the place of residence. More than 70% of cancer patients die in hospital.

Cancer registration is active, the doctors from the registry visiting each of many sources regularly to establish lists of new cases, and to fill out an epidemiological questionnaire. The lists from each of these sources are com-pared to ensure complete registration and eliminate errors, in particular, duplicate registrations. Cancers discovered by autopsy are registered. Death certificates are not used as a source, but serve only to verify the completeness of registration.

For each case of cancer registered, the identity and address of the patient are noted, and in a different file, the date of diagnosis, the method of diagnosis, the laboratory of pathology, the number of the pathological examination, the topography in ICD-O and ICD-9 and morphology coded to ICD-O, and the behaviour (benign, *in situ*, cancer, metastasis). The two sources where the most complete information was found are also noted, as well as the number of the medical file, the date of death, or that of the last information according to which the patient was still alive, and the cause of death.

The identity of the patients is used only to avoid registering more than once the same patient with the same cancer. This makes it necessary to bring together precise data on the identity of the patients. An identification number common to the identity file and the file of medical data is used, which permits the two files to be linked. The data are coded by the doctors who have visited the information sources. Morphology and topography are coded to ICD-O, and when the data are entered, the topography is automatically converted by a computer program to ICD-9.

Lesions or cancers diagnosed or discovered at the *in situ* stage and with histological verification are registered, but are not included in calculations of incidence.

Incidence can be calculated both by person and by tumour. If a person develops more than one primary cancer, each of the cancers is registered separately, while retaining the possibility of linking the cancers to the person in whom they have been registered. A tumour is not considered as a second primary cancer unless it is different at the three-digit level of the topographic code or unless the morphology is different.

For paired organs, with the exception of the ovary and testicle, two primary cancers are registered if they are discovered simultaneously or at an interval of several years in each of the organs. For the colon, different cancers are registered according to whether they appear in the ascending colon, the transverse colon or the descending colon.

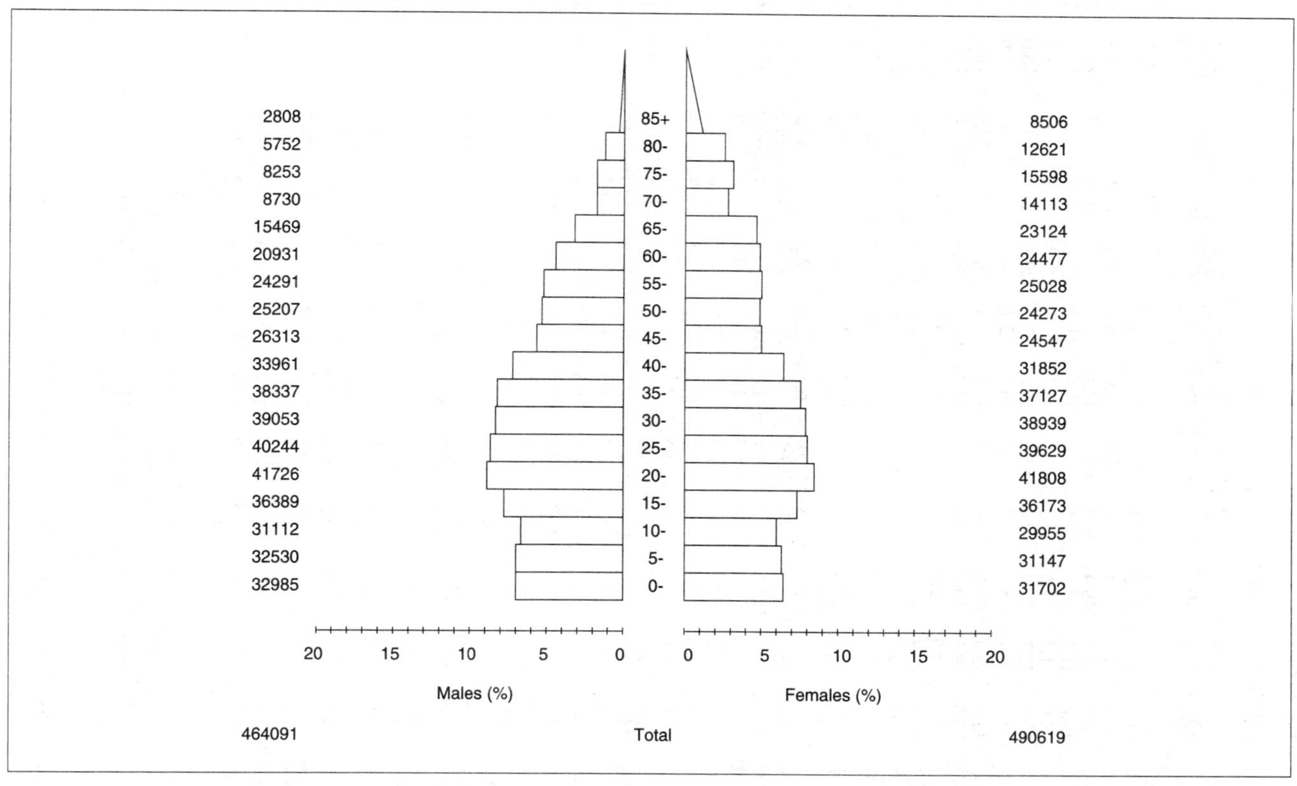

France, Bas-Rhin
Source of population: 1988–92
Census: Recensement de la population 1990, Population de la France, Départements, arrondissements, cantons, communes. Direction Générale des Collectivités Locales, Institut National de la Statistique et des Etudes Economiques.
Estimate: Population estimates provided by the official national department of demography (INSEE) were used for each of the years 1988-92 (Estimations de la Population, INSEE, 1996)

Notes to tables overleaf:
† 173 excludes basal cell carcinoma
† 188 does not include non-invasive tumours
Screening programmes in the area
Organised screening of the population aged 50-65 for breast cancer has been carried out since 1989 (20,000 examinations annually). Screening for cancer of other sites is opportunistic; 100,000 examinations for cervical cancer are carried out each year.

FRANCE, BAS-RHIN 1988-1992

ANNUAL INCIDENCE PER 100,000 BY AGE GROUP (YEARS) - MALE

SITE	ALL AGES	AGE UNK	0-	5-	10-	15-	20-	25-	30-	35-	40-	45-	50-	55-	60-	65-	70-	75-	80-	85+	CRUDE RATE	%	CR 64	CR 74	ASR (W)	ICD (9th)
Lip	18	0	-	-	-	-	-	-	-	0.5	-	-	2.4	2.5	3.8	-	2.3	7.3	10.4	-	0.8	0.2	0.05	0.06	**0.6**	*140*
Tongue	216	0	-	-	-	-	-	-	-	3.1	11.8	16.0	23.0	32.1	49.7	27.2	32.1	17.0	24.3	-	9.3	1.9	0.68	0.97	**8.0**	*141*
Salivary gland	25	0	-	-	-	-	-	-	-	0.5	0.6	1.5	2.4	1.6	2.9	3.9	6.9	9.7	10.4	-	1.1	0.2	0.05	0.10	**0.9**	*142*
Mouth	333	0	-	-	0.6	-	-	0.5	1.5	4.2	16.5	27.4	48.4	56.8	62.1	50.4	13.7	21.8	20.9	7.1	14.4	3.0	1.09	1.41	**12.4**	*143-5*
Oropharynx	317	0	-	-	-	0.5	-	-	1.5	2.6	11.8	31.2	42.8	67.5	56.4	31.0	41.2	17.0	10.4	-	13.7	2.8	1.07	1.43	**11.9**	*146*
Nasopharynx	30	0	-	-	2.6	-	-	0.5	1.0	-	0.6	1.5	1.6	4.1	4.8	5.2	2.3	7.3	-	-	1.3	0.3	0.08	0.12	**1.2**	*147*
Hypopharynx	372	0	-	-	-	-	-	-	-	0.5	3.1	13.5	32.7	52.4	79.0	53.5	55.6	43.5	29.1	20.9	7.1	16.0	3.3	1.17	1.67	**13.9**	*148*
Pharynx unspecified	83	0	-	-	-	-	-	-	-	0.5	3.5	9.1	8.7	17.3	15.3	10.3	13.7	4.8	-	-	3.6	0.7	0.27	0.39	**3.2**	*149*
Oesophagus	443	0	-	-	-	-	-	-	1.0	2.6	11.8	33.4	50.0	79.9	72.6	63.4	89.3	70.3	59.1	14.2	19.1	4.0	1.26	2.02	**16.3**	*150*
Stomach	358	0	-	-	-	-	-	-	0.5	5.2	3.5	9.1	16.7	37.1	44.0	75.0	98.5	128.4	139.1	163.8	15.4	3.2	0.58	1.45	**12.2**	*151*
Small intestine	30	0	-	-	-	-	-	0.5	-	-	0.6	3.0	2.4	3.3	4.8	2.6	9.2	7.3	3.5	14.2	1.3	0.3	0.07	0.13	**1.1**	*152*
Colon	885	0	-	-	-	-	-	0.5	2.0	4.7	11.2	16.7	35.7	79.0	127.1	205.6	261.2	327.2	354.7	327.6	38.1	8.0	1.38	3.72	**30.2**	*153*
Rectum	560	0	-	-	-	-	0.5	-	0.5	1.6	8.2	13.7	27.0	57.6	88.9	115.1	130.6	222.9	208.6	199.4	24.1	5.0	0.99	2.22	**19.0**	*154*
Liver	370	0	-	0.6	-	0.5	-	-	0.5	1.0	3.5	9.1	18.2	42.8	70.7	104.7	84.8	96.9	100.8	78.3	15.9	3.3	0.74	1.68	**13.1**	*155*
Gallbladder etc.	64	0	-	-	-	-	-	-	-	-	1.8	1.5	1.6	6.6	11.5	19.4	11.5	21.8	13.9	28.5	2.8	0.6	0.11	0.27	**2.2**	*156*
Pancreas	192	0	-	-	-	-	-	-	-	0.5	2.9	9.9	12.7	23.9	26.8	44.0	57.3	50.9	45.2	49.9	8.3	1.7	0.38	0.89	**6.9**	*157*
Nose, sinuses etc.	28	0	-	-	-	-	-	-	-	-	1.2	-	2.4	4.9	2.9	6.5	2.3	7.3	10.4	14.2	1.2	0.3	0.06	0.10	**0.9**	*160*
Larynx	310	0	-	-	-	-	-	-	0.5	3.1	6.5	25.8	35.7	48.6	57.3	60.8	48.1	43.6	20.9	14.2	13.4	2.8	0.89	1.43	**11.6**	*161*
Bronchus, lung	1875	0	-	-	-	-	0.5	0.5	3.6	12.0	34.2	76.0	123.8	271.7	328.7	391.8	490.3	470.1	351.2	306.2	80.8	16.8	4.25	8.66	**67.4**	*162*
Other thoracic organs	28	0	-	-	0.6	-	-	0.5	1.0	1.0	1.2	1.5	1.6	3.3	1.9	3.9	9.2	2.4	3.5	7.1	1.2	0.3	0.06	0.13	**1.0**	*163-4*
Bone	31	0	0.6	-	1.3	1.1	2.4	2.0	-	1.6	0.6	0.8	3.2	3.3	1.0	-	2.3	-	7.0	-	1.3	0.3	0.09	0.10	**1.2**	*170*
Connective tissue	49	0	2.4	0.6	-	-	1.9	-	1.0	2.6	0.6	2.3	2.4	3.3	1.0	9.1	11.5	7.3	20.9	-	2.1	0.4	0.09	0.19	**1.9**	*171*
Mesothelioma	17	0	-	-	-	-	-	-	-	-	0.6	0.8	-	1.6	3.8	9.1	2.3	2.4	-	-	0.7	0.2	0.03	0.09	**0.6**	*MES*
Kaposi's sarcoma	54	0	-	-	-	-	1.0	4.5	5.6	6.3	1.8	2.3	3.2	0.8	3.8	-	6.9	2.4	3.5	-	2.3	0.5	0.15	0.18	**1.9**	*KAP*
Melanoma of skin	184	0	-	-	-	-	3.4	4.5	4.1	2.6	14.7	11.4	19.0	13.2	17.2	20.7	27.5	41.2	31.3	21.4	7.9	1.7	0.45	0.69	**6.6**	*172*
†Other skin	485	0	-	-	-	-	0.5	1.0	2.0	1.6	2.4	7.6	9.5	24.7	53.5	85.3	169.5	230.2	264.3	370.3	20.9	-	0.51	1.79	**16.0**	*173*
Breast	36	0	-	-	-	-	-	0.5	0.5	-	-	3.0	1.6	1.6	10.5	6.5	9.2	4.8	10.4	7.1	1.6	0.3	0.09	0.17	**1.3**	*175*
Prostate	1502	0	-	-	0.5	-	-	-	-	-	1.2	4.6	16.7	73.3	172.9	285.7	565.9	790.0	1011.8	833.2	64.7	13.5	1.35	5.60	**48.1**	*185*
Testis	188	0	0.6	-	-	1.6	10.1	20.4	24.1	15.7	8.2	8.4	6.3	4.1	3.8	1.3	2.3	-	-	7.1	8.1	1.7	0.52	0.53	**6.8**	*186*
Penis	21	0	-	-	-	-	-	-	1.0	-	0.6	0.8	1.6	1.6	-	2.6	4.6	14.5	7.0	7.1	0.9	0.2	0.03	0.06	**0.7**	*187.1-.4*
Other male genital	7	0	-	-	1.3	-	-	0.5	-	0.5	-	-	-	0.8	-	-	2.3	2.4	-	-	0.3	0.1	0.02	0.03	**0.3**	*187.5-.9*
†Bladder	660	0	-	-	-	1.1	-	0.5	2.0	4.2	8.2	16.0	34.1	70.8	102.2	148.7	192.4	193.9	219.1	227.9	28.4	5.9	1.20	2.90	**23.1**	*188*
Kidney etc.	439	0	4.9	-	-	-	-	0.5	2.6	4.7	10.0	17.5	38.1	58.5	69.8	85.3	107.7	106.6	76.5	35.6	18.9	3.9	1.03	2.00	**16.1**	*189*
Eye	22	0	0.6	-	-	-	-	0.5	0.5	1.0	0.6	1.5	1.6	2.5	3.8	2.6	4.6	2.4	-	-	0.9	0.2	0.06	0.10	**0.9**	*190*
Brain, nervous system	127	0	3.0	4.9	-	1.6	1.9	1.5	2.6	4.7	5.3	6.8	10.3	13.2	12.4	16.8	20.6	17.0	-	7.1	5.5	1.1	0.34	0.53	**5.1**	*191-2*
Thyroid	36	0	-	-	-	-	1.0	1.0	0.5	2.1	0.6	3.8	3.2	1.6	3.8	3.9	2.3	12.1	-	14.2	1.6	0.3	0.09	0.12	**1.3**	*193*
Other endocrine	18	0	1.8	0.6	0.6	0.5	1.0	-	-	-	1.8	-	-	0.8	-	1.3	4.6	4.8	-	7.1	0.8	0.2	0.04	0.07	**0.8**	*194*
Hodgkin's disease	69	0	0.6	1.2	1.3	1.6	3.4	6.0	3.1	1.0	4.7	4.6	4.8	2.5	2.9	2.6	2.3	-	17.4	-	3.0	0.6	0.19	0.21	**2.7**	*201*
Non-Hodgkin lymphoma	342	0	1.8	1.8	0.6	3.3	4.3	5.0	2.6	7.3	13.5	9.1	19.8	32.9	33.4	51.7	82.5	80.0	121.7	85.5	14.7	3.1	0.68	1.35	**12.1**	*200,202*
Multiple myeloma	67	0	-	-	-	-	-	-	-	0.5	1.8	1.5	6.3	4.1	10.5	15.5	11.5	21.8	24.3	28.5	2.9	0.6	0.12	0.26	**2.3**	*203*
Lymphoid leukaemia	115	0	5.5	1.8	3.2	1.1	-	1.0	0.5	0.5	1.8	2.3	4.8	11.5	10.5	19.4	27.5	36.4	27.8	35.6	5.0	1.0	0.22	0.46	**4.5**	*204*
Myeloid leukaemia	98	0	-	-	-	0.5	2.9	2.5	2.6	3.1	1.8	5.3	3.2	5.8	7.6	12.9	27.5	41.2	17.4	14.2	4.2	0.9	0.18	0.38	**3.4**	*205*
Monocytic leukaemia	7	0	0.6	-	0.5	-	-	-	-	-	-	-	-	1.6	-	-	2.3	2.4	3.5	-	0.3	0.1	0.01	0.03	**0.3**	*206*
Other leukaemia	0	0	-	-	-	-	-	-	-	-	-	-	-	-	-	-	-	-	-	-	0.0	0.0	0.00	0.00	**0.0**	*207*
Leukaemia unspecified	14	0	1.2	-	-	-	-	-	-	-	-	-	-	0.8	0.8	1.0	-	2.3	7.3	17.4	-	0.6	0.1	0.02	0.03	**0.5**	*208*
Other and unspecified	488	0	1.2	-	-	0.5	-	1.0	1.5	3.7	11.8	20.5	24.6	65.0	85.0	93.1	119.1	138.1	100.8	121.1	21.0	4.4	1.07	2.14	**17.4**	*O&U*
All sites	11613	0	24.9	11.7	12.2	15.4	34.5	55.7	71.2	110.1	237.3	450.0	724.4	1319.8	1696.0	2150.1	2859.1	3322.4	3390.1	3055.1	500.5		23.82	48.86	**410.0**	*ALL*
All sites but 173	11128	0	24.9	11.7	12.2	15.4	34.0	54.7	69.1	108.5	235.0	442.4	714.9	1295.1	1642.5	2064.8	2689.6	3092.2	3125.9	2684.8	479.6	100.0	23.30	47.07	**394.0**	*ALLb*

Rate from 1 case   0.606   0.615   0.643   0.550   0.479   0.497   0.512   0.522   0.589   0.760   0.793   0.823   0.956   1.293   2.291   2.423   3.477   7.121

†Important: see notes on population page

FRANCE, BAS-RHIN 1988-1992

ANNUAL INCIDENCE PER 100,000 BY AGE GROUP (YEARS) - FEMALE

SITE	ALL AGES	AGE UNK	0-	5-	10-	15-	20-	25-	30-	35-	40-	45-	50-	55-	60-	65-	70-	75-	80-	85+	CRUDE RATE	%	CR 64	CR 74	ASR (W)	ICD (9th)
Lip	0	0	-	-	-	-	-	-	-	-	-	-	-	-	-	-	-	-	-	-	0.0	0.0	0.00	0.00	**0.0**	140
Tongue	35	0	-	-	-	-	-	-	0.5	-	0.6	1.6	3.3	6.4	4.9	2.6	4.3	3.8	4.8	2.4	1.4	0.4	0.09	0.12	**1.0**	141
Salivary gland	26	0	-	-	-	-	-	-	1.0	-	1.3	-	0.8	0.8	2.5	3.5	4.3	1.3	9.5	7.1	1.1	0.3	0.03	0.07	**0.6**	142
Mouth	36	0	-	-	-	-	-	-	0.5	0.5	0.6	1.6	5.8	4.8	6.5	2.6	1.4	1.3	3.2	7.1	1.5	0.4	0.10	0.12	**1.1**	143-5
Oropharynx	28	0	-	-	-	-	-	-	-	-	-	2.4	3.3	2.4	4.1	2.6	5.7	1.3	4.8	4.7	1.1	0.3	0.06	0.10	**0.8**	146
Nasopharynx	7	0	-	-	0.7	-	-	-	-	0.5	-	-	0.8	0.8	1.6	-	1.4	-	-	-	0.3	0.1	0.02	0.03	**0.3**	147
Hypopharynx	18	0	-	-	-	-	-	-	-	0.5	-	4.1	-	1.6	3.3	2.6	-	2.6	-	2.4	0.7	0.2	0.05	0.06	**0.6**	148
Pharynx unspecified	9	0	-	-	-	-	-	-	0.5	-	-	0.8	0.8	1.6	0.8	0.9	-	1.3	-	2.4	0.4	0.1	0.02	0.03	**0.3**	149
Oesophagus	48	0	-	-	-	-	-	-	0.5	0.5	-	0.8	2.5	6.4	6.5	5.2	7.1	7.7	9.5	7.1	2.0	0.6	0.09	0.15	**1.2**	150
Stomach	240	0	-	-	-	-	0.5	-	1.0	1.6	2.5	4.1	9.9	12.0	13.9	28.5	26.9	64.1	76.1	72.9	9.8	2.9	0.23	0.50	**4.9**	151
Small intestine	20	0	-	-	-	-	-	-	-	0.5	-	0.8	0.8	0.8	2.5	2.6	2.8	6.4	1.6	2.4	0.8	0.2	0.03	0.06	**0.5**	152
Colon	834	0	-	-	0.7	-	1.0	0.5	3.6	5.4	10.7	18.7	35.4	55.9	63.7	94.3	143.1	194.9	193.3	230.4	34.0	9.9	0.98	2.17	**18.8**	153
Rectum	390	0	-	-	-	-	0.5	-	1.0	2.2	5.7	9.8	8.2	28.8	34.3	61.4	65.2	78.2	103.0	72.9	15.9	4.6	0.45	1.09	**8.9**	154
Liver	87	0	1.3	-	-	-	0.5	-	-	1.1	1.9	1.6	4.1	4.8	6.5	13.0	14.2	12.8	23.8	18.8	3.5	1.0	0.11	0.24	**2.1**	155
Gallbladder etc.	136	0	-	-	-	-	-	0.5	-	-	1.3	0.8	2.5	4.8	11.4	13.8	26.9	26.9	46.0	56.4	5.5	1.6	0.11	0.31	**2.7**	156
Pancreas	171	0	-	-	-	-	-	-	-	0.5	0.6	6.5	4.1	12.0	14.7	22.5	28.3	42.3	41.2	42.3	7.0	2.0	0.19	0.45	**3.8**	157
Nose, sinuses etc.	7	0	-	-	-	-	1.0	-	-	-	-	0.8	-	0.8	0.9	-	-	-	-	4.7	0.3	0.1	0.01	0.02	**0.2**	160
Larynx	22	0	-	-	-	-	-	-	-	-	1.3	-	3.3	1.6	2.5	1.7	1.4	3.8	4.8	4.7	0.9	0.3	0.04	0.06	**0.6**	161
Bronchus, lung	274	0	-	-	0.7	-	-	1.0	0.5	3.2	5.7	8.1	16.5	25.6	27.8	46.7	39.7	46.2	38.0	40.0	11.2	3.3	0.45	0.88	**7.2**	162
Other thoracic organs	9	0	-	-	-	-	-	-	-	-	0.6	-	-	1.6	0.8	2.6	-	-	-	4.7	0.4	0.1	0.02	0.03	**0.2**	163-4
Bone	23	0	-	-	1.3	2.2	0.5	-	1.0	0.5	0.6	0.8	1.6	0.8	1.6	2.6	1.4	1.3	-	2.4	0.9	0.3	0.06	0.08	**0.8**	170
Connective tissue	55	0	0.6	0.6	0.7	0.6	1.4	-	1.5	2.2	2.5	0.8	2.5	4.8	1.6	7.8	8.5	6.4	1.6	9.4	2.2	0.7	0.10	0.18	**1.7**	171
Mesothelioma	5	0	-	-	-	-	-	-	-	0.5	-	0.8	-	1.6	0.8	-	-	-	-	-	0.2	0.1	0.02	0.02	**0.2**	MES
Kaposi's sarcoma	6	0	-	-	-	-	-	-	1.0	-	-	0.8	-	-	-	0.9	-	1.3	1.6	-	0.2	0.1	0.01	0.01	**0.2**	KAP
Melanoma of skin	253	0	-	-	0.7	1.1	2.9	4.5	8.2	15.1	9.4	13.9	22.2	17.6	16.3	22.5	29.8	24.4	20.6	25.9	10.3	3.0	0.56	0.82	**7.8**	172
†Other skin	391	0	-	-	-	1.1	0.5	2.0	2.1	-	2.5	8.1	11.5	10.4	24.5	23.4	53.8	91.0	136.3	204.5	15.9		0.31	0.70	**7.4**	173
Breast	2621	0	-	-	-	0.6	1.4	7.1	27.2	61.4	128.1	198.8	215.1	246.1	295.0	301.0	320.3	289.8	248.8	237.5	106.8	31.2	5.90	9.01	**78.8**	174
Uterus unspecified	22	0	-	-	-	-	0.5	-	-	0.5	-	0.8	3.3	2.4	0.8	1.7	5.7	2.6	1.6	4.7	0.9	0.3	0.04	0.08	**0.6**	179
Cervix uteri	317	0	-	-	-	-	1.4	6.6	13.4	22.1	22.6	19.6	22.2	25.6	24.5	19.9	25.5	29.5	19.0	21.2	12.9	3.8	0.79	1.02	**10.0**	180
Placenta	0	0	-	-	-	-	-	-	-	-	-	-	-	-	-	-	-	-	-	-	0.0	0.0	0.00	0.00	**0.0**	181
Corpus uteri	571	0	-	-	-	-	-	-	1.0	1.6	8.2	17.9	48.6	83.9	81.7	75.2	85.0	80.8	50.7	58.8	23.3	6.8	1.21	2.02	**16.1**	182
Ovary etc.	423	0	-	0.6	-	2.2	1.9	3.0	4.6	6.5	5.0	22.8	35.4	51.1	44.1	45.0	70.9	52.6	46.0	42.3	17.2	5.0	0.89	1.47	**12.3**	183
Other female genital	78	0	-	-	-	-	-	-	2.2	0.6	2.4	0.8	3.2	4.9	9.5	12.8	11.5	22.2	37.6		3.2	0.9	0.07	0.18	**1.6**	184
†Bladder	190	0	-	-	-	-	-	0.5	0.5	1.1	1.3	1.6	4.9	14.4	15.5	17.3	38.3	39.7	60.2	54.1	7.7	2.3	0.20	0.48	**4.0**	188
Kidney etc.	266	0	2.5	-	-	0.6	0.5	-	0.5	1.1	5.7	7.3	14.0	24.8	31.9	45.8	46.8	41.0	39.6	21.2	10.8	3.2	0.44	0.91	**7.3**	189
Eye	24	0	1.9	-	-	-	0.5	-	0.5	1.1	-	2.4	1.6	2.4	0.8	0.9	2.8	5.1	1.6	-	1.0	0.3	0.06	0.07	**0.9**	190
Brain, nervous system	117	0	2.5	3.2	0.7	1.7	1.0	2.5	3.1	4.3	3.8	4.1	7.4	12.8	13.1	9.5	7.1	14.1	4.8	2.4	4.8	1.4	0.30	0.38	**4.0**	191-2
Thyroid	85	0	-	-	1.3	-	1.4	2.0	7.7	1.6	3.1	6.5	4.9	4.0	4.9	5.2	9.9	3.8	15.8	4.7	3.5	1.0	0.19	0.26	**2.6**	193
Other endocrine	11	0	2.5	0.6	-	-	-	-	0.5	1.3	-	-	2.4	-	-	-	-	-	-	-	0.4	0.1	0.04	0.04	**0.6**	194
Hodgkin's disease	50	0	-	1.3	1.3	2.8	1.0	4.5	3.1	2.2	3.8	0.8	0.8	1.6	3.3	0.9	-	2.6	4.8	-	2.0	0.6	0.13	0.14	**1.8**	201
Non-Hodgkin lymphoma	324	0	1.3	0.6	1.3	1.7	0.5	2.5	5.1	3.8	8.8	10.6	17.3	13.6	25.3	40.7	46.8	68.0	52.3	72.9	13.2	3.9	0.46	0.90	**8.3**	200,202
Multiple myeloma	47	0	-	-	-	-	-	-	-	-	0.6	0.8	1.6	4.0	4.1	7.8	9.9	7.7	12.7	7.1	1.9	0.6	0.06	0.14	**1.1**	203
Lymphoid leukaemia	90	0	5.7	1.3	1.3	1.1	0.5	-	1.0	1.6	-	1.6	1.6	2.4	8.2	6.9	14.2	21.8	12.7	21.2	3.7	1.1	0.13	0.24	**2.7**	204
Myeloid leukaemia	68	0	-	-	1.3	-	0.5	-	-	0.5	2.5	-	4.1	1.6	6.5	10.4	14.2	10.3	11.1	18.8	2.8	0.8	0.09	0.21	**1.7**	205
Monocytic leukaemia	7	0	0.6	-	-	-	0.5	-	0.5	0.5	-	-	-	-	-	1.4	1.3	1.6	-	-	0.3	0.1	0.01	0.02	**0.2**	206
Other leukaemia	1	0	-	-	-	-	-	-	-	-	-	-	-	-	-	-	1.3	-	-	-	0.0	0.0	0.00	0.00	**0.0**	207
Leukaemia unspecified	9	0	-	-	-	-	-	-	0.5	0.5	-	-	-	0.8	-	1.7	2.8	1.3	-	2.4	0.4	0.1	0.01	0.03	**0.2**	208
Other and unspecified	328	0	3.8	0.6	-	-	-	0.5	1.0	2.2	3.1	10.6	9.9	21.6	27.8	37.2	62.4	62.8	84.0	79.9	13.4	3.9	0.41	0.90	**7.9**	O&U
All sites	8779	0	22.7	9.0	12.0	15.5	20.1	38.4	93.0	149.8	246.1	396.8	534.7	726.4	846.5	1001.5	1242.8	1366.8	1408.7	1511.8	357.9		15.55	26.78	**236.7**	ALL
All sites but 173	8388	0	22.7	9.0	12.0	14.4	19.6	36.3	90.9	149.8	243.6	388.6	523.2	716.0	822.0	978.2	1188.9	1275.8	1272.4	1307.2	341.9	100.0	15.24	26.08	**229.3**	ALLb

| Rate from 1 case | | | 0.631 | 0.642 | 0.668 | 0.553 | 0.478 | 0.505 | 0.514 | 0.539 | 0.628 | 0.815 | 0.824 | 0.799 | 0.817 | 0.865 | 1.417 | 1.282 | 1.585 | 2.351 | | | | | | |

†Important: see notes on population page

France, Calvados

There are two cancer registries in the Département of Calvados, both located in Caen. The general registry is situated in the Centre Régional de Lutte contre le Cancer, and the specialized digestive tumour registry in the University Hospital. The two registries are supported by INSERM (Institut National de la Santé et de la Recherche Médicale) and by the Ministry of Health. They also receive contributions from the National League against Cancer and from the European Union for special studies. They are affiliated to the French Association of Cancer Registries, FRANCIM, and to the EUROCARE network.

The Département of Calvados covers a surface area of 5548 km². Situated in Normandy, it includes parts of the Armorican Massif (Bocage) and of the Paris Basin (Bessin, Plain of Caen, Pays d'Auge). To the north is the coastline of the English Channel. The maximum altitude is 365 m above sea level. The département includes 635 rural communes (35% of the population) and 73 urban communes. There are 625 500 inhabitants, with 48.3% male. Foreigners account for 1.7% of the population. There is very little migration. 6.2% of the population is aged over 75 years. Among those employed, 7.7% are in agriculture, 22.2% in industry, 6.9% building and public works, 12.3% in commerce and 50.9% in service industries. In 1990 unemployment was 8.3%.

Registration has been carried on without interruption since 1978, using data from the private and public medical facilities in the département (22 general hospitals excluding psychiatric care, 1544 doctors including 719 specialists, and six pathology laboratories). Registration is active, and the medical and pathology records are consulted directly. Death certificates are also examined, but the cases for which this is the only source of information are not registered. Completeness is ensured by linking the information collected from the different sources. The index date is the date of first pathological diagnosis or, if this is not available, of the first diagnostic examination such as endoscopy, X-ray or biology. Multiple tumours are registered according to the rules recommended by IARC/IACR. The Digestive Registry routinely codes TNM stage and treatment. The two registries collect follow-up information at regular intervals from the treating physicians and from the municipal registry offices. A computer system common to the two registries permits grouping of the data and cross-linkage. Paper documentation is kept for each case.

In addition to analysis of incidence and trends, many studies are carried out: evolution of stage at diagnosis, evaluation of treatment, survival trends and rare tumours. Of particular interest are environmental factors in relation to oesophageal cancer, tumours of the oral cavity, exposure to herbal medicines, evaluation of treatment for colo-rectal cancer, and peritoneal and pleural mesotheliomas. A mass screening programme for colo-rectal cancer began in 1991, and the effects on the incidence of this cancer have become evident over the last two years.

J.F. Heron
M. Gignoux

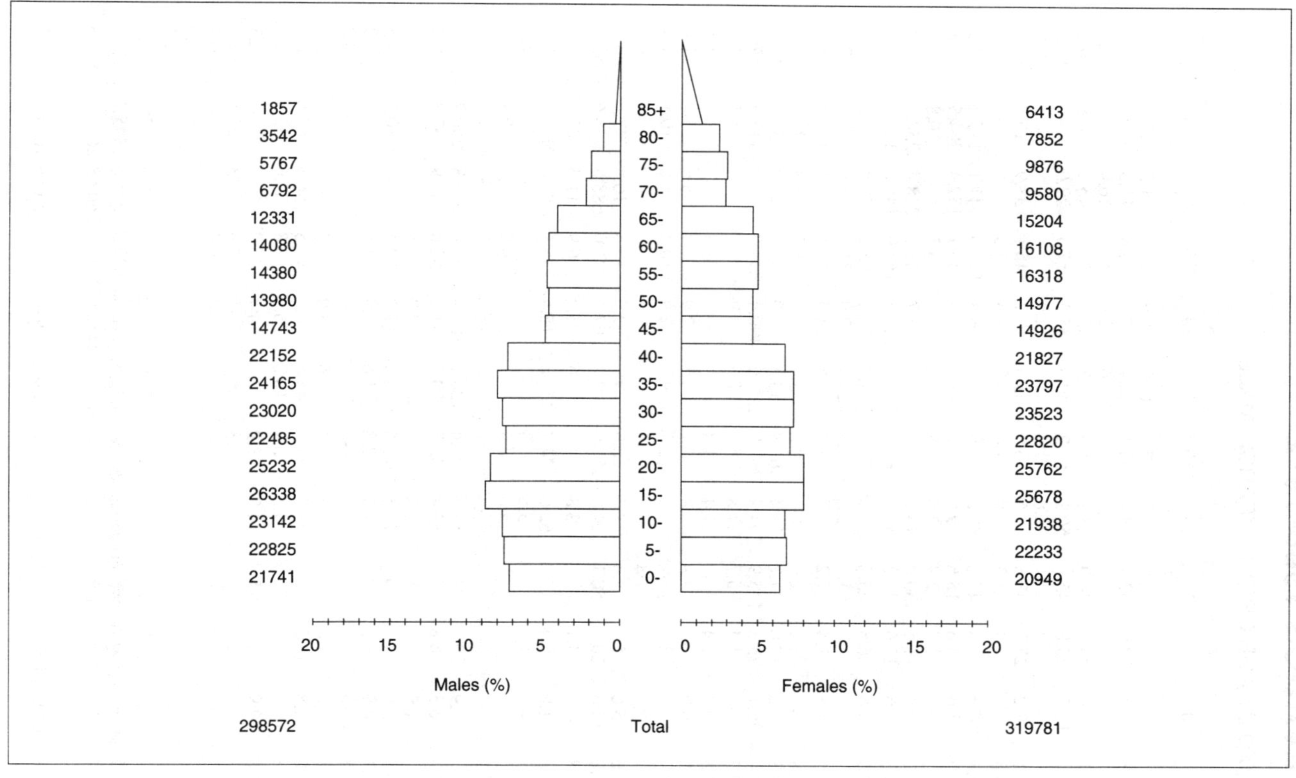

France, Calvados
Source of population: 1988–92
Census: Recensement de la population 1990, Population de la France, Départements, arrondissements, cantons, communes. Direction Générale des Collectivités Locales, Institut National de la Statistique et des Etudes Economiques.
Estimate: Population estimates provided by the official national department of demography (INSEE) were used for each of the years 1988-92 (Estimations de la Population, INSEE, 1996)

Notes to tables overleaf:
*†The data for leukaemia are incomplete and should not be used.
Screening programmes in the area
Screening programmes for large bowel cancer have been set up in different regions of the registration area over the years 1991 and 1992, aimed at the population aged 45-74.

* FRANCE, CALVADOS 1988-1992

ANNUAL INCIDENCE PER 100,000 BY AGE GROUP (YEARS) - MALE

SITE	ALL AGES	AGE UNK	0-	5-	10-	15-	20-	25-	30-	35-	40-	45-	50-	55-	60-	65-	70-	75-	80-	85+	CRUDE RATE	%	CR 64	CR 74	ASR (W)	ICD (9th)
Lip	32	0	-	-	-	-	-	-	-	-	-	-	2.9	4.2	7.1	13.0	5.9	27.7	11.3	21.5	2.1	0.5	0.07	0.16	**1.5**	140
Tongue	132	0	-	-	-	0.8	-	-	-	5.8	9.9	19.0	32.9	33.4	34.1	22.7	17.7	20.8	11.3	-	8.8	2.1	0.68	0.88	**7.8**	141
Salivary gland	9	0	-	-	-	0.8	-	0.9	-	-	-	-	2.8	-	1.6	2.9	-	16.9	-	-	0.6	0.1	0.02	0.04	**0.4**	142
Mouth	154	0	-	-	-	-	-	-	-	4.1	9.0	23.1	20.0	43.1	35.5	37.3	35.3	27.7	45.2	10.8	10.3	2.4	0.67	1.04	**8.7**	143-5
Oropharynx	199	0	-	-	-	-	-	-	-	5.0	11.7	25.8	45.8	50.1	58.2	50.3	35.3	17.3	22.6	-	13.3	3.1	0.98	1.41	**11.7**	146
Nasopharynx	9	0	-	-	-	0.8	-	-	-	-	-	2.7	-	2.8	1.4	1.6	2.9	-	10.8	-	0.6	0.1	0.04	0.06	**0.6**	147
Hypopharynx	262	0	-	-	-	-	-	-	-	4.1	17.2	27.1	48.6	69.5	73.9	63.3	67.7	45.1	33.9	10.8	17.5	4.1	1.20	1.86	**15.0**	148
Pharynx unspecified	15	0	-	-	-	-	-	-	-	0.8	-	1.4	4.3	2.8	1.4	4.9	8.8	3.5	-	-	1.0	0.2	0.05	0.12	**0.9**	149
Oesophagus	406	1	-	-	-	-	-	-	-	0.8	16.3	39.3	48.6	86.2	117.9	107.0	138.4	100.6	141.1	118.4	27.2	6.4	1.55	2.78	**22.3**	150
Stomach	266	2	-	-	-	-	-	-	0.9	5.0	3.6	13.6	18.6	19.5	42.6	77.8	144.3	149.1	152.4	204.5	17.8	4.2	0.52	1.64	**13.4**	151
Small intestine	17	0	-	-	-	-	-	-	-	-	-	2.7	2.9	2.8	2.8	3.2	14.7	3.5	-	10.8	1.1	0.3	0.06	0.15	**1.0**	152
Colon	401	7	-	-	-	-	-	1.8	1.7	0.8	9.9	9.5	30.0	43.1	82.4	123.3	173.7	201.1	248.4	258.4	26.9	6.3	0.91	2.42	**20.1**	153
Rectum	338	1	-	-	-	-	-	-	-	5.0	3.6	17.6	27.2	59.8	63.9	123.3	132.5	163.0	146.8	140.0	22.6	5.3	0.89	2.17	**17.3**	154
Liver	247	1	-	-	-	-	-	-	0.9	2.5	3.6	6.8	25.8	34.8	72.4	98.9	135.4	83.2	28.2	32.3	16.5	3.9	0.74	1.91	**13.3**	155
Gallbladder etc.	33	0	-	-	-	-	-	-	-	-	-	-	1.4	2.8	4.3	21.1	2.9	31.2	5.6	32.3	2.2	0.5	0.04	0.16	**1.5**	156
Pancreas	119	0	-	-	-	-	-	0.9	-	-	1.8	1.4	7.2	9.7	41.2	40.5	38.3	45.1	62.1	129.2	8.0	1.9	0.31	0.70	**6.0**	157
Nose, sinuses etc.	27	0	-	-	-	-	0.8	-	0.9	0.8	-	1.4	2.9	8.3	8.5	3.2	2.9	6.9	11.3	21.5	1.8	0.4	0.12	0.15	**1.5**	160
Larynx	214	0	-	-	-	-	-	-	0.9	3.3	7.2	19.0	37.2	58.4	66.8	50.3	53.0	52.0	28.2	32.3	14.3	3.4	0.96	1.48	**12.1**	161
Bronchus, lung	1005	0	-	-	-	-	-	-	0.9	9.9	36.1	73.3	145.9	204.4	267.0	293.6	400.4	294.7	271.0	118.4	67.3	15.8	3.69	7.16	**55.1**	162
Other thoracic organs	21	0	-	-	-	-	-	-	0.9	1.7	-	1.4	5.7	2.8	5.7	1.6	2.9	-	16.9	21.5	1.4	0.3	0.09	0.11	**1.2**	163-4
Bone	17	0	-	-	0.9	3.8	-	0.9	1.7	2.5	0.9	1.4	-	1.4	1.4	-	-	3.5	-	-	1.1	0.3	0.07	0.07	**1.0**	170
Connective tissue	27	0	1.8	0.9	-	0.8	0.8	-	0.9	2.5	0.9	-	2.9	2.8	7.1	6.5	2.9	6.9	5.6	-	1.8	0.4	0.11	0.15	**1.6**	171
Mesothelioma	21	0	-	-	-	-	-	-	-	1.7	-	2.7	-	1.4	5.7	9.7	2.9	10.4	5.6	10.8	1.4	0.3	0.06	0.12	**1.1**	MES
Kaposi's sarcoma	8	0	-	-	-	-	0.8	-	2.6	-	2.7	-	1.4	-	-	-	2.7	-	-	-	0.5	0.1	0.04	0.04	**0.5**	KAP
Melanoma of skin	58	1	-	-	-	0.8	2.4	1.8	4.3	5.0	3.6	5.4	4.3	8.3	8.5	9.7	2.9	10.4	16.9	43.1	3.9	0.9	0.23	0.29	**3.2**	172
Other skin	782	1	-	-	-	1.5	1.6	0.9	3.5	5.8	14.4	20.3	50.1	64.0	152.0	209.2	297.4	371.0	688.8	936.6	52.4	-	1.57	4.11	**38.2**	173
Breast	21	0	-	-	-	-	-	-	-	0.8	-	4.1	-	2.8	4.3	6.5	5.9	6.9	11.3	21.5	1.4	0.3	0.06	0.12	**1.1**	175
Prostate	1076	0	-	-	-	-	-	-	-	-	1.8	5.4	15.7	62.6	174.7	369.8	615.4	735.1	886.4	915.1	72.1	16.9	1.30	6.23	**50.5**	185
Testis	59	0	0.9	-	-	1.5	4.8	7.1	14.8	8.3	4.5	1.4	4.3	5.6	2.8	-	-	-	-	-	4.0	0.9	0.28	0.28	**3.5**	186
Penis	18	0	-	-	-	-	-	-	-	-	-	-	-	5.6	8.5	3.2	-	6.9	16.9	10.8	1.2	0.3	0.07	0.09	**0.9**	187.1-.4
Other male genital	2	0	-	-	-	0.8	-	-	0.8	-	-	-	-	-	-	-	-	-	-	-	0.1	0.0	0.01	0.01	**0.1**	187.5-.9
Bladder	469	0	0.9	-	-	0.8	0.8	-	2.6	-	9.9	20.3	32.9	83.4	99.4	128.1	188.4	256.6	225.8	290.7	31.4	7.4	1.26	2.84	**23.9**	188
Kidney etc.	148	0	3.7	-	-	-	1.6	-	-	3.3	6.3	6.8	14.3	33.4	32.7	50.3	41.2	52.0	33.9	32.3	9.9	2.3	0.51	0.97	**8.1**	189
Eye	13	0	0.9	-	-	-	-	-	-	-	1.8	-	1.4	2.8	-	4.9	2.9	10.4	-	-	0.9	0.2	0.03	0.07	**0.7**	190
Brain, nervous system	67	0	0.9	3.5	3.5	2.3	3.2	0.9	1.7	0.8	3.6	4.1	10.0	11.1	15.6	6.5	17.7	10.4	-	10.8	4.5	1.1	0.31	0.43	**4.2**	191-2
Thyroid	28	0	-	-	-	-	-	1.8	1.7	4.1	0.9	6.8	8.6	1.4	2.8	1.6	5.9	3.5	-	-	1.9	0.4	0.14	0.18	**1.8**	193
Other endocrine	3	0	0.9	-	-	0.8	-	-	0.8	-	-	-	-	-	-	-	-	-	-	-	0.2	0.0	0.01	0.01	**0.2**	194
Hodgkin's disease	34	0	-	-	-	3.8	4.0	3.6	3.5	4.1	3.6	1.4	-	1.4	1.4	1.6	5.9	3.5	-	-	2.3	0.5	0.13	0.17	**2.0**	201
Non-Hodgkin lymphoma	154	0	-	0.9	1.7	-	-	2.7	1.7	5.0	10.8	12.2	5.7	25.0	31.3	45.4	50.1	48.5	56.5	64.6	10.3	2.4	0.49	0.96	**8.2**	200,202
Multiple myeloma	42	0	-	-	-	-	-	-	-	0.8	-	-	2.9	4.2	5.7	16.2	26.5	20.8	22.6	32.3	2.8	0.7	0.07	0.28	**2.1**	203
†Lymphoid leukaemia	34	0	-	-	-	-	-	-	-	0.8	0.9	-	5.7	4.2	9.9	3.2	14.7	27.7	16.9	-	2.3	0.5	0.11	0.20	**1.7**	204
†Myeloid leukaemia	21	0	-	1.8	0.9	-	0.8	-	1.7	-	0.9	2.7	-	-	4.3	6.5	-	3.5	11.3	21.5	1.4	0.3	0.07	0.10	**1.2**	205
†Monocytic leukaemia	2	0	-	-	-	-	-	-	-	-	-	-	-	-	-	-	-	6.9	-	-	0.1	0.0	0.00	0.00	**0.1**	206
†Other leukaemia	0	0	-	-	-	-	-	-	-	-	-	-	-	-	-	-	-	-	-	-	0.0	0.0	0.00	0.00	**0.0**	207
†Leukaemia unspecified	1	0	-	-	-	-	-	-	-	-	-	-	-	1.4	-	-	-	-	-	-	0.1	0.0	0.01	0.01	**0.1**	208
Other and unspecified	121	0	-	-	-	-	-	-	0.9	1.7	8.1	10.9	25.8	22.3	19.9	25.9	53.0	31.2	39.5	32.3	8.1	1.9	0.45	0.84	**6.8**	O&U
All sites	7132	14	10.1	7.0	6.9	19.0	21.4	23.1	48.7	98.5	205.9	390.7	693.8	1086.2	1575.3	2043.5	2750.0	2899.0	3291.6	3595.7	477.7	-	20.97	44.99	**374.0**	ALL
All sites but 173	6350	13	10.1	7.0	6.9	17.5	19.8	22.2	45.2	92.7	191.4	370.3	643.8	1022.2	1423.3	1834.3	2452.6	2527.9	2602.8	2659.1	425.3	100.0	19.40	40.88	**335.8**	ALLb

Rate from 1 case   0.920 0.876 0.864 0.759 0.793 0.889 0.869 0.828 0.903 1.357 1.431 1.391 1.420 1.622 2.944 3.468 5.646 10.765

†Important: see notes on population page

* FRANCE, CALVADOS 1988-1992

ANNUAL INCIDENCE PER 100,000 BY AGE GROUP (YEARS) - FEMALE

SITE	ALL AGES	AGE UNK	0-	5-	10-	15-	20-	25-	30-	35-	40-	45-	50-	55-	60-	65-	70-	75-	80-	85+	CRUDE RATE	%	CR 64	CR 74	ASR (W)	ICD (9th)
Lip	9	0	-	-	-	-	-	-	-	-	-	-	-	-	2.5	1.3	2.1	2.0	5.1	6.2	0.6	0.2	0.01	0.03	0.3	140
Tongue	16	0	-	-	-	-	-	-	-	-	1.8	4.0	-	3.7	2.5	2.6	2.1	-	7.6	-	1.0	0.3	0.06	0.08	0.8	141
Salivary gland	9	0	-	-	-	-	-	-	-	-	0.9	1.3	-	-	1.2	1.3	2.1	2.0	5.1	3.1	0.6	0.2	0.02	0.03	0.3	142
Mouth	29	0	-	-	-	-	-	-	-	0.8	2.7	1.3	4.0	4.9	5.0	9.2	2.1	-	2.5	12.5	1.8	0.6	0.09	0.15	1.3	143-5
Oropharynx	16	0	-	-	-	-	-	-	-	-	-	4.0	2.7	4.9	2.5	2.6	-	-	2.5	6.2	1.0	0.3	0.07	0.08	0.8	146
Nasopharynx	3	0	-	-	0.9	-	-	-	-	-	-	-	-	-	-	-	2.1	2.0	-	-	0.2	0.1	0.00	0.01	0.1	147
Hypopharynx	4	0	-	-	-	-	-	-	-	-	-	1.3	1.3	-	1.2	1.3	-	-	-	-	0.3	0.1	0.02	0.03	0.2	148
Pharynx unspecified	1	0	-	-	-	-	-	-	-	-	-	-	-	-	-	1.3	-	-	-	-	0.1	0.0	0.00	0.01	0.0	149
Oesophagus	31	0	-	-	-	-	-	-	-	-	-	1.3	4.0	2.5	6.2	5.3	6.3	8.1	7.6	18.7	1.9	0.7	0.07	0.13	1.1	150
Stomach	175	3	-	-	-	-	-	-	0.9	-	3.7	2.7	5.3	11.0	16.1	22.4	27.1	79.0	119.7	71.7	10.9	3.8	0.20	0.45	4.8	151
Small intestine	24	0	-	-	0.9	-	-	-	-	-	-	1.3	1.3	4.9	2.5	3.9	8.4	4.0	2.5	15.6	1.5	0.5	0.05	0.12	0.9	152
Colon	441	4	-	-	-	-	-	-	4.3	4.2	7.3	16.1	18.7	30.6	50.9	82.9	112.7	145.8	152.8	243.2	27.6	9.5	0.67	1.65	14.4	153
Rectum	283	2	-	-	-	-	-	-	0.9	1.7	5.5	5.4	14.7	30.6	47.2	65.8	64.7	79.0	107.0	99.8	17.7	6.1	0.53	1.19	9.8	154
Liver	47	0	-	-	-	0.8	-	-	-	2.5	1.8	-	-	6.1	1.2	9.2	12.5	12.1	17.8	28.1	2.9	1.0	0.06	0.17	1.5	155
Gallbladder etc.	52	1	-	-	-	-	-	-	-	0.8	0.9	1.3	6.7	-	7.4	10.5	8.4	16.2	17.8	31.2	3.3	1.1	0.09	0.18	1.7	156
Pancreas	111	0	-	-	-	-	-	0.9	-	2.5	0.9	4.0	4.0	2.5	21.1	28.9	16.7	42.5	35.7	49.9	6.9	2.4	0.18	0.41	3.7	157
Nose, sinuses etc.	6	0	-	-	-	-	-	-	-	-	-	1.3	-	-	1.2	2.6	2.1	2.0	-	-	0.4	0.1	0.01	0.04	0.3	160
Larynx	14	0	-	-	-	-	-	-	-	-	0.9	2.7	-	3.7	-	2.6	6.3	-	-	9.4	0.9	0.3	0.04	0.08	0.6	161
Bronchus, lung	104	0	-	-	-	-	-	0.9	-	3.4	4.6	9.4	9.3	23.3	17.4	23.7	18.8	20.2	20.4	6.2	6.5	2.2	0.34	0.55	4.6	162
Other thoracic organs	11	0	1.0	-	-	-	-	-	0.9	-	-	-	-	1.2	2.5	1.3	2.1	2.0	5.1	3.1	0.7	0.2	0.03	0.04	0.5	163-4
Bone	17	0	-	-	-	2.3	-	1.8	3.4	-	1.8	-	2.7	-	2.5	-	-	2.0	-	3.1	1.1	0.4	0.07	0.07	0.9	170
Connective tissue	33	0	1.0	-	-	-	2.3	0.9	-	0.8	-	1.3	2.7	1.2	3.7	6.6	8.4	4.0	12.7	12.5	2.1	0.7	0.07	0.14	1.4	171
Mesothelioma	5	0	-	-	-	-	-	-	-	-	-	-	-	2.7	1.2	-	1.3	-	2.0	-	0.3	0.1	0.02	0.03	0.2	MES
Kaposi's sarcoma	3	0	-	-	-	-	-	-	1.7	-	-	-	-	-	-	1.3	-	-	-	-	0.2	0.1	0.01	0.02	0.1	KAP
Melanoma of skin	136	0	-	-	0.9	0.8	3.1	2.6	5.1	14.3	11.9	10.7	17.4	13.5	11.2	17.1	20.9	14.2	20.4	37.4	8.5	2.9	0.46	0.65	6.3	172
Other skin	724	2	-	-	-	-	-	-	3.4	8.4	12.8	18.8	34.7	28.2	69.5	93.4	162.8	245.0	326.0	552.0	45.3		0.88	2.17	21.2	173
Breast	1630	0	-	-	-	-	0.8	10.5	22.1	91.6	142.0	190.3	229.7	264.7	214.8	273.6	242.2	232.9	277.6	237.0	101.9	35.0	5.83	8.41	76.3	174
Uterus unspecified	8	0	-	-	-	-	-	-	-	-	-	-	-	1.2	1.2	1.3	6.3	2.0	-	3.1	0.5	0.2	0.01	0.05	0.3	179
Cervix uteri	222	0	-	-	-	-	-	6.1	13.6	21.0	22.0	20.1	21.4	20.8	22.3	34.2	43.8	22.3	43.3	28.1	13.9	4.8	0.74	1.13	10.4	180
Placenta	1	0	-	-	-	-	-	-	0.9	-	-	-	-	-	-	-	-	-	-	-	0.1	0.0	0.00	0.00	0.1	181
Corpus uteri	200	0	-	-	-	-	-	0.9	-	2.5	6.4	12.1	21.4	27.0	43.5	43.4	56.4	44.5	48.4	18.7	12.5	4.3	0.57	1.07	8.4	182
Ovary etc.	202	0	-	-	0.9	0.8	0.8	1.8	2.6	5.0	11.9	13.4	29.4	34.3	33.5	38.1	31.3	46.6	33.1	24.9	12.6	4.3	0.67	1.02	9.0	183
Other female genital	48	0	1.0	-	-	0.8	-	-	-	0.8	-	1.3	-	1.2	6.2	1.3	18.8	12.1	20.4	43.7	3.0	1.0	0.06	0.16	1.5	184
Bladder	118	0	1.0	-	-	-	-	-	-	-	-	-	5.3	9.8	12.4	27.6	35.5	38.5	50.9	56.1	7.4	2.5	0.14	0.46	3.7	188
Kidney etc.	87	0	1.0	-	-	-	0.8	1.8	-	3.4	2.7	2.7	8.0	11.0	13.7	14.5	25.1	22.3	22.9	15.6	5.4	1.9	0.22	0.42	3.6	189
Eye	6	0	-	-	-	-	-	0.9	-	-	-	1.3	-	1.2	1.2	-	-	-	-	6.2	0.4	0.1	0.02	0.02	0.3	190
Brain, nervous system	55	0	2.9	0.9	-	1.6	1.6	2.6	1.7	2.5	1.8	4.0	4.0	9.8	9.9	9.2	10.4	6.1	-	-	3.4	1.2	0.22	0.31	3.0	191-2
Thyroid	131	1	-	-	0.9	1.6	3.9	10.5	11.1	14.3	11.9	12.1	17.4	13.5	11.2	9.2	12.5	10.1	7.6	12.5	8.2	2.8	0.55	0.65	7.0	193
Other endocrine	7	0	-	-	-	-	-	1.8	0.9	-	0.9	1.3	-	-	1.2	-	2.1	-	-	-	0.4	0.2	0.03	0.04	0.4	194
Hodgkin's disease	35	0	-	-	0.9	3.1	2.3	9.6	4.3	1.7	1.8	1.3	-	1.2	-	1.3	4.2	2.0	-	3.1	2.2	0.8	0.13	0.16	2.1	201
Non-Hodgkin lymphoma	152	2	-	1.8	-	0.8	0.8	1.8	2.6	2.5	5.5	8.0	16.0	14.7	23.6	17.1	29.2	50.6	50.9	34.3	9.5	3.3	0.40	0.63	6.0	200,202
Multiple myeloma	39	0	-	-	-	-	-	-	0.9	-	-	-	8.0	3.7	6.2	7.9	10.4	18.2	7.6	3.1	2.4	0.8	0.09	0.19	1.5	203
†Lymphoid leukaemia	35	0	-	0.9	1.8	-	1.6	0.9	-	-	0.9	-	2.7	3.7	5.0	5.3	12.5	8.1	5.1	9.4	2.2	0.8	0.09	0.18	1.5	204
†Myeloid leukaemia	24	0	-	0.9	-	-	1.6	0.9	0.9	1.7	1.8	1.3	-	-	1.2	2.6	12.5	-	7.6	6.2	1.5	0.5	0.05	0.13	1.1	205
†Monocytic leukaemia	1	0	-	-	-	-	-	-	-	-	-	-	-	-	-	1.3	-	-	-	-	0.1	0.0	0.00	0.01	0.0	206
†Other leukaemia	2	0	-	-	-	-	-	-	0.9	-	-	-	-	-	1.2	-	-	-	-	-	0.1	0.0	0.01	0.01	0.1	207
†Leukaemia unspecified	2	0	-	-	-	-	-	-	-	-	-	-	-	-	-	1.3	2.1	-	-	-	0.1	0.0	0.00	0.02	0.1	208
Other and unspecified	72	0	-	-	-	-	-	-	-	1.7	1.8	4.0	2.7	7.4	11.2	15.8	10.4	22.3	38.2	15.6	4.5	1.5	0.14	0.27	2.5	O&U
All sites	5381	15	7.6	4.5	7.3	12.5	19.4	57.0	82.5	188.3	269.4	361.8	498.1	600.5	694.0	903.7	1054.3	1223.1	1482.3	1727.7	336.5		14.05	23.87	217.1	ALL
All sites but 173	4657	13	7.6	4.5	7.3	12.5	19.4	57.0	79.1	179.9	256.6	343.0	463.4	572.3	624.5	810.3	891.4	978.1	1156.3	1175.7	291.3	100.0	13.17	21.70	195.9	ALLb
Rate from 1 case			0.955	0.900	0.912	0.779	0.776	0.876	0.850	0.840	0.916	1.340	1.335	1.226	1.242	1.315	2.088	2.025	2.547	3.119						

†Important: see notes on population page

France, Doubs

The Cancer Registry of Doubs began its activities in 1976. Its main purpose is the collection of data on cancer incidence in the département, with special reference to urban and rural cancer distribution and analytical studies (case–control) using the data of the registry. The registry is partly supported by INSERM (Institut National de la Santé et de la Recherche Médicale) and the Ministry of Health. The cancer registry has received special grants to perform specific descriptive or analytical studies.

The registration area is the Doubs département, which covers 5260 km^2 and had a total population of 484 770 (321 282 in urban areas and 163 488 in rural areas) according to the 1990 census, of whom 216 468 (123 877 men and 92 591 women) were economically active. 9000 work in agriculture, 81 000 are labourers and 105 000 work in business, administrative, sales and transport sector.

There are 11 776 residents who work across the border in Switzerland and 34 937 foreigners who work in the département, mostly from north Africa. The main religion is Roman Catholic.

There are two industrial areas: one in Sochaux-Montbeliard, with a large automobile factory, and the other in Besançon, the main city, which has several small industries that produce little or no pollution.

There was about one physician per 780 inhabitants in 1990. All the population have health insurance. Nearly all Doubs inhabitants are treated in the département, although a few go to Switzerland which is on its eastern frontier.

The registry obtains morbidity data from pathology laboratories, hospitals and private clinic files and private specialist practitioners. However, it is difficult to convince some practitioners to submit data because of confidentiality and the absence of any specific law in France on this problem. Residents who are treated in a regional or a Parisian cancer institute are also registered.

Data collected on the report card include name, address, age, sex, source of information, basis of diagnosis (histological or, if not available, diagnosis by X-ray or by clinical or endoscopic examination), primary tumour site, tumour stage, details of histological diagnosis and name of the laboratory and the initial treatments. The index date is the day of diagnosis. Cards are returned either monthly or annually to the cancer registry, but more frequently registry staff visit all wards of the three hospitals or enquire from the private practitioners. Copies of death certificates are sent to the registry by the local Director of Health, but they are anonymous and are not used as sources of data. The autopsy rate is low and few data are obtained from autopsies. Information is stored using a binary code to ensure confidentiality. Access to information is controlled by passwords.

Checking for duplicates is done by hand and by computer on the basis of two index files: by name and by date of birth. Residence at index date is checked with the official registers of towns and villages to separate urban from rural areas. Follow-up of cases is done only for survival computation.

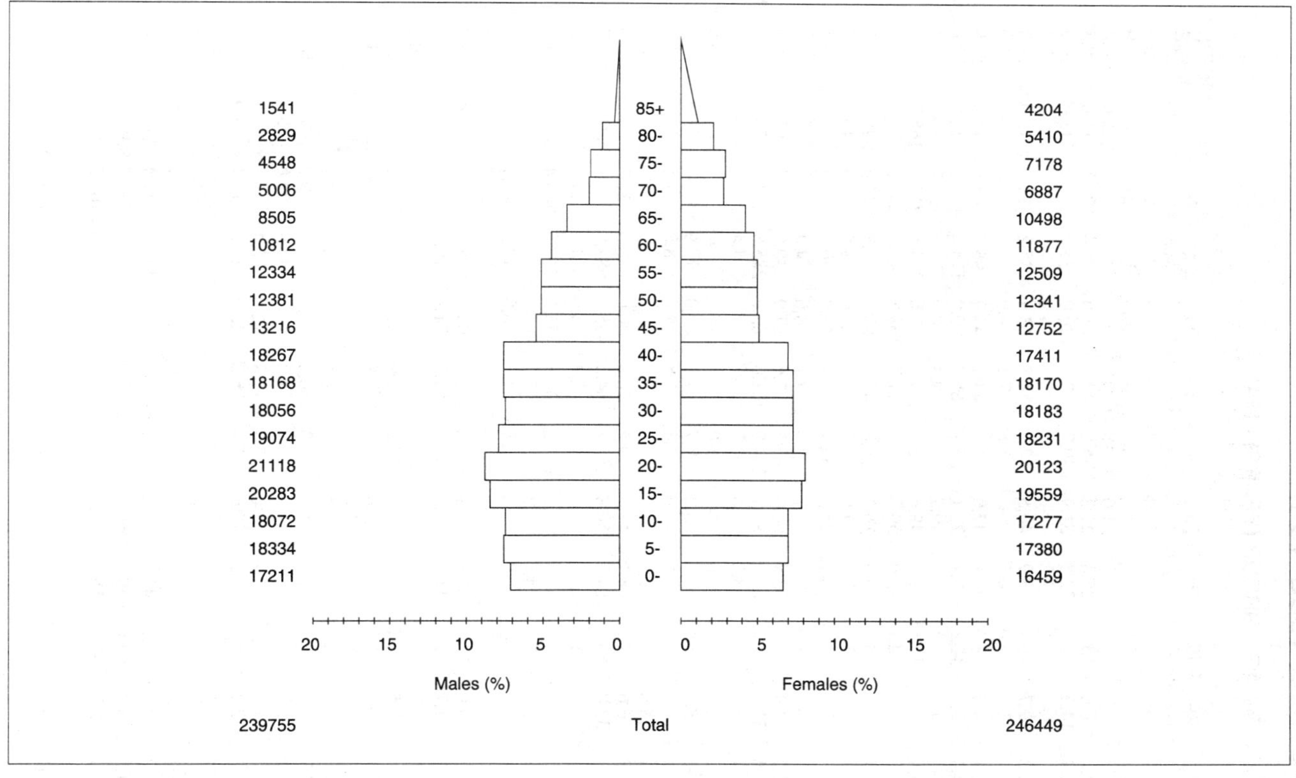

France, Doubs
Source of population: 1988–92
Census: Recensement de la population 1990, Population de la France, Départements, arrondissements, cantons, communes. Direction Générale des Collectivités Locales, Institut National de la Statistique et des Etudes Economiques.
Estimate: Population estimates provided by the official national department of demography (INSEE) were used for each of the years 1988-92 (Estimations de la Population, INSEE, 1996)

FRANCE, DOUBS 1988-1992

ANNUAL INCIDENCE PER 100,000 BY AGE GROUP (YEARS) - MALE

SITE	ALL AGES	AGE UNK	0-	5-	10-	15-	20-	25-	30-	35-	40-	45-	50-	55-	60-	65-	70-	75-	80-	85+	CRUDE RATE	%	CR 64	CR 74	ASR (W)	ICD (9th)
Lip	4	0	-	-	-	-	-	-	-	-	-	-	-	-	1.8	-	4.0	-	14.1	-	0.3	0.1	0.01	0.03	**0.2**	*140*
Tongue	71	1	-	-	-	-	0.9	-	-	7.7	3.3	7.6	11.3	21.1	20.3	14.1	36.0	17.6	21.2	13.0	5.9	1.5	0.37	0.62	**5.0**	*141*
Salivary gland	5	0	-	-	-	-	-	-	-	-	-	-	-	1.6	1.8	4.7	-	-	-	13.0	0.4	0.1	0.02	0.04	**0.3**	*142*
Mouth	105	0	-	-	-	-	-	1.1	2.2	6.6	13.6	25.8	29.2	35.1	49.4	28.0	4.4	28.3	13.0	8.8	2.2	0.57	0.96	**7.6**	*143-5*
Oropharynx	131	2	-	-	-	-	-	1.1	2.2	14.2	22.7	22.6	51.9	40.7	32.9	20.0	35.2	14.1	13.0	10.9	2.7	0.79	1.06	**9.3**	*146*
Nasopharynx	5	0	-	-	-	-	-	-	-	-	1.5	3.2	-	-	2.4	4.0	-	-	-	0.4	0.1	0.02	0.06	**0.4**	*147*
Hypopharynx	141	2	-	-	-	-	-	2.2	2.2	7.7	9.1	33.9	40.5	42.5	58.8	63.9	35.2	21.2	13.0	11.8	2.9	0.70	1.32	**10.0**	*148*
Pharynx unspecified	12	0	-	-	-	-	-	-	-	1.1	3.0	6.5	-	1.8	7.1	4.0	-	-	-	1.0	0.2	0.06	0.12	**0.9**	*149*
Oesophagus	165	1	-	-	-	-	-	-	1.1	4.4	13.6	29.1	47.0	64.7	44.7	47.9	96.7	63.6	77.8	13.8	3.4	0.80	1.27	**11.1**	*150*
Stomach	166	1	-	-	-	-	-	2.2	4.4	7.7	12.1	9.7	21.1	35.1	65.8	99.9	114.3	127.2	116.8	13.8	3.5	0.46	1.30	**10.7**	*151*
Small intestine	17	0	-	-	-	-	-	-	-	1.1	1.5	-	9.7	-	9.4	8.0	-	21.2	-	1.4	0.4	0.06	0.15	**1.1**	*152*
Colon	301	1	-	-	-	-	-	1.1	4.4	9.9	13.6	27.5	48.6	68.4	129.3	183.8	215.5	212.1	168.7	25.1	6.3	0.87	2.44	**19.5**	*153*
Rectum	264	0	-	-	-	-	-	2.2	5.5	5.5	12.1	21.0	50.3	86.9	91.7	163.8	145.1	240.3	77.8	22.0	5.5	0.92	2.20	**17.1**	*154*
Liver	98	0	-	-	-	-	-	1.1	1.1	-	3.0	6.5	16.2	38.8	42.3	63.9	74.8	42.4	25.9	8.2	2.0	0.33	0.87	**6.5**	*155*
Gallbladder etc.	20	0	-	-	-	-	-	1.1	-	1.1	3.0	-	4.9	3.7	-	12.0	8.8	35.3	13.0	1.7	0.4	0.07	0.13	**1.2**	*156*
Pancreas	78	0	-	-	-	-	-	-	-	2.2	7.6	8.1	25.9	35.1	25.9	40.0	30.8	21.2	-	6.5	1.6	0.39	0.72	**5.4**	*157*
Nose, sinuses etc.	14	0	-	-	-	-	-	-	-	-	1.5	1.6	3.2	7.4	7.1	8.0	4.4	-	-	1.2	0.3	0.07	0.14	**1.0**	*160*
Larynx	188	0	-	-	-	-	-	2.2	2.2	4.4	15.1	33.9	60.0	83.2	77.6	67.9	30.8	42.4	51.9	15.7	3.9	1.01	1.73	**13.3**	*161*
Bronchus, lung	735	2	-	-	-	-	-	5.5	17.6	31.8	72.6	105.0	189.7	234.9	301.0	363.6	285.8	254.5	77.8	61.3	15.3	3.29	6.63	**50.8**	*162*
Other thoracic organs	8	0	-	-	-	-	-	1.1	1.1	-	-	3.2	1.6	3.7	-	-	4.4	-	-	0.7	0.2	0.05	0.05	**0.6**	*163-4*
Bone	10	0	-	2.2	3.3	3.0	-	-	-	-	-	1.6	-	1.8	-	-	-	-	-	0.8	0.2	0.06	0.06	**0.9**	*170*
Connective tissue	38	0	4.6	1.1	3.3	-	-	-	2.2	-	3.3	3.0	8.1	3.2	3.7	7.1	24.0	17.6	-	13.0	3.2	0.8	0.16	0.32	**3.1**	*171*
Mesothelioma	22	0	-	-	-	-	-	-	-	-	-	1.5	6.5	1.6	7.4	11.8	12.0	8.8	7.1	13.0	1.8	0.5	0.08	0.20	**1.6**	*MES*
Kaposi's sarcoma	11	0	-	-	-	-	-	-	3.3	1.1	6.6	-	1.6	-	-	-	-	-	-	0.9	0.2	0.06	0.06	**0.7**	*KAP*
Melanoma of skin	67	2	-	-	1.1	2.0	3.8	3.1	3.3	3.3	6.6	7.6	8.1	11.4	9.2	18.8	20.0	8.8	21.2	38.9	5.6	1.4	0.31	0.51	**4.8**	*172*
Other skin	1015	57	-	-	-	1.0	1.9	5.2	11.1	17.6	32.8	63.6	84.0	150.8	253.4	364.5	455.5	584.8	749.3	804.4	84.7		3.29	7.64	**65.9**	*173*
Breast	7	0	-	-	-	-	-	-	-	-	-	1.5	-	1.8	2.4	4.0	4.4	14.1	-	0.6	0.1	0.02	0.05	**0.4**	*175*
Prostate	733	2	-	-	-	-	-	-	-	-	4.5	11.3	50.3	157.2	331.5	455.5	712.4	869.4	843.3	61.1	15.3	1.12	5.07	**44.0**	*185*
Testis	73	0	-	-	3.9	8.5	12.6	12.2	19.8	6.6	7.6	4.8	3.2	-	7.1	-	-	-	-	6.1	1.5	0.40	0.43	**5.4**	*186*
Penis	15	0	-	-	-	-	-	-	-	-	-	4.8	3.2	1.8	4.7	8.0	13.2	14.1	-	1.3	0.3	0.05	0.11	**0.9**	*187.1-.4*
Other male genital	4	0	-	-	-	-	-	-	-	-	-	-	1.8	-	-	-	-	21.2	-	0.3	0.1	0.01	0.01	**0.2**	*187.5-.9*
Bladder	398	4	-	-	1.0	0.9	-	1.1	1.1	9.9	24.2	54.9	55.1	127.6	152.8	199.8	268.2	219.1	272.4	33.2	8.3	1.39	3.17	**26.4**	*188*
Kidney etc.	129	0	1.2	2.2	-	-	-	-	-	1.1	7.7	9.1	11.3	27.6	40.7	54.1	71.9	79.2	35.3	25.9	10.8	2.7	0.50	1.13	**8.9**	*189*
Eye	7	0	2.3	-	1.1	-	-	1.0	-	-	-	-	3.2	-	-	4.0	-	-	-	0.6	0.1	0.04	0.06	**0.7**	*190*
Brain, nervous system	64	0	4.6	2.2	1.1	3.0	1.9	4.2	2.2	3.3	5.5	6.1	6.5	3.2	12.9	25.9	28.0	8.8	7.1	-	5.3	1.3	0.28	0.55	**5.1**	*191-2*
Thyroid	16	0	-	1.1	1.1	1.0	0.9	2.1	2.2	1.1	-	1.5	-	1.6	7.4	2.4	-	-	-	1.3	0.3	0.10	0.11	**1.3**	*193*
Other endocrine	4	0	-	-	1.1	1.0	-	-	-	-	-	-	1.6	1.6	-	-	-	-	-	0.3	0.1	0.03	0.03	**0.3**	*194*
Hodgkin's disease	29	0	-	-	1.1	3.0	2.8	3.1	8.9	3.3	-	3.0	-	3.2	-	4.7	-	4.4	7.1	2.4	0.6	0.14	0.17	**2.1**	*201*
Non-Hodgkin lymphoma	198	0	-	3.3	1.1	2.0	1.9	4.2	6.6	7.7	8.8	12.1	30.7	34.1	57.3	56.4	51.9	127.5	99.0	77.8	16.5	4.1	0.85	1.39	**13.3**	*200,202*
Multiple myeloma	60	0	-	-	-	-	-	-	-	1.1	5.5	3.0	-	11.4	22.2	21.2	12.0	44.0	63.6	25.9	5.0	1.2	0.22	0.38	**3.7**	*203*
Lymphoid leukaemia	43	0	5.8	2.2	2.2	2.0	1.9	1.0	-	-	1.1	9.1	3.2	1.6	7.4	11.8	12.0	26.4	-	13.0	3.6	0.9	0.19	0.31	**3.6**	*204*
Myeloid leukaemia	52	0	-	1.1	1.1	1.0	0.9	1.0	1.1	-	2.2	-	4.8	14.6	7.4	28.2	20.0	35.2	14.1	13.0	4.3	1.1	0.18	0.42	**3.5**	*205*
Monocytic leukaemia	1	0	-	-	-	-	0.9	-	-	-	-	-	-	-	-	-	-	-	-	0.1	0.0	0.00	0.00	**0.1**	*206*
Other leukaemia	1	0	-	-	-	-	-	-	-	-	-	-	1.6	-	-	-	-	-	-	0.1	0.0	0.01	0.01	**0.1**	*207*
Leukaemia unspecified	10	0	1.2	-	-	-	-	-	1.1	-	-	-	-	-	5.5	2.4	4.0	4.4	7.1	13.0	0.8	0.2	0.04	0.07	**0.7**	*208*
Other and unspecified	283	3	-	-	-	-	1.9	-	1.1	2.2	10.9	24.2	43.6	58.4	81.4	96.4	143.8	123.1	141.4	220.6	23.6	5.9	1.13	2.34	**19.2**	*O&U*
All sites	5818	78	19.8	15.3	17.7	23.7	29.4	37.7	77.5	114.5	208.0	395.0	639.7	1060.4	1614.9	2167.9	2744.7	3174.9	3449.5	3048.8	485.3		21.56	46.45	**389.1**	*ALL*
All sites but 173	4803	21	19.8	15.3	17.7	22.7	27.5	32.5	66.5	96.9	175.2	331.4	555.7	909.6	1361.5	1803.5	2289.3	2590.0	2700.2	2244.4	400.6	100.0	18.24	38.79	**323.1**	*ALLb*

| Rate from 1 case | | | 1.162 | 1.091 | 1.107 | 0.986 | 0.947 | 1.049 | 1.108 | 1.101 | 1.095 | 1.513 | 1.615 | 1.621 | 1.850 | 2.351 | 3.995 | 4.397 | 7.069 | 12.974 | | | | | | |

FRANCE, DOUBS 1988-1992

ANNUAL INCIDENCE PER 100,000 BY AGE GROUP (YEARS) - FEMALE

SITE	ALL AGES	AGE UNK	0-	5-	10-	15-	20-	25-	30-	35-	40-	45-	50-	55-	60-	65-	70-	75-	80-	85+	CRUDE RATE	%	CR 64	CR 74	ASR (W)	ICD (9th)
Lip	0	0	-	-	-	-	-	-	-	-	-	-	-	1.6	1.6	8.4	3.8	5.8	-	-	0.0	0.0	0.00	0.00	0.0	140
Tongue	16	0	-	-	-	-	-	-	-	-	-	-	-	1.6	1.6	8.4	3.8	5.8	-	11.1	9.5	1.3	0.4	0.06	0.11	0.8	141
Salivary gland	8	0	-	-	-	-	1.0	-	-	1.1	-	-	1.6	-	-	1.9	2.9	-	3.7	9.5	0.6	0.2	0.02	0.04	0.4	142
Mouth	25	0	-	-	-	-	-	-	-	-	-	4.7	6.5	4.8	3.4	5.7	11.6	11.1	3.7	4.8	2.0	0.7	0.10	0.18	1.5	143-5
Oropharynx	16	0	-	-	-	-	-	-	-	-	1.1	4.7	3.2	4.8	-	1.9	8.7	8.4	-	-	1.3	0.4	0.07	0.12	1.0	146
Nasopharynx	5	0	-	-	-	-	-	-	1.1	-	1.6	-	1.6	1.7	1.9	-	-	-	-	-	0.4	0.1	0.03	0.04	0.3	147
Hypopharynx	6	0	-	-	-	-	-	-	-	-	-	1.6	1.6	1.7	3.8	-	2.8	-	-	-	0.5	0.2	0.02	0.04	0.4	148
Pharynx unspecified	0	0	-	-	-	-	-	-	-	-	-	-	-	-	-	-	-	-	-	-	0.0	0.0	0.00	0.00	0.0	149
Oesophagus	26	0	-	-	-	-	-	-	-	1.1	1.1	3.1	4.9	1.6	5.1	11.4	5.8	8.4	7.4	9.5	2.1	0.7	0.08	0.17	1.5	150
Stomach	97	1	-	-	-	-	1.0	-	-	2.2	2.3	-	8.1	-	5.1	21.0	31.9	55.7	88.7	80.9	7.9	2.7	0.09	0.36	3.7	151
Small intestine	12	0	-	-	-	-	-	-	-	-	1.1	-	-	3.2	5.1	5.7	2.9	2.8	3.7	-	1.0	0.3	0.05	0.09	0.7	152
Colon	282	3	-	-	-	1.0	-	2.2	2.2	4.4	5.7	15.7	43.8	25.6	47.1	80.0	78.4	86.4	214.4	123.7	22.9	7.9	0.75	1.55	13.7	153
Rectum	200	1	-	-	-	-	-	-	-	3.3	4.6	9.4	17.8	32.0	42.1	51.4	63.9	97.5	73.9	123.7	16.2	5.6	0.55	1.13	9.7	154
Liver	32	0	-	-	-	-	1.0	-	-	1.1	3.4	-	1.6	6.4	5.1	7.6	14.5	16.7	7.4	9.5	2.6	0.9	0.09	0.20	1.7	155
Gallbladder etc.	44	0	-	-	-	-	-	1.1	-	1.1	3.1	-	8.0	6.7	5.7	26.1	16.7	37.0	14.3	3.6	1.2	0.10	0.26	2.0	156
Pancreas	42	0	-	-	-	-	-	1.1	-	-	3.1	1.6	3.2	10.1	22.9	14.5	19.5	14.8	9.5	3.4	1.2	0.10	0.28	2.2	157
Nose, sinuses etc.	3	0	-	-	-	-	-	-	-	-	-	-	-	1.7	1.9	-	-	-	4.8	0.2	0.1	0.01	0.02	0.1	160
Larynx	10	0	-	-	-	-	-	-	-	-	-	-	3.2	1.6	1.7	7.6	2.9	2.8	-	-	0.8	0.3	0.03	0.09	0.6	161
Bronchus, lung	114	0	-	-	-	1.0	-	-	3.3	4.4	6.9	6.3	13.0	30.4	25.3	30.5	34.8	36.2	33.3	19.0	9.3	3.2	0.45	0.78	6.5	162
Other thoracic organs	3	0	-	-	-	-	1.0	-	-	-	-	-	-	-	-	-	2.9	-	3.7	-	0.2	0.1	0.00	0.02	0.2	163-4
Bone	15	1	1.2	-	1.2	1.0	-	-	2.2	-	1.1	-	-	1.6	1.7	-	5.8	5.6	3.7	4.8	1.2	0.4	0.05	0.08	1.0	170
Connective tissue	29	1	2.4	-	-	1.0	-	1.1	2.2	2.2	3.4	4.7	3.2	3.2	1.7	3.8	5.8	5.6	3.7	9.5	2.4	0.8	0.13	0.18	2.0	171
Mesothelioma	6	0	-	-	-	-	-	-	-	-	-	-	-	1.6	1.7	5.7	-	-	3.7	-	0.5	0.2	0.02	0.04	0.3	MES
Kaposi's sarcoma	0	0	-	-	-	-	-	-	-	-	-	-	-	-	-	-	-	-	-	-	0.0	0.0	0.00	0.00	0.0	KAP
Melanoma of skin	136	5	-	-	-	-	4.0	11.0	14.3	9.9	14.9	14.1	13.0	17.6	26.9	13.3	23.2	27.9	25.9	28.5	11.0	3.8	0.65	0.84	8.6	172
Other skin	974	45	-	1.2	1.2	2.0	3.0	-	17.6	17.6	33.3	59.6	85.9	107.1	163.3	236.2	270.1	351.1	469.5	647.0	79.0		2.58	5.23	47.2	173
Breast	1095	11	-	-	-	-	1.0	4.4	19.8	50.6	114.9	191.3	207.4	201.5	217.2	224.8	238.1	225.7	262.5	275.9	88.9	30.7	5.09	7.43	67.3	174
Uterus unspecified	6	0	-	-	-	-	-	-	-	-	-	1.6	-	-	1.7	-	5.8	-	3.7	4.8	0.5	0.2	0.02	0.05	0.3	179
Cervix uteri	129	3	-	-	-	-	4.4	9.9	14.3	16.1	12.5	11.3	25.6	18.5	26.7	17.4	33.4	33.3	14.3		10.5	3.6	0.58	0.80	7.8	180
Placenta	5	0	-	-	-	-	2.0	2.2	-	-	1.1	-	-	-	-	-	-	-	-	-	0.4	0.1	0.03	0.03	0.4	181
Corpus uteri	176	7	-	-	-	-	-	-	-	3.3	8.0	7.8	21.1	35.2	53.9	49.5	58.1	52.9	55.5	33.3	14.3	4.9	0.67	1.23	9.8	182
Ovary etc.	137	3	-	-	-	-	1.0	4.4	4.4	2.2	11.5	12.5	27.6	28.8	25.3	32.4	17.4	39.0	44.4	28.5	11.1	3.8	0.60	0.86	8.1	183
Other female genital	47	1	-	-	-	-	-	-	-	-	-	3.1	3.2	3.2	3.4	9.5	8.7	33.4	37.0	38.1	3.8	1.3	0.07	0.16	1.8	184
Bladder	90	0	-	-	-	-	1.0	-	-	-	5.7	1.6	6.5	8.0	23.6	26.7	17.4	39.0	40.7	71.4	7.3	2.5	0.23	0.45	4.2	188
Kidney etc.	96	3	-	2.3	1.2	1.0	3.0	-	1.1	3.3	3.4	7.8	9.7	16.0	20.2	19.1	46.5	41.8	18.5	-	7.8	2.7	0.36	0.69	5.7	189
Eye	4	0	-	-	-	-	-	-	1.1	-	-	-	1.6	-	1.7	1.9	-	-	-	-	0.3	0.1	0.02	0.03	0.3	190
Brain, nervous system	62	0	1.2	4.6	-	-	2.0	-	1.1	3.3	4.6	15.7	4.9	4.8	13.5	17.1	20.3	8.4	11.1	4.8	5.0	1.7	0.28	0.47	4.3	191-2
Thyroid	78	0	-	-	-	3.1	4.0	4.4	7.7	7.7	3.4	18.8	11.3	4.8	11.8	9.5	14.5	19.5	3.7	14.3	6.3	2.2	0.39	0.51	5.3	193
Other endocrine	5	0	-	-	-	-	1.0	-	1.1	1.1	1.1	-	-	-	1.7	-	-	-	-	-	0.4	0.1	0.03	0.03	0.3	194
Hodgkin's disease	23	0	1.2	-	-	4.1	3.0	8.8	-	1.1	3.4	-	4.9	-	-	-	-	-	-	-	1.9	0.6	0.13	0.13	2.0	201
Non-Hodgkin lymphoma	159	1	1.2	-	-	1.0	5.0	4.4	3.3	5.5	9.2	12.5	19.4	11.2	25.3	45.7	26.1	50.2	73.9	85.6	12.9	4.5	0.49	0.85	8.5	200,202
Multiple myeloma	57	0	-	-	-	-	-	-	-	2.2	1.1	6.3	1.6	8.0	11.8	19.1	23.2	27.9	18.5	19.0	4.6	1.6	0.16	0.37	3.0	203
Lymphoid leukaemia	35	0	3.6	3.5	1.2	3.1	-	-	-	-	1.1	-	1.6	4.8	1.7	7.6	5.8	13.9	11.1	23.8	2.8	1.0	0.10	0.17	2.2	204
Myeloid leukaemia	44	0	1.2	1.2	2.3	-	1.0	1.1	1.1	2.2	3.4	6.3	3.2	1.6	1.7	11.4	5.8	22.3	18.5	14.3	3.6	1.2	0.13	0.22	2.6	205
Monocytic leukaemia	0	0	-	-	-	-	-	-	-	-	-	-	-	-	-	-	-	-	-	-	0.0	0.0	0.00	0.00	0.0	206
Other leukaemia	0	0	-	-	-	-	-	-	-	-	-	-	-	-	-	-	-	-	-	-	0.0	0.0	0.00	0.00	0.0	207
Leukaemia unspecified	6	0	-	-	-	-	-	-	-	1.1	-	-	1.6	3.2	-	-	2.9	2.8	-	-	0.5	0.2	0.03	0.04	0.4	208
Other and unspecified	188	1	3.6	-	1.2	-	1.0	3.3	3.3	1.1	12.6	12.5	16.2	24.0	28.6	38.1	63.9	91.9	77.6	85.6	15.3	5.3	0.54	1.05	9.8	O&U
All sites	4543	87	15.8	12.7	8.1	18.4	35.8	51.6	97.9	147.5	281.4	440.7	564.0	637.9	826.8	1063.1	1184.8	1457.2	1719.0	1822.1	368.7		16.00	27.46	250.0	ALL
All sites but 173	3569	42	15.8	11.5	6.9	16.4	32.8	51.6	80.3	129.9	248.1	381.1	478.1	530.8	663.5	826.8	914.8	1106.2	1249.5	1175.1	289.6	100.0	13.39	22.20	202.6	ALLb

Rate from 1 case   1.215 1.151 1.158 1.023 0.994 1.097 1.100 1.101 1.149 1.568 1.621 1.599 1.684 1.905 2.904 2.786 3.697 4.757

France, Haut-Rhin

The Haut-Rhin Cancer Registry is a general population-based registry. Created in 1989, it is administered by an association under a law specially constituted for the purpose. It was set up in order to obtain data on the burden of cancer in the area, so as to have a basis for evaluation of public health measures in the prevention, screening and treatment of cancer. It is financed entirely locally (local and regional groups, health insurance funds, the Anti-Cancer League).

The département of Haut-Rhin, an area of 3522 km², is situated in the north-east of France. It is bordered by the département of Bas-Rhin to the north (the département with which it constitutes the Alsace region), the département of the Vosges to the west, and the Franche-Comté region and Switzerland to the south. To the east, the Rhine separates Haut-Rhin from Germany. The altitude varies from 195 m on the Rhine to 1424 m in the Vosges mountains. The climate is semi-continental, with fairly cold winters and hot, dry summers. The conditions favour the vineyards of the lower slopes of the Vosges. The area has four geographical regions: the Vosges mountains (crystalline massif), the lower hills of the Vosges (wine and fruit cultivation), the plain of the Rhine (land of loess and former marshland), and the Alsatian Jura (limestone).

The population of Haut-Rhin is divided into 377 communes, of which 269 are rural with less than 1000 inhabitants. According to the 1990 census, the total population was 671 334 inhabitants (328 967 men and 342 367 women). Haut-Rhin had a higher proportion of economically active (aged 15–64) persons and a lower proportion aged over 65 years than France as a whole. 8.9% of the residents were foreign, of whom 72% were born outside metropolitan France. 26% of the population lived in rural communes and 52% in the 21 communes with more than 5000 inhabitants. The urban area of Mulhouse had 223 856 inhabitants. The average population density was 190 inhabitants per km², varying from 78 in the rural communes to 4885 in the commune of Mulhouse.

57.1% of the population is economically active. The unemployment rate is 4.4% among men and 10.8% among women. The industrial sector employs 35.3% of the active population (automobile, arms, chemical, textile, wood and paper, nuclear); the agricultural sector, 2.8% (market gardening, wine production, forestry), and the tertiary sector 54.6% (commerce, administration, education, health, transport). A special feature, related to the geographical situation of Haut-Rhin, is that 14% of the employed population resident in the département works in Switzerland or Germany.

With 141 general practitioners and 124 specialists per 100 000 inhabitants, the medical coverage of the Haut-Rhin population is below the national French average. The hospital infrastructure, public and private, comprises 1695 beds in medical departments, 1472 in surgery, and 362 in gynaecology and obstetrics. There are two radiotherapy departments, one in the south (Mulhouse), and the other in the north (Colmar). There is no specialized cancer centre in the département.

The registry collects information on all new cases of cancer occurring among the inhabitants of Haut-Rhin, including those diagnosed and treated elsewhere. Registration is active. The main sources of information are the pathology and cytology laboratories, and the services of radiotherapy, oncology, paediatrics and haematology. The medical information departments and medical records departments of the hospitals are also excellent sources of first notifications. Cases discovered at autopsy are registered, and identified as such. The data collected are systematically verified, completed or modified, using secondary sources (hospitalization services, treating physicians). The average number of sources per registered case is three. Death certificates are not used.

When data are entered, two distinct files are created: one contains only the nominative information and works with specially designed software, the other includes all the medical data concerning the case and uses the IARC CAN-REG software. A registration number is given to each case, and appears in both files. The software for the nominative information file includes a module for checking for duplication based on comparison of surname, forename, sex, date of birth and address. Systematic searches for homonyms are carried out regularly by comparing incidence dates and sites with the nominative information. ICD-O-1 is used for coding site and histology. The first three characters of the site code are used to define multiple primaries. The IARC/IACR rules for multiple primaries are used. The data are converted into ICD-9 to present the results.

The Haut-Rhin Cancer Registry, in its sixth year of existence, has not yet undertaken any survival studies. Its participation in collaborative studies is just beginning. An Information Letter describing the registry results is published regularly for physicians in the département.

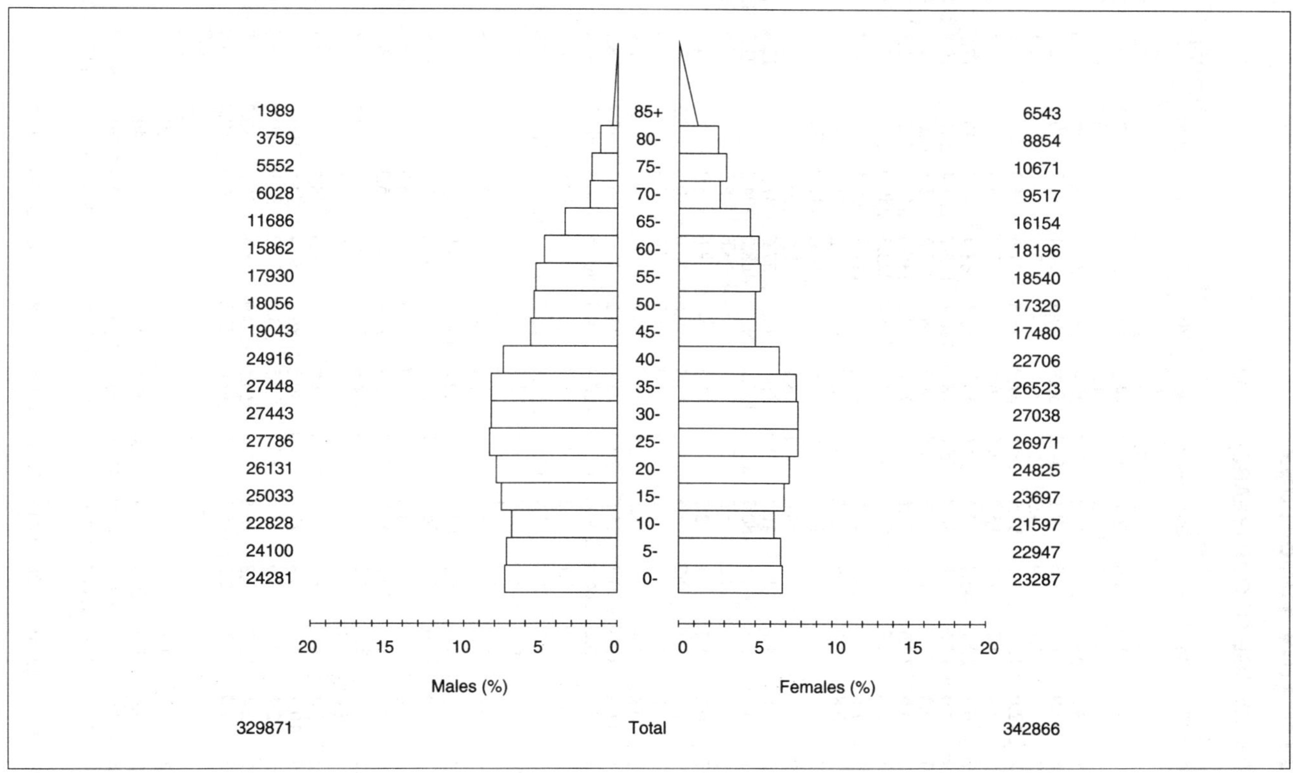

France, Haut-Rhin
Source of population: 1988–92
Census: Recensement de la population 1990, Population de la France, Départements, arrondissements, cantons, communes. Direction Générale des Collectivités Locales, Institut National de la Statistique et des Etudes Economiques.
Estimate: Population estimates provided by the official national department of demography (INSEE) were used for each of the years 1988-92 (Estimations de la Population, INSEE, 1996)

Notes to tables overleaf:
† 173 does not include basal cell carcinoma for the years 1988–90
† 188 does not include non-invasive tumours

FRANCE, HAUT-RHIN 1988-1992

ANNUAL INCIDENCE PER 100,000 BY AGE GROUP (YEARS) - MALE

SITE	ALL AGES	AGE UNK	0-	5-	10-	15-	20-	25-	30-	35-	40-	45-	50-	55-	60-	65-	70-	75-	80-	85+	CRUDE RATE	%	CR 64	CR 74	ASR (W)	ICD (9th)
Lip	17	0	-	-	-	-	-	-	-	-	-	-	3.3	3.3	1.3	3.4	10.0	7.2	16.0	-	1.0	0.2	0.04	0.11	**0.8**	*140*
Tongue	153	0	-	-	-	-	-	0.7	1.5	2.2	4.0	18.9	21.0	26.8	40.3	44.5	39.8	28.8	10.6	10.1	9.3	2.1	0.58	1.00	**7.9**	*141*
Salivary gland	11	0	-	-	-	-	-	-	-	-	-	-	1.1	4.5	2.5	1.7	-	-	-	30.2	0.7	0.1	0.04	0.05	**0.5**	*142*
Mouth	198	0	-	-	-	-	-	-	1.5	13.6	23.1	27.7	46.8	49.2	39.4	53.1	32.4	5.3	20.1	12.0	2.7	0.81	1.27	**10.2**	*143-5*
Oropharynx	230	0	-	-	-	-	-	0.7	3.6	16.9	27.3	36.6	59.1	54.2	35.9	49.8	14.4	31.9	20.1	13.9	3.1	0.99	1.42	**11.8**	*146*
Nasopharynx	18	0	-	-	0.9	-	-	-	-	0.7	-	2.1	8.9	3.3	2.5	-	-	3.6	-	-	1.1	0.2	0.09	N.09	**1.0**	*147*
Hypopharynx	204	0	-	-	-	-	-	-	-	2.2	12.0	16.8	32.1	53.5	60.5	47.9	26.5	21.6	16.0	-	12.4	2.8	0.89	1.26	**10.3**	*148*
Pharynx unspecified	42	0	-	-	-	-	-	-	-	-	2.4	3.2	11.1	13.4	8.8	6.8	-	7.2	5.3	-	2.5	0.6	0.19	0.23	**2.1**	*149*
Oesophagus	286	0	-	-	-	-	-	-	0.7	6.4	22.1	45.4	60.2	94.6	54.8	53.1	68.4	74.5	50.3	17.3	3.9	1.15	1.69	**14.2**	*150*
Stomach	326	0	-	-	-	-	-	-	2.2	2.9	4.0	12.6	18.8	36.8	65.6	78.7	126.1	165.7	223.4	281.5	19.8	4.4	0.71	1.74	**15.4**	*151*
Small intestine	21	0	-	-	-	-	-	-	-	1.5	0.8	-	1.1	3.3	7.6	1.7	6.6	7.2	5.3	20.1	1.3	0.3	0.07	0.11	**1.0**	*152*
Colon	595	0	-	-	-	-	0.8	0.7	0.7	2.2	5.6	12.6	38.8	78.1	104.6	178.0	268.7	335.0	345.8	392.1	36.1	8.0	1.22	3.45	**28.4**	*153*
Rectum	446	0	-	-	-	-	-	-	2.9	2.2	5.6	12.6	35.4	51.3	90.8	133.5	205.7	223.3	250.0	211.1	27.0	6.0	1.00	2.70	**21.5**	*154*
Liver	235	0	-	-	-	-	0.8	0.7	-	0.7	1.6	2.1	13.3	41.3	55.5	92.4	92.9	111.7	90.4	50.3	14.2	3.2	0.58	1.51	**11.4**	*155*
Gallbladder etc.	45	0	-	-	-	-	-	-	-	-	0.8	2.1	5.5	5.6	10.1	8.6	19.9	25.2	21.3	20.1	2.7	0.6	0.12	0.26	**2.2**	*156*
Pancreas	128	0	-	-	-	-	-	-	-	0.7	4.0	4.2	15.5	16.7	24.0	35.9	49.8	64.8	47.9	70.4	7.8	1.7	0.33	0.75	**6.3**	*157*
Nose, sinuses etc.	32	0	-	-	-	0.8	-	-	0.7	1.5	-	1.1	3.3	10.0	10.1	5.1	-	7.2	10.6	-	1.9	0.4	0.14	0.16	**1.5**	*160*
Larynx	205	0	-	-	-	-	-	-	0.7	2.2	5.6	14.7	42.1	41.3	49.2	51.3	43.1	57.6	37.2	-	12.4	2.8	0.78	1.25	**10.3**	*161*
Bronchus, lung	1174	0	-	-	-	-	0.8	-	1.5	5.1	24.1	57.8	108.5	180.7	302.6	397.0	441.3	468.2	324.5	231.2	71.2	15.9	3.41	7.60	**58.3**	*162*
Other thoracic organs	13	0	-	-	-	-	1.5	0.7	-	-	-	-	3.3	3.3	2.5	-	-	3.6	5.3	-	0.8	0.2	0.06	0.06	**0.6**	*163-4*
Bone	18	0	0.8	-	0.9	1.6	1.5	0.7	1.5	0.7	0.8	1.1	1.1	2.2	-	1.7	-	3.6	5.3	-	1.1	0.2	0.06	0.07	**1.0**	*170*
Connective tissue	51	0	2.5	0.8	2.6	0.8	2.3	-	0.7	2.9	1.6	1.1	2.2	4.5	6.3	15.4	6.6	18.0	10.6	30.2	3.1	0.7	0.14	0.25	**2.8**	*171*
Mesothelioma	12	0	-	-	-	-	-	-	-	0.7	0.8	1.1	-	1.1	2.5	3.4	3.3	7.2	5.3	-	0.7	0.2	0.03	0.06	**0.6**	*MES*
Kaposi's sarcoma	13	0	-	-	-	-	0.8	0.7	2.2	2.2	0.8	1.1	-	-	1.3	-	6.6	-	-	-	0.8	0.2	0.04	0.08	**0.7**	*KAP*
Melanoma of skin	134	0	-	-	-	1.6	3.8	5.0	5.8	1.5	11.2	10.5	13.3	15.6	30.3	25.7	23.2	32.4	5.3	40.2	8.1	1.8	0.49	0.74	**6.9**	*172*
†Other skin	997	0	-	-	-	-	0.8	2.9	7.3	8.7	23.3	45.2	66.5	106.0	153.8	282.4	394.8	565.5	638.4	603.3	60.4		2.07	5.46	**47.3**	*173*
Breast	7	0	-	-	-	-	-	-	0.7	-	-	-	1.1	2.2	-	1.7	-	-	10.6	-	0.4	0.1	0.02	0.03	**0.3**	*175*
Prostate	1122	0	-	-	-	-	-	-	-	-	-	1.1	21.0	66.9	176.5	352.5	570.7	785.2	1064.0	1065.8	68.0	15.2	1.33	5.94	**51.3**	*185*
Testis	150	0	0.8	-	-	4.0	18.4	23.8	25.5	16.0	8.0	6.3	3.3	6.7	2.5	1.7	3.3	-	5.3	-	9.1	2.0	0.58	0.60	**7.9**	*186*
Penis	21	0	-	-	-	-	-	-	-	0.7	-	-	4.4	1.1	5.0	8.6	-	10.8	16.0	-	1.3	0.3	0.06	0.10	**1.0**	*187.1-.4*
Other male genital	3	0	-	-	-	-	-	-	-	-	-	-	-	1.1	-	1.7	3.3	-	-	-	0.2	0.0	0.01	0.03	**0.2**	*187.5-.9*
†Bladder	447	0	-	-	-	-	0.8	0.7	1.5	2.9	3.2	17.9	32.1	60.2	94.6	142.0	159.3	176.5	255.4	321.7	27.1	6.0	1.07	2.58	**21.5**	*188*
Kidney etc.	262	0	1.6	-	0.9	0.8	-	0.7	-	5.1	5.6	11.6	25.5	54.7	68.1	71.9	86.3	61.2	95.8	30.2	15.9	3.5	0.87	1.66	**13.0**	*189*
Eye	11	0	-	-	-	0.8	-	-	-	0.7	0.8	-	4.5	1.3	1.7	3.3	-	5.3	-	-	0.7	0.1	0.04	0.07	**0.5**	*190*
Brain, nervous system	106	0	4.1	1.7	-	1.6	3.1	2.9	4.4	8.0	5.6	9.5	10.0	16.7	13.9	17.1	29.9	3.6	5.3	-	6.4	1.4	0.41	0.64	**5.8**	*191-2*
Thyroid	28	0	-	-	-	-	1.5	1.4	2.9	2.2	-	3.2	1.1	2.2	5.0	3.4	10.0	-	-	20.1	1.7	0.4	0.10	0.16	**1.5**	*193*
Other endocrine	13	0	1.6	-	-	-	-	0.7	-	-	1.6	1.1	2.2	2.2	2.5	-	-	3.6	-	-	0.8	0.2	0.06	0.06	**0.8**	*194*
Hodgkin's disease	39	0	-	0.8	1.8	0.8	3.1	7.2	2.2	2.2	3.2	4.2	1.1	-	3.8	1.7	-	3.6	5.3	-	2.4	0.5	0.15	0.16	**2.2**	*201*
Non-Hodgkin lymphoma	197	0	1.6	2.5	-	0.8	0.8	2.9	5.1	8.0	10.4	14.7	13.3	22.3	34.0	30.8	86.3	50.4	74.5	100.5	11.9	2.7	0.58	1.17	**10.1**	*200,202*
Multiple myeloma	62	0	-	-	-	-	-	-	-	1.5	2.4	2.1	8.9	5.6	17.7	20.5	3.3	25.2	31.9	20.1	3.8	0.8	0.19	0.31	**2.9**	*203*
Lymphoid leukaemia	75	0	3.3	3.3	0.9	4.0	1.5	-	0.7	0.7	2.4	3.2	7.8	5.6	12.6	10.3	19.9	28.8	26.6	40.2	4.5	1.0	0.23	0.38	**4.2**	*204*
Myeloid leukaemia	50	0	0.8	-	-	0.8	0.8	0.7	0.7	1.5	4.0	1.1	2.2	4.5	8.8	12.0	23.2	14.4	16.0	30.2	3.0	0.7	0.13	0.31	**2.6**	*205*
Monocytic leukaemia	0	0	-	-	-	-	-	-	-	-	-	-	-	-	-	-	-	-	-	-	0.0	0.0	0.00	0.00	**0.0**	*206*
Other leukaemia	3	0	-	-	-	-	0.8	-	-	-	0.8	-	-	1.3	-	-	-	-	-	-	0.2	0.0	0.01	0.01	**0.2**	*207*
Leukaemia unspecified	11	0	0.8	2.5	-	-	0.8	-	-	0.7	-	1.1	-	-	-	-	-	7.2	-	20.1	0.7	0.1	0.03	0.03	**0.7**	*208*
Other and unspecified	189	0	1.6	-	-	0.8	-	-	1.5	1.5	5.6	9.5	29.9	23.4	50.4	49.6	49.8	64.8	63.8	40.2	11.5	2.6	0.62	1.12	**9.5**	*O&U*
All sites	8400	0	19.8	11.6	7.9	19.2	44.4	53.3	73.6	98.4	199.9	379.1	720.0	1148.9	1728.6	2272.6	2969.4	3515.3	3862.3	3770.4	509.3		22.52	48.73	**410.8**	*ALL*
All sites but 173	7403	0	19.8	11.6	7.9	19.2	43.6	50.4	66.3	89.6	176.6	334.0	653.5	1042.9	1574.8	1990.3	2574.6	2949.9	3223.9	3167.1	448.8	100.0	20.45	43.28	**363.5**	*ALLb*

Rate from 1 case   0.824   0.830   0.876   0.799   0.765   0.720   0.729   0.729   0.803   1.050   1.108   1.115   1.261   1.711   3.318   3.602   5.320   10.054

†Important: see notes on population page

FRANCE, HAUT-RHIN 1988-1992

ANNUAL INCIDENCE PER 100,000 BY AGE GROUP (YEARS) - FEMALE

SITE	ALL AGES	AGE UNK	0-	5-	10-	15-	20-	25-	30-	35-	40-	45-	50-	55-	60-	65-	70-	75-	80-	85+	CRUDE RATE	%	CR 64	CR 74	ASR (W)	ICD (9th)
Lip	3	0	-	-	-	-	-	-	-	-	-	-	-	-	1.1	-	2.1	-	-	3.1	0.2	0.1	0.01	0.02	**0.1**	140
Tongue	19	0	-	-	-	-	0.8	-	-	1.5	0.9	1.1	3.5	2.2	2.2	1.2	2.1	5.6	-	6.1	1.1	0.3	0.06	0.08	**0.8**	141
Salivary gland	10	0	-	-	-	-	0.8	0.7	-	0.8	0.9	-	-	-	-	-	4.2	1.9	4.5	3.1	0.6	0.2	0.02	0.04	**0.4**	142
Mouth	27	0	-	-	-	-	-	0.7	-	-	-	3.4	5.8	2.2	5.5	1.2	4.2	3.7	4.5	12.2	1.6	0.5	0.09	0.12	**1.1**	143-5
Oropharynx	26	0	-	-	-	-	-	-	-	-	0.9	2.3	2.3	2.2	8.8	5.0	2.1	3.7	4.5	6.1	1.5	0.4	0.08	0.12	**1.0**	146
Nasopharynx	4	0	-	-	-	0.8	-	-	-	-	1.8	1.1	-	-	-	-	-	-	-	-	0.2	0.1	0.02	0.02	**0.3**	147
Hypopharynx	11	0	-	-	-	-	-	-	-	0.8	-	1.1	2.3	1.1	1.1	3.7	2.1	1.9	-	-	0.6	0.2	0.03	0.06	**0.5**	148
Pharynx unspecified	4	0	-	-	-	-	-	-	-	-	1.8	1.1	-	1.1	-	-	-	-	-	-	0.2	0.1	0.02	0.02	**0.2**	149
Oesophagus	38	0	-	-	-	-	-	-	-	-	-	1.1	6.9	1.1	8.8	6.2	6.3	5.6	18.1	9.2	2.2	0.6	0.09	0.15	**1.3**	150
Stomach	228	0	-	-	0.9	-	0.8	0.7	2.2	3.0	4.4	3.4	8.1	11.9	16.5	32.2	54.6	82.5	94.9	119.2	13.3	3.9	0.26	0.69	**6.5**	151
Small intestine	13	0	-	-	-	-	-	-	-	-	-	1.2	1.1	2.2	2.5	2.1	3.7	6.8	3.1	-	0.8	0.2	0.02	0.05	**0.4**	152
Colon	601	0	-	-	-	-	0.8	1.5	1.5	7.5	7.9	16.0	20.8	49.6	78.0	100.3	149.2	189.3	266.5	174.2	35.1	10.3	0.92	2.17	**18.4**	153
Rectum	343	0	-	-	-	-	-	1.5	1.5	2.3	4.4	9.2	24.2	27.0	46.2	73.0	84.1	82.5	101.6	143.7	20.0	5.9	0.58	1.37	**11.2**	154
Liver	39	0	-	-	-	-	0.8	0.7	-	-	-	1.1	1.2	5.4	3.3	7.4	6.3	9.4	15.8	18.3	2.3	0.7	0.06	0.13	**1.2**	155
Gallbladder etc.	110	0	-	-	-	-	-	-	-	-	-	1.1	4.6	6.5	14.3	28.5	31.5	30.0	33.9	52.0	6.4	1.9	0.13	0.43	**3.3**	156
Pancreas	97	0	-	-	-	-	0.8	-	-	-	1.8	2.3	9.2	7.6	7.7	21.0	23.1	28.1	40.7	27.5	5.7	1.7	0.15	0.37	**3.1**	157
Nose, sinuses etc.	5	0	-	-	-	-	0.8	-	0.7	-	-	-	-	-	-	2.1	-	2.3	3.1	-	0.3	0.1	0.01	0.02	**0.2**	160
Larynx	15	0	-	-	-	-	-	-	1.5	-	-	1.2	1.1	1.1	8.7	6.3	-	-	-	-	0.9	0.3	0.02	0.10	**0.6**	161
Bronchus, lung	168	0	-	-	-	-	-	-	-	2.3	4.4	6.9	17.3	25.9	39.6	34.7	44.1	24.4	24.8	18.3	9.8	2.9	0.48	0.88	**6.7**	162
Other thoracic organs	8	0	-	0.9	-	-	-	-	0.7	-	-	1.1	-	1.1	-	5.0	-	-	-	-	0.5	0.1	0.02	0.04	**0.4**	163-4
Bone	12	0	-	0.9	0.9	-	-	-	-	0.8	0.9	-	-	-	3.3	2.5	2.1	1.9	2.3	-	0.7	0.2	0.03	0.06	**0.5**	170
Connective tissue	40	0	-	-	0.9	0.8	1.6	1.5	1.5	1.5	1.8	2.3	2.3	1.1	5.5	8.7	10.5	5.6	6.8	-	2.3	0.7	0.10	0.20	**1.8**	171
Mesothelioma	5	0	-	-	-	-	-	-	-	-	-	-	-	2.2	1.1	1.2	-	1.9	-	-	0.3	0.1	0.02	0.02	**0.2**	MES
Kaposi's sarcoma	1	0	-	-	0.8	-	-	-	-	-	-	-	-	-	-	-	-	-	-	-	0.1	0.0	0.00	0.00	**0.1**	KAP
Melanoma of skin	148	0	-	-	1.9	0.8	7.3	3.7	7.4	7.5	14.1	11.4	17.3	10.8	16.5	14.9	16.8	20.6	20.3	15.3	8.6	2.5	0.49	0.65	**6.7**	172
†Other skin	1042	0	-	-	-	0.8	-	3.7	12.6	18.1	27.3	44.6	60.0	78.7	123.1	149.8	224.8	245.5	359.2	519.6	60.8		1.85	3.72	**33.4**	173
Breast	1922	0	-	-	-	-	1.6	8.9	29.6	51.3	119.8	189.9	255.2	258.9	294.6	300.9	319.4	322.4	311.7	195.6	112.1	32.8	6.05	9.15	**80.3**	174
Uterus unspecified	10	0	-	-	-	-	-	-	-	-	-	-	1.2	1.1	1.1	1.2	-	3.7	4.5	6.1	0.6	0.2	0.02	0.02	**0.3**	179
Cervix uteri	263	0	-	-	-	-	4.0	10.4	14.1	21.1	19.4	26.3	21.9	22.7	41.8	40.9	29.4	24.4	15.8	21.4	15.3	4.5	0.91	1.26	**11.9**	180
Placenta	4	0	-	-	-	-	-	2.2	-	0.8	-	-	-	-	-	-	-	-	-	-	0.2	0.1	0.01	0.01	**0.2**	181
Corpus uteri	393	0	-	-	-	0.8	0.8	0.7	3.0	0.8	7.9	12.6	48.5	74.4	63.8	83.0	69.3	84.3	65.5	67.2	22.9	6.7	1.07	1.83	**15.0**	182
Ovary etc.	254	0	-	-	2.5	2.4	3.0	3.0	9.8	17.6	29.7	27.7	35.6	35.2	43.3	46.2	16.9	38.4	27.5	14.8	4.3	0.83	1.28	**11.2**	183
Other female genital	62	0	-	-	-	0.8	1.5	-	-	-	2.3	-	3.2	5.5	9.9	10.5	22.5	33.9	27.5	3.6	1.1	0.07	0.17	**1.7**	184
†Bladder	112	0	-	-	-	-	-	-	-	0.8	-	4.6	5.4	13.2	16.1	42.0	31.9	52.0	52.0	6.5	1.9	0.12	0.41	**3.2**	188
Kidney etc.	159	0	2.6	0.9	-	-	-	0.7	1.5	0.8	2.6	6.9	8.1	23.7	19.8	29.7	35.7	54.4	33.9	30.6	9.3	2.7	0.34	0.66	**5.8**	189
Eye	8	0	0.9	-	-	-	-	-	-	1.5	-	-	1.1	-	5.0	-	-	-	-	-	0.5	0.1	0.02	0.04	**0.4**	190
Brain, nervous system	85	0	1.7	3.5	2.8	0.8	2.4	1.5	2.2	3.0	5.3	10.3	6.9	5.4	18.7	9.9	10.5	9.4	4.5	-	5.0	1.4	0.32	0.42	**4.4**	191-2
Thyroid	58	0	-	-	-	1.7	1.6	3.0	3.0	2.3	4.4	-	-	5.4	4.4	11.1	12.6	7.5	15.8	9.2	3.4	1.0	0.13	0.25	**2.3**	193
Other endocrine	7	0	0.9	-	-	1.7	-	0.7	0.7	-	-	1.1	-	-	1.1	-	-	-	-	-	0.4	0.1	0.03	0.03	**0.5**	194
Hodgkin's disease	38	0	-	-	1.9	2.5	4.0	5.2	3.0	4.5	0.9	2.3	4.6	-	-	2.5	-	-	2.3	3.1	2.2	0.6	0.14	0.16	**2.1**	201
Non-Hodgkin lymphoma	184	0	0.9	-	-	-	0.8	4.4	2.2	5.3	4.4	13.7	9.2	17.3	27.5	31.0	35.7	41.2	61.0	27.5	10.7	3.1	0.43	0.76	**6.8**	200,202
Multiple myeloma	70	0	-	-	-	-	-	-	-	-	0.9	1.1	1.2	10.8	13.2	11.1	6.3	24.4	20.3	33.6	4.1	1.2	0.14	0.22	**2.1**	203
Lymphoid leukaemia	61	0	4.3	0.9	0.9	-	0.8	0.7	0.7	-	-	1.1	3.5	7.6	7.7	6.2	14.7	20.6	15.8	9.2	3.6	1.0	0.14	0.25	**2.5**	204
Myeloid leukaemia	47	0	0.9	0.9	3.7	-	-	0.7	-	1.5	2.6	2.3	5.8	4.3	1.1	6.2	10.5	9.4	11.3	9.2	2.7	0.8	0.12	0.20	**2.1**	205
Monocytic leukaemia	6	0	-	-	-	-	0.8	-	0.7	-	-	-	-	1.1	2.2	1.2	-	-	-	-	0.3	0.1	0.02	0.03	**0.3**	206
Other leukaemia	0	0	-	-	-	-	-	-	-	-	-	-	-	-	-	-	-	-	-	-	0.0	0.0	0.00	0.00	**0.0**	207
Leukaemia unspecified	11	0	-	-	-	-	-	-	0.7	-	-	-	1.2	-	2.2	3.7	-	1.9	2.3	6.1	0.6	0.2	0.02	0.04	**0.4**	208
Other and unspecified	134	0	0.9	-	-	-	-	-	0.7	0.8	0.9	3.4	8.1	7.6	25.3	26.0	35.7	35.6	33.9	55.0	7.8	2.3	0.24	0.55	**4.5**	O&U
All sites	6905	0	12.9	7.8	13.9	14.3	34.6	58.6	94.7	150.1	259.8	414.2	595.8	724.9	963.9	1146.5	1359.6	1458.1	1730.3	1714.7	402.8		16.73	29.26	**258.2**	ALL
All sites but 173	5863	0	12.9	7.8	13.9	13.5	34.6	54.9	82.1	132.0	232.5	369.5	535.8	646.2	840.8	996.6	1134.7	1212.6	1371.1	1195.1	342.0	100.0	14.88	25.54	**224.7**	ALLb

Rate from 1 case			0.859	0.872	0.926	0.844	0.806	0.742	0.740	0.754	0.881	1.144	1.155	1.079	1.099	1.238	2.101	1.874	2.259	3.057

†Important: see notes on population page

France, Hérault

The Cancer Registry of the Hérault was created in 1983 in order to collect data on cancer at all sites. The general objective was to determine the annual incidence of cancer in the Hérault département, since population-based cancer registries were insufficient in the south of France. The registry is located in Montpellier, the capital of the département.

The Hérault département is part of the Languedoc Roussillon region and covers 6101 km^2 in the south of France near the Mediterrannean Sea (latitude 43° N, longitude 4° E).

In 1992, the population of Hérault comprised 818 281 inhabitants (48% males, 52% females), with a population density of 136 inhabitants per km^2. The birth rate was 12.4 per 1000 and the mortality rate 9.3 per 1000, the annual variation being + 1.49%. The population of the département lives in 344 communes. The number of hospital beds in 1992 was 9971, in 10 public hospitals and 52 private clinics. There were 1406 general practitioners in 1992 and 1617 specialists. In the town of Montpellier, there is a hospital specializing in cancer treatment.

Registration is active, in that doctors from the registry regularly visit each of the many sources of data to establish lists of new cases and to fill out epidemiological questionnaires for the medical files. Lists from each of these sources are then compared, so as to ensure complete registration and eliminate errors, especially duplicate registrations. Patients living in the Hérault département but treated in a regional or Parisian cancer institute are also included.

Death certificates are not used as a source. The data are coded after visiting the information sources, using the ICD-O morphology and topography codes, and are kept on computer files to be used for various studies.

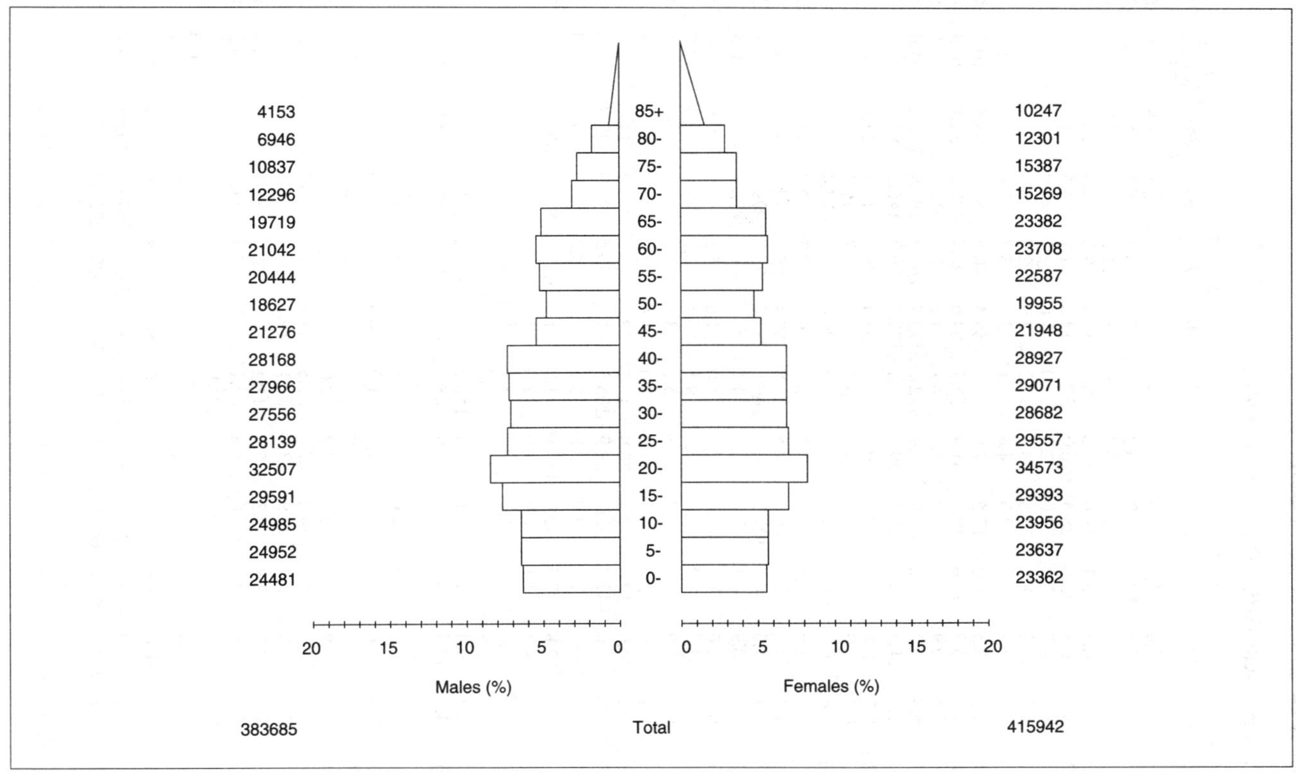

France, Hérault

Source of population: 1988–92

Census: Recensement de la population 1990, Population de la France, Départements, arrondissements, cantons, communes. Direction Générale des Collectivités Locales, Institut National de la Statistique et des Etudes Economiques.

Estimate: Population estimates provided by the official national department of demography (INSEE) were used for each of the years 1988-92 (Estimations de la Population, INSEE, 1996).

Notes to tables overleaf:

* The low rates for the leukaemias (combined with unlikely mortality/incidence ratios) and rather low rates generally, with a high level of histological verification, suggest under-registration.

† 188 does not include non-invasive tumours for the years 1988-90

* FRANCE, HERAULT 1988-1992

ANNUAL INCIDENCE PER 100,000 BY AGE GROUP (YEARS) - MALE

SITE	ALL AGES	AGE UNK	0-	5-	10-	15-	20-	25-	30-	35-	40-	45-	50-	55-	60-	65-	70-	75-	80-	85+	CRUDE RATE	%	CR 64	CR 74	ASR (W)	ICD (9th)
Lip	34	0	-	-	-	-	-	-	-	-	0.7	1.9	2.1	5.9	5.7	4.1	8.1	9.2	5.8	4.8	1.8	0.4	0.08	0.14	1.2	140
Tongue	109	0	-	-	-	-	-	0.7	0.7	0.7	6.4	7.5	19.3	14.7	16.2	12.2	21.1	20.3	5.8	4.8	5.7	1.4	0.33	0.50	4.2	141
Salivary gland	16	0	-	-	-	-	-	-	-	-	-	-	1.0	4.8	1.0	1.6	11.1	2.9	4.8	-	0.8	0.2	0.03	0.04	0.4	142
Mouth	126	0	-	-	-	-	-	-	-	4.3	5.7	6.6	16.1	19.6	27.6	16.2	19.5	9.2	14.4	14.4	6.6	1.6	0.40	0.58	4.8	143-5
Oropharynx	140	0	-	-	-	-	0.6	-	1.5	2.9	5.7	10.3	23.6	28.4	20.0	22.3	13.0	11.1	14.4	4.8	7.3	1.8	0.46	0.64	5.5	146
Nasopharynx	22	0	-	-	-	1.4	-	-	-	-	1.4	4.7	2.1	2.0	2.9	2.0	1.6	3.7	2.9	-	1.1	0.3	0.07	0.09	0.9	147
Hypopharynx	101	0	-	-	-	-	-	-	-	1.4	5.0	13.2	8.6	10.8	18.1	17.2	17.9	12.9	5.8	14.4	5.3	1.3	0.28	0.46	3.9	148
Pharynx unspecified	28	0	-	-	-	-	-	-	-	-	0.7	2.8	3.2	2.0	4.8	9.1	3.3	3.7	2.9	-	1.5	0.3	0.07	0.13	1.0	149
Oesophagus	194	0	-	-	-	-	-	-	0.7	1.4	5.0	8.5	15.0	17.6	27.6	37.5	45.5	40.6	54.7	38.5	10.1	2.4	0.38	0.79	6.4	150
Stomach	325	0	-	-	-	-	-	0.7	0.7	2.1	4.3	13.2	15.0	19.6	31.4	52.7	84.6	90.4	138.2	154.1	16.9	4.1	0.43	1.12	9.7	151
Small intestine	22	0	-	-	-	-	-	-	-	-	1.4	0.9	1.1	1.0	1.0	4.1	4.9	9.2	11.5	-	1.1	0.3	0.03	0.07	0.6	152
Colon	653	0	-	-	-	0.7	-	2.1	1.5	4.3	6.4	19.7	25.8	51.8	82.7	122.7	175.7	201.2	192.9	202.2	34.0	8.2	0.97	2.47	20.0	153
Rectum	470	0	-	-	-	-	-	-	0.7	1.4	6.4	11.3	22.5	29.3	59.9	97.4	125.2	129.2	146.8	183.0	24.5	5.9	0.66	1.77	14.3	154
Liver	123	0	-	-	-	-	-	-	1.5	0.7	0.7	2.8	6.4	9.8	20.0	29.4	37.4	29.5	17.3	24.1	6.4	1.5	0.21	0.54	4.0	155
Gallbladder etc.	47	0	-	-	-	-	-	-	-	-	0.7	1.9	2.1	3.9	2.9	5.1	14.6	27.7	17.3	-	2.4	0.6	0.06	0.16	1.3	156
Pancreas	92	0	-	-	-	-	-	-	-	0.7	2.8	0.9	6.4	11.7	14.3	19.3	26.0	20.3	14.4	9.6	4.8	1.2	0.18	0.41	3.1	157
Nose, sinuses etc.	33	0	-	-	-	-	0.6	-	-	-	-	1.9	4.3	2.0	5.7	6.1	9.8	3.7	2.9	14.4	1.7	0.4	0.07	0.15	1.2	160
Larynx	339	0	-	-	-	-	-	-	0.7	10.0	9.9	23.5	39.7	40.1	67.5	57.8	50.4	59.1	17.3	48.2	17.7	4.2	0.96	1.50	12.6	161
Bronchus, lung	1273	0	-	-	-	-	-	2.1	5.1	12.2	22.7	54.5	106.3	127.2	195.8	269.8	283.0	278.7	279.3	158.9	66.4	15.9	2.63	5.39	42.8	162
Other thoracic organs	15	0	-	-	-	-	1.2	0.7	0.7	0.7	0.7	0.9	1.1	2.0	-	4.1	-	-	2.9	-	0.8	0.2	0.04	0.06	0.6	163-4
Bone	31	0	-	-	3.2	-	1.8	-	-	2.9	0.7	5.6	1.1	1.0	2.9	1.0	1.6	5.5	2.9	9.6	1.6	0.4	0.10	0.11	1.4	170
Connective tissue	53	0	1.6	-	-	2.0	0.6	-	-	1.4	1.4	2.8	3.2	3.9	9.5	9.1	6.5	3.7	14.4	14.4	2.8	0.7	0.13	0.21	2.1	171
Mesothelioma	21	0	-	-	-	-	-	-	-	-	0.7	1.9	-	1.0	3.8	5.1	3.3	7.4	5.8	-	1.1	0.3	0.04	0.08	0.7	MES
Kaposi's sarcoma	53	0	-	-	-	-	-	7.1	6.5	3.6	7.1	3.8	2.1	3.9	1.9	2.0	1.6	3.7	5.8	-	2.8	0.7	0.18	0.20	2.3	KAP
Melanoma of skin	135	0	-	-	-	0.7	0.6	1.4	2.9	2.9	9.2	16.0	12.9	7.8	20.0	10.1	22.8	29.5	25.9	14.4	7.0	1.7	0.37	0.54	5.1	172
Other skin	695	0	-	-	-	-	0.6	1.4	2.2	1.4	2.8	5.6	17.2	35.2	59.9	105.5	164.3	280.5	322.5	447.8	36.2		0.63	1.98	18.7	173
Breast	19	0	-	-	-	-	-	-	-	-	-	-	1.1	2.0	3.8	5.1	1.6	9.2	-	4.8	1.0	0.2	0.03	0.07	0.6	175
Prostate	1526	0	-	-	-	-	-	-	-	-	-	2.8	7.5	50.9	137.8	271.8	501.0	607.1	800.4	654.9	79.5	19.1	1.00	4.86	39.6	185
Testis	56	0	1.6	-	-	0.7	2.5	7.1	10.2	2.9	5.0	4.7	1.1	2.9	1.0	2.0	3.3	-	-	-	2.9	0.7	0.20	0.22	2.7	186
Penis	23	0	-	-	-	-	0.6	-	-	0.7	-	-	-	1.0	2.9	4.1	11.4	9.2	2.9	-	1.2	0.3	0.03	0.10	0.7	187.1-.4
Other male genital	1	0	-	-	-	-	-	-	-	-	-	-	-	-	-	1.0	-	-	-	-	0.1	0.0	0.00	0.01	0.0	187.5-.9
†Bladder	612	0	-	-	-	-	-	-	0.7	-	5.7	9.4	19.3	41.1	67.5	156.2	138.3	164.2	241.8	240.8	31.9	7.7	0.72	2.19	17.8	188
Kidney etc.	274	0	-	0.8	0.8	-	0.6	-	2.2	3.6	4.3	10.3	20.4	27.4	39.9	68.0	60.2	55.4	48.9	28.9	14.3	3.4	0.55	1.19	9.3	189
Eye	5	0	0.8	-	-	-	-	-	-	-	-	-	1.1	1.0	-	-	-	1.8	2.9	-	0.3	0.1	0.01	0.01	0.2	190
Brain, nervous system	115	0	1.6	2.4	1.6	0.7	1.8	1.4	4.4	4.3	3.6	9.4	6.4	9.8	18.1	11.2	21.1	12.9	17.3	14.4	6.0	1.4	0.33	0.49	4.7	191-2
Thyroid	39	0	-	-	-	0.7	0.6	-	1.5	2.9	3.6	5.6	3.2	4.9	1.9	1.0	4.9	3.7	8.6	4.8	2.0	0.5	0.12	0.15	1.6	193
Other endocrine	8	0	-	-	-	-	-	-	-	0.7	-	-	-	1.9	-	3.3	3.7	2.9	-	-	0.4	0.1	0.01	0.03	0.2	194
Hodgkin's disease	63	0	2.5	0.8	0.8	1.4	3.7	4.3	6.5	6.4	3.6	2.8	5.4	2.0	4.8	2.0	1.6	3.7	2.9	-	3.3	0.8	0.22	0.24	3.0	201
Non-Hodgkin lymphoma	287	0	1.6	1.6	1.6	2.0	2.5	6.4	8.0	10.7	15.6	12.2	8.6	34.2	27.6	39.6	47.2	51.7	63.3	67.4	15.0	3.6	0.66	1.10	10.4	200,202
Multiple myeloma	68	0	-	-	-	-	-	-	-	-	2.1	2.8	5.4	4.9	7.6	10.1	19.5	25.8	11.5	19.3	3.5	0.8	0.11	0.26	2.2	203
Lymphoid leukaemia	65	0	2.5	-	-	0.7	1.2	-	-	-	1.4	3.8	3.2	8.8	5.7	11.2	11.4	16.6	17.3	9.6	3.4	0.8	0.14	0.25	2.4	204
Myeloid leukaemia	68	0	1.6	1.6	-	1.4	2.5	2.1	2.2	3.6	2.1	3.8	2.1	7.8	3.8	7.1	13.0	7.4	11.5	14.4	3.5	0.8	0.17	0.27	2.8	205
Monocytic leukaemia	1	0	-	-	-	-	-	-	-	-	-	-	-	-	-	-	1.0	-	-	-	0.1	0.0	0.00	0.01	0.0	206
Other leukaemia	0	0	-	-	-	-	-	-	-	-	-	-	-	-	-	-	-	-	-	-	0.0	0.0	0.00	0.00	0.0	207
Leukaemia unspecified	21	0	0.8	0.8	1.6	-	0.6	-	-	-	-	-	0.9	-	1.9	4.1	6.5	3.7	2.9	9.6	1.1	0.3	0.03	0.09	0.9	208
Other and unspecified	294	0	0.8	-	0.8	-	-	0.7	1.5	4.3	7.1	6.6	23.6	32.3	39.0	59.8	56.9	73.8	86.4	28.9	15.3	3.7	0.58	1.17	9.7	O&U
All sites	8695	0	15.5	8.0	10.4	12.2	22.8	38.4	62.4	95.1	162.6	298.0	466.0	683.8	1071.2	1578.1	2044.6	2351.1	2648.7	2465.5	453.2		14.73	32.85	277.5	ALL
All sites but 173	8000	0	15.5	8.0	10.4	12.2	22.1	37.0	60.2	93.7	159.8	292.3	448.8	648.6	1011.3	1472.7	1880.3	2070.6	2326.3	2017.6	417.0	100.0	14.10	30.86	258.8	ALLb

Rate from 1 case   0.817   0.802   0.800   0.676   0.615   0.711   0.726   0.715   0.710   0.940   1.074   0.978   0.950   1.014   1.627   1.845   2.879   4.815

†Important: see notes on population page

492

* FRANCE, HERAULT 1988-1992

ANNUAL INCIDENCE PER 100,000 BY AGE GROUP (YEARS) - FEMALE

SITE	ALL AGES	AGE UNK	0-	5-	10-	15-	20-	25-	30-	35-	40-	45-	50-	55-	60-	65-	70-	75-	80-	85+	CRUDE RATE	%	CR 64	CR 74	ASR (W)	ICD (9th)
Lip	6	0	-	-	-	-	-	-	-	-	-	-	-	0.9	-	0.9	1.3	-	1.6	3.9	0.3	0.1	0.00	0.02	**0.1**	*140*
Tongue	27	0	-	-	-	-	0.6	0.7	-	-	0.7	2.7	2.0	3.5	4.2	2.6	2.6	1.3	4.9	2.0	1.3	0.4	0.07	0.10	**0.9**	*141*
Salivary gland	10	0	-	-	-	-	-	0.7	0.7	-	1.4	-	-	2.7	0.8	-	1.3	-	1.6	-	0.5	0.2	0.03	0.04	**0.4**	*142*
Mouth	45	0	-	-	-	-	-	-	0.7	-	0.7	2.7	1.0	6.2	5.9	3.4	5.2	5.2	13.0	9.8	2.2	0.7	0.09	0.13	**1.2**	*143-5*
Oropharynx	19	0	-	-	-	-	-	0.7	-	-	0.7	1.8	4.0	2.7	5.9	0.9	-	-	-	-	0.9	0.3	0.08	0.08	**0.8**	*146*
Nasopharynx	5	0	-	-	0.7	1.2	-	-	0.7	-	-	-	-	-	-	0.9	-	-	-	-	0.2	0.1	0.01	0.02	**0.2**	*147*
Hypopharynx	4	0	-	-	-	-	-	-	-	-	-	-	1.0	1.8	-	-	-	-	1.3	-	-	0.2	0.1	0.01	0.01	**0.1**	*148*
Pharynx unspecified	5	0	-	-	-	-	-	-	-	-	0.7	-	-	0.9	-	0.9	1.3	-	-	2.0	0.2	0.1	0.01	0.02	**0.1**	*149*
Oesophagus	51	0	-	-	-	-	-	-	-	1.4	-	2.7	1.0	2.7	5.1	4.3	5.2	7.8	14.6	23.4	2.5	0.8	0.06	0.11	**1.1**	*150*
Stomach	192	0	-	-	-	-	-	-	1.4	2.1	2.8	1.8	8.0	4.4	11.8	24.0	39.3	48.1	56.9	46.8	9.2	2.9	0.16	0.48	**4.0**	*151*
Small intestine	25	0	-	-	-	-	-	-	-	-	-	0.9	1.0	4.4	1.7	1.7	6.5	5.2	-	9.8	1.2	0.4	0.04	0.08	**0.6**	*152*
Colon	589	0	-	0.8	-	-	-	0.7	1.4	0.7	8.3	22.8	22.0	40.7	38.8	75.3	91.7	130.0	134.9	179.6	28.3	8.9	0.68	1.52	**13.4**	*153*
Rectum	339	0	-	-	-	-	-	0.7	1.4	0.7	4.1	9.1	15.0	23.0	30.4	44.5	69.4	81.9	68.3	62.5	16.3	5.1	0.42	0.99	**8.1**	*154*
Liver	28	0	-	-	-	-	-	-	-	-	0.7	-	1.0	-	6.7	5.1	6.5	5.2	1.6	3.9	1.3	0.4	0.04	0.10	**0.7**	*155*
Gallbladder etc.	66	0	-	-	-	-	-	-	-	-	0.7	2.7	4.0	2.7	6.7	6.8	11.8	11.7	17.9	19.5	3.2	1.0	0.08	0.18	**1.5**	*156*
Pancreas	76	0	-	-	-	-	-	0.7	-	1.4	-	3.6	3.0	5.3	5.1	20.5	11.8	14.3	8.1	9.8	3.7	1.1	0.10	0.26	**2.0**	*157*
Nose, sinuses etc.	18	0	0.9	-	-	-	-	0.7	-	-	-	-	3.0	1.8	1.7	3.4	2.6	1.3	3.3	-	0.9	0.3	0.04	0.07	**0.6**	*160*
Larynx	21	0	-	-	-	-	-	-	-	0.7	2.8	2.7	3.0	-	4.2	1.7	1.3	-	3.3	-	1.0	0.3	0.07	0.08	**0.8**	*161*
Bronchus, lung	185	0	-	-	-	-	-	-	2.1	0.7	6.2	9.1	12.0	17.7	30.4	22.2	34.1	27.3	19.5	17.6	8.9	2.8	0.39	0.67	**5.4**	*162*
Other thoracic organs	4	0	-	-	-	-	-	-	0.7	0.7	-	-	-	-	-	0.9	-	1.3	-	-	0.2	0.1	0.01	0.01	**0.1**	*163-4*
Bone	25	0	0.9	-	1.7	1.4	1.2	1.4	0.7	1.4	1.4	0.9	-	1.8	0.8	2.6	-	-	4.9	2.0	1.2	0.4	0.07	0.08	**1.1**	*170*
Connective tissue	52	0	1.7	-	0.8	2.7	2.3	-	1.4	0.7	1.4	4.6	1.0	5.3	3.4	3.4	2.6	6.5	4.9	11.7	2.5	0.8	0.13	0.16	**1.9**	*171*
Mesothelioma	8	0	-	-	-	-	-	-	-	-	-	0.9	2.0	1.8	-	1.7	-	-	1.6	-	0.4	0.1	0.02	0.03	**0.3**	*MES*
Kaposi's sarcoma	5	0	-	-	-	-	-	-	0.7	-	-	-	-	2.7	-	0.9	-	-	-	-	0.2	0.1	0.02	0.02	**0.2**	*KAP*
Melanoma of skin	182	0	-	-	0.8	2.0	5.2	2.7	4.9	8.3	10.4	16.4	15.0	10.6	16.9	11.1	14.4	23.4	21.1	21.5	8.8	2.7	0.47	0.59	**6.2**	*172*
Other skin	407	0	-	-	-	-	-	0.7	1.4	3.4	2.1	3.6	8.0	13.3	16.0	43.6	47.2	80.6	123.6	244.0	19.6		0.24	0.70	**7.2**	*173*
Breast	2489	0	-	-	-	-	-	9.5	23.7	82.6	140.4	216.9	224.5	233.8	267.4	296.8	301.3	291.2	248.8	236.2	119.7	37.6	5.99	8.98	**80.1**	*174*
Uterus unspecified	9	0	-	-	-	-	-	-	0.7	-	-	1.8	1.0	0.9	1.7	0.9	-	-	-	2.0	0.4	0.1	0.03	0.03	**0.3**	*179*
Cervix uteri	379	0	-	-	-	-	2.3	8.8	31.4	28.9	36.0	30.1	34.1	23.9	28.7	28.2	27.5	18.2	30.9	15.6	18.2	5.7	1.12	1.40	**14.1**	*180*
Placenta	0	0	-	-	-	-	-	-	-	-	-	-	-	-	-	-	-	-	-	-	0.0	0.0	0.00	0.00	**0.0**	*181*
Corpus uteri	350	0	-	-	-	-	-	-	0.7	4.8	14.6	30.1	37.2	51.5	58.2	56.3	58.5	39.0	25.4	-	16.8	5.3	0.69	1.27	**10.0**	*182*
Ovary etc.	211	0	-	-	0.8	-	2.3	2.0	3.5	5.5	5.5	11.8	16.0	23.9	27.8	30.8	19.6	22.1	29.3	13.7	10.1	3.2	0.50	0.75	**6.6**	*183*
Other female genital	68	0	-	-	-	-	-	-	-	0.7	0.9	1.0	7.1	2.5	12.8	14.4	11.7	17.9	15.6	-	3.3	1.0	0.06	0.20	**1.5**	*184*
†Bladder	134	0	-	-	-	-	0.6	-	-	-	-	-	3.0	3.5	11.0	12.8	19.6	32.5	53.7	48.8	6.4	2.0	0.09	0.25	**2.4**	*188*
Kidney etc.	112	0	1.7	-	-	-	0.6	0.7	0.7	-	4.1	2.7	6.0	12.4	11.8	18.0	21.0	23.4	9.8	5.9	5.4	1.7	0.20	0.40	**3.3**	*189*
Eye	4	0	0.9	-	-	-	-	-	-	0.7	-	-	-	0.9	-	0.9	-	-	-	-	0.2	0.1	0.01	0.02	**0.2**	*190*
Brain, nervous system	91	0	2.6	-	-	1.4	1.2	0.7	4.2	2.1	2.8	2.7	11.0	10.6	6.7	13.7	13.1	7.8	3.3	3.9	4.4	1.4	0.23	0.36	**3.3**	*191-2*
Thyroid	123	0	-	-	-	2.0	0.6	6.8	10.5	6.2	6.9	14.6	9.0	9.7	9.3	8.6	9.2	7.8	8.1	-	5.9	1.9	0.38	0.47	**4.8**	*193*
Other endocrine	4	0	0.9	-	-	-	-	-	-	0.7	-	-	-	0.9	0.8	0.9	-	-	-	-	0.2	0.1	0.01	0.02	**0.2**	*194*
Hodgkin's disease	36	0	-	-	0.8	2.0	3.5	0.7	2.8	4.8	2.1	0.9	3.0	-	1.7	1.7	1.3	1.3	-	2.0	1.7	0.5	0.11	0.13	**1.5**	*201*
Non-Hodgkin lymphoma	251	0	1.7	-	-	2.0	-	4.7	4.2	2.8	4.1	10.0	12.0	12.4	19.4	30.8	51.1	53.3	50.4	31.2	12.1	3.8	0.37	0.78	**6.8**	*200,202*
Multiple myeloma	69	0	-	-	-	-	-	-	0.7	1.4	1.4	2.7	1.0	2.7	6.7	12.8	10.5	15.6	14.6	9.8	3.3	1.0	0.08	0.20	**1.7**	*203*
Lymphoid leukaemia	54	0	3.4	2.5	0.8	-	-	0.7	-	0.7	1.4	0.9	2.0	3.5	5.1	6.0	11.8	3.9	11.4	5.9	2.6	0.8	0.11	0.19	**2.0**	*204*
Myeloid leukaemia	33	0	0.9	-	1.7	-	-	-	1.4	0.7	2.1	-	3.0	3.5	1.7	1.7	6.5	5.2	4.9	2.0	1.6	0.5	0.07	0.12	**1.1**	*205*
Monocytic leukaemia	2	0	-	-	-	-	-	-	-	-	-	-	-	-	-	-	-	1.3	1.3	-	0.1	0.0	0.00	0.01	**0.0**	*206*
Other leukaemia	0	0	-	-	-	-	-	-	-	-	-	-	-	-	-	-	-	-	-	-	0.0	0.0	0.00	0.00	**0.0**	*207*
Leukaemia unspecified	18	0	0.9	0.8	-	0.7	1.2	-	0.7	0.7	-	0.9	-	-	1.7	3.4	1.3	2.6	-	2.0	0.9	0.3	0.04	0.06	**0.7**	*208*
Other and unspecified	203	0	1.7	2.5	-	-	-	-	2.8	6.2	2.1	3.6	5.0	15.9	21.1	20.5	28.8	57.2	29.3	42.9	9.8	3.1	0.30	0.55	**5.2**	*O&U*
All sites	7034	0	18.0	6.8	7.5	15.0	22.6	44.0	103.9	167.2	259.3	404.6	469.0	559.6	673.2	842.5	950.9	1065.8	1056.8	1132.0	338.2		13.75	22.72	**204.9**	*ALL*
All sites but 173	6627	0	18.0	6.8	7.5	15.0	22.6	43.3	102.5	163.7	257.2	400.9	461.0	546.3	657.2	798.9	903.8	985.2	933.2	888.0	318.6	100.0	13.51	22.02	**197.8**	*ALLb*
Rate from 1 case			0.856	0.846	0.835	0.680	0.578	0.677	0.697	0.688	0.691	0.911	1.002	0.885	0.844	0.855	1.310	1.300	1.626	1.952						

†Important: see notes on population page

France, Isère

The Isère Cancer Registry opened in the autumn of 1978 and published its first cancer incidence report in 1979. It has always received financial support from the Isère General Council. In 1992, the registry obtained support from the French Government, and especially from the Department of Health and the Institut National de la Santé et de la Recherche Médicale (INSERM). For the years 1988–92, the registry was staffed by two technicians who entered the data, one secretary, one statistician/programmer, one investigating physician and two medical epidemiologists.

Surrounded by the Alps to the east and by the Rhone valley to the north and west, the département of Isère covers 7431 km² (3500 of which are mountainous), making it the tenth largest département in France. It is situated at latitude 45°, with a minimum altitude of 191 metres, and maximum of 4102 metres (Ecrins mountain).

The population of the Isère was 1 016 000 in 1990, with a density of 137 persons per km². This population has increased by 1% a year; by 1993 the population was 1 045 000. As in the rest of France, the population of Isère has been ageing since 1982. At that time, 30% of the population was aged under 20 years, and 62% under 40 years. Eight years later, the population under 20 years represented only 28% and that under 40 years 59%.

Since the 1960s, the Rhone–Alpes region has had a higher proportion of foreigners than the rest of France. The proportion is even higher in Isère than elsewhere in the region, with 9.3% in 1968 in comparison to the regional proportion of 5.3%. However, in 1990, this had dropped to 7.9%. In 1990, there was a total of 33 700 (3.3%) foreigners born in the EU, with 1.3% Italians, 0.4% Spaniards and 1.3% Portuguese. Foreigners born outside the EU (4.6%) comprised 1.8% Algerians (18 000), 0.6% Moroccans (6200), 0.7% Tunisians (7428) and 0.7% Turks (6900).

In 1989, the département of Isère had 15 hospitals, one of which was a regional and university hospital, and nine private clinics. In 1990, there were 3186 doctors, 1770 of whom were general practitioners and 1416 specialists. Among these were 470 specialists of anatomical systems (dermatology, medical gynaecology, pneumology, etc.), 27 pathologists and 10 radiologists. There were 329 (23%) surgeons.

Data are obtained from some 80 sources of information in Isère and the surrounding départements, including pathology and cytology laboratories, health insurance companies, public and private radiotherapy units, medical and surgical departments of general hospitals and private clinics, as well as the administrative departments of hospitals, and, since 1992, medical information departments of several hospitals.

After each file has been created by technicians, it is checked and the medical information coded by doctors. This double checking, the multiple sources (1.7 sources per case) and computer-checked data entry all add to the completeness and quality of the data.

There is no active follow-up of the registered cases, except, from time to time, for specific survival studies. However, follow-up information on patients that is received is recorded, as is information obtained from death certificates. However, this cannot be considered as a comprehensive follow-up.

A cancer map (distribution of SIR in the 45 cantons of Isère) using data from 1979–84 showed an area of lower incidence along the north-western border of Isère which was interpreted as due to under-reporting. Over the period 1979–84, coverage was evaluated at 95%. Since then, efforts have been made to improve data collection, but no re-evaluation has yet been carried out.

In addition to preparing incidence data, the registry has carried out:

Evaluation of screening for breast, colon and cervix cancers, which began in 1990;

Analysis of different methods of diagnosis and treatment of breast and prostate cancers;

Surveillance of occupational cohorts (notably in the field of chemistry);

Case–control studies of brain tumours in adults

Evaluation of prevalence in collaboration with other French registries and with IARC.

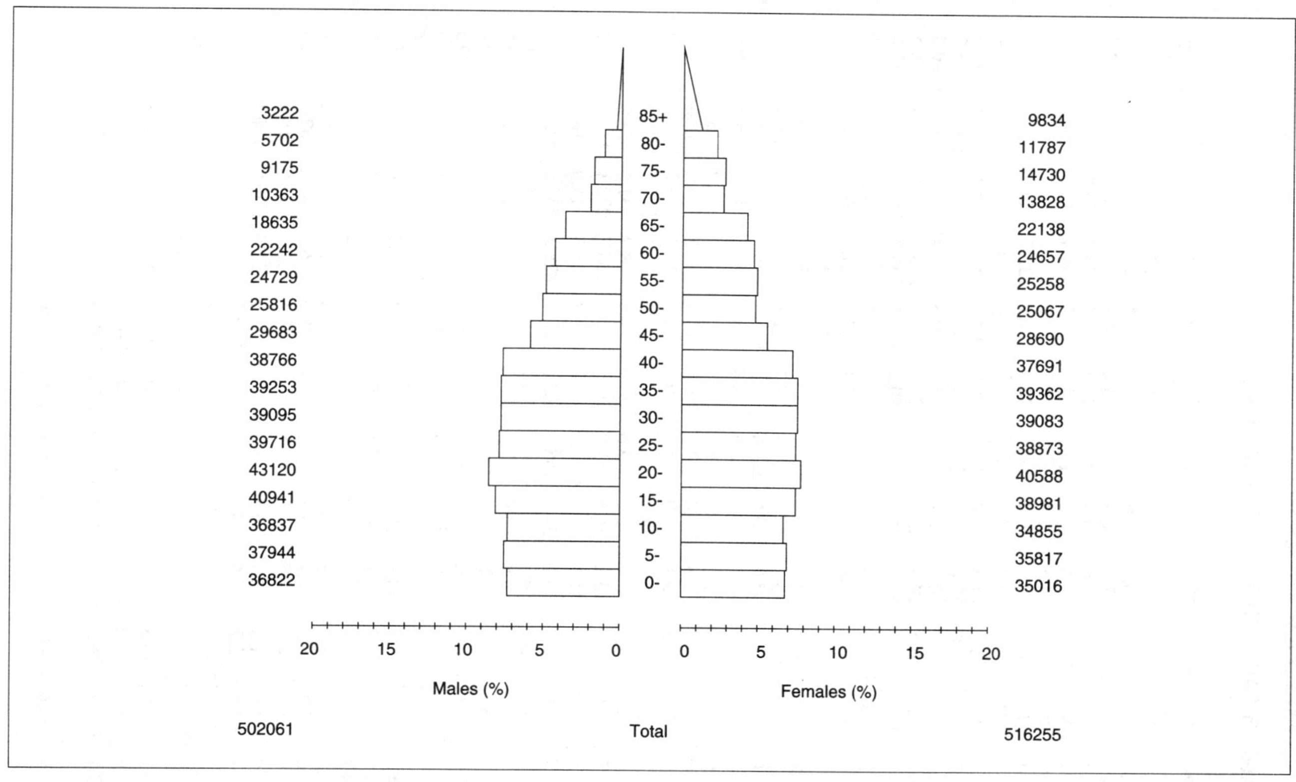

France, Isère
Source of population: 1988–92
Census: Recensement de la population 1990, Population de la France, Départements, arrondissements, cantons, communes. Direction Générale des Collectivités Locales, Institut National de la Statistique et des Etudes Economiques.
Estimate: Population estimates provided by the official national department of demography (INSEE) were used for each of the years 1988-92 (Estimations de la Population, INSEE, 1996)

Notes to tables overleaf:
† 173 does not include basal cell carcinoma
Screening programmes in the area
Since 1990, the population aged 50-69 has been screened for cervical, breast and large bowel cancer every two and a half years.

FRANCE, ISERE 1988-1992

ANNUAL INCIDENCE PER 100,000 BY AGE GROUP (YEARS) - MALE

SITE	ALL AGES	AGE UNK	0-	5-	10-	15-	20-	25-	30-	35-	40-	45-	50-	55-	60-	65-	70-	75-	80-	85+	CRUDE RATE	%	CR 64	CR 74	ASR (W)	ICD (9th)
Lip	24	0	-	-	-	-	-	-	0.5	-	0.5	2.7	0.8	2.4	2.7	1.1	3.9	10.9	-	18.6	1.0	0.3	0.05	0.07	**0.8**	140
Tongue	122	0	-	-	-	-	-	0.5	0.5	1.0	4.1	8.1	16.3	18.6	12.6	20.4	15.4	24.0	7.0	-	4.9	1.3	0.31	0.49	**4.1**	141
Salivary gland	11	0	-	-	-	-	-	0.5	0.5	-	-	1.5	0.8	-	3.2	3.9	-	3.5	-	-	0.4	0.1	0.02	0.05	**0.4**	142
Mouth	158	0	-	-	-	-	-	-	-	1.0	5.2	10.1	17.8	18.6	26.1	29.0	23.2	26.2	14.0	6.2	6.3	1.7	0.39	0.65	**5.4**	143-5
Oropharynx	175	0	-	-	-	-	0.5	-	-	3.6	8.3	12.1	19.4	16.2	19.8	34.3	32.8	24.0	17.5	6.2	7.0	1.9	0.40	0.73	**5.9**	146
Nasopharynx	18	0	-	-	0.5	-	0.9	0.5	-	1.5	0.5	-	1.5	2.4	0.9	3.2	1.9	-	-	-	0.7	0.2	0.04	0.07	**0.6**	147
Hypopharynx	194	0	-	-	-	-	-	-	-	1.0	4.1	16.8	20.1	29.9	36.0	26.8	17.4	32.7	24.6	-	7.7	2.1	0.54	0.76	**6.6**	148
Pharynx unspecified	29	0	-	-	-	-	-	-	-	0.5	0.5	2.0	5.4	3.2	2.7	4.3	11.6	-	-	-	1.2	0.3	0.07	0.15	**1.1**	149
Oesophagus	294	0	-	-	-	-	-	0.5	1.5	6.7	12.1	21.7	34.8	65.6	56.9	63.7	34.9	28.1	31.0	11.7	3.2	0.71	1.32	**10.0**	150
Stomach	381	0	-	-	-	-	0.5	-	3.1	3.6	8.3	8.8	17.0	25.9	51.3	71.9	86.8	124.3	129.8	130.4	15.2	4.1	0.59	1.39	**11.8**	151
Small intestine	21	0	-	-	-	-	-	-	-	-	-	0.8	2.4	2.7	4.3	9.6	4.4	7.0	-	0.8	0.2	0.03	0.10	**0.7**	152
Colon	715	0	-	-	-	0.5	-	0.5	2.6	4.1	7.2	20.9	24.8	45.3	89.0	127.7	218.1	233.2	273.6	316.6	28.5	7.8	0.97	2.70	**22.3**	153
Rectum	497	0	-	-	-	-	-	0.5	0.5	4.1	11.9	6.7	23.2	34.8	71.0	90.2	135.1	180.9	161.3	117.9	19.8	5.4	0.76	1.89	**15.4**	154
Liver	277	0	1.6	0.5	-	-	-	0.5	0.5	-	2.5	3.6	6.1	13.9	18.6	45.9	60.1	84.9	78.5	56.1	37.2	11.0	3.0	0.47	1.19	**9.1**	155
Gallbladder etc.	47	0	-	-	-	-	-	-	-	-	-	0.5	0.7	3.9	2.4	6.3	5.4	13.5	21.8	24.6	6.2	1.9	0.5	0.07	0.16	**1.4**	156
Pancreas	144	0	-	-	-	-	-	0.5	-	-	2.6	6.7	7.7	17.0	15.3	30.1	32.8	41.4	28.1	49.7	5.7	1.6	0.25	0.56	**4.6**	157
Nose, sinuses etc.	36	0	-	-	-	-	-	-	0.5	0.5	0.7	1.5	3.2	5.4	10.7	7.7	10.9	7.0	-	1.4	0.4	0.06	0.15	**1.1**	160
Larynx	288	0	-	-	-	-	-	-	0.5	3.1	5.7	12.1	25.6	42.9	56.6	53.7	52.1	21.8	42.1	24.8	11.5	3.1	0.73	1.26	**9.7**	161
Bronchus, lung	1532	0	-	-	-	-	0.5	-	1.0	6.1	29.4	53.2	93.0	170.6	235.6	317.7	411.0	368.4	280.6	186.2	61.0	16.6	2.95	6.59	**50.1**	162
Other thoracic organs	16	0	-	-	-	-	-	-	-	0.5	-	0.7	-	-	3.6	4.3	3.9	-	10.5	6.2	0.6	0.2	0.02	0.06	**0.5**	163-4
Bone	24	0	0.5	0.5	-	1.0	1.4	1.0	2.0	0.5	0.5	1.3	1.5	-	0.9	1.1	-	-	7.0	6.2	1.0	0.3	0.06	0.06	**0.9**	170
Connective tissue	49	0	1.1	-	0.5	1.0	0.5	-	1.5	1.0	2.6	2.0	1.5	2.4	2.7	6.4	15.4	8.7	3.5	18.6	2.0	0.5	0.08	0.19	**1.7**	171
Mesothelioma	48	0	-	-	-	-	-	0.5	-	0.5	2.1	1.3	3.1	4.9	7.2	9.7	5.8	15.3	10.5	-	1.9	0.5	0.10	0.18	**1.5**	MES
Kaposi's sarcoma	22	0	-	-	-	-	-	2.0	2.0	2.5	1.0	-	1.6	0.9	2.1	3.9	-	-	-	-	0.9	0.2	0.05	0.08	**0.7**	KAP
Melanoma of skin	124	0	-	0.5	0.5	-	0.9	2.0	3.1	5.1	6.2	4.7	12.4	12.1	12.6	12.9	13.5	8.7	31.6	24.8	4.9	1.3	0.30	0.43	**4.1**	172
†Other skin	452	0	-	-	-	-	0.5	0.5	1.5	0.5	4.1	4.7	13.2	18.6	45.9	75.1	110.0	165.7	270.1	372.4	18.0		0.45	1.37	**13.3**	173
Breast	31	0	-	-	-	-	-	-	-	0.5	0.5	-	1.5	-	4.5	5.4	5.8	15.3	14.0	18.6	1.2	0.3	0.04	0.09	**0.9**	175
Prostate	1642	0	-	-	-	-	-	-	-	0.5	2.1	6.1	13.2	54.2	158.3	302.6	584.7	828.3	852.3	993.2	65.4	17.8	1.17	5.61	**48.0**	185
Testis	103	0	0.5	-	-	3.9	3.7	11.6	7.2	7.1	8.3	5.4	0.8	2.4	4.5	1.1	-	-	3.5	-	4.1	1.1	0.28	0.28	**3.7**	186
Penis	19	0	-	-	-	-	-	-	-	-	-	-	0.8	4.0	1.8	3.2	1.9	6.5	10.5	6.2	0.8	0.2	0.03	0.06	**0.6**	187.1-.4
Other male genital	6	0	-	-	-	-	-	0.5	-	-	-	0.7	0.8	-	3.2	-	-	-	-	-	0.2	0.1	0.01	0.03	**0.2**	187.5-.9
Bladder	514	0	-	-	0.5	-	-	-	-	2.0	3.1	10.8	18.6	38.0	69.2	111.6	144.7	148.2	199.9	217.3	20.5	5.6	0.71	1.99	**16.0**	188
Kidney etc.	288	0	3.3	-	-	-	-	0.5	1.0	3.1	4.1	14.8	18.6	34.8	36.9	51.5	67.5	78.5	42.1	24.8	11.5	3.1	0.59	1.18	**9.6**	189
Eye	14	0	-	-	-	-	-	-	-	-	-	-	3.9	-	2.7	1.1	-	10.9	-	-	0.6	0.2	0.03	0.04	**0.4**	190
Brain, nervous system	150	0	1.6	2.6	3.3	2.0	2.8	2.5	4.6	4.6	5.2	6.1	10.1	10.5	17.1	21.5	17.4	8.7	14.0	12.4	6.0	1.6	0.36	0.56	**5.4**	191-2
Thyroid	47	0	-	-	-	-	-	1.0	2.6	2.0	4.6	2.7	3.1	4.0	1.8	6.4	5.8	4.4	3.5	-	1.9	0.5	0.11	0.17	**1.6**	193
Other endocrine	7	0	1.1	-	-	-	-	-	-	0.5	-	0.7	0.8	0.8	-	-	-	2.2	-	-	0.3	0.1	0.02	0.02	**0.3**	194
Hodgkin's disease	66	0	-	1.6	1.1	2.9	2.8	6.5	4.1	1.0	4.1	1.3	2.3	3.2	1.8	3.2	1.9	2.2	3.5	6.2	2.6	0.7	0.16	0.19	**2.4**	201
Non-Hodgkin lymphoma	320	0	4.3	1.6	1.6	1.5	1.9	2.5	5.1	5.6	16.0	16.2	20.1	17.8	29.7	49.4	38.6	76.3	91.2	62.1	12.7	3.5	0.62	1.06	**10.6**	200,202
Multiple myeloma	79	0	-	-	-	-	-	-	1.0	1.0	1.0	4.0	7.7	1.6	10.8	19.3	17.4	13.1	24.6	18.6	3.1	0.9	0.14	0.32	**2.6**	203
Lymphoid leukaemia	113	0	2.2	3.2	2.7	2.4	0.9	1.0	0.5	1.5	4.6	1.3	3.1	6.5	9.9	17.2	19.3	24.0	35.1	24.8	4.5	1.2	0.20	0.38	**3.9**	204
Myeloid leukaemia	120	0	0.5	0.5	-	1.5	1.9	1.5	2.6	3.1	2.6	2.7	4.6	8.9	11.7	17.2	23.2	28.3	38.6	37.2	4.8	1.3	0.21	0.41	**3.9**	205
Monocytic leukaemia	5	0	-	0.5	-	-	-	0.5	-	-	-	-	-	-	-	1.9	4.4	-	-	-	0.2	0.1	0.01	0.01	**0.2**	206
Other leukaemia	0	0	-	-	-	-	-	-	-	-	-	-	-	-	-	-	-	-	-	-	0.0	0.0	0.00	0.00	**0.0**	207
Leukaemia unspecified	9	0	-	-	-	-	-	-	-	0.5	-	-	-	-	-	-	3.2	1.9	4.4	7.0	0.4	0.1	0.00	0.03	**0.2**	208
Other and unspecified	432	0	1.1	-	0.5	-	-	0.5	2.0	5.1	3.6	13.5	20.9	42.9	56.6	90.2	106.1	100.3	126.3	142.8	17.2	4.7	0.73	1.72	**13.9**	O&U
All sites	9663	0	17.9	11.6	11.4	16.6	19.9	37.3	51.2	83.6	175.9	281.0	478.8	759.4	1236.4	1769.8	2416.1	2792.4	2904.1	2929.9	384.9		15.90	36.83	**308.2**	ALL
All sites but 173	9211	0	17.9	11.6	11.4	16.6	19.5	36.8	49.6	83.1	171.8	276.3	465.6	740.8	1190.5	1694.6	2306.1	2626.7	2634.1	2557.4	366.9	100.0	15.46	35.46	**294.9**	ALLb

Rate from 1 case   0.543   0.527   0.543   0.489   0.464   0.504   0.512   0.510   0.516   0.674   0.775   0.809   0.899   1.073   1.930   2.180   3.507   6.207

†Important: see notes on population page

FRANCE, ISERE 1988-1992

ANNUAL INCIDENCE PER 100,000 BY AGE GROUP (YEARS) - FEMALE

SITE	ALL AGES	AGE UNK	0-	5-	10-	15-	20-	25-	30-	35-	40-	45-	50-	55-	60-	65-	70-	75-	80-	85+	CRUDE RATE	%	CR 64	CR 74	ASR (W)	ICD (9th)
Lip	8	0	-	-	-	-	-	-	-	-	-	0.7	0.8	-	-	-	-	1.4	-	5.1	4.1	0.3	0.1	0.01	0.01	**0.2**	140
Tongue	27	0	-	-	-	-	-	0.5	1.0	0.5	0.5	-	1.6	1.6	4.9	0.9	-	6.8	8.5	2.0	1.0	0.3	0.05	0.06	**0.7**	141
Salivary gland	15	0	-	-	-	-	-	-	-	0.5	0.5	0.7	1.6	-	2.4	2.7	1.4	1.4	1.7	2.0	0.6	0.2	0.03	0.05	**0.4**	142
Mouth	37	0	-	-	-	-	-	-	-	1.5	-	2.8	1.6	2.4	2.4	4.5	10.1	4.1	6.8	6.1	1.4	0.5	0.05	0.13	**1.0**	143-5
Oropharynx	34	0	-	-	-	-	-	-	-	-	1.6	2.1	3.2	4.0	3.2	2.7	4.3	5.4	3.4	6.1	1.3	0.4	0.07	0.11	**0.9**	146
Nasopharynx	4	0	-	-	-	-	-	-	-	-	-	0.7	0.8	-	0.8	-	-	-	1.7	-	0.2	0.1	0.01	0.01	**0.1**	147
Hypopharynx	7	0	-	-	-	-	-	-	-	-	-	0.7	-	-	2.4	1.8	1.4	-	-	-	0.3	0.1	0.02	0.03	**0.2**	148
Pharynx unspecified	5	0	-	-	-	-	-	-	-	-	-	-	-	1.6	1.6	0.9	-	-	-	-	0.2	0.1	0.02	0.02	**0.2**	149
Oesophagus	41	0	-	-	-	-	-	-	-	1.0	-	-	1.6	7.1	2.4	9.0	5.8	5.4	6.8	6.1	1.6	0.5	0.06	0.13	**1.0**	150
Stomach	257	0	-	-	-	-	-	0.5	2.0	1.5	4.8	4.2	6.4	6.3	12.2	17.2	34.7	47.5	110.3	122.0	10.0	3.3	0.19	0.45	**4.7**	151
Small intestine	27	0	-	-	-	-	-	0.5	0.5	-	1.1	1.4	-	1.6	4.1	2.7	1.4	4.1	6.8	6.1	1.0	0.3	0.05	0.07	**0.7**	152
Colon	727	0	-	-	-	0.5	-	1.5	2.0	2.5	8.0	17.4	18.4	32.5	66.5	79.5	128.7	160.2	235.8	191.2	28.2	9.3	0.75	1.79	**15.5**	153
Rectum	425	0	-	-	-	-	-	-	1.0	2.5	4.8	9.8	12.0	34.0	41.4	58.7	78.1	73.3	103.5	105.8	16.5	5.4	0.53	1.21	**9.8**	154
Liver	37	0	-	-	-	-	-	-	-	-	1.1	1.4	1.6	3.2	2.4	5.4	7.2	8.1	3.4	10.2	1.4	0.5	0.05	0.11	**0.9**	155
Gallbladder etc.	60	0	-	-	-	-	-	-	-	0.5	0.5	0.7	-	2.4	1.6	10.8	18.8	9.5	8.5	30.5	2.3	0.8	0.03	0.18	**1.3**	156
Pancreas	113	0	-	-	-	-	0.5	-	-	1.0	1.6	2.1	6.4	8.7	4.9	19.9	33.3	16.3	18.7	22.4	4.4	1.4	0.13	0.39	**2.8**	157
Nose, sinuses etc.	13	0	-	-	-	0.5	-	-	-	-	0.5	0.7	-	0.8	0.8	0.9	1.4	5.4	1.7	2.0	0.5	0.2	0.02	0.03	**0.3**	160
Larynx	18	0	-	-	-	-	0.5	-	-	0.5	0.5	1.4	2.4	0.8	2.4	1.8	-	4.1	-	2.0	0.7	0.2	0.04	0.05	**0.5**	161
Bronchus, lung	213	0	-	-	-	-	-	0.5	1.5	2.5	3.7	8.4	9.6	18.2	19.5	39.8	36.2	42.1	32.2	14.2	8.3	2.7	0.32	0.70	**5.6**	162
Other thoracic organs	14	0	1.1	-	-	0.5	-	0.5	-	0.5	-	1.4	-	0.8	-	1.8	1.4	1.4	3.4	-	0.5	0.2	0.02	0.04	**0.5**	163-4
Bone	17	0	-	-	2.3	1.0	0.5	0.5	0.5	0.5	0.5	-	0.8	1.6	-	0.9	-	-	3.4	-	0.7	0.2	0.04	0.05	**0.6**	170
Connective tissue	61	0	2.9	-	0.6	-	1.0	-	2.0	2.5	1.6	2.8	4.0	4.8	2.4	7.2	5.8	2.7	11.9	4.1	2.4	0.8	0.12	0.19	**1.9**	171
Mesothelioma	7	0	-	-	-	-	-	-	-	-	-	-	0.8	1.6	0.8	-	1.4	1.4	1.7	-	0.3	0.1	0.02	0.02	**0.2**	MES
Kaposi's sarcoma	3	0	-	-	-	-	-	-	-	-	-	-	0.8	-	-	-	1.4	-	1.7	-	0.1	0.0	0.00	0.01	**0.1**	KAP
Melanoma of skin	201	0	0.6	0.6	-	1.5	3.0	3.1	6.7	6.6	14.9	14.6	17.6	13.5	12.2	11.7	15.9	10.9	22.1	20.3	7.8	2.6	0.47	0.61	**6.2**	172
†Other skin	308	0	-	0.6	-	1.0	1.5	1.0	-	2.5	3.2	6.3	7.2	11.1	11.4	28.9	30.4	61.1	91.6	185.1	11.9		0.23	0.52	**5.8**	173
Breast	2896	0	-	-	-	-	0.5	7.7	16.4	74.7	138.5	240.5	261.7	260.5	303.4	335.2	296.5	306.8	269.8	209.5	112.2	37.1	6.52	9.68	**85.9**	174
Uterus unspecified	25	0	-	-	-	-	-	-	0.5	-	-	2.1	0.8	2.4	2.4	3.6	1.4	1.4	11.9	2.0	1.0	0.3	0.04	0.07	**0.6**	179
Cervix uteri	329	0	-	-	-	-	2.0	5.1	8.7	11.7	19.6	20.2	17.6	22.2	34.1	30.7	41.9	33.9	28.8	24.4	12.7	4.2	0.71	1.07	**9.7**	180
Placenta	2	0	-	-	-	-	0.5	-	-	-	-	-	-	-	-	-	-	-	-	2.0	0.1	0.0	0.00	0.00	**0.0**	181
Corpus uteri	371	0	-	-	-	-	-	0.5	1.5	1.5	3.7	15.3	22.3	34.8	51.1	67.8	55.0	50.2	54.3	36.6	14.4	4.8	0.65	1.27	**10.0**	182
Ovary etc.	310	0	-	-	-	2.6	0.5	3.1	1.5	4.1	11.1	16.0	24.7	30.1	43.0	39.8	34.7	38.0	25.5	20.3	12.0	4.0	0.68	1.06	**9.1**	183
Other female genital	59	0	-	-	-	-	0.5	0.5	0.5	0.5	-	1.4	0.8	4.0	2.4	6.3	13.0	10.9	13.6	24.4	2.3	0.8	0.05	0.15	**1.3**	184
Bladder	140	0	-	-	-	-	0.5	-	-	0.5	-	2.1	2.4	4.8	8.1	15.4	18.8	40.7	56.0	46.8	5.4	1.8	0.09	0.26	**2.6**	188
Kidney etc.	143	0	1.1	-	0.6	0.5	0.5	-	2.0	1.5	2.7	4.9	8.8	14.3	13.8	16.3	31.8	19.0	25.5	8.1	5.5	1.8	0.25	0.49	**4.0**	189
Eye	17	0	2.3	-	-	-	-	-	-	0.5	-	-	0.8	1.6	3.2	1.8	1.4	2.7	-	-	0.7	0.2	0.04	0.06	**0.6**	190
Brain, nervous system	121	0	5.1	3.4	4.0	1.5	1.5	2.6	3.1	2.5	5.8	3.5	5.6	9.5	11.4	13.6	8.7	4.1	5.1	2.0	4.7	1.6	0.30	0.41	**4.4**	191-2
Thyroid	143	0	-	-	0.6	0.5	2.5	4.1	3.6	4.6	8.5	12.5	9.6	13.5	16.2	10.8	10.1	2.7	11.9	2.0	5.5	1.8	0.38	0.49	**4.7**	193
Other endocrine	15	0	3.4	1.1	0.6	-	-	-	0.5	0.5	-	-	0.8	-	-	1.8	-	-	1.7	-	0.6	0.2	0.03	0.04	**0.7**	194
Hodgkin's disease	36	0	-	-	0.6	2.1	3.9	-	1.5	2.0	1.6	0.7	1.6	0.8	0.8	3.6	2.9	1.4	1.7	-	1.4	0.5	0.08	0.11	**1.2**	201
Non-Hodgkin lymphoma	263	0	0.6	2.8	-	1.0	1.5	3.1	6.1	6.1	4.8	10.5	9.6	8.7	22.7	32.5	40.5	47.5	56.0	30.5	10.2	3.4	0.39	0.75	**6.9**	200,202
Multiple myeloma	90	0	-	-	-	-	0.5	-	-	1.0	2.7	0.7	4.8	10.3	9.7	11.7	14.5	13.6	11.9	20.3	3.5	1.2	0.15	0.28	**2.3**	203
Lymphoid leukaemia	70	0	5.1	2.8	1.1	1.0	0.5	-	-	0.5	0.5	2.1	2.4	1.6	5.7	7.2	7.2	6.8	10.2	20.3	2.7	0.9	0.12	0.19	**2.3**	204
Myeloid leukaemia	70	0	0.6	-	-	1.0	0.5	0.5	3.1	0.5	-	1.4	1.6	6.3	4.9	10.8	4.3	9.5	23.8	8.1	2.7	0.9	0.10	0.18	**1.7**	205
Monocytic leukaemia	3	0	0.6	-	-	-	-	-	-	0.5	-	-	-	-	-	-	1.4	-	-	-	0.1	0.0	0.01	0.01	**0.1**	206
Other leukaemia	0	0	-	-	-	-	-	-	-	-	-	-	-	-	-	-	-	-	-	-	0.0	0.0	0.00	0.00	**0.0**	207
Leukaemia unspecified	4	0	0.6	0.6	-	-	-	-	-	-	-	-	-	-	-	-	-	1.4	1.7	-	0.2	0.1	0.01	0.01	**0.1**	208
Other and unspecified	326	0	-	-	0.6	-	2.5	1.0	4.1	1.5	5.3	4.9	9.6	15.0	33.3	35.2	50.6	69.2	91.6	79.3	12.6	4.2	0.39	0.82	**7.3**	O&U
All sites	8112	0	24.0	11.7	10.9	15.4	25.1	37.0	70.6	142.3	254.2	419.0	484.3	598.6	768.9	954.0	1055.8	1131.0	1391.3	1279.2	314.3		14.31	24.36	**217.9**	ALL
All sites but 173	7804	0	24.0	11.2	10.9	14.4	23.7	36.0	70.6	139.7	251.0	412.7	477.1	587.5	757.6	925.1	1025.4	1069.9	1299.7	1094.1	302.3	100.0	14.08	23.83	**212.1**	ALLb

| Rate from 1 case | | | 0.571 | 0.558 | 0.574 | 0.513 | 0.493 | 0.514 | 0.512 | 0.508 | 0.531 | 0.697 | 0.798 | 0.792 | 0.811 | 0.903 | 1.446 | 1.358 | 1.697 | 2.034 |

†Important: see notes on population page

France, Somme

The Somme Cancer Registry has been recording all cancer cases occurring in the département since 1982. The two main sources of finance are the General Council of Somme and the departmental committee of the League against Cancer.

The Association for Epidemiological Research by Registries in Picardy, of which the Somme Cancer Registry is part, has been created with the aims of:

(1) assessing the incidence and prevalence rate in Picardy or in each département, of pathological conditions which constitute the main causes of morbidity and mortality;

(2) comparing the observed rates with those in other French départements or other countries;

(3) investigating the causes of geographical differences, particularly environmental and sociocultural factors.

The population of the département is 550 000, including 110 200 children. The urban/rural ratio for all ages was 1.38 in 1990. The département is considered as rural, although many industries have been established for a long time. The Amiens agglomeration contains 150 000 inhabitants, and one other town 30 000; the remaining towns have less than 10 000 inhabitants. 90% of the communes have less than 1000 inhabitants.

The collection of cases is largely active, and some 70 sources of information are used, visited annually by 3–6 physician inquirers, as well as four cancer institutes outside the département. The first data come from anatomo-pathology laboratories for about 75% of cases. The remainder are found by systematic investigation of medical or surgical records, or by reading operative reports. In some hospitals, newly created departments of medical information provide a complementary source of information.

There is about 92% of histological confirmation. Death certificates are not used in the absence of any other information on the patient, particularly if an initial date of diagnosis is lacking. In 1995, additional procedures were introduced to reduce the number of cases with death certificate only.

Follow up of patients is carried out only in connection with specific studies.

The registry annually publishes comparative and crude incidence rates. It has participated since 1990 in the FRANCIM network, of which an initial aim is to standardize coding practices within French registries. A secondary aim of the network is to work with the Institut National de la Santé et de la Recherche Médicale (INSERM) and IACR to publish incidence data and to start common studies. In addition, the Somme registry is involved in the EUROCARE working group, studying survival and therapeutic practices.

Since 1995, registry data have been available on the EUROCIM database, allowing mortality and incidence comparisons between European registries. Locally, the registry has monitored a programme for screening by mammography every three years in women aged 50–69 years old and prepares an annual report covering incidence of invasive and *in situ* cancers, spotting of false negatives, and the evolution of medical practices in breast cancer diagnosis and treatment.

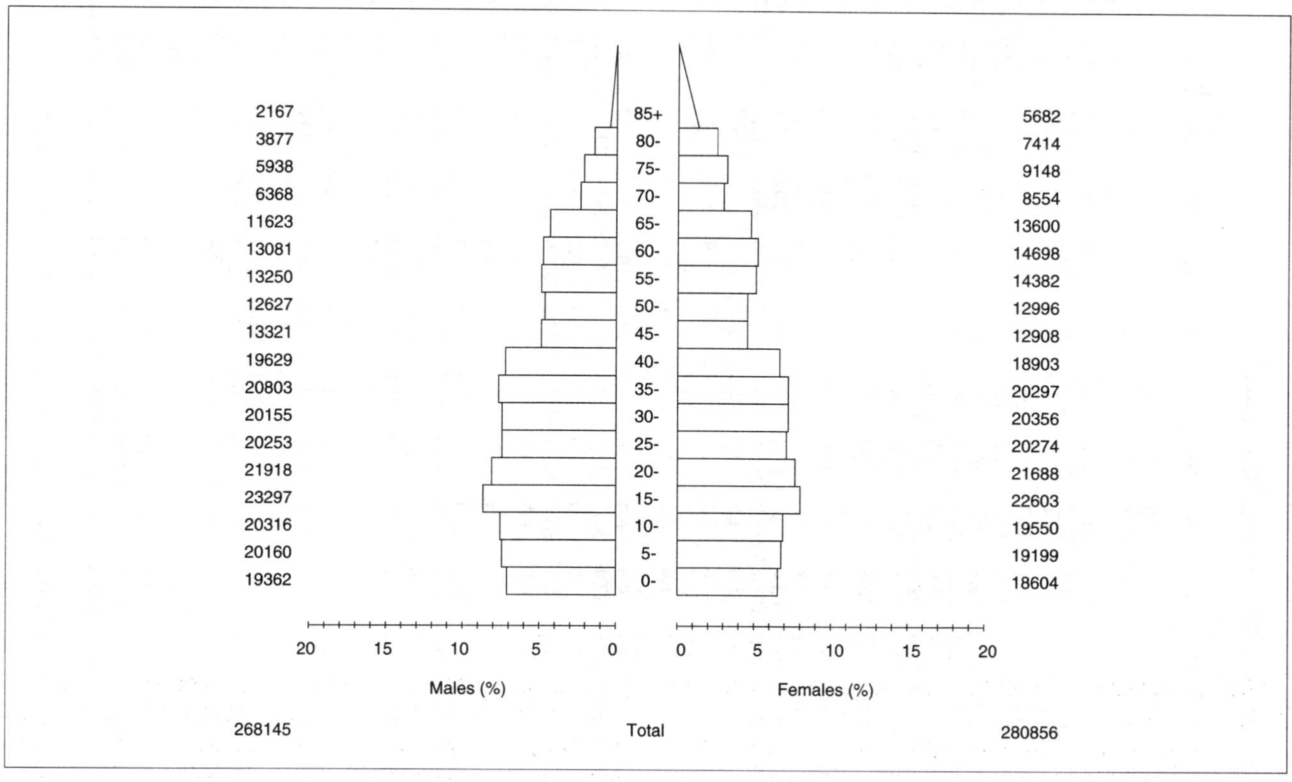

France, Somme

Source of population: 1988–92

Census: Recensement de la population 1990, Population de la France, Départements, arrondissements, cantons, communes. Direction Générale des Collectivités Locales, Institut National de la Statistique et des Etudes Economiques.

Estimate: Population estimates provided by the official national department of demography (INSEE) were used for each of the years 1988-92 (Estimations de la Population, INSEE, 1996)

Notes to tables overleaf

* The falls in rates for many sites since the period published previously, generally combined with high mortality/incidence ratios, indicate under-registration.

† 173 does not include basal cell carcinomas

Screening programmes in the area

5 000 screening examinations for breast cancer have been carried out annually in the population aged 50-69 since 1990.

* FRANCE, SOMME 1988-1992

ANNUAL INCIDENCE PER 100,000 BY AGE GROUP (YEARS) - MALE

SITE	ALL AGES	AGE UNK	0-	5-	10-	15-	20-	25-	30-	35-	40-	45-	50-	55-	60-	65-	70-	75-	80-	85+	CRUDE RATE	%	CR 64	CR 74	ASR (W)	ICD (9th)
Lip	42	0	-	-	-	-	-	-	-	-	1.0	1.5	4.8	7.5	9.2	20.6	-	23.6	30.9	9.2	3.1	0.8	0.12	0.22	**2.1**	140
Tongue	102	0	-	-	-	-	-	-	1.0	4.8	8.2	12.0	28.5	25.7	22.9	22.4	22.0	20.2	15.5	9.2	7.6	1.8	0.52	0.74	**6.4**	141
Salivary gland	11	0	-	-	1.0	-	-	1.0	-	1.0	-	-	-	-	3.1	5.2	6.3	3.4	-	-	0.8	0.2	0.03	0.09	**0.7**	142
Mouth	171	0	-	-	-	-	-	-	2.0	1.9	6.1	37.5	50.7	54.3	33.6	29.3	40.8	47.2	5.2	9.2	12.8	3.1	0.93	1.28	**11.1**	143-5
Oropharynx	211	0	-	-	-	-	-	-	-	6.7	16.3	30.0	44.3	78.5	58.1	49.9	25.1	30.3	10.3	18.5	15.7	3.8	1.17	1.55	**13.3**	146
Nasopharynx	9	0	-	-	1.0	-	0.9	-	-	-	1.0	-	-	1.5	3.1	1.7	3.1	3.4	-	-	0.7	0.2	0.04	0.06	**0.6**	147
Hypopharynx	172	0	-	-	-	-	-	-	-	4.8	10.2	18.0	34.8	51.3	71.9	36.1	44.0	20.2	5.2	-	12.8	3.1	0.96	1.36	**10.8**	148
Pharynx unspecified	54	0	-	-	-	-	-	-	-	1.9	5.1	7.5	17.4	13.6	15.3	10.3	9.4	6.7	5.2	-	4.0	1.0	0.30	0.40	**3.5**	149
Oesophagus	306	0	-	-	-	-	-	-	-	3.8	10.2	27.0	69.7	69.4	68.8	91.2	94.2	114.5	77.4	64.6	22.8	5.5	1.24	2.17	**18.0**	150
Stomach	197	0	-	-	-	-	-	-	-	1.0	3.1	9.0	12.7	21.1	38.2	44.7	91.1	171.8	118.6	101.5	14.7	3.5	0.43	1.10	**9.8**	151
Small intestine	9	0	-	-	-	-	-	-	-	1.0	-	1.5	1.6	3.0	1.5	1.7	-	3.4	-	9.2	0.7	0.2	0.04	0.05	**0.5**	152
Colon	391	0	-	-	-	-	-	1.0	2.0	4.8	7.1	15.0	28.5	45.3	84.1	137.7	172.7	198.7	247.6	193.8	29.2	7.0	0.94	2.49	**20.2**	153
Rectum	269	0	-	-	-	-	-	1.0	2.0	1.9	10.2	12.0	17.4	28.7	55.0	80.9	147.6	124.6	154.7	175.4	20.1	4.8	0.64	1.78	**14.1**	154
Liver	127	0	-	-	-	-	0.9	-	-	-	1.0	7.5	15.8	22.6	52.0	34.4	66.0	37.0	30.9	27.7	9.5	2.3	0.50	1.00	**7.4**	155
Gallbladder etc.	24	0	-	-	-	-	-	-	-	-	-	-	6.0	7.6	10.3	3.1	20.2	10.3	-	1.8	0.4	0.07	0.14	**1.2**	156
Pancreas	77	0	-	-	-	-	-	-	-	1.0	1.0	4.5	9.5	18.1	22.9	20.6	34.5	26.9	36.1	9.2	5.7	1.4	0.29	0.56	**4.3**	157
Nose, sinuses etc.	20	0	-	-	-	-	-	-	-	1.0	2.0	4.5	4.8	3.0	4.6	3.4	6.3	6.7	-	-	1.5	0.4	0.10	0.15	**1.3**	160
Larynx	237	0	-	-	-	-	-	-	-	3.8	10.2	30.0	63.4	69.4	68.8	53.3	53.4	57.3	20.6	27.7	17.7	4.3	1.23	1.76	**14.8**	161
Bronchus, lung	967	0	-	-	-	-	-	1.0	2.0	11.5	27.5	85.6	107.7	218.9	261.4	323.5	373.7	316.6	330.1	175.4	72.1	17.4	3.58	7.06	**55.1**	162
Other thoracic organs	17	0	-	-	-	-	-	1.0	1.0	-	-	-	1.6	1.5	4.6	5.2	3.1	10.1	-	27.7	1.3	0.3	0.05	0.09	**0.9**	163-4
Bone	8	0	-	-	-	2.6	-	-	-	-	-	-	1.6	1.5	-	1.7	3.1	3.4	-	-	0.6	0.1	0.03	0.05	**0.5**	170
Connective tissue	22	0	1.0	-	-	-	1.8	1.0	1.0	1.9	3.1	1.5	3.2	-	-	1.7	3.1	13.5	10.3	9.2	1.6	0.4	0.07	0.10	**1.3**	171
Mesothelioma	17	0	-	-	-	-	-	-	-	1.9	-	3.0	1.6	3.0	3.1	3.4	9.4	6.7	5.2	-	1.3	0.3	0.06	0.13	**1.0**	MES
Kaposi's sarcoma	8	0	-	-	-	-	-	-	1.0	1.0	-	3.0	-	1.5	-	-	3.1	3.4	-	9.2	0.6	0.1	0.03	0.05	**0.5**	KAP
Melanoma of skin	54	0	-	-	1.0	1.7	0.9	2.0	5.0	3.8	7.1	4.5	9.5	6.0	7.6	5.2	12.6	10.1	5.2	27.7	4.0	1.0	0.25	0.33	**3.4**	172
†Other skin	317	0	-	-	-	-	0.9	1.0	1.0	3.8	6.1	10.5	17.4	31.7	53.5	77.4	113.1	178.5	247.6	443.0	23.6		0.63	1.58	**15.5**	173
Breast	13	0	-	-	-	-	-	-	-	-	-	1.5	3.2	3.0	1.5	1.7	6.3	10.1	5.2	-	1.0	0.2	0.05	0.09	**0.7**	175
Prostate	779	0	-	-	-	-	-	-	-	-	-	3.0	6.3	63.4	116.2	297.7	402.0	545.6	624.1	655.3	58.1	14.0	0.94	4.44	**36.5**	185
Testis	55	0	-	1.0	1.0	-	9.1	6.9	6.0	11.5	7.1	3.0	4.8	4.5	4.6	-	-	-	-	-	4.1	1.0	0.30	0.30	**3.7**	186
Penis	6	0	-	-	-	-	-	-	-	1.0	-	1.5	-	-	-	1.7	-	3.4	-	9.2	0.4	0.1	0.02	0.03	**0.4**	187.1-.4
Other male genital	3	0	-	-	-	-	-	-	-	-	1.0	-	-	1.5	-	-	-	3.4	-	-	0.2	0.1	0.01	0.01	**0.2**	187.5-.9
Bladder	403	0	-	-	-	0.9	-	1.0	2.0	2.9	3.1	22.5	23.8	58.9	87.1	127.3	191.6	205.4	268.2	175.4	30.1	7.2	1.01	2.60	**20.9**	188
Kidney etc.	147	0	1.0	-	-	-	-	1.0	1.0	1.0	3.1	10.5	17.4	33.2	45.9	60.2	50.2	37.0	25.8	27.7	11.0	2.6	0.57	1.12	**8.6**	189
Eye	15	0	1.0	-	-	-	-	-	-	-	-	-	1.6	-	6.1	-	12.6	13.5	5.2	-	1.1	0.3	0.04	0.11	**0.9**	190
Brain, nervous system	91	0	2.1	3.0	2.0	3.4	1.8	4.9	5.0	2.9	5.1	9.0	11.1	12.1	19.9	20.6	15.7	20.2	10.3	9.2	6.8	1.6	0.41	0.59	**6.0**	191-2
Thyroid	12	0	-	-	-	-	-	1.0	1.0	1.0	-	-	-	6.0	3.1	3.4	-	3.4	-	-	0.9	0.2	0.06	0.08	**0.7**	193
Other endocrine	6	0	1.0	-	1.0	-	-	-	-	-	-	-	1.5	-	1.7	6.3	-	-	-	-	0.4	0.1	0.02	0.06	**0.5**	194
Hodgkin's disease	38	0	-	-	2.0	-	5.5	2.0	4.0	2.9	3.1	3.0	4.8	4.5	4.6	3.4	3.1	6.7	5.2	9.2	2.8	0.7	0.18	0.21	**2.5**	201
Non-Hodgkin lymphoma	144	0	-	1.0	1.0	2.6	-	3.0	6.0	8.7	6.1	10.5	15.8	22.6	30.6	34.4	53.4	33.7	41.3	73.8	10.7	2.6	0.54	0.98	**8.5**	200,202
Multiple myeloma	34	0	-	-	-	-	-	1.0	-	1.0	4.1	3.0	3.2	4.5	9.2	8.6	9.4	20.2	5.2	-	2.5	0.6	0.13	0.22	**1.9**	203
Lymphoid leukaemia	83	0	3.1	4.0	2.0	1.7	0.9	-	-	-	3.1	-	4.8	3.0	12.2	36.1	31.4	40.4	30.9	55.4	6.2	1.5	0.17	0.51	**4.8**	204
Myeloid leukaemia	43	0	3.1	-	-	0.9	0.9	3.0	2.0	2.9	2.0	1.5	1.6	1.5	4.6	6.9	9.4	20.2	30.9	27.7	3.2	0.8	0.12	0.20	**2.5**	205
Monocytic leukaemia	3	0	-	-	-	-	-	-	-	-	-	1.5	-	1.5	-	-	-	3.4	-	-	0.2	0.1	0.02	0.02	**0.2**	206
Other leukaemia	2	0	-	-	-	-	-	-	-	-	-	-	-	1.5	-	-	-	-	-	9.2	0.1	0.0	0.01	0.01	**0.1**	207
Leukaemia unspecified	4	0	-	-	-	-	-	-	-	1.0	-	-	1.6	1.5	-	-	1.7	-	-	-	0.3	0.1	0.02	0.03	**0.2**	208
Other and unspecified	169	0	1.0	-	-	-	-	1.0	2.0	2.9	7.1	13.5	15.8	24.1	52.0	55.1	50.2	53.9	98.0	27.7	12.6	3.0	0.60	1.12	**9.4**	O&U
All sites	5889	0	13.4	8.9	11.8	13.7	23.7	35.5	45.6	102.9	181.4	409.9	662.1	1032.4	1348.4	1732.7	2182.7	2478.8	2517.0	2427.3	439.2		19.45	39.03	**327.4**	ALL
All sites but 173	5572	0	13.4	8.9	11.8	13.7	22.8	34.6	44.7	99.0	175.2	399.4	644.6	1000.7	1294.9	1655.3	2069.7	2300.3	2269.4	1984.3	415.6	100.0	18.82	37.44	**311.9**	ALLb

Rate from 1 case	1.033	0.992	0.984	0.858	0.912	0.987	0.992	0.961	1.019	1.501	1.584	1.509	1.529	1.721	3.141	3.368	5.158	9.229

†Important: see notes on population page

* FRANCE, SOMME 1988-1992

ANNUAL INCIDENCE PER 100,000 BY AGE GROUP (YEARS) - FEMALE

SITE	ALL AGES	AGE UNK	0-	5-	10-	15-	20-	25-	30-	35-	40-	45-	50-	55-	60-	65-	70-	75-	80-	85+	CRUDE RATE	%	CR 64	CR 74	ASR (W)	ICD (9th)
Lip	5	0	-	-	-	-	-	-	-	-	-	-	-	-	-	-	-	6.6	2.7	3.5	0.4	0.1	0.00	0.00	0.1	140
Tongue	11	0	-	-	-	-	-	-	-	-	1.5	1.5	1.4	1.4	4.4	2.3	-	5.4	3.5	0.8	0.3	0.03	0.06	0.5	141
Salivary gland	4	0	-	-	-	-	-	-	-	-	-	1.5	-	1.4	-	2.3	-	2.7	-	0.3	0.1	0.01	0.03	0.2	142
Mouth	29	0	-	-	-	-	-	-	1.0	3.2	3.1	1.5	8.3	2.7	7.4	4.7	4.4	2.7	14.1	2.1	0.8	0.10	0.16	1.4	143-5
Oropharynx	14	0	-	-	-	-	-	1.0	-	2.1	1.5	3.1	2.8	1.4	2.9	-	4.4	-	3.5	1.0	0.4	0.06	0.07	0.7	146
Nasopharynx	3	0	-	-	-	-	-	1.0	-	-	-	1.4	-	1.5	-	-	-	-	-	0.2	0.1	0.01	0.02	0.2	147
Hypopharynx	7	0	-	-	-	-	-	-	-	1.1	1.5	1.5	1.4	2.7	-	2.3	-	-	-	0.5	0.2	0.04	0.05	0.4	148
Pharynx unspecified	1	0	-	-	-	-	-	-	-	-	1.5	-	-	-	-	-	-	-	-	0.1	0.0	0.01	0.01	0.1	149
Oesophagus	39	0	-	-	-	-	-	-	-	1.1	-	1.5	4.2	5.4	11.8	16.4	19.7	5.4	14.1	2.8	1.0	0.06	0.20	1.5	150
Stomach	132	0	-	-	-	-	-	1.0	1.0	1.1	1.5	4.6	8.3	16.3	19.1	32.7	50.3	64.7	116.2	9.4	3.5	0.17	0.43	4.1	151
Small intestine	14	0	-	-	-	-	-	-	-	-	1.5	1.5	1.4	1.4	1.5	2.3	2.2	13.5	7.0	1.0	0.4	0.03	0.05	0.5	152
Colon	331	0	-	-	-	-	2.9	3.9	4.2	4.6	27.7	30.6	57.1	72.1	86.5	107.1	161.8	140.8	23.6	8.8	0.66	1.45	12.3	153
Rectum	203	0	-	-	-	-	1.0	1.0	3.0	5.3	9.3	13.9	12.5	24.5	39.7	70.1	63.4	97.1	102.1	14.5	5.4	0.35	0.90	7.6	154
Liver	25	0	-	-	-	-	-	1.0	-	1.1	3.1	4.6	4.2	5.4	5.9	-	6.6	8.1	3.5	1.8	0.7	0.10	0.13	1.2	155
Gallbladder etc.	51	0	-	-	-	-	-	-	-	1.1	3.1	3.1	5.6	10.9	10.3	14.0	15.3	27.0	14.1	3.6	1.4	0.12	0.24	2.0	156
Pancreas	70	0	-	-	-	-	-	1.0	-	1.1	1.5	7.7	9.7	12.2	8.8	9.4	28.4	35.1	35.2	5.0	1.9	0.17	0.26	2.6	157
Nose, sinuses etc.	11	0	-	-	-	-	-	1.0	1.0	-	1.5	-	-	-	2.9	2.3	4.4	5.4	3.5	0.8	0.3	0.02	0.04	0.4	160
Larynx	21	0	-	-	-	-	-	-	1.0	1.1	7.7	1.5	2.8	-	7.4	2.3	4.4	5.4	3.5	1.5	0.6	0.07	0.12	1.1	161
Bronchus, lung	98	0	-	-	-	-	-	1.0	1.0	6.3	6.2	4.6	16.7	16.3	33.8	32.7	13.1	29.7	17.6	7.0	2.6	0.26	0.59	4.5	162
Other thoracic organs	4	0	-	-	-	-	-	-	-	-	3.1	-	-	-	-	2.3	-	2.7	-	0.3	0.1	0.02	0.03	0.2	163-4
Bone	7	0	-	1.0	1.0	0.9	-	-	-	-	1.1	-	-	-	-	-	4.7	2.2	-	0.5	0.2	0.02	0.04	0.5	170
Connective tissue	17	0	1.1	1.0	-	-	0.9	1.0	1.0	-	-	1.5	-	-	6.8	4.4	-	2.2	2.7	3.5	1.2	0.5	0.07	0.09	1.0	171
Mesothelioma	5	0	-	-	-	-	-	-	-	1.0	-	-	1.5	1.4	-	1.5	-	2.2	-	-	0.4	0.1	0.02	0.03	0.3	MES
Kaposi's sarcoma	1	0	-	-	-	-	-	1.0	-	-	-	-	-	-	-	-	-	-	-	-	0.1	0.0	0.00	0.00	0.1	KAP
Melanoma of skin	86	0	1.1	-	1.0	-	1.8	2.0	5.9	3.0	3.2	9.3	20.0	11.1	10.9	10.3	11.7	17.5	21.6	17.6	6.1	2.3	0.35	0.46	4.6	172
†Other skin	172	0	-	-	-	-	-	-	1.0	-	2.1	3.1	6.2	8.3	6.8	7.4	39.7	54.7	86.3	257.0	12.2		0.14	0.37	4.6	173
Breast	1241	0	-	-	-	-	0.9	12.8	34.4	63.1	122.7	187.5	195.4	219.7	231.3	245.6	208.1	185.8	151.0	137.3	88.4	33.0	5.34	7.61	68.2	174
Uterus unspecified	15	0	-	-	-	-	-	-	-	-	2.1	1.5	3.1	5.6	-	-	4.7	4.4	-	7.0	1.1	0.4	0.06	0.08	0.8	179
Cervix uteri	182	0	-	-	-	-	0.9	4.9	26.5	13.8	24.3	21.7	18.5	29.2	29.9	35.3	11.7	10.9	13.5	14.1	13.0	4.8	0.85	1.08	10.5	180
Placenta	1	0	-	-	-	-	-	1.0	-	-	-	-	-	-	-	-	-	-	-	-	0.1	0.0	0.00	0.00	0.1	181
Corpus uteri	195	0	-	-	-	-	-	-	-	2.0	5.3	6.2	20.0	33.4	54.4	66.2	56.1	37.2	37.8	24.6	13.9	5.2	0.61	1.22	9.1	182
Ovary etc.	203	0	-	-	1.0	-	3.7	3.9	1.0	4.9	6.3	20.1	32.3	30.6	34.0	48.5	42.1	56.8	45.9	24.6	14.5	5.4	0.69	1.14	10.1	183
Other female genital	25	0	-	-	-	-	-	1.0	-	-	1.1	-	3.1	1.4	4.1	8.8	2.3	2.2	5.4	24.6	1.8	0.7	0.05	0.11	1.0	184
Bladder	69	0	-	-	-	-	-	1.0	-	1.0	1.1	-	6.2	9.7	10.9	7.4	11.7	30.6	32.4	38.7	4.9	1.8	0.15	0.24	2.4	188
Kidney etc.	97	0	5.4	-	1.0	-	1.8	-	-	1.0	2.1	6.2	6.2	16.7	29.9	23.5	21.0	17.5	10.8	24.6	6.9	2.6	0.35	0.57	5.1	189
Eye	10	0	1.1	-	-	-	-	-	-	-	-	-	-	2.8	5.4	2.9	-	-	2.7	-	0.7	0.3	0.05	0.06	0.6	190
Brain, nervous system	59	0	2.1	2.1	-	3.5	0.9	1.0	2.9	3.9	2.1	6.2	4.6	8.3	13.6	13.2	9.4	4.4	2.7	3.5	4.2	1.6	0.26	0.37	3.6	191-2
Thyroid	54	0	-	-	0.9	1.8	4.9	6.9	3.0	4.2	6.2	3.1	9.7	8.2	1.5	18.7	-	8.1	3.5	3.8	1.4	0.24	0.35	3.2	193
Other endocrine	3	0	-	-	-	-	-	1.0	1.0	-	-	-	1.4	-	-	-	-	-	-	0.2	0.1	0.02	0.02	0.2	194
Hodgkin's disease	29	0	-	-	2.0	1.8	4.6	2.0	3.9	3.9	4.2	3.1	-	-	-	-	2.2	5.4	3.5	2.1	0.8	0.13	0.13	1.8	201
Non-Hodgkin lymphoma	123	0	-	-	1.0	0.9	0.9	1.0	1.0	2.0	-	3.1	7.7	15.3	25.9	29.4	32.7	45.9	27.0	49.3	8.8	3.3	0.29	0.60	5.1	200,202
Multiple myeloma	42	0	-	-	-	-	-	-	-	-	-	3.1	3.1	7.0	5.4	14.7	7.0	15.3	18.9	7.0	3.0	1.1	0.09	0.20	1.7	203
Lymphoid leukaemia	65	0	4.3	3.1	-	-	-	-	-	-	3.2	4.6	6.2	12.5	6.8	14.7	9.4	21.9	16.2	14.1	4.6	1.7	0.20	0.32	3.4	204
Myeloid leukaemia	33	0	-	-	1.0	0.9	0.9	1.0	-	-	3.2	1.5	3.1	2.8	6.8	7.4	4.7	4.4	5.4	17.6	2.3	0.9	0.11	0.17	1.6	205
Monocytic leukaemia	4	0	-	-	-	-	-	-	-	-	-	-	1.5	-	-	1.5	4.7	-	-	-	0.3	0.1	0.01	0.04	0.2	206
Other leukaemia	0	0	-	-	-	-	-	-	-	-	-	-	-	-	-	-	-	-	-	-	0.0	0.0	0.00	0.00	0.0	207
Leukaemia unspecified	3	0	-	1.0	-	-	-	-	-	-	-	-	-	-	-	1.5	-	-	-	3.5	0.2	0.1	0.01	0.01	0.2	208
Other and unspecified	121	0	-	-	1.0	-	0.9	-	-	2.0	1.1	6.2	12.3	7.0	15.0	32.4	14.0	65.6	45.9	45.8	8.6	3.2	0.23	0.46	4.6	O&U
All sites	3935	0	15.0	8.3	9.2	8.8	20.3	39.5	95.3	118.2	217.9	345.5	432.4	545.1	665.4	807.4	797.3	913.8	1008.8	1203.8	280.2		12.61	20.63	186.1	ALL
All sites but 173	3763	0	15.0	8.3	9.2	8.8	20.3	39.5	94.3	118.2	215.8	342.4	426.3	536.8	658.6	800.0	757.5	859.1	922.5	946.8	268.0	100.0	12.47	20.26	181.5	ALLb

		0-	5-	10-	15-	20-	25-	30-	35-	40-	45-	50-	55-	60-	65-	70-	75-	80-	85+
Rate from 1 case		1.075	1.042	1.023	0.885	0.922	0.986	0.982	0.985	1.058	1.549	1.539	1.391	1.361	1.471	2.338	2.186	2.697	3.520

†Important: see notes on population page

France, Tarn

When the Tarn Cancer Registry began its activities in 1981, the aim was to systematically record all new cancer cases within the département. At the time, there was no cancer registry in the south-west of France. The registry functions according to the French Association Law 1901, and is constituted of representatives from the medical, university and local authority communities both within the département and elsewhere in the Midi-Pyrenees region.

The Tarn is part of the Midi–Pyrenees region, covering an area of 5758 km². Most of the département is situated south of latitude 44° N and on longitude 2° E.

The département, with a population of 342 723 in 1990, is relatively urbanised and industrialised in comparison to neighbouring départements. The population overall is slowly increasing, but certain areas are undergoing quite a rapid increase while others are in recession. The population has been ageing rapidly during the 1980s due to the decreasing birth rate, which in 1990 was 9.6/1000. Many persons aged between 20 and 30 years left (representing a loss of nearly 15% of that age group between 1982 and 1990), while those migrating into the département are mainly aged between 30 and 45 years (representing about 5% of the population) and bring children with them.

In 1990, 42.2% (144 582 persons) of the population were employed. The development of services in the two main towns of Albi and Castres has helped to create employment, but the number of non-salaried workers has decreased. Farming still accounts for 3.4% of the population, and factory work for 13.4%.

The département is fairly autonomous as far as medical coverage for cancer patients is concerned. There were 930 doctors in 1990 (450 general practitioners and 476 specialists, including five pathologists and three radiotherapists. There are 4059 hospital beds divided between the 6 public and 16 private hospitals.

Registration is active: cases are by seven investigating physicians of the registry, who visit the different laboratories, private and public hospital services, administrative services and general practitioners at variable time intervals. As a certain number of cancer patients from the Tarn are treated in Toulouse, the Tarn Cancer Registry also investigates the major private clinics and the University Hospital Centre there. Cases treated at the regional 'Fight Against Cancer Centre' are also registered. In recent years, the search for cases in public hospitals has been simplified by the exis-

tence of medical information departments which provide lists of the cancer cases covered by the social welfare system in those establishments.

For each case, the investigating doctor fills in a medical/administrative form from the medical record. The names of the different doctors involved in the diagnosis and treatment of the patient, and in particular the general practitioner, are systematically noted so they may be contacted if necessary.

When the forms arrive in the registry, the secretaries first check the computer file to avoid duplicate registrations. The cases are then systematically verified from a second source by the registry physicians. If, after this verification, the information on a case is insufficient, a questionnaire is addressed to the treating physician. Cases which should not be registered are eliminated (metastasis from or recurrence of a cancer diagnosed before 1982, a patient not resident in the area covered by the registry).

The medical information on the cases is coded by the director of the registry, who is a physician. The diagnoses of cancer are coded to ICD-O and the TNM. The administrative information is coded by the secretaries. The data are then entered onto the registry computer, so creating a computer file which can be updated as additional information reaches the registry from other sources.

All invasive and *in situ* cancers are registered, except for basal cell carcinomas of the skin. For bladder, all diagnoses regardless of behaviour are registered and coded according to the rules of the European Network of Cancer Registries. Multiple primaries are registered according to the IARC/IACR rules with the exception of breast and colon cancers.

The registry carries out passive follow-up for all cases except for specific series entered into special studies. For the latter, follow-up is active via letters to the town halls where the patients were registered at birth and to the treating physicians.

In addition to basic descriptive epidemiology, the Tarn registry carries out, alone or in collaboration with other registries, such as FRANCIM (the association of French cancer registries), and European registries in general, studies including estimation of the incidence and prevalence of cancers in France, time trends, case–control studies and evaluation of diagnostic and therapeutic practices for certain sites.

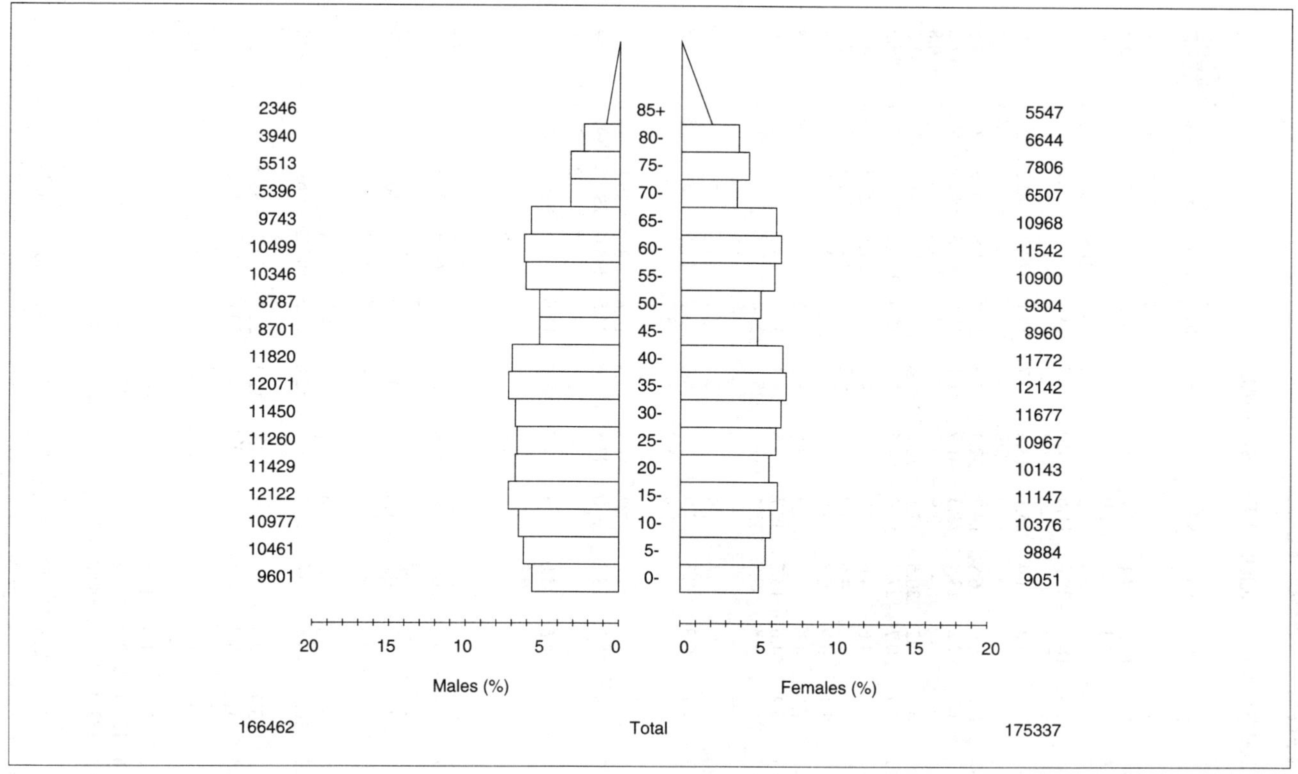

France, Tarn

Source of population: 1988–92

Census: Recensement de la population 1990, Population de la France, Départements, arrondissements, cantons, communes. Direction Générale des Collectivités Locales, Institut National de la Statistique et des Etudes Economiques.

Estimate: Population estimates provided by the official national department of demography (INSEE) were used for each of the years 1988-92 (Estimations de la Population, INSEE, 1996)

Notes to tables overleaf:

* The high ratios of mortality to incidence for several sites, such as stomach, lung, the leukaemias and lymphomas and childhood cancer in boys, suggest under-ascertainment.

† 173 does not include basal cell carcinomas

* FRANCE, TARN 1988-1992

ANNUAL INCIDENCE PER 100,000 BY AGE GROUP (YEARS) - MALE

SITE	ALL AGES	AGE UNK	0-	5-	10-	15-	20-	25-	30-	35-	40-	45-	50-	55-	60-	65-	70-	75-	80-	85+	CRUDE RATE	%	CR 64	CR 74	ASR (W)	ICD (9th)
Lip	55	0	-	-	-	-	-	-	-	-	-	-	11.4	9.7	1.9	20.5	18.5	36.3	71.1	42.6	6.6	1.3	0.11	0.31	2.9	140
Tongue	46	0	-	-	-	-	-	-	1.7	-	5.1	13.8	9.1	7.7	11.4	18.5	18.5	14.5	20.3	-	5.5	1.1	0.24	0.43	3.6	141
Salivary gland	8	0	-	-	-	-	3.5	-	-	1.7	-	2.3	-	1.9	-	4.1	-	-	5.1	-	1.0	0.2	0.05	0.07	0.7	142
Mouth	41	0	-	-	-	-	-	-	1.7	1.7	5.1	-	6.8	21.3	9.5	10.3	-	21.8	20.3	17.0	4.9	1.0	0.23	0.28	2.8	143-5
Oropharynx	62	0	-	-	-	-	-	-	-	3.3	6.8	18.4	25.0	11.6	21.0	26.7	14.8	7.3	5.1	-	7.4	1.5	0.43	0.64	5.5	146
Nasopharynx	8	0	-	-	-	-	-	1.8	1.7	-	1.7	2.3	-	-	5.7	-	-	3.6	-	-	1.0	0.2	0.07	0.07	0.8	147
Hypopharynx	65	0	-	-	-	-	-	-	-	-	-	9.2	11.4	25.1	13.3	26.7	37.1	29.0	10.2	25.6	7.8	1.6	0.30	0.61	4.7	148
Pharynx unspecified	3	0	-	-	-	-	-	-	-	-	-	-	-	-	3.8	-	-	-	-	8.5	0.4	0.1	0.02	0.02	0.2	149
Oesophagus	73	0	-	-	-	-	-	-	-	-	5.1	6.9	6.8	19.3	32.4	24.6	25.9	21.8	40.6	34.1	8.8	1.8	0.35	0.61	5.0	150
Stomach	143	0	-	-	-	-	-	-	-	1.7	1.7	9.2	13.7	21.3	41.9	41.1	81.5	65.3	142.1	85.2	17.2	3.4	0.45	1.06	8.6	151
Small intestine	7	0	-	-	-	-	-	-	-	-	-	-	-	3.9	3.8	-	3.7	3.6	-	8.5	0.8	0.2	0.04	0.06	0.5	152
Colon	313	0	-	-	-	-	-	-	5.2	9.9	6.8	9.2	20.5	27.1	76.2	131.4	166.8	232.2	198.0	179.0	37.6	7.5	0.77	2.27	18.5	153
Rectum	293	0	-	-	-	-	-	1.8	-	3.3	3.4	20.7	27.3	58.0	68.6	121.1	126.0	177.7	218.3	136.4	35.2	7.1	0.92	2.15	17.9	154
Liver	38	0	-	-	-	-	-	-	-	-	-	4.6	4.6	3.9	9.5	14.4	25.9	21.8	20.3	25.6	4.6	0.9	0.11	0.31	2.4	155
Gallbladder etc.	18	0	-	-	-	-	-	-	-	-	-	-	4.6	3.9	-	6.2	-	14.5	20.3	25.6	2.2	0.4	0.04	0.07	0.9	156
Pancreas	56	0	-	-	-	-	-	-	-	-	3.4	6.9	6.8	3.9	7.6	12.3	33.4	39.9	50.8	51.1	6.7	1.3	0.14	0.37	3.4	157
Nose, sinuses etc.	15	0	-	-	-	-	-	-	-	-	1.7	4.6	-	3.9	3.8	6.2	3.7	7.3	5.1	8.5	1.8	0.4	0.07	0.12	1.1	160
Larynx	88	0	-	-	-	-	-	-	1.7	3.3	3.4	4.6	13.7	36.7	43.8	14.4	33.4	18.1	20.3	68.2	10.6	2.1	0.54	0.77	6.4	161
Bronchus, lung	587	3	-	-	-	-	-	-	3.5	3.3	25.4	36.8	88.8	131.4	188.6	225.8	322.4	268.4	238.6	213.1	70.5	14.1	2.40	5.16	39.7	162
Other thoracic organs	5	0	-	-	-	-	-	-	1.7	1.7	-	-	-	-	3.8	-	-	3.6	-	-	0.6	0.1	0.04	0.04	0.4	163-4
Bone	13	0	2.1	1.9	1.8	3.3	-	-	1.7	5.0	-	-	-	1.9	-	-	3.7	3.6	5.1	-	1.6	0.3	0.09	0.11	1.5	170
Connective tissue	23	0	-	-	-	3.3	-	1.8	1.7	1.7	1.7	6.9	2.3	3.9	1.9	6.2	3.7	14.5	5.1	8.5	2.8	0.6	0.13	0.17	2.0	171
Mesothelioma	9	0	-	-	-	-	-	-	-	-	-	-	-	1.9	5.7	8.2	3.7	-	-	-	1.1	0.2	0.04	0.10	0.6	MES
Kaposi's sarcoma	1	0	-	-	-	-	-	-	-	-	1.7	-	-	-	-	-	-	-	-	-	0.1	0.0	0.01	0.01	0.1	KAP
Melanoma of skin	56	1	-	-	-	-	1.7	3.6	1.7	8.3	11.8	-	11.4	7.7	13.3	12.3	14.8	18.1	35.5	8.5	6.7	1.3	0.30	0.44	4.3	172
†Other skin	328	9	-	-	-	-	-	-	3.5	3.3	3.4	16.1	18.2	29.0	43.8	100.6	144.5	243.0	299.5	392.1	39.4		0.60	1.86	17.7	173
Breast	8	0	-	-	-	-	-	-	-	-	-	-	-	-	-	2.1	3.7	-	10.2	34.1	1.0	0.2	0.00	0.03	0.4	175
Prostate	1109	3	-	-	-	-	-	-	-	-	-	4.6	25.0	73.5	211.4	443.4	711.6	837.9	939.0	1022.8	133.2	26.7	1.58	7.37	58.8	185
Testis	24	0	-	-	-	3.3	7.0	5.3	8.7	5.0	-	4.6	4.6	-	-	2.1	3.7	-	5.1	-	2.9	0.6	0.19	0.22	2.8	186
Penis	10	0	-	-	-	-	-	-	-	-	-	-	-	1.9	8.2	3.7	3.6	10.2	8.5	1.2	0.2	0.01	0.07	0.5	187.1-.4		
Other male genital	2	0	-	-	-	-	-	-	-	-	-	-	-	1.9	2.1	-	-	-	-	-	0.2	0.0	0.01	0.02	0.1	187.5-.9
Bladder	401	0	-	-	-	-	-	-	-	3.3	10.2	27.6	45.5	52.2	118.1	133.4	203.8	246.7	294.4	221.6	48.2	9.7	1.28	2.97	24.7	188
Kidney etc.	115	0	-	-	-	-	-	-	-	1.7	5.1	9.2	6.8	32.9	41.9	26.7	66.7	65.3	55.8	42.6	13.8	2.8	0.49	0.95	7.6	189
Eye	9	0	-	-	1.8	-	1.7	-	-	-	1.7	-	2.3	-	-	-	3.7	7.3	-	17.0	1.1	0.2	0.04	0.06	0.8	190
Brain, nervous system	41	0	2.1	-	-	3.3	-	3.6	-	-	3.4	2.3	6.8	11.6	13.3	12.3	22.2	7.3	10.2	8.5	4.9	1.0	0.23	0.40	3.5	191-2
Thyroid	24	0	-	-	-	-	-	1.8	-	-	5.1	2.3	6.8	5.8	5.7	10.3	7.4	10.9	-	-	2.9	0.6	0.14	0.23	2.0	193
Other endocrine	1	0	-	-	-	-	-	-	-	-	-	-	-	-	-	2.1	-	-	-	-	0.1	0.0	0.00	0.01	0.1	194
Hodgkin's disease	20	0	-	-	-	1.6	3.5	7.1	3.5	1.7	3.4	2.3	-	3.9	3.8	-	3.7	7.3	-	-	2.4	0.5	0.15	0.17	2.1	201
Non-Hodgkin lymphoma	101	0	-	-	3.6	-	-	1.8	5.2	5.0	10.2	13.8	6.8	11.6	24.8	32.8	18.5	47.2	96.4	42.6	12.1	2.4	0.41	0.67	6.8	200,202
Multiple myeloma	28	0	-	-	-	-	-	-	-	-	-	2.3	-	7.7	9.5	10.3	11.1	18.1	20.3	8.5	3.4	0.7	0.10	0.20	1.7	203
Lymphoid leukaemia	47	0	4.2	1.9	-	1.6	3.5	1.8	1.7	-	3.4	2.3	2.3	11.6	3.8	12.3	22.2	14.5	35.5	34.1	5.6	1.1	0.19	0.36	3.7	204
Myeloid leukaemia	25	0	-	-	-	-	1.7	-	-	3.3	1.7	6.9	6.8	-	5.7	2.1	14.8	10.9	15.2	8.5	3.0	0.6	0.13	0.22	2.0	205
Monocytic leukaemia	2	0	-	-	-	-	-	1.8	-	-	-	-	-	-	-	2.1	-	-	-	-	0.2	0.0	0.01	0.02	0.2	206
Other leukaemia	0	0	-	-	-	-	-	-	-	-	-	-	-	-	-	-	-	-	-	-	0.0	0.0	0.00	0.00	0.0	207
Leukaemia unspecified	2	0	-	-	-	-	-	-	-	-	-	-	-	-	4.1	-	-	-	-	-	0.2	0.0	0.00	0.02	0.1	208
Other and unspecified	155	0	-	1.9	-	1.6	-	-	-	1.7	3.4	11.5	11.4	30.9	40.0	65.7	103.8	72.5	76.1	68.2	18.6	3.7	0.51	1.36	10.2	O&U
All sites	4478	16	8.3	5.7	7.3	18.1	22.7	32.0	45.4	69.6	135.4	262.0	407.4	676.6	1093.4	1603.1	2283.1	2615.4	2999.8	2855.2	538.0		13.97	33.47	280.3	ALL
All sites but 173	4150	7	8.3	5.7	7.3	18.1	22.7	32.0	41.9	66.3	132.0	245.9	389.2	647.6	1049.5	1502.5	2138.5	2372.3	2700.4	2463.1	498.6	100.0	13.36	31.59	262.6	ALLb
Rate from 1 case			2.083	1.912	1.822	1.650	1.750	1.776	1.747	1.657	1.692	2.298	2.276	1.933	1.905	2.053	3.706	3.627	5.076	8.523						

†Important: see notes on population page

* FRANCE, TARN 1988-1992

ANNUAL INCIDENCE PER 100,000 BY AGE GROUP (YEARS) - FEMALE

SITE	ALL AGES	AGE UNK	0-	5-	10-	15-	20-	25-	30-	35-	40-	45-	50-	55-	60-	65-	70-	75-	80-	85+	CRUDE RATE	%	CR 64	CR 74	ASR (W)	ICD (9th)
Lip	10	1	-	-	-	-	-	-	-	-	-	-	-	-	-	1.8	-	2.6	15.0	7.2	1.1	0.4	0.00	0.01	0.2	140
Tongue	9	0	-	-	-	-	-	-	-	-	1.7	-	2.1	1.8	3.5	-	-	5.1	3.0	3.6	1.0	0.3	0.05	0.05	0.5	141
Salivary gland	3	0	-	-	-	-	-	-	-	-	-	-	-	-	1.7	-	-	2.6	-	3.6	0.3	0.1	0.01	0.01	0.1	142
Mouth	9	0	-	-	-	-	-	-	-	-	-	2.2	-	-	3.6	-	-	2.6	6.0	10.8	1.0	0.3	0.01	0.03	0.4	143-5
Oropharynx	4	0	-	-	-	-	-	-	-	-	3.4	2.2	-	-	1.7	-	-	-	-	-	0.5	0.1	0.04	0.04	0.4	146
Nasopharynx	0	0	-	-	-	-	-	-	-	-	-	-	-	-	-	-	-	-	-	-	0.0	0.0	0.00	0.00	0.0	147
Hypopharynx	4	0	-	-	-	-	-	-	-	-	-	2.2	-	-	3.5	1.8	-	-	-	-	0.5	0.1	0.03	0.04	0.3	148
Pharynx unspecified	0	0	-	-	-	-	-	-	-	-	-	-	-	-	-	-	-	-	-	-	0.0	0.0	0.00	0.00	0.0	149
Oesophagus	10	0	-	-	-	-	-	-	-	-	-	-	4.3	3.7	3.5	3.6	-	-	6.0	-	1.1	0.4	0.06	0.08	0.6	150
Stomach	77	0	-	-	-	-	-	-	-	3.3	5.1	2.2	4.3	-	10.4	18.2	30.7	43.6	42.1	43.3	8.8	2.7	0.13	0.37	3.3	151
Small intestine	2	0	-	-	-	-	-	-	-	-	-	-	-	-	-	-	-	2.6	3.0	-	0.2	0.1	0.00	0.00	0.0	152
Colon	298	0	-	-	-	3.6	-	1.8	1.7	3.3	6.8	15.6	19.3	33.0	38.1	80.2	92.2	143.5	156.5	180.3	34.0	10.5	0.62	1.48	13.3	153
Rectum	205	0	-	-	-	-	-	-	-	1.6	8.5	13.4	30.1	18.3	34.7	63.8	58.4	99.9	99.3	82.9	23.4	7.2	0.53	1.14	10.0	154
Liver	14	0	-	-	-	-	-	-	-	-	-	2.2	-	5.5	-	7.3	6.1	-	9.0	3.6	1.6	0.5	0.04	0.11	0.8	155
Gallbladder etc.	42	0	-	-	-	-	-	-	-	3.3	1.7	2.2	-	5.5	5.2	9.1	21.5	5.1	27.1	32.4	4.8	1.5	0.09	0.24	1.9	156
Pancreas	32	0	-	-	-	-	-	-	-	1.6	-	-	2.1	9.2	5.2	5.5	3.1	17.9	18.1	18.0	3.6	1.1	0.09	0.13	1.4	157
Nose, sinuses etc.	6	0	-	-	-	-	-	-	-	-	-	-	-	3.7	-	1.8	-	-	6.0	3.6	0.7	0.2	0.02	0.03	0.2	160
Larynx	11	0	-	-	-	-	-	-	-	-	1.7	2.2	2.1	1.8	-	3.6	-	5.1	6.0	3.6	1.3	0.4	0.04	0.06	0.6	161
Bronchus, lung	60	0	-	-	-	-	-	1.8	3.4	-	5.1	-	10.7	9.2	10.4	10.9	18.4	25.6	30.1	21.6	6.8	2.1	0.20	0.35	3.2	162
Other thoracic organs	0	0	-	-	-	-	-	-	-	-	-	-	-	-	-	-	-	-	-	-	0.0	0.0	0.00	0.00	0.0	163-4
Bone	8	0	-	-	1.9	-	2.0	-	-	-	1.7	-	4.3	1.8	-	-	-	-	3.0	3.6	0.9	0.3	0.06	0.06	0.8	170
Connective tissue	18	0	2.2	-	-	3.6	-	1.8	-	-	-	-	4.3	-	1.7	5.5	-	7.7	6.0	10.8	2.1	0.6	0.07	0.10	1.3	171
Mesothelioma	1	0	-	-	-	-	-	-	-	-	-	-	-	-	-	1.8	-	-	-	-	0.1	0.0	0.00	0.01	0.1	MES
Kaposi's sarcoma	1	0	-	-	-	-	-	-	-	-	-	-	-	-	1.7	-	-	-	-	-	0.1	0.0	0.01	0.01	0.1	KAP
Melanoma of skin	86	0	-	-	-	1.8	3.9	5.5	8.6	11.5	5.1	15.6	17.2	12.8	15.6	16.4	24.6	12.8	15.0	25.2	9.8	3.0	0.49	0.69	6.7	172
†Other skin	229	5	-	-	-	-	2.0	-	-	-	6.8	4.5	2.1	14.7	20.8	25.5	52.2	115.3	129.4	277.6	26.1		0.26	0.66	7.5	173
Breast	905	0	-	-	-	-	2.0	7.3	22.3	64.2	117.2	154.0	189.1	170.6	206.2	215.2	236.7	235.7	222.7	176.7	103.2	31.9	4.66	6.92	62.3	174
Uterus unspecified	4	0	-	-	-	-	-	-	-	-	-	2.2	-	-	-	-	-	2.6	3.0	3.6	0.5	0.1	0.01	0.01	0.2	179
Cervix uteri	102	0	-	-	-	-	-	5.5	5.1	13.2	11.9	20.1	17.2	20.2	31.2	23.7	18.4	10.2	27.1	10.8	11.6	3.6	0.62	0.83	7.7	180
Placenta	0	0	-	-	-	-	-	-	-	-	-	-	-	-	-	-	-	-	-	-	0.0	0.0	0.00	0.00	0.0	181
Corpus uteri	167	0	-	-	-	-	-	-	-	1.6	5.1	11.2	27.9	44.0	57.2	58.4	46.1	46.1	54.2	18.0	19.0	5.9	0.74	1.26	10.0	182
Ovary etc.	131	0	-	-	-	1.8	-	3.6	3.4	8.2	5.1	11.2	30.1	27.5	32.9	38.3	43.0	43.6	24.1	18.0	14.9	4.6	0.62	1.03	8.7	183
Other female genital	35	0	-	2.0	-	-	-	1.8	-	-	-	-	8.6	12.8	5.2	5.5	6.1	10.2	12.0	21.6	4.0	1.2	0.15	0.21	2.1	184
Bladder	91	1	-	-	-	-	-	-	-	-	-	2.2	2.1	1.8	13.9	12.8	27.7	51.2	45.1	100.9	10.4	3.2	0.10	0.31	3.1	188
Kidney etc.	46	0	2.2	2.0	-	-	2.0	-	1.7	1.6	1.7	2.2	4.3	12.8	6.9	9.1	15.4	23.1	12.0	10.8	5.2	1.6	0.19	0.31	3.0	189
Eye	7	0	-	-	-	-	-	3.6	-	-	-	-	6.4	-	-	1.8	-	-	-	3.6	0.8	0.2	0.05	0.06	0.7	190
Brain, nervous system	28	0	4.4	-	1.9	1.8	-	1.8	-	3.3	1.7	4.5	2.1	5.5	-	9.1	9.2	7.7	6.0	3.6	3.2	1.0	0.14	0.23	2.5	191-2
Thyroid	79	0	-	-	1.9	-	2.0	7.3	8.6	6.6	17.0	22.3	23.6	18.3	6.9	20.1	9.2	7.7	3.0	3.6	9.0	2.8	0.57	0.72	7.3	193
Other endocrine	2	0	-	-	1.9	-	-	-	-	-	-	-	-	-	-	1.8	-	-	-	-	0.2	0.1	0.01	0.02	0.2	194
Hodgkin's disease	7	0	-	-	-	1.8	2.0	-	3.4	-	1.7	-	-	-	-	1.8	-	2.6	-	-	0.8	0.2	0.04	0.05	0.7	201
Non-Hodgkin lymphoma	103	0	-	-	1.9	1.8	-	3.6	1.7	-	8.5	2.2	12.9	9.2	10.4	25.5	40.0	51.2	48.2	43.3	11.7	3.6	0.26	0.59	5.3	200,202
Multiple myeloma	32	0	-	-	-	-	-	1.8	-	-	-	-	-	11.0	10.4	7.3	15.4	15.4	9.0	3.6	3.6	1.1	0.12	0.23	1.7	203
Lymphoid leukaemia	30	0	8.8	2.0	3.9	1.8	-	-	-	-	1.7	-	-	1.8	-	10.9	3.1	10.2	15.0	14.4	3.4	1.1	0.10	0.17	2.6	204
Myeloid leukaemia	32	0	-	-	1.9	-	2.0	1.8	1.7	1.6	1.7	2.2	-	9.2	6.9	5.5	6.1	17.9	9.0	3.6	3.6	1.1	0.15	0.20	2.1	205
Monocytic leukaemia	2	0	-	-	-	-	-	-	-	-	-	-	-	-	1.7	-	-	2.6	-	-	0.2	0.1	0.01	0.01	0.1	206
Other leukaemia	0	0	-	-	-	-	-	-	-	-	-	-	-	-	-	-	-	-	-	-	0.0	0.0	0.00	0.00	0.0	207
Leukaemia unspecified	5	0	-	-	-	-	-	-	-	-	-	-	-	-	-	-	-	5.1	3.0	7.2	0.6	0.2	0.00	0.00	0.1	208
Other and unspecified	123	0	2.2	2.0	-	-	-	-	-	3.3	-	6.7	10.7	20.2	19.1	29.2	18.4	48.7	78.3	79.3	14.0	4.3	0.32	0.56	5.7	O&U
All sites	3070	7	19.9	8.1	15.4	17.9	17.7	49.2	61.7	128.5	220.9	305.8	438.5	486.2	566.6	736.7	802.2	1083.7	1152.8	1254.6	350.2		11.71	19.42	180.0	ALL
All sites but 173	2841	2	19.9	8.1	15.4	17.9	15.8	49.2	61.7	128.5	214.1	301.3	436.3	471.5	545.8	711.1	749.9	968.4	1023.4	977.0	324.0	100.0	11.44	18.75	172.4	ALLb
Rate from 1 case			2.210	2.023	1.927	1.794	1.972	1.824	1.713	1.647	1.699	2.232	2.149	1.835	1.733	1.823	3.073	2.562	3.010	3.605						

†Important: see notes on population page

Germany, Federal States Berlin, Brandenburg, Mecklenburg-Vorpommern, Sachsen-Anhalt and Free States Sachsen and Thüringen

The former National Cancer Registry of the German Democratic Republic (GDR) has continued its work as the Common Cancer Registry of the Federal States of Berlin, Brandenburg, Mecklenburg-Vorpommern, Sachsen-Anhalt and the Free States of Sachsen and Thüringen (CCR). These states were constituted from the territory of the former GDR after the reunification of Germany in 1990. With effect from 1 January 1995, a nation-wide law on cancer registration, with a period of validity until 31 December 1999, requires all federal states to install population-based cancer registries.

The data in this volume relate only to the years 1988–89, during which the cancer-reporting system of the GDR was still in operation, and this is described below.

The registry covered the entire territory of the GDR. a total of 108 333 km^2 located between latitudes 50°10′ and 54°41′ N and longitudes 10°0′ and 15°10′ E. The maximum altitude is 1000 m. The population was 16 660 000 in 1987 (density 153 persons per km^2), with 58.8% of the population living in towns of more than 10 000 inhabitants. The population was stable with a high average level of education and was rather homogeneous. The GDR was highly industrialized, but there was a substantial agricultural and forestry sector. In the 1980s, pollution of air and water reached alarming levels. The mean emissions amounted to 51 tons of SO_2 and 22 tons of dust per square kilometre in 1987. About 45% of all rivers could not be used for the extraction of drinking water. Water pollution by nitrates was serious, especially in the southern part of the GDR.

An obligatory system of cancer case-reporting was established in 1953. This system was an integral element in a network of medical and social services for cancer patients, provided or coordinated by a Cancer Control Agency (CCA) in each of the 227 counties. The cancer registry was a branch of the Central Institute for Cancer Research of the Academy of Sciences of the GDR, whereas the CCAs were part of the local health services.

A physician who diagnosed a cancer case (including some benign tumours and carcinomas *in situ* but excluding basal cell carcinoma of the skin) had to send a report to the CCA in the patient's county of residence. The form was reviewed and a copy forwarded to the registry. Any subsequent course of treatment including that for recurrent or metastatic disease was similarly reported. Pathological institutes performing an autopsy on a deceased cancer patient had similarly to submit a report. If a diagnosis of cancer was found on a death certificate of a person not previously known to the CCA, the case was investigated and the required reporting forms were completed. The completeness of case reporting was estimated to be about 95%.

Cancer patient follow-up was reported annually by the physician responsible for the patient's after-care and might be supplemented by personal contact through the CCA staff and by consulting the official residency registers. The follow-up report was obligatory until five years after the initial treatment or the treatment of recurrent or metastatic disease.

Reporting forms were edited at the registry and selected information was coded by specially trained clerks. Anatomical site was coded by an internal code which could be translated by a computer program into ICD-8, ICD-9 or ICD-O. Histology was coded by a classification developed from the ICD-O morphology classification. Multiple neoplasms in the same patient were sequentially numbered, permitting identification of patients with previously reported cases and earlier diagnoses.

84% of male and 90% of female cases were histologically verified. The overall autopsy rate was about 25% and 55% for cancer cases. 5% of all cases were diagnosed at post mortem, and 5% of the diagnoses were revised at autopsy.

Reports submitted on each cancer patient registered since 1953 are stored by year of diagnosis and an identification number. Data for cancer cases since 1961 are available on a local PC network in the registry, and were updated regularly until 1989. Data input using personal computers started in 1988, using software developed in the registry. The data were checked for completeness, internal consistency and double registration. Errors were corrected immediately, or, if necessary, the CCA or the reporting physician was contacted.

The cancer registry data were used for health services planning, evaluation of medical services and for epidemiological research. A number of standard analyses of incidence data were prepared regularly.

Linkage with the NCR was used for cohort studies. The personal identification number included in the patient's record was particularly helpful for such studies. The registry data also provided material for case–control and clinical studies.

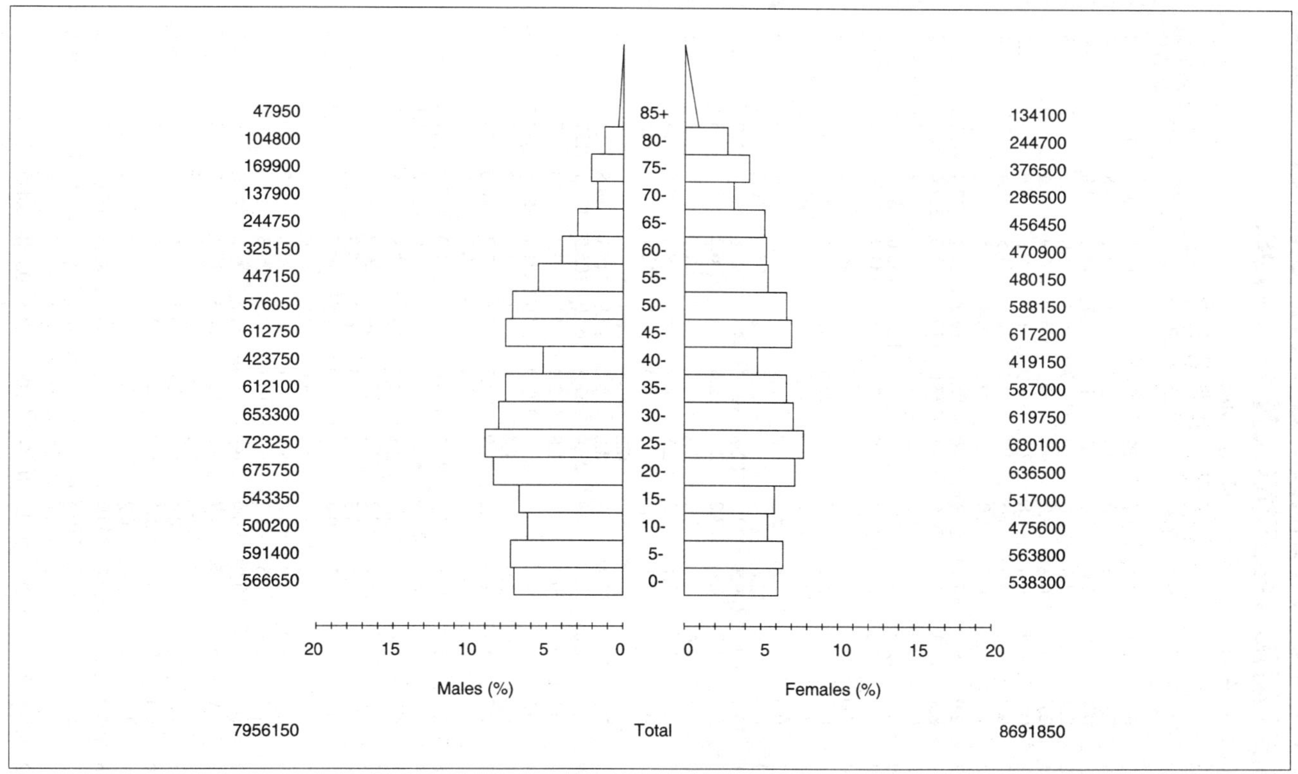

Germany, Federal States Berlin, Brandenburg, Mecklenburg-Vorpommern, Sachsen-Anhalt and Free States Sachsen and Thüringen
Source of population: average annual 1988–92
Notes to tables overleaf:
† 173 does not include basal cell carcinomas

Screening programmes in the area:
60-80% of the female population aged 20-65 have been covered by cervical cancer screening since 1968.

GERMANY, FEDERAL STATES BERLIN, BRANDENBURG, MECKLENBURG-VORPOMMERN, SACHSEN-ANHALT AND FREE STATES SACHSEN AND THURINGEN 1988-1989

ANNUAL INCIDENCE PER 100,000 BY AGE GROUP (YEARS) - MALE

SITE	ALL AGES	AGE UNK	0-	5-	10-	15-	20-	25-	30-	35-	40-	45-	50-	55-	60-	65-	70-	75-	80-	85+	CRUDE RATE	%	CR 64	CR 74	ASR (W)	ICD (9th)
Lip	317	0	-	-	-	-	-	-	0.1	0.1	0.2	1.1	3.4	3.1	6.8	9.0	13.8	15.9	16.7	17.7	2.0	0.6	0.07	0.19	**1.5**	*140*
Tongue	321	0	-	-	-	-	-	0.1	0.2	0.8	2.0	3.7	6.6	7.0	5.1	5.9	4.7	4.1	4.8	6.3	2.0	0.6	0.13	0.18	**1.6**	*141*
Salivary gland	94	0	-	-	0.1	-	0.1	-	0.2	0.3	0.4	0.5	1.0	1.1	1.7	1.4	4.7	3.2	4.8	2.1	0.6	0.2	0.03	0.06	**0.5**	*142*
Mouth	365	0	-	-	0.1	-	0.1	-	0.2	0.8	2.4	4.3	7.6	8.6	5.4	5.7	8.0	5.0	3.3	5.2	2.3	0.7	0.15	0.22	**1.8**	*143-5*
Oropharynx	342	0	-	-	-	-	-	-	0.4	0.4	2.6	4.6	6.2	6.9	6.2	6.5	6.5	5.9	4.3	1.0	2.1	0.7	0.14	0.20	**1.7**	*146*
Nasopharynx	80	0	-	-	0.1	0.1	0.1	0.1	0.1	0.2	0.9	0.9	0.8	1.8	2.0	1.0	1.5	0.9	1.0	-	0.5	0.2	0.04	0.05	**0.4**	*147*
Hypopharynx	223	0	-	-	-	-	-	0.1	0.1	0.2	0.9	3.8	4.9	5.6	4.3	2.7	2.5	1.5	1.4	2.1	1.4	0.4	0.10	0.13	**1.1**	*148*
Pharynx unspecified	26	0	-	-	-	-	-	-	0.2	0.2	-	0.2	0.2	1.0	0.3	0.2	0.4	1.5	-	-	0.2	0.1	0.01	0.01	**0.1**	*149*
Oesophagus	848	0	-	-	-	-	-	0.1	0.2	0.2	2.9	6.5	14.1	18.3	18.0	17.8	19.2	27.7	22.4	12.5	5.3	1.7	0.30	0.49	**4.1**	*150*
Stomach	4142	0	-	-	-	-	0.2	0.9	2.1	4.1	8.8	14.3	31.6	50.5	84.1	125.0	170.1	207.5	227.6	180.4	26.0	8.3	0.98	2.46	**20.1**	*151*
Small intestine	80	0	-	-	-	-	-	-	0.2	0.1	0.9	1.0	1.5	1.4	1.4	3.6	2.9	1.4	2.1	-	0.5	0.2	0.03	0.05	**0.4**	*152*
Colon	3201	0	-	-	0.1	0.2	0.9	1.8	3.0	8.0	12.9	23.8	45.0	64.9	91.9	120.7	153.6	169.4	144.9	20.1	6.4	0.80	1.87	**15.5**	*153*
Rectum	3181	0	-	-	-	-	0.1	0.6	1.3	2.0	8.7	14.2	26.9	46.7	70.0	92.1	124.7	147.7	135.0	123.0	20.0	6.4	0.85	1.94	**15.7**	*154*
Liver	1015	0	0.1	-	0.1	0.4	0.1	0.2	0.2	1.0	2.0	3.8	8.0	15.7	22.8	35.8	37.7	46.8	35.5	35.5	6.4	2.0	0.27	0.64	**5.1**	*155*
Gallbladder etc.	777	0	-	-	-	-	-	0.1	0.1	0.2	0.7	2.0	5.2	7.7	11.4	22.5	33.7	47.1	56.3	58.4	4.9	1.6	0.14	0.42	**3.6**	*156*
Pancreas	1501	0	-	-	-	-	0.1	-	0.5	1.3	3.7	7.8	13.6	21.2	32.3	41.1	55.8	73.6	65.8	54.2	9.4	3.0	0.40	0.89	**7.3**	*157*
Nose, sinuses etc.	126	0	-	-	0.1	0.1	0.1	0.1	0.2	0.2	0.5	0.6	1.8	2.2	2.0	2.9	1.8	4.4	6.2	5.2	0.8	0.3	0.04	0.06	**0.6**	*160*
Larynx	998	0	0.1	-	-	-	-	0.3	0.5	1.3	4.4	7.8	14.8	20.1	25.7	26.1	22.8	25.6	16.2	9.4	6.3	2.0	0.37	0.62	**5.1**	*161*
Bronchus, lung	11787	0	-	0.1	-	-	0.2	0.7	1.5	5.1	15.9	49.2	109.5	220.5	302.8	390.2	442.0	445.6	405.1	270.1	74.1	23.5	3.53	7.69	**59.2**	*162*
Other thoracic organs	144	0	-	-	-	0.3	0.1	0.1	0.3	0.2	0.2	1.0	2.0	2.2	2.3	2.5	4.0	6.2	5.7	3.1	0.9	0.3	0.04	0.08	**0.7**	*163-4*
Bone	243	0	0.2	0.3	0.9	1.3	1.0	1.0	0.7	1.0	1.5	1.6	1.2	2.3	2.8	3.9	8.3	7.7	4.3	4.2	1.5	0.5	0.08	0.14	**1.4**	*170*
Connective tissue	332	0	0.9	0.6	0.8	0.6	0.7	0.8	1.0	1.5	2.1	2.4	3.1	2.8	3.8	6.7	5.4	9.4	9.5	14.6	2.1	0.7	0.11	0.17	**1.8**	*171*
Mesothelioma	187	0	-	-	-	-	-	0.3	0.1	0.3	0.6	1.3	1.1	2.2	4.5	5.3	7.6	7.7	8.1	5.2	1.2	0.4	0.05	0.12	**0.9**	*MES*
Kaposi's sarcoma	5	0	-	-	-	-	-	-	-	-	0.1	-	-	0.1	0.2	-	0.4	-	0.5	-	0.0	0.0	0.00	0.00	**0.0**	*KAP*
Melanoma of skin	968	0	-	0.1	0.2	0.6	1.0	1.3	3.4	5.4	7.0	10.3	12.2	13.3	18.0	19.6	17.8	19.1	14.8	14.6	6.1	1.9	0.36	0.55	**5.0**	*172*
†Other skin	1543	0	-	-	-	0.1	0.2	0.3	0.5	0.9	1.3	2.0	7.1	8.9	21.4	37.8	64.9	105.9	131.7	187.7	9.7		0.21	0.73	**7.0**	*173*
Breast	103	0	-	-	-	-	0.1	0.1	0.2	0.2	0.5	0.8	0.7	1.6	1.8	2.9	3.3	3.2	3.3	7.3	0.6	0.2	0.03	0.06	**0.5**	*175*
Prostate	5017	0	-	-	-	-	-	-	-	-	0.2	2.4	9.3	30.1	85.2	173.9	297.0	371.7	382.6	333.7	31.5	10.0	0.64	2.99	**23.7**	*185*
Testis	1466	0	0.6	0.3	0.3	5.0	14.1	24.5	24.5	18.5	10.3	8.0	5.9	2.5	1.4	1.6	0.7	1.5	1.4	5.2	9.2	2.9	0.58	0.59	**7.9**	*186*
Penis	187	0	-	-	-	-	0.1	0.1	0.2	0.2	0.5	1.1	1.5	2.2	2.9	4.5	7.6	7.9	10.0	15.6	1.2	0.4	0.04	0.10	**0.9**	*187.1-.4*
Other male genital	16	0	0.1	0.1	-	-	-	-	0.1	-	0.1	0.2	-	-	0.8	0.4	-	0.3	1.0	-	0.1	0.0	0.01	0.01	**0.1**	*187.5-.9*
Bladder	3879	0	0.1	-	0.1	-	0.2	0.6	0.8	1.8	5.1	11.3	21.8	47.9	91.7	133.0	178.8	201.0	197.0	141.8	24.4	7.7	0.91	2.47	**19.2**	*188*
Kidney etc.	2706	0	1.6	0.7	0.2	0.3	0.2	0.2	1.5	3.4	10.5	19.8	36.2	50.9	63.7	65.8	84.1	73.0	65.8	51.1	17.0	5.4	0.95	1.70	**13.8**	*189*
Eye	161	0	1.1	0.1	0.1	-	-	0.1	0.2	0.2	0.9	1.1	1.6	3.4	2.5	4.5	2.2	3.8	4.8	4.2	1.0	0.3	0.06	0.09	**0.9**	*190*
Brain, nervous system	1209	0	3.3	4.3	2.9	2.5	2.7	2.9	4.1	5.1	6.8	11.5	13.5	17.2	22.1	20.2	14.1	10.9	15.3	11.5	7.6	2.4	0.49	0.67	**6.8**	*191-2*
Thyroid	243	0	-	0.1	-	0.5	0.2	0.6	0.5	1.6	1.2	2.0	2.5	3.5	4.2	4.5	6.9	5.9	6.2	3.1	1.5	0.5	0.08	0.14	**1.2**	*193*
Other endocrine	61	0	1.0	-	0.1	0.1	0.1	0.1	0.4	0.1	0.4	0.4	0.5	0.4	0.6	1.0	1.5	0.6	1.9	1.0	0.4	0.1	0.02	0.03	**0.4**	*194*
Hodgkin's disease	454	0	0.4	0.4	1.0	3.6	4.7	2.7	3.4	2.7	2.5	2.3	2.3	4.0	4.2	4.9	8.3	5.9	4.3	3.1	2.9	0.9	0.17	0.24	**2.6**	*201*
Non-Hodgkin lymphoma	1058	0	1.8	1.5	1.2	1.2	1.9	1.2	1.6	2.9	4.2	7.2	9.0	13.0	18.6	24.1	34.1	36.5	31.0	29.2	6.6	2.1	0.33	0.62	**5.6**	*200,202*
Multiple myeloma	437	0	-	-	-	-	-	0.1	0.1	0.4	1.1	2.1	3.6	7.2	10.6	13.1	19.9	20.3	11.0	9.4	2.7	0.9	0.13	0.29	**2.2**	*203*
Lymphoid leukaemia	610	0	4.0	2.7	1.7	1.6	0.6	0.4	0.4	0.7	0.5	3.6	4.2	6.9	6.9	12.9	23.2	23.0	22.4	16.7	3.8	1.2	0.17	0.35	**3.5**	*204*
Myeloid leukaemia	519	0	1.1	0.4	0.5	1.3	1.2	1.5	1.8	1.1	2.9	3.2	3.9	4.7	8.3	11.4	17.0	17.1	12.9	15.6	3.3	1.0	0.16	0.30	**2.8**	*205*
Monocytic leukaemia	15	0	0.1	-	-	-	-	-	0.1	0.1	-	-	0.2	-	0.2	-	0.7	1.2	1.4	-	0.1	0.0	0.00	0.01	**0.1**	*206*
Other leukaemia	27	0	-	-	-	0.1	-	0.1	0.1	0.1	-	0.3	0.2	0.4	0.3	1.0	0.7	0.6	1.0	-	0.2	0.1	0.01	0.02	**0.1**	*207*
Leukaemia unspecified	108	0	-	-	0.2	0.4	0.2	-	0.2	0.6	0.1	0.6	0.6	1.1	0.9	2.9	4.7	3.5	6.7	5.2	0.7	0.2	0.02	0.06	**0.5**	*208*
Other and unspecified	511	0	0.9	0.1	0.1	0.3	0.5	0.6	1.2	0.9	1.4	2.9	4.4	6.2	11.1	12.7	18.9	18.2	18.6	13.6	3.2	1.0	0.15	0.31	**2.6**	*O&U*
All sites	51633	0	17.1	11.7	10.8	20.2	31.4	43.7	56.7	71.6	127.3	238.4	429.8	719.8	1057.7	1450.3	1906.5	2182.5	2150.8	1826.9	324.5		14.18	30.96	**257.6**	*ALL*
All sites but 173	50090	0	17.1	11.7	10.8	20.1	31.2	43.4	56.2	70.7	126.0	236.4	422.7	710.8	1036.3	1412.5	1841.6	2076.5	2019.1	1639.2	314.8	100.0	13.97	30.24	**250.6**	*ALLb*

| Rate from 1 case | | | 0.088 | 0.085 | 0.100 | 0.092 | 0.074 | 0.069 | 0.077 | 0.082 | 0.118 | 0.082 | 0.087 | 0.112 | 0.154 | 0.204 | 0.363 | 0.294 | 0.477 | 1.043 |

†Important: see notes on population page

GERMANY, FEDERAL STATES BERLIN, BRANDENBURG, MECKLENBURG-VORPOMMERN, SACHSEN-ANHALT AND FREE STATES SACHSEN AND THURINGEN 1988-1989

ANNUAL INCIDENCE PER 100,000 BY AGE GROUP (YEARS) - FEMALE

SITE	ALL AGES	AGE UNK	0-	5-	10-	15-	20-	25-	30-	35-	40-	45-	50-	55-	60-	65-	70-	75-	80-	85+	CRUDE RATE	%	CR 64	CR 74	ASR (W)	ICD (9th)
Lip	71	0	-	-	-	-	-	-	-	-	0.1	0.1	-	0.2	0.4	2.0	1.2	2.1	3.1	2.6	0.4	0.1	0.00	0.02	0.2	140
Tongue	87	0	-	-	-	-	-	0.2	0.2	0.4	0.4	0.5	0.6	0.7	1.5	1.2	1.2	1.5	1.4	1.1	0.5	0.1	0.02	0.03	0.3	141
Salivary gland	95	0	-	-	0.1	-	-	0.1	0.1	0.3	0.1	0.5	0.6	0.9	1.1	1.2	1.2	1.7	1.8	5.6	0.5	0.2	0.02	0.03	0.3	142
Mouth	117	0	-	-	-	-	0.1	-	-	0.2	0.5	0.9	0.8	1.1	2.1	1.9	1.6	2.4	1.6	2.6	0.7	0.2	0.03	0.05	0.4	143-5
Oropharynx	88	0	-	-	-	-	-	-	-	0.1	0.1	0.6	1.1	0.7	1.3	1.6	1.7	1.3	1.4	1.9	0.5	0.2	0.02	0.04	0.3	146
Nasopharynx	33	0	-	0.1	-	0.1	0.1	0.1	0.1	0.2	0.1	0.3	-	0.2	0.5	0.1	0.5	1.1	0.2	0.4	0.2	0.1	0.01	0.01	0.1	147
Hypopharynx	27	0	-	-	-	-	-	-	-	-	-	0.2	0.7	0.5	0.2	-	0.2	0.5	0.8	-	0.2	0.0	0.01	0.01	0.1	148
Pharynx unspecified	6	0	-	-	-	-	-	-	-	-	-	0.1	-	0.2	-	-	-	0.4	-	-	0.0	0.0	0.00	0.00	0.0	149
Oesophagus	210	0	-	-	-	-	-	-	-	0.1	0.5	0.4	0.9	2.0	1.7	3.5	4.7	5.7	6.9	7.1	1.2	0.4	0.03	0.07	0.6	150
Stomach	3911	0	-	-	-	-	0.5	0.7	1.9	4.0	7.8	11.0	13.9	22.2	34.3	57.0	86.7	125.1	133.4	116.7	22.5	6.7	0.48	1.20	10.5	151
Small intestine	95	0	-	-	0.1	-	-	0.2	-	0.1	0.5	0.3	1.2	1.5	1.4	1.4	2.3	2.5	1.9	0.5	0.2	0.02	0.03	0.3	152
Colon	5063	0	-	-	-	-	0.2	1.0	2.5	3.1	7.8	10.5	21.0	35.1	51.4	86.9	116.4	147.9	159.6	135.3	29.1	8.7	0.66	1.68	13.9	153
Rectum	3526	0	-	-	-	0.1	0.1	0.4	1.0	2.3	6.1	11.0	16.4	27.1	39.4	65.3	75.7	93.4	105.6	81.7	20.3	6.1	0.52	1.22	10.1	154
Liver	811	0	0.2	0.1	0.1	0.1	-	0.1	0.6	0.6	1.2	1.9	3.9	5.6	9.3	15.0	16.8	22.3	23.9	18.6	4.7	1.4	0.12	0.28	2.3	155
Gallbladder etc.	2584	0	-	-	-	-	-	0.1	0.3	0.8	2.3	3.9	9.9	18.6	26.5	43.9	53.6	78.5	87.9	85.0	14.9	4.4	0.31	0.80	6.8	156
Pancreas	1685	0	-	-	-	0.1	0.1	0.1	0.4	0.7	1.4	4.2	5.1	10.4	17.1	27.3	42.9	49.3	56.8	51.8	9.7	2.9	0.20	0.55	4.5	157
Nose, sinuses etc.	76	0	-	-	-	-	0.1	0.1	-	0.3	0.1	0.1	0.3	0.8	0.5	0.8	1.9	2.8	1.4	1.5	0.1	0.1	0.01	0.01	0.2	160
Larynx	78	0	-	-	-	-	-	-	0.2	0.4	0.2	0.7	0.5	1.0	1.3	1.4	1.4	0.4	1.0	0.7	0.4	0.1	0.02	0.04	0.3	161
Bronchus, lung	2407	0	-	-	-	0.3	0.2	0.4	1.0	1.7	2.6	7.3	14.4	26.8	36.2	45.2	62.3	55.0	44.7	30.2	13.8	4.1	0.45	0.99	7.6	162
Other thoracic organs	104	0	-	-	-	0.1	0.2	0.2	-	0.1	0.4	0.2	1.0	0.7	0.7	2.0	1.6	2.5	1.6	3.7	0.6	0.2	0.02	0.04	0.3	163-4
Bone	237	0	0.2	0.1	0.9	1.1	1.2	0.7	0.6	0.5	0.8	0.9	0.5	2.6	2.2	2.5	3.3	4.8	3.7	3.4	1.4	0.4	0.06	0.09	1.0	170
Connective tissue	383	0	0.9	0.4	0.6	0.6	0.9	1.2	1.3	0.9	1.8	1.8	2.5	3.0	3.9	5.7	5.6	4.6	7.6	5.2	2.2	0.7	0.10	0.16	1.6	171
Mesothelioma	103	0	-	-	-	-	-	0.1	-	-	0.2	0.7	0.6	0.5	1.4	1.4	2.1	2.9	2.9	1.9	0.6	0.2	0.02	0.04	0.3	MES
Kaposi's sarcoma	4	0	-	-	-	-	-	-	0.1	-	-	0.1	0.1	-	-	-	0.1	-	-	0.0	0.0	0.00	0.0	KAP		
Melanoma of skin	1314	0	-	-	-	0.7	1.3	3.2	4.8	7.5	11.5	11.2	12.8	13.0	12.5	17.6	15.5	16.3	12.9	13.8	7.6	2.3	0.39	0.56	5.3	172
†Other skin	1337	0	-	0.2	0.1	-	0.2	0.1	0.2	0.9	0.5	2.2	3.0	4.3	6.4	11.8	23.0	41.0	64.6	105.9	7.7		0.09	0.26	2.9	173
Breast	13215	0	-	-	-	-	0.9	4.4	17.3	39.4	85.2	119.4	124.8	131.1	163.6	195.7	209.8	209.4	197.8	177.9	76.0	22.7	3.43	5.46	48.2	174
Uterus unspecified	45	0	-	-	-	-	-	0.1	0.1	0.1	-	0.3	0.5	0.6	0.4	0.5	0.9	2.0	1.5	0.3	0.1	0.01	0.01	0.1	179	
Cervix uteri	4722	0	-	-	-	0.1	7.2	34.8	53.0	50.3	39.8	35.8	31.5	34.3	35.9	41.6	45.4	35.5	26.0	22.4	27.2	8.1	1.61	2.05	21.2	180
Placenta	13	0	-	-	-	-	0.5	0.1	0.1	0.2	-	0.1	0.2	-	-	-	-	-	-	0.1	0.0	0.01	0.01	0.1	181	
Corpus uteri	4021	0	-	-	-	0.3	0.3	0.2	0.7	2.1	8.8	20.9	40.6	56.1	68.4	79.0	72.1	64.4	55.6	34.7	23.1	6.9	0.99	1.75	13.9	182
Ovary etc.	3356	0	0.2	0.1	0.2	1.0	1.7	2.1	3.6	5.5	12.6	23.4	33.3	43.3	47.6	56.6	55.1	50.6	45.0	35.8	19.3	5.8	0.87	1.43	12.2	183
Other female genital	762	0	0.2	-	-	0.1	0.2	0.1	0.7	0.4	0.6	2.6	2.4	4.0	7.3	12.9	16.2	20.3	26.2	28.7	4.4	1.3	0.09	0.24	2.1	184
Bladder	1294	0	-	0.1	-	-	-	0.1	0.2	0.4	0.5	2.4	4.1	8.7	15.5	23.4	28.3	42.6	39.4	30.6	7.4	2.2	0.16	0.42	3.4	188
Kidney etc.	1974	0	1.6	0.3	-	0.1	0.1	0.2	1.2	1.4	4.8	9.6	17.4	25.5	31.0	34.9	35.4	37.8	29.2	25.0	11.4	3.4	0.47	0.82	6.8	189
Eye	153	0	1.7	-	-	-	0.1	0.1	0.2	0.1	0.7	1.1	1.4	1.2	2.2	1.9	2.4	2.4	1.6	1.5	0.9	0.3	0.04	0.07	0.7	190
Brain, nervous system	812	0	2.0	2.2	3.3	1.6	2.6	2.3	2.6	3.4	3.9	5.2	9.4	10.0	9.7	12.3	5.8	4.1	1.4	1.5	4.7	1.4	0.29	0.38	4.0	191-2
Thyroid	656	0	0.1	0.1	0.2	1.4	1.3	1.7	2.9	3.8	4.5	5.4	4.3	4.5	7.8	7.8	7.2	9.4	9.4	6.7	3.8	1.1	0.19	0.26	2.7	193
Other endocrine	62	0	0.9	0.2	0.1	0.3	0.1	0.2	0.3	0.2	0.5	0.2	0.8	0.3	0.5	0.7	0.5	0.3	-	0.4	0.4	0.1	0.02	0.03	0.4	194
Hodgkin's disease	409	0	0.1	0.6	0.9	3.9	4.3	3.3	2.5	1.5	1.8	1.2	1.1	2.5	2.4	2.8	4.0	4.9	3.9	3.0	2.4	0.7	0.13	0.17	2.0	201
Non-Hodgkin lymphoma	1075	0	1.2	0.2	0.3	1.1	0.8	1.0	1.3	2.3	3.0	4.0	6.6	9.0	13.8	18.7	19.0	22.0	24.9	16.4	6.2	1.8	0.22	0.41	3.7	200,202
Multiple myeloma	480	0	-	-	-	-	-	-	-	0.2	0.8	1.2	2.7	4.6	7.5	10.2	10.5	12.9	10.0	3.7	2.8	0.8	0.09	0.19	1.5	203
Lymphoid leukaemia	483	0	4.2	2.3	0.6	0.6	0.2	0.1	0.2	0.3	1.0	1.1	2.1	4.0	3.8	6.9	10.3	8.9	11.0	9.3	2.8	0.8	0.10	0.19	2.0	204
Myeloid leukaemia	553	0	0.7	0.5	0.5	0.7	0.5	1.2	1.1	1.6	2.5	2.0	2.9	4.5	6.8	6.7	11.0	10.5	11.4	8.6	3.2	1.0	0.13	0.22	2.1	205
Monocytic leukaemia	22	0	0.2	-	0.1	-	-	-	-	-	0.1	0.1	0.2	0.3	0.1	0.3	0.2	0.3	0.4	1.1	0.1	0.0	0.01	0.01	0.1	206
Other leukaemia	39	0	0.1	0.1	-	-	-	-	0.1	-	0.2	0.2	0.6	0.3	0.5	1.0	1.2	0.6	-	0.2	0.1	0.01	0.02	0.1	207	
Leukaemia unspecified	113	0	0.2	0.1	0.1	-	0.2	0.1	0.3	0.3	0.4	0.4	0.5	1.0	0.8	1.3	2.3	2.8	2.7	2.2	0.7	0.2	0.02	0.04	0.4	208
Other and unspecified	783	0	1.1	0.2	0.1	0.3	0.2	0.2	0.3	0.5	1.2	2.5	4.2	7.2	8.7	12.6	16.6	17.7	22.3	20.9	4.5	1.3	0.13	0.28	2.4	O&U
All sites	59494	0	15.8	7.8	8.5	14.4	26.5	61.2	104.2	139.3	219.4	310.5	401.6	533.1	688.0	924.2	1076.3	1225.0	1248.3	1110.4	342.2		12.65	22.65	200.4	ALL
All sites but 173	58157	0	15.8	7.6	8.4	14.4	26.3	61.1	103.9	138.3	218.9	308.3	398.6	528.8	681.7	912.4	1053.2	1183.9	1183.7	1004.5	334.5	100.0	12.56	22.39	197.4	ALLb

Rate from 1 case: 0.093 0.089 0.105 0.097 0.079 0.074 0.081 0.085 0.119 0.081 0.085 0.104 0.106 0.109 0.174 0.133 0.204 0.373

†Important: see notes on population page

509

Germany, Saarland

The Saarland Cancer Registry was established in 1967. It is an integrated unit of the State Statistical Office and is based on the Saarland Law of Cancer Registration, which came into force in 1979. It is financed by the Government of Saarland and by regular subsidies from the German Federal Ministry of Health.

A Federal Law of Cancer Registration was enacted in Germany on 1 January 1995, which has fundamentally changed the preconditions of cancer registration in Germany. This requires all the federal states to establish population-based cancer registries for their territories until 1999. The rules of the new federal law require amendment of existing laws for cancer registration in some states, so that a new legal basis for registration of cancer cases in Saarland is in preparation and will probably come into force on 1 January 1998..

Located in the south-west of Germany between latitudes 49°38′ and 49°7′ N and longitudes 6°21′ and 7°34′ E, bordering France and Luxembourg, Saarland is the second smallest state in the Federal Republic. The area amounts to 2567 km² of hilly country with altitudes ranging from 150 to 695 m above sea-level. About 45.5% of the land is used for agricultural purposes, 33.4% is covered with forests, and the remaining 21.1% comprises housing and industrial areas, water, playing and recreation grounds, etc.

The population of the registration area is 1 080 000 (in 1992) (density 422 per km²) or 1.3% of the whole German population. Some 53.5% live in conurbations of more than 20 000 inhabitants. The overwhelming majority (72.7%) are Roman Catholic, with 21.7% Protestants and 5.6% other religions. The working population, 44.4% of the total, is employed in industry (41.1%), commerce and transport (18.9%), agriculture (1%), and other personal services.

The basic system of the cancer registry is a centralized registration of individual records including personal identifiers which do not require the consent of registered patients.

Notification is voluntary. Hospitals, physicians and persons acting on their behalf have a right, but not a duty, to report cancer cases without violating their professional obligations. The main suppliers of information are hospitals, outpatient departments, pathology and radiotherapy departments and private practitioners. To minimize underregistration, death certificates are also used as data sources.

There are 30 hospitals including four radiotherapeutic departments and seven institutes of pathology in the registration area. About 50% of all new reports of cases come from pathologists. Hospitals are visited periodically by registry staff. It is believed that registration, with the exception of basal skin cancers, is nearly total.

The first date of cancer diagnosis is taken as the index date for computing incidence and survival rates, without regard to the type of diagnostic verification. It may, but does not necessarily, coincide with the date of histological diagnosis.

Due to the highly restrictive legal framework, the follow-up of patients is largely passive. Though all physicians treating cancer patients are generally requested to report any serious change in the state of a patient's health, the registry is not allowed to conduct further enquiries. The files of the registered cases are linked annually with all death certificates, but there is no regular matching with migration data for people leaving the Saarland region.

The very stringent rules for processing, storage, evaluation and potential dissemination still hinder the use of personal data for epidemiological research. The new legal framework will provide new models and methods for more effective use while strictly securing confidentiality of personal information.

H. Ziegler
C. Stegmaier

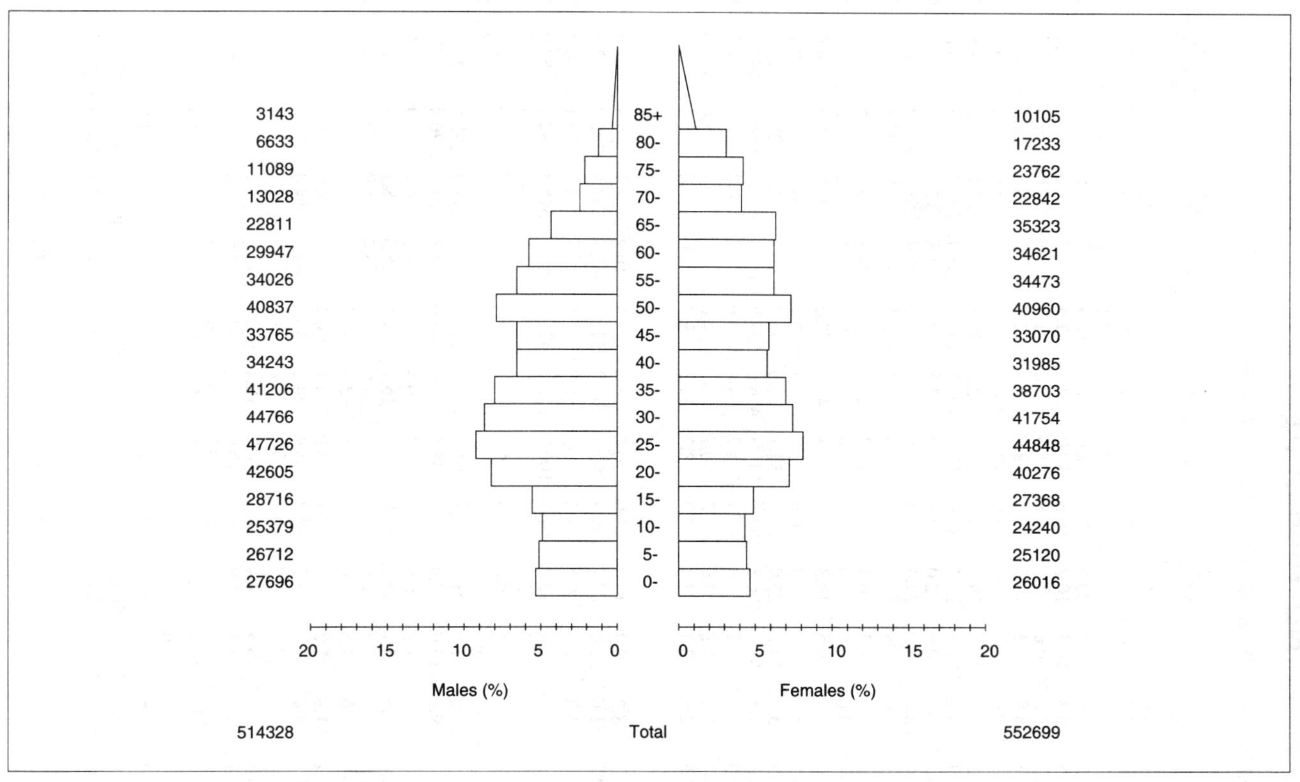

Germany, Saarland

Source of population: average annual 1988–92
Census: 1987 "Gemeindestatistik 1987, Bevölkerung und Erwerbstätigkeit, Ergebnisse der Volks- und Berufszählung am 25. Mai 1987
Einzelschriften zur Statistik des Saarlandes Nr. 75, Statistisches Amt des Saarlandes, Saarbrücken 1989, ISBN 3-88718-056-9, ISSN 0558-0838.
Estimate: The 1987 Census data are updated by current statistical records of births, deaths and migration to produce annual population figures.

Notes to tables overleaf:
+ The editors were unable to verify these data
† 163-164 includes mesothelioma of the pleura
† Mesothelioma not available separately
† Kaposi's sarcoma not available separately

Screening programmes in the area

Since 1971, women over age 30 have been screened annually for cervical cancer; women over age 20 were included in the screening programme in 1982. The population over age 30 has been screened annually for breast cancer, and the population over age 40 has been screened each year for prostate and large bowel cancer, since 1971.

+ GERMANY, SAARLAND 1988-1992

ANNUAL INCIDENCE PER 100,000 BY AGE GROUP (YEARS) - MALE

SITE	ALL AGES	AGE UNK	0-	5-	10-	15-	20-	25-	30-	35-	40-	45-	50-	55-	60-	65-	70-	75-	80-	85+	CRUDE RATE	%	CR 64	CR 74	ASR (W)	ICD (9th)
Lip	42	0	-	-	-	-	-	-	-	-	0.6	0.6	1.0	4.1	4.0	5.3	4.6	18.0	12.1	12.7	1.6	0.3	0.05	0.10	**1.0**	*140*
Tongue	147	0	-	-	-	-	-	0.4	-	3.9	5.3	13.0	12.2	13.5	14.7	21.0	10.7	5.4	6.0	6.4	5.7	1.2	0.32	0.47	**4.1**	*141*
Salivary gland	29	0	-	-	-	-	0.9	0.8	-	0.5	0.6	1.2	1.0	1.2	2.0	4.4	3.1	3.6	3.0	25.5	1.1	0.2	0.04	0.08	**0.8**	*142*
Mouth	195	0	-	-	-	-	-	-	-	5.3	7.6	14.8	20.6	22.9	22.0	12.3	16.9	7.2	6.0	6.4	7.6	1.6	0.47	0.61	**5.3**	*143-5*
Oropharynx	112	0	-	-	-	-	-	-	-	1.5	5.3	14.8	10.8	10.6	10.0	12.3	1.5	7.2	3.0	-	4.4	0.9	0.26	0.33	**3.1**	*146*
Nasopharynx	20	0	-	-	-	-	-	0.4	-	0.5	1.2	0.6	1.0	1.8	1.3	2.6	1.5	3.6	3.0	6.4	0.8	0.2	0.03	0.05	**0.5**	*147*
Hypopharynx	126	0	-	-	-	-	-	-	-	1.5	5.8	11.3	19.6	11.2	8.0	7.9	12.3	7.2	3.0	6.4	4.9	1.0	0.29	0.39	**3.5**	*148*
Pharynx unspecified	13	0	-	-	-	-	-	-	0.4	-	0.6	-	-	2.9	2.7	0.9	-	-	3.0	-	0.5	0.1	0.03	0.04	**0.3**	*149*
Oesophagus	248	1	-	-	-	-	-	-	-	1.5	4.7	16.6	19.1	24.1	25.4	32.4	35.3	18.0	27.1	70.0	9.6	2.0	0.46	0.80	**6.7**	*150*
Stomach	747	0	-	-	-	-	0.5	0.4	2.7	3.9	8.2	21.3	25.5	37.0	62.1	101.7	147.4	225.4	283.4	267.3	29.0	6.1	0.81	2.05	**18.5**	*151*
Small intestine	28	0	-	-	-	-	-	-	-	-	-	0.6	2.0	2.4	2.7	3.5	4.6	1.8	12.1	19.1	1.1	0.2	0.04	0.08	**0.7**	*152*
Colon	1031	0	-	-	-	0.7	-	0.4	2.2	4.4	8.8	13.0	27.4	69.4	82.8	154.3	222.6	299.4	358.8	470.9	40.1	8.4	1.05	2.93	**25.5**	*153*
Rectum	697	1	-	-	-	-	-	-	1.3	3.4	7.0	8.3	31.8	51.7	74.8	114.9	115.1	164.1	199.0	203.6	27.1	5.6	0.89	2.04	**17.3**	*154*
Liver	169	0	-	-	-	-	0.5	-	0.9	-	-	1.2	6.4	11.2	24.7	28.9	38.4	36.1	39.2	25.5	6.6	1.4	0.22	0.56	**4.2**	*155*
Gallbladder etc.	122	0	-	-	-	-	-	-	-	-	0.6	0.6	2.0	4.1	13.4	21.0	20.0	36.1	48.2	101.8	4.7	1.0	0.10	0.31	**3.0**	*156*
Pancreas	280	0	-	-	-	-	-	-	0.9	1.0	2.9	6.5	10.3	15.9	25.4	42.1	52.2	77.6	102.5	95.5	10.9	2.3	0.31	0.79	**6.9**	*157*
Nose, sinuses etc.	19	0	-	-	-	-	-	0.8	-	0.5	1.2	-	0.5	0.6	3.3	0.9	3.1	5.4	3.0	-	0.7	0.2	0.03	0.05	**0.5**	*160*
Larynx	313	0	-	-	-	-	-	-	-	1.9	5.3	14.2	25.0	37.0	34.1	38.6	43.0	32.5	51.3	25.5	12.2	2.5	0.59	1.00	**8.1**	*161*
Bronchus, lung	2799	1	-	-	-	0.7	-	0.4	0.4	8.3	24.5	58.6	106.3	183.4	341.3	486.6	587.9	616.8	654.3	636.3	108.8	22.7	3.62	9.00	**70.9**	*162*
†Other thoracic organs	45	0	-	-	-	-	0.5	0.4	0.4	1.0	-	1.2	2.4	2.4	4.7	4.4	4.6	16.2	6.0	19.1	1.7	0.4	0.06	0.11	**1.1**	*163-4*
Bone	26	0	-	-	1.6	1.4	1.9	0.4	0.4	-	1.2	1.8	2.0	1.2	0.7	-	4.6	-	-	6.4	1.0	0.2	0.06	0.09	**1.0**	*170*
Connective tissue	66	0	1.4	-	-	-	0.5	0.4	1.3	0.5	2.9	2.4	3.4	2.9	8.7	12.3	9.2	3.6	3.0	6.4	2.6	0.5	0.12	0.23	**1.9**	*171*
†Mesothelioma																										
†Kaposi's sarcoma																										
Melanoma of skin	215	2	-	-	-	-	0.9	2.9	3.6	6.3	8.2	8.9	15.7	15.9	20.0	25.4	21.5	19.8	21.1	25.5	8.4	1.7	0.42	0.65	**5.8**	*172*
Other skin	2390	10	-	0.7	0.8	0.7	0.9	4.2	9.4	9.7	31.0	58.6	89.1	139.9	202.4	340.2	546.5	597.0	690.5	922.7	92.9		2.75	7.20	**60.7**	*173*
Breast	17	0	-	-	-	-	-	-	-	-	1.2	1.2	0.5	1.2	-	0.9	1.5	5.4	6.0	19.1	0.7	0.1	0.02	0.03	**0.4**	*175*
Prostate	1491	1	-	-	-	-	-	-	-	-	-	4.7	13.2	61.1	106.9	228.8	426.7	568.1	645.3	782.7	58.0	12.1	0.93	4.21	**35.9**	*185*
Testis	189	1	0.7	-	-	5.6	10.3	17.6	16.1	16.5	7.0	5.3	5.4	4.7	1.3	1.8	-	-	-	6.4	7.3	1.5	0.46	0.46	**6.1**	*186*
Penis	34	0	-	-	-	-	-	-	-	-	-	0.6	1.8	0.5	0.6	6.0	5.3	6.1	7.2	3.0	25.5	1.3	0.3	0.05	0.10	**0.9**	*187.1-.4*
Other male genital	1	0	-	-	-	-	-	0.4	-	-	-	-	-	-	-	-	-	-	-	-	-	0.0	0.0	0.00	0.00	**0.0**	*187.5-.9*
Bladder	932	0	-	-	-	-	-	1.7	2.2	1.9	10.5	7.7	21.1	53.5	95.5	155.2	228.7	239.9	328.7	273.6	36.2	7.6	0.97	2.89	**23.1**	*188*
Kidney etc.	467	0	0.7	1.5	-	-	-	0.8	2.2	2.4	9.3	13.0	23.0	42.9	45.4	75.4	82.9	84.8	81.4	76.4	18.2	3.8	0.71	1.50	**12.2**	*189*
Eye	14	0	0.7	-	-	-	-	-	-	1.0	-	1.2	0.5	-	1.3	0.9	-	3.6	6.0	6.4	0.5	0.1	0.02	0.03	**0.4**	*190*
Brain, nervous system	187	0	2.9	3.0	1.6	3.5	0.5	3.4	5.4	2.4	5.3	4.7	10.8	11.8	18.7	16.7	27.6	25.3	18.1	12.7	7.3	1.5	0.37	0.59	**5.7**	*191-2*
Thyroid	70	0	-	-	-	-	0.5	1.3	1.8	2.9	4.1	2.4	2.9	2.4	9.3	7.0	7.7	5.4	6.0	19.1	2.7	0.6	0.14	0.21	**2.0**	*193*
Other endocrine	21	0	2.2	0.7	-	0.7	-	-	0.4	-	0.6	1.8	1.0	1.2	1.3	3.5	1.5	-	-	-	0.8	0.2	0.05	0.07	**0.9**	*194*
Hodgkin's disease	76	0	-	-	0.8	2.8	3.8	1.7	4.9	3.4	1.8	1.2	2.4	4.1	4.0	4.4	10.7	5.4	6.0	6.4	3.0	0.6	0.15	0.23	**2.3**	*201*
Non-Hodgkin lymphoma	328	1	2.9	2.2	4.7	1.4	1.4	3.4	2.2	6.3	8.8	11.8	13.7	18.2	31.4	34.2	56.8	48.7	84.4	70.0	12.8	2.7	0.54	1.00	**9.4**	*200,202*
Multiple myeloma	99	0	-	-	-	-	-	-	-	0.5	-	0.6	3.9	6.5	6.0	13.2	27.6	30.7	42.2	31.8	3.8	0.8	0.09	0.29	**2.4**	*203*
Lymphoid leukaemia	135	0	1.4	3.0	3.2	1.4	-	1.3	0.4	0.5	1.2	5.3	4.4	8.8	10.0	18.4	18.4	28.9	39.2	38.2	5.2	1.1	0.20	0.39	**4.0**	*204*
Myeloid leukaemia	160	0	1.4	-	-	-	0.9	1.3	2.7	3.4	4.7	5.3	5.9	8.2	10.0	21.9	32.2	32.5	36.2	38.2	6.2	1.3	0.22	0.49	**4.3**	*205*
Monocytic leukaemia	12	0	-	-	-	-	-	0.4	-	-	-	-	1.0	0.6	0.7	-	6.1	1.8	3.0	6.4	0.5	0.1	0.01	0.04	**0.3**	*206*
Other leukaemia	7	0	-	-	-	-	-	-	0.4	-	-	0.6	-	0.6	0.7	0.9	-	-	3.0	6.4	0.3	0.1	0.01	0.02	**0.2**	*207*
Leukaemia unspecified	16	0	-	-	-	-	-	-	0.4	-	-	0.6	-	-	-	2.6	4.6	3.6	9.0	19.1	0.6	0.1	0.01	0.04	**0.4**	*208*
Other and unspecified	595	0	-	-	-	0.7	0.5	-	1.3	3.9	7.6	9.5	17.6	40.0	57.4	80.7	98.2	147.9	229.2	311.8	23.1	4.8	0.69	1.59	**14.8**	*O&U*
All sites	14730	18	14.4	11.2	12.6	19.5	24.4	45.3	64.8	100.5	195.7	348.9	562.7	933.4	1397.1	2145.5	2944.2	3441.2	4085.6	4708.9	572.8		18.68	44.15	**377.4**	*ALL*
All sites but 173	12340	8	14.4	10.5	11.8	18.8	23.5	41.1	55.4	90.8	164.7	290.2	473.6	793.5	1194.8	1805.3	2397.8	2844.3	3395.1	3786.2	479.8	100.0	15.93	36.95	**316.6**	*ALLb*

Rate from 1 case   0.722   0.749   0.788   0.696   0.469   0.419   0.447   0.485   0.584   0.592   0.490   0.588   0.668   0.877   1.535   1.804   3.015   6.363

†Important: see notes on population page

+ GERMANY, SAARLAND 1988-1992

ANNUAL INCIDENCE PER 100,000 BY AGE GROUP (YEARS) - FEMALE

SITE	ALL AGES	AGE UNK	0-	5-	10-	15-	20-	25-	30-	35-	40-	45-	50-	55-	60-	65-	70-	75-	80-	85+	CRUDE RATE	%	CR 64	CR 74	ASR (W)	ICD (9th)
Lip	9	0	-	-	-	-	-	0.4	-	-	-	-	-	1.2	1.2	-	1.8	-	1.2	2.0	0.3	0.1	0.01	0.02	**0.2**	140
Tongue	29	0	-	-	-	-	-	-	-	-	-	3.0	1.0	1.7	1.2	0.6	4.4	2.5	4.6	7.9	1.0	0.2	0.03	0.06	**0.5**	141
Salivary gland	20	0	-	-	-	-	-	-	-	-	-	-	2.0	0.6	-	1.1	2.6	4.2	2.3	5.9	0.7	0.2	0.01	0.03	**0.3**	142
Mouth	50	0	-	-	-	0.7	-	-	-	0.5	2.5	2.4	3.9	2.3	4.0	3.4	2.6	5.0	5.8	2.0	1.8	0.4	0.08	0.11	**1.1**	143-5
Oropharynx	27	0	-	-	-	-	-	-	-	0.5	0.6	3.0	1.0	1.2	2.3	2.8	0.9	0.8	3.5	4.0	1.0	0.2	0.04	0.06	**0.6**	146
Nasopharynx	8	0	-	-	-	-	-	-	-	-	-	1.2	-	0.6	1.7	-	-	2.3	-	-	0.3	0.1	0.01	0.02	**0.2**	147
Hypopharynx	16	0	-	-	-	-	-	-	-	-	0.6	-	1.5	0.6	4.6	1.1	-	-	-	2.0	0.6	0.1	0.04	0.04	**0.4**	148
Pharynx unspecified	2	0	-	-	-	-	-	-	-	-	-	0.6	-	-	-	-	0.9	-	-	-	0.1	0.0	0.00	0.01	**0.1**	149
Oesophagus	53	0	-	-	-	-	-	-	-	0.5	-	-	1.5	4.1	4.0	2.3	7.9	5.9	7.0	17.8	1.9	0.4	0.05	0.10	**0.8**	150
Stomach	655	0	-	-	-	-	1.0	0.9	1.9	2.1	5.0	9.1	6.8	19.1	24.3	43.0	70.0	100.2	153.2	245.4	23.7	5.4	0.35	0.92	**9.0**	151
Small intestine	37	0	-	-	-	-	-	-	-	-	0.6	0.6	1.0	0.6	1.7	6.2	4.4	5.0	4.6	5.9	1.3	0.3	0.02	0.08	**0.6**	152
Colon	1385	0	-	1.6	0.8	-	1.5	3.1	1.0	3.1	13.8	12.7	30.8	40.6	83.2	97.4	155.9	202.8	298.3	387.9	50.1	11.4	0.96	2.23	**20.4**	153
Rectum	691	0	-	-	-	-	0.5	0.4	1.4	2.6	8.8	11.5	17.6	30.7	39.9	57.8	86.7	108.6	120.7	110.8	25.0	5.7	0.57	1.29	**10.9**	154
Liver	110	0	-	-	-	-	0.5	-	-	1.6	-	0.6	1.5	4.1	4.6	9.1	18.4	15.1	23.2	23.8	4.0	0.9	0.06	0.20	**1.6**	155
Gallbladder etc.	358	1	-	-	-	-	-	-	-	-	1.3	1.8	3.4	7.0	20.8	30.0	47.3	52.2	80.1	116.8	13.0	2.9	0.17	0.56	**4.8**	156
Pancreas	304	0	-	-	-	-	-	-	-	0.5	2.5	4.8	3.4	6.4	16.2	24.9	28.9	48.8	70.8	97.0	11.0	2.5	0.17	0.44	**4.2**	157
Nose, sinuses etc.	11	0	-	-	-	-	0.5	-	-	-	-	-	0.6	1.7	0.6	1.8	0.8	1.2	2.0	-	0.4	0.1	0.01	0.03	**0.2**	160
Larynx	33	0	-	-	-	-	-	0.4	-	0.5	1.9	2.4	0.5	1.7	2.3	4.0	3.5	2.5	1.2	2.0	1.2	0.3	0.05	0.09	**0.7**	161
Bronchus, lung	578	1	-	-	-	-	-	0.4	1.9	3.1	6.9	19.4	18.1	33.1	46.2	62.8	48.2	76.6	61.5	77.2	20.9	4.8	0.65	1.20	**10.3**	162
†Other thoracic organs	33	0	-	-	-	-	-	0.4	-	-	0.6	1.2	1.5	1.2	1.7	4.0	3.5	0.8	5.8	7.9	1.2	0.3	0.03	0.07	**0.6**	163-4
Bone	20	0	-	0.8	-	1.5	0.5	0.4	-	1.6	-	0.6	0.5	0.6	0.6	2.3	0.9	0.8	-	4.0	0.7	0.2	0.04	0.05	**0.6**	170
Connective tissue	66	0	2.3	0.8	0.8	0.7	0.5	0.9	1.4	1.6	3.1	-	2.4	2.9	4.0	6.8	6.1	1.7	7.0	4.0	2.4	0.5	0.11	0.17	**1.8**	171
†Mesothelioma																										
†Kaposi's sarcoma																										
Melanoma of skin	270	1	-	-	-	0.7	4.5	4.0	6.7	4.7	9.4	11.5	19.5	13.3	13.9	19.3	21.0	14.3	23.2	21.8	9.8	2.2	0.44	0.64	**6.1**	172
Other skin	2365	13	-	-	-	3.7	0.5	5.8	6.7	14.5	21.9	40.5	65.4	85.9	123.0	187.4	264.4	353.5	437.5	522.5	85.6		1.85	4.12	**36.9**	173
Breast	3031	1	-	-	-	0.7	1.5	4.0	21.6	57.4	100.7	147.0	148.4	181.6	195.3	244.6	284.6	273.5	289.0	338.4	109.7	24.9	4.29	6.94	**61.5**	174
Uterus unspecified	73	0	-	-	-	-	-	0.9	-	1.0	-	1.2	1.5	4.6	4.6	3.4	10.5	8.4	11.6	19.8	2.6	0.6	0.07	0.14	**1.2**	179
Cervix uteri	463	0	-	-	-	-	0.5	4.5	12.0	26.9	32.5	26.0	22.9	23.2	29.5	27.7	28.0	24.4	20.9	27.7	16.8	3.8	0.89	1.17	**11.4**	180
Placenta	6	0	-	-	-	-	-	0.9	1.0	0.5	0.6	-	-	-	-	-	-	-	-	-	0.2	0.0	0.01	0.01	**0.2**	181
Corpus uteri	729	0	-	-	-	-	-	-	-	1.0	7.5	11.5	26.9	48.2	54.9	80.4	97.2	90.1	80.1	67.3	26.4	6.0	0.75	1.64	**12.7**	182
Ovary etc.	514	0	-	-	-	2.2	0.5	1.8	2.9	4.7	6.3	13.3	20.5	33.6	32.9	56.1	58.7	44.6	49.9	79.2	18.6	4.2	0.59	1.17	**9.6**	183
Other female genital	144	0	-	-	-	-	-	-	2.4	0.5	0.6	1.2	3.9	4.6	4.6	9.1	21.0	21.0	25.5	47.5	5.2	1.2	0.09	0.24	**2.1**	184
Bladder	351	0	-	-	-	-	-	0.9	-	-	1.3	2.4	6.3	11.0	16.2	34.0	62.2	49.7	61.5	79.2	12.7	2.9	0.19	0.67	**5.2**	188
Kidney etc.	307	0	2.3	-	-	-	-	0.4	0.5	1.6	1.9	7.9	9.8	19.1	26.6	26.0	37.6	29.5	42.9	45.5	11.1	2.5	0.35	0.67	**5.6**	189
Eye	9	0	-	-	-	-	-	-	-	0.5	-	0.6	0.5	1.2	0.6	-	1.8	-	-	2.0	0.3	0.1	0.02	0.03	**0.2**	190
Brain, nervous system	191	0	4.6	4.8	1.7	0.7	2.0	4.5	1.4	5.2	8.8	5.4	7.3	10.4	13.9	18.1	12.3	13.5	8.1	-	6.9	1.6	0.35	0.51	**5.3**	191-2
Thyroid	155	0	-	-	-	1.5	2.0	2.2	3.4	6.2	3.1	7.9	7.3	5.8	12.1	9.1	7.9	13.5	9.3	23.8	5.6	1.3	0.26	0.34	**3.5**	193
Other endocrine	17	0	-	-	-	0.7	-	0.4	-	0.5	0.6	0.6	0.5	1.2	1.2	1.7	1.8	-	1.2	2.0	0.6	0.1	0.03	0.05	**0.4**	194
Hodgkin's disease	60	0	-	-	-	5.1	2.0	2.7	1.9	3.6	3.1	0.6	1.5	1.7	2.3	4.0	3.5	2.5	2.3	-	2.2	0.5	0.12	0.16	**1.9**	201
Non-Hodgkin lymphoma	303	1	2.3	-	0.8	-	3.0	1.3	3.4	2.6	5.6	7.9	10.7	15.7	17.9	24.3	27.1	39.6	42.9	33.6	11.0	2.5	0.36	0.62	**5.8**	200,202
Multiple myeloma	129	0	-	-	-	-	-	-	-	-	0.6	1.8	2.0	4.6	10.4	16.4	12.3	18.5	22.1	21.8	4.7	1.1	0.10	0.24	**2.0**	203
Lymphoid leukaemia	112	0	2.3	0.8	3.3	1.5	0.5	0.4	1.0	-	0.6	1.2	3.4	5.2	9.2	7.4	14.9	9.3	15.1	17.8	4.1	0.9	0.15	0.26	**2.6**	204
Myeloid leukaemia	124	0	0.8	-	0.8	1.5	0.5	1.8	1.9	1.0	3.1	5.4	3.4	4.1	6.9	5.7	11.4	17.7	20.9	13.9	4.5	1.0	0.16	0.24	**2.5**	205
Monocytic leukaemia	6	0	-	-	-	-	0.5	-	-	-	-	-	-	-	-	-	-	1.7	3.5	-	0.2	0.0	0.00	0.00	**0.1**	206
Other leukaemia	12	0	-	-	-	-	-	-	-	0.5	-	-	0.5	-	1.7	0.6	-	-	5.8	2.0	0.4	0.1	0.01	0.02	**0.2**	207
Leukaemia unspecified	34	0	0.8	-	-	-	-	-	-	-	-	-	-	0.6	1.2	0.6	6.1	5.9	7.0	17.8	1.2	0.3	0.01	0.05	**0.5**	208
Other and unspecified	616	1	-	-	-	-	1.0	0.9	1.0	0.5	5.6	9.7	9.8	18.6	26.0	40.8	62.2	98.5	125.3	233.5	22.3	5.1	0.37	0.88	**8.7**	O&U
All sites	14516	19	15.4	8.8	8.3	21.2	23.8	45.0	75.2	151.4	262.0	378.6	470.2	654.4	870.0	1178.3	1542.8	1764.1	2159.8	2743.2	525.3		14.94	28.56	**256.1**	ALL
All sites but 173	12151	6	15.4	8.8	8.3	17.5	23.3	39.2	68.5	136.9	240.1	338.1	404.8	568.6	746.9	990.8	1278.3	1410.6	1722.3	2220.7	439.7	100.0	13.09	24.44	**219.1**	ALLb

Rate from 1 case   0.769   0.796   0.825   0.731   0.497   0.446   0.479   0.517   0.625   0.605   0.488   0.580   0.578   0.566   0.876   0.842   1.161   1.979

†Important: see notes on population page

Iceland

The Icelandic Cancer Registry is population-based and covers the entire population of Iceland. It was founded in 1954, in order to conduct epidemiological research on cancer and facilitate such research, as well as to produce information to assist public health officials in planning both for prevention and treatment of cancer.

The Icelandic Cancer Society runs the registry and has done so from the beginning. In recent years the Society has received a subsidy for this purpose from the Icelandic government, in 1992 amounting to 15% of the cost of running the registry.

The area covered by the registry and the population is that of Iceland, which is an island in the north Atlantic situated between latitudes 64 and 68° N and longitudes 14 and 24° W. The total area is 103 000 km^2.

The population in 1990 was 127 895 males and 126 893 females. The population is Caucasian and the principal religion is Lutheran. Over half of the population lives in and around the capital Reykjavik, which is situated in the southwest of the island. Primary care medical facilities are spread around the country and the system is that of family practices. The principal treating hospitals for malignant diseases are in Reykjavik where all radiotherapy equipment is located, but surgery for malignant diseases is also performed in smaller hospitals in other parts of the country.

The sources of data for cancer registration are pathology and haematology laboratories, all hospital departments and health care stations. Registrations are also received from the practising specialists. All death certificates are seen by the cancer registry. Incomplete information is followed up by contact with the aforementioned institutions.

Registration is voluntary. The registry personnel do not make direct contact with patients but search for follow-up information from the reporting institutions and individuals.

Data are classified according to ICD and ICD-O. The principal classifications are ICD-7 and ICD-O-2 but tables can be produced in other classifications such as other ICD revisions and special classifications for childhood tumours. The data are published annually by the registry and regularly in *Cancer Incidence in Five Continents*, as well as in collaboration with the other Nordic cancer registries.

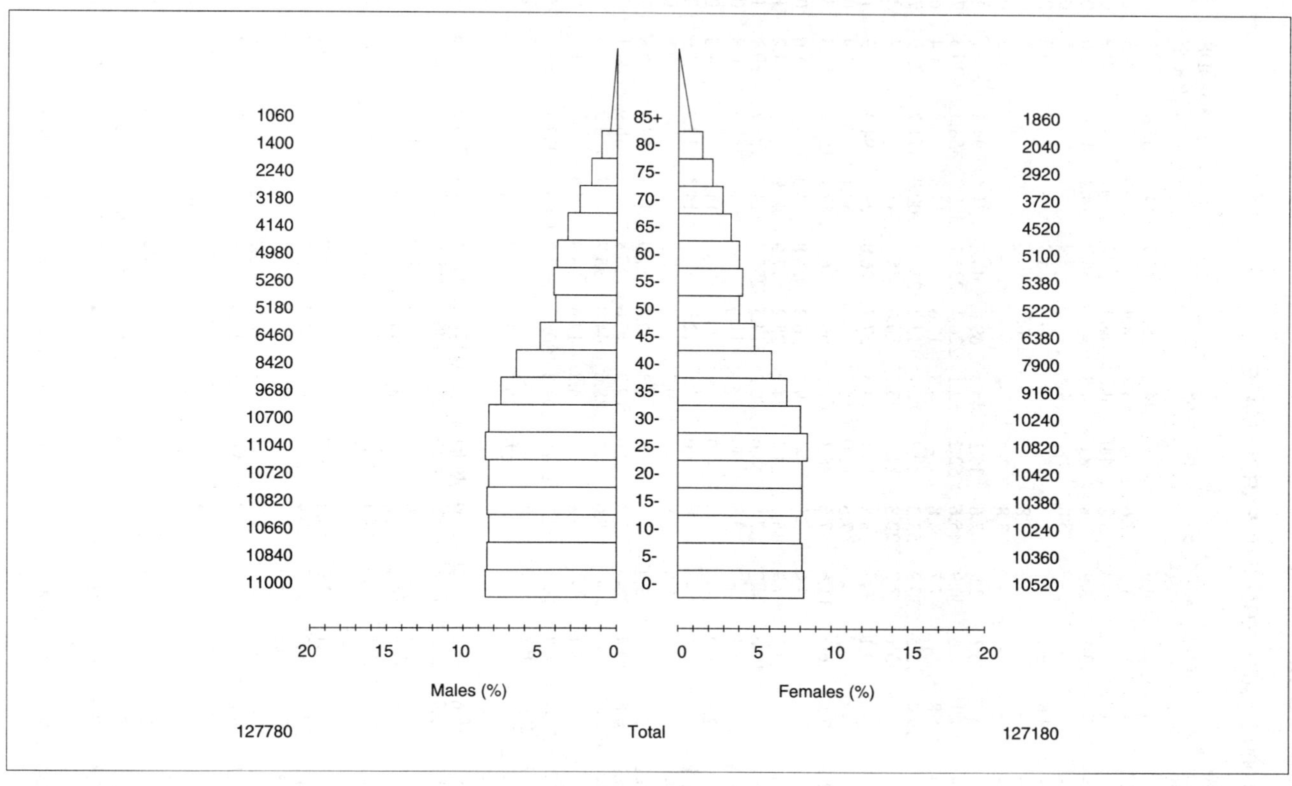

Iceland

Source of population: average annual 1988–92

The population-at-risk derives from the Icelandic National Roster, in operation since 1952 and regularly updated for births, deaths and migration.

Notes to tables overleaf:

† 173 does not include basal cell carcinoma

† 188 does not include non-invasive tumours

Screening programmes in the area

The population aged 20-69 has been screened for cervical cancer every two years since 1964.

Women between 40 and 69 have been screened for breast cancer by palpation every two years since 1973, with subsequent referral for mammography if indicated.

ICELAND 1988-1992

ANNUAL INCIDENCE PER 100,000 BY AGE GROUP (YEARS) - MALE

SITE	ALL AGES	AGE UNK	0-	5-	10-	15-	20-	25-	30-	35-	40-	45-	50-	55-	60-	65-	70-	75-	80-	85+	CRUDE RATE	%	CR 64	CR 74	ASR (W)	ICD (9th)
Lip	16	0	-	-	-	-	-	-	-	-	-	-	3.9	-	-	24.2	25.2	17.9	14.3	56.6	2.5	0.7	0.02	0.27	**2.0**	140
Tongue	8	0	-	-	-	-	-	-	-	2.1	-	-	3.9	7.6	-	4.8	18.9	-	-	-	1.3	0.4	0.07	0.19	**1.1**	141
Salivary gland	6	0	-	-	-	-	1.8	-	-	-	-	-	-	3.8	4.0	4.8	6.3	-	-	18.9	0.9	0.3	0.05	0.10	**0.8**	142
Mouth	13	0	-	-	-	1.8	-	-	-	-	-	3.1	3.9	3.8	8.0	4.8	-	35.7	14.3	18.9	2.0	0.6	0.10	0.13	**1.7**	143-5
Oropharynx	3	0	-	-	-	-	-	-	-	-	-	-	-	3.8	-	4.8	-	8.9	-	-	0.5	0.1	0.02	0.04	**0.4**	146
Nasopharynx	4	0	-	-	-	-	-	-	-	-	4.8	3.1	-	-	-	-	-	8.9	-	-	0.6	0.2	0.04	0.04	**0.6**	147
Hypopharynx	2	0	-	-	-	-	-	-	-	-	-	-	-	3.8	-	-	6.3	-	-	-	0.3	0.1	0.02	0.05	**0.3**	148
Pharynx unspecified	1	0	-	-	-	-	-	-	-	-	-	-	-	3.8	-	-	-	-	-	-	0.2	0.0	0.02	0.02	**0.2**	149
Oesophagus	49	0	-	-	-	-	-	-	-	-	-	3.1	3.9	7.6	36.1	48.3	69.2	44.6	71.4	94.3	7.7	2.3	0.25	0.84	**6.2**	150
Stomach	168	0	-	-	-	1.9	-	-	-	-	7.1	18.6	30.9	45.6	52.2	82.1	226.4	232.1	385.7	358.5	26.3	7.9	0.78	2.32	**20.2**	151
Small intestine	9	0	-	-	-	-	-	-	-	-	4.8	-	7.7	3.8	-	4.8	12.6	-	14.3	-	1.4	0.4	0.08	0.17	**1.3**	152
Colon	153	0	-	-	-	-	-	-	-	-	19.0	15.5	30.9	53.2	80.3	82.1	113.2	214.3	200.0	471.7	23.9	7.2	0.99	1.97	**19.2**	153
Rectum	47	0	-	-	-	-	-	-	-	-	-	3.1	7.7	22.8	24.1	43.5	56.6	35.7	42.9	132.1	7.4	2.2	0.29	0.79	**6.1**	154
Liver	25	0	-	-	-	-	-	-	-	-	-	3.1	-	3.8	16.1	14.5	37.7	26.8	28.6	94.3	3.9	1.2	0.11	0.38	**3.1**	155
Gallbladder etc.	12	0	-	-	-	-	-	-	-	-	-	-	-	7.6	12.0	14.5	-	57.1	-	-	1.9	0.6	0.10	0.17	**1.5**	156
Pancreas	66	0	-	-	-	-	-	1.8	1.9	2.1	2.4	6.2	11.6	7.6	28.1	67.6	56.6	116.1	57.1	150.9	10.3	3.1	0.31	0.93	**8.3**	157
Nose, sinuses etc.	10	0	-	-	-	-	-	-	-	-	2.4	-	3.9	-	-	9.7	6.3	26.8	14.3	18.9	1.6	0.5	0.03	0.11	**1.2**	160
Larynx	27	0	-	-	-	-	-	-	-	-	-	3.1	7.7	15.2	24.1	24.2	25.2	17.9	42.9	-	4.2	1.3	0.25	0.50	**3.8**	161
Bronchus, lung	250	0	-	-	-	-	-	-	-	4.1	2.4	18.6	34.7	87.5	148.6	280.2	314.5	285.7	314.3	188.7	39.1	11.7	1.48	4.45	**32.8**	162
Other thoracic organs	5	0	-	-	-	-	1.9	-	-	-	-	3.1	-	3.8	-	-	12.6	-	-	-	0.8	0.2	0.04	0.11	**0.7**	163-4
Bone	8	0	-	-	3.8	1.8	-	-	-	-	2.4	6.2	-	-	4.0	-	-	-	14.3	-	1.3	0.4	0.09	0.09	**1.3**	170
Connective tissue	12	0	3.6	-	-	-	-	-	3.7	2.1	-	-	-	-	8.0	4.8	12.6	-	14.3	18.9	1.9	0.6	0.09	0.17	**1.7**	171
Mesothelioma	5	0	-	-	-	-	-	-	-	-	-	-	3.9	3.8	-	9.7	-	8.9	-	-	0.8	0.2	0.04	0.09	**0.7**	MES
Kaposi's sarcoma	18	0	-	-	-	-	-	-	-	-	6.2	2.4	-	3.9	-	8.0	4.8	12.6	17.9	14.3	94.3	2.8	0.8	0.10	0.19	**2.1**	KAP
Melanoma of skin	26	0	-	-	1.9	-	-	1.8	1.9	6.2	4.8	12.4	-	3.8	12.0	19.3	12.6	26.8	-	18.9	4.1	1.2	0.22	0.38	**3.7**	172
†Other skin	40	0	-	1.8	-	3.7	1.8	-	-	-	-	-	7.6	16.1	38.6	44.0	35.7	71.4	113.2	6.3	0.16	0.57	**4.9**	173
Breast	7	0	-	-	-	-	-	-	-	-	-	3.1	-	3.8	-	4.8	12.6	8.9	14.3	-	1.1	0.3	0.03	0.12	**0.9**	175
Prostate	529	0	-	-	-	-	-	-	-	-	-	9.3	19.3	72.2	216.9	391.3	805.0	892.9	1200.0	1037.7	82.8	24.7	1.59	7.57	**61.0**	185
Testis	46	0	-	-	1.9	5.5	5.6	14.5	24.3	6.2	26.1	6.2	3.9	3.8	-	-	-	-	-	-	7.2	2.2	0.49	0.49	**6.4**	186
Penis	9	0	-	-	-	-	-	1.8	-	-	-	-	-	4.0	9.7	6.3	17.9	14.3	18.9	1.4	0.4	0.03	0.11	**1.1**	187.1-.4
Other male genital	0	0	-	-	-	-	-	-	-	-	-	-	-	-	-	-	-	-	-	-	0.0	0.0	0.00	0.00	**0.0**	187.5-.9
†Bladder	151	0	-	-	-	-	-	-	2.1	16.6	6.2	23.2	38.0	104.4	91.8	132.1	232.1	271.4	264.2	23.6	7.1	0.95	2.07	**18.7**	188
Kidney etc.	118	0	-	-	-	-	-	-	2.1	11.9	15.5	15.4	34.2	64.3	53.1	100.6	169.6	285.7	226.4	18.5	5.5	0.72	1.49	**14.3**	189
Eye	7	0	-	-	-	-	-	-	-	-	3.1	-	7.6	4.0	-	6.3	8.9	-	18.9	1.1	0.3	0.07	0.11	**1.0**	190
Brain, nervous system	63	0	3.6	1.8	7.5	1.8	3.7	1.8	3.7	12.4	9.5	21.7	15.4	26.6	20.1	24.2	37.7	17.9	42.9	18.9	9.9	2.9	0.65	0.96	**9.4**	191-2
Thyroid	44	0	-	-	-	-	3.7	1.8	1.9	2.1	7.1	15.5	11.6	11.4	24.1	14.5	31.4	53.6	28.6	56.6	6.9	2.1	0.40	0.63	**6.1**	193
Other endocrine	2	0	-	-	1.9	1.8	-	-	-	-	-	-	-	-	-	-	-	-	-	-	0.3	0.1	0.02	0.02	**0.3**	194
Hodgkin's disease	20	0	-	1.8	1.9	5.5	3.7	7.2	1.9	-	-	3.1	3.9	15.2	4.0	-	-	8.9	-	-	3.1	0.9	0.24	0.24	**3.1**	201
Non-Hodgkin lymphoma	62	0	-	-	-	-	-	1.8	3.7	4.1	9.5	6.2	34.7	30.4	28.1	29.0	37.7	53.6	71.4	75.5	9.7	2.9	0.59	0.93	**8.5**	200,202
Multiple myeloma	27	0	-	-	-	-	-	-	-	-	7.1	6.2	3.9	11.4	24.1	9.7	31.4	-	71.4	-	4.2	1.3	0.26	0.47	**3.7**	203
Lymphoid leukaemia	18	0	3.6	3.7	-	3.7	-	-	-	2.1	-	3.1	-	-	-	4.8	18.9	35.7	28.6	-	2.8	0.8	0.08	0.20	**2.5**	204
Myeloid leukaemia	22	0	1.8	-	1.9	1.8	-	3.6	-	2.1	4.8	-	3.9	3.8	4.0	4.8	12.6	26.8	42.9	37.7	3.4	1.0	0.14	0.23	**2.8**	205
Monocytic leukaemia	1	0	-	-	-	-	-	-	-	-	-	-	-	3.9	-	-	-	-	-	-	0.2	0.0	0.02	0.02	**0.2**	206
Other leukaemia	2	0	-	-	-	-	-	-	-	-	-	-	-	-	3.8	-	-	-	14.3	-	0.3	0.1	0.02	0.02	**0.2**	207
Leukaemia unspecified	2	0	-	-	-	-	-	-	-	-	2.4	-	-	-	-	-	-	-	-	18.9	0.3	0.1	0.01	0.01	**0.2**	208
Other and unspecified	66	0	-	-	-	-	-	-	1.9	-	2.4	3.1	15.4	22.8	32.1	19.3	62.9	71.4	157.1	226.4	10.3	3.1	0.39	0.80	**7.9**	O&U
All sites	2179	0	12.7	9.2	20.6	24.0	24.3	39.9	44.9	55.8	149.6	201.2	312.7	585.6	1012.0	1449.3	2364.8	2758.9	3614.3	3849.1	341.1		12.46	31.53	**273.9**	ALL
All sites but 173	2139	0	12.7	7.4	20.6	24.0	20.5	38.0	44.9	55.8	149.6	201.2	312.7	577.9	996.0	1410.6	2320.8	2723.2	3542.9	3735.8	334.8	100.0	12.31	30.96	**269.0**	ALLb

Rate from 1 case   1.818   1.845   1.876   1.848   1.866   1.812   1.869   2.066   2.375   3.096   3.861   3.802   4.016   4.831   6.289   8.929   14.286   18.868

†Important: see notes on population page

ICELAND 1988-1992

ANNUAL INCIDENCE PER 100,000 BY AGE GROUP (YEARS) - FEMALE

SITE	ALL AGES	AGE UNK	0-	5-	10-	15-	20-	25-	30-	35-	40-	45-	50-	55-	60-	65-	70-	75-	80-	85+	CRUDE RATE	%	CR 64	CR 74	ASR (W)	ICD (9th)
Lip	2	0	-	-	-	-	-	-	-	-	-	-	-	-	-	4.4	-	-	9.8	-	0.3	0.1	0.00	0.02	**0.2**	*140*
Tongue	5	0	-	-	-	-	-	-	-	-	-	-	-	-	3.9	4.4	5.4	-	19.6	-	0.8	0.3	0.02	0.07	**0.5**	*141*
Salivary gland	3	0	-	-	-	-	-	-	-	-	3.1	-	-	-	3.9	-	-	6.8	-	-	0.5	0.2	0.04	0.04	**0.4**	*142*
Mouth	12	0	-	-	-	-	-	-	-	-	-	-	3.8	7.4	-	13.3	5.4	20.5	9.8	10.8	1.9	0.6	0.06	0.15	**1.3**	*143-5*
Oropharynx	2	0	-	-	-	-	-	-	-	-	2.5	-	-	-	-	-	5.4	-	-	-	0.3	0.1	0.01	0.04	**0.3**	*146*
Nasopharynx	1	0	-	-	-	-	-	-	-	-	3.7	-	-	-	-	-	-	-	-	-	0.2	0.1	0.02	0.02	**0.1**	*147*
Hypopharynx	0	0	-	-	-	-	-	-	-	-	-	-	-	-	-	-	-	-	-	-	0.0	0.0	0.00	0.00	**0.0**	*148*
Pharynx unspecified	0	0	-	-	-	-	-	-	-	-	-	-	-	-	-	-	-	-	-	-	0.0	0.0	0.00	0.00	**0.0**	*149*
Oesophagus	21	0	-	-	-	-	-	-	-	-	-	3.1	3.8	-	7.8	4.4	32.3	27.4	29.4	32.3	3.3	1.1	0.07	0.26	**2.1**	*150*
Stomach	101	0	-	-	-	-	-	2.2	2.5	15.7	11.5	18.6	51.0	53.1	80.6	116.4	137.3	161.3	15.9	5.1	0.51	1.18	**10.4**	*151*
Small intestine	6	0	-	-	-	-	-	-	-	-	-	-	3.7	3.9	4.4	5.4	6.8	-	10.8	0.9	0.3	0.04	0.09	**0.7**	*152*
Colon	146	0	-	-	-	1.9	-	5.5	-	-	2.5	12.5	26.8	44.6	51.0	106.2	96.8	143.8	176.5	258.1	23.0	7.4	0.72	1.74	**15.4**	*153*
Rectum	55	0	-	-	-	-	-	1.8	-	-	2.5	-	3.8	22.3	27.5	31.0	32.3	75.3	98.0	53.8	8.6	2.8	0.29	0.61	**5.6**	*154*
Liver	9	0	-	-	-	-	-	-	-	-	6.3	-	-	3.9	4.4	10.8	-	9.8	21.5	1.4	0.5	0.05	0.13	**1.0**	*155*
Gallbladder etc.	16	0	-	-	-	-	-	-	-	-	3.1	3.8	-	-	4.4	16.1	20.5	39.2	32.3	2.5	0.8	0.03	0.14	**1.4**	*156*
Pancreas	61	0	-	-	-	-	-	-	4.4	2.5	-	3.8	26.0	35.3	31.0	32.3	68.5	78.4	107.5	9.6	3.1	0.36	0.68	**6.2**	*157*
Nose, sinuses etc.	4	0	-	-	-	-	-	-	-	-	-	3.8	11.2	-	-	-	-	-	-	0.6	0.2	0.07	0.07	**0.6**	*160*
Larynx	2	0	-	-	-	-	-	-	-	-	-	-	-	-	4.4	-	6.8	-	-	0.3	0.1	0.00	0.02	**0.2**	*161*
Bronchus, lung	213	0	-	-	-	-	1.8	2.0	6.6	7.6	28.2	84.3	104.1	105.9	146.0	150.5	226.0	127.5	129.0	33.5	10.8	1.70	3.18	**26.4**	*162*
Other thoracic organs	2	0	-	-	-	-	-	-	-	-	-	-	-	3.9	4.4	-	-	-	-	0.3	0.1	0.02	0.04	**0.3**	*163-4*
Bone	3	0	-	-	-	-	-	-	-	-	3.1	-	-	-	8.8	-	-	-	-	0.5	0.2	0.02	0.06	**0.5**	*170*
Connective tissue	9	0	-	-	-	1.9	-	-	-	5.1	3.1	-	-	-	4.4	-	6.8	19.6	10.8	1.4	0.5	0.05	0.07	**1.0**	*171*
Mesothelioma	0	0	-	-	-	-	-	-	-	-	-	-	-	-	-	-	-	-	-	0.0	0.0	0.00	0.00	**0.0**	*MES*
Kaposi's sarcoma	10	0	-	-	-	-	-	-	-	-	-	-	-	-	-	5.4	6.8	29.4	53.8	1.6	0.5	0.00	0.03	**0.6**	*KAP*
Melanoma of skin	53	0	-	-	-	-	1.8	-	10.9	15.2	18.8	23.0	7.4	35.3	13.3	16.1	47.9	29.4	21.5	8.3	2.7	0.56	0.71	**7.2**	*172*
†Other skin	45	0	-	-	-	-	-	2.0	2.2	2.5	9.4	7.7	14.9	3.9	4.4	32.3	41.1	49.0	150.5	7.1		0.21	0.40	**4.3**	*173*
Breast	576	0	-	-	-	-	5.5	9.8	59.0	144.3	175.5	249.0	252.8	305.9	323.0	258.1	253.4	294.1	311.8	90.6	29.2	6.01	8.91	**79.0**	*174*
Uterus unspecified	2	0	-	-	-	-	-	-	-	-	-	-	-	3.9	-	-	-	-	10.8	0.3	0.1	0.02	0.02	**0.2**	*179*
Cervix uteri	58	0	-	-	-	-	1.9	18.5	5.9	15.3	20.3	12.5	7.7	14.9	23.5	22.1	10.8	20.5	19.6	10.8	9.1	2.9	0.60	0.77	**8.0**	*180*
Placenta	0	0	-	-	-	-	-	-	-	-	-	-	-	-	-	-	-	-	-	0.0	0.0	0.00	0.00	**0.0**	*181*
Corpus uteri	105	0	-	-	-	-	-	-	6.6	-	34.5	38.3	59.5	78.4	75.2	69.9	47.9	58.8	21.5	16.5	5.3	1.09	1.81	**14.4**	*182*
Ovary etc.	89	0	-	-	-	1.9	-	2.0	2.2	7.6	12.5	38.3	29.7	70.6	35.4	32.3	82.2	78.4	96.8	14.0	4.5	0.82	1.16	**10.9**	*183*
Other female genital	14	0	-	-	-	-	-	-	-	-	6.3	3.8	-	11.8	4.4	10.8	6.8	19.6	21.5	2.2	0.7	0.11	0.19	**1.7**	*184*
†Bladder	45	0	-	-	-	1.9	-	-	2.2	-	-	7.7	11.2	35.3	31.0	32.3	47.9	58.8	32.3	7.1	2.3	0.29	0.61	**5.0**	*188*
Kidney etc.	66	0	-	-	-	1.9	-	-	-	7.6	6.3	19.2	26.0	31.4	57.5	48.4	82.2	19.6	43.0	10.4	3.4	0.46	0.99	**8.1**	*189*
Eye	3	0	3.8	-	-	-	-	-	2.0	2.2	5.1	9.4	3.8	22.3	3.9	26.5	-	-	10.8	0.5	0.2	0.02	0.02	**0.5**	*190*
Brain, nervous system	29	0	-	-	-	-	-	-	2.0	2.2	5.1	9.4	3.8	22.3	3.9	26.5	32.3	13.7	-	4.6	1.5	0.24	0.54	**3.9**	*191-2*
Thyroid	75	0	-	-	-	3.9	-	12.9	15.6	13.1	15.2	15.7	30.7	22.3	11.8	17.7	32.3	20.5	49.0	64.5	11.8	3.8	0.71	0.96	**9.8**	*193*
Other endocrine	5	0	1.9	-	2.0	-	-	-	-	-	-	-	3.8	-	3.9	4.4	-	-	-	0.8	0.3	0.06	0.08	**0.9**	*194*
Hodgkin's disease	8	0	-	-	-	1.9	1.9	1.8	5.9	-	-	3.1	-	-	3.9	-	-	-	-	1.3	0.4	0.09	0.09	**1.2**	*201*
Non-Hodgkin lymphoma	40	0	-	-	-	-	1.9	1.8	2.0	4.4	5.1	12.5	3.8	7.4	15.7	17.7	26.9	41.1	39.2	32.3	6.3	2.0	0.27	0.50	**4.7**	*200,202*
Multiple myeloma	20	0	-	-	-	-	-	-	-	-	2.5	3.1	3.8	3.7	19.6	8.8	5.4	20.5	19.6	32.3	3.1	1.0	0.16	0.24	**2.3**	*203*
Lymphoid leukaemia	16	0	3.8	1.9	2.0	-	-	-	-	-	2.5	-	3.8	3.7	3.9	8.8	10.8	-	-	43.0	2.5	0.8	0.11	0.21	**2.2**	*204*
Myeloid leukaemia	13	0	3.8	1.9	-	-	-	1.8	-	2.2	2.5	-	7.7	-	3.9	4.4	16.1	-	-	-	2.0	0.7	0.12	0.22	**2.1**	*205*
Monocytic leukaemia	0	0	-	-	-	-	-	-	-	-	-	-	-	-	-	-	-	-	-	0.0	0.0	0.00	0.00	**0.0**	*206*
Other leukaemia	2	0	-	-	-	-	-	-	-	-	-	-	-	-	-	-	6.8	-	10.8	0.3	0.1	0.00	0.00	**0.1**	*207*
Leukaemia unspecified	4	0	1.9	-	-	-	-	-	-	-	2.5	3.1	-	-	-	-	5.4	-	-	0.6	0.2	0.04	0.06	**0.7**	*208*
Other and unspecified	64	0	-	-	-	-	-	2.0	-	5.1	3.1	7.7	14.9	31.4	26.5	59.1	47.9	68.6	161.3	10.1	3.2	0.32	0.75	**6.5**	*O&U*
All sites	2015	0	15.2	3.9	3.9	7.7	13.4	53.6	48.8	133.2	263.3	404.4	605.4	732.3	996.1	1110.6	1177.4	1513.7	1588.2	1957.0	316.9		16.41	27.85	**248.7**	*ALL*
All sites but 173	1970	0	15.2	3.9	3.9	7.7	13.4	53.6	46.9	131.0	260.8	395.0	597.7	717.5	992.2	1106.2	1145.2	1472.6	1539.2	1806.5	309.8	100.0	16.19	27.45	**244.5**	*ALLb*

Rate from 1 case   1.901 1.931 1.953 1.927 1.919 1.848 1.953 2.183 2.532 3.135 3.831 3.717 3.922 4.425 5.376 6.849 9.804 10.753

†Important: see notes on population page

517

Ireland, Southern

The Southern Tumour Registry, founded in 1975, was the first cancer registry in the Republic of Ireland. This regional registry provided comprehensive population coverage from 1977 to 1991. In 1991 the Irish National Cancer Registry was set up by the Department of Health to provide population-based statistics for the entire country, and took over the functions and staff of the Southern Tumour Registry in November 1991, extending its coverage to the rest of the country in 1994.

The registry is administered by the National Cancer Registry Board, whose members are predominantly medical; University College, Cork, the Department of Health and the Irish Cancer Society are also represented. The national registry operates by active data collection, with 16 registration officers based throughout the country making regular returns of data to the central registry.

The data presented here apply to the area of the former Southern Tumour Registry, counties Cork and Kerry in the south-west of Ireland. The area covered, lying between latitudes 51°30′ and 52°35′ N and longitudes 7°50′ and 10°30′ W (12 155 km^2) is predominantly rural and has a long Atlantic coastline. The population at the 1991 census was 532 263 persons (43.8 per km^2). The one major urban centre, Cork city, has a population of 127 253, and a further 47 147 living in the suburbs. Only one other town has a population over 10 000. The west and south of the region is hilly and sparsely populated (density under 20 per km^2). 48% of the population lives in areas designated as rural (fewer than 1500 inhabitants). The climate is oceanic temperate with average temperatures of 6°C in winter and 15°C in summer. Typical annual rainfall ranges from 3000 mm in the west to 1000 mm in the east. The area is relatively free from environmental pollution. The lower Cork harbour area has a number of chemical and pharmaceutical plants.

The population is ethnically quite homogeneous and 95% Roman Catholic; 74% are over 15 years of age. 32% of the population was employed in 1991. The main areas of employment were: production industries, 22%; commerce, insurance, finance and business services, 19%; agriculture, fishery and forestry, 16%; professional services, 16%; building and construction, 8%; public administration, 6%; transport, communications and storage, 5%.

Cancers arising in Irish residents in the UK are reported by the UK registries, but recent Irish emigrants to the UK usually give UK addresses and so their cancers may not be reported to us.

The main treatment centre is Cork University Hospital (534 beds), which contains the regional radiotherapy service, with two full-time radiotherapist/oncologists. There is one medical oncologist in private practice in the region, but none in the public service. Oncology services are provided by surgical, radiotherapy and haematology consultants. A small number of patients (3%) have cancer treatment outside the area. There are no organized cancer screening programmes in the area.

Most notifications come from pathology services, which make copies of all reports of malignant disease available to the registry. Registry staff regularly examine outpatient records from the radiotherapy and haematology clinics. Some cases are also discovered from the computerized hospital inpatient diagnosis codes in all public hospitals. Registry staff have full access to medical records of hospital patients within the region. The registry also receives copies of death certificates of all patients dying of cancer in the region, and follows these up with local hospitals and general practitioners. Patients diagnosed or treated outside the area are reported to the registry from the hospital inpatient enquiry data.

Cancer registration is not legally or administratively mandatory, but the registry has the full co-operation of all medical personnel in the region. Three trained members of registry staff carry out active registration, using the sources listed above. Patients are not followed up except through death certificates.

Data were coded in ICD-O-1 in the period to which this report applies. The data are entered into a database at the registry and checked for duplication by use of the patients' names and variables such as date of birth, hospital medical record number and address. Consistency checks are run to identify unusual site/histology/age combinations, and all registrations of patients under 15 are examined individually. Second or subsequent tumours arising in the same person are treated as duplicates if this was the opinion of the consultant or pathologist, except that for skin cancers, only one melanoma, one squamous and one basal cell carcinoma are registered for each individual per lifetime.

Death certificates reporting cases not previously registered are followed up with the certifying doctor. If no supporting data are obtained, the death is not registered as a cancer case. These have amounted to 40 (2%) cases per year on average. The level of death certificate notification is 6%, but higher (8%) in Kerry. As the rate of incidence of many cancers appears lower in Kerry, this may represent a slightly lower level of ascertainment.

The data are presented in an annual report of cancer incidence. This report has also been used to examine time trends in cancer incidence and also in national cancer mortality. A volume *Cancer:the Irish experience* has been published, summarizing the data from 1977 to 1990, and looking at time trends, survival and geographical variation in incidence. The data have been widely used to extrapolate to national figures for planning purposes.

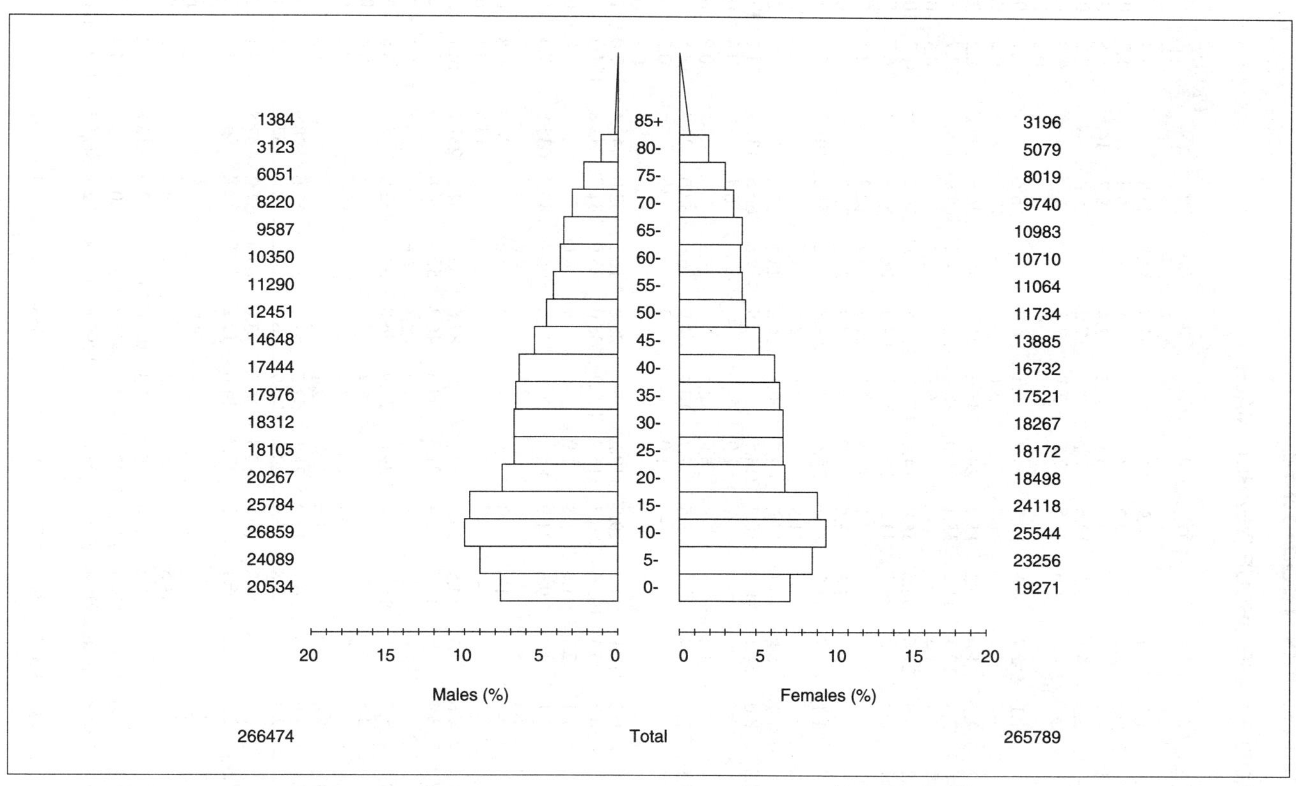

Ireland, Southern
Source of population: average annual 1988–92
Census: Census 86, Volume 2, Central Statistics Office, Ireland. Census 91, Volume 2, Central Statistics Office, Ireland.
Estimate: Linear interpolation/extrapolation

IRELAND, SOUTHERN 1988-1992

ANNUAL INCIDENCE PER 100,000 BY AGE GROUP (YEARS) - MALE

SITE	ALL AGES	AGE UNK	0-	5-	10-	15-	20-	25-	30-	35-	40-	45-	50-	55-	60-	65-	70-	75-	80-	85+	CRUDE RATE	%	CR 64	CR 74	ASR (W)	ICD (9th)
Lip	57	0	-	-	-	-	-	-	-	-	1.1	1.4	9.6	8.9	11.6	16.7	31.6	33.1	44.8	-	4.3	1.4	0.16	0.40	**3.1**	140
Tongue	22	0	-	-	-	-	-	1.1	-	-	-	2.7	4.8	3.5	7.7	6.3	7.3	9.9	6.4	-	1.7	0.5	0.10	0.17	**1.4**	141
Salivary gland	20	0	-	-	-	0.8	-	-	-	1.1	-	4.1	-	5.3	5.8	4.2	2.4	6.6	19.2	14.5	1.5	0.5	0.09	0.12	**1.2**	142
Mouth	36	0	-	-	-	-	-	-	-	-	2.3	4.1	9.6	10.6	7.7	8.3	17.0	3.3	19.2	-	2.7	0.9	0.17	0.30	**2.3**	143-5
Oropharynx	13	0	-	-	-	-	-	-	-	-	-	2.7	1.6	3.5	7.7	2.1	7.3	-	-	-	1.0	0.3	0.08	0.12	**0.9**	146
Nasopharynx	3	0	-	-	-	0.8	-	-	-	-	-	1.4	-	1.8	-	-	-	-	-	-	0.2	0.1	0.02	0.02	**0.2**	147
Hypopharynx	14	0	-	-	-	-	-	-	-	-	1.1	2.7	1.6	3.5	3.9	6.3	4.9	-	6.4	-	1.1	0.3	0.06	0.12	**0.9**	148
Pharynx unspecified	3	0	-	-	-	-	-	-	-	-	-	-	-	1.8	-	2.1	-	-	-	14.5	0.2	0.1	0.01	0.02	**0.2**	149
Oesophagus	109	0	-	-	-	-	-	-	-	1.1	2.3	1.4	19.3	15.9	29.0	45.9	41.4	36.4	76.8	101.2	8.2	2.6	0.34	0.78	**6.5**	150
Stomach	236	0	-	-	-	-	-	-	1.1	-	2.3	12.3	11.2	35.4	56.0	98.0	131.4	132.2	108.9	144.5	17.7	5.7	0.59	1.74	**13.3**	151
Small intestine	6	0	-	-	-	-	-	-	-	1.1	-	1.4	-	-	-	6.3	-	3.3	-	-	0.5	0.1	0.01	0.04	**0.4**	152
Colon	423	0	-	-	-	-	-	-	-	2.2	8.0	24.6	38.6	54.9	114.0	152.3	177.6	257.8	230.5	317.9	31.7	10.2	1.21	2.86	**24.2**	153
Rectum	222	0	-	-	-	-	-	1.1	-	1.1	6.9	8.2	24.1	44.3	59.9	85.5	104.6	112.4	83.3	86.7	16.7	5.4	0.73	1.68	**13.1**	154
Liver	28	0	1.0	-	-	-	-	-	-	-	-	-	-	7.1	13.5	2.1	21.9	13.2	12.8	-	2.1	0.7	0.11	0.23	**1.6**	155
Gallbladder etc.	34	0	-	-	-	-	-	-	-	2.2	-	-	1.6	3.5	7.7	4.2	24.3	23.1	32.0	14.5	2.6	0.8	0.08	0.22	**1.7**	156
Pancreas	137	0	-	-	-	-	1.0	-	-	-	1.1	-	2.7	11.2	21.3	38.6	48.0	63.3	99.2	51.2	101.2	10.3	3.3	0.38	0.94	**7.7**	157
Nose, sinuses etc.	5	0	-	-	-	-	-	-	-	-	-	-	-	1.8	-	-	4.9	3.3	-	-	0.4	0.1	0.01	0.04	**0.3**	160
Larynx	94	0	-	-	-	-	-	-	-	-	-	1.1	6.8	16.1	14.2	44.4	50.1	26.8	23.1	25.6	14.5	7.1	2.3	0.41	0.80	**6.1**	161
Bronchus, lung	721	0	-	-	-	-	2.0	-	-	3.3	8.0	34.1	40.2	118.7	214.5	342.1	330.9	419.8	262.6	187.9	54.1	17.5	2.10	5.47	**41.6**	162
Other thoracic organs	6	0	-	-	-	-	2.0	-	2.2	-	-	-	-	-	1.9	-	-	-	6.4	-	0.5	0.1	0.03	0.03	**0.4**	163-4
Bone	12	0	-	-	0.7	2.3	1.0	1.1	-	-	-	1.4	-	-	5.8	2.1	-	3.3	-	-	0.9	0.3	0.06	0.07	**0.9**	170
Connective tissue	33	0	2.9	-	0.7	0.8	1.0	1.1	-	1.1	2.3	1.4	-	3.5	7.7	10.4	4.9	6.6	32.0	28.9	2.5	0.8	0.11	0.19	**2.2**	171
Mesothelioma	3	0	-	-	-	-	-	-	-	-	-	-	-	-	1.9	-	4.9	-	-	-	0.2	0.1	0.01	0.03	**0.2**	MES
Kaposi's sarcoma	1	0	-	-	-	-	-	1.1	-	-	-	-	-	-	-	-	-	-	-	-	0.1	0.0	0.01	0.01	**0.1**	KAP
Melanoma of skin	93	0	-	-	-	-	1.0	5.5	10.9	5.6	9.2	10.9	11.2	19.5	19.3	8.3	26.8	16.5	32.0	43.4	7.0	2.3	0.47	0.64	**6.2**	172
Other skin	1389	0	1.0	-	0.7	0.8	3.0	3.3	9.8	22.3	36.7	75.1	107.6	180.7	316.9	442.3	635.0	823.0	787.7	1242.8	104.3		3.79	9.18	**79.0**	173
Breast	10	0	-	-	-	-	-	-	-	-	1.1	2.7	1.6	1.8	1.9	-	4.9	6.6	-	-	0.8	0.2	0.05	0.07	**0.6**	175
Prostate	631	0	-	-	-	-	-	-	-	-	1.1	4.1	9.6	31.9	85.0	189.8	333.3	594.9	685.2	635.8	47.4	15.3	0.66	3.27	**30.4**	185
Testis	46	0	1.9	-	-	3.1	9.9	7.7	8.7	6.7	3.4	4.1	-	-	-	2.1	-	3.3	6.4	-	3.5	1.1	0.23	0.24	**3.4**	186
Penis	11	0	-	-	-	-	-	1.1	-	-	-	-	1.6	1.8	1.9	4.2	2.4	6.6	-	28.9	0.8	0.3	0.03	0.07	**0.7**	187.1-.4
Other male genital	1	0	-	-	-	-	-	-	-	-	-	-	-	-	-	-	-	-	-	14.5	0.1	0.0	0.00	0.00	**0.1**	187.5-.9
Bladder	214	0	-	-	-	0.8	1.0	-	2.2	1.1	4.6	4.1	14.5	39.0	42.5	91.8	87.6	105.8	134.5	231.2	16.1	5.2	0.55	1.45	**12.2**	188
Kidney etc.	104	0	1.9	-	0.7	-	1.0	1.1	3.3	2.2	3.4	6.8	11.2	12.4	21.3	39.6	46.2	52.9	44.8	-	7.8	2.5	0.33	0.76	**6.2**	189
Eye	7	0	1.0	-	-	-	-	-	-	-	-	-	-	1.8	-	4.2	2.4	6.6	-	-	0.5	0.2	0.01	0.05	**0.4**	190
Brain, nervous system	117	0	3.9	0.8	1.5	3.1	3.0	-	7.6	7.8	5.7	9.6	16.1	23.0	29.0	20.9	26.8	39.7	32.0	14.5	8.8	2.8	0.56	0.79	**7.7**	191-2
Thyroid	8	0	-	-	-	-	-	1.1	-	-	2.3	-	-	-	-	4.2	7.3	-	-	-	0.6	0.2	0.02	0.07	**0.6**	193
Other endocrine	8	0	1.0	-	-	1.6	-	1.1	-	-	-	2.7	-	-	-	4.2	-	-	-	-	0.6	0.2	0.03	0.05	**0.6**	194
Hodgkin's disease	21	0	-	1.7	-	-	3.9	2.2	4.4	1.1	3.4	2.7	1.6	1.8	-	2.1	-	-	-	-	1.6	0.5	0.11	0.12	**1.6**	201
Non-Hodgkin lymphoma	142	0	-	1.7	1.5	2.3	3.0	3.3	5.5	10.0	8.0	6.8	20.9	15.9	25.1	52.2	51.1	36.4	57.6	28.9	10.7	3.4	0.52	1.04	**8.9**	200,202
Multiple myeloma	68	0	-	-	-	-	-	-	-	-	2.3	2.7	4.8	15.9	23.2	20.9	26.8	29.7	38.4	57.8	5.1	1.6	0.24	0.48	**4.0**	203
Lymphoid leukaemia	108	0	3.9	3.3	0.7	3.9	1.0	3.3	-	-	1.1	4.1	4.8	10.6	17.4	35.5	43.8	69.4	51.2	57.8	8.1	2.6	0.27	0.67	**6.4**	204
Myeloid leukaemia	55	0	1.0	0.8	0.7	1.6	2.0	-	2.2	4.5	2.3	5.5	6.4	5.3	7.7	14.6	12.2	16.5	12.8	86.7	4.1	1.3	0.20	0.33	**3.6**	205
Monocytic leukaemia	0	0	-	-	-	-	-	-	-	-	-	-	-	-	-	-	-	-	-	-	0.0	0.0	0.00	0.00	**0.0**	206
Other leukaemia	0	0	-	-	-	-	-	-	-	-	-	-	-	-	-	-	-	-	-	-	0.0	0.0	0.00	0.00	**0.0**	207
Leukaemia unspecified	20	0	-	-	-	-	-	1.1	-	1.1	-	-	1.6	-	-	3.9	4.2	7.3	23.1	6.4	28.9	1.5	0.5	0.04	0.10	**1.1**	208
Other and unspecified	229	0	1.9	-	-	-	-	1.1	2.2	3.3	3.4	1.4	11.2	26.6	58.0	56.3	104.6	175.2	172.9	216.8	17.2	5.5	0.55	1.35	**12.4**	O&U
All sites	5520	0	21.4	8.3	7.4	21.7	35.5	37.6	60.1	79.0	125.0	256.7	414.4	747.6	1292.8	1892.1	2425.8	3192.9	3080.4	3713.9	414.3		15.54	37.13	**316.6**	ALL
All sites but 173	4131	0	20.5	8.3	6.7	20.9	32.6	34.2	50.2	56.7	88.3	181.6	306.8	566.9	975.8	1449.9	1790.8	2369.9	2292.7	2471.1	310.0	100.0	11.75	27.95	**237.6**	ALLb
Rate from 1 case			0.974	0.830	0.745	0.776	0.987	1.105	1.092	1.113	1.147	1.365	1.606	1.771	1.932	2.086	2.433	3.305	6.404	14.451						

IRELAND, SOUTHERN 1988-1992

ANNUAL INCIDENCE PER 100,000 BY AGE GROUP (YEARS) - FEMALE

SITE	ALL AGES	AGE UNK	0-	5-	10-	15-	20-	25-	30-	35-	40-	45-	50-	55-	60-	65-	70-	75-	80-	85+	CRUDE RATE	%	CR 64	CR 74	ASR (W)	ICD (9th)
Lip	11	0	-	-	-	-	-	-	-	-	-	-	-	1.8	-	3.6	4.1	5.0	7.9	12.5	0.8	0.3	0.01	0.05	**0.4**	*140*
Tongue	12	0	-	-	-	-	-	-	-	-	-	4.3	1.7	-	3.7	3.6	2.1	2.5	-	12.5	0.9	0.3	0.05	0.08	**0.7**	*141*
Salivary gland	4	0	-	-	-	-	-	-	-	-	-	1.4	-	1.8	-	-	2.1	2.5	-	-	0.3	0.1	0.02	0.03	**0.2**	*142*
Mouth	13	0	-	-	-	-	-	-	-	-	-	-	-	1.8	-	9.1	6.2	5.0	3.9	6.3	1.0	0.3	0.01	0.09	**0.6**	*143-5*
Oropharynx	4	0	-	-	-	-	-	-	-	-	-	-	1.7	-	1.9	-	-	5.0	-	-	0.3	0.1	0.02	0.02	**0.2**	*146*
Nasopharynx	3	0	-	-	-	0.8	-	-	-	-	-	-	-	1.8	-	-	-	3.9	-	-	0.2	0.1	0.01	0.01	**0.2**	*147*
Hypopharynx	8	0	-	-	-	-	-	-	1.1	-	-	1.4	-	-	1.9	1.8	4.1	2.5	3.9	-	0.6	0.2	0.02	0.05	**0.4**	*148*
Pharynx unspecified	5	0	-	-	-	-	-	-	-	-	-	-	-	-	-	3.6	2.1	5.0	-	-	0.4	0.1	0.00	0.03	**0.2**	*149*
Oesophagus	88	0	-	-	-	-	-	-	-	-	-	1.4	1.7	5.4	9.3	27.3	41.1	57.4	66.9	18.8	6.6	2.2	0.09	0.43	**3.4**	*150*
Stomach	125	0	-	-	-	-	-	-	2.3	-	2.4	4.3	-	3.6	20.5	32.8	37.0	74.8	66.9	137.7	9.4	3.2	0.17	0.51	**5.0**	*151*
Small intestine	7	0	-	-	-	-	-	-	-	-	1.2	-	-	1.8	1.9	-	2.1	7.5	-	-	0.5	0.2	0.02	0.03	**0.3**	*152*
Colon	425	0	-	-	-	-	-	-	2.2	4.6	14.3	27.4	34.1	47.0	76.6	140.2	133.5	162.1	236.3	212.8	32.0	10.8	1.03	2.40	**20.3**	*153*
Rectum	150	0	-	-	-	-	-	-	1.1	4.6	3.6	13.0	11.9	18.1	28.0	36.4	45.2	72.3	90.6	43.8	11.3	3.8	0.40	0.81	**7.2**	*154*
Liver	11	0	-	-	-	-	-	-	-	-	-	-	-	-	-	3.6	4.1	7.5	7.9	12.5	0.8	0.3	0.00	0.04	**0.4**	*155*
Gallbladder etc.	54	0	-	-	-	-	-	-	-	1.1	-	1.4	1.7	9.0	11.2	20.0	20.5	32.4	7.9	25.0	4.1	1.4	0.12	0.33	**2.6**	*156*
Pancreas	101	0	-	-	-	-	1.1	-	-	-	2.4	4.3	5.1	9.0	22.4	23.7	32.9	47.4	39.4	106.4	7.6	2.6	0.22	0.50	**4.6**	*157*
Nose, sinuses etc.	6	0	-	-	-	-	1.1	-	-	-	-	-	-	1.9	1.8	2.1	-	7.9	-	-	0.5	0.2	0.01	0.03	**0.3**	*160*
Larynx	14	0	-	-	-	-	-	-	-	-	-	1.4	3.4	3.6	1.9	3.6	4.1	5.0	7.9	-	1.1	0.4	0.05	0.09	**0.8**	*161*
Bronchus, lung	294	0	-	-	-	-	-	-	1.1	-	1.2	8.6	10.2	52.4	69.1	105.6	127.3	142.2	118.1	43.8	22.1	7.5	0.71	1.88	**14.0**	*162*
Other thoracic organs	2	0	-	-	-	-	1.1	-	-	-	-	-	-	-	-	1.8	-	-	-	-	0.2	0.1	0.01	0.01	**0.1**	*163-4*
Bone	8	0	-	-	1.6	-	-	1.1	-	-	-	2.9	1.7	-	-	-	2.1	2.5	-	-	0.6	0.2	0.04	0.05	**0.6**	*170*
Connective tissue	22	0	2.1	-	0.8	1.7	-	-	2.2	-	2.4	1.4	3.4	1.8	1.9	3.6	4.1	7.5	3.9	-	1.7	0.6	0.09	0.13	**1.4**	*171*
Mesothelioma	1	0	-	-	-	-	-	-	-	-	-	-	-	-	-	-	-	2.1	-	-	0.1	0.0	0.00	0.01	**0.0**	*MES*
Kaposi's sarcoma	0	0	-	-	-	-	-	-	-	-	-	-	-	-	-	-	-	-	-	-	0.0	0.0	0.00	0.00	**0.0**	*KAP*
Melanoma of skin	174	0	-	-	0.8	2.5	3.2	7.7	13.1	9.1	22.7	27.4	18.7	14.5	43.0	31.0	20.5	32.4	39.4	62.6	13.1	4.4	0.81	1.07	**10.9**	*172*
Other skin	1145	0	2.1	-	1.6	0.8	2.2	4.4	12.0	18.3	49.0	59.1	98.9	137.4	211.0	265.9	381.9	468.9	626.1	619.5	86.2		2.98	6.22	**54.7**	*173*
Breast	1033	0	1.0	-	-	0.8	1.1	7.7	16.4	47.9	115.9	180.1	175.6	195.2	246.5	224.0	195.1	214.5	200.8	287.9	77.7	26.3	4.94	7.04	**64.2**	*174*
Uterus unspecified	7	0	-	-	-	-	-	-	-	-	-	-	1.7	-	1.9	-	6.2	2.5	3.9	-	0.5	0.2	0.02	0.05	**0.3**	*179*
Cervix uteri	95	0	-	-	-	-	-	1.1	5.5	12.0	18.3	9.6	13.0	18.7	7.2	18.7	9.1	18.5	15.0	-	7.1	2.4	0.52	0.66	**6.5**	*180*
Placenta	0	0	-	-	-	-	-	-	-	-	-	-	-	-	-	-	-	-	-	-	0.0	0.0	0.00	0.00	**0.0**	*181*
Corpus uteri	137	0	-	-	-	-	-	-	-	1.1	7.2	8.6	25.6	47.0	43.0	38.2	39.0	27.4	31.5	6.3	10.3	3.5	0.66	1.05	**8.3**	*182*
Ovary etc.	220	0	-	-	-	1.7	2.2	1.1	5.5	2.3	23.9	25.9	37.5	52.4	57.9	58.3	43.1	57.4	31.5	25.0	16.6	5.6	1.05	1.56	**13.6**	*183*
Other female genital	33	0	-	-	-	-	-	-	-	-	-	1.4	1.7	-	7.5	5.5	20.5	10.0	27.6	18.8	2.5	0.8	0.05	0.18	**1.4**	*184*
Bladder	86	0	2.1	-	-	-	-	1.1	-	2.3	2.4	4.3	5.1	7.2	13.1	20.0	24.6	49.9	47.3	43.8	6.5	2.2	0.19	0.41	**4.0**	*188*
Kidney etc.	68	0	4.2	0.9	-	-	-	1.1	-	4.6	-	7.2	10.2	3.6	13.1	10.9	16.4	34.9	19.7	31.3	5.1	1.7	0.22	0.36	**3.8**	*189*
Eye	7	0	2.1	-	-	-	-	-	-	-	-	-	-	3.6	-	1.8	2.1	-	3.9	-	0.5	0.2	0.03	0.05	**0.5**	*190*
Brain, nervous system	56	0	1.0	0.9	0.8	0.8	1.1	-	2.2	4.6	6.0	2.9	1.7	9.0	9.3	14.6	20.5	12.5	15.8	-	4.2	1.4	0.20	0.38	**3.3**	*191-2*
Thyroid	41	0	-	-	0.8	-	4.3	1.1	6.6	4.6	3.6	1.4	1.7	5.4	-	12.7	8.2	5.0	7.9	12.5	3.1	1.0	0.15	0.25	**2.5**	*193*
Other endocrine	9	0	2.1	-	-	0.8	-	-	2.2	-	-	1.4	-	-	3.7	-	2.1	-	-	-	0.7	0.2	0.05	0.06	**0.7**	*194*
Hodgkin's disease	27	0	-	-	-	1.7	5.4	1.1	5.5	-	3.6	2.9	3.4	3.6	1.9	1.8	2.1	5.0	-	-	2.0	0.7	0.14	0.16	**1.9**	*201*
Non-Hodgkin lymphoma	140	0	2.1	-	1.6	-	4.3	2.2	2.2	3.4	6.0	10.1	6.8	19.9	29.9	20.0	49.3	67.3	55.1	37.5	10.5	3.6	0.44	0.79	**7.3**	*200,202*
Multiple myeloma	66	0	-	-	-	-	-	-	-	-	-	-	8.5	7.2	7.5	27.3	30.8	29.9	19.7	37.5	5.0	1.7	0.12	0.41	**3.0**	*203*
Lymphoid leukaemia	53	0	8.3	5.2	0.8	-	-	-	-	1.1	-	4.3	-	3.6	3.7	5.5	16.4	24.9	31.5	6.3	4.0	1.3	0.14	0.24	**3.1**	*204*
Myeloid leukaemia	47	0	-	-	0.8	2.5	-	-	1.1	2.3	2.4	4.3	1.7	3.6	7.5	3.6	10.3	20.0	35.4	25.0	3.5	1.2	0.13	0.20	**2.2**	*205*
Monocytic leukaemia	0	0	-	-	-	-	-	-	-	-	-	-	-	-	-	-	-	-	-	-	0.0	0.0	0.00	0.00	**0.0**	*206*
Other leukaemia	0	0	-	-	-	-	-	-	-	-	-	-	-	-	-	-	-	-	-	-	0.0	0.0	0.00	0.00	**0.0**	*207*
Leukaemia unspecified	8	0	-	-	-	-	-	-	-	-	1.2	1.4	-	-	-	-	-	2.1	10.0	6.3	0.6	0.2	0.01	0.02	**0.3**	*208*
Other and unspecified	260	0	-	-	-	-	-	1.1	-	1.1	2.4	7.2	10.2	18.1	43.0	58.3	108.8	144.7	137.8	212.8	19.6	6.6	0.42	1.25	**10.8**	*O&U*
All sites	5080	0	27.0	6.9	9.4	14.1	28.1	35.2	86.5	133.6	283.3	436.4	504.5	697.8	1014.0	1231.0	1496.9	1878.0	2008.3	2065.1	382.3		16.38	30.02	**267.2**	*ALL*
All sites but 173	3935	0	24.9	6.9	7.8	13.3	25.9	30.8	74.5	115.3	234.3	377.4	405.7	560.4	803.0	965.1	1115.0	1409.2	1382.2	1445.6	296.1	100.0	13.40	23.80	**212.5**	*ALLb*
Rate from 1 case			1.038	0.860	0.783	0.829	1.081	1.101	1.095	1.141	1.195	1.440	1.704	1.808	1.867	1.821	2.053	2.494	3.938	6.258						

Italy, Ferrara Province

The Tumour Registry of Ferrara province began its activity in 1987. The aim was to evaluate tumour incidence and mortality in order to obtain deeper insight into etiological factors and possible preventive measures. Previous mortality data clearly indicated a high level of cancer in this area, especially for neoplasia strongly related to environmental risk factors.

The registry is located in the Pathology Department of Ferrara University and in recent years it has been supported by the Italian Cancer League and provincial Local Health Administration. The registration of incidence started in 1989 and since 1991 it has been extended to the whole province; in 1994 the registry received approval and support from Emilia Romagna Regional Health Care Service.

The Province of Ferrara is located in the area of the Po delta, between latitudes 44°32′ and 44°58′ N. It is bordered to the north by the Po river, to the east by the Adriatic Sea, to the south by the provinces of Ravenna and Bologna, and to the west by those of Modena and Mantova. The province has a total surface area of 2632 km^2 and lies close to sea level (maximum altitude 22 m) and mainly assigned to agriculture (81.6%). In 1991 the average temperature was 13.1°C (winter average +2.0°C, summer average +23.9°C) and the overall rainfall was 670 mm. The population was 360 763 at the 1991 census, with 26 municipalities ranging from Migliaro (2411) to Ferrara city (138 015). The level of employment was 43.0% (34.7% industry, 15.5% agriculture, 49.9% trade and services). Mechanical and chemical industries are present in the province; the main sources of air and water pollution are represented by industries, breeding, traffic, heating plants and agricultural chemical treatments.

The area covered by the registry has a range of diagnostic services and eight general hospitals with 2328 beds in 1991. In recent years, the population has shown a progressive decrease, mainly due to a fall in the birth rate; migration to other areas is minimal and immigration from other countries is still fairly rare.

Sources of cancer information for the registry are the diagnoses at discharge from regional hospitals and the database of the Institute of Pathology of Ferrara University (seat of the overall pathological diagnostic activity in the province); additional information is collected from general practitioners and other major oncological care services. Mortality data for all causes of death among the resident population are collected from public health services to identify cases not otherwise registered and for follow-up purposes. The official mortality statistics of the province for indices and comparisons are acquired from the Italian Institute of Statistics.

Data collection is voluntary and is performed both passively and actively; follow-up of patients for survival statistics is in progress through the linkage of mortality files and residence registries of municipalities and care units.

Reports are classified according to the ICD-O topography and morphology; ICD-9 is also applied. Data are stored in a computerized database and regular maintenance is carried out. Checking for duplication is carried out by sorting cases on name and date of birth. Error and consistency checks are performed by comparing data received from different sources of information and comparing patients' age, sex, site and morphology code of tumours.

All malignant tumours are recorded; *in situ* carcinomas and several benign and uncertain tumours are also collected, but not included in incidence statistics. Malignant tumours are defined as those coded from 140.0 to 208.9 in ICD-9 and those with code 3 or more in ICD-O 5th digit. The date of first hospital admission or the date of a previous histo-cytological diagnosis, if available, is assumed as the incidence date; for death-certificate-only cases, the incidence date is taken as the date of death. Multiple primaries are recorded according to the IARC rules.

Some local suspected etiological factors are currently being investigated. The role of fog, a characteristic climatic feature of the province, as an aggravating factor in air pollution, is also under consideration.

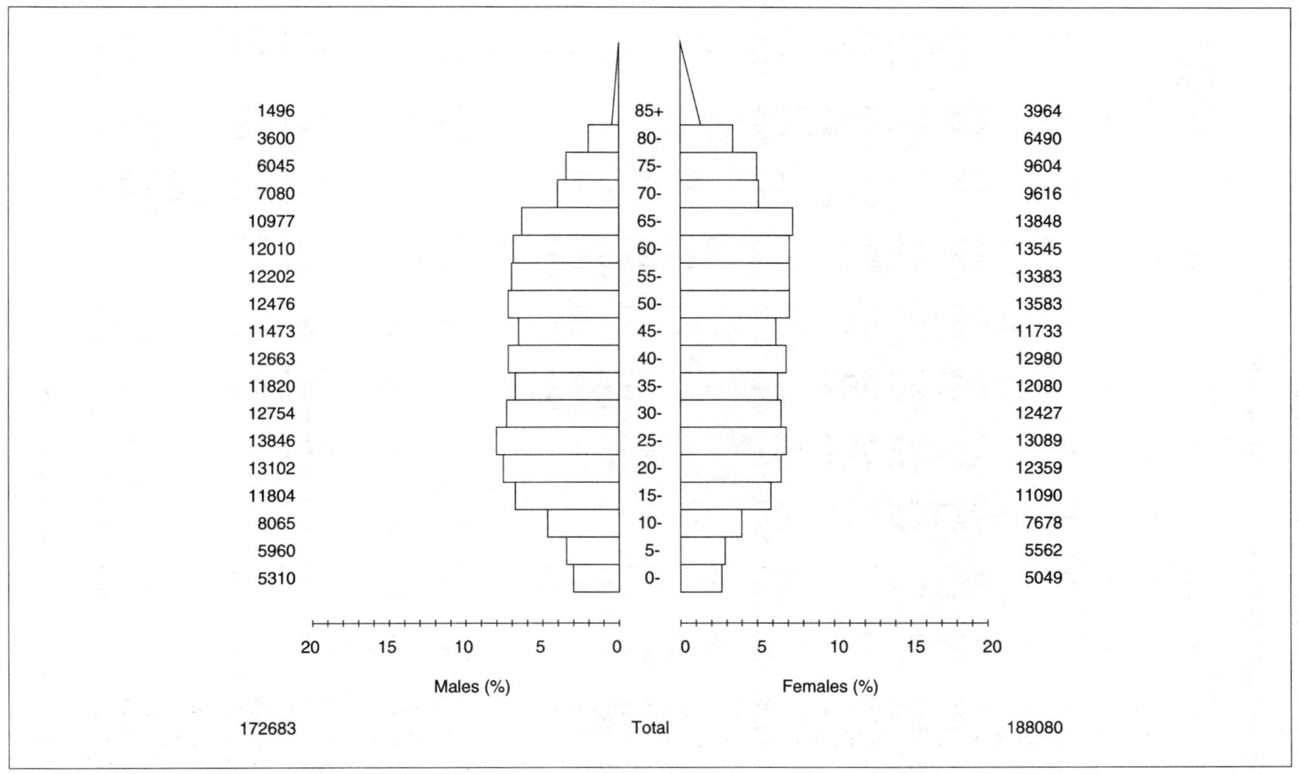

Italy, Ferrarra Province
Source of population: 1991
Census: Italian general census, 1991. Istituto Centrale di Statistica: "Popolazione e Abitazioni", Fascicolo 38, XIII Censimento Generale della Popolazione e delle Abitazioni 20 ottobre '91, Roma 1994

ITALY, FERRARA PROVINCE 1991-1992

ANNUAL INCIDENCE PER 100,000 BY AGE GROUP (YEARS) - MALE

SITE	ALL AGES	AGE UNK	0-	5-	10-	15-	20-	25-	30-	35-	40-	45-	50-	55-	60-	65-	70-	75-	80-	85+	CRUDE RATE	%	CR 64	CR 74	ASR (W)	ICD (9th)
Lip	9	0	-	-	-	-	-	-	-	-	-	-	-	12.3	8.3	9.1	7.1	8.3	-	-	2.6	0.4	0.10	0.18	1.3	140
Tongue	9	0	-	-	-	-	-	-	-	-	-	-	-	-	16.7	18.2	7.1	-	-	-	2.6	0.4	0.08	0.21	1.4	141
Salivary gland	4	0	-	-	-	-	-	-	-	-	-	4.4	-	-	-	-	7.1	8.3	13.9	-	1.2	0.2	0.02	0.06	0.6	142
Mouth	14	0	-	-	-	-	-	-	4.2	3.9	4.4	8.0	-	16.7	13.7	14.1	-	-	-	-	4.1	0.6	0.19	0.32	2.5	143-5
Oropharynx	10	0	-	-	-	-	-	-	-	-	13.1	4.0	4.1	4.2	9.1	7.1	-	13.9	-	-	2.9	0.5	0.13	0.21	1.8	146
Nasopharynx	3	0	-	-	-	-	-	-	-	-	-	-	-	4.1	-	4.6	-	8.3	-	-	0.9	0.1	0.02	0.04	0.4	147
Hypopharynx	3	0	-	-	-	-	-	-	-	-	-	-	-	-	-	13.7	-	-	-	-	0.9	0.1	0.00	0.07	0.4	148
Pharynx unspecified	2	0	-	-	-	-	-	-	-	-	-	-	-	-	8.3	-	-	-	-	-	0.6	0.1	0.04	0.04	0.3	149
Oesophagus	22	0	-	-	-	-	-	3.9	-	7.9	8.7	4.0	8.2	16.7	13.7	7.1	16.5	27.8	66.8	6.4	1.0	0.25	0.35	3.6	150
Stomach	142	0	-	-	-	-	-	-	-	15.8	13.1	28.1	20.5	62.4	123.0	169.5	173.7	375.0	300.8	41.1	6.4	0.70	2.16	18.6	151
Small intestine	7	0	-	-	-	-	-	-	-	-	-	-	4.1	16.7	9.1	-	-	-	-	2.0	0.3	0.10	0.15	1.1	152
Colon	203	0	-	-	-	-	-	-	8.5	19.7	13.1	40.1	49.2	149.9	150.3	268.4	239.9	319.4	401.1	58.8	9.2	1.40	3.50	28.3	153
Rectum	81	0	-	-	-	-	-	3.9	-	3.9	21.8	8.0	32.8	20.8	59.2	169.5	82.7	111.1	133.7	23.5	3.7	0.46	1.60	11.5	154
Liver	57	0	-	-	-	-	-	-	-	7.9	4.4	8.0	4.1	41.6	72.9	63.6	49.6	97.2	100.3	16.5	2.6	0.33	1.01	7.9	155
Gallbladder etc.	25	0	-	-	-	-	-	-	-	-	-	-	-	8.2	8.3	22.8	42.4	41.4	69.4	-	7.2	1.1	0.08	0.41	3.0	156
Pancreas	53	0	-	-	-	-	-	-	-	-	-	8.0	20.5	45.8	36.4	84.7	66.2	69.4	66.8	15.3	2.4	0.37	0.98	7.2	157
Nose, sinuses etc.	5	0	-	-	-	-	-	-	-	-	-	-	4.1	-	-	14.1	8.3	-	33.4	1.4	0.2	0.02	0.09	0.7	160
Larynx	66	0	-	-	-	-	-	-	4.2	-	4.4	44.1	32.8	45.8	63.8	77.7	33.1	55.6	33.4	19.1	3.0	0.66	1.36	10.1	161
Bronchus, lung	597	0	-	-	-	-	3.6	3.9	4.2	15.8	65.4	160.3	262.3	416.3	651.4	621.5	736.1	416.7	701.9	172.9	27.0	4.66	11.02	85.7	162
Other thoracic organs	3	0	-	-	-	-	3.8	-	-	-	-	-	-	4.2	4.6	-	-	-	-	0.9	0.1	0.04	0.06	0.6	163-4
Bone	5	0	-	-	-	-	3.8	-	-	-	-	4.0	-	-	9.1	-	8.3	-	-	1.4	0.2	0.04	0.08	0.9	170
Connective tissue	11	0	-	-	-	-	-	-	-	4.2	-	-	-	8.2	4.2	-	28.2	16.5	13.9	-	3.2	0.5	0.08	0.22	1.5	171
Mesothelioma	6	0	-	-	-	-	-	-	-	-	-	4.4	-	-	4.2	-	14.1	8.3	-	33.4	1.7	0.3	0.04	0.11	1.0	MES
Kaposi's sarcoma	16	0	-	-	-	-	-	-	-	3.9	13.1	4.0	8.2	8.3	-	14.1	33.1	13.9	-	4.6	0.7	0.19	0.26	2.6	KAP
Melanoma of skin	19	0	-	-	-	-	3.8	-	7.8	-	3.9	4.4	12.0	-	16.7	18.2	14.1	8.3	-	-	5.5	0.9	0.24	0.40	3.5	172
Other skin	371	0	-	-	-	-	-	3.6	3.9	25.4	19.7	82.8	44.1	127.0	170.7	323.4	452.0	537.6	555.6	534.8	107.4		2.39	6.26	51.9	173
Breast	7	0	-	-	-	-	-	-	-	-	-	-	4.0	-	-	4.6	14.1	16.5	13.9	-	2.0	0.3	0.02	0.11	0.9	175
Prostate	179	0	-	-	-	-	-	-	-	-	-	-	8.0	41.0	99.9	145.8	211.9	405.3	319.4	300.8	51.8	8.1	0.74	2.53	21.8	185
Testis	9	0	-	-	-	-	3.8	7.2	-	-	3.9	-	12.0	8.2	-	-	-	-	-	-	2.6	0.4	0.18	0.18	2.0	186
Penis	5	0	-	-	-	-	-	-	-	-	-	-	-	-	4.2	9.1	7.1	8.3	-	-	1.4	0.2	0.02	0.10	0.7	187.1-.4
Other male genital	0	0	-	-	-	-	-	-	-	-	-	-	-	-	-	-	-	-	-	-	0.0	0.0	0.00	0.00	0.0	187.5-.9
Bladder	233	0	-	-	-	-	-	7.8	4.2	15.8	26.1	16.0	57.4	166.5	236.9	282.5	289.5	361.1	300.8	67.5	10.5	1.47	4.07	32.0	188
Kidney etc.	105	0	-	-	-	-	-	-	16.9	7.9	13.1	40.1	36.9	70.8	100.2	105.9	91.0	111.1	133.7	30.4	4.7	0.93	1.96	15.8	189
Eye	4	0	-	-	-	4.2	-	-	-	-	-	-	-	4.2	4.6	-	8.3	-	-	1.2	0.2	0.04	0.06	0.8	190
Brain, nervous system	36	0	-	-	-	-	-	3.6	-	12.7	-	4.4	16.0	20.5	8.3	18.2	21.2	74.4	55.6	-	10.4	1.6	0.33	0.52	5.3	191-2
Thyroid	13	0	-	-	-	4.2	-	3.6	3.9	-	-	4.4	4.0	8.2	4.2	9.1	21.2	-	-	-	3.8	0.6	0.16	0.31	2.6	193
Other endocrine	1	0	-	-	-	4.2	-	-	-	-	-	-	-	-	-	-	-	-	-	-	0.3	0.0	0.02	0.02	0.4	194
Hodgkin's disease	14	0	9.4	-	-	8.5	7.6	3.6	-	8.5	3.9	-	-	4.1	8.3	4.6	7.1	-	-	-	4.1	0.6	0.27	0.33	4.3	201
Non-Hodgkin lymphoma	77	0	-	8.4	6.2	4.2	-	-	7.8	12.7	11.8	21.8	20.0	28.7	41.6	54.7	49.4	82.7	13.9	300.8	22.3	3.5	0.82	1.34	13.9	200,202
Multiple myeloma	32	0	-	-	-	-	-	-	-	-	-	-	8.0	4.1	16.7	22.8	35.3	33.1	83.3	167.1	9.3	1.4	0.14	0.43	4.2	203
Lymphoid leukaemia	24	0	-	8.4	6.2	4.2	-	3.6	-	4.2	3.9	-	-	4.1	8.3	22.8	28.2	16.5	41.7	33.4	6.9	1.1	0.22	0.47	4.8	204
Myeloid leukaemia	19	0	-	-	-	-	-	-	-	4.2	-	4.4	4.0	-	4.2	9.1	28.2	24.8	55.6	66.8	5.5	0.9	0.08	0.27	2.6	205
Monocytic leukaemia	0	0	-	-	-	-	-	-	-	-	-	-	-	-	-	-	-	-	-	-	0.0	0.0	0.00	0.00	0.0	206
Other leukaemia	0	0	-	-	-	-	-	-	-	-	-	-	-	-	-	-	-	-	-	-	0.0	0.0	0.00	0.00	0.0	207
Leukaemia unspecified	14	0	-	-	-	4.2	3.8	-	-	-	-	-	4.0	4.1	8.3	9.1	-	33.1	27.8	-	4.1	0.6	0.12	0.17	2.1	208
Other and unspecified	68	0	-	-	-	-	3.8	-	3.9	4.2	3.9	-	8.0	20.5	16.7	36.4	56.5	107.5	194.4	334.2	19.7	3.1	0.31	0.77	8.9	O&U
All sites	2583	0	9.4	16.8	12.4	33.9	30.5	28.9	47.0	118.4	154.0	331.2	521.0	848.2	1548.7	2313.9	2952.0	3275.4	3430.6	4044.1	747.9		18.50	44.83	371.3	ALL
All sites but 173	2212	0	9.4	16.8	12.4	33.9	30.5	25.3	43.1	93.1	134.2	248.4	476.9	721.2	1378.0	1990.5	2500.0	2737.8	2875.0	3509.4	640.5	100.0	16.12	38.57	319.4	ALLb

Rate from 1 case   9.416 8.389 6.200 4.236 3.816 3.611 3.920 4.230 3.949 4.358 4.008 4.098 4.163 4.555 7.062 8.271 13.889 33.422

ITALY, FERRARA PROVINCE 1991-1992

ANNUAL INCIDENCE PER 100,000 BY AGE GROUP (YEARS) - FEMALE

SITE	ALL AGES	AGE UNK	0-	5-	10-	15-	20-	25-	30-	35-	40-	45-	50-	55-	60-	65-	70-	75-	80-	85+	CRUDE RATE	%	CR 64	CR 74	ASR (W)	ICD (9th)
Lip	1	0	-	-	-	-	-	-	-	-	-	-	-	3.7	-	-	-	-	-	-	0.3	0.1	0.02	0.02	**0.1**	*140*
Tongue	2	0	-	-	-	-	-	-	-	-	-	-	-	-	-	-	5.2	5.2	-	-	0.5	0.1	0.00	0.03	**0.2**	*141*
Salivary gland	3	0	-	-	-	-	3.8	-	-	-	-	-	-	-	3.7	-	-	-	-	12.6	0.8	0.2	0.04	0.04	**0.5**	*142*
Mouth	9	0	-	-	-	-	-	-	-	-	-	-	-	7.5	3.7	3.6	15.6	10.4	-	-	2.4	0.5	0.06	0.15	**1.0**	*143-5*
Oropharynx	3	0	-	-	-	-	-	-	-	-	-	4.3	-	-	3.7	-	5.2	-	-	-	0.8	0.2	0.04	0.07	**0.5**	*146*
Nasopharynx	2	0	-	-	-	-	-	-	-	-	-	-	-	-	-	3.6	-	-	7.7	-	0.5	0.1	0.00	0.02	**0.1**	*147*
Hypopharynx	2	0	-	-	-	-	-	-	-	-	-	4.3	-	-	-	3.6	-	-	-	-	0.5	0.1	0.02	0.04	**0.4**	*148*
Pharynx unspecified	0	0	-	-	-	-	-	-	-	-	-	-	-	-	-	-	-	-	-	-	0.0	0.0	0.00	0.00	**0.0**	*149*
Oesophagus	6	0	-	-	-	-	-	-	-	-	-	-	7.4	-	-	3.6	-	15.6	-	-	1.6	0.3	0.04	0.05	**0.6**	*150*
Stomach	105	0	-	-	-	-	-	-	-	8.3	3.9	8.5	11.0	11.2	14.8	68.6	93.6	93.7	177.2	151.4	27.9	5.5	0.29	1.10	**9.3**	*151*
Small intestine	5	0	-	-	-	-	-	-	-	-	3.9	-	-	3.7	-	-	5.2	5.2	7.7	-	1.3	0.3	0.04	0.06	**0.6**	*152*
Colon	195	0	-	-	-	-	-	3.8	4.0	4.1	3.9	8.5	33.1	59.8	92.3	140.8	166.4	151.0	192.6	176.6	51.8	10.2	1.05	2.58	**20.2**	*153*
Rectum	58	0	-	-	-	-	-	-	-	4.1	-	17.0	11.0	11.2	18.5	46.9	10.4	46.9	92.4	75.7	15.4	3.0	0.31	0.60	**5.9**	*154*
Liver	34	0	-	-	-	-	-	-	-	-	4.3	-	7.5	7.4	14.4	31.2	26.0	61.6	75.7	-	9.0	1.8	0.10	0.32	**2.9**	*155*
Gallbladder etc.	35	0	-	-	-	-	-	-	-	7.7	8.5	-	3.7	7.5	11.1	25.3	26.0	26.0	23.1	63.1	9.3	1.8	0.19	0.45	**3.9**	*156*
Pancreas	70	0	-	-	-	-	-	-	-	3.9	-	-	14.7	18.7	25.8	21.7	46.8	67.7	138.7	88.3	18.6	3.7	0.32	0.66	**6.1**	*157*
Nose, sinuses etc.	1	0	-	-	-	-	-	-	-	-	-	-	-	-	-	3.6	-	-	-	-	0.3	0.1	0.00	0.02	**0.1**	*160*
Larynx	3	0	-	-	-	-	-	-	-	-	-	-	-	3.7	-	-	5.2	-	7.7	-	0.8	0.2	0.02	0.04	**0.3**	*161*
Bronchus, lung	130	0	-	-	-	4.5	-	-	-	-	3.9	17.0	25.8	56.0	59.1	86.7	104.0	104.1	92.4	126.1	34.6	6.8	0.83	1.78	**14.4**	*162*
Other thoracic organs	5	0	-	-	-	-	-	-	-	4.1	-	4.3	3.7	3.7	-	-	-	-	-	12.6	1.3	0.3	0.08	0.08	**0.9**	*163-4*
Bone	5	0	-	-	-	-	-	-	-	-	3.9	-	-	3.7	-	-	-	10.4	-	12.6	1.3	0.3	0.04	0.09	**0.7**	*170*
Connective tissue	10	0	-	-	-	-	-	-	-	-	3.9	-	-	-	11.1	7.2	-	10.4	7.7	12.6	2.7	0.5	0.07	0.11	**1.1**	*171*
Mesothelioma	0	0	-	-	-	-	-	-	-	-	-	-	-	-	-	-	-	-	-	-	0.0	0.0	0.00	0.00	**0.0**	*MES*
Kaposi's sarcoma	7	0	-	-	-	-	-	3.8	-	-	-	-	-	-	-	-	-	15.6	7.7	25.2	1.9	0.4	0.02	0.06	**0.6**	*KAP*
Melanoma of skin	28	0	9.9	-	-	4.5	4.0	3.8	4.0	8.3	3.9	12.8	-	11.2	29.5	10.8	-	5.2	-	25.2	7.4	1.5	0.46	0.51	**6.1**	*172*
Other skin	273	0	-	-	-	-	8.1	-	20.1	16.6	19.3	21.3	47.9	74.7	107.1	137.2	187.2	229.1	315.9	391.0	72.6		1.57	3.20	**28.6**	*173*
Breast	527	0	-	-	-	-	-	3.8	12.1	74.5	142.5	213.1	147.2	205.5	273.2	260.0	280.8	307.2	323.6	277.5	140.1	27.6	5.36	8.06	**72.8**	*174*
Uterus unspecified	4	0	-	-	-	-	-	-	-	-	-	-	-	-	3.7	5.2	5.2	7.7	-	-	1.1	0.2	0.02	0.04	**0.3**	*179*
Cervix uteri	47	0	-	-	-	-	-	4.0	16.6	11.6	17.0	18.4	26.2	11.1	28.9	20.8	15.6	23.1	25.2	-	12.5	2.5	0.52	0.77	**7.0**	*180*
Placenta	0	0	-	-	-	-	-	-	-	-	-	-	-	-	-	-	-	-	-	-	0.0	0.0	0.00	0.00	**0.0**	*181*
Corpus uteri	98	0	-	-	-	-	-	3.8	-	4.1	15.4	29.8	29.4	59.8	59.1	43.3	67.6	36.4	61.6	63.1	26.1	5.1	1.01	1.56	**13.1**	*182*
Ovary etc.	57	0	-	-	-	-	-	-	4.0	4.1	7.7	4.3	14.7	26.2	29.5	39.7	52.0	20.8	53.9	12.6	15.2	3.0	0.45	0.91	**6.9**	*183*
Other female genital	25	0	9.9	-	-	4.5	-	3.8	-	-	3.9	-	7.4	3.7	-	7.2	10.4	26.0	38.5	50.5	6.6	1.3	0.17	0.25	**3.8**	*184*
Bladder	46	0	-	-	-	-	-	-	-	-	-	4.3	-	7.5	7.4	25.3	67.6	52.1	38.5	75.7	12.2	2.4	0.10	0.56	**4.1**	*188*
Kidney etc.	57	0	-	-	-	-	-	-	-	3.9	-	-	14.7	18.7	22.1	18.1	46.8	72.9	69.3	50.5	15.2	3.0	0.30	0.62	**5.4**	*189*
Eye	6	0	-	-	-	-	-	-	-	-	-	-	7.4	3.7	3.7	3.6	5.2	-	-	-	1.6	0.3	0.07	0.12	**0.9**	*190*
Brain, nervous system	32	0	-	9.0	6.5	4.5	-	3.8	-	-	3.9	12.8	14.7	14.9	3.7	10.8	26.0	31.2	-	12.6	8.5	1.7	0.37	0.55	**5.9**	*191-2*
Thyroid	49	0	-	9.0	-	-	8.1	26.7	16.1	16.6	11.6	34.1	14.7	7.5	18.5	14.4	20.8	5.2	-	-	13.0	2.6	0.81	0.99	**11.1**	*193*
Other endocrine	2	0	-	-	-	-	-	-	-	-	-	4.3	-	-	3.7	-	-	-	-	-	0.5	0.1	0.04	0.04	**0.4**	*194*
Hodgkin's disease	13	0	-	-	-	-	4.0	15.3	4.0	-	-	-	-	3.7	7.4	7.2	-	-	7.7	12.6	3.5	0.7	0.17	0.21	**2.6**	*201*
Non-Hodgkin lymphoma	94	0	-	-	-	4.5	4.0	7.6	4.0	8.3	3.9	12.8	18.4	37.4	48.0	39.7	62.4	104.1	61.6	50.5	25.0	4.9	0.74	1.25	**11.5**	*200,202*
Multiple myeloma	31	0	-	-	-	-	-	-	-	-	-	-	3.7	7.5	22.1	18.1	10.4	20.8	53.9	50.5	8.2	1.6	0.17	0.31	**2.8**	*203*
Lymphoid leukaemia	25	0	-	-	6.5	-	-	-	4.0	-	-	4.3	-	3.7	7.4	7.2	31.2	10.4	46.2	37.8	6.6	1.3	0.13	0.32	**2.9**	*204*
Myeloid leukaemia	18	0	-	-	-	-	-	3.8	4.0	-	-	-	-	3.7	-	10.8	10.4	10.4	30.8	37.8	4.8	0.9	0.08	0.18	**1.9**	*205*
Monocytic leukaemia	3	0	-	-	-	-	-	-	-	-	-	-	-	-	3.7	-	-	5.2	5.2	-	0.8	0.2	0.02	0.04	**0.3**	*206*
Other leukaemia	1	0	-	-	-	-	-	-	-	-	-	-	-	-	-	-	-	5.2	-	-	0.3	0.1	0.00	0.03	**0.1**	*207*
Leukaemia unspecified	0	0	-	-	-	-	-	-	-	-	-	-	-	-	-	-	-	-	-	-	0.0	0.0	0.00	0.00	**0.0**	*208*
Other and unspecified	55	0	9.9	-	-	-	-	3.8	-	-	-	-	7.4	3.7	22.1	28.9	36.4	20.8	92.4	164.0	14.6	2.9	0.23	0.56	**6.0**	*O&U*
All sites	2182	0	29.7	18.0	13.0	22.5	28.3	87.9	80.5	169.7	261.9	447.5	460.1	713.6	937.6	1141.0	1476.7	1556.6	2041.6	2169.5	580.1		16.35	29.44	**264.9**	*ALL*
All sites but 173	1909	0	29.7	18.0	13.0	22.5	20.2	87.9	60.4	153.1	242.7	426.1	412.3	638.9	830.6	1003.8	1289.5	1327.6	1725.7	1778.5	507.5	100.0	14.78	26.24	**236.2**	*ALLb*
Rate from 1 case			9.903	8.990	6.512	4.509	4.046	3.820	4.023	4.139	3.852	4.261	3.681	3.736	3.691	3.611	5.200	5.206	7.704	12.614						

Italy, Florence

The Tuscany Cancer Registry is associated with the Epidemiology Unit of the Centre for the Study and Prevention of Cancer (CSPO) in Florence. The registry collects, registers and analyses information related to cases of cancer in residents of the province of Florence.

Collection and registration began on 1 January 1984 with a one-year experimental phase to evaluate feasibility. This first phase of identifying the sources of information, evaluating the quality of the baseline information, and defining the criteria for collection and registration, provided an archive of prevalent cases diagnosed before 1 January 1985.

The territory of the Tuscany Cancer Registry corresponds to the province of Florence excluding the municipality of Fucecchio (population 20 540 inhabitants). It is situated at 44° N and 11° E. The average temperature in the decade 1976–85 was 14.7°C in January and highest 33.7°C in July, and the average annual precipitation was 940 mm. The registry covers an area of 3815 km^2, with a population of 1 164 141 inhabitants according to the 1991 census (density 305 inhabitants per km^2). The province of Florence is one of the nine provinces of the region of Tuscany, bordered by the region of Emilia-Romagna to the north-east along the Apennines, by the province of Arezzo to the east, by the province of Siena to the south-east, by the province of Pisa to the south-west and west and by the province of Pistoia to the north-west. The territory is divided into 51 municipalities and 12 local health units (USL).

The only two municipalities with a population greater than 100 000 in 1991 were Prato (population 165 707) and Florence (population 403 294).

About 1% of the residents in the area are foreigners, of whom 38% come from other European countries, 33% from Asia and 14% from Africa and America respectively.

In 1991, 90% of residents aged 15–64 years were employed. In the decade 1961–71, the percentages in various employment categories were: 62% industrial, 22% commercial, 14% other activities and 0.6% agricultural. In 1991 these had changed to 49% industrial, 26% commercial, 25% other activities and 0.6% agricultural.

Industry in the province is concentrated mainly around the cities of Florence and Prato. Manufacturing is the most developed branch of the industrial sector, especially the textile industry. These activities are connected to the much larger fashion industry which occupies 40% of the industrial employees. The second largest branch is metallurgy and mechanical work which comprises 22% of the industrial employees.

In 1985, there were 6551 beds in public hospitals and 1328 beds in private hospitals, excluding chronic care and psychiatric institutions. There are 6.71 beds for every 1000 inhabitants.

Cases required to be reported to the registry comprise all malignant tumours, including those of the lymphatic and haematopoietic systems, and benign tumours of the central nervous system. Bladder papillomas and tumours of uncertain malignancy are also included.

The registry receives copies of cancer patient records from both public and private hospitals, which are then filed individually for each tumour case. Copies of all autopsy and cyto-histological referrals positive for neoplastic pathology are also received, from both the public and private pathology services. The information concerning each tumour, including personal identification and full clinical details, is coded and entered into the computer. The case is "closed" with the death of the patient, when the documentation is microfilmed and the originals are destroyed.

The Regional Mortality Registry receives death certificates (a copy of the National Institute of Statistics form) for all inhabitants of the province. Its files are periodically checked against the cancer registry records to identify cases not otherwise notified.

The Centre for the Study and Prevention of Cancer in Florence has provided screening in the province since 1980 for cancer of the uterine cervix (20–60 years) with 45% compliance. Since 1970, the centre has offered mammographic breast cancer screening for about 15% of women aged 40–70 years resident in rural municipalities of the province, with 55% compliance. Moreover, since 1990, women aged 50–69 years resident in the municipality of Florence (about 22% of the women of this age group resident in the province) have also been involved in a mammographic screening programme with about 60% compliance. The centre has run since 1982 a screening programme by haemoccult test for colorectal cancer involving about 12% of the resident population aged 40–70 years; the compliance is about 30%. Outpatient services for the early diagnosis of breast, cervix, gastrointestinal and prostate cancers are also active at the centre.

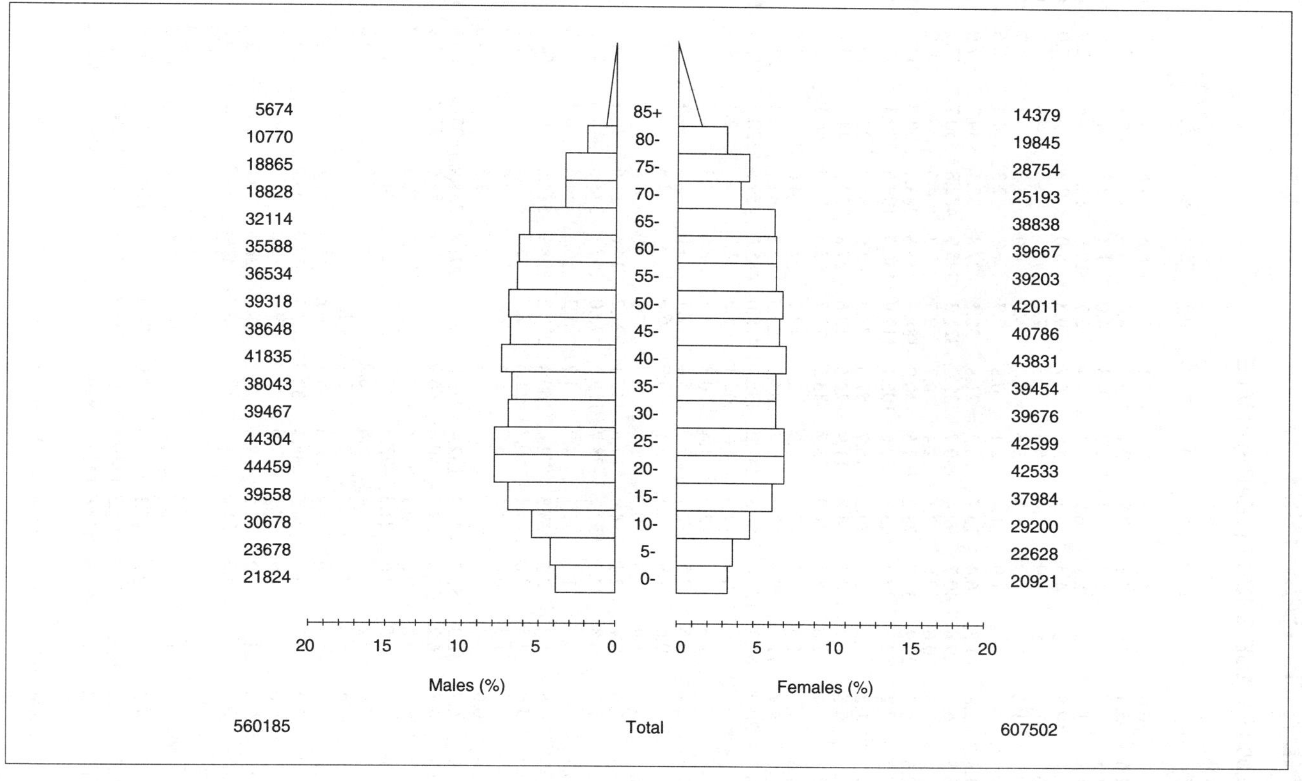

Italy, Florence

Source of population: average annual 1988–91

Census: 12 Censimento generale della popolazione, 25 ottobre 1981, Vol. II: Dati sulle caratteristiche strutturali della popolazione e delle abitazioni, ISTAT, Roma. 13 Censimento generale della popolazione, 20 ottobre 1991: Popolazione e abitazioni, ISTAT, Roma.

Estimate: Intercensal estimates based on the 1981 and 1991 censuses, taking into account births and deaths, and the migration rate for central Italy, provided by the National Institute of Health.

Notes to tables overleaf:

† 188 does not include non-invasive tumours

Screening programmes in the area

60 000 screening examinations for cervical cancer have been carried out each year in the population aged 25-69 since 1980. Breast cancer screening has been undertaken in some municipalities since 1970, with 10 000 examinations a year, and in the municipality of Florence since 1991, with 20 000 examinations a year.

ITALY, FLORENCE 1988-1991

ANNUAL INCIDENCE PER 100,000 BY AGE GROUP (YEARS) - MALE

SITE	ALL AGES	AGE UNK	0-	5-	10-	15-	20-	25-	30-	35-	40-	45-	50-	55-	60-	65-	70-	75-	80-	85+	CRUDE RATE	%	CR 64	CR 74	ASR (W)	ICD (9th)
Lip	26	0	-	-	-	-	-	-	-	-	0.6	0.6	1.3	2.1	0.7	5.4	1.3	6.6	4.6	13.2	1.2	0.2	0.03	0.06	0.6	140
Tongue	58	0	-	-	-	-	-	-	-	2.6	3.0	2.6	3.8	2.7	9.1	9.3	8.0	4.0	-	4.4	2.6	0.4	0.12	0.21	1.7	141
Salivary gland	23	0	-	-	-	-	-	0.6	1.3	-	2.6	1.3	2.1	2.8	0.8	4.0	1.3	2.3	4.4	1.0	0.2	0.05	0.08	0.7	142
Mouth	66	0	-	-	-	-	0.6	-	0.6	1.3	1.8	3.2	5.1	6.2	8.4	5.4	2.7	10.6	16.2	4.4	2.9	0.5	0.14	0.18	1.7	143-5
Oropharynx	45	0	-	-	-	-	-	-	-	-	0.6	1.9	4.5	4.1	3.5	4.7	9.3	8.0	9.3	-	2.0	0.3	0.07	0.14	1.1	146
Nasopharynx	33	0	-	-	-	0.6	-	0.6	1.3	0.7	1.8	1.9	1.9	3.4	5.6	2.3	2.7	-	-	4.4	1.5	0.3	0.09	0.11	1.0	147
Hypopharynx	39	0	-	-	-	-	-	-	0.6	0.7	1.2	1.9	1.3	5.5	5.6	5.4	4.0	4.0	2.3	-	1.7	0.3	0.08	0.13	1.1	148
Pharynx unspecified	13	0	-	-	-	-	-	-	-	-	-	1.9	1.4	2.1	0.8	2.7	-	-	2.3	4.4	0.6	0.1	0.03	0.04	0.3	149
Oesophagus	157	0	-	-	-	-	-	-	-	1.3	1.8	1.3	6.4	13.7	16.2	21.8	30.5	27.8	37.1	39.7	7.0	1.2	0.20	0.46	3.7	150
Stomach	1628	0	-	-	-	-	-	0.6	2.5	8.5	6.6	29.8	40.7	92.4	130.7	232.0	321.3	390.9	482.8	550.7	72.7	12.4	1.56	4.33	36.3	151
Small intestine	21	0	-	-	-	-	-	-	-	-	0.6	0.6	0.6	2.1	2.1	4.7	2.7	2.7	4.6	-	0.9	0.2	0.03	0.07	0.5	152
Colon	1068	0	-	-	-	-	0.6	0.6	0.6	2.6	8.4	23.9	33.7	73.2	107.5	188.5	246.5	283.2	290.8	47.7	8.1	1.26	2.90	24.5	153
Rectum	692	0	-	-	-	-	-	1.7	1.9	0.7	7.2	12.3	29.9	43.8	57.6	105.1	112.9	136.5	199.6	229.1	30.9	5.3	0.77	1.86	15.9	154
Liver	371	0	1.1	1.1	-	-	-	-	0.6	1.3	1.2	6.5	12.7	19.2	45.7	57.6	78.3	68.9	81.2	92.5	16.6	2.8	0.45	1.13	8.9	155
Gallbladder etc.	126	0	-	-	-	-	-	-	-	-	0.6	1.9	4.5	4.8	11.9	22.6	18.6	27.8	39.5	44.1	5.6	1.0	0.12	0.32	2.8	156
Pancreas	300	0	-	-	-	-	-	0.6	0.6	1.3	2.4	2.6	8.3	21.9	33.7	33.5	75.7	63.6	74.3	66.1	13.4	2.3	0.36	0.90	7.0	157
Nose, sinuses etc.	34	0	-	-	-	-	-	-	-	1.3	1.2	1.9	1.3	5.5	4.9	2.3	2.7	4.0	4.6	-	1.5	0.3	0.08	0.11	0.9	160
Larynx	480	0	-	-	-	-	-	-	0.6	-	8.4	17.5	25.4	52.7	59.7	84.9	50.5	74.2	62.7	26.4	21.4	3.7	0.82	1.50	12.1	161
Bronchus, lung	2592	0	-	-	-	-	1.1	2.5	10.5	20.9	62.7	121.4	184.8	297.2	432.1	478.0	485.0	459.6	330.4	115.7	19.7	3.51	8.06	62.6	162
Other thoracic organs	16	0	-	-	-	0.6	-	0.6	-	-	-	0.6	0.6	1.4	-	3.1	5.3	1.3	-	4.4	0.7	0.1	0.02	0.06	0.5	163-4
Bone	34	0	-	1.1	1.6	2.5	1.7	1.1	1.3	-	-	1.3	-	2.7	1.4	0.8	1.3	8.0	9.3	-	1.5	0.3	0.07	0.08	1.2	170
Connective tissue	47	0	-	1.1	0.8	-	1.1	-	1.3	1.3	2.4	0.6	2.5	2.1	7.0	5.4	2.7	4.0	9.3	4.4	2.1	0.4	0.10	0.14	1.4	171
Mesothelioma	21	0	-	-	-	-	-	-	-	-	-	0.6	1.9	2.1	2.1	3.9	6.6	-	2.3	-	0.9	0.2	0.03	0.09	0.6	MES
Kaposi's sarcoma	37	0	-	-	-	-	-	0.6	6.3	0.7	3.6	1.9	1.3	0.7	2.1	0.8	5.3	4.0	4.6	-	1.7	0.3	0.09	0.12	1.2	KAP
Melanoma of skin	184	0	-	-	0.6	2.2	3.4	8.2	3.3	9.6	9.1	12.1	14.4	17.6	17.1	21.2	14.6	11.6	26.4	8.2	1.4	0.40	0.59	5.5	172
Other skin	1061	0	-	-	-	0.6	0.6	1.7	5.7	4.6	7.2	16.8	27.3	52.7	78.7	159.6	170.0	257.1	343.5	418.6	47.3		0.98	2.63	23.5	173
Breast	27	0	-	-	-	-	-	-	-	0.7	-	-	1.3	2.1	4.9	4.7	1.3	5.3	4.6	4.4	1.2	0.2	0.04	0.07	0.6	175
Prostate	1231	0	-	-	-	-	-	-	-	-	0.6	1.3	12.1	23.3	72.4	160.4	272.2	398.9	524.6	590.4	54.9	9.4	0.55	2.71	24.4	185
Testis	82	0	1.1	-	0.8	1.3	6.7	6.8	8.2	3.9	3.6	4.5	3.8	4.1	0.7	1.6	2.7	5.3	2.3	-	3.7	0.6	0.23	0.25	3.2	186
Penis	29	0	-	-	-	-	-	-	-	-	-	1.3	0.6	2.1	3.5	5.4	6.6	4.0	7.0	-	1.3	0.2	0.04	0.10	0.7	187.1-.4
Other male genital	7	0	-	-	-	-	-	-	-	-	0.6	-	-	-	-	2.3	-	2.7	2.3	-	0.3	0.1	0.00	0.01	0.1	187.5-.9
†Bladder	1498	0	-	-	-	-	0.6	1.7	1.9	3.9	16.7	32.3	51.5	99.2	152.4	232.8	294.8	304.8	338.9	295.2	66.9	11.4	1.80	4.44	35.2	188
Kidney etc.	490	0	1.1	-	1.6	0.6	0.6	1.1	1.9	3.9	4.8	16.2	20.3	39.7	50.6	66.9	90.3	100.7	83.6	57.3	21.9	3.7	0.71	1.50	12.2	189
Eye	16	0	-	-	-	-	-	-	-	-	-	0.6	0.6	0.7	1.4	3.1	5.3	2.7	2.3	-	0.7	0.1	0.02	0.06	0.4	190
Brain, nervous system	231	0	5.7	5.3	0.8	0.6	0.6	2.3	3.2	5.9	3.6	6.5	14.6	23.3	23.2	23.4	21.2	38.4	34.8	17.6	10.3	1.8	0.48	0.70	7.1	191-2
Thyroid	68	0	-	-	0.8	0.6	1.7	4.5	1.9	2.6	2.4	3.2	4.5	3.4	5.6	6.2	4.0	6.6	7.0	-	3.0	0.5	0.16	0.21	2.2	193
Other endocrine	16	0	-	-	0.8	-	-	-	-	-	0.6	0.6	0.6	1.4	2.1	3.1	2.7	-	2.3	-	0.7	0.1	0.03	0.06	0.5	194
Hodgkin's disease	98	0	-	-	0.8	3.8	3.4	5.6	4.4	4.6	3.6	3.2	7.0	6.8	4.9	3.1	10.6	5.3	11.6	4.4	4.4	0.7	0.24	0.31	3.3	201
Non-Hodgkin lymphoma	346	0	1.1	2.1	1.6	3.2	2.8	5.6	5.1	9.9	7.2	9.7	15.3	24.6	36.5	32.7	63.7	49.0	53.4	39.7	15.4	2.6	0.62	1.11	9.8	200,202
Multiple myeloma	205	0	-	-	-	-	-	-	-	-	0.6	3.2	8.9	10.3	17.6	26.5	39.8	49.0	55.7	88.1	9.1	1.6	0.20	0.53	4.6	203
Lymphoid leukaemia	131	0	3.4	2.1	0.8	2.5	1.1	0.6	1.3	0.7	0.6	2.6	3.2	4.8	9.8	20.2	18.6	26.5	30.2	48.5	5.8	1.0	0.17	0.36	3.7	204
Myeloid leukaemia	139	0	-	1.1	-	0.6	0.6	2.8	3.2	0.7	3.6	7.1	4.5	11.6	9.1	17.1	13.3	30.5	30.2	13.2	6.2	1.1	0.22	0.38	3.7	205
Monocytic leukaemia	1	0	-	-	-	-	-	-	-	-	-	-	-	-	-	-	-	1.3	-	-	0.0	0.0	0.00	0.00	0.0	206
Other leukaemia	1	0	-	-	-	-	-	-	-	-	-	-	-	-	-	-	-	1.3	-	-	0.0	0.0	0.00	0.00	0.0	207
Leukaemia unspecified	44	0	-	-	-	1.3	1.1	-	-	-	1.3	-	2.7	1.4	5.4	10.6	8.0	16.2	17.6	2.0	0.3	0.04	0.12	1.1	208
Other and unspecified	368	0	-	-	-	0.6	0.6	-	1.3	0.7	4.2	7.8	9.5	15.1	39.3	42.0	70.4	63.6	120.7	193.9	16.4	2.8	0.39	0.96	8.5	O&U
All sites	14200	0	13.7	13.7	10.6	20.2	26.4	43.4	67.8	81.5	143.4	308.6	509.9	892.3	1349.5	2019.4	2534.7	2955.1	3474.7	3529.1	633.7		17.41	40.18	338.5	ALL
All sites but 173	13139	0	13.7	13.7	10.6	19.6	25.9	41.8	62.1	76.9	136.2	291.7	482.6	839.6	1270.8	1859.8	2364.8	2698.0	3131.2	3110.5	586.4	100.0	16.43	37.55	315.0	ALLb

Rate from 1 case   1.145 1.056 0.815 0.632 0.562 0.564 0.633 0.657 0.598 0.647 0.636 0.684 0.702 0.778 1.328 1.325 2.321 4.406

†Important: see notes on population page

ITALY, FLORENCE 1988-1991

ANNUAL INCIDENCE PER 100,000 BY AGE GROUP (YEARS) - FEMALE

SITE	ALL AGES	AGE UNK	0-	5-	10-	15-	20-	25-	30-	35-	40-	45-	50-	55-	60-	65-	70-	75-	80-	85+	CRUDE RATE	%	CR 64	CR 74	ASR (W)	ICD (9th)
Lip	7	0	-	-	-	-	-	-	-	-	-	-	-	0.6	-	0.6	2.0	-	1.3	3.5	0.3	0.1	0.00	0.02	**0.1**	140
Tongue	27	0	-	-	-	-	-	0.6	-	0.6	1.7	-	0.6	1.3	1.9	1.3	5.0	4.3	2.5	3.5	1.1	0.2	0.03	0.06	**0.6**	141
Salivary gland	17	0	-	-	-	-	1.2	0.6	0.6	-	-	-	0.6	0.6	2.5	0.6	1.0	1.7	1.3	3.5	0.7	0.2	0.03	0.04	**0.4**	142
Mouth	46	0	-	-	-	-	-	-	-	-	1.7	3.1	1.2	2.6	4.4	1.9	2.0	6.1	6.3	13.9	1.9	0.4	0.06	0.08	**0.9**	143-5
Oropharynx	17	0	-	-	-	-	-	0.6	-	-	-	0.6	1.8	0.6	1.9	1.9	2.0	-	1.3	3.5	0.7	0.2	0.03	0.05	**0.4**	146
Nasopharynx	15	0	-	-	-	0.7	-	-	1.3	-	-	0.6	0.6	1.3	1.9	1.3	1.0	0.9	1.3	-	0.6	0.1	0.03	0.04	**0.4**	147
Hypopharynx	6	0	-	-	-	-	-	-	-	-	0.6	-	0.6	0.6	-	0.6	-	-	-	3.5	0.2	0.1	0.01	0.01	**0.1**	148
Pharynx unspecified	5	0	-	-	-	-	-	-	-	-	-	-	-	-	-	0.6	1.0	-	1.3	3.5	0.2	0.0	0.00	0.01	**0.1**	149
Oesophagus	58	0	-	-	-	-	-	-	-	-	0.6	-	1.2	1.3	3.2	8.4	9.9	4.3	10.1	20.9	2.4	0.5	0.03	0.12	**0.9**	150
Stomach	1113	0	-	-	-	-	0.6	1.2	1.9	3.2	5.7	15.3	19.0	28.1	46.0	81.1	133.0	206.9	268.3	359.9	45.8	9.9	0.60	1.68	**15.9**	151
Small intestine	29	0	-	-	-	-	-	-	-	-	-	-	0.6	1.2	1.3	2.5	3.2	4.0	4.3	2.5	7.0	1.2	0.3	0.03	0.06	**0.5**	152
Colon	1199	0	-	-	-	0.7	-	0.6	1.9	7.6	13.1	24.5	32.7	53.6	71.2	104.3	159.8	194.8	216.7	257.3	49.3	10.6	1.03	2.35	**20.2**	153
Rectum	548	0	-	-	-	-	0.6	-	0.6	2.5	5.1	9.2	21.4	26.8	36.6	56.6	59.5	82.6	98.3	106.1	22.6	4.9	0.51	1.10	**9.4**	154
Liver	223	0	-	-	-	-	-	-	-	0.6	1.1	1.2	1.8	5.1	13.9	23.2	32.7	35.6	50.4	60.9	9.2	2.0	0.12	0.40	**3.3**	155
Gallbladder etc.	195	0	-	-	-	-	-	-	-	-	-	1.8	3.0	7.7	11.3	14.8	32.7	30.4	45.4	52.2	8.0	1.7	0.12	0.36	**2.9**	156
Pancreas	330	0	-	-	-	-	-	-	-	1.3	2.3	2.5	5.4	10.8	19.5	29.6	46.6	59.1	69.3	81.7	13.6	2.9	0.21	0.59	**5.0**	157
Nose, sinuses etc.	7	0	-	-	-	-	-	-	-	-	0.6	0.6	-	-	0.6	1.3	-	-	1.3	1.7	0.3	0.1	0.01	0.02	**0.1**	160
Larynx	48	0	-	-	-	-	-	-	-	-	0.6	0.6	1.8	1.2	1.9	2.5	8.4	5.0	8.7	5.0	3.5	2.0	0.4	0.04	0.11	**0.9**	161
Bronchus, lung	600	0	-	-	-	-	-	0.6	1.3	2.5	9.7	13.5	22.6	34.4	51.7	59.2	71.4	80.9	99.5	76.5	24.7	5.3	0.68	1.33	**11.1**	162
Other thoracic organs	15	0	-	-	0.9	-	-	-	-	-	-	1.2	0.6	0.6	-	0.6	5.0	1.7	1.3	1.7	0.6	0.1	0.02	0.04	**0.4**	163-4
Bone	23	0	-	-	3.4	0.7	0.6	0.6	-	0.6	0.6	-	0.6	0.6	1.3	2.6	1.0	1.7	1.3	3.5	0.9	0.2	0.04	0.06	**0.8**	170
Connective tissue	58	0	2.4	-	-	0.7	1.2	0.6	0.6	3.8	3.4	3.1	3.0	3.2	3.2	4.5	2.0	4.3	3.8	3.5	2.4	0.5	0.13	0.16	**1.8**	171
Mesothelioma	12	0	-	-	-	-	-	-	-	-	0.6	-	1.2	1.9	1.3	0.6	1.0	0.9	1.3	-	0.5	0.1	0.02	0.03	**0.3**	MES
Kaposi's sarcoma	10	0	-	-	-	-	-	-	-	-	-	-	0.6	-	0.6	0.6	3.0	2.6	-	1.7	0.4	0.1	0.01	0.02	**0.2**	KAP
Melanoma of skin	208	0	-	-	-	1.3	2.9	4.1	5.7	6.3	8.0	9.2	11.3	9.6	17.6	18.0	12.9	17.4	12.6	22.6	8.6	1.8	0.38	0.53	**5.2**	172
Other skin	717	0	-	-	-	-	0.6	0.6	5.0	4.4	7.4	9.8	22.0	26.1	35.9	53.4	78.4	122.6	154.9	191.3	29.5		0.56	1.22	**11.4**	173
Breast	2873	0	-	-	-	-	1.2	5.9	18.9	56.4	120.3	196.8	184.5	193.2	208.0	256.2	255.0	253.0	243.1	222.5	118.2	25.5	4.93	7.48	**67.0**	174
Uterus unspecified	42	0	-	-	-	-	-	-	0.6	-	-	1.2	0.6	0.6	3.8	3.2	3.0	5.2	7.6	19.1	1.7	0.4	0.03	0.07	**0.7**	179
Cervix uteri	253	0	-	-	-	-	1.8	1.8	3.8	12.0	15.4	12.9	13.7	16.6	11.3	19.3	24.8	24.3	18.9	15.6	10.4	2.2	0.45	0.67	**6.2**	180
Placenta	2	0	-	-	-	-	-	-	0.6	0.6	0.6	-	-	-	-	-	-	-	-	-	0.1	0.0	0.01	0.01	**0.1**	181
Corpus uteri	550	0	-	-	-	-	-	-	2.5	2.5	8.6	22.1	49.4	41.5	54.2	54.7	60.5	54.8	44.1	22.6	22.6	4.9	0.90	1.48	**12.2**	182
Ovary etc.	411	0	-	-	0.9	1.3	-	3.5	4.4	5.1	13.7	21.5	28.6	24.9	29.6	41.2	33.7	41.7	36.5	33.0	16.9	3.6	0.67	1.04	**9.4**	183
Other female genital	111	0	-	-	-	-	0.6	0.6	-	1.3	2.3	0.6	3.6	2.6	5.0	10.9	15.9	14.8	21.4	29.6	4.6	1.0	0.08	0.22	**1.9**	184
†Bladder	363	0	-	-	-	0.7	1.2	-	1.3	2.5	1.1	4.3	12.5	20.4	20.8	23.2	47.6	58.3	76.8	81.7	14.9	3.2	0.32	0.68	**6.0**	188
Kidney etc.	256	0	2.4	-	0.9	0.7	0.6	1.2	1.9	1.3	5.1	6.1	13.1	17.2	20.8	21.9	37.7	22.6	42.8	19.1	10.5	2.3	0.36	0.65	**5.6**	189
Eye	16	0	-	-	0.9	-	-	-	-	-	-	2.5	-	1.9	-	0.6	1.0	3.5	2.5	-	0.7	0.1	0.03	0.03	**0.4**	190
Brain, nervous system	204	0	2.4	2.2	2.6	2.6	1.8	2.3	1.3	3.8	2.9	5.5	11.9	10.8	18.9	17.4	21.8	27.0	15.1	8.7	8.4	1.8	0.34	0.54	**5.2**	191-2
Thyroid	154	0	-	-	-	2.0	1.8	3.5	8.2	5.1	12.0	9.8	10.1	8.9	7.6	9.7	3.0	7.0	12.6	8.7	6.3	1.4	0.34	0.41	**4.4**	193
Other endocrine	18	0	1.2	-	-	-	-	1.2	-	-	0.6	1.2	0.6	-	1.3	2.6	2.0	1.7	-	1.7	0.7	0.2	0.03	0.05	**0.6**	194
Hodgkin's disease	79	0	-	-	-	3.9	4.1	6.5	3.8	4.4	3.4	2.5	3.0	3.8	3.8	2.6	5.0	2.6	2.5	1.7	3.3	0.7	0.20	0.23	**2.7**	201
Non-Hodgkin lymphoma	294	0	1.2	-	-	2.6	0.6	2.3	3.2	6.3	7.4	8.6	8.9	17.2	21.4	23.2	37.7	38.3	45.4	20.9	12.1	2.6	0.40	0.70	**6.3**	200,202
Multiple myeloma	172	0	-	-	-	-	-	-	0.6	1.3	-	3.1	7.7	6.4	10.1	17.4	25.8	27.8	30.2	27.8	7.1	1.5	0.15	0.36	**2.9**	203
Lymphoid leukaemia	89	0	2.4	2.2	3.4	2.6	0.6	1.2	0.6	2.5	1.7	0.6	1.8	2.6	3.8	4.5	12.9	11.3	10.1	19.1	3.7	0.8	0.13	0.22	**2.5**	204
Myeloid leukaemia	114	0	2.4	2.2	0.9	0.7	1.2	0.6	1.9	3.8	1.1	1.2	3.6	5.7	5.7	10.3	13.9	16.5	15.1	12.2	4.7	1.0	0.15	0.28	**2.8**	205
Monocytic leukaemia	3	0	-	-	-	-	-	-	-	-	-	-	-	-	-	-	0.9	2.5	-	-	0.1	0.0	0.00	0.00	**0.0**	206
Other leukaemia	2	0	1.2	-	-	-	-	-	-	-	-	-	-	-	-	-	-	0.9	-	-	0.1	0.0	0.01	0.01	**0.2**	207
Leukaemia unspecified	27	0	-	-	0.9	0.7	-	-	-	-	-	-	0.6	-	0.6	0.6	4.0	6.1	5.0	12.2	1.1	0.2	0.01	0.04	**0.4**	208
Other and unspecified	434	0	1.2	-	-	-	-	1.8	0.6	2.5	1.1	8.0	6.0	15.3	17.6	33.5	45.6	58.3	107.1	170.4	17.9	3.8	0.27	0.67	**6.5**	O&U
All sites	12000	0	16.7	6.6	14.6	21.7	22.9	42.3	72.5	145.7	260.1	407.0	514.2	610.3	775.8	1032.5	1322.8	1548.4	1796.4	2013.4	493.8		14.55	26.33	**237.4**	ALL
All sites but 173	11283	0	16.7	6.6	14.6	21.7	22.3	41.7	67.4	141.3	252.7	397.2	492.1	584.1	739.9	979.1	1244.4	1425.9	1641.4	1822.1	464.3	100.0	13.99	25.11	**226.0**	ALLb
Rate from 1 case			1.195	1.105	0.856	0.658	0.588	0.587	0.630	0.634	0.570	0.613	0.595	0.638	0.630	0.644	0.992	0.869	1.260	1.739						

†Important: see notes on population page

Italy, Genoa

The Ligurian Tumour Registry belongs to the Health Councillorship of the region of Liguria and is part of the Tumour Registry Department of the National Institute for Cancer Research (IST) of Genoa

This department is engaged in the field of descriptive epidemiology and is functionally divided into two research units: the Tumour Registry and the Mortality Registry of the Region of Liguria.

The former was established in 1984, as the Genoa Tumour Registry. After two years of collection of prevalence data, production of incidence data was begun in 1986. Until 1992 incidence data covered only the population of the city of Genoa. In October 1993, the Liguria Region extended registration to the population of the province (940 443 inhabitants in January 1993). The three-year Cancer Plan of the Region of Liguria envisaged extension to the entire region (population 1 668 881 inhabitants in January 1993) from 1996.

Genoa, situated on the coast of the Gulf of Liguria, is the main city of the region of Liguria and one of the largest metropolitan areas in north-western Italy. While it stretches for 27 km along the coast, developed areas inland are limited to two narrow valleys. The Apennine mountain range creates a natural barrier which forces a sometimes difficult coexistence between residential and industrial areas. Thus, the inhabited area is only 73.5 km^2 out of a total of 239.6 km^2.

The population of Genoa on 31 December 1993 was 659 754 inhabitants, a significant decrease since the maximum attained in 1971 (842 114 inhabitants). The crude birth rate is only 6.5/1000, one of the lowest in Italy, whereas the death rate is 13.7/1000, one of the highest, due to the ageing of the population (median ages at death are 79 and 82 years for males and females, respectively). The decreasing trend in population is also related to short-range emigration, especially towards smaller towns situated along the coast.

During the 1980s Genoa was hit by a drastic decline in industrial activity, and subsequent economic recovery has thus far been poor.

As concerns air pollution, on the basis of criteria set by the province of Genoa, in 1993, warning levels were exceeded 25 times for NO_2 alone, 23 times for O_3 alone, twice for NO_2/O_3 together, 16 times for CO alone and twice for CO/NO_2 together.

As of December 1995, all cases of cancer among residents of the province of Genoa are collected by the registry staff through regular consultation of some 215 000 clinical records available each year from all public (17) and private (4) hospitals (outpatients included), and radiotherapy and anatomo-pathological departments throughout the territory. Further data are provided by the discharge records of the two main hospitals.

Another information source is the mortality registry, which, in addition to the principal cause of death, systematically codes data on any cancer mentioned on the death certificate and supplies the tumour registry with a copy of the certificate for each death from cancer. For cancer deaths not previously notified, the tumour registry attempts to trace information. Unsuccessful attempts are included among death-certificate-only cases.

The tumour registry records data on all malignant tumours, on carcinomas *in situ* and on other tumours of benign and uncertain nature of the urinary tract, brain and CNS and the liver. While all data pertinent to the above are registered, the only non-malignant tumours included in the incidence figures for malignant cancers are those for bladder. Multiple primary cancers (except for multiple skin cancers) are included as independent primary tumours.

Tumours are coded according to ICD-9 and ICD-O. The information recorded includes name, sex, place and date of birth, address, site, morphology and behaviour of the neoplasm, additional data on stage and grading of disease (such as p-TNM, Dukes, Clarks, etc., if recorded), and the source of notification.

To produce survival data, registry data are checked at least annually through record linkage with the data of the General Registry of Genoa and the mortality registry, providing information on vital status, migration and the cause of death of each recorded case.

The registry collaborates with all other Italian registries in research projects and publication of incidence, mortality and survival data. It contributes to the EUROCARE II project and to an analysis of cancer survival in Italy performed in conjunction with the Istituto Superiore di Sanità and the Istituto Nazionale Tumori of Milan.

The tumour registry also carries out two specific research programmes involving one or both registries, in collaboration with other regional and national bodies. These aim to produce national figures on incidence, mortality and survival in the elderly Italian population as a step towards validating a new instrument for standardized decision-making on whether to subject elderly patients to cancer therapy, and to assess cancer risk among the AIDS/HIV-positive subjects resident in the region of Liguria.

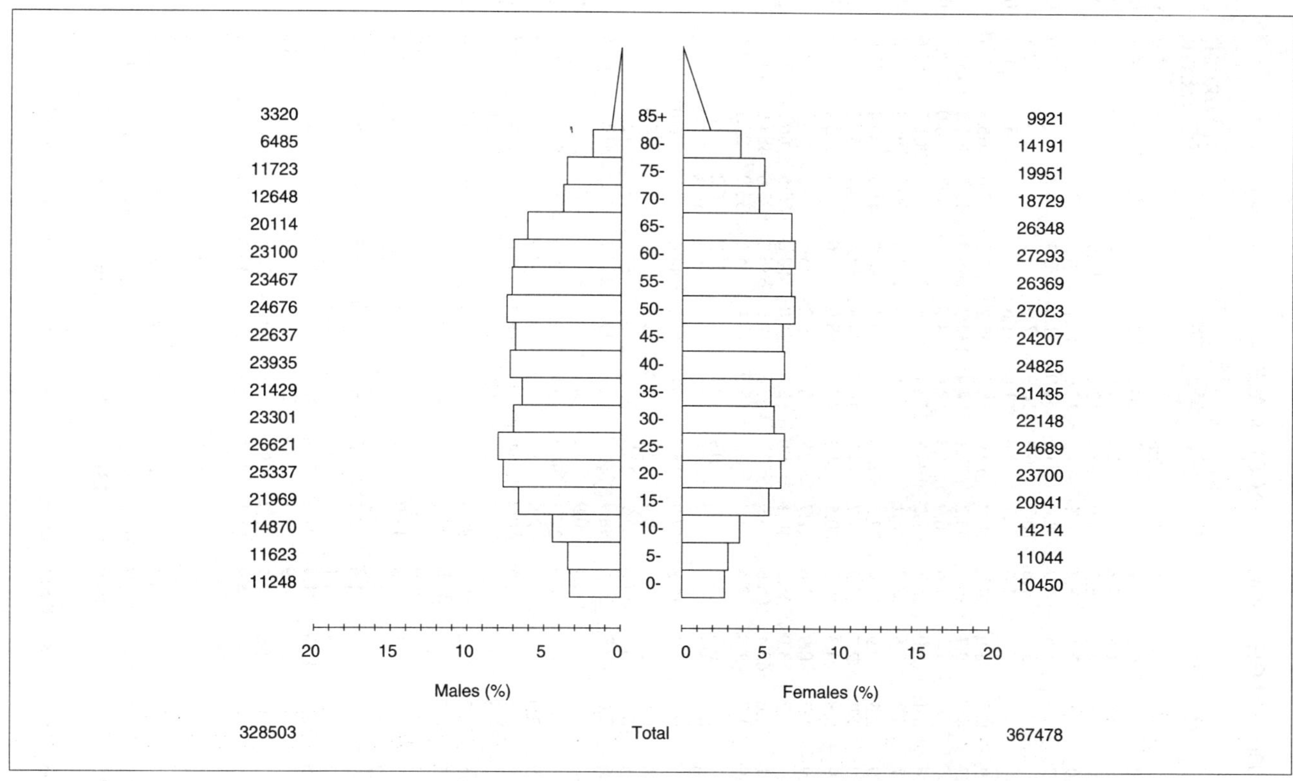

Italy, Genoa
Source of population: average annual 1988–92
Estimate: The population data are collected for ISTAT by the
Statistical Department of the Municipality of Genoa, using the
files of the official residents.

ITALY, GENOA 1988-1992

ANNUAL INCIDENCE PER 100,000 BY AGE GROUP (YEARS) - MALE

SITE	ALL AGES	AGE UNK	0-	5-	10-	15-	20-	25-	30-	35-	40-	45-	50-	55-	60-	65-	70-	75-	80-	85+	CRUDE RATE	%	CR 64	CR 74	ASR (W)	ICD (9th)
Lip	15	0	-	-	-	-	-	-	-	-	-	-	2.4	1.7	2.6	-	3.2	5.1	-	12.0	0.9	0.1	0.03	0.05	**0.5**	140
Tongue	72	0	-	-	-	-	-	0.8	-	0.9	1.7	6.2	4.9	6.0	11.3	10.9	22.1	8.5	15.4	-	4.4	0.7	0.16	0.32	**2.5**	141
Salivary gland	29	0	-	-	-	-	-	-	-	-	0.8	1.8	3.2	4.3	4.3	4.0	3.2	3.4	6.2	12.0	1.8	0.3	0.07	0.11	**1.0**	142
Mouth	70	0	-	-	-	-	-	0.9	0.9	1.7	4.4	6.5	6.0	10.4	12.7	12.9	12.7	11.9	9.3	18.1	4.3	0.7	0.15	0.28	**2.3**	143-5
Oropharynx	68	0	-	-	-	-	-	-	-	0.9	3.3	7.1	3.2	9.4	11.3	12.9	12.7	8.5	3.1	-	4.1	0.6	0.18	0.30	**2.4**	146
Nasopharynx	33	0	-	-	-	0.9	-	0.8	2.6	1.9	-	1.8	4.9	2.6	3.5	6.0	1.6	3.4	6.2	-	2.0	0.3	0.09	0.13	**1.3**	147
Hypopharynx	45	0	-	-	-	-	-	-	-	-	-	3.5	1.6	10.2	6.9	10.9	7.9	5.1	-	-	2.7	0.4	0.11	0.21	**1.5**	148
Pharynx unspecified	8	0	-	-	-	-	-	-	-	-	-	-	1.6	1.7	0.9	1.0	1.6	-	-	6.0	0.5	0.1	0.02	0.03	**0.3**	149
Oesophagus	126	0	-	-	-	-	-	-	-	0.9	0.8	8.0	4.1	10.2	19.0	18.9	33.2	22.2	37.0	66.3	7.7	1.2	0.22	0.48	**3.9**	150
Stomach	625	0	-	-	-	-	-	0.8	0.9	4.7	4.2	9.7	25.9	33.2	77.1	104.4	132.8	209.8	246.7	301.2	38.1	5.9	0.78	1.97	**17.6**	151
Small intestine	21	0	-	-	-	-	-	-	-	-	-	-	1.6	0.9	4.3	3.0	4.7	6.8	6.2	6.0	1.3	0.2	0.03	0.07	**0.6**	152
Colon	913	0	-	-	-	1.8	-	0.8	0.9	5.6	8.4	15.0	36.5	91.2	106.5	154.1	186.6	284.9	342.3	301.2	55.6	8.6	1.33	3.04	**26.2**	153
Rectum	456	0	-	-	-	-	-	-	0.9	3.7	4.2	8.8	22.7	28.1	57.1	75.6	115.4	124.5	166.5	198.8	27.8	4.3	0.63	1.58	**13.2**	154
Liver	371	0	-	-	-	-	-	0.8	-	1.9	2.5	0.9	15.4	37.5	46.8	83.5	79.1	88.7	141.9	90.4	22.6	3.5	0.53	1.34	**10.7**	155
Gallbladder etc.	123	0	-	-	-	-	-	-	-	1.9	1.7	2.7	3.2	1.7	14.7	19.9	34.8	32.4	70.9	54.2	7.5	1.2	0.13	0.40	**3.4**	156
Pancreas	277	0	-	-	-	-	-	-	-	1.9	5.8	13.3	10.5	20.5	24.2	48.7	68.0	83.6	92.5	102.4	16.9	2.6	0.38	0.96	**8.2**	157
Nose, sinuses etc.	27	0	-	1.7	-	-	-	-	-	1.9	1.7	0.9	1.6	1.7	1.7	8.9	3.2	5.1	3.1	-	1.6	0.3	0.06	0.12	**1.1**	160
Larynx	380	0	-	-	-	-	-	-	-	-	4.2	23.9	25.1	40.1	71.0	62.6	98.0	58.0	55.5	66.3	23.1	3.6	0.82	1.62	**12.4**	161
Bronchus, lung	2418	0	-	-	-	-	-	-	0.9	12.1	22.6	65.4	108.6	213.9	350.6	467.3	612.0	636.4	623.0	488.0	147.2	22.8	3.87	9.27	**72.2**	162
Other thoracic organs	68	0	-	-	-	-	-	-	0.9	1.9	1.7	1.8	2.4	4.3	2.6	8.9	17.4	25.6	33.9	24.1	4.1	0.6	0.08	0.21	**1.9**	163-4
Bone	19	0	-	-	-	1.8	-	1.5	0.9	-	-	0.9	3.2	-	0.9	-	4.7	1.7	6.2	-	1.2	0.2	0.05	0.08	**0.8**	170
Connective tissue	69	0	-	3.4	1.3	-	0.8	2.3	-	1.9	2.5	2.7	7.3	11.1	6.9	5.0	7.9	15.4	12.3	6.0	4.2	0.6	0.20	0.27	**2.8**	171
Mesothelioma	161	0	-	-	-	-	-	-	-	-	0.8	6.2	17.8	17.9	15.6	30.8	41.1	44.4	24.7	6.0	9.8	1.5	0.29	0.65	**5.0**	MES
Kaposi's sarcoma	47	0	-	-	-	0.9	0.8	1.5	5.1	5.6	0.8	2.7	3.2	0.9	2.6	7.0	9.5	8.5	-	6.0	2.9	0.4	0.12	0.20	**1.9**	KAP
Melanoma of skin	126	0	-	-	-	-	0.8	3.0	6.0	6.5	10.9	15.9	17.0	7.7	14.7	13.9	6.3	13.6	3.1	12.0	7.7	1.2	0.41	0.51	**5.2**	172
Other skin	1109	0	-	-	-	0.9	0.8	-	4.3	5.6	22.6	32.7	57.5	98.9	130.7	201.8	249.8	293.4	333.1	319.3	67.5		1.77	4.03	**33.4**	173
Breast	18	0	-	-	-	-	-	-	0.9	-	-	-	2.4	0.9	5.2	4.0	-	3.4	3.1	-	1.1	0.2	0.05	0.07	**0.6**	175
Prostate	965	0	-	-	-	-	-	-	-	-	-	4.4	4.9	21.3	96.1	168.0	267.2	406.0	478.0	524.1	58.8	9.1	0.63	2.81	**24.7**	185
Testis	79	0	1.8	-	-	3.6	7.1	5.3	18.9	14.9	2.5	1.8	4.1	2.6	1.7	2.0	1.6	3.4	-	-	4.8	0.7	0.32	0.34	**4.3**	186
Penis	22	0	-	-	-	-	-	-	-	-	0.8	-	1.6	0.9	0.9	4.0	3.2	3.4	15.4	24.1	1.3	0.2	0.02	0.06	**0.6**	187.1-.4
Other male genital	8	0	-	-	-	-	-	-	-	-	0.8	0.9	-	0.9	1.0	-	3.4	-	12.0	0.5	0.1	0.01	0.02	**0.3**	187.5-.9
Bladder	1281	0	-	-	-	-	0.8	-	6.9	5.6	24.2	36.2	68.1	98.0	152.4	238.6	322.6	336.1	404.0	295.2	78.0	12.1	1.96	4.77	**38.3**	188
Kidney etc.	344	0	1.8	-	-	-	-	-	-	6.5	5.8	8.8	21.9	34.1	56.3	58.7	79.1	76.8	70.9	60.2	20.9	3.2	0.68	1.36	**11.0**	189
Eye	10	0	3.6	-	-	-	0.8	-	-	-	-	-	1.6	-	-	1.0	3.2	1.7	3.1	-	0.6	0.1	0.03	0.05	**0.7**	190
Brain, nervous system	150	0	8.9	3.4	1.3	3.6	1.6	-	3.4	3.7	2.5	7.1	13.8	11.9	13.0	21.9	31.6	34.1	18.5	18.1	9.1	1.4	0.37	0.64	**6.5**	191-2
Thyroid	49	0	-	-	1.3	-	0.8	0.8	0.9	1.9	1.7	1.8	4.1	5.1	2.6	5.0	11.1	11.9	9.3	18.1	3.0	0.5	0.10	0.18	**1.8**	193
Other endocrine	14	0	3.6	-	-	-	-	-	0.9	-	1.7	-	1.6	0.9	-	1.0	4.7	1.7	-	6.0	0.9	0.1	0.04	0.07	**0.9**	194
Hodgkin's disease	72	0	-	-	2.7	4.6	7.1	3.8	7.7	4.7	4.2	1.8	4.1	5.1	6.9	7.0	4.7	1.7	-	-	4.4	0.7	0.26	0.32	**3.6**	201
Non-Hodgkin lymphoma	356	0	1.8	3.4	5.4	1.8	3.2	12.8	12.9	7.5	16.7	13.3	21.9	21.3	29.4	46.7	83.8	69.9	83.3	84.3	21.7	3.4	0.76	1.41	**13.2**	200,202
Multiple myeloma	132	0	-	-	-	-	-	-	0.9	-	-	2.7	4.9	9.4	13.9	23.9	26.9	40.9	49.3	84.3	8.0	1.2	0.16	0.41	**3.7**	203
Lymphoid leukaemia	102	0	5.3	1.7	4.0	-	0.8	0.8	0.9	3.7	-	1.8	4.1	7.7	8.7	16.9	14.2	34.1	30.8	36.1	6.2	1.0	0.20	0.35	**4.0**	204
Myeloid leukaemia	83	0	-	-	2.7	-	1.6	1.5	0.9	1.9	3.3	-	4.9	5.1	13.0	12.9	14.2	13.6	24.7	30.1	5.1	0.8	0.17	0.31	**2.9**	205
Monocytic leukaemia	0	0	-	-	-	-	-	-	-	-	-	-	-	-	-	-	-	-	-	-	0.0	0.0	0.00	0.00	**0.0**	206
Other leukaemia	1	0	-	-	-	-	-	-	-	-	-	-	-	-	-	-	-	1.7	-	-	0.1	0.0	0.00	0.00	**0.0**	207
Leukaemia unspecified	20	0	-	-	-	-	-	-	0.9	0.8	0.9	-	0.9	0.9	1.0	4.7	8.5	12.3	12.0	1.2	0.2	0.02	0.05	**0.6**	208
Other and unspecified	350	0	-	-	-	-	0.8	-	-	0.9	2.5	6.2	6.5	23.9	43.3	60.7	88.6	104.1	157.3	138.6	21.3	3.3	0.42	1.17	**9.8**	O&U
All sites	11732	0	26.7	13.8	18.8	20.0	27.6	36.8	79.0	112.9	170.5	323.4	562.5	910.2	1443.3	2049.3	2730.9	3157.9	3599.1	3439.8	714.3		18.73	42.63	**359.5**	ALL
All sites but 173	10623	0	26.7	13.8	18.8	19.1	26.8	36.8	74.7	107.3	147.9	290.7	504.9	811.4	1312.6	1847.5	2481.0	2864.5	3266.0	3120.5	646.8	100.0	16.96	38.60	**326.1**	ALLb

Rate from 1 case: 1.778 1.721 1.345 0.910 0.789 0.751 0.858 0.933 0.836 0.884 0.811 0.852 0.866 0.994 1.581 1.706 3.084 6.024

ITALY, GENOA 1988-1992

ANNUAL INCIDENCE PER 100,000 BY AGE GROUP (YEARS) - FEMALE

SITE	ALL AGES	AGE UNK	0-	5-	10-	15-	20-	25-	30-	35-	40-	45-	50-	55-	60-	65-	70-	75-	80-	85+	CRUDE RATE	%	CR 64	CR 74	ASR (W)	ICD (9th)
Lip	2	0	-	-	-	-	-	-	-	-	-	-	-	-	-	1.5	-	-	-	-	0.1	0.0	0.00	0.01	**0.0**	*140*
Tongue	37	0	-	-	-	-	-	-	-	-	0.8	-	3.0	0.8	3.7	5.3	3.2	3.0	8.5	14.1	2.0	0.4	0.04	0.08	**0.7**	*141*
Salivary gland	16	0	-	-	-	-	-	-	-	-	-	-	0.7	0.8	1.5	1.5	4.3	2.0	2.8	4.0	0.9	0.2	0.01	0.04	**0.3**	*142*
Mouth	40	0	-	-	-	-	-	-	-	-	-	0.8	-	2.3	3.7	4.6	5.3	5.0	12.7	12.1	2.2	0.4	0.03	0.08	**0.7**	*143-5*
Oropharynx	17	0	-	-	-	-	-	-	-	-	-	0.8	1.5	1.5	1.5	2.3	2.1	2.0	-	6.0	0.9	0.2	0.03	0.05	**0.4**	*146*
Nasopharynx	7	0	-	-	-	-	-	-	-	1.9	-	1.7	-	-	-	0.8	2.1	-	-	-	0.4	0.1	0.02	0.03	**0.3**	*147*
Hypopharynx	14	0	-	-	-	-	-	0.8	-	-	-	0.8	-	1.5	-	1.5	2.1	2.0	2.8	4.0	0.8	0.2	0.02	0.03	**0.3**	*148*
Pharynx unspecified	0	0	-	-	-	-	-	-	-	-	-	-	-	-	-	-	-	-	-	-	0.0	0.0	0.00	0.00	**0.0**	*149*
Oesophagus	49	0	-	-	-	-	-	-	-	-	0.8	1.7	2.2	-	5.9	3.0	1.1	12.0	14.1	16.1	2.7	0.5	0.05	0.07	**0.9**	*150*
Stomach	486	0	-	-	-	-	-	-	2.7	1.9	4.8	12.4	12.6	12.9	21.3	38.7	60.9	93.2	136.7	199.6	26.5	5.3	0.34	0.84	**8.3**	*151*
Small intestine	19	0	-	-	-	-	-	-	-	-	-	-	-	1.5	0.7	1.5	3.2	3.0	9.9	2.0	1.0	0.2	0.01	0.03	**0.3**	*152*
Colon	952	0	-	-	-	-	-	0.8	0.9	3.7	15.3	19.0	39.2	45.5	63.0	105.5	126.0	188.5	186.0	258.0	51.8	10.3	0.94	2.10	**18.5**	*153*
Rectum	441	0	-	-	-	-	-	1.6	-	1.9	3.2	8.3	20.0	24.3	36.6	49.3	54.5	79.2	94.4	104.8	24.0	4.8	0.48	1.00	**8.7**	*154*
Liver	198	0	-	-	-	-	0.8	-	-	0.9	-	2.5	5.9	4.6	11.0	20.5	32.0	42.1	43.7	68.5	10.8	2.1	0.13	0.39	**3.4**	*155*
Gallbladder etc.	228	0	-	-	-	-	-	-	-	-	2.4	0.8	5.2	7.6	16.1	22.8	24.6	53.1	56.4	78.6	12.4	2.5	0.16	0.40	**3.8**	*156*
Pancreas	306	0	-	-	-	-	-	-	-	-	0.8	0.8	8.9	11.4	25.6	27.3	48.1	71.2	74.7	74.6	16.7	3.3	0.24	0.61	**5.3**	*157*
Nose, sinuses etc.	19	0	-	-	-	-	0.8	-	-	-	-	0.8	0.7	0.8	1.5	0.8	5.3	5.0	1.4	2.0	1.0	0.2	0.02	0.05	**0.4**	*160*
Larynx	31	0	-	-	-	-	-	-	0.9	-	-	0.7	2.3	5.9	3.8	6.4	5.0	5.0	1.7	-	1.7	0.3	0.05	0.10	**0.7**	*161*
Bronchus, lung	475	0	-	-	-	-	-	1.6	0.9	2.8	4.0	9.1	21.5	29.6	38.1	64.5	83.3	78.2	88.8	58.5	25.9	5.1	0.54	1.28	**10.0**	*162*
Other thoracic organs	34	0	-	-	-	-	-	-	-	0.9	0.8	-	1.5	0.8	-	1.5	5.3	12.0	8.5	8.1	1.9	0.4	0.02	0.05	**0.6**	*163-4*
Bone	21	0	-	1.8	4.2	1.9	0.8	0.8	-	-	-	0.8	-	-	2.2	1.5	1.1	2.0	4.2	2.0	1.1	0.2	0.06	0.08	**1.1**	*170*
Connective tissue	62	0	1.9	1.8	-	-	0.8	2.4	0.9	0.9	1.6	0.8	3.0	5.3	7.3	7.6	6.4	6.0	7.0	6.0	3.4	0.7	0.13	0.20	**2.1**	*171*
Mesothelioma	40	0	-	-	-	-	-	-	-	0.9	-	2.5	3.0	3.0	2.9	3.0	5.3	9.0	7.0	2.0	2.2	0.4	0.06	0.10	**0.9**	*MES*
Kaposi's sarcoma	7	0	-	-	-	-	0.8	0.8	0.9	-	0.8	-	-	-	-	1.1	1.0	1.4	-	-	0.4	0.1	0.02	0.02	**0.3**	*KAP*
Melanoma of skin	165	0	-	-	-	1.0	5.1	5.7	6.3	9.3	11.3	13.2	14.1	12.9	11.0	12.1	8.5	12.0	15.5	12.1	9.0	1.8	0.45	0.55	**5.8**	*172*
Other skin	884	0	-	-	1.0	1.0	2.5	4.1	5.4	14.0	14.5	26.4	37.7	56.1	60.1	88.8	126.0	153.4	157.8	195.5	48.1		1.11	2.18	**19.3**	*173*
Breast	2608	0	-	-	-	-	0.8	6.5	31.6	49.5	133.7	193.3	197.6	221.5	243.3	246.7	284.1	297.7	281.9	266.1	141.9	28.2	5.39	8.04	**72.3**	*174*
Uterus unspecified	52	0	-	-	-	-	-	-	0.9	0.8	1.7	0.7	5.3	1.5	1.5	7.5	8.0	11.3	26.2	-	2.8	0.6	0.05	0.10	**1.0**	*179*
Cervix uteri	260	0	-	-	-	-	-	2.4	9.9	14.0	15.3	19.0	18.5	12.9	21.3	24.3	26.7	31.1	32.4	14.1	14.2	2.8	0.57	0.82	**7.8**	*180*
Placenta	1	0	-	-	-	-	-	-	-	-	-	0.8	-	-	-	-	-	-	-	-	0.1	0.0	0.00	0.00	**0.0**	*181*
Corpus uteri	347	0	-	-	-	-	-	-	0.9	1.9	2.4	17.4	28.1	29.6	33.0	44.0	49.1	46.1	45.1	32.3	18.9	3.8	0.57	1.03	**8.4**	*182*
Ovary etc.	360	0	-	-	1.0	-	0.8	4.1	3.6	6.5	10.5	24.8	22.9	29.6	39.6	27.3	40.6	52.1	45.1	34.3	19.6	3.9	0.72	1.06	**9.7**	*183*
Other female genital	111	0	-	-	-	-	-	-	0.9	-	0.8	4.4	4.6	7.3	7.6	8.5	23.1	32.4	46.4	-	6.0	1.2	0.09	0.17	**1.8**	*184*
Bladder	343	0	-	-	-	1.0	0.8	0.8	-	1.9	7.3	5.0	5.2	13.7	27.1	38.0	56.6	58.1	63.4	110.9	18.7	3.7	0.31	0.79	**6.7**	*188*
Kidney etc.	201	0	3.8	1.8	1.4	1.0	-	-	0.9	2.8	5.6	5.0	5.2	15.9	22.7	18.2	28.8	29.1	36.6	28.2	10.9	2.2	0.33	0.57	**5.3**	*189*
Eye	13	0	1.9	-	-	-	-	-	-	-	-	0.8	0.7	1.5	0.7	0.8	2.1	2.0	1.4	2.0	0.7	0.1	0.03	0.04	**0.5**	*190*
Brain, nervous system	139	0	1.9	-	-	1.0	-	0.8	1.8	3.7	4.0	6.6	7.4	9.1	5.9	25.0	20.3	19.0	14.1	12.1	7.6	1.5	0.21	0.44	**3.8**	*191-2*
Thyroid	121	0	-	-	-	1.0	5.1	0.8	4.5	8.4	6.4	4.1	11.8	5.3	5.9	9.9	10.7	14.0	14.1	16.1	6.6	1.3	0.27	0.37	**3.8**	*193*
Other endocrine	11	0	1.9	-	1.4	-	-	-	-	-	0.8	-	1.5	0.8	-	0.8	2.1	-	2.8	-	0.6	0.1	0.03	0.05	**0.6**	*194*
Hodgkin's disease	48	0	-	-	1.4	1.9	8.4	4.1	1.8	4.7	1.6	2.5	1.5	0.8	0.7	3.8	1.1	5.0	4.2	-	2.6	0.5	0.15	0.17	**2.3**	*201*
Non-Hodgkin lymphoma	308	0	1.9	-	-	-	0.8	7.3	5.4	5.6	9.7	9.9	10.4	12.1	27.1	38.0	40.6	42.1	57.8	46.4	16.8	3.3	0.45	0.84	**7.7**	*200,202*
Multiple myeloma	119	0	-	-	-	-	-	-	-	0.9	0.8	3.3	3.7	4.6	5.1	12.1	19.2	25.1	26.8	34.3	6.5	1.3	0.09	0.25	**2.2**	*203*
Lymphoid leukaemia	75	0	1.9	-	7.0	2.9	-	-	-	0.9	0.8	0.8	3.0	5.3	2.9	6.1	7.5	14.0	16.9	14.1	4.1	0.8	0.13	0.20	**2.4**	*204*
Myeloid leukaemia	92	0	1.9	-	2.8	1.0	-	1.6	2.7	1.9	-	3.3	5.2	3.0	10.3	8.3	12.8	10.0	12.7	20.2	5.0	1.0	0.17	0.27	**2.7**	*205*
Monocytic leukaemia	2	0	-	-	-	-	-	-	-	-	-	-	0.8	-	0.8	-	-	-	-	-	0.1	0.0	0.00	0.01	**0.1**	*206*
Other leukaemia	0	0	-	-	-	-	-	-	-	-	-	-	-	-	-	-	-	-	-	-	0.0	0.0	0.00	0.00	**0.0**	*207*
Leukaemia unspecified	18	0	-	-	-	-	-	-	-	-	-	-	-	-	0.7	1.5	1.1	3.0	8.5	10.1	1.0	0.2	0.00	0.02	**0.2**	*208*
Other and unspecified	345	0	-	-	-	-	0.8	-	0.9	-	2.4	0.8	8.1	12.1	20.5	24.3	47.0	68.2	104.3	133.1	18.8	3.7	0.23	0.59	**5.6**	*O&U*
All sites	10124	0	17.2	5.4	18.3	14.3	28.7	47.8	83.1	143.7	264.2	402.4	517.3	613.6	795.1	1008.8	1284.6	1587.9	1749.0	1975.6	551.0		14.76	26.22	**237.9**	*ALL*
All sites but 173	9240	0	17.2	5.4	18.3	13.4	26.2	43.7	77.7	129.7	249.7	375.9	479.6	557.5	735.0	920.0	1158.6	1434.5	1591.1	1780.1	502.9	100.0	13.65	24.04	**218.7**	*ALLb*
Rate from 1 case			1.914	1.811	1.407	0.955	0.844	0.810	0.903	0.933	0.806	0.826	0.740	0.758	0.733	0.759	1.068	1.002	1.409	2.016						

Italy, Latina Province

The Population Cancer Registry of Latina Province was established by initiative of the local section of the Italian League against Cancer and became one of the operational tools of the Regional Epidemiologic Observatory (OER) following *ad hoc* legislation of the Regional Government of Lazio. The Section of Epidemiology of the National Cancer Institute "Regina Elena" in Rome is the scientific reference centre for the registry.

The registry started data collection in the second half of 1981; official registration started on 1 January 1982. Resolutions of the regional government of Lazio have ensured the continuity of administrative support to the registry, allowing easy and efficient management of information, and requiring the mandatory reporting to the registry of each cancer case observed within the province.

Latina Province has a surface area of 2250 km^2, and is located between latitudes 40°47′ and 41°43′ N and longitudes 12°31′ and 13°37′ E. It is bordered by the provinces of Rome to the north and Frosinone to the east, by the Tyrrhenian Sea to the west and by the Campania Region to the south, along the Garigliano river. The Pontine Islands belong to the territory of the province. The Pontina plain, stretching between Terracina and Torre Astura, occupies about half of the surface of the province, being the result of land reclamation work carried out between 1926 and 1935. The remaining territory comprises the western ridges of the Aurunci and Lepini mountains; there is, in addition, a plain at the south-east border of the province (Plain of Fondi).

At the 20 October 1991 census, 476 282 inhabitants (234 926 males, 241 356 females) were resident in the province; the population density was 212 inhabitants per km^2. Due to the relatively recent formation of Latina Province, and as a consequence of heavy immigration in the 1930s (especially from the Veneto Region of northern Italy), at present only one third of the urban population was born in Latina. The agriculturally productive area is equivalent to 90.3% of the whole territory, and agriculture employs 20 801 persons (12.3% of the working population). Olive and fruit-tree plantations are predominant on the hills; on the plains plantations of vines and vegetables, cereals, sugar beet, hemp, tobacco and cotton are predominant. In recent years, the growing of exotic fruits and greenhouse activities have developed rapidly. The coastal area of Latina Province is one of the most important industrial districts of Lazio, involving 34% of the working population. The most developed branches of the industrial sector are: building, metallurgic, mechanical, extractive and chemical industries (58 068 workers). Fishing, tourism and tertiary industry contribute to the local economy (53.5%). In the territory of the province, since the 1960s, there have been two electronuclear power plants, both at present shut down.

Sources of information are the public and private hospitals of the province, the public diagnostic centres and the pathology laboratory. The registry routinely analyses patients' records from numerous extra-provincial hospitals, particularly from Rome. There are exchanges of information with other Italian cancer registries and with some foreign oncological institutions, such as the Institut Gustave Roussy in France.

The municipal mortality registries and the death certificates collected by the WHO MONICA project, performed by the Istituto Superiore di Sanità in a part of Latina Province, are checked periodically, together with the data available from the nominative registry of causes of death managed by the Epidemiological Observatory of the Lazio Region.

Individual collectors are responsible for collecting information on new cases and the death certificates for their own specific areas. Registration is mandatory, which facilitates the task of the data collectors as they have privileged access to the health and administrative services. The data collected are computerized, after being checked for completeness and accuracy. Death certificates are traced back and only those for which no further notification was found are registered as death-certificate-only cases.

Survival statistics at 31 December 1990 for cases registered over the period 1983–85 have been published.

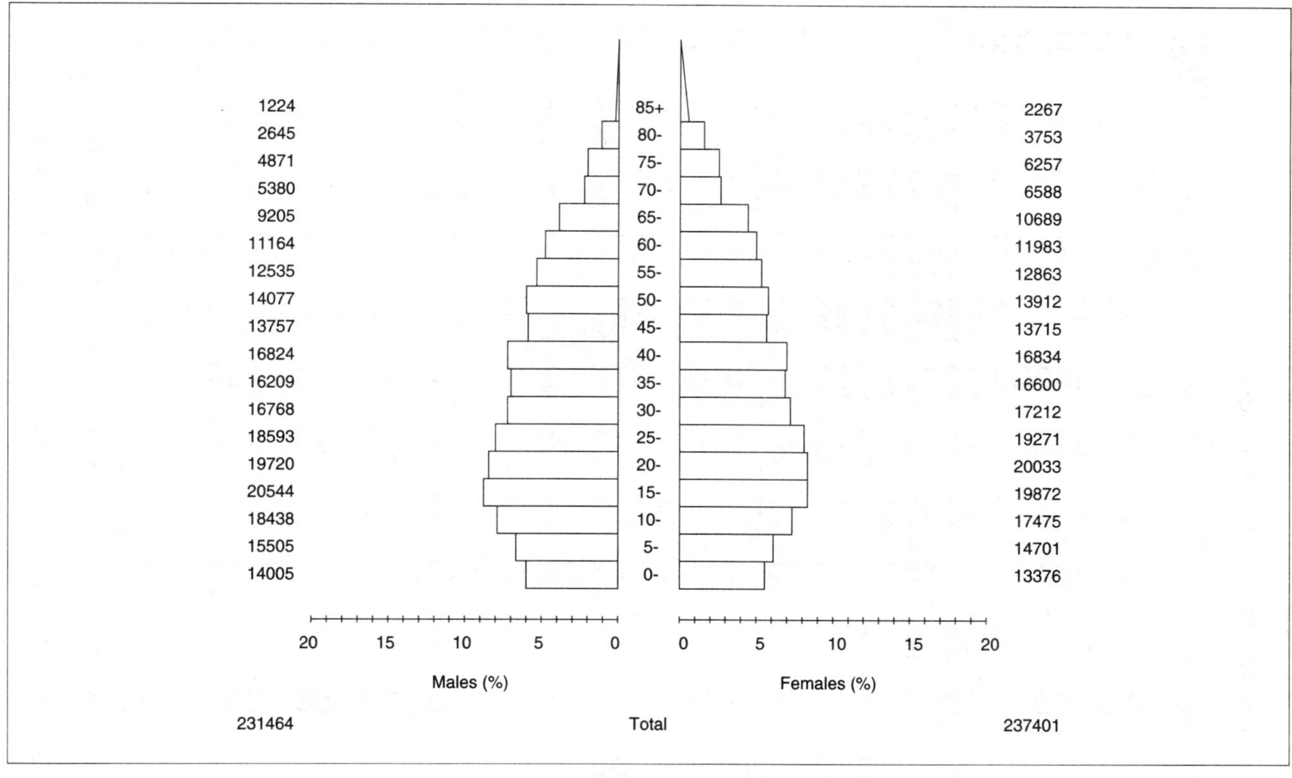

Italy, Latina
Source of population: average annual 1988–91
Estimate: The estimated populations are provided by the National Institute of Health.

Notes to tables overleaf:
* Incidence for a number of sites has increased more than would have been expected since the period reported in Volume VI.

* ITALY, LATINA 1988-1991

ANNUAL INCIDENCE PER 100,000 BY AGE GROUP (YEARS) - MALE

SITE	ALL AGES	AGE UNK	0-	5-	10-	15-	20-	25-	30-	35-	40-	45-	50-	55-	60-	65-	70-	75-	80-	85+	CRUDE RATE	%	CR 64	CR 74	ASR (W)	ICD (9th)
Lip	27	0	-	-	-	-	-	-	-	-	-	-	3.6	8.0	22.4	10.9	13.9	10.3	18.9	-	2.9	0.9	0.17	0.29	**2.2**	140
Tongue	15	0	-	-	-	-	-	-	-	-	1.5	3.6	3.6	4.0	9.0	5.4	9.3	-	-	-	1.6	0.5	0.11	0.18	**1.4**	141
Salivary gland	14	0	-	-	-	-	-	-	-	-	1.5	-	-	4.0	4.5	5.4	13.9	15.4	-	20.4	1.5	0.5	0.05	0.15	**1.1**	142
Mouth	13	0	-	-	-	-	1.3	-	-	-	-	5.5	1.8	6.0	6.7	2.7	4.6	-	-	-	1.4	0.4	0.11	0.14	**1.2**	143-5
Oropharynx	10	0	-	-	-	-	-	-	-	-	1.5	-	3.6	-	4.5	5.4	-	5.1	18.9	-	1.1	0.3	0.05	0.07	**0.8**	146
Nasopharynx	5	0	-	-	-	-	-	-	-	-	1.5	-	1.8	-	2.2	5.4	-	-	-	-	0.5	0.2	0.03	0.05	**0.4**	147
Hypopharynx	4	0	-	-	-	-	-	-	-	-	-	-	1.8	4.0	-	2.7	-	-	-	-	0.4	0.1	0.03	0.04	**0.3**	148
Pharynx unspecified	8	0	-	-	-	-	-	-	-	-	-	1.8	-	4.0	-	2.7	4.6	5.1	9.4	20.4	0.9	0.3	0.03	0.07	**0.6**	149
Oesophagus	31	0	-	-	-	-	-	-	-	-	-	5.5	1.8	6.0	20.2	10.9	23.2	-	37.8	40.8	3.3	1.0	0.17	0.34	**2.6**	150
Stomach	237	0	-	-	-	-	-	-	1.5	6.2	1.5	23.6	37.3	55.8	73.9	92.3	176.6	159.1	189.0	265.5	25.6	8.0	1.00	2.34	**19.2**	151
Small intestine	9	0	-	-	-	-	-	-	-	-	-	-	3.6	2.0	-	8.1	9.3	5.1	-	-	1.0	0.3	0.03	0.11	**0.7**	152
Colon	202	0	1.8	-	-	-	-	-	1.5	3.1	7.4	16.4	17.8	43.9	42.5	108.6	167.3	174.5	170.1	102.1	21.8	6.8	0.67	2.05	**16.0**	153
Rectum	131	0	-	-	-	-	-	-	-	1.5	-	18.2	17.8	23.9	58.2	40.7	65.0	138.6	122.8	61.3	14.1	4.4	0.60	1.13	**10.2**	154
Liver	103	0	-	-	-	1.2	-	-	-	1.5	4.5	3.6	14.2	17.9	22.4	51.6	92.9	92.4	94.5	40.8	11.1	3.5	0.33	1.05	**8.0**	155
Gallbladder etc.	42	0	-	-	-	-	-	-	-	-	-	1.8	3.6	16.0	26.9	16.3	23.2	25.7	-	61.3	4.5	1.4	0.24	0.44	**3.5**	156
Pancreas	67	0	-	-	-	1.2	-	-	-	1.5	-	1.8	12.4	19.9	35.8	16.3	55.8	41.1	47.2	-	7.2	2.3	0.36	0.72	**5.4**	157
Nose, sinuses etc.	5	0	-	-	-	1.2	-	-	-	1.5	-	-	1.8	-	2.2	2.7	-	-	-	-	0.5	0.2	0.03	0.05	**0.5**	160
Larynx	105	0	-	-	-	-	-	-	-	-	3.1	3.0	21.8	28.4	16.0	49.3	35.3	69.7	35.9	66.1	20.4	11.3	3.5	0.61	1.13	**8.9**	161
Bronchus, lung	830	0	-	-	-	-	-	4.5	12.3	11.9	50.9	90.6	163.5	318.0	507.9	543.6	600.4	652.0	367.6	89.6	27.9	3.26	8.52	**65.8**	162
Other thoracic organs	5	0	1.8	-	-	-	-	-	-	-	-	-	-	-	-	2.2	2.7	4.6	5.1	-	-	0.5	0.2	0.02	0.06	**0.5**	163-4
Bone	10	0	-	3.2	1.4	1.2	-	1.3	-	-	1.5	-	1.8	-	2.2	-	4.6	5.1	-	-	1.1	0.3	0.06	0.09	**1.1**	170
Connective tissue	16	0	3.6	-	-	1.2	1.3	-	1.5	3.1	3.0	-	-	-	2.2	5.4	18.6	-	-	-	1.7	0.5	0.08	0.20	**1.7**	171
Mesothelioma	3	0	-	-	-	-	-	-	-	-	-	-	1.8	2.0	-	-	-	-	9.4	-	0.3	0.1	0.02	0.02	**0.2**	MES
Kaposi's sarcoma	11	0	-	-	-	-	-	-	-	-	1.5	-	3.6	2.0	-	8.1	9.3	10.3	-	-	1.2	0.4	0.04	0.12	**0.9**	KAP
Melanoma of skin	36	0	-	-	-	1.2	1.3	1.3	4.5	7.7	7.4	5.5	7.1	4.0	9.0	8.1	13.9	5.1	-	-	3.9	1.2	0.24	0.36	**3.3**	172
Other skin	328	0	-	-	-	-	1.3	-	3.0	4.6	8.9	32.7	32.0	63.8	105.2	157.5	209.1	307.9	236.2	265.5	35.4		1.26	3.09	**25.9**	173
Breast	7	0	-	-	-	-	-	-	-	-	-	1.8	3.6	-	2.2	-	-	10.3	9.4	-	0.8	0.2	0.04	0.04	**0.5**	175
Prostate	173	0	-	-	-	-	-	-	-	-	1.5	1.8	7.1	12.0	42.5	86.9	153.3	164.2	292.9	285.9	18.7	5.8	0.32	1.53	**12.9**	185
Testis	22	0	-	-	1.2	2.5	8.1	8.9	1.5	5.9	-	-	-	-	2.7	4.6	-	-	-	-	2.4	0.7	0.14	0.18	**2.1**	186
Penis	13	0	-	-	-	-	-	-	-	-	3.6	5.3	-	-	2.2	8.1	9.3	-	18.9	-	1.4	0.4	0.06	0.14	**1.1**	187.1-.4
Other male genital	0	0	-	-	-	-	-	-	-	-	-	-	-	-	-	-	-	-	-	-	0.0	0.0	0.00	0.00	**0.0**	187.5-.9
Bladder	314	0	-	-	-	-	1.3	-	-	3.1	7.4	16.4	26.6	75.8	98.5	135.8	250.9	261.7	245.7	388.1	33.9	10.5	1.15	3.08	**24.9**	188
Kidney etc.	68	0	-	-	-	-	-	-	1.5	-	4.5	1.8	16.0	21.9	15.7	43.5	27.9	46.2	18.9	61.3	7.3	2.3	0.31	0.66	**5.5**	189
Eye	4	0	-	-	-	-	-	-	-	-	-	-	3.6	2.0	-	2.7	-	-	-	-	0.4	0.1	0.03	0.04	**0.3**	190
Brain, nervous system	80	0	3.6	3.2	2.7	1.2	-	2.7	1.5	12.3	8.9	16.4	10.7	14.0	22.4	40.7	27.9	5.1	18.9	-	8.6	2.7	0.50	0.84	**7.6**	191-2
Thyroid	24	0	-	-	-	-	-	5.4	3.0	3.1	4.5	3.6	3.6	4.0	9.0	2.7	9.3	-	-	-	2.6	0.8	0.18	0.24	**2.2**	193
Other endocrine	4	0	-	-	-	-	-	-	-	-	-	-	-	-	4.5	2.7	4.6	-	-	-	0.4	0.1	0.02	0.06	**0.4**	194
Hodgkin's disease	24	0	-	-	1.4	4.9	3.8	4.0	4.5	4.6	3.0	3.6	-	-	6.7	-	-	-	-	-	2.6	0.8	0.18	0.18	**2.4**	201
Non-Hodgkin lymphoma	79	0	-	-	-	3.7	2.5	5.4	4.5	4.6	3.0	12.7	19.5	12.0	26.9	32.6	13.9	41.1	18.9	20.4	8.5	2.7	0.47	0.71	**6.8**	200,202
Multiple myeloma	32	0	-	-	-	-	-	-	1.5	-	-	-	7.1	4.0	6.7	8.1	46.5	20.5	37.8	20.4	3.5	1.1	0.10	0.37	**2.5**	203
Lymphoid leukaemia	56	0	7.1	3.2	2.7	1.2	-	-	1.5	-	1.5	-	5.3	8.0	20.2	35.3	18.6	41.1	28.3	20.4	6.0	1.9	0.25	0.52	**5.2**	204
Myeloid leukaemia	48	0	-	-	-	1.2	2.5	1.3	4.5	-	3.0	3.6	1.8	8.0	17.9	16.3	32.5	41.1	18.9	20.4	5.2	1.6	0.22	0.46	**4.0**	205
Monocytic leukaemia	4	0	-	-	-	-	-	-	-	-	-	-	-	-	-	5.4	-	5.1	9.4	-	0.4	0.1	0.00	0.03	**0.3**	206
Other leukaemia	0	0	-	-	-	-	-	-	-	-	-	-	-	-	-	-	-	-	-	-	0.0	0.0	0.00	0.00	**0.0**	207
Leukaemia unspecified	10	0	-	1.6	-	-	3.8	-	1.5	1.5	-	-	1.8	-	2.2	-	-	5.1	9.4	-	1.1	0.3	0.06	0.06	**0.9**	208
Other and unspecified	76	0	1.8	1.6	-	-	-	-	-	3.1	3.0	5.5	10.7	21.9	13.4	24.4	51.1	61.6	75.6	81.7	8.2	2.6	0.30	0.68	**6.2**	O&U
All sites	3305	0	19.6	12.9	8.1	20.7	20.3	30.9	49.2	80.2	102.5	263.5	413.8	650.1	1110.7	1561.7	2183.8	2345.2	2475.7	2165.0	357.0		13.91	32.64	**268.4**	ALL
All sites but 173	2977	0	19.6	12.9	8.1	20.7	19.0	30.9	46.2	75.6	93.6	230.8	381.8	586.3	1005.4	1404.1	1974.7	2037.3	2239.4	1899.5	321.5	100.0	12.66	29.55	**242.5**	ALLb
Rate from 1 case			1.785	1.612	1.356	1.217	1.268	1.345	1.491	1.542	1.486	1.817	1.776	1.994	2.239	2.716	4.646	5.132	9.449	20.425						

* ITALY, LATINA 1988-1991

ANNUAL INCIDENCE PER 100,000 BY AGE GROUP (YEARS) - FEMALE

SITE	ALL AGES	AGE UNK	0-	5-	10-	15-	20-	25-	30-	35-	40-	45-	50-	55-	60-	65-	70-	75-	80-	85+	CRUDE RATE	%	CR 64	CR 74	ASR (W)	ICD (9th)
Lip	6	0	-	-	-	-	-	-	-	-	-	3.6	-	-	-	-	7.6	4.0	6.7	-	0.6	0.3	0.02	0.06	0.4	140
Tongue	3	0	-	-	-	-	-	-	-	-	-	-	-	-	-	-	3.8	8.0	-	-	0.3	0.1	0.00	0.02	0.2	141
Salivary gland	6	0	-	-	-	-	-	-	1.5	-	1.5	-	1.8	-	-	4.7	3.8	-	-	-	0.6	0.3	0.02	0.07	0.5	142
Mouth	5	0	-	-	-	-	-	-	-	-	1.5	-	-	-	2.1	-	3.8	-	6.7	11.0	0.5	0.2	0.02	0.04	0.3	143-5
Oropharynx	0	0	-	-	-	-	-	-	-	-	-	-	-	-	-	-	-	-	-	-	0.0	0.0	0.00	0.00	0.0	146
Nasopharynx	1	0	-	-	-	-	-	-	-	-	1.5	-	-	-	-	-	-	-	-	-	0.1	0.0	0.01	0.01	0.1	147
Hypopharynx	1	0	-	-	-	-	-	-	-	1.5	-	-	-	-	-	-	-	-	-	-	0.1	0.0	0.01	0.01	0.1	148
Pharynx unspecified	0	0	-	-	-	-	-	-	-	-	-	-	-	-	-	-	-	-	-	-	0.0	0.0	0.00	0.00	0.0	149
Oesophagus	7	0	-	-	-	-	-	-	-	-	-	1.8	-	-	4.2	-	-	4.0	20.0	-	0.7	0.3	0.03	0.03	0.4	150
Stomach	165	0	-	-	-	-	1.2	2.6	2.9	3.0	7.4	3.6	16.2	25.3	45.9	39.8	68.3	119.9	193.2	143.4	17.4	7.0	0.54	1.08	10.4	151
Small intestine	4	0	-	-	-	-	-	-	1.5	-	-	-	1.9	-	-	-	3.8	4.0	-	-	0.4	0.2	0.02	0.04	0.3	152
Colon	199	0	-	-	-	-	-	-	1.5	4.5	4.5	14.6	34.1	29.2	48.0	60.8	79.7	163.8	193.2	110.3	21.0	8.5	0.68	1.38	12.9	153
Rectum	104	0	-	-	-	1.3	-	-	2.9	3.0	7.4	16.4	16.2	15.5	14.6	25.7	49.3	59.9	113.2	55.1	11.0	4.4	0.39	0.76	7.1	154
Liver	76	0	-	1.7	-	-	-	-	-	4.5	1.5	3.6	1.8	11.7	16.7	21.0	41.7	67.9	73.3	66.2	8.0	3.2	0.21	0.52	4.8	155
Gallbladder etc.	83	0	-	-	-	-	-	-	-	-	-	3.6	7.2	11.7	41.7	32.7	41.7	51.9	46.6	66.2	8.7	3.5	0.32	0.69	5.6	156
Pancreas	62	0	-	-	-	-	-	-	-	-	5.5	5.4	-	16.7	30.4	19.0	44.0	99.9	44.1	-	6.5	2.6	0.14	0.38	3.7	157
Nose, sinuses etc.	1	0	-	-	-	-	-	-	-	-	-	-	-	-	-	-	3.8	-	-	-	0.1	0.0	0.00	0.02	0.1	160
Larynx	9	0	-	-	-	-	-	-	-	-	-	-	1.8	1.9	2.1	2.3	3.8	8.0	13.3	-	0.9	0.4	0.03	0.06	0.5	161
Bronchus, lung	135	0	-	-	-	-	-	1.3	1.5	1.5	3.0	10.9	19.8	35.0	27.1	39.8	79.7	99.9	73.3	88.2	14.2	5.7	0.50	1.10	9.2	162
Other thoracic organs	0	0	-	-	-	-	-	-	-	-	-	-	-	-	-	-	-	-	-	-	0.0	0.0	0.00	0.00	0.0	163-4
Bone	3	0	-	-	-	-	-	-	-	-	-	-	3.6	-	2.1	-	-	-	-	-	0.3	0.1	0.03	0.03	0.3	170
Connective tissue	14	0	-	-	-	-	2.5	-	2.9	1.5	3.0	5.5	-	5.8	-	-	-	4.0	-	-	1.5	0.6	0.11	0.11	1.2	171
Mesothelioma	2	0	-	-	-	-	-	-	-	-	1.5	-	-	-	-	-	-	4.0	-	-	0.2	0.1	0.01	0.01	0.1	MES
Kaposi's sarcoma	5	0	-	-	-	-	-	-	-	1.5	-	-	-	-	2.3	3.8	4.0	6.7	-	-	0.5	0.2	0.01	0.04	0.3	KAP
Melanoma of skin	36	0	-	-	-	1.3	-	-	4.4	1.5	10.4	3.6	5.4	1.9	12.5	7.0	19.0	16.0	-	-	3.8	1.5	0.21	0.34	2.9	172
Other skin	226	0	-	-	-	-	1.3	1.5	4.5	7.4	9.1	27.0	27.2	45.9	84.2	110.0	195.8	213.1	154.4	-	23.8		0.62	1.59	14.2	173
Breast	646	0	-	-	-	-	6.5	23.2	39.2	89.1	131.2	115.0	165.2	144.0	212.8	212.5	251.7	179.8	132.3		68.0	27.5	3.57	5.69	50.3	174
Uterus unspecified	23	0	-	-	-	-	-	-	-	3.0	3.6	1.8	1.9	4.2	9.4	11.4	12.0	20.0	22.1		2.4	1.0	0.07	0.18	1.6	179
Cervix uteri	80	0	-	-	-	-	2.6	4.4	9.0	7.4	16.4	9.0	23.3	20.9	18.7	34.2	20.0	26.6	22.1		8.4	3.4	0.46	0.73	6.3	180
Placenta	1	0	-	-	-	-	-	-	-	1.5	-	-	-	-	-	-	-	-	-		0.1	0.0	0.01	0.01	0.1	181
Corpus uteri	117	0	-	-	-	-	-	-	1.5	1.5	4.5	3.6	19.8	40.8	41.7	63.1	56.9	44.0	33.3	-	12.3	5.0	0.57	1.17	8.6	182
Ovary etc.	92	0	1.9	-	-	-	1.2	1.3	2.9	3.0	8.9	3.6	19.8	31.1	18.8	28.1	49.3	36.0	33.3	22.1	9.7	3.9	0.46	0.85	7.0	183
Other female genital	22	0	-	-	-	-	-	-	-	-	-	-	-	3.9	2.1	7.0	15.2	28.0	13.3	33.1	2.3	0.9	0.03	0.14	1.3	184
Bladder	47	0	-	-	-	1.3	-	-	-	1.5	-	1.5	3.6	3.6	7.8	8.3	28.1	19.0	20.0	40.0	44.1	4.9	2.0	0.14	0.37	3.2	188
Kidney etc.	25	0	1.9	-	-	-	-	-	-	-	-	4.5	3.6	5.4	5.8	18.8	-	3.8	4.0	13.3	-	2.6	1.1	0.20	0.22	2.1	189
Eye	4	0	-	-	-	-	-	-	-	1.5	-	-	-	1.9	-	2.3	-	4.0	-	-	0.4	0.2	0.02	0.03	0.3	190
Brain, nervous system	53	0	5.6	3.4	1.4	3.8	1.2	2.6	2.9	-	4.5	7.3	14.4	9.7	16.7	14.0	7.6	12.0	-	-	5.6	2.3	0.37	0.48	5.1	191-2
Thyroid	51	0	-	-	1.4	2.5	-	6.5	4.4	10.5	13.4	14.6	7.2	13.6	4.2	2.3	7.6	-	-	-	5.4	2.2	0.39	0.44	4.7	193
Other endocrine	2	0	1.9	-	-	-	-	-	-	-	-	1.8	-	-	-	-	-	-	-	-	0.2	0.1	0.02	0.02	0.3	194
Hodgkin's disease	23	0	-	-	1.4	2.5	3.7	6.5	-	3.0	4.5	1.8	1.8	3.9	2.1	-	-	13.3	-		2.4	1.0	0.16	0.16	2.1	201
Non-Hodgkin lymphoma	67	0	-	-	-	3.8	1.2	5.2	1.5	4.5	4.5	7.3	5.4	15.5	10.4	28.1	30.4	44.0	6.7	-	7.1	2.8	0.30	0.59	5.1	200,202
Multiple myeloma	31	0	-	-	-	-	-	-	-	-	4.5	3.6	-	3.9	6.3	14.0	7.6	36.0	20.0	11.0	3.3	1.3	0.09	0.20	2.0	203
Lymphoid leukaemia	40	0	5.6	3.4	2.9	1.3	-	-	-	-	1.5	-	1.8	3.9	14.6	18.7	19.0	24.0	6.7	11.0	4.2	1.7	0.17	0.36	3.6	204
Myeloid leukaemia	25	0	-	5.1	-	1.3	1.2	-	-	-	-	1.8	1.8	5.8	10.4	14.0	3.8	4.0	13.3	-	2.6	1.1	0.14	0.23	2.2	205
Monocytic leukaemia	0	0	-	-	-	-	-	-	-	-	-	-	-	-	-	-	-	-	-	-	0.0	0.0	0.00	0.00	0.0	206
Other leukaemia	0	0	-	-	-	-	-	-	-	-	-	-	-	-	-	-	-	-	-	-	0.0	0.0	0.00	0.00	0.0	207
Leukaemia unspecified	11	0	-	1.7	-	-	-	-	-	-	-	-	1.8	-	-	-	2.1	9.4	-	4.0	20.0	-	1.2	0.5	0.03	0.07	0.8	208
Other and unspecified	66	0	-	-	4.3	-	1.2	-	-	-	-	1.5	5.5	5.4	11.7	12.5	21.0	7.6	40.0	66.6	132.3	7.0	2.8	0.21	0.35	4.3	O&U
All sites	2579	0	16.8	15.3	11.4	18.9	13.7	36.3	62.5	99.4	204.9	293.5	352.2	517.0	617.5	842.0	1028.3	1442.4	1565.2	1168.9	271.6		11.30	20.65	186.8	ALL
All sites but 173	2353	0	16.8	15.3	11.4	18.9	13.7	35.0	61.0	94.9	197.5	284.3	325.2	489.8	571.6	757.8	918.3	1246.6	1352.1	1014.6	247.8	100.0	10.68	19.06	172.6	ALLb

Rate from 1 case: 1.869 1.701 1.431 1.258 1.248 1.297 1.452 1.506 1.485 1.823 1.797 1.944 2.086 2.339 3.795 3.996 6.660 11.028

Italy, Macerata Province

The Macerata Province Cancer Registry was created in 1991 on the initiative of the Hygiene, Health and Environmental Sciences Department of Camerino University, in central Italy (Marches Region). The objectives were to establish the annual incidence and mortality of cancer by site in the province and to monitor their evolution in order to assess risk factors related to the environment, socio-economic factors and occupation.

Collection and registration began on 1 January 1989 in some Local Health Units (LHUs) covering about 70 000 inhabitants, for a three-year experimental phase, with support from the Regional Health Administration. Since January 1991, the registry has covered 95% of the resident population of Macerata Province and since January 1995, registration has been extended to the whole province. The registry is financially supported and run by Camerino University and Macerata Province Section of the Italian League against Cancer. The staff includes an epidemiologist, a computer and coding practices expert and three part-time doctors, while a medical oncologist and a pathologist act as consultants.

The Province of Macerata (2774 km²) is situated between latitudes 42°45′ and 43°28′ N and longitudes 12°50′ and 13°45′ E. It is bordered by the Province of Ancona to the north, that of Ascoli Piceno to the south, that of Perugia (Umbria region) to the west, and the Adriatic Sea to the east.

The population was 295 481 (143 350 males and 152 131 females; density 106 persons per km²) at the 1991 census, distributed among 57 municipalities. The only municipalities with more than 30 000 inhabitants are Macerata (43 040) and Civitanova Marche (37 260), and many, mainly those located in mountains areas, have populations of less than 5000 (72% of all municipalities).

The province can be divided into three zones: a mountain zone (31.6% of municipalities) with low population density (19.1 inhabitants per km² in 1991), a high fraction of people engaged in services (52.2%) but relatively few in other sectors of economic activity, and a marked decrease in population (−16.9% between the 1971 and 1991 censuses); a coastal zone (5.3% of municipalities) bordering the Adriatic Sea, with high population density (530 inhabitants per km²), a low number of people engaged in agriculture (5.7%) and a high demographic increase (+15.6%); and a hill zone (63.1% of municipalities), with little population change (+2.3%) and characteristics intermediate between those of the other two zones. The population of the whole province is fairly stable (+3.2%), despite variations between the zones. In the same period there have been a decrease of 72% in the population employed in the agricultural sector (most marked in the hill zone) and an increase of 22% in the industrial sector.

Following the Regional Health Reform of 1980, the municipalities of the province have been grouped into six local health districts, three for those situated in the coastal and low hill zones and three for those in the high hill and mountain zones. In the province there are 1994 beds and 354 doctors in 12 hospitals of the National Health Service and 463 beds and 32 doctors in three private hospitals, excluding intensive care and psychiatric institutions. There are two hospital oncology services and two pathology departments, but neither hospitals nor departments for oncology. The nearest oncology hospital with radiotherapeutic facilities is outside Macerata Province, in Ancona, the capital of the Marches Region.

Information on cancer cases is based on active data collection by registry personnel. New cases of patients and outpatients are identified from clinical records of all public and private hospitals in the province. Records of cases are also supplied by the pathology departments of Ancona University and the hospital pathology services of the province, while preliminary information may be directly supplied by general practitioners or taken from the list of patients exempted from payment. Other sources of information include the Italian Association of Haematology and Paediatric Oncology, the Paediatric Clinic of Bologna University; the Cancer Registries of Varese and Romagna for patients admitted to hospitals in their zones; clinical records of Ancona LHUs for admissions to hospitals outside Macerata Province; and direct consultation with doctors involved in diagnosis.

The registry receives every three months from LHUs copies of all death certificates and from each municipality a list of all deaths at the end of each year.

The information concerning each tumour, including personal identification and full clinical details, is coded and entered in a computer database by the same operator. All malignant neoplasms are recorded. Carcinomas *in situ* and a number of other tumours of a benign or uncertain nature are recorded, as well as benign papillomas of the bladder, but they are excluded from the incidence calculation. Malignant tumours included in the incidence figures are defined as those coded in the 140–208 sections of ICD-9 and those for which the ICD-O behaviour code is 3. Multiple primaries occurring in the same patient are coded according to the IARC/IACR rules. The index date for incidence computation is the date of first diagnosis (histological if available) for patients or the date of death if no other information is available.

Franco Pannelli
Susanna Vitarelli

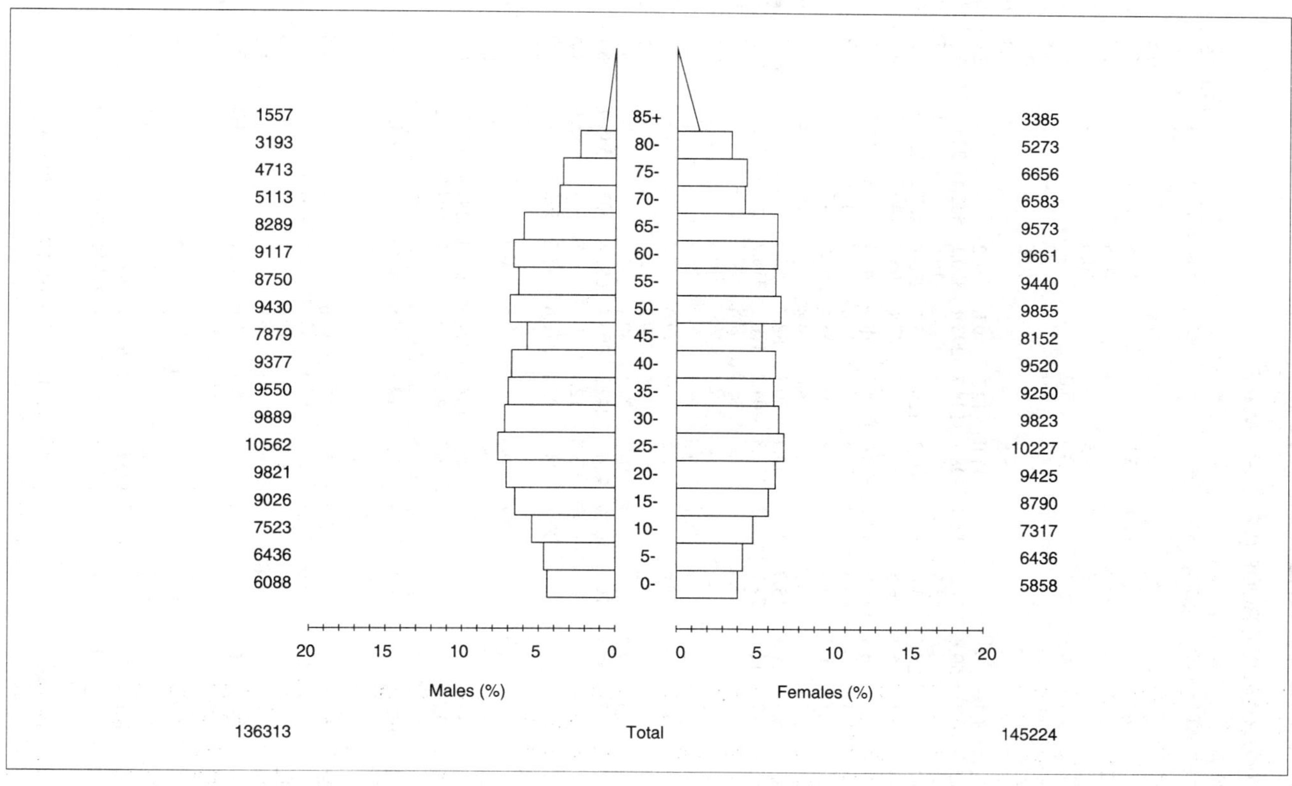

Italy, Macerata Province
Source of population: 1991
Census: 13° Censimento generale della popolazione e delle
abitazioni, 20 Ottobre 1991. Fascicolo provinciale Macerata,
Istituto Nazionale di Statistics (ISTAT), Roma, 1993.

ITALY, MACERATA PROVINCE 1991-1992

ANNUAL INCIDENCE PER 100,000 BY AGE GROUP (YEARS) - MALE

SITE	ALL AGES	AGE UNK	0-	5-	10-	15-	20-	25-	30-	35-	40-	45-	50-	55-	60-	65-	70-	75-	80-	85+	CRUDE RATE	%	CR 64	CR 74	ASR (W)	ICD (9th)
Lip	1	0	-	-	-	-	-	-	-	-	-	-	-	-	-	-	9.8	-	-	-	0.4	0.1	0.00	0.05	**0.2**	*140*
Tongue	7	0	-	-	-	-	-	-	-	-	10.7	-	-	11.4	5.5	-	-	10.6	15.7	-	2.6	0.5	0.14	0.14	**1.5**	*141*
Salivary gland	2	0	-	-	-	-	-	-	5.2	-	-	-	-	-	-	-	-	10.6	-	-	0.7	0.1	0.03	0.03	**0.4**	*142*
Mouth	2	0	-	-	-	-	-	-	-	-	-	-	-	5.5	-	-	-	10.6	-	-	0.7	0.1	0.03	0.03	**0.3**	*143-5*
Oropharynx	4	0	-	-	-	-	-	-	-	-	5.3	6.3	5.3	-	-	6.0	-	-	-	-	1.5	0.3	0.08	0.12	**1.1**	*146*
Nasopharynx	1	0	-	-	-	-	-	-	-	-	-	-	-	-	-	6.0	-	-	-	-	0.4	0.1	0.00	0.03	**0.2**	*147*
Hypopharynx	1	0	-	-	-	-	-	-	-	-	-	-	-	-	-	-	-	10.6	-	-	0.4	0.1	0.00	0.00	**0.1**	*148*
Pharynx unspecified	1	0	-	-	-	-	-	-	-	-	-	-	-	5.5	-	-	-	-	-	-	0.4	0.1	0.03	0.03	**0.2**	*149*
Oesophagus	8	0	-	-	-	-	-	-	-	5.3	-	-	11.0	12.1	9.8	21.2	-	-	-	-	2.9	0.6	0.08	0.19	**1.5**	*150*
Stomach	174	0	-	-	-	-	-	5.1	5.2	10.7	50.8	37.1	51.4	98.7	138.7	293.4	350.1	532.4	256.9	63.8	12.1	1.29	3.46	**29.6**	*151*
Small intestine	3	0	-	-	-	-	-	-	-	-	-	5.3	-	-	-	-	10.6	-	32.1	1.1	0.2	0.03	0.03	**0.5**	*152*
Colon	146	0	-	-	-	-	5.1	4.7	-	5.2	-	25.4	53.0	85.7	60.3	126.7	215.1	275.8	407.1	256.9	53.6	10.1	1.20	2.91	**25.3**	*153*
Rectum	81	0	-	-	-	-	-	-	5.1	-	10.7	6.3	26.5	5.7	65.8	138.7	127.1	95.5	140.9	160.6	29.7	5.6	0.60	1.93	**14.7**	*154*
Liver	36	0	-	-	-	-	-	-	-	-	6.3	15.9	17.1	38.4	54.3	48.9	42.4	31.3	64.2	13.2	2.5	0.39	0.90	**6.9**	*155*
Gallbladder etc.	16	0	-	-	-	-	-	-	-	5.3	-	10.6	11.4	16.5	-	19.6	21.2	47.0	32.1	5.9	1.1	0.22	0.32	**3.0**	*156*
Pancreas	40	0	-	-	-	-	-	-	-	5.3	6.3	15.9	5.7	49.4	60.3	68.5	53.0	47.0	-	14.7	2.8	0.41	1.06	**7.6**	*157*
Nose, sinuses etc.	6	0	-	-	-	-	-	-	-	-	-	-	16.5	6.0	9.8	-	15.7	-	2.2	0.4	0.08	0.16	**1.1**	*160*
Larynx	39	0	-	-	-	-	-	-	-	5.3	19.0	15.9	11.4	49.4	60.3	58.7	53.0	-	-	14.3	2.7	0.51	1.10	**8.2**	*161*
Bronchus, lung	255	0	-	-	-	-	-	-	5.2	10.7	12.7	74.2	154.3	230.3	404.2	420.5	318.3	281.9	289.0	93.5	17.7	2.44	6.56	**47.4**	*162*
Other thoracic organs	4	0	-	-	-	-	-	-	-	-	5.3	-	-	6.0	9.8	10.6	-	-	1.5	0.3	0.03	0.11	**0.7**	*163-4*
Bone	2	0	-	-	-	-	-	-	-	5.3	-	-	-	-	-	10.6	-	-	0.7	0.1	0.03	0.03	**0.4**	*170*
Connective tissue	10	0	-	-	-	-	-	-	-	5.3	12.7	-	5.7	5.5	18.1	-	21.2	-	-	3.7	0.7	0.15	0.24	**2.3**	*171*
Mesothelioma	8	0	-	-	-	-	-	-	-	-	-	10.6	-	5.5	-	19.6	21.2	15.7	-	2.9	0.6	0.08	0.18	**1.4**	*MES*
Kaposi's sarcoma	4	0	-	-	-	-	-	-	5.2	-	5.3	-	-	6.0	9.8	-	-	-	1.5	0.3	0.05	0.13	**1.0**	*KAP*
Melanoma of skin	27	0	-	-	-	-	-	-	5.2	10.7	12.7	21.2	17.1	16.5	24.1	39.1	42.4	-	-	9.9	1.9	0.42	0.73	**6.1**	*172*
Other skin	262	0	-	-	-	4.7	5.1	5.2	21.3	38.1	74.2	102.9	224.9	247.3	293.4	657.8	407.1	545.9	96.1	2.38	5.09	**46.0**	*173*
Breast	4	0	-	-	-	-	-	-	-	-	-	-	5.5	12.1	-	-	-	32.1	1.5	0.3	0.03	0.09	**0.7**	*175*
Prostate	177	0	-	-	-	-	-	-	-	-	5.3	17.1	98.7	199.1	371.6	371.3	595.1	353.2	64.9	12.3	0.61	3.46	**26.8**	*185*
Testis	10	0	-	-	-	-	5.1	4.7	10.1	10.5	5.3	6.3	5.3	-	-	6.0	-	-	-	3.7	0.7	0.24	0.27	**3.2**	*186*
Penis	6	0	-	-	-	-	-	-	-	-	-	6.3	-	5.7	5.5	6.0	9.8	10.6	-	2.2	0.4	0.09	0.17	**1.3**	*187.1-.4*
Other male genital	0	0	-	-	-	-	-	-	-	-	-	-	-	-	-	-	-	-	-	0.0	0.0	0.00	0.00	**0.0**	*187.5-.9*
Bladder	155	0	-	-	-	-	-	-	-	-	5.3	6.3	21.2	131.4	148.1	138.7	342.3	180.4	281.9	192.7	56.9	10.8	1.56	3.97	**28.1**	*188*
Kidney etc.	36	0	-	-	-	-	-	-	5.1	5.2	10.7	-	5.3	17.1	16.5	48.3	39.1	53.0	94.0	64.2	13.2	2.5	0.30	0.74	**6.4**	*189*
Eye	3	0	-	-	-	-	-	-	-	-	5.3	-	-	5.5	-	-	-	15.7	-	1.1	0.2	0.05	0.05	**0.6**	*190*
Brain, nervous system	24	0	-	-	-	11.1	-	-	5.1	5.2	10.7	-	26.5	11.4	27.4	12.1	9.8	10.6	-	64.2	8.8	1.7	0.49	0.60	**6.1**	*191-2*
Thyroid	3	0	-	-	-	-	-	4.7	-	5.2	-	-	5.7	-	-	-	-	-	-	1.1	0.2	0.08	0.08	**0.9**	*193*
Other endocrine	2	0	8.2	-	-	-	-	-	-	-	-	-	-	5.5	-	-	-	-	-	0.7	0.1	0.07	0.07	**1.2**	*194*
Hodgkin's disease	12	0	-	7.8	-	-	-	-	-	10.5	5.3	12.7	-	5.7	5.5	12.1	19.6	-	-	4.4	0.8	0.24	0.40	**3.7**	*201*
Non-Hodgkin lymphoma	40	0	-	-	-	5.5	-	-	5.1	-	-	12.7	15.9	17.1	49.4	60.3	58.7	31.8	31.3	-	14.7	2.8	0.53	1.12	**8.5**	*200,202*
Multiple myeloma	15	0	-	-	-	-	-	-	-	5.2	-	-	-	-	21.9	18.1	19.6	31.8	31.3	-	5.5	1.0	0.14	0.32	**2.6**	*203*
Lymphoid leukaemia	14	0	8.2	-	-	-	-	-	-	-	-	-	5.3	-	27.4	24.1	9.8	-	31.3	-	5.1	1.0	0.20	0.37	**3.4**	*204*
Myeloid leukaemia	14	0	-	-	-	5.5	-	-	5.1	-	-	-	6.3	-	5.7	-	18.1	19.6	21.2	15.7	64.2	5.1	1.0	0.11	0.30	**3.0**	*205*
Monocytic leukaemia	0	0	-	-	-	-	-	-	-	-	-	-	-	-	-	-	-	-	-	0.0	0.0	0.00	0.00	**0.0**	*206*
Other leukaemia	0	0	-	-	-	-	-	-	-	-	-	-	-	-	-	-	-	-	-	0.0	0.0	0.00	0.00	**0.0**	*207*
Leukaemia unspecified	8	0	8.2	-	-	-	-	-	-	-	5.3	-	10.6	-	5.5	6.0	-	21.2	-	-	2.9	0.6	0.15	0.18	**2.4**	*208*
Other and unspecified	40	0	8.2	-	-	-	-	-	-	5.2	-	-	15.9	17.1	27.4	42.2	58.7	53.0	78.3	128.5	14.7	2.8	0.37	0.87	**7.9**	*O&U*
All sites	1703	0	32.9	7.8	-	22.2	10.2	18.9	45.5	83.8	160.0	247.5	487.8	714.3	1354.6	1918.2	2611.0	2832.6	3116.2	2536.9	624.7		15.93	38.57	**314.8**	*ALL*
All sites but 173	1441	0	32.9	7.8	-	22.2	10.2	14.2	40.4	78.5	138.6	209.4	413.6	611.4	1129.8	1670.9	2317.6	2174.8	2709.1	1991.0	528.6	100.0	13.54	33.49	**268.7**	*ALLb*

Rate from 1 case: 8.213 7.769 6.646 5.540 5.091 4.734 5.056 5.236 5.332 6.346 5.302 5.714 5.484 6.032 9.779 10.609 15.659 32.113

ITALY, MACERATA PROVINCE 1991-1992

ANNUAL INCIDENCE PER 100,000 BY AGE GROUP (YEARS) - FEMALE

SITE	ALL AGES	AGE UNK	0-	5-	10-	15-	20-	25-	30-	35-	40-	45-	50-	55-	60-	65-	70-	75-	80-	85+	CRUDE RATE	%	CR 64	CR 74	ASR (W)	ICD (9th)
Lip	0	0	-	-	-	-	-	-	-	-	-	-	-	-	-	-	-	-	-	-	0.0	0.0	0.00	0.00	**0.0**	*140*
Tongue	3	0	-	-	-	-	-	-	-	-	-	-	-	-	5.2	-	-	15.0	-	-	1.0	0.3	0.03	0.03	**0.4**	*141*
Salivary gland	0	0	-	-	-	-	-	-	-	-	-	-	-	-	-	-	-	-	-	-	0.0	0.0	0.00	0.00	**0.0**	*142*
Mouth	4	0	-	-	-	-	-	-	-	-	-	-	-	5.3	-	-	15.2	7.5	-	-	1.4	0.3	0.03	0.10	**0.6**	*143-5*
Oropharynx	1	0	-	-	-	-	-	-	-	-	-	-	-	-	-	-	-	-	9.5	-	0.3	0.1	0.00	0.00	**0.0**	*146*
Nasopharynx	0	0	-	-	-	-	-	-	-	-	-	-	-	-	-	-	-	-	-	-	0.0	0.0	0.00	0.00	**0.0**	*147*
Hypopharynx	0	0	-	-	-	-	-	-	-	-	-	-	-	-	-	-	-	-	-	-	0.0	0.0	0.00	0.00	**0.0**	*148*
Pharynx unspecified	0	0	-	-	-	-	-	-	-	-	-	-	-	-	-	-	-	-	-	-	0.0	0.0	0.00	0.00	**0.0**	*149*
Oesophagus	5	0	-	-	-	-	-	-	-	-	-	-	-	5.3	-	5.2	7.6	-	19.0	-	1.7	0.4	0.03	0.09	**0.6**	*150*
Stomach	108	0	-	-	-	-	-	4.9	-	16.2	10.5	12.3	10.1	31.8	46.6	62.7	98.7	157.8	199.1	236.3	37.2	9.2	0.66	1.47	**14.0**	*151*
Small intestine	3	0	-	-	-	-	-	-	-	-	-	6.1	-	-	-	-	-	-	-	29.5	1.0	0.3	0.03	0.03	**0.5**	*152*
Colon	125	0	-	-	-	-	-	-	5.1	-	15.8	6.1	55.8	63.6	41.4	57.5	136.7	195.3	113.8	325.0	43.0	10.6	0.94	1.91	**17.2**	*153*
Rectum	51	0	-	-	-	-	-	-	-	-	-	12.3	15.2	31.8	15.5	26.1	60.8	82.6	85.3	59.1	17.6	4.3	0.37	0.81	**6.9**	*154*
Liver	21	0	-	-	-	-	-	-	-	-	-	-	15.2	21.2	5.2	10.4	22.8	22.5	19.0	44.3	7.2	1.8	0.21	0.37	**3.1**	*155*
Gallbladder etc.	12	0	-	-	-	-	-	-	-	-	-	-	5.1	5.3	5.2	10.4	22.8	15.0	9.5	14.8	4.1	1.0	0.08	0.24	**1.7**	*156*
Pancreas	34	0	-	-	-	-	-	-	-	-	5.3	6.1	5.1	21.2	25.9	20.9	15.2	37.6	85.3	29.5	11.7	2.9	0.32	0.50	**4.7**	*157*
Nose, sinuses etc.	0	0	-	-	-	-	-	-	-	-	-	-	-	-	-	-	-	-	-	-	0.0	0.0	0.00	0.00	**0.0**	*160*
Larynx	2	0	-	-	-	-	-	-	-	-	-	-	-	10.4	-	-	-	-	-	-	0.7	0.2	0.05	0.05	**0.4**	*161*
Bronchus, lung	43	0	-	-	-	-	-	-	-	5.4	5.3	18.4	10.1	10.6	36.2	73.1	15.2	37.6	28.4	44.3	14.8	3.6	0.43	0.87	**7.4**	*162*
Other thoracic organs	2	0	-	-	-	-	-	-	-	-	-	6.1	-	-	-	-	-	-	-	14.8	0.7	0.2	0.03	0.03	**0.4**	*163-4*
Bone	2	0	-	-	-	-	-	-	-	-	-	-	-	-	5.2	-	-	9.5	-	-	0.7	0.2	0.03	0.03	**0.3**	*170*
Connective tissue	13	0	-	7.8	-	-	-	-	-	-	-	-	5.1	5.3	5.2	10.4	7.6	22.5	19.0	14.8	4.5	1.1	0.12	0.21	**2.3**	*171*
Mesothelioma	2	0	-	-	-	-	-	-	-	-	-	-	-	-	-	-	7.6	7.5	-	-	0.7	0.2	0.00	0.04	**0.2**	*MES*
Kaposi's sarcoma	1	0	-	-	-	-	-	-	-	-	-	-	5.1	-	-	-	-	-	-	-	0.3	0.1	0.03	0.03	**0.3**	*KAP*
Melanoma of skin	24	0	-	-	-	-	-	-	5.1	-	26.3	6.1	10.1	5.3	20.7	15.7	15.2	22.5	19.0	-	8.3	2.0	0.37	0.52	**4.9**	*172*
Other skin	183	0	-	-	-	-	-	4.9	10.2	10.8	15.8	24.5	35.5	68.9	56.9	141.0	227.9	225.4	189.6	487.4	63.0		1.14	2.98	**25.3**	*173*
Breast	299	0	-	-	-	-	4.9	20.4	37.8	120.8	122.7	182.6	169.5	232.9	177.6	227.9	180.3	246.5	251.1	-	102.9	25.4	4.46	6.49	**57.9**	*174*
Uterus unspecified	13	0	-	-	-	-	-	-	-	5.4	-	12.3	-	5.3	-	15.7	7.6	22.5	9.5	14.8	4.5	1.1	0.11	0.23	**2.2**	*179*
Cervix uteri	12	0	-	-	-	-	-	-	-	16.2	15.8	-	-	-	10.4	10.4	-	7.5	9.5	-	4.1	1.0	0.21	0.26	**2.8**	*180*
Placenta	0	0	-	-	-	-	-	-	-	-	-	-	-	-	-	-	-	-	-	-	0.0	0.0	0.00	0.00	**0.0**	*181*
Corpus uteri	76	0	-	-	-	-	-	-	-	-	21.0	6.1	55.8	26.5	46.6	41.8	113.9	105.2	66.4	29.5	26.2	6.4	0.78	1.56	**12.4**	*182*
Ovary etc.	55	0	-	-	-	5.3	4.9	-	10.8	15.8	18.4	10.1	21.2	25.9	57.5	45.6	60.1	56.9	44.3	-	18.9	4.7	0.56	1.08	**9.6**	*183*
Other female genital	11	0	-	-	-	-	-	-	-	-	-	-	5.1	-	5.2	10.4	15.2	7.5	9.5	44.3	3.8	0.9	0.05	0.18	**1.4**	*184*
Bladder	25	0	-	-	-	-	-	-	-	5.4	-	-	5.1	10.6	-	5.2	15.2	67.6	66.4	29.5	8.6	2.1	0.11	0.21	**2.6**	*188*
Kidney etc.	23	0	-	-	-	-	-	-	-	-	-	12.3	-	15.9	5.2	10.4	45.6	30.0	19.0	44.3	7.9	2.0	0.17	0.45	**3.4**	*189*
Eye	2	0	-	-	-	-	-	-	-	-	-	-	5.1	-	5.2	-	-	-	-	-	0.7	0.2	0.05	0.05	**0.5**	*190*
Brain, nervous system	30	0	8.5	7.8	6.8	-	5.3	-	-	-	-	6.1	25.4	5.3	31.1	31.3	22.8	22.5	9.5	-	10.3	2.5	0.48	0.75	**7.6**	*191-2*
Thyroid	32	0	-	7.8	-	-	10.6	4.9	10.2	5.4	36.8	12.3	25.4	-	20.7	15.7	15.2	7.5	-	14.8	11.0	2.7	0.67	0.82	**8.9**	*193*
Other endocrine	2	0	-	-	-	-	-	-	-	-	-	-	-	-	-	5.2	-	7.5	-	-	0.7	0.2	0.00	0.03	**0.2**	*194*
Hodgkin's disease	12	0	-	-	6.8	-	5.3	9.8	5.1	-	5.3	-	-	-	-	-	22.8	15.0	-	14.8	4.1	1.0	0.16	0.28	**3.1**	*201*
Non-Hodgkin lymphoma	39	0	-	-	-	5.7	-	4.9	-	10.8	5.3	6.1	-	5.3	20.7	41.8	60.8	67.6	19.0	14.8	13.4	3.3	0.29	0.81	**6.6**	*200,202*
Multiple myeloma	19	0	-	-	-	-	-	-	-	-	5.3	-	-	5.3	15.5	26.1	30.4	37.6	-	-	6.5	1.6	0.13	0.41	**2.9**	*203*
Lymphoid leukaemia	11	0	8.5	-	6.8	-	-	-	-	-	-	-	5.1	-	5.2	5.2	22.8	7.5	19.0	-	3.8	0.9	0.13	0.27	**2.9**	*204*
Myeloid leukaemia	7	0	-	-	-	-	-	4.9	-	-	-	6.1	-	-	10.4	-	-	7.5	-	29.5	2.4	0.6	0.11	0.11	**1.4**	*205*
Monocytic leukaemia	1	0	-	-	-	-	-	-	-	-	-	-	-	-	-	-	-	-	9.5	-	0.3	0.1	0.00	0.00	**0.0**	*206*
Other leukaemia	0	0	-	-	-	-	-	-	-	-	-	-	-	-	-	-	-	-	-	-	0.0	0.0	0.00	0.00	**0.0**	*207*
Leukaemia unspecified	8	0	8.5	-	6.8	-	5.3	-	-	-	-	5.3	-	10.6	5.2	-	-	7.5	-	-	2.8	0.7	0.21	0.21	**3.1**	*208*
Other and unspecified	46	0	-	-	-	-	-	-	-	-	-	-	10.1	5.3	31.1	20.9	45.6	90.1	47.4	147.7	15.8	3.9	0.23	0.56	**5.4**	*O&U*
All sites	1362	0	25.6	23.3	27.3	5.7	31.8	44.0	56.0	124.3	309.9	300.5	502.3	556.1	750.4	908.8	1344.4	1600.1	1393.9	1979.3	468.9		13.79	25.05	**226.3**	*ALL*
All sites but 173	1179	0	25.6	23.3	27.3	5.7	31.8	39.1	45.8	113.5	294.1	276.0	466.8	487.3	693.5	767.8	1116.5	1374.7	1204.2	1491.9	405.9	100.0	12.65	22.07	**201.0**	*ALLb*
Rate from 1 case			8.535	7.769	6.833	5.688	5.305	4.889	5.090	5.405	5.252	6.133	5.074	5.297	5.175	5.223	7.595	7.512	9.482	14.771						

Italy, Modena

The Modena Cancer Registry was established in 1988. The registry is supported by the Italian League Against Cancer and by the Health Department of the Province of Modena.

The area covered by the registry is the whole province of Modena, which is one of the nine provinces of the region of Emilia Romagna in northern Italy. It borders the provinces of Bologna to the east, of Lucca and Pistoia along the Apennines to the south, of Reggio Emilia to the west and of Mantua and Ferrara to the north. It is located between latitudes 44° 06´ and 44° 57´ N and longitudes 10° 19´ and 11° 22´ E. The total area is 2690 km^2. The population on 31 December 1991 numbered 604 680 (density 224 inhabitants per km^2).

The province is divided into 47 municipalities, of which only two have 30 000–100 000 inhabitants and one more than 100 000. The only municipality with a population greater than 100 000 is Modena (177 501 inhabitants in 1991).

Spring and autumn weather is wet and mild, summer is dry and hot, while winter is wet and cold, with occasional snow. The relative humidity is fairly high.

The registry collects data relative to all malignant tumours diagnosed in residents of the province of Modena. Malignant tumours are coded according to ICD-9.

The registry staff collects a copy of the discharge form of each patient suffering from a malignant tumour from the general hospital's clinical files. Information is usually collected through meticulous examination of all admission and discharge forms. Information is also received from the Oncology Department and the Radiotherapy Institute of the University of Modena.

The registry staff also checks records at the Dermatology Department and the archives of private hospitals of the province. The pathology services of the University of Modena supply a list of all malignant tumours diagnosed histologically and their origin. In addition, the Public Health Services of the province supply a file stating whether death was or was not caused by cancer. All the information concerning a single tumour is coded, and entered into a computer.

Since 1994 information on survival of all cases of malignant tumours registered has been periodically brought up to date by the General Registries Offices of the various municipalities in the province, allowing the calculation of survival rates.

The registry staff periodically cross-check records on deaths from malignant tumours in the Province of Modena, in order to identify cases not previously reported.

All malignant tumours are recorded (ICD-9 codes 140–208). In addition, carcinoma *in situ* and other tumours of a benign or uncertain nature of the brain, liver, nervous system and bladder are registered, but only bladder papillomas are included in incidence figures. Tumours diagnosed with uncertain malignancy are registered but excluded from incidence data. Since 1994 the stage of breast and lung tumours has been consistently recorded.

Doubtful cases are periodically considered by a scientific committee of different specialists. Whenever new elements appear to confirm the malignancy of a tumour, the case is recoded and included among incident cases.

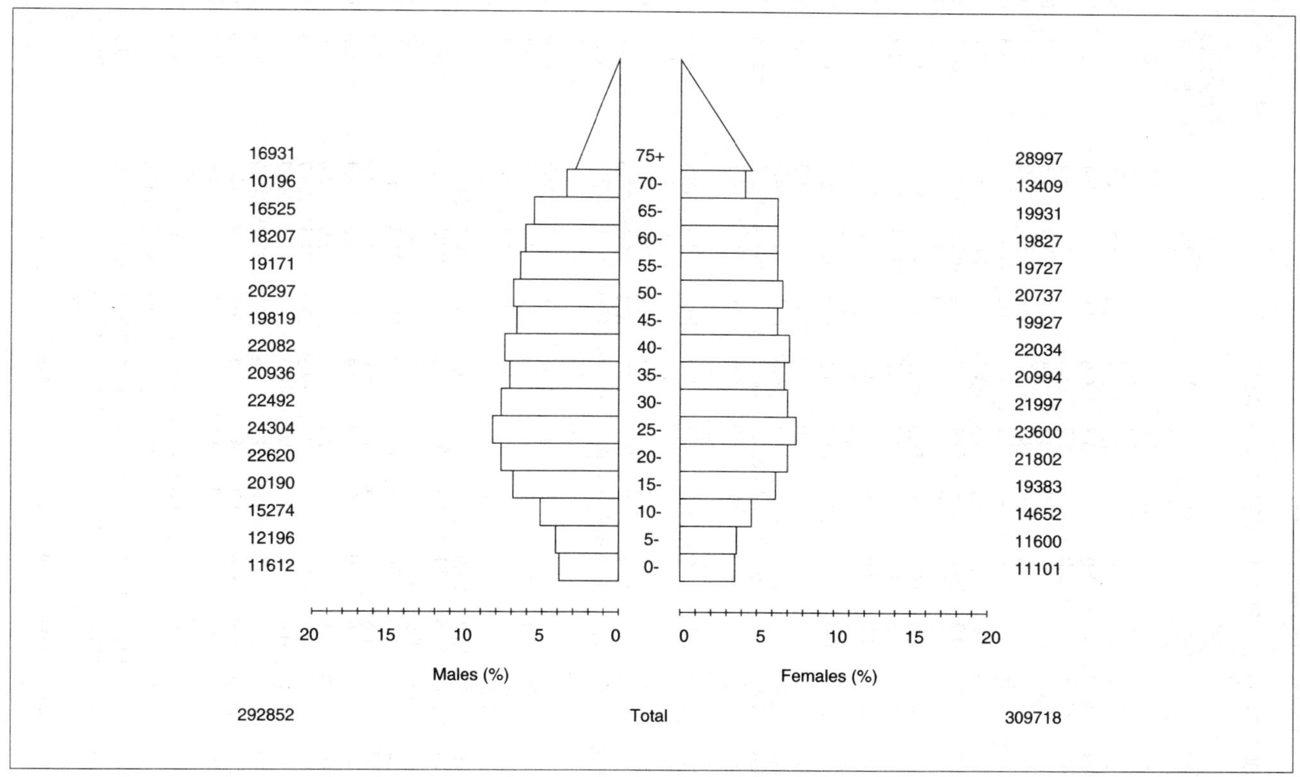

Italy, Modena
Source of population: average annual 1988–91
Screening programmes in the area:
The population aged 50-69 has been screened annually for
breast cancer since 1959.

ITALY, MODENA 1988-1992

ANNUAL INCIDENCE PER 100,000 BY AGE GROUP (YEARS) - MALE

SITE	ALL AGES	AGE UNK	0-	5-	10-	15-	20-	25-	30-	35-	40-	45-	50-	55-	60-	65-	70-	75+	CRUDE RATE	%	CR 64	CR 74	ASR (W)	ICD (9th)
Lip	6	0	-	-	-	-	-	-	-	-	-	-	1.0	1.0	-	-	-	4.7	0.4	0.1	0.01	0.01	0.2	140
Tongue	42	0	-	-	-	-	-	-	-	1.9	0.9	4.0	4.9	6.3	6.6	9.7	13.7	3.5	2.9	0.5	0.12	0.24	1.8	141
Salivary gland	16	0	-	-	-	-	-	-	-	-	-	1.0	1.0	1.0	3.3	2.4	2.0	8.3	1.1	0.2	0.03	0.05	0.6	142
Mouth	34	0	-	-	-	-	-	0.9	-	-	-	2.0	5.9	6.3	6.6	3.6	3.9	9.4	2.3	0.4	0.11	0.15	1.4	143-5
Oropharynx	34	0	-	-	-	-	-	-	-	-	-	2.0	3.0	8.3	3.3	14.5	5.9	3.5	2.3	0.4	0.08	0.19	1.4	146
Nasopharynx	17	0	-	-	-	-	-	-	-	1.0	0.9	1.0	2.0	2.1	4.4	2.4	2.0	3.5	1.2	0.2	0.06	0.08	0.7	147
Hypopharynx	34	0	-	-	-	-	-	-	-	-	2.7	4.0	3.9	8.3	7.7	6.1	3.9	1.2	2.3	0.4	0.13	0.18	1.5	148
Pharynx unspecified	4	0	-	-	-	-	-	-	-	-	-	-	2.1	1.1	1.2	-	-	-	0.3	0.1	0.02	0.02	0.2	149
Oesophagus	74	0	-	-	-	-	-	-	-	3.6	7.1	3.0	7.3	13.2	15.7	21.6	20.1		5.1	1.0	0.17	0.36	2.9	150
Stomach	651	0	-	-	-	-	-	0.8	1.8	2.9	10.9	20.2	30.5	51.1	86.8	131.9	162.8	309.5	44.5	8.4	1.02	2.50	22.7	151
Small intestine	17	0	-	-	-	-	-	0.8	-	1.0	0.9	-	1.0	2.1	3.3	2.4	3.9	4.7	1.2	0.2	0.05	0.08	0.7	152
Colon	589	0	-	-	-	-	0.9	0.8	3.6	4.8	10.0	14.1	29.6	53.2	96.7	113.8	170.6	239.8	40.2	7.6	1.07	2.49	21.2	153
Rectum	358	0	-	-	-	-	-	-	-	1.9	3.6	11.1	18.7	32.3	61.5	99.2	113.8	112.2	24.4	4.6	0.65	1.71	13.2	154
Liver	263	0	-	-	-	-	-	-	-	1.0	2.7	4.0	11.8	18.8	52.7	81.1	90.2	75.6	18.0	3.4	0.46	1.31	9.7	155
Gallbladder etc.	66	0	-	-	-	-	-	-	-	-	-	-	1.0	5.2	9.9	15.7	5.9	41.3	4.5	0.9	0.08	0.19	2.1	156
Pancreas	218	0	-	-	-	-	-	-	-	1.9	0.9	7.1	17.7	11.5	24.2	60.5	68.7	85.0	14.9	2.8	0.32	0.96	7.8	157
Nose, sinuses etc.	4	0	-	-	-	-	-	-	-	-	-	-	1.0	-	-	3.9	1.2		0.3	0.1	0.01	0.02	0.1	160
Larynx	282	0	-	-	-	-	-	0.8	-	2.9	3.6	15.1	20.7	34.4	64.8	77.5	70.6	54.3	19.3	3.6	0.71	1.45	11.2	161
Bronchus, lung	1821	0	-	-	-	0.9	-	1.8	4.8	19.9	59.5	84.7	214.9	404.2	492.6	486.4	492.6		124.4	23.5	3.95	8.85	68.6	162
Other thoracic organs	23	0	-	-	-	0.9	0.8	-	-	-	2.0	3.0	1.0	4.4	3.6	7.8	4.7		1.6	0.3	0.06	0.12	1.0	163-4
Bone	10	0	-	-	3.0	1.8	0.8	-	-	-	1.0	-	-	2.4	-	1.2			0.7	0.1	0.03	0.04	0.6	170
Connective tissue	58	0	1.7	1.6	-	1.0	-	0.8	1.8	1.0	2.7	2.0	6.9	2.1	8.8	10.9	7.8	18.9	4.0	0.7	0.15	0.25	2.6	171
Mesothelioma	13	0	-	-	-	-	-	-	-	-	0.9	2.0	1.0	1.0	1.1	6.1	2.0	1.2	0.9	0.2	0.03	0.07	0.6	MES
Kaposi's sarcoma	26	0	-	-	-	-	-	0.8	2.7	2.9	1.8	-	3.0	1.0	3.3	3.6	5.9	4.7	1.8	0.3	0.08	0.12	1.1	KAP
Melanoma of skin	100	0	-	-	-	-	0.9	1.6	2.7	6.7	4.5	11.1	10.8	10.4	7.7	12.1	25.5	23.6	6.8	1.3	0.28	0.47	4.3	172
Other skin	1185	0	1.7	-	-	-	0.9	2.5	4.4	5.7	22.6	40.4	72.9	99.1	159.3	239.6	351.1	487.9	80.9		2.05	5.00	42.8	173
Breast	9	0	-	-	-	-	-	-	-	-	-	-	1.0	1.0	4.4	3.6	-	-	0.6	0.1	0.03	0.05	0.4	175
Prostate	717	0	-	-	-	-	-	-	-	-	-	1.0	3.9	34.4	86.8	161.0	296.2	373.3	49.0	9.2	0.63	2.92	23.3	185
Testis	60	0	-	-	-	2.0	5.3	9.1	4.4	10.5	2.7	6.1	5.9	1.0	1.1	3.6	2.0	4.7	4.1	0.8	0.24	0.27	3.4	186
Penis	11	0	-	-	-	-	-	-	0.9	1.0	-	-	-	-	-	-	3.9	8.3	0.8	0.1	0.01	0.03	0.4	187.1-.4
Other male genital	4	0	-	-	-	-	-	-	-	1.0	-	-	1.0	-	1.1	-	-	1.2	0.3	0.1	0.02	0.02	0.2	187.5-.9
Bladder	816	0	3.4	-	-	1.0	1.8	0.8	3.6	7.6	10.9	28.3	53.2	89.7	139.5	206.9	219.7	245.7	55.7	10.5	1.70	3.83	31.1	188
Kidney etc.	292	0	1.7	-	-	-	-	0.9	-	5.7	3.6	7.1	11.8	36.5	61.5	66.6	90.2	81.5	19.9	3.8	0.64	1.43	11.2	189
Eye	14	0	1.7	-	-	-	-	-	-	-	0.9	1.0	-	-	6.6	4.8	-	1.2	1.0	0.2	0.05	0.08	0.8	190
Brain, nervous system	131	0	5.2	1.6	1.3	1.0	1.8	4.1	4.4	3.8	4.5	5.0	10.8	16.7	20.9	21.8	21.6	28.3	8.9	1.7	0.41	0.62	6.2	191-2
Thyroid	40	0	-	-	-	3.0	1.8	2.5	2.7	-	1.8	7.1	3.9	1.0	6.6	3.6	5.9	3.5	2.7	0.5	0.15	0.20	2.1	193
Other endocrine	19	0	1.7	-	-	-	0.9	-	-	-	3.6	1.0	2.0	2.1	4.4	1.2	2.0	2.4	1.3	0.2	0.08	0.09	1.0	194
Hodgkin's disease	42	0	-	1.6	-	4.0	0.9	4.9	3.6	3.8	3.6	6.1	3.0	2.1	2.2	2.4	2.0	2.4	2.9	0.5	0.18	0.20	2.5	201
Non-Hodgkin lymphoma	316	0	-	1.6	5.2	5.0	1.8	4.9	7.1	3.8	12.7	13.1	22.7	27.1	39.5	53.3	74.5	108.7	21.6	4.1	0.72	1.36	12.9	200,202
Multiple myeloma	102	0	-	-	-	-	-	-	-	1.0	0.9	1.0	3.9	8.3	16.5	26.6	29.4	41.3	7.0	1.3	0.16	0.44	3.6	203
Lymphoid leukaemia	89	0	-	1.6	2.6	1.0	-	-	0.9	1.0	-	2.0	3.0	11.5	6.6	15.7	27.5	40.2	6.1	1.1	0.15	0.37	3.4	204
Myeloid leukaemia	73	0	-	-	-	3.0	1.8	0.8	0.9	1.9	0.9	4.0	5.9	4.2	5.5	16.9	5.9	31.9	5.0	0.9	0.14	0.26	2.9	205
Monocytic leukaemia	7	0	-	-	1.3	-	-	-	-	-	-	-	1.0	1.0	-	2.4	-	2.4	0.5	0.1	0.02	0.03	0.3	206
Other leukaemia	1	0	-	-	-	-	-	-	-	-	-	-	-	-	-	-	2.0	-	0.1	0.0	0.00	0.01	0.0	207
Leukaemia unspecified	4	0	-	-	-	-	-	-	-	-	-	-	1.0	-	-	-	2.0	2.4	0.3	0.1	0.00	0.01	0.1	208
Other and unspecified	248	0	-	-	-	1.0	0.9	1.6	-	1.9	2.7	7.1	15.8	27.1	25.3	53.3	68.7	103.9	16.9	3.2	0.42	1.03	8.9	O&U
All sites	8940	0	17.2	8.2	10.5	24.8	23.0	39.5	48.9	83.1	142.2	300.7	487.7	846.1	1463.1	2052.5	2483.2	3096.0	610.5		17.47	40.15	335.5	ALL
All sites but 173	7755	0	15.5	8.2	10.5	24.8	22.1	37.0	44.5	77.4	119.6	260.4	414.8	746.9	1303.8	1812.9	2132.1	2608.2	529.6	100.0	15.43	35.15	292.7	ALLb

| Rate from 1 case | | | 1.722 | 1.640 | 1.309 | 0.991 | 0.884 | 0.823 | 0.889 | 0.955 | 0.906 | 1.009 | 0.985 | 1.043 | 1.098 | 1.210 | 1.961 | 1.181 |

ITALY, MODENA 1988-1992

ANNUAL INCIDENCE PER 100,000 BY AGE GROUP (YEARS) - FEMALE

SITE	ALL AGES	AGE UNK	0-	5-	10-	15-	20-	25-	30-	35-	40-	45-	50-	55-	60-	65-	70-	75+	CRUDE RATE	%	CR 64	CR 74	ASR (W)	ICD (9th)
Lip	0	0	-	-	-	-	-	-	-	-	-	-	-	-	-	-	-	-	0.0	0.0	0.00	0.00	0.0	140
Tongue	10	0	-	-	-	-	-	-	-	-	0.9	-	-	1.0	2.0	2.0	3.0	1.4	0.6	0.2	0.02	0.04	0.3	141
Salivary gland	9	0	-	-	-	-	-	-	-	-	-	-	1.0	-	1.0	2.0	1.5	2.8	0.6	0.1	0.01	0.03	0.2	142
Mouth	17	0	-	-	-	-	-	-	-	-	1.8	2.0	1.9	1.0	2.0	-	-	5.5	1.1	0.3	0.04	0.04	0.6	143-5
Oropharynx	7	0	-	-	-	-	-	-	-	-	-	-	1.9	1.0	-	-	3.0	1.4	0.5	0.1	0.01	0.03	0.2	146
Nasopharynx	5	0	-	-	-	-	-	-	1.8	-	-	-	1.0	-	-	2.0	-	-	0.3	0.1	0.01	0.02	0.2	147
Hypopharynx	6	0	-	-	-	-	-	-	-	-	-	1.0	-	-	2.0	-	1.5	1.4	0.4	0.1	0.02	0.02	0.2	148
Pharynx unspecified	0	0	-	-	-	-	-	-	-	-	-	-	-	-	-	-	-	-	0.0	0.0	0.00	0.00	0.0	149
Oesophagus	26	0	-	-	-	-	-	-	-	-	-	-	1.0	1.0	3.0	2.0	4.5	11.0	1.7	0.4	0.03	0.06	0.6	150
Stomach	478	0	-	-	-	-	0.9	-	1.8	4.8	8.2	4.0	18.3	21.3	45.4	55.2	94.0	175.2	30.9	7.2	0.52	1.27	11.8	151
Small intestine	24	0	-	-	-	-	-	-	-	-	-	2.0	-	3.0	4.0	2.0	6.0	6.2	1.5	0.4	0.05	0.09	0.7	152
Colon	599	0	-	-	-	-	0.9	2.5	1.8	5.7	6.4	24.1	28.9	50.7	62.5	87.3	135.7	162.8	38.7	9.1	0.92	2.03	17.1	153
Rectum	291	0	-	-	-	-	-	-	-	1.0	3.6	9.0	19.3	24.3	39.3	31.1	67.1	81.4	18.8	4.4	0.48	0.97	8.2	154
Liver	148	0	-	-	-	1.0	-	-	-	-	2.0	1.9	5.1	12.1	31.1	25.4	53.8		9.6	2.2	0.11	0.39	3.5	155
Gallbladder etc.	122	0	-	-	-	-	-	-	-	-	-	1.0	3.9	5.1	13.1	13.0	25.4	47.6	7.9	1.8	0.12	0.31	2.8	156
Pancreas	199	0	-	-	-	-	-	0.8	-	1.0	1.8	3.0	9.6	11.2	24.2	31.1	41.8	60.7	12.9	3.0	0.26	0.62	5.3	157
Nose, sinuses etc.	5	0	-	-	-	-	-	0.8	-	-	-	-	-	1.0	1.0	2.0	-	-	0.3	0.1	0.01	0.02	0.2	160
Larynx	18	0	-	-	-	-	-	-	-	-	-	-	1.9	1.0	2.0	9.0	3.0	1.4	1.2	0.3	0.02	0.08	0.6	161
Bronchus, lung	305	0	-	-	-	-	-	-	0.9	-	5.4	10.0	20.3	26.4	46.4	62.2	53.7	66.9	19.7	4.6	0.55	1.13	9.2	162
Other thoracic organs	11	0	-	-	-	-	-	-	-	-	-	1.0	1.0	1.0	-	1.0	4.5	2.8	0.7	0.2	0.01	0.04	0.3	163-4
Bone	11	0	-	-	2.7	1.0	1.8	-	-	-	-	-	1.0	2.0	1.0	-	1.5	0.7	0.7	0.2	0.05	0.06	0.7	170
Connective tissue	29	0	3.6	-	-	1.0	-	-	0.9	-	1.8	1.0	1.0	4.1	4.0	2.0	4.5	5.5	1.9	0.4	0.09	0.12	1.4	171
Mesothelioma	8	0	-	-	-	-	-	-	-	-	-	1.0	-	1.0	3.0	2.0	-	0.7	0.5	0.1	0.03	0.04	0.3	MES
Kaposi's sarcoma	6	0	-	-	-	-	-	-	-	-	-	-	-	-	-	2.0	1.5	2.1	0.4	0.1	0.00	0.00	0.1	KAP
Melanoma of skin	102	0	-	-	-	-	-	1.7	6.4	6.7	5.4	8.0	7.7	12.2	6.1	11.0	6.0	21.4	6.6	1.5	0.27	0.36	3.7	172
Other skin	759	0	-	-	-	-	2.8	2.5	6.4	10.5	16.3	30.1	38.6	40.6	64.6	108.4	134.2	238.0	49.0		1.06	2.27	21.0	173
Breast	1830	0	-	-	-	-	-	4.2	19.1	52.4	121.6	188.7	178.4	202.8	244.1	272.9	268.5	240.0	118.2	27.7	5.06	7.76	68.4	174
Uterus unspecified	14	0	-	-	-	-	-	-	-	1.0	-	-	1.0	1.0	2.0	1.0	1.5	4.8	0.9	0.2	0.02	0.04	0.4	179
Cervix uteri	151	0	-	-	-	-	-	3.4	5.5	6.7	10.9	12.0	13.5	18.2	18.2	18.1	22.4	18.6	9.8	2.3	0.44	0.64	5.9	180
Placenta	0	0	-	-	-	-	-	-	-	-	-	-	-	-	-	-	-	-	0.0	0.0	0.00	0.00	0.0	181
Corpus uteri	357	0	-	-	-	-	-	-	-	4.8	11.8	22.1	34.7	55.8	52.5	65.2	59.7	47.6	23.1	5.4	0.91	1.53	12.5	182
Ovary etc.	307	0	-	-	1.4	-	0.9	7.6	2.7	9.5	10.9	15.1	20.3	30.4	40.3	48.2	49.2	57.9	19.8	4.6	0.70	1.18	10.5	183
Other female genital	73	0	-	-	-	-	-	-	1.8	1.0	0.9	1.0	1.0	4.1	1.0	5.0	17.9	31.0	4.7	1.1	0.05	0.17	1.7	184
Bladder	189	0	-	-	-	2.1	1.8	0.8	-	1.9	3.6	3.0	8.7	14.2	23.2	33.1	29.8	52.4	12.2	2.9	0.30	0.61	5.5	188
Kidney etc.	182	0	3.6	-	-	-	-	-	1.8	1.0	4.5	10.0	9.6	14.2	34.3	35.1	29.8	33.8	11.8	2.8	0.40	0.72	6.2	189
Eye	7	0	1.8	-	-	-	-	-	-	-	0.9	-	-	-	1.0	1.0	-	2.1	0.5	0.1	0.02	0.02	0.4	190
Brain, nervous system	110	0	5.4	-	4.1	3.1	1.8	2.5	3.6	-	4.5	5.0	11.6	15.2	7.1	16.1	11.9	16.6	7.1	1.7	0.32	0.46	5.0	191-2
Thyroid	119	0	-	-	1.4	3.1	2.8	8.5	9.1	12.4	7.3	13.0	6.8	8.1	16.1	8.0	10.4	8.3	7.7	1.8	0.44	0.53	5.7	193
Other endocrine	13	0	-	-	-	1.0	-	-	-	-	0.9	2.0	1.0	-	3.0	3.0	-	1.4	0.8	0.2	0.04	0.05	0.6	194
Hodgkin's disease	42	0	-	-	4.1	3.1	2.8	4.2	2.7	1.0	4.5	1.0	-	1.0	3.0	3.0	4.5	5.5	2.7	0.6	0.14	0.17	2.2	201
Non-Hodgkin lymphoma	289	0	-	-	-	2.1	2.8	3.4	9.1	7.6	15.4	9.0	17.4	20.3	30.3	33.1	55.2	67.6	18.7	4.4	0.59	1.03	9.5	200,202
Multiple myeloma	96	0	-	-	-	-	-	-	-	-	-	-	3.9	10.1	9.1	12.0	25.4	30.3	6.2	1.5	0.12	0.30	2.4	203
Lymphoid leukaemia	68	0	9.0	-	4.1	1.0	-	0.8	0.9	-	-	2.0	3.9	7.1	6.1	14.0	7.5	13.1	4.4	1.0	0.17	0.28	3.3	204
Myeloid leukaemia	72	0	1.8	1.7	-	-	1.8	-	1.8	3.8	3.6	3.0	4.8	3.0	9.1	2.0	14.9	17.9	4.6	1.1	0.17	0.26	2.7	205
Monocytic leukaemia	3	0	-	-	-	-	-	-	-	-	-	-	-	-	1.0	-	1.5	0.7	0.2	0.0	0.01	0.01	0.1	206
Other leukaemia	0	0	-	-	-	-	-	-	-	-	-	-	-	-	-	-	-	-	0.0	0.0	0.00	0.00	0.0	207
Leukaemia unspecified	6	0	-	-	-	-	-	-	-	-	-	-	1.0	-	1.0	-	1.5	2.1	0.4	0.1	0.01	0.02	0.2	208
Other and unspecified	246	0	-	1.7	1.4	-	-	-	0.9	1.0	1.8	9.0	6.8	16.2	18.2	27.1	56.7	86.2	15.9	3.7	0.28	0.70	6.4	O&U
All sites	7369	0	25.2	3.4	19.1	18.6	21.1	44.1	79.1	133.4	255.1	395.4	484.1	635.7	859.4	1056.6	1285.6	1688.5	475.8		14.87	26.58	238.9	ALL
All sites but 173	6610	0	25.2	3.4	19.1	18.6	18.3	41.5	72.7	122.9	238.7	365.3	445.6	595.1	794.9	948.2	1151.4	1450.5	426.8	100.0	13.81	24.31	217.9	ALLb

Rate from 1 case: 1.802 1.724 1.365 1.032 0.917 0.847 0.909 0.953 0.908 1.004 0.964 1.014 1.009 1.003 1.491 0.690

Italy, Parma Province

The Parma Province Cancer Registry was founded in 1976 and began to operate in the Medical Oncology Division of the local Health District. Its objective is to estimate, for the population of the province of Parma, the incidence, mortality and survival of different forms of cancer, in relation to the primary site, sex, age and morphology; to compare its results with those of other tumour registries, and to formulate etiological hypotheses.

The registration of newly detected tumour cases is based upon reports from in- and outpatient departments in hospitals of the province of Parma and on histological reports from both public and private institutions. Other sources of information are the archives of autopsy reports, death certificates (some copies of which are received), procedures for reimbursement of care received abroad and other Italian cancer registries. Personal data are verified against the Health Service Registry.

The area of registration includes the whole province; the total area is 34 449 km^2 (44% mountains, 31% hills, 25% plains), subdivided into 47 municipalities. The highest point in the province is 1861 m above sea level and the lowest about 20 m.

The population covered by the registry was 390 634 in 1990 (188 005 males and 202 629 females), with a population density of 114 inhabitants per km^2. The area is predominantly urban and industrialized, with a major food-production industry. Significant migration abroad or to other parts of Italy occurs, and more local migration from the mountainous regions towards the city and the plains.

The province contains seven hospitals (one main general university hospital, three small public hospitals and three private hospitals). These allow the diagnosis and treatment of all cases of cancer in the province. Only a small minority turn to external health structures.

All malignant tumours, according to the categories 140–199 (ICD-O first edition) are registered and included in the incidence figures, as well as benign tumours and *in situ* carcinomas of transitional epithelium of the urinary tract (188 and 189). Benign intracranial tumours are registered but not included in the incidence statistics. This is the only exception to ICD rates.

The following data are recorded: personal data, date of first diagnosis (date of incidence is usually that of the histological report, where available; for cases without histological report the date of first discharge from the hospital is utilized).

Active retrieval of data on the vital status of patients and the cause of death, for survival evaluation, is carried out.

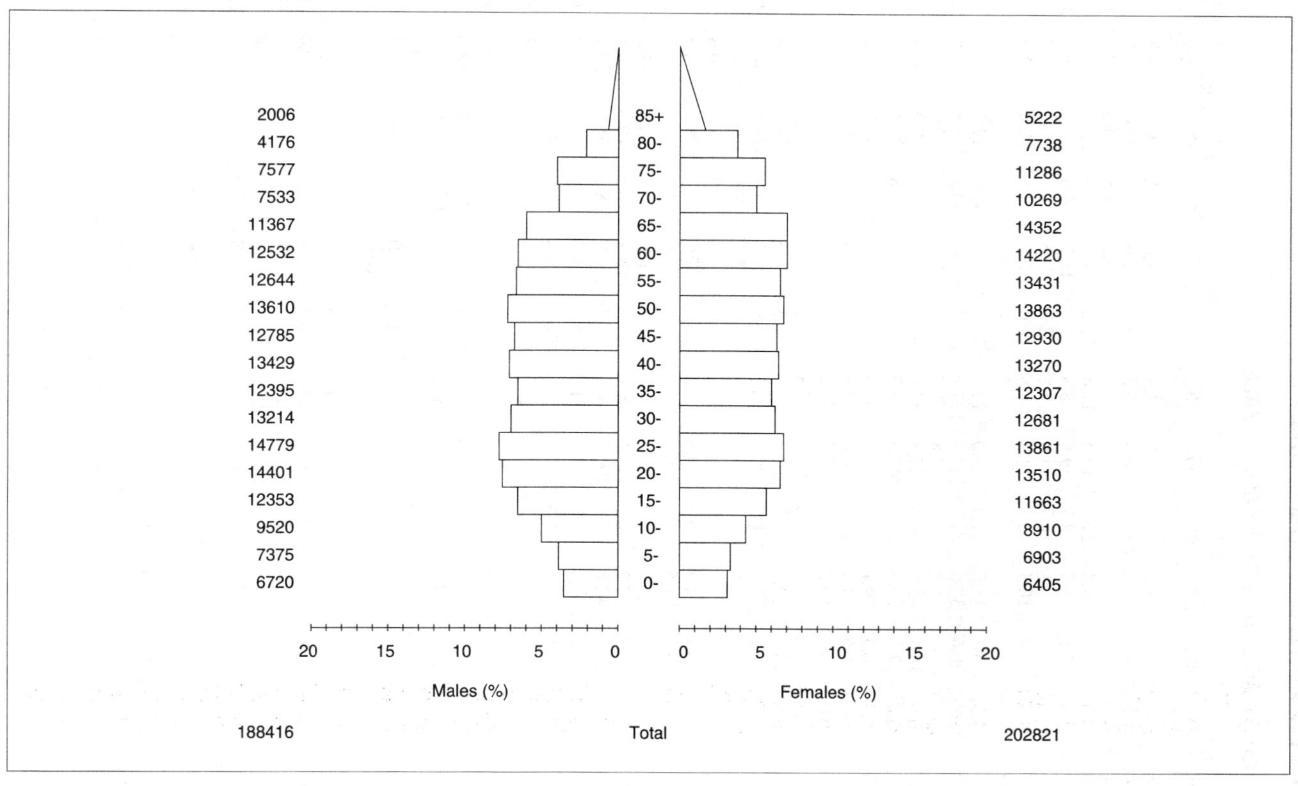

Italy, Parma Province
Source of population: average annual 1988–92
Census: 13° Censimento generale della popolazione e delle
abitazioni, 20 Ottobre 1991. Fascicolo provinciale Macerata,
Istituto Nazionale di Statistics (ISTAT), Roma, 1993.
Estimate: Intercensal.

ITALY, PARMA PROVINCE 1988-1992

ANNUAL INCIDENCE PER 100,000 BY AGE GROUP (YEARS) - MALE

SITE	ALL AGES	AGE UNK	0-	5-	10-	15-	20-	25-	30-	35-	40-	45-	50-	55-	60-	65-	70-	75-	80-	85+	CRUDE RATE	%	CR 64	CR 74	ASR (W)	ICD (9th)
Lip	12	0	-	-	-	-	-	-	-	-	-	-	1.5	1.6	3.2	1.8	-	2.6	19.2	19.9	1.3	0.2	0.03	0.04	**0.5**	140
Tongue	30	0	-	-	-	-	1.4	1.5	-	-	1.5	4.7	4.4	14.2	6.4	5.3	8.0	2.6	-	10.0	3.2	0.5	0.17	0.24	**2.0**	141
Salivary gland	5	0	-	-	-	-	-	-	-	-	-	1.6	-	-	-	-	-	5.3	4.8	10.0	0.5	0.1	0.01	0.01	**0.2**	142
Mouth	48	0	-	-	-	-	-	-	-	-	3.0	3.1	8.8	11.1	14.4	17.6	18.6	2.6	4.8	29.9	5.1	0.8	0.20	0.38	**2.9**	143-5
Oropharynx	28	0	-	-	-	-	-	-	-	-	3.0	3.1	5.9	4.7	9.6	8.8	-	13.2	4.8	-	3.0	0.5	0.13	0.18	**1.7**	146
Nasopharynx	12	0	-	-	-	-	-	1.4	-	-	-	-	-	4.7	1.6	8.8	2.7	2.6	-	-	1.3	0.2	0.04	0.10	**0.7**	147
Hypopharynx	41	0	-	-	-	-	-	-	1.5	-	4.5	4.7	10.3	7.9	11.2	8.8	10.6	10.6	4.8	10.0	4.4	0.7	0.20	0.30	**2.6**	148
Pharynx unspecified	1	0	-	-	-	-	-	-	-	1.6	-	-	-	-	-	-	-	-	-	-	0.1	0.0	0.01	0.01	**0.1**	149
Oesophagus	71	0	-	-	-	-	-	1.4	-	-	1.5	3.1	11.8	17.4	16.0	15.8	21.2	23.8	33.5	49.8	7.5	1.2	0.26	0.44	**3.9**	150
Stomach	714	0	-	-	-	-	-	-	4.5	6.5	8.9	26.6	33.8	82.2	129.3	197.1	300.0	364.2	560.3	478.5	75.8	12.2	1.46	3.94	**33.7**	151
Small intestine	10	0	-	-	-	-	-	-	-	1.6	-	-	-	1.6	4.8	1.8	-	7.9	-	10.0	1.1	0.2	0.04	0.05	**0.5**	152
Colon	488	0	-	-	-	-	1.4	1.4	1.5	8.1	10.4	14.1	42.6	69.6	97.3	132.0	191.1	227.0	292.1	358.9	51.8	8.3	1.23	2.85	**24.4**	153
Rectum	261	0	-	-	-	-	-	-	-	-	6.0	17.2	26.4	33.2	47.9	63.3	100.9	132.0	162.8	189.4	27.7	4.4	0.65	1.47	**13.0**	154
Liver	256	0	-	-	-	-	1.4	-	-	1.6	4.5	6.3	19.1	42.7	62.2	107.3	114.2	79.2	119.7	89.7	27.2	4.4	0.69	1.80	**13.3**	155
Gallbladder etc.	68	0	-	-	-	-	-	-	-	-	-	1.6	4.4	11.1	16.0	17.6	23.9	37.0	38.3	59.8	7.2	1.2	0.17	0.37	**3.3**	156
Pancreas	160	0	-	-	-	-	-	-	-	3.2	6.0	6.3	16.2	22.1	25.5	42.2	53.1	97.7	95.8	79.8	17.0	2.7	0.40	0.87	**7.8**	157
Nose, sinuses etc.	13	0	-	-	-	-	-	-	-	-	1.5	1.6	-	7.9	1.6	3.5	2.7	-	4.8	10.0	1.4	0.2	0.06	0.09	**0.8**	160
Larynx	194	0	-	-	-	-	-	-	-	-	6.0	14.1	32.3	49.0	52.7	58.1	87.6	44.9	47.9	19.9	20.6	3.3	0.77	1.50	**11.2**	161
Bronchus, lung	1229	0	-	-	-	-	1.4	-	-	-	17.9	50.1	91.1	188.2	349.5	462.7	469.9	543.7	454.9	428.7	130.5	20.9	3.49	8.15	**63.4**	162
Other thoracic organs	6	0	-	-	-	-	-	-	-	-	-	-	1.5	-	-	-	-	2.7	5.3	9.6	0.6	0.1	0.01	0.02	**0.2**	163-4
Bone	6	0	-	-	-	3.2	-	1.4	-	1.6	-	-	-	-	1.6	-	-	-	4.8	-	0.6	0.1	0.04	0.04	**0.6**	170
Connective tissue	27	0	-	-	-	3.2	-	1.4	-	-	-	3.1	4.4	6.3	4.8	8.8	5.3	7.9	-	19.9	2.9	0.5	0.12	0.19	**1.8**	171
Mesothelioma	16	0	-	-	-	-	-	-	-	-	1.5	3.1	1.5	4.7	6.4	1.8	-	7.9	4.8	-	1.7	0.3	0.09	0.09	**1.0**	MES
Kaposi's sarcoma	11	0	-	-	-	-	1.4	1.4	1.5	-	-	-	-	3.2	-	3.5	-	10.6	-	-	1.2	0.2	0.04	0.05	**0.6**	KAP
Melanoma of skin	61	0	-	-	-	-	6.8	3.0	6.5	4.5	4.7	10.3	6.3	17.6	10.6	21.2	15.8	4.8	10.0	6.5	1.0	0.30	0.46	**4.1**	172
Other skin	547	0	3.0	-	-	-	-	2.7	3.0	3.2	10.4	23.5	42.6	82.2	106.9	160.1	244.2	256.0	268.2	338.9	58.1		1.39	3.41	**28.0**	173
Breast	11	0	-	-	-	-	-	-	-	-	1.5	1.6	2.9	-	-	1.8	8.0	5.3	4.8	-	1.2	0.2	0.03	0.08	**0.6**	175
Prostate	515	0	-	-	-	-	-	-	-	-	-	1.6	10.3	39.5	67.0	147.8	254.9	348.4	431.0	378.8	54.7	8.8	0.59	2.61	**21.9**	185
Testis	51	0	-	-	3.2	13.9	4.1	13.6	12.9	7.4	6.3	4.4	3.2	1.6	3.5	2.7	2.6	-	-	-	5.4	0.9	0.35	0.38	**4.7**	186
Penis	13	0	-	-	-	-	-	-	-	-	-	1.6	-	1.6	-	7.0	-	7.9	4.8	29.9	1.4	0.2	0.02	0.05	**0.6**	187.1-.4
Other male genital	2	0	-	-	-	-	-	-	-	-	-	-	-	-	3.2	-	-	-	-	-	0.2	0.0	0.02	0.02	**0.1**	187.5-.9
Bladder	549	0	-	-	-	-	-	-	1.5	-	10.4	18.8	13.2	87.0	130.9	163.6	270.8	250.7	258.6	388.8	58.3	9.3	1.31	3.48	**27.3**	188
Kidney etc.	233	0	-	-	-	-	-	-	1.5	4.8	6.0	23.5	30.9	61.7	59.0	63.3	71.7	84.5	67.0	39.9	24.7	4.0	0.94	1.61	**13.2**	189
Eye	4	0	-	-	-	-	-	-	-	-	-	-	-	1.6	1.6	-	5.3	-	-	-	0.4	0.1	0.02	0.04	**0.2**	190
Brain, nervous system	99	0	3.0	2.7	8.4	3.2	-	-	4.5	1.6	10.4	3.1	4.4	11.1	31.9	33.4	31.9	37.0	14.4	-	10.5	1.7	0.42	0.75	**6.9**	191-2
Thyroid	31	0	-	-	-	-	2.8	4.1	1.5	3.2	3.0	4.7	2.9	-	6.4	5.3	10.6	10.6	4.8	-	3.3	0.5	0.14	0.22	**2.2**	193
Other endocrine	3	0	-	-	-	1.6	-	-	-	-	-	-	1.5	-	1.6	-	-	-	-	-	0.3	0.1	0.02	0.02	**0.3**	194
Hodgkin's disease	24	0	-	-	-	1.6	4.2	2.7	3.0	1.6	-	6.3	1.5	4.7	4.8	1.8	2.7	2.6	4.8	-	2.5	0.4	0.15	0.17	**2.0**	201
Non-Hodgkin lymphoma	192	0	-	-	2.1	3.2	5.6	2.7	9.1	8.1	10.4	15.6	22.0	28.5	51.1	52.8	53.1	52.8	52.7	89.7	20.4	3.3	0.79	1.32	**11.9**	200,202
Multiple myeloma	84	0	-	-	-	-	-	-	-	-	1.5	4.7	4.4	6.3	3.2	28.2	53.1	55.4	43.1	49.8	8.9	1.4	0.10	0.51	**3.9**	203
Lymphoid leukaemia	43	0	3.0	-	2.1	3.2	1.4	2.7	-	1.6	-	3.1	2.9	4.7	3.2	14.1	10.6	15.8	23.9	29.9	4.6	0.7	0.14	0.26	**3.0**	204
Myeloid leukaemia	50	0	-	-	2.1	-	-	-	1.5	1.6	1.5	-	2.9	3.2	14.4	3.5	21.2	23.8	38.3	59.8	5.3	0.9	0.14	0.26	**2.6**	205
Monocytic leukaemia	5	0	-	-	-	-	-	-	-	-	-	-	-	-	-	1.8	-	10.6	-	-	0.5	0.1	0.00	0.01	**0.2**	206
Other leukaemia	2	0	-	-	-	-	-	-	-	-	-	-	-	-	-	-	-	2.6	-	10.0	0.2	0.0	0.00	0.00	**0.1**	207
Leukaemia unspecified	26	0	-	-	-	-	-	-	-	-	-	1.6	4.4	7.9	4.8	3.5	2.7	18.5	19.2	-	2.8	0.4	0.09	0.12	**1.3**	208
Other and unspecified	167	0	-	-	-	-	-	-	-	-	4.5	9.4	4.4	28.5	27.1	42.2	50.4	97.7	110.1	169.5	17.7	2.8	0.37	0.83	**7.9**	O&U
All sites	6419	0	8.9	2.7	14.7	22.7	33.3	35.2	53.0	69.4	147.4	294.1	482.0	961.7	1398.0	1910.8	2527.3	2927.1	3217.9	3469.2	681.3		17.62	39.81	**333.1**	ALL
All sites but 173	5872	0	6.0	2.7	14.7	22.7	33.3	32.5	49.9	66.2	137.0	270.6	439.4	879.4	1291.1	1750.7	2283.1	2671.1	2949.8	3130.3	623.3	100.0	16.23	36.40	**305.1**	ALLb

| Rate from 1 case | | | 2.976 | 2.712 | 2.101 | 1.619 | 1.389 | 1.353 | 1.514 | 1.613 | 1.489 | 1.564 | 1.469 | 1.582 | 1.596 | 1.759 | 2.655 | 2.639 | 4.789 | 9.969 | | | | | | |

ITALY, PARMA PROVINCE 1988-1992

ANNUAL INCIDENCE PER 100,000 BY AGE GROUP (YEARS) - FEMALE

SITE	ALL AGES	AGE UNK	0-	5-	10-	15-	20-	25-	30-	35-	40-	45-	50-	55-	60-	65-	70-	75-	80-	85+	CRUDE RATE	%	CR 64	CR 74	ASR (W)	ICD (9th)
Lip	2	0	-	-	-	-	-	-	-	-	-	-	-	-	-	-	-	-	2.6	3.8	0.2	0.0	0.00	0.00	**0.0**	*140*
Tongue	10	0	-	-	-	-	-	1.6	-	1.5	-	1.4	3.0	-	-	2.8	-	5.3	-	-	1.0	0.2	0.04	0.05	**0.5**	*141*
Salivary gland	4	0	-	-	-	-	-	-	-	1.5	-	1.4	-	-	-	1.9	-	-	3.8	0.4	0.1	0.01	0.02	**0.2**	*142*
Mouth	14	0	-	-	-	-	-	-	-	-	-	-	1.5	1.4	2.8	3.9	7.1	10.3	-	1.4	0.3	0.01	0.05	**0.4**	*143-5*
Oropharynx	5	0	-	-	-	-	-	-	-	-	-	-	3.0	-	-	3.9	1.8	-	-	0.5	0.1	0.01	0.03	**0.2**	*146*
Nasopharynx	6	0	-	-	-	-	-	-	-	-	-	1.4	-	1.4	-	-	5.3	2.6	-	0.6	0.1	0.01	0.01	**0.2**	*147*
Hypopharynx	8	0	-	-	-	-	-	-	-	-	-	1.4	1.5	2.8	2.8	1.9	-	-	3.8	0.8	0.2	0.03	0.05	**0.4**	*148*
Pharynx unspecified	0	0	-	-	-	-	-	-	-	-	-	-	-	-	-	-	-	-	-	0.0	0.0	0.00	0.00	**0.0**	*149*
Oesophagus	19	0	-	-	-	-	-	-	-	-	3.0	-	-	3.0	4.2	7.0	-	-	10.3	11.5	1.9	0.4	0.05	0.09	**0.8**	*150*
Stomach	484	0	-	-	-	-	-	2.9	-	3.2	9.0	9.3	17.3	31.3	50.6	75.3	85.7	196.7	242.9	367.7	47.7	9.6	0.62	1.42	**14.7**	*151*
Small intestine	10	0	-	-	-	-	-	-	1.6	1.6	-	-	-	-	-	2.8	1.9	1.8	5.2	7.7	1.0	0.2	0.02	0.04	**0.4**	*152*
Colon	460	0	-	-	-	-	-	1.4	3.2	4.9	10.6	32.5	30.3	59.6	68.9	89.2	101.3	143.5	165.4	210.6	45.4	9.1	1.06	2.01	**17.8**	*153*
Rectum	243	0	-	-	-	-	-	-	-	3.2	4.5	13.9	11.5	25.3	36.6	44.6	66.2	70.9	126.6	88.1	24.0	4.8	0.48	1.03	**8.8**	*154*
Liver	131	0	-	-	-	-	-	1.4	1.6	1.6	1.5	-	4.3	13.4	22.5	47.4	29.2	42.5	33.6	49.8	12.9	2.6	0.23	0.61	**4.9**	*155*
Gallbladder etc.	102	0	-	-	-	-	-	-	-	-	-	4.6	5.8	10.4	9.8	15.3	23.4	33.7	69.8	46.0	10.1	2.0	0.15	0.35	**3.2**	*156*
Pancreas	176	0	-	-	-	-	-	-	-	3.2	1.5	1.5	5.8	14.9	18.3	29.3	48.7	54.9	93.0	122.6	17.4	3.5	0.23	0.62	**5.5**	*157*
Nose, sinuses etc.	8	0	-	-	-	-	-	-	-	-	-	-	2.9	1.5	-	4.2	1.9	-	2.6	-	0.8	0.2	0.02	0.05	**0.4**	*160*
Larynx	13	0	-	-	-	-	-	-	-	-	-	1.5	-	6.0	2.8	1.4	1.9	5.3	2.6	-	1.3	0.3	0.05	0.07	**0.6**	*161*
Bronchus, lung	299	0	-	-	-	-	1.5	-	1.6	4.9	4.5	9.3	26.0	38.7	45.0	82.2	93.5	88.6	69.8	95.7	29.5	5.9	0.66	1.54	**12.0**	*162*
Other thoracic organs	1	0	-	-	-	-	-	-	-	-	-	-	-	-	-	-	1.9	-	-	-	0.1	0.0	0.00	0.01	**0.0**	*163-4*
Bone	10	0	-	-	4.5	1.7	-	2.9	1.6	-	-	1.5	-	1.5	1.4	-	-	-	-	3.8	1.0	0.2	0.08	0.08	**1.1**	*170*
Connective tissue	30	0	-	-	-	-	-	1.4	-	3.2	-	3.1	-	4.5	11.3	7.0	7.8	1.8	5.2	7.7	3.0	0.6	0.12	0.19	**1.6**	*171*
Mesothelioma	5	0	-	-	-	-	-	-	-	-	-	-	-	-	1.4	2.8	-	3.5	-	-	0.5	0.1	0.01	0.02	**0.2**	*MES*
Kaposi's sarcoma	0	0	-	-	-	-	-	-	-	-	-	-	-	-	-	-	-	-	-	-	0.0	0.0	0.00	0.00	**0.0**	*KAP*
Melanoma of skin	77	0	-	-	-	-	3.0	4.3	4.7	6.5	12.1	15.5	15.9	3.0	8.4	11.1	9.7	14.2	12.9	7.7	7.6	1.5	0.37	0.47	**4.9**	*172*
Other skin	358	0	-	-	-	-	-	1.4	3.2	8.1	7.5	21.7	17.3	26.8	49.2	65.5	76.0	138.2	139.6	183.8	35.3		0.68	1.38	**12.9**	*173*
Breast	1353	0	-	-	-	-	1.5	11.5	26.8	52.0	141.7	247.5	212.1	205.5	227.8	252.2	194.7	264.0	279.1	214.5	133.4	26.8	5.63	7.87	**73.6**	*174*
Uterus unspecified	28	0	-	-	-	-	-	-	1.6	1.5	1.5	2.9	-	-	8.4	9.7	8.9	10.3	11.5	-	2.8	0.6	0.04	0.13	**1.1**	*179*
Cervix uteri	98	0	-	-	-	-	-	-	3.2	8.1	15.1	21.7	18.8	11.9	15.5	12.5	15.6	14.2	18.1	11.5	9.7	1.9	0.47	0.61	**5.9**	*180*
Placenta	2	0	-	-	-	-	-	1.4	-	-	1.5	-	-	-	-	-	-	-	-	-	0.2	0.0	0.01	0.01	**0.2**	*181*
Corpus uteri	250	0	-	-	-	-	-	-	-	4.9	12.1	20.1	56.3	37.2	56.3	51.6	68.2	44.3	36.2	42.1	24.7	5.0	0.93	1.53	**12.5**	*182*
Ovary etc.	200	0	-	-	2.2	1.7	1.5	2.9	3.2	6.5	9.0	15.5	27.4	26.8	42.2	43.2	38.9	58.5	36.2	30.6	19.7	4.0	0.69	1.11	**9.9**	*183*
Other female genital	59	0	-	-	-	-	-	-	-	-	1.5	1.5	-	4.5	2.8	8.4	33.1	10.6	31.0	42.1	5.8	1.2	0.05	0.26	**1.9**	*184*
Bladder	155	0	-	-	-	-	-	-	-	-	3.0	1.5	2.9	17.9	15.5	26.5	54.5	51.4	75.0	84.3	15.3	3.1	0.20	0.61	**4.9**	*188*
Kidney etc.	105	0	3.1	-	-	-	3.0	-	1.6	3.2	1.5	6.2	11.5	22.3	16.9	12.5	31.2	26.6	23.3	38.3	10.4	2.1	0.35	0.57	**5.1**	*189*
Eye	4	0	-	-	-	-	-	-	-	-	-	-	-	1.4	-	1.8	2.6	-	-	3.8	0.4	0.1	0.00	0.01	**0.1**	*190*
Brain, nervous system	71	0	3.1	2.9	2.2	1.7	-	-	3.2	1.6	1.5	3.1	5.8	6.0	19.7	15.3	21.4	12.4	23.3	3.8	7.0	1.4	0.25	0.44	**4.0**	*191-2*
Thyroid	49	0	-	-	2.2	-	1.5	2.9	9.5	9.7	4.5	4.6	4.3	7.4	4.2	8.4	7.8	8.9	-	3.8	4.8	1.0	0.25	0.34	**3.5**	*193*
Other endocrine	8	0	-	-	-	-	-	1.4	1.6	-	-	-	1.4	-	1.4	-	3.9	-	-	3.8	0.8	0.2	0.03	0.06	**0.5**	*194*
Hodgkin's disease	32	0	-	-	2.2	1.7	3.0	5.8	6.3	3.2	-	3.1	1.4	1.5	2.8	4.2	-	8.9	5.2	7.7	3.2	0.6	0.16	0.18	**2.3**	*201*
Non-Hodgkin lymphoma	187	0	-	-	2.2	1.7	1.5	4.3	-	11.4	3.0	12.4	18.8	20.8	23.9	40.4	40.9	46.1	75.0	57.4	18.4	3.7	0.50	0.91	**8.3**	*200,202*
Multiple myeloma	68	0	-	-	-	-	-	-	-	-	-	-	2.9	4.5	16.9	8.4	27.3	19.5	36.2	23.0	6.7	1.3	0.12	0.30	**2.3**	*203*
Lymphoid leukaemia	27	0	6.2	2.9	2.2	-	1.5	-	-	-	-	3.1	1.4	1.5	4.2	2.8	7.8	1.8	5.2	23.0	2.7	0.5	0.12	0.17	**2.2**	*204*
Myeloid leukaemia	57	0	-	2.9	-	1.7	-	-	-	3.2	3.0	1.5	-	10.4	8.4	2.8	13.6	21.3	31.0	15.3	5.6	1.1	0.16	0.24	**2.5**	*205*
Monocytic leukaemia	2	0	-	-	-	-	-	-	-	-	-	-	-	-	1.4	-	1.4	-	-	-	0.2	0.0	0.01	0.01	**0.1**	*206*
Other leukaemia	0	0	-	-	-	-	-	-	-	-	-	-	-	-	-	-	-	-	-	-	0.0	0.0	0.00	0.00	**0.0**	*207*
Leukaemia unspecified	22	0	-	-	2.2	-	-	-	1.6	-	-	-	-	1.5	1.4	2.8	9.7	7.1	7.8	15.3	2.2	0.4	0.03	0.10	**0.9**	*208*
Other and unspecified	146	0	-	-	-	-	-	1.4	-	-	3.0	3.1	2.9	7.4	14.1	19.5	23.4	51.4	87.9	134.0	14.4	2.9	0.16	0.37	**4.2**	*O&U*
All sites	5398	0	12.5	8.7	20.2	10.3	17.8	47.6	74.1	147.9	259.2	460.9	515.0	635.8	811.5	1015.9	1162.6	1472.5	1778.1	1980.1	532.3		15.11	26.00	**237.8**	*ALL*
All sites but 173	5040	0	12.5	8.7	20.2	10.3	17.8	46.2	71.0	139.7	251.7	439.3	497.7	609.0	762.3	950.4	1086.7	1334.3	1638.6	1796.2	497.0	100.0	14.43	24.62	**224.8**	*ALLb*
Rate from 1 case			3.122	2.897	2.245	1.715	1.480	1.443	1.577	1.625	1.507	1.547	1.443	1.489	1.406	1.394	1.947	1.772	2.585	3.830						

Italy, Ragusa Province

Ragusa Cancer Registry (RCR) was founded in 1979 by the head of the Department of Histopathology of Ospedali Riuniti Civile e M.P. Arezzo of Ragusa and by the director of the Institute of Hygiene of the University of Palermo. Population-based incidence data are available since 1981.

RCR is funded and supported by the Lega Italiana per la lotta contro i Tumori, by Regione Sicilia, by Provincia Regionale di Ragusa and by the Local Health Authority No 23. The staff consists of a part-time pathologist as Director, two part-time medically qualified epidemiologists, two full-time clerical officers and one full-time data entry clerk; there is a variable number of field work personnel, usually medical doctors trained by RCR and employed on a temporary basis.

The Registry covers the province of Ragusa and is located in south- eastern Sicily lying between 36°42 and 37°8′ N, and 14°9′ and 15° E, approximately in the geographical middle of the Mediterranean Sea. The area covers 1614 sq km, two-thirds consisting of highland, with elevation ranging between 500 and 975 metres, and one third of coastal plain. The climate has been classified as temperate Mediterranean with an average annual temperature of 16.9° and average annual precipitation of approximately 509 ml. In 1981 the province of Ragusa, which includes 12 Municipalities, had a population of 274 583 and in 1991 289 733 plus 2134 immigrants mostly from northern Africa. The 1991 Italian census showed only the city of Ragusa with a population exceeding 60 000 inhabitants. The area has been divided into three geographical districts for Health Service purposes.

Despite a decrease in the number of people involved in agricultural activities, patterns of work and employment opportunities in the period 1988-1992 reflect those reported in Volume VI of CI5, with farming, cattle-breeding and associated activities representing the main occupations; starting from the 1970s indoor vegetable growing by means of green-houses has been an important and common practice and has became the leading crop. As in the description reported in Volume VI of CI5, the province of Ragusa still has the highest per-capita-income and industrialisation rate in Sicily, but still these are still much lower than in the provinces of northern Italy.

From the Oncological and Epidemiological point of view the area covered by RCR is interesting for its geographical location (the southernmost population-based cancer registry in Europe), for the local dietary habits (Mediterranean diet) and in that the incidence of all sites of cancer (non-melanoma skin cancer excluded) is relatively low whereas mortality from the most preventable and curable tumours (cervix uteri, breast, thyroid, colon, haematological malignancies and paediatric tumours) is high compared to the Italian and Western European registries. Since the beginning RCR has adopted an active data collection method by involving field work personnel who abstract the required information onto the registration form; histological reports are systematically copied. Main sources of data are the medical records of all of departments of the six hospitals, the two local laboratories of pathology, the Computerised Axial Tomography Service and death certificates in which tumours are mentioned; data are also collected from a few of hospitals located in neighbouring counties and in northern Italy which are used to admit or to treat Ragusa residents (so called extra-territorial sources).

In order to detect those cases which are not traced from the main sources RCR uses some complementary sources such as the Health Insurance Office for patients' compensation funds, Health Authority Office for exemption from prescription and diagnostic charges and all of the other administrative bureaux which deal with cancer patients; these complementary sources, together with the involvement of the general practitioners, have been useful for detecting residents who were only treated in hospitals outside the county of Ragusa, for out-patients and for the patients never attending hospitals.

In the period 1988-1992 the management of the local Health System moderately improved compared to the previous five years of registration and the accessibility of medical records was also improved by the introduction of the hospital discharge form which is filled in and classified according to ICD rules by trained personnel and centrally stored. The improvement of the management of cancer patients led to an increase of thin-needle aspiration biopsies and bladder and gastric-intestinal endoscopies. These improvements made it possible to increase the percentage of cases with histological verification and to enrich each of the cancer notifications with better clinical details. Nevertheless, the Health Service development has been inadequate to the needs of the local population (as has been the case in the other areas of Southern Italy) and, for this reason, RCR has been very careful in checking for under-ascertainment.

For survival analysis purposes, since the 1st of January 1992 the Vital Statistics Office of the Local Health Authority provides copies of death certificates for all causes every three months (before that date RCR only used to collect the death certificates in which tumours were mentioned). Furthermore, the 12 Municipalities' Population Registers are routinely used for the verification of residence in the registry area of notified and recorded cases and for the date of death of those cases who died outside Ragusa county.

At RCR all of the items about the tumour (incidence date, most valid basis of diagnosis, topography, morphology, behaviour, multiple tumours) are inspected by a pathologist who is in charge of the classification and ICD-coding for all of the cases; after his final checking the cases are ready for the data entry. Physicians of cases with insufficient basic information for data entry are systematically contacted and, if necessary, further details sought from the complementary sources mentioned above.

Cancer research based on data collected by the Registry has formed an increasing part of RCR's activity and has led the RCR to be involved in several analytical studies; RCR is a collaborating centre for the following projects: the EPIC study (European Prospective Investigation into Cancer and Nutrition) co-ordinated by IARC with the creation of a "biological bank" in which blood samples from 10 000 subjects will be stored at Nitrogen Liquid temperature; the Eurocare project to compare cancer survival across Europe co-ordinated by the National Cancer Institute of Milan (IARC monograph No 132); Italian multicentre case-control study on the relationship between pesticides and haematological malignancies, co-ordinated by the Cancer Epidemiology Unit of the Turin University; the Helios case-control study on sunlight exposure and risk of non-melanoma skin cancer, co-ordinated by the Piedmont Cancer Registry; the BIOMED-Non Hodgkin Lymphomas study for the European descriptive and trend analysis of

NHL, co-ordinated by the Leukaemia Research Fund of Leeds University. Further, RCR has focused its interest on the techniques of case detection/registration and in the definition and management of multiple tumours.

Despite its small size we think that the information provided by RCR is of great value in issues concerning cancer causes and control both for Sicily and Southern Italy, regions where cancer epidemiology is very poor.

Lorenzo Gafá
Luigi Dardanoni
Rosario Tumino

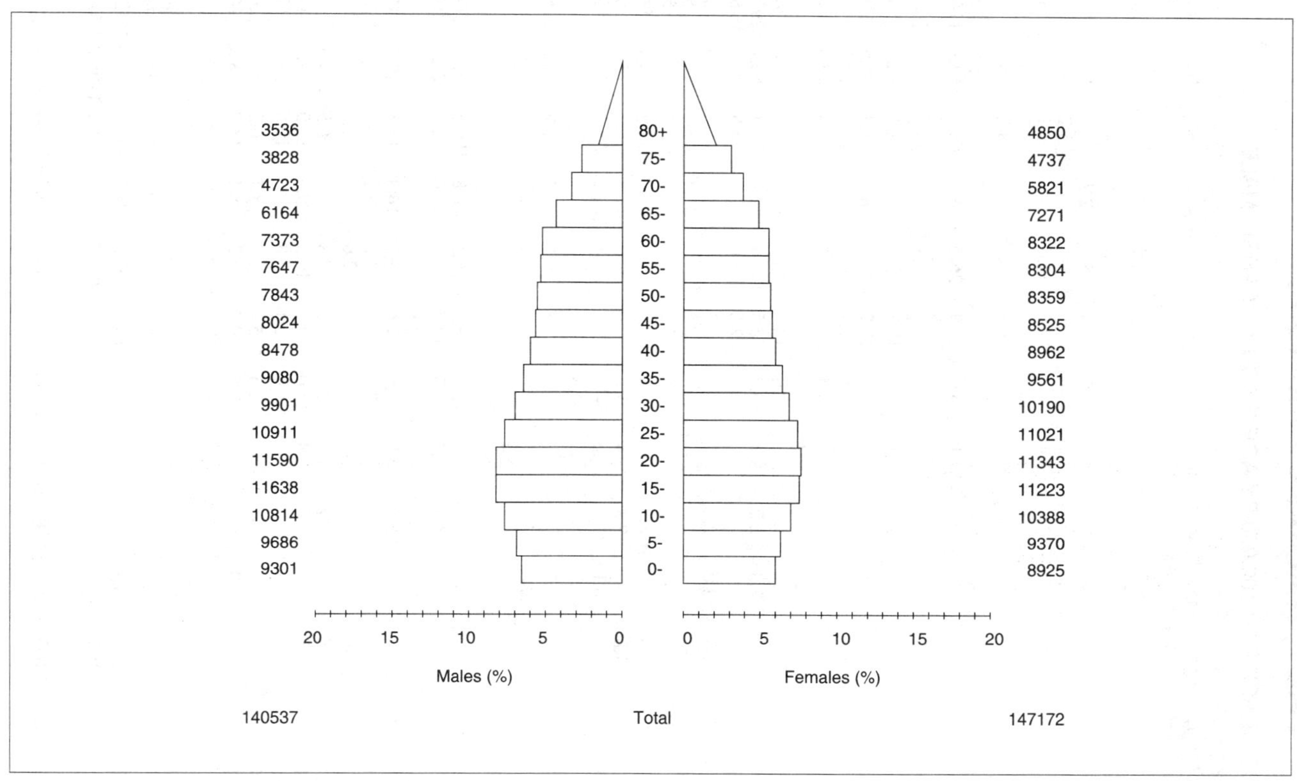

Italy, Ragusa
Source of population: average annual 1988–92
Census: 13th National Census 1991. Sistema Statistico Nazionale, Istituto Nazionale di Statistica (ISTAT), Rome.
Estimate: The 1988, 1989, 1990 and 1992 populations were estimated by the Istituto Superiore di Statistica on the basis of the 1991 Census.

Notes to tables overleaf:
† 188 does not include non-invasive tumours

ITALY, RAGUSA 1988-1992

ANNUAL INCIDENCE PER 100,000 BY AGE GROUP (YEARS) - MALE

SITE	ALL AGES	AGE UNK	0-	5-	10-	15-	20-	25-	30-	35-	40-	45-	50-	55-	60-	65-	70-	75-	80+	CRUDE RATE	%	CR 64	CR 74	ASR (W)	ICD (9th)
Lip	52	0	-	-	-	-	-	-	2.0	-	-	7.5	-	23.5	24.4	19.5	25.4	41.8	56.6	7.4	2.6	0.29	0.51	**4.6**	140
Tongue	12	0	-	-	-	-	-	-	-	-	4.7	-	2.5	7.8	-	-	12.7	15.7	-	1.7	0.6	0.08	0.14	**1.1**	141
Salivary gland	6	0	-	-	-	-	1.8	-	-	-	-	-	2.6	2.7	3.2	-	5.2	5.7	-	0.9	0.3	0.04	0.05	**0.6**	142
Mouth	10	0	-	-	-	-	-	-	-	-	-	2.5	2.5	5.2	2.7	-	12.7	10.4	-	1.4	0.5	0.06	0.13	**1.0**	143-5
Oropharynx	1	0	-	-	-	-	-	-	-	-	-	-	-	-	-	3.2	-	-	-	0.1	0.0	0.00	0.02	**0.1**	146
Nasopharynx	6	0	-	-	-	-	-	-	2.2	2.4	-	2.5	2.6	-	-	3.2	-	5.2	-	0.9	0.3	0.05	0.06	**0.7**	147
Hypopharynx	1	0	-	-	-	-	-	-	-	-	-	-	-	-	-	3.2	-	-	-	0.1	0.0	0.00	0.02	**0.1**	148
Pharynx unspecified	3	0	-	-	-	-	-	-	-	-	-	-	5.1	-	-	3.2	-	-	-	0.4	0.1	0.03	0.04	**0.4**	149
Oesophagus	13	0	-	-	-	-	-	-	-	-	-	-	-	2.7	13.0	8.5	10.4	22.6		1.8	0.6	0.01	0.12	**1.0**	150
Stomach	161	0	-	-	1.8	-	-	-	-	-	7.1	5.0	22.9	26.2	48.8	68.1	110.1	114.9	277.1	22.9	8.0	0.56	1.45	**13.2**	151
Small intestine	5	0	-	-	-	-	-	-	-	-	-	-	2.5	-	5.4	3.2	-	-	5.7	0.7	0.2	0.04	0.06	**0.5**	152
Colon	120	0	-	-	-	-	-	1.8	-	2.2	4.7	5.0	10.2	39.2	21.7	42.2	101.6	130.6	141.4	17.1	6.0	0.42	1.14	**9.8**	153
Rectum	115	0	-	-	-	-	-	-	2.0	2.2	7.1	7.5	15.3	23.5	46.1	68.1	38.1	120.2	124.4	16.4	5.7	0.52	1.05	**9.9**	154
Liver	101	0	-	-	-	-	-	-	-	-	-	7.5	10.2	23.5	38.0	38.9	101.6	99.3	90.5	14.4	5.0	0.40	1.10	**8.5**	155
Gallbladder etc.	44	0	-	-	-	-	-	1.8	-	-	-	2.5	12.7	10.5	19.0	22.7	12.7	41.8	45.2	6.3	2.2	0.23	0.41	**3.9**	156
Pancreas	73	0	-	-	-	-	-	-	-	4.4	-	2.5	-	15.7	24.4	61.6	29.6	62.7	96.2	10.4	3.6	0.24	0.69	**6.0**	157
Nose, sinuses etc.	3	0	-	-	-	-	-	-	-	-	2.4	-	-	5.2	-	-	-	-	-	0.4	0.1	0.04	0.04	**0.4**	160
Larynx	53	0	-	-	-	-	-	-	-	-	-	5.0	10.2	26.2	13.6	35.7	25.4	20.9	62.2	7.5	2.6	0.27	0.58	**4.8**	161
Bronchus, lung	421	0	-	-	-	-	-	-	2.0	2.2	9.4	39.9	76.5	138.6	184.4	275.8	266.7	292.6	248.9	59.9	21.0	2.27	4.98	**39.0**	162
Other thoracic organs	8	0	-	-	-	-	1.7	-	-	-	-	-	2.5	2.6	2.7	6.5	-	5.2	5.7	1.1	0.4	0.05	0.08	**0.8**	163-4
Bone	11	0	-	2.1	1.8	-	3.5	1.8	2.0	2.2	-	-	2.5	-	-	-	8.5	5.2	-	1.6	0.5	0.08	0.12	**1.4**	170
Connective tissue	11	0	-	2.1	-	1.7	-	-	-	-	-	-	2.5	-	2.7	3.2	-	5.2	28.3	1.6	0.5	0.05	0.06	**1.0**	171
Mesothelioma	5	0	-	-	-	-	1.7	-	-	-	-	2.5	2.5	-	-	3.2	-	5.2	-	0.7	0.2	0.03	0.05	**0.6**	MES
Kaposi's sarcoma	14	0	-	-	-	-	-	-	-	-	-	-	2.5	-	3.2	25.4	15.7	17.0		2.0	0.7	0.01	0.16	**1.1**	KAP
Melanoma of skin	40	0	-	-	-	-	1.8	-	-	2.2	2.4	7.5	7.6	18.3	16.3	16.2	12.7	20.9	33.9	5.7	2.0	0.28	0.43	**3.9**	172
Other skin	549	0	-	-	-	1.7	-	-	10.1	13.2	23.6	54.8	91.8	109.8	162.7	308.2	245.6	559.0	605.2	78.1		2.34	5.11	**47.6**	173
Breast	6	0	-	-	-	-	-	-	-	-	-	2.5	-	-	-	9.7	-	5.2	5.7	0.9	0.3	0.01	0.06	**0.6**	175
Prostate	170	0	-	-	1.8	-	-	-	-	-	-	-	2.5	10.5	24.4	77.9	118.6	250.8	311.1	24.2	8.5	0.20	1.18	**12.0**	185
Testis	8	0	-	-	-	-	-	1.8	2.0	4.4	-	2.5	-	2.6	2.7	-	-	5.2	-	1.1	0.4	0.08	0.08	**0.9**	186
Penis	6	0	-	-	-	-	-	-	-	-	2.4	-	2.5	-	-	-	-	-	22.6	0.9	0.3	0.02	0.02	**0.5**	187.1-.4
Other male genital	1	0	-	-	-	-	-	-	-	-	-	-	-	-	-	3.2	-	-	-	0.1	0.0	0.00	0.02	**0.1**	187.5-.9
†Bladder	170	0	-	-	-	-	-	-	-	-	-	12.5	15.3	26.2	48.8	100.6	101.6	172.4	243.2	24.2	8.5	0.51	1.52	**13.7**	188
Kidney etc.	46	0	-	2.1	-	-	-	-	-	-	4.4	2.4	7.5	12.7	5.2	13.6	32.4	25.4	20.9	39.6	6.5	2.3	0.24	0.53	**4.5**	189
Eye	3	0	-	-	-	-	-	-	2.0	-	-	2.5	2.5	-	-	-	-	-	-	0.4	0.1	0.04	0.04	**0.4**	190
Brain, nervous system	51	0	4.3	2.1	-	3.4	3.5	1.8	2.0	8.8	4.7	2.5	7.6	15.7	16.3	19.5	12.7	47.0	11.3	7.3	2.5	0.36	0.52	**5.6**	191-2
Thyroid	10	0	-	-	-	3.4	-	-	-	-	4.7	2.5	2.5	2.6	8.1	-	-	-	-	1.4	0.5	0.12	0.12	**1.3**	193
Other endocrine	3	0	-	-	-	-	-	-	-	-	-	-	-	2.6	-	6.5	-	-	-	0.4	0.1	0.01	0.05	**0.3**	194
Hodgkin's disease	20	0	-	2.1	1.8	1.7	1.7	5.5	2.0	2.2	7.1	2.5	2.5	7.8	-	6.5	4.2	-	-	2.8	1.0	0.19	0.24	**2.7**	201
Non-Hodgkin lymphoma	63	0	-	-	1.8	3.4	-	1.8	-	11.0	9.4	15.0	7.6	10.5	29.8	13.0	29.6	47.0	33.9	9.0	3.1	0.45	0.67	**6.5**	200,202
Multiple myeloma	36	0	-	-	-	-	-	-	-	-	-	5.0	5.1	7.8	-	19.5	33.9	15.7	67.9	5.1	1.8	0.09	0.36	**3.0**	203
Lymphoid leukaemia	30	0	4.3	6.2	1.8	3.4	-	1.8	-	-	-	2.5	5.1	-	8.1	6.5	12.7	26.1	28.3	4.3	1.5	0.17	0.26	**3.5**	204
Myeloid leukaemia	27	0	-	-	-	3.4	-	3.7	2.0	-	-	2.5	10.2	5.2	8.1	13.0	8.5	26.1	5.7	3.8	1.3	0.18	0.28	**2.8**	205
Monocytic leukaemia	0	0	-	-	-	-	-	-	-	-	-	-	-	-	-	-	-	-	-	0.0	0.0	0.00	0.00	**0.0**	206
Other leukaemia	0	0	-	-	-	-	-	-	-	-	-	-	-	-	-	-	-	-	-	0.0	0.0	0.00	0.00	**0.0**	207
Leukaemia unspecified	10	0	-	-	-	1.7	-	-	-	-	-	-	2.5	-	-	-	-	12.7	20.9	5.7	1.4	0.5	0.02	0.08	**0.8**	208
Other and unspecified	59	0	-	-	-	-	-	-	-	-	-	7.1	7.5	5.1	23.5	16.3	29.2	42.3	36.6	56.6	8.4	2.9	0.30	0.66	**5.4**	O&U
All sites	2557	0	8.6	16.5	11.1	24.1	12.1	25.7	28.3	61.7	101.4	221.8	364.6	601.5	794.7	1343.2	1439.6	2262.3	2698.0	363.9		11.36	25.27	**226.4**	ALL
All sites but 173	2008	0	8.6	16.5	11.1	22.3	12.1	25.7	18.2	48.5	77.8	167.0	272.8	491.7	632.0	1034.9	1194.0	1703.2	2092.8	285.8	100.0	9.02	20.17	**178.9**	ALLb

Rate from 1 case   2.150   2.065   1.849   1.719   1.726   1.833   2.020   2.203   2.359   2.492   2.550   2.615   2.712   3.244   4.234   5.225   5.656

†Important: see notes on population page

ITALY, RAGUSA 1988-1992

ANNUAL INCIDENCE PER 100,000 BY AGE GROUP (YEARS) - FEMALE

SITE	ALL AGES	AGE UNK	0-	5-	10-	15-	20-	25-	30-	35-	40-	45-	50-	55-	60-	65-	70-	75-	80+	CRUDE RATE	%	CR 64	CR 74	ASR (W)	ICD (9th)
Lip	8	0	-	-	-	-	-	-	2.1	-	2.3	-	-	4.8	-	-	8.4	8.2	1.1	0.5	0.05	0.05	**0.6**	140
Tongue	5	0	-	-	-	-	-	-	-	-	-	4.8	-	2.4	-	3.4	-	4.1	0.7	0.3	0.04	0.05	**0.4**	141
Salivary gland	6	0	-	-	1.9	-	-	-	-	-	2.3	-	-	-	2.8	3.4	8.4	-	0.8	0.4	0.02	0.05	**0.5**	142
Mouth	7	0	2.2	-	-	-	-	-	-	-	-	4.8	2.4	4.8	-	-	-	4.1	1.0	0.4	0.07	0.07	**0.8**	143-5
Oropharynx	1	0	-	-	-	-	-	-	-	-	-	2.4	-	-	-	-	-	-	0.1	0.1	0.01	0.01	**0.1**	146
Nasopharynx	3	0	-	-	-	-	-	1.8	-	-	-	-	-	2.4	-	3.4	-	-	0.4	0.2	0.02	0.04	**0.3**	147
Hypopharynx	0	0	-	-	-	-	-	-	-	-	-	-	-	-	-	-	-	-	0.0	0.0	0.00	0.00	**0.0**	148
Pharynx unspecified	0	0	-	-	-	-	-	-	-	-	-	-	-	-	-	-	-	-	0.0	0.0	0.00	0.00	**0.0**	149
Oesophagus	5	0	-	-	-	-	-	-	-	-	2.3	-	-	-	-	6.9	-	8.2	0.7	0.3	0.01	0.05	**0.4**	150
Stomach	100	0	-	-	-	-	-	-	2.0	-	2.2	4.7	12.0	9.6	28.8	30.3	24.0	84.4	152.6	13.6	5.8	0.30	0.57	**6.4**	151
Small intestine	4	0	-	-	-	-	-	-	-	-	-	2.3	-	-	-	3.4	4.2	-	0.5	0.2	0.02	0.04	**0.3**	152
Colon	148	0	-	-	-	-	-	7.9	2.1	4.5	21.1	9.6	14.5	33.6	52.3	85.9	92.9	173.2	20.1	8.6	0.47	1.16	**10.5**	153
Rectum	71	0	-	-	-	-	-	-	-	-	7.0	7.2	12.0	19.2	27.5	41.2	54.9	70.1	9.6	4.1	0.23	0.57	**4.9**	154
Liver	49	0	-	-	-	-	-	-	-	-	-	12.0	7.2	9.6	11.0	34.4	38.0	57.7	6.7	2.9	0.14	0.37	**3.2**	155
Gallbladder etc.	61	0	-	-	-	-	-	-	-	-	2.3	-	12.0	14.4	24.8	24.0	38.0	99.0	8.3	3.6	0.14	0.39	**3.8**	156
Pancreas	52	0	-	-	-	-	-	1.8	-	-	2.3	-	12.0	14.4	27.5	24.0	38.0	53.6	7.1	3.0	0.15	0.41	**3.6**	157
Nose, sinuses etc.	1	0	-	-	-	-	-	-	-	-	-	-	-	-	2.8	-	-	-	0.1	0.1	0.00	0.01	**0.1**	160
Larynx	4	0	-	-	-	-	-	-	-	2.2	-	-	-	2.4	-	-	8.4	-	0.5	0.2	0.02	0.02	**0.3**	161
Bronchus, lung	64	0	-	-	-	-	-	1.8	-	4.2	4.5	4.7	9.6	14.5	24.0	16.5	30.9	63.3	28.9	8.7	3.7	0.32	0.55	**5.0**	162
Other thoracic organs	4	0	2.2	-	-	1.8	-	-	-	-	2.2	-	-	-	2.4	-	-	-	0.5	0.2	0.04	0.04	**0.7**	163-4
Bone	6	0	-	-	-	1.8	1.8	-	-	-	-	-	-	2.4	-	5.5	3.4	-	0.8	0.4	0.03	0.07	**0.6**	170
Connective tissue	9	0	-	-	-	-	5.3	3.6	-	2.1	-	-	-	-	-	-	8.4	4.1	1.2	0.5	0.06	0.06	**1.0**	171
Mesothelioma	0	0	-	-	-	-	-	-	-	-	-	-	-	-	-	-	-	-	0.0	0.0	0.00	0.00	**0.0**	MES
Kaposi's sarcoma	6	0	-	-	-	-	-	-	-	-	-	-	-	-	2.8	3.4	8.4	8.2	0.8	0.4	0.00	0.03	**0.3**	KAP
Melanoma of skin	24	0	-	-	-	-	1.8	-	2.0	4.2	6.7	2.3	2.4	7.2	7.2	8.3	3.4	4.2	16.5	3.3	1.4	0.17	0.23	**2.3**	172
Other skin	304	0	-	-	-	1.8	-	1.8	3.9	12.6	26.8	32.8	38.3	53.0	86.5	121.0	127.1	181.5	288.7	41.3		1.29	2.53	**23.2**	173
Breast	473	0	-	-	-	-	-	7.3	21.6	35.6	98.2	93.8	107.7	125.2	158.6	165.0	158.0	190.0	177.3	64.3	27.6	3.24	4.85	**44.1**	174
Uterus unspecified	12	0	-	-	-	-	-	-	-	-	-	-	-	-	-	8.3	6.9	12.7	16.5	1.6	0.7	0.00	0.08	**0.7**	179
Cervix uteri	75	0	-	-	-	-	-	3.6	3.9	6.3	17.9	25.8	12.0	31.3	21.6	19.3	13.7	38.0	8.2	10.2	4.4	0.61	0.78	**7.6**	180
Placenta	0	0	-	-	-	-	-	-	-	-	-	-	-	-	-	-	-	-	0.0	0.0	0.00	0.00	**0.0**	181
Corpus uteri	130	0	-	-	-	-	-	1.8	-	-	-	11.7	23.9	53.0	50.5	60.5	61.8	105.5	24.7	17.7	7.6	0.70	1.32	**10.5**	182
Ovary etc.	81	0	-	-	-	-	-	1.8	-	6.3	4.5	9.4	16.7	26.5	33.6	24.8	37.8	38.0	41.2	11.0	4.7	0.49	0.81	**6.9**	183
Other female genital	14	0	-	-	-	-	-	-	-	-	2.2	-	2.4	-	2.4	5.5	6.9	16.9	12.4	1.9	0.8	0.04	0.10	**0.9**	184
†Bladder	25	0	-	-	-	-	-	-	-	-	2.2	-	-	2.4	11.0	30.9	16.9	24.7	3.4	1.5	0.02	0.23	**1.6**	188
Kidney etc.	24	0	6.7	-	-	-	-	-	-	2.1	-	-	7.2	-	4.8	11.0	13.7	21.1	8.2	3.3	1.4	0.10	0.23	**2.4**	189
Eye	0	0	-	-	-	-	-	-	-	-	-	-	-	-	-	-	-	-	0.0	0.0	0.00	0.00	**0.0**	190
Brain, nervous system	34	0	2.2	4.3	3.9	1.8	-	-	5.9	2.1	-	2.3	4.8	14.5	19.2	8.3	13.7	-	-	4.6	2.0	0.30	0.41	**3.9**	191-2
Thyroid	25	0	-	-	1.9	-	-	3.6	3.9	6.3	2.2	2.3	7.2	-	2.4	13.8	6.9	8.4	8.2	3.4	1.5	0.15	0.25	**2.5**	193
Other endocrine	3	0	-	-	-	-	1.8	-	-	-	-	-	-	-	-	3.4	-	-	0.4	0.2	0.02	0.04	**0.3**	194
Hodgkin's disease	18	0	-	-	-	1.8	5.3	3.6	2.0	4.2	2.2	-	-	7.2	2.8	6.9	4.2	-	2.4	1.1	0.14	0.19	**2.0**	201
Non-Hodgkin lymphoma	42	0	2.2	-	-	1.8	1.8	-	-	-	6.7	4.7	12.0	12.0	24.0	8.3	13.7	21.1	8.2	5.7	2.5	0.33	0.44	**4.1**	200,202
Multiple myeloma	21	0	-	-	-	-	-	-	-	-	2.2	-	2.4	4.8	4.8	8.3	13.7	12.7	20.6	2.9	1.2	0.07	0.18	**1.5**	203
Lymphoid leukaemia	26	0	4.5	2.1	-	1.8	1.8	-	2.0	2.1	-	-	-	2.4	12.0	2.8	13.7	16.9	16.5	3.5	1.5	0.14	0.23	**2.6**	204
Myeloid leukaemia	27	0	-	2.1	-	1.8	-	-	-	2.1	2.2	2.3	2.4	9.6	-	11.0	3.4	21.1	28.9	3.7	1.6	0.11	0.19	**2.2**	205
Monocytic leukaemia	1	0	-	-	-	-	-	-	-	-	-	-	-	-	-	-	4.2	-	0.1	0.1	0.00	0.00	**0.0**	206
Other leukaemia	0	0	-	-	-	-	-	-	-	-	-	-	-	-	-	-	-	-	0.0	0.0	0.00	0.00	**0.0**	207
Leukaemia unspecified	4	0	-	-	-	-	-	-	-	-	2.2	-	-	-	-	-	10.3	-	-	0.5	0.2	0.01	0.06	**0.3**	208
Other and unspecified	41	0	-	-	-	-	-	-	2.0	-	-	2.3	12.0	2.4	16.8	13.8	27.5	21.1	33.0	5.6	2.4	0.18	0.38	**3.1**	O&U
All sites	2018	0	20.2	8.5	7.7	14.3	17.6	34.5	56.9	94.1	191.9	241.6	313.4	433.5	620.0	706.9	865.7	1190.5	1406.2	274.2		10.27	18.13	**166.8**	ALL
All sites but 173	1714	0	20.2	8.5	7.7	12.5	17.6	32.7	53.0	81.6	165.1	208.8	275.1	380.5	533.5	585.8	738.6	1009.0	1117.5	232.9	100.0	8.98	15.61	**143.6**	ALLb

Rate from 1 case 2.241 2.134 1.925 1.782 1.763 1.815 1.963 2.092 2.232 2.346 2.392 2.408 2.403 2.750 3.435 4.222 4.124

†Important: see notes on population page

Italy, Romagna

The Cancer Registry of Romagna is a population-based cancer Registry, situated in the Division of Oncology of the Civil Hospital in Forli. It is the outcome of a research project of the Oncological Institute. Activity started on 1 January 1985, following a feasibility study.

The population covered corresponds, from January 1994, to the whole of Romagna, in the north-east of Italy, and numbers 957 639 inhabitants of Caucasian origin and Catholic religion.

The area covered is 4769 km^2. The territory consists of both rural and urban areas and, since January 1995, is subdivided into three districts (Ravenna, Forli, Rimini).

Romagna contains seven Local Health Units (LHU), in the districts of Ravenna, Forli and Rimini.

In the past a programme was developed to encourage women to present themselves for spontaneous breast and cervical examination. Since March 1996 population screening for cervical and breast cancer lesions has been carried out.

For both the districts of Forli and Ravenna, as in much of Italy, a progressive reduction in agricultural labour has taken place in favour of industry and more recently in services. In 1950, 53% of the inhabitants of the district of Forli and 60% of those of Ravenna were engaged in agriculture, while in 1980 these figures had fallen to 12% and 20% respectively. In Forli 24% of the population and in Ravenna 20% was employed in industry in 1950, and these rose to 37% and 35% in 1980. The service sector rose from 23% to 51% of the population in Forli, and from 20% to 45% of the population in Ravenna for the same years.

The data presented here for the four-year period 1989–92 relate to the whole districts of Forli and Ravenna (total population at 31 December 1992 of 602 444 inhabitants) and Cesena LHU (not included in the previous volume of this series), which is an area that is mainly rural and marine.

Notification of malignant cases of cancer comes from several different sources within the hospital and/or university structure at the regional and national level.

The reporting of cancer cases occurs through both compulsory procedures by administrative order and voluntary actions.

The information gathered is related to the patient (name, sex, date of birth) and to the tumour (incidence date, diagnosis modality, morphology, behaviour and source of information).

Follow-up is carried out on a passive basis for all cases. Information on date of death is obtained.

Multiple primaries are coded according to IARC rules and it is possible to retrieve information on subsequent or synchronous primaries in the same patient. The coding system used for morphology is ICD-O M-code, first edition.

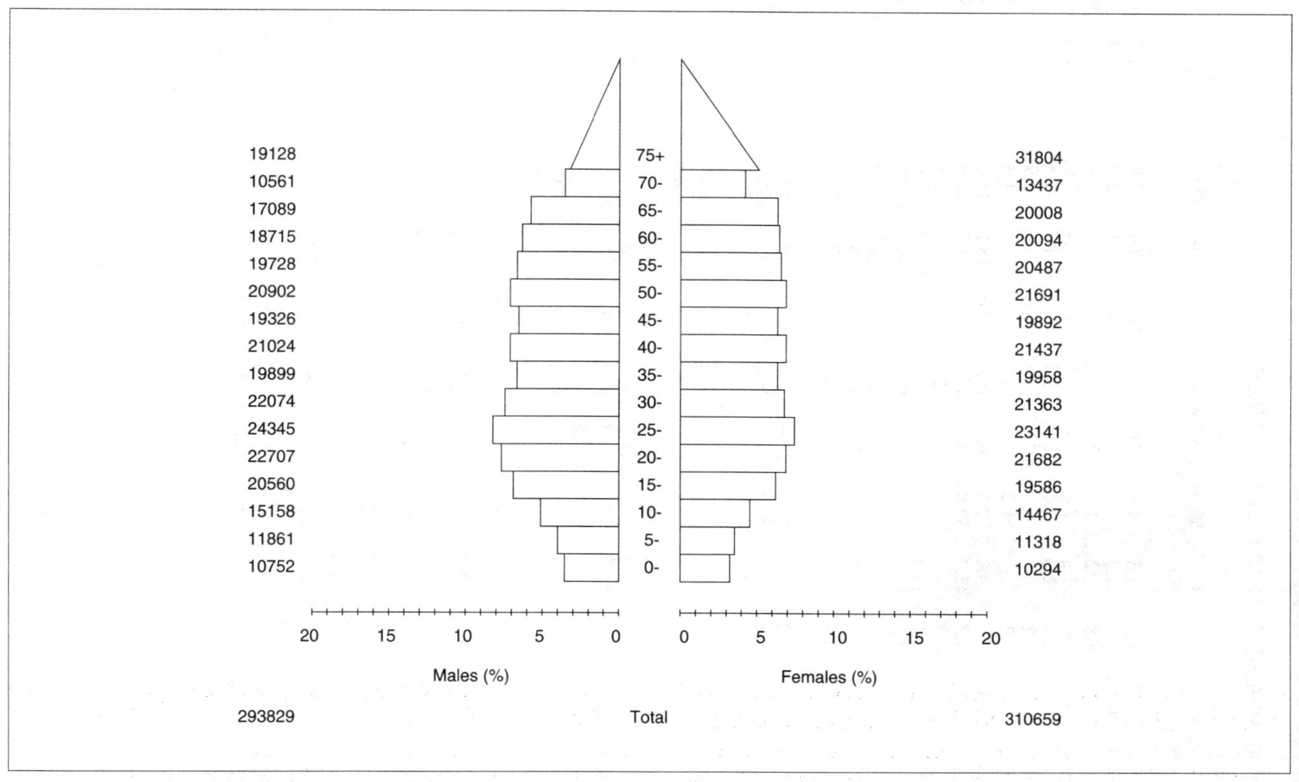

Italy, Romagna

Source of population: average annual 1989–92
Census: General Census 25 October 1981. Istituto Centrale di Statistica, Rome 1984. General Census 1991. Istituto Centrale di Statistica. Source: Chamber of Commerce
Estimate: The 1989 and 1990 population estimates were based on the 1981 Census and that for 1992 on the 1991 Census.

Notes to tables overleaf:

Note that the registration area is larger than that covered in Volume VI and rates are not comparable.

ITALY, ROMAGNA 1989-1992

ANNUAL INCIDENCE PER 100,000 BY AGE GROUP (YEARS) - MALE

SITE	ALL AGES	AGE UNK	0-	5-	10-	15-	20-	25-	30-	35-	40-	45-	50-	55-	60-	65-	70-	75+	CRUDE RATE	%	CR 64	CR 74	ASR (W)	ICD (9th)
Lip	1	0	-	-	-	-	-	-	-	-	-	-	-	-	-	-	2.4	-	0.1	0.0	0.00	0.01	0.0	140
Tongue	32	0	-	-	-	-	-	-	-	-	1.2	1.3	4.8	7.6	5.3	10.2	7.1	7.8	2.7	0.4	0.10	0.19	1.5	141
Salivary gland	20	0	-	-	-	-	-	1.0	-	1.3	-	1.3	4.8	5.1	1.3	4.4	7.1	2.6	1.7	0.3	0.07	0.13	1.1	142
Mouth	32	0	-	-	-	-	-	-	-	-	4.8	5.2	1.2	13.9	4.0	2.9	2.4	7.8	2.7	0.4	0.15	0.17	1.7	143-5
Oropharynx	24	0	-	-	-	-	-	-	-	-	-	1.3	2.4	5.1	10.7	7.3	2.4	3.9	2.0	0.3	0.10	0.15	1.2	146
Nasopharynx	20	0	-	2.1	1.6	-	-	-	-	-	2.4	2.6	2.4	2.5	2.7	7.3	4.7	1.3	1.7	0.3	0.08	0.14	1.3	147
Hypopharynx	14	0	-	-	-	-	-	-	-	-	1.2	-	-	3.8	1.3	8.8	-	3.9	1.2	0.2	0.03	0.08	0.6	148
Pharynx unspecified	5	0	-	-	-	-	-	-	-	-	1.2	-	1.2	1.3	1.3	-	-	1.3	0.4	0.1	0.02	0.02	0.3	149
Oesophagus	58	0	-	-	-	-	-	-	-	1.3	-	3.9	7.2	6.3	16.0	19.0	18.9	13.1	4.9	0.8	0.17	0.36	2.8	150
Stomach	933	0	-	-	-	-	1.1	1.0	3.4	7.5	14.3	45.3	59.8	95.0	146.9	212.1	324.3	467.9	79.4	13.1	1.87	4.55	39.3	151
Small intestine	18	0	-	-	-	-	-	-	-	-	-	-	-	-	5.3	5.9	-	13.1	1.5	0.3	0.03	0.06	0.7	152
Colon	528	0	-	-	-	-	-	1.0	1.1	2.5	13.1	19.4	43.1	58.3	78.8	168.2	151.5	232.6	44.9	7.4	1.09	2.69	22.6	153
Rectum	300	0	-	-	-	-	-	-	-	1.3	4.8	10.3	13.2	45.6	58.8	71.7	80.5	147.7	25.5	4.2	0.67	1.43	12.5	154
Liver	147	0	2.3	-	-	-	-	1.0	1.1	1.3	-	5.2	7.2	7.6	32.1	54.1	26.0	71.9	12.5	2.1	0.29	0.69	6.3	155
Gallbladder etc.	49	0	-	-	-	-	-	-	-	-	-	2.6	1.2	7.6	12.0	11.7	16.6	20.9	4.2	0.7	0.12	0.26	2.1	156
Pancreas	156	0	-	-	-	-	-	1.0	-	-	2.4	1.3	14.4	22.8	30.7	27.8	59.2	71.9	13.3	2.2	0.36	0.80	6.6	157
Nose, sinuses etc.	10	0	-	-	-	1.2	-	-	-	-	1.2	1.3	1.2	3.8	1.3	1.5	-	1.3	0.9	0.1	0.05	0.06	0.6	160
Larynx	207	0	-	-	-	-	-	-	-	-	1.2	9.1	17.9	32.9	57.4	67.3	59.2	57.5	17.6	2.9	0.59	1.23	9.5	161
Bronchus, lung	1485	0	-	-	-	-	-	1.0	-	6.3	17.8	54.3	87.3	182.5	360.7	526.6	494.7	478.4	126.3	20.8	3.55	8.66	66.1	162
Other thoracic organs	7	0	-	-	-	-	-	-	-	-	1.2	1.3	-	-	-	2.9	-	3.9	0.6	0.1	0.01	0.03	0.3	163-4
Bone	16	0	2.3	-	1.6	1.2	-	1.0	-	1.3	-	1.3	-	5.1	1.3	-	-	6.5	1.4	0.2	0.08	0.08	1.2	170
Connective tissue	36	0	2.3	2.1	3.3	1.2	2.2	-	-	2.5	-	1.3	4.8	3.8	1.3	7.3	7.1	13.1	3.1	0.5	0.12	0.20	2.4	171
Mesothelioma	27	0	-	-	-	-	-	-	-	-	-	1.3	3.6	7.6	5.3	7.3	7.1	6.5	2.3	0.4	0.09	0.16	1.3	MES
Kaposi's sarcoma	23	0	-	-	-	-	-	3.1	1.1	5.0	1.2	1.3	1.2	1.3	4.0	1.5	-	9.1	2.0	0.3	0.09	0.10	1.3	KAP
Melanoma of skin	109	0	-	-	-	1.2	3.3	4.1	4.5	7.5	7.1	10.3	17.9	15.2	14.7	17.6	18.9	24.8	9.3	1.5	0.43	0.61	6.0	172
Other skin	1376	0	-	2.1	3.3	2.4	2.2	6.2	4.5	23.9	26.2	53.0	95.7	160.9	233.8	361.3	478.1	582.9	117.1		3.07	7.27	60.5	173
Breast	17	0	-	-	-	-	-	-	-	-	-	-	3.6	2.5	2.7	2.9	7.1	6.5	1.4	0.2	0.04	0.09	0.7	175
Prostate	779	0	-	-	-	-	-	-	-	1.3	-	6.5	19.1	26.6	90.8	199.0	279.3	541.1	66.3	10.9	0.72	3.11	28.5	185
Testis	53	0	2.3	-	-	4.9	5.5	8.2	7.9	6.3	2.4	10.3	3.6	2.5	4.0	1.5	4.7	2.6	4.5	0.7	0.29	0.32	4.1	186
Penis	15	0	-	-	-	-	-	-	-	-	-	-	1.2	1.3	5.3	5.9	9.5	1.3	1.3	0.2	0.04	0.12	0.7	187.1-.4
Other male genital	3	0	-	-	-	-	-	-	-	-	-	-	1.2	-	-	1.5	2.4	-	0.3	0.0	0.01	0.03	0.2	187.5-.9
Bladder	740	0	-	-	-	1.2	-	-	2.3	6.3	4.8	23.3	50.2	103.9	163.0	210.7	232.0	290.1	63.0	10.4	1.77	3.99	32.3	188
Kidney etc.	285	0	-	-	-	1.2	-	2.1	3.4	2.5	5.9	12.9	23.9	44.4	77.5	70.2	94.7	79.7	24.2	4.0	0.87	1.69	13.4	189
Eye	10	0	-	-	-	-	-	-	-	-	-	1.3	-	1.3	4.0	1.5	2.4	3.9	0.9	0.1	0.03	0.05	0.5	190
Brain, nervous system	114	0	-	6.3	3.3	2.4	-	2.1	5.7	2.5	3.6	5.2	7.2	16.5	32.1	21.9	26.0	28.8	9.7	1.6	0.43	0.67	6.4	191-2
Thyroid	52	0	-	-	-	-	2.2	2.1	3.4	6.3	8.3	7.8	3.6	2.5	8.0	8.8	4.7	10.5	4.4	0.7	0.22	0.29	3.1	193
Other endocrine	5	0	2.3	-	-	-	-	-	-	-	1.2	1.3	1.2	-	-	1.5	-	-	0.4	0.1	0.03	0.04	0.5	194
Hodgkin's disease	36	0	2.3	2.1	-	3.6	1.1	4.1	6.8	2.5	3.6	1.3	2.4	3.8	1.3	2.9	7.1	3.9	3.1	0.5	0.17	0.23	2.7	201
Non-Hodgkin lymphoma	296	0	2.3	-	-	7.3	2.2	10.3	13.6	12.6	14.3	20.7	25.1	41.8	48.1	48.3	97.0	82.3	25.2	4.1	0.99	1.72	15.5	200,202
Multiple myeloma	97	0	-	-	-	-	-	-	-	-	2.4	2.6	9.6	6.3	18.7	26.3	21.3	51.0	8.3	1.4	0.20	0.44	4.0	203
Lymphoid leukaemia	100	0	4.7	-	1.6	-	-	1.0	2.3	3.8	1.2	2.6	8.4	7.6	13.4	32.2	28.4	40.5	8.5	1.4	0.23	0.54	5.0	204
Myeloid leukaemia	88	0	-	2.1	-	-	1.1	2.1	2.3	1.3	4.8	3.9	6.0	6.3	14.7	14.6	23.7	43.1	7.5	1.2	0.22	0.41	4.1	205
Monocytic leukaemia	3	0	-	-	-	-	-	-	-	-	-	-	-	1.3	-	1.5	-	1.3	0.3	0.0	0.01	0.01	0.1	206
Other leukaemia	1	0	-	-	-	-	-	-	-	-	-	-	-	-	-	1.5	-	-	0.1	0.0	0.00	0.01	0.0	207
Leukaemia unspecified	16	0	-	-	-	-	-	1.0	-	-	-	-	-	-	-	1.5	7.1	14.4	1.4	0.2	0.01	0.05	0.6	208
Other and unspecified	179	0	-	-	-	-	2.2	-	-	-	4.8	5.2	14.4	11.4	28.1	35.1	47.3	108.5	15.2	2.5	0.33	0.74	7.2	O&U
All sites	8522	0	20.9	16.9	14.8	28.0	23.1	53.4	63.4	106.8	158.2	338.9	572.9	975.7	1598.9	2293.8	2662.9	3561.5	725.1		19.86	44.64	379.1	ALL
All sites but 173	7146	0	20.9	14.8	11.5	25.5	20.9	47.2	58.9	82.9	132.0	285.9	477.2	814.8	1365.2	1932.5	2184.8	2978.6	608.0	100.0	16.79	37.38	318.7	ALLb

Rate from 1 case: 2.325 | 2.108 | 1.649 | 1.216 | 1.101 | 1.027 | 1.133 | 1.256 | 1.189 | 1.294 | 1.196 | 1.267 | 1.336 | 1.463 | 2.367 | 1.307

Important: see notes on population page

556

ITALY, ROMAGNA 1989-1992

ANNUAL INCIDENCE PER 100,000 BY AGE GROUP (YEARS) - FEMALE

SITE	ALL AGES	AGE UNK	0-	5-	10-	15-	20-	25-	30-	35-	40-	45-	50-	55-	60-	65-	70-	75+	CRUDE RATE	%	CR 64	CR 74	ASR (W)	ICD (9th)
Lip	1	0	-	-	-	-	-	-	-	-	-	-	-	-	1.2	-	-	-	0.1	0.0	0.01	0.01	**0.0**	*140*
Tongue	12	0	-	-	-	-	-	-	-	-	-	1.3	-	2.4	-	1.2	-	6.3	1.0	0.2	0.02	0.02	**0.3**	*141*
Salivary gland	15	0	-	-	-	1.3	-	-	-	-	1.2	-	1.2	3.7	2.5	2.5	9.3	-	1.2	0.3	0.05	0.11	**0.7**	*142*
Mouth	13	0	-	-	-	-	-	-	-	-	-	-	1.2	2.4	5.0	2.5	-	3.1	1.0	0.2	0.04	0.06	**0.5**	*143-5*
Oropharynx	3	0	-	-	-	-	-	-	-	-	-	-	1.2	-	-	-	-	1.6	0.2	0.1	0.01	0.01	**0.1**	*146*
Nasopharynx	7	0	-	-	-	-	-	-	-	-	-	-	1.2	2.4	1.2	-	-	2.4	0.6	0.1	0.02	0.02	**0.3**	*147*
Hypopharynx	2	0	-	-	-	-	-	-	-	-	-	-	-	-	-	-	1.9	0.8	0.2	0.0	0.00	0.01	**0.1**	*148*
Pharynx unspecified	1	0	-	-	-	-	-	-	-	-	-	1.3	-	-	-	-	-	-	0.1	0.0	0.01	0.01	**0.1**	*149*
Oesophagus	14	0	-	-	-	-	-	-	-	-	-	-	-	2.3	1.2	1.2	2.5	3.7	4.7	1.1	0.2	0.02	0.05	**0.5**	*150*
Stomach	786	0	-	-	-	-	-	2.2	2.3	11.3	14.0	20.1	19.6	51.3	67.2	117.5	174.9	349.0	63.3	13.3	0.94	2.40	**22.8**	*151*
Small intestine	19	0	-	-	-	-	1.2	-	-	-	-	1.3	3.5	2.4	2.5	1.2	3.7	5.5	1.5	0.3	0.05	0.08	**0.8**	*152*
Colon	567	0	-	-	-	-	-	-	1.2	7.5	7.0	31.4	35.7	45.1	74.6	95.0	128.4	201.2	45.6	9.6	1.01	2.13	**18.8**	*153*
Rectum	232	0	-	-	-	-	-	2.2	1.2	5.0	10.5	7.5	15.0	24.4	32.3	37.5	54.0	72.3	18.7	3.9	0.49	0.95	**8.3**	*154*
Liver	77	0	-	-	-	-	-	1.1	1.2	-	-	-	-	1.2	7.5	17.5	18.6	34.6	6.2	1.3	0.05	0.24	**2.1**	*155*
Gallbladder etc.	88	0	-	-	-	-	-	-	-	-	1.2	-	1.2	-	5.0	20.0	27.9	40.1	7.1	1.5	0.04	0.28	**2.3**	*156*
Pancreas	156	0	-	-	-	-	-	-	-	1.3	-	2.5	6.9	7.3	17.4	30.0	48.4	60.5	12.6	2.6	0.18	0.57	**4.6**	*157*
Nose, sinuses etc.	8	0	-	-	-	1.3	-	-	-	1.3	-	-	1.2	-	1.2	-	1.9	2.4	0.6	0.1	0.02	0.03	**0.4**	*160*
Larynx	17	0	-	-	-	-	-	-	1.2	-	2.3	1.3	1.2	1.2	6.2	1.2	3.7	2.4	1.4	0.3	0.07	0.09	**0.8**	*161*
Bronchus, lung	260	0	-	-	-	-	-	-	-	2.5	9.3	17.6	10.4	25.6	47.3	55.0	63.3	70.7	20.9	4.4	0.56	1.15	**9.5**	*162*
Other thoracic organs	12	0	-	-	-	-	-	-	1.2	-	2.3	1.3	-	-	3.7	1.2	-	3.1	1.0	0.2	0.04	0.05	**0.5**	*163-4*
Bone	16	0	-	-	1.7	1.3	1.2	1.1	2.3	-	-	2.5	2.3	2.4	-	-	-	3.1	1.3	0.3	0.07	0.07	**1.0**	*170*
Connective tissue	27	0	2.4	-	-	-	1.2	-	1.2	3.8	1.2	2.5	3.5	1.2	5.0	1.2	1.9	6.3	2.2	0.5	0.11	0.12	**1.5**	*171*
Mesothelioma	11	0	-	-	-	-	-	-	-	-	-	-	-	3.7	-	2.5	3.7	3.1	0.9	0.2	0.02	0.05	**0.4**	*MES*
Kaposi's sarcoma	12	0	-	-	-	-	2.3	-	2.3	-	-	-	-	-	-	-	1.9	5.5	1.0	0.2	0.02	0.03	**0.5**	*KAP*
Melanoma of skin	136	0	-	-	-	3.8	1.2	5.4	5.9	8.8	14.0	8.8	11.5	20.7	18.7	25.0	14.9	20.4	10.9	2.3	0.49	0.69	**6.7**	*172*
Other skin	1033	0	-	-	-	1.3	3.5	2.2	9.4	23.8	28.0	41.5	61.1	70.8	124.4	148.7	225.1	386.7	83.1		1.83	3.70	**34.3**	*173*
Breast	1454	0	-	-	-	-	-	5.4	22.2	60.1	108.5	165.9	191.3	224.5	225.2	232.4	251.2	239.7	117.0	24.5	5.02	7.43	**66.2**	*174*
Uterus unspecified	9	0	-	-	-	-	-	-	-	-	-	1.3	-	1.2	1.2	-	1.9	3.9	0.7	0.2	0.02	0.03	**0.3**	*179*
Cervix uteri	205	0	-	-	-	-	1.2	5.4	14.0	13.8	16.3	27.6	24.2	26.8	31.1	26.2	29.8	27.5	16.5	3.5	0.80	1.08	**10.3**	*180*
Placenta	0	0	-	-	-	-	-	-	-	-	-	-	-	-	-	-	-	-	0.0	0.0	0.00	0.00	**0.0**	*181*
Corpus uteri	283	0	-	-	-	-	-	1.1	1.2	6.3	9.3	12.6	34.6	47.6	51.0	60.0	68.8	49.5	22.8	4.8	0.82	1.46	**11.7**	*182*
Ovary etc.	205	0	-	-	1.3	2.3	3.2	1.2	1.3	12.8	16.3	20.7	29.3	32.3	27.5	48.4	44.8	-	16.5	3.5	0.60	0.98	**8.6**	*183*
Other female genital	37	0	-	-	-	-	-	-	-	1.3	1.2	-	-	3.7	1.2	7.5	7.4	16.5	3.0	0.6	0.04	0.11	**1.0**	*184*
Bladder	155	0	-	-	-	-	-	2.2	-	2.5	-	2.5	10.4	12.2	19.9	37.5	39.1	49.5	12.5	2.6	0.25	0.63	**5.2**	*188*
Kidney etc.	149	0	2.4	-	-	-	-	2.2	3.5	1.3	2.3	3.8	13.8	19.5	26.1	22.5	40.9	37.7	12.0	2.5	0.37	0.69	**5.9**	*189*
Eye	17	0	2.4	-	-	-	1.2	-	-	1.3	-	1.3	-	-	3.7	1.2	7.4	3.9	1.4	0.3	0.05	0.09	**0.9**	*190*
Brain, nervous system	107	0	9.7	2.2	1.7	1.3	-	2.2	2.3	3.8	4.7	6.3	6.9	13.4	8.7	17.5	16.7	29.1	8.6	1.8	0.32	0.49	**5.5**	*191-2*
Thyroid	153	0	-	-	1.7	2.6	4.6	9.7	12.9	22.5	14.0	20.1	21.9	23.2	10.0	12.5	18.6	11.0	12.3	2.6	0.72	0.87	**9.1**	*193*
Other endocrine	7	0	-	-	-	-	-	-	-	1.3	-	-	2.3	1.2	-	1.2	1.9	0.8	0.6	0.1	0.02	0.04	**0.3**	*194*
Hodgkin's disease	35	0	2.4	2.2	3.5	5.1	1.2	8.6	2.3	3.8	1.2	1.3	2.3	2.4	2.5	1.2	5.6	0.8	2.8	0.6	0.19	0.23	**3.1**	*201*
Non-Hodgkin lymphoma	201	0	-	2.2	-	2.6	-	9.7	4.7	5.0	5.8	7.5	13.8	18.3	23.6	30.0	50.2	57.4	16.2	3.4	0.47	0.87	**8.0**	*200,202*
Multiple myeloma	88	0	-	-	-	-	-	-	-	-	-	1.3	4.6	9.8	14.9	16.2	18.6	31.4	7.1	1.5	0.15	0.33	**2.8**	*203*
Lymphoid leukaemia	64	0	4.9	2.2	3.5	-	-	1.1	-	2.5	1.2	3.8	2.3	3.7	7.5	12.5	16.7	17.3	5.2	1.1	0.16	0.31	**3.3**	*204*
Myeloid leukaemia	56	0	-	-	-	1.3	2.3	2.2	-	-	3.5	2.5	3.5	3.7	2.5	10.0	14.9	17.3	4.5	0.9	0.11	0.23	**2.2**	*205*
Monocytic leukaemia	0	0	-	-	-	-	-	-	-	-	-	-	-	-	-	-	-	-	0.0	0.0	0.00	0.00	**0.0**	*206*
Other leukaemia	2	0	-	-	-	-	-	-	-	-	-	-	-	1.2	1.2	-	-	-	0.2	0.0	0.01	0.01	**0.1**	*207*
Leukaemia unspecified	12	0	-	2.2	-	-	-	-	-	2.5	-	-	1.2	1.2	-	-	1.9	4.7	1.0	0.2	0.04	0.04	**0.6**	*208*
Other and unspecified	192	0	-	-	-	-	-	-	-	-	2.3	5.0	5.8	13.4	17.4	21.2	50.2	88.0	15.5	3.2	0.22	0.58	**5.4**	*O&U*
All sites	6956	0	24.3	11.0	12.1	23.0	23.1	67.0	93.6	194.2	274.1	419.8	539.4	726.0	904.5	1099.5	1477.2	2017.0	559.8		16.56	29.44	**268.3**	*ALL*
All sites but 173	5923	0	24.3	11.0	12.1	21.7	19.6	64.8	84.3	170.4	246.1	378.3	478.3	655.3	780.1	950.8	1252.1	1630.3	476.6	100.0	14.73	25.75	**234.1**	*ALLb*

Rate from 1 case

			0-	5-	10-	15-	20-	25-	30-	35-	40-	45-	50-	55-	60-	65-	70-	75+
			2.429	2.209	1.728	1.276	1.153	1.080	1.170	1.253	1.166	1.257	1.153	1.220	1.244	1.249	1.860	0.786

Important: see notes on population page

Italy, Torino

Registration of cancer incidence in the population of Torino recommenced in 1985, following a period of cessation of activity by the Piedmont Cancer Registry. The registry is now supported by the Regional Health Administration and is run by the Epidemiology Unit of the local health authority.

The city of Turin, in the north-west of Italy, is the centre of a large industrial conurbation. The tumour registry covers the population of the city (996 700 inhabitants), where 45% of the active population works in industry. Mechanical (mainly car and truck), rubber, and electronic industries are the most important activities. The present composition of the population has been influenced by two important internal migrations: during the 1920s and 1930s from the east of Italy and during the 1950s and 1960s from the south of Italy. In 1985, 7.7% of the population between 25 and 74 years of age had been born in the east of Italy and 34.4% in the south.

In Turin there are 11 public hospitals and 7 private clinics; the total number of hospitals beds is about 7800. The registry can enter the National Health Service files to check names and other personal data, and receives copies of all death certificates from the Public Health Department. Two screening programmes started in 1992, biennial mammography in women aged 50–69 years and triennial Pap-testing in those aged 25–64 years, covering the same population. The registry contribution to screening programmes consists of case-interval finding and estimation of short-term indicators.

The main sources of data for the registry are hospital archives, pathological department archives, radiotherapy department archives and death certificates. In addition, the registry receives notification of Torino residents treated for cancer in some institutes outside the regional boundaries (e.g., the National Cancer Institute of Milan and Genoa). Indirect information indicates that 1–2% of incident cases have total or partial recourse to foreign hospitals (usually in France or Switzerland) for diagnosis or treatment or both. Some of these cases are identified by the registry from their reimbursement forms and are then included in the incidence, even on the basis of incomplete documentation (e.g., histology).

Registration is voluntary and almost completely active. The follow-up procedures include linkage with mortality data and active follow-up of patients at regular intervals (five years). All malignant tumours and also bladder papillomas are included in the tabulation of incidence data; carcinomas *in situ* and a number of other benign tumours (registered but not included in incidence data) are coded according to both ICD-9 and ICD-O. Storage of data is completed in two steps: (*a*) a 'working storage' in personal lap-top computers at the location of data collection (hospitals, laboratories, etc.) and (*b*) storage of the definitive file in a personal computer operating as central server. In both working and final storage, data are automatically checked for errors and inconsistencies. Multiple neoplasms are registered following the IARC/IACR recommendations.

Roberto Zanetti
Stefano Rosso

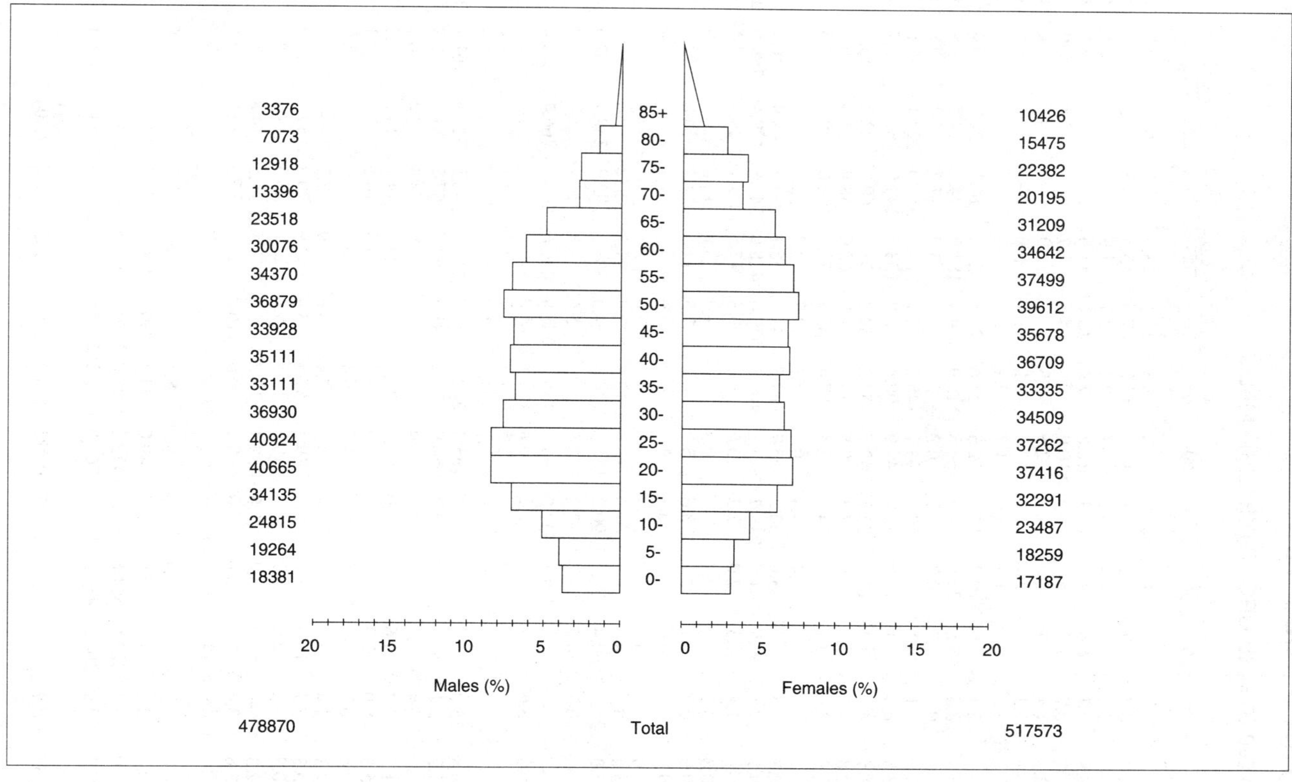

Italy, Torino
Source of population: average annual 1988–91
Source: The population for each year is based on the figures
at 31 December as derived from Offical Notification to the
Municipality of Turin.

ITALY, TORINO 1988-1991

ANNUAL INCIDENCE PER 100,000 BY AGE GROUP (YEARS) - MALE

SITE	ALL AGES	AGE UNK	0-	5-	10-	15-	20-	25-	30-	35-	40-	45-	50-	55-	60-	65-	70-	75-	80-	85+	CRUDE RATE	%	CR 64	CR 74	ASR (W)	ICD (9th)
Lip	39	0	-	-	-	-	-	-	-	-	-	-	1.4	2.9	5.8	8.5	13.1	13.5	7.1	14.8	2.0	0.4	0.05	0.16	1.2	140
Tongue	64	0	-	-	-	-	-	0.6	0.7	0.8	0.7	3.7	4.1	5.8	11.6	12.8	7.5	15.5	3.5	14.8	3.3	0.7	0.14	0.24	2.1	141
Salivary gland	15	0	-	-	-	-	0.6	-	-	1.4	-	1.4	0.7	1.7	2.1	3.7	1.9	7.1	-	0.8	0.2	0.03	0.06	0.5	142
Mouth	79	0	1.4	-	-	0.7	-	-	-	0.8	0.7	6.6	4.1	10.9	16.6	7.4	13.1	11.6	17.7	-	4.1	0.8	0.21	0.31	2.7	143-5
Oropharynx	58	0	-	-	-	-	-	-	-	-	0.7	1.5	6.1	10.9	10.0	9.6	5.6	7.7	7.1	7.4	3.0	0.6	0.15	0.22	1.8	146
Nasopharynx	27	0	-	-	-	-	-	0.6	1.4	2.3	1.4	0.7	2.0	4.4	2.5	5.3	-	1.9	-	-	1.4	0.3	0.08	0.10	1.0	147
Hypopharynx	34	0	-	-	-	-	-	-	-	-	1.4	1.5	2.7	3.6	7.5	8.5	3.7	3.9	-	-	1.8	0.4	0.08	0.14	1.1	148
Pharynx unspecified	13	0	-	-	-	-	-	-	-	-	-	-	1.4	3.6	1.7	2.1	3.7	-	-	-	0.7	0.1	0.03	0.06	0.4	149
Oesophagus	114	0	-	-	-	-	-	-	-	-	2.1	2.9	10.8	12.4	12.5	27.6	20.5	29.0	14.1	22.2	6.0	1.2	0.20	0.44	3.6	150
Stomach	573	0	-	-	-	-	-	1.2	2.0	5.3	8.5	8.8	25.8	47.3	62.3	115.9	134.4	181.9	194.4	214.7	29.9	6.0	0.81	2.06	17.3	151
Small intestine	15	0	-	-	-	-	-	-	-	-	0.7	0.7	0.7	0.7	0.8	2.1	-	3.9	17.7	7.4	0.8	0.2	0.02	0.03	0.4	152
Colon	796	0	-	-	-	-	0.6	-	0.7	4.5	7.1	25.1	35.2	59.6	93.1	145.6	212.7	224.5	357.0	222.1	41.6	8.3	1.13	2.92	23.9	153
Rectum	434	0	-	-	-	-	-	-	-	3.8	6.4	11.1	19.0	34.2	49.9	90.4	98.9	133.5	144.9	162.9	22.7	4.5	0.62	1.57	13.1	154
Liver	254	0	-	-	-	-	-	1.8	-	1.5	4.3	4.4	12.9	22.5	40.7	54.2	69.0	58.1	60.1	22.2	13.3	2.7	0.44	1.06	7.9	155
Gallbladder etc.	133	0	-	-	-	-	-	-	-	0.8	1.4	5.2	5.4	7.3	20.8	19.1	16.8	60.0	38.9	81.4	6.9	1.4	0.20	0.38	3.9	156
Pancreas	258	0	-	-	-	-	-	-	-	0.8	3.6	8.1	12.2	14.5	32.4	57.4	63.4	73.5	106.0	59.2	13.5	2.7	0.36	0.96	7.8	157
Nose, sinuses etc.	18	0	-	-	-	-	-	-	-	-	-	-	1.4	4.4	0.8	2.1	3.7	7.7	3.5	-	0.9	0.2	0.03	0.06	0.5	160
Larynx	323	0	-	-	-	-	-	-	-	0.8	2.8	11.1	23.0	50.2	55.7	64.8	42.9	56.1	49.5	44.4	16.9	3.4	0.72	1.26	10.1	161
Bronchus, lung	2099	0	-	-	1.0	0.7	0.6	0.6	1.4	9.1	17.1	56.7	91.5	219.7	344.1	409.3	530.0	478.0	547.8	429.4	109.6	22.0	3.71	8.41	65.0	162
Other thoracic organs	40	0	-	-	-	0.7	-	0.6	1.4	-	1.4	1.5	2.0	2.2	6.6	-	9.3	13.5	7.1	29.6	2.1	0.4	0.08	0.13	1.3	163-4
Bone	18	0	-	-	2.0	2.9	0.6	0.6	-	0.8	0.7	-	0.7	-	0.8	-	1.9	3.9	10.6	-	0.9	0.2	0.05	0.06	0.8	170
Connective tissue	47	0	1.4	-	1.0	1.5	0.6	-	1.4	0.8	0.7	0.7	2.7	3.6	5.0	6.4	7.5	11.6	14.1	14.8	2.5	0.5	0.10	0.17	1.7	171
Mesothelioma	28	0	-	-	-	-	-	-	-	0.8	-	0.7	1.4	5.1	4.2	4.3	5.6	5.8	7.1	-	1.5	0.3	0.06	0.11	0.9	MES
Kaposi's sarcoma	37	0	-	-	-	-	-	4.3	2.0	3.0	5.7	0.7	2.7	-	1.7	1.1	5.6	5.8	-	7.4	1.9	0.4	0.10	0.13	1.5	KAP
Melanoma of skin	117	0	-	-	-	0.6	-	2.7	3.0	6.4	8.8	9.5	5.8	16.6	13.8	22.4	21.3	28.3	7.4	6.1	1.2	0.27	0.45	3.9	172			
Other skin	1283	0	-	-	-	0.7	3.1	2.4	0.7	15.9	28.5	60.4	71.2	90.2	161.3	224.3	274.3	383.2	392.3	288.7	67.0		2.17	4.66	39.9	173
Breast	23	0	-	-	-	-	-	-	0.7	-	0.7	0.7	1.4	2.2	2.5	2.1	5.6	5.8	14.1	-	1.2	0.2	0.04	0.08	0.7	175
Prostate	850	0	-	-	-	-	-	-	-	-	-	-	8.1	32.0	69.8	156.3	251.9	429.6	505.4	466.4	44.4	8.9	0.55	2.59	23.4	185
Testis	72	0	-	-	-	4.4	5.5	4.9	10.2	6.8	3.6	3.7	4.7	2.2	0.8	1.1	1.9	-	7.1	-	3.8	0.8	0.23	0.25	3.1	186
Penis	23	0	-	-	-	-	-	-	-	-	-	3.7	0.7	-	2.5	7.4	3.7	5.8	7.1	-	1.2	0.2	0.03	0.09	0.7	187.1-.4
Other male genital	8	0	-	-	-	-	-	-	-	-	-	-	-	-	1.7	3.2	1.9	3.9	-	-	0.4	0.1	0.01	0.03	0.2	187.5-.9
Bladder	1171	0	1.4	-	-	-	0.6	-	2.0	6.8	15.0	31.7	53.6	99.7	165.4	249.8	283.7	292.2	342.8	318.4	61.1	12.3	1.88	4.55	36.2	188
Kidney etc.	348	0	1.4	-	-	-	-	-	0.7	1.5	2.1	11.1	23.0	32.7	54.9	71.2	91.4	67.7	67.2	81.4	18.2	3.6	0.64	1.45	11.1	189
Eye	13	0	-	-	-	-	0.6	-	-	-	0.7	-	-	2.2	0.8	2.1	-	5.8	3.5	7.4	0.7	0.1	0.02	0.03	0.4	190
Brain, nervous system	178	0	2.7	2.6	2.0	2.9	3.1	3.7	3.4	1.5	5.7	9.6	10.8	16.0	21.6	22.3	42.9	29.0	14.1	14.8	9.3	1.9	0.43	0.75	6.8	191-2
Thyroid	59	0	-	-	-	-	4.3	-	2.0	5.3	5.0	2.9	4.7	3.6	4.2	1.1	11.2	5.8	10.6	7.4	3.1	0.6	0.16	0.22	2.2	193
Other endocrine	19	0	2.7	-	-	-	-	-	-	0.8	0.7	-	1.4	0.7	1.7	6.4	3.7	3.9	-	-	1.0	0.2	0.04	0.09	0.9	194
Hodgkin's disease	74	0	-	1.3	1.0	4.4	6.8	4.3	6.8	2.3	1.4	3.7	1.4	5.8	3.3	7.4	5.6	3.9	7.1	-	3.9	0.8	0.21	0.28	3.2	201
Non-Hodgkin lymphoma	339	0	1.4	1.3	2.0	2.9	3.7	1.8	4.7	5.3	5.7	19.9	13.6	30.5	39.1	57.4	63.4	92.9	70.7	59.2	17.7	3.6	0.66	1.26	11.3	200,202
Multiple myeloma	90	0	-	-	-	-	-	-	-	0.8	1.4	2.9	4.7	5.8	10.8	13.8	29.9	23.2	28.3	44.4	4.7	0.9	0.13	0.35	2.8	203
Lymphoid leukaemia	98	0	10.9	3.9	-	1.5	0.6	0.6	0.7	2.3	-	2.2	3.4	5.8	9.1	13.8	26.1	27.1	31.8	14.8	5.1	1.0	0.20	0.40	4.4	204
Myeloid leukaemia	106	0	-	2.6	1.0	1.5	-	0.6	6.8	3.8	3.6	8.1	2.0	8.0	9.1	10.6	16.8	21.3	35.3	29.6	5.5	1.1	0.24	0.37	3.8	205
Monocytic leukaemia	5	0	1.4	1.3	-	-	-	-	-	-	-	-	-	-	-	-	-	1.9	3.5	7.4	0.3	0.1	0.01	0.01	0.4	206
Other leukaemia	1	0	-	-	-	-	-	-	-	-	-	-	-	-	0.8	-	-	-	-	-	0.1	0.0	0.00	0.00	0.0	207
Leukaemia unspecified	31	0	-	-	-	-	-	-	-	0.8	-	-	1.4	1.5	8.3	8.5	-	9.7	7.1	7.4	1.6	0.3	0.06	0.10	0.9	208
Other and unspecified	401	0	1.4	-	2.0	0.7	-	0.6	0.7	0.8	2.8	7.4	15.6	26.2	49.0	74.4	130.6	106.4	173.2	133.3	20.9	4.2	0.54	1.56	12.4	O&U
All sites	10825	0	25.8	13.0	12.1	25.6	32.0	29.3	52.8	92.9	152.4	328.6	501.6	897.6	1422.2	2003.8	2539.8	2943.5	3364.8	2843.0	565.1		17.93	40.65	339.6	ALL
All sites but 173	9542	0	25.8	13.0	12.1	24.9	28.9	26.9	52.1	77.0	123.9	268.2	430.5	807.4	1261.0	1779.5	2265.5	2560.3	2972.5	2554.2	498.1	100.0	15.76	35.98	299.7	ALLb

| Rate from 1 case | | | 1.360 | 1.298 | 1.007 | 0.732 | 0.615 | 0.611 | 0.677 | 0.755 | 0.712 | 0.737 | 0.678 | 0.727 | 0.831 | 1.063 | 1.866 | 1.935 | 3.534 | 7.404 | | | | | | |

ITALY, TORINO 1988-1991

ANNUAL INCIDENCE PER 100,000 BY AGE GROUP (YEARS) - FEMALE

SITE	ALL AGES	AGE UNK	0-	5-	10-	15-	20-	25-	30-	35-	40-	45-	50-	55-	60-	65-	70-	75-	80-	85+	CRUDE RATE	%	CR 64	CR 74	ASR (W)	ICD (9th)
Lip	7	0	-	-	-	-	-	-	-	-	-	-	-	-	-	2.4	1.2	-	3.2	2.4	0.3	0.1	0.00	0.02	0.1	140
Tongue	42	0	-	-	-	-	-	-	0.7	0.7	-	1.4	1.9	2.7	3.6	1.6	5.0	12.3	8.1	9.6	2.0	0.5	0.06	0.09	0.9	141
Salivary gland	15	0	-	-	-	-	-	-	0.7	-	0.7	-	-	1.3	1.4	0.8	-	5.6	3.2	2.4	0.7	0.2	0.02	0.02	0.3	142
Mouth	16	0	-	-	-	-	-	-	-	-	0.7	-	-	1.3	1.4	0.8	-	3.4	8.1	4.8	0.8	0.2	0.02	0.02	0.3	143-5
Oropharynx	21	0	1.5	-	-	-	-	-	-	1.5	0.7	0.7	-	0.7	2.9	-	5.0	2.2	4.8	4.8	1.0	0.2	0.04	0.06	0.7	146
Nasopharynx	7	0	-	-	-	-	-	-	-	-	-	0.7	0.6	1.3	-	0.8	1.2	1.1	-	-	0.3	0.1	0.01	0.02	0.2	147
Hypopharynx	9	0	-	-	-	-	-	-	0.7	-	-	0.7	0.6	-	0.7	-	3.7	-	3.2	-	0.4	0.1	0.01	0.03	0.2	148
Pharynx unspecified	0	0	-	-	-	-	-	-	-	-	-	-	-	-	-	-	-	-	-	-	0.0	0.0	0.00	0.00	0.0	149
Oesophagus	34	0	-	-	-	-	-	-	-	-	-	0.7	1.3	1.3	5.1	1.6	2.5	5.6	9.7	16.8	1.6	0.4	0.04	0.06	0.6	150
Stomach	454	0	-	-	-	-	-	1.3	1.4	5.2	4.8	9.8	11.4	20.7	24.5	38.5	63.1	92.7	132.5	179.8	21.9	5.3	0.40	0.90	8.7	151
Small intestine	19	0	-	-	-	-	-	-	-	-	-	0.7	1.9	-	2.9	0.8	2.5	1.1	8.1	4.8	0.9	0.2	0.03	0.04	0.4	152
Colon	783	0	-	-	-	-	-	1.3	2.2	3.0	10.2	15.4	29.0	36.7	59.2	92.9	121.3	156.4	185.8	203.8	37.8	9.2	0.79	1.86	16.0	153
Rectum	417	0	-	-	-	-	-	0.7	2.2	2.2	6.1	12.6	14.5	31.3	30.3	44.9	71.8	76.0	82.4	91.1	20.1	4.9	0.50	1.08	9.0	154
Liver	120	0	-	-	-	-	-	-	0.7	-	0.7	0.7	3.8	6.0	7.9	15.2	27.2	23.5	35.5	16.8	5.8	1.4	0.10	0.31	2.4	155
Gallbladder etc.	219	0	-	-	-	-	-	-	0.7	-	3.4	2.8	4.4	8.7	17.3	25.6	27.2	52.5	61.4	62.3	10.6	2.6	0.19	0.45	4.1	156
Pancreas	241	0	-	-	-	-	0.7	0.7	0.7	-	2.0	2.1	8.2	9.3	10.8	31.2	38.4	61.4	69.5	52.8	11.6	2.8	0.17	0.52	4.5	157
Nose, sinuses etc.	9	0	-	-	-	-	-	0.7	-	-	-	-	1.9	-	0.7	0.8	-	1.1	1.6	2.4	0.4	0.1	0.02	0.02	0.2	160
Larynx	27	0	-	-	-	-	-	0.7	-	-	0.7	0.7	0.6	3.3	2.9	4.0	7.4	3.4	-	-	1.3	0.3	0.04	0.10	0.7	161
Bronchus, lung	500	0	-	-	-	-	0.7	-	-	4.5	6.8	13.3	22.7	26.7	37.5	66.5	79.2	97.2	98.5	98.3	24.2	5.9	0.56	1.29	10.8	162
Other thoracic organs	24	0	-	-	-	-	-	-	-	1.5	-	0.7	1.9	2.0	1.4	-	6.2	3.4	3.2	7.2	1.2	0.3	0.04	0.07	0.6	163-4
Bone	17	0	-	-	1.1	-	0.7	-	1.4	1.5	0.7	-	-	0.7	0.7	0.8	1.2	1.1	4.8	4.8	0.8	0.2	0.03	0.04	0.5	170
Connective tissue	40	0	1.5	-	1.1	3.9	-	0.7	-	0.7	0.7	2.1	1.9	2.7	1.4	6.4	5.0	5.6	-	2.4	1.9	0.5	0.08	0.14	1.5	171
Mesothelioma	19	0	-	-	-	-	-	-	-	-	0.7	0.7	0.6	1.3	0.7	1.6	6.2	2.2	1.6	7.2	0.9	0.2	0.02	0.06	0.4	MES
Kaposi's sarcoma	9	0	-	-	-	-	-	0.7	-	-	-	1.4	-	0.7	-	-	2.5	-	1.6	4.8	0.4	0.1	0.01	0.03	0.2	KAP
Melanoma of skin	156	0	-	-	-	-	1.3	3.4	5.8	3.0	12.3	8.4	12.0	8.7	13.7	12.8	14.9	13.4	14.5	16.8	7.5	1.8	0.34	0.48	4.6	172
Other skin	1093	0	1.5	-	1.1	1.5	2.7	4.0	4.3	12.0	21.8	42.0	58.7	71.3	93.8	114.6	136.2	188.8	193.9	223.0	52.8		1.57	2.83	25.4	173
Breast	2426	0	-	-	-	-	2.7	6.0	22.5	52.5	100.1	169.6	173.6	196.7	221.6	265.1	236.4	291.5	253.6	254.2	117.2	28.5	4.73	7.23	64.9	174
Uterus unspecified	19	0	-	-	-	-	-	-	-	-	-	-	-	0.7	-	1.6	2.5	6.7	3.2	14.4	0.9	0.2	0.00	0.02	0.3	179
Cervix uteri	287	0	-	-	-	-	0.7	0.7	5.8	19.5	12.9	9.8	19.6	20.7	31.8	22.4	37.1	27.9	30.7	24.0	13.9	3.4	0.61	0.90	8.0	180
Placenta	1	0	-	-	-	-	-	-	-	-	0.7	-	-	-	-	-	-	-	-	-	0.0	0.0	0.00	0.00	0.0	181
Corpus uteri	439	0	-	-	-	-	0.7	0.7	0.7	2.2	6.1	20.3	36.0	43.3	46.2	58.5	59.4	57.0	48.5	16.8	21.2	5.2	0.78	1.37	11.1	182
Ovary etc.	334	0	-	-	2.1	0.8	0.7	0.7	2.9	4.5	8.9	21.0	28.4	27.3	30.3	37.6	45.8	40.2	19.4	38.4	16.1	3.9	0.64	1.06	9.1	183
Other female genital	84	0	-	-	-	-	-	-	-	-	-	0.7	1.3	2.7	4.3	7.2	17.3	20.1	17.8	45.6	4.1	1.0	0.04	0.17	1.5	184
Bladder	266	0	-	-	-	-	0.7	1.3	0.7	-	2.0	5.6	15.8	13.3	14.4	31.2	30.9	71.5	53.3	59.9	12.8	3.1	0.27	0.58	5.4	188
Kidney etc.	161	0	1.5	1.4	-	0.8	0.7	-	1.4	1.5	2.7	4.9	8.2	13.3	15.9	20.8	17.3	19.0	32.3	24.0	7.8	1.9	0.26	0.45	4.1	189
Eye	10	0	-	-	-	-	-	-	-	-	0.7	-	0.6	0.7	0.7	1.6	-	3.4	-	2.4	0.5	0.1	0.01	0.02	0.2	190
Brain, nervous system	145	0	1.5	2.7	4.3	-	0.7	1.3	-	4.5	4.1	3.5	4.4	12.7	15.9	16.0	22.3	22.3	17.8	2.4	7.0	1.7	0.28	0.47	4.3	191-2
Thyroid	135	0	-	-	-	3.9	2.7	3.4	5.8	6.0	10.2	7.7	6.9	9.3	5.8	8.8	9.9	14.5	16.2	9.6	6.5	1.6	0.31	0.40	4.3	193
Other endocrine	13	0	2.9	-	-	0.8	-	-	-	1.5	0.7	0.7	1.3	-	0.7	0.8	-	1.1	1.6	-	0.6	0.2	0.04	0.05	0.7	194
Hodgkin's disease	64	0	-	-	1.1	3.9	5.3	3.4	7.2	2.2	4.8	2.8	1.3	-	4.3	4.8	1.2	4.5	3.2	-	3.1	0.8	0.18	0.21	2.6	201
Non-Hodgkin lymphoma	271	0	1.5	-	1.1	0.8	0.7	4.7	5.1	3.0	9.5	10.5	13.9	16.7	28.9	36.0	30.9	34.6	29.1	33.6	13.1	3.2	0.48	0.82	7.3	200,202
Multiple myeloma	94	0	-	-	-	-	-	-	-	-	-	1.4	2.5	4.7	10.1	11.2	14.9	17.9	25.8	21.6	4.5	1.1	0.09	0.22	1.9	203
Lymphoid leukaemia	83	0	4.4	4.1	4.3	-	0.7	-	1.4	1.5	1.4	-	2.5	2.0	5.1	4.0	11.1	23.5	16.2	16.8	4.0	1.0	0.14	0.21	2.8	204
Myeloid leukaemia	90	0	-	-	-	1.5	0.7	2.0	2.2	1.5	2.7	4.9	1.9	4.0	7.9	7.2	7.4	21.2	11.3	16.8	4.3	1.1	0.15	0.22	2.3	205
Monocytic leukaemia	4	0	1.5	1.4	1.1	-	0.7	-	-	-	-	-	-	-	-	-	-	-	-	-	0.2	0.0	0.02	0.02	0.5	206
Other leukaemia	6	0	-	-	-	-	-	-	-	-	-	0.7	-	-	0.7	0.8	-	1.1	-	4.8	0.3	0.1	0.01	0.01	0.1	207
Leukaemia unspecified	13	0	-	-	-	-	-	-	-	0.7	-	0.7	-	-	1.4	1.6	1.2	-	6.5	4.8	0.6	0.2	0.01	0.03	0.3	208
Other and unspecified	374	0	1.5	-	-	-	-	-	1.4	3.0	-	9.1	10.1	10.7	20.2	28.8	50.8	74.8	129.2	167.8	18.1	4.4	0.28	0.68	6.8	O&U
All sites	9617	0	18.9	9.6	17.0	17.8	23.4	38.2	79.0	140.2	240.4	391.7	506.2	617.3	787.3	1031.0	1225.5	1562.6	1651.0	1776.8	464.5		14.44	25.72	232.1	ALL
All sites but 173	8524	0	17.5	9.6	16.0	16.3	20.7	34.2	74.6	128.2	218.6	349.7	447.5	546.0	693.5	916.4	1089.4	1373.8	1457.1	1553.8	411.7	100.0	12.86	22.89	206.6	ALLb
Rate from 1 case			1.455	1.369	1.064	0.774	0.668	0.671	0.724	0.750	0.681	0.701	0.631	0.667	0.722	0.801	1.238	1.117	1.615	2.398						

Italy, Trieste

The Tumour Registry of the province of Trieste was set up by the Regional County Council for Health of the region Friuli Venezia Giulia and it has functioned since 1 January 1984; the staff consists of one scientific coordinator, one director, two full-time doctors, one office worker and three fellowships.

The province of Trieste is part of the Italian region Friuli Venezia Giulia and covers 212 km^2; it is bordered by Slovenia to the north-east, the Adriatic Sea to the south-west and the province of Gorizia to the north-west. The area is closely circumscribed and highly populated. Most of the population lives in a single major conurbation. The inhabitants of Trieste numbered 261 825 on 20 October 1991, about 90% (231 100) living in the commune of Trieste and the rest in five minor communes. The average population density is 1271 inhabitants per km^2. The Trieste area has an old population (one out of four people aged 65 years or more). The present resident population appears to be particularly stable.

Within the province of Trieste there are four public hospitals, which provide for most of the health needs, one children's hospital and a few private clinics. There is only one department of surgical pathology and histology in the province. Pathology specimens from the hospital wards and the infant hospital, accounting for 83.8% of all admissions, as well as those from minor private centres in the area, are sent to this department. Therefore all histopathological reports concerning hospitalized patients are analysed and collected in the same department.

More than 10% of the hospitalizations of Trieste residents are in the hospital of the neighbouring province of Gorizia, from which the registry can obtain data. Thus information on over 95% of all admissions is available to the registry. In 1984 a computerized system was implemented and progressively developed for the collection of anatomo-pathological data from the main laboratories operating in the region Friuli Venezia Giulia. This allows information to be obtained about specimens for residents of the province of Trieste when collected in any hospital within the whole region.

Most of the residents who die undergo autopsy (about 70% of all deaths in the province). All the autopsy reports are available to the registry and are very important in the evaluation of the occurrence of malignant neoplasms which are difficult to diagnose because of the anatomical site, deceptive symptoms, rapid evolution or extreme old age of the patients.

The registry collects data on all malignant tumours, corresponding to categories 140–208 of ICD-9. The data on *in situ* carcinomas, severe dysplasia of the cervix uteri and benign tumours are also collected and registered.

The date of the patient's hospital admission at the first diagnosis of a neoplasm is considered the date of incidence; in the case of non-hospitalized patients, the date of the first morphological test positive for a neoplasm is taken. The remaining cases are inferred from the death certificates and autopsy reports.

The central medical archives of the Health District and the archives of the private clinics operating in the province can also provide the medical records needed to clarify any question of cancer care. Other sources of data are the General Register Offices and the registers of the patient's family doctor and, for death-certificate-only cases, the Regional Information System which has been recording all death reports for the whole Friuli Venezia Giulia region since 1989.

Access to the data bank of the register is strictly limited to the people working for the registry. An authorization to examine the paper files, which are still used alongside the computerized system, can be obtained for research purposes by request to the scientific coordinator.

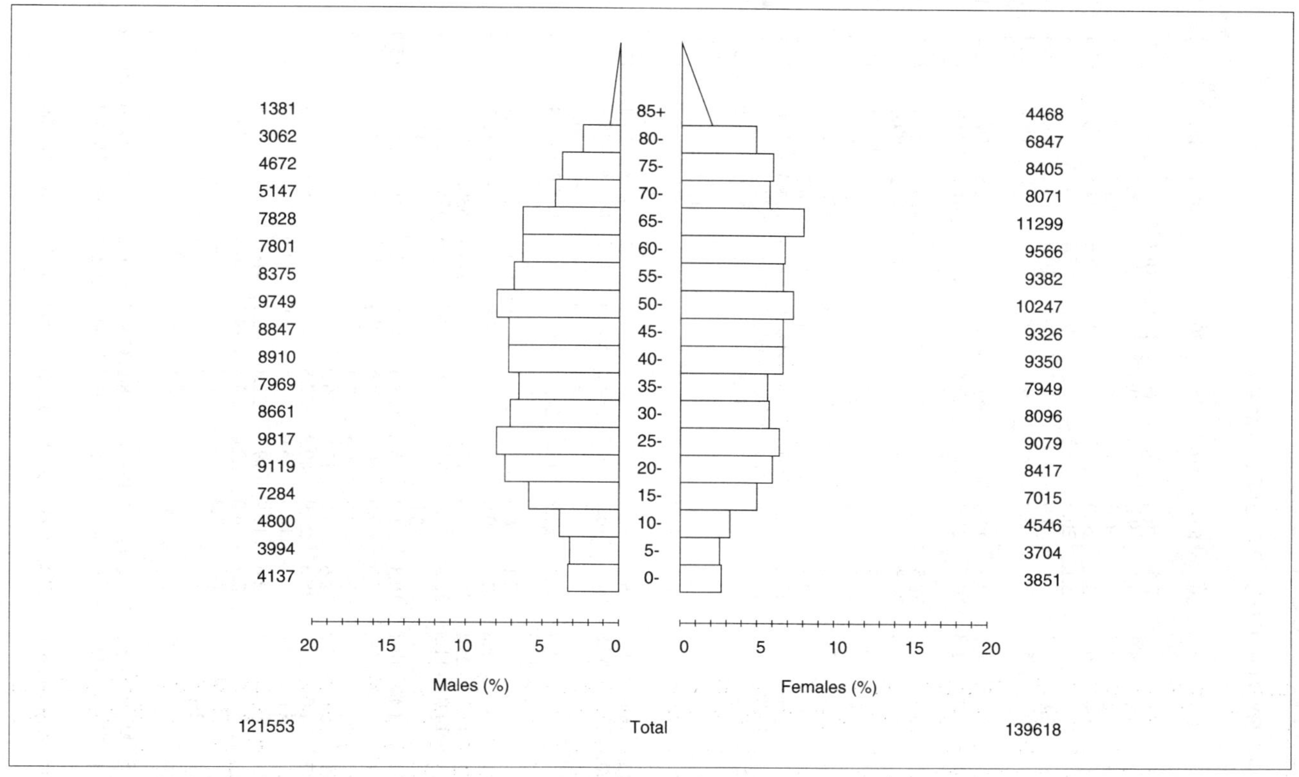

Italy, Trieste
Source of population: average annual 1989–92
Census: 13° Censimento generale della popolazione e delle
abitazioni, 20 Ottobre 1991. Fascicolo provinciale Macerata,
Istituto Nazionale di Statistics (ISTAT), Roma, 1993.
Estimate: The estimates for 1989, 1990 and 1992 were pro-
vided by the General Registry Office of the Communes.

ITALY, TRIESTE 1989-1992

ANNUAL INCIDENCE PER 100,000 BY AGE GROUP (YEARS) - MALE

SITE	ALL AGES	AGE UNK	0-	5-	10-	15-	20-	25-	30-	35-	40-	45-	50-	55-	60-	65-	70-	75-	80-	85+	CRUDE RATE	%	CR 64	CR 74	ASR (W)	ICD (9th)
Lip	17	0	-	-	-	-	-	-	2.9	3.1	-	-	2.6	6.0	3.2	6.4	29.1	16.1	-	-	3.5	0.4	0.09	0.27	**1.8**	140
Tongue	21	0	-	-	-	-	-	-	-	-	8.4	5.7	5.1	9.0	12.8	9.6	-	16.1	8.2	-	4.3	0.5	0.20	0.25	**2.5**	141
Salivary gland	12	0	-	-	-	3.4	-	-	-	-	5.6	2.8	-	6.0	6.4	3.2	9.7	-	8.2	-	2.5	0.3	0.12	0.19	**1.6**	142
Mouth	73	0	-	-	-	-	2.7	5.1	2.9	-	8.4	19.8	23.1	26.9	19.2	47.9	43.7	37.5	24.5	18.1	15.0	1.7	0.54	1.00	**8.4**	143-5
Oropharynx	21	0	-	-	-	-	-	-	-	-	-	5.7	5.1	20.9	19.2	3.2	9.7	5.4	-	-	4.3	0.5	0.25	0.32	**2.5**	146
Nasopharynx	8	0	-	-	-	-	-	-	-	-	2.8	2.8	-	3.0	-	6.4	-	10.7	-	18.1	1.6	0.2	0.04	0.08	**0.8**	147
Hypopharynx	14	0	-	-	-	-	-	-	-	-	-	5.7	2.6	3.0	16.0	9.6	-	-	8.2	18.1	2.9	0.3	0.14	0.18	**1.6**	148
Pharynx unspecified	0	0	-	-	-	-	-	-	-	-	-	-	-	-	-	-	-	-	-	-	0.0	0.0	0.00	0.00	**0.0**	149
Oesophagus	65	0	-	-	-	-	-	-	-	-	8.4	5.7	20.5	17.9	35.3	47.9	48.6	26.8	24.5	36.2	13.4	1.5	0.44	0.92	**7.0**	150
Stomach	206	0	-	-	-	-	2.7	-	2.9	6.3	8.4	11.3	10.3	26.9	80.1	89.4	145.7	208.7	261.2	506.8	42.4	4.7	0.74	1.92	**18.3**	151
Small intestine	10	0	-	-	-	-	-	-	-	-	5.6	-	-	-	3.2	12.8	4.9	10.7	-	-	2.1	0.2	0.04	0.13	**1.1**	152
Colon	341	0	-	-	-	-	-	-	-	3.1	16.8	17.0	38.5	95.5	131.4	201.2	233.1	337.1	416.3	271.5	70.1	7.8	1.51	3.68	**30.7**	153
Rectum	206	0	-	-	-	-	-	-	-	-	8.4	8.5	30.8	68.7	70.5	99.0	145.7	214.0	212.2	289.6	42.4	4.7	0.93	2.16	**18.7**	154
Liver	200	0	-	-	-	-	-	-	-	6.3	2.8	8.5	10.3	44.8	105.8	118.2	165.1	230.1	171.4	126.7	41.1	4.6	0.89	2.31	**18.2**	155
Gallbladder etc.	61	0	-	-	-	-	-	-	-	-	2.8	8.5	10.3	17.9	12.8	31.9	14.6	80.3	98.0	54.3	12.5	1.4	0.26	0.49	**5.2**	156
Pancreas	139	0	-	-	-	-	-	2.5	-	-	5.6	17.0	35.9	23.9	44.9	67.1	87.4	133.8	146.9	217.2	28.6	3.2	0.65	1.42	**13.0**	157
Nose, sinuses etc.	9	0	-	-	-	3.4	-	-	-	-	-	-	2.6	6.0	3.2	-	4.9	10.7	8.2	-	1.9	0.2	0.08	0.10	**1.0**	160
Larynx	156	0	-	-	-	-	-	-	-	-	16.8	22.6	43.6	56.7	70.5	70.3	116.6	85.6	114.3	144.8	32.1	3.6	1.05	1.99	**16.2**	161
Bronchus, lung	897	0	-	-	-	-	-	-	5.8	3.1	16.8	45.2	146.2	226.9	410.2	546.1	641.1	914.9	832.6	633.5	184.5	20.6	4.27	10.21	**82.7**	162
Other thoracic organs	29	0	-	-	-	-	2.7	5.1	5.8	-	5.6	5.7	5.1	-	12.8	12.8	-	21.4	40.8	18.1	6.0	0.7	0.21	0.28	**3.3**	163-4
Bone	4	0	-	-	-	6.9	-	-	-	-	-	-	-	3.2	-	-	5.4	-	-	-	0.8	0.1	0.05	0.05	**0.8**	170
Connective tissue	25	0	-	-	5.2	-	-	-	8.7	-	2.8	-	-	9.0	12.8	12.8	14.6	21.4	16.3	-	5.1	0.6	0.19	0.33	**3.0**	171
Mesothelioma	63	0	-	-	-	-	-	-	-	-	5.6	2.8	28.2	17.9	28.8	31.9	34.0	37.5	57.1	54.3	13.0	1.4	0.42	0.75	**6.4**	MES
Kaposi's sarcoma	6	0	-	-	-	-	-	-	-	-	-	-	-	-	-	6.4	-	10.7	16.3	-	1.2	0.1	0.00	0.03	**0.4**	KAP
Melanoma of skin	84	0	-	-	-	3.4	2.7	2.5	5.8	6.3	5.6	8.5	35.9	32.8	35.3	41.5	29.1	48.2	32.7	72.4	17.3	1.9	0.69	1.05	**9.7**	172
Other skin	723	0	-	-	5.2	6.9	-	7.6	8.7	22.0	33.7	67.8	94.9	176.1	250.0	364.0	544.0	781.2	693.8	724.0	148.7		3.36	7.90	**68.1**	173
Breast	10	0	-	-	-	-	-	-	2.9	-	-	-	-	-	6.4	14.6	10.7	-	36.2		2.1	0.2	0.01	0.12	**0.9**	175
Prostate	578	0	-	-	-	-	-	-	-	-	2.8	5.7	23.1	44.8	118.6	242.7	451.7	743.7	955.0	1610.9	118.9	13.2	0.97	4.45	**44.8**	185
Testis	20	0	-	-	-	6.9	-	-	5.8	-	5.6	11.3	5.1	6.0	6.4	9.6	4.9	-	-	-	4.1	0.5	0.24	0.31	**3.1**	186
Penis	12	0	-	-	-	-	-	-	-	-	-	-	5.1	6.0	3.2	-	14.6	5.4	16.3	18.1	2.5	0.3	0.07	0.14	**1.1**	187.1-.4
Other male genital	11	0	-	6.3	-	-	-	-	-	3.1	-	2.8	2.6	9.0	-	-	4.9	10.7	-	18.1	2.3	0.3	0.12	0.14	**1.8**	187.5-.9
Bladder	451	0	-	-	-	-	-	2.5	2.9	-	11.2	25.4	48.7	80.6	115.4	245.9	320.6	545.7	530.6	796.4	92.8	10.3	1.43	4.27	**38.7**	188
Kidney etc.	177	0	-	-	-	-	-	-	-	-	14.0	11.3	33.3	50.7	83.3	76.6	92.3	176.6	179.6	253.4	36.4	4.1	0.96	1.81	**16.6**	189
Eye	3	0	-	-	-	3.4	-	-	-	-	-	-	-	3.0	-	-	-	-	-	18.1	0.6	0.1	0.03	0.03	**0.5**	190
Brain, nervous system	73	0	6.0	-	10.4	-	8.2	2.5	-	9.4	8.4	14.1	10.3	11.9	25.6	38.3	48.6	42.8	49.0	54.3	15.0	1.7	0.54	0.97	**9.5**	191-2
Thyroid	20	0	-	-	-	-	-	-	2.9	3.1	-	-	2.6	9.0	6.4	9.6	19.4	10.7	16.3	18.1	4.1	0.5	0.12	0.26	**2.1**	193
Other endocrine	16	0	-	6.3	-	-	2.7	2.5	-	-	-	-	5.1	3.0	6.4	6.4	9.7	10.7	16.3	-	3.3	0.4	0.13	0.21	**2.3**	194
Hodgkin's disease	21	0	-	-	-	-	2.7	2.5	2.9	3.1	5.6	2.8	2.6	3.0	12.8	16.0	-	5.4	16.3	-	4.3	0.5	0.19	0.27	**2.7**	201
Non-Hodgkin lymphoma	131	0	-	-	-	6.9	8.2	7.6	2.9	15.7	14.0	33.9	25.6	23.9	60.9	57.5	92.3	64.2	89.8	54.3	26.9	3.0	1.00	1.75	**15.5**	200,202
Multiple myeloma	51	0	-	-	-	-	-	-	-	-	5.6	2.8	5.1	14.9	16.0	12.8	34.0	74.9	57.1	72.4	10.5	1.2	0.22	0.46	**4.5**	203
Lymphoid leukaemia	70	0	-	25.0	-	3.4	8.2	-	5.8	3.1	-	14.1	2.6	11.9	19.2	22.4	43.7	48.2	98.0	108.6	14.4	1.6	0.47	0.80	**9.3**	204
Myeloid leukaemia	39	0	-	-	-	-	-	-	5.8	3.1	5.6	-	7.7	6.0	22.4	25.5	29.1	26.8	8.2	36.2	8.0	0.9	0.25	0.53	**4.2**	205
Monocytic leukaemia	2	0	-	-	-	-	-	-	-	-	-	-	-	3.0	-	3.2	-	-	-	-	0.4	0.0	0.01	0.03	**0.2**	206
Other leukaemia	5	0	-	-	-	-	-	-	-	3.1	2.8	-	-	-	3.2	3.2	-	5.4	-	-	1.0	0.1	0.05	0.06	**0.6**	207
Leukaemia unspecified	6	0	-	-	-	-	-	-	-	3.1	-	-	-	-	3.2	3.2	4.9	10.7	-	-	1.2	0.1	0.03	0.07	**0.6**	208
Other and unspecified	0	0	-	-	-	-	-	-	-	-	-	-	-	-	-	-	-	-	-	-	0.0	0.0	0.00	0.00	**0.0**	O&U
All sites	5086	0	6.0	37.6	20.8	44.6	41.1	40.7	75.0	97.2	246.9	395.6	730.8	1182.1	1890.7	2618.6	3506.7	5056.2	5224.1	6298.6	1046.0		24.05	54.67	**482.1**	ALL
All sites but 173	4363	0	6.0	37.6	15.6	37.8	41.1	33.1	66.4	75.3	213.2	327.8	635.9	1005.9	1640.8	2254.5	2962.7	4275.0	4530.2	5574.7	897.3	100.0	20.68	46.77	**414.0**	ALLb
Rate from 1 case			6.043	6.259	5.208	3.432	2.741	2.546	2.886	3.137	2.806	2.826	2.564	2.985	3.205	3.193	4.857	5.350	8.163	18.100						

ITALY, TRIESTE 1989-1992

ANNUAL INCIDENCE PER 100,000 BY AGE GROUP (YEARS) - FEMALE

SITE	ALL AGES	AGE UNK	0-	5-	10-	15-	20-	25-	30-	35-	40-	45-	50-	55-	60-	65-	70-	75-	80-	85+	CRUDE RATE	%	CR 64	CR 74	ASR (W)	ICD (9th)
Lip	8	0	-	-	-	-	-	-	-	-	-	-	2.4	-	2.6	-	-	5.9	3.7	16.8	1.4	0.2	0.03	0.03	0.4	140
Tongue	10	0	-	-	-	-	-	-	-	3.1	2.7	2.7	4.9	5.3	2.6	2.2	-	-	-	5.6	1.8	0.3	0.11	0.12	1.2	141
Salivary gland	12	0	-	-	-	-	-	3.1	-	-	-	-	2.4	-	-	4.4	6.2	3.0	11.0	11.2	2.1	0.3	0.03	0.08	0.7	142
Mouth	28	0	-	-	-	3.6	-	-	-	-	5.3	-	9.8	8.0	10.5	13.3	-	3.0	18.3	11.2	5.0	0.8	0.19	0.25	2.4	143-5
Oropharynx	5	0	-	-	-	-	-	-	-	-	2.7	-	2.7	5.2	-	3.1	-	-	-	-	0.9	0.1	0.05	0.07	0.5	146
Nasopharynx	5	0	-	-	-	3.6	-	-	-	-	2.7	-	-	-	-	3.1	5.9	-	-	-	0.9	0.1	0.03	0.05	0.6	147
Hypopharynx	0	0	-	-	-	-	-	-	-	-	-	-	-	-	-	-	-	-	-	-	0.0	0.0	0.00	0.00	0.0	148
Pharynx unspecified	0	0	-	-	-	-	-	-	-	-	-	-	-	-	-	-	-	-	-	-	0.0	0.0	0.00	0.00	0.0	149
Oesophagus	24	0	-	-	-	-	-	-	-	-	-	-	4.9	5.3	7.8	6.6	6.2	8.9	18.3	22.4	4.3	0.7	0.09	0.15	1.4	150
Stomach	162	0	-	-	-	-	-	2.8	3.1	3.1	8.0	10.7	9.8	18.7	26.1	44.3	49.6	110.1	109.5	156.7	29.0	4.6	0.41	0.88	8.7	151
Small intestine	18	0	-	-	-	-	-	-	-	-	-	-	-	5.3	2.6	8.9	6.2	11.9	3.7	22.4	3.2	0.5	0.04	0.11	1.0	152
Colon	303	0	-	-	-	-	-	-	6.2	6.3	5.3	10.7	29.3	69.3	65.3	81.9	111.5	181.4	175.3	268.6	54.3	8.6	0.96	1.93	17.3	153
Rectum	149	0	-	-	-	-	-	-	3.1	-	5.3	5.4	9.8	40.0	23.5	62.0	58.8	65.4	69.4	156.7	26.7	4.2	0.44	1.04	8.7	154
Liver	71	0	-	-	-	-	-	-	-	-	-	8.0	7.3	-	10.5	33.2	24.8	44.6	32.9	78.3	12.7	2.0	0.13	0.42	3.8	155
Gallbladder etc.	116	0	-	-	-	-	-	-	-	-	-	-	7.3	8.0	18.3	17.7	34.1	89.2	98.6	151.1	20.8	3.3	0.17	0.43	4.8	156
Pancreas	144	0	-	-	-	-	-	-	-	-	-	2.7	2.4	10.7	26.1	33.2	74.3	98.2	124.1	123.1	25.8	4.1	0.21	0.75	6.5	157
Nose, sinuses etc.	5	0	-	-	-	-	-	-	-	-	-	-	2.4	-	-	2.2	-	5.9	3.7	-	0.9	0.1	0.01	0.02	0.3	160
Larynx	21	0	-	-	-	-	-	-	3.1	-	-	-	12.2	2.7	10.5	6.6	12.4	8.9	-	-	3.8	0.6	0.14	0.24	1.9	161
Bronchus, lung	239	0	-	-	-	-	-	-	3.1	3.1	10.7	13.4	26.8	34.6	52.3	108.4	127.0	124.9	102.2	134.3	42.8	6.8	0.72	1.90	14.9	162
Other thoracic organs	13	0	-	-	-	-	-	2.8	3.1	-	-	-	4.9	2.7	2.6	4.4	-	5.9	7.3	5.6	2.3	0.4	0.08	0.10	1.1	163-4
Bone	7	0	-	6.7	-	7.1	-	-	-	-	-	-	-	-	-	-	-	3.1	3.0	3.7	5.6	1.3	0.2	0.07	0.08	1.5	170
Connective tissue	10	0	-	6.7	-	-	-	-	-	-	-	-	2.7	2.4	-	2.6	2.2	3.1	3.0	11.0	-	1.8	0.3	0.07	0.10	1.3	171
Mesothelioma	6	0	-	-	-	-	-	-	-	-	-	-	2.7	-	2.7	5.2	2.2	-	-	3.7	-	1.1	0.2	0.05	0.06	0.6	MES
Kaposi's sarcoma	5	0	-	-	-	-	-	-	-	-	-	-	2.4	-	-	-	-	5.9	3.7	5.6	0.9	0.1	0.01	0.01	0.2	KAP
Melanoma of skin	96	0	-	-	-	3.6	5.9	16.5	3.1	18.9	16.0	18.8	31.7	16.0	7.8	22.1	27.9	41.6	21.9	33.6	17.2	2.7	0.69	0.94	10.0	172
Other skin	681	0	-	6.7	-	3.6	-	5.5	21.6	28.3	48.1	67.0	104.9	109.2	182.9	203.6	294.2	318.3	335.9	436.4	121.9		2.89	5.38	47.3	173
Breast	744	0	-	-	-	-	-	8.3	43.2	66.0	115.0	136.7	173.2	181.2	193.4	272.1	266.4	232.0	215.4	296.5	133.2	21.1	4.59	7.28	64.3	174
Uterus unspecified	16	0	-	-	-	-	-	-	-	-	-	-	-	-	2.7	2.6	6.6	3.1	5.9	18.3	16.8	2.9	0.5	0.03	0.08	0.7	179
Cervix uteri	134	0	-	-	-	-	3.0	13.8	12.4	12.6	24.1	32.2	29.3	24.0	41.8	33.2	34.1	56.5	36.5	39.2	24.0	3.8	0.96	1.30	12.9	180
Placenta	0	0	-	-	-	-	-	-	-	-	-	-	-	-	-	-	-	-	-	-	0.0	0.0	0.00	0.00	0.0	181
Corpus uteri	175	0	-	-	-	-	-	2.8	3.1	3.1	5.3	29.5	34.2	50.6	52.3	70.8	58.8	98.2	43.8	56.0	31.3	5.0	0.90	1.55	13.3	182
Ovary etc.	156	0	-	-	5.5	3.6	-	2.8	3.1	6.3	10.7	29.5	24.4	32.0	54.9	64.2	58.8	50.6	65.7	50.4	27.9	4.4	0.86	1.48	12.9	183
Other female genital	63	0	-	-	-	-	-	-	-	-	-	2.7	9.8	8.0	13.1	24.3	18.6	26.8	47.5	61.5	11.3	1.8	0.17	0.38	3.4	184
Bladder	160	0	6.5	-	-	-	-	-	3.1	3.1	-	8.0	14.6	21.3	26.1	59.7	58.8	101.1	98.6	128.7	28.6	4.5	0.41	1.01	9.4	188
Kidney etc.	107	0	-	6.7	-	-	3.0	-	-	3.1	5.3	2.7	17.1	26.6	20.9	26.6	40.3	44.6	62.1	106.3	19.2	3.0	0.43	0.76	7.2	189
Eye	4	0	-	-	-	-	-	-	-	-	-	-	-	-	-	2.2	-	-	7.3	5.6	0.7	0.1	0.00	0.01	0.1	190
Brain, nervous system	69	0	19.5	-	11.0	-	3.0	2.8	-	3.1	10.7	10.7	12.2	13.3	13.1	33.2	18.6	14.9	32.9	16.8	12.4	2.0	0.50	0.76	8.7	191-2
Thyroid	61	0	-	-	-	3.6	3.0	-	6.2	3.1	10.7	18.8	9.8	5.3	15.7	19.9	15.5	17.8	29.2	28.0	10.9	1.7	0.38	0.56	5.6	193
Other endocrine	30	0	-	-	-	-	3.0	-	3.1	6.3	2.7	10.7	12.2	2.7	5.2	13.3	3.1	5.9	11.0	5.6	5.4	0.9	0.23	0.31	3.1	194
Hodgkin's disease	25	0	-	-	-	3.6	-	5.5	3.1	6.3	8.0	-	2.4	-	2.6	11.1	9.3	14.9	3.7	-	4.5	0.7	0.16	0.26	2.7	201
Non-Hodgkin lymphoma	141	0	-	-	-	3.6	3.0	2.8	3.1	-	5.3	16.1	14.6	18.7	39.2	66.4	40.3	83.3	62.1	72.7	25.2	4.0	0.53	1.06	9.6	200,202
Multiple myeloma	69	0	-	-	-	-	-	-	-	-	-	8.0	2.4	8.0	15.7	24.3	24.8	32.7	54.8	61.5	12.4	2.0	0.17	0.42	3.7	203
Lymphoid leukaemia	59	0	6.5	-	-	-	-	-	-	-	-	-	12.2	5.3	7.8	19.9	24.8	32.7	40.2	50.4	10.6	1.7	0.16	0.38	3.8	204
Myeloid leukaemia	46	0	-	6.7	-	3.6	-	2.8	6.2	3.1	5.3	2.7	7.3	10.7	7.8	8.9	18.6	14.9	21.9	33.6	8.2	1.3	0.28	0.42	4.4	205
Monocytic leukaemia	0	0	-	-	-	-	-	-	-	-	-	-	-	-	-	-	-	-	-	-	0.0	0.0	0.00	0.00	0.0	206
Other leukaemia	4	0	-	-	-	-	-	-	-	-	-	-	-	-	-	2.6	-	3.1	-	3.7	5.6	0.7	0.1	0.01	0.03	0.2	207
Leukaemia unspecified	9	0	-	-	-	-	-	-	3.1	-	-	-	-	2.7	-	-	-	-	14.9	3.7	5.6	1.6	0.3	0.03	0.03	0.5	208
Other and unspecified	0	0	-	-	-	-	-	-	-	-	-	-	-	-	-	-	-	-	-	-	0.0	0.0	0.00	0.00	0.0	O&U
All sites	4210	0	32.5	33.7	16.5	39.2	23.8	68.8	138.9	179.3	304.8	461.0	653.8	751.4	980.0	1416.1	1542.5	1992.8	2015.4	2685.6	753.8		18.42	33.21	303.4	ALL
All sites but 173	3529	0	32.5	27.0	16.5	35.6	23.8	63.3	117.3	151.0	256.7	394.0	548.9	642.2	797.1	1212.5	1248.2	1674.5	1679.5	2249.2	631.9	100.0	15.53	27.83	256.1	ALLb
Rate from 1 case			6.491	6.749	5.499	3.564	2.970	2.754	3.088	3.145	2.674	2.680	2.440	2.665	2.613	2.213	3.097	2.974	3.651	5.595							

Italy, Varese Province

The Lombardy Cancer Registry (Registro Tumori della Lombardia), established in 1974, is supported by the Regional Health Authority and run by the Epidemiology Unit of the Milan National Cancer Institute. The main registry's staff comprises three epidemiologists, a computer expert and four clerks.

Varese Province is one of the northernmost in Italy and is located in the Lombardy Region. It is bordered to the north by Switzerland, to the west by Lake Verbano and by the Ticino River, which forms the border with the Piedmont Region, and to the south and east by two other provinces which are also part of the Lombardy Region. The northern part of the province is mountainous, whereas the southern part is flat.

The population has increased from 581 526 in 1961 to the present size of 797 039 (density 665 inhabitants per km^2). More than 30% of the residents in the area were born outside Lombardy. Considerable migrations occurred in the past, mainly from the east and south of Italy. The migrants tended to keep the distinct dietary and other cultural habits of their native regions.

The proportion of elderly people has increased as migration has diminished: the ratio of population aged over 64 years to children aged less than 6 years was 1.2 in 1961 and 1971 but was 2.8 in the 1991 census.

The proportion of active people working in industry is roughly 60% for males and 40% for females, with a considerable decrease since the 1971 census. Less than 1% of the active population is employed in agriculture.

The area is served by 11 public general hospitals, including one university teaching hospital with all facilities for diagnosis and treatment of cancer. There are also three private clinics. The total number of hospital beds is 5800 (7.3 per 1000 inhabitants).

All public and private hospitals in the province are requested to notify every admission for cancer, whether new or previously reported, using a unique form. However, difficulties in maintaining a purely passive system of notification, as well as the improvement of automated hospital discharge systems, have led on the one hand to an active search at many hospitals, and on the other hand to incorporation of information from automated systems into the registry's information flow. Files of the National Cancer Institute in Milan are also systematically scrutinized.

The surgical pathology departments of the province are also a systematic source of information for the registry. They are accessed automatically, and all cancer diagnoses are matched with existing files. For the attribution of morphology and for checking coherence with the site, the text diagnosis is used.

The registry receives, from the 141 municipalities of the province, transcripts of all notifications of death occurring both among residents and among the present population.

The search for cases treated outside the registry's information system and a check for completeness of hospital sources are made by matching files with the Regional Hospital Discharge Diagnosis information system, that records almost all discharges in Lombardy Region.

A link with the population files used by the National Health Service is systematically made when a patient's residence is unknown or in doubt.

All malignant tumours are recorded. *In situ* lesions and a number of neoplasms of uncertain behaviour are recorded as well, but are not included in incidence figures, except for urothelial neoplasms. With the above exception, tumours included in incidence are those coded under rubrics 140–208 of the ICD-9, and those for which the ICD-O behaviour digit is 3 or more. The index date for incidence is the date of first hospital admission at which diagnosis of malignancy was made. For cases never admitted and for cases first treated as outpatients, the index date is that of diagnosis (histological diagnosis if available). For cases first notified by a death certificate, trace-back was not performed.

Two large prospective studies are in progress in the registry area, one on diet, hormones and breast cancer, and one on diet and cancer; also case–control studies have been carried out, mainly on occupational determinants of cancer. The registry coordinates a European Concerted Action on the evaluation of care (EUROCARE) by using registry-based survival data.

The differences in lifestyle of migrants have allowed descriptive studies to be performed on variations in cancer risk by place of birth.

Paolo Crosignani
Franco Berrino
Giovanna Tagliabue
Gemma Gatta
Milena Sant
Daniele Speciale
Tiziana Codazzi
Anna Maghini
Andrea Tittarelli
Clotilde Vigano'

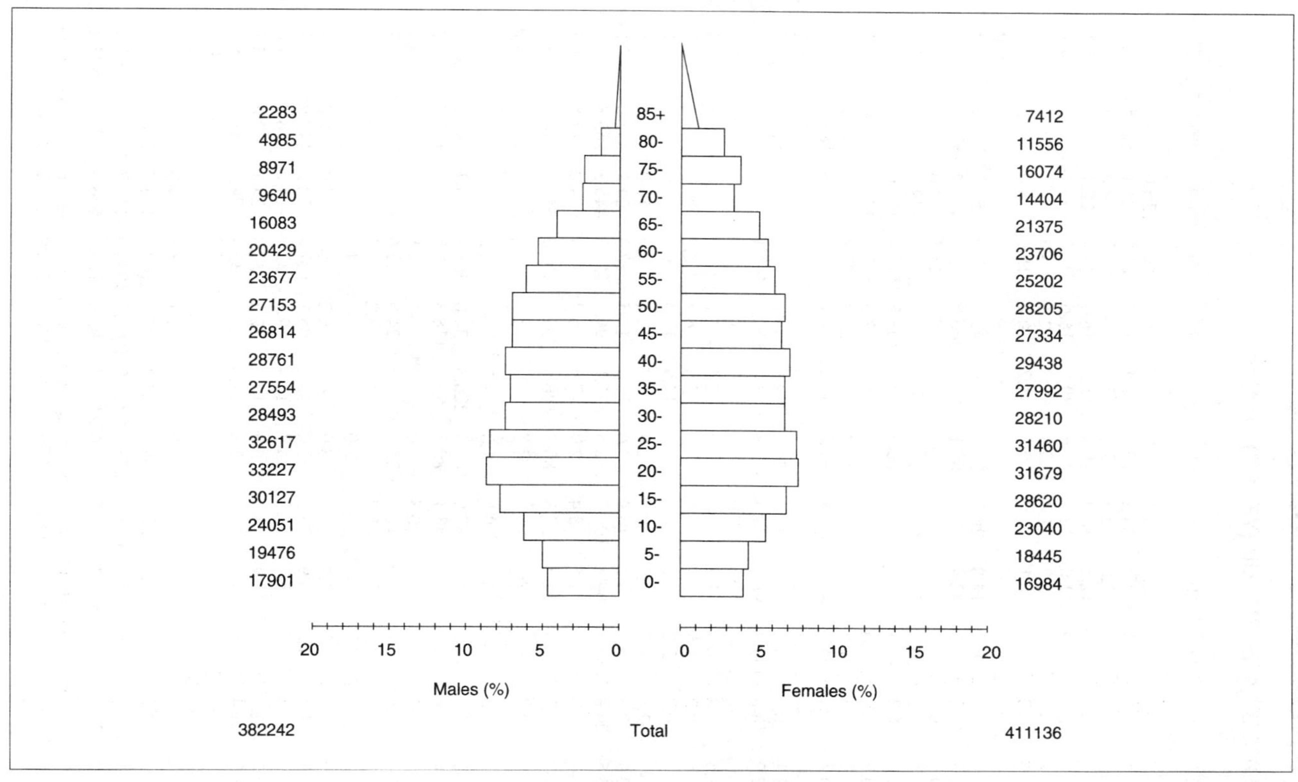

Italy, Varese Province

Source of population: average annual 1988–92
Estimate: The population was estimated at 1 July of each year using the 1981 and 1991 Censuses and making allowance for births, deaths and migration.

Screening programmes in the area

150 000 screening examinations for cervical cancer have been carried out each year since 1970 in the population over age 20.

ITALY, VARESE PROVINCE 1988-1992

ANNUAL INCIDENCE PER 100,000 BY AGE GROUP (YEARS) - MALE

SITE	ALL AGES	AGE UNK	0-	5-	10-	15-	20-	25-	30-	35-	40-	45-	50-	55-	60-	65-	70-	75-	80-	85+	CRUDE RATE	%	CR 64	CR 74	ASR (W)	ICD (9th)
Lip	36	0	-	-	-	-	-	-	-	-	-	0.7	2.2	2.5	8.8	8.7	6.2	6.7	16.0	26.3	1.9	0.4	0.07	0.15	1.3	140
Tongue	97	0	-	-	-	0.7	-	-	-	0.7	3.5	5.2	3.7	15.2	16.6	17.4	20.7	24.5	24.1	17.5	5.1	1.0	0.23	0.42	3.5	141
Salivary gland	18	0	-	-	-	-	0.6	0.7	0.7	0.7	-	1.5	2.5	2.9	3.7	-	4.5	4.0	-	0.9	0.2	0.05	0.07	0.6	142
Mouth	101	0	-	1.0	-	-	-	-	-	-	2.8	4.5	12.5	16.0	19.6	16.2	16.6	13.4	28.1	-	5.3	1.0	0.28	0.45	3.7	143-5
Oropharynx	99	0	-	-	-	-	-	-	-	-	2.8	3.0	11.0	13.5	17.6	29.8	16.6	22.3	-	-	5.2	1.0	0.24	0.47	3.6	146
Nasopharynx	26	0	-	-	-	-	0.6	1.2	0.7	0.7	0.7	2.2	2.2	1.7	5.9	3.7	2.1	4.5	-	-	1.4	0.3	0.08	0.11	1.0	147
Hypopharynx	65	0	-	-	-	-	-	-	-	-	0.7	3.7	8.1	11.0	9.8	11.2	10.4	15.6	8.0	17.5	3.4	0.6	0.17	0.27	2.3	148
Pharynx unspecified	0	0	-	-	-	-	-	-	-	-	-	-	-	-	-	-	-	-	-	-	0.0	0.0	0.00	0.00	0.0	149
Oesophagus	192	0	-	-	-	-	-	0.7	-	2.1	6.0	14.0	26.2	32.3	46.0	43.6	37.9	56.2	70.1		10.0	1.9	0.41	0.85	6.8	150
Stomach	786	0	-	-	-	-	-	0.6	0.7	6.5	13.2	17.2	32.4	45.6	89.1	150.5	246.9	312.1	413.2	534.4	41.1	7.8	1.03	3.01	26.6	151
Small intestine	21	0	-	-	-	-	-	-	-	-	0.7	0.7	-	-	3.4	-	6.2	8.3	11.1	4.0	-	1.1	0.2	0.02	0.10	0.7	152
Colon	802	0	-	-	-	0.7	-	-	2.1	5.1	11.1	26.9	39.8	62.5	97.9	170.4	186.7	307.6	349.0	516.9	42.0	8.0	1.23	3.02	27.4	153
Rectum	464	0	-	-	-	-	-	0.7	2.2	6.3	13.4	21.4	49.8	66.6	90.8	153.5	140.4	196.6	157.7		24.3	4.6	0.80	2.02	16.0	154
Liver	377	0	-	-	-	-	-	0.6	-	0.7	2.1	9.0	13.3	28.7	61.7	98.2	118.3	147.1	120.3	113.9	19.7	3.8	0.58	1.66	13.0	155
Gallbladder etc.	90	0	-	-	-	-	-	-	-	0.7	-	1.5	2.2	8.4	10.8	16.2	27.0	37.9	48.1	70.1	4.7	0.9	0.12	0.33	3.0	156
Pancreas	250	0	-	-	-	-	-	-	-	0.7	0.7	6.7	16.2	25.3	35.2	53.5	74.7	60.2	96.3	184.0	13.1	2.5	0.42	1.07	8.8	157
Nose, sinuses etc.	23	0	1.1	-	-	-	-	0.6	-	-	-	1.5	2.2	2.5	4.9	5.0	-	4.5	4.0	8.8	1.2	0.2	0.06	0.09	0.9	160
Larynx	353	0	-	-	-	-	-	-	-	2.2	0.7	9.0	28.0	45.6	74.4	79.6	85.1	78.0	64.2	113.9	18.5	3.5	0.80	1.62	12.7	161
Bronchus, lung	2202	0	-	-	-	0.7	1.2	0.6	3.5	2.9	18.8	55.9	98.7	254.3	427.8	543.4	620.3	604.1	605.7	499.3	115.2	22.0	4.32	10.14	77.6	162
Other thoracic organs	5	0	-	-	-	0.7	0.6	-	-	-	0.7	-	0.8	-	-	-	2.1	-	-	-	0.3	0.0	0.01	0.02	0.2	163-4
Bone	20	0	1.1	1.0	0.8	2.0	-	0.6	-	1.5	-	0.7	1.5	-	1.0	2.5	2.1	-	12.0	8.8	1.0	0.2	0.05	0.07	1.0	170
Connective tissue	40	0	2.2	1.0	-	0.7	0.6	0.6	0.7	1.5	0.7	1.5	3.7	3.4	7.8	2.5	6.2	2.2	20.1	-	2.1	0.4	0.12	0.17	1.7	171
Mesothelioma	40	0	-	-	-	-	-	-	-	-	0.7	2.2	2.2	1.7	8.8	14.9	10.4	6.7	4.0	8.8	2.1	0.4	0.08	0.20	1.5	MES
Kaposi's sarcoma	40	0	-	-	-	-	0.6	0.6	4.2	-	2.1	1.5	2.9	0.8	2.9	6.2	10.4	8.9	16.0	8.8	2.1	0.4	0.08	0.16	1.5	KAP
Melanoma of skin	135	0	-	-	-	-	0.6	2.5	6.3	2.9	9.7	8.2	9.6	16.9	17.6	17.4	14.5	22.3	24.1	35.0	7.1	1.3	0.37	0.53	5.1	172
Other skin	1293	0	1.1	-	2.5	2.7	1.8	3.1	5.6	6.5	20.9	37.3	64.1	104.7	162.5	271.1	396.3	461.5	445.3	665.8	67.7		2.06	5.40	45.3	173
Breast	28	0	-	-	-	-	-	-	0.7	-	-	-	1.5	3.4	2.9	7.5	6.2	13.4	4.0	17.5	1.5	0.3	0.04	0.11	1.0	175
Prostate	884	0	-	-	-	-	-	-	-	-	-	1.5	12.5	33.8	80.3	186.5	309.1	463.7	649.8	648.3	46.3	8.8	0.64	3.12	28.2	185
Testis	84	0	-	1.0	-	3.3	4.2	10.4	7.7	13.1	4.9	5.2	0.7	3.4	3.9	-	2.1	-	-	8.8	4.4	0.8	0.29	0.30	3.8	186
Penis	16	0	-	-	-	-	-	0.6	-	-	-	-	1.5	-	3.9	1.2	4.1	2.2	8.0	26.3	0.8	0.2	0.03	0.06	0.6	187.1-.4
Other male genital	5	0	-	-	-	-	-	-	-	-	-	0.7	0.8	1.0	1.2	-	2.2	-	-	-	0.3	0.0	0.01	0.02	0.2	187.5-.9
Bladder	1013	0	-	-	-	-	0.6	1.2	3.5	6.5	11.1	14.2	36.8	87.0	161.5	226.3	334.0	361.1	373.1	394.2	53.0	10.1	1.61	4.41	35.0	188
Kidney etc.	424	0	1.1	1.0	-	-	-	-	2.1	3.6	5.6	12.7	21.4	43.1	80.3	93.3	118.3	115.9	120.3	113.9	22.2	4.2	0.85	1.91	15.2	189
Eye	10	0	2.2	1.0	-	-	-	-	0.7	-	-	-	-	0.8	2.0	-	-	4.5	4.0	-	0.5	0.1	0.03	0.03	0.6	190
Brain, nervous system	150	0	2.2	3.1	3.3	1.3	3.0	3.1	3.5	4.4	4.9	9.7	9.6	16.9	25.5	17.4	24.9	15.6	24.1	-	7.8	1.5	0.45	0.66	6.3	191-2
Thyroid	46	0	-	-	0.8	-	1.2	-	4.2	2.2	2.8	3.7	3.7	5.9	3.9	1.2	6.2	6.7	8.0	-	2.4	0.5	0.14	0.18	1.8	193
Other endocrine	8	0	1.1	-	-	-	-	0.6	-	0.7	-	0.7	-	-	2.0	-	-	4.5	-	-	0.4	0.1	0.03	0.03	0.4	194
Hodgkin's disease	77	0	-	2.1	0.8	3.3	6.0	7.4	7.7	2.9	3.5	3.0	2.2	3.4	5.9	6.2	6.2	-	4.0	8.8	4.0	0.8	0.24	0.30	3.5	201
Non-Hodgkin lymphoma	365	0	4.5	1.0	1.7	0.7	2.4	9.2	9.1	8.7	11.1	14.2	19.9	24.5	39.2	72.1	85.1	107.0	72.2	148.9	19.1	3.6	0.73	1.52	13.9	200,202
Multiple myeloma	92	0	-	-	-	-	-	-	-	-	1.4	2.2	3.7	9.3	14.7	12.4	39.4	22.3	64.2	8.8	4.8	0.9	0.16	0.42	3.1	203
Lymphoid leukaemia	111	0	12.3	4.1	1.7	3.3	-	1.2	-	0.7	2.1	3.7	4.4	8.4	6.9	18.7	22.8	37.9	24.1	52.6	5.8	1.1	0.24	0.45	5.4	204
Myeloid leukaemia	103	0	2.2	1.0	0.8	1.3	0.6	1.8	2.1	1.5	1.4	4.5	4.4	11.8	7.8	17.4	24.9	33.4	24.1	43.8	5.4	1.0	0.21	0.42	4.0	205
Monocytic leukaemia	3	0	1.1	-	-	0.7	-	-	-	-	-	-	-	-	-	-	-	2.2	-	-	0.2	0.0	0.01	0.01	0.2	206
Other leukaemia	0	0	-	-	-	-	-	-	-	-	-	-	-	-	-	-	-	-	-	-	0.0	0.0	0.00	0.00	0.0	207
Leukaemia unspecified	11	0	-	-	-	-	-	-	-	-	-	0.7	-	-	1.0	3.7	2.1	8.9	4.0	-	0.6	0.1	0.01	0.04	0.3	208
Other and unspecified	306	0	-	-	-	-	-	-	-	-	4.2	3.0	8.8	22.8	48.0	62.2	97.5	100.3	168.5	210.2	16.0	3.1	0.43	1.23	10.4	O&U
All sites	11311	0	32.4	17.5	12.5	21.9	24.1	47.2	67.4	80.6	153.7	297.6	525.2	1018.7	1673.1	2392.5	3161.8	3636.0	4111.7	4739.4	591.8		19.86	47.63	399.9	ALL
All sites but 173	10018	0	31.3	17.5	10.0	19.3	22.3	44.1	61.8	74.0	132.8	260.3	461.1	914.0	1510.6	2121.4	2765.5	3174.5	3666.4	4073.6	524.2	100.0	17.79	42.23	354.6	ALLb

Rate from 1 case   1.117   1.027   0.832   0.664   0.602   0.613   0.702   0.726   0.695   0.746   0.737   0.845   0.979   1.244   2.075   2.229   4.011   8.760

ITALY, VARESE PROVINCE 1988-1992

ANNUAL INCIDENCE PER 100,000 BY AGE GROUP (YEARS) - FEMALE

SITE	ALL AGES	AGE UNK	0-	5-	10-	15-	20-	25-	30-	35-	40-	45-	50-	55-	60-	65-	70-	75-	80-	85+	CRUDE RATE	%	CR 64	CR 74	ASR (W)	ICD (9th)
Lip	0	0	-	-	-	-	-	-	-	-	-	-	-	-	-	-	-	-	-	-	0.0	0.0	0.00	0.00	0.0	140
Tongue	17	0	-	-	-	-	-	-	-	-	-	-	0.7	1.6	0.8	1.9	1.4	3.7	5.2	10.8	0.8	0.2	0.02	0.03	0.3	141
Salivary gland	19	0	-	-	-	-	-	-	-	-	-	0.7	-	1.6	2.5	1.9	1.4	3.7	8.7	5.4	0.9	0.2	0.02	0.04	0.4	142
Mouth	23	0	-	-	-	-	-	-	-	-	0.7	2.9	-	3.2	1.7	1.9	2.8	1.2	8.7	5.4	1.1	0.3	0.04	0.07	0.6	143-5
Oropharynx	12	0	-	-	-	-	-	-	-	0.7	-	1.5	-	0.8	-	0.9	2.8	1.2	6.9	-	0.6	0.1	0.01	0.03	0.3	146
Nasopharynx	12	0	-	-	-	-	0.6	-	-	-	0.7	0.7	0.7	1.6	2.5	0.9	-	2.5	-	-	0.6	0.1	0.03	0.04	0.4	147
Hypopharynx	9	0	-	-	-	-	-	-	-	0.7	0.7	-	0.7	-	1.7	1.9	-	1.2	1.7	-	0.4	0.1	0.02	0.03	0.3	148
Pharynx unspecified	2	0	-	-	-	-	-	-	-	-	-	-	-	-	0.8	-	-	-	-	2.7	0.1	0.0	0.00	0.00	0.0	149
Oesophagus	40	0	-	-	-	-	-	-	-	-	-	0.7	0.7	1.6	1.7	2.8	4.2	11.2	20.8	18.9	1.9	0.5	0.02	0.06	0.7	150
Stomach	636	0	-	-	-	-	-	1.3	2.1	5.7	7.5	14.6	14.9	17.5	34.6	54.3	101.4	171.7	211.1	315.7	30.9	7.4	0.49	1.27	12.7	151
Small intestine	14	0	-	-	-	-	-	-	-	-	-	-	1.4	2.4	-	0.9	2.8	5.0	1.7	2.7	0.7	0.2	0.02	0.04	0.3	152
Colon	825	0	-	-	-	-	0.6	1.9	2.1	5.0	16.3	17.6	33.3	56.3	61.6	97.3	119.4	176.7	235.4	280.6	40.1	9.6	0.97	2.06	18.7	153
Rectum	362	0	-	-	-	-	-	0.6	-	2.1	9.5	9.5	14.9	17.5	27.0	43.0	54.1	83.4	93.5	134.9	17.6	4.2	0.41	0.89	8.2	154
Liver	166	0	-	-	0.9	-	-	-	-	1.4	-	1.5	2.8	4.8	10.1	18.7	34.7	51.0	53.7	59.4	8.1	1.9	0.11	0.37	3.3	155
Gallbladder etc.	179	0	-	-	-	-	-	-	0.7	-	1.4	2.2	5.0	7.9	19.4	17.8	38.9	39.8	50.2	67.5	8.7	2.1	0.18	0.47	3.9	156
Pancreas	269	0	-	-	-	-	0.6	-	0.7	1.4	2.7	4.4	9.2	9.5	16.0	42.1	43.0	54.7	93.5	99.8	13.1	3.1	0.22	0.65	5.7	157
Nose, sinuses etc.	13	0	-	-	-	-	0.6	-	-	0.7	-	-	2.1	0.8	-	0.9	1.4	2.5	-	8.1	0.6	0.2	0.02	0.03	0.4	160
Larynx	23	0	-	-	-	-	-	-	-	1.4	-	-	1.4	3.2	4.2	0.9	2.8	2.5	3.5	8.1	1.1	0.3	0.05	0.07	0.6	161
Bronchus, lung	350	0	-	-	-	-	-	0.6	0.7	4.3	6.1	9.5	12.1	26.2	39.7	52.4	41.7	69.7	95.2	70.2	17.0	4.1	0.50	0.97	8.5	162
Other thoracic organs	10	0	-	-	-	-	0.6	-	-	0.7	0.7	0.7	-	0.8	0.8	-	-	1.2	3.5	2.7	0.5	0.1	0.02	0.02	0.3	163-4
Bone	19	0	-	-	-	1.4	-	0.6	-	-	0.7	0.7	1.4	-	3.4	0.9	1.4	3.7	1.7	5.4	0.9	0.2	0.04	0.05	0.6	170
Connective tissue	46	0	2.4	-	-	1.4	0.6	-	1.4	1.4	0.7	2.2	2.8	1.6	5.1	1.9	12.5	3.7	5.2	10.8	2.2	0.5	0.10	0.17	1.6	171
Mesothelioma	17	0	-	-	-	-	-	-	-	0.7	0.7	0.7	0.7	-	1.7	1.9	-	3.7	10.4	-	0.8	0.2	0.02	0.03	0.4	MES
Kaposi's sarcoma	10	0	-	-	-	-	-	-	0.7	-	-	-	-	-	-	1.9	-	1.2	6.9	5.4	0.5	0.1	0.00	0.01	0.2	KAP
Melanoma of skin	161	0	-	-	-	-	1.9	3.2	8.5	5.0	5.4	15.4	5.0	11.1	18.6	15.9	11.1	21.2	17.3	27.0	7.8	1.9	0.37	0.51	5.0	172
Other skin	1139	0	-	-	-	-	1.9	1.9	6.4	10.0	23.1	24.1	39.7	50.0	95.3	114.2	162.4	251.3	327.1	488.4	55.4		1.26	2.65	25.2	173
Breast	2497	0	-	-	-	-	1.3	7.6	21.3	57.9	123.0	170.5	221.9	211.1	237.1	268.5	344.3	298.6	325.4	364.3	121.5	28.9	5.26	8.32	73.5	174
Uterus unspecified	16	0	-	-	-	-	-	-	-	-	-	-	-	0.8	-	-	1.4	2.5	8.7	18.9	0.8	0.2	0.00	0.01	0.2	179
Cervix uteri	200	0	-	-	-	-	-	1.9	7.1	12.1	12.9	13.2	21.3	16.7	11.8	16.8	23.6	22.4	13.8	18.9	9.7	2.3	0.48	0.69	6.4	180
Placenta	1	0	-	-	-	-	-	-	-	0.7	-	-	-	-	-	-	-	-	-	-	0.0	0.0	0.00	0.00	0.0	181
Corpus uteri	460	0	-	-	-	-	1.3	-	0.7	4.3	7.5	19.0	36.2	34.9	68.3	68.3	70.8	65.9	84.8	32.4	22.4	5.3	0.86	1.56	12.6	182
Ovary etc.	354	0	-	-	0.9	2.1	1.9	2.5	3.5	5.7	8.8	22.7	29.1	30.9	34.6	45.8	34.7	57.2	53.7	37.8	17.2	4.1	0.71	1.12	10.2	183
Other female genital	79	0	-	-	-	-	-	-	-	0.7	1.4	0.7	2.8	0.8	5.9	5.6	11.1	19.9	36.3	32.4	3.8	0.9	0.06	0.15	1.5	184
Bladder	220	0	-	-	-	0.7	0.6	-	0.7	0.7	2.7	5.1	8.5	15.9	12.7	34.6	38.9	34.8	64.0	75.6	10.7	2.5	0.24	0.61	5.1	188
Kidney etc.	213	0	1.2	-	-	-	0.6	1.3	0.7	2.1	2.7	5.1	10.6	18.3	18.6	30.9	29.2	54.7	34.6	43.2	10.4	2.5	0.31	0.61	5.4	189
Eye	17	0	-	-	-	-	-	-	0.7	-	0.7	-	2.1	1.6	1.7	0.9	1.4	5.0	1.7	2.7	0.8	0.2	0.03	0.05	0.4	190
Brain, nervous system	135	0	2.4	2.2	1.7	1.4	1.3	2.5	1.4	0.7	5.4	8.8	5.7	12.7	12.7	21.5	8.3	22.4	12.1	13.5	6.6	1.6	0.29	0.44	4.5	191-2
Thyroid	172	0	-	-	-	1.4	1.9	5.1	16.3	10.0	4.8	14.6	9.2	8.7	16.9	14.0	11.1	17.4	8.7	24.3	8.4	2.0	0.44	0.57	5.9	193
Other endocrine	8	0	1.2	1.1	-	-	-	-	-	-	0.7	1.4	0.7	-	0.8	0.8	-	-	-	-	0.4	0.1	0.03	0.03	0.5	194
Hodgkin's disease	64	0	-	-	0.9	9.8	3.8	9.5	5.0	2.1	0.7	0.7	1.4	0.8	2.5	0.9	2.8	3.7	1.7	8.1	3.1	0.7	0.19	0.20	2.9	201
Non-Hodgkin lymphoma	382	0	2.4	-	0.9	0.7	1.3	3.2	4.3	6.4	10.2	15.4	19.9	21.4	36.3	41.2	48.6	77.1	81.3	91.7	18.6	4.4	0.61	1.06	10.1	200,202
Multiple myeloma	118	0	-	-	-	-	-	-	-	-	1.4	6.6	3.5	1.6	9.3	14.0	18.0	32.3	38.1	35.1	5.7	1.4	0.11	0.27	2.6	203
Lymphoid leukaemia	88	0	8.2	1.1	0.9	2.1	-	-	-	1.4	-	-	2.8	2.4	10.1	7.5	13.9	14.9	27.7	24.3	4.3	1.0	0.15	0.25	3.0	204
Myeloid leukaemia	105	0	-	1.1	0.9	1.4	0.6	3.8	2.8	2.9	1.4	4.4	7.1	8.7	5.9	11.2	9.7	18.7	13.8	21.6	5.1	1.2	0.20	0.31	3.2	205
Monocytic leukaemia	4	0	-	-	-	-	-	-	0.7	-	-	-	-	-	-	-	1.9	1.4	-	-	0.2	0.0	0.00	0.02	0.1	206
Other leukaemia	1	0	-	-	-	-	-	-	-	-	-	0.7	-	-	-	-	-	-	-	-	0.0	0.0	0.00	0.00	0.0	207
Leukaemia unspecified	9	0	-	-	-	-	-	-	-	-	-	-	-	-	0.8	0.9	-	3.7	3.5	5.4	0.4	0.1	0.00	0.01	0.1	208
Other and unspecified	252	0	-	-	-	-	-	-	1.4	0.7	0.7	0.7	7.8	7.1	15.2	17.8	31.9	57.2	88.3	188.9	12.3	2.9	0.17	0.42	4.6	O&U
All sites	9768	0	17.7	5.4	6.9	22.4	22.1	47.7	90.0	150.8	262.2	398.8	539.6	615.0	850.4	1079.8	1341.2	1776.7	2159.9	2668.6	475.2		15.15	27.25	251.7	ALL
All sites but 173	8629	0	17.7	5.4	6.9	22.4	20.2	45.8	83.7	140.8	239.1	374.6	499.9	565.0	755.1	965.6	1178.8	1525.4	1832.8	2180.2	419.8	100.0	13.88	24.60	226.5	ALLb

| Rate from 1 case | | | 1.178 | 1.084 | 0.868 | 0.699 | 0.631 | 0.636 | 0.709 | 0.714 | 0.679 | 0.732 | 0.709 | 0.794 | 0.844 | 0.936 | 1.388 | 1.244 | 1.731 | 2.698 |

Italy, Venetian Region

The Venetian Region (population 4 380 797 in 1991, 7.7% of the national population) is the largest in the north-east of Italy. The territory (18 364 km^2) of the region is subdivided into 36 Local Health Units (LHUs) which are in charge of all public health-related matters including the management of the 73 hospitals of the region.

In 1990 the government of the Venetian Region charged a Working Group of experts in the field of cancer epidemiology from the two Regional Oncological Centres of Padua and Verona with the task of exploring the feasibility of a cancer registration system at the regional level. The aim was to use the routinely computerized and coded diagnoses of cancer from pathology departments and hospitals, and from death certificates, after appropriate processing and quality control, to estimate cancer incidence.

Computerized files of hospital admissions and discharges since the mid-1980s exist, being stored and managed by a local information system in each LHU. These also include other individual information concerning all residents assisted by the national health insurance (comprising almost the whole population). Each individual is assigned a unique regional identification number.

Hospital diagnoses are coded according to the ICD revision operating at the time of the discharge. Histological diagnoses are computerized in several, but not all, LHUs. Diagnoses are mostly coded according to SNOMED or, in a few situations, to ICD-O-1.

The feasibility study started in the second half of 1990 and covered the period 1987–94 in terms of data collection. This period was chosen in relation to the availability of computerized data and the possibility of cross-linkage with the computerized files for a variable number of years (2 to 8) available before 1987. This allowed, at least in part, the exclusion of prevalent cases.

LHUs were selected according to two criteria: availability of computerized files and populations at higher risk of cancer according to cancer mortality.

The computerized population file of residents in the LHU was first linked to records of hospital discharges, pathology reports and death certificates of both the index LHU and of the other LHUs included in the network, thus allowing a search for cases diagnosed and/or treated outside the area of residence. Records from radiotherapy departments were also available. Since all the main hospital centres of the region are included in the network, the proportion of cases missed by the registry should be small and limited to patients with diagnosis and treatment completed outside the region.

All the histological and cytological diagnoses coded in SNOMED are transcoded through an *ad hoc* program into ICD codes. After various logical checks and quality controls, the data are processed by a program which assigns a three-digit cancer diagnosis (ICD-9) according to an algorithm which accepts:

(*a*) cancer cases with full concordance between two or more sources;

(*b*) histologically confirmed cases in the presence of other compatible hospital diagnosis (e.g., metastases or ill-defined);

(*c*) histologically confirmed skin cancer (ICD 173) unless in combination with skin melanoma (172);

(*d*) histologically confirmed benign, *in situ*, and uncertain behaviour tumours.

Diagnoses based on only one source are systematically rejected and checked unless based on pathology, as are multiple primary tumours. Manual checking is performed also for all discordant or incompatible diagnoses according to the criteria reported above.

Cases with a new diagnosis of cancer between 1 January 1987 and 31 December 1994 have been included in the incidence estimates. The earliest year for which computerized files were available was 1979 for hospital discharges and 1984 for pathology reports. Death certificates were available for residents who died during the study period.

The incident rates of cancer in the LHUs eventually included in the project concern a total population, at the 1991 census, of 1 449 513 (33.1% of the total regional population).

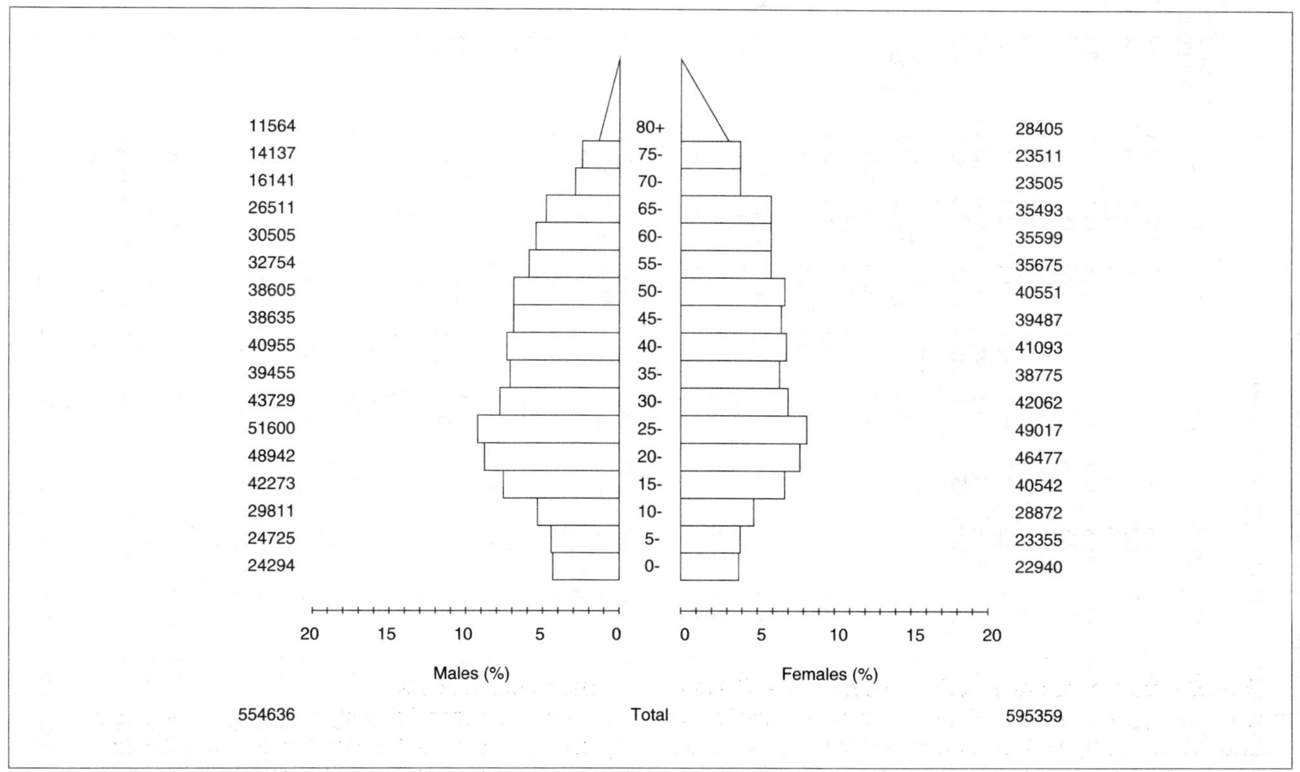

Italy, Venetian Region
Source of population: 1991
Census: 1991 Census. Department of Statistics of the
Venetian Region.

ITALY, VENETIAN REGION 1988-1992

ANNUAL INCIDENCE PER 100,000 BY AGE GROUP (YEARS) - MALE

SITE	ALL AGES	AGE UNK	0-	5-	10-	15-	20-	25-	30-	35-	40-	45-	50-	55-	60-	65-	70-	75-	80+	CRUDE RATE	%	CR 64	CR 74	ASR (W)	ICD (9th)
Lip	66	0	-	-	-	-	-	-	-	-	0.5	-	1.6	1.8	10.5	7.5	11.2	22.6	13.8	2.4	0.4	0.07	0.17	1.4	140
Tongue	150	0	-	-	-	-	-	-	0.5	3.5	2.4	6.2	6.2	19.5	21.0	18.1	18.6	8.5	6.9	5.4	1.0	0.30	0.48	3.8	141
Salivary gland	33	0	-	-	-	-	0.4	-	-	-	-	1.0	1.0	3.7	2.6	7.5	3.7	4.2	3.5	1.2	0.2	0.04	0.10	0.8	142
Mouth	196	0	-	-	-	-	-	-	2.0	2.9	5.2	15.5	21.4	24.9	30.9	18.6	14.1	12.1	7.1	1.3	0.36	0.61	4.8	143-5
Oropharynx	120	0	-	-	-	-	-	-	1.5	3.4	5.7	7.8	9.8	19.7	9.1	9.9	18.4	8.6	4.3	0.8	0.24	0.33	2.9	146
Nasopharynx	28	0	-	-	0.7	-	-	-	0.5	0.5	0.5	2.1	2.1	3.7	2.0	4.5	1.2	-	-	1.0	0.2	0.06	0.09	0.8	147
Hypopharynx	81	0	-	-	-	-	-	-	-	0.5	1.0	3.6	6.2	8.5	11.1	12.1	3.7	9.9	3.5	2.9	0.5	0.16	0.23	2.0	148
Pharynx unspecified	82	0	-	-	-	-	0.4	-	-	1.5	3.6	5.2	9.2	13.8	12.1	7.4	1.4	3.5	3.0	0.5	0.17	0.27	2.1	149
Oesophagus	418	0	-	-	-	-	-	-	0.5	4.4	8.8	30.6	40.3	49.2	44.5	55.8	75.0	58.8	15.1	2.7	0.67	1.17	9.7	150
Stomach	912	0	-	-	-	-	0.4	0.4	2.7	4.6	10.7	15.0	29.0	53.7	72.1	110.9	143.7	230.6	283.6	32.9	5.9	0.94	2.22	19.9	151
Small intestine	31	0	-	-	-	-	-	-	-	-	-	0.5	1.6	3.1	2.6	3.0	2.5	11.3	6.9	1.1	0.2	0.04	0.07	0.7	152
Colon	1013	0	-	-	-	-	0.8	0.8	2.3	8.1	10.7	8.3	32.6	58.0	82.6	145.6	193.3	246.2	247.3	36.5	6.6	1.02	2.72	22.3	153
Rectum	581	0	-	-	-	-	-	1.2	2.7	2.5	6.8	9.3	23.3	31.8	59.0	74.7	107.8	118.8	134.9	21.0	3.8	0.68	1.60	13.1	154
Liver	785	0	-	-	0.7	0.5	0.4	-	0.9	1.5	2.0	10.4	24.9	56.2	83.3	128.2	152.4	176.8	117.6	28.3	5.1	0.90	2.31	17.7	155
Gallbladder etc.	115	0	-	-	-	-	-	-	-	-	0.5	0.5	1.6	7.9	11.1	20.4	23.5	24.1	29.4	4.1	0.7	0.11	0.33	2.5	156
Pancreas	423	0	-	-	-	-	-	0.4	0.9	1.5	4.4	8.8	15.0	30.5	37.4	51.3	83.0	100.4	84.7	15.3	2.7	0.49	1.17	9.5	157
Nose, sinuses etc.	39	0	0.8	-	-	0.5	-	-	-	-	1.0	1.0	1.6	4.9	3.3	0.8	9.9	4.2	8.6	1.4	0.3	0.07	0.12	1.0	160
Larynx	688	0	-	-	-	-	-	-	0.5	2.5	6.8	17.6	40.4	69.6	100.3	99.6	76.8	83.5	62.3	24.8	4.5	1.19	2.07	16.4	161
Bronchus, lung	3568	0	-	-	-	-	-	-	0.4	3.7	7.6	18.6	51.8	120.2	276.6	438.0	553.7	712.5	626.7	520.6	128.7	23.1	4.58	10.91	81.9	162
Other thoracic organs	56	0	-	-	-	-	1.2	0.4	0.5	-	0.5	1.6	2.1	2.4	6.6	9.1	8.7	5.7	10.4	2.0	0.4	0.08	0.16	1.3	163-4
Bone	22	0	-	-	2.0	2.8	0.4	0.4	0.5	0.5	-	0.5	1.0	1.2	0.7	1.5	1.2	-	-	0.8	0.1	0.05	0.06	0.8	170
Connective tissue	119	0	1.6	0.8	2.0	0.9	1.2	0.4	2.7	2.5	2.9	6.2	2.6	8.5	10.5	7.5	11.2	17.0	20.8	4.3	0.8	0.22	0.31	3.3	171
Mesothelioma	50	0	-	-	-	-	-	-	-	0.5	0.5	2.1	3.1	3.7	5.9	6.8	2.5	11.3	6.9	1.8	0.3	0.08	0.13	1.2	MES
Kaposi's sarcoma	35	0	-	-	-	-	-	0.8	3.2	1.0	0.5	2.6	0.5	0.6	2.6	2.3	2.5	5.7	5.2	1.3	0.2	0.06	0.08	0.9	KAP
Melanoma of skin	244	0	-	-	0.9	1.2	2.7	4.6	6.1	9.8	13.5	10.4	15.9	18.4	27.2	19.8	36.8	20.8	8.8	1.6	0.42	0.65	6.1	172
Other skin	2272	0	-	-	0.9	4.5	2.7	7.3	15.2	27.3	49.2	94.8	143.5	182.9	304.0	373.0	507.9	510.2	81.9			2.64	6.03	51.2	173
Breast	36	0	-	-	-	-	-	0.5	-	0.5	1.6	1.6	3.1	5.2	4.5	5.0	4.2	3.5	1.3	0.2	0.06	0.11	0.9	175
Prostate	1325	0	-	-	-	-	-	-	0.5	-	4.7	9.8	36.6	85.9	168.2	296.1	434.3	581.1	47.8	8.6	0.69	3.01	26.8	185
Testis	109	0	0.8	-	-	1.9	4.5	7.8	9.1	9.1	6.3	3.1	1.6	2.4	3.3	2.3	-	1.4	-	3.9	0.7	0.25	0.26	3.3	186
Penis	24	0	-	-	-	-	-	-	-	-	0.5	-	0.5	1.8	2.6	3.0	8.7	-	6.9	0.9	0.2	0.03	0.09	0.6	187.1-.4
Other male genital	5	0	-	-	-	-	-	-	-	-	0.5	-	0.5	-	0.7	0.8	1.2	-	-	0.2	0.0	0.01	0.02	0.1	187.5-.9
Bladder	1356	0	-	-	-	0.5	-	1.6	1.4	4.6	7.8	17.6	42.0	75.1	138.3	202.2	262.7	312.7	299.2	48.9	8.8	1.44	3.77	30.1	188
Kidney etc.	670	0	0.8	-	0.7	-	0.8	1.6	3.2	4.1	10.7	17.1	31.6	44.6	76.1	89.8	90.5	120.3	112.4	24.2	4.3	0.96	1.86	15.7	189
Eye	18	0	-	-	-	-	-	-	-	-	1.0	0.5	0.5	-	-	3.0	5.0	7.1	1.7	0.6	0.1	0.01	0.05	0.4	190
Brain, nervous system	265	0	4.1	4.0	2.0	2.8	1.6	3.1	4.6	6.6	10.3	9.8	17.1	25.0	19.0	13.6	33.5	19.8	15.6	9.6	1.7	0.55	0.79	7.6	191-2
Thyroid	75	0	-	-	-	1.4	0.8	1.2	1.4	4.6	3.4	1.0	3.6	5.5	5.9	4.5	7.4	5.7	8.6	2.7	0.5	0.14	0.20	2.0	193
Other endocrine	25	0	1.6	-	-	-	0.8	-	-	0.5	0.5	-	0.5	2.4	2.6	1.5	1.2	4.2	6.9	0.9	0.2	0.05	0.06	0.7	194
Hodgkin's disease	129	0	0.8	1.6	2.0	6.2	5.3	4.7	5.5	3.0	5.4	7.8	5.2	4.3	3.3	4.5	5.0	9.9	3.5	4.7	0.8	0.27	0.32	4.0	201
Non-Hodgkin lymphoma	545	0	-	2.4	2.0	3.8	1.2	3.9	5.9	13.2	15.1	16.6	22.8	28.1	47.2	55.1	73.1	87.7	103.8	19.7	3.5	0.81	1.45	13.4	200,202
Multiple myeloma	143	0	-	-	-	-	-	-	-	1.5	1.0	3.1	6.2	9.8	13.8	13.6	27.3	35.4	31.1	5.2	0.9	0.18	0.38	3.2	203
Lymphoid leukaemia	151	0	7.4	3.2	0.7	2.8	2.5	1.6	-	0.5	1.5	2.6	2.6	6.1	13.1	8.3	22.3	34.0	41.5	5.4	1.0	0.22	0.38	4.5	204
Myeloid leukaemia	146	0	0.8	-	0.7	-	0.4	0.8	2.7	1.0	2.4	3.6	4.1	6.7	9.8	15.1	23.5	28.3	48.4	5.3	0.9	0.17	0.36	3.4	205
Monocytic leukaemia	8	0	-	-	-	-	-	-	0.5	-	-	-	1.0	-	0.7	1.5	1.2	1.4	-	0.3	0.1	0.01	0.02	0.2	206
Other leukaemia	5	0	-	-	-	-	-	-	-	-	-	-	0.5	-	-	1.5	-	1.4	1.7	0.2	0.0	0.00	0.01	0.1	207
Leukaemia unspecified	45	0	-	-	-	1.4	-	-	-	-	0.5	1.0	1.0	1.8	3.3	3.8	6.2	18.4	10.4	1.6	0.3	0.05	0.10	1.0	208
Other and unspecified	514	0	-	-	-	1.4	0.4	0.4	0.5	0.5	4.4	5.2	9.3	26.3	45.9	72.4	90.5	133.0	162.6	18.5	3.3	0.47	1.29	11.1	O&U
All sites	17721	0	18.9	12.1	13.4	28.9	29.4	36.8	69.1	112.0	191.4	330.3	642.9	1165.7	1748.6	2362.0	3014.7	3620.3	3619.9	639.0		22.00	48.88	407.0	ALL
All sites but 173	15449	0	18.9	12.1	13.4	27.9	24.9	34.1	61.7	96.8	164.1	281.1	548.1	1022.2	1565.6	2058.0	2641.7	3112.4	3109.7	557.1	100.0	19.36	42.85	355.9	ALLb

Rate from 1 case   0.823   0.809   0.671   0.473   0.409   0.388   0.457   0.507   0.488   0.518   0.518   0.611   0.656   0.754   1.239   1.415   1.730

ITALY, VENETIAN REGION 1988-1992

ANNUAL INCIDENCE PER 100,000 BY AGE GROUP (YEARS) - FEMALE

SITE	ALL AGES	AGE UNK	0-	5-	10-	15-	20-	25-	30-	35-	40-	45-	50-	55-	60-	65-	70-	75-	80+	CRUDE RATE	%	CR 64	CR 74	ASR (W)	ICD (9th)
Lip	15	0	-	-	-	-	-	-	-	-	-	-	0.6	1.7	1.1	0.9	1.7	4.2	0.5	0.1	0.01	0.02	0.2	140
Tongue	43	0	-	-	-	0.5	-	-	1.0	0.5	1.0	2.5	1.1	5.1	5.1	2.6	3.4	3.5	1.4	0.3	0.06	0.10	0.8	141
Salivary gland	19	0	-	-	-	-	-	0.5	0.5	-	0.5	0.5	1.1	0.6	1.7	0.9	2.6	3.5	0.6	0.1	0.02	0.03	0.3	142
Mouth	59	0	-	-	-	-	-	0.5	1.5	-	3.5	1.5	2.8	2.8	4.5	7.7	3.4	9.9	2.0	0.5	0.06	0.12	1.1	143-5
Oropharynx	28	0	-	-	-	-	-	-	-	1.5	0.5	3.0	2.8	2.8	0.6	1.7	0.9	2.8	0.9	0.2	0.05	0.06	0.6	146
Nasopharynx	14	0	-	-	-	0.5	-	0.4	-	-	0.5	-	2.2	1.1	0.6	1.7	1.7	-	0.5	0.1	0.02	0.04	0.3	147
Hypopharynx	9	0	-	-	-	-	-	-	-	-	0.5	-	0.6	1.7	0.6	1.7	-	0.7	0.3	0.1	0.01	0.03	0.2	148
Pharynx unspecified	22	0	-	-	-	0.5	-	-	-	-	0.5	2.0	1.7	2.8	1.7	1.7	0.9	1.4	0.7	0.2	0.04	0.05	0.5	149
Oesophagus	104	0	-	-	-	-	-	-	-	0.5	2.0	1.5	2.2	10.7	7.3	9.4	13.6	23.2	3.5	0.8	0.08	0.17	1.5	150
Stomach	644	0	-	-	-	-	0.4	1.9	2.6	5.8	7.6	13.8	16.3	30.3	38.3	68.9	108.9	154.2	21.6	5.0	0.39	0.93	8.8	151
Small intestine	35	0	-	-	-	-	-	-	1.0	1.0	0.5	1.5	1.1	2.8	1.1	2.6	4.3	7.0	1.2	0.3	0.04	0.06	0.6	152
Colon	1095	0	-	-	-	-	-	0.8	1.9	5.2	7.3	19.8	31.6	49.9	51.1	82.3	120.0	166.7	209.8	36.8	8.5	0.84	1.85	16.4	153
Rectum	509	0	-	-	-	-	-	0.4	0.5	2.6	2.9	11.1	14.3	26.9	27.5	41.1	61.3	55.3	97.2	17.1	4.0	0.43	0.94	7.9	154
Liver	350	0	-	-	0.7	-	-	-	1.4	-	1.9	3.5	6.4	10.1	20.2	26.5	47.6	59.5	66.9	11.8	2.7	0.22	0.59	5.0	155
Gallbladder etc.	236	0	-	-	-	-	-	-	-	-	1.0	3.5	5.4	7.8	11.8	16.9	25.5	45.9	47.2	7.9	1.8	0.15	0.36	3.3	156
Pancreas	449	0	-	-	-	-	0.4	-	-	2.1	1.0	3.5	12.3	7.8	25.3	37.8	66.4	74.0	83.8	15.1	3.5	0.26	0.78	6.4	157
Nose, sinuses etc.	6	0	-	-	-	-	-	-	-	-	-	0.5	-	-	-	1.7	0.9	1.4	0.2	0.0	0.00	0.01	0.1	160
Larynx	63	0	-	-	-	-	-	-	-	-	0.5	3.0	2.5	2.8	5.1	6.2	8.5	7.7	4.9	2.1	0.5	0.07	0.14	1.1	161
Bronchus, lung	854	0	0.9	-	-	0.5	-	0.4	-	3.1	2.9	13.2	17.8	44.8	66.9	90.2	114.0	112.3	107.0	28.7	6.6	0.75	1.77	13.9	162
Other thoracic organs	16	0	-	-	0.7	-	-	0.4	-	-	-	-	0.5	0.6	-	0.6	0.9	5.1	2.8	0.5	0.1	0.01	0.02	0.3	163-4
Bone	22	0	0.9	-	1.4	0.5	-	1.6	1.0	-	0.5	1.0	-	-	1.1	1.7	1.7	0.9	0.7	0.7	0.2	0.04	0.06	0.7	170
Connective tissue	90	0	-	-	0.7	-	0.4	0.8	1.0	1.0	1.9	2.0	5.4	5.6	6.2	6.8	6.8	6.8	9.9	3.0	0.7	0.13	0.19	1.8	171
Mesothelioma	23	0	-	-	-	-	-	-	-	-	0.5	0.5	-	1.0	0.6	2.2	2.8	1.7	3.4	2.1	0.8	0.2	0.02	0.05	0.4	MES
Kaposi's sarcoma	12	0	-	-	-	-	-	-	0.5	-	-	-	-	-	0.6	0.6	3.4	2.6	1.4	0.4	0.1	0.01	0.03	0.2	KAP
Melanoma of skin	298	0	-	-	0.7	1.0	5.2	6.1	7.1	9.8	11.2	18.7	13.8	17.4	18.5	12.4	15.3	12.8	19.0	10.0	2.3	0.55	0.69	7.0	172
Other skin	1750	0	-	0.9	-	2.0	4.3	3.3	8.1	15.0	24.8	40.0	55.2	60.5	96.1	150.5	160.0	262.9	278.8	58.8		1.55	3.10	28.3	173
Breast	3661	0	-	-	-	-	0.4	6.5	24.7	54.7	117.3	192.5	188.9	204.6	257.9	292.5	291.9	296.0	315.4	123.0	28.4	5.24	8.16	72.6	174
Uterus unspecified	125	0	-	-	-	-	-	0.4	2.4	3.1	4.4	3.0	4.9	3.9	6.7	8.5	14.5	11.9	16.2	4.2	1.0	0.14	0.26	2.3	179
Cervix uteri	258	0	-	-	-	-	0.9	2.4	6.2	6.2	16.1	13.7	7.4	11.2	16.3	14.7	23.0	22.1	15.5	8.7	2.0	0.40	0.59	5.5	180
Placenta	1	0	-	-	-	-	-	0.4	-	-	-	-	-	-	-	-	-	-	-	0.0	0.0	0.00	0.00	0.0	181
Corpus uteri	463	0	-	-	-	-	-	1.6	0.5	1.0	6.8	12.7	28.1	42.0	34.8	35.5	48.5	49.3	31.7	15.6	3.6	0.64	1.06	8.7	182
Ovary etc.	494	0	0.9	-	1.4	1.5	0.9	4.9	4.8	6.7	10.7	20.8	22.7	33.1	33.7	37.2	34.0	44.2	45.8	16.6	3.8	0.71	1.07	9.9	183
Other female genital	146	0	-	-	-	-	-	0.4	0.5	1.0	-	2.5	2.5	6.2	8.4	10.1	14.5	17.9	35.2	4.9	1.1	0.11	0.23	2.1	184
Bladder	372	0	-	-	-	-	-	0.8	1.0	1.0	2.4	4.1	9.4	14.6	19.1	29.9	50.2	62.9	62.0	12.5	2.9	0.26	0.66	5.5	188
Kidney etc.	308	0	1.7	-	-	-	-	0.4	0.5	2.1	2.9	4.1	10.9	12.3	27.5	31.6	34.9	35.7	38.0	10.3	2.4	0.31	0.64	5.3	189
Eye	16	0	-	-	-	-	-	-	-	-	-	0.5	1.0	1.1	0.6	0.6	0.9	4.3	2.1	0.5	0.1	0.02	0.02	0.2	190
Brain, nervous system	228	0	2.6	4.3	1.4	3.9	2.2	2.0	1.4	5.7	6.8	5.1	11.8	12.3	15.7	18.0	19.6	16.2	9.9	7.7	1.8	0.38	0.56	5.6	191-2
Thyroid	216	0	-	-	1.5	4.7	5.3	5.7	7.7	12.7	9.6	8.9	9.5	6.2	9.0	14.5	15.3	14.1	7.3	1.7	0.36	0.48	5.0	193
Other endocrine	16	0	1.7	-	-	-	0.4	-	0.5	1.0	0.5	-	1.7	1.1	-	0.9	-	2.1	0.5	0.1	0.03	0.04	0.5	194
Hodgkin's disease	117	0	-	0.9	4.2	5.4	3.9	6.1	5.2	3.1	3.4	6.1	2.5	5.6	1.7	2.3	5.1	4.3	4.2	3.9	0.9	0.24	0.28	3.5	201
Non-Hodgkin lymphoma	485	0	-	1.7	0.7	1.5	2.2	5.3	7.1	5.2	7.8	13.7	12.3	25.2	27.5	38.9	61.3	49.3	52.8	16.3	3.8	0.55	1.05	9.1	200,202
Multiple myeloma	178	0	-	-	-	-	-	-	-	-	1.0	1.0	4.4	9.0	7.9	13.5	28.9	32.3	27.5	6.0	1.4	0.12	0.33	2.6	203
Lymphoid leukaemia	138	0	3.5	2.6	3.5	2.0	0.4	-	0.5	0.5	1.5	1.5	3.9	2.2	5.6	7.3	15.3	23.8	22.5	4.6	1.1	0.14	0.25	2.9	204
Myeloid leukaemia	140	0	0.9	1.7	0.7	-	1.7	2.4	0.5	2.6	1.5	2.5	3.0	3.4	5.6	13.0	15.3	14.5	22.5	4.7	1.1	0.13	0.27	2.7	205
Monocytic leukaemia	6	0	0.9	-	-	-	-	-	-	-	-	-	-	0.6	0.6	-	-	0.9	1.4	0.2	0.0	0.01	0.02	0.2	206
Other leukaemia	4	0	-	-	-	-	-	-	-	-	-	-	0.5	0.6	-	-	-	0.9	0.7	0.1	0.0	0.01	0.01	0.1	207
Leukaemia unspecified	29	0	1.7	-	-	-	-	0.4	-	-	1.0	1.5	0.5	1.1	0.6	2.8	2.6	3.4	3.5	1.0	0.2	0.03	0.06	0.7	208
Other and unspecified	470	0	-	-	0.7	-	-	-	1.4	0.5	4.4	3.0	8.9	15.7	18.5	30.4	47.6	76.6	120.4	15.8	3.6	0.27	0.66	6.3	O&U
All sites	14636	0	15.7	12.0	16.6	21.2	27.5	54.7	86.5	147.5	267.2	435.1	525.3	683.4	891.0	1134.3	1457.6	1739.6	1987.0	491.7		15.92	28.88	258.9	ALL
All sites but 173	12886	0	15.7	11.1	16.6	19.2	23.2	51.4	78.5	132.6	242.4	395.1	470.0	622.8	795.0	983.9	1297.6	1476.8	1708.2	432.9	100.0	14.37	25.78	230.6	ALLb

Rate from 1 case			0.872	0.856	0.693	0.493	0.430	0.408	0.476	0.516	0.487	0.507	0.493	0.561	0.562	0.564	0.851	0.851	0.704

Latvia

Cancer registration in Latvia started in 1953 and covers the whole population of the country. Since 1979 computerized oncological data-processing and storage have been introduced. This cancer registration system developed according to the regulations of the Health Ministry of the Republic.

Latvia is one of the Baltic countries, with an area of about 64 600 km², located between latitudes 55°40´ and 58°05´ N and longitudes 20°58´ and 28°14´ E. The population of Latvia in 1990 was 2 625 000. Due to emigration of Soviet military personnel, the number of residents in 1992 decreased to 2 606 000. The main groups are Latvians (53%), Russians (34%), Belarusians (4.2%), Ukrainians (3.4%), Poles (2.2%), Lithuanians (1.3%) and Jews (0.6%). In 1992, 69% of the population resided in urban areas and 31% in rural areas. About 14% of the population is occupied in industry, and 8–9% in agriculture.

Since 1986 the birth rate has decreased, reaching 12/1000 in 1992. The average death rate in 1992 was 13.5/1000 and life expectancy at birth was 63.8 years for males and 74.8 years for females. Thus overall the population decreased by 0.1/1000 in 1991 and 1.5/1000 in 1992.

Malignancies are the second main cause of death in Latvia. The main problem for Latvian oncologists is an increasing number of advanced cancer cases, especially during the last 2–4 years. This seems to be connected to the transition from one form of social structure to another.

Every physician in a hospital, outpatient department, pathological or forensic medicine department is requested to report all new cancer cases to the Cancer Registry. Death certificates with a cancer diagnosis are regularly checked.

In 1993 the Latvian Cancer Registry group was organized, which carries out not only cancer registration but also epidemiological research and cancer prevention activities.

A. Stengrevics
A. Eglite
I. Rogovska
R. Suveizde

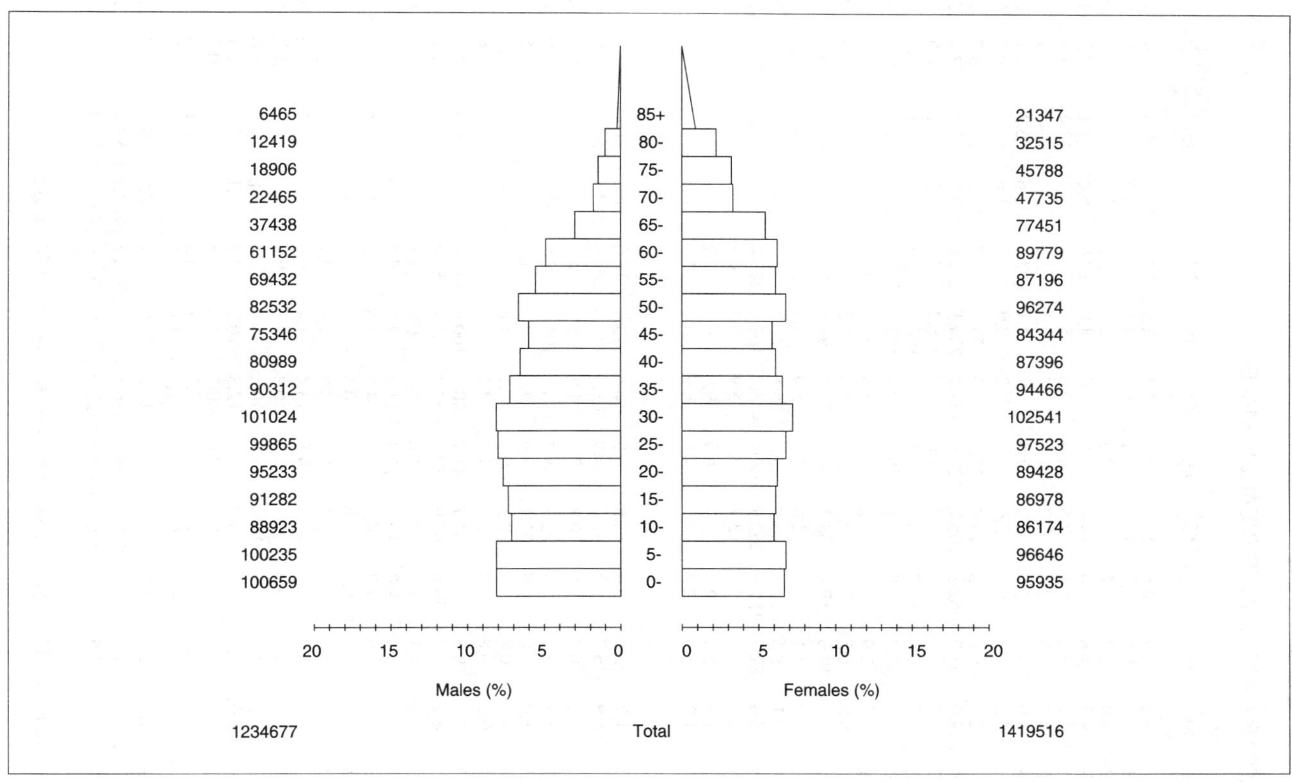

Latvia

Source of population: average annual 1988–92

Census: 1989 The Results of Census in Latvia, Year 1989. Latvian Republic's Committee of Statistics, Riga, 1992, p. 307.

Estimate: The populations for 1988, 1990, 1991 and 1992 are estimates based on the 1989 Census, making allowance for births and deaths and migration into and out of the registration area.

Notes to tables overleaf:

* The low level of histological verification implies lack of validity in the data.

+ The editors were unable to verify these data

† 163-164 includes mesothelioma of the pleura

† Mesothelioma not available separately

† Kaposi's sarcoma not available separately

† 188 does not include non-invasive tumours

Screening programmes in the area

The population aged 18-70 has been screened for cervical cancer since 1972. 678 959 examinations were carried out in 1988 (64.4% of the population-at-risk), in 1989 620 493 (59%), in 1990 549 920 (51.8%), in 1991 501 810 (47.4%) and in 1992 392 085 (37%).

+* LATVIA 1988-1992

ANNUAL INCIDENCE PER 100,000 BY AGE GROUP (YEARS) - MALE

SITE	ALL AGES	AGE UNK	0-	5-	10-	15-	20-	25-	30-	35-	40-	45-	50-	55-	60-	65-	70-	75-	80-	85+	CRUDE RATE	%	CR 64	CR 74	ASR (W)	ICD (9th)
Lip	208	0	-	-	-	-	-	-	0.6	-	1.2	2.9	4.8	10.1	12.8	14.4	28.5	22.2	19.3	9.3	3.4	1.2	0.16	0.38	**2.8**	*140*
Tongue	153	0	-	-	-	-	-	-	-	0.4	2.7	6.6	4.4	11.2	11.4	5.3	7.1	3.2	3.2	-	2.5	0.9	0.18	0.25	**2.1**	*141*
Salivary gland	43	0	-	0.2	-	-	-	-	0.4	0.7	1.0	0.8	1.7	0.6	2.0	3.7	2.7	3.2	3.2	-	0.7	0.3	0.04	0.07	**0.6**	*142*
Mouth	200	0	-	-	0.2	-	-	0.2	0.2	0.9	4.7	4.8	9.0	14.4	8.5	9.6	8.9	10.6	6.4	3.1	3.2	1.2	0.21	0.31	**2.7**	*143-5*
Oropharynx	114	0	-	-	-	-	0.2	-	-	0.4	1.7	3.2	5.1	7.5	4.6	9.6	5.3	3.2	-	12.4	1.8	0.7	0.11	0.19	**1.6**	*146*
Nasopharynx	58	0	-	-	-	-	-	0.4	0.4	0.2	1.2	1.3	2.9	3.7	1.6	2.7	4.5	3.2	-	-	0.9	0.3	0.06	0.09	**0.8**	*147*
Hypopharynx	132	0	-	-	-	-	-	-	-	0.4	3.0	4.2	5.8	6.9	7.5	6.9	7.1	7.4	1.6	6.2	2.1	0.8	0.14	0.21	**1.8**	*148*
Pharynx unspecified	25	0	-	-	-	-	-	-	-	-	0.2	-	0.7	2.0	2.0	3.2	0.9	-	1.6	-	0.4	0.1	0.02	0.05	**0.3**	*149*
Oesophagus	350	0	-	-	-	-	-	-	1.1	2.0	6.6	13.3	19.9	24.5	23.0	23.1	31.7	11.3	21.7	5.7	2.0	0.34	0.57	**4.7**	*150*
Stomach	2314	0	-	-	0.2	0.2	0.2	2.0	4.6	8.9	19.0	38.0	62.8	105.7	129.8	173.1	234.1	252.8	202.9	133.0	37.5	13.5	1.86	3.89	**31.1**	*151*
Small intestine	33	0	-	-	-	-	-	-	-	0.2	0.5	-	-	0.9	1.0	3.7	6.2	7.4	3.2	3.1	0.5	0.2	0.01	0.06	**0.5**	*152*
Colon	870	0	-	-	-	-	0.4	0.8	1.2	4.2	3.7	10.1	18.7	28.8	51.3	76.9	100.6	115.3	103.1	68.1	14.1	5.1	0.60	1.48	**11.7**	*153*
Rectum	781	0	-	-	-	-	0.2	0.4	1.4	2.4	3.2	7.2	16.0	28.5	46.1	59.3	102.4	107.9	119.2	37.1	12.7	4.5	0.53	1.34	**10.4**	*154*
Liver	300	0	0.4	0.2	-	0.4	0.2	0.4	0.4	0.4	2.0	2.9	5.1	11.2	20.6	27.8	40.1	30.7	25.8	12.4	4.9	1.7	0.22	0.56	**4.2**	*155*
Gallbladder etc.	60	0	-	-	-	-	-	-	-	0.7	0.5	0.5	1.9	2.3	3.6	4.8	6.2	5.3	8.1	-	1.0	0.3	0.05	0.10	**0.8**	*156*
Pancreas	853	0	-	-	-	-	-	0.6	1.0	1.6	6.9	14.6	19.4	33.1	51.3	70.0	90.8	93.1	82.1	95.9	13.8	5.0	0.64	1.45	**11.6**	*157*
Nose, sinuses etc.	47	0	-	-	-	-	-	0.2	0.6	0.4	1.0	1.1	0.5	2.6	1.3	5.9	0.9	1.1	6.4	3.1	0.8	0.3	0.04	0.07	**0.6**	*160*
Larynx	671	0	-	-	-	-	-	0.2	0.2	5.1	10.1	18.6	27.1	36.9	43.5	35.8	41.8	31.7	24.2	9.3	10.9	3.9	0.71	1.10	**9.0**	*161*
Bronchus, lung	4859	0	0.2	-	-	0.2	0.2	0.2	1.4	5.8	18.8	82.3	151.9	262.7	360.4	413.5	402.4	373.4	246.4	194.9	78.7	28.3	4.42	8.50	**65.5**	*162*
†Other thoracic organs	94	0	-	-	0.2	0.9	1.1	0.2	0.4	1.3	0.2	1.9	2.2	3.7	4.3	5.9	6.2	6.3	11.3	3.1	1.5	0.5	0.08	0.14	**1.3**	*163-4*
Bone	118	0	0.4	0.4	0.7	1.8	0.4	0.6	0.8	0.7	1.7	2.4	2.7	3.7	6.9	9.6	6.2	3.2	3.2	-	1.9	0.7	0.12	0.19	**1.7**	*170*
Connective tissue	117	0	1.0	0.4	0.4	0.9	0.6	0.6	0.4	1.1	1.2	3.5	2.4	5.5	4.6	6.9	6.2	5.3	8.1	-	1.9	0.7	0.11	0.18	**1.7**	*171*
†Mesothelioma																										
†Kaposi's sarcoma																										
Melanoma of skin	154	0	-	-	-	0.2	0.6	1.0	1.6	2.7	1.7	3.7	3.4	5.5	4.9	6.4	13.4	18.0	16.1	6.2	2.5	0.9	0.13	0.23	**2.1**	*172*
Other skin	1414	0	-	-	0.4	0.2	1.6	2.0	4.0	8.9	16.7	23.7	46.7	74.9	108.4	138.0	201.0	252.8	253.7	22.9		0.90	2.13	**18.7**	*173*
Breast	32	0	-	-	-	-	-	-	-	-	0.2	0.3	1.5	0.3	2.6	1.1	2.7	4.2	8.1	3.1	0.5	0.2	0.02	0.04	**0.4**	*175*
Prostate	1185	0	-	-	-	-	-	-	-	0.7	1.5	2.1	5.8	22.2	48.7	110.0	195.9	265.5	262.5	241.3	19.2	6.9	0.40	1.93	**15.8**	*185*
Testis	93	0	0.2	-	0.2	0.2	2.7	3.0	3.2	1.3	1.0	1.6	1.0	1.4	2.9	3.2	3.6	1.1	1.6	-	1.5	0.5	0.09	0.13	**1.4**	*186*
Penis	31	0	-	-	-	-	-	-	-	0.7	0.2	0.8	1.2	2.3	0.7	1.1	1.8	1.1	4.8	3.1	0.5	0.2	0.03	0.04	**0.4**	*187.1-.4*
Other male genital	39	0	-	-	-	-	0.8	0.8	-	0.7	0.2	0.8	1.0	1.7	1.6	2.1	-	3.2	-	6.2	0.4	0.2	0.04	0.05	**0.5**	*187.5-.9*
†Bladder	882	0	0.2	-	0.2	-	-	0.4	0.2	0.9	3.5	9.3	18.4	31.7	48.7	80.7	100.6	117.4	132.1	99.0	14.3	5.1	0.57	1.47	**11.8**	*188*
Kidney etc.	688	0	2.2	0.4	-	0.2	0.8	0.4	0.8	1.3	4.2	11.7	20.8	38.9	39.9	52.4	61.4	55.0	45.1	21.7	11.1	4.0	0.61	1.18	**9.4**	*189*
Eye	30	0	0.4	-	-	-	-	-	-	-	0.5	1.3	1.2	2.0	1.0	1.1	0.9	1.1	3.2	-	0.5	0.2	0.03	0.04	**0.4**	*190*
Brain, nervous system	278	0	1.2	1.4	0.9	0.7	1.1	2.4	2.4	2.9	5.2	6.9	9.0	16.1	12.4	11.2	8.9	6.3	1.6	-	4.5	1.6	0.31	0.41	**3.9**	*191-2*
Thyroid	70	0	-	-	-	0.2	0.2	0.2	0.6	1.1	1.0	1.9	1.7	4.0	2.6	4.8	4.5	3.2	1.6	3.1	1.1	0.4	0.07	0.11	**1.0**	*193*
Other endocrine	22	0	0.2	-	0.2	-	0.2	-	0.2	-	-	0.5	2.6	1.0	0.5	-	-	1.6	-	-	0.4	0.1	0.03	0.03	**0.3**	*194*
Hodgkin's disease	169	0	0.6	1.4	1.6	2.6	6.3	1.8	2.6	2.0	3.0	2.4	4.1	5.5	2.9	3.7	1.8	2.1	1.6	3.1	2.7	1.0	0.18	0.21	**2.6**	*201*
Non-Hodgkin lymphoma	247	0	1.0	1.6	2.9	2.2	1.7	1.0	0.8	1.3	1.7	3.2	5.6	11.5	9.8	13.4	21.4	16.9	12.9	9.3	4.0	1.4	0.22	0.40	**3.6**	*200,202*
Multiple myeloma	108	0	-	-	-	-	-	0.2	0.2	0.4	1.7	1.3	4.6	4.9	5.9	6.4	9.8	9.5	8.1	3.1	1.7	0.6	0.10	0.18	**1.4**	*203*
Lymphoid leukaemia	343	0	1.2	1.4	1.6	0.7	1.3	0.4	0.6	1.3	1.7	4.8	8.7	10.9	16.0	29.4	31.2	43.4	33.8	9.3	5.6	2.0	0.25	0.56	**4.8**	*204*
Myeloid leukaemia	147	0	0.4	0.4	0.2	-	0.6	0.4	1.8	2.9	2.0	3.7	3.2	4.3	3.9	12.3	10.7	12.7	8.1	3.1	2.4	0.9	0.12	0.23	**2.1**	*205*
Monocytic leukaemia	19	0	-	-	-	0.2	0.4	-	0.2	-	-	-	0.3	2.0	0.5	1.8	5.3	-	-	-	0.3	0.1	0.02	0.03	**0.3**	*206*
Other leukaemia	59	0	0.4	-	0.4	0.2	0.2	0.2	0.2	0.2	1.2	1.1	1.5	2.6	2.9	2.1	2.7	3.2	4.8	3.1	1.0	0.3	0.06	0.08	**0.8**	*207*
Leukaemia unspecified	21	0	0.2	0.2	-	-	0.6	-	0.2	-	1.0	-	0.2	0.3	1.0	1.1	1.8	2.1	-	-	0.3	0.1	0.02	0.03	**0.3**	*208*
Other and unspecified	178	0	0.4	0.2	-	0.2	0.8	1.0	0.4	0.9	1.5	2.4	3.9	5.8	8.8	12.8	24.0	20.1	12.9	9.3	2.9	1.0	0.13	0.32	**2.5**	*O&U*
All sites	18609	0	10.5	8.2	10.1	12.5	22.3	21.6	32.3	62.7	128.7	289.3	479.3	823.5	1095.0	1436.5	1769.0	1910.4	1703.8	1289.9	301.4		14.98	31.01	**251.7**	*ALL*
All sites but 173	17195	0	10.5	8.2	10.1	12.1	22.1	20.0	30.3	58.7	119.8	272.6	455.6	776.9	1020.1	1328.0	1631.0	1709.4	1451.0	1036.3	278.5	100.0	14.08	28.88	**233.0**	*ALLb*

Rate from 1 case 0.199 0.200 0.225 0.219 0.210 0.200 0.198 0.221 0.247 0.265 0.242 0.288 0.327 0.534 0.890 1.058 1.610 3.093

†Important: see notes on population page

+* LATVIA 1988-1992

ANNUAL INCIDENCE PER 100,000 BY AGE GROUP (YEARS) - FEMALE

SITE	ALL AGES	AGE UNK	0-	5-	10-	15-	20-	25-	30-	35-	40-	45-	50-	55-	60-	65-	70-	75-	80-	85+	CRUDE RATE	%	CR 64	CR 74	ASR (W)	ICD (9th)
Lip	49	0	-	-	-	-	-	-	-	0.2	0.5	0.2	0.2	0.7	0.7	1.3	1.7	4.8	8.0	4.7	0.7	0.3	0.01	0.03	0.3	140
Tongue	24	0	-	-	-	-	-	-	-	0.2	0.2	0.5	1.0	0.7	0.4	0.5	1.3	1.3	1.2	-	0.3	0.1	0.02	0.02	0.2	141
Salivary gland	39	0	-	-	-	-	0.2	-	0.2	0.4	0.2	0.2	0.8	0.7	0.9	1.0	0.8	4.4	1.8	2.8	0.5	0.2	0.02	0.03	0.3	142
Mouth	37	0	-	-	-	-	-	-	0.2	0.4	0.2	0.5	0.4	0.7	1.8	1.8	0.4	2.2	1.8	1.9	0.5	0.2	0.02	0.03	0.3	143-5
Oropharynx	11	0	0.2	-	-	-	-	-	-	-	0.2	-	-	0.2	1.1	0.8	-	-	-	-	0.2	0.1	0.01	0.01	0.1	146
Nasopharynx	20	0	-	-	-	-	-	-	-	0.2	-	0.7	0.6	0.2	0.4	0.8	0.8	1.3	0.6	0.9	0.3	0.1	0.01	0.02	0.2	147
Hypopharynx	10	0	-	-	-	-	-	-	0.2	-	-	0.6	-	0.2	0.3	0.8	0.4	-	0.9	0.1	0.1	0.01	0.01	0.1	148	
Pharynx unspecified	5	0	-	-	-	-	0.2	-	-	-	-	0.2	0.2	-	-	-	0.8	-	-	-	0.1	0.0	0.00	0.01	0.1	149
Oesophagus	96	0	-	-	-	-	-	-	-	-	0.2	0.7	1.2	1.8	2.5	3.6	5.4	8.3	8.0	7.5	1.4	0.6	0.03	0.08	0.7	150
Stomach	1810	0	-	-	0.2	-	0.7	0.2	3.1	8.0	14.4	16.8	26.6	37.4	54.4	82.1	87.6	129.3	113.8	69.3	25.5	10.5	0.81	1.66	14.1	151
Small intestine	26	0	-	-	-	-	0.2	-	-	-	0.2	0.2	0.5	0.2	1.0	2.9	2.6	0.6	1.9	0.4	0.2	0.01	0.03	0.2	152	
Colon	1182	0	-	-	-	-	0.4	0.2	2.1	4.0	5.9	10.4	17.9	22.9	36.3	53.2	75.8	72.1	80.0	45.0	16.7	6.9	0.50	1.15	9.1	153
Rectum	893	0	-	-	-	-	-	0.8	1.2	1.5	4.1	9.5	13.9	19.5	31.9	36.7	52.4	60.3	48.0	37.5	12.6	5.2	0.41	0.86	7.0	154
Liver	223	0	0.2	0.2	-	-	-	-	-	0.4	0.4	1.8	2.6	3.1	3.9	8.0	11.4	12.6	12.7	10.5	9.4	3.1	1.3	0.10	0.22	1.8	155
Gallbladder etc.	136	0	-	-	-	-	-	-	-	-	-	0.2	0.7	2.1	3.7	5.6	6.7	6.7	8.3	8.6	5.6	1.9	0.8	0.06	0.13	1.0	156
Pancreas	757	0	-	-	-	-	-	-	0.2	0.6	0.8	3.4	3.3	7.1	12.2	19.6	29.7	48.6	67.3	66.4	48.7	10.7	4.4	0.24	0.63	5.2	157
Nose, sinuses etc.	32	0	-	-	-	-	-	-	0.2	-	-	0.5	0.4	0.7	0.4	0.8	1.7	2.6	4.3	1.9	0.5	0.2	0.01	0.02	0.2	160	
Larynx	46	0	-	-	-	-	-	-	-	-	0.2	0.5	0.2	1.2	1.6	1.3	2.3	1.7	1.3	2.5	2.8	0.6	0.3	0.03	0.05	0.4	161
Bronchus, lung	924	0	-	-	-	0.2	0.2	0.6	0.8	1.9	2.1	5.5	8.9	20.2	37.0	51.1	54.0	62.9	46.1	29.0	13.0	5.4	0.39	0.91	7.1	162
†Other thoracic organs	61	0	0.2	-	0.2	0.2	0.7	-	0.4	-	0.7	1.2	0.8	1.8	1.1	2.8	2.5	2.2	2.5	1.9	0.9	0.4	0.04	0.06	0.6	163-4
Bone	85	0	0.4	0.2	0.7	0.9	0.9	0.4	0.2	1.1	1.4	2.1	0.6	0.9	1.8	1.8	5.0	2.2	4.3	1.9	1.2	0.5	0.06	0.09	1.0	170
Connective tissue	139	0	0.6	0.2	1.2	0.9	0.4	0.8	0.6	0.8	1.8	1.7	2.5	3.7	3.3	5.9	6.3	3.9	4.3	0.9	2.0	0.8	0.09	0.15	1.5	171
†Mesothelioma																										
†Kaposi's sarcoma																										
Melanoma of skin	317	0	-	-	-	0.2	1.6	1.6	1.8	3.4	5.9	5.0	8.1	7.1	7.1	9.8	9.6	14.4	13.5	10.3	4.5	1.8	0.21	0.31	3.0	172
Other skin	1869	0	-	-	0.2	-	-	1.0	2.5	5.5	8.9	15.4	27.2	39.2	49.2	84.4	107.3	118.4	130.4	122.7	26.3		0.75	1.70	14.1	173
Breast	3483	0	-	-	-	-	0.4	4.3	15.0	32.0	67.1	96.7	100.3	103.0	117.2	110.5	94.7	94.8	79.3	68.4	49.1	20.2	2.68	3.71	33.7	174
Uterus unspecified	3	0	-	-	-	-	-	-	-	-	0.2	-	-	-	-	0.3	-	-	-	-	0.9	0.0	0.0	0.00	0.00	0.0	179
Cervix uteri	985	0	-	-	-	-	0.7	4.3	8.8	8.0	13.7	21.3	27.2	31.9	36.3	28.7	28.1	30.6	23.4	8.4	13.9	5.7	0.76	1.05	9.5	180
Placenta	17	0	-	-	-	0.2	0.4	1.4	0.8	0.6	-	-	-	-	-	-	-	-	-	-	0.2	0.1	0.02	0.02	0.3	181
Corpus uteri	1567	0	-	-	-	-	0.2	0.8	2.0	4.2	11.9	27.7	48.2	58.9	66.6	66.9	52.4	51.5	32.6	18.7	22.1	9.1	1.10	1.70	14.1	182
Ovary etc.	1380	0	-	-	0.7	1.1	2.5	4.9	6.0	12.3	17.6	34.9	36.1	43.1	48.8	47.5	46.9	39.7	29.5	7.5	19.4	8.0	1.04	1.51	13.4	183
Other female genital	226	0	0.2	-	-	-	-	0.2	-	0.2	1.1	1.7	2.5	4.1	5.3	9.3	9.6	21.8	19.1	15.9	3.2	1.3	0.08	0.17	1.6	184
†Bladder	278	0	-	-	-	-	-	0.2	0.2	0.2	-	0.7	1.5	3.7	8.5	10.8	15.5	29.3	22.1	27.2	3.9	1.6	0.07	0.21	1.8	188
Kidney etc.	470	0	1.0	0.6	0.2	-	-	0.4	0.4	1.1	3.4	5.0	12.5	13.1	18.3	23.5	18.0	22.7	13.5	8.4	6.6	2.7	0.28	0.49	4.1	189
Eye	35	0	0.8	-	-	-	-	0.2	0.2	0.2	0.7	0.7	1.0	0.9	0.2	0.5	1.3	0.9	1.8	1.9	0.5	0.2	0.03	0.03	0.4	190
Brain, nervous system	248	0	1.5	0.8	0.9	0.9	0.7	1.8	2.5	2.3	3.2	5.9	6.0	7.1	10.7	8.3	3.4	1.7	1.2	-	3.5	1.4	0.22	0.28	2.8	191-2
Thyroid	245	0	-	-	-	0.2	1.1	2.1	2.3	3.2	5.3	4.3	3.3	8.7	7.8	5.2	9.6	8.3	4.9	1.9	3.5	1.4	0.19	0.27	2.5	193
Other endocrine	18	0	-	-	-	-	-	-	-	-	0.5	-	0.4	0.7	0.9	0.3	1.3	0.9	0.6	-	0.3	0.1	0.01	0.02	0.2	194
Hodgkin's disease	153	0	-	0.6	1.2	4.4	4.9	4.1	2.3	1.9	1.8	1.2	1.2	1.8	1.1	2.1	4.2	3.1	3.1	0.9	2.2	0.9	0.13	0.16	2.1	201
Non-Hodgkin lymphoma	223	0	0.4	0.8	0.9	2.1	1.6	1.2	1.4	1.7	0.9	2.8	4.2	5.5	7.8	7.5	8.0	8.7	6.8	1.9	3.1	1.3	0.16	0.23	2.3	200,202
Multiple myeloma	167	0	-	-	-	-	-	-	0.2	0.2	0.9	1.7	1.9	5.3	8.5	8.5	11.3	7.4	3.1	1.9	2.4	1.0	0.09	0.19	1.4	203
Lymphoid leukaemia	316	0	2.3	1.0	1.9	0.5	1.3	0.2	0.2	1.5	1.8	0.9	4.6	7.8	10.9	10.3	16.3	19.2	18.5	4.7	4.5	1.8	0.17	0.31	2.9	204
Myeloid leukaemia	187	0	-	0.6	0.5	0.7	0.7	0.2	1.8	1.3	2.5	2.6	2.5	5.7	4.0	7.5	8.0	7.9	8.0	3.7	2.6	1.1	0.12	0.19	1.8	205
Monocytic leukaemia	23	0	0.2	0.2	0.2	-	-	0.2	0.2	0.2	0.5	0.5	-	0.5	0.9	0.5	1.7	0.4	-	-	0.3	0.1	0.02	0.03	0.3	206
Other leukaemia	62	0	0.2	-	-	0.2	-	-	-	-	-	0.2	0.8	3.2	2.5	4.1	2.5	2.2	1.2	0.9	0.9	0.4	0.04	0.07	0.5	207
Leukaemia unspecified	21	0	-	-	0.2	-	0.2	-	0.2	-	-	0.6	0.5	0.4	-	1.3	1.3	1.2	2.8	0.3	0.1	0.01	0.02	0.2	208	
Other and unspecified	197	0	0.6	-	-	0.5	0.7	0.4	0.4	0.6	0.9	3.1	4.6	5.7	8.5	8.0	6.3	8.7	6.2	3.7	2.8	1.1	0.13	0.20	1.8	O&U
All sites	19095	0	9.0	5.4	9.3	13.3	21.0	33.0	59.1	101.2	187.0	290.2	385.4	491.5	630.4	750.1	827.1	944.3	833.4	587.4	269.0		11.18	19.07	166.0	ALL
All sites but 173	17226	0	9.0	5.4	9.1	13.3	21.0	32.0	56.6	95.7	178.0	274.8	358.1	452.3	581.2	665.7	719.8	826.0	703.0	464.7	242.7	100.0	10.43	17.36	151.9	ALLb

Rate from 1 case   0.208   0.207   0.232   0.230   0.224   0.205   0.195   0.212   0.229   0.237   0.208   0.229   0.223   0.258   0.419   0.437   0.615   0.937

†Important: see notes on population page

Malta

The Malta Cancer Registry has been in operation since 1984. Until 1990 it was predominantly a hospital-based registry recording data on cancer cases presenting at the major general hospital on the island of Malta, namely St Luke's Hospital. In 1991, the scope of the registry was widened to cover the whole resident population of the islands. The registry is part of the Department of Health Information which also houses other national registers, including the Mortality and Infectious Diseases registries.

The Maltese islands are an archipelago in the middle of the Mediterranean Sea. They are situated about 93 km south of Sicily, Italy and about 230 km north of the northern African coast. The total area of all the islands is 316 km^2. There are three inhabited islands, Malta (the largest), Gozo and Comino. The population of the Maltese islands at the end of 1994 was estimated to be 369 451. There is no clear distinction on the islands between urban and rural parts. However, the harbour area (centred around the capital Valletta) can be considered as the most urban, with much of the rest of Malta being suburban, and most of the northwest part and the whole of Gozo being rural.

The official languages are Maltese and English. Maltese is a semitic language written in Roman script, containing a vast number of loan-words mostly of Italian, French and English origin. Practically all Maltese are well conversant in English, and this is the language used most commonly to communicate with foreign visitors. Although quite a large number of foreigners are resident on the islands, one cannot speak of any distinct ethnic minority groups.

Malta was under the rule of many different nations until its independence in 1964. The last occupiers were the British, who governed Malta from 1800 to 1964. Previous occupiers included the French, the Knights of St John of Jerusalem, better known as the Knights of Malta, the Spanish, the Arabs and the Romans. The Maltese culture has a distinct Mediterranean nature, which reflects the occupation of the islands by all these nations.

Information is obtained by the registry from various sources. The main sources are the pathology laboratories of St Luke's Hospital and private laboratories. The registry's staff has access to histological, cytological, haematological and biochemical reports issued by these laboratories. Through the pathology department of St Luke's Hospital, the registry can also examine autopsy reports. Other sources include notification by medical practitioners, which has been statutory since 1957, and the mortality registry. Copies of all death certificates bearing a diagnosis of cancer, whether as the underlying cause of death or not, are passed to the cancer registry for investigation. The registry is also in close contact with the oncological department at Sir Paul Boffa Hospital, which is the only radiotherapy centre on the island. The oncologists regularly send lists of all patients referred to this unit. The hospital files of all cases which come in contact with the state-run hospital services are reviewed during registration to obtain the most detailed and accurate information possible about each case. The registry is tumour-based so that each tumour in a patient having more than one primary tumour is registered.

Until 1992, the data were classified according to the ICD-9 topographic coding system. No morphological coding was used. Since the beginning of 1993, the ICD-O-2 coding system has been used for both topography and morphology. Each Maltese resident has a unique personal identification number which is given at the Public Registry, either at birth or on immigration into the country. This number is used on most official documents. It is used to check for duplications, to trace the hospital notes, and to link incidence and mortality data. Annual reports with national incidence data were started in 1992 and mortality data were included in the reports from 1993.

The population at risk is taken as the mid-year population calculated from the population estimates published annually by the Central Office of Statistics. A national census is performed every 10 years; the last one was carried out in 1985 and the annual population figures are estimated from the censal population. The national Electoral Register which is updated every six months is used to establish the residence of the cancer patient at the time of diagnosis.

Miriam Dalmas

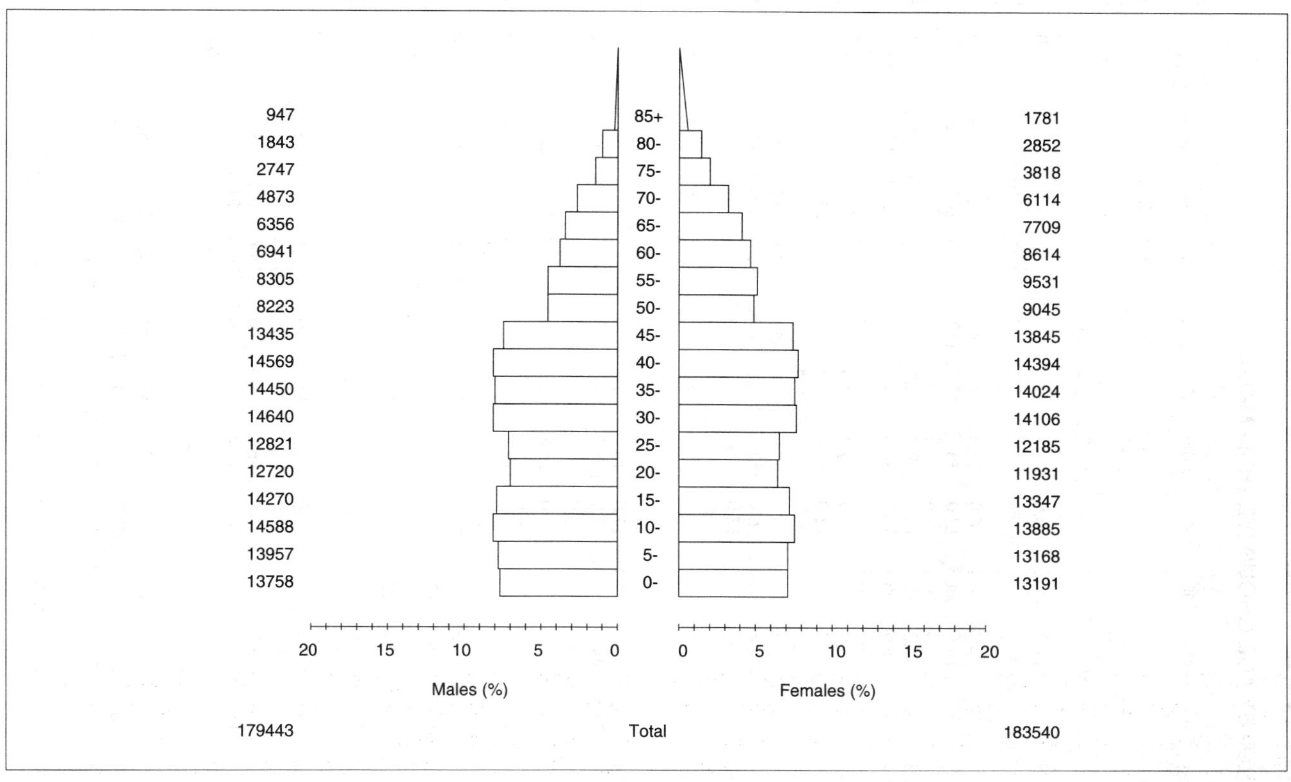

Malta

Source of population: average annual 1992–93

Census: 1985. Census 1985. Central Office of Statistics, Malta, 1985.

Estimate: The mid-year populations were calculated as the average of the end-year population estimates, for 1992 for the years 1991 and 1992 and for 1993 for 1992 and 1993, published by the Central Office of Statistics in the Demographic Reviews of the Maltese Islands. The population estimates are projected from the Census data. References: Demographic review of the Maltese Islands, 1992. Central Office of Statistics, Malta, 1994. Demographic review of the Maltese Islands, 1993. Central Office of Statistics, Malta, 1994.

Notes to tables overleaf:
+ The editors were unable to verify the 1992 data
† 163-164 includes mesothelioma of the pleura
† Mesothelioma not available separately
† Kaposi's sarcoma not available separately
† 188 does not include non-invasive tumours

+ MALTA 1992-1993

ANNUAL INCIDENCE PER 100,000 BY AGE GROUP (YEARS) - MALE

SITE	ALL AGES	AGE UNK	0-	5-	10-	15-	20-	25-	30-	35-	40-	45-	50-	55-	60-	65-	70-	75-	80-	85+	CRUDE RATE	%	CR 64	CR 74	ASR (W)	ICD (9th)
Lip	11	2	-	-	-	-	-	-	3.4	3.5	-	7.4	-	6.0	-	7.9	10.3	18.2	27.1	-	3.1	1.1	0.12	0.24	2.3	140
Tongue	4	0	-	-	-	-	-	-	3.4	-	-	-	-	-	-	-	30.8	-	-	-	1.1	0.4	0.02	0.17	0.8	141
Salivary gland	1	0	-	-	-	-	-	-	-	-	-	3.7	-	-	-	-	-	-	-	-	0.3	0.1	0.02	0.02	0.2	142
Mouth	6	0	-	-	-	-	-	-	-	-	-	-	6.1	-	7.2	7.9	30.8	-	-	-	1.7	0.6	0.07	0.26	1.4	143-5
Oropharynx	0	0	-	-	-	-	-	-	-	-	-	-	-	-	-	-	-	-	-	-	0.0	0.0	0.00	0.00	0.0	146
Nasopharynx	7	0	-	-	-	-	-	-	6.9	-	11.2	6.1	6.0	-	-	-	-	-	-	-	2.0	0.7	0.15	0.15	1.6	147
Hypopharynx	3	0	-	-	-	-	-	-	-	-	-	-	-	-	-	-	-	36.4	27.1	-	0.8	0.3	0.00	0.00	0.5	148
Pharynx unspecified	0	0	-	-	-	-	-	-	-	-	-	-	-	-	-	-	-	-	-	-	0.0	0.0	0.00	0.00	0.0	149
Oesophagus	14	0	-	-	-	-	-	-	-	-	-	-	6.1	6.0	21.6	31.5	41.0	-	27.1	-	3.9	1.4	0.17	0.53	3.3	150
Stomach	51	0	-	-	-	-	-	-	-	13.7	18.6	24.3	12.0	36.0	47.2	133.4	91.0	162.8	52.8	14.2	5.2	0.52	1.43	11.2	151
Small intestine	7	0	-	-	-	-	-	-	-	-	7.4	6.1	6.0	7.2	-	20.5	-	-	-	2.0	0.7	0.13	0.24	1.7	152
Colon	59	1	-	-	-	-	-	13.8	6.9	11.2	12.2	18.1	79.2	78.7	112.9	91.0	81.4	211.2	16.4	6.0	0.72	1.69	13.6	153
Rectum	42	0	-	-	-	-	-	-	3.5	3.4	18.6	6.1	30.1	36.0	55.1	51.3	91.0	135.6	105.6	11.7	4.3	0.49	1.02	9.3	154
Liver	8	0	-	-	-	-	-	-	-	-	-	6.1	-	-	23.6	30.8	18.2	-	-	2.2	0.8	0.03	0.30	1.8	155
Gallbladder etc.	4	0	-	-	-	-	-	-	-	-	-	-	-	6.0	7.2	7.9	-	18.2	-	1.1	0.4	0.07	0.11	0.9	156
Pancreas	47	0	-	-	-	-	-	-	-	-	-	3.7	12.2	12.0	21.6	78.7	82.1	145.6	244.2	211.2	13.1	4.8	0.25	1.05	9.9	157
Nose, sinuses etc.	4	0	-	3.6	-	-	-	3.9	-	-	-	-	-	-	-	7.9	-	-	52.8	1.1	0.4	0.04	0.08	1.2	160
Larynx	43	0	-	-	-	-	-	-	-	-	-	3.7	12.2	36.1	93.6	62.9	51.3	72.8	54.3	105.6	12.0	4.4	0.73	1.30	10.5	161
Bronchus, lung	208	4	-	-	-	-	-	-	-	-	17.2	18.6	85.1	126.4	252.1	346.1	287.3	491.4	406.9	528.0	58.0	21.3	2.55	5.78	48.2	162
†Other thoracic organs	4	0	-	-	-	-	-	-	-	-	-	-	-	12.0	-	-	10.3	-	27.1	-	1.1	0.4	0.06	0.11	0.8	163-4
Bone	2	0	-	-	-	-	-	-	3.4	-	-	-	-	-	-	-	10.3	-	-	-	0.6	0.2	0.02	0.07	0.4	170
Connective tissue	7	0	-	-	-	-	-	-	-	-	11.2	12.2	-	-	7.9	-	-	27.1	-	2.0	0.7	0.12	0.16	1.6	171
†Mesothelioma																										
†Kaposi's sarcoma																										
Melanoma of skin	10	1	-	-	-	-	-	3.9	-	6.9	-	-	6.1	12.0	14.4	7.9	-	-	-	2.8	1.0	0.24	0.28	2.6	172
Other skin	234	14	-	3.6	-	-	-	3.9	10.2	13.8	27.5	44.7	60.8	78.3	165.7	283.2	359.1	564.3	841.0	633.6	65.2		2.17	5.59	51.0	173
Breast	4	0	-	-	-	-	-	-	-	-	-	-	6.0	-	7.9	-	36.4	-	-	1.1	0.4	0.03	0.07	0.8	175
Prostate	109	2	-	-	-	-	-	-	-	-	-	6.1	6.0	64.8	102.3	287.3	364.0	624.0	633.6	30.4	11.2	0.39	2.38	22.3	185
Testis	12	0	-	-	3.5	11.8	3.9	6.8	10.4	-	-	6.0	-	-	-	-	-	52.8	3.3	1.2	0.21	0.21	3.1	186
Penis	7	0	-	-	-	-	3.5	-	-	-	-	6.0	14.4	-	10.3	18.2	-	52.8	2.0	0.7	0.12	0.17	1.7	187.1-.4
Other male genital	1	0	-	-	-	-	-	-	-	-	-	6.0	-	-	-	-	-	-	0.3	0.1	0.03	0.03	0.2	187.5-.9
†Bladder	122	1	-	-	-	-	-	-	-	17.2	18.6	36.5	66.2	108.0	149.5	277.0	145.6	434.1	475.2	34.0	12.5	1.24	3.39	27.2	188
Kidney etc.	24	0	3.6	-	-	-	-	3.4	-	10.3	3.7	18.2	6.0	14.4	39.3	30.8	54.6	27.1	-	6.7	2.5	0.30	0.65	5.7	189
Eye	1	0	3.6	-	-	-	-	-	-	-	-	-	-	-	-	-	-	-	-	0.3	0.1	0.02	0.02	0.4	190
Brain, nervous system	24	1	7.3	3.6	6.9	-	-	-	-	-	3.7	12.2	18.1	21.6	31.5	30.8	36.4	-	-	6.7	2.5	0.38	0.71	6.5	191-2
Thyroid	2	0	-	-	-	-	3.9	3.4	-	-	-	-	-	-	-	-	-	-	-	0.6	0.2	0.04	0.04	0.5	193
Other endocrine	1	0	3.6	-	-	-	-	-	-	-	-	-	-	-	-	-	-	-	-	0.3	0.1	0.02	0.02	0.4	194
Hodgkin's disease	7	0	-	-	3.4	3.5	3.9	-	-	-	10.3	-	-	-	-	7.9	-	-	-	2.0	0.7	0.11	0.15	1.8	201
Non-Hodgkin lymphoma	30	1	-	-	-	-	-	-	6.8	10.4	6.9	7.4	24.3	12.0	21.6	15.7	20.5	72.8	54.3	52.8	8.4	3.1	0.46	0.65	6.8	200,202
Multiple myeloma	10	0	-	-	-	-	-	-	-	-	-	11.2	-	6.0	-	23.6	20.5	18.2	-	-	2.8	1.0	0.09	0.31	2.2	203
Lymphoid leukaemia	18	0	7.3	-	-	-	-	-	3.4	-	-	3.7	-	-	36.0	7.9	10.3	54.6	81.4	52.8	5.0	1.8	0.25	0.34	4.4	204
Myeloid leukaemia	15	0	-	-	-	-	3.9	-	-	-	13.7	3.7	-	6.0	14.4	-	10.3	36.4	81.4	-	4.2	1.5	0.21	0.26	3.2	205
Monocytic leukaemia	0	0	-	-	-	-	-	-	-	-	-	-	-	-	-	-	-	-	-	0.0	0.0	0.00	0.00	0.0	206
Other leukaemia	0	0	-	-	-	-	-	-	-	-	-	-	-	-	-	-	-	-	-	0.0	0.0	0.00	0.00	0.0	207
Leukaemia unspecified	0	0	-	-	-	-	-	-	-	-	-	-	-	-	-	-	-	-	-	0.0	0.0	0.00	0.00	0.0	208
Other and unspecified	47	0	-	-	-	-	-	-	3.4	-	3.4	11.2	18.2	12.0	50.4	55.1	51.3	127.4	271.3	52.8	13.1	4.8	0.49	1.03	10.1	O&U
All sites	1210	27	25.4	10.7	10.3	7.0	19.7	19.5	47.8	72.7	130.4	223.3	377.0	523.7	1087.7	1494.5	2011.1	2602.8	3635.4	3273.5	337.1		13.07	31.00	272.3	ALL
All sites but 173	976	13	25.4	7.2	10.3	7.0	19.7	15.6	37.6	58.8	103.0	178.6	316.2	445.5	922.0	1211.4	1652.0	2038.6	2794.4	2639.9	271.9	100.0	10.88	25.39	221.2	ALLb

Rate from 1 case   3.634 3.582 3.427 3.504 3.931 3.900 3.415 3.460 3.432 3.721 6.081 6.020 7.203 7.866 10.261 18.202 27.130 52.798

†Important: see notes on population page

+ MALTA 1992-1993

ANNUAL INCIDENCE PER 100,000 BY AGE GROUP (YEARS) - FEMALE

SITE	ALL AGES	AGE UNK	0-	5-	10-	15-	20-	25-	30-	35-	40-	45-	50-	55-	60-	65-	70-	75-	80-	85+	CRUDE RATE	%	CR 64	CR 74	ASR (W)	ICD (9th)
Lip	0	0	-	-	-	-	-	-	-	-	-	-	-	-	-	-	-	-	-	-	0.0	0.0	0.00	0.00	0.0	140
Tongue	6	0	-	-	-	-	-	-	-	-	-	-	5.5	15.7	-	6.5	-	13.1	-	-	1.6	0.6	0.11	0.14	1.2	141
Salivary gland	5	0	-	-	3.6	-	-	-	-	-	-	-	-	-	-	19.5	-	-	-	28.1	1.4	0.5	0.02	0.12	1.0	142
Mouth	6	1	-	-	-	-	-	-	-	-	-	-	-	-	5.8	6.5	16.4	-	-	28.1	1.6	0.6	0.03	0.17	1.1	143-5
Oropharynx	1	0	-	-	-	-	-	-	-	-	-	-	-	-	-	-	-	-	17.5	-	0.3	0.1	0.00	0.00	0.1	146
Nasopharynx	5	0	-	-	-	-	4.2	-	-	-	10.4	-	-	-	-	6.5	-	-	-	-	1.4	0.5	0.07	0.11	1.2	147
Hypopharynx	0	0	-	-	-	-	-	-	-	-	-	-	-	-	-	-	-	-	-	-	0.0	0.0	0.00	0.00	0.0	148
Pharynx unspecified	0	0	-	-	-	-	-	-	-	-	-	-	-	-	-	-	-	-	-	-	0.0	0.0	0.00	0.00	0.0	149
Oesophagus	7	0	-	-	-	-	-	-	-	-	-	-	-	-	11.6	-	8.2	13.1	52.6	-	1.9	0.7	0.06	0.10	1.0	150
Stomach	36	0	-	-	-	-	-	-	-	-	3.5	-	5.5	15.7	29.0	38.9	49.1	78.6	105.2	56.1	9.8	3.5	0.27	0.71	6.0	151
Small intestine	2	0	-	-	-	-	-	-	-	-	-	-	-	5.8	6.5	-	-	-	-	-	0.5	0.2	0.03	0.06	0.4	152
Colon	68	1	-	-	-	-	-	-	3.5	3.6	13.9	14.4	16.6	36.7	52.2	45.4	98.1	144.0	105.2	56.1	18.5	6.6	0.72	1.44	12.3	153
Rectum	37	0	-	-	-	-	-	-	7.1	-	3.5	3.6	11.1	10.5	29.0	32.4	65.4	52.4	87.7	56.1	10.1	3.6	0.32	0.81	6.5	154
Liver	7	0	-	-	-	-	-	-	-	-	3.5	-	-	-	-	16.4	-	70.1	-	-	1.9	0.7	0.02	0.10	0.9	155
Gallbladder etc.	7	0	-	-	-	-	-	-	-	-	-	-	-	-	5.8	6.5	8.2	26.2	-	56.1	1.9	0.7	0.03	0.10	1.1	156
Pancreas	21	0	-	-	-	-	-	-	3.5	-	3.5	-	5.5	10.5	11.6	6.5	49.1	39.3	70.1	-	5.7	2.0	0.17	0.45	3.5	157
Nose, sinuses etc.	3	0	-	-	-	-	-	-	-	-	3.5	-	-	5.2	-	-	-	13.1	-	-	0.8	0.3	0.04	0.04	0.5	160
Larynx	2	0	-	-	-	-	-	-	-	3.6	-	-	-	-	5.8	-	-	-	-	-	0.5	0.2	0.05	0.05	0.4	161
Bronchus, lung	18	0	-	-	-	-	-	-	-	-	-	-	11.1	21.0	11.6	13.0	16.4	13.1	17.5	112.3	4.9	1.7	0.22	0.36	3.4	162
†Other thoracic organs	2	0	-	-	-	-	-	-	-	-	-	-	-	-	-	-	-	13.1	17.5	-	0.5	0.2	0.00	0.00	0.2	163-4
Bone	5	0	-	3.8	-	-	-	-	3.5	-	-	-	-	-	-	-	8.2	26.2	-	-	1.4	0.5	0.04	0.08	1.0	170
Connective tissue	8	0	-	-	-	-	4.1	-	-	6.9	3.6	5.5	-	5.8	-	-	13.1	-	28.1		2.2	0.8	0.13	0.13	1.7	171
†Mesothelioma																										
†Kaposi's sarcoma																										
Melanoma of skin	16	0	-	-	-	-	4.1	-	10.7	3.5	3.6	5.5	-	-	23.2	13.0	16.4	13.1	-	-	4.4	1.5	0.25	0.40	3.4	172
Other skin	127	9	-	-	-	-	-	-	17.7	3.6	20.8	10.8	60.8	36.7	58.0	84.3	122.7	157.1	315.6	477.3	34.6		1.12	2.24	22.1	173
Breast	397	5	-	-	-	-	-	12.3	10.6	46.3	138.9	177.0	293.0	209.8	267.0	240.0	343.4	379.7	420.8	365.0	108.1	38.4	5.85	8.80	79.9	174
Uterus unspecified	4	0	-	-	-	-	-	-	-	-	-	-	-	10.5	-	-	8.2	13.1	-	-	1.1	0.4	0.05	0.09	0.7	179
Cervix uteri	29	0	-	-	-	-	-	10.6	14.3	6.9	14.4	22.1	15.7	29.0	13.0	16.4	-	-	-	-	7.9	2.8	0.57	0.71	6.4	180
Placenta	0	0	-	-	-	-	-	-	-	-	-	-	-	-	-	-	-	-	-	-	0.0	0.0	0.00	0.00	0.0	181
Corpus uteri	81	0	-	-	-	-	-	-	7.1	3.6	10.4	18.1	33.2	47.2	116.1	90.8	130.8	26.2	52.6	-	22.1	7.8	1.18	2.29	16.4	182
Ovary etc.	58	0	-	-	-	-	-	8.2	7.1	14.3	17.4	10.8	22.1	62.9	40.6	51.9	40.9	39.3	35.1	28.1	15.8	5.6	0.92	1.38	12.0	183
Other female genital	7	0	-	-	-	-	-	-	-	-	3.5	-	-	-	5.8	-	16.4	26.2	17.5	-	1.9	0.7	0.05	0.13	1.1	184
†Bladder	28	0	-	-	-	-	-	-	3.5	-	-	-	5.5	5.2	17.4	38.9	24.5	78.6	52.6	112.3	7.6	2.7	0.16	0.48	4.7	188
Kidney etc.	11	0	-	-	-	-	-	-	-	-	-	7.2	-	-	11.6	13.0	16.4	13.1	35.1	-	3.0	1.1	0.09	0.24	1.9	189
Eye	0	0	-	-	-	-	-	-	-	-	-	-	-	-	-	-	-	-	-	-	0.0	0.0	0.00	0.00	0.0	190
Brain, nervous system	22	0	3.8	3.8	-	-	4.1	-	-	3.6	3.5	7.2	16.6	5.2	11.6	19.5	16.4	13.1	35.1	28.1	6.0	2.1	0.30	0.48	4.9	191-2
Thyroid	14	0	-	-	-	-	4.2	12.3	-	3.6	-	7.2	11.1	-	11.6	19.5	-	-	-	-	3.8	1.4	0.25	0.35	3.6	193
Other endocrine	2	0	-	-	-	-	-	-	-	3.6	-	3.6	-	-	-	-	-	-	-	-	0.5	0.2	0.04	0.04	0.4	194
Hodgkin's disease	10	0	-	-	-	-	8.4	4.1	-	-	-	-	-	-	5.8	-	24.5	13.1	17.5	28.1	2.7	1.0	0.09	0.21	2.1	201
Non-Hodgkin lymphoma	29	1	-	-	-	-	4.2	-	-	3.6	3.5	3.6	11.1	15.7	11.6	32.4	49.1	26.2	35.1	56.1	7.9	2.8	0.28	0.70	5.5	200,202
Multiple myeloma	13	0	-	-	-	-	-	-	-	-	-	-	3.6	5.5	5.8	32.4	8.2	52.4	-	-	3.5	1.3	0.07	0.28	2.4	203
Lymphoid leukaemia	9	0	3.8	-	-	-	-	-	7.1	-	3.6	-	10.5	-	-	8.2	13.1	17.5	-		2.5	0.9	0.13	0.17	1.9	204
Myeloid leukaemia	18	0	-	-	-	7.5	-	-	-	10.7	6.9	3.6	11.1	5.2	17.4	6.5	8.2	-	35.1	-	4.9	1.7	0.31	0.39	3.9	205
Monocytic leukaemia	0	0	-	-	-	-	-	-	-	-	-	-	-	-	-	-	-	-	-	-	0.0	0.0	0.00	0.00	0.0	206
Other leukaemia	0	0	-	-	-	-	-	-	-	-	-	-	-	-	-	-	-	-	-	-	0.0	0.0	0.00	0.00	0.0	207
Leukaemia unspecified	1	0	-	-	-	-	-	-	-	-	-	-	-	-	-	-	-	6.5	-	-	0.3	0.1	0.00	0.03	0.2	208
Other and unspecified	40	1	-	-	-	-	-	-	-	-	-	7.2	5.5	10.5	34.8	51.9	57.2	65.5	87.7	84.2	10.9	3.9	0.30	0.86	6.9	O&U
All sites	1162	18	7.6	7.6	3.6	7.5	21.0	49.2	74.4	128.4	264.0	307.0	563.8	550.8	841.6	901.5	1242.9	1374.9	1700.6	1600.2	316.5		14.35	25.25	224.2	ALL
All sites but 173	1035	9	7.6	7.6	3.6	7.5	21.0	49.2	56.7	124.8	243.1	296.1	503.0	514.1	783.6	817.2	1120.3	1217.8	1385.0	1123.0	281.9	100.0	13.20	22.98	202.0	ALLb

Rate from 1 case			3.790	3.797	3.601	3.746	4.191	4.103	3.544	3.565	3.474	3.611	5.528	5.246	5.804	6.486	8.177	13.094	17.532	28.074

†Important: see notes on population page

The Netherlands

In the mid-1980s, the existing cancer registry of the Eindhoven region was included in a new organizational set-up for a nationwide Netherlands Cancer Registry. Since 1 January 1989, all Dutch hospitals have been associated with one of the regional cancer registries and all registry data are submitted to the national database. The nine Comprehensive Cancer Centres are responsible for the collection of data at the regional level.

In 1989/1992, the average population of the Netherlands was 15.0 million. The Dutch territory covers 41 574 km^2, 7636 of which are water. The population density was 447 inhabitants per km^2 of land area in 1992. The western part of the country with three major cities, Amsterdam, the Hague and Rotterdam, had a population density exceeding 1000. More than 70% of the employed population in 1992 worked in services, a quarter in industry, while only 4.5% worked in agriculture. The Netherlands have a mixed Protestant/Roman Catholic population, the latter concentrated in the south. However, the percentage of non-religious people is considerable. During the last decades immigration changed the structure of the predominantly white population, especially in the larger cities. The non-Dutch population constituted 4.8% of the total population in 1992. The majority of the non-Dutch population consisted of Turks and Moroccans, most of whom were below the age of 55, as well as citizens of other countries of the European Union. Another 4.7% of the Dutch population in 1992 comprised ethnic minorities originating from the former Dutch colonies of Indonesia, Surinam (Hindustani, Creoles and Javanese) and the Netherlands Antilles.

Accessibility of medical care in the Netherlands is good as a result of the relatively short distances to a hospital and ample supply of various health services. In 1989/1992 life expectancy in the Netherlands was 74 years for males and 80 years for females. The majority of people were covered by the Sickness Benefit Fund, a compulsory social insurance policy for those with lower and intermediate incomes, while the others had private insurance. Virtually all specialized clinicians work in about 100 community hospitals, 8 university and 2 cancer hospitals. Radiotherapy is provided by the cancer hospitals and most university hospitals as well as by 10 regional institutes that serve combinations of community hospitals. The pathologists work in about 70 laboratories, which enter all diagnoses into a nationwide computer system, that also notifies the regional registries.

Since 1988 screening for cervix carcinoma has been carried out by general practitioners among women between 35 and 55 years of age, the exposure rates being less than 30%. However, numerous cervical smears are taken outside the programme. In 1990, a national breast cancer screening programme for women between 50 and 70 years of age was started and in 1992 15.2% of the women in this age group were screened. As of 1997 all women between 50 and 70 will be offered screening every two years.

With the consent of the specialists and institutes, data are collected from the medical records in the hospitals. The coding of data is performed by specially trained co-workers of the cancer registry. They receive lists of newly diagnosed cancer cases from the pathology and haematology departments in their hospital(s) on a regular basis. In addition, lists of hospitalized cancer patients are obtained from the medical records departments. Often, regional cancer registries use other notification sources, e.g., radiotherapy departments. Due to privacy regulations and the absence of a personal identification number, death certificates of the Central Bureau of Statistics cannot be used as an additional source of notification.

Topography and morphology are coded by means of ICD-O. Multiple tumours are recorded according to the following rules: two or more primary tumours are recorded when the interval is three months or more (except for bladder cancer), when they are of different histology with regard to the three-digit morphological code of ICD-O or when the site is different. Multiple tumours are also recognized in paired organs (excluding ovary) and in subsites of colon, rectum, skin, bone and soft tissue. However, incidence rates for this volume were calculated according to IARC/IACR rules. For the staging of tumours, the TNM classification is used. Autopsy data, including malignancies first discovered at autopsy, are included in the registry. All regional cancer registries apply consistency checks (range and cross-checks). An extensive control programme, e.g., for duplicate records, is also applied to the data submitted to the national data bank. For the privacy of those registered, legal and technical guidelines have been created which ensure adequate protection of registered patients and collaborating physicians.

O. Visser
R.A.M. Damhuis
R. Otter
J.W.W. Coebergh
M. Oostindiër
M.W.E. de Kok
C.H.F. Gimbrère
J.P. van Andel
L.J. Schouten

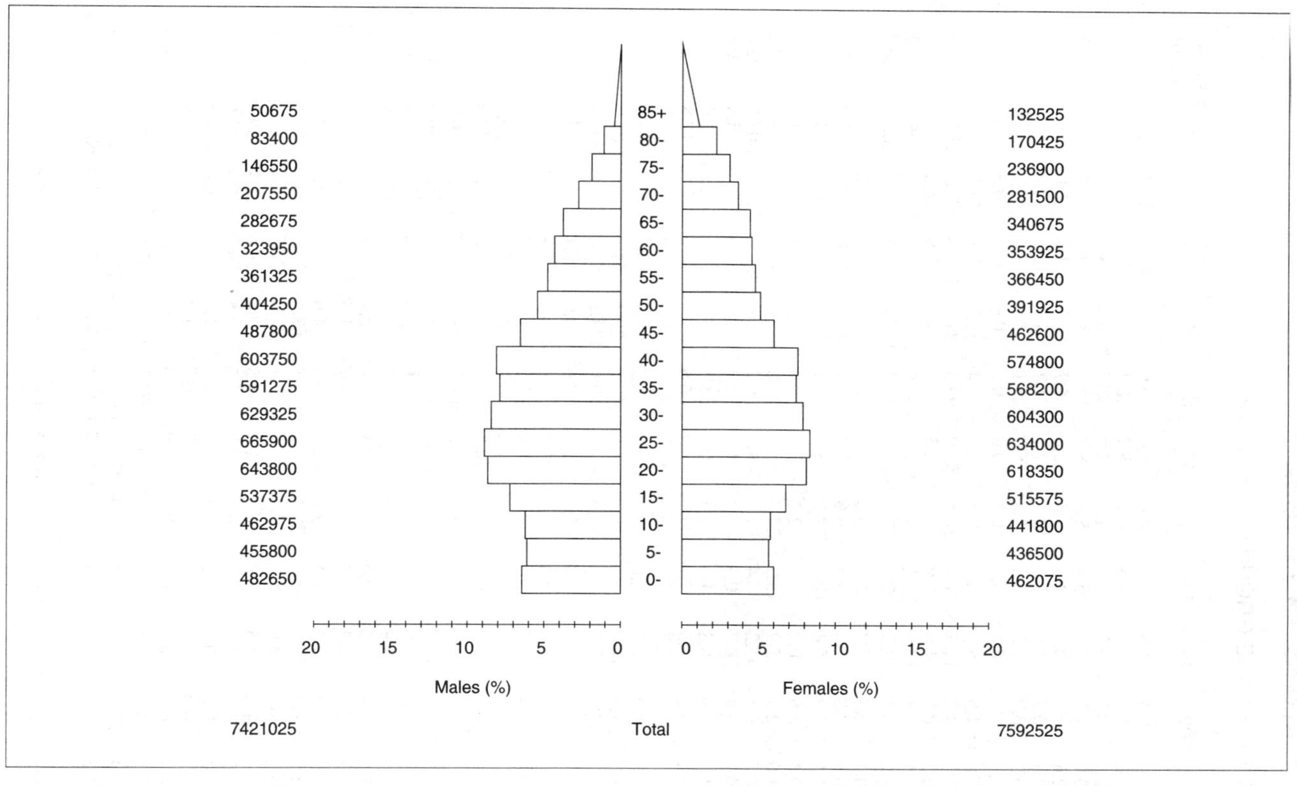

Netherlands

Source of population: average annual 1989–92

Census: Population data are collected from the Municipal Population Registers, which are assumed to be 100% complete. Information is collected and distributed by the Dutch Central Bureau of Statistics for 1 January of each calendar year.

Notes to tables overleaf:

† 173 does not include basal cell carcinomas

† 188 does not include non-invasive tumours

Screening programmes in the area

The population aged 35-55 has been screened for cervical cancer since 1989. Breast cancer screening commenced in 1991 in women aged 50-70 (147 959 examinations in 1991, 289 520 in 1992).

THE NETHERLANDS 1989-1992

ANNUAL INCIDENCE PER 100,000 BY AGE GROUP (YEARS) - MALE

SITE	ALL AGES	AGE UNK	0-	5-	10-	15-	20-	25-	30-	35-	40-	45-	50-	55-	60-	65-	70-	75-	80-	85+	CRUDE RATE	%	CR 64	CR 74	ASR (W)	ICD (9th)
Lip	688	0	-	-	-	0.0	-	0.0	0.4	0.4	0.4	1.3	2.9	4.6	6.6	10.6	11.3	17.1	20.7	24.7	2.3	0.6	0.08	0.19	1.7	140
Tongue	519	0	-	-	-	-	0.1	0.0	0.4	1.0	1.2	2.5	3.5	4.2	5.9	6.3	7.1	7.5	6.9	6.4	1.7	0.4	0.09	0.16	1.4	141
Salivary gland	223	0	-	-	0.2	0.1	-	0.2	0.3	0.1	0.5	0.7	0.8	1.5	2.9	2.7	3.0	4.8	3.6	3.5	0.8	0.2	0.04	0.07	0.6	142
Mouth	782	0	-	-	-	0.0	0.0	-	0.2	0.6	1.7	3.9	5.4	8.3	8.8	10.3	11.2	9.6	8.4	13.8	2.6	0.7	0.15	0.25	2.1	143-5
Oropharynx	487	0	-	0.1	-	-	0.0	-	0.1	0.6	1.2	2.7	3.8	4.8	5.8	6.7	6.9	4.8	6.0	1.0	1.6	0.4	0.09	0.16	1.3	146
Nasopharynx	198	0	0.1	-	0.1	0.1	0.0	0.1	0.3	0.3	0.7	1.0	1.7	2.1	2.1	1.7	1.8	2.0	1.2	3.0	0.7	0.2	0.04	0.06	0.5	147
Hypopharynx	391	0	-	-	-	-	-	-	-	0.2	0.7	2.2	3.3	3.0	5.2	5.1	5.8	4.6	5.1	4.4	1.3	0.3	0.07	0.13	1.1	148
Pharynx unspecified	27	0	-	-	-	-	-	-	-	-	0.1	0.1	0.3	0.2	0.5	0.6	0.7	0.3	-	0.1	0.0	0.00	0.01	0.1	149
Oesophagus	2076	0	-	-	-	-	0.0	0.0	0.1	0.8	1.9	5.9	8.3	17.4	22.5	33.4	39.3	41.1	51.3	48.8	7.0	1.8	0.28	0.65	5.2	150
Stomach	6394	0	-	-	-	-	0.1	0.4	1.1	2.5	4.3	11.3	21.4	38.5	55.9	93.3	131.5	173.5	223.3	212.1	21.5	5.5	0.68	1.80	15.4	151
Small intestine	261	0	-	-	-	0.0	0.0	-	0.2	0.2	0.5	1.0	0.9	1.7	2.5	4.2	4.0	5.8	6.3	5.4	0.9	0.2	0.04	0.08	0.7	152
Colon	9100	0	-	0.2	0.3	1.2	0.8	1.2	2.0	3.5	9.1	15.9	25.2	49.5	80.9	133.0	181.9	255.7	318.3	296.5	30.7	7.8	0.95	2.52	21.9	153
Rectum	5925	0	-	-	-	0.0	0.2	0.6	1.1	2.5	6.1	12.2	22.8	37.1	59.2	88.2	116.7	145.9	182.6	162.3	20.0	5.1	0.71	1.73	14.5	154
Liver	610	0	0.5	-	0.2	0.1	0.2	0.3	0.3	0.4	0.8	0.9	1.9	3.8	6.7	10.7	11.0	13.3	12.6	12.3	2.1	0.5	0.08	0.19	1.6	155
Gallbladder etc.	868	0	-	0.1	-	-	0.0	0.0	-	0.3	0.8	1.3	3.5	4.6	7.5	13.1	18.7	20.0	29.4	37.0	2.9	0.7	0.09	0.25	2.1	156
Pancreas	2762	0	-	-	0.1	0.0	0.1	0.2	0.2	1.1	1.9	5.4	10.0	17.0	28.9	43.3	59.3	66.7	84.2	68.1	9.3	2.4	0.32	0.84	6.8	157
Nose, sinuses etc.	316	0	0.1	0.2	-	-	0.0	0.1	0.2	0.3	0.5	0.8	1.6	2.2	3.5	3.7	7.3	5.5	7.2	4.4	1.1	0.3	0.05	0.10	0.8	160
Larynx	2426	0	-	-	-	-	-	-	0.1	1.0	2.7	5.9	13.3	22.8	33.9	38.6	44.6	41.8	35.4	33.1	8.2	2.1	0.40	0.81	6.3	161
Bronchus, lung	29631	0	-	-	0.1	-	0.0	0.4	1.2	4.5	16.1	41.2	88.4	197.3	344.1	509.2	713.0	800.1	705.3	407.5	99.8	25.5	3.47	9.58	73.0	162
Other thoracic organs	189	0	0.1	-	0.1	0.1	0.3	0.2	0.3	0.1	0.4	0.7	0.5	1.0	1.5	2.4	2.2	4.6	2.7	6.4	0.6	0.2	0.03	0.05	0.5	163-4
Bone	293	0	0.1	0.3	1.3	2.6	1.2	0.6	0.6	1.0	0.6	0.8	1.1	1.4	0.9	1.1	1.3	1.4	2.1	1.0	1.0	0.3	0.06	0.07	0.9	170
Connective tissue	926	0	1.2	0.5	0.7	1.3	1.2	1.8	1.4	2.4	3.0	3.3	3.7	4.2	6.9	6.6	11.1	12.3	18.3	17.8	3.1	0.8	0.16	0.25	2.6	171
Mesothelioma	1013	0	-	-	-	-	0.0	-	0.2	0.2	1.0	2.7	5.8	9.9	10.7	17.4	18.8	20.0	16.8	12.3	3.4	0.9	0.15	0.33	2.6	MES
Kaposi's sarcoma	448	0	-	-	-	-	0.2	1.9	3.1	3.8	4.2	2.5	2.0	0.7	0.5	0.8	0.7	0.3	3.5	1.5	0.4	0.09	0.10	1.2	KAP
Melanoma of skin	2554	0	-	0.1	0.1	1.2	3.1	4.9	6.4	9.2	11.9	14.6	15.7	16.7	17.9	19.6	20.1	21.5	21.6	26.1	8.6	2.2	0.51	0.71	6.9	172
†Other skin	6426	0	-	0.1	-	0.6	0.5	0.9	1.2	2.2	4.6	7.2	14.3	26.4	47.3	80.0	134.5	186.8	265.6	401.1	21.6		0.53	1.60	15.0	173
Breast	176	0	-	-	-	-	0.0	0.0	0.0	-	0.2	0.5	0.8	1.5	1.5	2.6	3.9	3.1	4.5	4.4	0.6	0.2	0.02	0.06	0.4	175
Prostate	17659	0	-	-	-	-	-	-	-	0.0	0.6	3.0	14.0	44.6	120.4	255.9	455.8	674.3	817.7	886.0	59.5	15.2	0.91	4.47	39.6	185
Testis	1389	0	0.8	0.1	0.3	2.9	7.3	10.1	10.2	9.0	4.9	4.5	3.6	2.8	1.9	1.5	1.6	1.7	1.5	-	4.7	1.2	0.29	0.31	4.0	186
Penis	303	0	-	-	-	-	-	-	0.1	0.2	0.5	0.8	1.7	1.7	1.5	3.4	4.9	8.0	9.6	20.2	1.0	0.3	0.03	0.07	0.7	187.1-.4
Other male genital	43	0	0.1	-	0.1	0.0	-	0.0	0.0	-	0.1	0.1	0.1	0.2	0.5	0.8	0.8	0.5	1.2	0.5	0.1	0.0	0.01	0.01	0.1	187.5-.9
†Bladder	6317	0	0.1	0.1	-	-	0.1	0.0	0.5	1.3	2.4	7.0	16.6	33.7	60.8	104.3	138.0	172.8	218.5	226.9	21.3	5.4	0.61	1.83	15.2	188
Kidney etc.	3939	0	2.0	0.5	0.2	0.0	0.2	0.5	0.5	2.2	4.7	11.9	18.6	30.6	42.7	62.1	71.7	85.5	77.6	50.8	13.3	3.4	0.57	1.24	10.2	189
Eye	280	0	1.5	0.1	0.1	-	0.1	0.2	0.1	0.5	1.0	0.8	1.2	1.3	2.4	3.6	3.6	3.4	5.1	4.9	0.9	0.2	0.05	0.08	0.8	190
Brain, nervous system	2005	0	3.7	4.0	3.3	1.7	2.4	2.7	3.8	4.1	5.9	8.3	11.3	12.5	17.2	21.0	16.7	17.7	14.1	6.9	6.8	1.7	0.41	0.59	6.0	191-2
Thyroid	341	0	-	-	-	0.2	0.5	0.6	1.0	1.4	1.4	1.5	2.0	2.3	2.1	2.4	3.4	3.4	5.1	2.0	1.1	0.3	0.06	0.09	0.9	193
Other endocrine	133	0	1.1	0.4	0.3	0.2	0.2	0.1	0.2	0.3	0.1	0.3	0.4	0.8	1.2	1.1	1.3	0.7	1.2	-	0.4	0.1	0.03	0.04	0.5	194
Hodgkin's disease	839	0	0.2	0.3	1.3	2.7	3.9	3.5	4.5	3.1	3.2	2.3	2.4	2.6	3.3	3.6	4.6	4.3	5.4	2.5	2.8	0.7	0.17	0.21	2.4	201
Non-Hodgkin lymphoma	4033	0	1.2	1.9	1.7	1.9	2.1	3.3	4.6	5.5	9.2	14.2	18.1	23.4	34.4	47.8	68.5	73.0	75.8	74.5	13.6	3.5	0.61	1.19	10.6	200,202
Multiple myeloma	1394	0	-	-	-	-	0.0	0.1	0.2	0.7	1.7	3.0	5.8	7.3	14.7	21.1	27.0	37.7	37.2	35.5	4.7	1.2	0.17	0.41	3.4	203
Lymphoid leukaemia	1290	0	4.7	3.2	1.6	2.1	0.7	0.4	0.5	0.9	1.0	1.5	3.8	6.3	9.7	14.8	20.8	26.6	28.2	39.5	4.3	1.1	0.18	0.36	3.8	204
Myeloid leukaemia	1210	0	0.7	0.5	0.4	0.6	0.9	0.9	1.0	2.2	1.9	3.1	5.4	6.8	9.7	15.2	17.5	24.7	29.7	31.6	4.1	1.0	0.17	0.33	3.2	205
Monocytic leukaemia	66	0	0.3	-	-	0.0	-	-	0.1	0.0	0.0	0.2	0.1	0.2	0.3	0.4	0.9	1.1	1.2	2.4	0.2	0.1	0.01	0.02	0.2	206
Other leukaemia	68	0	-	-	-	-	0.0	-	0.2	0.0	0.0	0.1	0.2	0.3	0.7	0.7	1.2	1.9	0.9	5.4	0.2	0.1	0.01	0.02	0.2	207
Leukaemia unspecified	128	0	0.4	0.1	0.2	0.0	0.0	0.1	0.1	0.2	0.1	0.1	0.2	0.5	0.9	1.3	2.0	2.9	5.7	3.9	0.4	0.1	0.02	0.03	0.3	208
Other and unspecified	5706	0	0.3	0.1	0.1	0.3	0.4	0.8	1.2	2.7	4.7	9.7	19.6	39.6	55.9	84.5	120.7	142.4	160.7	159.3	19.2	4.9	0.68	1.70	14.0	O&U
All sites	122852	0	19.0	12.8	12.6	20.1	27.3	37.3	50.0	73.4	120.7	220.7	388.1	700.4	1150.9	1791.1	2528.9	3153.4	3537.5	3369.0	413.9		14.17	35.77	303.4	ALL
All sites but 173	116426	0	19.0	12.7	12.6	19.5	26.7	36.4	48.7	71.2	116.2	213.6	373.8	674.0	1103.6	1711.1	2394.4	2966.6	3271.9	2967.9	392.2	100.0	13.64	34.17	288.4	ALLb

Rate from 10 cases   0.518   0.548   0.540   0.465   0.388   0.375   0.397   0.423   0.414   0.513   0.618   0.692   0.772   0.884   1.205   1.706   2.998   4.933

†Important: see notes on population page

THE NETHERLANDS 1989-1992

ANNUAL INCIDENCE PER 100,000 BY AGE GROUP (YEARS) - FEMALE

SITE	ALL AGES	AGE UNK	0-	5-	10-	15-	20-	25-	30-	35-	40-	45-	50-	55-	60-	65-	70-	75-	80-	85+	CRUDE RATE	%	CR 64	CR 74	ASR (W)	ICD (9th)
Lip	119	0	-	-	-	-	-	-	-	0.0	0.1	0.2	0.3	0.8	0.8	0.9	2.0	2.1	2.2	2.8	0.4	0.1	0.01	0.03	0.2	140
Tongue	357	0	-	-	-	-	0.2	0.1	0.2	0.4	0.9	1.2	1.5	3.1	2.8	2.9	3.6	5.2	3.4	6.2	1.2	0.3	0.05	0.08	0.8	141
Salivary gland	201	0	-	-	0.1	0.0	0.2	0.3	0.4	0.5	0.5	0.5	1.0	1.2	1.2	1.2	2.3	2.0	2.6	2.8	0.7	0.2	0.03	0.05	0.4	142
Mouth	498	0	0.1	-	-	-	0.1	0.1	0.2	0.4	1.1	2.4	3.1	3.8	4.0	3.8	4.0	5.5	6.3	10.0	1.6	0.5	0.08	0.12	1.1	143-5
Oropharynx	209	0	0.1	-	-	0.0	-	-	0.0	0.1	0.9	1.7	1.8	2.3	2.0	1.5	1.6	1.1	1.0	0.9	0.7	0.2	0.04	0.06	0.5	146
Nasopharynx	83	0	-	-	0.1	0.1	0.1	0.1	0.2	0.2	0.1	0.4	0.5	0.8	0.7	0.1	0.4	0.6	0.9	0.8	0.3	0.1	0.02	0.02	0.2	147
Hypopharynx	105	0	-	-	-	-	-	-	-	0.0	0.3	0.4	0.5	0.8	0.8	0.9	0.8	2.0	1.5	1.7	0.3	0.1	0.01	0.02	0.2	148
Pharynx unspecified	11	0	-	-	-	-	-	0.0	-	-	0.0	-	0.1	0.1	0.1	-	0.1	0.1	0.3	0.2	0.0	0.0	0.00	0.00	0.0	149
Oesophagus	1102	0	-	-	-	-	-	-	0.0	0.3	0.8	2.5	3.3	4.6	6.3	9.8	15.8	19.9	26.4	26.4	3.6	1.0	0.09	0.22	1.9	150
Stomach	3723	0	-	-	-	0.0	0.1	0.7	1.1	1.5	3.0	5.2	7.3	14.1	21.5	33.5	43.6	73.4	97.0	102.8	12.3	3.5	0.27	0.66	6.1	151
Small intestine	231	0	-	0.1	-	-	0.0	0.0	0.0	0.3	0.4	0.5	0.6	1.0	1.3	3.1	3.2	3.7	4.5	2.6	0.8	0.2	0.02	0.05	0.4	152
Colon	10804	0	-	0.2	0.8	1.6	1.7	1.5	2.2	3.7	8.3	15.4	28.4	45.0	70.9	106.8	148.7	208.6	236.8	232.4	35.6	10.2	0.90	2.18	18.9	153
Rectum	4773	0	-	-	-	0.0	0.2	0.2	0.9	1.8	4.0	8.6	17.0	24.6	37.3	52.4	67.0	80.8	89.9	84.5	15.7	4.5	0.47	1.07	8.9	154
Liver	336	0	0.2	-	-	0.0	0.1	0.3	0.0	0.3	0.7	0.4	1.0	1.1	2.3	3.0	5.2	5.7	6.2	5.8	1.1	0.3	0.03	0.07	0.6	155
Gallbladder etc.	1606	0	-	0.1	-	-	0.1	0.1	0.2	0.4	0.7	1.3	2.9	6.5	9.4	16.3	25.0	29.9	42.0	37.7	5.3	1.5	0.11	0.31	2.6	156
Pancreas	2651	0	-	-	0.1	-	0.1	0.2	0.2	0.7	1.9	3.9	6.1	12.5	20.2	26.3	38.3	50.1	56.0	56.6	8.7	2.5	0.23	0.55	4.6	157
Nose, sinuses etc.	153	0	-	-	-	-	0.0	0.2	-	0.3	0.3	0.4	0.6	0.8	1.3	1.2	2.0	2.0	2.9	1.7	0.5	0.1	0.02	0.04	0.3	160
Larynx	332	0	-	-	-	-	0.0	0.1	0.2	0.8	1.3	2.7	4.0	4.2	3.6	2.4	2.3	2.3	1.5	1.1	0.3	0.07	0.10	0.8	161
Bronchus, lung	5694	0	-	-	0.1	0.0	0.2	0.4	2.2	5.2	9.7	19.0	31.8	50.1	70.4	68.0	66.8	57.3	46.1	31.3	18.7	5.4	0.95	1.62	13.0	162
Other thoracic organs	75	0	-	-	-	-	0.0	0.1	0.2	0.2	0.3	0.2	0.1	0.5	0.4	0.8	1.2	0.7	0.4	0.6	0.2	0.1	0.01	0.02	0.2	163-4
Bone	225	0	0.1	0.4	1.3	1.3	0.7	0.6	0.7	0.4	0.5	0.6	0.4	0.8	0.8	1.2	1.2	1.3	0.9	1.5	0.7	0.2	0.04	0.05	0.7	170
Connective tissue	750	0	1.5	0.4	1.0	0.8	0.9	1.1	1.4	1.7	1.2	1.7	2.2	4.0	4.2	5.6	7.2	8.5	9.2	9.1	2.5	0.7	0.11	0.17	1.8	171
Mesothelioma	151	0	-	-	-	-	-	0.0	-	0.2	0.1	0.6	0.4	1.3	1.4	2.2	1.9	2.1	1.6	0.9	0.5	0.1	0.02	0.04	0.3	MES
Kaposi's sarcoma	16	0	-	-	-	-	-	-	0.1	-	0.1	-	0.1	0.1	-	0.1	0.1	0.3	0.1	0.6	0.1	0.0	0.00	0.00	0.0	KAP
Melanoma of skin	3852	0	0.1	0.1	0.2	2.2	6.4	9.9	12.4	14.9	18.1	21.0	19.9	21.9	21.5	22.0	20.8	20.2	22.9	24.0	12.7	3.6	0.74	0.96	9.8	172
†Other skin	3654	0	-	-	0.2	0.3	0.3	0.9	1.0	1.5	3.0	4.9	8.7	10.7	14.9	26.3	41.1	62.6	84.8	169.8	12.0		0.23	0.57	5.7	173
Breast	34939	0	-	-	-	0.0	1.2	7.9	31.2	65.6	126.3	185.5	219.9	233.2	274.6	327.6	322.7	340.5	355.6	306.2	115.0	32.9	5.73	8.98	79.6	174
Uterus unspecified	18	0	-	-	-	-	-	-	0.0	-	0.1	0.1	0.1	-	0.1	0.4	0.2	0.3	0.4	0.1	0.0	0.00	0.00	0.0	179
Cervix uteri	2939	0	-	-	-	0.1	1.2	4.7	13.1	19.3	14.7	13.7	12.8	11.3	15.0	18.7	21.5	18.0	19.4	12.1	9.7	2.8	0.53	0.73	7.1	180
Placenta	30	0	-	-	-	-	0.1	0.5	0.2	0.1	0.1	0.1	-	-	0.1	-	-	-	-	0.1	0.0	0.01	0.01	0.1	181
Corpus uteri	5129	0	-	-	-	-	0.1	0.1	0.5	2.2	6.0	10.4	28.3	42.7	50.9	59.3	71.0	67.3	60.3	53.6	16.9	4.8	0.71	1.36	10.8	182
Ovary etc.	5013	0	-	0.3	0.5	0.9	1.4	2.5	3.8	6.4	11.4	18.0	28.3	36.4	43.2	54.3	56.1	56.9	51.0	38.3	16.5	4.7	0.77	1.32	11.2	183
Other female genital	1115	0	-	-	-	-	0.1	0.3	0.7	0.7	0.9	1.3	3.5	4.6	6.1	9.1	14.5	21.1	28.9	25.7	3.7	1.0	0.09	0.21	1.9	184
†Bladder	1776	0	-	-	-	0.0	0.0	0.1	0.1	0.4	1.2	2.6	4.1	8.2	12.1	18.3	21.6	31.1	40.0	50.6	5.8	1.7	0.14	0.34	3.0	188
Kidney etc.	2552	0	1.6	0.9	-	-	0.1	0.4	0.5	1.0	2.4	5.9	9.6	17.2	22.9	29.9	34.7	39.4	35.2	30.2	8.4	2.4	0.31	0.63	5.3	189
Eye	238	0	1.5	0.1	-	-	0.0	0.1	0.2	0.3	0.5	0.7	0.8	1.6	2.3	2.4	2.7	2.5	1.5	0.9	0.8	0.2	0.04	0.07	0.7	190
Brain, nervous system	1464	0	2.5	2.9	1.8	1.7	2.1	2.4	2.8	3.0	3.8	5.3	8.1	8.1	10.9	11.7	11.1	10.4	9.7	3.2	4.8	1.4	0.28	0.39	4.1	191-2
Thyroid	892	0	-	0.1	0.2	0.8	1.8	2.2	2.6	3.3	3.8	4.1	3.6	2.7	5.2	6.6	6.9	5.7	7.3	5.7	2.9	0.8	0.15	0.22	2.2	193
Other endocrine	111	0	1.2	0.3	-	0.2	0.1	0.0	0.1	0.2	0.2	0.4	0.4	0.5	1.1	0.5	0.5	1.1	0.7	-	0.4	0.1	0.02	0.03	0.4	194
Hodgkin's disease	578	0	-	0.2	0.8	3.4	3.5	2.8	2.2	1.5	1.9	1.5	0.8	1.4	1.8	2.5	2.4	2.6	2.9	1.7	1.9	0.5	0.11	0.13	1.7	201
Non-Hodgkin lymphoma	3433	0	0.5	1.1	0.9	1.1	1.3	1.9	2.2	3.8	5.8	9.5	12.6	17.8	21.5	32.1	43.3	47.7	60.9	54.1	11.3	3.2	0.40	0.78	7.0	200,202
Multiple myeloma	1271	0	-	-	-	-	-	-	0.2	0.6	0.7	1.8	2.6	5.9	10.1	14.7	19.0	22.2	28.6	21.1	4.2	1.2	0.11	0.28	2.3	203
Lymphoid leukaemia	917	0	4.7	2.1	1.4	0.5	0.6	0.2	0.3	0.4	0.7	0.7	2.0	2.7	5.4	8.2	9.1	12.1	17.6	18.5	3.0	0.9	0.11	0.19	2.3	204
Myeloid leukaemia	969	0	0.3	0.3	0.8	0.5	0.8	1.3	1.2	1.8	1.8	2.2	2.7	5.5	5.7	7.7	10.3	14.2	14.5	13.4	3.2	0.9	0.12	0.21	2.1	205
Monocytic leukaemia	44	0	0.1	0.1	-	0.0	0.0	0.1	-	-	0.2	0.3	0.1	0.1	0.3	0.6	0.4	0.6	0.8	-	0.1	0.0	0.01	0.01	0.1	206
Other leukaemia	34	0	0.3	-	-	-	-	0.0	-	-	0.1	0.1	0.1	0.3	0.1	0.4	0.4	0.5	0.4	-	0.1	0.0	0.00	0.01	0.1	207
Leukaemia unspecified	99	0	0.5	0.1	0.1	0.1	0.1	0.0	0.1	0.0	0.2	0.2	0.1	0.1	0.6	0.5	0.7	1.2	2.1	3.2	0.3	0.1	0.01	0.02	0.2	208
Other and unspecified	4734	0	0.4	0.1	-	0.1	0.2	0.6	1.2	2.7	4.9	7.7	14.4	22.2	33.4	44.1	59.2	83.2	103.7	107.3	15.6	4.5	0.44	0.96	8.5	O&U
All sites	110006	0	15.5	9.6	10.2	16.5	26.3	44.9	87.0	148.3	245.5	366.2	497.1	639.4	824.0	1042.4	1214.7	1426.7	1589.6	1562.2	362.2		14.65	25.94	230.7	ALL
All sites but 173	106352	0	15.5	9.6	10.0	16.1	26.0	44.0	86.0	146.8	242.5	361.4	488.4	628.7	809.1	1016.1	1173.6	1364.1	1504.8	1392.4	350.2	100.0	14.42	25.37	225.0	ALLb

Rate from 10 cases   0.541   0.573   0.566   0.485   0.404   0.394   0.414   0.440   0.435   0.540   0.638   0.682   0.706   0.734   0.888   1.055   1.467   1.886

†Important: see notes on population page

Netherlands, Eindhoven

This regional registry began operation in 1955 as part of a programme for nationwide cancer registration. The original 13 participating hospitals have now been reduced to 8. The registry has always cooperated systematically with three pathology laboratories, which have a bank of paraffin-embedded blocks of biopsy specimens from all patients since the 1970s, and it has access to the medical records of most hospitals. The regional Department of Radiotherapy in Eindhoven, which has gradually extended service to all of these hospitals, was the basis of operation until 1983. The growing interest in oncology was formalized in 1979 by the establishment of a regional organization, the Cooperative Association of Hospitals in Oncology (SOOZ). In 1982 the Comprehensive Cancer Centre South (IKZ) was founded as a collaborative effort of 18 community hospitals and the radiotherapy institutes in Eindhoven and Tilburg, and one of its tasks is cancer registration. The registry now functions within the scope of a national scheme for cancer registration which was introduced in 1984 and has published information on cancer incidence since 1989.

Assessment of completeness and accuracy was carried out in the period 1980–83 with the support of the Department of Epidemiology of the Erasmus University, Rotterdam, and the National Institute of Health and Environmental Hygiene (RIVM). The database was computerized for patients registered since 1974. All data on patients registered during the period 1955–74 were fed into the computer during 1991. This has permitted extensive analyses of the incidence since 1960, e.g., for lung and breast cancer, both of which exhibited major changes. Incidence rates are available back to 1958 for most sites, including non-melanoma skin cancer. Using the municipal population registers, active follow-up with respect to vital status was performed in 1987, 1991 and 1994. The percentage of patients lost to follow-up declined from 5% to less than 1%. An overview of trends in incidence and survival of patients registered during the period 1955–94, with detailed information on uncommon tumours and stage since 1970, was published, including data on prevalence and co-morbidity. Cancer survival and patterns of care have also been studied within the framework of the EUROCARE study.

The registry serves an area of about 2500 km^2, which lies 20 to 50 m above sea level and includes almost one million inhabitants (6% of the 1990 Dutch population). Since 1988 another one million people have been added; their data are included in the national registry but not, for reasons of continuity, in this data-set. The population density is about 400 per km^2, roughly the national average; 47% of the population-at-risk live in urban, 43% in suburban and 10% in rural municipalities.

In the past 20 years an intensive pig and poultry breeding industry has been developed, now contributing considerably to acid rain and a rising nitrate level in ground water. The main industries produce electronic goods, cars and trucks, photocopiers, textiles and food products. The tobacco-processing industry, important in the Eindhoven area until the 1980s, had a marked effect on the incidence of lung cancer among males, whose prevalence of smoking was 95% in the 1950s; by contrast the prevalence of smoking and incidence of smoking-related cancers among females were very low until the 1970s. Zinc factories, situated along the border with Belgium since 1900, caused marked pollution of the soil with cadmium. Relatively high concentrations in the air of ozone, lead, nitrogen monoxide and sulfur dioxide, coming mainly from surrounding industrialized regions and automobile traffic, have been declining in the last decade.

Some 60% of the inhabitants are covered by Sickness Benefit Funds, a compulsory social insurance policy for people with low income; less than 1% of the population is uninsured. There is good access to clinical specialists, generally through general practitioners, one for every 2200 persons. The number of hospital beds has decreased from 5 to 3 per 1000 persons in the past 20 years, while the number of nursing home beds has increased markedly, as well as, more recently, home care provision. At the end of the 1980s the hospitals generally comprised 400 to 700 beds. During the period 1988–92 screening for cervical cancer among women 35–55 years of age received renewed attention; and biannual screening for breast cancer among women between 50 and 70 years started during 1992.

During the period 1988–92 the decentralized and active registration procedures remained largely unchanged; however coding was refined within the framework of the newly developed national registration. At the registration office data, coded according to ICD-9 and ICD-O and the TNM staging manuals, are entered directly into the computer (starting in 1986). Application of the recent IARC coding rules for multiple primaries results in slightly lower rates, for breast, lung and colorectal cancer also for the previous periods.

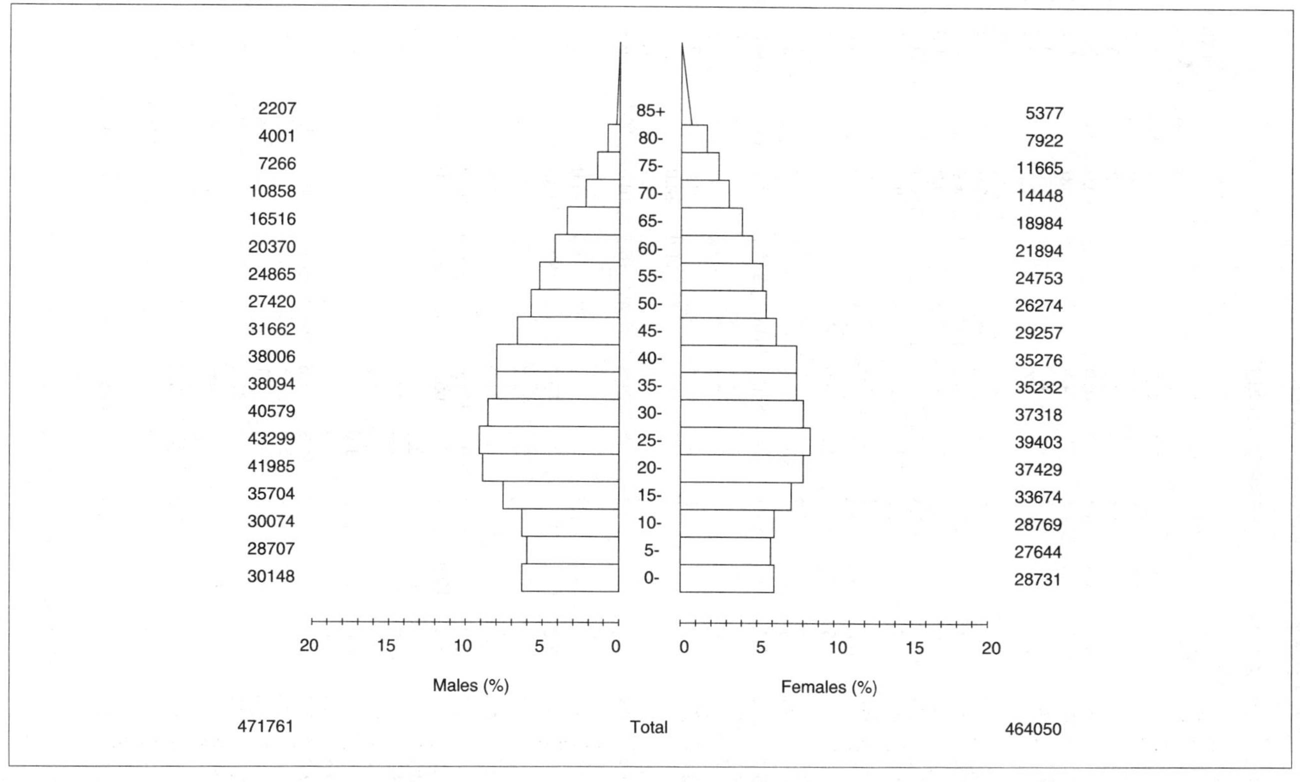

Netherlands, Eindhoven

Source of population: average annual 1988–92

Census: Population data are collected from the Municipal Population Registers, which are assumed to be 100% complete. Information is collected and distributed by the Dutch Central Bureau of Statistics for 1 January of each calendar year.

Notes to tables overleaf:

† 173 Diagnoses of basal cell carcinoma are collected in a core area of approximately 650,000 persons, and were calculated with a separate denominator:

Screening programmes in the area:

A screening programme for breast cancer started in 1992, to examine 80% of the female population aged 50-69 every two years.

Basal cell carcinoma	Male Age-specific rate	Female Age-specific rate
0-	-	-
5-	-	-
10-	-	-
15-	0.8	1.7
20-	2.0	-
25-	2.6	4.3
30-	9.0	15.3
35-	17.8	30.5
40-	42.0	45.5
45-	78.2	84.3
50-	115.2	76.0
55-	153.6	115.5
60-	203.2	159.9
65-	319.8	188.1
70-	399.4	253.1
75-	489.2	360.0
80-	509.9	394.6
85+	617.1	447.6
Crude rate	70.7	68.6
Cum 64	3.12	2.66
Cum 74	6.72	4.87
ASR World	57.4	44.4

NETHERLANDS, EINDHOVEN 1988-1992

ANNUAL INCIDENCE PER 100,000 BY AGE GROUP (YEARS) - MALE

SITE	ALL AGES	AGE UNK	0-	5-	10-	15-	20-	25-	30-	35-	40-	45-	50-	55-	60-	65-	70-	75-	80-	85+	CRUDE RATE	%	CR 64	CR 74	ASR (W)	ICD (9th)
Lip	68	0	-	-	-	-	-	-	-	0.5	-	1.3	2.2	3.2	5.9	15.7	23.9	30.3	45.0	54.4	2.9	0.8	0.07	0.26	**2.3**	*140*
Tongue	29	0	-	-	-	-	-	-	-	-	0.5	3.2	2.2	2.4	6.9	2.4	7.4	5.5	10.0	-	1.2	0.3	0.08	0.12	**1.0**	*141*
Salivary gland	13	0	-	-	-	-	-	1.0	0.5	1.1	-	-	2.4	1.0	2.4	-	2.8	5.0	-	-	0.6	0.2	0.03	0.04	**0.4**	*142*
Mouth	60	0	-	-	-	-	-	-	-	-	1.1	3.8	7.3	6.4	6.9	10.9	16.6	2.8	10.0	54.4	2.5	0.7	0.13	0.26	**2.2**	*143-5*
Oropharynx	33	0	-	0.7	-	-	-	-	-	0.5	0.5	1.3	2.9	2.4	7.9	4.8	9.2	8.3	5.0	-	1.4	0.4	0.08	0.15	**1.2**	*146*
Nasopharynx	14	0	-	-	-	-	-	-	-	1.1	0.5	1.9	1.5	1.6	1.0	1.2	3.7	-	-	-	0.6	0.2	0.04	0.06	**0.5**	*147*
Hypopharynx	18	0	-	-	-	-	-	-	-	0.5	-	1.3	-	4.8	2.9	3.6	3.7	-	5.0	-	0.8	0.2	0.05	0.08	**0.6**	*148*
Pharynx unspecified	1	0	-	-	-	-	-	-	-	-	-	-	-	-	-	-	1.8	-	-	-	0.0	0.0	0.00	0.01	**0.0**	*149*
Oesophagus	103	0	-	-	-	-	-	-	-	0.5	0.5	3.8	5.1	18.5	12.8	18.2	35.0	27.5	25.0	27.2	4.4	1.2	0.21	0.47	**3.6**	*150*
Stomach	498	0	-	-	-	-	-	0.9	2.0	2.6	4.7	11.4	21.2	42.6	54.0	96.9	158.4	211.9	254.9	262.8	21.1	5.7	0.70	1.97	**17.0**	*151*
Small intestine	24	0	-	-	-	-	-	-	-	-	-	1.9	1.5	0.8	2.9	6.1	9.2	5.5	10.0	9.1	1.0	0.3	0.04	0.11	**0.9**	*152*
Colon	686	0	-	-	-	0.6	1.4	0.9	3.0	3.2	8.4	15.2	27.0	64.3	105.1	153.8	167.6	291.8	234.9	299.0	29.1	7.9	1.14	2.75	**23.7**	*153*
Rectum	488	0	-	-	-	-	-	0.9	1.0	4.7	4.7	10.7	24.1	44.2	75.6	88.4	141.8	162.4	219.9	280.9	20.7	5.6	0.83	1.98	**17.0**	*154*
Liver	34	0	1.3	-	-	-	-	-	-	-	0.5	1.9	-	2.4	2.9	8.5	9.2	19.3	5.0	18.1	1.4	0.4	0.05	0.13	**1.3**	*155*
Gallbladder etc.	61	0	-	-	-	-	-	-	-	0.5	-	0.6	2.9	2.4	3.9	19.4	14.7	30.3	40.0	45.3	2.6	0.7	0.05	0.22	**2.1**	*156*
Pancreas	174	0	-	-	-	-	-	-	0.5	1.1	1.1	2.5	9.5	16.9	21.6	46.0	47.9	74.3	45.0	81.6	7.4	2.0	0.27	0.74	**6.0**	*157*
Nose, sinuses etc.	24	0	0.7	0.7	-	-	-	-	-	0.5	-	1.3	-	2.4	3.9	3.6	9.2	5.5	5.0	9.1	1.0	0.3	0.05	0.11	**0.9**	*160*
Larynx	232	0	-	-	-	-	-	-	-	-	2.1	2.1	6.3	15.3	28.2	35.3	65.4	55.3	71.6	35.0	45.3	9.8	2.7	0.45	1.05	**8.1**	*161*
Bronchus, lung	2359	0	-	-	0.7	-	-	0.5	0.5	5.3	13.2	32.2	92.6	218.8	378.0	570.3	814.1	955.1	854.7	498.4	100.0	27.2	3.71	10.63	**81.4**	*162*
Other thoracic organs	9	0	-	-	-	-	0.5	0.5	0.5	1.1	0.5	-	-	-	1.0	1.2	-	-	-	9.1	0.4	0.1	0.02	0.03	**0.3**	*163-4*
Bone	28	0	-	1.4	2.0	2.8	1.4	0.5	1.0	-	1.6	0.6	0.7	1.6	-	2.4	3.7	2.8	-	-	1.2	0.3	0.07	0.10	**1.2**	*170*
Connective tissue	67	0	2.0	-	1.3	1.7	1.0	0.5	1.5	3.2	2.1	1.9	2.2	5.6	9.8	8.5	9.2	13.8	10.0	9.1	2.8	0.8	0.16	0.25	**2.5**	*171*
Mesothelioma	45	0	-	-	-	-	-	-	0.5	-	1.1	-	3.6	10.5	5.9	8.5	5.5	11.0	20.0	-	1.9	0.5	0.11	0.18	**1.5**	*MES*
Kaposi's sarcoma	6	0	-	-	-	-	-	0.5	1.0	-	1.1	-	0.7	-	-	-	-	-	-	-	0.3	0.1	0.02	0.02	**0.2**	*KAP*
Melanoma of skin	161	0	-	-	-	-	2.9	4.6	5.9	7.4	8.4	12.0	11.7	12.9	11.8	21.8	18.4	16.5	10.0	36.2	6.8	1.9	0.39	0.59	**5.6**	*172*
†Other skin																										
Breast	16	0	-	-	-	-	-	-	1.0	0.5	0.5	-	0.7	1.6	2.0	1.2	3.7	5.5	5.0	9.1	0.7	0.2	0.03	0.06	**0.5**	*175*
Prostate	1053	0	-	-	-	-	-	-	-	-	-	3.2	16.8	48.3	132.5	219.2	405.2	580.8	734.8	643.3	44.6	12.2	1.00	4.13	**35.6**	*185*
Testis	103	0	-	-	-	2.8	8.6	11.1	7.4	6.3	4.2	5.1	3.6	1.6	2.0	3.6	1.8	-	-	-	4.4	1.2	0.26	0.29	**3.7**	*186*
Penis	21	0	-	-	-	-	-	0.5	0.5	-	-	0.6	2.2	0.8	2.9	1.2	3.7	2.8	25.0	18.1	0.9	0.2	0.04	0.06	**0.7**	*187.1-.4*
Other male genital	4	0	-	-	-	-	-	-	-	-	0.5	-	-	-	-	1.2	-	-	10.0	-	0.2	0.0	0.00	0.01	**0.1**	*187.5-.9*
Bladder	738	0	-	-	-	-	0.5	0.5	1.5	1.6	6.3	13.9	28.4	56.3	100.1	175.6	245.0	300.0	304.9	335.3	31.3	8.5	1.05	3.15	**25.5**	*188*
Kidney etc.	249	0	-	-	-	-	0.5	-	-	1.1	7.4	8.8	19.0	20.1	37.3	65.4	46.0	85.3	65.0	54.4	10.6	2.9	0.47	1.03	**8.7**	*189*
Eye	18	0	2.0	1.4	-	-	-	-	-	0.5	-	-	0.7	0.8	2.0	4.8	7.4	-	-	-	0.8	0.2	0.04	0.10	**0.8**	*190*
Brain, nervous system	131	0	3.3	5.6	3.3	1.1	1.4	7.9	3.0	3.2	2.1	10.7	10.2	10.5	8.8	12.1	16.6	5.5	-	9.1	5.6	1.5	0.36	0.50	**5.3**	*191-2*
Thyroid	23	0	-	-	-	0.6	-	0.9	1.5	2.1	-	1.3	2.2	3.2	2.0	1.2	-	2.8	-	-	1.0	0.3	0.07	0.07	**0.8**	*193*
Other endocrine	8	0	0.7	-	0.7	-	-	0.5	-	-	-	0.6	0.7	0.8	1.0	1.2	-	-	-	-	0.3	0.1	0.02	0.03	**0.4**	*194*
Hodgkin's disease	53	0	-	-	1.3	2.8	1.0	1.8	4.4	2.6	4.2	1.9	2.2	1.6	3.9	2.4	1.8	5.5	-	9.1	2.2	0.6	0.14	0.16	**1.9**	*201*
Non-Hodgkin lymphoma	279	0	1.3	2.8	-	2.2	2.9	2.8	4.4	7.9	5.3	16.4	10.9	16.1	35.3	43.6	68.2	101.8	40.0	72.5	11.8	3.2	0.54	1.10	**10.0**	*200,202*
Multiple myeloma	84	0	-	-	-	-	-	-	-	1.1	1.6	1.3	7.3	12.9	3.9	21.8	22.1	30.3	15.0	27.2	3.6	1.0	0.14	0.36	**2.9**	*203*
Lymphoid leukaemia	85	0	4.6	3.5	0.7	1.7	1.4	-	-	-	1.6	1.3	6.6	8.0	7.9	12.1	14.7	33.0	-	36.2	3.6	1.0	0.19	0.32	**3.5**	*204*
Myeloid leukaemia	72	0	0.7	-	0.7	0.6	-	1.4	0.5	2.1	1.6	1.9	6.6	5.6	2.9	12.1	16.6	33.0	20.0	9.1	3.1	0.8	0.12	0.27	**2.5**	*205*
Monocytic leukaemia	3	0	-	-	-	-	-	-	-	-	-	-	0.7	-	-	-	1.8	-	-	9.1	0.1	0.0	0.00	0.01	**0.1**	*206*
Other leukaemia	8	0	-	-	-	-	-	-	-	0.5	-	-	0.7	-	2.0	1.2	-	2.8	10.0	-	0.3	0.1	0.02	0.02	**0.3**	*207*
Leukaemia unspecified	3	0	-	-	-	-	0.5	0.5	-	-	-	-	-	-	-	1.2	-	-	-	-	0.1	0.0	0.00	0.01	**0.1**	*208*
Other and unspecified	475	0	2.0	-	-	-	2.4	1.8	1.0	3.7	3.2	13.3	27.0	50.7	56.0	111.4	125.3	145.9	209.9	135.9	20.1	5.5	0.80	1.99	**16.5**	*O&U*
All sites																										
All sites but 173	8661	0	18.6	16.0	10.6	16.8	26.2	38.8	43.4	68.8	92.1	195.2	380.7	734.3	1159.5	1852.7	2545.5	3283.7	3289.0	3108.0	367.2	100.0	14.01	36.00	**301.6**	*ALLb*

Rate from 1 case   0.663   0.697   0.665   0.560   0.476   0.462   0.493   0.525   0.526   0.632   0.729   0.804   0.982   1.211   1.842   2.752   4.999   9.061

†Important: see notes on population page

NETHERLANDS, EINDHOVEN 1988-1992

ANNUAL INCIDENCE PER 100,000 BY AGE GROUP (YEARS) - FEMALE

SITE	ALL AGES	AGE UNK	0-	5-	10-	15-	20-	25-	30-	35-	40-	45-	50-	55-	60-	65-	70-	75-	80-	85+	CRUDE RATE	%	CR 64	CR 74	ASR (W)	ICD (9th)
Lip	13	0	-	-	-	-	-	-	-	-	-	0.7	-	1.6	3.7	1.1	5.5	-	-	3.7	0.6	0.2	0.03	0.06	**0.4**	*140*
Tongue	22	0	-	-	-	-	-	0.5	-	1.1	2.1	-	2.4	-	3.2	6.9	5.1	2.5	3.7	0.9	0.3	0.03	0.08	**0.6**	*141*
Salivary gland	8	0	-	-	-	-	0.5	-	-	-	-	-	-	1.8	1.1	2.8	1.7	-	3.7	0.3	0.1	0.01	0.03	**0.2**	*142*
Mouth	34	0	-	-	-	-	0.5	1.0	0.5	0.6	0.6	0.7	0.8	5.7	4.6	5.3	4.2	6.9	2.5	3.7	1.5	0.5	0.07	0.12	**1.1**	*143-5*
Oropharynx	8	0	-	-	-	-	-	-	-	-	0.6	0.7	-	2.4	0.9	2.1	-	-	-	-	0.3	0.1	0.02	0.03	**0.3**	*146*
Nasopharynx	10	0	-	-	-	1.2	-	-	0.5	-	-	1.4	0.8	2.4	-	-	-	-	2.5	-	0.4	0.1	0.03	0.03	**0.4**	*147*
Hypopharynx	2	0	-	-	-	-	-	-	-	-	-	-	-	-	-	1.1	-	-	-	3.7	0.1	0.0	0.00	0.01	**0.1**	*148*
Pharynx unspecified	0	0	-	-	-	-	-	-	-	-	-	-	-	-	-	-	-	-	-	-	0.0	0.0	0.00	0.00	**0.0**	*149*
Oesophagus	42	0	-	-	-	-	-	-	-	-	0.6	-	2.3	1.6	5.5	5.3	9.7	12.0	15.1	18.6	1.8	0.6	0.05	0.12	**1.1**	*150*
Stomach	298	0	-	-	-	-	-	2.0	1.1	1.7	3.4	6.2	5.3	15.4	25.6	40.0	49.8	106.3	111.1	148.8	12.8	4.2	0.30	0.75	**7.4**	*151*
Small intestine	10	0	-	-	-	-	-	-	-	-	1.1	0.7	0.8	0.8	-	-	4.2	1.7	2.5	-	0.4	0.1	0.02	0.04	**0.3**	*152*
Colon	730	0	-	0.7	0.7	4.8	1.1	0.5	2.7	2.8	2.8	15.7	22.1	45.2	72.2	99.0	175.8	210.9	265.1	245.5	31.5	10.3	0.86	2.23	**19.1**	*153*
Rectum	353	0	-	-	-	-	-	-	-	-	4.0	13.7	19.0	29.9	43.8	61.1	66.4	82.3	118.7	55.8	15.2	5.0	0.55	1.19	**9.8**	*154*
Liver	16	0	-	0.7	-	-	-	0.5	0.5	-	0.6	-	-	-	0.9	2.1	8.3	3.4	2.5	-	0.7	0.2	0.02	0.07	**0.5**	*155*
Gallbladder etc.	108	0	-	-	-	-	1.1	-	-	-	-	0.7	2.3	5.7	8.2	12.6	40.1	20.6	60.6	33.5	4.7	1.5	0.09	0.35	**2.7**	*156*
Pancreas	150	0	-	-	-	-	-	-	-	-	1.1	2.1	9.1	11.3	20.1	19.0	34.6	44.6	40.4	44.6	6.5	2.1	0.22	0.49	**4.0**	*157*
Nose, sinuses etc.	9	0	-	-	-	-	0.5	-	-	0.6	-	0.7	-	-	0.9	-	4.2	1.7	2.5	-	0.4	0.1	0.01	0.03	**0.3**	*160*
Larynx	19	0	-	-	-	-	-	-	-	-	1.1	-	2.3	2.4	3.7	2.1	2.8	1.7	5.0	-	0.8	0.3	0.05	0.07	**0.6**	*161*
Bronchus, lung	361	0	-	-	-	-	-	1.0	0.5	7.4	7.4	13.0	32.7	46.1	62.1	69.5	49.8	30.9	45.4	26.0	15.6	5.1	0.85	1.45	**11.5**	*162*
Other thoracic organs	8	0	-	-	-	-	-	-	-	-	1.1	-	0.8	0.8	-	2.1	-	3.4	-	-	0.3	0.1	0.01	0.02	**0.2**	*163-4*
Bone	21	0	-	0.7	-	1.2	1.6	-	-	0.6	-	1.4	0.8	2.4	-	-	4.2	3.4	5.0	3.7	0.9	0.3	0.04	0.06	**0.7**	*170*
Connective tissue	32	0	0.7	-	1.4	1.2	1.1	-	0.5	2.3	0.6	2.1	0.8	4.0	1.8	3.2	1.4	3.4	-	7.4	1.4	0.4	0.08	0.10	**1.2**	*171*
Mesothelioma	11	0	-	-	-	-	-	-	-	-	-	-	-	1.6	0.9	4.2	1.4	5.1	-	-	0.5	0.2	0.01	0.04	**0.3**	*MES*
Kaposi's sarcoma	1	0	-	-	-	-	-	0.5	-	-	-	-	-	-	-	-	-	-	-	-	0.0	0.0	0.00	0.00	**0.0**	*KAP*
Melanoma of skin	248	0	0.7	-	0.7	1.8	5.9	13.2	13.9	13.1	14.2	19.8	15.2	21.8	10.0	12.6	15.2	13.7	22.7	18.6	10.7	3.5	0.65	0.79	**8.6**	*172*
†Other skin																										
Breast	2301	0	-	-	-	-	1.6	4.1	27.9	59.6	116.2	181.8	187.3	193.1	242.1	296.0	260.2	366.9	338.3	353.3	99.2	32.3	5.07	7.85	**71.6**	*174*
Uterus unspecified	0	0	-	-	-	-	-	-	-	-	-	-	-	-	-	-	-	-	-	-	0.0	0.0	0.00	0.00	**0.0**	*179*
Cervix uteri	196	0	-	-	-	-	0.5	4.1	8.0	22.1	15.3	13.0	12.2	10.5	11.0	12.6	16.6	15.4	17.7	22.3	8.4	2.8	0.48	0.63	**6.4**	*180*
Placenta	0	0	-	-	-	-	-	-	-	-	-	-	-	-	-	-	-	-	-	-	0.0	0.0	0.00	0.00	**0.0**	*181*
Corpus uteri	334	0	-	-	-	-	-	0.5	0.5	1.1	2.3	17.1	30.4	40.4	53.9	54.8	54.0	48.0	58.1	37.2	14.4	4.7	0.73	1.28	**10.3**	*182*
Ovary etc.	348	0	-	-	3.6	2.1	2.0	4.8	9.7	7.9	17.1	28.2	39.6	45.7	43.2	66.4	49.7	22.7	22.3	15.0	4.9	0.80	1.35	**11.2**	*183*
Other female genital	45	0	-	-	-	-	1.1	-	-	-	1.1	0.7	5.3	3.2	3.7	6.3	5.5	12.0	5.0	22.3	1.9	0.6	0.08	0.13	**1.3**	*184*
Bladder	202	0	-	-	-	-	-	-	1.1	0.6	1.7	6.2	6.1	25.0	21.9	33.7	37.4	58.3	48.0	44.6	8.7	2.8	0.31	0.67	**5.6**	*188*
Kidney etc.	149	0	0.7	-	-	0.6	-	0.5	-	0.6	1.7	6.2	3.8	13.7	17.4	25.3	40.1	34.3	35.3	18.6	6.4	2.1	0.23	0.55	**4.3**	*189*
Eye	15	0	2.8	-	-	-	-	0.5	-	0.6	0.7	-	-	1.1	5.5	-	5.0	-	-	-	0.6	0.2	0.03	0.06	**0.6**	*190*
Brain, nervous system	112	0	0.7	1.4	4.2	3.0	3.7	3.6	3.2	4.5	4.5	5.5	5.3	7.3	8.2	9.5	11.1	13.7	10.1	-	4.8	1.6	0.28	0.38	**4.1**	*191-2*
Thyroid	58	0	-	-	-	-	4.3	1.5	2.7	2.8	4.0	1.4	2.3	3.2	4.6	4.2	6.9	8.6	5.0	-	2.5	0.8	0.13	0.19	**1.9**	*193*
Other endocrine	11	0	2.1	-	-	-	-	-	-	1.1	1.1	1.4	0.8	-	-	-	-	1.7	-	-	0.5	0.2	0.03	0.03	**0.5**	*194*
Hodgkin's disease	36	0	-	-	0.7	1.8	3.7	2.5	1.1	0.6	4.0	0.7	0.8	-	0.9	3.2	2.8	-	5.0	-	1.6	0.5	0.08	0.11	**1.4**	*201*
Non-Hodgkin lymphoma	204	0	1.4	1.4	1.4	-	1.1	1.0	1.6	2.8	4.0	8.9	11.4	9.7	18.3	27.4	38.8	51.4	55.5	48.4	8.8	2.9	0.31	0.65	**6.0**	*200,202*
Multiple myeloma	82	0	-	-	-	-	-	-	0.5	-	1.1	2.1	2.3	3.2	11.9	16.9	19.4	20.6	22.7	18.6	3.5	1.2	0.11	0.29	**2.2**	*203*
Lymphoid leukaemia	60	0	2.8	1.4	2.8	0.6	0.5	0.5	1.1	-	0.6	1.4	1.5	4.0	3.7	8.4	5.5	15.4	17.7	11.2	2.6	0.8	0.10	0.17	**2.1**	*204*
Myeloid leukaemia	66	0	0.7	-	0.7	-	1.1	1.5	1.1	1.1	1.7	-	2.3	6.5	6.4	3.2	13.8	18.9	15.1	14.9	2.8	0.9	0.12	0.20	**1.9**	*205*
Monocytic leukaemia	2	0	-	-	-	-	-	-	-	-	-	-	0.8	-	-	-	-	2.5	-		0.1	0.0	0.00	0.00	**0.0**	*206*
Other leukaemia	3	0	0.7	-	-	-	-	-	-	-	0.7	-	0.8	-	-	-	-	-	-	-	0.1	0.0	0.01	0.01	**0.2**	*207*
Leukaemia unspecified	4	0	0.7	0.7	-	-	-	-	-	-	0.6	-	-	-	-	1.1	-	-	-	-	0.2	0.1	0.01	0.02	**0.2**	*208*
Other and unspecified	375	0	1.4	-	-	-	0.5	0.5	2.1	4.0	6.2	6.8	16.0	21.8	32.0	63.2	58.1	109.7	143.9	122.7	16.2	5.3	0.46	1.06	**9.8**	*O&U*
All sites																										
All sites but 173	7117	0	15.3	7.2	12.5	19.6	32.6	40.6	77.7	139.6	214.9	352.7	430.8	587.4	748.1	956.6	1129.6	1383.6	1512.2	1357.6	306.7	100.0	13.40	23.83	**212.8**	*ALLb*

Rate from 1 case			0.696	0.723	0.695	0.594	0.534	0.508	0.536	0.568	0.567	0.684	0.761	0.808	0.913	1.053	1.384	1.714	2.524	3.719

†Important: see notes on population page

Netherlands, Maastricht

The IKL Cancer Registry in the Province of Limburg was established in 1984 as part of the Comprehensive Cancer Centre Limburg. Within the structure of the centre, there is collaboration between hospitals, the University of Limburg and the Radiotherapy Institute of Limburg. Besides cancer registration, the centre is involved in cancer research and treatment and it coordinates regional activities on cancer prevention, screening (breast and cervical cancer), education and psychosocial care. The IKL Cancer Registry is one of nine regional cancer registries in the Netherlands that together represent the Netherlands national cancer registry.

The staff of the cancer registry comprises one physician specialized in epidemiology as head of the registry, one computer programmer and six tumour registrars. In addition, two consultants on cancer registration (from the field of epidemiology and radiotherapy) are available.

The area covered by the IKL Cancer Registry (1355 km^2) consists of the southern and middle parts of the province of Limburg in the south-east of the Netherlands. To the west, south and east, it is bordered by Belgium and Germany, while to the north is the area covered by the Eindhoven Cancer Registry. There are rural, urban and fairly heavily industrialized areas.

Population data are provided on an annual basis by the Dutch Central Bureau of Statistics. On 1 January 1991, the population at risk consisted of 848 937 inhabitants, of whom 420 018 were men and 428 919 women, living in 38 municipalities. In the southern part of Limburg, the population density was 938 per km^2, whereas in the middle part it was 325 per km^2. About 29% of the population were living in rural (non-urban) municipalities, 57% in sparsely and moderately urbanized municipalities and 14% in densely urbanized municipalities (classified according to the average address density).

Industrial activities in the region now include chemical, automobile, ceramic and cement industry. From 1919 to 1975 coal mining was a very important source of employment. In 1992, about 35% of the working population were employed in industry and less than 5% in agriculture. The large majority of the population are Catholics.

There is easy access to medical care in the Netherlands. About 60% of the population are covered for medical expenses by a government plan for people with lower incomes. The great majority of the remaining people are privately insured.

In the province of Limburg, there is about one general practitioner per 2300 inhabitants. Medical specialists usually work at the hospitals; they can be consulted after referral by a general practitioner. Almost all cancer patients are diagnosed and treated by medical specialists. In the IKL area, there are five general hospitals and one university hospital, with a total of 3800 beds. The area also has one radiotherapy institute.

Notification of cases to the cancer registry is voluntary. The cancer registry receives lists of newly diagnosed cases on a regular basis from the seven pathology departments in the region. In addition, lists of hospitalized cancer patients are provided by the medical records departments of all the notifying hospitals. Following such notification, the medical records of newly diagnosed patients (and tumours) are collected and the necessary information is abstracted by trained tumour registrars for the cancer registry. Death certificates cannot be used because of privacy regulations of the Dutch Central Bureau of Statistics. Tumour data are copied to registration forms at the hospitals and entered into the computer at the registration office. Identifying information is entered into a portable personal computer at the hospital. After encryption, these data are also sent to the registration office. This procedure provides better protection of the privacy of cancer patients. Patients treated at hospitals in other parts of the Netherlands are recorded by the other regional cancer registries and are submitted to the national cancer registry. From 1989 onwards, the information on these cases has been distributed by the national cancer registry and it is used to improve the completeness of case ascertainment.

Tumour data are coded according to ICD-O. Completeness of records, data consistency and the possibility of duplicate records are continuously and extensively checked by computer programs.

The completeness of registration within the IKL area has been investigated recently. The registry data were compared to data on cancer patients registered in a computerized network of general practitioners. Overall completeness was estimated to be 96% for the years 1988–90.

L.J. Schouten
P.A. van den Brandt
J.A.M. Huveneers
J.J. Jager
A.G. Koppejan-Rensenbrink

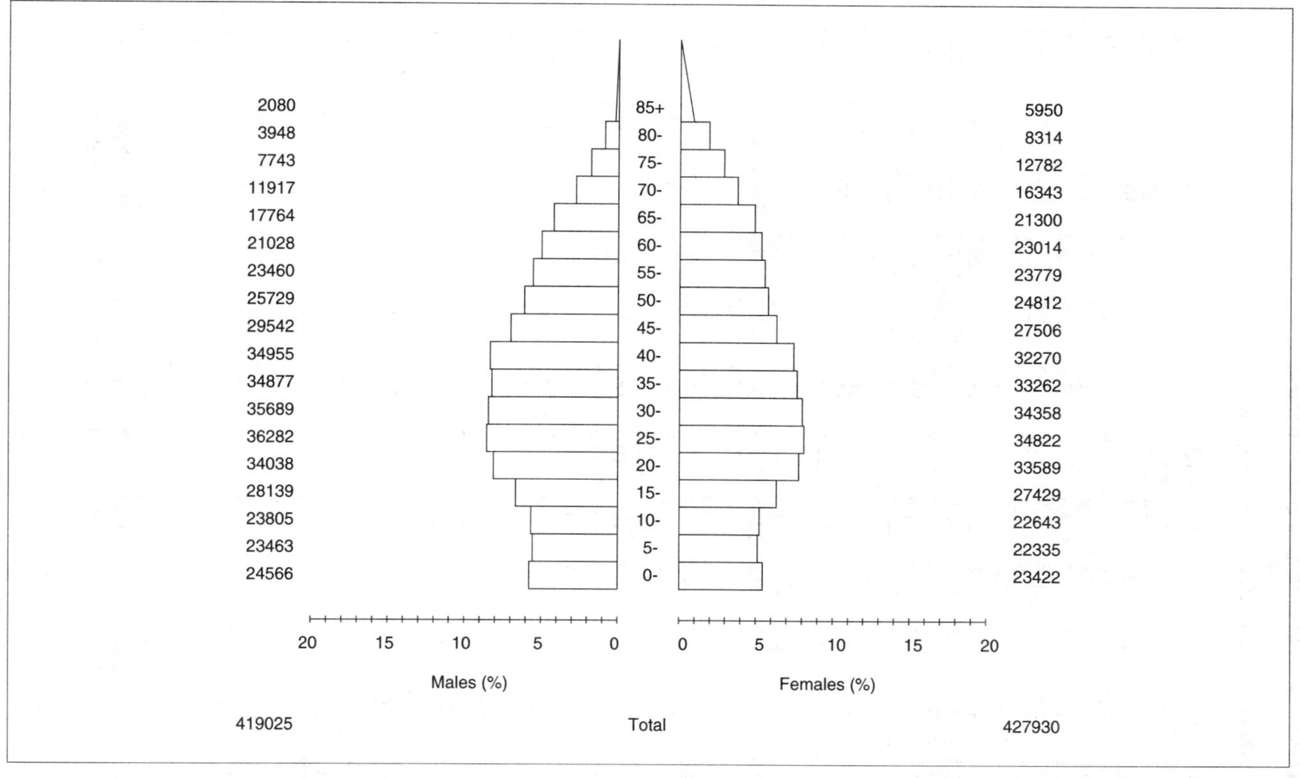

Netherlands, Maastricht

Source of population: average annual 1988–92

Census: Population data are collected from the Municipal Population Registers, which are assumed to be 100% complete. Information is collected and distributed by the Dutch Central Bureau of Statistics for 1 January of each calendar year.

Notes to tables overleaf:

† 173 does not include basal cell carcinomas
† 188 does not include non-invasive diagnoses

Screening programmes in the area:

A cervical screening programme started in 1990 for women aged 35-55; 9 000 examinations were carried out in 1990, 31 000 in 1991 and 37 000 in 1992. Women aged 50-70 have been screened since 1991 for breast cancer, with 12 050 examinations in 1991 and 29 311 in 1992.

NETHERLANDS, MAASTRICHT 1988-1992

ANNUAL INCIDENCE PER 100,000 BY AGE GROUP (YEARS) - MALE

SITE	ALL AGES	AGE UNK	0-	5-	10-	15-	20-	25-	30-	35-	40-	45-	50-	55-	60-	65-	70-	75-	80-	85+	CRUDE RATE	%	CR 64	CR 74	ASR (W)	ICD (9th)
Lip	28	0	-	-	-	-	-	-	-	-	-	0.7	0.8	3.4	2.9	6.8	6.7	7.7	25.3	9.6	1.3	0.3	0.04	0.11	0.9	140
Tongue	44	0	-	-	-	0.7	-	-	-	1.1	0.6	4.1	3.1	5.1	8.6	5.6	10.1	5.2	10.1	-	2.1	0.5	0.12	0.19	1.6	141
Salivary gland	12	0	-	-	-	-	-	0.6	-	-	0.6	0.7	1.6	-	1.9	1.1	5.0	2.6	-	-	0.6	0.1	0.03	0.06	0.4	142
Mouth	48	0	-	-	-	-	-	-	-	0.6	1.7	2.7	5.4	6.8	2.9	11.3	11.7	5.2	15.2	-	2.3	0.6	0.10	0.22	1.7	143-5
Oropharynx	32	0	-	-	-	-	-	-	-	1.1	1.1	3.4	4.7	2.6	1.9	5.6	8.4	5.2	-	-	1.5	0.4	0.07	0.14	1.1	146
Nasopharynx	16	0	-	-	-	-	-	-	-	-	0.6	1.4	0.8	1.7	1.0	4.5	6.7	-	5.1	-	0.8	0.2	0.03	0.08	0.6	147
Hypopharynx	35	0	-	-	-	-	-	-	-	0.6	1.7	3.4	3.9	5.1	3.8	6.8	5.0	5.2	-	-	1.7	0.4	0.09	0.15	1.2	148
Pharynx unspecified	4	0	-	-	-	-	-	-	-	-	-	-	-	-	1.9	1.1	-	-	5.1	-	0.2	0.0	0.01	0.02	0.1	149
Oesophagus	116	0	-	-	-	-	-	-	-	-	1.7	7.4	7.8	12.8	13.3	27.0	31.9	20.7	50.7	19.2	5.5	1.4	0.22	0.51	4.0	150
Stomach	459	0	-	-	-	-	0.6	-	2.2	2.3	5.1	11.5	18.7	35.0	46.6	105.8	152.7	162.7	207.7	201.9	21.9	5.4	0.61	1.90	15.4	151
Small intestine	25	0	-	-	-	-	-	-	1.1	0.6	0.6	-	0.8	2.6	1.9	7.9	5.0	7.7	10.1	-	1.2	0.3	0.04	0.10	0.8	152
Colon	659	0	-	-	-	0.7	-	0.6	0.6	2.9	6.3	12.2	27.2	41.8	68.5	150.9	204.7	299.6	324.2	288.4	31.5	7.8	0.80	2.58	21.9	153
Rectum	549	0	-	-	-	-	-	-	1.7	2.3	6.3	19.6	25.7	45.2	64.7	119.3	154.4	188.6	243.2	278.8	26.2	6.5	0.83	2.20	18.6	154
Liver	45	0	2.4	-	-	-	0.6	0.6	-	-	1.1	-	2.3	2.6	11.4	9.0	8.4	7.7	10.1	19.2	2.1	0.5	0.11	0.19	1.8	155
Gallbladder etc.	73	0	-	-	-	-	-	-	-	-	1.7	0.7	1.6	3.4	9.5	21.4	13.4	28.4	35.5	76.9	3.5	0.9	0.08	0.26	2.5	156
Pancreas	174	0	-	-	-	-	-	-	0.6	1.7	-	6.1	11.7	12.8	22.8	39.4	48.7	62.0	81.1	28.8	8.3	2.1	0.28	0.72	5.8	157
Nose, sinuses etc.	24	0	-	-	-	-	-	0.6	-	-	-	0.7	2.3	3.4	1.9	4.5	1.7	15.5	10.1	-	1.1	0.3	0.04	0.08	0.8	160
Larynx	193	0	-	-	-	-	-	-	-	1.1	4.0	8.8	11.7	13.6	36.1	41.7	65.4	46.5	20.3	38.5	9.2	2.3	0.38	0.91	6.7	161
Bronchus, lung	2395	0	-	-	-	-	0.6	1.1	2.9	18.9	44.7	102.6	199.5	353.8	556.2	807.2	973.8	754.8	471.1	114.3	28.3	3.62	10.44	80.1	162
Other thoracic organs	12	0	-	-	-	-	-	0.6	-	-	0.7	-	-	2.9	3.4	5.0	2.6	-	-	0.6	0.1	0.02	0.06	0.4	163-4
Bone	23	0	0.8	-	0.8	2.1	2.4	1.7	0.6	1.7	1.1	1.4	-	0.9	-	-	-	5.2	-	-	1.1	0.3	0.07	0.07	1.1	170
Connective tissue	63	0	0.8	1.7	0.8	-	1.8	1.1	2.8	2.3	1.1	6.8	4.7	0.9	3.8	7.9	8.4	10.3	20.3	19.2	3.0	0.7	0.14	0.22	2.5	171
Mesothelioma	85	0	-	-	-	-	-	-	-	-	0.6	3.4	6.2	19.6	13.3	16.9	16.8	15.5	5.1	19.2	4.1	1.0	0.22	0.38	3.0	MES
Kaposi's sarcoma	4	0	-	-	-	-	0.6	-	0.6	0.6	-	-	-	1.0	-	-	-	-	-	-	0.2	0.0	0.01	0.01	0.2	KAP
Melanoma of skin	142	0	-	-	0.8	0.7	2.9	4.4	3.9	7.5	5.7	10.8	10.1	10.2	10.5	18.0	23.5	12.9	30.4	38.5	6.8	1.7	0.34	0.55	5.2	172
†Other skin	351	0	-	-	0.8	-	-	1.7	3.4	0.6	2.9	6.1	9.3	25.6	33.3	66.4	90.6	170.5	207.7	278.8	16.8		0.42	1.20	11.7	173
Breast	14	0	-	-	-	-	-	-	-	-	-	-	1.6	1.7	1.9	1.1	6.7	2.6	10.1	-	0.7	0.2	0.03	0.07	0.5	175
Prostate	1101	0	-	-	-	-	-	-	-	-	1.1	4.1	12.4	36.7	114.1	253.3	386.0	625.1	673.8	807.6	52.5	13.0	0.84	4.04	35.9	185
Testis	88	0	-	-	0.8	5.7	8.8	7.7	11.2	4.0	5.1	4.1	2.3	2.6	-	1.1	-	2.6	-	-	4.2	1.0	0.26	0.27	3.7	186
Penis	18	0	-	-	-	-	-	-	-	-	-	1.4	1.6	-	1.9	1.1	6.7	2.6	15.2	28.8	0.9	0.2	0.02	0.06	0.6	187.1-.4
Other male genital	3	0	-	-	0.8	-	-	-	-	-	0.6	-	0.8	-	-	-	-	-	-	-	0.1	0.0	0.01	0.01	0.1	187.5-.9
†Bladder	346	0	-	-	-	-	-	-	-	0.6	2.9	3.4	13.2	23.0	44.7	72.1	112.4	139.5	187.4	211.5	16.5	4.1	0.44	1.36	11.6	188
Kidney etc.	327	0	0.8	-	-	-	-	-	1.1	1.7	2.9	19.6	17.1	43.5	42.8	67.6	78.9	82.7	106.4	86.5	15.6	3.9	0.65	1.38	11.3	189
Eye	20	0	1.6	-	-	-	-	-	-	1.1	0.6	-	0.8	-	1.9	3.4	6.7	5.2	10.1	9.6	1.0	0.2	0.03	0.08	0.8	190
Brain, nervous system	159	0	2.4	4.3	4.2	0.7	2.4	3.3	2.8	1.1	8.6	8.8	8.6	15.3	24.7	18.0	20.1	25.8	30.4	9.6	7.6	1.9	0.44	0.63	6.3	191-2
Thyroid	27	0	-	-	-	0.7	0.6	1.7	2.2	2.3	1.7	-	0.8	-	1.9	3.4	5.0	-	5.1	9.6	1.3	0.3	0.06	0.10	1.0	193
Other endocrine	10	0	0.8	-	0.8	-	-	-	0.6	0.6	-	0.7	0.8	2.6	-	1.1	-	-	-	-	0.5	0.1	0.03	0.04	0.5	194
Hodgkin's disease	56	0	-	-	2.5	1.4	4.7	3.3	2.8	4.6	2.3	1.4	-	1.7	3.8	3.4	11.7	2.6	-	9.6	2.7	0.7	0.14	0.22	2.3	201
Non-Hodgkin lymphoma	247	0	1.6	2.6	2.5	0.7	2.4	1.1	2.8	6.3	6.3	12.2	10.1	24.7	31.4	33.8	58.7	74.9	60.8	57.7	11.8	2.9	0.52	0.99	9.0	200,202
Multiple myeloma	92	0	-	-	-	-	-	-	-	-	0.6	1.7	3.4	5.4	6.0	14.3	20.3	20.1	38.7	45.6	-	4.4	1.1	0.16	0.36	3.0	203
Lymphoid leukaemia	97	0	4.9	4.3	2.5	0.7	-	-	1.7	2.9	0.6	0.7	5.4	6.8	7.6	21.4	18.5	7.7	40.5	76.9	4.6	1.1	0.19	0.39	4.2	204
Myeloid leukaemia	94	0	0.8	1.7	1.7	-	1.2	2.8	1.1	4.6	0.6	3.4	3.9	5.1	12.4	12.4	16.8	31.0	15.2	57.7	4.5	1.1	0.20	0.34	3.6	205
Monocytic leukaemia	1	0	-	-	-	-	-	-	-	-	-	-	-	-	1.0	-	-	-	-	-	0.0	0.0	0.00	0.00	0.0	206
Other leukaemia	1	0	-	-	-	-	-	-	-	-	-	-	0.9	-	-	-	-	-	-	-	0.0	0.0	0.00	0.00	0.0	207
Leukaemia unspecified	10	0	-	-	-	0.7	-	-	-	-	-	-	0.8	-	-	2.3	5.0	2.6	5.1	9.6	0.5	0.1	0.01	0.04	0.4	208
Other and unspecified	483	0	-	-	-	-	0.7	0.6	-	-	1.7	5.1	10.2	26.4	40.1	59.0	100.2	162.8	180.8	207.7	134.6	23.1	5.7	0.72	2.03	16.2	O&U
All sites	8805	0	17.1	14.5	19.3	15.6	28.8	32.0	44.8	61.9	104.1	230.2	374.7	664.9	1083.3	1854.3	2607.9	3285.5	3485.3	3297.8	420.3		13.46	35.77	301.2	ALL
All sites but 173	8454	0	17.1	14.5	18.5	15.6	28.8	30.3	41.5	61.4	101.3	224.1	365.3	639.4	1050.0	1787.8	2517.3	3115.1	3277.6	3018.9	403.5	100.0	13.04	34.56	289.4	ALLb

Rate from 1 case

| | | | 0.814 | 0.852 | 0.840 | 0.711 | 0.588 | 0.551 | 0.560 | 0.573 | 0.572 | 0.677 | 0.777 | 0.852 | 0.951 | 1.126 | 1.678 | 2.583 | 5.066 | 9.614 |

†Important: see notes on population page

NETHERLANDS, MAASTRICHT 1988-1992

ANNUAL INCIDENCE PER 100,000 BY AGE GROUP (YEARS) - FEMALE

SITE	ALL AGES	AGE UNK	0-	5-	10-	15-	20-	25-	30-	35-	40-	45-	50-	55-	60-	65-	70-	75-	80-	85+	CRUDE RATE	%	CR 64	CR 74	ASR (W)	ICD (9th)
Lip	6	0	-	-	-	-	-	-	-	-	-	-	0.8	-	0.9	-	2.4	-	2.4	3.4	0.3	0.1	0.01	0.02	**0.2**	140
Tongue	20	0	-	-	-	-	0.6	-	1.2	0.6	-	2.4	2.5	2.6	1.9	1.2	3.1	4.8	-	-	0.9	0.3	0.05	0.07	**0.6**	141
Salivary gland	15	0	-	-	-	-	-	-	0.6	-	0.6	0.7	0.8	2.5	1.7	-	2.4	1.6	4.8	3.4	0.7	0.2	0.03	0.05	**0.4**	142
Mouth	31	0	-	-	-	-	-	0.6	0.6	1.2	1.9	2.9	2.4	3.4	2.6	0.9	3.7	4.7	2.4	6.7	1.4	0.4	0.08	0.10	**1.0**	143-5
Oropharynx	21	0	-	-	-	-	-	-	-	0.6	2.9	2.4	1.7	4.3	3.8	-	-	2.4	3.4		1.0	0.3	0.06	0.08	**0.7**	146
Nasopharynx	2	0	-	-	-	-	-	-	-	0.7	-	-	0.9	-	-	-	-	-	-	-	0.1	0.0	0.01	0.01	**0.1**	147
Hypopharynx	2	0	-	-	-	-	-	-	-	-	-	0.8	-	0.9	-	-	-	-	-	-	0.1	0.0	0.01	0.01	**0.1**	148
Pharynx unspecified	2	0	-	-	-	-	-	-	-	-	-	-	-	-	-	-	-	3.1	-	-	0.1	0.0	0.00	0.00	**0.0**	149
Oesophagus	51	0	-	-	-	-	-	-	0.6	-	1.5	2.4	1.7	4.3	9.4	8.6	11.0	24.1	13.4		2.4	0.7	0.05	0.14	**1.2**	150
Stomach	282	0	-	-	-	-	0.6	1.2	1.8	5.0	1.5	10.5	10.1	21.7	31.0	58.7	87.6	108.2	114.3		13.2	3.8	0.26	0.71	**6.5**	151
Small intestine	23	0	-	-	-	0.7	-	-	-	-	1.2	2.2	1.6	1.7	1.7	4.7	1.2	4.7	2.4	3.4	1.1	0.3	0.05	0.08	**0.4**	152
Colon	729	0	-	-	1.8	-	-	1.1	0.6	1.8	8.7	14.5	29.8	37.8	66.0	100.5	146.8	237.8	206.9	215.1	34.1	9.7	0.81	2.05	**17.9**	153
Rectum	406	0	-	-	-	-	-	-	1.2	2.4	3.7	10.9	21.0	33.6	41.7	56.3	72.2	100.1	122.7	104.2	19.0	5.4	0.57	1.22	**10.4**	154
Liver	25	0	-	-	-	-	0.6	-	-	0.6	0.7	1.6	1.7	3.5	1.9	6.1	3.1	4.8	10.1		1.2	0.3	0.04	0.08	**0.7**	155
Gallbladder etc.	120	0	-	-	-	-	-	-	-	-	0.6	-	2.4	5.9	7.0	17.8	30.6	37.6	55.3	33.6	5.6	1.6	0.08	0.32	**2.6**	156
Pancreas	186	0	-	-	-	-	-	-	0.6	0.6	0.6	4.4	4.0	14.3	18.2	22.5	39.2	59.5	67.4	40.3	8.7	2.5	0.21	0.52	**4.5**	157
Nose, sinuses etc.	12	0	-	-	-	-	1.1	-	-	0.6	0.6	1.5	-	0.8	0.9	0.9	1.2	-	2.4	3.4	0.6	0.2	0.03	0.04	**0.4**	160
Larynx	23	0	-	-	-	-	-	-	-	0.6	0.6	0.7	1.6	3.4	4.3	5.6	-	1.6	4.8	-	1.1	0.3	0.06	0.08	**0.7**	161
Bronchus, lung	416	0	-	-	-	-	0.6	0.6	4.1	5.4	10.5	21.1	22.6	51.3	69.5	46.0	78.3	67.3	43.3	30.3	19.4	5.6	0.93	1.55	**12.5**	162
Other thoracic organs	4	0	-	-	-	-	-	-	-	-	0.6	-	-	-	-	0.9	-	1.6	-	3.4	0.2	0.1	0.00	0.01	**0.1**	163-4
Bone	15	0	-	-	2.6	1.5	-	0.6	-	1.2	0.6	1.5	0.8	-	0.9	-	1.2	1.6	-	-	0.7	0.2	0.05	0.05	**0.7**	170
Connective tissue	47	0	1.7	0.9	1.8	1.5	-	2.3	0.6	1.2	1.2	0.7	3.2	1.7	3.5	4.7	7.3	6.3	9.6	3.4	2.2	0.6	0.10	0.16	**1.8**	171
Mesothelioma	12	0	-	-	-	-	-	-	-	-	-	-	-	1.7	0.9	4.7	2.4	1.6	-	3.4	0.6	0.2	0.01	0.05	**0.3**	MES
Kaposi's sarcoma	0	0	-	-	-	-	-	-	-	-	-	-	-	-	-	-	-	-	-	-	0.0	0.0	0.00	0.00	**0.0**	KAP
Melanoma of skin	273	0	-	-	-	5.1	6.0	10.3	15.1	17.4	19.8	21.8	24.2	11.8	7.0	20.7	15.9	21.9	28.9	26.9	12.8	3.7	0.69	0.88	**9.6**	172
†Other skin	227	0	-	-	-	-	0.6	2.3	1.7	2.4	3.7	5.8	8.1	10.1	18.2	23.5	40.4	43.8	72.2	141.2	10.6		0.26	0.58	**5.6**	173
Breast	2351	0	-	-	-	-	-	6.9	24.4	58.9	115.9	167.2	195.1	228.8	275.5	270.4	302.3	306.7	348.8	252.1	109.9	31.4	5.36	8.23	**72.7**	174
Uterus unspecified	1	0	-	-	-	-	-	-	-	-	-	-	0.8	-	-	-	-	-	-	-	0.0	0.0	0.00	0.00	**0.0**	179
Cervix uteri	224	0	-	-	-	1.5	1.2	4.0	11.1	24.1	15.5	10.9	16.9	11.8	17.4	16.0	23.3	15.6	19.2	16.8	10.5	3.0	0.57	0.77	**7.5**	180
Placenta	0	0	-	-	-	-	-	-	-	-	-	-	-	-	-	-	-	-	-	-	0.0	0.0	0.00	0.00	**0.0**	181
Corpus uteri	366	0	-	-	-	-	-	-	-	1.8	3.7	5.8	34.7	40.4	50.4	59.2	69.8	62.6	69.8	37.0	17.1	4.9	0.68	1.33	**10.4**	182
Ovary etc.	347	0	-	0.9	-	2.2	1.2	1.7	2.3	6.0	8.7	19.6	17.7	32.8	39.1	51.6	68.5	53.2	50.5	37.0	16.2	4.6	0.66	1.26	**10.4**	183
Other female genital	78	0	-	-	-	-	-	0.6	1.2	1.2	-	2.2	6.4	1.7	6.1	2.8	13.5	29.7	31.3	23.5	3.6	1.0	0.10	0.18	**1.9**	184
†Bladder	86	0	-	-	-	-	-	-	-	-	1.2	1.5	2.4	2.5	12.2	11.3	14.7	26.6	33.7	23.5	4.0	1.2	0.10	0.23	**2.1**	188
Kidney etc.	186	0	0.9	0.9	-	-	-	0.6	0.6	0.6	3.1	5.1	4.0	12.6	22.6	46.0	33.0	37.6	28.9	37.0	8.7	2.5	0.25	0.65	**5.2**	189
Eye	13	0	-	-	-	-	-	-	-	-	1.2	0.7	-	1.7	0.9	0.9	1.2	3.1	2.4	6.7	0.6	0.2	0.02	0.03	**0.3**	190
Brain, nervous system	113	0	-	0.9	3.5	2.2	4.2	1.7	2.9	3.0	4.3	4.4	8.1	5.9	8.7	19.7	13.5	9.4	14.4	3.4	5.3	1.5	0.25	0.41	**4.0**	191-2
Thyroid	63	0	-	-	-	0.7	0.6	2.3	2.9	1.8	3.1	1.5	2.4	1.7	7.0	9.4	6.1	4.7	21.6	6.7	2.9	0.8	0.12	0.20	**1.9**	193
Other endocrine	7	0	1.7	-	-	-	-	-	-	-	1.2	-	-	-	0.8	0.9	0.9	-	-	-	0.3	0.1	0.02	0.03	**0.4**	194
Hodgkin's disease	45	0	-	-	0.9	2.2	3.0	1.7	4.1	3.6	1.2	1.5	1.6	0.8	2.6	1.9	6.1	1.6	2.4	3.4	2.1	0.6	0.12	0.16	**1.7**	201
Non-Hodgkin lymphoma	235	0	-	0.9	0.9	-	1.8	1.1	2.3	2.4	6.8	11.6	12.9	18.5	18.2	33.8	39.2	46.9	48.1	53.8	11.0	3.1	0.39	0.75	**6.7**	200,202
Multiple myeloma	75	0	-	-	-	-	-	-	-	-	-	0.7	4.8	5.0	6.1	13.1	12.2	21.9	28.9	16.8	3.5	1.0	0.08	0.21	**1.8**	203
Lymphoid leukaemia	81	0	3.4	4.5	1.8	0.7	0.6	0.6	0.6	-	0.6	0.7	1.6	4.2	7.8	5.6	11.0	17.2	24.1	40.3	3.8	1.1	0.14	0.22	**2.7**	204
Myeloid leukaemia	83	0	-	-	-	0.7	0.6	-	-	0.6	4.3	2.2	2.4	8.4	7.8	7.5	13.5	20.3	19.2	26.9	3.9	1.1	0.14	0.24	**2.2**	205
Monocytic leukaemia	8	0	-	-	-	-	-	-	-	-	-	0.7	0.8	0.8	-	0.9	1.2	3.1	-	3.4	0.4	0.1	0.01	0.02	**0.2**	206
Other leukaemia	1	0	-	-	-	-	-	-	-	-	0.6	-	-	-	-	-	-	-	-	-	0.0	0.0	0.00	0.00	**0.0**	207
Leukaemia unspecified	9	0	-	-	-	-	-	0.6	-	-	-	-	-	0.8	0.9	3.8	-	1.6	-	3.4	0.4	0.1	0.01	0.03	**0.3**	208
Other and unspecified	383	0	-	-	-	-	-	0.6	0.6	5.4	6.8	5.8	20.2	22.7	40.8	54.5	62.4	98.6	134.7	87.4	17.9	5.1	0.51	1.10	**9.7**	O&U
All sites	7705	0	7.7	9.0	13.2	19.0	21.4	41.9	79.2	149.1	239.2	338.1	476.4	599.7	808.2	967.1	1211.5	1459.8	1647.8	1442.0	360.1		14.01	24.90	**221.5**	ALL
All sites but 173	7478	0	7.7	9.0	13.2	19.0	20.8	39.6	77.4	146.7	235.5	332.3	468.3	589.6	789.9	943.7	1171.1	1416.0	1575.6	1300.8	349.5	100.0	13.75	24.32	**215.9**	ALLb

Rate from 1 case			0.854	0.895	0.883	0.729	0.595	0.574	0.582	0.601	0.620	0.727	0.806	0.841	0.869	0.939	1.224	1.565	2.406	3.361

†Important: see notes on population page

Norway

The Cancer Registry of Norway was initiated by the Norwegian Cancer Society and established in 1951 as a joint project of this society, the Ministry of Health and Social Affairs, the Norwegian Radium Hospital and the Central Bureau of Statistics. Since 1979 it has been the administrative and financial responsibility of the Ministry of Health and Social Affairs.

The registry is based on compulsory reporting of all new cases of cancer in the total population which have been diagnosed since 1953. It aims:

1. To collect data about all new cases of cancer in Norway in order to describe the distribution of this disease and any changes which may occur, as well as to analyse the survival of Norwegian cancer patients.

2. To act as adviser to the Director of Health and the regional cancer centres, etc., and particularly to interpret the need for prophylactic and curative measures against the cancer diseases in Norway as a basis for planning by the health authorities.

3. To conduct epidemiological cancer research, in particular (a) to point out possible endogenous and exogenous carcinogens, especially any that are linked to residence, occupation or lifestyle, and (b) to analyse the effects of prophylactic and curative measures against cancer in Norway.

4. To cooperate with other health and research institutes, and with other registries including cancer registries in other countries.

Norway has an area of 324 000 km^2, and lies between latitudes 57° and 71° N and longitudes 4° and 31° E. The total population is 4 200 000, most of whom are Caucasians, but approximately 0.5% are Lapps and 1% are foreign-born. In 1990 the main occupational areas for men over 15 years were: industry 21%, agriculture 8%, community 23% and other services 48%; the corresponding figures for women were: industry 9%, agriculture 4%, community 50% and other services 37%.

In 1990 there were approximately 16 hospital beds and 2.4 physicians per 1000 inhabitants. Surgical treatment of cancer is carried out both at general hospitals and at oncological centres. Each year the registry receives about 90 000 reports which consist of clinical forms, and copies of cytology, biopsy and autopsy reports from the Central Bureau of Statistics. At regular intervals, the registry materi-al is matched against all deaths in the country and the date and cause of death of cancer patients are recorded.

Primary tumours in different organs in one individual are classified as independent tumours. If multiple tumours occur with paired organs or other sites within the same three-digit ICD code (e.g., kidney, colon), the case is classified in such a way that it can be counted either as one primary cancer only or as the number of primaries that actually exist. A double coding system is also used for lymphomas. Lymphomas in, for instance, the tonsils or the stomach are coded both to the lymphoma site and to the specific organ site. The female breast is an exception because two primary cancers may be registered in one individual. For this publication, however, only one tumour is included for the same three-digit ICD-code. The site coding follows ICD-7 Morphology is coded according to the Manual of Tumour Nomenclature and Coding (MOTNAC) (1968) with modifications according to SNOMED (1979) and special up-to-date codes for the histology of lymphomas (with conversion possibilities to the official codes). From January 1993, all new cases are coded according to the ICD-O-2 classification.

As of 1995, the registry is responsible for organizing the nationwide mass screening for cervical cancer and from 1996 a pilot screening programme for breast cancer covering 50% of the female population aged 50–69 years.

The registry is organized as a multi-user on-line database. All reports are interpreted and, after coding, updated and processed. The database has information on more than 600 000 cancer cases (dating back to 1953) and two million individual reports (dating back to 1970). User-friendly software covering database utilities such as update and retrieval of individual patients, incidence and survival programs, has been developed.

Annual reports on cancer incidence and summary reports with more detailed information on incidence are published regularly. Reports covering survival, trends in incidence and geographical variation in incidence are published. In addition, the registry data are used in epidemiological studies of different cancer sites, on different causes of cancer (e.g., occupational, lifestyle) and on screening. The registry is linked with data on occupation and type of industry obtained at the censuses. A bank including 425 000 specimens of frozen serum is also available for research.

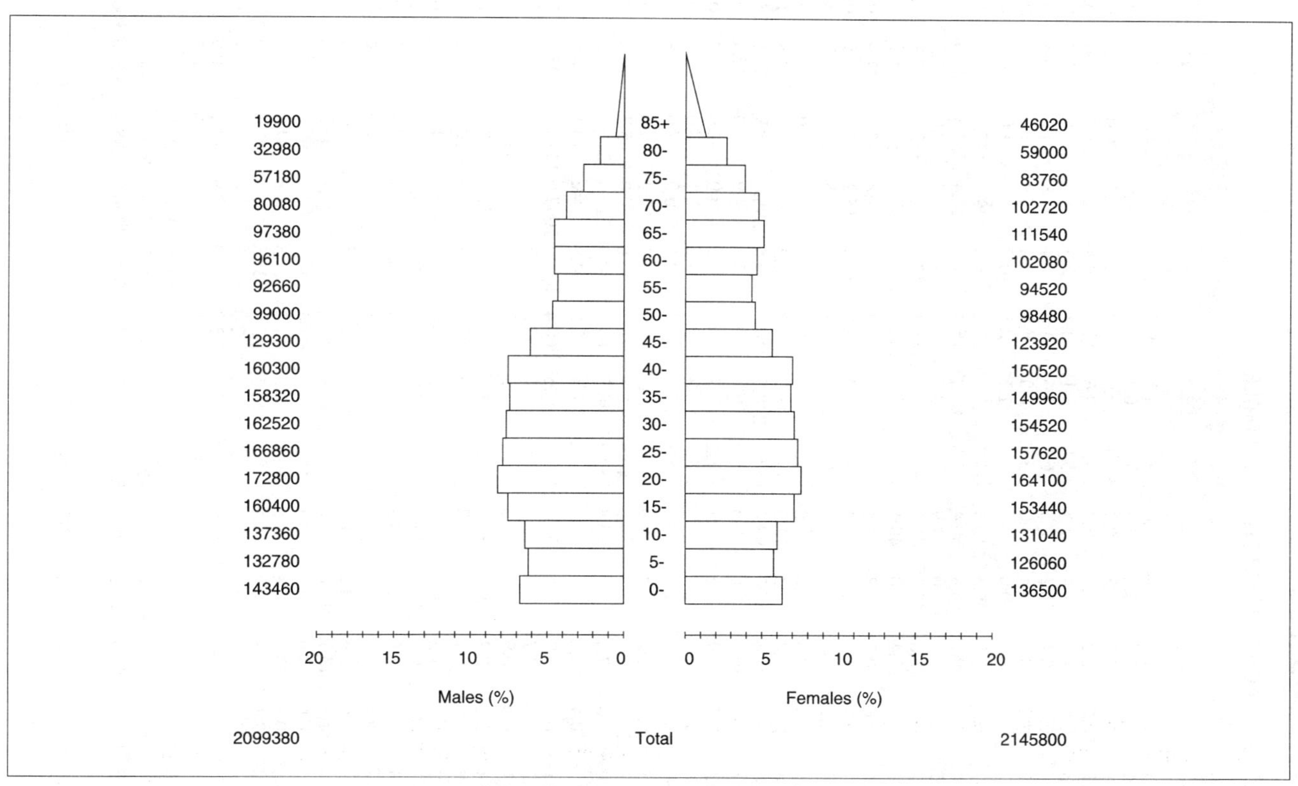

Norway
Source of population: average annual 1988–92
Census: Annual census
Notes to tables overleaf:
† 173 does not include basal cell carcinomas

NORWAY 1988-1992

ANNUAL INCIDENCE PER 100,000 BY AGE GROUP (YEARS) - MALE

SITE	ALL AGES	AGE UNK	0-	5-	10-	15-	20-	25-	30-	35-	40-	45-	50-	55-	60-	65-	70-	75-	80-	85+	CRUDE RATE	%	CR 64	CR 74	ASR (W)	ICD (9th)
Lip	402	0	-	-	-	-	-	-	-	0.5	1.0	1.2	3.4	5.0	8.9	14.6	19.2	24.8	25.5	38.2	3.8	0.9	0.10	0.27	**2.3**	140
Tongue	188	0	-	-	-	-	-	0.2	0.6	0.4	2.0	1.5	3.2	4.3	7.7	6.2	6.2	4.5	4.9	3.0	1.8	0.4	0.10	0.16	**1.3**	141
Salivary gland	101	0	-	-	-	0.2	0.3	0.2	0.6	0.1	1.0	0.3	1.2	0.9	2.1	2.9	4.0	5.2	4.2	6.0	1.0	0.2	0.04	0.07	**0.6**	142
Mouth	273	0	-	-	-	0.1	0.2	0.1	0.4	0.1	0.6	2.2	4.2	3.9	8.1	8.6	13.5	10.8	12.1	21.1	2.6	0.6	0.10	0.21	**1.7**	143-5
Oropharynx	110	0	-	-	-	-	-	-	-	0.3	0.5	1.2	1.4	4.5	5.0	3.1	3.7	2.8	1.8	3.0	1.0	0.2	0.06	0.10	**0.8**	146
Nasopharynx	45	0	-	-	0.1	0.1	0.1	-	0.1	-	0.1	0.2	1.2	1.5	0.6	1.6	1.0	2.4	1.8	1.0	0.4	0.1	0.02	0.03	**0.3**	147
Hypopharynx	130	0	-	-	-	-	-	0.1	-	0.1	0.4	0.8	1.4	3.0	5.8	6.0	4.5	5.2	4.9	1.0	1.2	0.3	0.06	0.11	**0.9**	148
Pharynx unspecified	15	0	-	-	-	-	-	-	-	-	0.1	-	0.6	-	-	1.2	0.5	0.7	-	1.0	0.1	0.0	0.00	0.01	**0.1**	149
Oesophagus	522	0	-	-	-	-	-	0.1	-	0.2	2.8	6.3	10.4	13.3	20.9	27.2	24.8	29.7	27.1	5.0	1.2	0.17	0.41	**3.2**	150
Stomach	2523	0	-	-	-	-	0.3	0.2	1.1	2.0	4.2	9.7	16.8	30.4	41.6	80.9	115.4	171.0	227.4	253.3	24.0	5.7	0.53	1.51	**13.6**	151
Small intestine	131	0	0.1	-	-	-	-	-	0.1	0.5	0.6	1.4	2.0	1.9	3.7	3.1	4.7	8.4	7.9	3.0	1.2	0.3	0.05	0.09	**0.8**	152
Colon	3973	1	-	-	-	0.1	0.3	0.7	1.6	3.7	6.0	18.6	32.1	46.2	82.0	136.6	181.3	252.2	316.6	352.8	37.8	9.0	0.96	2.55	**22.2**	153
Rectum	2764	0	-	-	-	-	-	0.2	1.1	2.3	3.6	12.4	24.0	40.1	62.9	92.0	140.1	178.0	190.4	187.9	26.3	6.3	0.73	1.89	**15.7**	154
Liver	305	0	0.6	-	-	-	0.2	0.5	-	0.6	0.6	0.9	1.8	4.5	6.2	9.4	14.2	18.5	21.8	27.1	2.9	0.7	0.08	0.20	**1.8**	155
Gallbladder etc.	204	0	-	-	-	-	-	0.2	0.4	0.4	0.4	0.5	1.1	1.0	2.4	4.0	7.0	7.5	14.0	15.2	21.1	1.9	0.5	0.05	0.12	**1.1**	156
Pancreas	1436	0	-	-	-	-	-	0.1	-	0.8	2.2	4.8	8.7	18.3	30.2	51.3	73.7	86.4	119.5	118.6	13.7	3.3	0.33	0.95	**7.9**	157
Nose, sinuses etc.	117	0	-	-	-	0.1	0.1	0.1	0.1	0.4	0.4	0.6	2.0	2.2	1.7	3.5	5.2	7.7	4.9	7.0	1.1	0.3	0.04	0.08	**0.7**	160
Larynx	502	0	-	-	-	-	-	-	0.1	0.4	0.6	2.8	5.3	11.9	17.1	18.7	25.2	26.2	18.2	15.1	4.8	1.1	0.19	0.41	**3.1**	161
Bronchus, lung	5782	1	-	-	0.1	0.1	-	0.4	0.5	3.0	8.0	24.4	47.3	98.4	162.1	240.5	316.4	329.5	298.4	185.9	55.1	13.1	1.72	4.51	**34.3**	162
Other thoracic organs	52	0	-	-	-	-	-	0.2	0.1	-	0.5	0.6	0.6	1.0	0.4	2.7	4.5	4.9	1.0	0.5	0.1	0.02	0.03	**0.3**	163-4
Bone	104	0	-	0.3	0.7	1.4	1.5	1.6	0.9	0.3	0.4	0.9	0.6	1.1	1.2	2.7	0.5	2.1	3.0	2.0	1.0	0.2	0.05	0.07	**0.9**	170
Connective tissue	179	0	2.0	0.6	1.0	0.6	0.7	1.1	1.0	0.9	2.0	1.7	0.8	2.4	3.1	2.7	5.0	4.2	6.1	7.0	1.7	0.4	0.09	0.13	**1.5**	171
Mesothelioma	198	0	-	-	-	-	-	-	-	0.6	0.5	2.4	3.7	5.8	7.4	10.7	10.1	10.9	7.0	1.9	0.4	0.07	0.16	**1.2**	MES
Kaposi's sarcoma	77	0	-	-	-	-	-	0.2	0.7	0.8	0.7	1.2	0.4	0.9	0.8	-	1.5	4.2	7.3	9.0	0.7	0.2	0.03	0.04	**0.5**	KAP
Melanoma of skin	1938	0	0.1	-	0.1	0.9	3.1	6.8	9.7	12.9	21.8	32.5	38.4	39.5	40.6	46.8	47.7	44.8	60.0	65.3	18.5	4.4	1.03	1.51	**14.1**	172
†Other skin	2050	0	-	-	0.3	0.2	0.8	0.2	1.4	2.0	3.0	7.3	8.3	15.8	32.9	48.7	89.4	140.3	216.5	315.6	19.5		0.36	1.05	**10.6**	173
Breast	71	0	-	-	-	-	-	-	-	-	0.4	0.2	1.0	0.9	1.2	2.3	2.5	4.9	4.2	10.1	0.7	0.2	0.02	0.04	**0.4**	175
Prostate	10014	0	0.3	-	-	-	-	0.1	-	0.1	0.5	3.2	17.0	51.4	140.9	306.6	560.4	813.9	1097.0	1118.6	95.4	22.7	1.07	5.40	**48.4**	185
Testis	927	0	1.4	0.2	0.6	6.1	13.1	20.1	22.3	16.2	11.2	9.7	7.9	5.0	4.6	2.7	2.2	1.7	4.2	2.0	8.8	2.1	0.59	0.62	**8.0**	186
Penis, other male genital	116	0	-	-	-	-	-	0.1	-	0.1	0.6	0.9	0.8	3.0	1.5	3.5	3.7	5.2	7.9	18.1	1.1	0.3	0.04	0.07	**0.7**	187
Bladder	3033	0	-	0.2	-	-	0.2	0.1	1.1	2.4	2.2	8.7	20.0	32.8	66.8	101.0	148.4	203.2	251.1	275.4	28.9	6.9	0.67	1.92	**16.6**	188
Kidney etc.	1496	0	0.7	0.5	0.1	0.1	-	0.2	0.4	1.9	4.6	10.1	12.9	25.7	36.8	53.6	71.7	80.8	94.6	69.3	14.3	3.4	0.47	1.10	**9.0**	189
Eye	118	0	1.7	0.2	-	-	0.2	0.6	0.8	0.5	1.2	0.8	1.3	2.5	3.3	4.5	3.8	4.9	4.0	1.1	0.3	0.05	0.09	**0.9**	190
Brain, nervous system	924	0	4.2	4.1	3.6	2.1	2.5	3.4	4.8	5.3	8.6	9.1	13.1	16.2	18.1	24.9	22.2	28.0	19.4	17.1	8.8	2.1	0.48	0.71	**7.3**	191-2
Thyroid	241	0	0.1	-	-	0.4	1.4	0.8	1.8	1.3	2.7	2.6	4.2	3.7	5.4	4.5	7.5	6.3	7.9	7.0	2.3	0.5	0.12	0.18	**1.7**	193
Other endocrine	65	0	0.6	0.5	0.4	0.4	0.2	-	0.4	0.4	0.9	0.5	1.6	-	1.9	1.0	1.7	1.4	-	1.0	0.6	0.1	0.04	0.05	**0.6**	194
Hodgkin's disease	260	0	0.1	0.3	0.1	2.5	3.8	4.0	2.5	2.9	2.6	2.6	2.8	1.7	3.3	3.1	4.5	3.5	2.4	4.0	2.5	0.6	0.15	0.18	**2.1**	201
Non-Hodgkin lymphoma	1531	0	0.6	1.2	1.2	2.5	2.4	3.1	4.6	6.8	11.2	13.1	19.6	21.6	33.1	41.9	56.2	67.5	83.1	63.3	14.6	3.5	0.60	1.10	**10.1**	200,202
Multiple myeloma	681	0	-	-	-	-	-	0.2	0.4	0.4	0.6	0.2	3.2	10.4	16.9	23.4	31.5	36.4	62.5	63.3	6.5	1.5	0.17	0.44	**3.8**	203
Lymphoid leukaemia	327	0	5.3	2.7	2.2	1.2	0.2	0.4	-	0.6	0.1	0.8	1.4	2.6	2.7	7.0	11.0	17.5	21.8	34.2	3.1	0.7	0.10	0.19	**2.5**	204
Myeloid leukaemia	437	0	1.3	0.2	0.1	0.5	0.8	1.2	1.7	2.0	2.1	2.8	4.2	4.1	8.1	12.1	13.0	24.5	32.1	27.1	4.2	1.0	0.15	0.27	**2.8**	205
Monocytic leukaemia	44	0	-	-	-	-	0.1	0.1	-	-	-	-	0.4	0.4	1.2	1.2	2.0	3.5	3.0	3.0	0.4	0.1	0.01	0.03	**0.2**	206
Other leukaemia	97	0	0.3	-	-	0.1	0.3	-	0.2	-	0.1	-	0.6	1.9	1.0	2.1	3.0	8.0	7.9	13.1	0.9	0.2	0.02	0.05	**0.6**	207
Leukaemia unspecified	16	0	0.1	-	-	-	-	-	-	-	0.1	-	-	0.4	1.0	0.5	0.7	1.2	1.0	-	0.2	0.0	0.00	0.01	**0.1**	208
Other and unspecified	1685	0	0.1	-	0.1	0.2	0.6	0.4	1.4	1.0	3.5	5.1	9.3	18.8	34.1	48.9	75.7	107.0	156.5	192.0	16.1	3.8	0.37	1.00	**9.2**	O&U
All sites	46204	2	19.5	10.7	11.1	20.3	33.7	47.7	62.9	74.7	114.2	204.2	336.6	555.1	929.2	1460.9	2143.6	2801.7	3475.4	3604.0	440.2		12.10	30.12	**266.4**	ALL
All sites but 173	44154	2	19.5	10.7	10.8	20.1	32.9	47.5	61.5	72.6	111.2	196.9	328.3	539.4	896.4	1412.2	2054.2	2661.4	3258.9	3288.4	420.6	100.0	11.74	29.07	**255.8**	ALLb
Rate from 1 case			0.139	0.151	0.146	0.125	0.116	0.120	0.123	0.126	0.125	0.155	0.202	0.216	0.208	0.205	0.250	0.350	0.606	1.005						

†Important: see notes on population page

NORWAY 1988-1992

ANNUAL INCIDENCE PER 100,000 BY AGE GROUP (YEARS) - FEMALE

SITE	ALL AGES	AGE UNK	0-	5-	10-	15-	20-	25-	30-	35-	40-	45-	50-	55-	60-	65-	70-	75-	80-	85+	CRUDE RATE	%	CR 64	CR 74	ASR (W)	ICD (9th)
Lip	108	0	-	-	-	-	-	-	-	0.1	0.1	1.0	1.2	1.5	1.6	2.2	3.5	4.8	6.1	4.8	1.0	0.3	0.03	0.06	0.5	140
Tongue	119	0	-	-	-	-	0.1	0.1	0.6	0.1	0.7	0.8	1.8	1.7	2.4	1.8	2.5	4.1	5.8	6.5	1.1	0.3	0.04	0.06	0.6	141
Salivary gland	69	0	-	-	-	0.1	0.4	0.1	0.3	0.3	0.3	0.5	1.0	1.3	1.2	1.8	1.8	2.6	1.0	2.2	0.6	0.2	0.03	0.04	0.4	142
Mouth	181	0	-	-	-	-	-	0.1	-	-	0.7	1.0	2.2	2.1	3.3	4.3	5.1	6.4	6.8	14.8	1.7	0.4	0.05	0.09	0.8	143-5
Oropharynx	31	0	-	-	-	-	-	-	-	0.1	-	1.2	0.6	0.8	0.9	1.4	1.0	0.3	-	0.3	0.1	0.01	0.03	0.2	146
Nasopharynx	13	0	-	-	-	-	-	-	-	0.1	0.5	-	-	-	0.4	0.4	1.0	-	0.4	0.1	0.0	0.00	0.01	0.1	147
Hypopharynx	31	0	-	-	-	-	-	-	-	0.3	0.3	0.4	1.1	1.0	0.5	0.8	0.5	0.7	1.7	0.3	0.1	0.02	0.02	0.2	148
Pharynx unspecified	4	0	-	-	-	-	-	-	-	-	-	-	-	0.2	-	0.4	0.2	-	-	0.0	0.0	0.00	0.00	0.0	149
Oesophagus	187	0	-	-	-	-	-	-	-	0.1	0.3	1.3	1.2	1.7	3.7	4.1	5.3	8.1	11.9	10.4	1.7	0.5	0.04	0.09	0.8	150
Stomach	1624	0	-	-	-	-	-	0.3	0.6	1.1	3.6	6.9	7.9	15.0	22.1	29.6	49.1	70.9	106.1	125.6	15.1	4.0	0.29	0.68	6.4	151
Small intestine	154	0	-	-	-	-	-	0.3	-	0.1	0.1	1.5	1.8	2.3	3.1	3.4	5.6	8.4	3.7	4.8	1.4	0.4	0.05	0.09	0.8	152
Colon	4475	0	-	-	0.3	0.1	-	0.9	1.3	4.5	7.7	16.9	31.3	51.4	76.0	102.4	148.6	184.1	245.1	280.3	41.7	11.0	0.95	2.21	19.1	153
Rectum	2277	0	0.1	-	-	-	0.1	0.4	0.4	2.5	5.0	10.2	21.1	25.6	41.9	55.2	82.4	90.7	103.7	127.3	21.2	5.6	0.54	1.23	10.3	154
Liver	230	0	0.4	-	0.5	-	0.1	0.4	0.1	0.1	0.1	1.5	1.4	1.9	3.7	5.4	7.2	10.0	11.9	12.6	2.1	0.6	0.05	0.11	1.1	155
Gallbladder etc.	315	0	-	-	-	-	-	-	0.1	0.3	0.4	0.5	2.0	4.2	3.9	8.1	10.9	11.9	19.3	20.9	2.9	0.8	0.06	0.15	1.3	156
Pancreas	1436	0	-	-	0.2	-	-	-	0.1	0.8	1.3	5.2	6.3	13.3	20.8	32.3	48.9	71.9	85.4	87.8	13.4	3.5	0.24	0.65	5.7	157
Nose, sinuses etc.	72	0	-	0.2	-	-	-	-	-	0.1	0.1	0.5	0.6	0.6	0.6	1.8	1.4	4.5	3.1	5.2	0.7	0.2	0.01	0.03	0.3	160
Larynx	60	0	-	-	-	0.1	0.1	-	0.1	0.1	-	0.6	0.4	0.8	2.0	1.4	1.8	1.9	1.7	2.6	0.6	0.1	0.02	0.04	0.3	161
Bronchus, lung	2340	0	-	-	-	-	-	0.3	0.4	2.7	6.6	13.7	24.8	47.6	69.6	74.8	83.1	79.0	62.0	52.2	21.8	5.7	0.83	1.62	12.6	162
Other thoracic organs	28	0	-	0.2	-	-	0.1	-	-	0.3	0.1	-	-	0.4	1.2	0.4	1.0	0.7	1.0	0.9	0.3	0.1	0.01	0.02	0.2	163-4
Bone	75	0	-	0.5	0.8	1.2	0.6	0.3	0.4	0.5	0.1	0.5	0.6	1.3	1.0	1.4	1.2	1.4	0.7	1.7	0.7	0.2	0.04	0.05	0.6	170
Connective tissue	188	0	1.5	0.2	0.5	0.9	0.9	0.5	0.8	1.3	1.7	1.8	1.2	1.7	1.6	3.9	4.5	5.3	4.4	6.1	1.8	0.5	0.07	0.11	1.3	171
Mesothelioma	43	0	-	-	-	-	-	-	-	0.1	0.1	0.5	0.6	0.2	0.6	1.1	2.1	1.4	1.7	1.3	0.4	0.1	0.01	0.03	0.2	MES
Kaposi's sarcoma	30	0	-	-	-	-	-	-	0.1	-	-	-	-	-	0.8	0.5	0.4	1.2	1.7	4.3	0.3	0.1	0.00	0.01	0.1	KAP
Melanoma of skin	2186	0	0.1	0.2	0.3	3.5	8.4	13.5	17.9	19.3	29.0	33.6	35.5	34.5	35.5	36.0	36.8	39.4	40.7	33.5	20.4	5.4	1.16	1.52	15.3	172
†Other skin	1721	0	-	-	0.2	0.7	0.6	1.0	1.8	2.0	4.5	6.9	11.8	9.9	18.6	27.4	50.2	63.3	109.2	173.0	16.0		0.29	0.68	6.7	173
Breast	9425	0	-	-	-	-	0.5	5.3	16.7	44.3	85.8	145.4	142.2	139.9	175.0	189.9	246.9	269.3	307.5	328.1	87.8	23.1	3.78	5.96	54.2	174
Uterus unspecified	28	0	-	-	-	-	-	-	-	0.1	-	-	0.4	-	0.2	0.8	0.7	1.0	6.1	0.3	0.1	0.00	0.01	0.1	179
Cervix uteri	1802	0	-	-	-	-	2.1	9.8	23.2	28.9	22.7	27.1	28.8	25.6	29.8	30.5	25.3	27.2	29.2	25.2	16.8	4.4	0.99	1.27	12.7	180
Placenta	27	0	-	-	-	0.1	0.9	1.3	0.8	-	0.3	0.2	-	-	-	-	-	-	-	-	0.3	0.1	0.02	0.02	0.3	181
Corpus uteri	2122	0	-	-	-	-	-	0.4	1.3	2.8	7.6	16.9	42.9	54.4	57.0	61.9	64.6	53.2	56.6	43.5	19.8	5.2	0.92	1.55	12.5	182
Ovary etc.	2214	0	0.6	0.2	0.3	0.5	2.3	3.0	4.8	6.0	16.2	27.0	37.4	47.8	45.1	53.1	53.9	60.9	64.4	56.9	20.6	5.4	0.96	1.49	13.3	183
Other female genital	394	0	-	-	-	-	-	0.1	0.3	1.5	1.6	2.6	0.8	3.4	6.1	7.2	13.2	13.8	18.0	35.6	3.7	1.0	0.08	0.18	1.7	184
Bladder	997	0	0.1	-	-	-	0.1	-	0.3	0.5	1.1	2.6	4.5	9.7	18.6	27.1	33.5	40.4	51.9	68.2	9.3	2.4	0.19	0.49	4.1	188
Kidney etc.	1056	0	1.8	0.5	-	-	0.2	0.6	0.6	1.2	2.5	4.7	8.9	14.2	20.8	27.6	39.1	42.5	46.4	36.9	9.8	2.6	0.28	0.61	5.2	189
Eye	120	0	1.9	0.3	-	-	-	0.5	0.1	0.5	0.5	0.8	1.2	1.5	1.8	1.4	2.9	4.3	5.8	3.0	1.1	0.3	0.05	0.07	0.8	190
Brain, nervous system	769	0	4.0	2.4	2.3	1.7	2.1	3.4	3.5	5.2	5.0	7.3	7.9	12.3	10.4	17.8	20.6	19.6	16.3	9.1	7.2	1.9	0.34	0.53	5.3	191-2
Thyroid	679	0	-	0.2	0.2	1.6	3.2	5.5	5.4	7.7	9.3	9.4	9.3	9.7	7.6	10.0	11.3	12.7	12.2	14.8	6.3	1.7	0.35	0.45	4.7	193
Other endocrine	66	0	1.9	0.2	0.3	0.3	0.4	0.3	0.3	0.1	0.8	0.5	0.6	0.8	0.4	1.3	1.2	1.4	0.7	0.4	0.6	0.2	0.03	0.05	0.6	194
Hodgkin's disease	178	0	-	0.5	0.2	2.6	3.2	2.7	1.4	1.3	1.1	1.1	1.4	1.3	1.4	1.6	2.1	3.6	2.4	3.9	1.7	0.4	0.09	0.11	1.4	201
Non-Hodgkin lymphoma	1342	1	0.4	0.6	0.5	0.9	1.1	1.8	2.8	5.3	8.0	9.7	16.2	17.1	23.5	27.8	40.5	50.1	49.8	51.3	12.5	3.3	0.44	0.78	7.1	200,202
Multiple myeloma	577	0	-	-	-	-	-	-	0.1	0.3	1.3	1.8	2.8	7.6	8.0	12.7	21.4	30.1	30.2	28.7	5.4	1.4	0.11	0.28	2.4	203
Lymphoid leukaemia	253	0	5.3	2.2	0.2	0.9	0.4	0.1	0.3	0.4	0.1	0.6	0.4	1.1	2.2	2.3	6.2	10.3	9.8	20.0	2.4	0.6	0.07	0.11	1.7	204
Myeloid leukaemia	369	0	1.3	-	0.5	0.7	0.6	1.1	0.9	2.0	2.0	2.6	3.2	4.9	4.5	5.9	8.6	14.6	14.6	18.7	3.4	0.9	0.12	0.19	2.0	205
Monocytic leukaemia	50	0	-	0.2	0.2	-	-	-	0.3	-	-	0.3	-	0.6	0.4	0.7	1.9	1.9	2.0	4.8	0.5	0.1	0.01	0.02	0.2	206
Other leukaemia	88	0	-	-	-	-	-	0.1	-	0.1	0.1	0.2	0.2	0.4	0.8	2.0	2.1	2.9	6.1	10.9	0.8	0.2	0.01	0.03	0.3	207
Leukaemia unspecified	13	0	-	0.2	-	-	-	-	-	-	-	-	0.2	0.2	0.2	0.4	0.4	0.5	0.7	0.4	0.1	0.0	0.00	0.01	0.1	208
Other and unspecified	1891	0	0.4	0.3	-	-	0.1	-	0.3	2.0	3.5	5.2	8.5	15.7	33.9	31.4	53.7	77.8	109.5	183.0	17.6	4.6	0.35	0.77	7.4	O&U
All sites	42457	1	19.9	8.7	7.0	15.9	28.5	54.1	88.3	147.0	232.9	371.9	474.2	589.5	764.3	913.8	1206.6	1412.6	1668.8	1930.5	395.7		14.01	24.61	223.9	ALL
All sites but 173	40736	1	19.9	8.7	6.9	15.3	27.9	53.0	86.5	145.0	228.4	364.9	462.4	579.6	745.7	886.3	1156.3	1349.3	1559.7	1757.5	379.7	100.0	13.72	23.93	217.1	ALLb

Rate from 1 case   0.146 0.159 0.153 0.130 0.122 0.127 0.129 0.133 0.133 0.161 0.203 0.212 0.196 0.179 0.195 0.239 0.339 0.435

†Important: see notes on population page

Poland, Cracow

In Poland, nationwide reporting of cancer has been compulsory by administrative order since 1952. However, with the resources available, it proved impossible to obtain data of uniformly good quality from the central registration scheme covering the whole country. To improve the quality of registration, a few selected areas of Poland were chosen, where reporting of cancer is based on active registration. One of those areas is Cracow City, where the Cancer Registry was established in 1965. The registry is housed in the Cracow Branch Centre of the Oncology Marie Sklodowska-Curie Memorial Institute.

Cracow City, the third largest town of Poland, is situated on the Vistula River at latitude 50°4′ N and longitude 19°58′ E, at 220 m above sea level. The surface area is 357km². The 1992 population was 750 540 and was homogeneously of Slav origin.

Cracow City is one of the biggest industrial (with metallurgical, electromechanical, chemical and food industries), cultural and educational centres of Poland. As the old capital of Poland it is also one of the main centres of tourism.

The main occupational groups in 1990 were: industry 29%; science and education 17.4%; construction 14.1%; health service 8.8%; transport and communication 6.4%; trade 4.6%.

Cracow City has a high level of air pollution, with an annual average of 53 µg/m³ particulates; 60.5 µg/m³ SO_2; 47.5 µg/m³ NO_2 and 1.75 µg/m³ fluorine (1990 data).

The number of physicians in 1990 was 2641 and the total number of hospital beds 8383, including 220 beds in the Cracow Branch Centre of the Oncology Maria Sklodowska-Curie Memorial Institute.

Because of its location, the registry has direct access to medical records of patients treated and followed in the Cancer Centre, who amount to about 50% of all patients with cancer in Cracow City; these include about 90% of all patients treated by radiotherapy and about 75% of patients who need complex treatment.

By administrative order, all hospitals and outpatient clinics have to report cancer cases to the registry. This information is completed and checked against data from pathology departments and death certificates. Cases are filed in alphabetical order by year, and new reports are checked there for duplicates. Patient follow-up is carried out by the registry through an annual check of medical records, death certificates and other information from local Vital Statistics Offices.

Since 1980, a Cancer Registry Report has been prepared each year to provide information about cancer incidence and mortality, methods of diagnosis and treatment in Cracow City and the rural Nowy Sacz Region. This report is sent to all doctors involved in cancer control. Information from Cracow Cancer Registry is also used to study trends in cancer incidence, mortality and survival. It is the only Polish population-based cancer registry participating in the EUROCARE study of cancer survival.

Since 1986, the registry data have been used to survey cancer patients about their smoking, drinking and nutrition habits, and also to evaluate occupational cancer risks.

J. Pawlega

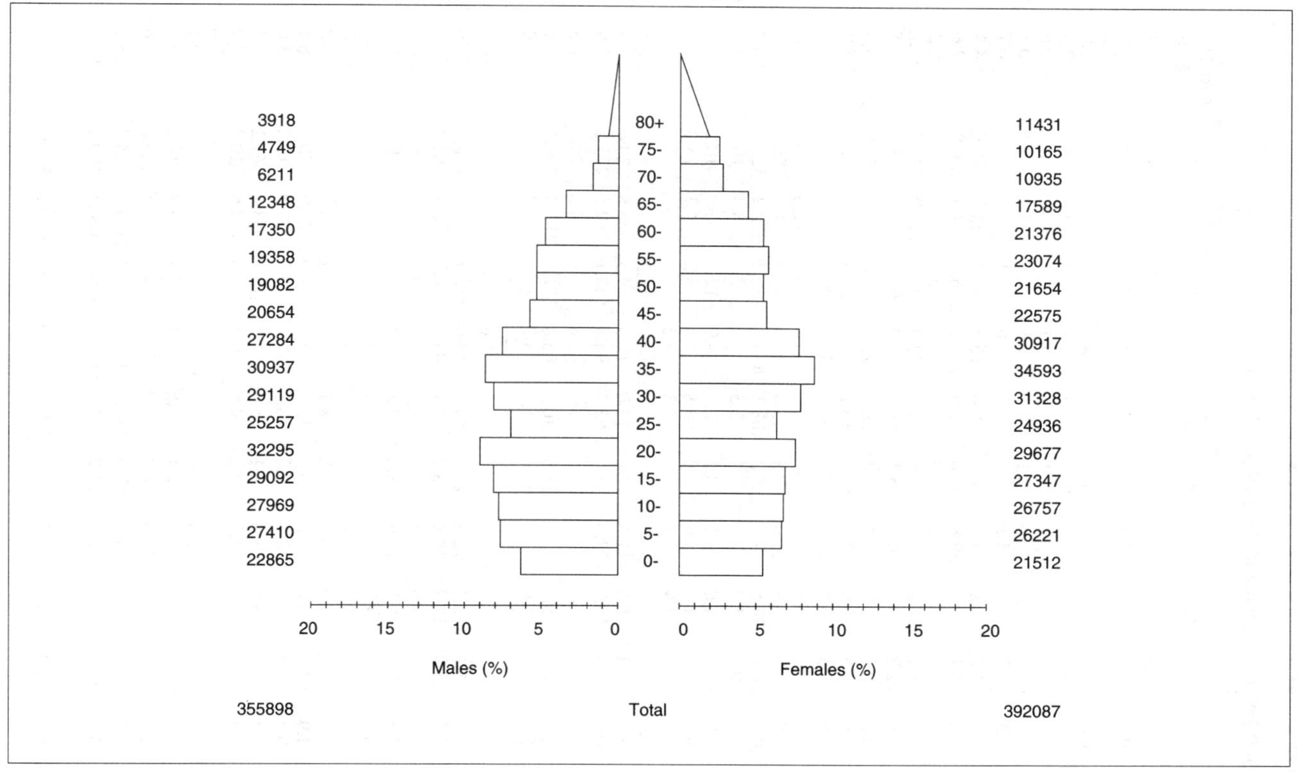

Poland, Cracow
Source of population: average annual 1988–92
Census: 6.12.1988 – Central Statistical Office
Estimate: The estimated population for each of the years 1989–92 was based on the 1988 Census, updated every three months by additions (births, returning residents) and deductions (deaths and departing residents).

Notes to tables overleaf:
* The high proportion of DCO diagnoses and low levels of morphological verification for several sites suggest under-ascertainment and problems of validity.
† 188 does not include non-invasive tumours

* POLAND, CRACOW 1988-1992

ANNUAL INCIDENCE PER 100,000 BY AGE GROUP (YEARS) - MALE

SITE	ALL AGES	AGE UNK	0-	5-	10-	15-	20-	25-	30-	35-	40-	45-	50-	55-	60-	65-	70-	75-	80+	CRUDE RATE	%	CR 64	CR 74	ASR (W)	ICD (9th)
Lip	32	0	-	-	-	-	-	-	-	-	1.5	1.9	-	2.1	6.9	4.9	12.9	12.6	51.0	1.8	0.6	0.06	0.15	1.6	140
Tongue	28	0	-	-	-	-	-	-	-	0.6	0.7	2.9	6.3	7.2	5.8	4.9	6.4	-	-	1.6	0.5	0.12	0.17	1.4	141
Salivary gland	17	0	-	-	-	-	-	-	-	0.6	1.5	-	5.2	-	5.8	3.2	-	8.4	-	1.0	0.3	0.07	0.08	0.8	142
Mouth	33	0	-	-	-	-	-	-	-	0.6	2.9	4.8	3.1	6.2	4.6	8.1	12.9	-	5.1	1.9	0.6	0.11	0.22	1.6	143-5
Oropharynx	41	0	-	-	-	-	-	-	-	-	0.7	1.9	4.2	11.4	11.5	8.1	9.7	8.4	15.3	2.3	0.8	0.15	0.24	2.0	146
Nasopharynx	11	0	-	-	-	-	-	0.8	-	-	-	1.0	2.1	3.1	-	3.2	-	-	10.2	0.6	0.2	0.03	0.05	0.5	147
Hypopharynx	6	0	-	-	-	-	-	-	-	-	-	1.0	-	2.1	-	1.6	-	4.2	5.1	0.3	0.1	0.02	0.02	0.3	148
Pharynx unspecified	12	0	-	-	-	-	-	-	-	1.3	0.7	-	3.1	3.1	1.2	1.6	3.2	-	-	0.7	0.2	0.05	0.07	0.6	149
Oesophagus	85	0	-	-	-	-	-	-	-	0.6	1.5	4.8	13.6	10.3	19.6	16.2	41.9	33.7	30.6	4.8	1.7	0.25	0.54	4.3	150
Stomach	438	1	-	-	-	-	-	-	1.4	2.6	4.4	9.7	39.8	63.0	79.5	126.3	186.8	227.4	290.9	24.6	8.5	1.00	2.57	21.5	151
Small intestine	5	0	-	-	-	-	-	-	-	-	1.5	-	-	1.0	-	-	6.4	-	-	0.3	0.1	0.01	0.04	0.3	152
Colon	234	0	-	-	-	-	-	-	0.7	0.6	8.1	6.8	11.5	28.9	54.2	72.9	93.4	117.9	132.7	13.1	4.6	0.55	1.39	11.4	153
Rectum	215	0	-	-	-	-	-	-	2.1	1.9	2.2	3.9	6.3	35.1	46.1	81.0	67.6	75.8	168.4	12.1	4.2	0.49	1.23	10.4	154
Liver	99	0	-	-	-	0.7	-	-	-	0.6	0.7	1.9	6.3	13.4	26.5	21.1	38.6	71.6	51.0	5.6	1.9	0.25	0.55	4.8	155
Gallbladder etc.	92	0	-	-	-	-	-	-	0.7	0.6	1.5	1.9	3.1	13.4	16.1	29.2	29.0	50.5	86.8	5.2	1.8	0.19	0.48	4.5	156
Pancreas	192	0	-	-	-	-	-	-	0.7	1.9	1.5	5.8	21.0	24.8	33.4	48.6	90.2	105.3	122.5	10.8	3.7	0.45	1.14	9.5	157
Nose, sinuses etc.	8	0	-	-	-	-	-	-	-	-	-	1.9	1.0	-	-	3.2	-	12.6	-	0.4	0.2	0.01	0.03	0.4	160
Larynx	194	0	-	-	-	-	-	-	-	1.9	9.5	20.3	21.0	40.3	45.0	48.6	41.9	21.1	56.1	10.9	3.8	0.69	1.14	9.4	161
Bronchus, lung	1605	0	-	-	-	-	0.6	0.8	4.1	10.3	26.4	76.5	152.0	286.2	408.1	474.5	486.2	602.2	525.7	90.2	31.3	4.82	9.63	77.8	162
Other thoracic organs	22	0	0.9	-	-	0.7	0.6	0.8	-	-	0.7	1.0	-	2.1	3.5	9.7	3.2	8.4	10.2	1.2	0.4	0.05	0.12	1.1	163-4
Bone	23	0	-	-	0.7	1.4	0.6	0.8	-	1.3	-	1.0	3.1	3.1	-	4.9	12.9	-	10.2	1.3	0.4	0.06	0.15	1.2	170
Connective tissue	26	0	-	-	-	1.4	0.6	2.4	0.7	0.6	0.7	1.9	1.0	1.0	5.8	4.9	3.2	4.2	15.3	1.5	0.5	0.08	0.12	1.3	171
Mesothelioma	9	0	-	-	-	-	-	0.8	-	-	-	1.9	1.0	-	2.3	3.2	-	-	5.1	0.5	0.2	0.03	0.05	0.5	MES
Kaposi's sarcoma	1	0	-	-	-	-	-	-	-	-	-	-	-	-	-	3.2	-	-	-	0.1	0.0	0.00	0.02	0.1	KAP
Melanoma of skin	89	0	-	-	-	-	0.6	2.4	-	3.9	7.3	6.8	11.5	12.4	15.0	14.6	19.3	29.5	20.4	5.0	1.7	0.30	0.47	4.3	172
Other skin	354	0	-	-	-	-	1.2	-	4.1	0.6	5.9	16.5	22.0	43.4	63.4	98.8	148.1	189.5	255.2	19.9		0.79	2.02	17.5	173
Breast	6	0	-	-	-	-	-	-	-	-	-	-	-	-	-	1.6	-	4.2	20.4	0.3	0.1	0.00	0.01	0.3	175
Prostate	266	0	-	-	-	-	1.2	0.8	-	-	0.7	5.8	2.1	15.5	40.3	85.8	151.3	185.3	306.2	14.9	5.2	0.33	1.52	13.4	185
Testis	53	0	-	-	-	0.7	4.3	7.9	8.9	5.8	5.9	1.0	-	1.2	3.2	-	4.2	-	-	3.0	1.0	0.18	0.19	2.5	186
Penis	9	0	-	-	-	-	-	-	-	1.3	-	1.9	2.1	1.0	-	-	3.2	4.2	-	0.5	0.2	0.03	0.05	0.4	187.1-.4
Other male genital	1	0	-	-	-	-	-	-	-	-	-	-	-	-	1.6	-	-	-	-	0.1	0.0	0.00	0.01	0.0	187.5-.9
†Bladder	242	0	-	-	-	-	-	-	-	-	5.1	5.8	12.6	22.7	59.9	68.0	112.7	147.4	158.2	13.6	4.7	0.53	1.43	11.9	188
Kidney etc.	234	0	1.7	-	0.7	-	-	2.4	0.7	2.6	5.9	19.4	28.3	38.2	61.1	43.7	54.7	88.4	66.3	13.1	4.6	0.80	1.30	11.5	189
Eye	9	0	-	-	-	-	-	-	-	-	-	1.0	1.0	-	3.5	3.2	3.2	-	5.1	0.5	0.2	0.03	0.06	0.5	190
Brain, nervous system	120	0	0.9	0.7	2.9	0.7	-	3.2	4.1	2.6	12.5	8.7	19.9	18.6	13.8	19.4	19.3	16.8	10.2	6.7	2.3	0.44	0.64	6.0	191-2
Thyroid	15	0	-	-	-	-	-	-	-	0.6	-	1.0	-	2.1	4.6	8.1	6.4	-	-	0.8	0.3	0.04	0.11	0.7	193
Other endocrine	9	0	-	-	1.4	-	-	-	-	0.6	-	1.0	1.0	-	-	6.5	-	-	-	0.5	0.2	0.02	0.05	0.5	194
Hodgkin's disease	54	0	-	0.7	2.1	0.7	1.2	2.4	6.2	3.9	2.2	1.9	5.2	7.2	8.1	1.6	9.7	4.2	-	3.0	1.1	0.21	0.27	2.6	201
Non-Hodgkin lymphoma	114	0	-	2.2	0.7	1.4	1.2	4.0	0.7	1.9	4.4	5.8	16.8	20.7	13.8	17.8	41.9	37.9	20.4	6.4	2.2	0.37	0.67	5.8	200,202
Multiple myeloma	54	0	-	-	-	-	-	-	0.7	0.6	2.2	1.0	2.1	7.2	8.1	19.4	29.0	37.9	10.2	3.0	1.1	0.11	0.35	2.6	203
Lymphoid leukaemia	63	0	4.4	2.2	2.9	1.4	-	-	1.4	-	-	3.9	1.0	3.1	5.8	16.2	12.9	33.7	61.2	3.5	1.2	0.13	0.28	3.5	204
Myeloid leukaemia	52	0	0.9	0.7	2.1	0.7	1.2	2.4	2.1	1.9	2.9	1.0	2.1	6.2	4.6	9.7	22.5	12.6	10.2	2.9	1.0	0.14	0.31	2.7	205
Monocytic leukaemia	0	0	-	-	-	-	-	-	-	-	-	-	-	-	-	-	-	-	-	0.0	0.0	0.00	0.00	0.0	206
Other leukaemia	2	0	-	-	-	-	-	-	-	-	-	1.0	1.0	-	-	-	-	-	-	0.1	0.0	0.01	0.01	0.1	207
Leukaemia unspecified	15	0	0.9	-	-	-	-	-	-	-	-	1.0	-	2.1	3.5	4.9	6.4	4.2	10.2	0.8	0.3	0.04	0.09	0.8	208
Other and unspecified	295	0	-	0.7	-	-	-	0.8	1.4	2.6	7.3	10.7	21.0	39.3	65.7	72.9	74.1	185.3	199.0	16.6	5.8	0.75	1.48	14.2	O&U
All sites	5484	1	9.6	7.3	13.6	9.6	13.6	32.5	40.5	55.6	129.0	247.9	454.9	797.6	1148.1	1477.1	1864.4	2349.8	2745.7	308.2		14.80	31.51	269.2	ALL
All sites but 173	5130	1	9.6	7.3	13.6	9.6	12.4	32.5	36.4	54.9	123.1	231.4	432.9	754.2	1084.7	1378.3	1716.3	2160.3	2490.6	288.3	100.0	14.02	29.49	251.7	ALLb

Rate from 1 case 0.875 0.730 0.715 0.687 0.619 0.792 0.687 0.646 0.733 0.968 1.048 1.033 1.153 1.620 3.220 4.211 5.104

†Important: see notes on population page

* POLAND, CRACOW 1988-1992

ANNUAL INCIDENCE PER 100,000 BY AGE GROUP (YEARS) - FEMALE

SITE	ALL AGES	AGE UNK	0-	5-	10-	15-	20-	25-	30-	35-	40-	45-	50-	55-	60-	65-	70-	75-	80+	CRUDE RATE	%	CR 64	CR 74	ASR (W)	ICD (9th)
Lip	8	0	-	-	-	-	-	-	-	-	-	0.9	-	-	-	-	3.7	5.9	3.5	0.4	0.1	0.00	0.02	**0.2**	*140*
Tongue	3	0	-	-	-	-	-	-	-	-	-	-	-	0.9	1.9	-	-	-	-	0.2	0.1	0.01	0.01	**0.1**	*141*
Salivary gland	12	0	-	-	-	-	-	-	-	-	-	1.8	0.9	0.9	0.9	3.4	3.7	-	3.5	0.6	0.2	0.02	0.06	**0.4**	*142*
Mouth	14	0	-	-	-	-	-	-	0.6	0.6	1.3	0.9	1.8	-	3.7	1.1	1.8	-	1.7	0.7	0.2	0.04	0.06	**0.5**	*143-5*
Oropharynx	11	0	-	-	-	-	0.7	0.8	0.6	-	-	-	-	0.9	1.9	3.4	-	2.0	1.7	0.6	0.2	0.02	0.04	**0.4**	*146*
Nasopharynx	12	0	-	-	-	-	-	-	0.6	1.2	3.9	-	-	-	0.9	1.1	1.8	-	-	0.6	0.2	0.03	0.05	**0.4**	*147*
Hypopharynx	6	0	-	-	-	-	-	-	-	-	-	-	0.9	-	1.9	2.3	-	2.0	-	0.3	0.1	0.01	0.03	**0.2**	*148*
Pharynx unspecified	3	0	-	-	-	-	-	-	-	-	-	-	-	-	-	-	3.7	-	1.7	0.2	0.1	0.00	0.02	**0.1**	*149*
Oesophagus	22	0	-	-	-	-	-	-	-	-	-	0.9	1.8	2.6	2.8	5.7	3.7	-	10.5	1.1	0.4	0.04	0.09	**0.7**	*150*
Stomach	283	1	-	-	-	-	-	-	1.9	2.3	5.2	5.3	6.5	19.9	22.5	42.1	67.7	80.7	161.0	14.4	5.0	0.32	0.87	**8.0**	*151*
Small intestine	9	0	-	-	-	-	-	-	-	-	-	-	-	1.7	1.9	2.3	1.8	2.0	1.7	0.5	0.2	0.02	0.04	**0.3**	*152*
Colon	274	0	-	-	-	-	-	-	1.9	4.6	3.2	8.0	11.1	30.3	36.5	40.9	71.3	63.0	98.0	14.0	4.8	0.48	1.04	**8.6**	*153*
Rectum	204	0	-	-	-	-	-	-	0.6	2.9	5.8	10.6	13.9	13.9	19.6	37.5	38.4	53.1	77.0	10.4	3.6	0.34	0.72	**6.4**	*154*
Liver	114	0	-	-	-	-	-	-	-	0.6	0.6	0.9	3.7	9.5	13.1	18.2	25.6	33.4	61.2	5.8	2.0	0.14	0.36	**3.2**	*155*
Gallbladder etc.	240	0	-	-	-	-	-	-	0.6	-	1.3	3.5	8.3	17.3	28.1	47.8	60.4	82.6	99.7	12.2	4.2	0.30	0.84	**7.0**	*156*
Pancreas	208	0	-	-	-	-	-	-	-	1.7	-	2.7	4.6	18.2	27.1	44.3	40.2	64.9	92.7	10.6	3.7	0.27	0.69	**6.0**	*157*
Nose, sinuses etc.	5	0	-	-	-	-	-	-	-	-	-	-	-	1.9	1.1	1.8	-	1.7		0.3	0.1	0.01	0.02	**0.2**	*160*
Larynx	28	0	-	-	-	-	-	-	-	0.6	0.9	2.8	1.7	7.5	5.7	5.5	5.9	3.5		1.4	0.5	0.07	0.12	**1.0**	*161*
Bronchus, lung	463	1	-	-	-	-	-	-	0.6	1.7	10.4	16.8	19.4	45.9	80.5	114.8	106.1	88.5	103.2	23.6	8.2	0.88	1.99	**15.3**	*162*
Other thoracic organs	13	0	-	-	-	-	-	-	-	-	-	-	0.9	-	1.9	2.3	1.8	7.9	5.2	0.7	0.2	0.01	0.03	**0.4**	*163-4*
Bone	19	0	-	0.8	2.2	-	-	-	0.6	-	-	-	0.9	3.5	0.9	2.3	5.5	5.9	-	1.0	0.3	0.04	0.08	**0.8**	*170*
Connective tissue	24	0	1.9	-	0.7	0.7	-	0.8	-	-	1.3	-	2.8	2.6	-	1.1	3.7	7.9	7.0	1.2	0.4	0.05	0.08	**1.0**	*171*
Mesothelioma	7	0	-	-	-	-	-	-	-	-	0.6	-	0.9	-	1.9	-	-	-	5.2	0.4	0.1	0.02	0.02	**0.2**	*MES*
Kaposi's sarcoma	0	0	-	-	-	-	-	-	-	-	-	-	-	-	-	-	-	-	-	0.0	0.0	0.00	0.00	**0.0**	*KAP*
Melanoma of skin	100	0	-	-	-	-	0.7	0.8	5.1	2.3	9.1	6.2	4.6	13.9	15.0	9.1	11.0	11.8	14.0	5.1	1.8	0.29	0.39	**3.6**	*172*
Other skin	335	0	-	-	-	-	2.0	0.8	1.9	2.3	11.0	14.2	14.8	31.2	29.0	51.2	80.5	86.6	131.2	17.1		0.54	1.19	**10.5**	*173*
Breast	1214	0	-	-	-	-	-	4.8	8.9	33.5	62.1	107.2	134.8	126.5	162.8	180.8	171.9	186.9	183.7	61.9	21.5	3.20	4.97	**44.0**	*174*
Uterus unspecified	23	0	-	-	-	-	-	-	-	0.6	0.6	-	1.8	-	1.9	3.4	1.8	2.0	21.0	1.2	0.4	0.02	0.05	**0.6**	*179*
Cervix uteri	550	0	-	-	-	0.7	-	2.4	19.2	28.9	43.3	57.6	42.5	60.7	73.9	51.2	58.5	64.9	50.7	28.1	9.7	1.65	2.19	**20.6**	*180*
Placenta	0	0	-	-	-	-	-	-	-	-	-	-	-	-	-	-	-	-	-	0.0	0.0	0.00	0.00	**0.0**	*181*
Corpus uteri	342	0	-	-	-	-	-	-	0.6	0.6	7.1	15.9	42.5	53.7	63.6	61.4	54.9	45.3	49.0	17.4	6.0	0.92	1.50	**12.2**	*182*
Ovary etc.	377	0	1.9	-	0.7	2.2	1.3	2.4	3.8	6.4	21.3	31.0	38.8	46.8	44.9	58.0	49.4	76.7	35.0	19.2	6.7	1.01	1.54	**14.0**	*183*
Other female genital	67	0	-	-	-	-	-	-	0.6	-	0.6	1.8	0.9	1.7	12.2	12.5	12.8	25.6	28.0	3.4	1.2	0.09	0.22	**2.0**	*184*
†Bladder	49	0	-	-	-	-	-	-	-	-	-	0.9	0.9	2.6	10.3	11.4	11.0	13.8	17.5	2.5	0.9	0.07	0.19	**1.5**	*188*
Kidney etc.	136	0	1.9	1.5	-	-	1.6	0.6	0.6	3.9	5.3	12.9	18.2	20.6	21.6	31.1	31.5	12.2		6.9	2.4	0.34	0.60	**5.0**	*189*
Eye	20	0	-	-	-	-	-	0.6	-	-	0.9	5.5	2.6	1.9	3.4	3.7	2.0	1.7		1.0	0.4	0.06	0.09	**0.8**	*190*
Brain, nervous system	82	0	2.8	2.3	0.7	0.7	2.7	0.8	0.6	1.7	7.1	3.5	6.5	10.4	5.6	10.2	9.1	15.7	5.2	4.2	1.5	0.23	0.32	**3.4**	*191-2*
Thyroid	63	0	-	-	-	0.7	0.7	0.8	1.3	0.6	4.5	6.2	5.5	4.3	5.6	5.7	9.1	15.7	14.0	3.2	1.1	0.15	0.23	**2.3**	*193*
Other endocrine	12	0	-	-	-	-	-	-	0.6	-	1.3	-	1.8	-	0.9	1.1	3.7	3.9	1.7	0.6	0.2	0.02	0.05	**0.4**	*194*
Hodgkin's disease	52	0	-	-	0.7	0.7	2.0	4.0	3.8	1.7	1.9	1.8	5.5	3.5	4.7	3.4	3.7	7.9	7.0	2.7	0.9	0.15	0.19	**2.1**	*201*
Non-Hodgkin lymphoma	75	0	0.9	-	-	2.2	0.7	0.8	1.3	1.7	1.9	0.9	5.5	8.7	6.5	14.8	11.0	19.7	14.0	3.8	1.3	0.16	0.28	**2.7**	*200,202*
Multiple myeloma	57	0	-	-	-	-	-	-	-	-	-	0.9	1.8	10.4	7.5	15.9	12.8	9.8	14.0	2.9	1.0	0.10	0.25	**1.8**	*203*
Lymphoid leukaemia	37	0	2.8	1.5	1.5	-	-	-	0.6	0.6	-	1.8	3.7	1.7	2.8	2.3	5.5	9.8	12.2	1.9	0.7	0.09	0.12	**1.6**	*204*
Myeloid leukaemia	54	0	0.9	2.3	-	2.2	-	1.6	-	0.6	2.6	3.5	2.8	5.2	0.9	6.8	9.1	15.7	12.2	2.8	1.0	0.11	0.19	**2.1**	*205*
Monocytic leukaemia	0	0	-	-	-	-	-	-	-	-	-	-	-	-	-	-	-	-	-	0.0	0.0	0.00	0.00	**0.0**	*206*
Other leukaemia	1	0	0.9	-	-	-	-	-	-	-	-	-	-	-	-	-	-	-	-	0.1	0.0	0.00	0.00	**0.1**	*207*
Leukaemia unspecified	17	0	-	-	-	-	-	-	-	-	-	-	0.9	-	-	1.9	2.3	3.7	9.8	8.7	0.9	0.3	0.01	0.04	**0.5**	*208*
Other and unspecified	345	0	1.9	-	-	-	-	0.8	3.2	-	7.1	10.6	18.5	18.2	30.9	59.1	89.6	120.0	136.5	17.6	6.1	0.46	1.20	**10.6**	*O&U*
All sites	5990	2	15.8	8.4	6.7	10.2	10.8	23.3	61.3	97.7	219.9	324.3	433.2	590.3	760.7	963.1	1091.9	1280.8	1509.8	305.5		12.82	23.10	**203.6**	*ALL*
All sites but 173	5655	2	15.8	8.4	6.7	10.2	8.8	22.5	59.4	95.4	208.9	310.1	418.4	559.1	731.7	911.9	1011.4	1194.3	1378.6	288.5	100.0	12.28	21.90	**193.1**	*ALLb*

Rate from 1 case   0.930 0.763 0.747 0.731 0.674 0.802 0.638 0.578 0.647 0.886 0.924 0.867 0.936 1.137 1.829 1.967 1.750

†Important: see notes on population page

Poland, Kielce

The Kielce Cancer Registry was established in 1962 by administrative order of the Ministry of Health. Until 1986, data were collected on special patient cards. Until 1988 the epidemiological staff was largely untrained and not supervised, so that the data available from this period are of limited use for cancer epidemiology.

The Holycross Cancer Registry was established in 1986, and all hospitals and outpatient clinics of the province were asked to collaborate with it so that full coverage of the population was achieved. In 1988 a team of highly educated workers was employed who started to pursue active follow-up and follow-back. Each year statisticians visit all hospitals and outpatient clinics in the province, checking the reporting of cancer cases. As a result, this cancer registry is now one of the best in Poland. It is a department of the Holycross Cancer Centre and its full name is Department of Epidemiology and Cancer Control – Regional Cancer Registry.

The main aims of the registry are to describe the incidence and major epidemiological characteristics of cancers occurring in Kielce Province and to promote and facilitate epidemiological research, to assess current and future needs for cancer care services, to support the implementation of preventive and other cancer control activities and to evaluate their effects. The data provided are used by the National Cancer Registry of Poland.

The registry staff consists of: a physician oncologist as head, working part-time, one biologist, one computer scientist and one statistician. In cases of uncertainty, the problem is always discussed with oncologists.

The registry covers the Province of Kielce (area 9211 km^2), one of 49 provinces in Poland, which is located in the central part of the country between latitudes 51°23′ and 50°13′ N and longitudes 21°41′ and 19°45′ E. The Holy Cross Mountains (about 600 m above sea level) are situated in the north of province. In the south is a fertile agricultural region. The Wisla (Vistula) river forms the province's south-eastern border.

The annual average temperature is 6.9°C (maximum 32.9°C and minimum −33.9°C). Annual rainfall amounts to about 565 mm.

The population of the province in 1992 was 1 135 607 (about 3% of the Polish population), with 49% males and 51% females (density 123.3 per km^2). 47% of the population lived in the towns and 53% in the country. The average age was 34 years. The working population was 198 978 (67% males and 33% females) and unemployment was 17%. The population was homogeneously of Slav origin and the great majority belonged to the Roman Catholic church.

The urban population includes 215 400 in Kielce city and about 160 000 in three cities in the north of the province where heavy metallurgical industry is located. About 30 km to the west of Kielce city, there is cement and lime industry. Of the working population, 39% were employed in heavy industry (cement, metallurgy, energy), 32% in light industry (cloth, leather, food) and 8% in construction. In villages about 74% of working people work in their own small farms with sizes varying from 2 to 10 ha, which account for about 80% of all farms.

Most air pollution is produced by the cement and metal industries and by coal combustion. According to 1993 data, air pollution consisted of dust (27 804 tonnes/y), SO_2 (15 680 tonnes/y), NO_x 6818 (tonnes/y), CO (4815 tonnes/y) and hydrocarbons (45 722 tonnes/y).

Surface and subterranean water was polluted by industrial wastes, domestic sewage, agricultural wastes (fertilizers and plant pesticides), erosion of the dumping grounds and oil-derivatives from petrol stations. Only 3.8% of the surface water fell in the first class for purity and up to 49% was out of class. None of the 11 water reservoirs was of first class purity and four of them were beyond class. Only 12% of subterranean water was in a permitted class, the rest having too low pH or elevated content of heavy metals, ammonia or nitrates.

In 1993 there were 2253 physicians in Kielce Province and 18 hospitals with a total of 6876 beds (60.1 per 10 000) and 161 outpatient clinics. Psychiatric centres are not included. There are no oncological beds or radiotherapy equipment in the province, so cancer patients have to travel about 150 km to the nearest oncological hospital. In 1983, construction of a 300-bed oncological hospital was started. There is an oncological outpatient clinic with a Department of Nuclear Medicine, Department of Biochemistry and Haematology and Department of Histopathology. In 1996 a radiotherapy department and an oncological ward with sixty beds will open.

The registry maintains two basic files: a computerized file containing the patient's serial number, sex, surname, name, date of birth, date of first cancer diagnosis, ICD code and year of death (if applicable); and a file containing cards of first and follow-up registration arranged according to information mentioned above.

By administrative order all doctors and medical centres are obliged to report all cases of cancer on a special cancer reporting card with information advised by IARC. Although cancer reporting is obligatory, it is often neglected and therefore reports received have to be completed and checked against data from the main Statistical Office, local civil departments and hospital data.

Stanislaw Góźdź

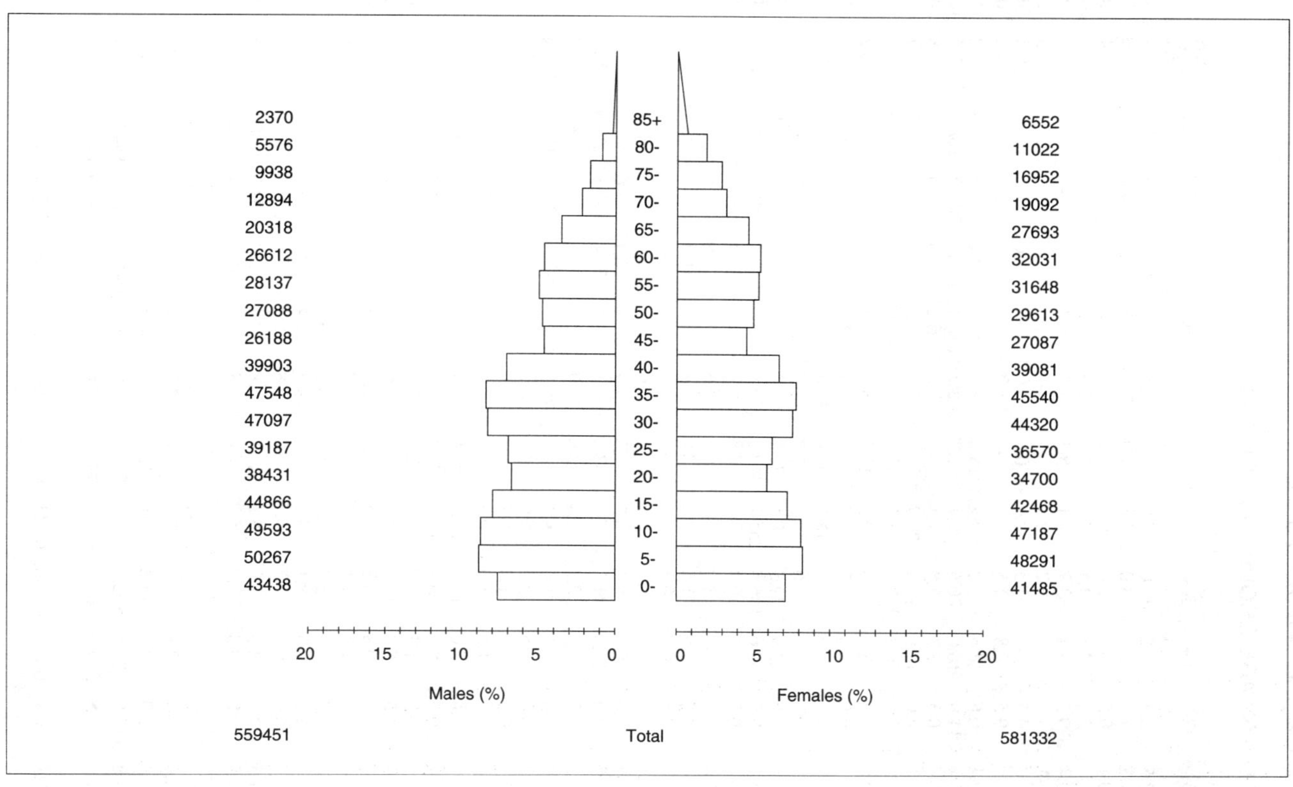

Poland, Kielce
Source of population: average annual 1988–92
Census: 6.12.1988 – Central Statistical Office
Notes to tables overleaf:
* The rather low incidence rates, combined with high ratios of
  mortality to incidence, suggest under-ascertainment
† 188 does not include the non-invasive tumours

* POLAND, KIELCE 1988-1992

ANNUAL INCIDENCE PER 100,000 BY AGE GROUP (YEARS) - MALE

SITE	ALL AGES	AGE UNK	0-	5-	10-	15-	20-	25-	30-	35-	40-	45-	50-	55-	60-	65-	70-	75-	80-	85+	CRUDE RATE	%	CR 64	CR 74	ASR (W)	ICD (9th)
Lip	214	0	-	-	-	-	-	-	0.8	2.5	2.5	7.6	14.0	27.0	31.6	25.6	41.9	44.3	43.0	42.2	7.7	3.0	0.43	0.77	6.3	140
Tongue	26	0	-	-	-	-	-	-	-	1.3	-	2.3	3.0	2.8	3.0	3.9	1.6	2.0	3.6	8.4	0.9	0.4	0.06	0.09	0.8	141
Salivary gland	10	0	-	-	-	-	-	-	0.4	0.5	-	3.0	0.7	1.5	-	1.6	-	-	-	-	0.4	0.1	0.03	0.04	0.3	142
Mouth	28	0	-	-	-	-	-	-	-	2.0	2.3	4.4	3.6	5.3	2.0	1.6	-	-	-	-	1.0	0.4	0.09	0.11	0.9	143-5
Oropharynx	30	0	-	-	-	-	-	-	-	0.4	0.5	3.1	3.7	2.1	5.3	4.9	6.2	-	-	-	1.1	0.4	0.08	0.13	1.0	146
Nasopharynx	8	0	-	-	-	-	-	-	0.4	-	-	-	2.2	2.1	-	-	1.6	-	-	-	0.3	0.1	0.02	0.03	0.3	147
Hypopharynx	9	0	-	-	-	-	-	-	-	-	0.5	-	1.5	2.1	0.8	1.0	-	2.0	-	-	0.3	0.1	0.02	0.03	0.3	148
Pharynx unspecified	6	0	-	-	-	-	-	-	-	-	0.5	0.8	1.5	-	-	1.0	-	-	3.6	-	0.2	0.1	0.01	0.02	0.2	149
Oesophagus	105	0	-	-	-	-	-	-	-	0.4	0.5	4.6	5.2	9.2	15.8	19.7	20.2	22.1	35.9	16.9	3.8	1.5	0.18	0.38	3.1	150
Stomach	761	0	-	-	-	-	-	0.5	0.8	3.4	11.0	16.0	40.6	71.1	97.7	142.7	178.4	173.1	200.9	168.7	27.2	10.8	1.21	2.81	22.1	151
Small intestine	23	0	-	-	-	-	-	1.0	-	-	0.5	2.3	3.0	2.1	-	2.0	6.2	6.0	3.6	-	0.8	0.3	0.04	0.09	0.7	152
Colon	271	0	-	-	-	-	-	1.0	1.3	2.1	4.0	11.5	18.5	22.7	37.6	47.2	51.2	54.3	68.1	33.7	9.7	3.8	0.49	0.99	8.0	153
Rectum	287	0	-	-	-	-	1.0	-	1.3	2.5	3.5	10.7	8.1	23.5	39.8	44.3	62.0	82.5	75.3	92.8	10.3	4.1	0.45	0.98	8.3	154
Liver	174	0	-	-	-	0.4	-	-	0.8	1.5	3.1	6.6	9.2	18.8	25.6	71.3	38.2	64.6	67.5	6.2	2.5	0.20	0.69	5.1	155	
Gallbladder etc.	87	0	-	-	-	-	-	0.5	-	-	0.5	2.3	3.7	6.4	8.3	10.8	24.8	30.2	32.3	50.6	3.1	1.2	0.11	0.29	2.5	156
Pancreas	245	0	-	-	-	-	-	0.5	0.8	2.9	5.0	11.5	15.5	15.6	31.6	46.3	46.5	62.4	35.9	59.1	8.8	3.5	0.42	0.88	7.3	157
Nose, sinuses etc.	19	0	-	-	-	-	-	-	0.8	-	1.0	-	3.0	-	2.3	1.0	4.7	-	7.2	16.9	0.7	0.3	0.04	0.06	0.6	160
Larynx	435	0	-	-	-	-	-	-	0.4	3.4	11.5	22.9	49.5	50.5	72.1	66.9	57.4	50.3	25.1	16.9	15.6	6.2	1.05	1.67	13.5	161
Bronchus, lung	2259	0	-	-	-	0.4	1.6	0.5	3.0	15.1	28.6	59.6	156.5	255.2	349.5	450.8	452.9	362.2	304.9	210.9	80.8	31.9	4.35	8.87	67.4	162
Other thoracic organs	30	0	0.5	-	-	-	0.5	-	-	-	0.5	0.8	0.7	3.6	0.8	6.9	4.7	14.1	7.2	-	1.1	0.4	0.04	0.09	0.9	163-4
Bone	33	0	-	0.8	0.8	1.8	0.5	0.5	-	0.4	-	-	3.7	-	5.3	2.0	7.8	4.0	3.6	-	1.2	0.5	0.07	0.12	1.1	170
Connective tissue	56	0	0.5	1.2	-	0.9	1.0	-	0.4	-	2.5	1.5	1.5	3.6	3.0	7.9	9.3	16.1	10.8	33.7	2.0	0.8	0.08	0.17	1.7	171
Mesothelioma	5	0	-	-	-	-	-	-	-	-	0.5	0.8	0.7	1.4	-	-	-	-	-	-	0.2	0.1	0.02	0.02	0.2	MES
Kaposi's sarcoma	1	0	-	-	-	-	-	-	-	-	-	-	-	-	1.0	-	-	-	-	-	0.0	0.0	0.00	0.00	0.0	KAP
Melanoma of skin	74	0	0.5	-	-	-	1.0	-	1.3	1.7	5.0	5.3	5.2	5.7	7.5	4.9	17.1	10.1	3.6	-	2.6	1.0	0.17	0.28	2.3	172
Other skin	628	0	-	-	-	-	0.5	-	1.3	3.8	7.0	14.5	41.3	47.6	83.4	107.3	139.6	138.8	197.3	210.9	22.5		1.00	2.23	18.4	173
Breast	12	0	-	-	-	-	-	-	-	-	0.5	-	0.7	1.4	3.0	1.0	3.1	-	-	8.4	0.4	0.2	0.03	0.05	0.4	175
Prostate	376	0	-	-	-	-	0.5	-	-	0.8	1.5	2.3	6.6	18.5	30.8	76.8	122.5	142.9	172.2	126.6	13.4	5.3	0.31	1.30	10.3	185
Testis	58	0	-	0.4	1.8	4.7	3.6	2.5	2.9	3.0	1.5	2.2	5.0	3.0	-	3.1	-	-	-	2.1	0.8	0.15	0.17	2.0	186	
Penis	8	0	-	-	-	-	-	-	1.3	0.5	-	1.5	0.7	-	-	1.6	-	-	-	0.3	0.1	0.02	0.03	0.2	187.1-.4	
Other male genital	17	0	-	-	-	-	-	0.4	0.4	0.5	1.5	3.0	0.7	1.5	3.0	1.6	-	3.6	-	0.6	0.2	0.04	0.06	0.5	187.5-.9	
†Bladder	377	0	-	-	-	-	-	-	1.7	2.1	2.5	7.6	19.2	27.0	58.6	66.9	65.1	108.7	125.5	101.2	13.5	5.3	0.59	1.25	10.8	188
Kidney etc.	203	0	0.5	0.8	0.4	0.4	-	-	0.4	0.8	6.5	9.2	16.2	24.9	33.1	35.4	24.8	30.2	7.2	-	7.3	2.9	0.47	0.77	6.3	189
Eye	16	0	0.9	-	-	-	0.5	-	0.4	-	-	1.5	0.7	-	2.3	3.9	1.6	2.0	-	-	0.6	0.2	0.03	0.06	0.6	190
Brain, nervous system	154	0	2.3	3.6	2.8	2.2	1.0	1.0	2.1	2.5	5.5	5.3	16.2	12.8	13.5	23.6	15.5	4.0	3.6	-	5.5	2.2	0.36	0.55	5.1	191-2
Thyroid	20	0	-	-	-	-	0.5	-	0.4	0.8	-	0.8	0.7	2.1	2.3	3.0	4.7	2.0	3.6	-	0.7	0.3	0.04	0.08	0.6	193
Other endocrine	17	0	-	1.2	-	0.4	-	0.5	0.8	0.4	-	1.5	1.5	0.7	2.3	1.0	-	-	-	-	0.6	0.2	0.05	0.05	0.6	194
Hodgkin's disease	76	0	0.5	2.0	0.4	1.8	2.6	2.0	3.4	3.8	1.5	5.3	5.2	2.1	4.5	3.9	6.2	6.0	7.2	-	2.7	1.1	0.18	0.23	2.5	201
Non-Hodgkin lymphoma	134	0	1.4	0.8	2.4	0.4	1.0	2.0	2.1	2.9	2.5	7.6	8.1	14.9	15.0	19.7	12.4	10.1	14.3	-	4.8	1.9	0.31	0.47	4.3	200,202
Multiple myeloma	45	0	-	-	-	-	-	-	0.8	-	-	0.8	3.7	5.7	6.0	9.8	15.5	2.0	-	-	1.6	0.6	0.09	0.21	1.4	203
Lymphoid leukaemia	106	0	3.7	2.4	2.0	1.3	0.5	1.5	-	1.3	1.5	2.3	2.2	5.0	12.8	12.8	17.1	20.1	32.3	8.4	3.8	1.5	0.18	0.33	3.4	204
Myeloid leukaemia	64	0	1.4	0.4	0.4	0.4	1.6	1.0	1.3	1.3	1.0	0.8	5.2	5.0	6.0	9.8	6.2	10.1	7.2	8.4	2.3	0.9	0.13	0.21	2.0	205
Monocytic leukaemia	0	0	-	-	-	-	-	-	-	-	-	-	-	-	-	-	-	-	-	-	0.0	0.0	0.00	0.00	0.0	206
Other leukaemia	3	0	-	-	-	0.4	-	-	-	-	-	-	0.7	-	-	-	2.0	-	-	0.1	0.0	0.01	0.01	0.1	207	
Leukaemia unspecified	14	0	0.5	-	-	-	-	0.5	-	0.8	-	0.8	-	0.7	0.8	2.0	1.6	4.0	3.6	8.4	0.5	0.2	0.02	0.04	0.4	208
Other and unspecified	175	0	-	-	-	0.4	1.0	1.0	0.8	1.3	2.0	2.3	13.3	17.8	15.8	27.6	38.8	50.3	32.3	59.1	6.3	2.5	0.28	0.61	5.2	O&U
All sites	7699	0	12.4	13.1	9.7	13.4	20.3	17.9	30.2	64.8	118.8	234.5	502.8	713.6	1031.8	1325.9	1549.5	1507.2	1538.7	1349.9	275.2		13.92	28.29	230.1	ALL
All sites but 173	7071	0	12.4	13.1	9.7	13.4	19.8	17.9	28.9	61.0	111.8	219.9	461.5	666.0	948.4	1218.6	1409.9	1368.4	1341.4	1139.0	252.8	100.0	12.92	26.06	211.7	ALLb

Rate from 1 case   0.460 0.398 0.403 0.446 0.520 0.510 0.425 0.421 0.501 0.764 0.738 0.711 0.752 0.984 1.551 2.012 3.587 8.437

†Important: see notes on population page

* POLAND, KIELCE 1988-1992

ANNUAL INCIDENCE PER 100,000 BY AGE GROUP (YEARS) - FEMALE

SITE	ALL AGES	AGE UNK	0-	5-	10-	15-	20-	25-	30-	35-	40-	45-	50-	55-	60-	65-	70-	75-	80-	85+	CRUDE RATE	%	CR 64	CR 74	ASR (W)	ICD (9th)
Lip	38	0	-	-	-	-	-	-	0.5	0.4	-	-	-	2.5	3.1	2.9	9.4	8.3	7.3	9.2	1.3	0.7	0.03	0.09	0.7	140
Tongue	8	0	-	-	-	-	-	-	-	-	-	1.5	-	0.6	1.2	1.4	1.0	-	-	-	0.3	0.1	0.02	0.03	0.2	141
Salivary gland	8	0	-	-	-	-	-	-	-	-	0.5	0.7	0.7	0.6	1.2	-	-	1.2	1.8	-	0.3	0.1	0.02	0.02	0.2	142
Mouth	5	0	-	-	-	-	-	-	-	-	-	0.7	1.4	-	0.6	-	-	1.2	-	-	0.2	0.1	0.01	0.01	0.1	143-5
Oropharynx	7	0	-	-	-	-	-	-	-	0.4	-	0.7	-	1.3	-	0.7	1.0	-	1.8	-	0.2	0.1	0.01	0.02	0.2	146
Nasopharynx	5	0	-	-	-	-	-	-	-	-	-	-	-	-	0.6	1.4	1.0	-	1.8	-	0.2	0.1	0.00	0.02	0.1	147
Hypopharynx	0	0	-	-	-	-	-	-	-	-	-	-	-	-	-	-	-	-	-	-	0.0	0.0	0.00	0.00	0.0	148
Pharynx unspecified	3	0	-	-	-	-	-	-	-	-	-	-	-	-	-	-	2.1	1.2	-	-	0.1	0.1	0.00	0.01	0.1	149
Oesophagus	30	0	-	-	-	-	0.6	-	-	-	0.5	0.7	0.7	0.6	1.2	1.4	7.3	7.1	12.7	3.1	1.0	0.6	0.02	0.07	0.6	150
Stomach	405	0	-	-	-	-	-	2.2	1.8	2.6	3.6	8.1	13.5	17.7	25.6	41.2	71.2	83.8	119.8	67.1	13.9	7.5	0.38	0.94	8.0	151
Small intestine	25	0	-	-	-	-	-	-	-	-	-	-	2.0	2.5	2.5	2.2	4.2	2.4	3.6	9.2	0.9	0.5	0.04	0.07	0.5	152
Colon	230	0	-	-	-	-	0.6	-	-	2.6	1.5	6.6	6.1	16.4	21.9	20.9	36.7	42.5	54.4	33.6	7.9	4.2	0.28	0.57	4.8	153
Rectum	262	0	-	-	-	-	-	0.5	0.5	1.8	3.6	5.9	10.1	17.7	29.3	28.2	29.3	56.6	38.1	45.8	9.0	4.8	0.35	0.63	5.6	154
Liver	180	0	0.5	-	0.4	-	-	-	0.9	0.9	1.0	1.5	4.1	5.7	16.2	12.3	24.1	61.3	49.0	30.5	6.2	3.3	0.16	0.34	3.3	155
Gallbladder etc.	242	0	-	-	-	-	0.6	-	-	0.4	1.0	5.9	8.8	12.6	20.0	18.8	37.7	50.7	76.2	54.9	8.3	4.5	0.25	0.53	4.7	156
Pancreas	227	0	-	-	-	-	-	-	-	0.4	0.5	2.2	6.1	16.4	21.2	28.9	46.1	36.6	36.3	54.9	7.8	4.2	0.23	0.61	4.6	157
Nose, sinuses etc.	14	0	-	-	-	-	-	-	-	-	-	1.4	1.3	1.9	0.7	3.1	1.2	3.6	-	0.5	0.3	0.02	0.04	0.3	160
Larynx	21	0	-	-	-	-	-	-	-	-	3.1	1.4	2.5	1.9	2.9	2.1	-	-	-	-	0.7	0.4	0.04	0.07	0.6	161
Bronchus, lung	310	0	-	-	-	0.5	0.6	-	2.3	2.2	7.7	12.6	11.5	24.0	26.8	31.8	50.3	54.3	30.8	39.7	10.7	5.7	0.44	0.85	7.0	162
Other thoracic organs	18	0	-	0.4	-	-	0.6	-	0.9	-	1.0	-	1.4	-	3.1	-	2.1	1.2	-	6.1	0.6	0.3	0.04	0.05	0.5	163-4
Bone	24	0	-	0.4	0.8	0.5	-	1.1	0.5	0.4	-	1.5	-	1.9	2.5	-	3.1	2.4	3.6	-	0.8	0.4	0.05	0.06	0.7	170
Connective tissue	46	0	-	0.4	0.4	-	1.7	0.5	0.9	0.4	0.5	3.0	-	3.2	4.4	2.9	3.1	7.1	3.6	15.3	1.6	0.8	0.08	0.11	1.2	171
Mesothelioma	6	0	-	-	-	-	-	-	-	0.4	-	0.7	0.7	-	0.6	0.7	-	1.2	-	-	0.2	0.1	0.01	0.02	0.2	MES
Kaposi's sarcoma	0	0	-	-	-	-	-	-	-	-	-	-	-	-	-	-	-	-	-	-	0.0	0.0	0.00	0.00	0.0	KAP
Melanoma of skin	92	0	-	-	-	-	-	1.6	0.9	4.0	6.1	3.7	4.1	5.7	6.9	10.1	10.5	7.1	9.1	-	3.2	1.7	0.16	0.27	2.3	172
Other skin	585	0	-	-	-	-	1.2	-	1.4	3.5	8.7	17.7	20.9	32.9	46.2	70.1	99.5	106.2	99.8	112.9	20.1		0.66	1.51	12.4	173
Breast	983	0	-	-	-	-	-	1.6	9.9	25.0	60.4	70.9	69.6	79.0	89.3	86.7	79.6	82.6	56.2	58.0	33.8	18.1	2.03	2.86	25.9	174
Uterus unspecified	14	0	-	-	-	-	-	-	-	-	0.5	2.2	-	1.3	0.6	0.7	2.1	3.5	-	3.1	0.5	0.3	0.02	0.04	0.4	179
Cervix uteri	567	0	-	-	-	-	1.2	6.0	22.1	27.2	37.4	35.4	43.2	38.5	41.2	39.7	26.2	42.5	18.1	15.3	19.5	10.4	1.26	1.59	15.6	180
Placenta	0	0	-	-	-	-	-	-	-	-	-	-	-	-	-	-	-	-	-	-	0.0	0.0	0.00	0.00	0.0	181
Corpus uteri	372	0	-	-	-	0.5	-	-	1.8	1.3	4.1	17.0	28.4	42.3	54.3	41.2	30.4	37.8	29.0	9.2	12.8	6.9	0.75	1.11	9.2	182
Ovary etc.	289	0	-	0.8	-	2.4	-	1.6	3.2	4.8	13.8	27.3	26.3	19.6	30.6	28.2	16.8	10.6	14.5	18.3	9.9	5.3	0.65	0.88	8.1	183
Other female genital	83	0	-	-	-	-	0.6	-	0.9	0.4	0.5	1.5	2.7	6.3	8.7	8.7	11.5	17.7	14.5	6.1	2.9	1.5	0.11	0.21	1.8	184
†Bladder	74	0	-	-	-	0.5	-	-	-	1.3	1.0	3.0	3.4	0.6	5.0	9.4	8.4	17.7	14.5	18.3	2.5	1.4	0.07	0.16	1.5	188
Kidney etc.	130	0	2.9	0.8	-	0.5	-	1.1	0.9	0.4	2.6	3.7	4.1	10.1	17.5	18.8	15.7	8.3	12.7	3.1	4.5	2.4	0.22	0.40	3.4	189
Eye	8	0	-	0.4	-	-	-	0.5	-	-	0.5	-	-	1.2	-	1.0	-	-	-	6.1	0.3	0.1	0.01	0.02	0.2	190
Brain, nervous system	124	0	2.4	2.5	1.3	2.4	0.6	2.2	2.7	4.8	3.1	8.9	10.1	8.2	9.4	7.2	8.4	1.2	3.6	3.1	4.3	2.3	0.29	0.37	3.9	191-2
Thyroid	39	0	-	-	-	0.5	0.6	-	0.5	0.9	1.0	1.5	4.1	3.2	1.9	2.2	3.1	5.9	7.3	3.1	1.3	0.7	0.07	0.10	1.0	193
Other endocrine	17	0	1.4	0.8	0.8	-	-	-	0.5	-	0.5	0.7	2.0	1.3	0.6	-	-	-	-	3.1	0.6	0.3	0.04	0.04	0.6	194
Hodgkin's disease	51	0	1.0	0.8	-	3.8	4.0	2.7	2.7	1.8	1.0	0.7	0.7	0.6	1.9	2.2	2.1	2.4	3.6	-	1.8	0.9	0.11	0.13	1.7	201
Non-Hodgkin lymphoma	87	0	0.5	-	-	0.9	1.2	1.6	0.9	1.3	1.0	3.0	9.5	7.0	9.4	6.5	5.2	13.0	5.4	-	3.0	1.6	0.18	0.24	2.3	200,202
Multiple myeloma	51	0	-	-	-	-	-	-	-	-	0.5	0.7	0.7	3.8	5.6	10.1	10.5	8.3	3.6	-	1.8	0.9	0.06	0.16	1.1	203
Lymphoid leukaemia	62	0	2.9	2.1	1.3	1.4	-	1.1	-	0.4	0.5	1.5	2.0	4.4	4.4	5.1	4.2	7.1	7.3	3.1	2.1	1.1	0.11	0.16	1.8	204
Myeloid leukaemia	67	0	1.0	-	1.3	-	1.2	0.5	0.9	2.2	1.0	3.0	4.1	7.0	6.2	3.6	7.3	4.7	3.6	3.1	2.3	1.2	0.14	0.20	1.9	205
Monocytic leukaemia	0	0	-	-	-	-	-	-	-	-	-	-	-	-	-	-	-	-	-	-	0.0	0.0	0.00	0.00	0.0	206
Other leukaemia	1	0	-	-	-	-	-	-	-	-	-	-	-	0.6	-	-	-	-	-	-	0.0	0.0	0.00	0.00	0.0	207
Leukaemia unspecified	10	0	-	-	-	-	-	-	-	-	-	-	-	-	0.6	0.6	2.9	1.0	-	1.8	6.1	0.3	0.2	0.01	0.03	0.2	208
Other and unspecified	194	0	0.5	0.4	-	0.5	-	-	-	0.9	3.6	4.4	4.1	9.5	23.1	21.7	19.9	40.1	38.1	42.7	6.7	3.6	0.23	0.44	4.0	O&U
All sites	6014	0	13.0	9.9	6.4	14.1	15.0	25.2	57.3	93.5	172.5	259.2	309.3	410.1	550.7	574.2	698.7	836.4	787.5	683.7	206.9		9.68	16.05	143.4	ALL
All sites but 173	5429	0	13.0	9.9	6.4	14.1	13.8	25.2	56.0	90.0	163.8	241.4	288.4	377.3	504.5	504.1	599.2	730.3	687.7	570.7	186.8	100.0	9.02	14.54	131.0	ALLb

Rate from 1 case			0.482	0.414	0.424	0.471	0.576	0.547	0.451	0.439	0.512	0.738	0.675	0.632	0.624	0.722	1.048	1.180	1.814	3.052

†Important: see notes on population page

Poland, Lower Silesia

The Lower Silesian Cancer Registry was established in 1962, when compulsory reporting of all cancer cases was introduced in Poland. The registry is a part of the Cancer Epidemiology Department of the Regional Cancer Centre in Wroclaw. Apart from six members of the medical administrative staff working on the quality and completeness of the data, a physician, a mathematician and a computer programmer are employed.

The registry covers the Lower Silesian region, in the south-western part of Poland, covering an area of 18 870 km^2. This region borders Germany to the west, the Czech Republic to the south, Upper Silesia in the east and Poznan province in the north (the latter two are Polish regions). The region is divided into four voivodships, surrounding the major cities of Wroclaw, Walbrzych, Jelenia Gora and Legnica.

Lower Silesia is a heavily urbanized region, with many industries. About 15% of the inhabitants are employed in industry. The region covers a plain and a submountainous area, the south border of which is formed by the Karkonosze Mountains.

In 1992 Lower Silesia had 2 915 769 inhabitants (48.7% males, 51.3% females), 70% of whom were living in cities and 30% in rural areas.

Almost all of the population of Lower Silesia is of Caucasian background; there are no data on ethnic groups. The great majority belong to the Roman Catholic church.

There are 6600 physicians in Lower Silesia, and they are compulsorily required to submit data concerning cancer cases to the registry. The registry also pursues active registration by checking hospital records and death certificates. Previously, the registry did not actively follow up patients, but it is now checking all those still alive.

Data on patients, including name, date of birth and ICD site code, have been computerized since 1984. Many checks are applied to eliminate duplicate registrations, to identify multiple primaries and to correct discrepancies of topography and morphology.

After a two-year period of verification, the information collected is analysed to give estimates of cancer incidence and mortality by site, standardized to the world population. Distribution of new cases by age and place as well as trends in changes are studied. Mapping is widely used for visualization of the data.

Jerzy Blaszczyk
Marek Pudelko

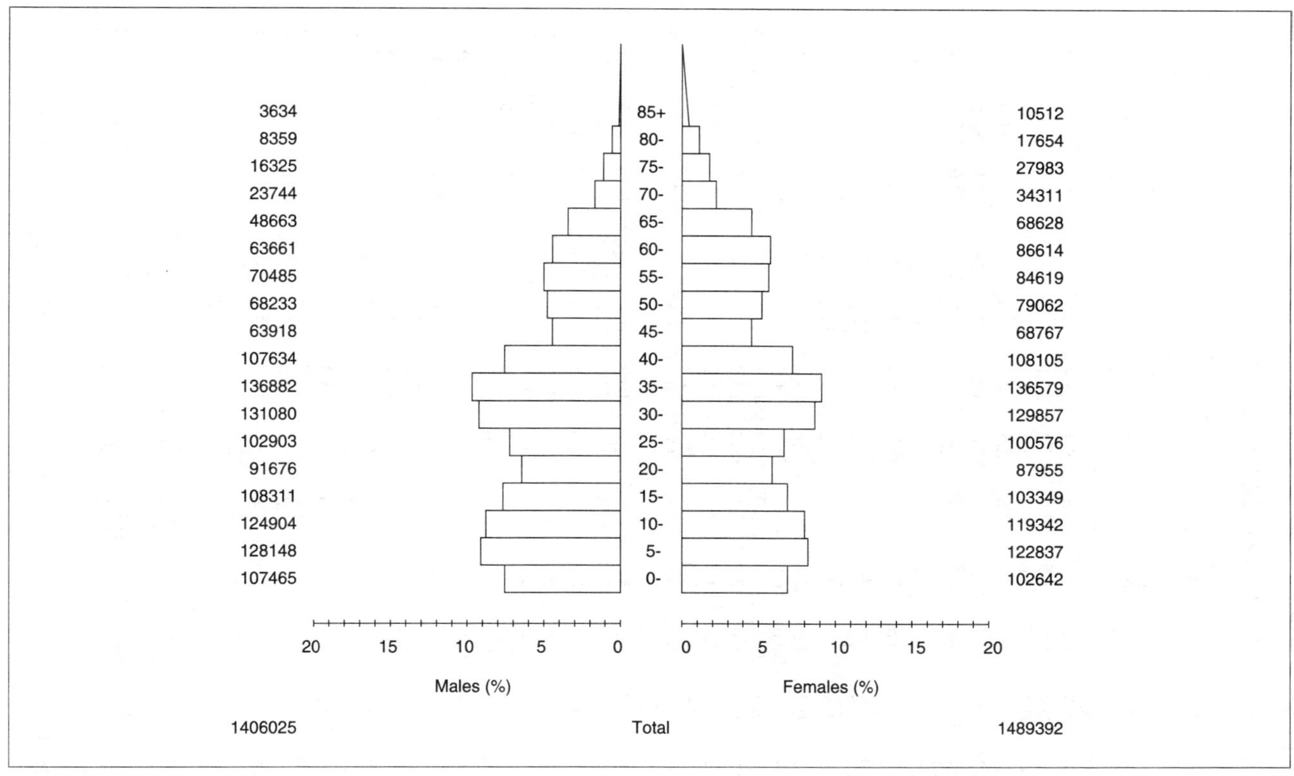

Poland, Lower Silesia
Source of population: average annual 1988–92
Census: National Population Count, 1988.
Estimate: The populations for 1989-92 were estimated on the basis of the 1988 Census, making allowance for births, deaths and migration.

Notes to tables overleaf:
* The low proportions of cases diagnosed histologically suggest lack of validity in the data.
† 188 does not include the non-invasive tumours

* POLAND, LOWER SILESIA 1988-1992

ANNUAL INCIDENCE PER 100,000 BY AGE GROUP (YEARS) - MALE

SITE	ALL AGES	AGE UNK	0-	5-	10-	15-	20-	25-	30-	35-	40-	45-	50-	55-	60-	65-	70-	75-	80-	85+	CRUDE RATE	%	CR 64	CR 74	ASR (W)	ICD (9th)
Lip	282	0	-	-	-	-	-	-	0.2	0.3	0.9	3.8	6.7	8.2	15.4	25.5	23.6	40.4	64.6	60.5	4.0	1.3	0.18	0.42	3.9	140
Tongue	127	0	-	-	-	-	-	-	0.3	0.3	2.4	3.8	6.7	7.4	6.0	7.4	4.2	4.9	7.2	-	1.8	0.6	0.13	0.19	1.7	141
Salivary gland	51	0	-	-	-	-	0.2	-	-	0.4	0.2	2.2	0.6	2.0	2.8	4.9	2.5	3.7	7.2	-	0.7	0.2	0.04	0.08	0.7	142
Mouth	165	0	-	-	-	0.2	-	-	0.2	1.2	3.9	6.6	6.7	7.9	9.4	8.6	7.6	-	4.8	-	2.3	0.8	0.18	0.26	2.2	143-5
Oropharynx	103	0	-	-	-	-	-	-	-	0.4	1.5	3.4	3.8	7.4	5.3	5.8	4.2	4.9	4.8	-	1.5	0.5	0.11	0.16	1.4	146
Nasopharynx	36	0	-	-	0.2	-	-	0.2	-	0.3	0.4	1.6	1.5	2.0	2.2	2.1	-	-	2.4	-	0.5	0.2	0.04	0.05	0.5	147
Hypopharynx	29	0	-	-	-	-	-	-	-	-	0.4	0.6	0.6	0.9	2.5	3.3	1.7	1.2	2.4	-	0.4	0.1	0.02	0.05	0.4	148
Pharynx unspecified	43	0	-	-	-	-	-	-	-	0.3	-	1.6	2.1	2.8	2.5	2.1	0.8	-	7.2	11.0	0.6	0.2	0.05	0.06	0.6	149
Oesophagus	430	0	-	-	-	-	0.2	-	-	0.3	1.7	6.9	17.0	22.7	27.6	31.2	37.1	35.5	33.5	38.5	6.1	2.0	0.38	0.72	5.8	150
Stomach	1839	0	-	0.2	-	0.2	0.2	0.4	1.5	4.1	12.3	23.8	35.8	67.2	103.0	146.7	196.3	253.6	308.6	225.6	26.2	8.4	1.24	2.96	24.7	151
Small intestine	29	0	-	-	-	-	-	-	0.2	0.1	-	0.6	-	1.1	2.2	3.3	0.8	2.5	4.8	5.5	0.4	0.1	0.02	0.04	0.4	152
Colon	897	0	-	-	-	0.4	-	0.6	1.2	3.2	5.2	11.0	25.8	29.5	52.5	72.7	95.2	101.7	134.0	60.5	12.8	4.1	0.65	1.49	12.0	153
Rectum	928	0	-	-	-	-	0.4	-	1.7	1.8	5.6	10.6	20.2	36.3	59.7	75.6	94.3	104.1	126.8	99.0	13.2	4.2	0.68	1.53	12.4	154
Liver	502	0	0.4	0.2	-	0.2	-	-	0.5	1.6	2.6	3.4	9.4	19.3	28.0	46.9	47.2	69.8	76.6	60.5	7.1	2.3	0.33	0.80	6.7	155
Gallbladder etc.	182	0	-	-	-	-	-	-	0.2	0.3	1.3	0.9	2.6	4.3	9.1	16.9	18.5	34.3	43.1	38.5	2.6	0.8	0.09	0.27	2.5	156
Pancreas	794	0	-	-	-	0.2	-	0.4	1.1	2.9	5.4	8.1	17.0	28.4	51.2	65.8	79.2	90.7	95.7	110.0	11.3	3.6	0.57	1.30	10.6	157
Nose, sinuses etc.	48	0	-	-	-	-	-	-	0.2	0.7	0.7	1.3	1.5	0.9	2.8	3.7	1.7	2.5	4.8	11.0	0.7	0.2	0.04	0.07	0.6	160
Larynx	1142	0	-	-	-	-	-	0.2	1.4	3.9	14.7	30.0	46.9	61.3	74.1	71.9	65.7	42.9	52.6	44.0	16.2	5.2	1.16	1.85	15.2	161
Bronchus, lung	7213	0	-	-	-	0.4	0.2	1.7	3.4	12.9	38.5	85.1	180.3	343.0	497.9	618.5	683.1	656.7	638.8	462.2	102.6	33.0	5.82	12.33	95.5	162
Other thoracic organs	193	0	0.6	0.2	0.3	0.4	0.7	0.6	1.1	0.6	0.6	1.6	3.2	5.1	13.2	14.8	17.7	25.7	19.1	16.5	2.7	0.9	0.14	0.30	2.6	163-4
Bone	126	0	-	0.2	1.0	2.6	1.3	0.8	0.6	1.2	2.6	2.5	1.2	3.1	6.6	5.3	4.2	6.1	2.4	5.5	1.8	0.6	0.12	0.17	1.7	170
Connective tissue	137	0	0.9	0.6	0.2	1.1	0.7	0.4	1.5	1.5	0.9	4.7	2.6	3.1	6.3	7.4	5.9	11.0	2.4	5.5	1.9	0.6	0.12	0.19	1.9	171
Mesothelioma	19	0	0.2	-	-	-	0.2	-	0.3	0.2	0.3	0.3	0.9	1.6	0.8	0.8	-	-	-	-	0.3	0.1	0.02	0.03	0.2	MES
Kaposi's sarcoma	1	0	-	-	-	-	-	-	-	-	-	-	0.3	-	-	-	-	-	-	-	0.0	0.0	0.00	0.00	0.0	KAP
Melanoma of skin	224	0	-	-	-	0.6	1.1	1.0	1.8	2.9	5.2	3.8	5.6	6.8	11.6	10.7	10.1	13.5	12.0	27.5	3.2	1.0	0.20	0.31	2.9	172
Other skin	936	0	0.2	-	-	-	1.1	1.0	1.7	2.3	7.8	13.1	19.3	30.4	47.4	75.6	87.6	111.5	198.6	154.1	13.3		0.62	1.44	12.7	173
Breast	28	0	-	-	-	-	-	-	-	0.1	0.2	0.9	0.6	0.6	1.6	2.5	3.4	1.2	2.4	11.0	0.4	0.1	0.02	0.05	0.4	175
Prostate	1110	0	-	-	-	-	-	-	0.3	0.1	0.6	2.8	5.6	19.0	51.8	100.3	196.3	257.3	251.2	286.1	15.8	5.1	0.40	1.88	15.5	185
Testis	204	0	0.6	0.2	0.2	1.5	4.8	6.0	7.2	5.4	3.0	2.2	2.6	1.1	0.9	0.8	4.2	6.1	2.4	11.0	2.9	0.9	0.18	0.20	2.6	186
Penis	70	0	-	0.2	-	-	-	-	0.3	0.9	1.3	0.3	2.1	2.8	4.1	4.1	5.1	3.7	2.4	16.5	1.0	0.3	0.06	0.11	0.9	187.1-.4
Other male genital	14	0	-	-	-	-	-	-	-	0.6	0.2	0.3	0.3	-	0.9	1.2	0.8	-	-	-	0.2	0.1	0.01	0.02	0.2	187.5-.9
†Bladder	1165	0	0.2	-	-	-	0.4	0.6	0.3	1.0	3.7	10.6	20.2	37.7	74.5	106.0	116.2	182.5	198.6	159.6	16.6	5.3	0.75	1.86	15.7	188
Kidney etc.	835	0	1.3	0.5	0.2	0.7	0.2	0.6	1.4	3.1	7.2	16.6	27.6	35.8	55.0	66.6	60.6	47.8	47.8	33.0	11.9	3.8	0.75	1.39	11.1	189
Eye	62	0	0.7	0.2	-	-	-	0.2	0.3	0.3	0.6	1.3	2.6	1.4	2.8	2.9	4.2	6.1	4.8	16.5	0.9	0.3	0.05	0.09	0.9	190
Brain, nervous system	509	0	2.0	4.1	2.4	3.0	3.3	2.5	4.4	5.6	8.0	12.2	17.9	18.7	17.9	18.1	24.4	8.6	-	-	7.2	2.3	0.51	0.72	6.9	191-2
Thyroid	61	0	-	0.2	-	0.4	0.4	0.2	0.5	0.6	0.7	1.6	2.1	2.0	3.8	2.5	3.4	3.7	-	-	0.9	0.3	0.06	0.09	0.8	193
Other endocrine	65	0	0.2	0.3	0.6	0.2	0.2	-	0.8	0.7	1.1	2.2	2.9	2.3	2.8	0.8	2.5	1.2	-	-	0.9	0.3	0.07	0.09	0.9	194
Hodgkin's disease	175	0	-	0.6	1.1	1.8	1.7	4.3	3.7	2.9	2.8	2.8	2.9	4.3	4.4	3.3	3.4	3.7	4.8	-	2.5	0.8	0.17	0.20	2.3	201
Non-Hodgkin lymphoma	369	0	0.7	1.7	1.6	2.2	1.5	2.3	1.4	2.0	4.5	7.2	6.7	11.6	15.1	25.9	27.8	28.2	23.9	11.0	5.2	1.7	0.29	0.56	5.0	200,202
Multiple myeloma	115	0	-	-	-	-	0.2	-	0.2	0.4	0.6	1.9	2.9	2.8	9.1	7.8	13.5	11.0	12.0	16.5	1.6	0.5	0.09	0.20	1.6	203
Lymphoid leukaemia	286	0	3.7	3.1	2.1	0.9	0.7	0.2	0.4	0.6	0.6	1.6	3.5	9.6	12.9	18.5	27.0	34.3	28.7	38.5	4.1	1.3	0.20	0.43	4.1	204
Myeloid leukaemia	197	0	0.4	0.6	1.0	0.6	1.3	0.6	1.2	1.3	2.4	1.6	3.2	4.3	12.3	10.7	13.5	24.5	19.1	16.5	2.8	0.9	0.15	0.27	2.6	205
Monocytic leukaemia	5	0	-	-	-	-	-	-	0.2	-	-	-	0.3	0.3	-	-	0.8	1.2	-	-	0.1	0.0	0.00	0.01	0.1	206
Other leukaemia	29	0	-	-	-	-	0.4	-	-	0.3	0.2	0.9	1.2	0.9	1.3	2.1	2.5	-	4.8	-	0.4	0.1	0.03	0.05	0.4	207
Leukaemia unspecified	39	0	0.7	0.2	0.2	-	-	0.3	0.3	-	-	1.5	0.9	0.6	3.7	3.4	4.9	-	11.0		0.6	0.2	0.02	0.06	0.6	208
Other and unspecified	985	0	1.1	0.8	0.5	0.7	1.1	0.8	2.1	2.9	6.1	12.2	24.6	34.9	53.4	76.0	96.0	123.7	102.9	176.1	14.0	4.5	0.71	1.57	13.5	O&U
All sites	22799	0	14.0	13.7	11.4	18.1	22.7	25.5	43.2	73.1	158.5	310.4	548.7	893.2	1366.3	1781.2	2099.0	2366.9	2559.9	2239.5	324.3		17.49	36.89	305.6	ALL
All sites but 173	21863	0	13.8	13.7	11.4	18.1	21.6	24.5	41.5	70.7	150.7	297.3	529.4	862.9	1318.8	1705.6	2011.4	2255.4	2361.4	2085.4	311.0	100.0	16.87	35.46	292.9	ALLb

Rate from 1 case: 0.186 0.156 0.160 0.185 0.218 0.194 0.153 0.146 0.186 0.313 0.293 0.284 0.314 0.411 0.842 1.225 2.392 5.502

†Important: see notes on population page

* POLAND, LOWER SILESIA 1988-1992

ANNUAL INCIDENCE PER 100,000 BY AGE GROUP (YEARS) - FEMALE

SITE	ALL AGES	AGE UNK	0-	5-	10-	15-	20-	25-	30-	35-	40-	45-	50-	55-	60-	65-	70-	75-	80-	85+	CRUDE RATE	%	CR 64	CR 74	ASR (W)	ICD (9th)
Lip	50	0	-	-	-	-	-	-	-	-	-	0.9	0.3	0.7	1.2	1.7	3.5	8.6	11.3	7.6	0.7	0.3	0.01	0.04	0.4	140
Tongue	37	0	-	-	-	0.2	-	-	0.3	-	0.4	-	1.0	1.4	1.2	1.5	2.3	3.6	-	5.7	0.5	0.2	0.02	0.04	0.4	141
Salivary gland	48	0	-	-	-	-	0.2	0.8	0.7	0.6	0.9	0.3	2.1	2.1	0.9	1.2	1.4	3.4	3.8	0.6	0.3	0.04	0.05	0.5	142
Mouth	58	0	-	0.2	-	-	0.2	0.2	0.2	0.7	0.7	1.5	2.0	2.1	0.7	3.5	2.3	0.7	3.4	-	0.8	0.3	0.04	0.07	0.6	143-5
Oropharynx	41	0	-	-	-	-	-	-	-	0.7	0.7	1.7	1.3	0.5	0.7	1.7	1.7	1.4	2.3	5.7	0.6	0.2	0.03	0.05	0.4	146
Nasopharynx	17	0	-	-	-	0.4	-	-	0.1	0.2	0.3	0.3	0.7	0.9	1.2	-	-	-	-	-	0.2	0.1	0.01	0.02	0.2	147
Hypopharynx	6	0	-	-	-	-	-	-	-	0.2	0.3	-	0.5	-	0.3	-	-	-	1.9	0.1	0.0	0.00	0.01	0.1	148
Pharynx unspecified	6	0	-	-	-	-	-	-	-	-	-	-	-	-	1.2	0.6	-	1.1	-	0.1	0.0	0.00	0.01	0.1	149
Oesophagus	101	0	-	-	-	-	-	-	0.2	-	0.2	0.6	1.3	2.8	4.2	4.4	5.8	8.6	21.5	11.4	1.4	0.5	0.05	0.10	0.9	150
Stomach	1113	0	-	-	-	-	0.2	1.0	1.8	4.0	6.5	9.3	11.4	19.9	33.9	53.6	102.6	127.9	128.0	138.9	14.9	5.8	0.44	1.22	10.4	151
Small intestine	25	0	-	-	-	-	-	-	-	-	0.2	0.6	0.5	1.7	0.7	0.3	0.6	4.3	-	3.8	0.3	0.1	0.02	0.02	0.2	152
Colon	992	0	-	-	-	0.4	-	0.2	2.3	2.6	5.6	8.7	16.9	26.7	36.0	54.2	69.9	87.2	95.2	91.3	13.3	5.2	0.50	1.12	9.4	153
Rectum	797	0	-	-	-	-	-	0.2	1.1	2.1	4.1	8.1	13.7	19.6	29.8	51.3	61.2	70.8	71.4	30.4	10.7	4.2	0.39	0.96	7.6	154
Liver	471	0	-	-	0.2	-	-	0.2	0.2	0.6	1.3	2.0	3.8	10.6	16.9	26.8	41.4	52.9	58.9	53.3	6.3	2.5	0.18	0.52	4.3	155
Gallbladder etc.	765	0	-	-	-	-	-	-	0.3	1.2	2.6	2.9	9.6	22.5	29.8	39.6	65.9	75.8	82.7	78.0	10.3	4.0	0.34	0.87	7.1	156
Pancreas	672	0	-	-	-	-	0.5	0.6	0.5	0.6	3.0	5.5	9.4	16.3	24.2	42.0	58.3	52.2	74.8	59.0	9.0	3.5	0.30	0.80	6.4	157
Nose, sinuses etc.	28	0	-	-	0.2	-	-	-	-	0.1	0.2	0.6	0.8	0.7	0.7	2.3	-	0.7	2.3	5.7	0.4	0.1	0.02	0.03	0.3	160
Larynx	158	0	-	-	-	-	-	-	0.2	0.9	4.1	2.9	5.1	6.6	6.9	6.7	2.9	5.7	2.3	5.7	2.1	0.8	0.13	0.18	1.6	161
Bronchus, lung	1696	0	-	-	-	0.2	0.2	1.4	1.4	4.2	10.4	15.1	30.6	52.5	71.1	101.4	115.4	117.9	143.9	98.9	22.8	8.8	0.94	2.02	16.2	162
Other thoracic organs	127	0	0.4	-	0.2	-	-	0.2	0.6	0.9	1.3	1.2	3.0	3.3	3.9	5.8	5.8	8.6	13.6	9.5	1.7	0.7	0.07	0.13	1.2	163-4
Bone	99	0	0.2	0.5	1.7	1.9	0.5	0.6	0.9	0.7	1.7	0.6	0.5	1.7	2.3	2.6	5.2	2.9	4.5	5.7	1.3	0.5	0.07	0.11	1.2	170
Connective tissue	138	0	0.4	0.8	0.7	0.8	0.7	1.2	1.7	1.2	1.5	3.5	1.8	2.8	3.5	4.4	2.3	9.3	4.5	9.5	1.9	0.7	0.10	0.14	1.6	171
Mesothelioma	7	0	-	-	-	-	-	-	0.2	-	0.2	-	0.3	-	0.7	-	0.6	-	-	-	0.1	0.0	0.01	0.01	0.1	MES
Kaposi's sarcoma	1	0	-	-	-	-	-	-	-	-	-	-	-	-	-	0.6	-	-	-	-	0.0	0.0	0.00	0.00	0.0	KAP
Melanoma of skin	277	0	0.2	-	0.2	0.8	1.1	1.4	2.6	4.4	2.4	7.6	5.1	7.3	8.5	9.0	15.2	10.7	6.8	13.3	3.7	1.4	0.21	0.33	3.0	172
Other skin	954	0	-	-	-	0.6	0.9	0.4	2.3	3.1	5.2	11.6	16.9	21.7	32.8	44.3	66.5	83.6	120.1	97.0	12.8		0.48	1.03	9.1	173
Breast	3148	0	-	-	-	-	0.7	5.2	13.2	30.3	60.1	92.2	90.3	87.9	111.3	129.4	134.1	112.9	114.4	76.1	42.3	16.4	2.46	3.77	33.4	174
Uterus unspecified	87	0	-	-	-	-	0.2	-	0.3	0.1	0.6	0.9	0.5	2.1	4.2	3.5	9.9	8.6	4.5	5.7	1.2	0.5	0.04	0.11	0.8	179
Cervix uteri	2028	0	-	-	-	-	3.0	12.1	22.3	38.4	51.6	57.9	42.0	40.4	57.7	64.4	71.7	53.6	52.1	32.3	27.2	10.6	1.63	2.31	21.8	180
Placenta	12	0	-	-	-	-	0.9	-	0.5	0.3	-	0.6	-	-	0.2	-	-	-	-	-	0.2	0.1	0.01	0.01	0.2	181
Corpus uteri	1112	0	-	-	-	-	0.2	0.2	0.6	2.8	7.2	19.2	42.5	48.7	53.8	56.0	50.7	38.6	37.4	17.1	14.9	5.8	0.88	1.41	11.4	182
Ovary etc.	1308	0	0.4	0.2	1.0	0.8	2.7	5.4	5.4	10.3	22.2	32.3	38.5	43.7	44.6	53.9	57.1	42.9	30.6	38.0	17.6	6.8	1.04	1.59	14.1	183
Other female genital	252	0	-	-	-	0.2	-	0.2	0.6	1.3	1.5	2.9	3.5	5.7	8.1	14.9	19.8	22.2	26.1	13.3	3.4	1.3	0.12	0.29	2.4	184
†Bladder	244	0	0.2	-	-	-	-	0.4	0.5	0.4	2.0	0.9	3.5	3.5	9.0	13.7	19.8	25.0	30.6	19.0	3.3	1.3	0.10	0.27	2.3	188
Kidney etc.	532	0	1.8	1.1	0.2	0.4	0.9	0.4	1.2	2.1	4.3	8.1	13.2	18.0	22.4	29.4	32.6	22.9	17.0	9.5	7.1	2.8	0.37	0.68	5.6	189
Eye	56	0	1.4	0.3	0.2	-	-	-	0.3	0.1	0.2	0.6	1.8	1.4	2.8	1.5	1.7	2.1	3.4	1.9	0.8	0.3	0.05	0.06	0.7	190
Brain, nervous system	485	0	3.3	2.6	2.8	3.3	2.7	3.8	2.8	5.1	6.5	10.2	12.4	16.8	15.5	13.4	11.1	6.4	3.4	-	6.5	2.5	0.44	0.56	5.8	191-2
Thyroid	206	0	-	-	0.2	0.4	1.4	1.8	2.5	1.8	2.4	5.8	5.3	5.9	6.9	6.1	6.4	4.3	7.9	11.4	2.8	1.1	0.17	0.23	2.3	193
Other endocrine	45	0	0.6	0.3	0.3	0.8	-	0.2	0.5	-	1.1	0.9	0.8	0.9	0.5	2.0	1.7	1.4	-	-	0.6	0.2	0.03	0.05	0.6	194
Hodgkin's disease	141	0	0.2	0.2	1.3	1.0	2.7	2.4	2.5	2.3	2.8	2.3	1.5	1.4	2.1	4.7	1.7	2.1	4.5	-	1.9	0.7	0.11	0.15	1.7	201
Non-Hodgkin lymphoma	265	0	0.4	1.0	0.2	1.2	1.4	1.2	1.7	2.9	2.6	4.1	6.1	4.3	8.3	11.4	13.4	16.4	13.6	7.6	3.6	1.4	0.18	0.30	2.8	200,202
Multiple myeloma	137	0	-	-	-	-	-	-	0.2	0.4	0.9	0.9	2.8	7.8	4.8	9.0	7.6	7.9	3.4	3.8	1.8	0.7	0.09	0.17	1.3	203
Lymphoid leukaemia	197	0	2.7	3.3	0.8	1.2	0.5	0.2	0.2	0.1	0.9	0.3	2.0	4.0	3.9	8.7	13.4	18.6	12.5	17.1	2.6	1.0	0.10	0.21	2.3	204
Myeloid leukaemia	193	0	1.0	1.0	0.3	1.0	1.1	1.6	1.1	1.3	1.9	1.5	3.0	4.3	6.7	9.3	9.9	6.4	13.6	3.8	2.6	1.0	0.13	0.22	2.1	205
Monocytic leukaemia	1	0	-	-	-	-	-	-	-	-	-	-	0.2	-	-	-	-	-	-	-	0.0	0.0	0.00	0.00	0.0	206
Other leukaemia	25	0	-	-	-	-	-	-	-	-	0.2	0.3	1.8	0.7	1.2	1.2	1.2	-	1.1	1.9	0.3	0.1	0.02	0.03	0.3	207
Leukaemia unspecified	35	0	-	-	0.2	0.4	-	-	0.2	0.1	0.2	-	1.5	0.9	1.2	1.5	1.7	2.1	2.3	1.9	0.5	0.2	0.02	0.04	0.4	208
Other and unspecified	948	0	1.2	0.2	0.2	0.6	0.9	1.0	0.9	2.5	4.8	9.6	11.4	23.4	31.6	45.2	69.4	83.6	115.5	137.0	12.7	4.9	0.44	1.01	9.1	O&U
All sites	20141	0	14.2	11.6	10.7	16.3	23.6	43.7	74.7	131.6	226.8	337.7	419.9	546.7	709.6	939.8	1167.0	1212.9	1345.8	1133.9	270.5		12.84	23.37	204.2	ALL
All sites but 173	19187	0	14.2	11.6	10.7	15.7	22.7	43.3	72.4	128.6	221.6	326.0	403.0	524.9	676.8	895.5	1100.5	1129.2	1225.7	1036.8	257.6	100.0	12.36	22.34	195.1	ALLb

| Rate from 1 case | | | 0.195 | 0.163 | 0.168 | 0.194 | 0.227 | 0.199 | 0.154 | 0.146 | 0.185 | 0.291 | 0.253 | 0.236 | 0.231 | 0.291 | 0.583 | 0.715 | 1.133 | 1.902 | | | | | | |

†Important: see notes on population page

Poland, Warsaw City

The Warsaw Cancer Registry was established in 1963 in collaboration with the National Cancer Institute, USA, to conduct comparative studies on the incidence of gastric cancer in Poland and among Americans of Polish origin. Later, these studies were extended to cancer of other organs, and registration now embraces all sites.

The Warsaw Cancer Registry is located in the Maria Sklodowska-Curie Memorial Cancer Centre and Institute of Oncology in Warsaw, which is responsible for the organization of epidemiological activities, scientific research and therapeutic services in relation to cancer for the whole country. The registry is sponsored by the Ministry of Health and Social Welfare.

From 1963 to 1988, the Warsaw Cancer Registry collected cancer reporting cards for the population of Warsaw which include selected municipalities of the provinces of Warsaw, Ciechanow, Plock and Siedlce. Since 1989 it has collected reporting cards for the population of the provinces of Warsaw, Ciechanow, Ostroleka, Plock, Radom and Siedlce, which altogether cover an area of 37 558 km^2, 12% of the total Polish territory. This area is inhabited by over five million people (13.5% of total Polish population).

Warsaw is the capital of Poland and the largest centre of the Metropolitan Province of Warsaw. It lies on the river Vistula, in the Mazovian Lowlands, in the eastern part of central Poland, at latitude 52°16′ N and longitude 20°59′ E. The average altitude is 100 m above sea level. The area for which data are presented here (Warsaw City) amounts to 485 km^2, with a population of 1 626 000.

The main branches of industry in Warsaw are the electromechanical, chemical, engineering, steel, printing, food, clothing, and transport industries.

The population is ethnically little differentiated, and mostly Roman Catholic.

Poland is divided into 11 regions, with regional oncological centres located in each which play the role of diagnostic and therapeutic centres. Nationwide supervision is performed by the Maria Sklodowska-Curie Memorial Cancer Centre and Institute of Oncology. Provincial oncological clinics provide oncological health services in each of 49 provinces. The number of oncologists in Poland is over 600, of whom 137 are in Warsaw. The number of oncological beds is over 5000, with a further 1000 under construction.

In Warsaw, specialized care of cancer patients is provided by the Maria Sklodowska-Curie Memorial Cancer Centre and Institute of Oncology, the Metropolitan Oncological Clinic and the Oncological Ward of the Grochowski Hospital, clinics of the Medical Academy, and the Institute of Mother and Child. Patients are also treated at all other hospital wards in Warsaw, district outpatient clinics and specialist centres (private and state-run), as well as cooperatives and foundations.

The recording and reporting of every case or suspected case of malignant neoplasm by all health service institutions and also by individual physicians has been compulsory in Poland since 1952. Individual doctors as well as medical centres are obliged to report all cases of malignant disease on a special reporting card for each case, which are routinely submitted to the registry.

The percentage of underregistration in Poland was estimated in 1992 at about 11%, but in Warsaw was only about 5%).

Cancer cases and related deaths are registered by opening a new type of cancer reporting card introduced in January 1989, and further processing through a computerized registration system. Apart from this, registration of new cancer cases diagnosed in Warsaw and Selected Rural Areas during the period 1963–88 has continued according to the old procedure.

The registry contains two basic files: an alphabetical computerized file by patients' names with cancer site, date of birth, date of first diagnosis and, if applicable, date of death; and a file containing cards of first and follow-up registration arranged by sex, site, year of registration and surname.

New notification cards are checked for consistency of their identification data. When more than one neoplasm is observed, with different histopathology, in the same person, a new card is prepared for each site. All entries are checked for duplication, unless there are multiple primaries.

Site coding is to ICD-9 and histology to MOTNAC.

The registry performs active follow-up of cancer patients. If no data about a cancer patient are available, information is requested from the Address Register. Information about cancer-related deaths recorded in Warsaw was taken from death certificates issued by the Central Statistical Office of Poland.

The data collected in registry have been used for:
• analysis of incidence and mortality by sex, age groups and site;
• analysis of trends of incidence and mortality by sex, age groups and site;
• analysis of clinical stages of some cancers;
• calculations and analysis of survival of cancer patients;
• analysis of methods and type of treatment, basis for diagnosis;
• detailed epidemiological studies for selected sites.

The data from database in Warsaw Registry are used in the EUROCIM and EUROCARE studies.

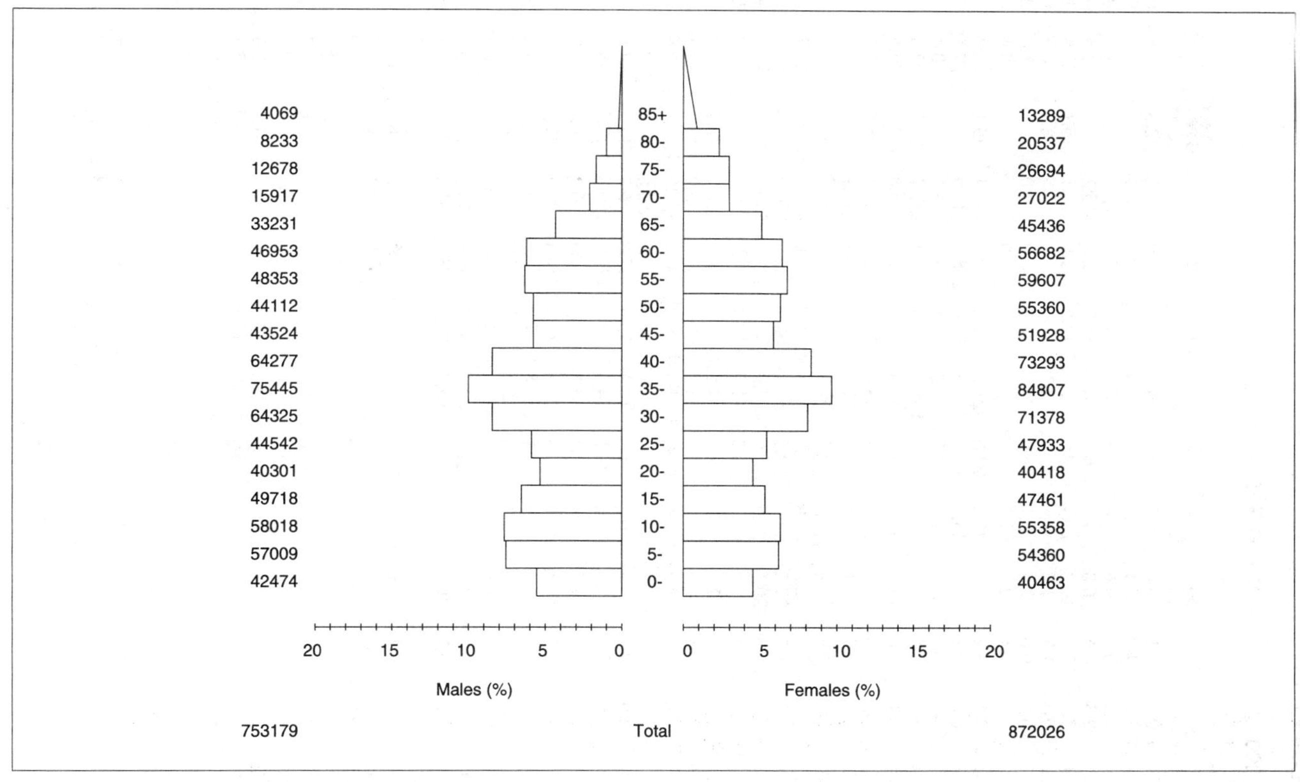

Poland, Warsaw City
Source of population: average annual 1988–92
Census: 1988 – Official Statistics Office
Estimate: Annual estimates are based on the 1988 Census, allowing for births and deaths.

Screening programmes in the area
Some 5 000 screening examinations for cervical cancer were performed annually during the period 1988-90 in women aged 30-60.

POLAND, WARSAW CITY 1989-1992

ANNUAL INCIDENCE PER 100,000 BY AGE GROUP (YEARS) - MALE

SITE	ALL AGES	AGE UNK	0-	5-	10-	15-	20-	25-	30-	35-	40-	45-	50-	55-	60-	65-	70-	75-	80-	85+	CRUDE RATE	%	CR 64	CR 74	ASR (W)	ICD (9th)
Lip	54	0	-	-	-	-	-	-	-	0.3	0.4	1.1	0.6	4.7	8.0	6.8	6.3	7.9	18.2	12.3	1.8	0.5	0.08	0.14	1.2	140
Tongue	68	0	-	-	-	-	-	-	-	0.3	0.8	4.0	5.1	5.7	9.1	10.5	6.3	2.0	6.1	-	2.3	0.6	0.12	0.21	1.6	141
Salivary gland	32	0	-	-	-	-	-	-	-	-	0.8	0.6	0.6	1.6	4.3	6.8	4.7	3.9	9.1	-	1.1	0.3	0.04	0.10	0.7	142
Mouth	75	0	-	-	-	-	-	-	-	0.3	2.3	4.6	6.8	9.3	6.4	6.8	4.7	2.0	15.2	-	2.5	0.7	0.15	0.21	1.8	143-5
Oropharynx	108	0	-	-	-	-	-	-	-	1.0	3.9	2.9	10.8	11.4	10.6	9.8	12.6	5.9	12.1	6.1	3.6	1.0	0.20	0.31	2.6	146
Nasopharynx	27	0	-	-	-	0.5	-	-	0.4	0.3	0.8	1.7	1.7	2.1	3.2	2.3	-	-	-	18.4	0.9	0.3	0.05	0.06	0.7	147
Hypopharynx	30	0	-	-	-	-	-	-	-	-	0.4	0.6	2.3	1.3	6.9	-	4.7	2.0	3.0	-	1.0	0.3	0.07	0.09	0.7	148
Pharynx unspecified	11	0	-	-	-	-	-	-	-	-	-	1.1	2.3	2.1	-	-	-	2.0	-	-	0.4	0.1	0.03	0.03	0.3	149
Oesophagus	206	0	-	-	-	-	-	-	-	1.0	3.1	3.4	14.7	22.2	24.0	21.8	18.8	29.6	33.4	49.1	6.8	1.9	0.34	0.55	4.8	150
Stomach	824	2	-	-	-	-	-	0.6	1.2	2.7	6.6	16.1	24.4	46.0	68.2	115.9	158.6	258.3	242.9	239.6	27.4	7.7	0.83	2.21	19.1	151
Small intestine	12	0	-	-	-	-	-	-	-	-	-	-	0.6	1.0	1.1	0.8	3.1	3.9	6.1	-	0.4	0.1	0.01	0.03	0.3	152
Colon	688	0	-	-	-	0.5	-	0.6	1.9	3.0	3.1	15.5	18.1	33.6	61.8	106.1	133.5	177.5	227.7	202.7	22.8	6.4	0.69	1.89	16.0	153
Rectum	498	0	-	-	-	-	-	1.1	0.4	1.0	3.1	4.6	17.6	35.7	45.8	83.5	77.0	110.4	170.0	110.6	16.5	4.7	0.55	1.35	11.3	154
Liver	216	0	-	-	0.4	0.5	0.6	-	-	0.7	1.2	0.6	1.7	14.0	21.3	36.9	55.0	43.4	66.8	55.3	7.2	2.0	0.20	0.66	5.0	155
Gallbladder etc.	180	0	-	-	-	-	0.6	-	-	0.3	1.2	1.7	5.1	7.2	19.2	21.1	31.4	55.2	88.1	49.1	6.0	1.7	0.18	0.44	4.1	156
Pancreas	333	0	-	-	-	-	-	-	-	0.7	6.6	8.0	10.2	18.1	30.3	46.6	77.0	65.1	97.2	86.0	11.1	3.1	0.37	0.99	7.9	157
Nose, sinuses etc.	35	0	-	-	-	-	-	-	0.4	0.3	-	2.3	2.3	1.6	1.6	6.8	1.6	7.9	9.1	12.3	1.2	0.3	0.04	0.08	0.8	160
Larynx	454	1	-	-	-	-	-	-	-	0.7	6.2	19.5	27.2	48.6	57.5	52.7	64.4	21.7	54.7	67.6	15.1	4.2	0.80	1.39	10.9	161
Bronchus, lung	2939	0	-	-	-	-	-	0.6	1.2	9.6	17.5	61.5	120.1	226.5	336.0	495.0	497.9	477.2	580.0	399.3	97.6	27.5	3.86	8.83	68.4	162
Other thoracic organs	55	0	-	-	-	-	-	0.6	0.4	-	0.8	2.3	2.8	3.1	4.3	11.3	9.4	7.9	9.1	-	1.8	0.5	0.07	0.17	1.3	163-4
Bone	36	0	-	0.9	1.7	1.0	0.6	-	0.4	0.3	0.8	1.1	1.1	2.6	2.7	1.5	3.1	-	12.1	6.1	1.2	0.3	0.07	0.09	1.0	170
Connective tissue	68	0	4.7	0.9	0.4	3.0	2.5	-	1.2	1.3	1.6	1.1	2.3	5.2	3.2	3.0	3.1	7.9	3.0	18.4	2.3	0.6	0.14	0.17	2.3	171
Mesothelioma	17	0	-	-	-	-	-	-	-	0.3	0.8	2.3	2.3	1.6	-	1.5	-	-	3.0	-	0.6	0.2	0.04	0.04	0.4	MES
Kaposi's sarcoma	2	0	-	-	-	-	-	-	-	-	-	-	-	-	-	-	-	2.0	3.0	-	0.1	0.0	0.00	0.00	0.0	KAP
Melanoma of skin	146	0	-	0.9	-	1.0	1.2	3.4	2.3	2.0	3.9	7.5	7.4	10.3	11.2	14.3	23.6	13.8	6.1	12.3	4.8	1.4	0.26	0.44	3.8	172
Other skin	554	0	-	-	-	-	-	1.1	1.6	3.3	3.9	5.2	15.3	25.3	42.1	74.5	139.8	124.2	230.8	227.3	18.4		0.49	1.56	12.9	173
Breast	28	0	-	-	-	-	-	-	0.8	-	-	1.1	1.1	1.6	2.1	3.8	4.7	7.9	6.1	6.1	0.9	0.3	0.03	0.08	0.7	175
Prostate	678	0	-	0.4	-	-	-	-	-	-	1.2	1.7	9.1	18.6	45.8	103.1	213.6	254.4	279.4	239.6	22.5	6.3	0.38	1.97	15.7	185
Testis	144	0	-	0.4	0.4	4.5	5.6	9.0	13.6	11.6	3.5	1.7	2.3	3.1	2.1	3.8	7.9	2.0	3.0	-	4.8	1.3	0.29	0.35	4.1	186
Penis	36	0	-	-	-	-	-	-	-	-	0.4	0.6	2.8	2.1	4.3	5.3	4.7	3.9	6.1	18.4	1.2	0.3	0.05	0.10	0.9	187.1-.4
Other male genital	4	0	-	-	-	-	-	-	-	-	0.8	-	0.6	-	-	-	-	1.6	-	-	0.1	0.0	0.01	0.01	0.1	187.5-.9
Bladder	573	0	-	-	-	-	-	-	0.4	1.0	2.3	5.2	14.7	26.4	63.9	100.1	98.9	144.0	179.2	178.1	19.0	5.4	0.57	1.56	13.1	188
Kidney etc.	544	0	2.4	0.9	0.4	-	0.6	-	1.2	2.3	7.8	16.7	30.0	43.4	60.7	82.8	83.2	76.9	36.4	73.7	18.1	5.1	0.83	1.66	13.3	189
Eye	22	0	1.2	0.9	-	-	-	-	-	0.7	-	0.6	1.7	1.6	3.2	0.8	1.6	2.0	-	-	0.7	0.2	0.05	0.06	0.7	190
Brain, nervous system	314	0	2.9	3.5	2.6	3.0	2.5	1.7	4.7	8.0	8.9	12.1	13.0	20.7	27.2	30.8	33.0	37.5	18.2	6.1	10.4	2.9	0.55	0.87	8.2	191-2
Thyroid	38	0	-	-	-	-	0.6	-	0.4	1.0	0.4	1.1	0.6	1.6	2.7	7.5	7.9	3.9	9.1	6.1	1.3	0.4	0.04	0.12	0.9	193
Other endocrine	26	0	-	0.4	0.4	0.5	-	-	0.4	0.3	0.8	1.1	-	2.1	0.5	6.0	6.3	-	-	-	0.9	0.2	0.03	0.09	0.7	194
Hodgkin's disease	72	0	-	0.4	1.3	2.0	2.5	3.9	3.1	2.3	2.3	2.3	3.4	4.1	1.1	4.5	3.1	5.9	3.0	-	2.4	0.7	0.14	0.18	2.1	201
Non-Hodgkin lymphoma	250	0	1.2	2.2	2.2	1.0	1.2	2.2	0.8	5.6	4.7	7.5	9.6	12.9	18.6	30.8	45.5	49.3	30.4	24.6	8.3	2.3	0.35	0.73	6.4	200,202
Multiple myeloma	87	0	-	-	-	-	-	-	-	0.3	-	1.1	2.3	7.2	9.6	14.3	9.4	23.7	27.3	12.3	2.9	0.8	0.10	0.22	1.9	203
Lymphoid leukaemia	111	0	4.1	3.5	0.9	2.0	0.6	1.1	-	1.0	0.8	2.3	1.1	4.1	3.7	12.8	17.3	31.6	21.3	61.4	3.7	1.0	0.13	0.28	3.3	204
Myeloid leukaemia	94	0	1.8	1.3	0.9	1.0	2.5	1.1	1.2	-	1.6	1.1	4.0	3.6	5.9	7.5	17.3	23.7	18.2	30.7	3.1	0.9	0.13	0.25	2.7	205
Monocytic leukaemia	0	0	-	-	-	-	-	-	-	-	-	-	-	-	-	-	-	-	-	-	0.0	0.0	0.00	0.00	0.0	206
Other leukaemia	1	0	-	-	-	-	-	-	-	-	-	-	0.6	-	-	-	-	-	-	-	0.0	0.0	0.00	0.00	0.0	207
Leukaemia unspecified	26	0	-	-	0.4	-	0.6	-	-	0.3	0.8	0.6	-	1.6	2.1	3.0	-	3.9	6.1	30.7	0.9	0.2	0.03	0.05	0.7	208
Other and unspecified	534	1	0.6	-	-	1.0	0.6	-	1.6	3.0	3.1	9.2	23.2	26.4	45.3	72.2	86.4	144.0	200.4	153.6	17.7	5.0	0.57	1.37	12.4	O&U
All sites	11250	4	18.8	16.7	12.1	21.6	23.0	26.9	39.3	66.9	108.9	235.5	423.4	723.3	1077.1	1625.0	1979.0	2246.0	2751.1	2414.2	373.4		13.97	32.00	267.9	ALL
All sites but 173	10696	4	18.8	16.7	12.1	21.6	23.0	25.8	37.7	63.6	105.0	230.3	408.1	698.0	1035.1	1550.5	1839.2	2121.8	2520.3	2186.9	355.0	100.0	13.48	30.44	254.9	ALLb
Rate from 1 case			0.589	0.439	0.431	0.503	0.620	0.561	0.389	0.331	0.389	0.574	0.567	0.517	0.532	0.752	1.571	1.972	3.037	6.143						

POLAND, WARSAW CITY 1989-1992

ANNUAL INCIDENCE PER 100,000 BY AGE GROUP (YEARS) - FEMALE

SITE	ALL AGES	AGE UNK	0-	5-	10-	15-	20-	25-	30-	35-	40-	45-	50-	55-	60-	65-	70-	75-	80-	85+	CRUDE RATE	%	CR 64	CR 74	ASR (W)	ICD (9th)
Lip	13	0	-	-	-	-	-	-	-	-	-	-	0.8	0.9	-	2.8	1.9	3.7	1.9	0.4	0.1	0.01	0.02	**0.2**	140
Tongue	34	0	-	-	-	-	-	-	0.3	0.3	1.0	1.4	0.8	2.2	3.9	2.8	1.9	6.1	5.6	1.0	0.3	0.03	0.06	**0.5**	141
Salivary gland	31	0	-	-	-	0.5	-	-	-	0.3	2.0	0.5	0.9	0.8	2.2	1.7	0.9	1.9	2.4	9.4	0.9	0.3	0.04	0.05	**0.5**	142
Mouth	23	0	-	-	-	-	-	0.5	-	-	0.3	0.5	0.9	1.3	0.9	1.7	2.8	1.9	1.2	7.5	0.7	0.2	0.02	0.04	**0.4**	143-5
Oropharynx	27	0	-	-	-	-	-	-	-	-	1.0	1.0	0.9	0.8	2.6	2.8	2.8	2.8	1.2	-	0.8	0.2	0.03	0.06	**0.5**	146
Nasopharynx	5	0	-	-	-	-	-	-	-	-	0.7	1.0	-	-	-	-	-	0.9	-	-	0.1	0.0	0.01	0.01	**0.1**	147
Hypopharynx	5	0	-	-	-	-	-	-	-	-	-	-	0.5	-	0.4	-	1.1	-	-	-	0.1	0.0	0.00	0.01	**0.1**	148
Pharynx unspecified	4	0	-	-	-	-	-	-	-	-	-	-	-	-	-	0.4	-	1.9	-	-	1.9	0.1	0.0	0.00	0.01	**0.1**	149
Oesophagus	85	0	-	-	-	-	-	-	-	-	0.7	1.4	0.5	2.5	7.5	3.3	6.5	9.4	23.1	26.3	2.4	0.7	0.06	0.11	**1.1**	150
Stomach	486	0	-	-	-	-	-	1.6	0.7	2.9	4.1	7.7	9.5	17.2	20.7	35.8	52.7	77.7	87.6	107.2	13.9	4.1	0.32	0.76	**6.9**	151
Small intestine	18	0	-	-	-	-	-	-	-	-	0.3	-	0.5	1.7	0.4	1.7	0.9	1.9	4.9	1.9	0.5	0.2	0.01	0.03	**0.2**	152
Colon	722	0	-	-	-	-	-	0.5	-	2.1	4.4	8.2	15.8	17.2	41.0	53.9	79.6	121.7	137.6	165.6	20.7	6.1	0.45	1.11	**10.0**	153
Rectum	470	0	-	-	-	-	-	-	1.1	1.5	3.8	5.3	11.3	25.6	25.1	39.1	46.3	74.0	75.5	65.8	13.5	4.0	0.37	0.79	**6.8**	154
Liver	220	1	-	-	-	-	-	-	-	0.9	1.0	1.9	3.6	5.5	12.3	19.8	19.4	30.0	51.1	54.6	6.3	1.9	0.13	0.32	**2.9**	155
Gallbladder etc.	556	0	-	-	-	-	-	-	0.4	0.6	0.7	1.9	8.6	20.1	33.5	54.5	54.6	78.7	113.2	129.8	15.9	4.7	0.33	0.87	**7.5**	156
Pancreas	363	0	-	-	-	-	-	-	0.4	1.2	2.4	2.9	5.0	11.3	16.3	40.2	35.2	61.8	63.3	77.1	10.4	3.1	0.20	0.57	**5.0**	157
Nose, sinuses etc.	13	0	-	-	-	-	-	-	-	-	-	1.0	0.5	0.4	1.8	1.1	-	-	2.4	1.9	0.4	0.1	0.02	0.02	**0.2**	160
Larynx	69	0	-	-	-	-	-	-	-	0.6	1.7	1.4	3.2	5.0	6.6	5.5	7.4	2.8	3.7	1.9	2.0	0.6	0.09	0.16	**1.2**	161
Bronchus, lung	1241	0	-	-	-	-	-	-	0.4	2.7	9.2	17.3	28.4	52.0	114.2	132.6	155.4	137.7	127.8	114.8	35.6	10.5	1.12	2.56	**19.5**	162
Other thoracic organs	48	1	-	-	-	-	-	-	0.4	0.3	0.3	1.0	2.3	1.7	2.6	3.9	6.5	3.7	3.7	11.3	1.4	0.4	0.04	0.10	**0.8**	163-4
Bone	31	0	0.6	0.9	1.4	1.1	0.6	-	1.1	-	1.0	-	1.4	1.3	1.3	0.6	0.9	3.7	1.2	-	0.9	0.3	0.05	0.06	**0.8**	170
Connective tissue	65	0	0.6	1.4	-	1.6	-	1.0	0.7	0.6	0.3	-	1.9	3.2	2.1	5.3	3.9	4.6	2.8	8.5	1.9	1.9	0.5	0.09	0.14	**1.4**	171
Mesothelioma	18	0	-	-	0.5	-	-	-	0.4	-	0.3	-	0.9	2.1	1.3	1.1	-	1.9	1.2	-	0.5	0.2	0.03	0.03	**0.3**	MES
Kaposi's sarcoma	1	0	-	-	-	-	-	-	-	-	-	-	-	-	-	-	-	0.9	-	-	0.0	0.0	0.00	0.00	**0.0**	KAP
Melanoma of skin	195	0	-	-	-	-	1.2	2.1	3.2	4.7	8.2	9.1	8.6	8.0	7.5	13.2	12.0	11.2	11.0	15.1	5.6	1.6	0.26	0.39	**3.7**	172
Other skin	683	0	-	-	-	-	1.9	0.5	-	3.2	6.5	6.7	13.1	26.0	40.6	58.3	71.2	98.3	125.4	114.8	19.6		0.49	1.14	**9.9**	173
Breast	2412	0	-	-	-	-	1.9	2.6	14.4	33.3	69.2	107.4	117.4	120.4	159.2	177.7	186.0	163.0	148.5	180.6	69.1	20.3	3.13	4.95	**43.2**	174
Uterus unspecified	28	0	-	-	-	-	-	-	-	-	0.3	-	0.5	-	1.8	2.2	0.9	3.7	7.3	13.2	0.8	0.2	0.01	0.03	**0.3**	179
Cervix uteri	812	0	-	-	-	-	2.5	2.1	13.7	20.9	44.0	37.1	32.1	41.9	39.7	49.5	38.9	45.0	41.4	24.5	23.3	6.8	1.17	1.61	**15.2**	180
Placenta	13	0	-	-	-	0.5	1.9	0.5	1.4	0.3	1.0	-	-	-	-	-	-	-	-	-	0.4	0.1	0.03	0.03	**0.4**	181
Corpus uteri	740	0	-	-	-	-	-	-	0.7	2.7	11.3	20.2	46.1	57.5	64.8	62.7	53.7	38.4	47.5	30.1	21.2	6.2	1.02	1.60	**13.0**	182
Ovary etc.	726	0	0.6	-	0.9	0.5	1.9	3.1	3.9	9.7	21.1	29.8	39.7	36.1	45.0	52.3	52.7	51.5	43.8	48.9	20.8	6.1	0.96	1.49	**13.3**	183
Other female genital	147	0	-	-	-	-	-	-	0.7	2.1	1.4	2.4	2.7	4.6	4.0	13.2	15.7	23.4	21.9	35.7	4.2	1.2	0.09	0.23	**2.1**	184
Bladder	205	0	0.6	-	-	-	-	-	0.4	0.3	1.0	1.4	4.5	4.6	12.8	28.6	18.5	22.5	34.1	41.4	5.9	1.7	0.13	0.36	**3.0**	188
Kidney etc.	368	0	1.9	0.5	-	-	-	-	1.1	1.2	3.1	5.3	12.2	22.2	26.0	39.1	38.9	37.5	39.0	24.5	10.6	3.1	0.37	0.76	**6.1**	189
Eye	22	0	0.6	-	-	-	-	-	0.7	0.3	0.3	1.4	0.5	2.1	-	1.1	1.9	0.9	3.7	-	0.6	0.2	0.03	0.04	**0.4**	190
Brain, nervous system	299	0	1.2	1.8	3.2	1.6	1.9	2.1	2.5	3.5	4.1	7.2	9.5	15.1	21.6	29.7	30.5	19.7	13.4	9.4	8.6	2.5	0.38	0.68	**5.9**	191-2
Thyroid	121	0	-	-	-	-	-	0.5	1.4	3.5	5.1	3.9	4.5	5.9	6.2	7.7	6.5	10.3	8.5	7.5	3.5	1.0	0.15	0.23	**2.1**	193
Other endocrine	36	0	0.6	-	-	-	-	1.0	1.1	0.3	1.4	1.0	0.5	1.7	3.1	2.2	1.9	-	6.1	-	1.0	0.3	0.05	0.07	**0.7**	194
Hodgkin's disease	61	0	-	0.5	1.4	4.7	1.9	2.1	2.8	2.4	1.0	2.4	0.5	1.7	2.2	0.6	2.8	0.9	1.2	1.9	1.7	0.5	0.12	0.13	**1.7**	201
Non-Hodgkin lymphoma	194	0	-	0.5	-	-	-	0.5	2.1	1.5	0.7	4.8	7.2	8.0	11.0	14.3	29.6	22.5	23.1	15.1	5.6	1.6	0.18	0.40	**3.2**	200,202
Multiple myeloma	117	1	-	-	-	-	-	-	-	-	1.0	1.4	3.2	6.3	8.8	10.5	13.9	18.7	14.6	3.8	3.4	1.0	0.10	0.23	**1.8**	203
Lymphoid leukaemia	90	0	4.3	3.7	0.9	1.1	0.6	-	0.4	0.6	0.7	-	0.9	1.7	2.6	3.9	10.2	14.0	8.5	24.5	2.6	0.8	0.09	0.16	**2.1**	204
Myeloid leukaemia	123	0	2.5	0.5	1.4	0.5	-	1.0	1.1	2.7	1.7	1.9	1.4	5.5	6.6	7.7	7.4	15.9	19.5	9.4	3.5	1.0	0.13	0.21	**2.3**	205
Monocytic leukaemia	0	0	-	-	-	-	-	-	-	-	-	-	-	-	-	-	-	-	-	-	0.0	0.0	0.00	0.00	**0.0**	206
Other leukaemia	5	0	-	-	-	-	-	-	-	0.3	-	-	-	0.4	0.4	-	0.9	-	1.2	-	0.1	0.0	0.01	0.01	**0.1**	207
Leukaemia unspecified	23	0	0.6	-	-	-	-	-	-	-	-	-	0.5	-	0.4	2.2	0.9	2.8	8.5	9.4	0.7	0.2	0.01	0.02	**0.3**	208
Other and unspecified	589	2	0.6	-	0.5	-	-	-	-	0.3	1.7	7.2	9.0	18.5	30.0	46.2	72.2	80.5	131.5	143.0	16.9	5.0	0.34	0.93	**8.1**	O&U
All sites	12557	5	14.8	9.7	9.9	12.1	16.1	21.9	56.4	107.6	219.7	307.2	412.7	558.7	793.9	1030.6	1150.9	1300.8	1479.0	1540.7	360.0		12.71	23.62	**206.1**	ALL
All sites but 173	11874	5	14.8	9.7	9.9	12.1	14.2	21.4	56.4	104.4	213.2	300.4	399.7	532.7	753.3	972.2	1079.6	1202.5	1353.6	1426.0	340.4	100.0	12.22	22.48	**196.2**	ALLb
Rate from 1 case			0.618	0.460	0.452	0.527	0.619	0.522	0.350	0.295	0.341	0.481	0.452	0.419	0.441	0.550	0.925	0.937	1.217	1.881						

Slovakia

Despite the introduction of compulsory notification of all cancer patients and deaths in Slovakia in 1952, underestimation of incident cases led to mortality/incidence ratios over 100 for most individual cancer sites, indicating approximately 30% undernotification of incident cases at the end of the 1960s. In 1976 a population-based pilot cancer registry covering about 2 million inhabitants in the western part of Slovakia, including its capital city of Bratislava, was established at the Department of Cancer Epidemiology of the Cancer Research Institute of the Slovak Academy of Sciences. The first data collected covered the decade 1968–77.

In 1980 the National Cancer Registry covering the whole territory of Slovakia was established in Bratislava. Until 1990 the data were stored on magnetic media and all computations and analyses were performed in the State Computer Centre located elsewhere. In 1990, the database was moved to Bratislava and all information is now stored, analysed and evaluated in the registry's own computer. The registry is situated in the National Cancer Institute in Bratislava.

The registry covers the entire Slovak Republic (until 1992 the eastern part of former Czechoslovakia). Administratively Slovakia is divided into 38 districts, including the major towns of Bratislava and Košice with about 430 000 and 230 000 inhabitants respectively. Nearly 13% of the population live in these two cities, about 10% in seven others with 50 000 to 100 000 inhabitants. 56% of the population live in villages and towns with 5000 to 50 000 inhabitants, the remainder in settlements with less than 5000 inhabitants.

About 48% of all employed persons in 1990 were women. Approximately 12.1% of persons of productive age were employed in agriculture, 33.2% in industry, 10.2% in building and the remainder in administration, health, culture and public services. Since the political changes in 1989, the number of employed persons has decreased gradually, mainly in industry, so that over 12% unemployment has been recorded recently. The majority of the population is of Slovak nationality, the second most numerous group being Hungarians (11%) living mainly in the southern parts of Slovakia.

A network of outpatient oncological clinics was established during 1976–85 throughout the country. More detailed notification forms were introduced in 1977 allowing the collection of the majority of core and optional items recommended for population-based cancer registries by WHO (1976) and IARC and IACR (1978). At the end of 1987 new notification forms fully adapted for use with computers were introduced. With the abolition of counties as territorial units in 1992, the outpatient oncological clinics at this level were eliminated, and the peripheral network of registration now consists of outpatient oncological clinics at the level of districts.

Physicians have three months to complete the notification form after the description of primary treatment is requested. In the district outpatient oncological clinics, the notification is revised and completed together with assessment of further information on persons dying from cancer. Active, life-long follow-up is also performed in district outpatient clinics. The registry is informed only of changes of permanent address, diagnosis and death of the patients. More active follow-up is not possible because of the limited resources of the registry.

In the registry each new notification is compared and checked with the main file of patients already registered. All notification forms are coded and rechecked before the data are stored in the computer. The proper registration of multiple primaries is ensured together with the elimination of repeatedly notified cases. All death certificates (not only those containing cancer as a main cause of death or accompanying disease) are regularly reviewed in the registry to ensure the inclusion of previously unregistered patients and complete the data on registered patients. Since 1990, the registry has received much complementary information from other documents accompanying the notification form (autopsy reports, discharge summary, operative report, hospital records, results of histology or cytology etc.).

Cases registered in the decade 1968–77 and completed after 1977 were coded using ICD-O classification only. Since 1978 the ICD-O classification for coding topography and morphology of tumours (including behaviour and histological grading) has been simultaneously used with ICD-9. Great attention is also paid to the development of cancer mortality statistics in the registry using the four-digit code of ICD-9 as well as to properly distinguishing persons dying from and with cancer, using all available information.

Annual reports from the registry with detailed data on cancer incidence have been published regularly since 1984. Data on cancer incidence for the period 1968–83 were published in 1988, replacing the lower and incomplete figures from the official cancer statistics. An atlas of cancer incidence and mortality (1975–84) was published in 1989.

The political changes in 1989 caused some problems in cancer notification and function of the registry, mainly during 1990–91. In recent years the financial situation of the registry and notification has gradually improved.

Environmental pollution is evident only in highly industrialized areas. About 226 000 tonnes of solid particulates were emitted into the ambient air annually in the whole country together with 447 000 tons of SO_2, 167 000 tons of CO and 166 000 tons of NO_x at the end of the 1980s. Among the regions with the highest air pollution are the conurbation of Bratislava (petroleum and chemical industry), upper Nitra (electricity-producing stations using coal with high arsenic content), the basin of Žiar (aluminium production) and the basin of Košice (steel and smelting industry).

I.Pleško

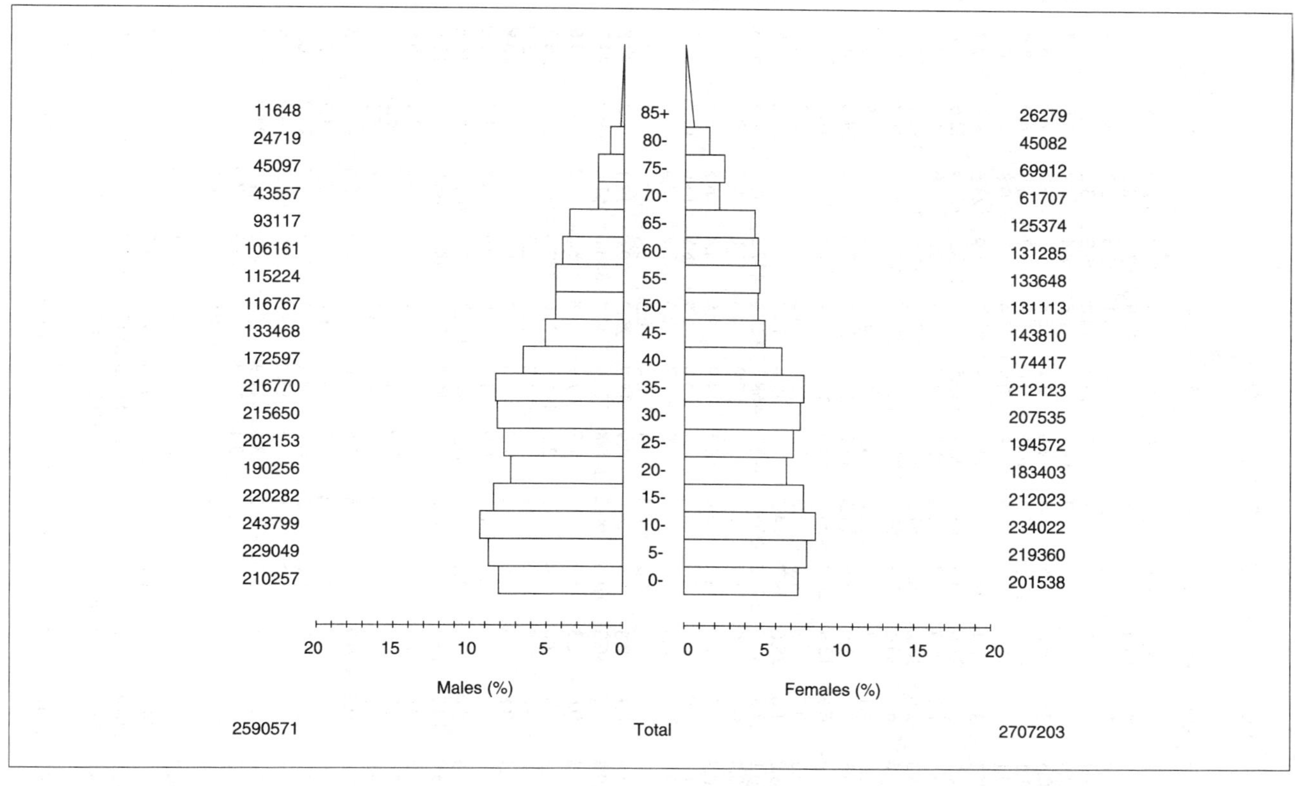

Slovakia

Source of population: average annual 1988–91
Census: Population of Czech and Slovak Federal Republic – Census 1991. Czech and Slovak Bureau of Statistics, Prague and Bratislava, 1992.
Estimate: The population data for each of the years 1988–90 were estimated on the basis of the 1980 census making allowance for births, deaths and migration. *References:* Age-structure of the population in 1988. Federal Bureau of Statistics, Prague, 1989. Age-structure of the population in 1989. Federal Bureau of Statistics, Prague, 1990. Age-structure of the population in 1990. Federal Bureau of Statistics, Prague, 1991.

Notes to data overleaf:
† 188 does not include the non-invasive tumours
Screening programmes in the area:
Screening programmes have been in operation since 1976 for cervical cancer (women over age 25, 350 000 examinations annually in recent years), breast cancer (women over age 35) and prostate cancer (men over age 55). The numbers of examinations each year for breast and prostate vary widely between different areas and hospitals. In 1987 a screening programme was set up for large bowel cancer in the population over age 35, but not many examinations take place.

SLOVAKIA 1988-1992

ANNUAL INCIDENCE PER 100,000 BY AGE GROUP (YEARS) - MALE

SITE	ALL AGES	AGE UNK	0-	5-	10-	15-	20-	25-	30-	35-	40-	45-	50-	55-	60-	65-	70-	75-	80-	85+	CRUDE RATE	%	CR 64	CR 74	ASR (W)	ICD (9th)
Lip	566	0	-	-	-	-	-	-	0.1	0.3	1.0	3.7	6.5	12.3	17.0	20.0	34.4	31.9	42.9	61.8	4.4	1.3	0.20	0.48	3.9	140
Tongue	674	0	-	-	-	-	-	0.1	0.8	3.2	9.5	15.9	23.3	16.3	17.1	13.3	11.9	7.1	8.1	10.3	5.2	1.5	0.43	0.56	5.1	141
Salivary gland	98	0	-	-	0.1	-	0.1	0.2	0.4	1.0	1.0	1.2	1.9	3.6	2.6	5.1	3.5	3.5	3.2	3.4	0.8	0.2	0.05	0.09	0.7	142
Mouth	710	0	-	-	0.1	-	0.1	-	0.6	3.4	9.5	16.3	23.8	19.3	19.2	15.7	13.8	6.2	3.2	1.7	5.5	1.6	0.46	0.61	5.4	143-5
Oropharynx	673	0	-	-	-	-	-	0.2	0.4	2.9	10.2	17.7	20.0	17.2	18.1	12.7	11.5	8.4	4.9	15.5	5.2	1.5	0.43	0.55	5.1	146
Nasopharynx	83	0	-	-	0.3	0.1	0.2	-	0.4	0.5	0.9	0.6	1.5	1.4	2.6	2.1	2.8	1.3	3.2	1.7	0.6	0.2	0.04	0.07	0.6	147
Hypopharynx	504	0	-	-	-	-	-	0.2	1.1	7.8	12.1	17.8	15.3	10.6	12.0	7.8	2.7	8.9	6.9	3.9	1.1	0.32	0.42	3.8	148
Pharynx unspecified	36	0	-	-	-	-	-	-	0.1	0.7	1.0	0.9	0.5	0.9	0.9	1.4	-	0.8	1.7	0.3	0.1	0.02	0.03	0.3	149
Oesophagus	1000	0	-	-	-	-	-	0.2	0.2	2.3	8.1	17.4	23.5	28.8	29.2	30.3	33.5	31.9	23.5	20.6	7.7	2.3	0.55	0.87	7.3	150
Stomach	3597	0	-	-	-	-	0.3	0.9	1.1	4.7	13.6	21.0	38.4	63.7	96.8	140.5	231.0	243.5	271.9	202.6	27.8	8.2	1.20	3.06	24.5	151
Small intestine	110	0	-	-	-	-	0.1	-	0.2	0.5	1.2	0.9	1.2	2.3	1.9	4.5	7.3	5.3	4.9	1.7	0.8	0.3	0.04	0.10	0.8	152
Colon	2903	0	-	-	-	0.5	0.4	1.2	1.7	4.3	8.6	16.2	30.5	57.3	88.0	116.2	187.8	180.9	173.1	151.1	22.4	6.6	1.04	2.56	20.0	153
Rectum	2984	0	-	-	-	-	0.1	0.9	1.3	2.6	6.3	20.4	37.3	58.1	91.6	123.5	171.7	177.8	204.7	171.7	23.0	6.8	1.09	2.57	20.6	154
Liver	1039	0	0.5	-	-	0.3	0.3	0.3	0.9	1.3	3.1	8.7	14.0	24.8	30.7	44.7	50.0	54.5	52.6	39.5	8.0	2.4	0.42	0.90	7.2	155
Gallbladder etc.	558	0	-	-	-	0.1	-	-	0.3	0.5	0.7	1.8	6.5	11.5	13.2	21.7	36.7	47.0	45.3	24.0	4.3	1.3	0.17	0.46	3.7	156
Pancreas	1544	0	-	-	-	-	0.1	0.6	0.7	3.0	6.6	12.9	20.7	34.4	45.8	57.6	81.7	87.8	94.7	51.5	11.9	3.5	0.62	1.32	10.7	157
Nose, sinuses etc.	97	0	-	-	0.1	0.1	0.1	0.1	0.3	0.3	0.7	1.5	1.0	2.3	2.3	3.7	3.2	2.7	4.9	6.9	0.7	0.2	0.04	0.08	0.7	160
Larynx	1525	0	-	-	-	-	-	0.1	0.5	3.8	11.6	25.6	39.7	44.3	53.7	49.4	43.2	26.2	28.3	29.2	11.8	3.5	0.90	1.36	11.3	161
Bronchus, lung	11110	0	-	-	0.1	0.4	0.6	2.3	10.1	31.2	85.7	198.2	296.1	413.0	468.7	535.4	437.3	441.8	324.5	85.8	25.3	5.19	10.21	79.1	162
Other thoracic organs	165	0	0.9	0.1	-	0.1	0.4	0.1	0.3	0.4	0.3	1.6	1.7	2.1	2.6	7.9	4.6	12.0	9.7	10.3	1.3	0.4	0.05	0.12	1.1	163-4
Bone	224	0	0.2	0.3	1.5	1.7	0.4	0.9	0.6	0.8	1.2	1.0	3.3	4.9	4.5	4.9	9.6	4.4	6.5	3.4	1.7	0.5	0.11	0.18	1.6	170
Connective tissue	302	0	1.5	0.5	0.2	0.4	0.3	1.6	1.3	1.4	3.0	3.1	3.9	4.9	7.9	5.6	6.4	8.9	14.6	13.7	2.3	0.7	0.15	0.21	2.2	171
Mesothelioma	46	0	-	-	0.1	-	-	-	MES	0.2	0.3	0.1	0.6	0.5	1.0	0.9	1.7	2.3	2.2	2.4	-	0.4	0.1	0.02	0.04	0.3	MES
Kaposi's sarcoma	11	0	-	-	-	-	-	-	0.1	-	-	-	0.2	0.5	0.4	0.4	0.5	0.4	-	-	0.1	0.0	0.01	Kap01	0.1	KAP
Melanoma of skin	621	0	-	0.1	-	0.1	0.8	1.8	1.9	4.9	6.1	7.5	8.4	14.1	14.9	18.7	23.0	20.0	12.1	17.2	4.8	1.4	0.30	0.51	4.4	172
Other skin	5796	0	0.1	-	0.1	0.4	0.5	1.3	5.4	10.3	18.7	36.3	61.5	100.2	148.8	220.4	344.4	383.6	461.2	449.9	44.7		1.92	4.74	39.4	173
Breast	72	0	-	-	-	-	-	-	-	0.3	0.6	1.3	1.4	1.9	1.7	1.9	2.8	3.5	3.2	-	0.6	0.2	0.04	0.06	0.5	175
Prostate	3452	0	-	-	-	-	-	-	-	0.1	0.7	3.6	8.4	31.2	72.2	144.8	276.0	362.3	430.4	317.7	26.7	7.9	0.58	2.68	22.0	185
Testis	660	0	0.8	0.2	0.3	3.5	10.0	13.7	14.7	8.8	6.6	2.5	1.7	1.2	1.3	1.5	1.4	2.7	3.2	3.4	5.1	1.5	0.33	0.34	4.6	186
Penis	108	0	-	-	-	-	-	0.1	0.1	0.4	0.8	1.3	1.9	1.9	1.5	4.3	2.3	8.0	5.7	10.3	0.8	0.2	0.04	0.07	0.7	187.1-.4
Other male genital	29	0	-	-	-	0.1	-	0.1	0.2	0.2	-	0.1	0.5	0.3	0.9	1.3	0.9	0.9	0.8	1.7	0.2	0.1	0.01	0.02	0.2	187.5-.9
†Bladder	2177	1	-	0.1	-	-	0.3	0.5	0.7	2.5	5.0	10.6	21.1	37.0	63.3	94.3	122.1	143.7	167.5	188.9	16.8	5.0	0.71	1.79	14.8	188
Kidney etc.	1502	0	1.9	0.1	0.2	0.3	0.2	0.6	1.8	3.0	10.1	16.3	25.0	37.0	50.7	56.7	71.2	44.8	46.9	25.8	11.6	3.4	0.74	1.37	10.9	189
Eye	112	0	1.0	-	-	0.2	0.2	-	0.3	0.2	0.6	1.0	2.4	2.1	4.0	3.2	3.2	3.1	3.2	1.7	0.9	0.3	0.06	0.09	0.9	190
Brain, nervous system	779	0	2.9	2.4	2.1	2.5	2.1	2.6	3.7	3.5	6.7	7.8	11.8	16.1	17.9	21.0	24.3	7.1	5.7	5.2	6.0	1.8	0.41	0.64	5.9	191-2
Thyroid	141	0	-	0.1	0.1	0.4	0.6	0.5	0.4	0.9	1.0	1.6	2.6	3.5	2.1	5.2	3.7	2.7	2.4	5.2	1.1	0.3	0.07	0.11	1.0	193
Other endocrine	61	0	0.2	0.1	0.1	0.3	0.2	-	-	0.3	0.2	0.9	1.4	1.4	1.5	2.4	1.4	0.9	0.8	-	0.5	0.1	0.03	0.05	0.5	194
Hodgkin's disease	308	0	0.7	1.2	0.8	2.7	3.7	1.9	1.9	3.0	2.3	2.7	2.1	2.8	3.0	3.4	6.0	8.4	7.3	1.7	2.4	0.7	0.14	0.19	2.2	201
Non-Hodgkin lymphoma	784	0	2.1	1.7	1.2	1.5	1.1	2.4	2.4	2.8	5.0	6.7	10.6	14.2	16.8	23.2	32.1	30.2	33.2	24.0	6.1	1.8	0.34	0.62	5.6	200,202
Multiple myeloma	371	0	-	-	-	-	-	-	0.1	0.6	1.7	2.2	4.5	6.9	11.3	17.2	23.4	20.0	22.7	6.9	2.9	0.8	0.14	0.34	2.6	203
Lymphoid leukaemia	702	1	5.9	3.1	1.7	0.9	0.7	0.7	0.4	0.6	0.9	3.1	5.8	9.2	13.8	21.9	43.6	43.5	41.3	24.0	5.4	1.6	0.23	0.56	5.2	204
Myeloid leukaemia	455	0	1.3	0.6	0.7	1.1	1.4	1.6	2.8	2.3	2.4	2.8	6.0	5.0	9.4	12.9	19.7	19.5	17.0	12.0	3.5	1.0	0.19	0.35	3.2	205
Monocytic leukaemia	12	0	-	0.1	-	0.1	-	0.1	-	-	-	0.6	-	0.2	-	-	0.9	0.4	0.8	-	0.1	0.0	0.01	0.01	0.1	206
Other leukaemia	6	0	0.1	-	-	0.1	0.1	-	-	-	-	0.3	-	-	-	-	0.5	-	-	-	0.0	0.0	0.00	0.01	0.1	207
Leukaemia unspecified	55	0	-	-	-	0.2	-	0.1	0.1	0.2	-	0.4	0.5	0.7	0.9	1.9	3.7	3.1	7.3	1.7	0.4	0.1	0.02	0.04	0.4	208
Other and unspecified	960	0	1.7	0.4	0.2	0.4	0.4	1.6	0.9	1.7	4.1	6.4	10.8	17.2	24.7	32.6	46.8	51.0	76.1	84.1	7.4	2.2	0.35	0.75	6.7	O&U
All sites	49722	2	21.7	11.1	9.8	17.8	25.8	37.2	52.3	94.3	210.4	403.2	704.3	1025.1	1432.2	1849.3	2547.0	2543.4	2802.7	2335.2	383.9		20.23	42.21	347.9	ALL
All sites but 173	43926	2	21.6	11.1	9.7	17.4	25.2	35.9	46.9	84.0	191.8	367.0	642.8	925.0	1283.3	1628.9	2202.6	2159.8	2341.5	1885.3	339.1	100.0	18.31	37.47	308.5	ALLb

Rate from 1 case   0.095   0.087   0.082   0.091   0.105   0.099   0.093   0.092   0.116   0.150   0.171   0.174   0.188   0.215   0.459   0.443   0.809   1.717

†Important: see notes on population page

SLOVAKIA 1988-1992

ANNUAL INCIDENCE PER 100,000 BY AGE GROUP (YEARS) - FEMALE

SITE	ALL AGES	UNK	0-	5-	10-	15-	20-	25-	30-	35-	40-	45-	50-	55-	60-	65-	70-	75-	80-	85+	CRUDE RATE	%	CR 64	CR 74	ASR (W)	ICD (9th)
Lip	150	0	-	-	-	-	-	-	-	-	0.2	0.1	0.8	1.0	2.6	2.7	8.1	9.7	9.8	15.2	1.1	0.4	0.02	0.08	**0.7**	*140*
Tongue	53	0	-	-	-	-	-	0.1	0.2	0.2	0.7	0.6	0.5	0.1	1.1	1.4	1.9	1.7	1.3	2.3	0.4	0.2	0.02	0.03	**0.3**	*141*
Salivary gland	63	0	-	-	-	-	0.2	-	-	0.3	0.1	0.7	0.8	1.0	0.6	1.3	1.9	2.0	5.3	2.3	0.5	0.2	0.02	0.03	**0.3**	*142*
Mouth	68	0	-	-	-	-	0.1	-	-	0.1	0.8	0.4	1.2	1.0	1.7	2.2	1.6	1.7	0.9	2.3	0.5	0.2	0.03	0.05	**0.4**	*143-5*
Oropharynx	44	0	-	-	-	0.1	-	-	0.1	0.1	0.2	1.0	0.5	0.4	0.9	1.3	0.3	1.4	1.8	1.5	0.3	0.1	0.02	0.02	**0.2**	*146*
Nasopharynx	48	0	0.1	-	0.1	0.2	0.1	-	0.1	0.4	0.3	0.4	0.9	0.6	1.1	0.8	0.3	1.7	0.9	0.8	0.4	0.1	0.02	0.03	**0.3**	*147*
Hypopharynx	14	0	-	-	-	-	-	-	-	-	0.1	0.1	-	0.3	0.5	0.3	-	0.9	0.9	-	0.1	0.0	0.01	0.01	**0.1**	*148*
Pharynx unspecified	4	0	-	-	-	-	-	-	-	0.1	-	-	-	-	-	0.2	-	-	0.4	0.8	0.0	0.0	0.00	0.00	**0.0**	*149*
Oesophagus	112	0	-	-	-	-	0.1	-	-	0.1	0.2	0.3	0.5	1.2	2.9	2.7	2.9	4.9	8.4	10.7	0.8	0.3	0.03	0.05	**0.5**	*150*
Stomach	2197	0	0.1	-	-	-	0.3	0.9	1.3	4.3	6.7	7.6	13.0	22.3	33.7	57.3	87.5	120.2	146.8	134.7	16.2	6.4	0.45	1.17	**10.3**	*151*
Small intestine	87	0	-	-	-	-	-	0.1	0.2	0.5	0.1	0.7	0.8	1.2	1.1	3.0	1.9	3.4	4.4	4.6	0.6	0.3	0.02	0.05	**0.4**	*152*
Colon	2512	0	-	-	0.1	0.4	0.2	0.4	2.3	4.2	6.8	12.8	24.6	35.0	46.8	74.3	99.8	111.0	121.6	108.8	18.6	7.4	0.67	1.54	**12.6**	*153*
Rectum	2162	0	-	-	-	-	0.1	0.8	1.1	3.1	6.1	12.4	19.8	28.9	44.2	60.8	91.1	90.1	111.4	95.9	16.0	6.3	0.58	1.34	**10.9**	*154*
Liver	620	0	0.4	0.1	-	0.1	0.4	0.3	0.4	0.8	1.3	1.9	3.8	7.8	13.7	18.2	25.3	29.8	29.3	31.2	4.6	1.8	0.15	0.37	**3.1**	*155*
Gallbladder etc.	1340	0	-	-	-	-	-	0.2	0.1	0.4	2.1	3.9	7.8	15.4	26.4	41.3	63.5	70.9	78.5	60.9	9.9	3.9	0.28	0.81	**6.4**	*156*
Pancreas	1134	0	-	-	-	0.1	0.1	-	0.2	0.8	2.2	4.5	4.9	13.6	23.0	38.1	45.1	61.2	55.0	61.6	8.4	3.3	0.25	0.66	**5.4**	*157*
Nose, sinuses etc.	51	0	-	-	-	-	0.1	0.1	-	-	0.2	0.3	0.5	1.0	0.9	1.0	1.6	2.9	0.9	4.6	0.4	0.1	0.02	0.03	**0.3**	*160*
Larynx	73	0	-	-	-	-	-	-	0.1	0.5	0.3	0.7	1.5	1.3	1.5	1.9	0.6	2.0	3.5	0.8	0.5	0.2	0.03	0.04	**0.4**	*161*
Bronchus, lung	1680	0	-	-	-	0.1	0.3	0.5	0.9	2.6	4.7	8.6	15.9	26.2	34.4	49.1	75.8	68.7	70.1	65.5	12.4	4.9	0.47	1.10	**8.7**	*162*
Other thoracic organs	111	0	0.7	-	0.2	-	0.1	0.3	0.3	0.3	0.5	0.6	0.9	1.3	2.0	2.2	4.9	2.9	5.3	3.8	0.8	0.3	0.04	0.07	**0.6**	*163-4*
Bone	176	0	-	0.5	0.8	0.8	0.7	0.5	0.6	0.8	0.9	1.4	1.7	1.9	3.5	2.2	5.5	5.4	4.0	3.0	1.3	0.5	0.07	0.11	**1.1**	*170*
Connective tissue	256	0	0.9	0.4	0.5	0.4	0.5	0.8	0.8	1.2	1.5	2.8	2.7	3.3	3.0	6.4	7.1	6.0	6.7	6.1	1.9	0.8	0.09	0.16	**1.6**	*171*
Mesothelioma	22	0	-	-	-	-	0.1	0.1	-	-	0.2	-	0.2	1.0	0.5	0.3	0.6	0.6	0.4	-	0.2	0.1	0.01	0.02	**0.1**	*MES*
Kaposi's sarcoma	1	0	-	-	-	-	-	-	-	-	-	-	-	-	-	-	-	-	0.4	-	0.0	0.0	0.00	0.00	**0.0**	*KAP*
Melanoma of skin	740	0	-	-	-	0.3	1.3	3.2	4.8	5.7	8.5	9.2	9.3	12.6	11.1	12.8	14.3	12.6	16.4	16.0	5.5	2.2	0.33	0.46	**4.4**	*172*
Other skin	5839	0	-	0.1	0.1	0.4	0.8	3.5	5.5	12.3	22.6	39.8	45.9	76.5	104.7	146.1	221.7	259.8	317.2	304.4	43.1		1.56	3.40	**29.3**	*173*
Breast	6591	0	-	-	-	0.3	0.9	3.2	15.5	32.7	58.9	102.2	99.8	116.0	131.8	140.1	174.7	165.6	146.0	131.7	48.7	19.3	2.81	4.38	**38.6**	*174*
Uterus unspecified	46	0	-	-	-	-	-	-	-	-	0.2	-	0.5	0.1	0.6	0.6	2.6	3.4	2.7	4.6	0.3	0.1	0.01	0.02	**0.2**	*179*
Cervix uteri	2627	0	-	-	-	0.1	1.4	11.5	22.2	39.1	43.1	39.9	30.2	32.0	39.0	36.1	37.6	27.2	29.7	16.0	19.4	7.7	1.29	1.66	**16.4**	*180*
Placenta	20	0	-	-	-	0.4	0.4	0.7	0.2	0.2	-	0.1	-	-	-	-	-	-	-	-	0.1	0.1	0.01	0.01	**0.2**	*181*
Corpus uteri	2736	0	-	-	0.1	0.2	0.3	0.6	1.6	4.3	12.0	29.5	49.7	66.0	74.3	75.9	84.3	54.1	51.5	36.5	20.2	8.0	1.19	1.99	**16.0**	*182*
Ovary etc.	1816	0	-	0.3	0.6	1.8	2.0	2.9	5.4	7.4	16.3	25.9	28.1	34.3	37.0	40.0	45.7	32.0	36.4	27.4	13.4	5.3	0.81	1.24	**10.9**	*183*
Other female genital	363	0	0.2	-	-	-	-	0.1	0.4	0.4	1.5	2.1	1.4	4.8	7.5	8.1	14.9	20.3	16.4	22.1	2.7	1.1	0.09	0.21	**1.8**	*184*
†Bladder	622	0	-	-	-	0.2	0.1	0.2	0.4	1.1	0.9	2.2	4.3	9.9	12.9	17.1	23.7	28.0	38.2	25.9	4.6	1.8	0.16	0.36	**3.0**	*188*
Kidney etc.	1044	0	1.7	0.4	-	0.2	-	0.4	1.3	2.3	4.1	8.6	12.8	19.5	26.5	29.4	34.7	32.6	25.7	23.6	7.7	3.1	0.39	0.71	**5.9**	*189*
Eye	132	0	1.2	0.1	-	0.2	-	0.2	0.5	0.4	0.9	1.0	1.2	2.1	2.3	3.2	3.6	3.4	3.1	3.0	1.0	0.4	0.05	0.08	**0.8**	*190*
Brain, nervous system	625	0	2.3	3.2	2.0	1.9	2.7	2.5	1.9	3.2	4.9	5.6	8.1	12.0	10.7	11.3	11.3	5.4	3.1	2.3	4.6	1.8	0.30	0.42	**4.3**	*191-2*
Thyroid	476	0	0.1	0.2	0.3	0.8	2.1	2.0	1.7	3.2	6.1	6.4	6.7	5.5	6.4	6.2	11.7	12.0	8.9	8.4	3.5	1.4	0.21	0.30	**2.9**	*193*
Other endocrine	63	0	0.5	-	0.2	0.2	0.1	-	0.2	0.3	0.6	1.4	0.2	0.6	1.1	1.6	1.3	1.1	1.3	-	0.5	0.2	0.03	0.04	**0.4**	*194*
Hodgkin's disease	244	0	0.2	0.8	1.3	3.0	3.9	2.7	1.9	1.4	1.5	0.8	2.4	1.6	1.1	0.6	3.6	4.3	1.3	2.3	1.8	0.7	0.11	0.13	**1.7**	*201*
Non-Hodgkin lymphoma	633	0	1.1	1.1	0.3	0.8	0.7	1.6	1.1	2.3	3.9	4.7	6.7	8.1	11.9	15.6	21.7	18.6	20.9	16.0	4.7	1.9	0.22	0.41	**3.6**	*200,202*
Multiple myeloma	375	0	-	-	-	-	-	-	0.3	0.3	1.0	2.6	2.6	4.8	8.4	13.9	17.8	13.2	13.8	13.7	2.8	1.1	0.10	0.26	**2.0**	*203*
Lymphoid leukaemia	442	0	4.3	1.3	1.8	1.1	0.2	0.3	0.4	0.3	0.5	1.8	3.5	3.7	5.8	10.4	16.9	19.7	14.6	13.7	3.3	1.3	0.12	0.26	**2.7**	*204*
Myeloid leukaemia	383	0	0.7	0.6	0.6	0.7	1.1	1.6	1.1	1.9	1.5	3.3	4.7	6.0	7.5	7.7	10.0	9.2	10.6	4.6	2.8	1.1	0.16	0.24	**2.3**	*205*
Monocytic leukaemia	10	0	-	-	-	0.1	0.1	-	-	-	-	0.1	0.3	-	-	-	0.6	0.3	0.9	-	0.1	0.0	0.00	0.01	**0.1**	*206*
Other leukaemia	11	0	0.1	-	-	-	-	0.1	-	-	0.1	-	-	-	0.3	0.5	0.6	0.3	-	-	0.1	0.0	0.00	0.01	**0.1**	*207*
Leukaemia unspecified	56	0	0.3	-	-	-	-	0.1	-	-	-	-	0.8	0.6	0.6	1.4	1.6	2.9	5.3	2.3	0.4	0.2	0.01	0.03	**0.3**	*208*
Other and unspecified	1081	0	2.1	0.2	0.2	0.3	0.2	0.4	0.8	1.6	2.5	4.0	7.5	9.6	15.1	24.6	45.4	48.3	81.6	85.2	8.0	3.2	0.22	0.57	**5.2**	*O&U*
All sites	39953	0	16.9	9.2	9.0	14.9	21.9	43.1	75.6	141.0	228.0	353.1	429.6	592.5	762.3	972.3	1327.9	1373.4	1513.7	1376.8	295.2		13.48	24.99	**217.7**	*ALL*
All sites but 173	34114	0	16.9	9.1	8.9	14.5	21.2	39.6	70.1	128.7	205.4	313.3	383.6	516.0	657.7	826.2	1106.2	1113.7	1196.5	1072.3	252.0	100.0	11.92	21.59	**188.5**	*ALLb*
Rate from 1 case			0.099	0.091	0.086	0.094	0.109	0.103	1.096	0.094	0.115	0.139	0.152	0.150	0.152	0.159	0.324	0.286	0.444	0.761						

†Important: see notes on population page

Slovenia

The Cancer Registry of Slovenia was founded in 1950 at the Institute of Oncology in Ljubljana, the capital of Slovenia, to collect, process and analyse data on cancer incidence and cancer patient survival. It was also to serve as a basis for planning and evaluation of cancer control programmes and services, as well as for epidemiological and clinical studies

The current staff comprises a full-time physician specialized in social medicine and trained in cancer epidemiology as head, one physician-junior researcher, four full-time tumour registrars (registered nurses), one PC-operator and a part-time ADP system engineer.

The registry covers the population of the entire Republic of Slovenia, which, until 1991, was one of the six republics of Yugoslavia. Its territory amounts to 20 255 km^2 and borders on Italy to the west, Austria to the north, Hungary to the north-east and Croatia to the south-east. Slovenia lies between latitudes 45°53′ and 46°25′ N and longitudes 13°23′ and 16°36′ E.

The population according to the 1991 census was 1 965 986, of whom 21% were younger than 15 years, and 12.2% older than 65 years. 87.8% of the population were Slovenians, 2.8% Croats and 2.4% Serbs. Approximately 50.5% of the population live in urban areas, but only 19% in conurbations of more than 100 000 inhabitants. In 1991, 47.4% of the male and 44.6% of the female population were economically active. Of these, 35.7% were employed in manufacturing, mining and electricity supply, 13% in agriculture and fishing, 5.5% in forestry and hunting, 4.6% in construction, 5.3% in transport and communications, 0.9% in trade, 3.2% in hotels, restaurants and travel agencies, 5.2% in crafts and personal service activities, 1.2% in community service activities, 5.6% in financial and business activities, 5.9% in education and culture, 6% in health and social work and 4.4% in public administration, funds, associations and organisations. 40 327 people (0.5% of the working population) were temporarily employed abroad. The traditional religion of Slovenia is Roman Catholic.

Basic health service is provided by 22 outpatient establishments. Since 1992 increasing numbers of general practitioners and specialists have opened private practices. In each of nine health regions, there is at least one general hospital, and in three of them one or two specialized hospitals as well. In Ljubljana, there is a clinical centre with specialized departments affiliated to the Medical Faculty of the University. The Institute of Oncology in Ljubljana is a comprehensive cancer centre, also affiliated to the University. Besides the clinical wards and the cancer registry, it has its own pathology and cytology departments, tumour biology department, epidemiology unit and documentation service. More than 50% of cancer patients in Slovenia are at some time admitted to the Institute. Except for skin cancer, radio-

therapy as well as the majority of cytotoxic drugs are given exclusively at the Institute.

In the registry, the patients are identified by their personal identification number and by unique registration numbers, and the particular patient's cancer by a unique registration number alone.

The main data sources are notifications from hospitals (inpatients and outpatients). These are filled in by doctors, nurses or clerical staff depending on the hospital. At the Institute, notifications are written by specially trained nurses. Other sources are autopsy protocols stating cancer diagnosis and notifications from regional health centres. Notification and follow-up of cancer patients are compulsory, and registration is mostly passive, but in some departments where reporting is incomplete or delayed it can also be active. Completeness of registration is improved by checking the hospital-discharge lists and by stimulating clinicians' interest through publications and workshops.

Death certificates have been one of the data sources since 1950, and are traced back. In 1991, 15% of the cases registered came from tracing back death certificate notifications.

The registration of non-melanoma skin cancer is incomplete due to underreporting of patients treated in surgical outpatient departments. The registration of multiple myeloma and chronic lymphatic leukemia is also incomplete.

Follow-up of registered cancer patients has been performed annually since 1950. Until 1990 inquiries were sent to regional health centres and/or local authorities if the registry had not already been informed about the vital and health status of the patient. Linkage with the Central Register of the Population via the personal identification numbers now allows automatic addition of vital status to the registry's database. Data protection laws are strictly respected.

The items collected regarding cancer are primary site, histology, stage (clinical and surgical), basis of diagnosis, treatment modality and tumour status at death. Primary cancer sites have been coded according to ICD-8 since 1968. Data from 1961–67 were recoded into the same revision in 1993. Histolological types have been coded according to ICD-O since 1983. Data are coded by specially trained registered nurses under a physician's supervision. Quality checks (error and consistency) and checks for duplication are made during the coding process and during the data input. For recording more than one neoplasm in one person, the IACR/IARC rules are respected.

Reports on cancer incidence have been published since the 1950s. The incidence data for 1957–1971 appeared in WHO periodicals. Since 1965, annual reports have been published in Slovene and English. An atlas of cancer incidence in Slovenia appeared in 1992, and *Cancer Patients Survival in Slovenia 1963-1990* in 1995.

The registry participates in several international research projects. National and international studies are performed with extra funds and external co-workers.

The data users are clinicians, epidemiologists, postgraduate students, candidates for doctoral or master's degrees, social medicine specialists as well as also ecologists and journalists.

Vera Pompe-Kirn

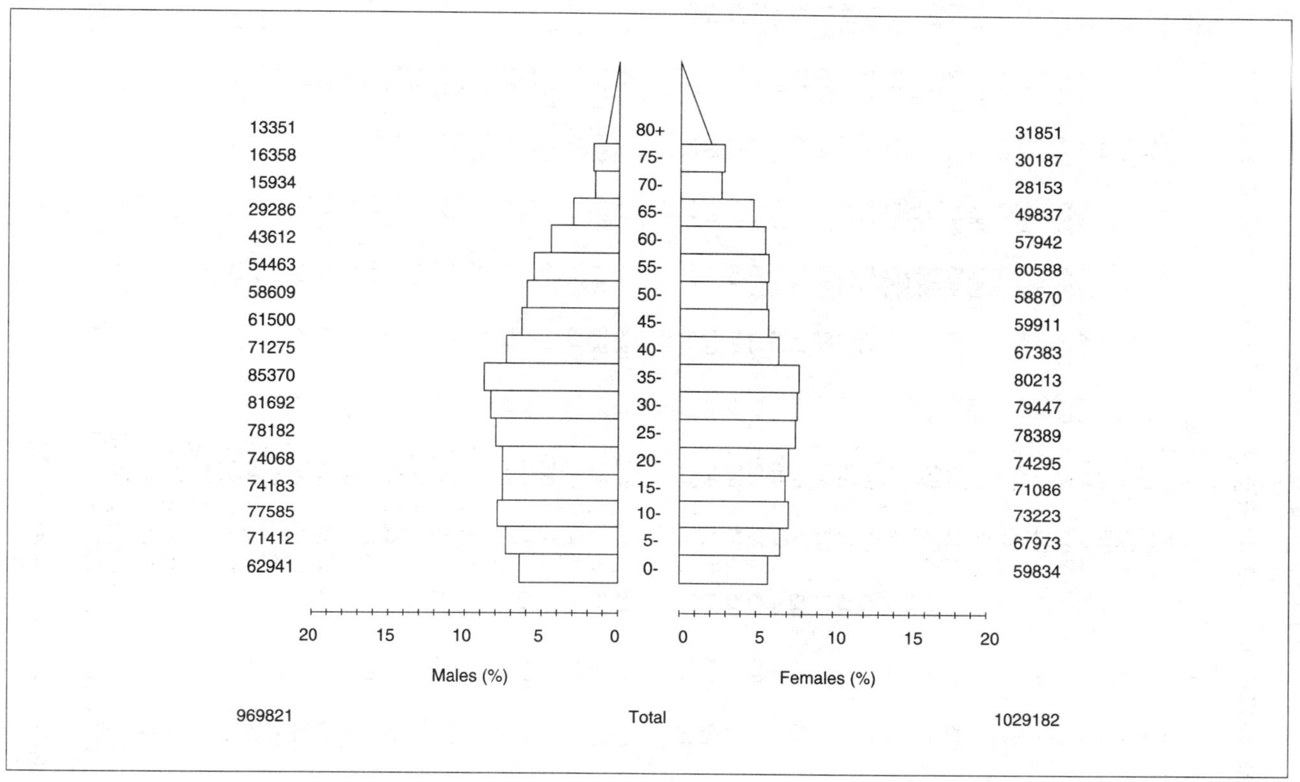

Slovenia
Source of population: average annual 1988–92
Census: Data for each year at 30 June are obtained from the Central Register of the Population of Slovenia.
Notes to tables overleaf:
† 188 does not include non-invasive tumours

Screening programmes in the area:
A pilot study of breast cancer screening was conducted in six communities, comprising 7% of the total female population aged 50-64, between 1988 and 1994.

SLOVENIA 1988-1992

ANNUAL INCIDENCE PER 100,000 BY AGE GROUP (YEARS) - MALE

SITE	ALL AGES	AGE UNK	0-	5-	10-	15-	20-	25-	30-	35-	40-	45-	50-	55-	60-	65-	70-	75-	80+	CRUDE RATE	%	CR 64	CR 74	ASR (W)	ICD (9th)
Lip	118	0	-	-	-	-	-	-	0.2	0.2	1.4	0.3	5.5	6.2	8.3	9.6	15.1	20.8	24.0	2.4	0.8	0.11	0.23	**2.0**	140
Tongue	198	0	-	-	-	-	-	-	0.5	1.2	2.5	6.2	9.2	17.3	16.5	18.4	16.3	7.3	10.5	4.1	1.3	0.27	0.44	**3.5**	141
Salivary gland	27	0	-	-	-	-	-	-	0.2	0.5	0.6	0.7	1.0	0.7	2.8	3.4	2.5	1.2	1.5	0.6	0.2	0.03	0.06	**0.5**	142
Mouth	288	0	-	-	-	-	-	0.5	-	1.9	6.2	9.8	21.8	25.0	21.6	21.2	7.5	6.1	7.5	5.9	1.9	0.43	0.58	**5.0**	143-5
Oropharynx	382	0	-	-	-	-	-	-	0.5	2.3	9.3	15.0	23.9	27.5	35.8	24.6	20.1	15.9	4.5	7.9	2.5	0.57	0.79	**6.7**	146
Nasopharynx	31	0	-	-	0.3	-	0.3	0.3	0.2	0.7	-	1.0	1.7	1.8	2.8	2.0	1.3	1.2	-	0.6	0.2	0.05	0.06	**0.5**	147
Hypopharynx	205	0	-	-	-	-	-	-	0.2	1.9	3.9	7.8	11.6	15.8	15.6	17.8	12.6	8.6	6.0	4.2	1.4	0.28	0.44	**3.6**	148
Pharynx unspecified	5	0	-	-	-	-	-	-	-	-	-	-	-	0.4	0.9	1.4	-	-	-	0.1	0.0	0.01	0.01	**0.1**	149
Oesophagus	393	0	-	-	-	-	-	-	-	0.2	3.6	8.1	15.4	28.6	32.6	42.3	28.9	44.0	58.4	8.1	2.6	0.44	0.80	**6.8**	150
Stomach	1525	0	-	-	-	0.5	0.5	0.8	2.2	4.5	10.7	17.6	40.3	64.6	113.7	170.0	246.0	256.7	301.1	31.4	10.1	1.28	3.36	**27.0**	151
Small intestine	14	0	-	-	-	-	-	0.3	0.2	0.2	-	-	0.3	0.7	1.4	2.0	1.3	-	1.5	0.3	0.1	0.02	0.03	**0.3**	152
Colon	899	0	-	-	-	-	-	0.5	1.7	4.0	5.6	12.7	22.9	37.8	60.5	96.3	140.6	173.6	175.3	18.5	5.9	0.73	1.91	**15.7**	153
Rectum	985	0	-	-	-	-	-	-	1.0	3.3	4.8	15.3	27.3	45.5	87.1	95.6	129.3	176.1	182.7	20.3	6.5	0.92	2.05	**17.2**	154
Liver	165	0	1.0	-	-	-	-	0.3	0.7	0.7	0.6	2.3	2.7	7.7	20.6	21.2	20.1	20.8	12.0	3.4	1.1	0.18	0.39	**3.0**	155
Gallbladder etc.	146	0	-	-	-	-	-	0.3	-	0.5	0.6	0.7	2.7	4.8	9.2	22.5	23.8	25.7	37.4	3.0	1.0	0.09	0.32	**2.6**	156
Pancreas	454	0	-	-	-	-	-	0.3	0.5	1.9	1.1	4.2	9.9	23.5	28.9	52.6	89.1	81.9	82.4	9.4	3.0	0.35	1.06	**8.1**	157
Nose, sinuses etc.	46	0	-	-	0.3	0.3	-	0.3	-	0.5	0.6	1.6	2.7	2.2	1.8	2.7	3.8	7.3	4.5	0.9	0.3	0.05	0.08	**0.8**	160
Larynx	521	0	-	-	-	-	-	-	-	4.0	6.7	12.4	24.2	42.6	42.2	49.2	46.4	30.6	43.4	10.7	3.4	0.66	1.14	**9.1**	161
Bronchus, lung	3681	0	-	-	-	-	0.3	1.5	2.4	7.7	25.5	52.7	112.3	238.3	393.0	440.5	435.5	375.3	365.5	75.9	24.3	4.17	8.55	**65.6**	162
Other thoracic organs	16	0	-	-	-	0.3	-	0.5	0.5	0.2	0.3	-	1.0	0.4	0.5	0.7	2.5	1.2	-	0.3	0.1	0.02	0.03	**0.3**	163-4
Bone	34	0	-	0.3	1.0	1.3	0.5	0.3	0.7	0.7	-	0.7	1.7	0.4	0.5	-	1.3	3.7	3.0	0.7	0.2	0.04	0.05	**0.6**	170
Connective tissue	89	0	3.2	0.3	0.8	1.1	1.4	0.8	0.5	1.6	1.4	2.3	2.0	4.4	2.8	3.4	8.8	1.2	7.5	1.8	0.6	0.11	0.17	**1.8**	171
Mesothelioma	43	0	-	-	-	-	-	-	0.2	-	-	2.6	2.0	4.4	2.8	2.7	1.3	3.7	3.0	0.9	0.3	0.06	0.08	**0.7**	MES
Kaposi's sarcoma	0	0	-	-	-	-	-	-	-	-	-	-	-	-	-	-	-	-	-	0.0	0.0	0.00	0.00	**0.0**	KAP
Melanoma of skin	267	0	-	-	-	0.3	1.9	1.8	2.0	5.6	5.1	8.5	9.6	11.0	16.5	19.8	25.1	23.2	21.0	5.5	1.8	0.31	0.54	**4.7**	172
Other skin	1243	0	-	-	-	0.3	1.4	0.3	1.5	3.3	9.5	19.5	34.1	48.1	84.4	115.4	188.3	229.8	299.6	25.6		1.01	2.53	**21.7**	173
Breast	28	0	-	-	-	-	0.3	-	-	-	0.3	0.3	0.3	1.1	2.8	2.7	3.8	8.6	1.5	0.6	0.2	0.03	0.06	**0.5**	175
Prostate	1210	0	-	-	-	-	-	-	-	0.2	0.3	1.3	7.5	20.6	49.1	130.4	234.7	355.8	524.3	25.0	8.0	0.39	2.22	**20.7**	185
Testis	238	0	0.6	-	-	2.2	10.8	13.3	9.1	9.4	6.7	4.6	1.7	2.2	3.2	0.7	1.3	1.2	-	4.9	1.6	0.32	0.33	**4.3**	186
Penis	41	0	-	-	-	-	-	-	-	0.2	0.6	0.7	1.4	2.6	0.9	3.4	6.3	7.3	10.5	0.8	0.3	0.03	0.08	**0.7**	187.1-.4
Other male genital	6	0	-	-	-	-	-	-	-	0.2	-	-	0.7	-	0.5	0.7	1.3	-	-	0.1	0.0	0.01	0.02	**0.1**	187.5-.9
†Bladder	580	0	-	-	-	0.3	-	-	0.2	1.2	0.6	5.2	12.3	21.3	40.8	66.9	82.8	112.5	173.8	12.0	3.8	0.41	1.16	**10.1**	188
Kidney etc.	385	0	1.3	0.3	-	-	0.5	0.5	0.2	1.2	5.6	8.5	14.3	17.3	26.1	49.2	47.7	47.7	43.4	7.9	2.5	0.38	0.86	**7.0**	189
Eye	37	0	1.0	-	-	-	-	0.3	-	0.2	0.8	0.3	0.7	2.2	2.3	4.1	2.5	6.1	3.0	0.8	0.2	0.04	0.07	**0.7**	190
Brain, nervous system	240	0	1.3	1.7	2.8	2.7	1.9	3.1	3.2	4.0	4.2	6.2	5.8	12.5	14.7	15.0	8.8	14.7	3.0	4.9	1.6	0.32	0.44	**4.4**	191-2
Thyroid	75	0	-	-	0.3	0.5	0.8	0.3	1.5	1.2	1.7	1.6	1.0	2.9	6.9	2.7	11.3	3.7	6.0	1.5	0.5	0.09	0.16	**1.4**	193
Other endocrine	12	0	-	-	0.3	-	-	-	-	0.7	0.3	-	0.7	1.5	-	-	1.3	-	-	0.2	0.1	0.02	0.02	**0.2**	194
Hodgkin's disease	112	0	1.0	1.7	1.5	2.7	3.5	1.8	2.4	2.3	2.5	1.3	3.1	3.7	2.3	2.7	3.8	2.4	1.5	2.3	0.7	0.15	0.18	**2.2**	201
Non-Hodgkin lymphoma	351	0	1.0	1.7	2.1	2.2	1.6	2.0	1.2	5.2	5.1	4.9	11.3	16.5	22.0	25.3	30.1	42.8	44.9	7.2	2.3	0.38	0.66	**6.3**	200,202
Multiple myeloma	133	0	-	-	-	-	-	0.3	-	0.2	0.3	1.0	3.1	8.4	15.6	9.6	23.8	15.9	22.5	2.7	0.9	0.14	0.31	**2.4**	203
Lymphoid leukaemia	219	0	4.4	3.1	1.0	1.6	0.8	0.3	0.7	0.9	2.2	2.3	5.8	7.0	10.1	19.8	22.6	30.6	41.9	4.5	1.4	0.20	0.41	**4.3**	204
Myeloid leukaemia	154	0	-	0.6	1.5	1.1	0.8	2.0	1.2	2.3	1.7	2.0	3.4	7.7	8.7	8.2	16.3	14.7	25.5	3.2	1.0	0.17	0.29	**2.8**	205
Monocytic leukaemia	10	0	-	-	-	-	-	-	-	0.2	-	-	0.3	-	0.5	1.4	1.3	2.4	3.0	0.2	0.1	0.01	0.02	**0.2**	206
Other leukaemia	0	0	-	-	-	-	-	-	-	-	-	-	-	-	-	-	-	-	-	0.0	0.0	0.00	0.00	**0.0**	207
Leukaemia unspecified	10	0	0.3	-	-	-	-	-	-	-	-	-	-	0.4	0.9	-	-	4.9	3.0	0.2	0.1	0.01	0.01	**0.2**	208
Other and unspecified	794	0	0.3	-	-	-	0.5	1.5	1.7	1.9	7.0	13.3	21.8	38.2	52.3	86.7	85.4	132.0	178.3	16.4	5.2	0.69	1.55	**13.8**	O&U
All sites	16410	0	15.3	9.5	11.9	17.3	27.8	33.8	37.7	79.2	139.7	255.0	481.2	825.9	1262.0	1664.9	2052.2	2319.2	2738.2	338.4		15.98	34.57	**290.2**	ALL
All sites but 173	15167	0	15.3	9.5	11.9	17.0	26.5	33.5	36.2	75.9	130.2	235.4	447.0	777.8	1177.7	1549.5	1863.9	2089.4	2438.7	312.8	100.0	14.97	32.04	**268.5**	ALLb

Rate from 1 case   0.318   0.280   0.258   0.270   0.270   0.256   0.245   0.234   0.281   0.325   0.341   0.367   0.459   0.683   1.255   1.223   1.498

†Important: see notes on population page

SLOVENIA 1988-1992

ANNUAL INCIDENCE PER 100,000 BY AGE GROUP (YEARS) - FEMALE

SITE	ALL AGES	AGE UNK	0-	5-	10-	15-	20-	25-	30-	35-	40-	45-	50-	55-	60-	65-	70-	75-	80+	CRUDE RATE	%	CR 64	CR 74	ASR (W)	ICD (9th)
Lip	30	0	-	-	-	-	-	-	0.3	0.2	-	0.3	0.3	0.7	1.4	1.2	1.4	4.6	5.0	0.6	0.2	0.02	0.03	0.3	140
Tongue	28	0	-	-	-	-	-	-	-	-	0.6	0.3	0.7	1.7	1.4	0.4	-	4.0	4.4	0.5	0.2	0.02	0.03	0.3	141
Salivary gland	17	0	-	-	-	0.3	-	-	0.3	0.2	0.3	0.7	-	0.7	0.3	0.4	2.1	2.0	0.6	0.3	0.1	0.01	0.03	0.2	142
Mouth	41	0	-	-	-	-	0.3	0.3	-	-	0.3	1.0	1.0	3.0	2.1	2.8	2.8	2.0	1.9	0.8	0.3	0.04	0.07	0.6	143-5
Oropharynx	27	0	-	-	-	-	-	-	-	-	0.3	1.3	0.3	0.3	2.8	2.0	0.7	0.7	3.1	0.5	0.2	0.03	0.04	0.4	146
Nasopharynx	12	0	-	-	0.3	-	-	-	0.3	-	0.3	1.0	-	1.0	-	-	0.7	0.7	0.6	0.2	0.1	0.01	0.02	0.2	147
Hypopharynx	11	0	-	-	-	-	-	-	-	-	-	-	1.0	1.0	0.3	1.2	-	0.7	-	0.2	0.1	0.01	0.02	0.1	148
Pharynx unspecified	1	0	-	-	-	-	-	-	-	-	-	-	-	-	-	-	-	-	0.6	0.0	0.0	0.00	0.00	0.0	149
Oesophagus	79	0	-	-	-	-	-	-	0.3	-	0.6	1.3	1.7	2.3	3.5	4.0	5.0	5.3	15.7	1.5	0.6	0.05	0.09	0.9	150
Stomach	1000	0	-	-	-	-	0.3	0.8	2.0	3.7	8.6	11.4	15.3	16.8	34.9	57.8	73.2	117.3	181.5	19.4	7.1	0.47	1.12	10.6	151
Small intestine	22	0	-	-	-	-	-	-	-	-	0.3	0.3	1.0	1.0	0.3	2.8	1.4	1.3	1.3	0.4	0.2	0.01	0.04	0.3	152
Colon	883	0	-	-	-	-	0.3	1.8	2.3	2.7	5.0	9.0	18.7	21.5	36.6	52.2	93.8	92.1	115.5	17.2	6.2	0.49	1.22	10.1	153
Rectum	868	0	-	-	-	-	-	0.5	1.0	2.2	3.9	9.7	14.3	29.4	38.7	56.6	78.9	84.8	118.0	16.9	6.1	0.50	1.18	9.8	154
Liver	80	0	0.7	-	-	-	-	-	0.3	-	0.3	1.0	1.7	3.6	3.8	6.0	3.6	8.0	8.8	1.6	0.6	0.06	0.10	1.0	155
Gallbladder etc.	380	0	-	-	-	-	-	-	-	0.2	1.8	2.7	3.7	8.9	15.2	24.9	34.1	53.0	58.4	7.4	2.7	0.16	0.46	4.0	156
Pancreas	472	0	-	-	-	-	-	-	-	1.0	1.8	2.7	6.5	10.6	22.4	27.7	43.3	55.0	78.5	9.2	3.3	0.22	0.58	5.0	157
Nose, sinuses etc.	31	0	-	-	-	-	-	-	-	0.2	0.6	0.3	0.3	0.3	2.0	0.7	0.8	2.1	4.0	3.8	0.6	0.2	0.02	0.04	0.4	160
Larynx	42	0	-	-	-	-	-	-	-	-	0.2	0.9	1.3	1.7	2.0	3.5	2.0	2.1	2.0	1.3	0.8	0.3	0.05	0.07	0.6	161
Bronchus, lung	741	0	-	-	-	-	-	-	0.3	0.8	2.2	7.4	10.7	18.3	29.0	38.3	56.2	63.9	62.3	59.0	14.4	5.2	0.54	1.14	9.1	162
Other thoracic organs	7	0	0.3	-	-	-	-	-	-	0.2	0.3	-	-	-	0.3	-	-	-	1.9	0.1	0.0	0.01	0.01	0.1	163-4
Bone	38	0	-	0.6	0.5	1.1	0.5	-	0.3	0.5	0.6	0.7	0.7	1.7	1.4	1.2	2.1	2.0	0.6	0.7	0.3	0.04	0.06	0.6	170
Connective tissue	81	0	1.7	0.3	1.4	0.6	0.5	0.3	1.0	1.0	1.5	1.7	1.7	2.0	1.7	2.4	6.4	4.6	5.7	1.6	0.6	0.08	0.12	1.3	171
Mesothelioma	18	0	-	-	-	-	0.5	-	-	-	-	-	1.7	-	1.4	1.6	0.7	-	1.3	0.3	0.1	0.02	0.03	0.3	MES
Kaposi's sarcoma	0	0	-	-	-	-	-	-	-	-	-	-	-	-	-	-	-	-	-	0.0	0.0	0.00	0.00	0.0	KAP
Melanoma of skin	371	0	-	-	0.3	0.8	1.1	2.0	7.3	8.0	11.0	9.7	14.9	15.5	11.7	13.2	19.2	17.2	10.7	7.2	2.6	0.41	0.57	5.4	172
Other skin	1457	0	-	0.3	-	-	0.5	1.8	2.8	5.2	10.1	13.7	22.4	37.6	51.1	89.9	122.2	183.5	212.9	28.3		0.73	1.79	15.9	173
Breast	3381	0	-	-	-	-	0.3	3.8	11.6	39.6	84.9	119.8	113.8	133.0	152.2	179.4	211.0	186.8	194.7	65.7	23.9	3.30	5.25	46.2	174
Uterus unspecified	72	0	-	-	-	-	0.3	-	-	-	0.9	0.7	2.0	2.3	2.8	2.0	3.6	6.0	16.3	1.4	0.5	0.04	0.07	0.8	179
Cervix uteri	836	0	-	-	-	-	1.1	10.0	20.9	25.9	31.5	25.7	19.0	29.0	29.0	30.1	29.1	30.5	20.7	16.2	5.9	0.96	1.26	12.4	180
Placenta	5	0	-	-	-	-	-	0.3	0.2	0.2	-	1.0	-	-	-	-	-	-	-	0.1	0.0	0.01	0.01	0.1	181
Corpus uteri	940	0	-	-	-	-	-	0.5	0.5	1.0	4.2	16.4	40.8	52.2	60.8	66.2	77.4	51.7	39.6	18.3	6.6	0.88	1.60	12.4	182
Ovary etc.	766	0	-	0.3	0.8	0.6	0.8	1.5	1.5	5.5	13.7	24.7	28.2	34.0	41.4	38.1	50.4	51.0	33.9	14.9	5.4	0.76	1.21	10.5	183
Other female genital	198	0	0.3	-	-	-	-	0.5	0.3	0.7	1.8	1.3	3.1	5.0	5.2	12.8	13.5	21.9	36.4	3.8	1.4	0.09	0.22	2.1	184
†Bladder	200	0	-	-	-	-	0.3	-	0.3	-	0.9	0.7	1.7	5.9	8.6	14.0	11.4	29.2	31.4	3.9	1.4	0.09	0.22	2.1	188
Kidney etc.	285	0	-	0.6	-	-	0.3	0.5	1.0	1.2	2.4	5.0	6.1	11.9	16.9	18.1	23.4	24.5	18.8	5.5	2.0	0.23	0.44	3.6	189
Eye	39	0	0.7	0.3	-	-	0.3	-	0.5	0.5	-	1.3	1.0	2.3	2.1	1.6	1.4	2.7	0.6	0.8	0.3	0.04	0.06	0.6	190
Brain, nervous system	198	0	1.3	2.9	1.1	0.3	1.3	1.0	2.3	2.2	4.2	5.0	8.5	6.6	12.1	10.4	5.0	4.6	1.9	3.8	1.4	0.24	0.32	3.2	191-2
Thyroid	186	0	-	-	0.3	0.6	1.3	3.3	2.5	4.0	4.5	3.7	4.4	5.0	6.9	10.8	9.2	4.0	11.9	3.6	1.3	0.18	0.28	2.7	193
Other endocrine	18	0	-	0.3	-	-	0.3	-	0.3	-	0.9	-	0.7	0.7	0.3	0.2	0.7	-	0.6	0.3	0.1	0.02	0.03	0.3	194
Hodgkin's disease	78	0	0.7	0.3	0.3	2.5	3.5	4.1	0.3	1.7	1.8	0.3	0.7	0.7	1.7	1.6	2.8	2.0	0.6	1.5	0.6	0.09	0.11	1.5	201
Non-Hodgkin lymphoma	323	0	-	0.3	0.3	1.1	1.1	1.3	1.8	2.2	4.5	5.7	5.4	10.6	11.7	23.3	24.9	25.2	29.5	6.3	2.3	0.23	0.47	4.1	200,202
Multiple myeloma	147	0	-	-	-	-	-	-	-	-	1.2	3.7	3.1	2.3	7.6	14.0	11.4	13.3	14.4	2.9	1.0	0.09	0.22	1.8	203
Lymphoid leukaemia	232	0	6.4	2.6	0.8	2.3	0.8	0.3	1.3	1.0	2.1	1.3	1.4	3.3	9.7	11.6	19.2	17.2	28.3	4.5	1.6	0.17	0.32	3.5	204
Myeloid leukaemia	141	0	1.3	-	1.1	0.3	1.1	1.0	1.8	1.2	1.5	4.3	4.1	4.0	3.8	4.4	10.7	10.6	10.7	2.7	1.0	0.13	0.20	2.1	205
Monocytic leukaemia	6	0	0.3	0.3	-	-	-	-	0.3	-	-	0.3	-	-	0.3	-	-	0.7	-	0.1	0.0	0.01	0.01	0.1	206
Other leukaemia	2	0	-	-	-	-	-	-	-	-	-	-	-	-	-	-	-	-	1.3	0.0	0.0	0.00	0.00	0.0	207
Leukaemia unspecified	7	0	-	-	-	-	-	-	-	-	-	-	0.3	-	0.3	-	2.1	0.7	0.6	0.1	0.0	0.00	0.01	0.1	208
Other and unspecified	809	0	1.0	-	-	-	0.3	0.8	1.8	1.5	3.6	5.0	10.9	20.1	27.6	44.9	68.2	102.7	141.9	15.7	5.7	0.36	0.93	8.5	O&U
All sites	15606	0	14.7	9.1	7.1	10.4	17.2	36.5	67.2	116.9	220.5	305.8	384.2	520.9	674.8	892.9	1135.2	1291.9	1525.2	303.3		11.93	22.07	195.9	ALL
All sites but 173	14149	0	14.7	8.8	7.1	10.4	16.7	34.7	64.4	111.7	210.4	292.1	361.8	483.3	623.7	803.0	1013.0	1108.4	1312.3	275.0	100.0	11.20	20.28	180.0	ALLb

Rate from 1 case: 0.334 0.294 0.273 0.281 0.269 0.255 0.252 0.249 0.297 0.334 0.340 0.330 0.345 0.401 0.710 0.662 0.628

†Important: see notes on population page

Spain, Albacete

The Cancer Registry of Albacete was created in February 1990 by the Consejeria de Salud de la Comunidad Autonoma de Castilla-La Mancha, and it belongs to the Regional Service of epidemiology, with the principal objective of analysing cancer incidence in the province. It is financed by the Comunidad Autonoma.

Albacete is situated in the Central Meseta in the southeast of Spain. The province consists of 86 municipalities, 67.5% of which have less than 2000 inhabitants and only 5.9% have more than 10 000. The climate is Mediterranean temperate with some continental features. The average total annual rainfall is approximately 275 mm.

The population of the province for 1991–92 was 342 223. The population density (23 inhabitants per km^2) is very low compared to that of the country as a whole.The age structure is similar to the rest of the Spanish population, with 21.2% under the age of 15 years and 13.8% above the age of 65 years. 15.3% of the population live in rural areas of less than 2000 inhabitants, 23.2% in semi-rural areas of 2000–10 000 inhabitants, and 61.5% in urban areas.

In 1991 the birth rate was 11.9 per 1000 and the fertility rate 50.4 per 1000; the average number of children per woman was 1.6.

The average annual employment rate is 50.8%, with 16.3% in agriculture, 22.7% in industry, 14.2% in construction and 46.8% in services. The unemployment rate is 17% of the active population.

Five hospital centres are located in the province, two of which are private surgical hospitals and three public general hospitals. There is one private pathology laboratory. There are 34 public primary care centres. Almost all of the population are covered by the public health system.

The numbers of health personnel per 10 000 inhabitants are: physicians 31.5, nurses 33.3, dental surgeons 1.8, and pharmacists 10.5.

Data for the registry are obtained from the General Hospital of Albacete (pathology and haematology laboratories, oncological and medical records departments); the Local Hospital of Hellin (pathology and haematology laboratories and medical records); the hospitals Virgen de Los Llanos, Santa Cristina and Virgen del Rosario, the Dr Iñiguez de Onzoño pathology laboratory, the Provincial Office of INSALUD, the regional mortality register and the National Institute of Statistics.

Data collection from these sources of information is active, carried out by the personnel of the registry from lists provided by the sources, and by consulting the files and clinical records concerned. The registry records cases voluntarily notified by physicians in the primary care services.

No active follow-up of cases is carried out. The registry has access to death certificates mentioning cancer for local residents who die in the Autonomous Community. Death certificates are traced back to find further information if the case is not already registered, and if no further information is found the case is registered as death certificate only. There is no personal contact with patients or their families.

All data are automatically processed using a system which includes checking for duplicate registrations by name, social security number and/or clinical record. Cases are coded by ICD-O topography and morphology. Multiple tumours are coded following the IARC/IACR recommendations. The CHECK program is used to detect errors and discrepancies in the data.

The cancer registry data are used to determine cancer incidence by site, sex and age. As the registry was created recently, it is not yet possible to analyse survival or trends.

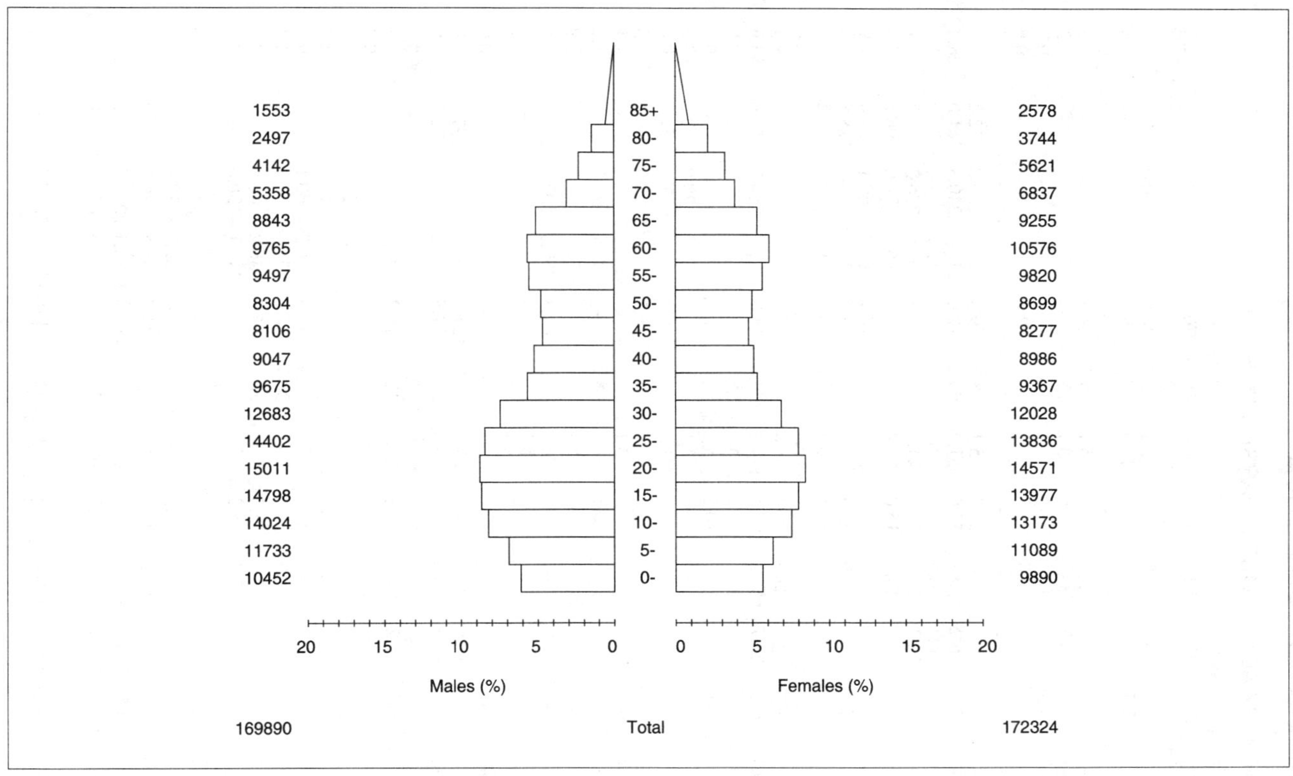

Spain, Albacete
Source of population: average annual 1991–92
Census: 1991. Instituto Nacional de Estadistica.
Estimate: The 1992 population was estimated by geometric interpolation, based on the 1986 and 1991 censuses. Servicio de Epidemiologia de la Comunidad Autonoma de Castilla La Mancha.
Notes to tables overleaf:
* There are indications of a degree of under-ascertainment, such as the high proportion of diagnoses based on a death certificate alone for sites such as liver and lung. It is probable that these are due to the inevitable problems in the early years of a registry functioning.
† 173 does not include basal cell or squamous cell carcinomas

* SPAIN, ALBACETE 1991-1992

ANNUAL INCIDENCE PER 100,000 BY AGE GROUP (YEARS) - MALE

SITE	ALL AGES	AGE UNK	0-	5-	10-	15-	20-	25-	30-	35-	40-	45-	50-	55-	60-	65-	70-	75-	80-	85+	CRUDE RATE	%	CR 64	CR 74	ASR (W)	ICD (9th)
Lip	12	0	-	-	-	-	-	-	-	-	-	6.2	12.0	5.3	5.1	5.7	28.0	-	40.0	32.2	3.5	1.1	0.14	0.31	**2.5**	140
Tongue	9	0	-	-	-	-	-	-	-	-	5.5	6.2	-	15.8	15.4	-	9.3	-	-	-	2.6	0.9	0.21	0.26	**2.1**	141
Salivary gland	2	0	-	-	-	-	-	-	-	-	-	-	12.0	-	-	-	-	-	-	-	0.6	0.2	0.06	0.06	**0.6**	142
Mouth	5	0	-	-	-	-	-	-	-	-	-	-	-	5.3	5.1	5.7	18.7	-	-	-	1.5	0.5	0.05	0.17	**1.0**	143-5
Oropharynx	4	0	-	-	-	-	-	-	3.9	-	-	6.2	-	-	5.1	5.7	-	-	-	-	1.2	0.4	0.08	0.10	**1.0**	146
Nasopharynx	1	0	-	-	-	-	-	-	-	-	5.5	-	-	-	-	-	-	-	-	-	0.3	0.1	0.03	0.03	**0.3**	147
Hypopharynx	3	0	-	-	-	-	-	-	-	-	-	-	6.0	5.3	-	-	9.3	-	-	-	0.9	0.3	0.06	0.10	**0.7**	148
Pharynx unspecified	1	0	-	-	-	-	-	-	-	-	-	6.2	-	-	-	-	-	-	-	-	0.3	0.1	0.03	0.03	**0.4**	149
Oesophagus	17	0	-	-	-	-	-	-	-	-	-	6.0	26.3	5.1	28.3	9.3	24.1	20.0	32.2	5.0	1.6	0.19	0.38	**3.1**	150
Stomach	96	0	-	-	-	-	-	-	-	-	5.5	6.2	60.2	52.6	51.2	96.1	112.0	217.3	240.3	161.0	28.3	9.1	0.88	1.92	**17.2**	151
Small intestine	4	0	-	-	-	-	-	-	-	-	-	6.2	6.0	-	-	-	-	12.1	-	32.2	1.2	0.4	0.06	0.06	**1.0**	152
Colon	58	0	-	-	-	-	-	3.9	-	-	-	12.3	24.1	15.8	41.0	56.5	93.3	96.6	220.3	32.2	17.1	5.5	0.49	1.23	**10.2**	153
Rectum	49	0	-	-	-	-	-	-	-	-	-	6.2	18.1	15.8	61.4	45.2	93.3	96.6	20.0	96.6	14.4	4.6	0.51	1.20	**9.1**	154
Liver	27	0	-	-	-	-	-	-	-	-	-	-	21.1	25.6	17.0	46.7	60.4	60.1	64.4	7.9	2.6	0.23	0.55	**4.5**	155
Gallbladder etc.	13	0	-	-	-	-	-	-	-	-	5.5	-	6.0	5.3	-	17.0	18.7	12.1	-	128.8	3.8	1.2	0.08	0.26	**2.5**	156
Pancreas	25	0	-	-	-	-	-	-	-	-	-	-	21.1	30.7	5.7	46.7	48.3	80.1	32.2	7.4	2.4	0.26	0.52	**4.2**	157
Nose, sinuses etc.	0	0	-	-	-	-	-	-	-	-	-	-	-	-	-	-	-	-	-	0.0	0.0	0.00	0.00	**0.0**	160
Larynx	62	0	-	-	-	-	-	-	-	5.2	5.5	12.3	54.2	47.4	35.8	90.5	93.3	84.5	-	-	18.2	5.9	0.80	1.72	**12.8**	161
Bronchus, lung	183	0	-	-	-	-	-	-	-	10.3	16.6	24.7	54.2	105.3	174.1	209.2	261.3	289.7	280.3	257.6	53.9	17.3	1.93	4.28	**34.1**	162
Other thoracic organs	2	0	-	-	-	-	-	-	-	-	-	-	-	5.1	5.7	-	-	-	-	0.6	0.2	0.03	0.05	**0.4**	163-4
Bone	3	0	-	-	-	-	-	-	-	-	-	-	-	10.5	5.1	-	-	-	-	-	0.9	0.3	0.08	0.08	**0.6**	170
Connective tissue	11	0	-	-	-	6.8	3.3	-	3.9	-	-	-	-	-	5.1	11.3	-	24.1	20.0	32.2	3.2	1.0	0.10	0.15	**2.2**	171
Mesothelioma	2	0	-	-	-	-	-	-	-	-	-	-	-	-	-	9.3	-	-	32.2	0.6	0.2	0.00	0.05	**0.3**	MES
Kaposi's sarcoma	5	0	-	-	-	-	-	-	3.9	-	-	-	-	-	5.7	18.7	-	20.0	-	1.5	0.5	0.02	0.14	**0.9**	KAP
Melanoma of skin	7	0	-	-	-	3.4	3.3	-	3.9	-	16.6	-	-	-	5.1	-	-	-	-	2.1	0.7	0.16	0.16	**2.0**	172
†Other skin	4	0	-	-	-	-	-	-	-	-	-	-	5.3	-	5.7	-	12.1	20.0	-	1.2	-	0.03	0.05	**0.6**	173
Breast	3	0	-	-	-	-	-	-	-	-	-	-	-	-	5.1	-	12.1	20.0	-	0.9	0.3	0.03	0.03	**0.4**	175
Prostate	138	1	-	-	-	-	-	-	-	-	-	42.1	56.3	90.5	261.3	350.0	600.7	482.9	40.6	13.1	0.50	2.27	**20.9**	185
Testis	6	0	-	-	-	-	6.7	6.9	3.9	-	-	-	-	5.1	-	-	-	-	-	1.8	0.6	0.11	0.11	**1.5**	186
Penis	5	0	-	-	-	-	-	-	-	-	-	-	5.3	5.1	5.7	-	12.1	20.0	-	1.5	0.5	0.05	0.08	**0.8**	187.1-.4
Other male genital	0	0	-	-	-	-	-	-	-	-	-	-	-	-	-	-	-	-	-	0.0	0.0	0.00	0.00	**0.0**	187.5-.9
Bladder	102	0	-	-	3.6	-	-	-	-	-	-	18.5	24.1	57.9	87.0	135.7	121.3	169.0	140.2	257.6	30.0	9.6	0.96	2.24	**18.6**	188
Kidney etc.	19	0	-	-	-	-	-	-	-	-	-	18.5	6.0	-	25.6	22.6	37.3	12.1	-	32.2	5.6	1.8	0.25	0.55	**4.1**	189
Eye	3	0	-	-	-	-	-	-	-	-	-	-	-	5.3	-	5.7	-	12.1	-	0.9	0.3	0.03	0.05	**0.5**	190
Brain, nervous system	25	0	4.8	-	-	6.8	-	3.5	-	-	5.5	6.2	24.1	15.8	20.5	22.6	18.7	24.1	-	-	7.4	2.4	0.44	0.64	**6.1**	191-2
Thyroid	1	0	-	-	-	-	-	-	-	-	-	-	-	-	-	5.7	-	-	-	0.3	0.1	0.00	0.03	**0.2**	193
Other endocrine	1	0	-	-	-	-	-	-	-	-	-	-	-	-	-	-	-	-	20.0	0.3	0.1	0.00	0.00	**0.1**	194
Hodgkin's disease	12	0	-	-	-	-	3.3	10.4	3.9	-	11.1	-	-	10.2	17.0	-	-	-	-	3.5	1.1	0.19	0.28	**2.9**	201
Non-Hodgkin lymphoma	32	0	-	-	-	-	-	3.5	7.9	-	5.5	6.2	-	21.1	30.7	33.9	37.3	36.2	60.1	32.2	9.4	3.0	0.37	0.73	**6.1**	200,202
Multiple myeloma	15	0	-	-	-	-	-	-	-	-	-	-	6.0	-	20.5	33.9	18.7	24.1	-	-	4.4	1.4	0.13	0.40	**2.8**	203
Lymphoid leukaemia	25	0	14.4	4.3	-	3.4	-	-	-	-	11.1	-	12.0	5.3	-	28.3	46.7	36.2	40.0	-	7.4	2.4	0.25	0.63	**6.3**	204
Myeloid leukaemia	9	0	-	-	-	-	-	-	-	-	-	5.5	6.2	12.0	5.3	-	5.7	-	12.1	20.0	32.2	2.6	0.9	0.15	0.17	**2.1**	205
Monocytic leukaemia	1	0	-	-	-	-	-	-	-	-	-	-	-	-	-	5.7	-	-	-	-	0.3	0.1	0.00	0.03	**0.2**	206
Other leukaemia	0	0	-	-	-	-	-	-	-	-	-	-	-	-	-	-	-	-	-	0.0	0.0	0.00	0.00	**0.0**	207
Leukaemia unspecified	4	0	-	-	-	-	-	-	3.9	-	-	6.2	-	-	-	-	-	12.1	20.0	-	1.2	0.4	0.05	0.05	**0.8**	208
Other and unspecified	55	0	9.6	-	-	-	-	-	3.9	-	-	6.2	18.1	21.1	61.4	62.2	74.7	96.6	80.1	32.2	16.2	5.2	0.60	1.29	**10.8**	O&U
All sites	1061	1	28.7	4.3	3.6	20.3	16.7	24.3	43.4	15.5	99.5	160.4	361.3	537.0	803.9	1085.5	1483.8	1786.4	2042.5	1803.0	312.2		10.60	23.46	**199.6**	ALL
All sites but 173	1057	1	28.7	4.3	3.6	20.3	16.7	24.3	43.4	15.5	99.5	160.4	361.3	531.7	803.9	1079.9	1483.8	1774.3	2022.4	1803.0	311.1	100.0	10.58	23.41	**199.0**	ALLb

Rate from 1 case   4.784   4.261   3.565   3.379   3.331   3.472   3.942   5.168   5.526   6.168   6.021   5.265   5.120   5.654   9.332   12.070   20.024   32.196

†Important: see notes on population page

* SPAIN, ALBACETE 1991-1992

ANNUAL INCIDENCE PER 100,000 BY AGE GROUP (YEARS) - FEMALE

SITE	ALL AGES	AGE UNK	0-	5-	10-	15-	20-	25-	30-	35-	40-	45-	50-	55-	60-	65-	70-	75-	80-	85+	CRUDE RATE	%	CR 64	CR 74	ASR (W)	ICD (9th)
Lip	4	0	-	-	-	-	-	-	-	-	-	-	-	-	-	-	-	8.9	-	58.2	1.2	0.5	0.00	0.00	**0.4**	*140*
Tongue	3	0	-	-	-	-	-	-	-	-	-	-	-	-	-	5.4	-	8.9	-	19.4	0.9	0.4	0.00	0.03	**0.3**	*141*
Salivary gland	3	0	-	-	-	-	-	-	-	-	-	-	-	-	-	-	14.6	8.9	-	-	0.9	0.4	0.00	0.07	**0.4**	*142*
Mouth	3	0	-	-	-	-	-	-	-	-	-	-	-	-	-	-	7.3	8.9	13.4	-	0.9	0.4	0.00	0.04	**0.3**	*143-5*
Oropharynx	0	0	-	-	-	-	-	-	-	-	-	-	-	-	-	-	-	-	-	-	0.0	0.0	0.00	0.00	**0.0**	*146*
Nasopharynx	1	0	-	-	-	-	-	-	-	-	-	-	-	5.1	-	-	-	-	-	-	0.3	0.1	0.03	0.03	**0.2**	*147*
Hypopharynx	0	0	-	-	-	-	-	-	-	-	-	-	-	-	-	-	-	-	-	-	0.0	0.0	0.00	0.00	**0.0**	*148*
Pharynx unspecified	0	0	-	-	-	-	-	-	-	-	-	-	-	-	-	-	-	-	-	-	0.0	0.0	0.00	0.00	**0.0**	*149*
Oesophagus	1	0	-	-	-	-	-	-	-	-	-	-	-	-	-	-	-	-	-	19.4	0.3	0.1	0.00	0.00	**0.1**	*150*
Stomach	57	0	-	-	-	-	-	-	-	-	16.7	-	17.2	5.1	42.5	10.8	65.8	124.5	173.6	58.2	16.5	7.3	0.41	0.79	**7.8**	*151*
Small intestine	1	0	-	-	-	-	-	-	-	-	-	-	-	-	-	-	-	-	13.4	-	0.3	0.1	0.00	0.00	**0.1**	*152*
Colon	61	0	-	-	-	-	-	-	-	-	5.6	-	23.0	15.3	37.8	64.8	73.1	71.2	120.2	116.4	17.7	7.8	0.41	1.10	**8.9**	*153*
Rectum	34	0	-	-	-	-	-	-	-	5.3	11.1	-	5.7	20.4	28.4	27.0	43.9	26.7	40.1	58.2	9.9	4.3	0.35	0.71	**5.7**	*154*
Liver	19	0	-	-	-	-	-	-	-	5.3	-	-	-	5.1	14.2	21.6	29.3	8.9	40.1	38.8	5.5	2.4	0.12	0.38	**2.8**	*155*
Gallbladder etc.	32	0	-	-	-	-	-	-	-	-	-	-	-	5.1	28.4	32.4	29.3	53.4	106.8	19.4	9.3	4.1	0.17	0.48	**4.1**	*156*
Pancreas	20	0	-	-	-	-	-	-	4.2	-	-	-	11.5	5.1	23.6	5.4	14.6	26.7	53.4	19.4	5.8	2.5	0.22	0.32	**3.1**	*157*
Nose, sinuses etc.	1	0	-	-	-	-	-	-	-	-	-	-	-	-	-	-	7.3	-	-	-	0.3	0.1	0.00	0.04	**0.1**	*160*
Larynx	0	0	-	-	-	-	-	-	-	-	-	-	-	-	-	-	-	-	-	-	0.0	0.0	0.00	0.00	**0.0**	*161*
Bronchus, lung	19	0	-	-	-	-	-	-	-	5.3	5.6	-	5.7	5.1	14.2	21.6	14.6	8.9	40.1	38.8	5.5	2.4	0.18	0.36	**3.1**	*162*
Other thoracic organs	0	0	-	-	-	-	-	-	-	-	-	-	-	-	-	-	-	-	-	-	0.0	0.0	0.00	0.00	**0.0**	*163-4*
Bone	6	0	-	4.5	7.6	3.6	3.4	-	-	-	-	-	-	-	-	-	-	-	-	19.4	1.7	0.8	0.10	0.10	**1.8**	*170*
Connective tissue	8	0	5.1	-	-	-	3.4	-	-	-	5.6	-	-	5.1	-	10.8	14.6	-	-	-	2.3	1.0	0.10	0.22	**2.0**	*171*
Mesothelioma	3	0	-	-	-	-	-	3.6	-	-	-	-	-	5.7	-	5.4	-	-	-	-	0.9	0.4	0.05	0.07	**0.7**	*MES*
Kaposi's sarcoma	1	0	-	-	-	-	-	-	-	-	-	-	-	-	-	5.4	-	-	-	-	0.3	0.1	0.00	0.03	**0.2**	*KAP*
Melanoma of skin	10	0	-	-	-	-	3.4	-	-	5.3	-	-	-	5.1	4.7	10.8	7.3	17.8	-	19.4	2.9	1.3	0.09	0.18	**1.7**	*172*
†Other skin	5	0	-	-	-	-	3.4	-	-	5.3	5.6	-	-	-	-	-	-	8.9	-	19.4	1.5		0.07	0.07	**1.1**	*173*
Breast	217	0	-	-	-	-	-	10.8	16.6	53.4	100.2	108.7	137.9	147.7	141.8	124.3	153.6	160.1	133.5	174.6	63.0	27.6	3.59	4.97	**46.0**	*174*
Uterus unspecified	9	0	-	-	-	-	-	-	-	-	-	-	11.5	5.1	4.7	-	14.6	8.9	13.4	19.4	2.6	1.1	0.11	0.18	**1.5**	*179*
Cervix uteri	24	0	-	-	-	-	-	-	3.6	5.3	33.4	12.1	17.2	10.2	23.6	10.8	14.6	-	-	-	7.0	3.1	0.53	0.65	**6.2**	*180*
Placenta	0	0	-	-	-	-	-	-	-	-	-	-	-	-	-	-	-	-	-	-	0.0	0.0	0.00	0.00	**0.0**	*181*
Corpus uteri	32	0	-	-	-	-	-	-	5.3	5.6	-	-	17.2	25.5	18.9	43.2	43.9	26.7	13.4	-	9.3	4.1	0.36	0.80	**5.8**	*182*
Ovary etc.	39	0	-	-	-	7.2	-	3.6	4.2	5.3	22.3	6.0	5.7	10.2	37.8	43.2	21.9	17.8	26.7	58.2	11.3	5.0	0.51	0.84	**7.7**	*183*
Other female genital	11	0	-	-	-	-	-	-	-	-	-	-	-	-	-	5.4	14.6	26.7	53.4	19.4	3.2	1.4	0.00	0.10	**1.1**	*184*
Bladder	12	0	-	-	-	-	-	-	-	-	-	-	-	-	14.2	21.6	7.3	8.9	26.7	19.4	3.5	1.5	0.07	0.22	**1.7**	*188*
Kidney etc.	13	0	-	4.5	-	-	-	-	-	-	-	-	-	10.2	14.2	10.8	14.6	17.8	-	19.4	3.8	1.7	0.14	0.27	**2.3**	*189*
Eye	1	0	5.1	-	-	-	-	-	-	-	-	-	-	-	-	-	-	-	-	-	0.3	0.1	0.03	0.03	**0.6**	*190*
Brain, nervous system	17	0	-	-	3.8	-	-	-	-	-	11.1	12.1	-	15.3	14.2	5.4	21.9	17.8	-	-	4.9	2.2	0.28	0.42	**3.7**	*191-2*
Thyroid	18	0	-	-	3.8	-	3.4	7.2	4.2	5.3	11.1	6.0	5.7	20.4	4.7	-	-	17.8	13.4	-	5.2	2.3	0.36	0.36	**4.3**	*193*
Other endocrine	0	0	-	-	-	-	-	-	-	-	-	-	-	-	-	-	-	-	-	-	0.0	0.0	0.00	0.00	**0.0**	*194*
Hodgkin's disease	4	0	-	-	-	3.6	3.4	-	-	-	5.6	6.0	-	-	-	-	-	-	-	-	1.2	0.5	0.09	0.09	**1.3**	*201*
Non-Hodgkin lymphoma	23	0	-	-	-	3.6	-	-	-	5.3	-	6.0	23.0	15.3	4.7	16.2	21.9	44.5	-	19.4	6.7	2.9	0.29	0.48	**4.4**	*200,202*
Multiple myeloma	17	0	-	-	-	-	-	-	-	5.3	-	-	11.5	5.1	9.5	16.2	29.3	17.8	-	38.8	4.9	2.2	0.16	0.38	**2.9**	*203*
Lymphoid leukaemia	11	0	5.1	-	-	-	-	3.4	-	-	-	6.0	-	-	-	16.2	-	26.7	-	38.8	3.2	1.4	0.07	0.15	**2.2**	*204*
Myeloid leukaemia	8	0	-	4.5	-	-	-	-	-	-	-	-	-	-	-	5.4	14.6	17.8	13.4	19.4	2.3	1.0	0.02	0.12	**1.2**	*205*
Monocytic leukaemia	1	0	-	-	-	-	-	-	-	-	-	-	-	-	-	-	-	-	13.4	-	0.3	0.1	0.00	0.00	**0.1**	*206*
Other leukaemia	0	0	-	-	-	-	-	-	-	-	-	-	-	-	-	-	-	-	-	-	0.0	0.0	0.00	0.00	**0.0**	*207*
Leukaemia unspecified	2	0	-	-	-	-	-	-	-	-	-	-	5.7	-	-	-	-	-	13.4	-	0.6	0.3	0.03	0.03	**0.4**	*208*
Other and unspecified	39	0	-	-	-	-	-	-	4.2	-	5.6	6.0	-	-	14.2	27.0	36.6	35.6	80.1	252.1	11.3	5.0	0.15	0.47	**5.1**	*O&U*
All sites	790	0	15.2	13.5	15.2	17.9	24.0	28.9	33.3	112.1	244.8	169.1	304.6	341.1	496.4	567.3	731.3	827.3	1001.5	1183.1	229.2		9.08	15.57	**143.5**	*ALL*
All sites but 173	785	0	15.2	13.5	15.2	17.9	20.6	28.9	33.3	106.8	239.2	169.1	304.6	341.1	496.4	567.3	731.3	818.4	1001.5	1163.7	227.8	100.0	9.01	15.50	**142.4**	*ALLb*

Rate from 1 case	5.056	4.509	3.795	3.577	3.431	3.614	4.157	5.338	5.564	6.041	5.747	5.092	4.727	5.402	7.313	8.895	13.353	19.395

†Important: see notes on population page

Spain, Asturias

The Principality of Asturias Tumour Registry began its activities in 1978, and its first results were published in 1982.

The area covered by the registry is the Autonomous Community of the Principality of Asturias, a region well defined both geographically and administratively, on the northern coastal strip of the Iberian Peninsula. It is situated between latitudes 42°54′ and 43°43′ N and longitudes 4°30′ and 7°10′ W. Its total area is 10 564 km². Asturias is a very hilly region, altitudes ranging from sea level to 2500 m. However, three quarters of its surface lies below 1000 m.

The climate is mild oceanic with abundant rainfall throughout the year, with an average annual relative humidity of 80% and average rainfall ranging from 800 to 1800 mm. The average annual temperature is 10°C.

According to the 1991 census, the population of Asturias was 1 093 937 inhabitants (48.3% males and 51.7% females), giving an average population density of 103.5 inhabitants per km². The occupational distribution by economic sector was: 11.3% in agriculture and fishing, 25.7% in industry (mainly iron and steel industry and coal-mining), 10.6% in building and 52.4% in services. The population is mainly of the Roman Catholic religion, and ethnically white, with virtually no migration.

The main objectives of the Asturias registry are to enumerate cases of malignant cancer and analyse incidence in the region, describing the distribution by site, sex, and age groups. Case collection is actively performed by the registry's staff, and all the centres, both public and private, where a tumour can be diagnosed or treated in the region, are information sources for the registry. Death certificates for all causes are available to the registry. Topographic site and morphology are both coded to ICD-O-1. For skin, only melanoma is registered, all other tumours for this site being collected but not tabulated, as is the case for all *in situ*, uncertain and benign diagnoses of brain tumours.

All the recommendations from IARC have been adopted by the registry.

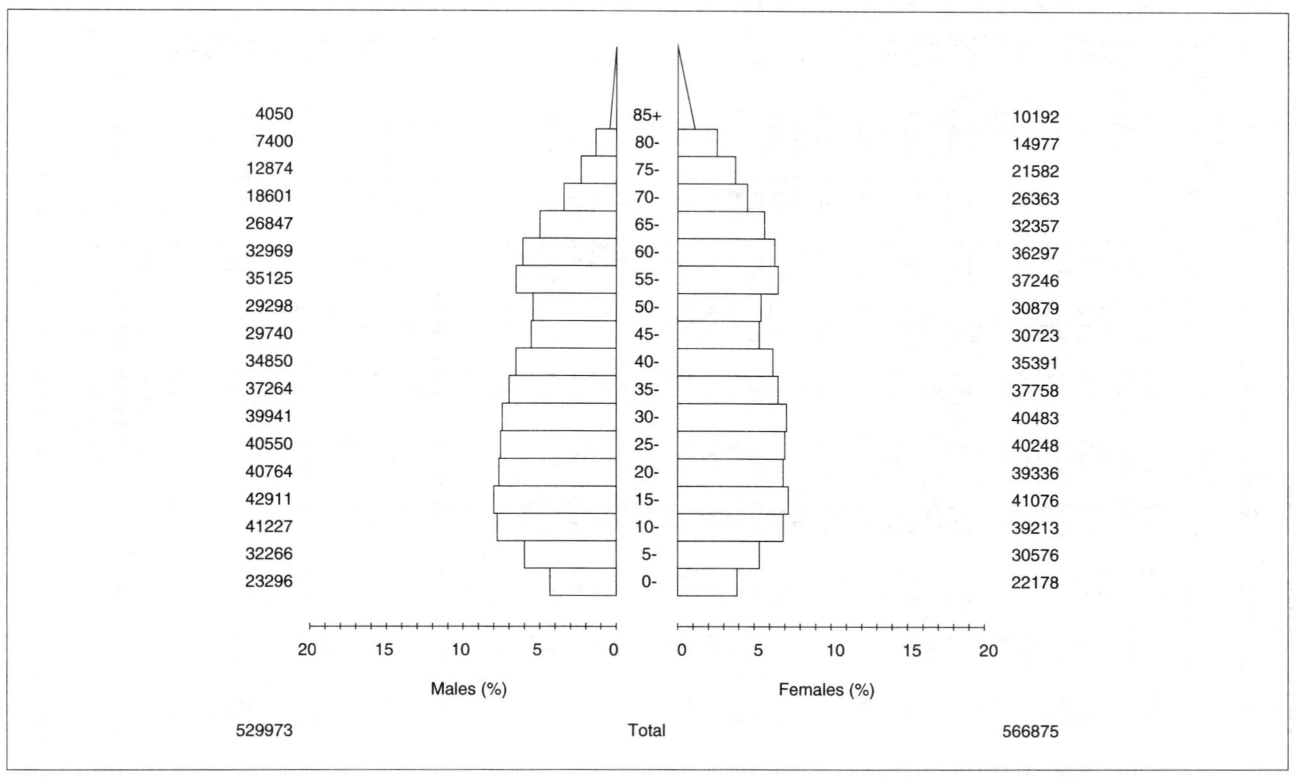

Spain, Asturias
Source of population: average annual 1988–92
Census: 1991
Notes to tables overleaf:
† 173 not available

SPAIN, ASTURIAS 1988-1991

ANNUAL INCIDENCE PER 100,000 BY AGE GROUP (YEARS) - MALE

SITE	ALL AGES	AGE UNK	0-	5-	10-	15-	20-	25-	30-	35-	40-	45-	50-	55-	60-	65-	70-	75-	80-	85+	CRUDE RATE	%	CR 64	CR 74	ASR (W)	ICD (9th)
Lip	82	1	-	-	-	-	-	-	-	1.3	0.7	1.7	6.0	5.7	11.4	14.0	10.8	25.2	16.9	30.9	3.9	0.9	0.14	0.26	2.4	140
Tongue	164	0	-	-	-	-	-	-	-	2.7	9.3	5.9	17.9	30.6	19.7	21.4	14.8	19.4	16.9	6.2	7.7	1.7	0.43	0.61	5.2	141
Salivary gland	23	0	-	-	-	-	-	-	-	-	0.7	0.8	2.6	4.3	2.3	-	4.0	3.9	13.5	-	1.1	0.2	0.05	0.07	0.7	142
Mouth	109	0	-	-	0.6	-	-	-	-	4.0	2.9	7.6	9.4	16.4	16.7	15.8	14.8	5.8	3.4	6.2	5.1	1.1	0.29	0.44	3.6	143-5
Oropharynx	126	0	-	-	-	-	-	-	1.3	4.0	10.8	8.4	10.2	14.9	22.0	10.2	14.8	15.5	-	6.2	5.9	1.3	0.36	0.48	4.2	146
Nasopharynx	43	0	-	0.8	-	-	-	0.6	-	2.0	0.7	1.7	4.3	9.3	4.5	3.7	4.0	7.8	-	-	2.0	0.4	0.12	0.16	1.4	147
Hypopharynx	129	0	-	-	-	-	-	-	-	0.7	3.6	15.1	14.5	19.2	15.2	18.6	14.8	13.6	10.1	-	6.1	1.3	0.34	0.51	4.3	148
Pharynx unspecified	48	0	-	-	-	-	-	-	-	2.0	2.9	2.5	3.4	7.1	5.3	7.4	5.4	3.9	6.8	6.2	2.3	0.5	0.12	0.18	1.5	149
Oesophagus	246	0	-	-	-	-	-	-	-	0.7	5.0	9.2	21.3	29.2	35.6	47.5	44.4	27.2	27.0	49.4	11.6	2.6	0.51	0.96	7.5	150
Stomach	669	6	-	-	-	-	-	-	1.9	6.0	10.8	17.7	22.2	39.1	72.0	114.5	146.5	217.5	202.7	216.0	31.6	7.0	0.86	2.17	18.5	151
Small intestine	33	1	-	-	-	-	-	-	-	1.3	1.4	-	2.6	0.7	3.0	5.6	8.1	7.8	6.8	12.3	1.6	0.3	0.05	0.12	1.0	152
Colon	619	7	-	-	-	-	-	1.2	1.9	3.4	5.7	9.2	28.2	42.0	61.4	121.1	112.9	168.9	243.2	228.4	29.2	6.5	0.77	1.96	17.0	153
Rectum	405	1	-	-	-	-	-	-	1.9	0.7	2.9	5.0	13.7	28.5	49.3	84.7	90.0	97.1	135.1	129.6	19.1	4.2	0.51	1.39	11.1	154
Liver	307	0	-	-	-	0.6	-	-	0.6	1.3	1.4	1.7	7.7	17.8	52.3	50.3	73.9	85.4	94.6	92.6	14.5	3.2	0.42	1.04	8.3	155
Gallbladder etc.	41	0	-	-	-	-	-	-	-	-	-	-	-	4.3	6.1	9.3	2.7	13.6	13.5	24.7	1.9	0.4	0.05	0.11	1.1	156
Pancreas	192	0	-	-	-	-	-	-	-	0.7	-	5.0	7.7	17.8	21.2	26.1	41.7	58.3	47.3	123.4	9.1	2.0	0.26	0.60	5.3	157
Nose, sinuses etc.	42	1	-	-	-	0.6	0.6	0.6	-	0.7	1.4	2.5	5.1	4.3	4.5	8.4	-	1.9	6.8	12.3	2.0	0.4	0.10	0.15	1.4	160
Larynx	511	3	-	-	-	0.6	-	-	0.6	6.0	15.1	22.7	42.7	54.8	93.3	74.5	67.2	75.7	74.3	55.6	24.1	5.3	1.18	1.90	15.8	161
Bronchus, lung	2256	11	-	-	-	0.6	-	-	5.0	12.7	25.1	51.3	100.7	179.4	288.9	418.1	509.4	627.2	493.2	450.6	106.4	23.5	3.33	7.99	63.5	162
Other thoracic organs	37	0	-	-	-	-	-	-	1.9	0.7	0.7	-	0.9	5.0	1.5	6.5	5.4	9.7	6.8	24.7	1.7	0.4	0.05	0.11	1.1	163-4
Bone	26	0	-	0.8	1.2	1.7	-	-	0.6	-	-	2.5	1.7	0.7	2.3	0.9	4.0	1.9	3.4	24.7	1.2	0.3	0.06	0.08	1.0	170
Connective tissue	58	0	-	1.5	0.6	0.6	0.6	1.2	1.3	2.7	5.0	0.8	2.6	4.3	3.0	5.6	8.1	13.6	10.1	12.3	2.7	0.6	0.12	0.19	2.0	171
Mesothelioma	10	0	-	-	-	0.6	-	-	0.6	0.7	-	-	-	0.7	2.3	0.9	1.3	1.9	-	-	0.5	0.1	0.02	0.04	0.3	MES
Kaposi's sarcoma	1	0	-	-	-	-	-	-	0.6	-	-	-	-	-	-	-	-	-	-	-	0.0	0.0	0.00	0.00	0.0	KAP
Melanoma of skin	65	5	-	-	0.6	-	0.6	0.6	-	1.3	2.2	2.5	8.5	6.4	3.8	4.7	9.4	11.7	13.5	18.5	3.1	0.7	0.14	0.22	2.1	172
†Other skin	17	0	-	-	-	-	-	-	-	-	0.7	-	-	2.1	1.5	0.9	6.7	5.8	6.8	-	0.8	-	0.02	0.06	0.4	173
Breast	17	0	-	-	-	-	-	-	-	1.3	-	-	2.6	1.4	2.3	0.9	-	1.9	10.1	12.3	0.8	0.2	0.04	0.04	0.5	175
Prostate	720	7	-	-	-	-	-	-	1.3	0.7	1.4	0.8	11.9	17.8	56.1	108.9	172.0	308.8	368.2	500.0	34.0	7.5	0.45	1.87	18.1	185
Testis	43	0	1.1	-	-	0.6	3.7	4.3	5.6	2.0	0.7	3.4	1.7	1.4	3.0	0.9	-	3.9	-	-	2.0	0.4	0.14	0.14	1.9	186
Penis	20	1	-	-	-	-	-	-	-	-	-	1.7	0.9	-	2.3	1.9	5.4	7.8	10.1	-	0.9	0.2	0.03	0.06	0.6	187.1-.4
Other male genital	1	0	-	-	-	-	-	-	-	0.7	-	-	-	-	-	-	-	-	-	-	0.0	0.0	0.00	0.00	0.0	187.5-.9
Bladder	979	10	-	-	-	-	1.8	1.2	5.0	2.7	11.5	16.8	45.2	58.4	94.0	182.5	221.8	293.2	310.8	327.1	46.2	10.2	1.20	3.24	27.1	188
Kidney etc.	247	1	1.1	-	0.6	0.6	-	-	0.6	4.0	8.6	5.9	17.9	14.9	29.6	50.3	45.7	54.4	40.5	49.4	11.7	2.6	0.42	0.90	7.5	189
Eye	16	1	1.1	-	-	-	-	0.6	-	-	-	-	1.7	2.8	1.5	1.9	2.7	-	-	6.2	0.8	0.2	0.04	0.07	0.6	190
Brain, nervous system	136	0	3.2	4.6	1.2	2.3	1.8	1.2	3.8	4.0	4.3	7.6	9.4	9.3	17.4	18.6	13.4	11.7	13.5	12.3	6.4	1.4	0.35	0.51	5.2	191-2
Thyroid	43	1	-	-	-	1.2	1.2	1.2	1.3	3.4	2.9	2.5	3.4	2.1	2.3	4.7	2.7	3.9	10.1	-	2.0	0.4	0.11	0.15	1.6	193
Other endocrine	17	0	3.2	3.1	0.6	-	-	0.6	-	0.7	-	-	-	0.7	1.5	1.9	-	1.9	3.4	-	0.8	0.2	0.05	0.06	1.0	194
Hodgkin's disease	83	2	-	0.8	4.2	4.1	3.7	4.9	5.0	6.7	2.9	2.5	3.4	5.0	3.8	6.5	2.7	1.9	3.4	-	3.9	0.9	0.24	0.29	3.4	201
Non-Hodgkin lymphoma	231	3	1.1	0.8	-	1.7	-	2.5	5.0	6.0	6.5	10.1	10.2	20.6	21.2	34.5	44.4	38.8	64.2	18.5	10.9	2.4	0.43	0.83	7.2	200,202
Multiple myeloma	83	2	-	-	-	-	-	-	-	-	1.4	1.7	2.6	5.7	13.6	9.3	25.5	15.5	23.6	24.7	3.9	0.9	0.13	0.31	2.3	203
Lymphoid leukaemia	140	6	4.3	4.6	1.2	1.7	3.7	-	1.3	-	0.7	2.5	2.6	7.1	18.2	14.0	25.5	27.2	37.2	67.9	6.6	1.5	0.25	0.46	4.9	204
Myeloid leukaemia	55	1	-	0.8	0.6	1.2	-	0.6	-	0.7	0.8	2.6	3.6	2.3	4.7	9.4	11.7	30.4	55.6	6.2	2.6	0.6	0.07	0.14	1.6	205
Monocytic leukaemia	4	0	-	-	-	-	-	-	-	-	-	-	-	-	1.5	-	-	-	3.4	6.2	0.2	0.0	0.01	0.01	0.1	206
Other leukaemia	0	0	-	-	-	-	-	-	-	-	-	-	-	-	-	-	-	-	-	-	0.0	0.0	0.00	0.00	0.0	207
Leukaemia unspecified	85	2	1.1	0.8	1.2	0.6	1.8	-	3.8	1.3	0.7	2.5	2.6	2.8	5.3	6.5	20.2	27.2	27.0	30.9	4.0	0.9	0.13	0.26	2.7	208
Other and unspecified	433	8	-	-	-	-	-	-	1.3	3.4	7.9	13.4	22.2	28.5	46.3	56.8	82.0	112.6	172.3	203.7	20.4	4.5	0.63	1.33	12.2	O&U
All sites	9612	81	16.1	18.6	12.7	18.6	19.6	21.0	52.6	92.6	159.3	246.3	474.4	726.7	1121.5	1575.6	1888.3	2442.9	2580.8	2845.5	453.4		15.03	32.49	279.5	ALL
All sites but 173	9595	81	16.1	18.6	12.7	18.6	19.6	21.0	52.6	92.6	158.5	246.3	474.4	724.6	1120.0	1574.6	1881.6	2437.0	2574.1	2845.5	452.6	100.0	15.00	32.43	279.1	ALLb
Rate from 1 case			1.073	0.775	0.606	0.583	0.613	0.617	0.626	0.671	0.717	0.841	0.853	0.712	0.758	0.931	1.344	1.942	3.378	6.172							

†Important: see notes on population page

SPAIN, ASTURIAS 1988-1991

ANNUAL INCIDENCE PER 100,000 BY AGE GROUP (YEARS) - FEMALE

SITE	ALL AGES	AGE UNK	0-	5-	10-	15-	20-	25-	30-	35-	40-	45-	50-	55-	60-	65-	70-	75-	80-	85+	CRUDE RATE	%	CR 64	CR 74	ASR (W)	ICD (9th)
Lip	15	0	-	-	-	-	-	-	-	-	-	-	-	-	-	1.5	3.8	1.2	5.0	12.3	0.7	0.2	0.00	0.03	**0.2**	140
Tongue	38	0	-	-	-	-	-	-	0.6	2.0	1.4	0.8	3.2	0.7	3.4	3.9	3.8	5.8	5.0	9.8	1.7	0.6	0.06	0.10	**0.9**	141
Salivary gland	18	0	-	0.8	-	0.6	0.6	0.6	1.2	3.3	-	-	-	-	0.7	2.3	0.9	1.2	1.7	-	0.8	0.3	0.04	0.06	**0.6**	142
Mouth	24	0	-	0.8	-	-	0.6	0.6	1.2	-	-	-	1.6	-	0.7	0.8	3.8	6.9	3.3	7.4	1.1	0.4	0.03	0.05	**0.6**	143-5
Oropharynx	9	0	-	-	-	-	-	-	-	0.7	-	1.6	0.8	-	0.7	-	2.8	1.2	-	-	0.4	0.1	0.02	0.03	**0.3**	146
Nasopharynx	18	0	-	-	-	-	-	-	1.2	-	-	-	2.4	4.0	2.1	1.5	0.9	1.2	-	-	0.8	0.3	0.05	0.06	**0.5**	147
Hypopharynx	5	0	-	-	-	-	-	-	-	-	-	-	-	-	-	-	0.7	-	1.2	3.3	2.5	0.2	0.1	0.00	0.00	**0.1**	148
Pharynx unspecified	7	0	-	-	-	-	-	-	0.6	0.7	-	-	-	-	-	-	-	4.6	1.7	-	0.3	0.1	0.01	0.01	**0.1**	149
Oesophagus	36	1	-	-	-	-	-	-	-	-	-	0.8	-	2.7	2.1	2.3	8.5	5.8	5.0	17.2	1.6	0.5	0.03	0.08	**0.7**	150
Stomach	496	1	-	-	-	-	1.9	1.2	1.9	2.0	2.8	1.6	13.0	13.4	25.5	37.9	89.1	101.9	153.6	201.1	21.9	7.2	0.32	0.95	**8.7**	151
Small intestine	21	1	-	-	-	-	-	-	-	-	0.7	1.6	0.8	2.7	2.1	0.8	2.8	4.6	1.7	2.5	0.9	0.3	0.04	0.06	**0.5**	152
Colon	532	8	-	-	-	-	0.6	0.6	1.2	4.6	10.6	11.4	18.6	28.9	37.9	58.7	81.6	76.4	128.5	142.3	23.5	7.8	0.58	1.29	**11.1**	153
Rectum	280	2	-	-	-	-	-	-	1.2	2.6	3.5	4.1	12.1	19.5	21.4	27.8	38.9	44.0	70.1	73.6	12.3	4.1	0.32	0.66	**5.7**	154
Liver	163	1	-	-	-	-	-	-	-	0.7	2.8	-	4.9	6.7	15.2	14.7	17.1	25.5	43.4	83.4	7.2	2.4	0.15	0.31	**3.0**	155
Gallbladder etc.	110	0	-	-	-	-	-	-	-	-	2.1	2.4	2.4	4.0	6.9	16.2	18.0	23.2	26.7	22.1	4.9	1.6	0.09	0.26	**2.2**	156
Pancreas	146	1	-	-	-	-	-	-	-	0.7	1.4	0.8	1.6	3.4	12.4	10.8	19.9	23.2	51.7	73.6	6.4	2.1	0.10	0.26	**2.5**	157
Nose, sinuses etc.	24	0	-	-	-	-	-	-	0.6	0.7	-	0.8	3.2	-	1.4	3.9	2.8	4.6	3.3	2.5	1.1	0.4	0.03	0.07	**0.6**	160
Larynx	17	0	-	-	-	-	-	-	-	-	0.7	-	-	1.3	1.4	0.8	2.8	3.5	5.0	4.9	0.7	0.2	0.02	0.04	**0.3**	161
Bronchus, lung	203	1	-	-	-	-	-	-	0.6	2.6	3.5	9.0	5.7	10.7	20.0	14.7	24.7	32.4	61.8	46.6	9.0	3.0	0.26	0.46	**4.3**	162
Other thoracic organs	22	0	-	-	-	-	-	-	-	-	0.7	-	4.0	0.7	0.7	3.1	1.9	2.3	10.0	-	1.0	0.3	0.03	0.06	**0.5**	163-4
Bone	21	0	-	1.6	-	2.4	-	-	0.6	-	0.7	-	-	1.3	1.4	2.3	-	2.3	1.7	7.4	0.9	0.3	0.04	0.05	**0.7**	170
Connective tissue	48	0	-	0.8	-	-	3.8	1.2	1.9	0.7	1.4	-	3.2	0.7	6.2	3.1	2.8	6.9	3.3	9.8	2.1	0.7	0.10	0.13	**1.4**	171
Mesothelioma	8	0	-	-	-	-	-	-	0.6	-	-	1.6	-	-	0.7	0.8	0.9	1.2	-	-	0.4	0.1	0.02	0.03	**0.2**	MES
Kaposi's sarcoma	1	0	-	-	-	-	-	-	-	-	-	-	-	-	-	-	-	1.7	-	-	0.0	0.0	0.00	0.00	**0.0**	KAP
Melanoma of skin	152	4	-	-	-	-	1.2	3.1	5.3	6.4	5.7	10.5	8.1	8.3	14.7	20.9	17.4	18.4	31.9	-	6.7	2.2	0.25	0.43	**3.9**	172
†Other skin	25	2	-	-	-	-	-	-	-	-	-	-	-	-	-	1.5	3.8	3.5	8.3	22.1	1.1		0.00	0.03	**0.3**	173
Breast	1695	20	-	-	-	-	1.3	5.0	14.8	45.0	93.2	105.8	129.5	126.9	143.9	161.5	171.6	178.4	207.0	208.5	74.8	24.7	3.37	5.05	**46.0**	174
Uterus unspecified	39	1	-	-	-	-	-	0.6	0.6	1.3	0.7	2.4	4.9	4.7	1.4	2.3	2.8	4.6	6.7	2.5	1.7	0.6	0.09	0.11	**1.1**	179
Cervix uteri	260	0	-	-	-	-	1.3	1.9	4.9	21.2	18.4	26.9	20.2	18.8	26.2	16.2	17.1	9.3	21.7	12.3	11.5	3.8	0.70	0.86	**8.4**	180
Placenta	2	0	-	-	-	-	-	0.6	0.6	-	-	-	-	-	-	-	-	-	-	-	0.1	0.0	0.01	0.01	**0.1**	181
Corpus uteri	437	4	-	-	-	-	-	-	3.7	2.0	7.1	13.8	39.7	49.7	56.5	53.3	51.2	47.5	40.1	9.8	19.3	6.4	0.87	1.40	**11.3**	182
Ovary etc.	345	2	-	0.8	0.6	1.2	-	1.2	3.7	4.0	12.7	18.7	23.5	30.9	38.6	27.8	34.1	47.5	40.1	39.2	15.2	5.0	0.68	1.00	**9.1**	183
Other female genital	101	1	1.1	-	-	-	-	0.6	-	0.7	1.4	-	1.6	2.7	5.5	13.9	9.5	16.2	31.7	49.1	4.5	1.5	0.07	0.19	**1.9**	184
Bladder	189	2	-	-	-	-	-	0.6	0.6	0.7	1.4	6.5	0.8	10.1	11.0	20.1	31.3	35.9	48.4	56.4	8.3	2.8	0.16	0.42	**3.6**	188
Kidney etc.	132	0	3.4	0.8	-	-	-	0.6	0.6	1.3	3.5	4.9	5.7	9.4	7.6	16.2	18.0	26.6	16.7	19.6	5.8	1.9	0.19	0.36	**3.4**	189
Eye	10	0	-	-	-	-	-	0.6	-	0.7	0.8	0.8	-	0.7	0.8	0.9	2.3	3.3	-	-	0.4	0.1	0.02	0.02	**0.2**	190
Brain, nervous system	109	0	2.3	1.6	1.3	2.4	0.6	-	-	3.3	3.5	4.9	6.5	9.4	9.0	14.7	9.5	12.7	8.3	4.9	4.8	1.6	0.22	0.34	**3.4**	191-2
Thyroid	156	1	-	-	0.6	1.2	4.4	4.3	6.8	7.9	4.9	9.8	14.6	5.4	8.3	7.0	17.1	17.4	15.0	17.2	6.9	2.3	0.34	0.46	**4.8**	193
Other endocrine	10	0	-	-	-	-	-	0.6	-	-	-	-	0.8	-	2.1	2.3	0.9	1.2	-	-	0.4	0.1	0.02	0.03	**0.3**	194
Hodgkin's disease	53	3	-	-	0.6	3.0	5.1	3.7	3.7	2.0	1.4	1.6	-	0.7	0.7	4.6	5.8	5.8	1.7	-	2.3	0.8	0.12	0.16	**2.0**	201
Non-Hodgkin lymphoma	240	7	1.1	2.5	1.3	0.6	0.6	1.9	3.7	2.0	3.5	9.0	13.0	14.8	17.2	24.0	32.2	38.2	38.4	31.9	10.6	3.5	0.37	0.66	**6.0**	200,202
Multiple myeloma	78	3	-	-	-	-	-	-	-	-	0.7	0.8	2.4	6.7	6.9	9.3	8.5	20.8	13.4	7.4	3.4	1.1	0.09	0.18	**1.6**	203
Lymphoid leukaemia	113	2	2.3	-	0.6	0.6	0.6	-	0.6	-	0.7	4.1	5.7	4.0	5.5	19.3	14.2	18.5	20.0	24.5	5.0	1.6	0.13	0.30	**2.7**	204
Myeloid leukaemia	53	0	-	-	0.6	0.6	0.6	0.6	1.2	3.3	0.7	2.4	3.2	2.0	5.5	4.6	2.8	8.1	6.7	7.4	2.3	0.8	0.10	0.14	**1.5**	205
Monocytic leukaemia	2	0	-	-	-	-	-	0.6	-	-	-	-	-	-	-	-	0.9	-	-	-	0.1	0.0	0.00	0.01	**0.1**	206
Other leukaemia	1	0	-	-	-	-	-	-	-	-	-	-	-	-	-	-	-	1.2	-	-	0.0	0.0	0.00	0.00	**0.0**	207
Leukaemia unspecified	70	2	1.1	-	1.3	0.6	1.9	0.6	0.6	1.3	-	2.4	1.6	2.0	4.8	8.5	4.7	10.4	11.7	24.5	3.1	1.0	0.09	0.16	**1.8**	208
Other and unspecified	348	3	-	-	-	0.6	-	1.2	1.2	2.6	4.9	8.1	13.0	14.1	21.4	27.8	35.1	56.8	111.8	152.1	15.3	5.1	0.34	0.66	**6.7**	O&U
All sites	6882	72	11.3	9.8	7.0	14.0	24.2	29.8	64.8	125.1	198.5	265.3	375.7	421.5	544.1	658.3	818.4	961.4	1256.9	1439.9	303.5		10.57	18.03	**166.1**	ALL
All sites but 173	6857	70	11.3	9.8	7.0	14.0	24.2	29.8	64.8	125.1	198.5	265.3	375.7	421.5	544.1	656.7	814.6	957.9	1248.6	1417.8	302.4	100.0	10.56	18.00	**165.8**	ALLb

Rate from 1 case   1.127   0.818   0.638   0.609   0.636   0.621   0.618   0.662   0.706   0.814   0.810   0.671   0.689   0.773   0.948   1.158   1.669   2.453

†Important: see notes on population page

Spain, Basque Country

The Registro de Cancer de Euskadi (Basque Country Cancer Registry) was founded in 1986 by the Department of Health of the Basque Government. Previously, there was a cancer registry in the province of Gipuzkoa, set up by the Oncological Institute of Gipuzkoa, and a pilot study in the rest of the province. The aim of the registry is to determine the incidence of malignant tumours in the Basque Country, so as to allow better planning of resources for oncology (prevention, care facilities, teaching) and to carry out epidemiological studies.

The registry personnel consists of the director, one junior doctor (half-time) and six full-time clerks, one of whom coordinates work in the field, for active case-finding. An agreement with the Oncological Institute of Gipuzkoa provides for data collection in this province to be carried out by their own personnel. There is an Advisory Committee composed of doctors who represent the different institutions, and a small sub-committee to resolve problems posed by individual cases. The Basque Institute of Statistics provides the population data for the Basque Country. The physical location, equipment and administrative personnel of the registry are provided by the Health Department. Confidentiality is assured by applying the rules proposed by IARC/IACR.

The area covered by the registry is the Autonomous Community of the Basque Country (Comunidad Autonoma del Pais Vasco; CAPV), situated in the north of Spain, between latitudes 43°27′ and 42°28′ N and longitudes 1°44′ and 3°26′ W, and bordered by the Pyrenees, France, Cantabrian Sea (Bay of Biscay) and other Spanish provinces. It consists of three provinces: Alava, Bizkaia and Gipuzkoa, with a total surface area of 7261 km^2 and 197 km of coastline. The climate is temperate and humid, with an average temperature of 15°C and humidity 70%. The territory is quite mountainous.

At the 1991 census, the total population was 2 104 041 (1 033 980 men and 1 070 061 women). The average density is 291.9 inhabitants per km^2 unequally distributed between the provinces: Alava 89.4/km^2, Bizkaia 521.2/km^2 and Gipuzkoa 338.7/km^2. Approximately 40% of the population is concentrated in four municipalities of more than 100 000 inhabitants and 26% live in rural areas (10 000 inhabitants or less). About 25% of the population is under 20 years old and 13% over age 65, the population of Alava being the youngest. The population is decreasing due to a fall in the birth rate and an increase in emigration. Life expectancy is 72.8 years for men and 81.5 years for women. The official languages are Basque and Spanish, and the majority of the population is of Roman Catholic religion.

In 1989, 53% of the active population was employed, 49.3% in the service sector, 41.3% in industry, 6.1% in building and 3.8% in agriculture and fishing.

Due to diminishing industrial activity, and the introduction of alternative energy sources such as gas, there has been a decrease in emissions of CO_2 and SO_2. There is no clear evidence of a decrease in river pollution.

In 1988 most of the health services administered by the Basque Health Service (Osakidetza), a public service which ensures health coverage of 99.7% of the Basque population, were transferred to CAPV. Since then, some changes have been made, one being the improvement of the health information system, which has had an effect on the cancer registry. There are 56 health centres, 18 of which belong to the Basque Health Service. The Oncological Institute of Gipuzkoa is a private centre dedicated to the diagnosis and treatment of cancer. There are 5982 physicians and 10 024 hospital beds (4.7 per 1000 inhabitants). There are no cancer screening programmes.

Data collection is both active and passive, always voluntary. The principal sources of information are all of the public and most of the private hospitals, the pathology laboratories, departments of oncology, haematology and paediatrics and medical records departments. Other sources of information used include municipal lists of inhabitants, health databases, social insurance, etc. The registry also receives death certificates mentioning cancer and uses them both as a source of information and for passive follow-up. Before accepting a case as a death-certificate-only diagnosis, an active search is carried out in the various data sources. Data are exchanged with other provinces, especially if there is a cancer registry.

Various quality control measures, both manual and mechanical, are carried out during data-processing. All malignant and *in situ* diagnoses are collected, but only malignant tumours are included in computing incidence. Multiple tumours are coded following the IARC/IACR recommendations. Basal and squamous cell cancers of the skin are not registered. The data are coded to ICD-O.

The information obtained is used to produce annual incidence reports and to answer numerous requests for data, mostly from research workers in the region. The data on cancer incidence serve as a basis for health planning. The registry has carried out and participated in a number of epidemiological studies.

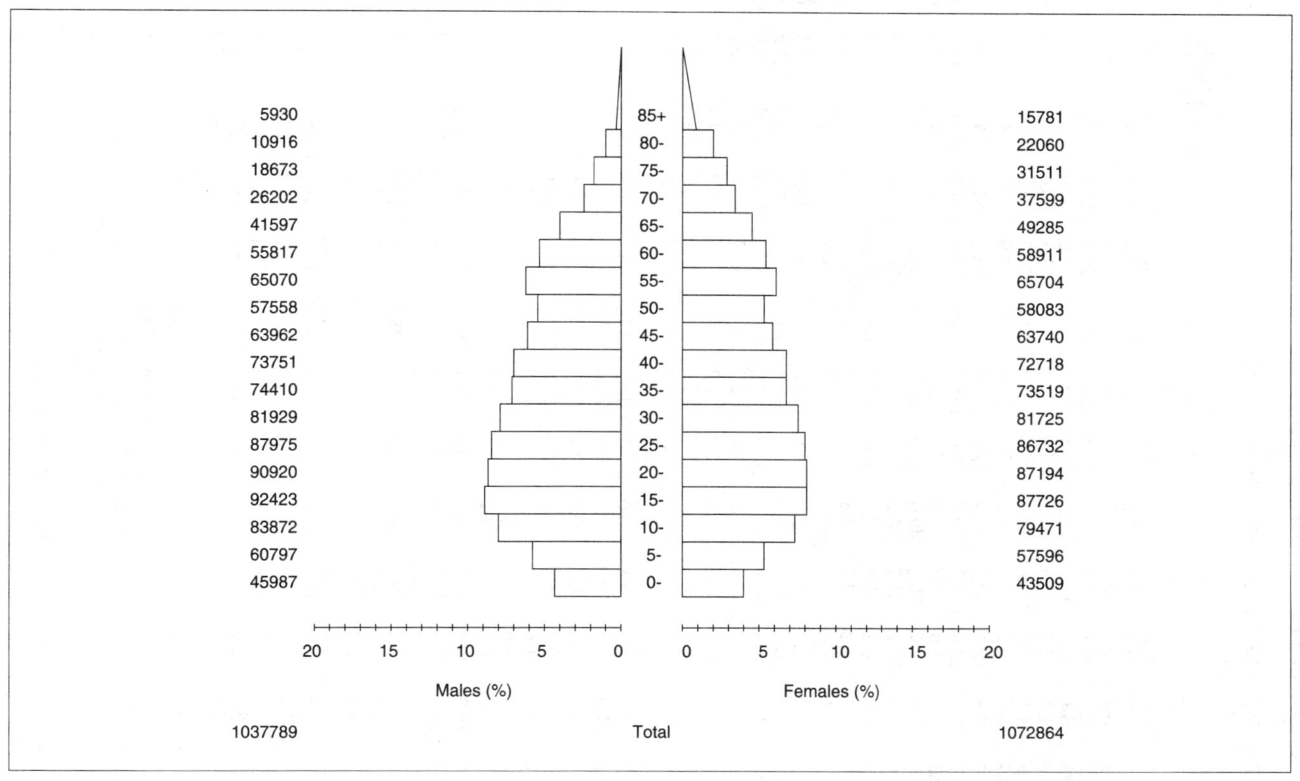

Spain, Basque Country

Source of population: average annual 1988–91
Census: 1991 General Census (March 1991)
Estimate: The 1988, 1989 and 1990 populations are estimates at 31 December of each year, based on the 1986 Municipality Census and the 1991 General Census. The 1991 population was estimated at 31 December 1991 on the basis of the 1991 General Census, taking into account births, deaths and migration.

Notes to tables overleaf:

† 173 does not include basal cell or squamous cell carcinomas

SPAIN, BASQUE COUNTRY 1988-1991

ANNUAL INCIDENCE PER 100,000 BY AGE GROUP (YEARS) - MALE

SITE	ALL AGES	AGE UNK	0-	5-	10-	15-	20-	25-	30-	35-	40-	45-	50-	55-	60-	65-	70-	75-	80-	85+	CRUDE RATE	%	CR 64	CR 74	ASR (W)	ICD (9th)
Lip	275	1	-	-	-	-	-	-	-	1.7	4.1	6.3	8.7	14.6	22.4	25.8	28.6	33.5	61.8	33.7	6.6	1.7	0.29	0.56	4.8	140
Tongue	252	0	-	-	-	-	-	0.3	0.3	3.4	6.8	9.0	13.9	14.2	25.1	18.6	17.2	21.4	11.5	8.4	6.1	1.5	0.36	0.54	4.7	141
Salivary gland	27	0	-	-	-	-	-	-	-	0.7	0.3	1.2	0.4	1.2	1.8	3.0	2.9	5.4	-	4.2	0.7	0.2	0.03	0.06	0.5	142
Mouth	263	0	-	-	-	-	-	0.3	0.6	2.7	6.1	9.4	15.2	14.2	23.3	25.8	21.0	16.1	18.3	4.2	6.3	1.6	0.36	0.59	4.9	143-5
Oropharynx	190	0	-	-	-	-	-	-	0.9	1.3	6.1	5.5	11.3	16.5	14.3	19.2	9.5	8.0	4.6	-	4.6	1.2	0.28	0.42	3.5	146
Nasopharynx	60	0	-	0.4	0.3	0.3	0.3	1.1	0.6	1.0	1.4	2.7	4.3	3.1	4.5	3.0	-	1.3	4.6	-	1.4	0.4	0.10	0.12	1.2	147
Hypopharynx	198	1	-	-	-	-	-	-	-	1.3	4.1	9.0	14.8	15.0	17.5	9.0	20.0	10.7	4.6	-	4.8	1.2	0.31	0.46	3.7	148
Pharynx unspecified	118	0	-	-	-	-	-	-	0.6	0.7	3.4	5.5	7.4	9.6	7.6	10.8	7.6	4.0	-	8.4	2.8	0.7	0.17	0.27	2.2	149
Oesophagus	534	0	-	-	-	-	-	-	-	1.7	5.8	18.0	30.0	41.9	38.1	45.1	55.3	48.2	64.1	25.3	12.9	3.2	0.68	1.18	9.6	150
Stomach	1398	0	-	-	-	-	-	0.9	2.1	6.7	18.6	25.4	34.7	70.7	86.0	135.2	174.6	245.0	311.5	274.0	33.7	8.5	1.23	2.78	24.2	151
Small intestine	46	0	-	-	-	-	-	-	0.3	0.3	0.3	1.6	1.7	2.7	2.2	3.6	4.8	6.7	4.6	21.1	1.1	0.3	0.05	0.09	0.8	152
Colon	988	2	-	-	0.3	0.3	-	3.1	5.0	7.5	12.9	20.8	40.0	62.7	102.8	155.5	192.8	187.8	219.2	23.8	6.0	0.76	2.06	17.1	153	
Rectum	768	1	-	-	-	0.3	-	-	0.9	4.0	7.5	12.1	21.7	34.2	54.2	79.3	110.7	108.4	144.3	193.9	18.5	4.7	0.68	1.63	13.5	154
Liver	462	0	0.5	-	-	0.5	0.5	0.3	1.2	1.7	6.3	12.2	17.7	32.7	63.7	65.8	83.0	64.1	71.7	11.1	2.8	0.37	1.02	8.1	155	
Gallbladder etc.	159	0	-	-	-	-	0.3	-	-	1.0	0.7	1.2	3.5	5.8	8.5	18.0	27.7	29.5	22.9	71.7	3.8	1.0	0.10	0.33	2.8	156
Pancreas	370	0	-	-	-	-	-	0.3	0.6	1.7	5.1	7.0	7.4	19.2	19.7	33.1	52.5	66.9	93.9	71.7	8.9	2.2	0.30	0.73	6.4	157
Nose, sinuses etc.	54	0	-	-	0.3	-	-	-	0.3	0.3	1.0	1.2	2.6	2.3	4.0	4.8	3.8	8.0	13.7	-	1.3	0.3	0.06	0.10	1.0	160
Larynx	986	2	-	-	-	-	-	0.3	1.2	4.7	15.9	36.3	54.7	70.3	87.8	96.8	84.0	65.6	32.1	33.7	23.8	6.0	1.36	2.26	18.2	161
Bronchus, lung	3027	2	-	-	-	0.3	-	0.3	6.1	12.4	31.2	45.3	99.9	153.7	229.8	352.2	404.5	421.7	483.2	333.0	72.9	18.3	2.90	6.68	53.1	162
Other thoracic organs	28	0	-	0.8	-	-	-	0.9	-	0.7	0.4	0.4	0.4	1.5	1.8	2.4	-	2.7	6.9	4.2	0.7	0.2	0.03	0.05	0.5	163-4
Bone	50	0	0.5	0.4	1.2	3.0	0.3	1.1	0.9	1.3	0.7	0.4	0.9	0.8	2.2	1.2	3.8	1.3	2.3	4.2	1.2	0.3	0.07	0.09	1.1	170
Connective tissue	103	0	1.1	0.4	1.2	0.3	1.1	2.3	0.9	1.7	2.4	1.2	3.9	4.6	2.2	5.4	9.5	10.7	11.5	29.5	2.5	0.6	0.12	0.19	2.1	171
Mesothelioma	27	0	-	-	-	-	-	-	-	-	-	-	1.7	0.4	2.2	3.0	6.7	2.7	6.9	-	0.7	0.2	0.02	0.07	0.5	MES
Kaposi's sarcoma	34	0	-	-	-	-	-	1.7	1.8	1.3	1.0	0.4	1.3	1.2	0.9	-	3.8	1.3	2.3	-	0.8	0.2	0.05	0.07	0.7	KAP
Melanoma of skin	160	0	-	-	-	-	1.4	2.0	2.1	5.7	5.4	4.3	4.8	10.0	2.2	13.2	17.2	8.0	16.0	8.4	3.9	1.0	0.19	0.34	3.0	172
†Other skin	29	0	-	-	-	-	0.5	-	0.3	2.0	1.0	1.6	0.9	-	0.9	0.6	1.9	4.0	-	12.6	0.7		0.04	0.05	0.6	173
Breast	23	0	-	-	-	-	-	-	-	-	0.3	-	0.4	1.5	1.8	1.8	2.9	5.4	6.9	-	0.6	0.1	0.02	0.04	0.4	175
Prostate	1285	2	-	-	-	-	-	-	-	-	0.8	6.9	18.1	50.6	128.6	222.3	338.7	568.0	661.8	31.0	7.8	0.38	2.14	21.0	185	
Testis	100	0	0.5	-	0.3	1.1	4.9	6.3	3.7	2.4	5.1	1.6	1.3	0.4	0.4	1.8	3.8	2.7	2.3	4.2	2.4	0.6	0.14	0.17	2.1	186
Penis	47	0	-	-	-	-	-	-	-	-	-	1.6	2.2	3.1	2.7	3.0	5.7	2.7	16.0	16.9	1.1	0.3	0.05	0.09	0.8	187.1-.4
Other male genital	13	0	-	-	-	0.3	-	-	-	-	-	-	0.8	1.2	1.8	1.2	-	-	-	4.2	0.3	0.1	0.02	0.03	0.2	187.5-.9
Bladder	1562	2	-	0.4	0.3	0.5	0.5	1.7	1.8	4.0	14.9	20.3	41.7	66.9	100.8	179.7	200.4	279.8	327.5	328.8	37.6	9.5	1.27	3.17	27.1	188
Kidney etc.	488	2	0.5	-	-	0.5	0.5	0.6	3.1	5.0	5.4	11.3	13.5	20.0	34.9	58.9	62.0	58.9	64.1	54.8	11.8	3.0	0.48	1.09	8.8	189
Eye	26	0	-	-	-	-	-	0.3	0.3	-	1.7	0.4	0.4	1.2	1.8	1.8	2.9	1.3	6.9	-	0.6	0.2	0.03	0.05	0.5	190
Brain, nervous system	312	0	3.8	2.5	1.8	2.2	1.6	2.8	3.4	5.0	5.1	7.8	9.1	16.9	16.6	24.6	28.6	29.5	20.6	16.9	7.5	1.9	0.39	0.66	6.3	191-2
Thyroid	43	0	-	-	0.5	0.5	1.4	0.3	0.7	1.0	2.0	1.7	1.2	0.9	1.8	3.8	6.7	4.6	-	1.0	0.3	0.05	0.08	0.8	193	
Other endocrine	14	0	2.2	-	-	-	-	-	0.3	-	0.3	0.4	2.2	-	0.4	-	1.0	-	-	-	0.3	0.1	0.03	0.03	0.5	194
Hodgkin's disease	147	0	0.5	0.8	1.5	1.9	4.9	4.5	4.0	4.4	3.4	4.3	6.1	2.7	4.5	4.2	4.8	9.4	-	4.2	3.5	0.9	0.22	0.26	3.1	201
Non-Hodgkin lymphoma	419	1	2.2	2.5	1.2	1.6	3.6	7.4	3.7	5.0	7.5	10.9	14.3	14.6	25.1	27.6	35.3	56.2	45.8	42.2	10.1	2.5	0.50	0.81	8.1	200,202
Multiple myeloma	116	0	-	-	-	-	-	-	0.3	-	2.0	2.0	3.5	2.3	3.6	9.0	21.0	25.4	32.1	50.6	2.8	0.7	0.07	0.22	2.0	203
Lymphoid leukaemia	185	1	8.2	5.3	2.4	1.6	1.6	0.9	0.3	2.4	1.0	2.0	3.9	5.8	8.5	7.8	21.9	20.1	32.1	37.9	4.5	1.1	0.22	0.37	4.4	204
Myeloid leukaemia	123	0	-	0.8	0.9	0.8	1.1	1.1	0.9	1.3	2.0	2.7	2.2	6.1	5.4	10.8	19.1	8.0	16.0	12.6	3.0	0.7	0.13	0.28	2.3	205
Monocytic leukaemia	8	0	-	-	-	0.3	-	-	-	-	0.3	-	-	-	0.9	-	-	1.3	2.3	8.4	0.2	0.0	0.01	0.01	0.1	206
Other leukaemia	4	0	-	-	-	-	-	-	-	-	-	-	-	-	0.6	-	-	2.7	2.3	-	0.1	0.0	0.00	0.00	0.1	207
Leukaemia unspecified	51	0	0.5	0.8	1.2	-	0.8	0.3	0.6	-	-	0.4	-	0.8	2.7	7.2	5.7	6.7	13.7	-	1.2	0.3	0.04	0.11	1.0	208
Other and unspecified	971	0	-	0.8	-	-	0.5	1.1	3.4	3.4	9.2	14.5	21.3	41.9	62.7	90.8	124.0	172.7	213.0	324.6	23.4	5.9	0.79	1.87	16.9	O&U
All sites	16543	17	20.7	16.0	12.5	16.2	25.6	40.1	51.0	98.8	196.6	307.6	509.9	769.5	1080.8	1637.1	2054.2	2435.3	2947.5	3001.3	398.5		15.74	34.22	295.3	ALL
All sites but 173	16514	17	20.7	16.0	12.5	16.2	25.0	40.1	50.7	96.8	195.6	306.0	509.0	769.5	1079.9	1636.5	2052.3	2431.3	2947.5	2988.7	397.8	100.0	15.71	34.17	294.7	ALLb

Rate from 1 case   0.544   0.411   0.298   0.270   0.275   0.284   0.305   0.336   0.339   0.391   0.434   0.384   0.448   0.601   0.954   1.339   2.290   4.215

†Important: see notes on population page

SPAIN, BASQUE COUNTRY 1988-1991

ANNUAL INCIDENCE PER 100,000 BY AGE GROUP (YEARS) - FEMALE

SITE	ALL AGES	AGE UNK	0-	5-	10-	15-	20-	25-	30-	35-	40-	45-	50-	55-	60-	65-	70-	75-	80-	85+	CRUDE RATE	%	CR 64	CR 74	ASR (W)	ICD (9th)
Lip	23	0	-	-	-	-	-	-	-	-	-	0.4	0.4	0.8	0.4	1.0	2.0	4.0	6.8	3.2	0.5	0.2	0.01	0.03	**0.3**	140
Tongue	33	0	-	-	-	-	-	-	-	0.7	-	0.4	0.9	2.7	1.7	1.5	0.7	5.6	4.5	3.2	0.8	0.3	0.03	0.04	**0.4**	141
Salivary gland	19	0	-	-	-	-	-	0.6	0.3	-	0.3	0.4	-	-	0.8	1.0	0.7	1.6	4.5	4.8	0.4	0.2	0.01	0.02	**0.2**	142
Mouth	43	0	-	-	-	-	0.3	-	0.3	0.3	-	0.8	1.7	1.1	1.3	1.5	4.7	6.3	6.8	6.3	1.0	0.4	0.03	0.06	**0.6**	143-5
Oropharynx	12	0	-	-	-	-	-	-	-	0.3	-	0.8	0.4	-	0.4	1.0	-	0.8	2.3	3.2	0.3	0.1	0.01	0.01	**0.2**	146
Nasopharynx	31	0	-	-	-	-	0.3	0.6	0.9	1.0	0.3	0.8	0.9	1.9	1.7	0.5	2.0	0.8	3.4	-	0.7	0.3	0.04	0.05	**0.5**	147
Hypopharynx	7	0	-	-	-	-	-	-	-	-	-	0.4	0.4	0.8	0.8	-	-	0.8	-	-	0.2	0.1	0.01	0.01	**0.1**	148
Pharynx unspecified	6	0	-	-	-	-	-	-	-	-	0.3	-	-	-	-	-	0.7	0.8	3.4	-	0.1	0.1	0.00	0.01	**0.1**	149
Oesophagus	52	0	-	-	-	-	-	-	-	-	0.3	1.2	0.9	1.5	0.4	1.5	3.3	7.9	13.6	17.4	1.2	0.5	0.02	0.05	**0.6**	150
Stomach	788	0	-	-	-	0.6	-	0.6	2.4	2.4	5.5	11.0	11.2	21.3	34.4	48.7	72.5	102.3	143.9	160.0	18.4	7.4	0.45	1.05	**9.6**	151
Small intestine	22	0	-	-	-	-	-	-	-	-	-	-	-	0.4	0.8	2.0	3.3	4.0	5.7	-	0.5	0.2	0.01	0.03	**0.2**	152
Colon	843	0	-	-	-	-	-	0.3	1.8	3.1	7.6	10.6	16.4	30.4	40.3	53.3	67.2	118.2	139.4	137.8	19.6	7.9	0.55	1.15	**10.6**	153
Rectum	480	1	-	-	-	-	-	0.3	1.5	2.0	4.1	7.1	8.6	20.9	22.9	36.5	51.9	52.4	62.3	58.6	11.2	4.5	0.34	0.78	**6.4**	154
Liver	164	0	0.6	0.4	-	-	-	-	-	-	0.7	0.8	0.9	3.8	8.5	13.7	15.3	26.2	22.7	36.4	3.8	1.5	0.08	0.22	**2.0**	155
Gallbladder etc.	263	0	-	-	-	-	-	-	0.3	-	1.0	2.0	0.9	3.8	8.9	19.8	28.6	45.2	56.7	50.7	6.1	2.5	0.08	0.33	**2.9**	156
Pancreas	327	0	-	-	-	-	0.3	-	1.2	0.3	1.7	1.6	4.7	8.4	11.5	19.3	35.2	50.8	63.5	65.0	7.6	3.1	0.15	0.42	**3.8**	157
Nose, sinuses etc.	14	0	-	-	0.3	-	-	-	-	-	0.3	-	-	-	0.8	-	2.7	1.6	1.1	4.8	0.3	0.1	0.01	0.02	**0.2**	160
Larynx	20	0	-	-	-	-	-	0.3	0.3	0.3	-	0.4	0.4	2.5	1.0	1.3	1.6	1.1	3.2	-	0.5	0.2	0.02	0.03	**0.3**	161
Bronchus, lung	248	0	-	-	-	0.3	-	-	1.2	2.0	4.8	5.5	7.3	6.5	11.9	15.2	21.3	29.4	29.5	34.9	5.8	2.3	0.20	0.38	**3.4**	162
Other thoracic organs	18	0	1.1	-	-	-	-	0.3	-	-	0.3	0.4	-	1.1	1.3	1.0	1.3	0.8	2.3	-	0.4	0.2	0.02	0.03	**0.4**	163-4
Bone	43	0	-	0.4	1.3	0.6	0.6	1.2	0.9	0.3	0.7	0.8	1.3	-	1.3	2.5	1.3	4.0	2.3	3.2	1.0	0.4	0.05	0.07	**0.8**	170
Connective tissue	84	1	0.6	0.9	-	0.3	0.6	1.4	0.6	2.4	1.4	2.4	2.6	2.7	2.5	3.6	5.3	10.3	3.4	4.8	2.0	0.8	0.09	0.14	**1.5**	171
Mesothelioma	13	0	-	-	-	-	-	-	-	0.7	-	-	-	0.8	1.3	1.0	1.3	0.8	1.1	-	0.3	0.1	0.01	0.03	**0.2**	MES
Kaposi's sarcoma	6	0	-	-	-	-	-	-	-	-	0.3	-	0.4	0.4	-	-	0.7	-	1.1	1.6	0.1	0.1	0.01	0.01	**0.1**	KAP
Melanoma of skin	242	1	0.6	-	0.3	0.9	3.7	3.7	6.7	3.1	7.2	7.1	6.5	9.9	11.0	8.1	13.3	11.9	12.5	17.4	5.6	2.3	0.30	0.41	**4.2**	172
†Other skin	22	0	-	-	-	-	0.6	-	-	1.0	0.3	0.8	0.4	0.4	-	0.5	2.0	2.4	3.4	3.2	0.5		0.02	0.03	**0.3**	173
Breast	2835	5	-	-	-	0.3	0.3	5.2	22.3	47.6	77.7	117.7	117.1	138.1	148.1	157.8	180.2	188.8	173.4	180.6	66.1	26.7	3.38	5.07	**45.8**	174
Uterus unspecified	47	0	-	-	-	-	-	0.6	-	0.3	-	1.6	0.9	0.8	1.7	3.6	2.0	4.0	5.7	19.0	1.1	0.4	0.03	0.06	**0.6**	179
Cervix uteri	349	0	-	-	-	-	0.6	1.7	8.3	6.1	15.8	10.6	18.1	16.4	17.0	15.7	14.0	19.0	13.6	15.8	8.1	3.3	0.47	0.62	**6.0**	180
Placenta	1	0	-	-	-	-	-	0.3	-	-	-	-	-	-	-	-	-	-	-	-	0.0	0.0	0.00	0.00	**0.0**	181
Corpus uteri	589	0	-	-	-	-	0.3	-	0.6	1.7	10.3	10.6	28.8	36.9	45.0	48.2	43.2	41.3	35.1	17.4	13.7	5.5	0.67	1.13	**9.1**	182
Ovary etc.	481	1	-	0.4	0.3	0.6	0.6	2.6	3.7	5.8	11.3	14.1	19.4	25.5	30.1	24.9	33.9	41.3	30.6	7.9	11.2	4.5	0.57	0.87	**7.7**	183
Other female genital	148	0	-	-	0.3	-	-	-	-	0.3	0.3	1.2	1.7	3.4	5.1	10.1	18.0	23.8	24.9	28.5	3.4	1.4	0.06	0.20	**1.7**	184
Bladder	234	1	0.6	-	-	-	0.3	-	0.9	0.3	0.7	2.7	4.7	6.1	9.8	12.7	25.3	37.3	34.0	44.4	5.5	2.2	0.13	0.32	**2.9**	188
Kidney etc.	222	0	0.6	-	-	-	0.6	0.6	0.9	0.7	2.4	2.0	9.5	8.0	14.4	13.2	19.3	23.0	27.2	23.8	5.2	2.1	0.20	0.36	**3.2**	189
Eye	18	0	0.6	-	-	-	-	-	-	-	-	0.4	0.9	1.9	0.4	-	0.7	4.0	1.1	1.6	0.4	0.2	0.02	0.02	**0.3**	190
Brain, nervous system	245	0	4.0	3.9	1.9	1.1	1.7	1.7	1.2	1.7	3.8	4.7	6.9	9.5	12.7	18.3	16.6	16.7	21.5	4.8	5.7	2.3	0.27	0.45	**4.5**	191-2
Thyroid	147	1	-	-	0.6	1.7	0.9	2.0	4.0	3.7	3.4	4.7	6.5	4.2	5.1	9.6	6.0	7.1	3.4	6.3	3.4	1.4	0.19	0.26	**2.6**	193
Other endocrine	12	0	1.7	0.4	-	-	-	-	-	-	-	0.8	0.4	0.8	-	0.5	-	0.8	-	1.6	0.3	0.1	0.02	0.02	**0.4**	194
Hodgkin's disease	93	0	-	0.9	0.9	3.7	3.2	3.5	2.4	1.0	2.1	2.4	0.9	1.1	1.3	2.5	4.0	4.8	3.4	1.6	2.2	0.9	0.12	0.15	**1.9**	201
Non-Hodgkin lymphoma	331	1	0.6	0.4	0.9	2.0	0.9	2.9	2.1	2.4	2.4	4.3	9.9	12.2	21.2	18.3	40.6	30.9	21.5	20.6	7.7	3.1	0.31	0.61	**5.1**	200,202
Multiple myeloma	141	0	-	-	-	-	-	-	0.3	-	-	0.8	2.2	2.3	6.8	12.7	18.0	23.8	22.7	14.3	3.3	1.3	0.06	0.21	**1.7**	203
Lymphoid leukaemia	117	0	4.6	1.7	1.9	1.1	0.3	-	0.3	1.0	0.3	0.8	1.3	2.3	3.4	6.1	10.6	13.5	11.3	23.8	2.7	1.1	0.10	0.18	**2.2**	204
Myeloid leukaemia	85	0	-	0.4	0.6	0.9	0.9	2.3	0.3	-	2.4	2.0	0.9	1.9	3.4	5.1	8.0	5.6	10.2	3.2	2.0	0.8	0.08	0.14	**1.4**	205
Monocytic leukaemia	6	0	-	-	-	-	-	-	-	-	-	0.4	0.4	0.4	0.4	1.0	-	-	-	-	0.1	0.1	0.01	0.01	**0.1**	206
Other leukaemia	1	0	-	-	-	-	-	-	-	-	-	-	-	-	-	-	-	0.8	-	-	0.0	0.0	0.00	0.00	**0.0**	207
Leukaemia unspecified	56	0	1.7	-	-	-	0.3	-	1.2	0.3	0.3	0.4	0.4	2.3	1.3	3.6	3.3	5.6	5.7	17.4	1.3	0.5	0.04	0.08	**0.9**	208
Other and unspecified	677	2	1.7	-	-	-	0.3	0.9	1.8	0.7	3.4	4.7	13.3	13.3	26.7	30.9	52.5	92.0	134.9	212.3	15.8	6.4	0.34	0.75	**7.9**	O&U
All sites	10658	14	19.0	10.0	9.4	14.0	17.2	33.4	69.1	93.9	174.3	241.6	311.2	407.1	521.5	629.0	834.5	1074.2	1177.5	1264.2	248.4		9.62	16.95	**155.6**	ALL
All sites but 173	10636	14	19.0	10.0	9.4	14.0	16.6	33.4	69.1	92.8	174.0	240.8	310.8	406.7	521.5	628.5	832.5	1071.8	1174.1	1261.0	247.8	100.0	9.60	16.92	**155.3**	ALLb

Rate from 1 case   0.575   0.434   0.315   0.285   0.287   0.288   0.306   0.340   0.344   0.392   0.430   0.380   0.424   0.507   0.665   0.793   1.133   1.584

†Important: see notes on population page

Spain, Granada

The Cancer Registry of Granada began its activities in 1985. It is a project financed by the Regional Health Ministry of the Andalusian Government and is carried out in the Andalusian School of Public Health, Granada. The registry's main objective is to determine the incidence of cancer, thus facilitating the gathering of information for further studies. In addition, it contributes to the assessment of needs for cancer services and the implementation of preventive measures.

The registry personnel consist of two physicians (one of them part-time), a nurse and an administrative assistant. At present, two other physicians collaborate in the tasks of the registry as well as in research projects.

The area covered by the registry is the province of Granada, situated in southern Spain within the Andalusian Region. It lies between latitudes 38°5′ and 36°42′ N, and covers 12 531 km². The province has 71 km of coast along the Mediterranean; a large part of its territory is mountainous and one of the highest summits of Spain is to be found there (Mulhacén, 3478 m).

At the 1991 census, the province had a population of 790 515 (387 553 men and 402 962 women), 13% of them aged 65 years or more. The province is divided into 168 municipalities: there is one urban centre, Granada, with approximately 250 000 inhabitants, and 13 other centres have more than 10 000 inhabitants, the rest of the population living in smaller municipalities. The population is ethnically very homogeneous. It is one of the Spanish provinces with the lowest incomes per inhabitant, an important factor influencing migratory movements from 1950 to 1970, which have since stabilized.

The economically active population is divided as follows: 15% are employed in agriculture, 26% in industry and building, and 59% in services. Industrial activity is limited to light industry, particularly food and wood processing. There are a wealth of mineral deposits, mainly iron and lead, but they are not sufficiently exploited and employ only a small part of the population.

The area contains five public (3336 beds) and three private (396 beds) hospitals. 99% of the population is covered by social security and has free access to public hospitalization. Private hospitals serve a small part of the population. Diagnosis and treatment of cancer are available within the province, so few cancer cases are diagnosed outside.

The basic information sources of the registry include all the hospitals (public and private) of the province. Within these hospitals, the data are obtained mainly from the admission services, general history archives, pathology, radiotherapy, oncology and haematology departments. Information about primary care is limited and can only be obtained from a few health centres. Notification is voluntary, and the collection of cases by the registry is active in the large majority of sources.

Another source of information is the death certificates which must be produced for all deceased person. Because of confidentiality requirements existing in Spain, no access to them is possible at the Statistics Institute where they are centralized. They must be obtained from the civil registry of each municipality by the registry's personnel (coverage of this source is about 90%).

No active follow-up of cases is carried out except for selected tumours within specific studies. In the rest of the cases, it is only through consultation of the death certificates that registered cases are known to have died.

Data are coded to ICD-O-1 and the rules used for coding multiple tumours are those proposed by IARC/IACR. Data-processing is carried out on a personal computer and quality control of the data is ensured through the IARC-CHECK program and other specific computer programs developed in the registry.

The information obtained has been used to determine cancer incidence. Due to the registry's relatively short period of existence, it is still difficult to evaluate trends. Two etiological studies on lip cancer and skin cancer were conducted recently. The registry is participating in the multicentre European Prospective Investigation into Cancer and Nutrition (EPIC). Studies on survival and care of patients with cancer are also being carried out for some specific tumours within the framework of the EUROCARE Study

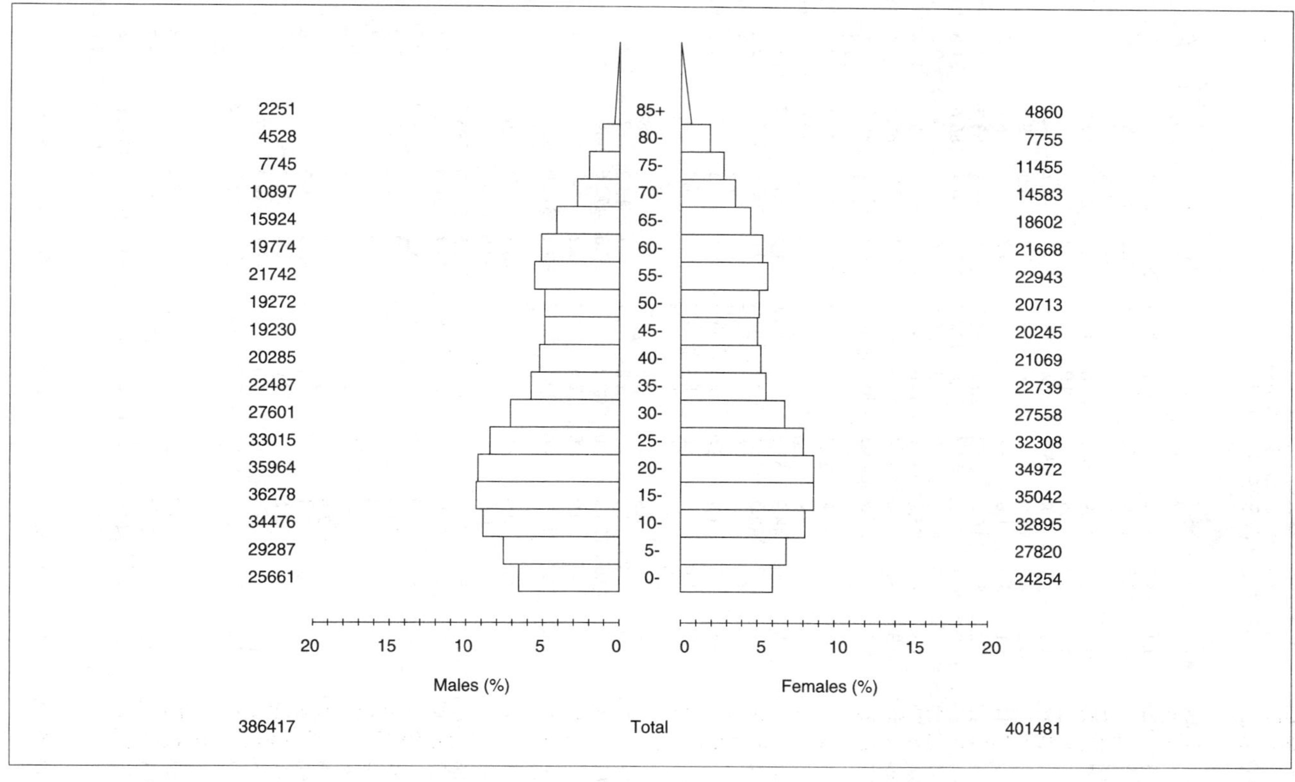

Spain, Granada
Source of population: average annual 1988–92
Census: 1991. Instituto Nacional de Estadistica. Poblaciones de derecho y hecho de los municipios españoles. Censo de Población 1991. Madrid, INE, 1993.

Estimate: The populations for 1988, 1989, 1990 and 1992 are estimated by intercensal interpolation taking into account the censuses of population held in 1981 and 1991 as well as the Municipal Census (Padrón) held in 1986.

SPAIN, GRANADA 1988-1992

ANNUAL INCIDENCE PER 100,000 BY AGE GROUP (YEARS) - MALE

SITE	ALL AGES	AGE UNK	0-	5-	10-	15-	20-	25-	30-	35-	40-	45-	50-	55-	60-	65-	70-	75-	80-	85+	CRUDE RATE	%	CR 64	CR 74	ASR (W)	ICD (9th)
Lip	300	0	-	-	-	-	1.1	1.8	3.6	5.3	12.8	10.4	33.2	33.1	46.5	74.1	71.6	59.4	83.9	62.2	15.5	5.1	0.74	1.47	**12.0**	140
Tongue	70	0	-	-	-	-	-	-	0.7	0.9	3.9	3.1	12.5	11.0	19.2	8.8	7.3	5.2	17.7	8.9	3.6	1.2	0.26	0.34	**2.9**	141
Salivary gland	14	0	-	-	-	-	-	-	-	0.9	-	-	-	2.8	3.0	1.3	5.5	-	8.8	8.9	0.7	0.2	0.03	0.07	**0.5**	142
Mouth	94	0	-	-	-	-	-	0.6	-	2.7	5.9	9.4	10.4	13.8	14.2	17.6	11.0	20.7	26.5	17.8	4.9	1.6	0.28	0.43	**3.9**	143-5
Oropharynx	30	0	-	-	-	-	-	-	-	-	2.0	3.1	4.2	5.5	2.0	10.0	3.7	7.7	-	-	1.6	0.5	0.08	0.15	**1.3**	146
Nasopharynx	29	0	-	-	-	-	1.1	-	0.7	0.9	1.0	3.1	2.1	2.8	5.1	5.0	3.7	10.3	4.4	-	1.5	0.5	0.08	0.13	**1.2**	147
Hypopharynx	53	0	-	-	-	-	-	-	-	-	3.9	4.2	9.3	11.0	7.1	12.6	3.7	5.2	8.8	8.9	2.7	0.9	0.18	0.26	**2.3**	148
Pharynx unspecified	24	0	-	-	-	-	-	-	-	0.9	1.0	2.1	4.2	1.8	6.1	2.5	5.5	5.2	-	8.9	1.2	0.4	0.08	0.12	**1.0**	149
Oesophagus	95	0	-	-	-	-	-	-	-	1.8	1.0	6.2	8.3	16.6	15.2	20.1	14.7	18.1	35.3	53.3	4.9	1.6	0.25	0.42	**3.7**	150
Stomach	418	0	-	-	-	-	-	-	-	4.4	8.9	19.8	20.8	44.2	60.7	71.6	130.3	152.3	216.4	186.6	21.6	7.0	0.79	1.80	**15.5**	151
Small intestine	11	0	-	-	-	-	-	-	-	-	1.0	-	1.0	-	3.0	2.5	5.5	2.6	-	-	0.6	0.2	0.03	0.07	**0.4**	152
Colon	279	0	-	-	-	-	2.2	0.6	2.2	4.4	7.9	7.3	8.3	25.8	36.4	54.0	99.1	121.4	97.2	115.5	14.4	4.7	0.48	1.24	**10.3**	153
Rectum	238	1	-	-	-	-	1.1	0.6	-	0.9	3.9	7.3	13.5	15.6	38.4	65.3	66.1	87.8	97.2	88.8	12.3	4.0	0.41	1.07	**8.8**	154
Liver	196	0	-	-	-	-	-	-	0.7	2.7	3.9	5.2	7.3	17.5	28.3	50.2	56.9	82.6	75.1	80.0	10.1	3.3	0.33	0.86	**7.2**	155
Gallbladder etc.	82	0	-	-	-	-	-	0.6	-	-	-	2.1	4.2	6.4	7.1	18.8	33.0	46.5	35.3	17.8	4.2	1.4	0.10	0.36	**2.9**	156
Pancreas	138	0	-	-	-	-	-	-	-	2.7	1.0	7.3	9.3	13.8	23.3	35.2	31.2	54.2	26.5	71.1	7.1	2.3	0.29	0.62	**5.3**	157
Nose, sinuses etc.	20	0	-	-	-	-	-	0.6	-	-	-	2.1	2.1	1.8	2.0	2.5	11.0	2.6	-	17.8	1.0	0.3	0.04	0.11	**0.8**	160
Larynx	335	0	-	-	-	-	-	-	0.7	4.4	9.9	25.0	41.5	48.8	65.7	77.9	66.1	54.2	66.2	26.7	17.3	5.6	0.98	1.70	**13.7**	161
Bronchus, lung	1201	0	-	-	-	-	-	0.6	2.9	6.2	16.8	43.7	67.5	145.3	222.5	300.2	341.4	379.6	340.1	337.6	62.2	20.2	2.53	5.74	**45.3**	162
Other thoracic organs	11	0	0.8	-	0.6	1.1	-	0.7	-	-	-	1.0	-	1.0	-	5.5	-	4.4	-	-	0.6	0.2	0.03	0.05	**0.5**	163-4
Bone	21	0	-	0.7	1.2	1.7	0.6	-	-	0.9	-	2.1	-	1.8	4.0	1.3	1.8	5.2	4.4	-	1.1	0.4	0.06	0.08	**0.9**	170
Connective tissue	30	0	1.6	0.7	1.2	1.1	0.6	0.6	0.7	-	1.0	3.1	1.0	2.8	4.0	1.3	1.8	10.3	4.4	8.9	1.6	0.5	0.09	0.11	**1.4**	171
Mesothelioma	7	0	-	-	-	-	-	-	-	-	-	1.0	1.0	-	2.0	1.3	3.7	-	-	-	0.4	0.1	0.02	0.05	**0.3**	MES
Kaposi's sarcoma	12	0	-	-	-	-	1.1	0.6	0.7	-	1.0	1.0	-	0.9	1.0	2.5	1.8	-	-	8.9	0.6	0.2	0.03	0.05	**0.5**	KAP
Melanoma of skin	74	0	-	-	-	0.6	0.6	1.2	8.7	3.6	3.0	-	7.3	10.1	9.1	8.8	14.7	7.7	13.2	17.8	3.8	1.2	0.23	0.34	**3.1**	172
Other skin	1207	0	-	-	-	-	0.6	2.4	9.4	14.2	20.7	38.5	79.9	123.3	175.0	300.2	323.0	410.6	472.6	444.2	62.5		2.32	5.44	**45.3**	173
Breast	8	0	-	-	-	-	-	-	-	-	-	-	-	0.9	1.0	2.5	3.7	5.2	-	-	0.4	0.1	0.01	0.04	**0.3**	175
Prostate	454	0	-	-	-	-	-	-	-	-	1.0	1.0	3.1	17.5	49.6	90.4	156.0	289.2	318.0	355.4	23.5	7.7	0.36	1.59	**15.1**	185
Testis	32	0	0.8	-	0.6	1.7	4.4	3.6	2.9	0.9	3.9	3.1	-	-	-	1.8	-	-	-	-	1.7	0.5	0.11	0.12	**1.6**	186
Penis	27	0	-	-	-	-	-	-	0.7	-	1.0	1.0	1.0	0.9	3.0	3.8	11.0	10.3	13.2	26.7	1.4	0.5	0.04	0.11	**1.0**	187.1-.4
Other male genital	4	0	-	-	-	-	-	-	-	-	-	-	-	0.9	1.0	1.3	-	2.6	-	-	0.2	0.1	0.01	0.02	**0.1**	187.5-.9
Bladder	646	0	-	-	0.6	-	0.6	1.2	3.6	3.6	10.8	13.5	25.9	74.5	90.0	146.9	211.1	268.5	247.3	195.5	33.4	10.9	1.12	2.91	**23.5**	188
Kidney etc.	110	0	3.9	0.7	-	-	-	-	0.7	2.7	1.0	5.2	10.4	14.7	9.1	23.9	45.9	20.7	26.5	8.9	5.7	1.9	0.24	0.59	**4.6**	189
Eye	9	0	-	0.7	-	-	-	0.6	-	-	-	-	1.0	0.9	1.0	-	1.8	5.2	-	8.9	0.5	0.2	0.02	0.03	**0.4**	190
Brain, nervous system	139	0	3.9	2.7	1.2	1.1	1.7	1.8	2.9	2.7	5.9	9.4	14.5	17.5	18.2	17.6	33.0	20.7	22.1	17.8	7.2	2.3	0.42	0.67	**6.2**	191-2
Thyroid	24	0	-	-	-	-	1.1	0.6	0.7	4.4	1.0	-	1.0	4.6	4.0	1.3	3.7	2.6	-	-	1.2	0.4	0.09	0.11	**1.0**	193
Other endocrine	6	0	0.8	0.7	-	-	-	0.6	-	-	-	-	1.0	-	1.0	1.3	-	-	-	-	0.3	0.1	0.02	0.03	**0.3**	194
Hodgkin's disease	44	0	-	1.4	2.3	1.1	2.8	4.2	1.4	1.8	3.0	3.1	3.1	2.8	3.0	2.5	1.8	2.6	4.4	-	2.3	0.7	0.15	0.17	**2.1**	201
Non-Hodgkin lymphoma	127	0	2.3	2.0	0.6	1.7	1.1	3.6	2.9	3.6	8.9	8.3	10.4	6.4	20.2	25.1	14.7	20.7	39.7	17.8	6.6	2.1	0.36	0.56	**5.6**	200,202
Multiple myeloma	63	0	-	-	-	-	-	0.6	-	0.9	1.0	1.0	6.2	5.5	12.1	12.6	14.7	28.4	26.5	-	3.3	1.1	0.14	0.27	**2.3**	203
Lymphoid leukaemia	78	0	4.7	0.7	1.2	1.1	2.8	0.6	0.7	1.8	1.0	1.0	1.0	5.5	8.1	11.3	25.7	18.1	39.7	17.8	4.0	1.3	0.15	0.34	**3.3**	204
Myeloid leukaemia	63	0	-	0.7	0.6	-	1.1	0.6	1.4	0.9	-	4.2	5.2	5.5	7.1	21.4	11.0	12.9	13.2	17.8	3.3	1.1	0.14	0.30	**2.6**	205
Monocytic leukaemia	3	0	-	-	-	-	-	-	-	-	1.0	-	-	-	1.3	1.8	-	-	-	-	0.2	0.1	0.00	0.02	**0.1**	206
Other leukaemia	2	0	-	-	-	-	-	-	-	-	-	1.0	-	-	1.8	-	-	-	-	-	0.1	0.0	0.01	0.01	**0.1**	207
Leukaemia unspecified	16	0	-	-	-	-	-	-	-	0.9	1.0	-	1.0	0.9	2.0	2.5	3.7	7.7	13.2	-	0.8	0.3	0.03	0.06	**0.6**	208
Other and unspecified	294	0	-	-	-	-	0.6	0.6	0.7	1.8	10.8	7.3	16.6	24.8	41.5	65.3	108.3	85.2	123.7	133.3	15.2	5.0	0.52	1.39	**11.1**	O&U
All sites	7138	1	18.7	10.9	9.9	11.0	25.0	29.1	50.7	83.6	161.7	267.3	451.4	740.5	1074.1	1576.2	1971.1	2349.8	2526.3	2390.0	369.4		14.67	32.41	**273.3**	ALL
All sites but 173	5931	1	18.7	10.9	9.9	11.0	24.5	26.7	41.3	69.4	141.0	228.8	371.5	617.2	899.1	1276.0	1648.1	1939.2	2053.7	1945.8	307.0	100.0	12.35	26.98	**228.0**	ALLb

			0-	5-	10-	15-	20-	25-	30-	35-	40-	45-	50-	55-	60-	65-	70-	75-	80-	85+
Rate from 1 case			0.779	0.683	0.580	0.551	0.556	0.606	0.725	0.889	0.986	1.040	1.038	0.920	1.011	1.256	1.835	2.582	4.417	8.885

SPAIN, GRANADA 1988-1992

ANNUAL INCIDENCE PER 100,000 BY AGE GROUP (YEARS) - FEMALE

SITE	ALL AGES	AGE UNK	0-	5-	10-	15-	20-	25-	30-	35-	40-	45-	50-	55-	60-	65-	70-	75-	80-	85+	CRUDE RATE	%	CR 64	CR 74	ASR (W)	ICD (9th)
Lip	28	0	-	-	-	-	-	-	-	-	0.9	-	1.0	0.9	5.5	2.2	2.7	12.2	12.9	12.3	1.4	0.7	0.04	0.07	**0.7**	140
Tongue	16	0	-	-	-	-	-	0.6	1.5	-	-	-	1.9	0.9	4.6	3.2	1.4	-	-	4.1	0.8	0.4	0.05	0.07	**0.6**	141
Salivary gland	11	0	-	-	0.6	0.6	-	0.6	0.7	-	0.9	1.0	-	-	-	1.1	-	1.7	7.7	-	0.5	0.3	0.02	0.03	**0.4**	142
Mouth	30	0	-	-	-	-	0.6	0.6	-	-	-	3.0	1.0	4.4	2.8	6.5	5.5	3.5	10.3	-	1.5	0.7	0.06	0.12	**1.0**	143-5
Oropharynx	0	0	-	-	-	-	-	-	-	-	-	-	-	-	-	-	-	-	-	-	0.0	0.0	0.00	0.00	**0.0**	146
Nasopharynx	8	0	-	-	-	-	0.6	-	-	0.9	-	-	1.0	0.9	0.9	1.1	-	1.7	2.6	-	0.4	0.2	0.02	0.03	**0.3**	147
Hypopharynx	0	0	-	-	-	-	-	-	-	-	-	-	-	-	-	-	-	-	-	-	0.0	0.0	0.00	0.00	**0.0**	148
Pharynx unspecified	2	0	-	-	-	-	-	-	-	-	-	-	-	0.9	-	1.1	-	-	-	-	0.1	0.0	0.00	0.01	**0.1**	149
Oesophagus	19	0	-	-	-	-	-	-	-	-	0.9	-	-	3.5	1.8	1.1	4.1	7.0	5.2	8.2	0.9	0.5	0.03	0.06	**0.5**	150
Stomach	250	0	-	-	-	-	-	1.2	2.9	4.4	7.6	7.9	9.7	14.8	17.5	28.0	48.0	83.8	95.4	127.6	12.5	6.0	0.33	0.71	**7.0**	151
Small intestine	9	0	-	-	-	-	-	-	-	-	-	1.0	-	1.7	0.9	2.2	1.4	3.5	-	-	0.4	0.2	0.02	0.04	**0.3**	152
Colon	296	0	-	-	0.6	-	0.6	1.9	1.5	5.3	12.3	7.9	17.4	17.4	34.2	44.1	50.7	89.0	79.9	111.1	14.7	7.2	0.49	0.97	**9.0**	153
Rectum	184	0	-	-	-	0.6	-	-	2.2	2.6	2.8	4.0	12.6	20.9	21.2	30.1	35.7	52.4	43.8	37.0	9.2	4.4	0.33	0.66	**5.6**	154
Liver	136	0	-	-	-	0.6	-	-	-	-	-	1.0	3.9	6.1	12.0	17.2	28.8	34.9	67.1	111.1	6.8	3.3	0.12	0.35	**3.4**	155
Gallbladder etc.	177	0	-	-	-	-	-	-	-	-	-	-	6.8	15.7	17.5	29.0	45.3	52.4	61.9	78.2	8.8	4.3	0.20	0.57	**4.7**	156
Pancreas	121	0	-	-	-	-	-	0.6	0.7	-	-	3.0	3.9	10.5	14.8	15.1	19.2	43.6	67.1	20.6	6.0	2.9	0.17	0.34	**3.2**	157
Nose, sinuses etc.	5	0	-	-	-	-	-	-	-	-	-	-	-	-	-	1.1	-	3.5	-	8.2	0.2	0.1	0.00	0.01	**0.1**	160
Larynx	5	0	-	-	-	-	-	-	-	-	-	-	1.0	-	-	-	-	-	2.6	12.3	0.2	0.1	0.00	0.00	**0.1**	161
Bronchus, lung	92	0	-	-	-	-	0.6	-	-	0.9	-	2.0	6.8	11.3	10.2	10.8	23.3	22.7	23.2	32.9	4.6	2.2	0.16	0.33	**2.7**	162
Other thoracic organs	7	0	2.5	-	-	-	-	-	-	-	-	-	-	2.6	-	1.1	-	-	-	-	0.3	0.2	0.03	0.03	**0.4**	163-4
Bone	17	0	-	0.7	2.4	1.1	0.6	1.2	-	-	-	-	-	-	1.8	1.1	1.4	1.7	2.6	4.1	0.8	0.4	0.04	0.05	**0.7**	170
Connective tissue	33	0	0.8	0.7	-	1.1	-	1.2	2.2	0.9	-	1.0	2.9	1.7	4.6	2.2	1.4	8.7	7.7	4.1	1.6	0.8	0.09	0.10	**1.3**	171
Mesothelioma	4	0	-	-	-	-	-	-	-	-	-	-	-	0.9	2.2	-	1.7	-	-	-	0.2	0.1	0.00	0.02	**0.1**	MES
Kaposi's sarcoma	1	0	-	-	-	-	-	-	-	-	-	-	-	0.9	-	-	-	-	-	-	0.0	0.0	0.00	0.00	**0.0**	KAP
Melanoma of skin	93	0	-	0.7	-	-	1.1	2.5	2.2	3.5	8.5	10.9	11.6	12.2	12.0	7.5	4.1	5.2	5.2	20.6	4.6	2.2	0.33	0.38	**3.9**	172
Other skin	900	0	-	-	1.7	1.7	2.5	6.5	8.8	16.1	33.6	54.1	72.4	83.1	127.9	170.1	214.7	371.4	333.3	44.8		1.40	2.89	**26.2**	173
Breast	973	1	-	-	-	0.6	0.6	8.0	18.1	43.1	73.1	92.9	99.5	106.3	129.2	117.2	133.0	125.7	100.6	123.5	48.5	23.5	2.86	4.11	**37.4**	174
Uterus unspecified	10	0	-	-	-	-	0.6	-	-	-	-	-	-	-	1.1	-	3.5	5.2	16.5	0.5	0.2	0.00	0.01	**0.2**	179
Cervix uteri	146	0	-	-	-	0.6	1.9	5.1	9.7	11.4	9.9	13.5	11.3	22.2	10.8	26.1	19.2	15.5	20.6	7.3	3.5	0.43	0.61	**5.6**	180
Placenta	2	0	-	-	-	-	0.6	-	0.9	-	-	-	-	-	-	-	-	-	-	0.1	0.0	0.01	0.01	**0.1**	181
Corpus uteri	271	0	-	-	-	-	-	1.2	0.7	4.4	3.8	10.9	23.2	40.1	36.0	55.9	50.7	41.9	38.7	45.3	13.5	6.5	0.60	1.13	**9.0**	182
Ovary etc.	177	0	-	1.4	-	1.1	0.6	0.6	2.9	6.2	9.5	14.8	13.5	20.9	21.2	23.7	30.2	21.0	41.3	8.2	8.8	4.3	0.46	0.73	**6.5**	183
Other female genital	66	0	0.8	-	-	-	-	-	-	-	-	-	2.9	5.2	5.5	14.0	15.1	15.7	30.9	20.6	3.3	1.6	0.07	0.22	**1.8**	184
Bladder	111	0	-	-	-	-	-	0.6	-	1.8	1.9	1.0	2.9	5.2	6.5	15.1	27.4	38.4	41.3	70.0	5.5	2.7	0.10	0.31	**2.9**	188
Kidney etc.	72	0	1.6	-	-	-	0.6	-	0.7	0.9	-	4.0	7.7	8.7	6.5	11.8	11.0	17.5	12.9	16.5	3.6	1.7	0.15	0.27	**2.5**	189
Eye	5	0	-	-	-	-	-	-	-	-	-	1.0	-	-	3.2	1.4	-	-	-	-	0.2	0.1	0.00	0.03	**0.2**	190
Brain, nervous system	102	0	3.3	1.4	1.8	-	2.3	0.6	2.2	1.8	1.9	5.9	10.6	7.8	12.9	18.3	13.7	15.7	7.7	8.2	5.1	2.5	0.26	0.42	**4.1**	191-2
Thyroid	67	0	-	-	0.6	2.3	4.0	3.7	3.6	7.0	3.8	5.9	1.9	7.8	0.9	8.6	8.2	-	-	-	3.3	1.6	0.21	0.29	**3.0**	193
Other endocrine	8	0	2.5	-	-	0.6	0.6	0.6	0.7	-	-	-	1.0	0.9	-	-	-	-	-	-	0.4	0.2	0.03	0.03	**0.5**	194
Hodgkin's disease	32	0	-	0.7	-	1.1	3.4	3.7	2.9	0.9	-	1.0	1.9	2.6	0.9	2.2	-	1.7	-	8.2	1.6	0.8	0.10	0.11	**1.4**	201
Non-Hodgkin lymphoma	117	0	1.6	1.4	1.2	1.1	1.1	1.9	2.2	3.5	5.7	3.0	6.8	7.8	12.9	17.2	26.1	26.2	5.2	24.7	5.8	2.8	0.25	0.47	**4.3**	200,202
Multiple myeloma	55	0	-	-	-	-	-	-	-	-	-	4.0	2.9	4.4	11.1	11.8	8.2	10.5	18.1	4.1	2.7	1.3	0.11	0.21	**1.7**	203
Lymphoid leukaemia	54	0	5.8	2.9	3.0	1.7	0.6	0.6	0.7	1.8	-	-	2.9	1.7	2.8	5.4	12.3	3.5	12.9	4.1	2.7	1.3	0.12	0.21	**2.5**	204
Myeloid leukaemia	48	0	0.8	-	-	-	-	2.5	0.7	-	3.0	3.9	3.5	7.4	4.3	6.9	19.2	-	8.2	2.4	1.2	0.11	0.17	**1.7**	205
Monocytic leukaemia	5	0	-	-	-	-	-	0.6	-	-	0.9	1.0	-	-	1.1	1.4	-	-	-	0.2	0.1	0.01	0.03	**0.2**	206
Other leukaemia	2	0	0.8	-	-	-	-	-	-	-	-	-	0.9	-	-	-	-	-	-	0.1	0.0	0.01	0.01	**0.1**	207
Leukaemia unspecified	27	0	-	-	-	0.6	-	0.6	0.7	-	2.8	1.0	1.0	-	2.8	-	6.9	7.0	12.9	8.2	1.3	0.7	0.05	0.08	**0.8**	208
Other and unspecified	245	0	0.8	-	-	-	-	0.6	1.5	1.8	1.9	2.0	4.8	14.8	21.2	22.6	53.5	80.3	113.5	164.6	12.2	5.9	0.25	0.63	**6.2**	O&U
All sites	5039	1	21.4	10.1	10.3	14.3	20.0	42.1	63.1	111.7	167.1	237.1	336.0	449.8	546.4	679.5	875.0	1091.2	1322.9	1477.4	251.0		10.15	17.92	**165.0**	ALL
All sites but 173	4139	1	21.4	10.1	10.3	12.6	18.3	39.6	56.6	102.9	150.9	203.5	281.9	377.4	463.4	551.5	704.9	876.4	951.6	1144.0	206.2	100.0	8.75	15.03	**138.8**	ALLb

Rate from 1 case   0.825 0.719 0.608 0.571 0.572 0.619 0.726 0.880 0.949 0.988 0.966 0.872 0.923 1.075 1.371 1.746 2.579 4.115

Spain, Mallorca

The Cancer Registry of Mallorca (Majorca) began its activities in 1982 under the auspices of the Consell Insular de Mallorca. It initially functioned as a specialized registry for colo-rectal cancer, providing a basis for a variety of clinical and epidemiological research activities. In 1989, the registry extended its coverage to all types of cancer and became population-based. It operates within a Cancer Epidemiology Unit, which has as its main objective the descriptive epidemiology of cancer, to contribute to the elucidation of causal factors and to support planning and prevention activities.

The Unitat d'Epidemiologia i Registre de Càncer de Mallorca has been supported and financed by the following institutions: the Consell Insular de Mallorca, the Conselleria de Sanitat del Govern Balear, the Insalud, the Universitat de les Illes Balears and the Junta Provincial de Baleares de la Asociación Española contra el Cáncer. The Grup d'Estudi del Cáncer Colo-rectal (colo-rectal cancer study group), a private non-profitmaking organization, is in charge of the project.

The registry personnel consists of a director (part-time), an epidemiologist, an oncologist, a physician and two secretaries (full time) and another doctor and two auxiliaries (part-time). The oncologist coordinates the work of the registry, and a doctor, a secretary and the two auxiliaries work exclusively on collecting and processing the data. Advice is available from the oncologists and pathologists of the island, the Cancer Registry of Tarragona and the Institut Catalá d'Oncologia.

The population covered by the registry is that permanently resident in Mallorca, the largest and central island in the Balearic Archipelago. Coverage of the rest of the archipelago came into effect in 1993.

Mallorca is situated in the Mediterranean Sea, 200 km from the Spanish coast, between 39°15′ and 39°57′ N. Its total area is 3625 km. In 1990, the population comprised 284 922 males and 296 462 females. This population is relatively stable, with 72% of the population born locally, 25% in other regions of Spain (who migrated mainly in the 1960s) and 3% foreigners. Around 6 000 000 tourists visit Mallorca every year.

Among the employed population, 4% belong to the primary sector, 28% to the secondary sector and 66% to the services sector.

Around half of the population is concentrated in Palma de Mallorca, the capital, which is the only municipality with more than 100 000 inhabitants. Given the small distance to the capital from any part of the island, the types of occupation and geographical factors, Mallorca may be considered an entirely urban area. It is also considered as a single area in terms of health care, and most of the public and private hospitals are situated in Palma. There are 1729 beds in the public sector (of which 520 are psychiatric) and 752 beds in the private sector. There are 3.4 beds per 1000 inhabitants, excluding the beds for psychiatric patients). There are 2.86 doctors and 2.96 nurses per 1000 inhabitants.

Mallorca has six pathology laboratories (three public and three private), three radiotherapy services (one public and two private), five oncology services (two public and three private) and four haematology laboratories (two public and two private). All provide information to the registry. The medical records departments of the private and public hospitals also collaborate, as do physicians and specialists who are asked to provide missing information.

Notification of cancer is voluntary. For 1988–92, 30% of the cases were notified using automated medical information systems and 70% through active collection. The registry does not have access to death statistics for reasons of confidentiality, but information on death certificates is actively collected in all the municipalities. This transcription of causes of death from a document which is not 'official' could result in errors, but where possible, the cause of death is checked against information in the registry and the clinical history.

The definition of a registrable case refers to tumours and not patients, and multiple tumours are coded following the IARC/IACR rules. Squamous cell and basal cell carcinomas of skin are recorded only once, and the morphology code of the tumour diagnosed first is assigned. The registry records invasive and *in situ* diagnoses, excluding those which are benign and of uncertain behaviour. Uncertain tumours of the central nervous system are always registered when detected through the death certificate alone.

The individual records are checked for inconsistencies and duplicates, and then processed by computer. The software performs logical controls to detect possible errors and duplicates.

During the period 1988–92, 61 (0.6%) of cases were excluded as it could not be confirmed that they were resident on the island and 35 (0.35%) were lacking adequate information on items such as site and date of diagnosis. Some cases who were temporary residents might not be included in the census population, which may have led to small errors in the incidence data.

The creation of the general population-based registry has improved coverage and timeliness in the colo-rectal programme. Other indicators, such as percentage of histological verification, proportion first notified by death certificates, percentage of DCO, and the number of notifications per case confirm this conclusion.

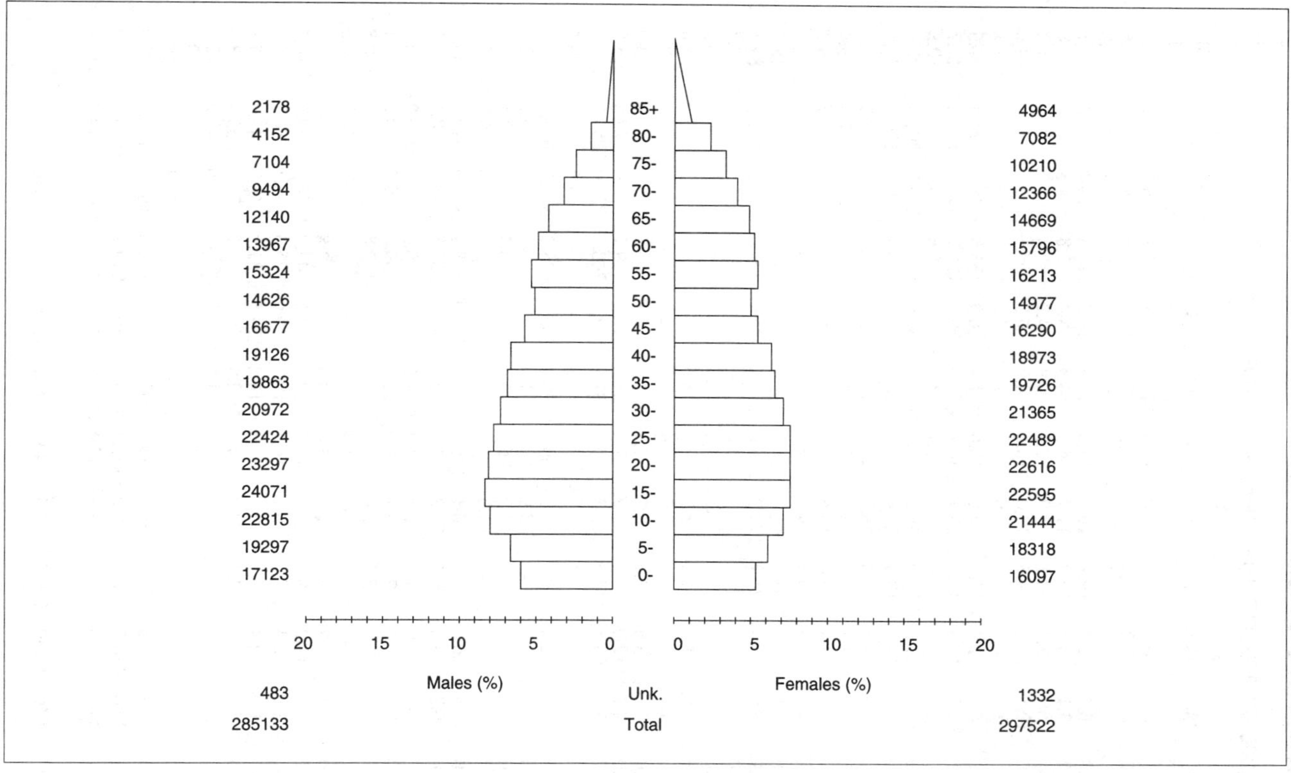

Spain, Mallorca

Source of population: average annual 1988–92
Census: 1991
Estimate: The 1988, 1989 and 1990 populations were calculated by linear interpolation between the 1986 and the 1991 Censuses, taking into consideration births, deaths and migration. The 1991 population was based on the 1991 Census, corrected by the post-censal rectifications up to 1 January 1992, and applying the age-structure of the 1991 Census. The 1992 population was estimated by a projection of the previous years based on the hypothesis of a null migratory flow. *Reference:* L'experenca de vida a les Balears. Institut Balear d'Estadistica, 1995.

Notes to tables overleaf:
† 173 does not include basal cell or squamous cell carcinomas

SPAIN, MALLORCA 1988-1992

ANNUAL INCIDENCE PER 100,000 BY AGE GROUP (YEARS) - MALE

SITE	ALL AGES	AGE UNK	0-	5-	10-	15-	20-	25-	30-	35-	40-	45-	50-	55-	60-	65-	70-	75-	80-	85+	CRUDE RATE	%	CR 64	CR 74	ASR (W)	ICD (9th)
Lip	122	1	-	-	-	-	-	-	1.0	-	4.2	10.8	12.3	20.9	18.6	42.8	21.1	59.1	38.5	36.7	8.6	2.0	0.34	0.66	5.9	140
Tongue	51	1	-	-	-	-	-	-	-	1.0	4.2	7.2	10.9	5.2	15.8	9.9	10.5	11.3	4.8	-	3.6	0.9	0.23	0.33	2.8	141
Salivary gland	12	0	-	-	-	-	-	-	-	-	1.2	1.4	-	-	6.6	2.1	8.4	4.8	9.2		0.8	0.2	0.01	0.06	0.5	142
Mouth	87	1	-	-	-	-	-	-	1.0	3.0	6.3	12.0	19.1	19.6	15.8	16.5	16.9	11.3	14.4	9.2	6.1	1.5	0.39	0.56	4.8	143-5
Oropharynx	54	0	-	-	-	-	-	-	-	4.0	3.1	6.0	10.9	11.7	14.3	14.8	8.4	2.8	4.8	-	3.8	0.9	0.25	0.37	3.0	146
Nasopharynx	17	0	-	1.0	-	-	-	-	1.0	-	-	2.4	4.1	3.9	2.9	4.9	4.2	-	-	-	1.2	0.3	0.08	0.12	1.0	147
Hypopharynx	66	0	-	-	-	-	-	-	-	4.0	10.5	13.2	9.6	17.0	18.6	4.9	6.3	5.6	-	-	4.6	1.1	0.36	0.42	3.9	148
Pharynx unspecified	16	0	-	-	-	-	-	-	-	1.0	6.0	2.7	2.6	4.3	1.6	4.2	-	-	-	-	1.1	0.3	0.08	0.11	1.0	149
Oesophagus	108	0	-	-	-	-	-	-	2.0	6.3	12.0	17.8	17.0	18.6	21.4	16.9	33.8	48.2	73.4		7.6	1.8	0.37	0.56	5.5	150
Stomach	252	0	-	-	-	-	-	1.8	-	9.1	3.1	15.6	13.7	28.7	40.1	67.5	99.0	126.7	96.3	110.2	17.7	4.2	0.56	1.39	11.6	151
Small intestine	12	0	-	-	-	-	-	-	-	-	1.0	-	1.4	-	5.7	3.3	-	5.6	9.6	-	0.8	0.2	0.04	0.06	0.6	152
Colon	405	0	-	-	-	-	0.9	0.9	2.9	7.0	11.5	21.6	15.0	39.2	85.9	108.7	130.6	191.4	216.7	201.9	28.4	6.8	0.92	2.12	18.4	153
Rectum	285	0	-	-	-	-	-	0.9	1.9	2.0	12.5	18.0	10.9	27.4	51.5	80.7	101.1	146.4	130.0	110.2	20.0	4.8	0.63	1.54	13.0	154
Liver	147	0	-	-	-	-	0.9	-	1.9	-	1.0	7.2	9.6	26.1	48.7	42.8	46.3	36.6	48.2	45.9	10.3	2.5	0.48	0.92	7.2	155
Gallbladder etc.	48	0	-	-	-	-	-	-	1.0	1.0	1.0	2.4	-	3.9	11.5	13.2	21.1	16.9	24.1	27.5	3.4	0.8	0.10	0.28	2.2	156
Pancreas	133	0	-	-	-	-	-	-	1.0	-	3.1	8.4	15.0	19.6	18.6	41.2	35.8	39.4	110.8	36.7	9.3	2.2	0.33	0.71	6.1	157
Nose, sinuses etc.	15	0	-	-	-	-	-	-	1.0	-	-	1.2	2.7	3.9	5.7	1.6	-	2.8	9.6	-	1.1	0.3	0.07	0.08	0.8	160
Larynx	259	0	-	-	-	-	-	-	1.9	4.0	12.5	25.2	35.6	61.3	74.5	69.2	50.6	59.1	19.3	36.7	18.2	4.3	1.08	1.67	13.8	161
Bronchus, lung	1271	0	-	-	-	-	-	-	5.7	16.1	35.6	74.4	121.7	174.9	295.0	377.2	446.6	444.8	390.1	403.9	89.1	21.3	3.62	7.74	61.4	162
Other thoracic organs	10	0	1.2	-	-	-	-	-	1.0	2.0	-	1.2	-	-	4.3	-	-	2.8	4.8	-	0.7	0.2	0.05	0.05	0.6	163-4
Bone	11	0	-	-	1.8	2.5	0.9	-	-	-	-	-	-	1.4	-	4.2	5.6	-	-	0.8	0.2	0.03	0.05	0.6	170
Connective tissue	28	0	1.2	-	1.8	0.8	2.6	-	1.0	-	1.0	1.2	1.4	1.3	1.4	6.6	6.3	11.3	19.3	-	2.0	0.5	0.07	0.13	1.5	171
Mesothelioma	6	0	-	-	-	-	-	0.9	-	-	1.0	-	-	1.3	1.4	1.6	2.1	-	-	-	0.4	0.1	0.02	0.04	0.3	MES
Kaposi's sarcoma	43	0	-	-	-	0.8	2.6	4.5	12.4	3.0	6.3	3.6	4.1	3.9	1.4	1.6	2.1	-	-	-	3.0	0.7	0.21	0.23	2.7	KAP
Melanoma of skin	69	0	-	-	-	-	1.7	2.7	1.9	3.0	4.2	12.0	8.2	5.2	7.2	21.4	10.5	19.7	9.6	27.5	4.8	1.2	0.23	0.39	3.8	172
†Other skin	1928	71	-	-	0.9	2.5	3.4	8.9	16.2	23.2	49.1	93.5	144.9	232.3	350.8	487.6	577.2	760.1	915.0	1055.6	135.2		4.81	10.33	89.7	173
Breast	5	0	-	-	-	-	-	-	-	-	-	1.4	-	-	3.3	-	-	9.6	-	-	0.4	0.1	0.01	0.02	0.2	175
Prostate	605	4	-	-	-	-	-	-	-	-	-	2.4	9.6	30.0	60.1	120.3	263.3	408.2	524.9	688.5	42.4	10.1	0.51	2.44	23.4	185
Testis	28	0	-	-	-	0.8	4.3	5.4	4.8	3.0	3.1	-	3.9	-	1.6	-	-	-	-	9.2	2.0	0.5	0.13	0.13	1.8	186
Penis	24	1	-	-	-	-	-	-	-	1.0	-	-	3.9	5.7	6.6	6.3	8.4	9.6	27.5	1.7	0.4	0.06	0.12	1.1	187.1-.4
Other male genital	3	0	-	-	-	-	-	-	-	-	-	-	1.3	-	-	-	-	4.8	9.2	0.2	0.1	0.01	0.01	0.1	187.5-.9
Bladder	791	5	-	-	-	0.8	-	1.8	2.9	6.0	11.5	30.0	49.2	90.1	176.1	227.3	334.9	318.1	317.9	312.1	55.5	13.2	1.85	4.68	36.4	188
Kidney etc.	130	0	1.2	1.0	-	-	0.9	1.8	-	2.0	6.3	8.4	9.6	22.2	21.5	36.2	46.3	53.5	28.9	18.4	9.1	2.2	0.37	0.79	6.5	189
Eye	9	0	1.2	-	-	-	-	-	-	-	-	-	1.4	2.6	1.4	1.6	-	5.6	-	9.2	0.6	0.2	0.03	0.04	0.5	190
Brain, nervous system	115	0	2.3	3.1	3.5	1.7	-	2.7	1.0	5.0	7.3	9.6	12.3	13.1	20.0	21.4	35.8	39.4	9.6	9.2	8.1	1.9	0.41	0.69	6.4	191-2
Thyroid	12	0	-	-	0.9	-	-	0.9	-	-	-	1.0	1.2	5.5	2.6	-	-	2.1	2.8	-	0.8	0.2	0.06	0.07	0.7	193
Other endocrine	4	0	3.5	-	-	-	-	-	-	-	-	-	-	1.4	-	-	-	-	-	-	0.3	0.1	0.02	0.02	0.5	194
Hodgkin's disease	37	0	1.2	1.0	-	3.3	3.4	3.6	2.9	7.0	3.1	1.2	4.1	2.6	1.4	3.3	-	2.8	-	-	2.6	0.6	0.17	0.19	2.5	201
Non-Hodgkin lymphoma	150	0	2.3	1.0	0.9	4.2	5.2	1.8	3.8	10.1	9.4	13.2	9.6	13.1	12.9	37.9	42.1	47.9	48.2	27.5	10.5	2.5	0.44	0.84	7.9	200,202
Multiple myeloma	66	0	-	-	-	-	-	-	1.0	-	1.0	2.4	2.7	9.1	14.3	19.8	19.0	25.3	43.3	36.7	4.6	1.1	0.15	0.35	3.0	203
Lymphoid leukaemia	76	0	3.5	5.2	3.5	1.7	0.9	-	-	-	1.0	2.4	-	2.6	10.0	14.8	29.5	31.0	48.2	45.9	5.3	1.3	0.15	0.38	4.0	204
Myeloid leukaemia	54	0	1.2	-	0.9	-	0.9	0.9	4.8	1.0	2.1	-	4.1	7.8	4.3	4.9	19.0	19.7	24.1	55.1	3.8	0.9	0.14	0.26	2.6	205
Monocytic leukaemia	4	0	-	-	-	-	-	-	-	-	-	-	-	-	-	1.6	-	-	9.6	9.2	0.3	0.1	0.00	0.01	0.1	206
Other leukaemia	0	0	-	-	-	-	-	-	-	-	-	-	-	-	-	-	-	-	-	-	0.0	0.0	0.00	0.00	0.0	207
Leukaemia unspecified	9	0	1.2	-	-	-	-	-	-	-	-	-	1.4	-	-	-	2.1	2.8	14.4	18.4	0.6	0.2	0.01	0.02	0.4	208
Other and unspecified	326	0	-	-	-	0.8	-	-	1.9	6.0	5.2	9.6	24.6	56.1	54.4	95.5	111.6	112.6	168.6	174.4	22.9	5.5	0.79	1.83	15.0	O&U
All sites	7903	84	19.9	12.4	14.0	19.9	28.3	39.2	75.3	125.9	230.0	436.5	608.5	988.0	1497.7	2044.4	2536.2	3079.7	3380.9	3635.0	554.3		20.70	43.85	375.9	ALL
All sites but 173	5975	13	19.9	12.4	13.1	17.4	24.9	30.3	59.1	102.7	180.9	343.0	463.5	755.7	1146.9	1556.8	1959.0	2319.6	2465.8	2579.4	419.1	100.0	15.88	33.50	286.1	ALLb

Rate from 1 case: 1.168 1.036 0.877 0.831 0.858 0.892 0.954 1.007 1.046 1.199 1.367 1.305 1.432 1.647 2.107 2.815 4.816 9.179

†Important: see notes on population page

SPAIN, MALLORCA 1988-1992

ANNUAL INCIDENCE PER 100,000 BY AGE GROUP (YEARS) - FEMALE

SITE	ALL AGES	AGE UNK	0-	5-	10-	15-	20-	25-	30-	35-	40-	45-	50-	55-	60-	65-	70-	75-	80-	85+	CRUDE RATE	%	CR 64	CR 74	ASR (W)	ICD (9th)
Lip	14	0	-	-	-	-	-	-	-	-	2.1	-	1.2	1.3	2.7	-	7.8	5.6	8.1	0.9	0.3	0.02	0.04	**0.5**	*140*
Tongue	13	0	-	-	-	-	-	1.0	-	1.2	4.0	-	1.3	1.4	-	3.9	5.6	8.1	0.9	0.3	0.04	0.04	**0.5**	*141*
Salivary gland	4	0	-	-	-	-	-	-	-	-	-	1.2	-	1.2	-	1.4	-	-	-	4.0	0.3	0.1	0.01	0.02	**0.2**	*142*
Mouth	17	0	-	-	-	-	-	-	-	-	1.1	-	1.3	2.5	3.8	1.4	6.5	2.0	2.8	12.1	1.1	0.4	0.04	0.08	**0.6**	*143-5*
Oropharynx	6	0	-	-	-	-	-	-	1.0	-	-	-	1.2	2.5	-	1.6	-	-	4.0	0.4	0.1	0.02	0.03	**0.3**	*146*
Nasopharynx	6	0	-	-	-	-	-	-	1.0	1.1	1.2	-	-	-	4.1	-	-	-	-	-	0.4	0.1	0.02	0.03	**0.3**	*147*
Hypopharynx	1	0	-	-	-	-	-	-	-	-	-	-	1.2	-	-	-	-	-	-	-	0.1	0.0	0.01	0.01	**0.0**	*148*
Pharynx unspecified	3	0	-	-	-	-	-	-	-	-	-	-	-	1.3	-	1.6	2.0	-	-	0.2	0.1	0.01	0.01	**0.1**	*149*
Oesophagus	16	0	-	-	-	-	-	-	-	1.0	1.1	-	2.7	-	2.5	1.4	-	3.9	5.6	20.1	1.1	0.4	0.04	0.04	**0.6**	*150*
Stomach	176	0	-	-	-	-	0.9	0.9	1.9	4.1	3.2	8.6	14.7	16.0	17.7	16.4	43.7	68.6	70.6	84.6	11.8	4.1	0.34	0.64	**6.1**	*151*
Small intestine	12	0	-	-	-	-	-	-	-	-	1.1	1.2	1.3	-	1.3	-	3.2	5.9	8.5	-	0.8	0.3	0.02	0.04	**0.4**	*152*
Colon	425	0	-	-	-	-	0.9	1.8	6.6	4.1	5.3	28.2	32.0	32.1	55.7	77.7	111.6	146.9	115.8	189.3	28.6	10.0	0.83	1.78	**15.5**	*153*
Rectum	223	0	-	-	-	-	-	-	0.9	3.0	5.3	3.7	10.7	22.2	41.8	32.7	55.0	60.7	113.0	92.7	15.0	5.2	0.44	0.88	**7.6**	*154*
Liver	80	0	-	-	-	-	-	-	-	-	2.7	6.2	10.1	13.6	16.2	35.3	22.6	76.5	5.4	1.9	0.09	0.24	**2.4**	*155*
Gallbladder etc.	113	0	-	-	-	-	-	-	0.9	-	1.1	-	2.7	1.2	12.7	17.7	37.2	49.0	64.9	56.4	7.6	2.6	0.09	0.37	**3.2**	*156*
Pancreas	100	0	-	-	-	-	-	0.9	-	-	1.0	2.1	2.5	2.7	9.9	10.1	15.0	35.6	25.5	50.8	48.3	6.7	2.3	0.15	0.40	**3.3**	*157*
Nose, sinuses etc.	4	0	-	-	-	-	-	-	-	-	-	1.2	-	1.3	2.7	-	-	-	-	0.3	0.1	0.01	0.03	**0.2**	*160*
Larynx	7	0	-	-	-	-	-	-	-	-	2.5	1.3	1.2	2.5	-	1.6	-	-	-	0.5	0.2	0.04	0.05	**0.4**	*161*
Bronchus, lung	111	0	-	-	-	-	-	0.9	2.8	3.0	4.2	4.9	5.3	17.3	11.4	23.2	29.1	47.0	22.6	8.1	7.5	2.6	0.25	0.51	**4.3**	*162*
Other thoracic organs	6	0	1.2	-	-	-	-	-	-	2.0	1.1	-	1.3	-	-	-	-	-	2.8	-	0.4	0.1	0.03	0.03	**0.4**	*163-4*
Bone	9	0	-	1.1	2.8	-	-	0.9	0.9	-	-	1.2	-	1.2	-	-	-	-	-	4.0	0.6	0.2	0.04	0.04	**0.6**	*170*
Connective tissue	29	0	-	2.2	-	0.9	0.9	1.8	1.9	3.0	2.1	-	-	1.2	3.8	5.5	8.1	3.9	-	4.0	1.9	0.7	0.09	0.16	**1.5**	*171*
Mesothelioma	6	0	-	-	-	-	-	-	-	-	-	-	-	1.2	1.3	1.4	3.2	2.0	-	-	0.4	0.1	0.01	0.04	**0.2**	*MES*
Kaposi's sarcoma	3	0	-	-	-	-	0.9	-	-	-	1.1	-	-	-	1.3	-	-	-	-	0.2	0.1	0.02	0.02	**0.2**	*KAP*
Melanoma of skin	85	2	-	-	-	0.9	1.8	2.7	2.8	8.1	7.4	7.4	4.0	2.5	10.1	16.4	16.2	5.9	14.1	40.3	5.7	2.0	0.24	0.41	**3.9**	*172*
†Other skin	1654	74	1.2	-	1.9	-	3.5	14.2	18.7	38.5	46.4	95.8	102.8	134.5	207.6	260.4	349.3	466.2	581.7	709.0	111.2		3.48	6.67	**61.2**	*173*
Breast	1084	2	-	-	-	-	0.9	5.3	32.8	51.7	89.6	119.1	126.9	153.0	167.1	170.4	207.0	170.4	211.8	165.2	72.9	25.4	3.74	5.63	**50.2**	*174*
Uterus unspecified	20	0	-	-	-	-	-	-	-	-	-	-	1.3	1.2	2.5	-	4.9	5.9	16.9	16.1	1.3	0.5	0.03	0.05	**0.5**	*179*
Cervix uteri	247	1	-	-	-	-	4.4	9.8	19.7	24.3	27.4	44.2	33.4	22.2	26.6	31.4	29.1	19.6	11.3	16.1	16.6	5.8	1.06	1.37	**13.6**	*180*
Placenta	0	0	-	-	-	-	-	-	-	-	-	-	-	-	-	-	-	-	-	-	0.0	0.0	0.00	0.00	**0.0**	*181*
Corpus uteri	270	1	-	-	-	-	-	0.9	0.9	2.0	9.5	23.3	34.7	50.6	49.4	64.1	67.9	54.8	22.6	24.2	18.1	6.3	0.86	1.52	**12.1**	*182*
Ovary etc.	162	0	-	-	0.9	-	0.9	1.8	2.8	2.0	11.6	19.6	25.4	23.4	30.4	31.4	37.2	9.8	14.1	32.2	10.9	3.8	0.59	0.94	**7.9**	*183*
Other female genital	76	0	-	-	-	-	-	0.9	1.0	-	1.2	1.3	4.9	7.6	9.5	22.6	27.4	36.7	56.4	5.1	1.8	0.09	0.25	**2.2**	*184*
Bladder	128	1	-	-	-	-	-	-	0.9	1.0	1.1	3.7	6.7	9.9	8.9	17.7	35.6	54.8	67.8	56.4	8.6	3.0	0.16	0.43	**3.9**	*188*
Kidney etc.	56	0	5.0	-	-	-	-	-	-	1.0	1.1	1.2	-	4.9	16.5	9.5	12.9	17.6	11.3	16.1	3.8	1.3	0.15	0.26	**2.5**	*189*
Eye	8	0	2.5	-	-	-	-	-	-	-	-	1.2	-	-	-	2.7	3.2	-	-	4.0	0.5	0.2	0.02	0.05	**0.5**	*190*
Brain, nervous system	96	0	1.2	-	6.5	3.5	1.8	2.7	2.8	4.1	4.2	8.6	5.3	8.6	16.5	16.4	22.6	13.7	5.6	8.1	6.5	2.3	0.33	0.52	**5.0**	*191-2*
Thyroid	58	0	-	-	2.7	3.5	1.8	4.7	8.1	10.5	7.4	-	6.2	6.3	5.5	3.2	2.0	2.8	8.1	3.9	1.4	0.26	0.30	**3.3**	*193*
Other endocrine	5	0	1.2	-	-	-	-	0.9	-	3.0	-	-	-	-	-	-	-	-	-	0.3	0.1	0.03	0.03	**0.4**	*194*
Hodgkin's disease	28	0	-	-	3.5	3.5	3.6	5.6	2.0	-	-	2.5	2.7	-	1.3	2.7	-	-	2.8	-	1.9	0.7	0.12	0.14	**1.8**	*201*
Non-Hodgkin lymphoma	120	0	1.2	-	0.9	1.8	0.9	2.8	4.1	5.3	3.7	13.4	9.9	17.7	23.2	25.9	27.4	42.4	24.2	8.1	2.8	0.31	0.55	**5.0**	*200,202*
Multiple myeloma	61	0	-	-	-	-	-	-	-	-	2.5	4.0	6.2	13.9	13.6	14.6	23.5	16.9	12.1	4.1	1.4	0.13	0.27	**2.2**	*203*
Lymphoid leukaemia	40	0	5.0	1.1	1.9	0.9	-	-	1.9	-	2.1	-	5.3	4.9	1.3	4.1	8.1	9.8	5.6	16.1	2.7	0.9	0.12	0.18	**2.2**	*204*
Myeloid leukaemia	52	0	1.2	1.1	0.9	1.8	-	1.8	0.9	4.1	3.2	7.4	4.0	6.2	5.1	1.4	9.7	5.9	16.9	12.1	3.5	1.2	0.19	0.24	**2.7**	*205*
Monocytic leukaemia	5	0	-	-	-	-	0.9	0.9	-	-	-	-	-	1.3	-	-	2.0	2.8	-	0.3	0.1	0.02	0.02	**0.2**	*206*
Other leukaemia	2	0	-	-	-	-	-	-	-	-	-	-	-	-	-	1.6	-	2.8	-	0.1	0.0	0.00	0.01	**0.0**	*207*
Leukaemia unspecified	18	0	-	-	-	-	-	-	-	-	-	-	1.3	1.2	2.5	1.4	3.2	-	16.9	20.1	1.2	0.4	0.03	0.05	**0.5**	*208*
Other and unspecified	260	0	-	-	-	-	-	0.9	2.8	1.0	4.2	4.9	12.0	17.3	26.6	49.1	69.5	82.3	132.7	141.0	17.5	6.1	0.35	0.94	**8.3**	*O&U*
All sites	5919	81	19.9	5.5	14.9	15.0	27.4	54.2	117.0	180.5	255.1	411.3	467.4	584.7	802.7	948.9	1298.7	1463.2	1728.2	1998.1	397.9		14.98	26.38	**239.8**	*ALL*
All sites but 173	4265	7	18.6	5.5	13.1	15.0	23.9	40.0	98.3	141.9	208.7	315.5	364.5	450.3	595.1	688.5	949.3	997.0	1146.5	1289.1	286.7	100.0	11.47	19.67	**178.4**	*ALLb*

Rate from 1 case			1.242	1.092	0.933	0.885	0.884	0.889	0.936	1.014	1.054	1.228	1.335	1.234	1.266	1.363	1.617	1.959	2.824	4.028

†Important: see notes on population page

Spain, Murcia

The Murcia Cancer Registry (Registro de Cáncer de Murcia) was established in 1981 as a project of the Consejería de Sanidad y Política Social of the region of Murcia, developed by the Department of Epidemiology. Its main purpose is to estimate cancer incidence in the region. In addition, the registry participates in planning and evaluation of cancer control programmes as well as in epidemiological studies.

The registry covers the whole region of Murcia, one of the 17 autonomous communities of Spain. This region is situated in the south-east, between latitudes 38°45′ and 37°23′ N and longitudes 3°03′ and 1°20′ E. The total area is 11 317 km^2, with an average density of 94.4 inhabitants per km^2. The region is divided into 45 municipalities. Approximately 54% of the population live in three municipalities with more than 50 000 inhabitants, while 10% live in rural areas (less than 10 000 inhabitants). The main cities are Murcia (the capital, 328 000 inhabitants) and Cartagena (168 023).

The population (1991) was 1 055 000, of whom 22.7% are children. Nearly 15% of the working population is employed in agriculture, although the proportion has been decreasing, 54% work in services and 31% in industry and construction. The region has an important food-processing industry. Mediterranean diet (high consumption of vegetables, fruits, legumes and olive oil) is very common. The prevalence of smoking in 1992 was 54% in males and 31% in females, with an increasing trend for women and a decreasing one for men. During the 1970s and early 80s, the city of Cartagena had severe air pollution problems, mostly due to industrial emissions.

Primary health care and hospital treatment are provided free of charge to every member of the population through the National Health Service. The region is divided in six health districts, each with at least one public hospital. There are nine public hospitals and 14 private hospitals, with a total of 3797 beds, 72% of which belong to public hospitals, although practically all private beds may be used by the public health service by agreement. The hospital located in the capital has the regional radiotherapy unit.

A regional law makes the supply of information compulsory, when required, by professionals and health centres diagnosing, treating and following up cancer patients. Its main objective is to protect notifying people from lawsuits related to confidentiality.

Information is principally collected by registry personnel. The identification of new cases is done mainly through the pathology, haematology, oncology, radiotherapy, outpatient clinics and clinical departments of public hospitals. Registry staff abstract medical records to complete cancer data. In private hospitals the main sources of information are pathology laboratories and medical records departments. In order to identify cancer patients who are treated outside the region, the registry receives notifications from the National Registry for Childhood Cancer as well as from the social security reimbursement service which refunds expenses for treatment in hospitals outside the region of Murcia.

When cancer is mentioned on a death certificate, and the registry has no information on the case, the main files of the principal hospitals are searched through. If the case is not found, the certifying physician is questioned. If the information gathered is sufficient to register the case, it is registered as a death certificate notification (DCN). If no other information is available apart from that on the certificate, the case is accepted as a death-certificate-only (DCO) case. Both DCO and DCN, among other indicators, are used for monitoring quality control. Based on numbers of DCN and the observed mortality:incidence ratio in the same period, the global completeness of registration appears to be around 91%.

The registry has participated in two multicentric case–control studies, one on human papillomavirus and cervical cancer carried out in Colombia and Spain and another on non-melanoma skin cancer in four Mediterranean countries. It is also involved in the European Prospective Investigation into Cancer and Nutrition (EPIC), coordinated by IARC.

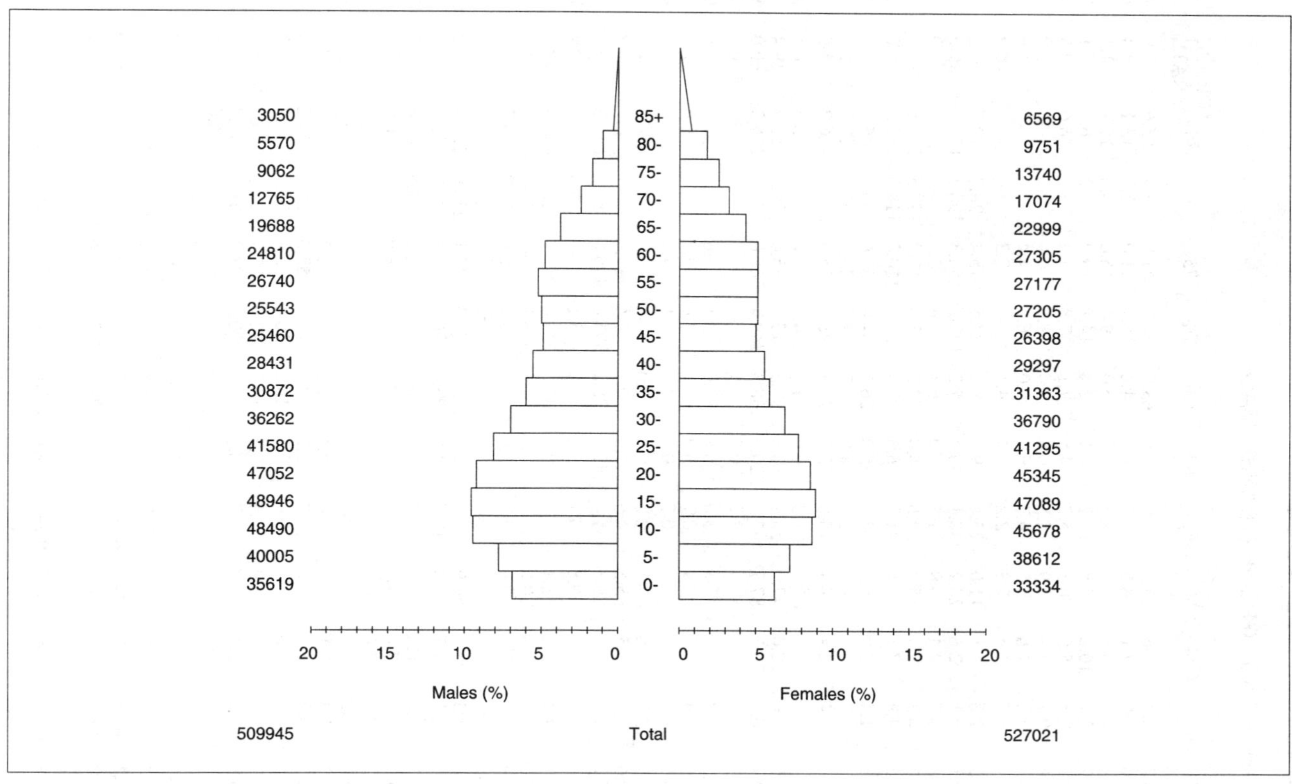

Spain, Murcia
Source of population: average annual 1988–92
Census: 1991. Centro Regional de Estadística de Murcia.
Censo de Población y vivienda de 1991. Región de Murcia.
Murcia: Consejería de Economía. Hacienda y Fomento.
Comunidad Autónoma de la Región de Murcia, 1993.

Estimate: The populations for 1988, 1989, 1990 and 1992 were estimates. *Reference:* Dirección General de Salud y Consumo, Servicio de Epidemiología. Proyecciones de población de derecho en la Región de Murcia y sus Areas de Salud, por grupos de edad y sexo. 1986-2000. Murcia: Consejería de Sanidad y Asuntos Sociales, 1995.

SPAIN, MURCIA 1988-1992

ANNUAL INCIDENCE PER 100,000 BY AGE GROUP (YEARS) - MALE

SITE	ALL AGES	AGE UNK	0-	5-	10-	15-	20-	25-	30-	35-	40-	45-	50-	55-	60-	65-	70-	75-	80-	85+	CRUDE RATE	%	CR 64	CR 74	ASR (W)	ICD (9th)
Lip	352	7	-	-	-	-	0.4	1.0	2.8	4.5	13.4	8.6	25.1	41.9	47.6	63.0	50.1	61.8	75.4	65.6	13.8	4.4	0.74	1.32	11.1	140
Tongue	112	1	-	-	-	-	-	0.5	1.1	2.6	5.6	7.1	8.6	17.2	16.9	14.2	14.1	11.0	7.2	13.1	4.4	1.4	0.30	0.44	3.8	141
Salivary gland	28	0	-	-	-	-	-	-	-	0.7	0.8	0.8	2.2	5.6	2.0	9.4	6.6	3.6	19.7	1.1	0.3	0.05	0.11	0.9	142
Mouth	104	0	-	-	-	-	-	0.5	-	3.2	2.1	10.2	7.8	14.2	16.1	12.2	14.1	19.9	7.2	6.6	4.1	1.3	0.27	0.40	3.5	143-5
Oropharynx	64	0	-	-	-	0.4	-	-	-	1.3	2.8	5.5	6.3	5.2	14.5	7.1	7.8	4.4	7.2	6.6	2.5	0.8	0.18	0.25	2.2	146
Nasopharynx	26	1	-	-	-	-	-	0.5	0.6	0.6	0.7	2.4	3.9	4.5	0.8	3.0	1.6	4.4	-	-	1.0	0.3	0.07	0.10	0.9	147
Hypopharynx	42	0	-	-	-	-	-	-	0.6	-	4.2	1.6	5.5	6.7	6.4	3.0	6.3	4.4	-	-	1.6	0.5	0.13	0.17	1.4	148
Pharynx unspecified	22	0	-	-	-	-	-	-	-	3.5	1.6	2.3	2.2	2.4	4.1	-	2.2	3.6	-	0.9	0.3	0.06	0.08	0.8	149	
Oesophagus	140	0	-	-	-	-	-	1.1	1.3	2.8	7.1	11.0	25.4	19.3	18.3	23.5	15.4	28.7	19.7	5.5	1.7	0.34	0.55	4.5	150
Stomach	501	0	-	-	-	-	-	0.5	-	7.1	9.1	12.6	28.2	38.1	56.4	77.2	133.2	152.3	190.3	131.1	19.6	6.2	0.76	1.81	15.1	151
Small intestine	26	0	-	-	-	-	-	0.5	0.6	-	0.7	2.4	3.9	1.5	4.0	6.1	1.6	2.2	-	-	1.0	0.3	0.07	0.11	0.9	152
Colon	469	1	-	-	-	-	-	1.4	2.2	2.6	6.3	7.9	15.7	39.6	58.0	79.2	103.4	147.9	179.5	209.8	18.4	5.8	0.67	1.59	13.8	153
Rectum	397	1	-	-	-	-	-	0.6	3.2	4.9	7.1	19.6	41.9	36.3	87.4	89.3	110.3	118.5	144.2	15.6	4.9	0.57	1.45	11.9	154	
Liver	168	0	1.7	-	-	-	0.9	-	-	1.3	1.4	3.9	6.3	7.5	25.0	26.4	54.8	59.6	35.9	45.9	6.6	2.1	0.24	0.65	5.2	155
Gallbladder etc.	70	0	-	-	-	-	-	0.5	-	-	0.7	0.8	-	5.2	8.9	15.2	12.5	28.7	35.9	19.7	2.7	0.9	0.08	0.22	2.0	156
Pancreas	141	0	-	-	-	-	-	-	-	1.3	1.4	2.4	4.7	15.0	25.0	25.4	28.2	35.3	50.3	26.2	5.5	1.7	0.25	0.52	4.2	157	
Nose, sinuses etc.	13	0	0.6	-	-	-	-	-	-	-	-	-	-	1.5	1.6	1.0	4.7	2.2	7.2	6.6	0.5	0.2	0.02	0.05	0.4	160
Larynx	495	2	-	-	-	-	-	1.7	4.5	8.4	22.0	47.0	53.1	83.8	97.5	75.2	75.0	79.0	52.4	19.4	6.1	1.11	1.97	15.9	161	
Bronchus, lung	1531	1	-	-	-	0.4	-	1.7	9.1	26.7	39.3	87.7	147.3	220.9	338.3	349.4	368.6	305.2	216.3	60.0	18.9	2.67	6.11	47.2	162	
Other thoracic organs	9	0	1.7	-	-	-	0.4	-	-	-	-	-	-	2.2	0.8	-	-	3.6	-	0.4	0.1	0.03	0.03	0.4	163-4	
Bone	40	0	-	0.5	2.9	3.3	1.7	1.0	1.1	1.3	-	1.6	-	3.0	0.8	1.0	3.1	6.6	3.6	-	1.6	0.5	0.09	0.11	1.4	170
Connective tissue	56	0	2.2	-	1.2	1.2	0.9	1.4	1.7	0.6	1.4	1.6	3.9	0.7	3.2	7.1	7.8	13.2	14.4	6.6	2.2	0.7	0.10	0.18	2.0	171
Mesothelioma	14	0	-	-	-	-	-	-	-	0.6	-	0.8	-	0.7	0.8	4.1	3.1	4.4	7.2	-	0.5	0.2	0.01	0.05	0.4	MES	
Kaposi's sarcoma	32	0	-	-	-	-	0.9	2.9	4.4	3.5	1.6	-	2.2	0.8	1.0	-	-	7.2	-	1.3	0.4	0.09	0.09	1.1	KAP	
Melanoma of skin	85	0	-	-	0.4	0.4	0.9	2.9	1.7	0.6	3.5	5.5	5.5	4.5	11.3	9.1	9.4	19.9	28.7	-	3.3	1.1	0.19	0.28	2.8	172
Other skin	1914	58	-	-	0.4	0.8	3.4	5.3	8.8	16.2	31.7	58.1	89.3	135.4	247.5	335.2	394.8	496.6	581.6	675.2	75.1	-	3.08	6.84	58.4	173	
Breast	10	0	-	-	-	-	-	-	0.6	-	-	-	0.8	0.7	1.6	2.0	3.1	-	3.6	-	0.4	0.1	0.02	0.04	0.3	175	
Prostate	699	8	-	-	-	-	-	-	-	-	1.4	0.8	3.1	9.0	50.0	135.1	214.6	342.1	420.0	445.8	27.4	8.7	0.33	2.09	19.0	185
Testis	32	0	0.6	-	0.4	2.0	3.8	2.4	0.6	2.6	1.4	0.8	0.8	-	-	3.1	-	-	-	-	1.3	0.4	0.08	0.09	1.2	186
Penis	38	0	-	-	-	-	-	1.0	0.6	1.9	-	2.4	0.8	3.7	1.6	4.1	9.4	6.6	18.0	19.7	1.5	0.5	0.06	0.13	1.2	187.1-.4
Other male genital	1	0	-	-	-	-	-	-	-	-	-	-	-	-	-	-	-	2.2	-	-	0.0	0.0	0.00	0.00	0.0	187.5-.9	
Bladder	1025	4	-	-	0.4	-	0.4	2.9	1.7	2.6	11.3	26.7	50.9	83.0	112.9	192.0	277.3	342.1	272.9	281.9	40.2	12.7	1.47	3.82	30.8	188
Kidney etc.	131	0	0.6	0.5	-	0.4	0.4	-	0.6	0.6	2.1	4.7	6.3	12.7	21.0	23.4	26.6	28.7	35.9	13.1	5.1	1.6	0.25	0.50	4.1	189	
Eye	18	2	1.1	1.0	-	-	-	-	0.6	-	1.4	0.8	-	0.7	-	3.0	1.6	2.2	3.6	6.6	0.7	0.2	0.03	0.06	0.7	190
Brain, nervous system	181	0	5.1	1.0	2.9	2.5	1.7	3.4	4.4	4.5	7.0	9.4	14.1	15.0	21.8	23.4	14.1	19.9	7.2	6.6	7.1	2.2	0.46	0.65	6.5	191-2
Thyroid	33	0	-	0.5	-	-	1.7	1.4	1.7	1.3	2.1	2.4	0.8	2.2	2.4	3.0	4.7	-	3.6	-	1.3	0.4	0.08	0.12	1.2	193
Other endocrine	10	1	1.7	-	-	-	0.4	-	-	0.6	0.7	-	-	0.7	0.8	-	-	-	-	6.6	0.4	0.1	0.03	0.03	0.5	194	
Hodgkin's disease	50	0	-	0.5	0.4	2.9	2.1	1.9	3.3	3.2	1.4	3.1	2.3	3.0	2.4	2.0	3.1	2.2	-	-	2.0	0.6	0.13	0.16	1.8	201
Non-Hodgkin lymphoma	228	2	2.2	4.0	1.2	-	2.1	3.8	1.7	5.2	4.9	11.8	18.8	15.7	32.2	28.4	26.6	53.0	25.1	26.2	8.9	2.8	0.52	0.80	7.8	200,202
Multiple myeloma	82	2	-	-	-	-	-	-	1.1	-	0.7	1.6	-	9.0	12.1	15.2	20.4	15.4	35.9	19.7	3.2	1.0	0.13	0.31	2.4	203	
Lymphoid leukaemia	96	0	6.2	2.5	1.2	0.8	-	0.5	-	1.9	0.7	0.8	3.9	7.5	9.7	14.2	12.5	22.1	21.5	26.2	3.8	1.2	0.18	0.31	3.4	204
Myeloid leukaemia	111	0	1.7	1.5	1.2	0.8	0.4	1.0	3.3	5.8	4.2	3.1	3.9	3.7	8.1	14.2	20.4	28.7	18.0	45.9	4.4	1.4	0.19	0.37	3.7	205
Monocytic leukaemia	2	0	-	-	-	-	-	-	-	-	-	-	-	-	-	1.0	-	-	-	6.6	0.1	0.0	0.00	0.01	0.1	206
Other leukaemia	2	0	-	-	-	-	-	-	-	-	-	-	-	-	-	-	-	4.4	-	-	0.1	0.0	0.00	0.00	0.0	207
Leukaemia unspecified	17	0	0.6	0.5	-	-	-	0.5	-	-	-	-	-	-	3.2	-	3.1	6.6	10.8	13.1	0.7	0.2	0.02	0.04	0.5	208	
Other and unspecified	377	3	0.6	-	0.4	-	0.9	-	-	3.2	5.6	12.6	20.4	30.7	37.9	59.9	98.7	117.0	114.9	131.1	14.8	4.7	0.57	1.36	11.5	O&U	
All sites	9994	94	26.4	12.5	13.2	15.9	23.4	37.5	50.2	97.2	180.8	293.0	509.7	816.7	1232.6	1759.4	2137.0	2646.2	2771.6	2714.0	392.0		16.70	36.37	309.0	ALL
All sites but 173	8080	36	26.4	12.5	12.8	15.1	20.0	32.2	41.4	81.0	149.1	234.9	420.5	681.4	985.1	1424.2	1742.2	2149.6	2190.0	2038.8	316.9	100.0	13.62	29.52	250.5	ALLb

Rate from 1 case: 0.561 0.500 0.412 0.409 0.425 0.481 0.552 0.648 0.703 0.786 0.783 0.748 0.806 1.016 1.567 2.207 3.590 6.556

SPAIN, MURCIA 1988-1992

ANNUAL INCIDENCE PER 100,000 BY AGE GROUP (YEARS) - FEMALE

SITE	ALL AGES	AGE UNK	0-	5-	10-	15-	20-	25-	30-	35-	40-	45-	50-	55-	60-	65-	70-	75-	80-	85+	CRUDE RATE	%	CR 64	CR 74	ASR (W)	ICD (9th)
Lip	19	1	-	-	0.4	-	-	-	-	-	0.7	0.8	-	0.7	2.2	2.6	3.5	2.9	4.1	3.0	0.7	0.3	0.03	0.06	**0.5**	*140*
Tongue	32	0	-	-	-	-	-	-	-	1.3	-	0.8	2.2	2.2	1.5	3.5	7.0	7.3	8.2	6.1	1.2	0.6	0.04	0.09	**0.8**	*141*
Salivary gland	18	1	-	-	-	-	-	-	-	0.6	0.7	-	-	2.2	1.5	1.7	2.3	1.5	2.1	12.2	0.7	0.3	0.03	0.05	**0.4**	*142*
Mouth	28	1	-	-	0.4	-	-	0.5	-	-	-	2.3	-	2.9	1.5	2.6	3.5	4.4	12.3	3.0	1.1	0.5	0.04	0.07	**0.7**	*143-5*
Oropharynx	4	0	-	-	-	-	-	-	-	-	-	-	-	2.2	-	-	-	2.1	-	0.2	0.1	0.01	0.01	**0.1**	*146*
Nasopharynx	5	0	-	-	-	-	-	-	-	-	-	0.8	-	1.5	-	-	1.2	-	-	3.0	0.2	0.1	0.01	0.02	**0.1**	*147*
Hypopharynx	1	0	-	-	-	-	-	-	-	-	-	-	-	-	-	-	-	-	2.1	-	0.0	0.0	0.00	0.00	**0.0**	*148*
Pharynx unspecified	4	0	-	-	-	-	-	-	-	-	-	-	-	-	0.7	-	-	1.5	4.1	-	0.2	0.1	0.00	0.00	**0.1**	*149*
Oesophagus	22	0	-	-	-	-	-	0.5	-	-	-	0.8	0.7	-	0.7	2.6	1.2	8.7	10.3	9.1	0.8	0.4	0.01	0.03	**0.4**	*150*
Stomach	329	1	-	-	-	-	-	0.5	1.6	1.3	4.8	9.1	13.2	16.2	24.9	24.3	57.4	90.2	104.6	118.7	12.5	5.8	0.36	0.77	**7.3**	*151*
Small intestine	8	0	-	-	-	-	-	-	-	-	-	-	-	2.2	1.5	-	-	2.9	-	3.0	0.3	0.1	0.02	0.02	**0.2**	*152*
Colon	453	4	-	-	-	-	0.9	1.0	1.6	2.6	10.9	12.9	19.1	23.5	43.2	49.6	70.3	106.3	116.9	124.8	17.2	7.9	0.58	1.19	**10.7**	*153*
Rectum	332	1	-	-	-	-	0.4	-	1.1	2.6	6.1	5.3	16.2	19.1	28.6	52.2	44.5	85.9	88.2	63.9	12.6	5.8	0.40	0.88	**7.8**	*154*
Liver	78	0	1.2	-	-	0.4	-	-	0.5	1.3	0.7	-	10.3	5.9	4.3	15.2	13.1	24.6	30.4	-	3.0	1.4	0.10	0.20	**1.8**	*155*
Gallbladder etc.	167	0	-	-	-	-	-	-	-	-	0.7	1.5	3.7	7.4	16.8	18.3	29.3	49.5	59.5	51.8	6.3	2.9	0.15	0.39	**3.5**	*156*
Pancreas	110	2	-	-	-	-	-	-	-	-	-	1.5	2.2	1.5	8.1	18.3	17.6	30.6	39.0	42.6	4.2	1.9	0.07	0.25	**2.2**	*157*
Nose, sinuses etc.	11	0	-	-	-	-	-	-	-	-	-	2.3	-	-	1.5	1.7	1.2	2.9	2.1	-	0.4	0.2	0.02	0.03	**0.3**	*160*
Larynx	7	0	-	-	-	-	-	0.5	0.6	0.7	-	0.7	-	0.7	0.9	-	-	1.5	-	-	0.3	0.1	0.02	0.02	**0.2**	*161*
Bronchus, lung	146	0	0.6	-	-	-	-	-	0.5	0.6	2.0	6.8	3.7	9.6	16.1	13.0	38.7	24.7	30.8	33.5	5.5	2.6	0.20	0.46	**3.6**	*162*
Other thoracic organs	1	0	-	-	-	-	-	-	-	-	-	-	-	-	-	-	-	1.5	-	-	0.0	0.0	0.00	0.00	**0.0**	*163-4*
Bone	15	0	0.6	0.5	0.9	0.4	0.9	0.5	-	0.7	-	-	-	1.5	-	1.2	1.5	2.1	3.0	-	0.6	0.3	0.03	0.04	**0.5**	*170*
Connective tissue	54	0	1.2	1.0	1.3	-	0.4	1.5	1.1	0.6	3.4	1.5	-	2.9	5.1	4.3	8.2	8.7	4.1	6.1	2.0	0.9	0.10	0.16	**1.7**	*171*
Mesothelioma	5	0	-	-	-	-	-	-	-	-	-	-	0.7	2.2	-	-	-	1.5	-	-	0.2	0.1	0.01	0.01	**0.1**	*MES*
Kaposi's sarcoma	1	0	-	-	-	-	-	0.5	-	-	-	-	-	-	-	-	-	-	-	-	0.0	0.0	0.00	0.00	**0.0**	*KAP*
Melanoma of skin	149	0	0.6	-	-	0.4	0.9	3.4	4.9	5.7	8.2	10.6	9.6	5.2	8.8	9.6	19.9	14.6	26.7	33.5	5.7	2.6	0.29	0.44	**4.4**	*172*
Other skin	1506	47	-	-	0.4	1.3	0.9	3.9	6.0	17.9	20.5	32.6	47.0	84.6	119.4	167.0	212.0	301.3	469.7	554.1	57.2		1.73	3.68	**34.1**	*173*
Breast	1479	4	-	-	-	-	0.4	7.7	21.7	47.8	77.1	93.2	125.0	136.9	147.2	155.7	166.3	174.7	133.3	134.0	56.1	25.9	3.29	4.91	**43.9**	*174*
Uterus unspecified	20	0	-	-	-	-	-	-	-	-	-	-	2.2	0.7	1.5	1.7	2.3	5.8	8.2	6.1	0.8	0.4	0.02	0.04	**0.4**	*179*
Cervix uteri	236	1	-	-	-	-	-	2.4	5.4	10.2	15.0	15.2	14.7	19.9	25.6	26.1	28.1	21.8	14.4	12.2	9.0	4.1	0.54	0.82	**7.2**	*180*
Placenta	1	0	-	-	-	-	-	-	-	-	0.7	-	-	-	-	-	-	-	-	-	0.0	0.0	0.00	0.00	**0.0**	*181*
Corpus uteri	377	0	-	-	-	-	-	1.0	0.5	1.9	5.5	19.7	29.4	50.0	57.9	64.4	45.7	37.8	14.4	12.2	14.3	6.6	0.83	1.38	**10.9**	*182*
Ovary etc.	254	1	-	-	1.3	1.3	0.4	2.9	3.3	2.6	5.5	9.8	17.6	28.0	30.8	41.7	31.6	26.2	16.4	12.2	9.6	4.4	0.52	0.89	**7.3**	*183*
Other female genital	70	0	-	-	-	-	-	-	0.5	-	-	0.8	5.1	2.9	5.1	4.3	17.6	21.8	12.3	27.4	2.7	1.2	0.07	0.18	**1.6**	*184*
Bladder	142	1	-	-	-	-	-	-	1.1	-	-	2.3	3.7	8.1	15.4	15.7	34.0	26.2	34.9	51.8	5.4	2.5	0.15	0.40	**3.2**	*188*
Kidney etc.	68	0	1.2	-	-	0.4	0.4	0.5	-	-	2.0	1.5	3.7	4.4	10.3	6.1	14.1	7.3	8.2	15.2	2.6	1.2	0.12	0.22	**1.9**	*189*
Eye	5	0	1.2	-	-	-	-	-	-	-	-	-	-	0.7	-	-	-	1.5	-	-	0.2	0.1	0.01	0.01	**0.2**	*190*
Brain, nervous system	111	0	3.6	4.7	3.1	2.1	1.8	0.5	1.1	3.8	1.4	3.8	5.1	5.9	16.1	9.6	8.2	10.2	2.1	3.0	4.2	1.9	0.26	0.35	**3.9**	*191-2*
Thyroid	123	0	-	-	0.9	2.5	1.3	3.4	8.2	10.8	8.2	12.9	8.8	4.4	5.9	6.1	2.3	8.7	4.1	3.0	4.7	2.2	0.34	0.38	**4.3**	*193*
Other endocrine	11	0	1.2	0.5	-	0.4	0.9	0.5	0.5	0.6	-	-	-	0.7	-	-	-	1.5	-	-	0.4	0.2	0.03	0.03	**0.5**	*194*
Hodgkin's disease	32	0	-	-	0.4	1.7	0.9	4.4	2.2	1.3	0.7	-	0.7	-	1.5	2.6	3.5	-	-	-	1.2	0.6	0.07	0.10	**1.1**	*201*
Non-Hodgkin lymphoma	173	1	0.6	0.5	0.9	-	1.3	1.9	2.7	3.2	7.5	3.0	10.3	15.5	13.9	22.6	35.1	16.0	24.6	9.1	6.6	3.0	0.31	0.60	**4.9**	*200,202*
Multiple myeloma	96	1	-	-	-	-	-	-	0.5	-	-	2.3	4.4	7.4	7.3	20.9	14.1	23.3	16.4	15.2	3.6	1.7	0.11	0.29	**2.3**	*203*
Lymphoid leukaemia	84	5	4.8	3.6	1.8	1.3	-	1.0	-	-	-	-	3.7	3.7	4.4	12.2	5.9	13.1	18.5	6.1	3.2	1.5	0.13	0.22	**2.7**	*204*
Myeloid leukaemia	80	1	1.2	1.0	1.3	-	0.4	-	1.1	1.3	3.4	0.8	5.9	4.4	6.6	4.3	8.2	18.9	16.4	15.2	3.0	1.4	0.14	0.20	**2.2**	*205*
Monocytic leukaemia	1	0	-	-	-	-	-	-	-	-	-	-	-	-	-	-	-	-	2.1	-	0.0	0.0	0.00	0.00	**0.0**	*206*
Other leukaemia	5	0	-	-	-	-	-	-	-	-	-	0.7	-	-	-	-	-	2.9	4.1	-	0.2	0.1	0.00	0.00	**0.1**	*207*
Leukaemia unspecified	16	0	-	-	-	-	-	-	-	-	0.7	-	-	0.7	1.5	0.9	5.9	2.9	4.1	6.1	0.6	0.3	0.01	0.05	**0.4**	*208*
Other and unspecified	331	2	1.2	-	0.4	0.4	2.2	0.5	1.6	1.3	2.0	6.1	9.6	15.5	27.1	35.7	57.4	74.2	75.9	164.4	12.6	5.8	0.34	0.81	**7.5**	*O&U*
All sites	7220	75	19.2	11.9	13.6	12.7	14.6	39.2	68.0	119.9	189.8	260.6	369.8	503.4	671.7	807.0	1014.4	1257.6	1423.4	1595.4	274.0		11.59	20.79	**188.1**	*ALL*
All sites but 173	5714	28	19.2	11.9	13.1	11.5	13.7	35.4	62.0	102.0	169.3	228.0	322.7	418.7	552.3	640.0	802.4	956.3	953.7	1041.3	216.8	100.0	9.85	17.09	**153.8**	*ALLb*

	0-	5-	10-	15-	20-	25-	30-	35-	40-	45-	50-	55-	60-	65-	70-	75-	80-	85+
Rate from 1 case	0.600	0.518	0.438	0.425	0.441	0.484	0.544	0.638	0.683	0.758	0.735	0.736	0.732	0.870	1.171	1.456	2.051	3.045

Spain, Navarra

The population-based cancer registry of Navarra started its activities in 1970 as a result of a collaboration between the Spanish Association Against Cancer and the Public Health Institute of Navarra. The main objective is to study the incidence and describe the characteristics of tumours occurring in Navarra. In addition, the registry promotes and facilitates epidemiological research, health services planning and preventive activities.

The registry staff comprises an epidemiologist (part-time), a nurse and a social worker (full-time) who carry out the collection and coding of the information, in addition to an administrative assistant who records and processes the data. A pathologist collaborates with the registry as an external consultant.

The registry covers the whole area of the Autonomous Community of Navarra, one of the 17 autonomous communities in Spain. Situated in the north of the peninsula, Navarra borders on France to the north (the Pyrenees), the Autonomous Community of Aragón to the east, the Autonomous Community of La Rioja to the south, and the Autonomous Community of the Basque Country to the west. Its total area is 10 491 km^2. In 1992, 88% of the population had access to a chlorinated drinking water supply, including 100% of municipalities of more than 2000 inhabitants.

According the 1991 census, Navarra had 523 563 inhabitants (49.5 inhabitants per km^2). Approximately 50% lived within the region around Pamplona. 49.6% were males, with 17.3% under 14 years old and 15.5% over age 65. The population growth was 0.2–0.3% in 1991. Population ageing is mainly due to a decline in birth rate, which fell from 17.9 in 1975 to 8.9 in 1991. The adjusted mortality rates were 923 per 100 000 inhabitants in males and 533 in females during 1985–89. In 1989, life expectancy was 75 years for males and 82 years for females.

Castilian and Euskera are both official languages, but their prevalence varies geographically. The population is ethnically homogeneous, and mainly Catholic. According to 1991 data, illiteracy was 1% and, within those over 16 years old, 41% have an educational level higher than primary studies. The activity rate was 49.4% and the unemployment rate 10.6%. 51.6% of the active population worked in services and only 7.2% in the primary sector. The main industrial activities are those related to car manufacturing. During the last decade there was no major migration, although within the province, the main feature is a spatial redistribution which has led to a demographic concentration in and around Pamplona.

99% of the population is covered by the national health service. Health assistance in Navarra is based on several basic health zones aggregated into three health areas. Access to the health system is either through primary-level assistance within a basic zone (Centros de Salud and Consultorios) or through emergency systems of both primary or secondary (specialized) levels.

Cancer control activities include the promotion of healthy lifestyles (nutrition, tobacco consumption prevention), occupational health checks for all those production processes related to carcinogenic substances, hepatitis B vaccination in children and young population, breast cancer screening in women between 45 and 64 years old, vaginal smears in high-risk women and *ad hoc* advice to the population.

Patients with a suspected tumour diagnosis undergo all the necessary tests to confirm the diagnosis and are treated and followed by public network assistance services and/or by private services.

The main sources of information for the registry are the departments of pathology, haematology, radiotherapy and oncology, as well as all the clinical records services in public and private hospitals. Incidence data are complemented with mortality data from the Mortality Registry through a systematic search to complete mainly the cause and date of death.

Cancer notification is not mandatory. Data collection on tumour cases is active with a systematic search in the hospital services mentioned above. Follow-up of cases is performed through examination of medical records and death certificates and never through direct contact with the patients.

Data for the 1987–91 period were coded following ICD-9 for tumour site and ICD-O-1 for histological code. Multiple primary tumours are coded applying the rules suggested by IARC/IACR.

Data are collected and recorded using individual protocols before computerization. Duplicate checks and quality controls are run periodically to detect possible mistakes and inconsistencies. Data are stored in registry specific personal computers with access controls.

A breast cancer screening programme started in 1990 and its target population is all women in the province aged between 45 and 64 years.

The registry usually publishes incidence reports based on five-year periods. It has participated in two case–control studies on cervix and larynx cancers, and is participating in the European Prospective Study into Cancer and Nutrition (EPIC). The registry is also developing other studies of trends for specific sites and of childhood cancer.

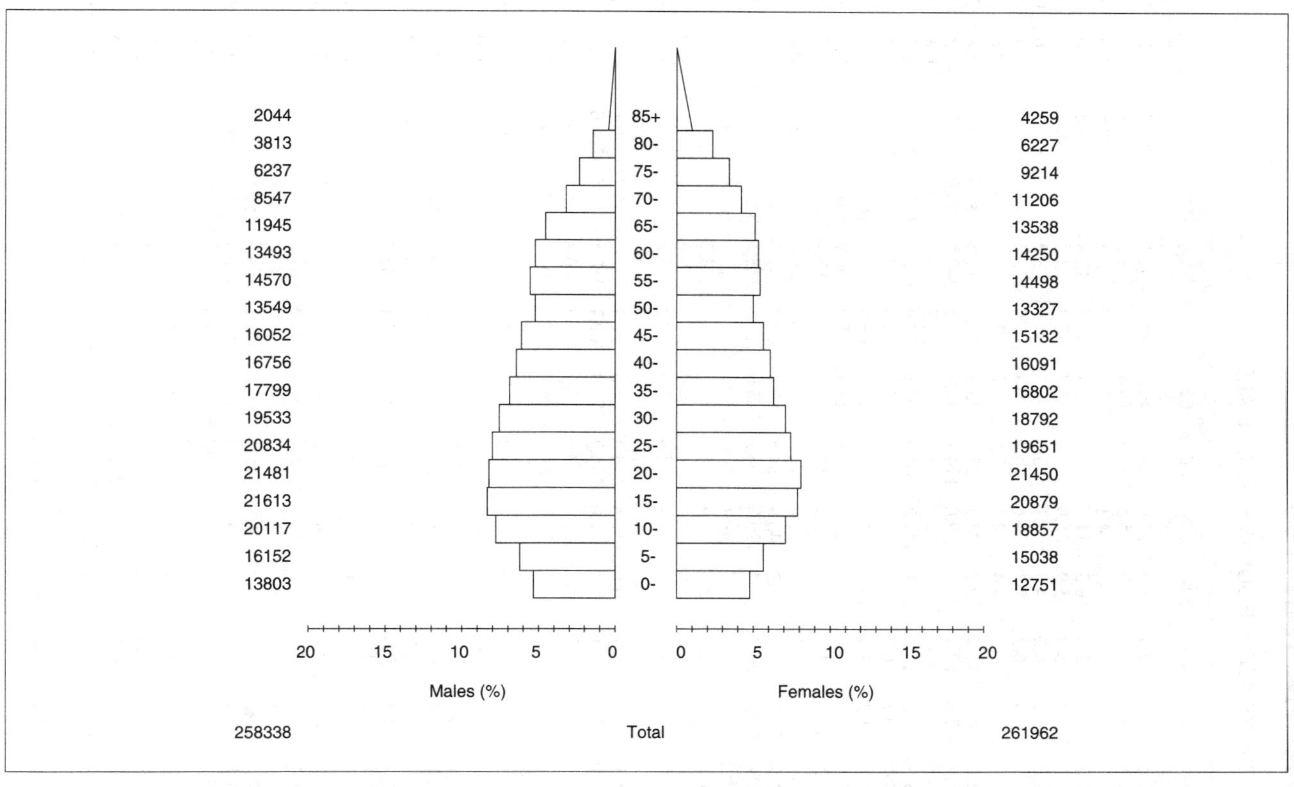

Spain, Navarra
Source of population:
Census: Instituto Nacional de Estadistica. Poblaciones de derecho y hecho de los municipios españoles. Censo de Población 1991. Madrid, INE, 1993. Municipal Census (padrón) held in 1986.
Estimate: The population was estimated by linear interpolation between the 1986 and 1991 official figures.

Screening programmes in the area:
28 000 breast cancer screening examinations are carried out annually in the population aged 45-64.

SPAIN, NAVARRA 1987-1991

ANNUAL INCIDENCE PER 100,000 BY AGE GROUP (YEARS) - MALE

SITE	ALL AGES	AGE UNK	0-	5-	10-	15-	20-	25-	30-	35-	40-	45-	50-	55-	60-	65-	70-	75-	80-	85+	CRUDE RATE	%	CR 64	CR 74	ASR (W)	ICD (9th)
Lip	127	0	-	-	-	-	-	-	-	2.2	6.0	2.5	13.3	22.0	29.6	40.2	49.1	32.1	57.7	68.5	9.8	2.3	0.38	0.82	**6.5**	*140*
Tongue	39	0	-	-	-	-	-	-	-	1.1	6.0	1.2	5.9	5.5	13.3	18.4	7.0	3.2	-	-	3.0	0.7	0.17	0.29	**2.3**	*141*
Salivary gland	13	0	-	-	-	-	-	-	-	-	-	-	-	4.1	-	5.0	7.0	3.2	10.5	9.8	1.0	0.2	0.02	0.08	**0.6**	*142*
Mouth	64	0	-	-	-	-	-	-	-	2.2	4.8	12.5	10.3	11.0	22.2	8.4	16.4	12.8	5.2	9.8	5.0	1.2	0.32	0.44	**3.8**	*143-5*
Oropharynx	29	0	-	-	-	-	-	-	-	2.2	1.2	5.0	5.9	6.9	8.9	6.7	2.3	3.2	5.2	-	2.2	0.5	0.15	0.20	**1.7**	*146*
Nasopharynx	21	0	-	-	-	0.9	-	-	1.0	2.2	1.2	6.2	4.4	4.1	3.0	3.3	-	3.2	-	-	1.6	0.4	0.12	0.13	**1.4**	*147*
Hypopharynx	35	0	-	-	-	-	-	-	1.0	-	4.8	6.2	7.4	9.6	4.4	8.4	7.0	6.4	-	-	2.7	0.6	0.17	0.24	**2.1**	*148*
Pharynx unspecified	10	0	-	-	-	-	-	-	-	-	-	-	4.4	4.1	1.5	1.7	2.3	3.2	-	-	0.8	0.2	0.05	0.07	**0.6**	*149*
Oesophagus	126	1	-	-	-	-	-	-	1.0	2.2	4.8	12.5	19.2	37.1	25.2	45.2	23.4	12.8	31.5	39.1	9.8	2.3	0.51	0.86	**7.0**	*150*
Stomach	520	0	-	-	-	-	0.9	1.0	4.1	7.9	17.9	22.4	41.3	59.0	114.1	127.2	173.2	240.5	340.9	352.2	40.3	9.6	1.34	2.85	**25.4**	*151*
Small intestine	5	0	-	-	-	-	-	-	-	-	-	-	-	-	3.0	-	4.7	-	5.2	-	0.4	0.1	0.01	0.04	**0.2**	*152*
Colon	345	1	-	-	-	-	-	-	3.1	5.6	1.2	11.2	22.1	41.2	62.3	100.5	133.4	182.8	183.6	293.5	26.7	6.4	0.74	1.91	**16.5**	*153*
Rectum	267	0	-	-	-	-	-	1.9	1.0	3.4	10.7	6.2	23.6	34.3	45.9	77.0	72.5	153.9	167.8	176.1	20.7	4.9	0.64	1.38	**12.8**	*154*
Liver	177	0	-	-	-	-	-	1.9	-	1.1	1.2	3.7	14.8	22.0	41.5	46.9	65.5	80.2	104.9	146.8	13.7	3.3	0.43	0.99	**8.6**	*155*
Gallbladder etc.	68	0	-	-	-	-	-	-	-	1.1	1.2	-	-	12.4	8.9	18.4	25.7	60.9	47.2	9.8	5.3	1.3	0.12	0.34	**3.0**	*156*
Pancreas	135	1	-	-	-	-	0.9	-	1.0	2.2	10.7	1.2	8.9	15.1	19.3	43.5	46.8	83.4	68.2	48.9	10.5	2.5	0.30	0.75	**6.5**	*157*
Nose, sinuses etc.	10	0	-	-	-	-	-	-	-	-	2.4	1.2	-	1.4	-	3.3	-	6.4	5.2	9.8	0.8	0.2	0.03	0.04	**0.5**	*160*
Larynx	276	1	-	-	-	-	1.0	2.0	4.5	22.7	31.1	41.3	43.9	84.5	80.4	67.9	57.7	47.2	29.4		21.4	5.1	1.16	1.90	**15.7**	*161*
Bronchus, lung	826	3	-	-	-	-	0.9	1.9	3.1	7.9	27.5	24.9	69.4	126.3	194.2	283.0	327.6	333.5	335.7	195.7	63.9	15.2	2.29	5.35	**41.5**	*162*
Other thoracic organs	8	0	-	-	-	-	-	1.0	1.0	-	-	3.7	-	2.7	-	-	-	-	5.2	-	0.6	0.1	0.04	0.04	**0.5**	*163-4*
Bone	22	0	-	-	1.0	4.6	0.9	1.9	1.0	1.1	-	1.2	3.0	1.4	4.4	1.7	2.3	3.2	-	9.8	1.7	0.4	0.10	0.12	**1.5**	*170*
Connective tissue	26	0	1.4	-	-	-	0.9	-	1.0	-	3.6	3.7	3.0	4.1	-	10.0	7.0	9.6	-	-	2.0	0.5	0.09	0.17	**1.6**	*171*
Mesothelioma	10	0	-	-	-	-	-	-	-	-	-	1.2	-	1.4	5.9	3.3	3.2	3.2	-	-	0.8	0.2	0.04	0.07	**0.5**	*MES*
Kaposi's sarcoma	6	0	-	-	-	-	0.9	1.0	-	-	2.4	1.2	-	-	-	2.3	-	-	-		0.5	0.1	0.03	0.04	**0.4**	*KAP*
Melanoma of skin	58	0	-	-	1.0	0.9	0.9	1.0	3.1	4.5	3.6	8.7	3.0	12.4	4.4	5.0	21.1	22.4	15.7	9.8	4.5	1.1	0.22	0.35	**3.3**	*172*
Other skin	1034	9	-	-	-	0.9	3.7	1.9	5.1	13.5	32.2	51.1	84.1	151.0	195.7	277.9	369.7	410.5	566.5	724.0	80.0		2.72	5.99	**51.5**	*173*
Breast	11	0	-	-	-	-	-	-	-	1.1	-	1.2	-	1.4	3.0	-	2.3	6.4	15.7	-	0.9	0.2	0.03	0.05	**0.5**	*175*
Prostate	641	0	-	-	-	-	-	-	-	-	1.2	1.2	11.8	32.9	86.0	184.2	287.8	506.7	550.7	518.5	49.6	11.8	0.67	3.03	**27.2**	*185*
Testis	31	0	-	-	0.9	10.2	5.8	6.1	3.4	1.2	1.2	1.5	-	1.7	-	-	-	-	-		2.4	0.6	0.15	0.16	**2.2**	*186*
Penis	19	1	-	-	-	0.9	1.0	-	-	-	-	1.5	6.9	4.4	-	7.0	6.4	5.2	9.8		1.5	0.3	0.08	0.11	**1.0**	*187.1-.4*
Other male genital	0	0	-	-	-	-	-	-	-	-	-	-	-	-	-	-	-	-	-	-	0.0	0.0	0.00	0.00	**0.0**	*187.5-.9*
Bladder	557	1	-	-	1.0	1.9	0.9	1.9	5.1	4.5	16.7	16.2	45.8	79.6	129.0	159.1	196.6	279.0	215.1	303.3	43.1	10.3	1.52	3.30	**27.8**	*188*
Kidney etc.	157	0	1.4	-	-	-	-	-	-	1.1	2.4	10.0	17.7	28.8	31.1	45.2	65.5	60.9	68.2	39.1	12.2	2.9	0.46	1.02	**8.1**	*189*
Eye	12	0	2.9	-	-	-	-	-	-	-	-	1.2	-	2.7	3.0	1.7	4.7	3.2	5.2	-	0.9	0.2	0.05	0.08	**0.9**	*190*
Brain, nervous system	148	0	1.4	3.7	4.0	0.9	0.9	1.9	2.0	5.6	8.4	2.5	23.6	24.7	32.6	31.8	35.1	57.7	47.2	29.4	11.5	2.7	0.56	0.90	**8.4**	*191-2*
Thyroid	36	0	-	-	2.0	0.9	4.7	1.0	3.1	3.4	6.0	1.2	1.5	1.4	4.4	5.0	4.7	9.6	10.5	-	2.8	0.7	0.15	0.20	**2.2**	*193*
Other endocrine	9	0	1.4	-	1.0	0.9	-	-	-	-	-	-	1.5	1.4	5.9	-	-	-	-	-	0.7	0.2	0.06	0.06	**0.7**	*194*
Hodgkin's disease	39	0	-	1.2	1.0	0.9	0.9	6.7	-	1.1	6.0	2.5	4.4	4.1	3.0	6.7	11.7	6.4	5.2	-	3.0	0.7	0.16	0.25	**2.5**	*201*
Non-Hodgkin lymphoma	149	0	2.9	3.7	4.0	3.7	3.7	5.8	5.1	4.5	7.2	8.7	17.7	16.5	23.7	30.1	32.8	67.3	36.7	39.1	11.5	2.7	0.54	0.85	**8.8**	*200,202*
Multiple myeloma	48	0	-	-	-	-	-	-	1.0	-	2.4	-	4.4	8.2	11.9	16.7	9.4	28.9	26.2	-	3.7	0.9	0.14	0.27	**2.3**	*203*
Lymphoid leukaemia	65	0	7.2	-	2.0	-	-	-	-	1.1	1.2	1.2	3.0	6.9	16.3	10.0	21.1	25.7	52.5	39.1	5.0	1.2	0.19	0.35	**3.8**	*204*
Myeloid leukaemia	44	1	1.4	-	-	-	-	-	1.0	3.4	2.4	2.5	7.4	4.1	5.9	15.1	11.7	6.4	10.5	39.1	3.4	0.8	0.14	0.28	**2.6**	*205*
Monocytic leukaemia	4	0	-	-	-	-	-	-	-	-	-	-	-	-	3.0	-	2.3	3.2	-	-	0.3	0.1	0.01	0.03	**0.2**	*206*
Other leukaemia	1	0	-	-	-	-	-	-	-	-	-	-	-	-	1.5	-	-	-	-	-	0.1	0.0	0.01	0.01	**0.1**	*207*
Leukaemia unspecified	25	0	-	1.2	-	-	0.9	-	3.1	1.1	2.4	-	4.4	2.7	-	1.7	7.0	-	21.0	39.1	1.9	0.5	0.08	0.12	**1.4**	*208*
Other and unspecified	212	0	-	-	-	-	0.9	1.0	1.0	3.4	7.2	5.0	19.2	17.8	32.6	60.3	98.3	80.2	141.6	176.1	16.4	3.9	0.44	1.23	**10.3**	*O&U*
All sites	6465	19	20.3	9.9	16.9	17.6	34.4	39.4	56.3	98.9	230.4	274.1	550.6	873.0	1289.5	1784.8	2234.7	2876.4	3215.3	3365.6	500.5		17.61	37.76	**326.9**	*ALL*
All sites but 173	5431	10	20.3	9.9	16.9	16.7	30.7	37.4	51.2	85.4	198.1	223.0	466.4	722.0	1093.9	1506.9	1864.9	2465.9	2648.8	2641.6	420.4	100.0	14.89	31.78	**275.4**	*ALLb*

| Rate from 1 case | | | 1.449 | 1.238 | 0.994 | 0.925 | 0.931 | 0.960 | 1.024 | 1.124 | 1.194 | 1.246 | 1.476 | 1.373 | 1.482 | 1.674 | 2.340 | 3.207 | 5.245 | 9.784 | | | | | | |

SPAIN, NAVARRA 1987-1991

ANNUAL INCIDENCE PER 100,000 BY AGE GROUP (YEARS) - FEMALE

SITE	ALL AGES	AGE UNK	0-	5-	10-	15-	20-	25-	30-	35-	40-	45-	50-	55-	60-	65-	70-	75-	80-	85+	CRUDE RATE	%	CR 64	CR 74	ASR (W)	ICD (9th)
Lip	6	0	-	-	-	-	-	1.0	-	-	-	-	1.5	-	-	-	-	2.2	3.2	14.1	0.5	0.2	0.01	0.01	**0.2**	*140*
Tongue	15	0	-	-	-	-	-	1.0	-	-	-	1.3	-	2.8	2.8	5.9	3.6	2.2	3.2	4.7	1.1	0.4	0.04	0.09	**0.7**	*141*
Salivary gland	7	0	-	-	-	1.0	-	-	-	1.2	-	-	-	1.4	1.4	-	-	-	9.6	-	0.5	0.2	0.02	0.02	**0.3**	*142*
Mouth	7	0	-	-	-	-	-	-	-	-	-	-	1.5	4.1	-	1.5	1.8	-	3.2	-	0.5	0.2	0.03	0.04	**0.3**	*143-5*
Oropharynx	3	0	-	-	-	-	-	-	-	-	-	-	1.5	-	-	-	3.6	-	-	-	0.2	0.1	0.01	0.03	**0.1**	*146*
Nasopharynx	3	0	-	-	1.1	-	-	-	-	-	-	-	-	-	-	-	1.8	-	-	4.7	0.2	0.1	0.01	0.01	**0.2**	*147*
Hypopharynx	0	0	-	-	-	-	-	-	-	-	-	-	-	-	-	-	-	-	-	-	0.0	0.0	0.00	0.00	**0.0**	*148*
Pharynx unspecified	1	0	-	-	-	-	-	-	-	-	-	-	-	-	-	-	-	-	-	4.7	0.1	0.0	0.00	0.00	**0.0**	*149*
Oesophagus	18	0	-	-	-	-	-	-	-	1.2	1.2	1.3	1.5	1.4	1.4	3.0	1.8	4.3	16.1	9.4	1.4	0.5	0.04	0.06	**0.7**	*150*
Stomach	294	0	-	-	-	-	-	2.1	7.1	6.2	9.3	18.0	17.9	22.5	68.0	64.3	138.9	176.6	150.3	22.4	7.4	0.42	1.08	**10.3**	*151*
Small intestine	9	0	-	-	-	-	-	-	-	-	1.2	1.3	1.5	1.4	-	-	1.8	8.7	-	-	0.7	0.2	0.03	0.04	**0.4**	*152*
Colon	331	0	-	-	-	0.9	1.0	4.3	6.0	6.2	5.3	21.0	44.1	53.3	66.5	103.5	95.5	150.9	155.0	25.3	8.4	0.71	1.56	**13.0**	*153*
Rectum	162	0	-	-	1.0	0.9	1.0	-	2.4	1.2	10.6	9.0	20.7	23.9	34.0	46.4	71.6	51.4	56.4	12.4	4.1	0.35	0.76	**6.5**	*154*
Liver	110	0	-	-	-	-	-	-	-	1.2	-	3.0	5.5	11.2	16.3	33.9	45.6	93.1	70.4	8.4	2.8	0.10	0.36	**3.3**	*155*
Gallbladder etc.	113	1	-	-	-	-	-	-	-	-	-	1.5	12.4	11.2	26.6	26.8	45.6	70.7	84.5	8.6	2.9	0.13	0.40	**3.6**	*156*
Pancreas	114	0	-	-	-	-	-	1.1	-	1.2	2.6	10.5	5.5	11.2	22.2	23.2	43.4	86.7	75.1	8.7	2.9	0.16	0.39	**3.9**	*157*
Nose, sinuses etc.	6	0	-	-	-	-	-	-	-	-	-	-	2.8	2.8	1.5	-	-	-	4.7	0.5	0.2	0.03	0.04	**0.3**	*160*
Larynx	6	0	-	-	-	-	-	-	-	1.2	-	1.5	-	1.5	1.8	4.3	-	-	-	0.5	0.2	0.01	0.03	**0.3**	*161*
Bronchus, lung	82	0	-	-	-	-	2.0	-	7.1	1.2	1.3	4.5	4.1	7.0	22.2	41.0	23.9	19.3	28.2	6.3	2.1	0.14	0.45	**3.4**	*162*
Other thoracic organs	7	0	-	-	-	-	-	-	1.2	-	2.6	-	-	-	3.0	-	4.3	-	-	0.5	0.2	0.02	0.03	**0.4**	*163-4*
Bone	11	0	-	-	2.1	-	0.9	-	-	-	-	-	1.4	1.4	1.5	3.6	2.2	3.2	4.7	0.8	0.3	0.03	0.05	**0.6**	*170*
Connective tissue	24	0	-	1.3	-	1.9	0.9	-	-	-	2.5	1.3	3.0	6.9	2.8	4.4	5.4	2.2	3.2	-	1.8	0.6	0.10	0.15	**1.4**	*171*
Mesothelioma	15	0	-	-	-	-	-	-	-	-	2.5	-	3.0	2.8	1.4	3.0	7.1	2.2	3.2	-	1.1	0.4	0.05	0.10	**0.7**	*MES*
Kaposi's sarcoma	3	0	-	-	-	-	-	1.1	-	-	-	-	-	-	-	-	2.2	-	4.7	0.2	0.1	0.01	Ka0.01	**0.1**	*KAP*
Melanoma of skin	68	0	-	-	-	-	3.7	4.1	5.3	6.0	6.2	4.0	3.0	11.0	5.6	10.3	8.9	17.4	6.4	28.2	5.2	1.7	0.24	0.34	**3.6**	*172*
Other skin	777	4	-	-	2.9	1.9	3.1	3.2	23.8	33.6	44.9	45.0	86.9	119.3	131.5	203.5	264.8	279.4	427.3	59.3		1.83	3.52	**31.8**	*173*
Breast	1156	0	-	-	-	-	8.1	18.1	51.2	113.1	170.5	172.6	202.8	233.0	199.4	192.8	206.2	205.5	178.4	88.3	29.2	4.85	6.81	**61.7**	*174*
Uterus unspecified	31	0	-	-	-	-	-	-	-	1.2	1.3	3.0	4.1	2.8	4.4	7.1	2.2	28.9	23.5	2.4	0.8	0.06	0.12	**1.1**	*179*
Cervix uteri	82	0	-	-	1.0	-	4.1	3.2	8.3	12.4	5.3	10.5	9.7	18.2	10.3	19.6	13.0	3.2	4.7	6.3	2.1	0.36	0.51	**4.7**	*180*
Placenta	3	0	-	-	-	-	-	1.1	-	1.3	1.5	-	-	-	-	-	-	-	-	0.2	0.1	0.02	0.02	**0.2**	*181*
Corpus uteri	226	0	-	-	-	-	-	-	6.0	12.4	21.1	33.0	56.6	50.5	45.8	66.0	36.9	25.7	14.1	17.3	5.7	0.90	1.46	**11.6**	*182*
Ovary etc.	161	0	-	-	1.9	4.7	3.1	3.2	3.6	9.9	11.9	19.5	24.8	35.1	28.1	33.9	36.9	32.1	32.9	12.3	4.1	0.59	0.90	**8.1**	*183*
Other female genital	43	0	-	-	-	-	-	-	-	2.5	1.3	1.5	2.8	4.2	8.9	1.8	19.5	32.1	37.6	3.3	1.1	0.06	0.11	**1.4**	*184*
Bladder	91	0	-	-	-	-	-	1.0	-	2.4	1.2	4.0	3.0	11.0	9.8	17.7	25.0	28.2	48.2	61.0	6.9	2.3	0.16	0.38	**3.4**	*188*
Kidney etc.	71	0	4.7	-	-	-	-	-	1.1	2.4	2.5	1.3	3.0	4.1	19.6	17.7	16.1	21.7	16.1	32.9	5.4	1.8	0.19	0.36	**3.4**	*189*
Eye	7	0	1.6	-	-	-	-	-	1.1	-	-	-	-	1.4	-	1.5	1.8	2.2	-	4.7	0.5	0.2	0.02	0.04	**0.4**	*190*
Brain, nervous system	89	0	3.1	-	1.1	1.9	1.9	5.1	3.2	2.4	3.7	6.6	13.5	11.0	7.0	16.3	17.8	26.0	16.1	18.8	6.8	2.2	0.30	0.47	**4.8**	*191-2*
Thyroid	111	0	-	-	3.2	3.8	2.8	7.1	8.5	11.9	17.4	9.3	16.5	15.2	7.0	10.3	17.8	17.4	9.6	-	8.5	2.8	0.51	0.65	**6.9**	*193*
Other endocrine	4	0	1.6	-	-	-	-	-	-	-	1.2	-	-	-	-	3.0	-	-	-	-	0.3	0.1	0.01	0.03	**0.4**	*194*
Hodgkin's disease	33	1	-	-	1.9	1.9	5.1	3.2	4.8	1.2	2.6	3.0	4.1	-	1.5	1.8	6.5	6.4	4.7	2.5	0.8	0.14	0.16	**2.0**	*201*
Non-Hodgkin lymphoma	117	1	-	1.3	-	1.0	-	2.0	1.1	3.6	8.7	9.3	13.5	4.1	18.2	22.2	35.7	47.8	25.7	18.8	8.9	3.0	0.32	0.61	**5.4**	*200,202*
Multiple myeloma	52	0	-	-	-	-	-	-	1.1	1.2	-	-	1.5	4.1	7.0	7.4	16.1	26.0	35.3	18.8	4.0	1.3	0.07	0.19	**1.7**	*203*
Lymphoid leukaemia	41	0	4.7	1.3	-	-	-	1.0	-	1.2	-	-	4.5	2.8	5.6	5.9	8.9	17.4	22.5	9.4	3.1	1.0	0.11	0.18	**2.1**	*204*
Myeloid leukaemia	26	0	-	-	2.1	-	0.9	-	1.1	1.2	2.5	5.3	1.5	-	4.2	5.9	1.8	8.7	6.4	-	2.0	0.7	0.09	0.13	**1.4**	*205*
Monocytic leukaemia	2	0	-	-	-	-	-	-	-	-	-	-	-	-	-	3.0	-	-	-	-	0.2	0.1	0.00	0.01	**0.1**	*206*
Other leukaemia	1	0	-	-	-	-	-	-	-	1.2	-	-	-	-	-	-	-	-	-	-	0.1	0.0	0.01	0.01	**0.1**	*207*
Leukaemia unspecified	17	0	1.6	-	-	-	-	-	-	-	1.2	2.6	1.5	1.4	1.4	1.5	1.8	13.0	6.4	-	1.3	0.4	0.05	0.07	**0.9**	*208*
Other and unspecified	180	1	-	-	-	-	2.0	-	2.4	3.7	4.0	10.5	13.8	19.6	25.1	46.4	67.3	109.2	140.9	13.7	4.5	0.28	0.64	**6.3**	*O&U*
All sites	4736	8	17.3	4.0	9.5	18.2	21.4	50.9	62.8	159.5	261.0	343.6	444.2	607.0	722.8	858.3	1095.8	1378.3	1609.0	1728.1	361.6		13.63	23.42	**214.3**	*ALL*
All sites but 173	3959	4	17.3	4.0	9.5	15.3	19.6	47.8	59.6	135.7	227.5	298.7	399.2	520.1	603.5	726.8	892.4	1113.5	1329.6	1300.8	302.3	100.0	11.80	19.90	**182.4**	*ALLb*

Rate from 1 case | | | 1.568 | 1.330 | 1.061 | 0.958 | 0.932 | 1.018 | 1.064 | 1.190 | 1.243 | 1.322 | 1.501 | 1.380 | 1.404 | 1.477 | 1.785 | 2.171 | 3.212 | 4.696

Spain, Tarragona

The Cancer Registry of Tarragona contains population-based cancer incidence data from 1980. It is administratively part of the Tarragona Cancer League, which receives financial support for the registry from the Department of Health of the Catalan Government. The registry also receives support from the provincial administration for epidemiological research.

The registry produces incidence and survival cancer statistics for the area and describes their major epidemiological characteristics and their evolution. It also promotes epidemiological research, assesses current and future needs for cancer care services, supports the implementation of preventive and other cancer control activities and evaluates their effects.

The registry staff includes a director, two epidemiologists, one technical member and one secretary. There are also one part-time computer assistant and two part-time data collectors. Several oncologists, pathologists, computer scientists, epidemiologists and other specialists act as external collaborators.

The registry covers the Province of Tarragona, which is located in the south of Catalonia in the north-west of Spain, between latitudes 40°32′ and 41°35′ N. The surface area is 6283 km^2, with 216 km of coastline along the Mediterranean Sea. The annual average minimal and maximal temperatures are 12.4°C and 21.1°C. Annual rainfall amounts to about 430 mm. 80% of the population live at altitudes below 200 m above sea level. In 1990 the population comprised 267 235 men and 272 139 women. The two largest towns (109 747 and 86 913 inhabitants respectively) together make up a conurbation which includes several other smaller towns. Thirty other towns have 3000 to 30 000 inhabitants and 148 villages less than 3000 inhabitants.

There is now little migration, although approximately a third of the population was born in other parts of Spain and migrated between the 1950s and 1970s. Roman Catholicism is the major religion. The official languages are Catalan and Spanish.

In 1990 the active population was 218 700: 139 900 men (63.5%) and 79 800 women (36.5%). The working population was 195 400 (89.3% of the active population), of whom 12.3% worked in the agricultural sector, 23.5% in the industrial sector, 13.7% in the building sector and 50.5% in the services sector. In the industrial sector, over 20 000 employees work in the metal industry and over 9000 in the chemical industry. A major petrochemical complex including two refineries, located in the principal conurbation, has been running since the early 1970s, and employs about 7000 workers. There are two nuclear sites, one with two nuclear power stations and the other with one functioning and another closed.

98% of the population is covered by the National Health Service and normally uses its services. In 1990 the number of physicians was 1763. In the period 1988–92 there were eight public hospitals (1695 beds) and eight private ones (422 beds) in the area. Psychiatric centres are not included. One public hospital has an oncology department with high-energy radiotherapy equipment. This department had an average of 30 beds in the period 1988–92. Some cancer patients are transferred to hospitals in Barcelona, which is located 100 km from Tarragona. Although most of these patients are diagnosed in the province, the hospitals located outside the area are also covered by the registry.

The registry also obtains data from 11 pathology services, nine of which are in the province (5 public and 5 private) and one in Barcelona. The registry receives copies of all death certificates of people living in the province. Cases notified from a death certificate are systematically traced and if no further information is obtained, are registered as death-certificate-only cases.

Notification of cancer is voluntary. Registration is active for the sources mentioned, except for death certificates. The registry records malignant tumours whether *in situ* or invasive (behaviour categories 2, 3, 6 and 9 of ICD-O) and includes tumours of the nervous system of undetermined nature. Bladder papillomas, if histologically verified, are not registered. The registry employs a set of rules for the inclusion and coding of multiple primaries which are more liberal than those of IARC/IACR, but it is able to distinguish between those cases which according to IARC/IACR rules would be included as multiple neoplasms and those which would not. The results presented here follow the IARC/IACR rules.

A first check for duplicates is manual, based on the name. A second check is computerized using name, birth date, places of birth and residence, personal identity number and social security number. On-line checks are made when entering the data in the computer to detect errors and inconsistencies.

Recent efforts to improve the completeness and the accuracy of registration with more sources of information have reduced the percentages of death-certificate-only registrations from 7% (male) and 6% (female) in Volume VI to 2.9% and 3.5% respectively in Volume VII. A semi-independent case-ascertainment study estimated the overall completeness for the period 1985–89 as 95.2%.

J.Galceran
J.Borràs

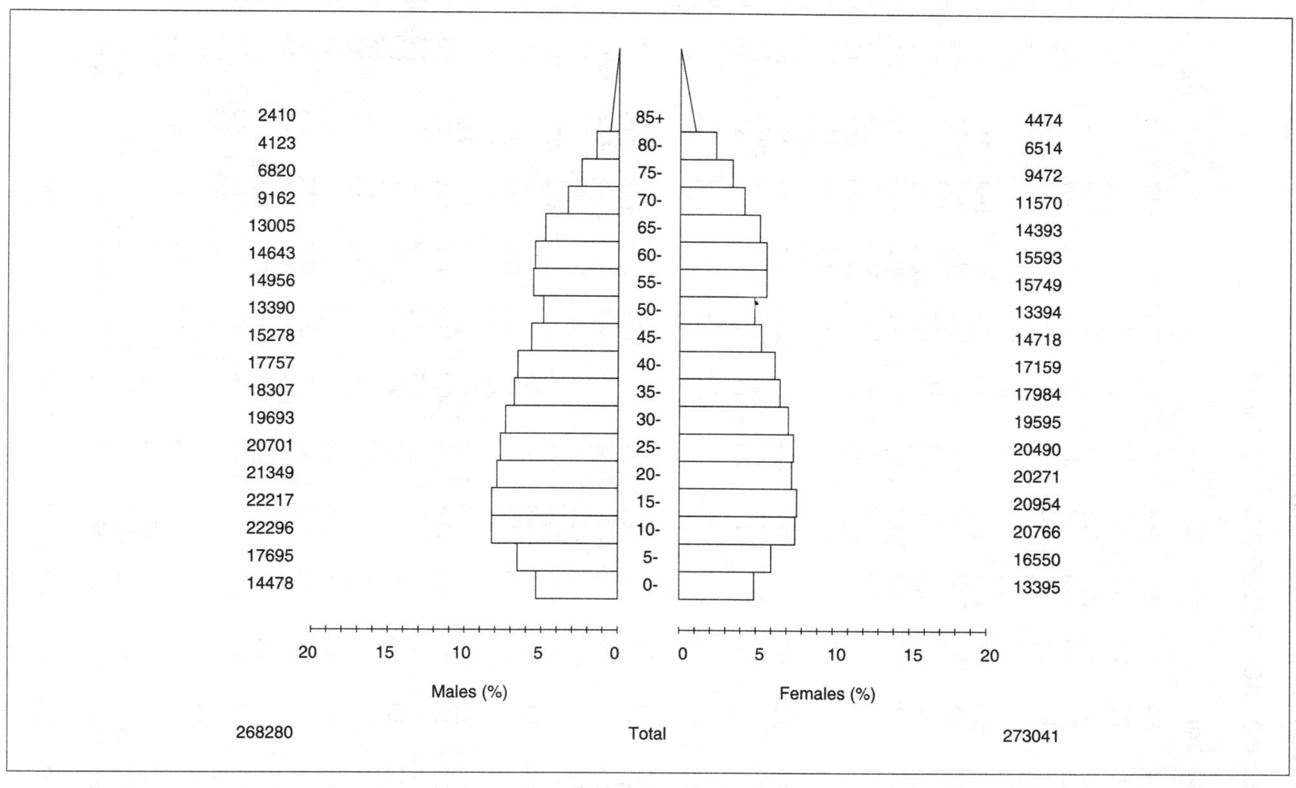

Spain, Tarragona

Source of population: average annual 1988–92

*Census:*1986 and 1991. The methodology used for carrying out the 1991 Census count is given in: Statistics Canada, *Population Estimation Methods.* Demography Division Statistics, Canada, 1987.

Estimate: The populations for 1988, 1989 and 1990 are intercensal stimates, based on the 1986 and 1991 Censuses and taking into account births, deaths and migration. The 1991 and 1992 populations are postcensal estimates, taking into account births, deaths and migration.

Screening programmes in the area

There were no population-based screening programmes in the area during the period, but an annual average of approximately 20 000 cytological examinations for cervical cancer were carried out.

SPAIN, TARRAGONA 1988-1992

ANNUAL INCIDENCE PER 100,000 BY AGE GROUP (YEARS) - MALE

SITE	ALL AGES	AGE UNK	0-	5-	10-	15-	20-	25-	30-	35-	40-	45-	50-	55-	60-	65-	70-	75-	80-	85+	CRUDE RATE	%	CR 64	CR 74	ASR (W)	ICD (9th)
Lip	129	3	-	-	-	-	1.9	-	-	1.1	3.4	6.5	29.9	13.4	21.9	38.4	37.1	38.1	43.7	41.5	9.6	2.5	0.40	0.79	**6.6**	140
Tongue	58	0	-	-	-	-	-	-	1.0	1.1	4.5	5.2	9.0	12.0	9.6	21.5	6.5	14.7	-	33.2	4.3	1.1	0.21	0.35	**3.1**	141
Salivary gland	14	0	-	-	-	-	-	-	-	-	1.1	1.3	4.5	2.7	-	3.1	8.7	-	4.9	-	1.0	0.3	0.05	0.11	**0.8**	142
Mouth	59	0	-	-	-	-	-	-	-	3.3	-	5.2	10.5	24.1	5.5	12.3	17.5	11.7	14.6	-	4.4	1.2	0.24	0.39	**3.1**	143-5
Oropharynx	35	0	-	-	-	-	-	-	-	1.1	5.6	2.6	6.0	8.0	8.2	7.7	4.4	8.8	4.9	-	2.6	0.7	0.16	0.22	**1.9**	146
Nasopharynx	15	0	-	-	-	0.9	-	2.9	-	-	3.4	1.3	1.5	2.7	1.4	1.5	-	-	9.7	-	1.1	0.3	0.07	0.08	**0.9**	147
Hypopharynx	33	0	-	-	-	-	-	-	-	1.1	3.4	9.2	4.5	5.3	9.6	3.1	4.4	2.9	-	24.9	2.5	0.6	0.17	0.20	**2.0**	148
Pharynx unspecified	3	0	-	-	-	-	-	-	-	1.1	-	-	1.5	-	1.4	-	-	-	-	-	0.2	0.1	0.02	0.02	**0.2**	149
Oesophagus	111	0	-	-	-	-	-	-	-	2.2	5.6	10.5	13.4	25.4	21.9	30.8	28.4	35.2	19.4	24.9	8.3	2.2	0.39	0.69	**5.7**	150
Stomach	298	3	-	-	-	-	-	1.0	2.0	5.5	6.8	15.7	13.4	34.8	41.0	81.5	115.7	137.8	140.7	182.5	22.2	5.8	0.61	1.60	**13.5**	151
Small intestine	12	0	-	-	-	-	-	-	-	-	-	1.3	-	2.7	4.1	4.6	4.4	-	4.9	-	0.9	0.2	0.04	0.09	**0.6**	152
Colon	415	2	-	-	-	-	-	-	6.1	7.6	9.0	14.4	20.9	46.8	75.1	113.8	139.7	202.3	223.1	199.1	30.9	8.1	0.90	2.18	**18.6**	153
Rectum	277	2	-	-	-	-	0.9	-	2.0	1.1	1.1	10.5	13.4	41.5	46.4	66.1	122.2	120.2	145.5	149.3	20.6	5.4	0.59	1.54	**12.3**	154
Liver	106	0	1.4	-	0.9	-	-	-	1.0	-	1.1	1.3	11.9	12.0	23.2	33.8	30.6	44.0	48.5	49.8	7.9	2.1	0.26	0.59	**5.0**	155
Gallbladder etc.	43	1	-	-	-	-	-	-	-	-	-	-	-	2.7	9.6	6.2	17.5	14.7	67.9	16.6	3.2	0.8	0.06	0.18	**1.6**	156
Pancreas	90	0	-	-	-	-	-	1.0	-	-	1.1	3.9	4.5	12.0	16.4	29.2	37.1	38.1	29.1	49.8	6.7	1.8	0.19	0.53	**4.1**	157
Nose, sinuses etc.	8	0	-	-	-	-	-	-	-	-	1.3	-	2.7	1.4	3.1	-	2.9	-	-	8.3	0.6	0.2	0.03	0.04	**0.4**	160
Larynx	218	0	-	-	-	-	0.9	-	1.0	4.4	9.0	20.9	35.8	36.1	51.9	72.3	65.5	41.1	24.3	24.9	16.3	4.3	0.80	1.49	**11.6**	161
Bronchus, lung	879	0	-	-	-	-	-	1.9	2.0	8.7	22.5	44.5	106.0	125.7	170.7	290.7	364.5	275.6	232.8	207.4	65.5	17.2	2.41	5.69	**42.9**	162
Other thoracic organs	12	0	-	-	-	-	-	1.0	1.0	-	2.3	-	-	1.3	4.1	1.5	4.4	-	-	8.3	0.9	0.2	0.05	0.08	**0.7**	163-4
Bone	11	0	-	-	-	2.7	-	1.0	1.0	-	-	-	-	-	-	4.6	2.2	-	9.7	-	0.8	0.2	0.02	0.06	**0.6**	170
Connective tissue	32	0	1.4	-	0.9	1.8	1.9	-	2.0	2.2	1.1	1.3	6.0	2.7	1.4	7.7	2.2	5.9	19.4	8.3	2.4	0.6	0.11	0.16	**1.9**	171
Mesothelioma	3	0	-	-	-	-	-	-	-	-	-	-	-	1.3	1.4	1.5	-	-	-	-	0.2	0.1	0.01	0.02	**0.2**	MES
Kaposi's sarcoma	14	0	-	-	-	-	-	3.9	2.0	1.1	3.4	2.6	-	1.3	-	-	2.2	-	-	-	1.0	0.3	0.07	0.08	**1.0**	KAP
Melanoma of skin	66	2	-	-	-	0.9	0.9	2.9	2.0	3.3	2.3	6.5	6.0	5.3	16.4	10.8	13.1	23.5	14.6	24.9	4.9	1.3	0.24	0.36	**3.5**	172
Other skin	1345	63	-	1.1	-	-	0.9	1.9	7.1	21.8	31.5	72.0	89.6	167.1	236.3	362.9	438.7	489.7	601.5	680.3	100.3		3.30	7.51	**62.8**	173
Breast	17	0	-	-	-	-	-	-	1.0	1.1	-	-	-	2.7	-	4.6	6.5	14.7	4.9	8.3	1.3	0.3	0.02	0.08	**0.7**	175
Prostate	551	2	-	-	-	-	-	-	-	-	-	2.6	11.9	20.1	57.4	141.5	218.3	392.9	480.2	472.9	41.1	10.8	0.46	2.27	**21.2**	185
Testis	27	0	-	1.1	-	2.7	2.8	5.8	4.1	4.4	1.1	2.6	1.5	1.3	-	1.5	-	-	-	-	2.0	0.5	0.14	0.14	**1.9**	186
Penis	29	0	-	-	-	-	-	-	-	-	-	1.3	3.0	5.3	5.5	3.1	10.9	17.6	9.7	24.9	2.2	0.6	0.08	0.15	**1.3**	187.1-.4
Other male genital	4	0	-	-	-	-	-	-	-	-	-	-	-	-	-	4.6	2.2	-	-	-	0.3	0.1	0.00	0.03	**0.2**	187.5-.9
Bladder	659	5	-	-	-	-	1.9	1.9	3.0	4.4	7.9	28.8	47.8	90.9	109.3	213.8	270.7	269.8	223.1	273.8	49.1	12.9	1.49	3.93	**30.6**	188
Kidney etc.	125	0	2.8	-	-	-	-	-	3.0	2.2	2.3	2.6	9.0	17.4	21.9	40.0	41.5	49.8	58.2	41.5	9.3	2.4	0.31	0.71	**6.0**	189
Eye	8	0	1.4	-	-	-	-	1.0	1.0	-	-	-	-	-	2.7	1.5	2.2	2.9	-	-	0.6	0.2	0.03	0.05	**0.5**	190
Brain, nervous system	80	0	1.4	3.4	0.9	1.8	3.7	-	2.0	3.3	3.4	2.6	4.5	10.7	19.1	29.2	24.0	8.8	4.9	-	6.0	1.6	0.28	0.55	**4.6**	191-2
Thyroid	12	0	-	-	-	-	-	1.0	-	1.1	1.1	-	3.0	-	1.4	6.2	-	4.9	-	8.3	0.9	0.2	0.04	0.07	**0.7**	193
Other endocrine	9	0	-	-	0.9	0.9	0.9	-	1.0	-	1.1	-	-	-	-	3.1	-	2.9	4.9	-	0.7	0.2	0.02	0.04	**0.5**	194
Hodgkin's disease	42	0	1.4	1.1	2.7	2.7	4.7	4.8	3.0	1.1	2.3	2.6	3.0	6.7	6.8	-	4.4	-	-	16.6	3.1	0.8	0.21	0.24	**2.9**	201
Non-Hodgkin lymphoma	106	0	-	2.3	0.9	1.8	0.9	4.8	6.1	5.5	9.0	10.5	3.0	13.4	13.7	23.1	13.1	52.8	29.1	8.3	7.9	2.1	0.36	0.54	**5.7**	200,202
Multiple myeloma	66	0	-	-	-	-	-	-	-	1.1	1.1	1.3	3.0	9.4	16.4	16.9	19.6	29.3	34.0	41.5	4.9	1.3	0.16	0.34	**3.0**	203
Lymphoid leukaemia	74	1	4.1	2.3	1.8	1.8	1.9	1.0	-	-	-	1.3	6.0	12.0	6.8	21.5	28.4	14.7	34.0	24.9	5.5	1.4	0.20	0.45	**4.1**	204
Myeloid leukaemia	57	0	1.4	1.1	0.9	0.9	0.9	1.9	1.0	5.5	2.3	2.6	3.0	2.7	10.9	15.4	8.7	23.5	24.3	8.3	4.2	1.1	0.18	0.30	**3.1**	205
Monocytic leukaemia	3	0	-	-	-	-	-	-	-	-	-	-	-	-	-	-	2.2	-	4.9	8.3	0.2	0.1	0.00	0.01	**0.1**	206
Other leukaemia	1	0	-	-	-	-	-	-	-	-	1.1	-	-	-	-	-	-	-	-	-	0.1	0.0	0.01	0.01	**0.1**	207
Leukaemia unspecified	19	0	-	-	-	-	-	-	-	-	-	-	-	-	6.8	10.8	2.2	8.8	4.9	16.6	1.4	0.4	0.03	0.10	**0.8**	208
Other and unspecified	289	1	1.4	-	0.9	-	0.9	-	4.1	2.2	6.8	19.6	25.4	42.8	34.1	69.2	100.4	114.4	169.8	157.6	21.5	5.6	0.69	1.54	**13.5**	O&U
All sites	6464	85	16.6	12.4	10.8	18.9	26.2	39.6	59.9	98.3	157.7	316.8	512.3	825.0	1091.3	1814.7	2222.0	2510.0	2750.4	2845.5	481.9		16.14	36.59	**307.4**	ALL
All sites but 173	5119	22	16.6	11.3	10.8	18.9	25.3	37.7	52.8	76.5	126.1	244.8	422.7	657.9	855.0	1451.7	1783.3	2020.3	2148.9	2165.3	381.6	100.0	12.84	29.08	**244.5**	ALLb
Rate from 1 case			1.381	1.130	0.897	0.900	0.937	0.966	1.016	1.092	1.126	1.309	1.494	1.337	1.366	1.538	2.183	2.932	4.851	8.296						

SPAIN, TARRAGONA 1988-1992

ANNUAL INCIDENCE PER 100,000 BY AGE GROUP (YEARS) - FEMALE

SITE	ALL AGES	AGE UNK	0-	5-	10-	15-	20-	25-	30-	35-	40-	45-	50-	55-	60-	65-	70-	75-	80-	85+	CRUDE RATE	%	CR 64	CR 74	ASR (W)	ICD (9th)
Lip	16	1	-	-	-	-	-	-	-	-	-	-	1.5	1.3	2.6	-	1.7	8.4	12.3	8.9	1.2	0.4	0.03	0.04	0.5	140
Tongue	14	1	-	-	-	-	1.0	-	-	1.1	-	-	-	2.5	1.3	2.8	1.7	6.3	3.1	4.5	1.0	0.4	0.03	0.06	0.6	141
Salivary gland	6	0	-	-	-	-	-	-	-	1.1	-	-	-	-	1.4	1.7	4.2	3.1	-	-	0.4	0.2	0.01	0.02	0.2	142
Mouth	14	0	-	-	-	-	-	-	-	1.1	-	1.4	4.5	1.3	-	5.6	3.5	-	6.1	-	1.0	0.4	0.04	0.09	0.7	143-5
Oropharynx	2	0	-	-	-	-	-	-	-	-	-	-	-	-	-	-	-	-	6.1	-	0.1	0.1	0.00	0.00	0.0	146
Nasopharynx	1	0	-	-	-	-	-	-	-	-	-	-	-	-	-	1.4	-	-	-	-	0.1	0.0	0.00	0.01	0.0	147
Hypopharynx	1	0	-	-	-	-	-	-	-	-	-	-	-	1.3	-	-	-	-	-	-	0.1	0.0	0.01	0.01	0.1	148
Pharynx unspecified	1	0	-	-	-	-	-	-	-	-	-	-	-	-	-	-	1.7	-	-	-	0.1	0.0	0.00	0.00	0.0	149
Oesophagus	7	0	-	-	-	-	-	-	-	-	-	-	-	1.3	1.3	-	1.7	2.1	3.1	8.9	0.5	0.2	0.01	0.02	0.2	150
Stomach	180	1	-	-	-	-	-	2.0	-	3.3	9.3	4.1	3.0	16.5	19.2	27.8	41.5	69.7	95.2	111.7	13.2	4.8	0.29	0.64	6.2	151
Small intestine	4	0	-	-	-	-	-	-	-	-	-	-	-	1.3	4.2	-	-	-	-	-	0.3	0.1	0.01	0.03	0.2	152
Colon	390	0	-	-	-	-	1.0	6.1	2.2	9.3	13.6	31.4	30.5	41.0	61.1	122.7	154.1	190.3	160.9	-	28.6	10.3	0.68	1.59	14.0	153
Rectum	164	0	-	-	-	1.0	1.0	1.0	-	1.2	6.8	10.5	22.9	21.8	34.7	34.6	50.7	73.7	89.4	-	12.0	4.4	0.33	0.68	6.1	154
Liver	64	0	-	-	-	-	-	-	-	2.7	1.5	3.8	9.0	12.5	19.0	33.8	24.6	31.3	-	-	4.7	1.7	0.08	0.24	2.1	155
Gallbladder etc.	86	1	-	-	-	-	-	-	-	1.1	-	1.4	1.5	1.3	16.7	16.7	19.0	27.4	61.4	53.6	6.3	2.3	0.11	0.29	2.7	156
Pancreas	93	0	-	-	-	-	-	1.0	-	-	2.3	2.7	4.5	5.1	9.0	15.3	25.9	27.4	52.2	80.5	6.8	2.5	0.12	0.33	3.1	157
Nose, sinuses etc.	2	0	-	-	-	-	-	-	-	-	-	-	-	-	-	1.4	-	-	3.1	-	0.1	0.1	0.00	0.01	0.1	160
Larynx	3	0	-	-	-	-	-	1.0	-	-	-	1.4	-	-	-	-	2.1	-	-	-	0.2	0.1	0.01	0.01	0.2	161
Bronchus, lung	72	0	-	-	-	-	-	-	1.0	-	1.2	8.2	11.9	7.6	6.4	16.7	19.0	16.9	24.6	26.8	5.3	1.9	0.18	0.36	3.1	162
Other thoracic organs	10	1	-	-	-	-	-	-	-	1.1	-	-	-	3.0	-	1.4	5.2	2.1	3.1	-	0.7	0.3	0.02	0.06	0.4	163-4
Bone	16	0	-	-	-	1.9	3.9	1.0	1.0	1.1	-	-	-	-	-	1.4	3.5	2.1	6.1	4.5	1.2	0.4	0.04	0.07	0.9	170
Connective tissue	28	0	-	-	-	1.0	-	-	6.1	1.1	4.7	-	3.0	-	3.8	2.8	3.5	4.2	3.1	17.9	2.1	0.7	0.10	0.13	1.4	171
Mesothelioma	2	0	-	-	-	-	-	-	-	-	-	-	-	1.3	-	1.4	-	-	-	-	0.1	0.1	0.01	0.01	0.1	MES
Kaposi's sarcoma	1	0	-	-	-	-	-	-	-	-	-	-	-	-	-	-	-	-	-	3.1	0.1	0.0	0.00	0.00	0.0	KAP
Melanoma of skin	63	1	-	-	1.0	-	2.0	2.9	1.0	4.4	4.7	6.8	6.0	8.9	6.4	8.3	10.4	8.4	21.5	13.4	4.6	1.7	0.22	0.32	3.2	172
Other skin	1014	51	-	1.2	-	4.8	3.0	11.7	9.2	23.4	35.0	43.5	71.7	83.8	147.5	155.6	261.0	287.2	374.6	446.9	74.3		2.29	4.48	40.1	173
Breast	1043	10	-	-	-	-	-	7.8	26.5	62.3	93.2	114.1	128.4	135.9	143.7	205.6	197.1	196.4	239.5	183.2	76.4	27.7	3.59	5.63	50.7	174
Uterus unspecified	5	0	-	-	-	-	-	-	-	-	-	-	-	2.5	-	1.4	1.7	-	-	4.5	0.4	0.1	0.01	0.03	0.2	179
Cervix uteri	172	2	-	-	-	-	-	3.9	10.2	16.7	22.1	25.8	19.4	33.0	20.5	19.5	27.7	12.7	6.1	44.7	12.6	4.6	0.77	1.01	9.5	180
Placenta	1	0	-	-	-	-	1.0	-	-	-	-	-	-	-	-	-	-	-	-	-	0.1	0.0	0.00	0.00	0.1	181
Corpus uteri	254	4	-	-	-	-	-	-	1.0	1.1	10.5	16.3	26.9	64.8	64.1	55.6	39.8	50.7	52.2	17.9	18.6	6.7	0.94	1.42	11.7	182
Ovary etc.	144	0	-	1.2	1.9	1.0	1.0	5.9	-	5.6	11.7	16.3	17.9	19.0	19.2	30.6	25.9	29.6	27.6	17.9	10.5	3.8	0.50	0.79	7.3	183
Other female genital	63	0	-	-	-	-	-	-	-	1.1	1.2	2.7	-	2.5	9.0	8.3	22.5	29.6	27.6	35.8	4.6	1.7	0.08	0.24	2.1	184
Bladder	120	1	-	-	-	-	-	1.0	-	1.1	-	4.1	1.5	11.4	18.0	27.8	36.3	44.3	61.4	35.8	8.8	3.2	0.19	0.51	4.2	188
Kidney etc.	59	0	-	-	-	-	-	-	1.0	1.1	2.3	4.1	6.0	1.3	9.0	18.1	10.4	21.1	15.4	26.8	4.3	1.6	0.12	0.27	2.4	189
Eye	8	0	3.0	-	-	-	-	-	-	-	-	1.4	-	1.3	1.4	1.7	-	-	-	8.9	0.6	0.2	0.03	0.04	0.6	190
Brain, nervous system	73	0	4.5	1.2	-	1.9	2.0	1.0	2.0	2.2	3.5	5.4	9.0	14.0	7.7	22.2	12.1	8.4	6.1	4.5	5.3	1.9	0.27	0.44	4.2	191-2
Thyroid	62	0	-	-	1.0	1.9	4.9	5.9	3.1	7.8	7.0	4.1	3.0	6.3	11.5	2.8	6.9	10.6	3.1	4.5	4.5	1.6	0.28	0.33	3.7	193
Other endocrine	10	0	6.0	-	-	-	-	2.0	-	-	-	-	-	-	1.3	3.8	-	-	-	-	0.7	0.3	0.07	0.07	1.1	194
Hodgkin's disease	17	0	-	1.2	2.9	1.9	-	1.0	2.0	-	1.2	-	-	-	1.3	2.8	1.7	4.2	-	4.5	1.2	0.5	0.06	0.08	1.1	201
Non-Hodgkin lymphoma	122	1	1.5	1.2	-	-	1.0	1.0	2.0	3.3	7.0	12.2	13.4	11.4	10.3	27.8	29.4	33.8	36.8	26.8	8.9	3.2	0.32	0.61	5.6	200,202
Multiple myeloma	56	0	-	-	-	-	-	-	-	-	-	1.2	1.4	3.0	1.3	14.1	11.1	25.9	19.0	21.5	4.5	4.1	1.5	0.10	0.29	2.1	203
Lymphoid leukaemia	40	0	6.0	2.4	1.0	1.0	-	-	-	-	-	1.4	-	6.3	3.8	6.9	6.9	16.9	15.4	4.5	2.9	1.1	0.11	0.18	2.2	204
Myeloid leukaemia	36	0	1.5	2.4	-	-	-	-	-	3.3	3.5	4.1	1.5	1.3	3.8	8.3	8.6	14.8	3.1	-	2.6	1.0	0.11	0.19	1.9	205
Monocytic leukaemia	3	0	-	-	-	-	-	-	-	-	-	-	-	-	-	-	-	2.1	3.1	4.5	0.2	0.1	0.00	0.00	0.1	206
Other leukaemia	0	0	-	-	-	-	-	-	-	-	-	-	-	-	-	-	-	-	-	-	0.0	0.0	0.00	0.00	0.0	207
Leukaemia unspecified	12	0	-	-	-	-	-	-	-	-	-	1.2	-	1.5	1.3	-	-	4.2	5.2	2.1	4.5	0.9	0.3	0.02	0.07	0.5	208
Other and unspecified	229	0	1.5	-	-	1.0	-	2.0	1.0	4.4	8.2	4.1	13.4	15.2	30.8	32.0	38.0	90.8	128.9	156.4	16.8	6.1	0.41	0.76	8.1	O&U
All sites	4783	75	23.9	10.9	7.7	16.2	19.7	53.7	74.5	151.2	241.3	309.8	398.7	518.1	659.3	858.7	1075.2	1294.3	1621.0	1649.2	350.3		12.62	22.45	205.4	ALL
All sites but 173	3769	24	23.9	9.7	7.7	11.5	16.8	42.0	65.3	127.9	206.3	266.3	327.0	434.3	511.8	703.1	814.1	1007.1	1246.5	1202.3	276.1	100.0	10.32	17.95	165.1	ALLb

Rate from 1 case — 0-: 1.493 | 5-: 1.208 | 10-: 0.963 | 15-: 0.954 | 20-: 0.987 | 25-: 0.976 | 30-: 1.021 | 35-: 1.112 | 40-: 1.166 | 45-: 1.359 | 50-: 1.493 | 55-: 1.270 | 60-: 1.283 | 65-: 1.390 | 70-: 1.729 | 75-: 2.111 | 80-: 3.070 | 85+: 4.469

Spain, Zaragoza

The Cancer Registry of Zaragoza began its activities in 1960, sponsored by the Spanish Association Against Cancer. It published its data for the first time in 1966, referring to the period 1960–64 and since then has reported data regularly. It was the first population-based cancer registry established in Spain and its main aim was to determine cancer incidence by age, sex, site, etc.

Since 1985, the registry has depended entirely upon the General Public Health Headquarters of the Government of Aragon, a region that includes Zaragoza. The registry staff consists of an epidemiologist and two clerks for coding, checking and computing; year by year, clerks for collecting cases from hospitals are engaged.

The area covered is the province of Zaragoza, in the north-east of the peninsula, with an area of 17 194 km^2. It lies between 75 and 1100 m above sea level.

The province has 833 275 inhabitants (407 739 males and 425 536 females) according to an inter-censal estimation for 1 July 1988. The overall population density is 48 inhabitants per km^2, but three quarters of the population live in the city of Zaragoza, which, furthermore, has the highest population growth. Birth rates have fallen during the last two decades.The majority of the population are Roman Catholic, of Mediterranean origin, and speak Castilian. 75% were born in the province, and only 0.2% were born outside Spain.

The economically active population amounts to 40%, while unemployment reached 15% in 1988. The distribution of the active population is as follows: agriculture 9.5%, industry 26.5%, building 7.4%, services 48.7%. The main industrial activities are shoe-manufacturing, wood and furniture, stationery and car-manufacturing.

All hospital centres but one are located in the city of Zaragoza. 80% of the hospital beds belong to public centres, and 20% to the private sector. This facilitates the task of cancer registration, but the greatest advantage lies in the low rate of hospital migration: only 3% of patients seek treatment outside the province of Zaragoza.

Information is obtained through documents and never by personal interviews with the patients. There are three hospital-based cancer registries created in 1980 (Miguel Servet Hospital), 1988 (University Hospital Centre) and 1989 (Provincial Hospital). The Cancer Registry of Zaragoza and the National Registry of Childhood Tumours (directed by Dr R. Peris) operate an agreement for the exchange of information. Some general practitioners who work in rural areas voluntarily send notifications to the registry. Further information is actively gathered from the departments of pathology, haematology/oncology, radiotherapy, clinical history, central filing, etc. A military hospital has been incorporated as a new information source for the registry for the latest period. Its specific contribution to incidence figures (with no other source of information) is about 40 cases per year.

The registry does not perform active follow-up but it keeps track of the evolution of the disease through hospital information, and, in case of death, from death certificates. According to a study carried out by the registry, and based on information from 1983, the coincidence between death certificate diagnosis and hospital information was 73% at the three-digit level of ICD-O.

After collection, forms are verified to assess whether core variables are stated, patients and diseases comply with our case definition and cases were previously registered. A first check for duplicates is done manually. After manual coding, the information is entered with a specially designed computer program. Coding and computing errors are checked by case listing, and further checking for duplicates is carried out by means of computer tools. There are inconsistency checks: sex vs. site, age vs. site, age vs. morphology, and site vs. histology. For the data presented in this volume, the recommendations of the IARC/IACR Working Group on multiple tumours, with the groups of "different" tumours suggested by Berg, have been followed.

The registry has taken part in several observational studies, some coordinated by IARC. Projects are in progress, with the support of Regional and National Health Research Funds, to study survival and trends of cancer in Zaragoza. The registry databank is often used by postgraduates for their doctoral theses or other studies. Access to registry data is limited by regulations.

Alberto Vergara

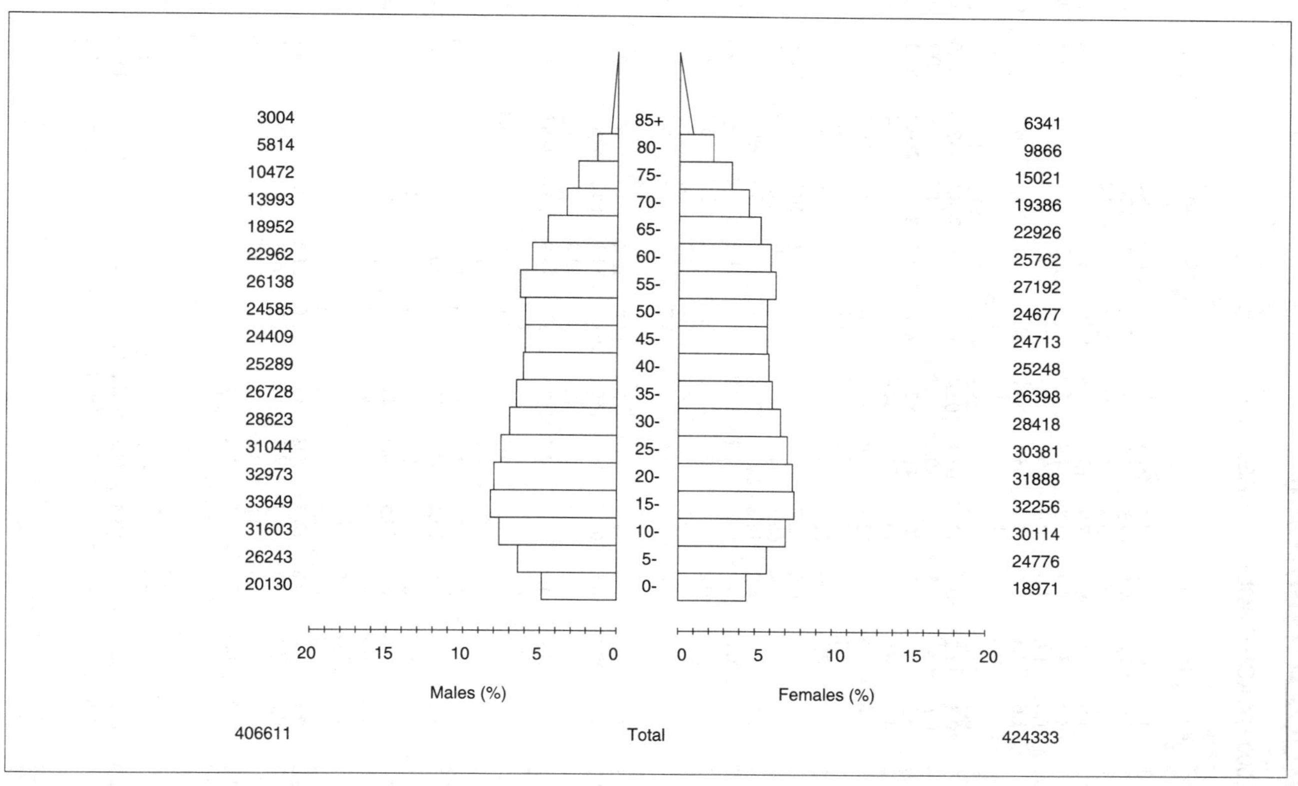

Spain, Zaragoza

Source of population: average annual 1986–90
Census: 1986. Instituto Nacional de Estadistica. Padrón Municipal de habitantes a 1 de Abril de 1986. Madrid, 1988.
Estimate: The populations for each of the years 1987, 1988, 1989 and 1990 were intercensal estimates based on the 1986 (Padrón) and 1991 Censuses, produced by interpolation using a polynomic regression model. *Reference:* Aikin, M., Dunn, C.N. & Flood, T.J. Estimation of Population Denominators for Public Health Studies at the Tract, Gender, and Age-Specific Level. Am. J. Public Health, **81**: 918-920, 1991.

Notes to tables overleaf:
† 188 does not include non-invasive tumours

SPAIN, ZARAGOZA 1986-1990

ANNUAL INCIDENCE PER 100,000 BY AGE GROUP (YEARS) - MALE

SITE	ALL AGES	AGE UNK	0-	5-	10-	15-	20-	25-	30-	35-	40-	45-	50-	55-	60-	65-	70-	75-	80-	85+	CRUDE RATE	%	CR 64	CR 74	ASR (W)	ICD (9th)
Lip	203	1	-	-	-	-	-	-	-	3.0	4.0	4.1	11.4	19.9	34.8	34.8	37.2	51.6	48.2	53.3	10.0	2.6	0.39	0.75	**6.3**	140
Tongue	82	0	-	-	-	-	0.6	-	2.1	1.5	4.0	7.4	4.1	15.3	9.6	10.6	7.1	13.4	13.8	-	4.0	1.1	0.22	0.31	**2.8**	141
Salivary gland	22	0	-	-	-	-	-	-	0.7	1.5	0.8	1.6	-	0.8	3.5	5.3	2.9	1.9	3.4	13.3	1.1	0.3	0.04	0.09	**0.8**	142
Mouth	77	0	-	-	-	-	-	-	0.7	0.7	4.0	6.6	8.1	7.7	15.7	11.6	11.4	5.7	6.9	-	3.8	1.0	0.22	0.33	**2.7**	143-5
Oropharynx	37	0	-	-	-	-	-	-	0.7	-	3.2	3.3	4.9	6.9	4.4	4.2	-	5.7	3.4	-	1.8	0.5	0.12	0.14	**1.3**	146
Nasopharynx	21	0	-	-	-	-	-	-	0.7	-	1.6	1.6	1.6	2.3	0.9	6.3	1.4	-	10.3	-	1.0	0.3	0.04	0.08	**0.7**	147
Hypopharynx	33	0	-	-	-	-	-	-	-	1.6	3.3	8.1	3.1	3.5	4.2	4.3	-	3.4	6.7	1.6	0.4	0.10	0.14	**1.2**	148
Pharynx unspecified	5	0	-	-	-	-	-	-	-	-	0.8	-	1.5	-	1.1	-	1.9	-	-		0.2	0.1	0.01	0.02	**0.2**	149
Oesophagus	163	0	-	-	-	-	-	-	-	1.5	6.3	11.5	19.5	24.5	19.2	25.3	17.2	28.6	27.5	13.3	8.0	2.1	0.41	0.62	**5.5**	150
Stomach	670	2	-	-	-	-	0.6	1.3	3.5	1.5	10.3	17.2	30.1	42.8	67.1	103.4	160.1	215.8	278.6	332.8	33.0	8.7	0.87	2.20	**19.6**	151
Small intestine	9	0	-	-	-	-	-	-	-	-	0.8	-	0.8	-	0.9	2.1	-	5.7	3.4	-	0.4	0.1	0.01	0.02	**0.3**	152
Colon	450	1	-	-	-	-	-	1.3	2.1	3.0	6.3	5.7	19.5	26.8	41.8	82.3	98.6	139.4	220.1	226.3	22.1	5.8	0.53	1.44	**12.9**	153
Rectum	382	1	-	-	-	-	-	-	0.7	3.0	4.0	6.6	13.8	19.9	54.9	64.4	94.3	118.4	147.9	166.4	18.8	4.9	0.52	1.31	**11.1**	154
Liver	184	0	1.0	-	1.9	-	0.6	-	-	1.5	1.6	1.6	9.8	12.2	20.9	29.5	41.4	59.2	79.1	66.6	9.1	2.4	0.26	0.61	**5.5**	155
Gallbladder etc.	85	0	-	-	-	-	-	-	-	-	-	4.1	1.6	5.4	7.8	12.7	25.7	28.6	27.5	59.9	4.2	1.1	0.09	0.29	**2.5**	156
Pancreas	196	0	-	-	-	-	-	0.6	1.4	1.5	0.8	4.1	10.6	27.5	20.9	33.8	38.6	47.7	55.0	79.9	9.6	2.5	0.34	0.70	**5.9**	157
Nose, sinuses etc.	19	0	-	-	-	-	-	-	-	1.6	0.8	2.3	1.7	2.1	4.3	5.7	10.3	-	0.9	0.2	0.03	0.06	**0.6**	160
Larynx	508	0	-	-	-	-	-	-	0.7	3.0	12.7	28.7	46.4	65.8	94.1	106.6	84.3	45.8	44.7	26.6	25.0	6.6	1.26	2.21	**17.1**	161
Bronchus, lung	1572	4	-	-	-	-	0.6	-	2.8	10.5	22.9	42.6	86.2	114.8	229.1	322.9	367.3	376.2	443.7	399.4	77.3	20.3	2.55	6.01	**48.0**	162
Other thoracic organs	10	0	-	-	-	0.6	0.6	-	-	0.7	-	0.8	-	-	0.9	3.2	1.4	1.9	-	-	0.5	0.1	0.02	0.04	**0.4**	163-4
Bone	22	0	1.0	1.5	-	1.2	-	-	-	1.5	2.4	-	0.8	-	0.9	4.2	2.9	3.8	3.4	6.7	1.1	0.3	0.05	0.08	**1.0**	170
Connective tissue	44	0	1.0	-	-	1.2	1.2	1.9	1.4	2.2	-	3.3	1.6	3.8	6.1	4.2	7.1	3.8	-	13.3	2.2	0.6	0.12	0.18	**1.7**	171
Mesothelioma	25	1	-	-	-	-	-	-	-	-	0.8	2.5	1.6	3.1	2.6	3.2	5.7	5.7	-	6.7	1.2	0.3	0.05	0.10	**0.8**	MES
Kaposi's sarcoma	3	0	-	-	-	-	-	-	1.3	-	-	-	-	-	-	1.3	-	-	3.4	-	0.1	0.0	0.01	0.01	**0.1**	KAP
Melanoma of skin	69	0	-	-	-	0.6	0.6	1.9	0.7	1.5	1.6	2.5	4.9	8.4	6.1	8.4	12.9	13.4	24.1	6.7	3.4	0.9	0.14	0.25	**2.3**	172
Other skin	858	7	-	0.8	-	-	0.6	2.6	1.4	4.5	11.1	22.1	36.6	63.5	88.8	159.3	161.5	252.1	354.3	446.0	42.2		1.17	2.79	**25.3**	173
Breast	6	0	-	-	-	-	-	-	-	-	-	-	-	1.5	-	2.1	-	3.8	-	-	0.3	0.1	0.01	0.02	**0.2**	175
Prostate	747	4	-	-	-	-	-	-	-	-	2.4	1.6	4.9	19.9	52.3	112.9	188.7	318.9	454.0	718.9	36.7	9.7	0.41	1.92	**19.7**	185
Testis	34	1	-	-	-	0.6	4.9	3.2	1.4	3.7	4.7	0.8	0.8	2.3	-	1.4	-	-	-	-	1.7	0.4	0.12	0.12	**1.5**	186
Penis	22	0	-	-	-	-	-	-	-	-	-	-	0.8	0.8	3.5	2.1	7.1	1.9	20.6	13.3	1.1	0.3	0.03	0.07	**0.6**	187.1-.4
Other male genital	4	0	-	0.8	-	-	-	-	-	-	-	-	-	-	0.9	-	1.9	3.4	-	0.2	0.1	0.01	0.01	**0.1**	187.5-.9
†Bladder	763	4	-	-	-	0.6	-	-	2.1	2.2	11.9	13.1	22.8	52.0	91.5	158.3	168.6	219.6	278.6	372.8	37.5	9.9	0.99	2.63	**22.4**	188
Kidney etc.	201	1	-	0.8	0.6	-	-	-	2.8	1.5	1.6	5.7	10.6	19.1	30.5	36.9	44.3	40.1	68.8	20.0	9.9	2.6	0.37	0.78	**6.2**	189
Eye	16	0	-	0.8	-	-	-	0.6	-	0.7	-	0.8	0.8	0.8	2.6	3.2	2.9	1.9	3.4	-	0.8	0.2	0.04	0.07	**0.6**	190
Brain, nervous system	165	1	2.0	2.3	5.1	1.8	1.8	1.9	2.1	3.0	7.1	4.1	8.1	24.5	18.3	23.2	22.9	24.8	20.6	6.7	8.1	2.1	0.41	0.64	**6.1**	191-2
Thyroid	25	0	-	-	-	-	1.2	1.9	-	-	1.6	0.8	4.1	1.5	1.7	1.1	2.9	5.7	3.4	6.7	1.2	0.3	0.06	0.08	**0.9**	193
Other endocrine	13	0	4.0	-	-	0.6	-	-	-	-	-	0.8	0.8	2.3	1.7	-	1.4	-	-	-	0.6	0.2	0.05	0.06	**0.8**	194
Hodgkin's disease	53	0	-	-	-	0.6	1.2	5.2	2.8	4.5	2.4	7.4	0.8	4.6	4.4	5.3	1.4	-	3.4	6.7	2.6	0.7	0.17	0.20	**2.2**	201
Non-Hodgkin lymphoma	195	2	4.0	1.5	3.2	2.4	2.4	1.3	1.4	5.2	7.1	7.4	9.8	10.7	21.8	30.6	28.6	51.6	24.1	73.2	9.6	2.5	0.39	0.69	**7.0**	200,202
Multiple myeloma	77	0	-	-	-	-	-	-	-	0.7	0.8	1.6	3.3	5.4	13.1	13.7	17.2	19.1	24.1	33.3	3.8	1.0	0.12	0.28	**2.3**	203
Lymphoid leukaemia	74	0	5.0	4.6	3.2	-	0.6	1.3	-	-	0.8	-	2.4	3.8	4.4	8.4	18.6	19.1	24.1	20.0	3.6	1.0	0.13	0.27	**3.0**	204
Myeloid leukaemia	75	0	2.0	-	1.3	2.4	2.4	-	2.1	2.2	4.7	0.8	2.4	3.1	5.2	9.5	12.9	22.9	13.8	20.0	3.7	1.0	0.14	0.26	**2.7**	205
Monocytic leukaemia	2	0	-	-	0.6	-	-	-	-	-	-	-	-	-	-	1.1	-	-	-	-	0.1	0.0	0.00	0.01	**0.1**	206
Other leukaemia	1	0	-	-	-	-	-	-	-	-	-	-	-	-	-	-	-	1.9	-	-	0.0	0.0	0.00	0.00	**0.0**	207
Leukaemia unspecified	9	0	-	-	-	-	-	0.6	0.2	-	-	-	0.8	-	-	-	2.9	5.7	-	6.7	0.4	0.1	0.01	0.03	**0.3**	208
Other and unspecified	367	1	-	-	-	-	0.6	1.3	0.7	4.5	7.1	8.2	12.2	23.0	36.6	55.9	90.0	116.5	158.2	179.7	18.1	4.7	0.47	1.20	**10.7**	O&U
All sites	8598	31	19.9	13.0	15.8	12.5	20.6	28.3	35.6	71.1	152.6	236.8	408.4	653.4	1024.3	1510.1	1799.4	2287.9	2913.5	3401.7	422.9		13.51	30.12	**264.1**	ALL
All sites but 173	7740	24	19.9	12.2	15.8	12.5	20.0	25.8	34.2	66.6	141.6	214.7	371.8	589.9	935.5	1350.7	1637.9	2035.8	2559.2	2955.7	380.7	100.0	12.34	27.33	**238.8**	ALLb

Rate from 1 case — 0.994 0.762 0.633 0.594 0.607 0.644 0.699 0.748 0.791 0.819 0.813 0.765 0.871 1.055 1.429 1.910 3.440 6.657

†Important: see notes on population page

SPAIN, ZARAGOZA 1986-1990

ANNUAL INCIDENCE PER 100,000 BY AGE GROUP (YEARS) - FEMALE

SITE	ALL AGES	AGE UNK	0-	5-	10-	15-	20-	25-	30-	35-	40-	45-	50-	55-	60-	65-	70-	75-	80-	85+	CRUDE RATE	%	CR 64	CR 74	ASR (W)	ICD (9th)
Lip	8	1	-	-	-	-	-	-	-	-	-	-	-	0.7	-	1.7	-	-	4.1	6.3	0.4	0.1	0.00	0.01	0.2	140
Tongue	14	0	-	-	-	-	-	-	-	-	0.8	0.8	-	0.7	0.8	1.7	3.1	2.7	4.1	3.2	0.7	0.3	0.02	0.04	0.3	141
Salivary gland	8	0	-	-	-	-	-	-	-	-	-	-	0.8	-	0.8	0.9	1.0	1.3	4.1	3.2	0.4	0.1	0.01	0.02	0.2	142
Mouth	10	0	-	-	-	-	-	-	-	-	-	-	-	1.6	0.9	2.1	1.3	4.1	6.3	0.5	0.2	0.01	0.02	0.2	143-5
Oropharynx	6	0	-	-	-	-	-	-	-	-	-	0.8	-	-	-	0.9	1.0	1.3	2.0	3.2	0.3	0.1	0.00	0.01	0.1	146
Nasopharynx	9	0	-	-	-	-	-	0.7	-	-	0.8	1.6	0.7	1.6	-	-	1.3	-	3.2	0.4	0.2	0.03	0.03	0.3	147
Hypopharynx	0	0	-	-	-	-	-	-	-	-	-	-	-	-	-	-	-	-	-	-	0.0	0.0	0.00	0.00	0.0	148
Pharynx unspecified	1	0	-	-	-	-	-	-	-	-	0.8	-	-	-	-	-	-	-	-	-	0.0	0.0	0.00	0.00	0.0	149
Oesophagus	24	0	-	-	-	-	-	-	0.7	-	-	-	-	2.2	2.3	0.9	2.1	2.7	10.1	22.1	1.1	0.4	0.03	0.04	0.5	150
Stomach	428	1	-	-	-	-	-	-	1.4	-	3.2	10.5	9.7	16.9	21.0	42.7	45.4	113.2	186.5	239.7	20.2	7.8	0.31	0.76	8.4	151
Small intestine	7	0	-	-	-	-	-	-	-	-	-	-	-	0.9	4.1	1.3	-	3.2	0.3	0.1	0.00	0.02	0.1	152
Colon	458	1	-	-	-	-	0.6	3.3	3.5	1.5	4.8	7.3	21.1	19.1	40.4	41.9	70.2	109.2	129.7	198.7	21.6	8.4	0.51	1.07	10.2	153
Rectum	273	1	-	-	-	-	-	0.7	2.8	2.3	0.8	7.3	13.8	19.1	20.2	42.7	36.1	53.3	79.1	69.4	12.9	5.0	0.34	0.73	6.4	154
Liver	106	1	1.1	-	-	-	1.9	1.3	0.7	-	-	0.8	0.8	3.7	6.2	10.5	13.4	22.6	36.5	72.5	5.0	1.9	0.08	0.20	2.3	155
Gallbladder etc.	150	0	-	-	-	-	-	-	-	-	-	-	-	5.9	7.0	14.0	32.0	53.3	48.6	69.4	7.1	2.7	0.06	0.29	2.7	156
Pancreas	169	1	-	-	-	-	-	-	-	-	-	3.2	4.9	4.4	17.1	10.5	30.9	53.3	54.7	66.2	8.0	3.1	0.15	0.36	3.4	157
Nose, sinuses etc.	11	0	-	-	-	-	-	-	-	-	-	0.8	0.7	-	0.9	2.1	2.7	6.1	3.2	0.5	0.2	0.01	0.02	0.2	160
Larynx	5	0	-	-	-	-	-	-	-	-	-	-	-	1.7	-	2.7	-	3.2	0.2	0.1	0.00	0.01	0.1	161
Bronchus, lung	116	0	-	-	-	-	0.6	0.7	-	0.8	1.6	2.4	3.2	7.4	10.9	13.1	21.7	18.6	38.5	34.7	5.5	2.1	0.14	0.31	2.7	162
Other thoracic organs	14	0	-	-	-	0.6	0.6	-	1.4	-	2.4	-	-	0.7	0.8	0.9	-	4.1	6.3	0.7	0.3	0.03	0.04	0.5	163-4
Bone	20	0	-	-	0.7	0.6	1.3	-	-	0.8	-	0.8	4.1	0.7	-	3.5	2.1	1.3	-	3.2	0.9	0.4	0.04	0.07	0.7	170
Connective tissue	30	0	1.1	-	0.7	1.9	0.6	0.7	-	1.5	0.8	0.8	1.6	2.2	1.6	0.9	3.1	5.3	4.1	6.3	1.4	0.5	0.07	0.09	1.1	171
Mesothelioma	6	0	-	-	-	-	-	-	-	-	-	0.8	-	-	2.6	1.0	1.3	-	-	0.3	0.1	0.00	0.02	0.2	MES
Kaposi's sarcoma	1	0	-	-	-	-	-	-	-	-	-	-	-	-	-	-	-	2.0	-	0.0	0.0	0.00	0.00	0.0	KAP
Melanoma of skin	106	0	-	-	-	0.6	0.6	1.3	3.5	6.1	6.3	6.5	5.7	6.6	9.3	7.9	13.4	17.3	16.2	6.3	5.0	1.9	0.23	0.34	3.3	172
Other skin	565	5	-	-	-	-	0.6	1.3	2.8	6.8	7.9	12.1	17.0	19.1	34.9	66.3	59.8	138.5	170.3	331.1	26.6		0.52	1.15	12.1	173
Breast	1347	8	-	-	-	-	-	3.9	19.7	34.9	80.0	92.3	94.8	125.0	146.7	150.0	135.1	155.8	158.1	220.8	63.5	24.7	3.00	4.44	40.4	174
Uterus unspecified	39	0	-	-	-	-	-	-	0.8	-	-	1.6	0.7	3.9	5.2	6.2	6.7	18.2	12.6	1.8	0.7	0.03	0.09	0.8	179
Cervix uteri	146	1	-	-	-	-	0.6	1.3	4.2	6.8	7.9	11.3	13.0	13.2	19.4	11.3	12.4	12.0	18.2	3.2	6.9	2.7	0.39	0.51	4.8	180
Placenta	0	0	-	-	-	-	-	-	-	-	-	-	-	-	-	-	-	-	-	-	0.0	0.0	0.00	0.00	0.0	181
Corpus uteri	312	3	-	-	0.6	-	-	-	3.8	6.3	11.3	24.3	32.4	47.4	40.1	45.4	35.9	36.5	34.7	14.7	5.7	0.64	1.07	8.7	182
Ovary etc.	273	0	-	0.7	0.6	0.6	2.0	2.8	4.5	8.7	18.6	21.9	28.7	25.6	38.4	27.9	30.6	30.4	47.3	12.9	5.0	0.57	0.90	8.1	183
Other female genital	103	0	-	-	-	-	-	0.7	-	1.6	1.6	2.4	5.1	8.5	12.2	17.5	29.3	28.4	31.5	4.9	1.9	0.10	0.25	2.2	184
†Bladder	125	0	-	-	-	-	-	0.7	0.8	1.6	0.8	4.9	7.4	7.0	13.1	22.7	29.3	36.5	56.8	5.9	2.3	0.12	0.29	2.7	188
Kidney etc.	100	2	1.1	-	-	-	-	0.7	1.4	1.5	1.6	0.8	7.3	9.6	7.0	12.2	14.4	16.0	18.2	28.4	4.7	1.8	0.16	0.29	2.6	189
Eye	10	0	2.1	0.8	-	-	-	-	-	-	-	0.8	0.8	0.7	0.8	0.9	-	-	2.0	3.2	0.5	0.2	0.03	0.03	0.5	190
Brain, nervous system	123	0	2.1	2.4	1.3	2.5	0.6	1.3	1.4	3.8	4.0	7.3	8.9	5.9	17.1	14.8	8.3	14.6	12.2	15.8	5.8	2.3	0.29	0.41	4.2	191-2
Thyroid	83	1	-	-	0.7	1.9	1.9	2.6	7.7	3.8	7.9	4.0	5.7	5.9	5.4	1.7	4.1	8.0	8.1	6.3	3.9	1.5	0.24	0.27	3.1	193
Other endocrine	12	0	1.1	-	-	0.6	-	0.7	0.8	-	-	-	2.3	0.9	2.1	1.3	-	3.2	0.6	0.2	0.03	0.04	0.5	194
Hodgkin's disease	42	0	-	-	2.7	0.6	1.3	5.9	2.1	3.0	2.4	-	1.6	-	1.6	2.6	1.0	6.7	2.0	2.0	0.8	0.11	0.12	1.7	201
Non-Hodgkin lymphoma	172	0	2.1	2.4	-	0.6	1.9	0.7	4.2	3.0	3.2	6.5	8.9	16.2	22.5	18.3	18.6	26.6	24.3	22.1	8.1	3.2	0.36	0.55	5.2	200,202
Multiple myeloma	89	0	-	-	-	-	-	-	-	-	0.8	1.6	2.4	2.2	6.2	13.1	17.5	22.6	26.4	31.5	4.2	1.6	0.07	0.22	1.9	203
Lymphoid leukaemia	65	0	3.2	2.4	2.0	1.9	0.6	0.7	-	0.8	1.6	1.6	0.8	2.9	3.9	5.2	7.2	14.6	14.2	15.8	3.1	1.2	0.11	0.17	2.2	204
Myeloid leukaemia	86	0	2.1	0.8	1.3	1.2	1.3	2.6	1.4	1.5	3.2	3.2	2.4	5.1	9.3	7.9	8.3	13.3	8.1	25.2	4.1	1.6	0.18	0.26	2.8	205
Monocytic leukaemia	3	0	-	-	-	-	-	0.7	-	-	-	-	-	-	2.1	-	-	-	0.1	0.1	0.00	0.01	0.1	206
Other leukaemia	3	0	-	-	-	-	-	-	-	-	-	-	-	1.7	1.0	-	-	-	0.1	0.1	0.00	0.01	0.1	207
Leukaemia unspecified	16	0	-	-	-	-	0.7	0.7	-	-	-	-	-	1.6	0.9	3.1	4.0	6.1	6.3	0.8	0.3	0.01	0.03	0.3	208
Other and unspecified	328	1	1.1	0.8	-	-	0.6	1.3	0.7	2.3	4.0	7.3	8.1	9.6	29.5	33.2	38.2	78.6	115.5	164.0	15.5	6.0	0.33	0.68	7.1	O&U
All sites	6022	27	16.9	9.7	10.0	13.6	16.9	32.9	66.9	91.7	164.0	223.4	295.8	381.7	541.9	651.7	737.6	1110.4	1368.3	1895.4	283.8		9.37	16.35	156.0	ALL
All sites but 173	5457	22	16.9	9.7	10.0	13.6	16.3	31.6	64.0	84.9	156.0	211.2	278.8	362.6	506.9	585.4	677.8	971.9	1198.0	1564.3	257.2	100.0	8.85	15.19	143.9	ALLb

| Rate from 1 case | | | 1.054 | 0.807 | 0.664 | 0.620 | 0.627 | 0.658 | 0.704 | 0.758 | 0.792 | 0.809 | 0.810 | 0.736 | 0.776 | 0.872 | 1.032 | 1.331 | 2.027 | 3.154 |

†Important: see notes on population page

Sweden

The Swedish Cancer Registry was founded in 1958 and is tumour-based. It is organized within the Centre for Epidemiology at the National Board of Health and Welfare and is financed by the government.

The registry covers the population of the whole of Sweden. The country is surrounded to the north and west by Norway, to the east by Finland and to the east, south and west by the Baltic Sea. Sweden is located between latitudes 55°20′ and 69°4′ N and longitudes 10°58′ and 24°10′ E. The total registration area is 449 964 km².

In 1990 the population of Sweden was 8 558 834. Virtually the whole population is Caucasian and Protestant. The main occupations of the economically active population on 1 November 1990 were services 37%, manufacturing 20% and commerce 14%. The unemployment of the labour force was 1.5%. In December 1990, 5.6% of the population were foreigners. The main immigration groups were from the Nordic countries, the rest of Europe and from Asia. The total number of hospital beds of all kinds was 98 009. The total number of doctors in practice in the registration area was 21 700 (253 per 100 000 inhabitants).

The registration of newly detected tumour cases is based upon compulsory reports from all physicians responsible for in- and outpatient departments in hospitals, in both public and private administration. In Sweden nearly every cancer case is sooner or later seen at a hospital for in- or outpatient care. Hospital and forensic pathologists give independent compulsory reports for every cancer diagnosis made from surgical biopsies, cytological specimens and autopsies. Reporting is also compulsory for pathologists working in private laboratories.

The registration of new cancer reports and the major work of checking and correction is performed by six regional cancer registries covering the whole country. These registries are associated with the oncological centres in each medical region of Sweden. The regionalization implies a close contact between the registry and the reporting physician, which in turn simplifies the task of correcting and checking the material. The regional registries annually send information about newly registered cases and corrections concerning those previously reported to the National Cancer Registry. The overall reporting to the registry is estimated to be 96% of all diagnosed cases.

The data in the registry are supplemented with information on cause and date of death by computerized linking with the Cause of Death Registry at Statistics Sweden. The Swedish Cancer Registry does not use information on cancers based on death certificates only, the reason being that the data on death certificates in many instances are uncertain. In 1990, there were 1507 persons in the Cause of Death Registry with cancer stated as underlying cause of death who were not on file in the Cancer Registry. The commonest cancer sites were bronchus/lung, pancreas, liver, prostate and colon. 90% of these did not have an autopsy and 81% were over 70 years of age. According to the Cause of Death Registry, cancer caused approximately 22% of all deaths in the country in 1990.

Besides cases of cancer and malignant lymphoma, histologically benign hormonally active endocrine tumours (except adenomas of the thyroid gland), non-invasive urinary tract papillomas, and benign intracranial and intraspinal tumours are included in reports on incidence. Basal cell carcinomas of the skin are excluded. Reports are received on a variety of benign and potentially malignant tumours; these are registered separately and not included in the incidence figures. Precancerous lesions, such as carcinoma *in situ* of the cervix uteri, are reported but computed separately. Likewise, hydatidiform moles are reported but registered separately.

Primary tumours in different organs in one individual are classified as independent tumours. If multiple tumours occur within paired organs, or in other sites, the case is classified in such a way that it is possible to count the case as one primary cancer only, as well as the number of primaries that actually exist.

The only follow-up undertaken by the registry is estimation of survival time.

Lotti Barlow

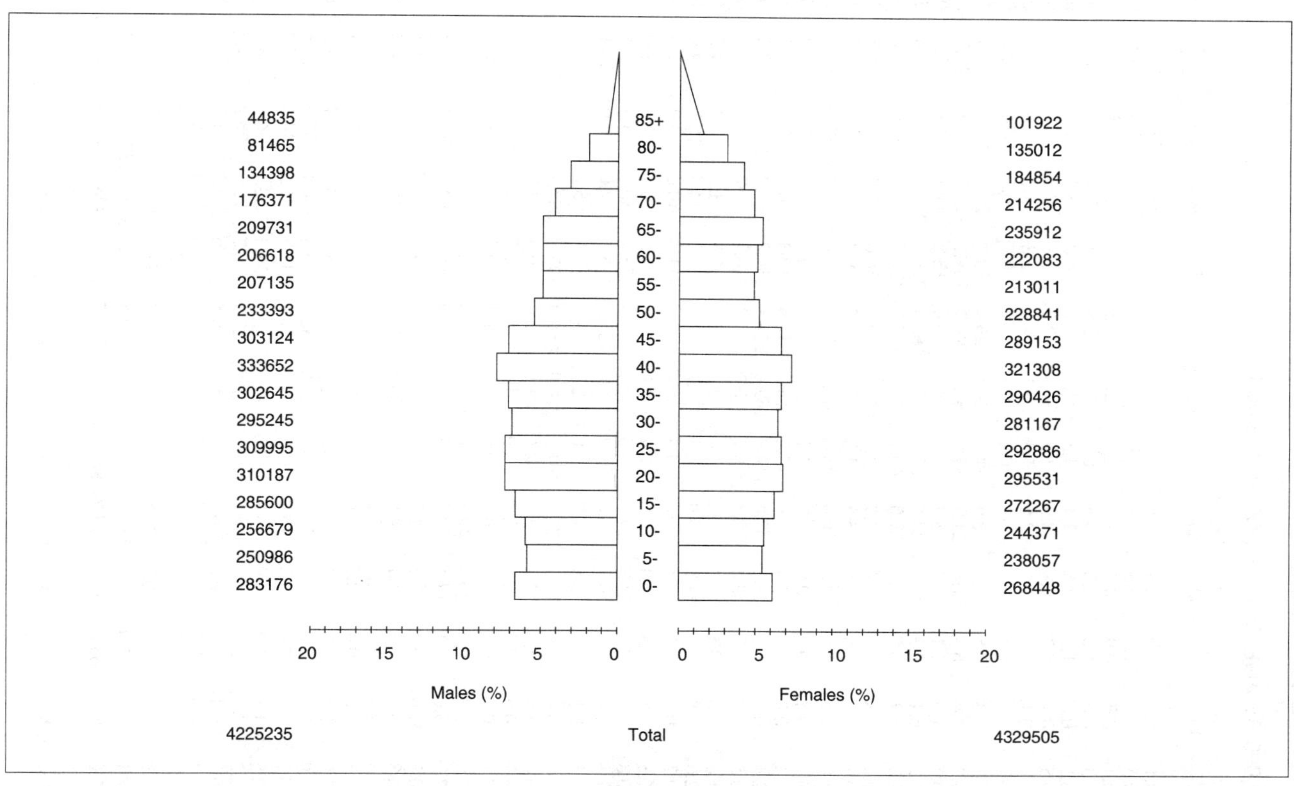

Sweden
Source of population: 1988–92
Notes to tables overleaf:
† 173 does not include basal cell carcinomas
Screening programmes in the area:
Cervical cancer screening began in the mid–60s, covering women aged 25-54. Screening for breast cancer began in some areas in the mid–80s with further areas joining in 1990, covering the population aged 40-69.

SWEDEN 1988-1992

ANNUAL INCIDENCE PER 100,000 BY AGE GROUP (YEARS) - MALE

SITE	ALL AGES	AGE UNK	0-	5-	10-	15-	20-	25-	30-	35-	40-	45-	50-	55-	60-	65-	70-	75-	80-	85+	CRUDE RATE	%	CR 64	CR 74	ASR (W)	ICD (9th)
Lip	686	0	-	-	-	-	-	-	-	0.1	0.3	1.7	2.3	3.8	5.3	8.6	13.5	22.0	25.3	32.1	3.2	0.7	0.07	0.18	1.6	140
Tongue	324	0	-	-	-	-	-	0.5	0.3	0.5	1.0	1.5	2.5	3.1	4.4	5.1	5.1	4.0	5.4	5.4	1.5	0.3	0.07	0.12	1.0	141
Salivary gland	210	0	-	-	-	-	0.2	0.2	0.5	0.4	0.7	0.9	0.8	1.2	2.4	2.5	3.5	4.2	5.2	6.2	1.0	0.2	0.04	0.07	0.6	142
Mouth	502	0	-	-	-	0.1	0.1	0.1	0.2	0.3	0.6	1.6	3.2	4.5	8.2	7.2	8.8	10.4	9.1	12.0	2.4	0.5	0.09	0.17	1.5	143-5
Oropharynx	274	0	-	-	-	-	-	-	-	0.1	0.6	1.3	2.5	3.4	4.5	4.6	4.6	4.0	3.2	1.8	1.3	0.3	0.06	0.11	0.9	146
Nasopharynx	123	0	0.1	-	-	0.1	-	0.1	0.1	0.5	0.4	0.7	0.8	0.9	1.3	1.6	2.0	1.8	2.2	2.7	0.6	0.1	0.02	0.04	0.4	147
Hypopharynx	277	0	-	-	-	-	-	-	0.1	-	0.1	1.1	1.6	2.6	5.3	5.1	4.6	5.8	3.7	3.6	1.3	0.3	0.05	0.10	0.8	148
Pharynx unspecified	14	0	-	-	-	-	-	-	-	-	-	0.1	-	-	0.1	0.4	-	0.7	0.5	0.4	0.1	0.0	0.00	0.00	0.0	149
Oesophagus	1172	0	-	-	-	-	-	-	-	0.1	0.4	2.8	3.2	8.9	14.7	20.5	26.4	30.4	28.5	32.6	5.5	1.3	0.15	0.38	3.1	150
Stomach	4497	0	-	-	-	-	0.1	0.3	0.8	1.2	4.4	6.3	11.8	21.9	37.6	61.1	99.7	134.2	173.3	183.3	21.3	4.8	0.42	1.23	10.7	151
Small intestine	498	0	-	-	-	-	0.1	0.1	0.4	0.7	1.0	1.1	1.9	3.7	5.7	8.5	9.0	13.2	11.5	9.8	2.4	0.5	0.07	0.16	1.3	152
Colon	7307	0	-	0.1	0.2	0.7	0.7	1.4	1.4	3.2	6.1	9.9	21.5	34.5	67.3	95.6	162.5	216.1	267.6	294.9	34.6	7.8	0.73	2.02	17.7	153
Rectum	4779	0	-	-	-	0.1	0.3	0.6	0.8	2.2	3.4	6.7	17.9	29.0	49.7	73.1	108.1	132.7	143.4	153.0	22.6	5.1	0.55	1.46	12.1	154
Liver	1377	0	0.8	0.2	-	0.2	0.1	0.1	0.5	0.4	0.8	1.5	2.9	7.9	12.6	21.6	29.1	36.0	57.0	46.8	6.5	1.5	0.14	0.39	3.4	155
Gallbladder etc.	1031	0	0.1	-	-	-	-	-	0.2	0.2	1.0	1.5	2.5	5.5	11.8	15.5	22.7	29.2	31.7	40.1	4.9	1.1	0.11	0.30	2.6	156
Pancreas	2765	0	-	0.1	-	-	0.2	0.4	0.3	1.0	2.6	5.9	9.2	16.6	28.4	44.3	62.7	75.6	79.8	80.3	13.1	3.0	0.32	0.86	7.0	157
Nose, sinuses etc.	216	0	-	-	0.1	0.1	-	0.1	0.3	0.1	0.4	0.9	0.9	1.7	2.1	3.1	4.6	4.3	5.6	5.4	1.0	0.2	0.03	0.07	0.6	160
Larynx	907	0	-	-	-	-	0.1	0.1	0.1	0.3	0.8	1.9	4.4	9.9	13.0	16.0	16.9	19.8	20.9	13.8	4.3	1.0	0.15	0.32	2.5	161
Bronchus, lung	8977	0	-	-	-	0.1	0.2	0.2	0.7	2.4	6.7	16.6	35.6	67.4	114.3	169.6	211.5	216.8	207.0	142.7	42.5	9.6	1.22	3.13	23.9	162
Other thoracic organs	57	0	0.1	-	-	0.2	0.1	0.1	0.3	0.5	-	0.3	0.2	0.3	0.7	0.7	0.8	0.3	1.2	-	0.3	0.1	0.01	0.02	0.2	163-4
Bone	243	0	0.2	0.8	1.2	2.8	1.2	0.6	0.5	1.0	1.0	0.5	0.4	1.2	1.4	2.3	2.6	2.2	1.2	1.3	1.2	0.3	0.06	0.09	1.1	170
Connective tissue	846	0	2.0	0.5	0.8	0.8	1.4	1.2	1.6	2.6	2.8	3.4	4.2	5.0	6.1	8.1	12.5	18.9	14.5	18.7	4.0	0.9	0.16	0.27	2.8	171
Mesothelioma	423	0	-	-	-	-	-	0.1	-	0.2	0.5	1.6	2.6	2.8	4.4	6.4	8.6	11.5	10.6	8.0	2.0	0.5	0.06	0.14	1.1	MES
Kaposi's sarcoma	210	0	-	-	-	0.1	0.1	1.0	1.7	1.5	1.1	0.8	0.8	0.6	0.4	1.0	1.5	4.5	6.1	7.6	1.0	0.2	0.04	0.05	0.6	KAP
Melanoma of skin	3463	0	-	0.1	0.3	1.8	2.6	5.5	5.9	10.8	12.8	20.2	24.7	27.4	34.6	44.4	53.5	53.7	50.6	45.9	16.4	3.7	0.73	1.22	11.0	172
†Other skin	5505	0	-	-	-	0.1	-	-	0.4	1.1	2.4	4.0	10.7	16.6	29.2	57.0	105.8	176.9	272.0	426.0	26.1		0.32	1.14	11.9	173
Breast	158	0	-	-	-	-	-	-	-	0.1	0.1	0.5	0.5	1.7	2.0	2.7	3.3	2.1	5.6	4.0	0.7	0.2	0.02	0.05	0.4	175
Prostate	25253	0	-	-	-	-	-	-	-	0.6	3.3	20.5	72.1	191.5	370.3	656.0	897.6	1053.7	997.9	119.5	27.1	1.44	6.57	55.3	185
Testis	1077	0	0.6	0.1	0.3	2.5	9.7	14.1	12.4	10.4	6.5	5.3	2.7	3.0	2.6	1.3	1.4	0.9	1.2	1.8	5.1	1.2	0.35	0.36	4.8	186
Penis	271	0	-	-	-	-	-	-	0.2	0.7	0.5	0.7	1.4	2.2	1.9	4.1	4.3	6.5	7.9	10.3	1.3	0.3	0.04	0.08	0.7	187.1-.4
Other male genital	57	0	0.1	-	-	0.1	-	-	0.1	0.1	0.1	0.1	0.1	0.4	0.8	0.8	1.4	0.7	2.0	1.3	0.3	0.1	0.01	0.02	0.2	187.5-.9
Bladder	6973	0	-	-	-	-	0.2	0.8	0.6	2.0	6.3	10.0	20.9	43.7	71.0	107.1	151.4	202.4	224.9	221.7	33.0	7.5	0.78	2.07	17.3	188
Kidney etc.	3745	0	1.8	0.6	0.1	0.1	0.3	0.1	0.5	2.2	5.0	8.1	17.1	29.8	44.7	59.5	81.9	86.8	94.8	75.4	17.7	4.0	0.55	1.26	10.3	189
Eye	238	0	0.7	0.2	-	-	0.1	0.1	0.3	0.3	1.0	0.7	1.5	1.5	2.4	3.6	4.8	4.0	3.7	3.1	1.1	0.3	0.04	0.09	0.8	190
Brain, nervous system	1735	0	3.3	4.3	3.0	2.8	2.8	3.7	5.1	6.3	6.5	8.5	11.1	14.9	18.8	20.5	21.5	15.2	10.8	8.5	8.2	1.9	0.46	0.67	6.6	191-2
Thyroid	438	0	-	-	-	0.4	0.5	0.5	1.2	1.3	2.3	2.5	2.5	3.4	4.1	5.2	7.4	6.1	5.9	6.2	2.1	0.5	0.09	0.16	1.4	193
Other endocrine	84	0	0.4	0.2	0.2	0.1	0.1	0.2	0.1	0.2	0.2	0.4	0.7	0.6	0.5	0.5	1.1	1.5	1.2	1.3	0.4	0.1	0.02	0.03	0.3	194
Hodgkin's disease	539	0	0.1	0.8	1.1	2.7	2.8	3.2	3.0	2.3	2.2	2.2	2.2	3.2	3.8	2.8	4.5	4.2	5.6	6.7	2.6	0.6	0.15	0.18	2.2	201
Non-Hodgkin lymphoma	3713	0	1.6	2.2	1.2	1.3	1.6	2.3	3.0	5.0	7.9	15.0	17.7	27.1	36.2	52.0	68.3	76.9	90.1	87.0	17.6	4.0	0.61	1.21	10.8	200,202
Multiple myeloma	1520	0	-	-	-	-	-	-	0.3	0.9	1.4	2.6	4.5	10.2	14.5	24.7	31.9	45.2	46.2	44.2	7.2	1.6	0.17	0.45	3.8	203
Lymphoid leukaemia	1345	0	5.1	4.1	2.0	2.1	0.7	0.6	0.8	0.5	1.1	2.2	4.0	5.7	10.0	17.7	23.8	37.5	33.1	36.1	6.4	1.4	0.19	0.40	4.3	204
Myeloid leukaemia	998	0	1.1	0.6	0.6	0.8	0.9	1.4	1.8	2.2	2.3	3.4	4.1	6.1	8.3	12.0	17.9	20.7	22.8	25.9	4.7	1.1	0.17	0.32	3.0	205
Monocytic leukaemia	36	0	-	-	-	-	-	0.1	-	0.1	0.1	0.1	0.2	0.2	0.3	0.3	0.8	0.6	1.7	1.3	0.2	0.0	0.00	0.01	0.1	206
Other leukaemia	277	0	-	-	-	-	-	0.1	0.3	0.3	0.4	0.7	1.5	1.9	2.8	4.3	5.2	7.6	7.1	6.2	1.3	0.3	0.04	0.09	0.7	207
Leukaemia unspecified	147	0	-	-	0.2	0.1	0.2	-	0.1	0.1	0.1	0.5	0.3	0.4	0.9	1.5	2.7	3.9	5.4	10.3	0.7	0.2	0.01	0.04	0.4	208
Other and unspecified	3454	0	-	-	0.1	0.3	0.3	0.5	1.4	1.9	2.6	5.7	10.7	22.8	35.0	52.5	72.2	92.9	110.0	122.7	16.3	3.7	0.41	1.03	8.8	O&U
All sites	98741	0	18.1	14.7	11.3	20.4	27.8	40.5	48.2	68.1	98.7	167.0	293.0	531.3	917.3	1427.6	2142.5	2742.6	3170.7	3246.5	467.4		11.28	29.13	252.7	ALL
All sites but 173	93236	0	18.1	14.7	11.3	20.3	27.8	40.5	47.8	67.0	96.3	163.0	282.3	514.7	888.1	1370.6	2036.7	2565.7	2898.7	2820.5	441.3	100.0	10.96	28.00	240.7	ALLb

Rate from 10 cases   0.706   0.797   0.779   0.700   0.645   0.645   0.677   0.661   0.599   0.660   0.857   0.966   0.968   0.954   1.134   1.488   2.455   4.461

†Important: see notes on population page

SWEDEN 1988-1992

ANNUAL INCIDENCE PER 100,000 BY AGE GROUP (YEARS) - FEMALE

SITE	ALL AGES	AGE UNK	0-	5-	10-	15-	20-	25-	30-	35-	40-	45-	50-	55-	60-	65-	70-	75-	80-	85+	CRUDE RATE	%	CR 64	CR 74	ASR (W)	ICD (9th)
Lip	194	0	0.1	-	-	-	-	-	-	0.1	0.4	0.7	1.0	0.8	1.4	1.6	2.2	3.2	5.2	6.3	0.9	0.2	0.02	0.04	**0.4**	*140*
Tongue	260	0	-	-	-	-	0.3	0.1	0.2	0.3	0.7	1.0	1.3	2.1	2.0	2.2	2.5	4.5	4.7	7.1	1.2	0.3	0.04	0.06	**0.6**	*141*
Salivary gland	228	0	-	-	-	0.2	0.4	-	0.4	0.3	0.6	1.1	1.2	1.3	1.3	2.5	3.1	4.3	3.4	3.3	1.1	0.2	0.03	0.06	**0.6**	*142*
Mouth	367	0	0.1	-	-	-	0.1	0.1	0.4	0.3	0.4	0.6	1.4	2.8	2.6	4.7	5.0	6.1	7.6	9.4	1.7	0.4	0.04	0.09	**0.8**	*143-5*
Oropharynx	121	0	-	-	-	-	-	-	0.1	0.1	0.2	1.0	0.6	1.7	1.4	1.8	1.2	1.5	1.3	0.4	0.6	0.1	0.03	0.04	**0.3**	*146*
Nasopharynx	55	0	-	-	-	-	0.1	-	0.1	0.1	0.4	0.2	0.4	0.3	0.6	0.8	0.3	1.2	0.4	0.4	0.3	0.1	0.01	0.02	**0.2**	*147*
Hypopharynx	59	0	-	-	-	-	-	-	-	-	0.1	0.1	0.3	0.5	0.7	0.6	0.7	1.2	1.6	0.6	0.3	0.1	0.01	0.01	**0.1**	*148*
Pharynx unspecified	1	0	-	-	-	-	-	-	-	-	-	-	-	-	-	-	-	-	-	0.2	0.0	0.0	0.00	0.00	**0.0**	*149*
Oesophagus	549	0	-	-	0.1	-	-	0.1	-	0.1	0.1	0.8	1.6	2.5	4.1	6.0	7.5	11.7	15.1	15.9	2.5	0.6	0.05	0.11	**1.0**	*150*
Stomach	2896	0	-	-	-	-	0.1	0.4	0.8	1.8	2.2	5.0	7.8	10.7	20.8	28.0	42.0	58.5	78.1	90.5	13.4	3.2	0.25	0.60	**5.4**	*151*
Small intestine	427	0	-	-	-	0.1	0.1	-	0.1	0.4	0.4	1.4	1.3	2.5	4.3	5.5	6.1	7.0	8.4	9.8	2.0	0.5	0.05	0.11	**0.9**	*152*
Colon	8166	0	-	-	1.2	1.4	2.2	1.6	2.1	4.3	6.2	11.1	23.2	40.0	56.4	88.8	119.1	172.7	210.1	209.6	37.7	8.9	0.75	1.79	**15.9**	*153*
Rectum	4037	0	-	-	-	-	0.1	0.3	1.1	1.7	4.1	6.5	16.0	24.3	33.1	46.0	61.0	79.2	88.4	97.1	18.6	4.4	0.44	0.97	**8.3**	*154*
Liver	916	0	0.6	0.1	-	0.1	0.1	0.2	0.1	0.6	0.7	1.7	1.6	3.9	5.7	10.6	14.5	19.5	20.6	26.5	4.2	1.0	0.08	0.20	**1.8**	*155*
Gallbladder etc.	2166	0	-	-	-	-	0.1	-	0.1	0.2	0.9	3.3	6.4	10.1	17.9	24.8	32.5	42.4	57.3	58.7	10.0	2.4	0.19	0.48	**4.1**	*156*
Pancreas	3048	0	-	-	0.1	0.1	0.1	0.1	0.4	0.7	1.8	4.3	7.6	14.6	21.9	34.3	50.8	64.2	75.1	79.1	14.1	3.3	0.26	0.68	**5.8**	*157*
Nose, sinuses etc.	129	0	-	-	-	-	-	0.1	0.1	0.1	0.1	0.1	0.6	0.8	0.9	1.6	1.2	2.3	3.7	2.9	0.6	0.1	0.02	0.03	**0.3**	*160*
Larynx	129	0	-	-	-	-	-	0.1	-	0.2	0.3	0.3	1.4	1.4	1.9	1.9	1.3	1.4	0.9	1.4	0.6	0.1	0.03	0.04	**0.4**	*161*
Bronchus, lung	4343	0	-	-	-	0.1	0.1	0.4	1.3	3.0	7.2	15.7	24.1	35.6	53.6	63.9	71.7	60.3	53.9	46.7	20.1	4.7	0.71	1.38	**10.9**	*162*
Other thoracic organs	29	0	-	-	-	-	-	0.1	0.1	0.1	0.1	0.1	0.3	0.2	0.5	0.3	0.3	0.4	0.1	-	0.1	0.0	0.01	0.01	**0.1**	*163-4*
Bone	171	0	0.4	0.5	0.8	0.7	0.9	0.3	0.4	0.3	0.6	0.5	0.9	0.6	1.3	1.4	1.6	1.3	1.3	2.2	0.8	0.2	0.04	0.06	**0.7**	*170*
Connective tissue	700	0	2.1	0.4	0.6	1.0	1.1	1.8	1.5	1.7	1.4	3.4	3.4	2.7	3.8	6.6	8.1	10.2	10.7	9.2	3.2	0.8	0.12	0.20	**2.1**	*171*
Mesothelioma	87	0	-	-	-	-	-	-	0.1	-	-	0.2	0.3	0.3	0.8	0.9	1.3	2.2	1.9	1.8	0.4	0.1	0.01	0.02	**0.2**	*MES*
Kaposi's sarcoma	45	0	-	-	-	-	-	-	0.1	-	-	0.1	-	0.1	0.1	0.7	0.2	0.9	1.3	2.7	0.2	0.0	0.00	0.01	**0.1**	*KAP*
Melanoma of skin	3543	0	-	0.1	0.6	2.1	6.4	10.2	11.5	14.9	20.0	23.1	20.8	22.0	29.4	29.2	31.9	32.9	37.9	35.9	16.4	3.9	0.81	1.11	**11.1**	*172*
†Other skin	3371	0	-	-	0.2	0.1	-	0.2	0.5	1.1	1.4	4.0	6.3	10.2	15.0	22.6	41.1	64.5	100.6	182.9	15.6		0.20	0.51	**5.3**	*173*
Breast	26459	0	-	-	-	-	0.7	4.6	19.4	46.6	101.9	172.4	202.2	229.6	273.6	317.6	311.4	284.1	329.9	308.3	122.2	28.8	5.25	8.40	**72.9**	*174*
Uterus unspecified	590	0	-	-	-	-	-	0.1	0.6	0.5	2.2	3.3	4.4	5.1	4.7	8.0	7.8	6.6	7.6	9.0	2.7	0.6	0.10	0.18	**1.5**	*179*
Cervix uteri	2462	0	-	-	-	-	1.8	7.6	14.9	17.8	16.9	15.8	14.8	13.9	15.3	19.9	19.3	24.7	18.4	14.5	11.4	2.7	0.59	0.79	**8.0**	*180*
Placenta	28	0	-	-	-	0.1	0.5	0.4	0.2	0.1	0.1	0.1	0.4	-	-	-	0.1	-	-	-	0.1	0.0	0.01	0.01	**0.1**	*181*
Corpus uteri	5113	0	-	-	-	-	-	0.1	0.6	1.3	4.2	14.2	36.9	54.6	72.4	79.1	72.1	69.7	61.0	47.7	23.6	5.6	0.92	1.68	**13.2**	*182*
Ovary etc.	4755	0	0.1	0.1	0.2	1.2	1.8	2.1	3.6	7.7	13.5	24.2	37.8	42.4	52.5	59.9	62.4	57.8	52.3	42.4	22.0	5.2	0.94	1.55	**13.2**	*183*
Other female genital	890	0	-	-	0.1	0.1	-	0.3	0.3	1.0	1.4	2.6	1.7	3.8	5.7	8.2	12.6	20.6	22.4	21.2	4.1	1.0	0.09	0.19	**1.7**	*184*
Bladder	2317	0	0.1	-	0.1	-	0.3	0.5	0.8	1.4	2.2	3.7	6.4	12.8	19.1	25.9	34.5	43.3	58.5	57.3	10.7	2.5	0.24	0.54	**4.6**	*188*
Kidney etc.	2764	0	2.5	0.6	0.2	0.3	0.3	0.3	0.6	1.2	2.7	5.0	10.8	21.4	23.6	36.9	47.9	50.1	44.7	47.1	12.8	3.0	0.35	0.77	**6.4**	*189*
Eye	236	0	1.4	0.1	-	-	0.2	0.2	0.6	0.6	0.6	0.6	1.2	1.6	2.3	2.9	2.0	3.7	3.0	3.5	1.1	0.3	0.04	0.07	**0.7**	*190*
Brain, nervous system	1435	0	5.3	4.4	3.8	2.2	2.0	2.9	3.9	4.5	6.0	5.5	8.0	10.1	12.9	15.8	13.9	11.3	8.0	6.1	6.6	1.6	0.36	0.51	**5.5**	*191-2*
Thyroid	1135	0	0.1	0.1	0.7	1.8	2.6	3.3	6.0	4.8	5.8	5.9	6.0	6.1	7.9	8.6	9.2	12.6	13.3	10.8	5.2	1.2	0.25	0.34	**3.6**	*193*
Other endocrine	86	0	0.4	0.3	-	-	0.1	0.1	0.1	0.2	0.1	0.5	0.3	0.3	1.3	0.6	1.2	1.0	0.9	0.6	0.4	0.1	0.02	0.03	**0.3**	*194*
Hodgkin's disease	394	0	-	0.6	0.8	2.6	3.1	2.5	2.2	1.9	1.1	0.9	1.1	0.9	2.0	2.5	3.0	2.7	3.4	3.1	1.8	0.4	0.10	0.13	**1.5**	*201*
Non-Hodgkin lymphoma	2990	0	1.0	0.6	0.8	0.7	1.7	2.1	3.6	4.2	8.1	12.1	18.5	24.3	32.3	46.3	55.1	55.6	54.9	13.8	3.3	0.39	0.79	**6.9**	*200,202*
Multiple myeloma	1245	0	-	-	-	-	-	0.1	0.1	0.2	1.1	1.9	3.0	5.8	8.5	15.3	22.6	27.8	28.9	25.5	5.8	1.4	0.10	0.29	**2.4**	*203*
Lymphoid leukaemia	883	0	5.8	2.4	2.4	0.7	0.5	0.1	0.3	0.3	0.7	1.5	2.7	3.6	4.5	7.4	11.7	16.9	16.9	17.3	4.1	1.0	0.13	0.22	**2.7**	*204*
Myeloid leukaemia	916	0	0.7	0.4	0.6	0.7	0.9	1.6	1.4	1.7	2.4	3.0	4.5	4.1	6.5	11.1	10.0	14.4	15.6	15.3	4.2	1.0	0.14	0.25	**2.4**	*205*
Monocytic leukaemia	31	0	-	-	-	0.1	-	0.1	-	0.1	-	0.1	0.1	0.1	0.1	0.4	0.3	0.8	0.6	0.8	0.1	0.0	0.00	0.01	**0.1**	*206*
Other leukaemia	318	0	0.1	-	-	0.1	-	0.1	0.2	0.1	0.6	0.6	0.5	1.3	2.3	4.1	5.0	8.4	6.4	4.7	1.5	0.3	0.03	0.07	**0.6**	*207*
Leukaemia unspecified	112	0	0.2	0.1	-	0.1	0.1	-	0.1	0.1	0.1	-	0.3	0.2	0.8	0.6	1.6	1.7	3.4	4.7	0.5	0.1	0.01	0.02	**0.2**	*208*
Other and unspecified	4052	0	0.1	0.1	-	-	0.3	0.5	0.8	1.6	4.1	7.3	12.6	20.7	30.8	46.5	60.7	80.0	98.5	102.6	18.7	4.4	0.39	0.93	**8.0**	*O&U*
All sites	95248	0	21.1	10.7	13.2	16.5	27.8	45.3	79.7	129.7	222.1	363.3	497.9	649.1	852.4	1090.6	1262.7	1446.4	1639.0	1698.0	440.0		14.64	26.41	**233.9**	*ALL*
All sites but 173	91877	0	21.1	10.7	13.0	16.5	27.8	45.1	79.2	128.6	220.7	359.3	491.6	638.8	837.3	1068.0	1221.6	1381.9	1538.4	1515.1	424.4	100.0	14.45	25.90	**228.5**	*ALLb*
Rate from 10 cases			0.745	0.840	0.818	0.735	0.677	0.683	0.711	0.689	0.622	0.692	0.874	0.939	0.901	0.848	0.933	1.082	1.481	1.962						

†Important: see notes on population page

Switzerland, Basel

The Cancer Registry of Basel-City and Basel-Country was established in 1969 by the cancer league of these two cantons. Collection of population-based data started in 1970. The aim is to add a German-speaking predominantly urban region to the association of nine Swiss population-based cancer registries covering 57% of the resident population of Switzerland.

The registry is located in the Department of Pathology of the University of Basel. In addition to a part-time pathologist, the staff comprises two full-time tumour registrars. Computerized registration is undertaken in collaboration with the computer department of the canton of Basel-City. Financial support comes from the cantonal governments of Basel-City and Basel-Country, a substantial contribution being supplied by the Federal Government of Switzerland.

The registration area is situated in the north-west of Switzerland, bordering France and Germany, at latitude 47°30′ N and longitude 7°40′ E. The area is 465 km^2, the highest point being 1169 m and the lowest 244 m above sea level.

The population at risk comprises 429 000 residents, 16% of whom are 65 years old or older and 19% less than 20. 19% of the population are foreigners, almost exclusively Caucasian, with the majority coming from Italy, Spain and Germany. 85% of the total population live in the conurbation of Basel. 41% of the inhabitants are Protestants, 30% Roman Catholics, 29% other denominations or of no religion. Employment distribution is: 2% in agriculture and forestry, 30% in industry and 61% in the service sector, 5% unknown and 2% unemployed, according to the 1990 census.

Air pollution has been measured in the Basel area for over 10 years. The mean SO$_2$ values per year have been below the recommended limit (30 pg/m^3) since 1988, but NO$_2$ values have not yet come down to the recommended limit (30 pg/m^3). The ozone exposure is very much higher than the recommendation (more than 120 pg/m^3 for only one hour per year).

Out of the 5459 hospital beds (12 per 1000 residents) 71% are located in eight central hospitals, the rest being distributed among six private hospitals. There is no separate specialized clinic treating cancer patients only. Outpatient care is provided by 970 practising physicians (450 residents per physician).

Information on new cancers is sent to the registry on a voluntary basis by two pathology departments, two other hospital-based and two additional private pathology laboratories and three haematology laboratories. Treating physicians are asked for additional information routinely (response-rate over 90%). Some of them use the registry standard form for tumour documentation in their medical records. Linkage of different sources of information is performed manually using an index file containing accession number, name, maiden name, christian name, date of birth and place of residence. Since 1987 patient data have been entered directly into a personal computer, the paper document being filed and automated coding performed by the computer. Date of death is supplied by the official population registries. 50% of deceased cancer patients have an autopsy. Death certificates are not used for case-finding. The cancer registry personnel has no direct contact with patients. All of the population-based cancer registries in Switzerland have permission from a Central Governmental Commission for Data Protection in Medical Research to receive non-anonymized data on cancer patients.

The data are transferred to standard forms ordered alphabetically (1970–78) or according to the accession number (1979–). The following data are coded for every tumour and transferred to magnetic tape (since 1981): personal identification number, tumours occurring before the registry was started, basis of diagnosis, date of diagnosis, topography (ICD-O-1), histology (ICD-O-1), tumour stage at diagnosis (TNM and pT, pN, pM, in addition in breast cancer the tumour diameter in mm, the number of axillary nodes and the number of metastatic nodes, in malignant melanoma the tumour thickness in mm are registered), first treatment, treating physician and/or hospital, and date of death. Checking for duplicate registration is done by comparing every new item of information manually with the index file. Consistency checks (age–histology, sex–site and histology, site and histology) are performed for selected combinations. Multiple tumours in the same person are registered if the 4th digit of localization is different, if tumours occur in the following paired organs: breast, lung, testis, kidney, ureter, eye, adrenal glands; or if histology is different according to ICD-O-1. For multiple basal cell cancer of the skin, only the first recognized tumour is counted.

Annual incidence data by sex, age, site and morphology, as well as comparisons between the data of the nine Swiss cancer registries, are produced routinely. Descriptive epidemiological studies have been undertaken, in collaboration with the Basel Registry for Tumours in Families, the Swiss Association of Cancer Registries, the Swiss Institute for Applied Cancer Research and IARC.

J. Torhorst

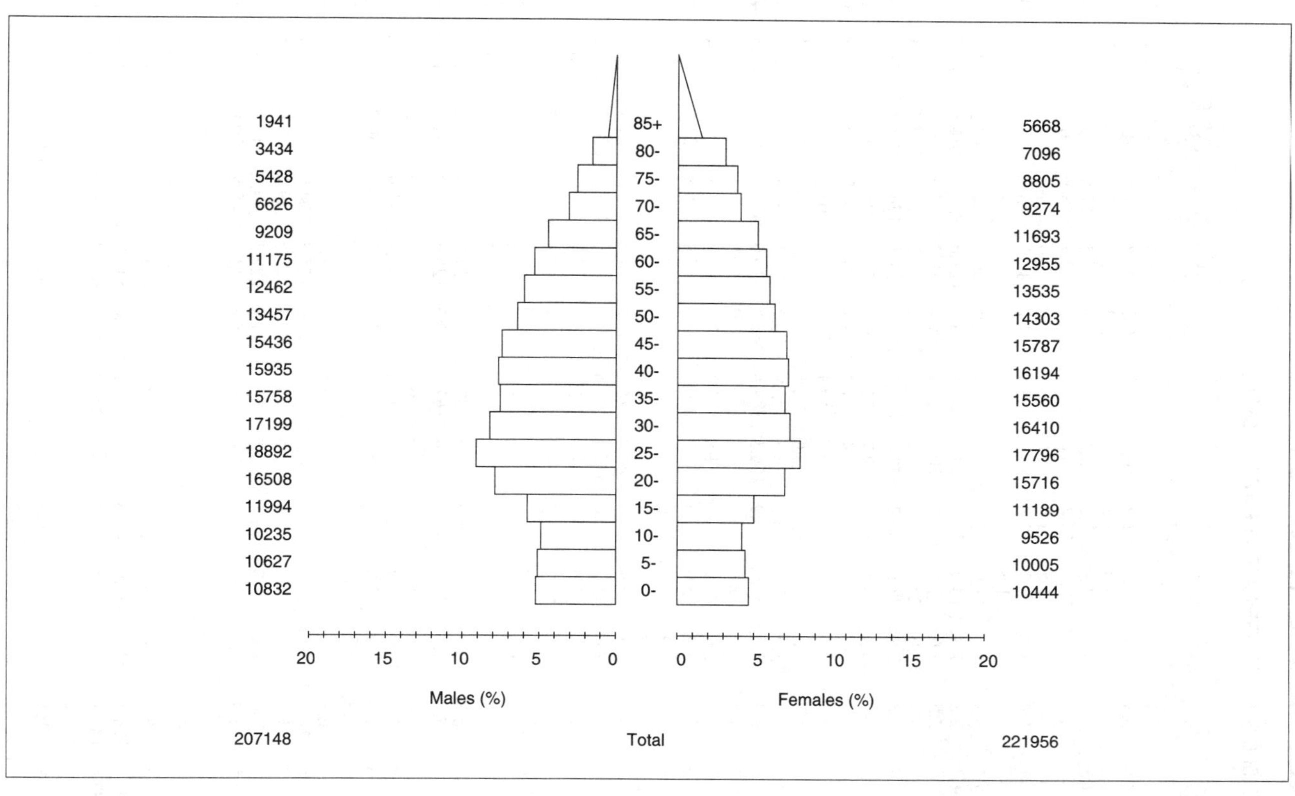

Switzerland, Basel
Source of population: average annual 1988–92
Census: 1990. 'Eidgenòssische Volkszàhlung' 1990. Bundesamt für Statistik, Schweiz.
Estimate: 1988–92. Kantonale Bevölkerungs-Fortschreiburg Statistische Amter, Kanton Basel-Stadt, Kanton Basel-Lancschaft.
Notes to tables overleaf:
* The very high level of histological verification, although this may be related to the high proportion of cancer deaths autopsied (see Table 5.1), suggests some under-registration, as do the lack of diagnoses based on a death certificate alone and some high mortality:incidence ratios,
† 188 does not include non-invasive tumours

* SWITZERLAND, BASEL 1988-1992

ANNUAL INCIDENCE PER 100,000 BY AGE GROUP (YEARS) - MALE

SITE	ALL AGES	AGE UNK	0-	5-	10-	15-	20-	25-	30-	35-	40-	45-	50-	55-	60-	65-	70-	75-	80-	85+	CRUDE RATE	%	CR 64	CR 74	ASR (W)	ICD (9th)
Lip	11	0	-	-	-	-	-	-	-	1.3	2.5	-	-	-	3.6	4.3	-	7.4	5.8	10.3	1.1	0.2	0.04	0.06	**0.7**	*140*
Tongue	46	0	-	-	-	-	-	-	-	2.5	3.8	6.5	11.9	11.2	16.1	2.2	6.0	25.8	5.8	10.3	4.4	1.0	0.26	0.30	**3.0**	*141*
Salivary gland	10	0	-	-	-	-	-	1.1	-	1.3	-	-	3.0	1.6	-	-	3.0	11.1	5.8	-	1.0	0.2	0.03	0.05	**0.6**	*142*
Mouth	45	0	-	-	-	-	-	-	2.3	1.3	-	9.1	22.3	3.2	5.4	10.9	9.1	7.4	11.6	30.9	4.3	0.9	0.22	0.32	**3.0**	*143-5*
Oropharynx	37	0	-	-	-	-	-	-	-	-	3.8	2.6	10.4	14.4	5.4	15.2	9.1	3.7	5.8	10.3	3.6	0.8	0.18	0.30	**2.4**	*146*
Nasopharynx	5	0	-	-	-	-	-	-	-	-	-	-	1.5	1.6	1.8	-	-	7.4	-	-	0.5	0.1	0.02	0.02	**0.3**	*147*
Hypopharynx	34	0	-	-	-	-	-	-	-	-	1.3	3.9	5.9	12.8	14.3	6.5	9.1	11.1	5.8	-	3.3	0.7	0.19	0.27	**2.2**	*148*
Pharynx unspecified	1	0	-	-	-	-	-	-	-	-	-	-	1.5	-	-	-	-	-	-	-	0.1	0.0	0.01	0.01	**0.1**	*149*
Oesophagus	89	0	-	-	-	-	-	-	-	2.5	2.5	6.5	11.9	22.5	17.9	30.4	48.3	40.5	34.9	10.3	8.6	1.8	0.32	0.71	**5.4**	*150*
Stomach	196	0	-	-	-	-	-	-	2.3	1.3	3.8	7.8	14.9	22.5	44.7	69.5	90.5	121.6	139.8	164.8	18.9	4.1	0.49	1.29	**11.0**	*151*
Small intestine	37	0	-	-	-	-	-	-	-	-	2.5	2.6	1.5	6.4	10.7	10.9	15.1	18.4	23.3	30.9	3.6	0.8	0.12	0.25	**2.1**	*152*
Colon	371	0	-	-	-	-	1.2	-	1.2	-	3.8	13.0	22.3	51.4	75.2	117.3	205.2	213.7	314.5	339.9	35.8	7.7	0.84	2.45	**20.4**	*153*
Rectum	285	0	-	-	-	-	-	-	1.2	3.8	8.8	7.8	23.8	36.9	73.4	104.2	153.9	151.1	174.7	185.4	27.5	5.9	0.78	2.07	**16.4**	*154*
Liver	92	0	-	-	-	-	-	1.1	1.2	-	-	6.5	4.5	17.7	19.7	32.6	36.2	58.9	75.7	41.2	8.9	1.9	0.25	0.60	**5.1**	*155*
Gallbladder etc.	28	0	-	-	-	-	-	-	-	-	-	-	-	6.4	5.4	4.3	9.1	25.8	40.8	20.6	2.7	0.6	0.06	0.13	**1.3**	*156*
Pancreas	109	0	-	-	-	-	-	1.1	-	1.3	1.3	-	11.9	11.2	26.8	30.4	48.3	95.8	64.1	92.7	10.5	2.3	0.27	0.66	**6.0**	*157*
Nose, sinuses etc.	14	0	-	-	-	-	-	1.1	1.2	1.3	1.3	-	1.5	3.2	3.6	6.5	-	3.7	-	10.3	1.4	0.3	0.07	0.10	**0.9**	*160*
Larynx	71	0	-	-	-	-	-	-	-	1.3	1.3	3.9	7.4	16.0	23.3	23.9	30.2	22.1	52.4	20.6	6.9	1.5	0.27	0.54	**4.2**	*161*
Bronchus, lung	842	0	-	-	-	-	1.2	1.1	1.2	6.3	6.3	35.0	63.9	146.0	254.1	388.8	368.2	420.0	419.3	401.7	81.3	17.4	2.58	6.36	**49.6**	*162*
Other thoracic organs	4	0	-	-	-	-	-	-	-	-	1.3	-	1.5	-	-	-	6.0	-	-	-	0.4	0.1	0.01	0.04	**0.3**	*163-4*
Bone	15	0	-	-	3.9	1.7	-	-	1.2	1.3	-	2.6	5.9	-	1.8	2.2	3.0	-	5.8	-	1.4	0.3	0.09	0.12	**1.3**	*170*
Connective tissue	27	0	-	-	-	3.3	1.2	-	-	1.3	3.8	3.9	3.0	1.6	7.2	6.5	6.0	7.4	5.8	20.6	2.6	0.6	0.13	0.19	**2.0**	*171*
Mesothelioma	29	0	-	-	-	-	-	-	-	-	-	2.6	3.0	4.8	5.4	6.5	12.1	29.5	17.5	10.3	2.8	0.6	0.08	0.17	**1.6**	*MES*
Kaposi's sarcoma	12	0	-	-	-	-	1.2	2.1	3.5	2.5	1.3	3.9	-	-	-	-	-	-	-	-	1.2	0.2	0.07	0.07	**0.9**	*KAP*
Melanoma of skin	172	0	-	-	-	-	3.6	4.2	8.1	7.6	18.8	10.4	14.9	17.7	41.2	36.9	69.4	114.2	46.6	61.8	16.6	3.6	0.63	1.16	**10.6**	*172*
Other skin	1545	0	-	-	-	-	3.6	5.3	20.9	29.2	60.2	92.0	141.2	200.6	345.4	477.8	639.9	880.6	1112.3	1050.7	149.2		4.49	10.08	**88.5**	*173*
Breast	8	0	-	-	-	-	-	-	-	1.3	1.3	1.5	-	1.8	2.2	3.0	7.4	-	-	-	0.8	0.2	0.03	0.06	**0.5**	*175*
Prostate	1008	0	-	-	-	-	-	-	-	-	-	2.6	19.3	57.8	141.4	312.7	558.4	957.9	995.8	1215.5	97.3	20.9	1.11	5.46	**50.3**	*185*
Testis	111	0	-	-	-	-	20.6	23.3	24.4	21.6	15.1	11.7	8.9	3.2	5.4	-	3.0	-	5.8	-	10.7	2.3	0.67	0.69	**8.8**	*186*
Penis	11	0	-	-	-	-	-	-	-	-	-	1.3	-	3.2	3.6	6.5	3.0	3.7	-	10.3	1.1	0.2	0.04	0.09	**0.7**	*187.1-.4*
Other male genital	2	0	-	-	-	-	-	-	-	-	-	-	-	-	-	-	3.0	3.7	-	-	0.2	0.0	0.00	0.02	**0.1**	*187.5-.9*
†Bladder	214	0	-	-	-	-	-	-	-	-	6.3	6.5	19.3	28.9	37.6	97.7	72.4	121.6	151.4	247.2	20.7	4.4	0.49	1.34	**12.0**	*188*
Kidney etc.	196	0	-	-	-	-	1.2	1.1	2.3	-	7.5	9.1	23.8	44.9	39.4	67.3	81.5	125.3	93.2	51.5	18.9	4.1	0.65	1.39	**11.5**	*189*
Eye	15	0	3.7	-	-	-	1.2	-	-	1.3	-	-	1.5	1.6	3.6	6.5	-	3.7	11.6	10.3	1.4	0.3	0.06	0.10	**1.2**	*190*
Brain, nervous system	104	0	5.5	1.9	7.8	1.7	2.4	3.2	1.2	2.5	7.5	13.0	11.9	24.1	34.0	13.0	33.2	36.8	11.6	-	10.0	2.2	0.58	0.81	**8.0**	*191-2*
Thyroid	26	0	-	-	-	-	1.2	1.1	2.3	1.3	1.3	3.9	3.0	-	5.4	8.7	12.1	3.7	-	30.9	2.5	0.5	0.10	0.20	**1.8**	*193*
Other endocrine	8	0	1.8	-	2.0	-	1.2	-	-	1.3	1.3	1.5	-	-	4.3	-	-	-	-	-	0.8	0.2	0.05	0.07	**0.9**	*194*
Hodgkin's disease	30	0	-	-	2.0	1.7	7.3	3.2	2.3	1.3	6.3	-	3.0	1.6	3.6	6.5	6.0	3.7	-	-	2.9	0.6	0.16	0.22	**2.5**	*201*
Non-Hodgkin lymphoma	235	0	1.8	3.8	3.9	5.0	3.6	1.1	9.3	7.6	18.8	9.1	17.8	22.5	64.4	63.0	93.6	125.3	104.8	133.9	22.7	4.9	0.84	1.63	**15.0**	*200,202*
Multiple myeloma	47	0	-	-	-	-	-	-	-	1.3	1.3	-	7.4	9.6	12.5	10.9	21.1	29.5	29.1	20.6	4.5	1.0	0.16	0.32	**2.7**	*203*
Lymphoid leukaemia	52	0	5.5	-	2.0	1.7	1.2	1.1	2.3	-	-	2.6	3.0	6.4	12.5	15.2	27.2	22.1	29.1	10.3	5.0	1.1	0.19	0.40	**3.8**	*204*
Myeloid leukaemia	43	0	3.7	-	-	-	1.2	2.1	1.2	2.5	1.3	2.6	-	11.2	5.4	8.7	15.1	11.1	40.8	30.9	4.2	0.9	0.16	0.27	**2.9**	*205*
Monocytic leukaemia	0	0	-	-	-	-	-	-	-	-	-	-	-	-	-	-	-	-	-	-	0.0	0.0	0.00	0.00	**0.0**	*206*
Other leukaemia	0	0	-	-	-	-	-	-	-	-	-	-	-	-	-	-	-	-	-	-	0.0	0.0	0.00	0.00	**0.0**	*207*
Leukaemia unspecified	5	0	-	-	-	-	-	-	-	-	-	-	-	1.5	-	1.8	-	3.0	3.7	5.8	0.5	0.1	0.02	0.03	**0.3**	*208*
Other and unspecified	132	0	-	-	-	-	-	-	1.2	1.3	2.5	7.8	8.9	22.5	37.6	52.1	42.3	81.1	69.9	92.7	12.7	2.7	0.41	0.88	**7.6**	*O&U*
All sites	6374	0	22.2	5.6	21.5	15.0	53.3	52.9	90.7	106.6	198.3	292.8	521.6	847.3	1412.1	2063.2	2755.6	3817.0	4117.2	4377.8	615.4		18.20	42.29	**370.4**	*ALL*
All sites but 173	4829	0	22.2	5.6	21.5	15.0	49.7	47.6	69.8	77.4	138.1	200.8	380.4	646.7	1066.6	1585.4	2115.8	2936.4	3004.9	3327.2	466.2	100.0	13.71	32.21	**281.9**	*ALLb*

Rate from 1 case

	0-	5-	10-	15-	20-	25-	30-	35-	40-	45-	50-	55-	60-	65-	70-	75-	80-	85+
	1.846	1.882	1.954	1.667	1.212	1.059	1.163	1.269	1.255	1.296	1.486	1.605	1.790	2.172	3.018	3.684	5.823	10.301

†Important: see notes on population page

* SWITZERLAND, BASEL 1988-1992

ANNUAL INCIDENCE PER 100,000 BY AGE GROUP (YEARS) - FEMALE

SITE	ALL AGES	AGE UNK	0-	5-	10-	15-	20-	25-	30-	35-	40-	45-	50-	55-	60-	65-	70-	75-	80-	85+	CRUDE RATE	%	CR 64	CR 74	ASR (W)	ICD (9th)
Lip	1	0	-	-	-	-	-	-	-	-	-	-	-	-	-	-	-	-	2.8	-	0.1	0.0	0.00	0.00	**0.0**	140
Tongue	12	0	-	-	-	-	-	-	-	-	2.5	-	5.6	-	-	1.7	-	9.1	-	3.5	1.1	0.3	0.04	0.05	**0.6**	141
Salivary gland	5	0	-	-	-	-	-	-	-	-	1.2	-	-	1.5	1.5	-	-	-	5.6	-	0.5	0.1	0.02	0.02	**0.2**	142
Mouth	15	0	-	-	-	-	-	1.3	-	-	-	-	7.4	1.5	1.7	4.3	6.8	2.8	3.5		1.4	0.3	0.05	0.08	**0.7**	143-5
Oropharynx	7	0	-	-	-	-	-	-	-	-	-	-	5.6	3.0	1.5	-	-	-	-	-	0.6	0.2	0.05	0.05	**0.5**	146
Nasopharynx	1	0	-	-	-	-	-	-	-	-	-	-	-	-	1.5	-	-	-	-	-	0.1	0.0	0.01	0.01	**0.1**	147
Hypopharynx	7	0	-	-	-	-	-	-	-	-	-	-	2.8	-	1.5	3.4	4.3	-	-	-	0.6	0.2	0.02	0.06	**0.4**	148
Pharynx unspecified	0	0	-	-	-	-	-	-	-	-	-	-	-	-	-	-	-	-	-	-	0.0	0.0	0.00	0.00	**0.0**	149
Oesophagus	33	0	-	-	-	-	-	-	-	-	2.5	1.3	4.2	10.3	3.1	3.4	6.5	9.1	14.1	14.1	3.0	0.7	0.11	0.16	**1.4**	150
Stomach	148	0	-	-	-	-	-	1.1	2.4	1.3	2.5	2.5	2.8	8.9	23.2	18.8	45.3	52.2	78.9	120.0	13.3	3.3	0.22	0.54	**5.0**	151
Small intestine	24	0	-	-	-	-	-	-	-	-	1.2	1.3	1.4	4.4	1.5	3.4	10.8	9.1	5.6	14.1	2.2	0.5	0.05	0.12	**1.0**	152
Colon	401	0	-	-	-	-	1.3	-	2.4	2.6	7.4	11.4	14.0	31.0	58.7	87.2	131.5	165.8	166.3	239.9	36.1	9.0	0.64	1.74	**14.8**	153
Rectum	241	0	-	-	-	-	-	-	-	3.9	2.5	8.9	16.8	31.0	27.8	51.3	79.8	84.0	129.6	98.8	21.7	5.4	0.45	1.11	**9.2**	154
Liver	28	0	-	-	-	-	1.1	-	-	-	-	3.0	4.6	5.1	6.5	11.4	11.3	24.7		2.5	0.6	0.04	0.10	**1.0**	155
Gallbladder etc.	60	0	-	-	-	-	-	-	-	-	1.2	1.3	2.8	4.4	6.2	8.6	19.4	27.3	33.8	38.8	5.4	1.3	0.08	0.22	**2.0**	156
Pancreas	115	0	-	-	-	-	-	-	-	-	1.2	3.8	8.4	16.3	20.1	20.5	43.1	31.8	47.9	63.5	10.4	2.6	0.25	0.57	**4.5**	157
Nose, sinuses etc.	5	0	-	-	-	-	-	-	-	-	1.2	-	-	-	3.4	-	2.3	2.8	-		0.5	0.1	0.01	0.02	**0.2**	160
Larynx	10	0	-	-	-	-	-	-	-	-	1.2	1.3	-	3.0	-	1.7	8.6	2.3	-	-	0.9	0.2	0.03	0.08	**0.5**	161
Bronchus, lung	261	0	-	-	-	1.8	1.3	-	-	3.9	7.4	16.5	18.2	31.0	75.6	58.2	71.2	95.4	70.5	70.6	23.5	5.9	0.78	1.42	**11.9**	162
Other thoracic organs	2	0	-	-	-	-	-	-	-	-	-	-	-	-	-	1.7	-	-	2.8	-	0.2	0.0	0.00	0.01	**0.1**	163-4
Bone	15	0	1.9	2.0	4.2	1.8	-	-	1.2	3.9	-	1.3	-	1.5	-	1.7	-	-	2.8	7.1	1.4	0.3	0.09	0.10	**1.5**	170
Connective tissue	30	0	-	-	2.1	1.8	2.5	1.1	1.2	1.3	-	1.3	1.4	3.0	1.5	3.4	8.6	4.5	5.6	28.2	2.7	0.7	0.09	0.15	**1.6**	171
Mesothelioma	7	0	-	-	-	-	-	-	1.2	-	-	-	-	1.5	1.5	-	4.3	-	5.6	-	0.6	0.2	0.02	0.04	**0.3**	MES
Kaposi's sarcoma	1	0	-	-	-	-	-	-	1.2	-	-	-	-	-	-	-	-	-	-	-	0.1	0.0	0.01	0.01	**0.1**	KAP
Melanoma of skin	164	0	-	-	-	3.6	5.1	9.0	9.8	11.6	16.1	11.4	22.4	23.6	13.9	20.5	23.7	36.3	50.7	45.9	14.8	3.7	0.63	0.85	**8.9**	172
Other skin	1384	0	1.9	-	-	1.8	3.8	6.7	12.2	41.1	46.9	98.8	90.9	153.7	199.1	304.4	388.1	438.4	569.3	578.6	124.7		3.29	6.75	**58.9**	173
Breast	1417	0	-	-	-	-	-	3.4	14.6	59.1	87.7	179.9	197.2	221.6	248.5	319.8	312.7	365.7	324.1	292.8	127.7	31.9	5.06	8.22	**72.0**	174
Uterus unspecified	0	0	-	-	-	-	-	-	-	-	-	-	-	-	-	-	-	-	-	-	0.0	0.0	0.00	0.00	**0.0**	179
Cervix uteri	98	0	-	-	-	-	1.3	1.1	4.9	10.3	11.1	11.4	15.4	8.9	7.7	20.5	28.0	27.3	14.1	7.1	8.8	2.2	0.36	0.60	**5.4**	180
Placenta	0	0	-	-	-	-	-	-	-	-	-	-	-	-	-	-	-	-	-	-	0.0	0.0	0.00	0.00	**0.0**	181
Corpus uteri	260	0	-	-	-	-	-	-	3.7	-	4.9	11.4	15.4	38.4	67.9	83.8	75.5	70.4	87.4	60.0	23.4	5.8	0.71	1.51	**11.7**	182
Ovary etc.	199	0	-	-	2.1	-	-	4.5	4.9	5.1	14.8	13.9	15.4	26.6	41.7	44.5	64.7	63.6	39.5	31.8	17.9	4.5	0.65	1.19	**10.0**	183
Other female genital	57	0	-	-	-	-	-	1.1	-	2.6	2.5	3.8	4.2	3.0	7.7	20.5	8.6	22.7	19.7	21.2	5.1	1.3	0.12	0.27	**2.5**	184
†Bladder	102	0	-	-	-	-	-	-	-	1.3	2.5	3.8	2.8	4.4	17.0	18.8	23.7	43.2	62.0	60.0	9.2	2.3	0.16	0.37	**3.5**	188
Kidney etc.	118	0	1.9	2.0	-	1.8	-	-	-	1.3	4.9	7.6	11.2	10.3	27.8	20.5	38.8	47.7	39.5	21.2	10.6	2.7	0.34	0.64	**5.7**	189
Eye	13	0	3.8	-	-	-	-	-	-	-	1.3	4.2	1.5	1.5	1.7	2.2	4.5	2.8	-	-	1.2	0.3	0.06	0.08	**1.0**	190
Brain, nervous system	69	0	3.8	-	2.1	1.8	1.3	2.2	2.4	1.3	7.4	2.5	8.4	8.9	13.9	13.7	12.9	25.0	11.3	3.5	6.2	1.6	0.28	0.41	**4.2**	191-2
Thyroid	63	0	-	-	2.1	1.8	2.5	6.7	7.3	1.3	1.2	3.8	7.0	5.9	9.3	12.0	8.6	15.9	11.3	17.6	5.7	1.4	0.24	0.35	**3.7**	193
Other endocrine	9	0	1.9	-	-	-	-	-	1.2	-	-	1.3	1.4	1.5	-	1.7	-	2.3	5.6	-	0.8	0.2	0.04	0.04	**0.6**	194
Hodgkin's disease	29	0	-	-	2.1	5.4	6.4	2.2	2.4	1.3	2.5	1.3	1.4	4.4	1.5	3.4	2.2	4.5	-	7.1	2.6	0.7	0.15	0.18	**2.3**	201
Non-Hodgkin lymphoma	176	0	-	-	-	-	2.5	2.2	4.9	2.6	4.9	7.6	16.8	22.2	12.4	41.0	45.3	54.5	64.8	102.3	15.9	4.0	0.38	0.81	**7.3**	200,202
Multiple myeloma	32	0	-	-	-	-	-	-	-	-	1.2	1.3	1.4	5.9	3.1	8.6	10.8	9.1	14.1	14.1	2.9	0.7	0.06	0.16	**1.3**	203
Lymphoid leukaemia	31	0	1.9	-	-	1.8	-	1.1	1.2	-	1.2	1.3	2.8	3.0	7.7	8.6	6.5	4.5	8.5	10.6	2.8	0.7	0.11	0.19	**1.8**	204
Myeloid leukaemia	48	0	-	2.0	-	-	1.3	-	3.7	3.9	1.2	2.5	2.8	1.5	7.7	13.7	12.9	11.4	16.9	14.1	4.3	1.1	0.13	0.27	**2.4**	205
Monocytic leukaemia	1	0	-	-	-	-	-	-	-	-	-	1.3	-	-	-	-	-	-	-	-	0.1	0.0	0.01	0.01	**0.1**	206
Other leukaemia	0	0	-	-	-	-	-	-	-	-	-	-	-	-	-	-	-	-	-	-	0.0	0.0	0.00	0.00	**0.0**	207
Leukaemia unspecified	3	0	-	-	-	-	-	-	-	-	-	-	-	-	-	-	-	6.8	-	-	0.3	0.1	0.00	0.00	**0.1**	208
Other and unspecified	129	0	1.9	-	-	-	-	1.1	-	-	2.5	2.5	12.6	8.9	26.2	35.9	34.5	59.1	50.7	35.3	11.6	2.9	0.28	0.63	**5.4**	O&U
All sites	5831	0	19.1	6.0	14.7	23.2	29.3	45.0	82.9	160.7	245.8	419.3	517.4	715.2	946.3	1269.1	1544.0	1823.8	1981.3	2049.9	525.4		16.12	30.19	**266.4**	ALL
All sites but 173	4447	0	17.2	6.0	14.7	21.4	25.5	38.2	70.7	119.5	198.8	320.5	426.5	561.5	747.2	964.6	1155.8	1385.5	1412.0	1471.3	400.7	100.0	12.84	23.44	**207.6**	ALLb

Rate from 1 case   1.915   1.999   2.099   1.787   1.273   1.124   1.219   1.285   1.235   1.267   1.398   1.478   1.544   1.710   2.156   2.271   2.818   3.528

†Important: see notes on population page

Switzerland, Geneva

The Geneva Cancer Registry was founded in 1969 and started recording cases in 1970. Since 1991, the Registry has been attached directly to the Public Health Service of the Canton of Geneva, which provides most of the budget. Additional funds are obtained from the Federal Ministry of Health, through the Swiss Association of Cancer Registries, which aims at standardizing definitions, codes and procedures as well as carrying out collaborative studies, mainly descriptive.

The Canton of Geneva is situated at the extreme west of Switzerland. It has a total area of 282 km^2, of which Lake Geneva occupies 36 km^2. The climate is temperate with average temperatures varying from 0.3°C in January to 22°C in August, and the annual rainfall amounts to 931 mm (1992). Air quality is fairly good: the highest annual average pollutant concentrations observed are 16 µg/m^3 for SO_2, 74 µg/m^3 for NO, 65 µg/m^3 for NO_2, 64 µg/m^3 for O_3 and 1.5 mg/m^3 for CO (1992).

At 31 December 1992, the population of the canton was 387 000, of whom 13.6% were aged 65 or more and only 21.2% younger than 20 years. This structure is due not only to the joint effects of a low fertility rate and an increase in life expectancy, but also reflects a fairly heavy immigration (often temporary) at the ages of economic activity. This immigration comes traditionally from Latin countries. Due to a restrictive policy in granting Swiss nationality, the proportion of the resident population considered as foreign remains high, at 37.1%, of which 7.1% were Italian, 6.3% Portuguese, 5.8% Spanish and 4.6% French.

The majority of the population is Christian, with 48% of Roman Catholics and 23% Protestants.

The active population is concentrated in the administrative and service sectors (80.9%), with production workers comprising most of the remaining population (17.9%); agricultural workers are few (<2%), due to the small amount of cultivated land and the high degree of agricultural mechanization (1991 figures).

The hospital facilities for acute illness comprise one general public university hospital with nearly 1500 beds (1992) and some smaller private hospitals and clinics. Cancer patients are also treated at two other university hospitals, namely a geriatric institution (300 beds) and a hospital for chronic affections (300 beds). No hospital, either public or private, has beds reserved specifically for cancer patients.

Biopsies are mainly carried out at the central laboratory or in other specialized services of the public hospital. There are three private pathology laboratories, which provide records to the registry or permit systematic consultation of them. Haematological examinations are carried out in several private laboratories. Autopsies are performed at the university hospitals and the necropsy rate is estimated at 24% of the deceased residents.

Data collection for the registry is undertaken by examining the university hospital records of the various services concerned, as well as by a questionnaire sent to private practitioners. The response rate of the latter is more than 90%.

The registry has access to all death certificates in the canton which, in addition to clinical records, permit a continuous follow-up. In addition to this passive follow-up, the registry also undertakes active follow-up of all cases on a five-year basis from the date of diagnosis. This follow-up is facilitated by direct access to the Cantonal Office of Population registry. In the case of death, the primary cause is recorded and re-examined, as well as the possible presence of a tumour, clinical or confirmed, at the time of death.

As an indicator of reliability of the data, a very low percentage of cases (<1%) is recorded from death certificates only. In addition, the low rate of cases found at autopsy (2.2%) compared with the total number of cases confirmed histologically suggests that most cases are identified during the lifetime of the patient.

There is no systematic screening programme in the canton, for either breast or cervical cancer. Nonetheless spontaneous screening is well accepted in the population, with mean annual screening rates of about 40% for Pap-tests (women aged 15 years and above) and about 15% for mammographic screening (woman aged 50–69 years) (1991–93 data).

In addition to the processing and publication of routine incidence and survival data, the registry initiates or participates in analytical epidemiological investigations. Several case–control and cohort studies have been undertaken for etiological or evaluative purposes.

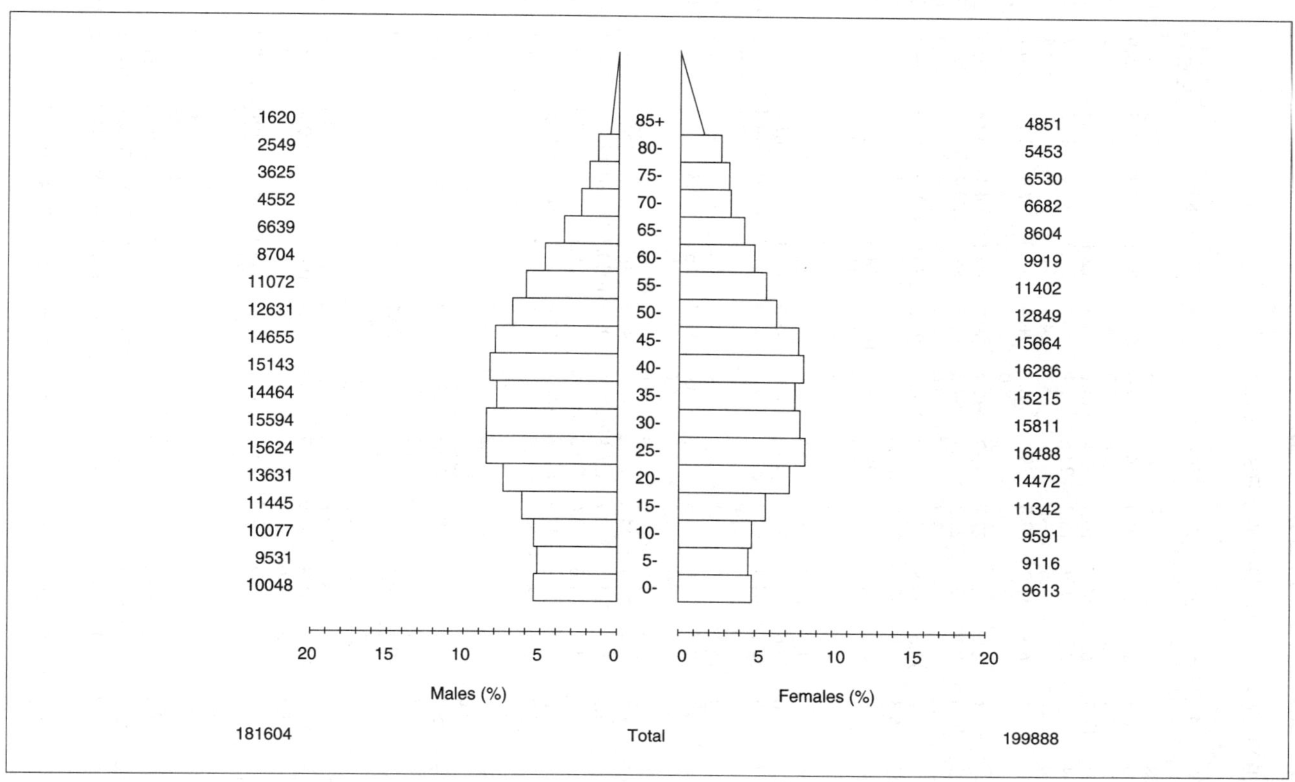

Switzerland, Geneva
Source of population: 1988
Estimate: The population for 1988 is an official inter-Census estimate supplied by the Office Cantonal de Population, Geneva.

Screening programmes in the area
9 500 breast cancer screening examinations have been carried out annually in the population aged 30-89 since 1991.

SWITZERLAND, GENEVA 1988-1992

ANNUAL INCIDENCE PER 100,000 BY AGE GROUP (YEARS) - MALE

SITE	ALL AGES	AGE UNK	0-	5-	10-	15-	20-	25-	30-	35-	40-	45-	50-	55-	60-	65-	70-	75-	80-	85+	CRUDE RATE	%	CR 64	CR 74	ASR (W)	ICD (9th)
Lip	20	0	-	-	-	-	-	1.3	1.3	2.8	1.3	-	11.1	1.8	6.9	6.0	-	-	7.8	12.3	2.2	0.5	0.13	0.16	**1.6**	*140*
Tongue	51	0	-	-	-	1.5	-	-	5.5	6.6	1.4	22.2	9.0	16.1	9.0	22.0	22.1	7.8	12.3	5.6	1.2	0.31	0.47	**4.1**	*141*
Salivary gland	11	0	-	-	-	-	-	-	-	1.3	1.4	-	-	4.6	12.0	8.8	-	-	12.3	1.2	0.3	0.04	0.14	**0.9**	*142*
Mouth	59	0	-	-	-	-	-	-	1.4	11.9	6.8	14.2	16.3	18.4	15.1	4.4	22.1	23.5	61.7	6.5	1.3	0.34	0.44	**4.5**	*143-5*
Oropharynx	70	0	-	-	-	-	-	-	1.4	6.6	12.3	26.9	16.3	27.6	21.1	-	27.6	31.4	12.3	7.7	1.6	0.46	0.56	**5.4**	*146*
Nasopharynx	4	0	-	-	-	1.7	-	-	1.4	-	-	1.6	-	-	-	4.4	-	-	-	0.4	0.1	0.02	0.05	**0.4**	*147*
Hypopharynx	61	0	-	-	-	-	-	-	-	1.3	6.8	14.2	23.5	39.1	18.1	26.4	11.0	7.8	12.3	6.7	1.4	0.42	0.65	**5.0**	*148*
Pharynx unspecified	1	0	-	-	-	-	-	-	-	-	-	-	-	3.0	-	-	-	-	-	0.1	0.0	0.00	0.02	**0.1**	*149*
Oesophagus	95	0	-	-	-	-	-	-	-	5.3	2.7	14.2	27.1	43.7	39.2	39.5	44.1	94.1	49.4	10.5	2.2	0.47	0.86	**7.1**	*150*
Stomach	165	0	-	-	-	1.5	1.3	-	4.1	10.6	9.6	22.2	25.3	39.1	84.3	101.1	88.3	180.4	123.4	18.2	3.8	0.57	1.49	**12.3**	*151*
Small intestine	9	0	-	-	-	-	-	-	-	-	-	-	1.8	2.3	6.0	4.4	5.5	23.5	-	1.0	0.2	0.02	0.07	**0.6**	*152*
Colon	357	0	-	-	-	-	-	2.6	1.4	7.9	13.6	34.8	59.6	64.3	120.5	290.0	286.9	455.0	481.4	39.3	8.1	0.92	2.97	**25.2**	*153*
Rectum	166	0	-	-	-	-	-	3.8	4.1	5.3	6.8	12.7	23.5	62.0	84.3	79.1	137.9	133.4	185.1	18.3	3.8	0.59	1.41	**12.3**	*154*
Liver	149	0	-	-	-	-	-	1.3	-	2.6	4.1	14.2	27.1	48.3	78.3	101.1	154.5	86.3	123.4	16.4	3.4	0.49	1.38	**11.2**	*155*
Gallbladder etc.	27	0	-	-	-	-	-	-	1.4	-	-	-	1.8	2.3	3.0	17.6	38.6	70.6	37.0	3.0	0.6	0.03	0.13	**1.6**	*156*
Pancreas	125	0	-	-	-	-	-	1.3	-	4.0	5.5	12.7	23.5	32.2	60.2	92.3	110.3	125.5	61.7	13.8	2.8	0.40	1.16	**9.2**	*157*
Nose, sinuses etc.	10	0	-	-	-	-	-	1.3	-	-	1.4	4.7	1.8	2.3	-	-	11.0	-	12.3	1.1	0.2	0.06	0.06	**0.7**	*160*
Larynx	109	0	-	-	-	-	-	-	1.4	6.6	13.6	22.2	34.3	46.0	39.2	48.3	44.1	23.5	61.7	12.0	2.5	0.62	1.06	**8.6**	*161*
Bronchus, lung	696	0	-	-	-	-	-	2.6	9.7	22.5	34.1	83.9	146.3	291.8	361.5	408.6	391.7	455.0	518.4	76.6	15.9	2.95	6.80	**53.7**	*162*
Other thoracic organs	2	0	-	-	-	-	-	-	-	-	-	-	1.8	-	-	-	-	-	12.3	0.2	0.0	0.01	0.01	**0.1**	*163-4*
Bone	12	0	-	-	-	3.5	4.4	1.3	1.3	-	1.3	2.7	-	-	2.3	3.0	-	-	-	1.3	0.3	0.08	0.10	**1.3**	*170*
Connective tissue	20	0	2.0	-	-	1.7	-	1.3	1.3	-	-	2.7	1.6	1.8	6.9	3.0	13.2	16.6	7.8	12.3	2.2	0.5	0.10	0.18	**1.8**	*171*
Mesothelioma	9	0	-	-	-	-	-	-	-	-	-	-	-	7.2	2.3	6.0	4.4	5.5	-	1.0	0.2	0.05	0.10	**0.7**	*MES*
Kaposi's sarcoma	64	0	-	-	-	-	2.9	11.5	12.8	11.1	13.2	15.0	4.7	10.8	2.3	6.0	4.4	-	-	12.3	7.0	1.5	0.42	0.47	**5.4**	*KAP*
Melanoma of skin	130	0	-	-	4.0	1.7	1.5	6.4	9.0	9.7	11.9	10.9	23.7	25.3	41.4	30.1	52.7	60.7	62.8	24.7	14.3	3.0	0.73	1.14	**10.5**	*172*
Other skin	1468	0	-	-	-	3.5	5.9	6.4	20.5	29.0	64.7	96.9	201.1	263.7	438.9	608.5	799.6	1020.7	1161.0	1468.8	161.7		5.65	12.69	**109.7**	*173*
Breast	8	0	-	-	-	-	-	-	-	-	1.4	1.6	3.6	2.3	3.0	-	5.5	-	12.3	0.9	0.2	0.04	0.06	**0.6**	*175*
Prostate	708	0	-	-	-	-	-	-	-	-	2.6	2.7	15.8	45.2	135.6	349.4	553.6	789.0	941.3	1296.0	78.0	16.1	1.01	5.52	**49.0**	*185*
Testis	81	0	-	-	-	3.5	11.7	29.4	12.8	19.4	13.2	6.8	6.3	5.4	2.3	-	-	5.5	-	-	8.9	1.8	0.55	0.55	**7.4**	*186*
Penis	15	0	-	-	-	-	-	-	-	-	1.3	-	1.6	3.6	2.3	6.0	8.8	11.0	15.7	24.7	1.7	0.3	0.04	0.12	**1.1**	*187.1-.4*
Other male genital	7	0	-	-	-	-	-	-	-	-	-	1.4	-	-	2.3	6.0	4.4	5.5	-	12.3	0.8	0.2	0.02	0.07	**0.6**	*187.5-.9*
Bladder	443	0	-	-	-	-	1.5	-	-	2.8	7.9	19.1	47.5	88.5	131.0	213.9	259.2	397.2	423.6	345.6	48.8	10.1	1.49	3.86	**32.5**	*188*
Kidney etc.	133	0	-	-	-	-	-	-	-	1.4	5.3	10.9	3.2	19.9	25.3	114.5	83.5	88.3	133.4	74.1	14.6	3.0	0.33	1.32	**10.0**	*189*
Eye	9	0	-	-	-	-	-	-	-	-	1.3	1.4	-	3.6	4.6	3.0	-	5.5	7.8	-	1.0	0.2	0.05	0.07	**0.7**	*190*
Brain, nervous system	73	0	-	2.1	-	1.7	2.9	3.8	3.8	4.1	4.0	10.9	6.3	10.8	27.6	24.1	35.1	38.6	23.5	12.3	8.0	1.7	0.39	0.69	**6.1**	*191-2*
Thyroid	12	0	-	-	-	-	-	1.3	-	1.4	1.3	4.1	1.6	-	4.6	6.0	4.4	-	-	-	1.3	0.3	0.07	0.12	**1.0**	*193*
Other endocrine	5	0	2.0	-	-	-	-	-	-	-	-	-	-	1.8	-	-	4.4	-	15.7	-	0.6	0.1	0.02	0.04	**0.5**	*194*
Hodgkin's disease	31	0	-	-	-	3.5	1.5	5.1	2.6	2.8	2.6	1.4	4.7	3.6	11.5	6.0	4.4	11.0	-	24.7	3.4	0.7	0.20	0.25	**2.7**	*201*
Non-Hodgkin lymphoma	165	0	2.0	-	2.0	5.2	10.3	3.8	9.0	8.3	11.9	16.4	15.8	37.9	43.7	66.3	35.1	104.8	47.1	135.8	18.2	3.8	0.83	1.34	**13.5**	*200,202*
Multiple myeloma	47	0	-	-	-	-	-	-	-	-	1.3	5.5	1.6	9.0	11.5	6.0	48.3	44.1	15.7	98.7	5.2	1.1	0.14	0.42	**3.5**	*203*
Lymphoid leukaemia	63	0	10.0	-	4.0	5.2	1.5	-	-	-	1.4	7.9	7.2	9.2	18.1	57.1	33.1	54.9	74.1	6.9	1.4	0.23	0.61	**5.9**	*204*
Myeloid leukaemia	57	0	-	2.1	-	1.5	-	2.6	2.8	1.3	5.5	1.6	7.2	9.2	30.1	48.3	27.6	70.6	24.7	6.3	1.3	0.17	0.56	**4.4**	*205*
Monocytic leukaemia	0	0	-	-	-	-	-	-	-	-	-	-	-	-	-	-	-	-	-	0.0	0.0	0.00	0.00	**0.0**	*206*
Other leukaemia	0	0	-	-	-	-	-	-	-	-	-	-	-	-	-	-	-	-	-	0.0	0.0	0.00	0.00	**0.0**	*207*
Leukaemia unspecified	3	0	-	-	-	-	-	-	-	-	-	1.6	-	-	-	-	-	7.8	12.3	0.3	0.1	0.01	0.01	**0.2**	*208*
Other and unspecified	108	0	2.0	-	-	-	-	2.6	-	2.8	1.3	8.2	17.4	9.0	43.7	24.1	61.5	71.7	78.4	197.5	11.9	2.5	0.43	0.86	**8.2**	*O&U*
All sites	5858	0	17.9	4.2	9.9	31.5	48.4	75.5	89.8	130.0	240.4	345.3	677.7	1006.1	1707.3	2494.3	3330.4	4137.9	4792.9	5652.9	645.1		21.92	51.04	**442.0**	*ALL*
All sites but 173	4390	0	17.9	4.2	9.9	28.0	42.6	69.1	69.3	100.9	175.7	248.4	476.6	742.4	1268.4	1885.8	2530.8	3117.2	3631.9	4184.2	483.5	100.0	16.27	38.35	**332.3**	*ALLb*

Rate from 1 case: 1.990 2.098 1.985 1.747 1.467 1.280 1.283 1.383 1.321 1.365 1.583 1.806 2.298 3.012 4.394 5.517 7.844 12.343

SWITZERLAND, GENEVA 1988-1992

ANNUAL INCIDENCE PER 100,000 BY AGE GROUP (YEARS) - FEMALE

SITE	ALL AGES	AGE UNK	0-	5-	10-	15-	20-	25-	30-	35-	40-	45-	50-	55-	60-	65-	70-	75-	80-	85+	CRUDE RATE	%	CR 64	CR 74	ASR (W)	ICD (9th)
Lip	5	0	-	-	-	-	-	-	-	-	-	-	3.1	-	2.0	-	-	6.1	-	-	0.5	0.1	0.03	0.03	0.3	140
Tongue	22	0	2.1	-	-	-	-	1.2	1.3	-	-	2.6	3.1	3.5	2.0	2.3	9.0	12.3	7.3	8.2	2.2	0.5	0.08	0.14	1.4	141
Salivary gland	7	0	-	-	-	-	-	-	-	-	-	-	1.6	-	-	2.3	6.0	3.1	3.7	4.1	0.7	0.2	0.01	0.05	0.3	142
Mouth	26	0	-	-	-	-	-	-	1.3	-	-	1.3	6.2	12.3	10.1	-	-	6.1	7.3	16.5	2.6	0.6	0.16	0.16	1.5	143-5
Oropharynx	22	0	-	-	-	-	-	-	-	1.3	4.9	2.6	6.2	3.5	10.1	4.6	3.0	-	-	4.1	2.2	0.5	0.14	0.18	1.6	146
Nasopharynx	4	0	-	-	-	-	-	-	1.3	-	-	1.3	-	1.8	-	2.3	-	-	-	-	0.4	0.1	0.02	0.03	0.3	147
Hypopharynx	10	0	-	-	-	-	-	-	-	-	-	2.6	1.6	1.8	4.0	2.3	3.0	-	3.7	4.1	1.0	0.2	0.05	0.08	0.6	148
Pharynx unspecified	4	0	-	-	-	-	-	-	-	-	-	3.8	-	-	-	2.3	-	-	-	-	0.4	0.1	0.02	0.03	0.3	149
Oesophagus	27	0	-	-	-	-	-	-	-	-	1.2	1.3	3.1	3.5	2.0	9.3	18.0	9.2	11.0	16.5	2.7	0.7	0.06	0.19	1.4	150
Stomach	124	0	-	-	-	-	-	1.2	2.5	3.9	1.2	3.8	9.3	8.8	18.1	27.9	35.9	55.1	99.0	103.1	12.4	3.0	0.24	0.56	5.4	151
Small intestine	10	0	-	-	-	-	-	-	-	-	-	-	-	1.8	2.0	2.3	6.0	3.1	11.0	4.1	1.0	0.2	0.02	0.06	0.4	152
Colon	352	0	-	-	-	-	-	-	2.5	2.6	6.1	6.4	20.2	38.6	56.5	74.4	143.7	171.5	231.0	313.3	35.2	8.6	0.66	1.76	15.4	153
Rectum	139	0	-	-	-	-	-	-	-	-	4.9	5.1	14.0	19.3	26.2	48.8	50.9	58.2	88.0	70.1	13.9	3.4	0.35	0.85	7.0	154
Liver	29	0	-	-	-	-	2.4	-	-	1.2	1.3	3.1	7.0	4.0	9.3	12.0	3.1	11.0	20.6	2.9	0.7	0.10	0.20	1.6	155
Gallbladder etc.	61	0	-	-	-	-	-	-	-	-	1.2	-	-	-	4.0	16.3	18.0	45.9	55.0	61.8	6.1	1.5	0.03	0.20	2.1	156
Pancreas	140	0	-	-	-	-	-	-	1.3	1.2	2.6	6.2	8.8	36.3	34.9	56.9	67.4	91.7	115.4	14.0	3.4	0.28	0.74	6.3	157
Nose, sinuses etc.	9	0	-	-	-	-	-	-	-	-	2.6	-	2.0	4.6	6.0	3.1	3.7	-	0.9	0.2	0.02	0.08	0.5	160
Larynx	13	0	-	-	-	-	-	-	1.3	-	3.1	3.5	10.1	4.6	3.0	-	-	-	1.3	0.3	0.09	0.13	1.0	161
Bronchus, lung	268	0	-	-	-	-	1.4	1.2	1.3	3.9	6.1	17.9	18.7	43.9	56.5	102.3	86.8	140.9	135.7	90.7	26.8	6.5	0.75	1.70	14.3	162
Other thoracic organs	4	0	-	-	-	-	-	-	-	-	-	-	-	1.8	4.0	2.3	-	-	-	-	0.4	0.1	0.03	0.04	0.3	163-4
Bone	4	0	-	-	-	-	1.4	-	1.3	-	-	-	-	-	-	-	-	6.1	-	-	0.4	0.1	0.01	0.01	0.2	170
Connective tissue	27	0	2.1	2.2	-	3.5	2.8	-	-	2.6	2.5	-	1.6	1.8	4.0	4.6	18.0	3.1	3.7	12.4	2.7	0.7	0.11	0.23	2.2	171
Mesothelioma	10	0	-	-	-	-	-	-	1.3	-	1.3	3.1	-	2.0	2.3	6.0	-	3.7	4.1	1.0	0.2	0.04	0.08	0.6	MES
Kaposi's sarcoma	3	0	-	-	-	-	-	-	-	-	1.2	-	-	-	-	-	-	3.1	-	4.1	0.3	0.1	0.01	0.01	0.1	KAP
Melanoma of skin	158	0	-	-	-	5.3	4.1	10.9	3.8	19.7	17.2	21.7	37.4	21.0	30.2	23.2	23.9	24.5	33.0	33.0	15.8	3.9	0.86	1.09	11.1	172
Other skin	1500	0	-	-	-	-	6.9	9.7	22.8	47.3	105.6	130.2	174.3	192.9	241.9	346.3	529.8	545.1	707.8	849.2	150.1		4.66	9.04	80.0	173
Breast	1269	0	-	-	-	-	4.1	6.1	21.5	42.1	109.3	181.3	249.0	256.1	274.2	285.9	311.3	343.0	385.1	391.6	127.0	30.9	5.72	8.70	77.8	174
Uterus unspecified	7	0	-	-	-	-	-	-	-	-	-	-	-	1.8	-	-	-	-	11.0	12.4	0.7	0.2	0.01	0.01	0.2	179
Cervix uteri	91	0	-	-	-	-	-	3.6	7.6	9.2	8.6	14.0	14.0	15.8	14.1	25.6	21.0	21.4	18.3	8.2	9.1	2.2	0.43	0.67	6.1	180
Placenta	3	0	-	-	-	1.8	-	-	-	1.3	-	-	1.6	-	-	-	-	-	-	-	0.3	0.1	0.02	0.02	0.3	181
Corpus uteri	214	0	-	-	-	-	-	-	1.3	3.9	4.9	12.8	28.0	31.6	70.6	93.0	86.8	64.3	55.0	82.4	21.4	5.2	0.77	1.66	12.7	182
Ovary etc.	201	0	-	-	-	-	1.4	2.4	1.3	2.6	11.1	20.4	24.9	47.4	52.4	48.8	62.9	88.8	55.0	61.8	20.1	4.9	0.82	1.38	11.9	183
Other female genital	33	0	-	-	-	-	-	-	1.3	1.3	1.2	-	3.1	-	4.0	7.0	12.0	21.4	14.7	33.0	3.3	0.8	0.05	0.15	1.4	184
Bladder	132	0	-	-	-	-	-	2.4	-	2.6	-	3.8	6.2	22.8	16.1	51.1	50.9	39.8	80.7	107.2	13.2	3.2	0.27	0.78	6.3	188
Kidney etc.	85	0	-	-	-	-	-	-	1.3	4.9	5.1	4.7	15.8	12.1	11.6	44.9	39.8	51.3	45.3	8.5	2.1	0.22	0.50	4.2	189
Eye	8	0	-	-	-	-	-	-	-	1.2	2.6	2.6	-	-	4.0	-	-	6.1	-	4.1	0.8	0.2	0.04	0.04	0.5	190
Brain, nervous system	58	0	2.1	4.4	-	-	1.4	2.4	-	5.3	2.5	5.1	10.9	7.0	16.1	11.6	3.0	24.5	25.7	8.2	5.8	1.4	0.29	0.36	4.1	191-2
Thyroid	58	0	-	-	2.1	1.8	4.1	3.6	7.6	5.3	11.1	3.8	7.8	8.8	-	20.9	18.0	3.1	3.7	4.1	5.8	1.4	0.28	0.47	4.4	193
Other endocrine	11	0	-	-	-	-	1.4	-	-	1.3	-	1.3	3.1	-	4.0	-	6.0	-	3.7	4.1	1.1	0.3	0.06	0.09	0.7	194
Hodgkin's disease	20	0	-	-	-	3.5	4.1	3.6	3.8	1.3	-	-	-	-	4.0	4.6	6.0	3.1	-	4.1	2.0	0.5	0.10	0.16	1.7	201
Non-Hodgkin lymphoma	153	0	-	-	4.2	-	1.4	2.4	5.1	3.9	4.9	14.0	12.5	24.6	18.1	41.8	35.9	49.0	69.7	123.7	15.3	3.7	0.46	0.84	8.1	200,202
Multiple myeloma	46	0	-	-	-	-	-	1.2	-	-	1.2	6.4	3.1	7.0	4.0	13.9	21.0	27.6	25.7	8.2	4.6	1.1	0.11	0.29	2.4	203
Lymphoid leukaemia	47	0	10.4	2.2	-	-	-	2.4	1.3	-	2.5	1.3	-	3.5	8.1	11.6	6.0	24.5	18.3	37.1	4.7	1.1	0.16	0.25	3.4	204
Myeloid leukaemia	49	0	-	-	-	-	-	1.2	3.8	5.3	3.7	2.6	3.1	3.5	4.0	9.3	9.0	24.5	36.7	20.6	4.9	1.2	0.14	0.23	2.5	205
Monocytic leukaemia	2	0	-	-	-	-	-	-	-	-	-	-	-	-	-	-	3.0	-	-	4.1	0.2	0.0	0.00	0.01	0.1	206
Other leukaemia	0	0	-	-	-	-	-	-	-	-	-	-	-	-	-	-	-	-	-	-	0.0	0.0	0.00	0.00	0.0	207
Leukaemia unspecified	3	0	-	-	-	-	-	-	-	-	-	-	-	-	-	-	-	-	-	12.4	0.3	0.1	0.00	0.00	0.1	208
Other and unspecified	134	0	-	-	2.1	-	-	-	-	1.3	-	8.9	15.6	15.8	8.1	27.9	29.9	49.0	84.4	169.0	13.4	3.3	0.26	0.55	5.7	O&U
All sites	5602	0	16.6	8.8	8.3	15.9	34.5	58.2	93.6	172.2	321.7	491.5	703.5	836.7	1042.4	1394.6	1762.9	1996.8	2446.2	2877.3	560.5		19.02	34.81	311.2	ALL
All sites but 173	4102	0	16.6	8.8	8.3	15.9	27.6	48.5	70.8	124.9	216.1	361.3	529.2	643.7	800.4	1048.3	1233.1	1451.6	1738.4	2028.1	410.4	100.0	14.36	25.77	231.2	ALLb

| Rate from 1 case | | | 2.080 | 2.194 | 2.085 | 1.763 | 1.382 | 1.213 | 1.265 | 1.314 | 1.228 | 1.277 | 1.556 | 1.754 | 2.016 | 2.324 | 2.993 | 3.063 | 3.667 | 4.122 |

Switzerland, Graubünden

The Graubünden Cancer Registry was founded in 1989 by the local cancer league to collect population-based data in an alpine region of Switzerland. Since 1993 the registry has been a member of the Association of Swiss Cancer Registries. It forms part of the Department of Pathology of the main hospital in Chur. It is financed by the local government and the Federal Government of Switzerland.

The Graubünden canton (one of 26 cantons in Switzerland), located in the eastern end of Switzerland at latitude 46°30′ N and longitude 9°30′ E, is bordered to the north by Austria, to the east and south by Italy and to the west by the cantons of Glarus, Tessin and Uri. Of the total surface area of the canton (7106 km^2, the largest canton of Switzerland), 90% lies over 1200 m above sea level. The highest point is 4049 m and the lowest 275 m.

The population (according to the federal census of 1990) comprises 87 372 females and 86 518 males, living in 243 communities. About 19% of the inhabitants live in the main city of Chur and 81% in rural regions. The proportion aged 0–19 years was 24.6 % (compared with 22.9% for Switzerland as a whole), while 14.8 % was older than 65 years (Switzerland: 14.4 %). Foreigners, mainly from Italy and ex-Yugoslavia, accounted for 13.3% of residents.

In 1990 the main occupational groups were agriculture 6.0%, industry 26.3% and services 64.5% (compared with 4.1%, 30.7% and 61.6% for Switzerland as a whole). The language groups were German, 65.3%; Reto-Romanic, 17.1%; Italian, 11% and others 6.6%.

Within the registry, two data managers and one pathologist are responsible for the computer-assisted on-line registration of about 85% of cases diagnosed in the Department of Pathology. Notification of cancer cases is voluntary. Additional cases are notified by the cancer registries of Zürich, St Gallen and Basel, which supply pathological reports. To improve completeness of registration, the registry staff periodically searches the medical records of 16 clinical departments of seven hospitals and the statistical reports of 10 departments of four hospitals in the canton.

There are 322 private practitioners (1 per 540 population) who give, if necessary, additional information on a voluntary basis by completing a malignancy report.

The registry collects all malignant tumours including all basal cell carcinomas of the skin, carcinomas *in situ* and all papillary tumours of the bladder with behaviour codes of 2 or higher, but these are all eliminated for presentations of data. The autopsy rate is about 15%.

The Federal Statistical Office periodically supplies death certificates. Complete data for each patient (including scanned reports) are stored in a personal computer that allows extraction of information about multiple tumours, plausibilities, double registrations and incidence rates. Double tumours are eliminated according to the criteria of IARC.

J. Allemann

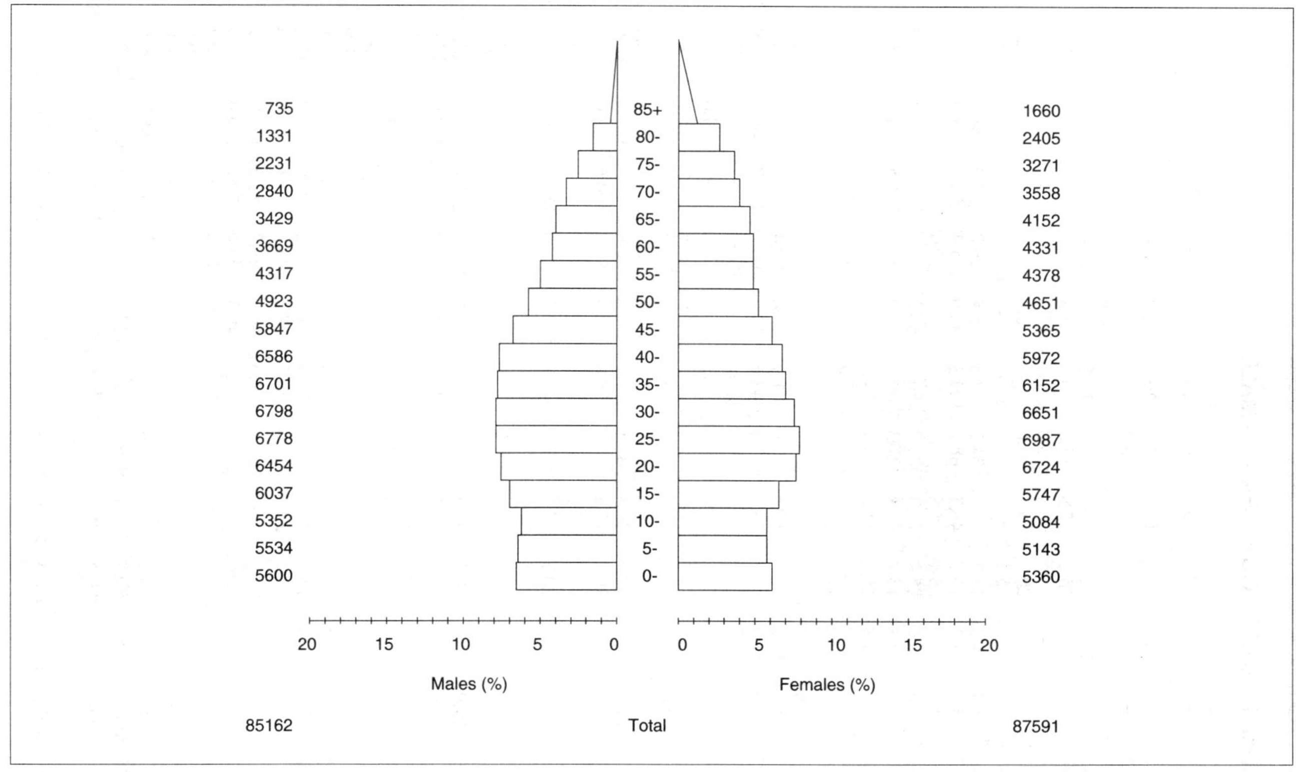

Switzerland, Graubunden
Source of population: average annual 1989–92
Census: 1990. Recensement fédéral de la population suisse, Décembre 1990. Population résidante selon le canton et les groupes d'ages en 1990. Annuaire statistique de la Suisse, Office fédéral de la statistique, Berne, 1993, pp 48-49.
Estimate: The mid-year populations were estimated for the years 1989, 1991 and 1992.

Notes to tables overleaf:
† 188 does not include the non-invasive tumours

SWITZERLAND, GRAUBUNDEN 1989-1992

ANNUAL INCIDENCE PER 100,000 BY AGE GROUP (YEARS) - MALE

SITE	ALL AGES	AGE UNK	0-	5-	10-	15-	20-	25-	30-	35-	40-	45-	50-	55-	60-	65-	70-	75-	80-	85+	CRUDE RATE	%	CR 64	CR 74	ASR (W)	ICD (9th)
Lip	16	0	-	-	-	-	-	-	-	3.7	-	4.3	-	11.6	6.8	29.2	8.8	56.0	-	34.0	4.7	1.1	0.13	0.32	3.0	140
Tongue	4	0	-	-	-	-	-	-	-	3.7	-	-	-	13.6	7.3	-	-	-	-	-	1.2	0.3	0.09	0.12	1.0	141
Salivary gland	3	0	-	-	-	-	-	-	-	-	-	-	-	-	-	-	8.8	-	18.8	34.0	0.9	0.2	0.00	0.04	0.4	142
Mouth	10	0	-	-	-	-	-	-	-	-	-	21.4	-	-	6.8	14.6	-	22.4	-	-	2.9	0.7	0.14	0.21	2.2	143-5
Oropharynx	7	0	-	-	-	-	-	-	-	-	-	-	15.2	5.8	13.6	-	8.8	-	-	-	2.1	0.5	0.17	0.22	1.7	146
Nasopharynx	4	0	-	-	-	-	-	-	-	-	-	-	-	-	6.8	-	17.6	-	18.8	-	1.2	0.3	0.03	0.12	0.7	147
Hypopharynx	8	0	-	-	-	-	-	-	-	-	-	-	20.3	5.8	13.6	-	8.8	-	-	-	2.3	0.6	0.20	0.24	2.0	148
Pharynx unspecified	1	0	-	-	-	-	-	-	-	-	-	-	5.1	-	-	-	-	-	-	-	0.3	0.1	0.03	0.03	0.3	149
Oesophagus	26	0	-	-	-	-	-	-	-	-	3.8	4.3	15.2	-	34.1	7.3	26.4	56.0	93.9	68.0	7.6	1.8	0.29	0.46	4.7	150
Stomach	88	0	-	-	-	-	-	-	7.4	3.7	3.8	17.1	15.2	46.3	68.1	109.3	132.0	134.4	206.6	204.0	25.8	6.2	0.81	2.02	16.6	151
Small intestine	6	0	-	-	-	-	-	3.7	-	-	-	-	5.1	5.8	-	7.3	-	22.4	-	-	1.8	0.4	0.07	0.11	1.2	152
Colon	109	0	-	-	-	-	-	-	-	-	7.6	8.6	25.4	75.3	81.8	80.2	167.2	134.4	375.6	442.0	32.0	7.7	0.99	2.23	19.7	153
Rectum	51	0	-	-	-	-	-	3.7	3.7	-	17.1	15.2	34.7	27.3	43.7	88.0	78.4	131.5	68.0	15.0	3.6	0.51	1.17	9.6	154
Liver	21	0	-	-	4.1	-	-	-	-	-	-	4.3	15.2	11.6	20.4	29.2	35.2	11.2	37.6	-	6.2	1.5	0.28	0.60	4.6	155
Gall bladder etc.	10	0	-	-	-	-	-	-	-	-	-	-	-	-	6.8	7.3	-	33.6	56.3	68.0	2.9	0.7	0.03	0.07	1.4	156
Pancreas	57	0	-	-	-	-	-	-	-	-	-	21.4	15.2	23.2	40.9	43.7	70.4	123.2	187.8	136.0	16.7	4.0	0.50	1.07	10.2	157
Nose, sinuses etc.	1	0	-	-	-	-	-	-	-	3.8	-	-	-	-	-	-	-	-	-	-	0.3	0.1	0.02	0.02	0.2	160
Larynx	23	0	-	-	-	-	-	-	3.7	3.8	12.8	-	17.4	40.9	21.9	17.6	22.4	37.6	-	-	6.8	1.6	0.39	0.59	5.0	161
Bronchus, lung	255	0	-	-	4.1	-	3.7	-	3.7	7.6	59.9	91.4	173.7	177.2	342.6	413.6	403.3	431.9	306.0	74.9	18.1	2.61	6.39	49.8	162
Other thoracic organs	1	0	-	-	-	-	-	-	-	-	4.3	-	-	-	-	-	-	-	-	-	0.3	0.1	0.02	0.02	0.3	163-4
Bone	4	0	-	-	-	3.9	-	3.7	-	-	-	-	-	-	7.3	-	-	-	34.0	1.2	0.3	0.04	0.07	0.9	170
Connective tissue	10	0	-	4.5	-	-	-	3.7	-	-	-	-	-	5.8	-	-	17.6	22.4	37.6	34.0	2.9	0.7	0.07	0.16	1.9	171
Mesothelioma	10	0	-	-	-	-	-	-	-	-	3.8	8.6	-	5.8	-	14.6	17.6	22.4	-	-	2.9	0.7	0.09	0.25	2.0	MES
Kaposi's sarcoma	1	0	-	-	-	-	-	3.7	-	-	-	-	-	-	3.7	-	-	-	-	-	0.3	0.1	0.02	0.02	0.3	KAP
Melanoma of skin	36	0	-	-	4.1	-	-	-	-	-	11.4	34.2	10.2	40.5	34.1	14.6	8.8	44.8	-	102.0	10.6	2.6	0.67	0.79	8.2	172
Other skin	116	0	-	-	-	-	-	-	-	-	-	8.6	20.3	23.2	81.8	94.8	158.4	291.3	300.5	714.0	34.1		0.67	1.93	19.7	173
Breast	2	0	-	-	-	-	-	-	-	-	-	-	-	5.8	-	-	8.8	-	-	-	0.6	0.1	0.03	0.07	0.4	175
Prostate	299	0	-	-	-	-	-	-	-	-	-	4.3	20.3	75.3	163.5	349.9	519.2	885.0	788.7	986.1	87.8	21.2	1.32	5.66	49.4	185
Testis	36	0	4.5	-	-	8.3	19.4	51.6	11.0	3.7	19.0	4.3	20.3	-	-	-	-	-	-	-	10.6	2.6	0.71	0.71	10.3	186
Penis	1	0	-	-	-	-	-	-	-	-	-	-	-	-	6.8	-	-	-	-	-	0.3	0.1	0.03	0.03	0.3	187.1-.4
Other male genital	0	0	-	-	-	-	-	-	-	-	-	-	-	-	-	-	-	-	-	-	0.0	0.0	0.00	0.00	0.0	187.5-.9
†Bladder	83	0	-	-	-	-	-	3.7	-	-	19.0	-	10.2	46.3	68.1	65.6	132.0	201.6	206.6	136.0	24.4	5.9	0.74	1.72	14.9	188
Kidney etc.	43	0	4.5	-	-	-	-	-	-	-	7.6	-	15.2	52.1	34.1	51.0	52.8	56.0	37.6	102.0	12.6	3.1	0.57	1.09	9.0	189
Eye	3	0	-	-	-	-	-	-	-	3.7	-	-	-	11.6	-	-	-	-	-	-	0.9	0.2	0.08	0.08	0.7	190
Brain, nervous system	21	0	-	-	-	4.1	3.9	-	-	7.5	-	4.3	15.2	23.2	20.4	7.3	35.2	-	-	34.0	6.2	1.5	0.39	0.61	5.0	191-2
Thyroid	2	0	-	-	-	4.1	-	3.7	-	-	-	-	-	-	-	-	-	-	-	-	0.6	0.1	0.04	0.04	0.7	193
Other endocrine	0	0	-	-	-	-	-	-	-	-	-	-	-	-	-	-	-	-	-	-	0.0	0.0	0.00	0.00	0.0	194
Hodgkin's disease	14	0	-	4.5	4.7	8.3	-	3.7	3.7	3.7	3.8	4.3	-	11.6	6.8	7.3	-	11.2	-	-	4.1	1.0	0.28	0.31	3.9	201
Non-Hodgkin lymphoma	39	0	-	-	-	-	-	3.7	3.7	3.7	7.6	8.6	15.2	23.2	13.6	21.9	61.6	67.2	93.9	68.0	11.4	2.8	0.40	0.81	7.3	200,202
Multiple myeloma	23	0	-	-	-	-	-	-	-	-	-	4.3	5.1	23.2	13.6	43.7	17.6	44.8	18.8	68.0	6.8	1.6	0.23	0.54	4.5	203
Lymphoid leukaemia	28	0	-	9.0	4.7	4.1	3.9	-	-	-	-	4.3	-	-	20.4	14.6	44.0	67.2	56.3	102.0	8.2	2.0	0.23	0.53	5.9	204
Myeloid leukaemia	19	0	-	-	-	-	3.9	-	3.7	7.5	-	-	-	-	13.6	-	26.4	33.6	56.3	136.0	5.6	1.3	0.14	0.28	3.3	205
Monocytic leukaemia	1	0	-	-	-	-	-	-	-	-	-	-	-	-	-	-	-	11.2	-	-	0.3	0.1	0.00	0.00	0.1	206
Other leukaemia	0	0	-	-	-	-	-	-	-	-	-	-	-	-	-	-	-	-	-	-	0.0	0.0	0.00	0.00	0.0	207
Leukaemia unspecified	0	0	-	-	-	-	-	-	-	-	-	-	-	-	-	-	-	-	-	-	0.0	0.0	0.00	0.00	0.0	208
Other and unspecified	32	0	-	-	-	-	-	3.7	-	3.7	3.8	-	10.2	11.6	20.4	36.4	35.2	67.2	93.9	68.0	9.4	2.3	0.27	0.63	5.8	O&U
All sites	1524	0	8.9	18.1	9.3	41.4	34.9	84.8	36.8	56.0	106.3	260.8	380.8	770.1	1056.1	1472.5	2138.5	2923.7	3286.4	3944.2	447.4		14.32	32.38	289.0	ALL
All sites but 173	1408	0	8.9	18.1	9.3	41.4	34.9	84.8	36.8	56.0	106.3	252.2	360.5	746.9	974.4	1377.8	1980.1	2632.5	2985.9	3230.2	413.3	100.0	13.65	30.44	269.3	ALLb

Rate from 1 case   4.464 4.518 4.671 4.141 3.874 3.688 3.677 3.731 3.796 4.275 5.078 5.790 6.814 7.290 8.800 11.202 18.779 34.002

†Important: see notes on population page

SWITZERLAND, GRAUBUNDEN 1989-1992

ANNUAL INCIDENCE PER 100,000 BY AGE GROUP (YEARS) - FEMALE

SITE	ALL AGES	AGE UNK	0-	5-	10-	15-	20-	25-	30-	35-	40-	45-	50-	55-	60-	65-	70-	75-	80-	85+	CRUDE RATE	%	CR 64	CR 74	ASR (W)	ICD (9th)
Lip	6	0	-	-	-	-	-	-	-	-	-	4.7	-	-	5.8	-	7.0	-	20.8	15.1	1.7	0.5	0.05	0.09	**0.8**	*140*
Tongue	4	0	-	-	-	-	-	-	-	-	-	-	10.8	5.7	-	6.0	-	-	-	-	1.1	0.3	0.08	0.11	**0.9**	*141*
Salivary gland	5	0	-	-	4.9	-	-	-	-	-	-	-	-	-	-	-	7.0	15.3	-	15.1	1.4	0.4	0.02	0.06	**0.8**	*142*
Mouth	1	0	-	-	-	-	-	-	-	-	-	-	-	-	-	-	-	-	-	15.1	0.3	0.1	0.00	0.00	**0.1**	*143-5*
Oropharynx	2	0	-	-	-	-	-	-	-	-	-	-	-	5.7	-	-	-	7.6	-	-	0.6	0.2	0.03	0.03	**0.3**	*146*
Nasopharynx	2	0	-	-	-	-	-	-	-	-	4.2	-	5.4	-	-	-	-	-	-	-	0.6	0.2	0.05	0.05	**0.5**	*147*
Hypopharynx	0	0	-	-	-	-	-	-	-	-	-	-	-	-	-	-	-	-	-	-	0.0	0.0	0.00	0.00	**0.0**	*148*
Pharynx unspecified	0	0	-	-	-	-	-	-	-	-	-	-	-	-	-	-	-	-	-	-	0.0	0.0	0.00	0.00	**0.0**	*149*
Oesophagus	6	0	-	-	-	-	-	-	-	-	-	-	-	-	6.0	7.0	15.3	10.4	15.1		1.7	0.5	0.00	0.07	**0.6**	*150*
Stomach	56	0	-	-	-	-	-	-	7.5	-	4.2	4.7	-	5.7	40.4	30.1	63.2	99.3	103.9	105.4	16.0	4.6	0.31	0.78	**7.0**	*151*
Small intestine	2	0	-	-	-	-	-	-	-	-	-	-	-	-	-	7.0	-	-	15.1		0.6	0.2	0.00	0.04	**0.2**	*152*
Colon	119	0	-	-	-	-	3.7	-	7.5	4.1	4.2	23.3	32.3	45.7	23.1	102.4	147.5	152.8	218.2	180.7	34.0	9.7	0.72	1.97	**16.5**	*153*
Rectum	46	0	-	-	-	-	-	-	-	4.1	-	14.0	5.4	51.4	17.3	36.1	28.1	53.5	72.7	75.3	13.1	3.8	0.46	0.78	**7.0**	*154*
Liver	16	0	-	-	-	-	-	-	-	-	4.2	-	5.4	5.7	11.5	12.0	14.1	15.3	20.8	45.2	4.6	1.3	0.13	0.26	**2.3**	*155*
Gallbladder etc.	22	0	-	-	-	-	-	-	-	-	-	-	9.3	-	-	17.3	6.0	35.1	45.9	52.0	-	6.3	1.8	0.13	0.34	**2.9**	*156*
Pancreas	49	0	-	-	-	-	-	-	-	4.1	-	4.7	21.5	11.4	28.9	36.1	42.2	84.1	103.9	45.2	14.0	4.0	0.35	0.74	**6.7**	*157*
Nose, sinuses etc.	1	0	-	-	-	-	-	-	-	-	-	-	-	-	-	-	-	7.6	-	-	0.3	0.1	0.00	0.00	**0.1**	*160*
Larynx	3	0	-	-	-	-	-	-	-	-	-	-	5.4	5.7	-	6.0	-	-	-	-	0.9	0.2	0.06	0.09	**0.7**	*161*
Bronchus, lung	58	0	-	-	-	-	-	-	3.8	-	8.4	14.0	26.9	28.6	63.5	30.1	42.2	61.1	83.1	60.2	16.6	4.7	0.73	1.09	**9.7**	*162*
Other thoracic organs	1	0	-	-	-	-	-	-	-	-	-	-	-	-	-	-	-	7.6	-	-	0.3	0.1	0.00	0.00	**0.1**	*163-4*
Bone	7	0	-	-	4.9	8.7	3.7	3.6	-	-	-	4.7	-	-	-	-	-	-	-	15.1	2.0	0.6	0.13	0.13	**2.2**	*170*
Connective tissue	7	0	-	-	-	-	-	-	-	-	-	-	-	17.1	-	6.0	14.1	-	10.4	-	2.0	0.6	0.09	0.19	**1.2**	*171*
Mesothelioma	0	0	-	-	-	-	-	-	-	-	-	-	-	-	-	-	-	-	-	-	0.0	0.0	0.00	0.00	**0.0**	*MES*
Kaposi's sarcoma	0	0	-	-	-	-	-	-	-	-	-	-	-	-	-	-	-	-	-	-	0.0	0.0	0.00	0.00	**0.0**	*KAP*
Melanoma of skin	50	0	-	-	-	-	3.7	14.3	15.0	20.3	12.6	23.3	-	40.0	34.6	18.1	14.1	45.9	20.8	30.1	14.3	4.1	0.82	0.98	**10.2**	*172*
Other skin	87	0	-	-	-	-	-	-	-	-	-	-	5.4	5.7	17.3	60.2	28.1	175.8	176.7	421.7	24.8		0.14	0.58	**8.3**	*173*
Breast	353	0	-	-	-	-	-	3.6	30.1	44.7	92.1	167.7	225.8	194.1	155.8	240.8	252.9	328.6	311.8	346.4	100.7	28.9	4.57	7.04	**64.5**	*174*
Uterus unspecified	4	0	-	-	-	-	-	-	-	-	-	-	5.4	-	5.8	-	-	7.6	10.4	-	1.1	0.3	0.06	0.06	**0.6**	*179*
Cervix uteri	43	0	-	-	-	-	-	7.2	22.6	28.4	20.9	32.6	16.1	22.8	11.5	6.0	14.1	-	10.4	45.2	12.3	3.5	0.81	0.91	**9.8**	*180*
Placenta	1	0	-	-	-	-	-	3.6	-	-	-	-	-	-	-	-	-	-	-	-	0.3	0.1	0.02	0.02	**0.3**	*181*
Corpus uteri	53	0	-	-	-	-	-	-	-	-	-	9.3	43.0	79.9	34.6	36.1	35.1	53.5	41.6	15.1	15.1	4.3	0.83	1.19	**9.9**	*182*
Ovary etc.	72	0	-	-	-	-	-	7.2	3.8	-	4.2	4.7	21.5	28.6	40.4	66.2	70.3	107.0	62.4	150.6	20.5	5.9	0.55	1.23	**10.7**	*183*
Other female genital	12	0	-	-	-	-	-	-	-	-	-	-	-	11.4	5.8	-	14.1	22.9	31.2	15.1	3.4	1.0	0.09	0.16	**1.4**	*184*
†Bladder	24	0	-	-	-	-	-	-	3.8	4.1	-	-	-	5.7	11.5	6.0	35.1	22.9	20.8	120.5	6.8	2.0	0.13	0.33	**3.0**	*188*
Kidney etc.	36	0	-	-	-	-	-	-	3.8	-	4.2	-	26.9	5.7	57.7	24.1	21.1	68.8	10.4	15.1	10.3	2.9	0.49	0.72	**6.3**	*189*
Eye	4	0	-	-	-	-	-	3.6	-	-	-	-	5.4	-	5.8	6.0	-	-	-	-	1.1	0.3	0.07	0.10	**1.0**	*190*
Brain, nervous system	12	0	-	-	-	-	-	3.6	3.8	-	4.2	4.7	5.4	-	23.1	-	7.0	7.6	10.4	-	3.4	1.0	0.22	0.26	**2.5**	*191-2*
Thyroid	18	0	-	-	4.9	-	3.7	7.2	-	-	-	-	-	5.7	11.5	12.0	14.1	38.2	10.4	15.1	5.1	1.5	0.17	0.30	**3.2**	*193*
Other endocrine	3	0	4.7	-	-	-	-	-	-	-	-	-	-	-	-	6.0	-	7.6	-	-	0.9	0.2	0.02	0.05	**0.8**	*194*
Hodgkin's disease	6	0	-	-	-	-	3.7	-	-	-	-	-	5.4	5.7	-	6.0	-	7.6	10.4	-	1.7	0.5	0.07	0.10	**1.1**	*201*
Non-Hodgkin lymphoma	29	0	-	-	-	-	3.7	3.6	-	-	8.4	4.7	5.4	28.6	17.3	24.1	21.1	30.6	20.8	30.1	8.3	2.4	0.36	0.58	**5.2**	*200,202*
Multiple myeloma	22	0	-	-	-	-	-	-	-	-	-	4.7	16.1	-	5.8	6.0	21.1	68.8	20.8	30.1	6.3	1.8	0.13	0.27	**2.9**	*203*
Lymphoid leukaemia	11	0	4.7	-	-	-	-	-	-	-	-	-	5.4	5.7	5.8	12.0	7.0	22.9	10.4	-	3.1	0.9	0.11	0.20	**2.1**	*204*
Myeloid leukaemia	16	0	-	4.9	-	4.3	-	3.6	-	4.1	4.2	-	10.8	5.7	5.8	-	7.0	22.9	31.2	-	4.6	1.3	0.22	0.25	**3.2**	*205*
Monocytic leukaemia	1	0	-	-	-	-	-	-	-	-	-	-	-	-	-	-	-	-	-	15.1	0.3	0.1	0.00	0.00	**0.1**	*206*
Other leukaemia	0	0	-	-	-	-	-	-	-	-	-	-	-	-	-	-	-	-	-	-	0.0	0.0	0.00	0.00	**0.0**	*207*
Leukaemia unspecified	1	0	-	-	-	-	-	-	-	-	-	-	-	-	-	-	-	-	-	15.1	0.3	0.1	0.00	0.00	**0.1**	*208*
Other and unspecified	38	0	-	-	-	-	-	-	-	-	-	4.7	5.4	-	11.5	30.1	21.1	22.9	83.1	225.9	10.8	3.1	0.11	0.36	**4.1**	*O&U*
All sites	1309	0	9.3	4.9	14.8	13.0	22.3	60.8	101.5	113.8	175.8	335.5	516.0	628.1	669.5	836.9	997.6	1627.7	1590.1	2093.4	373.6		13.33	22.50	**211.8**	*ALL*
All sites but 173	1222	0	9.3	4.9	14.8	13.0	22.3	60.8	101.5	113.8	175.8	335.5	510.6	622.4	652.2	776.7	969.5	1451.9	1413.4	1671.7	348.8	100.0	13.18	21.92	**203.5**	*ALLb*

Rate from 1 case			4.664	4.861	4.917	4.350	3.718	3.578	3.759	4.064	4.186	4.660	5.375	5.710	5.771	6.021	7.025	7.642	10.393	15.060

†Important: see notes on population page

Switzerland, Neuchâtel

The Cancer Registry of the Swiss French-speaking canton of Neuchâtel, the "Registre Neuchâtelois des tumeurs", was established in 1972. Costs are shared between the local Public Health Department and the League Against Cancer, a substantial contribution being also supplied by the Swiss Federal Government. Although the scientific supervision of the registry is shared with that of the registry in the neighbouring Vaud canton, the Neuchâtel registry maintains structural and administrative independence. The computer department at the University of Neuchâtel has provided support and expertise in setting up a uniform and structured database for the Neuchâtel data file.

The registry, which covers the whole of the canton (800 km^2 with about 160 000 inhabitants), is located in the western part of Switzerland, sharing half of its frontier with France. The canton is a mainly rural region with only two cities of approximately 40 000 inhabitants. In the absence of heavy industry, watchmaking and microtechniques are the main activities.

Almost all the population is of Caucasian origin; 45% are Protestant and 36% Roman Catholic. Foreigners, predominantly of Mediterranean origin, account for about 20% of residents. In 1990, the main occupational sectors in the canton of Neuchâtel were: industry 39%, agriculture 4%, and services 57%.

In 1990, the region covered by the registry had about 1100 hospital beds available for diagnosis and treatment (i.e., about 7 beds per 1000 population). In the same year there were about 300 hospital and privately practising physicians (one medical doctor per 530 population).

The bulk of information is provided by the local Institute of Pathology through biopsy–cytology and autopsy reports. Notification is based on voluntary agreement between the recording medical institutions of the canton and the registry. Other sources of information are the departments of oncology and haematology, which also centralize diagnostic and therapeutic procedures for malignant haematological disorders.

Information on residents diagnosed or treated outside hospital, elsewhere in Switzerland or in other countries is supplied by the neighbouring cantonal tumour registries of Vaud and Geneva (mostly upper aero-digestive tract, skin and childhood cancer cases) and general practitioners.

Further information is abstracted and systematically checked by the registry staff from hospital charts. Specific to, and one of the strengths of the registry is the routine integration of an abstract of the medical record in the registry data file. All death certificates are checked annually against the registry files. Death-certificate-only cases account for 2% of the total registered cases. Passive follow-up is recorded, each subsequent item of information being used to complete the record of an already registered case.

All relevant information is manually scrutinized before being interactively introduced into the computer of the Department of Informatics and Statistics of the University of Neuchâtel. Sophisticated automated verifications and analyses are performed on stored data in batch mode using *ad hoc* programs by the Vaud Cancer Registry on the computer of the University of Lausanne.

The registry is patient-based and if multiple primary tumours are diagnosed in the same person each is recorded separately, except for non-melanomatous skin tumours which are classified by the site of the first recognized primary. However, for the present volume, multiple tumours were classified as independent primaries according to the rules proposed by the IARC and IACR, except for squamous- and basal-cell carcinomas of the skin, which were considered different primaries.

Apart from providing routine annual incidence and mortality data by sex, age and primary site, and data for local planning purposes, the registry is engaged in (mostly) descriptive epidemiological studies in collaboration with the Vaud Cancer Registry and the other Swiss population-based registries, which are coordinated by the Swiss Association of Cancer Registries and are a constituent part of the Swiss Institute for Applied Cancer Research.

F Levi
P Siegenthaler

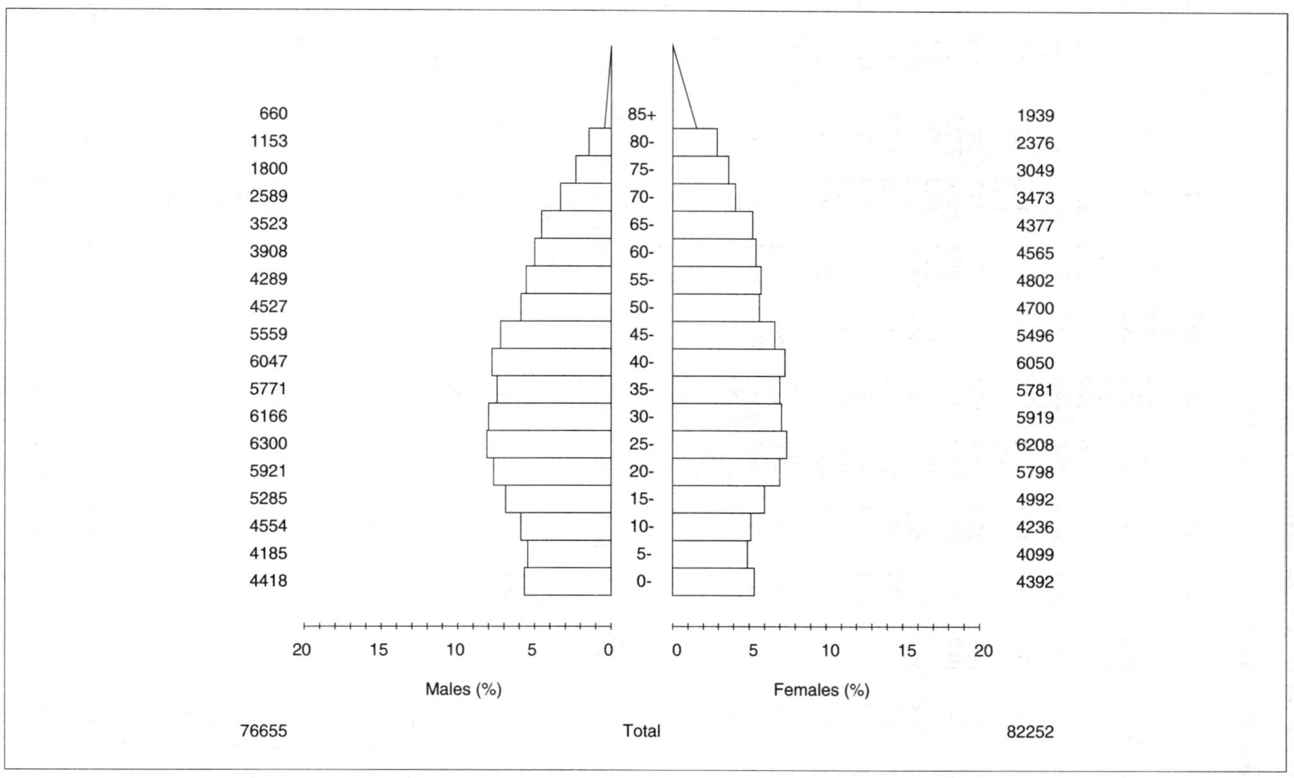

Switzerland, Neuchâtel
Source of population: average annual 1988–92
Census: December 1990. Recensement fédéral de la population suisse, Décembre 1990. Population résidante selon le canton et les groupes d'ages en 1990. Annuaire statistique de la Suisse, Office fédéral de la statistique, Berne, 1993, pp 48-49.
Estimate: The 1988, 1989, 1991 and 1992 populations are mid-year Federal and Cantonal estimates using the classical interpolation method, based on official numbers of births, deaths, immigration and emigration.

Notes to tables overleaf:
† 188 does not include non-invasive tumours

SWITZERLAND, NEUCHATEL 1988-1992

ANNUAL INCIDENCE PER 100,000 BY AGE GROUP (YEARS) - MALE

SITE	ALL AGES	AGE UNK	0-	5-	10-	15-	20-	25-	30-	35-	40-	45-	50-	55-	60-	65-	70-	75-	80-	85+	CRUDE RATE	%	CR 64	CR 74	ASR (W)	ICD (9th)
Lip	9	0	-	-	-	-	-	-	-	-	-	-	4.4	-	5.1	11.4	7.7	22.2	-	60.6	2.3	0.5	0.05	0.14	1.4	140
Tongue	20	0	-	-	-	-	-	-	-	-	9.9	10.8	-	18.7	10.2	22.7	15.4	22.2	-	-	5.2	1.1	0.25	0.44	3.6	141
Salivary gland	2	0	-	-	-	-	-	-	-	-	-	-	4.4	-	5.7	-	-	-	-	-	0.5	0.1	0.02	0.05	0.4	142
Mouth	29	0	-	-	-	-	-	-	-	-	6.6	10.8	22.1	23.3	25.6	17.0	7.7	22.2	52.0	-	7.6	1.7	0.44	0.57	5.3	143-5
Oropharynx	24	0	-	-	-	-	-	-	-	-	3.3	18.0	4.4	18.7	35.8	28.4	7.7	-	-	-	6.3	1.4	0.40	0.58	4.7	146
Nasopharynx	2	0	-	-	-	-	3.4	-	-	-	-	-	4.4	-	-	-	-	-	-	-	0.5	0.1	0.04	0.04	0.5	147
Hypopharynx	22	0	-	-	-	-	-	-	-	-	-	7.2	4.4	18.7	15.4	17.0	54.1	-	17.3	30.3	5.7	1.3	0.23	0.58	3.8	148
Pharynx unspecified	3	0	-	-	-	-	-	-	-	-	-	-	4.4	-	5.1	-	-	-	17.3	-	0.8	0.2	0.05	0.05	0.5	149
Oesophagus	38	0	-	-	-	-	-	-	-	-	3.3	14.4	13.3	23.3	25.6	51.1	7.7	77.7	34.7	30.3	9.9	2.2	0.40	0.69	6.5	150
Stomach	81	0	-	-	-	-	-	-	-	10.4	-	10.8	8.8	32.6	81.9	34.1	92.7	88.8	260.0	272.7	21.1	4.6	0.72	1.36	12.7	151
Small intestine	8	0	-	-	-	-	-	-	-	-	-	-	-	10.2	-	15.4	22.2	17.3	30.3	-	2.1	0.5	0.05	0.13	1.2	152
Colon	136	0	-	-	-	-	3.4	3.2	-	-	6.6	21.6	17.7	56.0	71.6	124.9	146.8	299.9	277.3	363.6	35.5	7.8	0.90	2.26	21.1	153
Rectum	89	0	-	-	-	-	-	-	-	-	3.3	7.2	17.7	37.3	92.1	68.1	131.3	100.0	121.3	333.3	23.2	5.1	0.79	1.79	14.6	154
Liver	45	0	-	-	-	-	-	-	3.2	-	3.3	-	13.3	18.7	40.9	17.0	54.1	133.3	86.7	30.3	11.7	2.6	0.40	0.75	6.9	155
Gallbladder etc.	11	0	-	-	-	-	-	-	-	-	-	-	-	9.3	10.2	11.4	15.4	11.1	34.7	-	2.9	0.6	0.10	0.23	1.7	156
Pancreas	47	0	-	-	-	-	-	-	-	3.5	3.3	-	30.9	14.0	46.1	39.7	54.1	55.5	86.7	60.6	12.3	2.7	0.49	0.96	7.9	157
Nose, sinuses etc.	4	0	-	-	-	-	-	-	-	-	-	-	4.4	-	10.2	-	-	11.1	-	-	1.0	0.2	0.07	0.07	0.7	160
Larynx	32	0	-	-	-	-	-	-	-	-	6.6	7.2	13.3	18.7	35.8	34.1	30.9	44.4	-	-	8.3	1.8	0.41	0.73	5.8	161
Bronchus, lung	360	0	-	-	-	-	-	-	-	6.9	26.5	61.2	106.0	191.2	286.6	431.5	471.2	388.7	433.4	454.5	93.9	20.6	3.39	7.90	60.8	162
Other thoracic organs	6	0	4.5	-	-	-	3.4	3.2	-	-	-	-	-	4.7	-	5.7	-	-	17.3	-	1.6	0.3	0.08	0.11	1.5	163-4
Bone	2	0	-	-	-	-	-	-	-	-	-	-	-	-	-	-	-	22.2	-	-	0.5	0.1	0.00	0.00	0.2	170
Connective tissue	3	0	-	-	-	-	-	-	-	-	3.3	-	-	-	-	5.7	-	-	17.3	-	0.8	0.2	0.02	0.04	0.5	171
Mesothelioma	7	0	-	-	-	-	-	-	-	-	3.3	-	-	-	10.2	11.4	7.7	11.1	-	-	1.8	0.4	0.07	0.16	1.2	MES
Kaposi's sarcoma	8	0	-	-	-	-	-	-	6.5	6.9	9.9	-	4.4	-	-	-	-	-	-	-	2.1	0.5	0.14	0.14	1.6	KAP
Melanoma of skin	60	0	9.1	-	-	-	3.4	-	6.5	3.5	23.2	3.6	17.7	56.0	30.7	51.1	46.3	55.5	34.7	60.6	15.7	3.4	0.77	1.25	11.4	172
Other skin	529	0	-	-	-	-	-	3.2	13.0	17.3	59.5	57.6	123.7	191.2	271.2	493.9	726.1	921.8	1074.7	1121.2	138.0		3.68	9.78	83.3	173
Breast	2	0	-	-	-	-	-	-	-	-	-	-	-	-	5.7	-	-	17.3	-	-	0.5	0.1	0.00	0.03	0.3	175
Prostate	298	0	-	-	-	-	-	-	-	-	-	-	22.1	65.3	107.5	278.2	502.1	744.1	849.4	848.5	77.7	17.1	0.97	4.88	42.3	185
Testis	41	0	-	-	-	-	10.1	34.9	22.7	38.1	3.3	3.6	8.8	18.7	-	-	7.7	-	-	-	10.7	2.4	0.70	0.74	9.0	186
Penis	10	0	-	-	-	-	-	-	-	-	3.3	-	4.4	4.7	-	11.4	23.2	11.1	-	30.3	2.6	0.6	0.06	0.23	1.7	187.1-.4
Other male genital	3	0	-	-	-	-	-	-	-	-	-	-	-	-	5.7	-	11.1	-	30.3	-	0.8	0.2	0.00	0.03	0.4	187.5-.9
†Bladder	95	0	-	-	-	-	-	-	3.5	-	7.2	13.3	37.3	46.1	68.1	108.1	255.4	225.3	303.0		24.8	5.4	0.54	1.42	14.0	188
Kidney etc.	54	0	-	-	-	-	-	-	-	-	9.9	14.4	17.7	23.3	30.7	39.7	61.8	88.8	121.3	60.6	14.1	3.1	0.48	0.99	8.7	189
Eye	3	0	4.5	-	-	-	-	-	-	-	-	-	-	4.7	-	-	7.7	-	-	-	0.8	0.2	0.05	0.08	0.9	190
Brain, nervous system	26	0	-	-	-	7.6	-	6.3	3.2	3.5	13.2	10.8	17.7	9.3	-	11.4	15.4	22.2	17.3	-	6.8	1.5	0.36	0.49	5.2	191-2
Thyroid	2	0	-	-	-	-	-	-	-	-	-	-	-	4.7	-	-	7.7	-	-	-	0.5	0.1	0.02	0.06	0.3	193
Other endocrine	1	0	-	-	-	-	-	-	-	-	-	-	-	5.1	-	-	-	-	-	-	0.3	0.1	0.03	0.03	0.2	194
Hodgkin's disease	11	0	-	-	4.4	-	3.4	3.2	-	6.9	3.3	3.6	-	4.7	-	5.7	-	11.1	-	30.3	2.9	0.6	0.15	0.18	2.4	201
Non-Hodgkin lymphoma	55	0	4.5	-	-	-	-	6.3	9.7	10.4	6.6	14.4	13.3	23.3	40.9	22.7	69.5	44.4	69.3	90.9	14.3	3.2	0.65	1.11	10.1	200,202
Multiple myeloma	11	0	-	-	-	-	-	-	-	-	-	-	4.4	9.3	-	11.4	23.2	-	52.0	-	2.9	0.6	0.07	0.24	1.7	203
Lymphoid leukaemia	25	0	-	-	4.4	7.6	-	-	-	-	-	-	4.7	20.5	22.7	23.2	44.4	-	181.8		6.5	1.4	0.19	0.41	4.6	204
Myeloid leukaemia	16	0	-	-	4.4	-	-	3.2	-	-	-	-	4.4	9.3	5.1	11.4	30.9	22.2	34.7	17.3	4.2	0.9	0.13	0.34	2.8	205
Monocytic leukaemia	1	0	-	-	-	-	-	-	-	-	-	-	-	-	-	-	-	-	17.3	-	0.3	0.1	0.00	0.00	0.1	206
Other leukaemia	1	0	-	-	-	-	-	-	-	-	-	-	-	-	-	-	-	7.7	-	-	0.3	0.1	0.00	0.04	0.2	207
Leukaemia unspecified	2	0	-	-	-	-	-	-	-	-	-	-	-	-	-	-	-	-	34.7	-	0.5	0.1	0.00	0.00	0.2	208
Other and unspecified	39	0	-	4.8	-	-	-	-	-	-	6.6	-	-	9.3	10.2	45.4	46.3	111.1	69.3	121.2	10.2	2.2	0.15	0.61	6.0	O&U
All sites	2273	0	22.6	4.8	13.2	15.1	27.0	63.5	64.9	110.9	218.3	284.2	525.6	960.6	1386.8	2021.0	2827.1	3676.1	4090.8	4545.5	593.0		18.49	42.73	371.0	ALL
All sites but 173	1744	0	22.6	4.8	13.2	15.1	27.0	60.3	51.9	93.6	158.7	226.6	402.0	769.4	1115.6	1527.1	2101.0	2754.3	3016.1	3424.2	455.0	100.0	14.80	32.95	287.7	ALLb

| Rate from 1 case | | | 4.526 | 4.779 | 4.392 | 3.784 | 3.377 | 3.174 | 3.243 | 3.465 | 3.307 | 3.597 | 4.417 | 4.663 | 5.117 | 5.677 | 7.724 | 11.106 | 17.334 | 30.303 |

†Important: see notes on population page

SWITZERLAND, NEUCHATEL 1988-1992

ANNUAL INCIDENCE PER 100,000 BY AGE GROUP (YEARS) - FEMALE

SITE	ALL AGES	AGE UNK	0-	5-	10-	15-	20-	25-	30-	35-	40-	45-	50-	55-	60-	65-	70-	75-	80-	85+	CRUDE RATE	%	CR 64	CR 74	ASR (W)	ICD (9th)
Lip	3	0	-	-	-	-	-	-	-	-	3.3	-	-	-	4.4	-	-	-	8.4	-	0.7	0.2	0.04	0.04	0.4	140
Tongue	6	0	-	-	-	-	-	-	-	3.5	-	-	-	-	13.1	4.6	-	6.6	-	-	1.5	0.4	0.08	0.11	0.9	141
Salivary gland	3	0	-	-	-	-	-	-	-	-	-	-	-	-	-	-	-	6.6	16.8	-	0.7	0.2	0.00	0.00	0.1	142
Mouth	9	0	-	-	-	-	-	-	-	-	-	3.6	4.3	12.5	8.8	-	5.8	6.6	-	-	2.2	0.6	0.15	0.17	1.5	143-5
Oropharynx	6	0	-	-	-	-	-	-	-	-	-	-	8.5	4.2	8.8	-	5.8	-	-	-	1.5	0.4	0.11	0.14	1.1	146
Nasopharynx	2	0	-	-	-	-	-	-	3.4	-	-	-	-	-	-	4.6	-	-	-	-	0.5	0.1	0.02	0.04	0.3	147
Hypopharynx	2	0	-	-	-	-	-	-	-	3.5	-	-	4.3	-	-	-	-	-	-	-	0.5	0.1	0.04	0.04	0.4	148
Pharynx unspecified	2	0	-	-	-	-	-	-	3.4	-	-	-	-	4.2	-	-	-	-	-	-	0.5	0.1	0.04	0.04	0.4	149
Oesophagus	19	0	-	-	-	-	-	-	-	-	3.6	-	8.3	4.4	18.3	-	26.2	8.4	61.9	4.6	1.2	0.08	0.17	1.9	150
Stomach	57	0	-	-	-	-	-	3.2	-	10.4	3.3	3.6	-	8.3	4.4	32.0	34.6	105.0	117.8	51.6	13.9	3.6	0.17	0.50	5.4	151
Small intestine	4	0	-	-	-	-	-	-	-	-	-	-	4.3	-	-	4.6	-	6.6	8.4	-	1.0	0.3	0.02	0.04	0.5	152
Colon	129	0	-	-	-	-	-	-	6.8	13.8	13.2	7.3	29.8	29.2	30.7	105.1	103.7	144.3	151.5	154.7	31.4	8.3	0.65	1.70	14.5	153
Rectum	72	0	-	-	-	-	-	3.2	-	10.4	3.3	7.3	17.0	20.8	21.9	54.8	46.1	85.3	58.9	113.4	17.5	4.6	0.42	0.92	8.4	154
Liver	8	0	-	-	-	-	-	-	-	-	-	-	8.8	4.6	-	13.1	16.8	10.3	1.9	0.5	0.04	0.07	0.8	155
Gallbladder etc.	23	0	-	-	-	-	-	-	-	-	-	4.3	4.2	13.1	9.1	23.0	59.0	8.4	20.6	5.6	1.5	0.11	0.27	2.4	156
Pancreas	42	0	-	-	-	-	-	-	-	-	-	4.3	-	17.5	36.5	40.3	39.4	58.9	92.8	10.2	2.7	0.11	0.49	4.0	157
Nose, sinuses etc.	3	0	-	-	-	-	-	-	-	1.9	-	-	-	-	-	9.1	-	6.6	-	-	0.7	0.2	0.00	0.05	0.3	160
Larynx	6	0	-	-	-	-	-	-	-	-	-	-	-	-	13.1	4.6	5.8	-	-	-	1.5	0.4	0.08	0.13	1.0	161
Bronchus, lung	87	0	-	-	-	-	-	-	6.9	9.9	14.6	38.3	12.5	39.4	91.4	80.6	111.5	25.2	30.9	21.2	5.6	0.61	1.47	11.6	162
Other thoracic organs	1	0	-	-	-	-	-	-	-	4.4	-	-	-	4.4	-	-	-	-	-	0.2	0.1	0.02	0.02	0.2	163-4
Bone	2	0	-	-	4.7	-	-	-	-	-	3.3	-	-	-	-	-	-	-	-	-	0.5	0.1	0.04	0.04	0.6	170
Connective tissue	4	0	-	-	-	-	-	-	3.4	-	-	-	-	-	-	4.6	5.8	6.6	-	-	1.0	0.3	0.02	0.07	0.5	171
Mesothelioma	1	0	-	-	-	-	-	-	-	-	-	-	-	4.2	-	-	-	-	-	-	0.2	0.1	0.02	0.02	0.2	MES
Kaposi's sarcoma	0	0	-	-	-	-	-	-	-	-	-	-	-	-	-	-	-	-	-	-	0.0	0.0	0.00	0.00	0.0	KAP
Melanoma of skin	63	0	-	-	4.7	-	3.4	16.1	20.3	10.4	13.2	21.8	17.0	16.7	13.1	18.3	57.6	19.7	42.1	41.3	15.3	4.0	0.68	1.06	10.3	172
Other skin	479	0	-	-	-	-	3.4	12.9	27.0	17.3	66.1	72.8	89.4	141.6	179.6	237.6	305.2	465.7	656.3	732.3	116.5	-	3.05	5.76	54.4	173
Breast	497	0	-	-	-	-	6.9	12.9	10.1	31.1	109.1	229.2	187.2	208.2	245.3	237.6	287.9	400.1	403.9	226.9	120.8	31.8	5.20	7.83	71.9	174
Uterus unspecified	4	0	-	-	-	-	-	-	-	-	-	-	-	-	4.4	-	5.8	6.6	-	10.3	1.0	0.3	0.02	0.05	0.4	179
Cervix uteri	57	0	-	-	-	-	6.4	16.9	6.9	19.8	18.2	8.5	16.7	48.2	22.8	34.6	19.7	25.2	30.9	13.9	3.6	0.71	1.00	9.1	180
Placenta	1	0	-	-	-	-	3.2	-	-	-	-	-	-	-	-	-	-	-	-	0.2	0.1	0.02	0.02	0.3	181
Corpus uteri	87	0	-	-	-	-	-	-	3.5	3.3	7.3	17.0	33.3	70.1	59.4	74.9	78.7	101.0	51.6	21.2	5.6	0.67	1.34	10.7	182
Ovary etc.	83	0	-	-	-	-	-	3.4	6.9	16.5	14.6	29.8	20.8	52.6	54.8	69.1	78.7	25.2	82.5	20.2	5.3	0.72	1.34	11.3	183
Other female genital	14	0	-	-	-	-	-	-	-	-	-	-	-	8.8	4.6	23.0	19.7	25.2	10.3	3.4	0.9	0.04	0.18	1.3	184
†Bladder	27	0	-	-	-	-	-	-	-	-	3.6	-	12.5	8.8	18.3	23.0	32.8	25.2	51.6	6.6	1.7	0.12	0.33	2.8	188
Kidney etc.	40	0	-	-	-	-	-	3.2	-	9.9	7.3	4.3	8.3	21.9	32.0	28.8	59.0	33.7	10.3	9.7	2.6	0.27	0.58	5.1	189
Eye	5	0	4.6	-	-	-	-	3.4	-	-	-	-	-	4.4	-	-	6.6	8.4	-	1.2	0.3	0.06	0.06	1.0	190
Brain, nervous system	25	0	4.6	9.8	-	-	-	-	-	3.5	3.3	-	4.3	4.2	13.1	22.8	28.8	32.8	-	-	6.1	1.6	0.21	0.47	4.4	191-2
Thyroid	17	0	-	-	-	4.0	-	6.4	-	-	16.5	-	-	4.2	13.1	9.1	5.8	6.6	8.4	-	4.1	1.1	0.22	0.30	3.1	193
Other endocrine	1	0	4.6	-	-	-	-	-	-	-	-	-	-	-	-	-	-	-	-	-	0.2	0.1	0.02	0.02	0.5	194
Hodgkin's disease	6	0	-	-	-	4.0	-	-	-	3.4	-	3.3	-	-	-	4.4	4.6	-	6.6	-	-	1.5	0.4	0.08	0.10	1.1	201
Non-Hodgkin lymphoma	45	0	-	-	-	-	-	-	-	13.8	6.6	3.6	-	20.8	17.5	32.0	34.6	45.9	25.2	61.9	10.9	2.9	0.31	0.64	5.5	200,202
Multiple myeloma	13	0	-	-	-	-	-	-	-	-	-	-	4.2	8.8	13.7	-	13.1	16.8	30.9	3.2	0.8	0.06	0.13	1.3	203
Lymphoid leukaemia	9	0	-	-	-	-	-	-	-	-	-	4.3	-	-	13.7	5.8	6.6	8.4	20.6	2.2	0.6	0.02	0.12	0.9	204
Myeloid leukaemia	16	0	-	-	-	-	-	-	3.4	6.9	-	4.3	-	8.8	-	28.8	6.6	8.4	30.9	3.9	1.0	0.12	0.26	2.0	205
Monocytic leukaemia	1	0	-	-	-	-	-	-	-	-	5.8	-	-	-	-	-	5.8	-	-	-	0.2	0.1	0.00	0.03	0.1	206
Other leukaemia	0	0	-	-	-	-	-	-	-	-	-	-	-	-	-	-	-	-	-	-	0.0	0.0	0.00	0.00	0.0	207
Leukaemia unspecified	2	0	-	-	-	-	-	-	-	-	-	-	-	-	-	-	-	13.1	-	-	0.5	0.1	0.00	0.00	0.1	208
Other and unspecified	58	0	-	-	-	-	-	-	-	-	3.3	7.3	17.0	12.5	-	27.4	74.9	39.4	109.4	103.1	14.1	3.7	0.20	0.71	5.8	O&U
All sites	2041	0	13.7	9.8	9.4	8.0	13.8	67.7	104.7	148.8	310.7	425.7	497.8	612.2	915.7	1192.4	1445.4	1981.0	2002.7	2031.8	496.2		15.69	28.88	260.8	ALL
All sites but 173	1562	0	13.7	9.8	9.4	8.0	10.3	54.8	77.7	131.5	244.6	352.9	408.5	470.6	736.0	954.8	1140.2	1515.3	1346.3	1299.5	379.8	100.0	12.64	23.11	206.3	ALLb

Rate from 1 case   4.553 4.879 4.721 4.006 3.449 3.222 3.379 3.459 3.306 3.638 4.255 4.165 4.381 4.569 5.759 6.560 8.415 10.314

†Important: see notes on population page

Switzerland, St Gall-Appenzell

The cancer registry was founded by the Regional Cancer League in 1960 at the department of pathology in the non-university central hospital of St Gall. It was hospital-based until 1980, when it became population-based. The sponsoring bodies are the Regional Cancer League and the three cantons covered by the registry, and it is also subsidized by the Federal Government. At present the registry has four full-time positions. In addition it has access to external data management resources.

The registry covers the three cantons of St Gall, Appenzell AR and Appenzell IR in the north-eastern part of Switzerland, a total area of 2430 km². It extends between latitudes 46°52′ and 47°30′ N; the lowest point is 396 m and the highest 3247 m above sea level.

The registry covers the entire resident population, amounting to 482 000 in 1990 (mid-year estimate). Of this total, 87% belong to the canton of St Gall. Major parts of the area are rural. There is one city with 75 000 inhabitants. The proportion of employed persons working in agriculture was 5.3% in 1990, above the Swiss average of 4.2%. Important industries are production of textiles, metal machines and vehicles, and construction, which are relatively broadly distributed over much of the region. In 1990 the per capita income was 86% of Swiss average in St Gall, 84% in Appenzell AR, and only 73% in Appenzell IR. Five sixths of the population are Swiss, the others mainly of European origin. 56% are Roman Catholics and 33% Protestants.

In 1990 there were 1060 active physicians (1 per 465 inhabitants). About 2500 public hospital beds were available in acute hospitals. The central hospital in the city of St Gall with 850 beds is well equipped. There is a special clinic for oncology and a public outpatient clinic for cancer patients that takes care of patients referred to them by general practitioners and other clinics. In addition there are some five consultant oncologists. For inpatient care patients are usually referred to a hospital within their region. Most cancer patients are treated at the central hospital or in one of the 11 peripheral acute hospitals within the region at least at one time during their disease, although for neoplasms of central nervous system, patients may be referred to the neighbouring canton of Zürich, and neoplasms of the haematological system are often diagnosed and treated outside hospital. Some people in areas adjacent to the urbanized canton of Zürich seek care there.

There are no population-based cancer screening programmes in this region. Screening is performed as an individual initiative and seems to be popular and effective for cervical carcinoma, for which 80% of cancers registered were *in situ* carcinomas (not counted in our incidence data). Early detection of breast cancer, on the other hand, could be improved.

Reporting of cancer cases is voluntary. A new law on data protection in Switzerland allowing data collection by institutions like cancer registries, has led to improved collaboration with the registry. The most important data source is passive collection of reports from the central pathology laboratory. In addition, the registry staff actively collect data in selected other pathology laboratories and in all regional acute hospitals. In the central hospital, the departments of oncology, haematology, radiotherapy, neurosurgery and paediatrics are actively scrutinized. There is a routine exchange of information with cancer registries covering two neighbouring cantons, including the city of Zürich. Active case ascertainment has also been organized with consultant oncologists in the region. Finally all death certificates with a cancer diagnosis are scrutinized, and if necessary additional information is sought, usually by mailed questionnaire to the treating physician or by looking at the case notes in hospitals. The registry had to temporarily stop active follow-up of patients, for capacity reasons. Limited follow-up is still performed by checking death certificates.

All tumours that meet the international criteria for a new primary also meet the registry criteria. On the other hand the registry accepts some tumours that do not fulfil the international criteria. The data presented here include only the cases meeting the international criteria.

Reports are usually checked within a few days after receipt. If a patient has not yet been registered or if a registered patient has developed a new tumour, basic information such as name, sex, exact date of birth, address, reporting physician, date of onset and character of tumour is put into the computer by clerical staff. Names and dates of birth are checked in order to find duplicates. In doubt a physician is asked for advice. Three months after receipt of the first report a physician looks at the file and decides whether additional information needs to be sought. Addresses are checked with official population control offices. Cases are finally coded and closed by a physician only about two years after onset.

Several plausibility checks, i.e. logical sequence of dates, validity of codes, compatibility of sex with diagnosis are done by the computer. The coding is visually checked on the screen and, after completion of a case, on the case printout. There is no routine checking of the plausibility of morphology by topography, or topography and morphology by age.

Analysis of the registry's data has taken place mainly in joint studies of the Association of Swiss Cancer Registries, e.g., on time trends of incidence of lung cancer, cutaneous melanoma and breast cancer. For the latter disease, a joint study was performed on stage distribution and survival.

I wish to thank the Cancer Registry of Zurich and its Head, Dr G. Schüler, for their support to our work. Of special value is the help they provided to us in dealing with processing information from death certificates.

T. Fisch

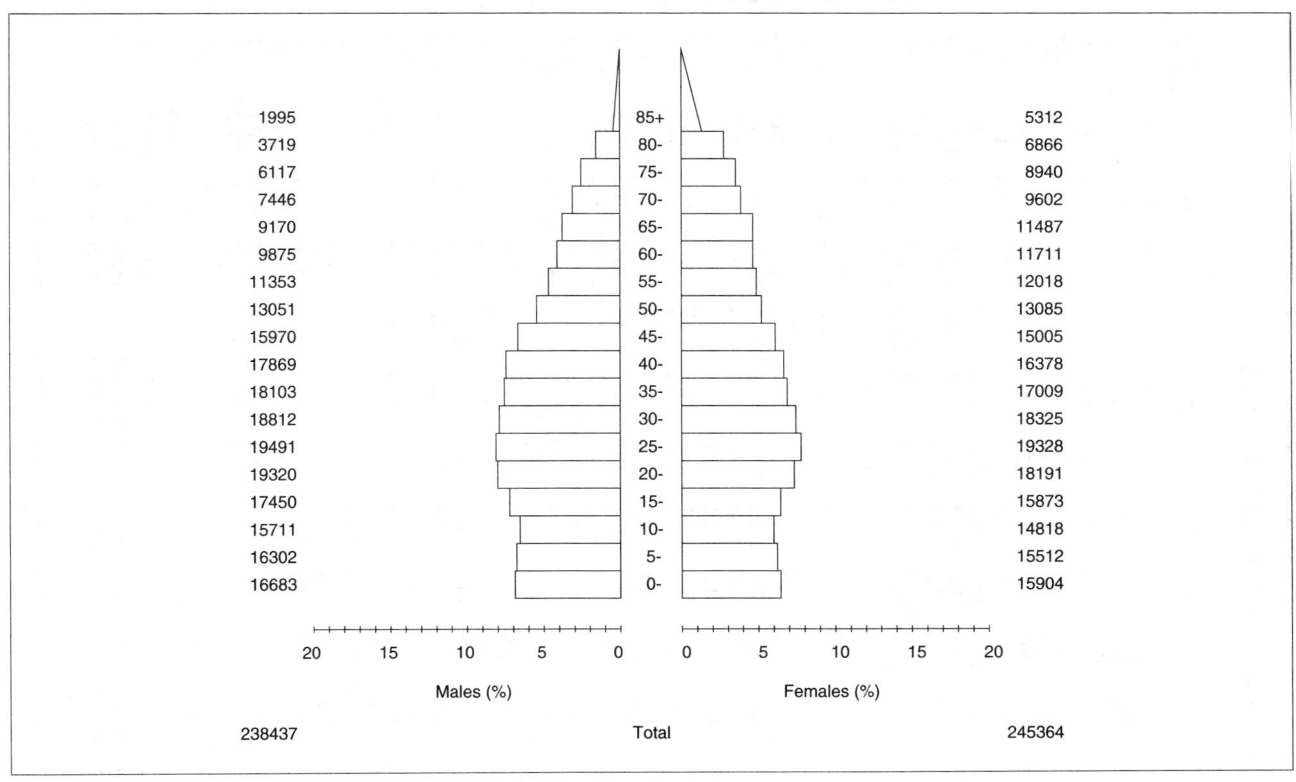

Switzerland, St Gall-Appenzell
Source of population: average annual 1988–92
Census: 1990. Bundesamt für Statistik (Federal Office of Statistics, Switzerland)
Estimate: The mid-year estimates for the years 1988, 1989, 1991 and 1992 were provided by the Bundesamt für Statistik (Federal Office of Statistics, Switzerland)

Notes to tables overleaf:
† 188 does not include non-invasive tumours

SWITZERLAND, ST GALL-APPENZELL 1988-1992

ANNUAL INCIDENCE PER 100,000 BY AGE GROUP (YEARS) - MALE

SITE	ALL AGES	AGE UNK	0-	5-	10-	15-	20-	25-	30-	35-	40-	45-	50-	55-	60-	65-	70-	75-	80-	85+	CRUDE RATE	%	CR 64	CR 74	ASR (W)	ICD (9th)
Lip	28	0	-	-	-	-	-	-	-	3.3	1.1	-	3.1	-	2.0	15.3	8.1	9.8	21.5	40.1	2.3	0.6	0.05	0.16	**1.5**	*140*
Tongue	29	0	-	-	-	-	-	-	-	-	2.2	6.3	3.1	1.8	4.1	8.7	8.1	19.6	10.8	20.1	2.4	0.6	0.09	0.17	**1.7**	*141*
Salivary gland	6	0	-	-	-	-	-	-	-	-	1.1	1.3	-	1.8	-	-	-	3.3	-	20.1	0.5	0.1	0.02	0.02	**0.3**	*142*
Mouth	45	0	-	-	-	-	-	-	1.1	1.1	6.7	6.3	4.6	10.6	16.2	17.4	2.7	9.8	5.4	20.1	3.8	0.9	0.23	0.33	**3.0**	*143-5*
Oropharynx	35	0	-	-	-	-	-	-	-	-	2.2	5.0	10.7	8.8	6.1	6.5	5.4	6.5	32.3	10.0	2.9	0.7	0.16	0.22	**2.1**	*146*
Nasopharynx	8	0	-	-	-	-	1.0	-	-	-	2.2	1.3	1.5	-	2.2	-	6.5	-	-	-	0.7	0.2	0.03	0.04	**0.5**	*147*
Hypopharynx	30	0	-	-	-	-	-	-	-	1.1	1.1	5.0	7.7	5.3	12.2	-	13.4	9.8	-	20.1	2.5	0.6	0.16	0.23	**2.0**	*148*
Pharynx unspecified	5	0	-	-	-	-	-	-	-	-	-	-	-	1.8	2.0	-	-	3.3	5.4	10.0	0.4	0.1	0.02	0.02	**0.3**	*149*
Oesophagus	92	0	-	-	-	-	-	-	-	-	4.5	11.3	10.7	19.4	20.3	19.6	43.0	26.2	48.4	90.2	7.7	1.9	0.33	0.64	**5.5**	*150*
Stomach	230	0	-	-	-	-	-	-	1.1	2.2	9.0	7.5	9.2	31.7	52.7	65.4	96.7	163.5	166.7	160.4	19.3	4.8	0.57	1.38	**12.2**	*151*
Small intestine	18	0	-	-	-	-	-	-	-	-	3.4	-	3.1	1.8	4.1	8.7	5.4	9.8	-	10.0	1.5	0.4	0.06	0.13	**1.1**	*152*
Colon	317	0	-	-	-	-	1.0	-	2.2	7.8	3.8	13.8	28.2	64.8	100.3	163.8	206.0	247.4	310.8	26.6	6.6	0.61	1.93	**16.5**	*153*
Rectum	254	0	-	-	-	-	1.0	2.1	2.2	-	16.3	24.5	37.0	52.7	72.0	131.6	147.1	134.4	210.5	21.3	5.3	0.68	1.70	**14.1**	*154*
Liver	95	0	-	-	-	-	-	-	-	-	3.4	2.5	7.7	29.9	26.3	30.5	40.3	39.2	53.8	40.1	8.0	2.0	0.35	0.70	**5.6**	*155*
Gallbladder etc.	34	0	-	-	-	-	-	-	-	-	-	2.5	-	7.0	6.1	15.3	16.1	13.1	26.9	30.1	2.9	0.7	0.08	0.24	**1.9**	*156*
Pancreas	166	0	-	-	-	-	-	-	1.1	1.1	5.6	5.0	4.6	33.5	38.5	39.3	88.6	104.6	102.2	120.3	13.9	3.4	0.45	1.09	**9.0**	*157*
Nose, sinuses etc.	15	0	-	-	-	1.1	-	-	-	1.1	1.1	1.3	1.5	-	2.0	6.5	8.1	-	5.4	20.1	1.3	0.3	0.04	0.11	**1.0**	*160*
Larynx	59	0	-	-	-	-	-	-	-	-	2.2	3.4	2.5	7.7	24.7	16.2	17.4	24.2	16.3	5.4	4.9	1.2	0.28	0.49	**3.8**	*161*
Bronchus, lung	844	0	-	-	-	-	-	-	2.1	5.5	22.4	35.1	56.7	179.7	253.2	340.2	359.9	425.0	424.8	260.7	70.8	17.5	2.77	6.27	**49.1**	*162*
Other thoracic organs	17	0	-	-	-	1.1	-	1.0	-	-	3.4	1.3	4.6	1.8	-	4.4	5.4	3.3	5.4	10.0	1.4	0.4	0.07	0.11	**1.1**	*163-4*
Bone	17	0	-	1.2	5.1	2.3	2.1	2.1	1.1	-	1.1	-	1.5	3.5	2.0	-	-	-	-	-	1.4	0.4	0.11	0.11	**1.5**	*170*
Connective tissue	38	0	1.2	-	1.3	1.1	2.1	-	1.1	-	-	5.0	7.7	1.8	12.2	2.2	10.7	22.9	10.8	20.1	3.2	0.8	0.17	0.23	**2.5**	*171*
Mesothelioma	32	0	-	-	-	-	-	-	-	-	1.1	3.8	4.6	5.3	10.1	6.5	18.8	19.6	-	10.0	2.7	0.7	0.12	0.25	**2.0**	*MES*
Kaposi's sarcoma	12	0	-	-	-	-	-	3.1	-	4.4	1.1	1.3	1.5	3.5	-	-	-	-	-	-	1.0	0.2	0.07	0.07	**0.9**	*KAP*
Melanoma of skin	128	0	-	-	1.1	3.1	2.1	6.4	7.7	9.0	11.3	15.3	21.1	28.4	37.1	48.3	49.0	21.5	20.1	10.7	2.6	0.53	0.95	**8.1**	*172*
Other skin	1019	0	-	-	-	-	1.0	5.1	10.6	16.6	38.1	55.1	91.9	133.9	216.7	290.1	411.0	513.3	747.5	852.1	85.5		2.85	6.35	**56.4**	*173*
Breast	6	0	-	-	-	-	-	-	-	-	-	-	3.1	1.8	-	2.2	2.7	-	5.4	-	0.5	0.1	0.02	0.05	**0.4**	*175*
Prostate	1093	0	-	-	-	-	-	-	-	-	-	1.3	15.3	70.5	196.5	364.2	639.3	817.4	1032.5	982.5	91.7	22.6	1.42	6.43	**53.5**	*185*
Testis	140	0	-	-	-	3.4	12.4	32.8	33.0	27.6	17.9	7.5	4.6	8.8	4.1	6.5	2.7	3.3	-	-	11.7	2.9	0.76	0.81	**10.1**	*186*
Penis	17	0	-	-	-	-	-	-	-	1.1	1.1	2.5	-	-	4.1	8.7	-	6.5	10.8	30.1	1.4	0.4	0.04	0.09	**1.0**	*187.1-.4*
Other male genital	4	0	-	-	1.3	-	-	-	-	-	-	-	-	-	2.0	-	2.7	3.3	-	-	0.3	0.1	0.02	0.03	**0.3**	*187.5-.9*
†Bladder	210	0	-	-	-	-	-	-	1.1	2.2	4.5	3.8	19.9	8.8	40.5	65.4	110.1	127.5	193.6	160.4	17.6	4.3	0.40	1.28	**10.9**	*188*
Kidney etc.	170	0	-	-	-	1.1	-	-	-	1.1	2.2	11.3	23.0	19.4	34.4	69.8	69.8	85.0	96.8	120.3	14.3	3.5	0.46	1.16	**9.7**	*189*
Eye	7	0	-	1.2	-	-	-	-	-	1.1	-	-	-	-	4.1	-	-	6.5	5.4	-	0.6	0.1	0.03	0.03	**0.4**	*190*
Brain, nervous system	84	0	1.2	7.4	2.5	-	4.1	3.1	5.3	4.4	4.5	7.5	4.6	12.3	16.2	28.4	24.2	16.3	16.1	10.0	7.0	1.7	0.37	0.63	**6.0**	*191-2*
Thyroid	25	0	-	-	-	-	2.1	-	3.2	1.1	2.2	2.5	3.1	-	4.1	6.5	5.4	6.5	5.4	30.1	2.1	0.5	0.09	0.15	**1.6**	*193*
Other endocrine	2	0	1.2	-	-	-	-	-	-	-	-	-	-	1.8	-	-	-	-	-	-	0.2	0.0	0.01	0.01	**0.2**	*194*
Hodgkin's disease	31	0	-	-	-	1.1	6.2	4.1	2.1	5.5	4.5	-	3.1	5.3	2.0	2.2	-	3.3	-	10.0	2.6	0.6	0.17	0.18	**2.2**	*201*
Non-Hodgkin lymphoma	161	0	2.4	3.7	-	1.1	4.1	5.1	3.2	2.2	10.1	17.5	10.7	15.9	24.3	56.7	61.8	55.6	69.9	110.3	13.5	3.3	0.50	1.09	**10.0**	*200,202*
Multiple myeloma	67	0	-	-	-	-	-	-	-	1.1	3.4	3.8	3.1	10.6	20.3	21.8	24.2	39.2	26.9	60.2	5.6	1.4	0.21	0.44	**3.8**	*203*
Lymphoid leukaemia	74	0	8.4	3.7	1.3	2.3	3.1	-	1.1	1.1	2.2	-	-	12.3	18.2	21.8	24.2	22.9	43.0	40.1	6.2	1.5	0.27	0.50	**5.2**	*204*
Myeloid leukaemia	66	0	-	2.5	1.3	4.6	1.0	2.1	4.3	2.2	-	5.0	6.1	8.8	8.1	13.1	10.7	26.2	43.0	70.2	5.5	1.4	0.23	0.35	**4.1**	*205*
Monocytic leukaemia	2	0	-	-	-	-	-	-	-	-	-	-	-	-	-	-	-	3.3	5.4	-	0.2	0.0	0.00	0.00	**0.1**	*206*
Other leukaemia	3	0	-	-	-	1.1	-	-	-	-	-	-	-	-	-	-	-	-	10.8	-	0.3	0.1	0.01	0.01	**0.2**	*207*
Leukaemia unspecified	6	0	1.2	-	-	-	-	-	-	-	-	-	-	1.5	-	4.1	-	-	3.3	-	10.0	0.5	0.1	0.03	0.03	**0.5**	*208*
Other and unspecified	110	0	-	-	-	1.1	-	1.0	2.1	2.2	-	2.5	7.7	12.3	14.2	32.7	53.7	62.1	80.7	140.4	9.2	2.3	0.22	0.65	**5.8**	*O&U*
All sites	5851	0	15.6	19.6	12.7	22.9	42.4	63.6	81.9	103.8	183.6	255.5	403.0	782.1	1245.5	1805.8	2541.0	3115.9	3721.4	4100.3	490.8		16.16	37.90	**329.5**	*ALL*
All sites but 173	4832	0	15.6	19.6	12.7	22.9	41.4	58.5	71.2	87.3	145.5	200.4	311.1	648.3	1028.8	1515.7	2130.0	2602.6	2973.9	3248.1	405.3	100.0	13.32	31.55	**273.1**	*ALLb*

Rate from 1 case 1.199 1.227 1.273 1.146 1.035 1.026 1.063 1.105 1.119 1.252 1.532 1.762 2.025 2.181 2.686 3.270 5.378 10.025

†Important: see notes on population page

SWITZERLAND, ST GALL-APPENZELL 1988-1992

ANNUAL INCIDENCE PER 100,000 BY AGE GROUP (YEARS) - FEMALE

SITE	ALL AGES	AGE UNK	0-	5-	10-	15-	20-	25-	30-	35-	40-	45-	50-	55-	60-	65-	70-	75-	80-	85+	CRUDE RATE	%	CR 64	CR 74	ASR (W)	ICD (9th)
Lip	6	0	-	-	-	-	-	-	-	-	-	-	-	-	5.1	-	6.2	-	-	-	0.5	0.1	0.03	0.06	**0.3**	140
Tongue	13	0	-	-	-	-	-	-	1.2	-	2.7	3.1	5.0	-	1.7	4.2	2.2	-	3.8	1.1	0.3	0.06	0.09	**0.8**	141
Salivary gland	8	0	-	-	-	-	2.2	-	-	-	2.7	-	-	1.7	-	2.1	2.2	-	3.8	0.7	0.2	0.03	0.04	**0.5**	142
Mouth	16	0	-	-	-	-	-	1.0	-	-	4.0	6.1	3.3	-	3.5	2.1	-	-	11.3	1.3	0.4	0.07	0.10	**1.0**	143-5
Oropharynx	5	0	-	-	-	-	-	-	-	-	-	-	-	1.7	-	-	6.7	2.9	-		0.4	0.1	0.01	0.01	**0.1**	146
Nasopharynx	3	0	-	-	-	-	-	-	1.1	-	-	-	1.5	1.7	-	-	-	-	-	-	0.2	0.1	0.02	0.02	**0.2**	147
Hypopharynx	0	0	-	-	-	-	-	-	-	-	-	-	-	-	-	-	-	-	-	-	0.0	0.0	0.00	0.00	**0.0**	148
Pharynx unspecified	0	0	-	-	-	-	-	-	-	-	-	-	-	-	-	-	-	-	-	-	0.0	0.0	0.00	0.00	**0.0**	149
Oesophagus	24	0	-	-	-	-	-	-	1.1	-	-	-	-	3.4	1.7	8.3	8.9	17.5	22.6	2.0	0.6	0.02	0.07	**0.7**	150
Stomach	164	0	-	-	-	-	-	-	2.2	3.5	1.2	4.0	4.6	20.0	12.0	33.1	45.8	62.6	81.6	135.5	13.4	4.1	0.24	0.63	**5.8**	151
Small intestine	18	0	-	-	-	-	-	-	-	-	1.2	-	-	1.7	6.8	3.5	-	8.9	11.7	7.5	1.5	0.4	0.05	0.07	**0.7**	152
Colon	314	0	-	-	-	-	-	2.1	-	1.2	8.5	8.0	21.4	34.9	35.9	62.7	114.6	107.4	183.5	150.6	25.6	7.8	0.56	1.45	**12.0**	153
Rectum	176	0	-	-	-	-	-	1.0	1.1	2.4	6.1	10.7	16.8	30.0	20.5	52.2	43.7	55.9	52.4	90.3	14.3	4.4	0.44	0.92	**7.9**	154
Liver	31	0	-	-	-	1.3	-	-	1.1	-	-	-	3.1	1.7	1.7	8.7	14.6	11.2	17.5	7.5	2.5	0.8	0.04	0.16	**1.3**	155
Gallbladder etc.	91	0	-	-	-	-	-	-	-	-	1.2	-	3.1	10.0	10.2	15.7	25.0	58.2	32.0	67.8	7.4	2.3	0.12	0.33	**3.1**	156
Pancreas	180	0	-	-	-	-	-	-	-	-	2.4	1.2	8.0	7.6	16.6	22.2	41.8	43.7	69.3	107.8	112.9	14.7	4.5	0.29	0.72	**6.6**	157
Nose, sinuses etc.	8	0	-	-	-	-	-	-	-	1.2	-	1.3	-	-	1.7	-	2.1	2.2	2.9	7.5	0.7	0.2	0.02	0.03	**0.3**	160
Larynx	5	0	-	-	-	-	-	-	-	-	-	-	-	1.7	-	3.5	-	2.2	2.9	-	0.4	0.1	0.01	0.03	**0.2**	161
Bronchus, lung	161	0	-	-	-	-	-	1.0	-	4.7	9.8	9.3	24.5	25.0	44.4	38.3	47.9	49.2	29.1	26.4	13.1	4.0	0.59	1.02	**8.4**	162
Other thoracic organs	5	0	-	-	-	-	-	-	1.1	-	-	2.7	-	1.7	-	1.7	-	-	-	-	0.4	0.1	0.03	0.04	**0.3**	163-4
Bone	15	0	-	-	-	5.0	2.2	-	-	-	1.2	-	-	1.7	1.7	3.5	-	2.2	8.7	-	1.2	0.4	0.06	0.08	**1.0**	170
Connective tissue	32	0	-	-	1.3	-	1.1	-	2.2	-	3.7	1.3	3.1	1.7	5.1	13.9	2.1	11.2	2.9	11.3	2.6	0.8	0.10	0.18	**1.7**	171
Mesothelioma	1	0	-	-	-	-	-	-	-	-	-	-	-	-	-	-	-	-	2.9	-	0.1	0.0	0.00	0.00	**0.0**	MES
Kaposi's sarcoma	0	0	-	-	-	-	-	-	-	-	-	-	-	-	-	-	-	-	-	-	0.0	0.0	0.00	0.00	**0.0**	KAP
Melanoma of skin	178	0	-	-	-	1.3	3.3	9.3	9.8	3.5	12.2	17.3	35.2	25.0	35.9	26.1	39.6	40.3	32.0	30.1	14.5	4.4	0.76	1.09	**10.2**	172
Other skin	976	0	-	-	-	1.3	-	4.1	8.7	24.7	28.1	44.0	77.9	106.5	140.0	193.2	258.3	335.5	410.7	613.6	79.6		2.18	4.43	**40.0**	173
Breast	1093	0	-	-	-	-	-	2.1	12.0	37.6	90.4	139.9	174.2	159.7	204.9	186.3	224.9	241.6	358.3	350.1	89.1	27.3	4.10	6.16	**56.3**	174
Uterus unspecified	7	0	-	-	-	-	-	-	-	-	-	-	-	-	-	5.2	4.2	2.2	-	3.8	0.6	0.2	0.00	0.05	**0.3**	179
Cervix uteri	147	0	-	-	-	-	-	6.2	10.9	20.0	17.1	18.7	13.8	13.3	34.2	27.9	22.9	11.2	37.9	15.1	12.0	3.7	0.67	0.92	**8.8**	180
Placenta	2	0	-	-	-	-	-	1.0	1.1	-	-	-	-	-	-	-	-	-	-	-	0.2	0.0	0.01	0.01	**0.1**	181
Corpus uteri	234	0	-	-	-	-	-	-	-	-	4.9	6.7	39.7	56.6	52.9	64.4	64.6	82.8	43.7	52.7	19.1	5.8	0.80	1.45	**11.6**	182
Ovary etc.	237	0	-	-	5.0	4.4	5.2	1.1	3.5	12.2	16.0	27.5	48.3	52.9	52.2	54.2	55.9	67.0	60.2	19.3	5.9	0.88	1.41	**12.5**	183
Other female genital	50	0	-	-	-	-	-	-	3.3	1.2	-	-	1.5	5.0	10.2	8.7	18.7	24.6	23.3	11.3	4.1	1.2	0.11	0.24	**2.0**	184
†Bladder	70	0	-	-	-	-	-	-	-	-	1.2	-	-	5.0	5.1	19.2	25.0	38.0	40.8	33.9	5.7	1.7	0.06	0.28	**2.3**	188
Kidney etc.	97	0	1.3	-	-	-	-	1.0	2.2	3.5	2.4	6.7	6.1	10.0	22.2	26.1	31.2	33.6	29.1	18.8	7.9	2.4	0.28	0.56	**4.7**	189
Eye	5	0	-	-	-	-	-	-	-	-	-	-	-	-	-	5.2	4.2	-	-	-	0.4	0.1	0.00	0.05	**0.2**	190
Brain, nervous system	67	0	3.8	2.6	1.3	1.3	3.3	2.1	4.4	4.7	4.9	2.7	9.2	5.0	13.7	12.2	14.6	15.7	5.8	3.8	5.5	1.7	0.29	0.43	**4.4**	191-2
Thyroid	83	0	-	-	-	1.3	2.2	3.1	12.0	4.7	8.5	6.7	7.6	5.0	10.2	10.4	20.8	15.7	23.3	18.8	6.8	2.1	0.31	0.46	**4.5**	193
Other endocrine	3	0	1.3	-	-	-	-	-	-	1.2	-	-	-	-	-	-	2.2	-	-	0.2	0.1	0.01	0.01	**0.2**	194
Hodgkin's disease	28	0	-	-	2.7	2.5	6.6	4.1	4.4	2.4	1.2	1.3	3.1	1.7	1.7	-	2.2	-	3.8	2.3	0.7	0.16	0.16	**2.2**	201
Non-Hodgkin lymphoma	146	0	3.8	-	-	2.5	1.1	3.1	5.5	2.4	4.9	8.0	12.2	11.6	34.2	20.9	39.6	53.7	58.3	37.6	11.9	3.6	0.45	0.75	**7.1**	200,202
Multiple myeloma	59	0	-	-	-	-	-	-	-	-	-	4.0	9.2	5.0	6.8	12.2	25.0	20.1	26.2	22.6	4.8	1.5	0.12	0.31	**2.5**	203
Lymphoid leukaemia	46	0	3.8	1.3	2.7	-	1.1	-	-	-	1.2	1.3	3.1	5.0	6.8	15.7	14.6	8.9	20.4	3.8	3.7	1.1	0.13	0.28	**2.7**	204
Myeloid leukaemia	50	0	-	-	-	-	-	-	1.1	2.4	-	5.3	6.1	8.3	5.1	7.0	12.5	13.4	20.4	30.1	4.1	1.2	0.14	0.24	**2.2**	205
Monocytic leukaemia	2	0	-	1.3	-	-	-	-	-	-	-	-	-	-	-	-	-	-	3.8	0.2	0.0	0.01	0.01	**0.1**	206
Other leukaemia	1	0	-	-	-	-	-	-	-	-	-	-	-	-	-	-	2.1	-	-	0.1	0.0	0.00	0.01	**0.0**	207
Leukaemia unspecified	3	0	1.3	-	-	-	-	-	-	-	-	-	-	1.7	-	-	2.1	-	-	0.2	0.1	0.01	0.03	**0.3**	208
Other and unspecified	117	0	-	-	-	-	-	1.0	1.1	2.4	3.7	2.7	4.6	8.3	15.4	17.4	27.1	40.3	81.6	82.8	9.5	2.9	0.20	0.42	**4.1**	O&U
All sites	4977	0	15.1	5.2	8.1	21.4	27.5	47.6	87.3	131.7	225.9	335.9	525.8	637.3	826.5	995.8	1268.4	1498.8	1835.0	2055.4	405.7		14.48	25.80	**232.4**	ALL
All sites but 173	4001	0	15.1	5.2	8.1	20.2	27.5	43.5	78.6	107.0	197.8	291.9	447.8	530.8	686.5	802.6	1010.1	1163.2	1424.3	1441.8	326.1	100.0	12.30	21.36	**192.4**	ALLb

Rate from 1 case			1.257	1.289	1.350	1.260	1.099	1.035	1.091	1.176	1.221	1.333	1.528	1.664	1.708	1.741	2.083	2.237	2.913	3.764

†Important: see notes on population page

Switzerland, Valais

The Valais Cancer Registry commenced activity on 1 January 1989. It is situated in Sion, capital of the Canton of Valais, and attached to the Central Institute of Valais hospitals, where several medical examination departments are grouped including the only histo- and cyto-pathology services in the canton. This institute provides part of the financial support for the registry, the rest coming from the League Against Cancer of the canton and the Swiss Federal Government.

The registry has a pathologist, an assistant physician in charge of the routine functioning of the registry, a consultant medical epidemiologist and two secretaries, all part-time.

The canton of Valais, with an area of 5255 km^2, is the third largest of the Swiss cantons. Agricultural land and Alpine pastures represent 21.7% of the surface and forests 22.2%, while 53.6% consists of unproductive mountainous terrain. There is some 200 km of border with Italy to the south and some 80 km with France to the west. The highest point is at 4634 m (Pic Dufour, the highest summit in Switzerland) and the lowest at 372 m on the edge of Lake Geneva. The river Rhone crosses the canton from east to west for 114 km in a valley with a maximum width of 6 km, where the towns of the canton (with 36% of the population) and the majority of the economic activity are located.

The resident population of the canton, according to the 1990 census, numbers 250 000, mostly of Caucasian origin. The proportions of age-groups 0–19 and 20–39 years are slightly above the Swiss average. The majority of the population (59.7%) is French-speaking, but about 30% living in the east of the canton speak German. In 1992 15.6% of the population was foreign, the majority being Portuguese or Italian. Most of the population (88.5%) are of Roman Catholic religion, and 5.5% are Protestant.

The tertiary sector employs 60.8% of the population active in 1990, reflecting the importance of tourism in the economy. The secondary sector (31.2%) is represented mainly by construction, followed by chemical, metallurgical and wood industries. The economic share of the primary sector has greatly diminished from over 40% in 1950 to 3.4% in 1990. Only 2.9% of the active population is now employed in agriculture, but the canton is an important producer of wine, fruit and vegetables.

The climate is sunnier than in the rest of Switzerland, particularly in autumn and winter, when there is practically never any fog. In Sion, the average temperature is between −2 and +2°C in January and 18 and 22°C in July.

Emissions of NO_2 in Sion exceeded permitted levels as an annual average in 1993, but elsewhere were below the permitted level. The ozone levels were above 100 μg/m^3 for about half of the year, principally in summer. Emissions of SO_2 never exceeded the maximum permitted level in any part of the territory.

There are six regional hospitals and two private clinics for general medicine, with a total of 1209 beds, as well as geriatric, psychiatric and pneumology services with a total of 727 beds.. There is no specialized oncological service, but an oncologist and two onco-haematological specialists share the consultations and supervision of treatment. There is a radiotherapy service at Sion hospital. In 1992 there were 434 doctors in the canton (1 per 605 inhabitants).

Most biopsies from the seven intensive care hospitals and one private clinic are sent to the Institute, and constitute the main source of data on incident cases (75%); other sources are the medical records of these hospitals (a little under 10% of cases). For patients who need to be treated outside the canton, data are provided either by the registries of Basel, Geneva, Vaud and Zurich or by the medical records of the university hospital of Bern. Doctors diagnosing and/or treating cases of cancer provide complementary information on occupation, the symptoms and examinations leading to diagnosis, antecedents and therapy. The response rate is over 80%.

Access to the records of hospital patients is greatly facilitated by the provision of annual lists of the cancer cases treated at each hospital, coded according to ICD-9.

An extract from the file of the Federal Office of Statistics containing the annual mortality data for Valais, produced on the basis of the death certificates, enables the registry to keep its files up to date and, using a methodology which is partly computerised, to establish the DCO diagnoses - an annual average of 1.6% over five years. Active follow-up is carried out by sending forms to the services responsible for monitoring inhabitants in 163 municipalities, from which it is possible to obtain confirmation of residence, dates of death and, where appropriate, dates of departure abroad or to other cantons. The anonymous data file is checked for coherence and validity using the IARC CHECK program.

The registry has no personal contact with the patients and ensures that rules of strict confidentiality are respected, but has an authorization permitting it to consult medical records as necessary

The data are used to compare annual incidence with those of neighbouring registries, to identify population groups at high risk of cancer, to formulate hypotheses on possible exposures to risk factors, and to evaluate the efficacy of treatment.

F. Joris
F. Faggiano
D. de Weck

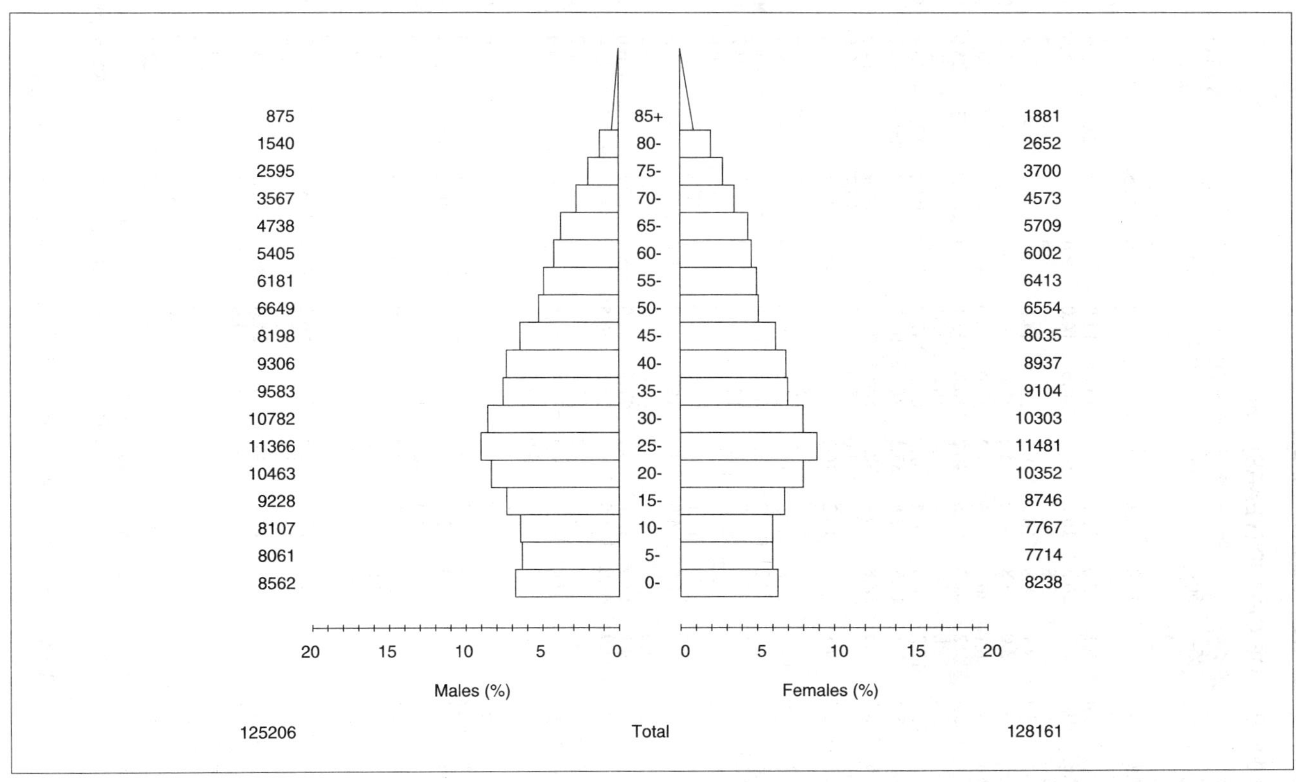

Switzerland, Valais

Source of population: average annual 1989–92
Census: 1990 Swiss Federal Census (recensement fédéral de la population). Federal Office of Statistics, Bern.
Estimate: The 1989 population was estimated at the end of the year on the basis of the 1980 Census, taking into account births, deaths and migration. The 1991 and 1992 populations were estimated at the end of each year based on the 1990 Census, updated by births, deaths and migration.

Notes to tables overleaf:
† 188 does not include non-invasive tumours

SWITZERLAND, VALAIS 1989-1992

ANNUAL INCIDENCE PER 100,000 BY AGE GROUP (YEARS) - MALE

SITE	ALL AGES	AGE UNK	0-	5-	10-	15-	20-	25-	30-	35-	40-	45-	50-	55-	60-	65-	70-	75-	80-	85+	CRUDE RATE	%	CR 64	CR 74	ASR (W)	ICD (9th)
Lip	3	0	-	-	-	-	-	-	-	-	-	-	-	-	-	5.3	-	19.3	-	-	0.6	0.2	0.00	0.03	**0.4**	140
Tongue	19	0	-	-	-	-	-	-	-	7.8	-	9.1	15.0	8.1	9.2	-	14.0	9.6	32.5	-	3.8	1.0	0.25	0.32	**3.0**	141
Salivary gland	1	0	-	-	-	-	-	-	-	-	-	-	-	-	-	-	7.0	-	-	-	0.2	0.1	0.00	0.04	**0.1**	142
Mouth	25	0	-	-	-	-	-	-	-	-	13.4	6.1	15.0	16.2	13.9	15.8	14.0	-	16.2	28.6	5.0	1.3	0.32	0.47	**4.1**	143-5
Oropharynx	28	0	-	-	-	-	-	-	2.3	2.6	10.7	6.1	26.3	16.2	18.5	10.6	14.0	9.6	-	-	5.6	1.4	0.41	0.54	**4.7**	146
Nasopharynx	4	0	-	-	-	-	-	-	2.3	2.6	-	-	3.8	-	-	-	-	9.6	-	-	0.8	0.2	0.04	0.04	**0.6**	147
Hypopharynx	26	0	-	-	-	-	-	-	-	-	5.4	9.1	18.8	16.2	18.5	26.4	14.0	9.6	-	-	5.2	1.3	0.34	0.54	**4.4**	148
Pharynx unspecified	6	0	-	-	-	-	-	-	-	-	-	3.0	3.8	4.0	4.6	10.6	-	-	-	-	1.2	0.3	0.08	0.13	**1.0**	149
Oesophagus	48	0	-	-	-	-	-	-	-	2.6	-	6.1	30.1	28.3	27.7	58.0	28.0	38.5	81.2	-	9.6	2.4	0.47	0.90	**7.4**	150
Stomach	123	0	-	-	-	-	-	-	9.3	-	10.7	12.2	41.4	56.6	46.2	110.8	133.1	211.9	162.3	114.3	24.6	6.3	0.88	2.10	**17.6**	151
Small intestine	6	0	-	-	-	-	-	-	-	-	5.4	3.0	-	-	-	10.6	-	9.6	-	-	1.2	0.3	0.04	0.09	**0.9**	152
Colon	134	0	-	-	-	-	-	-	2.3	2.6	13.4	12.2	48.9	40.4	87.9	63.3	147.2	202.3	292.2	257.1	26.8	6.8	1.04	2.09	**19.0**	153
Rectum	91	0	-	-	-	-	-	-	2.3	5.2	5.4	9.1	18.8	52.6	55.5	84.4	105.1	106.0	64.9	200.0	18.2	4.6	0.74	1.69	**13.6**	154
Liver	71	0	8.8	-	-	-	2.4	-	2.3	2.6	2.7	3.0	18.8	40.4	32.4	68.6	77.1	125.2	64.9	-	14.2	3.6	0.57	1.30	**10.9**	155
Gallbladder etc.	10	0	-	-	-	-	-	-	-	-	-	-	-	-	4.6	5.3	14.0	48.2	16.2	-	2.0	0.5	0.02	0.12	**1.2**	156
Pancreas	59	0	-	-	-	-	-	-	-	2.6	2.7	9.1	-	16.2	46.2	58.0	91.1	57.8	97.4	114.3	11.8	3.0	0.38	1.13	**8.6**	157
Nose, sinuses etc.	3	0	-	-	-	-	-	-	-	-	-	-	-	-	-	5.3	-	9.6	-	28.6	0.6	0.2	0.00	0.03	**0.4**	160
Larynx	42	0	-	-	-	-	-	-	-	-	2.7	15.2	18.8	52.6	32.4	26.4	14.0	28.9	16.2	-	8.4	2.1	0.61	0.81	**6.9**	161
Bronchus, lung	319	0	-	-	-	-	-	-	2.3	2.6	21.5	42.7	90.2	109.2	208.1	369.3	462.5	356.5	324.7	171.4	63.7	16.2	2.38	6.54	**47.7**	162
Other thoracic organs	11	0	-	-	-	-	2.4	-	-	2.6	-	6.1	-	4.0	-	5.3	7.0	28.9	16.2	-	2.2	0.6	0.08	0.14	**1.5**	163-4
Bone	3	0	-	-	-	-	-	-	-	2.6	2.7	-	-	-	-	-	-	-	16.2	-	0.6	0.2	0.03	0.03	**0.4**	170
Connective tissue	13	0	-	-	-	-	-	-	-	-	2.7	6.1	-	12.1	-	5.3	7.0	28.9	16.2	28.6	2.6	0.7	0.10	0.17	**1.8**	171
Mesothelioma	11	0	-	-	-	-	-	-	-	-	-	3.0	7.5	4.0	9.2	15.8	7.0	9.6	-	-	2.2	0.6	0.12	0.23	**1.8**	MES
Kaposi's sarcoma	2	0	-	-	-	-	-	-	-	-	2.7	3.0	-	-	-	-	-	-	-	-	0.4	0.1	0.03	0.03	**0.3**	KAP
Melanoma of skin	33	0	-	-	-	-	-	2.2	2.3	-	8.1	9.1	15.0	12.1	23.1	21.1	28.0	28.9	16.2	28.6	6.6	1.7	0.36	0.61	**5.2**	172
Other skin	488	0	2.9	-	-	-	4.8	4.4	13.9	18.3	37.6	57.9	109.0	133.5	305.2	353.5	476.5	905.6	746.8	971.4	97.4		3.44	7.59	**69.5**	173
Breast	6	0	-	-	-	-	-	-	-	-	-	-	-	4.0	9.2	5.3	7.0	-	16.2	-	1.2	0.3	0.07	0.13	**0.9**	175
Prostate	350	0	-	-	-	-	-	-	-	2.6	5.4	-	7.5	56.6	180.4	311.3	539.6	722.5	892.9	742.9	69.9	17.8	1.26	5.52	**45.9**	185
Testis	43	0	-	-	-	5.4	16.7	19.8	20.9	13.0	13.4	6.1	3.8	-	4.6	10.6	-	-	-	-	8.6	2.2	0.52	0.57	**7.3**	186
Penis	2	0	-	-	-	-	-	-	-	-	-	3.0	-	-	-	-	-	-	16.2	-	0.4	0.1	0.02	0.02	**0.3**	187.1-.4
Other male genital	3	0	-	-	-	-	-	-	-	-	-	-	-	-	-	5.3	14.0	-	-	-	0.6	0.2	0.00	0.10	**0.4**	187.5-.9
†Bladder	94	0	-	-	-	-	-	-	-	5.2	10.7	6.1	22.6	28.3	74.0	100.2	126.1	154.1	48.7	28.6	18.8	4.8	0.73	1.87	**14.0**	188
Kidney etc.	67	0	-	-	-	-	-	-	-	2.6	5.4	24.4	11.3	32.4	46.2	89.7	70.1	38.5	16.2	85.7	13.4	3.4	0.61	1.41	**10.6**	189
Eye	9	0	-	-	-	-	-	-	-	-	-	3.0	-	4.0	4.6	10.6	21.0	9.6	-	-	1.8	0.5	0.06	0.22	**1.4**	190
Brain, nervous system	24	0	-	6.2	-	2.7	2.4	-	2.3	7.8	5.4	-	3.8	8.1	9.2	5.3	28.0	19.3	32.5	-	4.8	1.2	0.24	0.41	**3.9**	191-2
Thyroid	10	0	-	-	-	-	4.8	2.2	-	5.2	-	-	3.8	-	4.6	5.3	14.0	-	-	-	2.0	0.5	0.10	0.20	**1.7**	193
Other endocrine	0	0	-	-	-	-	-	-	-	-	-	-	-	-	-	-	-	-	-	-	0.0	0.0	0.00	0.00	**0.0**	194
Hodgkin's disease	10	0	-	-	-	-	-	2.2	2.3	5.2	-	6.1	-	-	9.2	-	14.0	-	-	-	2.0	0.5	0.13	0.20	**1.6**	201
Non-Hodgkin lymphoma	60	0	-	-	-	2.7	-	4.4	9.3	7.8	18.8	3.0	22.6	12.1	18.5	31.7	56.1	48.2	113.6	85.7	12.0	3.0	0.50	0.93	**8.8**	200,202
Multiple myeloma	33	0	-	-	-	-	-	-	-	-	-	2.7	-	16.2	23.1	36.9	7.0	57.8	97.4	85.7	6.6	1.7	0.21	0.43	**4.5**	203
Lymphoid leukaemia	27	0	2.9	9.3	9.3	2.7	4.8	-	-	-	-	-	-	12.1	4.6	5.3	21.0	48.2	32.5	57.1	5.4	1.4	0.23	0.36	**4.9**	204
Myeloid leukaemia	17	0	-	-	-	-	-	-	-	-	5.4	3.0	-	8.1	-	15.8	14.0	28.9	32.5	57.1	3.4	0.9	0.08	0.23	**2.3**	205
Monocytic leukaemia	1	0	-	-	-	-	-	-	-	-	-	-	-	-	-	-	-	-	16.2	-	0.2	0.1	0.00	0.00	**0.1**	206
Other leukaemia	4	0	2.9	-	-	-	2.4	-	-	-	-	-	-	-	-	-	7.0	-	16.2	-	0.8	0.2	0.03	0.06	**0.8**	207
Leukaemia unspecified	5	0	-	-	-	-	-	-	-	-	-	-	-	-	4.0	4.6	5.3	7.0	-	16.2	1.0	0.3	0.04	0.10	**0.7**	208
Other and unspecified	112	0	2.9	-	3.1	-	-	-	-	5.2	8.1	9.1	33.8	56.6	60.1	47.5	154.2	125.2	276.0	142.9	22.4	5.7	0.90	1.90	**16.2**	O&U
All sites	2456	0	20.4	15.5	12.3	13.5	40.6	35.2	74.2	109.6	223.0	295.8	590.3	865.5	1396.7	2015.4	2761.0	3506.7	3603.9	3228.6	490.4		18.46	42.35	**359.5**	ALL
All sites but 173	1968	0	17.5	15.5	12.3	13.5	35.8	30.8	60.3	91.3	185.4	237.9	481.3	732.0	1091.4	1661.9	2284.5	2601.2	2857.1	2257.1	392.9	100.0	15.03	34.76	**289.9**	ALLb

Rate from 1 case

		0-	5-	10-	15-	20-	25-	30-	35-	40-	45-	50-	55-	60-	65-	70-	75-	80-	85+
		2.920	3.101	3.084	2.709	2.389	2.199	2.319	2.609	2.686	3.050	3.760	4.044	4.625	5.276	7.008	9.634	16.234	28.571

†Important: see notes on population page

SWITZERLAND, VALAIS 1989-1992

ANNUAL INCIDENCE PER 100,000 BY AGE GROUP (YEARS) - FEMALE

SITE	ALL AGES	AGE UNK	0-	5-	10-	15-	20-	25-	30-	35-	40-	45-	50-	55-	60-	65-	70-	75-	80-	85+	CRUDE RATE	%	CR 64	CR 74	ASR (W)	ICD (9th)
Lip	2	0	-	-	-	-	-	-	-	-	-	-	-	-	-	-	-	-	18.9	-	0.4	0.1	0.00	0.00	**0.1**	140
Tongue	6	0	-	-	-	-	-	-	-	-	-	-	-	3.9	8.3	4.4	-	13.5	-	-	1.2	0.4	0.06	0.08	**0.8**	141
Salivary gland	2	0	-	-	-	-	-	-	-	-	-	-	3.8	-	4.2	-	-	-	-	-	0.4	0.1	0.04	0.04	**0.4**	142
Mouth	5	0	-	-	-	-	-	-	-	-	-	3.1	-	-	8.3	-	5.5	6.8	-	-	1.0	0.3	0.06	0.08	**0.7**	143-5
Oropharynx	2	0	-	-	-	-	-	-	-	-	-	3.1	-	-	4.2	-	-	-	-	-	0.4	0.1	0.04	0.04	**0.4**	146
Nasopharynx	1	0	-	-	-	-	-	-	-	-	-	-	-	-	-	4.4	-	-	-	-	0.2	0.1	0.00	0.02	**0.1**	147
Hypopharynx	2	0	-	-	-	-	-	-	-	-	-	-	-	-	-	4.4	5.5	-	-	-	0.4	0.1	0.00	0.05	**0.2**	148
Pharynx unspecified	0	0	-	-	-	-	-	-	-	-	-	-	-	-	-	-	-	-	-	-	0.0	0.0	0.00	0.00	**0.0**	149
Oesophagus	10	0	-	-	-	-	-	-	-	-	-	-	3.8	-	-	-	16.4	13.5	18.9	26.6	2.0	0.6	0.02	0.10	**0.9**	150
Stomach	75	0	-	-	-	-	-	-	-	2.7	5.6	9.3	19.1	35.1	12.5	52.5	43.7	67.6	113.1	132.9	14.6	4.7	0.42	0.90	**8.3**	151
Small intestine	4	0	-	-	-	-	-	-	-	-	-	-	-	3.9	4.2	4.4	5.5	-	-	-	0.8	0.3	0.04	0.09	**0.6**	152
Colon	116	0	-	-	-	-	4.8	-	4.9	-	16.8	9.3	15.3	42.9	70.8	65.7	120.3	101.3	94.3	119.6	22.6	7.3	0.82	1.75	**14.0**	153
Rectum	62	0	-	-	-	-	-	-	-	2.7	5.6	9.3	3.8	39.0	25.0	30.7	54.7	33.8	113.1	66.4	12.1	3.9	0.43	0.85	**7.1**	154
Liver	19	0	-	-	-	-	-	-	2.4	-	-	-	3.8	11.7	4.2	8.8	10.9	13.5	9.4	79.7	3.7	1.2	0.11	0.21	**2.0**	155
Gallbladder etc.	28	0	-	-	-	-	-	-	-	2.7	2.8	3.1	-	-	8.3	26.3	27.3	47.3	37.7	13.3	5.5	1.8	0.08	0.35	**2.9**	156
Pancreas	59	0	-	-	-	-	-	-	-	2.7	2.8	6.2	3.8	7.8	29.2	26.3	10.9	108.1	103.7	132.9	11.5	3.7	0.26	0.45	**5.6**	157
Nose, sinuses etc.	6	0	-	-	-	-	-	-	-	-	-	3.8	7.8	-	4.4	5.5	6.8	-	-	-	1.2	0.4	0.06	0.11	**0.8**	160
Larynx	8	0	-	-	-	-	-	-	-	-	5.6	-	3.8	-	4.2	13.1	-	6.8	-	-	1.6	0.5	0.07	0.13	**1.2**	161
Bronchus, lung	71	0	-	-	-	-	-	-	2.4	2.7	5.6	18.7	30.5	31.2	62.5	52.5	54.7	20.3	28.3	26.6	13.8	4.5	0.77	1.30	**10.2**	162
Other thoracic organs	5	0	3.0	-	-	-	-	2.2	-	-	-	6.2	-	-	-	-	-	6.8	-	-	1.0	0.3	0.06	0.06	**1.0**	163-4
Bone	2	0	-	-	-	-	-	-	-	2.7	-	-	-	-	-	-	-	6.8	-	-	0.4	0.1	0.01	0.01	**0.2**	170
Connective tissue	21	0	-	3.2	3.2	-	4.8	2.2	-	-	2.8	3.1	7.6	7.8	4.2	17.5	-	6.8	28.3	13.3	4.1	1.3	0.19	0.28	**3.2**	171
Mesothelioma	2	0	-	-	-	-	-	-	-	-	-	-	-	-	4.2	4.4	-	-	-	-	0.4	0.1	0.02	0.04	**0.3**	MES
Kaposi's sarcoma	1	0	-	-	-	-	-	-	2.4	-	-	-	-	-	-	-	-	-	-	-	0.2	0.1	0.01	0.01	**0.1**	KAP
Melanoma of skin	63	0	-	-	-	2.9	2.4	6.5	9.7	8.2	11.2	15.6	3.8	42.9	12.5	35.0	32.8	20.3	75.4	26.6	12.3	4.0	0.58	0.92	**8.5**	172
Other skin	430	0	-	-	-	-	-	4.4	12.1	19.2	47.6	49.8	87.7	85.8	179.1	275.9	300.6	378.3	546.8	837.1	83.9		2.43	5.31	**48.0**	173
Breast	474	0	-	-	-	-	2.4	2.2	21.8	57.7	117.5	183.6	156.4	214.4	212.4	227.7	256.9	283.7	254.5	345.5	92.5	29.9	4.84	7.26	**65.9**	174
Uterus unspecified	5	0	-	-	-	-	-	-	-	-	-	-	3.8	-	4.2	-	-	6.8	9.4	13.3	1.0	0.3	0.04	0.04	**0.5**	179
Cervix uteri	45	0	-	-	-	-	-	4.4	7.3	24.7	14.0	-	22.9	15.6	20.8	26.3	16.4	13.5	-	-	8.8	2.8	0.55	0.76	**7.0**	180
Placenta	0	0	-	-	-	-	-	-	-	-	-	-	-	-	-	-	-	-	-	-	0.0	0.0	0.00	0.00	**0.0**	181
Corpus uteri	75	0	-	-	-	-	-	-	2.7	5.6	9.3	30.5	46.8	45.8	35.0	71.1	54.0	37.7	66.4	-	14.6	4.7	0.70	1.23	**9.8**	182
Ovary etc.	80	0	-	-	3.2	-	-	2.2	7.3	11.0	14.0	21.8	22.9	42.9	33.3	30.7	49.2	60.8	56.6	39.9	15.6	5.1	0.79	1.19	**10.9**	183
Other female genital	12	0	-	-	-	-	-	-	2.7	-	-	-	-	3.9	4.2	17.5	-	13.5	9.4	26.6	2.3	0.8	0.05	0.14	**1.3**	184
†Bladder	27	0	-	-	-	-	2.2	-	-	-	-	-	-	23.4	8.3	17.5	27.3	27.0	28.3	26.6	5.3	1.7	0.17	0.39	**3.1**	188
Kidney etc.	49	0	3.0	-	-	-	-	-	-	-	5.6	9.3	7.6	19.5	33.3	30.7	32.8	60.8	47.1	13.3	9.6	3.1	0.39	0.71	**6.2**	189
Eye	7	0	-	-	-	-	-	-	-	-	-	3.1	3.8	3.9	4.2	4.4	-	6.8	-	13.3	1.4	0.4	0.07	0.10	**1.0**	190
Brain, nervous system	20	0	-	3.2	-	2.9	-	2.2	-	-	-	9.3	11.4	11.7	4.2	-	10.9	20.3	9.4	13.3	3.9	1.3	0.22	0.28	**3.1**	191-2
Thyroid	23	0	-	-	-	-	2.4	6.5	4.9	2.7	-	6.2	7.6	11.7	4.2	13.1	-	6.8	28.3	13.3	4.5	1.5	0.23	0.30	**3.2**	193
Other endocrine	3	0	3.0	-	-	-	-	-	-	2.7	-	-	-	-	4.2	-	-	-	-	-	0.6	0.2	0.05	0.05	**0.7**	194
Hodgkin's disease	15	0	-	-	-	11.4	4.8	-	4.9	5.5	2.8	-	-	-	-	8.8	-	-	9.4	13.3	2.9	0.9	0.15	0.19	**2.6**	201
Non-Hodgkin lymphoma	42	0	-	3.2	3.2	2.9	4.8	4.4	2.4	-	2.8	6.2	7.6	19.5	20.8	13.1	32.8	27.0	47.1	13.3	8.2	2.7	0.39	0.62	**5.9**	200,202
Multiple myeloma	21	0	-	-	-	-	-	-	-	-	-	3.1	-	3.9	8.3	21.9	16.4	13.5	47.1	26.6	4.1	1.3	0.08	0.27	**2.2**	203
Lymphoid leukaemia	17	0	3.0	3.2	3.2	-	2.4	-	-	2.7	-	-	-	7.8	4.2	8.8	16.4	6.8	18.9	13.3	3.3	1.1	0.13	0.26	**2.6**	204
Myeloid leukaemia	14	0	3.0	-	-	-	-	-	-	2.7	2.8	3.1	-	-	8.3	4.4	5.5	6.8	28.3	26.6	2.7	0.9	0.10	0.15	**1.8**	205
Monocytic leukaemia	0	0	-	-	-	-	-	-	-	-	-	-	-	-	-	-	-	-	-	-	0.0	0.0	0.00	0.00	**0.0**	206
Other leukaemia	1	0	-	-	-	-	-	-	-	-	-	-	-	-	-	-	-	5.5	-	-	0.2	0.1	0.00	0.03	**0.1**	207
Leukaemia unspecified	3	0	-	-	-	-	-	-	-	-	-	-	-	-	-	4.2	-	6.8	9.4	-	0.6	0.2	0.02	0.02	**0.3**	208
Other and unspecified	78	0	-	-	-	2.9	-	-	-	-	5.6	-	7.6	15.6	12.5	43.8	38.3	94.6	141.4	265.7	15.2	4.9	0.22	0.63	**7.2**	O&U
All sites	2013	0	15.2	13.0	12.9	22.9	29.0	39.2	82.5	159.3	276.9	392.0	473.0	760.1	883.0	1134.1	1273.6	1567.2	1970.2	2405.0	392.6		15.79	27.83	**252.8**	ALL
All sites but 173	1583	0	15.2	13.0	12.9	22.9	29.0	34.8	70.4	140.0	229.4	342.2	385.2	674.4	703.9	858.3	973.0	1188.9	1423.5	1567.9	308.8	100.0	13.37	22.52	**204.8**	ALLb
Rate from 1 case			3.035	3.241	3.218	2.858	2.415	2.178	2.426	2.746	2.797	3.111	3.814	3.898	4.165	4.379	5.466	6.755	9.427	13.287						

†Important: see notes on population page

Switzerland, Vaud

The Registre Vaudois des Tumeurs began operation in January 1972 and population-based data have been available since 1973. The Vaud registry forms part of the Cancer Epidemiology Unit at the Social and Preventive Medicine Institute of the University of Lausanne. Its main financial support comes from the Public Health Department of the Canton of Vaud; substantial contributions are also supplied by the Swiss Federal Government, the Swiss and Vaud Cancer Leagues and the Swiss Research Foundation.

In addition to the director, the staff comprises one part-time medical associate, one part-time computer programmer and 3.5 clerks. The director is also in charge of the administrative and scientific supervision of the cantonal registry of Neuchâtel(see above).

The registry covers the entire canton of Vaud, which is the fourth largest (surface area 3219 km^2) of the 26 Swiss cantons and third in number of inhabitants (about 575 000 in 1990). It is situated between latitudes 46°58′ and 46°11′ N and longitudes 7°15′ and 6°3′ E. The population density (166 per km^2) slightly exceeds the mean for the whole country. In December 1990, foreigners accounted for about 23% of residents. Between 1950 and 1974 there was a considerable influx of immigrant workers. In 1990 the main occupations were: industry 25%, agriculture and fishing 5% and services 70%.

A declining birth rate (from 25 per 1000 at the beginning of the century to 7 per 1000 in 1992) and increasing longevity are the main causes of ageing of the Vaud population. In December 1990, 23% of the population was 0–19 years old, while 15% was aged 65 years and older. Although Lausanne, the capital and its suburbs represent only 4% (115 km^2) of the canton in area, about a third of the total population resides there.

In 1992, there were about 2900 public hospital beds (about five beds per 1000 population) and about 2700 hospital doctors and private practitioners (one medical doctor per 220 population) in the canton. About 15% of all deceased undergo a post-mortem examination.

The health care system is insurance-based, but practically the whole population enjoys access to medical care. Except for a pilot study on breast cancer mammography screening targeting 12 000 women aged 50–69 years, there is no organized screening, but for cervical cancer, spontaneous attendance is high, about 65% of women reporting a screening during the previous three years.

The registry is tumour-based and multiple primaries occurring in the same subject are classified as independent if so specified by pathological report and, for the present volume, according to the rules established by IARC and IACR. However, for skin cancers, squamous- and basal-cell carcinomas have been considered different primaries.

Notification is based on a voluntary agreement between the medical institutions of the canton and the registry. All hospitals, pathological laboratories and most practitioners are asked to report all new or past cases of cancer on pre-paid-postage notification forms. The main sources of notification are the University Pathological Department of Lausanne and three major private pathology laboratories which perform the majority of histological examinations. Most cases are notified repeatedly and from different institutions. The information recorded includes name, sex, nationality, marital status, place of residence, site and morphology (ICD-O-1 coding) and, for colorectum, gynaecological sites and melanomas of the skin, stage of the tumour and identification code of the source of notification. The date of histological or clinical diagnosis is taken as the date of onset.

All relevant information is checked manually by the registry staff and then coded before being interactively entered into the computer of the University Hospital. A first series of automatic checks on data is carried out by the computer at this stage. Moreover, data are transferred to the computer of the University of Lausanne, where more specialized checks and analyses are performed.

Annual incidence data by sex, age, site and morphology are routinely produced. Passive and active follow-up information is recorded. Identification data on all deaths in the canton of Vaud as well as on cancer deaths are available. Information from death certificates is added to the morbidity file. Death-certificate-only cases contribute less than 2% and pathological confirmation is performed in about 95% of cases.

The registry is engaged in both descriptive and analytical epidemiological research, its data being used for population-based case–control studies on ENT, colorectal, breast, endometrial and thyroid cancers.

The canton provides a favourable environment for non-melanocytic skin cancer registration, since traditionally most cutaneous lesions are surgically resected and examined by a pathologist.

The registry participates in the implementation and evaluation of mammographic cancer screening in the Vaud population.

Fabio Levi
Van-Cong Te
Lalao Randimbison

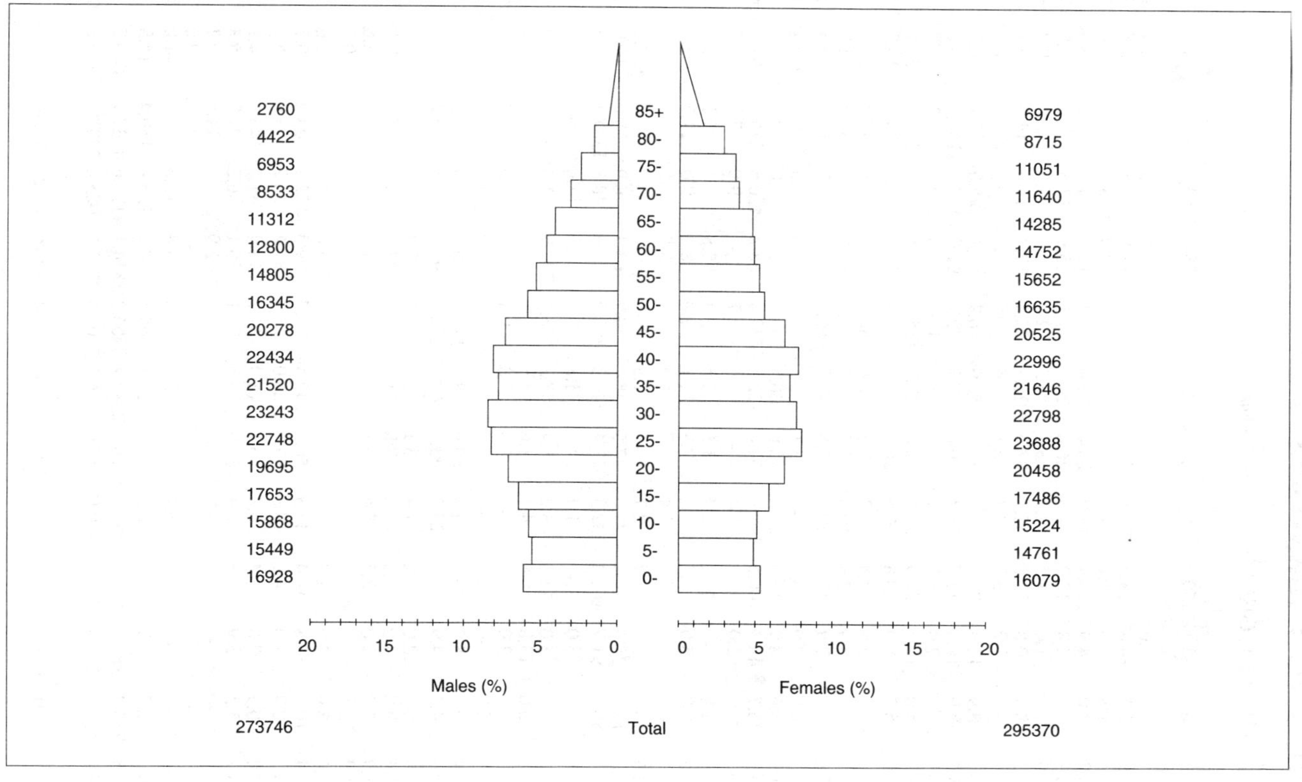

Switzerland, Vaud

Source of population: average annual 1988–92

Census: December 1990. Recensement fédéral de la population suisse, Décembre 1990. Population résidante selon le canton et les groupes d'ages en 1990. Annuaire statistique de la Suisse, Office fédéral de la statistique, Berne, 1993, pp 48-49.

Estimate: The 1988, 1989, 1991 and 1992 populations are mid-year Federal and Cantonal estimates using the classical interpolation method, based on official numbers of births, deaths, immigration and emigration.

Notes to tables overleaf:

† 188 does not include non-invasive tumours

SWITZERLAND, VAUD 1988-1992

ANNUAL INCIDENCE PER 100,000 BY AGE GROUP (YEARS) - MALE

SITE	ALL AGES	AGE UNK	0-	5-	10-	15-	20-	25-	30-	35-	40-	45-	50-	55-	60-	65-	70-	75-	80-	85+	CRUDE RATE	%	CR 64	CR 74	ASR (W)	ICD (9th)
Lip	19	0	-	-	-	-	-	-	-	-	-	1.0	-	1.4	1.6	7.1	11.7	14.4	9.0	-	1.4	0.3	0.02	0.11	**0.8**	140
Tongue	89	0	-	-	-	-	-	-	-	0.9	2.7	14.8	13.5	20.3	23.4	17.7	28.1	11.5	4.5	14.5	6.5	1.4	0.38	0.61	**4.8**	141
Salivary gland	19	0	-	-	-	-	-	0.9	-	-	1.8	-	1.2	4.1	-	8.8	4.7	2.9	18.1	-	1.4	0.3	0.04	0.11	**0.9**	142
Mouth	77	0	-	-	-	1.1	-	-	-	0.9	8.0	4.9	14.7	18.9	23.4	12.4	16.4	11.5	4.5	7.2	5.6	1.2	0.36	0.50	**4.2**	143-5
Oropharynx	105	0	-	-	-	-	-	-	-	0.9	7.1	14.8	12.2	24.3	26.6	24.8	21.1	25.9	13.6	7.2	7.7	1.6	0.43	0.66	**5.5**	146
Nasopharynx	12	0	-	-	-	-	1.0	-	-	0.9	-	1.0	1.2	2.7	3.1	3.5	2.3	-	4.5	-	0.9	0.2	0.05	0.08	**0.7**	147
Hypopharynx	125	0	-	-	-	-	-	-	-	-	8.9	10.8	22.0	35.1	37.5	26.5	23.4	17.3	13.6	14.5	9.1	1.9	0.57	0.82	**6.8**	148
Pharynx unspecified	11	0	-	-	-	-	-	-	-	-	-	1.0	3.7	2.7	3.1	1.8	-	5.8	-	-	0.8	0.2	0.05	0.06	**0.6**	149
Oesophagus	195	0	-	-	-	-	-	-	0.9	-	8.9	11.8	28.1	35.1	34.4	56.6	46.9	60.4	95.0	50.7	14.2	3.0	0.60	1.11	**9.5**	150
Stomach	227	0	-	-	-	-	1.0	-	1.7	5.6	8.9	10.8	13.5	29.7	40.6	47.7	72.7	92.0	117.6	159.4	16.6	3.5	0.56	1.16	**10.4**	151
Small intestine	26	0	-	-	-	-	-	-	-	-	-	2.0	3.7	4.1	-	8.8	11.7	5.8	22.6	7.2	1.9	0.4	0.05	0.15	**1.2**	152
Colon	481	0	-	-	-	1.1	-	0.9	2.6	3.7	8.0	17.8	26.9	56.7	100.0	127.3	154.7	207.1	312.1	275.4	35.1	7.3	1.09	2.50	**21.6**	153
Rectum	269	0	-	-	-	-	-	-	0.9	0.9	6.2	8.9	20.8	36.5	56.2	77.8	84.4	123.7	140.2	123.2	19.7	4.1	0.65	1.46	**12.3**	154
Liver	150	0	-	1.3	-	-	-	-	0.9	-	-	7.9	4.9	20.3	29.7	56.6	60.9	54.7	90.5	36.2	11.0	2.3	0.32	0.91	**7.0**	155
Gallbladder etc.	53	0	-	-	-	-	-	-	-	-	-	3.9	2.4	10.8	6.2	17.7	11.7	31.6	18.1	36.2	3.9	0.8	0.12	0.26	**2.4**	156
Pancreas	199	0	-	-	-	-	-	-	-	2.8	1.8	7.9	17.1	29.7	37.5	47.7	86.7	74.8	90.5	115.9	14.5	3.0	0.48	1.16	**9.2**	157
Nose, sinuses etc.	10	0	-	-	-	-	-	-	-	-	0.9	2.0	-	-	3.1	-	2.3	8.6	4.5	-	0.7	0.2	0.03	0.04	**0.5**	160
Larynx	126	0	-	-	-	-	-	-	-	-	1.9	3.6	8.9	13.5	32.4	40.6	26.5	35.2	40.3	9.0	29.0	9.2	1.9	0.50	0.81	**6.5**	161
Bronchus, lung	1256	0	-	-	-	1.1	2.0	1.8	2.6	6.5	26.7	48.3	106.5	191.8	332.8	422.5	438.3	468.8	420.6	275.4	91.8	19.1	3.60	7.90	**61.4**	162
Other thoracic organs	9	0	-	-	-	-	1.0	-	-	-	-	2.0	-	1.4	-	-	4.7	-	9.0	7.2	0.7	0.1	0.02	0.05	**0.4**	163-4
Bone	16	0	-	1.3	-	2.3	1.0	-	-	-	1.8	-	1.2	2.7	1.6	3.5	2.3	5.8	-	7.2	1.2	0.2	0.06	0.09	**1.0**	170
Connective tissue	45	0	4.7	1.3	-	2.3	2.0	0.9	1.7	1.9	0.9	3.0	3.7	-	7.8	14.1	7.0	8.6	9.0	21.7	3.3	0.7	0.15	0.26	**2.9**	171
Mesothelioma	18	0	-	-	-	-	-	-	-	-	0.9	3.9	3.7	1.4	4.7	5.3	-	5.8	4.5	-	1.3	0.3	0.07	0.10	**1.0**	MES
Kaposi's sarcoma	51	0	-	-	-	3.0	7.9	8.6	4.6	10.7	5.9	3.7	2.7	-	1.8	-	-	-	-	-	3.7	0.8	0.24	0.24	**3.0**	KAP
Melanoma of skin	233	0	-	-	1.3	-	7.1	5.3	7.7	13.0	12.5	25.6	26.9	23.0	37.5	35.4	60.9	63.3	76.9	58.0	17.0	3.6	0.80	1.28	**12.0**	172
Other skin	2208	0	-	-	-	2.3	5.1	4.4	21.5	28.8	55.3	91.7	160.3	232.3	373.4	546.3	803.9	1026.9	1148.8	1304.3	161.3		4.88	11.63	**100.0**	173
Breast	15	0	-	-	-	-	-	-	-	-	-	3.0	-	1.4	4.7	1.8	4.7	5.8	13.6	-	1.1	0.2	0.04	0.08	**0.7**	175
Prostate	1149	0	-	-	-	-	-	-	-	-	-	3.0	11.0	43.2	148.4	348.3	478.1	793.9	891.0	985.5	83.9	17.5	1.03	5.16	**45.7**	185
Testis	146	0	1.2	-	1.3	5.7	12.2	32.5	19.8	19.5	16.0	13.8	8.6	4.1	1.6	3.5	2.3	-	-	-	10.7	2.2	0.68	0.71	**9.3**	186
Penis	16	0	-	-	-	-	-	0.9	-	-	-	3.0	-	-	1.6	1.8	9.4	8.6	9.0	7.2	1.2	0.2	0.03	0.08	**0.7**	187.1-.4
Other male genital	5	0	-	-	1.3	-	-	-	-	0.9	-	1.2	-	-	-	-	-	2.9	4.5	-	0.4	0.1	0.02	0.02	**0.3**	187.5-.9
†Bladder	327	0	-	-	-	-	-	-	-	1.9	0.9	5.9	13.5	44.6	60.9	88.4	112.5	210.0	176.4	181.2	23.9	5.0	0.64	1.64	**14.2**	188
Kidney etc.	190	0	1.2	-	-	-	-	1.8	0.9	0.9	4.5	4.9	13.5	25.7	43.7	60.1	72.7	92.0	49.8	65.2	13.9	2.9	0.48	1.15	**9.2**	189
Eye	14	0	2.4	-	-	-	-	-	-	-	0.9	2.0	1.2	1.4	3.1	5.3	2.3	2.9	-	-	1.0	0.2	0.05	0.09	**0.9**	190
Brain, nervous system	99	0	1.2	3.9	1.3	1.1	3.0	2.6	5.2	7.4	9.8	4.9	7.3	17.6	7.8	21.2	23.4	23.0	9.0	7.2	7.2	1.5	0.37	0.59	**5.6**	191-2
Thyroid	35	0	-	-	-	-	1.0	2.6	1.7	1.9	2.7	3.0	3.7	5.4	3.1	3.5	4.7	11.5	13.6	7.2	2.6	0.5	0.13	0.17	**1.8**	193
Other endocrine	7	0	-	1.3	-	2.3	-	-	-	1.9	-	-	1.2	-	-	-	2.3	-	-	-	0.5	0.1	0.03	0.04	**0.6**	194
Hodgkin's disease	35	0	-	-	6.3	1.1	4.1	5.3	1.7	1.9	3.6	3.9	1.2	-	-	5.3	-	5.8	4.5	-	2.6	0.5	0.15	0.17	**2.4**	201
Non-Hodgkin lymphoma	284	0	-	3.9	2.5	1.1	7.1	5.3	9.5	8.4	10.7	13.8	18.4	47.3	56.2	42.4	72.7	109.3	122.1	94.2	20.7	4.3	0.92	1.50	**14.2**	200,202
Multiple myeloma	69	0	-	-	-	-	-	-	-	0.9	0.9	1.0	4.9	10.8	9.4	23.0	23.4	37.4	36.2	29.0	5.0	1.1	0.14	0.37	**3.1**	203
Lymphoid leukaemia	56	0	3.5	-	-	2.3	1.0	0.9	-	2.8	0.9	2.0	2.4	6.8	6.2	15.9	11.7	14.4	31.7	43.5	4.1	0.9	0.14	0.28	**3.0**	204
Myeloid leukaemia	73	0	3.5	1.3	-	-	3.0	0.9	2.6	3.7	5.3	3.9	7.3	6.8	10.9	5.3	21.1	20.1	36.2	21.7	5.3	1.1	0.25	0.38	**4.0**	205
Monocytic leukaemia	3	0	-	-	-	-	-	-	-	-	-	-	-	-	-	-	-	2.9	-	14.5	0.2	0.0	0.00	0.00	**0.1**	206
Other leukaemia	0	0	-	-	-	-	-	-	-	-	-	-	-	-	-	-	-	-	-	-	0.0	0.0	0.00	0.00	**0.0**	207
Leukaemia unspecified	14	0	1.2	-	-	1.1	1.0	-	-	-	-	-	-	1.4	-	3.5	7.0	5.8	13.6	-	1.0	0.2	0.02	0.08	**0.8**	208
Other and unspecified	203	0	2.4	-	-	-	1.0	-	1.7	0.9	2.7	4.9	11.0	16.2	43.7	54.8	65.6	100.7	126.6	130.4	14.8	3.1	0.42	1.03	**9.2**	O&U
All sites	8769	0	21.3	14.2	13.9	24.9	56.9	73.9	92.9	125.5	235.4	383.7	611.8	1052.3	1626.5	2282.4	2906.3	3814.1	4174.6	4137.7	640.7		21.66	47.61	**412.2**	ALL
All sites but 173	6561	0	21.3	14.2	13.9	22.7	51.8	69.5	71.4	96.7	180.1	291.9	451.5	820.0	1253.0	1736.1	2102.4	2787.2	3025.8	2833.3	479.3	100.0	16.79	35.98	**312.2**	ALLb

Rate from 1 case: 1.181 1.295 1.260 1.133 1.015 0.879 0.860 0.929 0.891 0.986 1.224 1.351 1.562 1.768 2.344 2.876 4.523 7.246

†Important: see notes on population page

SWITZERLAND, VAUD 1988-1992

ANNUAL INCIDENCE PER 100,000 BY AGE GROUP (YEARS) - FEMALE

SITE	ALL AGES	AGE UNK	0-	5-	10-	15-	20-	25-	30-	35-	40-	45-	50-	55-	60-	65-	70-	75-	80-	85+	CRUDE RATE	%	CR 64	CR 74	ASR (W)	ICD (9th)
Lip	2	0	-	-	-	-	-	-	-	-	-	-	-	-	-	-	-	-	-	5.7	0.1	0.0	0.00	0.00	**0.0**	*140*
Tongue	31	0	-	-	-	-	-	-	-	1.8	1.7	1.0	7.2	3.8	4.1	9.8	1.7	3.6	2.3	8.6	2.1	0.5	0.10	0.16	**1.4**	*141*
Salivary gland	7	0	-	-	-	-	-	-	-	-	0.9	1.9	1.2	-	-	-	1.7	-	2.3	2.9	0.5	0.1	0.02	0.03	**0.3**	*142*
Mouth	34	0	-	-	-	-	1.0	-	-	-	2.6	-	4.8	3.8	5.4	2.8	1.7	10.9	4.6	22.9	2.3	0.6	0.09	0.11	**1.2**	*143-5*
Oropharynx	20	0	-	-	-	-	-	-	-	-	-	1.9	3.6	1.3	9.5	1.4	3.4	1.8	4.6	2.9	1.4	0.3	0.08	0.11	**0.9**	*146*
Nasopharynx	2	0	-	-	1.3	-	-	-	-	-	1.2	-	-	-	-	-	-	-	-	-	0.1	0.0	0.01	0.01	**0.2**	*147*
Hypopharynx	21	0	-	-	-	-	-	-	-	0.9	1.7	4.9	3.6	3.8	4.1	1.4	-	3.6	2.3	-	1.4	0.4	0.10	0.10	**1.0**	*148*
Pharynx unspecified	2	0	-	-	-	-	-	-	-	-	-	1.0	-	1.3	-	-	-	-	-	-	0.1	0.0	0.01	0.01	**0.1**	*149*
Oesophagus	68	0	-	-	-	-	-	-	-	-	0.9	1.0	3.6	5.1	9.5	11.2	17.2	12.7	34.4	34.4	4.6	1.2	0.10	0.24	**2.0**	*150*
Stomach	143	0	-	-	-	-	-	0.8	1.8	2.8	0.9	3.9	3.6	8.9	13.6	22.4	41.2	47.1	66.6	48.7	9.7	2.5	0.18	0.50	**4.2**	*151*
Small intestine	23	0	-	-	-	-	-	-	0.9	1.7	1.0	-	2.6	4.1	7.0	5.2	-	9.2	5.7	1.6	0.4	0.05	0.11	**0.9**	*152*
Colon	484	0	-	-	-	-	-	2.6	2.8	7.8	7.8	16.8	38.3	42.0	79.8	147.8	139.3	204.2	220.6	32.8	8.3	0.59	1.73	**14.2**	*153*
Rectum	247	0	-	-	-	-	-	0.9	7.4	2.6	4.9	15.6	29.4	38.0	47.6	65.3	77.8	50.5	83.1	16.7	4.2	0.49	1.06	**8.6**	*154*
Liver	33	0	1.2	-	-	-	-	-	-	-	0.9	-	2.4	-	2.7	1.4	18.9	18.1	6.9	5.7	2.2	0.6	0.04	0.14	**1.1**	*155*
Gallbladder etc.	86	0	-	-	-	-	-	-	-	-	-	1.0	1.2	7.7	12.2	15.4	24.1	18.1	36.7	51.6	5.8	1.5	0.11	0.31	**2.5**	*156*
Pancreas	199	0	-	-	-	-	-	-	-	0.9	2.6	1.0	12.0	16.6	24.4	33.6	44.7	56.1	75.7	111.8	13.5	3.4	0.29	0.68	**5.9**	*157*
Nose, sinuses etc.	15	0	-	-	-	-	-	0.8	-	-	-	-	1.3	4.1	-	3.4	5.4	6.9	5.7	1.0	0.3	0.03	0.05	**0.5**	*160*
Larynx	19	0	-	-	-	1.1	-	-	1.8	1.8	-	-	-	5.4	5.6	3.4	1.8	4.6	2.9	1.3	0.3	0.05	0.10	**0.8**	*161*
Bronchus, lung	318	0	-	-	-	-	0.8	4.4	2.8	10.4	19.5	38.5	34.5	59.7	65.8	55.0	83.2	64.3	60.2	21.5	5.5	0.85	1.46	**12.5**	*162*
Other thoracic organs	5	0	-	-	-	-	-	-	-	-	-	1.2	-	-	-	1.7	1.8	4.6	-	0.3	0.1	0.01	0.01	**0.1**	*163-4*
Bone	7	0	-	-	-	-	1.0	-	-	-	-	2.4	1.3	-	-	1.7	1.8	2.3	-	0.5	0.1	0.02	0.03	**0.3**	*170*
Connective tissue	49	0	2.5	-	-	1.1	1.0	0.8	1.8	1.8	3.5	1.9	3.6	8.9	5.4	4.2	1.7	7.2	11.5	20.1	3.3	0.8	0.16	0.19	**2.2**	*171*
Mesothelioma	7	0	-	-	-	-	-	-	-	-	-	-	-	-	2.7	2.8	3.4	-	2.9	0.5	0.1	0.01	0.04	**0.3**	*MES*
Kaposi's sarcoma	6	0	-	-	-	-	1.0	0.8	1.8	-	-	-	1.2	-	1.4	-	-	-	-	0.4	0.1	0.02	0.03	**0.4**	*KAP*
Melanoma of skin	272	0	-	-	-	3.4	5.9	6.8	13.2	17.6	21.7	26.3	25.2	31.9	28.5	49.0	41.2	29.0	41.3	25.8	18.4	4.7	0.90	1.35	**12.6**	*172*
Other skin	2170	0	-	-	-	4.6	5.9	11.8	25.4	36.0	83.5	108.2	143.1	226.2	277.9	324.8	427.8	537.5	711.4	808.1	146.9		4.61	8.38	**75.6**	*173*
Breast	1831	0	-	-	-	-	1.0	6.8	21.9	62.8	111.3	200.7	236.8	251.7	248.1	292.6	274.9	329.4	362.6	312.3	124.0	31.4	5.71	8.54	**77.2**	*174*
Uterus unspecified	5	0	-	-	-	-	-	-	-	-	-	-	-	-	-	1.4	-	1.8	2.3	5.7	0.3	0.1	0.00	0.01	**0.1**	*179*
Cervix uteri	140	0	-	-	-	-	1.0	3.4	6.1	9.2	13.0	13.6	9.6	14.1	17.6	25.2	30.9	10.9	16.1	22.9	9.5	2.4	0.44	0.72	**6.3**	*180*
Placenta	1	0	-	-	-	-	1.0	-	-	-	-	-	-	-	-	-	-	-	-	-	0.1	0.0	0.00	0.00	**0.1**	*181*
Corpus uteri	342	0	-	-	-	-	-	-	1.8	-	7.8	9.7	24.0	49.8	84.1	78.4	89.3	74.2	75.7	51.6	23.2	5.9	0.89	1.73	**13.2**	*182*
Ovary etc.	248	0	-	-	-	-	2.0	2.5	0.9	0.9	5.2	11.7	22.8	42.2	47.4	40.6	55.0	56.1	64.3	45.8	16.8	4.3	0.68	1.16	**9.6**	*183*
Other female genital	64	0	-	-	-	-	-	-	1.8	1.7	3.9	6.0	8.9	1.4	2.8	5.2	19.9	32.1	37.3	4.3	1.1	0.12	0.16	**1.9**	*184*
†Bladder	99	0	-	-	-	-	-	-	-	-	-	1.0	2.4	8.7	17.6	18.2	22.3	27.1	48.2	40.1	6.7	1.7	0.15	0.35	**2.9**	*188*
Kidney etc.	123	0	2.5	2.7	-	-	-	-	0.9	1.8	1.7	5.8	6.0	23.0	19.0	29.4	24.1	23.5	39.0	17.2	8.3	2.1	0.32	0.58	**5.0**	*189*
Eye	23	0	1.2	1.4	-	-	1.0	0.8	0.9	1.8	0.9	-	2.4	1.3	1.4	4.2	6.9	-	6.9	2.9	1.6	0.4	0.07	0.12	**1.2**	*190*
Brain, nervous system	88	0	-	2.7	2.6	2.3	2.0	0.8	2.6	2.8	2.6	9.7	10.8	11.5	14.9	11.2	15.5	12.7	16.1	-	6.0	1.5	0.33	0.46	**4.5**	*191-2*
Thyroid	90	0	-	-	-	-	5.9	8.4	4.4	5.5	8.7	3.9	7.2	3.8	8.1	8.4	10.3	9.0	13.8	31.5	6.1	1.5	0.28	0.37	**4.1**	*193*
Other endocrine	3	0	-	-	-	-	-	-	-	-	0.9	-	-	2.6	-	-	-	-	-	-	0.2	0.1	0.02	0.02	**0.2**	*194*
Hodgkin's disease	32	0	-	-	3.9	2.3	4.9	3.4	1.8	2.8	1.7	2.9	2.4	1.3	1.4	1.4	1.7	1.8	-	2.9	2.2	0.5	0.14	0.16	**2.1**	*201*
Non-Hodgkin lymphoma	229	0	-	-	1.3	1.1	1.0	1.7	2.6	3.7	7.0	10.7	15.6	16.6	38.0	32.2	51.5	76.0	78.0	43.0	15.5	3.9	0.50	0.92	**8.2**	*200,202*
Multiple myeloma	77	0	-	-	-	-	-	-	-	-	0.9	1.7	1.0	3.6	7.7	16.3	11.2	22.3	23.5	20.7	25.8	5.2	1.3	0.16	0.32	**2.6**	*203*
Lymphoid leukaemia	44	0	3.7	2.7	1.3	1.1	1.0	-	0.9	-	-	-	2.4	-	2.7	7.0	5.2	12.7	11.5	31.5	3.0	0.8	0.08	0.14	**2.0**	*204*
Myeloid leukaemia	55	0	-	-	1.3	-	1.0	1.7	0.9	-	1.7	2.9	1.2	2.6	8.1	9.8	15.5	12.7	16.1	17.2	3.7	0.9	0.11	0.23	**2.0**	*205*
Monocytic leukaemia	3	0	-	-	-	-	-	-	-	-	0.9	-	-	-	1.4	-	-	-	2.9	0.2	0.1	0.01	0.01	**0.1**	*206*
Other leukaemia	1	0	-	-	-	-	-	-	-	-	-	-	-	-	1.4	-	-	-	-	0.1	0.0	0.01	0.01	**0.1**	*207*
Leukaemia unspecified	10	0	-	-	-	-	-	-	-	-	-	-	-	-	1.4	2.8	-	3.6	11.5	-	0.7	0.2	0.01	0.02	**0.2**	*208*
Other and unspecified	224	0	1.2	-	-	-	-	0.8	0.9	3.7	2.6	5.8	6.0	10.2	19.0	32.2	44.7	67.0	103.3	143.3	15.2	3.8	0.25	0.64	**6.2**	*O&U*
All sites	8002	0	12.4	9.5	11.8	17.2	37.1	53.2	100.0	175.5	313.1	470.6	651.6	883.0	1102.2	1296.4	1587.6	1818.7	2265.0	2364.0	541.8		19.19	33.61	**299.8**	*ALL*
All sites but 173	5832	0	12.4	9.5	11.8	12.6	31.3	41.4	74.6	139.5	229.6	362.5	508.5	656.8	824.3	971.6	1159.8	1281.3	1553.6	1556.0	394.9	100.0	14.57	25.23	**224.2**	*ALLb*

Rate from 1 case			1.244	1.355	1.314	1.144	0.978	0.844	0.877	0.924	0.870	0.974	1.202	1.278	1.356	1.400	1.718	1.810	2.295	2.865

†Important: see notes on population page

Switzerland, Zürich

The cancer registry of the canton of Zürich was founded in 1980 with the primary aim of establishing the incidence of cancer in this canton and to serve as a basis for epidemiological and clinico-pathological cancer research. It is affiliated to the Department of Pathology of the University of Zürich. The Institute of Social and Preventive Medicine of the University actively collaborates, especially in the analysis of incidence and mortality data. Funding is supplied by the canton, the Cantonal Cancer Society and a Swiss federal grant to the Association of Swiss Cancer Registries.

A medical epidemiologist, a data manager, and 3–4 tumour registrars form the staff of the registry. Processing and analysis of data are handled by the medical epidemiologist and an expert medical geographer. Since 1993, a new data-processing system has been introduced.

The canton of Zürich is located in the German-speaking part of the Mittelland plateau, where more than half of the Swiss population live, between latitudes 47°42′ and 47°10′ N and longitudes 8°21′ and 8°59′ E, with an area of 1729 km^2 and altitudes ranging from 332 to 1293 m above sea level. Air pollution is generally not serious, except for NO_2 and ozone. Mean annual levels of NO_2 reached a maximum in 1986/87 and have been decreasing since then, but in 1992 the recommended limit was still exceeded in industrial and densely populated areas of the canton, while ozone levels exceed the recommended maximum level everywhere in the canton for 3–7 months in summer.

The population of the canton increased by 5% between 1980 and 1990; at the end of 1992, there were 1 158 000 residents (561 000 males, 597 000 females), or 16.8% of the total Swiss population. The population is almost completely Caucasian; foreigners (mostly from Italy and ex-Yugoslavia) accounted for about 20%. In Zürich City, the largest town of Switzerland, the population decreased between 1962 and 1985, then stabilized, with an increasing proportion of foreigners (25% at the end of 1992). In 1990, 31% of the cantonal population lived in the City of Zürich, another 7.5% in Winterthur, a focus of Switzerland's machine industry. The Zürich Metropolitan Area has expanded to the neighbouring areas of Aargau and Schwyz not covered by the Zürich Cancer Registry. Areas that are mainly rural account for less than 10% of the total population of the canton.

The industrial sector is decreasing (32.1% in 1991) in favour of services (66.5 % in 1991). In 1990 agriculture and forestry accounted for 2.2%. In 1991 the non-agricultural workforce was distributed between manufacturing, 21.7%; construction, 10.3%; commerce and catering, 24.0%; transport and communication, 8.5%; banking, insurance and consulting, 20.4%.

The medical system is well developed. The number of physicians in private practice is increasing by about 3% per annum and attained 2126 (i.e., 1 per 553 inhabitants) at the end of 1992. The number of hospital physicians is fairly stable (1339, including 882 residents). Overall, there was 1 physician per 286 population. There were about 6000 beds for acute care within 28 public and 6 private hospitals; affiliated to these hospitals were 19 long-term care departments with nearly 1000 beds. Another 2900 beds were located in 23 long-term care facilities. In addition there were about 2600 beds in psychiatric hospitals, many dedicated to elderly people.

The main sources of information are the medical records of the public hospitals and the histology and autopsy reports of the four public institutes of pathology in the canton (including the section of dermatopathology), as well as some private histopathology laboratories. These services also provide other microscopic confirmation of malignancy (cytology, haematology). Most of these files are abstracted in an active manner by the staff of the registry. Unclear diagnoses are discussed and reviewed with the help of the contributing pathologists. The autopsy rate has decreased since the late 1980s (in 1988–92 it averaged 28% of all cancer deaths). All autopsies are checked by the registry for mention of tumours. Additional information is obtained from questionnaires sent to private practitioners. The coverage of incidence is estimated to be almost complete for Zürich City (95%) and about 90% for the rest of the canton.

Each patient has a unique identification number; each tumour is separately recorded. Multiple tumours are thus easily identifiable. Regarding multiple primaries, it has always been the practice of the registry to count in its incidence rates only one tumour for each tumour-type within a three-digit tumour site of ICD-9. Follow-up is mainly passive. New information concerning already registered cases is systematically used for correcting and updating demographic and diagnostic variables. Special attention is paid to malignant melanoma (Zürich is a high-incidence area); a population-based multivariate analysis of its survival has been performed. For urothelial tumours (bladder, ureter, renal pelvis) intraepithelial cancers are included in the incidence. Squamous and basal cell carcinomas of the skin are usually not registered, except for rare cases which have metastasized or led to death.

The registry has elaborated the comprehensive 'Atlas of Cancer Mortality in Switzerland 1970–1990' (Basel 1997: Birkhäuser); based on case-by-case matching, incident cases from the registry have been used to evaluate the quality of diagnoses on death certificates.

Georges Schüler

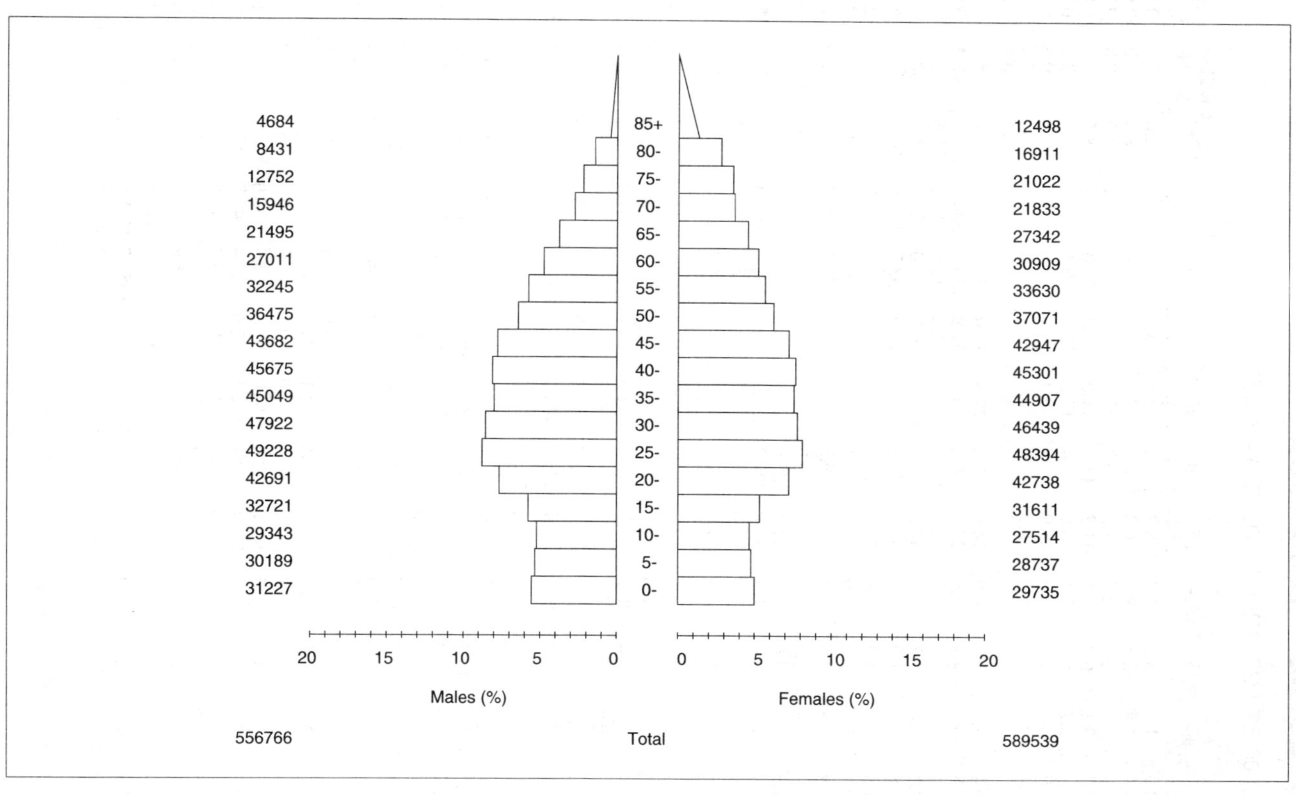

Switzerland, Zurich
Source of population: average annual 1988–92
Census: 1990. 'Eidgenòssische Volkszàhlung' 1990.
Bundesamt für Statistik, Schweiz.
Estimate: 1988–92. Kantonale Bevölkerungs-Fortschreiburg
Statistische Amter.

Notes to tables overleaf:
† 173 does not include basal cell or squamous cell carcinomas

SWITZERLAND, ZURICH 1988-1992

ANNUAL INCIDENCE PER 100,000 BY AGE GROUP (YEARS) - MALE

SITE	ALL AGES	AGE UNK	0-	5-	10-	15-	20-	25-	30-	35-	40-	45-	50-	55-	60-	65-	70-	75-	80-	85+	CRUDE RATE	%	CR 64	CR 74	ASR (W)	ICD (9th)
Lip	60	0	-	-	-	-	-	-	-	0.9	1.3	3.2	3.3	6.2	4.4	2.8	6.3	9.4	14.2	25.6	2.2	0.5	0.10	0.14	**1.4**	*140*
Tongue	83	0	-	-	-	0.6	-	0.4	-	0.4	1.8	2.7	9.3	6.2	8.9	7.4	15.1	7.8	9.5	8.5	3.0	0.6	0.15	0.26	**2.1**	*141*
Salivary gland	22	0	-	-	-	0.6	-	-	-	-	-	-	2.2	1.2	0.7	5.6	3.8	3.1	2.4	8.5	0.8	0.2	0.02	0.07	**0.6**	*142*
Mouth	103	0	-	-	-	-	-	-	-	2.7	3.1	6.9	5.5	11.2	11.1	14.0	5.0	11.0	9.5	8.5	3.7	0.8	0.20	0.30	**2.6**	*143-5*
Oropharynx	90	0	-	-	-	-	-	-	-	-	2.2	5.0	7.1	5.0	7.4	19.5	12.5	9.4	14.2	-	3.2	0.7	0.13	0.29	**2.3**	*146*
Nasopharynx	14	0	-	-	-	-	-	0.4	-	0.9	0.4	1.4	0.5	1.9	0.7	0.9	-	-	2.4	-	0.5	0.1	0.03	0.04	**0.4**	*147*
Hypopharynx	67	0	-	-	-	-	-	-	0.4	0.4	2.6	4.1	5.5	6.2	4.4	10.2	11.3	4.7	2.4	-	2.4	0.5	0.12	0.23	**1.7**	*148*
Pharynx unspecified	2	0	-	-	-	-	-	-	-	-	-	0.9	-	-	-	-	-	-	-	-	0.1	0.0	0.00	0.00	**0.1**	*149*
Oesophagus	146	0	-	-	-	-	-	-	-	0.4	3.5	3.7	9.9	14.9	17.8	22.3	10.0	23.5	16.6	38.4	5.2	1.1	0.25	0.41	**3.6**	*150*
Stomach	513	0	-	-	-	-	-	0.9	-	1.7	1.8	3.9	4.1	23.0	26.1	39.2	60.5	92.8	133.3	208.7	153.7	18.4	3.9	0.50	1.27	**11.3**	*151*
Small intestine	63	0	-	-	-	-	-	-	-	0.4	-	-	0.5	2.2	2.5	8.9	12.1	10.0	12.5	14.2	25.6	2.3	0.5	0.07	0.18	**1.5**	*152*
Colon	846	0	-	-	-	0.6	0.9	0.4	1.3	3.1	7.4	13.7	20.3	40.3	63.7	132.1	156.8	196.0	322.6	294.6	30.4	6.5	0.76	2.20	**19.0**	*153*
Rectum	596	0	-	-	-	-	-	-	1.7	1.8	5.3	11.0	20.3	32.3	56.3	68.9	112.9	153.7	185.0	200.7	21.4	4.6	0.64	1.55	**13.5**	*154*
Liver	258	0	-	-	-	-	-	-	0.4	1.8	3.5	2.7	6.6	14.9	27.4	33.5	56.4	53.3	94.9	47.0	9.3	2.0	0.29	0.74	**5.9**	*155*
Gallbladder etc.	108	0	-	-	-	-	-	-	-	0.4	1.3	2.7	4.9	3.1	8.1	17.7	22.6	20.4	21.3	59.8	3.9	0.8	0.10	0.30	**2.6**	*156*
Pancreas	330	0	-	-	-	-	-	-	-	0.9	4.4	5.5	9.3	14.9	19.3	52.1	65.2	86.3	97.3	149.4	11.9	2.5	0.27	0.86	**7.4**	*157*
Nose, sinuses etc.	23	0	0.6	-	-	-	-	-	-	-	0.4	1.4	-	3.1	0.7	4.7	5.0	4.7	-	-	0.8	0.2	0.03	0.08	**0.6**	*160*
Larynx	162	0	-	-	-	-	-	-	-	1.3	1.8	4.6	7.7	17.4	25.9	26.1	18.8	20.4	9.5	34.2	5.8	1.2	0.29	0.52	**4.2**	*161*
Bronchus, lung	1992	0	-	-	-	-	0.5	1.2	1.7	2.7	12.7	29.8	70.2	142.0	224.3	337.7	396.3	442.3	448.3	316.0	71.6	15.2	2.43	6.10	**47.4**	*162*
Other thoracic organs	25	0	-	-	-	-	-	0.4	-	0.4	1.3	0.9	1.6	0.6	-	3.7	6.3	3.1	4.7	4.3	0.9	0.2	0.03	0.08	**0.6**	*163-4*
Bone	49	0	-	2.0	0.7	3.1	-	1.2	0.8	1.8	2.2	1.8	2.7	1.2	2.2	3.7	2.5	6.3	4.7	-	1.8	0.4	0.10	0.13	**1.6**	*170*
Connective tissue	92	0	-	-	0.7	-	-	1.2	2.9	1.3	2.2	2.7	1.6	7.4	5.9	5.6	3.8	28.2	16.6	42.7	3.3	0.7	0.13	0.18	**2.1**	*171*
Mesothelioma	59	0	-	-	-	-	-	-	-	-	0.9	3.2	2.2	4.3	4.4	7.4	16.3	7.8	11.9	8.5	2.1	0.5	0.08	0.19	**1.4**	*MES*
Kaposi's sarcoma	145	0	-	-	-	-	0.9	6.9	8.3	14.2	10.9	11.4	6.0	3.1	-	1.9	1.3	1.6	7.1	4.3	5.2	1.1	0.31	0.33	**3.9**	*KAP*
Melanoma of skin	540	0	-	-	-	1.2	4.7	7.3	10.9	11.1	11.8	23.4	30.2	36.0	43.7	54.9	64.0	84.7	64.0	76.9	19.4	4.1	0.90	1.50	**13.7**	*172*
†Other skin	41	0	-	-	0.7	-	0.5	0.4	0.4	-	0.9	0.9	1.1	1.9	3.0	2.8	7.5	9.4	11.9	17.1	1.5	-	0.05	0.10	**1.0**	*173*
Breast	14	0	-	-	-	-	-	-	-	-	-	-	1.1	-	2.2	2.8	2.5	-	2.4	12.8	0.5	0.1	0.02	0.04	**0.4**	*175*
Prostate	3089	0	-	-	-	-	-	-	-	-	0.4	5.5	19.7	79.4	208.1	442.0	765.1	1064.9	1285.7	1387.7	111.0	23.6	1.57	7.60	**65.4**	*185*
Testis	301	0	0.6	-	-	5.5	16.4	23.6	26.3	26.6	14.9	8.7	4.4	4.3	1.5	1.9	2.5	-	-	4.3	10.8	2.3	0.66	0.69	**8.9**	*186*
Penis	42	0	-	-	-	-	-	-	-	-	0.9	0.5	0.5	1.2	3.7	3.7	7.5	12.5	19.0	21.3	1.5	0.3	0.03	0.09	**0.9**	*187.1-.4*
Other male genital	6	0	-	-	-	-	-	-	-	0.4	-	-	1.1	0.6	0.7	-	-	-	-	4.3	0.2	0.0	0.01	0.01	**0.2**	*187.5-.9*
Bladder	976	0	-	-	-	-	0.5	0.8	0.8	1.8	5.3	13.7	29.6	50.2	90.3	156.3	195.7	243.1	301.3	264.7	35.1	7.5	0.97	2.73	**22.4**	*188*
Kidney etc.	442	0	-	1.3	-	-	-	0.8	1.7	2.7	6.6	6.0	11.5	25.4	47.4	65.1	100.3	103.5	104.4	59.8	15.9	3.4	0.52	1.34	**10.5**	*189*
Eye	31	0	2.6	0.7	0.7	-	0.5	0.8	0.4	1.8	0.4	0.9	1.1	1.9	0.7	1.9	2.5	3.1	4.7	-	1.1	0.2	0.06	0.08	**1.1**	*190*
Brain, nervous system	239	0	3.8	5.3	2.0	4.3	1.4	4.1	3.3	5.3	8.8	9.2	11.5	15.5	13.3	18.6	31.4	23.5	30.8	21.3	8.6	1.8	0.44	0.69	**7.0**	*191-2*
Thyroid	97	0	-	-	0.7	1.2	1.4	0.4	3.8	2.7	1.8	4.6	4.4	6.8	6.7	11.2	7.5	6.3	21.3	8.5	3.5	0.7	0.17	0.27	**2.5**	*193*
Other endocrine	9	0	1.3	-	-	-	-	-	0.4	-	-	-	2.7	-	0.7	-	-	-	-	-	0.3	0.1	0.03	0.03	**0.3**	*194*
Hodgkin's disease	98	0	-	0.7	2.0	3.1	4.7	5.3	6.7	3.6	7.4	1.4	1.6	3.7	1.5	0.9	3.8	6.3	2.4	8.5	3.5	0.8	0.21	0.23	**3.0**	*201*
Non-Hodgkin lymphoma	522	0	2.6	1.3	2.0	1.8	2.3	7.3	8.3	13.8	12.7	14.7	18.6	21.7	35.5	52.1	74.0	92.5	147.1	93.9	18.8	4.0	0.71	1.34	**12.9**	*200,202*
Multiple myeloma	152	0	-	-	-	-	-	-	-	0.4	0.9	1.8	1.4	2.2	8.1	14.1	27.0	20.1	31.4	59.3	68.3	5.5	1.2	0.14	0.38	**3.4**	*203*
Lymphoid leukaemia	141	0	7.7	4.0	3.4	0.6	-	0.8	-	-	1.3	1.8	0.5	6.8	7.4	14.9	25.1	34.5	38.0	51.2	5.1	1.1	0.17	0.37	**4.3**	*204*
Myeloid leukaemia	143	0	2.6	-	0.7	1.2	1.9	1.6	0.4	3.1	3.1	2.3	6.0	7.4	8.1	12.1	22.6	20.4	42.7	51.2	5.1	1.1	0.19	0.37	**3.7**	*205*
Monocytic leukaemia	22	0	-	-	-	-	-	0.4	-	0.4	-	-	0.5	0.6	2.2	1.9	6.3	4.7	11.9	-	0.8	0.2	0.02	0.06	**0.5**	*206*
Other leukaemia	8	0	-	-	-	-	-	-	-	-	0.9	0.9	-	-	0.7	1.9	-	-	-	4.3	0.3	0.1	0.01	0.02	**0.2**	*207*
Leukaemia unspecified	3	0	-	-	-	-	-	0.4	-	-	-	-	-	-	0.7	-	-	1.6	-	-	0.1	0.0	0.01	0.01	**0.1**	*208*
Other and unspecified	343	0	0.6	-	-	0.6	0.5	0.8	1.7	0.4	4.4	8.2	8.8	24.8	25.2	38.1	56.4	75.3	121.0	128.1	12.3	2.6	0.38	0.85	**7.8**	*O&U*
All sites	13107	0	22.4	15.2	13.6	24.4	37.9	67.0	85.1	111.9	156.3	228.0	379.4	662.4	1059.6	1760.4	2425.6	3056.7	3785.9	3714.8	470.8		14.32	35.25	**308.2**	*ALL*
All sites but 173	13066	0	22.4	15.2	13.0	24.4	37.5	66.6	84.7	111.9	155.4	227.1	378.3	660.6	1056.6	1757.6	2418.1	3047.3	3774.1	3697.7	469.3	100.0	14.27	35.15	**307.2**	*ALLb*

Rate from 1 case   0.640   0.662   0.682   0.611   0.468   0.406   0.417   0.444   0.438   0.458   0.548   0.620   0.740   0.930   1.254   1.568   2.372   4.270

†Important: see notes on population page

SWITZERLAND, ZURICH 1988-1992

ANNUAL INCIDENCE PER 100,000 BY AGE GROUP (YEARS) - FEMALE

SITE	ALL AGES	AGE UNK	0-	5-	10-	15-	20-	25-	30-	35-	40-	45-	50-	55-	60-	65-	70-	75-	80-	85+	CRUDE RATE	%	CR 64	CR 74	ASR (W)	ICD (9th)
Lip	30	0	-	-	-	-	-	-	-	-	-	0.5	-	1.9	1.5	4.6	6.7	8.3	8.0	1.0	0.3	0.01	0.04	**0.4**	*140*
Tongue	34	0	-	-	-	-	-	0.4	0.4	1.8	1.9	1.6	3.0	2.6	2.2	0.9	1.0	5.9	3.2	1.2	0.3	0.06	0.07	**0.7**	*141*
Salivary gland	16	0	-	-	-	-	-	-	-	0.4	-	0.5	1.2	1.9	0.7	1.8	2.9	3.5	-	0.5	0.1	0.02	0.03	**0.3**	*142*
Mouth	40	0	-	-	-	-	-	-	0.4	1.3	2.3	1.1	3.6	1.9	1.5	2.7	2.9	9.5	6.4	1.4	0.4	0.05	0.07	**0.7**	*143-5*
Oropharynx	27	0	-	-	-	-	-	-	-	-	0.4	2.8	1.1	3.0	-	2.9	5.5	1.9	-	1.6	0.9	0.2	0.04	0.08	**0.6**	*146*
Nasopharynx	6	0	-	-	-	-	-	0.4	-	-	-	1.1	0.6	-	0.7	-	1.0	-	-	-	0.2	0.1	0.01	0.01	**0.1**	*147*
Hypopharynx	11	0	-	-	-	-	-	-	-	0.4	1.4	1.6	1.8	-	-	-	1.0	-	-	-	0.4	0.1	0.03	0.03	**0.3**	*148*
Pharynx unspecified	1	0	-	-	-	-	-	-	-	-	-	-	-	-	-	-	-	-	-	1.6	0.0	0.0	0.00	0.00	**0.0**	*149*
Oesophagus	67	0	-	-	-	-	-	-	-	-	0.9	2.3	1.6	5.9	4.5	5.1	5.5	7.6	13.0	12.8	2.3	0.6	0.08	0.13	**1.2**	*150*
Stomach	342	0	-	-	-	-	-	0.8	0.4	2.2	1.8	4.2	10.8	9.5	16.2	21.9	31.1	59.0	76.9	110.4	11.6	3.0	0.23	0.50	**5.0**	*151*
Small intestine	41	0	-	-	-	-	-	-	0.4	1.8	-	1.4	1.6	-	1.3	3.7	6.4	4.8	8.3	6.4	1.4	0.4	0.03	0.08	**0.7**	*152*
Colon	847	0	-	-	-	-	0.5	1.7	1.3	2.7	7.1	9.8	20.5	33.9	46.6	69.5	106.3	137.0	197.5	171.2	28.7	7.5	0.62	1.50	**13.1**	*153*
Rectum	526	0	-	-	-	-	-	-	0.9	3.1	6.2	7.9	15.6	20.8	39.5	45.4	71.4	77.1	91.1	100.8	17.8	4.7	0.47	1.05	**8.8**	*154*
Liver	89	0	-	-	-	-	-	-	0.4	1.3	0.4	1.9	1.6	4.2	5.2	8.0	8.2	16.2	14.2	20.8	3.0	0.8	0.08	0.16	**1.4**	*155*
Gallbladder etc.	189	0	-	-	-	-	-	-	0.4	-	0.4	0.4	1.4	1.1	4.2	10.4	23.4	21.1	34.2	33.1	62.4	6.4	1.7	0.09	0.31	**2.7**	*156*
Pancreas	378	0	-	-	-	-	-	-	-	0.4	0.9	1.9	4.3	11.3	20.7	28.5	61.4	66.6	88.7	97.6	12.8	3.3	0.20	0.65	**5.4**	*157*
Nose, sinuses etc.	6	0	-	-	-	-	-	-	-	0.4	0.9	0.5	-	0.6	-	-	1.0	-	-	0.2	0.1	0.01	0.01	**0.1**	*160*
Larynx	18	0	-	-	-	-	-	-	-	0.9	0.5	-	1.2	1.9	0.7	2.7	2.9	1.2	3.2	0.6	0.2	0.02	0.04	**0.3**	*161*
Bronchus, lung	565	0	-	-	-	-	-	0.8	0.4	3.6	7.5	21.0	24.8	38.7	45.3	59.2	55.9	70.4	71.0	56.0	19.2	5.0	0.71	1.29	**10.8**	*162*
Other thoracic organs	12	0	-	-	-	-	0.5	-	-	0.4	-	0.9	0.5	0.6	-	0.7	-	2.9	1.2	1.6	0.4	0.1	0.01	0.02	**0.2**	*163-4*
Bone	34	0	0.7	-	-	2.5	0.5	0.8	-	0.9	1.3	-	1.6	0.6	1.3	2.2	1.8	3.8	2.4	6.4	1.2	0.3	0.05	0.07	**0.9**	*170*
Connective tissue	92	0	2.0	0.7	0.7	0.6	2.3	1.2	2.2	1.3	1.8	2.8	2.2	4.8	6.5	4.4	7.3	12.4	5.9	9.6	3.1	0.8	0.15	0.20	**2.2**	*171*
Mesothelioma	9	0	-	-	-	-	-	-	-	0.4	-	1.1	0.6	2.6	-	-	-	-	1.2	-	0.3	0.1	0.02	0.02	**0.2**	*MES*
Kaposi's sarcoma	4	0	-	-	-	-	-	-	1.3	-	0.4	-	-	-	-	-	-	-	-	-	0.1	0.0	0.01	0.01	**0.1**	*KAP*
Melanoma of skin	583	0	-	-	0.7	0.6	8.0	14.1	19.8	16.0	17.2	25.6	30.2	22.6	34.3	37.3	43.1	45.7	35.5	49.6	19.8	5.2	0.95	1.35	**13.3**	*172*
†Other skin	38	0	-	0.7	0.7	-	-	1.2	0.4	-	0.4	1.4	-	1.2	3.2	2.9	2.7	3.8	4.7	9.6	1.3		0.05	0.08	**0.8**	*173*
Breast	3193	0	-	-	-	-	1.9	4.5	16.4	52.6	104.2	160.7	174.8	188.5	225.8	277.2	272.1	293.0	330.0	300.8	108.3	28.3	4.65	7.39	**65.7**	*174*
Uterus unspecified	9	0	-	-	-	-	-	-	-	-	-	-	0.5	-	1.3	1.5	-	1.0	1.2	3.2	0.3	0.1	0.01	0.02	**0.2**	*179*
Cervix uteri	302	0	-	-	-	-	0.5	5.0	12.5	13.4	15.0	15.8	8.1	13.1	17.5	19.0	18.3	21.9	23.7	14.4	10.2	2.7	0.50	0.69	**6.8**	*180*
Placenta	2	0	-	-	-	-	-	0.4	0.4	-	-	-	-	-	-	-	-	-	-	-	0.1	0.0	0.00	0.00	**0.1**	*181*
Corpus uteri	775	0	-	-	-	-	-	0.4	0.4	2.2	6.6	13.0	31.8	62.4	70.5	100.9	107.2	85.6	80.4	62.4	26.3	6.9	0.94	1.98	**15.0**	*182*
Ovary etc.	531	0	-	0.7	0.7	1.9	3.7	0.8	2.2	4.9	10.2	23.8	26.4	24.4	47.9	50.5	51.3	59.0	67.4	28.8	18.0	4.7	0.74	1.25	**11.0**	*183*
Other female genital	108	0	-	-	-	0.6	0.5	-	0.4	0.4	2.2	-	2.7	7.1	4.5	7.3	12.8	15.2	21.3	27.2	3.7	1.0	0.09	0.19	**1.8**	*184*
Bladder	358	0	-	-	-	-	0.5	-	0.4	1.3	0.4	3.7	10.3	14.9	14.9	41.0	44.9	62.8	72.1	72.0	12.1	3.2	0.23	0.66	**5.6**	*188*
Kidney etc.	247	0	2.0	0.7	-	-	-	-	0.4	2.2	0.4	5.1	2.7	11.9	23.9	26.3	40.3	31.4	39.0	27.2	8.4	2.2	0.25	0.58	**4.6**	*189*
Eye	38	0	1.3	-	-	-	-	0.4	-	0.4	0.9	0.9	3.8	3.6	2.6	2.9	2.7	2.9	2.4	1.6	1.3	0.3	0.07	0.10	**1.0**	*190*
Brain, nervous system	177	0	3.4	2.1	2.2	3.2	3.3	4.1	3.9	4.0	4.9	4.2	4.3	10.1	10.4	15.4	15.6	14.3	11.8	3.2	6.0	1.6	0.30	0.45	**4.7**	*191-2*
Thyroid	210	0	-	-	0.7	1.9	2.8	3.7	10.3	4.5	8.8	5.6	5.9	9.5	8.4	13.9	17.4	21.9	14.2	19.2	7.1	1.9	0.31	0.47	**4.7**	*193*
Other endocrine	17	0	2.7	0.7	-	-	-	0.4	1.3	0.4	-	0.5	-	-	-	2.2	1.8	1.0	-	-	0.6	0.2	0.03	0.05	**0.7**	*194*
Hodgkin's disease	76	0	-	0.7	2.2	3.2	3.7	2.5	6.0	1.8	1.8	0.9	0.5	3.0	1.9	3.7	2.7	2.9	4.7	8.0	2.6	0.7	0.14	0.17	**2.2**	*201*
Non-Hodgkin lymphoma	460	0	0.7	1.4	-	2.5	2.3	4.1	2.2	4.9	5.3	8.4	12.9	22.0	34.3	38.8	44.0	63.7	69.8	81.6	15.6	4.1	0.51	0.92	**8.5**	*200,202*
Multiple myeloma	147	0	-	-	-	-	-	-	-	0.9	0.9	1.4	3.2	5.9	8.4	14.6	22.0	24.7	28.4	27.2	5.0	1.3	0.10	0.29	**2.3**	*203*
Lymphoid leukaemia	126	0	6.1	4.2	-	-	0.5	0.4	0.4	0.4	1.3	-	2.7	4.2	6.5	11.7	19.2	16.2	13.0	27.2	4.3	1.1	0.13	0.29	**3.0**	*204*
Myeloid leukaemia	107	0	0.7	-	0.7	-	0.5	-	0.4	0.9	1.3	2.3	3.8	1.8	5.2	7.3	10.1	20.0	22.5	22.4	3.6	0.9	0.09	0.17	**1.8**	*205*
Monocytic leukaemia	15	0	-	-	-	-	-	-	-	-	0.4	-	0.5	1.1	0.6	1.3	1.5	0.9	1.0	2.4	0.5	0.1	0.02	0.03	**0.3**	*206*
Other leukaemia	5	0	-	-	-	-	-	0.4	-	-	-	-	0.5	-	-	-	1.8	1.0	-	-	0.2	0.0	0.00	0.01	**0.1**	*207*
Leukaemia unspecified	11	0	-	-	-	-	-	-	-	-	0.9	-	-	-	-	-	0.7	3.7	1.0	3.5	-	0.4	0.1	0.00	0.03	**0.2**	*208*
Other and unspecified	410	0	-	-	-	-	-	-	-	1.8	2.6	7.9	8.1	11.3	18.8	25.6	44.0	57.1	110.0	134.4	13.9	3.6	0.25	0.60	**5.8**	*O&U*
All sites	11329	0	19.5	11.8	8.7	17.1	31.8	48.4	86.1	133.2	219.9	346.9	430.0	567.3	752.5	984.6	1173.4	1359.5	1590.6	1603.4	384.3		13.37	24.16	**216.3**	*ALL*
All sites but 173	11291	0	19.5	11.1	8.0	17.1	31.8	47.1	85.7	133.2	219.4	345.5	430.0	566.2	749.3	981.6	1170.7	1355.7	1585.9	1593.8	383.0	100.0	13.32	24.08	**215.5**	*ALLb*

Rate from 1 case	0.673	0.696	0.727	0.633	0.468	0.413	0.431	0.445	0.441	0.466	0.540	0.595	0.647	0.731	0.916	0.951	1.183	1.600

†Important: see notes on population page

UK, England and Wales

Cancer registration in England and Wales during 1988–92 was conducted by 12 independent regional registries, which collect data on cancers incident in residents of their areas, and submit notification of registrations, with a standard data set, to the National Registry at the Office of National Statistics (ONS), formerly the Office of Population Censuses and Surveys. A national registry has existed since 1945, although it did not then cover the whole of England and Wales. Complete geographical national coverage (but not 100% completeness of registration) was achieved in 1962. The current person-based database at ONS holds data from 1971 onwards.

England and Wales lie between latitudes 49°58′ and 55°33′ N and longitudes 6°30′ W and 1°31′ E, and have a combined area of 151 207 km². The population live mainly at low altitudes; the highest point is 1085 m above sea level.

The registry covers a population of 50 million; registrations are included in the present data-set only for residents of England and Wales. About 35% of the population live in metropolitan areas, with a further 34% in smaller urban districts (cities, industrial areas, new towns, resort and retirement areas), 20% in mixed urban/rural areas. Data from the 1991 census indicated that 94% of the population described themselves as white, 1.7% as Indian, 1.2% as either Pakistani or Bangladeshi, 0.3% as Chinese (with 0.4% in other Asian groups), 1% as Black Caribbean, 0.4% as Black Africans (with 0.4% in other Black groups), and 0.6% as belonging to other ethnic groups. The most common occupations in the male population are: craft and related occupations (24%), managers and administrators (19%), and plant and machine operators (15%). Among females, the most common occupations are clerical and secretarial (28%), personal and protective service (13%) and managers and administrators(12%).

Cancer registration in England and Wales was voluntary until 1993, when a compulsory (but not statutory) "minimum data" was established in the National Health Service (this does not cover the private sector, although there is close cooperation with the Independent Healthcare Association). The methods of registration and the completeness and accuracy of registration vary between regional registries. Each registry has, since 1971, received notification from national death registration at ONS of all deaths in residents of their region where the death certificate mentioned cancer, enabling the registry to identify cases not previously known to them. Most of the registries use hospital records staff to collect data, and some use specially employed peripatetic data collectors and information from other sources including coroners, pathology laboratories and private nursing homes. When histological confirmation is not available, cancers are registered on the basis of clinical diagnosis alone.

The registries supply to ONS on magnetic media most or all of a common minimum data-set including identifying code, usual residence, birthplace, date of birth, sex, occupation, occupational status and industry, primary tumour site, histology, anniversary data and date of death. Some registries collect much further information, which is not forwarded to ONS. At ONS, data quality checks are undertaken, the results of which are fed back to the registries.

Since 1971, cancer registrations have been recorded in the National Health Service Central Register (NHSCR) maintained by ONS, which includes almost all of the population of England and Wales. Deaths in England and Wales are also recorded in this register, and linkage of cancer registrations and deaths allows routine follow-up of survival of cancer patients (one registry also conducts direct patient follow-up). The process of recording cancers at NHSCR also enables elimination of duplicate registrations from the national file and identification of multiple primary tumours.

ONS publishes routine data annually on cancer registrations in England and Wales and periodically on survival. *Ad hoc* analyses of the data are also performed by ONS and by other research workers, and are published in scientific journals or in ONS publications. Data are also used to answer enquiries from Parliament, the public, health administrators etc., and are supplied to specialist registries. In addition, recording of cancer registrations on the NHSCR enables cohort studies to be undertaken with cancer as an outcome under investigation; over 150 such studies are now in progress.

A review of the operation of national cancer registration and its future direction was carried out during the period covered. Key recommendations were for the formation of a national steering committee and clearer responsibility in the National Health Service for provision of registration data, for national measures to improve registration of private patients (an increasing difficulty), for computerized links to pathology laboratories in all regions, for an increased range of variables to be collected, and for improved quality control and access to the data for users. Much progress has been made in implementing these recommendations and ONS has redeveloped its computer system to provide efficient processing and a person-based database (data from 1971).

Mike Quinn

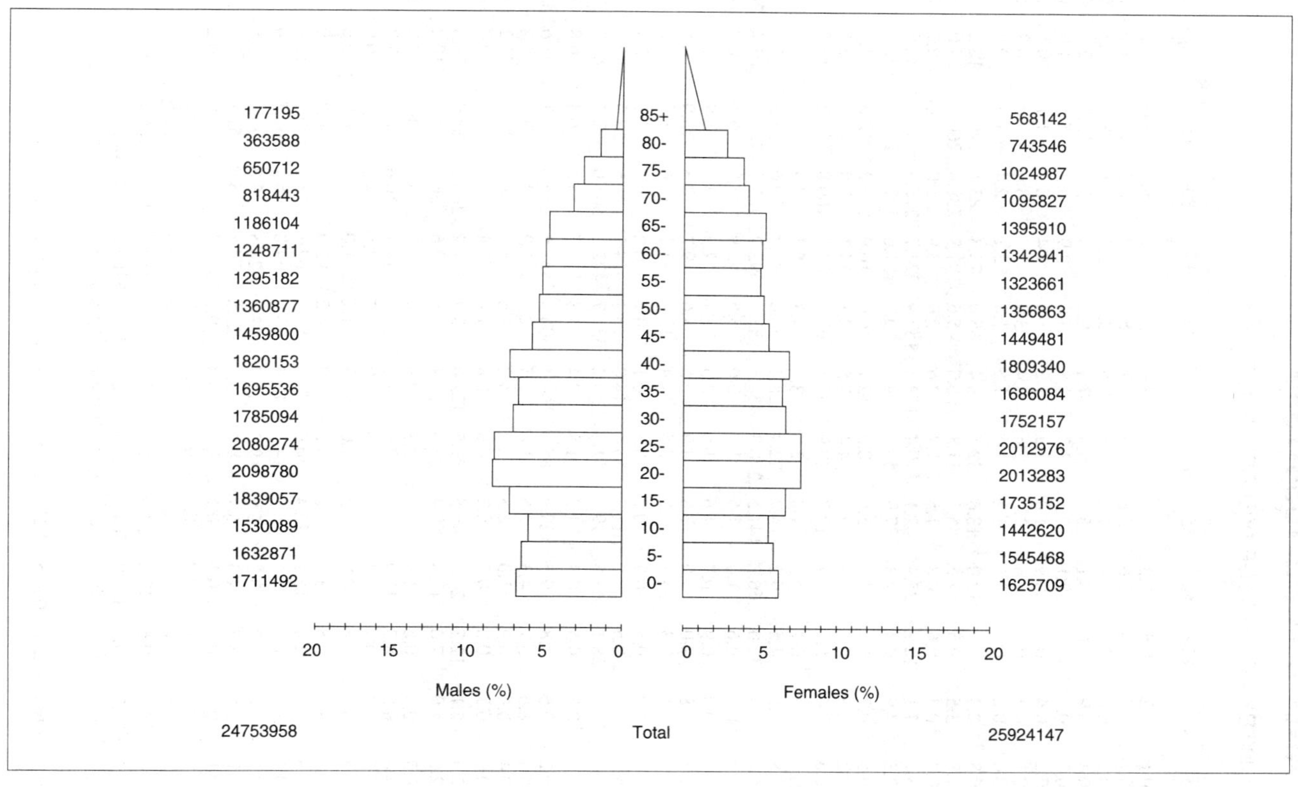

UK, England and Wales

Source of population: average annual 1988–90.

Census: 1991 Census: Usual Residence, Great Britain, OPCS. London: HMSO, 1993.

Estimate: The population estimates are derived from the Census counts. Data for the years 1988–90 were derived from the 1981 Census and subsequently adjusted to take account of the 1991 Census. Reference: OPCS Monitor, PP1 94/1

Notes to tables overleaf:

* As the national data set comprises contributions from all regional registries it necessarily includes material from those with problems of completeness and/or validity. Basis of diagnosis and DCO diagnoses are not available.

+ The editors were unable to verify these data.

*+ UK, ENGLAND AND WALES 1988-1990

ANNUAL INCIDENCE PER 100,000 BY AGE GROUP (YEARS) - MALE

SITE	ALL AGES	AGE UNK	0-	5-	10-	15-	20-	25-	30-	35-	40-	45-	50-	55-	60-	65-	70-	75-	80-	85+	CRUDE RATE	%	CR 64	CR 74	ASR (W)	ICD (9th)
Lip	543	0	-	-	-	0.0	0.0	0.0	0.0	0.1	0.2	0.4	0.8	1.0	1.6	2.9	3.8	4.4	5.8	5.6	0.7	0.2	0.02	0.05	**0.5**	*140*
Tongue	1267	2	-	-	-	0.0	0.1	0.1	0.3	0.7	1.3	1.6	2.6	3.8	4.6	5.7	6.6	6.9	6.7	10.5	1.7	0.4	0.08	0.14	**1.2**	*141*
Salivary gland	575	0	0.0	-	0.0	0.1	0.1	0.2	0.2	0.2	0.4	0.6	1.1	1.2	1.6	2.6	3.3	3.3	5.1	8.1	0.8	0.2	0.03	0.06	**0.5**	*142*
Mouth	1604	2	-	-	-	0.0	0.0	0.0	0.2	0.4	0.9	2.6	4.1	5.4	5.8	7.4	8.5	8.5	9.4	13.2	2.2	0.5	0.10	0.18	**1.5**	*143-5*
Oropharynx	769	0	-	-	-	0.0	-	0.0	0.1	0.3	0.7	1.4	2.1	2.5	3.3	3.8	3.0	2.9	4.2	5.5	1.0	0.2	0.05	0.09	**0.7**	*146*
Nasopharynx	350	0	0.0	0.0	0.1	0.3	0.1	0.1	0.2	0.2	0.4	0.6	0.9	1.0	1.3	1.2	1.5	1.4	0.8	1.1	0.5	0.1	0.03	0.04	**0.4**	*147*
Hypopharynx	674	0	-	-	-	-	-	-	0.0	0.1	0.3	0.7	1.4	2.4	2.6	3.4	3.8	3.7	3.9	7.0	0.9	0.2	0.04	0.07	**0.6**	*148*
Pharynx unspecified	330	0	0.0	0.0	0.0	-	-	0.1	0.0	0.2	0.4	0.6	1.2	1.4	1.6	2.1	2.4	1.5	0.4	0.1	0.02	0.04	**0.3**	*149*
Oesophagus	9055	0	-	-	0.0	0.0	0.0	0.2	0.3	0.8	2.3	5.9	12.0	18.6	32.5	48.4	65.0	73.3	83.1	96.7	12.2	2.9	0.36	0.93	**7.6**	*150*
Stomach	20053	6	0.0	-	0.0	0.1	0.1	0.4	0.9	1.8	3.5	9.5	17.6	35.1	61.8	100.0	145.6	191.8	238.8	260.9	27.0	6.5	0.65	1.88	**16.1**	*151*
Small intestine	531	0	0.0	-	-	0.1	-	0.0	0.1	0.2	0.3	0.6	0.8	1.5	1.7	2.6	2.9	3.9	5.0	3.6	0.7	0.2	0.03	0.05	**0.5**	*152*
Colon	23731	15	0.0	0.0	0.2	0.1	0.3	0.6	1.3	3.1	7.1	12.9	25.4	42.1	70.4	112.8	157.9	224.7	276.9	348.8	32.0	7.6	0.82	2.17	**19.3**	*153*
Rectum	17577	9	0.1	-	-	0.1	0.2	0.3	0.9	2.3	4.9	10.3	22.3	37.9	58.6	89.1	119.7	151.6	172.4	211.4	23.7	5.7	0.69	1.73	**14.6**	*154*
Liver	2320	1	0.2	0.1	0.1	0.1	0.1	0.3	0.3	0.5	0.7	1.4	2.5	5.6	8.6	12.7	16.0	16.9	17.2	22.6	3.1	0.7	0.10	0.25	**2.0**	*155*
Gallbladder etc.	1533	1	0.1	-	-	-	0.0	0.0	0.1	0.2	0.5	0.7	1.6	2.9	4.4	7.5	10.8	14.1	17.8	20.3	2.1	0.5	0.05	0.14	**1.2**	*156*
Pancreas	9049	2	0.1	-	-	-	0.1	0.2	0.4	0.6	2.4	5.3	9.7	17.7	29.9	43.5	62.3	84.3	100.8	110.2	12.2	2.9	0.33	0.86	**7.4**	*157*
Nose, sinuses etc.	705	0	0.1	0.1	0.1	0.0	0.0	0.0	0.1	0.2	0.3	0.7	1.2	1.8	2.4	3.3	4.8	5.3	4.4	4.9	0.9	0.2	0.04	0.08	**0.6**	*160*
Larynx	5002	6	0.0	-	0.0	-	-	0.1	0.2	0.8	1.6	4.6	9.2	14.7	22.4	28.4	30.6	30.7	29.6	33.3	6.7	1.6	0.27	0.56	**4.5**	*161*
Bronchus, lung	76751	21	0.0	0.0	0.0	0.1	0.2	0.2	1.0	4.1	11.9	32.0	66.2	141.5	278.3	432.6	587.4	692.2	767.7	762.2	103.4	24.7	2.68	7.78	**62.4**	*162*
Other thoracic organs	619	0	0.1	0.0	0.0	0.1	0.1	0.2	0.2	0.4	0.4	0.6	1.0	1.5	1.8	3.0	3.5	3.9	3.9	5.1	0.8	0.2	0.03	0.06	**0.6**	*163-4*
Bone	861	0	0.2	0.6	1.5	1.5	1.0	1.0	0.6	0.7	0.8	0.9	0.7	1.6	1.5	2.3	2.1	2.5	3.9	5.8	1.2	0.3	0.06	0.08	**1.0**	*170*
Connective tissue	1861	3	1.2	0.4	0.4	0.9	0.7	0.9	1.4	1.5	1.8	2.0	3.0	3.8	4.9	6.5	8.6	9.2	12.3	13.0	2.5	0.6	0.11	0.19	**1.9**	*171*
Mesothelioma	2089	0	-	-	0.0	-	-	0.0	0.0	0.3	1.1	2.3	4.4	6.8	8.8	11.4	12.3	13.1	11.6	8.7	2.8	0.7	0.12	0.24	**1.9**	*MES*
Kaposi's sarcoma	321	0	-	-	-	-	0.2	0.7	1.2	1.4	1.0	0.5	0.3	0.2	0.3	0.1	0.1	0.2	0.2	1.1	0.4	0.1	0.03	0.03	**0.4**	*KAP*
Melanoma of skin	4547	5	0.1	0.1	0.3	0.7	1.4	2.8	4.2	5.5	7.5	8.5	9.8	11.3	13.0	14.0	16.4	18.1	18.6	27.5	6.1	1.5	0.33	0.48	**4.6**	*172*
Other skin	50011	40	0.2	0.0	0.3	0.5	1.2	2.7	5.7	10.0	20.4	38.1	62.5	99.5	151.6	234.2	334.7	422.1	506.0	692.1	67.3		1.96	4.81	**42.0**	*173*
Breast	600	0	-	-	-	-	0.0	0.0	0.1	0.1	0.3	0.5	0.8	1.3	1.8	2.4	4.3	5.7	5.8	6.4	0.8	0.2	0.02	0.06	**0.5**	*175*
Prostate	38317	13	0.0	0.0	0.0	0.0	0.1	0.0	0.1	0.2	0.5	1.8	9.5	29.9	85.4	164.4	306.3	461.6	635.6	771.1	51.6	12.3	0.64	2.99	**28.0**	*185*
Testis	3859	2	0.6	0.1	0.2	2.3	7.6	11.5	12.5	10.8	8.6	5.7	4.3	2.6	1.8	1.5	2.3	1.9	2.6	7.1	5.2	1.2	0.34	0.36	**4.6**	*186*
Penis	904	0	-	-	-	-	0.0	0.1	0.1	0.4	0.6	0.9	1.0	2.3	2.2	4.2	4.6	8.1	8.6	13.2	1.2	0.3	0.04	0.08	**0.8**	*187.1-.4*
Other male genital	173	0	-	-	-	0.0	0.0	0.0	-	0.0	0.1	0.2	0.1	0.2	0.6	0.8	1.4	1.4	1.7	2.3	0.2	0.1	0.01	0.02	**0.1**	*187.5-.9*
Bladder	24741	10	0.2	0.0	0.1	0.1	0.3	0.6	1.4	2.5	5.1	12.3	24.5	46.5	81.5	122.0	178.7	217.2	268.3	354.0	33.3	8.0	0.88	2.38	**20.3**	*188*
Kidney etc.	7566	3	1.9	0.3	0.0	0.1	0.1	0.3	0.9	2.0	4.0	7.0	13.8	20.4	28.6	36.1	46.6	49.6	56.1	58.3	10.2	2.4	0.40	0.81	**6.9**	*189*
Eye	671	0	0.9	0.1	0.0	0.0	0.1	0.1	0.3	0.5	0.5	0.8	1.4	1.5	2.3	2.6	3.4	3.1	3.6	4.1	0.9	0.2	0.04	0.07	**0.7**	*190*
Brain, nervous system	5733	1	3.0	3.0	2.2	2.1	2.2	2.7	3.9	4.6	6.5	8.7	12.0	16.1	20.9	21.9	21.7	17.7	10.6	10.7	7.7	1.8	0.44	0.66	**6.3**	*191-2*
Thyroid	702	0	0.0	0.0	0.1	0.1	0.3	0.4	0.7	0.7	0.9	0.7	1.4	1.5	2.0	2.9	3.3	2.5	4.1	4.3	0.9	0.2	0.04	0.08	**0.7**	*193*
Other endocrine	442	1	1.6	0.3	0.2	0.2	0.2	0.1	0.3	0.3	0.5	0.4	0.8	0.9	1.0	1.3	1.1	1.0	1.7	0.9	0.6	0.1	0.03	0.05	**0.6**	*194*
Hodgkin's disease	2149	2	0.1	0.6	0.9	3.0	4.0	4.6	3.5	2.8	3.3	2.5	3.5	3.0	3.0	3.9	4.2	2.9	3.2	6.8	2.9	0.7	0.17	0.22	**2.5**	*201*
Non-Hodgkin lymphoma	10124	8	1.2	1.2	1.3	1.8	2.3	3.3	4.0	6.6	9.1	12.4	16.7	22.4	30.6	41.8	54.1	62.1	68.1	79.2	13.6	3.3	0.57	1.05	**9.6**	*200,202*
Multiple myeloma	4146	0	-	-	-	-	0.1	0.1	0.2	0.4	1.0	2.1	5.4	8.7	14.4	19.4	26.6	34.8	46.7	61.7	5.6	1.3	0.16	0.39	**3.4**	*203*
Lymphoid leukaemia	4105	3	5.8	3.1	1.8	1.8	1.0	0.6	0.5	0.7	1.0	1.9	3.2	5.9	9.3	15.4	22.7	28.5	39.3	68.5	5.5	1.3	0.18	0.37	**4.2**	*204*
Myeloid leukaemia	3799	0	1.0	0.6	0.6	0.7	1.0	1.3	1.5	1.9	2.5	3.2	4.3	6.1	9.4	15.1	21.6	28.8	35.0	52.1	5.1	1.2	0.17	0.35	**3.5**	*205*
Monocytic leukaemia	123	0	0.1	-	0.0	-	0.0	0.1	0.0	0.1	0.0	0.1	0.0	0.1	0.3	0.4	0.6	1.3	1.4	1.7	0.2	0.0	0.01	0.01	**0.1**	*206*
Other leukaemia	74	0	0.1	-	0.0	0.1	0.0	0.1	0.0	0.0	0.0	0.0	0.1	0.0	0.2	0.2	0.4	0.6	0.4	0.2	0.1	0.0	0.00	0.01	**0.1**	*207*
Leukaemia unspecified	517	0	0.4	0.1	0.2	0.1	0.1	0.1	0.1	0.2	0.1	0.2	0.3	0.4	1.3	1.9	2.9	4.6	5.5	12.6	0.7	0.2	0.02	0.04	**0.5**	*208*
Other and unspecified	19047	9	0.4	-	0.0	0.3	0.5	0.9	1.2	3.0	4.7	9.6	18.2	31.9	56.2	92.8	125.2	182.3	227.2	286.1	25.6	6.1	0.63	1.73	**15.4**	*O&U*
All sites	360520	165	19.8	10.9	11.0	17.4	26.2	38.0	51.3	74.3	122.2	216.5	384.9	664.2	1127.7	1732.3	2445.3	3106.7	3733.8	4482.1	485.5		13.83	34.72	**303.1**	*ALL*
All sites but 173	310509	125	19.6	10.9	10.7	16.9	25.0	35.3	45.6	64.2	101.7	178.4	322.5	564.7	976.1	1498.1	2110.6	2684.6	3227.8	3790.0	418.1	100.0	11.86	29.91	**261.1**	*ALLb*

| Rate from 10 cases | | | 0.195 | 0.204 | 0.218 | 0.181 | 0.159 | 0.160 | 0.187 | 0.197 | 0.183 | 0.228 | 0.245 | 0.257 | 0.267 | 0.281 | 0.407 | 0.512 | 0.917 | 1.881 | | | | | | |

*+ UK, ENGLAND AND WALES 1988-1990

ANNUAL INCIDENCE PER 100,000 BY AGE GROUP (YEARS) - FEMALE

SITE	ALL AGES	AGE UNK	0-	5-	10-	15-	20-	25-	30-	35-	40-	45-	50-	55-	60-	65-	70-	75-	80-	85+	CRUDE RATE	%	CR 64	CR 74	ASR (W)	ICD (9th)
Lip	157	0	-	-	-	-	-	0.0	-	-	0.1	0.0	0.2	0.3	0.1	0.5	0.6	0.9	1.0	1.8	0.2	0.0	0.00	0.01	0.1	140
Tongue	764	1	0.0	-	-	0.0	0.0	0.0	0.2	0.3	0.4	0.6	1.0	1.6	2.0	2.7	3.9	3.0	4.2	4.4	1.0	0.2	0.03	0.06	0.5	141
Salivary gland	521	1	-	-	0.1	0.1	0.1	0.2	0.2	0.4	0.5	0.4	0.5	1.3	1.0	1.8	1.6	1.8	2.4	4.0	0.7	0.2	0.02	0.04	0.4	142
Mouth	1015	1	0.0	0.0	0.0	0.0	0.1	-	0.2	0.3	0.6	0.8	1.4	1.8	3.2	3.8	4.1	4.6	5.2	6.0	1.3	0.3	0.04	0.08	0.7	143-5
Oropharynx	331	0	-	-	-	-	-	-	0.0	0.1	0.2	0.4	0.7	0.6	1.2	1.7	1.4	1.1	1.0	1.1	0.4	0.1	0.02	0.03	0.3	146
Nasopharynx	191	0	0.1	0.0	0.1	0.0	0.1	0.1	0.1	0.2	0.2	0.3	0.2	0.4	0.6	0.5	0.8	0.4	0.7	0.5	0.2	0.1	0.01	0.02	0.2	147
Hypopharynx	413	1	-	-	-	-	-	0.0	-	0.1	0.2	0.3	0.5	0.8	1.3	1.7	1.9	2.0	2.2	1.9	0.5	0.1	0.02	0.03	0.3	148
Pharynx unspecified	188	0	-	-	-	-	0.0	-	0.0	0.0	0.0	0.2	0.3	0.3	0.7	0.7	0.8	0.7	1.1	0.9	0.2	0.1	0.01	0.02	0.1	149
Oesophagus	6531	3	0.0	-	-	-	-	0.0	0.2	0.4	0.8	2.0	4.8	8.2	13.9	19.8	29.4	40.3	53.0	63.0	8.4	2.1	0.15	0.40	3.5	150
Stomach	12541	3	-	-	0.0	0.0	0.1	0.2	0.5	1.1	2.1	3.0	6.3	11.8	20.5	35.7	52.9	79.5	112.9	143.0	16.1	3.9	0.23	0.67	6.3	151
Small intestine	580	0	0.0	-	-	-	0.0	0.0	0.1	0.1	0.3	0.5	0.7	1.2	1.5	2.1	2.3	3.1	3.4	3.4	0.7	0.2	0.02	0.04	0.4	152
Colon	28073	14	0.0	0.0	0.0	0.1	0.3	0.6	1.2	2.7	7.1	12.0	22.5	38.1	58.2	87.2	121.1	165.0	210.9	276.0	36.1	8.8	0.71	1.76	15.6	153
Rectum	13781	3	0.0	-	-	0.0	0.1	0.2	0.9	1.7	3.7	7.4	14.3	21.5	32.4	45.7	61.1	77.1	94.5	114.9	17.7	4.3	0.41	0.95	8.1	154
Liver	1474	0	0.2	0.1	0.0	0.2	0.2	0.1	0.2	0.4	0.4	1.1	1.3	2.9	3.1	4.4	6.3	7.7	9.5	11.2	1.9	0.5	0.05	0.11	1.0	155
Gallbladder etc.	2226	0	0.0	-	-	-	0.0	-	0.1	0.1	0.6	0.9	1.7	3.1	4.6	7.4	9.7	13.4	18.5	18.1	2.9	0.7	0.06	0.14	1.2	156
Pancreas	9604	0	-	0.0	0.0	-	0.1	0.1	0.2	0.6	1.4	3.5	6.6	12.6	21.9	30.6	45.8	58.1	74.2	84.3	12.3	3.0	0.24	0.62	5.3	157
Nose, sinuses etc.	498	1	0.0	0.0	0.0	0.0	-	0.0	0.1	0.2	0.3	0.4	0.5	0.9	1.3	1.5	2.0	2.4	3.0	3.1	0.6	0.2	0.02	0.04	0.3	160
Larynx	1106	0	-	-	-	-	-	0.0	0.1	0.1	0.5	0.9	1.5	3.3	4.0	5.6	4.9	4.4	4.2	3.1	1.4	0.3	0.05	0.10	0.8	161
Bronchus, lung	34917	10	0.1	0.0	0.0	0.1	0.1	0.3	1.0	2.5	7.9	16.4	31.6	62.4	123.9	163.7	186.1	182.9	170.0	140.9	44.9	11.0	1.23	2.98	22.8	162
Other thoracic organs	381	0	0.1	-	0.1	0.0	0.0	0.0	0.2	0.1	0.2	0.3	0.6	0.6	1.2	1.4	1.6	1.8	1.3	1.9	0.5	0.1	0.02	0.03	0.3	163-4
Bone	673	0	0.2	0.5	1.3	1.1	0.5	0.5	0.5	0.5	0.6	0.5	0.6	0.7	0.8	1.3	1.9	1.5	2.7	2.8	0.9	0.2	0.04	0.06	0.7	170
Connective tissue	1694	0	0.9	0.4	0.6	0.9	0.8	0.9	1.0	1.1	1.6	1.9	2.3	2.8	3.8	4.0	4.8	5.9	7.1	9.1	2.2	0.5	0.10	0.14	1.5	171
Mesothelioma	378	0	-	-	-	-	-	0.0	0.0	0.0	0.1	0.3	0.4	0.7	0.9	1.1	1.8	2.1	1.7	1.0	0.8	0.5	0.1	0.02	0.04	0.3	MES
Kaposi's sarcoma	16	0	-	-	-	-	-	0.0	-	0.0	-	0.0	-	-	0.0	0.0	-	0.1	0.1	0.2	0.0	0.0	0.00	0.00	0.0	KAP
Melanoma of skin	7160	6	0.1	0.1	0.2	1.3	3.3	5.2	7.6	9.3	11.6	14.1	13.3	13.8	16.2	17.2	18.3	18.7	16.7	24.8	9.2	2.3	0.48	0.66	6.6	172
Other skin	46567	45	0.2	0.1	0.4	0.8	1.5	3.6	6.6	12.4	21.9	33.5	51.6	67.8	95.7	145.6	207.2	255.6	298.8	378.1	59.9		1.48	3.25	28.6	173
Breast	84649	52	0.1	-	-	0.2	1.3	7.5	23.4	55.0	101.8	156.9	190.7	221.5	261.9	250.7	271.5	269.5	285.5	381.8	108.8	26.6	5.10	7.72	68.8	174
Uterus unspecified	1176	0	-	-	-	0.0	0.1	0.1	0.2	0.4	0.7	1.0	2.0	2.7	3.0	3.5	4.6	5.2	5.9	8.7	1.5	0.4	0.05	0.09	0.8	179
Cervix uteri	13000	6	0.0	0.0	-	0.2	2.3	10.1	22.4	29.2	24.8	24.1	24.2	25.0	28.0	31.7	32.6	24.4	21.7	26.6	16.7	4.1	0.95	1.27	12.5	180
Placenta	20	0	-	-	-	0.1	0.0	0.1	0.1	0.1	0.0	-	-	-	-	-	-	-	-	-	0.0	0.0	0.00	0.00	0.0	181
Corpus uteri	11369	3	0.0	-	-	0.0	0.0	0.1	0.8	2.3	4.9	11.0	25.4	37.6	41.9	43.1	44.8	43.1	39.9	43.7	14.6	3.6	0.62	1.06	8.6	182
Ovary etc.	15483	7	0.2	0.1	0.6	1.1	1.4	2.6	3.5	6.8	12.1	21.1	33.6	41.3	50.7	54.8	56.8	54.7	52.9	56.6	19.9	4.9	0.88	1.43	12.4	183
Other female genital	3319	2	0.1	0.0	0.0	0.0	0.1	0.4	0.5	0.8	1.3	1.9	2.9	3.8	5.9	9.6	13.4	19.0	25.8	32.2	4.3	1.0	0.09	0.20	1.9	184
Bladder	9897	7	0.1	0.0	0.0	0.1	0.2	0.3	0.5	1.2	2.0	3.3	8.7	14.4	23.3	35.2	45.3	57.2	68.7	81.4	12.7	3.1	0.27	0.67	5.7	188
Kidney etc.	4510	0	1.8	0.4	0.1	0.2	0.1	0.2	0.6	1.2	1.9	3.6	5.9	8.8	13.3	17.2	19.4	21.8	22.4	20.9	5.8	1.4	0.19	0.37	3.3	189
Eye	699	0	0.9	0.1	0.1	0.1	0.1	0.2	0.3	0.4	0.6	0.9	1.3	1.4	1.8	2.1	2.3	2.2	2.5	2.8	0.9	0.2	0.04	0.06	0.6	190
Brain, nervous system	4454	1	2.7	2.6	1.7	1.6	1.6	2.1	2.9	3.7	4.9	5.5	7.9	12.1	12.8	14.9	13.2	10.9	7.4	5.5	5.7	1.4	0.31	0.45	4.5	191-2
Thyroid	1913	2	0.0	0.0	0.2	0.6	1.2	1.9	2.5	2.6	2.5	2.9	3.1	3.1	3.5	4.6	5.1	5.3	5.2	7.0	2.5	0.6	0.12	0.17	1.7	193
Other endocrine	413	0	1.4	0.5	0.1	0.1	0.2	0.2	0.3	0.4	0.4	0.4	0.7	0.7	0.9	1.0	0.9	0.7	0.5	0.7	0.5	0.1	0.03	0.04	0.5	194
Hodgkin's disease	1564	0	0.0	0.3	0.7	3.0	4.1	3.1	2.6	2.4	1.3	1.2	1.4	2.0	1.8	2.1	2.1	2.7	2.2	2.8	2.0	0.5	0.12	0.14	1.8	201
Non-Hodgkin lymphoma	8828	6	0.7	0.5	0.5	1.0	1.2	1.5	2.3	3.8	6.2	8.3	11.7	17.3	20.4	29.7	37.0	42.7	43.9	45.7	11.4	2.8	0.38	0.71	6.3	200,202
Multiple myeloma	4036	3	-	-	-	-	-	0.0	0.1	0.3	0.8	1.8	3.4	6.0	9.6	13.6	19.3	24.1	27.3	33.4	5.2	1.3	0.11	0.27	2.3	203
Lymphoid leukaemia	3002	1	5.2	2.2	1.4	0.7	0.4	0.4	0.6	0.4	0.6	1.0	1.8	2.7	4.3	6.8	10.4	15.0	19.7	29.2	3.9	0.9	0.11	0.19	2.4	204
Myeloid leukaemia	3489	1	0.8	0.5	0.6	0.7	0.8	1.2	1.5	1.3	2.3	2.6	4.0	5.3	6.5	9.5	12.6	16.6	20.2	26.3	4.5	1.1	0.14	0.25	2.5	205
Monocytic leukaemia	124	0	0.1	-	-	0.0	0.0	0.0	0.0	-	0.1	0.1	0.1	0.2	0.4	0.1	0.6	0.5	0.9	1.2	0.2	0.0	0.00	0.01	0.1	206
Other leukaemia	58	0	0.1	0.0	0.0	-	0.0	0.0	-	0.0	0.0	0.0	0.0	0.0	0.1	0.1	0.3	0.2	0.6	0.4	0.1	0.0	0.00	0.00	0.0	207
Leukaemia unspecified	489	0	0.3	0.1	0.1	0.1	0.1	0.0	0.1	0.1	0.1	0.2	0.2	0.6	0.7	0.8	1.8	2.4	3.3	7.3	0.6	0.2	0.01	0.03	0.3	208
Other and unspecified	20270	5	0.5	0.1	0.1	0.2	0.3	0.6	1.2	2.0	4.5	8.3	14.0	26.0	43.1	64.8	86.1	116.6	153.5	205.7	26.1	6.4	0.50	1.26	11.2	O&U
All sites	364542	185	17.0	9.0	9.4	14.6	23.5	45.0	87.5	148.9	237.3	358.4	509.0	692.2	948.1	1184.6	1452.8	1668.4	1909.7	2319.4	468.7		15.51	28.70	254.1	ALL
All sites but 173	317975	140	16.9	8.9	9.0	13.8	22.0	41.4	80.9	136.5	215.4	324.9	457.4	624.4	852.4	1039.0	1245.5	1412.8	1610.9	1941.3	408.9	100.0	14.03	25.45	225.5	ALLb
Rate from 10 cases			0.205	0.216	0.231	0.192	0.166	0.166	0.190	0.198	0.184	0.230	0.246	0.252	0.248	0.239	0.304	0.325	0.448	0.587						

UK, England, Birmingham and West Midlands

Cancer registration in Birmingham dates back to 1936. Based originally on a single hospital in the city, its scope was gradually extended until by 1957 it included the whole region. The outer boundaries of the West Midlands Region remained unchanged during a major reorganization of local government areas in 1974 and a reorganization of health authority boundaries accompanying the replacement of Regional Health Authorities with Regional Offices in April 1996. The region spans an area of 13 014 km^2 and lies between latitudes 52°8′ and 53°0′ N and longitudes 1°10′ and 3°3′ W.

The registration area covered in 1990 a population of 5 200 000 people (11% of the total of 47.8 million in England). There are marked differences in population density across the region, with very densely populated urban areas such as the Birmingham/Black Country conurbation, Coventry and Stoke on Trent, contrasting markedly with more sparsely populated rural areas in Hereford, Shropshire and parts of Worcestershire and South Staffordshire. The region includes a sizeable proportion of members of ethnic groups other than the indigenous English and Irish, due to immigration from the Indian subcontinent and Africa of Asians, and of West Indians from the Caribbean. The 1991 census provided, for the first time, information about the ethnic composition of the population in terms of a self-assessed definition of ethnic group, as opposed to the country of origin data collected previously. These data indicate that non-white residents make up 8% of the total West Midlands population and that, of these, 24% are Black Caribbean, African or other black origin, 37% are of Indian origin, 23% are of Pakistani origin and 10% are of other Asian origin. Some districts within the West Midlands have a high proportion of ethnic minority groups. For example in West Birmingham over 11% of the population is Black Caribbean, 14% Indian, nearly 7% Pakistani and 3% Bangladeshi. Other districts with large ethnic minorities include Wolverhampton, Sandwell, East and South Birmingham and Coventry.

Cases are mainly registered following receipt of notification forms onto which clerical staff at individual hospitals extract specified items from hospital inpatient and outpatient records, radiotherapy notes and histopathology reports. These forms are usually sent to the registry accompanied by copies of relevant histopathology reports and clinical case notes, such as radiotherapy reports. The information collected includes patient demographic details (name, date of birth, sex, residence, marital status, occupation etc.), tumour characteristics (size, extent, nodes, metastases, stage etc.) and details of the clinicians and hospitals involved in treatment and the nature of the treatment given. Copies of death certificates are routinely received from the Office of National Statistics (ONS; formerly OPCS) for all cases where cancer is mentioned either as a cause of death or as present at the time of death. If no further information is received after six months, additional details are sought from Family Health Service Authorities (to whom all general practitioner records are returned after a patient's death) and hospitals contacted to obtain relevant admission and treatment details. Non-cancer deaths are provided routinely by the National Health Service Central Register where all registered cancer patients are flagged. Active follow-up of patients is carried out for specific research studies but not on a routine basis.

In 1994, in conjunction with the introduction of a new Sun microcomputer and an Oracle relational database, the registry's existing tumour-based records were converted to a patient-based system in which all patients have a unique identifier and individual patients can have several tumours each with a unique tumour number. This has increased the ease and speed with which registrations can be made and has facilitated the implementation of more complex validation and data-quality checks in line with those recommended by IARC and ONS.

The registry's database is used for routine data provision and for clinical audit and research purposes. Studies are undertaken by the in-house research and information team together with external collaborators from hospitals, teaching establishments and district health authorities. The registry is also involved in the EUROCARE study of cancer survival and contributes data to EUROCIM. The incorporation of the National Breast and Cervical Screening Quality Assurance Services within the existing structure in April 1996 has allowed the synergistic combination of registration and screening databases. The first major outcome of this has been the establishment of a routine system for obtaining breast screening histories for all women in the screening age band, including the determination of interval cancer rates and rates in non-attenders. The merger has also led to a change of name for the registry, which has become the West Midlands Cancer Intelligence Unit.

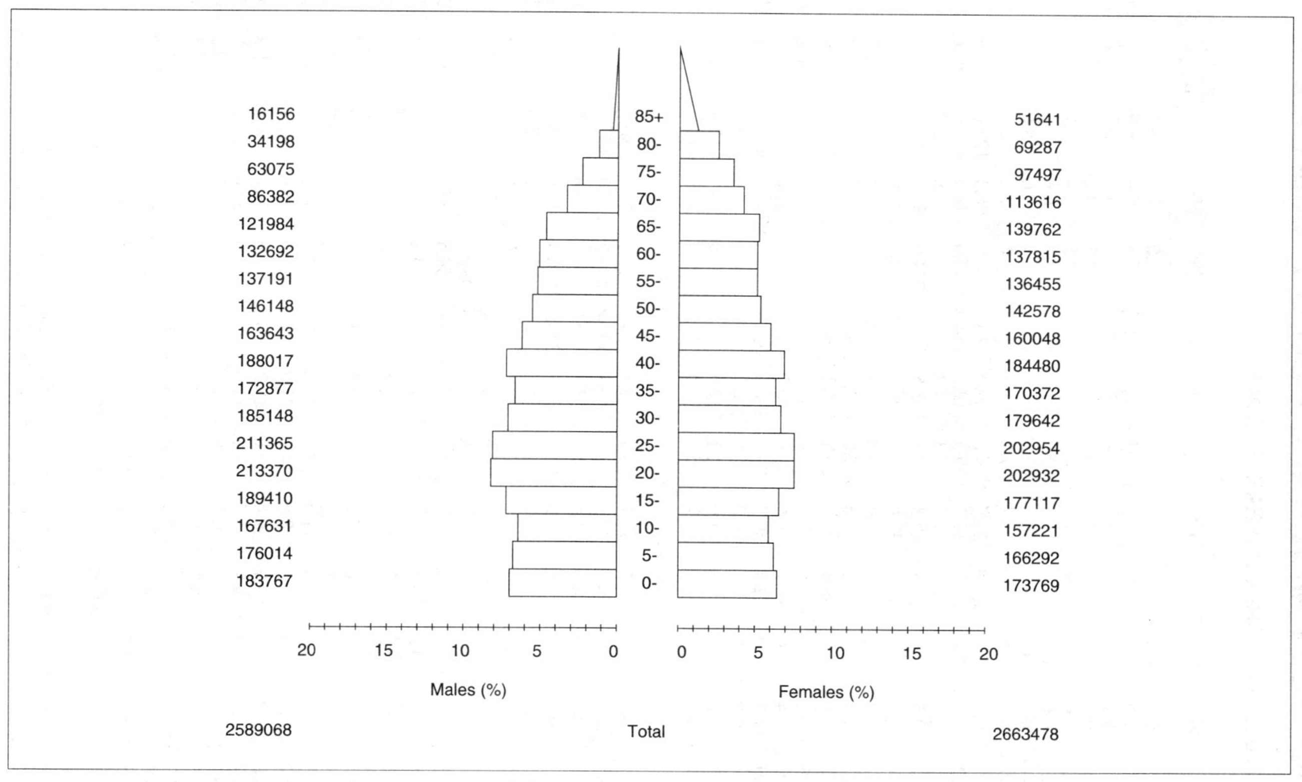

UK, England, West Midlands
Source of population: average annual 1988–1992
Census: 1991 Census: Usual Residence, Great Britain, OPCS. London: HMSO, 1993.
Estimate: The population for each year are OPCS (ONS) estimates modified on the basis of the 1991 Census.
Notes to data overleaf:
* Because neither histology nor basis of diagnosis were systematically recorded by the registry during the period, the editors were unable to evaluate the validity of these data.
+ The editors were unable to verify these data
† 163-164 includes mesothelioma of the pleura
† Mesothelioma not available seperately
† Kaposi's sarcoma not available seperately

Screening programmes in the area:
Women aged 20-64 have been screened since the 1960s for cervical cancer at 3 or 5 yearly intervals, and breast cancer screening commenced during the period 1988-91 for women aged 50-64, at 3 yearly intervals.

*+ UK, ENGLAND, BIRMINGHAM AND WEST MIDLANDS REGION 1988-1992

ANNUAL INCIDENCE PER 100,000 BY AGE GROUP (YEARS) - MALE

SITE	ALL AGES	AGE UNK	0-	5-	10-	15-	20-	25-	30-	35-	40-	45-	50-	55-	60-	65-	70-	75-	80-	85+	CRUDE RATE	%	CR 64	CR 74	ASR (W)	ICD (9th)
Lip	31	0	-	-	-	-	-	-	-	-	0.1	0.1	0.5	0.6	0.5	0.7	2.1	1.0	1.2	-	0.2	0.1	0.01	0.02	**0.2**	*140*
Tongue	241	0	-	-	-	-	0.1	0.5	0.2	0.8	1.6	2.8	2.5	4.2	4.7	6.1	6.7	7.9	6.4	9.9	1.9	0.4	0.09	0.15	**1.3**	*141*
Salivary gland	79	0	-	-	0.1	-	-	0.1	0.1	0.2	0.1	0.5	1.5	1.3	1.4	1.3	1.9	4.1	4.7	3.7	0.6	0.1	0.03	0.04	**0.4**	*142*
Mouth	320	0	-	-	-	-	-	-	0.3	0.8	0.7	3.9	4.8	5.2	8.1	10.2	7.6	8.6	9.4	9.9	2.5	0.6	0.12	0.21	**1.8**	*143-5*
Oropharynx	149	0	-	-	-	0.1	-	-	-	0.2	1.0	2.1	1.9	1.9	4.5	3.8	4.9	3.5	2.9	3.7	1.2	0.3	0.06	0.10	**0.8**	*146*
Nasopharynx	67	0	-	0.3	0.1	0.2	0.3	-	0.1	0.3	0.6	0.4	1.2	1.3	0.9	1.1	1.2	2.5	0.6	-	0.5	0.1	0.03	0.04	**0.4**	*147*
Hypopharynx	142	0	-	-	-	-	-	-	0.2	-	0.1	0.5	2.3	2.5	2.7	4.9	4.4	5.7	7.0	5.0	1.1	0.2	0.04	0.09	**0.7**	*148*
Pharynx unspecified	53	0	-	-	-	-	-	-	-	0.1	0.1	0.5	0.3	0.7	1.8	1.3	1.9	1.6	3.5	1.2	0.4	0.1	0.02	0.03	**0.3**	*149*
Oesophagus	1889	0	-	-	-	-	0.1	0.1	0.2	0.6	2.7	8.1	14.9	24.5	39.6	60.0	80.8	84.7	98.3	122.6	14.6	3.3	0.45	1.16	**9.4**	*150*
Stomach	3769	0	-	-	0.1	-	-	0.7	0.9	1.9	4.0	8.8	20.1	39.2	69.5	112.6	154.4	215.0	288.3	278.5	29.1	6.5	0.73	2.06	**17.8**	*151*
Small intestine	143	0	0.1	-	-	-	-	-	0.3	0.1	0.6	0.5	1.8	1.7	2.3	4.9	5.1	6.7	5.8	6.2	1.1	0.2	0.04	0.09	**0.7**	*152*
Colon	4912	0	0.1	-	0.1	0.3	0.2	1.1	1.4	5.1	9.5	17.1	30.4	49.3	89.1	138.5	203.1	274.9	333.9	366.4	37.9	8.5	1.02	2.73	**23.7**	*153*
Rectum	3539	0	-	-	-	-	0.3	0.8	1.2	2.7	5.9	13.2	29.4	45.6	71.6	106.2	148.9	166.1	200.0	211.7	27.3	6.1	0.85	2.13	**17.5**	*154*
Liver	344	0	0.4	0.1	0.1	0.1	0.4	0.2	0.8	0.7	0.9	2.0	3.0	6.0	5.9	10.5	10.9	14.6	15.2	11.1	2.7	0.6	0.10	0.21	**1.8**	*155*
Gallbladder etc.	416	0	-	-	-	-	-	0.1	0.1	0.2	1.2	1.7	3.1	3.5	7.8	12.0	18.5	20.9	24.6	33.4	3.2	0.7	0.09	0.24	**2.0**	*156*
Pancreas	1542	0	-	-	-	-	-	0.1	0.2	0.4	0.5	2.0	5.3	9.4	16.9	30.1	45.1	63.0	87.8	104.1	101.5	11.9	2.7	0.32	0.87	**7.4**	*157*
Nose, sinuses etc.	108	0	0.1	-	-	-	-	0.2	0.2	0.5	0.9	0.9	1.5	1.2	2.1	3.8	2.5	3.8	2.9	-	0.8	0.2	0.04	0.07	**0.6**	*160*
Larynx	943	0	-	-	-	-	-	-	0.2	0.9	2.4	5.0	10.7	16.6	22.6	30.7	38.4	31.7	31.6	24.8	7.3	1.6	0.29	0.64	**4.9**	*161*
Bronchus, lung	13780	0	-	-	-	-	0.1	0.3	0.8	4.0	11.4	29.9	72.4	150.2	289.2	490.9	634.2	722.9	786.6	675.9	106.4	23.9	2.79	8.42	**65.9**	*162*
†Other thoracic organs	306	0	0.3	-	-	0.2	0.4	-	0.1	0.3	0.9	3.4	3.4	5.0	6.6	8.7	9.0	11.1	9.4	13.6	2.4	0.5	0.10	0.19	**1.7**	*163-4*
Bone	277	0	0.4	2.8	4.9	5.1	2.8	1.4	0.9	1.5	1.8	1.5	0.8	1.9	1.1	2.6	1.4	1.9	4.7	2.5	2.1	0.5	0.13	0.15	**2.2**	*170*
Connective tissue	426	0	0.7	0.3	0.5	1.4	1.3	1.7	1.9	3.1	2.7	3.2	4.1	5.7	5.3	7.5	13.4	9.5	12.9	14.9	3.3	0.7	0.16	0.26	**2.5**	*171*
†Mesothelioma																										
†Kaposi's sarcoma																										
Melanoma of skin	771	0	0.1	-	-	0.5	1.2	2.1	3.6	4.4	6.5	10.3	11.2	11.2	13.1	12.1	14.6	20.0	25.1	30.9	6.0	1.3	0.32	0.45	**4.5**	*172*
Other skin	10802	0	0.2	0.1	0.2	0.5	1.4	2.5	6.3	14.8	26.2	53.5	80.7	130.8	197.1	284.1	432.5	529.5	689.5	787.3	83.4		2.57	6.16	**53.5**	*173*
Breast	104	0	-	-	-	-	-	-	0.1	0.2	0.2	0.4	0.8	1.6	1.5	3.0	6.0	4.1	5.8	2.5	0.8	0.2	0.02	0.07	**0.5**	*175*
Prostate	7229	0	-	-	0.1	0.1	-	-	-	-	0.4	3.3	11.8	31.5	91.5	185.3	359.6	550.4	717.6	793.5	55.8	12.5	0.69	3.42	**31.6**	*185*
Testis	664	0	0.8	-	-	1.7	8.2	12.5	13.3	9.3	8.4	5.5	4.1	3.2	2.1	1.6	2.1	1.6	1.8	2.5	5.1	1.2	0.34	0.36	**4.6**	*186*
Penis	177	0	-	-	-	-	-	0.1	0.2	0.3	1.0	0.7	2.5	4.1	2.0	3.3	5.6	8.6	7.6	16.1	1.4	0.3	0.05	0.10	**0.9**	*187.1-.4*
Other male genital	30	0	-	-	-	-	0.2	-	0.1	-	0.1	0.1	-	0.1	0.6	0.8	1.6	1.3	1.8	1.2	0.2	0.1	0.01	0.02	**0.1**	*187.5-.9*
Bladder	4498	0	0.2	-	-	0.2	0.5	0.3	1.3	3.0	6.4	12.8	28.6	51.9	87.6	133.5	184.1	258.1	271.4	309.5	34.7	7.8	0.96	2.55	**21.7**	*188*
Kidney etc.	1395	0	2.3	0.5	0.1	-	0.1	0.2	1.2	2.5	4.0	7.0	16.0	21.7	31.8	37.1	51.6	54.5	55.6	55.7	10.8	2.4	0.44	0.88	**7.4**	*189*
Eye	91	0	1.4	0.3	0.1	-	0.2	-	0.1	0.5	0.5	0.5	0.8	1.3	1.4	1.1	2.5	3.2	3.5	-	0.7	0.2	0.04	0.05	**0.6**	*190*
Brain, nervous system	998	0	3.3	3.1	3.2	2.2	2.6	3.7	4.0	4.9	7.2	9.8	11.8	14.7	18.5	18.2	22.5	20.0	6.4	8.7	7.7	1.7	0.44	0.65	**6.4**	*191-2*
Thyroid	137	0	-	-	-	0.3	0.6	0.4	0.9	1.3	1.0	0.7	1.8	2.2	1.5	3.0	3.5	3.5	3.5	2.5	1.1	0.2	0.05	0.08	**0.8**	*193*
Other endocrine	153	0	2.5	0.3	0.4	0.1	0.6	0.6	0.5	0.8	0.7	1.6	1.6	2.6	2.4	2.3	1.2	2.2	1.8	5.0	1.2	0.3	0.07	0.09	**1.1**	*194*
Hodgkin's disease	397	0	0.1	1.2	1.2	3.4	3.9	5.3	3.3	2.8	3.1	3.4	3.1	3.8	3.5	3.3	5.8	1.6	4.7	3.7	3.1	0.7	0.19	0.24	**2.8**	*201*
Non-Hodgkin lymphoma	1563	0	1.6	1.0	1.1	2.5	2.1	2.6	2.8	6.5	7.4	12.1	15.5	21.9	27.9	38.0	47.0	53.3	65.5	52.0	12.1	2.7	0.53	0.95	**8.7**	*200,202*
Multiple myeloma	749	0	-	-	-	-	-	-	0.1	0.2	1.5	2.1	5.3	8.6	14.5	21.0	27.3	45.3	38.6	81.7	5.8	1.3	0.16	0.40	**3.7**	*203*
Lymphoid leukaemia	747	0	7.3	3.2	1.4	2.0	0.7	0.8	0.8	0.8	1.7	2.9	3.7	9.0	9.6	15.2	23.2	31.4	36.8	54.5	5.8	1.3	0.22	0.41	**4.6**	*204*
Myeloid leukaemia	615	0	0.9	0.3	0.6	1.2	1.2	1.4	1.1	2.7	2.8	3.4	4.4	5.7	7.1	14.6	19.2	32.0	31.6	34.7	4.8	1.1	0.16	0.33	**3.3**	*205*
Monocytic leukaemia	29	0	-	-	0.1	-	0.1	-	-	-	0.1	-	-	0.1	0.9	1.0	0.7	1.6	1.2	3.7	0.2	0.1	0.01	0.02	**0.2**	*206*
Other leukaemia	14	0	0.1	-	-	-	-	-	-	-	0.1	-	0.1	0.3	-	0.7	0.7	0.6	-	-	0.1	0.0	0.00	0.01	**0.1**	*207*
Leukaemia unspecified	152	0	0.7	0.1	0.1	0.2	0.1	0.1	0.2	0.3	0.5	1.0	0.7	1.2	2.3	3.1	5.6	6.7	13.5	8.7	1.2	0.3	0.04	0.08	**0.8**	*208*
Other and unspecified	3628	0	0.2	0.1	0.4	1.0	1.0	1.1	0.5	3.0	6.1	11.1	20.9	34.6	69.3	99.8	144.9	210.2	252.6	286.0	28.0	6.3	0.75	1.97	**17.5**	*O&U*
All sites	68419	0	23.8	14.0	15.0	23.3	30.6	40.9	50.8	82.9	136.9	253.6	445.7	747.1	1253.6	1945.5	2775.8	3526.2	4189.7	4436.6	528.5		15.59	39.20	**339.5**	*ALL*
All sites but 173	57617	0	23.6	13.9	14.8	22.8	29.2	38.4	44.5	68.1	110.7	200.1	365.0	616.4	1056.4	1661.4	2343.3	2996.7	3500.2	3649.3	445.1	100.0	13.02	33.04	**286.0**	*ALLb*

| Rate from 1 case | | | 0.109 | 0.114 | 0.119 | 0.106 | 0.094 | 0.095 | 0.108 | 0.116 | 0.106 | 0.122 | 0.137 | 0.146 | 0.151 | 0.164 | 0.232 | 0.317 | 0.585 | 1.238 |

†Important: see notes on population page

*+ UK, ENGLAND, BIRMINGHAM AND WEST MIDLANDS REGION 1988-1992

ANNUAL INCIDENCE PER 100,000 BY AGE GROUP (YEARS) - FEMALE

SITE	ALL AGES	AGE UNK	0-	5-	10-	15-	20-	25-	30-	35-	40-	45-	50-	55-	60-	65-	70-	75-	80-	85+	CRUDE RATE	%	CR 64	CR 74	ASR (W)	ICD (9th)
Lip	11	0	-	-	-	-	-	-	-	-	-	-	0.1	0.1	0.1	-	0.2	0.4	0.3	1.5	0.1	0.0	0.00	0.00	**0.0**	140
Tongue	127	0	-	-	-	0.1	-	-	0.1	0.4	0.5	0.6	0.8	2.1	1.6	2.0	3.9	2.3	5.2	6.2	1.0	0.2	0.03	0.06	**0.5**	141
Salivary gland	63	0	-	-	-	0.2	0.1	0.1	0.1	0.1	0.2	0.1	0.4	1.0	0.9	0.9	0.9	1.8	2.6	3.5	0.5	0.1	0.02	0.03	**0.3**	142
Mouth	169	0	-	-	-	-	0.1	-	0.1	0.2	0.3	1.0	1.7	2.6	1.9	2.7	5.1	5.3	6.9	5.0	1.3	0.3	0.04	0.08	**0.7**	143-5
Oropharynx	44	0	-	-	-	-	-	-	-	0.1	-	0.2	0.4	1.0	0.9	1.6	1.4	0.2	0.9	0.8	0.3	0.1	0.01	0.03	**0.2**	146
Nasopharynx	31	0	0.1	-	-	0.1	0.3	-	-	0.1	0.2	0.2	0.3	0.7	0.4	0.4	0.5	0.8	0.3	-	0.2	0.1	0.01	0.02	**0.2**	147
Hypopharynx	72	0	-	-	-	-	-	0.1	-	0.1	0.1	0.5	1.0	0.6	1.5	1.9	2.6	2.1	1.4	0.4	0.5	0.1	0.02	0.04	**0.3**	148
Pharynx unspecified	26	0	-	-	-	-	0.1	-	-	-	-	-	-	0.4	0.4	0.7	0.5	0.4	1.4	1.5	0.2	0.0	0.00	0.01	**0.1**	149
Oesophagus	1271	0	-	-	-	-	-	0.2	0.2	0.5	0.9	3.1	6.9	10.6	16.0	23.2	35.2	45.9	65.2	72.4	9.5	2.2	0.19	0.48	**4.2**	150
Stomach	2263	0	0.1	-	-	-	0.2	0.2	0.9	1.3	3.6	4.1	7.0	12.0	23.7	38.1	56.9	89.8	127.0	159.2	17.0	4.0	0.27	0.74	**7.0**	151
Small intestine	105	0	-	-	-	-	-	-	0.2	0.1	0.3	-	0.4	1.2	1.6	2.3	3.3	2.5	4.9	5.0	0.8	0.2	0.02	0.05	**0.4**	152
Colon	5212	0	-	-	-	-	0.3	0.8	0.8	4.0	8.0	15.7	23.6	43.2	70.5	106.0	142.1	183.4	240.2	285.4	39.1	9.2	0.83	2.08	**18.0**	153
Rectum	2438	0	-	-	-	-	-	0.4	1.0	1.6	5.3	9.1	16.6	22.4	34.5	51.1	62.3	84.9	106.2	111.2	18.3	4.3	0.45	1.02	**8.9**	154
Liver	162	0	0.2	0.2	0.3	0.2	0.2	0.2	0.1	0.2	0.1	0.4	1.0	2.5	2.8	3.4	4.2	3.7	5.5	5.8	1.2	0.3	0.04	0.08	**0.7**	155
Gallbladder etc.	519	0	-	-	-	-	-	0.1	-	0.1	0.7	2.1	3.1	4.0	7.5	10.4	13.7	21.1	20.2	26.7	3.9	0.9	0.09	0.21	**1.8**	156
Pancreas	1558	0	-	-	-	-	0.3	0.4	0.2	0.5	1.0	3.2	5.9	12.6	22.6	29.8	43.8	59.3	72.5	88.7	11.7	2.7	0.23	0.60	**5.2**	157
Nose, sinuses etc.	95	0	0.1	-	0.1	-	-	-	0.4	0.4	0.3	0.1	1.0	0.9	1.3	1.9	1.6	2.7	2.6	6.2	0.7	0.2	0.02	0.04	**0.4**	160
Larynx	191	0	-	-	-	0.1	-	-	-	0.1	0.7	1.1	1.4	4.3	3.9	6.3	4.6	4.7	3.5	1.2	1.4	0.3	0.06	0.11	**0.9**	161
Bronchus, lung	5447	0	-	-	-	-	-	0.3	0.7	2.5	6.9	15.9	29.0	56.9	117.8	156.1	182.0	175.6	158.8	111.5	40.9	9.6	1.15	2.84	**21.5**	162
†Other thoracic organs	86	0	0.1	-	-	-	0.1	-	-	-	0.2	0.2	0.8	1.3	2.0	2.9	2.5	2.1	1.2	1.2	0.6	0.2	0.02	0.05	**0.4**	163-4
Bone	218	0	-	1.4	4.6	3.8	2.5	1.3	0.6	1.4	1.2	0.9	1.4	0.4	1.3	1.7	1.6	1.6	2.3	1.5	1.6	0.4	0.10	0.12	**1.7**	170
Connective tissue	410	0	0.3	0.6	0.3	1.4	2.2	2.1	1.6	2.9	2.7	3.6	3.2	4.1	5.4	7.4	4.9	6.4	8.1	9.7	3.1	0.7	0.15	0.21	**2.2**	171
†Mesothelioma																										
†Kaposi's sarcoma																										
Melanoma of skin	1111	0	0.2	-	0.4	1.5	3.1	4.2	6.5	9.0	13.2	13.0	12.5	12.6	14.4	12.6	17.1	19.7	14.7	20.1	8.3	2.0	0.45	0.60	**6.1**	172
Other skin	10046	0	0.9	-	0.5	0.8	2.2	4.4	9.0	16.9	30.5	46.7	68.0	90.0	128.6	180.9	268.4	346.7	404.4	470.5	75.4		1.99	4.24	**37.7**	173
Breast	15779	0	0.2	-	-	0.1	0.9	8.2	28.3	63.2	110.3	181.6	230.6	254.0	309.8	267.6	284.6	300.5	317.8	331.9	118.5	27.8	5.94	8.70	**77.8**	174
Uterus unspecified	257	0	-	-	-	-	0.2	-	0.3	1.1	1.5	1.7	2.8	3.1	3.0	5.6	4.8	6.2	7.2	12.4	1.9	0.5	0.07	0.12	**1.1**	179
Cervix uteri	2306	0	-	-	-	0.2	4.1	15.3	32.4	38.5	27.1	23.2	22.3	25.5	26.4	27.2	26.1	20.3	17.6	15.1	17.3	4.1	1.08	1.34	**13.7**	180
Placenta	9	0	-	-	-	0.2	-	0.4	0.1	0.1	0.1	-	-	-	-	-	-	-	-	-	0.1	0.0	0.00	0.00	**0.1**	181
Corpus uteri	2241	0	-	-	-	-	-	0.1	0.9	2.0	4.0	12.6	30.0	44.6	53.7	51.2	52.6	49.2	49.6	46.5	16.8	4.0	0.74	1.26	**10.2**	182
Ovary etc.	2935	0	0.2	0.1	0.8	1.0	2.1	3.6	4.3	10.0	14.7	21.0	37.6	48.8	59.2	58.5	61.8	63.0	60.0	56.9	22.0	5.2	1.02	1.62	**14.1**	183
Other female genital	621	0	0.1	-	-	0.1	0.1	0.7	1.2	2.1	2.4	2.1	3.5	4.4	5.9	8.7	16.0	24.6	22.8	37.2	4.7	1.1	0.11	0.24	**2.3**	184
Bladder	1673	0	0.3	-	-	-	0.1	0.3	0.6	1.2	1.6	4.2	10.4	16.4	25.0	37.2	45.1	58.3	63.2	87.1	12.6	3.0	0.30	0.71	**6.1**	188
Kidney etc.	764	0	0.9	0.5	-	0.1	0.1	0.2	0.8	0.8	3.4	4.0	7.0	11.3	13.8	18.5	18.1	16.8	25.1	18.6	5.7	1.3	0.21	0.40	**3.4**	189
Eye	104	0	1.5	0.4	-	-	-	-	0.2	0.2	0.4	0.6	0.6	1.6	1.0	1.6	2.1	2.9	2.9	2.3	0.8	0.2	0.03	0.05	**0.6**	190
Brain, nervous system	695	0	3.5	2.6	2.8	2.3	1.9	3.0	3.6	3.2	4.1	5.5	9.0	10.3	9.0	12.7	10.6	8.6	4.3	3.5	5.2	1.2	0.30	0.42	**4.4**	191-2
Thyroid	360	0	0.1	0.1	-	0.7	1.1	1.4	2.0	3.3	3.5	2.9	3.6	3.5	4.5	4.0	6.2	8.0	6.4	8.1	2.7	0.6	0.13	0.18	**1.9**	193
Other endocrine	145	0	1.2	0.7	0.3	0.1	0.4	0.7	0.7	0.8	0.8	1.5	2.2	2.3	1.3	2.6	1.6	0.6	0.6	3.9	1.1	0.3	0.06	0.09	**1.0**	194
Hodgkin's disease	260	0	-	-	0.9	4.1	4.9	3.0	3.5	1.8	0.9	1.1	1.5	1.6	1.7	2.1	1.2	2.1	1.4	1.2	2.0	0.5	0.12	0.14	**1.8**	201
Non-Hodgkin lymphoma	1388	0	0.6	0.5	1.0	1.5	1.5	1.8	2.6	3.9	6.4	8.1	13.2	14.9	19.2	27.3	35.0	42.5	39.5	32.1	10.4	2.4	0.38	0.69	**6.2**	200,202
Multiple myeloma	653	0	-	-	-	-	-	-	0.2	0.8	1.0	2.9	2.5	4.7	10.2	16.7	16.5	22.6	27.7	29.0	4.9	1.2	0.11	0.28	**2.4**	203
Lymphoid leukaemia	486	0	3.7	2.6	1.1	0.6	0.4	0.6	0.3	0.7	0.7	1.4	2.2	3.1	3.6	7.7	10.7	13.7	22.8	22.8	3.6	0.9	0.11	0.20	**2.3**	204
Myeloid leukaemia	538	0	1.2	1.1	0.5	0.6	0.6	1.1	1.1	1.3	2.4	2.7	3.5	3.5	7.1	9.7	11.4	16.6	15.9	23.6	4.0	0.9	0.13	0.24	**2.4**	205
Monocytic leukaemia	24	0	0.1	-	-	-	-	-	-	0.1	0.1	-	-	0.3	-	0.3	0.9	0.2	1.7	1.9	0.2	0.0	0.00	0.01	**0.1**	206
Other leukaemia	8	0	0.1	-	-	-	-	-	-	-	-	-	-	-	0.1	-	0.6	0.3	0.8	0.8	0.1	0.0	0.00	0.00	**0.0**	207
Leukaemia unspecified	113	0	0.8	0.1	-	0.1	0.1	-	0.1	0.1	0.4	0.4	0.3	0.9	1.6	1.6	2.3	3.3	4.3	7.7	0.8	0.2	0.02	0.04	**0.5**	208
Other and unspecified	3680	0	0.6	-	-	0.5	0.6	1.1	1.9	2.2	6.6	8.7	17.1	31.7	47.7	74.3	103.0	131.3	161.6	199.8	27.6	6.5	0.59	1.48	**12.9**	O&U
All sites	66714	0	17.3	11.1	13.5	20.3	30.6	56.1	107.5	180.0	269.3	408.6	586.6	774.0	1065.5	1279.6	1570.0	1855.2	2109.2	2338.0	501.0		17.70	31.95	**284.6**	ALL
All sites but 173	56668	0	16.3	11.1	13.0	19.5	28.4	51.6	98.5	163.1	238.8	361.9	518.6	684.0	936.9	1098.7	1301.6	1508.6	1704.8	1867.5	425.5	100.0	15.71	27.71	**246.8**	ALLb
Rate from 10 cases			1.151	1.203	1.272	1.129	0.986	0.985	1.113	1.174	1.084	1.250	1.403	1.466	1.451	1.431	1.760	2.051	2.887	3.873						

†Important: see notes on population page

UK, England, East Anglia

The East Anglian Cancer Registry was officially created in 1989 by amalgamation of the cancer registration bureaux in Cambridge, Norwich and Ipswich. However, data are available for the whole of the East Anglian Region from these bureaux from 1961. In 1994 the East Anglian and Oxford Regional Health Authorities (RHA) were merged, but the registries stayed separate, although there is increasing coordination of activities between the two. At the time of the merger, the county of Bedfordshire was transferred from North Thames RHA to the new Anglia and Oxford RHA, and from 1996 the East Anglian Registry data will include those from Bedfordshire. The current population served is approximately 2.1 million and the new county will raise this to 2.5 million.

The registry is based in Addenbrooke's Hospital, Cambridge, but registration staff continue to work in the other two original bureaux in Norwich and Ipswich. The analytical staff, who, together with registry staff, form the Cancer Intelligence Unit, work in the Institute of Public Health, adjacent to Addenbrooke's Hospital.

The three bureaux are all based on radiotherapy units, so the bulk of the data can be extracted from records by trained clerks. Registry staff visit other hospitals where cancer patients are treated and data are occasionally sent from private hospitals and Family Health Service Authorities (general practitioner records).

The bulk of the data come from pathology laboratories on paper copies of reports. Data are also abstracted from clinical records and from death notifications which are sent regularly from the Office for National Statistics. After the initial registration, patients are actively followed to determine vital status at three years and at five-yearly intervals until death.

The initial registration data are recorded on paper, and when complete they are transferred to the registry computer network.

The computer network has been developed since 1989 and is based entirely on personal computers. There is a secure link between the cancer registry network and the Medical School network that allows access to software not purchased solely for the registry.

Although the cancer registry data go back to 1961, only data from 1971 are fully computerized. However, living cases from that first decade, plus records from patients who developed a second primary at a subsequent date, are currently being added.

The current data set includes all items on the National Minimum Dataset, plus information on stage for 18 main cancer sites, vital status at follow-up and cause of death. The registry data can be combined with other morbidity and mortality data available in the Institute of Public Health.

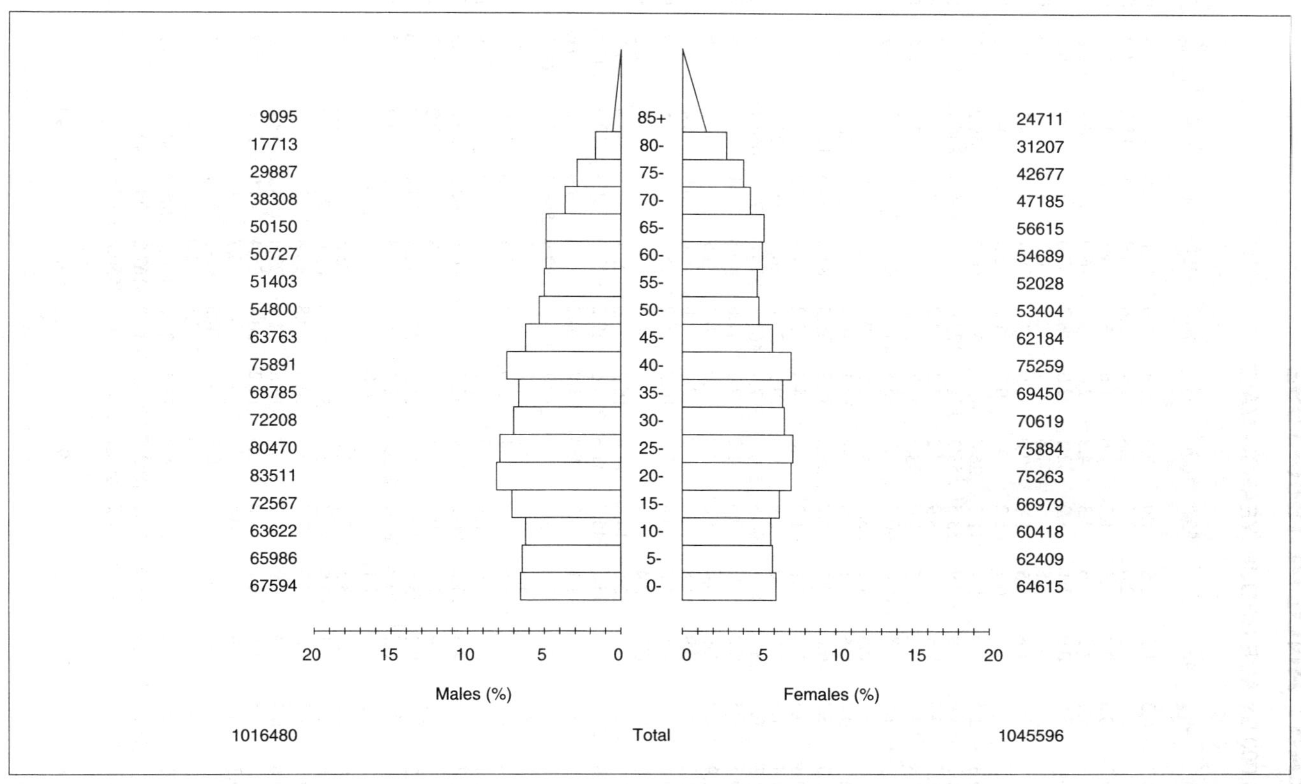

UK, England and Wales, East Anglia

Source of population: average annual 1988–92

Census: 1991 Census: Usual Residence, Great Britain, OPCS. London: HMSO, 1993.

Estimate: The estimated populations for 1988, 1989 and 1990 were projected back from the 1991 Census. That for 1992 is a mid-year estimated provided by the Office for National Statistics.

Notes to tables overleaf:

* The data in the tables of indices of data quality relate to one year only (1992). The low level of diagnoses based on a death certificate alone, combined with a low percentage of histological verification in general and some high mortality:incidence ratios, indicates under-ascertainment of cases.

† 188 does not include non-invasive tumours

* UK, ENGLAND, EAST ANGLIA 1988-1992

ANNUAL INCIDENCE PER 100,000 BY AGE GROUP (YEARS) - MALE

SITE	ALL AGES	AGE UNK	0-	5-	10-	15-	20-	25-	30-	35-	40-	45-	50-	55-	60-	65-	70-	75-	80-	85+	CRUDE RATE	%	CR 64	CR 74	ASR (W)	ICD (9th)
Lip	129	0	-	-	-	-	-	-	-	0.3	0.3	1.3	2.6	1.9	7.5	10.8	11.0	14.1	15.8	19.8	2.5	0.6	0.07	0.18	1.5	140
Tongue	61	0	-	-	-	-	-	-	0.3	0.6	0.3	1.3	2.6	3.9	2.8	2.4	2.6	6.0	3.4	13.2	1.2	0.3	0.06	0.08	0.8	141
Salivary gland	33	0	-	-	0.3	-	-	-	-	0.3	0.5	0.3	0.4	1.2	1.6	1.6	3.7	3.3	3.4	2.2	0.6	0.2	0.02	0.05	0.4	142
Mouth	83	0	-	-	-	-	-	-	0.6	-	1.1	2.2	2.6	4.3	4.3	2.4	6.3	6.0	11.3	8.8	1.6	0.4	0.07	0.12	1.1	143-5
Oropharynx	36	0	-	-	-	-	-	-	-	-	0.5	0.9	1.1	1.2	2.4	2.0	3.7	2.0	3.4	2.2	0.7	0.2	0.03	0.06	0.5	146
Nasopharynx	16	0	-	-	-	-	-	-	0.3	-	-	-	1.5	-	1.6	0.4	2.1	0.7	1.1	-	0.3	0.1	0.02	0.03	0.2	147
Hypopharynx	47	0	-	-	-	-	-	-	-	-	-	1.6	1.5	1.2	2.0	2.8	3.7	5.4	2.3	13.2	0.9	0.2	0.03	0.06	0.6	148
Pharynx unspecified	13	0	-	-	-	-	-	-	-	-	-	-	0.7	1.2	-	0.8	1.6	1.3	1.1	-	0.3	0.1	0.01	0.02	0.2	149
Oesophagus	548	0	-	-	-	-	-	-	0.3	0.3	2.4	5.0	8.4	11.7	26.4	43.1	51.7	60.2	82.4	68.2	10.8	2.6	0.27	0.75	6.1	150
Stomach	1322	0	-	-	-	-	-	0.2	0.8	1.5	3.4	6.9	17.9	33.5	53.2	101.3	129.0	145.9	195.3	255.1	26.0	6.2	0.59	1.74	14.5	151
Small intestine	56	0	-	-	-	-	-	-	-	1.5	0.5	0.9	-	3.9	3.2	3.2	4.2	4.7	5.6	-	1.1	0.3	0.05	0.09	0.7	152
Colon	1828	0	-	-	-	-	0.2	0.5	0.3	5.8	7.9	12.2	29.6	51.0	83.2	107.7	165.0	219.5	281.1	327.6	36.0	8.6	0.95	2.32	20.2	153
Rectum	1307	0	-	-	-	-	-	-	0.8	2.6	4.5	8.8	18.6	40.9	57.2	95.3	114.9	145.2	197.6	215.5	25.7	6.2	0.67	1.72	14.5	154
Liver	90	0	-	-	-	0.3	0.2	-	0.3	-	-	0.9	1.1	3.1	5.1	8.0	10.4	8.0	6.8	4.4	1.8	0.4	0.06	0.15	1.1	155
Gallbladder etc.	137	0	-	-	-	-	-	-	0.3	0.3	0.8	0.6	1.1	3.9	3.9	10.4	10.4	18.7	23.7	26.4	2.7	0.6	0.05	0.16	1.4	156
Pancreas	569	0	-	-	-	-	-	-	0.3	0.3	3.2	6.0	9.1	8.2	26.8	30.3	58.5	83.6	65.5	112.1	11.2	2.7	0.27	0.71	6.2	157
Nose, sinuses etc.	57	0	0.3	-	0.3	-	-	-	0.3	0.3	0.3	1.3	1.1	1.2	2.0	4.8	5.2	4.0	7.9	4.4	1.1	0.3	0.03	0.08	0.7	160
Larynx	264	0	-	-	-	-	-	0.2	0.3	0.9	1.3	1.9	4.0	8.9	19.3	19.1	26.6	26.1	18.1	24.2	5.2	1.2	0.18	0.41	3.2	161
Bronchus, lung	4513	0	-	-	-	-	-	-	0.8	2.3	9.8	23.8	40.1	94.5	210.1	337.4	467.3	576.8	675.2	664.1	88.8	21.3	1.91	5.93	48.3	162
Other thoracic organs	21	0	-	0.3	-	-	-	0.2	0.3	0.3	0.3	0.3	-	0.4	1.2	2.0	1.6	1.3	1.1	-	0.4	0.1	0.02	0.03	0.3	163-4
Bone	40	0	0.3	0.3	1.6	1.1	0.7	0.2	0.8	0.9	0.3	0.6	0.4	1.6	0.8	1.2	0.5	2.7	-	2.2	0.8	0.2	0.05	0.06	0.7	170
Connective tissue	125	0	0.9	0.9	1.3	0.8	0.2	0.5	-	1.2	1.3	0.9	1.8	3.5	4.7	7.2	8.9	9.4	16.9	15.4	2.5	0.6	0.09	0.17	1.7	171
Mesothelioma	147	0	-	-	-	-	-	-	-	0.6	1.1	4.1	1.8	5.8	5.5	10.8	16.2	16.1	10.2	6.6	2.9	0.7	0.09	0.23	1.8	MES
Kaposi's sarcoma	9	0	-	-	-	-	-	0.2	0.6	0.6	0.3	0.3	0.4	-	-	-	0.5	-	-	-	0.2	0.0	0.01	0.01	0.2	KAP
Melanoma of skin	399	0	-	-	0.6	0.6	1.4	4.0	5.5	7.3	12.1	9.1	12.8	14.4	15.4	16.7	18.8	22.1	18.1	33.0	7.9	1.9	0.42	0.59	5.8	172
Other skin	5475	0	-	-	-	1.4	1.9	3.2	5.3	16.6	34.0	64.9	93.1	145.9	241.3	334.6	489.2	617.0	781.3	890.6	107.7		3.04	7.16	62.3	173
Breast	30	0	-	-	-	-	-	-	-	-	0.3	-	1.1	0.8	0.4	1.2	4.2	2.0	9.0	2.2	0.6	0.1	0.01	0.04	0.3	175
Prostate	3551	0	-	-	-	-	-	-	-	-	0.3	2.5	9.5	33.5	89.9	210.2	351.4	582.9	806.2	917.0	69.9	16.7	0.68	3.49	33.4	185
Testis	300	0	0.6	0.3	-	2.8	5.3	14.7	17.2	13.1	9.8	8.2	4.7	3.1	0.8	1.2	2.6	0.7	3.4	2.2	5.9	1.4	0.40	0.42	5.3	186
Penis, other male genital	84	0	-	-	-	-	-	0.2	0.3	0.6	0.8	0.6	1.5	1.6	5.1	3.6	6.8	11.4	11.3	11.0	1.7	0.4	0.05	0.11	1.0	187
†Bladder	1297	0	-	-	-	-	0.2	-	0.6	1.7	1.8	6.3	17.2	26.8	56.4	89.7	113.3	167.3	215.7	261.7	25.5	6.1	0.56	1.57	13.8	188
Kidney etc.	532	0	2.1	0.3	-	-	-	-	1.4	1.7	4.7	7.5	14.6	20.2	28.4	32.7	40.2	46.8	62.1	50.6	10.5	2.5	0.40	0.77	6.7	189
Eye	38	0	0.3	-	-	-	0.5	1.0	0.3	-	0.3	0.9	1.1	0.8	1.6	2.4	1.0	3.3	3.4	2.2	0.7	0.2	0.03	0.05	0.5	190
Brain, nervous system	438	0	4.4	3.0	1.9	2.2	1.7	2.2	3.6	3.5	7.4	10.0	13.1	12.1	17.0	24.3	25.1	30.8	27.1	19.8	8.6	2.1	0.41	0.66	6.6	191-2
Thyroid	61	0	-	-	-	-	0.5	1.0	0.6	0.9	1.1	1.3	0.7	1.2	2.0	2.4	6.8	3.3	6.8	4.4	1.2	0.3	0.05	0.09	0.8	193
Other endocrine	24	0	3.3	-	-	-	0.2	-	0.3	0.3	0.3	-	1.1	-	-	0.8	1.0	1.3	-	-	0.5	0.1	0.03	0.04	0.6	194
Hodgkin's disease	137	0	-	0.3	0.3	3.9	3.1	4.7	3.3	3.8	2.6	2.8	3.3	2.7	2.8	3.2	3.7	3.3	1.1	2.2	2.7	0.6	0.17	0.20	2.4	201
Non-Hodgkin lymphoma	798	0	1.2	3.0	1.6	1.7	1.7	3.5	5.0	7.6	10.8	10.4	17.5	23.3	35.9	53.8	55.3	68.9	71.1	61.6	15.7	3.8	0.62	1.16	10.5	200,202
Multiple myeloma	315	0	-	-	-	-	-	0.2	0.3	0.3	1.1	1.6	3.3	7.0	15.8	20.3	29.8	36.8	53.1	57.2	6.2	1.5	0.15	0.40	3.4	203
Lymphoid leukaemia	254	0	5.3	1.2	1.3	1.1	1.0	-	0.6	0.6	0.3	1.9	2.9	4.7	9.9	12.8	21.4	29.4	28.2	48.4	5.0	1.2	0.15	0.32	3.5	204
Myeloid leukaemia	263	0	1.2	-	-	0.6	0.7	0.7	1.9	1.5	1.8	4.1	4.7	7.0	8.3	13.2	20.4	25.4	44.0	39.6	5.2	1.2	0.16	0.33	3.2	205
Monocytic leukaemia	9	0	-	-	-	-	-	-	-	0.3	-	0.9	-	0.8	-	-	-	0.7	1.1	2.2	0.2	0.0	0.01	0.01	0.1	206
Other leukaemia	4	0	-	-	-	-	-	-	-	-	-	-	-	-	0.8	-	0.5	-	1.1	-	0.1	0.0	0.00	0.01	0.0	207
Leukaemia unspecified	12	0	0.3	-	-	-	-	-	-	0.3	-	-	-	-	0.4	-	2.1	2.0	-	4.4	0.2	0.1	0.00	0.02	0.2	208
Other and unspecified	1226	0	-	-	-	-	0.5	0.2	0.6	1.2	4.0	5.6	15.3	24.5	46.9	73.4	120.6	150.6	205.5	303.5	24.1	5.8	0.49	1.46	13.0	O&U
All sites	26698	0	20.1	9.7	9.1	16.3	20.1	38.0	53.7	81.4	133.1	220.8	365.7	617.1	1103.5	1701.3	2419.3	3167.2	3978.9	4499.1	525.3		13.44	34.05	300.3	ALL
All sites but 173	21223	0	20.1	9.7	9.1	14.9	18.2	34.8	48.5	64.8	99.1	155.9	272.6	471.2	862.2	1366.7	1930.1	2550.2	3197.5	3608.5	417.6	100.0	10.41	26.89	238.0	ALLb
Rate from 1 case			0.296	0.303	0.314	0.276	0.239	0.249	0.277	0.291	0.264	0.314	0.365	0.389	0.394	0.399	0.522	0.669	1.129	2.199						

†Important: see notes on population page

* UK, ENGLAND, EAST ANGLIA 1988-1992

ANNUAL INCIDENCE PER 100,000 BY AGE GROUP (YEARS) - FEMALE

SITE	ALL AGES	AGE UNK	0-	5-	10-	15-	20-	25-	30-	35-	40-	45-	50-	55-	60-	65-	70-	75-	80-	85+	CRUDE RATE	%	CR 64	CR 74	ASR (W)	ICD (9th)
Lip	22	0	-	-	-	-	-	0.3	-	-	0.3	-	-	0.8	0.4	1.4	0.8	3.3	1.3	1.6	0.4	0.1	0.01	0.02	0.2	140
Tongue	54	0	-	-	-	-	-	0.3	0.3	0.3	1.1	0.6	0.7	2.3	0.4	1.4	4.2	2.8	5.1	6.5	1.0	0.3	0.03	0.06	0.5	141
Salivary gland	25	0	-	-	-	0.3	0.5	-	0.6	-	0.3	-	0.4	0.8	0.7	1.8	1.3	0.5	1.9	1.6	0.5	0.1	0.02	0.03	0.3	142
Mouth	66	0	-	-	-	0.3	-	-	0.3	-	0.3	0.6	0.4	2.7	3.7	2.8	4.7	4.7	4.5	5.7	1.3	0.3	0.04	0.08	0.6	143-5
Oropharynx	21	0	-	-	-	-	-	-	-	-	-	1.0	-	1.5	1.8	0.7	0.4	-	0.6	4.0	0.4	0.1	0.02	0.03	0.2	146
Nasopharynx	16	0	0.3	-	-	-	-	-	0.9	0.3	0.6	-	0.4	1.1	0.4	0.4	0.5	0.6	0.8	0.3	0.1	0.02	0.02	0.2	147
Hypopharynx	38	0	-	-	-	-	-	-	-	0.3	0.3	0.4	0.8	4.4	2.5	1.3	2.3	0.6	4.0	0.7	0.2	0.03	0.05	0.4	148
Pharynx unspecified	11	0	-	-	-	-	-	-	-	-	-	-	1.5	-	0.7	-	-	0.5	1.3	1.6	0.2	0.1	0.01	0.01	0.1	149
Oesophagus	393	0	-	-	-	-	-	0.3	-	0.3	0.5	1.0	3.0	6.9	11.3	13.8	23.3	40.8	50.6	55.8	7.5	1.8	0.12	0.30	2.8	150
Stomach	660	0	-	-	-	-	-	-	-	1.4	1.6	3.5	2.2	6.2	13.2	26.5	47.0	59.0	85.2	109.3	12.6	3.1	0.14	0.51	4.6	151
Small intestine	52	0	-	-	-	-	-	0.3	-	0.3	-	1.0	0.7	1.5	1.1	1.4	4.2	3.7	7.7	4.0	1.0	0.2	0.02	0.05	0.4	152
Colon	2096	0	-	-	-	-	-	0.3	1.4	3.7	7.7	12.9	25.8	43.1	64.7	92.6	120.8	181.8	236.5	280.0	40.1	9.8	0.80	1.86	16.8	153
Rectum	1006	0	-	-	-	-	-	0.3	0.6	1.4	3.5	9.3	16.1	22.3	38.4	57.6	60.2	81.1	99.3	94.7	19.2	4.7	0.46	1.05	8.9	154
Liver	45	0	-	-	-	-	0.5	-	-	-	0.3	0.7	1.9	1.1	2.5	3.0	4.2	3.2	3.2	0.9	0.2	0.02	0.05	0.4	155
Gallbladder etc.	168	0	-	-	-	-	-	-	-	0.3	1.3	1.3	1.5	2.3	5.9	8.1	10.2	13.1	18.6	22.7	3.2	0.8	0.06	0.15	1.4	156
Pancreas	637	0	-	-	0.3	-	-	-	0.3	0.3	2.9	1.9	4.5	11.9	21.6	31.1	38.6	52.0	84.6	75.3	12.2	3.0	0.22	0.57	4.9	157
Nose, sinuses etc.	31	0	-	-	-	-	0.3	-	-	0.6	-	-	-	1.2	1.1	1.4	1.7	1.4	3.8	4.0	0.6	0.1	0.02	0.03	0.3	160
Larynx	60	0	-	-	-	-	-	-	0.3	-	0.3	1.0	0.7	1.9	2.6	4.9	3.8	2.8	5.1	3.2	1.1	0.3	0.03	0.08	0.6	161
Bronchus, lung	1917	0	-	-	-	-	-	0.3	-	1.7	5.0	12.2	19.1	43.4	86.3	128.2	146.7	162.6	153.8	127.1	36.7	8.9	0.84	2.21	17.1	162
Other thoracic organs	15	0	-	-	-	0.3	-	-	-	0.3	0.5	-	-	-	0.7	0.7	0.4	0.9	1.3	1.6	0.3	0.1	0.01	0.01	0.2	163-4
Bone	31	0	-	-	1.7	1.2	0.3	0.5	-	-	0.3	-	0.4	0.4	0.4	2.1	1.7	-	1.9	1.6	0.6	0.1	0.03	0.04	0.5	170
Connective tissue	139	0	0.6	1.3	0.7	0.9	0.5	1.8	0.8	1.2	0.8	1.9	2.6	3.5	7.3	6.0	4.2	8.0	9.0	7.3	2.7	0.6	0.12	0.17	1.8	171
Mesothelioma	27	0	-	-	-	-	-	0.3	0.3	-	0.3	0.3	0.7	1.2	0.4	1.4	3.0	1.9	1.3	-	0.5	0.1	0.02	0.04	0.3	MES
Kaposi's sarcoma	2	0	-	-	-	-	-	-	-	-	-	-	-	-	-	0.4	0.4	-	-	-	0.0	0.0	0.00	0.00	0.0	KAP
Melanoma of skin	576	0	-	0.3	-	1.2	2.4	5.5	7.6	11.5	15.4	14.5	15.7	15.4	21.2	24.4	17.0	27.2	16.0	31.6	11.0	2.7	0.55	0.76	7.5	172
Other skin	4483	0	0.6	0.3	-	0.6	2.1	5.0	11.0	17.0	34.0	47.9	71.2	100.7	139.3	207.7	266.6	363.7	406.3	498.6	85.7		2.15	4.52	40.2	173
Breast	6346	0	-	-	-	-	1.1	4.2	26.6	53.0	103.6	172.1	221.3	267.5	331.3	258.9	290.3	294.3	312.1	321.3	121.4	29.6	5.90	8.65	76.4	174
Uterus unspecified	30	0	-	-	-	0.3	-	-	-	-	0.3	0.6	-	-	0.4	1.1	0.8	2.3	2.6	8.9	0.6	0.1	0.01	0.02	0.2	179
Cervix uteri	742	0	-	-	-	-	1.3	10.5	17.3	23.6	26.0	20.3	18.4	15.0	21.2	27.2	23.7	29.1	21.8	14.6	14.2	3.5	0.77	1.02	10.3	180
Placenta	1	0	-	-	-	-	-	-	0.3	-	-	-	-	-	-	-	-	-	-	-	0.0	0.0	0.00	0.00	0.0	181
Corpus uteri	928	0	-	-	-	-	0.5	-	0.3	2.9	6.6	13.2	34.8	45.4	49.7	52.3	48.7	55.3	47.4	38.0	17.8	4.3	0.77	1.27	10.5	182
Ovary etc.	1078	0	-	-	0.3	0.6	1.9	1.1	4.2	4.0	10.4	22.2	40.1	43.8	52.3	49.5	58.5	60.5	54.5	57.5	20.6	5.0	0.90	1.44	12.4	183
Other female genital	216	0	-	-	-	-	-	0.3	-	0.3	0.8	1.6	3.4	3.1	3.7	11.0	14.4	18.3	28.8	24.3	4.1	1.0	0.07	0.19	1.7	184
†Bladder	461	0	-	-	-	-	-	-	0.3	0.9	-	1.9	6.0	6.5	10.6	22.3	29.7	39.4	54.5	70.4	8.8	2.1	0.13	0.39	3.4	188
Kidney etc.	242	0	2.2	0.3	-	-	0.8	0.5	0.6	1.4	1.1	3.2	3.7	6.2	10.2	12.4	11.9	20.6	17.9	15.4	4.6	1.1	0.15	0.27	2.6	189
Eye	36	0	-	-	-	-	-	-	-	-	0.8	-	1.5	0.8	1.8	2.1	1.7	1.9	2.6	3.2	0.7	0.2	0.02	0.04	0.4	190
Brain, nervous system	332	0	3.7	2.6	2.0	0.6	1.1	1.6	2.3	2.3	4.5	7.7	5.2	11.5	13.2	15.9	19.1	13.1	17.9	8.9	6.4	1.5	0.29	0.47	4.5	191-2
Thyroid	134	0	-	-	0.3	0.6	1.6	3.4	3.7	1.7	2.7	2.6	3.7	3.8	5.1	3.5	3.0	3.7	7.7	3.2	2.6	0.6	0.15	0.18	1.9	193
Other endocrine	12	0	1.5	0.3	-	0.3	-	-	-	-	-	-	-	-	0.4	0.7	-	0.5	-	0.8	0.2	0.1	0.01	0.02	0.3	194
Hodgkin's disease	106	0	-	0.3	0.7	3.6	4.3	1.8	3.1	0.9	2.7	1.3	1.9	0.8	1.1	2.5	3.4	3.7	2.6	2.4	2.0	0.5	0.11	0.14	1.7	201
Non-Hodgkin lymphoma	676	0	1.5	1.3	1.0	1.5	0.5	1.3	3.7	3.7	7.2	9.6	9.4	21.5	16.1	30.7	44.9	58.6	40.4	51.0	12.9	3.2	0.39	0.77	7.0	200,202
Multiple myeloma	264	0	-	-	-	-	-	-	-	-	0.8	1.6	2.2	6.5	6.6	14.1	17.8	22.0	32.7	28.3	5.0	1.2	0.09	0.25	2.1	203
Lymphoid leukaemia	150	0	4.0	1.6	1.7	0.6	-	-	0.8	0.6	0.3	-	1.9	1.9	3.7	3.9	7.6	14.1	14.1	14.6	2.9	0.7	0.09	0.14	1.8	204
Myeloid leukaemia	245	0	0.3	-	-	0.6	1.6	2.1	1.1	2.3	1.1	3.5	3.7	4.2	5.1	9.2	13.1	17.8	21.1	30.8	4.7	1.1	0.13	0.24	2.4	205
Monocytic leukaemia	7	0	-	-	-	-	-	-	-	-	-	-	-	-	0.4	-	0.4	0.9	1.3	0.8	0.1	0.0	0.00	0.00	0.0	206
Other leukaemia	1	0	-	-	-	-	-	-	-	-	-	-	-	-	-	0.4	-	-	-	-	0.0	0.0	0.00	0.00	0.0	207
Leukaemia unspecified	24	0	0.3	-	-	-	-	0.3	0.3	-	0.3	-	0.4	-	0.4	0.7	1.7	2.8	0.6	4.0	0.5	0.1	0.01	0.02	0.2	208
Other and unspecified	1310	0	0.9	-	-	-	-	0.8	0.6	1.4	5.6	7.4	11.6	23.8	41.0	54.4	81.0	108.7	148.0	194.2	25.1	6.1	0.47	1.14	10.3	O&U
All sites	25932	0	16.1	8.3	8.6	13.4	21.3	42.7	88.6	140.2	251.1	381.1	537.8	735.4	1004.2	1194.4	1437.3	1786.4	2029.0	2238.7	496.0		16.24	29.40	261.8	ALL
All sites but 173	21449	0	15.5	8.0	8.6	12.8	19.1	37.7	77.6	123.3	217.1	333.2	466.6	634.7	864.9	986.7	1170.7	1422.8	1622.7	1740.1	410.3	100.0	14.10	24.88	221.6	ALLb

Rate from 1 case   0.310   0.321   0.331   0.299   0.266   0.264   0.283   0.288   0.266   0.322   0.375   0.384   0.366   0.353   0.424   0.469   0.641   0.809

†Important: see notes on population page

UK, England, Merseyside and Cheshire

The registry was founded in 1944 as the Liverpool Clinical Cancer Registry, with the primary objective of registering all cases of malignancy occurring in the area served by the Liverpool Radium Institute. It extended its coverage to the surrounding area and since 1974 has collected data on all cancers occurring in residents of Merseyside and Cheshire wherever treated, and on residents of other regions treated in Merseyside and Cheshire hospitals. The registry also collects data for Isle of Man residents on behalf of their local government. The data presented here cover the population of Merseyside and Cheshire, as in the previous volume of this series. In 1994 the name of the registry changed from the Mersey Regional Registry to the Merseyside and Cheshire Cancer Registry.

In 1990 new posts of epidemiologist and systems analyst were added to the existing positions of a manager and eight registration officers. The Medical Director of the registry is a Clinical Senior Lecturer in the Department of Public Health Medicine in the University of Liverpool.

Population centres in the registration area include the city of Liverpool; industrial towns such as Birkenhead (previously shipbuilding), Runcorn (chemicals), St Helens (glass); the retirement coastal town of Southport; and the rural towns of Cheshire. Over the past 15 years, there has been a fall in the population living in the large metropolitan area of Merseyside and an increase in the more rural area of Cheshire. Merseyside has particularly high unemployment rates, while those of Cheshire are below the national rate. Both have experienced a drop in GDP per head, from quite a high level in Cheshire but from an already low level in Merseyside. The proportion of ethnic minorities is lower than the national average, and the majority of these segments of the population are concentrated in Liverpool.

Local cancer services are being re-organized into specialist cancer centres (with full radiotherapy and oncology facilities) and cancer units in a 'hub and spoke' arrangement, to achieve the most effective concentration of expertise and also obtain the closer involvement of primary care.

The most important source of notification of new cases of cancer is pathology reports, copies of which are routinely sent to the registry. All cases are followed up by trained registration officers who abstract relevant clinical information from hospital case records. Notifications are also received from the Office for National Statistics, which sends death certificates for people who have died of cancer. Full registration information for these cases is sought from the hospital or certifying doctor. The local specialist centres for oncology also supply notifications. Details of Merseyside and Cheshire residents whose cancers are diagnosed elsewhere are supplied by the local registry. Cases registered during life are flagged at the National Health Service Central Register so that the cancer registry is informed when these cases die.

Substantial improvements have been made to the registry's computer system since 1988. Data are held on a dedicated relational person-based system. Each tumour is allocated a tumour number in addition to the patient's unique identifier. Validation checks within the system were extended in 1994 to improve the quality of data at inputting. The registry has embarked upon a rolling programme of quality assurance focusing on the ascertainment, completeness, timeliness and validity of data. All postgraduate researchers contribute to data 'housekeeping', and several projects have explored different aspects of data quality. Data are coded in ICD-O and kept securely and released in a controlled manner, in accordance with ethical and data protection conventions. Regular back-ups are taken of the data and kept both locally and off-site.

In addition to the personal details of the patient, information is recorded about the tumour, its clinical management and about the outcome of the patient. The data items held extend beyond the minimum data-set required nationally. The registry is an active member of the UK Association of Cancer Registries,and has its own programme of research as well as undertaking research in partnership with clinical and other academic and service colleagues.

Publications include specialist reports on geographical variations (1990), lung cancer (1993), breast cancer (1994) and skin cancer (1994), in addition to regular five-year incidence reports. As well as responding to about 60 *ad hoc* enquiries each year, in 1995 the registry provided analyses to support the planning of local cancer services.

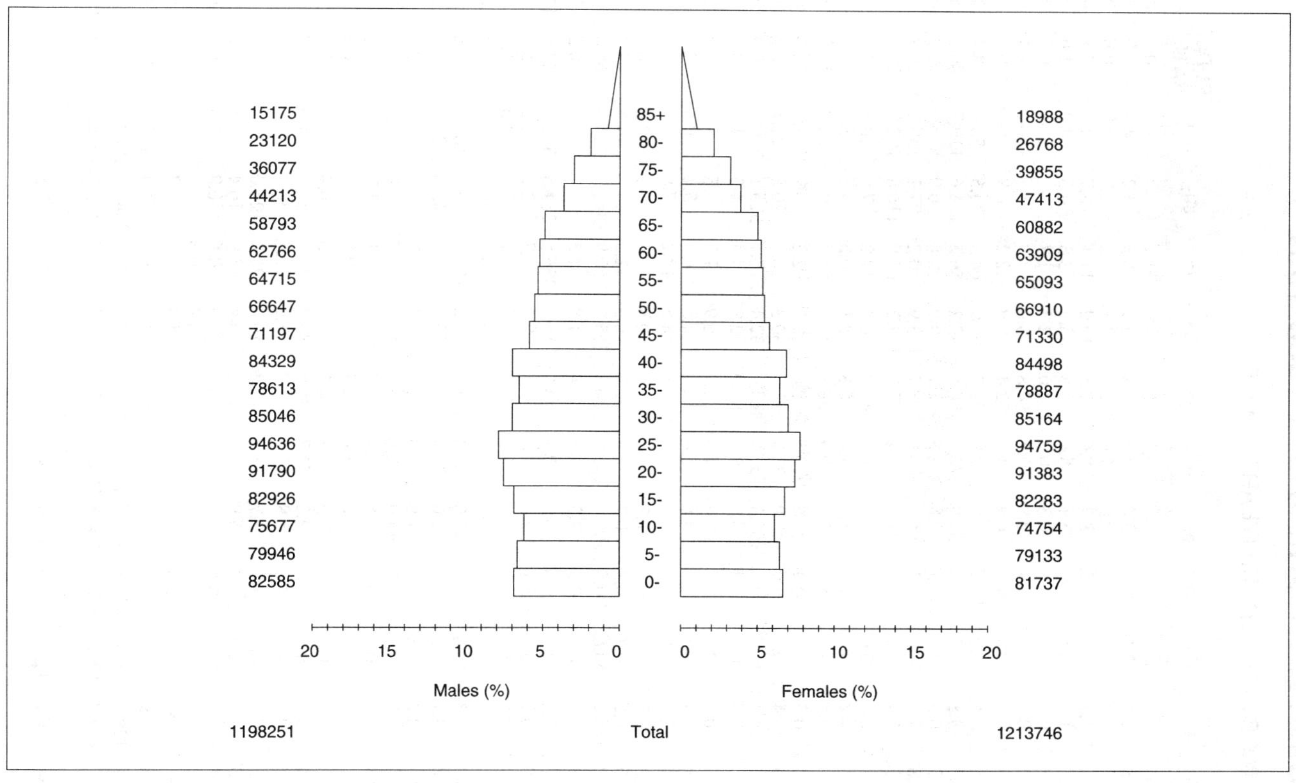

UK, England and Wales, Merseyside and Cheshire
Source of population: average annual 1988–92
Census: 1991 Census: Usual Residence, Great Britain, OPCS. London: HMSO, 1993.
Notes to tables overleaf:
* The low rates for a number of sites, associated with declines in incidence since the period published in the previous volume and high mortality:incidence ratios, indicate under-ascertainment of cases.

Note: In earlier volumes of Cancer Incidence in Five Continents this entry appeared as UK, England, Mersey Region. In 1994 the name of the Registry changed to the Merseyside and Cheshire Cancer Registry reflecting the merger of the former Mersey and North Western regions to create the new North West region. The area covered by Merseyside and Cheshire remains the same as previously.

Screening programmes in the area:
A cervical cancer screening programme started in 1988 for females aged 20-64, examined every three to five years. Women aged 50-64 have been screened for breast cancer since 1990 and are examined every three years.

* UK, ENGLAND, MERSEYSIDE AND CHESHIRE 1988-1992

ANNUAL INCIDENCE PER 100,000 BY AGE GROUP (YEARS) - MALE

SITE	ALL AGES	AGE UNK	0-	5-	10-	15-	20-	25-	30-	35-	40-	45-	50-	55-	60-	65-	70-	75-	80-	85+	CRUDE RATE	%	CR 64	CR 74	ASR (W)	ICD (9th)
Lip	7	0	-	-	-	-	-	-	-	-	-	-	0.3	-	0.3	0.7	-	1.1	-	1.3	0.1	0.0	0.00	0.01	0.1	140
Tongue	121	0	-	-	-	-	-	-	0.2	0.8	2.4	3.1	2.4	5.6	5.4	5.4	5.9	8.3	5.2	4.0	2.0	0.5	0.10	0.16	1.4	141
Salivary gland	34	0	-	-	-	-	0.4	-	0.5	0.3	0.2	0.3	-	0.6	1.0	2.7	2.3	2.2	1.7	4.0	0.6	0.1	0.02	0.04	0.3	142
Mouth	187	0	-	-	-	-	-	0.2	-	-	1.7	5.1	8.7	8.7	8.6	7.5	10.0	11.1	8.7	4.0	3.1	0.8	0.16	0.25	2.1	143-5
Oropharynx	97	0	-	-	-	-	-	-	0.2	0.8	1.4	2.5	3.9	3.1	5.4	5.8	3.2	3.3	4.3	4.0	1.6	0.4	0.09	0.13	1.1	146
Nasopharynx	28	0	-	-	0.3	0.2	-	0.2	-	0.5	0.2	1.1	1.5	0.3	0.3	1.0	2.3	1.7	-	-	0.5	0.1	0.02	0.04	0.4	147
Hypopharynx	83	0	-	-	-	-	-	-	0.2	0.3	0.5	1.4	3.9	2.8	5.7	4.8	5.0	3.9	1.7	-	1.4	0.3	0.07	0.12	1.0	148
Pharynx unspecified	32	0	-	-	-	-	-	-	0.2	0.3	0.7	0.8	0.9	0.9	1.3	2.4	0.9	2.2	0.9	-	0.5	0.1	0.03	0.04	0.4	149
Oesophagus	800	0	-	-	-	-	-	-	0.7	1.5	2.4	7.9	13.8	17.0	37.9	50.7	62.9	64.3	73.5	58.0	13.4	3.3	0.41	0.97	7.7	150
Stomach	1597	0	-	-	-	-	0.2	-	0.9	1.3	3.8	9.0	20.4	39.9	72.3	100.4	140.2	156.3	124.6	110.7	26.7	6.6	0.74	1.94	15.0	151
Small intestine	44	0	-	-	-	-	-	-	0.5	0.3	0.5	0.3	1.5	2.8	2.5	2.7	0.9	2.8	0.9	-	0.7	0.2	0.04	0.06	0.5	152
Colon	1784	0	-	-	0.3	-	0.2	0.4	1.6	1.8	7.4	14.6	22.2	45.7	81.6	98.7	133.9	150.2	197.2	158.2	29.8	7.4	0.88	2.04	16.7	153
Rectum	1322	0	-	-	-	-	0.2	0.2	0.7	2.3	5.9	11.5	25.2	41.4	53.2	77.2	102.2	105.9	116.8	102.8	22.1	5.5	0.70	1.60	12.8	154
Liver	192	0	0.2	-	0.3	0.2	-	0.8	0.5	1.0	0.5	0.6	3.3	5.9	9.2	11.9	16.3	12.2	7.8	18.5	3.2	0.8	0.11	0.25	2.0	155
Gallbladder etc.	111	0	-	-	-	-	-	0.2	-	-	0.2	0.8	1.5	1.5	4.8	5.8	8.1	10.5	14.7	13.2	1.9	0.5	0.05	0.12	1.0	156
Pancreas	672	0	-	-	-	-	0.2	0.2	0.2	0.8	3.6	4.8	8.4	21.0	30.9	38.1	52.9	58.2	70.9	32.9	11.2	2.8	0.35	0.81	6.4	157
Nose, sinuses etc.	41	0	-	-	-	-	-	-	0.5	-	0.5	1.4	0.9	0.6	2.5	2.0	2.7	2.2	0.9	2.6	0.7	0.2	0.03	0.06	0.5	160
Larynx	440	0	-	-	-	-	-	-	-	0.5	1.4	6.5	6.9	17.9	25.8	30.3	30.3	28.3	20.8	21.1	7.3	1.8	0.30	0.60	4.6	161
Bronchus, lung	6590	0	-	-	0.3	-	0.2	0.2	3.3	5.3	16.4	41.0	90.3	168.4	337.4	464.0	532.4	577.1	525.1	320.3	110.0	27.3	3.31	8.30	63.3	162
Other thoracic organs	46	0	0.2	-	-	-	-	0.4	-	0.3	0.5	0.6	1.2	0.9	2.9	1.0	2.3	4.4	4.3	1.3	0.8	0.2	0.03	0.05	0.5	163-4
Bone	54	0	-	0.5	0.5	2.4	0.9	0.8	-	1.3	0.7	0.6	0.6	0.3	1.3	1.7	0.9	1.7	3.5	1.3	0.9	0.2	0.05	0.06	0.8	170
Connective tissue	130	0	2.2	0.8	-	0.7	-	0.2	0.7	0.8	1.4	2.5	2.7	4.3	5.4	6.1	4.5	6.1	5.2	10.5	2.2	0.5	0.11	0.16	1.7	171
Mesothelioma	217	0	-	-	-	-	-	0.2	-	-	1.4	2.5	6.0	8.7	12.4	13.3	18.5	12.2	7.8	4.0	3.6	0.9	0.16	0.32	2.3	MES
Kaposi's sarcoma	11	0	-	-	-	-	0.2	-	0.2	0.3	0.5	-	-	0.3	0.3	-	0.5	-	0.9	2.6	0.2	0.0	0.01	0.01	0.1	KAP
Melanoma of skin	283	0	-	-	0.5	0.4	3.2	3.5	4.6	4.5	6.7	6.9	10.2	10.2	12.6	6.3	11.6	14.7	14.5	4.7	1.2	0.25	0.35	3.4	172
Other skin	3941	0	0.2	-	0.5	0.4	4.2	5.9	12.2	24.9	50.6	70.5	100.7	159.6	220.8	265.5	350.9	341.7	305.8	65.8		2.15	4.58	38.7	173
Breast	31	0	-	-	-	-	-	-	0.3	-	0.6	0.3	2.5	1.3	1.4	1.8	3.3	-	1.3	0.5	0.1	0.02	0.04	0.3	175
Prostate	2671	0	-	-	-	0.2	-	-	0.5	-	0.2	2.2	9.6	30.3	77.1	144.2	254.7	336.5	381.5	332.1	44.6	11.1	0.60	2.60	21.3	185
Testis	344	0	0.7	-	0.3	2.9	7.6	14.8	12.7	14.0	10.9	5.9	5.7	2.5	2.2	1.4	0.5	1.7	2.6	2.6	5.7	1.4	0.40	0.41	5.3	186
Penis	63	0	-	-	-	-	-	0.6	-	-	0.5	1.4	0.6	1.9	1.9	4.4	3.2	6.7	3.5	4.0	1.1	0.3	0.03	0.07	0.6	187.1-.4
Other male genital	9	0	-	-	-	-	-	-	-	-	-	-	-	0.3	0.3	0.9	0.6	0.9	4.0	4.0	0.2	0.0	0.00	0.01	0.1	187.5-.9
Bladder	1903	0	-	-	-	-	0.2	0.8	1.2	3.8	4.3	14.6	24.3	43.0	87.3	121.1	150.6	156.3	186.0	168.7	31.8	7.9	0.90	2.26	17.9	188
Kidney etc.	561	0	1.5	0.3	-	-	-	-	0.5	1.8	4.7	6.5	11.1	22.6	26.4	33.3	35.3	36.0	45.0	21.1	9.4	2.3	0.38	0.72	5.9	189
Eye	35	0	0.5	-	-	-	-	-	-	0.5	0.2	0.8	0.3	1.9	1.9	2.7	1.4	1.7	-	-	0.6	0.1	0.03	0.05	0.4	190
Brain, nervous system	495	0	5.1	2.0	2.9	2.9	3.1	1.5	4.0	4.3	5.7	9.3	14.1	18.9	22.0	24.2	18.5	17.7	6.9	2.6	8.3	2.1	0.48	0.69	6.8	191-2
Thyroid	44	0	-	-	-	-	1.3	0.4	0.5	0.8	0.5	0.6	0.3	1.5	1.9	2.0	0.9	1.1	1.7	4.0	0.7	0.2	0.04	0.05	0.5	193
Other endocrine	20	0	1.2	-	-	-	0.2	0.2	-	-	0.2	-	0.6	0.3	1.0	1.4	0.5	0.6	-	-	0.3	0.1	0.02	0.03	0.3	194
Hodgkin's disease	136	0	-	0.5	0.8	2.9	4.4	2.5	3.1	2.8	3.3	0.8	1.5	2.5	4.1	4.1	2.7	0.6	0.9	-	2.3	0.6	0.15	0.18	2.1	201
Non-Hodgkin lymphoma	614	0	1.0	0.3	2.1	2.4	1.7	1.5	4.2	6.4	5.0	9.6	15.6	19.2	21.7	28.9	35.7	35.5	38.1	31.6	10.2	2.5	0.45	0.78	7.0	200,202
Multiple myeloma	252	0	-	-	-	-	-	-	-	0.3	0.9	2.5	4.8	5.9	11.2	16.0	14.9	20.5	30.3	21.1	4.2	1.0	0.13	0.28	2.4	203
Lymphoid leukaemia	218	0	3.4	1.8	0.3	0.7	0.7	0.8	-	0.3	0.7	0.8	1.2	3.7	8.0	10.2	10.9	20.0	26.0	23.7	3.6	0.9	0.11	0.22	2.4	204
Myeloid leukaemia	239	0	0.5	0.5	0.5	1.7	0.7	1.1	1.6	1.3	3.1	2.0	6.0	5.9	7.3	11.2	15.4	13.9	16.4	17.1	4.0	1.0	0.16	0.29	2.7	205
Monocytic leukaemia	8	0	0.2	-	-	-	-	-	-	-	-	-	0.3	-	0.3	0.9	0.6	0.9	1.3	0.1	0.0	0.00	0.01	0.1	206
Other leukaemia	6	0	-	-	-	-	-	-	-	-	-	-	0.3	-	0.7	0.9	0.6	-	-	0.1	0.0	0.00	0.01	0.1	207
Leukaemia unspecified	26	0	-	0.3	-	-	-	-	0.2	-	-	-	0.3	0.6	1.0	0.7	1.4	4.4	1.7	4.0	0.4	0.1	0.01	0.02	0.2	208
Other and unspecified	1528	0	0.2	0.3	-	0.7	0.4	0.6	1.2	2.8	5.9	7.3	26.1	33.1	58.0	92.2	121.2	146.4	151.4	127.8	25.5	6.3	0.68	1.75	14.2	O&U
All sites	28067	0	17.2	7.0	8.5	19.1	23.7	36.6	50.3	76.1	129.7	241.0	426.7	705.5	1213.4	1668.2	2083.1	2393.2	2447.2	1962.4	468.5		14.77	33.53	275.7	ALL
All sites but 173	24126	0	17.0	7.0	8.5	18.6	23.3	32.3	44.4	63.9	104.8	190.5	356.2	604.8	1053.7	1447.4	1817.5	2042.3	2105.5	1656.7	402.7	100.0	12.62	28.95	237.0	ALLb

Rate from 1 case 0.242 0.250 0.264 0.241 0.218 0.211 0.235 0.254 0.237 0.281 0.300 0.309 0.319 0.340 0.452 0.554 0.865 1.318

* UK, ENGLAND, MERSEYSIDE AND CHESHIRE 1988-1992

ANNUAL INCIDENCE PER 100,000 BY AGE GROUP (YEARS) - FEMALE

SITE	ALL AGES	AGE UNK	0-	5-	10-	15-	20-	25-	30-	35-	40-	45-	50-	55-	60-	65-	70-	75-	80-	85+	CRUDE RATE	%	CR 64	CR 74	ASR (W)	ICD (9th)
Lip	5	0	-	-	-	-	-	-	-	-	-	-	-	-	-	-	-	-	0.7	4.2	0.1	0.0	0.00	0.00	**0.0**	*140*
Tongue	51	0	-	-	-	-	-	-	-	-	0.7	-	1.2	1.5	0.6	3.6	2.5	3.5	3.7	8.4	0.8	0.2	0.02	0.05	**0.4**	*141*
Salivary gland	38	0	-	-	-	-	-	-	-	-	0.2	0.3	1.2	0.9	-	1.0	0.4	4.0	3.0	13.7	0.6	0.2	0.01	0.02	**0.3**	*142*
Mouth	97	0	-	-	-	-	-	-	0.2	0.3	0.9	1.1	1.8	1.8	4.4	5.3	4.2	5.5	9.0	12.6	1.6	0.4	0.05	0.10	**0.9**	*143-5*
Oropharynx	31	0	-	-	-	-	0.2	-	-	0.3	0.2	0.8	0.9	0.6	0.9	3.0	0.8	2.0	0.7	1.1	0.5	0.1	0.02	0.04	**0.3**	*146*
Nasopharynx	24	0	-	-	-	-	-	-	0.8	0.2	0.8	1.2	0.3	0.3	2.0	1.3	-	1.5	-	-	0.4	0.1	0.02	0.03	**0.3**	*147*
Hypopharynx	46	0	-	-	-	-	-	-	-	-	0.6	0.9	2.5	1.9	2.0	2.1	4.0	4.5	2.1	0.8	0.2	0.03	0.05	**0.4**	*148*
Pharynx unspecified	16	0	-	-	-	-	-	-	-	-	-	0.3	0.3	0.6	0.6	-	0.4	2.0	3.7	-	0.3	0.1	0.01	Ph.01	**0.1**	*149*
Oesophagus	556	0	-	-	-	-	-	-	-	0.8	0.5	2.2	5.1	8.6	15.3	26.6	35.9	53.7	70.2	86.4	9.2	2.3	0.16	0.47	**4.3**	*150*
Stomach	1130	0	-	-	-	-	-	-	0.2	0.8	2.1	2.5	8.1	13.2	21.9	40.7	73.0	115.4	171.1	223.3	18.6	4.6	0.24	0.81	**8.0**	*151*
Small intestine	42	0	-	-	-	-	-	-	-	-	-	-	0.9	0.9	2.5	0.7	3.4	3.5	4.5	5.3	0.7	0.2	0.02	0.04	**0.4**	*152*
Colon	2086	0	-	-	-	0.5	-	0.4	0.9	3.8	6.6	14.3	23.3	35.3	54.8	92.6	119.8	186.7	267.5	337.0	34.4	8.4	0.70	1.76	**16.5**	*153*
Rectum	1051	0	-	-	-	-	0.2	-	0.7	2.3	2.8	7.3	17.9	16.3	28.2	50.9	64.5	98.4	105.3	160.1	17.3	4.3	0.38	0.96	**8.6**	*154*
Liver	107	0	-	-	-	0.2	-	0.2	0.2	0.3	0.2	1.1	1.5	4.0	3.8	4.9	3.8	11.5	6.0	13.7	1.8	0.4	0.06	0.10	**1.0**	*155*
Gallbladder etc.	167	0	-	-	-	-	-	-	-	0.8	0.5	0.6	2.7	2.2	4.4	7.2	10.5	15.6	20.2	26.3	2.8	0.7	0.06	0.14	**1.3**	*156*
Pancreas	708	0	-	-	-	-	0.2	-	-	1.0	0.9	3.1	8.1	13.8	20.7	31.2	48.9	57.2	88.9	111.6	11.7	2.9	0.24	0.64	**5.6**	*157*
Nose, sinuses etc.	50	0	-	-	-	0.2	-	0.2	-	-	0.2	0.6	1.2	0.9	0.9	3.0	4.6	2.5	3.0	6.3	0.8	0.2	0.02	0.06	**0.5**	*160*
Larynx	109	0	-	-	-	-	-	-	0.5	0.3	0.7	0.6	2.7	3.1	4.1	8.5	9.7	5.0	6.0	2.1	1.8	0.4	0.06	0.15	**1.1**	*161*
Bronchus, lung	3460	0	-	-	-	-	0.2	0.8	1.9	2.5	9.2	22.4	43.9	76.8	169.6	225.4	256.0	268.5	248.8	229.6	57.0	14.0	1.64	4.04	**31.3**	*162*
Other thoracic organs	31	0	-	-	-	-	-	0.2	-	0.3	-	-	0.3	0.9	0.6	3.3	-	4.0	1.5	3.2	0.5	0.1	0.01	0.03	**0.3**	*163-4*
Bone	29	0	0.2	0.3	0.5	-	0.4	0.2	0.2	-	0.2	-	-	0.3	1.6	0.3	0.4	1.5	2.2	6.3	0.5	0.1	0.02	0.02	**0.3**	*170*
Connective tissue	104	0	1.0	0.3	0.3	0.5	1.3	-	0.7	2.0	0.7	0.8	2.1	2.5	3.1	3.3	7.2	4.0	4.5	7.4	1.7	0.4	0.08	0.13	**1.2**	*171*
Mesothelioma	19	0	-	-	-	-	-	-	-	-	-	-	0.9	-	0.6	1.3	2.1	1.0	1.5	1.1	0.3	0.1	0.01	0.02	**0.2**	*MES*
Kaposi's sarcoma	1	0	-	-	-	-	-	-	-	-	-	-	-	-	-	-	-	-	0.7	-	0.0	0.0	0.00	0.00	**0.0**	*KAP*
Melanoma of skin	383	0	0.2	0.3	-	-	3.1	4.4	6.3	4.6	7.6	9.3	7.8	10.4	13.8	10.8	11.8	17.1	15.7	16.9	6.3	1.6	0.34	0.45	**4.6**	*172*
Other skin	4203	0	0.2	-	0.5	0.2	2.8	4.4	10.6	18.8	27.0	44.9	67.0	79.3	116.4	161.6	260.3	331.2	452.8	571.9	69.3		1.86	3.97	**36.4**	*173*
Breast	6197	0	-	-	-	-	1.3	7.4	23.5	54.0	99.6	161.5	189.8	216.0	261.6	231.6	237.5	282.0	322.0	432.9	102.1	25.1	5.07	7.42	**67.9**	*174*
Uterus unspecified	24	0	-	-	-	-	-	-	-	-	-	-	0.6	0.6	1.3	0.7	1.3	0.5	3.0	6.3	0.4	0.1	0.01	0.02	**0.2**	*179*
Cervix uteri	1133	0	-	-	-	-	2.4	11.2	33.6	28.4	29.6	26.6	30.5	24.9	28.8	37.4	31.2	29.6	35.9	25.3	18.7	4.6	1.08	1.42	**14.2**	*180*
Placenta	0	0	-	-	-	-	-	-	-	-	-	-	-	-	-	-	-	-	-	-	0.0	0.0	0.00	0.00	**0.0**	*181*
Corpus uteri	903	0	-	-	-	-	0.4	0.7	3.3	8.0	10.9	24.2	34.1	45.4	48.6	43.9	59.2	43.3	49.5	14.9	3.7	0.64	1.10	**9.2**	*182*
Ovary etc.	1076	0	-	0.3	-	0.7	1.3	1.5	3.8	3.5	10.9	19.9	35.3	37.5	47.9	48.6	51.5	53.2	62.8	62.1	17.7	4.4	0.81	1.31	**11.4**	*183*
Other female genital	219	0	0.2	-	-	-	0.2	-	0.5	1.0	0.7	0.8	1.8	2.8	5.6	7.2	11.4	19.6	34.4	40.0	3.6	0.9	0.07	0.16	**1.7**	*184*
Bladder	811	0	-	-	-	-	0.4	0.6	0.7	1.3	2.6	3.4	9.9	15.7	33.5	38.1	52.7	71.3	77.7	102.2	13.4	3.3	0.34	0.79	**6.8**	*188*
Kidney etc.	328	0	1.5	0.5	0.3	-	0.4	-	0.5	0.3	1.7	2.5	6.9	6.5	12.8	18.4	23.6	21.6	28.4	21.1	5.4	1.3	0.17	0.38	**3.2**	*189*
Eye	27	0	0.2	-	-	-	0.4	-	0.5	0.3	0.2	0.3	-	1.2	1.3	1.3	0.4	2.0	2.2	1.1	0.4	0.1	0.02	0.03	**0.3**	*190*
Brain, nervous system	412	0	3.7	1.8	1.9	2.9	2.6	1.7	3.5	4.8	8.0	5.9	10.2	14.7	16.6	18.4	13.9	14.1	4.5	4.2	6.8	1.7	0.39	0.55	**5.5**	*191-2*
Thyroid	109	0	-	-	-	0.2	1.3	1.7	0.7	1.0	1.4	2.2	3.6	2.8	1.6	3.6	5.1	3.0	6.7	9.5	1.8	0.4	0.08	0.13	**1.3**	*193*
Other endocrine	26	0	1.2	0.3	-	0.5	-	-	0.7	0.3	-	1.1	-	-	0.9	1.3	-	1.5	-	-	0.4	0.1	0.02	0.03	**0.4**	*194*
Hodgkin's disease	108	0	-	0.3	0.5	1.9	5.5	1.9	1.6	2.0	1.2	1.4	0.6	1.5	1.9	3.6	0.8	3.0	2.2	3.2	1.8	0.4	0.10	0.12	**1.6**	*201*
Non-Hodgkin lymphoma	591	0	0.2	1.0	0.5	0.5	0.9	1.3	2.1	2.0	3.3	8.7	11.4	15.7	18.2	25.0	32.9	47.2	52.3	47.4	9.7	2.4	0.33	0.62	**5.7**	*200,202*
Multiple myeloma	248	0	-	-	-	-	-	0.2	-	-	1.2	1.4	0.9	4.9	7.5	11.8	15.6	26.1	26.9	34.8	4.1	1.0	0.08	0.22	**2.0**	*203*
Lymphoid leukaemia	173	0	4.2	1.0	1.3	1.0	0.4	0.4	0.5	0.3	0.9	2.0	1.5	1.8	2.8	6.2	7.6	9.0	13.4	33.7	2.9	0.7	0.09	0.16	**2.0**	*204*
Myeloid leukaemia	202	0	0.5	-	0.5	0.7	0.9	1.1	1.2	1.3	2.1	1.7	3.0	3.7	5.3	6.6	10.1	18.1	16.4	21.1	3.3	0.8	0.11	0.19	**2.0**	*205*
Monocytic leukaemia	12	0	-	-	-	-	0.2	-	-	-	-	-	0.3	-	0.3	-	0.4	1.5	1.5	3.2	0.2	0.0	0.00	0.01	**0.1**	*206*
Other leukaemia	5	0	-	-	-	-	-	-	-	-	-	-	0.3	-	-	-	0.5	0.7	2.1	0.1	0.0	0.00	0.00	**0.0**	*207*
Leukaemia unspecified	28	0	-	-	-	-	-	-	-	-	0.2	0.3	-	-	0.9	1.0	1.3	2.0	3.0	9.5	0.5	0.1	0.01	0.02	**0.2**	*208*
Other and unspecified	1729	0	1.0	-	0.3	0.2	0.7	0.4	0.9	3.5	4.3	9.3	15.2	24.6	48.2	71.6	102.9	144.0	231.6	321.2	28.5	7.0	0.54	1.42	**13.4**	*O&U*
All sites	28905	0	14.4	5.8	6.7	10.5	27.1	40.7	97.5	146.5	237.9	373.5	546.7	685.8	1013.3	1270.3	1567.9	2006.7	2466.4	3080.8	476.3		16.03	30.22	**273.2**	*ALL*
All sites but 173	24702	0	14.2	5.8	6.2	10.2	24.3	36.3	86.9	127.8	210.9	328.6	479.7	606.5	896.9	1108.7	1307.6	1675.5	2013.6	2508.9	407.0	100.0	14.17	26.25	**236.8**	*ALLb*
Rate from 1 case			0.245	0.253	0.268	0.243	0.219	0.211	0.235	0.254	0.237	0.280	0.299	0.307	0.313	0.329	0.422	0.502	0.747	1.053						

UK, England, North Western

The North Western Regional Cancer Registry was founded in 1962. It is part of the Centre for Cancer Epidemiology at the Christie Hospital in Manchester, which is the principal cancer centre serving the region.

The registry collects data on all residents of the North Western Health Region who develop cancer. The region comprises the counties of Greater Manchester and Lancashire, South Cumbria and a small part of Derbyshire. It covers an area of 4500 km^2 and has a population of four million. Of this population, 65% reside in the conurbation of Greater Manchester. The remainder of the region is of mixed urban–industrial and rural character. Eleven per cent of the population, including a high proportion of elderly retired residents, live in areas adjoining the coast.

The vast majority of patients receive their hospital care in National Health Service hospitals, but the private sector is growing. All hospitals notify the registry on a special form of all cases of cancer diagnosed in patients admitted to their hospital. The registries of other regions send notifications concerning residents of the North Western Region who are treated in hospitals outside the region. The registry also receives information from the special registers which operate in the region: the Children's Tumour Registry, the Ovarian Tumour Register and the Adult Leukaemia Register. The registry has links with all laboratories in the region so that copies of pathology reports are sent directly to the registry. The registry receives copies of the death certificates of all regional residents whose certificates mention cancer. The registry collects further information on cases identified by a death certificate who have not already been registered.

Follow-up of cases is through the statutory registration of deaths. All registered patients are flagged at the National Health Service Central Register, which notifies the registry of the death of flagged patients.

All addresses are assigned post-codes and all information is put on computer and submitted to validation and consistency checks. Diagnostic details are entered on the computer, which then automatically codes them to ICD-O. Two or more neoplasms may be separately registered in the same person if the neoplasms are in different sites or are in the same site with different histology.

A number of reports have been published in which registry data were used to examine variations in cancer incidence and survival within the North Western Region. Registry data are used to plan and evaluate cancer services, including the breast and cervical screening programmes. Several research studies, both national and international, have used registry data. These include studies on second malignancies after treatment for a first malignancy, studies on familial cancers and lymphoid malignancies.

The Centre for Cancer Epidemiology has undertaken a series of population-based surveys of the management of different malignancies, which have also provided the means and opportunity to confirm the completeness and quality of cancer registration.

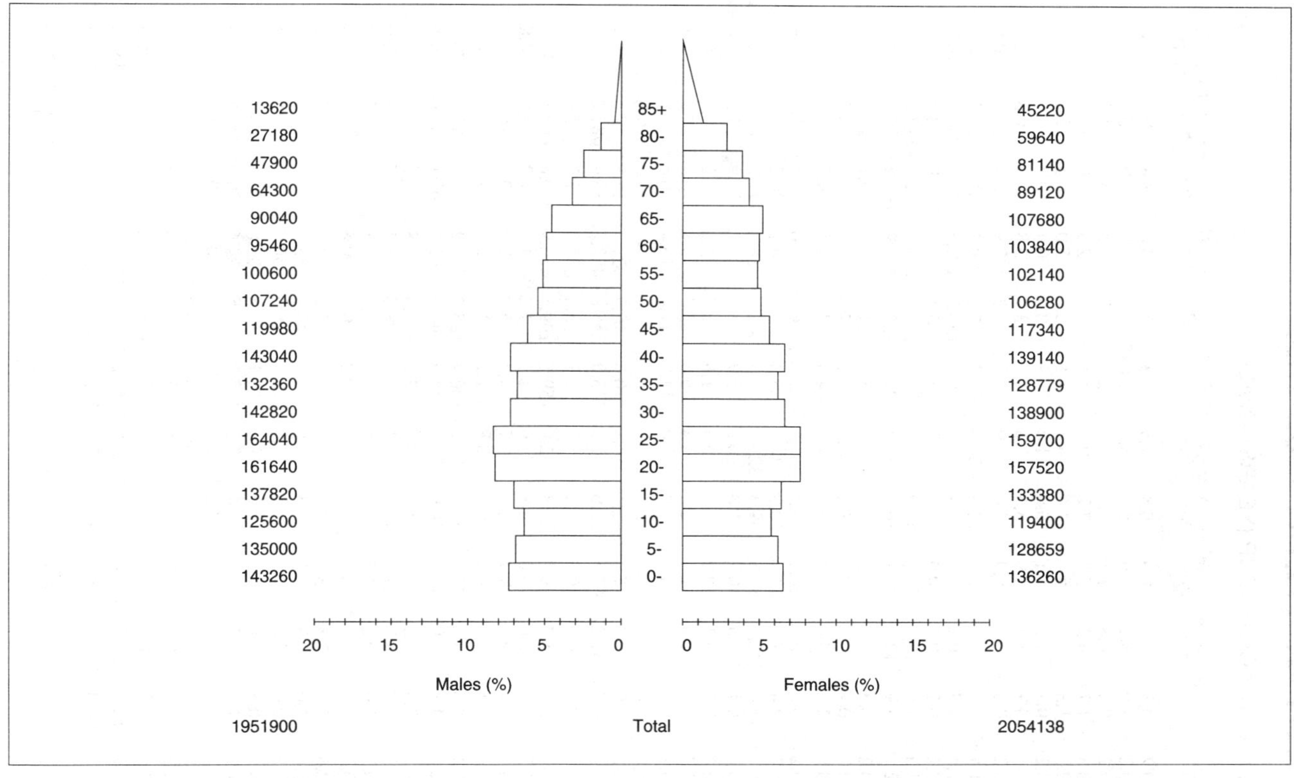

UK, England and Wales, North Western

Source of population: average annual 1988–92

Estimate: Resident population for the North Western Regional Health Authority, using the Registrar General's mid-year estimates (1981 series), updated annually starting with figures derived from the 1981 Census and allowing for births, deaths and migration. Adjustments are made for changes such as stationed armed forces, prisoners and boarding school children. Figures are unit estimates to the nearest hundred.

Notes to tables overleaf:

* The low level of histological verification indicates possible lack of validity in the data.

Screening programmes in the area:

Since 1964 the population aged 18-55 has been screened for cervical cancer every 3 to 5 years, on a recall basis. Similarly, the population aged 50-64 has been screened every 3 years for breast cancer on a recall basis since 1988.

* UK, ENGLAND, NORTH WESTERN 1988-1992

ANNUAL INCIDENCE PER 100,000 BY AGE GROUP (YEARS) - MALE

SITE	ALL AGES	AGE UNK	0-	5-	10-	15-	20-	25-	30-	35-	40-	45-	50-	55-	60-	65-	70-	75-	80-	85+	CRUDE RATE	%	CR 64	CR 74	ASR (W)	ICD (9th)
Lip	60	0	-	-	-	-	-	0.1	-	0.2	0.3	0.2	0.9	0.8	1.5	1.3	2.5	4.6	8.8	2.9	0.6	0.1	0.02	0.04	0.4	140
Tongue	199	0	-	-	0.2	-	0.1	0.4	0.8	0.2	2.0	3.2	3.9	5.4	5.0	7.6	4.7	8.8	5.9	5.9	2.0	0.5	0.11	0.17	1.5	141
Salivary gland	65	0	-	-	-	-	0.1	0.2	0.1	0.2	0.4	0.8	1.1	0.8	2.3	2.9	2.2	1.3	5.2	1.5	0.7	0.2	0.03	0.06	0.5	142
Mouth	305	0	-	-	-	0.1	0.1	-	0.1	0.3	1.7	4.2	5.2	7.2	9.4	11.1	15.2	12.5	11.0	14.7	3.1	0.7	0.14	0.27	2.2	143-5
Oropharynx	172	0	-	-	-	-	-	-	0.4	0.3	1.3	1.7	5.0	4.4	4.4	7.1	6.2	5.0	6.6	7.3	1.8	0.4	0.09	0.15	1.3	146
Nasopharynx	40	0	-	-	0.2	0.1	0.1	0.2	0.1	0.2	0.7	1.2	1.1	0.6	1.0	0.9	0.3	0.4	0.7	-	0.4	0.1	0.03	0.03	0.3	147
Hypopharynx	124	0	-	-	-	-	-	-	-	-	0.7	1.7	1.9	3.6	3.6	4.7	3.7	5.8	7.4	10.3	1.3	0.3	0.06	0.10	0.9	148
Pharynx unspecified	61	0	-	-	-	0.1	-	-	-	0.2	0.3	-	0.9	2.6	2.9	2.2	1.2	2.9	2.9	-	0.6	0.1	0.04	0.05	0.4	149
Oesophagus	1384	0	-	-	-	-	-	0.2	0.4	1.4	3.1	6.5	16.6	22.3	36.9	63.3	67.5	99.4	101.5	79.3	14.2	3.4	0.44	1.09	9.0	150
Stomach	2608	0	-	-	-	-	0.2	0.1	0.8	1.4	4.3	10.7	15.1	33.4	72.7	98.8	136.2	204.6	245.8	281.9	26.7	6.3	0.69	1.87	16.4	151
Small intestine	70	0	-	-	-	0.1	-	-	-	0.2	0.7	0.3	0.9	1.2	2.7	2.0	3.1	4.6	2.9	4.4	0.7	0.2	0.03	0.06	0.5	152
Colon	3043	0	-	-	-	-	0.2	0.7	1.0	3.0	7.6	10.2	23.1	40.0	74.8	121.1	158.0	244.3	262.7	317.2	31.2	7.4	0.80	2.20	19.3	153
Rectum	2372	0	-	-	-	-	-	0.2	0.8	2.1	4.9	12.7	24.1	36.8	71.4	102.2	122.2	142.4	197.2	179.1	24.3	5.8	0.77	1.89	15.6	154
Liver	354	0	0.7	0.1	-	-	0.1	0.1	0.6	0.2	0.3	1.3	3.0	5.2	11.1	15.3	21.2	23.4	19.1	25.0	3.6	0.9	0.11	0.30	2.4	155
Gallbladder etc.	173	0	0.1	-	-	-	-	-	-	0.2	0.4	0.7	0.9	3.8	4.2	8.2	7.5	10.9	16.2	16.2	1.8	0.4	0.05	0.13	1.1	156
Pancreas	1158	0	-	-	-	-	-	0.1	0.1	-	0.6	2.8	5.0	9.3	19.7	31.0	44.0	62.5	82.7	104.5	96.9	11.9	2.8	0.34	0.88	7.4	157
Nose, sinuses etc.	83	0	0.1	-	-	0.1	0.1	0.1	0.1	0.2	0.6	0.5	1.2	3.4	3.1	4.7	4.6	3.7	1.5	0.9	0.2	0.03	0.07	0.6	160
Larynx	810	0	-	-	-	-	-	0.1	0.1	1.2	2.4	7.8	14.0	20.9	30.8	35.3	33.0	34.2	30.2	30.8	8.3	2.0	0.39	0.73	5.8	161
Bronchus, lung	10979	0	-	-	-	-	0.1	0.1	1.0	5.7	15.4	42.0	84.5	169.4	329.4	484.5	647.3	788.7	779.2	709.3	112.5	26.7	3.24	8.90	70.8	162
Other thoracic organs	59	0	-	-	-	0.1	-	0.2	0.4	0.2	0.1	0.5	0.9	1.0	0.8	2.9	3.4	2.1	2.9	1.5	0.6	0.1	0.02	0.05	0.4	163-4
Bone	73	0	-	0.1	0.5	1.3	1.1	-	0.8	0.3	0.7	0.3	0.7	0.8	0.4	1.6	2.5	2.9	2.2	1.5	0.7	0.2	0.04	0.06	0.6	170
Connective tissue	174	0	0.4	0.3	0.3	1.5	0.4	0.6	0.8	1.7	1.0	1.0	2.4	2.2	3.4	5.6	5.3	5.8	10.3	13.2	1.8	0.4	0.08	0.13	1.4	171
Mesothelioma	272	0	-	-	-	-	-	-	-	0.2	0.6	2.5	4.8	7.0	8.0	14.9	11.8	15.4	6.6	2.9	2.8	0.7	0.11	0.25	1.9	MES
Kaposi's sarcoma	27	0	-	-	-	-	-	0.7	1.4	0.8	0.6	-	-	0.2	-	-	-	-	-	1.5	0.3	0.1	0.02	0.02	0.2	KAP
Melanoma of skin	475	0	-	0.3	0.5	0.9	1.7	2.8	2.1	6.2	4.9	7.3	7.3	7.4	11.3	10.0	10.3	21.3	15.5	17.6	4.9	1.2	0.26	0.36	3.7	172
Other skin	6117	0	0.1	-	-	-	0.9	2.4	5.6	8.0	16.4	32.2	62.5	95.6	142.5	213.0	295.8	452.2	536.4	687.2	62.7		1.83	4.37	39.6	173
Breast	70	0	-	-	-	-	-	0.1	-	-	0.1	0.5	0.9	1.2	1.7	3.1	3.4	5.0	3.7	5.9	0.7	0.2	0.02	0.06	0.5	175
Prostate	4614	0	0.1	-	-	-	0.1	-	-	-	0.1	1.7	9.9	26.8	82.8	159.5	299.5	458.9	579.8	660.8	47.3	11.2	0.61	2.90	26.6	185
Testis	466	0	0.8	-	-	1.7	5.4	10.5	12.5	11.5	6.3	6.0	6.0	2.8	1.9	1.1	1.2	1.3	2.2	2.9	4.8	1.1	0.33	0.34	4.3	186
Penis	127	0	-	-	-	-	0.1	0.1	-	0.5	0.4	0.5	1.1	2.0	2.7	4.7	5.9	9.2	10.3	16.2	1.3	0.3	0.04	0.09	0.8	187.1-.4
Other male genital	32	0	-	-	-	-	-	-	-	-	0.1	0.2	0.2	0.2	0.8	1.1	1.6	2.1	4.4	4.4	0.3	0.1	0.01	0.02	0.2	187.5-.9
Bladder	3277	0	-	0.1	-	-	0.1	0.6	2.4	1.4	5.6	13.8	22.2	46.9	83.2	138.4	185.7	232.2	289.2	293.7	33.6	8.0	0.88	2.50	20.9	188
Kidney etc.	955	0	2.4	-	-	-	0.2	0.5	1.0	2.0	4.1	7.0	11.2	18.9	32.1	34.9	47.3	45.5	61.1	47.0	9.8	2.3	0.40	0.81	6.8	189
Eye	72	0	1.0	0.1	-	0.1	-	0.4	0.3	0.2	0.8	1.2	0.7	1.2	0.8	2.2	2.5	3.8	1.5	1.5	0.7	0.2	0.03	0.06	0.6	190
Brain, nervous system	675	0	2.2	3.7	1.6	1.9	3.2	2.1	2.5	4.2	5.7	8.7	11.0	14.1	19.1	17.8	23.6	15.4	8.8	4.4	6.9	1.6	0.40	0.61	5.7	191-2
Thyroid	92	0	-	-	0.2	0.3	0.1	0.4	1.0	0.2	1.0	0.2	1.7	1.4	1.5	4.4	3.1	3.3	5.2	1.5	0.9	0.2	0.04	0.08	0.7	193
Other endocrine	32	0	1.4	0.4	0.2	0.1	0.4	0.1	-	0.3	-	-	0.7	-	0.6	0.2	0.3	0.8	-	-	0.3	0.1	0.02	0.02	0.4	194
Hodgkin's disease	276	0	0.1	1.2	0.6	2.5	4.8	4.5	3.1	2.6	3.6	2.8	3.4	2.2	3.6	4.0	2.2	4.6	3.7	1.5	2.8	0.7	0.17	0.21	2.5	201
Non-Hodgkin lymphoma	1158	0	0.6	0.4	0.6	0.6	2.2	3.3	4.2	5.4	6.0	9.3	15.3	23.3	30.6	40.0	43.9	55.5	69.2	58.7	11.9	2.8	0.51	0.93	8.4	200,202
Multiple myeloma	445	0	-	-	-	-	-	0.1	0.4	0.3	0.4	2.2	3.4	8.0	11.9	18.9	19.3	30.9	42.7	42.6	4.6	1.1	0.13	0.32	2.9	203
Lymphoid leukaemia	478	0	5.0	2.7	2.4	1.3	0.7	0.5	0.4	0.5	0.3	0.8	2.1	4.2	9.0	15.1	19.3	33.8	35.3	63.1	4.9	1.2	0.15	0.32	3.7	204
Myeloid leukaemia	441	0	1.1	0.7	0.3	0.9	0.9	1.5	1.5	1.2	1.7	3.2	3.5	6.4	7.1	15.3	21.5	24.6	30.9	39.6	4.5	1.1	0.15	0.33	3.2	205
Monocytic leukaemia	7	0	-	-	-	-	-	-	-	-	-	-	0.2	0.2	0.2	-	0.8	0.7	1.5	0.1	0.0	0.00	0.00	0.0	206
Other leukaemia	6	0	-	-	-	-	-	-	-	-	-	0.2	-	0.2	0.4	0.6	-	-	-	0.1	0.0	0.00	0.01	0.0	207
Leukaemia unspecified	54	0	-	0.1	0.3	0.3	-	0.1	0.1	0.3	-	0.2	0.2	-	0.4	2.4	2.8	4.6	5.2	4.4	0.6	0.1	0.01	0.04	0.4	208
Other and unspecified	2763	0	0.3	-	0.2	0.4	0.6	1.0	1.4	2.4	6.2	8.8	26.5	33.2	68.7	118.2	145.9	191.2	231.8	308.4	28.3	6.7	0.75	2.07	17.8	O&U
All sites	47297	0	16.6	10.5	8.0	14.7	24.6	35.5	48.6	67.4	116.3	221.4	411.0	685.9	1223.8	1845.2	2457.9	3304.4	3771.2	4067.5	484.6		14.42	35.94	310.8	ALL
All sites but 173	41180	0	16.5	10.5	8.0	14.7	23.8	33.0	43.0	59.4	100.0	189.2	348.6	590.3	1081.3	1632.2	2162.1	2852.2	3234.7	3380.3	421.9	100.0	12.59	31.56	271.2	ALLb

| Rate from 1 case | | | | | | | 0.140 | 0.148 | 0.159 | 0.145 | 0.124 | 0.122 | 0.140 | 0.151 | 0.140 | 0.167 | 0.186 | 0.199 | 0.210 | 0.222 | 0.311 | 0.418 | 0.736 | 1.468 | | |

* UK, ENGLAND, NORTH WESTERN 1988-1992

ANNUAL INCIDENCE PER 100,000 BY AGE GROUP (YEARS) - FEMALE

SITE	ALL AGES	AGE UNK	0-	5-	10-	15-	20-	25-	30-	35-	40-	45-	50-	55-	60-	65-	70-	75-	80-	85+	CRUDE RATE	%	CR 64	CR 74	ASR (W)	ICD (9th)
Lip	19	0	-	-	-	-	-	-	-	-	0.1	-	0.2	0.2	0.2	0.2	1.1	0.7	1.0	1.3	0.2	0.0	0.00	0.01	0.1	140
Tongue	95	0	-	-	-	-	-	0.3	0.1	0.3	0.3	0.5	0.9	2.2	2.3	2.4	3.1	2.5	3.0	4.9	0.9	0.2	0.03	0.06	0.5	141
Salivary gland	54	0	-	-	-	-	0.1	0.1	-	0.5	0.4	-	0.4	0.8	0.4	2.2	1.6	3.0	2.0	0.4	0.5	0.1	0.01	0.03	0.3	142
Mouth	136	0	-	-	-	-	0.1	-	0.4	0.8	0.3	1.2	1.5	1.6	3.3	5.0	3.6	4.7	4.7	4.0	1.3	0.3	0.05	0.09	0.8	143-5
Oropharynx	69	0	-	-	-	-	-	-	-	0.5	-	1.2	1.5	1.4	1.5	1.7	1.3	2.2	2.7	1.8	0.7	0.2	0.03	0.05	0.4	146
Nasopharynx	21	0	-	-	-	-	-	0.1	-	-	0.1	0.7	0.6	0.2	0.6	0.4	0.2	0.2	1.3	-	0.2	0.0	0.01	0.01	0.1	147
Hypopharynx	65	0	-	-	-	-	-	-	-	-	0.1	0.7	1.1	0.6	2.1	1.9	2.2	1.7	1.3	4.0	0.6	0.2	0.02	0.04	0.4	148
Pharynx unspecified	37	0	-	-	-	-	-	-	-	-	0.3	0.5	0.6	0.4	0.6	0.7	0.7	1.5	2.0	2.2	0.4	0.1	0.01	0.02	0.2	149
Oesophagus	961	0	-	-	-	-	-	-	0.1	0.2	1.4	2.7	4.1	8.2	18.5	21.7	32.3	46.6	58.0	66.3	9.4	2.3	0.18	0.45	3.9	150
Stomach	1845	0	-	-	-	-	-	0.5	0.7	0.6	2.3	3.2	7.0	13.1	22.7	36.2	56.6	97.9	125.4	157.9	18.0	4.4	0.25	0.71	6.8	151
Small intestine	79	0	-	-	-	-	-	0.1	0.1	0.2	0.3	0.2	0.8	0.6	2.1	1.9	3.4	3.5	3.0	3.1	0.8	0.2	0.02	0.05	0.4	152
Colon	3555	0	-	-	-	0.1	-	0.8	0.7	2.0	6.5	11.4	23.0	38.0	54.1	83.4	121.2	167.6	212.3	229.5	34.6	8.4	0.68	1.71	15.0	153
Rectum	1754	0	-	-	-	-	0.1	0.5	1.2	1.1	3.0	9.0	13.7	20.2	31.0	43.5	55.4	76.4	93.2	112.3	17.1	4.1	0.40	0.89	7.8	154
Liver	243	0	0.3	0.2	-	0.3	-	-	0.1	0.2	0.6	1.7	0.6	3.1	2.9	5.4	7.6	13.8	10.4	16.8	2.4	0.6	0.05	0.11	1.1	155
Gallbladder etc.	304	0	-	-	-	-	-	-	-	-	0.9	0.7	1.3	2.7	5.6	7.2	10.1	12.6	22.1	19.0	3.0	0.7	0.06	0.14	1.2	156
Pancreas	1235	0	-	-	-	-	-	-	0.3	0.9	1.1	3.4	9.4	12.5	22.5	31.4	38.8	60.6	71.1	74.3	12.0	2.9	0.25	0.60	5.3	157
Nose, sinuses etc.	72	0	0.1	-	-	-	-	-	-	-	0.3	1.2	0.9	0.8	0.8	1.7	2.9	2.5	3.7	2.7	0.7	0.2	0.02	0.04	0.4	160
Larynx	189	0	-	-	-	-	-	-	0.3	0.2	0.7	1.0	1.9	3.7	4.4	7.6	5.8	6.4	6.7	4.4	1.8	0.4	0.06	0.13	1.0	161
Bronchus, lung	5486	0	0.1	-	-	0.1	0.3	0.4	1.0	3.6	11.2	24.9	39.5	75.4	142.1	209.1	231.8	199.9	189.1	158.3	53.4	12.9	1.49	3.70	27.8	162
Other thoracic organs	41	0	0.3	-	-	-	0.3	-	-	-	0.3	0.3	0.2	1.0	1.2	1.7	1.8	0.2	0.7	0.4	0.4	0.1	0.02	0.03	0.3	163-4
Bone	66	0	-	0.5	1.0	0.9	0.6	0.1	0.1	0.5	0.4	0.5	0.2	0.2	0.8	0.6	1.3	1.7	2.3	2.7	0.6	0.2	0.03	0.04	0.5	170
Connective tissue	157	0	1.3	0.5	0.5	0.6	0.9	0.4	0.4	0.6	0.7	1.2	1.1	2.0	1.9	2.8	2.9	6.7	5.0	5.7	1.5	0.4	0.06	0.09	1.1	171
Mesothelioma	64	0	-	-	-	-	-	-	-	-	0.3	0.7	0.8	1.2	2.1	3.2	2.0	2.0	0.7	0.4	0.6	0.2	0.03	0.05	0.4	MES
Kaposi's sarcoma	2	0	-	-	-	-	-	0.1	-	-	-	-	-	-	-	-	-	-	-	0.4	0.0	0.0	0.00	0.00	0.0	KAP
Melanoma of skin	802	1	-	0.3	0.2	1.0	4.1	5.5	7.3	10.4	9.8	11.6	10.5	10.4	13.1	13.2	12.6	16.3	17.8	16.8	7.8	1.9	0.42	0.55	5.7	172
Other skin	6694	0	-	-	0.3	1.0	0.8	2.3	6.2	10.4	17.0	32.4	48.4	71.5	100.3	155.5	205.3	297.0	369.9	460.0	65.2		1.45	3.26	29.5	173
Breast	10917	0	-	-	-	-	0.9	7.0	25.9	53.7	105.9	160.7	189.1	230.5	258.7	246.7	248.4	261.8	289.1	337.9	106.3	25.7	5.16	7.64	68.6	174
Uterus unspecified	226	0	-	-	-	-	-	0.4	0.1	0.3	1.0	0.9	1.5	3.3	3.7	8.2	4.9	8.4	9.4	15.9	2.2	0.5	0.06	0.12	1.1	179
Cervix uteri	1923	0	-	-	-	0.3	2.8	9.6	27.2	31.8	27.9	29.0	29.9	31.1	31.4	37.3	32.8	31.3	22.8	18.1	18.7	4.5	1.11	1.46	14.3	180
Placenta	2	0	-	-	-	-	0.1	-	-	-	0.1	-	-	-	-	-	-	-	-	-	0.0	0.0	0.00	0.00	0.0	181
Corpus uteri	1160	0	-	-	-	0.1	-	-	0.4	0.6	3.2	10.4	18.6	31.5	30.6	37.0	34.6	34.8	31.5	27.4	11.3	2.7	0.48	0.84	6.8	182
Ovary etc.	1851	1	0.1	-	-	0.6	1.0	1.8	3.3	6.1	10.3	19.4	26.9	40.9	45.6	49.8	55.7	54.0	46.9	49.1	18.0	4.4	0.78	1.31	11.1	183
Other female genital	465	0	0.1	-	-	-	0.1	0.4	1.4	1.4	1.6	1.5	2.6	5.7	6.5	8.2	12.3	21.0	30.5	30.5	4.5	1.1	0.11	0.21	2.0	184
Bladder	1435	0	-	-	-	-	0.4	0.4	0.6	0.6	2.3	4.4	10.4	13.9	29.9	39.6	50.5	66.6	74.8	73.9	14.0	3.4	0.31	0.76	6.4	188
Kidney etc.	676	0	1.6	0.5	0.2	-	0.3	0.1	0.7	1.2	2.2	4.3	7.7	11.9	14.4	16.9	22.9	27.6	24.5	22.1	6.6	1.6	0.23	0.42	3.7	189
Eye	74	0	2.1	0.2	-	-	0.1	0.1	0.1	0.3	0.6	1.0	1.3	0.8	1.3	1.5	1.1	2.5	1.0	-	0.7	0.2	0.04	0.05	0.7	190
Brain, nervous system	489	0	2.2	3.3	2.2	1.5	1.8	1.9	2.6	2.8	3.9	3.9	6.4	10.2	12.3	11.5	11.7	8.1	4.7	1.8	4.8	1.2	0.27	0.39	3.9	191-2
Thyroid	245	0	-	-	0.2	0.6	1.7	1.9	1.7	3.7	2.7	3.9	2.8	2.9	3.7	2.2	5.2	4.7	6.0	5.7	2.4	0.6	0.13	0.17	1.8	193
Other endocrine	28	0	1.3	0.3	-	-	-	-	0.1	0.3	0.3	0.3	0.2	0.4	-	-	0.7	0.7	-	0.4	0.3	0.1	0.02	0.02	0.3	194
Hodgkin's disease	200	0	-	-	1.0	2.1	3.7	2.9	2.4	3.1	2.4	1.2	1.5	1.6	1.5	2.2	2.7	2.0	2.3	1.8	1.9	0.5	0.12	0.14	1.7	201
Non-Hodgkin lymphoma	1039	0	0.3	-	0.5	0.3	1.4	1.8	3.5	1.7	5.2	7.0	11.5	13.7	24.1	28.6	32.5	33.8	42.3	34.1	10.1	2.5	0.35	0.66	5.7	200,202
Multiple myeloma	499	0	-	-	-	-	-	-	-	0.5	0.9	1.7	3.6	4.7	9.6	13.9	17.7	22.7	26.5	27.4	4.9	1.2	0.10	0.26	2.2	203
Lymphoid leukaemia	347	0	3.2	1.6	1.0	0.4	0.5	0.5	0.6	0.3	0.6	1.2	0.9	2.0	3.9	5.4	8.1	15.3	21.8	23.9	3.4	0.8	0.08	0.15	1.9	204
Myeloid leukaemia	431	0	0.7	0.5	0.8	1.0	0.8	1.3	1.2	2.5	2.9	2.2	4.7	2.3	5.0	8.9	11.2	15.8	20.5	23.0	4.2	1.0	0.13	0.23	2.4	205
Monocytic leukaemia	4	0	-	-	-	-	-	-	-	-	-	-	-	-	0.2	0.2	0.2	-	-	0.4	0.0	0.0	0.00	0.00	0.0	206
Other leukaemia	1	0	-	-	-	-	-	-	-	-	-	-	-	-	-	0.2	-	-	-	-	0.0	0.0	0.00	0.00	0.0	207
Leukaemia unspecified	54	0	0.1	-	0.2	-	0.1	0.1	-	-	0.3	-	0.2	0.6	0.6	0.4	2.0	1.5	2.0	8.0	0.5	0.1	0.01	0.02	0.2	208
Other and unspecified	2989	0	0.4	0.2	-	0.1	0.4	0.1	1.2	2.3	5.9	8.4	19.6	29.4	51.6	67.6	106.8	130.1	160.6	220.3	29.1	7.0	0.60	1.47	12.8	O&U
All sites	49100	2	14.5	7.8	8.0	11.4	23.2	41.3	92.4	146.1	238.6	372.4	509.6	709.2	971.9	1226.4	1468.1	1770.5	2026.8	2271.6	478.1		15.73	29.21	258.5	ALL
All sites but 173	42406	2	14.5	7.8	7.7	10.3	22.5	39.1	86.2	135.7	221.6	340.0	461.2	637.8	871.5	1071.0	1262.8	1473.5	1656.9	1811.6	412.9	100.0	14.28	25.95	229.0	ALLb
Rate from 1 case			0.147	0.155	0.167	0.150	0.127	0.125	0.144	0.155	0.144	0.170	0.188	0.196	0.193	0.186	0.224	0.246	0.335	0.442						

UK, England, Oxford Region

Cancer registration data have been collected on a regional basis since 1952. The Oxford Cancer Registry is now part of the Oxford Cancer Intelligence Unit. This Unit is responsible not only for cancer registration, but also for providing a cancer information service, managing the work on quality assurance and evaluation of the breast and cervical screening programmes in the Region and undertaking and contributing to programmes of clinical audit and research.

The Oxford Region consists of the counties of Berkshire, Buckinghamshire, Northamptonshire and Oxfordshire in central England, and covers a population of about 2 600 000, with a slight excess of females, mainly in the 85+-year age bracket. Around 14% of the population is aged under 10 years, about 17% between 20 and 30 years and nearly 6% 75 years or over. Berkshire has a population of 758 000, Buckinghamshire 645 000, Northamptonshire 590 200 and Oxfordshire 587 100. Berkshire has more residents from African, Caribbean, Indian, Pakistani, Bangladeshi, Chinese, Asian or other minority groups, which account for 7.6% of its population, than the other counties.

The registry collects data on patients who are resident in or treated within the region. Cases are notified by histopathology and cytopathology laboratories and medical records departments. Death certificates relating to the region's resident population, where cancer is mentioned, are also passed to the registry from the Office of National Statistics. In addition, all registered cancer patients are flagged on the National Health Service Central Register to ensure that the local registry is informed of deaths among the registered population, including those from causes other than cancer and those occurring outside the region. There is collaboration with specialist registers (e.g., Childhood Cancer Research Group, Oxford Regional Leukaemia Register) and directly with clinicians to collect certain types of data.

The registry collects data on all malignant tumours, *in situ* neoplasms and certain benign tumours. An abstract of each tumour record is passed to the Office of National Statistics for inclusion in the National Cancer Registration Scheme. Information on non-residents treated within the Oxford Region is passed to the appropriate regional registry.

The process of registration was entirely manual until 1992, when a minicomputer system was installed. Initially, the registry continued to receive paper copies of histopathology and cytopathology reports from contributing hospitals and all data were manually entered on the system. Currently electronic versions of pathology reports (abstracted by identifying all cancer SNOMED codes) with demographic details separately identified are received from all laboratories. Electronic downloads from Casemix/Patient Administration Systems are received from all provider sites. Record-matching software is used to distinguish new registrations from amendments or non-registrable cases. Demographic details of new registrations are added automatically to the file. Clerks then add the diagnosis and treatment details.

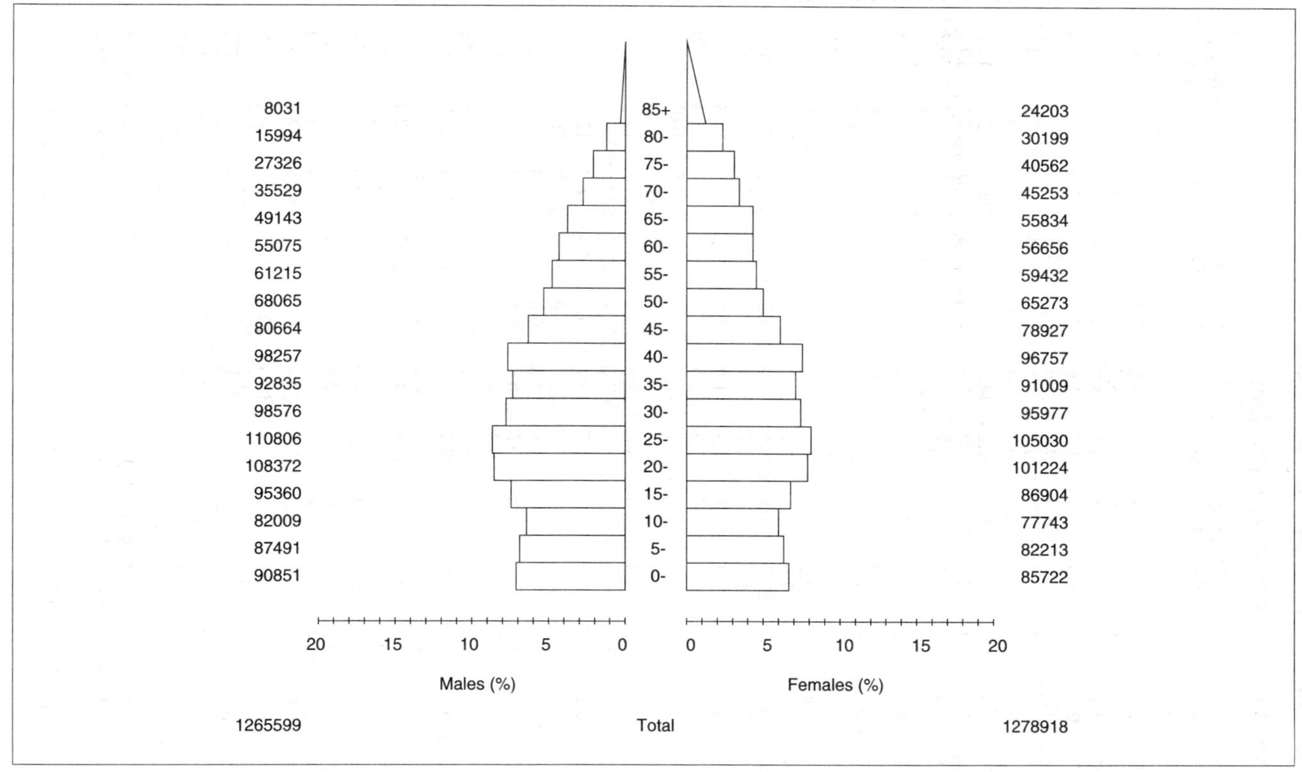

UK, England and Wales, Oxford Region
Source of population: average annual 1988–92
Estimate: The populations for 1988–91 are those published in OPCS PE81-91 (3) Annual Population Estimates Mid–81-Mid 1991 (1991 Boundaries). The 1992 estimate is published in OPCS PE92 (3) Population Estimates Mid–92.

Screening programmes in the area:
In figures giving a point estimate estimate for 1990/91 (Source: KC61 & 62), 260 788 examinations for cervical cancer are carried out annually in the population over age 20, screened every 3 to 5 years, and 38 079 breast cancer examinations in the population over age 50, screened every 2 to 3 years.

UK, ENGLAND, OXFORD REGION 1988-1992

ANNUAL INCIDENCE PER 100,000 BY AGE GROUP (YEARS) - MALE

SITE	ALL AGES	AGE UNK	0-	5-	10-	15-	20-	25-	30-	35-	40-	45-	50-	55-	60-	65-	70-	75-	80-	85+	CRUDE RATE	%	CR 64	CR 74	ASR (W)	ICD (9th)
Lip	61	0	-	-	-	-	0.2	0.2	-	0.2	-	0.5	1.2	1.0	2.9	3.3	3.9	8.8	12.5	10.0	1.0	0.3	0.03	0.07	0.7	140
Tongue	95	0	-	-	-	0.2	-	0.7	-	0.9	1.4	-	3.5	2.9	3.3	6.5	7.3	6.6	6.3	14.9	1.5	0.4	0.06	0.13	1.2	141
Salivary gland	52	0	-	-	-	-	0.2	-	-	-	0.4	0.5	0.9	1.6	2.9	3.7	1.1	7.3	11.3	2.5	0.8	0.2	0.03	0.06	0.6	142
Mouth	92	0	-	-	-	-	0.2	0.2	0.2	0.9	0.6	1.7	3.5	3.3	5.1	5.7	3.9	4.4	12.5	5.0	1.5	0.4	0.08	0.13	1.1	143-5
Oropharynx	40	0	-	-	-	-	-	-	0.2	0.2	0.2	1.0	1.5	1.3	3.3	1.6	2.3	0.7	7.5	-	0.6	0.2	0.04	0.06	0.5	146
Nasopharynx	20	0	-	-	-	0.4	-	0.2	0.2	0.4	0.2	-	0.3	1.3	0.4	1.6	0.6	1.5	-	-	0.3	0.1	0.02	0.03	0.3	147
Hypopharynx	43	0	-	-	-	-	-	-	-	-	-	0.2	0.9	2.0	0.7	4.5	3.9	4.4	5.0	7.5	0.7	0.2	0.02	0.06	0.5	148
Pharynx unspecified	16	0	-	-	-	-	-	-	-	-	-	0.2	0.2	-	0.3	0.7	2.4	0.6	2.2	1.3	-	0.3	0.1	0.01	0.02	0.2	149
Oesophagus	645	0	-	-	-	-	-	0.2	0.2	0.4	2.4	5.0	9.4	18.9	31.2	44.0	56.3	79.0	102.5	87.2	10.2	2.8	0.34	0.84	7.2	150
Stomach	1246	0	-	-	-	-	-	0.2	0.6	0.9	4.3	6.7	12.6	26.1	55.9	83.8	134.0	154.4	210.1	224.1	19.7	5.4	0.54	1.63	13.6	151
Small intestine	42	0	-	-	-	-	-	-	-	0.4	0.6	0.5	0.6	0.7	2.9	3.3	2.8	0.7	8.8	5.0	0.7	0.2	0.03	0.06	0.5	152
Colon	1845	0	-	0.2	0.7	0.4	0.7	0.5	1.0	1.7	7.9	13.9	27.3	45.4	82.4	120.5	173.9	218.8	270.1	361.1	29.2	8.0	0.91	2.38	20.6	153
Rectum	1299	1	-	-	-	-	0.2	0.2	1.2	1.9	4.1	11.2	23.5	37.6	53.0	93.6	123.8	152.2	172.6	196.7	20.5	5.6	0.66	1.75	14.6	154
Liver	145	1	-	-	0.5	-	-	0.5	0.4	0.2	0.2	0.7	2.6	2.6	5.4	9.0	19.1	13.9	22.5	17.4	2.3	0.6	0.07	0.21	1.6	155
Gallbladder etc.	97	0	-	-	-	-	0.2	0.2	-	-	0.2	0.7	1.5	2.9	4.4	4.9	9.0	13.9	12.5	19.9	1.5	0.4	0.05	0.12	1.1	156
Pancreas	669	0	-	-	-	-	-	-	0.8	1.1	1.8	5.7	9.7	19.3	31.2	40.7	63.6	77.6	106.3	114.6	10.6	2.9	0.35	0.87	7.4	157
Nose, sinuses etc.	53	0	-	-	-	-	-	0.2	0.2	-	0.8	0.5	1.2	1.6	1.5	3.7	5.6	4.4	5.0	7.5	0.8	0.2	0.03	0.08	0.6	160
Larynx	288	0	-	-	-	-	-	-	-	0.6	1.2	3.2	7.6	11.1	17.1	18.7	24.8	25.6	25.0	34.9	4.6	1.3	0.20	0.42	3.4	161
Bronchus, lung	5076	0	-	-	-	0.2	0.2	0.2	1.0	4.1	6.9	25.8	54.7	108.5	228.4	383.0	527.5	682.9	845.3	689.8	80.2	22.1	2.15	6.70	55.1	162
Other thoracic organs	21	0	0.2	-	-	-	-	-	-	0.6	0.2	1.0	0.9	-	0.7	1.6	-	1.5	1.3	-	0.3	0.1	0.02	0.03	0.3	163-4
Bone	65	0	0.9	-	1.5	2.3	1.1	1.1	0.2	0.4	0.6	0.7	0.3	2.3	1.5	1.2	1.7	1.5	-	7.5	1.0	0.3	0.06	0.08	1.0	170
Connective tissue	183	0	1.5	0.5	0.7	1.5	0.2	0.7	3.2	2.2	3.5	2.0	2.9	6.2	7.3	6.5	7.3	9.5	10.0	22.4	2.9	0.8	0.16	0.23	2.4	171
Mesothelioma	150	0	-	-	-	-	-	-	-	0.2	1.0	3.5	5.6	7.5	6.5	12.6	9.6	8.8	7.5	10.0	2.4	0.7	0.12	0.23	1.9	MES
Kaposi's sarcoma	12	0	-	-	-	-	-	0.2	0.6	0.4	1.2	-	-	-	-	-	-	-	-	-	0.2	0.1	0.01	0.01	0.2	KAP
Melanoma of skin	452	1	-	-	0.2	1.5	1.7	3.6	5.7	8.2	8.3	11.2	10.3	16.0	15.6	18.3	23.6	19.0	21.3	12.5	7.1	2.0	0.41	0.62	5.8	172
Other skin	6160	50	-	-	1.0	1.8	4.2	9.3	17.2	30.9	63.5	91.4	150.3	236.4	367.1	551.7	709.9	927.8	1299.9	97.3		3.06	7.69	68.7	173
Breast	54	0	-	-	-	-	-	-	-	-	0.2	0.7	0.9	2.3	2.2	4.1	3.4	4.4	8.8	12.5	0.9	0.2	0.03	0.07	0.6	175
Prostate	3239	1	-	-	-	-	-	-	0.2	-	1.0	2.7	8.8	33.3	89.7	188.4	358.0	550.4	769.0	936.3	51.2	14.1	0.68	3.41	32.5	185
Testis	420	0	0.4	-	0.7	3.1	9.2	15.5	14.0	15.1	12.2	5.0	4.7	3.3	1.8	2.8	0.6	3.7	1.3	-	6.6	1.8	0.43	0.44	5.7	186
Penis	72	0	-	-	-	-	-	0.4	-	0.6	0.6	1.2	1.5	2.6	0.4	6.1	5.1	8.8	7.5	7.5	1.1	0.3	0.04	0.09	0.8	187.1-.4
Other male genital	11	0	-	-	-	-	-	-	-	-	-	0.2	0.6	0.3	0.4	0.8	0.6	1.5	-	2.5	0.2	0.0	0.01	0.01	0.1	187.5-.9
Bladder	1843	1	-	-	-	-	0.2	0.7	2.4	2.2	3.9	12.1	27.0	51.3	75.2	124.1	176.8	230.5	268.8	353.6	29.1	8.0	0.88	2.38	20.4	188
Kidney etc.	628	0	4.8	0.7	-	-	0.2	0.5	0.8	2.8	5.1	6.4	10.9	24.2	30.1	39.1	50.7	68.1	57.5	29.9	9.9	2.7	0.43	0.88	7.6	189
Eye	46	0	0.9	0.2	-	-	-	0.2	0.6	-	1.0	1.5	0.9	1.3	2.2	0.8	2.3	2.2	5.0	-	0.7	0.2	0.04	0.06	0.6	190
Brain, nervous system	491	0	2.6	5.0	2.7	2.5	2.0	2.7	2.8	4.1	6.3	8.2	13.5	11.8	22.5	24.8	27.0	31.5	10.0	17.4	7.8	2.1	0.43	0.69	6.7	191-2
Thyroid	60	0	-	-	0.4	0.9	0.5	0.2	1.5	0.8	0.7	2.4	1.6	-	4.1	3.4	1.5	3.8	2.5	0.9	0.3	0.05	0.08	0.8	193	
Other endocrine	44	0	2.0	0.2	0.7	0.4	-	0.2	0.2	0.2	0.6	0.5	0.6	1.0	1.5	1.6	1.1	1.5	3.8	2.5	0.7	0.2	0.04	0.05	0.7	194
Hodgkin's disease	179	0	-	0.2	0.2	2.5	5.9	5.2	3.9	3.0	2.8	3.2	2.4	2.9	2.9	2.8	3.9	2.2	-	5.0	2.8	0.8	0.18	0.21	2.5	201
Non-Hodgkin lymphoma	849	0	1.1	1.4	0.7	1.7	1.5	4.3	4.9	5.4	9.0	14.4	24.7	28.8	31.6	41.1	51.2	73.2	73.8	84.7	13.4	3.7	0.65	1.11	10.4	200,202
Multiple myeloma	357	0	-	-	-	-	-	-	0.6	1.1	1.8	2.2	6.5	10.5	17.4	20.8	30.4	43.2	62.5	37.4	5.6	1.6	0.20	0.46	3.9	203
Lymphoid leukaemia	303	0	7.5	4.1	2.4	2.1	1.1	0.4	0.8	0.2	0.8	0.5	2.9	6.2	9.1	13.8	23.1	21.2	40.0	54.8	4.8	1.3	0.19	0.38	4.3	204
Myeloid leukaemia	353	0	2.0	0.5	0.7	0.2	2.0	1.8	1.4	2.8	3.5	2.7	4.1	5.6	11.3	21.2	24.8	34.4	48.8	62.3	5.6	1.5	0.19	0.42	4.2	205
Monocytic leukaemia	33	0	0.4	0.2	-	0.4	0.2	-	0.2	-	0.2	0.2	-	0.3	1.1	0.8	3.4	5.9	2.5	5.0	0.5	0.1	0.02	0.04	0.4	206
Other leukaemia	8	0	0.2	-	0.2	0.2	-	-	-	-	-	0.2	-	0.3	-	0.4	0.6	-	1.3	-	0.1	0.0	0.01	0.01	0.1	207
Leukaemia unspecified	28	0	-	-	-	-	0.2	-	-	-	-	-	0.6	0.3	1.1	1.6	0.6	3.7	7.5	12.5	0.4	0.1	0.01	0.02	0.3	208
Other and unspecified	1276	0	0.4	-	-	0.4	0.6	0.4	1.4	3.9	3.5	9.4	10.6	27.4	42.5	81.8	119.9	159.6	241.3	311.3	20.2	5.5	0.50	1.51	13.8	O&U
All sites	29161	55	25.1	13.3	12.2	21.6	30.8	46.0	59.4	86.2	132.7	232.3	397.3	686.1	1143.5	1822.8	2644.6	3456.7	4417.7	5087.5	460.8		14.46	36.84	327.5	ALL
All sites but 173	23001	5	25.1	13.3	12.2	20.6	29.0	41.9	50.1	68.9	101.8	168.8	305.9	535.8	907.1	1455.7	2092.9	2746.8	3489.9	3787.6	363.5	100.0	11.40	29.15	258.8	ALLb

Rate from 1 case: 0.220 0.229 0.244 0.210 0.185 0.180 0.203 0.215 0.204 0.248 0.294 0.327 0.363 0.407 0.563 0.732 1.250 2.490

UK, ENGLAND, OXFORD REGION 1988-1992

ANNUAL INCIDENCE PER 100,000 BY AGE GROUP (YEARS) - FEMALE

SITE	ALL AGES	AGE UNK	0-	5-	10-	15-	20-	25-	30-	35-	40-	45-	50-	55-	60-	65-	70-	75-	80-	85+	CRUDE RATE	%	CR 64	CR 74	ASR (W)	ICD (9th)
Lip	23	0	-	-	-	-	-	-	-	-	0.2	0.3	0.3	0.7	0.4	0.7	1.3	2.0	2.6	3.3	0.4	0.1	0.01	0.02	**0.2**	140
Tongue	54	0	-	-	-	-	-	-	0.2	0.2	0.2	0.5	0.9	2.0	0.7	3.9	2.7	2.5	6.0	5.8	0.8	0.2	0.02	0.06	**0.5**	141
Salivary gland	39	0	-	-	-	-	0.2	-	0.2	0.2	0.6	0.5	0.6	1.3	1.8	1.4	1.8	2.0	2.6	3.3	0.6	0.2	0.03	0.04	**0.4**	142
Mouth	71	0	-	-	-	-	-	0.2	0.4	-	0.8	1.3	1.5	2.4	2.5	3.2	3.1	3.5	5.3	7.4	1.1	0.3	0.05	0.08	**0.7**	143-5
Oropharynx	22	0	-	-	-	-	-	-	-	-	-	-	1.5	0.3	0.7	2.1	0.4	2.0	1.3	0.8	0.3	0.1	0.01	0.03	**0.2**	146
Nasopharynx	13	0	-	-	-	-	-	0.2	-	-	0.2	-	-	0.3	0.4	0.4	1.3	0.5	2.0	0.8	0.2	0.1	0.01	0.01	**0.1**	147
Hypopharynx	25	0	-	-	-	-	-	-	-	-	0.2	0.5	-	0.3	0.7	2.1	1.3	1.0	2.0	4.1	0.4	0.1	0.01	0.03	**0.2**	148
Pharynx unspecified	11	0	-	-	-	-	-	-	-	0.2	-	-	-	0.3	0.7	0.4	2.2	-	0.7	-	0.2	0.0	0.01	0.02	**0.1**	149
Oesophagus	453	0	-	-	-	-	-	-	-	-	0.8	1.8	4.0	5.4	12.7	20.4	38.4	41.4	56.3	52.9	7.1	1.9	0.12	0.42	**3.4**	150
Stomach	681	1	-	-	-	-	-	-	0.2	0.4	1.7	3.5	3.4	13.1	18.7	29.4	42.9	59.2	82.1	106.6	10.6	2.8	0.21	0.57	**5.1**	151
Small intestine	55	0	-	-	-	-	-	0.2	0.2	0.2	0.2	0.5	1.2	1.7	1.4	2.9	4.4	3.9	4.0	3.3	0.9	0.2	0.03	0.06	**0.5**	152
Colon	2130	1	-	-	0.3	0.5	1.0	1.5	1.7	4.4	7.4	10.6	25.7	41.1	66.0	91.0	135.2	172.1	235.1	289.2	33.3	8.7	0.80	1.93	**17.1**	153
Rectum	994	0	-	-	-	-	-	-	0.6	1.1	4.3	7.3	15.0	22.2	32.1	49.1	64.5	77.4	88.1	129.7	15.5	4.1	0.41	0.98	**8.4**	154
Liver	111	0	0.5	0.2	-	0.2	0.2	-	-	0.2	0.6	1.5	0.9	2.0	4.6	2.9	6.6	7.9	12.6	13.2	1.7	0.5	0.06	0.10	**1.0**	155
Gallbladder etc.	158	0	0.2	-	-	-	-	-	-	0.2	0.4	-	0.6	3.7	5.3	5.7	9.3	14.8	26.5	15.7	2.5	0.6	0.05	0.13	**1.2**	156
Pancreas	760	0	-	-	0.3	-	0.2	0.2	0.2	1.1	1.7	5.1	6.1	12.8	24.7	31.5	51.3	73.5	88.1	90.1	11.9	3.1	0.26	0.68	**5.9**	157
Nose, sinuses etc.	36	0	-	-	0.3	-	-	-	0.2	0.2	0.8	0.3	0.7	2.8	1.8	-	1.5	3.3	5.0	-	0.6	0.1	0.03	0.04	**0.4**	160
Larynx	57	0	-	-	-	-	0.2	-	-	-	0.2	0.3	1.8	-	3.5	4.3	4.9	3.5	4.0	1.7	0.9	0.2	0.03	0.08	**0.6**	161
Bronchus, lung	2225	1	-	-	-	0.5	-	0.2	0.6	2.4	7.0	15.0	27.0	47.8	102.0	137.5	162.6	208.6	169.5	135.5	34.8	9.1	1.01	2.51	**19.9**	162
Other thoracic organs	22	0	-	-	-	-	-	-	-	0.2	0.2	0.3	0.3	0.3	0.4	0.7	3.5	3.0	-	-	0.3	0.1	0.01	0.03	**0.2**	163-4
Bone	45	0	-	0.2	2.1	0.5	0.2	0.6	0.6	0.9	0.2	1.0	0.6	0.7	0.7	0.7	1.3	1.5	2.0	0.8	0.7	0.2	0.04	0.05	**0.6**	170
Connective tissue	136	0	0.5	1.2	0.3	0.9	1.2	1.1	0.6	0.7	1.9	2.5	3.4	1.7	2.5	5.4	5.3	8.4	6.0	9.1	2.1	0.6	0.09	0.15	**1.6**	171
Mesothelioma	22	0	-	-	-	-	-	-	-	0.2	0.4	-	0.6	0.3	1.4	1.8	1.8	1.0	-	0.8	0.3	0.1	0.01	0.03	**0.2**	MES
Kaposi's sarcoma	2	0	-	-	-	-	-	-	-	-	-	-	-	-	-	-	-	0.4	-	0.7	0.0	0.0	0.00	0.00	**0.0**	KAP
Melanoma of skin	660	3	-	-	1.0	0.5	4.3	5.7	9.2	14.3	13.2	17.7	12.9	11.8	19.1	21.1	18.1	29.1	25.2	23.1	10.3	2.7	0.55	0.75	**7.6**	172
Other skin	5004	36	0.2	0.2	0.3	1.2	3.2	4.6	10.2	25.9	40.5	50.7	72.9	106.3	137.3	187.0	289.9	403.3	480.1	572.7	78.3		2.28	4.69	**42.8**	173
Breast	7328	3	0.2	-	-	-	2.2	9.5	23.8	61.3	115.8	201.5	230.4	263.5	300.4	288.0	316.0	321.5	326.5	384.2	114.6	30.0	6.05	9.07	**80.9**	174
Uterus unspecified	16	0	-	-	-	-	-	-	-	-	0.4	0.3	0.3	1.3	0.4	-	0.4	1.0	0.7	2.5	0.3	0.1	0.01	0.02	**0.2**	179
Cervix uteri	794	0	-	-	-	-	1.6	7.8	20.0	24.8	18.0	14.4	15.6	14.5	19.1	27.9	32.3	19.2	21.2	17.4	12.4	3.2	0.68	0.98	**9.4**	180
Placenta	4	0	-	-	-	-	0.2	0.4	0.2	-	-	-	-	-	-	-	-	-	-	-	0.1	0.0	0.00	0.00	**0.1**	181
Corpus uteri	957	0	-	-	-	-	-	-	0.4	1.5	6.0	10.6	27.9	42.1	51.5	54.4	52.6	59.2	52.3	37.2	15.0	3.9	0.70	1.24	**10.0**	182
Ovary etc.	1218	1	-	0.2	-	1.6	0.8	2.3	3.3	7.7	12.2	23.6	31.3	49.1	51.9	61.6	80.4	54.7	49.7	45.4	19.0	5.0	0.92	1.63	**13.3**	183
Other female genital	249	0	0.5	-	-	-	-	-	0.8	1.1	1.7	1.8	1.5	2.4	7.1	11.8	13.3	18.7	27.8	39.7	3.9	1.0	0.08	0.21	**2.0**	184
Bladder	676	0	-	-	-	0.2	0.2	0.2	0.2	0.2	1.4	2.3	7.4	11.8	26.5	33.3	41.5	57.7	68.9	93.4	10.6	2.8	0.25	0.63	**5.4**	188
Kidney etc.	355	0	1.4	0.5	0.8	0.5	0.2	0.6	1.0	1.5	1.9	4.3	6.4	10.8	14.1	17.9	21.2	25.1	21.2	21.5	5.6	1.5	0.22	0.42	**3.7**	189
Eye	61	0	1.2	0.2	-	-	0.2	0.6	0.2	0.7	0.6	1.0	1.5	1.7	2.5	1.8	2.2	2.0	2.0	5.0	1.0	0.2	0.05	0.07	**0.8**	190
Brain, nervous system	443	0	2.6	2.7	1.3	1.6	1.8	2.7	6.0	4.0	5.2	5.6	10.7	15.1	16.2	19.3	19.9	14.8	15.2	11.6	6.9	1.8	0.38	0.57	**5.5**	191-2
Thyroid	196	0	-	-	-	0.7	1.6	3.6	4.4	3.1	3.7	5.1	4.9	3.0	2.1	2.9	5.7	9.4	6.0	10.7	3.1	0.8	0.16	0.20	**2.3**	193
Other endocrine	38	0	2.1	0.5	-	0.2	1.0	0.2	-	0.2	0.4	0.5	0.3	1.0	1.1	0.4	1.3	0.5	1.3	0.8	0.6	0.2	0.04	0.05	**0.6**	194
Hodgkin's disease	167	0	-	0.2	0.8	2.8	6.9	4.4	3.1	4.2	1.4	2.0	0.3	2.0	2.5	2.9	3.5	3.5	4.6	-	2.6	0.7	0.15	0.19	**2.3**	201
Non-Hodgkin lymphoma	654	0	0.9	0.2	0.8	1.2	1.4	2.1	1.7	4.0	5.0	9.4	16.2	19.9	19.8	25.1	41.5	42.4	43.7	43.0	10.2	2.7	0.41	0.75	**6.6**	200,202
Multiple myeloma	343	1	-	-	-	-	-	0.2	-	0.2	0.8	0.8	4.6	7.4	12.7	20.4	22.1	32.0	31.1	33.9	5.4	1.4	0.13	0.35	**2.9**	203
Lymphoid leukaemia	229	0	6.3	2.2	1.3	2.1	1.4	0.4	1.3	0.2	0.8	-	1.5	3.7	3.9	7.2	12.4	11.3	16.6	29.7	3.6	0.9	0.13	0.22	**2.7**	204
Myeloid leukaemia	327	0	0.7	0.7	0.3	0.9	2.4	2.5	2.9	0.9	3.9	4.8	2.5	5.7	8.1	9.7	15.0	21.2	26.5	35.5	5.1	1.3	0.18	0.30	**3.2**	205
Monocytic leukaemia	12	0	-	-	-	-	-	-	-	-	0.4	0.3	0.3	0.3	0.7	-	0.4	1.0	1.3	-	0.2	0.0	0.01	0.01	**0.1**	206
Other leukaemia	5	0	-	0.2	0.3	-	-	-	0.2	-	-	0.3	-	-	-	-	-	0.5	-	0.8	0.1	0.0	0.00	0.00	**0.1**	207
Leukaemia unspecified	25	0	-	-	0.3	-	-	-	0.2	-	-	-	-	0.7	-	0.4	-	3.5	2.6	5.0	0.4	0.1	0.01	0.01	**0.2**	208
Other and unspecified	1553	1	1.2	-	-	-	0.2	1.0	1.9	1.8	3.7	8.9	15.3	25.6	45.9	65.2	92.8	134.1	173.5	238.8	24.3	6.4	0.53	1.32	**12.1**	O&U
All sites	29459	49	18.4	9.7	10.0	15.9	32.6	52.9	96.3	170.5	266.6	418.9	560.7	760.9	1029.4	1257.6	1630.8	1956.5	2198.7	2531.1	460.7		17.24	31.71	**283.2**	ALL
All sites but 173	24455	13	18.2	9.5	9.8	14.7	29.4	48.4	86.1	144.6	226.1	368.2	487.8	654.5	892.0	1070.7	1340.9	1553.2	1718.6	1958.4	382.4	100.0	14.95	27.02	**240.3**	ALLb

Rate from 1 case			0.233	0.243	0.257	0.230	0.198	0.190	0.208	0.220	0.207	0.253	0.306	0.336	0.353	0.358	0.442	0.493	0.662	0.826						

UK, England, South Thames

The registry was founded in 1958 as the South Metropolitan Cancer Registry, became population-based in 1960 and was renamed the South Thames Cancer Registry in 1974. Until 1984 it covered the South East and South West Thames Regional Health Authority areas, with a population of 6 780 000. In 1985 the registry expanded to include the two North Thames Health Regions, becoming the Thames Cancer Registry and covering, in 1990, a population of 13 950 000. Data in this volume, as in previous volumes, covers the South Thames regions only.

The Thames Cancer Registry is funded by the District Health Authorities which constitute the North and South Thames Health Regions. The registry moved location in 1996 and is now situated on the Guys Hospital campus at London Bridge, and is managed by UMDS, the United Medical and Dental Schools of Guys and St Thomas.

Although there is little heavy industry in the registration area, most of the population live in urban areas. The most common occupations are in local and national government, finance and commerce. A wide variety of races is represented in the population of the area, especially in Greater London. While the registry population includes some of the most affluent in the United Kingdom, there are pockets of extreme poverty, especially in the Greater London area.

The majority of cancer patients are treated within the National Health Service, but an increasing number receive at least part of their care in the private sector. It is believed that most private patients with cancer are registered, but the level of detail obtained may be lower than that for NHS patients.

Data are collected by a team of peripatetic tumour registrars employed by the registry, who abstract details from hospital medical records. Various sources of information are used, including hospital information systems, medical secretaries, outpatient departments, pathology departments and radiotherapy units. Information on new cancer cases is increasingly sent directly to the Registry on magnetic media from various hospitals.

Completeness of ascertainment is estimated at over 90% within three years of the initial diagnosis. Completeness is estimated by comparison with previous years' registrations, by comparison with independent case series, and using a semi-empirical method developed at the Thames Registry.

The registry installed a new computer system in October 1994, based on special software developed by a commercial company and designed to increase the accessibility of the database, which now holds records of over 1 million tumours. This system retained the previous one's user-friendly interface for manual data input from registration forms, and added a much improved patient search, and numerous cross-field validation checks. It continues the automatic coding system introduced at the registry in 1982.

Data-entry operators enter text and this is coded by the computer from dictionary tables. SNOMED2 terms and codes are used by the system to store the diagnosis, and these are translated to the relevant version of ICD. A wide range of consistency checks between data items is carried out by the computer system at the time of data entry. Quality assurance procedures are currently being extended, to include regular retrospective checks on the quality of the data stored and regular checks on the quality and consistency of the work of all staff involved in collecting and processing the data.

Each patient registered has a unique identification number. This number has a subscript which indicates how many primary cancers the patient has. The registry uses the rules for registering multiple primaries agreed between the Registries of England and Wales and the Office for National Statistics.

Basal cell carcinomas of the skin (M809–811) are included in this data-set presented in this volume, but the registry ceased to register these tumours on 1 April 1993.

The registry does not carry out active follow-up. All patients registered are flagged on the NHS Central Register (NHSCR) so that the registry is notified if they die. The registry is also notified of all cancer deaths occurring within its area, whether the patients are flagged at NHSCR or not.

Registrations based on a death certificate only (DCOs) are created if the patients' case notes cannot be traced. The proportion of such registrations rose in 1983 when cuts in resources limited the tracing of case notes through hospitals or general practitioners for patients identified from death certificates. Efforts have been made to reduce the death-certificate-only rate for 1990 onwards by tracing records held by Family Health Service Authorities. A special study has shown that in 92.6% of cases the cancer site on the death certificate had the correct three-digit ICD site code, while 4% of the patients were found not to have been suffering from a registrable neoplasm.

The reorganisation of the NHS and of cancer services in particular has increased substantially the demand for our cancer information service. The registry now employs three full time staff to handle the production of reports and answer queries from medical staff and researchers both within the region and nationally.

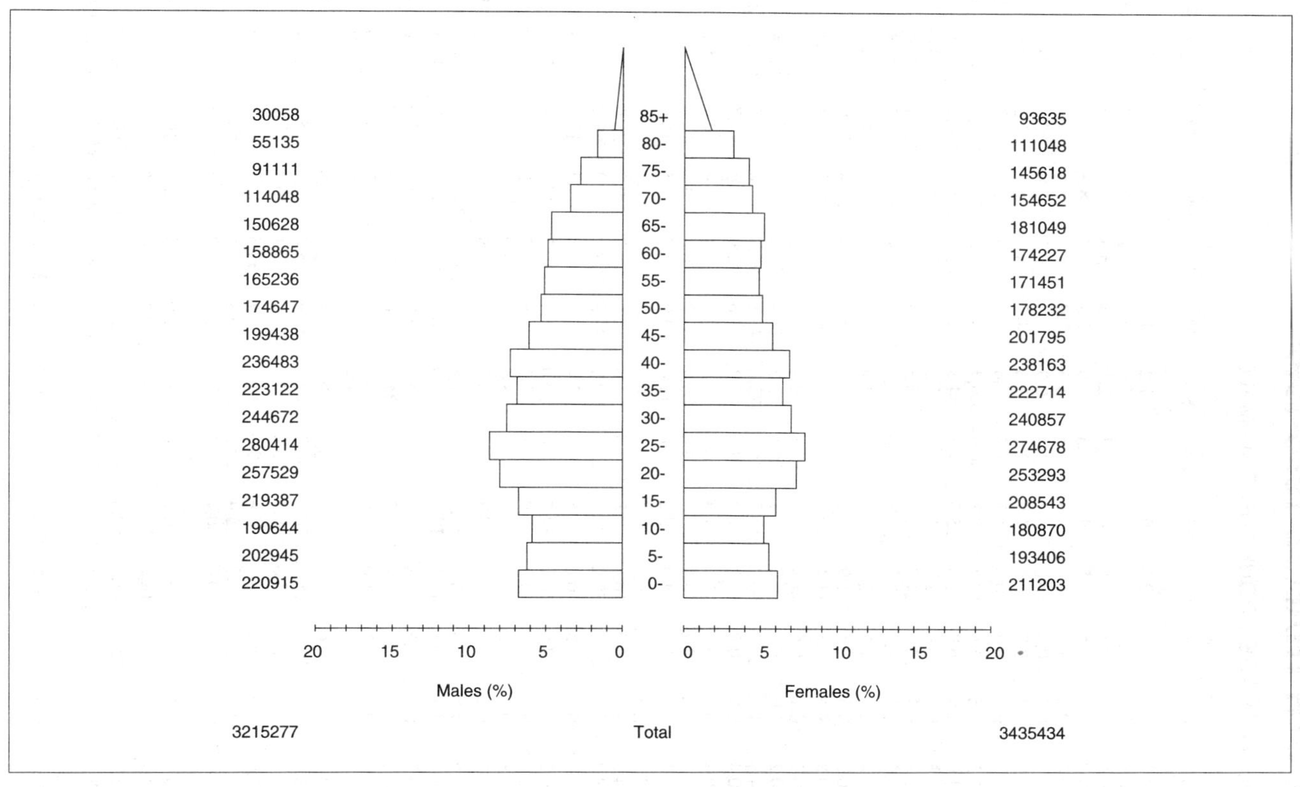

UK, England and Wales, South Thames
Source of population: average annual 1988–92
Census: 1991 Census: Usual Residence, Great Britain, OPCS. London: HMSO, 1993.
Estimate: The 1988, 1989 and 1990 populations were estimated on the basis of the 1981 Census, making allowance for births, deaths and migration. The 1992 estimate was based on the 1991 Census.
Notes to tables overleaf:
* The very high proportion of cases based on a death certificate alone, a low rate of histological verification for several sites (even allowing for the DCO diagnoses at the same site), and some rates lower than would be expected, indicate under-registration. These data are included for their historic interest.

Screening programmes in the area:
The population aged 20-64 has been screened every 3 to 5 years for cervical cancer since 1966. In 1988 a breast cancer screening programme was established for women aged 50-64, with 3-yearly examinations. There are small research projects screening for other types of cancer within the area.

* UK, ENGLAND, SOUTH THAMES 1988-1992

ANNUAL INCIDENCE PER 100,000 BY AGE GROUP (YEARS) - MALE

SITE	ALL AGES	AGE UNK	0-	5-	10-	15-	20-	25-	30-	35-	40-	45-	50-	55-	60-	65-	70-	75-	80-	85+	CRUDE RATE	%	CR 64	CR 74	ASR (W)	ICD (9th)
Lip	46	0	-	-	-	-	-	-	-	0.2	-	0.2	0.6	0.6	0.6	1.2	1.1	1.1	1.5	2.0	0.3	0.1	0.01	0.02	0.2	140
Tongue	242	0	-	-	-	-	0.2	0.1	0.2	0.8	1.1	1.1	2.5	3.3	4.0	4.6	5.3	6.1	5.8	8.0	1.5	0.4	0.07	0.12	1.0	141
Salivary gland	122	0	0.1	-	0.1	-	-	0.2	0.4	0.4	0.7	0.3	0.8	0.5	1.4	2.1	3.5	3.3	4.4	8.0	0.8	0.2	0.02	0.05	0.5	142
Mouth	285	0	-	-	-	-	0.2	0.1	-	0.2	1.0	1.5	2.5	4.1	5.3	4.9	6.8	9.2	8.3	9.3	1.8	0.4	0.07	0.13	1.1	143-5
Oropharynx	167	0	-	-	-	-	-	0.1	0.1	0.4	0.8	1.3	1.7	3.9	1.5	3.5	3.0	3.7	5.4	3.3	1.0	0.2	0.05	0.08	0.7	146
Nasopharynx	73	0	-	0.2	-	-	0.2	0.1	0.2	0.5	0.3	0.5	0.8	1.1	1.3	0.9	1.2	0.7	1.8	0.7	0.5	0.1	0.03	0.04	0.3	147
Hypopharynx	129	0	-	-	-	-	-	-	-	0.1	0.3	0.7	0.5	1.9	2.1	2.4	4.2	4.4	5.1	3.3	0.8	0.2	0.03	0.06	0.5	148
Pharynx unspecified	67	0	-	-	-	-	-	-	-	-	0.1	0.3	0.5	1.1	1.3	1.6	2.3	1.5	2.5	0.7	0.4	0.1	0.02	0.04	0.3	149
Oesophagus	2038	0	-	-	-	0.1	-	0.1	0.2	1.3	1.6	5.6	10.3	18.3	30.6	46.2	58.9	76.8	90.0	118.4	12.7	3.0	0.34	0.87	7.4	150
Stomach	3900	0	-	-	-	0.2	-	0.2	0.6	1.6	2.9	6.9	13.4	25.5	47.8	84.3	122.9	163.3	221.6	244.9	24.3	5.7	0.50	1.53	13.3	151
Small intestine	103	0	-	-	-	-	-	0.1	0.2	0.3	0.3	0.6	1.3	1.3	0.6	2.3	3.5	3.5	1.8	1.3	0.6	0.2	0.02	0.05	0.4	152
Colon	5175	0	-	-	0.2	0.2	-	0.6	1.1	2.3	6.4	12.5	24.2	42.5	66.7	103.3	142.9	211.8	286.6	321.4	32.2	7.6	0.78	2.01	18.1	153
Rectum	3504	0	-	-	-	-	0.1	0.3	1.3	1.6	5.5	9.1	17.5	32.7	49.6	71.0	105.2	135.4	158.9	200.9	21.8	5.2	0.59	1.47	12.6	154
Liver	544	0	0.3	-	0.2	-	0.5	0.1	0.5	0.4	0.8	1.3	2.3	5.6	7.9	13.9	18.6	17.6	21.4	13.3	3.4	0.8	0.10	0.26	2.1	155
Gallbladder etc.	310	0	-	-	-	-	-	-	-	0.3	0.3	0.5	1.9	2.5	3.1	7.0	8.4	11.9	21.4	14.6	1.9	0.5	0.04	0.12	1.1	156
Pancreas	2197	0	-	-	-	-	0.1	0.1	0.4	0.8	2.5	5.8	11.1	19.9	31.6	44.6	64.9	91.1	99.4	124.4	13.7	3.2	0.36	0.91	7.9	157
Nose, sinuses etc.	159	0	-	0.1	0.2	-	0.1	0.1	0.2	0.2	0.1	0.5	1.4	2.1	3.1	2.4	4.2	5.5	5.4	5.3	1.0	0.2	0.04	0.07	0.6	160
Larynx	890	0	-	-	-	-	-	0.1	0.2	1.0	4.7	6.0	9.7	16.5	19.5	27.4	28.8	30.1	31.9	5.5	1.3	0.19	0.42	3.4	161
Bronchus, lung	16156	0	0.1	-	-	-	0.2	0.1	1.0	4.4	11.2	28.0	60.8	114.7	226.0	373.0	543.1	697.4	803.8	734.6	100.5	23.8	2.23	6.81	56.1	162
Other thoracic organs	153	0	0.1	-	0.1	0.3	-	0.4	0.1	0.4	0.5	0.8	1.3	2.2	2.3	2.7	4.6	2.9	3.6	4.7	1.0	0.2	0.04	0.08	0.7	163-4
Bone	174	0	0.1	0.6	2.0	1.3	1.2	1.5	0.5	0.4	0.9	0.3	1.4	1.3	0.9	1.5	2.5	0.4	2.9	4.7	1.1	0.3	0.06	0.08	1.0	170
Connective tissue	378	0	1.1	0.4	0.5	0.7	0.6	1.1	1.2	1.3	2.2	2.2	3.3	3.1	3.0	5.8	7.2	8.6	9.8	12.0	2.4	0.6	0.10	0.17	1.8	171
Mesothelioma	522	0	-	-	-	-	-	-	0.1	0.1	1.3	2.6	4.9	8.2	8.8	11.4	13.0	18.0	14.5	10.6	3.2	0.8	0.13	0.25	2.1	MES
Kaposi's sarcoma	201	0	-	-	-	-	0.2	1.7	3.9	5.4	2.5	2.1	0.7	0.4	0.5	0.3	-	-	-	-	1.3	0.3	0.09	0.09	1.1	KAP
Melanoma of skin	1013	0	-	-	0.1	0.7	1.9	2.7	4.7	4.6	8.1	8.0	10.5	9.8	12.8	15.0	15.6	18.7	20.3	26.6	6.3	1.5	0.32	0.47	4.6	172
Other skin	9812	0	0.1	-	-	0.1	1.2	2.0	4.1	8.2	15.9	28.2	50.2	77.7	122.0	190.9	292.2	398.4	484.3	568.2	61.0		1.55	3.96	35.0	173
Breast	162	0	-	-	-	-	0.1	-	0.2	-	0.3	0.5	0.8	1.5	2.0	2.4	4.0	6.8	8.7	13.3	1.0	0.2	0.03	0.06	0.6	175
Prostate	9529	0	-	-	-	-	0.1	-	0.1	0.2	0.5	2.6	10.1	32.7	88.4	169.6	307.4	486.2	697.2	842.4	59.3	14.0	0.67	3.06	29.3	185
Testis	898	0	0.3	0.3	0.1	2.4	8.3	12.8	13.1	11.9	9.4	6.6	4.2	2.9	1.1	1.7	1.6	2.2	1.5	2.0	5.6	1.3	0.37	0.38	4.9	186
Penis	171	0	-	-	-	-	-	0.1	0.2	0.3	0.7	1.8	0.6	1.1	2.3	3.5	3.5	5.0	9.4	8.0	1.1	0.3	0.03	0.07	0.7	187.1-.4
Other male genital	33	0	-	-	-	0.1	-	-	-	0.1	0.2	-	0.2	0.4	0.4	0.7	0.7	0.9	1.8	2.0	0.2	0.0	0.01	0.01	0.1	187.5-.9
Bladder	5587	0	0.1	-	-	-	0.2	0.3	1.1	2.6	5.6	10.3	20.2	39.9	78.2	109.8	171.2	235.1	295.3	368.0	34.8	8.2	0.79	2.20	19.3	188
Kidney etc.	1656	0	1.3	0.3	0.1	0.1	0.1	0.4	0.7	1.8	3.8	5.8	12.1	17.6	27.4	34.0	46.1	52.7	65.7	59.2	10.3	2.4	0.36	0.76	6.5	189
Eye	171	0	1.3	0.4	-	0.1	0.2	0.1	0.4	0.3	0.3	0.6	1.8	1.9	2.9	3.7	3.2	2.4	5.4	2.0	1.1	0.3	0.05	0.09	0.8	190
Brain, nervous system	1281	0	2.8	2.7	1.9	1.6	2.5	2.9	4.7	4.8	6.8	7.6	13.1	18.9	19.3	24.3	22.6	17.1	9.4	6.0	8.0	1.9	0.45	0.68	6.4	191-2
Thyroid	154	0	-	-	0.2	-	0.4	0.6	1.0	0.9	0.4	0.6	0.6	1.0	1.6	2.8	3.3	2.1	2.9	2.2	1.0	0.2	0.05	0.07	0.7	193
Other endocrine	118	0	1.8	0.1	0.4	0.5	0.3	0.3	0.2	0.4	0.6	0.5	0.3	0.7	1.3	1.9	2.3	1.8	2.2	0.7	0.7	0.2	0.04	0.06	0.7	194
Hodgkin's disease	474	0	0.2	0.1	1.0	3.1	4.3	4.6	4.0	2.8	3.0	2.6	3.0	3.1	3.0	5.3	3.2	3.5	3.6	3.3	2.9	0.7	0.17	0.22	2.6	201
Non-Hodgkin lymphoma	2475	0	0.4	1.5	1.2	1.9	3.4	4.4	6.0	8.6	10.8	14.9	15.5	24.8	31.7	42.5	55.6	65.0	84.9	75.2	15.4	3.6	0.63	1.12	10.4	200,202
Multiple myeloma	943	0	-	-	-	-	-	-	0.1	0.4	1.2	2.0	5.6	8.4	15.0	19.3	26.3	35.1	45.7	57.2	5.9	1.4	0.16	0.39	3.4	203
Lymphoid leukaemia	897	0	5.8	3.4	1.5	1.9	1.1	0.4	0.3	0.9	1.0	1.8	3.4	5.9	9.3	15.3	16.7	30.3	37.7	63.2	5.6	1.3	0.18	0.34	4.1	204
Myeloid leukaemia	867	0	1.3	0.6	0.7	0.5	1.3	1.3	1.6	1.5	2.7	3.4	3.8	5.4	10.2	13.3	19.8	30.1	40.6	50.6	5.4	1.3	0.17	0.34	3.5	205
Monocytic leukaemia	25	0	0.1	-	-	-	-	-	-	-	-	0.1	0.2	0.1	0.1	0.8	0.4	0.9	2.2	0.7	0.2	0.0	0.00	0.01	0.1	206
Other leukaemia	10	0	0.1	-	-	-	-	-	0.1	-	-	-	-	0.4	0.4	-	0.4	-	-	0.1	0.0	0.00	0.00	0.0	207
Leukaemia unspecified	118	0	0.5	-	0.2	0.2	0.1	0.1	0.1	0.3	0.3	0.4	0.3	0.2	0.8	2.3	1.9	5.3	5.4	10.6	0.7	0.2	0.02	0.04	0.5	208
Other and unspecified	3757	0	0.3	-	-	0.1	0.4	0.7	1.2	2.4	4.1	7.7	14.4	28.4	42.7	70.1	107.0	164.0	217.6	256.8	23.4	5.5	0.51	1.40	12.9	O&U
All sites	77686	0	17.9	10.6	10.8	16.1	29.2	40.7	55.7	76.3	119.8	195.7	343.0	589.6	990.6	1540.3	2257.8	3067.7	3847.2	4298.4	483.2		12.48	31.47	281.2	ALL
All sites but 173	67874	0	17.8	10.6	10.8	16.0	28.0	38.7	51.7	68.1	103.9	167.6	292.8	511.9	868.7	1349.4	1965.6	2669.3	3363.0	3730.1	422.2	100.0	10.93	27.51	246.2	ALLb

| Rate from 10 cases | | | 0.905 | 0.985 | 1.049 | 0.912 | 0.777 | 0.713 | 0.817 | 0.896 | 0.846 | 1.003 | 1.145 | 1.210 | 1.259 | 1.328 | 1.754 | 2.195 | 3.627 | 6.654 | | | | | | |

* UK, ENGLAND, SOUTH THAMES 1988-1992

ANNUAL INCIDENCE PER 100,000 BY AGE GROUP (YEARS) - FEMALE

SITE	ALL AGES	AGE UNK	0-	5-	10-	15-	20-	25-	30-	35-	40-	45-	50-	55-	60-	65-	70-	75-	80-	85+	CRUDE RATE	%	CR 64	CR 74	ASR (W)	ICD (9th)
Lip	25	0	-	-	-	-	-	-	-	-	0.1	-	-	0.3	0.2	0.1	0.3	0.5	0.9	1.5	0.1	0.0	0.00	0.01	0.1	140
Tongue	185	0	0.1	-	-	0.1	0.1	0.1	0.2	0.1	0.8	1.0	0.7	1.2	2.0	2.2	3.8	4.5	4.3	4.3	1.1	0.3	0.03	0.06	0.5	141
Salivary gland	125	0	-	-	0.1	0.1	-	0.1	0.1	0.1	0.8	0.6	0.7	0.9	1.5	2.1	1.7	2.1	1.8	4.5	0.7	0.2	0.02	0.04	0.4	142
Mouth	233	0	-	-	-	-	0.1	-	0.2	0.2	0.3	1.4	0.8	1.7	3.0	3.9	3.9	5.1	5.6	6.4	1.4	0.3	0.04	0.08	0.7	143-5
Oropharynx	81	0	-	-	-	-	-	-	0.3	0.3	0.5	0.8	0.7	1.3	1.9	1.6	1.1	0.4	1.3	0.5	0.1	0.02	0.04	0.3	146
Nasopharynx	40	0	-	0.1	-	0.1	-	0.2	0.1	0.2	-	0.5	0.3	0.1	0.5	0.4	0.6	0.4	0.7	0.6	0.2	0.1	0.01	0.02	0.2	147
Hypopharynx	91	0	-	-	-	-	-	-	-	0.1	0.1	0.2	1.0	1.0	0.7	2.2	2.1	1.4	2.5	0.6	0.5	0.1	0.02	0.04	0.3	148
Pharynx unspecified	31	0	-	-	-	-	-	-	-	-	-	0.1	0.3	0.1	0.6	0.4	0.3	0.4	1.3	1.1	0.2	0.0	0.01	0.01	0.1	149
Oesophagus	1467	0	-	-	-	-	-	0.1	0.2	0.2	0.7	1.7	4.7	7.6	12.9	17.5	26.5	40.4	51.5	58.5	8.5	2.0	0.14	0.36	3.2	150
Stomach	2532	0	-	-	-	-	0.1	0.2	0.5	0.8	1.6	2.7	3.9	8.3	16.9	28.3	42.7	67.6	99.1	125.2	14.7	3.5	0.17	0.53	5.1	151
Small intestine	117	0	-	-	-	-	0.1	-	0.2	0.1	0.2	0.3	0.7	1.3	0.9	2.1	1.3	2.5	3.1	4.1	0.7	0.2	0.02	0.04	0.3	152
Colon	6513	0	-	-	-	-	0.2	0.1	0.7	2.9	5.2	11.6	21.4	36.6	61.5	81.1	116.8	164.4	204.4	273.2	37.9	9.0	0.70	1.69	15.0	153
Rectum	2993	0	-	-	-	-	0.2	0.3	1.3	1.7	3.8	6.7	12.0	20.8	28.8	39.2	56.1	75.8	83.2	106.8	17.4	4.1	0.38	0.85	7.4	154
Liver	353	0	-	-	-	0.2	0.3	0.3	0.2	0.4	0.4	0.6	1.1	2.9	3.4	5.0	5.4	9.2	7.9	13.2	2.1	0.5	0.05	0.10	0.9	155
Gallbladder etc.	447	0	-	-	-	-	-	-	0.2	0.3	0.1	0.4	1.2	2.8	4.4	6.1	6.9	11.0	14.9	19.7	2.6	0.6	0.05	0.11	1.0	156
Pancreas	2441	0	-	0.1	-	0.1	-	-	0.2	0.8	1.7	3.5	7.5	12.9	21.6	30.2	50.7	63.9	81.8	90.1	14.2	3.4	0.24	0.65	5.6	157
Nose, sinuses etc.	92	0	0.1	0.2	-	-	0.1	0.1	-	0.2	0.2	0.1	0.3	0.9	0.9	1.2	1.8	2.3	2.3	1.7	0.5	0.1	0.02	0.03	0.3	160
Larynx	220	0	-	-	-	-	-	-	0.1	-	0.4	0.4	0.9	2.6	3.6	4.0	4.0	4.3	5.2	4.7	1.3	0.3	0.04	0.08	0.6	161
Bronchus, lung	8094	0	-	-	0.1	-	-	0.4	1.2	1.9	7.7	14.7	27.8	51.8	103.1	155.4	187.6	195.6	206.6	169.6	47.1	11.2	1.04	2.76	21.4	162
Other thoracic organs	104	0	0.3	-	0.2	0.1	0.1	0.1	0.3	-	0.3	0.4	0.8	0.8	1.1	1.3	2.5	1.6	1.6	1.5	0.6	0.1	0.02	0.04	0.4	163-4
Bone	139	0	0.1	0.3	1.4	0.9	0.9	0.7	0.5	0.9	0.8	0.6	0.3	0.9	1.1	0.6	0.9	1.0	1.8	2.3	0.8	0.2	0.05	0.05	0.7	170
Connective tissue	366	0	0.9	0.4	0.4	1.1	0.7	0.7	1.0	0.9	1.2	1.8	1.9	2.0	3.9	4.1	4.1	4.8	7.7	10.7	2.1	0.5	0.08	0.13	1.4	171
Mesothelioma	113	0	-	-	-	-	-	-	-	0.2	0.5	0.8	0.9	0.9	1.3	2.7	2.6	1.6	2.0	0.6	0.7	0.2	0.02	0.05	0.4	MES
Kaposi's sarcoma	7	0	-	-	-	-	0.1	0.1	-	0.2	-	0.1	-	0.1	-	-	-	-	-	-	0.0	0.0	0.00	0.00	0.0	KAP
Melanoma of skin	1622	0	-	-	0.4	1.2	3.8	5.4	7.9	8.3	9.7	12.8	11.8	12.7	18.9	17.7	22.1	19.4	17.3	22.4	9.4	2.2	0.46	0.66	6.4	172
Other skin	8921	0	-	0.1	-	0.5	0.8	3.1	5.8	9.6	18.2	27.2	38.6	49.0	72.1	117.0	160.1	216.3	265.8	310.8	51.9		1.12	2.51	22.5	173
Breast	19976	0	-	-	-	-	1.3	7.4	23.2	54.7	106.3	156.4	205.5	242.4	283.4	248.6	254.2	281.6	313.0	372.3	116.3	27.6	5.40	7.92	71.2	174
Uterus unspecified	9	0	-	-	-	-	-	-	-	-	-	-	0.1	0.2	0.2	0.1	0.1	-	0.2	0.2	0.1	0.0	0.00	0.00	0.0	179
Cervix uteri	2171	0	-	-	-	0.1	1.4	7.3	15.4	23.3	17.9	20.3	17.4	17.4	20.2	20.3	22.4	21.7	18.6	19.2	12.6	3.0	0.70	0.92	9.2	180
Placenta	3	0	-	-	-	-	-	0.1	0.2	-	-	-	-	-	-	-	-	-	-	-	0.0	0.0	0.00	0.00	0.0	181
Corpus uteri	2666	0	-	-	-	-	0.1	-	1.2	2.2	4.9	10.5	25.0	39.1	40.5	44.0	42.3	42.4	45.7	56.4	15.5	3.7	0.62	1.05	8.7	182
Ovary etc.	3790	0	-	-	0.2	1.2	1.4	2.1	3.7	6.5	13.6	23.6	37.4	40.8	52.2	62.0	59.7	62.1	60.2	56.8	22.1	5.2	0.91	1.52	13.1	183
Other female genital	647	0	0.1	-	-	-	0.1	0.3	0.6	1.3	0.9	1.8	2.9	3.0	3.9	6.6	8.9	15.0	24.5	28.0	3.8	0.9	0.07	0.15	1.5	184
Bladder	2231	0	-	-	-	0.1	0.1	0.2	0.2	0.2	0.9	1.6	3.2	6.8	11.3	20.9	29.4	42.8	52.5	76.7	89.3	13.0	3.1	0.23	0.59	5.1	188
Kidney etc.	1044	0	1.9	0.3	0.1	0.1	0.2	0.4	0.6	0.7	2.0	2.5	5.7	9.1	12.5	16.6	19.9	21.7	24.1	24.1	6.1	1.4	0.18	0.36	3.2	189
Eye	181	0	1.4	-	0.1	0.2	0.1	0.2	0.5	0.4	0.5	1.3	1.2	2.1	2.0	2.5	2.5	1.6	3.1	2.6	1.1	0.3	0.05	0.08	0.8	190
Brain, nervous system	999	0	2.6	1.7	2.2	2.2	1.6	2.3	2.7	4.0	5.7	7.3	8.6	11.2	12.6	13.8	11.6	10.7	8.8	3.6	5.8	1.4	0.32	0.45	4.6	191-2
Thyroid	425	0	-	-	0.2	0.3	1.7	1.7	2.5	2.2	2.4	2.7	3.4	2.4	3.4	3.8	4.9	6.5	4.9	7.9	2.5	0.6	0.12	0.16	1.7	193
Other endocrine	82	0	1.5	0.3	0.1	0.2	0.2	0.1	0.2	0.6	0.8	0.3	0.3	0.2	0.5	1.2	0.9	0.7	0.4	0.2	0.5	0.1	0.03	0.04	0.5	194
Hodgkin's disease	346	0	-	0.4	1.0	2.2	5.1	3.7	2.9	2.0	1.6	1.2	1.0	1.6	1.5	2.7	1.3	2.5	2.5	1.1	2.0	0.5	0.12	0.14	1.8	201
Non-Hodgkin lymphoma	2186	0	0.8	0.4	0.2	0.6	1.4	2.8	2.2	4.8	6.5	9.0	15.1	17.5	21.9	29.3	37.8	48.1	50.4	42.5	12.7	3.0	0.42	0.75	6.8	200,202
Multiple myeloma	955	0	-	-	-	-	-	0.1	-	0.2	0.6	1.5	3.9	7.0	10.9	12.5	19.1	27.2	25.8	29.5	5.6	1.3	0.12	0.28	2.4	203
Lymphoid leukaemia	699	0	4.7	2.0	1.5	0.8	0.3	0.4	0.5	0.6	0.3	1.7	2.2	3.7	4.4	6.3	8.1	14.1	22.0	27.8	4.1	1.0	0.12	0.19	2.4	204
Myeloid leukaemia	849	0	1.0	0.6	0.8	0.4	0.7	1.7	1.7	1.8	2.0	3.7	4.4	6.2	6.2	7.5	14.4	15.7	23.2	25.2	4.9	1.2	0.16	0.27	2.7	205
Monocytic leukaemia	13	0	-	-	-	-	-	-	-	-	0.1	-	-	-	-	-	0.8	-	0.4	0.9	0.1	0.0	0.00	0.00	0.0	206
Other leukaemia	8	0	0.2	-	-	-	-	-	-	-	-	-	-	-	-	0.1	-	-	0.9	-	0.0	0.0	0.00	0.00	0.0	207
Leukaemia unspecified	121	0	0.3	0.1	-	0.1	-	-	0.2	-	0.1	0.3	0.6	0.6	1.3	2.3	2.7	3.8	6.2	0.7	0.2	0.01	0.03	0.3	208
Other and unspecified	4463	0	0.7	0.1	-	0.1	0.3	0.5	1.1	1.3	3.8	5.7	11.0	20.3	35.0	54.8	77.2	111.1	153.6	209.5	26.0	6.2	0.40	1.06	9.8	O&U
All sites	81216	0	16.6	7.1	9.3	12.7	23.5	43.5	79.9	137.8	226.3	343.2	493.1	657.4	898.9	1089.8	1337.6	1635.0	1936.5	2238.7	472.8		14.75	26.88	240.9	ALL
All sites but 173	72295	0	16.6	7.0	9.3	12.2	22.7	40.5	74.1	128.1	208.1	316.1	454.5	608.5	826.9	972.8	1177.5	1418.6	1670.6	1927.9	420.9	100.0	13.62	24.37	218.3	ALLb

Rate from 10 cases

	0-	5-	10-	15-	20-	25-	30-	35-	40-	45-	50-	55-	60-	65-	70-	75-	80-	85+
	0.947	1.034	1.106	0.959	0.790	0.728	0.830	0.898	0.840	0.991	1.122	1.167	1.148	1.105	1.293	1.373	1.801	2.136

UK, England, South Western

During the reporting period 1988–92, the registry was funded and supported by the South-Western Regional Health Authority but managed as part of the Cancer Epidemiology Unit of the Department of Epidemiology and Public Health Medicine, University of Bristol.

Until 1981, separate registries were maintained in Bristol and Plymouth. These have been merged and since then the present registry has provided a service to the whole of the South Western Region. The registry covers the counties of Gloucestershire, Avon, Somerset, Devon and Cornwall, which comprise a peninsula between the Bristol Channel to the north and the English Channel to the south. The region is about 320 km long, lying between latitudes 40°55′ and 52° N and longitudes 2° and 6°21′ W, and the total area is about 17 000 km², with a population of over three million. The resident population is relatively stable, although the counties of Devon and Cornwall in particular attract a large number of visitors in the summer and a high proportion of elderly people who move to the area on retirement.

Data acquisition by the registry is largely dependent on links with hospital-based, patient-related information systems. Since 1991 these links have been upgraded and data from all parts of the region have been received on magnetic media; more recently data have been transmitted across the regional data network. Additional links have been established with a number of histopathology systems to receive data, although these have provided mainly paper outputs. Pilot projects have been run to receive data electronically and to include automatic mapping of SNOMED topography codes to ICD codes.

Computerized data are available back to 1971. Data from earlier years, going back to 1945, are held in manual files. There is no active follow-up of patients by the registry but the Office of National Statistics regularly supplies details of patients who die of cancer and have been resident in the region, or patients registered in the region and who died of other causes.

The registry database is patient-based and a separate information database has been established holding anonymized records for all tumours. These records are held on a separate computer for analysis and information purposes. The information database is updated regularly each month from the cancer register. The cancer registry data-set has been expanded to allow the support of clinical trials and the monitoring and evaluation of screening programmes across the region. The unit has had a major role in the specification and development of clinical audit support systems throughout the region, facilitating the comparative evaluation of outcomes of treatment and care, and has been involved in the development of programmes of multi-disciplinary training and quality enhancement in all areas of cancer control. The Cancer Epidemiology Unit takes an active part in the research activities of the Department. A cancer clinical practice unit has also been established and together these constitute the core of the Regional Cancer Organization.

Recently the registry has undergone a substantial reorganization. The South West and Wessex regions have been merged to create the new South & West region. With the abolition of Regional Health Authorities, funding is now from District Health Authorities overseen by the Regional Office of the National Health Service Executive and is divided between the Bristol and Winchester sites. A single Medical Director has been appointed to manage the harmonization of data collection and processing across these two sites. Joint publications are now produced to support the planning and redevelopment of cancer services throughout the new, enlarged region.

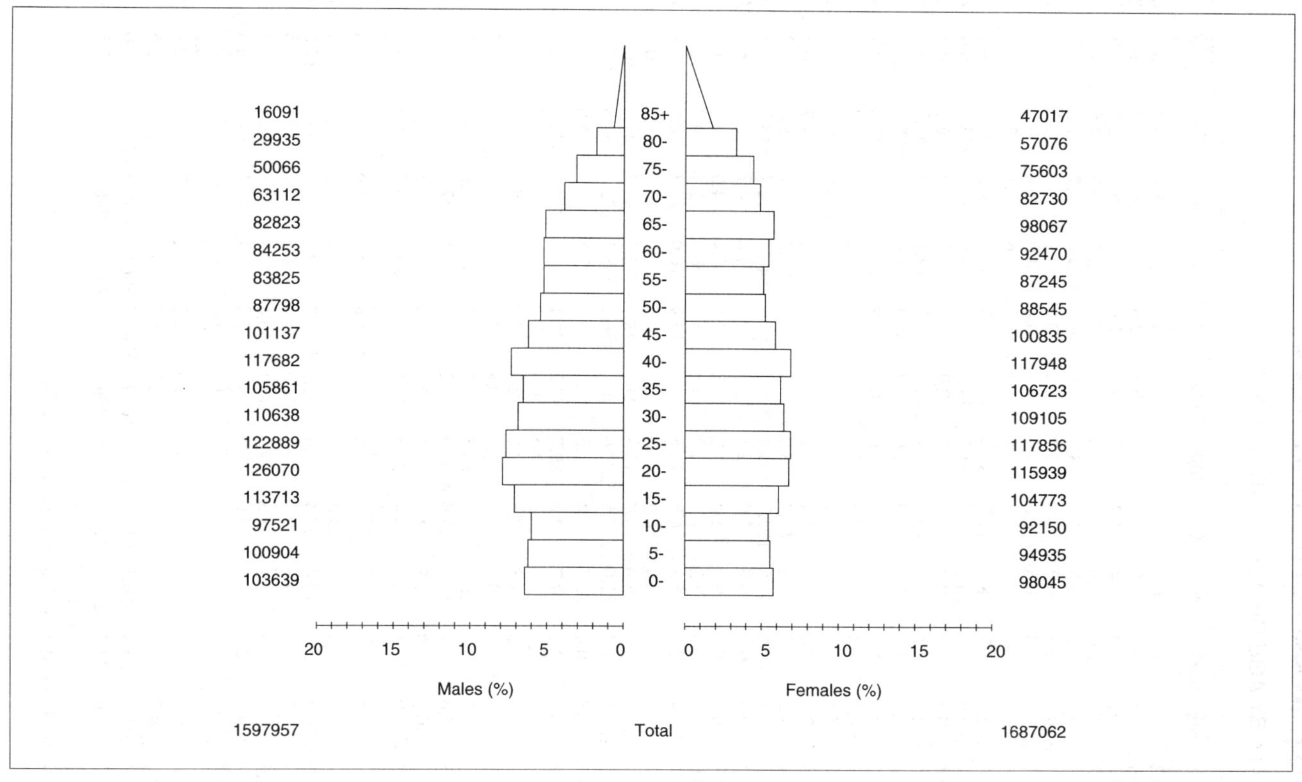

UK, England and Wales, South Western
Source of population: average annual 1988–92
Census: 1991 Census: Usual Residence, Great Britain, OPCS. London: HMSO, 1993.
Estimate: The data for 1988, 1989, 1990 and 1992 were intercensal estimates provided by the Office of Population Censuses and Surveys (OPCS).
Screening programmes in the area
A screening programme for cervical cancer started in 1985 in the population aged 20/25-64 (depending on the district); 200 000 to 230 000 examinations are carried out annually. Screening for breast cancer commenced in Cornwall in 1989 in the age-group 50-64 and the programme has since been extended elsewhere, now comprising some 620 000 to 630 000 examinations annually.

UK, ENGLAND, SOUTH WESTERN 1988-1992

ANNUAL INCIDENCE PER 100,000 BY AGE GROUP (YEARS) - MALE

SITE	ALL AGES	AGE UNK	0-	5-	10-	15-	20-	25-	30-	35-	40-	45-	50-	55-	60-	65-	70-	75-	80-	85+	CRUDE RATE	%	CR 64	CR 74	ASR (W)	ICD (9th)
Lip	72	0	-	-	-	-	-	-	-	0.2	-	1.2	0.2	2.4	1.4	3.1	3.5	5.2	5.3	3.7	0.9	0.2	0.03	0.06	**0.5**	140
Tongue	123	0	-	-	-	-	-	-	-	0.6	0.8	0.8	2.5	3.1	3.3	5.3	7.6	5.2	6.0	6.2	1.5	0.4	0.06	0.12	**0.9**	141
Salivary gland	69	0	0.2	-	-	-	-	0.2	-	0.4	0.2	1.0	1.4	1.2	1.9	3.1	1.9	3.2	5.3	6.2	0.9	0.2	0.03	0.06	**0.5**	142
Mouth	117	0	-	-	-	-	-	-	-	0.2	0.2	2.0	0.9	4.8	3.8	6.5	5.4	2.4	6.0	7.5	1.5	0.3	0.06	0.12	**0.9**	143-5
Oropharynx	62	0	-	-	-	-	-	-	-	-	0.3	0.6	0.5	2.1	3.3	1.4	3.5	4.0	2.7	1.2	0.8	0.2	0.03	0.06	**0.5**	146
Nasopharynx	29	0	0.2	-	-	-	0.3	0.2	-	-	0.2	0.4	0.2	1.7	0.9	1.0	0.6	1.2	-	1.2	0.4	0.1	0.02	0.03	**0.3**	147
Hypopharynx	56	0	-	-	-	-	-	-	-	-	-	0.8	0.5	1.0	1.4	3.1	3.8	4.0	1.3	3.7	0.7	0.2	0.02	0.05	**0.4**	148
Pharynx unspecified	24	0	-	-	-	-	-	-	-	-	0.2	-	-	0.7	0.7	1.4	1.3	1.6	0.7	2.5	0.3	0.1	0.01	0.02	**0.2**	149
Oesophagus	1084	0	-	-	-	-	-	0.2	-	0.6	2.2	5.7	8.2	17.7	35.4	47.6	67.8	69.9	78.8	93.2	13.6	3.2	0.35	0.93	**7.4**	150
Stomach	2127	0	-	-	-	-	0.2	0.2	0.4	1.3	3.9	8.1	13.7	31.3	51.7	78.5	118.5	169.4	221.1	234.9	26.6	6.2	0.55	1.54	**13.6**	151
Small intestine	72	0	-	-	-	-	-	-	-	0.2	0.3	0.6	0.9	1.7	1.7	2.9	1.9	5.2	8.0	6.2	0.9	0.2	0.03	0.05	**0.5**	152
Colon	2930	0	-	-	-	0.2	0.2	0.8	1.3	2.5	7.5	12.5	23.0	40.3	75.7	112.3	159.7	212.1	281.9	354.2	36.7	8.6	0.82	2.18	**19.2**	153
Rectum	2074	0	-	-	-	-	-	0.3	0.5	1.1	4.1	9.9	25.5	37.9	62.0	87.4	105.8	147.0	157.7	195.1	26.0	6.1	0.71	1.67	**14.2**	154
Liver	219	0	0.2	0.2	0.2	0.2	-	0.3	0.2	0.6	0.7	1.0	1.4	3.6	6.6	10.4	10.8	14.8	15.4	17.4	2.7	0.6	0.08	0.18	**1.6**	155
Gallbladder etc.	169	0	-	-	-	-	-	-	-	-	0.7	1.0	1.8	2.1	3.8	7.7	7.9	13.2	17.4	13.7	2.1	0.5	0.05	0.13	**1.1**	156
Pancreas	1103	0	-	-	-	-	-	-	0.4	1.1	2.5	4.9	10.7	19.1	24.7	43.9	63.1	76.7	102.9	120.6	13.8	3.2	0.32	0.85	**7.3**	157
Nose, sinuses etc.	62	0	-	-	-	-	-	0.2	-	0.4	0.5	0.8	0.5	1.4	1.2	1.7	5.1	4.0	3.3	1.2	0.8	0.2	0.02	0.06	**0.5**	160
Larynx	458	0	-	-	-	-	-	-	-	0.4	1.2	5.5	3.2	10.3	18.3	23.4	24.7	28.8	16.7	18.6	5.7	1.3	0.19	0.43	**3.4**	161
Bronchus, lung	7222	0	-	-	-	0.3	0.2	0.3	0.4	1.9	8.7	25.5	48.5	102.8	199.4	315.4	454.1	540.9	622.7	643.8	90.4	21.1	1.94	5.79	**47.0**	162
Other thoracic organs	81	0	-	-	-	0.2	0.2	0.3	0.2	0.4	0.3	0.6	0.7	1.0	2.1	5.3	2.5	4.8	4.7	5.0	1.0	0.2	0.03	0.07	**0.6**	163-4
Bone	89	0	0.2	0.4	1.2	1.8	1.1	1.0	0.5	0.8	0.3	0.8	0.9	1.4	1.2	1.7	2.5	2.4	4.0	2.5	1.1	0.3	0.06	0.08	**1.0**	170
Connective tissue	170	0	0.8	0.6	0.4	1.1	0.6	0.2	0.7	0.6	1.2	2.0	3.2	2.4	4.3	4.8	5.7	8.4	11.4	9.9	2.1	0.5	0.09	0.14	**1.5**	171
Mesothelioma	308	0	-	-	-	-	-	-	-	0.2	1.4	2.6	6.2	6.7	13.8	11.8	13.9	16.0	16.7	18.6	3.9	0.9	0.15	0.28	**2.3**	MES
Kaposi's sarcoma	23	0	-	-	-	-	0.2	0.3	1.1	0.9	0.5	0.6	0.5	0.2	-	-	-	-	-	-	0.3	0.1	0.02	0.02	**0.3**	KAP
Melanoma of skin	828	0	-	0.4	0.2	0.7	2.5	3.9	6.1	8.7	12.7	15.4	18.9	15.7	18.5	22.7	25.7	30.8	32.7	24.9	10.4	2.4	0.52	0.76	**7.3**	172
Other skin	7945	0	0.4	-	0.2	1.1	1.0	4.1	9.2	15.7	25.5	49.4	82.0	126.5	209.6	306.9	426.2	538.1	672.1	781.8	99.4		2.62	6.29	**54.5**	173
Breast	78	0	-	-	-	-	-	-	-	0.2	0.8	0.4	0.7	1.4	1.2	2.9	5.1	7.6	3.3	5.0	1.0	0.2	0.02	0.06	**0.5**	175
Prostate	5634	0	-	0.2	-	-	-	-	-	0.2	0.8	2.6	7.7	34.6	89.7	192.2	338.1	542.5	724.2	934.6	70.5	16.5	0.68	3.33	**31.8**	185
Testis	445	0	0.4	-	0.2	2.1	9.2	11.6	16.3	13.0	9.5	5.9	3.6	3.1	2.4	0.7	1.9	0.8	1.3	5.0	5.6	1.3	0.39	0.40	**5.1**	186
Penis	102	0	-	-	-	-	0.2	0.2	0.2	0.2	0.2	0.8	1.8	2.6	2.6	2.9	2.9	7.6	8.7	12.4	1.3	0.3	0.04	0.07	**0.7**	187.1-.4
Other male genital	18	0	-	-	-	-	-	-	-	-	-	0.2	-	0.7	0.7	0.6	1.2	2.7	2.5	0.2	0.1	0.00	0.01	**0.1**	187.5-.9
Bladder	2969	0	-	-	-	-	0.2	1.0	1.6	3.0	4.9	13.6	26.7	44.4	80.5	116.2	171.1	207.7	272.6	308.2	37.2	8.7	0.88	2.32	**19.7**	188
Kidney etc.	890	0	1.5	-	-	-	0.2	0.2	1.3	2.8	4.6	9.7	13.7	18.4	31.6	36.2	39.0	47.1	52.8	52.2	11.1	2.6	0.42	0.80	**6.9**	189
Eye	77	0	1.0	0.2	0.2	-	0.2	0.2	-	0.6	0.3	1.0	1.8	1.7	2.1	2.7	1.9	3.2	2.7	6.2	1.0	0.2	0.05	0.07	**0.7**	190
Brain, nervous system	686	0	2.7	3.6	2.1	3.2	2.9	2.8	5.1	4.0	5.9	11.1	12.3	13.4	22.3	21.5	25.4	20.4	13.4	8.7	8.6	2.0	0.46	0.69	**6.7**	191-2
Thyroid	82	0	-	0.2	-	0.2	0.5	0.8	0.4	0.6	1.0	1.2	1.4	2.1	0.2	3.6	4.4	2.0	0.7	5.0	1.0	0.2	0.04	0.07	**0.7**	193
Other endocrine	48	0	1.5	0.2	0.6	-	0.3	0.2	0.4	-	0.2	0.8	1.4	0.7	0.7	1.0	1.6	0.4	2.0	1.2	0.6	0.1	0.03	0.05	**0.6**	194
Hodgkin's disease	228	0	0.2	0.2	1.4	2.8	5.2	2.9	4.5	2.8	3.7	2.8	4.6	2.4	1.9	3.9	3.8	2.4	2.0	1.2	2.9	0.7	0.18	0.22	**2.5**	201
Non-Hodgkin lymphoma	1405	0	1.5	1.4	2.5	2.6	2.4	3.7	3.8	7.9	10.4	13.1	19.4	27.4	35.4	51.7	62.7	79.5	79.5	69.6	17.6	4.1	0.66	1.23	**11.2**	200,202
Multiple myeloma	518	0	-	-	-	-	0.2	-	0.4	0.4	1.2	2.8	4.8	9.3	16.4	21.5	31.1	34.8	33.4	48.5	6.5	1.5	0.18	0.44	**3.6**	203
Lymphoid leukaemia	601	0	7.5	3.2	1.4	1.2	1.3	0.8	0.9	0.4	1.2	3.0	4.1	8.6	9.0	17.1	30.4	42.7	48.1	64.6	7.5	1.8	0.21	0.45	**5.0**	204
Myeloid leukaemia	501	0	1.0	0.2	0.6	1.6	1.4	1.6	0.9	1.7	3.4	2.6	3.2	6.0	8.5	15.0	26.0	34.4	40.1	64.6	6.3	1.5	0.16	0.37	**3.7**	205
Monocytic leukaemia	34	0	0.2	-	-	-	0.2	0.7	0.2	0.2	-	0.4	-	-	0.7	1.0	1.0	3.2	3.3	1.2	0.4	0.1	0.01	0.02	**0.3**	206
Other leukaemia	6	0	-	-	-	-	0.2	-	-	-	-	-	-	-	0.5	0.3	0.4	0.7	-	0.1	0.0	0.00	0.00	**0.0**	207
Leukaemia unspecified	67	0	0.8	-	0.2	-	-	-	0.2	0.2	-	0.2	-	0.7	0.5	1.4	2.5	5.2	12.7	9.9	0.8	0.2	0.01	0.03	**0.5**	208
Other and unspecified	199	0	0.6	-	-	-	0.3	-	0.2	0.2	0.7	1.4	1.4	3.8	4.7	8.7	8.2	9.6	19.4	29.8	2.5	0.6	0.07	0.15	**1.4**	O&U
All sites	42104	0	20.8	10.9	11.5	18.8	31.1	38.7	57.1	76.9	125.1	226.8	364.5	619.6	1058.0	1610.9	2281.6	2961.7	3618.5	4204.6	527.0		13.30	32.76	**289.1**	ALL
All sites but 173	34159	0	20.5	10.9	11.3	17.8	30.1	34.7	47.9	61.2	99.6	177.4	282.5	493.2	848.4	1304.0	1855.4	2423.6	2946.3	3422.9	427.5	100.0	10.68	26.47	**234.6**	ALLb

Rate from 1 case   0.193   0.198   0.205   0.176   0.159   0.163   0.181   0.189   0.170   0.198   0.228   0.239   0.237   0.241   0.317   0.399   0.668   1.243

UK, ENGLAND, SOUTH WESTERN 1988-1992

ANNUAL INCIDENCE PER 100,000 BY AGE GROUP (YEARS) - FEMALE

SITE	ALL AGES	AGE UNK	0-	5-	10-	15-	20-	25-	30-	35-	40-	45-	50-	55-	60-	65-	70-	75-	80-	85+	CRUDE RATE	%	CR 64	CR 74	ASR (W)	ICD (9th)
Lip	24	0	-	-	-	-	-	-	-	0.2	0.2	-	0.2	0.2	0.2	0.6	-	1.3	1.8	2.6	0.3	0.1	0.01	0.01	0.1	140
Tongue	97	0	-	-	-	-	-	-	0.5	0.4	0.3	0.8	0.7	1.4	1.5	2.4	4.1	2.9	5.6	6.0	1.1	0.3	0.03	0.06	0.5	141
Salivary gland	64	0	-	-	0.2	-	0.2	0.2	0.2	0.2	0.5	0.4	0.7	1.1	1.1	1.8	2.7	1.9	2.1	3.4	0.8	0.2	0.02	0.05	0.4	142
Mouth	85	0	-	-	0.2	-	-	-	0.2	0.2	0.2	0.6	0.9	1.1	1.5	2.7	3.4	4.5	2.5	4.7	1.0	0.2	0.02	0.05	0.5	143-5
Oropharynx	18	0	-	-	-	-	-	-	-	-	0.2	-	0.7	-	0.2	1.8	0.2	0.3	-	0.9	0.2	0.1	0.01	0.02	0.1	146
Nasopharynx	11	0	-	-	-	-	-	-	-	0.2	0.2	-	-	0.2	0.6	0.2	-	0.3	1.1	-	0.1	0.0	0.01	0.01	0.1	147
Hypopharynx	39	0	-	-	-	-	-	-	-	-	-	0.2	0.2	0.5	1.3	1.4	1.7	2.1	1.4	1.3	0.5	0.1	0.01	0.03	0.2	148
Pharynx unspecified	17	0	-	-	-	-	-	-	-	0.2	0.2	-	0.7	0.4	0.4	1.0	0.3	0.4	0.9	0.2	0.0	0.01	0.01	0.1	149
Oesophagus	897	0	-	-	-	-	-	-	0.2	0.4	0.3	3.0	3.8	6.2	11.0	25.5	30.9	48.4	59.2	75.3	10.6	2.5	0.12	0.41	3.7	150
Stomach	1302	0	0.2	-	0.2	-	0.2	0.5	0.2	1.3	1.7	2.0	5.2	10.8	14.9	25.7	40.6	58.5	103.4	135.7	15.4	3.6	0.19	0.52	5.1	151
Small intestine	75	0	-	-	-	-	-	-	0.2	-	0.3	0.6	0.2	0.7	0.9	2.9	3.1	2.9	4.9	3.8	0.9	0.2	0.01	0.04	0.4	152
Colon	3637	0	-	-	-	-	0.5	0.7	1.5	1.7	8.5	11.5	19.7	39.2	65.1	89.1	131.3	166.1	230.2	289.7	43.1	10.2	0.74	1.84	16.2	153
Rectum	1845	0	-	-	-	-	0.3	-	0.9	2.6	4.6	6.9	15.8	27.5	38.3	47.5	61.9	85.7	103.7	121.7	21.9	5.2	0.49	1.03	9.0	154
Liver	157	0	-	-	-	-	0.2	0.2	0.2	0.4	0.3	0.8	0.7	2.3	2.4	4.3	5.6	8.2	8.8	9.4	1.9	0.4	0.04	0.09	0.8	155
Gallbladder etc.	246	0	-	-	-	-	0.2	-	-	0.2	0.2	0.6	1.4	2.5	4.1	5.3	9.7	12.4	16.8	18.3	2.9	0.7	0.05	0.12	1.1	156
Pancreas	1121	0	-	-	-	-	0.2	0.2	0.2	0.2	1.9	4.0	7.0	11.5	14.9	27.9	40.6	51.6	79.9	88.5	13.3	3.1	0.20	0.54	4.8	157
Nose, sinuses etc.	52	0	-	-	-	-	-	-	-	-	0.3	-	0.5	1.4	1.5	1.8	1.0	2.4	2.1	3.0	0.6	0.1	0.02	0.03	0.3	160
Larynx	86	0	-	-	-	-	-	-	-	-	0.3	0.6	1.4	1.8	1.9	3.3	4.6	3.4	1.4	2.6	1.0	0.2	0.03	0.07	0.5	161
Bronchus, lung	3340	0	-	-	-	-	0.2	0.3	0.4	1.9	6.3	11.7	22.1	45.2	83.9	122.4	142.9	173.5	150.3	114.9	39.6	9.3	0.86	2.19	17.1	162
Other thoracic organs	41	0	-	-	-	0.2	-	0.2	-	0.2	0.2	0.4	0.2	0.7	0.4	0.6	1.2	3.4	2.5	0.9	0.5	0.1	0.01	0.02	0.2	163-4
Bone	52	0	-	0.8	0.7	0.6	-	0.7	-	0.4	0.2	1.0	0.7	1.4	0.2	0.8	1.2	1.1	1.8	0.9	0.6	0.1	0.03	0.04	0.5	170
Connective tissue	156	0	1.4	0.6	0.7	0.6	0.3	1.0	0.5	1.1	0.8	1.6	1.8	1.1	2.8	2.9	5.3	5.3	4.9	6.0	1.8	0.4	0.07	0.11	1.2	171
Mesothelioma	45	0	-	-	-	-	-	-	-	-	0.3	0.2	0.7	2.1	0.6	1.6	2.4	0.8	1.1	1.3	0.5	0.1	0.02	0.04	0.3	MES
Kaposi's sarcoma	0	0	-	-	-	-	-	-	-	-	-	-	-	-	-	-	-	-	-	-	0.0	0.0	0.00	0.00	0.0	KAP
Melanoma of skin	1268	0	0.2	-	-	1.7	4.7	8.8	13.0	12.2	18.1	23.6	23.3	20.9	24.7	28.3	30.5	25.9	31.9	23.4	15.0	3.5	0.76	1.05	10.3	172
Other skin	6847	0	0.2	0.2	0.9	1.3	1.7	4.8	10.4	15.6	33.1	50.2	72.7	92.6	129.1	173.1	226.0	300.5	353.9	406.2	81.2		2.06	4.06	36.3	173
Breast	10500	0	-	-	-	-	0.3	7.1	21.3	56.2	103.4	154.9	217.5	254.7	297.8	259.8	260.1	288.9	297.1	386.2	124.5	29.3	5.57	8.17	73.0	174
Uterus unspecified	200	0	-	-	-	-	0.2	-	-	0.4	0.3	1.4	2.9	4.4	5.0	2.7	6.0	9.0	7.0	17.4	2.4	0.6	0.07	0.12	1.1	179
Cervix uteri	1200	0	-	-	-	-	2.8	10.7	19.1	24.0	21.7	22.4	14.9	17.2	22.5	23.7	24.9	21.2	18.6	21.7	14.2	3.4	0.78	1.02	10.3	180
Placenta	2	0	-	-	-	-	-	0.3	-	-	-	-	-	-	-	-	-	-	-	-	0.0	0.0	0.00	0.00	0.0	181
Corpus uteri	1454	0	-	-	-	0.2	-	0.3	0.5	2.1	5.4	12.9	27.3	45.2	46.3	46.5	45.9	41.8	47.3	41.3	17.2	4.1	0.70	1.16	9.5	182
Ovary etc.	1762	0	0.4	-	0.7	1.0	2.6	3.6	3.3	5.6	9.7	19.8	34.1	38.7	48.4	53.8	49.8	53.4	61.7	50.6	20.9	4.9	0.84	1.36	11.9	183
Other female genital	364	0	0.2	-	-	-	-	0.2	0.7	1.5	1.0	2.4	3.8	3.0	5.6	8.6	10.4	18.3	20.3	27.2	4.3	1.0	0.09	0.19	1.8	184
Bladder	1075	0	-	0.2	-	0.2	-	0.2	0.2	1.7	0.8	3.0	7.0	13.8	17.5	29.6	43.3	51.1	63.8	72.7	12.7	3.0	0.22	0.59	4.9	188
Kidney etc.	523	0	2.7	0.4	0.4	0.4	0.3	0.5	1.3	1.9	2.7	3.4	6.6	7.1	10.6	15.9	18.1	20.4	23.5	18.3	6.2	1.5	0.19	0.36	3.3	189
Eye	77	0	0.4	-	-	0.2	0.2	0.2	0.7	0.4	0.5	1.4	0.7	0.5	0.9	1.6	2.7	3.2	3.2	3.0	0.9	0.2	0.03	0.05	0.5	190
Brain, nervous system	508	0	2.0	4.0	2.6	1.3	1.6	2.0	4.4	3.4	4.2	5.8	6.8	9.6	13.0	12.4	12.6	14.5	11.6	4.3	6.0	1.4	0.30	0.43	4.4	191-2
Thyroid	249	0	-	-	0.6	1.9	2.5	2.6	3.9	2.9	3.0	3.2	3.4	3.0	5.3	6.5	5.8	4.9	8.9	3.0	0.7	0.14	0.19	2.0	193
Other endocrine	38	0	0.8	0.2	0.2	-	-	-	-	0.4	0.5	0.8	0.2	0.9	0.4	-	1.9	0.8	1.1	0.9	0.5	0.1	0.02	0.03	0.4	194
Hodgkin's disease	145	0	-	0.2	0.2	3.2	3.3	4.1	2.6	2.4	1.0	1.2	1.6	1.4	0.9	0.6	2.7	1.6	1.4	1.3	1.7	0.4	0.11	0.13	1.6	201
Non-Hodgkin lymphoma	1242	0	0.4	1.1	0.4	1.1	1.2	1.5	3.1	4.1	8.1	9.9	14.2	19.9	26.2	33.7	46.4	51.6	48.7	47.6	14.7	3.5	0.46	0.86	7.5	200,202
Multiple myeloma	524	0	-	-	-	-	-	-	0.2	0.6	1.0	1.8	3.2	6.6	8.7	14.1	23.4	27.2	31.5	26.8	6.2	1.5	0.11	0.30	2.4	203
Lymphoid leukaemia	441	0	5.5	3.8	2.0	0.6	0.5	0.2	0.4	0.4	1.2	1.4	2.3	3.4	7.6	12.2	11.1	18.3	23.1	25.9	5.2	1.2	0.15	0.26	3.1	204
Myeloid leukaemia	439	0	1.0	0.4	0.9	1.1	0.3	1.2	1.1	0.6	1.9	1.6	4.3	4.8	7.1	10.0	13.3	19.6	22.4	29.8	5.2	1.2	0.13	0.25	2.5	205
Monocytic leukaemia	25	0	-	-	-	0.2	0.2	-	-	0.2	0.2	0.2	0.5	-	0.6	0.2	1.2	1.1	1.4	0.4	0.3	0.1	0.01	0.02	0.2	206
Other leukaemia	7	0	-	-	-	-	-	-	-	-	0.2	-	-	0.2	0.2	0.2	0.3	0.4	-	-	0.1	0.0	0.00	0.01	0.0	207
Leukaemia unspecified	64	0	-	-	0.2	-	0.2	-	0.2	0.2	-	0.2	0.5	0.2	0.9	0.4	1.5	1.9	4.6	10.2	0.8	0.2	0.01	0.02	0.3	208
Other and unspecified	278	0	0.6	-	0.2	-	0.2	-	0.2	0.2	0.3	0.8	1.6	1.8	2.6	6.7	6.5	15.6	17.2	29.8	3.3	0.8	0.04	0.11	1.2	O&U
All sites	42639	0	16.1	12.0	10.6	14.5	24.3	51.9	90.6	149.0	246.4	368.9	533.5	710.0	929.6	1112.5	1340.5	1629.0	1882.0	2145.2	505.5		15.79	28.05	251.7	ALL
All sites but 173	35792	0	15.9	11.8	9.8	13.2	22.6	47.2	80.1	133.4	213.3	318.7	460.8	617.3	800.5	939.4	1114.5	1328.5	1528.1	1738.9	424.3	100.0	13.72	23.99	215.3	ALLb

Rate from 1 case   0.204   0.211   0.217   0.191   0.172   0.170   0.183   0.187   0.170   0.198   0.226   0.229   0.216   0.204   0.242   0.265   0.350   0.425

UK, England, Wessex

Cancer registration data for residents of the Wessex region is available from 1973 when the Wessex Regional Cancer Registry was established by separating from the Thames Cancer Registry.

The registry covers the counties of Dorset, Wiltshire, Hampshire and the Isle of Wight; an area of 10 700 km^2, with a population of 3 150 000. It lies between latitudes 50°30′ and 51°30′ N and longitudes 0°30′ and 5°30′ W. 55% of the population live in large towns or cities and the remainder in rural areas. The coastal area attracts a comparatively elderly population.

Information on registrations comes from hospital in-patient records, pathology laboratories and death certificates. In 1986 a system to accept data on electronic media was introduced and this has been extended such that new data are received in this way from all the hospitals in the area and all the pathology laboratory computer systems.

Where the data cannot be processed automatically because of apparent inconsistencies or inaccuracies, the records are verified by registry staff before being added to the register. Information is obtained from both National Health Service and private hospitals.

The data items recorded include: patient identification (name, age, sex, residence etc.), the hospital where treated, tumour details (site, histology and morphology). Some information about surgical treatment is available and expanded information on treatment is now being added.

The Wessex Cancer Register is the main work of the Wessex Cancer Intelligence Unit, but other staff are involved in the quality assurance and evaluation of the breast and cervical screening programmes, support for regional clinical audit programmes and a modest amount of epidemiological research. There are particular interests in colorectal and breast cancers.

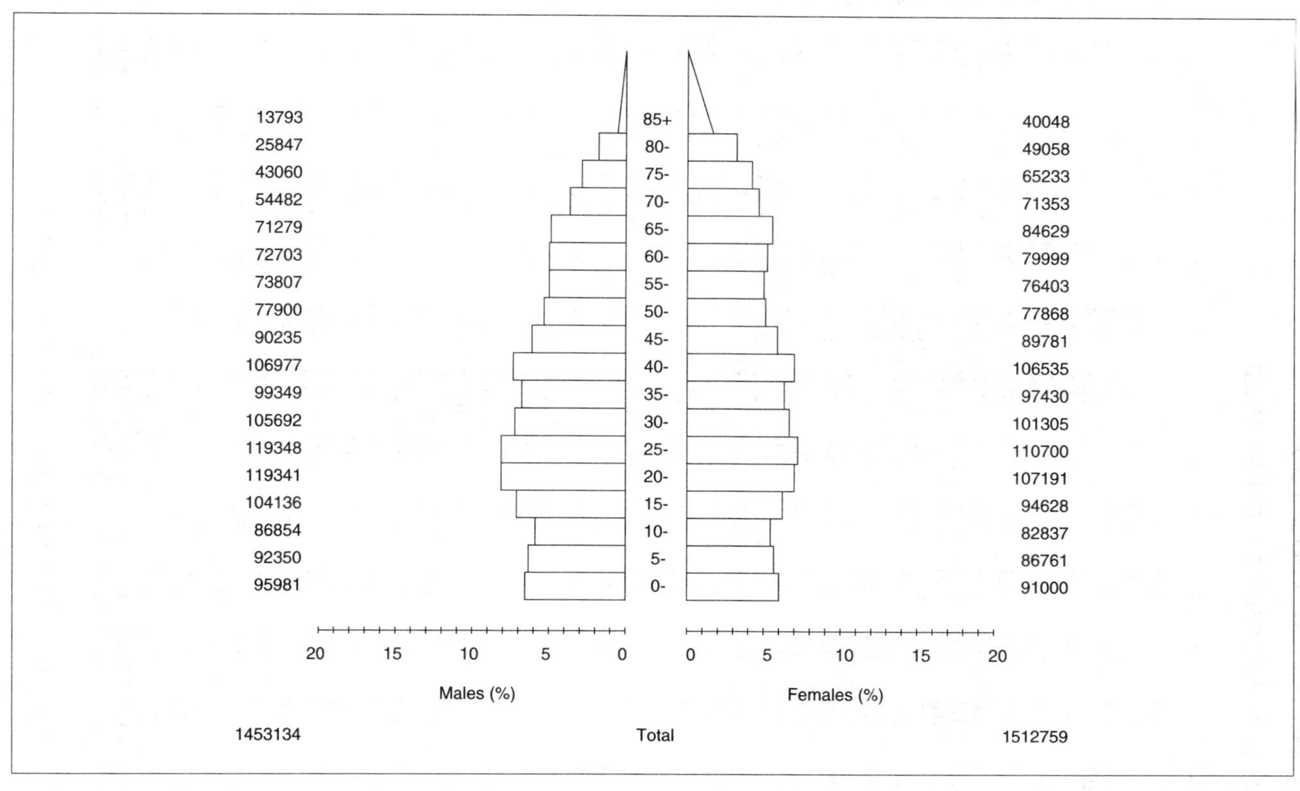

UK, England, Wessex

Source of population: average annual 1988–92

Census: 1991 Census: Usual Residence, Great Britain, OPCS. London: HMSO, 1993.

Estimate: The population data for each of the five years were derived from the OPCS updated Census data in 1993, based on the 1991 Census.

Notes to tables overleaf:

† 173 includes basal and squamous cell carcinomas for 1988 only.

Screening programmes in the area:

The population aged 25-64 has been screened every five years for cervical cancer since 1986. Screening for breast cancer in women aged 50-64 (by invitation with an examination every three years) commenced in 1988.

UK, ENGLAND, WESSEX 1988-1992

ANNUAL INCIDENCE PER 100,000 BY AGE GROUP (YEARS) - MALE

SITE	ALL AGES	AGE UNK	0-	5-	10-	15-	20-	25-	30-	35-	40-	45-	50-	55-	60-	65-	70-	75-	80-	85+	CRUDE RATE	%	CR 64	CR 74	ASR (W)	ICD (9th)
Lip	73	0	-	-	-	0.4	-	0.2	0.2	-	0.6	-	1.5	0.5	1.1	2.2	7.3	5.1	7.0	8.7	1.0	0.2	0.02	0.07	**0.6**	*140*
Tongue	121	0	-	-	-	-	-	0.3	0.6	-	0.6	0.2	2.6	1.9	4.7	8.4	6.2	7.4	6.2	10.2	1.7	0.4	0.05	0.13	**1.0**	*141*
Salivary gland	76	0	-	-	-	-	0.2	-	0.2	0.6	0.4	0.9	0.3	1.6	1.7	3.6	4.4	5.1	7.0	10.2	1.0	0.2	0.03	0.07	**0.6**	*142*
Mouth	138	0	-	-	-	-	0.2	-	0.2	0.2	-	1.8	3.1	4.9	4.4	7.6	7.0	7.4	6.2	16.0	1.9	0.4	0.07	0.15	**1.2**	*143-5*
Oropharynx	52	0	-	-	-	-	-	-	0.2	-	0.4	0.9	1.5	1.9	2.5	3.1	2.2	0.5	2.3	2.9	0.7	0.2	0.04	0.06	**0.5**	*146*
Nasopharynx	38	0	-	-	-	-	0.2	0.7	0.8	0.2	0.7	0.4	0.8	0.8	1.4	1.4	0.7	1.4	-	1.5	0.5	0.1	0.03	0.04	**0.4**	*147*
Hypopharynx	51	0	-	-	-	-	-	-	-	-	-	0.7	0.5	1.9	1.4	1.7	3.7	4.2	3.9	5.8	0.7	0.2	0.02	0.05	**0.4**	*148*
Pharynx unspecified	41	0	-	-	-	-	-	-	-	-	0.2	0.7	1.3	0.3	1.9	0.8	2.6	2.8	3.9	4.4	0.6	0.1	0.02	0.04	**0.3**	*149*
Oesophagus	1022	0	-	-	0.2	0.2	-	0.2	0.6	1.0	2.6	6.6	11.0	23.0	31.1	48.0	60.2	73.4	109.9	132.0	14.1	3.0	0.38	0.92	**8.0**	*150*
Stomach	1802	0	-	0.2	-	-	-	0.7	0.8	1.6	1.7	8.2	15.7	26.6	49.2	74.9	114.9	175.6	206.6	255.2	24.8	5.3	0.52	1.47	**13.2**	*151*
Small intestine	77	0	-	-	-	-	-	0.2	-	0.4	0.6	0.9	1.0	1.9	2.5	4.5	5.5	2.3	6.2	4.4	1.1	0.2	0.04	0.09	**0.7**	*152*
Colon	2984	0	-	-	-	-	0.3	0.2	1.5	3.8	6.7	12.4	30.6	45.8	80.6	134.1	186.5	267.5	336.6	411.8	41.1	8.8	0.91	2.51	**22.3**	*153*
Rectum	1733	0	-	-	-	0.2	0.2	-	0.9	1.8	4.9	9.8	17.7	37.9	50.6	77.4	116.7	137.5	171.8	205.9	23.9	5.1	0.62	1.59	**13.4**	*154*
Liver	257	0	0.6	-	0.2	0.2	0.2	0.2	-	0.6	0.4	0.4	2.3	5.7	6.9	14.9	17.6	14.4	24.0	36.3	3.5	0.8	0.09	0.25	**2.1**	*155*
Gallbladder etc.	140	0	-	-	-	-	-	-	0.2	-	0.2	0.7	1.5	1.9	5.0	4.8	5.9	13.5	20.1	23.2	1.9	0.4	0.05	0.10	**1.0**	*156*
Pancreas	899	0	0.2	-	-	-	0.2	0.2	0.4	0.8	2.2	3.8	8.2	13.0	24.5	37.9	60.2	80.8	93.6	142.1	12.4	2.7	0.27	0.76	**6.7**	*157*
Nose, sinuses etc.	69	0	-	-	-	-	-	-	-	-	0.6	1.1	1.8	2.2	0.6	2.0	5.9	4.6	4.6	7.3	0.9	0.2	0.03	0.07	**0.6**	*160*
Larynx	451	0	0.2	-	0.2	-	-	-	0.6	1.1	4.0	8.9	19.0	25.5	30.5	26.5	28.6	30.5	6.2	1.3	0.21	0.49	**3.8**	*161*
Bronchus, lung	6841	0	-	-	-	-	0.2	0.3	0.6	5.6	7.5	25.3	53.1	116.2	201.9	334.2	487.9	580.1	734.3	819.3	94.2	20.2	2.05	6.16	**51.1**	*162*
Other thoracic organs	72	0	0.2	-	-	-	0.3	-	0.6	-	0.4	0.4	0.8	2.2	1.9	2.5	6.6	6.5	1.5	1.5	1.0	0.2	0.03	0.08	**0.6**	*163-4*
Bone	92	0	-	0.4	0.2	1.5	0.3	0.7	0.8	0.2	0.9	1.3	1.0	1.6	3.0	3.6	1.5	5.1	4.6	5.8	1.3	0.3	0.06	0.09	**1.0**	*170*
Connective tissue	233	0	0.6	0.4	0.5	1.2	0.7	1.0	1.7	1.4	2.2	2.7	4.4	4.1	3.9	8.7	10.3	12.1	15.5	27.6	3.2	0.7	0.12	0.22	**2.2**	*171*
Mesothelioma	389	0	-	-	0.2	-	-	-	-	0.2	1.1	3.1	6.4	11.4	16.8	20.5	26.1	27.4	15.5	23.2	5.4	1.1	0.20	0.43	**3.3**	*MES*
Kaposi's sarcoma	11	0	-	-	0.2	-	0.2	0.3	0.2	0.2	0.4	0.2	0.3	-	-	-	-	0.8	-	-	0.2	0.0	0.01	0.01	**0.1**	*KAP*
Melanoma of skin	665	0	0.2	-	0.5	1.3	1.8	2.5	6.1	7.6	7.5	14.4	13.4	18.7	22.6	21.3	20.6	25.5	25.5	45.0	9.2	2.0	0.48	0.69	**6.6**	*172*
†Other skin	2731	0	-	-	0.2	1.3	1.0	0.5	3.0	6.8	10.3	18.6	27.7	50.9	71.0	108.3	176.2	222.5	281.6	379.9	37.6		0.96	2.38	**21.2**	*173*
Breast	78	0	-	-	-	-	-	-	-	0.2	-	0.7	0.3	1.1	1.7	3.4	4.8	8.4	8.5	13.1	1.1	0.2	0.02	0.06	**0.6**	*175*
Prostate	5254	0	0.2	-	-	-	0.2	-	-	0.2	0.7	2.0	8.2	26.6	89.1	180.4	359.4	595.9	843.4	1144.1	72.3	15.5	0.64	3.34	**33.7**	*185*
Testis	447	0	0.8	0.2	-	2.1	8.0	13.9	14.8	11.3	9.0	8.6	6.4	4.3	3.6	2.2	2.9	0.9	3.1	4.4	6.2	1.3	0.42	0.44	**5.5**	*186*
Penis	110	0	-	-	-	-	-	-	0.2	1.0	0.7	1.6	0.8	1.6	2.2	4.2	5.5	8.4	12.4	17.4	1.5	0.3	0.04	0.09	**0.9**	*187.1-.4*
Other male genital	22	0	-	-	-	-	-	-	-	0.2	-	-	0.3	0.3	0.8	1.4	1.8	0.5	2.3	2.9	0.3	0.1	0.01	0.02	**0.2**	*187.5-.9*
Bladder	3100	0	0.2	0.2	-	0.6	0.8	0.8	2.3	2.2	5.8	16.0	26.2	49.6	98.2	142.0	203.0	251.7	331.2	417.6	42.7	9.1	1.01	2.74	**23.6**	*188*
Kidney etc.	816	0	2.5	1.1	-	0.6	0.7	0.7	1.1	2.2	3.6	9.8	14.6	21.1	27.2	38.4	45.5	48.8	58.0	47.9	11.2	2.4	0.43	0.85	**7.3**	*189*
Eye	82	0	0.2	0.2	0.2	0.2	0.2	0.2	0.4	-	0.6	0.9	0.8	1.1	3.9	2.2	2.9	7.4	6.2	8.7	1.1	0.2	0.04	0.07	**0.7**	*190*
Brain, nervous system	608	0	4.0	3.2	2.5	1.7	1.8	2.7	3.6	4.2	6.2	9.8	11.8	15.7	20.6	24.4	24.2	21.4	18.6	11.6	8.4	1.8	0.44	0.68	**6.6**	*191-2*
Thyroid	72	0	-	-	-	0.2	0.5	0.2	0.4	0.8	1.7	1.1	0.8	1.1	3.0	2.8	2.6	2.8	3.1	2.9	1.0	0.2	0.05	0.08	**0.7**	*193*
Other endocrine	49	0	2.3	0.2	-	0.4	0.2	0.3	0.2	0.6	0.7	0.2	0.5	0.8	0.8	0.8	2.2	1.9	0.8	1.5	0.7	0.1	0.04	0.05	**0.7**	*194*
Hodgkin's disease	212	0	-	0.4	0.9	3.5	4.7	5.5	4.2	2.2	1.7	3.1	3.3	3.0	2.5	3.9	3.3	4.2	2.3	4.4	2.9	0.6	0.17	0.21	**2.6**	*201*
Non-Hodgkin lymphoma	1331	0	1.9	1.3	1.4	1.2	3.0	2.8	5.5	4.6	9.3	16.4	18.5	30.1	41.0	48.0	76.0	85.9	101.4	97.2	18.3	3.9	0.68	1.30	**11.8**	*200,202*
Multiple myeloma	562	0	-	0.2	-	-	0.2	-	0.8	0.6	1.9	3.1	6.7	12.7	15.7	23.8	34.1	43.2	61.1	71.1	7.7	1.7	0.21	0.50	**4.4**	*203*
Lymphoid leukaemia	502	0	6.7	3.9	2.1	1.7	1.8	1.2	0.6	1.2	1.7	2.9	3.6	6.5	11.6	14.9	25.3	34.4	51.8	60.9	6.9	1.5	0.23	0.43	**4.9**	*204*
Myeloid leukaemia	534	0	1.3	0.6	1.4	0.2	1.3	1.8	1.9	2.8	3.4	3.1	5.9	9.8	12.9	18.2	29.7	40.4	53.4	50.8	7.3	1.6	0.23	0.47	**4.6**	*205*
Monocytic leukaemia	11	0	-	-	-	-	-	-	-	-	-	-	0.3	0.5	0.3	-	-	1.9	0.8	2.9	0.2	0.0	0.01	0.01	**0.1**	*206*
Other leukaemia	11	0	-	-	-	-	-	-	-	-	-	-	0.3	0.3	0.3	0.8	0.4	1.4	-	1.5	0.2	0.0	0.00	0.01	**0.1**	*207*
Leukaemia unspecified	53	0	0.2	-	-	-	0.2	-	0.2	0.2	0.2	-	0.3	0.8	1.4	2.2	2.6	4.2	3.1	16.0	0.7	0.2	0.02	0.04	**0.4**	*208*
Other and unspecified	1735	0	1.3	0.4	-	0.4	0.3	0.7	0.9	2.0	3.7	8.0	14.4	23.0	45.9	68.2	113.8	139.8	219.0	294.4	23.9	5.1	0.51	1.42	**13.0**	*O&U*
All sites	36647	0	23.5	13.2	11.1	19.0	29.8	38.9	56.2	70.5	104.9	206.6	340.2	595.9	992.5	1534.5	2307.2	3012.5	3898.2	4880.7	504.4		12.51	31.72	**285.4**	*ALL*
All sites but 173	33916	0	23.5	13.2	10.8	17.7	28.8	38.4	53.2	63.6	94.6	188.0	312.5	544.9	921.6	1426.2	2131.0	2790.0	3616.6	4500.8	466.8	100.0	11.55	29.34	**264.2**	*ALLb*
Rate from 1 case			0.208	0.217	0.230	0.192	0.168	0.168	0.189	0.201	0.187	0.222	0.257	0.271	0.275	0.281	0.367	0.464	0.774	1.450						

†Important: see notes on population page

UK, ENGLAND, WESSEX 1988-1992

ANNUAL INCIDENCE PER 100,000 BY AGE GROUP (YEARS) - FEMALE

SITE	ALL AGES	AGE UNK	0-	5-	10-	15-	20-	25-	30-	35-	40-	45-	50-	55-	60-	65-	70-	75-	80-	85+	CRUDE RATE	%	CR 64	CR 74	ASR (W)	ICD (9th)
Lip	27	0	-	-	-	-	-	-	-	-	0.2	-	0.3	-	0.5	0.9	1.4	2.8	0.4	2.0	0.4	0.1	0.00	0.02	**0.1**	*140*
Tongue	110	0	-	-	-	-	0.4	-	0.4	0.6	0.4	1.3	1.3	1.3	2.5	5.0	3.9	4.6	4.1	7.5	1.5	0.3	0.04	0.09	**0.7**	*141*
Salivary gland	66	0	-	-	0.2	0.2	-	0.2	0.6	0.2	0.4	0.4	0.8	1.0	2.0	2.4	2.2	1.5	3.7	4.0	0.9	0.2	0.03	0.05	**0.5**	*142*
Mouth	110	0	-	-	-	0.2	0.4	-	0.4	-	0.4	0.7	1.3	1.8	1.8	4.5	5.3	3.4	5.3	9.5	1.5	0.3	0.03	0.08	**0.7**	*143-5*
Oropharynx	22	0	-	-	-	-	-	-	-	-	0.4	-	-	0.3	0.8	1.4	1.1	-	2.0	0.5	0.3	0.1	0.01	0.02	**0.1**	*146*
Nasopharynx	20	0	-	0.2	-	-	-	-	0.2	0.2	-	0.7	-	-	1.3	0.7	0.6	0.6	0.4	0.5	0.3	0.1	0.01	0.02	**0.2**	*147*
Hypopharynx	43	0	-	-	-	-	-	-	-	-	0.2	0.2	0.5	0.3	-	1.7	2.0	3.1	2.9	3.5	0.6	0.1	0.01	0.02	**0.2**	*148*
Pharynx unspecified	21	0	-	-	-	-	-	-	-	-	-	0.4	-	0.5	0.5	0.5	1.1	1.5	0.4	1.5	0.3	0.1	0.01	0.02	**0.1**	*149*
Oesophagus	710	0	-	-	-	-	0.2	-	0.6	0.9	2.5	4.4	6.8	14.3	19.4	24.7	40.2	55.9	75.9	9.4	2.0	0.15	0.37	**3.5**	*150*
Stomach	1081	0	-	-	-	-	-	0.2	0.2	1.0	1.9	3.1	4.1	9.7	9.5	22.2	39.2	66.2	96.6	135.8	14.3	3.0	0.15	0.46	**4.6**	*151*
Small intestine	89	0	-	-	-	-	-	0.2	0.2	0.4	-	1.3	1.3	3.5	2.8	4.8	3.7	3.7	2.5	1.2	0.3	0.04	0.08	**0.6**	*152*
Colon	3630	0	-	-	0.5	-	0.4	0.5	1.6	3.7	8.1	13.8	29.3	45.3	74.8	104.2	148.0	192.8	254.8	341.1	48.0	10.2	0.89	2.15	**19.0**	*153*
Rectum	1433	0	-	-	-	0.2	-	-	0.8	0.8	3.6	4.7	12.8	20.9	25.5	45.8	63.9	74.2	95.4	126.8	18.9	4.0	0.35	0.90	**7.6**	*154*
Liver	163	0	0.7	-	0.2	-	0.2	0.2	-	0.4	0.4	0.7	2.8	1.8	4.3	5.7	6.7	6.4	8.2	13.0	2.2	0.5	0.06	0.12	**1.1**	*155*
Gallbladder etc.	174	0	-	-	-	-	-	-	-	-	0.4	0.2	1.8	2.1	3.3	6.9	6.2	7.7	16.7	13.0	2.3	0.5	0.04	0.10	**0.9**	*156*
Pancreas	999	0	0.2	-	-	-	0.4	-	-	0.4	1.3	3.3	5.7	10.2	19.5	29.3	45.1	58.3	73.4	88.9	13.2	2.8	0.21	0.58	**5.0**	*157*
Nose, sinuses etc.	51	0	-	-	-	-	0.2	0.4	0.2	-	-	0.4	-	1.0	2.0	1.9	1.1	3.1	1.6	3.5	0.7	0.1	0.02	0.04	**0.3**	*160*
Larynx	78	0	-	-	-	-	-	-	-	-	-	0.2	1.5	2.4	1.5	3.3	3.9	3.7	4.1	3.0	1.0	0.2	0.03	0.06	**0.5**	*161*
Bronchus, lung	3111	0	-	-	-	0.6	0.4	0.4	1.0	1.4	6.2	15.4	21.3	43.7	80.3	129.0	162.6	166.5	183.0	150.3	41.1	8.8	0.85	2.31	**18.0**	*162*
Other thoracic organs	49	0	-	-	-	-	0.2	-	0.2	0.4	0.8	0.9	-	0.8	1.0	1.9	1.7	1.8	2.0	2.5	0.6	0.1	0.02	0.04	**0.4**	*163-4*
Bone	81	0	0.7	-	1.4	1.9	0.7	0.5	0.6	0.2	0.6	0.4	0.8	0.8	1.5	1.7	1.7	2.8	3.7	2.0	1.1	0.2	0.05	0.07	**0.9**	*170*
Connective tissue	208	0	0.9	0.5	-	1.1	0.9	0.9	1.2	1.4	2.1	3.1	3.3	2.6	4.0	4.5	5.6	9.8	9.4	8.0	2.7	0.6	0.11	0.16	**1.7**	*171*
Mesothelioma	39	0	-	-	-	-	-	-	-	-	0.2	0.4	0.8	0.3	1.5	0.9	2.8	2.8	1.2	-	0.5	0.1	0.02	0.03	**0.3**	*MES*
Kaposi's sarcoma	0	0	-	-	-	-	-	-	-	-	-	-	-	-	-	-	-	-	-	-	0.0	0.0	0.00	0.00	**0.0**	*KAP*
Melanoma of skin	1146	0	-	0.5	0.2	3.0	5.8	5.8	11.8	15.8	17.5	21.4	19.5	22.0	25.0	30.0	33.1	32.2	25.7	33.5	15.2	3.2	0.74	1.06	**10.3**	*172*
†Other skin	2246	0	0.7	0.5	0.7	1.5	1.1	3.1	3.4	4.7	11.3	18.7	26.5	26.7	46.0	59.1	89.1	110.1	148.0	172.3	29.7		0.72	1.46	**13.4**	*173*
Breast	9633	0	-	-	-	-	0.4	1.7	7.6	23.1	50.9	96.3	163.1	219.3	249.5	302.0	278.6	287.9	325.0	335.5	432.5	127.4	27.2	5.57	8.40	**75.0**	*174*
Uterus unspecified	179	0	-	-	-	-	0.4	-	0.4	0.8	0.6	1.8	4.1	2.4	1.3	4.3	5.9	6.7	9.8	22.5	2.4	0.5	0.06	0.11	**1.1**	*179*
Cervix uteri	1197	0	-	-	-	0.4	2.6	11.7	21.5	27.7	24.2	21.4	22.1	21.7	22.5	28.4	23.0	28.5	23.2	18.0	15.8	3.4	0.88	1.14	**11.6**	*180*
Placenta	4	0	-	-	-	0.2	-	0.2	-	0.4	-	-	-	-	-	-	-	-	-	-	0.1	0.0	0.00	0.00	**0.1**	*181*
Corpus uteri	1326	0	-	-	-	-	-	0.5	0.8	1.6	4.1	10.9	24.4	42.7	49.5	47.7	58.9	52.1	47.7	42.4	17.5	3.7	0.67	1.21	**9.6**	*182*
Ovary etc.	1679	0	0.2	0.9	0.2	1.1	1.3	2.0	4.7	6.0	12.0	17.4	33.1	51.3	53.8	58.8	58.6	65.6	57.5	50.9	22.2	4.7	0.92	1.51	**12.9**	*183*
Other female genital	367	0	-	-	-	-	-	0.5	0.8	0.8	1.1	2.2	2.8	3.1	8.3	11.1	10.7	16.2	23.6	43.9	4.9	1.0	0.10	0.21	**2.0**	*184*
Bladder	1262	0	-	0.2	0.2	0.4	0.6	1.1	0.6	2.1	3.0	4.0	10.5	16.2	30.0	43.2	51.6	65.9	80.3	99.9	16.7	3.6	0.34	0.82	**7.1**	*188*
Kidney etc.	522	0	1.5	0.2	-	-	0.7	0.5	0.2	1.0	2.1	5.6	5.9	11.0	17.0	18.0	19.1	23.9	24.1	25.5	6.9	1.5	0.23	0.41	**3.7**	*189*
Eye	65	0	0.2	-	-	0.2	-	-	0.4	0.6	0.9	-	1.5	1.8	1.8	1.4	1.7	2.8	3.3	2.0	0.9	0.2	0.04	0.05	**0.5**	*190*
Brain, nervous system	512	0	1.8	3.5	1.9	1.7	1.5	3.3	2.0	4.3	5.4	6.2	9.2	14.4	17.3	15.8	17.4	13.2	6.5	5.5	6.8	1.4	0.36	0.53	**5.1**	*191-2*
Thyroid	243	0	-	-	-	1.1	0.7	2.0	3.6	3.5	3.4	4.0	4.6	4.7	4.5	5.2	6.2	9.8	5.3	4.5	3.2	0.7	0.16	0.22	**2.2**	*193*
Other endocrine	58	0	1.3	1.2	0.5	-	0.2	0.2	1.0	0.2	0.4	0.7	1.3	1.3	0.3	1.7	1.4	1.8	-	1.5	0.8	0.2	0.04	0.06	**0.7**	*194*
Hodgkin's disease	186	0	-	0.5	0.7	3.0	6.7	4.5	2.4	2.5	2.3	2.0	1.5	1.6	1.8	2.1	1.7	4.0	2.9	3.5	2.5	0.5	0.15	0.17	**2.2**	*201*
Non-Hodgkin lymphoma	1210	0	0.7	-	0.5	1.3	1.3	2.3	1.6	3.1	7.5	10.9	14.6	20.9	29.0	39.2	49.1	57.6	63.6	64.4	16.0	3.4	0.47	0.91	**8.0**	*200,202*
Multiple myeloma	544	0	-	-	-	-	-	-	0.2	0.6	0.9	2.7	4.9	5.2	10.8	20.1	21.3	29.1	37.5	46.4	7.2	1.5	0.13	0.33	**2.9**	*203*
Lymphoid leukaemia	440	0	4.4	2.8	1.4	1.3	0.6	-	0.6	0.6	0.6	0.9	2.1	4.2	6.0	12.3	15.7	19.6	31.0	41.9	5.8	1.2	0.13	0.27	**3.0**	*204*
Myeloid leukaemia	447	0	1.1	0.5	1.0	0.8	1.3	0.9	2.4	1.6	2.1	1.1	6.4	6.0	10.3	10.6	14.6	19.9	26.1	34.5	5.9	1.3	0.18	0.30	**3.0**	*205*
Monocytic leukaemia	16	0	-	-	-	-	-	-	0.2	-	0.4	-	0.3	0.5	-	0.3	0.6	1.2	2.0	0.2	0.0	0.01	0.01	**0.1**	*206*
Other leukaemia	7	0	-	-	-	-	-	-	-	-	0.2	-	-	-	-	0.6	-	0.4	1.5	0.1	0.0	0.00	0.00	**0.0**	*207*
Leukaemia unspecified	39	0	-	-	-	-	0.4	-	-	-	-	-	0.5	0.5	0.3	0.2	0.6	2.8	2.9	6.5	0.5	0.1	0.01	0.01	**0.2**	*208*
Other and unspecified	2078	0	0.7	-	0.7	-	1.1	0.5	1.8	2.7	4.7	8.0	13.6	21.5	33.5	55.5	83.2	105.8	160.2	220.2	27.5	5.9	0.44	1.14	**10.5**	*O&U*
All sites	37721	0	14.9	11.3	10.6	20.5	32.1	50.4	90.6	143.7	228.7	357.8	522.7	684.0	926.5	1140.0	1386.9	1650.7	1945.0	2371.1	498.7		15.47	28.10	**252.1**	*ALL*
All sites but 173	35475	0	14.3	10.8	9.9	19.0	31.0	47.3	87.3	139.0	217.4	339.0	496.2	657.3	880.5	1081.0	1297.8	1540.6	1797.0	2198.9	469.0	100.0	14.75	26.64	**238.7**	*ALLb*

Rate from 1 case 0.220 0.2310 0.241 0.211 0.187 0.181 0.197 0.205 0.188 0.223 0.257 0.262 0.250 0.236 0.280 0.307 0.408 0.499

†Important: see notes on population page

UK, England, Yorkshire

The Yorkshire Cancer Registry was established in 1957 and now forms part of the Yorkshire Cancer Organization, located on the site of the Yorkshire Regional Centre for Cancer Treatment at Cookridge Hospital, Leeds. It currently employs 27 staff, approximately 50% of whom are involved in data collection and 50% in information, clinical audit and research.

The registry covers an area of approximately 13 700 km^2, extending from the northern edge of the North Yorkshire Moors to the borders of Lincolnshire in the south, Flamborough Head in the east and the Pennines in the west. It comprises seven Health Districts which form part of the Northern and Yorkshire Regional Health Authority. In 1974 the boundaries were redefined as part of the national reorganization of Health Authorities. The resident population of 3 600 000 constitutes 7.2% of the population of England and Wales. There are marked differences in population density, with some 60% of the population living in 15% of the area. The latter area includes the densely populated urban areas of Leeds and Bradford, while North Yorkshire and East Yorkshire are relatively sparsely populated. Indian, Pakistani and Bangladeshi ethnic groups form 3.5% of the total population (1991 census).

The age structure is not significantly different from that of England and Wales as a whole. However, the percentage of 0–14-year-olds is slightly higher and that of males over 65 years is lower.

Traditional industries include shipping, fishing, textile and clothing manufacture, steel production and coal mining.

The vast majority of patients receive their hospital care in National Health Service (NHS) hospitals, but the private sector is growing. 19 000 NHS beds are available and the region is served by approximately 3500 medical and dental staff. Nationally, a re-organization of cancer services has begun, following the report of an Expert Advisory Group on Cancer to the Chief Medical Officers of England and Wales.

Cancer registration in Yorkshire, as in the rest of the UK, is a mandatory requirement and cases diagnosed in hospitals (inpatient and outpatient) are notified directly. All pathology laboratories throughout the region routinely send copies of pathology reports and these act as a cross-reference to information received directly. Yorkshire residents treated outside the region are notified by other cancer registries. Notification also comes from Breast Screening Units and hospices. Cases are registered by registry staff who visit the hospitals and abstract treatment details from the hospital case notes following primary notification. Copies of death certificates are routinely received from the Office for National Statistics for all cases where cancer is a cause of death. When this information is the first notification of cancer, the registry sends an enquiry to the hospital where the patient died, or to the doctor if the patient did not die in hospital. Primary registration is carried out from a death certificate only if no other information can be obtained.

When the cause of death is non-malignant, the registry is notified by the National Health Service Central Register, where all registered cancer patients are flagged.

Registration details include the personal details of the patient, method of diagnosis, anatomical site and morphology, stage of disease at presentation and initial treatment administered. Religion and occupation are also recorded.

The registry operates an advanced computer system, with data being entered at up to 15 terminals. Incoming data are linked to existing data for the same patient and new cases are assigned an accession number by the computer. All data items are encoded by the computer using look-up dictionaries. The system also automatically generates a general practitioner's enquiry letter, a cancer registration document and a follow-up enquiry letter where necessary. At the point of entry, data are validated using the Office for National Statistics edit procedures. The system is also capable of identifying duplicate registrations and a record link allows the automatic identification of patients with multiple primaries. Data are regularly exchanged with local specialist tumour registries to ensure complete ascertainment.

The registry regularly produces reports and actively promotes the use of the data which it holds. A statistical report on incidence, mortality, treatment and survival of all cases is published every five years; site-specific reports are produced on an occasional basis. Registry information will also be available as a PC-based user-friendly database (Quickdata) and at a site on the worldwide web (http://www.yco.leeds.ac.uk). Current research projects include an evaluation of the breast screening programme and a study of treatment variation, delay in referral and effect on outcome for the 17 most common cancer sites.

Lesley Rider

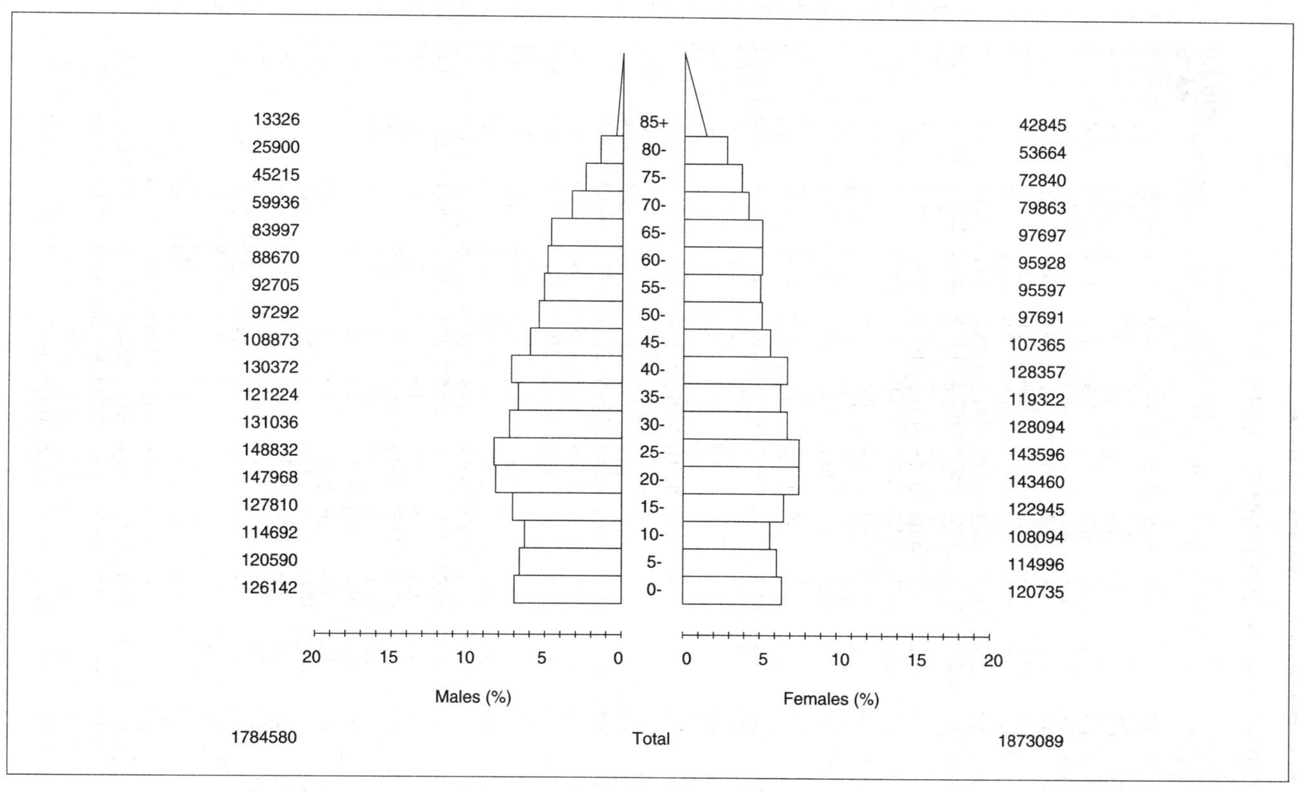

UK, England, Yorkshire
Source of population: average annual 1988–92
Census: 1991 Census: Usual Residence, Great Britain, OPCS. London: HMSO, 1993.
Estimate: The populations for 1988, 1989 and 1990 are mid-year estimates based on the 1981 Census, and that for 1992 is a mid-year estimate based on the 1991 Census (OPCS).

Screening programmes in the area:
During the period women aged 20-64 were screened for cervical cancer (240,000 examinations performed in 1994), and women aged 50-64 for breast cancer (the number of examinations annually rising from 6,000 in 1988 to 60,000 in 1992).

UK, ENGLAND, YORKSHIRE 1988-1992

ANNUAL INCIDENCE PER 100,000 BY AGE GROUP (YEARS) - MALE

SITE	ALL AGES	AGE UNK	0-	5-	10-	15-	20-	25-	30-	35-	40-	45-	50-	55-	60-	65-	70-	75-	80-	85+	CRUDE RATE	%	CR 64	CR 74	ASR (W)	ICD (9th)
Lip	65	0	-	-	-	-	-	-	-	-	0.5	0.4	0.8	1.1	1.1	3.8	4.0	3.5	3.9	7.5	0.7	0.2	0.02	0.06	0.5	140
Tongue	165	0	-	-	-	-	-	-	0.3	1.3	0.9	2.4	4.1	3.7	5.6	4.8	6.0	8.8	8.5	7.5	1.8	0.4	0.09	0.15	1.3	141
Salivary gland	77	0	-	-	-	-	0.1	0.5	0.2	0.2	0.2	0.7	1.6	0.9	1.6	4.5	4.3	1.8	5.4	4.5	0.9	0.2	0.03	0.07	0.6	142
Mouth	233	0	-	-	-	-	-	-	0.5	0.5	1.1	3.5	6.4	6.7	7.0	7.9	8.7	12.4	8.5	15.0	2.6	0.6	0.13	0.21	1.8	143-5
Oropharynx	96	0	-	-	-	-	-	-	0.3	0.5	0.9	1.7	1.9	2.6	2.3	4.3	3.7	4.4	3.9	1.5	1.1	0.2	0.05	0.09	0.8	146
Nasopharynx	48	0	-	0.2	0.2	0.6	-	-	-	-	0.8	1.1	1.6	1.5	0.2	2.1	0.7	0.4	1.5	1.5	0.5	0.1	0.03	0.05	0.4	147
Hypopharynx	76	0	-	-	-	-	-	-	-	-	0.3	0.7	1.0	1.7	4.1	4.8	2.0	1.3	3.9	7.5	0.9	0.2	0.04	0.07	0.6	148
Pharynx unspecified	44	0	-	-	-	-	-	-	-	-	-	0.7	1.0	1.1	2.3	1.9	2.0	1.8	1.5	-	0.5	0.1	0.03	0.05	0.4	149
Oesophagus	997	0	-	-	-	-	-	0.5	-	1.2	2.3	5.1	11.5	20.7	30.7	44.3	55.4	68.6	70.3	85.5	11.2	2.6	0.36	0.86	7.1	150
Stomach	2399	0	-	-	0.2	0.2	0.1	0.5	1.1	2.8	4.1	12.7	22.8	38.2	62.9	101.2	141.5	186.2	228.6	208.6	26.9	6.2	0.73	1.94	16.4	151
Small intestine	81	0	-	-	-	-	-	-	-	-	0.2	0.7	1.0	1.7	2.9	3.8	4.7	4.0	6.2	4.5	0.9	0.2	0.03	0.08	0.6	152
Colon	2830	0	-	-	-	0.3	0.4	0.5	1.7	2.6	6.9	12.1	28.2	44.4	75.6	106.2	165.2	234.9	257.1	300.2	31.7	7.4	0.86	2.22	19.3	153
Rectum	2173	0	-	-	-	-	0.1	0.1	0.9	2.0	4.0	12.9	21.2	39.7	65.4	91.9	116.8	170.7	173.7	199.6	24.4	5.6	0.73	1.77	15.1	154
Liver	241	0	-	0.2	0.2	-	-	0.1	-	0.2	0.5	1.3	1.6	5.0	9.0	8.6	16.0	19.5	13.9	15.0	2.7	0.6	0.09	0.21	1.7	155
Gallbladder etc.	155	0	-	-	-	-	-	-	0.2	-	0.2	1.4	3.0	5.4	7.4	8.7	11.5	14.7	9.0	1.7	0.4	0.05	0.13	1.1	156
Pancreas	982	0	-	-	-	-	-	-	0.2	0.5	2.5	4.4	10.5	13.4	30.7	42.1	60.7	74.3	82.6	82.5	11.0	2.6	0.31	0.82	6.8	157
Nose, sinuses etc.	80	0	-	0.2	-	-	0.1	-	0.2	0.2	0.2	0.4	1.2	2.8	2.3	3.1	2.0	7.5	4.6	3.0	0.9	0.2	0.04	0.06	0.6	160
Larynx	627	0	-	-	-	-	-	-	0.2	1.2	1.5	4.2	11.3	14.0	22.3	34.3	36.7	30.5	26.3	15.0	7.0	1.6	0.27	0.63	4.7	161
Bronchus, lung	9380	0	-	-	-	0.2	0.3	0.5	1.4	2.8	13.5	28.5	77.7	144.8	293.0	442.9	610.3	713.0	749.0	727.9	105.1	24.4	2.81	8.08	64.3	162
Other thoracic organs	45	0	-	-	-	0.2	-	0.1	-	0.3	0.5	0.2	1.0	1.3	1.4	2.1	2.0	0.4	2.3	1.5	0.5	0.1	0.02	0.05	0.4	163-4
Bone	72	0	-	1.0	1.2	0.9	0.7	0.4	0.5	0.5	0.8	0.6	0.4	0.9	2.0	1.7	1.0	1.3	2.3	-	0.8	0.2	0.05	0.06	0.7	170
Connective tissue	223	0	1.3	0.3	0.5	0.9	1.2	0.7	1.1	2.1	2.1	2.0	3.1	4.1	3.8	6.9	8.3	9.3	10.0	9.0	2.5	0.6	0.12	0.19	1.9	171
Mesothelioma	263	0	-	-	-	-	-	-	-	0.5	1.4	2.2	4.5	10.8	9.0	10.5	11.0	14.2	10.0	7.5	2.9	0.7	0.14	0.25	2.0	MES
Kaposi's sarcoma	12	0	-	-	-	-	-	0.3	-	0.2	0.3	0.3	0.4	0.2	-	-	0.2	-	0.4	-	0.1	0.0	0.01	0.01	0.1	KAP
Melanoma of skin	492	0	-	-	-	0.2	0.9	2.3	3.4	6.1	6.1	6.6	10.7	12.5	10.8	12.6	15.7	15.0	21.6	18.0	5.5	1.3	0.30	0.44	4.1	172
Other skin	6558	0	-	-	0.3	0.6	1.6	3.1	4.6	10.1	21.5	34.7	65.8	104.2	157.4	269.8	364.4	475.5	609.3	760.9	73.5		2.02	5.19	45.5	173
Breast	75	0	0.2	-	-	-	-	0.1	-	0.3	0.6	0.2	0.8	-	1.8	2.4	6.7	6.2	4.6	6.0	0.8	0.2	0.02	0.07	0.5	175
Prostate	4866	0	-	-	-	-	-	-	-	-	0.2	0.6	0.9	8.2	33.2	82.8	181.4	319.0	524.2	693.4	741.4	54.5	12.6	0.63	3.13	29.4	185
Testis	455	0	0.5	0.3	0.2	2.5	6.5	11.4	12.1	10.6	9.4	7.2	3.9	1.5	2.7	1.2	0.3	2.2	3.9	4.5	5.1	1.2	0.34	0.35	4.6	186
Penis	130	0	-	-	-	-	-	0.1	-	0.2	0.3	1.5	1.2	1.9	4.1	5.5	7.7	7.5	10.8	12.0	1.5	0.3	0.05	0.11	0.9	187.1-.4
Other male genital	22	0	-	-	-	-	-	0.1	-	-	0.2	0.2	0.6	-	0.5	1.3	1.8	2.3	1.5	0.2	0.1	0.01	0.02	0.2	187.5-.9
Bladder	3672	0	-	-	-	0.2	0.1	0.7	1.4	3.5	8.6	15.1	33.5	64.1	100.8	155.5	216.9	272.0	325.1	376.7	41.2	9.5	1.14	3.00	25.3	188
Kidney etc.	943	0	1.6	0.3	-	0.2	-	0.5	0.6	2.1	3.4	8.3	15.0	23.7	29.8	39.5	47.4	50.4	54.1	52.5	10.6	2.5	0.43	0.86	7.2	189
Eye	72	0	1.1	0.2	-	-	-	-	0.9	0.7	-	0.6	1.9	1.5	1.1	2.6	2.7	2.2	3.1	3.0	0.8	0.2	0.04	0.07	0.7	190
Brain, nervous system	650	0	2.9	3.0	2.1	1.9	1.5	3.2	4.4	4.5	5.2	9.4	13.2	15.7	20.3	18.6	19.4	13.3	12.4	7.5	7.3	1.7	0.44	0.63	6.1	191-2
Thyroid	89	0	-	0.2	0.2	-	0.5	0.4	1.2	0.5	0.9	1.7	2.1	1.7	1.8	2.6	1.3	1.8	3.9	6.0	1.0	0.2	0.06	0.08	0.8	193
Other endocrine	49	0	1.6	0.3	0.2	0.2	0.3	0.3	0.5	0.2	0.5	0.2	0.2	0.6	1.1	2.4	1.3	-	-	0.5	0.1	0.03	0.04	0.5	194
Hodgkin's disease	254	0	0.2	1.0	1.4	2.7	3.8	3.9	3.7	3.8	4.3	2.4	3.1	2.6	2.3	4.5	2.7	3.1	3.9	1.5	2.8	0.7	0.17	0.21	2.5	201
Non-Hodgkin lymphoma	1223	0	1.7	2.0	2.1	2.2	1.2	2.4	3.1	6.3	8.7	10.8	18.9	21.4	29.5	44.8	57.4	67.2	64.1	84.0	13.7	3.2	0.55	1.06	9.7	200,202
Multiple myeloma	546	0	-	-	-	-	-	0.1	0.3	0.5	2.5	2.6	7.6	8.0	13.3	23.6	29.0	38.0	46.3	67.5	6.1	1.4	0.17	0.44	3.8	203
Lymphoid leukaemia	513	0	6.2	3.5	1.6	1.4	0.3	0.7	0.2	1.0	2.5	2.8	3.9	8.2	11.7	16.2	17.0	33.2	33.2	66.0	5.7	1.3	0.22	0.38	4.5	204
Myeloid leukaemia	444	0	1.4	1.3	1.0	0.5	0.8	1.2	2.6	2.1	3.1	1.8	2.7	8.6	9.2	13.3	18.0	32.7	23.9	51.0	5.0	1.2	0.18	0.34	3.5	205
Monocytic leukaemia	9	0	-	-	-	-	-	-	-	-	0.2	0.4	-	0.5	0.3	0.9	-	1.5	0.1	0.0	0.00	0.01	0.1	206
Other leukaemia	8	0	0.3	-	-	-	-	-	-	-	-	-	0.5	0.5	0.3	0.4	-	-	0.1	0.0	0.00	0.01	0.1	207
Leukaemia unspecified	47	0	0.2	-	-	-	0.1	-	0.2	-	-	-	0.2	-	1.8	0.2	3.3	4.0	6.2	10.5	0.5	0.1	0.01	0.03	0.3	208
Other and unspecified	2559	0	0.3	-	-	0.3	0.1	1.2	1.7	3.5	5.8	10.5	17.9	39.5	65.6	103.8	140.5	208.3	267.9	273.1	28.7	6.6	0.73	1.95	17.3	O&U
All sites	45040	0	19.3	13.9	11.3	16.0	21.2	36.0	49.1	75.6	129.3	216.4	428.0	713.0	1189.6	1843.2	2543.4	3342.2	3878.7	4259.3	504.8		14.59	36.53	316.8	ALL
All sites but 173	38482	0	19.3	13.9	11.0	15.3	19.6	32.9	44.6	65.5	107.8	181.7	362.2	608.8	1032.1	1573.4	2179.0	2866.7	3269.4	3498.4	431.3	100.0	12.57	31.34	271.3	ALLb

Rate from 1 case   0.159 0.166 0.174 0.156 0.135 0.134 0.153 0.165 0.153 0.184 0.206 0.216 0.226 0.238 0.334 0.442 0.772 1.501

UK, ENGLAND, YORKSHIRE 1988-1992

ANNUAL INCIDENCE PER 100,000 BY AGE GROUP (YEARS) - FEMALE

SITE	ALL AGES	AGE UNK	0-	5-	10-	15-	20-	25-	30-	35-	40-	45-	50-	55-	60-	65-	70-	75-	80-	85+	CRUDE RATE	%	CR 64	CR 74	ASR (W)	ICD (9th)
Lip	21	0	-	-	-	-	-	-	-	0.2	-	0.2	0.2	0.2	-	0.8	0.8	0.5	1.1	2.3	0.2	0.1	0.00	0.01	0.1	140
Tongue	95	0	0.2	-	-	-	-	0.1	0.5	0.5	0.6	0.4	0.6	1.9	1.7	2.9	3.0	3.3	2.6	7.5	1.0	0.2	0.03	0.06	0.6	141
Salivary gland	57	0	0.2	-	0.4	-	-	0.4	0.2	0.7	-	-	1.0	0.2	0.8	1.8	2.0	1.6	1.9	3.7	0.6	0.1	0.02	0.04	0.4	142
Mouth	132	0	-	-	-	-	-	-	0.2	0.2	0.3	1.5	0.6	2.1	5.0	3.3	5.3	4.1	5.2	7.9	1.4	0.3	0.05	0.09	0.8	143-5
Oropharynx	36	0	-	-	-	-	-	-	-	-	0.8	0.2	0.4	0.6	0.6	1.2	1.3	0.8	1.5	1.9	0.4	0.1	0.01	0.03	0.2	146
Nasopharynx	13	0	-	-	-	0.2	-	-	-	-	-	0.4	0.4	0.2	-	0.4	0.8	0.3	-	0.5	0.1	0.0	0.01	0.01	0.1	147
Hypopharynx	49	0	-	-	-	-	-	-	-	0.2	0.5	-	0.6	0.4	0.8	2.0	2.0	1.6	2.6	2.3	0.5	0.1	0.01	0.03	0.3	148
Pharynx unspecified	20	0	-	-	-	-	-	-	0.2	-	-	-	-	0.8	0.6	0.8	0.5	0.3	1.1	0.9	0.2	0.1	0.01	0.01	0.1	149
Oesophagus	712	0	-	-	-	-	-	-	0.2	0.3	0.3	1.1	4.7	8.6	13.6	18.0	23.3	43.9	44.0	52.7	7.6	1.8	0.14	0.35	3.2	150
Stomach	1580	0	-	-	-	-	0.1	0.1	1.2	0.8	3.0	4.7	7.4	13.6	19.8	36.0	59.1	77.2	122.6	141.4	16.9	4.0	0.25	0.73	6.7	151
Small intestine	90	0	-	-	-	-	-	0.3	0.2	0.3	0.3	0.6	0.8	1.3	2.1	3.3	2.8	4.4	3.4	3.7	1.0	0.2	0.03	0.06	0.5	152
Colon	3282	0	-	-	-	0.2	-	0.6	1.1	2.7	8.3	11.0	19.0	38.9	59.2	81.7	128.7	157.1	199.0	261.4	35.0	8.4	0.70	1.76	15.2	153
Rectum	1756	0	-	-	-	-	-	0.1	0.9	1.3	3.9	6.9	11.5	25.7	32.5	55.1	62.9	80.5	102.1	120.0	18.7	4.5	0.41	1.00	8.5	154
Liver	199	0	0.3	-	-	0.2	0.1	0.1	-	0.3	0.6	1.7	1.8	2.5	3.8	5.1	6.0	7.1	16.0	12.6	2.1	0.5	0.05	0.11	1.0	155
Gallbladder etc.	243	0	-	-	-	-	-	-	-	0.2	0.8	0.6	2.3	1.5	4.6	6.1	9.0	13.7	18.6	13.1	2.6	0.6	0.05	0.12	1.1	156
Pancreas	1112	0	-	-	-	-	-	-	-	1.2	1.7	3.9	7.6	10.7	19.4	28.3	43.3	57.4	73.8	81.2	11.9	2.8	0.22	0.58	5.1	157
Nose, sinuses etc.	57	0	-	-	-	0.2	-	-	0.2	0.2	0.3	0.2	0.2	0.2	0.6	2.3	1.8	2.2	4.5	3.7	0.6	0.1	0.01	0.03	0.3	160
Larynx	156	0	-	-	-	-	-	-	-	0.2	0.6	0.7	0.6	4.2	6.5	5.9	6.8	5.8	3.0	3.7	1.7	0.4	0.06	0.13	1.0	161
Bronchus, lung	4511	0	-	-	-	-	-	0.3	1.1	2.2	7.9	16.0	38.1	65.9	139.9	181.8	203.3	193.0	174.8	143.8	48.2	11.6	1.36	3.28	24.8	162
Other thoracic organs	45	0	-	-	-	-	0.1	-	-	0.2	0.7	0.2	1.0	2.5	0.6	1.3	1.4	1.5	1.9	0.5	0.1	0.02	0.03	0.3	163-4
Bone	53	0	0.2	0.3	1.1	1.6	0.4	0.4	0.2	-	0.2	0.4	0.8	-	0.6	1.2	1.0	1.1	-	1.4	0.6	0.1	0.03	0.04	0.5	170
Connective tissue	190	0	1.3	0.2	0.4	0.7	1.0	0.4	0.6	0.3	2.3	2.4	1.6	3.8	3.5	3.1	5.8	4.9	8.2	4.7	2.0	0.5	0.09	0.14	1.4	171
Mesothelioma	65	0	-	-	-	-	-	-	-	-	0.7	1.0	0.8	2.1	2.3	4.3	2.5	1.9	-	0.7	0.2	0.02	0.06	0.4	MES
Kaposi's sarcoma	4	0	-	-	-	-	-	-	0.3	-	-	-	-	-	-	-	-	0.4	0.5	0.0	0.0	0.00	0.00	0.0	KAP
Melanoma of skin	867	0	0.2	-	0.2	1.1	2.8	4.0	9.2	9.4	11.5	11.4	17.6	16.9	15.0	17.2	17.8	18.1	16.8	25.2	9.3	2.2	0.50	0.67	6.6	172
Other skin	6304	0	0.2	-	0.4	0.3	1.4	3.8	5.6	15.4	23.2	38.4	51.8	78.2	106.5	166.4	216.1	297.6	343.2	448.1	67.3		1.63	3.54	31.7	173
Breast	9968	0	-	-	-	0.2	1.7	7.9	24.5	56.3	100.5	156.3	198.8	238.5	263.7	240.7	251.2	255.1	277.3	323.5	106.4	25.5	5.24	7.70	68.9	174
Uterus unspecified	197	0	-	-	-	-	-	-	-	0.8	0.9	2.2	3.3	4.8	5.0	3.5	6.3	7.1	7.5	10.7	2.1	0.5	0.09	0.13	1.2	179
Cervix uteri	1752	0	-	-	0.2	2.6	12.7	28.3	41.6	34.0	23.8	24.2	25.3	33.4	30.3	33.3	28.0	17.1	17.7	18.7	4.5	1.13	1.45	14.5	180
Placenta	5	0	-	-	0.2	0.3	-	0.3	-	-	-	-	-	-	-	-	-	-	-	0.1	0.0	0.00	0.00	0.1	181
Corpus uteri	1282	0	-	-	0.2	-	0.3	0.2	2.2	5.1	12.1	18.8	33.9	38.2	42.0	46.1	42.8	42.1	33.6	13.7	3.3	0.55	0.99	8.0	182
Ovary etc.	1782	0	-	-	0.4	0.5	1.0	1.8	2.3	4.4	15.0	23.3	33.0	37.9	50.0	55.1	54.1	52.2	49.6	49.0	19.0	4.6	0.85	1.39	11.9	183
Other female genital	435	0	-	-	-	0.1	0.6	0.5	0.7	1.7	1.5	2.7	3.1	3.5	11.7	17.5	18.9	33.9	33.6	4.6	1.1	0.07	0.22	1.9	184
Bladder	1459	0	0.2	-	-	0.2	0.1	0.4	0.5	0.8	3.0	5.4	8.4	16.7	29.4	43.4	54.8	75.2	85.3	93.8	15.6	3.7	0.33	0.82	7.0	188
Kidney etc.	597	0	2.5	0.9	-	-	0.1	-	1.6	3.0	2.2	5.8	8.0	8.6	17.3	17.0	18.5	22.8	22.4	18.7	6.4	1.5	0.25	0.43	3.9	189
Eye	92	0	1.3	-	-	-	-	0.1	0.2	0.3	0.5	1.1	1.6	2.1	1.7	2.5	2.8	3.0	3.4	0.9	1.0	0.2	0.04	0.07	0.7	190
Brain, nervous system	480	0	2.7	3.1	1.9	1.1	1.0	1.8	3.7	2.0	2.8	6.5	5.7	9.2	11.0	16.4	12.3	9.3	7.5	5.6	5.1	1.2	0.26	0.41	4.0	191-2
Thyroid	223	0	-	-	0.2	0.8	1.4	1.8	2.7	3.5	2.6	2.2	3.9	2.5	2.9	3.9	3.0	6.9	4.8	6.1	2.4	0.6	0.12	0.16	1.7	193
Other endocrine	44	0	1.8	0.5	0.2	0.2	0.4	-	0.3	0.2	0.2	0.6	0.6	0.4	0.2	0.2	0.3	1.4	0.7	1.4	0.5	0.1	0.03	0.03	0.5	194
Hodgkin's disease	193	0	0.2	0.2	0.6	3.9	4.0	3.1	2.0	2.2	1.2	1.5	1.6	3.6	1.7	1.8	2.3	2.5	3.4	0.9	2.1	0.5	0.13	0.15	1.9	201
Non-Hodgkin lymphoma	996	0	0.8	0.7	1.1	0.3	1.0	0.7	3.1	2.7	4.7	7.1	11.5	15.1	20.0	28.3	35.3	41.2	45.8	40.6	10.6	2.6	0.34	0.66	5.9	200,202
Multiple myeloma	515	0	-	-	-	-	-	0.1	-	0.3	0.6	1.7	4.5	6.5	10.2	11.9	20.0	26.4	35.0	32.2	5.5	1.3	0.12	0.28	2.4	203
Lymphoid leukaemia	337	0	6.3	2.1	1.3	0.8	0.1	0.1	0.5	0.3	0.8	1.1	1.8	2.7	5.2	8.0	8.5	15.1	14.9	19.6	3.6	0.9	0.12	0.20	2.5	204
Myeloid leukaemia	386	0	1.0	0.2	0.6	0.5	1.3	0.8	1.6	0.7	2.5	3.0	2.7	4.8	6.7	9.0	12.5	14.0	19.8	21.5	4.1	1.0	0.13	0.24	2.3	205
Monocytic leukaemia	7	0	-	-	-	-	-	-	-	-	-	-	-	0.2	0.4	-	-	0.8	-	0.5	0.1	0.0	0.00	0.00	0.0	206
Other leukaemia	3	0	-	-	-	-	-	-	-	-	-	-	-	0.2	-	-	0.3	-	-	0.5	0.0	0.0	0.00	0.00	0.0	207
Leukaemia unspecified	38	0	-	-	-	-	-	-	-	-	-	-	-	0.6	0.2	0.8	1.0	2.7	2.2	4.7	0.4	0.1	0.00	0.01	0.1	208
Other and unspecified	2911	0	0.7	0.2	0.4	0.3	0.8	0.3	1.2	2.8	5.9	9.7	16.0	34.5	54.8	75.1	113.9	123.0	190.1	230.1	31.1	7.5	0.64	1.58	13.7	O&U
All sites	45351	0	19.9	8.3	8.9	13.7	22.0	43.3	95.1	161.4	251.5	368.8	516.9	731.6	997.4	1229.1	1502.6	1729.0	2012.5	2291.5	484.2		16.19	29.85	263.8	ALL
All sites but 173	39047	0	19.7	8.3	8.5	13.3	20.6	39.6	89.5	146.0	228.3	330.5	465.1	653.4	890.9	1062.7	1286.5	1431.4	1669.3	1843.4	416.9	100.0	14.57	26.31	232.1	ALLb
Rate from 1 case			0.166	0.174	0.185	0.163	0.139	0.139	0.156	0.167	0.156	0.186	0.205	0.209	0.208	0.205	0.250	0.275	0.373	0.467						

UK, Scotland

Cancer registration in Scotland has evolved from a system initiated in 1936 by the Radium Commission aimed at facilitating follow-up, a function now undertaken through hospitals and general practitioners. The national scheme was reorganized in 1959 and is now mainly statistical and research-orientated. There are five regional registries that are run as separate organizations, each with its own director and data collection staff. National coordination is carried out by the Information & Statistics Division (ISD) of the Common Services Agency for the National Health Service in Scotland, which is also responsible for analysis of the national data.

Scotland lies between latitudes 54°38′ and 60°51′ N and longitudes 1°45′ and 7°40′ W. It covers an area of 77 179 km², and few parts of the country are more than 64 km from the sea.

The population covered is over five million, of whom 90% were born in Scotland and 7% elsewhere in the United Kingdom (England, Wales, Northern Ireland). 0.6% were born in Europe, 0.2% in India or Bangladesh, 0.2% in Africa or the Caribbean and 2.2% in the rest of the world.

The distribution of the workforce in Scotland in 1991 showed 34% of the employed population to be working in public administration and other services, 9.8% in manufacturing, 21.2% in distribution, hotels and catering, 7.6% in metal goods, engineering and vehicles industries, 10.4% in banking, finance and insurance, 5.8% in construction, 5.6% in transport and communication, 2.9% in energy and water supplies, 1.9% in metals, minerals and chemicals, and 1.4% in agriculture, forestry and fishing.

Cancer registration in Scotland is voluntary. Data are derived mainly from hospital inpatient sources and only a small proportion comes from outpatient departments. Some pathology departments now supply computerized data from histopathology and cytopathology systems. The registries which were computerized in 1990/91 supply a minimum data set to ISD (submitted on floppy disc) comprising cancer registration number, name of hospital, case reference number, patient's name, maiden surname, date of birth, sex and marital status, postcode, NHS number, date treatment commenced, tumour type and site, indication of the presence of multiple tumours, histological verification of the tumour, and date of death.

Some registries collect other information, which is not forwarded to ISD. The national data are stored on a mainframe computer after validity and feasibility checks have been made. Data on the computer file at the National Register go back to 1958, and complete national coverage is held from 1968. Registrations are included in this dataset only for residents of Scotland (subject to a six-month residence rule).

Death information is added to the national database routinely from information received from the General Register Office (Scotland). This is received quarterly on tape and the relevant information is sent to the regional registries on diskette with an accompanying print. In this way, survival information can be produced without need for an active follow-up system.

ISD publishes data regularly on incidence, and periodically on survival. *Ad hoc* analyses of the data are carried out in response to enquiries from clinicians, research workers, members of the public, the Scottish Office Department of Health and any other interested bodies. ISD is involved in several major studies, and the data are used increasingly in the investigation of possible environmental hazards. The registration data are also used for planning, management, clinical audit and research.

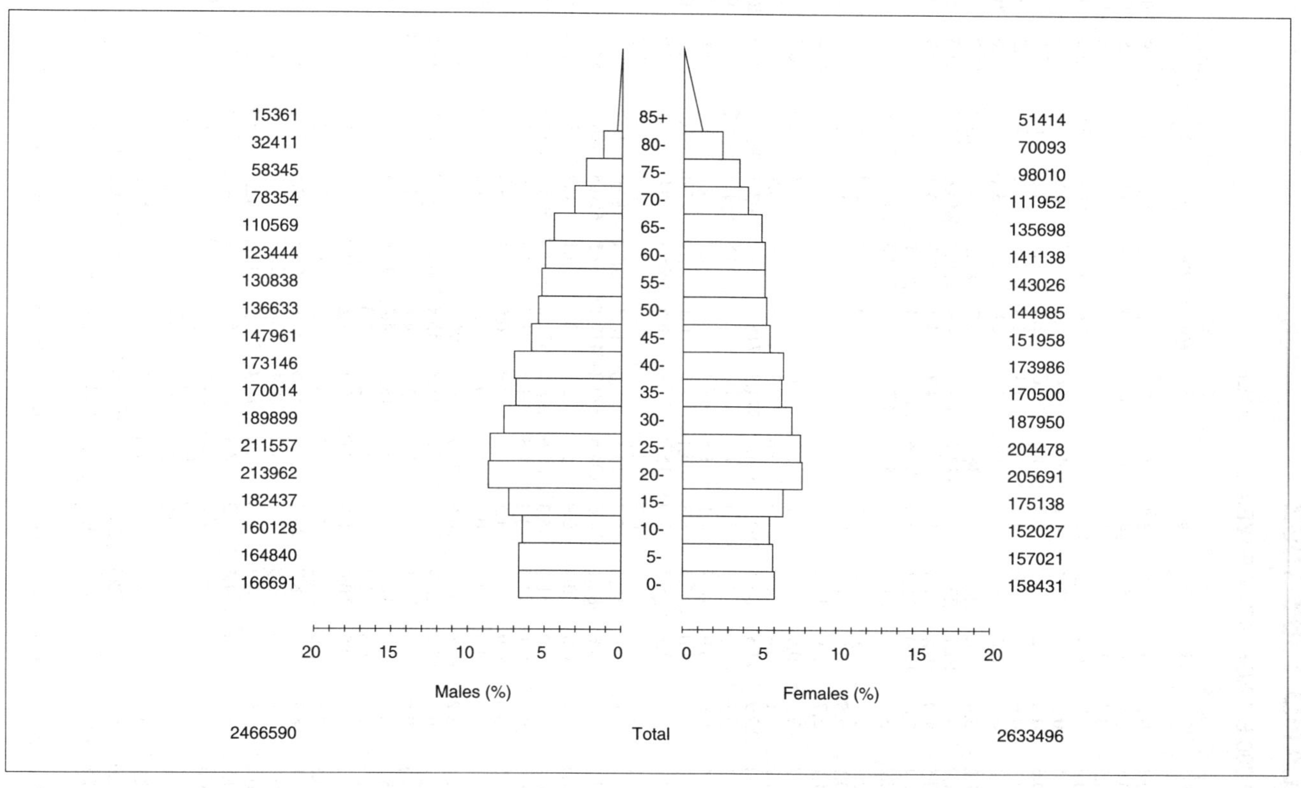

UK, Scotland

Source of population: average annual 1988–92
Census: 1991 Census: Usual Residence, Great Britain, OPCS. London: HMSO, 1993.
Estimate: The estimates for 1988, 1989, 1990 and 1992 were revised to be consistent with the final Census results for 1991.

Screening programmes in the area:

Women aged 21-60 have been screened for cervical cancer since the mid–60s (567,136 examinations in 1990). A breast cancer screening programme was set up in 1988 for women aged 50-64 (approximately 10 700 examinations annually).

UK, SCOTLAND 1988-1992

ANNUAL INCIDENCE PER 100,000 BY AGE GROUP (YEARS) - MALE

SITE	ALL AGES	AGE UNK	0-	5-	10-	15-	20-	25-	30-	35-	40-	45-	50-	55-	60-	65-	70-	75-	80-	85+	CRUDE RATE	%	CR 64	CR 74	ASR (W)	ICD (9th)
Lip	232	0	-	-	-	-	0.1	0.2	0.1	0.4	0.8	0.8	1.5	3.8	4.4	6.3	8.2	12.0	21.6	16.9	1.9	0.4	0.06	0.13	**1.2**	140
Tongue	314	0	-	-	-	-	0.1	0.2	0.2	0.6	1.4	3.9	5.3	4.9	6.8	10.9	12.0	7.9	8.0	13.0	2.5	0.6	0.12	0.23	**1.9**	141
Salivary gland	116	0	-	-	-	0.1	0.2	0.1	0.2	0.5	0.7	0.8	1.5	1.7	1.5	3.6	3.3	4.1	8.0	7.8	0.9	0.2	0.04	0.07	**0.7**	142
Mouth	475	0	-	-	-	-	0.1	0.1	0.3	0.6	1.7	6.4	7.2	11.8	10.7	15.4	14.0	13.0	11.1	19.5	3.9	0.8	0.19	0.34	**2.8**	143-5
Oropharynx	178	0	-	-	-	-	-	0.1	-	0.1	0.3	2.0	3.8	4.1	4.7	5.4	4.8	5.5	4.9	3.9	1.4	0.3	0.08	0.13	**1.1**	146
Nasopharynx	72	0	-	-	-	-	-	0.1	0.2	0.6	0.6	1.2	0.7	0.9	1.6	2.0	2.3	2.4	0.6	1.3	0.6	0.1	0.03	0.05	**0.4**	147
Hypopharynx	153	0	-	-	-	-	-	-	0.1	0.1	0.6	1.6	2.0	3.2	4.2	5.4	4.6	3.8	6.2	5.2	1.2	0.3	0.06	0.11	**0.9**	148
Pharynx unspecified	79	0	-	-	-	-	0.1	-	-	0.4	0.3	0.8	1.5	1.5	1.8	2.7	2.8	1.0	3.1	1.3	0.6	0.1	0.03	0.06	**0.5**	149
Oesophagus	1731	0	-	-	-	-	-	0.1	0.2	1.2	3.9	6.6	20.3	27.4	36.1	64.8	69.7	80.2	86.4	115.9	14.0	3.0	0.48	1.15	**9.4**	150
Stomach	3388	0	-	-	0.1	-	-	0.4	1.5	1.9	4.6	10.4	22.1	43.1	72.1	108.2	151.6	199.2	230.8	274.7	27.5	5.9	0.78	2.08	**17.7**	151
Small intestine	114	0	-	-	-	0.3	-	0.3	-	0.5	1.0	0.4	1.3	1.7	1.6	4.3	4.3	2.7	4.3	7.8	0.9	0.2	0.04	0.08	**0.7**	152
Colon	4588	0	-	-	-	0.3	0.5	0.7	1.3	4.4	7.4	16.0	31.3	56.9	84.6	140.7	202.4	282.1	348.0	359.3	37.2	8.1	1.02	2.73	**23.7**	153
Rectum	2668	0	0.1	-	-	-	-	0.4	0.7	2.2	5.7	11.5	21.2	37.3	56.1	87.7	117.2	132.0	169.1	214.8	21.6	4.7	0.68	1.70	**14.3**	154
Liver	577	0	0.2	-	-	-	0.2	-	0.4	0.4	1.2	1.4	3.2	7.5	13.4	18.5	28.8	33.6	29.0	41.7	4.7	1.0	0.14	0.38	**3.1**	155
Gallbladder etc.	278	0	-	-	-	0.1	-	0.1	0.2	0.1	0.6	0.9	1.5	2.8	4.7	9.0	10.5	18.5	21.0	32.5	2.3	0.5	0.05	0.15	**1.4**	156
Pancreas	1533	0	-	-	-	0.1	0.2	-	0.1	1.1	2.7	5.9	12.0	19.3	35.0	44.1	65.1	96.3	97.5	118.5	12.4	2.7	0.38	0.93	**8.1**	157
Nose, sinuses etc.	84	0	0.1	-	0.1	-	-	0.2	0.2	0.2	0.9	2.3	1.7	1.3	2.0	2.8	1.4	3.7	2.6	0.7	0.1	0.04	0.06	**0.5**	160
Larynx	1078	0	-	-	-	-	-	-	1.2	2.1	10.8	14.9	29.6	40.3	38.8	35.0	30.9	22.1	8.7	1.9	0.40	0.80	**6.2**	161
Bronchus, lung	15212	0	-	-	-	0.1	0.2	0.8	1.4	4.4	15.9	43.5	89.1	194.7	373.9	574.3	716.2	820.6	903.4	860.6	123.3	26.7	3.62	10.07	**79.8**	162
Other thoracic organs	64	0	0.1	-	-	-	0.1	-	0.3	0.1	0.1	-	0.3	1.5	1.1	1.6	2.6	3.8	1.9	6.5	0.5	0.1	0.02	0.04	**0.4**	163-4
Bone	122	0	0.1	0.7	1.4	1.9	0.7	0.7	0.4	0.6	0.6	0.9	0.7	1.1	1.5	1.4	1.5	1.7	4.9	3.9	1.0	0.2	0.06	0.07	**0.9**	170
Connective tissue	285	0	0.8	0.5	0.2	1.2	0.5	0.9	1.1	1.9	1.5	2.0	2.9	4.3	4.1	7.1	6.1	7.9	15.4	10.4	2.3	0.5	0.11	0.18	**1.8**	171
Mesothelioma	570	0	-	-	-	-	-	-	-	0.1	0.8	3.1	5.7	7.9	15.6	19.9	26.5	25.4	29.0	22.1	4.6	1.0	0.17	0.40	**3.1**	MES
Kaposi's sarcoma	40	0	-	-	-	-	0.1	0.6	0.5	1.2	1.2	0.5	-	0.2	0.2	-	0.3	0.6	-	-	0.3	0.1	0.02	0.02	**0.3**	KAP
Melanoma of skin	969	0	-	0.2	0.4	1.3	2.7	4.0	4.4	7.1	9.5	10.3	12.6	15.7	16.5	17.0	18.6	26.1	30.9	48.2	7.9	1.7	0.42	0.60	**6.0**	172
Other skin	10185	0	-	-	0.5	0.5	1.8	4.1	7.7	14.2	26.3	46.6	81.1	124.6	204.6	299.2	417.1	562.5	690.5	868.4	82.6		2.56	6.14	**54.2**	173
Breast	74	0	-	-	-	-	-	-	-	0.4	0.2	0.5	0.4	0.9	1.5	2.7	2.6	3.1	6.2	3.9	0.6	0.1	0.02	0.05	**0.4**	175
Prostate	6552	0	0.1	-	-	-	0.1	0.2	-	0.1	1.0	3.2	11.0	35.3	88.6	198.4	332.6	510.4	695.4	839.8	53.1	11.5	0.70	3.35	**31.2**	185
Testis	802	0	1.0	0.1	0.2	2.3	9.0	13.3	17.2	16.1	10.5	8.1	4.0	3.2	1.6	1.8	1.8	0.3	1.9	3.9	6.5	1.4	0.43	0.45	**5.8**	186
Penis	171	0	-	-	-	-	-	0.1	0.2	1.2	0.5	0.9	2.3	1.5	3.7	4.9	6.6	5.1	9.9	18.2	1.4	0.3	0.05	0.11	**1.0**	187.1-.4
Other male genital	39	0	-	0.1	-	-	-	-	0.1	-	-	0.3	0.3	0.3	1.5	0.7	1.0	1.7	4.9	1.3	0.3	0.1	0.01	0.02	**0.2**	187.5-.9
Bladder	4351	0	-	-	-	0.3	0.5	0.9	0.8	2.6	8.2	15.1	33.7	54.6	94.9	134.4	195.0	243.4	299.9	317.7	35.3	7.6	1.06	2.71	**22.9**	188
Kidney etc.	1417	0	1.8	0.2	-	-	0.3	0.2	0.4	2.2	4.5	10.8	13.9	22.2	34.8	45.8	55.4	60.3	58.0	75.5	11.5	2.5	0.46	0.96	**8.1**	189
Eye	161	0	1.1	0.2	-	-	0.2	0.6	0.3	0.8	0.8	2.3	1.6	2.3	3.9	2.9	4.6	4.1	4.3	6.5	1.3	0.3	0.07	0.11	**1.1**	190
Brain, nervous system	920	0	3.0	2.5	3.1	2.4	2.3	2.6	3.4	5.2	6.7	7.3	10.5	16.5	19.9	18.3	24.8	20.6	9.3	13.0	7.5	1.6	0.43	0.64	**6.2**	191-2
Thyroid	148	0	-	-	-	0.1	0.5	0.5	0.7	1.9	1.3	1.6	1.8	2.0	2.4	2.9	4.3	2.7	3.7	5.2	1.2	0.3	0.06	0.10	**0.9**	193
Other endocrine	68	0	1.9	0.1	0.5	0.8	0.2	0.4	-	0.1	0.7	0.5	0.6	0.2	0.6	0.4	1.8	0.7	1.2	1.3	0.6	0.1	0.03	0.04	**0.6**	194
Hodgkin's disease	368	0	0.1	0.2	1.4	2.1	5.1	5.0	3.2	3.8	2.8	2.0	3.2	2.9	3.7	3.3	5.6	5.5	2.5	2.6	3.0	0.6	0.18	0.22	**2.6**	201
Non-Hodgkin lymphoma	1607	0	0.6	1.1	1.7	1.2	1.8	3.3	4.5	6.8	8.7	11.8	18.7	23.4	28.4	39.6	53.9	63.8	72.8	79.4	13.0	2.8	0.56	1.03	**9.4**	200,202
Multiple myeloma	681	0	-	-	-	0.1	-	-	0.1	0.2	1.4	2.8	4.5	7.8	13.1	20.1	35.2	38.7	51.8	45.6	5.5	1.2	0.15	0.43	**3.5**	203
Lymphoid leukaemia	705	0	7.7	3.8	1.7	2.5	0.5	0.5	0.6	0.4	0.5	2.4	3.2	8.6	10.4	18.3	25.3	28.8	42.6	48.2	5.7	1.2	0.21	0.43	**4.7**	204
Myeloid leukaemia	562	0	0.7	0.7	-	0.7	1.2	2.0	1.1	1.4	3.9	3.0	4.1	4.3	8.9	16.1	15.8	29.1	34.6	37.8	4.6	1.0	0.16	0.32	**3.2**	205
Monocytic leukaemia	18	0	0.1	-	-	0.1	0.1	-	-	0.1	-	-	-	0.2	0.3	0.4	0.8	1.0	1.2	1.3	0.1	0.0	0.00	0.01	**0.1**	206
Other leukaemia	9	0	-	-	-	-	-	-	-	-	-	-	-	0.3	0.3	0.4	0.5	0.3	-	-	0.1	0.0	0.00	0.01	**0.0**	207
Leukaemia unspecified	78	0	0.1	0.1	0.1	-	-	-	0.1	-	0.1	-	0.1	0.9	1.3	2.4	2.8	5.5	6.2	10.4	0.6	0.1	0.01	0.04	**0.4**	208
Other and unspecified	3295	0	0.5	-	0.4	0.1	0.7	0.6	0.7	2.9	5.3	9.9	18.3	37.8	61.6	102.2	147.8	195.7	251.8	322.9	26.7	5.8	0.69	1.94	**17.1**	O&U
All sites	67131	0	20.3	10.8	12.0	18.7	29.8	43.8	55.1	92.0	148.8	272.2	478.5	826.1	1369.2	2107.6	2850.1	3599.9	4318.9	4913.7	544.3		16.89	41.68	**360.4**	ALL
All sites but 173	56946	0	20.3	10.8	11.5	18.2	28.0	39.7	47.4	77.8	122.4	225.6	397.4	701.5	1164.6	1808.5	2433.0	3037.4	3628.4	4045.3	461.7	100.0	14.33	35.53	**306.2**	ALLb

Rate from 1 case   0.120 0.121 0.125 0.110 0.093 0.095 0.105 0.118 0.116 0.135 0.146 0.153 0.162 0.181 0.255 0.343 0.617 1.302

UK, SCOTLAND 1988-1992

ANNUAL INCIDENCE PER 100,000 BY AGE GROUP (YEARS) - FEMALE

SITE	ALL AGES	AGE UNK	0-	5-	10-	15-	20-	25-	30-	35-	40-	45-	50-	55-	60-	65-	70-	75-	80-	85+	CRUDE RATE	%	CR 64	CR 74	ASR (W)	ICD (9th)
Lip	76	0	-	-	-	-	0.1	-	0.2	0.1	-	0.1	0.4	0.1	0.7	1.9	2.0	2.9	2.6	5.8	0.6	0.1	0.01	0.03	0.3	140
Tongue	162	0	-	-	-	0.1	-	0.1	0.3	0.4	0.1	1.1	0.8	3.1	2.4	3.1	2.5	4.7	5.1	9.3	1.2	0.3	0.04	0.07	0.7	141
Salivary gland	111	0	-	-	-	0.2	-	0.1	0.3	1.1	0.5	0.3	0.7	1.0	2.3	1.3	1.8	3.7	2.3	6.6	0.8	0.2	0.03	0.05	0.5	142
Mouth	306	0	-	-	-	0.1	0.2	0.1	0.2	0.2	0.9	2.1	3.2	5.5	6.5	5.6	7.3	5.9	7.7	12.1	2.3	0.5	0.10	0.16	1.4	143-5
Oropharynx	71	0	0.1	-	-	-	-	-	-	-	0.3	0.5	1.4	1.5	1.4	1.2	2.1	1.0	0.9	1.6	0.5	0.1	0.03	0.04	0.4	146
Nasopharynx	29	0	-	-	-	0.1	0.1	0.1	-	0.4	0.2	0.1	0.4	0.3	0.6	0.4	0.4	0.8	0.3	0.4	0.2	0.0	0.01	0.02	0.2	147
Hypopharynx	68	0	-	-	-	-	-	-	0.1	-	-	0.1	-	0.3	1.5	1.7	1.5	2.1	1.8	2.6	0.4	0.5	0.1	0.02	0.04	0.3	148
Pharynx unspecified	33	0	-	-	-	-	-	0.1	-	0.1	0.1	-	0.1	0.3	1.0	1.3	0.7	0.4	0.9	0.8	0.3	0.1	0.01	0.02	0.1	149
Oesophagus	1481	0	-	-	-	-	-	-	0.3	0.2	1.5	3.9	5.8	13.1	19.1	29.2	44.5	49.6	72.2	85.2	11.2	2.5	0.22	0.59	5.0	150
Stomach	2330	0	-	-	0.1	-	-	0.3	0.9	1.5	2.0	3.8	8.3	18.2	28.1	38.3	64.1	88.8	131.3	138.9	17.7	3.9	0.32	0.83	7.5	151
Small intestine	105	0	-	-	-	-	-	0.1	-	-	0.1	0.5	1.0	1.4	1.3	2.5	2.7	3.5	4.6	3.1	0.8	0.2	0.02	0.05	0.4	152
Colon	5588	0	-	0.1	-	0.6	0.7	1.4	1.7	3.4	8.7	15.3	29.7	48.2	75.8	108.8	139.5	206.7	257.9	308.5	42.4	9.3	0.93	2.17	19.4	153
Rectum	2292	0	-	-	-	-	0.1	0.2	0.4	2.9	4.0	7.5	12.3	23.1	34.9	49.1	60.2	71.8	95.6	121.0	17.4	3.8	0.43	0.97	8.3	154
Liver	365	0	0.3	0.1	0.1	-	0.1	0.1	0.1	0.7	0.5	0.8	1.9	3.4	5.2	9.0	8.0	11.8	15.4	19.1	2.8	0.6	0.07	0.15	1.4	155
Gallbladder etc.	468	0	-	-	-	-	-	-	-	0.5	0.7	0.9	2.1	4.5	5.7	8.4	9.3	17.1	26.3	30.7	3.6	0.8	0.07	0.16	1.5	156
Pancreas	1599	0	0.1	-	-	-	0.1	0.1	0.2	0.9	1.5	3.8	6.9	12.0	24.4	31.2	47.3	55.9	75.6	85.6	12.1	2.7	0.25	0.64	5.5	157
Nose, sinuses etc.	75	0	-	-	-	-	0.2	0.1	0.1	0.2	0.2	0.5	0.8	1.0	1.1	1.3	2.0	2.0	2.0	1.9	0.6	0.1	0.02	0.04	0.3	160
Larynx	285	0	-	-	-	-	-	-	0.1	0.1	0.9	2.1	3.2	5.9	6.5	6.2	8.4	5.7	6.8	2.7	2.2	0.5	0.09	0.17	1.3	161
Bronchus, lung	8442	0	-	-	-	0.3	0.2	0.3	0.7	5.2	10.1	27.8	52.8	98.6	168.2	248.1	281.0	260.4	227.1	187.1	64.1	14.1	1.82	4.47	33.7	162
Other thoracic organs	43	0	-	-	-	-	-	0.1	-	0.2	-	0.5	-	0.4	0.4	1.0	1.4	1.0	1.7	1.6	0.3	0.1	0.01	0.02	0.2	163-4
Bone	95	0	0.1	0.3	0.8	0.9	0.4	0.7	0.4	0.6	0.8	0.1	0.8	1.0	0.6	1.5	0.7	1.2	1.7	2.7	0.7	0.2	0.04	0.05	0.6	170
Connective tissue	229	0	0.4	0.5	0.8	0.5	0.6	0.7	1.0	1.1	1.0	1.6	1.8	2.4	2.8	3.8	3.6	6.5	4.3	6.6	1.7	0.4	0.08	0.11	1.2	171
Mesothelioma	87	0	-	-	-	-	-	-	-	-	0.1	1.1	0.3	0.7	1.1	2.8	3.2	2.9	2.6	1.2	0.7	0.1	0.02	0.05	0.4	MES
Kaposi's sarcoma	4	0	-	-	-	-	-	-	-	-	-	-	-	-	0.3	-	0.4	-	-	-	0.0	0.0	0.00	0.00	0.0	KAP
Melanoma of skin	1524	0	0.1	0.4	0.3	3.0	4.9	8.9	9.6	12.6	13.3	17.4	15.0	15.5	16.4	19.7	24.1	24.7	31.4	27.2	11.6	2.5	0.59	0.81	8.3	172
Other skin	9982	0	-	-	-	0.8	2.3	4.6	8.9	15.8	31.4	46.3	64.4	81.8	115.1	180.7	235.6	347.1	422.3	571.8	75.8		1.86	3.94	36.4	173
Breast	14825	0	-	-	-	-	0.8	7.0	28.2	53.6	109.3	168.9	221.5	248.5	271.5	247.5	244.4	280.8	299.3	396.0	112.6	24.7	5.55	8.01	72.7	174
Uterus unspecified	222	0	-	-	-	-	-	0.2	-	0.1	0.7	1.1	2.6	2.5	4.0	3.4	5.0	8.0	6.6	10.5	1.7	0.4	0.06	0.10	0.9	179
Cervix uteri	2183	0	-	-	-	0.1	2.1	10.7	24.4	28.2	28.7	28.6	23.3	26.4	24.5	31.0	27.2	21.4	21.4	16.3	16.6	3.6	0.98	1.28	12.7	180
Placenta	6	0	-	-	-	-	0.2	0.2	-	0.2	-	-	-	-	-	-	-	-	-	-	0.0	0.0	0.00	0.00	0.0	181
Corpus uteri	1594	0	-	-	-	0.1	0.2	0.2	0.5	1.5	4.9	11.2	22.5	35.4	32.6	33.3	34.8	37.1	31.4	32.7	12.1	2.7	0.55	0.89	7.4	182
Ovary etc.	2844	0	-	0.1	0.7	0.8	1.2	2.6	4.9	5.4	16.8	23.6	33.9	42.9	50.0	60.6	62.5	73.3	61.9	51.3	21.6	4.7	0.91	1.53	13.3	183
Other female genital	546	0	0.1	-	-	-	0.3	0.4	0.7	1.4	2.5	1.6	3.3	3.8	5.4	9.0	16.1	18.0	22.5	30.3	4.1	0.9	0.10	0.22	2.0	184
Bladder	1995	0	-	-	-	-	0.2	0.3	0.6	1.1	1.8	6.3	13.4	19.3	30.9	45.4	55.6	66.5	81.6	88.3	15.2	3.3	0.37	0.87	7.3	188
Kidney etc.	1047	0	1.9	0.5	0.1	-	0.1	0.3	0.5	1.5	2.1	5.9	9.1	13.4	17.6	23.1	27.5	30.2	33.4	31.1	8.0	1.7	0.27	0.52	4.5	189
Eye	165	0	1.3	0.3	-	-	0.2	0.2	0.5	0.6	0.5	1.2	1.2	2.0	2.3	3.1	3.0	5.1	2.6	5.8	1.3	0.3	0.05	0.08	0.9	190
Brain, nervous system	740	0	3.9	3.3	2.8	1.7	1.1	3.0	3.6	4.1	3.9	5.0	7.3	9.5	11.5	14.3	11.4	12.0	8.6	4.7	5.6	1.2	0.30	0.43	4.6	191-2
Thyroid	358	0	-	-	0.3	0.5	1.4	2.2	2.6	2.9	3.3	4.7	3.7	2.2	4.1	3.8	5.7	5.9	6.8	7.0	2.7	0.6	0.14	0.19	2.0	193
Other endocrine	73	0	1.3	-	0.3	0.8	-	0.4	-	0.5	0.6	0.5	0.6	1.1	0.9	1.0	0.5	0.6	0.9	1.2	0.6	0.1	0.03	0.04	0.5	194
Hodgkin's disease	285	0	-	0.1	1.8	3.2	3.5	2.9	3.1	2.1	1.6	0.8	2.2	1.8	2.3	2.4	3.4	3.3	2.0	2.3	2.2	0.5	0.13	0.16	1.9	201
Non-Hodgkin lymphoma	1758	0	0.5	0.6	0.4	0.8	1.9	1.5	1.9	4.3	7.1	7.4	14.6	17.6	29.0	34.0	46.4	53.1	56.5	56.4	13.4	2.9	0.44	0.84	7.4	200,202
Multiple myeloma	714	0	-	-	-	-	-	0.1	-	0.1	0.8	1.3	4.1	6.4	8.8	15.9	20.2	29.6	29.7	33.8	5.4	1.2	0.11	0.29	2.5	203
Lymphoid leukaemia	485	0	5.7	1.7	1.6	1.1	0.2	0.2	0.2	0.1	0.8	1.2	2.9	2.7	5.7	6.6	12.3	14.7	16.5	22.6	3.7	0.8	0.12	0.21	2.5	204
Myeloid leukaemia	553	0	0.5	0.1	0.8	0.7	1.0	2.1	1.5	1.8	2.9	2.8	4.4	4.3	5.1	10.0	10.7	13.9	20.8	24.1	4.2	0.9	0.14	0.24	2.5	205
Monocytic leukaemia	14	0	0.1	-	-	-	-	-	0.1	0.1	0.1	0.1	-	-	0.1	0.4	0.2	0.2	0.3	0.8	0.1	0.0	0.00	0.01	0.1	206
Other leukaemia	5	0	0.1	-	-	-	-	-	-	-	-	-	-	-	-	0.1	0.2	0.2	0.3	-	0.0	0.0	0.00	0.00	0.0	207
Leukaemia unspecified	100	0	-	-	0.1	-	0.1	-	0.2	0.1	-	0.1	0.1	0.4	0.6	1.5	1.3	4.9	5.7	9.7	0.8	0.2	0.01	0.02	0.3	208
Other and unspecified	3703	0	0.6	0.1	-	0.2	0.2	0.9	0.9	2.7	4.1	10.5	16.1	28.0	47.2	64.6	98.1	125.5	186.9	245.1	28.1	6.2	0.56	1.37	12.4	O&U
All sites	70065	0	17.2	8.3	10.9	16.7	24.5	53.5	100.0	160.7	271.9	420.9	601.4	812.7	1077.5	1369.1	1641.6	1982.2	2296.6	2702.0	532.1		17.88	32.93	293.2	ALL
All sites but 173	60083	0	17.2	8.3	10.9	15.9	22.2	48.9	91.1	144.9	240.5	374.6	537.0	730.9	962.5	1188.4	1406.0	1635.1	1874.4	2130.1	456.3	100.0	16.02	29.00	256.8	ALLb
Rate from 1 case			0.126	0.127	0.132	0.114	0.097	0.098	0.106	0.117	0.115	0.132	0.138	0.140	0.142	0.147	0.179	0.204	0.285	0.389						

UK, Scotland, West

Cancer registration in the West of Scotland commenced in 1958 and is carried out on behalf of the six West of Scotland Health Boards (Greater Glasgow, Argyll and Clyde, Lanarkshire, Ayrshire and Arran, Dumfries and Galloway and Forth Valley) by the West of Scotland Cancer Surveillance Unit. The Unit is a constituent member of Glasgow Regional Cancer Institutes, which in turn is a member of the European Organisation of Cancer Institutes and the UICC. The Unit was designated as a Collaborating Centre for Community Cancer Care by WHO Regional Office for Europe in 1987. The staffing comprises a medically qualified director, one principal epidemiologist, one statistician, one information systems analyst and six registration officers (one part-time).

The area covered by the registry is 22 972 km^2 and lies between latitudes 54° and 57° N and longitudes 3° and 7° W. The population resident in the area is 2 716 900 (estimated at June 1991). One third of these are resident within the Greater Glasgow Health Board area. The majority of the population live in the conurbation encompassing the city of Glasgow and extending west along the Clyde estuary and east through the Central Belt. Apart from several smaller urban areas, the remaining area is largely rural. Only Glasgow has an established and significant immigrant (Asian) population.

Both active and passive techniques of registration are applied. Primarily the registry is reliant on notification of cancer cases by hospital medical records' staff. These may originate from any of the 141 hospitals in the registry region. Cases from all general hospitals in Glasgow (approximately 38% of annual registered cases) are received in a computer-readable format. Pathology data are received in the same format from some Glasgow hospitals. Registration staff make regular visits to hospitals in order to verify case details and to validate the diagnosis of cases based solely on the Registrar General's death certificates. Despite such efforts, a small number (approximately 5%) are registered as death certificate only.

The registry is responsible for the classification, coding, verification and validation of all data received.

The registry operates a PC network which supports a MUMPS-based registration database, as used in four of the five Scottish registries. This application is patient-based and facilitates recording of multiple primaries. The system allows on-line access to all registry data since 1958, and is used by statistical staff to identify and extract cases for surveys and studies. Data received on diskette are automatically linked to existing registry cases to identify possible duplicate and multiple primary registrations.

The cancer registry plays an important role in cancer control activities by provision of local data for primary and secondary preventive programmes, for public and professional education and for the interpretation of local cancer hazards.

The Cancer Surveillance Unit undertakes epidemiological studies based on the cancer registry data. Recent work has concentrated on examining variations in survival in order to provide evidence on how patient outcomes can be improved. Publications have appeared demonstrating the benefit of multi-disciplinary management in ovarian cancer and the advantage to be gained by specialist care in breast cancer. A linkage of the cancer registry has been set up with the Renfrew/Paisley General Population Survey, established as the third largest prospective cohort study in the world with cancer incidence as an endpoint.

C.R. Gillis
D.J. Hole
A. Graham
D.W. Lamont
K. Campbell

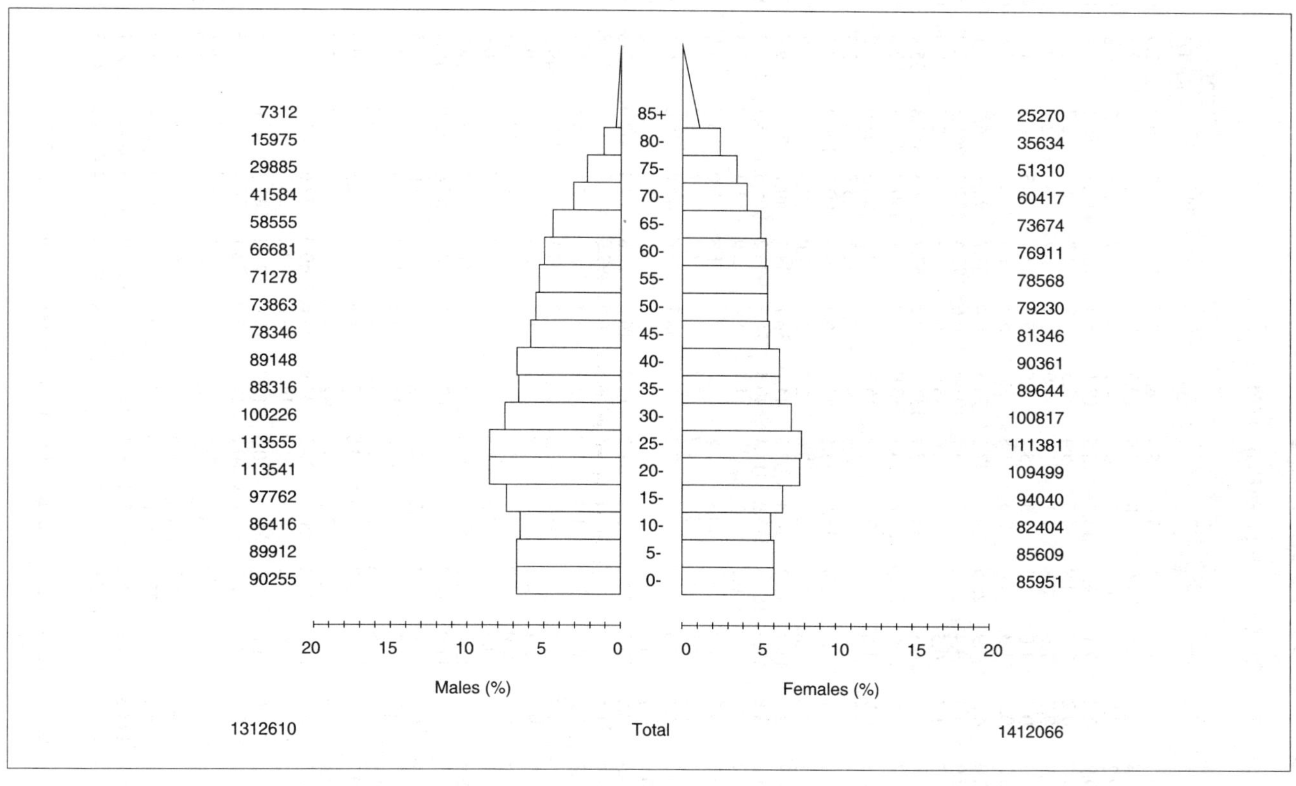

UK, Scotland, West

Source of population: average annual 1988–92

Census: 1991 Census: Usual Residence, Great Britain, OPCS. London: HMSO, 1993.

Estimate: The estimates for 1988, 1989, 1990 and 1992 were revised to be consistent with the final Census results for 1991.

Screening programmes in the area:

Women aged 21-60 have been screened for cervical cancer since the mid–60s, and breast cancer screening was established in 1988 for women aged 50-64.

UK, SCOTLAND, WEST 1988-1992

ANNUAL INCIDENCE PER 100,000 BY AGE GROUP (YEARS) - MALE

SITE	ALL AGES	AGE UNK	0-	5-	10-	15-	20-	25-	30-	35-	40-	45-	50-	55-	60-	65-	70-	75-	80-	85+	CRUDE RATE	%	CR 64	CR 74	ASR (W)	ICD (9th)
Lip	125	0	-	-	-	-	0.2	-	-	0.5	0.7	1.3	1.4	3.6	5.4	6.8	9.6	10.7	22.5	10.9	1.9	0.4	0.06	0.15	1.3	140
Tongue	174	0	-	-	-	-	-	0.2	0.4	0.5	1.6	6.1	4.6	4.8	8.4	10.6	10.1	8.7	5.0	19.1	2.7	0.6	0.13	0.24	2.0	141
Salivary gland	54	0	-	-	-	-	0.4	-	-	0.2	0.9	-	0.8	1.4	0.9	4.1	3.8	4.7	8.8	5.5	0.8	0.2	0.02	0.06	0.5	142
Mouth	291	0	-	-	-	-	0.2	0.2	-	0.9	2.2	7.1	9.7	13.7	13.5	17.1	15.4	10.7	16.3	16.4	4.4	0.9	0.24	0.40	3.3	143-5
Oropharynx	95	0	-	-	-	-	-	-	-	-	0.2	2.0	4.9	4.5	5.4	5.5	3.8	4.7	2.5	2.7	1.4	0.3	0.09	0.13	1.1	146
Nasopharynx	38	0	-	-	-	-	-	-	0.4	0.5	0.7	1.0	0.8	1.1	1.2	2.0	2.4	2.7	-	2.7	0.6	0.1	0.03	0.05	0.4	147
Hypopharynx	86	0	-	-	-	-	-	-	-	-	0.7	1.0	1.9	2.8	5.4	5.5	5.3	5.4	7.5	8.2	1.3	0.3	0.06	0.11	0.9	148
Pharynx unspecified	53	0	-	-	-	-	-	-	-	0.5	0.2	1.3	1.4	2.5	1.8	3.4	5.3	1.3	2.5	-	0.8	0.2	0.04	0.08	0.6	149
Oesophagus	1059	0	-	-	-	-	-	-	0.4	2.0	4.5	7.9	25.5	29.2	47.1	76.5	78.4	87.7	92.6	136.8	16.1	3.4	0.58	1.36	11.1	150
Stomach	1763	0	-	-	0.2	-	-	0.4	1.2	2.0	4.3	9.4	25.2	44.1	63.3	108.6	160.6	193.4	237.9	265.3	26.9	5.7	0.75	2.10	17.5	151
Small intestine	59	0	-	-	-	0.6	-	0.5	-	0.5	1.3	0.5	0.8	1.4	0.6	5.5	5.3	1.3	3.8	2.7	0.9	0.2	0.03	0.09	0.7	152
Colon	2356	0	-	-	-	0.6	0.5	0.9	1.8	3.8	7.6	16.3	33.3	54.7	77.7	137.6	210.2	267.7	344.3	352.8	35.9	7.6	0.99	2.73	23.4	153
Rectum	1363	0	-	-	-	-	-	0.4	0.2	2.7	6.1	11.0	22.2	36.8	56.1	83.0	116.9	125.1	150.2	232.5	20.8	4.4	0.68	1.68	14.0	154
Liver	282	0	0.2	-	-	-	0.2	-	0.4	0.5	0.9	1.5	3.2	7.6	13.2	15.7	25.0	39.5	22.5	21.9	4.3	0.9	0.14	0.34	2.8	155
Gallbladder etc.	151	0	-	-	-	0.2	-	-	0.4	-	0.7	1.0	1.4	2.2	4.5	9.2	9.6	22.1	23.8	38.3	2.3	0.5	0.05	0.15	1.5	156
Pancreas	818	0	-	-	-	0.2	0.4	-	-	0.9	3.1	5.9	11.4	18.8	38.1	44.4	66.4	100.4	100.2	109.4	12.5	2.7	0.39	0.95	8.2	157
Nose, sinuses etc.	43	0	0.2	-	-	-	-	-	0.2	0.5	0.4	0.8	1.6	2.0	0.6	2.7	2.4	2.0	2.5	2.7	0.7	0.1	0.03	0.06	0.5	160
Larynx	630	0	-	-	-	-	-	-	-	0.9	2.7	11.7	18.7	24.4	33.3	44.1	36.1	38.1	40.1	21.9	9.6	2.0	0.46	0.86	6.9	161
Bronchus, lung	8877	0	-	-	-	0.2	0.4	1.2	1.6	4.8	18.8	47.0	101.8	215.2	415.1	640.4	774.3	926.2	995.3	1036.7	135.3	28.8	4.03	11.10	88.9	162
Other thoracic organs	18	0	0.2	-	-	-	0.2	-	0.2	0.2	-	-	0.5	-	-	1.4	1.4	2.0	1.3	2.7	0.3	0.1	0.01	0.02	0.2	163-4
Bone	67	0	-	0.4	1.9	2.5	1.1	0.7	-	0.7	0.2	1.0	0.5	0.8	1.8	1.4	1.9	1.3	5.0	5.5	1.0	0.2	0.06	0.07	1.0	170
Connective tissue	146	0	0.7	0.4	0.2	1.0	0.5	1.2	0.4	1.4	1.1	2.6	2.4	4.5	4.8	7.2	7.2	8.7	11.3	8.2	2.2	0.5	0.11	0.18	1.7	171
Mesothelioma	422	0	-	-	-	-	-	-	-	0.2	1.1	2.6	6.8	8.4	22.2	31.8	36.1	40.8	43.8	35.6	6.4	1.4	0.21	0.55	4.3	MES
Kaposi's sarcoma	12	0	-	-	-	-	0.2	0.2	0.2	0.5	0.7	0.8	-	-	-	-	-	1.3	-	-	0.2	0.0	0.01	0.01	0.2	KAP
Melanoma of skin	509	0	-	0.4	0.2	1.4	1.8	4.2	4.2	6.3	9.0	10.5	14.1	15.4	19.2	17.8	16.8	22.8	· 30.0	52.0	7.8	1.7	0.43	0.61	6.1	172
Other skin	4580	0	-	-	0.2	0.2	0.5	2.1	6.4	11.8	21.8	43.7	63.1	110.8	182.1	254.8	354.5	499.9	597.2	735.8	69.8		2.21	5.26	46.5	173
Breast	45	0	-	-	-	-	-	-	-	0.7	0.2	0.8	-	1.4	1.2	3.1	3.4	3.3	7.5	5.5	0.7	0.1	0.02	0.05	0.5	175
Prostate	3233	0	0.2	-	-	-	0.2	0.2	-	-	0.9	3.8	10.6	35.4	79.5	196.4	322.2	470.5	681.0	790.5	49.3	10.5	0.65	3.25	29.9	185
Testis	397	0	0.9	-	-	2.5	9.5	13.4	14.6	14.7	9.2	7.4	4.1	2.5	1.8	2.0	1.4	0.7	2.5	2.7	6.0	1.3	0.40	0.42	5.4	186
Penis	84	0	-	-	-	-	-	-	-	1.6	0.2	1.0	3.0	1.1	3.0	4.4	4.3	7.4	8.8	19.1	1.3	0.3	0.05	0.09	0.9	187.1-.4
Other male genital	24	0	-	-	-	-	-	-	0.2	-	-	0.3	0.5	0.3	1.5	0.7	1.0	2.0	7.5	2.7	0.4	0.1	0.01	0.02	0.2	187.5-.9
Bladder	2281	0	-	-	-	0.2	0.4	1.4	0.8	2.9	7.9	13.5	32.2	60.9	96.9	132.2	194.8	241.6	306.7	295.4	34.8	7.4	1.09	2.72	22.9	188
Kidney etc.	718	0	1.8	-	-	-	0.2	0.2	0.4	2.3	4.0	11.0	12.7	19.6	32.1	42.0	60.1	60.2	57.6	73.9	10.9	2.3	0.42	0.93	7.7	189
Eye	96	0	0.9	0.4	-	-	0.4	0.9	0.4	0.9	0.9	2.8	2.4	2.0	4.5	2.7	4.3	4.7	5.0	8.2	1.5	0.3	0.08	0.12	1.2	190
Brain, nervous system	472	0	2.0	2.2	3.2	2.9	2.5	2.3	3.2	5.7	6.7	7.7	8.1	16.3	19.8	18.4	23.1	19.4	6.3	19.1	7.2	1.5	0.41	0.62	6.0	191-2
Thyroid	75	0	-	-	-	-	0.4	0.2	0.6	1.6	1.3	1.5	1.6	1.7	2.4	3.4	4.8	2.7	3.8	8.2	1.1	0.2	0.06	0.10	0.9	193
Other endocrine	38	0	2.7	0.2	0.7	0.4	0.4	0.2	-	0.2	0.7	0.3	0.8	-	0.6	0.3	1.9	-	2.5	-	0.6	0.1	0.04	0.05	0.7	194
Hodgkin's disease	179	0	-	0.4	1.4	2.0	4.9	5.5	3.0	3.4	2.5	1.8	2.4	2.2	3.6	2.7	4.3	4.7	-	2.7	2.7	0.6	0.17	0.20	2.4	201
Non-Hodgkin lymphoma	783	0	0.7	1.3	0.9	1.4	1.9	2.3	4.0	6.6	8.5	11.0	15.4	20.5	30.3	35.9	48.6	60.9	72.6	62.9	11.9	2.5	0.52	0.95	8.7	200,202
Multiple myeloma	350	0	-	-	-	0.2	-	-	0.2	-	1.6	3.6	5.1	7.9	12.0	16.7	33.2	42.2	51.3	49.2	5.3	1.1	0.15	0.40	3.5	203
Lymphoid leukaemia	351	0	7.8	4.7	1.9	2.5	0.5	0.5	0.6	0.2	0.9	1.8	3.5	5.3	10.5	14.7	25.0	29.4	41.3	41.0	5.3	1.1	0.20	0.40	4.5	204
Myeloid leukaemia	294	0	0.9	0.7	-	0.4	1.4	2.1	1.0	1.1	5.2	2.0	2.7	4.8	10.2	19.1	15.9	26.1	28.8	32.8	4.5	1.0	0.16	0.34	3.2	205
Monocytic leukaemia	6	0	0.2	-	-	-	0.2	-	-	-	-	-	-	-	0.3	-	0.7	1.3	2.7	0.1	0.0	0.00	0.00	0.1	206
Other leukaemia	2	0	-	-	-	-	-	-	-	-	-	-	-	0.3	-	0.3	-	-	-	-	0.0	0.0	0.00	0.00	0.0	207
Leukaemia unspecified	46	0	-	-	-	-	-	-	-	-	-	-	-	0.3	1.4	1.5	2.7	3.8	6.0	6.3	13.7	0.7	0.1	0.02	0.05	0.4	208
Other and unspecified	1836	0	0.4	-	-	-	0.7	0.5	0.8	3.6	6.1	11.2	22.5	41.0	72.9	107.9	160.2	210.8	242.9	289.9	28.0	6.0	0.80	2.14	18.3	O&U
All sites	35381	0	19.7	11.3	10.9	19.4	29.8	41.7	48.1	88.1	148.3	275.4	486.0	835.3	1406.1	2142.9	2871.2	3621.2	4301.6	4846.8	539.1		17.10	42.17	363.2	ALL
All sites but 173	30801	0	19.7	11.3	10.6	19.2	29.2	39.6	41.7	76.3	126.5	231.8	422.9	724.5	1224.0	1888.1	2516.8	3121.3	3704.4	4111.1	469.3	100.0	14.89	36.91	316.6	ALLb

Rate from 1 case   0.222   0.222   0.231   0.205   0.176   0.176   0.200   0.226   0.224   0.255   0.271   0.281   0.300   0.342   0.481   0.669   1.252   2.735

UK, SCOTLAND, WEST 1988-1992

ANNUAL INCIDENCE PER 100,000 BY AGE GROUP (YEARS) - FEMALE

SITE	ALL AGES	AGE UNK	0-	5-	10-	15-	20-	25-	30-	35-	40-	45-	50-	55-	60-	65-	70-	75-	80-	85+	CRUDE RATE	%	CR 64	CR 74	ASR (W)	ICD (9th)
Lip	54	0	-	-	-	-	0.2	-	0.4	-	-	-	0.3	-	0.5	2.7	2.6	3.1	4.5	11.1	0.8	0.2	0.01	0.03	**0.3**	140
Tongue	91	0	-	-	-	0.2	-	-	-	0.4	0.2	1.2	1.3	3.3	3.1	2.7	2.3	4.7	5.1	11.1	1.3	0.3	0.05	0.07	**0.7**	141
Salivary gland	58	0	-	-	-	-	-	-	-	1.1	0.7	0.2	0.5	0.5	2.3	1.4	2.0	4.3	1.7	8.7	0.8	0.2	0.03	0.04	**0.4**	142
Mouth	164	0	-	-	-	0.2	0.2	-	0.4	0.4	1.3	2.5	3.0	6.6	6.0	5.4	6.6	4.7	6.2	14.2	2.3	0.5	0.10	0.16	**1.4**	143-5
Oropharynx	39	0	-	-	-	-	-	-	-	-	0.4	0.2	1.5	1.8	1.0	1.1	2.3	1.6	1.1	1.6	0.6	0.1	0.03	0.04	**0.3**	146
Nasopharynx	13	0	-	-	-	0.2	0.2	-	-	0.4	0.4	-	0.3	-	0.8	-	0.3	-	0.6	0.8	0.2	0.0	0.01	0.01	**0.1**	147
Hypopharynx	44	0	-	-	-	-	-	-	-	-	0.2	-	0.3	2.0	2.1	2.4	2.3	1.6	3.4	-	0.6	0.1	0.02	0.05	**0.3**	148
Pharynx unspecified	22	0	-	-	-	-	-	0.2	-	0.2	0.2	-	0.3	0.3	1.3	1.1	0.7	0.8	1.1	1.6	0.3	0.1	0.01	0.02	**0.2**	149
Oesophagus	837	0	-	-	-	-	-	-	0.2	0.4	2.0	3.7	6.3	13.5	17.9	31.8	46.0	49.5	90.9	93.4	11.9	2.6	0.22	0.61	**5.2**	150
Stomach	1229	0	-	-	-	-	-	0.2	1.0	1.6	1.5	3.9	7.8	20.1	29.1	41.0	60.9	85.0	133.0	143.3	17.4	3.8	0.33	0.84	**7.5**	151
Small intestine	60	0	-	-	-	-	-	-	-	-	0.2	0.7	1.0	2.3	1.0	2.7	2.6	2.7	4.5	4.7	0.8	0.2	0.03	0.05	**0.4**	152
Colon	2754	0	-	0.2	-	0.6	0.9	1.4	2.2	2.2	8.2	14.5	28.3	44.0	71.0	98.3	137.0	193.7	225.1	307.1	39.0	8.6	0.87	2.04	**18.2**	153
Rectum	1173	0	-	-	-	-	0.2	0.2	0.2	2.2	4.0	4.9	12.1	23.7	34.8	46.7	54.0	70.9	93.2	129.8	16.6	3.7	0.41	0.91	**8.0**	154
Liver	192	0	0.5	0.2	-	-	-	0.2	0.2	0.9	0.4	1.2	2.0	3.6	5.7	7.9	9.8	10.9	13.5	15.8	2.7	0.6	0.07	0.16	**1.4**	155
Gallbladder etc.	249	0	-	-	-	-	-	-	-	-	0.2	0.4	1.2	3.3	4.1	6.8	8.7	9.9	17.2	22.5	31.7	3.5	0.8	0.08	0.17	**1.6**	156
Pancreas	834	0	0.2	-	-	-	-	-	-	0.2	0.9	2.2	3.9	6.6	10.4	22.1	32.8	46.7	58.1	67.9	93.4	11.8	2.6	0.23	0.63	**5.4**	157
Nose, sinuses etc.	37	0	-	-	-	-	0.4	-	-	0.4	0.2	-	0.8	0.5	1.0	0.8	3.0	1.9	2.2	1.6	0.5	0.1	0.02	0.04	**0.3**	160
Larynx	168	0	-	-	-	-	-	0.2	-	-	0.9	3.0	3.5	6.1	6.8	7.6	9.9	7.0	5.1	1.6	2.4	0.5	0.10	0.19	**1.5**	161
Bronchus, lung	5086	0	-	-	-	0.6	0.2	0.2	0.8	6.9	11.3	32.7	62.9	122.7	185.1	284.2	307.2	283.4	250.3	214.5	72.0	15.9	2.12	5.07	**38.5**	162
Other thoracic organs	16	0	-	-	-	-	-	0.2	-	0.2	-	0.5	-	0.3	-	1.1	0.7	1.2	0.6	0.8	0.2	0.0	0.01	0.01	**0.1**	163-4
Bone	58	0	-	0.5	1.0	0.9	0.7	0.5	0.4	0.7	0.9	0.2	1.0	1.5	0.8	0.5	0.3	1.6	3.4	4.0	0.8	0.2	0.05	0.05	**0.7**	170
Connective tissue	123	0	0.2	0.5	1.2	0.4	0.7	1.1	1.4	1.1	1.3	0.7	1.8	2.5	2.3	4.1	4.3	5.1	3.4	7.1	1.7	0.4	0.08	0.12	**1.2**	171
Mesothelioma	55	0	-	-	-	-	-	-	-	-	0.2	1.2	-	1.0	1.0	3.5	3.6	3.5	4.5	-	0.8	0.2	0.02	0.05	**0.4**	MES
Kaposi's sarcoma	1	0	-	-	-	-	-	-	-	-	-	-	-	-	0.3	-	-	-	-	-	0.0	0.0	0.00	0.00	**0.0**	KAP
Melanoma of skin	773	0	0.2	0.5	0.2	3.0	4.0	8.4	7.9	12.5	12.4	14.5	13.1	15.3	14.0	20.1	23.5	28.1	28.1	33.2	10.9	2.4	0.53	0.75	**7.7**	172
Other skin	4617	0	-	-	-	0.4	1.8	3.4	6.5	13.6	23.7	39.1	55.8	67.7	101.4	160.2	206.9	307.9	383.9	522.4	65.4		1.57	3.40	**31.5**	173
Breast	7772	0	-	-	-	-	0.9	6.8	26.8	49.8	102.0	166.2	212.8	247.7	273.6	245.4	240.7	267.4	304.2	401.3	110.1	24.2	5.43	7.86	**71.2**	174
Uterus unspecified	160	0	-	-	-	-	-	0.4	-	0.2	0.4	1.0	3.5	4.3	5.7	4.3	7.3	10.5	7.9	15.0	2.3	0.5	0.08	0.14	**1.2**	179
Cervix uteri	1177	0	-	-	0.2	2.2	8.8	22.6	27.2	29.2	29.3	24.7	27.0	24.2	33.4	32.1	21.4	16.8	20.6	16.7	3.7	0.98	1.30	**12.7**	180
Placenta	3	0	-	-	-	-	0.2	0.2	-	0.2	-	-	-	-	-	-	-	-	-	-	0.0	0.0	0.00	0.00	**0.0**	181
Corpus uteri	761	0	-	-	-	-	0.2	0.4	0.6	1.1	3.1	10.3	17.2	31.8	28.1	29.9	32.4	33.1	30.9	35.6	10.8	2.4	0.46	0.78	**6.4**	182
Ovary etc.	1466	0	-	0.2	0.2	0.4	0.4	1.8	4.8	3.6	14.6	23.4	31.0	40.5	46.8	55.4	65.9	78.7	61.2	57.8	20.8	4.6	0.84	1.44	**12.4**	183
Other female genital	260	0	0.2	-	-	-	-	0.5	0.2	1.3	2.4	1.5	2.3	4.6	5.7	7.1	14.2	17.9	20.2	25.3	3.7	0.8	0.09	0.20	**1.8**	184
Bladder	1077	0	-	-	-	-	-	0.5	0.8	1.3	2.2	7.6	14.4	19.3	28.9	45.6	55.9	67.8	88.7	87.1	15.3	3.4	0.38	0.88	**7.5**	188
Kidney etc.	520	0	2.3	0.2	-	-	-	-	0.8	1.8	2.2	5.7	8.8	10.4	18.2	22.0	26.2	28.1	28.6	27.7	7.4	1.6	0.25	0.49	**4.3**	189
Eye	83	0	0.7	0.2	-	-	0.4	-	0.4	0.9	0.4	0.7	1.8	1.8	1.8	2.7	3.6	5.1	1.7	6.3	1.2	0.3	0.05	0.08	**0.8**	190
Brain, nervous system	382	0	3.7	3.5	2.4	1.9	1.1	2.2	3.2	2.7	3.3	4.7	7.3	8.9	11.2	15.7	12.2	11.3	6.7	7.1	5.4	1.2	0.28	0.42	**4.3**	191-2
Thyroid	167	0	-	0.2	0.2	0.4	0.5	2.0	1.8	2.9	2.7	3.4	3.0	1.8	4.7	3.5	4.6	5.1	7.9	8.7	2.4	0.5	0.12	0.16	**1.7**	193
Other endocrine	38	0	1.2	-	0.2	0.9	-	0.2	-	0.4	0.7	0.2	0.8	1.3	0.8	1.1	0.3	0.8	0.6	1.6	0.5	0.1	0.03	0.04	**0.5**	194
Hodgkin's disease	149	0	-	-	2.2	2.3	4.6	2.9	2.0	2.2	2.0	0.2	2.8	1.5	2.6	3.0	2.6	2.3	2.2	1.6	2.1	0.5	0.13	0.15	**1.9**	201
Non-Hodgkin lymphoma	894	0	0.2	0.2	0.5	0.9	1.6	1.4	2.0	3.6	6.0	5.9	14.4	13.0	29.1	33.1	47.7	52.2	50.5	64.9	12.7	2.8	0.39	0.80	**6.9**	200,202
Multiple myeloma	356	0	-	-	-	-	-	-	-	-	0.4	1.2	3.0	6.1	9.9	13.8	20.5	27.7	29.2	30.9	5.0	1.1	0.10	0.28	**2.3**	203
Lymphoid leukaemia	254	0	5.4	0.9	1.9	1.3	0.2	0.2	-	0.2	0.9	1.5	2.3	2.8	6.5	6.0	9.9	14.4	16.3	29.3	3.6	0.8	0.12	0.20	**2.4**	204
Myeloid leukaemia	277	0	0.7	0.2	-	0.6	1.3	2.7	1.4	1.6	3.1	2.0	3.5	4.1	4.9	10.0	12.9	12.1	17.4	19.8	3.9	0.9	0.13	0.25	**2.4**	205
Monocytic leukaemia	4	0	-	-	-	-	-	-	-	-	0.2	-	-	-	0.3	-	-	-	0.6	0.8	0.1	0.0	0.00	0.00	**0.0**	206
Other leukaemia	2	0	-	-	-	-	-	-	-	-	-	-	-	-	-	0.3	-	0.4	-	-	0.0	0.0	0.00	0.00	**0.0**	207
Leukaemia unspecified	71	0	-	-	0.2	-	0.2	-	0.4	0.2	-	0.2	-	0.8	0.8	2.2	2.3	6.2	6.7	12.7	1.0	0.2	0.01	0.04	**0.4**	208
Other and unspecified	2050	0	0.5	-	-	0.2	-	1.1	1.2	2.7	4.4	10.6	17.9	30.0	46.8	67.1	103.3	130.6	207.7	258.8	29.0	6.4	0.58	1.43	**13.0**	O&U
All sites	36670	0	16.1	7.5	10.4	15.7	23.2	47.9	90.9	150.6	253.9	405.9	585.1	811.5	1069.0	1372.3	1638.6	1941.5	2261.3	2766.1	519.4		17.44	32.49	**287.8**	ALL
All sites but 173	32053	0	16.1	7.5	10.4	15.3	21.4	44.5	84.3	137.0	230.2	366.8	529.3	743.8	967.6	1212.1	1431.7	1633.6	1877.4	2243.8	454.0	100.0	15.87	29.09	**256.2**	ALLb

Rate from 1 case	0.233	0.234	0.243	0.213	0.183	0.180	0.199	0.223	0.221	0.246	0.252	0.255	0.260	0.271	0.331	0.390	0.561	0.791

Yugoslavia, Vojvodina

The population-based Cancer Registry of Vojvodina was founded at the Institute of Oncology in Sremska Kamenica in 1966 to provide information on cancer incidence, as a basis for planning and evaluation of cancer services and for scientific and educational work. The registry was moved to the Institute of Public Health in 1975, becoming part of the Section of non-communicable diseases. It was moved again to the Institute of Oncology in 1990, as a part of the Department of Epidemiology. The registry employs three doctors specialized in epidemiology, two of whom are university teachers, two nurses, one computer operator and a part-time engineer.

The registry covers the population of the whole territory of Province of Vojvodina, which is a part of the Republic of Yugoslavia. Lying between latitudes 44°40′ and 46°10′ N, it borders Romania to the east, Hungary to the north and Croatia to the west. The total registration area covers 21 506 km^2, divided into 46 municipalities.

The population according to the 1991 census comprised a total of 2 013 890 inhabitants (980 732 males and 1 033 158 females). The main population subgroups are Serbs 57%, Hungarians 17%, Yugoslavs 9%, Croats 4%, Slovaks 3%. The main occupation is industry, which employs 40%, followed by agriculture with 11%.

The population of Vojvodina is relatively old, with 12% older than 65. From 1989 there is evidence of negative population growth. Refugees from ex-Yugoslav Republics are not included in such figures, nor in the registry data.

In 1991, a 13-digit identification number was introduced which included the date of birth. Linkage between the cancer registry files and the Population Registry should provide information on vital status of cancer patients, but not all inhabitants have introduced the identification number in their personal documentation, in particular the elderly who form the majority of registered patients.

Basic health services are provided by outpatient establishments where general practitioners and specialists work. Besides these, there are one university clinic, nine general hospitals, ten specialized hospitals and eight maternity hospitals with a total of 12 381 hospital beds (1989). In 1989 there were 4145 doctors of all specialities in Vojvodina.

Private practice was established recently, with outpatient clinics and hospitals as well. In Novi Sad, the capital of Vojvodina, the medical faculty of the university comprises institutes and clinics as a comprehensive health, scientific and education centre for the province. The Institute of Oncology in Sremska Kamenica is a comprehensive cancer centre as well as a scientific and educational institution for the Province of Vojvodina. There are eight oncology dispensaries in Vojvodina dealing with preventive and curative work in oncology, in a good relationship with the Institute of Oncology and the cancer registry.

The general process of registration is the same across the whole territory of the province. A doctor who detects a cancer patient must send a notification card to the oncology dispensary for the region of residence of the patient or directly to the registry.

The major sources of data are the first and subsequent reports of malignancy, reports from pathology and cytology laboratories, reports from radiotherapy departments, and death certificates. If necessary, other documentation can be used such as hospital discharge reports.

All data are coded according to standard international classifications, including ICD-9 for site and ICD-O for histology.

Checking the data of the statistics department, which is responsible for registering cancer deaths, is carried out once a year for all cancer deaths from the previous year.

Information about cancer incidence and mortality is sent to the Ministry of Health and Federal Institute of Public Health annually.

Registry data have been used in a number of national epidemiological studies, research and education.

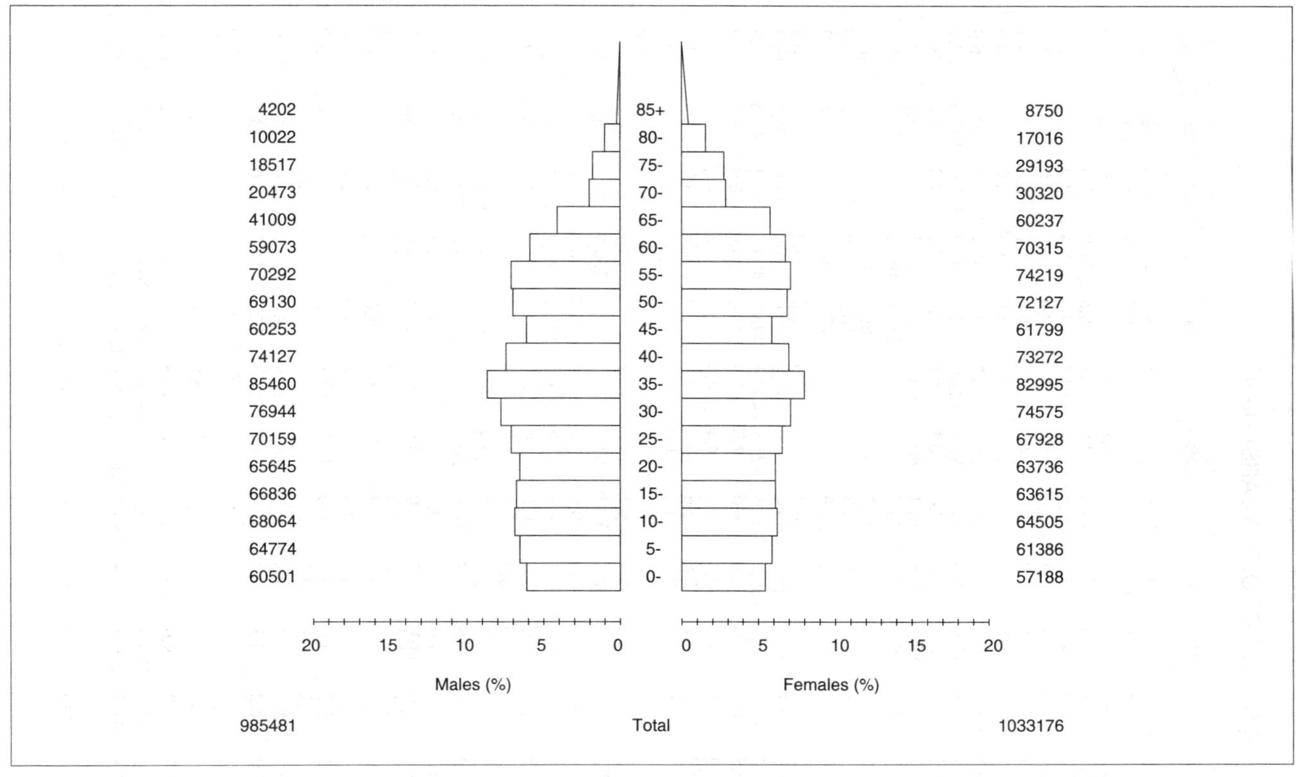

Yugoslavia, Vojvodina
Source of population: average annual 1988–92
Census: 1991
Estimate: The estimated populations for 1988, 1989, 1990 and 1992 are based on the official data of the Department of Demographic Statistics. Refugees from ex-Yugoslav Republics are not included.

Notes to tables overleaf:
* The high proportion of cases based on a death certificate alone, with a low level of histological verification, indicates under-ascertainment.
Screening programmes in the area:
The population over age 40 was screened every three years for large bowel cancer between 1981 and 1989.

* YUGOSLAVIA, VOJVODINA 1988-1992

ANNUAL INCIDENCE PER 100,000 BY AGE GROUP (YEARS) - MALE

SITE	ALL AGES	AGE UNK	0-	5-	10-	15-	20-	25-	30-	35-	40-	45-	50-	55-	60-	65-	70-	75-	80-	85+	CRUDE RATE	%	CR 64	CR 74	ASR (W)	ICD (9th)
Lip	280	0	-	-	-	-	-	-	0.3	0.9	2.2	3.3	9.3	14.8	15.9	16.6	18.6	44.3	41.9	52.4	5.7	1.6	0.23	0.41	**3.9**	*140*
Tongue	207	0	-	-	-	-	-	0.3	-	0.9	3.8	5.3	11.0	10.0	13.5	11.7	20.5	9.7	8.0	4.8	4.2	1.2	0.22	0.39	**3.0**	*141*
Salivary gland	42	0	0.3	-	-	-	-	-	-	0.2	-	0.3	1.7	1.7	3.4	5.4	1.0	3.2	4.0	-	0.9	0.2	0.04	0.07	**0.6**	*142*
Mouth	163	0	-	-	-	-	-	-	0.5	0.9	2.7	4.6	7.2	10.8	9.8	9.8	8.8	11.9	2.0	-	3.3	1.0	0.18	0.28	**2.3**	*143-5*
Oropharynx	142	0	-	-	-	-	0.3	-	0.3	0.2	1.9	4.0	7.5	8.8	9.1	10.2	8.8	5.4	2.0	-	2.9	0.8	0.16	0.26	**2.0**	*146*
Nasopharynx	52	0	-	-	-	-	-	0.6	-	0.5	1.3	1.3	1.7	2.6	5.8	1.5	2.9	-	2.0	-	1.1	0.3	0.07	0.09	**0.8**	*147*
Hypopharynx	201	0	-	-	-	-	-	-	-	0.7	1.3	5.6	8.7	13.7	14.6	12.2	16.6	9.7	8.0	-	4.1	1.2	0.22	0.37	**2.9**	*148*
Pharynx unspecified	24	0	-	-	-	-	-	-	-	-	-	0.3	1.4	2.0	2.0	0.5	2.0	1.1	2.0	-	0.5	0.1	0.03	0.04	**0.3**	*149*
Oesophagus	340	0	-	-	-	-	-	-	0.3	0.2	1.3	6.0	7.8	20.8	24.4	30.2	27.4	42.1	20.0	19.0	6.9	2.0	0.30	0.59	**4.7**	*150*
Stomach	1463	0	-	-	-	0.3	0.3	1.4	2.3	4.7	9.7	18.6	33.6	65.4	87.7	121.9	174.9	184.7	197.6	147.5	29.7	8.6	1.12	2.60	**20.8**	*151*
Small intestine	51	0	-	-	-	-	-	-	0.5	0.5	0.8	0.7	1.2	2.0	2.4	5.4	2.9	7.6	4.0	4.8	1.0	0.3	0.04	0.08	**0.7**	*152*
Colon	981	0	-	-	-	-	0.9	2.0	2.6	5.1	5.1	15.3	24.6	36.4	60.9	90.2	93.8	114.5	135.7	123.7	19.9	5.7	0.77	1.69	**14.1**	*153*
Rectum	1020	0	-	-	-	0.3	-	1.1	2.3	4.2	5.7	10.0	19.4	36.7	57.2	84.9	134.8	163.1	151.7	157.1	20.7	6.0	0.68	1.78	**14.6**	*154*
Liver	536	0	-	-	0.3	0.3	0.3	-	0.5	2.1	3.0	4.3	10.1	22.2	34.2	54.1	66.4	67.0	69.8	38.1	10.9	3.1	0.39	0.99	**7.6**	*155*
Gallbladder etc.	181	0	-	-	-	-	-	-	0.3	0.2	0.3	2.7	4.9	5.7	11.8	14.1	20.5	25.9	35.9	28.6	3.7	1.1	0.13	0.30	**2.6**	*156*
Pancreas	529	0	-	-	-	-	-	0.3	0.8	1.4	3.2	6.6	18.8	23.9	32.2	38.5	47.9	70.2	79.8	47.6	10.7	3.1	0.44	0.87	**7.4**	*157*
Nose, sinuses etc.	19	0	-	-	-	-	-	-	0.2	0.3	0.2	1.0	0.3	0.3	0.2	0.5	2.0	3.2	-	-	0.4	0.1	0.02	0.03	**0.3**	*160*
Larynx	802	0	-	-	-	-	-	0.3	0.8	2.8	9.2	18.3	30.7	50.9	57.9	52.2	43.0	51.8	43.9	95.2	16.3	4.7	0.85	1.33	**11.4**	*161*
Bronchus, lung	5064	0	-	-	-	-	0.6	0.6	3.9	15.2	46.9	79.7	169.2	268.6	375.5	432.6	428.9	409.3	341.2	247.5	102.8	29.6	4.80	9.11	**71.7**	*162*
Other thoracic organs	107	0	0.3	-	-	-	0.3	0.3	-	0.5	0.5	2.0	2.9	4.0	7.4	8.3	15.6	10.8	6.0	9.5	2.2	0.6	0.09	0.21	**1.6**	*163-4*
Bone	98	0	-	0.3	0.3	1.8	1.5	1.1	0.8	1.9	0.5	1.3	2.6	4.0	4.4	4.9	9.8	5.4	6.0	-	2.0	0.6	0.10	0.18	**1.6**	*170*
Connective tissue	93	0	1.3	0.3	0.3	-	-	1.1	1.3	0.7	1.3	3.7	2.6	2.6	4.4	7.3	2.9	7.6	4.0	4.8	1.9	0.5	0.10	0.15	**1.5**	*171*
Mesothelioma	9	0	-	-	-	-	-	-	-	-	0.5	0.3	0.6	0.3	1.0	-	-	-	-	-	0.2	0.1	0.01	0.01	**0.1**	*MES*
Kaposi's sarcoma	0	0	-	-	-	-	-	-	-	-	-	-	-	-	-	-	-	-	-	-	0.0	0.0	0.00	Kapo.01	**0.0**	*KAP*
Melanoma of skin	191	0	-	0.3	0.3	0.6	-	1.4	2.9	4.0	1.9	4.6	7.5	5.4	8.8	10.7	11.7	15.1	20.0	19.0	3.9	1.1	0.19	0.30	**2.9**	*172*
Other skin	1479	0	-	-	-	0.3	0.6	0.3	2.3	7.3	10.8	21.6	38.8	51.5	85.7	122.4	149.5	200.9	209.5	318.9	30.0		1.10	2.45	**21.4**	*173*
Breast	35	0	-	-	-	-	-	-	-	-	0.3	1.3	1.2	0.9	1.0	2.9	3.9	6.5	4.0	9.5	0.7	0.2	0.02	0.06	**0.5**	*175*
Prostate	1036	0	-	-	0.3	0.3	0.3	-	-	0.7	0.3	2.0	5.5	15.1	37.9	101.9	171.9	259.2	311.3	276.0	21.0	6.1	0.31	1.68	**14.7**	*185*
Testis	143	0	-	0.3	0.6	1.5	5.5	6.8	7.8	4.4	2.7	3.0	1.4	0.6	2.0	0.5	3.9	4.3	4.0	4.8	2.9	0.8	0.18	0.21	**2.6**	*186*
Penis, other male genital	46	0	-	-	-	-	-	-	0.3	-	-	1.0	0.9	2.0	2.7	1.0	8.8	7.6	6.0	14.3	0.9	0.3	0.03	0.08	**0.7**	*187*
Bladder	821	0	-	-	-	-	-	0.6	1.0	2.8	4.3	6.3	15.0	31.9	52.8	71.7	85.0	123.1	145.7	128.5	16.7	4.8	0.57	1.36	**11.5**	*188*
Kidney etc.	315	0	1.7	-	-	0.6	-	-	0.3	2.3	2.2	6.6	10.7	14.8	20.0	24.4	29.3	24.8	22.0	33.3	6.4	1.8	0.30	0.56	**4.7**	*189*
Eye	37	0	0.3	0.3	-	-	-	0.3	0.5	0.5	0.8	1.0	0.3	0.3	2.4	2.9	4.9	1.1	4.0	4.8	0.8	0.2	0.03	0.07	**0.6**	*190*
Brain, nervous system	369	0	2.0	1.5	2.4	2.1	2.7	2.6	3.9	4.4	5.9	11.9	14.2	15.9	20.0	19.0	19.5	8.6	2.0	4.8	7.5	2.2	0.45	0.64	**6.0**	*191-2*
Thyroid	45	0	-	-	-	-	-	0.9	0.3	0.7	1.1	0.7	2.3	0.6	2.0	3.9	2.9	4.3	2.0	-	0.9	0.3	0.04	0.07	**0.7**	*193*
Other endocrine	26	0	0.3	-	-	-	0.3	-	0.3	0.2	-	-	0.6	1.4	2.7	1.5	2.0	-	4.0	-	0.5	0.2	0.03	0.05	**0.4**	*194*
Hodgkin's disease	145	0	-	0.9	0.3	3.3	2.4	2.6	3.1	3.3	4.3	3.7	3.8	4.0	4.1	3.9	5.9	5.4	4.0	-	2.9	0.8	0.18	0.23	**2.5**	*201*
Non-Hodgkin lymphoma	248	0	0.7	1.5	1.2	1.8	0.6	2.0	2.1	2.3	5.7	4.0	8.7	8.0	12.5	13.7	19.5	15.1	20.0	19.0	5.0	1.5	0.26	0.42	**4.0**	*200,202*
Multiple myeloma	63	0	-	-	-	-	-	-	0.3	0.2	0.3	1.3	2.6	2.8	4.4	3.9	9.8	4.3	4.0	-	1.3	0.4	0.06	0.13	**0.9**	*203*
Lymphoid leukaemia	288	0	3.3	1.9	1.8	2.4	1.2	0.6	0.5	0.7	2.2	3.0	7.8	9.7	16.3	19.5	26.4	28.1	49.9	14.3	5.8	1.7	0.26	0.49	**4.6**	*204*
Myeloid leukaemia	190	0	1.0	0.6	0.3	0.9	1.5	2.3	1.3	3.0	2.2	3.7	4.9	7.4	11.2	11.2	12.7	14.0	6.0	14.3	3.9	1.1	0.20	0.32	**3.0**	*205*
Monocytic leukaemia	0	0	-	-	-	-	-	-	-	-	-	-	-	-	-	-	-	-	-	-	0.0	0.0	0.00	0.00	**0.0**	*206*
Other leukaemia	0	0	-	-	-	-	-	-	-	-	-	-	-	-	-	-	-	-	-	-	0.0	0.0	0.00	0.00	**0.0**	*207*
Leukaemia unspecified	31	0	0.3	-	-	0.6	-	-	-	-	-	0.3	1.2	1.1	1.4	2.9	5.9	1.1	4.0	-	0.6	0.2	0.02	0.07	**0.5**	*208*
Other and unspecified	670	0	1.3	0.3	0.3	-	1.2	1.1	1.8	3.5	5.9	9.6	23.4	25.3	37.6	47.3	60.6	64.8	115.7	119.0	13.6	3.9	0.56	1.10	**9.8**	*O&U*
All sites	18582	0	12.9	8.3	8.2	17.1	20.7	30.5	46.0	84.7	152.4	280.8	528.6	806.6	1163.0	1478.2	1783.8	2037.0	2103.3	1960.8	377.1		15.80	32.11	**268.5**	*ALL*
All sites but 173	17103	0	12.9	8.3	8.2	16.8	20.1	30.2	43.7	77.5	141.6	259.2	489.8	755.1	1077.3	1355.8	1634.3	1836.1	1893.8	1641.9	347.1	100.0	14.70	29.65	**247.2**	*ALLb*

| Rate from 1 case | | | | 0.331 | 0.309 | 0.294 | 0.299 | 0.305 | 0.285 | 0.260 | 0.234 | 0.270 | 0.332 | 0.289 | 0.285 | 0.339 | 0.488 | 0.977 | 1.080 | 1.996 | 4.759 |

* YUGOSLAVIA, VOJVODINA 1988-1992

ANNUAL INCIDENCE PER 100,000 BY AGE GROUP (YEARS) - FEMALE

SITE	ALL AGES	AGE UNK	0-	5-	10-	15-	20-	25-	30-	35-	40-	45-	50-	55-	60-	65-	70-	75-	80-	85+	CRUDE RATE	%	CR 64	CR 74	ASR (W)	ICD (9th)
Lip	77	0	-	-	-	-	-	-	0.3	-	-	0.6	2.2	1.9	2.0	4.3	6.6	8.2	9.4	20.6	1.5	0.5	0.04	0.09	**0.8**	140
Tongue	28	0	-	-	-	0.3	0.3	-	-	0.5	-	0.6	0.3	0.5	0.6	2.0	1.3	2.1	4.7	4.6	0.5	0.2	0.02	0.03	**0.3**	141
Salivary gland	35	0	-	-	-	-	-	-	-	0.2	0.5	0.3	1.9	1.1	1.1	2.3	2.0	0.7	3.5	4.6	0.7	0.2	0.03	0.05	**0.4**	142
Mouth	24	0	-	-	-	0.3	-	0.3	-	0.2	-	0.3	0.3	1.1	1.4	0.7	0.7	3.4	1.2	2.3	0.5	0.2	0.02	0.03	**0.3**	143-5
Oropharynx	26	0	-	-	-	0.3	-	-	-	-	0.5	1.3	-	1.1	1.1	1.0	3.3	1.4	1.2	-	0.5	0.2	0.02	0.04	**0.3**	146
Nasopharynx	20	0	-	-	-	-	0.3	-	-	0.2	0.5	0.3	0.8	0.3	0.3	1.3	2.0	2.1	-	-	0.4	0.1	0.01	0.03	**0.3**	147
Hypopharynx	19	0	-	-	-	-	-	-	0.5	-	0.3	-	0.6	1.1	-	1.0	2.6	0.7	-	4.6	0.4	0.1	0.01	0.03	**0.2**	148
Pharynx unspecified	2	0	-	-	-	-	-	-	-	-	-	-	0.3	0.3	-	-	-	-	-	-	0.0	0.0	0.00	0.00	**0.0**	149
Oesophagus	63	0	-	-	-	-	-	-	-	-	0.5	1.0	1.4	1.3	1.4	3.7	4.6	8.9	7.1	13.7	1.2	0.4	0.03	0.07	**0.7**	150
Stomach	852	0	-	-	-	-	-	2.4	3.0	4.1	7.6	10.0	15.0	25.3	35.3	50.1	77.8	68.5	105.8	59.4	16.5	5.7	0.51	1.15	**9.4**	151
Small intestine	33	0	-	-	-	-	-	-	0.3	-	0.3	1.0	-	0.8	1.1	3.0	2.0	2.1	5.9	2.3	0.6	0.2	0.02	0.04	**0.4**	152
Colon	952	0	-	-	-	-	0.6	0.9	1.1	4.1	6.6	15.2	19.1	32.6	39.0	57.8	73.9	78.1	105.8	86.9	18.4	6.3	0.60	1.25	**10.5**	153
Rectum	854	0	-	-	-	0.3	-	0.6	1.9	2.4	4.4	11.3	15.3	24.3	40.4	58.1	71.9	73.3	78.7	86.9	16.5	5.7	0.50	1.15	**9.4**	154
Liver	461	0	-	-	-	-	0.6	-	0.3	1.0	1.6	2.3	4.7	11.0	19.1	32.9	46.2	55.5	52.9	48.0	8.9	3.1	0.20	0.60	**4.8**	155
Gallbladder etc.	515	0	-	-	-	-	-	-	-	1.2	1.1	4.9	8.3	15.4	22.5	37.5	44.2	52.1	59.9	41.1	10.0	3.4	0.27	0.68	**5.4**	156
Pancreas	444	0	-	-	-	-	0.3	-	-	0.2	2.2	2.9	8.0	13.5	21.3	27.9	36.3	44.5	55.2	45.7	8.6	3.0	0.24	0.56	**4.7**	157
Nose, sinuses etc.	21	0	-	-	-	-	0.3	-	0.3	-	0.3	0.3	0.6	0.3	0.3	0.7	1.3	3.4	-	9.1	0.4	0.1	0.01	0.02	**0.3**	160
Larynx	60	0	-	-	-	-	-	-	-	-	0.8	0.3	2.2	2.2	5.1	1.7	4.6	4.8	3.5	-	1.2	0.4	0.05	0.08	**0.7**	161
Bronchus, lung	945	0	-	-	-	-	-	1.2	2.1	3.9	9.3	13.6	24.1	31.8	44.1	55.4	69.9	81.5	70.5	66.3	18.3	6.3	0.65	1.28	**10.6**	162
Other thoracic organs	53	0	-	-	-	-	-	-	-	0.2	0.5	1.3	1.4	2.7	1.7	2.7	4.6	4.1	3.5	2.3	1.0	0.4	0.04	0.08	**0.6**	163-4
Bone	66	0	-	-	0.3	0.9	-	0.6	0.3	0.5	0.3	-	1.9	3.5	3.1	2.7	2.6	4.8	3.5	6.9	1.3	0.4	0.06	0.08	**0.8**	170
Connective tissue	75	0	0.3	0.3	0.3	0.3	0.6	0.3	0.8	1.0	1.6	0.3	2.8	2.2	2.8	2.3	4.6	3.4	4.7	6.9	1.5	0.5	0.07	0.10	**1.0**	171
Mesothelioma	13	0	-	-	-	-	-	-	-	-	0.3	-	0.6	0.3	0.6	1.3	1.3	0.7	-	-	0.3	0.1	0.01	0.02	**0.2**	MES
Kaposi's sarcoma	0	0	-	-	-	-	-	-	-	-	-	-	-	-	-	-	-	-	-	-	0.0	0.0	0.00	0.00	**0.0**	KAP
Melanoma of skin	270	0	-	-	-	0.3	0.6	1.2	5.4	3.4	8.2	7.4	5.8	7.8	7.7	6.3	13.9	16.4	21.2	38.9	5.2	1.8	0.24	0.34	**3.5**	172
Other skin	1532	0	-	0.3	0.3	0.3	1.3	1.8	3.2	7.0	13.6	23.0	29.9	40.2	58.3	79.7	126.6	142.5	193.9	205.7	29.7		0.90	1.93	**16.9**	173
Breast	3503	0	-	-	-	-	0.6	4.1	14.5	37.6	73.4	116.2	118.7	142.8	149.9	157.4	152.4	178.8	158.7	144.0	67.8	23.3	3.29	4.84	**43.6**	174
Uterus unspecified	141	0	-	-	-	-	0.6	-	0.5	1.4	-	0.6	2.2	4.0	5.7	8.3	15.2	14.4	14.1	11.4	2.7	0.9	0.08	0.19	**1.5**	179
Cervix uteri	1339	0	-	-	-	0.3	1.6	4.7	15.3	27.7	40.7	41.1	49.1	47.2	48.4	49.1	54.7	41.8	45.8	36.6	25.9	8.9	1.38	1.90	**17.7**	180
Placenta	10	0	-	-	-	0.6	0.3	-	0.3	0.5	0.3	-	0.8	-	-	-	-	-	-	-	0.2	0.1	0.01	0.01	**0.2**	181
Corpus uteri	806	0	-	-	-	-	-	0.3	0.8	2.7	4.4	11.7	23.8	32.6	50.6	52.1	59.4	45.2	32.9	29.7	15.6	5.4	0.63	1.19	**9.2**	182
Ovary etc.	709	0	-	-	0.9	1.6	1.6	3.2	3.5	6.3	8.5	20.4	22.5	29.4	37.3	31.5	36.9	38.4	18.8	18.3	13.7	4.7	0.68	1.02	**9.0**	183
Other female genital	170	0	-	-	-	-	0.3	0.3	1.6	1.0	0.5	2.3	1.7	2.4	6.3	8.0	15.2	24.0	24.7	20.6	3.3	1.1	0.08	0.20	**1.8**	184
Bladder	251	0	-	0.3	-	-	-	0.3	0.5	0.7	1.4	1.3	2.5	8.6	10.5	13.9	19.1	27.4	38.8	29.7	4.9	1.7	0.13	0.30	**2.6**	188
Kidney etc.	254	0	0.7	0.3	-	-	0.3	1.2	0.5	1.0	1.4	3.6	8.0	10.0	11.9	16.9	19.1	15.1	11.8	9.1	4.9	1.7	0.19	0.37	**3.0**	189
Eye	29	0	1.0	-	-	-	-	0.3	0.3	-	-	-	0.8	1.9	0.6	1.0	3.3	-	1.2	6.9	0.6	0.2	0.02	0.05	**0.4**	190
Brain, nervous system	288	0	0.3	2.9	0.6	0.9	1.9	2.9	3.0	4.6	4.9	5.8	10.3	13.2	11.4	12.6	9.2	6.9	3.5	-	5.6	1.9	0.31	0.42	**4.1**	191-2
Thyroid	131	0	-	-	-	0.3	1.3	0.6	3.5	1.2	5.7	4.5	3.6	3.8	3.4	2.7	6.6	6.2	2.4	6.9	2.5	0.9	0.14	0.19	**1.9**	193
Other endocrine	28	0	-	-	-	-	0.9	0.6	0.5	0.2	0.3	-	0.8	1.3	1.1	-	0.7	1.4	3.5	2.3	0.5	0.2	0.03	0.03	**0.4**	194
Hodgkin's disease	78	0	-	-	0.6	1.6	1.9	2.1	1.3	2.2	1.4	1.0	2.5	1.1	1.4	2.3	2.6	2.7	3.5	-	1.5	0.5	0.08	0.11	**1.3**	201
Non-Hodgkin lymphoma	224	0	0.7	1.0	0.9	0.6	1.3	0.3	1.3	2.4	3.0	4.9	5.8	5.9	10.8	10.0	11.9	12.3	18.8	11.4	4.3	1.5	0.19	0.30	**2.9**	200,202
Multiple myeloma	87	0	-	-	-	-	-	-	-	0.2	0.8	1.0	2.2	2.2	6.0	5.6	7.3	6.2	7.1	-	1.7	0.6	0.06	0.13	**1.0**	203
Lymphoid leukaemia	161	0	1.4	2.0	1.9	1.3	0.9	-	0.5	0.5	1.4	1.3	2.5	4.6	8.0	7.6	9.2	12.3	16.5	4.6	3.1	1.1	0.13	0.22	**2.2**	204
Myeloid leukaemia	145	0	0.7	0.3	0.3	0.9	0.6	1.2	1.1	1.4	2.5	4.9	3.9	4.3	6.5	5.6	7.3	8.9	3.5	2.3	2.8	1.0	0.14	0.21	**2.0**	205
Monocytic leukaemia	0	0	-	-	-	-	-	-	-	-	-	-	-	-	-	-	-	-	-	-	0.0	0.0	0.00	0.00	**0.0**	206
Other leukaemia	3	0	-	-	-	-	-	-	-	-	-	-	-	0.3	-	0.7	-	-	-	-	0.1	0.0	0.00	0.00	**0.0**	207
Leukaemia unspecified	21	0	-	-	-	-	-	-	-	-	0.3	1.3	-	0.5	0.9	1.7	2.0	1.4	1.2	-	0.4	0.1	0.01	0.03	**0.3**	208
Other and unspecified	734	0	0.7	-	0.3	0.9	0.6	0.6	1.1	4.8	2.5	6.5	10.3	16.4	24.7	42.2	64.0	67.8	123.4	132.6	14.2	4.9	0.35	0.88	**7.8**	O&U
All sites	16552	0	5.9	7.5	6.5	12.3	19.8	31.8	69.5	126.5	214.3	326.5	419.5	554.6	706.0	865.2	1100.9	1174.9	1322.3	1222.8	320.4		12.50	22.33	**195.3**	ALL
All sites but 173	15020	0	5.9	7.2	6.2	11.9	18.5	30.0	66.2	119.5	200.6	303.6	389.6	514.4	647.6	785.6	974.3	1032.4	1128.3	1017.1	290.8	100.0	11.61	20.41	**178.4**	ALLb

| Rate from 1 case | | | 0.350 | 0.326 | 0.310 | 0.314 | 0.314 | 0.294 | 0.268 | 0.241 | 0.273 | 0.324 | 0.277 | 0.269 | 0.284 | 0.332 | 0.660 | 0.685 | 1.175 | 2.286 | | | | | | |

Australian Capital Territory

The Australian Capital Territory (ACT) Cancer Registry was established under the Public Health (Cancer Reporting) Regulations gazetted in 1994, to receive notifications of cancer in the ACT. The Department of Health and Community Care administers the registry. The New South Wales (NSW) Cancer Registry has been recording the incidence of cancer in the ACT since 1972 on a voluntary notification basis, and continues to process all notifications received by the ACT registry. This arrangement is necessary because of the large overlap of patients who use both ACT and NSW health services. Since the regulations came into effect in July 1994, all hospitals, nursing homes and pathology laboratories in the ACT have been required by law to notify the ACT registry when they diagnose or treat a person with cancer. The NSW Cancer Registry routinely follows up missing patient information from notifying institutions. Mortality data are supplied on a regular basis from the ACT Registrar of Births, Deaths and Marriages.

The Australian Capital Territory is the capital of Australia and is almost 2400 km^2 in area. 53% of the territory is devoted to national parks or reserves, 23% to agriculture (mainly sheep and cattle grazing), 14% urban development and 7% plantation forest. The ACT has a continental climate, characterized by a marked variation in temperature between seasons, with warm to hot summers and cold winters.

At June 1994 the ACT population was 300 867 persons. In 1994 the crude birth rate was 14.8 and the crude death rate 3.7 per 1000 population. Infant mortality was 4.3 per 1000 live births, compared with the national rate of 6.9. At the 1991 Census of Population and Housing, 75% of the population of the ACT reported their birthplace as Australia, 15% the United Kingdom, USA, New Zealand, Canada or other European countries, and 5% Asia.

In 1994 there were 130 700 wage and salary earners employed in the ACT, of whom 43% were employed in the private sector and the remaining 57% in the public sector. Almost one quarter of persons employed in the ACT were in the government administration and defence industry. A further 13% were employed in retailing, 10% in property and business services, 9% in education and 8% in health and community services.

The ACT is serviced by three public hospitals and six private hospitals. The Canberra Hospital is the major regional hospital and provides specialist cancer treatment supported by multi-disciplinary teams. It also includes a bone marrow transplant unit. Some chemotherapy is also provided at Calvary Public and Private Hospitals, and John James Hospital.

Information from the registry is used to monitor the incidence of cancer in the ACT population, compare local and national trends, assist in planning services within the ACT, for example screening programmes, and assist with research to determine causes of cancer and the level of risk from environmental hazards.

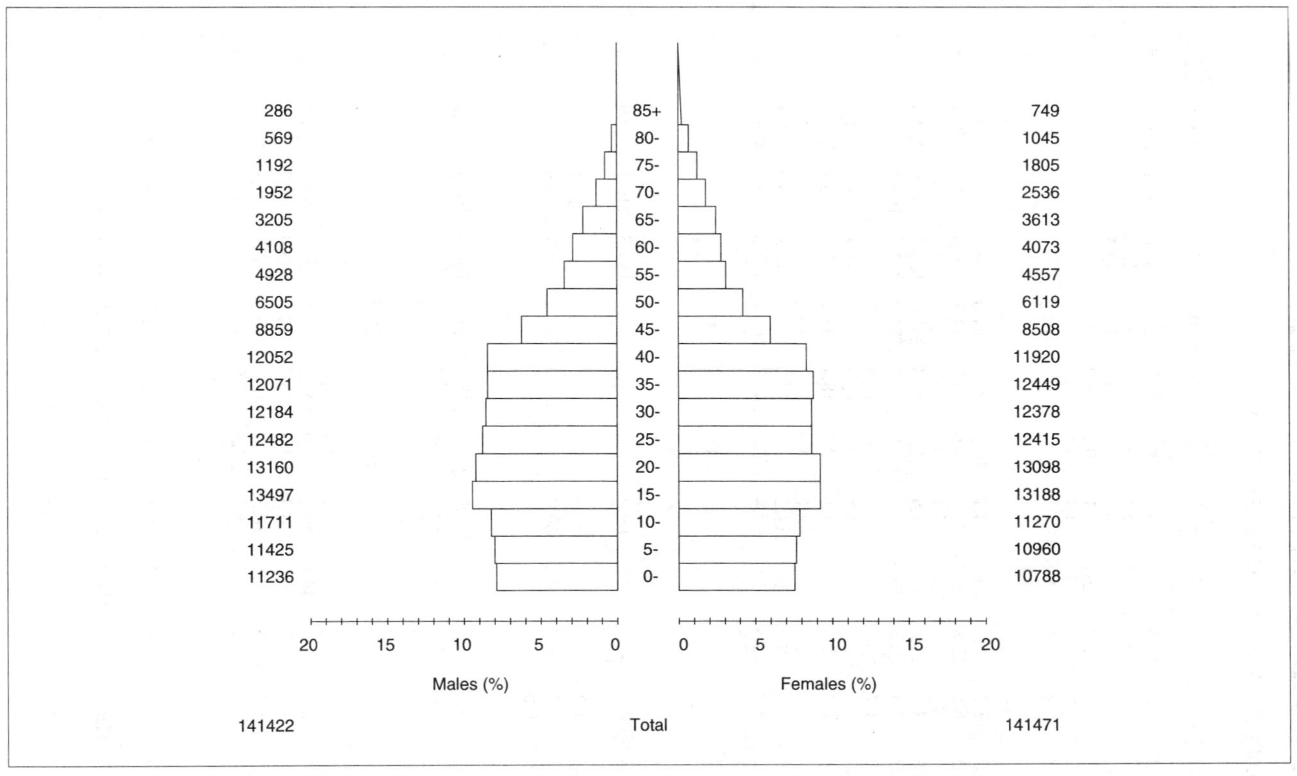

Australian Capital Territory
Source of population: average annual 1988–92
Census: 1991. Census count by usual place of residence, adjusted for under-enumeration and for Australian residents temporarily overseas.
Estimate: The populations for the years 1988, 1989 and 1990 were intercensal estimates, initially obtained from the 1986 Census by advancing age and allowing for births, deaths and migration, and adjusted in the light of the 1991 Census to give correct final results in each age and sex group. The 1992 population was a postcensal estimate calculated by advancing age from the 1991 Census, and allowing for births, deaths and migration.

Notes to tables overleaf:
† Kaposi's sarcoma is under-reported in this volume because cases of skin cancer (ICD-9 173) were not provided.
† 173 not available
† 188 does not include non-invasive tumours

AUSTRALIAN CAPITAL TERRITORY 1988-1992

ANNUAL INCIDENCE PER 100,000 BY AGE GROUP (YEARS) - MALE

SITE	ALL AGES	AGE UNK	0-	5-	10-	15-	20-	25-	30-	35-	40-	45-	50-	55-	60-	65-	70-	75-	80-	85+	CRUDE RATE	%	CR 64	CR 74	ASR (W)	ICD (9th)
Lip	57	0	-	-	-	-	-	1.6	6.6	13.3	11.6	13.5	12.3	8.1	9.7	43.7	61.5	100.6	35.1	209.8	8.1	3.4	0.38	0.91	8.9	140
Tongue	13	0	-	-	-	-	-	-	-	1.7	1.7	4.5	3.1	4.1	9.7	6.2	30.7	16.8	-	-	1.8	0.8	0.12	0.31	2.1	141
Salivary gland	7	0	-	-	-	-	-	1.6	-	1.7	-	3.1	-	-	6.2	10.2	33.5	-	-	-	1.0	0.4	0.03	0.11	1.1	142
Mouth	9	0	-	-	-	-	-	-	1.6	1.7	-	2.3	3.1	4.1	9.7	6.2	10.2	-	-	-	1.3	0.5	0.11	0.19	1.4	143-5
Oropharynx	3	0	-	-	-	-	-	-	-	-	1.7	-	-	4.1	4.9	-	-	-	-	-	0.4	0.2	0.05	0.05	0.5	146
Nasopharynx	7	0	-	-	-	-	-	1.6	-	1.7	3.3	2.3	3.1	-	-	-	10.2	-	-	-	1.0	0.4	0.06	0.11	0.9	147
Hypopharynx	4	0	-	-	-	-	-	-	-	-	-	-	3.1	-	14.6	-	-	-	-	-	0.6	0.2	0.09	0.09	0.7	148
Pharynx unspecified	1	0	-	-	-	-	-	-	-	-	-	-	-	-	-	6.2	-	-	-	-	0.1	0.1	0.00	0.03	0.2	149
Oesophagus	27	0	-	-	-	-	-	-	1.6	1.7	1.7	4.5	6.1	4.1	19.5	25.0	41.0	33.5	-	349.7	3.8	1.6	0.20	0.53	5.5	150
Stomach	57	0	-	-	-	-	-	-	1.6	3.3	6.6	15.8	15.4	20.3	14.6	43.7	71.7	100.6	281.0	139.9	8.1	3.4	0.39	0.97	9.7	151
Small intestine	4	0	-	-	-	-	-	-	-	-	-	2.3	3.1	4.1	-	6.2	-	-	-	-	0.6	0.2	0.05	0.08	0.6	152
Colon	165	0	-	-	-	-	-	3.2	-	6.6	8.3	22.6	61.5	101.5	121.7	193.4	235.6	167.7	245.9	209.8	23.3	9.7	1.63	3.77	29.0	153
Rectum	94	0	-	-	-	-	-	-	3.3	1.7	8.3	2.3	30.7	52.8	77.9	68.6	184.4	234.8	105.4	-	13.3	5.5	0.88	2.15	16.3	154
Liver	14	0	-	-	-	-	-	1.6	1.7	1.7	-	-	-	29.2	12.5	20.5	-	-	69.9	2.0	0.8	0.17	0.34	2.6	155
Gallbladder etc.	9	0	-	-	-	-	-	-	-	-	-	3.1	4.1	9.7	12.5	-	16.8	35.1	69.9	1.3	0.5	0.08	0.15	1.8	156
Pancreas	32	0	-	-	-	-	-	-	-	-	1.7	2.3	9.2	4.1	29.2	18.7	71.7	67.1	70.2	279.7	4.5	1.9	0.23	0.68	6.4	157
Nose, sinuses etc.	7	0	-	-	-	-	-	-	-	1.7	-	2.3	3.1	8.1	4.9	-	10.2	-	-	-	1.0	0.4	0.10	0.15	1.1	160
Larynx	26	0	-	-	-	1.5	-	-	-	-	-	9.0	6.1	12.2	29.2	25.0	20.5	16.8	70.2	69.9	3.7	1.5	0.29	0.52	4.7	161
Bronchus, lung	213	0	-	-	-	-	-	-	1.6	-	5.0	24.8	36.9	97.4	155.8	243.3	368.7	587.0	456.6	489.5	30.1	12.6	1.61	4.67	39.1	162
Other thoracic organs	5	0	1.8	-	-	-	-	1.6	-	1.7	-	2.3	-	-	-	10.2	-	-	-	-	0.7	0.3	0.04	0.09	0.8	163-4
Bone	11	0	-	3.5	3.4	3.0	-	-	1.6	1.7	-	-	-	-	4.9	6.2	10.2	-	-	-	1.6	0.6	0.09	0.17	1.7	170
Connective tissue	12	0	-	1.8	-	-	3.0	1.6	1.6	-	-	2.3	6.1	-	4.9	6.2	-	33.5	-	-	1.7	0.7	0.11	0.14	1.8	171
Mesothelioma	3	0	-	-	-	-	-	-	-	-	-	-	-	-	9.7	6.2	-	-	-	-	0.4	0.2	0.05	0.08	0.6	MES
†Kaposi's sarcoma	5	0	-	-	-	-	-	1.6	3.3	-	1.7	-	-	4.1	-	-	-	-	-	-	0.7	0.3	0.05	0.05	0.6	KAP
Melanoma of skin †Other skin	196	0	-	-	-	5.9	3.0	16.0	19.7	29.8	34.8	47.4	64.6	69.0	63.3	131.0	174.1	184.5	210.7	139.9	27.7	11.6	1.77	3.29	29.5	172
Breast	3	0	-	-	-	-	-	-	-	-	1.7	-	-	-	4.9	-	-	-	35.1	-	0.4	0.2	0.03	0.03	0.5	175
Prostate	252	0	-	-	-	1.5	-	-	-	-	1.7	6.8	9.2	60.9	155.8	318.2	522.3	754.7	1018.6	1468.5	35.6	14.9	1.18	5.38	49.7	185
Testis	29	0	1.8	-	-	4.4	-	12.8	6.6	9.9	6.6	2.3	6.1	-	-	-	-	-	-	-	4.1	1.7	0.25	0.25	3.5	186
Penis	3	0	-	-	-	-	-	-	-	-	-	-	-	-	6.2	10.2	-	-	69.9	0.4	0.2	0.00	0.08	0.7	187.1-.4
Other male genital	0	0	-	-	-	-	-	-	-	-	-	-	-	-	-	-	-	-	-	0.0	0.0	0.00	0.00	0.0	187.5-.9
†Bladder	48	0	-	-	-	-	1.5	-	-	-	5.0	2.3	9.2	8.1	43.8	43.7	92.2	134.2	105.4	139.9	6.8	2.8	0.35	1.03	8.8	188
Kidney etc.	61	0	1.8	1.8	-	-	-	-	1.6	1.7	3.3	11.3	12.3	16.2	34.1	87.3	102.4	100.6	175.6	-	8.6	3.6	0.42	1.37	10.6	189
Eye	8	0	-	-	-	-	-	-	1.6	1.7	-	2.3	-	8.1	9.7	-	10.2	-	-	-	1.1	0.5	0.12	0.17	1.3	190
Brain, nervous system	40	0	3.6	3.5	5.1	3.0	1.5	3.2	3.3	9.9	5.0	6.8	15.4	8.1	29.2	-	16.8	-	-	-	5.7	2.4	0.49	0.49	5.8	191-2
Thyroid	12	0	-	-	-	-	-	1.6	1.6	1.7	-	4.5	-	-	19.5	6.2	20.5	-	-	-	1.7	0.7	0.14	0.28	2.0	193
Other endocrine	3	0	1.8	-	-	1.5	1.5	-	-	-	-	-	-	-	-	-	-	-	-	-	0.4	0.2	0.02	0.02	0.5	194
Hodgkin's disease	11	0	-	-	-	1.5	4.6	1.6	-	-	-	4.5	-	4.1	4.9	6.2	-	-	-	69.9	1.6	0.6	0.11	0.14	1.8	201
Non-Hodgkin lymphoma	89	0	5.3	-	-	3.0	1.5	6.4	4.9	9.9	10.0	18.1	46.1	40.6	38.9	31.2	81.9	100.6	70.2	139.9	12.6	5.2	0.92	1.49	14.2	200,202
Multiple myeloma	30	0	-	-	-	-	-	-	-	-	1.7	2.3	6.1	20.3	14.6	43.7	30.7	83.9	70.2	69.9	4.2	1.8	0.22	0.60	5.4	203
Lymphoid leukaemia	30	0	10.7	-	-	3.0	-	1.6	-	-	1.7	4.5	9.2	16.2	4.9	18.7	30.7	16.8	35.1	139.9	4.2	1.8	0.26	0.51	5.6	204
Myeloid leukaemia	28	0	1.8	-	1.7	1.5	3.0	1.6	-	1.7	-	4.5	6.1	4.1	24.3	25.0	20.5	33.5	105.4	-	4.0	1.7	0.25	0.48	4.7	205
Monocytic leukaemia	0	0	-	-	-	-	-	-	-	-	-	-	-	-	-	-	-	-	-	-	0.0	0.0	0.00	0.00	0.0	206
Other leukaemia	1	0	1.8	-	-	-	-	-	-	-	-	-	-	-	-	-	-	-	-	-	0.1	0.1	0.01	0.01	0.2	207
Leukaemia unspecified	0	0	-	-	-	-	-	-	-	-	-	-	-	-	-	-	-	-	-	-	0.0	0.0	0.00	0.00	0.0	208
Other and unspecified	67	0	1.8	-	-	-	-	-	-	5.0	3.3	6.8	18.4	28.4	43.8	56.1	71.7	201.2	175.6	209.8	9.5	4.0	0.54	1.18	12.0	O&U
All sites																										
All sites but 173	1696	0	32.0	10.5	10.2	29.6	19.8	56.1	65.7	109.3	129.4	237.0	412.0	616.9	1051.5	1509.8	2335.1	3035.4	3301.7	4335.7	239.8	100.0	13.90	33.12	294.9	ALLb

Rate from 1 case

1.780 1.751 1.708 1.482 1.520 1.602 1.641 1.657 1.659 2.257 3.074 4.058 4.868 6.239 10.242 16.770 35.125 69.930

†Important: see notes on population page

AUSTRALIAN CAPITAL TERRITORY 1988-1992

ANNUAL INCIDENCE PER 100,000 BY AGE GROUP (YEARS) - FEMALE

SITE	ALL AGES	AGE UNK	0-	5-	10-	15-	20-	25-	30-	35-	40-	45-	50-	55-	60-	65-	70-	75-	80-	85+	CRUDE RATE	%	CR 64	CR 74	ASR (W)	ICD (9th)
Lip	11	0	-	-	-	-	-	-	-	-	1.7	2.4	-	4.4	-	5.5	7.9	11.1	76.5	26.7	1.6	0.7	0.04	0.11	**1.4**	140
Tongue	6	0	-	-	-	-	1.5	-	-	-	-	-	3.3	4.4	9.8	-	-	-	-	19.1	-	0.8	0.4	0.10	0.10	**0.9**	141
Salivary gland	3	0	-	-	-	-	-	-	-	-	3.4	-	-	-	-	5.5	-	-	-	-	0.4	0.2	0.02	0.04	**0.4**	142
Mouth	8	0	-	-	-	-	-	-	-	-	-	-	-	4.4	9.8	5.5	15.8	11.1	19.1	-	1.1	0.5	0.07	0.18	**1.3**	143-5
Oropharynx	1	0	-	-	-	-	-	-	-	-	-	-	-	-	4.9	-	-	-	-	-	0.1	0.1	0.02	0.02	**0.2**	146
Nasopharynx	2	0	-	-	-	-	-	-	-	-	-	-	-	4.4	-	5.5	-	-	-	-	0.3	0.1	0.02	0.05	**0.3**	147
Hypopharynx	0	0	-	-	-	-	-	-	-	-	-	-	-	-	-	-	-	-	-	-	0.0	0.0	0.00	0.00	**0.0**	148
Pharynx unspecified	0	0	-	-	-	-	-	-	-	-	-	-	-	-	-	-	-	-	-	-	0.0	0.0	0.00	0.00	**0.0**	149
Oesophagus	13	0	-	-	-	-	-	-	-	-	-	-	-	4.4	4.9	27.7	15.8	11.1	19.1	53.3	1.8	0.8	0.05	0.26	**2.0**	150
Stomach	40	0	-	-	-	-	-	-	-	4.8	5.0	14.1	19.6	-	-	22.1	23.7	66.5	76.5	133.4	5.7	2.5	0.22	0.45	**5.3**	151
Small intestine	7	0	-	-	-	-	-	-	-	1.6	-	-	3.3	4.4	4.9	11.1	7.9	-	-	-	1.0	0.4	0.07	0.17	**1.1**	152
Colon	136	0	-	-	-	-	-	-	-	3.2	6.7	16.5	45.8	35.1	78.6	116.2	181.4	188.3	286.9	240.1	19.2	8.6	0.93	2.42	**20.0**	153
Rectum	74	0	-	-	-	-	-	-	-	1.6	6.7	7.1	16.3	26.3	49.1	49.8	134.1	155.1	76.5	26.7	10.5	4.7	0.54	1.46	**11.0**	154
Liver	6	0	-	-	-	-	-	-	-	1.6	-	-	3.3	-	9.8	5.5	7.9	-	-	-	0.8	0.4	0.07	0.14	**1.0**	155
Gallbladder etc.	13	0	-	-	-	-	-	1.6	-	-	-	-	-	8.8	4.9	-	7.9	33.2	19.1	106.7	1.8	0.8	0.08	0.12	**1.8**	156
Pancreas	31	0	-	-	-	-	-	-	-	-	-	4.7	6.5	17.6	9.8	27.7	15.8	88.6	57.4	80.0	4.4	2.0	0.19	0.41	**4.4**	157
Nose, sinuses etc.	1	0	-	-	-	-	-	-	-	-	-	-	-	4.4	-	-	-	-	-	-	0.1	0.1	0.02	0.02	**0.2**	160
Larynx	2	0	-	-	-	-	-	-	-	-	-	-	-	-	4.9	5.5	-	-	-	-	0.3	0.1	0.02	0.05	**0.4**	161
Bronchus, lung	94	0	-	-	-	-	-	-	-	3.2	5.0	11.8	9.8	35.1	73.6	88.6	102.5	199.4	172.1	53.3	13.3	5.9	0.69	1.65	**13.9**	162
Other thoracic organs	1	0	-	-	-	-	-	-	-	-	-	-	-	-	4.9	-	-	-	-	-	0.1	0.1	0.02	0.02	**0.2**	163-4
Bone	5	0	-	1.8	-	1.5	-	-	-	-	1.7	2.4	-	-	-	5.5	-	-	-	-	0.7	0.3	0.04	0.06	**0.7**	170
Connective tissue	7	0	3.7	-	-	1.5	-	-	-	1.6	-	-	-	4.4	4.9	-	-	-	19.1	-	1.0	0.4	0.08	0.08	**1.1**	171
Mesothelioma	1	0	-	-	-	-	-	-	-	-	-	-	-	-	-	-	-	-	19.1	-	0.1	0.1	0.00	0.00	**0.1**	MES
†Kaposi's sarcoma	0	0	-	-	-	-	-	-	-	-	-	-	-	-	-	-	-	-	-	-	0.0	0.0	0.00	0.00	**0.0**	KAP
Melanoma of skin	173	0	-	-	-	6.1	18.3	30.6	19.4	27.3	38.6	37.6	62.1	74.6	49.1	33.2	71.0	55.4	19.1	80.0	24.5	10.9	1.82	2.34	**23.4**	172
†Other skin																										
Breast	461	0	-	-	-	-	-	9.7	12.9	46.6	122.5	166.9	156.9	219.4	279.9	276.8	197.2	265.9	267.7	160.0	65.2	29.1	5.07	7.44	**66.6**	174
Uterus unspecified	5	0	-	-	-	-	-	-	-	-	1.7	-	3.3	-	4.9	5.5	-	11.1	-	-	0.7	0.3	0.05	0.08	**0.7**	179
Cervix uteri	76	0	-	-	-	-	-	3.2	21.0	9.6	13.4	21.2	32.7	21.9	14.7	72.0	23.7	22.2	38.2	-	10.7	4.8	0.69	1.17	**10.3**	180
Placenta	1	0	-	-	-	1.5	-	-	-	-	-	-	-	-	-	-	-	-	-	-	0.1	0.1	0.01	0.01	**0.1**	181
Corpus uteri	46	0	-	-	-	-	-	1.6	-	-	1.7	11.8	19.6	35.1	44.2	38.7	31.5	33.2	-	53.3	6.5	2.9	0.57	0.92	**7.5**	182
Ovary etc.	57	0	-	-	-	1.5	-	-	6.5	1.6	11.7	16.5	19.6	21.9	34.4	49.8	7.9	66.5	57.4	-	8.1	3.6	0.57	0.86	**8.1**	183
Other female genital	11	0	1.9	-	-	-	-	-	-	1.6	1.7	2.4	3.3	-	4.9	-	23.7	11.1	19.1	-	1.6	0.7	0.08	0.20	**1.6**	184
†Bladder	14	0	-	-	-	-	-	-	-	-	-	-	3.3	8.8	14.7	11.1	23.7	33.2	-	-	2.0	0.9	0.13	0.31	**2.2**	188
Kidney etc.	25	0	1.9	1.8	1.8	-	-	1.6	-	-	-	-	9.8	4.4	14.7	27.7	15.8	33.2	38.2	53.3	3.5	1.6	0.18	0.40	**3.9**	189
Eye	8	0	-	-	-	-	-	-	-	1.6	-	2.4	-	-	5.5	7.9	33.2	19.1	-	-	1.1	0.5	0.02	0.09	**1.0**	190
Brain, nervous system	36	0	-	5.5	-	1.5	-	6.4	1.6	3.2	5.0	7.1	13.1	21.9	9.8	16.6	15.8	-	19.1	53.3	5.1	2.3	0.38	0.54	**5.3**	191-2
Thyroid	14	0	-	-	1.8	-	4.6	1.6	1.6	1.6	-	2.4	-	4.4	4.9	5.5	7.9	11.1	19.1	-	2.0	0.9	0.11	0.18	**1.9**	193
Other endocrine	3	0	-	1.8	-	-	-	-	-	-	4.7	-	-	-	-	-	-	-	-	-	0.4	0.2	0.03	0.03	**0.5**	194
Hodgkin's disease	8	0	-	-	-	1.5	3.1	1.6	1.6	1.6	-	3.3	-	-	-	-	-	11.1	-	-	1.1	0.5	0.06	0.06	**1.0**	201
Non-Hodgkin lymphoma	66	0	-	1.8	-	-	-	1.6	4.8	6.4	6.7	9.4	13.1	26.3	58.9	44.3	39.4	22.2	95.6	186.7	9.3	4.2	0.65	1.06	**9.8**	200,202
Multiple myeloma	27	0	-	-	-	-	-	-	-	1.6	1.7	7.1	-	8.8	29.5	22.1	15.8	33.2	95.6	-	3.8	1.7	0.24	0.43	**3.9**	203
Lymphoid leukaemia	12	0	3.7	-	-	-	-	-	-	-	-	-	9.8	4.4	9.8	11.1	7.9	-	-	26.7	1.7	0.8	0.14	0.23	**2.1**	204
Myeloid leukaemia	18	0	1.9	-	-	-	-	1.6	1.6	-	3.4	2.4	-	8.8	-	16.6	15.8	22.2	57.4	-	2.5	1.1	0.10	0.26	**2.5**	205
Monocytic leukaemia	0	0	-	-	-	-	-	-	-	-	-	-	-	-	-	-	-	-	-	-	0.0	0.0	0.00	0.00	**0.0**	206
Other leukaemia	0	0	-	-	-	-	-	-	-	-	-	-	-	-	-	-	-	-	-	-	0.0	0.0	0.00	0.00	**0.0**	207
Leukaemia unspecified	1	0	-	-	-	-	-	-	-	-	-	-	-	-	-	-	-	-	11.1	-	0.1	0.1	0.00	0.00	**0.1**	208
Other and unspecified	59	0	-	-	-	-	-	1.6	-	1.6	3.4	2.4	19.6	21.9	49.1	49.8	71.0	77.6	57.4	133.4	8.3	3.7	0.50	1.10	**9.0**	O&U
All sites																										
All sites but 173	1583	0	13.0	12.8	3.5	15.2	27.5	62.8	71.1	122.1	241.6	352.6	477.1	640.7	898.5	1068.4	1096.2	1517.8	1663.8	1467.1	223.8	100.0	14.69	25.52	**229.2**	ALLb

Rate from 1 case	0-	5-	10-	15-	20-	25-	30-	35-	40-	45-	50-	55-	60-	65-	70-	75-	80-	85+
	1.854	1.825	1.774	1.517	1.527	1.611	1.616	1.606	1.678	2.351	3.268	4.388	4.910	5.536	7.886	11.079	19.124	26.674

†Important: see notes on population page

Australia, New South Wales

The New South Wales Central Cancer Registry was established in 1971 to collect cancer statistics for the State from January 1972. This was achieved by altering the Public Health Act to require notification of cancer by hospitals and radiotherapy departments. A further modification in 1985 made notification by pathologists and out-patient departments obligatory. The registry was part of the NSW Health Department until 1986, when it was transferred to the NSW Cancer Council, although still funded by the Department of Health.

The region covered by the registry is the State of New South Wales (NSW), one of six federated states of Australia, situated between 28 and 38° S and 141 and 154° E. The area of NSW is 801 400 km^2 excluding the Australian Capital Territory which is bordered on all sides by NSW. The climate is temperate. Geographically, there are four main zones, extending from north to south: the coastal zone, the tablelands, the western slopes of the tablelands and the western plains that occupy two thirds of the area of the State.

At the 1991 census, the population of NSW was 5 898 731, of whom 67% live in the urban conurbation of Newcastle, Sydney and Wollongong. About 25% were migrants, coming principally from the United Kingdom and the Republic of Ireland (6%), southern Europe (4%), other Europe (2.5%), southeast Asia (2.6%), north-east Asia (1.9%), Middle East (1.9%) and New Zealand (1.5%).

The majority of the employed labour force was in wholesale and retail trade, community services and manufacturing, with only about 5% in agriculture and mining. Of the labour force, 12.1% were managers, 19.5% professionals, 13.5% trades persons, 15.8% clerks, 13.6% service workers, 6.9% factory workers and 12.2 % labourers. The unemployment rate in July 1991 was 8.8%.

The two most common religious affiliations were Catholic and Anglican, with just under 30% each, and other Christian about 20%. Non-Christians include Jews, Moslem, Buddhist and Hindu.

Cancer is treated in a wide range of hospitals. About 10 independent departments of radiation oncology are associated with major hospitals. Teaching hospitals maintain consultant cancer clinics in large country regions with regular visits by specialists.

The primary source of cancer data is the compulsory notification form or an alternative electronic notification completed by hospital staff for each cancer case in every public and private hospital. In addition, each radiotherapy and out-patient department must notify the first attendance per annum of each cancer case. The registry has developed systems for matching new notifications with cases already registered. Pathology reports confirming or diagnosing invasive cancer are received from all public and private histopathology laboratories and some haematology departments. The pathology report is particularly important and is used by the registry to improve consistency of coding.

Copies of death certificates are received fortnightly for deaths from all causes registered in NSW. A supplementary coded list of deaths mentioning cancer is received annually and is used to identify any cases not known to the registry. If no further information about such cases can be obtained, they are registered as "death certificate only" (DCO). During most of the period covered by the data reported here, the date of diagnosis for DCO cases was inferred from information given on the death certificate.

The registry is currently matching all cancer cases not known to be dead against a complete file of deaths in NSW since 1972 from any cause. These data will be used for survival analysis.

Paper notifications, pathology reports and death certificates not yet entered on the computer database are linked manually and an interactive search on name (including similar-sounding names) and sex is carried out to determine whether or not the person is already registered. For the cancers tabulated here, data were entered interactively or in batches. A computer matching program is run regularly to detect double registrations, including name changes or errors in identifying data.

Registration, classification of non-medical data and the keeping of manual and some computer systems are the responsibility of clerical staff. Disease classification—topography, morphology, behaviour, degree of spread at first presentation and date of diagnosis—is done by medical coding staff, who seek advice from specialist pathologists and clinicians as necessary. Additional information is often sought from treating doctors.

Analyses of the records of the registry are used to produce descriptive statistics based on age, sex, country of birth and geographical sub-region, for research, teaching, to respond to *ad hoc* requests from community, educational and industrial sources and to provide data for the planning and evaluation of cancer services.

Current programmes include contribution to the Australian Mesothelioma Surveillance programme, the Australian Paediatric Cancer Registry and studies of prostate and breast cancers and cancers associated with AIDS. The registry serves as a source of case follow-up for institutions and research workers.

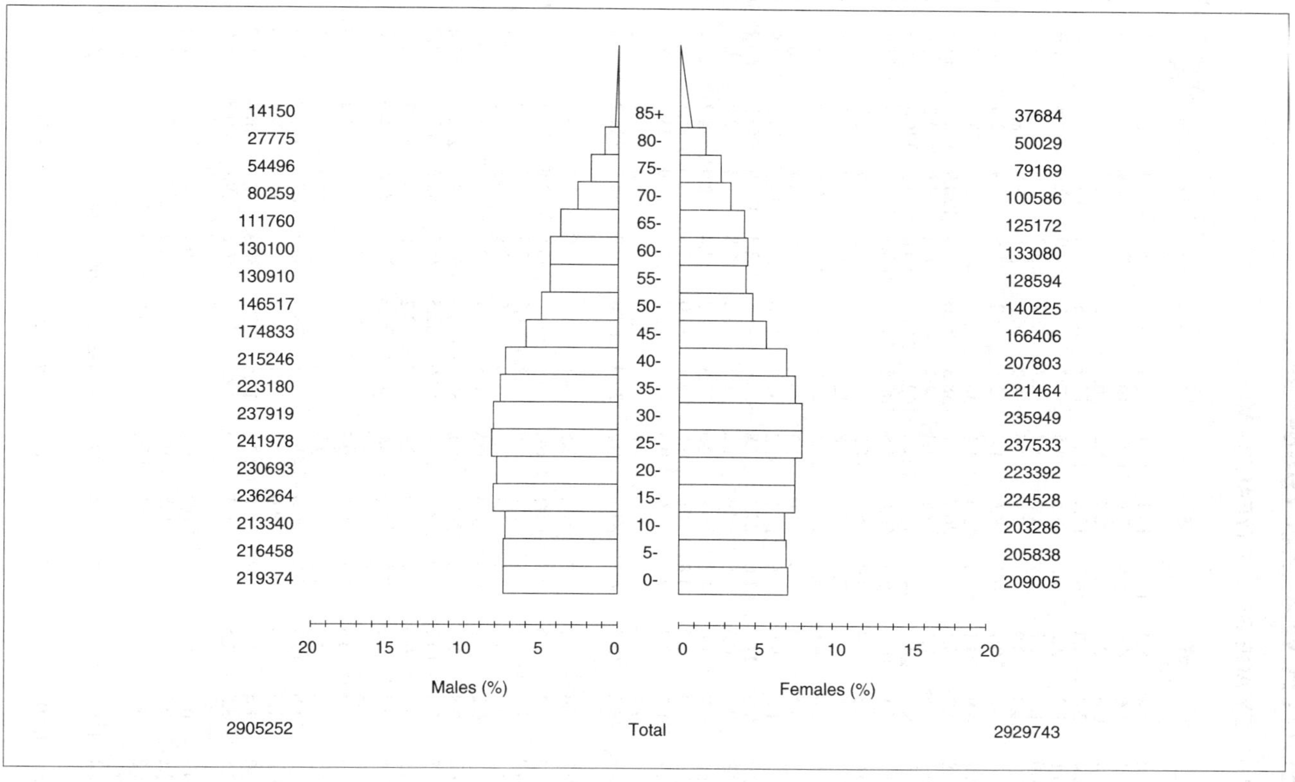

Australia, New South Wales

Source of population: average annual 1988–92

Census: 1991. Census count by usual place of residence, adjusted for under-enumeration and for Australian residents temporarily overseas.

Estimate: The populations for each of the years 1988, 1989 and 1990 were intercensal estimates, initially obtained from the 1986 Census by advancing age and allowing for births, deaths and migration and adjusted in the light of the 1991 Census to give correct final results in each sex and age-group.

Notes to tables overleaf:

† Kaposi's sarcoma is under-reported in this volume because cases of skin cancer (ICD-9 173) were not provided.

† 173 not available

† 188 does not include non-invasive tumours

AUSTRALIA, NEW SOUTH WALES 1988-1992

ANNUAL INCIDENCE PER 100,000 BY AGE GROUP (YEARS) - MALE

SITE	ALL AGES	AGE UNK	0-	5-	10-	15-	20-	25-	30-	35-	40-	45-	50-	55-	60-	65-	70-	75-	80-	85+	CRUDE RATE	%	CR 64	CR 74	ASR (W)	ICD (9th)
Lip	913	0	0.1	-	0.2	0.3	0.8	2.1	2.7	4.0	4.4	8.4	11.2	13.1	16.1	21.3	26.9	32.3	43.9	36.7	6.3	1.5	0.32	0.56	**5.1**	*140*
Tongue	383	0	-	-	-	-	0.2	0.4	0.3	0.4	1.6	4.0	5.5	7.9	11.7	10.7	12.7	7.7	7.9	7.1	2.6	0.6	0.16	0.28	**2.2**	*141*
Salivary gland	206	0	-	-	-	0.1	0.3	0.2	0.3	0.4	0.6	0.9	1.5	2.4	5.2	6.3	6.2	9.2	16.6	11.3	1.4	0.3	0.06	0.12	**1.1**	*142*
Mouth	498	0	-	-	-	-	0.2	0.1	0.4	2.0	3.8	6.7	12.4	17.2	15.2	14.5	12.8	10.1	2.8	3.4	0.8	0.21	0.36	**2.8**	*143-5*
Oropharynx	275	0	-	-	-	-	-	-	0.1	0.1	1.2	3.2	5.2	7.5	8.5	7.7	7.7	4.0	2.9	1.4	1.9	0.5	0.13	0.21	**1.6**	*146*
Nasopharynx	162	0	0.1	-	0.1	-	0.4	0.6	0.9	1.0	1.7	1.7	1.8	1.5	4.2	2.7	2.7	3.7	3.6	2.8	1.1	0.3	0.07	0.10	**0.9**	*147*
Hypopharynx	249	0	-	-	-	-	-	-	-	0.1	0.3	0.9	2.3	7.3	10.6	8.9	6.5	5.1	5.0	8.5	1.7	0.4	0.11	0.18	**1.4**	*148*
Pharynx unspecified	52	0	-	0.1	-	-	-	-	-	-	-	0.1	0.5	0.6	1.8	2.1	2.2	1.5	2.9	1.4	0.4	0.1	0.02	0.04	**0.3**	*149*
Oesophagus	834	0	-	-	-	-	-	-	0.1	0.4	0.9	3.1	7.6	13.4	21.1	30.2	37.4	42.2	41.0	28.3	5.7	1.4	0.23	0.57	**4.5**	*150*
Stomach	1931	0	-	-	-	-	-	0.1	0.8	1.8	4.3	8.1	12.7	26.7	38.7	58.3	82.0	117.8	128.9	152.6	13.3	3.2	0.47	1.17	**10.1**	*151*
Small intestine	148	0	-	-	-	-	-	-	-	0.3	0.5	1.1	1.2	2.1	4.3	4.5	5.5	6.2	8.6	4.2	1.0	0.2	0.05	0.10	**0.8**	*152*
Colon	5312	0	-	-	0.1	0.2	0.5	1.0	2.8	3.0	8.4	24.1	48.5	76.8	129.4	162.0	215.6	280.0	326.2	336.4	36.6	8.9	1.47	3.36	**28.4**	*153*
Rectum	3405	0	-	-	-	0.1	-	0.3	1.0	2.1	6.1	16.9	36.0	60.0	85.5	105.8	132.6	163.3	160.6	207.8	23.4	5.7	1.04	2.23	**18.5**	*154*
Liver	449	0	0.1	-	0.1	0.2	-	0.2	0.8	0.9	1.3	2.4	4.0	6.3	11.2	16.5	17.9	19.5	13.7	12.7	3.1	0.8	0.14	0.31	**2.5**	*155*
Gallbladder etc.	366	0	-	-	-	-	-	0.1	0.1	0.4	0.5	1.5	2.2	4.0	6.8	12.3	19.7	19.8	22.3	31.1	2.5	0.6	0.08	0.24	**1.9**	*156*
Pancreas	1309	0	-	-	0.1	-	-	0.2	0.3	1.0	2.0	4.6	10.1	17.1	29.1	36.0	58.3	69.7	99.4	130.0	9.0	2.2	0.32	0.79	**6.9**	*157*
Nose, sinuses etc.	126	0	-	-	-	0.1	0.1	0.1	0.2	0.3	0.3	0.9	2.0	2.0	2.2	3.2	3.5	5.9	9.4	5.7	0.9	0.2	0.04	0.07	**0.7**	*160*
Larynx	1007	0	-	-	-	-	-	-	0.2	0.6	1.8	5.0	12.6	22.0	31.2	37.4	32.6	34.9	33.8	19.8	6.9	1.7	0.37	0.72	**5.6**	*161*
Bronchus, lung	8816	0	-	-	-	0.1	0.3	0.2	0.4	2.4	9.5	27.7	61.6	129.1	227.8	334.6	396.5	472.3	470.9	356.2	60.7	14.8	2.30	5.95	**46.6**	*162*
Other thoracic organs	72	0	0.1	-	-	0.2	0.4	0.3	0.3	0.3	0.1	0.6	0.8	0.6	1.2	1.4	3.2	1.8	1.4	2.8	0.5	0.1	0.02	0.05	**0.4**	*163-4*
Bone	162	0	0.3	0.4	1.0	2.4	0.6	0.3	0.9	1.0	0.7	1.0	1.4	0.8	2.0	2.3	1.7	4.4	2.9	4.2	1.1	0.3	0.06	0.08	**1.0**	*170*
Connective tissue	431	0	1.4	0.5	0.4	1.0	1.0	1.2	1.7	2.3	1.9	2.2	4.8	4.6	6.8	8.1	14.0	15.4	18.0	11.3	3.0	0.7	0.15	0.26	**2.5**	*171*
Mesothelioma	454	0	-	-	-	-	-	-	-	0.1	1.2	2.4	3.5	7.0	9.8	15.0	22.7	22.4	20.9	25.4	3.1	0.8	0.12	0.31	**2.4**	*MES*
†Kaposi's sarcoma	453	0	-	-	0.1	-	0.8	6.0	9.2	8.2	7.1	5.7	2.6	1.2	0.6	0.2	0.7	1.1	1.4	4.2	3.1	0.8	0.21	0.21	**2.6**	*KAP*
Melanoma of skin	5865	6	0.3	0.2	0.9	4.7	9.4	18.1	22.9	31.5	43.2	45.6	64.3	84.5	110.7	129.0	167.0	170.3	174.3	185.2	40.4	9.8	2.18	3.67	**33.1**	*172*
†Other skin																										
Breast	126	0	-	-	-	-	-	-	0.1	0.3	0.4	0.5	0.8	1.2	2.8	4.1	5.7	7.0	7.2	9.9	0.9	0.2	0.03	0.08	**0.7**	*175*
Prostate	10870	0	-	-	-	-	-	-	-	0.3	1.4	2.6	16.2	64.3	166.3	373.3	597.8	885.6	1062.8	1177.3	74.8	18.2	1.26	6.11	**53.5**	*185*
Testis	770	0	0.5	0.1	0.2	3.5	6.9	14.5	12.8	10.0	7.2	5.3	2.9	2.7	2.9	1.4	1.5	1.1	0.7	2.8	5.3	1.3	0.35	0.36	**4.7**	*186*
Penis	66	0	-	-	-	-	-	-	-	0.1	0.7	0.2	0.4	1.4	1.7	1.4	1.5	2.9	4.3	7.1	0.5	0.1	0.02	0.04	**0.4**	*187.1-.4*
Other male genital	24	0	-	-	-	-	-	-	-	0.1	0.2	0.1	0.3	0.3	0.5	0.5	0.7	2.2	-	1.4	0.2	0.0	0.01	0.01	**0.1**	*187.5-.9*
†Bladder	2525	0	-	-	-	-	0.4	0.5	0.9	1.4	2.8	7.2	15.3	29.6	49.8	87.2	116.6	150.1	182.2	207.8	17.4	4.2	0.54	1.56	**13.2**	*188*
Kidney etc.	1695	0	1.5	0.2	-	0.2	0.4	0.4	1.3	3.5	5.4	10.2	16.0	29.3	38.4	50.6	62.5	76.7	80.6	69.3	11.7	2.8	0.53	1.10	**9.3**	*189*
Eye	163	0	1.9	-	-	0.1	0.3	0.7	0.3	0.8	0.7	0.9	1.1	4.0	2.9	2.7	3.2	4.0	4.3	4.2	1.1	0.3	0.07	0.10	**1.0**	*190*
Brain, nervous system	1131	0	3.5	3.0	2.6	2.3	2.8	2.7	3.4	5.8	6.4	7.8	10.5	15.3	22.0	26.3	26.2	30.1	23.8	15.5	7.8	1.9	0.44	0.70	**6.8**	*191-2*
Thyroid	281	0	0.1	-	0.3	0.5	0.4	1.8	1.5	1.9	2.8	3.1	3.8	3.1	4.2	4.7	6.0	4.8	4.3	5.7	1.9	0.5	0.12	0.17	**1.7**	*193*
Other endocrine	74	0	1.4	0.7	0.4	0.3	0.4	0.3	0.2	0.3	0.3	0.6	0.4	0.5	0.3	0.5	1.0	1.1	2.2	1.4	0.5	0.1	0.03	0.04	**0.5**	*194*
Hodgkin's disease	339	0	0.6	0.8	1.1	2.6	2.9	3.6	2.0	2.2	2.3	2.7	2.2	2.4	2.8	2.5	3.5	4.0	10.1	4.2	2.3	0.6	0.14	0.17	**2.1**	*201*
Non-Hodgkin lymphoma	2371	1	1.3	2.4	1.5	1.6	2.3	4.0	8.0	9.8	11.9	17.7	22.9	29.9	41.0	51.5	78.0	95.8	107.3	127.2	16.3	4.0	0.77	1.42	**13.3**	*200,202*
Multiple myeloma	658	0	-	-	-	-	-	0.2	0.3	0.6	1.7	3.4	6.6	9.0	14.1	18.1	30.2	30.8	46.8	39.6	4.5	1.1	0.18	0.42	**3.5**	*203*
Lymphoid leukaemia	775	0	6.7	3.5	2.0	2.2	0.9	0.9	0.3	0.8	1.4	1.7	4.0	10.7	12.3	19.5	23.7	30.8	38.9	46.6	5.3	1.3	0.24	0.45	**4.8**	*204*
Myeloid leukaemia	864	0	1.5	0.9	0.6	1.6	1.4	1.8	2.3	2.5	3.5	4.5	5.7	6.1	12.8	19.5	32.1	36.3	69.8	60.8	5.9	1.4	0.23	0.48	**4.8**	*205*
Monocytic leukaemia	18	0	0.2	-	0.2	-	0.1	-	0.1	-	-	0.1	0.1	-	0.4	0.2	0.4	2.9	2.8		0.1	0.0	0.00	0.01	**0.1**	*206*
Other leukaemia	18	0	0.1	-	-	-	-	-	0.1	0.1	0.1	0.1	-	0.3	0.3	0.7	0.7	0.7	-	-	0.1	0.0	0.01	0.01	**0.1**	*207*
Leukaemia unspecified	103	0	0.1	-	-	0.3	0.1	-	0.2	0.1	0.2	0.1	0.8	0.8	0.8	2.7	4.2	8.1	9.4	12.7	0.7	0.2	0.02	0.05	**0.5**	*208*
Other and unspecified	2872	2	0.7	-	0.1	0.1	0.5	0.9	0.8	1.8	4.6	7.0	19.7	39.3	60.1	90.4	118.9	173.2	211.7	230.4	19.8	4.8	0.68	1.73	**15.1**	*O&U*
All sites																										
All sites but 173	59621	9	22.2	12.8	11.9	24.4	34.8	63.9	80.4	105.4	155.1	251.9	440.2	761.4	1229.7	1789.9	2404.7	3069.2	3495.8	3616.8	410.4	100.0	15.97	36.95	**320.4**	*ALLb*

Rate from 1 case: 0.091 0.092 0.094 0.085 0.087 0.083 0.084 0.090 0.093 0.114 0.137 0.153 0.154 0.179 0.249 0.367 0.720 1.413

†Important: see notes on population page

AUSTRALIA, NEW SOUTH WALES 1988-1992

ANNUAL INCIDENCE PER 100,000 BY AGE GROUP (YEARS) - FEMALE

SITE	ALL AGES	AGE UNK	0-	5-	10-	15-	20-	25-	30-	35-	40-	45-	50-	55-	60-	65-	70-	75-	80-	85+	CRUDE RATE	%	CR 64	CR 74	ASR (W)	ICD (9th)
Lip	319	0	-	-	-	-	0.2	0.2	0.6	1.4	1.4	2.2	1.7	3.7	4.2	5.3	8.9	10.9	14.8	20.2	2.2	0.6	0.08	0.15	1.4	140
Tongue	215	0	-	-	-	-	0.1	0.2	0.3	0.4	0.4	1.2	2.1	3.3	4.1	6.2	6.2	7.3	7.6	5.3	1.5	0.4	0.06	0.12	1.0	141
Salivary gland	105	0	-	-	0.2	0.1	0.1	0.3	0.3	0.4	0.6	0.5	1.1	1.4	1.5	2.4	1.6	2.8	3.6	4.8	0.7	0.2	0.03	0.05	0.5	142
Mouth	258	0	-	-	-	-	-	0.1	-	0.5	0.8	1.7	2.7	3.7	6.5	6.9	7.2	7.3	8.4	7.4	1.8	0.5	0.08	0.15	1.2	143-5
Oropharynx	84	0	-	-	-	-	-	-	-	0.3	0.3	0.5	0.7	1.6	1.5	2.4	4.0	2.3	1.2	1.1	0.6	0.2	0.02	0.06	0.4	146
Nasopharynx	54	0	-	-	-	0.3	-	0.2	0.3	0.2	0.4	0.6	0.7	1.2	1.1	1.1	0.6	0.8	-	1.1	0.4	0.1	0.02	0.03	0.3	147
Hypopharynx	35	0	-	-	-	-	-	-	-	-	0.1	0.1	-	1.1	1.1	1.0	1.0	1.5	0.8	-	0.2	0.1	0.01	0.02	0.2	148
Pharynx unspecified	16	0	-	-	-	-	-	-	-	-	-	-	-	0.2	0.3	1.1	0.2	0.8	0.4	0.5	0.1	0.0	0.00	0.01	0.1	149
Oesophagus	524	0	0.1	-	-	-	-	0.1	0.1	0.2	0.3	1.0	0.9	3.6	9.9	13.4	17.7	18.2	36.4	40.9	3.6	1.1	0.08	0.24	2.0	150
Stomach	1070	0	-	-	-	-	0.2	0.7	0.8	2.2	2.0	3.1	6.3	7.3	14.0	21.1	36.4	46.7	60.4	76.4	7.3	2.2	0.18	0.47	4.2	151
Small intestine	121	0	-	-	-	-	-	-	0.2	0.2	0.7	0.8	1.7	1.7	1.8	3.2	3.0	4.5	4.0	2.7	0.8	0.2	0.04	0.07	0.6	152
Colon	4881	0	-	0.1	-	0.2	0.3	1.0	2.5	5.3	10.7	23.1	43.9	62.4	82.5	111.5	148.1	183.4	228.3	251.6	33.3	9.8	1.16	2.46	21.2	153
Rectum	2171	0	-	-	-	0.1	0.3	0.4	1.5	2.6	4.8	11.8	21.1	29.7	38.9	53.4	67.8	72.2	92.7	93.4	14.8	4.4	0.56	1.16	9.7	154
Liver	118	0	-	-	0.1	-	0.2	0.3	0.1	0.3	0.2	0.5	0.7	1.4	2.9	2.7	3.4	3.0	3.2	7.4	0.8	0.2	0.03	0.06	0.6	155
Gallbladder etc.	472	0	-	-	-	0.1	-	0.1	0.3	0.4	0.9	1.9	3.1	4.8	5.6	12.6	15.5	22.2	26.8	19.1	3.2	1.0	0.09	0.23	1.9	156
Pancreas	1224	0	-	-	0.1	0.1	0.3	0.2	0.3	0.8	1.2	2.8	5.6	13.2	18.6	29.6	43.3	52.8	71.2	69.5	8.4	2.5	0.22	0.58	4.9	157
Nose, sinuses etc.	57	0	-	-	-	0.1	0.1	0.2	0.2	0.3	0.4	0.2	0.3	0.6	1.1	0.8	2.2	1.5	2.0	1.1	0.4	0.1	0.02	0.03	0.3	160
Larynx	122	0	-	-	-	-	-	-	-	0.1	0.1	0.6	1.0	2.3	3.8	4.6	3.0	4.0	2.4	1.1	0.8	0.2	0.04	0.08	0.6	161
Bronchus, lung	3271	0	-	0.1	-	-	0.3	-	1.5	2.4	7.8	18.1	26.4	42.8	71.8	86.0	121.3	124.0	111.9	70.6	22.3	6.6	0.86	1.89	14.9	162
Other thoracic organs	38	0	0.2	0.1	0.1	0.1	-	0.1	-	0.1	0.3	0.1	0.3	0.9	0.5	0.2	1.0	0.8	1.6	1.6	0.3	0.1	0.01	0.02	0.2	163-4
Bone	101	0	0.5	0.2	0.7	1.1	0.6	0.4	0.7	0.6	1.0	0.2	0.4	0.6	0.3	0.8	0.6	0.8	4.0	3.2	0.7	0.2	0.04	0.04	0.6	170
Connective tissue	315	0	1.5	0.8	0.7	0.5	0.8	0.7	1.4	1.0	1.2	1.8	2.3	2.5	3.9	3.8	8.2	9.1	8.8	13.8	2.2	0.6	0.09	0.15	1.7	171
Mesothelioma	62	0	-	-	-	-	-	0.3	-	0.2	0.3	0.1	0.4	1.2	1.5	2.2	1.8	1.0	1.6	0.5	0.4	0.1	0.02	0.04	0.3	MES
†Kaposi's sarcoma	10	0	-	-	-	-	-	-	0.1	0.1	-	-	0.1	-	-	0.3	0.2	0.5	-	1.1	0.1	0.0	0.00	0.00	0.0	KAP
Melanoma of skin	4762	3	-	0.1	0.9	6.2	14.0	21.7	28.2	37.0	40.9	51.9	45.8	59.1	66.0	71.9	76.8	89.7	75.2	77.5	32.5	9.6	1.86	2.60	25.7	172
†Other skin																										
Breast	12880	0	-	-	-	-	1.2	5.8	25.3	59.2	112.2	173.2	188.4	200.3	223.6	245.7	265.4	274.3	277.0	259.0	87.9	25.9	4.95	7.50	67.2	174
Uterus unspecified	95	0	-	-	-	-	0.1	-	-	0.3	0.8	0.8	1.6	0.9	1.5	1.8	2.4	1.5	2.4	7.4	0.6	0.2	0.03	0.05	0.5	179
Cervix uteri	1817	0	0.1	-	-	0.4	1.3	7.7	16.1	20.1	20.8	20.9	18.8	21.9	23.6	26.4	23.9	25.0	20.8	20.2	12.4	3.7	0.76	1.01	9.9	180
Placenta	21	0	-	-	-	0.1	0.6	0.3	0.6	0.2	0.1	-	-	-	-	-	-	-	-	-	0.1	0.0	0.01	0.01	0.1	181
Corpus uteri	1754	0	-	-	-	-	0.1	0.3	0.8	2.4	5.6	9.4	24.1	39.2	45.4	45.2	50.9	44.2	38.0	23.9	12.0	3.5	0.64	1.12	8.8	182
Ovary etc.	1654	0	0.1	0.1	0.6	1.0	1.3	1.3	2.5	4.8	6.7	15.0	24.7	24.9	30.1	38.3	43.1	42.4	36.4	41.4	11.3	3.3	0.57	0.97	8.4	183
Other female genital	374	0	-	-	-	-	-	0.5	0.4	1.1	1.4	1.9	3.3	3.1	5.6	9.3	7.6	13.9	15.6	26.5	2.6	0.8	0.09	0.17	1.6	184
†Bladder	930	0	0.1	-	-	-	0.1	0.2	0.6	0.3	1.3	2.9	5.3	9.8	13.2	24.6	29.8	40.2	49.2	55.2	6.3	1.9	0.17	0.44	3.8	188
Kidney etc.	1281	0	2.6	0.4	-	0.2	0.4	0.3	0.6	1.3	3.8	6.9	11.3	17.1	27.2	32.6	39.6	44.5	48.4	28.1	8.7	2.6	0.36	0.72	6.1	189
Eye	164	0	1.5	-	0.1	-	-	0.4	0.3	0.6	0.6	1.1	2.0	2.5	2.3	3.4	3.6	4.0	3.2	4.2	1.1	0.3	0.06	0.09	0.9	190
Brain, nervous system	873	0	3.3	2.5	2.9	2.4	2.0	2.0	2.8	3.5	4.8	5.5	6.7	10.0	15.6	15.8	18.3	20.0	18.0	6.9	6.0	1.8	0.32	0.49	5.0	191-2
Thyroid	777	0	-	-	0.4	1.3	4.7	6.1	9.8	7.9	7.6	8.3	8.0	7.0	6.6	6.7	6.4	7.8	7.2	6.9	5.3	1.6	0.34	0.40	4.5	193
Other endocrine	65	0	2.4	0.5	0.1	-	-	0.1	0.3	0.1	0.2	0.2	0.1	0.6	1.1	0.6	0.8	0.5	0.4	0.5	0.4	0.1	0.03	0.04	0.5	194
Hodgkin's disease	248	0	0.1	0.1	0.6	1.7	3.0	2.6	2.3	1.5	0.9	0.6	1.4	1.2	2.7	2.1	4.0	3.5	4.0	2.7	1.7	0.5	0.09	0.12	1.4	201
Non-Hodgkin lymphoma	1853	0	1.1	0.9	0.3	0.9	1.1	2.1	3.1	4.9	7.5	9.1	15.7	24.3	28.0	40.4	55.1	69.2	67.6	60.5	12.6	3.7	0.49	0.97	8.6	200,202
Multiple myeloma	584	0	-	-	-	-	0.1	0.1	0.2	0.6	1.1	1.7	3.7	5.9	9.9	14.4	17.7	28.3	30.4	27.1	4.0	1.2	0.12	0.28	2.4	203
Lymphoid leukaemia	553	0	6.5	2.6	2.2	0.9	0.6	0.5	0.3	0.5	0.9	1.3	3.3	2.2	7.5	11.8	11.9	17.9	20.4	21.2	3.8	1.1	0.15	0.27	3.1	204
Myeloid leukaemia	591	0	0.8	0.7	0.8	0.7	0.5	1.1	1.6	2.1	3.1	3.2	4.1	4.8	5.7	9.6	16.5	21.0	21.2	33.4	4.0	1.2	0.15	0.28	2.8	205
Monocytic leukaemia	24	0	0.5	-	-	-	-	-	-	-	0.2	0.1	-	-	-	0.6	-	1.3	1.6	1.6	0.2	0.0	0.00	0.01	0.1	206
Other leukaemia	8	0	-	-	-	0.1	-	-	0.1	-	0.1	0.1	-	-	-	-	-	0.8	-	0.5	0.1	0.0	0.00	0.00	0.0	207
Leukaemia unspecified	83	0	0.1	-	-	-	0.1	-	-	-	-	-	0.1	0.5	1.5	1.1	3.4	3.0	7.2	6.9	0.6	0.2	0.01	0.03	0.3	208
Other and unspecified	2637	0	0.5	-	-	0.2	0.1	0.7	1.3	3.3	5.0	7.9	16.0	21.6	35.5	53.5	81.5	118.2	151.9	196.9	18.0	5.3	0.46	1.14	10.4	O&U
All sites																										
All sites but 173	49671	3	21.8	9.1	10.6	18.6	34.4	59.2	108.3	171.6	261.1	395.2	508.0	648.2	829.6	1028.5	1261.6	1449.8	1587.9	1602.8	339.1	100.0	15.38	26.83	240.9	ALLb

Rate from 1 case   0.096   0.097   0.098   0.089   0.089   0.084   0.085   0.090   0.096   0.120   0.143   0.156   0.150   0.160   0.199   0.253   0.340   0.531

†Important: see notes on population page

Australia, South Australia

The registry started in 1976, on a voluntary basis, but since 1977 notification of cancer has been a statutory obligation for all hospitals and pathology laboratories in South Australia.

South Australia is one of the six federated states of Australia and is situated between 26 and 38° S and 129 and 141° E. The state covers a total area of 984 375 km². Approximately one third of this area has no significant economic use and over one half is devoted to extensive pastoral pursuits.

The total population of South Australia was 1 382 550 persons at the 1986 census. Approximately 99% of the population live south of the 32nd parallel.

The primary objective of the registry is to describe the nature and extent of cancer in South Australia, to monitor cancer incidence, mortality and survival, and to evaluate spatial and subpopulation differences. Registry publications on cancer in South Australia have been well received locally, interstate and overseas.

The system of notification varies between hospitals depending on hospital size, staffing and types of record systems; in general the responsibility lies with medical records officers in public hospitals and managers in private institutions. The multiple notifications received are linked and a file is created for each patient.

Checks are available to the registry from death certification and pathology listings. Cases from such sources that are not reported by hospitals are followed up. Two or more primary sites are registered as two or more cancer cases but as one death.

The items on the notification form are divisible into two sections:

(1) patient identification: cancer registration number, name, sex, date of birth, race and occupation;

(2) medical history: primary site, histology, cause and date of death, TNM staging for melanoma and cancer of the breast.

The registry staff regularly visit or write to all hospitals to obtain information on inadequately reported cases and cases not reported but picked up from pathology laboratory reports. An annual cross linkage checks cancer registry live cases with the Registrar of Deaths' main death file to see whether any cancer cases have died of a condition other than cancer.

An analysis of survival has provided valuable information for the entire South Australian community, which should serve as a standard comparison for intra-hospital survival studies. The data are now sufficient for five-year relative survival rates to be calculated. The rates are based on the proportion of survivors from 1977 in the patient group, as related to the proportion of survivors in a similar group of people without the disease.

Special liaison has been established with the hospital departments to facilitate the follow-up of patients by clinicians to evaluate treatment outcomes.

Evaluation has been made of the effects of cancer control programmes on the early detection of breast cancer by breast self-examination, e.g. smoking control, cervical screening and early detection therapy.

The registry is being utilized increasingly in the investigation of environmental problems, and studies are regularly being carried out to determine whether any areas are exposed to a higher risk of cancer.

Information is being provided to the National Malignant Mesothelioma Project, National Paediatric Cancer Registry, and the National Clearing House.

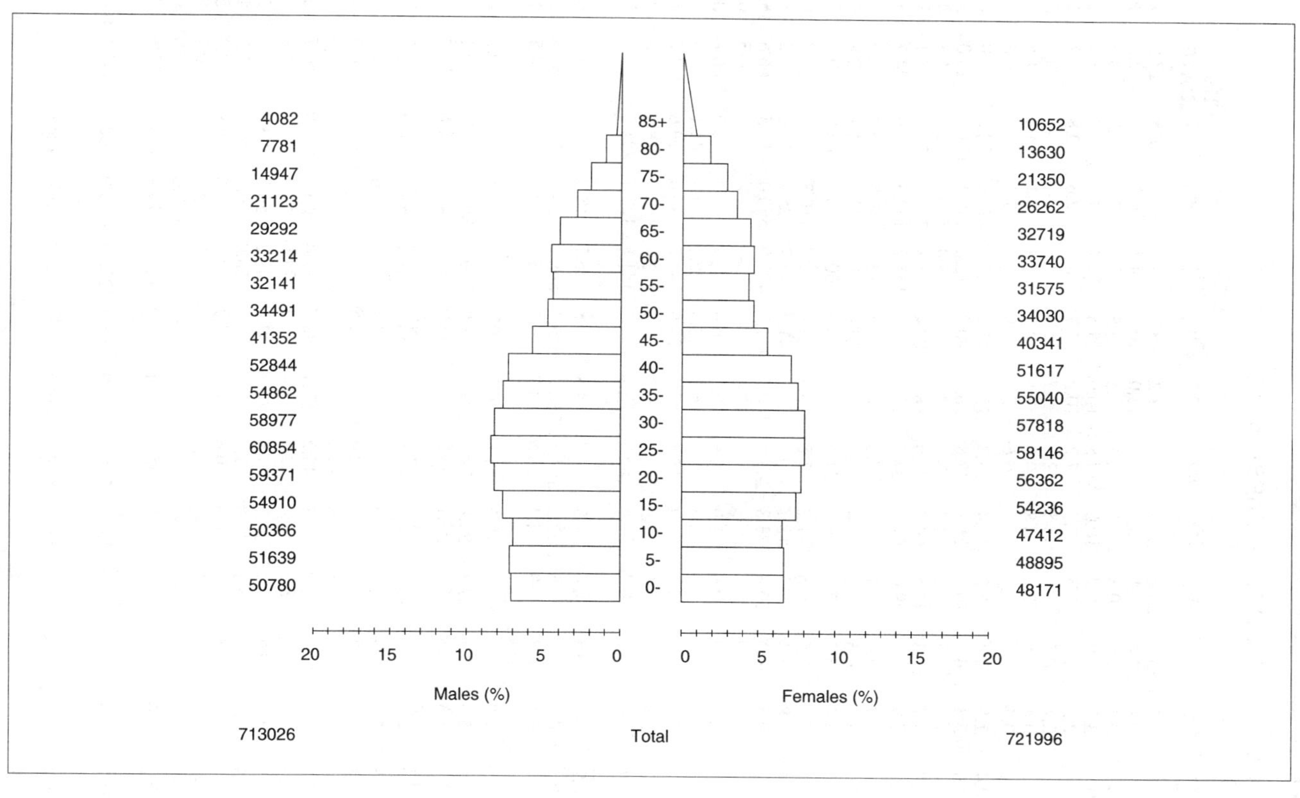

South Australia
Source of population: average annual 1988–92
Estimate: Intercensal
Notes to tables overleaf:
† Kaposi's sarcoma is under-reported in this volume because
   cases of skin cancer (ICD-9 173) were not provided.
† 173 not available

SOUTH AUSTRALIA 1988-1992

ANNUAL INCIDENCE PER 100,000 BY AGE GROUP (YEARS) - MALE

SITE	ALL AGES	AGE UNK	0-	5-	10-	15-	20-	25-	30-	35-	40-	45-	50-	55-	60-	65-	70-	75-	80-	85+	CRUDE RATE	%	CR 64	CR 74	ASR (W)	ICD (9th)
Lip	607	0	-	-	-	1.5	3.4	6.6	8.1	14.2	17.4	23.7	33.6	29.9	39.1	51.2	68.2	68.2	87.4	58.8	17.0	3.9	0.89	1.48	13.5	140
Tongue	83	0	-	-	-	-	0.3	-	-	-	1.1	2.4	4.1	8.1	7.8	13.0	10.4	9.4	10.3	-	2.3	0.5	0.12	0.24	1.8	141
Salivary gland	33	0	-	-	-	-	-	0.3	0.7	-	0.4	1.0	0.6	3.1	2.4	1.4	8.5	2.7	5.1	9.8	0.9	0.2	0.04	0.09	0.7	142
Mouth	111	0	-	-	-	-	-	-	0.3	0.7	3.0	1.9	8.7	10.0	14.5	10.9	8.5	10.7	7.7	24.5	3.1	0.7	0.20	0.29	2.5	143-5
Oropharynx	78	0	-	-	-	-	-	-	-	0.4	2.3	1.5	3.5	7.5	7.2	10.2	5.7	18.7	2.6	9.8	2.2	0.5	0.11	0.19	1.7	146
Nasopharynx	18	0	-	-	-	-	-	-	-	-	0.4	0.5	-	2.5	2.4	2.7	1.9	2.7	-	-	0.5	0.1	0.03	0.05	0.4	147
Hypopharynx	58	0	-	-	-	-	-	-	-	-	0.4	1.5	2.3	6.8	9.0	7.5	4.7	6.7	5.1	4.9	1.6	0.4	0.10	0.16	1.3	148
Pharynx unspecified	12	0	-	-	-	-	-	-	-	-	0.4	-	1.2	-	0.6	2.0	1.9	-	7.7	-	0.3	0.1	0.01	0.03	0.2	149
Oesophagus	209	0	-	-	-	-	-	-	0.3	0.4	1.5	2.4	5.2	12.4	15.7	25.9	41.7	28.1	72.0	58.8	5.9	1.3	0.19	0.53	4.2	150
Stomach	533	0	-	-	-	-	-	0.7	0.7	3.6	5.3	4.8	10.4	21.8	48.8	58.7	90.9	112.4	149.1	181.3	15.0	3.4	0.48	1.23	10.6	151
Small intestine	46	0	-	-	-	-	-	-	-	-	1.1	1.5	1.7	4.4	3.0	4.1	8.5	8.0	-	19.6	1.3	0.3	0.06	0.12	1.0	152
Colon	1358	0	-	-	-	0.4	-	1.0	1.0	4.7	8.7	29.5	47.5	69.7	100.0	158.4	207.4	323.8	347.0	323.3	38.1	8.6	1.31	3.14	27.4	153
Rectum	863	0	-	-	-	-	0.3	-	1.0	4.0	7.9	15.0	29.0	61.0	84.3	92.2	140.1	155.2	177.3	196.0	24.2	5.5	1.01	2.17	18.0	154
Liver	102	0	-	-	-	-	0.3	0.3	0.7	-	1.9	2.4	4.1	6.8	7.8	10.9	16.1	13.4	30.8	9.8	2.9	0.6	0.12	0.26	2.1	155
Gallbladder etc.	99	0	-	-	-	-	-	-	-	-	0.4	0.5	1.2	4.4	6.0	6.1	24.6	28.1	33.4	44.1	2.8	0.6	0.06	0.22	1.9	156
Pancreas	339	0	-	-	-	-	0.3	-	0.3	1.5	3.4	5.3	7.0	16.2	31.9	43.7	48.3	60.2	105.4	102.9	9.5	2.2	0.33	0.79	6.8	157
Nose, sinuses etc.	25	0	-	-	0.4	-	0.3	-	-	-	0.4	0.5	0.6	1.2	1.8	3.4	2.8	2.7	10.3	4.9	0.7	0.2	0.03	0.06	0.5	160
Larynx	221	0	-	-	-	-	-	-	0.3	0.4	0.8	3.4	9.3	18.7	30.1	28.7	41.7	18.7	25.7	19.6	6.2	1.4	0.31	0.67	4.8	161
Bronchus, lung	2375	0	-	-	-	-	-	0.3	1.0	2.2	9.5	26.6	56.8	123.8	241.5	340.7	411.9	475.0	550.0	411.5	66.6	15.1	2.31	6.07	47.9	162
Other thoracic organs	10	0	-	-	-	-	0.7	-	-	1.5	0.4	1.0	-	-	-	0.7	-	-	-	-	0.3	0.1	0.02	0.02	0.2	163-4
Bone	28	0	-	0.4	0.4	1.1	0.3	0.3	0.7	1.1	0.8	1.0	0.6	1.9	0.6	2.0	0.9	2.7	-	4.9	0.8	0.2	0.05	0.06	0.7	170
Connective tissue	117	0	1.6	0.8	-	1.5	0.7	1.0	1.4	1.5	4.2	2.9	2.9	5.6	8.4	6.1	13.3	20.1	5.1	44.1	3.3	0.7	0.16	0.26	2.7	171
Mesothelioma	167	0	-	-	-	-	0.3	-	-	0.4	1.1	2.4	4.1	11.2	18.1	15.0	24.6	48.2	36.0	19.6	4.7	1.1	0.19	0.39	3.3	MES
†Kaposi's sarcoma	27	0	-	-	-	-	-	0.7	2.4	1.8	0.8	1.0	1.2	1.2	-	0.7	1.9	2.7	-	-	0.8	0.2	0.04	0.06	0.6	KAP
Melanoma of skin	1218	0	-	-	1.6	6.9	10.1	15.4	18.7	23.7	39.0	54.2	60.3	71.6	87.9	73.1	105.1	141.8	123.4	225.3	34.2	7.7	1.95	2.84	27.8	172
†Other skin																										
Breast	38	0	-	-	0.4	-	-	-	0.3	0.7	-	0.5	0.6	1.9	4.8	4.8	2.8	6.7	12.9	4.9	1.1	0.2	0.05	0.08	0.8	175
Prostate	2904	0	-	-	-	-	-	-	-	0.4	0.4	2.9	14.5	57.2	191.5	368.0	585.1	868.4	1053.8	1200.2	81.5	18.4	1.33	6.10	53.6	185
Testis	162	0	1.2	-	-	1.5	5.4	11.8	9.8	8.7	6.4	6.3	2.9	4.4	0.6	0.7	0.9	5.4	2.6	-	4.5	1.0	0.30	0.30	4.0	186
Penis	16	0	-	-	-	-	0.3	-	-	-	-	0.5	1.2	1.2	1.2	0.7	2.8	1.3	5.1	4.9	0.4	0.1	0.02	0.04	0.4	187.1-.4
Other male genital	8	0	-	-	-	-	-	-	-	-	-	-	0.6	1.8	0.7	0.9	-	5.1	-	-	0.2	0.1	0.01	0.02	0.2	187.5-.9
Bladder	1042	0	-	-	0.4	-	0.3	1.3	2.4	5.1	5.3	13.1	27.8	39.8	79.5	122.9	178.9	239.5	303.3	313.5	29.2	6.6	0.88	2.38	20.6	188
Kidney etc.	403	0	0.8	-	-	-	-	-	0.7	2.9	8.3	7.3	16.2	26.1	34.9	51.2	53.0	83.0	48.8	68.6	11.3	2.6	0.49	1.01	8.5	189
Eye	40	0	0.8	-	0.4	-	-	0.7	0.3	0.4	0.4	-	1.2	1.2	4.2	6.1	4.7	5.4	2.6	9.8	1.1	0.3	0.05	0.10	0.9	190
Brain, nervous system	264	0	2.4	2.7	2.4	2.5	1.3	3.0	4.4	1.5	5.3	9.7	16.2	9.3	17.5	21.8	29.4	34.8	28.3	9.8	7.4	1.7	0.39	0.65	6.3	191-2
Thyroid	70	0	-	-	-	0.4	0.7	1.3	2.0	2.6	2.3	5.8	1.2	6.2	4.2	4.1	3.8	2.7	2.6	-	2.0	0.4	0.13	0.17	1.7	193
Other endocrine	23	0	1.2	-	0.4	0.4	1.3	0.3	-	0.7	-	0.5	-	-	2.4	2.0	2.8	-	-	-	0.6	0.1	0.04	0.06	0.6	194
Hodgkin's disease	71	0	-	0.4	1.6	2.9	2.7	4.3	2.4	1.8	1.1	1.9	0.6	1.9	4.2	1.4	2.8	-	2.6	4.9	2.0	0.5	0.13	0.15	1.8	201
Non-Hodgkin lymphoma	594	0	1.2	1.5	0.8	2.2	1.3	1.6	6.1	5.8	14.4	14.5	22.0	26.1	45.2	57.4	80.5	112.4	100.2	102.9	16.7	3.8	0.71	1.40	12.7	200,202
Multiple myeloma	233	0	-	-	-	-	-	-	0.3	0.4	1.1	2.4	3.5	10.0	22.3	31.4	31.2	74.9	51.4	44.1	6.5	1.5	0.20	0.51	4.5	203
Lymphoid leukaemia	323	0	7.5	1.5	2.0	1.8	1.0	-	0.7	1.5	2.6	5.3	8.7	13.1	31.9	36.2	43.6	48.2	56.5	83.3	9.1	2.0	0.39	0.79	7.5	204
Myeloid leukaemia	260	0	1.6	0.4	0.8	0.4	0.7	1.3	2.4	2.6	3.8	3.9	8.1	10.0	17.5	23.2	39.8	58.9	59.1	58.8	7.3	1.6	0.27	0.58	5.4	205
Monocytic leukaemia	12	0	-	-	-	0.4	-	-	0.3	-	0.4	0.5	-	0.6	0.6	0.7	0.9	2.7	2.6	4.9	0.3	0.1	0.01	0.02	0.3	206
Other leukaemia	7	0	-	-	-	-	-	-	-	-	-	-	1.2	-	0.6	0.7	-	2.7	2.6	-	0.2	0.0	0.01	0.01	0.1	207
Leukaemia unspecified	1	0	-	-	-	-	-	-	-	-	-	-	-	-	-	-	-	-	2.6	-	0.0	0.0	0.00	0.00	0.0	208
Other and unspecified	553	0	-	-	-	-	0.3	0.3	0.3	0.7	2.6	5.8	14.5	21.8	45.8	72.4	89.9	115.1	179.9	176.4	15.5	3.5	0.46	1.27	11.0	O&U
All sites / All sites but 173	15761	0	18.1	7.7	11.5	23.7	32.7	52.6	70.2	97.7	166.9	267.5	436.0	731.1	1279.6	1775.9	2443.7	3222.0	3713.9	3860.3	442.1	100.0	15.98	37.07	323.5	ALLb

Rate from 1 case: 0.394 (0-) 0.387 (5-) 0.397 (10-) 0.364 (15-) 0.337 (20-) 0.329 (25-) 0.339 (30-) 0.365 (35-) 0.378 (40-) 0.484 (45-) 0.580 (50-) 0.622 (55-) 0.602 (60-) 0.683 (65-) 0.947 (70-) 1.338 (75-) 2.570 (80-) 4.899 (85+)

†Important: see notes on population page

SOUTH AUSTRALIA 1988-1992

ANNUAL INCIDENCE PER 100,000 BY AGE GROUP (YEARS) - FEMALE

SITE	ALL AGES	AGE UNK	0-	5-	10-	15-	20-	25-	30-	35-	40-	45-	50-	55-	60-	65-	70-	75-	80-	85+	CRUDE RATE	%	CR 64	CR 74	ASR (W)	ICD (9th)
Lip	200	0	-	-	-	-	-	1.4	3.1	2.5	2.7	3.0	5.9	5.1	10.1	15.9	13.7	32.8	42.6	45.1	5.5	1.5	0.17	0.32	**3.2**	140
Tongue	36	0	-	-	-	-	0.4	-	0.3	-	0.4	0.5	0.6	2.5	1.8	4.9	3.0	5.6	5.9	3.8	1.0	0.3	0.03	0.07	**0.6**	141
Salivary gland	28	0	-	-	0.8	0.4	-	0.3	0.3	0.4	0.4	0.5	1.2	-	2.4	1.8	3.8	1.9	4.4	1.9	0.8	0.2	0.03	0.06	**0.6**	142
Mouth	77	0	-	-	0.4	-	0.4	-	0.3	0.4	0.8	0.5	1.2	3.8	5.3	8.6	9.9	13.1	7.3	13.1	2.1	0.6	0.07	0.16	**1.3**	143-5
Oropharynx	20	0	-	-	-	-	-	-	-	-	0.4	0.5	-	0.6	3.0	3.1	1.5	1.9	1.5	3.8	0.6	0.1	0.02	0.05	**0.4**	146
Nasopharynx	4	0	-	-	-	-	-	0.3	0.4	-	-	-	-	-	-	1.2	-	-	-	-	0.1	0.0	0.00	0.01	**0.1**	147
Hypopharynx	8	0	-	-	-	-	-	0.3	-	-	0.5	-	-	-	1.8	0.8	0.9	1.5	-	-	0.2	0.1	0.00	0.02	**0.1**	148
Pharynx unspecified	3	0	-	-	-	-	-	-	-	-	0.5	-	-	-	-	0.6	-	0.9	-	-	0.1	0.0	0.00	0.01	**0.1**	149
Oesophagus	125	0	-	-	-	-	-	-	-	-	1.0	2.4	3.8	8.9	16.5	16.8	20.6	23.5	20.7		3.5	0.9	0.08	0.25	**1.9**	150
Stomach	288	0	-	-	-	-	-	-	0.3	2.2	1.5	2.5	5.3	7.6	18.4	23.8	29.7	36.5	82.2	88.2	8.0	2.1	0.19	0.46	**4.2**	151
Small intestine	25	0	-	-	-	-	-	-	-	-	-	1.8	1.3	1.8	3.1	3.0	2.8	4.4	3.8	0.7	0.2	0.02	0.05	**0.4**	152
Colon	1374	0	-	-	1.7	0.4	1.1	1.0	2.1	2.5	11.6	24.3	42.9	72.2	92.5	113.7	151.5	212.6	248.0	276.0	38.1	10.2	1.26	2.59	**22.7**	153
Rectum	673	0	-	-	-	-	-	0.7	1.7	4.0	5.8	10.4	20.6	41.8	48.6	59.3	83.0	86.2	114.5	112.6	18.6	5.0	0.67	1.38	**11.5**	154
Liver	37	0	1.7	-	-	-	-	0.3	-	0.7	0.4	0.5	1.8	2.5	3.0	1.8	2.3	6.6	4.4	-	1.0	0.3	0.05	0.07	**0.8**	155
Gallbladder etc.	198	0	-	-	-	-	-	-	-	0.4	1.2	2.0	5.9	10.1	7.1	20.2	31.2	33.7	32.3	37.5	5.5	1.5	0.13	0.39	**3.1**	156
Pancreas	323	0	-	-	-	-	-	0.7	0.3	0.4	0.8	1.5	4.7	8.9	23.7	27.5	41.9	42.2	76.3	103.3	8.9	2.4	0.20	0.55	**4.8**	157
Nose, sinuses etc.	12	0	-	-	-	-	-	0.3	-	-	-	0.6	0.6	1.8	1.8	0.8	0.9	1.5	-	-	0.3	0.1	0.02	0.03	**0.2**	160
Larynx	26	0	-	-	-	-	-	-	-	-	1.0	1.8	3.6	2.4	4.6	1.9	2.9	-	-	-	0.7	0.2	0.03	0.07	**0.5**	161
Bronchus, lung	867	0	-	-	-	-	0.3	1.7	2.5	5.4	17.4	25.3	45.0	77.1	94.7	121.1	130.2	105.6	67.6		24.0	6.5	0.87	1.95	**15.2**	162
Other thoracic organs	8	0	-	-	-	-	-	-	-	-	0.8	0.5	-	0.6	0.6	1.2	-	0.9	-	-	0.2	0.1	0.01	0.02	**0.2**	163-4
Bone	28	0	0.4	-	0.4	1.5	0.7	1.0	0.7	1.1	1.5	-	-	-	1.2	-	-	2.8	2.9	1.9	0.8	0.2	0.04	0.04	**0.7**	170
Connective tissue	79	0	-	-	1.3	2.6	1.1	1.4	0.3	1.8	2.3	2.0	2.4	3.2	3.0	1.8	4.6	12.2	7.3	9.4	2.2	0.6	0.11	0.14	**1.6**	171
Mesothelioma	25	0	-	-	-	-	-	-	0.3	0.7	0.4	0.5	1.2	2.5	3.0	0.6	1.5	2.8	2.9	1.9	0.7	0.2	0.04	0.05	**0.5**	MES
†Kaposi's sarcoma	1	0	-	-	-	-	-	-	-	0.4	-	-	-	-	-	-	-	-	-	-	0.0	0.0	0.00	0.00	**0.0**	KAP
Melanoma of skin	1177	0	-	0.4	2.5	3.3	12.4	19.6	26.3	38.9	43.4	46.6	52.3	51.9	60.5	74.0	70.1	89.0	80.7	82.6	32.6	8.8	1.79	2.51	**24.9**	172
†Other skin																										
Breast	3341	0	-	-	-	-	1.4	5.8	26.3	57.0	105.4	175.5	192.2	218.5	234.7	254.9	246.7	264.2	294.9	317.3	92.5	24.9	5.08	7.59	**68.5**	174
Uterus unspecified	0	0	-	-	-	-	-	-	-	-	-	-	-	-	-	-	-	-	-	-	0.0	0.0	0.00	0.00	**0.0**	179
Cervix uteri	390	0	-	-	-	-	1.4	10.7	16.9	17.4	23.6	20.3	14.1	8.9	16.0	24.5	16.0	11.2	7.3	24.4	10.8	2.9	0.65	0.85	**8.7**	180
Placenta	3	0	-	-	-	-	-	-	0.7	0.4	-	-	-	-	-	-	-	-	-	-	0.1	0.0	0.01	0.01	**0.1**	181
Corpus uteri	556	0	-	-	-	-	-	0.3	1.4	3.3	9.3	16.9	34.1	37.4	53.3	55.6	50.3	52.5	55.8	48.8	15.4	4.1	0.78	1.31	**10.9**	182
Ovary etc.	480	0	0.4	0.4	0.4	1.1	0.7	2.1	4.2	5.5	7.0	15.4	27.0	32.9	42.1	37.3	41.1	47.8	47.0	43.2	13.3	3.6	0.70	1.09	**9.6**	183
Other female genital	102	0	-	-	-	-	-	0.3	1.0	0.4	1.9	3.5	1.8	2.5	4.7	3.1	11.4	14.1	24.9	33.8	2.8	0.8	0.08	0.15	**1.6**	184
Bladder	374	0	-	-	-	0.4	-	0.3	2.1	0.7	1.9	4.0	9.4	13.9	26.7	36.7	38.8	65.6	60.2	86.4	10.4	2.8	0.30	0.67	**5.9**	188
Kidney etc.	258	0	2.9	0.4	0.4	0.4	-	-	1.0	2.5	2.3	4.0	5.9	14.6	19.0	28.7	31.2	29.0	36.7	28.2	7.1	1.9	0.27	0.57	**4.8**	189
Eye	32	0	0.8	-	-	-	-	1.4	0.7	0.4	0.8	0.5	1.8	3.2	1.8	1.8	0.8	1.9	1.5	3.8	0.9	0.2	0.06	0.07	**0.8**	190
Brain, nervous system	251	0	2.9	4.1	3.4	2.6	2.8	1.4	4.5	5.1	3.9	5.9	8.2	11.4	14.8	15.9	19.8	25.3	27.9	5.6	7.0	1.9	0.36	0.53	**5.5**	191-2
Thyroid	148	0	-	-	-	0.7	3.9	2.4	8.0	6.2	2.7	5.9	5.9	7.0	9.5	6.1	4.6	6.6	7.3	7.5	4.1	1.1	0.26	0.31	**3.3**	193
Other endocrine	11	0	0.8	0.4	0.8	-	-	0.3	-	-	-	0.5	-	-	-	1.2	-	0.9	1.5	-	0.3	0.1	0.01	0.02	**0.3**	194
Hodgkin's disease	67	0	-	-	1.3	3.3	2.5	2.8	2.4	1.5	1.5	1.5	1.8	0.6	3.0	1.8	3.0	0.9	2.9	5.6	1.9	0.5	0.11	0.13	**1.6**	201
Non-Hodgkin lymphoma	498	0	0.4	0.4	0.8	1.5	1.1	2.1	3.1	4.0	12.8	8.4	17.6	20.9	29.0	44.6	62.4	72.1	57.2	52.6	13.8	3.7	0.51	1.05	**9.0**	200,202
Multiple myeloma	178	0	-	-	-	-	-	-	-	-	0.7	0.4	2.0	2.4	7.0	8.3	23.2	24.4	30.0	35.2	4.9	1.3	0.10	0.34	**2.7**	203
Lymphoid leukaemia	258	0	5.8	3.3	1.7	2.2	0.7	0.7	0.7	0.4	0.8	4.0	4.7	8.2	14.8	22.6	27.4	45.0	49.9	15.0	7.1	1.9	0.24	0.49	**5.0**	204
Myeloid leukaemia	195	0	1.2	0.4	0.4	1.8	2.5	1.7	1.0	2.9	3.1	4.0	4.7	5.7	8.3	11.0	12.2	21.5	33.7	65.7	5.4	1.5	0.19	0.31	**3.5**	205
Monocytic leukaemia	6	0	0.4	-	-	-	-	-	-	-	-	0.5	-	0.6	1.2	-	-	-	-	1.9	0.2	0.0	0.01	0.01	**0.2**	206
Other leukaemia	5	0	0.4	-	-	-	-	-	-	-	0.5	0.6	0.6	-	0.6	-	-	-	-	-	0.1	0.0	0.01	0.01	**0.2**	207
Leukaemia unspecified	4	0	0.4	-	-	-	-	-	-	-	-	-	-	-	-	-	-	-	1.5	3.8	0.1	0.0	0.00	0.00	**0.1**	208
Other and unspecified	610	0	-	-	-	-	-	0.7	-	1.1	2.3	6.9	10.6	20.9	34.4	55.0	70.1	87.1	155.5	178.4	16.9	4.5	0.38	1.01	**9.0**	O&U
All sites																										
All sites but 173	13409	0	18.7	9.8	16.5	22.1	33.0	59.8	113.1	168.6	259.6	396.1	520.1	679.7	898.6	1105.1	1255.0	1514.7	1753.5	1824.9	371.4	100.0	15.98	27.78	**250.8**	ALLb

Rate from 1 case

	0-	5-	10-	15-	20-	25-	30-	35-	40-	45-	50-	55-	60-	65-	70-	75-	80-	85+
	0.415	0.409	0.422	0.369	0.355	0.344	0.346	0.363	0.387	0.496	0.588	0.633	0.593	0.611	0.762	0.937	1.467	1.877

†Important: see notes on population page

Australia, Tasmania

The Tasmanian Cancer Registry was established in 1977, as a population-based registry covering the whole state. It was set up to provide the State Government with accurate cancer incidence and mortality statistics and the capacity to monitor cancer trends. In July 1988 responsibility for the operation of the cancer registry was transferred from the Department of Health Services to the Menzies Centre for Population Health Research which is affiliated to the University of Tasmania in Hobart. The State Government Department of Community and Health Services provides an annual grant to cover salaries, while the Menzies Centre provides housing, administrative, biostatistics, computing and other relevant services.

Tasmania, the smallest state of Australia, is an island of 68 300 km^2, about 0.9% of the total area of Australia. It lies between 40°38´ and 43°39´ S, and has a temperate climate. The principal industries are pulp and paper, metal refining, vegetable processing, farming and wine growing. There is a small chemical industry. Hydroelectric stations provide nearly all the electricity. Wood fires for home heating produce smoke in populated areas during the winter, but there is otherwise little air pollution. Some heavy metal pollution of river waters occurs in certain areas.

At the 1991 census, Tasmania had a population of 452 837 persons (50.3% female and 49.7% male), 75% of whom live in urban centres (localities with 1000 or more persons). In 1991 the median age of the population was 32.6 years, a significant rise from 27.4 years in 1976. There were 7703 people of aboriginal descent in Tasmania and 1245 descendants of Torres Strait Islanders. 89.2% of the population was born in Australia. The biggest group of migrants (5.3%) came from the United Kingdom. Data on religious affiliation is not recorded in the registry, but limited information on racial origin has been recorded since 1991. Occupation is recorded where available but not actively sought for every case.

The registry depended on voluntary notification between 1978 and 1992; since December 1992 cancer has been a notifiable disease. The registry is assisted by an Advisory Committee and a Data Release Committee. The registry staff comprises a non medical registrar, two clerks and a part-time clerical assistant. The registry has access to a biostatistician and a computer consultant. The medical director of the registry is the Director of the Menzies Centre for Population Health Research.

Tasmania is well served by oncology services. The three main population regions each have a public hospital system as well as several private hospitals. There are two radiation oncology units in the state.

All the pathology laboratories in the state send the registry copies of histopathological and cytology reports. Discharge summaries are supplied by the two radiation oncology clinics. Private and public hospitals notify cancer to the registry upon discharge of patients. Public hospitals provide annual computerized listings of cancer cases diagnosed during the previous calendar year. Copies of death certificates of people dying in Tasmania of all causes are received by the registry. Since 1994, listings from breast and cervix cancer screening programmes have been available to check against registry records.

In 1991 new cancer registration software was installed. Incoming paper is date stamped and checked against the computer database. If the case is already on the database any extra information is added. If the case is not on computer, a record and index card is generated and the record filed away pending disease coding and entry on to the computer.

The registry collects all pathology reports of non-melanoma skin cancers, but since 1988 no longer reports incidence.

The registry has no direct contact with patients. Follow-up is principally through death certificates, electoral rolls and annual computer listings of public hospital in-patients. Occasionally active follow-up is undertaken by means of a search of medical records or letters to medical practitioners. All Australian registries exchange details of cancer patients who have a residential address in another state. In addition, the National Cancer Statistics Clearing House in Canberra collates all state and territory data and checks for duplicate registrations. It is believed that registration is close to 100%, due to complete cooperation of pathology laboratories and hospitals. In addition, the small population of the state permits quite extensive follow-up of individual cases.

Cases are not accepted at the registry on the basis of a death certificate only. Each death certificate is researched until the time and place of diagnosis is ascertained. A significant minority of these turn out to be cases diagnosed in another State, or cases diagnosed in the years prior to 1978. These early cases are added to the data-base so that Tasmanian cancer mortality statistics can be accurately calculated.

Cancer registry data have formed the basis for a number of descriptive publications, and are used by medical practitioners making presentations at a conference, tertiary students carrying out assignments and health service organizations requiring data for planning purposes. A major user is now the Cancer Screening and Prevention Unit , where the breast and cervix screening programmes are conducted.

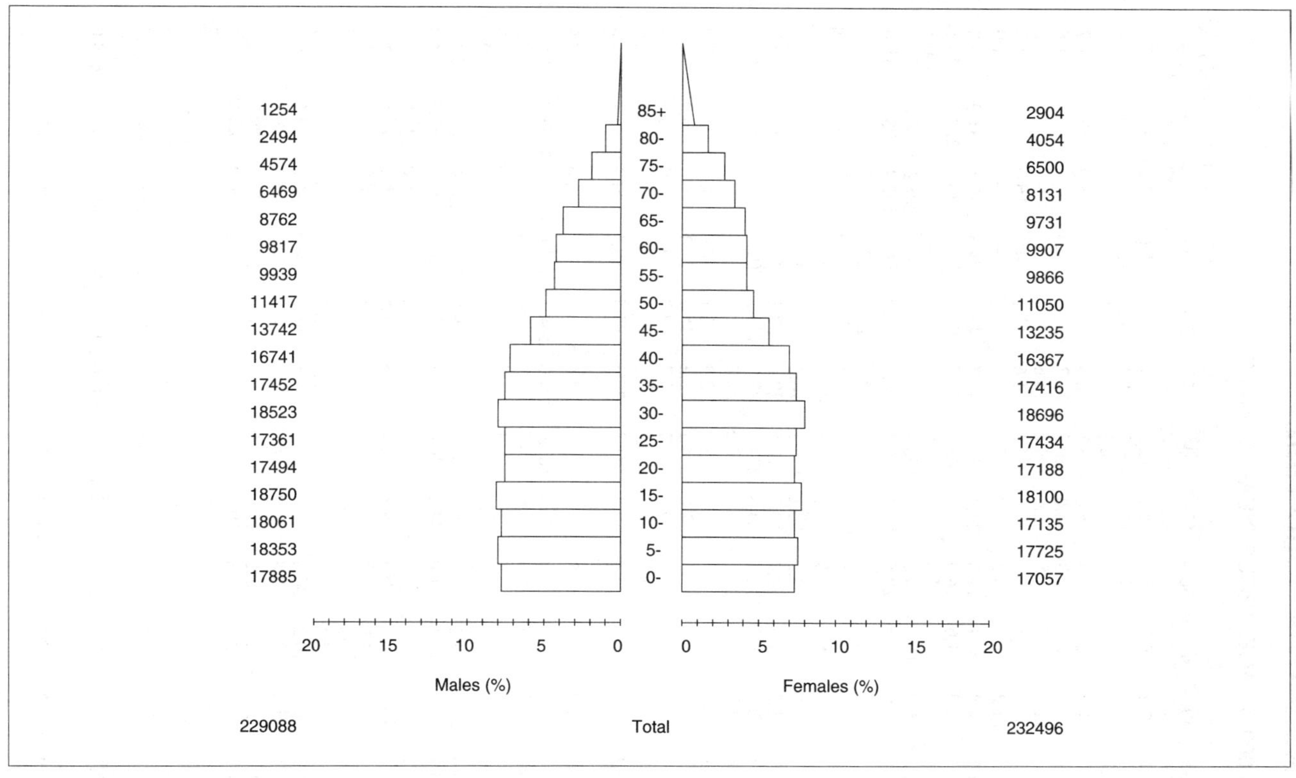

Australia, Tasmania
Source of population: average annual 1988–92
Census: 1986, 1991.
Estimate: The populations for each of the years 1988–92 were intercensal estimates, initially obtained from the 1986 Census by advancing age and allowing for migration, births and deaths. They have not been adjusted in the light of the 1991 Census. Ref.: Australian Bureau of Statistics No. 3204.6, 1988-92.

Notes to tables overleaf:
† Kaposi's sarcoma is under-reported in this volume because cases of skin cancer (ICD-9 173) were not provided.
† 173 not available
† 188 does not include the non-invasive tumours

AUSTRALIA, TASMANIA 1988-1992

ANNUAL INCIDENCE PER 100,000 BY AGE GROUP (YEARS) - MALE

SITE	ALL AGES	AGE UNK	0-	5-	10-	15-	20-	25-	30-	35-	40-	45-	50-	55-	60-	65-	70-	75-	80-	85+	CRUDE RATE	%	CR 64	CR 74	ASR (W)	ICD (9th)
Lip	89	0	-	-	-	-	-	2.3	-	4.6	7.2	8.7	15.8	18.1	18.3	41.1	34.0	35.0	32.1	47.8	7.8	1.9	0.37	0.75	6.3	140
Tongue	31	0	-	-	-	-	-	1.2	-	1.1	-	1.5	14.0	14.1	6.1	11.4	6.2	13.1	-	-	2.7	0.7	0.19	0.28	2.4	141
Salivary gland	5	0	-	-	-	-	-	-	-	-	-	-	-	-	4.1	-	9.3	-	-	-	0.4	0.1	0.02	0.07	0.3	142
Mouth	19	0	-	-	-	-	-	-	-	1.2	2.9	3.5	6.0	8.1	2.3	9.3	4.4	8.0	15.9	-	1.7	0.4	0.11	0.17	1.4	143-5
Oropharynx	21	0	-	-	-	-	-	1.1	-	1.2	2.9	1.8	8.0	10.2	13.7	-	4.4	-	-	-	1.8	0.4	0.13	0.19	1.6	146
Nasopharynx	10	0	-	-	-	-	-	1.1	-	2.4	1.5	1.8	2.0	4.1	4.6	-	-	-	-	-	0.9	0.2	0.06	0.09	0.8	147
Hypopharynx	13	0	-	-	-	-	-	-	-	-	1.5	-	8.0	4.1	4.6	3.1	4.4	16.0	-	-	1.1	0.3	0.07	0.11	0.9	148
Pharynx unspecified	12	0	-	-	-	-	-	-	-	1.2	2.9	5.3	2.0	2.0	9.1	-	-	-	-	-	1.0	0.3	0.07	0.11	0.9	149
Oesophagus	103	0	-	-	-	-	-	-	-	1.1	4.8	4.4	14.0	26.2	32.6	45.7	43.3	74.3	40.1	31.9	9.0	2.2	0.42	0.86	7.0	150
Stomach	173	0	-	-	-	-	-	1.2	1.1	1.1	6.0	14.6	14.0	26.2	38.7	52.5	95.8	139.9	120.3	223.3	15.1	3.7	0.51	1.26	11.4	151
Small intestine	4	0	-	-	-	-	-	-	-	-	-	-	1.8	-	2.0	4.6	-	-	-	-	0.3	0.1	0.02	0.04	0.3	152
Colon	447	0	-	-	1.1	1.1	1.1	-	1.1	1.1	6.0	16.0	64.8	90.5	150.8	207.7	197.9	244.9	288.6	366.8	39.0	9.6	1.67	3.70	30.5	153
Rectum	225	0	-	-	-	-	-	1.2	1.1	6.9	6.0	11.6	29.8	58.4	59.1	100.4	102.0	96.2	192.4	95.7	19.6	4.8	0.87	1.88	15.3	154
Liver	32	0	1.1	-	-	-	-	-	-	-	-	2.9	3.5	6.0	12.2	9.1	24.7	17.5	8.0	15.9	2.8	0.7	0.13	0.30	2.3	155
Gallbladder etc.	24	0	-	-	-	-	-	-	1.1	-	-	-	3.5	4.0	10.2	2.3	9.3	21.9	8.0	63.8	2.1	0.5	0.09	0.15	1.6	156
Pancreas	93	0	-	-	-	-	-	-	-	2.3	3.6	5.8	3.5	8.0	18.3	45.7	46.4	83.1	64.1	111.6	8.1	2.0	0.21	0.67	5.9	157
Nose, sinuses etc.	29	0	-	-	-	-	-	-	-	-	1.2	2.9	5.3	10.1	4.1	16.0	12.4	17.5	8.0	-	2.5	0.6	0.12	0.26	2.0	160
Larynx	65	0	-	-	-	-	-	-	-	-	1.2	1.5	8.8	10.1	28.5	29.7	37.1	43.7	24.1	15.9	5.7	1.4	0.25	0.58	4.4	161
Bronchus, lung	751	0	-	-	-	-	-	1.2	1.1	2.3	10.8	26.2	70.1	124.8	224.1	383.5	445.2	502.8	505.1	287.1	65.6	16.1	2.30	6.45	49.4	162
Other thoracic organs	6	0	-	-	-	1.1	-	-	-	-	1.2	2.9	-	-	2.0	2.3	-	-	-	-	0.5	0.1	0.04	0.05	0.5	163-4
Bone	10	0	-	-	-	2.1	-	-	1.1	1.1	-	1.5	-	-	2.0	2.3	3.1	4.4	8.0	-	0.9	0.2	0.04	0.07	0.7	170
Connective tissue	28	0	2.2	1.1	1.1	1.1	1.1	1.2	2.2	-	1.2	-	5.3	2.0	4.1	2.3	15.5	13.1	16.0	15.9	2.4	0.6	0.11	0.20	2.1	171
Mesothelioma	19	0	-	-	-	-	-	-	-	-	-	-	-	4.0	8.1	13.7	9.3	4.4	8.0	31.9	1.7	0.4	0.06	0.18	1.3	MES
†Kaposi's sarcoma	2	0	-	-	-	-	-	1.2	-	-	-	-	1.8	-	-	-	-	-	-	-	0.2	0.0	0.01	0.01	0.2	KAP
Melanoma of skin	328	0	-	-	-	6.4	10.3	17.3	37.8	33.2	29.9	39.3	33.3	42.3	71.3	75.3	80.4	118.1	120.3	95.7	28.6	7.0	1.60	2.38	23.5	172
†Other skin																										
Breast	6	0	-	-	-	-	-	-	-	-	1.2	-	1.8	-	-	4.6	3.1	-	8.0	-	0.5	0.1	0.01	0.05	0.4	175
Prostate	859	0	-	-	-	-	-	-	-	-	2.4	10.2	15.8	70.4	165.0	299.0	544.1	822.0	1194.7	1291.9	75.0	18.4	1.32	5.53	51.5	185
Testis	63	0	2.2	-	-	-	3.4	11.5	18.4	10.3	9.6	8.7	5.3	2.0	6.1	-	-	4.4	-	-	5.5	1.3	0.39	0.39	4.9	186
Penis	7	0	-	-	-	-	-	-	-	-	1.2	-	1.8	-	6.1	2.3	-	4.4	-	-	0.6	0.1	0.05	0.06	0.5	187.1-.4
Other male genital	1	0	-	-	-	-	-	-	-	-	-	-	-	-	-	2.3	-	-	-	-	0.1	0.0	0.00	0.01	0.1	187.5-.9
†Bladder	267	0	1.1	-	-	-	-	1.1	1.2	1.1	3.4	1.2	13.1	21.0	36.2	59.1	116.4	129.8	231.7	256.6	207.3	23.3	5.7	0.69	1.92	17.0	188
Kidney etc.	149	0	-	-	-	-	-	-	1.1	3.4	8.4	13.1	21.0	34.2	30.6	50.2	61.8	126.8	96.2	31.9	13.0	3.2	0.56	1.12	9.9	189
Eye	11	0	2.2	-	-	-	-	-	-	1.1	-	-	-	-	4.1	4.6	6.2	-	8.0	15.9	1.0	0.2	0.04	0.09	0.9	190
Brain, nervous system	100	0	1.1	3.3	5.5	2.1	2.3	2.3	4.3	11.5	10.8	8.7	10.5	24.1	12.2	22.8	27.8	21.9	56.1	15.9	8.7	2.1	0.49	0.75	7.4	191-2
Thyroid	21	0	-	-	-	-	1.1	-	-	1.1	3.6	5.8	3.5	2.0	-	9.1	3.1	13.1	8.0	-	1.8	0.4	0.09	0.15	1.5	193
Other endocrine	5	0	1.1	-	1.1	1.1	-	2.3	-	-	-	-	-	-	-	-	-	-	-	-	0.4	0.1	0.03	0.03	0.5	194
Hodgkin's disease	20	0	1.1	-	-	1.1	3.4	1.2	2.2	1.1	-	4.4	-	2.0	2.0	2.3	6.2	8.7	8.0	-	1.7	0.4	0.09	0.13	1.5	201
Non-Hodgkin lymphoma	186	0	-	-	1.1	5.3	-	3.5	5.4	9.2	10.8	10.2	36.8	26.2	61.1	54.8	68.0	74.3	96.2	143.5	16.2	4.0	0.85	1.46	13.3	200,202
Multiple myeloma	60	0	-	-	-	-	-	-	-	1.1	1.2	2.9	8.8	8.0	18.3	22.8	30.9	30.6	48.1	79.7	5.2	1.3	0.20	0.47	4.1	203
Lymphoid leukaemia	89	0	7.8	3.3	3.3	-	2.3	1.2	-	1.1	2.4	4.4	1.8	12.1	12.2	38.8	58.7	26.2	56.1	79.7	7.8	1.9	0.26	0.75	6.7	204
Myeloid leukaemia	61	0	1.1	-	-	-	2.3	1.2	4.3	1.1	1.2	2.9	8.8	10.1	8.1	22.8	15.5	21.9	96.2	47.8	5.3	1.3	0.21	0.40	4.1	205
Monocytic leukaemia	2	0	-	-	-	-	-	-	1.1	-	-	-	-	-	3.1	-	-	-	-	-	0.2	0.0	0.01	0.02	0.1	206
Other leukaemia	1	0	-	-	-	-	-	-	-	-	-	1.8	-	-	-	-	-	-	-	-	0.1	0.0	0.01	0.01	0.1	207
Leukaemia unspecified	6	0	-	-	-	-	-	-	-	-	-	1.8	2.0	2.0	4.6	-	4.4	-	-	-	0.5	0.1	0.03	0.05	0.4	208
Other and unspecified	221	0	-	-	-	-	-	1.2	3.2	-	6.0	4.4	14.0	52.3	48.9	63.9	126.8	139.9	208.5	382.8	19.3	4.7	0.65	1.60	14.5	O&U
All sites																										
All sites but 173	4674	0	21.2	7.6	13.3	21.3	28.6	51.8	89.6	99.7	144.6	240.1	455.4	752.5	1161.2	1801.0	2269.2	2973.3	3608.1	3716.1	408.0	100.0	15.44	35.79	312.4	ALLb

Rate from 1 case: 1.118 1.090 1.107 1.067 1.143 1.152 1.080 1.146 1.195 1.455 1.752 2.012 2.037 2.283 3.092 4.373 8.018 15.949

†Important: see notes on population page

AUSTRALIA, TASMANIA 1988-1992

ANNUAL INCIDENCE PER 100,000 BY AGE GROUP (YEARS) - FEMALE

SITE	ALL AGES	AGE UNK	0-	5-	10-	15-	20-	25-	30-	35-	40-	45-	50-	55-	60-	65-	70-	75-	80-	85+	CRUDE RATE	%	CR 64	CR 74	ASR (W)	ICD (9th)
Lip	25	0	-	-	-	-	-	-	-	-	-	-	1.8	4.1	6.1	2.1	7.4	18.5	19.7	34.4	2.2	0.7	0.06	0.11	1.2	140
Tongue	12	0	-	-	-	-	-	-	-	-	-	-	1.8	6.1	8.1	-	4.9	6.2	-	-	1.0	0.3	0.08	0.10	0.8	141
Salivary gland	8	0	-	-	-	-	-	-	-	-	-	1.5	1.8	2.0	-	4.1	4.9	-	4.9	-	0.7	0.2	0.03	0.07	0.5	142
Mouth	20	0	-	-	-	-	-	-	-	-	1.2	-	-	4.1	6.1	14.4	9.8	-	4.9	13.8	1.7	0.5	0.06	0.18	1.2	143-5
Oropharynx	5	0	-	-	-	-	-	-	-	-	-	-	1.8	2.0	2.0	-	4.9	-	-	-	0.4	0.1	0.03	0.05	0.4	146
Nasopharynx	5	0	-	-	-	1.1	1.2	-	-	-	-	-	-	2.0	-	-	-	3.1	4.9	-	0.4	0.1	0.02	0.02	0.3	147
Hypopharynx	1	0	-	-	-	-	-	-	-	-	-	-	-	-	-	2.1	-	-	-	-	0.1	0.0	0.00	0.01	0.1	148
Pharynx unspecified	2	0	-	-	-	-	-	-	-	-	-	-	-	-	-	2.1	2.5	-	-	-	0.2	0.1	0.00	0.02	0.1	149
Oesophagus	70	0	-	-	-	-	-	-	-	-	-	-	3.6	10.1	16.1	20.6	34.4	21.5	78.9	55.1	6.0	1.8	0.15	0.42	3.4	150
Stomach	95	0	-	-	-	-	1.2	2.3	1.1	2.3	2.4	3.0	3.6	14.2	12.1	18.5	44.3	36.9	74.0	110.2	8.2	2.5	0.21	0.52	4.8	151
Small intestine	5	0	-	-	-	-	-	-	-	-	-	-	1.8	-	4.0	-	2.5	3.1	-	-	0.4	0.1	0.03	0.04	0.3	152
Colon	417	0	-	-	-	-	1.2	-	2.1	5.7	11.0	24.2	50.7	68.9	76.7	115.1	155.0	221.5	222.0	330.5	35.9	10.9	1.20	2.55	22.6	153
Rectum	189	0	-	-	-	-	-	1.1	6.9	6.1	7.6	21.7	26.4	52.5	82.2	59.0	73.8	83.9	110.2	16.3	4.9	0.61	1.32	10.9	154
Liver	6	0	-	-	-	-	-	1.1	-	-	-	-	1.8	-	-	4.9	3.1	-	6.9		0.5	0.2	0.01	0.04	0.3	155
Gallbladder etc.	38	0	-	-	-	-	-	-	1.1	-	-	5.4	2.0	10.1	14.4	22.1	18.5	14.8	20.7	3.3	1.0	0.09	0.28	2.1	156
Pancreas	94	0	-	-	-	-	-	-	2.3	2.4	6.0	1.8	18.2	4.0	26.7	46.7	52.3	74.0	68.9	8.1	2.4	0.17	0.54	4.6	157
Nose, sinuses etc.	6	0	-	-	-	-	-	-	1.2	-	1.8	-	2.0	6.2	-	-	-	-	-	0.5	0.2	0.03	0.06	0.4	160
Larynx	6	0	-	-	-	-	-	-	1.2	-	-	2.0	4.1	-	-	-	-	13.8		0.5	0.2	0.02	0.02	0.3	161
Bronchus, lung	298	0	-	-	-	-	-	-	3.4	18.3	24.2	39.8	62.8	96.9	131.5	100.8	86.1	93.7	75.7	25.6	7.8	1.23	2.39	18.8	162
Other thoracic organs	3	0	1.2	-	-	-	-	-	-	1.5	-	-	-	-	-	-	-	6.9		0.3	0.1	0.01	0.01	0.3	163-4
Bone	7	0	-	-	-	1.1	-	1.1	1.1	-	-	-	4.1	-	2.1	2.5	-	-		0.6	0.2	0.04	0.06	0.5	170
Connective tissue	30	0	1.2	-	2.3	-	3.5	-	1.1	6.1	4.5	5.4	4.1	8.1	2.1	2.5	6.2	-	13.8	2.6	0.8	0.18	0.20	2.3	171
Mesothelioma	2	0	-	-	-	-	-	1.1	-	-	-	-	-	-	-	2.5	-	-		0.2	0.1	0.01	0.02	0.1	MES
†Kaposi's sarcoma	1	0	-	-	-	-	-	-	-	-	-	-	-	-	-	-	4.9	-		0.1	0.0	0.00	0.00	0.0	KAP
Melanoma of skin	337	0	-	-	1.2	2.2	16.3	26.4	33.2	28.7	46.4	37.8	45.2	50.7	40.4	71.9	46.7	76.9	88.8	75.7	29.0	8.8	1.64	2.24	23.1	172
†Other skin																										
Breast	877	0	-	-	-	-	8.0	20.3	45.9	97.8	139.0	164.7	154.1	189.8	211.7	201.7	261.5	296.0	330.5	75.4	22.8	4.10	6.16	56.9	174
Uterus unspecified	0	0	-	-	-	-	-	-	-	-	-	-	-	-	-	-	-	-	-	0.0	0.0	0.00	0.00	0.0	179
Cervix uteri	153	0	-	-	1.1	3.5	12.6	16.0	17.2	15.9	19.6	21.7	18.2	26.2	34.9	34.4	27.7	19.7	27.5	13.2	4.0	0.76	1.11	10.6	180
Placenta	0	0	-	-	-	-	-	-	-	-	-	-	-	-	-	-	-	-	-	0.0	0.0	0.00	0.00	0.0	181
Corpus uteri	165	0	-	-	-	-	-	2.1	-	4.9	4.5	39.8	52.7	50.5	39.1	73.8	36.9	69.1	55.1	14.2	4.3	0.77	1.34	10.4	182
Ovary etc.	127	0	-	2.3	-	1.1	3.5	1.1	-	10.3	6.1	21.2	12.7	26.4	36.3	24.7	34.4	49.2	14.8	62.0	10.9	3.3	0.60	0.90	8.4	183
Other female genital	33	0	-	-	-	1.2	-	-	-	2.4	1.5	3.6	8.1	8.1	6.2	12.3	12.3	24.7	13.8	2.8	0.9	0.12	0.22	1.9	184
†Bladder	87	0	-	-	-	-	-	-	1.1	4.9	6.0	10.9	10.1	10.1	20.6	41.8	36.9	74.0	55.1	7.5	2.3	0.22	0.53	4.5	188
Kidney etc.	68	0	2.3	-	-	-	-	1.1	-	1.1	1.2	4.5	5.4	6.1	18.2	22.6	27.1	43.1	14.8	41.3	5.8	1.8	0.20	0.45	4.0	189
Eye	5	0	-	-	-	-	-	-	-	1.2	-	1.8	-	2.0	2.1	-	3.1	-	-	0.4	0.1	0.03	0.04	0.3	190
Brain, nervous system	69	0	1.2	1.1	3.5	-	5.8	2.3	4.3	3.4	7.3	3.0	9.0	14.2	16.1	12.3	14.8	24.6	9.9	-	5.9	1.8	0.36	0.49	4.9	191-2
Thyroid	43	0	-	-	1.1	3.5	1.1	4.3	10.3	7.3	6.0	7.2	4.1	2.0	-	9.8	3.1	14.8		3.7	1.1	0.24	0.28	3.1	193
Other endocrine	4	0	2.3	-	-	-	-	-	-	-	1.5	-	-	-	-	2.5	-	-		0.3	0.1	0.02	0.03	0.4	194
Hodgkin's disease	27	0	-	-	2.3	5.5	3.5	1.1	5.3	1.1	2.4	-	6.1	2.0	8.2	-	-	-	-	2.3	0.7	0.15	0.19	2.2	201
Non-Hodgkin lymphoma	147	0	1.2	1.1	1.2	1.1	-	1.1	5.3	8.0	8.6	9.1	23.5	30.4	30.3	49.3	59.0	43.1	49.3	13.8	12.6	3.8	0.60	1.15	9.4	200,202
Multiple myeloma	40	0	-	-	-	-	-	-	-	1.1	-	1.5	1.8	4.1	8.1	18.5	22.1	15.4	29.6	13.8	3.4	1.0	0.08	0.29	2.1	203
Lymphoid leukaemia	52	0	2.3	2.3	-	-	-	1.1	-	-	1.2	-	1.8	4.1	16.1	20.6	27.1	18.5	24.7	20.7	4.5	1.4	0.14	0.38	3.1	204
Myeloid leukaemia	59	0	-	3.4	1.2	1.1	-	3.4	1.1	1.1	3.7	-	7.2	2.0	16.1	10.3	27.1	18.5	24.7	41.3	5.1	1.5	0.20	0.39	3.6	205
Monocytic leukaemia	1	0	-	-	-	-	-	-	-	-	-	-	-	-	-	-	-	4.9	-	0.1	0.0	0.00	0.00	0.0	206
Other leukaemia	1	0	-	-	1.2	-	-	-	-	-	-	-	-	-	-	-	-	-		0.1	0.0	0.01	0.01	0.1	207
Leukaemia unspecified	2	0	-	-	-	-	-	-	-	-	-	-	-	-	-	-	2.5	3.1	-	0.2	0.1	0.00	0.01	0.1	208
Other and unspecified	199	0	-	-	-	-	-	1.1	2.3	6.1	3.0	5.4	16.2	32.3	65.8	66.4	138.1	138.5	206.6	17.1	5.2	0.33	0.99	9.4	O&U
All sites																										
All sites but 173	3841	0	11.7	10.2	12.8	15.5	44.2	61.9	100.6	156.2	267.6	330.9	506.8	640.5	809.5	1066.7	1215.1	1363.0	1578.5	1817.8	330.4	100.0	14.84	26.25	235.0	ALLb

Rate from 1 case   1.173 1.128 1.167 1.105 1.164 1.147 1.070 1.148 1.222 1.511 1.810 2.027 2.019 2.055 2.460 3.077 4.933 6.886

†Important: see notes on population page

Australia, Victoria

In 1940, the Anti-Cancer Council of Victoria established the first cancer registry in Australia. By 1958 ten major teaching hospitals in Melbourne were contributing information to the registry on a voluntary basis. During the late 1970s registration was expanded to include other voluntary notifiers, particularly pathologists. In December 1981 notification of cancer became compulsory for all hospitals and pathology laboratories.

The registry covers the State of Victoria, the second most populous state in the Australian Commonwealth. Victoria is situated in the south-eastern corner of Australia between 35° and 39° S and 141° and 150° E. It is bounded to the north by New South Wales and to the west by South Australia. Its land area is 227 600 km^2 (3% of the area of Australia) and it has 1800 km of coastline. The Great Dividing Range which runs east–west across the state ensures that the southern half of the state receives much more rain than the north. The ocean to the south has a moderating effect on extremes of temperature, but in summer, the temperature may rise above 35°C with a strong northerly wind.

The population in 1991 comprised 4 420 373 persons, of whom 21% were children under 15 years and 11% aged 65 years or more. Almost three quarters live in the Melbourne Metropolitan Area. The average population density is 19.4 persons per km^2, ranging from less than 2 in the Wimmera to over 400 in the Melbourne Statistical Division.

At the 1991 census, 1 114 184 persons were described as being overseas-born. Of these, 21% were from Great Britain, 9% from Italy, 6% from Greece, 6% from Yugoslavia, 4% from Viet Nam, and most of the remainder from other European countries and the USSR, Malaysia, China or India. Almost 70% of Victorians were Christians (28% Catholic) and less than 1% each of Muslim, Jewish, Buddhist, Hindu and other religious denominations; one third of Victorians had no stated religion.

The employed population in 1991 was 1 972 100. Of these 24% worked in public administration, defence and community services, 20% in wholesale and retail trades, 19% in manufacturing, 12% in finance and business services, 7% each in construction, transport and communication, and recreation and personal services, and 5% in agriculture, forestry and fishing. Unemployment was 9.7%. Primary industries include mining, forestry and agriculture. Most secondary industries are concentrated in and around Melbourne, except for steel mills and smelters.

Victoria's medical care system is a mix of private and public sectors. In 1990 there were 154 public hospitals with several specialist oncology units, and one large hospital dedicated to cancer treatment, with a total of 14 891 public hospital beds. In addition, 116 private hospitals contained 6265 beds.

The registry receives reports from all hospitals and pathology laboratories in Victoria, increasingly in electronic form, and exchanges reports on non-residents with neighbouring states. Other data sources include death certificates, supplied on magnetic tape by the Registrar of Births, Deaths and Marriages. Some active follow-up is pursued for cases in specialist sub-registers, e.g. for *in-situ* and small invasive breast cancers, CNS neoplasms, childhood cancers and prostate cancers.

The minimum data-set includes identifiers for the patient, notifier and doctor, the patient's country of birth, vital status and date of last contact, date of diagnosis, basis of diagnosis, tumour topography (ICD-9) and morphology (ICD-O). No information is recorded on occupation or treatment. Each subsequent registration for the same tumour is added to a further registration file where the notifier, admission date and treating doctor are recorded. The registry records every primary tumour (including *in situ* forms) diagnosed in an individual, including each of several multiple melanomas, but follows IARC conventions for reporting multiple tumours as incident cases.

The data are rigorously checked for validity and consistency at input by the computer and routine checks are regularly run on the entire file. Data quality is assured by matching pathology reports with hospital registrations. A consultant pathologist advises on coding matters. For death-certificate-only registrations, a letter is sent to the doctor signing the death certificate to confirm the diagnosis; the registry does not contact patients directly.

The registry produces regular statistical reports and occasional overviews of its accumulated data, as well as a regular pamphlet called CANSTAT containing a digest of cancer facts and figures. Within the Anti-Cancer Council, registry data are used to assess cancer incidence and trends, particularly with regard to cancers targeted by prevention programmes, e.g. skin, lung, breast and cervix. The registry also facilitates cancer management surveys by identifying random samples of patients and sending their treating doctors questionnaires regarding their patterns of care for individual patients. The registry is also used to follow up cancer events in cohort studies, to identify cases for case–control studies and to confirm the occurrence of cancer in population-based studies of familial cancer of the breast, bowel and prostate.

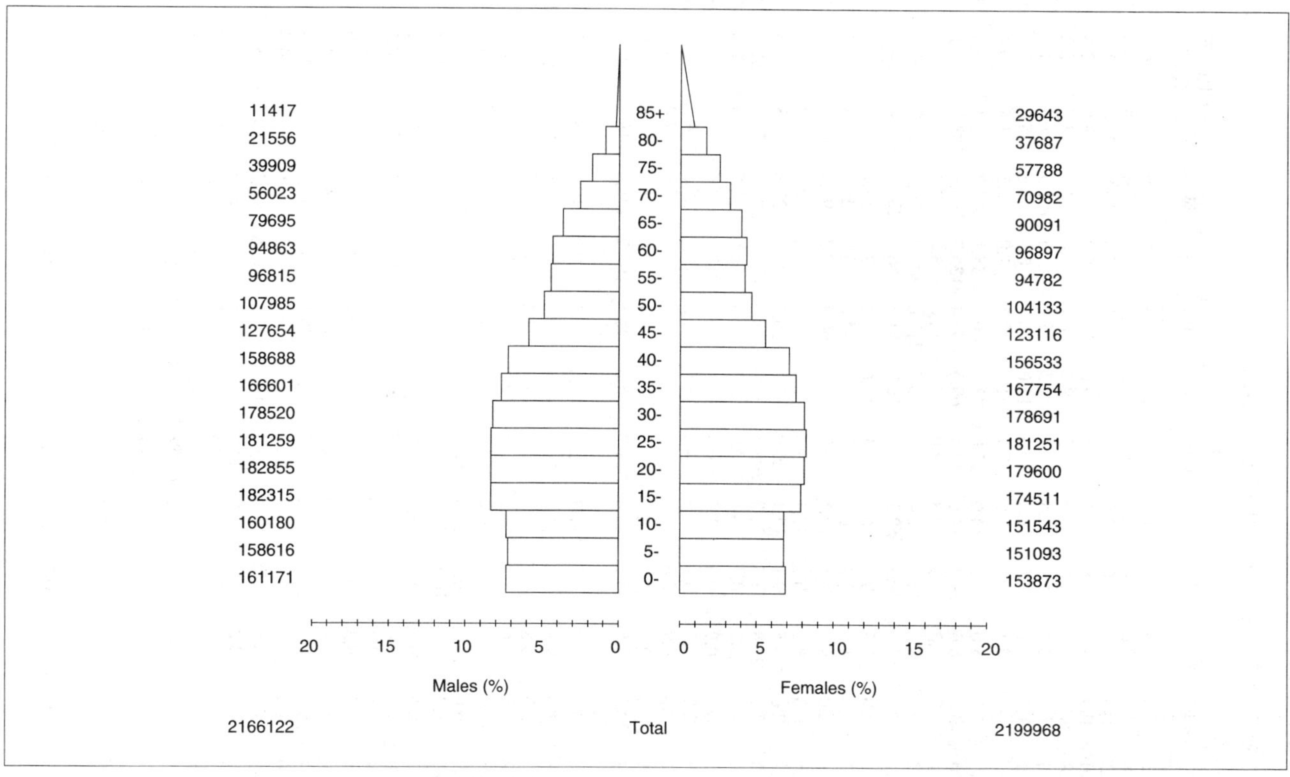

Australia, Victoria

Source of population: average annual 1988–92

Census: 1991. Final estimates from Australian Bureau of Statistics, Estimated Resident Population by Sex and Age, States and Territories of Australia (Catalogue No. 3201.0, released January 1994). The estimates by age at the date of the Census are derived from the census counts, adjusting for under-enumeration and for the number of Australian residents estimated to have been temporarily overseas at the time of the census.

Estimate: Post-censal age distributions are obtained by advancing age, subtracting deaths and adding births and net estimated interstate and overseas migration. After each Census final estimates for the preceding intercensal period are provided by incorporating an additional adjustment (inter-censal discrepancy) to ensure that the total intercensal increase at each age agrees with the differences between the estimated resident population at the two respective Census dates.

Notes to data overleaf:

† Kaposi's sarcoma is under-reported in this volume because cases of skin cancer (ICD-9 173) were not provided.

† 173 not available

Screening programmes in the area

The population over age 20 has been screened for cervical cancer since 1965. In 1994 562 000 women were examined. A breast cancer screening programme commenced in 1990 for women over age 40, with active recruitment of women aged 40-69. 116 335 examinations were carried out in 1994.

AUSTRALIA, VICTORIA 1988-1992

ANNUAL INCIDENCE PER 100,000 BY AGE GROUP (YEARS) - MALE

SITE	ALL AGES	AGE UNK	0-	5-	10-	15-	20-	25-	30-	35-	40-	45-	50-	55-	60-	65-	70-	75-	80-	85+	CRUDE RATE	%	CR 64	CR 74	ASR (W)	ICD (9th)
Lip	668	0	-	-	-	0.1	0.1	0.7	2.0	4.3	3.5	6.6	10.0	11.6	18.3	28.1	31.4	33.6	39.0	52.6	6.2	1.6	0.29	0.58	5.0	140
Tongue	273	0	-	0.1	-	-	0.1	0.2	0.7	0.8	3.2	3.8	5.0	8.3	8.6	9.3	11.4	8.5	7.4	8.8	2.5	0.6	0.15	0.26	2.1	141
Salivary gland	152	0	-	-	-	0.2	0.1	0.2	0.2	0.2	0.5	0.5	2.0	3.5	5.3	4.5	7.1	7.5	15.8	22.8	1.4	0.4	0.06	0.12	1.1	142
Mouth	307	0	-	-	0.1	-	0.1	0.1	0.1	1.0	0.9	3.8	5.6	7.2	13.3	15.6	10.7	15.0	11.1	3.5	2.8	0.7	0.16	0.29	2.4	143-5
Oropharynx	242	0	-	-	-	-	-	-	0.3	0.8	1.8	3.0	4.6	8.5	9.5	9.5	10.4	7.0	4.6	3.5	2.2	0.6	0.14	0.24	1.9	146
Nasopharynx	103	0	-	-	-	0.2	0.1	0.1	0.9	0.8	1.5	2.4	1.9	2.5	2.1	2.3	2.9	2.5	1.9	1.8	1.0	0.2	0.06	0.09	0.8	147
Hypopharynx	208	0	-	-	-	-	-	-	-	0.2	1.0	1.1	4.1	7.6	10.5	11.0	6.1	6.5	4.6	5.3	1.9	0.5	0.12	0.21	1.6	148
Pharynx unspecified	48	0	-	-	-	-	-	0.1	-	-	-	0.5	0.6	1.9	2.7	1.5	2.5	1.0	2.8	1.8	0.4	0.1	0.03	0.05	0.4	149
Oesophagus	735	0	-	-	-	-	-	0.1	0.1	0.6	1.1	5.0	7.2	14.0	25.9	33.1	40.7	55.1	60.3	63.1	6.8	1.7	0.27	0.64	5.4	150
Stomach	1631	0	-	-	-	0.2	-	0.4	1.0	2.6	3.8	8.6	19.3	24.0	43.9	69.5	96.4	125.3	166.1	183.9	15.1	3.9	0.52	1.35	11.7	151
Small intestine	93	0	-	-	-	-	0.1	-	0.1	0.1	0.3	1.3	0.9	2.3	3.0	5.3	4.6	3.0	7.4	3.5	0.9	0.2	0.04	0.09	0.7	152
Colon	3834	0	-	-	0.1	-	0.3	0.8	1.3	5.2	9.5	18.3	32.2	62.4	112.6	176.7	219.6	303.2	370.2	425.7	35.4	9.1	1.21	3.19	27.5	153
Rectum	2610	0	-	-	-	-	-	0.2	1.2	3.7	7.4	14.4	34.3	59.7	86.2	110.9	151.7	168.4	202.3	194.4	24.1	6.2	1.04	2.35	19.2	154
Liver	401	0	0.2	-	0.1	0.1	0.2	-	0.8	0.7	1.0	1.6	5.4	6.6	17.1	16.6	23.2	22.6	37.1	7.0	3.7	1.0	0.17	0.37	3.0	155
Gallbladder etc.	307	0	-	-	-	-	-	-	0.3	0.2	1.1	1.3	3.3	6.6	9.1	12.5	14.6	23.6	25.1	47.3	2.8	0.7	0.11	0.25	2.2	156
Pancreas	954	0	-	-	-	-	-	0.1	-	0.2	1.1	2.0	4.5	7.8	12.6	25.3	43.2	60.7	79.7	97.4	119.1	8.8	2.3	0.27	0.79	6.8	157
Nose, sinuses etc.	96	0	-	-	-	-	-	-	-	0.5	0.3	0.8	0.7	2.9	3.4	5.3	3.9	2.5	8.4	8.8	0.9	0.2	0.04	0.09	0.7	160
Larynx	623	0	-	-	-	-	0.1	0.2	-	0.2	2.0	4.5	9.1	17.1	29.9	31.1	25.3	31.1	28.8	19.3	5.8	1.5	0.32	0.60	4.8	161
Bronchus, lung	6374	0	-	-	-	-	0.4	0.3	1.0	3.2	7.7	24.8	53.5	120.0	208.5	335.0	408.0	471.6	524.2	471.2	58.9	15.1	2.10	5.81	46.0	162
Other thoracic organs	65	0	0.2	-	0.1	0.1	0.2	0.3	0.4	0.4	0.6	0.2	0.4	-	0.6	2.5	4.3	2.5	6.5	7.0	0.6	0.2	0.02	0.05	0.5	163-4
Bone	132	0	0.1	0.6	1.2	1.9	2.3	1.3	1.0	1.0	0.8	0.9	0.6	1.7	0.8	1.5	1.8	3.0	4.6	-	1.2	0.3	0.07	0.09	1.1	170
Connective tissue	323	0	0.5	0.8	0.5	0.9	0.8	1.7	1.5	2.5	2.9	2.7	3.0	3.9	4.2	8.0	12.5	19.0	28.8	24.5	3.0	0.8	0.13	0.23	2.4	171
Mesothelioma	249	0	-	-	-	-	-	-	-	0.1	0.6	0.9	2.6	5.0	8.2	13.6	14.3	24.1	13.0	7.0	2.3	0.6	0.09	0.23	1.8	MES
†Kaposi's sarcoma	219	0	-	-	-	-	0.3	3.6	4.5	5.5	4.4	2.2	1.7	2.1	0.6	1.8	1.1	3.0	4.6	8.8	2.0	0.5	0.12	0.14	1.7	KAP
Melanoma of skin	2905	0	-	-	0.4	4.9	8.2	12.0	16.8	24.4	29.2	39.5	45.7	48.3	71.9	75.8	92.5	109.7	138.2	148.9	26.8	6.9	1.51	2.35	22.4	172
†Other skin																										
Breast	79	0	-	-	-	-	-	-	0.1	-	0.4	0.3	0.6	1.7	2.3	3.5	3.2	7.0	10.2	5.3	0.7	0.2	0.03	0.06	0.6	175
Prostate	7086	0	-	-	-	-	-	0.1	-	-	1.0	2.8	12.8	51.4	129.0	318.5	511.6	756.7	1055.8	1364.6	65.4	16.8	0.99	5.14	47.6	185
Testis	558	0	0.6	0.1	0.1	2.0	6.5	12.0	14.8	9.0	8.3	5.8	3.0	2.7	2.3	1.0	1.4	1.5	1.9	3.5	5.2	1.3	0.34	0.35	4.5	186
Penis	71	0	-	-	-	-	-	-	0.1	0.2	0.3	0.6	1.3	1.9	0.8	2.5	2.9	5.0	7.4	10.5	0.7	0.2	0.03	0.05	0.5	187.1-.4
Other male genital	16	0	-	-	-	-	-	0.1	-	-	-	-	0.6	0.2	0.4	0.3	1.8	1.0	-	1.8	0.1	0.0	0.01	0.02	0.1	187.5-.9
Bladder	2587	0	0.4	-	0.1	0.1	0.7	1.1	1.6	2.9	6.0	11.9	20.7	40.5	66.6	99.1	151.4	235.0	282.0	329.3	23.9	6.1	0.76	2.02	18.3	188
Kidney etc.	1162	0	1.5	0.3	-	-	0.3	0.3	0.8	3.7	6.2	11.3	14.1	22.3	30.6	49.2	68.2	74.7	77.9	59.6	10.7	2.8	0.46	1.04	8.7	189
Eye	122	0	1.4	-	-	0.1	0.2	-	0.3	0.7	0.6	0.5	1.3	1.7	1.9	4.5	7.9	8.0	5.6	8.8	1.1	0.3	0.04	0.11	1.0	190
Brain, nervous system	879	0	2.2	1.8	2.6	2.1	2.2	2.8	5.2	6.0	7.1	8.6	10.9	15.1	23.8	25.8	31.1	37.1	30.6	22.8	8.1	2.1	0.45	0.74	7.0	191-2
Thyroid	176	0	0.1	0.1	0.1	0.2	0.9	0.7	1.6	1.4	1.5	2.7	1.9	3.5	3.4	5.3	4.6	8.0	5.6	5.3	1.6	0.4	0.09	0.14	1.4	193
Other endocrine	57	0	1.4	0.4	0.2	0.8	0.3	0.4	0.3	0.4	0.5	0.5	0.2	-	0.4	0.8	0.7	2.5	0.9	-	0.5	0.1	0.03	0.04	0.5	194
Hodgkin's disease	279	0	0.2	0.6	1.7	2.2	4.4	2.3	2.6	2.8	2.9	2.5	3.1	3.7	3.2	3.5	5.0	4.0	5.6	-	2.6	0.7	0.16	0.20	2.3	201
Non-Hodgkin lymphoma	1815	0	2.1	1.4	1.4	2.0	1.2	4.1	7.5	9.2	15.0	19.3	20.0	30.0	44.5	62.2	78.9	96.7	114.1	131.4	16.8	4.3	0.79	1.49	13.8	200,202
Multiple myeloma	476	0	-	-	-	-	0.1	-	0.1	0.6	1.4	3.0	4.8	8.3	12.6	16.8	29.3	38.1	52.0	56.1	4.4	1.1	0.15	0.39	3.4	203
Lymphoid leukaemia	598	0	7.4	6.2	2.2	2.3	1.9	0.9	0.9	0.5	1.1	3.1	3.9	5.0	13.7	19.1	19.6	32.6	45.5	50.8	5.5	1.4	0.25	0.44	5.2	204
Myeloid leukaemia	542	0	1.1	1.3	0.5	1.1	0.9	1.1	1.7	2.0	1.5	2.2	5.4	7.9	11.4	17.1	29.6	45.1	35.3	57.8	5.0	1.3	0.19	0.42	4.1	205
Monocytic leukaemia	22	0	0.4	0.3	-	-	-	-	-	-	-	-	0.4	0.4	0.4	-	0.7	0.5	3.7	7.0	0.2	0.1	0.01	0.01	0.2	206
Other leukaemia	10	0	0.2	-	-	-	-	0.1	-	-	-	-	-	-	0.8	-	0.5	2.8	-	0.1	0.0	0.00	0.01	0.1	207
Leukaemia unspecified	63	0	-	-	-	-	-	-	-	-	0.3	-	0.7	0.6	0.8	0.8	4.6	7.0	10.2	15.8	0.6	0.1	0.01	0.04	0.4	208
Other and unspecified	1997	0	0.9	0.3	-	0.1	0.4	0.7	1.0	2.2	4.7	8.9	18.5	30.4	55.2	88.8	106.0	158.9	218.0	252.3	18.4	4.7	0.62	1.59	14.3	O&U
All sites																										
All sites but 173	42147	0	21.1	14.1	11.7	21.6	33.6	49.4	73.2	102.0	145.8	236.9	385.4	667.3	1125.2	1743.6	2316.2	3048.9	3775.1	4221.7	389.1	100.0	14.44	34.74	307.1	ALLb

Rate from 1 case   0.124   0.126   0.125   0.110   0.109   0.110   0.112   0.120   0.126   0.157   0.185   0.207   0.211   0.251   0.357   0.501   0.928   1.752

†Important: see notes on population page

AUSTRALIA, VICTORIA 1988-1992

ANNUAL INCIDENCE PER 100,000 BY AGE GROUP (YEARS) - FEMALE

SITE	ALL AGES	AGE UNK	0-	5-	10-	15-	20-	25-	30-	35-	40-	45-	50-	55-	60-	65-	70-	75-	80-	85+	CRUDE RATE	%	CR 64	CR 74	ASR (W)	ICD (9th)
Lip	243	0	-	-	-	-	0.1	0.2	0.4	1.1	1.1	1.6	1.9	2.5	4.7	7.5	8.5	14.9	12.7	21.6	2.2	0.7	0.07	0.15	1.4	140
Tongue	134	0	-	-	-	0.2	-	0.3	0.3	-	0.5	1.0	1.7	2.5	3.9	4.9	4.8	4.5	6.4	8.1	1.2	0.4	0.05	0.10	0.9	141
Salivary gland	77	0	-	-	-	0.1	-	0.2	0.4	0.4	0.8	1.0	1.0	0.8	1.9	1.8	2.0	2.8	2.1	6.7	0.7	0.2	0.03	0.05	0.5	142
Mouth	192	0	-	-	-	0.1	0.2	0.3	-	0.2	1.3	1.1	2.1	2.5	5.0	5.1	8.2	11.8	8.0	12.8	1.7	0.5	0.06	0.13	1.2	143-5
Oropharynx	63	0	-	-	-	-	-	-	-	0.2	0.5	0.5	1.0	1.1	2.7	2.7	2.0	3.1	0.5	1.3	0.6	0.2	0.03	0.05	0.4	146
Nasopharynx	34	0	-	0.3	-	0.1	0.2	0.1	0.3	0.2	0.4	0.8	0.4	0.4	0.2	0.7	-	1.7	0.5	0.7	0.3	0.1	0.02	0.02	0.3	147
Hypopharynx	30	0	-	-	-	-	-	-	-	-	0.4	0.2	0.4	0.4	0.8	1.3	1.4	0.7	1.6	1.3	0.3	0.1	0.01	0.02	0.2	148
Pharynx unspecified	18	0	-	-	-	0.1	-	-	-	-	-	-	-	0.4	0.2	1.3	1.7	-	1.1	-	0.2	0.0	0.00	0.02	0.1	149
Oesophagus	460	0	-	-	-	-	-	0.1	-	0.2	0.4	0.6	1.9	5.1	10.5	14.2	23.4	23.9	35.6	55.3	4.2	1.2	0.09	0.28	2.4	150
Stomach	930	0	-	-	0.1	-	-	0.9	0.9	1.5	3.6	3.7	7.7	9.7	15.1	23.8	36.9	57.8	70.6	102.6	8.5	2.5	0.22	0.52	4.9	151
Small intestine	87	0	-	-	-	-	-	-	-	0.2	0.1	0.5	1.3	1.7	1.4	4.2	3.9	4.5	4.2	3.4	0.8	0.2	0.03	0.07	0.5	152
Colon	4038	0	-	-	-	0.1	0.1	1.7	2.4	6.1	12.3	18.4	34.2	67.1	85.2	133.6	173.0	214.6	273.8	323.2	36.7	10.8	1.14	2.67	22.9	153
Rectum	1876	0	-	-	-	-	0.2	0.3	1.5	2.9	5.7	11.4	22.5	32.3	42.1	60.8	75.8	101.1	112.0	134.3	17.1	5.0	0.59	1.28	11.0	154
Liver	115	0	-	0.1	-	0.1	-	0.2	0.1	0.5	0.4	1.1	0.8	1.9	2.3	3.8	6.2	6.9	3.7	4.0	1.0	0.3	0.04	0.09	0.7	155
Gallbladder etc.	408	0	-	-	-	-	-	-	-	0.1	1.0	1.1	2.5	7.2	10.1	13.1	15.8	22.5	30.2	39.8	3.7	1.1	0.11	0.25	2.2	156
Pancreas	878	0	-	-	-	-	-	-	0.2	0.4	0.5	1.6	4.4	8.9	15.9	27.3	42.0	55.7	81.2	88.4	8.0	2.4	0.16	0.51	4.4	157
Nose, sinuses etc.	45	0	-	-	-	-	-	-	-	0.4	0.3	0.5	0.6	0.6	0.8	1.1	1.1	3.1	1.1	4.7	0.4	0.1	0.02	0.03	0.3	160
Larynx	88	0	-	-	-	-	-	-	-	0.2	0.1	0.3	1.3	2.3	2.5	3.6	5.1	3.8	3.2	1.3	0.8	0.2	0.03	0.08	0.6	161
Bronchus, lung	2552	0	-	-	0.1	0.2	0.6	0.2	0.9	2.1	6.1	11.7	25.2	47.1	82.8	103.5	133.6	127.4	105.1	91.1	23.2	6.9	0.88	2.07	15.8	162
Other thoracic organs	38	0	0.1	-	0.1	-	-	0.1	0.2	0.2	0.3	0.3	1.0	0.2	0.6	1.3	1.4	1.0	1.6	0.7	0.3	0.1	0.02	0.03	0.3	163-4
Bone	91	0	0.3	0.8	1.5	1.0	0.6	0.3	0.4	0.7	1.0	1.0	-	0.6	0.2	1.3	1.4	1.7	4.8	1.3	0.8	0.2	0.04	0.06	0.7	170
Connective tissue	216	0	0.6	0.5	1.1	0.5	1.2	0.8	0.6	1.2	1.1	2.4	1.2	3.4	4.3	3.1	6.8	9.0	8.0	10.8	2.0	0.6	0.09	0.14	1.5	171
Mesothelioma	40	0	-	-	-	-	-	-	-	0.1	0.3	0.3	1.2	0.6	0.6	0.7	3.7	1.4	1.1	0.7	0.4	0.1	0.02	0.04	0.3	MES
†Kaposi's sarcoma	22	0	-	-	0.1	-	-	0.1	0.1	-	0.2	-	-	0.4	0.7	0.8	1.0	1.6	2.7	0.2	0.1	0.00	Kap0.01	0.1	KAP
Melanoma of skin	2818	0	-	0.3	0.5	4.5	12.4	15.6	21.0	27.9	33.3	38.3	39.4	44.1	51.8	61.0	65.1	68.9	70.6	66.8	25.6	7.6	1.45	2.08	20.3	172
†Other skin																										
Breast	9579	0	-	-	-	-	0.7	6.7	25.7	52.6	110.4	162.3	185.9	193.7	222.5	252.9	269.4	292.4	326.4	309.7	87.1	25.7	4.80	7.41	66.7	174
Uterus unspecified	0	0	-	-	-	-	-	-	-	-	-	-	-	-	-	-	-	-	-	-	0.0	0.0	0.00	0.00	0.0	179
Cervix uteri	1291	0	-	-	-	-	1.3	6.8	15.7	22.7	20.4	20.6	14.0	20.7	19.8	23.1	26.8	22.8	21.2	18.9	11.7	3.5	0.71	0.96	9.4	180
Placenta	11	0	-	-	-	-	0.2	0.3	0.2	0.5	-	-	-	-	-	-	-	-	-	-	0.1	0.0	0.01	0.01	0.1	181
Corpus uteri	1531	0	-	-	-	-	-	0.1	1.1	2.9	4.9	12.3	28.2	41.8	46.4	57.3	60.0	51.9	50.9	64.1	13.9	4.1	0.69	1.28	10.2	182
Ovary etc.	1408	0	-	0.1	0.5	1.1	1.7	2.1	4.1	5.0	8.9	14.1	22.1	29.1	38.8	51.5	47.3	44.6	43.5	47.9	12.8	3.8	0.64	1.13	9.6	183
Other female genital	303	0	0.1	-	-	0.1	0.1	0.2	0.8	0.8	1.3	2.9	2.1	2.7	3.7	6.4	10.1	18.7	24.9	32.4	2.8	0.8	0.07	0.16	1.6	184
Bladder	895	0	-	-	-	-	0.1	0.3	0.8	1.1	2.0	4.5	8.5	14.6	18.2	25.1	38.3	46.4	67.9	80.3	8.1	2.4	0.25	0.57	5.0	188
Kidney etc.	747	0	2.1	0.8	-	0.1	0.3	0.4	0.4	0.8	3.8	8.3	8.6	13.5	21.5	18.0	26.8	44.3	35.6	27.7	6.8	2.0	0.30	0.53	4.9	189
Eye	109	0	1.3	0.1	-	0.1	-	0.1	-	0.2	1.0	1.1	1.2	1.7	2.3	2.2	3.4	4.5	5.8	5.4	1.0	0.3	0.05	0.07	0.8	190
Brain, nervous system	659	0	2.6	3.0	1.8	0.9	2.1	3.0	4.8	3.5	4.7	6.5	9.2	8.2	14.2	14.4	18.6	20.1	18.6	12.8	6.0	1.8	0.32	0.49	5.0	191-2
Thyroid	404	0	-	-	0.1	0.3	3.1	3.3	4.4	4.9	5.2	6.5	6.9	5.7	4.7	4.7	6.2	9.0	8.5	6.7	3.7	1.1	0.23	0.28	3.0	193
Other endocrine	28	0	1.2	0.1	-	0.1	-	0.1	0.1	-	0.1	0.2	0.6	-	-	0.7	1.1	0.3	0.5	0.7	0.3	0.1	0.01	0.02	0.3	194
Hodgkin's disease	215	0	-	-	0.4	3.7	4.6	2.5	2.6	2.1	1.3	1.5	0.6	1.1	1.7	2.7	2.8	3.5	2.7	2.0	2.0	0.6	0.11	0.14	1.7	201
Non-Hodgkin lymphoma	1421	0	0.8	0.5	0.7	1.3	1.1	3.3	2.5	5.4	7.0	10.1	16.7	28.1	31.0	44.6	59.7	60.2	66.9	59.4	12.9	3.8	0.54	1.06	9.1	200,202
Multiple myeloma	446	0	-	-	-	-	-	0.2	0.2	0.2	0.9	1.5	2.9	6.1	12.4	12.9	20.0	29.1	33.4	29.7	4.1	1.2	0.12	0.29	2.5	203
Lymphoid leukaemia	362	0	4.4	3.0	1.6	1.6	0.7	0.4	0.4	0.6	0.3	0.8	1.9	3.4	4.1	7.3	12.4	15.9	23.9	26.3	3.3	1.0	0.12	0.22	2.6	204
Myeloid leukaemia	445	0	0.8	0.1	0.4	1.0	1.3	1.8	1.9	1.9	2.8	3.1	3.1	4.2	6.2	10.4	12.7	20.8	27.6	36.4	4.0	1.2	0.14	0.26	2.7	205
Monocytic leukaemia	19	0	0.4	0.1	-	-	0.2	-	0.1	-	0.3	-	-	-	0.2	0.4	-	1.0	2.1	0.7	0.2	0.1	0.01	0.01	0.1	206
Other leukaemia	11	0	0.3	0.1	-	-	-	-	-	0.1	-	0.2	0.4	-	0.2	0.3	-	-	0.7	0.1	0.1	0.0	0.01	0.01	0.1	207
Leukaemia unspecified	53	0	-	-	-	-	0.1	-	0.2	-	0.3	0.5	0.2	0.2	0.4	0.9	2.0	2.4	6.4	7.4	0.5	0.1	0.01	0.02	0.3	208
Other and unspecified	1815	0	1.2	0.1	0.3	-	0.3	0.8	1.3	3.2	5.4	8.3	11.3	21.1	27.9	55.3	69.3	109.7	148.6	185.5	16.5	4.9	0.41	1.03	9.7	O&U
All sites																										
All sites but 173	37245	0	16.1	10.3	9.2	17.6	33.6	54.1	97.4	155.6	252.6	365.0	477.9	639.4	822.1	1073.4	1311.6	1541.5	1756.5	1938.4	338.6	100.0	14.75	26.68	239.3	ALLb

Rate from 1 case   0.130   0.132   0.132   0.115   0.111   0.110   0.112   0.119   0.128   0.162   0.192   0.211   0.206   0.222   0.282   0.346   0.531   0.675

†Important: see notes on population page

Western Australia

Reporting of cancer in Western Australia became a statutory obligation in August 1981 with the establishment of the population-based Western Australian Cancer Registry.

The registry covers the entire State of Western Australia, an area of 2 525 500 km^2, almost one third of the total area of Australia. The state lies between latitude 13 and 35° S and longitude 113 and 129° E and extends approximately 2400 km from north to south. The northern third of the state lies within the tropics where desert or near desert conditions prevail and population density is sparse. Population distribution overall is extremely uneven, 73% of the population living in the metropolitan area of the capital city Perth, in the south of the state.

The Western Australian population of 1 636 783 at the June 1991 census was 9.5% of the total population of Australia. The mining boom of the 1960s brought a rapid expansion in population and Western Australia now has a high proportion of migrant inhabitants: 69% of the population were born in Australia, 22% in New Zealand and 18% in Europe (including the UK). It is estimated that 2.6% of the population are Aboriginals, for whom life expectancy is between 15 and 20 years less, on average, than for non-Aboriginal persons. Religious freedom is practised in Western Australia, 70% of the population declaring themselves to be Christian.

Employment is dominated by four major classes of industry which employ 58% of the workforce (18% community services, 16% retail trade, 12% finance and 12% manufacturing). 7% of all workers are employed in agriculture, 7% in building and construction and 4% in the mining industry.

From a largely rural-based economy before the 1960s, the state has diversified and is now a leading producer of several key minerals. Heavy manufacturing industry is relatively insignificant, but light manufacturing industry is widespread. As a result of favourable climatic conditions, air pollution is not a major problem and the lack of heavy manufacturing industry ensures that water pollution is minimal. These issues have, however, become subjects of greater concern in recent years.

Cancer therapy is concentrated in the Perth metropolitan area, the major (government-operated) teaching hospitals and several private clinics acting as referral centres for country areas. The large area of the state and the consequent difficulties in providing access to treatment and other support services in rural areas continue to entail significant expenditure within the health sector.

Notifications are received from all pathologists and radiotherapists across the state. For the period covered by the data presented here, all malignancies were subject to reporting, except that malignant melanoma was the only primary cutaneous neoplasm to be reported. Following recent legislative changes, primary basal cell and squamous cell carcinomas are now the only skin malignancies not reported, and reporting of all intracranial neoplasms—including benign tumours—is now mandatory.

Registry staff have access to medical records departments of major public hospitals to allow collection of additional data when necessary; enquiries are also made of private pathology laboratories and medical practitioners in case of need. Mortality information is routinely searched for outcomes of known cases, and additional cases are recorded and subjected to the routine enquiry process, when a death certificate indicates a cancer in an individual previously unknown to the registry. Search and matching routines are now fully computerized.

Data recorded for each tumour include basis of diagnosis, address at diagnosis, and diagnosis date. For each cancer, site and histology are coded using ICD-O codes. Demographic details such as date of birth, sex, address, country of birth and occupation are recorded, in addition to details of place, date and cause of death when available. For selected cancers, additional data (such as level and depth for melanomas) are stored in linked ancillary data files. Data entry, maintenance and analysis take place on a microcomputer network with a facility for multi-user simultaneous access. A variety of software including EPI5, EGRET, Excel and SPSS is used for statistical analyses of the data.

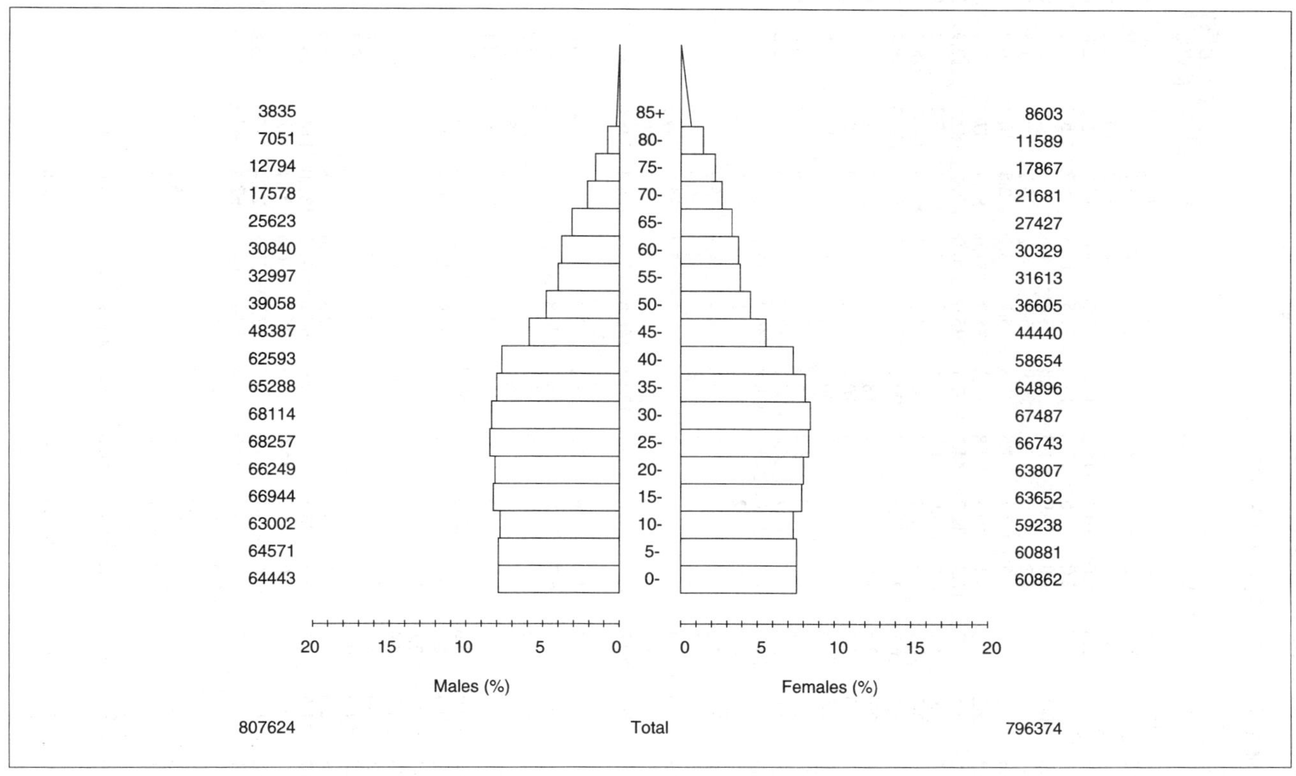

Western Australia

Source of population: average annual 1988–92
Census: 1991. Australian Bureau of Statistics, Estimated Resident Population
Estimate: The Australian Bureau of Statistics provides official estimates of the population each year, based on the Census counts.

Notes to tables overleaf:

† Kaposi's sarcoma is under-reported in this volume because cases of skin cancer (ICD-9 173) were not provided.

† 173 not available

† 188 does not include non-invasive tumours

Screening programmes in the area

Women over age 40 have been screened for breast cancer since 1989; 55 000 examinations are carried out each year. The age-group 20-79 has been screened for cervical cancer since 1992, with 20 000 annual examinations.

WESTERN AUSTRALIA 1988-1992

ANNUAL INCIDENCE PER 100,000 BY AGE GROUP (YEARS) - MALE

SITE	ALL AGES	AGE UNK	0-	5-	10-	15-	20-	25-	30-	35-	40-	45-	50-	55-	60-	65-	70-	75-	80-	85+	CRUDE RATE	%	CR 64	CR 74	ASR (W)	ICD (9th)
Lip	397	1	-	-	-	0.3	1.8	6.7	8.2	9.8	10.2	15.3	16.9	20.0	25.9	32.8	39.8	42.2	48.2	52.1	9.8	2.8	0.58	0.94	**8.7**	140
Tongue	122	0	-	-	-	-	-	-	0.3	1.2	0.6	3.3	7.2	12.7	13.0	21.1	14.8	14.1	5.7	5.2	3.0	0.9	0.19	0.37	**2.8**	141
Salivary gland	50	0	-	-	-	0.3	0.3	-	0.3	1.2	0.3	-	1.5	2.4	2.6	5.5	9.1	4.7	31.2	10.4	1.2	0.4	0.04	0.12	**1.0**	142
Mouth	113	0	-	-	-	-	-	-	0.6	0.9	1.3	2.5	5.6	10.3	15.6	14.8	17.1	9.4	14.2	5.2	2.8	0.8	0.18	0.34	**2.6**	143-5
Oropharynx	83	0	-	-	-	-	-	-	-	-	1.3	1.7	2.0	5.5	13.6	14.8	12.5	12.5	5.7	5.2	2.1	0.6	0.12	0.26	**1.9**	146
Nasopharynx	26	0	-	-	-	-	-	-	1.2	0.3	0.6	2.1	1.0	3.0	1.3	0.8	3.4	1.6	-	-	0.6	0.2	0.05	0.07	**0.6**	147
Hypopharynx	59	0	-	-	-	-	-	-	-	-	1.2	4.1	7.9	7.1	10.9	5.7	4.7	5.7	-	-	1.5	0.4	0.10	0.18	**1.4**	148
Pharynx unspecified	38	0	-	-	-	-	-	-	0.3	-	1.2	1.5	2.4	4.5	7.8	5.7	3.1	2.8	10.4	-	0.9	0.3	0.05	0.12	**0.9**	149
Oesophagus	212	0	-	-	-	-	-	-	-	0.3	2.2	2.9	5.1	10.3	20.8	34.3	35.3	51.6	53.9	57.4	5.2	1.5	0.21	0.56	**4.6**	150
Stomach	521	0	-	-	-	-	-	0.3	1.5	1.8	3.8	8.7	12.3	32.7	44.7	67.1	95.6	100.0	170.2	182.5	12.9	3.7	0.53	1.34	**11.4**	151
Small intestine	47	0	-	-	-	0.3	0.3	-	0.3	0.6	0.6	1.7	0.5	3.6	1.9	5.5	8.0	14.1	5.7	5.2	1.2	0.3	0.05	0.12	**1.0**	152
Colon	1158	0	-	-	-	-	0.3	1.5	1.5	4.0	7.7	20.7	39.9	69.1	104.4	144.4	204.8	264.2	295.0	359.8	28.7	8.1	1.24	2.99	**25.4**	153
Rectum	757	0	-	-	-	-	-	0.3	1.2	3.7	8.3	16.9	34.8	46.7	64.2	99.1	129.7	153.2	158.8	177.3	18.7	5.3	0.88	2.02	**16.8**	154
Liver	112	0	-	-	-	-	-	0.3	1.2	0.6	2.9	2.5	1.0	4.8	8.4	18.7	19.3	15.6	28.4	31.3	2.8	0.8	0.11	0.30	**2.4**	155
Gallbladder etc.	84	0	-	-	-	-	-	-	-	0.3	0.3	1.2	1.0	3.6	4.5	10.9	18.2	29.7	31.2	20.9	2.1	0.6	0.06	0.20	**1.7**	156
Pancreas	265	0	-	-	-	-	0.3	-	0.3	0.9	1.0	3.3	9.2	12.7	24.0	40.6	52.3	71.9	31.2	93.9	6.6	1.9	0.26	0.72	**5.9**	157
Nose, sinuses etc.	32	0	-	-	-	-	0.3	-	-	-	-	1.2	1.0	3.0	3.2	5.5	2.3	7.8	2.8	5.2	0.8	0.2	0.04	0.08	**0.7**	160
Larynx	210	0	-	-	-	-	-	-	-	0.3	1.0	3.7	13.3	12.7	24.0	35.1	33.0	37.5	28.4	26.1	5.2	1.5	0.28	0.62	**4.8**	161
Bronchus, lung	2172	0	0.3	-	-	-	0.3	0.3	0.9	1.8	10.2	21.9	64.0	120.0	243.2	320.8	436.9	486.1	513.4	469.3	53.8	15.2	2.31	6.10	**48.0**	162
Other thoracic organs	18	0	0.3	-	-	-	-	-	0.3	0.6	0.3	0.8	2.0	1.2	1.3	1.6	1.1	-	-	-	0.4	0.1	0.03	0.05	**0.4**	163-4
Bone	51	0	0.6	-	0.6	1.2	2.4	1.2	1.2	0.9	0.3	1.2	1.0	1.2	3.2	2.3	3.4	4.7	5.7	-	1.3	0.4	0.08	0.10	**1.2**	170
Connective tissue	87	0	-	0.3	1.0	0.6	0.9	1.8	1.8	1.5	0.3	1.2	4.1	3.6	5.2	7.0	6.8	14.1	19.9	20.9	2.2	0.6	0.11	0.18	**1.9**	171
Mesothelioma	183	0	-	-	-	-	0.3	0.3	0.6	0.3	2.6	5.4	7.2	17.0	21.4	23.4	19.3	25.0	34.0	36.5	4.5	1.3	0.27	0.49	**4.2**	MES
†Kaposi's sarcoma	32	0	-	-	-	-	0.3	0.6	0.9	3.1	1.3	1.2	0.5	0.6	0.6	-	-	4.7	2.8	10.4	0.8	0.2	0.05	0.05	**0.6**	KAP
Melanoma of skin	1456	1	0.3	0.3	1.0	4.8	10.0	18.5	26.7	33.1	38.7	50.8	60.4	78.2	100.5	122.5	146.8	159.4	184.4	208.6	36.1	10.2	2.12	3.46	**32.2**	172
†Other skin																										
Breast	18	0	-	-	-	-	-	-	-	-	-	0.4	1.0	0.6	2.6	3.1	2.3	3.1	5.7	-	0.4	0.1	0.02	0.05	**0.4**	175
Prostate	2534	0	-	-	-	-	0.3	-	-	-	1.0	2.5	16.9	58.8	165.4	349.7	576.8	861.3	1052.2	1366.1	62.8	17.8	1.22	5.86	**52.8**	185
Testis	175	0	-	-	-	1.8	5.7	11.1	10.6	9.2	6.4	4.5	1.0	2.4	1.9	2.3	-	-	2.8	10.4	4.3	1.2	0.27	0.29	**3.7**	186
Penis	17	0	-	-	-	-	-	-	-	-	-	0.8	-	1.2	1.9	2.3	1.1	4.7	5.7	5.2	0.4	0.1	0.02	0.04	**0.4**	187.1-.4
Other male genital	4	0	-	-	-	-	-	-	-	-	-	-	-	0.6	-	-	2.3	-	-	5.2	0.1	0.0	0.00	0.01	**0.1**	187.5-.9
†Bladder	450	0	0.3	-	-	-	-	-	0.3	1.2	0.6	5.8	8.7	20.6	44.1	53.9	91.0	107.9	167.3	166.8	11.1	3.2	0.41	1.13	**9.7**	188
Kidney etc.	371	0	1.2	0.3	-	-	-	0.3	1.8	2.1	5.4	6.6	16.4	25.5	35.7	43.7	64.9	53.1	70.9	93.9	9.2	2.6	0.48	1.02	**8.4**	189
Eye	35	0	0.6	-	0.3	-	-	-	-	0.3	0.6	0.8	2.6	1.8	3.2	3.9	1.1	7.8	8.5	-	0.9	0.2	0.05	0.08	**0.8**	190
Brain, nervous system	285	0	3.4	3.7	1.9	2.4	3.6	2.3	2.9	5.8	4.2	7.4	14.8	17.6	18.8	21.9	22.8	28.1	25.5	31.3	7.1	2.0	0.44	0.67	**6.7**	191-2
Thyroid	74	0	-	-	-	-	1.8	1.2	1.2	1.5	3.8	2.1	5.1	-	6.5	5.5	4.6	7.8	-	10.4	1.8	0.5	0.12	0.17	**1.7**	193
Other endocrine	19	0	2.2	-	0.3	0.6	-	-	0.6	0.3	1.0	0.4	0.5	0.6	-	-	-	-	-	-	0.5	0.1	0.03	0.03	**0.5**	194
Hodgkin's disease	92	0	-	0.6	1.9	3.3	2.1	4.7	3.2	2.5	2.6	2.5	0.5	3.0	1.3	3.9	2.3	1.6	2.8	-	2.3	0.6	0.14	0.17	**2.1**	201
Non-Hodgkin lymphoma	545	1	0.3	1.5	0.6	0.6	3.3	2.3	5.6	6.7	11.5	11.6	16.4	26.1	27.2	57.0	95.6	101.6	139.0	114.7	13.5	3.8	0.57	1.33	**11.8**	200,202
Multiple myeloma	141	0	-	-	-	-	-	-	-	0.3	0.6	1.2	5.6	6.1	15.6	9.4	25.0	40.6	51.1	62.6	3.5	1.0	0.15	0.32	**3.0**	203
Lymphoid leukaemia	153	0	5.9	2.8	1.9	0.9	0.6	0.6	0.9	0.6	1.0	4.1	2.6	6.1	11.0	10.1	13.7	25.0	28.4	57.4	3.8	1.1	0.19	0.31	**3.8**	204
Myeloid leukaemia	203	0	1.2	0.6	0.3	1.5	1.5	0.3	1.8	2.1	1.9	3.3	4.1	4.8	12.3	14.8	34.1	61.0	62.4	67.8	5.0	1.4	0.18	0.42	**4.3**	205
Monocytic leukaemia	12	0	0.6	-	0.3	-	-	0.3	-	-	-	-	0.5	1.2	-	0.8	1.1	3.1	2.8	-	0.3	0.1	0.01	0.02	**0.3**	206
Other leukaemia	7	0	0.3	-	-	-	-	-	0.3	0.3	-	-	-	0.6	-	0.8	-	3.1	-	-	0.2	0.0	0.01	0.01	**0.2**	207
Leukaemia unspecified	26	0	0.3	-	-	-	0.6	-	-	0.3	-	-	0.5	1.2	2.6	3.1	2.3	9.4	5.7	-	0.6	0.2	0.03	0.06	**0.6**	208
Other and unspecified	801	0	1.2	-	-	-	0.3	1.2	5.0	6.1	7.7	10.3	23.6	52.1	70.0	91.3	139.9	151.6	224.1	260.7	19.8	5.6	0.89	2.04	**17.6**	O&U
All sites																										
All sites but 173	14247	3	19.2	10.2	10.2	18.5	37.4	56.3	83.1	106.9	144.1	237.2	418.4	716.4	1179.6	1725.0	2401.8	3002.8	3533.9	4046.1	352.8	100.0	15.19	35.83	**312.2**	ALLb

Rate from 1 case | | | 0.310 | 0.310 | 0.317 | 0.299 | 0.302 | 0.293 | 0.294 | 0.306 | 0.320 | 0.413 | 0.512 | 0.606 | 0.648 | 0.781 | 1.138 | 1.563 | 2.836 | 5.214

†Important: see notes on population page

WESTERN AUSTRALIA 1988-1992

ANNUAL INCIDENCE PER 100,000 BY AGE GROUP (YEARS) - FEMALE

SITE	ALL AGES	AGE UNK	0-	5-	10-	15-	20-	25-	30-	35-	40-	45-	50-	55-	60-	65-	70-	75-	80-	85+	CRUDE RATE	%	CR 64	CR 74	ASR (W)	ICD (9th)
Lip	112	0	-	-	-	-	-	1.2	1.2	1.2	1.0	1.8	2.7	5.7	9.2	7.3	12.9	20.1	20.7	25.6	2.8	0.9	0.12	0.22	**2.1**	*140*
Tongue	41	0	-	-	-	-	0.3	-	0.6	1.2	-	0.5	2.2	3.8	2.6	2.2	4.6	4.5	3.5	11.6	1.0	0.3	0.06	0.09	**0.8**	*141*
Salivary gland	33	0	-	-	-	0.3	-	-	-	-	1.0	0.9	-	1.9	4.0	3.6	2.8	5.6	1.7	9.3	0.8	0.3	0.04	0.07	**0.7**	*142*
Mouth	55	0	-	-	-	-	-	-	0.6	-	0.7	0.9	0.5	5.1	4.0	8.0	6.5	3.4	13.8	11.6	1.4	0.4	0.06	0.13	**1.0**	*143-5*
Oropharynx	20	0	-	-	-	-	-	-	-	-	0.7	0.5	1.1	2.5	0.7	2.2	1.8	4.5	-	2.3	0.5	0.2	0.03	0.05	**0.4**	*146*
Nasopharynx	7	0	-	0.3	-	-	-	0.3	-	-	0.3	-	0.5	1.3	-	-	-	1.1	-	-	0.2	0.1	0.01	0.01	**0.2**	*147*
Hypopharynx	9	0	-	-	-	-	-	-	-	0.3	-	0.5	-	-	1.3	0.7	2.8	1.1	-	-	0.2	0.1	0.01	0.03	**0.2**	*148*
Pharynx unspecified	7	0	-	-	-	-	-	-	-	-	-	-	-	0.6	0.7	0.7	0.9	3.4	-	-	0.2	0.1	0.01	0.01	**0.1**	*149*
Oesophagus	103	0	-	-	-	-	-	-	-	-	-	0.5	4.9	2.5	8.6	8.8	11.1	20.1	38.0	27.9	2.6	0.8	0.08	0.18	**1.7**	*150*
Stomach	296	0	-	-	-	-	0.3	-	1.5	1.2	2.7	4.1	9.3	12.0	14.5	26.3	39.7	47.0	72.5	111.6	7.4	2.3	0.23	0.56	**5.1**	*151*
Small intestine	27	0	-	-	-	-	-	-	0.9	0.6	-	0.5	1.6	2.5	2.0	1.5	1.8	3.4	5.2	2.3	0.7	0.2	0.04	0.06	**0.5**	*152*
Colon	1190	0	-	-	-	-	0.3	0.3	2.4	4.9	11.3	17.6	43.2	58.8	83.1	132.7	151.3	199.2	241.6	302.2	29.9	9.4	1.11	2.53	**21.8**	*153*
Rectum	570	0	-	-	-	-	0.3	1.2	0.9	3.4	3.1	14.0	15.8	36.7	42.2	62.0	83.9	95.1	84.6	116.2	14.3	4.5	0.59	1.32	**10.8**	*154*
Liver	50	0	-	-	0.3	-	-	-	-	-	0.9	0.3	0.9	1.6	2.5	3.3	2.9	5.5	11.2	17.3	2.3	1.3	0.4	0.05	0.09	**0.9**	*155*
Gallbladder etc.	99	0	-	-	-	-	-	-	0.3	-	1.8	2.7	4.4	7.9	8.0	11.1	26.9	22.4	23.2	2.5	0.8	0.09	0.18	**1.7**	*156*
Pancreas	257	0	-	-	-	0.3	-	-	0.9	1.4	1.8	6.0	13.3	13.8	23.3	49.8	43.7	56.9	79.0	6.5	2.0	0.19	0.55	**4.5**	*157*
Nose, sinuses etc.	12	0	-	-	-	-	-	-	-	0.3	-	-	1.1	-	0.7	1.5	-	2.2	6.9	-	0.3	0.1	0.01	0.02	**0.2**	*160*
Larynx	26	0	-	-	-	-	-	-	-	-	-	0.5	0.5	1.9	3.3	6.6	4.6	1.1	1.7	-	0.7	0.2	0.03	0.09	**0.6**	*161*
Bronchus, lung	912	0	-	-	0.3	-	0.3	0.3	1.5	2.2	5.8	14.4	29.5	39.9	87.0	118.1	152.2	180.2	117.3	100.0	22.9	7.2	0.91	2.26	**17.5**	*162*
Other thoracic organs	4	0	0.3	-	-	-	-	-	-	-	-	-	0.5	0.6	-	-	-	-	-	2.3	0.1	0.0	0.01	0.01	**0.1**	*163-4*
Bone	40	0	-	0.7	0.3	1.6	1.3	1.2	0.9	0.9	0.7	0.9	2.2	1.3	1.3	-	1.8	2.2	-	4.6	1.0	0.3	0.07	0.08	**0.9**	*170*
Connective tissue	59	1	1.3	-	0.7	1.3	-	-	0.3	1.8	0.7	0.9	1.1	3.2	2.0	3.6	5.5	6.7	10.4	9.3	1.5	0.5	0.07	0.11	**1.2**	*171*
Mesothelioma	25	0	-	-	-	-	-	-	0.6	0.3	-	2.3	1.6	-	2.0	0.7	1.8	1.1	8.6	4.6	0.6	0.2	0.03	0.05	**0.5**	*MES*
†Kaposi's sarcoma	2	0	-	-	-	-	-	-	-	-	-	-	-	-	0.7	-	-	1.1	-	-	0.1	0.0	0.00	0.00	**0.0**	*KAP*
Melanoma of skin	1159	1	-	0.3	1.4	5.0	14.1	20.7	24.9	33.0	35.5	49.1	56.3	63.3	65.3	64.2	78.4	78.4	81.1	62.8	29.1	9.2	1.85	2.56	**24.9**	*172*
†Other skin																										
Breast	3462	0	-	-	-	-	1.6	8.7	26.4	56.1	114.6	184.1	208.7	198.7	261.1	256.0	292.4	310.1	333.1	423.1	86.9	27.4	5.30	8.04	**72.9**	*174*
Uterus unspecified	3	0	-	-	-	-	-	-	-	-	-	0.5	-	-	-	0.7	-	1.1	-	-	0.1	0.0	0.00	0.01	**0.1**	*179*
Cervix uteri	553	0	-	-	0.6	1.6	9.9	18.4	21.0	30.0	26.1	25.7	27.2	19.1	27.0	30.4	21.3	25.9	32.5	13.9	4.4	0.90	1.18	**11.8**	*180*
Placenta	0	0	-	-	-	-	-	-	-	-	-	-	-	-	-	-	-	-	-	-	0.0	0.0	0.00	0.00	**0.0**	*181*
Corpus uteri	519	0	-	-	0.6	-	0.6	1.2	2.2	5.5	14.0	25.1	31.0	58.0	64.2	72.0	58.2	70.8	34.9	13.0	4.1	0.69	1.37	**10.8**	*182*
Ovary etc.	407	0	-	-	0.7	0.9	1.9	0.9	2.7	3.4	7.8	15.8	15.3	27.8	35.6	44.5	37.8	49.3	46.6	37.2	10.2	3.2	0.56	0.98	**8.5**	*183*
Other female genital	75	0	-	-	-	-	-	0.6	0.3	0.7	1.8	2.2	5.7	5.3	7.3	9.2	11.2	12.1	18.6	1.9	0.6	0.08	0.17	**1.4**	*184*
†Bladder	141	0	-	-	-	-	-	-	0.3	-	0.3	1.4	3.8	4.4	7.9	12.4	20.3	30.2	29.3	62.8	3.5	1.1	0.09	0.25	**2.3**	*188*
Kidney etc.	254	0	1.6	1.3	0.3	0.3	-	0.9	0.9	2.2	2.0	4.5	8.7	14.6	17.1	22.6	36.0	38.1	46.6	41.8	6.4	2.0	0.27	0.57	**5.0**	*189*
Eye	33	0	0.7	0.3	-	-	-	-	-	0.3	1.4	1.4	1.1	1.9	1.3	2.9	3.7	3.4	5.2	2.3	0.8	0.3	0.04	0.07	**0.7**	*190*
Brain, nervous system	246	0	2.3	4.3	2.0	0.9	3.8	1.5	3.0	4.9	5.5	5.0	8.2	13.9	16.5	13.1	26.8	25.7	19.0	9.3	6.2	1.9	0.36	0.56	**5.4**	*191-2*
Thyroid	206	0	-	-	0.3	1.3	1.9	4.8	8.0	8.0	7.2	8.1	10.9	10.8	9.2	9.5	6.5	10.1	8.6	4.6	5.2	1.6	0.35	0.43	**4.5**	*193*
Other endocrine	16	0	0.7	-	0.3	0.3	-	-	0.3	0.6	0.7	-	0.5	-	1.3	0.7	1.8	-	1.7	-	0.4	0.1	0.02	0.04	**0.4**	*194*
Hodgkin's disease	65	0	-	-	0.7	1.3	3.1	3.0	1.5	2.2	0.7	1.8	0.5	0.6	2.0	2.9	2.8	7.8	1.7	2.3	1.6	0.5	0.09	0.12	**1.4**	*201*
Non-Hodgkin lymphoma	428	0	1.0	1.0	0.3	-	1.6	2.4	1.5	3.7	10.2	7.7	16.4	19.0	30.3	40.1	55.3	60.4	79.4	53.5	10.7	3.4	0.48	0.95	**8.3**	*200,202*
Multiple myeloma	119	0	-	-	-	-	-	-	-	0.3	0.3	0.9	3.8	5.1	12.5	11.7	23.1	21.3	22.4	18.6	3.0	0.9	0.11	0.29	**2.2**	*203*
Lymphoid leukaemia	100	0	4.9	1.3	0.3	0.9	0.6	0.9	1.2	-	0.7	1.4	1.6	1.9	5.9	8.0	8.3	13.4	17.3	13.9	2.5	0.8	0.11	0.19	**2.2**	*204*
Myeloid leukaemia	143	0	1.0	0.7	0.3	0.3	1.6	0.9	0.9	2.2	1.7	2.7	2.2	7.0	8.6	10.9	12.9	17.9	22.4	48.8	3.6	1.1	0.15	0.27	**2.7**	*205*
Monocytic leukaemia	4	0	0.3	-	0.3	0.3	-	-	-	-	-	-	-	-	-	-	1.1	-	-	-	0.1	0.0	0.00	0.00	**0.1**	*206*
Other leukaemia	2	0	-	-	0.3	-	-	-	-	-	-	-	-	-	-	-	0.9	-	-	-	0.1	0.0	0.00	0.01	**0.0**	*207*
Leukaemia unspecified	22	0	-	-	-	-	-	0.3	-	0.3	-	-	0.5	-	-	1.3	2.2	3.7	3.4	8.6	4.6	0.6	0.2	0.01	0.04	**0.4**	*208*
Other and unspecified	716	0	0.7	-	0.3	0.3	1.3	1.5	1.5	3.7	5.8	11.7	14.2	25.3	49.5	63.4	84.9	126.5	174.3	253.4	18.0	5.7	0.58	1.32	**12.4**	*O&U*
All sites	12629	2	14.8	10.2	9.5	16.7	35.7	61.4	104.3	164.9	260.2	402.3	534.9	658.6	902.8	1085.1	1359.7	1573.8	1729.1	1971.4	317.2	100.0	15.88	28.11	**252.0**	*ALLb*
All sites but 173																										

Rate from 1 case			0.329	0.329	0.338	0.314	0.313	0.300	0.296	0.308	0.341	0.450	0.546	0.633	0.659	0.729	0.922	1.119	1.726	2.325

†Important: see notes on population page

French Polynesia

The eighth regional conference of Directors of Health of the countries in the South Pacific Commission, held in 1979 in Apia (Western Samoa), recommended that a cancer registry be established in each country of the region. At that time, only two island countries already had such a registry, Papua New Guinea (since 1958) and Fiji (since 1965). French Polynesia, as well as American Samoa and New Caledonia, immediately declared an interest in adopting a common notification system for cancer. Other countries in the region followed.

Collection of data on cancer began in French Polynesia in 1981, with the technical assistance of the South Pacific Commission, the University of Southern California and Los Angeles and of the Center for Research on Cancer of the University of Hawaii. The registry is administered by the Health Ministry under the administrative responsibility of the Director.

The registry covers the whole of French Polynesia, consisting of 188 main islands divided into five archipelagos, corresponding to a land surface area of 4000 km², but spread out over a maritime area equivalent to the size of Europe.

The 219 521 inhabitants (September 1996) are concentrated on the island of Tahiti, where the town of Papeete is the only true agglomeration in the country. The population is young, with approximately one person in two aged under 20. The birth rate was 23.5 per 1000 in 1994, and the crude mortality rate was 4.9 per 1000 live births. Infant mortality was 9.4 per 1000. Life expectancy at birth is around 68.4 years for men and 72.8 years for women.

According to the latest census (1988), the population is made up of: Polynesians and assimilated groups, 83%; Europeans and assimilated, 12%; Asiatics and assimilated, 4%; others, 1%. The majority of the population is Christian, with a preponderance of Protestants. 54.1% of the population was economically active in 1994.

The health system in Polynesia includes, in Tahiti, a well equipped hospital centre with 388 beds, two private clinics with 81 and 112 beds, a medical–obstetric hospital administered by the Ministry of Health with 28 beds and 13 public dispensaries, also administered by the Ministry of Health. In 1996 there were 141 medical practitioners (96 doctors per 100 000 inhabitants) in Tahiti. In the islands, there are a few medical practitioners in Moorea and in the islands of Sous Le Vent. The Ministry of Health administers a hospital with 93 beds and a surgical department in Uturoa (Raiatea), and a smaller hospital (28 beds) but also equipped for surgery at Taiohae (Marquises Nord). There is a hospital of 25 beds without surgical facilities in Moorea and there are medical centres, some equipped with a few beds, for example Mataura at Australes (14 beds) and Atuona at Marquises Sud (18 beds). Certain islands which do not have a doctor have a nurse, some have only a health post, and some have no health facilities.

Treatment of a cancer patient, once the diagnosis has been confirmed by one of the two pathology laboratories in the territory, or in the case of a strong diagnostic suspicion, usually entails transfer to France or New Zealand. Only simple chemotherapeutic protocols and surgical treatment of certain tumours are carried out locally.

Notification of cancer cases is in principle based on voluntary notification by doctors. However, the number of spontaneous notifications remains very low, and the registry also undertakes active collection of the results from the two pathology laboratories and of cytological examinations from the laboratories of medical biology as well as consultation of the registry of persons evacuated for health reasons to France or New Zealand; death certificates are also used as a source of information. Medical practitioners remain reticent about the nominative declaration of cancer cases and do not authorize the registry to have access to the hospital records or to consult with the patients concerned. Follow-up of cases is limited to recording date of death.

For these reasons, the use of the registry's data is at present limited to descriptive analysis of the distribution by sex and age of the principle cancers in French Polynesia.

The data are coded to ICD-O. Two distinct tumours in a single individual are counted as two cancers. The basic data in the registry are analysed annually (numbers of cases and distribution). A compilation of results for five years is carried out at regular intervals.

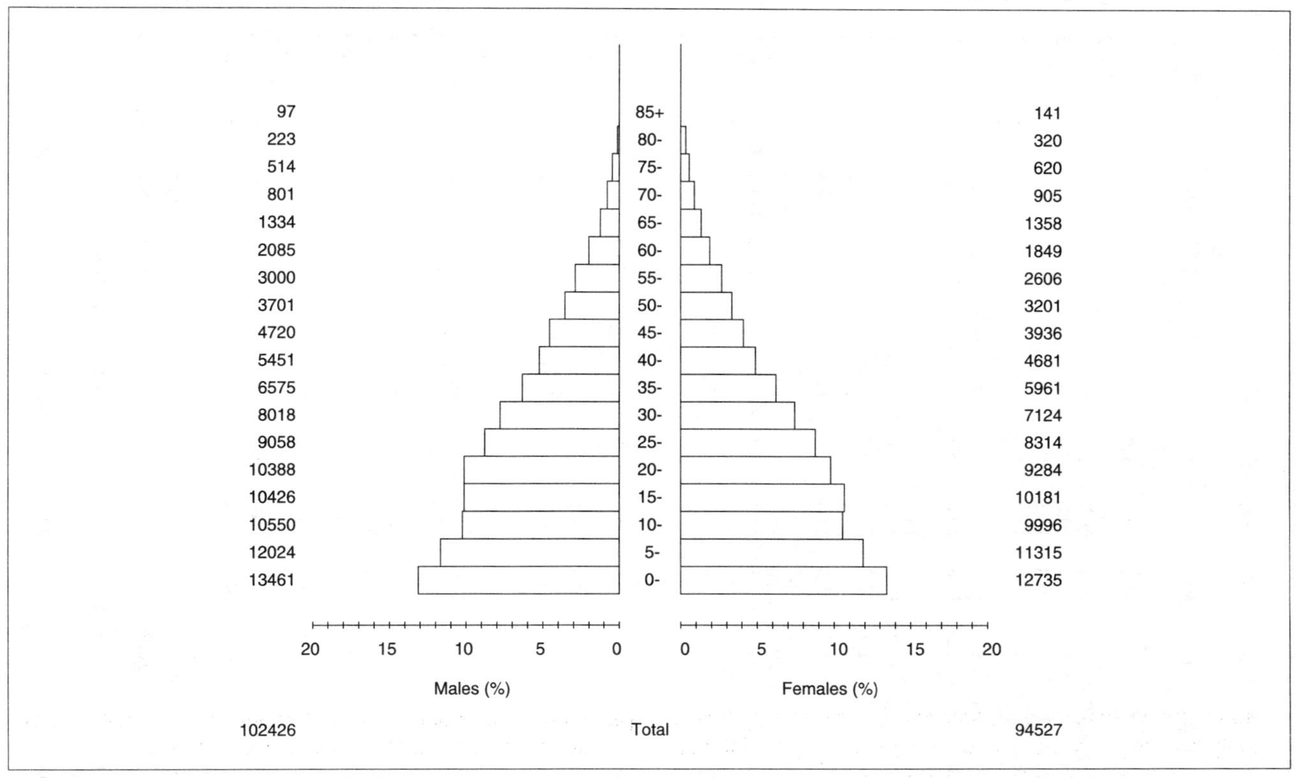

French Polynesia
Source of population: average annual 1988–92
Census: 6 September 1988, Recensement Général de la Population de Polynésie Française, Institut Territorial de la Statistique.
Estimate: The populations for 1989, 1990, 1991 and 1992 are estimates based on the 1988 Census, taking births and deaths into account, and considering migration as nul.
Notes to tables overleaf:
* The high proportion of diagnoses based on a death certificate alone, and irregular registration by year, indicate under-ascertainment.

† Kaposi's sarcoma is under-reported in this volume because cases of skin cancer (ICD-9 173) were not provided.
† 173 not available
† 188 does not include non-invasive tumours

* FRENCH POLYNESIA 1988-1992

ANNUAL INCIDENCE PER 100,000 BY AGE GROUP (YEARS) - MALE

SITE	ALL AGES	AGE UNK	0-	5-	10-	15-	20-	25-	30-	35-	40-	45-	50-	55-	60-	65-	70-	75-	80-	85+	CRUDE RATE	%	CR 64	CR 74	ASR (W)	ICD (9th)
Lip	0	0	-	-	-	-	-	-	-	-	-	-	-	-	-	-	-	-	-	-	0.0	0.0	0.00	0.00	0.0	140
Tongue	11	0	-	-	-	-	-	-	-	-	-	8.5	16.2	20.0	28.8	-	-	-	-	-	2.1	1.5	0.37	0.37	3.3	141
Salivary gland	1	0	-	-	-	1.9	-	-	-	-	-	-	-	-	-	-	-	-	-	-	0.2	0.1	0.01	0.01	0.2	142
Mouth	15	0	-	-	-	1.9	2.2	-	-	-	3.7	-	16.2	26.7	28.8	30.0	-	-	-	-	2.9	2.0	0.40	0.55	4.5	143-5
Oropharynx	13	0	-	-	-	-	-	2.5	3.0	7.3	16.9	-	20.0	9.6	-	25.0	-	-	-	-	2.5	1.7	0.30	0.42	3.5	146
Nasopharynx	9	0	-	-	-	-	-	-	3.0	3.7	4.2	10.8	13.3	19.2	-	-	-	-	-	-	1.8	1.2	0.27	0.27	2.5	147
Hypopharynx	13	0	-	-	-	-	-	-	3.0	7.3	4.2	21.6	13.3	19.2	15.0	-	-	-	-	-	2.5	1.7	0.34	0.42	3.7	148
Pharynx unspecified	8	0	-	-	-	-	-	-	-	-	3.7	8.5	-	26.7	9.6	-	-	-	-	-	1.6	1.1	0.24	0.24	2.2	149
Oesophagus	20	1	-	-	-	-	-	-	3.0	7.3	4.2	16.2	6.7	38.4	45.0	99.9	-	-	-	-	3.9	2.7	0.40	1.16	7.2	150
Stomach	29	0	-	-	-	-	-	2.5	3.0	3.7	8.5	10.8	20.0	28.8	45.0	174.8	116.7	269.1	-	-	5.7	3.9	0.39	1.49	10.9	151
Small intestine	2	0	-	-	-	1.9	-	-	-	-	-	-	5.4	-	-	-	-	-	-	-	0.4	0.3	0.04	0.04	0.4	152
Colon	26	1	-	-	-	1.9	-	-	-	-	7.3	8.5	10.8	13.3	48.0	104.9	74.9	38.9	-	-	5.1	3.5	0.47	1.40	9.5	153
Rectum	26	1	-	-	-	-	-	-	3.0	7.3	12.7	16.2	33.3	28.8	30.0	74.9	116.7	-	-	-	5.1	3.5	0.53	1.07	8.6	154
Liver	37	0	-	3.3	1.9	-	-	2.5	6.1	-	21.2	27.0	26.7	86.3	30.0	99.9	77.8	-	-	-	7.2	5.0	0.88	1.52	11.8	155
Gallbladder etc.	9	1	-	-	-	-	-	-	-	-	-	13.3	9.6	15.0	25.0	77.8	89.7	-	-	-	1.8	1.2	0.13	0.35	3.5	156
Pancreas	13	0	-	1.7	-	-	-	-	-	3.0	-	4.2	5.4	13.3	9.6	30.0	-	77.8	179.4	-	2.5	1.7	0.19	0.34	4.4	157
Nose, sinuses etc.	6	0	-	-	-	-	-	-	-	-	8.5	5.4	-	19.2	15.0	-	-	-	-	-	1.2	0.8	0.17	0.24	2.0	160
Larynx	29	0	-	-	-	-	2.2	2.5	-	7.3	29.7	21.6	46.7	28.8	30.0	-	77.8	-	-	-	5.7	3.9	0.69	0.84	8.3	161
Bronchus, lung	202	2	-	-	-	-	-	-	6.1	25.7	55.1	135.1	253.3	374.1	479.8	524.3	700.4	179.4	618.6	-	39.4	27.2	4.29	9.36	73.7	162
Other thoracic organs	7	0	1.5	-	-	-	2.2	-	-	-	4.2	-	13.3	-	15.0	-	-	89.7	-	-	1.4	0.9	0.11	0.18	2.0	163-4
Bone	8	1	1.5	-	1.9	-	1.9	-	-	-	-	5.4	6.7	-	15.0	25.0	-	-	-	-	1.6	1.1	0.10	0.33	2.3	170
Connective tissue	6	0	-	-	-	-	1.9	-	-	-	8.5	-	20.0	-	-	-	-	-	-	-	1.2	0.8	0.15	0.15	1.5	171
Mesothelioma	1	0	-	-	-	-	-	2.2	-	-	-	-	-	-	-	-	-	-	-	-	0.2	0.1	0.01	0.01	0.2	MES
†Kaposi's sarcoma	0	0	-	-	-	-	-	-	-	-	-	-	-	-	-	-	-	-	-	-	0.0	0.0	0.00	0.00	0.0	KAP
Melanoma of skin †Other skin	11	1	-	-	-	-	1.9	-	2.5	-	-	8.5	-	13.3	9.6	-	49.9	38.9	-	-	2.1	1.5	0.20	0.47	3.4	172
Breast	6	0	-	-	-	-	-	-	-	-	3.7	8.5	5.4	6.7	9.6	-	-	-	-	-	1.2	0.8	0.17	0.17	1.6	175
Prostate	52	2	-	-	-	-	-	-	-	-	-	4.2	5.4	26.7	57.6	179.9	174.8	466.9	358.7	618.6	10.2	7.0	0.49	2.33	23.2	185
Testis	9	0	-	-	-	-	1.9	8.8	5.0	-	3.7	4.2	-	-	-	-	-	-	-	-	1.8	1.2	0.12	0.12	1.6	186
Penis	0	0	-	-	-	-	-	-	-	-	-	-	-	-	-	-	-	-	-	-	0.0	0.0	0.00	0.00	0.0	187.1-.4
Other male genital	0	0	-	-	-	-	-	-	-	-	-	-	-	-	-	-	-	-	-	-	0.0	0.0	0.00	0.00	0.0	187.5-.9
†Bladder	19	0	-	-	-	-	-	-	-	-	-	-	21.6	-	19.2	60.0	124.8	116.7	-	206.2	3.7	2.6	0.20	1.13	8.3	188
Kidney etc.	19	0	3.0	-	3.8	-	-	-	-	9.1	-	-	16.2	13.3	28.8	45.0	-	38.9	-	-	3.7	2.6	0.37	0.60	5.5	189
Eye	1	0	-	-	-	-	1.9	-	-	-	-	-	-	-	-	-	-	-	-	-	0.2	0.1	0.01	0.01	0.2	190
Brain, nervous system	13	0	1.5	8.3	-	-	3.9	-	-	-	-	-	5.4	6.7	19.2	15.0	-	-	-	-	2.5	1.7	0.22	0.30	3.1	191-2
Thyroid	10	0	-	-	-	-	-	-	-	6.1	3.7	-	5.4	26.7	-	-	49.9	-	-	-	2.0	1.3	0.21	0.46	2.9	193
Other endocrine	4	0	3.0	1.7	-	-	-	-	-	-	-	4.2	-	-	-	-	-	-	-	-	0.8	0.5	0.04	0.04	0.8	194
Hodgkin's disease	7	0	1.5	1.7	-	1.9	1.9	4.4	2.5	-	-	-	-	-	-	-	-	-	-	-	1.4	0.9	0.07	0.07	1.2	201
Non-Hodgkin lymphoma	14	1	-	5.0	-	-	-	2.2	-	-	3.7	4.2	5.4	13.3	19.2	30.0	-	-	-	-	2.7	1.9	0.29	0.45	3.9	200,202
Multiple myeloma	7	0	-	-	-	-	-	-	2.5	-	-	4.2	10.8	6.7	19.2	-	-	-	-	-	1.4	0.9	0.22	0.22	2.0	203
Lymphoid leukaemia	7	0	3.0	1.7	1.9	-	-	-	-	-	-	-	-	-	28.8	-	-	-	-	-	1.4	0.9	0.18	0.18	1.8	204
Myeloid leukaemia	15	0	3.0	1.7	-	7.7	3.9	-	2.5	-	3.7	4.2	10.8	-	-	-	25.0	-	-	-	2.9	2.0	0.19	0.31	3.2	205
Monocytic leukaemia	1	0	-	-	-	1.9	-	-	-	-	-	-	-	-	-	-	-	-	-	-	0.2	0.1	0.01	0.01	0.2	206
Other leukaemia	1	0	1.5	-	-	-	-	-	-	-	-	-	-	-	-	-	-	-	-	-	0.2	0.1	0.01	0.01	0.2	207
Leukaemia unspecified	12	0	1.5	-	1.9	-	-	2.2	2.5	-	-	-	5.4	-	19.2	45.0	-	38.9	89.7	-	2.3	1.6	0.16	0.39	3.9	208
Other and unspecified	45	3	-	-	-	-	-	-	-	3.0	7.3	16.9	21.6	33.3	38.4	104.9	74.9	311.3	358.7	-	8.8	6.0	0.65	1.61	16.2	O&U
All sites																										
All sites but 173	744	14	20.8	25.0	11.4	15.3	23.1	26.5	27.4	51.7	110.1	266.9	437.7	733.3	1055.2	1379.3	1623.0	2295.7	1614.3	1443.3	145.3	100.0	14.29	29.59	248.9	ALLb

Rate from 1 case   1.486   1.663   1.896   1.918   1.925   2.208   2.494   3.042   3.669   4.237   5.404   6.667   9.592   14.993   24.969   38.911   89.686   206.186

†Important: see notes on population page

* FRENCH POLYNESIA 1988-1992

ANNUAL INCIDENCE PER 100,000 BY AGE GROUP (YEARS) - FEMALE

SITE	ALL AGES	AGE UNK	0-	5-	10-	15-	20-	25-	30-	35-	40-	45-	50-	55-	60-	65-	70-	75-	80-	85+	CRUDE RATE	%	CR 64	CR 74	ASR (W)	ICD (9th)
Lip	0	0	-	-	-	-	-	-	-	-	-	-	-	-	-	-	-	-	-	-	0.0	0.0	0.00	0.00	**0.0**	*140*
Tongue	3	0	-	-	-	-	-	-	-	3.4	-	-	-	-	10.8	14.7	-	-	-	-	0.6	0.4	0.07	0.14	**1.1**	*141*
Salivary gland	1	0	-	-	-	-	-	-	-	-	4.3	-	-	-	-	-	-	-	-	-	0.2	0.1	0.02	0.02	**0.3**	*142*
Mouth	8	0	-	-	-	-	-	-	-	-	8.5	-	18.7	7.7	10.8	14.7	-	-	-	-	1.7	1.0	0.23	0.30	**2.6**	*143-5*
Oropharynx	2	0	-	-	-	-	-	-	-	-	-	5.1	-	-	10.8	-	-	-	-	-	0.4	0.3	0.08	0.08	**0.7**	*146*
Nasopharynx	2	0	-	-	-	-	-	-	-	-	4.3	5.1	-	-	-	-	-	-	-	-	0.4	0.3	0.05	0.05	**0.6**	*147*
Hypopharynx	2	0	-	-	-	-	-	-	-	-	-	-	12.5	-	-	-	-	-	-	-	0.4	0.3	0.06	0.06	**0.6**	*148*
Pharynx unspecified	1	0	-	-	-	-	-	-	-	-	-	-	-	7.7	-	-	-	-	-	-	0.2	0.1	0.04	0.04	**0.3**	*149*
Oesophagus	4	0	-	-	-	-	-	-	-	-	-	-	12.5	-	-	14.7	22.1	-	-	-	0.8	0.5	0.06	0.25	**1.5**	*150*
Stomach	21	0	-	-	-	-	-	-	-	-	4.3	5.1	12.5	30.7	32.4	29.5	66.3	129.0	62.5	-	4.4	2.7	0.42	0.90	**7.5**	*151*
Small intestine	3	0	-	-	-	-	-	-	-	-	-	-	6.2	-	-	14.7	-	-	62.5	-	0.6	0.4	0.03	0.10	**1.1**	*152*
Colon	14	0	-	-	-	-	2.2	-	-	-	4.3	10.2	6.2	23.0	32.4	-	44.2	-	62.5	-	3.0	1.8	0.39	0.61	**4.8**	*153*
Rectum	12	1	-	-	-	-	-	-	-	3.4	4.3	10.2	6.2	7.7	21.6	-	22.1	64.5	-	-	2.5	1.5	0.29	0.41	**4.0**	*154*
Liver	12	0	1.6	-	-	-	-	-	-	-	8.5	15.2	12.5	-	10.8	-	-	32.3	125.0	-	2.5	1.5	0.24	0.24	**3.6**	*155*
Gallbladder etc.	5	0	-	-	-	-	-	-	2.8	-	4.3	5.1	-	-	-	-	44.2	-	-	-	1.1	0.6	0.06	0.28	**1.6**	*156*
Pancreas	9	1	-	-	-	-	-	-	-	-	-	5.1	-	7.7	10.8	29.5	44.2	32.3	-	-	1.9	1.1	0.13	0.55	**3.5**	*157*
Nose, sinuses etc.	3	0	-	-	-	2.0	-	-	-	-	-	5.1	-	-	-	14.7	-	-	-	-	0.6	0.4	0.04	0.11	**0.9**	*160*
Larynx	5	0	-	-	-	-	-	-	2.8	-	-	-	6.2	-	10.8	14.7	-	32.3	-	-	1.1	0.6	0.10	0.17	**1.7**	*161*
Bronchus, lung	75	6	-	-	-	-	-	-	2.8	3.4	8.5	20.3	56.2	115.1	108.2	147.3	176.8	193.5	-	425.5	15.9	9.5	1.71	3.47	**28.1**	*162*
Other thoracic organs	5	1	-	-	-	-	-	-	-	-	-	5.1	-	-	-	14.7	22.1	32.3	-	-	1.1	0.6	0.03	0.26	**1.9**	*163-4*
Bone	7	0	-	-	2.0	2.0	-	-	-	-	-	15.2	-	-	-	-	-	32.3	62.5	-	1.5	0.9	0.10	0.10	**1.9**	*170*
Connective tissue	4	0	-	1.8	-	-	-	-	-	-	4.3	-	-	7.7	-	14.7	-	-	-	-	0.8	0.5	0.07	0.14	**1.2**	*171*
Mesothelioma	0	0	-	-	-	-	-	-	-	-	-	-	-	-	-	-	-	-	-	-	0.0	0.0	0.00	0.00	**0.0**	*MES*
†Kaposi's sarcoma	0	0	-	-	-	-	-	-	-	-	-	-	-	-	-	-	-	-	-	-	0.0	0.0	0.00	0.00	**0.0**	*KAP*
Melanoma of skin	19	1	-	-	-	-	2.2	7.2	5.6	3.4	12.8	15.2	6.2	15.3	-	-	-	32.3	62.5	-	4.0	2.4	0.36	0.36	**4.8**	*172*
†Other skin																										
Breast	204	5	-	-	-	-	2.2	4.8	28.1	33.6	98.3	193.1	212.4	130.5	183.9	235.6	265.2	322.6	437.5	283.7	43.2	25.9	4.55	7.11	**65.7**	*174*
Uterus unspecified	23	1	-	-	-	-	-	-	5.6	-	4.3	5.1	12.5	38.4	21.6	29.5	88.4	64.5	-	141.8	4.9	2.9	0.46	1.07	**8.3**	*179*
Cervix uteri	91	4	-	-	-	-	-	2.4	14.0	26.8	51.3	91.5	87.5	92.1	75.7	73.6	66.3	64.5	-	-	19.3	11.5	2.31	3.04	**27.7**	*180*
Placenta	0	0	-	-	-	-	-	-	-	-	-	-	-	-	-	-	-	-	-	-	0.0	0.0	0.00	0.00	**0.0**	*181*
Corpus uteri	31	3	-	-	-	-	-	-	2.8	16.8	8.5	15.2	37.5	7.7	64.9	-	22.1	96.8	-	-	6.6	3.9	0.85	0.97	**9.7**	*182*
Ovary etc.	34	2	-	-	-	-	2.2	2.4	2.8	6.7	8.5	15.2	50.0	23.0	75.7	29.5	-	-	125.0	-	7.2	4.3	0.99	1.15	**11.0**	*183*
Other female genital	13	0	-	-	-	-	-	-	-	6.7	4.3	10.2	18.7	7.7	-	14.7	22.1	-	62.5	141.8	2.8	1.6	0.24	0.42	**4.4**	*184*
†Bladder	6	0	-	-	-	-	-	-	-	3.4	-	-	-	7.7	-	14.7	-	64.5	62.5	-	1.3	0.8	0.06	0.13	**1.9**	*188*
Kidney etc.	6	0	3.1	-	-	-	2.2	-	-	-	-	-	10.2	-	7.7	-	-	-	-	-	1.3	0.8	0.12	0.12	**1.5**	*189*
Eye	0	0	-	-	-	-	-	-	-	-	-	-	-	-	-	-	-	-	-	-	0.0	0.0	0.00	0.00	**0.0**	*190*
Brain, nervous system	16	0	1.6	1.8	-	-	2.2	2.4	5.6	-	4.3	15.2	-	7.7	10.8	44.2	-	32.3	-	-	3.4	2.0	0.26	0.48	**4.6**	*191-2*
Thyroid	57	0	-	-	-	2.0	6.5	14.4	16.8	3.4	34.2	35.6	37.5	76.7	21.6	58.9	22.1	32.3	62.5	-	12.1	7.2	1.24	1.65	**15.9**	*193*
Other endocrine	4	0	-	-	-	2.0	-	7.2	-	-	-	-	-	-	-	-	-	-	-	-	0.8	0.5	0.05	0.05	**0.8**	*194*
Hodgkin's disease	4	0	-	-	-	-	2.2	-	-	3.4	4.3	-	-	-	10.8	-	-	-	-	-	0.8	0.5	0.10	0.10	**1.1**	*201*
Non-Hodgkin lymphoma	15	0	3.1	-	-	-	4.3	-	-	6.7	4.3	-	6.2	15.3	10.8	14.7	44.2	32.3	-	-	3.2	1.9	0.25	0.55	**4.4**	*200,202*
Multiple myeloma	7	0	-	-	-	-	-	-	-	-	8.5	-	-	7.7	10.8	14.7	-	64.5	-	-	1.5	0.9	0.14	0.21	**2.3**	*203*
Lymphoid leukaemia	7	0	1.6	-	2.0	-	-	2.4	-	-	4.3	-	-	-	-	44.2	-	-	-	-	1.5	0.9	0.05	0.27	**2.1**	*204*
Myeloid leukaemia	10	0	1.6	1.8	-	-	8.6	-	-	-	-	-	-	6.2	-	-	-	32.3	125.0	-	2.1	1.3	0.09	0.09	**2.3**	*205*
Monocytic leukaemia	2	0	1.6	-	-	-	-	-	-	-	-	-	-	-	-	-	-	-	62.5	-	0.4	0.3	0.01	0.01	**0.5**	*206*
Other leukaemia	1	0	-	-	-	-	-	-	-	-	4.3	-	-	-	-	-	-	-	-	-	0.2	0.1	0.02	0.02	**0.3**	*207*
Leukaemia unspecified	6	0	1.6	-	2.0	-	-	-	-	-	-	-	-	15.3	10.8	-	22.1	-	-	-	1.3	0.8	0.15	0.26	**1.9**	*208*
Other and unspecified	35	1	3.1	3.5	-	-	-	2.4	-	-	4.3	15.2	6.2	23.0	32.4	117.8	44.2	193.5	62.5	141.8	7.4	4.4	0.46	1.30	**12.4**	*O&U*
All sites																										
All sites but 173	789	26	18.8	8.8	6.0	7.9	34.5	45.7	89.8	120.8	311.9	528.5	631.1	683.0	789.6	1016.2	1038.7	1580.6	1437.5	1134.8	166.9	100.0	16.94	27.56	**252.6**	*ALLb*
Rate from 1 case			1.570	1.768	2.001	1.964	2.154	2.406	2.807	3.355	4.273	5.081	6.248	7.675	10.817	14.728	22.099	32.258	62.500	141.844						

†Important: see notes on population page

New Zealand

The New Zealand Registry was established in 1948. It is located in the New Zealand Health Information Service (NZHIS), of the New Zealand Ministry of Health, Wellington. The registry was initially clinically oriented, only patients admitted to hospital for treatment being registered, but in 1972 became population-based.

New Zealand is situated in the south Pacific Ocean, 1600 km south-east of Australia. It is a long mountainous country surrounded by a large expanse of ocean. The total land area (including offshore islands) is 270 534 km^2.

The total population of New Zealand in 1991 was 3 373 926, of whom children aged under 15 years comprised about 23%. Within the New Zealand population there are population sub-groups with significantly different age structures. Ethnic groups such as Maori and Pacific Islands Polynesians have more youthful populations, containing proportionately twice as many children under the age of 15 as the rest of the population. In 1993, 21% of employed persons were engaged in the wholesale, retail, restaurant and hotel industries, 28% in community, social and personal services, 16% in manufacturing, 11% in business and financial services and 11% in agriculture, hunting, fishing and forestry.

Since 1972, case notification has been based on compulsory reporting of all cases treated in publicly funded hospitals and voluntary reporting of cases treated in private hospitals. In addition, the registry receives a copy of every death certificate or autopsy report with a mention of cancer. An overall case ascertainment level of greater than 90% is achieved, but there is probably significant under-reporting of early-stage melanomas of the skin treated other than in hospitals.

In the period 1988–93, the registry experienced difficulty in obtaining complete data about morphological type, with the result that a high proportion of cases were coded as not stated. Because of this, histology has not been included in the data-set for this volume. In 1994 legislation was introduced changing the method of reporting to notification by pathology laboratories.

Information is held on computer files and most editing functions are computerized, although duplication is prevented by manual means. Multiple primary tumours in one individual are registered and cross-referenced.

Data on cancer incidence and mortality are routinely published in annual reports, the latest being data for 1992.

All of the records included in this study are coded using the International Classification of Diseases, Ninth Revision-CM (topography).

James Fraser
Brenda Wordsworth

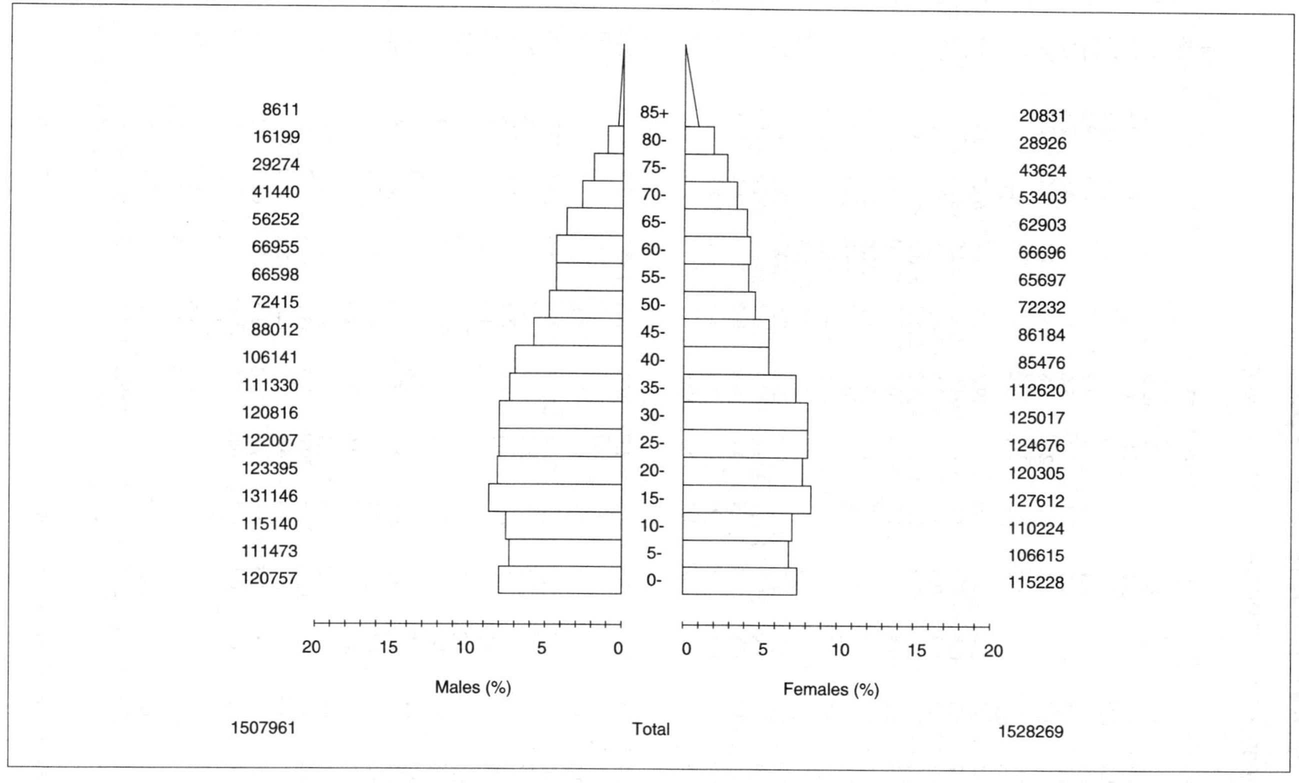

New Zealand: Non-Maori
Source of population: average annual 1988–92
Statistics New Zealand
Notes to tables overleaf:
+ The editors were unable to verify these data
† 163-164 includes mesothelioma of the pleura
† Mesothelioma not available separately
† Kaposi's sarcoma not available separately
† 173 does not include basal cell or squamous cell carcinoma
† 188 does not include non-invasive diagnoses

+ NEW ZEALAND: NON-MAORI 1988-1992

ANNUAL INCIDENCE PER 100,000 BY AGE GROUP (YEARS) - MALE

SITE	ALL AGES	AGE UNK	0-	5-	10-	15-	20-	25-	30-	35-	40-	45-	50-	55-	60-	65-	70-	75-	80-	85+	CRUDE RATE	%	CR 64	CR 74	ASR (W)	ICD (9th)
Lip	324	0	-	-	-	0.2	1.5	0.8	2.6	2.0	3.6	5.5	5.0	5.4	9.9	13.9	23.2	30.7	27.2	37.2	4.3	1.1	0.18	0.37	**3.4**	*140*
Tongue	134	0	-	-	0.2	0.2	-	0.2	0.7	0.2	1.5	1.1	3.6	4.5	7.8	6.4	8.2	8.2	9.9	9.3	1.8	0.5	0.10	0.17	**1.5**	*141*
Salivary gland	117	0	-	-	-	-	-	0.5	0.3	0.5	0.9	0.9	1.1	2.7	3.6	7.5	7.2	12.3	13.6	23.2	1.6	0.4	0.05	0.13	**1.2**	*142*
Mouth	170	0	-	-	-	-	-	-	-	0.5	0.9	1.6	4.1	6.6	11.4	9.2	9.7	15.7	8.6	9.3	2.3	0.6	0.13	0.22	**1.8**	*143-5*
Oropharynx	77	0	-	-	-	-	-	-	-	0.2	1.1	0.7	1.7	3.3	5.1	3.6	4.3	6.1	4.9	2.3	1.0	0.3	0.06	0.10	**0.8**	*146*
Nasopharynx	56	0	0.2	0.2	-	-	0.3	0.5	0.7	0.5	1.5	1.4	1.4	1.2	2.1	2.8	-	1.4	1.2	2.3	0.7	0.2	0.05	0.06	**0.7**	*147*
Hypopharynx	80	0	-	-	-	-	-	-	-	0.4	-	0.7	1.4	3.3	3.9	7.8	6.8	6.1	1.2	-	1.1	0.3	0.05	0.12	**0.9**	*148*
Pharynx unspecified	24	0	-	-	-	-	-	-	-	-	0.2	-	0.3	1.5	1.2	2.5	1.4	-	2.5	2.3	0.3	0.1	0.02	0.04	**0.3**	*149*
Oesophagus	515	0	-	-	-	-	-	0.2	0.4	0.9	3.4	6.9	12.0	24.8	39.5	41.5	38.9	66.7	83.6	6.8	1.8	0.24	0.65	**5.3**	*150*
Stomach	1134	0	-	-	-	-	0.3	-	0.7	2.7	1.3	6.8	8.6	22.2	41.8	64.0	100.9	132.5	181.5	234.6	15.0	4.0	0.42	1.25	**11.0**	*151*
Small intestine	71	0	-	-	-	-	-	-	-	0.2	0.4	0.7	0.8	3.0	4.5	2.5	4.3	6.1	9.9	9.3	0.9	0.2	0.05	0.08	**0.7**	*152*
Colon	3045	1	-	-	0.2	0.2	0.2	1.1	2.2	4.0	9.2	23.2	55.2	92.5	132.0	179.2	224.9	300.6	360.5	455.2	40.4	10.6	1.60	3.62	**31.2**	*153*
Rectum	1955	0	-	-	-	-	0.2	0.8	1.2	2.5	6.0	16.4	35.6	54.7	89.3	136.5	140.4	179.0	216.1	236.9	25.9	6.8	1.03	2.42	**20.1**	*154*
Liver	275	0	0.8	0.2	-	0.3	0.5	-	1.3	1.1	1.9	1.4	5.0	7.8	11.1	15.3	22.2	21.9	24.7	27.9	3.6	1.0	0.16	0.34	**2.9**	*155*
Gallbladder etc.	137	1	-	-	-	-	-	0.2	0.3	0.5	0.4	0.2	0.8	3.3	4.5	10.3	7.7	19.8	14.8	27.9	1.8	0.5	0.05	0.14	**1.3**	*156*
Pancreas	742	0	-	-	-	0.2	-	-	0.3	1.3	2.8	2.5	7.5	16.8	27.5	46.6	69.0	75.2	118.5	118.4	9.8	2.6	0.29	0.87	**7.3**	*157*
Nose, sinuses etc.	56	0	-	-	-	0.2	0.2	0.3	0.2	-	0.8	0.7	0.8	0.6	2.7	2.1	2.9	8.2	4.9	4.6	0.7	0.2	0.03	0.06	**0.6**	*160*
Larynx	384	0	-	-	-	-	-	-	-	0.4	0.6	3.2	7.7	14.7	19.4	29.2	28.5	30.7	38.3	13.9	5.1	1.3	0.23	0.52	**4.0**	*161*
Bronchus, lung	4691	0	-	-	0.2	-	0.2	0.5	0.3	0.9	7.9	18.9	50.5	107.8	209.1	327.8	412.2	541.1	591.4	615.4	62.2	16.4	1.98	5.68	**46.5**	*162*
†Other thoracic organs	145	0	0.2	-	-	0.3	0.3	0.3	0.3	0.5	0.8	1.8	2.5	7.5	4.8	8.9	9.7	12.3	6.2	11.6	1.9	0.5	0.10	0.19	**1.6**	*163-4*
Bone	119	0	-	-	2.3	3.1	2.4	1.3	1.2	1.3	0.8	0.5	1.1	0.9	4.2	1.4	1.4	4.8	8.6	2.3	1.6	0.4	0.09	0.11	**1.4**	*170*
Connective tissue	246	0	1.0	0.5	0.7	0.9	1.3	1.1	3.1	3.8	2.1	3.2	2.5	4.8	5.7	10.0	8.7	18.4	22.2	27.9	3.3	0.9	0.15	0.25	**2.7**	*171*
†Mesothelioma																										
†Kaposi's sarcoma																										
Melanoma of skin	2298	0	0.2	0.2	0.9.	3.4	7.3	14.3	23.3	24.1	32.8	37.9	48.6	48.7	82.7	93.5	115.8	138.7	176.5	132.4	30.5	8.0	1.62	2.67	**25.0**	*172*
†Other skin	1	0	-	-	-	-	-	-	-	-	-	-	-	0.3	-	-	-	-	-	-	0.0		0.00	0.00	**0.0**	*173*
Breast	67	0	-	-	-	0.2	0.2	0.7	0.2	0.2	0.2	0.5	1.4	2.1	1.5	3.9	5.8	6.1	6.2	4.6	0.9	0.2	0.03	0.08	**0.7**	*175*
Prostate	4192	0	-	-	-	0.2	-	-	-	0.2	0.6	1.8	12.7	33.6	91.4	203.4	396.7	703.0	918.5	1272.7	55.6	14.6	0.70	3.70	**37.8**	*185*
Testis	479	0	0.7	-	0.3	2.0	8.9	11.6	16.1	14.4	10.0	7.7	5.5	3.6	3.0	3.2	4.3	4.1	-	9.3	6.4	1.7	0.42	0.46	**5.6**	*186*
Penis	48	0	-	-	-	-	-	0.2	0.2	-	0.4	0.2	0.6	0.6	1.5	1.4	3.4	6.1	8.6	16.3	0.6	0.2	0.02	0.04	**0.5**	*187.1-.4*
Other male genital	12	0	-	0.2	-	-	-	-	0.2	-	-	0.2	0.3	-	0.3	-	1.0	0.7	3.7	2.3	0.2	0.0	0.01	0.01	**0.1**	*187.5-.9*
†Bladder	1446	0	0.2	-	-	-	0.3	1.1	0.7	1.3	3.0	7.0	12.2	27.3	46.3	84.3	132.2	175.6	240.7	290.3	19.2	5.0	0.50	1.58	**14.0**	*188*
Kidney etc.	679	0	1.7	0.2	-	0.3	0.2	0.2	0.8	1.6	5.1	4.8	13.8	21.3	26.6	42.3	49.2	56.0	72.8	69.7	9.0	2.4	0.38	0.84	**7.1**	*189*
Eye	106	0	2.6	0.4	0.2	0.2	0.2	-	0.2	0.5	1.3	1.6	1.4	1.5	2.7	5.0	8.2	6.1	7.4	4.6	1.4	0.4	0.06	0.13	**1.3**	*190*
Brain, nervous system	617	0	4.5	3.4	3.3	1.7	2.3	2.8	4.0	4.1	5.5	9.8	14.6	16.8	24.8	25.6	29.9	25.3	24.7	18.6	8.2	2.2	0.49	0.77	**7.4**	*191-2*
Thyroid	112	0	-	-	0.2	0.5	0.2	1.1	1.3	2.0	1.5	1.1	2.2	2.1	1.8	6.4	4.3	7.5	7.4	7.0	1.5	0.4	0.07	0.12	**1.2**	*193*
Other endocrine	51	0	1.7	0.4	0.9	0.2	0.3	0.3	0.3	0.2	0.6	0.2	0.8	0.9	0.6	1.8	1.4	4.1	-	-	0.7	0.2	0.04	0.05	**0.7**	*194*
Hodgkin's disease	157	0	-	0.5	1.6	1.7	1.9	3.0	2.0	2.7	1.9	2.5	2.2	1.8	2.1	5.0	4.3	4.1	4.9	4.6	2.1	0.5	0.12	0.17	**1.9**	*201*
Non-Hodgkin lymphoma	969	0	1.3	1.4	1.2	1.5	1.6	3.1	4.3	5.4	9.6	9.5	15.7	31.5	29.0	42.7	63.2	86.8	96.3	99.9	12.9	3.4	0.58	1.11	**10.3**	*200,202*
Multiple myeloma	411	0	-	-	0.2	0.2	-	0.2	0.3	0.9	0.9	3.6	5.5	5.4	14.9	22.4	32.3	45.8	63.0	102.2	5.5	1.4	0.16	0.43	**4.1**	*203*
Lymphoid leukaemia	471	0	7.0	3.4	1.9	2.3	1.5	0.8	1.0	0.4	0.9	1.6	2.5	6.0	11.6	19.2	33.8	46.5	61.7	92.9	6.2	1.6	0.20	0.47	**5.3**	*204*
Myeloid leukaemia	442	0	0.8	0.5	1.4	1.1	1.9	1.5	2.8	1.6	3.6	3.9	6.1	6.6	10.2	19.6	29.0	43.0	56.8	79.0	5.9	1.5	0.21	0.45	**4.6**	*205*
Monocytic leukaemia	10	0	-	-	-	-	-	-	-	0.2	-	-	-	-	-	1.9	0.7	-	1.2	7.0	0.1	0.0	0.00	0.01	**0.1**	*206*
Other leukaemia	11	0	-	-	0.3	0.2	-	-	0.2	-	-	-	0.3	-	0.3	0.7	1.0	-	1.2	-	0.1	0.0	0.01	0.01	**0.1**	*207*
Leukaemia unspecified	55	0	0.5	0.2	-	-	-	-	0.2	-	-	-	-	0.6	1.8	2.5	3.9	4.8	13.6	20.9	0.7	0.2	0.02	0.05	**0.6**	*208*
Other and unspecified	1518	1	0.5	0.2	0.2	0.2	0.6	1.5	1.2	2.7	4.1	9.8	14.1	31.2	55.0	80.0	124.5	156.5	265.4	336.7	20.1	5.3	0.61	1.63	**15.0**	*O&U*
All sites	28649	3	23.7	11.8	16.0	20.4	34.7	50.0	74.7	86.1	127.6	198.4	364.6	618.9	1034.4	1589.6	2181.4	2991.7	3764.3	4526.3	380.0		13.31	32.16	**290.4**	*ALL*
All sites but 173	28648	3	23.7	11.8	16.0	20.4	34.7	50.0	74.7	86.1	127.6	198.4	364.6	618.9	1034.1	1589.6	2181.4	2991.7	3764.3	4526.3	380.0	100.0	13.31	32.16	**290.3**	*ALLb*

| Rate from 1 case | | | 0.166 | 0.179 | 0.174 | 0.153 | 0.162 | 0.164 | 0.166 | 0.180 | 0.188 | 0.227 | 0.276 | 0.300 | 0.299 | 0.356 | 0.483 | 0.683 | 1.235 | 2.322 | | | | | | |

†Important: see notes on population page

+ NEW ZEALAND: NON-MAORI 1988-1992

ANNUAL INCIDENCE PER 100,000 BY AGE GROUP (YEARS) - FEMALE

SITE	ALL AGES	AGE UNK	0-	5-	10-	15-	20-	25-	30-	35-	40-	45-	50-	55-	60-	65-	70-	75-	80-	85+	CRUDE RATE	%	CR 64	CR 74	ASR (W)	ICD (9th)
Lip	115	0	0.2	-	-	-	0.2	0.2	0.2	0.4	0.9	1.4	1.7	1.8	3.3	3.5	6.4	7.8	11.1	14.4	1.5	0.4	0.05	0.10	**0.9**	*140*
Tongue	90	0	-	-	-	-	-	0.2	0.3	0.4	0.2	0.7	1.9	2.4	2.1	2.9	5.2	3.7	9.0	14.4	1.2	0.3	0.04	0.08	**0.7**	*141*
Salivary gland	57	0	-	-	0.2	0.2	0.2	0.5	0.5	0.2	1.4	0.7	0.8	0.9	1.8	2.5	1.9	1.8	3.5	3.8	0.7	0.2	0.04	0.06	**0.6**	*142*
Mouth	99	0	-	-	-	-	-	-	-	-	0.5	1.2	1.7	1.8	4.5	3.5	4.5	3.7	7.6	22.1	1.3	0.3	0.05	0.09	**0.8**	*143-5*
Oropharynx	41	0	-	-	-	-	-	0.2	-	0.2	0.7	-	1.4	0.6	2.1	1.6	1.1	3.7	0.7	4.8	0.5	0.1	0.03	0.04	**0.4**	*146*
Nasopharynx	26	0	-	0.2	-	-	0.2	-	0.3	-	0.5	0.2	0.8	0.3	1.5	1.3	-	1.8	-	1.9	0.3	0.1	0.02	0.03	**0.3**	*147*
Hypopharynx	29	0	-	-	-	-	-	-	-	-	-	0.2	1.1	-	0.9	1.3	1.9	1.4	4.1	2.9	0.4	0.1	0.01	0.03	**0.2**	*148*
Pharynx unspecified	6	0	-	-	0.2	0.2	-	-	-	0.2	-	-	0.3	-	-	-	-	-	0.7	1.0	0.1	0.0	0.00	0.00	**0.1**	*149*
Oesophagus	338	0	-	-	-	-	-	-	0.2	-	0.9	0.9	3.6	4.6	8.4	13.7	16.1	31.6	38.7	59.5	4.4	1.1	0.09	0.24	**2.4**	*150*
Stomach	666	0	-	-	0.3	0.3	0.5	1.4	1.6	2.6	5.1	6.1	9.1	14.7	25.1	30.7	55.0	78.8	107.5	8.7	2.2	0.21	0.49	**4.8**	*151*
Small intestine	69	0	-	-	-	0.2	0.2	0.2	0.2	0.5	0.7	0.7	1.1	0.9	0.9	3.2	4.1	6.0	2.8	7.7	0.9	0.2	0.03	0.06	**0.6**	*152*
Colon	3650	0	0.2	-	0.2	1.1	0.5	1.0	2.9	4.8	16.8	27.8	55.1	86.8	123.5	158.0	202.6	259.5	334.0	395.6	47.8	12.3	1.60	3.41	**29.6**	*153*
Rectum	1362	0	-	-	-	-	-	0.5	0.3	3.2	5.8	11.4	23.0	30.1	51.9	60.4	70.4	95.4	120.3	144.0	17.8	4.6	0.63	1.29	**11.2**	*154*
Liver	160	0	0.3	0.2	0.2	0.3	0.2	-	0.3	0.2	1.9	1.2	1.7	3.7	3.9	5.7	10.1	7.8	15.9	20.2	2.1	0.5	0.07	0.15	**1.3**	*155*
Gallbladder etc.	186	1	-	-	-	-	-	-	0.2	0.2	0.5	1.9	1.9	2.1	3.9	8.6	11.2	15.1	24.2	20.2	2.4	0.6	0.05	0.15	**1.4**	*156*
Pancreas	626	0	-	-	-	-	-	0.2	0.2	0.9	1.2	3.7	6.6	11.9	13.8	25.8	39.7	50.4	63.6	96.0	8.2	2.1	0.19	0.52	**4.6**	*157*
Nose, sinuses etc.	54	0	0.2	-	0.2	-	-	0.2	0.2	0.7	0.7	0.5	0.3	0.9	1.5	3.5	3.0	2.8	3.5	1.9	0.7	0.2	0.03	0.06	**0.5**	*160*
Larynx	65	0	-	-	-	-	-	0.2	0.2	0.2	0.2	0.2	1.7	1.8	2.1	3.5	5.6	4.1	2.8	1.9	0.9	0.2	0.03	0.08	**0.6**	*161*
Bronchus, lung	2113	0	0.5	-	-	0.2	0.2	0.5	2.1	3.4	9.4	16.0	27.4	54.5	84.0	122.7	150.2	139.4	125.1	128.7	27.7	7.1	0.99	2.35	**18.2**	*162*
†Other thoracic organs	48	0	-	-	-	-	-	-	0.2	0.5	0.2	0.2	1.4	0.9	0.9	2.9	2.6	2.8	3.5	3.8	0.6	0.2	0.02	0.05	**0.4**	*163-4*
Bone	79	0	0.3	0.6	1.5	1.4	0.8	1.0	0.3	0.4	0.5	0.7	0.8	0.9	0.6	2.2	1.9	2.8	4.1	4.8	1.0	0.3	0.05	0.07	**0.9**	*170*
Connective tissue	183	0	1.2	0.2	0.2	1.4	0.8	0.6	1.1	0.7	2.3	1.6	1.9	2.1	3.9	7.3	6.0	12.4	13.1	15.4	2.4	0.6	0.09	0.16	**1.7**	*171*
†Mesothelioma																										
†Kaposi's sarcoma																										
Melanoma of skin	2803	1	0.5	0.8	1.1	3.3	13.6	23.6	31.2	40.5	62.9	56.4	64.0	59.1	81.0	86.2	79.8	94.4	85.0	92.2	36.7	9.4	2.19	3.02	**29.8**	*172*
†Other skin	0	0	-	-	-	-	-	-	-	-	-	-	-	-	-	-	-	-	-	-	0.0	0.0	0.00	0.00	**0.0**	*173*
Breast	7604	1	0.2	-	-	-	1.3	7.1	24.8	61.6	140.2	189.8	226.8	220.4	258.5	279.5	298.1	298.5	322.2	416.7	99.5	25.6	5.65	8.54	**77.2**	*174*
Uterus unspecified	8	0	-	-	-	-	-	-	-	-	0.2	0.2	-	-	0.3	0.6	0.4	0.5	-	1.0	0.1	0.0	0.00	0.01	**0.1**	*179*
Cervix uteri	1073	0	-	-	-	0.5	2.7	8.8	17.1	27.0	33.7	26.0	21.9	24.7	24.3	27.0	24.0	19.7	24.9	14.4	14.0	3.6	0.93	1.19	**11.9**	*180*
Placenta	35	0	-	-	-	0.3	1.2	1.4	1.0	0.9	0.5	0.5	0.6	-	-	-	-	-	-	-	0.5	0.1	0.03	0.03	**0.4**	*181*
Corpus uteri	999	0	-	-	-	-	0.2	0.2	1.8	1.6	6.6	10.7	24.4	38.1	43.8	49.3	52.8	51.8	50.5	59.5	13.1	3.4	0.64	1.15	**9.4**	*182*
Ovary etc.	1125	0	-	0.4	1.3	1.3	2.0	2.9	4.0	7.1	15.9	17.4	27.4	26.2	44.4	46.4	46.8	56.6	62.2	49.9	14.7	3.8	0.75	1.22	**11.0**	*183*
Other female genital	313	0	0.2	-	-	0.2	0.3	0.8	1.6	2.0	4.0	1.9	4.2	4.0	7.8	16.2	11.6	19.7	22.8	44.2	4.1	1.1	0.13	0.27	**2.6**	*184*
†Bladder	538	0	-	-	-	-	-	0.3	0.2	1.2	1.6	3.0	5.5	9.1	17.7	21.6	30.3	35.8	57.4	85.4	7.0	1.8	0.19	0.45	**4.1**	*188*
Kidney etc.	489	0	2.8	0.9	0.2	0.2	0.7	1.0	1.1	1.8	2.8	4.9	4.2	13.4	15.3	20.0	22.8	38.5	32.5	39.4	6.4	1.6	0.25	0.46	**4.4**	*189*
Eye	69	0	1.2	0.4	0.4	-	0.2	0.3	0.3	0.7	1.2	0.5	0.8	3.0	1.5	1.3	3.0	3.7	1.4	1.9	0.9	0.2	0.05	0.07	**0.8**	*190*
Brain, nervous system	450	0	3.1	4.1	3.1	0.8	1.8	2.1	3.0	2.7	6.1	3.2	10.0	14.3	12.6	19.4	15.7	15.6	10.4	12.5	5.9	1.5	0.33	0.51	**5.1**	*191-2*
Thyroid	315	0	-	0.2	-	0.9	3.3	3.8	4.6	3.2	6.1	5.8	6.1	8.2	8.4	9.2	9.7	6.0	8.3	8.6	4.1	1.1	0.25	0.35	**3.4**	*193*
Other endocrine	57	0	1.4	0.6	0.5	-	0.3	0.3	0.8	0.2	1.4	0.5	0.6	1.2	1.8	1.6	0.4	1.8	1.4	1.0	0.7	0.2	0.05	0.06	**0.7**	*194*
Hodgkin's disease	115	0	-	0.2	0.5	2.0	2.5	1.9	2.1	1.1	1.6	0.7	1.4	1.2	2.4	1.6	3.7	0.9	4.1	1.9	1.5	0.4	0.09	0.12	**1.3**	*201*
Non-Hodgkin lymphoma	845	0	1.0	1.5	0.4	0.5	1.8	1.9	2.1	3.6	7.3	10.4	13.8	16.7	24.3	30.5	46.8	56.4	68.4	62.4	11.1	2.8	0.43	0.81	**7.5**	*200,202*
Multiple myeloma	337	1	-	-	-	-	-	-	0.6	0.5	0.7	2.8	4.7	5.5	11.1	14.6	24.3	27.0	27.7	30.7	4.4	1.1	0.13	0.33	**2.7**	*203*
Lymphoid leukaemia	355	0	6.4	3.8	1.1	0.8	1.3	0.8	0.3	0.7	0.9	1.2	3.6	4.6	6.3	11.1	14.6	21.1	36.0	36.5	4.6	1.2	0.16	0.29	**3.5**	*204*
Myeloid leukaemia	346	0	0.5	0.4	0.4	1.1	1.0	2.1	1.9	2.3	2.1	4.4	6.4	6.1	7.2	9.2	14.2	19.3	29.0	40.3	4.5	1.2	0.18	0.30	**3.1**	*205*
Monocytic leukaemia	8	0	-	-	-	-	-	-	-	-	-	0.2	-	-	-	0.3	1.5	0.5	-	1.0	0.1	0.0	0.00	0.01	**0.1**	*206*
Other leukaemia	7	0	0.2	-	-	-	-	0.2	0.2	-	-	-	-	0.3	-	-	0.9	0.7	-	-	0.1	0.0	0.00	0.00	**0.1**	*207*
Leukaemia unspecified	45	0	0.2	-	-	-	-	0.2	-	-	0.2	-	0.6	0.6	0.6	1.9	2.2	1.8	4.8	12.5	0.6	0.2	0.01	0.03	**0.3**	*208*
Other and unspecified	1735	1	0.2	-	0.2	0.5	0.2	0.5	1.8	3.6	7.0	9.7	17.2	29.8	48.6	68.4	100.4	107.3	169.4	324.5	22.7	5.8	0.60	1.44	**13.1**	*O&U*
All sites	29733	5	20.8	14.3	11.6	17.4	37.9	65.8	111.3	180.6	351.0	426.5	586.2	704.4	948.2	1175.1	1378.6	1586.7	1886.2	2408.9	389.1	100.0	17.38	30.15	**274.6**	*ALL*
All sites but 173	29733	5	20.8	14.3	11.6	17.4	37.9	65.8	111.3	180.6	351.0	426.5	586.2	704.4	948.2	1175.1	1378.6	1586.7	1886.2	2408.9	389.1	100.0	17.38	30.15	**274.6**	*ALLb*

Rate from 1 case		0.174	0.188	0.181	0.157	0.166	0.160	0.160	0.178	0.234	0.232	0.277	0.304	0.299	0.318	0.374	0.458	0.691	0.960

†Important: see notes on population page

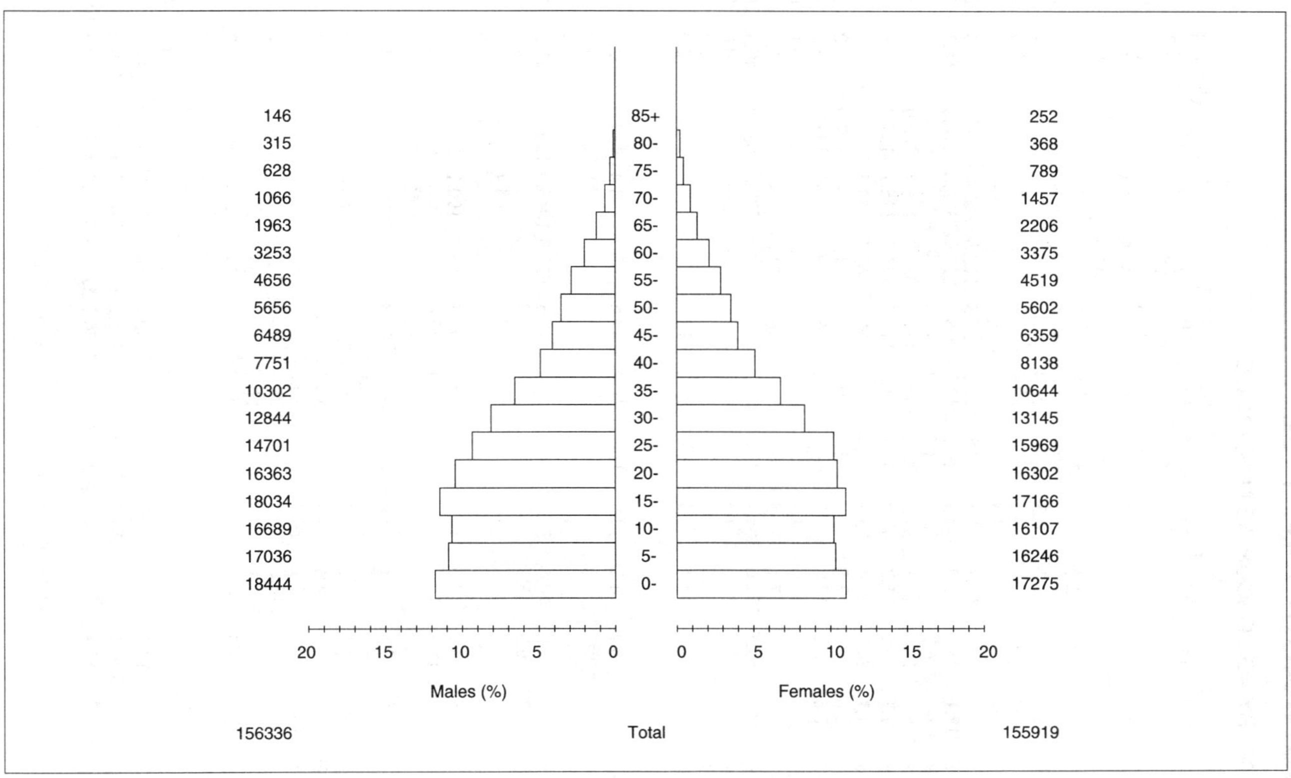

New Zealand: Maori
Source of population: average annual 1988–92
Statistics New Zealand
Notes to tables overleaf:
+ The editors were unable to verify these data
† 163-164 includes mesothelioma of the pleura
† Mesothelioma not available separately
† Kaposi's sarcoma not available separately
† 173 does not include basal cell or squamous cell carcinoma
† 188 does not include non-invasive diagnoses

+ NEW ZEALAND: MAORI 1988-1992

ANNUAL INCIDENCE PER 100,000 BY AGE GROUP (YEARS) - MALE

SITE	ALL AGES	AGE UNK	0-	5-	10-	15-	20-	25-	30-	35-	40-	45-	50-	55-	60-	65-	70-	75-	80-	85+	CRUDE RATE	%	CR 64	CR 74	ASR (W)	ICD (9th)
Lip	2	0	-	-	-	-	-	-	-	-	-	-	-	-	-	10.2	18.8	-	-	-	0.3	0.1	0.00	0.14	0.7	140
Tongue	11	0	-	-	-	-	-	-	-	1.9	2.6	-	3.5	17.2	-	20.4	-	31.8	63.4	-	1.4	0.7	0.13	0.23	2.4	141
Salivary gland	3	0	-	-	-	-	-	1.4	-	-	-	-	-	-	6.1	-	-	31.8	-	-	0.4	0.2	0.04	0.04	0.7	142
Mouth	14	0	-	-	-	-	-	-	-	-	-	3.1	7.1	-	43.0	30.6	18.8	-	-	-	1.8	0.9	0.27	0.51	3.6	143-5
Oropharynx	5	0	-	-	-	-	-	-	1.6	-	-	-	7.1	-	6.1	-	18.8	-	-	-	0.6	0.3	0.07	0.17	1.1	146
Nasopharynx	11	0	-	-	-	1.1	-	-	3.1	1.9	2.6	3.1	7.1	4.3	-	20.4	-	-	-	-	1.4	0.7	0.12	0.22	1.9	147
Hypopharynx	3	0	-	-	-	-	-	-	-	-	-	-	-	-	6.1	20.4	-	-	-	-	0.4	0.2	0.03	0.13	0.9	148
Pharynx unspecified	2	0	1.1	-	-	-	-	-	-	-	-	-	-	-	-	4.3	-	-	-	-	-	0.3	0.1	0.03	0.03	0.3	149
Oesophagus	34	0	-	-	-	-	-	-	-	-	-	-	14.1	21.5	30.7	122.2	56.3	127.3	63.4	-	4.3	2.3	0.33	1.22	9.2	150
Stomach	111	0	-	-	-	-	1.2	1.4	4.7	9.7	18.1	15.4	38.9	42.9	129.1	213.9	206.3	222.9	380.2	274.0	14.2	7.5	1.31	3.41	27.9	151
Small intestine	9	0	-	-	-	-	-	-	-	1.9	-	6.2	-	-	18.4	20.4	18.8	-	-	-	1.2	0.6	0.13	0.33	2.2	152
Colon	79	0	-	-	-	1.1	2.4	1.4	3.1	3.9	5.2	18.5	14.1	51.5	49.2	132.4	131.3	382.0	126.7	684.9	10.1	5.3	0.75	2.07	21.5	153
Rectum	53	0	-	-	-	-	-	2.7	1.6	3.9	7.7	9.2	21.2	42.9	36.9	71.3	112.5	127.3	126.7	137.0	6.8	3.6	0.63	1.55	12.8	154
Liver	61	0	1.1	-	1.2	-	1.2	-	-	11.6	7.7	24.7	42.4	25.8	73.8	40.7	75.0	63.7	63.4	-	7.8	4.1	0.95	1.53	12.8	155
Gallbladder etc.	8	0	-	-	-	-	-	-	-	-	2.6	3.1	3.5	-	6.1	20.4	-	31.8	-	137.0	1.0	0.5	0.08	0.18	2.4	156
Pancreas	38	0	-	-	-	-	-	-	-	5.8	2.6	6.2	17.7	8.6	61.5	61.1	56.3	159.2	-	137.0	4.9	2.6	0.51	1.10	9.8	157
Nose, sinuses etc.	1	0	-	-	-	-	-	-	-	-	-	-	-	4.3	-	-	-	-	-	-	0.1	0.1	0.02	0.02	0.2	160
Larynx	13	0	-	-	-	-	-	-	-	-	-	3.1	7.1	21.5	6.1	-	56.3	31.8	-	-	1.7	0.9	0.19	0.47	3.1	161
Bronchus, lung	387	0	-	-	-	-	-	-	-	1.9	20.6	55.5	152.0	365.1	448.8	621.3	1068.8	859.6	570.3	684.9	49.5	26.1	5.22	13.67	99.7	162
†Other thoracic organs	5	0	1.1	-	-	-	-	1.4	-	-	-	3.1	-	4.3	-	10.2	-	-	-	-	0.6	0.3	0.05	0.10	0.9	163-4
Bone	15	0	-	-	-	5.5	7.3	1.4	-	1.9	-	-	-	-	-	20.4	-	-	-	-	1.9	1.0	0.08	0.18	1.9	170
Connective tissue	16	0	-	3.5	1.2	-	-	1.4	1.6	3.9	-	-	14.1	4.3	6.1	10.2	18.8	-	-	-	2.0	1.1	0.18	0.33	2.7	171
†Mesothelioma																										
†Kaposi's sarcoma																										
Melanoma of skin	21	0	-	-	-	-	-	2.7	1.6	-	-	6.2	14.1	12.9	12.3	10.2	37.5	63.7	63.4	137.0	2.7	1.4	0.25	0.49	5.1	172
†Other skin	0	0	-	-	-	-	-	-	-	-	-	-	-	-	-	-	-	-	-	-	0.0	0.0	0.00	0.00	0.0	173
Breast	3	0	-	-	-	-	-	1.4	-	1.9	-	-	-	4.3	-	-	-	-	-	-	0.4	0.2	0.04	0.04	0.4	175
Prostate	135	0	-	-	-	-	-	-	-	1.9	-	6.2	10.6	38.7	110.7	244.4	412.5	923.3	1013.9	1506.8	17.3	9.1	0.84	4.13	44.4	185
Testis	61	0	3.3	-	-	1.1	13.4	34.0	15.6	7.8	7.7	6.2	3.5	-	-	-	18.8	-	-	-	7.8	4.1	0.46	0.56	7.1	186
Penis	1	0	-	-	-	-	-	-	-	-	-	-	-	-	-	-	-	-	63.4	-	0.1	0.1	0.00	0.00	0.3	187.1-.4
Other male genital	0	0	-	-	-	-	-	-	-	-	-	-	-	-	-	-	-	-	-	-	0.0	0.0	0.00	0.00	0.0	187.5-.9
†Bladder	37	0	-	-	-	1.1	-	-	-	1.9	2.6	3.1	10.6	17.2	43.0	71.3	93.8	63.7	190.1	274.0	4.7	2.5	0.40	1.22	10.5	188
Kidney etc.	36	0	2.2	1.2	-	-	-	-	1.6	-	5.2	15.4	17.7	34.4	36.9	20.4	75.0	-	-	-	4.6	2.4	0.57	1.05	7.6	189
Eye	1	0	-	-	-	-	-	-	-	-	-	-	-	-	6.1	-	-	-	-	-	0.1	0.1	0.03	0.03	0.2	190
Brain, nervous system	30	0	1.1	7.0	3.6	-	1.2	5.4	1.6	-	2.6	3.1	7.1	8.6	18.4	40.7	18.8	-	-	-	3.8	2.0	0.30	0.60	5.2	191-2
Thyroid	8	0	-	-	-	-	-	1.4	-	1.9	-	6.2	7.1	-	-	20.4	-	-	-	-	1.0	0.5	0.08	0.18	1.6	193
Other endocrine	9	0	-	-	-	2.2	-	-	3.1	-	-	3.1	-	4.3	6.1	10.2	-	-	63.4	-	1.2	0.6	0.09	0.15	1.6	194
Hodgkin's disease	11	0	-	1.2	-	-	1.2	5.4	-	1.9	-	3.1	3.5	4.3	-	10.2	-	-	-	-	1.4	0.7	0.10	0.15	1.6	201
Non-Hodgkin lymphoma	44	0	-	1.2	3.6	2.2	2.4	2.7	3.1	5.8	10.3	9.2	7.1	34.4	30.7	10.2	56.3	95.5	-	-	5.6	3.0	0.56	0.90	8.1	200,202
Multiple myeloma	25	0	-	-	-	-	-	-	1.6	-	5.2	3.1	10.6	21.5	49.2	20.4	56.3	-	-	-	3.2	1.7	0.46	0.84	5.7	203
Lymphoid leukaemia	26	0	4.3	7.0	1.2	5.5	-	2.7	-	-	-	-	7.1	8.6	6.1	20.4	-	31.8	-	-	3.3	1.8	0.21	0.32	3.9	204
Myeloid leukaemia	33	0	1.1	1.2	-	-	3.7	8.2	1.6	1.9	2.6	12.3	10.6	4.3	12.3	40.7	-	127.3	-	137.0	4.2	2.2	0.30	0.50	6.7	205
Monocytic leukaemia	0	0	-	-	-	-	-	-	-	-	-	-	-	-	-	-	-	-	-	-	0.0	0.0	0.00	0.00	0.0	206
Other leukaemia	3	0	-	-	1.2	-	-	-	-	-	-	2.6	-	-	-	10.2	-	-	-	-	0.4	0.2	0.02	0.07	0.6	207
Leukaemia unspecified	4	0	-	-	-	-	-	-	-	-	-	-	-	4.3	6.1	10.2	-	31.8	-	-	0.5	0.3	0.05	0.10	1.0	208
Other and unspecified	113	0	-	-	-	3.3	-	4.1	3.1	9.7	10.3	12.3	63.6	38.7	61.5	264.8	150.0	318.4	316.9	821.9	14.5	7.6	1.03	3.11	29.8	O&U
All sites	1482	0	15.2	22.3	12.0	23.3	34.2	78.9	48.3	83.5	118.7	240.4	523.3	854.7	1328.0	2251.0	2775.2	3724.9	3105.2	4931.5	189.6		16.91	42.04	359.7	ALL
All sites but 173	1482	0	15.2	22.3	12.0	23.3	34.2	78.9	48.3	83.5	118.7	240.4	523.3	854.7	1328.0	2251.0	2775.2	3724.9	3105.2	4931.5	189.6	100.0	16.91	42.04	359.7	ALLb

Rate from 1 case   1.084   1.174   1.198   1.109   1.222   1.360   1.557   1.941   2.580   3.082   3.536   4.295   6.148   10.185   18.751   31.837   63.371   136.986

†Important: see notes on population page

+ NEW ZEALAND: MAORI 1988-1992

ANNUAL INCIDENCE PER 100,000 BY AGE GROUP (YEARS) - FEMALE

SITE	ALL AGES	AGE UNK	0-	5-	10-	15-	20-	25-	30-	35-	40-	45-	50-	55-	60-	65-	70-	75-	80-	85+	CRUDE RATE	%	CR 64	CR 74	ASR (W)	ICD (9th)
Lip	0	0	-	-	-	-	-	-	-	-	-	-	-	-	-	-	-	-	-	-	0.0	0.0	0.00	0.00	0.0	140
Tongue	5	0	-	-	-	-	-	-	-	-	-	6.3	7.1	-	-	9.1	-	-	-	-	0.6	0.3	0.07	0.11	1.0	141
Salivary gland	7	0	-	-	-	-	-	1.3	-	-	2.5	6.3	3.6	4.4	-	9.1	-	-	-	-	0.9	0.4	0.09	0.14	1.3	142
Mouth	6	0	-	-	-	-	-	-	1.5	-	2.5	3.1	3.6	-	-	-	27.4	-	-	-	0.8	0.3	0.05	0.19	1.2	143-5
Oropharynx	2	0	-	-	-	-	-	-	-	-	-	3.1	3.6	-	-	-	-	-	-	-	0.3	0.1	0.03	0.03	0.4	146
Nasopharynx	2	0	1.2	-	-	-	-	-	-	-	-	-	-	4.4	-	-	-	-	-	-	0.3	0.1	0.03	0.03	0.3	147
Hypopharynx	0	0	-	-	-	-	-	-	-	-	-	-	-	-	-	-	-	-	-	-	0.0	0.0	0.00	0.00	0.0	148
Pharynx unspecified	0	0	-	-	-	-	-	-	-	-	-	-	-	-	-	-	-	-	-	-	0.0	0.0	0.00	0.00	0.0	149
Oesophagus	9	0	-	-	-	-	-	-	-	-	-	3.1	-	4.4	23.7	-	13.7	-	108.5	-	1.2	0.5	0.16	0.22	2.1	150
Stomach	73	0	-	-	-	-	-	1.3	9.1	13.2	9.8	28.3	35.7	57.5	29.6	63.5	41.2	202.6	-	-	9.4	4.2	0.92	1.45	13.7	151
Small intestine	4	0	-	-	-	-	-	-	-	-	-	-	-	5.9	27.2	-	-	-	-	0.5	0.2	0.03	0.17	1.1	152
Colon	70	0	-	-	-	1.2	2.5	-	3.0	1.9	4.9	6.3	17.9	48.7	41.5	108.8	96.0	253.3	271.1	237.5	9.0	4.0	0.64	1.66	16.0	153
Rectum	42	0	-	-	-	-	-	-	-	7.5	12.3	3.1	14.3	17.7	41.5	54.4	41.2	76.0	216.9	79.2	5.4	2.4	0.48	0.96	9.2	154
Liver	17	0	-	-	-	-	-	-	-	1.9	4.9	-	7.1	17.7	5.9	45.3	13.7	25.3	-	-	2.2	1.0	0.19	0.48	3.6	155
Gallbladder etc.	6	0	-	-	-	-	-	-	1.5	1.9	-	-	-	11.8	9.1	-	-	54.2	-	-	0.8	0.3	0.08	0.12	1.2	156
Pancreas	29	0	-	-	-	-	-	-	3.0	1.9	-	6.3	3.6	8.9	47.4	27.2	68.6	76.0	54.2	79.2	3.7	1.7	0.36	0.83	6.7	157
Nose, sinuses etc.	0	0	-	-	-	-	-	-	-	-	-	-	-	-	-	-	-	-	-	-	0.0	0.0	0.00	0.00	0.0	160
Larynx	5	0	-	-	-	-	-	-	-	-	-	-	3.6	-	11.8	-	27.4	-	-	-	0.6	0.3	0.08	0.21	1.2	161
Bronchus, lung	326	0	-	-	-	-	-	-	3.0	15.0	27.0	97.5	157.1	212.4	325.8	562.1	384.1	658.6	216.9	554.2	41.8	18.8	4.19	8.92	72.9	162
†Other thoracic organs	1	0	-	-	-	-	-	-	-	-	-	-	-	-	-	-	13.7	-	-	-	0.1	0.1	0.00	0.07	0.3	163-4
Bone	7	0	-	-	1.2	2.3	-	1.3	1.5	3.8	-	-	-	-	-	-	-	-	-	-	0.9	0.4	0.05	0.05	0.7	170
Connective tissue	17	0	2.3	-	3.7	-	-	2.5	4.6	1.9	-	-	7.1	4.4	5.9	18.1	-	-	-	-	2.2	1.0	0.16	0.25	2.5	171
†Mesothelioma																										
†Kaposi's sarcoma																										
Melanoma of skin	20	1	-	-	-	-	-	2.5	4.6	1.9	9.8	3.1	14.3	-	5.9	18.1	-	-	-	79.2	2.6	1.2	0.22	0.32	3.4	172
†Other skin	0	0	-	-	-	-	-	-	-	-	-	-	-	-	-	-	-	-	-	-	0.0	0.0	0.00	0.00	0.0	173
Breast	411	0	-	-	-	1.2	2.5	8.8	36.5	67.6	132.7	195.0	214.2	177.0	248.8	253.8	356.7	531.9	325.4	158.4	52.7	23.7	5.42	8.47	77.1	174
Uterus unspecified	0	0	-	-	-	-	-	-	-	-	-	-	-	-	-	-	-	-	-	-	0.0	0.0	0.00	0.00	0.0	179
Cervix uteri	193	0	-	-	-	-	-	13.8	22.8	65.8	83.6	69.2	82.1	66.4	94.8	126.9	54.9	50.7	54.2	79.2	24.8	11.1	2.49	3.40	32.2	180
Placenta	3	0	-	-	-	-	-	-	3.0	1.9	-	-	-	-	-	-	-	-	-	-	0.4	0.2	0.02	0.02	0.3	181
Corpus uteri	75	0	-	-	-	-	-	-	1.5	5.6	9.8	18.9	42.8	62.0	65.2	90.7	82.3	177.3	54.2	-	9.6	4.3	1.03	1.89	15.8	182
Ovary etc.	68	0	-	-	-	4.7	1.2	1.3	12.2	13.2	12.3	18.9	28.6	26.6	47.4	81.6	54.9	25.3	-	-	8.7	3.9	0.83	1.51	12.2	183
Other female genital	17	0	-	-	-	-	-	1.3	1.5	1.9	9.8	-	14.3	13.3	5.9	9.1	-	25.3	-	-	2.2	1.0	0.24	0.29	2.9	184
†Bladder	10	0	-	-	-	-	-	-	-	-	-	-	3.6	17.7	5.9	-	27.4	25.3	54.2	-	1.3	0.6	0.14	0.27	2.2	188
Kidney etc.	19	0	-	1.2	-	-	1.2	1.3	3.0	1.9	2.5	-	3.6	17.7	-	9.1	27.4	76.0	54.2	-	2.4	1.1	0.16	0.34	3.5	189
Eye	2	0	1.2	1.2	-	-	-	-	-	-	-	-	-	-	-	-	-	-	-	-	0.3	0.1	0.01	0.01	0.3	190
Brain, nervous system	27	0	-	3.7	3.7	2.3	1.2	1.3	3.0	3.8	4.9	15.7	14.3	-	5.9	-	13.7	-	-	-	3.5	1.6	0.30	0.37	4.0	191-2
Thyroid	43	0	-	-	1.2	-	6.1	10.0	3.0	5.6	9.8	6.3	21.4	31.0	5.9	18.1	27.4	-	-	-	5.5	2.5	0.50	0.73	6.5	193
Other endocrine	7	0	1.2	-	-	-	-	-	-	3.8	-	3.1	-	8.9	5.9	-	-	-	-	-	0.9	0.4	0.11	0.11	1.1	194
Hodgkin's disease	4	0	-	1.2	-	-	1.2	-	-	-	-	-	3.6	4.4	-	-	-	-	-	-	0.5	0.2	0.05	0.05	0.6	201
Non-Hodgkin lymphoma	35	0	1.2	-	2.5	1.2	1.2	-	3.0	1.9	4.9	9.4	25.0	13.3	23.7	18.1	27.4	76.0	-	79.2	4.5	2.0	0.44	0.66	6.7	200,202
Multiple myeloma	26	0	-	-	-	-	-	-	-	1.9	-	-	25.0	22.1	5.9	45.3	27.4	50.7	108.5	79.2	3.3	1.5	0.27	0.64	5.8	203
Lymphoid leukaemia	10	0	3.5	2.5	-	-	1.2	-	-	-	-	3.1	3.6	4.4	-	-	-	25.3	-	-	1.3	0.6	0.09	0.09	1.6	204
Myeloid leukaemia	30	0	1.2	-	2.5	4.7	1.2	-	9.1	3.8	9.8	9.4	7.1	4.4	11.8	-	-	-	54.2	79.2	3.8	1.7	0.33	0.33	4.5	205
Monocytic leukaemia	2	0	-	-	-	-	-	1.3	-	-	-	-	-	-	-	-	13.7	-	-	-	0.3	0.1	0.01	0.07	0.4	206
Other leukaemia	1	0	1.2	-	-	-	-	-	-	-	-	-	-	-	-	-	-	-	-	-	0.1	0.1	0.01	0.01	0.1	207
Leukaemia unspecified	5	0	-	-	-	-	1.2	-	-	-	-	-	-	-	-	-	-	25.3	108.5	79.2	0.6	0.3	0.01	0.01	1.3	208
Other and unspecified	98	0	-	-	-	1.2	-	3.8	4.6	1.9	9.8	18.9	32.1	70.8	118.5	172.2	68.6	101.3	108.5	395.9	12.6	5.7	1.31	2.51	21.8	O&U
All sites	1734	1	12.7	9.8	14.9	18.6	20.9	51.3	135.4	231.1	363.7	534.6	799.7	920.6	1202.7	1776.8	1509.1	2482.3	1843.8	1979.4	222.4		21.59	38.03	339.7	ALL
All sites but 173	1734	1	12.7	9.8	14.9	18.6	20.9	51.3	135.4	231.1	363.7	534.6	799.7	920.6	1202.7	1776.8	1509.1	2482.3	1843.8	1979.4	222.4	100.0	21.59	38.03	339.7	ALLb

Rate from 1 case: 1.158 1.231 1.242 1.165 1.227 1.252 1.521 1.879 2.457 3.145 3.570 4.426 5.925 9.065 13.719 25.329 54.230 79.177

†Important: see notes on population page

USA, Hawaii

The Hawaii Tumor Registry, which has been in operation since 1960, is a state-wide registry designed to monitor trends in cancer incidence and survival and to promote research in cancer etiology, prevention and control. The registry has been associated with the US Surveillance, Epidemiology, and End Results (SEER) Program since 1973, and receives its financial support from the US National Cancer Institute and the State of Hawaii.

The State of Hawaii, comprising the populated islands of Oahu, Maui, Hawaii, Molokai, Lanai, Kauai and Niihau, lies in the northern Pacific Ocean, 3861 km from San Francisco, California, and is geographically part of Oceania. It lies between latitudes 18°55′ and 22°15′ N and longitudes 154°50′ and 160°30′ W, the total registration area being 16 638 km². Of the total population, 71.3% live in conurbations of more than 100 000 (City of Honolulu and Kailua Kaneohe); 86.5% live in urban and 13.5% in rural areas.

The most striking feature of cancer incidence and survival in Hawaii is the degree of variation between the different ethnic groups. Accordingly, the Hawaii data for this monograph are presented in five ethnic tabulations (white, Chinese, Japanese, Filipino, Hawaiian) to permit comparisons within Hawaii, as well as with other registries.

Only 23% of the population is of Caucasian origin. Japanese comprise 20%, constituting by far the largest concentration of Japanese in the SEER Program. Other major groups are Filipinos (11%), Chinese (5%) and native Hawaiians (a Polynesian population) (19%). Other South Pacific islander groups (especially Samoans) and other Asian groups (especially Koreans and Vietnamese) are found in increasing numbers (4%). In addition, persons of mixed racial ancestry account for 18% of the population. Emigration rates are low, especially among non-whites; in an analysis of emigration rates from a large population cohort, only 10% of the cohort had left the state after 15 years.

Cases are identified through all hospitals in the state, private pathology laboratories and clinics, and through computer searches of the death files in the Department of Health. Tumour registrars are supported by the large hospitals and report all incident cases to the registry. Staff members of the registry visit each of the smaller hospitals and other facilities periodically to review medical records and identify new cases. Increasingly, cancer cases are being identified in non-hospital facilities. Quality checks on the completeness of case ascertainment, data abstraction and follow-up are performed regularly by both the National Cancer Institute and the registry. In addition, the Hawaii Oncology Data Management Association, comprising over 20 cancer registrars, most of whom are certified, provides a series of educational programmes for all hospital registrars and registry staff.

A special problem with the generation of population estimates in Hawaii is the inadequacy of the census data; the ethnic classification is too crude for Hawaii's population and the race definitions have been inconsistent over time. In order to maintain consistency in the temporal trends for cancer in the state, and to provide more correct estimates of the ethnic distribution of the population, the Health Surveillance Program of the Hawaii Department of Health began to develop separate population estimates from the US census based on an annual random household interview survey. Information from that survey is used to recompute the ethnic distributions within the census marginal totals by sex and age, according to the original census criteria on ethnicity. These recomputed estimates are the basis for the incidence rates in this monograph.

Squamous and basal-cell carcinomas of the skin are the only cancers for which data are not routinely collected. In addition to identifying all incident cases the registry collects information on various demographic characteristics, diagnostic procedures, clinical findings, treatment, histology, and staging. Follow-up information is obtained annually

Statistical data are released on request to qualified individuals and agencies, including local hospitals, physicians, educators, researchers and health-care providers. A special commission comprising eight physicians representing the Department of Health, Hawaii Medical Association, American Cancer Society (Hawaii Division), and the University of Hawaii Medical School oversees the release of all confidential information and sets the policy in this regard. The data in the registry are especially valuable as a resource for epidemiological research in the ethnically-diverse population of Hawaii.

Marc T. Goodman
Laurence N. Kolonel
Marilyn C. Hurst

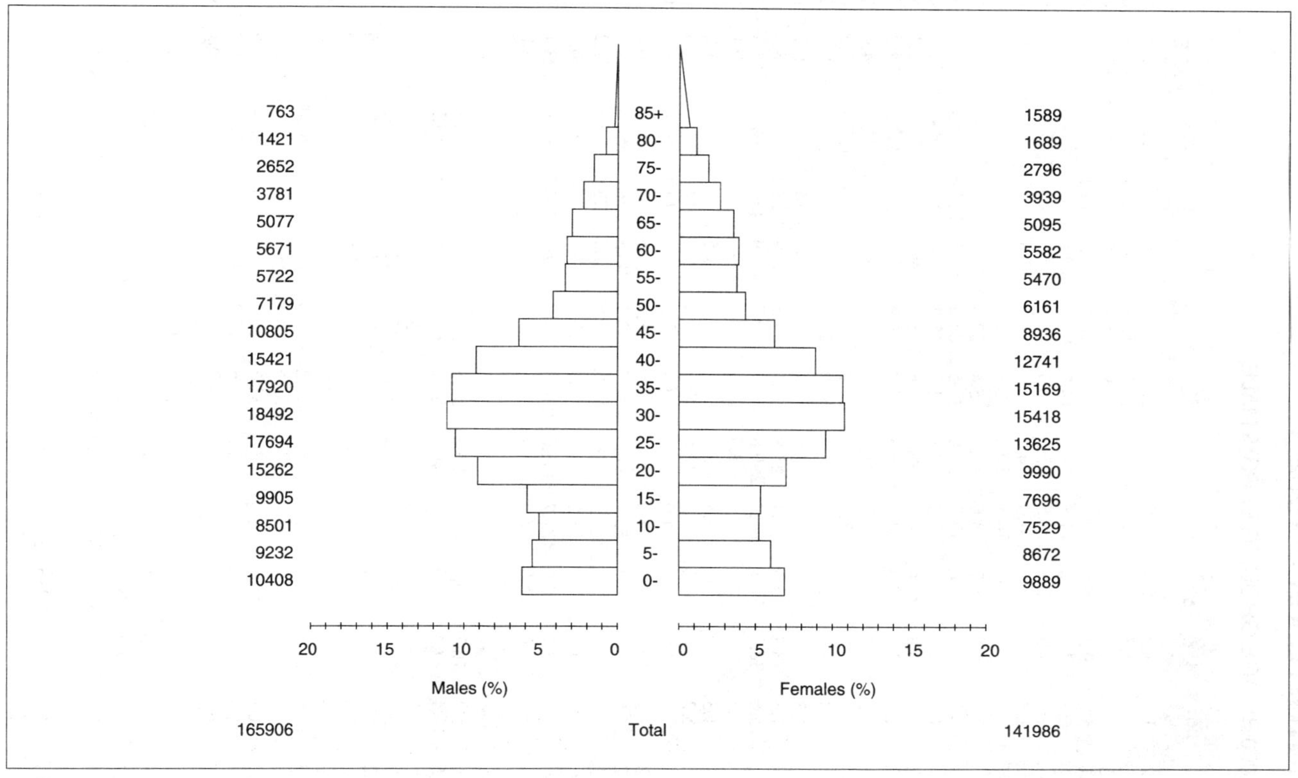

USA, Hawaii: White

Source of population: average annual 1988–92

Estimate: The Health Surveillance Program of the Hawaii Department of Health conducts an annual random survey of approximately 2% of households statewide. The populations for the different ethnic groups are derived by apportioning the census sex-age counts by the race distributions for each sex-age group as determined by the annual Health Surveillance Program survey. The ethnic distributions can vary substantially from year to year, especially among small groups, making it necessary to smooth the yearly estimates.

Notes to tables overleaf:

† 173 does not include basal cell or squamous cell carcinoma

USA, HAWAII: WHITE 1988-1992

ANNUAL INCIDENCE PER 100,000 BY AGE GROUP (YEARS) - MALE

SITE	ALL AGES	AGE UNK	0-	5-	10-	15-	20-	25-	30-	35-	40-	45-	50-	55-	60-	65-	70-	75-	80-	85+	CRUDE RATE	%	CR 64	CR 74	ASR (W)	ICD (9th)
Lip	18	0	-	-	-	-	-	-	1.1	2.2	1.3	1.9	2.8	7.0	3.5	19.7	5.3	7.5	-	52.4	2.2	0.5	0.10	0.22	**2.0**	140
Tongue	24	0	-	-	-	-	-	1.1	-	-	-	3.7	-	21.0	10.6	27.6	15.9	-	28.1	-	2.9	0.7	0.18	0.40	**2.9**	141
Salivary gland	7	0	-	-	-	-	-	-	-	3.3	-	-	-	-	7.9	5.3	7.5	-	-	-	0.8	0.2	0.02	0.08	**0.6**	142
Mouth	28	0	-	-	-	-	1.3	-	-	1.1	5.2	9.3	5.6	10.5	14.1	15.8	10.6	7.5	14.1	-	3.4	0.8	0.24	0.37	**3.1**	143-5
Oropharynx	33	0	-	-	-	-	-	-	-	-	6.5	7.4	5.6	17.5	21.2	19.7	21.2	15.1	-	-	4.0	0.9	0.29	0.49	**3.8**	146
Nasopharynx	8	0	-	-	-	-	-	-	-	-	-	1.9	2.8	10.5	3.5	3.9	-	7.5	-	-	1.0	0.2	0.09	0.11	**1.0**	147
Hypopharynx	17	0	-	-	-	-	-	-	-	-	1.3	1.9	-	7.0	24.7	7.9	15.9	7.5	-	-	2.0	0.5	0.17	0.29	**2.1**	148
Pharynx unspecified	9	0	-	-	-	2.0	-	-	-	-	-	-	-	10.5	10.6	3.9	5.3	-	-	-	1.1	0.2	0.12	0.16	**1.2**	149
Oesophagus	40	0	-	-	-	-	-	-	-	-	2.6	5.6	16.7	3.5	14.1	35.4	37.0	60.3	-	-	4.8	1.1	0.21	0.57	**4.4**	150
Stomach	72	0	-	-	-	-	-	-	1.1	-	3.9	5.6	5.6	17.5	38.8	31.5	84.6	60.3	126.6	157.3	8.7	2.0	0.36	0.94	**7.8**	151
Small intestine	13	0	-	-	-	-	-	-	-	1.1	1.3	1.9	-	3.5	7.1	11.8	15.9	-	14.1	-	1.6	0.4	0.07	0.21	**1.4**	152
Colon	293	0	-	-	-	-	-	-	5.4	2.2	5.2	14.8	72.4	76.9	130.5	220.6	275.0	309.2	309.5	471.8	35.3	8.0	1.54	4.02	**32.7**	153
Rectum	124	0	-	-	-	-	-	-	-	2.2	2.6	3.7	27.9	34.9	70.5	67.0	126.9	120.6	154.7	262.1	14.9	3.4	0.71	1.68	**14.0**	154
Liver	41	0	1.9	-	-	-	-	2.3	-	-	1.3	5.6	-	7.0	21.2	35.4	26.4	45.2	56.3	52.4	4.9	1.1	0.20	0.51	**4.5**	155
Gallbladder etc.	13	0	-	-	-	-	-	-	-	-	-	-	-	3.5	3.5	7.9	10.6	7.5	-	157.3	1.6	0.4	0.04	0.13	**1.6**	156
Pancreas	78	0	-	-	-	-	-	1.1	-	-	1.3	1.9	8.4	21.0	31.7	67.0	79.3	98.0	112.5	104.8	9.4	2.1	0.33	1.06	**8.5**	157
Nose, sinuses etc.	6	0	-	-	-	-	-	-	-	-	1.3	-	-	7.0	3.5	-	5.3	-	14.1	-	0.7	0.2	0.06	0.09	**0.7**	160
Larynx	70	0	-	-	-	-	-	-	-	-	1.3	3.7	5.6	52.4	45.8	55.1	63.5	67.9	28.1	-	8.4	1.9	0.54	1.14	**8.3**	161
Bronchus, lung	525	0	-	-	-	-	-	-	3.2	2.2	15.6	38.9	128.1	181.7	299.8	405.7	470.7	542.9	450.1	209.7	63.3	14.3	3.35	7.73	**59.6**	162
Other thoracic organs	1	0	-	-	-	-	-	-	-	-	-	-	-	-	3.5	-	-	-	-	-	0.1	0.0	0.02	0.02	**0.1**	163-4
Bone	10	0	-	-	-	-	-	2.3	1.1	1.1	1.3	1.9	-	3.5	3.5	-	5.3	7.5	-	-	1.2	0.3	0.07	0.10	**1.0**	170
Connective tissue	27	0	1.9	-	-	-	-	-	3.2	3.3	5.2	5.6	5.6	3.5	10.6	7.9	10.6	15.1	14.1	-	3.3	0.7	0.19	0.29	**2.8**	171
Mesothelioma	16	0	-	-	-	-	-	-	-	-	-	1.9	-	14.0	14.1	3.9	5.3	15.1	14.1	52.4	1.9	0.4	0.15	0.20	**1.9**	MES
Kaposi's sarcoma	90	0	-	-	-	-	1.3	7.9	21.6	22.3	28.5	16.7	11.1	7.0	3.5	3.9	5.3	15.1	-	-	10.8	2.5	0.60	0.65	**7.4**	KAP
Melanoma of skin	187	0	-	-	-	-	3.9	6.8	11.9	21.2	24.6	38.9	55.7	52.4	60.0	82.7	63.5	90.5	126.6	52.4	22.5	5.1	1.38	2.11	**19.5**	172
†Other skin	10	0	-	-	-	-	-	1.1	1.1	1.1	-	-	-	-	-	3.9	10.6	7.5	28.1	26.2	1.2		0.02	0.09	**0.9**	173
Breast	7	0	-	-	-	-	-	-	-	-	-	1.9	-	3.5	-	3.9	10.6	7.5	-	26.2	0.8	0.2	0.03	0.10	**0.8**	175
Prostate	1021	0	-	-	-	-	-	-	-	-	-	3.7	52.9	181.7	395.0	878.3	1295.7	1447.7	1744.3	1363.0	123.1	27.9	3.17	14.04	**108.2**	185
Testis	66	0	-	-	-	6.1	15.7	10.2	15.1	17.9	5.2	5.6	5.6	3.5	7.1	-	-	-	-	-	8.0	1.8	0.46	0.46	**5.9**	186
Penis	2	0	-	-	-	-	-	-	-	-	-	-	-	-	3.9	-	-	7.5	-	-	0.2	0.1	0.00	0.02	**0.2**	187.1-.4
Other male genital	0	0	-	-	-	-	-	-	-	-	-	-	-	-	-	-	-	-	-	-	0.0	0.0	0.00	0.00	**0.0**	187.5-.9
Bladder	226	0	-	-	-	-	-	-	-	5.6	5.2	16.7	16.7	66.4	105.8	153.6	222.1	256.4	407.9	235.9	27.2	6.2	1.08	2.96	**24.2**	188
Kidney etc.	107	0	7.7	-	-	-	-	1.1	1.1	4.5	10.4	7.4	13.9	38.4	49.4	59.1	63.5	105.6	112.5	157.3	12.9	2.9	0.67	1.28	**12.1**	189
Eye	5	0	-	-	-	-	-	-	-	-	1.1	1.3	-	-	7.0	-	-	5.3	-	-	0.6	0.1	0.05	0.07	**0.5**	190
Brain, nervous system	71	0	9.6	6.5	4.7	2.0	5.2	6.8	2.2	2.2	5.2	11.1	8.4	10.5	28.2	31.5	26.4	52.8	28.1	-	8.6	1.9	0.51	0.80	**8.7**	191-2
Thyroid	30	0	-	-	-	-	2.6	2.3	-	2.2	5.2	3.7	11.1	7.0	21.2	7.9	10.6	15.1	-	-	3.6	0.8	0.28	0.37	**3.3**	193
Other endocrine	4	0	-	2.2	-	-	1.3	-	-	-	1.3	-	-	-	-	-	-	7.5	-	-	0.5	0.1	0.02	0.02	**0.5**	194
Hodgkin's disease	30	0	-	-	-	2.0	3.9	4.5	8.7	5.6	3.9	3.7	2.8	7.0	-	3.9	-	-	-	-	3.6	0.8	0.21	0.23	**2.7**	201
Non-Hodgkin lymphoma	140	0	1.9	-	-	-	-	3.4	10.8	8.9	15.6	25.9	33.4	73.4	42.3	51.2	79.3	75.4	98.5	52.4	16.9	3.8	1.08	1.73	**15.1**	200,202
Multiple myeloma	31	0	-	-	-	-	-	-	-	-	-	3.7	-	24.5	10.6	31.5	26.4	37.7	14.1	-	3.7	0.8	0.19	0.48	**3.5**	203
Lymphoid leukaemia	41	0	3.8	6.5	-	-	2.6	3.4	1.1	2.2	1.3	1.9	13.9	7.0	7.1	31.5	26.4	7.5	14.1	52.4	4.9	1.1	0.25	0.54	**5.1**	204
Myeloid leukaemia	39	0	-	-	4.7	-	2.6	1.1	2.2	2.2	1.3	1.9	5.6	7.0	10.6	27.6	15.9	37.7	42.2	78.6	4.7	1.1	0.20	0.41	**4.3**	205
Monocytic leukaemia	1	0	-	-	-	-	-	-	-	-	-	-	-	-	-	3.9	-	-	-	-	0.1	0.0	0.00	0.02	**0.1**	206
Other leukaemia	2	0	-	-	-	-	-	-	-	-	-	-	-	-	-	-	10.6	-	-	-	0.2	0.1	0.00	0.05	**0.2**	207
Leukaemia unspecified	8	0	-	-	-	-	-	-	-	-	-	-	-	-	3.5	11.8	10.6	7.5	14.1	-	1.0	0.2	0.02	0.13	**0.9**	208
Other and unspecified	80	0	-	-	-	-	1.3	1.1	2.2	1.1	5.2	5.6	11.1	21.0	14.1	51.2	89.9	67.9	140.7	131.1	9.6	2.2	0.31	1.02	**8.4**	O&U
All sites	3671	0	26.9	15.2	9.4	12.1	41.9	56.5	93.0	117.2	171.2	264.7	529.3	1031.0	1544.6	2497.1	3268.5	3649.5	4107.5	3695.9	442.5		19.57	48.39	**398.6**	ALL
All sites but 173	3661	0	26.9	15.2	9.4	12.1	41.9	55.4	91.9	116.1	171.2	264.7	529.3	1031.0	1544.6	2493.2	3257.9	3642.0	4079.3	3669.7	441.3	100.0	19.55	48.30	**397.7**	ALLb
Rate from 1 case			1.922	2.166	2.353	2.019	1.310	1.130	1.082	1.116	1.297	1.851	2.786	3.495	3.527	3.939	5.289	7.540	14.067	26.212						

†Important: see notes on population page

USA, HAWAII: WHITE 1988-1992

ANNUAL INCIDENCE PER 100,000 BY AGE GROUP (YEARS) - FEMALE

SITE	ALL AGES	AGE UNK	0-	5-	10-	15-	20-	25-	30-	35-	40-	45-	50-	55-	60-	65-	70-	75-	80-	85+	CRUDE RATE	%	CR 64	CR 74	ASR (W)	ICD (9th)
Lip	6	0	-	-	-	-	-	-	-	-	-	-	-	-	-	7.9	10.2	-	11.8	12.6	0.8	0.2	0.00	0.09	0.6	140
Tongue	10	0	-	-	-	-	-	1.3	1.3	-	-	-	-	3.6	3.9	15.2	21.5	-	-	1.4	0.4	0.03	0.13	0.9	141
Salivary gland	4	0	2.0	-	-	-	-	-	-	-	2.2	-	-	-	3.9	5.1	-	-	-	0.6	0.1	0.02	0.07	0.6	142
Mouth	22	0	-	-	-	-	-	1.3	3.1	4.5	-	11.0	3.6	3.9	15.2	42.9	35.5	-	3.1	0.8	0.12	0.21	2.1	143-5
Oropharynx	4	0	-	-	-	-	-	-	-	2.2	-	-	3.6	3.9	-	7.2	-	-	-	0.6	0.1	0.03	0.05	0.5	146
Nasopharynx	2	0	-	-	-	-	-	-	-	-	-	-	-	3.9	5.1	-	-	-	0.3	0.1	0.00	0.05	0.2	147
Hypopharynx	7	0	-	-	-	-	-	-	1.6	-	-	3.7	-	3.9	20.3	-	-	-	1.0	0.3	0.03	0.15	0.8	148
Pharynx unspecified	3	0	-	-	-	-	-	-	-	-	-	-	3.6	3.9	-	7.2	-	-	0.4	0.1	0.02	0.04	0.3	149
Oesophagus	16	0	-	-	-	-	-	-	-	3.1	-	6.5	3.7	17.9	7.9	20.3	-	-	-	2.3	0.6	0.16	0.30	2.0	150
Stomach	45	0	-	-	-	-	-	-	-	1.6	4.5	13.0	14.6	10.7	7.9	25.4	78.7	71.0	88.1	6.3	1.7	0.22	0.39	4.4	151
Small intestine	5	0	-	-	-	-	-	1.3	-	-	-	-	-	3.6	-	10.2	7.2	-	-	0.7	0.2	0.02	0.08	0.5	152
Colon	235	0	-	-	-	-	-	1.3	6.6	7.8	22.4	29.2	58.5	82.4	113.8	177.7	243.1	521.0	302.0	33.1	8.7	1.04	2.50	22.9	153
Rectum	79	0	-	-	-	-	-	1.3	-	3.1	13.4	13.0	14.6	21.5	58.9	45.7	114.4	130.2	62.9	11.1	2.9	0.33	0.86	8.0	154
Liver	14	0	-	-	-	-	-	-	-	-	-	-	3.7	14.3	3.9	15.2	21.5	11.8	12.6	2.0	0.5	0.09	0.19	1.5	155
Gallbladder etc.	21	0	-	-	-	-	-	-	-	3.1	-	3.2	-	14.3	7.9	10.2	28.6	23.7	50.3	3.0	0.8	0.10	0.19	2.0	156
Pancreas	57	0	-	-	-	-	-	-	1.3	-	-	9.7	11.0	21.5	51.0	45.7	64.4	82.9	75.5	8.0	2.1	0.22	0.70	5.7	157
Nose, sinuses etc.	5	0	-	-	-	-	-	-	-	-	3.2	-	-	3.9	5.1	14.3	-	-	0.7	0.2	0.02	0.06	0.5	160
Larynx	12	0	-	-	-	-	-	-	-	-	-	-	3.7	3.6	7.9	15.2	28.6	11.8	-	1.7	0.4	0.04	0.15	1.2	161
Bronchus, lung	340	0	-	-	-	-	-	1.5	2.6	6.6	14.1	33.6	64.9	113.3	193.5	239.5	324.9	328.9	296.0	88.1	47.9	12.6	2.15	4.97	37.9	162
Other thoracic organs	1	0	-	-	-	-	-	-	-	-	-	-	-	3.7	-	-	-	-	-	0.1	0.0	0.02	0.02	0.1	163-4
Bone	3	0	-	-	-	2.0	-	1.3	-	-	-	-	-	-	-	-	-	-	0.4	0.1	0.03	0.03	0.4	170
Connective tissue	16	0	-	-	2.7	-	1.5	1.3	2.6	3.1	-	9.7	3.7	7.2	7.9	-	-	11.8	-	2.3	0.6	0.16	0.20	2.0	171
Mesothelioma	2	0	-	-	-	-	-	-	-	-	-	-	3.7	-	-	-	7.2	-	-	0.3	0.1	0.02	0.02	0.2	MES
Kaposi's sarcoma	1	0	-	-	-	-	-	1.3	-	-	-	-	-	-	-	-	-	-	0.1	0.0	0.01	0.01	0.1	KAP
Melanoma of skin	115	0	-	-	-	-	6.0	13.2	15.6	30.3	23.5	31.3	22.7	29.3	25.1	19.6	20.3	28.6	23.7	25.2	16.2	4.3	0.99	1.18	12.4	172
†Other skin	9	0	-	-	-	-	-	-	-	-	-	4.5	3.2	7.3	7.2	-	-	7.2	-	12.6	1.3		0.11	0.11	1.1	173
Breast	856	0	-	-	-	-	2.0	7.3	18.2	64.6	147.6	203.7	243.5	314.4	311.7	427.9	492.5	579.2	485.4	327.2	120.6	31.8	6.56	11.17	96.5	174
Uterus unspecified	1	0	-	-	-	-	-	-	-	-	2.2	-	-	-	-	-	-	-	-	0.1	0.0	0.01	0.01	0.1	179
Cervix uteri	97	0	-	-	-	-	2.0	20.5	11.7	19.8	14.1	24.6	19.5	11.0	28.7	31.4	20.3	28.6	35.5	25.2	13.7	3.6	0.76	1.02	10.5	180
Placenta	1	0	-	-	-	-	-	1.5	-	1.3	-	-	-	-	-	-	-	-	-	0.1	0.0	0.01	0.01	0.1	181
Corpus uteri	141	0	-	-	-	-	-	1.5	-	7.9	15.7	17.9	32.5	29.3	71.6	109.9	116.8	100.1	94.7	62.9	19.9	5.2	0.88	2.02	15.7	182
Ovary etc.	122	0	-	-	5.2	-	4.4	7.8	7.9	12.6	35.8	45.4	43.9	43.0	39.3	66.0	50.1	106.6	50.3	17.2	4.5	1.03	1.56	14.2	183
Other female genital	18	0	-	-	-	-	4.0	-	-	-	3.1	2.2	-	3.7	3.6	7.9	15.2	21.5	11.8	25.2	2.5	0.7	0.08	0.20	1.9	184
Bladder	55	0	-	-	-	-	-	-	1.3	1.3	1.6	6.7	13.0	18.3	21.5	23.6	66.0	42.9	82.9	25.2	7.7	2.0	0.32	0.77	5.9	188
Kidney etc.	35	0	-	-	-	-	-	1.5	-	1.3	4.7	2.2	16.2	-	21.5	11.8	25.4	57.2	23.7	-	4.9	1.3	0.24	0.42	3.8	189
Eye	2	0	2.0	-	-	-	-	-	-	-	-	-	-	-	3.6	-	-	-	-	0.3	0.1	0.03	0.03	0.4	190
Brain, nervous system	34	0	8.1	2.3	2.7	2.6	4.0	-	1.3	4.0	4.7	11.2	-	7.3	10.7	3.9	10.2	7.2	23.7	25.2	4.8	1.3	0.29	0.36	4.6	191-2
Thyroid	64	0	-	-	-	10.4	10.0	10.3	9.1	11.9	12.6	11.2	13.0	14.6	3.6	15.7	15.2	7.2	11.8	12.6	9.0	2.4	0.53	0.69	7.6	193
Other endocrine	2	0	2.0	-	-	-	-	-	-	-	1.6	-	-	-	-	-	-	-	-	0.3	0.1	0.02	0.02	0.3	194
Hodgkin's disease	22	0	-	-	2.7	5.2	2.0	13.2	1.3	-	3.1	-	-	10.7	3.9	5.1	-	-	12.6	3.1	0.8	0.19	0.24	2.9	201
Non-Hodgkin lymphoma	67	0	-	-	-	-	2.0	-	1.3	2.6	7.8	4.5	6.5	18.3	21.5	47.1	55.8	50.1	106.6	50.3	9.4	2.5	0.32	0.84	6.9	200,202
Multiple myeloma	19	0	-	-	-	-	-	-	-	1.3	1.6	-	7.3	3.6	15.7	20.3	21.5	11.8	2.5	2.7	0.7	0.07	0.25	1.9	203
Lymphoid leukaemia	26	0	6.1	2.3	-	-	-	-	1.3	-	1.6	2.2	3.2	7.3	7.2	7.9	10.2	21.5	23.7	62.9	3.7	1.0	0.16	0.25	3.1	204
Myeloid leukaemia	14	0	-	-	-	-	-	2.9	1.3	1.3	1.6	-	-	7.3	-	3.9	5.1	-	47.4	12.6	2.0	0.5	0.07	0.12	1.3	205
Monocytic leukaemia	2	0	-	-	-	-	-	-	-	-	-	-	-	-	3.6	-	-	7.2	-	-	0.3	0.1	0.02	0.02	0.2	206
Other leukaemia	0	0	-	-	-	-	-	-	-	-	-	-	-	-	-	-	-	-	-	0.0	0.0	0.00	0.00	0.0	207
Leukaemia unspecified	2	0	-	-	-	-	-	-	-	-	-	-	-	-	-	-	10.2	-	-	0.3	0.1	0.00	0.05	0.2	208
Other and unspecified	86	0	-	-	-	-	-	-	-	-	3.1	4.5	13.0	18.3	39.4	51.0	86.3	71.5	142.1	125.8	12.1	3.2	0.39	1.08	8.7	O&U
All sites	2700	0	20.2	4.6	8.0	23.4	34.0	77.8	81.7	175.4	301.4	447.6	584.3	789.8	1042.5	1366.0	1807.4	2116.7	2439.0	1573.1	380.3		17.95	33.82	295.9	ALL
All sites but 173	2691	0	20.2	4.6	8.0	23.4	34.0	77.8	81.7	175.4	301.4	443.1	581.1	782.4	1035.3	1366.0	1807.4	2109.6	2439.0	1560.5	379.0	100.0	17.84	33.71	294.7	ALLb

Rate from 1 case   2.022   2.306   2.656   2.599   2.002   1.468   1.297   1.318   1.570   2.238   3.246   3.656   3.582   3.925   5.077   7.151   11.840   12.585

†Important: see notes on population page

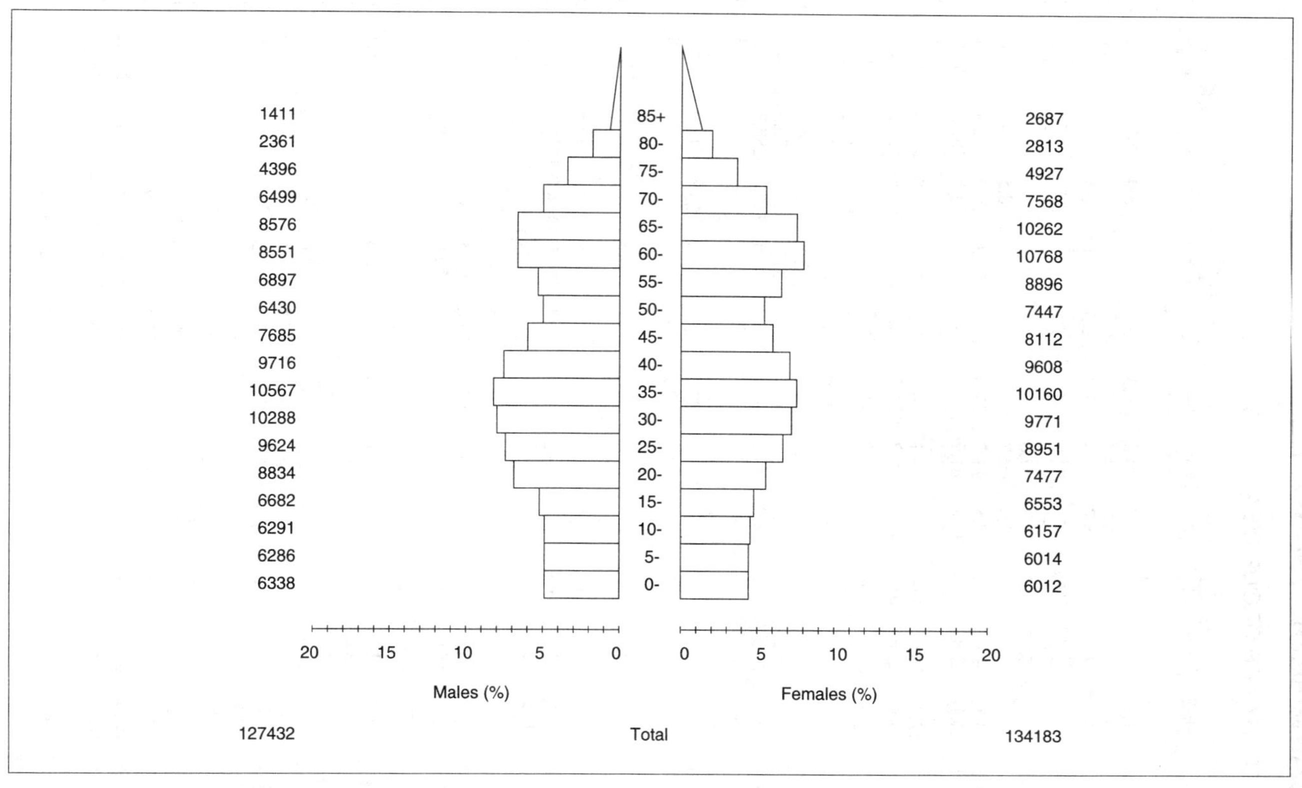

USA, Hawaii: Japanese

Source of population: average annual 1988–92

Estimate: The Health Surveillance Program of the Hawaii Department of Health conducts an annual random survey of approximately 2% of households statewide. The populations for the different ethnic groups are derived by apportioning the census sex-age counts by the race distributions for each sex-age group as determined by the annual Health Surveillance Program survey. The ethnic distributions can vary substantially from year to year, especially among small groups, making it necessary to smooth the yearly estimates.

Notes to tables overleaf:

† 173 does not include basal cell or squamous cell carcinoma

USA, HAWAII: JAPANESE 1988-1992

ANNUAL INCIDENCE PER 100,000 BY AGE GROUP (YEARS) - MALE

SITE	ALL AGES	AGE UNK	0-	5-	10-	15-	20-	25-	30-	35-	40-	45-	50-	55-	60-	65-	70-	75-	80-	85+	CRUDE RATE	%	CR 64	CR 74	ASR (W)	ICD (9th)
Lip	1	0	-	-	-	-	-	-	-	-	-	-	3.1	-	-	-	-	-	-	-	0.2	0.0	0.02	0.02	**0.2**	*140*
Tongue	21	0	-	-	-	-	-	-	-	-	4.1	-	-	5.8	14.0	9.3	6.2	9.1	16.9	14.2	3.3	0.6	0.12	0.20	**1.7**	*141*
Salivary gland	9	0	-	-	-	-	1.9	-	-	-	-	-	-	5.8	4.7	2.3	6.2	4.5	-	-	1.4	0.3	0.06	0.10	**0.8**	*142*
Mouth	20	0	-	-	-	-	-	-	-	-	-	2.6	-	8.7	9.4	11.7	12.3	9.1	8.5	-	3.1	0.6	0.10	0.22	**1.6**	*143-5*
Oropharynx	8	0	-	-	-	-	-	-	-	-	-	2.6	-	-	-	9.3	6.2	4.5	-	-	1.3	0.2	0.01	0.09	**0.6**	*146*
Nasopharynx	12	0	-	-	-	3.0	-	-	1.9	-	-	2.6	-	-	7.0	4.7	6.2	9.1	-	-	1.9	0.3	0.07	0.13	**1.2**	*147*
Hypopharynx	21	0	-	-	-	-	-	-	-	-	-	5.2	6.2	2.9	7.0	9.3	21.5	9.1	-	-	3.3	0.6	0.11	0.26	**1.8**	*148*
Pharynx unspecified	4	0	-	-	-	-	-	-	-	-	-	-	-	2.9	2.3	2.3	-	-	8.5	-	0.6	0.1	0.03	0.04	**0.3**	*149*
Oesophagus	47	0	-	-	-	-	-	-	-	1.9	4.1	2.6	3.1	14.5	11.7	37.3	18.5	22.7	16.9	42.5	7.4	1.4	0.19	0.47	**3.7**	*150*
Stomach	319	0	-	-	-	-	-	-	-	1.9	4.1	13.0	9.3	34.8	81.9	125.9	246.2	259.3	313.3	467.5	50.1	9.3	0.73	2.59	**21.5**	*151*
Small intestine	8	0	-	-	-	-	-	-	-	-	-	-	3.1	2.9	2.3	-	15.4	-	-	-	1.3	0.2	0.04	0.12	**0.7**	*152*
Colon	462	0	-	-	-	-	2.3	-	-	3.8	12.4	26.0	40.4	89.9	173.1	214.5	289.3	332.1	304.9	425.0	72.5	13.4	1.74	4.26	**34.4**	*153*
Rectum	235	0	-	-	-	-	-	-	-	7.6	14.4	15.6	40.4	55.1	98.2	121.3	116.9	150.1	101.6	127.5	36.9	6.8	1.16	2.35	**19.0**	*154*
Liver	63	0	-	-	-	-	-	1.9	-	-	4.1	-	6.2	20.3	35.1	28.0	30.8	40.9	33.9	14.2	9.9	1.8	0.34	0.63	**5.0**	*155*
Gallbladder etc.	33	0	-	-	-	-	-	-	-	-	2.1	-	6.2	8.7	4.7	18.7	15.4	13.6	67.7	14.2	5.2	1.0	0.11	0.28	**2.4**	*156*
Pancreas	84	0	-	-	-	-	-	-	3.8	2.1	-	9.3	5.8	21.1	42.0	70.8	68.2	67.7	42.5	13.2	2.4	0.21	0.77	**5.8**	*157*
Nose, sinuses etc.	11	0	-	-	-	-	-	-	-	-	2.1	-	-	-	9.4	-	6.2	13.6	-	-	1.7	0.3	0.06	0.09	**0.8**	*160*
Larynx	31	0	-	-	-	-	-	-	-	-	-	5.2	-	2.9	9.4	18.7	12.3	31.8	25.4	28.3	4.9	0.9	0.09	0.24	**2.2**	*161*
Bronchus, lung	456	0	-	-	-	-	-	-	3.9	1.9	16.5	26.0	43.5	89.9	140.3	256.5	317.0	286.6	287.9	283.3	71.6	13.2	1.61	4.48	**34.0**	*162*
Other thoracic organs	2	0	-	-	-	-	-	-	-	-	-	-	-	-	2.3	-	3.1	-	-	-	0.3	0.1	0.01	0.03	**0.2**	*163-4*
Bone	3	0	-	-	-	6.0	-	-	-	-	-	-	-	-	2.3	-	-	-	-	-	0.5	0.1	0.04	0.04	**0.6**	*170*
Connective tissue	14	0	-	3.2	-	-	-	-	-	1.9	-	-	-	2.9	-	2.3	9.2	13.6	25.4	14.2	2.2	0.4	0.04	0.10	**1.1**	*171*
Mesothelioma	3	0	-	-	-	-	-	-	-	-	-	2.6	-	-	2.3	2.3	-	-	-	-	0.5	0.1	0.02	0.04	**0.3**	*MES*
Kaposi's sarcoma	6	0	-	-	-	-	-	4.2	5.8	-	2.1	-	-	-	-	-	-	-	-	-	0.9	0.2	0.06	0.06	**0.8**	*KAP*
Melanoma of skin	3	0	-	-	-	-	-	-	-	-	-	2.6	-	-	-	2.3	-	4.5	-	-	0.5	0.1	0.01	0.02	**0.3**	*172*
†Other skin	8	0	-	-	-	-	-	-	5.8	1.9	-	-	-	-	2.3	4.7	3.1	-	-	-	1.3		0.05	0.09	**0.8**	*173*
Breast	6	0	-	-	-	-	-	-	-	-	-	-	3.1	2.9	-	2.3	-	9.1	-	14.2	0.9	0.2	0.03	0.04	**0.5**	*175*
Prostate	1029	0	-	-	-	-	-	-	-	-	2.1	-	15.6	92.8	196.5	438.4	772.4	1109.9	1134.7	1275.0	161.5	29.8	1.53	7.59	**64.2**	*185*
Testis	20	0	3.2	-	-	9.1	4.2	7.8	5.7	6.2	2.6	3.1	-	2.3	-	-	-	-	-	-	3.1	0.6	0.22	0.22	**3.0**	*186*
Penis	0	0	-	-	-	-	-	-	-	-	-	-	-	-	-	-	-	-	-	-	0.0	0.0	0.00	0.00	**0.0**	*187.1-.4*
Other male genital	5	0	-	-	-	-	-	-	-	-	-	-	-	-	-	4.7	6.2	4.5	-	-	0.8	0.1	0.00	0.05	**0.3**	*187.5-.9*
Bladder	140	0	-	-	-	2.3	-	1.9	1.9	4.1	10.4	21.8	34.8	35.1	65.3	70.8	86.4	135.5	155.8	22.0	4.1	0.56	1.24	**10.9**	*188*
Kidney etc.	91	0	-	-	-	-	-	-	1.9	2.1	15.6	12.4	23.2	21.1	42.0	61.5	50.0	50.8	99.2	14.3	2.6	0.38	0.90	**7.3**	*189*
Eye	1	0	3.2	-	-	-	-	-	-	-	-	-	-	-	-	-	-	-	-	-	0.2	0.0	0.02	0.02	**0.4**	*190*
Brain, nervous system	19	0	3.2	-	-	3.0	-	-	1.9	-	6.2	-	3.1	5.8	-	9.3	9.2	13.6	-	-	3.0	0.6	0.12	0.21	**2.1**	*191-2*
Thyroid	21	0	-	-	-	-	2.3	2.1	1.9	-	6.2	2.6	-	-	7.0	4.7	12.3	13.6	16.9	-	3.3	0.6	0.11	0.20	**1.9**	*193*
Other endocrine	2	0	-	-	-	-	-	-	-	-	-	2.6	3.1	-	-	-	-	-	-	-	0.3	0.1	0.03	0.03	**0.3**	*194*
Hodgkin's disease	9	0	-	-	-	-	-	-	-	-	2.1	2.6	3.1	2.9	-	2.3	3.1	9.1	8.5	-	1.4	0.3	0.05	0.08	**0.8**	*201*
Non-Hodgkin lymphoma	98	0	-	3.2	3.2	3.0	-	-	7.8	5.7	2.1	10.4	15.6	14.5	21.1	56.0	43.1	54.6	50.8	113.3	15.4	2.8	0.43	0.93	**8.5**	*200,202*
Multiple myeloma	22	0	-	-	-	-	-	-	-	-	-	2.6	-	8.7	11.7	14.0	18.5	4.5	-	-	3.5	0.6	0.11	0.28	**1.8**	*203*
Lymphoid leukaemia	13	0	-	6.4	-	-	-	1.9	1.9	-	-	-	-	2.9	7.0	2.3	3.1	4.5	-	28.3	2.0	0.4	0.10	0.13	**1.6**	*204*
Myeloid leukaemia	25	0	3.2	-	-	3.0	-	2.1	-	3.8	2.1	5.2	-	-	14.0	7.0	12.3	18.2	-	-	3.9	0.7	0.17	0.26	**2.7**	*205*
Monocytic leukaemia	1	0	-	-	-	-	-	-	-	-	-	-	-	-	2.3	-	-	-	-	-	0.2	0.0	0.01	0.01	**0.1**	*206*
Other leukaemia	3	0	-	-	3.2	-	-	-	-	-	-	-	-	2.9	2.3	-	-	-	-	-	0.5	0.1	0.04	0.04	**0.5**	*207*
Leukaemia unspecified	9	0	-	-	-	-	-	-	-	-	2.1	2.6	-	-	2.3	4.7	3.1	4.5	-	28.3	1.4	0.3	0.03	0.07	**0.8**	*208*
Other and unspecified	58	0	-	-	-	-	-	-	-	1.9	2.1	-	12.4	8.7	16.4	21.0	21.5	50.0	59.3	113.3	9.1	1.7	0.21	0.42	**4.3**	*O&U*
All sites	3456	0	12.6	12.7	6.4	18.0	15.8	12.5	44.7	47.3	105.0	163.9	264.4	553.8	980.0	1597.3	2249.5	2715.7	2735.2	3314.9	542.4		11.19	30.42	**253.8**	*ALL*
All sites but 173	3448	0	12.6	12.7	6.4	18.0	15.8	12.5	38.9	45.4	105.0	163.9	264.4	553.8	977.7	1592.7	2246.4	2715.7	2735.2	3314.9	541.1	100.0	11.14	30.33	**253.0**	*ALLb*

Rate from 1 case   3.155   3.182   3.179   2.993   2.264   2.078   1.944   1.893   2.058   2.602   3.110   2.900   2.339   2.332   3.077   4.549   8.468   14.166

†Important: see notes on population page

USA, HAWAII: JAPANESE 1988-1992

ANNUAL INCIDENCE PER 100,000 BY AGE GROUP (YEARS) - FEMALE

SITE	ALL AGES	AGE UNK	0-	5-	10-	15-	20-	25-	30-	35-	40-	45-	50-	55-	60-	65-	70-	75-	80-	85+	CRUDE RATE	%	CR 64	CR 74	ASR (W)	ICD (9th)
Lip	0	0	-	-	-	-	-	-	-	-	-	-	-	-	-	-	-	-	-	-	0.0	0.0	0.00	0.00	0.0	140
Tongue	13	0	-	-	-	-	-	-	-	-	2.1	-	-	4.5	-	5.8	2.6	16.2	14.2	-	1.9	0.5	0.03	0.08	0.8	141
Salivary gland	7	0	-	-	-	-	-	-	-	-	-	-	-	4.5	5.6	-	5.3	-	-	-	1.0	0.3	0.05	0.08	0.5	142
Mouth	10	0	-	-	-	-	-	-	-	-	-	-	2.7	2.2	3.7	-	5.3	8.1	-	14.9	1.5	0.4	0.04	0.07	0.6	143-5
Oropharynx	3	0	-	-	-	-	-	-	-	-	-	-	-	-	3.7	-	-	4.1	-	-	0.4	0.1	0.02	0.02	0.2	146
Nasopharynx	2	0	-	-	-	-	-	-	-	-	-	-	-	2.2	-	-	-	4.1	-	-	0.3	0.1	0.01	0.01	0.1	147
Hypopharynx	0	0	-	-	-	-	-	-	-	-	-	-	-	-	-	-	-	-	-	-	0.0	0.0	0.00	0.00	0.0	148
Pharynx unspecified	0	0	-	-	-	-	-	-	-	-	-	-	-	-	-	-	-	-	-	-	0.0	0.0	0.00	0.00	0.0	149
Oesophagus	9	0	-	-	-	-	-	-	-	-	2.1	-	-	2.2	-	3.9	5.3	-	7.1	14.9	1.3	0.3	0.02	0.07	0.5	150
Stomach	196	0	-	-	-	-	-	-	-	3.9	2.1	4.9	18.8	20.2	31.6	56.5	66.1	162.4	184.9	282.8	29.2	7.2	0.41	1.02	10.6	151
Small intestine	4	0	-	-	-	-	-	-	-	-	-	-	2.7	-	-	-	-	4.1	-	14.9	0.6	0.1	0.01	0.01	0.2	152
Colon	351	0	-	-	-	-	-	2.2	-	5.9	6.2	29.6	51.0	62.9	104.0	111.1	142.7	182.7	305.7	223.3	52.3	12.9	1.31	2.58	22.6	153
Rectum	115	0	-	-	-	-	-	-	-	2.0	4.2	7.4	24.2	27.0	40.9	39.0	42.3	48.7	71.1	59.5	17.1	4.2	0.53	0.93	7.9	154
Liver	34	0	-	-	-	-	-	-	-	-	-	2.5	2.7	-	9.3	9.7	10.6	32.5	28.4	44.7	5.1	1.3	0.07	0.17	1.8	155
Gallbladder etc.	38	0	-	-	-	-	-	-	-	-	2.1	-	-	-	11.1	7.8	15.9	40.6	28.4	52.1	5.7	1.4	0.07	0.18	1.9	156
Pancreas	101	0	-	-	-	-	-	-	-	-	4.2	2.5	5.4	15.7	27.9	31.2	47.6	93.4	49.8	74.4	15.1	3.7	0.28	0.67	5.9	157
Nose, sinuses etc.	5	0	-	-	-	-	-	-	-	-	-	2.5	2.7	-	-	-	12.2	-	-	-	0.7	0.2	0.03	0.03	0.4	160
Larynx	3	0	-	-	-	-	-	-	-	-	-	2.7	-	-	-	1.9	2.6	-	-	-	0.4	0.1	0.01	0.04	0.2	161
Bronchus, lung	176	0	-	-	-	-	-	-	2.0	-	4.2	2.5	26.9	27.0	53.9	79.9	89.8	81.2	56.9	134.0	26.2	6.5	0.58	1.43	11.1	162
Other thoracic organs	7	0	-	-	-	-	-	-	-	-	2.1	-	5.4	-	-	1.9	-	4.1	-	14.9	1.0	0.3	0.04	0.05	0.6	163-4
Bone	5	0	-	3.3	3.2	-	-	-	-	2.0	-	-	-	-	1.9	-	2.6	-	-	-	0.7	0.2	0.05	0.07	0.9	170
Connective tissue	12	0	-	-	-	-	-	-	-	-	-	-	5.4	2.2	1.9	3.9	-	8.1	14.2	14.9	1.8	0.4	0.05	0.07	0.8	171
Mesothelioma	0	0	-	-	-	-	-	-	-	-	-	-	-	-	-	-	-	-	-	-	0.0	0.0	0.00	0.00	0.0	MES
Kaposi's sarcoma	0	0	-	-	-	-	-	-	-	-	-	-	-	-	-	-	-	-	-	-	0.0	0.0	0.00	0.00	0.0	KAP
Melanoma of skin	4	0	-	-	-	-	-	-	-	2.0	-	-	-	2.2	1.9	-	2.6	-	-	-	0.6	0.1	0.03	0.04	0.3	172
†Other skin	12	0	-	-	-	-	-	2.2	-	-	-	-	5.4	2.2	3.7	1.9	-	12.2	7.1	7.4	1.8		0.07	0.08	0.9	173
Breast	903	0	-	-	-	-	-	-	18.4	80.7	118.6	197.2	153.1	213.6	267.4	294.3	351.5	320.7	263.1	148.9	134.6	33.3	5.25	8.47	72.9	174
Uterus unspecified	4	0	-	-	-	-	-	-	-	-	2.1	-	2.7	2.2	-	1.9	-	-	-	-	0.6	0.1	0.04	0.04	0.4	179
Cervix uteri	61	0	-	-	-	-	4.5	10.2	21.7	18.7	17.3	10.7	18.0	1.9	9.7	7.9	4.1	7.1	29.8		9.1	2.3	0.51	0.60	6.4	180
Placenta	1	0	-	-	-	-	-	-	2.1	-	-	-	-	-	-	-	-	-	-	-	0.1	0.0	0.01	0.01	0.1	181
Corpus uteri	166	0	-	-	-	-	2.2	14.3	11.8	18.7	39.4	45.7	42.7	42.7	39.0	52.9	64.9	71.1	14.9		24.7	6.1	1.09	1.55	14.2	182
Ovary etc.	95	0	-	-	6.1	-	8.2	5.9	4.2	17.3	21.5	33.7	22.3	37.0	21.1	40.6	14.2	22.3		14.2	3.5	0.60	0.89	8.1	183
Other female genital	13	0	-	-	-	-	-	-	-	-	-	2.7	-	5.6	1.9	-	8.1	21.3	22.3	1.9	0.5	0.04	0.05	0.7	184
Bladder	50	0	-	-	-	-	2.2	-	2.0	-	4.9	8.1	9.0	14.9	11.7	5.3	24.4	35.5	89.3	7.5	1.8	0.21	0.29	3.3	188
Kidney etc.	38	0	-	-	-	-	-	-	2.0	2.1	-	-	6.7	3.7	11.7	26.4	20.3	49.8	22.3	5.7	1.4	0.07	0.26	2.1	189
Eye	1	0	-	-	-	-	-	-	-	-	-	-	1.9	-	-	-	-	-	-	0.1	0.0	0.01	0.01	0.1	190
Brain, nervous system	11	0	3.3	-	-	-	-	-	2.0	2.0	2.1	2.5	-	2.2	3.7	-	2.6	8.1	-	-	1.6	0.4	0.09	0.10	1.3	191-2
Thyroid	63	0	-	-	-	-	2.7	6.7	8.2	2.0	4.2	12.3	18.8	15.7	13.0	11.7	23.8	12.2	28.4	29.8	9.4	2.3	0.42	0.60	5.7	193
Other endocrine	2	0	-	-	-	-	-	-	-	-	-	2.5	2.7	-	-	-	-	-	-	0.3	0.1	0.03	0.03	0.3	194
Hodgkin's disease	11	0	-	-	-	5.3	4.5	4.1	-	-	-	-	1.9	1.9	5.3	-	-	7.4	1.6	0.4	0.08	0.12	1.3	201	
Non-Hodgkin lymphoma	91	0	-	-	3.2	-	-	2.0	2.0	6.2	17.3	5.4	6.7	22.3	31.2	44.9	56.8	56.9	44.7	13.6	3.4	0.33	0.71	6.3	200,202
Multiple myeloma	13	0	-	-	-	-	-	-	-	-	2.5	2.7	-	-	5.3	20.3	7.1	22.3	1.9	0.5	0.05	0.05	0.7	203	
Lymphoid leukaemia	10	0	6.7	10.0	-	-	-	-	-	2.0	2.1	-	2.7	-	1.9	-	-	-	7.4	1.5	0.4	0.13	0.13	2.3	204	
Myeloid leukaemia	21	0	-	-	-	3.1	2.7	-	4.1	-	-	-	2.7	6.7	1.9	1.9	13.2	12.2	7.1	14.9	3.1	0.8	0.11	0.18	1.8	205
Monocytic leukaemia	1	0	-	-	-	-	-	-	-	-	-	-	-	-	-	-	-	4.1	-	0.1	0.0	0.00	0.00	0.0	206
Other leukaemia	0	0	-	-	-	-	-	-	-	-	-	-	-	-	-	-	-	-	-	0.0	0.0	0.00	0.00	0.0	207
Leukaemia unspecified	3	0	-	-	-	-	-	-	-	-	2.1	-	-	-	-	-	-	-	14.9	0.4	0.1	0.01	0.01	0.2	208
Other and unspecified	58	0	-	-	-	-	-	-	-	-	2.1	4.9	2.7	6.7	5.6	11.7	23.8	36.5	71.1	104.2	8.6	2.1	0.11	0.29	3.1	O&U
All sites	2723	0	10.0	13.3	6.5	9.2	10.7	24.6	73.7	147.6	214.4	369.8	437.7	539.6	711.3	820.5	1025.3	1347.7	1400.6	1548.1	405.8		12.84	22.07	200.4	ALL
All sites but 173	2711	0	10.0	13.3	6.5	9.2	10.7	22.3	73.7	147.6	214.4	369.8	432.3	537.3	707.6	818.5	1025.3	1335.5	1393.5	1540.6	404.1	100.0	12.77	21.99	199.4	ALLb

Rate from 1 case 3.326 3.325 3.248 3.052 2.675 2.234 2.047 1.969 2.081 2.465 2.685 2.248 1.857 1.949 2.643 4.059 7.110 7.443

†Important: see notes on population page

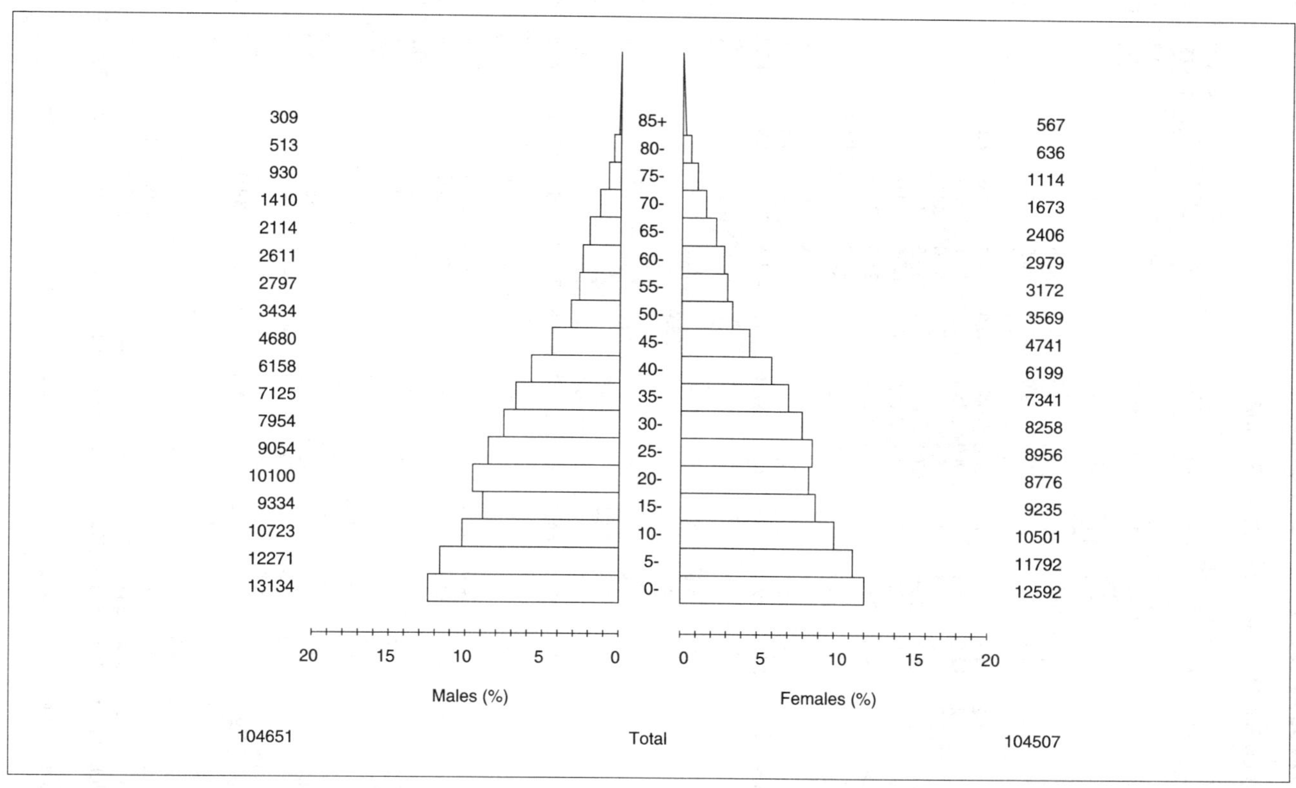

USA, Hawaii: Hawaiian

Source of population: average annual 1988–92

Estimate: The Health Surveillance Program of the Hawaii Department of Health conducts an annual random survey of approximately 2% of households statewide. The populations for the different ethnic groups are derived by apportioning the census sex-age counts by the race distributions for each sex-age group as determined by the annual Health Surveillance Program survey. The ethnic distributions can vary substantially from year to year, especially among small groups, making it necessary to smooth the yearly estimates.

Notes to tables overleaf:

† 173 does not include basal cell or squamous cell carcinoma

USA, HAWAII: HAWAIIAN 1988-1992

ANNUAL INCIDENCE PER 100,000 BY AGE GROUP (YEARS) - MALE

SITE	ALL AGES	AGE UNK	0-	5-	10-	15-	20-	25-	30-	35-	40-	45-	50-	55-	60-	65-	70-	75-	80-	85+	CRUDE RATE	%	CR 64	CR 74	ASR (W)	ICD (9th)
Lip	1	0	-	-	-	-	-	-	2.5	-	-	-	-	-	-	-	-	-	-	-	0.2	0.1	0.01	0.01	0.2	140
Tongue	7	0	-	-	-	-	-	-	-	-	3.2	8.5	-	7.2	7.7	18.9	-	-	-	-	1.3	0.7	0.13	0.23	1.9	141
Salivary gland	4	0	-	-	-	-	2.0	-	-	-	-	-	11.6	-	-	9.5	-	-	-	-	0.8	0.4	0.07	0.12	1.0	142
Mouth	9	0	-	-	-	-	-	-	-	-	-	4.3	5.8	14.3	23.0	9.5	14.2	-	-	-	1.7	0.9	0.24	0.36	2.6	143-5
Oropharynx	4	0	-	-	-	-	-	-	-	-	3.2	-	-	7.2	7.7	9.5	-	-	-	-	0.8	0.4	0.09	0.14	1.1	146
Nasopharynx	9	0	-	-	-	-	2.0	-	-	-	3.2	4.3	-	7.2	15.3	9.5	-	43.0	-	-	1.7	0.9	0.16	0.21	2.2	147
Hypopharynx	9	0	-	-	-	-	-	-	-	-	-	4.3	-	-	30.6	18.9	14.2	21.5	-	-	1.7	0.9	0.17	0.34	2.5	148
Pharynx unspecified	2	0	-	-	-	-	-	-	-	-	-	-	-	-	-	-	14.2	21.5	-	-	0.4	0.2	0.00	0.07	0.5	149
Oesophagus	28	0	-	-	1.9	-	-	-	-	2.8	3.2	4.3	5.8	7.2	53.6	56.7	70.9	21.5	77.9	64.6	5.4	2.7	0.39	1.03	7.6	150
Stomach	57	0	-	-	-	-	-	-	-	-	3.2	12.8	17.5	21.5	68.9	75.7	198.5	215.1	194.9	64.6	10.9	5.4	0.62	1.99	15.1	151
Small intestine	9	0	-	-	-	-	-	-	-	-	3.2	-	5.8	7.2	15.3	-	14.2	43.0	39.0	-	1.7	0.9	0.16	0.23	2.3	152
Colon	74	0	-	-	-	-	2.0	-	2.5	5.6	13.0	29.9	46.6	64.4	107.2	94.6	113.4	150.5	39.0	129.1	14.1	7.1	1.36	2.40	19.9	153
Rectum	50	0	-	-	-	-	-	-	-	-	6.5	12.8	29.1	57.2	68.9	141.9	56.7	64.5	39.0	-	9.6	4.8	0.87	1.87	13.9	154
Liver	25	0	-	-	-	-	-	-	-	2.8	6.5	4.3	23.3	35.8	46.0	28.4	14.2	21.5	39.0	-	4.8	2.4	0.59	0.81	6.8	155
Gallbladder etc.	7	0	-	-	-	-	-	-	-	-	-	-	5.8	-	-	28.4	14.2	21.5	-	64.6	1.3	0.7	0.03	0.24	2.0	156
Pancreas	33	0	-	-	-	-	-	-	2.5	-	3.2	4.3	29.1	21.5	7.7	85.1	85.1	129.0	-	-	6.3	3.2	0.34	1.19	8.8	157
Nose, sinuses etc.	4	0	-	-	-	-	-	-	2.5	-	-	-	5.8	-	7.7	-	-	21.5	-	-	0.8	0.4	0.08	0.08	1.0	160
Larynx	13	0	-	-	-	-	-	-	-	-	-	4.3	17.5	14.3	30.6	-	28.4	-	-	64.6	2.5	1.2	0.33	0.48	3.8	161
Bronchus, lung	261	0	-	-	-	-	-	-	2.5	5.6	13.0	64.1	139.8	300.3	413.6	482.4	524.6	451.6	311.8	129.1	49.9	24.9	4.69	9.73	72.3	162
Other thoracic organs	2	0	-	-	-	-	-	2.2	-	-	-	-	-	-	-	9.5	-	-	-	-	0.4	0.2	0.01	0.06	0.5	163-4
Bone	5	0	-	-	-	6.4	-	-	-	-	3.2	-	-	-	-	9.5	-	-	-	-	1.0	0.5	0.05	0.10	1.1	170
Connective tissue	13	0	-	-	-	8.6	-	-	2.5	-	6.5	4.3	5.8	14.3	7.7	-	-	21.5	-	-	2.5	1.2	0.25	0.25	3.0	171
Mesothelioma	5	0	-	-	-	-	-	-	-	-	-	-	5.8	-	7.7	9.5	28.4	-	-	-	1.0	0.5	0.07	0.26	1.4	MES
Kaposi's sarcoma	12	0	-	-	-	-	2.0	-	7.5	8.4	6.5	8.5	-	-	-	-	-	39.0	-	-	2.3	1.1	0.16	0.16	2.2	KAP
Melanoma of skin	3	0	-	-	-	-	-	-	-	-	-	-	5.8	-	7.7	-	14.2	-	-	-	0.6	0.3	0.07	0.14	0.9	172
†Other skin	6	0	-	-	-	-	-	4.4	-	-	-	-	5.8	14.3	-	9.5	-	-	-	-	1.1		0.12	0.17	1.5	173
Breast	2	0	-	-	-	-	-	-	2.5	-	-	-	-	-	-	9.5	-	-	-	-	0.4	0.2	0.01	0.06	0.4	175
Prostate	156	0	-	-	-	-	-	-	-	-	-	4.3	34.9	64.4	145.5	245.9	538.8	731.2	350.7	903.8	29.8	14.9	1.25	5.17	42.1	185
Testis	20	0	3.0	-	-	2.1	4.0	13.3	15.1	-	9.7	-	-	-	-	-	-	-	-	-	3.8	1.9	0.24	0.24	3.4	186
Penis	1	0	-	-	-	-	-	-	-	-	-	-	-	-	9.5	-	-	-	-	-	0.2	0.1	0.00	0.05	0.3	187.1-.4
Other male genital	0	0	-	-	-	-	-	-	-	-	-	-	-	-	-	-	-	-	-	-	0.0	0.0	0.00	0.00	0.0	187.5-.9
Bladder	16	0	-	-	-	-	-	-	-	5.6	3.2	-	5.8	14.3	-	28.4	28.4	21.5	116.9	64.6	3.1	1.5	0.14	0.43	3.9	188
Kidney etc.	31	0	-	-	-	-	-	-	-	-	-	-	40.8	42.9	38.3	28.4	42.5	107.5	39.0	64.6	5.9	3.0	0.61	0.96	8.6	189
Eye	1	0	-	-	-	-	-	-	-	-	-	-	-	-	7.7	-	-	-	-	-	0.2	0.1	0.04	0.04	0.3	190
Brain, nervous system	19	0	4.6	4.9	3.7	-	-	-	7.5	2.8	3.2	8.5	-	7.2	7.7	9.5	-	-	39.0	-	3.6	1.8	0.25	0.30	3.8	191-2
Thyroid	13	0	-	-	-	-	2.0	2.2	5.0	5.6	-	4.3	-	14.3	7.7	18.9	14.2	-	-	-	2.5	1.2	0.21	0.37	3.0	193
Other endocrine	6	0	6.1	-	-	-	-	-	-	-	3.2	-	-	7.2	-	-	-	-	-	-	1.1	0.6	0.08	0.08	1.2	194
Hodgkin's disease	4	0	-	-	-	-	4.0	-	-	-	3.2	-	-	-	7.7	-	-	-	-	-	0.8	0.4	0.07	0.07	0.8	201
Non-Hodgkin lymphoma	45	0	-	1.6	1.9	2.1	2.0	2.2	7.5	14.0	3.2	17.1	34.9	7.2	46.0	37.8	99.2	43.0	39.0	-	8.6	4.3	0.70	1.38	11.0	200,202
Multiple myeloma	15	0	-	-	-	-	-	-	-	-	3.2	4.3	5.8	14.3	30.6	28.4	14.2	43.0	-	-	2.9	1.4	0.29	0.50	4.1	203
Lymphoid leukaemia	11	0	7.6	3.3	-	-	2.0	-	-	-	-	-	5.8	-	15.3	-	-	-	-	-	2.1	1.1	0.17	0.17	2.3	204
Myeloid leukaemia	22	0	-	1.6	-	-	-	4.4	2.5	-	9.7	4.3	29.1	7.2	7.7	28.4	28.4	21.5	39.0	-	4.2	2.1	0.33	0.62	5.4	205
Monocytic leukaemia	3	0	1.5	-	-	-	-	-	-	-	-	-	-	7.2	-	-	21.5	-	-	-	0.6	0.3	0.04	0.04	0.7	206
Other leukaemia	1	0	-	-	-	-	-	-	-	-	-	-	-	-	14.2	-	-	-	-	-	0.2	0.1	0.00	0.07	0.3	207
Leukaemia unspecified	4	0	-	-	-	-	-	2.2	-	-	-	4.3	-	-	-	-	43.0	-	-	-	0.8	0.4	0.03	0.03	0.9	208
Other and unspecified	31	0	1.5	-	-	-	-	-	2.5	2.8	-	17.1	11.6	7.2	15.3	75.7	28.4	107.5	116.9	64.6	5.9	3.0	0.29	0.81	7.8	O&U
All sites	1053	0	24.4	11.4	7.5	19.3	21.8	30.9	65.4	56.1	116.9	235.0	535.8	786.5	1256.1	1626.8	2013.3	2387.1	1519.9	1613.9	201.2		15.84	34.04	276.2	ALL
All sites but 173	1047	0	24.4	11.4	7.5	19.3	21.8	26.5	65.4	56.1	116.9	235.0	530.0	772.2	1256.1	1617.3	2013.3	2387.1	1519.9	1613.9	200.1	100.0	15.71	33.87	274.7	ALLb

Rate from 1 case   1.523   1.630   1.865   2.143   1.980   2.209   2.514   2.807   3.248   4.273   5.824   7.150   7.659   9.458   14.178   21.505   38.971   64.558

†Important: see notes on population page

USA, HAWAII: HAWAIIAN 1988-1992

ANNUAL INCIDENCE PER 100,000 BY AGE GROUP (YEARS) - FEMALE

SITE	ALL AGES	AGE UNK	0-	5-	10-	15-	20-	25-	30-	35-	40-	45-	50-	55-	60-	65-	70-	75-	80-	85+	CRUDE RATE	%	CR 64	CR 74	ASR (W)	ICD (9th)
Lip	0	0	-	-	-	-	-	-	-	-	-	-	-	-	-	-	-	-	-	-	0.0	0.0	0.00	0.00	**0.0**	*140*
Tongue	6	0	-	-	-	-	2.3	-	2.4	-	-	-	-	-	-	-	8.3	12.0	35.9	-	-	1.1	0.5	0.02	0.12	**1.2**	*141*
Salivary gland	0	0	-	-	-	-	-	-	-	-	-	-	-	-	-	-	-	-	-	-	0.0	0.0	0.00	0.00	**0.0**	*142*
Mouth	4	0	-	-	-	-	-	-	-	-	-	-	-	-	6.7	8.3	12.0	-	31.4	-	0.8	0.3	0.03	0.13	**0.9**	*143-5*
Oropharynx	2	0	-	-	-	-	-	-	-	-	-	-	5.6	6.3	-	-	-	-	-	-	0.4	0.2	0.06	0.06	**0.5**	*146*
Nasopharynx	2	0	-	-	-	-	-	-	2.4	-	-	-	-	-	6.7	-	-	-	-	-	0.4	0.2	0.05	0.05	**0.4**	*147*
Hypopharynx	1	0	-	-	-	-	-	-	-	-	-	-	-	6.3	-	-	-	-	-	-	0.2	0.1	0.03	0.03	**0.3**	*148*
Pharynx unspecified	0	0	-	-	-	-	-	-	-	-	-	-	-	-	-	-	-	-	-	-	0.0	0.0	0.00	0.00	**0.0**	*149*
Oesophagus	5	0	-	-	-	-	-	-	-	-	-	4.2	-	6.3	6.7	-	23.9	-	-	-	1.0	0.4	0.09	0.21	**1.3**	*150*
Stomach	46	0	-	-	-	-	-	-	2.4	5.4	9.7	8.4	28.0	25.2	47.0	49.9	47.8	125.6	62.9	105.8	8.8	4.0	0.63	1.12	**10.4**	*151*
Small intestine	6	0	-	-	-	-	-	-	-	-	3.2	-	5.6	12.6	-	-	23.9	-	-	-	1.1	0.5	0.11	0.23	**1.5**	*152*
Colon	71	0	-	-	1.9	-	-	-	-	-	3.2	21.1	28.0	75.7	60.4	91.4	131.5	89.7	188.7	176.4	13.6	6.2	0.95	2.07	**16.6**	*153*
Rectum	34	0	-	-	-	-	-	-	-	5.4	-	21.1	22.4	18.9	40.3	33.2	59.8	53.8	-	70.5	6.5	3.0	0.54	1.01	**8.2**	*154*
Liver	11	0	1.6	-	-	-	-	2.2	-	2.7	-	4.2	5.6	6.3	13.4	16.6	12.0	-	-	-	2.1	1.0	0.18	0.32	**2.6**	*155*
Gallbladder etc.	6	0	-	-	-	-	-	-	-	2.7	-	-	5.6	-	20.1	-	-	-	-	35.3	1.1	0.5	0.14	0.14	**1.4**	*156*
Pancreas	32	0	-	-	-	-	-	-	-	2.7	6.5	21.1	16.8	25.2	20.1	16.6	35.9	35.9	94.3	141.1	6.1	2.8	0.46	0.72	**7.2**	*157*
Nose, sinuses etc.	6	0	-	-	1.9	2.2	-	-	2.4	2.7	-	-	-	-	6.7	-	-	17.9	-	-	1.1	0.5	0.08	0.08	**1.1**	*160*
Larynx	3	0	-	-	-	-	-	-	-	-	-	-	-	-	-	8.3	-	35.9	-	-	0.6	0.3	0.00	0.04	**0.6**	*161*
Bronchus, lung	145	0	-	-	-	-	-	2.2	-	8.2	12.9	21.1	72.8	176.5	154.4	207.8	310.8	179.4	157.2	70.5	27.7	12.7	2.24	4.83	**35.0**	*162*
Other thoracic organs	2	0	3.2	-	-	-	-	-	-	-	-	-	-	-	-	-	-	-	-	-	0.4	0.2	0.02	0.02	**0.4**	*163-4*
Bone	3	0	-	-	1.9	2.2	-	-	-	-	-	-	-	-	-	-	-	17.9	-	-	0.6	0.3	0.02	0.02	**0.5**	*170*
Connective tissue	12	0	-	-	1.9	2.2	-	-	2.4	5.4	3.2	-	11.2	6.3	6.7	-	-	17.9	31.4	-	2.3	1.0	0.20	0.20	**2.4**	*171*
Mesothelioma	0	0	-	-	-	-	-	-	-	-	-	-	-	-	-	-	-	-	-	-	0.0	0.0	0.00	0.00	**0.0**	*MES*
Kaposi's sarcoma	0	0	-	-	-	-	-	-	-	-	-	-	-	-	-	-	-	-	-	-	0.0	0.0	0.00	0.00	**0.0**	*KAP*
Melanoma of skin	5	0	-	-	-	-	-	-	-	-	3.2	4.2	-	12.6	6.7	-	-	-	-	-	1.0	0.4	0.13	0.13	**1.2**	*172*
†Other skin	4	0	-	-	-	-	-	2.2	-	-	-	-	-	-	-	8.3	12.0	17.9	-	-	0.8		0.01	0.11	**0.8**	*173*
Breast	360	0	-	-	-	-	-	2.2	21.8	65.4	116.1	198.3	235.3	321.6	268.5	324.2	418.4	376.7	345.9	141.1	68.9	31.4	6.15	9.86	**83.9**	*174*
Uterus unspecified	0	0	-	-	-	-	-	-	-	-	-	-	-	-	-	-	-	-	-	-	0.0	0.0	0.00	0.00	**0.0**	*179*
Cervix uteri	41	0	-	-	-	-	2.3	-	14.5	27.2	9.7	12.7	28.0	6.3	13.4	49.9	35.9	-	31.4	-	7.8	3.6	0.57	1.00	**8.6**	*180*
Placenta	0	0	-	-	-	-	-	-	-	-	-	-	-	-	-	-	-	-	-	-	0.0	0.0	0.00	0.00	**0.0**	*181*
Corpus uteri	91	0	-	-	-	-	-	6.7	7.3	13.6	41.9	33.7	61.6	56.7	73.8	91.4	59.8	107.6	157.2	35.3	17.4	7.9	1.48	2.23	**20.6**	*182*
Ovary etc.	36	0	-	-	-	6.5	-	2.2	4.8	-	6.5	8.4	16.8	31.5	26.8	66.5	35.9	17.9	62.9	-	6.9	3.1	0.52	1.03	**8.3**	*183*
Other female genital	8	0	-	-	-	-	-	-	-	-	-	-	22.4	-	-	8.3	-	35.9	31.4	-	1.5	0.7	0.11	0.15	**1.9**	*184*
Bladder	14	0	-	-	-	-	-	2.2	-	-	-	-	-	6.3	13.4	24.9	47.8	-	31.4	70.5	2.7	1.2	0.11	0.47	**3.2**	*188*
Kidney etc.	13	0	-	-	-	-	-	-	2.4	-	6.5	4.2	-	25.2	26.8	-	-	-	-	35.3	2.5	1.1	0.33	0.33	**3.0**	*189*
Eye	5	0	7.9	-	-	-	-	-	-	-	-	-	-	-	-	-	-	-	-	-	1.0	0.4	0.04	0.04	**1.0**	*190*
Brain, nervous system	15	0	-	1.7	5.7	-	2.3	2.2	4.8	-	3.2	-	-	6.3	6.7	-	23.9	-	31.4	35.3	2.9	1.3	0.17	0.28	**2.9**	*191-2*
Thyroid	42	0	-	-	1.9	2.2	6.8	4.5	12.1	8.2	19.4	21.1	28.0	25.2	26.8	24.9	-	-	-	-	8.0	3.7	0.78	0.91	**9.1**	*193*
Other endocrine	1	0	1.6	-	-	-	-	-	-	-	-	-	-	-	-	-	-	-	-	-	0.2	0.1	0.01	0.01	**0.2**	*194*
Hodgkin's disease	11	0	-	-	-	2.2	2.3	13.4	2.4	2.7	3.2	-	-	-	-	-	-	-	-	-	2.1	1.0	0.13	0.13	**2.0**	*201*
Non-Hodgkin lymphoma	23	0	-	-	-	2.2	2.3	-	-	2.7	3.2	4.2	-	25.2	-	33.2	47.8	17.9	62.9	105.8	4.4	2.0	0.20	0.60	**5.0**	*200,202*
Multiple myeloma	18	0	-	-	-	-	-	-	-	-	3.2	4.2	11.2	12.6	6.7	16.6	71.7	35.9	31.4	-	3.4	1.6	0.19	0.63	**4.2**	*203*
Lymphoid leukaemia	17	0	6.4	5.1	1.9	-	2.3	-	-	-	-	-	12.7	-	-	6.7	16.6	23.9	-	-	3.3	1.5	0.17	0.38	**3.6**	*204*
Myeloid leukaemia	11	0	-	1.7	-	4.3	2.3	-	-	-	-	-	8.4	5.6	-	13.4	8.3	-	17.9	-	2.1	1.0	0.18	0.22	**2.5**	*205*
Monocytic leukaemia	1	0	-	-	-	-	-	-	-	-	-	4.2	-	-	-	-	-	-	-	-	0.2	0.1	0.02	0.02	**0.3**	*206*
Other leukaemia	0	0	-	-	-	-	-	-	-	-	-	-	-	-	-	-	-	-	-	-	0.0	0.0	0.00	0.00	**0.0**	*207*
Leukaemia unspecified	1	0	-	-	-	-	-	-	-	-	-	-	-	-	-	8.3	-	-	-	-	0.2	0.1	0.00	0.04	**0.2**	*208*
Other and unspecified	35	0	-	-	-	-	-	-	-	-	6.5	29.5	22.4	12.6	13.4	41.6	12.0	107.6	157.2	35.3	6.7	3.1	0.42	0.69	**7.8**	*O&U*
All sites	1149	0	20.6	8.5	17.1	23.8	22.8	40.2	82.3	155.3	261.3	447.1	633.1	907.9	892.7	1163.7	1458.3	1345.5	1509.4	1058.2	219.9		17.56	30.67	**262.9**	*ALL*
All sites but 173	1145	0	20.6	8.5	17.1	23.8	22.8	38.0	82.3	155.3	261.3	447.1	633.1	907.9	892.7	1155.3	1446.3	1327.6	1509.4	1058.2	219.1	100.0	17.55	30.56	**262.0**	*ALLb*
Rate from 1 case			1.588	1.696	1.904	2.165	2.279	2.233	2.422	2.724	3.226	4.218	5.603	6.305	6.712	8.312	11.953	17.940	31.447	35.273						

†Important: see notes on population page

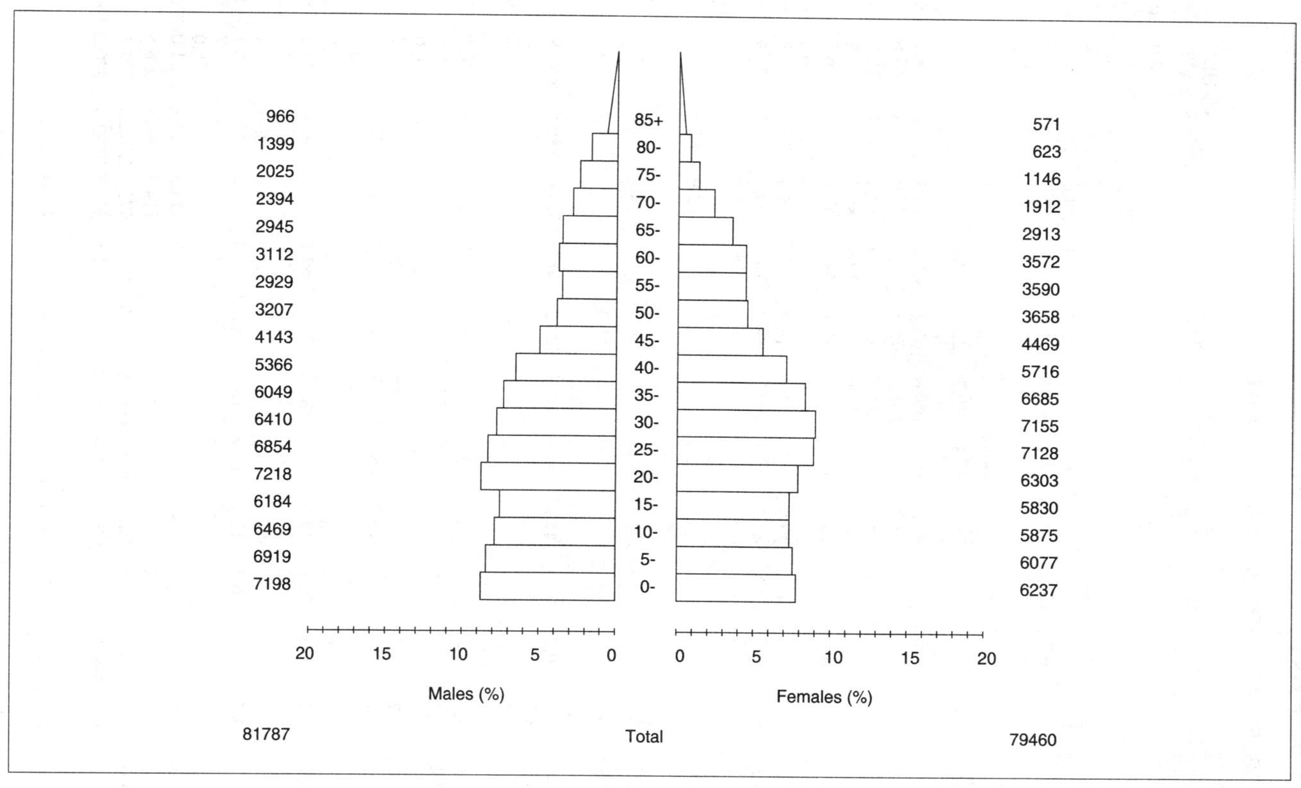

USA, Hawaii: Filipino

Source of population: average annual 1988–92

Estimate: The Health Surveillance Program of the Hawaii Department of Health conducts an annual random survey of approximately 2% of households statewide. The populations for the different ethnic groups are derived by apportioning the census sex-age counts by the race distributions for each sex-age group as determined by the annual Health Surveillance Program survey. The ethnic distributions can vary substantially from year to year, especially among small groups, making it necessary to smooth the yearly estimates.

Notes to tables overleaf:

† 173 does not include basal cell or squamous cell carcinoma

USA, HAWAII: FILIPINO 1988-1992

ANNUAL INCIDENCE PER 100,000 BY AGE GROUP (YEARS) - MALE

S I T E	ALL AGES	AGE UNK	0-	5-	10-	15-	20-	25-	30-	35-	40-	45-	50-	55-	60-	65-	70-	75-	80-	85+	CRUDE RATE	%	CR 64	CR 74	ASR (W)	ICD (9th)
Lip	0	0	-	-	-	-	-	-	-	-	-	-	-	-	-	-	-	-	-	-	0.0	0.0	0.00	0.00	0.0	140
Tongue	5	0	-	-	-	-	-	-	-	-	-	-	-	-	6.4	6.8	-	-	42.9	-	1.2	0.4	0.03	0.07	0.7	141
Salivary gland	3	0	-	-	-	-	2.8	2.9	-	-	-	-	-	-	-	-	-	-	14.3	-	0.7	0.2	0.03	0.03	0.5	142
Mouth	9	0	-	-	-	-	-	-	-	-	-	4.8	-	-	6.4	6.8	-	29.6	-	62.1	2.2	0.7	0.06	0.09	1.4	143-5
Oropharynx	8	0	-	-	-	-	-	-	-	-	3.7	-	-	-	6.4	-	16.7	9.9	28.6	20.7	2.0	0.6	0.05	0.13	1.2	146
Nasopharynx	14	0	-	-	-	-	-	-	3.1	-	-	9.7	12.5	20.5	12.9	6.8	8.4	9.9	14.3	-	3.4	1.1	0.29	0.37	3.3	147
Hypopharynx	3	0	-	-	-	-	-	-	-	-	-	4.8	-	6.8	-	-	-	-	14.3	-	0.7	0.2	0.06	0.06	0.6	148
Pharynx unspecified	2	0	-	-	-	-	-	-	-	-	-	-	-	-	-	-	-	9.9	14.3	-	0.5	0.2	0.00	0.00	0.2	149
Oesophagus	21	0	-	-	-	-	-	-	-	3.3	-	-	-	34.1	19.3	-	16.7	39.5	57.2	41.4	5.1	1.6	0.28	0.37	3.6	150
Stomach	40	0	-	-	-	-	-	-	6.6	3.7	-	31.2	13.7	32.1	40.7	33.4	79.0	42.9	82.7	9.8	3.1	0.44	0.81	7.3	151
Small intestine	3	0	-	-	-	-	-	-	-	-	-	-	-	-	-	16.7	-	14.3	-	0.7	0.2	0.00	0.08	0.4	152
Colon	115	0	-	-	-	-	-	-	6.6	11.2	4.8	24.9	54.6	57.8	108.6	100.2	266.7	314.5	227.6	28.1	8.8	0.80	1.84	17.7	153
Rectum	76	0	-	-	-	-	-	3.1	6.6	7.5	-	37.4	13.7	64.3	101.9	75.2	118.5	142.9	144.8	18.6	5.8	0.66	1.55	13.2	154
Liver	49	0	2.8	-	-	-	-	2.9	3.1	13.2	7.5	4.8	12.5	34.1	38.6	40.7	33.4	59.3	114.4	41.4	12.0	3.7	0.60	0.97	9.1	155
Gallbladder etc.	13	0	-	-	-	-	-	-	-	-	-	-	-	6.8	-	13.6	-	19.8	85.8	41.4	3.2	1.0	0.03	0.10	1.5	156
Pancreas	27	0	-	-	-	-	-	-	-	-	-	4.8	6.2	13.7	19.3	34.0	25.1	49.4	57.2	62.1	6.6	2.1	0.22	0.52	4.5	157
Nose, sinuses etc.	2	0	-	-	-	-	-	-	-	-	-	-	-	-	6.4	-	-	-	14.3	-	0.5	0.2	0.03	0.03	0.3	160
Larynx	12	0	-	-	-	-	-	-	-	-	-	-	6.2	27.3	6.4	13.6	16.7	-	14.3	20.7	2.9	0.9	0.20	0.35	2.6	161
Bronchus, lung	202	0	-	-	-	-	2.8	-	-	3.3	11.2	29.0	93.5	184.4	237.8	203.7	284.0	276.5	200.1	124.1	49.4	15.4	2.81	5.25	40.6	162
Other thoracic organs	3	0	-	-	-	-	2.8	-	-	-	-	4.8	-	-	-	-	-	-	14.3	-	0.7	0.2	0.04	0.04	0.6	163-4
Bone	7	0	-	-	-	9.7	2.8	-	-	-	3.7	-	-	-	12.9	-	-	-	-	-	1.7	0.5	0.15	0.15	1.8	170
Connective tissue	14	0	-	-	-	-	2.8	-	3.1	-	3.7	-	6.2	-	12.9	6.8	8.4	-	42.9	62.1	3.4	1.1	0.14	0.22	2.4	171
Mesothelioma	5	0	-	-	-	-	-	-	-	-	-	-	-	13.7	6.4	13.6	-	-	-	-	1.2	0.4	0.10	0.17	1.2	MES
Kaposi's sarcoma	9	0	-	-	-	-	-	-	6.2	16.5	3.7	-	-	-	-	-	-	-	14.3	-	2.2	0.7	0.13	0.13	1.7	KAP
Melanoma of skin	5	0	-	-	-	-	2.8	-	-	-	-	-	-	-	-	-	-	-	42.9	20.7	1.2	0.4	0.01	0.01	0.5	172
†Other skin	3	0	-	-	3.1	-	-	-	-	3.3	-	-	-	-	-	-	8.4	-	-	-	0.7		0.03	0.07	0.6	173
Breast	1	0	-	-	-	-	-	-	-	-	-	-	-	-	-	6.8	-	-	-	-	0.2	0.1	0.00	0.03	0.2	175
Prostate	380	0	-	-	-	-	-	-	-	-	-	9.7	12.5	41.0	186.4	332.7	384.3	948.1	1529.4	889.5	92.9	29.0	1.25	4.83	49.5	185
Testis	9	0	-	-	-	-	2.8	11.7	3.1	6.6	3.7	-	-	-	-	-	-	-	-	-	2.2	0.7	0.14	0.14	2.0	186
Penis	7	0	-	-	-	-	-	6.2	-	3.7	3.7	4.8	-	-	12.9	-	-	9.9	-	-	1.7	0.5	0.14	0.14	1.5	187.1-.4
Other male genital	0	0	-	-	-	-	-	-	-	-	-	-	-	-	-	-	-	-	-	-	0.0	0.0	0.00	0.00	0.0	187.5-.9
Bladder	33	0	-	-	-	-	2.9	3.1	3.3	3.7	4.8	18.7	6.8	12.9	27.2	25.1	39.5	128.6	41.4	-	8.1	2.5	0.28	0.54	5.4	188
Kidney etc.	25	0	-	-	-	-	-	-	6.6	-	-	-	6.2	20.5	12.9	40.7	25.1	19.8	85.8	-	6.1	1.9	0.23	0.56	4.4	189
Eye	0	0	-	-	-	-	-	-	-	-	-	-	-	-	-	-	-	-	-	-	0.0	0.0	0.00	0.00	0.0	190
Brain, nervous system	11	0	2.8	-	-	-	-	2.9	3.1	6.6	3.7	4.8	6.2	-	-	13.6	-	9.9	-	-	2.7	0.8	0.15	0.22	2.5	191-2
Thyroid	26	0	-	-	-	-	2.8	5.8	3.1	3.3	3.7	-	6.2	13.7	45.0	6.8	16.7	9.9	57.2	41.4	6.4	2.0	0.42	0.54	5.1	193
Other endocrine	2	0	-	-	3.1	3.2	-	-	-	-	-	-	-	-	-	-	-	-	-	-	0.5	0.2	0.03	0.03	0.6	194
Hodgkin's disease	4	0	-	-	-	6.5	-	-	-	-	4.8	-	-	6.8	-	-	-	-	-	-	1.0	0.3	0.09	0.09	1.1	201
Non-Hodgkin lymphoma	62	0	-	-	3.1	-	-	-	5.8	6.2	9.9	3.7	9.7	18.7	13.7	38.6	81.5	75.2	142.9	41.4	15.2	4.7	0.55	1.33	11.1	200,202
Multiple myeloma	21	0	-	-	-	-	-	-	-	-	-	-	-	6.2	-	6.4	40.7	19.8	100.1	20.7	5.1	1.6	0.06	0.39	3.1	203
Lymphoid leukaemia	14	0	11.1	5.8	-	-	-	-	-	-	-	-	-	-	-	6.4	-	-	39.5	28.6	20.7	3.4	1.1	0.12	0.12	2.8	204
Myeloid leukaemia	25	0	-	-	3.1	-	2.8	-	3.1	-	7.5	-	6.2	13.7	12.9	13.6	8.4	59.3	71.5	20.7	6.1	1.9	0.25	0.36	4.1	205
Monocytic leukaemia	3	0	2.8	-	-	-	-	-	2.8	-	-	-	-	-	-	-	-	9.9	-	-	0.7	0.2	0.03	0.03	0.7	206
Other leukaemia	0	0	-	-	-	-	-	-	-	-	-	-	-	-	-	-	-	-	-	-	0.0	0.0	0.00	0.00	0.0	207
Leukaemia unspecified	4	0	-	-	-	-	-	-	3.1	-	-	-	-	-	-	-	-	9.9	14.3	20.7	1.0	0.3	0.02	0.02	0.5	208
Other and unspecified	36	0	-	-	-	3.2	-	-	-	-	3.7	-	12.5	6.8	19.3	27.2	16.7	69.1	114.4	144.8	8.8	2.7	0.23	0.45	5.3	O&U
All sites	1313	0	19.4	5.8	12.4	22.6	27.7	35.0	49.9	95.9	89.4	106.2	324.2	546.2	899.6	1188.3	1219.6	2281.5	3573.5	2192.8	321.1		11.17	23.21	217.3	ALL
All sites but 173	1310	0	19.4	5.8	9.3	22.6	27.7	35.0	49.9	92.6	89.4	106.2	324.2	546.2	899.6	1188.3	1211.3	2281.5	3573.5	2192.8	320.3	100.0	11.14	23.14	216.7	ALLb

| Rate from 1 case | | | 2.778 | 2.890 | 3.091 | 3.234 | 2.771 | 2.918 | 3.120 | 3.306 | 3.727 | 4.827 | 6.235 | 6.828 | 6.426 | 6.790 | 8.354 | 9.877 | 14.294 | 20.687 |

†Important: see notes on population page

USA, HAWAII: FILIPINO 1988-1992

ANNUAL INCIDENCE PER 100,000 BY AGE GROUP (YEARS) - FEMALE

SITE	ALL AGES	AGE UNK	0-	5-	10-	15-	20-	25-	30-	35-	40-	45-	50-	55-	60-	65-	70-	75-	80-	85+	CRUDE RATE	%	CR 64	CR 74	ASR (W)	ICD (9th)
Lip	0	0	-	-	-	-	-	-	-	-	-	-	-	-	-	-	-	-	-	-	0.0	0.0	0.00	0.00	0.0	140
Tongue	9	0	-	-	-	-	-	-	-	-	3.5	4.5	5.5	-	5.6	-	10.5	17.5	32.1	70.0	2.3	1.0	0.10	0.15	1.9	141
Salivary gland	5	0	-	-	-	-	-	-	-	-	7.0	-	-	11.1	-	-	-	17.5	-	-	1.3	0.5	0.09	0.09	1.0	142
Mouth	8	0	-	-	-	-	-	2.8	-	-	-	-	5.5	5.6	5.6	6.9	10.5	-	-	70.0	2.0	0.9	0.10	0.18	1.7	143-5
Oropharynx	3	0	-	-	-	-	-	2.8	-	-	-	-	-	-	-	6.9	-	-	-	35.0	0.8	0.3	0.01	0.05	0.6	146
Nasopharynx	5	0	-	-	-	-	-	2.8	-	-	-	-	10.9	5.6	5.6	-	-	-	-	-	1.3	0.5	0.12	0.12	1.2	147
Hypopharynx	4	0	-	-	-	-	-	-	-	-	-	-	5.5	-	5.6	-	-	17.5	32.1	-	1.0	0.4	0.06	0.06	0.8	148
Pharynx unspecified	0	0	-	-	-	-	-	-	-	-	-	-	-	-	-	-	-	-	-	-	0.0	0.0	0.00	0.00	0.0	149
Oesophagus	4	0	-	-	-	-	-	-	-	-	-	-	-	5.6	-	-	10.5	-	64.2	-	1.0	0.4	0.03	0.08	0.8	150
Stomach	32	0	-	-	-	-	-	-	-	3.0	10.5	8.9	16.4	11.1	22.4	48.1	52.3	34.9	96.2	-	8.1	3.5	0.36	0.86	6.8	151
Small intestine	2	0	-	-	-	-	-	-	-	-	-	-	-	5.6	-	-	10.5	-	-	-	0.5	0.2	0.03	0.08	0.4	152
Colon	63	0	-	-	-	-	-	-	-	9.0	7.0	22.4	43.7	16.7	16.8	68.7	94.1	122.2	256.7	175.1	15.9	6.8	0.58	1.39	13.2	153
Rectum	33	0	-	-	-	-	-	-	-	-	-	13.4	16.4	39.0	22.4	34.3	41.8	52.4	96.2	35.0	8.3	3.6	0.46	0.84	7.1	154
Liver	9	0	-	-	-	-	-	-	-	-	-	-	-	-	11.2	20.6	10.5	34.9	-	35.0	2.3	1.0	0.06	0.21	1.8	155
Gallbladder etc.	6	0	-	-	-	-	-	-	-	-	-	4.5	-	-	11.2	-	-	17.5	32.1	35.0	1.5	0.6	0.08	0.08	1.2	156
Pancreas	18	0	3.2	-	-	-	-	-	-	-	-	-	16.4	5.6	22.4	27.5	31.4	17.5	32.1	-	4.5	1.9	0.24	0.53	4.1	157
Nose, sinuses etc.	3	0	-	-	-	-	-	-	-	-	-	4.5	-	-	11.2	-	-	-	-	-	0.8	0.3	0.08	0.08	0.7	160
Larynx	2	0	-	-	-	-	-	-	-	-	-	-	-	5.6	5.6	-	-	-	-	-	0.5	0.2	0.06	0.06	0.4	161
Bronchus, lung	83	0	-	-	-	-	-	-	-	9.0	7.0	17.9	38.3	89.1	67.2	103.0	83.7	192.0	32.1	140.1	20.9	9.0	1.14	2.08	17.7	162
Other thoracic organs	4	0	-	-	-	-	-	-	2.8	-	-	4.5	-	5.6	-	-	-	-	32.1	-	1.0	0.4	0.06	0.06	0.8	163-4
Bone	1	0	-	-	-	3.4	-	-	-	-	-	-	-	-	-	-	-	-	-	-	0.3	0.1	0.02	0.02	0.3	170
Connective tissue	8	0	3.2	-	-	-	-	2.8	2.8	-	7.0	-	-	5.6	5.6	6.9	-	-	-	-	2.0	0.9	0.13	0.17	1.8	171
Mesothelioma	0	0	-	-	-	-	-	-	-	-	-	-	-	-	-	-	-	-	-	-	0.0	0.0	0.00	0.00	0.0	MES
Kaposi's sarcoma	0	0	-	-	-	-	-	-	-	-	-	-	-	-	-	-	-	-	-	-	0.0	0.0	0.00	0.00	0.0	KAP
Melanoma of skin	3	0	-	-	-	-	-	-	2.8	-	-	-	-	-	5.6	6.9	-	-	-	-	0.8	0.3	0.04	0.08	0.6	172
†Other skin	1	0	-	-	-	-	-	-	-	-	3.5	-	-	-	-	-	-	-	-	-	0.3		0.02	0.02	0.2	173
Breast	259	0	-	-	-	-	-	2.8	25.2	62.8	125.9	179.0	136.7	211.7	201.5	137.3	136.0	209.4	192.5	70.0	65.2	28.0	4.73	6.09	57.4	174
Uterus unspecified	2	0	-	-	-	-	-	-	-	-	-	-	-	5.6	-	6.9	-	-	-	-	0.5	0.2	0.03	0.06	0.4	179
Cervix uteri	33	0	-	-	-	-	-	19.6	12.0	28.0	13.4	5.5	16.7	16.8	13.7	10.5	-	-	32.1	-	8.3	3.6	0.56	0.68	6.8	180
Placenta	1	0	-	-	-	-	-	-	-	-	3.5	-	-	-	-	-	-	-	-	-	0.3	0.1	0.02	0.02	0.2	181
Corpus uteri	50	0	-	-	-	-	-	2.8	2.8	6.0	21.0	-	38.3	83.6	28.0	34.3	52.3	34.9	-	35.0	12.6	5.4	0.91	1.35	11.0	182
Ovary etc.	35	0	-	-	6.8	3.4	3.2	-	5.6	9.0	3.5	13.4	38.3	16.7	22.4	13.7	41.8	17.5	32.1	-	8.8	3.8	0.61	0.89	8.1	183
Other female genital	5	0	-	-	-	-	-	5.6	-	-	-	-	-	-	-	-	-	34.9	-	35.0	1.3	0.5	0.03	0.03	1.0	184
Bladder	13	0	-	-	-	-	-	-	-	3.0	3.5	4.5	5.5	5.6	11.2	6.9	20.9	-	32.1	70.0	3.3	1.4	0.17	0.30	2.7	188
Kidney etc.	8	0	-	-	-	-	-	-	2.8	-	10.5	-	-	-	11.2	13.7	-	-	-	-	2.0	0.9	0.12	0.19	1.7	189
Eye	1	0	3.2	-	-	-	-	-	-	-	-	-	-	-	-	-	-	-	-	-	0.3	0.1	0.02	0.02	0.4	190
Brain, nervous system	7	0	6.4	3.3	-	-	-	-	-	-	-	-	-	5.5	-	11.2	6.9	-	-	-	1.8	0.8	0.13	0.17	2.0	191-2
Thyroid	115	0	-	-	3.4	6.9	12.7	14.0	28.0	50.9	45.5	40.3	98.4	61.3	39.2	54.9	62.8	52.4	32.1	-	28.9	12.4	2.00	2.59	25.5	193
Other endocrine	1	0	-	-	-	-	-	-	-	-	-	-	-	-	-	-	-	17.5	-	-	0.3	0.1	0.00	0.00	0.2	194
Hodgkin's disease	5	0	-	-	-	-	6.3	-	2.8	3.0	-	-	-	-	5.6	-	-	-	-	-	1.3	0.5	0.09	0.09	1.1	201
Non-Hodgkin lymphoma	37	0	-	-	-	6.9	3.2	2.8	-	6.0	14.0	-	-	27.9	44.8	34.3	41.8	17.5	64.2	70.0	9.3	4.0	0.53	0.91	7.9	200,202
Multiple myeloma	8	0	-	-	-	-	-	-	-	-	-	-	-	16.7	11.2	13.7	-	-	32.1	-	2.0	0.9	0.14	0.21	1.7	203
Lymphoid leukaemia	3	0	3.2	3.3	-	-	-	-	-	-	-	3.5	-	-	-	-	-	-	-	-	0.8	0.3	0.05	0.05	0.9	204
Myeloid leukaemia	18	0	3.2	-	-	3.4	6.3	2.8	2.8	-	3.5	8.9	-	16.7	5.6	6.9	20.9	-	32.1	35.0	4.5	1.9	0.27	0.41	4.2	205
Monocytic leukaemia	0	0	-	-	-	-	-	-	-	-	-	-	-	-	-	-	-	-	-	-	0.0	0.0	0.00	0.00	0.0	206
Other leukaemia	0	0	-	-	-	-	-	-	-	-	-	-	-	-	-	-	-	-	-	-	0.0	0.0	0.00	0.00	0.0	207
Leukaemia unspecified	4	0	-	-	-	-	-	2.8	-	-	-	-	-	5.6	-	-	10.5	-	32.1	-	1.0	0.4	0.04	0.09	0.8	208
Other and unspecified	16	0	-	-	-	-	-	-	-	-	-	-	5.5	11.1	11.2	34.3	10.5	52.4	32.1	35.0	4.0	1.7	0.14	0.36	3.3	O&U
All sites	927	0	22.4	6.6	10.2	24.0	31.7	44.9	97.8	173.5	307.9	340.1	492.1	685.2	649.4	707.1	763.5	959.9	1219.1	945.4	233.3		14.43	21.78	202.6	ALL
All sites but 173	926	0	22.4	6.6	10.2	24.0	31.7	44.9	97.8	173.5	304.4	340.1	492.1	685.2	649.4	707.1	763.5	959.9	1219.1	945.4	233.1	100.0	14.41	21.76	202.4	ALLb
Rate from 1 case			3.207	3.291	3.404	3.430	3.173	2.806	2.795	2.992	3.498	4.474	5.467	5.570	5.598	6.865	10.459	17.452	32.082	35.014						

†Important: see notes on population page

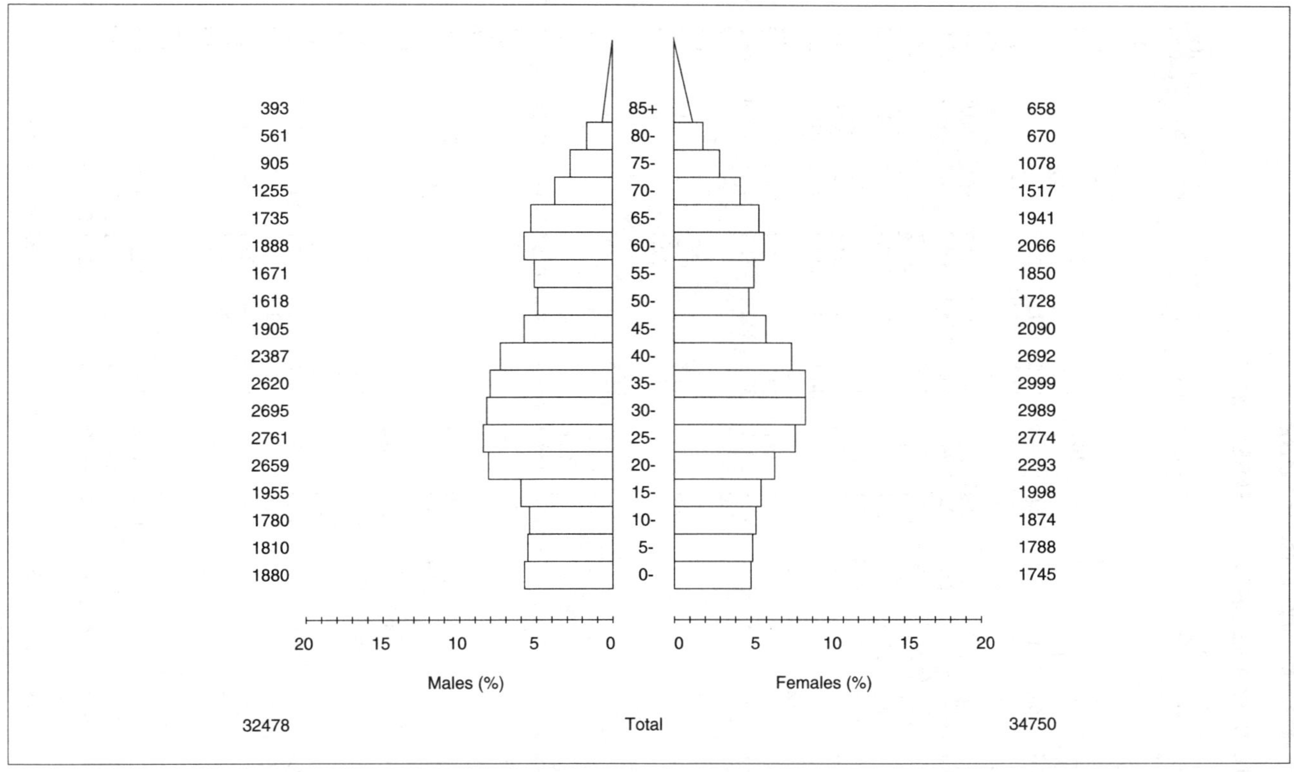

USA, Hawaii: Chinese

Source of population: average annual 1988–92

Estimate: The Health Surveillance Program of the Hawaii Department of Health conducts an annual random survey of approximately 2% of households statewide. The populations for the different ethnic groups are derived by apportioning the census sex-age counts by the race distributions for each sex-age group as determined by the annual Health Surveillance Program survey. The ethnic distributions can vary substantially from year to year, especially among small groups, making it necessary to smooth the yearly estimates.

Notes to tables overleaf:

† 173 does not include basal cell or squamous cell carcinoma

USA, HAWAII: CHINESE 1988-1992

ANNUAL INCIDENCE PER 100,000 BY AGE GROUP (YEARS) - MALE

SITE	ALL AGES	AGE UNK	0-	5-	10-	15-	20-	25-	30-	35-	40-	45-	50-	55-	60-	65-	70-	75-	80-	85+	CRUDE RATE	%	CR 64	CR 74	ASR (W)	ICD (9th)
Lip	0	0	-	-	-	-	-	-	-	-	-	-	-	-	-	-	-	-	-	-	0.0	0.0	0.00	0.00	0.0	140
Tongue	2	0	-	-	-	-	-	-	7.4	-	-	-	-	-	-	-	-	-	35.6	-	1.2	0.3	0.04	0.04	0.6	141
Salivary gland	1	0	-	-	-	-	-	-	-	-	-	-	12.4	-	-	-	-	-	-	-	0.6	0.1	0.06	0.06	0.6	142
Mouth	3	0	-	-	-	-	-	-	-	-	-	-	12.4	-	10.6	-	-	22.1	-	-	1.8	0.4	0.11	0.11	1.3	143-5
Oropharynx	2	0	-	-	-	-	-	-	-	-	-	10.5	-	-	-	-	-	-	35.6	-	1.2	0.3	0.05	0.05	0.8	146
Nasopharynx	13	0	-	-	-	-	-	-	-	7.6	16.8	21.0	-	12.0	31.8	11.5	31.9	22.1	-	-	8.0	1.8	0.45	0.66	5.7	147
Hypopharynx	3	0	-	-	-	-	-	-	-	-	-	-	-	-	-	11.5	31.9	-	-	-	1.8	0.4	0.00	0.22	1.0	148
Pharynx unspecified	0	0	-	-	-	-	-	-	-	-	-	-	-	-	-	-	-	-	-	-	0.0	0.0	0.00	0.00	0.0	149
Oesophagus	13	0	-	-	-	-	-	-	-	-	-	-	-	23.9	31.8	34.6	15.9	44.2	35.6	50.9	8.0	1.8	0.28	0.53	4.5	150
Stomach	34	0	-	-	-	-	-	7.2	-	7.6	-	-	24.7	12.0	74.1	80.7	143.4	66.3	71.2	50.9	20.9	4.8	0.63	1.75	12.3	151
Small intestine	1	0	-	-	-	-	-	-	-	-	-	-	-	-	-	11.5	-	-	-	-	0.6	0.1	0.00	0.06	0.3	152
Colon	71	0	-	-	-	-	-	7.2	14.8	-	16.8	-	37.1	35.9	63.5	103.7	223.1	309.2	356.0	356.1	43.7	9.9	0.88	2.51	22.5	153
Rectum	35	0	-	-	-	-	-	-	-	-	-	8.4	31.5	-	35.9	31.8	69.1	127.5	110.4	106.8	152.6	21.5	4.9	0.54	1.52	12.1	154
Liver	27	0	-	-	-	-	-	-	-	-	16.8	21.0	12.4	35.9	63.5	46.1	47.8	88.3	35.6	50.9	16.6	3.8	0.75	1.22	10.5	155
Gallbladder etc.	8	0	-	-	-	-	-	-	-	7.6	-	-	-	-	10.6	23.0	15.9	44.2	-	50.9	4.9	1.1	0.09	0.29	2.6	156
Pancreas	20	0	-	-	-	-	-	-	-	-	-	-	-	-	21.2	46.1	79.7	110.4	71.2	101.7	12.3	2.8	0.11	0.73	5.8	157
Nose, sinuses etc.	1	0	-	-	-	-	-	-	-	-	8.4	-	-	-	-	-	-	-	-	-	0.6	0.1	0.04	0.04	0.5	160
Larynx	6	0	-	-	-	-	-	-	-	-	-	-	-	12.0	10.6	23.0	-	22.1	35.6	-	3.7	0.8	0.11	0.23	2.0	161
Bronchus, lung	111	0	-	-	-	-	-	-	7.4	15.3	-	31.5	37.1	83.8	201.2	230.5	302.8	485.9	249.2	406.9	68.3	15.5	1.88	4.55	37.6	162
Other thoracic organs	2	0	-	-	-	-	7.5	-	-	-	-	-	12.0	-	-	-	-	-	-	-	1.2	0.3	0.10	0.10	1.1	163-4
Bone	1	0	-	-	-	-	-	-	-	-	8.4	-	-	-	-	-	-	-	-	-	0.6	0.1	0.04	0.04	0.5	170
Connective tissue	5	0	-	-	-	-	-	-	-	-	-	10.5	-	12.0	10.6	11.5	-	-	-	50.9	3.1	0.7	0.17	0.22	2.1	171
Mesothelioma	3	0	-	-	-	-	-	-	-	-	-	-	-	-	23.0	-	22.1	-	-	-	1.8	0.4	0.00	0.12	0.9	MES
Kaposi's sarcoma	5	0	-	-	-	-	-	-	7.4	-	25.1	-	-	-	15.9	-	-	-	-	-	3.1	0.7	0.16	0.24	2.3	KAP
Melanoma of skin	2	0	-	-	-	-	-	-	-	7.6	-	-	-	-	11.5	-	-	-	-	-	1.2	0.3	0.04	0.10	0.8	172
†Other skin	1	0	-	-	-	-	7.5	-	-	-	-	-	-	-	-	-	-	-	-	-	0.6		0.04	0.04	0.6	173
Breast	1	0	-	-	-	-	-	-	-	-	-	-	-	-	10.6	-	-	-	-	-	0.6	0.1	0.05	0.05	0.4	175
Prostate	213	0	-	-	-	-	-	-	-	-	-	-	-	59.8	158.9	668.4	749.0	1015.9	818.8	966.4	131.1	29.8	1.09	8.18	62.9	185
Testis	5	0	-	-	-	-	14.5	14.8	-	-	10.5	-	-	-	-	-	-	-	-	-	3.1	0.7	0.20	0.20	2.7	186
Penis	0	0	-	-	-	-	-	-	-	-	-	-	-	-	-	-	-	-	-	-	0.0	0.0	0.00	0.00	0.0	187.1-.4
Other male genital	0	0	-	-	-	-	-	-	-	-	-	-	-	-	-	-	-	-	-	-	0.0	0.0	0.00	0.00	0.0	187.5-.9
Bladder	29	0	-	-	-	-	-	-	-	-	-	-	12.4	35.9	31.8	57.6	111.6	110.4	35.6	203.5	17.9	4.1	0.40	1.25	9.6	188
Kidney etc.	15	0	-	-	-	-	-	-	-	-	-	-	24.7	23.9	21.2	34.6	47.8	-	35.6	101.7	9.2	2.1	0.35	0.76	5.7	189
Eye	1	0	-	-	-	-	-	-	-	-	8.4	-	-	-	-	-	-	-	-	-	0.6	0.1	0.04	0.04	0.5	190
Brain, nervous system	6	0	-	-	-	-	-	-	-	-	8.4	21.0	-	-	10.6	23.0	-	-	-	-	3.7	0.8	0.20	0.32	2.9	191-2
Thyroid	6	0	-	-	-	-	-	-	7.4	-	8.4	-	12.4	12.0	-	11.5	-	22.1	-	-	3.7	0.8	0.20	0.26	2.6	193
Other endocrine	0	0	-	-	-	-	-	-	-	-	-	-	-	-	-	-	-	-	-	-	0.0	0.0	0.00	0.00	0.0	194
Hodgkin's disease	1	0	-	-	-	-	-	-	-	-	-	-	-	12.0	-	-	-	-	-	-	0.6	0.1	0.06	0.06	0.5	201
Non-Hodgkin lymphoma	33	0	-	-	-	-	-	7.2	-	7.6	-	10.5	49.4	35.9	53.0	57.6	111.6	22.1	142.4	50.9	20.3	4.6	0.82	1.66	12.8	200,202
Multiple myeloma	6	0	-	-	-	-	-	-	-	-	-	-	-	12.0	-	11.5	63.7	-	-	-	3.7	0.8	0.06	0.44	2.1	203
Lymphoid leukaemia	3	0	-	-	-	-	-	-	-	-	-	-	-	-	-	11.5	-	22.1	-	50.9	1.8	0.4	0.00	0.06	0.8	204
Myeloid leukaemia	7	0	10.6	-	-	-	-	14.5	-	-	8.4	-	-	12.0	-	-	15.9	22.1	-	-	4.3	1.0	0.23	0.31	4.0	205
Monocytic leukaemia	2	0	-	-	-	-	-	-	-	-	-	-	-	-	-	-	-	44.2	-	-	1.2	0.3	0.00	0.00	0.4	206
Other leukaemia	0	0	-	-	-	-	-	-	-	-	-	-	-	-	-	-	-	-	-	-	0.0	0.0	0.00	0.00	0.0	207
Leukaemia unspecified	0	0	-	-	-	-	-	-	-	-	-	-	-	-	-	-	-	-	-	-	0.0	0.0	0.00	0.00	0.0	208
Other and unspecified	17	0	-	-	-	-	-	-	-	-	16.8	10.5	-	12.0	10.6	46.1	47.8	22.1	106.8	50.9	10.5	2.4	0.25	0.72	5.9	O&U
All sites	715	0	10.6	-	-	-	15.0	50.7	59.4	53.4	150.8	178.4	234.7	490.7	857.9	1659.4	2183.3	2628.1	2171.6	2695.8	440.2		10.51	29.72	242.8	ALL
All sites but 173	714	0	10.6	-	-	-	7.5	50.7	59.4	53.4	150.8	178.4	234.7	490.7	857.9	1659.4	2183.3	2628.1	2171.6	2695.8	439.6	100.0	10.47	29.68	242.2	ALLb

Rate from 1 case   10.638 11.047 11.233 10.228 7.522 7.242 7.421 7.633 8.379 10.494 12.355 11.969 10.591 11.523 15.936 22.085 35.600 50.865

†Important: see notes on population page

USA, HAWAII: CHINESE 1988-1992

ANNUAL INCIDENCE PER 100,000 BY AGE GROUP (YEARS) - FEMALE

SITE	ALL AGES	AGE UNK	0-	5-	10-	15-	20-	25-	30-	35-	40-	45-	50-	55-	60-	65-	70-	75-	80-	85+	CRUDE RATE	%	CR 64	CR 74	ASR (W)	ICD (9th)
Lip	0	0	-	-	-	-	-	-	-	-	-	-	-	-	-	-	-	-	-	-	0.0	0.0	0.00	0.00	0.0	140
Tongue	4	0	-	-	-	-	-	-	-	-	-	-	-	-	9.7	30.9	-	-	-	-	2.3	0.7	0.05	0.20	1.3	141
Salivary gland	3	0	-	-	-	-	-	-	-	-	-	-	11.6	10.8	9.7	-	-	-	-	-	1.7	0.5	0.16	0.16	1.4	142
Mouth	1	0	-	-	-	-	-	-	-	-	-	-	-	-	-	10.3	-	-	-	-	0.6	0.2	0.00	0.05	0.3	143-5
Oropharynx	0	0	-	-	-	-	-	-	-	-	-	-	-	-	-	-	-	-	-	-	0.0	0.0	0.00	0.00	0.0	146
Nasopharynx	9	0	-	-	-	-	-	7.2	-	-	14.9	-	-	10.8	19.4	20.6	13.2	-	-	-	5.2	1.6	0.26	0.43	3.6	147
Hypopharynx	1	0	-	-	-	-	-	-	-	-	-	-	11.6	-	-	-	-	-	-	-	0.6	0.2	0.06	0.06	0.6	148
Pharynx unspecified	0	0	-	-	-	-	-	-	-	-	-	-	-	-	-	-	-	-	-	-	0.0	0.0	0.00	0.00	0.0	149
Oesophagus	0	0	-	-	-	-	-	-	-	-	-	-	-	-	-	-	-	-	-	-	0.0	0.0	0.00	0.00	0.0	150
Stomach	18	0	-	-	-	-	-	-	-	-	7.4	-	-	21.6	29.0	30.9	39.5	37.1	29.8	91.2	10.4	3.2	0.29	0.64	5.2	151
Small intestine	4	0	-	-	-	-	-	-	-	-	-	-	-	-	-	10.3	-	18.5	29.8	30.4	2.3	0.7	0.00	0.05	0.8	152
Colon	68	0	-	-	-	-	-	7.2	-	6.7	-	9.6	23.1	32.4	77.4	113.3	105.4	259.6	149.2	425.5	39.1	12.2	0.78	1.88	18.1	153
Rectum	21	0	-	-	-	-	-	-	-	-	-	-	23.1	21.6	29.0	41.2	52.7	18.5	89.5	60.8	12.1	3.8	0.37	0.84	6.4	154
Liver	9	0	-	-	-	-	-	-	-	-	-	19.1	-	10.8	19.4	10.3	13.2	-	-	60.8	5.2	1.6	0.25	0.36	3.2	155
Gallbladder etc.	10	0	-	-	-	-	-	-	-	-	-	-	11.6	21.6	9.7	20.6	26.4	37.1	-	-	5.8	1.8	0.21	0.45	3.3	156
Pancreas	17	0	-	-	-	-	-	-	-	-	-	-	11.6	-	9.7	20.6	26.4	111.3	119.4	30.4	9.8	3.1	0.11	0.34	4.0	157
Nose, sinuses etc.	2	0	-	-	-	-	-	-	6.7	-	-	-	-	-	-	-	-	29.8	-	-	1.2	0.4	0.03	0.03	0.6	160
Larynx	0	0	-	-	-	-	-	-	-	-	-	-	-	-	-	-	-	-	-	-	0.0	0.0	0.00	0.00	0.0	161
Bronchus, lung	68	0	-	-	-	-	-	-	-	-	7.4	9.6	23.1	75.7	48.4	123.6	184.5	259.6	149.2	212.8	39.1	12.2	0.82	2.36	18.9	162
Other thoracic organs	0	0	-	-	-	-	-	-	-	-	-	-	-	-	-	-	-	-	-	-	0.0	0.0	0.00	0.00	0.0	163-4
Bone	0	0	-	-	-	-	-	-	-	-	-	-	-	-	-	-	-	-	-	-	0.0	0.0	0.00	0.00	0.0	170
Connective tissue	5	0	-	11.2	-	-	-	-	-	-	-	-	-	10.8	-	-	13.2	18.5	-	30.4	2.9	0.9	0.11	0.18	2.2	171
Mesothelioma	0	0	-	-	-	-	-	-	-	-	-	-	-	-	-	-	-	-	-	-	0.0	0.0	0.00	0.00	0.0	MES
Kaposi's sarcoma	0	0	-	-	-	-	-	-	-	-	-	-	-	-	-	-	-	-	-	-	0.0	0.0	0.00	0.00	0.0	KAP
Melanoma of skin	2	0	-	-	-	-	-	-	-	-	-	-	11.6	-	-	-	-	-	-	30.4	1.2	0.4	0.06	0.06	0.7	172
†Other skin	0	0	-	-	-	-	-	-	-	-	-	-	-	-	-	-	-	-	-	-	0.0	0.0	0.00	0.00	0.0	173
Breast	159	0	-	-	-	10.0	-	14.4	33.4	53.3	96.6	95.7	115.7	183.8	222.7	247.3	224.1	278.1	238.7	182.4	91.5	28.6	4.13	6.48	57.6	174
Uterus unspecified	1	0	-	-	-	-	-	-	-	-	-	-	-	-	10.3	-	-	-	-	-	0.6	0.2	0.00	0.05	0.3	179
Cervix uteri	10	0	-	-	-	-	-	-	-	20.0	14.9	19.1	23.1	-	-	-	-	-	29.8	-	5.8	1.8	0.39	0.39	4.5	180
Placenta	0	0	-	-	-	-	-	-	-	-	-	-	-	-	-	-	-	-	-	-	0.0	0.0	0.00	0.00	0.0	181
Corpus uteri	34	0	-	-	-	-	-	7.2	-	6.7	7.4	19.1	57.9	86.5	58.1	72.1	13.2	18.5	29.8	-	19.6	6.1	1.21	1.64	14.0	182
Ovary etc.	18	0	-	-	-	-	-	-	13.4	13.3	7.4	-	23.1	21.6	29.0	20.6	13.2	37.1	-	30.4	10.4	3.2	0.54	0.71	6.6	183
Other female genital	2	0	-	-	-	-	-	-	-	-	-	-	-	-	-	10.3	13.2	-	-	-	1.2	0.4	0.00	0.12	0.6	184
Bladder	9	0	-	-	-	-	-	-	6.7	-	-	-	11.6	10.8	-	-	39.5	37.1	29.8	-	5.2	1.6	0.15	0.34	2.7	188
Kidney etc.	5	0	-	-	-	-	-	-	-	-	-	-	-	-	19.4	-	26.4	-	-	30.4	2.9	0.9	0.10	0.23	1.5	189
Eye	0	0	-	-	-	-	-	-	-	-	-	-	-	-	-	-	-	-	-	-	0.0	0.0	0.00	0.00	0.0	190
Brain, nervous system	1	0	-	-	-	-	-	-	-	-	-	-	-	-	-	10.3	-	-	-	-	0.6	0.2	0.00	0.05	0.3	191-2
Thyroid	25	0	-	-	-	10.0	-	7.2	13.4	20.0	22.3	-	11.6	32.4	9.7	20.6	52.7	37.1	29.8	30.4	14.4	4.5	0.63	1.00	9.4	193
Other endocrine	1	0	-	-	-	-	-	-	-	-	-	-	-	10.8	-	-	-	-	-	-	0.6	0.2	0.05	0.05	0.4	194
Hodgkin's disease	1	0	-	-	-	-	-	-	-	-	-	-	-	-	-	-	-	29.8	-	-	0.6	0.2	0.00	0.00	0.1	201
Non-Hodgkin lymphoma	24	0	-	-	-	-	8.7	-	13.4	-	14.9	19.1	23.1	10.8	29.0	41.2	-	55.6	89.5	30.4	13.8	4.3	0.60	0.80	8.7	200,202
Multiple myeloma	2	0	-	-	-	-	-	-	-	-	-	-	-	-	-	-	-	37.1	-	-	1.2	0.4	0.00	0.00	0.4	203
Lymphoid leukaemia	1	0	-	-	-	-	-	-	-	-	-	-	-	-	-	-	-	18.5	-	-	0.6	0.2	0.00	0.00	0.2	204
Myeloid leukaemia	1	0	-	-	-	-	-	-	-	-	7.4	-	-	-	-	-	-	-	-	-	0.6	0.2	0.04	0.04	0.4	205
Monocytic leukaemia	2	0	-	-	-	-	-	-	-	6.7	-	-	-	-	-	10.3	-	-	-	-	1.2	0.4	0.03	0.08	0.7	206
Other leukaemia	0	0	-	-	-	-	-	-	-	-	-	-	-	-	-	-	-	-	-	-	0.0	0.0	0.00	0.00	0.0	207
Leukaemia unspecified	1	0	-	-	-	-	-	-	-	-	-	-	-	-	-	10.3	-	-	-	-	0.6	0.2	0.00	0.05	0.3	208
Other and unspecified	17	0	-	-	-	-	-	-	6.7	-	-	9.6	-	10.8	-	-	39.5	111.3	29.8	121.6	9.8	3.1	0.14	0.33	4.1	O&U
All sites	556	0	-	11.2	-	20.0	8.7	43.2	93.7	126.7	200.5	200.9	393.4	583.7	629.2	886.1	896.3	1390.7	1104.1	1398.2	319.9		11.56	20.47	183.5	ALL
All sites but 173	556	0	-	11.2	-	20.0	8.7	43.2	93.7	126.7	200.5	200.9	393.4	583.7	629.2	886.1	896.3	1390.7	1104.1	1398.2	319.9	100.0	11.56	20.47	183.5	ALLb

Rate from 1 case

11.460 11.184 10.670 10.008 8.720 7.208 6.690 6.668 7.427 9.566 11.571 10.810 9.681 10.304 13.180 18.543 29.842 30.395

†Important: see notes on population page

AGE-STANDARDIZED INCIDENCE RATES AND STANDARD ERRORS (per 100,000)

AGE-STANDARDIZED INCIDENCE
RATES AND STANDARD ERRORS (per 100,000)
Lip (ICD-9 140)

AFRICA	MALE		FEMALE	
*Algeria, Setif	2.3	0.56	0,1	0,10
*France, La Reunion	0,5	0,21	0,2	0,12
*Mali, Bamako	0,2	0,18	0,3	0,20
*Uganda, Kyadondo	0,4	0,44	-	-
*Zimbabwe, Harare: African	-	-	-	-
*Zimbabwe, Harare: European	1,0	1,00	-	-

AMERICA, CENTRAL AND SOUTH	MALE		FEMALE		
*Argentina, Concordia	1,8	0,80	0,3	0,27	
*Brazil, Belem	1.3	0.41	0,1	0,11	
*Brazil, Goiania	2.2	0.48	0,5	0,22	f
*Brazil, Porto Alegre	1.2	0.31	0,1	0,05	m
Colombia, Cali	0,3	0,13	0,1	0,06	m
*Costa Rica	1.3	0.17	0,5	0.10	
*Ecuador, Quito	0,2	0,11	-	-	
*Peru, Lima	0.3	0.09	0,2	0,06	
Peru, Trujillo	1,0	0,48	0,3	0,23	
US, Puerto Rico	0.6	0.09	0,2	0.05	
*Uruguay, Montevideo	0.9	0.20	0,1	0,06	

AMERICA, NORTH	MALE		FEMALE	
Canada	3.3	0.06	0.5	0.02
Canada, Alberta	4.7	0.27	0.9	0.11
Canada, British Columbia	1.7	0.13	0.3	0.05
Canada, Manitoba	6.2	0.42	0.9	0.15
Canada, New Brunswick	3.0	0.37	0.2	0,09
Canada, Newfoundland	12.7	0.91	0.8	0.24
Canada, Northwest Territories	1,0	0,96	-	-
Canada, Nova Scotia	3.5	0.35	0,2	0,09
Canada, Ontario	3.1	0.10	0.6	0.04
Canada, Prince Edward Island	7.6	1.35	0,2	0,17
Canada, Quebec	1.9	0.10	0.2	0.03
Canada, Saskatchewan	7.9	0.50	0.6	0.12
Canada, Yukon	2,0	1,26	1,6	1,62
US, Cent. Calif.: Non-Hisp. White	3.0	0.26	0.3	0.08
US, Cent. Calif.: Hispanic	1.4	0.38	0,1	0,10
US, Los Angeles: Non-Hisp. White	1.7	0.11	0.3	0.05
US, Los Angeles: Hispanic White	0.6	0.13	0,1	0,05
US, Los Angeles: Black	-	-	0,0	0,04
US, Los Angeles: Chinese	0,1	0,11	0,1	0,09
US, Los Angeles: Filipino	0,3	0,24	-	-
US, Los Angeles: Korean	0,2	0,25	-	-
US, Los Angeles: Japanese	-	-	-	-
US, San Francisco: Non-Hisp. White	1.8	0.16	0.3	0.06
US, San Francisco: Hispanic White	0,5	0,23	0,1	0,10
US, San Francisco: Black	0,2	0,15	-	-
US, San Francisco: Chinese	-	-	0,1	0,08
US, San Francisco: Filipino	-	-	0,5	0,32
US, San Francisco: Japanese	-	-	0,8	0,76
US, Connecticut: White	0.4	0.06	0,1	0.03
US, Connecticut: Black	-	-	-	-
US, Atlanta: White	1.2	0.19	0,1	0,05
US, Atlanta: Black	-	-	0,1	0,07
US, Iowa	3.6	0.20	0.4	0.06

	MALE		FEMALE	
US, Central Louisiana: White	2.6	0.63	0,1	0,12
US, Central Louisiana: Black	-	-	-	-
US, New Orleans: White	1.2	0.24	0,1	0,06
US, New Orleans: Black	0,3	0,22	-	-
US, Detroit: White	0.9	0.10	0.1	0.03
US, Detroit: Black	-	-	0,1	0,04
US, New Mexico: Non-Hisp. White	4.4	0.41	0.6	0.14
US, New Mexico: Hispanic White	1.7	0.38	0,2	0,10
US, New Mexico: American Indian	1,7	0,89	0,3	0,30
US, Utah	4.1	0.32	0.7	0.12
US, Seattle	1.9	0.14	0.3	0.05
US, SEER: White	1.9	0.06	0.3	0.02
US, SEER: Black	0,0	0,03	0,0	0,02

ASIA	MALE		FEMALE	
*China, Qidong	0,1	0,06	0,1	0,05
China, Shanghai	0.1	0.03	0.0	0.01
China, Tianjin	0.1	0.04	0,1	0,03
Hong Kong	0.1	0.02	0,0	0,01
*India, Bangalore	0.2	0.05	0.2	0.05
*India, Barshi, Paranda and Bhum	0,3	0,20	-	-
India, Bombay	0.4	0.05	0.3	0.05
*India, Karunagappally	0,6	0,44	1,0	0,57
India, Madras	0.4	0.08	0.5	0.09
*India, Trivandrum	1,1	0,45	-	-
Israel: All Jews	3.3	0.18	0.9	0.09
Jews born in Israel	4.8	0.70	1.6	0.39
Jews born in America or Europe	3.8	0.31	0.9	0.13
Jews born in Africa or Asia	1.5	0.25	0.5	0.12
Non-Jews	1.5	0.38	0.9	0.30
Japan, Hiroshima	0,0	0,03	0,0	0,03
Japan, Miyagi	0.2	0.05	0,1	0,03
Japan, Nagasaki	0,1	0,04	-	-
Japan, Osaka	0.0	0.01	0.0	0.01
*Japan, Saga	0,1	0,04	0,0	0,01
Japan, Yamagata	0,1	0,03	0,1	0,03
*Korea, Kangwha	-	-	0,2	0,18
*Kuwait: Non-Kuwaitis	0,7	0,48	0,1	0,06
*Kuwait: Kuwaitis	0,5	0,31	-	-
*Philippines, Manila	0,1	0,04	0,1	0,04
Singapore: Chinese	0,0	0,02	-	-
Singapore: Malay	-	-	-	-
Singapore: Indian	-	-	0,9	0,67
Thailand, Chiang Mai	0.2	0.08	0.4	0.12
*Thailand, Khon Kaen	0.3	0,14	2.7	0.37
*Viet Nam, Hanoi	0,1	0,07	0,2	0,09

* IMPORTANT-SEE NOTES ON POPULATION PAGE

AGE-STANDARDIZED INCIDENCE
RATES AND STANDARD ERRORS (per 100,000)
Lip (ICD-9 140) (contd)

EUROPE	MALE		FEMALE	
Austria, Tyrol	0,4	0,14	-	-
*Belarus	5.8	0.15	0.8	0.04
*Croatia	3.0	0.17	0.6	0.06
Czech Republic	1.6	0.07	0.3	0.03
Denmark	2.7	0.12	0.3	0.04
Estonia	2.3	0.24	0.3	0.06
Finland	3.5	0.14	0.6	0.05
France, Bas-Rhin	0.6	0.14	-	-
*France, Calvados	1.5	0.28	0,3	0,10
France, Doubs	0,2	0,12	-	-
France, Haut-Rhin	0.8	0.20	0,1	0,06
*France, Herault	1.2	0.21	0,1	0,05
France, Isere	0.8	0.16	0,2	0,07
*France, Somme	2.1	0.34	0,1	0,04
*France, Tarn	2.9	0.44	0.2	0.08
Germany, Eastern States	1.5	0.09	0.2	0.02
Germany, Saarland	1.0	0.16	0,2	0,06
Iceland	2.0	0.50	0,2	0,14
Ireland, Southern	3.1	0.44	0.4	0.14
Italy, Ferrara	1,3	0,45	0,1	0,15
Italy, Florence	0.6	0.12	0,1	0,04
Italy, Genoa	0.5	0.12	0,0	0,03
*Italy, Latina	2.2	0.43	0,4	0,20
Italy, Macerata	0,2	0,20	-	-
Italy, Modena	0,2	0,08	-	-
Italy, Parma	0.5	0.17	0,0	0,02
Italy, Ragusa	4.6	0.66	0,6	0,25
Italy, Romagna	0,0	0,05	0,0	0,05
Italy, Torino	1.2	0.19	0,1	0,05
Italy, Trieste	1.8	0.46	0,4	0,17
Italy, Varese	1.3	0.22	-	-
Italy, Veneto	1.4	0.18	0.2	0.06
*Latvia	2.8	0.20	0.3	0.05
Malta	2.3	0.77	-	- m
The Netherlands	1.7	0.07	0.2	0.02
The Netherlands, Eindhoven	2.3	0.29	0.4	0.12
The Netherlands, Maastricht	0.9	0.18	0,2	0,07
Norway	2.3	0.12	0.5	0.06
*Poland, Cracow	1.6	0.29	0,2	0,09
*Poland, Kielce	6.3	0.44	0.7	0.12
*Poland, Lower Silesia	3.9	0.24	0.4	0.07
Poland, Warsaw City	1.2	0.17	0.2	0.05
Slovakia	3.9	0.17	0.7	0.06
Slovenia	2.0	0.19	0.3	0.06
*Spain, Albacete	2.5	0.76	0,4	0,19
Spain, Asturias	2.4	0.27	0.2	0.06
Spain, Basque Country	4.8	0.30	0.3	0.06
Spain, Granada	12.0	0.71	0.7	0.15
Spain, Mallorca	5.9	0.56	0.5	0.14
Spain, Murcia	11.1	0.61	0.5	0.12
Spain, Navarra	6.5	0.60	0,2	0,09
Spain, Tarragona	6.6	0.61	0.5	0.14
Spain, Zaragoza	6.3	0.45	0,2	0,06 f

	MALE		FEMALE	
Sweden	1.6	0.07	0.4	0.03
*Switzerland, Basel	0.7	0.21	0,0	0,01
Switzerland, Geneva	1.6	0.36	0,3	0,14
Switzerland, Graubunden	3.0	0.78	0.8	0,40
Switzerland, Neuchatel	1,4	0,49	0.4	0,27
Switzerland, St Gall-Appenzell	1.5	0.30	0,3	0,14
Switzerland, Valais	0,4	0,21	0,1	0,07
Switzerland, Vaud	0.8	0.19	0,0	0,02
Switzerland, Zurich	1.4	0.19	0.4	0.08
*UK, England and Wales	0.5	0.02	0.1	0.01
*UK, East Anglia	1.5	0.14	0.2	0.05
*UK, Mersey	0,1	0,03	0,0	0,01
*UK, North Western	0.4	0.05	0.1	0.02
UK, Oxford	0.7	0.09	0.2	0.04
*UK, South Thames	0.2	0.03	0.1	0.01
UK, South Western	0.5	0.06	0.1	0.03
UK, Wessex	0.6	0.07	0.1	0.03
*UK, West Midlands	0.2	0.03	0.0	0.01
UK, Yorkshire	0.5	0.06	0.1	0.03
UK, Scotland	1.2	0.08	0.3	0.03
UK, Scotland, West	1.3	0.12	0.3	0.05
*Yugoslavia, Vojvodina	3.9	0.24	0.8	0.10

OCEANIA	MALE		FEMALE	
Australian Capital Territory	8.9	1.26	1.4	0.42
Australia, New South Wales	5.1	0.17	1.4	0.08
South Australia	13.5	0.56	3.2	0.25
Australia, Tasmania	6.3	0.68	1.2	0.26
Australia, Victoria	5.0	0.20	1.4	0.10
Western Australia	8.7	0.44	2.1	0.21
*French Polynesia	-	-	-	-
New Zealand: Non-Maori	3.4	0.19	0.9	0.10
New Zealand: Maori	0,7	0,48	-	-
US, Hawaii: White	2.0	0.48	0,6	0,24
US, Hawaii: Japanese	0,2	0,16	-	-
US, Hawaii: Hawaiian	0,2	0,15	-	-
US, Hawaii: Filipino	-	-	-	-
US, Hawaii: Chinese	-	-	-	-

* IMPORTANT-SEE NOTES ON POPULATION PAGE

AGE-STANDARDIZED INCIDENCE
RATES AND STANDARD ERRORS (per 100,000)
Tongue (ICD-9 141)

	MALE		FEMALE		
AFRICA					
*Algeria, Setif	0,6	0,30	0,1	0,07	
*France, La Reunion	5.4	0.69	0,4	0,18	
*Mali, Bamako	0,5	0,28	0,3	0,19	
*Uganda, Kyadondo	0,2	0,13	0,2	0,20	
*Zimbabwe, Harare: African	1,1	0,55	-	-	
*Zimbabwe, Harare: European	2,9	1,46	5,7	2,54	f
AMERICA, CENTRAL AND SOUTH					
*Argentina, Concordia	2,7	0,90	0,3	0,29	
*Brazil, Belem	4.0	0.73	1.7	0.38	
*Brazil, Goiania	2.9	0.55	0.2	0,10	
*Brazil, Porto Alegre	4.6	0.57	0.7	0.18	
Colombia, Cali	1.2	0.24	1.0	0.19	
*Costa Rica	1.1	0.16	0.6	0.11	
*Ecuador, Quito	0,4	0,17	0,2	0,11	m
*Peru, Lima	0.5	0.11	0.5	0.11	
Peru, Trujillo	0,7	0,43	0,1	0,13	
US, Puerto Rico	4.1	0.24	0.8	0.10	
*Uruguay, Montevideo	2.9	0.35	0.5	0.12	
AMERICA, NORTH					
Canada	2.2	0.05	0.8	0.03	
Canada, Alberta	1.5	0.15	0.7	0.10	
Canada, British Columbia	2.2	0.15	1.0	0.09	
Canada, Manitoba	2.0	0.25	1.0	0.18	
Canada, New Brunswick	2.1	0.32	0.4	0.13	
Canada, Newfoundland	1.4	0.31	0.6	0.18	
Canada, Northwest Territories	1,1	0,83	1,1	0,79	
Canada, Nova Scotia	2.2	0.30	0.6	0.13	
Canada, Ontario	2.4	0.09	0.8	0.05	
Canada, Prince Edward Island	3.2	0.96	0.8	0.46	
Canada, Quebec	2.3	0.11	0.6	0.05	
Canada, Saskatchewan	1.4	0.23	0.5	0.13	
Canada, Yukon	-	-	3,1	2,19	
US, Cent. Calif.: Non-Hisp. White	2.5	0.25	1.3	0.17	
US, Cent. Calif.: Hispanic	1.7	0.42	0,7	0,26	
US, Los Angeles: Non-Hisp. White	3.0	0.16	1.3	0.10	
US, Los Angeles: Hispanic White	1.4	0.19	0.6	0.11	
US, Los Angeles: Black	3.9	0.42	0.7	0.15	
US, Los Angeles: Chinese	0,7	0,33	0,6	0,30	
US, Los Angeles: Filipino	0,4	0,31	0,9	0,37	
US, Los Angeles: Korean	1,1	0,65	0,1	0,15	
US, Los Angeles: Japanese	1,2	0,49	1,2	0,48	
US, San Francisco: Non-Hisp. White	3.1	0.21	1.7	0.15	
US, San Francisco: Hispanic White	2.1	0.49	0.6	0.25	
US, San Francisco: Black	4.4	0.69	0.7	0.25	
US, San Francisco: Chinese	0.9	0.29	0.7	0.27	
US, San Francisco: Filipino	1,4	0,62	0,7	0,45	
US, San Francisco: Japanese	0,6	0,62	1,7	0,85	
US, Connecticut: White	2.8	0.18	1.1	0.10	
US, Connecticut: Black	6.0	1.08	1.6	0.49	
US, Atlanta: White	1.7	0.22	0.9	0.14	
US, Atlanta: Black	4.2	0.67	0.9	0.27	
US, Iowa	1.7	0.14	0.9	0.10	

	MALE		FEMALE		
US, Central Louisiana: White	2.8	0.67	1,0	0,36	
US, Central Louisiana: Black	4,3	1,81	-	-	
US, New Orleans: White	2.5	0.37	1.0	0.20	
US, New Orleans: Black	2.8	0.64	0,7	0,28	
US, Detroit: White	3.2	0.19	1.1	0.11	
US, Detroit: Black	4.9	0.50	1.2	0.22	
US, New Mexico: Non-Hisp. White	2.4	0.33	0.9	0.18	
US, New Mexico: Hispanic White	1.9	0.41	0,1	0,10	
US, New Mexico: American Indian	0,5	0,51	0,5	0,47	
US, Utah	1.7	0.22	1.0	0.16	
US, Seattle	2.6	0.17	1.2	0.11	
US, SEER: White	2.5	0.07	1.1	0.04	
US, SEER: Black	4.5	0.31	1.1	0.13	
ASIA					
*China, Qidong	0,1	0,06	0,2	0,06	
China, Shanghai	0.7	0.06	0.5	0.05	
China, Tianjin	0.5	0.07	0.5	0.07	
Hong Kong	2.1	0.12	1.2	0.09	
*India, Bangalore	3.5	0.24	1.2	0.14	
*India, Barshi, Paranda and Bhum	2.3	0.52	0,3	0,19	
India, Bombay	6.5	0.23	2.3	0.14	
*India, Karunagappally	5.4	1.29	3.7	0.99	
India, Madras	5.8	0.31	1.9	0.18	
*India, Trivandrum	4.4	0.82	1.8	0.48	
Israel: All Jews	0.8	0.09	0.6	0.07	
Jews born in Israel	1.1	0.38	0,5	0,21	
Jews born in America or Europe	0.9	0.16	0.5	0.09	
Jews born in Africa or Asia	0.8	0.15	0.5	0.12	
Non-Jews	0,2	0,16	0,4	0,20	
Japan, Hiroshima	2.0	0.26	0.8	0.15	
Japan, Miyagi	1.6	0.15	0.7	0.09	
Japan, Nagasaki	1.5	0.17	0.7	0.11	
Japan, Osaka	1.6	0.08	0.7	0.05	
*Japan, Saga	1.2	0.20	0.6	0.15	
Japan, Yamagata	0.4	0.09	0.4	0.08	
*Korea, Kangwha	0,7	0,49	0,3	0,26	
*Kuwait: Non-Kuwaitis	0.7	0.47	0,5	0,35	
*Kuwait: Kuwaitis	0,2	0,21	0,3	0,21	
*Philippines, Manila	2.6	0.25	2.1	0.20	
Singapore: Chinese	1.3	0.18	0.7	0.11	
Singapore: Malay	0,4	0,21	0,2	0,17	
Singapore: Indian	2.8	0.76	0,6	0,41	
Thailand, Chiang Mai	2.0	0.26	1.2	0.20	
*Thailand, Khon Kaen	1.0	0.23	0.8	0.18	
*Viet Nam, Hanoi	0.8	0.21	1.0	0.21	m

* IMPORTANT-SEE NOTES ON POPULATION PAGE

EUROPE	MALE		FEMALE	
Austria, Tyrol	1.6	0.31	0,2	0,10
*Belarus	2.6	0.10	0.2	0.03
*Croatia	3.6	0.18	0.4	0.06
Czech Republic	2.1	0.08	0.4	0.03
Denmark	1.2	0.08	0.5	0.05
Estonia	2.5	0.24	0.4	0.07
Finland	1.0	0.07	0.6	0.05
France, Bas-Rhin	8.0	0.55	1.0	0.18
*France, Calvados	7.8	0.69	0.8	0.21
France, Doubs	5.0	0.60	0.8	0.22
France, Haut-Rhin	7.9	0.65	0.8	0.19
*France, Herault	4.2	0.42	0.9	0.19
France, Isere	4.1	0.38	0.7	0.14
*France, Somme	6.4	0.65	0.5	0.17
*France, Tarn	3.6	0.58	0,5	0,20
Germany, Eastern States	1.6	0.09	0.3	0.04
Germany, Saarland	4.1	0.34	0.5	0.11
Iceland	1,1	0,41	0,5	0,24
Ireland, Southern	1.4	0.31	0.7	0.23
Italy, Ferrara	1,4	0,45	0,2	0,12
Italy, Florence	1.7	0.22	0.6	0.12
Italy, Genoa	2.5	0.30	0.7	0.14
*Italy, Latina	1.4	0.35	0,2	0,09
Italy, Macerata	1,5	0,61	0,4	0,23
Italy, Modena	1.8	0.29	0.3	0.11
Italy, Parma	2.0	0.38	0.5	0.18
Italy, Ragusa	1.1	0.34	0,4	0,21
Italy, Romagna	1.5	0.28	0.3	0.12
Italy, Torino	2.1	0.27	0.9	0.15
Italy, Trieste	2.5	0.57	1.2	0.39
Italy, Varese	3.5	0.36	0.3	0.09
Italy, Veneto	3.8	0.31	0.8	0.14
*Latvia	2.1	0.17	0.2	0.05
Malta	0,8	0,41	1,2	0,51
The Netherlands	1.4	0.06	0.8	0.04
The Netherlands, Eindhoven	1.0	0.19	0.6	0.14
The Netherlands, Maastricht	1.6	0.24	0.6	0.15
Norway	1.3	0.10	0.6	0.07
*Poland, Cracow	1.4	0.26	0,1	0,06
*Poland, Kielce	0.8	0.17	0,2	0,08
*Poland, Lower Silesia	1.7	0.15	0.4	0.06
Poland, Warsaw City	1.6	0.20	0.5	0.10
Slovakia	5.1	0.20	0.3	0.04
Slovenia	3.5	0.25	0.3	0.06
*Spain, Albacete	2,1	0,74	0,3	0,21
Spain, Asturias	5.2	0.42	0.9	0.17
Spain, Basque Country	4.7	0.30	0.4	0.08
Spain, Granada	2.9	0.36	0.6	0.15
Spain, Mallorca	2.8	0.41	0.5	0.17
Spain, Murcia	3.8	0.36	0.8	0.15
Spain, Navarra	2.3	0.37	0.7	0.19
Spain, Tarragona	3.1	0.42	0.6	0.17
Spain, Zaragoza	2.8	0.32	0.3	0.10

	MALE		FEMALE	
Sweden	1.0	0.06	0.6	0.04
*Switzerland, Basel	3.0	0.45	0.6	0.19
Switzerland, Geneva	4.1	0.58	1.4	0.37
Switzerland, Graubunden	1.0	0.50	0,9	0,48
Switzerland, Neuchatel	3.6	0.82	0,9	0,40
Switzerland, St Gall-Appenzell	1.7	0.33	0.8	0.22
Switzerland, Valais	3.0	0.71	0,8	0,33
Switzerland, Vaud	4.8	0.52	1.4	0.26
Switzerland, Zurich	2.1	0.24	0.7	0.13
*UK, England and Wales	1.2	0.03	0.5	0.02
*UK, East Anglia	0.8	0.11	0.5	0.08
*UK, Mersey	1.4	0.13	0.4	0.07
*UK, North Western	1.5	0.11	0.5	0.06
UK, Oxford	1.2	0.12	0.5	0.07
*UK, South Thames	1.0	0.07	0.5	0.05
UK, South Western	0.9	0.09	0.5	0.06
UK, Wessex	1.0	0.10	0.7	0.08
*UK, West Midlands	1.3	0.09	0.5	0.05
UK, Yorkshire	1.3	0.11	0.6	0.06
UK, Scotland	1.9	0.11	0.7	0.06
UK, Scotland, West	2.0	0.16	0.7	0.08
*Yugoslavia, Vojvodina	3.0	0.22	0.3	0.07

OCEANIA	MALE		FEMALE	
Australian Capital Territory	2.1	0.61	0,9	0,40
Australia, New South Wales	2.2	0.11	1.0	0.07
South Australia	1.8	0.20	0.6	0.11
Australia, Tasmania	2.4	0.43	0.8	0.25
Australia, Victoria	2.1	0.13	0.9	0.08
Western Australia	2.8	0.26	0.8	0.13
*French Polynesia	3.3	1.00	1,1	0,65
New Zealand: Non-Maori	1.5	0.13	0.7	0.08
New Zealand: Maori	2.4	0.76	1,0	0,46
US, Hawaii: White	2.9	0.59	0.9	0.30
US, Hawaii: Japanese	1.7	0.39	0.8	0.23
US, Hawaii: Hawaiian	1,9	0,71	1,2	0,49
US, Hawaii: Filipino	0,7	0,35	1,9	0,63
US, Hawaii: Chinese	0,6	0,48	1,3	0,66

* IMPORTANT-SEE NOTES ON POPULATION PAGE

AGE-STANDARDIZED INCIDENCE
RATES AND STANDARD ERRORS (per 100,000)
Salivary gland (ICD-9 142)

	MALE		FEMALE	
AFRICA				
*Algeria, Setif	0,2	0,16	-	-
*France, La Reunion	0,3	0,16	0,2	0,12
*Mali, Bamako	-	-	0,4	0,23
*Uganda, Kyadondo	0,3	0,22	0,8	0,39
*Zimbabwe, Harare: African	0,9	0,51	0,4	0,44
*Zimbabwe, Harare: European	-	-	-	-
AMERICA, CENTRAL AND SOUTH				
*Argentina, Concordia	1,0	0,60	0,8	0,48
*Brazil, Belem	0,9	0,32	0,6	0,24 f
*Brazil, Goiania	1.0	0.33	0,6	0,22
*Brazil, Porto Alegre	0,6	0,22	0.6	0.16
Colombia, Cali	0.6	0.19	0.5	0.14 mf
*Costa Rica	0.4	0.09	0.5	0.11
*Ecuador, Quito	0,5	0,17	0,3	0,12
*Peru, Lima	0.6	0.13	0.5	0.11
Peru, Trujillo	-	-	0,5	0,31
US, Puerto Rico	0.4	0.08	0.4	0.07
*Uruguay, Montevideo	1.0	0.21	0.4	0.11
AMERICA, NORTH				
Canada	0.8	0.03	0.5	0.03
Canada, Alberta	0.6	0.10	0.5	0.08
Canada, British Columbia	0.7	0.08	0.5	0.07
Canada, Manitoba	0.7	0.15	0.5	0.13
Canada, New Brunswick	0.6	0.17	0.3	0,12
Canada, Newfoundland	0.7	0.22	0.4	0,18
Canada, Northwest Territories	4.2	1.48	2,0	1,28
Canada, Nova Scotia	0.8	0.17	0.4	0.11
Canada, Ontario	0.8	0.05	0.6	0.04
Canada, Prince Edward Island	0,9	0,54	0,3	0,31
Canada, Quebec	0.9	0.07	0.5	0.05
Canada, Saskatchewan	0.6	0.14	0.6	0.15
Canada, Yukon	0,8	0,82	-	-
US, Cent. Calif.: Non-Hisp. White	1.0	0.16	0.5	0.09
US, Cent. Calif.: Hispanic	0,4	0,16	0.7	0.23
US, Los Angeles: Non-Hisp. White	1.0	0.09	0.7	0.08
US, Los Angeles: Hispanic White	0.4	0.09	0.4	0.09
US, Los Angeles: Black	0.9	0.20	0.4	0.12
US, Los Angeles: Chinese	0,8	0,36	0,4	0,25
US, Los Angeles: Filipino	0,4	0,26	1,0	0,41
US, Los Angeles: Korean	-	-	-	-
US, Los Angeles: Japanese	0,4	0,28	-	-
US, San Francisco: Non-Hisp. White	1.2	0.13	0.6	0.09
US, San Francisco: Hispanic White	1,0	0,34	0,6	0,21
US, San Francisco: Black	1.1	0.32	0,5	0,22
US, San Francisco: Chinese	0,8	0,34	0,3	0,18
US, San Francisco: Filipino	0,9	0,44	1,5	0,55
US, San Francisco: Japanese	-	-	1,4	0,81
US, Connecticut: White	1.1	0.10	0.8	0.10
US, Connecticut: Black	0,6	0,35	1,0	0,37
US, Atlanta: White	0.9	0.15	0.4	0.10
US, Atlanta: Black	1.1	0.37	0.9	0.26
US, Iowa	0.8	0.10	0.6	0.08
US, Central Louisiana: White	0,6	0,27	0,2	0,16
US, Central Louisiana: Black	0,4	0,40	0,7	0,69
US, New Orleans: White	1.3	0.26	0.7	0.18
US, New Orleans: Black	1.2	0.39	0,7	0,26
US, Detroit: White	0.9	0.10	0.8	0.09
US, Detroit: Black	0.7	0.18	0.4	0.12
US, New Mexico: Non-Hisp. White	1.0	0.19	0.5	0.13
US, New Mexico: Hispanic White	0,2	0,11	0,4	0,16
US, New Mexico: American Indian	-	-	0,3	0,25
US, Utah	1.0	0.16	0.5	0.11
US, Seattle	0.9	0.10	0.7	0.08
US, SEER: White	1.0	0.04	0.7	0.03
US, SEER: Black	0.9	0.13	0.7	0.10
ASIA				
*China, Qidong	0.4	0.11	0,1	0,04
China, Shanghai	0.5	0.05	0.4	0.04
China, Tianjin	0.4	0.06	0.3	0.06
Hong Kong	0.7	0.07	0.6	0.07
*India, Bangalore	0.6	0.10	0.4	0.08
*India, Barshi, Paranda and Bhum	0.5	0,23	0,1	0,06
India, Bombay	0.6	0.07	0.3	0.05
*India, Karunagappally	0,6	0,43	-	-
India, Madras	0.5	0.10	0.4	0.08
*India, Trivandrum	-	-	0,7	0,29
Israel: All Jews	0.7	0.09	0.5	0.07
Jews born in Israel	0.3	0.11	0.9	0.27
Jews born in America or Europe	0.9	0.15	0.3	0.08
Jews born in Africa or Asia	0.6	0.14	0.5	0.17
Non-Jews	0,2	0,12	0,2	0,09
Japan, Hiroshima	0.8	0.16	0,2	0,09
Japan, Miyagi	0.5	0.08	0.3	0.07
Japan, Nagasaki	0.4	0.09	0.4	0.09
Japan, Osaka	0.4	0.04	0.2	0.03
*Japan, Saga	0.5	0.13	0,3	0,10
Japan, Yamagata	0.5	0.11	0.2	0.05
*Korea, Kangwha	1,6	0,71	-	-
*Kuwait: Non-Kuwaitis	0,7	0,48	0,2	0,09
*Kuwait: Kuwaitis	0,4	0,25	0,8	0,38
*Philippines, Manila	1.2	0.16	1.0	0.14
Singapore: Chinese	0.6	0.11	0.6	0.11
Singapore: Malay	0,6	0,28	0,2	0,17
Singapore: Indian	0.3	0.22	1,3	0,88
Thailand, Chiang Mai	0.4	0.11	0.5	0.13
*Thailand, Khon Kaen	0,3	0,12	0,3	0,10
*Viet Nam, Hanoi	0.7	0.18	0.5	0.14

* IMPORTANT-SEE NOTES ON POPULATION PAGE

EUROPE	MALE		FEMALE	
Austria, Tyrol	0.5	0.16	0,4	0,14
*Belarus	0.8	0.06	0.3	0.03
*Croatia	1.4	0.11	0.5	0.06
Czech Republic	0.9	0.05	0.5	0.04
Denmark	0.6	0.06	0.4	0.05
Estonia	0.5	0.11	0.5	0.09
Finland	0.6	0.06	0.5	0.05
France, Bas-Rhin	0.9	0.18	0.6	0.13
*France, Calvados	0,4	0,16	0,3	0,13
France, Doubs	0,3	0,15	0,4	0,16
France, Haut-Rhin	0.5	0.16	0.4	0.13
*France, Herault	0.4	0.12	0.4	0.12
France, Isere	0.4	0.11	0.4	0.12
*France, Somme	0.7	0.20	0,2	0,12
*France, Tarn	0,7	0,29	0,1	0,08
Germany, Eastern States	0.5	0.05	0.3	0.03
Germany, Saarland	0.8	0.16	0.3	0.07
Iceland	0,8	0,34	0,4	0,25
Ireland, Southern	1.2	0.29	0,2	0,12
Italy, Ferrara	0,6	0,32	0,5	0,35
Italy, Florence	0.7	0.15	0.4	0.12
Italy, Genoa	1.0	0.19	0.3	0.09
*Italy, Latina	1.1	0.31	0,5	0,20
Italy, Macerata	0,4	0,33	-	-
Italy, Modena	0.6	0.15	0,2	0,09
Italy, Parma	0,2	0,12	0,2	0,12
Italy, Ragusa	0,6	0,24	0,5	0,25
Italy, Romagna	1.1	0.24	0.7	0.21
Italy, Torino	0.5	0.13	0.3	0.09
Italy, Trieste	1.6	0.52	0.7	0.26
Italy, Varese	0.6	0.16	0.4	0.10
Italy, Veneto	0.8	0.14	0.3	0.08
*Latvia	0.6	0.09	0.3	0.05
Malta	0,2	0,22	1,0	0,49
The Netherlands	0.6	0.04	0.4	0.03
The Netherlands, Eindhoven	0.4	0.12	0,2	0,09
The Netherlands, Maastricht	0.4	0.13	0.4	0.12
Norway	0.6	0.07	0.4	0.05
*Poland, Cracow	0.8	0.19	0.4	0.13
*Poland, Kielce	0.3	0.10	0,2	0,08
*Poland, Lower Silesia	0.7	0.10	0.5	0.07
Poland, Warsaw City	0.7	0.13	0.5	0.10
Slovakia	0.7	0.07	0.3	0.04
Slovenia	0.5	0.09	0.2	0.06
*Spain, Albacete	0,6	0,43	0,4	0,23
Spain, Asturias	0.7	0.15	0.6	0.17
Spain, Basque Country	0.5	0.10	0.2	0.06
Spain, Granada	0.5	0.14	0.4	0.14
Spain, Mallorca	0.5	0.16	0,2	0,10
Spain, Murcia	0.9	0.17	0.4	0.11
Spain, Navarra	0.6	0.17	0,3	0,14
Spain, Tarragona	0.8	0.21	0,2	0,09
Spain, Zaragoza	0.8	0.17	0,2	0,07

	MALE		FEMALE	
Sweden	0.6	0.04	0.6	0.04
*Switzerland, Basel	0.6	0.19	0,2	0,11
Switzerland, Geneva	0.9	0.29	0,3	0,14
Switzerland, Graubunden	0,4	0,26	0,8	0,48
Switzerland, Neuchatel	0,4	0,28	0,1	0,09
Switzerland, St Gall-Appenzell	0,3	0,15	0,5	0,19
Switzerland, Valais	0,1	0,14	0,4	0,25
Switzerland, Vaud	0.9	0.21	0,3	0,12
Switzerland, Zurich	0.6	0.13	0.3	0.08
*UK, England and Wales	0.5	0.02	0.4	0.02
*UK, East Anglia	0.4	0.08	0.3	0.07
*UK, Mersey	0.3	0.06	0.3	0.05
*UK, North Western	0.5	0.06	0.3	0.04
UK, Oxford	0.6	0.08	0.4	0.07
*UK, South Thames	0.5	0.05	0.4	0.04
UK, South Western	0.5	0.07	0.4	0.06
UK, Wessex	0.6	0.07	0.5	0.07
*UK, West Midlands	0.4	0.05	0.3	0.04
UK, Yorkshire	0.6	0.07	0.4	0.06
UK, Scotland	0.7	0.06	0.5	0.05
UK, Scotland, West	0.5	0.08	0.4	0.06
*Yugoslavia, Vojvodina	0.6	0.10	0.4	0.07

OCEANIA

	MALE		FEMALE	
Australian Capital Territory	1,1	0,42	0,4	0,22
Australia, New South Wales	1.1	0.08	0.5	0.05
South Australia	0.7	0.13	0.6	0.12
Australia, Tasmania	0,3	0,16	0,5	0,19
Australia, Victoria	1.1	0.09	0.5	0.06
Western Australia	1.0	0.15	0.7	0.12
*French Polynesia	0,2	0,15	0,3	0,26
New Zealand: Non-Maori	1.2	0.11	0.6	0.08
New Zealand: Maori	0,7	0,42	1,3	0,49
US, Hawaii: White	0,6	0,24	0,6	0,32
US, Hawaii: Japanese	0,8	0,27	0,5	0,20
US, Hawaii: Hawaiian	1,0	0,52	-	-
US, Hawaii: Filipino	0,5	0,33	1,0	0,47
US, Hawaii: Chinese	0,6	0,62	1,4	0,82

* IMPORTANT-SEE NOTES ON POPULATION PAGE

AGE-STANDARDIZED INCIDENCE
RATES AND STANDARD ERRORS (per 100,000)
Mouth (ICD-9 143-5)

	MALE		FEMALE	
AFRICA				
*Algeria, Setif	0,5	0,25	0,2	0,13
*France, La Reunion	6.2	0.75	0,6	0,22
*Mali, Bamako	0,3	0,19	0,3	0,18
*Uganda, Kyadondo	1,0	0,56	1,7	0,75 f
*Zimbabwe, Harare: African	0,5	0,28	0,3	0,21 m
*Zimbabwe, Harare: European	2,4	1,76	0,9	0,87
AMERICA, CENTRAL AND SOUTH				
*Argentina, Concordia	2,4	0,92	0,6	0,43
*Brazil, Belem	5.5	0.84	2.0	0.40
*Brazil, Goiania	3.4	0.59	1.4	0.35
*Brazil, Porto Alegre	3.7	0.51	0.6	0.17
Colombia, Cali	2.3	0.34	1.4	0.24 m
*Costa Rica	0.8	0.13	0.6	0.11
*Ecuador, Quito	0.7	0.21	0,2	0,10
*Peru, Lima	0.5	0.11	0.6	0.12
Peru, Trujillo	1,3	0,57	0,4	0,26
US, Puerto Rico	4.2	0.24	1.4	0.12
*Uruguay, Montevideo	2.7	0.33	0.9	0.15
AMERICA, NORTH				
Canada	2.7	0.06	1.2	0.04
Canada, Alberta	2.0	0.18	1.2	0.14
Canada, British Columbia	3.0	0.17	1.4	0.11
Canada, Manitoba	2.5	0.29	1.2	0.18
Canada, New Brunswick	2.4	0.35	1.0	0.22
Canada, Newfoundland	2.0	0.38	0.6	0.19
Canada, Northwest Territories	0,8	0,79	-	-
Canada, Nova Scotia	3.3	0.36	1.1	0.20
Canada, Ontario	2.7	0.10	1.4	0.06
Canada, Prince Edward Island	2.9	0.88	2,3	0,83
Canada, Quebec	2.8	0.12	0.8	0.06
Canada, Saskatchewan	1.4	0.23	1.1	0.19
Canada, Yukon	9,0	3,09	1,6	1,62
US, Cent. Calif.: Non-Hisp. White	2.9	0.27	1.5	0.17
US, Cent. Calif.: Hispanic	1.2	0.35	0,6	0,23
US, Los Angeles: Non-Hisp. White	3.0	0.16	1.9	0.12
US, Los Angeles: Hispanic White	1.4	0.19	0.5	0.09
US, Los Angeles: Black	4.4	0.46	1.5	0.23
US, Los Angeles: Chinese	0,7	0,39	0,1	0,09
US, Los Angeles: Filipino	0,8	0,44	0,4	0,23
US, Los Angeles: Korean	0,4	0,42	0,2	0,17
US, Los Angeles: Japanese	0,8	0,39	1,3	0,53
US, San Francisco: Non-Hisp. White	3.2	0.21	2.1	0.16
US, San Francisco: Hispanic White	1.7	0.44	1.0	0.30
US, San Francisco: Black	4.4	0.69	1.8	0.41
US, San Francisco: Chinese	1.4	0.40	0,6	0,30
US, San Francisco: Filipino	1,0	0,56	1,7	0,57
US, San Francisco: Japanese	2,3	1,65	1,0	0,78
US, Connecticut: White	3.4	0.19	1.5	0.12
US, Connecticut: Black	6.8	1.16	1.7	0.51
US, Atlanta: White	3.5	0.31	1.9	0.21
US, Atlanta: Black	4.9	0.74	2.0	0.39
US, Iowa	2.9	0.19	1.3	0.12

	MALE		FEMALE	
US, Central Louisiana: White	1,0	0,39	0.9	0.34
US, Central Louisiana: Black	1,8	1,08	1,5	0,93
US, New Orleans: White	3.7	0.46	1.6	0.26
US, New Orleans: Black	5.1	0.86	1.0	0.30
US, Detroit: White	3.6	0.21	1.7	0.13
US, Detroit: Black	6.2	0.56	2.2	0.29
US, New Mexico: Non-Hisp. White	2.3	0.30	1.4	0.24
US, New Mexico: Hispanic White	2.0	0.41	0.3	0,15
US, New Mexico: American Indian	0,9	0,68	0,4	0,39
US, Utah	1.8	0.22	0.9	0.14
US, Seattle	2.7	0.17	1.9	0.14
US, SEER: White	3.0	0.07	1.6	0.05
US, SEER: Black	5.4	0.33	1.9	0.18
ASIA				
*China, Qidong	0,3	0,09	0,2	0,09
China, Shanghai	1.0	0.07	0.8	0.06
China, Tianjin	0.8	0.09	0.4	0.07
Hong Kong	1.9	0.11	0.8	0.07
*India, Bangalore	2.8	0.21	8.9	0.39
*India, Barshi, Paranda and Bhum	3.8	0.67	0,8	0,31
India, Bombay	6.2	0.22	4.6	0.20
*India, Karunagappally	7.0	1.48	6.3	1.43
India, Madras	7.5	0.36	8.2	0.38
*India, Trivandrum	10.8	1.29	5.9	0.91
Israel: All Jews	0.8	0.09	0.6	0.07
Jews born in Israel	1.1	0.35	1.0	0.35
Jews born in America or Europe	0.8	0.17	0.5	0.10
Jews born in Africa or Asia	0.9	0.16	0.7	0.29
Non-Jews	0.5	0,24	0.5	0,20
Japan, Hiroshima	1.6	0.23	0.7	0.13
Japan, Miyagi	0.9	0.11	0.5	0.08
Japan, Nagasaki	1.9	0.19	0.6	0.10
Japan, Osaka	1.4	0.07	0.6	0.05
*Japan, Saga	1.5	0.22	0.6	0.13
Japan, Yamagata	0.8	0.12	0.3	0.06
*Korea, Kangwha	0,6	0,43	0,7	0,43
*Kuwait: Non-Kuwaitis	0.5	0.23	0,8	0,48
*Kuwait: Kuwaitis	0,6	0,36	0,7	0,36
*Philippines, Manila	3.1	0.27	3.2	0.25
Singapore: Chinese	1.6	0.20	0.6	0,11
Singapore: Malay	1,1	0,43	0,4	0,26
Singapore: Indian	3.7	0.82	3.6	1.15
Thailand, Chiang Mai	2.5	0.29	2.0	0.25
*Thailand, Khon Kaen	1.7	0.30	3.0	0.37
*Viet Nam, Hanoi	1.1	0.22	1.1	0.20

* IMPORTANT-SEE NOTES ON POPULATION PAGE

EUROPE	MALE		FEMALE	
Austria, Tyrol	3.9	0.48	1.2	0.25
*Belarus	3.6	0.12	0.4	0.03
*Croatia	3.1	0.17	0.4	0.05
Czech Republic	2.2	0.09	0.4	0.03
Denmark	2.6	0.12	1.3	0.09
Estonia	4.1	0.31	0.5	0.09
Finland	1.0	0.08	0.7	0.05
France, Bas-Rhin	12.4	0.69	1.1	0.20
*France, Calvados	8.7	0.72	1.3	0.25
France, Doubs	7.6	0.75	1.5	0.32
France, Haut-Rhin	10.2	0.73	1.1	0.23
*France, Herault	4.8	0.44	1.2	0.20
France, Isere	5.4	0.43	1.0	0.17
*France, Somme	11.1	0.88	1.4	0.28
*France, Tarn	2.8	0.47	0,4	0,16
Germany, Eastern States	1.8	0.10	0.4	0.04
Germany, Saarland	5.3	0.39	1.1	0.17
Iceland	1.7	0.49	1.3	0.41
Ireland, Southern	2.3	0.40	0.6	0.17
Italy, Ferrara	2.5	0.69	1,0	0,34
Italy, Florence	1.7	0.22	0.9	0.15
Italy, Genoa	2.3	0.29	0.7	0.13
*Italy, Latina	1.2	0.34	0,3	0,16
Italy, Macerata	0,3	0.24	0,6	0,31
Italy, Modena	1.4	0.24	0.6	0.16
Italy, Parma	2.9	0.43	0.4	0.12
Italy, Ragusa	1.0	0.32	0,8	0,36
Italy, Romagna	1.7	0.31	0.5	0.15
Italy, Torino	2.7	0.34	0.3	0.08
Italy, Trieste	8.4	1.04	2.4	0.57
Italy, Varese	3.7	0.38	0.6	0.14
Italy, Veneto	4.8	0.35	1.1	0.15
*Latvia	2.7	0.19	0.3	0.05
Malta	1,4	0,60	1,1	0,49
The Netherlands	2.1	0.08	1.1	0.05
The Netherlands, Eindhoven	2.2	0.29	1.1	0.19
The Netherlands, Maastricht	1.7	0.24	1.0	0.19
Norway	1.7	0.11	0.8	0.07
*Poland, Cracow	1.6	0.29	0.5	0.15
*Poland, Kielce	0.9	0.18	0,1	0,07
*Poland, Lower Silesia	2.2	0.17	0.6	0.09
Poland, Warsaw City	1.8	0.21	0.4	0.09
Slovakia	5.4	0.20	0.4	0.05
Slovenia	5.0	0.30	0.6	0.09
*Spain, Albacete	1,0	0,43	0,3	0,18
Spain, Asturias	3.6	0.35	0.6	0.15
Spain, Basque Country	4.9	0.30	0.6	0.09
Spain, Granada	3.9	0.42	1.0	0.20
Spain, Mallorca	4.8	0.53	0.6	0.17
Spain, Murcia	3.5	0.35	0.7	0.15
Spain, Navarra	3.8	0.49	0,3	0,14
Spain, Tarragona	3.1	0.42	0.7	0.20
Spain, Zaragoza	2.7	0.32	0.2	0.07

	MALE		FEMALE	
Sweden	1.5	0.07	0.8	0.05
*Switzerland, Basel	3.0	0.46	0.7	0.19
Switzerland, Geneva	4.5	0.59	1.5	0.33
Switzerland, Graubunden	2.2	0.72	0,1	0,08
Switzerland, Neuchatel	5.3	1.00	1,5	0,51
Switzerland, St Gall-Appenzell	3.0	0.46	1.0	0.26
Switzerland, Valais	4.1	0.83	0,7	0,33
Switzerland, Vaud	4.2	0.49	1.2	0.24
Switzerland, Zurich	2.6	0.26	0.7	0.13
*UK, England and Wales	1.5	0.04	0.7	0.02
*UK, East Anglia	1.1	0.12	0.6	0.09
*UK, Mersey	2.1	0.16	0.9	0.10
*UK, North Western	2.2	0.13	0.8	0.07
UK, Oxford	1.1	0.12	0.7	0.09
*UK, South Thames	1.1	0.07	0.7	0.05
UK, South Western	0.9	0.09	0.5	0.06
UK, Wessex	1.2	0.11	0.7	0.08
*UK, West Midlands	1.8	0.10	0.7	0.06
UK, Yorkshire	1.8	0.13	0.8	0.07
UK, Scotland	2.8	0.13	1.4	0.08
UK, Scotland, West	3.3	0.20	1.4	0.12
*Yugoslavia, Vojvodina	2.3	0.18	0.3	0.06

OCEANIA	MALE		FEMALE	
Australian Capital Territory	1,4	0,49	1,3	0,45
Australia, New South Wales	2.8	0.13	1.2	0.08
South Australia	2.5	0.25	1.3	0.16
Australia, Tasmania	1.4	0.33	1.2	0.28
Australia, Victoria	2.4	0.14	1.2	0.09
Western Australia	2.6	0.25	1.0	0.15
*French Polynesia	4.5	1.21	2,6	0,95
New Zealand: Non-Maori	1.8	0.14	0.8	0.09
New Zealand: Maori	3.6	0.97	1,2	0,50
US, Hawaii: White	3.1	0.61	2.1	0.48
US, Hawaii: Japanese	1.6	0.38	0.6	0.22
US, Hawaii: Hawaiian	2,6	0.87	0.9	0,46
US, Hawaii: Filipino	1,4	0,50	1,7	0,61
US, Hawaii: Chinese	1,3	0,78	0,3	0,31

* IMPORTANT-SEE NOTES ON POPULATION PAGE

AGE-STANDARDIZED INCIDENCE
RATES AND STANDARD ERRORS (per 100,000)
Oropharynx (ICD-9 146)

	MALE		FEMALE	
AFRICA				
*Algeria, Setif	0,6	0,27	0,2	0,11
*France, La Reunion	8.0	0.85	0,4	0,17
*Mali, Bamako	0,3	0,21	0,1	0,07
*Uganda, Kyadondo	0,7	0,37	0,6	0,37
*Zimbabwe, Harare: African	-	-	-	-
*Zimbabwe, Harare: European	-	-	1,0	1,00
AMERICA, CENTRAL AND SOUTH				
*Argentina, Concordia	2,0	0,83	0,3	0,32
*Brazil, Belem	2.1	0.49	0,6	0,23
*Brazil, Goiania	1.2	0.33	0,6	0,23
*Brazil, Porto Alegre	4.0	0.53	0,3	0,12
Colombia, Cali	0.9	0.20	0.4	0.13
*Costa Rica	0.8	0.14	0.4	0.09
*Ecuador, Quito	0,2	0,10	0,1	0,06
*Peru, Lima	0,2	0,07	0,2	0,06
Peru, Trujillo	1,1	0,58	-	-
US, Puerto Rico	3.2	0.22	0.5	0.07
*Uruguay, Montevideo	3.3	0.38	0.2	0.08
AMERICA, NORTH				
Canada	1.5	0.04	0.5	0.02
Canada, Alberta	1.0	0.13	0.3	0.07
Canada, British Columbia	1.6	0.13	0.5	0.07
Canada, Manitoba	2.0	0.25	0.4	0.11
Canada, New Brunswick	1.5	0.28	0.5	0,15
Canada, Newfoundland	1.4	0.31	0.5	0,18
Canada, Northwest Territories	1,2	0,96	-	-
Canada, Nova Scotia	1.6	0.25	0.5	0.14
Canada, Ontario	1.4	0.07	0.5	0.04
Canada, Prince Edward Island	0,9	0,50	0,2	0,23
Canada, Quebec	1.7	0.09	0.5	0.05
Canada, Saskatchewan	0.7	0.16	0.3	0,09
Canada, Yukon	0,8	0,82	2,0	1,45
US, Cent. Calif.: Non-Hisp. White	1.7	0.21	0.6	0.11
US, Cent. Calif.: Hispanic	0,6	0,22	0,2	0,12
US, Los Angeles: Non-Hisp. White	1.7	0.12	0.9	0.08
US, Los Angeles: Hispanic White	1.1	0.17	0.2	0.06
US, Los Angeles: Black	2.7	0.36	1.0	0.19
US, Los Angeles: Chinese	0,2	0,20	0.3	0,18
US, Los Angeles: Filipino	1,1	0,50	0,1	0,10
US, Los Angeles: Korean	0,9	0,56	-	-
US, Los Angeles: Japanese	0,4	0,27	0,1	0,15
US, San Francisco: Non-Hisp. White	2.0	0.17	1.0	0.11
US, San Francisco: Hispanic White	1.7	0.44	0,5	0,24
US, San Francisco: Black	3.9	0.65	0.9	0.28
US, San Francisco: Chinese	0,4	0,24	0,1	0,09
US, San Francisco: Filipino	1,2	0,61	0,5	0,28
US, San Francisco: Japanese	-	-	-	-
US, Connecticut: White	1.9	0.15	0.8	0.09
US, Connecticut: Black	5.7	1.07	1,2	0,44
US, Atlanta: White	1.6	0.21	0.7	0.13
US, Atlanta: Black	2.9	0.55	1.0	0.28
US, Iowa	1.4	0.13	0.6	0.08

	MALE		FEMALE	
US, Central Louisiana: White	0,8	0,35	0,7	0,32
US, Central Louisiana: Black	4,3	1,79	-	-
US, New Orleans: White	1.8	0.33	0.4	0.14
US, New Orleans: Black	3.3	0.68	0.4	0.18
US, Detroit: White	2.0	0.15	0.7	0.08
US, Detroit: Black	3.7	0.44	1.0	0.19
US, New Mexico: Non-Hisp. White	1.4	0.24	0.4	0.12
US, New Mexico: Hispanic White	1.1	0.31	0.2	0,13
US, New Mexico: American Indian	-	-	-	-
US, Utah	0.7	0.14	0.2	0,07
US, Seattle	1.2	0.11	0.7	0.08
US, SEER: White	1.6	0.06	0.6	0.03
US, SEER: Black	3.6	0.28	1.0	0.13
ASIA				
*China, Qidong	0,0	0,04	0,1	0,05
China, Shanghai	0.3	0.04	0.1	0.02
China, Tianjin	0.3	0.05	0.2	0.05
Hong Kong	0.9	0.08	0.2	0.04
*India, Bangalore	2.2	0.19	0.5	0.10
*India, Barshi, Paranda and Bhum	0,8	0,31	0,1	0,11
India, Bombay	3.5	0.17	0.5	0.07
*India, Karunagappally	2,7	0,90	-	-
India, Madras	2.7	0.22	0.5	0.09
*India, Trivandrum	3.2	0.71	0,4	0,22
Israel: All Jews	0.3	0.05	0.1	0.03
Jews born in Israel	0,1	0,10	0,0	0,01
Jews born in America or Europe	0.2	0.07	0,1	0,05
Jews born in Africa or Asia	0.3	0.10	0,1	0,05
Non-Jews	0,1	0,13	-	-
Japan, Hiroshima	0.7	0.16	0,1	0,05
Japan, Miyagi	0.4	0.07	0,0	0,02
Japan, Nagasaki	0.5	0.10	0,1	0,03
Japan, Osaka	0.7	0.05	0.1	0.02
*Japan, Saga	0.6	0.14	0,1	0,07
Japan, Yamagata	0,1	0,05	0,0	0,02
*Korea, Kangwha	1,0	0,61	-	-
*Kuwait: Non-Kuwaitis	1,3	1,22	-	-
*Kuwait: Kuwaitis	0,3	0,20	0,8	0,46
*Philippines, Manila	1.0	0.15	0.7	0.11
Singapore: Chinese	0.9	0.15	0.2	0.06
Singapore: Malay	0,9	0,38	0,2	0,19
Singapore: Indian	1,3	0,50	1,1	0,67
Thailand, Chiang Mai	1.6	0.22	0.9	0.17
*Thailand, Khon Kaen	0.7	0.18	0.2	0,10
*Viet Nam, Hanoi	0.8	0.19	0,2	0,09

f

* IMPORTANT-SEE NOTES ON POPULATION PAGE

EUROPE	MALE		FEMALE	
Austria, Tyrol	2.2	0.36	0.7	0.19
*Belarus	1.6	0.08	0.1	0.02
*Croatia	2.9	0.16	0.3	0.05
Czech Republic	2.1	0.08	0.3	0.03
Denmark	1.7	0.10	0.6	0.06
Estonia	3.1	0.27	0.2	0.06
Finland	0.4	0.05	0.1	0.02
France, Bas-Rhin	11.9	0.68	0.8	0.17
*France, Calvados	11.7	0.84	0.8	0.22
France, Doubs	9.3	0.83	1.0	0.27
France, Haut-Rhin	11.8	0.78	1.0	0.22
*France, Herault	5.5	0.48	0.8	0.18
France, Isere	5.9	0.45	0.9	0.17
*France, Somme	13.3	0.94	0.7	0.22
*France, Tarn	5.5	0.73	0,4	0,21
Germany, Eastern States	1.7	0.10	0.3	0.03
Germany, Saarland	3.1	0.30	0.6	0.12
Iceland	0,4	0,23	0,3	0,19
Ireland, Southern	0.9	0.25	0,2	0,12
Italy, Ferrara	1.8	0.60	0,5	0,31
Italy, Florence	1.1	0.18	0.4	0.10
Italy, Genoa	2.4	0.30	0.4	0.11
*Italy, Latina	0.8	0.25	-	-
Italy, Macerata	1,1	0,59	0,0	0,05
Italy, Modena	1.4	0.24	0,2	0,09
Italy, Parma	1.7	0.33	0,2	0,10
Italy, Ragusa	0,1	0,10	0,1	0,12
Italy, Romagna	1.2	0.25	0,1	0,06
Italy, Torino	1.8	0.24	0.7	0.21
Italy, Trieste	2.5	0.57	0,5	0,25
Italy, Varese	3.6	0.37	0.3	0.10
Italy, Veneto	2.9	0.27	0.6	0.12
*Latvia	1.6	0.15	0.1	0.04
Malta	-	-	0,1	0,09
The Netherlands	1.3	0.06	0.5	0.04
The Netherlands, Eindhoven	1.2	0.21	0.3	0.10
The Netherlands, Maastricht	1.1	0.20	0.7	0.16
Norway	0.8	0.08	0.2	0.04
*Poland, Cracow	2.0	0.31	0.4	0.13
*Poland, Kielce	1.0	0.18	0,2	0,07
*Poland, Lower Silesia	1.4	0.14	0.4	0.07
Poland, Warsaw City	2.6	0.25	0.5	0.10
Slovakia	5.1	0.20	0.2	0.04
Slovenia	6.7	0.35	0.4	0.07
*Spain, Albacete	1,0	0,51	-	-
Spain, Asturias	4.2	0.39	0,3	0,10
Spain, Basque Country	3.5	0.26	0.2	0.05
Spain, Granada	1.3	0.24	-	-
Spain, Mallorca	3.0	0.42	0,3	0,11
Spain, Murcia	2.2	0.28	0,1	0,05
Spain, Navarra	1.7	0.33	0,1	0,09
Spain, Tarragona	1.9	0.34	0,0	0,02
Spain, Zaragoza	1.3	0.22	0,1	0,06

	MALE		FEMALE	
Sweden	0.9	0.05	0.3	0.03
*Switzerland, Basel	2.4	0.41	0,5	0,17
Switzerland, Geneva	5.4	0.66	1.6	0.35
Switzerland, Graubunden	1,7	0,65	0,3	0,24
Switzerland, Neuchatel	4.7	0.96	1,1	0,44
Switzerland, St Gall-Appenzell	2.1	0.38	0,1	0,08
Switzerland, Valais	4.7	0.90	0,4	0,25
Switzerland, Vaud	5.5	0.55	0.9	0.21
Switzerland, Zurich	2.3	0.25	0.6	0.12
*UK, England and Wales	0.7	0.03	0.3	0.02
*UK, East Anglia	0.5	0.08	0.2	0.06
*UK, Mersey	1.1	0.12	0.3	0.06
*UK, North Western	1.3	0.10	0.4	0.06
UK, Oxford	0.5	0.08	0.2	0.05
*UK, South Thames	0.7	0.06	0.3	0.04
UK, South Western	0.5	0.06	0.1	0.03
UK, Wessex	0.5	0.07	0.1	0.03
*UK, West Midlands	0.8	0.07	0.2	0.03
UK, Yorkshire	0.8	0.08	0.2	0.04
UK, Scotland	1.1	0.08	0.4	0.05
UK, Scotland, West	1.1	0.11	0.3	0.06
*Yugoslavia, Vojvodina	2.0	0.18	0.3	0.07

OCEANIA	MALE		FEMALE	
Australian Capital Territory	0,5	0,27	0,2	0,20
Australia, New South Wales	1.6	0.10	0.4	0.05
South Australia	1.7	0.19	0.4	0.09
Australia, Tasmania	1.6	0.35	0,4	0,16
Australia, Victoria	1.9	0.12	0.4	0.06
Western Australia	1.9	0.21	0.4	0.10
*French Polynesia	3.5	1.01	0,7	0,53
New Zealand: Non-Maori	0.8	0.10	0.4	0.06
New Zealand: Maori	1,1	0,52	0,4	0,26
US, Hawaii: White	3.8	0.68	0.5	0,24
US, Hawaii: Japanese	0,6	0,23	0,2	0,11
US, Hawaii: Hawaiian	1,1	0,54	0,5	0,38
US, Hawaii: Filipino	1,2	0,45	0,6	0,35
US, Hawaii: Chinese	0,8	0,65	-	-

* IMPORTANT-SEE NOTES ON POPULATION PAGE

AGE-STANDARDIZED INCIDENCE RATES AND STANDARD ERRORS (per 100,000)
Nasopharynx (ICD-9 147)

	MALE		FEMALE	
AFRICA				
*Algeria, Setif	8.0	0.95	2.7	0.44
*France, La Reunion	0,6	0,21	0,2	0,12
*Mali, Bamako	0,1	0,13	-	-
*Uganda, Kyadondo	0,9	0,35	0,5	0,24
*Zimbabwe, Harare: African	2.0	0.75	0,9	0,56
*Zimbabwe, Harare: European	-	-	3,1	2,22
AMERICA, CENTRAL AND SOUTH				
*Argentina, Concordia	-	-	0,6	0,43
*Brazil, Belem	0,5	0,23	0,1	0,08
*Brazil, Goiania	0,4	0,15	0,2	0,11
*Brazil, Porto Alegre	0,4	0,17	0,1	0,05 m
Colombia, Cali	0,3	0,11	0,2	0,08
*Costa Rica	0.7	0.11	0.2	0.06
*Ecuador, Quito	0,1	0,06	-	- m
*Peru, Lima	0,2	0,07	0,1	0,05
Peru, Trujillo	0,3	0,30	-	-
US, Puerto Rico	0.6	0.10	0.1	0.04
*Uruguay, Montevideo	0.7	0.18	0,3	0,12
AMERICA, NORTH				
Canada	0.8	0.03	0.3	0.02
Canada, Alberta	0.9	0.12	0.2	0.06
Canada, British Columbia	1.0	0.10	0.5	0.07
Canada, Manitoba	0.5	0.13	0.4	0.10
Canada, New Brunswick	0.6	0.17	0,3	0,12
Canada, Newfoundland	1.0	0.26	0,5	0,19
Canada, Northwest Territories	8.2	2.26	5,1	1,88
Canada, Nova Scotia	0,1	0,07	0,1	0,08
Canada, Ontario	0.9	0.06	0.4	0.04
Canada, Prince Edward Island	0,7	0,44	0,1	0,10
Canada, Quebec	0.6	0.06	0.2	0.03
Canada, Saskatchewan	0.6	0.15	0,1	0,06
Canada, Yukon	-	-	-	-
US, Cent. Calif.: Non-Hisp. White	0.7	0.13	0.3	0.10
US, Cent. Calif.: Hispanic	0,4	0,18	0,1	0,11
US, Los Angeles: Non-Hisp. White	0.5	0.07	0.2	0.05
US, Los Angeles: Hispanic White	0.5	0.11	0.2	0,06
US, Los Angeles: Black	1.0	0.21	0.2	0,08
US, Los Angeles: Chinese	9.8	1.27	2.8	0.62
US, Los Angeles: Filipino	3.8	0.86	0,3	0,22
US, Los Angeles: Korean	0,2	0,25	0,2	0,24
US, Los Angeles: Japanese	0,2	0,21	0,3	0,23
US, San Francisco: Non-Hisp. White	0.6	0.11	0.2	0.06
US, San Francisco: Hispanic White	0,4	0,21	0,1	0,07
US, San Francisco: Black	0,7	0,28	0,2	0,15
US, San Francisco: Chinese	11.6	1.24	3.8	0.68
US, San Francisco: Filipino	4.2	1.01	1,0	0,46
US, San Francisco: Japanese	-	-	-	-
US, Connecticut: White	0.7	0.09	0.2	0.04
US, Connecticut: Black	1,1	0,45	0,4	0,21
US, Atlanta: White	0.5	0.12	0.3	0.08
US, Atlanta: Black	1.3	0.34	0,2	0,12
US, Iowa	0.4	0.07	0.2	0.05

	MALE		FEMALE	
US, Central Louisiana: White	0,3	0,24	0,2	0,18
US, Central Louisiana: Black	1,4	1,02	-	-
US, New Orleans: White	0.8	0.21	0.6	0.17
US, New Orleans: Black	1.2	0.38	0,4	0,19
US, Detroit: White	0.6	0.08	0.2	0.04
US, Detroit: Black	0.5	0.15	0,2	0,08
US, New Mexico: Non-Hisp. White	0,2	0,10	0,2	0,09
US, New Mexico: Hispanic White	0,2	0,13	0,3	0,15
US, New Mexico: American Indian	-	-	0,9	0,67
US, Utah	0,2	0,08	0,1	0,06
US, Seattle	0.6	0.08	0.4	0.06
US, SEER: White	0.5	0.03	0.2	0.02
US, SEER: Black	0.9	0.13	0.2	0.06
ASIA				
*China, Qidong	1.9	0.25	1.1	0.18
China, Shanghai	4.5	0.15	1.8	0.10
China, Tianjin	1.6	0.13	0.6	0.08
Hong Kong	24.3	0.40	9.5	0.26
*India, Bangalore	0.3	0.07	0.2	0.06
*India, Barshi, Paranda and Bhum	-	-	-	-
India, Bombay	0.7	0.07	0.3	0.04
*India, Karunagappally	1,8	0,72	0,9	0,50
India, Madras	0.9	0.12	0.3	0.07
*India, Trivandrum	0,5	0,28	0,5	0,25
Israel: All Jews	1.1	0.11	0.4	0.06
Jews born in Israel	0.6	0.16	0.6	0.21
Jews born in America or Europe	0.6	0.13	0.2	0.07
Jews born in Africa or Asia	2.1	0.66	0.5	0.13
Non-Jews	0.9	0.29	0,1	0,05
Japan, Hiroshima	0.5	0.13	0,3	0,09
Japan, Miyagi	0.6	0.09	0.1	0.04
Japan, Nagasaki	0.5	0.11	0.2	0.06
Japan, Osaka	0.6	0.05	0.2	0.03
*Japan, Saga	0.5	0.14	0,1	0,06
Japan, Yamagata	0.4	0.10	0,1	0,05
*Korea, Kangwha	0,7	0,47	0,3	0,30
*Kuwait: Non-Kuwaitis	1.2	0.50	0,1	0,11
*Kuwait: Kuwaitis	2.3	0.59	0,6	0,25
*Philippines, Manila	7.6	0.38	3.7	0.25
Singapore: Chinese	18.5	0.62	7.3	0.37
Singapore: Malay	6.5	0.97	2.0	0.49
Singapore: Indian	0,5	0,34	0,5	0,52
Thailand, Chiang Mai	2.6	0.28	1.5	0.22
*Thailand, Khon Kaen	2.6	0.34	0.9	0.19
*Viet Nam, Hanoi	10.3	0.66	4.8	0.44

* IMPORTANT-SEE NOTES ON POPULATION PAGE

EUROPE	MALE		FEMALE	
Austria, Tyrol	0.7	0.20	0,1	0,08
*Belarus	0.7	0.05	0.2	0.02
*Croatia	0.7	0.08	0.2	0.04
Czech Republic	0.6	0.05	0.2	0.03
Denmark	0.3	0.05	0.2	0.04
Estonia	0.5	0.11	0.2	0.06
Finland	0.3	0.04	0.1	0.02
France, Bas-Rhin	1.2	0.22	0,3	0,10
*France, Calvados	0,6	0,19	0,1	0,09
France, Doubs	0,4	0,18	0,3	0,16
France, Haut-Rhin	1.0	0.23	0,3	0,13
*France, Herault	0.9	0.21	0,2	0,10
France, Isere	0.6	0.15	0,1	0,07
*France, Somme	0,6	0,19	0,2	0,09
*France, Tarn	0,8	0,28	-	-
Germany, Eastern States	0.4	0.05	0.1	0.03
Germany, Saarland	0.5	0.12	0.2	0.06
Iceland	0,6	0,29	0,1	0,15
Ireland, Southern	0,2	0,13	0,2	0,11
Italy, Ferrara	0,4	0,23	0,1	0,11
Italy, Florence	1.0	0.19	0.4	0.11
Italy, Genoa	1.3	0.24	0,3	0,11
*Italy, Latina	0,4	0,19	0,1	0,09
Italy, Macerata	0,2	0,18	-	-
Italy, Modena	0.7	0.18	0,2	0,10
Italy, Parma	0.7	0.21	0,2	0,10
Italy, Ragusa	0,7	0,28	0,3	0,19
Italy, Romagna	1.3	0.35	0,3	0,11
Italy, Torino	1.0	0.19	0,2	0,07
Italy, Trieste	0,8	0,32	0,6	0,37
Italy, Varese	1.0	0.20	0.4	0.12
Italy, Veneto	0.8	0.15	0.3	0.09
*Latvia	0.8	0.10	0.2	0.04
Malta	1,6	0,62	1,2	0,53
The Netherlands	0.5	0.04	0.2	0.02
The Netherlands, Eindhoven	0.5	0.13	0.4	0.12
The Netherlands, Maastricht	0.6	0.14	0,1	0,06
Norway	0.3	0.05	0.1	0.02
*Poland, Cracow	0.5	0.17	0.4	0.13
*Poland, Kielce	0,3	0,09	0,1	0,05
*Poland, Lower Silesia	0.5	0.08	0.2	0.05
Poland, Warsaw City	0.7	0.14	0,1	0,05
Slovakia	0.6	0.07	0.3	0.04
Slovenia	0.5	0.10	0.2	0.06
*Spain, Albacete	0,3	0,33	0,2	0,20
Spain, Asturias	1.4	0.23	0.5	0.13
Spain, Basque Country	1.2	0.16	0.5	0.10
Spain, Granada	1.2	0.23	0,3	0,11
Spain, Mallorca	1.0	0.25	0,3	0,13
Spain, Murcia	0.9	0.18	0,1	0,07
Spain, Navarra	1.4	0.30	0,2	0,10
Spain, Tarragona	0.9	0.25	0,0	0,04
Spain, Zaragoza	0.7	0.16	0,3	0,10

	MALE		FEMALE	
Sweden	0.4	0.04	0.2	0.02
*Switzerland, Basel	0,3	0,13	0,1	0,06
Switzerland, Geneva	0,4	0,21	0,3	0,15
Switzerland, Graubunden	0,7	0,38	0,5	0,37
Switzerland, Neuchatel	0,5	0,35	0,3	0,24
Switzerland, St Gall-Appenzell	0,5	0,18	0,2	0,12
Switzerland, Valais	0,6	0,30	0,1	0,13
Switzerland, Vaud	0.7	0.20	0,2	0,13
Switzerland, Zurich	0.4	0.10	0,1	0,06
*UK, England and Wales	0.4	0.02	0.2	0.01
*UK, East Anglia	0.2	0.06	0.2	0.07
*UK, Mersey	0.4	0.07	0.3	0.06
*UK, North Western	0.3	0.06	0.1	0.03
UK, Oxford	0.3	0.06	0.1	0.03
*UK, South Thames	0.3	0.04	0.2	0.03
UK, South Western	0.3	0.05	0.1	0.02
UK, Wessex	0.4	0.07	0.2	0.05
*UK, West Midlands	0.4	0.05	0.2	0.03
UK, Yorkshire	0.4	0.07	0.1	0.03
UK, Scotland	0.4	0.05	0.2	0.03
UK, Scotland, West	0.4	0.07	0.1	0.04
*Yugoslavia, Vojvodina	0.8	0.11	0.3	0.06

OCEANIA

	MALE		FEMALE	
Australian Capital Territory	0,9	0,36	0,3	0,24
Australia, New South Wales	0.9	0.07	0.3	0.04
South Australia	0.4	0.09	0,1	0,04
Australia, Tasmania	0.8	0.24	0,3	0,16
Australia, Victoria	0.8	0.08	0.3	0.05
Western Australia	0.6	0.12	0,2	0,06
*French Polynesia	2,5	0,85	0,6	0,40
New Zealand: Non-Maori	0.7	0.09	0.3	0.06
New Zealand: Maori	1.9	0.61	0,3	0,23
US, Hawaii: White	1,0	0,36	0,2	0,16
US, Hawaii: Japanese	1.2	0.40	0,1	0,10
US, Hawaii: Hawaiian	2,2	0,76	0,4	0,31
US, Hawaii: Filipino	3.3	0.92	1,2	0,55
US, Hawaii: Chinese	5.7	1.63	3,6	1,22

* IMPORTANT-SEE NOTES ON POPULATION PAGE

AGE-STANDARDIZED INCIDENCE
RATES AND STANDARD ERRORS (per 100,000)
Hypopharynx (ICD-9 148)

	MALE		FEMALE		
AFRICA					
*Algeria, Setif	-	-	-	-	
*France, La Reunion	4.7	0.65	0,3	0,17	
*Mali, Bamako	-	-	-	-	
*Uganda, Kyadondo	0,4	0,35	0,5	0,33	
*Zimbabwe, Harare: African	0,2	0,17	0,4	0,44	
*Zimbabwe, Harare: European	-	-	-	-	
AMERICA, CENTRAL AND SOUTH					
*Argentina, Concordia	2,5	0,97	0,3	0,27	
*Brazil, Belem	1.9	0.48	-	-	m
*Brazil, Goiania	1.5	0.40	0,1	0,05	
*Brazil, Porto Alegre	2.4	0.41	0,1	0,08	
Colombia, Cali	0.6	0.16	0,0	0,00	f
*Costa Rica	0.7	0.13	0,1	0,05	
*Ecuador, Quito	-	-	-	-	
*Peru, Lima	0.3	0.08	0,1	0,05	
Peru, Trujillo	0,6	0,45	-	-	
US, Puerto Rico	3.1	0.21	0.3	0.05	
*Uruguay, Montevideo	3.3	0.37	0,2	0,08	
AMERICA, NORTH					
Canada	1.2	0.04	0.2	0.02	
Canada, Alberta	0.9	0.12	0.2	0.05	
Canada, British Columbia	1.2	0.11	0.2	0.04	
Canada, Manitoba	1.5	0.22	0.3	0.09	
Canada, New Brunswick	1.1	0.24	0,2	0,11	
Canada, Newfoundland	1.0	0.27	0,3	0,14	
Canada, Northwest Territories	-	-	-	-	
Canada, Nova Scotia	1.9	0.28	0,3	0,10	
Canada, Ontario	1.1	0.06	0.3	0.03	
Canada, Prince Edward Island	2,6	0,87	0,1	0,10	
Canada, Quebec	1.5	0.09	0.2	0.03	
Canada, Saskatchewan	1.0	0.19	0,2	0,08	
Canada, Yukon	-	-	1,4	1,39	
US, Cent. Calif.: Non-Hisp. White	1.0	0.15	0.3	0.08	
US, Cent. Calif.: Hispanic	0,7	0,25	0,1	0,10	
US, Los Angeles: Non-Hisp. White	1.3	0.10	0.4	0.06	
US, Los Angeles: Hispanic White	0.6	0.13	0,0	0,02	
US, Los Angeles: Black	1.7	0.28	0,2	0,09	
US, Los Angeles: Chinese	0.9	0,35	-	-	
US, Los Angeles: Filipino	0,1	0,13	-	-	
US, Los Angeles: Korean	1,0	0,56	-	-	
US, Los Angeles: Japanese	0,4	0,32	-	-	
US, San Francisco: Non-Hisp. White	1.8	0.16	0.5	0.08	
US, San Francisco: Hispanic White	1.8	0.46	0,1	0,09	
US, San Francisco: Black	2.8	0.55	0,7	0,27	
US, San Francisco: Chinese	0,4	0,22	-	-	
US, San Francisco: Filipino	-	-	0,4	0,31	
US, San Francisco: Japanese	0,6	0,62	-	-	
US, Connecticut: White	1.4	0.12	0.5	0.07	
US, Connecticut: Black	3.4	0.83	0,7	0,31	
US, Atlanta: White	1.4	0.20	0.3	0.08	
US, Atlanta: Black	2.5	0.52	0.8	0.24	
US, Iowa	1.4	0.13	0.2	0.05	

	MALE		FEMALE	
US, Central Louisiana: White	0,9	0,36	-	-
US, Central Louisiana: Black	4,8	1,83	0,4	0,41
US, New Orleans: White	1.3	0.27	0,2	0,09
US, New Orleans: Black	2.4	0.58	0,2	0,13
US, Detroit: White	1.6	0.13	0.3	0.06
US, Detroit: Black	3.5	0.42	0,3	0,12
US, New Mexico: Non-Hisp. White	0.7	0.16	0,2	0,08
US, New Mexico: Hispanic White	0,7	0,26	-	-
US, New Mexico: American Indian	-	-	-	-
US, Utah	0.5	0.12	0,1	0,05
US, Seattle	1.2	0.11	0.4	0.06
US, SEER: White	1.3	0.05	0.3	0.02
US, SEER: Black	3.0	0.25	0.5	0.09
ASIA				
*China, Qidong	0,1	0,06	-	-
China, Shanghai	0.1	0.03	0.0	0.01
China, Tianjin	0.2	0.04	0,0	0,02
Hong Kong	1.6	0.10	0.1	0.03
*India, Bangalore	5.8	0.31	1.1	0.13
*India, Barshi, Paranda and Bhum	6.7	0.91	0,5	0,24
India, Bombay	8.3	0.27	2.0	0.13
*India, Karunagappally	2.8	0.90	0,6	0,43
India, Madras	6.5	0.34	2.4	0.19
*India, Trivandrum	2.0	0.58	0,7	0,31
Israel: All Jews	0.2	0.04	0,0	0,01
Jews born in Israel	0,1	0,06	-	-
Jews born in America or Europe	0.1	0.04	0,0	0,02
Jews born in Africa or Asia	0,2	0,08	0,0	0,03
Non-Jews	0,1	0,07	0,2	0,15
Japan, Hiroshima	1.2	0.20	0,1	0,06
Japan, Miyagi	0.9	0.11	0.2	0.05
Japan, Nagasaki	0.8	0.12	0,1	0,04
Japan, Osaka	1.2	0.07	0.2	0.02
*Japan, Saga	0.7	0.15	0,1	0,06
Japan, Yamagata	0.7	0.11	0,1	0,05
*Korea, Kangwha	0,3	0,31	-	-
*Kuwait: Non-Kuwaitis	0,1	0,05	-	-
*Kuwait: Kuwaitis	0,9	0,41	1,4	0,56
*Philippines, Manila	0.3	0.08	0,1	0,04
Singapore: Chinese	1.7	0.20	0,1	0,04
Singapore: Malay	0,2	0,16	0,3	0,24
Singapore: Indian	1,4	0,51	0,9	0,56
Thailand, Chiang Mai	2.4	0.28	0.6	0.14
*Thailand, Khon Kaen	0.5	0.16	0,0	0,03
*Viet Nam, Hanoi	1.2	0.24	0.4	0.12

* IMPORTANT-SEE NOTES ON POPULATION PAGE

AGE-STANDARDIZED INCIDENCE
RATES AND STANDARD ERRORS (per 100,000)
Hypopharynx (ICD-9 148) (contd)

EUROPE	MALE		FEMALE	
Austria, Tyrol	1.5	0.30	0,3	0,11
*Belarus	2.0	0.09	0.0	0.01
*Croatia	4.4	0.20	0.3	0.05
Czech Republic	1.1	0.06	0.1	0.02
Denmark	0.7	0.07	0.2	0.03
Estonia	1.9	0.22	0,1	0,04
Finland	0.5	0.05	0.1	0.02
France, Bas-Rhin	13.9	0.73	0.6	0.15
*France, Calvados	15.0	0.94	0,2	0,12
France, Doubs	10.0	0.86	0,4	0,15
France, Haut-Rhin	10.3	0.73	0.5	0.15
*France, Herault	3.9	0.40	0,1	0,07
France, Isere	6.6	0.48	0,2	0,08
*France, Somme	10.8	0.84	0,4	0,17
*France, Tarn	4.7	0.62	0,3	0,17
Germany, Eastern States	1.1	0.08	0.1	0.02
Germany, Saarland	3.5	0.31	0.4	0.09
Iceland	0,3	0,20	-	-
Ireland, Southern	0.9	0.25	0,4	0,16
Italy, Ferrara	0,4	0,24	0,4	0,28
Italy, Florence	1.1	0.18	0,1	0,06
Italy, Genoa	1.5	0.23	0.3	0.10
*Italy, Latina	0,3	0,17	0,1	0,09
Italy, Macerata	0,1	0,11	-	-
Italy, Modena	1.5	0.27	0,2	0,09
Italy, Parma	2.6	0.42	0,4	0,14
Italy, Ragusa	0,1	0,10	-	-
Italy, Romagna	0.6	0.17	0,1	0,04
Italy, Torino	1.1	0.19	0,2	0,09
Italy, Trieste	1.6	0.46	-	-
Italy, Varese	2.3	0.29	0.3	0,09
Italy, Veneto	2.0	0.22	0,2	0,06
*Latvia	1.8	0.16	0.1	0.03
Malta	0,5	0,29	-	-
The Netherlands	1.1	0.05	0.2	0.02
The Netherlands, Eindhoven	0.6	0.15	0,1	0,04
The Netherlands, Maastricht	1.2	0.21	0,1	0,05
Norway	0.9	0.08	0.2	0.04
*Poland, Cracow	0,3	0,12	0,2	0,09
*Poland, Kielce	0,3	0,09	-	-
*Poland, Lower Silesia	0.4	0.07	0,1	0,03
Poland, Warsaw City	0.7	0.13	0,1	0,04
Slovakia	3.8	0.17	0.1	0.02
Slovenia	3.6	0.25	0.1	0.05
*Spain, Albacete	0,7	0,41	-	-
Spain, Asturias	4.3	0.39	0,1	0,03
Spain, Basque Country	3.7	0.27	0,1	0,05
Spain, Granada	2.3	0.32	-	-
Spain, Mallorca	3.9	0.49	0,0	0,05
Spain, Murcia	1.4	0.23	0,0	0,01
Spain, Navarra	2.1	0.36	-	-
Spain, Tarragona	2.0	0.35	0,1	0,05
Spain, Zaragoza	1.2	0.22	-	-

	MALE		FEMALE	
Sweden	0.8	0.05	0.1	0.02
*Switzerland, Basel	2.2	0.39	0,4	0,15
Switzerland, Geneva	5.0	0.64	0.6	0.21
Switzerland, Graubunden	2,0	0,70	-	-
Switzerland, Neuchatel	3.8	0.83	0,4	0,30
Switzerland, St Gall-Appenzell	2.0	0.37	-	-
Switzerland, Valais	4.4	0.86	0,2	0,17
Switzerland, Vaud	6.8	0.61	1.0	0.24
Switzerland, Zurich	1.7	0.22	0.3	0.08
*UK, England and Wales	0.6	0.02	0.3	0.02
*UK, East Anglia	0.6	0.09	0.4	0.07
*UK, Mersey	1.0	0.11	0.4	0.07
*UK, North Western	0.9	0.08	0.4	0.05
UK, Oxford	0.5	0.08	0.2	0.05
*UK, South Thames	0.5	0.05	0.3	0.03
UK, South Western	0.4	0.06	0.2	0.04
UK, Wessex	0.4	0.06	0.2	0.04
*UK, West Midlands	0.7	0.06	0.3	0.04
UK, Yorkshire	0.6	0.07	0.3	0.04
UK, Scotland	0.9	0.07	0.3	0.04
UK, Scotland, West	0.9	0.10	0.3	0.06
*Yugoslavia, Vojvodina	2.9	0.21	0.2	0.05

OCEANIA

	MALE		FEMALE	
Australian Capital Territory	0,7	0,37	-	-
Australia, New South Wales	1.4	0.09	0.2	0.03
South Australia	1.3	0.17	0,1	0,05
Australia, Tasmania	0.9	0.26	0,1	0,06
Australia, Victoria	1.6	0.11	0.2	0.04
Western Australia	1.4	0.18	0.2	0,06
*French Polynesia	3.7	1.06	0,6	0,44
New Zealand: Non-Maori	0.9	0.10	0.2	0.05
New Zealand: Maori	0,9	0,50	-	-
US, Hawaii: White	2.1	0.51	0.8	0,29
US, Hawaii: Japanese	1.8	0.43	-	-
US, Hawaii: Hawaiian	2,5	0,85	0,3	0,25
US, Hawaii: Filipino	0,6	0,40	0.8	0,43
US, Hawaii: Chinese	1,0	0,57	0,6	0,58

* IMPORTANT-SEE NOTES ON POPULATION PAGE

AFRICA	MALE		FEMALE	
*Algeria, Setif	0,1	0,08	0,0	0,03
*France, La Reunion	1.2	0.33	0,1	0,10
*Mali, Bamako	0,4	0,20	-	-
*Uganda, Kyadondo	0,5	0,28	-	-
*Zimbabwe, Harare: African	0,4	0,34	0,6	0,44
*Zimbabwe, Harare: European	-	-	-	-

AMERICA, CENTRAL AND SOUTH	MALE		FEMALE	
*Argentina, Concordia	1,0	0,60	-	-
*Brazil, Belem	0,5	0,24	0,3	0,15
*Brazil, Goiania	0,3	0,15	-	-
*Brazil, Porto Alegre	1.2	0.28	0,1	0,06
Colombia, Cali	0,1	0,05	0,1	0,04
*Costa Rica	0.4	0.09	0.2	0.06
*Ecuador, Quito	0,2	0,11	0,0	0,00
*Peru, Lima	-	-	0,0	0,02
Peru, Trujillo	0,3	0,23	0,2	0,20
US, Puerto Rico	0.6	0.09	0.1	0.03
*Uruguay, Montevideo	1.0	0.20	0,0	0,02

AMERICA, NORTH	MALE		FEMALE	
Canada	0.6	0.03	0.2	0.01
Canada, Alberta	0.3	0.07	0,1	0,04
Canada, British Columbia	0.4	0.06	0.1	0.02
Canada, Manitoba	0.5	0.12	0,1	0,06
Canada, New Brunswick	0,1	0,05	0,1	0,08
Canada, Newfoundland	0.7	0.23	0,1	0,06
Canada, Northwest Territories	1,0	0,96	-	-
Canada, Nova Scotia	0.7	0.17	0.4	0.13
Canada, Ontario	0.6	0.05	0.2	0.02
Canada, Prince Edward Island	0,3	0,26	-	-
Canada, Quebec	0.8	0.06	0.2	0.03
Canada, Saskatchewan	0.3	0.11	0,1	0,05
Canada, Yukon	2,9	2,03	1,3	0,92
US, Cent. Calif.: Non-Hisp. White	0.3	0.08	0,1	0,04
US, Cent. Calif.: Hispanic	0,3	0,17	-	-
US, Los Angeles: Non-Hisp. White	0.4	0.06	0.2	0.04
US, Los Angeles: Hispanic White	0,2	0,08	0,1	0,04
US, Los Angeles: Black	0.9	0.21	0,2	0,09
US, Los Angeles: Chinese	0,1	0,11	0,1	0,14
US, Los Angeles: Filipino	0,5	0,32	-	-
US, Los Angeles: Korean	0,3	0,35	-	-
US, Los Angeles: Japanese	0,2	0,22	0,2	0,16
US, San Francisco: Non-Hisp. White	0.3	0.06	0.2	0.05
US, San Francisco: Hispanic White	0,2	0,17	-	-
US, San Francisco: Black	0,6	0,27	0,3	0,17
US, San Francisco: Chinese	0,2	0,11	-	-
US, San Francisco: Filipino	-	-	-	-
US, San Francisco: Japanese	-	-	-	-
US, Connecticut: White	0.3	0.06	0.2	0.05
US, Connecticut: Black	1,3	0,52	0,5	0,27
US, Atlanta: White	0.5	0.11	0.4	0.09
US, Atlanta: Black	1.5	0.41	0,6	0,22
US, Iowa	0.5	0.08	0.1	0.03

	MALE		FEMALE	
US, Central Louisiana: White	1,2	0,43	0,2	0,20
US, Central Louisiana: Black	-	-	0,7	0,73
US, New Orleans: White	1.1	0.24	0,3	0,12
US, New Orleans: Black	0,8	0,33	0,4	0,20
US, Detroit: White	0.5	0.07	0.1	0.03
US, Detroit: Black	1.1	0.24	0,3	0,10
US, New Mexico: Non-Hisp. White	0.5	0.14	0,1	0,04
US, New Mexico: Hispanic White	0,4	0,19	-	-
US, New Mexico: American Indian	-	-	-	-
US, Utah	0,1	0,06	0,1	0,05
US, Seattle	0.5	0.08	0.3	0.05
US, SEER: White	0.4	0.03	0.2	0.02
US, SEER: Black	1.1	0.15	0.3	0.07

ASIA	MALE		FEMALE	
*China, Qidong	0,1	0,04	-	-
China, Shanghai	0.1	0.02	0,0	0,01
China, Tianjin	0,0	0,01	-	-
Hong Kong	0.1	0.03	0,0	0,01
*India, Bangalore	0.5	0.09	0.4	0.08
*India, Barshi, Paranda and Bhum	0,6	0,26	-	-
India, Bombay	1.8	0.13	0.7	0.08
*India, Karunagappally	0,6	0,41	-	-
India, Madras	1.1	0.14	0.3	0.07
*India, Trivandrum	0,3	0,18	-	-
Israel: All Jews	0,1	0,03	-	-
Jews born in Israel	0,0	0,01	-	-
Jews born in America or Europe	0,1	0,05	-	-
Jews born in Africa or Asia	0,1	0,04	-	-
Non-Jews	-	-	-	-
Japan, Hiroshima	0,3	0,09	0,1	0,04
Japan, Miyagi	0.2	0.05	0,0	0,02
Japan, Nagasaki	0,1	0,05	0,1	0,04
Japan, Osaka	0.1	0.02	0.0	0.01
*Japan, Saga	0,1	0,04	0,0	0,01
Japan, Yamagata	0,2	0,06	0,1	0,03
*Korea, Kangwha	-	-	0,2	0,24
*Kuwait: Non-Kuwaitis	0,0	0,02	-	-
*Kuwait: Kuwaitis	-	-	-	-
*Philippines, Manila	1.5	0.19	1.0	0.14
Singapore: Chinese	0,2	0,06	0,0	0,01
Singapore: Malay	-	-	-	-
Singapore: Indian	0,2	0,15	-	-
Thailand, Chiang Mai	0,3	0,09	0,1	0,05
*Thailand, Khon Kaen	0,1	0,06	0,0	0,03
*Viet Nam, Hanoi	0.5	0.14	0,1	0,05

f China, Tianjin

* IMPORTANT-SEE NOTES ON POPULATION PAGE

AGE-STANDARDIZED INCIDENCE
RATES AND STANDARD ERRORS (per 100,000)
Pharynx unspecified (ICD-9 149) (contd)

EUROPE	MALE		FEMALE	
Austria, Tyrol	0,2	0,11	0,1	0,07
*Belarus	0.6	0.05	0.1	0.01
*Croatia	0.4	0.06	0,0	0,02
Czech Republic	0.1	0.02	0,0	0,01
Denmark	0.1	0.02	0,0	0,02
Estonia	0,2	0,07	0,0	0,02
Finland	0.1	0.03	0,0	0,01
France, Bas-Rhin	3.2	0.35	0,3	0,10
*France, Calvados	0.9	0.23	0,0	0,04
France, Doubs	0.9	0.27	-	-
France, Haut-Rhin	2.1	0.32	0,2	0,11
*France, Herault	1.0	0.20	0,1	0,07
France, Isere	1.1	0.20	0,2	0,07
*France, Somme	3.5	0.49	0,1	0,09
*France, Tarn	0,2	0,12	-	-
Germany, Eastern States	0.1	0.02	0,0	0,01
Germany, Saarland	0.3	0.09	0,1	0,04
Iceland	0,2	0,15	-	-
Ireland, Southern	0,2	0,12	0,2	0,09
Italy, Ferrara	0,3	0,24	-	-
Italy, Florence	0.3	0.10	0,1	0,03
Italy, Genoa	0,3	0,10	-	-
*Italy, Latina	0,6	0,23	-	-
Italy, Macerata	0,2	0,22	-	-
Italy, Modena	0,2	0,08	-	-
Italy, Parma	0,1	0,10	-	-
Italy, Ragusa	0,4	0,20	-	-
Italy, Romagna	0,3	0,12	0,1	0,08
Italy, Torino	0.4	0.12	-	-
Italy, Trieste	-	-	-	-
Italy, Varese	-	-	0,0	0,04
Italy, Veneto	2.1	0.23	0.5	0.10
*Latvia	0.3	0.07	0,1	0,03
Malta	-	-	-	-
The Netherlands	0.1	0.01	0.0	0.01
The Netherlands, Eindhoven	0,0	0,04	-	-
The Netherlands, Maastricht	0,1	0,07	0,0	0,02
Norway	0.1	0.03	0,0	0,01
*Poland, Cracow	0.6	0.16	0,1	0,05
*Poland, Kielce	0,2	0,08	0,1	0,03
*Poland, Lower Silesia	0.6	0.09	0,1	0,02
Poland, Warsaw City	0.3	0.09	0,1	0,03
Slovakia	0.3	0.05	0,0	0,01
Slovenia	0,1	0,04	0,0	0,01
*Spain, Albacete	0,4	0,37	-	-
Spain, Asturias	1.5	0.23	0,1	0,06
Spain, Basque Country	2.2	0.21	0,1	0,03
Spain, Granada	1.0	0.22	0,1	0,05
Spain, Mallorca	1.0	0.25	0,1	0,06
Spain, Murcia	0.8	0.17	0,1	0,04
Spain, Navarra	0.6	0.19	0,0	0,02
Spain, Tarragona	0,2	0,11	0,0	0,03
Spain, Zaragoza	0,2	0,08	0,0	0,05

	MALE		FEMALE	
Sweden	0.0	0.01	0,0	0,00
*Switzerland, Basel	0,1	0,07	-	-
Switzerland, Geneva	0,1	0,09	0,3	0,15
Switzerland, Graubunden	0,3	0,25	-	-
Switzerland, Neuchatel	0,5	0,31	0,4	0,26
Switzerland, St Gall-Appenzell	0,3	0,13	-	-
Switzerland, Valais	1,0	0,42	-	-
Switzerland, Vaud	0.6	0.18	0,1	0,08
Switzerland, Zurich	0,1	0,04	0,0	0,01
*UK, England and Wales	0.3	0.02	0.1	0.01
*UK, East Anglia	0.2	0.05	0.1	0.04
*UK, Mersey	0.4	0.07	0.1	0.04
*UK, North Western	0.4	0.06	0.2	0.04
UK, Oxford	0.2	0.05	0.1	0.04
*UK, South Thames	0.3	0.03	0.1	0.02
UK, South Western	0.2	0.04	0.1	0.03
UK, Wessex	0.3	0.06	0.1	0.03
*UK, West Midlands	0.3	0.04	0.1	0.02
UK, Yorkshire	0.4	0.05	0.1	0.03
UK, Scotland	0.5	0.05	0.1	0.03
UK, Scotland, West	0.6	0.08	0.2	0.04
*Yugoslavia, Vojvodina	0.3	0.07	0,0	0,02

OCEANIA	MALE		FEMALE	
Australian Capital Territory	0,2	0,19	-	-
Australia, New South Wales	0.3	0.04	0.1	0.02
South Australia	0.2	0.07	0,1	0,04
Australia, Tasmania	0.9	0.27	0,1	0,08
Australia, Victoria	0.4	0.06	0.1	0.03
Western Australia	0.9	0.15	0,1	0,05
*French Polynesia	2,2	0,78	0,3	0,31
New Zealand: Non-Maori	0.3	0.05	0,1	0,03
New Zealand: Maori	0,3	0,22	-	-
US, Hawaii: White	1,2	0,42	0,3	0,20
US, Hawaii: Japanese	0,3	0,17	-	-
US, Hawaii: Hawaiian	0,5	0,36	-	-
US, Hawaii: Filipino	0,2	0,12	-	-
US, Hawaii: Chinese	-	-	-	-

* IMPORTANT-SEE NOTES ON POPULATION PAGE

AGE-STANDARDIZED INCIDENCE
RATES AND STANDARD ERRORS (per 100,000)
Oesophagus (ICD-9 150)

	MALE		FEMALE	
AFRICA				
*Algeria, Setif	1,2	0,43	0,3	0,16
*France, La Reunion	22.1	1.43	1.6	0.34
*Mali, Bamako	1.7	0.51	0,6	0,27
*Uganda, Kyadondo	18.2	2.44	8.7	1.51
*Zimbabwe, Harare: African	30.4	2.84	8.0	1.79
*Zimbabwe, Harare: European	2,4	1,37	1,5	0,87
AMERICA, CENTRAL AND SOUTH				
*Argentina, Concordia	17.5	2.52	3.7	1.08
*Brazil, Belem	6.3	0.86	1.5	0.36
*Brazil, Goiania	9.3	1.01	1.9	0.41
*Brazil, Porto Alegre	18.9	1.18	4.1	0.43
Colombia, Cali	3.9	0.44	2.3	0.30
*Costa Rica	4.0	0.30	1.4	0.17
*Ecuador, Quito	3.1	0.45	1.1	0.22
*Peru, Lima	1.8	0.21	0.6	0.13
Peru, Trujillo	3.3	0.88	0,7	0,40
US, Puerto Rico	9.0	0.35	2.2	0.15
*Uruguay, Montevideo	11.9	0.69	3.4	0.30
AMERICA, NORTH				
Canada	4.1	0.07	1.3	0.04
Canada, Alberta	2.6	0.20	1.0	0.12
Canada, British Columbia	4.3	0.20	1.6	0.11
Canada, Manitoba	3.8	0.33	1.3	0.17
Canada, New Brunswick	3.6	0.41	0.9	0.18
Canada, Newfoundland	4.1	0.52	1.0	0.24
Canada, Northwest Territories	3,3	1,69	5,5	2,38
Canada, Nova Scotia	4.0	0.38	1.2	0.18
Canada, Ontario	4.5	0.12	1.4	0.06
Canada, Prince Edward Island	4.5	1.01	0,4	0,29
Canada, Quebec	4.0	0.14	1.0	0.06
Canada, Saskatchewan	3.5	0.33	1.1	0.17
Canada, Yukon	6,3	2,60	-	-
US, Cent. Calif.: Non-Hisp. White	4.0	0.31	1.0	0.13
US, Cent. Calif.: Hispanic	2.4	0.49	0,5	0,21
US, Los Angeles: Non-Hisp. White	3.7	0.17	1.6	0.10
US, Los Angeles: Hispanic White	3.7	0.32	0.6	0.11
US, Los Angeles: Black	9.2	0.66	3.3	0.35
US, Los Angeles: Chinese	4.0	0.84	1.0	0,33
US, Los Angeles: Filipino	2,1	0,72	-	-
US, Los Angeles: Korean	6.0	1.72	0,3	0,30
US, Los Angeles: Japanese	5.8	1.15	1.0	0,44
US, San Francisco: Non-Hisp. White	4.5	0.25	1.5	0.13
US, San Francisco: Hispanic White	3.5	0.65	0,5	0,21
US, San Francisco: Black	11.5	1.09	3.8	0.58
US, San Francisco: Chinese	3.7	0.66	0,8	0,29
US, San Francisco: Filipino	2.7	0.83	0,2	0,20
US, San Francisco: Japanese	9.6	2.66	0,4	0,40
US, Connecticut: White	5.3	0.24	1.4	0.11
US, Connecticut: Black	20.1	2.02	3.9	0.78
US, Atlanta: White	4.1	0.34	1.2	0.17
US, Atlanta: Black	14.7	1.29	4.9	0.63
US, Iowa	4.1	0.22	0.8	0.09

	MALE		FEMALE	
US, Central Louisiana: White	3.8	0.76	0,7	0,31
US, Central Louisiana: Black	14.0	3.19	2,3	1,11
US, New Orleans: White	5.9	0.56	1.4	0.23
US, New Orleans: Black	11.1	1.24	2.6	0.51
US, Detroit: White	4.9	0.23	1.3	0.11
US, Detroit: Black	13.7	0.82	3.5	0.36
US, New Mexico: Non-Hisp. White	3.8	0.39	1.2	0.19
US, New Mexico: Hispanic White	2.3	0.43	0,4	0,15
US, New Mexico: American Indian	2,3	1,08	0,2	0,19
US, Utah	2.6	0.27	0.5	0.11
US, Seattle	4.9	0.23	1.6	0.12
US, SEER: White	4.5	0.09	1.2	0.04
US, SEER: Black	13.8	0.53	3.9	0.25
ASIA				
*China, Qidong	11.5	0.63	4.6	0.36
China, Shanghai	12.5	0.24	4.8	0.14
China, Tianjin	14.0	0.39	6.2	0.25
Hong Kong	14.2	0.31	3.2	0.14
*India, Bangalore	8.8	0.38	8.5	0.38
*India, Barshi, Paranda and Bhum	5.8	0.83	1.9	0.48
India, Bombay	10.8	0.32	8.3	0.28
*India, Karunagappally	6.8	1.43	3.3	1.00
India, Madras	10.5	0.43	7.0	0.35
*India, Trivandrum	4.6	0.83	1.3	0.42
Israel: All Jews	1.7	0.12	1.1	0.09
Jews born in Israel	1.8	0.50	1.1	0.37
Jews born in America or Europe	1.7	0.17	0.9	0.11
Jews born in Africa or Asia	1.5	0.20	1.3	0.18
Non-Jews	0,5	0,22	0,2	0,12
Japan, Hiroshima	10.7	0.61	1.7	0.21
Japan, Miyagi	14.0	0.43	2.2	0.15
Japan, Nagasaki	8.7	0.39	1.1	0.12
Japan, Osaka	9.1	0.19	1.6	0.07
*Japan, Saga	7.0	0.46	0.8	0.13
Japan, Yamagata	11.0	0.46	1.6	0.15
*Korea, Kangwha	10.2	1.82	0,5	0,36
*Kuwait: Non-Kuwaitis	2.0	1.02	0,6	0,39
*Kuwait: Kuwaitis	1,7	0,58	2.5	0.80
*Philippines, Manila	3.1	0.28	1.6	0.18
Singapore: Chinese	8.6	0.46	2.2	0.20
Singapore: Malay	1,1	0,45	0,7	0,36
Singapore: Indian	5.6	1.07	3.9	1.17
Thailand, Chiang Mai	2.3	0.27	1.5	0.23
*Thailand, Khon Kaen	1.5	0.27	0.5	0.15
*Viet Nam, Hanoi	2.2	0.32	0.6	0.15

* IMPORTANT-SEE NOTES ON POPULATION PAGE

AGE-STANDARDIZED INCIDENCE RATES AND STANDARD ERRORS (per 100,000)
Oesophagus (ICD-9 150) (contd)

EUROPE	MALE		FEMALE	
Austria, Tyrol	4.2	0.49	0.5	0.15
*Belarus	5.8	0.15	0.6	0.04
*Croatia	6.1	0.23	0.8	0.07
Czech Republic	4.2	0.12	0.5	0.03
Denmark	4.8	0.16	1.4	0.08
Estonia	5.6	0.37	0.7	0.10
Finland	3.5	0.14	1.7	0.08
France, Bas-Rhin	16.3	0.79	1.2	0.19
*France, Calvados	22.3	1.14	1.1	0.23
France, Doubs	11.1	0.89	1.5	0.31
France, Haut-Rhin	14.2	0.85	1.3	0.24
*France, Herault	6.4	0.49	1.1	0.19
France, Isere	10.0	0.59	1.0	0.17
*France, Somme	18.0	1.06	1.5	0.26
*France, Tarn	5.0	0.62	0.6	0.22
Germany, Eastern States	4.1	0.15	0.6	0.04
Germany, Saarland	6.7	0.43	0.8	0.13
Iceland	6.2	0.92	2.1	0.49
Ireland, Southern	6.5	0.65	3.4	0.40
Italy, Ferrara	3.6	0.82	0,6	0,30
Italy, Florence	3.7	0.31	0.9	0.13
Italy, Genoa	3.9	0.37	0.9	0.15
*Italy, Latina	2.6	0.48	0,4	0,18
Italy, Macerata	1,5	0,57	0,6	0,31
Italy, Modena	2.9	0.35	0.6	0.13
Italy, Parma	3.9	0.49	0.8	0.21
Italy, Ragusa	1.0	0.29	0,4	0,18
Italy, Romagna	2.8	0.38	0.5	0.14
Italy, Torino	3.6	0.34	0.6	0.12
Italy, Trieste	7.0	0.90	1.4	0.34
Italy, Varese	6.8	0.50	0.7	0.13
Italy, Veneto	9.7	0.48	1.5	0.17
*Latvia	4.7	0.25	0.7	0.07
Malta	3.3	0.90	1,0	0,42
The Netherlands	5.2	0.12	1.9	0.06
The Netherlands, Eindhoven	3.6	0.36	1.1	0.18
The Netherlands, Maastricht	4.0	0.37	1.2	0.19
Norway	3.2	0.15	0.8	0.07
*Poland, Cracow	4.3	0.47	0.7	0.16
*Poland, Kielce	3.1	0.31	0.6	0.12
*Poland, Lower Silesia	5.8	0.29	0.9	0.09
Poland, Warsaw City	4.8	0.34	1.1	0.13
Slovakia	7.3	0.24	0.5	0.05
Slovenia	6.8	0.35	0.9	0.11
*Spain, Albacete	3.1	0.77	0,1	0,10
Spain, Asturias	7.5	0.49	0.7	0.12
Spain, Basque Country	9.6	0.42	0.6	0.09
Spain, Granada	3.7	0.40	0.5	0.13
Spain, Mallorca	5.5	0.55	0.6	0.16
Spain, Murcia	4.5	0.39	0.4	0.10
Spain, Navarra	7.0	0.64	0.7	0.19
Spain, Tarragona	5.7	0.56	0,2	0,09
Spain, Zaragoza	5.5	0.44	0.5	0.11

	MALE		FEMALE	
Sweden	3.1	0.10	1.0	0.05
*Switzerland, Basel	5.4	0.59	1.4	0.28
Switzerland, Geneva	7.1	0.75	1.4	0.29
Switzerland, Graubunden	4.7	0.99	0,6	0,27
Switzerland, Neuchatel	6.5	1.08	1.9	0.49
Switzerland, St Gall-Appenzell	5.5	0.59	0.7	0.17
Switzerland, Valais	7.4	1.09	0.9	0.31
Switzerland, Vaud	9.5	0.70	2.0	0.28
Switzerland, Zurich	3.6	0.31	1.2	0.16
*UK, England and Wales	7.6	0.08	3.5	0.05
*UK, East Anglia	6.1	0.28	2.8	0.17
*UK, Mersey	7.7	0.29	4.3	0.20
*UK, North Western	9.0	0.25	3.9	0.15
UK, Oxford	7.2	0.29	3.4	0.18
*UK, South Thames	7.4	0.17	3.2	0.10
UK, South Western	7.4	0.24	3.7	0.15
UK, Wessex	8.0	0.27	3.5	0.16
*UK, West Midlands	9.4	0.22	4.2	0.14
UK, Yorkshire	7.1	0.23	3.2	0.14
UK, Scotland	9.4	0.23	5.0	0.15
UK, Scotland, West	11.1	0.35	5.2	0.20
*Yugoslavia, Vojvodina	4.7	0.26	0.7	0.09

OCEANIA	MALE		FEMALE	
Australian Capital Territory	5.5	1.13	2.0	0.56
Australia, New South Wales	4.5	0.16	2.0	0.10
South Australia	4.2	0.30	1.9	0.19
Australia, Tasmania	7.0	0.71	3.4	0.45
Australia, Victoria	5.4	0.20	2.4	0.12
Western Australia	4.6	0.32	1.7	0.19
*French Polynesia	7.2	1.72	1,5	0,77
New Zealand: Non-Maori	5.3	0.24	2.4	0.14
New Zealand: Maori	9.2	1.62	2,1	0,72
US, Hawaii: White	4.4	0.72	2.0	0.51
US, Hawaii: Japanese	3.7	0.58	0,5	0,20
US, Hawaii: Hawaiian	7.6	1.45	1,3	0,56
US, Hawaii: Filipino	3.6	0.86	0,8	0,38
US, Hawaii: Chinese	4.5	1.28	-	-

* IMPORTANT-SEE NOTES ON POPULATION PAGE

AGE-STANDARDIZED INCIDENCE
RATES AND STANDARD ERRORS (per 100,000)
Stomach (ICD-9 151)

	MALE		FEMALE	
AFRICA				
*Algeria, Setif	14.4	1.41	3.5	0.54
*France, La Reunion	22.2	1.46	8.3	0.78
*Mali, Bamako	19.6	1.72	11.1	1.27
*Uganda, Kyadondo	5.4	1.29	3.2	0.86
*Zimbabwe, Harare: African	13.8	1.97	18.4	2.77
*Zimbabwe, Harare: European	8,3	2,84	6,3	2,28
AMERICA, CENTRAL AND SOUTH				
*Argentina, Concordia	24.2	2.95	9.9	1.70
*Brazil, Belem	42.0	2.32	16.0	1.16
*Brazil, Goiania	19.2	1.47	10.6	0.96
*Brazil, Porto Alegre	27.9	1.45	8.9	0.65
Colombia, Cali	33.3	1.26	19.3	0.86
*Costa Rica	51.5	1.08	22.7	0.67
*Ecuador, Quito	32.2	1.46	19.5	0.98
*Peru, Lima	19.1	0.70	13.7	0.57
Peru, Trujillo	31.1	2.85	20.1	2.01
US, Puerto Rico	13.6	0.41	6.1	0.26
*Uruguay, Montevideo	19.3	0.88	9.0	0.49
AMERICA, NORTH				
Canada	10.6	0.11	4.5	0.07
Canada, Alberta	9.8	0.39	4.0	0.23
Canada, British Columbia	9.2	0.29	3.9	0.18
Canada, Manitoba	11.1	0.56	4.4	0.33
Canada, New Brunswick	10.8	0.69	4.5	0.42
Canada, Newfoundland	18.5	1.09	7.9	0.68
Canada, Northwest Territories	18.8	3.66	4,7	1,82
Canada, Nova Scotia	12.0	0.65	5.1	0.38
Canada, Ontario	9.9	0.18	4.2	0.11
Canada, Prince Edward Island	11.7	1.66	5.4	1.07
Canada, Quebec	12.1	0.24	5.2	0.14
Canada, Saskatchewan	8.7	0.49	3.7	0.32
Canada, Yukon	5,8	2,32	4,6	2,49
US, Cent. Calif.: Non-Hisp. White	6.9	0.38	2.9	0.23
US, Cent. Calif.: Hispanic	9.9	0.99	6.5	0.77
US, Los Angeles: Non-Hisp. White	7.6	0.24	3.2	0.14
US, Los Angeles: Hispanic White	11.8	0.56	6.9	0.36
US, Los Angeles: Black	13.6	0.79	5.9	0.43
US, Los Angeles: Chinese	11.7	1.38	7.6	1.03
US, Los Angeles: Filipino	6.8	1.14	4.0	0.83
US, Los Angeles: Korean	35.5	3.64	16.2	1.98
US, Los Angeles: Japanese	21.2	2.18	12.0	1.45
US, San Francisco: Non-Hisp. White	7.9	0.32	3.0	0.18
US, San Francisco: Hispanic White	12.6	1.21	4.8	0.63
US, San Francisco: Black	15.4	1.24	7.6	0.75
US, San Francisco: Chinese	10.9	1.14	6.9	0.87
US, San Francisco: Filipino	6.5	1.25	4.2	0.95
US, San Francisco: Japanese	26.4	4.67	11.8	2.48
US, Connecticut: White	9.2	0.30	3.8	0.17
US, Connecticut: Black	13.2	1.66	6.7	0.98
US, Atlanta: White	5.2	0.38	2.3	0.22
US, Atlanta: Black	13.4	1.23	5.0	0.59
US, Iowa	6.6	0.27	2.2	0.14

	MALE		FEMALE	
US, Central Louisiana: White	6.0	0.96	2.2	0.48
US, Central Louisiana: Black	14.4	2.97	5.5	1.68
US, New Orleans: White	7.4	0.62	2.9	0.35
US, New Orleans: Black	16.8	1.48	6.4	0.73
US, Detroit: White	8.5	0.30	3.5	0.17
US, Detroit: Black	14.9	0.83	5.6	0.43
US, New Mexico: Non-Hisp. White	5.4	0.45	2.5	0.29
US, New Mexico: Hispanic White	12.7	1.01	6.3	0.67
US, New Mexico: American Indian	9.2	2.09	7.8	1.66
US, Utah	5.6	0.38	2.9	0.26
US, Seattle	7.5	0.28	3.0	0.16
US, SEER: White	7.5	0.11	3.1	0.06
US, SEER: Black	14.5	0.54	5.9	0.29
ASIA				
*China, Qidong	42.7	1.21	20.7	0.77
China, Shanghai	46.5	0.46	21.0	0.29
China, Tianjin	29.8	0.56	11.4	0.34
Hong Kong	19.4	0.36	9.5	0.24
*India, Bangalore	10.3	0.41	5.1	0.29
*India, Barshi, Paranda and Bhum	0,8	0,30	0,9	0,32
India, Bombay	7.7	0.26	3.8	0.18
*India, Karunagappally	6.2	1.35	3.1	0.99
India, Madras	15.9	0.53	7.0	0.35
*India, Trivandrum	6.8	1.03	2.5	0.59
Israel: All Jews	13.0	0.35	6.2	0.23
Jews born in Israel	8.9	1.06	6.0	0.85
Jews born in America or Europe	15.2	0.56	6.9	0.36
Jews born in Africa or Asia	10.2	0.55	5.6	0.47
Non-Jews	6.8	0.86	3.2	0.53
Japan, Hiroshima	83.1	1.69	35.9	1.00
Japan, Miyagi	82.7	1.05	32.8	0.61
Japan, Nagasaki	71.0	1.13	31.3	0.68
Japan, Osaka	65.0	0.51	27.3	0.29
*Japan, Saga	70.7	1.48	28.1	0.85
Japan, Yamagata	95.5	1.39	40.1	0.83
*Korea, Kangwha	65.9	4.68	25.0	2.72
*Kuwait: Non-Kuwaitis	10.1	2.43	2.3	0.72
*Kuwait: Kuwaitis	4.1	0.87	4.8	1.04
*Philippines, Manila	11.1	0.53	6.4	0.35
Singapore: Chinese	29.3	0.85	13.6	0.51
Singapore: Malay	8.7	1.16	5.5	0.95
Singapore: Indian	10.3	1.44	7.9	1.88
Thailand, Chiang Mai	7.5	0.49	4.9	0.40
*Thailand, Khon Kaen	4.1	0.47	2.1	0.30
*Viet Nam, Hanoi	20.9	0.97	10.4	0.62

* IMPORTANT-SEE NOTES ON POPULATION PAGE

AGE-STANDARDIZED INCIDENCE
RATES AND STANDARD ERRORS (per 100,000)
Stomach (ICD-9 151) (contd)

EUROPE	MALE		FEMALE	
Austria, Tyrol	26.3	1.21	15.7	0.78
*Belarus	46.8	0.44	20.1	0.23
*Croatia	28.1	0.50	11.5	0.27
Czech Republic	19.5	0.25	9.2	0.14
Denmark	9.0	0.22	4.7	0.15
Estonia	34.0	0.91	16.6	0.51
Finland	16.6	0.30	9.2	0.19
France, Bas-Rhin	12.2	0.66	4.9	0.36
*France, Calvados	13.4	0.85	4.8	0.43
France, Doubs	10.7	0.86	3.7	0.43
France, Haut-Rhin	15.4	0.88	6.5	0.49
*France, Herault	9.7	0.58	4.0	0.34
France, Isere	11.8	0.62	4.7	0.34
*France, Somme	9.8	0.73	4.1	0.42
*France, Tarn	8.6	0.79	3.3	0.45
Germany, Eastern States	20.1	0.33	10.5	0.19
Germany, Saarland	18.5	0.70	9.0	0.40
Iceland	20.2	1.63	10.4	1.14
Ireland, Southern	13.3	0.90	5.0	0.49
Italy, Ferrara	18.6	1.66	9.3	1.05
Italy, Florence	36.3	0.95	15.9	0.56
Italy, Genoa	17.6	0.74	8.3	0.45
*Italy, Latina	19.2	1.28	10.4	0.86
Italy, Macerata	29.6	2.46	14.0	1.60
Italy, Modena	22.7	0.93	11.8	0.61
Italy, Parma	33.7	1.35	14.7	0.80
Italy, Ragusa	13.2	1.10	6.4	0.71
Italy, Romagna	39.3	1.36	22.8	0.94
Italy, Torino	17.3	0.74	8.7	0.46
Italy, Trieste	18.3	1.37	8.7	0.87
Italy, Varese	26.6	0.98	12.7	0.58
Italy, Veneto	19.9	0.68	8.8	0.39
*Latvia	31.1	0.66	14.1	0.35
Malta	11.2	1.60	6.0	1.05
The Netherlands	15.4	0.20	6.1	0.11
The Netherlands, Eindhoven	17.0	0.77	7.4	0.45
The Netherlands, Maastricht	15.4	0.73	6.5	0.42
Norway	13.6	0.29	6.4	0.19
*Poland, Cracow	21.5	1.04	8.0	0.50
*Poland, Kielce	22.1	0.82	8.0	0.43
*Poland, Lower Silesia	24.7	0.59	10.4	0.32
Poland, Warsaw City	19.1	0.68	6.9	0.34
Slovakia	24.5	0.42	10.3	0.23
Slovenia	27.0	0.71	10.6	0.36
*Spain, Albacete	17.2	1.85	7.8	1.18
Spain, Asturias	18.5	0.75	8.7	0.44
Spain, Basque Country	24.2	0.66	9.6	0.37
Spain, Granada	15.5	0.79	7.0	0.49
Spain, Mallorca	11.6	0.76	6.1	0.52
Spain, Murcia	15.1	0.69	7.3	0.44
Spain, Navarra	25.4	1.16	10.3	0.68
Spain, Tarragona	13.5	0.82	6.2	0.52
Spain, Zaragoza	19.6	0.79	8.4	0.45

	MALE		FEMALE	
Sweden	10.7	0.17	5.4	0.12
*Switzerland, Basel	11.0	0.81	5.0	0.48
Switzerland, Geneva	12.3	0.99	5.4	0.57
Switzerland, Graubunden	16.6	1.85	7.0	1.07
Switzerland, Neuchatel	12.7	1.47	5.4	0.83
Switzerland, St Gall-Appenzell	12.2	0.85	5.8	0.52
Switzerland, Valais	17.6	1.63	8.3	1.04
Switzerland, Vaud	10.4	0.72	4.2	0.41
Switzerland, Zurich	11.3	0.52	5.0	0.31
*UK, England and Wales	16.1	0.12	6.3	0.07
*UK, East Anglia	14.5	0.42	4.6	0.21
*UK, Mersey	15.0	0.40	8.0	0.26
*UK, North Western	16.4	0.33	6.8	0.19
UK, Oxford	13.6	0.40	5.1	0.22
*UK, South Thames	13.3	0.23	5.1	0.12
UK, South Western	13.6	0.31	5.1	0.17
UK, Wessex	13.2	0.33	4.6	0.17
*UK, West Midlands	17.8	0.30	7.0	0.17
UK, Yorkshire	16.4	0.35	6.7	0.20
UK, Scotland	17.7	0.31	7.5	0.18
UK, Scotland, West	17.5	0.43	7.5	0.24
*Yugoslavia, Vojvodina	20.8	0.56	9.4	0.34

OCEANIA	MALE		FEMALE	
Australian Capital Territory	9.7	1.33	5.3	0.85
Australia, New South Wales	10.1	0.24	4.2	0.14
South Australia	10.6	0.47	4.2	0.27
Australia, Tasmania	11.4	0.89	4.8	0.53
Australia, Victoria	11.7	0.30	4.9	0.18
Western Australia	11.4	0.51	5.1	0.32
*French Polynesia	10.9	2.11	7.5	1.67
New Zealand: Non-Maori	11.0	0.34	4.8	0.21
New Zealand: Maori	27.9	2.85	13.7	1.68
US, Hawaii: White	7.8	0.95	4.4	0.69
US, Hawaii: Japanese	21.5	1.27	10.6	0.84
US, Hawaii: Hawaiian	15.1	2.03	10.4	1.56
US, Hawaii: Filipino	7.3	1.26	6.8	1.22
US, Hawaii: Chinese	12.3	2.20	5.2	1.30

* IMPORTANT-SEE NOTES ON POPULATION PAGE

AFRICA

	MALE		FEMALE	
*Algeria, Setif	0,4	0,22	-	-
*France, La Reunion	1.0	0.32	1.0	0.28
*Mali, Bamako	0,6	0,32	-	-
*Uganda, Kyadondo	0,2	0,18	0,3	0,23
*Zimbabwe, Harare: African	0,1	0,10	0,5	0,55
*Zimbabwe, Harare: European	1,8	1,24	-	-

AMERICA, CENTRAL AND SOUTH

	MALE		FEMALE	
*Argentina, Concordia	0,9	0,67	1,1	0,55
*Brazil, Belem	0,7	0,25	0,3	0,18 f
*Brazil, Goiania	0,5	0,23	1.0	0.28
*Brazil, Porto Alegre	1.4	0.33	0.7	0.18
Colombia, Cali	0.4	0.14	0.8	0.18
*Costa Rica	0.6	0.11	0.5	0.10
*Ecuador, Quito	0.7	0.22	0.8	0.21
*Peru, Lima	0.5	0.11	0.4	0.10
Peru, Trujillo	1,5	0,64	0,8	0,42 m
US, Puerto Rico	0.8	0.10	0.6	0.08
*Uruguay, Montevideo	0.6	0.16	0.3	0.10

AMERICA, NORTH

	MALE		FEMALE	
Canada	0.9	0.03	0.7	0.03
Canada, Alberta	0.8	0.11	0.9	0.11
Canada, British Columbia	0.7	0.08	0.5	0.06
Canada, Manitoba	0.8	0.14	0.5	0.11
Canada, New Brunswick	0.6	0.17	0.4	0.14
Canada, Newfoundland	0.7	0.21	0.6	0.21
Canada, Northwest Territories	1,5	1,10	-	-
Canada, Nova Scotia	1.0	0.19	1.0	0.19
Canada, Ontario	1.0	0.06	0.7	0.04
Canada, Prince Edward Island	0,6	0,34	0,7	0,43
Canada, Quebec	0.8	0.06	0.6	0.05
Canada, Saskatchewan	1.0	0.18	0.8	0.15
Canada, Yukon	-	-	-	-
US, Cent. Calif.: Non-Hisp. White	1.2	0.17	0.7	0.12
US, Cent. Calif.: Hispanic	0,5	0,21	0.8	0.26
US, Los Angeles: Non-Hisp. White	1.3	0.10	0.9	0.08
US, Los Angeles: Hispanic White	0.7	0.14	0.5	0.10
US, Los Angeles: Black	1.7	0.28	1.3	0.21
US, Los Angeles: Chinese	0.3	0,20	0,1	0,14
US, Los Angeles: Filipino	0,6	0,33	0,2	0,14
US, Los Angeles: Korean	0,8	0,55	0,9	0,46
US, Los Angeles: Japanese	0,4	0,31	0,1	0,09
US, San Francisco: Non-Hisp. White	1.1	0.12	0.6	0.09
US, San Francisco: Hispanic White	0,8	0,29	0,5	0,20
US, San Francisco: Black	2.1	0.46	1.0	0.29
US, San Francisco: Chinese	0,7	0,26	0,5	0,28
US, San Francisco: Filipino	0,5	0,35	-	-
US, San Francisco: Japanese	-	-	-	-
US, Connecticut: White	1.0	0.10	0.9	0.09
US, Connecticut: Black	1,3	0,51	1.5	0.46
US, Atlanta: White	1.3	0.19	0.8	0.13
US, Atlanta: Black	1.9	0.46	1.4	0.33
US, Iowa	1.1	0.11	0.9	0.10

	MALE		FEMALE	
US, Central Louisiana: White	0.6	0.30	0.5	0.24
US, Central Louisiana: Black	1,2	0,89	-	-
US, New Orleans: White	1.5	0.29	0.6	0.16
US, New Orleans: Black	1,2	0,42	1.6	0.38
US, Detroit: White	1.4	0.13	0.8	0.09
US, Detroit: Black	2.5	0.34	1.2	0.20
US, New Mexico: Non-Hisp. White	1.5	0.25	0.8	0.16
US, New Mexico: Hispanic White	0.8	0.26	0,6	0,21
US, New Mexico: American Indian	0,6	0,56	-	-
US, Utah	0.9	0.15	0.8	0.14
US, Seattle	1.2	0.11	0.8	0.09
US, SEER: White	1.2	0.05	0.8	0.04
US, SEER: Black	2.1	0.20	1.2	0.14

ASIA

	MALE		FEMALE	
*China, Qidong	0.5	0.13	0.4	0.09
China, Shanghai	0.7	0.06	0.4	0.04
China, Tianjin	0.5	0.07	0.4	0.06
Hong Kong	1.0	0.08	0.7	0.07
*India, Bangalore	0,1	0,03	0,1	0,03
*India, Barshi, Paranda and Bhum	0,1	0,12	-	-
India, Bombay	0.4	0.06	0.2	0.04
*India, Karunagappally	0,6	0,40	-	-
India, Madras	0.1	0.04	0,1	0,04
*India, Trivandrum	0,1	0,13	0,1	0,12
Israel: All Jews	0.7	0.09	0.5	0.07
Jews born in Israel	0,4	0,20	0,3	0,20
Jews born in America or Europe	0.7	0.15	0.7	0.14
Jews born in Africa or Asia	0.7	0.15	0.3	0.08
Non-Jews	0,3	0,20	0,4	0,19
Japan, Hiroshima	0.5	0.13	0.3	0.10
Japan, Miyagi	0.5	0.08	0.3	0.06
Japan, Nagasaki	0.7	0.11	0.3	0.06
Japan, Osaka	0.6	0.05	0.3	0.03
*Japan, Saga	0.5	0.13	0.4	0.10
Japan, Yamagata	0.5	0.12	0.2	0.05
*Korea, Kangwha	0,6	0,43	0,9	0,53
*Kuwait: Non-Kuwaitis	-	-	0,1	0,10
*Kuwait: Kuwaitis	0,4	0,26	0,4	0,26
*Philippines, Manila	0.5	0.10	0.3	0.07
Singapore: Chinese	0.5	0.11	0.4	0.09
Singapore: Malay	0,3	0,23	0,3	0,24
Singapore: Indian	0,4	0,29	0,1	0,15
Thailand, Chiang Mai	0.4	0.11	0,1	0,06
*Thailand, Khon Kaen	0,1	0,07	0,1	0,07
*Viet Nam, Hanoi	0,1	0,07	-	-

* IMPORTANT-SEE NOTES ON POPULATION PAGE

EUROPE	MALE		FEMALE	
Austria, Tyrol	0.8	0.21	0,3	0,11
*Belarus	0.3	0.04	0.2	0.03
*Croatia	0.4	0.06	0.3	0.05
Czech Republic	0.5	0.04	0.3	0.03
Denmark	0.7	0.06	0.5	0.05
Estonia	0.5	0.11	0.2	0.06
Finland	1.0	0.07	0.7	0.06
France, Bas-Rhin	1.1	0.21	0.5	0.13
*France, Calvados	1.0	0.25	0.9	0.21
France, Doubs	1.1	0.27	0.7	0.20
France, Haut-Rhin	1.0	0.22	0.4	0.12
*France, Herault	0.6	0.15	0.6	0.14
France, Isere	0.7	0.15	0.7	0.14
*France, Somme	0,5	0,19	0.5	0.16
*France, Tarn	0,5	0,18	0,0	0,03
Germany, Eastern States	0.4	0.05	0.3	0.03
Germany, Saarland	0.7	0.14	0.6	0.11
Iceland	1,3	0,44	0,7	0,29
Ireland, Southern	0,4	0,15	0,3	0,14
Italy, Ferrara	1,1	0,42	0,6	0,30
Italy, Florence	0.5	0.12	0.5	0.11
Italy, Genoa	0.6	0.14	0.3	0.08
*Italy, Latina	0,7	0,25	0,3	0,14
Italy, Macerata	0.5	0.33	0.5	0.38
Italy, Modena	0.7	0.17	0.7	0.16
Italy, Parma	0.5	0.18	0.4	0.16
Italy, Ragusa	0,5	0,23	0.3	0,19
Italy, Romagna	0.7	0.16	0.8	0.20
Italy, Torino	0.4	0.11	0.4	0.10
Italy, Trieste	1.1	0.35	1.0	0.26
Italy, Varese	0.7	0.16	0.3	0.09
Italy, Veneto	0.7	0.12	0.6	0.11
*Latvia	0.5	0.08	0.2	0.04
Malta	1,7	0,65	0,4	0,30
The Netherlands	0.7	0.04	0.4	0.03
The Netherlands, Eindhoven	0.9	0.18	0.3	0.10
The Netherlands, Maastricht	0.8	0.16	0.7	0.16
Norway	0.8	0.08	0.8	0.07
*Poland, Cracow	0,3	0,12	0,3	0,10
*Poland, Kielce	0.7	0.16	0.5	0.11
*Poland, Lower Silesia	0.4	0.07	0.2	0.05
Poland, Warsaw City	0.3	0.08	0.2	0.06
Slovakia	0.8	0.07	0.4	0.05
Slovenia	0.3	0.07	0.3	0.06
*Spain, Albacete	1,0	0,52	0,1	0,07
Spain, Asturias	1.0	0.18	0.5	0.13
Spain, Basque Country	0.8	0.13	0.2	0.06
Spain, Granada	0.4	0.14	0.3	0,10
Spain, Mallorca	0.6	0.17	0.4	0.14
Spain, Murcia	0.9	0.18	0.2	0,07
Spain, Navarra	0,2	0,11	0,4	0,15
Spain, Tarragona	0.6	0.18	0.2	0,09
Spain, Zaragoza	0,3	0,09	0,1	0,05

	MALE		FEMALE	
Sweden	1.3	0.06	0.9	0.05
*Switzerland, Basel	2.1	0.37	1.0	0.22
Switzerland, Geneva	0,6	0,21	0.4	0.16
Switzerland, Graubunden	1,2	0,53	0,2	0,16
Switzerland, Neuchatel	1,2	0,43	0,5	0,26
Switzerland, St Gall-Appenzell	1.1	0.27	0.7	0.19
Switzerland, Valais	0,9	0,38	0,6	0,29
Switzerland, Vaud	1.2	0.24	0.9	0.20
Switzerland, Zurich	1.5	0.20	0.7	0.12
*UK, England and Wales	0.5	0.02	0.4	0.02
*UK, East Anglia	0.7	0.10	0.4	0.07
*UK, Mersey	0.5	0.08	0.4	0.06
*UK, North Western	0.5	0.06	0.4	0.05
UK, Oxford	0.5	0.08	0.5	0.08
*UK, South Thames	0.4	0.04	0.3	0.03
UK, South Western	0.5	0.06	0.4	0.05
UK, Wessex	0.7	0.08	0.6	0.08
*UK, West Midlands	0.7	0.06	0.4	0.04
UK, Yorkshire	0.6	0.07	0.5	0.06
UK, Scotland	0.7	0.06	0.4	0.04
UK, Scotland, West	0.7	0.09	0.4	0.06
*Yugoslavia, Vojvodina	0.7	0.10	0.4	0.07

OCEANIA

	MALE		FEMALE	
Australian Capital Territory	0,6	0,32	1,1	0,43
Australia, New South Wales	0.8	0.07	0.6	0.06
South Australia	1.0	0.15	0.4	0.09
Australia, Tasmania	0,3	0,15	0,3	0,16
Australia, Victoria	0.7	0.07	0.5	0.06
Western Australia	1.0	0.15	0.5	0.11
*French Polynesia	0,4	0,32	1,1	0,62
New Zealand: Non-Maori	0.7	0.09	0.6	0.08
New Zealand: Maori	2,2	0,77	1,1	0,53
US, Hawaii: White	1.4	0.40	0,5	0,23
US, Hawaii: Japanese	0,7	0,26	0,2	0,15
US, Hawaii: Hawaiian	2,3	0,78	1,5	0,60
US, Hawaii: Filipino	0,4	0,25	0,4	0,31
US, Hawaii: Chinese	0,3	0,35	0,8	0,42

* IMPORTANT-SEE NOTES ON POPULATION PAGE

AGE-STANDARDIZED INCIDENCE
RATES AND STANDARD ERRORS (per 100,000)
Colon (ICD-9 153)

AFRICA	MALE		FEMALE	
*Algeria, Setif	0,4	0,24	0,6	0,22
*France, La Reunion	6.9	0.82	5.5	0.64
*Mali, Bamako	3.1	0.69	1.4	0.44
*Uganda, Kyadondo	3.2	0.96	3.4	0.89
*Zimbabwe, Harare: African	6.6	1.33	3.0	1.01
*Zimbabwe, Harare: European	17.8	4.11	14.1	3.33

AMERICA, CENTRAL AND SOUTH

	MALE		FEMALE	
*Argentina, Concordia	17.2	2.54	15.3	2.10
*Brazil, Belem	4.5	0.75	3.9	0.58
*Brazil, Goiania	5.8	0.81	9.0	0.90
*Brazil, Porto Alegre	15.7	1.09	13.7	0.80
Colombia, Cali	6.6	0.56	6.3	0.49
*Costa Rica	6.0	0.36	6.5	0.36
*Ecuador, Quito	3.9	0.50	5.7	0.54
*Peru, Lima	5.6	0.38	5.3	0.35
Peru, Trujillo	4.4	1.01	5.0	1.07
US, Puerto Rico	14.8	0.45	12.1	0.38
*Uruguay, Montevideo	23.6	0.96	18.0	0.70

AMERICA, NORTH

	MALE		FEMALE	
Canada	26.9	0.18	21.3	0.15
Canada, Alberta	22.2	0.58	16.2	0.47
Canada, British Columbia	20.7	0.43	17.7	0.38
Canada, Manitoba	27.1	0.87	23.4	0.78
Canada, New Brunswick	28.1	1.12	22.6	0.94
Canada, Newfoundland	31.4	1.43	28.1	1.32
Canada, Northwest Territories	8.1	2.48	13.7	3.55
Canada, Nova Scotia	31.1	1.05	25.2	0.87
Canada, Ontario	30.1	0.31	22.8	0.25
Canada, Prince Edward Island	27.8	2.63	23.7	2.22
Canada, Quebec	26.4	0.36	21.1	0.29
Canada, Saskatchewan	22.8	0.82	19.1	0.73
Canada, Yukon	15.3	4.28	8,7	3,35
US, Cent. Calif.: Non-Hisp. White	24.4	0.71	19.5	0.58
US, Cent. Calif.: Hispanic	17.0	1.31	10.4	0.98
US, Los Angeles: Non-Hisp. White	28.9	0.46	20.6	0.35
US, Los Angeles: Hispanic White	17.1	0.68	11.8	0.47
US, Los Angeles: Black	34.8	1.27	26.5	0.94
US, Los Angeles: Chinese	18.3	1.74	12.3	1.31
US, Los Angeles: Filipino	14.4	1.77	8.1	1.13
US, Los Angeles: Korean	14.1	2.29	8.2	1.42
US, Los Angeles: Japanese	26.7	2.38	20.6	1.85
US, San Francisco: Non-Hisp. White	28.3	0.60	20.7	0.47
US, San Francisco: Hispanic White	21.4	1.58	15.5	1.15
US, San Francisco: Black	33.8	1.83	27.9	1.46
US, San Francisco: Chinese	20.0	1.51	21.1	1.56
US, San Francisco: Filipino	19.0	2.23	8.9	1.35
US, San Francisco: Japanese	26.1	4.27	27.0	3.71
US, Connecticut: White	30.4	0.54	21.6	0.41
US, Connecticut: Black	30.9	2.52	25.2	1.88
US, Atlanta: White	27.0	0.87	20.0	0.64
US, Atlanta: Black	32.4	1.93	26.2	1.38
US, Iowa	30.7	0.57	25.1	0.47

	MALE		FEMALE	
US, Central Louisiana: White	28.1	1.98	19.0	1.47
US, Central Louisiana: Black	27.9	4.28	25.0	3.50
US, New Orleans: White	29.1	1.21	23.2	0.93
US, New Orleans: Black	31.4	2.04	25.8	1.53
US, Detroit: White	30.5	0.57	20.5	0.41
US, Detroit: Black	35.0	1.26	27.9	0.98
US, New Mexico: Non-Hisp. White	23.1	0.91	17.5	0.73
US, New Mexico: Hispanic White	20.0	1.29	14.2	0.98
US, New Mexico: American Indian	9.7	2.00	7.1	1.60
US, Utah	21.7	0.73	15.8	0.58
US, Seattle	26.5	0.52	20.2	0.42
US, SEER: White	28.1	0.22	20.8	0.17
US, SEER: Black	33.6	0.81	26.8	0.63

ASIA

	MALE		FEMALE	
*China, Qidong	2.1	0.27	2.0	0.24
China, Shanghai	12.2	0.24	10.8	0.21
China, Tianjin	5.6	0.24	4.9	0.22
Hong Kong	22.5	0.39	18.8	0.34
*India, Bangalore	2.4	0.20	2.0	0.18
*India, Barshi, Paranda and Bhum	0,7	0,28	0,4	0,22
India, Bombay	3.7	0.18	3.0	0.17
*India, Karunagappally	1,5	0,73	1,3	0,61
India, Madras	1.8	0.17	1.3	0.15
*India, Trivandrum	2.4	0.59	1,0	0,36
Israel: All Jews	24.9	0.48	19.9	0.41
Jews born in Israel	23.9	1.87	20.2	1.49
Jews born in America or Europe	30.2	0.76	23.0	0.65
Jews born in Africa or Asia	15.7	0.73	14.1	0.63
Non-Jews	6.2	0.81	6.1	0.75
Japan, Hiroshima	31.6	1.05	18.2	0.70
Japan, Miyagi	24.9	0.58	15.7	0.42
Japan, Nagasaki	25.7	0.68	15.7	0.47
Japan, Osaka	20.7	0.29	13.1	0.20
*Japan, Saga	19.3	0.77	12.8	0.56
Japan, Yamagata	21.3	0.65	16.1	0.52
*Korea, Kangwha	4.5	1.21	2,3	0,88
*Kuwait: Non-Kuwaitis	9.3	2.40	2.2	0.75
*Kuwait: Kuwaitis	3.5	0.77	4.8	1.03
*Philippines, Manila	11.0	0.52	8.9	0.41
Singapore: Chinese	24.2	0.76	21.0	0.64
Singapore: Malay	11.2	1.32	6.6	0.99
Singapore: Indian	7.6	1.31	4.7	1.29
Thailand, Chiang Mai	4.2	0.36	3.7	0.34
*Thailand, Khon Kaen	4.9	0.49	3.3	0.37
*Viet Nam, Hanoi	5.2	0.48	2.9	0.33

* IMPORTANT-SEE NOTES ON POPULATION PAGE

EUROPE	MALE		FEMALE	
Austria, Tyrol	20.5	1.07	16.7	0.82
*Belarus	9.8	0.20	7.6	0.14
*Croatia	12.8	0.34	8.9	0.24
Czech Republic	24.0	0.28	15.7	0.19
Denmark	20.6	0.33	19.9	0.30
Estonia	14.1	0.59	11.4	0.41
Finland	12.8	0.26	11.6	0.22
France, Bas-Rhin	30.2	1.05	18.8	0.73
*France, Calvados	20.1	1.04	14.4	0.78
France, Doubs	19.5	1.16	13.7	0.91
France, Haut-Rhin	28.4	1.20	18.4	0.84
*France, Herault	20.0	0.83	13.4	0.64
France, Isere	22.3	0.85	15.5	0.65
*France, Somme	20.2	1.07	12.3	0.77
*France, Tarn	18.5	1.13	13.3	0.94
Germany, Eastern States	15.5	0.29	13.9	0.22
Germany, Saarland	25.5	0.81	20.4	0.63
Iceland	19.2	1.61	15.4	1.39
Ireland, Southern	24.2	1.23	20.3	1.09
Italy, Ferrara	28.3	2.09	20.2	1.61
Italy, Florence	24.5	0.79	20.2	0.67
Italy, Genoa	26.2	0.91	18.5	0.70
*Italy, Latina	16.0	1.16	12.9	0.97
Italy, Macerata	25.3	2.28	17.2	1.76
Italy, Modena	21.2	0.91	17.1	0.78
Italy, Parma	24.4	1.18	17.8	0.98
Italy, Ragusa	9.8	0.94	10.5	0.94
Italy, Romagna	22.6	1.03	18.8	0.90
Italy, Torino	23.9	0.88	16.0	0.63
Italy, Trieste	30.7	1.78	17.3	1.20
Italy, Varese	27.4	1.00	18.7	0.73
Italy, Veneto	22.3	0.72	16.4	0.55
*Latvia	11.7	0.41	9.1	0.28
Malta	13.6	1.82	12.3	1.55
The Netherlands	21.9	0.24	18.9	0.20
The Netherlands, Eindhoven	23.7	0.91	19.1	0.75
The Netherlands, Maastricht	21.9	0.86	17.9	0.71
Norway	22.2	0.38	19.1	0.34
*Poland, Cracow	11.4	0.75	8.6	0.54
*Poland, Kielce	8.0	0.50	4.8	0.34
*Poland, Lower Silesia	12.0	0.41	9.4	0.31
Poland, Warsaw City	16.0	0.63	10.0	0.40
Slovakia	20.0	0.38	12.6	0.27
Slovenia	15.7	0.54	10.1	0.36
*Spain, Albacete	10.2	1.43	8.9	1.24
Spain, Asturias	17.0	0.71	11.1	0.54
Spain, Basque Country	17.1	0.55	10.6	0.39
Spain, Granada	10.3	0.64	9.0	0.57
Spain, Mallorca	18.4	0.95	15.5	0.84
Spain, Murcia	13.8	0.65	10.7	0.55
Spain, Navarra	16.5	0.92	13.0	0.79
Spain, Tarragona	18.6	0.96	14.0	0.80
Spain, Zaragoza	12.9	0.64	10.2	0.53

	MALE		FEMALE	
Sweden	17.7	0.22	15.9	0.21
*Switzerland, Basel	20.4	1.10	14.8	0.84
Switzerland, Geneva	25.2	1.38	15.4	0.94
Switzerland, Graubunden	19.7	1.99	16.5	1.73
Switzerland, Neuchatel	21.1	1.87	14.5	1.44
Switzerland, St Gall-Appenzell	16.5	0.98	12.0	0.78
Switzerland, Valais	19.0	1.70	14.0	1.39
Switzerland, Vaud	21.6	1.04	14.2	0.74
Switzerland, Zurich	19.0	0.68	13.1	0.51
*UK, England and Wales	19.3	0.13	15.6	0.11
*UK, East Anglia	20.2	0.50	16.8	0.43
*UK, Mersey	16.7	0.42	16.5	0.40
*UK, North Western	19.3	0.36	15.0	0.29
UK, Oxford	20.6	0.50	17.1	0.42
*UK, South Thames	18.1	0.27	15.0	0.22
UK, South Western	19.2	0.38	16.2	0.32
UK, Wessex	22.3	0.43	19.0	0.38
*UK, West Midlands	23.7	0.35	18.0	0.28
UK, Yorkshire	19.3	0.38	15.2	0.31
UK, Scotland	23.7	0.36	19.4	0.29
UK, Scotland, West	23.4	0.50	18.2	0.39
*Yugoslavia, Vojvodina	14.1	0.46	10.5	0.36

OCEANIA

	MALE		FEMALE	
Australian Capital Territory	29.0	2.30	20.0	1.76
Australia, New South Wales	28.4	0.40	21.2	0.33
South Australia	27.4	0.77	22.7	0.67
Australia, Tasmania	30.5	1.48	22.6	1.20
Australia, Victoria	27.5	0.45	22.9	0.39
Western Australia	25.4	0.76	21.8	0.67
*French Polynesia	9.5	1.97	4.8	1.31
New Zealand: Non-Maori	31.2	0.58	29.6	0.54
New Zealand: Maori	21.5	2.69	16.0	1.99
US, Hawaii: White	32.7	1.96	22.9	1.58
US, Hawaii: Japanese	34.4	1.72	22.6	1.33
US, Hawaii: Hawaiian	19.9	2.34	16.6	1.99
US, Hawaii: Filipino	17.7	1.84	13.2	1.68
US, Hawaii: Chinese	22.5	2.85	18.1	2.40

* IMPORTANT-SEE NOTES ON POPULATION PAGE

AGE-STANDARDIZED INCIDENCE
RATES AND STANDARD ERRORS (per 100,000)
Rectum (ICD-9 154)

AFRICA	MALE		FEMALE	
*Algeria, Setif	2.6	0.57	2.3	0.46
*France, La Reunion	5.8	0.74	4.3	0.56
*Mali, Bamako	2.9	0.62	0,7	0,28
*Uganda, Kyadondo	4.3	1.19	1.8	0.61
*Zimbabwe, Harare: African	3.8	0.91	2.6	0.96
*Zimbabwe, Harare: European	22.4	4.84	7.4	2.56

AMERICA, CENTRAL AND SOUTH	MALE		FEMALE	
*Argentina, Concordia	9.0	1.78	4.5	1.17
*Brazil, Belem	2.8	0.57	4.7	0.63
*Brazil, Goiania	4.6	0.72	5.3	0.68
*Brazil, Porto Alegre	12.4	0.96	6.9	0.57
Colombia, Cali	5.4	0.50	4.5	0.42
*Costa Rica	4.8	0.33	4.0	0.28
*Ecuador, Quito	3.4	0.45	4.0	0.45
*Peru, Lima	3.3	0.29	3.3	0.28
Peru, Trujillo	3.8	0.98	4.2	0.93
US, Puerto Rico	8.5	0.34	6.1	0.27
*Uruguay, Montevideo	12.5	0.70	7.7	0.48

AMERICA, NORTH	MALE		FEMALE	
Canada	16.1	0.14	9.2	0.10
Canada, Alberta	15.7	0.49	8.7	0.35
Canada, British Columbia	16.4	0.39	9.9	0.30
Canada, Manitoba	16.0	0.69	9.2	0.49
Canada, New Brunswick	16.3	0.88	9.6	0.63
Canada, Newfoundland	15.9	1.02	10.2	0.81
Canada, Northwest Territories	16.5	3.66	9.1	2.61
Canada, Nova Scotia	16.7	0.78	9.8	0.56
Canada, Ontario	15.0	0.22	8.3	0.15
Canada, Prince Edward Island	12.6	1.73	10.3	1.57
Canada, Quebec	18.0	0.30	10.2	0.20
Canada, Saskatchewan	14.3	0.66	8.3	0.49
Canada, Yukon	33.7	6.86	14.4	4.19
US, Cent. Calif.: Non-Hisp. White	14.8	0.57	8.2	0.39
US, Cent. Calif.: Hispanic	12.5	1.12	6.9	0.81
US, Los Angeles: Non-Hisp. White	13.6	0.32	9.1	0.25
US, Los Angeles: Hispanic White	9.5	0.50	6.3	0.35
US, Los Angeles: Black	13.1	0.78	10.1	0.58
US, Los Angeles: Chinese	8.3	1.14	7.1	1.01
US, Los Angeles: Filipino	9.0	1.38	6.4	0.98
US, Los Angeles: Korean	8.1	1.64	6.9	1.34
US, Los Angeles: Japanese	15.2	1.76	10.6	1.39
US, San Francisco: Non-Hisp. White	15.0	0.45	9.0	0.32
US, San Francisco: Hispanic White	13.6	1.25	7.1	0.80
US, San Francisco: Black	13.0	1.14	8.5	0.82
US, San Francisco: Chinese	12.7	1.22	10.0	1.05
US, San Francisco: Filipino	11.8	1.77	8.6	1.29
US, San Francisco: Japanese	19.3	3.69	8.4	1.95
US, Connecticut: White	16.1	0.40	9.4	0.28
US, Connecticut: Black	12.1	1.59	9.0	1.15
US, Atlanta: White	11.5	0.57	7.9	0.41
US, Atlanta: Black	11.2	1.12	8.8	0.82
US, Iowa	14.3	0.39	8.7	0.29

	MALE		FEMALE	
US, Central Louisiana: White	12.3	1.34	6.4	0.87
US, Central Louisiana: Black	10.6	2.77	4.6	1.45
US, New Orleans: White	14.3	0.86	7.7	0.56
US, New Orleans: Black	11.2	1.22	7.2	0.81
US, Detroit: White	15.9	0.41	9.7	0.30
US, Detroit: Black	13.4	0.80	8.7	0.55
US, New Mexico: Non-Hisp. White	11.3	0.65	7.1	0.49
US, New Mexico: Hispanic White	13.5	1.06	6.3	0.67
US, New Mexico: American Indian	4.8	1.44	4.9	1.35
US, Utah	11.4	0.54	6.7	0.39
US, Seattle	13.6	0.38	8.8	0.29
US, SEER: White	14.3	0.16	8.7	0.11
US, SEER: Black	12.8	0.51	8.5	0.36

ASIA	MALE		FEMALE	
*China, Qidong	7.4	0.51	7.0	0.45
China, Shanghai	9.3	0.21	7.3	0.18
China, Tianjin	6.2	0.26	5.6	0.23
Hong Kong	12.6	0.29	9.2	0.24
*India, Bangalore	3.1	0.22	2.8	0.21
*India, Barshi, Paranda and Bhum	2.6	0.55	1.1	0.34
India, Bombay	3.9	0.19	2.7	0.15
*India, Karunagappally	1,6	0,67	0,3	0,31
India, Madras	3.8	0.26	2.8	0.22
*India, Trivandrum	3.0	0.68	2.3	0.55
Israel: All Jews	14.4	0.37	11.4	0.31
Jews born in Israel	10.7	1.15	10.9	1.08
Jews born in America or Europe	16.6	0.59	12.8	0.50
Jews born in Africa or Asia	11.6	0.58	8.9	0.52
Non-Jews	3.1	0.59	3.2	0.55
Japan, Hiroshima	19.4	0.82	9.7	0.52
Japan, Miyagi	16.7	0.47	9.0	0.32
Japan, Nagasaki	18.0	0.57	9.5	0.37
Japan, Osaka	13.5	0.23	6.8	0.15
*Japan, Saga	11.6	0.61	6.7	0.41
Japan, Yamagata	16.2	0.57	9.3	0.41
*Korea, Kangwha	8.3	1.68	5.3	1.23
*Kuwait: Non-Kuwaitis	3.6	1.19	2.3	0.84
*Kuwait: Kuwaitis	3.9	0.85	1.9	0.61
*Philippines, Manila	7.7	0.43	5.9	0.33
Singapore: Chinese	18.0	0.66	10.3	0.45
Singapore: Malay	7.8	1.09	7.7	1.13
Singapore: Indian	6.0	1.09	6.6	1.73
Thailand, Chiang Mai	3.1	0.31	2.8	0.30
*Thailand, Khon Kaen	3.0	0.39	1.9	0.29
*Viet Nam, Hanoi	4.3	0.45	2.5	0.30

* IMPORTANT-SEE NOTES ON POPULATION PAGE

AGE-STANDARDIZED INCIDENCE
RATES AND STANDARD ERRORS (per 100,000)
Rectum (ICD-9 154) (contd)

EUROPE	MALE		FEMALE	
Austria, Tyrol	14.8	0.92	8.9	0.61
*Belarus	12.3	0.23	8.3	0.15
*Croatia	13.4	0.35	8.3	0.23
Czech Republic	24.2	0.28	11.6	0.17
Denmark	17.0	0.30	10.4	0.22
Estonia	11.5	0.53	7.5	0.33
Finland	10.5	0.24	6.6	0.16
France, Bas-Rhin	19.0	0.83	8.9	0.50
*France, Calvados	17.3	0.97	9.8	0.65
France, Doubs	17.1	1.09	9.7	0.75
France, Haut-Rhin	21.5	1.05	11.2	0.67
*France, Herault	14.3	0.70	8.1	0.50
France, Isere	15.4	0.71	9.8	0.52
*France, Somme	14.1	0.90	7.6	0.61
*France, Tarn	17.9	1.14	10.0	0.84
Germany, Eastern States	15.7	0.29	10.1	0.19
Germany, Saarland	17.3	0.67	10.9	0.47
Iceland	6.1	0.92	5.6	0.82
Ireland, Southern	13.1	0.91	7.2	0.65
Italy, Ferrara	11.5	1.35	5.9	0.92
Italy, Florence	15.9	0.64	9.4	0.46
Italy, Genoa	13.2	0.65	8.7	0.48
*Italy, Latina	10.2	0.92	7.1	0.74
Italy, Macerata	14.7	1.72	6.9	1.13
Italy, Modena	13.2	0.72	8.2	0.54
Italy, Parma	13.0	0.86	8.8	0.66
Italy, Ragusa	9.9	0.98	4.9	0.63
Italy, Romagna	12.5	0.76	8.3	0.62
Italy, Torino	13.1	0.65	9.0	0.49
Italy, Trieste	18.7	1.38	8.7	0.84
Italy, Varese	16.0	0.76	8.2	0.48
Italy, Veneto	13.1	0.56	7.9	0.39
*Latvia	10.4	0.38	7.0	0.25
Malta	9.3	1.46	6.5	1.11
The Netherlands	14.5	0.19	8.9	0.14
The Netherlands, Eindhoven	17.0	0.78	9.8	0.55
The Netherlands, Maastricht	18.6	0.81	10.4	0.55
Norway	15.7	0.32	10.3	0.25
*Poland, Cracow	10.4	0.72	6.4	0.48
*Poland, Kielce	8.3	0.51	5.6	0.37
*Poland, Lower Silesia	12.4	0.42	7.6	0.28
Poland, Warsaw City	11.3	0.52	6.8	0.34
Slovakia	20.6	0.39	10.9	0.25
Slovenia	17.2	0.56	9.8	0.35
*Spain, Albacete	9.1	1.35	5.7	1.06
Spain, Asturias	11.1	0.57	5.7	0.38
Spain, Basque Country	13.5	0.50	6.4	0.31
Spain, Granada	8.8	0.59	5.6	0.44
Spain, Mallorca	13.0	0.80	7.6	0.57
Spain, Murcia	11.9	0.61	7.8	0.46
Spain, Navarra	12.8	0.82	6.5	0.57
Spain, Tarragona	12.3	0.78	6.1	0.53
Spain, Zaragoza	11.1	0.59	6.4	0.43

	MALE		FEMALE	
Sweden	12.1	0.19	8.3	0.15
*Switzerland, Basel	16.4	1.00	9.2	0.67
Switzerland, Geneva	12.3	0.98	7.0	0.66
Switzerland, Graubunden	9.6	1.41	7.0	1.17
Switzerland, Neuchatel	14.6	1.59	8.4	1.11
Switzerland, St Gall-Appenzell	14.1	0.93	7.9	0.66
Switzerland, Valais	13.6	1.45	7.1	0.97
Switzerland, Vaud	12.3	0.79	8.6	0.61
Switzerland, Zurich	13.5	0.57	8.8	0.43
*UK, England and Wales	14.6	0.12	8.1	0.08
*UK, East Anglia	14.5	0.43	8.9	0.32
*UK, Mersey	12.8	0.37	8.6	0.29
*UK, North Western	15.6	0.33	7.8	0.22
UK, Oxford	14.6	0.42	8.4	0.30
*UK, South Thames	12.6	0.23	7.4	0.16
UK, South Western	14.2	0.33	9.0	0.25
UK, Wessex	13.4	0.34	7.6	0.24
*UK, West Midlands	17.5	0.30	8.9	0.20
UK, Yorkshire	15.1	0.34	8.5	0.23
UK, Scotland	14.3	0.29	8.3	0.20
UK, Scotland, West	14.0	0.39	8.0	0.26
*Yugoslavia, Vojvodina	14.6	0.47	9.4	0.33

OCEANIA

	MALE		FEMALE	
Australian Capital Territory	16.3	1.71	11.0	1.31
Australia, New South Wales	18.5	0.32	9.7	0.22
South Australia	18.0	0.63	11.5	0.48
Australia, Tasmania	15.3	1.04	10.9	0.85
Australia, Victoria	19.2	0.38	11.0	0.27
Western Australia	16.8	0.62	10.8	0.48
*French Polynesia	8.6	1.79	4.0	1.23
New Zealand: Non-Maori	20.1	0.47	11.2	0.33
New Zealand: Maori	12.8	1.91	9.2	1.47
US, Hawaii: White	14.0	1.29	8.0	0.94
US, Hawaii: Japanese	19.0	1.33	7.9	0.81
US, Hawaii: Hawaiian	13.9	1.98	8.2	1.42
US, Hawaii: Filipino	13.2	1.65	7.1	1.25
US, Hawaii: Chinese	12.1	2.18	6.4	1.52

* IMPORTANT-SEE NOTES ON POPULATION PAGE

AGE-STANDARDIZED INCIDENCE
RATES AND STANDARD ERRORS (per 100,000)
Large bowel (ICD-9 153-4)

AFRICA	MALE		FEMALE	
*Algeria, Setif	3.1	0.62	2.9	0.51
*France, La Reunion	12.7	1.10	9.8	0.86
*Mali, Bamako	6.0	0.93	2.1	0.52
*Uganda, Kyadondo	7.5	1.54	5.1	1.08
*Zimbabwe, Harare: African	10.4	1.61	5.6	1.39
*Zimbabwe, Harare: European	40.2	6.35	21.5	4.20

AMERICA, CENTRAL AND SOUTH	MALE		FEMALE	
*Argentina, Concordia	26.2	3.11	19.8	2.40
*Brazil, Belem	7.3	0.94	8.6	0.86
*Brazil, Goiania	10.4	1.08	14.4	1.13
*Brazil, Porto Alegre	28.1	1.45	20.6	0.98
Colombia, Cali	11.9	0.75	10.8	0.64
*Costa Rica	10.8	0.49	10.5	0.46
*Ecuador, Quito	7.3	0.68	9.6	0.70
*Peru, Lima	8.8	0.48	8.6	0.45
Peru, Trujillo	8.1	1.40	9.2	1.42
US, Puerto Rico	23.3	0.57	18.2	0.46
*Uruguay, Montevideo	36.0	1.19	25.7	0.85

AMERICA, NORTH	MALE		FEMALE	
Canada	43.0	0.23	30.5	0.18
Canada, Alberta	37.8	0.76	25.0	0.58
Canada, British Columbia	37.1	0.58	27.5	0.48
Canada, Manitoba	43.1	1.11	32.5	0.92
Canada, New Brunswick	44.4	1.42	32.2	1.13
Canada, Newfoundland	47.3	1.76	38.3	1.55
Canada, Northwest Territories	24.7	4.42	22.8	4.41
Canada, Nova Scotia	47.8	1.31	35.0	1.03
Canada, Ontario	45.1	0.38	31.1	0.29
Canada, Prince Edward Island	40.4	3.15	34.0	2.72
Canada, Quebec	44.4	0.47	31.3	0.35
Canada, Saskatchewan	37.1	1.05	27.4	0.88
Canada, Yukon	49.0	8.09	23.1	5.36
US, Cent. Calif.: Non-Hisp. White	39.3	0.91	27.7	0.70
US, Cent. Calif.: Hispanic	29.5	1.73	17.3	1.27
US, Los Angeles: Non-Hisp. White	42.5	0.56	29.7	0.43
US, Los Angeles: Hispanic White	26.6	0.84	18.2	0.59
US, Los Angeles: Black	47.9	1.49	36.5	1.11
US, Los Angeles: Chinese	26.6	2.08	19.4	1.65
US, Los Angeles: Filipino	23.4	2.24	14.5	1.50
US, Los Angeles: Korean	22.3	2.81	15.1	1.95
US, Los Angeles: Japanese	42.0	2.96	31.2	2.31
US, San Francisco: Non-Hisp. White	43.3	0.75	29.6	0.57
US, San Francisco: Hispanic White	35.0	2.02	22.6	1.40
US, San Francisco: Black	46.8	2.16	36.4	1.67
US, San Francisco: Chinese	32.6	1.94	31.1	1.88
US, San Francisco: Filipino	30.8	2.85	17.5	1.87
US, San Francisco: Japanese	45.4	5.65	35.4	4.19
US, Connecticut: White	46.5	0.68	31.0	0.50
US, Connecticut: Black	42.9	2.98	34.1	2.20
US, Atlanta: White	38.5	1.04	27.9	0.77
US, Atlanta: Black	43.7	2.24	35.0	1.60
US, Iowa	44.9	0.69	33.7	0.55

	MALE		FEMALE	
US, Central Louisiana: White	40.4	2.39	25.4	1.71
US, Central Louisiana: Black	38.5	5.10	29.6	3.79
US, New Orleans: White	43.5	1.49	31.0	1.09
US, New Orleans: Black	42.6	2.38	33.0	1.73
US, Detroit: White	46.5	0.70	30.1	0.51
US, Detroit: Black	48.3	1.49	36.6	1.12
US, New Mexico: Non-Hisp. White	34.4	1.12	24.6	0.88
US, New Mexico: Hispanic White	33.5	1.67	20.4	1.19
US, New Mexico: American Indian	14.5	2.47	12.0	2.09
US, Utah	33.1	0.91	22.5	0.70
US, Seattle	40.1	0.64	29.1	0.51
US, SEER: White	42.4	0.27	29.5	0.20
US, SEER: Black	46.4	0.96	35.3	0.72

ASIA	MALE		FEMALE	
*China, Qidong	9.5	0.57	9.0	0.51
China, Shanghai	21.5	0.32	18.1	0.28
China, Tianjin	11.7	0.35	10.4	0.32
Hong Kong	35.1	0.49	28.0	0.42
*India, Bangalore	5.5	0.30	4.8	0.28
*India, Barshi, Paranda and Bhum	3.3	0.62	1.5	0.40
India, Bombay	7.6	0.26	5.6	0.23
*India, Karunagappally	3.1	0.97	1,7	0,68
India, Madras	5.6	0.31	4.1	0.27
*India, Trivandrum	5.4	0.90	3.3	0.65
Israel: All Jews	39.2	0.60	31.3	0.51
Jews born in Israel	34.7	2.19	31.1	1.84
Jews born in America or Europe	46.8	0.96	35.8	0.82
Jews born in Africa or Asia	27.3	0.93	23.0	0.82
Non-Jews	9.3	1.00	9.4	0.93
Japan, Hiroshima	51.0	1.33	27.9	0.88
Japan, Miyagi	41.5	0.75	24.8	0.52
Japan, Nagasaki	43.7	0.89	25.2	0.60
Japan, Osaka	34.2	0.37	19.9	0.25
*Japan, Saga	30.9	0.98	19.5	0.70
Japan, Yamagata	37.5	0.87	25.4	0.66
*Korea, Kangwha	12.8	2.07	7.6	1.51
*Kuwait: Non-Kuwaitis	13.0	2.68	4.5	1.13
*Kuwait: Kuwaitis	7.4	1.15	6.7	1.19
*Philippines, Manila	18.7	0.68	14.8	0.53
Singapore: Chinese	42.2	1.01	31.2	0.78
Singapore: Malay	19.0	1.71	14.3	1.51
Singapore: Indian	13.6	1.70	11.3	2.15
Thailand, Chiang Mai	7.2	0.48	6.5	0.46
*Thailand, Khon Kaen	7.9	0.63	5.2	0.47
*Viet Nam, Hanoi	9.6	0.66	5.4	0.45

* IMPORTANT-SEE NOTES ON POPULATION PAGE

AGE-STANDARDIZED INCIDENCE
RATES AND STANDARD ERRORS (per 100,000)
Large bowel (ICD-9 153-4) (contd)

EUROPE	MALE		FEMALE	
Austria, Tyrol	35.3	1.42	25.6	1.02
*Belarus	22.1	0.30	15.9	0.20
*Croatia	26.2	0.49	17.1	0.34
Czech Republic	48.2	0.39	27.3	0.26
Denmark	37.7	0.44	30.3	0.37
Estonia	25.7	0.79	18.9	0.53
Finland	23.2	0.35	18.2	0.27
France, Bas-Rhin	49.2	1.34	27.7	0.89
*France, Calvados	37.4	1.42	24.2	1.02
France, Doubs	36.6	1.59	23.4	1.19
France, Haut-Rhin	49.9	1.59	29.6	1.08
*France, Herault	34.2	1.08	21.4	0.81
France, Isere	37.7	1.11	25.3	0.83
*France, Somme	34.3	1.40	19.9	0.98
*France, Tarn	36.4	1.61	23.3	1.26
Germany, Eastern States	31.2	0.41	24.0	0.29
Germany, Saarland	42.8	1.05	31.4	0.79
Iceland	25.3	1.86	21.0	1.62
Ireland, Southern	37.3	1.53	27.5	1.27
Italy, Ferrara	39.9	2.49	26.1	1.85
Italy, Florence	40.4	1.01	29.6	0.81
Italy, Genoa	39.4	1.12	27.2	0.85
*Italy, Latina	26.2	1.48	20.0	1.22
Italy, Macerata	40.0	2.85	24.1	2.09
Italy, Modena	34.4	1.16	25.4	0.95
Italy, Parma	37.3	1.46	26.6	1.18
Italy, Ragusa	19.8	1.36	15.4	1.13
Italy, Romagna	35.1	1.28	27.1	1.09
Italy, Torino	37.1	1.09	25.0	0.80
Italy, Trieste	49.4	2.26	26.0	1.47
Italy, Varese	43.5	1.26	26.9	0.87
Italy, Veneto	35.4	0.91	24.3	0.68
*Latvia	22.1	0.56	16.1	0.38
Malta	22.9	2.33	18.8	1.91
The Netherlands	36.4	0.30	27.8	0.25
The Netherlands, Eindhoven	40.7	1.20	28.9	0.93
The Netherlands, Maastricht	40.5	1.18	28.3	0.90
Norway	38.0	0.49	29.4	0.42
*Poland, Cracow	21.8	1.04	15.0	0.72
*Poland, Kielce	16.4	0.71	10.3	0.50
*Poland, Lower Silesia	24.4	0.58	17.0	0.41
Poland, Warsaw City	27.3	0.81	16.8	0.52
Slovakia	40.6	0.54	23.6	0.37
Slovenia	32.9	0.78	19.9	0.50
*Spain, Albacete	19.4	1.97	14.6	1.63
Spain, Asturias	28.1	0.91	16.8	0.66
Spain, Basque Country	30.6	0.74	16.9	0.50
Spain, Granada	19.1	0.87	14.6	0.72
Spain, Mallorca	31.3	1.25	23.1	1.01
Spain, Murcia	25.8	0.89	18.5	0.71
Spain, Navarra	29.3	1.23	19.5	0.97
Spain, Tarragona	30.9	1.23	20.0	0.95
Spain, Zaragoza	24.1	0.87	16.6	0.68

	MALE		FEMALE	
Sweden	29.8	0.29	24.1	0.26
*Switzerland, Basel	36.8	1.49	24.0	1.08
Switzerland, Geneva	37.5	1.69	22.4	1.15
Switzerland, Graubunden	29.3	2.44	23.6	2.08
Switzerland, Neuchatel	35.7	2.46	22.9	1.82
Switzerland, St Gall-Appenzell	30.6	1.35	19.9	1.03
Switzerland, Valais	32.6	2.24	21.1	1.70
Switzerland, Vaud	34.0	1.30	22.8	0.96
Switzerland, Zurich	32.5	0.89	21.9	0.66
*UK, England and Wales	33.9	0.17	23.7	0.13
*UK, East Anglia	34.8	0.66	25.6	0.54
*UK, Mersey	29.5	0.56	25.1	0.49
*UK, North Western	34.9	0.49	22.8	0.36
UK, Oxford	35.2	0.65	25.4	0.51
*UK, South Thames	30.8	0.35	22.5	0.28
UK, South Western	33.4	0.50	25.2	0.41
UK, Wessex	35.7	0.55	26.6	0.45
*UK, West Midlands	41.2	0.46	26.9	0.35
UK, Yorkshire	34.5	0.51	23.7	0.39
UK, Scotland	38.0	0.46	27.7	0.35
UK, Scotland, West	37.4	0.63	26.2	0.47
*Yugoslavia, Vojvodina	28.7	0.66	19.9	0.49

OCEANIA	MALE		FEMALE	
Australian Capital Territory	45.3	2.87	31.0	2.19
Australia, New South Wales	46.9	0.51	30.9	0.40
South Australia	45.4	0.99	34.2	0.83
Australia, Tasmania	45.8	1.81	33.5	1.47
Australia, Victoria	46.7	0.59	33.9	0.48
Western Australia	42.2	0.98	32.6	0.83
*French Polynesia	18.1	2.66	8.7	1.79
New Zealand: Non-Maori	51.3	0.74	40.8	0.63
New Zealand: Maori	34.3	3.30	25.2	2.47
US, Hawaii: White	46.7	2.34	30.9	1.84
US, Hawaii: Japanese	53.5	2.17	30.5	1.56
US, Hawaii: Hawaiian	33.8	3.06	24.7	2.44
US, Hawaii: Filipino	30.9	2.47	20.3	2.10
US, Hawaii: Chinese	34.7	3.58	24.5	2.84

* IMPORTANT-SEE NOTES ON POPULATION PAGE

AGE-STANDARDIZED INCIDENCE
RATES AND STANDARD ERRORS (per 100,000)
Liver (ICD-9 155)

AFRICA	MALE		FEMALE	
*Algeria, Setif	5.1	0.83	2.2	0.46
*France, La Reunion	2.7	0.50	1.6	0.35
*Mali, Bamako	51.1	2.67	17.5	1.53
*Uganda, Kyadondo	9.9	1.61	4.7	1.09
*Zimbabwe, Harare: African	34.6	2.96	19.2	2.66
*Zimbabwe, Harare: European	12.9	3.51	4,7	1,73

AMERICA, CENTRAL AND SOUTH	MALE		FEMALE	
*Argentina, Concordia	1,3	0,76	0,7	0,48
*Brazil, Belem	0,7	0,26	0,5	0,23
*Brazil, Goiania	4.5	0.71	2.9	0.51
*Brazil, Porto Alegre	8.3	0.78	3.5	0.40
Colombia, Cali	2.6	0.35	2.2	0.29
*Costa Rica	6.6	0.38	3.7	0.27
*Ecuador, Quito	2.9	0.42	2.8	0.37
*Peru, Lima	3.4	0.29	3.4	0.28
Peru, Trujillo	7.2	1.30	5.9	1.05
US, Puerto Rico	4.0	0.23	1.6	0.13
*Uruguay, Montevideo	1.6	0.26	0.8	0.16

AMERICA, NORTH	MALE		FEMALE	
Canada	3.1	0.06	1.2	0.04
Canada, Alberta	2.9	0.21	1.0	0.11
Canada, British Columbia	3.2	0.18	1.4	0.12
Canada, Manitoba	2.8	0.29	1.1	0.18
Canada, New Brunswick	1.9	0.30	0.9	0.19
Canada, Newfoundland	1.0	0.27	0.6	0.19
Canada, Northwest Territories	4,4	1,65	-	-
Canada, Nova Scotia	1.6	0.24	1.1	0.19
Canada, Ontario	3.1	0.10	1.2	0.06
Canada, Prince Edward Island	0,7	0,39	0,3	0,15
Canada, Quebec	3.7	0.14	1.5	0.08
Canada, Saskatchewan	1.9	0.24	0.8	0.15
Canada, Yukon	-	-	1,0	1,03
US, Cent. Calif.: Non-Hisp. White	2.7	0.25	1.3	0.16
US, Cent. Calif.: Hispanic	5.4	0.73	3.4	0.56
US, Los Angeles: Non-Hisp. White	2.9	0.15	1.1	0.09
US, Los Angeles: Hispanic White	6.5	0.41	2.2	0.20
US, Los Angeles: Black	5.1	0.49	2.2	0.28
US, Los Angeles: Chinese	16.1	1.63	4.4	0.82
US, Los Angeles: Filipino	9.5	1.40	3.5	0.83
US, Los Angeles: Korean	23.9	2.85	5.5	1.15
US, Los Angeles: Japanese	5.8	1.13	3.3	0.76
US, San Francisco: Non-Hisp. White	3.0	0.21	1.2	0.13
US, San Francisco: Hispanic White	6.7	0.87	2.5	0.46
US, San Francisco: Black	8.1	0.92	2.1	0.42
US, San Francisco: Chinese	20.5	1.61	6.0	0.85
US, San Francisco: Filipino	11.0	1.76	4.2	0.94
US, San Francisco: Japanese	5,7	2,03	2,1	0,95
US, Connecticut: White	3.3	0.19	1.1	0.10
US, Connecticut: Black	6.9	1.16	1.4	0.46
US, Atlanta: White	3.0	0.30	1.0	0.16
US, Atlanta: Black	3.2	0.57	1.6	0.34
US, Iowa	2.4	0.17	1.0	0.10

	MALE		FEMALE	
US, Central Louisiana: White	2.1	0.55	1.3	0.44
US, Central Louisiana: Black	5,0	1,86	0,8	0,60
US, New Orleans: White	3.6	0.43	1.0	0.19
US, New Orleans: Black	7.9	1.05	2.2	0.47
US, Detroit: White	3.1	0.19	1.3	0.11
US, Detroit: Black	7.0	0.58	2.4	0.29
US, New Mexico: Non-Hisp. White	2.3	0.28	1.1	0.21
US, New Mexico: Hispanic White	4.5	0.60	2.1	0.38
US, New Mexico: American Indian	10.6	2.28	2,2	0,86
US, Utah	2.0	0.22	1.2	0.16
US, Seattle	3.5	0.19	1.4	0.12
US, SEER: White	3.0	0.07	1.2	0.04
US, SEER: Black	6.5	0.36	2.0	0.17

ASIA	MALE		FEMALE	
*China, Qidong	72.1	1.53	19.1	0.77
China, Shanghai	28.2	0.36	9.8	0.20
China, Tianjin	22.7	0.49	8.9	0.30
Hong Kong	36.2	0.49	9.5	0.24
*India, Bangalore	2.7	0.21	1.3	0.15
*India, Barshi, Paranda and Bhum	1.8	0.46	0,7	0,27
India, Bombay	3.9	0.19	1.9	0.13
*India, Karunagappally	2,7	0,91	1,7	0,72
India, Madras	2.5	0.21	0.5	0.09
*India, Trivandrum	3.1	0.67	1,1	0,38
Israel: All Jews	3.2	0.18	1.6	0.11
Jews born in Israel	1.3	0.39	1.4	0.43
Jews born in America or Europe	3.5	0.27	1.5	0.20
Jews born in Africa or Asia	3.3	0.31	2.1	0.24
Non-Jews	2.6	0.49	1.4	0.35
Japan, Hiroshima	45.5	1.26	11.4	0.56
Japan, Miyagi	15.4	0.46	5.4	0.24
Japan, Nagasaki	33.3	0.79	8.1	0.34
Japan, Osaka	46.7	0.43	11.5	0.19
*Japan, Saga	41.0	1.14	11.3	0.51
Japan, Yamagata	14.8	0.54	5.0	0.28
*Korea, Kangwha	27.7	3.03	7.7	1.46
*Kuwait: Non-Kuwaitis	7.3	1.64	3,1	1,13
*Kuwait: Kuwaitis	7.3	1.19	3.5	0.91
*Philippines, Manila	23.9	0.73	8.0	0.39
Singapore: Chinese	22.1	0.73	5.8	0.34
Singapore: Malay	11.6	1.33	3.9	0.79
Singapore: Indian	6.3	1.01	2,8	1,23
Thailand, Chiang Mai	20.1	0.80	9.7	0.57
*Thailand, Khon Kaen	97.4	2.19	39.0	1.31
*Viet Nam, Hanoi	20.3	0.94	4.9	0.43

* IMPORTANT-SEE NOTES ON POPULATION PAGE

EUROPE	MALE		FEMALE	
Austria, Tyrol	4.2	0.48	2.0	0.29
*Belarus	4.1	0.13	1.9	0.07
*Croatia	4.7	0.21	2.5	0.13
Czech Republic	6.6	0.15	2.7	0.08
Denmark	3.7	0.14	2.0	0.10
Estonia	4.2	0.32	1.9	0.17
Finland	4.8	0.16	2.7	0.10
France, Bas-Rhin	13.1	0.70	2.1	0.26
*France, Calvados	13.3	0.86	1.5	0.25
France, Doubs	6.5	0.67	1.7	0.31
France, Haut-Rhin	11.4	0.76	1.2	0.22
*France, Herault	4.0	0.38	0.7	0.15
France, Isere	9.1	0.56	0.9	0.16
*France, Somme	7.4	0.67	1.2	0.27
*France, Tarn	2.4	0.43	0.8	0.23
Germany, Eastern States	5.1	0.17	2.3	0.09
Germany, Saarland	4.2	0.33	1.6	0.17
Iceland	3.1	0.63	1,0	0,38
Ireland, Southern	1.6	0.33	0.4	0.12
Italy, Ferrara	7.9	1.10	2.9	0.56
Italy, Florence	8.9	0.50	3.3	0.25
Italy, Genoa	10.7	0.58	3.4	0.29
*Italy, Latina	8.0	0.81	4.8	0.59
Italy, Macerata	6.9	1.20	3.1	0.76
Italy, Modena	9.7	0.61	3.5	0.33
Italy, Parma	13.3	0.88	4.9	0.48
Italy, Ragusa	8.5	0.89	3.2	0.50
Italy, Romagna	6.3	0.60	2.1	0.27
Italy, Torino	7.9	0.51	2.4	0.24
Italy, Trieste	18.2	1.37	3.8	0.54
Italy, Varese	13.0	0.69	3.3	0.29
Italy, Veneto	17.7	0.64	5.0	0.30
*Latvia	4.2	0.25	1.8	0.13
Malta	1,8	0,65	0,9	0,36
The Netherlands	1.6	0.07	0.6	0.04
The Netherlands, Eindhoven	1.3	0.23	0.5	0.13
The Netherlands, Maastricht	1.8	0.29	0.7	0.15
Norway	1.8	0.11	1.1	0.09
*Poland, Cracow	4.8	0.49	3.2	0.32
*Poland, Kielce	5.1	0.39	3.3	0.27
*Poland, Lower Silesia	6.7	0.30	4.3	0.20
Poland, Warsaw City	5.0	0.35	2.9	0.22
Slovakia	7.2	0.23	3.1	0.13
Slovenia	3.0	0.24	1.0	0.12
*Spain, Albacete	4.5	0.90	2.8	0.69
Spain, Asturias	8.3	0.49	3.0	0.26
Spain, Basque Country	8.1	0.39	2.0	0.18
Spain, Granada	7.2	0.53	3.4	0.31
Spain, Mallorca	7.2	0.61	2.4	0.29
Spain, Murcia	5.2	0.41	1.8	0.23
Spain, Navarra	8.6	0.67	3.3	0.35
Spain, Tarragona	5.0	0.52	2.1	0.29
Spain, Zaragoza	5.5	0.43	2.3	0.27

	MALE		FEMALE	
Sweden	3.4	0.10	1.8	0.07
*Switzerland, Basel	5.1	0.56	1.0	0.21
Switzerland, Geneva	11.2	0.94	1.6	0.34
Switzerland, Graubunden	4.6	1.04	2.3	0.66
Switzerland, Neuchatel	6.9	1.08	0,8	0,31
Switzerland, St Gall-Appenzell	5.6	0.60	1.3	0.26
Switzerland, Valais	10.9	1.37	2.0	0.50
Switzerland, Vaud	7.0	0.60	1.1	0.24
Switzerland, Zurich	5.9	0.38	1.4	0.17
*UK, England and Wales	2.0	0.04	1.0	0.03
*UK, East Anglia	1.1	0.12	0.4	0.07
*UK, Mersey	2.0	0.15	1.0	0.10
*UK, North Western	2.4	0.13	1.1	0.08
UK, Oxford	1.6	0.14	1.0	0.11
*UK, South Thames	2.1	0.09	0.9	0.06
UK, South Western	1.6	0.11	0.8	0.07
UK, Wessex	2.1	0.14	1.1	0.10
*UK, West Midlands	1.8	0.10	0.7	0.06
UK, Yorkshire	1.7	0.12	1.0	0.09
UK, Scotland	3.1	0.13	1.4	0.08
UK, Scotland, West	2.8	0.17	1.4	0.12
*Yugoslavia, Vojvodina	7.6	0.34	4.8	0.23

OCEANIA

	MALE		FEMALE	
Australian Capital Territory	2.6	0.73	1,0	0,41
Australia, New South Wales	2.5	0.12	0.6	0.05
South Australia	2.1	0.22	0.8	0.15
Australia, Tasmania	2.3	0.42	0,3	0,14
Australia, Victoria	3.0	0.15	0.7	0.07
Western Australia	2.4	0.23	0.9	0.13
*French Polynesia	11.8	2.04	3.6	1.06
New Zealand: Non-Maori	2.9	0.18	1.3	0.12
New Zealand: Maori	12.8	1.73	3.6	0.90
US, Hawaii: White	4.5	0.74	1.5	0.41
US, Hawaii: Japanese	5.0	0.67	1.8	0.35
US, Hawaii: Hawaiian	6.8	1.37	2.6	0.79
US, Hawaii: Filipino	9.1	1.41	1,8	0,60
US, Hawaii: Chinese	10.5	2.13	3,2	1,16

* IMPORTANT-SEE NOTES ON POPULATION PAGE

AGE-STANDARDIZED INCIDENCE
RATES AND STANDARD ERRORS (per 100,000)
Gallbladder etc. (ICD-9 156)

AFRICA	MALE		FEMALE	
*Algeria, Setif	3.6	0.72	10.2	0.95
*France, La Reunion	1.3	0.36	2.6	0.43
*Mali, Bamako	0,2	0,19	-	-
*Uganda, Kyadondo	-	-	-	-
*Zimbabwe, Harare: African	0,5	0,41	0,8	0,63
*Zimbabwe, Harare: European	-	-	-	-

AMERICA, CENTRAL AND SOUTH	MALE		FEMALE	
*Argentina, Concordia	3.7	1.15	4.7	1.18
*Brazil, Belem	1.7	0.46	3.1	0.53
*Brazil, Goiania	2.1	0.50	4.6	0.65
*Brazil, Porto Alegre	2.0	0.39	6.9	0.56
Colombia, Cali	3.9	0.43	8.3	0.56
*Costa Rica	2.6	0.24	5.3	0.33
*Ecuador, Quito	5.5	0.59	8.6	0.67
*Peru, Lima	2.0	0.22	4.3	0.32
Peru, Trujillo	3.8	0.98	9.3	1.41
US, Puerto Rico	1.4	0.14	2.3	0.16
*Uruguay, Montevideo	2.9	0.33	4.2	0.34

AMERICA, NORTH	MALE		FEMALE	
Canada	1.8	0.05	2.1	0.05
Canada, Alberta	1.5	0.15	1.9	0.16
Canada, British Columbia	1.8	0.13	1.9	0.12
Canada, Manitoba	2.1	0.24	2.0	0.21
Canada, New Brunswick	1.1	0.21	1.6	0.26
Canada, Newfoundland	1.0	0.24	2.4	0.39
Canada, Northwest Territories	2,9	1,39	4,0	1,89
Canada, Nova Scotia	1.2	0.20	1.7	0.23
Canada, Ontario	1.8	0.07	2.0	0.07
Canada, Prince Edward Island	2.1	0.69	1.6	0.61
Canada, Quebec	2.2	0.10	2.3	0.09
Canada, Saskatchewan	1.7	0.21	2.2	0.24
Canada, Yukon	3,5	2,05	2,4	1,68
US, Cent. Calif.: Non-Hisp. White	1.5	0.18	1.2	0.14
US, Cent. Calif.: Hispanic	2.9	0.55	4.8	0.67
US, Los Angeles: Non-Hisp. White	1.5	0.10	1.3	0.09
US, Los Angeles: Hispanic White	2.1	0.24	4.2	0.28
US, Los Angeles: Black	1.5	0.27	1.4	0.21
US, Los Angeles: Chinese	1.9	0.53	2.1	0.52
US, Los Angeles: Filipino	1,6	0,55	1.9	0.57
US, Los Angeles: Korean	2,7	0,97	6.3	1.33
US, Los Angeles: Japanese	2.7	0.77	1.8	0.60
US, San Francisco: Non-Hisp. White	1.4	0.14	1.3	0.12
US, San Francisco: Hispanic White	1.9	0.45	1.7	0.37
US, San Francisco: Black	1.0	0.32	1.0	0.27
US, San Francisco: Chinese	2.4	0.52	2.1	0.47
US, San Francisco: Filipino	2.1	0.70	2.5	0.72
US, San Francisco: Japanese	2,8	1,44	3,2	1,16
US, Connecticut: White	1.5	0.12	1.6	0.11
US, Connecticut: Black	2.6	0.74	1.6	0.48
US, Atlanta: White	1.6	0.22	1.2	0.16
US, Atlanta: Black	1.7	0.45	1.5	0.33
US, Iowa	1.5	0.12	1.8	0.12

	MALE		FEMALE	
US, Central Louisiana: White	1.6	0.43	1.7	0.43
US, Central Louisiana: Black	1,8	1,10	1,4	0,86
US, New Orleans: White	1.7	0.30	1.3	0.23
US, New Orleans: Black	1.2	0.38	2.4	0.47
US, Detroit: White	1.6	0.13	2.1	0.13
US, Detroit: Black	1.2	0.22	1.7	0.24
US, New Mexico: Non-Hisp. White	1.1	0.20	1.1	0.17
US, New Mexico: Hispanic White	1.6	0.35	4.8	0.59
US, New Mexico: American Indian	4.9	1.52	12.5	2.20
US, Utah	0.8	0.14	1.7	0.19
US, Seattle	1.6	0.12	1.5	0.11
US, SEER: White	1.4	0.05	1.7	0.05
US, SEER: Black	1.4	0.16	1.5	0.15

ASIA	MALE		FEMALE	
*China, Qidong	1.4	0.22	1.1	0.18
China, Shanghai	2.5	0.11	3.6	0.12
China, Tianjin	2.4	0.16	1.9	0.14
Hong Kong	3.6	0.16	2.7	0.12
*India, Bangalore	0.5	0.09	0.7	0.11
*India, Barshi, Paranda and Bhum	0,1	0,12	0,2	0,15
India, Bombay	1.8	0.13	2.7	0.15
*India, Karunagappally	-	-	-	-
India, Madras	0.5	0.09	0.5	0.09
*India, Trivandrum	0,2	0,15	0,6	0,29
Israel: All Jews	1.6	0.12	2.4	0.14
Jews born in Israel	1.1	0.36	0.9	0.31
Jews born in America or Europe	1.4	0.15	2.6	0.20
Jews born in Africa or Asia	1.8	0.23	2.4	0.25
Non-Jews	1.5	0.41	3.2	0.56
Japan, Hiroshima	6.1	0.46	5.9	0.39
Japan, Miyagi	7.9	0.32	6.8	0.26
Japan, Nagasaki	7.7	0.36	7.1	0.30
Japan, Osaka	6.2	0.16	6.0	0.13
*Japan, Saga	7.7	0.48	7.8	0.42
Japan, Yamagata	6.7	0.35	6.9	0.31
*Korea, Kangwha	4.8	1.49	3.8	0.97
*Kuwait: Non-Kuwaitis	1.6	0.79	3.3	1.07
*Kuwait: Kuwaitis	1.9	0.62	1,4	0,54
*Philippines, Manila	1.4	0.19	1.6	0.18
Singapore: Chinese	1.7	0.20	1.9	0.19
Singapore: Malay	1.7	0.52	2.0	0.57
Singapore: Indian	1,2	0,42	1,4	0,63
Thailand, Chiang Mai	3.3	0.33	3.0	0.32
*Thailand, Khon Kaen	1.8	0.30	2.1	0.32
*Viet Nam, Hanoi	0,3	0,12	0,1	0,07

* IMPORTANT-SEE NOTES ON POPULATION PAGE

EUROPE	MALE		FEMALE	
Austria, Tyrol	3.0	0.41	2.6	0.30
*Belarus	1.0	0.06	1.2	0.06
*Croatia	2.1	0.13	3.1	0.14
Czech Republic	4.6	0.12	7.1	0.13
Denmark	1.8	0.10	2.3	0.10
Estonia	1.3	0.17	1.8	0.16
Finland	2.1	0.11	3.4	0.11
France, Bas-Rhin	2.2	0.29	2.7	0.26
*France, Calvados	1.5	0.27	1.7	0.28
France, Doubs	1.2	0.29	2.0	0.34
France, Haut-Rhin	2.2	0.34	3.3	0.35
*France, Herault	1.3	0.21	1.5	0.22
France, Isere	1.4	0.21	1.3	0.18
*France, Somme	1.2	0.25	2.0	0.32
*France, Tarn	0.9	0.25	1.9	0.36
Germany, Eastern States	3.6	0.14	6.8	0.15
Germany, Saarland	3.0	0.28	4.8	0.29
Iceland	1.5	0.46	1.4	0.40
Ireland, Southern	1.7	0.31	2.6	0.38
Italy, Ferrara	3.0	0.62	3.9	0.75
Italy, Florence	2.8	0.26	2.9	0.24
Italy, Genoa	3.4	0.33	3.8	0.29
*Italy, Latina	3.5	0.55	5.6	0.64
Italy, Macerata	3.0	0.80	1.7	0.54
Italy, Modena	2.1	0.26	2.8	0.29
Italy, Parma	3.3	0.42	3.2	0.38
Italy, Ragusa	3.9	0.62	3.8	0.52
Italy, Romagna	2.1	0.31	2.3	0.27
Italy, Torino	3.9	0.35	4.1	0.31
Italy, Trieste	5.2	0.73	4.8	0.54
Italy, Varese	3.0	0.33	3.9	0.32
Italy, Veneto	2.5	0.24	3.3	0.24
*Latvia	0.8	0.10	1.0	0.09
Malta	0,9	0,48	1,1	0,44
The Netherlands	2.1	0.07	2.6	0.07
The Netherlands, Eindhoven	2.1	0.27	2.7	0.27
The Netherlands, Maastricht	2.5	0.30	2.6	0.26
Norway	1.1	0.09	1.3	0.08
*Poland, Cracow	4.5	0.47	7.0	0.48
*Poland, Kielce	2.5	0.28	4.7	0.33
*Poland, Lower Silesia	2.5	0.19	7.1	0.26
Poland, Warsaw City	4.1	0.31	7.5	0.34
Slovakia	3.7	0.16	6.4	0.19
Slovenia	2.6	0.22	4.0	0.22
*Spain, Albacete	2.5	0.72	4.1	0.77
Spain, Asturias	1.1	0.17	2.2	0.23
Spain, Basque Country	2.8	0.23	2.9	0.19
Spain, Granada	2.9	0.33	4.7	0.37
Spain, Mallorca	2.2	0.33	3.2	0.33
Spain, Murcia	2.0	0.24	3.5	0.29
Spain, Navarra	3.0	0.37	3.6	0.38
Spain, Tarragona	1.6	0.26	2.7	0.33
Spain, Zaragoza	2.5	0.28	2.7	0.23

	MALE		FEMALE	
Sweden	2.6	0.09	4.1	0.10
*Switzerland, Basel	1.3	0.27	2.0	0.30
Switzerland, Geneva	1.6	0.33	2.1	0.32
Switzerland, Graubunden	1.4	0.49	2.9	0.70
Switzerland, Neuchatel	1.7	0.54	2.4	0.55
Switzerland, St Gall-Appenzell	1.9	0.34	3.1	0.37
Switzerland, Valais	1.2	0.39	2.9	0.60
Switzerland, Vaud	2.4	0.34	2.5	0.31
Switzerland, Zurich	2.6	0.25	2.7	0.23
*UK, England and Wales	1.2	0.03	1.2	0.03
*UK, East Anglia	1.4	0.13	1.4	0.12
*UK, Mersey	1.0	0.10	1.3	0.11
*UK, North Western	1.1	0.09	1.2	0.08
UK, Oxford	1.1	0.11	1.2	0.11
*UK, South Thames	1.1	0.06	1.0	0.06
UK, South Western	1.1	0.09	1.1	0.08
UK, Wessex	1.0	0.09	0.9	0.08
*UK, West Midlands	2.0	0.10	1.8	0.09
UK, Yorkshire	1.1	0.09	1.1	0.08
UK, Scotland	1.4	0.09	1.5	0.08
UK, Scotland, West	1.5	0.13	1.6	0.11
*Yugoslavia, Vojvodina	2.6	0.20	5.4	0.25

OCEANIA

	MALE		FEMALE		
Australian Capital Territory	1,8	0,61	1.8	0.51	
Australia, New South Wales	1.9	0.10	1.9	0.10	
South Australia	1.9	0.19	3.1	0.24	
Australia, Tasmania	1.6	0.34	2.1	0.36	
Australia, Victoria	2.2	0.13	2.2	0.12	
Western Australia	1.7	0.19	1.7	0.19	
*French Polynesia	3,5	1,26	1,6	0,76	m
New Zealand: Non-Maori	1.3	0.12	1.4	0.11	
New Zealand: Maori	2,4	0,95	1,2	0,53	
US, Hawaii: White	1.6	0.45	2.0	0.47	
US, Hawaii: Japanese	2.4	0.45	1.9	0.33	
US, Hawaii: Hawaiian	2,0	0,75	1,4	0,59	
US, Hawaii: Filipino	1.5	0.48	1,2	0,51	
US, Hawaii: Chinese	2,6	0,94	3.3	1.12	

* IMPORTANT-SEE NOTES ON POPULATION PAGE

AGE-STANDARDIZED INCIDENCE
RATES AND STANDARD ERRORS (per 100,000)
Pancreas (ICD-9 157)

AFRICA	MALE		FEMALE	
*Algeria, Setif	1.8	0.51	0,7	0,26
*France, La Reunion	2.8	0.52	1.9	0.38
*Mali, Bamako	2.4	0.61	0,8	0,36
*Uganda, Kyadondo	1,4	0,64	0,7	0,38
*Zimbabwe, Harare: African	5.9	1.21	8.0	1.84
*Zimbabwe, Harare: European	4,2	1,90	6,1	2,29

AMERICA, CENTRAL AND SOUTH				
*Argentina, Concordia	8.3	1.79	5.1	1.16
*Brazil, Belem	5.5	0.82	2.2	0.42
*Brazil, Goiania	4.6	0.73	4.0	0.60
*Brazil, Porto Alegre	9.0	0.80	6.3	0.54
Colombia, Cali	5.4	0.51	3.8	0.37
*Costa Rica	6.1	0.37	5.2	0.32
*Ecuador, Quito	3.8	0.49	4.4	0.49
*Peru, Lima	3.0	0.28	3.6	0.30
Peru, Trujillo	5.6	1.25	3.0	0.81
US, Puerto Rico	5.3	0.27	3.0	0.18
*Uruguay, Montevideo	8.6	0.58	5.9	0.40

AMERICA, NORTH				
Canada	7.7	0.10	5.5	0.07
Canada, Alberta	8.7	0.36	5.7	0.28
Canada, British Columbia	6.8	0.25	5.1	0.20
Canada, Manitoba	7.6	0.46	5.7	0.38
Canada, New Brunswick	7.3	0.57	4.4	0.41
Canada, Newfoundland	4.3	0.54	3.0	0.44
Canada, Northwest Territories	7.2	2.34	4,9	1,89
Canada, Nova Scotia	8.9	0.58	5.7	0.41
Canada, Ontario	7.5	0.16	5.5	0.12
Canada, Prince Edward Island	10.6	1.60	6.5	1.16
Canada, Quebec	8.6	0.21	5.7	0.15
Canada, Saskatchewan	6.5	0.44	5.3	0.37
Canada, Yukon	4,1	2,13	4,6	2,69
US, Cent. Calif.: Non-Hisp. White	7.6	0.40	5.5	0.31
US, Cent. Calif.: Hispanic	7.1	0.85	5.7	0.72
US, Los Angeles: Non-Hisp. White	8.1	0.25	5.6	0.19
US, Los Angeles: Hispanic White	7.2	0.44	5.2	0.32
US, Los Angeles: Black	10.5	0.70	8.2	0.51
US, Los Angeles: Chinese	3.9	0.80	2.5	0.59
US, Los Angeles: Filipino	4.2	0.90	5.4	0.99
US, Los Angeles: Korean	4.8	1.31	5.4	1.19
US, Los Angeles: Japanese	7.5	1.23	6.4	1.05
US, San Francisco: Non-Hisp. White	8.0	0.32	6.2	0.26
US, San Francisco: Hispanic White	6.3	0.84	5.3	0.67
US, San Francisco: Black	13.1	1.16	11.0	0.92
US, San Francisco: Chinese	6.1	0.83	4.9	0.72
US, San Francisco: Filipino	5.9	1.20	5.2	1.04
US, San Francisco: Japanese	7.7	2.38	3,6	1,26
US, Connecticut: White	7.9	0.28	5.9	0.22
US, Connecticut: Black	8.3	1.31	8.0	1.06
US, Atlanta: White	7.4	0.46	4.6	0.31
US, Atlanta: Black	10.5	1.11	8.9	0.81
US, Iowa	7.5	0.28	5.2	0.21

	MALE		FEMALE	
US, Central Louisiana: White	8.0	1.06	6.6	0.90
US, Central Louisiana: Black	20.8	3.64	8.0	1.86
US, New Orleans: White	9.1	0.68	6.2	0.47
US, New Orleans: Black	9.2	1.09	9.3	0.91
US, Detroit: White	8.5	0.30	5.8	0.22
US, Detroit: Black	12.9	0.78	9.2	0.55
US, New Mexico: Non-Hisp. White	8.2	0.55	5.2	0.40
US, New Mexico: Hispanic White	7.7	0.79	5.2	0.59
US, New Mexico: American Indian	6.7	1.73	6.2	1.52
US, Utah	5.9	0.39	4.4	0.30
US, Seattle	7.3	0.28	6.6	0.24
US, SEER: White	7.7	0.11	5.7	0.09
US, SEER: Black	11.8	0.49	9.3	0.37

ASIA				
*China, Qidong	7.0	0.49	4.8	0.37
China, Shanghai	6.3	0.17	4.1	0.13
China, Tianjin	5.4	0.24	3.4	0.18
Hong Kong	4.0	0.16	2.9	0.13
*India, Bangalore	1.5	0.16	0.9	0.12
*India, Barshi, Paranda and Bhum	0,5	0,24	0,2	0,16
India, Bombay	2.3	0.14	1.8	0.13
*India, Karunagappally	2,1	0,96	0,2	0,20
India, Madras	1.4	0.15	0.7	0.11
*India, Trivandrum	2.4	0.60	1,1	0,38
Israel: All Jews	7.2	0.26	5.7	0.21
Jews born in Israel	7.0	0.95	5.3	0.77
Jews born in America or Europe	8.0	0.40	5.9	0.31
Jews born in Africa or Asia	5.8	0.41	4.8	0.35
Non-Jews	4.0	0.67	2.9	0.53
Japan, Hiroshima	9.0	0.56	5.7	0.38
Japan, Miyagi	10.9	0.38	5.5	0.24
Japan, Nagasaki	9.0	0.40	4.8	0.24
Japan, Osaka	9.6	0.20	5.4	0.13
*Japan, Saga	9.5	0.53	5.5	0.34
Japan, Yamagata	9.5	0.43	4.7	0.26
*Korea, Kangwha	7.2	1.75	2.7	0.82
*Kuwait: Non-Kuwaitis	7.5	1.98	3.0	1.02
*Kuwait: Kuwaitis	4.8	0.96	3.5	0.94
*Philippines, Manila	4.7	0.34	3.3	0.26
Singapore: Chinese	4.9	0.34	3.3	0.25
Singapore: Malay	2.0	0.56	1,2	0,43
Singapore: Indian	1,7	0,57	1.5	0,79
Thailand, Chiang Mai	2.7	0.29	2.4	0.28
*Thailand, Khon Kaen	0.9	0.21	0.7	0.17
*Viet Nam, Hanoi	2.0	0.30	0.8	0.18

m

* IMPORTANT-SEE NOTES ON POPULATION PAGE

EUROPE	MALE		FEMALE	
Austria, Tyrol	7.0	0.63	5.7	0.45
*Belarus	8.6	0.19	3.6	0.09
*Croatia	9.0	0.28	5.0	0.18
Czech Republic	11.4	0.19	6.5	0.12
Denmark	7.8	0.20	6.4	0.17
Estonia	10.7	0.52	5.7	0.29
Finland	9.5	0.22	7.0	0.16
France, Bas-Rhin	6.9	0.51	3.8	0.33
*France, Calvados	6.0	0.57	3.7	0.40
France, Doubs	5.4	0.62	2.2	0.36
France, Haut-Rhin	6.3	0.57	3.1	0.35
*France, Herault	3.1	0.33	2.0	0.25
France, Isere	4.6	0.39	2.8	0.29
*France, Somme	4.3	0.51	2.6	0.36
*France, Tarn	3.4	0.51	1.4	0.29
Germany, Eastern States	7.3	0.20	4.5	0.12
Germany, Saarland	6.9	0.42	4.2	0.28
Iceland	8.3	1.05	6.2	0.87
Ireland, Southern	7.7	0.69	4.6	0.50
Italy, Ferrara	7.2	1.02	6.1	0.84
Italy, Florence	7.0	0.42	5.0	0.31
Italy, Genoa	8.2	0.52	5.3	0.34
*Italy, Latina	5.4	0.67	3.7	0.50
Italy, Macerata	7.6	1.27	4.7	0.95
Italy, Modena	7.8	0.55	5.3	0.42
Italy, Parma	7.8	0.67	5.5	0.49
Italy, Ragusa	6.0	0.74	3.6	0.53
Italy, Romagna	6.6	0.55	4.6	0.42
Italy, Torino	7.8	0.50	4.5	0.33
Italy, Trieste	13.0	1.19	6.5	0.64
Italy, Varese	8.8	0.57	5.7	0.39
Italy, Veneto	9.5	0.47	6.4	0.33
*Latvia	11.6	0.40	5.2	0.21
Malta	9.9	1.48	3.5	0.80
The Netherlands	6.8	0.13	4.6	0.10
The Netherlands, Eindhoven	6.0	0.46	4.0	0.35
The Netherlands, Maastricht	5.8	0.45	4.5	0.35
Norway	7.9	0.22	5.7	0.18
*Poland, Cracow	9.5	0.69	6.0	0.44
*Poland, Kielce	7.3	0.48	4.6	0.32
*Poland, Lower Silesia	10.6	0.39	6.4	0.25
Poland, Warsaw City	7.9	0.44	5.0	0.28
Slovakia	10.7	0.28	5.4	0.17
Slovenia	8.1	0.39	5.0	0.25
*Spain, Albacete	4.2	0.87	3.1	0.75
Spain, Asturias	5.3	0.40	2.5	0.23
Spain, Basque Country	6.4	0.34	3.8	0.23
Spain, Granada	5.3	0.47	3.2	0.32
Spain, Mallorca	6.1	0.56	3.3	0.36
Spain, Murcia	4.2	0.36	2.2	0.23
Spain, Navarra	6.5	0.59	3.9	0.41
Spain, Tarragona	4.1	0.45	3.1	0.36
Spain, Zaragoza	5.9	0.44	3.4	0.29

	MALE		FEMALE		
Sweden	7.0	0.14	5.8	0.12	
*Switzerland, Basel	6.0	0.60	4.5	0.47	
Switzerland, Geneva	9.2	0.85	6.3	0.61	
Switzerland, Graubunden	10.2	1.44	6.7	1.10	
Switzerland, Neuchatel	7.9	1.19	4.0	0.69	
Switzerland, St Gall-Appenzell	9.0	0.74	6.6	0.57	
Switzerland, Valais	8.6	1.14	5.6	0.82	
Switzerland, Vaud	9.2	0.68	5.9	0.48	
Switzerland, Zurich	7.4	0.42	5.4	0.31	
*UK, England and Wales	7.4	0.08	5.3	0.06	
*UK, East Anglia	6.2	0.28	4.9	0.23	
*UK, Mersey	6.4	0.26	5.6	0.23	
*UK, North Western	7.4	0.23	5.3	0.17	
UK, Oxford	7.4	0.30	5.9	0.24	
*UK, South Thames	7.9	0.18	5.6	0.13	
UK, South Western	7.3	0.23	4.8	0.17	
UK, Wessex	6.7	0.24	5.0	0.19	
*UK, West Midlands	7.4	0.19	5.2	0.15	
UK, Yorkshire	6.8	0.23	5.1	0.18	
UK, Scotland	8.1	0.21	5.5	0.15	
UK, Scotland, West	8.2	0.30	5.4	0.21	
*Yugoslavia, Vojvodina	7.4	0.33	4.7	0.23	

OCEANIA	MALE		FEMALE		
Australian Capital Territory	6.4	1.19	4.4	0.81	
Australia, New South Wales	6.9	0.20	4.9	0.15	
South Australia	6.8	0.38	4.8	0.29	
Australia, Tasmania	5.9	0.63	4.6	0.52	
Australia, Victoria	6.8	0.22	4.4	0.16	
Western Australia	5.9	0.37	4.5	0.30	
*French Polynesia	4.4	1.26	3,5	1,26	f
New Zealand: Non-Maori	7.3	0.27	4.6	0.20	
New Zealand: Maori	9.8	1.71	6.7	1.29	
US, Hawaii: White	8.5	0.98	5.7	0.80	
US, Hawaii: Japanese	5.8	0.67	5.9	0.63	
US, Hawaii: Hawaiian	8.8	1.54	7.2	1.30	
US, Hawaii: Filipino	4.5	0.96	4.1	0.99	
US, Hawaii: Chinese	5.8	1.33	4.0	1.06	

* IMPORTANT-SEE NOTES ON POPULATION PAGE

AGE-STANDARDIZED INCIDENCE
RATES AND STANDARD ERRORS (per 100,000)
Nose, sinuses etc. (ICD-9 160)

	MALE		FEMALE	
AFRICA				
*Algeria, Setif	0,6	0,29	0,4	0,18
*France, La Reunion	1.0	0.31	0,2	0,14
*Mali, Bamako	0,7	0,33	0,4	0,23
*Uganda, Kyadondo	1,5	0,72	0,3	0,14 m
*Zimbabwe, Harare: African	1,4	0,58	1,4	0,77
*Zimbabwe, Harare: European	3,1	1,85	1,0	0,71
AMERICA, CENTRAL AND SOUTH				
*Argentina, Concordia	1,7	0,85	0,4	0,36
*Brazil, Belem	0,6	0,26	0,2	0,12
*Brazil, Goiania	0,7	0,27	0,4	0,17
*Brazil, Porto Alegre	0,3	0,13	0,3	0,12
Colombia, Cali	1.1	0.23	0.8	0.18
*Costa Rica	0.5	0.10	0.2	0,06
*Ecuador, Quito	0,4	0,16	0,4	0,13
*Peru, Lima	0.9	0.14	0.4	0.10
Peru, Trujillo	0,5	0,37	0,5	0,33
US, Puerto Rico	0.7	0.10	0.3	0.05
*Uruguay, Montevideo	0.8	0.19	0.4	0.11
AMERICA, NORTH				
Canada	0.6	0.03	0.4	0.02
Canada, Alberta	0.6	0.10	0.4	0.07
Canada, British Columbia	0.6	0.08	0.5	0.07
Canada, Manitoba	0.3	0.10	0.2	0.08
Canada, New Brunswick	0.6	0.16	0.4	0.15
Canada, Newfoundland	0.8	0.25	0.4	0,16
Canada, Northwest Territories	0,5	0,48	-	-
Canada, Nova Scotia	0.7	0.16	0.4	0.12
Canada, Ontario	0.7	0.05	0.4	0.03
Canada, Prince Edward Island	1,0	0,59	-	-
Canada, Quebec	0.6	0.05	0.4	0.04
Canada, Saskatchewan	0.6	0.14	0.2	0.06
Canada, Yukon	-	-	-	-
US, Cent. Calif.: Non-Hisp. White	0.8	0.14	0.4	0.08
US, Cent. Calif.: Hispanic	0,3	0,15	-	-
US, Los Angeles: Non-Hisp. White	0.7	0.07	0.3	0.05
US, Los Angeles: Hispanic White	0.5	0.11	0.5	0.10
US, Los Angeles: Black	1.0	0.21	0.3	0.11
US, Los Angeles: Chinese	0,4	0,25	0,2	0,15
US, Los Angeles: Filipino	0,4	0,28	0,7	0,36
US, Los Angeles: Korean	-	-	0,2	0,24
US, Los Angeles: Japanese	0,3	0,33	-	-
US, San Francisco: Non-Hisp. White	0.6	0.10	0.2	0.05
US, San Francisco: Hispanic White	0,6	0,25	0,6	0,23
US, San Francisco: Black	0,5	0,22	0,3	0,16
US, San Francisco: Chinese	0,9	0,36	0,4	0,23
US, San Francisco: Filipino	0,9	0,49	0,4	0,25
US, San Francisco: Japanese	0,8	0,76	-	-
US, Connecticut: White	0.5	0.07	0.4	0.06
US, Connecticut: Black	0,6	0,35	0,6	0,26
US, Atlanta: White	0.7	0.13	0.4	0.10
US, Atlanta: Black	0,8	0,30	0,3	0,14
US, Iowa	0.6	0.09	0.4	0.06

	MALE		FEMALE	
US, Central Louisiana: White	0.3	0,22	0,3	0,20
US, Central Louisiana: Black	0,3	0,27	0,4	0,37
US, New Orleans: White	0.7	0.20	0.2	0,09
US, New Orleans: Black	1.4	0.41	0.8	0,29
US, Detroit: White	0.7	0.09	0.4	0.06
US, Detroit: Black	0,4	0,13	0.8	0.18
US, New Mexico: Non-Hisp. White	0.5	0.14	0.7	0.16
US, New Mexico: Hispanic White	0,7	0,22	0,2	0,13
US, New Mexico: American Indian	0,3	0,32	1,5	0,70
US, Utah	0.4	0.10	0.4	0.10
US, Seattle	0.7	0.09	0.3	0.05
US, SEER: White	0.6	0.03	0.4	0.02
US, SEER: Black	0.5	0.10	0.5	0.09
ASIA				
*China, Qidong	0.3	0.09	0.2	0,08
China, Shanghai	0.7	0.06	0.4	0.04
China, Tianjin	0.6	0.08	0.4	0.06
Hong Kong	0.9	0.08	0.4	0.05
*India, Bangalore	0.7	0.10	0.6	0.10
*India, Barshi, Paranda and Bhum	0.3	0,19	0,2	0,16
India, Bombay	1.0	0.09	0.7	0.08
*India, Karunagappally	0,6	0,43	0,2	0,21
India, Madras	0.9	0.13	0.7	0.11
*India, Trivandrum	0.9	0,39	0,7	0,30
Israel: All Jews	0.4	0.06	0.4	0.06
Jews born in Israel	0,3	0,22	0,4	0,19
Jews born in America or Europe	0.3	0.09	0.3	0.08
Jews born in Africa or Asia	1.0	0.51	0.2	0,08
Non-Jews	0,3	0,15	0,2	0,14
Japan, Hiroshima	1.1	0.19	0.4	0.11
Japan, Miyagi	1.4	0.14	0.7	0.09
Japan, Nagasaki	1.2	0.14	0.5	0.09
Japan, Osaka	0.9	0.06	0.5	0.04
*Japan, Saga	1.4	0.21	0.5	0.11
Japan, Yamagata	1.3	0.17	0.2	0.05
*Korea, Kangwha	-	-	0,3	0,28
*Kuwait: Non-Kuwaitis	1,5	1,00	0,1	0,06
*Kuwait: Kuwaitis	-	-	0,5	0,29
*Philippines, Manila	1.5	0.18	0.9	0.12
Singapore: Chinese	0,9	0,14	0,4	0,09
Singapore: Malay	0,5	0,26	1,0	0,40
Singapore: Indian	0,8	0,38	0,5	0,40
Thailand, Chiang Mai	1.0	0.18	0.6	0.14
*Thailand, Khon Kaen	0.4	0.14	0,4	0,12
*Viet Nam, Hanoi	1.1	0.21	1.0	0.19

* IMPORTANT-SEE NOTES ON POPULATION PAGE

AGE-STANDARDIZED INCIDENCE
RATES AND STANDARD ERRORS (per 100,000)
Nose, sinuses etc. (ICD-9 160) (contd)

EUROPE	MALE		FEMALE	
Austria, Tyrol	0,2	0,10	0,3	0,13
*Belarus	0.6	0.05	0.3	0.03
*Croatia	0.5	0.07	0.3	0.04
Czech Republic	0.5	0.04	0.3	0.03
Denmark	0.9	0.07	0.5	0.05
Estonia	0.7	0.13	0.4	0.09
Finland	0.6	0.06	0.2	0.03
France, Bas-Rhin	0.9	0.18	0.2	0,08
*France, Calvados	1.5	0.29	0.3	0,12
France, Doubs	1.0	0.27	0,1	0,09
France, Haut-Rhin	1.5	0.27	0.2	0,09
*France, Herault	1.2	0.22	0.6	0.17
France, Isere	1.1	0.19	0.3	0.10
*France, Somme	1.3	0.30	0.4	0.15
*France, Tarn	1.1	0.31	0.2	0,12
Germany, Eastern States	0.6	0.06	0.2	0.03
Germany, Saarland	0.5	0.12	0.2	0.07
Iceland	1.2	0.39	0,6	0,32
Ireland, Southern	0.3	0,12	0.3	0,14
Italy, Ferrara	0,7	0,32	0,1	0,11
Italy, Florence	0.9	0.17	0,1	0,06
Italy, Genoa	1.1	0.25	0.4	0.12
*Italy, Latina	0,5	0,21	0,1	0,08
Italy, Macerata	1,1	0,47	-	-
Italy, Modena	0,1	0,07	0,2	0,10
Italy, Parma	0.8	0.23	0,4	0,14
Italy, Ragusa	0,4	0,20	0,1	0,08
Italy, Romagna	0.6	0.20	0,4	0,16
Italy, Torino	0.5	0.12	0,2	0,09
Italy, Trieste	1,0	0,42	0,3	0,15
Italy, Varese	0.9	0.22	0.4	0.11
Italy, Veneto	1.0	0.18	0,1	0,04
*Latvia	0.6	0.09	0.2	0.04
Malta	1,2	0,59	0.5	0,32
The Netherlands	0.8	0.05	0.3	0.03
The Netherlands, Eindhoven	0.9	0.20	0.3	0,09
The Netherlands, Maastricht	0.8	0.16	0.4	0.12
Norway	0.7	0.07	0.3	0.04
*Poland, Cracow	0,4	0,14	0,2	0,07
*Poland, Kielce	0.6	0.14	0.3	0.09
*Poland, Lower Silesia	0.6	0.10	0.3	0.06
Poland, Warsaw City	0.8	0.15	0.2	0.07
Slovakia	0.7	0.07	0.3	0.04
Slovenia	0.8	0.12	0.4	0.07
*Spain, Albacete	-	-	0,1	0,15
Spain, Asturias	1.4	0.23	0.6	0.13
Spain, Basque Country	1.0	0.13	0.2	0.05
Spain, Granada	0.8	0.19	0,1	0,05
Spain, Mallorca	0.8	0.21	0,2	0,11
Spain, Murcia	0.4	0.12	0.3	0.10
Spain, Navarra	0.5	0.17	0.3	0,12
Spain, Tarragona	0,4	0,15	0,1	0,04
Spain, Zaragoza	0.6	0.13	0.2	0.07

	MALE		FEMALE	
Sweden	0.6	0.04	0.3	0.03
*Switzerland, Basel	0.9	0.25	0,2	0,11
Switzerland, Geneva	0.7	0.23	0,5	0,19
Switzerland, Graubunden	0,2	0,23	0,1	0,08
Switzerland, Neuchatel	0,7	0,38	0,3	0,20
Switzerland, St Gall-Appenzell	1.0	0.25	0,3	0,14
Switzerland, Valais	0,4	0,23	0,8	0,34
Switzerland, Vaud	0.5	0.15	0.5	0.14
Switzerland, Zurich	0.6	0.14	0,1	0,06
*UK, England and Wales	0.6	0.03	0.3	0.02
*UK, East Anglia	0.7	0.10	0.3	0.06
*UK, Mersey	0.5	0.08	0.5	0.07
*UK, North Western	0.6	0.07	0.4	0.05
UK, Oxford	0.6	0.09	0.4	0.07
*UK, South Thames	0.6	0.05	0.3	0.04
UK, South Western	0.5	0.06	0.3	0.05
UK, Wessex	0.6	0.07	0.3	0.06
*UK, West Midlands	0.6	0.06	0.4	0.05
UK, Yorkshire	0.6	0.07	0.3	0.04
UK, Scotland	0.5	0.06	0.3	0.04
UK, Scotland, West	0.5	0.08	0.3	0.05
*Yugoslavia, Vojvodina	0.3	0.07	0.3	0.06

OCEANIA	MALE		FEMALE	
Australian Capital Territory	1,1	0,43	0,2	0,18
Australia, New South Wales	0.7	0.06	0.3	0.04
South Australia	0.5	0.11	0.2	0.07
Australia, Tasmania	2.0	0.38	0,4	0,18
Australia, Victoria	0.7	0.08	0.3	0.04
Western Australia	0.7	0.13	0.2	0.06
*French Polynesia	2,0	0,84	0,9	0,57
New Zealand: Non-Maori	0.6	0.08	0.5	0.07
New Zealand: Maori	0,2	0,17	-	-
US, Hawaii: White	0,7	0,28	0,5	0,25
US, Hawaii: Japanese	0.8	0.26	0,4	0,21
US, Hawaii: Hawaiian	1,0	0,50	1,1	0,47
US, Hawaii: Filipino	0,3	0,27	0,7	0,42
US, Hawaii: Chinese	0,5	0,50	0,6	0,43

* IMPORTANT-SEE NOTES ON POPULATION PAGE

AGE-STANDARDIZED INCIDENCE
RATES AND STANDARD ERRORS (per 100,000)
Larynx (ICD-9 161)

	MALE		FEMALE	
AFRICA				
*Algeria, Setif	5.7	0.89	0,2	0,14
*France, La Reunion	8.3	0.88	0,3	0,13
*Mali, Bamako	2.3	0.62	0,7	0,33
*Uganda, Kyadondo	0,8	0,37	1,8	0,76
*Zimbabwe, Harare: African	4.5	1.08	1,0	0,70
*Zimbabwe, Harare: European	9.9	3.01	0,0	0,00 f
AMERICA, CENTRAL AND SOUTH				
*Argentina, Concordia	8.6	1.78	1,8	0,74
*Brazil, Belem	8.7	1.07	0,5	0,20 mf
*Brazil, Goiania	7.7	0.91	1.1	0.31
*Brazil, Porto Alegre	10.5	0.87	1.3	0.25
Colombia, Cali	5.2	0.50	1.1	0.22 f
*Costa Rica	4.0	0.30	0.6	0.11
*Ecuador, Quito	1.5	0.30	0,2	0,10
*Peru, Lima	2.4	0.25	0.4	0.10
Peru, Trujillo	2,2	0,78	0,3	0,18
US, Puerto Rico	5.8	0.29	0.8	0.10
*Uruguay, Montevideo	12.2	0.71	1.0	0.19
AMERICA, NORTH				
Canada	6.3	0.09	1.2	0.04
Canada, Alberta	4.3	0.26	0.8	0.11
Canada, British Columbia	4.8	0.22	0.9	0.09
Canada, Manitoba	4.3	0.37	0.9	0.17
Canada, New Brunswick	7.3	0.60	0.9	0.20
Canada, Newfoundland	5.8	0.63	0,5	0,20
Canada, Northwest Territories	2,5	1,29	1,1	1,12
Canada, Nova Scotia	6.6	0.50	0.9	0.18
Canada, Ontario	5.6	0.14	1.0	0.06
Canada, Prince Edward Island	5.8	1.25	0,5	0,32
Canada, Quebec	9.1	0.21	1.9	0.09
Canada, Saskatchewan	4.3	0.38	0.8	0.16
Canada, Yukon	4,2	2,19	-	-
US, Cent. Calif.: Non-Hisp. White	5.9	0.37	1.4	0.17
US, Cent. Calif.: Hispanic	3.9	0.63	0,2	0,13
US, Los Angeles: Non-Hisp. White	6.1	0.22	1.3	0.10
US, Los Angeles: Hispanic White	4.1	0.33	0.4	0.09
US, Los Angeles: Black	9.9	0.68	1.8	0.26
US, Los Angeles: Chinese	1,5	0,52	0,1	0,13
US, Los Angeles: Filipino	2.6	0.74	0,8	0,35
US, Los Angeles: Korean	5.5	1.34	1,0	0,52
US, Los Angeles: Japanese	1,1	0,45	0,2	0,17
US, San Francisco: Non-Hisp. White	6.0	0.29	1.4	0.14
US, San Francisco: Hispanic White	3.5	0.65	0,7	0,26
US, San Francisco: Black	9.4	0.99	2.1	0.43
US, San Francisco: Chinese	2.8	0.57	0,3	0,19
US, San Francisco: Filipino	1,5	0,65	0,7	0,38
US, San Francisco: Japanese	2,9	1,44	0,4	0,42
US, Connecticut: White	6.5	0.26	1.7	0.13
US, Connecticut: Black	10.4	1.46	1.9	0.54
US, Atlanta: White	7.4	0.46	1.7	0.20
US, Atlanta: Black	11.2	1.12	2.3	0.42
US, Iowa	6.5	0.28	1.3	0.12

	MALE		FEMALE	
US, Central Louisiana: White	8.4	1.12	2.1	0.56
US, Central Louisiana: Black	7.0	2.23	1,7	0,98
US, New Orleans: White	9.4	0.72	2.8	0.36
US, New Orleans: Black	11.1	1.23	2.1	0.46
US, Detroit: White	8.3	0.31	1.6	0.13
US, Detroit: Black	12.3	0.78	2.9	0.34
US, New Mexico: Non-Hisp. White	4.6	0.43	1.3	0.21
US, New Mexico: Hispanic White	3.9	0.58	0.7	0.22
US, New Mexico: American Indian	0,8	0,57	-	-
US, Utah	3.4	0.30	0.4	0.10
US, Seattle	5.5	0.25	1.2	0.11
US, SEER: White	6.3	0.11	1.4	0.05
US, SEER: Black	11.0	0.48	2.4	0.20
ASIA				
*China, Qidong	0.7	0.16	0,1	0,04
China, Shanghai	3.3	0.12	0.4	0.04
China, Tianjin	3.3	0.19	1.7	0.13
Hong Kong	7.7	0.23	0.8	0.07
*India, Bangalore	4.3	0.27	0.6	0.10
*India, Barshi, Paranda and Bhum	2.5	0.56	-	-
India, Bombay	8.2	0.27	1.4	0.11
*India, Karunagappally	5.1	1.23	-	-
India, Madras	5.1	0.30	0.6	0.10
*India, Trivandrum	5.5	0.95	0,4	0,24
Israel: All Jews	4.7	0.22	0.7	0.08
Jews born in Israel	3.6	0.61	0.7	0.22
Jews born in America or Europe	4.4	0.32	0.8	0.13
Jews born in Africa or Asia	5.3	0.40	0.6	0.12
Non-Jews	3.7	0.62	-	-
Japan, Hiroshima	3.9	0.37	0.3	0.09
Japan, Miyagi	3.5	0.21	0.2	0.04
Japan, Nagasaki	3.5	0.25	0.2	0.05
Japan, Osaka	3.4	0.12	0.3	0.03
*Japan, Saga	3.8	0.34	0,2	0,07
Japan, Yamagata	2.6	0.23	0,1	0,03
*Korea, Kangwha	1,4	0,70	0,3	0,26
*Kuwait: Non-Kuwaitis	6.9	2.04	0,1	0,10
*Kuwait: Kuwaitis	2.5	0.66	0,9	0,44
*Philippines, Manila	5.6	0.37	0.9	0.13
Singapore: Chinese	5.5	0.37	0.7	0.12
Singapore: Malay	2.5	0.65	0,9	0,42
Singapore: Indian	4.3	0.89	1,3	0,74
Thailand, Chiang Mai	5.3	0.42	1.8	0.25
*Thailand, Khon Kaen	1.2	0.26	0,2	0,10
*Viet Nam, Hanoi	0.8	0.19	0,1	0,05

* IMPORTANT-SEE NOTES ON POPULATION PAGE

AGE-STANDARDIZED INCIDENCE
RATES AND STANDARD ERRORS (per 100,000)
Larynx (ICD-9 161) (contd)

EUROPE	MALE		FEMALE	
Austria, Tyrol	7.7	0.67	0,3	0,14
*Belarus	10.5	0.20	0.3	0.03
*Croatia	13.1	0.34	0.6	0.07
Czech Republic	7.4	0.16	0.4	0.03
Denmark	5.5	0.18	1.1	0.08
Estonia	9.1	0.47	0.4	0.09
Finland	3.3	0.13	0.3	0.04
France, Bas-Rhin	11.6	0.67	0.6	0.13
*France, Calvados	12.1	0.84	0.6	0.18
France, Doubs	13.3	0.98	0.6	0.20
France, Haut-Rhin	10.3	0.73	0.6	0.16
*France, Herault	12.6	0.71	0.8	0.18
France, Isere	9.7	0.58	0.5	0.13
*France, Somme	14.8	0.99	1.1	0.28
*France, Tarn	6.4	0.72	0.6	0.23
Germany, Eastern States	5.1	0.17	0.3	0.04
Germany, Saarland	8.1	0.47	0.7	0.14
Iceland	3.8	0.75	0,2	0,15
Ireland, Southern	6.1	0.65	0.8	0.22
Italy, Ferrara	10.1	1.28	0,3	0,19
Italy, Florence	12.1	0.57	0.9	0.14
Italy, Genoa	12.4	0.66	0.7	0.14
*Italy, Latina	8.9	0.89	0,5	0,19
Italy, Macerata	8.2	1.38	0,4	0,29
Italy, Modena	11.2	0.68	0.6	0.14
Italy, Parma	11.2	0.83	0.6	0.18
Italy, Ragusa	4.8	0.69	0,3	0,18
Italy, Romagna	9.5	0.68	0.8	0.21
Italy, Torino	10.1	0.57	0.7	0.15
Italy, Trieste	16.2	1.37	1.9	0.44
Italy, Varese	12.7	0.69	0.6	0.14
Italy, Veneto	16.4	0.64	1.1	0.15
*Latvia	9.0	0.35	0.4	0.06
Malta	10.5	1.62	0,4	0,32
The Netherlands	6.3	0.13	0.8	0.05
The Netherlands, Eindhoven	8.1	0.54	0.6	0.14
The Netherlands, Maastricht	6.7	0.49	0.7	0.15
Norway	3.1	0.15	0.3	0.05
*Poland, Cracow	9.4	0.68	1.0	0.19
*Poland, Kielce	13.5	0.66	0.6	0.12
*Poland, Lower Silesia	15.2	0.46	1.6	0.13
Poland, Warsaw City	10.9	0.52	1.2	0.15
Slovakia	11.3	0.29	0.4	0.05
Slovenia	9.1	0.41	0.6	0.09
*Spain, Albacete	12.8	1.70	-	-
Spain, Asturias	15.8	0.72	0.3	0.09
Spain, Basque Country	18.2	0.59	0.3	0.07
Spain, Granada	13.7	0.77	0,1	0,06
Spain, Mallorca	13.8	0.88	0,4	0,15
Spain, Murcia	15.9	0.73	0,2	0,08
Spain, Navarra	15.7	0.97	0,3	0,12
Spain, Tarragona	11.6	0.81	0,2	0,11
Spain, Zaragoza	17.1	0.78	0,1	0,04

	MALE		FEMALE	
Sweden	2.5	0.09	0.4	0.04
*Switzerland, Basel	4.2	0.52	0.5	0.17
Switzerland, Geneva	8.6	0.84	1.0	0.27
Switzerland, Graubunden	5.0	1.07	0,7	0,40
Switzerland, Neuchatel	5.8	1.03	1,0	0,40
Switzerland, St Gall-Appenzell	3.8	0.51	0,2	0,10
Switzerland, Valais	6.9	1.07	1,2	0,42
Switzerland, Vaud	6.5	0.60	0.8	0.21
Switzerland, Zurich	4.2	0.33	0.3	0.09
*UK, England and Wales	4.5	0.07	0.8	0.03
*UK, East Anglia	3.2	0.21	0.6	0.09
*UK, Mersey	4.6	0.23	1.1	0.11
*UK, North Western	5.8	0.21	1.0	0.08
UK, Oxford	3.4	0.21	0.6	0.08
*UK, South Thames	3.4	0.12	0.6	0.05
UK, South Western	3.4	0.17	0.5	0.06
UK, Wessex	3.8	0.19	0.5	0.06
*UK, West Midlands	4.9	0.16	0.9	0.07
UK, Yorkshire	4.7	0.19	1.0	0.08
UK, Scotland	6.2	0.19	1.3	0.08
UK, Scotland, West	6.9	0.28	1.5	0.12
*Yugoslavia, Vojvodina	11.4	0.41	0.7	0.09

OCEANIA	MALE		FEMALE	
Australian Capital Territory	4.7	0.94	0,4	0,26
Australia, New South Wales	5.6	0.18	0.6	0.06
South Australia	4.8	0.33	0.5	0.11
Australia, Tasmania	4.4	0.56	0.3	0,15
Australia, Victoria	4.8	0.19	0.6	0.06
Western Australia	4.8	0.33	0.6	0.11
*French Polynesia	8.3	1.59	1,7	0,78
New Zealand: Non-Maori	4.0	0.21	0.6	0.08
New Zealand: Maori	3.1	0.91	1,2	0,54
US, Hawaii: White	8.3	1.01	1.2	0.35
US, Hawaii: Japanese	2.2	0.43	0,2	0,16
US, Hawaii: Hawaiian	3.8	1.06	0,6	0,36
US, Hawaii: Filipino	2.6	0.79	0,4	0,32
US, Hawaii: Chinese	2,0	0,85	-	-

AGE-STANDARDIZED INCIDENCE
RATES AND STANDARD ERRORS (per 100,000)
Bronchus, lung (ICD-9 162)

AFRICA	MALE		FEMALE	
*Algeria, Setif	28.1	1.98	2.9	0.51
*France, La Reunion	34.5	1.83	3.3	0.50
*Mali, Bamako	5.3	0.89	1.5	0.46
*Uganda, Kyadondo	4.2	1.11	0,4	0,29
*Zimbabwe, Harare: African	24.9	2.53	7.3	1.75
*Zimbabwe, Harare: European	36.0	5.72	18.1	3.91

AMERICA, CENTRAL AND SOUTH	MALE		FEMALE	
*Argentina, Concordia	55.5	4.45	8.1	1.58
*Brazil, Belem	28.6	1.86	7.2	0.79
*Brazil, Goiania	21.3	1.55	9.7	0.93
*Brazil, Porto Alegre	67.5	2.22	14.4	0.83
Colombia, Cali	24.4	1.09	9.5	0.61
*Costa Rica	15.6	0.60	5.4	0.33
*Ecuador, Quito	10.1	0.80	3.6	0.42
*Peru, Lima	15.9	0.64	6.3	0.39
Peru, Trujillo	11.9	1.78	4.1	0.90
US, Puerto Rico	19.1	0.51	6.6	0.28
*Uruguay, Montevideo	70.6	1.71	7.5	0.49

AMERICA, NORTH	MALE		FEMALE	
Canada	65.4	0.28	28.0	0.18
Canada, Alberta	50.0	0.88	24.6	0.61
Canada, British Columbia	54.9	0.71	31.1	0.53
Canada, Manitoba	58.4	1.30	28.3	0.89
Canada, New Brunswick	72.9	1.84	27.5	1.12
Canada, Newfoundland	57.0	1.95	14.1	0.97
Canada, Northwest Territories	90.3	8.30	65.6	7.61
Canada, Nova Scotia	74.6	1.64	32.4	1.07
Canada, Ontario	62.2	0.45	28.2	0.29
Canada, Prince Edward Island	59.8	3.91	36.6	3.12
Canada, Quebec	82.5	0.64	27.9	0.35
Canada, Saskatchewan	53.0	1.28	23.9	0.88
Canada, Yukon	68.1	8.46	47.6	7.89
US, Cent. Calif.: Non-Hisp. White	71.1	1.26	39.5	0.90
US, Cent. Calif.: Hispanic	34.5	1.88	15.4	1.21
US, Los Angeles: Non-Hisp. White	59.7	0.68	38.6	0.52
US, Los Angeles: Hispanic White	31.0	0.92	14.5	0.54
US, Los Angeles: Black	88.7	2.04	35.4	1.13
US, Los Angeles: Chinese	36.5	2.46	16.4	1.50
US, Los Angeles: Filipino	44.9	3.14	12.3	1.39
US, Los Angeles: Korean	36.7	3.64	12.3	1.75
US, Los Angeles: Japanese	31.2	2.56	12.6	1.55
US, San Francisco: Non-Hisp. White	58.6	0.90	40.4	0.71
US, San Francisco: Hispanic White	37.2	2.11	22.9	1.44
US, San Francisco: Black	101.5	3.26	44.3	1.94
US, San Francisco: Chinese	39.4	2.13	24.0	1.64
US, San Francisco: Filipino	46.8	3.61	15.9	1.79
US, San Francisco: Japanese	35.7	4.96	15.1	2.77
US, Connecticut: White	62.1	0.80	35.2	0.57
US, Connecticut: Black	86.2	4.23	33.2	2.24
US, Atlanta: White	72.4	1.43	35.5	0.91
US, Atlanta: Black	97.3	3.34	29.8	1.54
US, Iowa	65.9	0.85	28.6	0.55

	MALE		FEMALE	
US, Central Louisiana: White	77.4	3.37	27.3	1.88
US, Central Louisiana: Black	105.6	8.45	27.1	3.64
US, New Orleans: White	84.0	2.08	41.2	1.34
US, New Orleans: Black	110.8	3.88	36.9	1.88
US, Detroit: White	74.6	0.90	40.2	0.62
US, Detroit: Black	103.2	2.21	42.0	1.25
US, New Mexico: Non-Hisp. White	52.5	1.39	28.8	1.00
US, New Mexico: Hispanic White	27.5	1.51	13.8	1.00
US, New Mexico: American Indian	10.3	2.18	4.0	1.22
US, Utah	29.8	0.88	13.1	0.57
US, Seattle	63.2	0.82	37.6	0.61
US, SEER: White	61.3	0.33	33.8	0.23
US, SEER: Black	99.1	1.42	38.5	0.78

ASIA	MALE		FEMALE	
*China, Qidong	35.0	1.10	11.0	0.57
China, Shanghai	56.1	0.50	18.2	0.27
China, Tianjin	55.9	0.77	37.0	0.60
Hong Kong	74.7	0.71	30.7	0.43
*India, Bangalore	8.1	0.37	1.7	0.17
*India, Barshi, Paranda and Bhum	1.3	0.38	0,3	0,19
India, Bombay	14.5	0.36	3.7	0.19
*India, Karunagappally	17.0	2.29	2.6	0.82
India, Madras	12.6	0.47	2.4	0.20
*India, Trivandrum	10.6	1.30	1.9	0.51
Israel: All Jews	27.0	0.52	9.2	0.28
Jews born in Israel	22.6	1.62	10.7	1.04
Jews born in America or Europe	26.5	0.76	10.7	0.44
Jews born in Africa or Asia	27.8	0.91	5.4	0.40
Non-Jews	29.1	1.81	3.7	0.60
Japan, Hiroshima	39.6	1.17	11.7	0.56
Japan, Miyagi	39.6	0.72	10.3	0.33
Japan, Nagasaki	41.7	0.84	12.1	0.40
Japan, Osaka	43.5	0.42	12.4	0.19
*Japan, Saga	39.2	1.07	9.8	0.48
Japan, Yamagata	35.9	0.82	8.3	0.36
*Korea, Kangwha	33.8	3.42	8.4	1.52
*Kuwait: Non-Kuwaitis	35.3	4.50	10.3	1.92
*Kuwait: Kuwaitis	20.3	1.96	9.2	1.50
*Philippines, Manila	58.7	1.18	16.8	0.56
Singapore: Chinese	62.7	1.25	19.6	0.61
Singapore: Malay	37.2	2.46	9.6	1.26
Singapore: Indian	14.3	1.64	3.5	1.17
Thailand, Chiang Mai	36.0	1.08	30.3	1.00
*Thailand, Khon Kaen	17.0	0.93	5.3	0.47
*Viet Nam, Hanoi	34.9	1.26	6.3	0.49

f

EUROPE	MALE		FEMALE	
Austria, Tyrol	54.7	1.76	11.3	0.72
*Belarus	66.8	0.52	6.0	0.12
*Croatia	72.5	0.80	9.7	0.26
Czech Republic	77.8	0.50	10.1	0.16
Denmark	51.9	0.53	25.4	0.37
Estonia	75.7	1.36	8.3	0.36
Finland	54.3	0.54	8.2	0.19
France, Bas-Rhin	67.4	1.59	7.2	0.47
*France, Calvados	55.1	1.78	4.6	0.49
France, Doubs	50.8	1.91	6.5	0.64
France, Haut-Rhin	58.3	1.73	6.7	0.54
*France, Herault	42.8	1.26	5.4	0.43
France, Isere	50.1	1.30	5.6	0.41
*France, Somme	55.1	1.84	4.5	0.49
*France, Tarn	39.7	1.76	3.2	0.49
Germany, Eastern States	59.2	0.57	7.6	0.17
Germany, Saarland	70.9	1.37	10.3	0.47
Iceland	32.8	2.13	26.4	1.92
Ireland, Southern	41.6	1.61	14.0	0.89
Italy, Ferrara	85.7	3.65	14.4	1.42
Italy, Florence	62.6	1.28	11.1	0.51
Italy, Genoa	72.2	1.53	10.0	0.52
*Italy, Latina	65.8	2.34	9.2	0.83
Italy, Macerata	47.4	3.09	7.4	1.25
Italy, Modena	68.6	1.65	9.2	0.57
Italy, Parma	63.4	1.91	12.0	0.79
Italy, Ragusa	39.0	1.97	5.0	0.67
Italy, Romagna	66.1	1.78	9.5	0.66
Italy, Torino	65.0	1.45	10.8	0.53
Italy, Trieste	82.7	2.93	14.9	1.13
Italy, Varese	77.6	1.69	8.5	0.50
Italy, Veneto	81.9	1.39	13.9	0.52
*Latvia	65.5	0.95	7.1	0.25
Malta	48.2	3.44	3.4	0.82
The Netherlands	73.0	0.43	13.0	0.18
The Netherlands, Eindhoven	81.4	1.69	11.5	0.62
The Netherlands, Maastricht	80.1	1.65	12.5	0.64
Norway	34.3	0.48	12.6	0.29
*Poland, Cracow	77.8	1.96	15.3	0.74
*Poland, Kielce	67.4	1.44	7.0	0.43
*Poland, Lower Silesia	95.5	1.15	16.2	0.41
Poland, Warsaw City	68.4	1.29	19.5	0.58
Slovakia	79.1	0.77	8.7	0.22
Slovenia	65.6	1.10	9.1	0.35
*Spain, Albacete	34.1	2.63	3.1	0.80
Spain, Asturias	63.5	1.38	4.3	0.34
Spain, Basque Country	53.1	0.98	3.4	0.24
Spain, Granada	45.3	1.34	2.7	0.30
Spain, Mallorca	61.4	1.79	4.3	0.44
Spain, Murcia	47.2	1.23	3.6	0.32
Spain, Navarra	41.5	1.49	3.4	0.41
Spain, Tarragona	42.9	1.51	3.1	0.41
Spain, Zaragoza	48.0	1.25	2.7	0.27

	MALE		FEMALE	
Sweden	23.9	0.27	10.9	0.18
*Switzerland, Basel	49.6	1.76	11.9	0.82
Switzerland, Geneva	53.7	2.08	14.3	0.96
Switzerland, Graubunden	49.8	3.26	9.7	1.41
Switzerland, Neuchatel	60.8	3.28	11.6	1.35
Switzerland, St Gall-Appenzell	49.1	1.77	8.4	0.72
Switzerland, Valais	47.7	2.73	10.2	1.25
Switzerland, Vaud	61.4	1.79	12.5	0.77
Switzerland, Zurich	47.4	1.09	10.8	0.49
*UK, England and Wales	62.4	0.23	22.8	0.14
*UK, East Anglia	48.3	0.76	17.1	0.44
*UK, Mersey	63.3	0.82	31.3	0.57
*UK, North Western	70.8	0.70	27.8	0.42
UK, Oxford	55.1	0.80	19.9	0.46
*UK, South Thames	56.1	0.47	21.4	0.27
UK, South Western	47.0	0.59	17.1	0.34
UK, Wessex	51.1	0.66	18.0	0.37
*UK, West Midlands	65.9	0.58	21.5	0.32
UK, Yorkshire	64.3	0.69	24.8	0.41
UK, Scotland	79.8	0.67	33.7	0.40
UK, Scotland, West	88.9	0.97	38.5	0.58
*Yugoslavia, Vojvodina	71.7	1.03	10.6	0.36

OCEANIA

	MALE		FEMALE	
Australian Capital Territory	39.1	2.74	13.9	1.47
Australia, New South Wales	46.6	0.51	14.9	0.28
South Australia	47.9	1.01	15.2	0.56
Australia, Tasmania	49.4	1.85	18.8	1.15
Australia, Victoria	46.0	0.59	15.8	0.33
Western Australia	48.0	1.05	17.5	0.61
*French Polynesia	73.7	5.49	28.1	3.50
New Zealand: Non-Maori	46.5	0.70	18.2	0.43
New Zealand: Maori	99.7	5.37	72.9	4.15
US, Hawaii: White	59.6	2.66	37.9	2.14
US, Hawaii: Japanese	34.0	1.70	11.1	0.90
US, Hawaii: Hawaiian	72.3	4.51	35.0	2.93
US, Hawaii: Filipino	40.6	3.04	17.7	1.97
US, Hawaii: Chinese	37.6	3.75	18.9	2.48

* IMPORTANT-SEE NOTES ON POPULATION PAGE

AGE-STANDARDIZED INCIDENCE
RATES AND STANDARD ERRORS (per 100,000)
Other thoracic organs (ICD-9 163-4)

	MALE		FEMALE	
AFRICA				
*Algeria, Setif	1,0	0,39	0,4	0,19
*France, La Reunion	1.4	0.37	0.8	0.24
*Mali, Bamako	-	-	-	-
*Uganda, Kyadondo	0,3	0,29	0,4	0,29 f
*Zimbabwe, Harare: African	0,2	0,14	0,4	0,27
*Zimbabwe, Harare: European	-	-	-	-
AMERICA, CENTRAL AND SOUTH				
*Argentina, Concordia	2,1	0,85	2.9	0.95
*Brazil, Belem	0.9	0.34	0,6	0,35 mf
*Brazil, Goiania	0.9	0.30	0,4	0,18
*Brazil, Porto Alegre	1.2	0.29	0.8	0.20
Colombia, Cali	0.7	0.18	0.4	0.13
*Costa Rica	0.4	0.08	0,1	0,05
*Ecuador, Quito	-	-	-	-
*Peru, Lima	0.5	0.11	0.2	0.08
Peru, Trujillo	0,5	0,29	0,4	0,26
US, Puerto Rico	0.5	0.08	0.2	0.05
*Uruguay, Montevideo	1.0	0.22	0.3	0.09
AMERICA, NORTH				
Canada	0.6	0.03	0.4	0.02
Canada, Alberta	0.4	0.08	0.2	0.06
Canada, British Columbia	0.5	0.08	0.3	0.06
Canada, Manitoba	0.5	0.12	0.4	0.13
Canada, New Brunswick	0,4	0,14	0,3	0,11
Canada, Newfoundland	0,2	0,10	0,0	0,03
Canada, Northwest Territories	0,3	0,26	-	-
Canada, Nova Scotia	0.7	0.15	0.2	0,10
Canada, Ontario	0.7	0.05	0.4	0.04
Canada, Prince Edward Island	1,1	0,57	0,5	0,38
Canada, Quebec	0.9	0.07	0.5	0.05
Canada, Saskatchewan	0.4	0.12	0.4	0.12
Canada, Yukon	-	-	-	-
US, Cent. Calif.: Non-Hisp. White	0.3	0.09	0.2	0.07
US, Cent. Calif.: Hispanic	0,2	0,13	0,3	0,16
US, Los Angeles: Non-Hisp. White	0.5	0.07	0.2	0.05
US, Los Angeles: Hispanic White	0.4	0.08	0.2	0.06
US, Los Angeles: Black	0.5	0.16	0.2	0,09
US, Los Angeles: Chinese	0,7	0,34	-	-
US, Los Angeles: Filipino	0,2	0,21	-	-
US, Los Angeles: Korean	-	-	0,2	0,17
US, Los Angeles: Japanese	0,3	0,26	-	-
US, San Francisco: Non-Hisp. White	0.4	0.09	0,1	0,03
US, San Francisco: Hispanic White	0,4	0,19	0,1	0,11
US, San Francisco: Black	0,4	0,19	0,3	0,16
US, San Francisco: Chinese	0,9	0,35	0,1	0,11
US, San Francisco: Filipino	0,8	0,44	0,1	0,13
US, San Francisco: Japanese	-	-	-	-
US, Connecticut: White	0.5	0.08	0.3	0.07
US, Connecticut: Black	0,7	0,32	0,5	0,28
US, Atlanta: White	0.4	0.11	0.3	0.10
US, Atlanta: Black	0.9	0.28	0,4	0,17
US, Iowa	0.3	0.07	0.2	0.05

	MALE		FEMALE	
US, Central Louisiana: White	0,6	0,28	0,4	0,21
US, Central Louisiana: Black	-	-	0,4	0,37
US, New Orleans: White	0.7	0.21	0.5	0.17
US, New Orleans: Black	0.4	0,22	0.2	0,14
US, Detroit: White	0.3	0.06	0.2	0.06
US, Detroit: Black	0.4	0,14	0.2	0,08
US, New Mexico: Non-Hisp. White	0.5	0.16	0.3	0,13
US, New Mexico: Hispanic White	0.8	0.26	0.4	0,17
US, New Mexico: American Indian	-	-	-	-
US, Utah	0.5	0.11	0.3	0.08
US, Seattle	0.4	0.07	0.2	0.05
US, SEER: White	0.4	0.03	0.2	0.02
US, SEER: Black	0.5	0.10	0.3	0.07
ASIA				
†*China, Qidong	0.7	0.15	0.3	0.11
† China, Shanghai	1.2	0.08	0.7	0.06
China, Tianjin	0.9	0.10	0.5	0.07
Hong Kong	0.4	0.05	0.2	0.03
*India, Bangalore	0.5	0.09	0.4	0.08
*India, Barshi, Paranda and Bhum	-	-	-	-
India, Bombay	0.4	0.06	0.3	0.05
*India, Karunagappally	-	-	-	-
India, Madras	0.1	0.04	0,1	0,03
*India, Trivandrum	0,1	0,10	0,1	0,09
Israel: All Jews	0.5	0.07	0.4	0.06
Jews born in Israel	0.8	0.27	0.4	0.12
Jews born in America or Europe	0.4	0.13	0.3	0.09
Jews born in Africa or Asia	0.2	0,07	0.2	0,09
Non-Jews	0.3	0,18	0.1	0,08
Japan, Hiroshima	1.3	0.24	0.6	0.15
Japan, Miyagi	0.6	0.10	0.3	0.06
Japan, Nagasaki	0.6	0.12	0.3	0.09
Japan, Osaka	0.6	0.06	0.4	0.04
†*Japan, Saga	0.9	0.21	0.5	0.11
Japan, Yamagata	0.6	0.12	0.1	0,03
*Korea, Kangwha	-	-	0,8	0,49
*Kuwait: Non-Kuwaitis	0,3	0,10	0,7	0,45
*Kuwait: Kuwaitis	0,5	0,26	0,3	0,26
*Philippines, Manila	0.4	0.09	0.2	0.05
Singapore: Chinese	0.7	0.12	0.5	0.10
Singapore: Malay	0.6	0.27	0.5	0.26
Singapore: Indian	0.2	0,19	0.1	0,12
Thailand, Chiang Mai	0.1	0,04	0.1	0,05
*Thailand, Khon Kaen	0,3	0,10	0,1	0,06
*Viet Nam, Hanoi	2.1	0.31	0.8	0.18

* IMPORTANT-SEE NOTES ON POPULATION PAGE

EUROPE	MALE		FEMALE	
Austria, Tyrol	0.6	0.20	0.5	0.14
*Belarus	0.8	0.06	0.3	0.03
*Croatia	0.8	0.09	0.4	0.07
Czech Republic	1.0	0.06	0.5	0.04
Denmark	0.6	0.06	0.3	0.05
Estonia	0.6	0.13	0.4	0.09
Finland	0.5	0.05	0.2	0.03
France, Bas-Rhin	1.0	0.20	0,2	0,08
*France, Calvados	1.2	0.26	0.5	0.17
France, Doubs	0,6	0,20	0,2	0,10
France, Haut-Rhin	0.6	0.18	0,4	0,15
*France, Herault	0.6	0.16	0,1	0,07
France, Isere	0.5	0.13	0.5	0.15
*France, Somme	0.9	0.23	0,2	0,14
*France, Tarn	0,4	0,18	-	-
Germany, Eastern States	0.7	0.06	0.3	0.04
† Germany, Saarland	1.1	0.17	0.6	0.12
Iceland	0,7	0,33	0,3	0,20
Ireland, Southern	0,4	0,17	0,1	0,10
Italy, Ferrara	0,6	0,37	0,9	0,43
Italy, Florence	0.5	0.12	0.4	0.11
Italy, Genoa	1.9	0.25	0.6	0.12
*Italy, Latina	0,5	0,27	-	-
Italy, Macerata	0,7	0,39	0,4	0,38
Italy, Modena	1.0	0.21	0.3	0.11
Italy, Parma	0,2	0,10	0,0	0,04
Italy, Ragusa	0,8	0,29	0,7	0,35
Italy, Romagna	0,3	0,13	0.5	0.17
Italy, Torino	1.3	0.22	0.6	0.13
Italy, Trieste	3.3	0.68	1.1	0.38
Italy, Varese	0,2	0,10	0.3	0.10
Italy, Veneto	1.3	0.18	0.3	0.09
†*Latvia	1.3	0.14	0.6	0.08
† Malta	0,8	0,42	0,2	0,16
The Netherlands	0.5	0.04	0.2	0.02
The Netherlands, Eindhoven	0,3	0,11	0,2	0,09
The Netherlands, Maastricht	0.4	0.12	0,1	0,05
Norway	0.3	0.04	0.2	0.03
*Poland, Cracow	1.1	0.25	0.4	0.11
*Poland, Kielce	0.9	0.16	0.5	0.12
*Poland, Lower Silesia	2.6	0.19	1.2	0.12
Poland, Warsaw City	1.3	0.19	0.8	0.12
Slovakia	1.1	0.09	0.6	0.07
Slovenia	0.3	0.07	0,1	0,05
*Spain, Albacete	0,4	0,27	-	-
Spain, Asturias	1.1	0.18	0.5	0.12
Spain, Basque Country	0.5	0.11	0.4	0.12
Spain, Granada	0.5	0.16	0,4	0,18
Spain, Mallorca	0.6	0.22	0,4	0,20
Spain, Murcia	0,4	0,14	0,0	0,01
Spain, Navarra	0,5	0,18	0,4	0,15
Spain, Tarragona	0.7	0.20	0.4	0.16
Spain, Zaragoza	0.4	0.12	0.5	0.14

	MALE		FEMALE		
Sweden	0.2	0.03	0.1	0.02	
*Switzerland, Basel	0,3	0,14	0,1	0,05	
Switzerland, Geneva	0,1	0,10	0,3	0,15	
Switzerland, Graubunden	0,3	0,26	0,1	0,08	
Switzerland, Neuchatel	1,5	0,71	0,2	0,18	
Switzerland, St Gall-Appenzell	1.1	0.28	0,3	0,16	
Switzerland, Valais	1.5	0.48	1,0	0,49	
Switzerland, Vaud	0,4	0,15	0,1	0,07	
Switzerland, Zurich	0.6	0.13	0.2	0.08	
*UK, England and Wales	0.6	0.02	0.3	0.02	
*UK, East Anglia	0.3	0.07	0.2	0.05	
*UK, Mersey	0.5	0.08	0.3	0.05	
*UK, North Western	0.4	0.06	0.3	0.05	
UK, Oxford	0.3	0.06	0.2	0.05	
*UK, South Thames	0.7	0.06	0.4	0.04	
UK, South Western	0.6	0.07	0.2	0.04	
UK, Wessex	0.6	0.08	0.4	0.06	
†*UK, West Midlands	1.7	0.10	0.4	0.05	
UK, Yorkshire	0.4	0.06	0.3	0.05	
UK, Scotland	0.4	0.05	0.2	0.03	
UK, Scotland, West	0.2	0.05	0.1	0.04	
*Yugoslavia, Vojvodina	1.6	0.16	0.6	0.09	

OCEANIA	MALE		FEMALE		
Australian Capital Territory	0,8	0,36	0,2	0,20	
Australia, New South Wales	0.4	0.05	0.2	0.04	
South Australia	0.2	0.08	0.2	0,06	
Australia, Tasmania	0,5	0,20	0,3	0,17	
Australia, Victoria	0,5	0.06	0.3	0.05	
Western Australia	0.4	0.10	0,1	0,06	
*French Polynesia	2,0	0,82	1,9	0,96	f
† New Zealand: Non-Maori	1.6	0.13	0.4	0.06	
† New Zealand: Maori	0,9	0,43	0,3	0,27	
US, Hawaii: White	0,1	0,14	0,1	0,15	
US, Hawaii: Japanese	0,2	0,11	0,6	0,24	
US, Hawaii: Hawaiian	0,5	0,33	0,4	0,27	
US, Hawaii: Filipino	0,6	0,37	0,8	0,42	
US, Hawaii: Chinese	1,1	0,77	-	-	

* IMPORTANT-SEE NOTES ON POPULATION PAGE

AGE-STANDARDIZED INCIDENCE
RATES AND STANDARD ERRORS (per 100,000)
Kaposi's sarcoma

	MALE		FEMALE	
AFRICA				
*Algeria, Setif	-	-	-	-
*France, La Reunion	0,3	0,15	-	-
*Mali, Bamako	2.1	0.51	0,3	0,21
*Uganda, Kyadondo	43.5	2.58	18.0	1.45
*Zimbabwe, Harare: African	24.6	1.53	7.9	0.93
*Zimbabwe, Harare: European	3,0	2,15	-	-
AMERICA, CENTRAL AND SOUTH				
*Argentina, Concordia	0,3	0,30	-	-
*Brazil, Belem	0,1	0,13	-	-
*Brazil, Goiania	0.7	0.24	-	-
*Brazil, Porto Alegre	1.5	0.29	0,1	0,05
Colombia, Cali	0,2	0,08	0,1	0,05
*Costa Rica	0.4	0.09	0,1	0,04
*Ecuador, Quito	0,1	0,07	0,1	0,08
*Peru, Lima	0.4	0.10	0,1	0,04
Peru, Trujillo	0,3	0,29	0,3	0,33
US, Puerto Rico	3.3	0.23	0.3	0.05
*Uruguay, Montevideo	0,3	0,13	0,0	0,03
AMERICA, NORTH				
† Canada	0.3	0.02	0.0	0.00
† Canada, Alberta	-	-	-	-
† Canada, British Columbia	0,0	0,01	-	-
† Canada, Manitoba	0,0	0,02	0,0	0,01
† Canada, New Brunswick	-	-	-	-
† Canada, Newfoundland	-	-	-	-
† Canada, Northwest Territories	-	-	-	-
† Canada, Nova Scotia	-	-	-	-
† Canada, Ontario	0.5	0.04	0,0	0,01
† Canada, Prince Edward Island	-	-	-	-
† Canada, Quebec	0.3	0.03	0,0	0,01
† Canada, Saskatchewan	0,1	0,04	0,0	0,03
† Canada, Yukon	-	-	-	-
US, Cent. Calif.: Non-Hisp. White	1.6	0.21	0,1	0,03
US, Cent. Calif.: Hispanic	1.4	0.30	0,1	0,05
US, Los Angeles: Non-Hisp. White	14.5	0.35	0.1	0.03
US, Los Angeles: Hispanic White	8.1	0.33	0.2	0.06
US, Los Angeles: Black	9.0	0.56	0,2	0,08
US, Los Angeles: Chinese	0,8	0,34	-	-
US, Los Angeles: Filipino	2.4	0.60	-	-
US, Los Angeles: Korean	0,6	0,43	-	-
US, Los Angeles: Japanese	3.2	0.91	-	-
US, San Francisco: Non-Hisp. White	33.5	0.67	0.1	0.04
US, San Francisco: Hispanic White	19.9	1.19	0,1	0,07
US, San Francisco: Black	21.5	1.32	0,1	0,07
US, San Francisco: Chinese	1.8	0.49	-	-
US, San Francisco: Filipino	4.8	1.04	-	-
US, San Francisco: Japanese	5,7	2,10	-	-
US, Connecticut: White	2.4	0.17	0.1	0.03
US, Connecticut: Black	4.0	0.78	0,3	0,21
US, Atlanta: White	9.3	0.43	0,1	0,05
US, Atlanta: Black	4.4	0.48	0,1	0,07
US, Iowa	0.5	0.08	0,0	0,01

	MALE		FEMALE	
US, Central Louisiana: White	0,6	0,29	0,1	0,06
US, Central Louisiana: Black	0,4	0,36	0,8	0,63
US, New Orleans: White	10.0	0.74	0,2	0,11
US, New Orleans: Black	3.1	0.58	0,2	0,12
US, Detroit: White	2.1	0.15	0.1	0.03
US, Detroit: Black	3.3	0.38	0.3	0.10
US, New Mexico: Non-Hisp. White	2.8	0.35	0,0	0,02
US, New Mexico: Hispanic White	2.5	0.41	0,2	0,09
US, New Mexico: American Indian	0,5	0,35	-	-
US, Utah	1.0	0.15	0,0	0,02
US, Seattle	4.7	0.21	0,0	0,02
US, SEER: White	7.6	0.11	0.1	0.01
US, SEER: Black	7.0	0.32	0.2	0.05
ASIA				
*China, Qidong				
China, Shanghai				
China, Tianjin	-	-	-	-
Hong Kong	0,0	0,01	-	-
f *India, Bangalore	-	-	-	-
*India, Barshi, Paranda and Bhum	-	-	-	-
India, Bombay	-	-	0,0	0,01
*India, Karunagappally	-	-	-	-
India, Madras	-	-	-	-
*India, Trivandrum	-	-	-	-
Israel: All Jews	2.7	0.16	0.8	0.08
Jews born in Israel	2.3	0.51	0,6	0,27
Jews born in America or Europe	1.9	0.21	1.1	0.22
Jews born in Africa or Asia	3.7	0.33	1.0	0.15
Non-Jews	0,7	0,29	0,3	0,17
Japan, Hiroshima	-	-	-	-
Japan, Miyagi	-	-	-	-
Japan, Nagasaki	-	-	-	-
Japan, Osaka	0,0	0,01	-	-
*Japan, Saga				
Japan, Yamagata	-	-	-	-
*Korea, Kangwha	0,4	0,38	-	-
*Kuwait: Non-Kuwaitis	0,1	0,08	0,1	0,15
*Kuwait: Kuwaitis	0,5	0,29	0,1	0,07
*Philippines, Manila	0,1	0,03	-	-
Singapore: Chinese	0,1	0,05	-	-
Singapore: Malay	-	-	-	-
Singapore: Indian	0,3	0,21	-	-
Thailand, Chiang Mai	0,0	0,02	-	-
*Thailand, Khon Kaen	-	-	-	-
*Viet Nam, Hanoi	0,0	0,04	-	-

* IMPORTANT-SEE NOTES ON POPULATION PAGE

AGE-STANDARDIZED INCIDENCE
RATES AND STANDARD ERRORS (per 100,000)
Kaposi's sarcoma (contd)

EUROPE	MALE		FEMALE	
Austria, Tyrol	-	-	-	-
*Belarus	0.1	0.02	0.0	0.01
*Croatia	0,0	0,01	-	-
Czech Republic	0.1	0.02	0.0	0.01
Denmark	0.8	0.07	0,0	0,00
Estonia	0,0	0,03	0,0	0,02
Finland	0.4	0.05	0.1	0.01
France, Bas-Rhin	1.9	0.26	0,2	0,07
*France, Calvados	0,5	0,16	0,1	0,08
France, Doubs	0.7	0.22	-	-
France, Haut-Rhin	0.7	0.19	0,1	0,08
*France, Herault	2.3	0.33	0,2	0,08
France, Isere	0.7	0.16	0,1	0,05
*France, Somme	0,5	0,19	0,1	0,08
*France, Tarn	0,1	0,10	0,1	0,07
Germany, Eastern States	0,0	0,01	0,0	0,01
Germany, Saarland				
Iceland	2.1	0.52	0.6	0.20
Ireland, Southern	0,1	0,09	-	-
Italy, Ferrara	2.6	0.69	0,6	0,33
Italy, Florence	1.2	0.20	0.2	0.06
Italy, Genoa	1.9	0.30	0,3	0,12
*Italy, Latina	0.9	0.27	0,3	0,15
Italy, Macerata	1,0	0,49	0,3	0,25
Italy, Modena	1.1	0.23	0,1	0,06
Italy, Parma	0.6	0.22	-	-
Italy, Ragusa	1.1	0.30	0,3	0,14
Italy, Romagna	1.3	0.28	0.5	0.17
Italy, Torino	1.5	0.25	0,2	0,09
Italy, Trieste	0,4	0,17	0,2	0,13
Italy, Varese	1.5	0.24	0.2	0.06
Italy, Veneto	0.9	0.15	0.2	0.06
*Latvia				
Malta				
The Netherlands	1.2	0.06	0.0	0.01
The Netherlands, Eindhoven	0,2	0,08	0,0	0,03
The Netherlands, Maastricht	0,2	0,08	-	-
Norway	0.5	0.06	0.1	0.02
*Poland, Cracow	0,1	0,06	-	-
*Poland, Kielce	0,0	0,03	-	-
*Poland, Lower Silesia	0,0	0,01	0,0	0,01
Poland, Warsaw City	0,0	0,02	0,0	0,01
Slovakia	0.1	0.02	0,0	0,00
Slovenia	-	-	-	-
*Spain, Albacete	0,9	0,41	0,2	0,16
Spain, Asturias	0,0	0,04	0,0	0,01
Spain, Basque Country	0.7	0.11	0,1	0,04
Spain, Granada	0.5	0.16	0,0	0,03
Spain, Mallorca	2.7	0.41	0,2	0,11
Spain, Murcia	1.1	0.20	0,0	0,04
Spain, Navarra	0,4	0,17	0,1	0,07
Spain, Tarragona	1.0	0.26	0,0	0,02
Spain, Zaragoza	0,1	0,07	0,0	0,01

	MALE		FEMALE	
Sweden	0.6	0.05	0.1	0.01
*Switzerland, Basel	0.9	0.27	0,1	0,07
Switzerland, Geneva	5.4	0.68	0,1	0,08
Switzerland, Graubunden	0,3	0,30	-	-
Switzerland, Neuchatel	1,6	0,57	-	-
Switzerland, St Gall-Appenzell	0.9	0.25	-	-
Switzerland, Valais	0,3	0,24	0,1	0,15
Switzerland, Vaud	3.0	0.43	0,4	0,15
Switzerland, Zurich	3.9	0.33	0,1	0,05
*UK, England and Wales	0.4	0.02	0.0	0.00
*UK, East Anglia	0,2	0,05	0,0	0,02
*UK, Mersey	0.1	0.04	0,0	0,00
*UK, North Western	0.2	0.05	0,0	0,01
UK, Oxford	0.2	0.04	0,0	0,01
*UK, South Thames	1.1	0.08	0,0	0,01
UK, South Western	0.3	0.05	-	-
UK, Wessex	0.1	0.04	-	-
*UK, West Midlands				
UK, Yorkshire	0.1	0.03	0,0	0,01
UK, Scotland	0.3	0.04	0,0	0,01
UK, Scotland, West	0.2	0.05	0,0	0,01
*Yugoslavia, Vojvodina	-	-	-	-

OCEANIA

	MALE		FEMALE	
† Australian Capital Territory	0,6	0,27	-	-
† Australia, New South Wales	2.6	0.12	0.0	0.01
† South Australia	0.6	0.12	0,0	0,02
† Australia, Tasmania	0,2	0,13	0,0	0,02
† Australia, Victoria	1.7	0.11	0.1	0.03
† Western Australia	0.6	0.12	0,0	0,03
†*French Polynesia	-	-	-	-
New Zealand: Non-Maori				
New Zealand: Maori				
US, Hawaii: White	7.4	0.81	0,1	0,08
US, Hawaii: Japanese	0.8	0.33	-	-
US, Hawaii: Hawaiian	2.2	0.65	-	-
US, Hawaii: Filipino	1,7	0,57	-	-
US, Hawaii: Chinese	2,3	1,03	-	-

* IMPORTANT-SEE NOTES ON POPULATION PAGE

AGE-STANDARDIZED INCIDENCE
RATES AND STANDARD ERRORS (per 100,000)
Mesothelioma

	MALE		FEMALE	
AFRICA				
*Algeria, Setif	-	-	-	-
*France, La Reunion	0,5	0,22	0,2	0,10
*Mali, Bamako	-	-	-	-
*Uganda, Kyadondo	-	-	-	-
*Zimbabwe, Harare: African	-	-	-	-
*Zimbabwe, Harare: European	1,0	1,00	-	-
AMERICA, CENTRAL AND SOUTH				
*Argentina, Concordia	-	-	0,9	0,53
*Brazil, Belem	-	-	0,1	0,05
*Brazil, Goiania	0,1	0,13	-	-
*Brazil, Porto Alegre	-	-	-	-
Colombia, Cali	0,0	0,05	0,0	0,04
*Costa Rica	0,1	0,05	0,1	0,04
*Ecuador, Quito	-	-	-	-
*Peru, Lima	0.3	0.08	0,0	0,02
Peru, Trujillo	-	-	-	-
US, Puerto Rico	0.3	0.06	0.1	0.03
*Uruguay, Montevideo	0.5	0.15	0,3	0,10
AMERICA, NORTH				
Canada	1.1	0.04	0.2	0.02
Canada, Alberta	1.1	0.13	0.2	0.06
Canada, British Columbia	1.2	0.11	0.2	0.05
Canada, Manitoba	1.4	0.21	0.2	0.07
Canada, New Brunswick	0.7	0.18	0.1	0,05
Canada, Newfoundland	0.8	0.25	0.1	0,07
Canada, Northwest Territories	-	-	-	-
Canada, Nova Scotia	1.1	0.20	0.2	0,07
Canada, Ontario	1.0	0.06	0.2	0.03
Canada, Prince Edward Island	0.5	0,38	-	-
Canada, Quebec	1.5	0.09	0.3	0.04
Canada, Saskatchewan	0.7	0.15	0.2	0,08
Canada, Yukon	-	-	-	-
US, Cent. Calif.: Non-Hisp. White	1.3	0.17	0.4	0.08
US, Cent. Calif.: Hispanic	1.5	0.38	0.4	0,19
US, Los Angeles: Non-Hisp. White	1.2	0.09	0.3	0.05
US, Los Angeles: Hispanic White	1.2	0.18	0.2	0.06
US, Los Angeles: Black	0.7	0.18	0.2	0,08
US, Los Angeles: Chinese	0.1	0,11	-	-
US, Los Angeles: Filipino	0.1	0,13	0.2	0,16
US, Los Angeles: Korean	-	-	-	-
US, Los Angeles: Japanese	0.4	0,28	0.2	0,17
US, San Francisco: Non-Hisp. White	1.9	0.16	0.3	0.06
US, San Francisco: Hispanic White	2.0	0.49	0.5	0,23
US, San Francisco: Black	1.3	0.35	0.2	0,12
US, San Francisco: Chinese	0.5	0,23	-	-
US, San Francisco: Filipino	0.9	0,47	0.2	0,19
US, San Francisco: Japanese	0.6	0,62	-	-
US, Connecticut: White	1.0	0.10	0.3	0.06
US, Connecticut: Black	0.6	0,36	-	-
US, Atlanta: White	0.9	0.15	0.2	0.07
US, Atlanta: Black	0.7	0,26	0.1	0,09
US, Iowa	1.0	0.10	0.2	0.04

	MALE		FEMALE	
US, Central Louisiana: White	0,8	0,35	-	-
US, Central Louisiana: Black	-	-	-	-
US, New Orleans: White	2.4	0.35	0.7	0.19
US, New Orleans: Black	2.0	0.52	0.3	0,18
US, Detroit: White	1.2	0.11	0.2	0.05
US, Detroit: Black	0.6	0.16	0.3	0,10
US, New Mexico: Non-Hisp. White	1.4	0.23	0.4	0.11
US, New Mexico: Hispanic White	1.5	0.35	0.2	0,11
US, New Mexico: American Indian	0,8	0,58	0,5	0,47
US, Utah	1.0	0.16	0.3	0.08
US, Seattle	2.1	0.15	0.4	0.06
US, SEER: White	1.4	0.05	0.3	0.02
US, SEER: Black	0.8	0.13	0.2	0.06
ASIA				
*China, Qidong				
China, Shanghai				
China, Tianjin	0.2	0.04	0.2	0.04
Hong Kong	0,1	0,02	0.1	0.02
*India, Bangalore	0,2	0,05	0,0	0,01
*India, Barshi, Paranda and Bhum	-	-	-	-
India, Bombay	0.1	0.02	0,0	0,02
*India, Karunagappally	-	-	-	-
India, Madras	0,1	0,03	0,0	0,03
*India, Trivandrum	-	-	0,1	0,07
Israel: All Jews	0.4	0.07	0.2	0.04
Jews born in Israel	0,4	0,18	-	-
Jews born in America or Europe	0.6	0.13	0.3	0.08
Jews born in Africa or Asia	0.3	0,09	0.1	0,06
Non-Jews	0.1	0,13	0.4	0,17
Japan, Hiroshima	0.4	0.12	0.1	0,06
Japan, Miyagi	0.2	0.05	0.0	0,02
Japan, Nagasaki	0.4	0.09	0.1	0,04
Japan, Osaka	0.4	0.04	0.2	0.02
*Japan, Saga				
Japan, Yamagata	0,0	0,02	0,0	0,03
*Korea, Kangwha	-	-	-	-
*Kuwait: Non-Kuwaitis	0,2	0,10	0,1	0,04
*Kuwait: Kuwaitis	0,6	0,33	-	-
*Philippines, Manila	0,0	0,03	0,1	0,03
Singapore: Chinese	0,1	0,04	0,0	0,03
Singapore: Malay	-	-	-	-
Singapore: Indian	0,1	0,15	-	-
Thailand, Chiang Mai	0,0	0,02	-	-
*Thailand, Khon Kaen	0,0	0,02	-	-
*Viet Nam, Hanoi	0,2	0,11	0,2	0,08

* IMPORTANT-SEE NOTES ON POPULATION PAGE

AGE-STANDARDIZED INCIDENCE
RATES AND STANDARD ERRORS (per 100,000)
Mesothelioma (contd)

EUROPE

	MALE		FEMALE	
Austria, Tyrol	0,5	0,17	0,3	0,11
*Belarus	0.2	0.03	0.2	0.02
*Croatia	0.6	0.07	0.1	0.03
Czech Republic	0.4	0.04	0.3	0.03
Denmark	1.4	0.09	0.3	0.04
Estonia	0.5	0.10	0.2	0.07
Finland	1.0	0.08	0.4	0.04
France, Bas-Rhin	0.6	0.16	0,2	0,08
*France, Calvados	1.1	0.24	0,2	0,12
France, Doubs	1.6	0.34	0,3	0,14
France, Haut-Rhin	0.6	0.17	0,2	0,09
*France, Herault	0.7	0.15	0,3	0,11
France, Isere	1.5	0.22	0,2	0,08
*France, Somme	1.0	0.25	0,3	0,12
*France, Tarn	0,6	0,21	0,1	0,05
Germany, Eastern States	0.9	0.07	0.3	0.03
Germany, Saarland				
Iceland	0,7	0,33	-	-
Ireland, Southern	0,2	0,10	0,0	0,04
Italy, Ferrara	1,0	0,41	-	-
Italy, Florence	0.6	0.12	0.3	0.08
Italy, Genoa	5.0	0.41	0.9	0.17
*Italy, Latina	0,2	0,13	0,1	0,10
Italy, Macerata	1,4	0,54	0,2	0,17
Italy, Modena	0.6	0.16	0.3	0,11
Italy, Parma	1.0	0.25	0,2	0,09
Italy, Ragusa	0,6	0,26	-	-
Italy, Romagna	1.3	0.25	0.4	0.12
Italy, Torino	0.9	0.17	0.4	0.11
Italy, Trieste	6.4	0.84	0,6	0,25
Italy, Varese	1.5	0.24	0.4	0.11
Italy, Veneto	1.2	0.17	0.4	0.09
*Latvia				
Malta				
The Netherlands	2.6	0.08	0.3	0.03
The Netherlands, Eindhoven	1.5	0.23	0.3	0.10
The Netherlands, Maastricht	3.0	0.33	0.3	0.10
Norway	1.2	0.09	0.2	0.04
*Poland, Cracow	0,5	0,16	0,2	0,09
*Poland, Kielce	0,2	0,08	0,2	0,07
*Poland, Lower Silesia	0.2	0.06	0,1	0,03
Poland, Warsaw City	0.4	0.11	0.3	0.08
Slovakia	0.3	0.05	0.1	0.03
Slovenia	0.7	0.11	0.3	0.06
*Spain, Albacete	0,3	0,25	0,7	0,44
Spain, Asturias	0.3	0.11	0,2	0,09
Spain, Basque Country	0.5	0.09	0.2	0.06
Spain, Granada	0,3	0,12	0,1	0,06
Spain, Mallorca	0,3	0,14	0,2	0,10
Spain, Murcia	0.4	0.11	0,1	0,06
Spain, Navarra	0.5	0.18	0.7	0.20
Spain, Tarragona	0,2	0,09	0,1	0,07
Spain, Zaragoza	0.8	0.18	0,2	0,07

	MALE		FEMALE	
Sweden	1.1	0.06	0.2	0.02
*Switzerland, Basel	1.6	0.31	0,3	0,13
Switzerland, Geneva	0,7	0,24	0.6	0.21
Switzerland, Graubunden	2.0	0.65	-	-
Switzerland, Neuchatel	1,2	0,47	0,2	0,17
Switzerland, St Gall-Appenzell	2.0	0.36	0,0	0,01
Switzerland, Valais	1.8	0.55	0,3	0,21
Switzerland, Vaud	1.0	0.23	0,3	0,11
Switzerland, Zurich	1.4	0.19	0,2	0,07
*UK, England and Wales	1.9	0.04	0.3	0.02
*UK, East Anglia	1.8	0.15	0.3	0.06
*UK, Mersey	2.3	0.17	0.2	0.04
*UK, North Western	1.9	0.12	0.4	0.05
UK, Oxford	1.9	0.16	0.2	0.05
*UK, South Thames	2.1	0.10	0.4	0.04
UK, South Western	2.3	0.14	0.3	0.05
UK, Wessex	3.3	0.18	0.3	0.05
*UK, West Midlands				
UK, Yorkshire	2.0	0.13	0.4	0.05
UK, Scotland	3.1	0.13	0.4	0.04
UK, Scotland, West	4.3	0.21	0.4	0.06
*Yugoslavia, Vojvodina	0,1	0,04	0.2	0.04

OCEANIA

	MALE		FEMALE	
Australian Capital Territory	0,6	0,33	0,1	0,10
Australia, New South Wales	2.4	0.12	0.3	0.04
South Australia	3.3	0.27	0.5	0.11
Australia, Tasmania	1.3	0.31	0,1	0,08
Australia, Victoria	1.8	0.12	0.3	0.04
Western Australia	4.2	0.31	0.5	0.10
*French Polynesia	0,2	0,18	-	-
New Zealand: Non-Maori				
New Zealand: Maori				
US, Hawaii: White	1.9	0.50	0,2	0,16
US, Hawaii: Japanese	0,3	0,20	-	-
US, Hawaii: Hawaiian	1,4	0,65	-	-
US, Hawaii: Filipino	1,2	0,55	-	-
US, Hawaii: Chinese	0,9	0,54	-	-

* IMPORTANT-SEE NOTES ON POPULATION PAGE

AGE-STANDARDIZED INCIDENCE
RATES AND STANDARD ERRORS (per 100,000)
Bone (ICD-9 170)

	MALE		FEMALE	
AFRICA				
*Algeria, Setif	2.0	0.50	0.7	0.22
*France, La Reunion	1.2	0.30	0.8	0.23
*Mali, Bamako	0,8	0,33	1.0	0.39
*Uganda, Kyadondo	2.3	0.81	0.6	0,27
*Zimbabwe, Harare: African	1.4	0.52	0,9	0,43
*Zimbabwe, Harare: European	0,9	0,90	-	-
AMERICA, CENTRAL AND SOUTH				
*Argentina, Concordia	1,7	0,72	1,6	0,70
*Brazil, Belem	2.6	0.49	1.5	0.34 f
*Brazil, Goiania	1.1	0.26	1.1	0.24
*Brazil, Porto Alegre	3.6	0.49	1.9	0.31
Colombia, Cali	1.2	0.20	0.7	0.15
*Costa Rica	0.7	0.11	0.6	0.10
*Ecuador, Quito	0.9	0.19	0.8	0.16
*Peru, Lima	1.0	0.14	1.0	0.14
Peru, Trujillo	1,0	0,43	0,6	0,25 m
US, Puerto Rico	0.7	0.10	0.6	0.09
*Uruguay, Montevideo	1.0	0.22	0.8	0.18
AMERICA, NORTH				
Canada	1.1	0.04	0.9	0.04
Canada, Alberta	1.0	0.13	0.7	0.11
Canada, British Columbia	0.8	0.10	0.8	0.10
Canada, Manitoba	1.0	0.19	0.7	0.17
Canada, New Brunswick	0.9	0.22	0.5	0.18
Canada, Newfoundland	0.7	0.21	0.5	0.18
Canada, Northwest Territories	0,7	0,48	0.7	0.48
Canada, Nova Scotia	0.9	0.19	1.0	0.20
Canada, Ontario	1.1	0.07	0.9	0.06
Canada, Prince Edward Island	1,0	0,54	0,5	0,40
Canada, Quebec	1.4	0.09	1.1	0.08
Canada, Saskatchewan	0.8	0.18	0.8	0.18
Canada, Yukon	-	-	-	-
US, Cent. Calif.: Non-Hisp. White	1.2	0.19	1.0	0.18
US, Cent. Calif.: Hispanic	0.6	0.21	0.7	0.21
US, Los Angeles: Non-Hisp. White	1.1	0.12	0.9	0.12
US, Los Angeles: Hispanic White	0.9	0.11	0.9	0.12
US, Los Angeles: Black	0.9	0.20	0,2	0,09
US, Los Angeles: Chinese	0,2	0,17	0.3	0,21
US, Los Angeles: Filipino	0,5	0,32	0.6	0,30
US, Los Angeles: Korean	1.0	0,59	0,2	0,24
US, Los Angeles: Japanese	0,3	0,32	-	-
US, San Francisco: Non-Hisp. White	0.9	0.14	0.7	0.13
US, San Francisco: Hispanic White	0.9	0.29	0,5	0,20
US, San Francisco: Black	0,6	0,24	0,5	0,19
US, San Francisco: Chinese	0.9	0.44	0.3	0,24
US, San Francisco: Filipino	0,4	0,31	0.9	0,46
US, San Francisco: Japanese	0,6	0,57	-	-
US, Connecticut: White	0.9	0.11	0.7	0.10
US, Connecticut: Black	0,8	0,38	0,2	0,15
US, Atlanta: White	0.7	0.13	0.6	0.14
US, Atlanta: Black	0,7	0,24	0.8	0.24
US, Iowa	1.0	0.12	0.9	0.11

	MALE		FEMALE	
US, Central Louisiana: White	0,7	0,36	1,0	0,42
US, Central Louisiana: Black	-	-	0,5	0,46
US, New Orleans: White	1.0	0.27	0,4	0,16
US, New Orleans: Black	0,8	0,30	0,4	0,20
US, Detroit: White	1.1	0.13	0.7	0.10
US, Detroit: Black	0.5	0.16	0.7	0.17
US, New Mexico: Non-Hisp. White	0.9	0.23	0.8	0.23
US, New Mexico: Hispanic White	1.1	0.28	0.9	0.25
US, New Mexico: American Indian	0,3	0,27	0,7	0,53
US, Utah	1.3	0.18	0.7	0.13
US, Seattle	1.0	0.12	0.9	0.11
US, SEER: White	1.0	0.05	0.8	0.04
US, SEER: Black	0.6	0.10	0.7	0.11
ASIA				
*China, Qidong	1.6	0.23	1.1	0.19
China, Shanghai	1.6	0.10	1.3	0.08
China, Tianjin	2.0	0.15	1.8	0.14
Hong Kong	1.1	0.09	0.9	0.08
*India, Bangalore	1.0	0.11	0.9	0.11
*India, Barshi, Paranda and Bhum	0,3	0,18	0,5	0,24
India, Bombay	0.8	0.07	0.6	0.06
*India, Karunagappally	0,6	0,44	0,2	0,21
India, Madras	1.0	0.10	0.4	0.06
*India, Trivandrum	0,5	0,24	0,4	0,20
Israel: All Jews	1.4	0.12	0.9	0.10
Jews born in Israel	1.4	0.28	1.2	0.25
Jews born in America or Europe	1.3	0.30	0.5	0.14
Jews born in Africa or Asia	0.8	0.17	1.2	0.63
Non-Jews	0.9	0.26	0,3	0,11
Japan, Hiroshima	0.6	0.15	0.5	0.13
Japan, Miyagi	0.7	0.11	0.6	0.11
Japan, Nagasaki	0.6	0.14	0.5	0.11
Japan, Osaka	0.6	0.05	0.5	0.05
*Japan, Saga	0.6	0.16	0.5	0.15
Japan, Yamagata	0.3	0.11	0.4	0.12
*Korea, Kangwha	2,7	1,01	0,8	0,55
*Kuwait: Non-Kuwaitis	1.0	0.30	0,3	0,14
*Kuwait: Kuwaitis	0,7	0,28	0.8	0.32
*Philippines, Manila	1.5	0.17	1.1	0.13
Singapore: Chinese	0.8	0.12	0.9	0.13
Singapore: Malay	0,7	0,28	0,6	0,28
Singapore: Indian	1,8	0,66	0,5	0,34
Thailand, Chiang Mai	0.6	0.14	0.6	0.13
*Thailand, Khon Kaen	1.2	0.24	1.7	0.27
*Viet Nam, Hanoi	2.1	0.29	0.9	0.18

AGE-STANDARDIZED INCIDENCE
RATES AND STANDARD ERRORS (per 100,000)
Bone (ICD-9 170) (contd)

EUROPE	MALE		FEMALE	
Austria, Tyrol	1.4	0.29	0.9	0.24
*Belarus	2.3	0.10	1.3	0.07
*Croatia	1.7	0.14	1.2	0.11
Czech Republic	1.1	0.06	0.7	0.05
Denmark	1.0	0.09	0.6	0.07
Estonia	0.7	0.13	0.8	0.14
Finland	0.9	0.08	0.7	0.07
France, Bas-Rhin	1.2	0.23	0.8	0.19
*France, Calvados	1.0	0.25	0.9	0.24
France, Doubs	0.9	0.30	1.0	0.29
France, Haut-Rhin	1.0	0.25	0.5	0.17
*France, Herault	1.4	0.26	1.1	0.24
France, Isere	0.9	0.18	0.6	0.16
*France, Somme	0,5	0,19	0,5	0,19
*France, Tarn	1.5	0.47	0,8	0,31
Germany, Eastern States	1.4	0.09	1.0	0.07
Germany, Saarland	1.0	0.20	0.6	0.16
Iceland	1,3	0,45	0,5	0,27
Ireland, Southern	0.9	0.25	0,6	0,21
Italy, Ferrara	0,9	0,42	0,7	0,32
Italy, Florence	1.2	0.24	0.8	0.20
Italy, Genoa	0.8	0.20	1.1	0.33
*Italy, Latina	1.1	0.35	0,3	0,15
Italy, Macerata	0,4	0,34	0,3	0,21
Italy, Modena	0.6	0.21	0.7	0.24
Italy, Parma	0,6	0,26	1.1	0.40
Italy, Ragusa	1.4	0.44	0,6	0,27
Italy, Romagna	1.2	0.38	1.0	0.29
Italy, Torino	0.8	0.22	0.5	0.16
Italy, Trieste	0,8	0,46	1,5	0,82
Italy, Varese	1.0	0.25	0.6	0.15
Italy, Veneto	0.8	0.18	0.7	0.18
*Latvia	1.7	0.16	1.0	0.11
Malta	0,4	0,29	1,0	0,50
The Netherlands	0.9	0.06	0.7	0.05
The Netherlands, Eindhoven	1.2	0.23	0.7	0.17
The Netherlands, Maastricht	1.1	0.23	0.7	0.20
Norway	0.9	0.09	0.6	0.08
*Poland, Cracow	1.2	0.26	0.8	0.19
*Poland, Kielce	1.1	0.19	0.7	0.15
*Poland, Lower Silesia	1.7	0.16	1.2	0.12
Poland, Warsaw City	1.0	0.18	0.8	0.17
Slovakia	1.6	0.11	1.1	0.08
Slovenia	0.6	0.11	0.6	0.11
*Spain, Albacete	0,6	0,36	1,8	0,79
Spain, Asturias	1.0	0.21	0.7	0.18
Spain, Basque Country	1.1	0.17	0.8	0.13
Spain, Granada	0.9	0.21	0.7	0.19
Spain, Mallorca	0.6	0.21	0,6	0,22
Spain, Murcia	1.4	0.22	0.5	0.14
Spain, Navarra	1.5	0.33	0.6	0.19
Spain, Tarragona	0.6	0.20	0.9	0.24
Spain, Zaragoza	1.0	0.23	0.7	0.17

	MALE		FEMALE		
Sweden	1.1	0.07	0.7	0.06	
*Switzerland, Basel	1.3	0.38	1.5	0.48	
Switzerland, Geneva	1.3	0.38	0,2	0,14	
Switzerland, Graubunden	0,9	0,47	2,2	0,87	
Switzerland, Neuchatel	0,2	0,16	0,6	0,47	
Switzerland, St Gall-Appenzell	1.5	0.38	1.0	0.30	
Switzerland, Valais	0,4	0,24	0,2	0,18	
Switzerland, Vaud	1.0	0.27	0,3	0,13	
Switzerland, Zurich	1.6	0.24	0.9	0.18	
*UK, England and Wales	1.0	0.04	0.7	0.03	
*UK, East Anglia	0.7	0.12	0.5	0.10	
*UK, Mersey	0.8	0.12	0.3	0.07	
*UK, North Western	0.6	0.08	0.5	0.07	
UK, Oxford	1.0	0.13	0.6	0.10	
*UK, South Thames	1.0	0.08	0.7	0.07	
UK, South Western	1.0	0.11	0.5	0.08	
UK, Wessex	1.0	0.11	0.9	0.11	
*UK, West Midlands	2.2	0.14	1.7	0.12	
UK, Yorkshire	0.7	0.09	0.5	0.08	
UK, Scotland	0.9	0.09	0.6	0.07	
UK, Scotland, West	1.0	0.12	0.7	0.10	
*Yugoslavia, Vojvodina	1.6	0.17	0.8	0.11	

OCEANIA	MALE		FEMALE		
Australian Capital Territory	1.7	0.53	0,7	0,33	
Australia, New South Wales	1.0	0.08	0.6	0.07	
South Australia	0.7	0.14	0.7	0.14	
Australia, Tasmania	0.7	0.23	0,5	0,20	
Australia, Victoria	1.1	0.10	0.7	0.08	
Western Australia	1.2	0.17	0.9	0.15	
*French Polynesia	2,3	0,94	1,9	0,74	m
New Zealand: Non-Maori	1.4	0.13	0.9	0.11	
New Zealand: Maori	1.9	0.57	0.7	0,28	
US, Hawaii: White	1.0	0.32	0,4	0,23	
US, Hawaii: Japanese	0,6	0,39	0,9	0,47	
US, Hawaii: Hawaiian	1,1	0,48	0,5	0,32	
US, Hawaii: Filipino	1,8	0,70	0,3	0,31	
US, Hawaii: Chinese	0,5	0,50	-	-	

* IMPORTANT-SEE NOTES ON POPULATION PAGE

AGE-STANDARDIZED INCIDENCE
RATES AND STANDARD ERRORS (per 100,000)
Connective tissue (ICD-9 171)

	MALE		FEMALE		
AFRICA					
*Algeria, Setif	0,4	0,16	0,4	0,15	
*France, La Reunion	1.2	0.32	1.1	0.29	
*Mali, Bamako	0,4	0,19	0,4	0,26	
*Uganda, Kyadondo	1.6	0.59	1.2	0.40	
*Zimbabwe, Harare: African	1.1	0.29	1.9	0.80	f
*Zimbabwe, Harare: European	6,9	3,03	1,8	1,79	
AMERICA, CENTRAL AND SOUTH					
*Argentina, Concordia	1,3	0,67	2,0	0,77	
*Brazil, Belem	1.9	0.48	2.0	0.37	m
*Brazil, Goiania	1.3	0.35	2.4	0.43	
*Brazil, Porto Alegre	2.8	0.46	2.1	0.33	
Colombia, Cali	2.4	0.34	2.4	0.29	m
*Costa Rica	1.6	0.17	1.3	0.15	
*Ecuador, Quito	2.8	0.38	1.7	0.27	
*Peru, Lima	1.7	0.20	2.1	0.21	
Peru, Trujillo	1,5	0,58	1,2	0,50	
US, Puerto Rico	1.5	0.15	1.0	0.11	
*Uruguay, Montevideo	2.9	0.37	2.7	0.33	
AMERICA, NORTH					
Canada	2.2	0.05	1.6	0.05	
Canada, Alberta	1.7	0.17	1.4	0.15	
Canada, British Columbia	1.9	0.14	1.5	0.14	
Canada, Manitoba	1.8	0.24	1.4	0.22	
Canada, New Brunswick	1.9	0.31	1.7	0.28	
Canada, Newfoundland	2.5	0.42	1.3	0.29	
Canada, Northwest Territories	1,8	1,08	0,2	0,24	
Canada, Nova Scotia	2.4	0.31	2.6	0.32	
Canada, Ontario	2.3	0.09	1.7	0.08	
Canada, Prince Edward Island	3.1	0.95	0,9	0,45	
Canada, Quebec	2.3	0.11	1.7	0.09	
Canada, Saskatchewan	2.3	0.30	1.5	0.24	
Canada, Yukon	-	-	1,4	0,82	
US, Cent. Calif.: Non-Hisp. White	2.2	0.24	2.0	0.23	
US, Cent. Calif.: Hispanic	2.0	0.42	1.6	0.35	
US, Los Angeles: Non-Hisp. White	2.8	0.16	2.0	0.14	
US, Los Angeles: Hispanic White	2.0	0.20	1.5	0.16	
US, Los Angeles: Black	2.2	0.31	1.9	0.27	
US, Los Angeles: Chinese	1,8	0,61	1,1	0,40	
US, Los Angeles: Filipino	2.2	0.68	2.5	0.69	
US, Los Angeles: Korean	2,2	0,88	1,4	0,68	
US, Los Angeles: Japanese	1,3	0,53	1,7	0,86	
US, San Francisco: Non-Hisp. White	2.4	0.21	1.6	0.16	
US, San Francisco: Hispanic White	2.4	0.50	1.5	0.36	
US, San Francisco: Black	3.4	0.58	1.8	0.40	
US, San Francisco: Chinese	1.7	0.52	1.3	0.45	
US, San Francisco: Filipino	0,9	0,43	1,0	0,45	
US, San Francisco: Japanese	3,5	2,32	2,5	2,10	
US, Connecticut: White	2.3	0.17	1.5	0.13	
US, Connecticut: Black	3.9	0.86	2.5	0.60	
US, Atlanta: White	2.5	0.28	1.5	0.21	
US, Atlanta: Black	2.0	0.44	1.9	0.36	
US, Iowa	2.5	0.18	1.9	0.15	

	MALE		FEMALE	
US, Central Louisiana: White	2.3	0.61	1.8	0.57
US, Central Louisiana: Black	2,6	1,34	3,1	1,16
US, New Orleans: White	2.7	0.42	2.1	0.33
US, New Orleans: Black	2.7	0.58	1.3	0.36
US, Detroit: White	2.3	0.17	1.7	0.15
US, Detroit: Black	2.1	0.31	1.5	0.23
US, New Mexico: Non-Hisp. White	2.8	0.36	2.0	0.31
US, New Mexico: Hispanic White	1.8	0.38	1.7	0.35
US, New Mexico: American Indian	1,9	0,92	2,1	0,81
US, Utah	2.0	0.22	1.7	0.20
US, Seattle	2.5	0.17	2.0	0.15
US, SEER: White	2.4	0.07	1.7	0.06
US, SEER: Black	2.5	0.22	1.8	0.17
ASIA				
*China, Qidong	0,3	0,10	0,2	0,07
China, Shanghai	1.7	0.10	1.3	0.09
China, Tianjin	1.2	0.12	0.9	0.10
Hong Kong	2.2	0.12	2.1	0.12
*India, Bangalore	0.9	0.11	0.9	0.11
*India, Barshi, Paranda and Bhum	0,5	0,22	0,2	0,16
India, Bombay	1.3	0.10	1.0	0.09
*India, Karunagappally	1,4	0,63	0,5	0,40
India, Madras	1.0	0.12	1.0	0.12
*India, Trivandrum	1.4	0.44	0,7	0,30
Israel: All Jews	2.8	0.17	2.2	0.15
Jews born in Israel	3.2	0.50	1.5	0.33
Jews born in America or Europe	2.6	0.32	2.8	0.38
Jews born in Africa or Asia	1.9	0.27	2.6	0.83
Non-Jews	1.2	0.30	0.9	0.26
Japan, Hiroshima	1.2	0.21	1.2	0.23
Japan, Miyagi	1.6	0.18	1.0	0.14
Japan, Nagasaki	1.3	0.19	0.9	0.15
Japan, Osaka	1.1	0.08	0.9	0.08
*Japan, Saga	0.6	0.16	0.3	0.11
Japan, Yamagata	0.7	0.14	0.4	0.11
*Korea, Kangwha	-	-	-	-
*Kuwait: Non-Kuwaitis	1.6	0.38	0,9	0,44
*Kuwait: Kuwaitis	0,8	0,31	0,9	0,34
*Philippines, Manila	2.6	0.23	2.1	0.19
Singapore: Chinese	1.7	0.19	1.2	0.16
Singapore: Malay	1.8	0.52	1.1	0.34
Singapore: Indian	0,7	0,38	0,4	0,30
Thailand, Chiang Mai	0.5	0.11	0.7	0.16
*Thailand, Khon Kaen	0.9	0.18	0.7	0.16
*Viet Nam, Hanoi	2.3	0.32	1.3	0.21

* IMPORTANT-SEE NOTES ON POPULATION PAGE

EUROPE	MALE		FEMALE	
Austria, Tyrol	2.9	0.46	2.2	0.35
*Belarus	2.4	0.10	1.8	0.08
*Croatia	1.3	0.12	1.2	0.11
Czech Republic	2.2	0.09	1.7	0.08
Denmark	2.1	0.12	1.6	0.11
Estonia	2.3	0.25	2.1	0.21
Finland	2.4	0.12	2.0	0.11
France, Bas-Rhin	1.9	0.28	1.7	0.25
*France, Calvados	1.6	0.32	1.4	0.27
France, Doubs	3.1	0.52	2.0	0.41
France, Haut-Rhin	2.8	0.41	1.8	0.30
*France, Herault	2.1	0.31	1.9	0.31
France, Isere	1.7	0.25	1.9	0.27
*France, Somme	1.3	0.30	1.0	0.27
*France, Tarn	2.0	0.46	1.3	0.43
Germany, Eastern States	1.8	0.10	1.6	0.09
Germany, Saarland	1.9	0.26	1.8	0.27
Iceland	1.7	0.50	1,0	0,37
Ireland, Southern	2.2	0.40	1.4	0.33
Italy, Ferrara	1.5	0.49	1.1	0.39
Italy, Florence	1.4	0.23	1.8	0.30
Italy, Genoa	2.8	0.41	2.1	0.38
*Italy, Latina	1.7	0.46	1.2	0.34
Italy, Macerata	2.3	0.78	2.3	0.92
Italy, Modena	2.6	0.41	1.4	0.37
Italy, Parma	1.8	0.38	1.6	0.32
Italy, Ragusa	1.0	0.35	1,0	0,35
Italy, Romagna	2.4	0.51	1.5	0.40
Italy, Torino	1.7	0.30	1.5	0.30
Italy, Trieste	3.0	0.73	1.3	0.72
Italy, Varese	1.7	0.32	1.6	0.30
Italy, Veneto	3.3	0.33	1.8	0.21
*Latvia	1.7	0.16	1.5	0.14
Malta	1,6	0,64	1,7	0,64
The Netherlands	2.6	0.09	1.8	0.08
The Netherlands, Eindhoven	2.5	0.32	1.2	0.22
The Netherlands, Maastricht	2.5	0.33	1.8	0.30
Norway	1.5	0.12	1.3	0.11
*Poland, Cracow	1.3	0.26	1.0	0.24
*Poland, Kielce	1.7	0.24	1.2	0.19
*Poland, Lower Silesia	1.9	0.17	1.6	0.14
Poland, Warsaw City	2.3	0.31	1.4	0.20
Slovakia	2.2	0.13	1.6	0.10
Slovenia	1.8	0.21	1.3	0.16
*Spain, Albacete	2.2	0.69	2,0	0,83
Spain, Asturias	2.0	0.28	1.4	0.24
Spain, Basque Country	2.1	0.22	1.5	0.18
Spain, Granada	1.4	0.27	1.3	0.24
Spain, Mallorca	1.5	0.31	1.5	0.31
Spain, Murcia	2.0	0.27	1.7	0.25
Spain, Navarra	1.6	0.34	1.4	0.31
Spain, Tarragona	1.9	0.37	1.4	0.29
Spain, Zaragoza	1.7	0.28	1.1	0.23

	MALE		FEMALE	
Sweden	2.8	0.11	2.1	0.10
*Switzerland, Basel	2.0	0.40	1.6	0.37
Switzerland, Geneva	1.8	0.44	2.2	0.52
Switzerland, Graubunden	1.9	0.69	1,2	0,48
Switzerland, Neuchatel	0,5	0,28	0,5	0,28
Switzerland, St Gall-Appenzell	2.5	0.43	1.7	0.33
Switzerland, Valais	1.8	0.52	3.2	0.77
Switzerland, Vaud	2.9	0.48	2.2	0.38
Switzerland, Zurich	2.1	0.23	2.2	0.28
*UK, England and Wales	1.9	0.05	1.5	0.04
*UK, East Anglia	1.7	0.17	1.8	0.18
*UK, Mersey	1.7	0.16	1.2	0.14
*UK, North Western	1.4	0.11	1.1	0.10
UK, Oxford	2.4	0.19	1.6	0.15
*UK, South Thames	1.8	0.10	1.4	0.09
UK, South Western	1.5	0.13	1.2	0.12
UK, Wessex	2.2	0.16	1.7	0.14
*UK, West Midlands	2.5	0.13	2.2	0.12
UK, Yorkshire	1.9	0.14	1.4	0.12
UK, Scotland	1.8	0.11	1.2	0.09
UK, Scotland, West	1.7	0.15	1.2	0.13
*Yugoslavia, Vojvodina	1.5	0.17	1.0	0.13

OCEANIA

	MALE		FEMALE	
Australian Capital Territory	1.8	0.53	1,1	0,45
Australia, New South Wales	2.5	0.12	1.7	0.10
South Australia	2.7	0.26	1.6	0.20
Australia, Tasmania	2.1	0.42	2.3	0.45
Australia, Victoria	2.4	0.14	1.5	0.11
Western Australia	1.9	0.21	1.2	0.17
*French Polynesia	1,5	0,61	1,2	0,62
New Zealand: Non-Maori	2.7	0.18	1.7	0.14
New Zealand: Maori	2.7	0.74	2.5	0.66
US, Hawaii: White	2.8	0.57	2.0	0.53
US, Hawaii: Japanese	1.1	0.40	0.8	0.26
US, Hawaii: Hawaiian	3.0	0.84	2.4	0.73
US, Hawaii: Filipino	2.4	0.69	1,8	0,68
US, Hawaii: Chinese	2,1	0,99	2,2	1,25

* IMPORTANT-SEE NOTES ON POPULATION PAGE

AGE-STANDARDIZED INCIDENCE
RATES AND STANDARD ERRORS (per 100,000)
Melanoma of skin (ICD-9 172)

	MALE		FEMALE	
AFRICA				
*Algeria, Setif	0,1	0,08	0,1	0,07
*France, La Reunion	1.4	0.36	2.3	0.39
*Mali, Bamako	0,5	0,27	1,1	0,42
*Uganda, Kyadondo	1,3	0,66	1,1	0,52 m
*Zimbabwe, Harare: African	1.8	0.61	3.8	1.21
*Zimbabwe, Harare: European	18.6	4.38	15.0	3.97
AMERICA, CENTRAL AND SOUTH				
*Argentina, Concordia	1,2	0,62	2,3	0,84
*Brazil, Belem	1.4	0.38	0.9	0.27
*Brazil, Goiania	3.2	0.56	1.9	0.41
*Brazil, Porto Alegre	5.3	0.61	5.0	0.51 f
Colombia, Cali	2.7	0.36	3.1	0.34 m
*Costa Rica	2.1	0.21	1.8	0.19
*Ecuador, Quito	3.3	0.45	3.7	0.43
*Peru, Lima	1.7	0.21	1.5	0.18
Peru, Trujillo	3.1	0.99	1,7	0,61 m
US, Puerto Rico	1.4	0.14	1.1	0.11
*Uruguay, Montevideo	3.8	0.41	2.5	0.31
AMERICA, NORTH				
Canada	7.7	0.10	6.9	0.09
Canada, Alberta	7.5	0.34	7.5	0.33
Canada, British Columbia	9.9	0.32	10.2	0.32
Canada, Manitoba	7.1	0.48	7.0	0.47
Canada, New Brunswick	8.8	0.65	8.1	0.62
Canada, Newfoundland	3.9	0.52	5.2	0.58
Canada, Northwest Territories	1,4	0,83	1,9	1,13
Canada, Nova Scotia	9.6	0.61	9.3	0.58
Canada, Ontario	9.6	0.18	8.0	0.16
Canada, Prince Edward Island	8.8	1.52	9.4	1.61
Canada, Quebec	3.7	0.14	3.3	0.12
Canada, Saskatchewan	8.0	0.53	7.6	0.52
Canada, Yukon	5,1	1,79	6.9	2.21
US, Cent. Calif.: Non-Hisp. White	12.1	0.54	8.6	0.45
US, Cent. Calif.: Hispanic	3.0	0.53	2.9	0.49
US, Los Angeles: Non-Hisp. White	16.0	0.37	11.3	0.32
US, Los Angeles: Hispanic White	2.0	0.22	2.2	0.20
US, Los Angeles: Black	0.8	0.19	0.6	0.14
US, Los Angeles: Chinese	-	-	0,6	0,30
US, Los Angeles: Filipino	0,8	0,40	0,1	0,11
US, Los Angeles: Korean	-	-	0,4	0,30
US, Los Angeles: Japanese	0,9	0,41	0,8	0,43
US, San Francisco: Non-Hisp. White	16.4	0.49	11.9	0.41
US, San Francisco: Hispanic White	3.1	0.58	4.8	0.63
US, San Francisco: Black	0,7	0,26	0,6	0,22
US, San Francisco: Chinese	0,1	0,11	0,4	0,24
US, San Francisco: Filipino	1,1	0,56	0,9	0,42
US, San Francisco: Japanese	0,6	0,56	0,7	0,69
US, Connecticut: White	13.8	0.39	11.2	0.35
US, Connecticut: Black	1,6	0,58	1,0	0,37
US, Atlanta: White	17.1	0.67	12.0	0.52
US, Atlanta: Black	0,9	0,32	0,4	0,15
US, Iowa	9.9	0.35	8.4	0.32

	MALE		FEMALE	
US, Central Louisiana: White	9.9	1.27	7.5	1.03
US, Central Louisiana: Black	-	-	1,1	0,80
US, New Orleans: White	7.1	0.64	4.0	0.46
US, New Orleans: Black	0.9	0,34	0,1	0,06
US, Detroit: White	11.2	0.36	7.3	0.29
US, Detroit: Black	0.6	0.16	0.3	0.10
US, New Mexico: Non-Hisp. White	16.8	0.84	12.5	0.74
US, New Mexico: Hispanic White	2.7	0.45	3.3	0.49
US, New Mexico: American Indian	1,4	0,77	0,7	0,41
US, Utah	13.3	0.59	11.0	0.51
US, Seattle	12.2	0.36	10.7	0.33
US, SEER: White	13.1	0.16	10.2	0.13
US, SEER: Black	0.7	0.12	0.5	0.08
ASIA				
*China, Qidong	0.4	0.12	0.3	0.08
China, Shanghai	0.3	0.04	0.3	0.03
China, Tianjin	0.4	0.07	0.3	0.05
Hong Kong	1.0	0.08	0.7	0.07
*India, Bangalore	0.3	0.07	0.2	0.06
*India, Barshi, Paranda and Bhum	-	-	0,1	0,12
India, Bombay	0.4	0.06	0.3	0.06
*India, Karunagappally	0,9	0,50	-	-
India, Madras	0.4	0.09	0.3	0.07
*India, Trivandrum	0,3	0,23	0,1	0,13
Israel: All Jews	9.6	0.32	9.8	0.31
Jews born in Israel	15.7	1.02	14.9	0.96
Jews born in America or Europe	11.3	0.63	12.0	0.67
Jews born in Africa or Asia	2.6	0.31	2.5	0.32
Non-Jews	0.7	0.22	0,7	0,24
Japan, Hiroshima	0.5	0.13	0.5	0.12
Japan, Miyagi	0.6	0.09	0.2	0.05
Japan, Nagasaki	0.5	0.11	0.4	0.08
Japan, Osaka	0.2	0.03	0.2	0.03
*Japan, Saga	0.6	0.16	0.5	0.11
Japan, Yamagata	0.4	0.10	0.3	0.07
*Korea, Kangwha	0,3	0,27	0,2	0,18
*Kuwait: Non-Kuwaitis	1.0	0.52	1,8	0,91
*Kuwait: Kuwaitis	0,4	0,28	0,3	0,26
*Philippines, Manila	0.7	0.13	0.6	0.10
Singapore: Chinese	0.6	0.12	0.6	0.10
Singapore: Malay	0,1	0,07	0,2	0,16
Singapore: Indian	-	-	-	-
Thailand, Chiang Mai	0.6	0.14	0.5	0.12
*Thailand, Khon Kaen	0,4	0,14	0.6	0.16
*Viet Nam, Hanoi	0.3	0.11	0,3	0,11

* IMPORTANT-SEE NOTES ON POPULATION PAGE

EUROPE	MALE		FEMALE	
Austria, Tyrol	12.4	0.84	15.6	0.91
*Belarus	1.9	0.09	2.3	0.08
*Croatia	3.1	0.17	2.9	0.15
Czech Republic	6.5	0.15	6.1	0.14
Denmark	8.8	0.23	11.7	0.27
Estonia	3.6	0.30	4.1	0.28
Finland	7.8	0.21	6.7	0.19
France, Bas-Rhin	6.6	0.50	7.8	0.52
*France, Calvados	3.2	0.43	6.3	0.59
France, Doubs	4.8	0.61	8.6	0.79
France, Haut-Rhin	6.9	0.60	6.7	0.58
*France, Herault	5.1	0.46	6.2	0.51
France, Isere	4.1	0.38	6.2	0.46
*France, Somme	3.4	0.47	4.6	0.55
*France, Tarn	4.3	0.63	6.7	0.81
Germany, Eastern States	5.0	0.16	5.3	0.16
Germany, Saarland	5.8	0.41	6.1	0.41
Iceland	3.7	0.73	7.2	1.04
Ireland, Southern	6.2	0.66	10.9	0.88
Italy, Ferrara	3.5	0.83	6.1	1.58
Italy, Florence	5.5	0.42	5.2	0.40
Italy, Genoa	5.2	0.48	5.8	0.51
*Italy, Latina	3.3	0.55	2.9	0.50
Italy, Macerata	6.1	1.23	4.9	1.10
Italy, Modena	4.3	0.45	3.7	0.41
Italy, Parma	4.1	0.56	4.9	0.63
Italy, Ragusa	3.9	0.65	2.3	0.49
Italy, Romagna	6.0	0.60	6.7	0.64
Italy, Torino	3.9	0.37	4.6	0.40
Italy, Trieste	9.7	1.13	10.0	1.22
Italy, Varese	5.1	0.44	5.0	0.43
Italy, Veneto	6.1	0.40	7.0	0.43
*Latvia	2.1	0.17	3.0	0.18
Malta	2.6	0.87	3.4	0.88
The Netherlands	6.9	0.14	9.8	0.16
The Netherlands, Eindhoven	5.6	0.44	8.6	0.56
The Netherlands, Maastricht	5.2	0.44	9.6	0.61
Norway	14.1	0.33	15.3	0.35
*Poland, Cracow	4.3	0.46	3.6	0.37
*Poland, Kielce	2.3	0.28	2.3	0.26
*Poland, Lower Silesia	2.9	0.20	3.0	0.19
Poland, Warsaw City	3.8	0.33	3.7	0.28
Slovakia	4.4	0.18	4.4	0.17
Slovenia	4.7	0.29	5.4	0.29
*Spain, Albacete	2,0	0,77	1.7	0.60
Spain, Asturias	2.1	0.29	3.9	0.35
Spain, Basque Country	3.0	0.24	4.2	0.29
Spain, Granada	3.1	0.37	3.9	0.42
Spain, Mallorca	3.8	0.47	3.9	0.47
Spain, Murcia	2.8	0.31	4.4	0.39
Spain, Navarra	3.3	0.44	3.6	0.47
Spain, Tarragona	3.5	0.46	3.2	0.44
Spain, Zaragoza	2.3	0.28	3.3	0.35

	MALE		FEMALE	
Sweden	11.0	0.20	11.1	0.20
*Switzerland, Basel	10.6	0.84	8.9	0.78
Switzerland, Geneva	10.5	0.95	11.1	0.94
Switzerland, Graubunden	8.2	1.40	10.2	1.54
Switzerland, Neuchatel	11.4	1.58	10.3	1.43
Switzerland, St Gall-Appenzell	8.1	0.74	10.2	0.82
Switzerland, Valais	5.2	0.92	8.5	1.13
Switzerland, Vaud	12.0	0.81	12.6	0.82
Switzerland, Zurich	13.7	0.60	13.3	0.58
*UK, England and Wales	4.6	0.07	6.6	0.08
*UK, East Anglia	5.8	0.30	7.5	0.34
*UK, Mersey	3.4	0.21	4.6	0.25
*UK, North Western	3.7	0.18	5.7	0.22
UK, Oxford	5.8	0.28	7.6	0.32
*UK, South Thames	4.6	0.15	6.4	0.18
UK, South Western	7.3	0.27	10.3	0.32
UK, Wessex	6.6	0.27	10.3	0.34
*UK, West Midlands	4.5	0.17	6.1	0.20
UK, Yorkshire	4.1	0.19	6.6	0.24
UK, Scotland	6.0	0.20	8.3	0.23
UK, Scotland, West	6.1	0.28	7.7	0.30
*Yugoslavia, Vojvodina	2.9	0.21	3.5	0.22

OCEANIA	MALE		FEMALE	
Australian Capital Territory	29.5	2.19	23.4	1.82
Australia, New South Wales	33.1	0.44	25.7	0.39
South Australia	27.8	0.81	24.9	0.76
Australia, Tasmania	23.5	1.33	23.1	1.31
Australia, Victoria	22.4	0.42	20.3	0.40
Western Australia	32.2	0.86	24.9	0.75
*French Polynesia	3.4	1.16	4.8	1.16
New Zealand: Non-Maori	25.0	0.53	29.8	0.59
New Zealand: Maori	5.1	1.26	3.4	0.86
US, Hawaii: White	19.5	1.48	12.4	1.20
US, Hawaii: Japanese	0,3	0,18	0,3	0,17
US, Hawaii: Hawaiian	0,9	0,51	1,2	0,55
US, Hawaii: Filipino	0,5	0,27	0,6	0,35
US, Hawaii: Chinese	0,8	0,57	0,7	0,60

* IMPORTANT-SEE NOTES ON POPULATION PAGE

AFRICA	MALE		FEMALE	
*Algeria, Setif	3.9	0.73	1.8	0.40
†*France, La Reunion	10.2	0.99	7.2	0.73
*Mali, Bamako	5.0	0.87	2.6	0.62
*Uganda, Kyadondo	3.1	0.97	1.0	0.45
*Zimbabwe, Harare: African	4.0	1.11	4.3	1.38
*Zimbabwe, Harare: European	535.4	24.37	343.0	19.48

AMERICA, CENTRAL AND SOUTH

	MALE		FEMALE	
*Argentina, Concordia	48.6	4.29	32.1	3.00
*Brazil, Belem	34.9	2.10	21.9	1.35
*Brazil, Goiania	123.2	3.72	104.4	3.04
*Brazil, Porto Alegre	53.9	2.14	32.4	1.33 mf
Colombia, Cali	-	-	0,0	0,03
*Costa Rica	41.3	0.97	37.9	0.87
*Ecuador, Quito	21.9	1.16	22.5	1.06
*Peru, Lima	10.3	0.52	8.5	0.45
Peru, Trujillo	18.6	2.21	15.9	1.81
† US, Puerto Rico	0.3	0.06	0.4	0.07
*Uruguay, Montevideo	17.6	0.84	9.5	0.53

AMERICA, NORTH

	MALE		FEMALE	
Canada				
Canada, Alberta				
Canada, British Columbia				
Canada, Manitoba				
Canada, New Brunswick				
Canada, Newfoundland				
Canada, Northwest Territories				
Canada, Nova Scotia				
Canada, Ontario				
Canada, Prince Edward Island				
Canada, Quebec				
Canada, Saskatchewan				
Canada, Yukon				
† US, Cent. Calif.: Non-Hisp. White	1.0	0.15	0.6	0.12
† US, Cent. Calif.: Hispanic	0,3	0,14	0,4	0,16
† US, Los Angeles: Non-Hisp. White	1.1	0.10	0.8	0.08
† US, Los Angeles: Hispanic White	0.4	0.09	0.6	0.10
† US, Los Angeles: Black	0.8	0.19	0.8	0.17
† US, Los Angeles: Chinese	0,4	0,27	0.3	0,22
† US, Los Angeles: Filipino	0,3	0,22	0.3	0,20
† US, Los Angeles: Korean	-	-	0,1	0,15
† US, Los Angeles: Japanese	0,4	0,28	0.6	0,29
† US, San Francisco: Non-Hisp. White	1.0	0.12	0.9	0.11
† US, San Francisco: Hispanic White	0,4	0,19	0.5	0,20
† US, San Francisco: Black	0.8	0.26	1.1	0.31
† US, San Francisco: Chinese	0,2	0,17	0,1	0,10
† US, San Francisco: Filipino	-	-	0,4	0,32
† US, San Francisco: Japanese	-	-	-	-
† US, Connecticut: White	0.8	0.09	0.6	0.08
† US, Connecticut: Black	0,8	0,33	0.8	0,31
† US, Atlanta: White	1.0	0.16	0.4	0.10
† US, Atlanta: Black	0,5	0,16	0.9	0.22
† US, Iowa	0.9	0.10	0.5	0.08

	MALE		FEMALE	
† US, Central Louisiana: White	0,5	0,28	0,8	0,36
† US, Central Louisiana: Black	-	-	0,9	0,71
† US, New Orleans: White	0.5	0.16	0.6	0.17
† US, New Orleans: Black	0,4	0,21	0.8	0,27
† US, Detroit: White	0.7	0.09	0.7	0.08
† US, Detroit: Black	0.9	0.20	0.9	0.19
† US, New Mexico: Non-Hisp. White	1.4	0.23	1.1	0.22
† US, New Mexico: Hispanic White	1.0	0.29	0.8	0.24
† US, New Mexico: American Indian	-	-	0,2	0,20
† US, Utah	0.8	0.14	0.9	0.15
† US, Seattle	1.0	0.10	0.9	0.10
† US, SEER: White	0.9	0.04	0.7	0.03
† US, SEER: Black	0.7	0.11	1.0	0.12

ASIA

	MALE		FEMALE	
*China, Qidong	1.4	0.23	1.1	0.16
China, Shanghai	1.7	0.09	1.1	0.07
China, Tianjin	0.8	0.10	0.8	0.09
Hong Kong	5.6	0.20	4.4	0.17
*India, Bangalore	1.5	0.15	1.4	0.15
*India, Barshi, Paranda and Bhum	1.4	0.40	1.1	0.34
India, Bombay	1.7	0.12	1.2	0.10
*India, Karunagappally	2,4	0,81	2.7	0.86
India, Madras	1.7	0.17	1.1	0.14
*India, Trivandrum	1,1	0,39	1,1	0,39
Israel: All Jews	2.9	0.17	2.8	0.16
Jews born in Israel	3.6	0.60	4.2	0.60
Jews born in America or Europe	3.6	0.34	3.2	0.30
Jews born in Africa or Asia	1.6	0.25	1.1	0.18
Non-Jews	0,5	0,20	0,6	0,21
Japan, Hiroshima	5.2	0.42	3.9	0.33
Japan, Miyagi	2.6	0.19	1.7	0.14
Japan, Nagasaki	5.2	0.31	3.7	0.22
Japan, Osaka	1.2	0.07	0.8	0.05
*Japan, Saga	2.6	0.28	1.0	0.14
Japan, Yamagata	1.1	0.15	1.1	0.13
*Korea, Kangwha	2,5	0,94	0,5	0,38
*Kuwait: Non-Kuwaitis	5.9	1.79	3.3	0.97
*Kuwait: Kuwaitis	2.7	0.70	1,6	0,58
*Philippines, Manila	2.6	0.25	1.8	0.18
Singapore: Chinese	9.1	0.47	8.0	0.38
Singapore: Malay	4.2	0.78	3.5	0.75
Singapore: Indian	3.4	0.93	4.4	1.33
Thailand, Chiang Mai	4.2	0.37	3.0	0.31
*Thailand, Khon Kaen	3.9	0.46	3.4	0.38
*Viet Nam, Hanoi	2.9	0.38	2.4	0.31

* IMPORTANT-SEE NOTES ON POPULATION PAGE

AGE-STANDARDIZED INCIDENCE
RATES AND STANDARD ERRORS (per 100,000)
Other skin (ICD-9 173) (contd)

EUROPE	MALE		FEMALE	
Austria, Tyrol	22.4	1.12	14.9	0.78
*Belarus	20.3	0.29	16.3	0.20
*Croatia	1.0	0.10	0.8	0.06
Czech Republic	55.8	0.42	36.6	0.30
Denmark	53.1	0.53	43.3	0.47
Estonia	19.6	0.69	16.9	0.51
Finland	54.6	0.54	48.2	0.44
† France, Bas-Rhin	16.0	0.75	7.4	0.44
*France, Calvados	38.2	1.42	21.2	0.92
France, Doubs	65.9	2.19	47.2	1.71
† France, Haut-Rhin	47.3	1.54	33.4	1.17
*France, Herault	18.7	0.75	7.2	0.42
† France, Isere	13.3	0.65	5.8	0.38
†*France, Somme	15.5	0.92	4.6	0.42
†*France, Tarn	17.7	1.09	7.5	0.63
† Germany, Eastern States	7.0	0.19	2.9	0.09
Germany, Saarland	60.7	1.28	36.9	0.87
† Iceland	4.9	0.80	4.3	0.72
Ireland, Southern	79.0	2.22	54.7	1.79
Italy, Ferrara	51.9	2.86	28.6	2.00
Italy, Florence	23.5	0.76	11.4	0.49
Italy, Genoa	33.4	1.05	19.3	0.76
*Italy, Latina	25.9	1.47	14.2	1.00
Italy, Macerata	46.0	3.05	25.3	2.16
Italy, Modena	42.8	1.31	21.0	0.87
Italy, Parma	28.0	1.31	12.9	0.82
Italy, Ragusa	47.6	2.14	23.2	1.45
Italy, Romagna	60.5	1.73	34.3	1.23
Italy, Torino	39.9	1.15	25.4	0.87
Italy, Trieste	68.1	2.76	47.3	2.27
Italy, Varese	45.3	1.30	25.2	0.84
Italy, Veneto	51.2	1.10	28.3	0.76
*Latvia	18.7	0.51	14.1	0.35
Malta	51.0	3.52	22.1	2.13
† The Netherlands	15.0	0.19	5.7	0.11
† The Netherlands, Eindhoven	-	-	-	-
† The Netherlands, Maastricht	11.7	0.64	5.6	0.40
† Norway	10.6	0.25	6.7	0.19
*Poland, Cracow	17.5	0.94	10.5	0.60
*Poland, Kielce	18.4	0.75	12.4	0.55
*Poland, Lower Silesia	12.7	0.43	9.1	0.31
Poland, Warsaw City	12.9	0.57	9.9	0.41
Slovakia	39.4	0.53	29.3	0.41
Slovenia	21.7	0.63	15.9	0.45
†*Spain, Albacete	0,6	0,31	1,1	0,55
† Spain, Asturias	0.4	0.11	0.3	0.07
† Spain, Basque Country	0.6	0.11	0.3	0.08
Spain, Granada	45.3	1.34	26.2	0.95
† Spain, Mallorca	89.7	2.17	61.2	1.73
Spain, Murcia	58.4	1.39	34.1	0.97
Spain, Navarra	51.5	1.67	31.8	1.28
Spain, Tarragona	62.8	1.84	40.1	1.45
Spain, Zaragoza	25.3	0.90	12.1	0.57

	MALE		FEMALE	
† Sweden	11.9	0.17	5.3	0.11
*Switzerland, Basel	88.5	2.34	58.9	1.80
Switzerland, Geneva	109.7	2.94	80.0	2.28
Switzerland, Graubunden	19.7	1.94	8.3	1.01
Switzerland, Neuchatel	83.3	3.74	54.4	2.84
Switzerland, St Gall-Appenzell	56.4	1.86	40.0	1.47
Switzerland, Valais	69.5	3.25	48.0	2.52
Switzerland, Vaud	100.0	2.23	75.6	1.84
† Switzerland, Zurich	1.0	0.16	0.8	0.16
*UK, England and Wales	42.0	0.20	28.6	0.15
*UK, East Anglia	62.3	0.90	40.2	0.70
*UK, Mersey	38.7	0.66	36.4	0.62
*UK, North Western	39.6	0.53	29.5	0.42
UK, Oxford	68.7	0.91	42.8	0.68
*UK, South Thames	35.0	0.37	22.5	0.29
UK, South Western	54.5	0.65	36.3	0.52
† UK, Wessex	21.2	0.43	13.4	0.34
*UK, West Midlands	53.5	0.53	37.7	0.43
UK, Yorkshire	45.5	0.59	31.7	0.46
UK, Scotland	54.2	0.56	36.4	0.42
UK, Scotland, West	46.5	0.71	31.5	0.52
*Yugoslavia, Vojvodina	21.4	0.57	16.9	0.45

OCEANIA

	MALE		FEMALE	
Australian Capital Territory				
Australia, New South Wales				
South Australia				
Australia, Tasmania				
Australia, Victoria				
Western Australia				
*French Polynesia				
† New Zealand: Non-Maori	0,0	0,01	-	-
† New Zealand: Maori	-	-	-	-
† US, Hawaii: White	0.9	0.29	1,1	0,39
† US, Hawaii: Japanese	0,8	0,28	0.9	0.31
† US, Hawaii: Hawaiian	1,5	0,63	0,8	0,43
† US, Hawaii: Filipino	0,6	0,38	0,2	0,21
† US, Hawaii: Chinese	0,6	0,60	-	-

* IMPORTANT-SEE NOTES ON POPULATION PAGE

AGE-STANDARDIZED INCIDENCE
RATES AND STANDARD ERRORS (per 100,000)
Breast (ICD-9 174/175)

	MALE		FEMALE	
AFRICA				
*Algeria, Setif	0,3	0,22	9.5	0.89
*France, La Reunion	0,5	0,21	29.4	1.51
*Mali, Bamako	0,5	0,30	10.2	1.15
*Uganda, Kyadondo	1,4	0,69	20.7	2.17 m
*Zimbabwe, Harare: African	0,6	0,26	20.4	2.41
*Zimbabwe, Harare: European	-	-	127.7	11.80
AMERICA, CENTRAL AND SOUTH				
*Argentina, Concordia	0,4	0,36	60.2	4.26
*Brazil, Belem	0,8	0,29	30.2	1.58
*Brazil, Goiania	0,2	0,15	40.4	1.79
*Brazil, Porto Alegre	0,4	0,20	62.0	1.76 m
Colombia, Cali	0,2	0,10	38.8	1.21
*Costa Rica	0.3	0.08	28.8	0.76
*Ecuador, Quito	0,3	0,14	26.8	1.15 m
*Peru, Lima	0,2	0,07	32.3	0.85
Peru, Trujillo	0,3	0,29	29.7	2.45
US, Puerto Rico	0.3	0.07	45.7	0.76
*Uruguay, Montevideo	0.7	0.16	92.6	1.77
AMERICA, NORTH				
Canada	0.6	0.03	76.8	0.30
Canada, Alberta	0.5	0.09	78.0	1.09
Canada, British Columbia	0.4	0.06	84.3	0.90
Canada, Manitoba	0.6	0.13	79.3	1.54
Canada, New Brunswick	0.6	0.16	73.3	1.82
Canada, Newfoundland	0.6	0.19	62.6	2.03
Canada, Northwest Territories	1,4	1,05	58.1	6.62
Canada, Nova Scotia	0.4	0.11	77.8	1.67
Canada, Ontario	0.6	0.04	78.1	0.50
Canada, Prince Edward Island	0.8	0,45	79.2	4.54
Canada, Quebec	0.7	0.06	71.7	0.56
Canada, Saskatchewan	0.6	0.14	77.9	1.62
Canada, Yukon	1,2	1,21	74.7	9.17
US, Cent. Calif.: Non-Hisp. White	0.4	0.10	86.2	1.37
US, Cent. Calif.: Hispanic	0.6	0,25	53.6	2.21
US, Los Angeles: Non-Hisp. White	0.9	0.08	103.7	0.90
US, Los Angeles: Hispanic White	0.3	0.09	57.4	1.05
US, Los Angeles: Black	0.5	0.16	80.9	1.70
US, Los Angeles: Chinese	0,2	0,19	36.8	2.34
US, Los Angeles: Filipino	-	-	69.3	3.25
US, Los Angeles: Korean	-	-	21.4	2.21
US, Los Angeles: Japanese	0,6	0,33	63.0	3.66
US, San Francisco: Non-Hisp. White	0.9	0.11	103.3	1.17
US, San Francisco: Hispanic White	0,8	0,31	70.8	2.56
US, San Francisco: Black	1.2	0.35	83.7	2.67
US, San Francisco: Chinese	0.3	0,18	55.2	2.68
US, San Francisco: Filipino	0,5	0,37	65.3	3.64
US, San Francisco: Japanese	-	-	68.4	6.01
US, Connecticut: White	0.8	0.09	93.3	0.96
US, Connecticut: Black	1,3	0,54	84.5	3.50
US, Atlanta: White	0.4	0.10	89.9	1.43
US, Atlanta: Black	1.5	0.41	72.3	2.25
US, Iowa	0.6	0.08	85.3	0.98

	MALE		FEMALE	
US, Central Louisiana: White	0,7	0,33	62.3	2.95
US, Central Louisiana: Black	1,1	0,82	58.1	5.55
US, New Orleans: White	0.7	0.19	87.0	2.03
US, New Orleans: Black	1,0	0,35	84.9	2.88
US, Detroit: White	0.8	0.09	91.9	0.97
US, Detroit: Black	0.9	0.21	80.8	1.74
US, New Mexico: Non-Hisp. White	0.5	0.13	86.3	1.81
US, New Mexico: Hispanic White	0.3	0,16	61.3	2.15
US, New Mexico: American Indian	0,6	0,60	28.3	3.26
US, Utah	0.7	0.14	75.8	1.37
US, Seattle	0.8	0.09	92.5	0.97
US, SEER: White	0.7	0.04	90.7	0.39
US, SEER: Black	1.2	0.15	79.3	1.11
ASIA				
*China, Qidong	0,1	0,05	11.2	0.60
China, Shanghai	0.4	0.04	26.5	0.36
China, Tianjin	0.3	0.06	24.6	0.50
Hong Kong	0.3	0.05	34.0	0.48
*India, Bangalore	0.3	0.06	21.3	0.59
*India, Barshi, Paranda and Bhum	-	-	8.7	0.99
India, Bombay	0.6	0.07	28.2	0.48
*India, Karunagappally	-	-	15.1	2.10
India, Madras	0.3	0.07	23.5	0.62
*India, Trivandrum	0,5	0,28	18.8	1.53
Israel: All Jews	1.2	0.11	77.4	0.87
Jews born in Israel	1.9	0.50	90.5	2.65
Jews born in America or Europe	1.2	0.17	87.9	1.55
Jews born in Africa or Asia	0.9	0.16	56.4	1.31
Non-Jews	0,6	0,28	21.3	1.36
Japan, Hiroshima	0,3	0,10	33.4	0.99
Japan, Miyagi	0.3	0.06	31.1	0.65
Japan, Nagasaki	0,1	0,04	27.1	0.71
Japan, Osaka	0.1	0.02	24.3	0.28
*Japan, Saga	0,2	0,09	19.1	0.79
Japan, Yamagata	0,2	0,07	22.7	0.73
*Korea, Kangwha	0,3	0,31	7.1	1.51
*Kuwait: Non-Kuwaitis	0,2	0,08	34.8	2.66
*Kuwait: Kuwaitis	-	-	32.8	2.49
*Philippines, Manila	0.9	0.15	47.7	0.88
Singapore: Chinese	0,1	0,05	39.5	0.87
Singapore: Malay	0,4	0,26	33.9	2.21
Singapore: Indian	0,2	0,17	31.9	3.30
Thailand, Chiang Mai	0,1	0,04	14.6	0.69
*Thailand, Khon Kaen	-	-	8.4	0.56
*Viet Nam, Hanoi	0.5	0.15	18.2	0.83

* IMPORTANT-SEE NOTES ON POPULATION PAGE

EUROPE	MALE		FEMALE	
Austria, Tyrol	0,3	0,13	64.9	1.78
*Belarus	0.3	0.04	29.6	0.30
*Croatia	0.5	0.07	37.2	0.54
Czech Republic	0.5	0.04	45.1	0.35
Denmark	0.5	0.05	73.3	0.64
Estonia	0.5	0.10	36.5	0.82
Finland	0.3	0.04	65.0	0.56
France, Bas-Rhin	1.3	0.23	78.8	1.64
*France, Calvados	1.1	0.25	76.3	2.03
France, Doubs	0,4	0,17	67.3	2.17
France, Haut-Rhin	0,3	0,11	80.3	1.96
*France, Herault	0.6	0.14	80.1	1.75
France, Isere	0.9	0.17	85.9	1.68
*France, Somme	0.7	0.22	68.2	2.07
*France, Tarn	0,4	0,13	62.3	2.33
Germany, Eastern States	0.5	0.05	48.2	0.45
Germany, Saarland	0.4	0.11	61.5	1.23
Iceland	0,9	0,35	79.0	3.45
Ireland, Southern	0.6	0.21	64.2	2.11
Italy, Ferrara	0,9	0,34	72.8	3.54
Italy, Florence	0.6	0.13	67.0	1.36
Italy, Genoa	0.6	0.14	72.3	1.59
*Italy, Latina	0,5	0,21	50.3	2.04
Italy, Macerata	0,7	0,37	57.9	3.71
Italy, Modena	0,4	0,13	68.4	1.72
Italy, Parma	0.6	0.20	73.6	2.25
Italy, Ragusa	0,6	0,24	44.1	2.15
Italy, Romagna	0.7	0.19	66.2	1.89
Italy, Torino	0.7	0.15	64.9	1.42
Italy, Trieste	0.9	0.31	64.3	2.73
Italy, Varese	1.0	0.19	73.5	1.57
Italy, Veneto	0.9	0.15	72.6	1.29
*Latvia	0.4	0.07	33.7	0.60
Malta	0,8	0,42	79.9	4.16
The Netherlands	0.4	0.03	79.6	0.45
The Netherlands, Eindhoven	0.5	0.14	71.6	1.54
The Netherlands, Maastricht	0.5	0.13	72.7	1.57
Norway	0.4	0.05	54.2	0.63
*Poland, Cracow	0,3	0,12	44.0	1.31
*Poland, Kielce	0.4	0.11	25.9	0.87
*Poland, Lower Silesia	0.4	0.08	33.4	0.62
Poland, Warsaw City	0.7	0.13	43.2	0.92
Slovakia	0.5	0.06	38.6	0.49
Slovenia	0.5	0.09	46.2	0.83
*Spain, Albacete	0,4	0,26	46.0	3.39
Spain, Asturias	0.5	0.13	46.0	1.23
Spain, Basque Country	0.4	0.08	45.8	0.90
Spain, Granada	0,3	0,10	37.4	1.27
Spain, Mallorca	0,2	0,10	50.2	1.64
Spain, Murcia	0.3	0.10	43.9	1.20
Spain, Navarra	0.5	0.16	61.7	1.94
Spain, Tarragona	0.7	0.18	50.7	1.71
Spain, Zaragoza	0,2	0,07	40.4	1.19

	MALE		FEMALE	
Sweden	0.4	0.04	72.9	0.49
*Switzerland, Basel	0,5	0,18	72.0	2.07
Switzerland, Geneva	0,6	0,22	77.8	2.33
Switzerland, Graubunden	0,4	0,29	64.5	3.75
Switzerland, Neuchatel	0,3	0,19	71.9	3.52
Switzerland, St Gall-Appenzell	0,4	0,16	56.3	1.88
Switzerland, Valais	0,9	0,38	65.9	3.18
Switzerland, Vaud	0.7	0.19	77.2	1.95
Switzerland, Zurich	0.4	0.10	65.7	1.24
*UK, England and Wales	0.5	0.02	68.8	0.26
*UK, East Anglia	0.3	0.06	76.4	1.05
*UK, Mersey	0.3	0.06	67.9	0.92
*UK, North Western	0.5	0.06	68.6	0.72
UK, Oxford	0.6	0.09	80.9	1.01
*UK, South Thames	0.6	0.05	71.2	0.56
UK, South Western	0.5	0.06	73.0	0.80
UK, Wessex	0.6	0.07	75.0	0.86
*UK, West Midlands	0.5	0.05	77.8	0.67
UK, Yorkshire	0.5	0.06	68.9	0.76
UK, Scotland	0.4	0.05	72.7	0.65
UK, Scotland, West	0.5	0.07	71.2	0.87
*Yugoslavia, Vojvodina	0.5	0.09	43.6	0.77

OCEANIA

	MALE		FEMALE	
Australian Capital Territory	0,5	0,28	66.6	3.19
Australia, New South Wales	0.7	0.06	67.2	0.62
South Australia	0.8	0.13	68.5	1.26
Australia, Tasmania	0,4	0,17	56.9	2.03
Australia, Victoria	0.6	0.06	66.7	0.72
Western Australia	0.4	0.10	72.9	1.29
*French Polynesia	1,6	0,68	65.7	4.82
New Zealand: Non-Maori	0.7	0.09	77.2	0.94
New Zealand: Maori	0,4	0,23	77.1	3.97
US, Hawaii: White	0,8	0,30	96.5	3.43
US, Hawaii: Japanese	0,5	0,23	72.9	2.65
US, Hawaii: Hawaiian	0,4	0,32	83.9	4.49
US, Hawaii: Filipino	0,2	0,20	57.4	3.61
US, Hawaii: Chinese	0,4	0,42	57.6	4.87

* IMPORTANT-SEE NOTES ON POPULATION PAGE

AGE-STANDARDIZED INCIDENCE
RATES AND STANDARD ERRORS (per 100,000)
Uterus (ICD-9 179)

	MALE	FEMALE
AFRICA		
*Algeria, Setif	0,1	0,09
*France, La Reunion	1.3	0.32
*Mali, Bamako	2.3	0.51
*Uganda, Kyadondo	0,9	0,54
*Zimbabwe, Harare: African	1,4	0,59
*Zimbabwe, Harare: European	1,9	1,49
AMERICA, CENTRAL AND SOUTH		
*Argentina, Concordia	4.3	1.16
*Brazil, Belem	2.0	0.39
*Brazil, Goiania	2.0	0.40
*Brazil, Porto Alegre	9.0	0.67
Colombia, Cali	0.8	0.17
*Costa Rica	0.9	0.13
*Ecuador, Quito	2.5	0.35
*Peru, Lima	0.7	0.13
Peru, Trujillo	0,9	0,41
US, Puerto Rico	0.5	0.07
*Uruguay, Montevideo	1.2	0.20
AMERICA, NORTH		
Canada	0.5	0.02
Canada, Alberta	0.4	0.08
Canada, British Columbia	0.3	0.05
Canada, Manitoba	0.6	0.13
Canada, New Brunswick	0.3	0.11
Canada, Newfoundland	0.9	0.25
Canada, Northwest Territories	1,1	0,85
Canada, Nova Scotia	0.3	0.11
Canada, Ontario	0.4	0.03
Canada, Prince Edward Island	1,1	0,53
Canada, Quebec	0.9	0.06
Canada, Saskatchewan	0.2	0.08
Canada, Yukon	-	-
US, Cent. Calif.: Non-Hisp. White	0.2	0.05
US, Cent. Calif.: Hispanic	0,1	0,08
US, Los Angeles: Non-Hisp. White	0.2	0.03
US, Los Angeles: Hispanic White	0,1	0,05
US, Los Angeles: Black	0.3	0.11
US, Los Angeles: Chinese	0.3	0.20
US, Los Angeles: Filipino	-	-
US, Los Angeles: Korean	0.2	0,17
US, Los Angeles: Japanese	-	-
US, San Francisco: Non-Hisp. White	0.1	0.03
US, San Francisco: Hispanic White	0,2	0,14
US, San Francisco: Black	1.0	0.28
US, San Francisco: Chinese	0,6	0,27
US, San Francisco: Filipino	0,2	0,22
US, San Francisco: Japanese	-	-
US, Connecticut: White	0.5	0.07
US, Connecticut: Black	1,2	0,42
US, Atlanta: White	0,1	0,04
US, Atlanta: Black	0.6	0,21
US, Iowa	0.2	0.05

	MALE	FEMALE
US, Central Louisiana: White	0,2	0,09
US, Central Louisiana: Black	2,4	1,06
US, New Orleans: White	0.7	0.17
US, New Orleans: Black	0.9	0.29
US, Detroit: White	0.2	0.05
US, Detroit: Black	0.4	0.11
US, New Mexico: Non-Hisp. White	0.3	0.10
US, New Mexico: Hispanic White	0,3	0,14
US, New Mexico: American Indian	0,3	0,30
US, Utah	0.2	0.06
US, Seattle	0,1	0,02
US, SEER: White	0.2	0.02
US, SEER: Black	0.6	0.09
ASIA		
*China, Qidong	1.0	0.18
China, Shanghai	0.6	0.05
China, Tianjin	0.9	0.09
Hong Kong	0.2	0.04
*India, Bangalore	0.3	0.07
*India, Barshi, Paranda and Bhum	-	-
India, Bombay	1.3	0.11
*India, Karunagappally	-	-
India, Madras	0.4	0.08
*India, Trivandrum	0,4	0,22
Israel: All Jews	0.6	0.07
Jews born in Israel	0,3	0,11
Jews born in America or Europe	0.8	0.15
Jews born in Africa or Asia	0.4	0.10
Non-Jews	0,1	0,07
Japan, Hiroshima	0.7	0.13
Japan, Miyagi	0.5	0.07
Japan, Nagasaki	0.7	0.10
Japan, Osaka	1.2	0.06
*Japan, Saga	1.3	0.18
Japan, Yamagata	0.6	0.09
*Korea, Kangwha	0,3	0,30
*Kuwait: Non-Kuwaitis	0,3	0,34
*Kuwait: Kuwaitis	0,1	0,15
*Philippines, Manila	3.6	0.24
Singapore: Chinese	-	-
Singapore: Malay	-	-
Singapore: Indian	-	-
Thailand, Chiang Mai	-	-
*Thailand, Khon Kaen	0,2	0,08
*Viet Nam, Hanoi	0,2	0,10

* IMPORTANT-SEE NOTES ON POPULATION PAGE

EUROPE	MALE	FEMALE
Austria, Tyrol	0.9	0.18
*Belarus	0.1	0.02
*Croatia	1.6	0.10
Czech Republic	0.1	0.02
Denmark	0.5	0.05
Estonia	-	-
Finland	0.2	0.03
France, Bas-Rhin	0.6	0.15
*France, Calvados	0,3	0,11
France, Doubs	0,3	0,15
France, Haut-Rhin	0.3	0.10
*France, Herault	0,3	0,12
France, Isere	0.6	0.14
*France, Somme	0.8	0.22
*France, Tarn	0,2	0,14
Germany, Eastern States	0.1	0.02
Germany, Saarland	1.2	0.16
Iceland	0,2	0,17
Ireland, Southern	0,3	0,14
Italy, Ferrara	0,3	0,19
Italy, Florence	0.7	0.12
Italy, Genoa	1.0	0.16
*Italy, Latina	1.6	0.34
Italy, Macerata	2.2	0.74
Italy, Modena	0.4	0.12
Italy, Parma	1.1	0.24
Italy, Ragusa	0.7	0.20
Italy, Romagna	0,3	0,11
Italy, Torino	0.3	0.07
Italy, Trieste	0.7	0.21
Italy, Varese	0.2	0.06
Italy, Veneto	2.3	0.23
*Latvia	0,0	0,02
Malta	0,7	0,36
The Netherlands	0.0	0.01
The Netherlands, Eindhoven	-	-
The Netherlands, Maastricht	0,0	0,04
Norway	0.1	0.02
*Poland, Cracow	0.6	0.14
*Poland, Kielce	0.4	0.10
*Poland, Lower Silesia	0.8	0.09
Poland, Warsaw City	0.3	0.07
Slovakia	0.2	0.03
Slovenia	0.8	0.10
*Spain, Albacete	1,5	0,55
Spain, Asturias	1.1	0.19
Spain, Basque Country	0.6	0.10
Spain, Granada	0.2	0.08
Spain, Mallorca	0.5	0.14
Spain, Murcia	0.4	0.10
Spain, Navarra	1.1	0.23
Spain, Tarragona	0.2	0,09
Spain, Zaragoza	0.8	0.14

	MALE	FEMALE
Sweden	1.5	0.07
*Switzerland, Basel	-	-
Switzerland, Geneva	0,2	0,08
Switzerland, Graubunden	0,6	0,37
Switzerland, Neuchatel	0,4	0,23
Switzerland, St Gall-Appenzell	0,3	0,11
Switzerland, Valais	0,5	0,27
Switzerland, Vaud	0,1	0,05
Switzerland, Zurich	0,2	0,06
*UK, England and Wales	0.8	0.03
*UK, East Anglia	0.2	0.05
*UK, Mersey	0.2	0.05
*UK, North Western	1.1	0.08
UK, Oxford	0.2	0.04
*UK, South Thames	0,0	0,01
UK, South Western	1.1	0.09
UK, Wessex	1.1	0.10
*UK, West Midlands	1.1	0.08
UK, Yorkshire	1.2	0.10
UK, Scotland	0.9	0.07
UK, Scotland, West	1.2	0.11
*Yugoslavia, Vojvodina	1.5	0.13

OCEANIA	MALE	FEMALE
Australian Capital Territory	0,7	0,34
Australia, New South Wales	0.5	0.05
South Australia	-	-
Australia, Tasmania	-	-
Australia, Victoria	-	-
Western Australia	0,1	0,04
*French Polynesia	8.3	1.85
New Zealand: Non-Maori	0,1	0,03
New Zealand: Maori	-	-
US, Hawaii: White	0,1	0,13
US, Hawaii: Japanese	0,4	0,21
US, Hawaii: Hawaiian	-	-
US, Hawaii: Filipino	0,4	0,30
US, Hawaii: Chinese	0,3	0,31

* IMPORTANT-SEE NOTES ON POPULATION PAGE

AGE-STANDARDIZED INCIDENCE RATES AND STANDARD ERRORS (per 100,000)
Cervix uteri (ICD-9 180)

AFRICA

	MALE		FEMALE	
*Algeria, Setif			13.9	*1.10*
*France, La Reunion			24.7	*1.37*
*Mali, Bamako			23.5	*1.67*
*Uganda, Kyadondo			40.8	*3.02*
*Zimbabwe, Harare: African			67.2	*4.81*
*Zimbabwe, Harare: European			10.4	*3.50*

AMERICA, CENTRAL AND SOUTH

	MALE		FEMALE	
*Argentina, Concordia			32.0	*3.12*
*Brazil, Belem			64.8	*2.23*
*Brazil, Goiania			37.1	*1.73*
*Brazil, Porto Alegre			22.1	*1.02*
Colombia, Cali			34.4	*1.12*
*Costa Rica			24.5	*0.68*
*Ecuador, Quito			31.7	*1.25*
*Peru, Lima			27.3	*0.78*
Peru, Trujillo			53.5	*3.27*
US, Puerto Rico			9.8	*0.35*
*Uruguay, Montevideo			19.3	*0.88*

AMERICA, NORTH

	MALE		FEMALE	
Canada			7.8	*0.10*
Canada, Alberta			8.4	*0.35*
Canada, British Columbia			6.7	*0.26*
Canada, Manitoba			8.1	*0.50*
Canada, New Brunswick			7.3	*0.58*
Canada, Newfoundland			11.3	*0.85*
Canada, Northwest Territories			13.9	*2.78*
Canada, Nova Scotia			10.7	*0.62*
Canada, Ontario			8.4	*0.16*
Canada, Prince Edward Island			9.9	*1.64*
Canada, Quebec			6.7	*0.17*
Canada, Saskatchewan			7.7	*0.53*
Canada, Yukon			13.4	*3.78*
US, Cent. Calif.: Non-Hisp. White			7.8	*0.43*
US, Cent. Calif.: Hispanic			17.1	*1.19*
US, Los Angeles: Non-Hisp. White			7.2	*0.25*
US, Los Angeles: Hispanic White			17.9	*0.55*
US, Los Angeles: Black			11.6	*0.63*
US, Los Angeles: Chinese			7.7	*1.09*
US, Los Angeles: Filipino			8.6	*1.15*
US, Los Angeles: Korean			13.4	*1.79*
US, Los Angeles: Japanese			4.1	*0.94*
US, San Francisco: Non-Hisp. White			6.2	*0.29*
US, San Francisco: Hispanic White			12.9	*1.06*
US, San Francisco: Black			10.5	*0.92*
US, San Francisco: Chinese			6.0	*0.85*
US, San Francisco: Filipino			9.7	*1.41*
US, San Francisco: Japanese			5.9	*1.81*
US, Connecticut: White			7.0	*0.28*
US, Connecticut: Black			13.2	*1.36*
US, Atlanta: White			7.0	*0.39*
US, Atlanta: Black			12.0	*0.90*
US, Iowa			8.2	*0.32*
US, Central Louisiana: White			7.2	*1.05*
US, Central Louisiana: Black			11.0	*2.30*
US, New Orleans: White			6.7	*0.59*
US, New Orleans: Black			14.8	*1.17*
US, Detroit: White			7.9	*0.30*
US, Detroit: Black			12.7	*0.68*
US, New Mexico: Non-Hisp. White			9.1	*0.62*
US, New Mexico: Hispanic White			9.7	*0.83*
US, New Mexico: American Indian			8.8	*1.73*
US, Utah			7.7	*0.43*
US, Seattle			7.6	*0.28*
US, SEER: White			7.5	*0.12*
US, SEER: Black			12.0	*0.42*

ASIA

	MALE		FEMALE	
*China, Qidong			2.6	*0.28*
China, Shanghai			3.3	*0.11*
China, Tianjin			4.4	*0.21*
Hong Kong			15.3	*0.33*
*India, Bangalore			27.2	*0.67*
*India, Barshi, Paranda and Bhum			27.4	*1.74*
India, Bombay			20.2	*0.40*
*India, Karunagappally			15.7	*2.20*
India, Madras			38.9	*0.79*
*India, Trivandrum			15.9	*1.44*
Israel: All Jews			5.3	*0.23*
Jews born in Israel			6.3	*0.61*
Jews born in America or Europe			4.1	*0.38*
Jews born in Africa or Asia			6.1	*0.50*
Non-Jews			3.0	*0.49*
Japan, Hiroshima			12.6	*0.60*
Japan, Miyagi			6.4	*0.29*
Japan, Nagasaki			11.3	*0.46*
Japan, Osaka			9.2	*0.18*
*Japan, Saga			7.2	*0.48*
Japan, Yamagata			5.5	*0.35*
*Korea, Kangwha			21.8	*2.65*
*Kuwait: Non-Kuwaitis			5.4	*0.98*
*Kuwait: Kuwaitis			7.6	*1.23*
*Philippines, Manila			21.6	*0.59*
Singapore: Chinese			16.3	*0.56*
Singapore: Malay			11.1	*1.29*
Singapore: Indian			8.6	*1.65*
Thailand, Chiang Mai			25.6	*0.90*
*Thailand, Khon Kaen			18.8	*0.85*
*Viet Nam, Hanoi			6.1	*0.48*

* IMPORTANT-SEE NOTES ON POPULATION PAGE

AGE-STANDARDIZED INCIDENCE
RATES AND STANDARD ERRORS (per 100,000)
Cervix uteri (ICD-9 180) (contd)

EUROPE	MALE	FEMALE
Austria, Tyrol	17.7	0.96
*Belarus	11.2	0.19
*Croatia	11.6	0.31
Czech Republic	16.4	0.23
Denmark	15.2	0.31
Estonia	14.1	0.52
Finland	3.6	0.13
France, Bas-Rhin	10.0	0.59
*France, Calvados	10.4	0.74
France, Doubs	7.8	0.73
France, Haut-Rhin	11.9	0.77
*France, Herault	14.1	0.76
France, Isere	9.7	0.56
*France, Somme	10.5	0.81
*France, Tarn	7.7	0.84
Germany, Eastern States	21.2	0.32
Germany, Saarland	11.4	0.57
Iceland	8.0	1.08
Ireland, Southern	6.5	0.68
Italy, Ferrara	7.0	1.13
Italy, Florence	6.2	0.43
Italy, Genoa	7.8	0.55
*Italy, Latina	6.3	0.73
Italy, Macerata	2.8	0.87
Italy, Modena	5.9	0.51
Italy, Parma	5.9	0.66
Italy, Ragusa	7.6	0.92
Italy, Romagna	10.3	0.78
Italy, Torino	8.0	0.51
Italy, Trieste	12.9	1.31
Italy, Varese	6.4	0.48
Italy, Veneto	5.5	0.37
*Latvia	9.5	0.32
Malta	6.4	1.20
The Netherlands	7.1	0.14
The Netherlands, Eindhoven	6.4	0.47
The Netherlands, Maastricht	7.5	0.52
Norway	12.7	0.32
*Poland, Cracow	20.6	0.90
*Poland, Kielce	15.6	0.68
*Poland, Lower Silesia	21.8	0.50
Poland, Warsaw City	15.2	0.56
Slovakia	16.4	0.33
Slovenia	12.4	0.44
*Spain, Albacete	6.2	1.31
Spain, Asturias	8.4	0.56
Spain, Basque Country	6.0	0.33
Spain, Granada	5.6	0.49
Spain, Mallorca	13.6	0.90
Spain, Murcia	7.2	0.49
Spain, Navarra	4.7	0.54
Spain, Tarragona	9.5	0.77
Spain, Zaragoza	4.8	0.42

	MALE	FEMALE
Sweden	8.0	0.17
*Switzerland, Basel	5.4	0.59
Switzerland, Geneva	6.1	0.66
Switzerland, Graubunden	9.8	1.54
Switzerland, Neuchatel	9.1	1.28
Switzerland, St Gall-Appenzell	8.8	0.76
Switzerland, Valais	7.0	1.05
Switzerland, Vaud	6.3	0.56
Switzerland, Zurich	6.8	0.41
*UK, England and Wales	12.5	0.12
*UK, East Anglia	10.3	0.40
*UK, Mersey	14.2	0.44
*UK, North Western	14.3	0.34
UK, Oxford	9.4	0.35
*UK, South Thames	9.2	0.21
UK, South Western	10.3	0.32
UK, Wessex	11.6	0.36
*UK, West Midlands	13.7	0.30
UK, Yorkshire	14.5	0.36
UK, Scotland	12.7	0.28
UK, Scotland, West	12.7	0.39
*Yugoslavia, Vojvodina	17.7	0.50

OCEANIA	MALE	FEMALE
Australian Capital Territory	10.3	1.22
Australia, New South Wales	9.9	0.24
South Australia	8.7	0.45
Australia, Tasmania	10.6	0.89
Australia, Victoria	9.4	0.27
Western Australia	11.8	0.51
*French Polynesia	27.7	3.06
New Zealand: Non-Maori	11.9	0.38
New Zealand: Maori	32.2	2.45
US, Hawaii: White	10.5	1.11
US, Hawaii: Japanese	6.4	0.87
US, Hawaii: Hawaiian	8.6	1.38
US, Hawaii: Filipino	6.8	1.19
US, Hawaii: Chinese	4.5	1.49

* IMPORTANT-SEE NOTES ON POPULATION PAGE

AGE-STANDARDIZED INCIDENCE
RATES AND STANDARD ERRORS (per 100,000)
Placenta (ICD-9 181)

	MALE	FEMALE		MALE	FEMALE
AFRICA			US, Central Louisiana: White	-	-
*Algeria, Setif	-	-	US, Central Louisiana: Black	-	-
*France, La Reunion	0,1	0,09	US, New Orleans: White	0,1	0,09
*Mali, Bamako	0,1	0,08	US, New Orleans: Black	0,2	0,13
*Uganda, Kyadondo	0,8	0,33	US, Detroit: White	0,0	0,02
*Zimbabwe, Harare: African	0.8	0.26	US, Detroit: Black	0,1	0,06
*Zimbabwe, Harare: European	-	-	US, New Mexico: Non-Hisp. White	-	-
			US, New Mexico: Hispanic White	0,1	0,09
			US, New Mexico: American Indian	-	-
AMERICA, CENTRAL AND SOUTH			US, Utah	0,2	0,06
*Argentina, Concordia	-	-	US, Seattle	0.1	0.04
*Brazil, Belem	0.4	0.15 f	US, SEER: White	0.1	0.01
*Brazil, Goiania	-	-	US, SEER: Black	0,1	0,03
*Brazil, Porto Alegre	0,0	0,04			
Colombia, Cali	0.2	0.07	**ASIA**		
*Costa Rica	0.2	0.06	*China, Qidong	0.4	0.11
*Ecuador, Quito	0.3	0.09	China, Shanghai	0.1	0.02
*Peru, Lima	0.6	0.09	China, Tianjin	0.5	0.07
Peru, Trujillo	0,1	0,10	Hong Kong	0,0	0,02
US, Puerto Rico	0,1	0,03	*India, Bangalore	0,0	0,02
*Uruguay, Montevideo	0,1	0,06	*India, Barshi, Paranda and Bhum	-	-
			India, Bombay	0.2	0.03
AMERICA, NORTH			*India, Karunagappally	-	-
Canada	0.0	0.01	India, Madras	0.2	0.04
Canada, Alberta	0,0	0,02	*India, Trivandrum	-	-
Canada, British Columbia	0,0	0,02	Israel: All Jews	0.1	0.04
Canada, Manitoba	-	-	Jews born in Israel	0,1	0,05
Canada, New Brunswick	0,1	0,05	Jews born in America or Europe	0,1	0,06
Canada, Newfoundland	-	-	Jews born in Africa or Asia	0,3	0,15
Canada, Northwest Territories	1,1	0,79	Non-Jews	0,1	0,07
Canada, Nova Scotia	-	-	Japan, Hiroshima	0,0	0,03
Canada, Ontario	0.0	0.01	Japan, Miyagi	0,1	0,05
Canada, Prince Edward Island	0,3	0,30	Japan, Nagasaki	0,1	0,05
Canada, Quebec	0.1	0.02	Japan, Osaka	0.1	0.02
Canada, Saskatchewan	-	-	*Japan, Saga	0,1	0,05
Canada, Yukon	-	-	Japan, Yamagata	0,1	0,05
US, Cent. Calif.: Non-Hisp. White	0,1	0,05	*Korea, Kangwha	-	-
US, Cent. Calif.: Hispanic	0,1	0,07	*Kuwait: Non-Kuwaitis	0,2	0,12
US, Los Angeles: Non-Hisp. White	0,0	0,02	*Kuwait: Kuwaitis	0,7	0,29
US, Los Angeles: Hispanic White	0,1	0,04	*Philippines, Manila	0.4	0.06
US, Los Angeles: Black	0,1	0,04	Singapore: Chinese	0,1	0,03
US, Los Angeles: Chinese	-	-	Singapore: Malay	0,1	0,11
US, Los Angeles: Filipino	-	-	Singapore: Indian	-	-
US, Los Angeles: Korean	-	-	Thailand, Chiang Mai	0,2	0,08
US, Los Angeles: Japanese	-	-	*Thailand, Khon Kaen	0.3	0.10
US, San Francisco: Non-Hisp. White	0,2	0,07	*Viet Nam, Hanoi	1.8	0.24
US, San Francisco: Hispanic White	0,1	0,08			
US, San Francisco: Black	0,1	0,07			
US, San Francisco: Chinese	-	-			
US, San Francisco: Filipino	0,2	0,22			
US, San Francisco: Japanese	-	-			
US, Connecticut: White	0,0	0,02			
US, Connecticut: Black	0,1	0,10			
US, Atlanta: White	0,1	0,04			
US, Atlanta: Black	0,1	0,07			
US, Iowa	0,1	0,03			

* IMPORTANT-SEE NOTES ON POPULATION PAGE

EUROPE	MALE	FEMALE
Austria, Tyrol	-	-
*Belarus	0.1	0.02
*Croatia	0,1	0,03
Czech Republic	0.1	0.02
Denmark	0,1	0,02
Estonia	0.3	0.09
Finland	0.1	0.02
France, Bas-Rhin	-	-
*France, Calvados	0,1	0,05
France, Doubs	0,4	0,18
France, Haut-Rhin	0,2	0,11
*France, Herault	-	-
France, Isere	0,0	0,04
*France, Somme	0,1	0,08
*France, Tarn	-	-
Germany, Eastern States	0.1	0.02
Germany, Saarland	0,2	0,08
Iceland	-	-
Ireland, Southern	-	-
Italy, Ferrara	-	-
Italy, Florence	0,1	0,05
Italy, Genoa	0,0	0,05
*Italy, Latina	0,1	0,09
Italy, Macerata	-	-
Italy, Modena	-	-
Italy, Parma	0,2	0,15
Italy, Ragusa	-	-
Italy, Romagna	-	-
Italy, Torino	0,0	0,04
Italy, Trieste	-	-
Italy, Varese	0,0	0,04
Italy, Veneto	0,0	0,03
*Latvia	0.3	0.06
Malta	-	-
The Netherlands	0.1	0.02
The Netherlands, Eindhoven	-	-
The Netherlands, Maastricht	-	-
Norway	0.3	0.05
*Poland, Cracow	-	-
*Poland, Kielce	-	-
*Poland, Lower Silesia	0.2	0.05
Poland, Warsaw City	0.4	0.12
Slovakia	0.2	0.04
Slovenia	0,1	0,04
*Spain, Albacete	-	-
Spain, Asturias	0,1	0,06
Spain, Basque Country	0,0	0,02
Spain, Granada	0,1	0,07
Spain, Mallorca	-	-
Spain, Murcia	0,0	0,04
Spain, Navarra	0,2	0,13
Spain, Tarragona	0,1	0,08
Spain, Zaragoza	-	-

	MALE	FEMALE
Sweden	0.1	0.03
*Switzerland, Basel	-	-
Switzerland, Geneva	0,3	0,19
Switzerland, Graubunden	0,3	0,29
Switzerland, Neuchatel	0,3	0,26
Switzerland, St Gall-Appenzell	0,1	0,11
Switzerland, Valais	-	-
Switzerland, Vaud	0,1	0,08
Switzerland, Zurich	0,1	0,04
*UK, England and Wales	0.0	0.01
*UK, East Anglia	0,0	0,02
*UK, Mersey	-	-
*UK, North Western	0.0	0.01
UK, Oxford	0.1	0.03
*UK, South Thames	0.0	0.01
UK, South Western	0.0	0.02
UK, Wessex	0.1	0.03
*UK, West Midlands	0.1	0.02
UK, Yorkshire	0.1	0.03
UK, Scotland	0.0	0.02
UK, Scotland, West	0.0	0.02
*Yugoslavia, Vojvodina	0.2	0.06

OCEANIA	MALE	FEMALE
Australian Capital Territory	0,1	0,14
Australia, New South Wales	0.1	0.03
South Australia	0,1	0,04
Australia, Tasmania	-	-
Australia, Victoria	0.1	0.03
Western Australia	-	-
*French Polynesia	-	-
New Zealand: Non-Maori	0.4	0.07
New Zealand: Maori	0,3	0,17
US, Hawaii: White	0,1	0,08
US, Hawaii: Japanese	0,1	0,12
US, Hawaii: Hawaiian	-	-
US, Hawaii: Filipino	0,2	0,21
US, Hawaii: Chinese	-	-

* IMPORTANT-SEE NOTES ON POPULATION PAGE

AGE-STANDARDIZED INCIDENCE
RATES AND STANDARD ERRORS (per 100,000)
Corpus uteri (ICD-9 182)

	MALE	FEMALE		MALE	FEMALE
AFRICA			US, Central Louisiana: White	8.5	1.05
*Algeria, Setif	1.2	0.34	US, Central Louisiana: Black	9.2	2.16
*France, La Reunion	3.3	0.49	US, New Orleans: White	9.3	0.66
*Mali, Bamako	1,0	0,35	US, New Orleans: Black	9.0	0.92
*Uganda, Kyadondo	5.0	1.11	US, Detroit: White	19.6	0.44
*Zimbabwe, Harare: African	4.3	1.20	US, Detroit: Black	11.6	0.65
*Zimbabwe, Harare: European	9.8	2.93	US, New Mexico: Non-Hisp. White	15.8	0.76
			US, New Mexico: Hispanic White	9.4	0.83
AMERICA, CENTRAL AND SOUTH			US, New Mexico: American Indian	9.3	1.93
*Argentina, Concordia	8.5	1.62	US, Utah	19.0	0.69
*Brazil, Belem	1.9	0.40	US, Seattle	19.6	0.44
*Brazil, Goiania	4.3	0.63	US, SEER: White	18.2	0.17
*Brazil, Porto Alegre	6.2	0.55	US, SEER: Black	11.4	0.42
Colombia, Cali	6.5	0.51			
*Costa Rica	4.4	0.31	**ASIA**		
*Ecuador, Quito	5.3	0.53	*China, Qidong	0.6	0.13
*Peru, Lima	4.3	0.32	China, Shanghai	3.7	0.13
Peru, Trujillo	2.9	0.78	China, Tianjin	2.7	0.16
US, Puerto Rico	8.6	0.33	Hong Kong	7.0	0.23
*Uruguay, Montevideo	12.8	0.63	*India, Bangalore	1.9	0.18
			*India, Barshi, Paranda and Bhum	0,3	0,19
AMERICA, NORTH			India, Bombay	2.5	0.15
Canada	14.3	0.13	*India, Karunagappally	1,2	0,62
Canada, Alberta	15.2	0.48	India, Madras	2.2	0.20
Canada, British Columbia	14.0	0.36	*India, Trivandrum	2.1	0.53
Canada, Manitoba	17.0	0.71	Israel: All Jews	10.8	0.32
Canada, New Brunswick	12.0	0.72	Jews born in Israel	15.0	1.23
Canada, Newfoundland	13.2	0.95	Jews born in America or Europe	12.6	0.54
Canada, Northwest Territories	6,1	2,07	Jews born in Africa or Asia	7.5	0.46
Canada, Nova Scotia	13.7	0.70	Non-Jews	4.9	0.68
Canada, Ontario	14.9	0.21	Japan, Hiroshima	5.0	0.38
Canada, Prince Edward Island	10.9	1.59	Japan, Miyagi	4.1	0.23
Canada, Quebec	13.4	0.24	Japan, Nagasaki	4.2	0.28
Canada, Saskatchewan	13.6	0.67	Japan, Osaka	3.0	0.10
Canada, Yukon	20.3	5.37	*Japan, Saga	2.3	0.26
US, Cent. Calif.: Non-Hisp. White	16.7	0.59	Japan, Yamagata	3.2	0.26
US, Cent. Calif.: Hispanic	12.7	1.09	*Korea, Kangwha	0,3	0,28
US, Los Angeles: Non-Hisp. White	20.2	0.38	*Kuwait: Non-Kuwaitis	4.5	1.22
US, Los Angeles: Hispanic White	11.5	0.48	*Kuwait: Kuwaitis	2.4	0.69
US, Los Angeles: Black	10.7	0.61	*Philippines, Manila	5.7	0.31
US, Los Angeles: Chinese	7.0	1.06	Singapore: Chinese	7.0	0.38
US, Los Angeles: Filipino	11.4	1.36	Singapore: Malay	5.1	0.87
US, Los Angeles: Korean	2.6	0.83	Singapore: Indian	6.2	1.55
US, Los Angeles: Japanese	8.1	1.24	Thailand, Chiang Mai	3.5	0.34
US, San Francisco: Non-Hisp. White	18.8	0.49	*Thailand, Khon Kaen	2.0	0.28
US, San Francisco: Hispanic White	13.5	1.12	*Viet Nam, Hanoi	1.5	0.24
US, San Francisco: Black	11.4	0.98			
US, San Francisco: Chinese	11.3	1.22			
US, San Francisco: Filipino	9.5	1.39			
US, San Francisco: Japanese	16.5	2.96			
US, Connecticut: White	18.4	0.42			
US, Connecticut: Black	12.5	1.37			
US, Atlanta: White	15.4	0.60			
US, Atlanta: Black	10.6	0.89			
US, Iowa	17.7	0.44			

* IMPORTANT-SEE NOTES ON POPULATION PAGE

EUROPE	MALE	FEMALE
Austria, Tyrol	13.0	0.79
*Belarus	10.6	0.17
*Croatia	10.0	0.27
Czech Republic	17.7	0.22
Denmark	14.7	0.28
Estonia	12.9	0.47
Finland	12.9	0.24
France, Bas-Rhin	16.1	0.72
*France, Calvados	8.4	0.64
France, Doubs	9.8	0.80
France, Haut-Rhin	15.0	0.81
*France, Herault	10.0	0.59
France, Isere	10.0	0.55
*France, Somme	9.1	0.70
*France, Tarn	10.0	0.86
Germany, Eastern States	13.9	0.23
Germany, Saarland	12.7	0.51
Iceland	14.4	1.47
Ireland, Southern	8.3	0.75
Italy, Ferrara	13.1	1.46
Italy, Florence	12.2	0.56
Italy, Genoa	8.4	0.50
*Italy, Latina	8.6	0.81
Italy, Macerata	12.4	1.58
Italy, Modena	12.5	0.71
Italy, Parma	12.5	0.87
Italy, Ragusa	10.5	0.98
Italy, Romagna	11.7	0.75
Italy, Torino	11.1	0.56
Italy, Trieste	13.3	1.16
Italy, Varese	12.6	0.63
Italy, Veneto	8.7	0.43
*Latvia	14.1	0.37
Malta	16.4	1.86
The Netherlands	10.8	0.16
The Netherlands, Eindhoven	10.3	0.58
The Netherlands, Maastricht	10.4	0.57
Norway	12.5	0.30
*Poland, Cracow	12.2	0.68
*Poland, Kielce	9.2	0.50
*Poland, Lower Silesia	11.4	0.35
Poland, Warsaw City	13.0	0.50
Slovakia	16.0	0.32
Slovenia	12.4	0.42
*Spain, Albacete	5.8	1.09
Spain, Asturias	11.3	0.58
Spain, Basque Country	9.1	0.39
Spain, Granada	9.0	0.58
Spain, Mallorca	12.1	0.78
Spain, Murcia	10.9	0.58
Spain, Navarra	11.6	0.81
Spain, Tarragona	11.7	0.79
Spain, Zaragoza	8.7	0.52

	MALE	FEMALE
Sweden	13.2	0.20
*Switzerland, Basel	11.7	0.79
Switzerland, Geneva	12.7	0.93
Switzerland, Graubunden	9.9	1.46
Switzerland, Neuchatel	10.7	1.25
Switzerland, St Gall-Appenzell	11.6	0.83
Switzerland, Valais	9.8	1.20
Switzerland, Vaud	13.2	0.78
Switzerland, Zurich	15.0	0.58
*UK, England and Wales	8.6	0.09
*UK, East Anglia	10.5	0.38
*UK, Mersey	9.2	0.33
*UK, North Western	6.8	0.22
UK, Oxford	10.0	0.35
*UK, South Thames	8.7	0.19
UK, South Western	9.5	0.28
UK, Wessex	9.6	0.29
*UK, West Midlands	10.2	0.23
UK, Yorkshire	8.0	0.25
UK, Scotland	7.4	0.20
UK, Scotland, West	6.4	0.25
*Yugoslavia, Vojvodina	9.2	0.33

OCEANIA

	MALE	FEMALE
Australian Capital Territory	7.5	1.12
Australia, New South Wales	8.8	0.22
South Australia	10.9	0.49
Australia, Tasmania	10.4	0.86
Australia, Victoria	10.2	0.28
Western Australia	10.8	0.49
*French Polynesia	9.7	1.90
New Zealand: Non-Maori	9.4	0.32
New Zealand: Maori	15.8	1.87
US, Hawaii: White	15.7	1.37
US, Hawaii: Japanese	14.2	1.21
US, Hawaii: Hawaiian	20.6	2.20
US, Hawaii: Filipino	11.0	1.56
US, Hawaii: Chinese	14.0	2.49

* IMPORTANT-SEE NOTES ON POPULATION PAGE

AGE-STANDARDIZED INCIDENCE
RATES AND STANDARD ERRORS (per 100,000)
Ovary etc. (ICD-9 183)

	MALE	FEMALE
AFRICA		
*Algeria, Setif	1.2	0.32
*France, La Reunion	5.3	0.64
*Mali, Bamako	0.7	0.23
*Uganda, Kyadondo	6.6	1.20
*Zimbabwe, Harare: African	8.0	1.63
*Zimbabwe, Harare: European	14.1	4.07
AMERICA, CENTRAL AND SOUTH		
*Argentina, Concordia	7.6	1.53
*Brazil, Belem	4.5	0.60
*Brazil, Goiania	5.7	0.69
*Brazil, Porto Alegre	8.4	0.65
Colombia, Cali	8.9	0.57
*Costa Rica	5.9	0.34
*Ecuador, Quito	6.3	0.55
*Peru, Lima	6.0	0.36
Peru, Trujillo	7.6	1.24
US, Puerto Rico	5.2	0.25
*Uruguay, Montevideo	9.8	0.60
AMERICA, NORTH		
Canada	10.5	0.11
Canada, Alberta	10.5	0.40
Canada, British Columbia	10.5	0.32
Canada, Manitoba	10.0	0.55
Canada, New Brunswick	8.7	0.63
Canada, Newfoundland	9.8	0.82
Canada, Northwest Territories	8.6	2.46
Canada, Nova Scotia	10.1	0.60
Canada, Ontario	11.1	0.19
Canada, Prince Edward Island	8.4	1.52
Canada, Quebec	9.9	0.21
Canada, Saskatchewan	10.6	0.61
Canada, Yukon	19.9	5.14
US, Cent. Calif.: Non-Hisp. White	11.2	0.50
US, Cent. Calif.: Hispanic	9.3	0.91
US, Los Angeles: Non-Hisp. White	13.1	0.32
US, Los Angeles: Hispanic White	9.0	0.41
US, Los Angeles: Black	8.1	0.53
US, Los Angeles: Chinese	6.6	1.00
US, Los Angeles: Filipino	9.9	1.30
US, Los Angeles: Korean	4.9	1.13
US, Los Angeles: Japanese	8.7	1.36
US, San Francisco: Non-Hisp. White	13.2	0.42
US, San Francisco: Hispanic White	9.9	0.97
US, San Francisco: Black	9.5	0.89
US, San Francisco: Chinese	7.8	1.01
US, San Francisco: Filipino	7.4	1.26
US, San Francisco: Japanese	7.4	1.91
US, Connecticut: White	11.6	0.34
US, Connecticut: Black	7.0	1.03
US, Atlanta: White	11.5	0.51
US, Atlanta: Black	7.8	0.76
US, Iowa	12.0	0.37

	MALE	FEMALE
US, Central Louisiana: White	9.3	1.13
US, Central Louisiana: Black	8.2	2.08
US, New Orleans: White	11.2	0.74
US, New Orleans: Black	7.6	0.86
US, Detroit: White	12.4	0.36
US, Detroit: Black	8.0	0.53
US, New Mexico: Non-Hisp. White	11.0	0.65
US, New Mexico: Hispanic White	8.6	0.80
US, New Mexico: American Indian	12.9	2.23
US, Utah	10.3	0.51
US, Seattle	11.9	0.34
US, SEER: White	11.9	0.14
US, SEER: Black	8.1	0.35
ASIA		
*China, Qidong	1.2	0.19
China, Shanghai	5.8	0.17
China, Tianjin	5.3	0.23
Hong Kong	7.4	0.23
*India, Bangalore	4.3	0.26
*India, Barshi, Paranda and Bhum	1.2	0.36
India, Bombay	7.2	0.24
*India, Karunagappally	2,0	0,76
India, Madras	5.7	0.30
*India, Trivandrum	4.2	0.73
Israel: All Jews	11.6	0.34
Jews born in Israel	12.3	0.97
Jews born in America or Europe	13.5	0.60
Jews born in Africa or Asia	7.3	0.46
Non-Jews	3.0	0.52
Japan, Hiroshima	6.6	0.45
Japan, Miyagi	6.1	0.29
Japan, Nagasaki	6.7	0.37
Japan, Osaka	5.6	0.14
*Japan, Saga	5.2	0.41
Japan, Yamagata	4.9	0.34
*Korea, Kangwha	2,8	1,01
*Kuwait: Non-Kuwaitis	7.8	1.55
*Kuwait: Kuwaitis	4.7	1.02
*Philippines, Manila	9.4	0.39
Singapore: Chinese	10.7	0.46
Singapore: Malay	9.9	1.16
Singapore: Indian	7.5	1.52
Thailand, Chiang Mai	4.4	0.37
*Thailand, Khon Kaen	4.4	0.41
*Viet Nam, Hanoi	2.9	0.32

* IMPORTANT-SEE NOTES ON POPULATION PAGE

EUROPE	MALE	FEMALE
Austria, Tyrol	15.1	0.85
*Belarus	10.7	0.18
*Croatia	10.3	0.28
Czech Republic	13.3	0.20
Denmark	14.0	0.28
Estonia	12.5	0.47
Finland	10.9	0.23
France, Bas-Rhin	12.3	0.64
*France, Calvados	9.0	0.68
France, Doubs	8.1	0.74
France, Haut-Rhin	11.2	0.74
*France, Herault	6.6	0.50
France, Isere	9.1	0.55
*France, Somme	10.1	0.77
*France, Tarn	8.7	0.85
Germany, Eastern States	12.2	0.23
Germany, Saarland	9.6	0.47
Iceland	10.9	1.25
Ireland, Southern	13.6	0.97
Italy, Ferrara	6.9	1.01
Italy, Florence	9.4	0.51
Italy, Genoa	9.7	0.58
*Italy, Latina	7.0	0.76
Italy, Macerata	9.6	1.50
Italy, Modena	10.5	0.67
Italy, Parma	9.9	0.81
Italy, Ragusa	6.9	0.81
Italy, Romagna	8.6	0.67
Italy, Torino	9.1	0.54
Italy, Trieste	12.9	1.28
Italy, Varese	10.2	0.59
Italy, Veneto	9.9	0.49
*Latvia	13.4	0.38
Malta	12.0	1.61
The Netherlands	11.2	0.17
The Netherlands, Eindhoven	11.2	0.62
The Netherlands, Maastricht	10.4	0.59
Norway	13.3	0.32
*Poland, Cracow	14.0	0.75
*Poland, Kielce	8.1	0.50
*Poland, Lower Silesia	14.1	0.40
Poland, Warsaw City	13.3	0.53
Slovakia	10.9	0.27
Slovenia	10.5	0.40
*Spain, Albacete	7.7	1.35
Spain, Asturias	9.1	0.54
Spain, Basque Country	7.7	0.37
Spain, Granada	6.5	0.52
Spain, Mallorca	7.9	0.66
Spain, Murcia	7.3	0.48
Spain, Navarra	8.1	0.69
Spain, Tarragona	7.3	0.67
Spain, Zaragoza	8.1	0.53

	MALE	FEMALE
Sweden	13.2	0.21
*Switzerland, Basel	10.0	0.78
Switzerland, Geneva	11.9	0.90
Switzerland, Graubunden	10.7	1.41
Switzerland, Neuchatel	11.3	1.34
Switzerland, St Gall-Appenzell	12.5	0.89
Switzerland, Valais	10.9	1.29
Switzerland, Vaud	9.6	0.67
Switzerland, Zurich	11.0	0.52
*UK, England and Wales	12.4	0.11
*UK, East Anglia	12.4	0.42
*UK, Mersey	11.4	0.37
*UK, North Western	11.1	0.28
UK, Oxford	13.3	0.41
*UK, South Thames	13.1	0.24
UK, South Western	11.9	0.32
UK, Wessex	12.9	0.35
*UK, West Midlands	14.1	0.28
UK, Yorkshire	11.9	0.31
UK, Scotland	13.3	0.27
UK, Scotland, West	12.4	0.35
*Yugoslavia, Vojvodina	9.0	0.35

OCEANIA	MALE	FEMALE
Australian Capital Territory	8.1	1.11
Australia, New South Wales	8.4	0.22
South Australia	9.6	0.47
Australia, Tasmania	8.4	0.79
Australia, Victoria	9.6	0.27
Western Australia	8.5	0.44
*French Polynesia	11.0	2.00
New Zealand: Non-Maori	11.0	0.35
New Zealand: Maori	12.2	1.57
US, Hawaii: White	14.2	1.35
US, Hawaii: Japanese	8.1	0.94
US, Hawaii: Hawaiian	8.3	1.41
US, Hawaii: Filipino	8.1	1.40
US, Hawaii: Chinese	6.6	1.64

* IMPORTANT-SEE NOTES ON POPULATION PAGE

AGE-STANDARDIZED INCIDENCE
RATES AND STANDARD ERRORS (per 100,000)
Other female genital (ICD-9 184)

	MALE	FEMALE
AFRICA		
*Algeria, Setif	0,6	0,21
*France, La Reunion	1.4	0.32
*Mali, Bamako	0,6	0,20
*Uganda, Kyadondo	1.2	0.47
*Zimbabwe, Harare: African	1,1	0,78
*Zimbabwe, Harare: European	0,9	0,87
AMERICA, CENTRAL AND SOUTH		
*Argentina, Concordia	3.7	1.04
*Brazil, Belem	1.3	0.31
*Brazil, Goiania	2.3	0.45
*Brazil, Porto Alegre	3.6	0.42
Colombia, Cali	2.0	0.28
*Costa Rica	1.6	0.18
*Ecuador, Quito	0.7	0.20
*Peru, Lima	1.4	0.18
Peru, Trujillo	3.4	0.84
US, Puerto Rico	2.3	0.16
*Uruguay, Montevideo	2.2	0.26
AMERICA, NORTH		
Canada	1.9	0.04
Canada, Alberta	1.8	0.16
Canada, British Columbia	1.6	0.12
Canada, Manitoba	2.4	0.26
Canada, New Brunswick	2.0	0.29
Canada, Newfoundland	2.0	0.35
Canada, Northwest Territories	0,7	0,70
Canada, Nova Scotia	2.5	0.28
Canada, Ontario	2.0	0.08
Canada, Prince Edward Island	3.1	0.88
Canada, Quebec	1.6	0.08
Canada, Saskatchewan	1.5	0.22
Canada, Yukon	0,4	0,41
US, Cent. Calif.: Non-Hisp. White	1.8	0.19
US, Cent. Calif.: Hispanic	2.3	0.46
US, Los Angeles: Non-Hisp. White	1.9	0.12
US, Los Angeles: Hispanic White	1.5	0.17
US, Los Angeles: Black	1.6	0.24
US, Los Angeles: Chinese	0,4	0,21
US, Los Angeles: Filipino	1,1	0,50
US, Los Angeles: Korean	0,7	0,52
US, Los Angeles: Japanese	0,8	0,42
US, San Francisco: Non-Hisp. White	1.8	0.15
US, San Francisco: Hispanic White	1.3	0.33
US, San Francisco: Black	1.6	0.37
US, San Francisco: Chinese	0,6	0,26
US, San Francisco: Filipino	1,4	0,54
US, San Francisco: Japanese	-	-
US, Connecticut: White	1.8	0.12
US, Connecticut: Black	1.5	0.45
US, Atlanta: White	2.1	0.21
US, Atlanta: Black	2.3	0.40
US, Iowa	2.1	0.14

	MALE	FEMALE
US, Central Louisiana: White	1.7	0.49
US, Central Louisiana: Black	2,0	0,94
US, New Orleans: White	1.9	0.29
US, New Orleans: Black	2.7	0.53
US, Detroit: White	2.2	0.15
US, Detroit: Black	2.0	0.27
US, New Mexico: Non-Hisp. White	2.1	0.27
US, New Mexico: Hispanic White	1.2	0.28
US, New Mexico: American Indian	1,0	0,54
US, Utah	1.6	0.19
US, Seattle	2.1	0.14
US, SEER: White	2.0	0.05
US, SEER: Black	2.0	0.17
ASIA		
*China, Qidong	0,0	0,03
China, Shanghai	0.5	0.04
China, Tianjin	0.5	0.07
Hong Kong	1.1	0.08
*India, Bangalore	1.4	0.16
*India, Barshi, Paranda and Bhum	0,9	0,34
India, Bombay	1.5	0.12
*India, Karunagappally	0,6	0,45
India, Madras	1.9	0.18
*India, Trivandrum	0,8	0,33
Israel: All Jews	1.6	0.11
Jews born in Israel	1.7	0.49
Jews born in America or Europe	1.7	0.20
Jews born in Africa or Asia	1.5	0.20
Non-Jews	0,7	0,26
Japan, Hiroshima	0.9	0.16
Japan, Miyagi	0.4	0.06
Japan, Nagasaki	0.5	0.08
Japan, Osaka	0.4	0.04
*Japan, Saga	0.5	0.12
Japan, Yamagata	0.3	0.07
*Korea, Kangwha	0,3	0,26
*Kuwait: Non-Kuwaitis	0,8	0,60
*Kuwait: Kuwaitis	0,7	0,43
*Philippines, Manila	1.1	0.14
Singapore: Chinese	1.0	0.14
Singapore: Malay	0,6	0,30
Singapore: Indian	0,5	0,37
Thailand, Chiang Mai	1.2	0.19
*Thailand, Khon Kaen	0.8	0.18
*Viet Nam, Hanoi	1.6	0.24

* IMPORTANT-SEE NOTES ON POPULATION PAGE

EUROPE	MALE	FEMALE
Austria, Tyrol	2.6	0.34
*Belarus	1.8	0.07
*Croatia	1.6	0.10
Czech Republic	2.2	0.07
Denmark	2.1	0.10
Estonia	1.9	0.16
Finland	1.8	0.09
France, Bas-Rhin	1.6	0.21
*France, Calvados	1.5	0.26
France, Doubs	1.8	0.31
France, Haut-Rhin	1.7	0.25
*France, Herault	1.5	0.20
France, Isere	1.3	0.19
*France, Somme	1.0	0.23
*France, Tarn	1.9	0.38
Germany, Eastern States	2.1	0.09
Germany, Saarland	2.1	0.20
Iceland	1.7	0.49
Ireland, Southern	1.4	0.27
Italy, Ferrara	3.8	1.38
Italy, Florence	1.9	0.21
Italy, Genoa	1.8	0.21
*Italy, Latina	1.3	0.28
Italy, Macerata	1.4	0.48
Italy, Modena	1.7	0.22
Italy, Parma	1.9	0.28
Italy, Ragusa	0.9	0.28
Italy, Romagna	1.0	0.20
Italy, Torino	1.5	0.18
Italy, Trieste	3.4	0.52
Italy, Varese	1.5	0.20
Italy, Veneto	2.1	0.20
*Latvia	1.6	0.12
Malta	1,1	0,44
The Netherlands	1.9	0.06
The Netherlands, Eindhoven	1.3	0.20
The Netherlands, Maastricht	1.9	0.23
Norway	1.7	0.10
*Poland, Cracow	2.0	0.25
*Poland, Kielce	1.8	0.21
*Poland, Lower Silesia	2.4	0.16
Poland, Warsaw City	2.1	0.19
Slovakia	1.8	0.10
Slovenia	2.1	0.16
*Spain, Albacete	1.1	0.35
Spain, Asturias	1.9	0.24
Spain, Basque Country	1.7	0.15
Spain, Granada	1.8	0.25
Spain, Mallorca	2.2	0.29
Spain, Murcia	1.6	0.20
Spain, Navarra	1.4	0.25
Spain, Tarragona	2.1	0.29
Spain, Zaragoza	2.2	0.24

	MALE	FEMALE
Sweden	1.7	0.07
*Switzerland, Basel	2.5	0.37
Switzerland, Geneva	1.4	0.29
Switzerland, Graubunden	1.4	0.48
Switzerland, Neuchatel	1.3	0.39
Switzerland, St Gall-Appenzell	2.0	0.32
Switzerland, Valais	1.3	0.41
Switzerland, Vaud	1.9	0.28
Switzerland, Zurich	1.8	0.19
*UK, England and Wales	1.9	0.04
*UK, East Anglia	1.7	0.14
*UK, Mersey	1.7	0.13
*UK, North Western	2.0	0.11
UK, Oxford	2.0	0.14
*UK, South Thames	1.5	0.07
UK, South Western	1.8	0.12
UK, Wessex	2.0	0.12
*UK, West Midlands	2.3	0.10
UK, Yorkshire	1.9	0.11
UK, Scotland	2.0	0.10
UK, Scotland, West	1.8	0.13
*Yugoslavia, Vojvodina	1.8	0.15

OCEANIA	MALE	FEMALE
Australian Capital Territory	1.6	0.50
Australia, New South Wales	1.6	0.09
South Australia	1.6	0.17
Australia, Tasmania	1.9	0.36
Australia, Victoria	1.6	0.10
Western Australia	1.4	0.17
*French Polynesia	4.4	1.31
New Zealand: Non-Maori	2.6	0.16
New Zealand: Maori	2.9	0.73
US, Hawaii: White	1.9	0.46
US, Hawaii: Japanese	0.7	0.22
US, Hawaii: Hawaiian	1,9	0,68
US, Hawaii: Filipino	1,0	0,44
US, Hawaii: Chinese	0,6	0,41

* IMPORTANT-SEE NOTES ON POPULATION PAGE

AGE-STANDARDIZED INCIDENCE
RATES AND STANDARD ERRORS (per 100,000)
Prostate (ICD-9 185)

	MALE	FEMALE
AFRICA		
*Algeria, Setif	1.8	0.53
*France, La Reunion	23.6	1.55
*Mali, Bamako	5.4	0.96
*Uganda, Kyadondo	27.7	3.12
*Zimbabwe, Harare: African	29.2	3.07
*Zimbabwe, Harare: European	55.7	7.03
AMERICA, CENTRAL AND SOUTH		
*Argentina, Concordia	16.2	2.40
*Brazil, Belem	17.9	1.66
*Brazil, Goiania	35.2	2.08
*Brazil, Porto Alegre	42.8	1.86
Colombia, Cali	32.7	1.30
*Costa Rica	27.0	0.79
*Ecuador, Quito	22.4	1.18
*Peru, Lima	19.4	0.71
Peru, Trujillo	21.8	2.37
US, Puerto Rico	54.7	0.82
*Uruguay, Montevideo	32.6	1.09
AMERICA, NORTH		
Canada	64.7	0.27
Canada, Alberta	63.4	0.97
Canada, British Columbia	84.9	0.86
Canada, Manitoba	77.3	1.40
Canada, New Brunswick	69.2	1.70
Canada, Newfoundland	40.6	1.57
Canada, Northwest Territories	19.3	3.97
Canada, Nova Scotia	59.0	1.38
Canada, Ontario	63.0	0.44
Canada, Prince Edward Island	70.9	4.03
Canada, Quebec	56.2	0.52
Canada, Saskatchewan	66.8	1.32
Canada, Yukon	64.7	9.03
US, Cent. Calif.: Non-Hisp. White	91.9	1.34
US, Cent. Calif.: Hispanic	67.4	2.65
US, Los Angeles: Non-Hisp. White	96.3	0.82
US, Los Angeles: Hispanic White	60.4	1.30
US, Los Angeles: Black	130.6	2.47
US, Los Angeles: Chinese	20.2	1.79
US, Los Angeles: Filipino	46.1	3.06
US, Los Angeles: Korean	10.2	1.99
US, Los Angeles: Japanese	47.2	3.00
US, San Francisco: Non-Hisp. White	95.9	1.10
US, San Francisco: Hispanic White	68.5	2.89
US, San Francisco: Black	127.6	3.54
US, San Francisco: Chinese	26.0	1.63
US, San Francisco: Filipino	53.0	3.65
US, San Francisco: Japanese	43.1	5.41
US, Connecticut: White	79.1	0.85
US, Connecticut: Black	119.7	5.08
US, Atlanta: White	111.2	1.78
US, Atlanta: Black	142.3	4.11
US, Iowa	86.4	0.91

	MALE	FEMALE
US, Central Louisiana: White	64.8	2.89
US, Central Louisiana: Black	80.2	6.74
US, New Orleans: White	84.5	2.02
US, New Orleans: Black	96.4	3.49
US, Detroit: White	108.2	1.05
US, Detroit: Black	141.5	2.47
US, New Mexico: Non-Hisp. White	112.4	1.94
US, New Mexico: Hispanic White	74.1	2.44
US, New Mexico: American Indian	36.8	4.07
US, Utah	115.9	1.68
US, Seattle	131.5	1.15
US, SEER: White	100.8	0.40
US, SEER: Black	137.0	1.64
ASIA		
*China, Qidong	0.5	0.13
China, Shanghai	2.3	0.10
China, Tianjin	1.9	0.16
Hong Kong	7.9	0.24
*India, Bangalore	4.7	0.28
*India, Barshi, Paranda and Bhum	1.4	0.42
India, Bombay	7.9	0.30
*India, Karunagappally	3.9	1.07
India, Madras	3.6	0.28
*India, Trivandrum	7.3	1.13
Israel: All Jews	23.9	0.45
Jews born in Israel	32.9	2.25
Jews born in America or Europe	23.4	0.59
Jews born in Africa or Asia	23.2	0.81
Non-Jews	10.4	1.12
Japan, Hiroshima	10.9	0.62
Japan, Miyagi	9.0	0.34
Japan, Nagasaki	9.1	0.38
Japan, Osaka	6.8	0.17
*Japan, Saga	6.7	0.42
Japan, Yamagata	7.9	0.37
*Korea, Kangwha	0,9	0,52
*Kuwait: Non-Kuwaitis	18.3	3.64
*Kuwait: Kuwaitis	6.5	1.13
*Philippines, Manila	17.6	0.71
Singapore: Chinese	9.8	0.49
Singapore: Malay	9.1	1.25
Singapore: Indian	6.5	1.17
Thailand, Chiang Mai	4.1	0.37
*Thailand, Khon Kaen	2.8	0.41
*Viet Nam, Hanoi	1.2	0.24

m

* IMPORTANT-SEE NOTES ON POPULATION PAGE

EUROPE	MALE	FEMALE
Austria, Tyrol	51.6	1.66
*Belarus	12.2	0.23
*Croatia	17.5	0.41
Czech Republic	24.1	0.27
Denmark	31.0	0.38
Estonia	21.6	0.73
Finland	41.3	0.46
France, Bas-Rhin	48.1	1.30
*France, Calvados	50.5	1.59
France, Doubs	44.0	1.69
France, Haut-Rhin	51.3	1.59
*France, Herault	39.6	1.07
France, Isere	48.0	1.22
*France, Somme	36.5	1.36
*France, Tarn	58.8	1.89
Germany, Eastern States	23.7	0.36
Germany, Saarland	35.9	0.96
Iceland	61.0	2.75
Ireland, Southern	30.4	1.28
Italy, Ferrara	21.8	1.71
Italy, Florence	24.4	0.73
Italy, Genoa	24.7	0.83
*Italy, Latina	12.9	1.02
Italy, Macerata	26.8	2.13
Italy, Modena	23.3	0.90
Italy, Parma	21.9	1.03
Italy, Ragusa	12.0	0.96
Italy, Romagna	28.5	1.07
Italy, Torino	23.4	0.83
Italy, Trieste	44.8	1.99
Italy, Varese	28.2	0.99
Italy, Veneto	26.8	0.76
*Latvia	15.8	0.47
Malta	22.3	2.21
The Netherlands	39.6	0.31
The Netherlands, Eindhoven	35.6	1.11
The Netherlands, Maastricht	35.9	1.10
Norway	48.4	0.51
*Poland, Cracow	13.4	0.83
*Poland, Kielce	10.3	0.55
*Poland, Lower Silesia	15.5	0.48
Poland, Warsaw City	15.7	0.62
Slovakia	22.0	0.39
Slovenia	20.7	0.61
*Spain, Albacete	20.9	1.85
Spain, Asturias	18.1	0.70
Spain, Basque Country	21.0	0.60
Spain, Granada	15.1	0.73
Spain, Mallorca	23.4	1.00
Spain, Murcia	19.0	0.74
Spain, Navarra	27.2	1.11
Spain, Tarragona	21.2	0.94
Spain, Zaragoza	19.7	0.75

	MALE	FEMALE
Sweden	55.3	0.37
*Switzerland, Basel	50.3	1.65
Switzerland, Geneva	49.0	1.91
Switzerland, Graubunden	49.4	3.02
Switzerland, Neuchatel	42.3	2.53
Switzerland, St Gall-Appenzell	53.5	1.72
Switzerland, Valais	45.9	2.54
Switzerland, Vaud	45.7	1.42
Switzerland, Zurich	65.4	1.23
*UK, England and Wales	28.0	0.15
*UK, East Anglia	33.4	0.59
*UK, Mersey	21.3	0.44
*UK, North Western	26.6	0.41
UK, Oxford	32.5	0.59
*UK, South Thames	29.3	0.32
UK, South Western	31.8	0.45
UK, Wessex	33.7	0.49
*UK, West Midlands	31.6	0.39
UK, Yorkshire	29.4	0.44
UK, Scotland	31.2	0.40
UK, Scotland, West	29.9	0.54
*Yugoslavia, Vojvodina	14.7	0.47

OCEANIA	MALE	FEMALE
Australian Capital Territory	49.7	3.23
Australia, New South Wales	53.5	0.53
South Australia	53.6	1.02
Australia, Tasmania	51.5	1.82
Australia, Victoria	47.6	0.58
Western Australia	52.8	1.07
*French Polynesia	23.2	3.49
New Zealand: Non-Maori	37.8	0.60
New Zealand: Maori	44.4	4.07
US, Hawaii: White	108.2	3.48
US, Hawaii: Japanese	64.2	2.09
US, Hawaii: Hawaiian	42.1	3.41
US, Hawaii: Filipino	49.5	2.83
US, Hawaii: Chinese	62.9	4.44

* IMPORTANT-SEE NOTES ON POPULATION PAGE

AGE-STANDARDIZED INCIDENCE
RATES AND STANDARD ERRORS (per 100,000)
Testis (ICD-9 186)

	MALE	FEMALE
AFRICA		
*Algeria, Setif	0,2	0,18
*France, La Reunion	1.1	0.25
*Mali, Bamako	0,4	0,22
*Uganda, Kyadondo	0,7	0,47
*Zimbabwe, Harare: African	0,6	0,38
*Zimbabwe, Harare: European	-	-
AMERICA, CENTRAL AND SOUTH		
*Argentina, Concordia	2,9	0,96
*Brazil, Belem	1.3	0.35
*Brazil, Goiania	1.3	0.33
*Brazil, Porto Alegre	3.1	0.43
Colombia, Cali	1.7	0.22
*Costa Rica	2.1	0.17
*Ecuador, Quito	3.5	0.35
*Peru, Lima	2.9	0.22
Peru, Trujillo	2.3	0.57
US, Puerto Rico	1.3	0.14
*Uruguay, Montevideo	4.8	0.50
AMERICA, NORTH		
Canada	3.8	0.07
Canada, Alberta	4.1	0.24
Canada, British Columbia	4.2	0.21
Canada, Manitoba	4.0	0.36
Canada, New Brunswick	2.7	0.37
Canada, Newfoundland	2.4	0.38
Canada, Northwest Territories	4.3	1.12
Canada, Nova Scotia	4.0	0.39
Canada, Ontario	4.1	0.12
Canada, Prince Edward Island	2,6	0,87
Canada, Quebec	3.1	0.13
Canada, Saskatchewan	3.5	0.37
Canada, Yukon	9.2	2.17
US, Cent. Calif.: Non-Hisp. White	5.0	0.37
US, Cent. Calif.: Hispanic	2.6	0.37
US, Los Angeles: Non-Hisp. White	5.8	0.24
US, Los Angeles: Hispanic White	3.0	0.19
US, Los Angeles: Black	1.1	0.19
US, Los Angeles: Chinese	1,0	0,46
US, Los Angeles: Filipino	1,1	0,45
US, Los Angeles: Korean	0,8	0,50
US, Los Angeles: Japanese	0,9	0,44
US, San Francisco: Non-Hisp. White	6.7	0.33
US, San Francisco: Hispanic White	3.5	0.48
US, San Francisco: Black	0.9	0.28
US, San Francisco: Chinese	2.0	0.52
US, San Francisco: Filipino	1,5	0,58
US, San Francisco: Japanese	6,1	2,19
US, Connecticut: White	5.3	0.26
US, Connecticut: Black	0,7	0,33
US, Atlanta: White	4.7	0.33
US, Atlanta: Black	0.6	0.19
US, Iowa	4.5	0.25

	MALE	FEMALE
US, Central Louisiana: White	2.9	0.66
US, Central Louisiana: Black	0.9	0.91
US, New Orleans: White	5.0	0.54
US, New Orleans: Black	1.3	0.38
US, Detroit: White	5.4	0.26
US, Detroit: Black	0.7	0.17
US, New Mexico: Non-Hisp. White	5.7	0.54
US, New Mexico: Hispanic White	4.4	0.55
US, New Mexico: American Indian	2.8	0.91
US, Utah	5.4	0.35
US, Seattle	5.1	0.23
US, SEER: White	5.4	0.10
US, SEER: Black	0.7	0.11
ASIA		
*China, Qidong	0,2	0,08
China, Shanghai	0.7	0.06
China, Tianjin	0.5	0.08
Hong Kong	1.3	0.09
*India, Bangalore	0.5	0.07
*India, Barshi, Paranda and Bhum	0,3	0,19
India, Bombay	0.9	0.07
*India, Karunagappally	0,5	0,36
India, Madras	0.7	0.09
*India, Trivandrum	0,4	0,20
Israel: All Jews	3.0	0.18
Jews born in Israel	3.3	0.32
Jews born in America or Europe	4.0	0.48
Jews born in Africa or Asia	1.2	0.36
Non-Jews	0.8	0.22
Japan, Hiroshima	1.7	0.26
Japan, Miyagi	1.6	0.18
Japan, Nagasaki	0.9	0.18
Japan, Osaka	1.4	0.08
*Japan, Saga	0.9	0.22
Japan, Yamagata	1.3	0.23
*Korea, Kangwha	0,3	0,31
*Kuwait: Non-Kuwaitis	1.5	0,51
*Kuwait: Kuwaitis	0,8	0,29
*Philippines, Manila	0.7	0.10
Singapore: Chinese	0.9	0.14
Singapore: Malay	1,0	0,35
Singapore: Indian	2.0	0.59
Thailand, Chiang Mai	0.5	0.12
*Thailand, Khon Kaen	0.6	0.14
*Viet Nam, Hanoi	0.7	0.16

* IMPORTANT-SEE NOTES ON POPULATION PAGE

AGE-STANDARDIZED INCIDENCE
RATES AND STANDARD ERRORS (per 100,000)
Testis (ICD-9 186) (contd)

EUROPE	MALE	FEMALE
Austria, Tyrol	6.3 0.60	
*Belarus	1.3 0.07	
*Croatia	2.5 0.16	
Czech Republic	5.2 0.14	
Denmark	9.2 0.26	
Estonia	1.6 0.20	
Finland	2.5 0.13	
France, Bas-Rhin	6.8 0.50	
*France, Calvados	3.5 0.46	
France, Doubs	5.4 0.64	
France, Haut-Rhin	7.9 0.65	
*France, Herault	2.7 0.37	
France, Isere	3.7 0.37	
*France, Somme	3.7 0.51	
*France, Tarn	2.8 0.58	
Germany, Eastern States	7.9 0.21	
Germany, Saarland	6.1 0.46	
Iceland	6.4 0.95	
Ireland, Southern	3.4 0.52	
Italy, Ferrara	2,0 0,70	
Italy, Florence	3.2 0.37	
Italy, Genoa	4.3 0.52	
*Italy, Latina	2.1 0.45	
Italy, Macerata	3.2 1.02	
Italy, Modena	3.4 0.45	
Italy, Parma	4.7 0.68	
Italy, Ragusa	0,9 0,34	
Italy, Romagna	4.1 0.61	
Italy, Torino	3.1 0.38	
Italy, Trieste	3.1 0.74	
Italy, Varese	3.8 0.43	
Italy, Veneto	3.3 0.33	
*Latvia	1.4 0.14	
Malta	3.1 0.91	
The Netherlands	4.0 0.11	
The Netherlands, Eindhoven	3.7 0.37	
The Netherlands, Maastricht	3.7 0.40	
Norway	8.0 0.27	
*Poland, Cracow	2.5 0.35	
*Poland, Kielce	2.0 0.26	
*Poland, Lower Silesia	2.6 0.19	
Poland, Warsaw City	4.1 0.37	
Slovakia	4.6 0.18	
Slovenia	4.3 0.29	
*Spain, Albacete	1,5 0,63	
Spain, Asturias	1.9 0.30	
Spain, Basque Country	2.1 0.22	
Spain, Granada	1.6 0.29	
Spain, Mallorca	1.8 0.33	
Spain, Murcia	1.2 0.22	
Spain, Navarra	2.2 0.40	
Spain, Tarragona	1.9 0.38	
Spain, Zaragoza	1.5 0.27	

	MALE	FEMALE
Sweden	4.8 0.15	
*Switzerland, Basel	8.8 0.84	
Switzerland, Geneva	7.4 0.84	
Switzerland, Graubunden	10.3 1.74	
Switzerland, Neuchatel	9.0 1.42	
Switzerland, St Gall-Appenzell	10.1 0.86	
Switzerland, Valais	7.3 1.13	
Switzerland, Vaud	9.3 0.79	
Switzerland, Zurich	8.9 0.53	
*UK, England and Wales	4.6 0.08	
*UK, East Anglia	5.3 0.31	
*UK, Mersey	5.3 0.29	
*UK, North Western	4.3 0.20	
UK, Oxford	5.7 0.28	
*UK, South Thames	4.9 0.17	
UK, South Western	5.1 0.25	
UK, Wessex	5.5 0.26	
*UK, West Midlands	4.6 0.18	
UK, Yorkshire	4.6 0.22	
UK, Scotland	5.8 0.21	
UK, Scotland, West	5.4 0.27	
*Yugoslavia, Vojvodina	2.6 0.23	

OCEANIA	MALE	FEMALE
Australian Capital Territory	3.5 0.66	
Australia, New South Wales	4.7 0.17	
South Australia	4.0 0.32	
Australia, Tasmania	4.9 0.63	
Australia, Victoria	4.5 0.19	
Western Australia	3.7 0.28	
*French Polynesia	1,6 0,55	
New Zealand: Non-Maori	5.6 0.26	
New Zealand: Maori	7.1 0.96	
US, Hawaii: White	5.9 0.77	
US, Hawaii: Japanese	3.0 0.73	
US, Hawaii: Hawaiian	3.4 0.77	
US, Hawaii: Filipino	2,0 0,66	
US, Hawaii: Chinese	2,7 1,21	

* IMPORTANT-SEE NOTES ON POPULATION PAGE

AGE-STANDARDIZED INCIDENCE
RATES AND STANDARD ERRORS (per 100,000)
Penis, other male genital (ICD-9 187)

	MALE	FEMALE		MALE	FEMALE
AFRICA			US, Central Louisiana: White	0,2	0,12
*Algeria, Setif	0,2	0,16	US, Central Louisiana: Black	3,5	1,54
*France, La Reunion	1.3	0.35	US, New Orleans: White	0.6	0.18
*Mali, Bamako	0,5	0,29	US, New Orleans: Black	1.7	0.49
*Uganda, Kyadondo	3.7	1.04	US, Detroit: White	0.6	0.08
*Zimbabwe, Harare: African	2.8	0.91	US, Detroit: Black	0.7	0.19
*Zimbabwe, Harare: European	0,9	0,90	US, New Mexico: Non-Hisp. White	0.8	0.17
			US, New Mexico: Hispanic White	1.2	0.31
			US, New Mexico: American Indian	0,5	0,48
AMERICA, CENTRAL AND SOUTH			US, Utah	0.5	0.11
*Argentina, Concordia	0,6	0,40	US, Seattle	0.6	0.08
*Brazil, Belem	2.7	0.52	US, SEER: White	0.7	0.03
*Brazil, Goiania	2.1	0.48	US, SEER: Black	0.9	0.13
*Brazil, Porto Alegre	1.3	0.32			
Colombia, Cali	1.2	0.24	**ASIA**		
*Costa Rica	1.4	0.17	*China, Qidong	0.5	0.14
*Ecuador, Quito	0.6	0.19	China, Shanghai	0.5	0.05
*Peru, Lima	0.8	0.14	China, Tianjin	0.4	0.06
Peru, Trujillo	1,5	0,59	Hong Kong	0.6	0.06
US, Puerto Rico	2.5	0.18	*India, Bangalore	1.6	0.16
*Uruguay, Montevideo	0.9	0.20	*India, Barshi, Paranda and Bhum	3.9	0.66
			India, Bombay	1.6	0.12
AMERICA, NORTH			*India, Karunagappally	1,2	0,61
Canada	0.8	0.03	India, Madras	3.1	0.23
Canada, Alberta	0.7	0.10	*India, Trivandrum	1,3	0,46
Canada, British Columbia	0.7	0.08	Israel: All Jews	0.2	0.05
Canada, Manitoba	0.8	0.15	Jews born in Israel	0,1	0,05
Canada, New Brunswick	1.0	0.21	Jews born in America or Europe	0.2	0.07
Canada, Newfoundland	0.9	0.24	Jews born in Africa or Asia	0,2	0,08
Canada, Northwest Territories	0,5	0,54	Non-Jews	-	-
Canada, Nova Scotia	1.0	0.19	Japan, Hiroshima	0.6	0.14
Canada, Ontario	0.9	0.05	Japan, Miyagi	0.5	0.08
Canada, Prince Edward Island	1,4	0,58	Japan, Nagasaki	0.7	0.10
Canada, Quebec	0.7	0.06	Japan, Osaka	0.3	0.04
Canada, Saskatchewan	1.1	0.19	*Japan, Saga	0,1	0,06
Canada, Yukon	0,8	0,82	Japan, Yamagata	0.2	0.07
US, Cent. Calif.: Non-Hisp. White	0.9	0.14	*Korea, Kangwha	0,6	0,42
US, Cent. Calif.: Hispanic	1.3	0.35	*Kuwait: Non-Kuwaitis	0,2	0,11
US, Los Angeles: Non-Hisp. White	0.7	0.08	*Kuwait: Kuwaitis	-	-
US, Los Angeles: Hispanic White	1.0	0.16	*Philippines, Manila	0.7	0.12
US, Los Angeles: Black	1.1	0.22	Singapore: Chinese	1.0	0.15
US, Los Angeles: Chinese	0,4	0,26	Singapore: Malay	-	-
US, Los Angeles: Filipino	-	-	Singapore: Indian	1,0	0,42
US, Los Angeles: Korean	0,3	0,31	Thailand, Chiang Mai	2.4	0.27
US, Los Angeles: Japanese	0,2	0,18	*Thailand, Khon Kaen	1.8	0.29
US, San Francisco: Non-Hisp. White	0.6	0.10	*Viet Nam, Hanoi	2.3	0.32
US, San Francisco: Hispanic White	1.1	0.35			
US, San Francisco: Black	0,7	0,25			
US, San Francisco: Chinese	0,5	0,24			
US, San Francisco: Filipino	0,3	0,21			
US, San Francisco: Japanese	0,6	0,57			
US, Connecticut: White	0.6	0.08			
US, Connecticut: Black	1,4	0,54			
US, Atlanta: White	0.6	0.13			
US, Atlanta: Black	1.6	0.43			
US, Iowa	0.9	0.11			

* IMPORTANT-SEE NOTES ON POPULATION PAGE

AGE-STANDARDIZED INCIDENCE
RATES AND STANDARD ERRORS (per 100,000)
Penis, other male genital (ICD-9 187) (contd)

EUROPE	MALE	FEMALE
Austria, Tyrol	0.6	*0.18*
*Belarus	0.7	*0.05*
*Croatia	0.6	*0.08*
Czech Republic	0.9	*0.05*
Denmark	0.9	*0.07*
Estonia	1.0	*0.15*
Finland	0.5	*0.05*
France, Bas-Rhin	1.0	*0.19*
*France, Calvados	1.0	*0.23*
France, Doubs	1.1	*0.27*
France, Haut-Rhin	1.1	*0.23*
*France, Herault	0.7	*0.16*
France, Isere	0.8	*0.16*
*France, Somme	0,5	*0,18*
*France, Tarn	0.7	*0.20*
Germany, Eastern States	1.0	*0.07*
Germany, Saarland	1.0	*0.16*
Iceland	1,1	*0,37*
Ireland, Southern	0.8	*0.23*
Italy, Ferrara	0,7	*0,30*
Italy, Florence	0.8	*0.15*
Italy, Genoa	0.9	*0.17*
*Italy, Latina	1.1	*0.31*
Italy, Macerata	1,3	*0,57*
Italy, Modena	0.5	*0.15*
Italy, Parma	0.7	*0.21*
Italy, Ragusa	0,6	*0,24*
Italy, Romagna	0.9	*0.21*
Italy, Torino	1.0	*0.18*
Italy, Trieste	2.9	*0.81*
Italy, Varese	0.8	*0.17*
Italy, Veneto	0.7	*0.13*
*Latvia	0.9	*0.11*
Malta	1,9	*0,69*
The Netherlands	0.8	*0.05*
The Netherlands, Eindhoven	0.8	*0.17*
The Netherlands, Maastricht	0.8	*0.18*
Norway	0.7	*0.07*
*Poland, Cracow	0.5	*0.16*
*Poland, Kielce	0.8	*0.16*
*Poland, Lower Silesia	1.1	*0.12*
Poland, Warsaw City	1.0	*0.16*
Slovakia	0.9	*0.08*
Slovenia	0.8	*0.12*
*Spain, Albacete	0,8	*0,37*
Spain, Asturias	0.6	*0.14*
Spain, Basque Country	1.1	*0.14*
Spain, Granada	1.2	*0.21*
Spain, Mallorca	1.2	*0.24*
Spain, Murcia	1.2	*0.20*
Spain, Navarra	1.0	*0.25*
Spain, Tarragona	1.5	*0.27*
Spain, Zaragoza	0.8	*0.16*

	MALE	FEMALE
Sweden	0.9	*0.05*
*Switzerland, Basel	0.8	*0.22*
Switzerland, Geneva	1.6	*0.36*
Switzerland, Graubunden	0,3	*0,27*
Switzerland, Neuchatel	2.1	*0.59*
Switzerland, St Gall-Appenzell	1.3	*0.29*
Switzerland, Valais	0,7	*0,32*
Switzerland, Vaud	1.0	*0.24*
Switzerland, Zurich	1.1	*0.16*
*UK, England and Wales	0.9	*0.03*
*UK, East Anglia	1.0	*0.11*
*UK, Mersey	0.7	*0.09*
*UK, North Western	1.0	*0.08*
UK, Oxford	1.0	*0.11*
*UK, South Thames	0.8	*0.06*
UK, South Western	0.8	*0.08*
UK, Wessex	1.0	*0.10*
*UK, West Midlands	1.1	*0.08*
UK, Yorkshire	1.1	*0.09*
UK, Scotland	1.2	*0.08*
UK, Scotland, West	1.2	*0.11*
*Yugoslavia, Vojvodina	0.7	*0.11*

OCEANIA

	MALE	FEMALE
Australian Capital Territory	0,7	*0,45*
Australia, New South Wales	0.5	*0.05*
South Australia	0.5	*0.11*
Australia, Tasmania	0,6	*0,21*
Australia, Victoria	0.6	*0.07*
Western Australia	0.5	*0.10*
*French Polynesia	-	-
New Zealand: Non-Maori	0.6	*0.08*
New Zealand: Maori	0,3	*0,32*
US, Hawaii: White	0,2	*0,14*
US, Hawaii: Japanese	0,3	*0,14*
US, Hawaii: Hawaiian	0,3	*0,28*
US, Hawaii: Filipino	1,5	*0,59*
US, Hawaii: Chinese	-	-

* IMPORTANT-SEE NOTES ON POPULATION PAGE

AGE-STANDARDIZED INCIDENCE
RATES AND STANDARD ERRORS (per 100,000)
Bladder (ICD-9 188)

AFRICA	MALE		FEMALE	
†*Algeria, Setif	1.8	0.51	0,1	0,07
†*France, La Reunion	9.4	0.96	1.8	0.35
†*Mali, Bamako	10.6	1.29	2.3	0.50
†*Uganda, Kyadondo	2.4	0.84	0,6	0,43
†*Zimbabwe, Harare: African	13.2	1.88	12.5	2.17
†*Zimbabwe, Harare: European	27.4	5.02	7.8	2.59

AMERICA, CENTRAL AND SOUTH

	MALE		FEMALE	
†*Argentina, Concordia	9.1	1.81	3.9	1.07
†*Brazil, Belem	3.0	0.64	1.2	0.32
†*Brazil, Goiania	11.0	1.15	2.6	0.49
†*Brazil, Porto Alegre	18.6	1.22	3.4	0.40
† Colombia, Cali	7.4	0.61	2.7	0.33
†*Costa Rica	6.6	0.39	1.6	0.18
†*Ecuador, Quito	5.1	0.57	1.5	0.27
†*Peru, Lima	5.5	0.38	1.7	0.20
† Peru, Trujillo	2.8	0.82	0,7	0,43
† US, Puerto Rico	8.5	0.33	2.7	0.17
†*Uruguay, Montevideo	19.7	0.88	3.7	0.31

AMERICA, NORTH

	MALE		FEMALE	
† Canada	18.7	0.15	5.0	0.07
Canada, Alberta	17.6	0.52	5.1	0.27
Canada, British Columbia	11.3	0.32	3.0	0.15
Canada, Manitoba	17.5	0.69	5.3	0.37
Canada, New Brunswick	22.6	1.01	6.0	0.50
† Canada, Newfoundland	20.7	1.14	5.1	0.55
† Canada, Northwest Territories	7.9	2.44	1,7	1,20
Canada, Nova Scotia	21.7	0.87	6.2	0.45
† Canada, Ontario	17.8	0.24	4.8	0.11
Canada, Prince Edward Island	14.2	1.80	5.7	1.12
Canada, Quebec	23.6	0.34	5.8	0.15
Canada, Saskatchewan	19.5	0.76	5.6	0.41
Canada, Yukon	18.4	4.85	-	-
US, Cent. Calif.: Non-Hisp. White	17.7	0.61	3.9	0.27
US, Cent. Calif.: Hispanic	8.3	0.93	2.8	0.53
US, Los Angeles: Non-Hisp. White	17.1	0.35	4.2	0.16
US, Los Angeles: Hispanic White	8.3	0.47	2.5	0.22
US, Los Angeles: Black	9.1	0.64	3.5	0.33
US, Los Angeles: Chinese	7.4	1.08	2.1	0.58
US, Los Angeles: Filipino	5.5	1.11	1,0	0,42
US, Los Angeles: Korean	5.4	1.39	2,0	0,71
US, Los Angeles: Japanese	6.5	1.19	1.6	0.51
US, San Francisco: Non-Hisp. White	24.5	0.57	6.5	0.27
US, San Francisco: Hispanic White	10.4	1.11	2.0	0.41
US, San Francisco: Black	10.8	1.04	4.3	0.58
US, San Francisco: Chinese	9.1	1.02	3.0	0.54
US, San Francisco: Filipino	8.2	1.47	2.3	0.72
US, San Francisco: Japanese	11.7	2.91	3,4	1,22
US, Connecticut: White	28.4	0.53	7.6	0.26
US, Connecticut: Black	12.7	1.64	4.4	0.78
US, Atlanta: White	22.7	0.80	5.4	0.34
US, Atlanta: Black	9.6	1.03	3.5	0.49
US, Iowa	22.9	0.49	5.7	0.23

		MALE		FEMALE	
	US, Central Louisiana: White	21.5	1.76	3.5	0.61
	US, Central Louisiana: Black	14.3	3.03	3.5	1.23
	US, New Orleans: White	27.2	1.16	7.4	0.55
	US, New Orleans: Black	13.5	1.31	3.9	0.58
f	US, Detroit: White	27.4	0.54	7.1	0.25
	US, Detroit: Black	11.7	0.72	4.2	0.37
	US, New Mexico: Non-Hisp. White	23.2	0.91	5.4	0.41
	US, New Mexico: Hispanic White	10.7	0.94	3.1	0.46
	US, New Mexico: American Indian	2,6	1,01	0,6	0,44
	US, Utah	16.2	0.63	3.3	0.27
	US, Seattle	23.1	0.49	6.1	0.24
	US, SEER: White	24.0	0.20	6.2	0.09
f	US, SEER: Black	11.1	0.47	4.3	0.24

ASIA

	MALE		FEMALE	
†*China, Qidong	4.0	0.37	0.7	0.14
† China, Shanghai	6.9	0.18	1.8	0.08
† China, Tianjin	6.3	0.26	2.0	0.14
Hong Kong	14.5	0.32	4.3	0.16
*India, Bangalore	3.3	0.23	0.8	0.11
*India, Barshi, Paranda and Bhum	1,0	0,35	-	-
† India, Bombay	4.8	0.22	1.2	0.11
†*India, Karunagappally	2,6	0,88	0,5	0,32
† India, Madras	2.8	0.23	1.0	0.13
†*India, Trivandrum	2.6	0.67	0,3	0,21
Israel: All Jews	25.2	0.49	5.3	0.21
Jews born in Israel	22.5	1.68	4.7	0.70
Jews born in America or Europe	27.5	0.77	6.2	0.35
Jews born in Africa or Asia	21.5	0.80	4.0	0.32
Non-Jews	13.1	1.22	1.4	0.35
Japan, Hiroshima	12.9	0.67	2.8	0.27
† Japan, Miyagi	9.0	0.35	2.5	0.16
† Japan, Nagasaki	11.2	0.44	2.3	0.17
† Japan, Osaka	7.4	0.17	1.8	0.07
†*Japan, Saga	7.7	0.49	1.5	0.17
† Japan, Yamagata	7.4	0.37	1.7	0.16
†*Korea, Kangwha	3.1	0.99	1,3	0,63
*Kuwait: Non-Kuwaitis	17.5	3.29	4.2	1.25
*Kuwait: Kuwaitis	7.0	1.13	2.5	0.81
†*Philippines, Manila	4.9	0.36	1.5	0.17
† Singapore: Chinese	7.7	0.43	2.0	0.20
† Singapore: Malay	7.1	1.08	0,8	0,37
† Singapore: Indian	4.2	0.98	0,9	0,61
† Thailand, Chiang Mai	5.3	0.42	2.5	0.29
†*Thailand, Khon Kaen	3.2	0.41	0.5	0.15
†*Viet Nam, Hanoi	1.7	0.28	0,2	0,09

* IMPORTANT-SEE NOTES ON POPULATION PAGE

AGE-STANDARDIZED INCIDENCE
RATES AND STANDARD ERRORS (per 100,000)
Bladder (ICD-9 188) (contd)

EUROPE	MALE		FEMALE	
Austria, Tyrol	28.3	1.26	6.6	0.52
*Belarus	12.4	0.23	1.4	0.06
†*Croatia	11.7	0.33	2.5	0.13
† Czech Republic	15.4	0.22	3.2	0.09
Denmark	27.9	0.38	7.7	0.19
† Estonia	11.2	0.52	2.0	0.16
Finland	15.2	0.28	3.1	0.11
† France, Bas-Rhin	23.1	0.92	4.0	0.33
*France, Calvados	23.9	1.14	3.7	0.39
France, Doubs	26.4	1.36	4.2	0.49
† France, Haut-Rhin	21.5	1.04	3.2	0.34
†*France, Herault	17.8	0.76	2.4	0.24
France, Isere	16.0	0.73	2.6	0.25
*France, Somme	20.9	1.09	2.4	0.34
*France, Tarn	24.7	1.35	3.1	0.40
Germany, Eastern States	19.2	0.32	3.4	0.11
Germany, Saarland	23.1	0.78	5.2	0.30
† Iceland	18.7	1.59	5.0	0.81
Ireland, Southern	12.2	0.87	4.0	0.49
Italy, Ferrara	32.0	2.20	4.1	0.66
† Italy, Florence	35.2	0.95	6.0	0.36
Italy, Genoa	38.3	1.12	6.7	0.42
*Italy, Latina	24.9	1.44	3.2	0.48
Italy, Macerata	28.1	2.36	2.6	0.64
Italy, Modena	31.1	1.15	5.5	0.45
Italy, Parma	27.3	1.23	4.9	0.46
† Italy, Ragusa	13.7	1.11	1.6	0.34
Italy, Romagna	32.3	1.24	5.2	0.47
Italy, Torino	36.2	1.09	5.4	0.37
Italy, Trieste	38.7	1.96	9.4	1.14
Italy, Varese	35.0	1.13	5.1	0.38
Italy, Veneto	30.1	0.84	5.5	0.32
†*Latvia	11.8	0.41	1.8	0.12
† Malta	27.2	2.53	4.7	0.92
† The Netherlands	15.2	0.20	3.0	0.08
The Netherlands, Eindhoven	25.5	0.95	5.6	0.41
† The Netherlands, Maastricht	11.6	0.63	2.1	0.24
Norway	16.6	0.32	4.1	0.15
†*Poland, Cracow	11.9	0.78	1.5	0.22
†*Poland, Kielce	10.8	0.57	1.5	0.20
†*Poland, Lower Silesia	15.7	0.47	2.3	0.15
Poland, Warsaw City	13.1	0.56	3.0	0.23
† Slovakia	14.8	0.33	3.0	0.13
† Slovenia	10.1	0.43	2.1	0.15
*Spain, Albacete	18.6	1.92	1.7	0.51
Spain, Asturias	27.1	0.90	3.6	0.30
Spain, Basque Country	27.1	0.70	2.9	0.21
Spain, Granada	23.5	0.95	2.9	0.30
Spain, Mallorca	36.4	1.35	3.9	0.39
Spain, Murcia	30.8	0.99	3.2	0.29
Spain, Navarra	27.8	1.22	3.4	0.40
Spain, Tarragona	30.6	1.24	4.2	0.42
† Spain, Zaragoza	22.4	0.84	2.7	0.26

	MALE		FEMALE	
Sweden	17.3	0.22	4.6	0.11
†*Switzerland, Basel	12.0	0.85	3.5	0.41
Switzerland, Geneva	32.5	1.59	6.3	0.62
† Switzerland, Graubunden	14.9	1.73	3.0	0.68
† Switzerland, Neuchatel	14.0	1.49	2.8	0.60
† Switzerland, St Gall-Appenzell	10.9	0.80	2.3	0.31
† Switzerland, Valais	14.0	1.48	3.1	0.63
† Switzerland, Vaud	14.2	0.82	2.9	0.34
Switzerland, Zurich	22.4	0.74	5.6	0.33
*UK, England and Wales	20.3	0.13	5.7	0.07
†*UK, East Anglia	13.8	0.41	3.4	0.19
*UK, Mersey	17.9	0.44	6.8	0.26
*UK, North Western	20.9	0.38	6.4	0.19
UK, Oxford	20.4	0.49	5.4	0.24
*UK, South Thames	19.3	0.27	5.1	0.13
UK, South Western	19.7	0.39	4.9	0.18
UK, Wessex	23.6	0.45	7.1	0.24
*UK, West Midlands	21.7	0.34	6.1	0.17
UK, Yorkshire	25.3	0.43	7.0	0.21
UK, Scotland	22.9	0.36	7.3	0.18
UK, Scotland, West	22.9	0.49	7.5	0.25
*Yugoslavia, Vojvodina	11.5	0.41	2.6	0.17

OCEANIA

	MALE		FEMALE	
† Australian Capital Territory	8.8	1.31	2.2	0.61
† Australia, New South Wales	13.2	0.27	3.8	0.13
South Australia	20.6	0.66	5.9	0.34
† Australia, Tasmania	17.0	1.08	4.5	0.53
Australia, Victoria	18.3	0.37	5.0	0.18
† Western Australia	9.7	0.47	2.3	0.21
†*French Polynesia	8.3	2.04	1,9	0,80
† New Zealand: Non-Maori	14.0	0.38	4.1	0.19
† New Zealand: Maori	10.5	1.88	2.2	0.71
US, Hawaii: White	24.2	1.66	5.9	0.83
US, Hawaii: Japanese	10.9	1.00	3.3	0.53
US, Hawaii: Hawaiian	3.9	1.00	3.2	0.86
US, Hawaii: Filipino	5.4	1.06	2.7	0.77
US, Hawaii: Chinese	9.6	1.86	2,7	0,99

* IMPORTANT-SEE NOTES ON POPULATION PAGE

AGE-STANDARDIZED INCIDENCE
RATES AND STANDARD ERRORS (per 100,000)
Kidney etc. (ICD-9 189)

AFRICA	MALE		FEMALE	
*Algeria, Setif	0,4	0,21	0,3	0,13
*France, La Reunion	2.5	0.48	1.6	0.36
*Mali, Bamako	1.5	0.40	1.6	0.42
*Uganda, Kyadondo	1.0	0.48	2.0	0.62
*Zimbabwe, Harare: African	1.7	0.58	0,7	0,26
*Zimbabwe, Harare: European	2,9	1,66	2,7	1,69

AMERICA, CENTRAL AND SOUTH	MALE		FEMALE	
*Argentina, Concordia	3,2	1,13	3.3	1.00
*Brazil, Belem	2.3	0.51	1.5	0.32
*Brazil, Goiania	3.2	0.59	2.6	0.45
*Brazil, Porto Alegre	10.2	0.87	4.0	0.46
Colombia, Cali	2.5	0.33	1.5	0.24
*Costa Rica	3.3	0.27	2.2	0.21
*Ecuador, Quito	2.6	0.41	1.3	0.26
*Peru, Lima	3.4	0.30	2.0	0.21
Peru, Trujillo	3.2	0.91	3.3	0.82
US, Puerto Rico	4.0	0.24	2.4	0.17
*Uruguay, Montevideo	10.6	0.67	3.8	0.35

AMERICA, NORTH	MALE		FEMALE	
Canada	11.1	0.12	5.9	0.08
Canada, Alberta	11.4	0.42	5.9	0.30
Canada, British Columbia	9.6	0.31	4.6	0.21
Canada, Manitoba	10.7	0.58	6.0	0.42
Canada, New Brunswick	10.3	0.70	6.5	0.54
Canada, Newfoundland	10.0	0.83	6.5	0.67
Canada, Northwest Territories	11.2	2.86	7.8	2.49
Canada, Nova Scotia	13.6	0.72	6.7	0.48
Canada, Ontario	11.2	0.20	5.8	0.14
Canada, Prince Edward Island	12.8	1.86	3.7	0.87
Canada, Quebec	11.7	0.24	6.3	0.17
Canada, Saskatchewan	11.8	0.62	6.1	0.44
Canada, Yukon	6,8	2,66	5,8	2,71
US, Cent. Calif.: Non-Hisp. White	10.1	0.49	5.8	0.35
US, Cent. Calif.: Hispanic	11.6	1.07	5.8	0.72
US, Los Angeles: Non-Hisp. White	10.1	0.29	4.9	0.20
US, Los Angeles: Hispanic White	9.2	0.49	4.8	0.30
US, Los Angeles: Black	10.9	0.71	5.9	0.46
US, Los Angeles: Chinese	4.4	0.83	1.8	0.52
US, Los Angeles: Filipino	6.6	1.25	2.7	0.67
US, Los Angeles: Korean	6.1	1.44	4.2	1.12
US, Los Angeles: Japanese	4.5	1.01	2.2	0.63
US, San Francisco: Non-Hisp. White	9.9	0.38	4.7	0.25
US, San Francisco: Hispanic White	10.5	1.11	5.6	0.72
US, San Francisco: Black	10.0	1.00	6.3	0.75
US, San Francisco: Chinese	3.4	0.64	2.7	0.55
US, San Francisco: Filipino	6.5	1.33	2.6	0.71
US, San Francisco: Japanese	6,8	2,71	1,2	0,71
US, Connecticut: White	11.8	0.36	5.9	0.25
US, Connecticut: Black	11.2	1.50	5.2	0.85
US, Atlanta: White	10.6	0.55	4.9	0.35
US, Atlanta: Black	13.6	1.18	5.3	0.64
US, Iowa	10.6	0.36	6.1	0.26

	MALE		FEMALE	
US, Central Louisiana: White	8.3	1.09	4.3	0.80
US, Central Louisiana: Black	14.3	3.13	4.7	1.59
US, New Orleans: White	14.9	0.91	7.2	0.59
US, New Orleans: Black	12.0	1.27	7.1	0.81
US, Detroit: White	12.9	0.38	6.4	0.26
US, Detroit: Black	12.2	0.77	6.2	0.48
US, New Mexico: Non-Hisp. White	8.5	0.58	4.8	0.46
US, New Mexico: Hispanic White	10.1	0.93	5.4	0.64
US, New Mexico: American Indian	13.6	2.61	7.6	1.70
US, Utah	8.3	0.47	4.1	0.32
US, Seattle	10.3	0.34	5.5	0.24
US, SEER: White	10.8	0.14	5.5	0.10
US, SEER: Black	11.8	0.49	5.9	0.30

ASIA	MALE		FEMALE	
*China, Qidong	0.5	0.13	0.5	0.13
China, Shanghai	2.9	0.12	1.6	0.09
China, Tianjin	3.5	0.20	1.7	0.13
Hong Kong	3.8	0.16	2.3	0.12
*India, Bangalore	1.2	0.14	0.7	0.10
*India, Barshi, Paranda and Bhum	0,4	0,20	0,1	0,09
India, Bombay	2.0	0.13	0.9	0.09
*India, Karunagappally	0,9	0,52	-	-
India, Madras	1.0	0.12	0.7	0.11
*India, Trivandrum	0,5	0,25	0,3	0,16
Israel: All Jews	10.4	0.32	5.4	0.22
Jews born in Israel	9.3	1.04	5.2	0.77
Jews born in America or Europe	13.1	0.55	7.8	0.80
Jews born in Africa or Asia	6.1	0.42	3.5	0.33
Non-Jews	3.3	0.60	1.8	0.40
Japan, Hiroshima	7.8	0.52	3.2	0.32
Japan, Miyagi	6.5	0.30	2.5	0.18
Japan, Nagasaki	6.1	0.34	2.3	0.20
Japan, Osaka	5.5	0.15	1.9	0.08
*Japan, Saga	4.9	0.40	1.9	0.22
Japan, Yamagata	4.7	0.31	1.8	0.17
*Korea, Kangwha	1,8	0,81	1,2	0,63
*Kuwait: Non-Kuwaitis	4.9	1.44	3.3	1.08
*Kuwait: Kuwaitis	2.1	0.61	1.9	0.63
*Philippines, Manila	4.0	0.30	2.6	0.21
Singapore: Chinese	4.3	0.32	2.2	0.22
Singapore: Malay	2.4	0.58	0,9	0,35
Singapore: Indian	3.1	0.77	3,0	1,06
Thailand, Chiang Mai	1.6	0.22	1.5	0.22
*Thailand, Khon Kaen	1.2	0.23	0.7	0.16
*Viet Nam, Hanoi	0.6	0.16	0.4	0.11

* IMPORTANT-SEE NOTES ON POPULATION PAGE

AGE-STANDARDIZED INCIDENCE
RATES AND STANDARD ERRORS (per 100,000)
Kidney etc. (ICD-9 189) (contd)

EUROPE	MALE		FEMALE	
Austria, Tyrol	14.6	0.92	7.3	0.59
*Belarus	7.7	0.18	3.9	0.11
*Croatia	6.8	0.26	3.9	0.18
Czech Republic	16.9	0.24	8.5	0.15
Denmark	8.9	0.22	5.7	0.18
Estonia	11.4	0.53	6.0	0.33
Finland	12.1	0.26	6.7	0.18
France, Bas-Rhin	16.1	0.79	7.3	0.49
*France, Calvados	8.1	0.69	3.6	0.42
France, Doubs	8.9	0.80	5.7	0.63
France, Haut-Rhin	13.0	0.82	5.8	0.51
*France, Herault	9.3	0.59	3.3	0.35
France, Isere	9.6	0.58	4.0	0.36
*France, Somme	8.6	0.73	5.1	0.58
*France, Tarn	7.6	0.76	3.0	0.55
Germany, Eastern States	13.8	0.28	6.8	0.17
Germany, Saarland	12.2	0.58	5.6	0.37
Iceland	14.3	1.38	8.1	1.05
Ireland, Southern	6.2	0.64	3.8	0.52
Italy, Ferrara	15.8	1.62	5.4	0.81
Italy, Florence	12.2	0.59	5.6	0.42
Italy, Genoa	11.0	0.64	5.3	0.54
*Italy, Latina	5.5	0.68	2.1	0.46
Italy, Macerata	6.4	1.15	3.4	0.82
Italy, Modena	11.2	0.69	6.2	0.56
Italy, Parma	13.2	0.92	5.1	0.65
Italy, Ragusa	4.5	0.71	2.4	0.59
Italy, Romagna	13.4	0.83	5.9	0.59
Italy, Torino	11.1	0.62	4.1	0.40
Italy, Trieste	16.6	1.34	7.2	1.03
Italy, Varese	15.2	0.76	5.4	0.42
Italy, Veneto	15.7	0.62	5.3	0.35
*Latvia	9.4	0.37	4.1	0.20
Malta	5.7	1.20	1.9	0.60
The Netherlands	10.2	0.17	5.3	0.12
The Netherlands, Eindhoven	8.7	0.55	4.3	0.37
The Netherlands, Maastricht	11.3	0.64	5.2	0.41
Norway	9.0	0.25	5.2	0.19
*Poland, Cracow	11.5	0.76	5.0	0.46
*Poland, Kielce	6.3	0.45	3.4	0.32
*Poland, Lower Silesia	11.1	0.39	5.6	0.25
Poland, Warsaw City	13.3	0.59	6.1	0.35
Slovakia	10.9	0.29	5.9	0.19
Slovenia	7.0	0.36	3.6	0.22
*Spain, Albacete	4.1	1.00	2.3	0.72
Spain, Asturias	7.5	0.50	3.4	0.38
Spain, Basque Country	8.8	0.41	3.2	0.23
Spain, Granada	4.6	0.46	2.5	0.32
Spain, Mallorca	6.5	0.60	2.5	0.41
Spain, Murcia	4.1	0.37	1.9	0.25
Spain, Navarra	8.1	0.68	3.4	0.50
Spain, Tarragona	6.0	0.58	2.4	0.35
Spain, Zaragoza	6.2	0.46	2.6	0.30

	MALE		FEMALE	
Sweden	10.3	0.18	6.4	0.14
*Switzerland, Basel	11.5	0.85	5.7	0.63
Switzerland, Geneva	10.0	0.90	4.2	0.50
Switzerland, Graubunden	9.0	1.46	6.3	1.14
Switzerland, Neuchatel	8.7	1.23	5.1	0.88
Switzerland, St Gall-Appenzell	9.7	0.78	4.7	0.53
Switzerland, Valais	10.6	1.31	6.2	0.98
Switzerland, Vaud	9.2	0.69	5.0	0.53
Switzerland, Zurich	10.5	0.52	4.6	0.34
*UK, England and Wales	6.9	0.08	3.3	0.06
*UK, East Anglia	6.7	0.31	2.6	0.20
*UK, Mersey	5.9	0.27	3.2	0.20
*UK, North Western	6.8	0.23	3.7	0.17
UK, Oxford	7.6	0.32	3.7	0.22
*UK, South Thames	6.5	0.17	3.2	0.12
UK, South Western	6.9	0.25	3.3	0.18
UK, Wessex	7.3	0.28	3.7	0.19
*UK, West Midlands	7.4	0.21	3.4	0.14
UK, Yorkshire	7.2	0.25	3.9	0.18
UK, Scotland	8.1	0.22	4.5	0.16
UK, Scotland, West	7.7	0.30	4.3	0.21
*Yugoslavia, Vojvodina	4.7	0.28	3.0	0.20

OCEANIA	MALE		FEMALE	
Australian Capital Territory	10.6	1.38	3.9	0.79
Australia, New South Wales	9.3	0.23	6.1	0.18
South Australia	8.5	0.44	4.8	0.33
Australia, Tasmania	9.9	0.83	4.0	0.53
Australia, Victoria	8.7	0.26	4.9	0.19
Western Australia	8.4	0.44	5.0	0.33
*French Polynesia	5.5	1.34	1,5	0,62
New Zealand: Non-Maori	7.1	0.28	4.4	0.22
New Zealand: Maori	7.6	1.33	3.5	0.86
US, Hawaii: White	12.1	1.22	3.8	0.68
US, Hawaii: Japanese	7.3	0.83	2.1	0.37
US, Hawaii: Hawaiian	8.6	1.55	3.0	0.86
US, Hawaii: Filipino	4.4	0.96	1,7	0,59
US, Hawaii: Chinese	5.7	1.55	1,5	0,68

* IMPORTANT-SEE NOTES ON POPULATION PAGE

AGE-STANDARDIZED INCIDENCE
RATES AND STANDARD ERRORS (per 100,000)
Eye (ICD-9 190)

	MALE		FEMALE		
AFRICA					
*Algeria, Setif	0,2	0,16	0,1	0,06	
*France, La Reunion	0,5	0,22	0,4	0,19	
*Mali, Bamako	1.2	0.36	1.0	0.31	
*Uganda, Kyadondo	2.3	0.53	1.8	0.43	
*Zimbabwe, Harare: African	0.9	0.38	0,4	0,18	f
*Zimbabwe, Harare: European	4,1	2,63	-	-	
AMERICA, CENTRAL AND SOUTH					
*Argentina, Concordia	1,0	0,59	1,0	0,57	
*Brazil, Belem	0.8	0.28	0.6	0.19	
*Brazil, Goiania	0,5	0,22	0.8	0.24	
*Brazil, Porto Alegre	0.7	0.25	0.5	0.18	mf
Colombia, Cali	0.6	0.16	0.9	0.20	mf
*Costa Rica	0.8	0.12	0.4	0.08	
*Ecuador, Quito	0.8	0.21	0.9	0.20	
*Peru, Lima	0.6	0.12	0.5	0.10	
Peru, Trujillo	1,5	0,53	0,9	0,49	f
US, Puerto Rico	0.6	0.10	0.3	0.06	
*Uruguay, Montevideo	0,4	0,15	0,3	0,13	
AMERICA, NORTH					
Canada	0.9	0.04	0.7	0.03	
Canada, Alberta	0.9	0.12	0.8	0.11	
Canada, British Columbia	0.9	0.10	0.8	0.10	
Canada, Manitoba	0.7	0.15	1.1	0.20	
Canada, New Brunswick	0.5	0.16	0.5	0.17	
Canada, Newfoundland	0,4	0,16	0,3	0,13	
Canada, Northwest Territories	0,5	0,52	0,4	0,35	
Canada, Nova Scotia	1.0	0.22	0.8	0.18	
Canada, Ontario	1.0	0.06	0.7	0.05	
Canada, Prince Edward Island	1,7	0,76	0,5	0,34	
Canada, Quebec	0.9	0.07	0.6	0.06	
Canada, Saskatchewan	1.4	0.22	0.6	0.15	
Canada, Yukon	0,8	0,80	-	-	
US, Cent. Calif.: Non-Hisp. White	1.1	0.18	0.5	0.11	
US, Cent. Calif.: Hispanic	0.6	0.21	0,5	0,19	
US, Los Angeles: Non-Hisp. White	0.9	0.10	0.8	0.10	
US, Los Angeles: Hispanic White	0.5	0.10	0.3	0.07	
US, Los Angeles: Black	0,3	0,11	0,3	0,11	
US, Los Angeles: Chinese	-	-	0,1	0,11	
US, Los Angeles: Filipino	-	-	-	-	
US, Los Angeles: Korean	-	-	-	-	
US, Los Angeles: Japanese	-	-	0,2	0,22	
US, San Francisco: Non-Hisp. White	0.8	0.12	0.7	0.12	
US, San Francisco: Hispanic White	0,5	0,22	0,7	0,25	
US, San Francisco: Black	0,5	0,22	0,3	0,18	
US, San Francisco: Chinese	-	-	0,2	0,17	
US, San Francisco: Filipino	-	-	-	-	
US, San Francisco: Japanese	-	-	0,5	0,47	
US, Connecticut: White	0.5	0.08	0.5	0.08	
US, Connecticut: Black	0,2	0,17	0,2	0,17	
US, Atlanta: White	1.0	0.17	0.6	0.13	
US, Atlanta: Black	0,7	0,27	0,2	0,11	
US, Iowa	0.9	0.11	0.8	0.11	

	MALE		FEMALE	
US, Central Louisiana: White	0,6	0,33	0,5	0,25
US, Central Louisiana: Black	0,6	0,58	-	-
US, New Orleans: White	0.9	0.24	0.9	0.23
US, New Orleans: Black	0,2	0,15	-	-
US, Detroit: White	0.7	0.10	0.5	0.08
US, Detroit: Black	0,2	0,11	0,3	0,11
US, New Mexico: Non-Hisp. White	0.8	0.20	0.6	0.17
US, New Mexico: Hispanic White	0,6	0,22	0,2	0,12
US, New Mexico: American Indian	0,5	0,35	0,3	0,28
US, Utah	0.9	0.15	0.4	0.10
US, Seattle	0.9	0.11	0.6	0.09
US, SEER: White	0.8	0.04	0.6	0.04
US, SEER: Black	0.4	0.08	0.3	0.07
ASIA				
*China, Qidong	0,1	0,08	0,1	0,06
China, Shanghai	0.2	0.04	0.2	0.04
China, Tianjin	0.2	0.05	0.1	0.04
Hong Kong	0.3	0.06	0.4	0.07
*India, Bangalore	0.2	0.05	0.3	0.06
*India, Barshi, Paranda and Bhum	-	-	0,1	0,11
India, Bombay	0.2	0.04	0.2	0.03
*India, Karunagappally	-	-	-	-
India, Madras	0.4	0.08	0.4	0.07
*India, Trivandrum	0,1	0,12	0,2	0,17
Israel: All Jews	0.8	0.09	0.7	0.08
Jews born in Israel	1.1	0.33	0.6	0.21
Jews born in America or Europe	0.7	0.12	0.9	0.24
Jews born in Africa or Asia	3.0	2.61	0.3	0.10
Non-Jews	0.7	0.23	0.5	0.19
Japan, Hiroshima	0,4	0,16	0,1	0,08
Japan, Miyagi	0.2	0.07	0,1	0,05
Japan, Nagasaki	0.4	0.13	0,2	0,10
Japan, Osaka	0.2	0.04	0.1	0.03
*Japan, Saga	0,2	0,14	0,0	0,03
Japan, Yamagata	-	-	0,0	0,01
*Korea, Kangwha	-	-	-	-
*Kuwait: Non-Kuwaitis	-	-	-	-
*Kuwait: Kuwaitis	0,2	0,17	0,1	0,07
*Philippines, Manila	0.6	0.09	0.4	0.07
Singapore: Chinese	0.4	0.11	0.3	0.10
Singapore: Malay	0,3	0,26	0,3	0,19
Singapore: Indian	-	-	0,5	0,50
Thailand, Chiang Mai	0,2	0,09	0,2	0,08
*Thailand, Khon Kaen	0,4	0,14	0,4	0,12
*Viet Nam, Hanoi	0.8	0.18	0.5	0.14

* IMPORTANT-SEE NOTES ON POPULATION PAGE

EUROPE	MALE		FEMALE	
Austria, Tyrol	1.1	0.28	0.7	0.19
*Belarus	0.7	0.06	0.6	0.04
*Croatia	0.7	0.09	0.6	0.08
Czech Republic	0.7	0.05	0.6	0.05
Denmark	1.0	0.09	0.9	0.08
Estonia	0.9	0.15	0.6	0.12
Finland	1.0	0.08	0.9	0.07
France, Bas-Rhin	0.9	0.19	0.9	0.20
*France, Calvados	0.7	0.21	0,3	0,13
France, Doubs	0,7	0.27	0,3	0,14
France, Haut-Rhin	0.5	0.17	0,4	0,15
*France, Herault	0,2	0,12	0,2	0,12
France, Isere	0.4	0.12	0.6	0.17
*France, Somme	0.9	0.24	0.6	0.20
*France, Tarn	0,8	0,29	0,7	0,28
Germany, Eastern States	0.9	0.07	0.7	0.07
Germany, Saarland	0.4	0.13	0,2	0,07
Iceland	1,0	0,37	0,5	0,33
Ireland, Southern	0,4	0,18	0,5	0,22
Italy, Ferrara	0,8	0,45	0,9	0,37
Italy, Florence	0.4	0.10	0.4	0.12
Italy, Genoa	0.7	0.32	0.5	0.25
*Italy, Latina	0,3	0,17	0,3	0,14
Italy, Macerata	0,6	0,40	0,5	0,33
Italy, Modena	0.8	0.26	0,4	0,23
Italy, Parma	0,2	0,12	0,1	0,05
Italy, Ragusa	0,4	0,23	-	-
Italy, Romagna	0.5	0.15	0.9	0.35
Italy, Torino	0.4	0.11	0.2	0.08
Italy, Trieste	0.5	0,34	0,1	0,08
Italy, Varese	0.6	0.23	0.4	0.12
Italy, Veneto	0.4	0.10	0.2	0.07
*Latvia	0.4	0.08	0.4	0.08
Malta	0,4	0,44	-	-
The Netherlands	0.8	0.05	0.7	0.05
The Netherlands, Eindhoven	0.8	0.21	0.6	0.19
The Netherlands, Maastricht	0.8	0.20	0.3	0.10
Norway	0.9	0.09	0.8	0.09
*Poland, Cracow	0,5	0,15	0.8	0.17
*Poland, Kielce	0.6	0.15	0,2	0,08
*Poland, Lower Silesia	0.9	0.12	0.7	0.10
Poland, Warsaw City	0.7	0.16	0.4	0.11
Slovakia	0.9	0.08	0.8	0.08
Slovenia	0.7	0.12	0.6	0.11
*Spain, Albacete	0,5	0,30	0,6	0,61
Spain, Asturias	0.6	0.19	0.2	0.09
Spain, Basque Country	0.5	0.09	0.3	0.09
Spain, Granada	0,4	0,13	0,2	0,09
Spain, Mallorca	0,5	0,20	0,5	0,24
Spain, Murcia	0.7	0.19	0,2	0,11 m
Spain, Navarra	0.9	0.30	0,4	0,22
Spain, Tarragona	0,5	0,22	0,6	0,28
Spain, Zaragoza	0.6	0.16	0.5	0.21

	MALE		FEMALE	
Sweden	0.8	0.06	0.7	0.06
*Switzerland, Basel	1.2	0.39	1.0	0.37
Switzerland, Geneva	0,7	0,23	0,5	0,18
Switzerland, Graubunden	0,7	0,40	1,0	0,49
Switzerland, Neuchatel	0,9	0,59	1,0	0,61
Switzerland, St Gall-Appenzell	0,4	0,19	0,2	0,11
Switzerland, Valais	1,4	0,46	1,0	0,39
Switzerland, Vaud	0.9	0.28	1.2	0.29
Switzerland, Zurich	1.1	0.22	1.0	0.18
*UK, England and Wales	0.7	0.03	0.6	0.03
*UK, East Anglia	0.5	0.10	0.4	0.07
*UK, Mersey	0.4	0.08	0.3	0.06
*UK, North Western	0.6	0.08	0.7	0.09
UK, Oxford	0.6	0.10	0.8	0.11
*UK, South Thames	0.8	0.07	0.8	0.07
UK, South Western	0.7	0.09	0.5	0.07
UK, Wessex	0.7	0.09	0.5	0.07
*UK, West Midlands	0.6	0.07	0.6	0.07
UK, Yorkshire	0.7	0.08	0.7	0.09
UK, Scotland	1.1	0.09	0.9	0.08
UK, Scotland, West	1.2	0.13	0.8	0.10
*Yugoslavia, Vojvodina	0.6	0.11	0.4	0.10

OCEANIA

	MALE		FEMALE	
Australian Capital Territory	1,3	0,46	1,0	0,36
Australia, New South Wales	1.0	0.09	0.9	0.08
South Australia	0.9	0.15	0.8	0.14
Australia, Tasmania	0.9	0.28	0.3	0,16
Australia, Victoria	1.0	0.09	0.8	0.08
Western Australia	0.8	0.14	0.7	0.13
*French Polynesia	0,2	0,15	-	-
New Zealand: Non-Maori	1.3	0.13	0.8	0.10
New Zealand: Maori	0,2	0,25	0,3	0,19
US, Hawaii: White	0,5	0,25	0,4	0,28
US, Hawaii: Japanese	0,4	0,38	0,1	0,07
US, Hawaii: Hawaiian	0,3	0,31	1,0	0,43
US, Hawaii: Filipino	-	-	0,4	0,38
US, Hawaii: Chinese	0,5	0,50	-	-

* IMPORTANT-SEE NOTES ON POPULATION PAGE

AGE-STANDARDIZED INCIDENCE
RATES AND STANDARD ERRORS (per 100,000)
Brain, nervous system (ICD-9 191-2)

	MALE		FEMALE	
AFRICA				
*Algeria, Setif	1.6	0.47	0.6	0.20
*France, La Reunion	2.1	0.42	2.0	0.37
*Mali, Bamako	0,5	0,28	0,2	0,09
*Uganda, Kyadondo	0,5	0,36	0,3	0,25
*Zimbabwe, Harare: African	2.4	0.57	1.2	0.42
*Zimbabwe, Harare: European	14.8	4.78	11.4	4.03
AMERICA, CENTRAL AND SOUTH				
*Argentina, Concordia	3.3	1.04	1,3	0,61
*Brazil, Belem	3.4	0.60	1.8	0.32
*Brazil, Goiania	7.2	0.79	4.8	0.61
*Brazil, Porto Alegre	4.6	0.57	2.6	0.36
Colombia, Cali	4.4	0.41	3.5	0.35
*Costa Rica	5.1	0.31	3.9	0.26
*Ecuador, Quito	2.8	0.38	1.9	0.29
*Peru, Lima	3.1	0.26	2.6	0.23
Peru, Trujillo	2.3	0.66	1.6	0.52
US, Puerto Rico	3.5	0.23	2.5	0.19
*Uruguay, Montevideo	6.6	0.56	5.3	0.47
AMERICA, NORTH				
Canada	7.0	0.10	5.0	0.08
Canada, Alberta	6.7	0.33	4.6	0.27
Canada, British Columbia	6.3	0.27	4.3	0.23
Canada, Manitoba	7.0	0.50	4.7	0.41
Canada, New Brunswick	6.6	0.59	5.0	0.51
Canada, Newfoundland	5.2	0.62	3.2	0.50
Canada, Northwest Territories	5.2	1.68	3,3	1,48
Canada, Nova Scotia	6.1	0.51	3.8	0.39
Canada, Ontario	7.4	0.17	5.4	0.14
Canada, Prince Edward Island	6.7	1.41	5.1	1.17
Canada, Quebec	7.3	0.20	5.2	0.17
Canada, Saskatchewan	6.2	0.49	3.9	0.39
Canada, Yukon	11.6	2.97	1,1	1,13
US, Cent. Calif.: Non-Hisp. White	7.2	0.44	5.3	0.38
US, Cent. Calif.: Hispanic	5.6	0.67	3.6	0.53
US, Los Angeles: Non-Hisp. White	7.8	0.29	5.1	0.24
US, Los Angeles: Hispanic White	4.7	0.31	3.6	0.25
US, Los Angeles: Black	4.5	0.44	3.2	0.36
US, Los Angeles: Chinese	2.3	0.61	1,1	0,41
US, Los Angeles: Filipino	4.1	0.95	2.2	0.62
US, Los Angeles: Korean	1,4	0,64	1,9	0,74
US, Los Angeles: Japanese	1,4	0,58	1,1	0,43
US, San Francisco: Non-Hisp. White	7.5	0.37	5.5	0.32
US, San Francisco: Hispanic White	7.1	0.87	4.0	0.58
US, San Francisco: Black	5.5	0.77	3.0	0.55
US, San Francisco: Chinese	3.4	0.76	3.1	0.72
US, San Francisco: Filipino	5.4	1.23	3.0	0.85
US, San Francisco: Japanese	2,8	1,42	1,9	1,18
US, Connecticut: White	7.4	0.31	4.7	0.25
US, Connecticut: Black	3.6	0.80	2.2	0.57
US, Atlanta: White	7.3	0.46	5.8	0.41
US, Atlanta: Black	3.6	0.56	3.6	0.50
US, Iowa	7.0	0.31	4.9	0.26

	MALE		FEMALE	
US, Central Louisiana: White	6.1	1.00	5.1	0.89
US, Central Louisiana: Black	1,5	0,87	2,0	1,00
US, New Orleans: White	5.9	0.61	4.1	0.55
US, New Orleans: Black	4.6	0.77	2.8	0.53
US, Detroit: White	7.5	0.32	5.0	0.26
US, Detroit: Black	3.9	0.43	3.7	0.40
US, New Mexico: Non-Hisp. White	6.3	0.56	4.4	0.46
US, New Mexico: Hispanic White	4.0	0.57	3.5	0.51
US, New Mexico: American Indian	3,5	1,22	1,8	0,68
US, Utah	6.5	0.40	5.5	0.37
US, Seattle	7.6	0.30	5.1	0.24
US, SEER: White	7.3	0.12	5.1	0.10
US, SEER: Black	4.1	0.28	3.2	0.23
ASIA				
*China, Qidong	3.2	0.34	2.0	0.27
† China, Shanghai	5.6	0.18	4.7	0.16
China, Tianjin	5.1	0.24	4.8	0.22
Hong Kong	4.3	0.18	3.4	0.16
*India, Bangalore	3.1	0.20	1.6	0.15
*India, Barshi, Paranda and Bhum	0,4	0,19	0,2	0,14
India, Bombay	3.3	0.15	2.2	0.13
*India, Karunagappally	2,3	0,77	2,4	0,87
India, Madras	2.2	0.17	1.1	0.12
*India, Trivandrum	2.6	0.62	1.8	0.47
Israel: All Jews	5.7	0.25	4.3	0.21
Jews born in Israel	6.0	0.67	4.3	0.51
Jews born in America or Europe	6.6	0.68	4.9	0.68
Jews born in Africa or Asia	3.5	0.35	3.4	0.95
Non-Jews	2.6	0.48	2.4	0.42
Japan, Hiroshima	2.2	0.29	2.0	0.29
Japan, Miyagi	2.4	0.21	1.8	0.19
Japan, Nagasaki	2.9	0.27	2.2	0.26
Japan, Osaka	3.0	0.12	2.2	0.11
*Japan, Saga	2.6	0.33	2.3	0.35
Japan, Yamagata	1.8	0.24	1.7	0.24
*Korea, Kangwha	3,8	1,42	1,8	0,76
*Kuwait: Non-Kuwaitis	2.8	0.51	2.8	0.76
*Kuwait: Kuwaitis	3.7	0.73	2.9	0.70
*Philippines, Manila	2.6	0.22	2.0	0.17
Singapore: Chinese	2.3	0.23	1.8	0.19
Singapore: Malay	1.6	0.41	1,1	0,37
Singapore: Indian	1,9	0,64	2,4	0,94
Thailand, Chiang Mai	2.0	0.25	1.8	0.25
*Thailand, Khon Kaen	2.7	0.33	2.3	0.29
*Viet Nam, Hanoi	1.3	0.23	0.9	0.17

* IMPORTANT-SEE NOTES ON POPULATION PAGE

EUROPE	MALE		FEMALE	
Austria, Tyrol	5.3	0.59	5.0	0.57
*Belarus	3.9	0.13	2.8	0.10
*Croatia	8.5	0.30	6.3	0.25
Czech Republic	5.0	0.14	3.8	0.12
Denmark	6.8	0.23	5.0	0.20
Estonia	5.4	0.37	4.3	0.33
Finland	7.5	0.23	5.8	0.20
France, Bas-Rhin	5.1	0.47	4.0	0.40
*France, Calvados	4.2	0.52	3.0	0.44
France, Doubs	5.1	0.65	4.3	0.58
France, Haut-Rhin	5.8	0.58	4.4	0.51
*France, Herault	4.7	0.47	3.3	0.39
France, Isere	5.4	0.45	4.4	0.43
*France, Somme	6.0	0.65	3.6	0.50
*France, Tarn	3.5	0.60	2.5	0.58
Germany, Eastern States	5.5	0.19	4.0	0.15
Germany, Saarland	5.7	0.46	5.3	0.46
Iceland	9.4	1.21	3.9	0.75
Ireland, Southern	7.7	0.74	3.3	0.46
Italy, Ferrara	5.3	0.95	5.9	1.42
Italy, Florence	7.1	0.57	5.2	0.46
Italy, Genoa	6.5	0.71	3.8	0.42
*Italy, Latina	7.6	0.88	5.1	0.76
Italy, Macerata	6.1	1.33	7.6	1.79
Italy, Modena	6.2	0.64	5.0	0.61
Italy, Parma	6.9	0.85	4.0	0.68
Italy, Ragusa	5.6	0.85	3.9	0.72
Italy, Romagna	6.4	0.69	5.5	0.79
Italy, Torino	6.8	0.57	4.3	0.46
Italy, Trieste	9.5	1.41	8.7	1.72
Italy, Varese	6.3	0.55	4.5	0.46
Italy, Veneto	7.6	0.52	5.6	0.44
*Latvia	3.9	0.24	2.8	0.19
Malta	6.5	1.39	4.9	1.11
The Netherlands	6.0	0.14	4.1	0.12
The Netherlands, Eindhoven	5.3	0.49	4.1	0.41
The Netherlands, Maastricht	6.3	0.53	4.0	0.41
Norway	7.3	0.26	5.3	0.22
*Poland, Cracow	6.0	0.55	3.4	0.41
*Poland, Kielce	5.1	0.42	3.9	0.37
*Poland, Lower Silesia	6.9	0.31	5.8	0.28
Poland, Warsaw City	8.2	0.49	5.9	0.38
Slovakia	5.9	0.21	4.3	0.18
Slovenia	4.4	0.30	3.2	0.24
*Spain, Albacete	6.1	1.31	3.7	0.97
Spain, Asturias	5.2	0.50	3.4	0.39
Spain, Basque Country	6.3	0.38	4.5	0.34
Spain, Granada	6.2	0.55	4.1	0.44
Spain, Mallorca	6.4	0.64	5.0	0.55
Spain, Murcia	6.5	0.50	3.9	0.39
Spain, Navarra	8.4	0.74	4.8	0.59
Spain, Tarragona	4.6	0.55	4.2	0.56
Spain, Zaragoza	6.1	0.51	4.2	0.44

	MALE		FEMALE	
Sweden	6.6	0.17	5.5	0.16
*Switzerland, Basel	8.0	0.87	4.2	0.62
Switzerland, Geneva	6.1	0.74	4.1	0.63
Switzerland, Graubunden	5.0	1.11	2.5	0.77
Switzerland, Neuchatel	5.2	1.07	4.4	1.10
Switzerland, St Gall-Appenzell	6.0	0.69	4.4	0.60
Switzerland, Valais	3.9	0.85	3.1	0.75
Switzerland, Vaud	5.6	0.60	4.5	0.53
Switzerland, Zurich	7.0	0.50	4.7	0.41
*UK, England and Wales	6.3	0.09	4.5	0.07
*UK, East Anglia	6.6	0.34	4.5	0.29
*UK, Mersey	6.8	0.32	5.5	0.29
*UK, North Western	5.7	0.23	3.9	0.19
UK, Oxford	6.7	0.32	5.5	0.28
*UK, South Thames	6.4	0.19	4.6	0.16
UK, South Western	6.7	0.27	4.4	0.23
UK, Wessex	6.6	0.29	5.1	0.25
*UK, West Midlands	6.4	0.21	4.4	0.18
UK, Yorkshire	6.1	0.25	4.0	0.21
UK, Scotland	6.2	0.21	4.6	0.19
UK, Scotland, West	6.0	0.29	4.3	0.25
*Yugoslavia, Vojvodina	6.0	0.33	4.1	0.26

OCEANIA

	MALE		FEMALE	
Australian Capital Territory	5.8	0.95	5.3	0.90
Australia, New South Wales	6.8	0.21	5.0	0.18
South Australia	6.3	0.40	5.5	0.38
Australia, Tasmania	7.4	0.76	4.9	0.62
Australia, Victoria	7.0	0.24	5.0	0.21
Western Australia	6.7	0.41	5.4	0.36
*French Polynesia	3.1	0.93	4.6	1.23
New Zealand: Non-Maori	7.4	0.31	5.1	0.26
New Zealand: Maori	5.2	1.04	4.0	0.80
US, Hawaii: White	8.7	1.11	4.6	0.87
US, Hawaii: Japanese	2.1	0.60	1.3	0.50
US, Hawaii: Hawaiian	3.8	0.89	2.9	0.75
US, Hawaii: Filipino	2.5	0.78	2,0	0,79
US, Hawaii: Chinese	2,9	1,21	0,3	0,31

* IMPORTANT-SEE NOTES ON POPULATION PAGE

AGE-STANDARDIZED INCIDENCE
RATES AND STANDARD ERRORS (per 100,000)
Thyroid (ICD-9 193)

AFRICA	MALE		FEMALE	
*Algeria, Setif	0,3	0,20	0,7	0,23
*France, La Reunion	0.8	0.27	1.7	0.35
*Mali, Bamako	0,2	0,12	1.7	0.46
*Uganda, Kyadondo	0,7	0,40	3.4	0.99 f
*Zimbabwe, Harare: African	1,2	0,51	5.3	1.40
*Zimbabwe, Harare: European	-	-	2,2	1,62

AMERICA, CENTRAL AND SOUTH	MALE		FEMALE	
*Argentina, Concordia	-	-	1,8	0,75
*Brazil, Belem	0,3	0,20	1.2	0.30 mf
*Brazil, Goiania	1.0	0.30	4.3	0.56
*Brazil, Porto Alegre	1.2	0.28	2.9	0.38
Colombia, Cali	2.1	0.30	6.7	0.47
*Costa Rica	1.4	0.16	5.2	0.31
*Ecuador, Quito	2.4	0.36	7.4	0.57
*Peru, Lima	1.1	0.16	4.9	0.32
Peru, Trujillo	2.3	0.76	5.4	1.02
US, Puerto Rico	1.0	0.12	3.4	0.21
*Uruguay, Montevideo	1.2	0.23	4.4	0.42

AMERICA, NORTH	MALE		FEMALE	
Canada	1.8	0.05	4.9	0.08
Canada, Alberta	2.1	0.17	5.4	0.28
Canada, British Columbia	1.4	0.12	4.3	0.21
Canada, Manitoba	1.9	0.25	4.7	0.40
Canada, New Brunswick	1.4	0.26	4.3	0.47
Canada, Newfoundland	1.6	0.32	4.1	0.53
Canada, Northwest Territories	2,1	1,23	2,8	1,16
Canada, Nova Scotia	1.3	0.23	4.1	0.40
Canada, Ontario	2.0	0.08	5.9	0.14
Canada, Prince Edward Island	1,4	0,67	3.5	0.96
Canada, Quebec	1.5	0.09	4.0	0.14
Canada, Saskatchewan	2.6	0.31	4.1	0.40
Canada, Yukon	0,7	0,73	4,4	1,84
US, Cent. Calif.: Non-Hisp. White	2.4	0.25	4.6	0.34
US, Cent. Calif.: Hispanic	1.4	0.34	5.9	0.65
US, Los Angeles: Non-Hisp. White	2.8	0.16	6.6	0.25
US, Los Angeles: Hispanic White	1.7	0.19	5.4	0.29
US, Los Angeles: Black	1.0	0.21	3.0	0.32
US, Los Angeles: Chinese	1.5	0.47	3.5	0.71
US, Los Angeles: Filipino	4.0	0.89	11.2	1.32
US, Los Angeles: Korean	1,4	0,57	4.8	1.08
US, Los Angeles: Japanese	1,1	0,55	3.8	0.91
US, San Francisco: Non-Hisp. White	2.5	0.19	6.8	0.34
US, San Francisco: Hispanic White	2.7	0.51	7.5	0.77
US, San Francisco: Black	1.1	0.33	2.9	0.49
US, San Francisco: Chinese	2.3	0.53	7.1	1.02
US, San Francisco: Filipino	3.4	0.92	10.6	1.45
US, San Francisco: Japanese	2,6	1,56	7.4	2.15
US, Connecticut: White	2.4	0.17	4.8	0.24
US, Connecticut: Black	1,2	0,46	4.0	0.74
US, Atlanta: White	2.3	0.24	6.5	0.39
US, Atlanta: Black	2.0	0.48	3.4	0.47
US, Iowa	2.6	0.18	6.5	0.29

	MALE		FEMALE	
US, Central Louisiana: White	1,1	0,43	4.1	0.80
US, Central Louisiana: Black	1,7	1,19	2,0	0,98
US, New Orleans: White	2.3	0.37	6.3	0.59
US, New Orleans: Black	0,6	0,29	4.3	0.63
US, Detroit: White	2.6	0.17	6.7	0.28
US, Detroit: Black	1.6	0.28	3.3	0.35
US, New Mexico: Non-Hisp. White	2.8	0.35	6.6	0.55
US, New Mexico: Hispanic White	1.9	0.40	8.2	0.76
US, New Mexico: American Indian	1,3	0,81	4.0	1.19
US, Utah	2.9	0.27	8.1	0.45
US, Seattle	2.1	0.15	6.2	0.26
US, SEER: White	2.5	0.07	6.4	0.11
US, SEER: Black	1.4	0.17	3.3	0.22

ASIA	MALE		FEMALE	
*China, Qidong	0,1	0,06	0.5	0.12
China, Shanghai	1.0	0.07	3.0	0.12
China, Tianjin	0.8	0.09	2.0	0.14
Hong Kong	2.0	0.12	7.1	0.22
*India, Bangalore	1.1	0.13	3.2	0.22
*India, Barshi, Paranda and Bhum	0,5	0,23	0,2	0,16
India, Bombay	0.8	0.08	2.1	0.13
*India, Karunagappally	2,2	0,84	3.9	1.04 m
India, Madras	0.8	0.12	1.6	0.16
*India, Trivandrum	2.0	0.49	3.9	0.64
Israel: All Jews	2.7	0.17	7.7	0.28
Jews born in Israel	2.9	0.44	7.4	0.62
Jews born in America or Europe	2.5	0.29	7.4	0.54
Jews born in Africa or Asia	2.9	0.47	9.2	1.07
Non-Jews	1.3	0.32	4.1	0.56
Japan, Hiroshima	2.9	0.31	9.4	0.53
Japan, Miyagi	1.5	0.15	9.0	0.35
Japan, Nagasaki	1.4	0.17	6.7	0.36
Japan, Osaka	1.1	0.07	3.5	0.11
*Japan, Saga	1.0	0.18	2.6	0.29
Japan, Yamagata	1.0	0.16	5.7	0.38
*Korea, Kangwha	0,6	0,44	6.0	1.49
*Kuwait: Non-Kuwaitis	4.8	1.69	6.6	1.10
*Kuwait: Kuwaitis	2.0	0.56	6.1	1.00
*Philippines, Manila	2.9	0.25	8.7	0.36
Singapore: Chinese	2.0	0.21	6.0	0.33
Singapore: Malay	1.3	0.40	6.5	0.90
Singapore: Indian	0,9	0,40	2.9	0.84
Thailand, Chiang Mai	1.1	0.19	2.5	0.28
*Thailand, Khon Kaen	1.0	0.22	3.5	0.36
*Viet Nam, Hanoi	1.2	0.22	3.1	0.33

* IMPORTANT-SEE NOTES ON POPULATION PAGE

EUROPE

	MALE		FEMALE	
Austria, Tyrol	2.5	0.38	7.8	0.63
*Belarus	1.5	0.08	3.7	0.11
*Croatia	1.1	0.10	4.2	0.19
Czech Republic	1.3	0.06	3.0	0.10
Denmark	0.8	0.07	2.1	0.11
Estonia	0.7	0.13	2.5	0.22
Finland	1.8	0.10	6.4	0.19
France, Bas-Rhin	1.3	0.22	2.6	0.31
*France, Calvados	1.8	0.34	7.0	0.64
France, Doubs	1.3	0.32	5.3	0.63
France, Haut-Rhin	1.5	0.28	2.3	0.32
*France, Herault	1.6	0.27	4.8	0.46
France, Isere	1.6	0.23	4.7	0.40
*France, Somme	0.7	0.20	3.2	0.45
*France, Tarn	2.0	0.42	7.3	0.87
Germany, Eastern States	1.2	0.08	2.7	0.11
Germany, Saarland	2.0	0.24	3.5	0.31
Iceland	6.1	0.94	9.8	1.19
Ireland, Southern	0,5	0,18	2.5	0.41
Italy, Ferrara	2.6	0.76	11.1	1.79
Italy, Florence	2.2	0.28	4.4	0.38
Italy, Genoa	1.8	0.28	3.8	0.40
*Italy, Latina	2.2	0.46	4.7	0.67
Italy, Macerata	0,9	0,54	8.9	1.73
Italy, Modena	2.1	0.35	5.7	0.56
Italy, Parma	2.2	0.42	3.5	0.55
Italy, Ragusa	1.3	0.42	2.5	0.54
Italy, Romagna	3.1	0.44	9.1	0.79
Italy, Torino	2.2	0.30	4.3	0.41
Italy, Trieste	2.1	0.49	5.6	0.88
Italy, Varese	1.8	0.27	5.9	0.48
Italy, Veneto	2.0	0.23	5.0	0.37
*Latvia	1.0	0.12	2.5	0.17
Malta	0,5	0,37	3.6	0.97
The Netherlands	0.9	0.05	2.2	0.08
The Netherlands, Eindhoven	0.8	0.17	1.9	0.26
The Netherlands, Maastricht	1.0	0.20	1.9	0.26
Norway	1.7	0.12	4.7	0.20
*Poland, Cracow	0.7	0.19	2.3	0.30
*Poland, Kielce	0.6	0.14	1.0	0.17
*Poland, Lower Silesia	0.8	0.11	2.3	0.17
Poland, Warsaw City	0.9	0.15	2.1	0.20
Slovakia	1.0	0.09	2.9	0.14
Slovenia	1.4	0.16	2.7	0.21
*Spain, Albacete	0,2	0,17	4.3	1.09
Spain, Asturias	1.6	0.25	4.8	0.43
Spain, Basque Country	0.8	0.13	2.6	0.23
Spain, Granada	1.0	0.22	3.0	0.37
Spain, Mallorca	0.7	0.22	3.3	0.45
Spain, Murcia	1.2	0.21	4.3	0.40
Spain, Navarra	2.2	0.38	6.9	0.68
Spain, Tarragona	0.7	0.20	3.7	0.49
Spain, Zaragoza	0.9	0.19	3.1	0.36

	MALE		FEMALE	
Sweden	1.4	0.07	3.6	0.12
*Switzerland, Basel	1.8	0.35	3.7	0.53
Switzerland, Geneva	1.0	0.30	4.4	0.61
Switzerland, Graubunden	0,7	0,48	3.2	0.87
Switzerland, Neuchatel	0,3	0,24	3.1	0.80
Switzerland, St Gall-Appenzell	1.6	0.32	4.5	0.54
Switzerland, Valais	1.7	0.54	3.2	0.71
Switzerland, Vaud	1.8	0.31	4.1	0.47
Switzerland, Zurich	2.5	0.27	4.7	0.35
*UK, England and Wales	0.7	0.03	1.7	0.04
*UK, East Anglia	0.8	0.11	1.9	0.18
*UK, Mersey	0.5	0.09	1.3	0.13
*UK, North Western	0.7	0.07	1.8	0.12
UK, Oxford	0.8	0.10	2.3	0.17
*UK, South Thames	0.7	0.06	1.7	0.09
UK, South Western	0.7	0.09	2.0	0.14
UK, Wessex	0.7	0.09	2.2	0.16
*UK, West Midlands	0.8	0.07	1.9	0.11
UK, Yorkshire	0.8	0.09	1.7	0.13
UK, Scotland	0.9	0.08	2.0	0.11
UK, Scotland, West	0.9	0.10	1.7	0.14
*Yugoslavia, Vojvodina	0.7	0.10	1.9	0.17

OCEANIA

	MALE		FEMALE	
Australian Capital Territory	2.0	0.59	1.9	0.52
Australia, New South Wales	1.7	0.10	4.5	0.16
South Australia	1.7	0.20	3.3	0.28
Australia, Tasmania	1.5	0.33	3.1	0.48
Australia, Victoria	1.4	0.10	3.0	0.16
Western Australia	1.7	0.19	4.5	0.32
*French Polynesia	2.9	0.99	15.9	2.19
New Zealand: Non-Maori	1.2	0.12	3.4	0.20
New Zealand: Maori	1,6	0,59	6.5	1.06
US, Hawaii: White	3.3	0.63	7.6	1.01
US, Hawaii: Japanese	1.9	0.45	5.7	0.80
US, Hawaii: Hawaiian	3.0	0.85	9.1	1.44
US, Hawaii: Filipino	5.1	1.07	25.5	2.41
US, Hawaii: Chinese	2,6	1,11	9.4	2.04

* IMPORTANT-SEE NOTES ON POPULATION PAGE

AGE-STANDARDIZED INCIDENCE
RATES AND STANDARD ERRORS (per 100,000)
Other endocrine (ICD-9 194)

AFRICA	MALE		FEMALE	
*Algeria, Setif	-	-	-	-
*France, La Reunion	0,2	0,12	0,4	0,19
*Mali, Bamako	0,1	0,08	0,4	0,26
*Uganda, Kyadondo	0,1	0,06	0,2	0,24
*Zimbabwe, Harare: African	-	-	0,1	0,09
*Zimbabwe, Harare: European	-	-	-	-

AMERICA, CENTRAL AND SOUTH	MALE		FEMALE	
*Argentina, Concordia	-	-	-	-
*Brazil, Belem	0,2	0,09	0,0	0,05
*Brazil, Goiania	0,6	0,19	0,8	0,23
*Brazil, Porto Alegre	0,6	0,22	0,6	0,18 m
Colombia, Cali	0,2	0,09	0,2	0,07
*Costa Rica	0.3	0.08	0.1	0.05
*Ecuador, Quito	0,0	0,03	0,1	0,07
*Peru, Lima	0,1	0,05	0,1	0,05
Peru, Trujillo	0,2	0,22	-	-
US, Puerto Rico	0.1	0.05	0.2	0.06
*Uruguay, Montevideo	0,4	0,14	0,3	0,14

AMERICA, NORTH	MALE		FEMALE	
Canada	0.6	0.03	0.6	0.03
Canada, Alberta	0.3	0.07	0.4	0.08
Canada, British Columbia	0.3	0.06	0.4	0.08
Canada, Manitoba	0.6	0.15	0.4	0.13
Canada, New Brunswick	0.9	0.25	0.3	0,14
Canada, Newfoundland	0,1	0,07	0,2	0,12
Canada, Northwest Territories	0,7	0,48	0,4	0,35
Canada, Nova Scotia	0,4	0,15	0,1	0,08
Canada, Ontario	0.7	0.06	0.6	0.05
Canada, Prince Edward Island	0,2	0,24	-	-
Canada, Quebec	0.8	0.08	0.8	0.08
Canada, Saskatchewan	0,3	0,10	0.5	0.14
Canada, Yukon	-	-	-	-
US, Cent. Calif.: Non-Hisp. White	0.7	0.15	0.3	0.10
US, Cent. Calif.: Hispanic	0,4	0,13	0,2	0,09
US, Los Angeles: Non-Hisp. White	0.7	0.11	0.4	0.08
US, Los Angeles: Hispanic White	0.4	0.08	0.3	0.07
US, Los Angeles: Black	0.4	0.13	0.4	0,13
US, Los Angeles: Chinese	0,4	0,27	-	-
US, Los Angeles: Filipino	0,2	0,23	-	-
US, Los Angeles: Korean	-	-	-	-
US, Los Angeles: Japanese	0,2	0,17	0,7	0,71
US, San Francisco: Non-Hisp. White	0.6	0.13	0.4	0.10
US, San Francisco: Hispanic White	0,5	0,22	0,3	0,16
US, San Francisco: Black	0,4	0,19	0,4	0,21
US, San Francisco: Chinese	1,0	0,44	0,2	0,14
US, San Francisco: Filipino	0,6	0,42	0,2	0,22
US, San Francisco: Japanese	0,5	0,53	-	-
US, Connecticut: White	0.4	0.08	0.2	0.06
US, Connecticut: Black	0,4	0,25	0,3	0,25
US, Atlanta: White	0.3	0,11	0.4	0.12
US, Atlanta: Black	0.3	0,14	0.2	0,14
US, Iowa	0.4	0.09	0.5	0.09

	MALE		FEMALE	
US, Central Louisiana: White	0,4	0,31	0,5	0,33
US, Central Louisiana: Black	-	-	0,2	0,22
US, New Orleans: White	0,2	0,11	0.6	0.21
US, New Orleans: Black	0,4	0,24	0,6	0,23
US, Detroit: White	0.5	0.10	0.4	0.08
US, Detroit: Black	0,3	0,12	0.4	0.13
US, New Mexico: Non-Hisp. White	0,4	0,15	0,4	0,18
US, New Mexico: Hispanic White	0,5	0,20	0,2	0,10
US, New Mexico: American Indian	-	-	0,8	0,60
US, Utah	0.3	0.09	0.4	0.11
US, Seattle	0.4	0.08	0.3	0.07
US, SEER: White	0.5	0.03	0.4	0.03
US, SEER: Black	0.3	0.08	0.4	0.08

ASIA	MALE		FEMALE	
*China, Qidong	0,1	0,07	0,1	0,05
China, Shanghai	1.0	0.08	1.7	0.10
China, Tianjin	0.7	0.08	0.6	0.07
Hong Kong	0.8	0.08	0.8	0.08
*India, Bangalore	0,0	0,02	0,1	0,03
*India, Barshi, Paranda and Bhum	-	-	-	-
India, Bombay	0.2	0.03	0.1	0.02
*India, Karunagappally	0,3	0,31	-	-
India, Madras	0.2	0.05	0,1	0,04
*India, Trivandrum	0,1	0,12	-	-
Israel: All Jews	0.5	0.07	0.5	0.07
Jews born in Israel	0.5	0.22	0.4	0.08
Jews born in America or Europe	0.3	0.08	0.5	0.17
Jews born in Africa or Asia	0,3	0,15	0,0	0,03
Non-Jews	0,4	0,15	0,5	0,18
Japan, Hiroshima	0.5	0.16	0.5	0.18
Japan, Miyagi	0.5	0.12	0.7	0.15
Japan, Nagasaki	0.6	0.16	0.2	0,08
Japan, Osaka	0.7	0.07	0.5	0.06
*Japan, Saga	0,3	0,13	0,1	0,06
Japan, Yamagata	0,2	0,08	0,2	0,12
*Korea, Kangwha	-	-	-	-
*Kuwait: Non-Kuwaitis	0,2	0,10	0,4	0,15
*Kuwait: Kuwaitis	0,3	0,22	0,5	0,21
*Philippines, Manila	0.2	0.05	0.1	0.04
Singapore: Chinese	0.6	0.12	0.4	0.10
Singapore: Malay	0,5	0,23	0,4	0,25
Singapore: Indian	-	-	-	-
Thailand, Chiang Mai	0,1	0,04	0,1	0,06
*Thailand, Khon Kaen	0,2	0,07	0,2	0,08
*Viet Nam, Hanoi	0,1	0,07	0,1	0,04

* IMPORTANT-SEE NOTES ON POPULATION PAGE

EUROPE	MALE		FEMALE	
Austria, Tyrol	0.9	0.25	0.5	0.18
*Belarus	0.2	0.03	0.1	0.02
*Croatia	0.6	0.08	0.7	0.10
Czech Republic	0.5	0.05	0.4	0.04
Denmark	0.4	0.06	0.3	0.05
Estonia	0.4	0.10	0,1	0,05
Finland	0.4	0.05	0.3	0.04
France, Bas-Rhin	0.8	0.20	0.6	0.18
*France, Calvados	0.2	0,14	0,4	0,16
France, Doubs	0.3	0,17	0.3	0,16
France, Haut-Rhin	0.8	0.22	0.5	0,19
*France, Herault	0.2	0,09	0.2	0,12
France, Isere	0.3	0,12	0.7	0.21
*France, Somme	0.5	0,19	0.2	0,10
*France, Tarn	0,1	0,06	0.2	0,18
Germany, Eastern States	0.4	0.05	0.4	0.05
Germany, Saarland	0.9	0.21	0.4	0.12
Iceland	0.3	0,24	0.9	0,40
Ireland, Southern	0,6	0,23	0.7	0,26
Italy, Ferrara	0,4	0,38	0.4	0,30
Italy, Florence	0.5	0.13	0.6	0.18
Italy, Genoa	0.9	0.33	0.6	0.28
*Italy, Latina	0,4	0,18	0.3	0,25
Italy, Macerata	1,2	1,01	0.2	0,17
Italy, Modena	1.0	0.29	0.6	0.17
Italy, Parma	0.3	0,18	0.5	0,19
Italy, Ragusa	0.3	0,17	0.3	0,19
Italy, Romagna	0.5	0,31	0.3	0,13
Italy, Torino	0.9	0.27	0.7	0.28
Italy, Trieste	2.3	0.78	3.1	0.66
Italy, Varese	0,4	0,17	0.5	0,20
Italy, Veneto	0.7	0.18	0.5	0.17
*Latvia	0.3	0.06	0.2	0.04
Malta	0,4	0,44	0.4	0,30
The Netherlands	0.5	0.04	0.4	0.04
The Netherlands, Eindhoven	0,4	0,13	0.5	0.18
The Netherlands, Maastricht	0.5	0.16	0.4	0,16
Norway	0.6	0.08	0.6	0.09
*Poland, Cracow	0.5	0,16	0.4	0.12
*Poland, Kielce	0.6	0.15	0.6	0.16
*Poland, Lower Silesia	0.9	0.11	0.6	0.09
Poland, Warsaw City	0.7	0.14	0.7	0.14
Slovakia	0.5	0.06	0.4	0.06
Slovenia	0.2	0.06	0.3	0.07
*Spain, Albacete	0,1	0,10	-	-
Spain, Asturias	1.0	0.29	0.3	0.09
Spain, Basque Country	0.5	0.15	0.4	0.14
Spain, Granada	0.3	0,15	0.5	0,20
Spain, Mallorca	0.5	0.25	0.4	0,20
Spain, Murcia	0.5	0.16	0.5	0.15
Spain, Navarra	0,7	0,26	0.4	0,21
Spain, Tarragona	0,5	0,18	1.1	0.39
Spain, Zaragoza	0.8	0.26	0.5	0.17

	MALE		FEMALE	
Sweden	0.3	0.04	0.3	0.04
*Switzerland, Basel	0,9	0,34	0,6	0,28
Switzerland, Geneva	0,5	0,27	0.7	0.24
Switzerland, Graubunden	-	-	0,8	0,59
Switzerland, Neuchatel	0,2	0,20	0,5	0,55
Switzerland, St Gall-Appenzell	0,2	0,16	0,2	0,17
Switzerland, Valais	-	-	0,7	0,43
Switzerland, Vaud	0,6	0,22	0,2	0,09
Switzerland, Zurich	0,3	0,13	0.7	0.19
*UK, England and Wales	0.6	0.03	0.5	0.03
*UK, East Anglia	0.6	0.13	0.3	0.10
*UK, Mersey	0.3	0.08	0.4	0.09
*UK, North Western	0.4	0.07	0.3	0.06
UK, Oxford	0.7	0.12	0.6	0.11
*UK, South Thames	0.7	0.07	0.5	0.06
UK, South Western	0.6	0.09	0.4	0.07
UK, Wessex	0.7	0.11	0.7	0.11
*UK, West Midlands	1.1	0.10	1.0	0.09
UK, Yorkshire	0.5	0.08	0.5	0.09
UK, Scotland	0.6	0.08	0.5	0.07
UK, Scotland, West	0.7	0.12	0.5	0.09
*Yugoslavia, Vojvodina	0.4	0.08	0.4	0.08

OCEANIA

	MALE		FEMALE	
Australian Capital Territory	0,5	0,28	0,5	0,27
Australia, New South Wales	0.5	0.07	0.5	0.07
South Australia	0.6	0.14	0.3	0.11
Australia, Tasmania	0,5	0,23	0,4	0,22
Australia, Victoria	0.5	0.08	0.3	0.06
Western Australia	0.5	0.13	0.4	0.10
*French Polynesia	0,8	0,39	0,8	0,38
New Zealand: Non-Maori	0.7	0.10	0.7	0.10
New Zealand: Maori	1,6	0,60	1,1	0,45
US, Hawaii: White	0,5	0,26	0.3	0,26
US, Hawaii: Japanese	0.3	0,22	0,3	0,20
US, Hawaii: Hawaiian	1,2	0,50	0,2	0,19
US, Hawaii: Filipino	0,6	0,40	0,2	0,17
US, Hawaii: Chinese	-	-	0,4	0,43

* IMPORTANT-SEE NOTES ON POPULATION PAGE

AGE-STANDARDIZED INCIDENCE
RATES AND STANDARD ERRORS (per 100,000)
Non-Hodgkin lymphomas (ICD-9 200+202)

AFRICA	MALE		FEMALE	
*Algeria, Setif	6.3	0.87	2.7	0.48
*France, La Reunion	4.8	0.64	3.7	0.51
*Mali, Bamako	2.6	0.59	0.8	0.31
*Uganda, Kyadondo	3.5	0.67	2.2	0.48
*Zimbabwe, Harare: African	4.7	0.77	4.0	1.19
*Zimbabwe, Harare: European	4,1	2,08	3,9	2,07 m

AMERICA, CENTRAL AND SOUTH	MALE		FEMALE	
*Argentina, Concordia	3.6	1.09	3.5	1.05
*Brazil, Belem	4.2	0.64	2.1	0.40
*Brazil, Goiania	5.1	0.71	3.4	0.53
*Brazil, Porto Alegre	8.4	0.77	6.4	0.56
Colombia, Cali	7.9	0.59	6.0	0.48
*Costa Rica	6.1	0.35	3.6	0.26
*Ecuador, Quito	8.2	0.67	6.0	0.54
*Peru, Lima	7.1	0.41	5.8	0.36
Peru, Trujillo	9.3	1.52	5.2	1.04
US, Puerto Rico	7.8	0.33	5.0	0.25
*Uruguay, Montevideo	10.3	0.68	7.5	0.51

AMERICA, NORTH	MALE		FEMALE	
Canada	13.1	0.13	9.0	0.10
Canada, Alberta	11.7	0.43	8.4	0.35
Canada, British Columbia	13.0	0.36	8.5	0.28
Canada, Manitoba	14.4	0.67	10.7	0.55
Canada, New Brunswick	12.6	0.77	8.2	0.59
Canada, Newfoundland	8.4	0.76	5.9	0.64
Canada, Northwest Territories	8.7	2.38	10.5	2.78
Canada, Nova Scotia	12.3	0.69	8.8	0.57
Canada, Ontario	13.4	0.21	9.3	0.17
Canada, Prince Edward Island	11.2	1.79	11.0	1.67
Canada, Quebec	13.5	0.26	9.1	0.20
Canada, Saskatchewan	12.9	0.66	9.5	0.55
Canada, Yukon	5,9	2,26	6,2	2,93
US, Cent. Calif.: Non-Hisp. White	13.2	0.55	8.9	0.43
US, Cent. Calif.: Hispanic	10.5	0.99	8.6	0.88
US, Los Angeles: Non-Hisp. White	18.5	0.40	9.8	0.27
US, Los Angeles: Hispanic White	11.7	0.51	7.1	0.37
US, Los Angeles: Black	10.6	0.68	6.0	0.46
US, Los Angeles: Chinese	7.6	1.10	5.0	0.88
US, Los Angeles: Filipino	10.5	1.44	7.0	1.05
US, Los Angeles: Korean	5.0	1.21	4.3	1.03
US, Los Angeles: Japanese	12.6	1.76	5.8	1.08
US, San Francisco: Non-Hisp. White	25.0	0.59	10.0	0.36
US, San Francisco: Hispanic White	20.8	1.45	11.0	1.01
US, San Francisco: Black	14.0	1.15	7.3	0.76
US, San Francisco: Chinese	10.8	1.16	6.9	0.98
US, San Francisco: Filipino	11.0	1.68	8.4	1.33
US, San Francisco: Japanese	10.0	2.74	10.3	2.21
US, Connecticut: White	15.0	0.41	10.6	0.32
US, Connecticut: Black	13.2	1.52	9.2	1.15
US, Atlanta: White	14.6	0.62	10.3	0.48
US, Atlanta: Black	10.2	0.96	6.7	0.71
US, Iowa	14.6	0.41	10.4	0.33

	MALE		FEMALE	
US, Central Louisiana: White	13.4	1.38	8.5	1.08
US, Central Louisiana: Black	8.8	2.54	4.9	1.55
US, New Orleans: White	15.7	0.93	9.2	0.64
US, New Orleans: Black	9.4	1.11	5.5	0.72
US, Detroit: White	15.3	0.42	10.4	0.32
US, Detroit: Black	12.9	0.78	6.7	0.49
US, New Mexico: Non-Hisp. White	12.1	0.71	8.3	0.54
US, New Mexico: Hispanic White	9.0	0.85	5.6	0.63
US, New Mexico: American Indian	3.8	1.28	4.1	1.24
US, Utah	13.3	0.58	9.3	0.46
US, Seattle	16.0	0.41	10.0	0.31
US, SEER: White	16.3	0.17	10.1	0.13
US, SEER: Black	12.3	0.47	7.0	0.33

ASIA	MALE		FEMALE	
*China, Qidong	3.7	0.37	1.8	0.23
China, Shanghai	4.3	0.15	2.5	0.12
China, Tianjin	4.5	0.23	2.6	0.16
Hong Kong	8.7	0.24	6.2	0.20
*India, Bangalore	3.7	0.23	2.1	0.18
*India, Barshi, Paranda and Bhum	1,0	0,33	0,6	0,27
India, Bombay	4.1	0.18	2.7	0.15
*India, Karunagappally	5.1	1.22	1,1	0,56
India, Madras	3.7	0.23	2.0	0.17
*India, Trivandrum	4.5	0.81	2.1	0.52
Israel: All Jews	12.6	0.36	10.4	0.31
Jews born in Israel	13.5	1.11	11.1	0.98
Jews born in America or Europe	12.8	0.73	9.9	0.48
Jews born in Africa or Asia	10.4	0.85	8.9	0.64
Non-Jews	8.3	0.86	6.5	0.74
Japan, Hiroshima	8.6	0.56	4.4	0.36
Japan, Miyagi	6.5	0.32	4.2	0.23
Japan, Nagasaki	13.5	0.52	7.1	0.34
Japan, Osaka	6.1	0.16	3.6	0.12
*Japan, Saga	8.8	0.57	3.3	0.31
Japan, Yamagata	4.8	0.34	2.6	0.26
*Korea, Kangwha	2,9	0,96	1,9	0,83
*Kuwait: Non-Kuwaitis	9.4	1.86	6.7	1.40
*Kuwait: Kuwaitis	5.5	0.88	7.1	1.22
*Philippines, Manila	5.7	0.35	3.6	0.25
Singapore: Chinese	6.1	0.37	4.5	0.30
Singapore: Malay	6.9	0.99	5.6	0.89
Singapore: Indian	3.9	0.90	2.9	1.01
Thailand, Chiang Mai	3.8	0.34	2.6	0.29
*Thailand, Khon Kaen	2.7	0.35	1.8	0.27
*Viet Nam, Hanoi	6.3	0.52	2.8	0.32

* IMPORTANT-SEE NOTES ON POPULATION PAGE

EUROPE	MALE		FEMALE	
Austria, Tyrol	7.6	0.66	7.5	0.59
*Belarus	3.2	0.12	1.8	0.07
*Croatia	5.3	0.23	3.8	0.18
Czech Republic	7.0	0.16	4.4	0.11
Denmark	9.8	0.24	6.5	0.19
Estonia	4.5	0.34	2.5	0.22
Finland	10.5	0.25	7.8	0.19
France, Bas-Rhin	12.1	0.68	8.3	0.52
*France, Calvados	8.2	0.68	6.0	0.55
France, Doubs	13.3	0.97	8.5	0.75
France, Haut-Rhin	10.1	0.74	6.8	0.56
*France, Herault	10.4	0.66	6.8	0.50
France, Isere	10.6	0.61	6.9	0.47
*France, Somme	8.5	0.73	5.1	0.51
*France, Tarn	6.8	0.77	5.3	0.64
Germany, Eastern States	5.6	0.18	3.7	0.13
Germany, Saarland	9.4	0.56	5.8	0.40
Iceland	8.5	1.12	4.7	0.80
Ireland, Southern	8.9	0.77	7.3	0.68
Italy, Ferrara	13.9	1.82	11.5	1.38
Italy, Florence	9.8	0.58	6.3	0.43
Italy, Genoa	13.2	0.81	7.7	0.55
*Italy, Latina	6.8	0.78	5.1	0.65
Italy, Macerata	8.5	1.43	6.6	1.23
Italy, Modena	12.9	0.79	9.5	0.63
Italy, Parma	11.9	0.93	8.3	0.74
Italy, Ragusa	6.5	0.87	4.1	0.69
Italy, Romagna	15.5	0.98	8.0	0.67
Italy, Torino	11.3	0.66	7.3	0.51
Italy, Trieste	15.5	1.47	9.6	1.00
Italy, Varese	13.9	0.77	10.1	0.59
Italy, Veneto	13.4	0.60	9.1	0.46
*Latvia	3.6	0.24	2.3	0.17
Malta	6.8	1.30	5.5	1.08
The Netherlands	10.6	0.17	7.0	0.13
The Netherlands, Eindhoven	10.0	0.61	6.0	0.45
The Netherlands, Maastricht	9.0	0.59	6.7	0.47
Norway	10.1	0.27	7.1	0.22
*Poland, Cracow	5.8	0.55	2.7	0.33
*Poland, Kielce	4.3	0.38	2.3	0.27
*Poland, Lower Silesia	5.0	0.27	2.8	0.18
Poland, Warsaw City	6.4	0.42	3.2	0.25
Slovakia	5.6	0.21	3.6	0.15
Slovenia	6.3	0.34	4.1	0.24
*Spain, Albacete	6.1	1.13	4.4	1.01
Spain, Asturias	7.2	0.51	6.0	0.47
Spain, Basque Country	8.1	0.42	5.1	0.30
Spain, Granada	5.6	0.52	4.3	0.43
Spain, Mallorca	7.9	0.69	5.0	0.51
Spain, Murcia	7.8	0.53	4.9	0.39
Spain, Navarra	8.8	0.77	5.4	0.56
Spain, Tarragona	5.7	0.59	5.6	0.58
Spain, Zaragoza	7.0	0.56	5.2	0.45

	MALE		FEMALE	
Sweden	10.8	0.19	6.9	0.15
*Switzerland, Basel	15.0	1.06	7.3	0.63
Switzerland, Geneva	13.5	1.09	8.1	0.76
Switzerland, Graubunden	7.3	1.23	5.2	1.05
Switzerland, Neuchatel	10.1	1.44	5.5	0.91
Switzerland, St Gall-Appenzell	10.0	0.83	7.1	0.69
Switzerland, Valais	8.8	1.17	5.9	1.00
Switzerland, Vaud	14.2	0.89	8.2	0.62
Switzerland, Zurich	12.9	0.60	8.5	0.46
*UK, England and Wales	9.6	0.10	6.3	0.08
*UK, East Anglia	10.5	0.40	7.0	0.32
*UK, Mersey	7.0	0.30	5.7	0.26
*UK, North Western	8.4	0.26	5.7	0.20
UK, Oxford	10.4	0.37	6.6	0.29
*UK, South Thames	10.4	0.22	6.8	0.17
UK, South Western	11.2	0.32	7.5	0.25
UK, Wessex	11.8	0.35	8.0	0.27
*UK, West Midlands	8.7	0.23	6.2	0.19
UK, Yorkshire	9.7	0.29	5.9	0.21
UK, Scotland	9.4	0.24	7.4	0.20
UK, Scotland, West	8.7	0.32	6.9	0.26
*Yugoslavia, Vojvodina	4.0	0.26	2.9	0.21

OCEANIA

	MALE		FEMALE	
Australian Capital Territory	14.2	1.57	9.8	1.24
Australia, New South Wales	13.3	0.28	8.6	0.21
South Australia	12.7	0.54	9.0	0.44
Australia, Tasmania	13.3	1.00	9.4	0.82
Australia, Victoria	13.8	0.33	9.1	0.26
Western Australia	11.8	0.51	8.3	0.43
*French Polynesia	3.9	1.15	4.4	1.20
New Zealand: Non-Maori	10.3	0.34	7.5	0.28
New Zealand: Maori	8.1	1.34	6.7	1.20
US, Hawaii: White	15.1	1.33	6.9	0.88
US, Hawaii: Japanese	8.5	0.99	6.3	0.76
US, Hawaii: Hawaiian	11.0	1.68	5.0	1.05
US, Hawaii: Filipino	11.1	1.52	7.9	1.31
US, Hawaii: Chinese	12.8	2.37	8.7	1.94

* IMPORTANT-SEE NOTES ON POPULATION PAGE

AGE-STANDARDIZED INCIDENCE
RATES AND STANDARD ERRORS (per 100,000)
Hodgkin's disease (ICD-9 201)

	MALE		FEMALE	
AFRICA				
*Algeria, Setif	2.2	0.41	1.4	0.29
*France, La Reunion	1.0	0.27	0.6	0.20
*Mali, Bamako	1.0	0.23	0,4	0,20
*Uganda, Kyadondo	0,9	0,57	0,2	0,10
*Zimbabwe, Harare: African	1.0	0.30	0,6	0,30
*Zimbabwe, Harare: European	-	-	4,3	2,82
AMERICA, CENTRAL AND SOUTH				
*Argentina, Concordia	1,2	0,60	0,7	0,47
*Brazil, Belem	2.5	0.50	1.0	0.26
*Brazil, Goiania	2.3	0.42	1.9	0.36
*Brazil, Porto Alegre	2.5	0.42	1.1	0.24 mf
Colombia, Cali	1.9	0.26	0.9	0.18 f
*Costa Rica	2.6	0.21	1.4	0.15
*Ecuador, Quito	1.5	0.28	1.3	0.23
*Peru, Lima	1.0	0.14	0.8	0.13
Peru, Trujillo	0,9	0,35	0,1	0,10
US, Puerto Rico	2.2	0.18	1.7	0.15
*Uruguay, Montevideo	3.4	0.42	2.2	0.31
AMERICA, NORTH				
Canada	2.9	0.06	2.3	0.06
Canada, Alberta	2.7	0.20	1.8	0.17
Canada, British Columbia	2.2	0.16	2.1	0.16
Canada, Manitoba	2.5	0.29	1.6	0.24
Canada, New Brunswick	2.5	0.36	2.1	0.32
Canada, Newfoundland	1.8	0.34	2.1	0.37
Canada, Northwest Territories	0,2	0,21	0,3	0,29
Canada, Nova Scotia	2.8	0.34	2.3	0.31
Canada, Ontario	3.1	0.11	2.5	0.10
Canada, Prince Edward Island	2,4	0,82	1,5	0,64
Canada, Quebec	3.2	0.13	2.6	0.12
Canada, Saskatchewan	2.7	0.33	1.6	0.25
Canada, Yukon	7,9	2,93	4,1	1,71
US, Cent. Calif.: Non-Hisp. White	2.7	0.28	2.4	0.27
US, Cent. Calif.: Hispanic	1.8	0.35	1.5	0.34
US, Los Angeles: Non-Hisp. White	3.3	0.19	2.5	0.17
US, Los Angeles: Hispanic White	2.1	0.20	1.5	0.15
US, Los Angeles: Black	2.0	0.28	1.7	0.24
US, Los Angeles: Chinese	0.5	0.28	0.5	0,24
US, Los Angeles: Filipino	1,5	0,53	0,9	0,43
US, Los Angeles: Korean	0,2	0,21	0,2	0,24
US, Los Angeles: Japanese	0,3	0,25	0,3	0,21
US, San Francisco: Non-Hisp. White	4.3	0.29	3.2	0.26
US, San Francisco: Hispanic White	2.1	0.41	1.8	0.38
US, San Francisco: Black	3.0	0.53	2.1	0.43
US, San Francisco: Chinese	1,1	0,43	0,7	0,34
US, San Francisco: Filipino	1,2	0,56	0,7	0,36
US, San Francisco: Japanese	2,1	1,21	0,4	0,40
US, Connecticut: White	4.1	0.23	3.6	0.22
US, Connecticut: Black	2.0	0.57	1.9	0.52
US, Atlanta: White	2.8	0.27	2.4	0.25
US, Atlanta: Black	2.1	0.40	1.6	0.30
US, Iowa	3.1	0.21	2.6	0.20

	MALE		FEMALE	
US, Central Louisiana: White	1.7	0.54	2.1	0.59
US, Central Louisiana: Black	2,2	1,17	0,6	0,60
US, New Orleans: White	3.5	0.47	2.8	0.45
US, New Orleans: Black	1.8	0.45	1.5	0.37
US, Detroit: White	3.7	0.22	2.9	0.20
US, Detroit: Black	2.9	0.37	1.9	0.28
US, New Mexico: Non-Hisp. White	3.0	0.40	2.2	0.35
US, New Mexico: Hispanic White	2.4	0.42	1.4	0.31
US, New Mexico: American Indian	0,3	0,27	0,2	0,24
US, Utah	2.0	0.22	2.0	0.21
US, Seattle	3.1	0.19	2.4	0.17
US, SEER: White	3.4	0.08	2.7	0.08
US, SEER: Black	2.5	0.20	2.0	0.17
ASIA				
*China, Qidong	0,1	0,04	0,0	0,02
China, Shanghai	0.4	0.05	0.3	0.04
China, Tianjin	0.3	0.06	0.3	0.06
Hong Kong	0.6	0.07	0.3	0.04
*India, Bangalore	1.3	0.13	0.6	0.10
*India, Barshi, Paranda and Bhum	0,4	0,19	-	-
India, Bombay	1.3	0.09	0.6	0.07
*India, Karunagappally	0,8	0,47	0,3	0,35
India, Madras	1.3	0.13	0.6	0.09
*India, Trivandrum	0,7	0,30	0,4	0,21
Israel: All Jews	2.9	0.18	2.8	0.17
Jews born in Israel	3.2	0.35	2.9	0.27
Jews born in America or Europe	3.0	0.46	3.1	0.43
Jews born in Africa or Asia	1.8	0.35	1.1	0.23
Non-Jews	2.4	0.37	1.6	0.34
Japan, Hiroshima	0,3	0,10	0.4	0.12
Japan, Miyagi	0.4	0.08	0.2	0.06
Japan, Nagasaki	0.3	0.08	0.1	0,05
Japan, Osaka	0.5	0.05	0.2	0.03
*Japan, Saga	0,1	0,08	0,2	0,08
Japan, Yamagata	0,1	0,07	0,0	0,03
*Korea, Kangwha	0,4	0,40	-	-
*Kuwait: Non-Kuwaitis	2.0	0.32	2.1	0.64
*Kuwait: Kuwaitis	4.0	0.73	2.0	0.61
*Philippines, Manila	0.9	0.13	0.4	0.07
Singapore: Chinese	0.5	0.10	0.3	0.08
Singapore: Malay	1.4	0.43	0,3	0,21
Singapore: Indian	1,2	0,53	0,6	0,45
Thailand, Chiang Mai	1.2	0.18	0.4	0.11
*Thailand, Khon Kaen	0.4	0.12	0.5	0.14
*Viet Nam, Hanoi	1.7	0.26	0.9	0.18

* IMPORTANT-SEE NOTES ON POPULATION PAGE

AGE-STANDARDIZED INCIDENCE
RATES AND STANDARD ERRORS (per 100,000)
Hodgkin's disease (ICD-9 201) (contd)

EUROPE	MALE		FEMALE	
Austria, Tyrol	2.6	0.40	1.9	0.33
*Belarus	3.3	0.12	2.5	0.10
*Croatia	1.7	0.14	1.3	0.12
Czech Republic	3.0	0.11	2.4	0.10
Denmark	2.9	0.14	1.6	0.11
Estonia	2.7	0.27	1.6	0.21
Finland	2.4	0.12	1.8	0.11
France, Bas-Rhin	2.7	0.33	1.8	0.27
*France, Calvados	2.0	0.35	2.1	0.36
France, Doubs	2.1	0.40	2.0	0.42
France, Haut-Rhin	2.2	0.35	2.1	0.35
*France, Herault	3.0	0.40	1.5	0.27
France, Isere	2.4	0.30	1.2	0.21
*France, Somme	2.5	0.41	1.8	0.36
*France, Tarn	2.1	0.50	0,7	0,29
Germany, Eastern States	2.6	0.13	2.0	0.11
Germany, Saarland	2.3	0.28	1.9	0.27
Iceland	3.1	0.70	1,2	0,42
Ireland, Southern	1.6	0.34	1.9	0.38
Italy, Ferrara	4.3	1.46	2.6	0.79
Italy, Florence	3.3	0.36	2.7	0.33
Italy, Genoa	3.6	0.46	2.3	0.37
*Italy, Latina	2.4	0.49	2.1	0.46
Italy, Macerata	3.7	1.20	3.1	1.07
Italy, Modena	2.5	0.41	2.2	0.39
Italy, Parma	2.0	0.42	2.3	0.49
Italy, Ragusa	2.7	0.61	2.0	0.50
Italy, Romagna	2.7	0.53	3.1	0.60
Italy, Torino	3.2	0.40	2.6	0.36
Italy, Trieste	2.7	0.62	2.7	0.67
Italy, Varese	3.5	0.42	2.9	0.38
Italy, Veneto	4.0	0.38	3.5	0.35
*Latvia	2.6	0.20	2.1	0.18
Malta	1,8	0,69	2.1	0.71
The Netherlands	2.4	0.09	1.7	0.07
The Netherlands, Eindhoven	1.9	0.27	1.4	0.23
The Netherlands, Maastricht	2.3	0.32	1.7	0.27
Norway	2.1	0.14	1.4	0.11
*Poland, Cracow	2.6	0.36	2.1	0.31
*Poland, Kielce	2.5	0.30	1.7	0.26
*Poland, Lower Silesia	2.3	0.18	1.7	0.15
Poland, Warsaw City	2.1	0.26	1.7	0.24
Slovakia	2.2	0.13	1.7	0.11
Slovenia	2.2	0.21	1.5	0.18
*Spain, Albacete	2.9	0.87	1,3	0,65
Spain, Asturias	3.4	0.39	2.0	0.30
Spain, Basque Country	3.1	0.26	1.9	0.20
Spain, Granada	2.1	0.32	1.4	0.25
Spain, Mallorca	2.5	0.42	1.8	0.34
Spain, Murcia	1.8	0.26	1.1	0.20
Spain, Navarra	2.5	0.42	2.0	0.38
Spain, Tarragona	2.9	0.47	1.1	0.28
Spain, Zaragoza	2.2	0.31	1.7	0.28

	MALE		FEMALE	
Sweden	2.2	0.10	1.5	0.09
*Switzerland, Basel	2.5	0.47	2.3	0.49
Switzerland, Geneva	2.7	0.51	1.7	0.41
Switzerland, Graubunden	3.9	1.10	1,1	0,50
Switzerland, Neuchatel	2.4	0.75	1,1	0,51
Switzerland, St Gall-Appenzell	2.2	0.41	2.2	0.44
Switzerland, Valais	1.6	0.52	2.6	0.71
Switzerland, Vaud	2.4	0.43	2.1	0.40
Switzerland, Zurich	3.0	0.32	2.2	0.28
*UK, England and Wales	2.5	0.06	1.8	0.05
*UK, East Anglia	2.4	0.21	1.7	0.19
*UK, Mersey	2.1	0.18	1.6	0.16
*UK, North Western	2.5	0.16	1.7	0.13
UK, Oxford	2.5	0.19	2.3	0.19
*UK, South Thames	2.6	0.12	1.8	0.10
UK, South Western	2.5	0.17	1.6	0.14
UK, Wessex	2.6	0.18	2.2	0.17
*UK, West Midlands	2.8	0.14	1.8	0.12
UK, Yorkshire	2.5	0.16	1.9	0.14
UK, Scotland	2.6	0.14	1.9	0.12
UK, Scotland, West	2.4	0.18	1.9	0.16
*Yugoslavia, Vojvodina	2.5	0.22	1.3	0.15

OCEANIA

	MALE		FEMALE	
Australian Capital Territory	1.8	0.58	1,0	0,35
Australia, New South Wales	2.1	0.12	1.4	0.10
South Australia	1.8	0.22	1.6	0.21
Australia, Tasmania	1.5	0.36	2.2	0.43
Australia, Victoria	2.3	0.14	1.7	0.12
Western Australia	2.1	0.22	1.4	0.18
*French Polynesia	1,2	0,44	1,1	0,57
New Zealand: Non-Maori	1.9	0.15	1.3	0.13
New Zealand: Maori	1.6	0.52	0,6	0,30
US, Hawaii: White	2.7	0.52	2.9	0.66
US, Hawaii: Japanese	0,8	0,30	1.3	0.45
US, Hawaii: Hawaiian	0,8	0,43	2.0	0.59
US, Hawaii: Filipino	1,1	0,57	1,1	0,49
US, Hawaii: Chinese	0,5	0,48	0,1	0,15

* IMPORTANT-SEE NOTES ON POPULATION PAGE

	MALE		FEMALE	
AFRICA				
*Algeria, Setif	0,3	0,19	0,4	0,19
*France, La Reunion	3.1	0.55	3.1	0.47
*Mali, Bamako	-	-	-	-
*Uganda, Kyadondo	0,7	0,47	0,7	0,49
*Zimbabwe, Harare: African	2.7	0.71	4.1	1.28
*Zimbabwe, Harare: European	1,5	1,03	1,0	0,71
AMERICA, CENTRAL AND SOUTH				
*Argentina, Concordia	-	-	0,3	0,29
*Brazil, Belem	0,7	0,27	0,4	0,22
*Brazil, Goiania	1.3	0.39	1.5	0.38
*Brazil, Porto Alegre	2.5	0.42	1.8	0.29
Colombia, Cali	2.3	0.33	1.6	0.25
*Costa Rica	2.5	0.24	1.6	0.18
*Ecuador, Quito	1.7	0.34	1.0	0.22
*Peru, Lima	1.5	0.20	0.9	0.15
Peru, Trujillo	2.6	0.82	1,5	0,57
US, Puerto Rico	3.0	0.20	2.0	0.15
*Uruguay, Montevideo	2.3	0.31	1.9	0.23
AMERICA, NORTH				
Canada	4.0	0.07	2.7	0.05
Canada, Alberta	3.9	0.24	2.5	0.19
Canada, British Columbia	3.6	0.18	2.3	0.13
Canada, Manitoba	4.3	0.34	2.8	0.25
Canada, New Brunswick	3.9	0.42	2.6	0.33
Canada, Newfoundland	2.7	0.42	2.3	0.38
Canada, Northwest Territories	3,2	1,61	1,8	1,31
Canada, Nova Scotia	3.1	0.33	2.6	0.30
Canada, Ontario	4.4	0.12	3.0	0.09
Canada, Prince Edward Island	4.4	1.03	3.2	0.87
Canada, Quebec	3.9	0.14	2.6	0.10
Canada, Saskatchewan	4.2	0.36	2.0	0.23
Canada, Yukon	5,2	2,35	4,5	2,23
US, Cent. Calif.: Non-Hisp. White	3.6	0.29	2.6	0.22
US, Cent. Calif.: Hispanic	3.5	0.60	2.9	0.52
US, Los Angeles: Non-Hisp. White	3.5	0.16	2.4	0.12
US, Los Angeles: Hispanic White	3.7	0.31	2.5	0.22
US, Los Angeles: Black	9.5	0.66	5.0	0.41
US, Los Angeles: Chinese	1.8	0.57	1,0	0,37
US, Los Angeles: Filipino	2.7	0.72	1.6	0.48
US, Los Angeles: Korean	1,6	0,97	0,8	0,42
US, Los Angeles: Japanese	0,5	0,31	0,5	0,29
US, San Francisco: Non-Hisp. White	4.0	0.23	2.4	0.16
US, San Francisco: Hispanic White	4.3	0.71	2.3	0.45
US, San Francisco: Black	9.5	0.97	6.4	0.72
US, San Francisco: Chinese	1.3	0.40	2.0	0.47
US, San Francisco: Filipino	4.9	1.15	2.3	0.70
US, San Francisco: Japanese	2,4	1,44	0,6	0,58
US, Connecticut: White	3.5	0.19	2.3	0.14
US, Connecticut: Black	7.0	1.21	4.3	0.81
US, Atlanta: White	4.0	0.33	2.2	0.22
US, Atlanta: Black	8.2	0.98	6.1	0.66
US, Iowa	4.3	0.21	2.8	0.16

	MALE		FEMALE	
US, Central Louisiana: White	2.5	0.60	2.6	0.55
US, Central Louisiana: Black	6.2	2.04	3,4	1,27
US, New Orleans: White	3.2	0.40	1.7	0.25
US, New Orleans: Black	8.7	1.08	5.5	0.71
US, Detroit: White	4.2	0.21	2.7	0.15
US, Detroit: Black	8.7	0.64	6.4	0.47
US, New Mexico: Non-Hisp. White	3.4	0.35	2.4	0.27
US, New Mexico: Hispanic White	2.8	0.47	2.7	0.45
US, New Mexico: American Indian	2,7	1,05	3.5	1.15
US, Utah	4.0	0.32	2.2	0.22
US, Seattle	4.2	0.21	3.0	0.17
US, SEER: White	3.9	0.08	2.5	0.06
US, SEER: Black	8.6	0.41	6.1	0.30
ASIA				
*China, Qidong	1.3	0.21	0.5	0.12
China, Shanghai	0.7	0.06	0.5	0.04
China, Tianjin	0.5	0.07	0.3	0.06
Hong Kong	1.7	0.11	1.6	0.10
*India, Bangalore	0.7	0.11	0.6	0.10
*India, Barshi, Paranda and Bhum	0,1	0,11	0,1	0,12
India, Bombay	1.2	0.10	0.9	0.09
*India, Karunagappally	0,6	0,40	1,4	0,61
India, Madras	0.8	0.12	0.4	0.08
*India, Trivandrum	2.6	0.63	0,4	0,22
Israel: All Jews	2.4	0.15	1.9	0.13
Jews born in Israel	3.0	0.62	1.8	0.45
Jews born in America or Europe	2.2	0.19	1.8	0.20
Jews born in Africa or Asia	2.4	0.27	2.3	0.25
Non-Jews	2.1	0.47	1.6	0.39
Japan, Hiroshima	1.8	0.26	1.1	0.18
Japan, Miyagi	1.5	0.14	1.4	0.12
Japan, Nagasaki	1.6	0.17	1.2	0.13
Japan, Osaka	1.6	0.08	1.0	0.06
*Japan, Saga	1.9	0.24	1.1	0.16
Japan, Yamagata	1.9	0.19	0.9	0.11
*Korea, Kangwha	0,6	0,43	1,2	0,60
*Kuwait: Non-Kuwaitis	3.9	1.44	2,0	0,78
*Kuwait: Kuwaitis	1,2	0,48	1,4	0,54
*Philippines, Manila	1.0	0.15	0.6	0.10
Singapore: Chinese	1.2	0.17	0.8	0.12
Singapore: Malay	2.8	0.65	1.9	0.55
Singapore: Indian	1.6	0.51	1,0	0,64
Thailand, Chiang Mai	0.4	0.11	0.3	0.10
*Thailand, Khon Kaen	0,2	0,11	0,1	0,06
*Viet Nam, Hanoi	0,1	0,08	-	-

f

* IMPORTANT-SEE NOTES ON POPULATION PAGE

AGE-STANDARDIZED INCIDENCE
RATES AND STANDARD ERRORS (per 100,000)
Multiple myeloma (ICD-9 203) (contd)

EUROPE	MALE		FEMALE	
Austria, Tyrol	3.5	0.46	2.5	0.33
*Belarus	1.0	0.07	0.8	0.05
*Croatia	1.8	0.13	1.7	0.11
Czech Republic	2.6	0.09	2.0	0.07
Denmark	3.2	0.13	2.2	0.10
Estonia	1.7	0.20	1.2	0.14
Finland	3.5	0.14	2.5	0.10
France, Bas-Rhin	2.3	0.29	1.1	0.18
*France, Calvados	2.1	0.33	1.5	0.27
France, Doubs	3.7	0.49	3.0	0.42
France, Haut-Rhin	2.9	0.38	2.1	0.28
*France, Herault	2.2	0.28	1.7	0.23
France, Isere	2.6	0.30	2.3	0.26
*France, Somme	1.9	0.35	1.7	0.30
*France, Tarn	1.7	0.34	1.7	0.34
Germany, Eastern States	2.2	0.11	1.5	0.07
Germany, Saarland	2.4	0.25	2.0	0.19
Iceland	3.7	0.73	2.3	0.56
Ireland, Southern	4.0	0.51	3.0	0.41
Italy, Ferrara	4.2	0.78	2.8	0.57
Italy, Florence	4.6	0.34	2.9	0.25
Italy, Genoa	3.7	0.34	2.2	0.24
*Italy, Latina	2.5	0.46	2.0	0.38
Italy, Macerata	2.6	0.72	2.9	0.72
Italy, Modena	3.6	0.37	2.4	0.27
Italy, Parma	3.9	0.46	2.3	0.31
Italy, Ragusa	3.0	0.52	1.5	0.35
Italy, Romagna	4.0	0.43	2.8	0.33
Italy, Torino	2.8	0.31	1.9	0.21
Italy, Trieste	4.5	0.68	3.7	0.54
Italy, Varese	3.1	0.33	2.6	0.27
Italy, Veneto	3.2	0.27	2.6	0.21
*Latvia	1.4	0.14	1.4	0.11
Malta	2.2	0.70	2.4	0.68
The Netherlands	3.4	0.09	2.3	0.07
The Netherlands, Eindhoven	2.9	0.32	2.2	0.26
The Netherlands, Maastricht	3.0	0.32	1.8	0.22
Norway	3.8	0.16	2.4	0.12
*Poland, Cracow	2.6	0.36	1.8	0.25
*Poland, Kielce	1.4	0.21	1.1	0.16
*Poland, Lower Silesia	1.6	0.15	1.3	0.12
Poland, Warsaw City	1.9	0.21	1.8	0.18
Slovakia	2.6	0.14	2.0	0.11
Slovenia	2.4	0.21	1.8	0.15
*Spain, Albacete	2.8	0.73	2.9	0.76
Spain, Asturias	2.3	0.27	1.6	0.20
Spain, Basque Country	2.0	0.19	1.7	0.15
Spain, Granada	2.3	0.30	1.7	0.25
Spain, Mallorca	3.0	0.38	2.2	0.31
Spain, Murcia	2.4	0.27	2.3	0.25
Spain, Navarra	2.3	0.35	1.7	0.27
Spain, Tarragona	3.0	0.38	2.1	0.30
Spain, Zaragoza	2.3	0.27	1.9	0.22

	MALE		FEMALE	
Sweden	3.8	0.10	2.4	0.08
*Switzerland, Basel	2.7	0.41	1.3	0.25
Switzerland, Geneva	3.5	0.52	2.4	0.39
Switzerland, Graubunden	4.5	0.98	2.9	0.71
Switzerland, Neuchatel	1.7	0.52	1.3	0.41
Switzerland, St Gall-Appenzell	3.8	0.49	2.5	0.37
Switzerland, Valais	4.5	0.81	2.2	0.52
Switzerland, Vaud	3.1	0.39	2.6	0.33
Switzerland, Zurich	3.4	0.29	2.3	0.21
*UK, England and Wales	3.4	0.06	2.3	0.04
*UK, East Anglia	3.4	0.20	2.1	0.15
*UK, Mersey	2.4	0.16	2.0	0.14
*UK, North Western	2.9	0.14	2.2	0.11
UK, Oxford	3.9	0.22	2.9	0.17
*UK, South Thames	3.4	0.12	2.4	0.09
UK, South Western	3.6	0.17	2.4	0.13
UK, Wessex	4.4	0.20	2.9	0.15
*UK, West Midlands	3.7	0.14	2.4	0.10
UK, Yorkshire	3.8	0.17	2.4	0.12
UK, Scotland	3.5	0.14	2.5	0.10
UK, Scotland, West	3.5	0.19	2.3	0.13
*Yugoslavia, Vojvodina	0.9	0.12	1.0	0.11

OCEANIA	MALE		FEMALE	
Australian Capital Territory	5.4	1.01	3.9	0.78
Australia, New South Wales	3.5	0.14	2.4	0.11
South Australia	4.5	0.30	2.7	0.22
Australia, Tasmania	4.1	0.54	2.1	0.36
Australia, Victoria	3.4	0.16	2.5	0.13
Western Australia	3.0	0.26	2.2	0.22
*French Polynesia	2,0	0,77	2,3	0,90
New Zealand: Non-Maori	4.1	0.21	2.7	0.16
New Zealand: Maori	5.7	1.19	5.8	1.18
US, Hawaii: White	3.5	0.65	1.9	0.45
US, Hawaii: Japanese	1.8	0.40	0.7	0.24
US, Hawaii: Hawaiian	4.1	1.07	4.2	1.01
US, Hawaii: Filipino	3.1	0.75	1,7	0,60
US, Hawaii: Chinese	2,1	0,87	0,4	0,26

* IMPORTANT-SEE NOTES ON POPULATION PAGE

AGE-STANDARDIZED INCIDENCE
RATES AND STANDARD ERRORS (per 100,000)
Lymphoid leukaemia (ICD-9 204)

AFRICA	MALE		FEMALE		
*Algeria, Setif	2.9	0.56	1.3	0.29	
*France, La Reunion	1.7	0.38	1.7	0.37	
*Mali, Bamako	-	-	-	-	
*Uganda, Kyadondo	0,2	0,14	0,1	0,08	
*Zimbabwe, Harare: African	2.5	0.74	2.2	0.82	
*Zimbabwe, Harare: European	1,7	1,24	0,9	0,87	

AMERICA, CENTRAL AND SOUTH					
*Argentina, Concordia	1,8	0,80	1,8	0,72	
*Brazil, Belem	1.0	0.25	0.9	0.25	mf
*Brazil, Goiania	2.3	0.44	1.4	0.32	
*Brazil, Porto Alegre	3.0	0.51	2.0	0.34	mf
Colombia, Cali	2.1	0.28	2.2	0.26	
*Costa Rica	4.0	0.26	2.8	0.21	
*Ecuador, Quito	2.5	0.32	2.4	0.31	
*Peru, Lima	1.9	0.20	1.5	0.16	
Peru, Trujillo	1.6	0.52	1.7	0.53	
US, Puerto Rico	2.5	0.20	2.1	0.19	
*Uruguay, Montevideo	3.1	0.39	2.0	0.29	

AMERICA, NORTH	MALE		FEMALE		
Canada	5.7	0.09	3.4	0.07	
Canada, Alberta	5.1	0.29	3.4	0.24	
Canada, British Columbia	4.4	0.23	3.0	0.21	
Canada, Manitoba	4.9	0.41	3.0	0.34	
Canada, New Brunswick	3.7	0.46	3.0	0.44	
Canada, Newfoundland	2.8	0.49	2.4	0.48	
Canada, Northwest Territories	1,8	0,92	1,1	0,61	
Canada, Nova Scotia	3.9	0.42	2.6	0.37	
Canada, Ontario	6.4	0.16	3.7	0.12	
Canada, Prince Edward Island	5.2	1.24	2,6	0,97	
Canada, Quebec	6.3	0.19	3.3	0.14	
Canada, Saskatchewan	8.0	0.54	4.8	0.43	
Canada, Yukon	9.6	2.97	11.1	3.57	
US, Cent. Calif.: Non-Hisp. White	4.5	0.34	3.1	0.29	
US, Cent. Calif.: Hispanic	5.1	0.62	3.2	0.47	
US, Los Angeles: Non-Hisp. White	5.6	0.25	3.3	0.19	
US, Los Angeles: Hispanic White	4.2	0.28	3.0	0.22	
US, Los Angeles: Black	4.6	0.46	1.8	0.26	
US, Los Angeles: Chinese	1,7	0,57	1.9	0.63	
US, Los Angeles: Filipino	3.4	0.89	3.0	0.92	
US, Los Angeles: Korean	1,7	0,84	1,7	0,78	
US, Los Angeles: Japanese	1,3	0,94	3,8	1,57	
US, San Francisco: Non-Hisp. White	5.4	0.33	2.8	0.25	
US, San Francisco: Hispanic White	3.6	0.59	3.4	0.55	
US, San Francisco: Black	4.6	0.69	3.2	0.55	
US, San Francisco: Chinese	4.4	0.95	1,2	0,46	
US, San Francisco: Filipino	3.3	0.97	3.2	0.99	
US, San Francisco: Japanese	1,8	1,79	0,5	0,46	
US, Connecticut: White	4.9	0.26	2.9	0.20	
US, Connecticut: Black	3.4	0.80	2.9	0.65	
US, Atlanta: White	4.3	0.37	2.7	0.29	
US, Atlanta: Black	4.2	0.67	2.3	0.40	
US, Iowa	6.8	0.30	3.6	0.22	

	MALE		FEMALE	
US, Central Louisiana: White	3.0	0.69	2.0	0.52
US, Central Louisiana: Black	3,8	1,38	0,7	0,53
US, New Orleans: White	4.8	0.60	3.2	0.49
US, New Orleans: Black	3.7	0.71	2.0	0.45
US, Detroit: White	6.3	0.29	3.4	0.21
US, Detroit: Black	3.8	0.43	2.7	0.32
US, New Mexico: Non-Hisp. White	6.0	0.55	3.3	0.41
US, New Mexico: Hispanic White	5.2	0.64	1.9	0.38
US, New Mexico: American Indian	2.7	0.87	2,3	0,81
US, Utah	4.4	0.33	2.9	0.26
US, Seattle	5.7	0.26	3.1	0.20
US, SEER: White	5.6	0.11	3.2	0.08
US, SEER: Black	4.0	0.28	2.6	0.20

ASIA				
*China, Qidong	1.1	0.20	0.7	0.16
China, Shanghai	1.5	0.11	1.1	0.09
China, Tianjin	1.3	0.14	0.7	0.11
Hong Kong	2.4	0.15	1.6	0.12
*India, Bangalore	1.1	0.12	0.7	0.10
*India, Barshi, Paranda and Bhum	0,7	0,24	0,5	0,20
India, Bombay	1.6	0.10	1.1	0.09
*India, Karunagappally	1,3	0,56	1,0	0,52
India, Madras	1.4	0.13	0.8	0.10
*India, Trivandrum	2.1	0.51	1.1	0.33
Israel: All Jews	3.5	0.19	2.0	0.13
Jews born in Israel	2.9	0.45	2.2	0.46
Jews born in America or Europe	4.8	0.78	2.6	0.65
Jews born in Africa or Asia	3.3	0.88	4.9	2.88
Non-Jews	2.7	0.44	1.3	0.31
Japan, Hiroshima	1.8	0.27	0.9	0.21
Japan, Miyagi	2.3	0.24	1.3	0.17
Japan, Nagasaki	2.0	0.27	1.5	0.25
Japan, Osaka	2.0	0.11	1.6	0.10
*Japan, Saga	4.6	0.46	2.7	0.35
Japan, Yamagata	1.3	0.23	1.0	0.21
*Korea, Kangwha	2,4	1,29	0,7	0,47
*Kuwait: Non-Kuwaitis	4.6	1.18	3.6	1.00
*Kuwait: Kuwaitis	1.2	0.36	1.3	0.35
*Philippines, Manila	2.0	0.17	1.4	0.12
Singapore: Chinese	2.3	0.24	1.8	0.22
Singapore: Malay	1.9	0.48	1.1	0.34
Singapore: Indian	1,4	0,56	2,0	1,00
Thailand, Chiang Mai	1.2	0.22	0.7	0.16
*Thailand, Khon Kaen	1.2	0.21	0.8	0.16
*Viet Nam, Hanoi	0.7	0.15	0.5	0.12

* IMPORTANT-SEE NOTES ON POPULATION PAGE

AGE-STANDARDIZED INCIDENCE
RATES AND STANDARD ERRORS (per 100,000)
Lymphoid leukaemia (ICD-9 204) (contd)

EUROPE	MALE		FEMALE	
Austria, Tyrol	5.9	0.63	3.0	0.45
*Belarus	6.0	0.16	3.0	0.10
*Croatia	4.8	0.24	2.7	0.17
Czech Republic	5.4	0.14	2.8	0.10
Denmark	5.2	0.20	2.9	0.16
Estonia	5.4	0.37	3.0	0.26
Finland	4.0	0.17	2.8	0.15
France, Bas-Rhin	4.5	0.45	2.7	0.34
†*France, Calvados	1.7	0.30	1.5	0.29
France, Doubs	3.6	0.57	2.2	0.44
France, Haut-Rhin	4.2	0.50	2.5	0.38
*France, Herault	2.4	0.33	2.0	0.33
France, Isere	3.9	0.39	2.3	0.32
*France, Somme	4.8	0.56	3.4	0.49
*France, Tarn	3.7	0.65	2.6	0.67
Germany, Eastern States	3.5	0.15	2.0	0.11
Germany, Saarland	4.0	0.39	2.6	0.32
Iceland	2.5	0.62	2.2	0.59
Ireland, Southern	6.4	0.66	3.1	0.50
Italy, Ferrara	4.8	1.29	2.9	0.80
Italy, Florence	3.7	0.41	2.5	0.38
Italy, Genoa	4.0	0.55	2.4	0.43
*Italy, Latina	5.2	0.76	3.6	0.64
Italy, Macerata	3.4	1.21	2.9	1.28
Italy, Modena	3.4	0.41	3.3	0.59
Italy, Parma	3.0	0.59	2.2	0.68
Italy, Ragusa	3.5	0.72	2.6	0.60
Italy, Romagna	5.0	0.62	3.3	0.61
Italy, Torino	4.4	0.60	2.8	0.47
Italy, Trieste	9.3	1.57	3.8	0.91
Italy, Varese	5.4	0.62	3.0	0.46
Italy, Veneto	4.5	0.45	2.9	0.35
*Latvia	4.8	0.27	2.9	0.19
Malta	4.4	1.10	1,9	0,70
The Netherlands	3.8	0.12	2.3	0.09
The Netherlands, Eindhoven	3.5	0.41	2.1	0.31
The Netherlands, Maastricht	4.2	0.47	2.7	0.38
Norway	2.5	0.16	1.7	0.14
*Poland, Cracow	3.5	0.47	1.6	0.30
*Poland, Kielce	3.4	0.34	1.8	0.26
*Poland, Lower Silesia	4.1	0.25	2.3	0.17
Poland, Warsaw City	3.3	0.35	2.1	0.28
Slovakia	5.2	0.20	2.7	0.14
Slovenia	4.3	0.30	3.5	0.27
*Spain, Albacete	6.3	1.45	2.2	0.83
Spain, Asturias	4.9	0.49	2.7	0.33
Spain, Basque Country	4.4	0.38	2.2	0.26
Spain, Granada	3.3	0.40	2.5	0.39
Spain, Mallorca	4.0	0.52	2.2	0.42
Spain, Murcia	3.4	0.37	2.7	0.35
Spain, Navarra	3.8	0.55	2.1	0.44
Spain, Tarragona	4.1	0.54	2.2	0.47
Spain, Zaragoza	3.0	0.42	2.2	0.35

	MALE		FEMALE	
Sweden	4.3	0.14	2.7	0.12
*Switzerland, Basel	3.8	0.62	1.8	0.40
Switzerland, Geneva	5.9	0.85	3.4	0.69
Switzerland, Graubunden	5.9	1.24	2.1	0.77
Switzerland, Neuchatel	4.6	0.98	0,9	0,36
Switzerland, St Gall-Appenzell	5.2	0.67	2.7	0.47
Switzerland, Valais	4.9	1.04	2.6	0.74
Switzerland, Vaud	3.0	0.45	2.0	0.41
Switzerland, Zurich	4.3	0.43	3.0	0.35
*UK, England and Wales	4.2	0.07	2.4	0.06
*UK, East Anglia	3.5	0.25	1.8	0.20
*UK, Mersey	2.4	0.19	2.0	0.19
*UK, North Western	3.7	0.19	1.9	0.13
UK, Oxford	4.3	0.27	2.7	0.22
*UK, South Thames	4.1	0.16	2.4	0.12
UK, South Western	5.0	0.24	3.1	0.20
UK, Wessex	4.9	0.26	3.0	0.20
*UK, West Midlands	4.6	0.19	2.3	0.13
UK, Yorkshire	4.5	0.22	2.5	0.17
UK, Scotland	4.7	0.20	2.5	0.15
UK, Scotland, West	4.5	0.27	2.4	0.20
*Yugoslavia, Vojvodina	4.6	0.29	2.2	0.20

OCEANIA	MALE		FEMALE	
Australian Capital Territory	5.6	1.06	2.1	0.62
Australia, New South Wales	4.8	0.18	3.1	0.15
South Australia	7.5	0.44	5.0	0.36
Australia, Tasmania	6.7	0.74	3.1	0.48
Australia, Victoria	5.2	0.22	2.6	0.16
Western Australia	3.8	0.32	2.2	0.25
*French Polynesia	1,8	0,75	2,1	0,87
New Zealand: Non-Maori	5.3	0.26	3.5	0.21
New Zealand: Maori	3.9	0.84	1.6	0.51
US, Hawaii: White	5.1	0.84	3.1	0.68
US, Hawaii: Japanese	1.6	0.54	2.3	0.84
US, Hawaii: Hawaiian	2.3	0.72	3.6	0.89
US, Hawaii: Filipino	2.8	0.86	0,9	0,55
US, Hawaii: Chinese	0,8	0,48	0,2	0,19

* IMPORTANT-SEE NOTES ON POPULATION PAGE

AGE-STANDARDIZED INCIDENCE
RATES AND STANDARD ERRORS (per 100,000)
Myeloid leukaemia (ICD-9 205)

AFRICA	MALE		FEMALE	
*Algeria, Setif	2.0	0.45	1.7	0.35
*France, La Reunion	3.3	0.54	2.7	0.44
*Mali, Bamako	0,1	0,10	1.1	0.37
*Uganda, Kyadondo	0,2	0,19	0,6	0,37
*Zimbabwe, Harare: African	2.7	0.58	2.5	0.83
*Zimbabwe, Harare: European	4,4	1,99	2,5	1,50

AMERICA, CENTRAL AND SOUTH				
*Argentina, Concordia	0,3	0,27	0,3	0,29
*Brazil, Belem	2.0	0.44	1.0	0.25
*Brazil, Goiania	2.0	0.41	1.7	0.34
*Brazil, Porto Alegre	2.8	0.46	2.7	0.38 mf
Colombia, Cali	2.0	0.28	1.9	0.25
*Costa Rica	2.8	0.23	2.5	0.21
*Ecuador, Quito	3.8	0.45	2.3	0.31
*Peru, Lima	1.7	0.19	1.9	0.20
Peru, Trujillo	2.0	0.68	3.1	0.81
US, Puerto Rico	3.1	0.21	2.1	0.17
*Uruguay, Montevideo	3.0	0.37	2.0	0.26

AMERICA, NORTH				
Canada	3.7	0.07	2.5	0.06
Canada, Alberta	3.1	0.21	2.1	0.17
Canada, British Columbia	3.0	0.18	2.2	0.15
Canada, Manitoba	4.2	0.37	2.5	0.27
Canada, New Brunswick	2.9	0.37	1.9	0.28
Canada, Newfoundland	3.1	0.45	2.9	0.46
Canada, Northwest Territories	2,1	1,00	1,4	0,69
Canada, Nova Scotia	2.3	0.29	2.0	0.26
Canada, Ontario	4.6	0.12	3.1	0.10
Canada, Prince Edward Island	2.6	0.82	2.5	0.79
Canada, Quebec	3.2	0.13	2.2	0.10
Canada, Saskatchewan	3.6	0.35	2.1	0.26
Canada, Yukon	1,8	1,31	0,7	0,65
US, Cent. Calif.: Non-Hisp. White	4.4	0.33	2.8	0.26
US, Cent. Calif.: Hispanic	3.3	0.52	1.7	0.36
US, Los Angeles: Non-Hisp. White	4.8	0.21	3.2	0.17
US, Los Angeles: Hispanic White	3.3	0.27	2.7	0.21
US, Los Angeles: Black	4.4	0.44	3.0	0.32
US, Los Angeles: Chinese	4.0	0.79	2.0	0.57
US, Los Angeles: Filipino	6.7	1.17	3.0	0.71
US, Los Angeles: Korean	1,7	0,67	1,9	0,67
US, Los Angeles: Japanese	4.8	1.12	3.3	1.10
US, San Francisco: Non-Hisp. White	4.5	0.26	2.7	0.20
US, San Francisco: Hispanic White	4.1	0.67	4.0	0.61
US, San Francisco: Black	3.6	0.59	1.8	0.39
US, San Francisco: Chinese	2.9	0.68	3.1	0.70
US, San Francisco: Filipino	4.9	1.17	3.6	0.89
US, San Francisco: Japanese	3,9	1,75	1,4	0,84
US, Connecticut: White	3.7	0.20	2.5	0.16
US, Connecticut: Black	3.4	0.79	2.7	0.63
US, Atlanta: White	3.7	0.32	2.6	0.24
US, Atlanta: Black	3.2	0.56	2.8	0.45
US, Iowa	4.1	0.22	2.9	0.18

	MALE		FEMALE	
US, Central Louisiana: White	3.3	0.67	2.1	0.46
US, Central Louisiana: Black	3,2	1,51	0,6	0,33
US, New Orleans: White	3.6	0.44	3.1	0.41
US, New Orleans: Black	3.6	0.68	2.3	0.47
US, Detroit: White	4.7	0.23	3.3	0.19
US, Detroit: Black	4.5	0.46	2.8	0.32
US, New Mexico: Non-Hisp. White	4.2	0.42	2.9	0.34
US, New Mexico: Hispanic White	3.5	0.53	2.4	0.41
US, New Mexico: American Indian	2,7	1,03	1,3	0,59
US, Utah	3.4	0.29	2.5	0.23
US, Seattle	3.9	0.20	2.7	0.17
US, SEER: White	4.1	0.09	2.7	0.07
US, SEER: Black	3.9	0.27	2.7	0.20

ASIA				
*China, Qidong	1.8	0.26	1.8	0.26
China, Shanghai	1.7	0.10	1.3	0.09
China, Tianjin	1.8	0.15	1.4	0.13
Hong Kong	3.4	0.15	2.5	0.13
*India, Bangalore	1.9	0.16	1.6	0.15
*India, Barshi, Paranda and Bhum	1.1	0.34	0,4	0,20
India, Bombay	2.0	0.11	1.5	0.10
*India, Karunagappally	2,0	0,75	0,6	0,43
India, Madras	1.3	0.14	1.0	0.12
*India, Trivandrum	0,9	0,31	1.7	0.45
Israel: All Jews	2.7	0.17	2.1	0.14
Jews born in Israel	3.2	0.59	2.8	0.49
Jews born in America or Europe	3.8	0.58	2.7	0.50
Jews born in Africa or Asia	2.8	0.57	2.1	0.40
Non-Jews	2.0	0.44	2.0	0.37
Japan, Hiroshima	3.5	0.35	2.1	0.27
Japan, Miyagi	2.9	0.21	1.5	0.15
Japan, Nagasaki	2.6	0.24	2.2	0.22
Japan, Osaka	2.7	0.11	1.6	0.08
*Japan, Saga	3.5	0.37	1.9	0.26
Japan, Yamagata	2.4	0.24	1.6	0.21
*Korea, Kangwha	2,6	0,98	1,3	0,65
*Kuwait: Non-Kuwaitis	1.9	0.41	1.3	0.43
*Kuwait: Kuwaitis	2.3	0.55	2.7	0.76
*Philippines, Manila	2.1	0.19	1.7	0.16
Singapore: Chinese	3.3	0.27	2.0	0.20
Singapore: Malay	3.6	0.71	3.1	0.67
Singapore: Indian	1,5	0,50	2.9	0.95
Thailand, Chiang Mai	2.6	0.27	2.7	0.31
*Thailand, Khon Kaen	1.4	0.24	1.5	0.24
*Viet Nam, Hanoi	1.4	0.22	1.3	0.22

* IMPORTANT-SEE NOTES ON POPULATION PAGE

EUROPE	MALE		FEMALE	
Austria, Tyrol	3.1	0.43	2.5	0.35
*Belarus	2.4	0.10	1.7	0.07
*Croatia	3.0	0.18	2.5	0.15
Czech Republic	3.0	0.10	2.4	0.09
Denmark	4.1	0.16	2.9	0.14
Estonia	2.5	0.25	1.8	0.19
Finland	2.7	0.13	2.1	0.11
France, Bas-Rhin	3.4	0.36	1.7	0.23
†*France, Calvados	1.2	0.27	1.1	0.24
France, Doubs	3.5	0.50	2.6	0.44
France, Haut-Rhin	2.6	0.37	2.1	0.34
*France, Herault	2.8	0.37	1.1	0.23
France, Isere	3.9	0.36	1.7	0.23
*France, Somme	2.5	0.41	1.6	0.31
*France, Tarn	2.0	0.44	2.1	0.44
Germany, Eastern States	2.8	0.13	2.1	0.10
Germany, Saarland	4.3	0.36	2.5	0.28
Iceland	2.8	0.63	2.1	0.59
Ireland, Southern	3.6	0.50	2.2	0.37
Italy, Ferrara	2.6	0.64	1.9	0.54
Italy, Florence	3.7	0.34	2.8	0.36
Italy, Genoa	2.9	0.36	2.7	0.41
*Italy, Latina	4.0	0.58	2.2	0.47
Italy, Macerata	3.0	0.89	1,4	0,63
Italy, Modena	2.9	0.37	2.7	0.42
Italy, Parma	2.6	0.41	2.5	0.47
Italy, Ragusa	2.8	0.56	2.2	0.48
Italy, Romagna	4.1	0.50	2.2	0.35
Italy, Torino	3.8	0.41	2.3	0.28
Italy, Trieste	4.2	0.71	4.4	0.98
Italy, Varese	4.0	0.44	3.2	0.35
Italy, Veneto	3.4	0.30	2.7	0.28
*Latvia	2.1	0.17	1.8	0.14
Malta	3.2	0.84	3.9	0.97
The Netherlands	3.2	0.09	2.1	0.07
The Netherlands, Eindhoven	2.5	0.30	1.9	0.26
The Netherlands, Maastricht	3.6	0.39	2.2	0.26
Norway	2.8	0.14	2.0	0.13
*Poland, Cracow	2.7	0.39	2.1	0.32
*Poland, Kielce	2.0	0.26	1.9	0.24
*Poland, Lower Silesia	2.6	0.19	2.1	0.16
Poland, Warsaw City	2.7	0.30	2.3	0.25
Slovakia	3.2	0.16	2.3	0.12
Slovenia	2.8	0.23	2.1	0.19
*Spain, Albacete	2,1	0,74	1,2	0,55
Spain, Asturias	1.6	0.24	1.5	0.23
Spain, Basque Country	2.3	0.22	1.4	0.16
Spain, Granada	2.6	0.33	1.7	0.27
Spain, Mallorca	2.6	0.38	2.7	0.42
Spain, Murcia	3.7	0.37	2.2	0.27
Spain, Navarra	2.6	0.42	1.4	0.31
Spain, Tarragona	3.1	0.45	1.9	0.38
Spain, Zaragoza	2.7	0.35	2.8	0.36

	MALE		FEMALE	
Sweden	3.0	0.11	2.4	0.10
*Switzerland, Basel	2.9	0.50	2.4	0.41
Switzerland, Geneva	4.4	0.62	2.5	0.40
Switzerland, Graubunden	3.3	0.82	3.2	0.94
Switzerland, Neuchatel	2.8	0.76	2.0	0.56
Switzerland, St Gall-Appenzell	4.1	0.55	2.2	0.36
Switzerland, Valais	2.3	0.58	1.8	0.57
Switzerland, Vaud	4.0	0.51	2.0	0.32
Switzerland, Zurich	3.7	0.34	1.8	0.21
*UK, England and Wales	3.5	0.06	2.5	0.05
*UK, East Anglia	3.2	0.22	2.4	0.18
*UK, Mersey	2.7	0.19	2.0	0.16
*UK, North Western	3.2	0.16	2.4	0.14
UK, Oxford	4.2	0.24	3.2	0.20
*UK, South Thames	3.5	0.13	2.7	0.11
UK, South Western	3.7	0.18	2.5	0.15
UK, Wessex	4.6	0.22	3.0	0.18
*UK, West Midlands	3.3	0.14	2.4	0.12
UK, Yorkshire	3.5	0.18	2.3	0.14
UK, Scotland	3.2	0.14	2.5	0.12
UK, Scotland, West	3.2	0.20	2.4	0.16
*Yugoslavia, Vojvodina	3.0	0.23	2.0	0.18

OCEANIA	MALE		FEMALE	
Australian Capital Territory	4.7	0.90	2.5	0.60
Australia, New South Wales	4.8	0.17	2.8	0.12
South Australia	5.4	0.35	3.5	0.28
Australia, Tasmania	4.1	0.54	3.6	0.51
Australia, Victoria	4.1	0.18	2.7	0.14
Western Australia	4.3	0.31	2.7	0.25
*French Polynesia	3.2	0.89	2.3	0.76
New Zealand: Non-Maori	4.6	0.23	3.1	0.18
New Zealand: Maori	6.7	1.34	4.5	0.90
US, Hawaii: White	4.3	0.72	1.3	0.37
US, Hawaii: Japanese	2.7	0.65	1.8	0.47
US, Hawaii: Hawaiian	5.4	1.17	2.5	0.76
US, Hawaii: Filipino	4.1	0.92	4.2	1.01
US, Hawaii: Chinese	4,0	1,71	0,4	0,45

* IMPORTANT-SEE NOTES ON POPULATION PAGE

AGE-STANDARDIZED INCIDENCE
RATES AND STANDARD ERRORS (per 100,000)
Monocytic leukaemia (ICD-9 206)

	MALE		FEMALE	
AFRICA				
*Algeria, Setif	-	-	-	-
*France, La Reunion	-	-	0,1	0,09
*Mali, Bamako	-	-	-	-
*Uganda, Kyadondo	-	-	-	-
*Zimbabwe, Harare: African	-	-	-	-
*Zimbabwe, Harare: European	-	-	-	-
AMERICA, CENTRAL AND SOUTH				
*Argentina, Concordia	-	-	-	-
*Brazil, Belem	-	-	-	-
*Brazil, Goiania	0,2	0,11	0,1	0,05
*Brazil, Porto Alegre	0,2	0,13	-	-
Colombia, Cali	0,1	0,06	0,0	0,04
*Costa Rica	0,1	0,04	0,1	0,04
*Ecuador, Quito	0,2	0,12	0,1	0,07
*Peru, Lima	0,1	0,05	0,0	0,01
Peru, Trujillo	0,1	0,14	0,2	0,16
US, Puerto Rico	0,1	0,03	0,1	0,03
*Uruguay, Montevideo	-	-	0,0	0,03
AMERICA, NORTH				
Canada	0.2	0.02	0.1	0.01
Canada, Alberta	0.2	0.06	0,1	0,03
Canada, British Columbia	0.2	0.05	0.1	0.03
Canada, Manitoba	0,2	0,08	0,1	0,04
Canada, New Brunswick	0,1	0,06	0,1	0,07
Canada, Newfoundland	0,1	0,07	-	-
Canada, Northwest Territories	-	-	0,7	0,50
Canada, Nova Scotia	0.4	0.11	0,3	0,09
Canada, Ontario	0.1	0.02	0.1	0.02
Canada, Prince Edward Island	0,3	0,34	-	-
Canada, Quebec	0.2	0.03	0.2	0.03
Canada, Saskatchewan	0.4	0.11	0,2	0,09
Canada, Yukon	1,1	0,76	-	-
US, Cent. Calif.: Non-Hisp. White	0.2	0.06	0,1	0,05
US, Cent. Calif.: Hispanic	0,3	0,17	0,1	0,11
US, Los Angeles: Non-Hisp. White	0.2	0.04	0.1	0.03
US, Los Angeles: Hispanic White	0.2	0.06	0,1	0,03
US, Los Angeles: Black	0,2	0,10	0,0	0,05
US, Los Angeles: Chinese	0,2	0,19	0,2	0,23
US, Los Angeles: Filipino	-	-	0,3	0,30
US, Los Angeles: Korean	-	-	-	-
US, Los Angeles: Japanese	0,3	0,33	-	-
US, San Francisco: Non-Hisp. White	0.3	0.07	0.1	0.05
US, San Francisco: Hispanic White	-	-	-	-
US, San Francisco: Black	0,3	0,16	0,3	0,18
US, San Francisco: Chinese	-	-	-	-
US, San Francisco: Filipino	0,4	0,32	0,2	0,22
US, San Francisco: Japanese	-	-	-	-
US, Connecticut: White	0.3	0.06	0.2	0.05
US, Connecticut: Black	0,2	0,23	-	-
US, Atlanta: White	0,2	0,07	0.2	0.07
US, Atlanta: Black	-	-	-	-
US, Iowa	0.2	0.05	0.2	0.05

	MALE		FEMALE	
US, Central Louisiana: White	-	-	0,1	0,09
US, Central Louisiana: Black	-	-	-	-
US, New Orleans: White	0,4	0,16	0,3	0,16
US, New Orleans: Black	0,2	0,14	0,2	0,13
US, Detroit: White	0.4	0.07	0.2	0.04
US, Detroit: Black	0,3	0,11	0,1	0,05
US, New Mexico: Non-Hisp. White	0,2	0,09	0,2	0,12
US, New Mexico: Hispanic White	0,2	0,13	0,3	0,14
US, New Mexico: American Indian	-	-	-	-
US, Utah	0,1	0,06	0,1	0,04
US, Seattle	0.2	0.05	0.1	0.04
US, SEER: White	0.2	0.02	0.2	0.02
US, SEER: Black	0.2	0.06	0,1	0,04
ASIA				
*China, Qidong	-	-	0,0	0,02
China, Shanghai	0.6	0.06	0.4	0.04
China, Tianjin	0.2	0.04	0.2	0.05
Hong Kong	0,0	0,02	0,1	0,02
*India, Bangalore	0,0	0,02	0,0	0,01
*India, Barshi, Paranda and Bhum	-	-	-	-
India, Bombay	0,0	0,01	0,0	0,01
*India, Karunagappally	-	-	-	-
India, Madras	0,1	0,03	0,0	0,03
*India, Trivandrum	-	-	-	-
Israel: All Jews	0.3	0.05	0.2	0.05
Jews born in Israel	0,1	0,08	0,1	0,05
Jews born in America or Europe	0.5	0.21	0.2	0.06
Jews born in Africa or Asia	0,3	0,09	0,1	0,04
Non-Jews	-	-	-	-
Japan, Hiroshima	0,1	0,08	0,1	0,04
Japan, Miyagi	0,1	0,03	0.1	0.05
Japan, Nagasaki	0,1	0,06	0,1	0,03
Japan, Osaka	0.3	0.04	0.1	0.02
*Japan, Saga	0,0	0,04	-	-
Japan, Yamagata	0,1	0,05	0,2	0,06
*Korea, Kangwha	-	-	-	-
*Kuwait: Non-Kuwaitis	0,1	0,05	-	-
*Kuwait: Kuwaitis	0,1	0,06	-	-
*Philippines, Manila	0,1	0,05	0,1	0,03
Singapore: Chinese	0,0	0,02	-	-
Singapore: Malay	0,2	0,17	-	-
Singapore: Indian	-	-	-	-
Thailand, Chiang Mai	-	-	0,0	0,04
*Thailand, Khon Kaen	0,0	0,03	0,1	0,05
*Viet Nam, Hanoi	0,1	0,06	0,0	0,03

* IMPORTANT-SEE NOTES ON POPULATION PAGE

AGE-STANDARDIZED INCIDENCE
RATES AND STANDARD ERRORS (per 100,000)
Monocytic leukaemia (ICD-9 206) (contd)

EUROPE	MALE		FEMALE	
Austria, Tyrol	0,2	0,10	0,1	0,06
*Belarus	0.1	0.02	0.1	0.01
*Croatia	0,0	0,01	0,0	0,01
Czech Republic	0.2	0.03	0.1	0.02
Denmark	0.1	0.02	0,0	0,01
Estonia	0,1	0,06	0,0	0,04
Finland	0.1	0.03	0.1	0.01
France, Bas-Rhin	0,3	0,11	0,2	0,10
†*France, Calvados	0,1	0,05	0,0	0,04
France, Doubs	0,1	0,08	-	-
France, Haut-Rhin	-	-	0,3	0,12
*France, Herault	0,0	0,03	0,0	0,03
France, Isere	0,2	0,08	0,1	0,08
*France, Somme	0,2	0,11	0,2	0,11
*France, Tarn	0,2	0,15	0,1	0,07
Germany, Eastern States	0.1	0.02	0.1	0.02
Germany, Saarland	0.3	0.09	0,1	0,04
Iceland	0,2	0,19	-	-
Ireland, Southern	-	-	-	-
Italy, Ferrara	-	-	0,3	0,19
Italy, Florence	0,0	0,01	0,0	0,01
Italy, Genoa	-	-	0,1	0,04
*Italy, Latina	0,3	0,13	-	-
Italy, Macerata	-	-	0,0	0,05
Italy, Modena	0,3	0,15	0,1	0,05
Italy, Parma	0,2	0,07	0,1	0,09
Italy, Ragusa	-	-	0,0	0,04
Italy, Romagna	0,1	0,07	-	-
Italy, Torino	0,4	0,21	0,5	0,25
Italy, Trieste	0,2	0,15	-	-
Italy, Varese	0,2	0,15	0,1	0,06
Italy, Veneto	0,2	0,07	0,2	0,11
*Latvia	0.3	0.06	0.3	0.06
Malta	-	-	-	-
The Netherlands	0.2	0.02	0.1	0.02
The Netherlands, Eindhoven	0,1	0,07	0,0	0,03
The Netherlands, Maastricht	0,0	0,04	0,2	0,08
Norway	0.2	0.04	0.2	0.04
*Poland, Cracow	-	-	-	-
*Poland, Kielce	-	-	-	-
*Poland, Lower Silesia	0,1	0,03	0,0	0,01
Poland, Warsaw City	-	-	-	-
Slovakia	0.1	0.03	0.1	0.02
Slovenia	0.2	0.06	0,1	0,06
*Spain, Albacete	0,2	0,17	0,1	0,07
Spain, Asturias	0,1	0,06	0,1	0,04
Spain, Basque Country	0,1	0,05	0,1	0,04
Spain, Granada	0,1	0,08	0,2	0,10
Spain, Mallorca	0,1	0,08	0,2	0,11
Spain, Murcia	0,1	0,04	0,0	0,01
Spain, Navarra	0,2	0,10	0,1	0,06
Spain, Tarragona	0,1	0,06	0,1	0,03
Spain, Zaragoza	0,1	0,07	0,1	0,05

	MALE		FEMALE	
Sweden	0.1	0.02	0.1	0.02
*Switzerland, Basel	-	-	0,1	0,08
Switzerland, Geneva	-	-	0,1	0,06
Switzerland, Graubunden	0,1	0,11	0,1	0,08
Switzerland, Neuchatel	0,1	0,09	0,1	0,12
Switzerland, St Gall-Appenzell	0,1	0,04	0,1	0,13
Switzerland, Valais	0,1	0,08	-	-
Switzerland, Vaud	0,1	0,06	0,1	0,08
Switzerland, Zurich	0.5	0.11	0.3	0.08
*UK, England and Wales	0.1	0.01	0.1	0.01
*UK, East Anglia	0,1	0,05	0,0	0,02
*UK, Mersey	0,1	0,04	0.1	0.03
*UK, North Western	0,0	0,02	0,0	0,01
UK, Oxford	0.4	0.08	0.1	0.04
*UK, South Thames	0.1	0.02	0.0	0.01
UK, South Western	0.3	0.05	0.2	0.04
UK, Wessex	0.1	0.03	0.1	0.03
*UK, West Midlands	0.2	0.03	0.1	0.02
UK, Yorkshire	0,1	0,02	0,0	0,02
UK, Scotland	0.1	0.03	0.1	0.02
UK, Scotland, West	0,1	0,04	0,0	0,02
*Yugoslavia, Vojvodina	-	-	-	-

OCEANIA	MALE		FEMALE	
Australian Capital Territory	-	-	-	-
Australia, New South Wales	0.1	0.03	0.1	0.03
South Australia	0.3	0.08	0,2	0,07
Australia, Tasmania	0,1	0,09	0,0	0,02
Australia, Victoria	0.2	0.04	0.1	0.04
Western Australia	0.3	0.09	0,1	0,06
*French Polynesia	0,2	0,17	0,5	0,36
New Zealand: Non-Maori	0.1	0.03	0,1	0,02
New Zealand: Maori	-	-	0,4	0,29
US, Hawaii: White	0,1	0,12	0,2	0,16
US, Hawaii: Japanese	0,1	0,09	0,0	0,04
US, Hawaii: Hawaiian	0,7	0,40	0,3	0,25
US, Hawaii: Filipino	0,7	0,41	-	-
US, Hawaii: Chinese	0,4	0,31	0,7	0,51

* IMPORTANT-SEE NOTES ON POPULATION PAGE

	MALE		FEMALE	
AFRICA				
*Algeria, Setif	-	-	-	-
*France, La Reunion	0,3	0,16	0,1	0,05
*Mali, Bamako	-	-	-	-
*Uganda, Kyadondo	-	-	-	-
*Zimbabwe, Harare: African	-	-	-	-
*Zimbabwe, Harare: European	0,7	0,73	-	-
AMERICA, CENTRAL AND SOUTH				
*Argentina, Concordia	-	-	-	-
*Brazil, Belem	-	-	-	-
*Brazil, Goiania	-	-	-	-
*Brazil, Porto Alegre	-	-	0,0	0,05
Colombia, Cali	0,1	0,05	-	-
*Costa Rica	-	-	0,0	0,01
*Ecuador, Quito	-	-	-	-
*Peru, Lima	0,0	0,02	-	-
Peru, Trujillo	-	-	-	-
US, Puerto Rico	0,1	0,03	0,0	0,02
*Uruguay, Montevideo	-	-	-	-
AMERICA, NORTH				
Canada	0.2	0.02	0.1	0.01
Canada, Alberta	0,0	0,02	0,1	0,04
Canada, British Columbia	0,1	0,03	0,0	0,01
Canada, Manitoba	0,1	0,06	0,0	0,03
Canada, New Brunswick	-	-	0,1	0,07
Canada, Newfoundland	0,1	0,06	0,0	0,03
Canada, Northwest Territories	0,3	0,34	-	-
Canada, Nova Scotia	0,1	0,05	0,0	0,04
Canada, Ontario	0.2	0.03	0.1	0.02
Canada, Prince Edward Island	0,3	0,26	-	-
Canada, Quebec	0.3	0.04	0.3	0.04
Canada, Saskatchewan	0,1	0,06	0,1	0,07
Canada, Yukon	-	-	-	-
US, Cent. Calif.: Non-Hisp. White	0,0	0,03	0,1	0,06
US, Cent. Calif.: Hispanic	0,1	0,06	0,3	0,16
US, Los Angeles: Non-Hisp. White	0.1	0.03	0.1	0.04
US, Los Angeles: Hispanic White	0,1	0,04	0,0	0,03
US, Los Angeles: Black	0,1	0,05	-	-
US, Los Angeles: Chinese	0,3	0,23	-	-
US, Los Angeles: Filipino	-	-	0,2	0,22
US, Los Angeles: Korean	-	-	-	-
US, Los Angeles: Japanese	0,6	0,41	-	-
US, San Francisco: Non-Hisp. White	0,1	0,03	0,1	0,05
US, San Francisco: Hispanic White	-	-	0,1	0,10
US, San Francisco: Black	0,1	0,09	0,0	0,04
US, San Francisco: Chinese	-	-	-	-
US, San Francisco: Filipino	0,4	0,33	0,1	0,14
US, San Francisco: Japanese	-	-	-	-
US, Connecticut: White	0.1	0.03	0.1	0.02
US, Connecticut: Black	-	-	0,1	0,09
US, Atlanta: White	0,1	0,05	0,1	0,07
US, Atlanta: Black	0,1	0,05	-	-
US, Iowa	0,1	0,04	0,1	0,04

	MALE		FEMALE	
US, Central Louisiana: White	-	-	0,0	0,04
US, Central Louisiana: Black	-	-	0,4	0,37
US, New Orleans: White	0,1	0,07	0,1	0,07
US, New Orleans: Black	0,1	0,12	0,1	0,05
US, Detroit: White	0.2	0.05	0.1	0.03
US, Detroit: Black	0.4	0.14	0,1	0,04
US, New Mexico: Non-Hisp. White	0,1	0,05	-	-
US, New Mexico: Hispanic White	0,1	0,10	0,1	0,07
US, New Mexico: American Indian	-	-	-	-
US, Utah	0,0	0,02	0,1	0,04
US, Seattle	0.2	0.05	0.1	0.03
US, SEER: White	0.1	0.02	0.1	0.01
US, SEER: Black	0.2	0.07	0,0	0,02
ASIA				
*China, Qidong	0,1	0,04	0,1	0,06
China, Shanghai	0.1	0.02	0.1	0.02
China, Tianjin	0.1	0.04	0.1	0.04
Hong Kong	0,0	0,02	0,0	0,01
*India, Bangalore	0,0	0,01	0,0	0,02
*India, Barshi, Paranda and Bhum	-	-	-	-
India, Bombay	0.1	0.02	0,0	0,01
*India, Karunagappally	-	-	-	-
India, Madras	-	-	0,0	0,01
*India, Trivandrum	0,1	0,07	-	-
Israel: All Jews	0.1	0.04	0,0	0,02
Jews born in Israel	0,3	0,21	0,1	0,09
Jews born in America or Europe	0.2	0.05	0,1	0,04
Jews born in Africa or Asia	0,1	0,05	0,0	0,03
Non-Jews	0,2	0,14	0,0	0,04
Japan, Hiroshima	-	-	0,0	0,03
Japan, Miyagi	0.2	0.06	0,1	0,05
Japan, Nagasaki	0,1	0,04	0,2	0,09
Japan, Osaka	0.1	0.02	0.1	0.02
*Japan, Saga	0,1	0,08	0,1	0,10
Japan, Yamagata	0,1	0,04	0,1	0,03
*Korea, Kangwha	0,4	0,36	-	-
*Kuwait: Non-Kuwaitis	-	-	-	-
*Kuwait: Kuwaitis	-	-	0,0	0,05
*Philippines, Manila	0,0	0,01	0,0	0,02
Singapore: Chinese	-	-	0,0	0,03
Singapore: Malay	0,1	0,10	-	-
Singapore: Indian	-	-	0,2	0,19
Thailand, Chiang Mai	-	-	0,0	0,03
*Thailand, Khon Kaen	-	-	-	-
*Viet Nam, Hanoi	0,1	0,04	0,0	0,04

* IMPORTANT-SEE NOTES ON POPULATION PAGE

EUROPE	MALE		FEMALE	
Austria, Tyrol	-	-	0,0	0,04
*Belarus	0.2	0.03	0.2	0.02
*Croatia	0,0	0,02	0,0	0,01
Czech Republic	0.2	0.03	0.1	0.02
Denmark	0,0	0,02	0.0	0.01
Estonia	0.3	0.10	0.2	0.05
Finland	0.1	0.02	0.0	0.01
France, Bas-Rhin	-	-	0,0	0,01
†*France, Calvados	-	-	0,1	0,07
France, Doubs	0,1	0,06	-	-
France, Haut-Rhin	0,2	0,09	-	-
*France, Herault	-	-	-	-
France, Isere	-	-	-	-
*France, Somme	0,1	0,08	-	-
*France, Tarn	-	-	-	-
Germany, Eastern States	0.1	0.03	0.1	0.02
Germany, Saarland	0,2	0,07	0.2	0.06
Iceland	0,2	0,17	0,1	0,07
Ireland, Southern	-	-	-	-
Italy, Ferrara	-	-	0,1	0,10
Italy, Florence	0,0	0,01	0,2	0,14
Italy, Genoa	0,0	0,02	-	-
*Italy, Latina	-	-	-	-
Italy, Macerata	-	-	-	-
Italy, Modena	0,0	0,04	-	-
Italy, Parma	0,1	0,06	-	-
Italy, Ragusa	-	-	-	-
Italy, Romagna	0,0	0,04	0,1	0,07
Italy, Torino	0,0	0,03	0,1	0,06
Italy, Trieste	0,6	0,30	0,2	0,13
Italy, Varese	-	-	0,0	0,04
Italy, Veneto	0,1	0,05	0,1	0,04
*Latvia	0.8	0.11	0.5	0.07
Malta	-	-	-	-
The Netherlands	0.2	0.02	0.1	0.02
The Netherlands, Eindhoven	0,3	0,09	0,2	0,10
The Netherlands, Maastricht	0,0	0,03	0,0	0,04
Norway	0.6	0.06	0.3	0.04
*Poland, Cracow	0,1	0,08	0,1	0,11
*Poland, Kielce	0,1	0,05	0,0	0,03
*Poland, Lower Silesia	0.4	0.08	0.3	0.05
Poland, Warsaw City	0,0	0,03	0,1	0,04
Slovakia	0,1	0,02	0.1	0.02
Slovenia	-	-	0,0	0,01
*Spain, Albacete	-	-	-	-
Spain, Asturias	-	-	0,0	0,01
Spain, Basque Country	0,1	0,03	0,0	0,01
Spain, Granada	0,1	0,07	0,1	0,10
Spain, Mallorca	-	-	0,0	0,04
Spain, Murcia	0,0	0,03	0,1	0,04
Spain, Navarra	0,1	0,06	0,1	0,07
Spain, Tarragona	0,1	0,07	-	-
Spain, Zaragoza	0,0	0,02	0,1	0,04

	MALE		FEMALE	
Sweden	0.7	0.05	0.6	0.04
*Switzerland, Basel	-	-	-	-
Switzerland, Geneva	-	-	-	-
Switzerland, Graubunden	-	-	-	-
Switzerland, Neuchatel	0,2	0,15	-	-
Switzerland, St Gall-Appenzell	0,2	0,11	0,0	0,04
Switzerland, Valais	0,8	0,43	0,1	0,11
Switzerland, Vaud	-	-	0,1	0,05
Switzerland, Zurich	0,2	0,08	0,1	0,05
*UK, England and Wales	0.1	0.01	0.0	0.01
*UK, East Anglia	0,0	0,03	0,0	0,01
*UK, Mersey	0,1	0,02	0,0	0,02
*UK, North Western	0,0	0,02	0,0	0,00
UK, Oxford	0,1	0,05	0,1	0,04
*UK, South Thames	0.0	0.02	0,0	0,02
UK, South Western	0,0	0,02	0,0	0,02
UK, Wessex	0.1	0.03	0,0	0,01
*UK, West Midlands	0.1	0.02	0,0	0,02
UK, Yorkshire	0,1	0,03	0,0	0,01
UK, Scotland	0,0	0,02	0,0	0,02
UK, Scotland, West	0,0	0,02	0,0	0,01
*Yugoslavia, Vojvodina	-	-	0,0	0,02

OCEANIA	MALE		FEMALE	
Australian Capital Territory	0,2	0,21	-	-
Australia, New South Wales	0.1	0.02	0,0	0,01
South Australia	0,1	0,06	0,2	0,07
Australia, Tasmania	0,1	0,09	0,1	0,11
Australia, Victoria	0.1	0.03	0.1	0.03
Western Australia	0,2	0,06	0,0	0,04
*French Polynesia	0,2	0,18	0,3	0,26
New Zealand: Non-Maori	0.1	0.04	0,1	0,03
New Zealand: Maori	0,6	0,36	0,1	0,14
US, Hawaii: White	0,2	0,15	-	-
US, Hawaii: Japanese	0,5	0,32	-	-
US, Hawaii: Hawaiian	0,3	0,28	-	-
US, Hawaii: Filipino	-	-	-	-
US, Hawaii: Chinese	-	-	-	-

* IMPORTANT-SEE NOTES ON POPULATION PAGE

AGE-STANDARDIZED INCIDENCE
RATES AND STANDARD ERRORS (per 100,000)
Leukaemia, unspecified (ICD-9 208)

	MALE		FEMALE	
AFRICA				
*Algeria, Setif	1.3	0.37	0.7	0.22
*France, La Reunion	0,2	0,14	0,1	0,08
*Mali, Bamako	0.8	0.28	0.8	0.27
*Uganda, Kyadondo	0,3	0,14	0,5	0,25
*Zimbabwe, Harare: African	0,6	0,42	-	-
*Zimbabwe, Harare: European	1,0	0,97	-	-
AMERICA, CENTRAL AND SOUTH				
*Argentina, Concordia	1,0	0,61	1,2	0,57
*Brazil, Belem	0.7	0.22	0.8	0.22
*Brazil, Goiania	1.3	0.35	1.0	0.30
*Brazil, Porto Alegre	1.2	0.31	1.1	0.25 m
Colombia, Cali	2.0	0.29	1.3	0.20
*Costa Rica	0.9	0.14	0.8	0.12
*Ecuador, Quito	1.7	0.30	1.0	0.21
*Peru, Lima	0.6	0.12	0.4	0.10
Peru, Trujillo	1,1	0,50	0,3	0,21
US, Puerto Rico	0.9	0.11	0.4	0.07
*Uruguay, Montevideo	1.5	0.25	1.2	0.21
AMERICA, NORTH				
Canada	1.0	0.03	0.7	0.03
Canada, Alberta	0.4	0.08	0.3	0.06
Canada, British Columbia	0.7	0.08	0.5	0.06
Canada, Manitoba	0.4	0.10	0.2	0.07
Canada, New Brunswick	1.4	0.26	0.8	0.18
Canada, Newfoundland	0,5	0,20	0,3	0,13
Canada, Northwest Territories	0,3	0,34	0,6	0,64
Canada, Nova Scotia	2.3	0.29	1.1	0.18
Canada, Ontario	1.0	0.06	0.7	0.04
Canada, Prince Edward Island	0,4	0,26	0,1	0,08
Canada, Quebec	1.2	0.08	0.9	0.07
Canada, Saskatchewan	0.5	0.12	0.3	0.09
Canada, Yukon	-	-	-	-
US, Cent. Calif.: Non-Hisp. White	0.7	0.12	0.3	0.07
US, Cent. Calif.: Hispanic	0,5	0,20	0,4	0,18
US, Los Angeles: Non-Hisp. White	0.6	0.07	0.4	0.06
US, Los Angeles: Hispanic White	0.7	0.13	0.3	0.07
US, Los Angeles: Black	0.5	0.16	0.5	0.14
US, Los Angeles: Chinese	-	-	0,4	0,22
US, Los Angeles: Filipino	1,2	0,51	0,4	0,25
US, Los Angeles: Korean	1,2	0,60	0,3	0,30
US, Los Angeles: Japanese	0,2	0,17	-	-
US, San Francisco: Non-Hisp. White	0.5	0.09	0.3	0.06
US, San Francisco: Hispanic White	0,5	0,22	0,3	0,15
US, San Francisco: Black	0,6	0,24	0,3	0,14
US, San Francisco: Chinese	0,3	0,18	0,4	0,20
US, San Francisco: Filipino	0,7	0,44	1,3	0,66
US, San Francisco: Japanese	-	-	-	-
US, Connecticut: White	1.0	0.11	0.6	0.07
US, Connecticut: Black	0,7	0,36	0,6	0,33
US, Atlanta: White	0.5	0.12	0,1	0,05
US, Atlanta: Black	1.1	0.36	0,2	0,12
US, Iowa	0.8	0.10	0.4	0.06

	MALE		FEMALE	
US, Central Louisiana: White	0,8	0,37	0,1	0,08
US, Central Louisiana: Black	1,4	1,03	-	-
US, New Orleans: White	0.7	0.19	0.6	0.20
US, New Orleans: Black	1.8	0.49	0.4	0.18
US, Detroit: White	1.1	0.11	0.7	0.08
US, Detroit: Black	0.6	0.16	0.5	0.13
US, New Mexico: Non-Hisp. White	0.8	0.17	0.8	0.17
US, New Mexico: Hispanic White	0.3	0.15	0.8	0.24
US, New Mexico: American Indian	0.6	0.43	-	-
US, Utah	0.9	0.14	0.3	0.08
US, Seattle	0.9	0.10	0.5	0.07
US, SEER: White	0.8	0.04	0.5	0.03
US, SEER: Black	0.8	0.12	0.4	0.08
ASIA				
*China, Qidong	0.9	0.18	0.7	0.17
China, Shanghai	1.0	0.08	0.8	0.07
China, Tianjin	1.6	0.14	1.6	0.14
Hong Kong	0.9	0.08	0.7	0.07
*India, Bangalore	0.5	0.08	0.5	0.09
*India, Barshi, Paranda and Bhum	0,1	0,07	-	-
India, Bombay	0.4	0.05	0.4	0.05
*India, Karunagappally	0,4	0,31	0,2	0,22
India, Madras	0.2	0.04	0.2	0.05
*India, Trivandrum	0,2	0,14	0,5	0,28
Israel: All Jews	0.7	0.08	0.5	0.06
Jews born in Israel	0.6	0.26	0.2	0,14
Jews born in America or Europe	0.7	0.13	0.5	0.08
Jews born in Africa or Asia	0.6	0.13	0.4	0.11
Non-Jews	1.1	0.35	1.1	0.31
Japan, Hiroshima	0.5	0.14	0.2	0,06
Japan, Miyagi	0.6	0.10	0.2	0.05
Japan, Nagasaki	1.0	0.15	0.3	0.07
Japan, Osaka	0.7	0.06	0.4	0.04
*Japan, Saga	0.5	0.15	0.5	0.14
Japan, Yamagata	0.5	0.10	0.5	0.12
*Korea, Kangwha	2,0	1,22	0,5	0,33
*Kuwait: Non-Kuwaitis	0,3	0,12	1,4	0,76
*Kuwait: Kuwaitis	1.6	0.49	0,6	0,37
*Philippines, Manila	1.6	0.16	1.9	0.16
Singapore: Chinese	0.3	0.09	0.3	0.08
Singapore: Malay	0,6	0,29	0,1	0,11
Singapore: Indian	0,1	0,14	0,3	0,28
Thailand, Chiang Mai	0.8	0.16	0.9	0.18
*Thailand, Khon Kaen	1.2	0.22	1.1	0.19
*Viet Nam, Hanoi	1.3	0.22	1.4	0.22

f

* IMPORTANT-SEE NOTES ON POPULATION PAGE

EUROPE	MALE		FEMALE	
Austria, Tyrol	0,4	0,14	0,2	0,08
*Belarus	1.2	0.07	0.9	0.05
*Croatia	0.7	0.08	0.4	0.06
Czech Republic	0.5	0.04	0.3	0.03
Denmark	0.2	0.04	0.2	0.03
Estonia	0.5	0.11	0.7	0.13
Finland	0.2	0.04	0.2	0.03
France, Bas-Rhin	0.5	0.14	0,2	0,08
†*France, Calvados	0,1	0,06	0,1	0,06
France, Doubs	0.7	0.24	0,4	0,15
France, Haut-Rhin	0.7	0.22	0.4	0.12
*France, Herault	0.9	0.21	0.7	0.20
France, Isere	0,2	0,08	0,1	0,09
*France, Somme	0,2	0,13	0,2	0,11
*France, Tarn	0,1	0,09	0,1	0,05
Germany, Eastern States	0.5	0.06	0.4	0.04
Germany, Saarland	0.4	0.11	0.5	0.12
Iceland	0,2	0,17	0,7	0,29
Ireland, Southern	1.1	0.25	0,3	0,13
Italy, Ferrara	2.1	0.66	-	-
Italy, Florence	1.1	0.18	0.4	0.12
Italy, Genoa	0.6	0.14	0.2	0.06
*Italy, Latina	0.9	0.31	0.8	0.27
Italy, Macerata	2,4	1,15	3,1	1,36
Italy, Modena	0,1	0,07	0,2	0,07
Italy, Parma	1.3	0.27	0.9	0.27
Italy, Ragusa	0.8	0.29	0.3	0,18
Italy, Romagna	0.6	0.15	0.6	0.26
Italy, Torino	0.9	0.17	0.3	0.09
Italy, Trieste	0,6	0,28	0,5	0,26
Italy, Varese	0.3	0.11	0,1	0,05
Italy, Veneto	1.0	0.16	0.7	0.18
*Latvia	0.3	0.07	0.2	0.04
Malta	-	-	0,2	0,19
The Netherlands	0.3	0.03	0.2	0.03
The Netherlands, Eindhoven	0,1	0,06	0,2	0,12
The Netherlands, Maastricht	0.4	0.12	0.3	0,09
Norway	0.1	0.03	0.1	0.02
*Poland, Cracow	0.8	0.22	0.5	0.12
*Poland, Kielce	0.4	0.12	0.2	0.06
*Poland, Lower Silesia	0.6	0.10	0.4	0.06
Poland, Warsaw City	0.7	0.13	0.3	0.09
Slovakia	0.4	0.05	0.3	0.04
Slovenia	0.2	0.06	0,1	0,03
*Spain, Albacete	0,8	0,47	0,4	0,30
Spain, Asturias	2.7	0.33	1.8	0.28
Spain, Basque Country	1.0	0.15	0.9	0.16
Spain, Granada	0.6	0.15	0.8	0.18
Spain, Mallorca	0,4	0,18	0.5	0.14
Spain, Murcia	0.5	0.14	0.4	0.09
Spain, Navarra	1.4	0.30	0.9	0.27
Spain, Tarragona	0.8	0.20	0.5	0.15
Spain, Zaragoza	0,3	0,10	0.3	0.10

	MALE		FEMALE	
Sweden	0.4	0.03	0.2	0.03
*Switzerland, Basel	0,3	0,13	0,1	0,04
Switzerland, Geneva	0,2	0,11	0,1	0,04
Switzerland, Graubunden	-	-	0,1	0,08
Switzerland, Neuchatel	0,2	0,12	0,1	0,09
Switzerland, St Gall-Appenzell	0,5	0,21	0,3	0,17
Switzerland, Valais	0,7	0,33	0,3	0,19
Switzerland, Vaud	0.8	0.24	0.2	0.09
Switzerland, Zurich	0,1	0,05	0.2	0.06
*UK, England and Wales	0.5	0.02	0.3	0.02
*UK, East Anglia	0.2	0.05	0.2	0.06
*UK, Mersey	0.2	0.05	0.2	0.04
*UK, North Western	0.4	0.05	0.2	0.04
UK, Oxford	0.3	0.06	0.2	0.04
*UK, South Thames	0.5	0.05	0.3	0.04
UK, South Western	0.5	0.07	0.3	0.04
UK, Wessex	0.4	0.06	0.2	0.04
*UK, West Midlands	0.8	0.07	0.5	0.06
UK, Yorkshire	0.3	0.05	0.1	0.03
UK, Scotland	0.4	0.05	0.3	0.03
UK, Scotland, West	0.4	0.07	0.4	0.06
*Yugoslavia, Vojvodina	0.5	0.10	0.3	0.06

OCEANIA

	MALE		FEMALE	
Australian Capital Territory	-	-	0,1	0,11
Australia, New South Wales	0.5	0.05	0.3	0.04
South Australia	0.0	0,01	0,1	0,05
Australia, Tasmania	0,4	0,18	0,1	0,06
Australia, Victoria	0.4	0.06	0.3	0.04
Western Australia	0.6	0.11	0.4	0.08
*French Polynesia	3.9	1.20	1,9	0,80
New Zealand: Non-Maori	0.6	0.08	0.3	0.06
New Zealand: Maori	1,0	0,53	1,3	0,61
US, Hawaii: White	0,9	0,31	0,2	0,14
US, Hawaii: Japanese	0,8	0,27	0,2	0,14
US, Hawaii: Hawaiian	0,9	0,44	0,2	0,25
US, Hawaii: Filipino	0,5	0,25	0,8	0,41
US, Hawaii: Chinese	-	-	0,3	0,31

* IMPORTANT-SEE NOTES ON POPULATION PAGE

AGE-STANDARDIZED INCIDENCE
RATES AND STANDARD ERRORS (per 100,000)
All leukaemias (ICD-9 204-8)

	MALE		FEMALE	
AFRICA				
*Algeria, Setif	6.2	0.81	3.8	0.51
*France, La Reunion	5.5	0.69	4.6	0.59
*Mali, Bamako	1.0	0.30	1.9	0.46
*Uganda, Kyadondo	0.7	0.27	1.2	0.45
*Zimbabwe, Harare: African	5.7	1.03	4.8	1.17
*Zimbabwe, Harare: European	7,8	2,64	3,4	1,73
AMERICA, CENTRAL AND SOUTH				
*Argentina, Concordia	3,1	1,04	3.3	0.96
*Brazil, Belem	3.8	0.57	2.7	0.42
*Brazil, Goiania	5.8	0.70	4.1	0.55
*Brazil, Porto Alegre	7.3	0.76	5.9	0.56 mf
Colombia, Cali	6.2	0.50	5.4	0.42
*Costa Rica	7.8	0.38	6.3	0.32
*Ecuador, Quito	8.1	0.64	5.9	0.49
*Peru, Lima	4.4	0.30	3.8	0.27
Peru, Trujillo	4.9	1.00	5.2	1.00
US, Puerto Rico	6.6	0.31	4.8	0.26
*Uruguay, Montevideo	7.5	0.59	5.2	0.45
AMERICA, NORTH				
Canada	10.7	0.12	6.9	0.10
Canada, Alberta	8.8	0.38	6.1	0.31
Canada, British Columbia	8.4	0.31	5.8	0.26
Canada, Manitoba	9.8	0.57	5.9	0.45
Canada, New Brunswick	8.2	0.65	5.9	0.56
Canada, Newfoundland	6.6	0.70	5.6	0.68
Canada, Northwest Territories	4.6	1.44	3.8	1.23
Canada, Nova Scotia	8.9	0.61	6.0	0.50
Canada, Ontario	12.3	0.21	7.8	0.16
Canada, Prince Edward Island	8.8	1.57	5.2	1.26
Canada, Quebec	11.1	0.25	6.9	0.19
Canada, Saskatchewan	12.5	0.67	7.5	0.52
Canada, Yukon	12.5	3.34	11.7	3.62
US, Cent. Calif.: Non-Hisp. White	9.7	0.49	6.5	0.40
US, Cent. Calif.: Hispanic	9.3	0.86	5.8	0.65
US, Los Angeles: Non-Hisp. White	11.3	0.34	7.2	0.27
US, Los Angeles: Hispanic White	8.5	0.41	6.1	0.31
US, Los Angeles: Black	9.9	0.67	5.4	0.44
US, Los Angeles: Chinese	6.1	1.01	4.5	0.91
US, Los Angeles: Filipino	11.4	1.56	6.9	1.24
US, Los Angeles: Korean	4.6	1.23	3.9	1.07
US, Los Angeles: Japanese	7.2	1.57	7.0	1.91
US, San Francisco: Non-Hisp. White	10.8	0.44	6.1	0.33
US, San Francisco: Hispanic White	8.1	0.92	7.8	0.84
US, San Francisco: Black	9.1	0.95	5.7	0.71
US, San Francisco: Chinese	7.7	1.18	4.7	0.86
US, San Francisco: Filipino	9.8	1.64	8.4	1.51
US, San Francisco: Japanese	5,7	2,50	1,9	0,95
US, Connecticut: White	10.0	0.35	6.3	0.28
US, Connecticut: Black	7.7	1.20	6.3	0.97
US, Atlanta: White	8.9	0.51	5.7	0.39
US, Atlanta: Black	8.7	0.94	5.3	0.62
US, Iowa	12.1	0.39	7.2	0.29

	MALE		FEMALE	
US, Central Louisiana: White	7.2	1.03	4.3	0.70
US, Central Louisiana: Black	8.4	2.29	1,6	0,73
US, New Orleans: White	9.6	0.79	7.2	0.69
US, New Orleans: Black	9.4	1.11	4.9	0.69
US, Detroit: White	12.7	0.40	7.7	0.30
US, Detroit: Black	9.6	0.67	6.2	0.48
US, New Mexico: Non-Hisp. White	11.3	0.72	7.2	0.57
US, New Mexico: Hispanic White	9.3	0.86	5.4	0.63
US, New Mexico: American Indian	6.1	1.41	3.5	1.00
US, Utah	8.8	0.47	5.9	0.36
US, Seattle	10.9	0.36	6.6	0.27
US, SEER: White	10.9	0.15	6.7	0.11
US, SEER: Black	9.1	0.42	5.9	0.30
ASIA				
*China, Qidong	3.8	0.38	3.4	0.36
China, Shanghai	4.9	0.18	3.7	0.15
China, Tianjin	4.9	0.25	3.9	0.23
Hong Kong	6.8	0.23	4.9	0.20
*India, Bangalore	3.5	0.21	2.8	0.20
*India, Barshi, Paranda and Bhum	1.8	0.42	0.9	0.28
India, Bombay	4.1	0.16	3.0	0.15
*India, Karunagappally	3.6	0.99	1,9	0,71
India, Madras	3.0	0.19	2.0	0.17
*India, Trivandrum	3.2	0.62	3.3	0.62
Israel: All Jews	7.3	0.27	4.9	0.21
Jews born in Israel	7.1	0.82	5.4	0.69
Jews born in America or Europe	9.9	1.00	6.1	0.83
Jews born in Africa or Asia	7.0	1.06	7.5	2.93
Non-Jews	6.0	0.72	4.4	0.58
Japan, Hiroshima	5.8	0.47	3.3	0.35
Japan, Miyagi	6.0	0.34	3.3	0.24
Japan, Nagasaki	5.7	0.40	4.2	0.35
Japan, Osaka	5.8	0.17	3.8	0.14
*Japan, Saga	8.8	0.62	5.2	0.47
Japan, Yamagata	4.4	0.36	3.4	0.33
*Korea, Kangwha	7.4	2.07	2,4	0,87
*Kuwait: Non-Kuwaitis	6.8	1.26	6.3	1.33
*Kuwait: Kuwaitis	5.1	0.82	4.6	0.92
*Philippines, Manila	5.8	0.31	5.1	0.26
Singapore: Chinese	6.0	0.37	4.2	0.31
Singapore: Malay	6.4	0.92	4.3	0.76
Singapore: Indian	3.0	0.76	5.4	1.43
Thailand, Chiang Mai	4.7	0.38	4.5	0.39
*Thailand, Khon Kaen	3.9	0.39	3.5	0.35
*Viet Nam, Hanoi	3.6	0.35	3.3	0.33

* IMPORTANT-SEE NOTES ON POPULATION PAGE

EUROPE	MALE		FEMALE	
Austria, Tyrol	9.6	0.78	5.7	0.58
*Belarus	9.9	0.20	5.9	0.14
*Croatia	8.6	0.31	5.6	0.23
Czech Republic	9.3	0.19	5.7	0.14
Denmark	9.6	0.26	6.0	0.21
Estonia	8.8	0.48	5.7	0.35
Finland	7.1	0.22	5.1	0.19
France, Bas-Rhin	8.7	0.60	4.9	0.43
†*France, Calvados	3.0	0.41	2.8	0.39
France, Doubs	8.0	0.80	5.1	0.64
France, Haut-Rhin	7.6	0.67	5.2	0.54
*France, Herault	6.0	0.54	3.8	0.45
France, Isere	8.2	0.54	4.3	0.41
*France, Somme	7.8	0.72	5.4	0.60
*France, Tarn	6.1	0.81	4.9	0.81
Germany, Eastern States	7.0	0.21	4.7	0.16
Germany, Saarland	9.3	0.55	5.8	0.44
Iceland	5.9	0.93	5.0	0.91
Ireland, Southern	11.1	0.86	5.7	0.64
Italy, Ferrara	9.6	1.59	5.2	0.99
Italy, Florence	8.5	0.56	5.9	0.55
Italy, Genoa	7.5	0.67	5.4	0.60
*Italy, Latina	10.3	1.01	6.5	0.84
Italy, Macerata	8.8	1.89	7.4	1.97
Italy, Modena	6.8	0.58	6.3	0.73
Italy, Parma	7.0	0.77	5.7	0.87
Italy, Ragusa	7.1	0.96	5.1	0.79
Italy, Romagna	9.8	0.81	6.2	0.75
Italy, Torino	9.6	0.78	6.0	0.61
Italy, Trieste	15.0	1.78	9.0	1.37
Italy, Varese	10.0	0.78	6.5	0.59
Italy, Veneto	9.2	0.57	6.5	0.50
*Latvia	8.3	0.35	5.6	0.26
Malta	7.6	1.38	6.0	1.21
The Netherlands	7.7	0.16	4.8	0.13
The Netherlands, Eindhoven	6.5	0.52	4.4	0.43
The Netherlands, Maastricht	8.2	0.62	5.5	0.48
Norway	6.2	0.23	4.3	0.20
*Poland, Cracow	7.2	0.65	4.3	0.47
*Poland, Kielce	6.0	0.45	3.9	0.36
*Poland, Lower Silesia	7.8	0.34	5.0	0.25
Poland, Warsaw City	6.7	0.48	4.7	0.39
Slovakia	8.9	0.26	5.4	0.19
Slovenia	7.4	0.39	5.8	0.34
*Spain, Albacete	9.3	1.70	3.9	1.04
Spain, Asturias	9.3	0.64	6.1	0.49
Spain, Basque Country	8.0	0.47	4.6	0.35
Spain, Granada	6.7	0.55	5.4	0.53
Spain, Mallorca	7.2	0.67	5.6	0.62
Spain, Murcia	7.8	0.55	5.3	0.45
Spain, Navarra	8.0	0.77	4.6	0.61
Spain, Tarragona	8.2	0.74	4.7	0.62
Spain, Zaragoza	6.2	0.56	5.6	0.52

	MALE		FEMALE	
Sweden	8.6	0.19	6.1	0.16
*Switzerland, Basel	6.9	0.81	4.4	0.58
Switzerland, Geneva	10.5	1.06	6.0	0.80
Switzerland, Graubunden	9.3	1.49	5.4	1.22
Switzerland, Neuchatel	7.8	1.26	3.2	0.68
Switzerland, St Gall-Appenzell	10.0	0.90	5.3	0.63
Switzerland, Valais	8.8	1.31	4.8	0.96
Switzerland, Vaud	7.8	0.72	4.4	0.53
Switzerland, Zurich	8.8	0.56	5.4	0.43
*UK, England and Wales	8.4	0.10	5.4	0.08
*UK, East Anglia	7.0	0.34	4.5	0.28
*UK, Mersey	5.5	0.28	4.3	0.25
*UK, North Western	7.3	0.26	4.6	0.20
UK, Oxford	9.3	0.37	6.3	0.31
*UK, South Thames	8.1	0.21	5.4	0.17
UK, South Western	9.4	0.31	6.1	0.26
UK, Wessex	10.1	0.34	6.3	0.27
*UK, West Midlands	9.0	0.25	5.3	0.19
UK, Yorkshire	8.4	0.29	5.0	0.23
UK, Scotland	8.5	0.25	5.4	0.20
UK, Scotland, West	8.3	0.34	5.3	0.26
*Yugoslavia, Vojvodina	8.2	0.39	4.5	0.28

OCEANIA

	MALE		FEMALE	
Australian Capital Territory	10.5	1.41	4.7	0.87
Australia, New South Wales	10.4	0.26	6.3	0.20
South Australia	13.3	0.57	8.9	0.47
Australia, Tasmania	11.4	0.94	7.0	0.71
Australia, Victoria	10.0	0.30	5.8	0.22
Western Australia	9.2	0.47	5.5	0.36
*French Polynesia	9.3	1.69	7.1	1.48
New Zealand: Non-Maori	10.7	0.36	7.0	0.29
New Zealand: Maori	12.2	1.71	7.8	1.24
US, Hawaii: White	10.6	1.17	4.8	0.80
US, Hawaii: Japanese	5.6	0.95	4.3	0.97
US, Hawaii: Hawaiian	9.5	1.53	6.6	1.23
US, Hawaii: Filipino	8.1	1.35	5.9	1.22
US, Hawaii: Chinese	5.2	1.81	1,6	0,76

* IMPORTANT-SEE NOTES ON POPULATION PAGE

AGE-STANDARDIZED INCIDENCE
RATES AND STANDARD ERRORS (per 100,000)
Other and Unspecified

AFRICA	MALE		FEMALE	
*Algeria, Setif	5.7	0.87	2.5	0.46
*France, La Reunion	8.0	0.87	4.4	0.59
*Mali, Bamako	3.5	0.74	2.7	0.60
*Uganda, Kyadondo	6.6	1.35	5.9	1.22 m
*Zimbabwe, Harare: African	7.2	1.37	6.5	1.54
*Zimbabwe, Harare: European	15.4	3.72	8.7	2.64

AMERICA, CENTRAL AND SOUTH	MALE		FEMALE	
*Argentina, Concordia	32.5	3.43	20.4	2.44
*Brazil, Belem	14.0	1.31	9.2	0.90 f
*Brazil, Goiania	13.4	1.22	9.1	0.89
*Brazil, Porto Alegre	15.5	1.08	11.7	0.73
Colombia, Cali	10.7	0.72	12.0	0.69
*Costa Rica	10.0	0.47	8.3	0.41
*Ecuador, Quito	7.1	0.66	9.3	0.68
*Peru, Lima	6.7	0.42	6.6	0.39
Peru, Trujillo	6.7	1.23	8.4	1.34
US, Puerto Rico	8.5	0.34	5.9	0.26
*Uruguay, Montevideo	25.3	1.01	15.2	0.64

AMERICA, NORTH	MALE		FEMALE	
Canada	12.0	0.12	8.6	0.09
Canada, Alberta	10.4	0.40	8.8	0.34
Canada, British Columbia	10.4	0.31	9.1	0.28
Canada, Manitoba	10.2	0.54	8.8	0.47
Canada, New Brunswick	10.5	0.69	8.9	0.59
Canada, Newfoundland	10.7	0.83	10.3	0.80
Canada, Northwest Territories	10.2	2.88	10.9	3.01
Canada, Nova Scotia	14.9	0.73	10.4	0.58
Canada, Ontario	14.3	0.21	8.6	0.15
Canada, Prince Edward Island	11.8	1.70	6.7	1.07
Canada, Quebec	10.9	0.23	8.2	0.18
Canada, Saskatchewan	7.9	0.47	6.9	0.43
Canada, Yukon	18.3	4.58	25.6	5.98
US, Cent. Calif.: Non-Hisp. White	11.5	0.50	7.3	0.36
US, Cent. Calif.: Hispanic	9.3	0.96	7.3	0.82
US, Los Angeles: Non-Hisp. White	11.0	0.29	9.0	0.24
US, Los Angeles: Hispanic White	8.9	0.49	7.3	0.37
US, Los Angeles: Black	14.7	0.82	9.9	0.59
US, Los Angeles: Chinese	8.4	1.23	6.0	0.91
US, Los Angeles: Filipino	7.3	1.20	5.7	1.06
US, Los Angeles: Korean	5.5	1.30	6.6	1.28
US, Los Angeles: Japanese	5.0	1.08	4.6	0.92
US, San Francisco: Non-Hisp. White	9.9	0.37	8.6	0.31
US, San Francisco: Hispanic White	7.6	0.94	6.9	0.77
US, San Francisco: Black	15.7	1.28	11.2	0.93
US, San Francisco: Chinese	7.3	0.91	7.2	0.90
US, San Francisco: Filipino	8.2	1.48	6.1	1.12
US, San Francisco: Japanese	4,6	1,74	5.3	1.55
US, Connecticut: White	10.6	0.33	7.8	0.25
US, Connecticut: Black	14.0	1.70	11.0	1.25
US, Atlanta: White	9.0	0.50	6.5	0.38
US, Atlanta: Black	18.3	1.44	10.3	0.85
US, Iowa	8.4	0.30	6.2	0.23

	MALE		FEMALE	
US, Central Louisiana: White	12.8	1.36	7.6	0.95
US, Central Louisiana: Black	19.6	3.50	9.6	2.23
US, New Orleans: White	11.0	0.75	7.2	0.53
US, New Orleans: Black	16.4	1.48	11.3	1.01
US, Detroit: White	9.3	0.32	7.1	0.25
US, Detroit: Black	12.0	0.75	8.7	0.55
US, New Mexico: Non-Hisp. White	10.4	0.63	6.7	0.46
US, New Mexico: Hispanic White	8.9	0.84	6.1	0.63
US, New Mexico: American Indian	8.1	1.91	7.7	1.68
US, Utah	8.2	0.45	6.8	0.38
US, Seattle	8.0	0.29	6.6	0.24
US, SEER: White	9.2	0.13	7.1	0.10
US, SEER: Black	14.1	0.53	9.7	0.37

ASIA	MALE		FEMALE	
*China, Qidong	0.9	0.17	0.8	0.16
China, Shanghai	6.6	0.18	4.8	0.14
China, Tianjin	4.7	0.23	4.6	0.22
Hong Kong	14.9	0.32	9.9	0.25
*India, Bangalore	12.0	0.44	9.5	0.40
*India, Barshi, Paranda and Bhum	6.7	0.90	4.3	0.70
India, Bombay	9.4	0.29	6.8	0.25
*India, Karunagappally	15.2	2.16	7.7	1.50
India, Madras	9.5	0.41	7.1	0.34
*India, Trivandrum	15.5	1.56	6.7	0.93
Israel: All Jews	13.5	0.36	11.7	0.31
Jews born in Israel	11.0	1.11	10.6	1.08
Jews born in America or Europe	14.2	0.58	13.0	0.52
Jews born in Africa or Asia	12.9	0.61	9.4	0.50
Non-Jews	10.3	1.06	6.9	0.80
Japan, Hiroshima	4.1	0.38	2.6	0.26
Japan, Miyagi	3.6	0.24	2.4	0.17
Japan, Nagasaki	3.5	0.25	2.1	0.17
Japan, Osaka	4.2	0.13	2.9	0.10
*Japan, Saga	3.0	0.31	2.5	0.28
Japan, Yamagata	4.0	0.29	2.6	0.20
*Korea, Kangwha	4.0	1.18	1,1	0,56
*Kuwait: Non-Kuwaitis	5.8	1.60	5.0	1.28
*Kuwait: Kuwaitis	6.4	1.08	7.4	1.32
*Philippines, Manila	12.1	0.53	8.8	0.40
Singapore: Chinese	7.6	0.43	5.6	0.33
Singapore: Malay	5.9	0.95	4.7	0.88
Singapore: Indian	4.4	0.92	4.0	1.32
Thailand, Chiang Mai	17.4	0.74	16.7	0.74
*Thailand, Khon Kaen	23.3	1.06	14.0	0.78
*Viet Nam, Hanoi	5.4	0.49	3.5	0.37

* IMPORTANT-SEE NOTES ON POPULATION PAGE

EUROPE	MALE		FEMALE	
Austria, Tyrol	6.2	0.59	6.0	0.49
*Belarus	5.5	0.15	2.7	0.09
*Croatia	14.0	0.36	9.7	0.25
Czech Republic	9.9	0.18	7.2	0.13
Denmark	12.5	0.26	11.0	0.23
Estonia	7.2	0.42	3.0	0.22
Finland	5.7	0.17	5.0	0.13
France, Bas-Rhin	17.4	0.81	7.9	0.50
*France, Calvados	6.8	0.63	2.5	0.33
France, Doubs	19.2	1.18	9.8	0.80
France, Haut-Rhin	9.5	0.70	4.5	0.43
*France, Herault	9.7	0.60	5.2	0.43
France, Isere	13.9	0.68	7.3	0.45
*France, Somme	9.4	0.76	4.6	0.48
*France, Tarn	10.2	0.89	5.7	0.67
Germany, Eastern States	2.6	0.12	2.4	0.10
Germany, Saarland	14.8	0.62	8.7	0.40
Iceland	7.9	1.02	6.5	0.88
Ireland, Southern	12.4	0.87	10.8	0.74
Italy, Ferrara	8.9	1.16	6.0	1.41
Italy, Florence	8.5	0.47	6.5	0.39
Italy, Genoa	9.8	0.55	5.6	0.35
*Italy, Latina	6.2	0.74	4.3	0.57
Italy, Macerata	7.9	1.53	5.4	0.89
Italy, Modena	8.9	0.59	6.4	0.49
Italy, Parma	7.9	0.66	4.2	0.42
Italy, Ragusa	5.4	0.73	3.1	0.52
Italy, Romagna	7.2	0.58	5.4	0.45
Italy, Torino	12.4	0.66	6.8	0.43
Italy, Trieste	-	-	-	-
Italy, Varese	10.4	0.61	4.6	0.33
Italy, Veneto	11.1	0.50	6.3	0.33
*Latvia	2.5	0.19	1.8	0.14
Malta	10.1	1.51	6.9	1.15
The Netherlands	14.0	0.19	8.5	0.14
The Netherlands, Eindhoven	16.5	0.77	9.8	0.54
The Netherlands, Maastricht	16.2	0.75	9.7	0.53
Norway	9.2	0.24	7.4	0.20
*Poland, Cracow	14.2	0.84	10.6	0.61
*Poland, Kielce	5.2	0.40	4.0	0.31
*Poland, Lower Silesia	13.5	0.44	9.1	0.31
Poland, Warsaw City	12.4	0.55	8.1	0.37
Slovakia	6.7	0.22	5.2	0.17
Slovenia	13.8	0.50	8.5	0.33
*Spain, Albacete	10.8	1.61	5.1	0.91
Spain, Asturias	12.2	0.62	6.7	0.42
Spain, Basque Country	16.9	0.55	7.9	0.35
Spain, Granada	11.1	0.67	6.2	0.43
Spain, Mallorca	15.0	0.87	8.3	0.57
Spain, Murcia	11.5	0.61	7.5	0.45
Spain, Navarra	10.3	0.73	6.3	0.53
Spain, Tarragona	13.5	0.85	8.1	0.62
Spain, Zaragoza	10.7	0.58	7.1	0.46

	MALE		FEMALE	
Sweden	8.8	0.16	8.0	0.15
*Switzerland, Basel	7.6	0.69	5.4	0.56
Switzerland, Geneva	8.2	0.83	5.7	0.59
Switzerland, Graubunden	5.8	1.09	4.1	0.78
Switzerland, Neuchatel	6.0	1.04	5.8	0.87
Switzerland, St Gall-Appenzell	5.8	0.59	4.1	0.45
Switzerland, Valais	16.2	1.60	7.2	0.90
Switzerland, Vaud	9.2	0.69	6.2	0.50
Switzerland, Zurich	7.8	0.44	5.8	0.33
*UK, England and Wales	15.4	0.12	11.2	0.09
*UK, East Anglia	13.0	0.39	10.3	0.34
*UK, Mersey	14.2	0.39	13.4	0.36
*UK, North Western	17.8	0.35	12.8	0.27
UK, Oxford	13.8	0.40	12.1	0.35
*UK, South Thames	12.9	0.22	9.8	0.18
UK, South Western	1.4	0.11	1.2	0.09
UK, Wessex	13.0	0.33	10.5	0.28
*UK, West Midlands	17.5	0.30	12.9	0.24
UK, Yorkshire	17.3	0.36	13.7	0.30
UK, Scotland	17.1	0.31	12.4	0.23
UK, Scotland, West	18.3	0.44	13.0	0.32
*Yugoslavia, Vojvodina	9.8	0.39	7.8	0.31

OCEANIA	MALE		FEMALE	
Australian Capital Territory	12.0	1.51	9.0	1.20
Australia, New South Wales	15.1	0.29	10.4	0.22
South Australia	11.0	0.48	9.0	0.40
Australia, Tasmania	14.5	1.00	9.4	0.72
Australia, Victoria	14.3	0.33	9.7	0.25
Western Australia	17.6	0.63	12.4	0.50
*French Polynesia	16.2	2.58	12.4	2.22
New Zealand: Non-Maori	15.0	0.40	13.1	0.35
New Zealand: Maori	29.8	3.11	21.8	2.29
US, Hawaii: White	8.4	0.96	8.7	0.99
US, Hawaii: Japanese	4.3	0.61	3.1	0.46
US, Hawaii: Hawaiian	7.8	1.43	7.8	1.35
US, Hawaii: Filipino	5.3	1.00	3.3	0.82
US, Hawaii: Chinese	5.9	1.52	4.1	1.10

* IMPORTANT-SEE NOTES ON POPULATION PAGE

AGE-STANDARDIZED INCIDENCE
RATES AND STANDARD ERRORS (per 100,000)
All sites

	MALE		FEMALE	
AFRICA				
*Algeria, Setif	111.0	3.83	69.2	2.41
*France, La Reunion	216.2	4.52	135.4	3.19
*Mali, Bamako	129.5	4.32	92.8	3.45
*Uganda, Kyadondo	158.2	6.38	146.6	5.59
*Zimbabwe, Harare: African	238.5	7.58	236.2	9.09
*Zimbabwe, Harare: European	825.4	29.67	640.2	26.27
AMERICA, CENTRAL AND SOUTH				
*Argentina, Concordia	293.5	10.32	256.0	8.72
*Brazil, Belem	218.4	5.19	199.4	4.01
*Brazil, Goiania	314.1	5.89	292.0	4.98
*Brazil, Porto Alegre	380.4	5.38	264.0	3.61
Colombia, Cali	187.6	2.98	202.5	2.76
*Costa Rica	232.5	2.27	201.7	1.98
*Ecuador, Quito	165.8	3.18	191.0	3.06
*Peru, Lima	134.1	1.83	159.7	1.90
Peru, Trujillo	168.3	6.50	205.9	6.47
US, Puerto Rico	212.8	1.69	152.2	1.37
*Uruguay, Montevideo	334.2	3.70	264.7	2.96
AMERICA, NORTH				
Canada				
Canada, Alberta				
Canada, British Columbia				
Canada, Manitoba				
Canada, New Brunswick				
Canada, Newfoundland				
Canada, Northwest Territories				
Canada, Nova Scotia				
Canada, Ontario				
Canada, Prince Edward Island				
Canada, Quebec				
Canada, Saskatchewan				
Canada, Yukon				
US, Cent. Calif.: Non-Hisp. White	351.8	2.79	271.2	2.40
US, Cent. Calif.: Hispanic	246.2	4.93	203.3	4.26
US, Los Angeles: Non-Hisp. White	374.5	1.71	304.3	1.53
US, Los Angeles: Hispanic White	239.7	2.47	200.0	1.93
US, Los Angeles: Black	425.8	4.43	262.4	3.03
US, Los Angeles: Chinese	182.2	5.48	144.8	4.60
US, Los Angeles: Filipino	211.1	6.64	189.2	5.55
US, Los Angeles: Korean	188.8	8.23	138.1	5.88
US, Los Angeles: Japanese	216.7	6.85	187.6	6.30
US, San Francisco: Non-Hisp. White	409.0	2.37	306.3	2.01
US, San Francisco: Hispanic White	295.0	5.74	231.7	4.55
US, San Francisco: Black	466.3	6.83	287.1	4.88
US, San Francisco: Chinese	218.3	5.14	204.3	5.03
US, San Francisco: Filipino	240.7	7.95	199.2	6.43
US, San Francisco: Japanese	250.3	13.77	211.2	10.57
US, Connecticut: White	357.5	1.92	290.0	1.68
US, Connecticut: Black	426.0	9.37	274.0	6.31
US, Atlanta: White	385.0	3.27	273.6	2.50
US, Atlanta: Black	450.5	7.13	253.7	4.29
US, Iowa	349.1	1.96	271.2	1.71

	MALE		FEMALE	
US, Central Louisiana: White	318.4	6.76	215.2	5.37
US, Central Louisiana: Black	391.9	15.95	210.4	10.28
US, New Orleans: White	389.9	4.52	273.2	3.57
US, New Orleans: Black	418.2	7.43	271.8	5.07
US, Detroit: White	402.0	2.10	294.2	1.71
US, Detroit: Black	465.1	4.63	279.4	3.19
US, New Mexico: Non-Hisp. White	355.3	3.66	262.1	3.14
US, New Mexico: Hispanic White	255.0	4.55	195.7	3.77
US, New Mexico: American Indian	151.3	8.22	147.8	7.36
US, Utah	308.7	2.78	229.2	2.34
US, Seattle	395.5	2.03	290.6	1.69
US, SEER: White	371.7	0.80	281.6	0.68
US, SEER: Black	455.3	3.00	272.6	2.04
ASIA				
*China, Qidong	207.1	2.65	102.9	1.77
China, Shanghai	230.5	1.05	154.3	0.83
China, Tianjin	190.0	1.43	149.9	1.23
Hong Kong	307.2	1.45	215.5	1.19
*India, Bangalore	99.8	1.26	119.5	1.40
*India, Barshi, Paranda and Bhum	51.8	2.46	55.0	2.48
India, Bombay	133.1	1.08	126.6	1.04
*India, Karunagappally	110.4	5.76	82.5	4.93
India, Madras	118.2	1.42	130.9	1.46
*India, Trivandrum	109.2	4.10	87.1	3.34
Israel: All Jews	238.5	1.52	242.1	1.50
Jews born in Israel	235.5	5.20	265.6	4.80
Jews born in America or Europe	259.1	2.72	271.5	2.89
Jews born in Africa or Asia	199.7	3.88	186.2	4.10
Non-Jews	128.3	3.68	95.0	2.87
Japan, Hiroshima	327.5	3.38	198.9	2.39
Japan, Miyagi	278.5	1.96	171.6	1.45
Japan, Nagasaki	293.2	2.32	177.8	1.71
Japan, Osaka	274.0	1.06	155.5	0.72
*Japan, Saga	269.4	2.93	144.9	2.01
Japan, Yamagata	261.6	2.30	153.8	1.72
*Korea, Kangwha	201.7	8.46	110.7	5.81
*Kuwait: Non-Kuwaitis	178.6	9.61	129.1	5.92
*Kuwait: Kuwaitis	106.7	4.32	127.3	5.12
*Philippines, Manila	215.1	2.25	195.6	1.83
Singapore: Chinese	267.1	2.53	202.5	1.98
Singapore: Malay	148.8	4.78	136.5	4.50
Singapore: Indian	108.9	4.66	127.1	6.86
Thailand, Chiang Mai	148.4	2.18	155.6	2.25
*Thailand, Khon Kaen	190.6	3.06	132.4	2.35
*Viet Nam, Hanoi	145.6	2.54	91.8	1.85

* IMPORTANT-SEE NOTES ON POPULATION PAGE

EUROPE	MALE		FEMALE	
Austria, Tyrol	335.4	4.37	267.4	3.54
*Belarus	276.0	1.06	165.0	0.69
*Croatia	272.7	1.59	172.9	1.14
Czech Republic	360.8	1.09	248.7	0.82
Denmark	327.0	1.35	304.9	1.29
Estonia	289.4	2.66	189.2	1.81
Finland	305.6	1.29	252.3	1.07
France, Bas-Rhin	410.0	3.91	236.7	2.78
*France, Calvados	374.0	4.57	217.1	3.29
France, Doubs	389.1	5.28	250.0	4.08
France, Haut-Rhin	410.8	4.60	258.2	3.42
*France, Herault	277.5	3.18	204.9	2.76
France, Isere	308.2	3.21	217.9	2.63
*France, Somme	327.4	4.45	186.1	3.29
*France, Tarn	280.3	4.60	179.8	3.89
Germany, Eastern States	256.3	1.19	200.4	0.91
Germany, Saarland	377.4	3.21	256.1	2.44
Iceland	273.9	6.09	248.7	5.93
Ireland, Southern	316.6	4.47	267.2	4.11
Italy, Ferrara	371.3	7.87	264.9	6.87
Italy, Florence	338.5	3.04	237.4	2.51
Italy, Genoa	359.5	3.61	237.9	2.86
*Italy, Latina	268.4	4.80	186.8	3.88
Italy, Macerata	314.8	8.32	226.3	7.28
Italy, Modena	335.5	3.75	238.9	3.19
Italy, Parma	333.1	4.50	237.8	3.89
Italy, Ragusa	226.4	4.74	166.8	4.05
Italy, Romagna	379.1	4.42	268.3	3.77
Italy, Torino	339.6	3.44	232.1	2.70
Italy, Trieste	482.1	7.47	303.4	6.08
Italy, Varese	399.9	3.91	251.7	2.86
Italy, Veneto	407.0	3.16	258.9	2.41
*Latvia	251.7	1.88	166.0	1.29
Malta	272.3	8.11	224.2	6.89
The Netherlands	303.4	0.89	230.7	0.76
The Netherlands, Eindhoven	301.6	3.29	212.8	2.65
The Netherlands, Maastricht	301.2	3.28	221.5	2.70
Norway	266.4	1.33	223.9	1.26
*Poland, Cracow	269.2	3.68	203.6	2.77
*Poland, Kielce	230.1	2.68	143.4	1.98
*Poland, Lower Silesia	305.6	2.07	204.2	1.50
Poland, Warsaw City	267.9	2.61	206.1	1.99
Slovakia	347.9	1.60	217.7	1.15
Slovenia	290.2	2.32	195.9	1.67
*Spain, Albacete	199.6	6.52	143.5	5.71
Spain, Asturias	279.5	3.00	166.1	2.29
Spain, Basque Country	295.3	2.36	155.6	1.65
Spain, Granada	273.3	3.35	165.0	2.54
Spain, Mallorca	375.9	4.45	239.8	3.50
Spain, Murcia	309.0	3.19	188.1	2.39
Spain, Navarra	326.9	4.26	214.3	3.48
Spain, Tarragona	307.4	4.05	205.4	3.37
Spain, Zaragoza	264.1	3.00	156.0	2.27

	MALE		FEMALE	
Sweden	252.7	0.88	233.9	0.87
*Switzerland, Basel	370.4	4.88	266.4	3.97
Switzerland, Geneva	442.0	5.97	311.2	4.62
Switzerland, Graubunden	289.0	7.85	211.8	6.62
Switzerland, Neuchatel	371.0	8.10	260.8	6.51
Switzerland, St Gall-Appenzell	329.5	4.56	232.4	3.73
Switzerland, Valais	359.5	7.49	252.8	6.09
Switzerland, Vaud	412.2	4.63	299.8	3.77
Switzerland, Zurich	308.2	2.82	216.3	2.26
*UK, England and Wales	303.1	0.53	254.1	0.48
*UK, East Anglia	300.3	1.97	261.8	1.87
*UK, Mersey	275.7	1.76	273.2	1.76
*UK, North Western	310.8	1.49	258.5	1.34
UK, Oxford	327.5	1.99	283.2	1.83
*UK, South Thames	281.2	1.08	240.9	0.99
UK, South Western	289.1	1.52	251.7	1.44
UK, Wessex	285.4	1.61	252.1	1.53
*UK, West Midlands	339.5	1.35	284.6	1.23
UK, Yorkshire	316.8	1.57	263.8	1.42
UK, Scotland	360.4	1.45	293.2	1.25
UK, Scotland, West	363.2	2.00	287.8	1.68
*Yugoslavia, Vojvodina	268.5	2.03	195.3	1.60

OCEANIA

	MALE		FEMALE	
Australian Capital Territory				
Australia, New South Wales				
South Australia				
Australia, Tasmania				
Australia, Victoria				
Western Australia				
*French Polynesia				
New Zealand: Non-Maori	290.4	1.77	274.6	1.72
New Zealand: Maori	359.7	10.25	339.7	8.57
US, Hawaii: White	398.6	6.79	295.9	5.97
US, Hawaii: Japanese	253.8	4.72	200.4	4.35
US, Hawaii: Hawaiian	276.2	8.64	262.9	7.88
US, Hawaii: Filipino	217.3	6.63	202.6	6.75
US, Hawaii: Chinese	242.8	9.62	183.5	8.46

* IMPORTANT-SEE NOTES ON POPULATION PAGE

AGE-STANDARDIZED INCIDENCE
RATES AND STANDARD ERRORS (per 100,000)
All sites but 173

	MALE		FEMALE	
AFRICA				
*Algeria, Setif	107.1	3.76	67.4	2.38
*France, La Reunion	206.0	4.41	128.2	3.10
*Mali, Bamako	124.5	4.24	90.2	3.39
*Uganda, Kyadondo	155.2	6.31	145.5	5.57
*Zimbabwe, Harare: African	234.6	7.50	231.9	8.98
*Zimbabwe, Harare: European	290.6	17.01	297.5	17.64
AMERICA, CENTRAL AND SOUTH				
*Argentina, Concordia	244.9	9.38	223.9	8.19
*Brazil, Belem	183.5	4.74	177.5	3.77
*Brazil, Goiania	190.9	4.57	187.6	3.94
*Brazil, Porto Alegre	326.4	4.94	231.5	3.35
Colombia, Cali	187.6	2.98	202.5	2.76
*Costa Rica	191.2	2.05	163.8	1.78
*Ecuador, Quito	143.9	2.95	168.5	2.87
*Peru, Lima	123.8	1.76	151.2	1.85
Peru, Trujillo	149.8	6.11	190.0	6.21
US, Puerto Rico	212.5	1.69	151.8	1.36
*Uruguay, Montevideo	316.6	3.61	255.2	2.91
AMERICA, NORTH				
Canada	322.1	0.63	252.8	0.54
Canada, Alberta	288.0	2.10	243.5	1.90
Canada, British Columbia	307.0	1.70	254.4	1.55
Canada, Manitoba	324.6	3.05	261.3	2.75
Canada, New Brunswick	327.9	3.87	241.6	3.27
Canada, Newfoundland	282.0	4.30	225.1	3.84
Canada, Northwest Territories	257.8	13.69	252.5	14.05
Canada, Nova Scotia	337.6	3.50	268.4	3.06
Canada, Ontario	325.7	1.03	261.1	0.89
Canada, Prince Edward Island	322.4	8.99	260.4	8.06
Canada, Quebec	339.8	1.30	244.4	1.03
Canada, Saskatchewan	298.5	3.02	239.8	2.80
Canada, Yukon	325.7	19.05	294.8	18.97
US, Cent. Calif.: Non-Hisp. White	350.9	2.78	270.7	2.40
US, Cent. Calif.: Hispanic	245.9	4.93	202.8	4.26
US, Los Angeles: Non-Hisp. White	373.4	1.71	303.5	1.53
US, Los Angeles: Hispanic White	239.4	2.47	199.4	1.93
US, Los Angeles: Black	424.9	4.43	261.5	3.03
US, Los Angeles: Chinese	181.8	5.47	144.5	4.60
US, Los Angeles: Filipino	210.8	6.63	188.9	5.54
US, Los Angeles: Korean	188.8	8.23	138.0	5.88
US, Los Angeles: Japanese	216.3	6.84	187.1	6.29
US, San Francisco: Non-Hisp. White	407.9	2.37	305.4	2.01
US, San Francisco: Hispanic White	294.6	5.74	231.1	4.55
US, San Francisco: Black	465.4	6.83	286.0	4.87
US, San Francisco: Chinese	218.0	5.14	204.2	5.03
US, San Francisco: Filipino	240.7	7.95	198.8	6.42
US, San Francisco: Japanese	250.3	13.77	211.2	10.57
US, Connecticut: White	356.7	1.92	289.4	1.68
US, Connecticut: Black	425.2	9.36	273.2	6.30
US, Atlanta: White	384.0	3.27	273.2	2.50
US, Atlanta: Black	450.1	7.13	252.8	4.29
US, Iowa	348.2	1.95	270.7	1.71

	MALE		FEMALE	
US, Central Louisiana: White	317.9	6.75	214.4	5.35
US, Central Louisiana: Black	391.9	15.95	209.6	10.25
US, New Orleans: White	389.4	4.52	272.6	3.56
US, New Orleans: Black	417.9	7.43	271.0	5.06
US, Detroit: White	401.3	2.09	293.6	1.71
US, Detroit: Black	464.2	4.63	278.4	3.19
US, New Mexico: Non-Hisp. White	354.0	3.65	261.0	3.14
US, New Mexico: Hispanic White	254.0	4.54	194.9	3.76
US, New Mexico: American Indian	151.3	8.22	147.6	7.36
US, Utah	307.8	2.77	228.3	2.34
US, Seattle	394.6	2.03	289.6	1.69
US, SEER: White	370.9	0.80	280.9	0.68
US, SEER: Black	454.5	3.00	271.6	2.04
ASIA				
*China, Qidong	205.7	2.63	101.9	1.76
China, Shanghai	228.8	1.04	153.2	0.83
China, Tianjin	189.2	1.43	149.2	1.22
Hong Kong	301.7	1.43	211.1	1.18
*India, Bangalore	98.3	1.25	118.1	1.39
*India, Barshi, Paranda and Bhum	50.4	2.42	53.9	2.45
India, Bombay	131.4	1.07	125.4	1.03
*India, Karunagappally	108.0	5.70	79.8	4.86
India, Madras	116.5	1.41	129.8	1.46
*India, Trivandrum	108.1	4.08	86.0	3.31
Israel: All Jews	235.6	1.51	239.3	1.49
Jews born in Israel	231.9	5.17	261.4	4.76
Jews born in America or Europe	255.5	2.70	268.3	2.87
Jews born in Africa or Asia	198.1	3.87	185.1	4.09
Non-Jews	127.7	3.67	94.4	2.87
Japan, Hiroshima	322.3	3.35	195.0	2.37
Japan, Miyagi	275.9	1.95	169.9	1.45
Japan, Nagasaki	288.0	2.30	174.0	1.70
Japan, Osaka	272.8	1.05	154.8	0.72
*Japan, Saga	266.8	2.91	144.0	2.01
Japan, Yamagata	260.6	2.29	152.8	1.71
*Korea, Kangwha	199.2	8.40	110.2	5.80
*Kuwait: Non-Kuwaitis	172.7	9.44	125.8	5.84
*Kuwait: Kuwaitis	103.9	4.26	125.8	5.09
*Philippines, Manila	212.5	2.23	193.8	1.82
Singapore: Chinese	258.0	2.48	194.6	1.95
Singapore: Malay	144.6	4.72	133.0	4.44
Singapore: Indian	105.5	4.56	122.7	6.73
Thailand, Chiang Mai	144.2	2.15	152.6	2.23
*Thailand, Khon Kaen	186.8	3.02	129.0	2.31
*Viet Nam, Hanoi	142.7	2.51	89.4	1.83

* IMPORTANT-SEE NOTES ON POPULATION PAGE

AGE-STANDARDIZED INCIDENCE
RATES AND STANDARD ERRORS (per 100,000)
All sites but 173 (contd)

EUROPE

	MALE		FEMALE	
Austria, Tyrol	313.1	4.22	252.5	3.45
*Belarus	255.7	1.02	148.7	0.66
*Croatia	271.6	1.59	172.1	1.14
Czech Republic	305.0	1.00	212.0	0.76
Denmark	273.9	1.24	261.6	1.20
Estonia	269.8	2.57	172.3	1.74
Finland	251.0	1.18	204.1	0.98
France, Bas-Rhin	394.0	3.84	229.3	2.74
*France, Calvados	335.8	4.34	195.9	3.16
France, Doubs	323.1	4.80	202.6	3.69
France, Haut-Rhin	363.5	4.33	224.7	3.21
*France, Herault	258.8	3.09	197.8	2.72
France, Isere	294.9	3.15	212.1	2.60
*France, Somme	311.9	4.35	181.5	3.27
*France, Tarn	262.6	4.47	172.2	3.83
Germany, Eastern States	249.3	1.17	197.4	0.91
Germany, Saarland	316.6	2.95	219.1	2.28
Iceland	269.0	6.04	244.5	5.88
Ireland, Southern	237.6	3.88	212.5	3.70
Italy, Ferrara	319.4	7.33	236.2	6.57
Italy, Florence	315.0	2.94	226.0	2.47
Italy, Genoa	326.1	3.45	218.7	2.76
*Italy, Latina	242.5	4.57	172.6	3.75
Italy, Macerata	268.7	7.75	201.0	6.96
Italy, Modena	292.7	3.51	217.9	3.07
Italy, Parma	305.1	4.31	224.8	3.80
Italy, Ragusa	178.9	4.23	143.6	3.78
Italy, Romagna	318.7	4.07	234.1	3.56
Italy, Torino	299.7	3.24	206.6	2.55
Italy, Trieste	414.0	6.94	256.1	5.64
Italy, Varese	354.6	3.69	226.5	2.73
Italy, Veneto	355.9	2.96	230.6	2.29
*Latvia	233.0	1.81	151.9	1.24
Malta	221.2	7.31	202.0	6.54
The Netherlands	288.4	0.87	225.0	0.75
The Netherlands, Eindhoven	301.6	3.29	212.8	2.65
The Netherlands, Maastricht	289.4	3.22	215.9	2.67
Norway	255.8	1.31	217.1	1.24
*Poland, Cracow	251.7	3.56	193.1	2.71
*Poland, Kielce	211.7	2.57	131.0	1.91
*Poland, Lower Silesia	292.9	2.03	195.1	1.46
Poland, Warsaw City	254.9	2.55	196.2	1.95
Slovakia	308.5	1.51	188.5	1.08
Slovenia	268.5	2.23	180.0	1.61
*Spain, Albacete	199.0	6.51	142.4	5.68
Spain, Asturias	279.1	3.00	165.8	2.29
Spain, Basque Country	294.7	2.35	155.3	1.65
Spain, Granada	228.0	3.07	138.8	2.35
Spain, Mallorca	286.2	3.88	178.4	3.03
Spain, Murcia	250.5	2.87	153.8	2.19
Spain, Navarra	275.4	3.92	182.4	3.23
Spain, Tarragona	244.5	3.61	165.1	3.04
Spain, Zaragoza	238.8	2.86	143.9	2.20

	MALE		FEMALE	
Sweden	240.7	0.86	228.5	0.87
*Switzerland, Basel	281.9	4.28	207.6	3.54
Switzerland, Geneva	332.3	5.19	231.2	4.02
Switzerland, Graubunden	269.3	7.60	203.5	6.54
Switzerland, Neuchatel	287.7	7.18	206.3	5.85
Switzerland, St Gall-Appenzell	273.1	4.16	192.4	3.43
Switzerland, Valais	289.9	6.74	204.8	5.55
Switzerland, Vaud	312.2	4.06	224.2	3.29
Switzerland, Zurich	307.2	2.81	215.5	2.26
*UK, England and Wales	261.1	0.49	225.5	0.46
*UK, East Anglia	238.0	1.75	221.6	1.74
*UK, Mersey	237.0	1.64	236.8	1.65
*UK, North Western	271.2	1.40	229.0	1.27
UK, Oxford	258.8	1.77	240.3	1.69
*UK, South Thames	246.2	1.01	218.3	0.95
UK, South Western	234.6	1.38	215.3	1.34
UK, Wessex	264.2	1.55	238.7	1.49
*UK, West Midlands	286.0	1.24	246.8	1.16
UK, Yorkshire	271.3	1.45	232.1	1.34
UK, Scotland	306.2	1.33	256.8	1.17
UK, Scotland, West	316.6	1.87	256.2	1.59
*Yugoslavia, Vojvodina	247.2	1.95	178.4	1.53

OCEANIA

	MALE		FEMALE	
Australian Capital Territory	294.9	7.42	229.2	5.91
Australia, New South Wales	320.4	1.34	240.9	1.15
South Australia	323.5	2.66	250.8	2.34
Australia, Tasmania	312.4	4.71	235.0	4.06
Australia, Victoria	307.1	1.53	239.3	1.33
Western Australia	312.2	2.66	252.0	2.36
*French Polynesia	248.9	9.83	252.6	9.52
New Zealand: Non-Maori	290.3	1.77	274.6	1.72
New Zealand: Maori	359.7	10.25	339.7	8.57
US, Hawaii: White	397.7	6.79	294.7	5.95
US, Hawaii: Japanese	253.0	4.72	199.4	4.34
US, Hawaii: Hawaiian	274.7	8.62	262.0	7.87
US, Hawaii: Filipino	216.7	6.62	202.4	6.75
US, Hawaii: Chinese	242.2	9.60	183.5	8.46

* IMPORTANT-SEE NOTES ON POPULATION PAGE

AGE-STANDARDIZED(WORLD) INCIDENCE RATES (FOUR DIGIT RUBRICS)

AGE-STANDARDIZED (WORLD) INCIDENCE RATES (FOUR DIGIT RUBRICS)

	141.0 M	141.0 F	Tongue 141.1-6 M	141.1-6 F	141.8-9 M	141.8-9 F	142.0 M	142.0 F	Salivary gland 142.1-2 M	142.1-2 F	142.8-9 M	142.8-9 F	Gum 143 M	143 F	Floor 144 M	144 F
AFRICA																
*Algeria, Setif	0,1	-	-	-	0,6	0,1	0,2	-	-	-	-	-	0,1	0,2	-	-
*France, La Reunion	2.1	0,1	2.8	0,3	0,5	-	0,1	0,1	0,2	0,1	0,1	-	0,6	0,1	2.8	0,1
*Mali, Bamako	-	-	0,2	-	0,3	0,3	-	0,2	-	-	-	0,2	0,2	0,0	-	-
*Uganda, Kyadondo	-	-	-	-	0,2	0,2	0,0	0,6	0,1	-	0,2	0,2	0,4	-	-	0,2
*Zimbabwe, Harare: African	0,3	-	-	-	0,8	-	0,4	-	0,1	-	0,4	0,4	-	-	0,1	0,2
*Zimbabwe, Harare: European	0,7	-	-	-	2,2	5,7	-	-	-	-	-	-	-	-	1,5	-
AMERICA, CENTRAL AND SOUTH																
*Argentina, Concordia	-	-	0,6	-	2,0	0,3	0,3	0,3	0,3	-	0,4	0,5	-	-	0,3	0,3
*Brazil, Belem	1.4	0,8	0,3	0,1	2.4	0,9	0,7	0,6	0,2	-	-	-	0,6	0,5	0,8	0,3
*Brazil, Goiania	1.1	-	0,1	-	1.7	0,2	0,5	0,6	0,0	-	0,5	-	0,3	0,2	0,6	0,2
*Brazil, Porto Alegre	1.4	0,1	0,1	-	3.2	0,7	0,5	0,4	0,1	-	0,1	0,1	0,2	-	0,3	0,1
Colombia, Cali	0,4	0,2	0,2	0,1	0,6	0,7	0,4	0,3	0,2	0,2	0,1	-	0,2	0,2	0,5	0,2
*Costa Rica	0.5	0.2	0.2	0,1	0.4	0.3	0.3	0.3	0,1	0,1	0,0	0,1	0,1	0,1	0.2	0,0
*Ecuador, Quito	0,1	-	-	-	0,3	0,2	0,4	0,3	0,0	-	0,1	-	0,2	0,1	0,0	-
*Peru, Lima	0,1	0,0	-	0,0	0.4	0.5	0.5	0.3	0,1	0,2	0,0	0,0	0.2	0.3	0,1	0,0
Peru, Trujillo	-	-	-	-	0,7	0,1	-	-	-	-	-	0,5	0,6	0,2	0,3	-
US, Puerto Rico	2.4	0.4	0.9	0.3	0.7	0,1	0.3	0.3	0,1	0,1	-	-	0.5	0.3	1.2	0.3
*Uruguay, Montevideo	1.5	0,2	0,2	0,1	1.2	0.3	0.8	0.2	0,2	0,1	0,1	0,1	0,1	0,1	0.9	0.2
AMERICA, NORTH																
Canada	0.8	0.2	0.9	0.3	0.5	0.2	0.6	0.4	0.2	0.1	0.0	0.0	0.3	0.2	1.1	0.4
Canada, Alberta	0.6	0.2	0.6	0.4	0.3	0.2	0.5	0.3	0,1	0,1	0,0	0,0	0.2	0.1	0.8	0.4
Canada, British Columbia	0.9	0.2	1.1	0.6	0.3	0.2	0.5	0.4	0.2	0.1	0,0	0,0	0.3	0.2	1.3	0.5
Canada, Manitoba	0.6	0.3	0.7	0.2	0.7	0.5	0.6	0.4	0,1	0,1	0,1	0,1	0.3	0.3	1.3	0.5
Canada, New Brunswick	0.8	0.2	0.6	0.2	0.6	0,0	0.5	0.3	0,1	0,1	-	-	0.2	0.2	0.9	0,3
Canada, Newfoundland	0,6	0,1	0,1	0,1	0.7	0,4	0.4	0.2	0,1	0,1	0,2	0,1	0,1	0,0	0.8	-
Canada, Northwest Territories	-	-	0,3	0,7	0.8	0,4	3,4	1,7	0,8	0,3	-	-	-	-	-	-
Canada, Nova Scotia	0.9	0.3	0.8	0.3	0.5	0,1	0.5	0.3	0.2	0,0	0,1	0,0	0.5	0,1	1.2	0.3
Canada, Ontario	0.9	0.3	1.1	0.4	0.4	0.2	0.6	0.4	0.2	0.1	0.0	0.0	0.4	0.2	1.1	0.4
Canada, Prince Edward Island	1,6	0,2	0,5	-	1,1	0,7	0,9	0,3	-	-	-	-	0,5	0,3	1,2	0,6
Canada, Quebec	0.8	0.2	0.5	0.2	1.0	0.2	0.7	0.4	0.2	0.1	0,0	0,0	0.3	0.2	1.3	0.3
Canada, Saskatchewan	0.4	0,1	0.8	0.4	0.2	0,0	0.5	0.5	0,0	0,1	-	0,1	0.2	0.2	0.6	0.4
Canada, Yukon	-	-	-	-	-	3,1	-	-	0,8	-	-	-	-	-	6,8	-
US, Cent. Calif.: Non-Hisp. White	1.2	0.4	0.9	0.6	0.4	0.3	0.8	0.4	0,1	0,1	0,1	-	0.4	0.2	1.1	0.6
US, Cent. Calif.: Hispanic	0,8	0.2	0,4	0,3	0.4	0.2	0.3	0.5	0,1	0,2	-	0,0	-	0,1	0,5	0.2
US, Los Angeles: Non-Hisp. White	1.5	0.5	1.0	0.6	0.4	0.2	0.8	0.5	0.2	0.1	0,0	0,0	0.5	0.3	1.2	0.6
US, Los Angeles: Hispanic White	0.9	0,1	0.3	0.3	0.2	0.2	0.3	0.4	0,1	0,0	0,0	0,0	0,1	0,1	0.6	0,0
US, Los Angeles: Black	2.4	0.4	0.9	0.2	0.6	0,1	0.6	0.3	0.2	0,1	0,1	0,0	0.3	0.2	2.2	0.5
US, Los Angeles: Chinese	0,1	0.3	0,3	-	0.3	0.3	0.6	0.4	0.2	-	-	-	-	-	-	-
US, Los Angeles: Filipino	0,4	0,4	-	0,2	-	0,3	0,1	1,0	0,3	-	-	-	0,1	-	0,7	-
US, Los Angeles: Korean	0,7	0,1	-	-	0,4	-	-	-	-	-	-	-	-	-	-	-
US, Los Angeles: Japanese	0,7	0,4	0,2	0,8	0,4	-	0,2	-	0,2	-	-	-	-	0,2	0,4	0,6
US, San Francisco: Non-Hisp. White	1.5	0.8	1.3	0.6	0.4	0.3	1.0	0.5	0.2	0.1	0,1	0,1	0.4	0.3	1.3	0.6
US, San Francisco: Hispanic White	1,0	0,1	0.8	0.5	0.2	-	0.5	0.5	0.3	0,1	0,1	-	-	0,1	0.8	0.5
US, San Francisco: Black	2.9	0.3	0.9	0.2	0.6	0.3	0.8	0.3	0.3	0,1	-	0,1	0.2	0.3	1.8	0,7
US, San Francisco: Chinese	0.4	0,1	0,4	0.6	0,1	-	0.6	0,1	0.2	0.2	-	-	-	-	0.2	0.2
US, San Francisco: Filipino	0,9	0.2	0,2	0,4	0.2	0,2	0.4	1,1	0.5	0,4	-	-	-	0,6	0.3	-
US, San Francisco: Japanese	-	0,4	0,6	0,9	-	0,4	-	1,0	-	0,5	-	-	1,2	0,3	-	-
US, Connecticut: White	1.5	0.5	0.8	0.4	0.5	0.2	0.9	0.7	0.1	0.1	0,0	0,1	0.4	0.3	1.4	0.5
US, Connecticut: Black	3.3	0.8	1.3	0,4	1,4	0,4	0.4	0,7	0.2	0,3	-	-	0.4	0.4	3.2	0.2
US, Atlanta: White	1.0	0.4	0.4	0.3	0.4	0.2	0.6	0.3	0.3	0,1	0,0	0,0	0.4	0.2	1.2	0.6
US, Atlanta: Black	3.1	0.4	0.6	0.3	0.5	0.2	1,0	0.7	0,1	0,1	-	0,1	0.2	0.1	2.6	0.8
US, Iowa	0.7	0.3	0.7	0.4	0.3	0.2	0.6	0.4	0.2	0.2	0,1	-	0.4	0.2	1.3	0.3
US, Central Louisiana: White	1,2	0,4	0,6	0,4	1,0	0,2	0,2	0,2	0,4	-	-	-	0,1	0,4	0,4	0,1
US, Central Louisiana: Black	2,4	-	1,5	-	0,5	-	0,4	0,7	-	-	-	-	-	0,7	0,8	0,6
US, New Orleans: White	1.1	0.2	0.8	0.3	0.7	0.5	0.9	0.4	0.2	0,1	0.2	0,2	0.5	0,1	1.5	0.4
US, New Orleans: Black	1.7	0.3	0.3	0.2	0.8	0.2	0.9	0.5	0.3	0,1	-	-	0,1	-	2.9	0.5
US, Detroit: White	1.5	0.5	1.1	0.4	0.6	0.2	0.7	0.6	0.2	0.2	0,0	0,0	0.4	0.2	1.7	0.6
US, Detroit: Black	3.2	0.7	1.0	0.3	0.8	0.2	0.4	0.3	0.3	0,1	0,1	0,0	0.4	0.2	2.9	0.7
US, New Mexico: Non-Hisp. White	1.2	0.4	0.9	0.3	0.4	0.2	0.8	0.5	0,1	-	0,1	0,0	0.4	0.2	1.0	0.6
US, New Mexico: Hispanic White	0.9	0,0	0,5	-	0,5	0,1	0.2	0.2	-	0,1	-	0,1	0,1	-	1.3	0,0
US, New Mexico: American Indian	-	-	-	0,5	0,5	-	-	0,3	-	-	-	-	-	-	0,3	0,4
US, Utah	0.9	0.2	0.3	0.4	0.5	0.3	0.9	0.3	0,1	0,1	0,0	0,0	0.2	0.1	1.0	0.3
US, Seattle	0.9	0.4	1.3	0.6	0.4	0.2	0.7	0.5	0.1	0.2	0,0	0,0	0.3	0.2	1.1	0.6
US, SEER: White	1.2	0.4	0.9	0.4	0.4	0.2	0.7	0.4	0.2	0.1	0.0	0.0	0.4	0.2	1.3	0.5
US, SEER: Black	2.9	0.6	0.9	0.3	0.7	0.2	0.6	0.5	0.2	0.1	0,0	0,0	0.3	0.2	2.5	0.7

AGE-STANDARDIZED (WORLD) INCIDENCE RATES (FOUR DIGIT RUBRICS)

Tongue: 141.0, 141.1-6, 141.8-9 · 142.0 · Salivary gland: 142.1-2, 142.8-9 · Gum: 143 · Floor: 144

	141.0 M	141.0 F	141.1-6 M	141.1-6 F	141.8-9 M	141.8-9 F	142.0 M	142.0 F	142.1-2 M	142.1-2 F	142.8-9 M	142.8-9 F	143 M	143 F	144 M	144 F
ASIA																
*China, Qidong	-	-	0,0	-	0,1	0,2	0,3	0,0	0,1	-	0,0	0,0	0,1	0,2	0,0	-
China, Shanghai	0.1	0.1	0.3	0.2	0.3	0.2	0.3	0.3	0.1	0.1	0.0	0.0	0.3	0.2	0.1	0.0
China, Tianjin	0,0	0,1	0.1	0.1	0.3	0.3	0.2	0.1	0,1	0,1	0,1	0,0	0.4	0.2	0,1	0,0
Hong Kong																
*India, Bangalore	2.2	0.3	0.3	0.2	1.0	0.7	0.5	0.2	0,1	0,1	0,0	0,1	0.7	2.1	0.4	0,1
*India, Barshi, Paranda and Bhum	1.2	0,1	0,2	-	0,8	0,2	0,5	0,1	-	-	-	-	1.4	-	0,1	-
India, Bombay	4.1	0.7	1.2	0.8	1.2	0.8	0.5	0.3	0.1	0,0	0.1	0,0	1.5	1.3	0.6	0.1
*India, Karunagappally	1,6	0,2	1,1	2,1	2,7	1,4	-	-	-	-	0,6	-	0,6	1,5	0,3	0,3
India, Madras	2.9	0.4	1.3	1.1	1.6	0.5	0.4	0.4	0,1	0,0	0.0	0,0	1.0	1.6	0.7	0,1
*India, Trivandrum	1,3	0,1	2.5	1.4	0.7	0,3	-	0,6	-	-	-	0,1	2.6	1.9	0,7	-
Israel: All Jews	0.1	0,1	0.1	0,1	0.5	0.4	0.6	0.4	0.1	0,1	0,1	0,0	0.2	0.1	0.1	0.1
Jews born in Israel	0,1	0,1	0,2	0,2	0,8	0,2	0,2	0,7	0,0	0,2	0,0	0,1	0,2	0,4	0,3	0,1
Jews born in America or Europe	0,2	0,0	0,1	0,1	0.5	0.4	0.7	0.3	0,1	0,0	0,1	0,0	0,1	0.2	0,1	0,1
Jews born in Africa or Asia	0,1	0,1	0,1	-	0.5	0.4	0.5	0.3	0,1	0,1	0,0	0,1	0.3	0,0	0,2	0,0
Non-Jews	-	0,2	-	0,1	0,2	0,2	0,1	0,1	-	-	0,1	0,0	0,2	0,2	0,1	-
Japan, Hiroshima	0.2	0.1	0.7	0.2	1.1	0.4	0.4	0.1	0.3	0.1	-	-	0,3	0.1	0.7	0,1
Japan, Miyagi	0.1	-	0.1	0,0	1.5	0.7	0.3	0.2	0.2	0,0	-	0,0	0.3	0.3	0.2	0,0
Japan, Nagasaki	0.1	0.1	0.3	0.2	1.1	0.5	0.3	0.2	0,1	0,1	0.0	0,0	0.5	0.2	0.6	0.1
Japan, Osaka	0.1	0,0	0.4	0.2	1.1	0.5	0.3	0.1	0.1	0.1	0.0	0,0	0.5	0.3	0.4	0.1
*Japan, Saga																
Japan, Yamagata																
*Korea, Kangwha	0,4	-	-	-	0,3	0,3	1,0	-	0,3	-	0,3	-	0,6	-	-	-
*Kuwait: Non-Kuwaitis	0,1	0,1	0,6	0,4	0,1	-	0,6	0,1	-	0,0	0,1	-	0,1	0,1	0,0	-
*Kuwait: Kuwaitis	-	-	0,2	0,3	-	-	0,2	0,2	0,2	0,1	-	0,5	-	0,1	-	0,1
*Philippines, Manila	0.5	0.5	0,0	0,0	2.1	1.6	0.8	0.5	0.2	0.3	0.2	0.2	0.7	0.6	0.6	0.4
Singapore: Chinese	0.3	0,0	0,0	0,0	1.1	0.6	0.4	0.4	0,2	0,1	0,1	0,0	0,0	0,1	0.5	0,1
Singapore: Malay	-	-	-	-	0,4	0,2	0,6	0,1	-	0,2	-	-	-	-	0,3	-
Singapore: Indian	0,4	-	-	-	2.4	0,6	0,1	0,9	0,2	0,4	-	-	0,1	0,2	0,5	0,8
Thailand, Chiang Mai	1.0	0.8	0.4	0,2	0.5	0,2	0,1	0,2	0,2	0,1	0,1	0,1	0.8	0.6	0,2	0,2
*Thailand, Khon Kaen	0,4	0,1	0,0	0,1	0.7	0.7	0,1	0,2	0,1	0,1	0,1	-	0.6	0.6	0,2	0,3
*Viet Nam, Hanoi	0,0	0,1	-	0,1	0.8	0.8	0.6	0.4	0,1	0,1	0,0	0,0	0.5	0.3	0,0	0,1
EUROPE																
Austria, Tyrol	0.6	0,1	0,3	0,1	0.7	0,1	0,4	0,2	-	0,2	0,1	0,1	0.8	0,4	1.2	0,3
*Belarus																
*Croatia	1.4	0.1	0,0	0,0	2.2	0.3	0.7	0.3	0.7	0.2	0.0	0,0	0.6	0.2	1.1	0,0
Czech Republic	0.8	0.1	1.1	0.2	0.2	0.0	0.6	0.4	0.2	0.1	0.1	0,0	0.4	0.1	1.1	0.1
Denmark	0.3	0.1	0.1	0.1	0.8	0.3	0.4	0.3	0.2	0.1	0.0	0,0	0.2	0.1	0.8	0.3
Estonia	0.7	0,0	1.0	0.2	0.8	0.1	0.4	0.4	0,1	0,1	-	-	0.5	0,1	2.2	0.2
Finland																
France, Bas-Rhin	3.8	0,3	2.7	0.5	1.6	0,2	0.6	0.4	0,1	0,1	0,1	0,1	0.8	0,1	6.3	0.4
*France, Calvados	3.5	0,2	3.2	0.5	1.1	0,0	0,3	0,3	0,1	-	-	-	0,4	0,1	3.7	0.5
France, Doubs	2.2	0,1	2.0	0.5	0.7	0,2	0,2	0,2	0,1	0,2	-	-	0.5	0,3	3.3	0,5
France, Haut-Rhin	3.3	0,3	2.6	0,2	2.0	0,3	0,4	0,2	0,0	0,1	0,0	-	0.8	0,2	4.4	0,4
*France, Herault	1.3	0,3	0.8	0,2	2.1	0.4	0.4	0,2	0,1	0,1	-	0,1	0.4	0.3	1.8	0,1
France, Isere	1.5	0,1	1.3	0.3	1.3	0.3	0.4	0.3	-	0,1	-	-	0.6	0.2	2.5	0.3
*France, Somme	3.0	0,1	1.7	0,2	1.6	0,2	0.6	0,2	0,1	-	-	0,1	1.5	0.3	4.7	0.5
*France, Tarn	1.4	0,2	2.1	0,3	0,1	0,1	0,7	0,1	0,1	-	0,0	0,0	0,2	0,0	0.8	0,1
Germany, Eastern States	0.6	0.1	0.9	0.2	0.1	0,0	0.4	0.2	0.1	0.1	0.0	0,0	0.2	0.1	0.9	0.1
Germany, Saarland	1.3	0.3	1.5	0,1	1.2	0,1	0.6	0.2	0,1	0,0	0.2	0,1	0.5	0.2	3.4	0.5
Iceland	0,4	-	-	0,0	0,7	0,4	0,4	0,4	0,5	-	-	-	0,8	0,6	0.3	0,1
Ireland, Southern	0,2	0,1	0,1	0,2	1.1	0.4	0.7	0.2	0.2	0,0	0.3	-	0,4	0,1	1.2	0,2
Italy, Ferrara	0,4	-	-	-	0,9	0,2	0,4	0,4	0,1	-	-	0,1	0,3	0,1	0,7	0,4
Italy, Florence	0.4	0.2	0.5	0.2	0.7	0.2	0.6	0.3	0,1	0,1	-	0,0	0,0	0,1	0.4	0.3
Italy, Genoa	0.7	0,1	0.6	0,3	1.2	0,4	0.7	0.3	0,1	-	0,1	-	0,1	0.2	0.9	0,1
*Italy, Latina	0,2	-	0,1	0,1	1.1	0,0	1.0	0,3	-	0,1	0,1	0,1	-	-	0,2	0,1
Italy, Macerata	0,3	-	0,3	0,1	0,9	0,3	0,4	-	-	-	-	-	-	-	-	-
Italy, Modena	0.8	0,0	0.4	0,1	0.5	0.2	0.5	0.2	0,0	0,0	-	-	0.2	0,1	0.5	0,3
Italy, Parma	0.5	0.2	0.7	0.2	0.9	0.1	0.1	0.2	0.1	-	-	-	0,1	-	1.1	0,1
Italy, Ragusa	0.5	0.1	0,4	0,2	0.2	0.1	0.4	0.4	0.2	0.1	-	-	0.2	0.2	0.1	-
Italy, Romagna	0.8	0.1	0,3	0,0	0.4	0,2	0.6	0.5	0.2	0.1	0.2	0,1	0.3	0,1	0.6	0,2
Italy, Torino	0.7	0.2	0.5	0,2	0.9	0.5	0.4	0.2	0,1	0,1	-	-	0.2	0,0	1.2	-
Italy, Trieste	0,7	-	0,2	0,0	1.6	1,1	0,7	0.4	0.3	0,0	0.6	0,3	0.3	-	0,3	-
Italy, Varese	1.1	0,1	2.1	0.2	0,3	0,0	0.6	0.3	0,1	0,1	-	-	0.3	0,1	1.7	0,2
Italy, Veneto	0.7	0.2	0.6	0,1	2.4	0.5	0.5	0.2	0,1	0,1	0.2	0,1	0.2	0,1	0.9	0,1
*Latvia	1.2	0.1	0.4	0,1	0.4	0,0	0.5	0.2	0,1	0,1	0,0	0,0	0.3	0,0	1.6	0.1
Malta	-	-	0,4	0,2	0,4	1,0	0,2	0,9	-	0,2	-	-	0,2	-	0,2	0,4

AGE-STANDARDIZED (WORLD) INCIDENCE RATES (FOUR DIGIT RUBRICS)

	Tongue 141.0		141.1-6		141.8-9		142.0		Salivary gland 142.1-2		142.8-9		Gum 143		Floor 144	
	M	F	M	F	M	F	M	F	M	F	M	F	M	F	M	F
The Netherlands	0.4	0.1	0.8	0.5	0.1	0.1	0.5	0.3	0.1	0.1	0,0	0,0	0.3	0.2	1.0	0.4
The Netherlands, Eindhoven	0,3	0,1	0.6	0.4	0,2	0,2	0.3	0.2	0,1	0,0	-	0,0	0.3	0.2	1.1	0,3
The Netherlands, Maastricht	0.4	0,1	1.0	0.4	0,2	0,0	0.3	0.4	0,1	0,0	0,0	0,0	0.3	0.2	0.9	0.5
Norway																
*Poland, Cracow	-	-	-	-	1.4	0,1	0,3	0,2	-	0,0	0.5	0,2	0.2	0,1	0.9	0,1
*Poland, Kielce	0,1	-	0,0	-	0.7	0,2	0,1	0,1	-	0,0	0,2	0,1	0,1	0,1	0.6	0,0
*Poland, Lower Silesia	0,1	-	0,0	-	1.5	0.4	0.5	0.3	0,1	0,1	0,1	0,1	0.3	0,1	1.3	0.2
Poland, Warsaw City	0,2	0,1	0,0	-	1.5	0.5	0.5	0.3	0,1	0,1	0,1	0,1	0.4	0,2	1.1	0,1
Slovakia	2.0	0.1	2.5	0.2	0.5	0,0	0.5	0.2	0.2	0.1	0,0	0,0	0.8	0.1	3.2	0.1
Slovenia	1.2	0,1	1.8	0.1	0.5	0,0	0.4	0.2	-	-	0,0	0,0	0.4	0,1	3.0	0.2
*Spain, Albacete	1,0	-	0,4	0,1	0,7	0,3	0,6	0,4	-	-	-	-	-	0,1	0,2	-
Spain, Asturias	1.7	0,1	0.9	0.3	2.6	0.6	0.4	0.6	0,1	0,0	0,2	0,1	0.4	0,1	1.9	0.2
Spain, Basque Country	1.9	0,1	1.7	0.3	1.0	0,1	0.3	0.2	0,1	0,0	0,0	0,0	0.4	0,1	2.3	0,1
Spain, Granada	1.1	0,1	0.6	0,2	1.2	0,3	0.4	0.4	0,1	-	-	-	0.5	0,3	1.8	0,3
Spain, Mallorca	0.9	0,1	1.2	0,4	0.6	0,1	0.5	0,1	-	0,0	0,0	-	0.6	0,1	1.5	0,3
Spain, Murcia	1.2	0,1	1.8	0.5	0.7	0.2	0.8	0.3	0,0	0,0	0,0	0,1	0.4	0,2	1.7	0,1
Spain, Navarra	0,5	0,1	1.2	0.5	0.6	0,1	0.6	0.3	-	-	0,0	0,1	0,2	-	2.4	0,1
Spain, Tarragona	0.9	0,2	0.6	0,2	1.6	0,1	0.5	0,1	0.2	0,1	-	0,0	0,2	0,2	1.6	-
Spain, Zaragoza	1.0	0,0	0.9	0,2	0.8	0,1	0.7	0,1	0,0	0,1	0,1	0,0	0,2	0,0	1.5	0,0
Sweden	0.3	0.1	0.3	0.2	0.4	0.3	0.4	0.4	0.1	0.1	0.1	0.1	0.3	0.2	0.5	0.1
*Switzerland, Basel	1.2	0.2	1.4	0.2	0.4	0,2	0.4	0.2	0,1	-	-	-	0,4	0,2	1.1	0,1
Switzerland, Geneva	1.4	0,2	2.0	0.8	0,7	0,4	0.5	0.3	0.4	0,1	-	-	0,4	0,2	1.9	0,3
Switzerland, Graubunden	0,4	0,9	0.5	-	-	-	0,4	0,8	-	-	-	-	0.8	0,1	0.9	-
Switzerland, Neuchatel	2.4	0.5	0,9	0,4	0.3	-	0,4	0,1	-	0,0	-	0,0	1,3	0,5	2.8	0,6
Switzerland, St Gall-Appenzell	0.7	0.3	0.8	0.4	0.2	0,1	0.2	0.5	0,1	-	-	-	0.7	0,2	1.3	0,3
Switzerland, Valais	1,0	0,5	1,4	0,1	0,6	0,1	0,1	0,4	-	-	-	-	-	0,2	2.4	-
Switzerland, Vaud	1.9	0,3	2.8	1.0	0,1	0,1	0.8	0.2	0,0	0,1	-	-	0.6	0,2	1.8	0.5
Switzerland, Zurich	1.0	0.2	1.1	0.4	0,1	0,1	0.5	0.3	0,0	0,0	0,0	-	0.4	0.3	1.3	0,2
*UK, England and Wales	0.2	0.1	0.2	0.1	0.8	0.4	0.4	0.3	0.1	0.1	0.0	0.0	0.2	0.1	0.6	0.2
*UK, East Anglia																
*UK, Mersey	0.3	0,1	0.3	0.1	0.7	0.2	0.3	0.2	0,1	0,0	0,0	0,0	0.1	0.1	0.9	0.3
*UK, North Western	0.3	0.1	0.2	0.1	1.0	0.4	0.3	0.2	0,1	0.1	0.1	0,0	0.2	0.1	0.9	0.2
UK, Oxford	0.2	0,0	0.2	0.2	0.8	0.3	0.5	0.3	0.1	0.1	0.0	0.0	0.1	0.1	0.3	0.1
*UK, South Thames	0.2	0.1	0.1	0.0	0.8	0.4	0.4	0.3	0.1	0.1	0.0	0.0	0.2	0.1	0.5	0.2
UK, South Western	0.2	0,1	0.4	0.2	0.4	0.2	0.4	0.3	0.1	0.1	0,1	0,0	0.1	0.1	0.3	0.1
UK, Wessex	0.2	0.1	0.2	0.1	0.6	0.5	0.4	0.4	0.1	0.1	0.1	0,1	0.1	0.1	0.3	0.2
*UK, West Midlands	0.5	0.1	0.5	0.3	0.4	0.1	0.4	0.2	0.0	0.0	0.0	-	0.2	0.1	0.7	0.2
UK, Yorkshire	0.2	0.1	0.2	0.1	0.9	0.4	0.5	0.3	0.1	0.1	0.0	0.0	0.2	0.1	0.9	0.2
UK, Scotland	0.4	0.1	0.5	0.2	1.0	0.4	0.4	0.3	0.1	0.1	0.1	0.0	0.2	0.2	1.4	0.5
UK, Scotland, West	0.4	0.1	0.3	0.1	1.3	0.5	0.3	0.3	0,1	0.1	0.1	0,0	0.2	0.2	1.6	0.5
*Yugoslavia, Vojvodina																

OCEANIA

	Tongue 141.0		141.1-6		141.8-9		142.0		Salivary gland 142.1-2		142.8-9		Gum 143		Floor 144	
	M	F	M	F	M	F	M	F	M	F	M	F	M	F	M	F
Australian Capital Territory	0,6	0,5	0,3	0,2	1,3	0,3	0,6	0,2	0,4	-	0,1	0,2	0,2	-	0,5	0,7
Australia, New South Wales	0.6	0.2	0.5	0.3	1.1	0.5	0.9	0.4	0.1	0.1	0,0	0,0	0.3	0.2	1.2	0.4
South Australia	0.5	0,0	0.6	0.3	0.8	0.3	0.6	0.4	0,1	0,1	0,0	0,0	0.3	0.2	1.2	0.4
Australia, Tasmania	0,6	0,2	0.7	0,3	1.1	0,3	0,3	0,5	-	-	-	-	0,1	0,2	0,5	0,3
Australia, Victoria	0.6	0.2	0.4	0.2	1.1	0.5	0.9	0.3	0.2	0.1	0.1	0,0	0.1	0.1	1.3	0.4
Western Australia	0.5	0,1	0,1	0,1	2.2	0.6	0.9	0.5	0,1	0,1	0,0	-	0,2	0.2	1.4	0.3
*French Polynesia	0,8	-	0,9	0,4	1,6	0,6	0,2	0,3	-	-	-	-	-	0,4	3.2	0,9
New Zealand: Non-Maori	0.5	0.1	0.7	0.4	0.3	0.2	1.0	0.5	0.2	0,1	0,0	0,0	0.2	0.1	1.0	0.3
New Zealand: Maori	0,3	-	0,3	0,6	1,7	0,5	0,6	1,3	0,1	-	-	-	0,7	0,2	1,5	0,3
US, Hawaii: White	1.6	0,1	1.0	0.6	0.3	0.2	0.6	0.6	-	-	-	-	-	0,7	2.0	0,9
US, Hawaii: Japanese	0.5	0.2	0.8	0.5	0.4	0,1	0.5	0.3	0.2	0.2	-	0,1	0.4	0.2	0,4	0,1
US, Hawaii: Hawaiian	0.5	0.4	1.1	0.6	0.3	0.2	1.0	-	-	-	-	-	-	-	1,5	0,7
US, Hawaii: Filipino	0,1	0,8	0.5	0,8	0.1	0,2	0.5	0,8	-	0,2	-	-	0.4	0,2	0.6	0,5
US, Hawaii: Chinese	0,2	-	-	0,7	0.4	0.6	-	1,4	-	-	0,6	-	0,4	-	-	-

AGE-STANDARDIZED (WORLD) INCIDENCE RATES (FOUR DIGIT RUBRICS)

| | Other parts of mouth | | | | | | Oropharynx | | | | | | Hypopharynx | | | |
| | 145.0-1,6 | | 145.2-5 | | 145.8-9 | | 146.0 | | 146.1-7 | | 146.8-9 | | 148.1 | | 148.0,2-9 | |
AFRICA	M	F	M	F	M	F	M	F	M	F	M	F	M	F	M	F
*Algeria, Setif	0,1	-	0,2	-	0,2	-	0,3	0,2	0,3	-	-	-	-	-	-	-
*France, La Reunion	0,5	-	1.7	0,3	0,5	0,1	3.6	0,1	3.9	0,3	0,5	-	3.6	0,3	1.1	0,1
*Mali, Bamako	-	-	-	-	0,2	0,2	0,3	0,1	-	-	-	-	-	-	-	-
*Uganda, Kyadondo	0,1	0,2	0,2	0,8	0,3	0,4	0,7	0,6	-	-	-	-	-	-	0,4	0,5
*Zimbabwe, Harare: African	0,1	-	0,2	-	-	0,1	-	-	-	-	-	-	-	0,4	0,2	-
*Zimbabwe, Harare: European	-	-	1,0	0,9	-	-	-	1,0	-	-	-	-	-	-	-	-

AMERICA, CENTRAL AND SOUTH

	145.0-1,6		145.2-5		145.8-9		146.0		146.1-7		146.8-9		148.1		148.0,2-9	
	M	F	M	F	M	F	M	F	M	F	M	F	M	F	M	F
*Argentina, Concordia	0,2	-	1,8	0,3	-	-	1,3	0,3	0,7	-	-	-	0,7	-	1,8	0,3
*Brazil, Belem	0,5	0,2	2.4	0,8	1,2	0,2	1.8	0,5	-	0,1	0,3	0,1	0,3	-	1.6	-
*Brazil, Goiania	0,0	0,3	1.2	0,4	1.3	0,3	0,4	0,4	0,1	-	0,7	0,2	0,2	-	1.3	0,1
*Brazil, Porto Alegre	0,2	0,0	1.2	0,1	1.8	0,3	1.0	0,1	0,2	-	2.8	0,2	0,3	0,1	2.1	0,1
Colombia, Cali	0,1	0,3	0.8	0,6	0.7	0,1	0.6	0,3	0,0	-	0,2	0,0	0,4	-	0,1	-
*Costa Rica	0,0	0,1	0.2	0,1	0.2	0,2	0.8	0,4	0,0	0,0	-	-	0.3	0,0	0.4	0,1
*Ecuador, Quito	0,0	0,1	0.2	0,1	0.1	0,0	0.1	0,1	-	-	0,0	0,0	-	-	-	-
*Peru, Lima	0,0	0,0	0,1	0,1	0,0	0,1	0,1	0,1	-	-	0,1	0,0	0,0	-	0,2	0,1
Peru, Trujillo	-	-	0,4	0,2	-	-	1,1	-	-	-	-	-	-	-	0,6	-
US, Puerto Rico	0.4	0.2	1.7	0,4	0.4	0,1	1.8	0,3	0.9	0,1	0.5	0,0	2.3	0,2	0.8	0,1
*Uruguay, Montevideo	0,3	0,1	0.5	0,2	0.9	0,1	1.9	0,2	0.5	-	0.9	0,0	1.8	0,1	1.4	0,1

AMERICA, NORTH

	145.0-1,6		145.2-5		145.8-9		146.0		146.1-7		146.8-9		148.1		148.0,2-9	
	M	F	M	F	M	F	M	F	M	F	M	F	M	F	M	F
Canada	0.5	0.2	0.5	0.3	0.1	0.1	0.7	0.3	0.5	0.2	0.2	0.1	0.8	0.1	0.4	0.1
Canada, Alberta	0.6	0.4	0.3	0.2	0.1	0.1	0.6	0.2	0.4	0.1	0.0	-	0.5	0.1	0.4	0.0
Canada, British Columbia	0.6	0.3	0.7	0.3	0.0	0.0	0.7	0.3	0.8	0.2	0.2	0.0	0.8	0.1	0.4	0.1
Canada, Manitoba	0.4	0.1	0.3	0.2	0.2	0.1	0.9	0.2	0.9	0.2	0.2	0.1	1.0	0.1	0.5	0.2
Canada, New Brunswick	0.7	0.2	0.2	0,1	0.3	0,1	0.9	0.2	0.4	0,1	0.2	0,1	0.7	0,1	0.4	0,1
Canada, Newfoundland	0,3	0,2	0,6	0,2	0,3	0,2	0.8	0,2	0,1	0,1	0,4	0,1	0.8	0,0	0,2	0,3
Canada, Northwest Territories	0.8	-	-	-	-	-	0,3	-	-	-	0,9	-	-	-	-	-
Canada, Nova Scotia	0.6	0.3	0.9	0.3	0.2	0,0	0.5	0,1	0.9	0,3	0,1	0,1	1.6	0,2	0.4	0,0
Canada, Ontario	0.6	0.3	0.6	0.4	0.1	0.1	0.6	0.3	0.6	0.2	0.2	0.1	0.8	0.2	0.3	0.1
Canada, Prince Edward Island	0,3	0,6	0,6	0,8	0,3	-	-	-	0,9	0,2	-	-	2,1	0,1	0,4	-
Canada, Quebec	0.4	0.1	0.6	0.2	0.2	0.1	1.0	0.3	0.4	0.1	0.4	0.1	1.0	0.1	0.5	0.1
Canada, Saskatchewan	0.3	0.2	0.3	0.2	0.0	0.1	0.2	0.1	0.4	0.2	0.1	0.0	0.6	0.1	0.5	0.1
Canada, Yukon	2,2	-	-	1,6	-	-	-	1,0	-	1,1	0,8	-	-	1,4	-	-
US, Cent. Calif.: Non-Hisp. White	0.7	0.3	0.6	0.3	0.1	0,1	0.7	0.3	0.9	0.3	0.2	0,1	0.7	0,1	0.3	0.2
US, Cent. Calif.: Hispanic	0,2	0,2	0,4	0,1	-	-	0,2	-	0,4	0,1	-	0,1	0,3	0,1	0,3	-
US, Los Angeles: Non-Hisp. White	0.6	0.4	0.7	0.5	0.1	0.1	0.6	0.4	0.9	0.4	0.3	0.2	0.7	0.2	0.6	0.2
US, Los Angeles: Hispanic White	0.3	0,1	0.3	0.2	0.1	0,1	0.3	0,0	0.6	0,1	0.2	0,0	0.2	0,0	0.4	-
US, Los Angeles: Black	0,4	0,1	1.2	0,6	0,3	0,1	1.1	0,3	1.3	0,6	0,4	0,2	1.1	0,1	0.5	0,1
US, Los Angeles: Chinese	0,1	0,1	0,6	-	-	-	-	-	0,2	0,1	-	0,2	0,5	-	0,4	-
US, Los Angeles: Filipino	-	0,3	-	0,1	-	-	0,6	-	0,2	0,1	0,3	-	0,1	-	-	-
US, Los Angeles: Korean	-	-	0,4	0,2	-	-	0,9	-	-	-	-	-	1,0	-	-	-
US, Los Angeles: Japanese	0,2	0,2	0,2	0,3	-	-	-	-	0,4	0,1	-	-	-	-	0,4	-
US, San Francisco: Non-Hisp. White	0.7	0.4	0.7	0.7	0.1	0.1	0.8	0.3	1.0	0.5	0.2	0.2	1.2	0.3	0.6	0.2
US, San Francisco: Hispanic White	0,5	0,1	0,3	0,3	0,1	-	0,4	0,1	1.1	0,4	0,1	-	1.3	0,1	0.5	-
US, San Francisco: Black	0,7	0,3	1.8	0,5	-	-	1.0	0,3	2.3	0,4	0,6	0,2	1.8	0,4	1.0	0,3
US, San Francisco: Chinese	0,4	0,3	0,7	0,1	0,1	-	0,3	0,1	0,1	-	-	-	0,2	-	0,2	-
US, San Francisco: Filipino	0,3	0,6	0,3	0,5	0,1	-	0,9	0,3	0,3	0,1	-	-	-	0,2	-	0,2
US, San Francisco: Japanese	-	-	1,2	0,7	-	-	-	-	-	-	-	-	0,6	-	-	-
US, Connecticut: White	0.7	0.3	0.7	0.4	0.2	0.1	0.6	0.3	1.0	0.4	0.3	0.1	0.9	0.3	0.5	0.2
US, Connecticut: Black	0.8	0,1	2.1	0,9	0,4	0,2	3.0	0,6	1.3	0,7	1,4	-	2.6	0,5	0.8	0,2
US, Atlanta: White	0.8	0.6	0.8	0.4	0.4	0.2	0.7	0.4	0.6	0.2	0.3	0,1	1.0	0,1	0.3	0,1
US, Atlanta: Black	0.5	0.3	1.6	0,6	0,1	0,2	1.2	0,4	1.7	0,4	0,1	0,2	1.6	0,5	0.9	0,3
US, Iowa	0.5	0.4	0.5	0.4	0.1	0,0	0.4	0.3	0.9	0.3	0.1	0,0	0.9	0.2	0.5	0,1
US, Central Louisiana: White	0,1	0,3	0.3	0,1	-	0,1	0.5	0,2	0,3	0,5	-	-	0.9	-	-	-
US, Central Louisiana: Black	-	0,2	1,1	-	-	-	1,9	-	1,8	-	0,6	-	3,8	0,4	1,0	-
US, New Orleans: White	0.9	0.4	0.7	0.5	0.2	0,1	1.0	0.2	0.6	0,1	0.2	0,1	1.0	0,1	0.3	0,1
US, New Orleans: Black	0,2	0,4	1.1	0,1	0,6	-	1.5	0,2	1.3	0,0	0.5	0,1	2.2	-	0,2	0,2
US, Detroit: White	0.6	0.3	0.6	0.4	0.3	0.1	1.0	0.3	0.9	0.4	0.1	0,0	1.1	0.2	0.4	0.1
US, Detroit: Black	0.6	0.4	1.9	0,7	0,4	0,2	1.8	0,5	1.3	0,4	0.5	0,1	2.4	0,2	1.1	0,1
US, New Mexico: Non-Hisp. White	0,3	0,2	0.4	0,4	0,1	0,2	0.5	0,2	0.9	0,2	0,0	-	0.6	0,1	0,1	0,0
US, New Mexico: Hispanic White	0,1	0,1	0,4	0,1	0,1	0,1	0,1	-	0.9	0,2	0,1	-	0,7	-	-	-
US, New Mexico: American Indian	0,6	-	-	-	-	-	-	-	-	-	-	-	-	-	-	-
US, Utah	0.3	0,1	0.3	0.3	0,0	0,1	0.3	0,1	0.4	0,1	0,0	0,0	0.4	0,0	0,1	0,1
US, Seattle	0.7	0.6	0.6	0.4	0.1	0.1	0.4	0.3	0.7	0.3	0.1	0,1	0.7	0.3	0.4	0.1
US, SEER: White	0.6	0.4	0.6	0.4	0.2	0.1	0.6	0.2	0.8	0.3	0.2	0.1	0.9	0.2	0.4	0.1
US, SEER: Black	0.6	0.3	1.7	0,6	0,2	0,1	1.5	0,4	1.6	0,4	0.5	0,1	2.0	0,3	1.0	0,2

AGE-STANDARDIZED (WORLD) INCIDENCE RATES (FOUR DIGIT RUBRICS)

| | Other parts of mouth | | | | | | | | Oropharynx | | | | Hypopharynx | | | |
| | 145.0-1,6 | | 145.2-5 | | 145.8-9 | | 146.0 | | 146.1-7 | | 146.8-9 | | 148.1 | | 148.0,2-9 | |
ASIA	M	F	M	F	M	F	M	F	M	F	M	F	M	F	M	F
*China, Qidong	-	-	0,0	0,0	0,1	-	-	0,1	-	-	0,0	0,0	-	-	0,1	-
China, Shanghai	0.2	0.2	0.3	0.3	0.1	0.1	0.2	0.1	0.1	0,0	0,0	0,0	0,0	0,0	0.1	0,0
China, Tianjin	0,0	0,0	0.2	0,1	0.1	0.1	0,0	0,0	0,0	0,0	0.2	0.1	0,1	0,0	0.1	0,0
Hong Kong																
*India, Bangalore	1.1	6.1	0.6	0.4	0,0	0.2	1.2	0.4	0.8	0,0	0.2	0,1	4.7	0.5	1.1	0.6
*India, Barshi, Paranda and Bhum	1.9	0,6	0,4	0,2	-	-	0,5	0,1	0,3	-	-	-	4.8	0.5	1.9	-
India, Bombay	2.8	2.7	1.0	0.4	0.3	0.2	2.5	0.4	0.7	0,1	0.2	0,1	6.6	1.0	1.8	1.1
*India, Karunagappally	4.4	3.3	1,2	0,9	0,6	-	0,6	-	0,6	-	1,5	-	2,0	-	0,8	0,6
India, Madras	4.3	5.9	1.4	0.5	0.1	0,1	1.4	0.3	0.6	0,1	0.7	0,1	2.6	0.6	3.9	1.9
*India, Trivandrum	5.7	3.7	1.6	0,3	0,1	-	1,3	0,4	0,3	-	1.6	-	1.6	0,1	0,3	0,6
Israel: All Jews	0.1	0.1	0.2	0.2	0.1	0.1	0.1	0,1	0,1	0,0	0,0	0,0	0,1	0,0	0.2	0,0
Jews born in Israel	0,2	0,1	0,3	0,3	0,1	0,1	0,1	0,0	-	-	-	-	-	-	0,1	-
Jews born in America or Europe	0,2	0,1	0,3	0,0	0,1	0,1	0,1	0,0	0,1	0,0	0,0	0,0	0,1	0,0	0,1	0,0
Jews born in Africa or Asia	0,1	0,1	0,2	0.5	0,1	0,0	0,2	0,1	0,1	-	0,0	0,0	0,1	-	0,2	0,0
Non-Jews	0,1	0,2	0,1	-	-	0,0	0,1	-	-	-	-	-	0,1	-	-	0,2
Japan, Hiroshima	0,0	0,1	0.3	0,1	0.3	0.2	0.3	0,1	-	-	0.5	-	0,0	-	1.2	0,1
Japan, Miyagi	0,1	0,1	0.2	0,1	0.1	0,0	0.1	0,0	-	-	0.2	0,0	-	-	0.9	0.2
Japan, Nagasaki	0,0	0,1	0.4	0,1	0.3	0.1	0.3	0,1	-	-	0.2	0,0	-	-	0.8	0,1
Japan, Osaka	0.2	0.1	0.2	0,1	0.1	0.0	0.3	0.1	0.1	0,0	0.3	0.1	0.3	0,0	0.9	0.1
*Japan, Saga																
Japan, Yamagata																
*Korea, Kangwha	-	-	-	-	-	0,7	-	-	0,3	-	0,7	-	-	-	0,3	-
*Kuwait: Non-Kuwaitis	0,3	0,7	0,1	-	0,1	-	1,3	-	0,0	-	-	-	0,1	-	0,0	-
*Kuwait: Kuwaitis	0,4	0,3	-	-	0,2	0,2	0,1	0,5	0,1	0,3	-	-	0,9	0,3	-	1,1
*Philippines, Manila	0.6	0.5	0.8	1.4	0.4	0.3	0.8	0.6	0,0	0,0	0.2	0,0	0,0	-	0.2	0,1
Singapore: Chinese	0.5	0.2	0.5	0.2	0,1	0,0	0.7	0.2	0,1	-	0,1	0,1	1.1	0,1	0.5	0,0
Singapore: Malay	0,4	0,3	0,4	-	-	0,2	0,9	0,2	-	-	-	-	0,2	-	-	0,3
Singapore: Indian	1.9	2,1	1,2	0,4	-	0,2	1,0	0,3	-	-	0,3	0,9	1,1	0,7	0,3	0,3
Thailand, Chiang Mai	0.6	0.9	0.7	0,2	0.3	0,1	1.2	0.8	0,1	0,1	0.3	0,1	1.9	0.3	0.6	0,2
*Thailand, Khon Kaen	0,4	1.7	0,4	0,2	-	0,1	0.5	0,2	-	-	0,1	-	0,4	-	0,1	0,0
*Viet Nam, Hanoi	0,2	0,3	0,0	0,1	0.3	0,3	0.5	0,2	0,1	-	0,2	-	-	-	1.2	0.4
EUROPE																
Austria, Tyrol	0,1	0,1	0,1	0,2	1.6	0,1	0.7	0.4	0.7	0,1	0.7	0,2	0.9	0,1	0.6	0,2
*Belarus																
*Croatia	0.6	0.1	0.5	0,1	0.3	0,0	1.7	0.2	0.2	0,0	1.0	0.1	0.2	0,0	4.2	0.3
Czech Republic	0.2	0.1	0.3	0.1	0.1	0.0	1.5	0.2	0.5	0.1	0.2	0,0	0.4	0,0	0.6	0.1
Denmark	0.2	0.1	0.3	0.2	1.1	0.6	1.1	0.4	0.1	0.1	0.5	0.2	0.2	0,0	0.5	0.1
Estonia	0.3	0,1	0.5	0,0	0.6	0,0	0.4	0,0	1.3	0,1	1.4	0,1	1.2	0,0	0.8	0,0
Finland																
France, Bas-Rhin	1.8	0.2	3.3	0.3	0.2	0,1	2.8	0.2	6.9	0.5	2.3	0,1	10.0	0.3	3.9	0,3
*France, Calvados	1.8	0.2	2.7	0,4	0.1	0,1	2.9	0.4	7.4	0.4	1.4	-	11.1	0.2	3.9	-
France, Doubs	0.8	0.2	1.8	0,4	1.1	0,1	3.2	0.5	4.9	0.4	1.1	0,1	7.9	0.2	2.1	0.2
France, Haut-Rhin	1.4	0.2	2.9	0.3	0.7	0,0	3.6	0.2	6.5	0.7	1.6	0,1	8.1	0.5	2.2	-
*France, Herault	0.2	0.3	0.8	0.2	1.5	0.2	3.5	0.5	1.6	0.3	0.3	0,1	2.9	0,0	1.0	0,1
France, Isere	0.9	0.3	1.2	0.2	0.2	0,0	2.1	0.5	2.5	0.3	1.3	0,2	5.1	0.2	1.5	0,0
*France, Somme	1.7	0.1	2.7	0,5	0.5	0,0	4.1	0.4	5.9	0.4	3.4	-	7.4	0.3	3.5	0,1
*France, Tarn	0,6	0,2	1.2	-	-	-	1.8	0,1	3.4	0.2	0.3	0,1	3.4	0.3	1.3	-
Germany, Eastern States	0.2	0.1	0.4	0.1	0.1	0.0	1.4	0.3	0.1	0,0	0.2	0.0	0.1	0,0	1.1	0.1
Germany, Saarland	0,2	0,1	1.1	0.2	0.2	0,1	2.2	0.5	0.6	0,1	0.4	0,0	1.1	0,1	2.3	0.3
Iceland	0.2	0.3	0,1	-	0.3	0.2	0.2	0.3	-	-	0.2	-	-	-	0.3	-
Ireland, Southern	0.1	0.0	0,4	0.2	0.2	-	0.8	0.1	0,1	-	-	0.1	0.6	0.2	0.3	0,2
Italy, Ferrara	0.5	0.4	0.3	0.1	0.7	0,1	1.5	0.4	-	-	0.3	0.1	0.3	-	0.1	0.4
Italy, Florence	0.1	0.1	0.2	0,1	0.9	0.3	0.6	0,1	0.2	0,0	0.3	0.2	0.5	-	0.5	0.1
Italy, Genoa	0.4	0.2	0.5	0,1	0.5	0.2	1.3	0.3	0.9	0,1	0.2	0,0	0.7	0,1	0.8	0.2
*Italy, Latina	0,5	-	0.2	0,1	0.3	0,1	0.7	-	-	-	0,0	-	0,1	-	0.3	0,1
Italy, Macerata	-	0,2	0.2	-	0,1	0.4	0.9	0,0	-	-	0.3	-	-	-	0,1	-
Italy, Modena	0.2	0.1	0.3	0,1	0.1	0,0	0.9	0.2	0.2	0,0	0.2	-	0.6	0,0	0.9	0.2
Italy, Parma	0.5	0.1	0.4	0,1	0.8	0,1	1.2	0,1	0,1	-	0.4	0,1	1.6	0.3	1.0	0,1
Italy, Ragusa	0.1	0.1	0.2	0,1	0.4	0.5	0.1	-	-	-	-	0,1	0,1	-	-	-
Italy, Romagna	0.2	0.1	0.3	0,0	0.3	0,1	0.8	0,1	0.2	-	0.2	-	0.5	0,0	0.1	0,0
Italy, Torino	0.3	0.1	0.3	0,1	0.7	0,1	0.9	0.2	0.3	0,3	0.7	0.2	0.8	0,1	0.3	0.2
Italy, Trieste	0.6	0.7	0.8	0,4	6.3	1.4	0.9	0.2	0.3	-	1.3	0,3	1.0	-	0.6	-
Italy, Varese	0.8	0.2	0.8	0,1	0,0	-	1.0	0,1	1.8	0,1	0.8	0,1	1.4	0,1	0.9	0,1
Italy, Veneto	0.3	0,1	0.6	0,2	2.7	0.6	1.5	0.5	0.4	0,0	1.0	0,0	1.0	0,1	1.0	0,1
*Latvia	0.2	0,1	0.4	0.1	0.2	0,0	0.9	0,1	0.4	0,0	0.3	0,0	0,1	-	1.7	0.1
Malta	0,5	0,7	0,5	-	-	-	-	0,1	-	-	-	-	0,5	-	-	0.1

AGE-STANDARDIZED (WORLD) INCIDENCE RATES (FOUR DIGIT RUBRICS)

| | Other parts of mouth | | | | | | Oropharynx | | | | | | Hypopharynx | | | |
| | 145.0-1,6 | | 145.2-5 | | 145.8-9 | | 146.0 | | 146.1-7 | | 146.8-9 | | 148.1 | | 148.0,2-9 | |
	M	F	M	F	M	F	M	F	M	F	M	F	M	F	M	F
The Netherlands	0.4	0.2	0.3	0.2	0.1	0.1	0.5	0.3	0.5	0.2	0.3	0.1	0.7	0.1	0.3	0.1
The Netherlands, Eindhoven	0.4	0,2	0,3	0,2	0,1	0,1	0.4	0,0	0.5	0,1	0,3	0,2	0.3	0,0	0,3	0,0
The Netherlands, Maastricht	0.3	0,1	0,1	0,1	0,1	0,0	0.4	0,3	0.5	0,3	0,2	0,1	1.0	0,1	0,3	-
Norway																
*Poland, Cracow	0,1	0,1	0,2	0,1	0,3	0,1	0.4	0,3	0,1	-	1.5	0,1	-	-	0,3	0,2
*Poland, Kielce	0,1	-	0,1	0,1	0,0	-	0.3	0,1	0,1	0,0	0.6	0,0	-	-	0,3	-
*Poland, Lower Silesia	0.1	0.1	0.4	0.1	0.0	0.0	1.2	0.4	0.1	-	0,1	-	0,0	-	0.4	0,1
Poland, Warsaw City	0,0	0,0	0,2	0,1	0,1	0,0	1.0	0.3	-	0,0	1.6	0.2	0.2	0,0	0.5	0,1
Slovakia	0.5	0.1	0.8	0.1	0.1	0,0	2.7	0.1	1.7	0.1	0.7	0,0	1.4	0,0	2.5	0.1
Slovenia	0.8	0,1	0.4	0,1	0.4	0,1	1.1	0.2	-	-	5.6	0.2	2.4	0,1	1.2	0,1
*Spain, Albacete	0,4	-	0,4	-	-	0,2	0,4	-	-	-	0,5	-	0,4	-	0,3	-
Spain, Asturias	0.5	0,0	0.6	0,1	0,2	0,1	1.5	0,1	0.5	-	2.2	0,2	3.6	0,0	0.7	0,0
Spain, Basque Country	0.9	0.2	0.7	0,1	0.5	0,1	2.0	0,1	0.8	0,0	0.7	0,0	2.8	0,1	0.9	0,0
Spain, Granada	0.7	0.1	0.5	0,1	0.5	0,2	0.6	-	0,4	-	0,2	-	1.4	-	0.8	-
Spain, Mallorca	0.9	0,1	0.7	0,1	1.1	0,1	1.3	0,1	1.1	0,1	0.6	0,1	2.2	0,0	1.7	-
Spain, Murcia	0.7	0.2	0.3	0,1	0.4	0,1	1.7	0,1	0.3	-	0,2	-	0.9	0,0	0.5	-
Spain, Navarra	0.7	0.2	0,4	0,0	0,1	0,0	0.8	0,0	0,5	-	0,5	0,1	1.0	-	1.1	-
Spain, Tarragona	0.5	0,1	0.5	0,2	0,3	0,2	1.1	0,0	0.7	0,0	0,1	-	1.6	-	0,3	0,1
Spain, Zaragoza	0,3	0,1	0,3	0,0	0.4	0,0	0.9	0,1	0,2	-	0,3	-	0.8	-	0.4	-
Sweden	0.2	0.1	0.2	0.2	0.3	0.1	0.7	0.3	-	-	0.2	0.1	0.1	0,0	0.7	0.1
*Switzerland, Basel	0,5	0,1	0.8	0,2	0,3	0,2	1.4	0.2	0,5	-	0,5	0,3	0.6	0,2	1.6	0,2
Switzerland, Geneva	0,6	0,3	1.4	0,5	0,2	0,2	1.6	0.7	2.3	0,4	1.6	0,5	3.4	0,4	1.6	0,2
Switzerland, Graubunden	-	-	0,5	-	-	-	-	-	1,7	0,2	-	0,1	0,5	-	1,4	-
Switzerland, Neuchatel	0,3	-	0,6	0,3	0,2	0,2	1,8	0,6	2.0	0,5	0,9	-	3.2	-	0,6	0,4
Switzerland, St Gall-Appenzell	0,1	0,1	0.7	0,2	0,2	0,1	0.7	0,1	0,2	0,0	1.3	0,0	0,4	-	1.6	-
Switzerland, Valais	0.5	0.5	0,8	-	0,4	-	2.0	0,4	2.0	-	0,7	-	1,5	0,1	2.9	0,1
Switzerland, Vaud	0.7	0.2	0.8	0,2	0,2	0,1	2.1	0.5	3.0	0,3	0,4	0,1	4.0	0.5	2.7	0.5
Switzerland, Zurich	0.3	0.1	0.5	0,1	0,0	0,0	1.2	0.4	0.8	0,2	0,3	0,0	1.1	0,2	0.7	0,1
*UK, England and Wales	0.2	0.1	0.3	0.1	0.2	0.1	0.5	0.2	0.1	0.0	0.2	0.0	0.4	0.1	0.2	0.2
*UK, East Anglia																
*UK, Mersey	0.4	0.3	0.5	0,1	0.2	0.1	0.7	0.3	0.3	0,1	0.1	0,0	0.6	0.1	0.4	0.3
*UK, North Western	0.3	0.1	0.4	0.1	0.4	0.1	0.8	0.2	0.1	0.1	0.4	0.1	0.6	0.1	0.2	0.2
UK, Oxford	0.2	0.1	0.3	0.1	0.2	0.2	0.3	0.2	0,1	-	0.1	0,0	0.4	0.1	0,1	0.2
*UK, South Thames	0.2	0.1	0.2	0.1	0.1	0.1	0.5	0.2	0.1	0,0	0.1	0.0	0.4	0.1	0.1	0.2
UK, South Western	0.2	0.1	0.3	0.1	0.1	0.0	0.3	0.1	0.1	0,0	0.1	0,0	0.2	0.1	0.2	0.1
UK, Wessex	0.2	0.1	0.3	0.2	0.2	0.1	0.3	0.1	0.1	0,0	0.1	0,0	0.3	0,0	0.2	0.2
*UK, West Midlands	0.3	0.2	0.4	0.1	0.1	0.1	0.6	0.1	0.1	0,0	0.1	0.1	0.6	0.1	0.2	0.2
UK, Yorkshire	0.3	0.2	0.3	0.2	0.1	0.0	0.6	0.2	0,1	0,0	0.1	0,0	0.5	0.1	0.1	0.2
UK, Scotland	0.5	0.2	0.6	0.4	0.2	0.1	0.6	0.1	0.3	0.1	0.2	0.1	0.6	0.1	0.3	0.1
UK, Scotland, West	0.5	0.2	0.7	0.3	0.3	0.1	0.7	0.2	0.2	0.1	0.2	0,1	0.6	0.2	0.3	0.2
*Yugoslavia, Vojvodina																

OCEANIA

| | Other parts of mouth | | | | | | Oropharynx | | | | | | Hypopharynx | | | |
| | 145.0-1,6 | | 145.2-5 | | 145.8-9 | | 146.0 | | 146.1-7 | | 146.8-9 | | 148.1 | | 148.0,2-9 | |
	M	F	M	F	M	F	M	F	M	F	M	F	M	F	M	F
Australian Capital Territory	0,2	0,4	0,6	0,1	-	-	0,1	-	-	0,2	0,4	-	0,7	-	-	-
Australia, New South Wales	0.4	0.2	0.8	0.3	0.2	0.1	0.7	0.2	0.6	0.1	0.3	0.1	1.2	0.1	0.2	0.0
South Australia	0.3	0.2	0.5	0.3	0.3	0.3	1.0	0.2	0.6	0.1	0.1	0,0	1.1	0.1	0.2	0,1
Australia, Tasmania	0,1	0,2	0,4	0,3	0,3	0,2	0.8	0.2	0,4	0,1	0,4	-	0.8	0,1	0,1	-
Australia, Victoria	0.3	0.3	0.5	0.3	0.1	0.1	0.7	0.2	0.8	0.1	0.5	0.1	1.4	0.1	0.2	0.1
Western Australia	0.3	0.2	0.5	0.2	0.3	0,1	1.3	0.3	0.3	0.1	0.3	0,1	1.2	0.1	0.2	0,1
*French Polynesia	0,3	-	0,7	1,0	0,4	0,3	2.8	0,7	0,1	-	0,5	-	1,2	0,3	2,5	0,3
New Zealand: Non-Maori	0.3	0.2	0.3	0.1	0.1	0,0	0.5	0.2	0.3	0,0	0.1	0.1	0.7	0.1	0.2	0.1
New Zealand: Maori	0,6	-	0,2	0,7	0,6	-	0,6	0,2	0,5	0,2	-	-	0,9	-	-	-
US, Hawaii: White	0,2	0,2	0,9	0,3	0,1	-	2.0	-	1.6	0,3	0,3	0,2	1.5	0,4	0,6	0,4
US, Hawaii: Japanese	0,3	0,1	0,5	0,2	-	-	0,3	0,1	0,1	0,1	0,2	-	1.1	-	0,7	-
US, Hawaii: Hawaiian	0,3	0,2	0,5	-	0,3	-	0,5	0,3	0,3	-	0,3	0,3	2,0	-	0,6	0,3
US, Hawaii: Filipino	0,2	0,4	0,2	0,4	-	0,2	0,3	0,4	0,8	-	0,1	0,2	0,6	0,3	-	0,5
US, Hawaii: Chinese	0,8	0,3	-	-	-	-	0,2	-	-	-	0,6	-	0,3	0,6	0,7	-

AGE-STANDARDIZED (WORLD) INCIDENCE RATES (FOUR DIGIT RUBRICS)

| | Oesophagus | | | | | | | | | Stomach | | | | | | |
| | 150.0,3 | | 150.1,4 | | 150.2,5 | | 150.8-9 | | 151.0 | | 151.1-2 | | 151.3-6 | | 151.8-9 | |
AFRICA	M	F	M	F	M	F	M	F	M	F	M	F	M	F	M	F
*Algeria, Setif	-	-	-	-	-	-	1,2	0,3	-	-	0,4	0,1	0,2	-	13.9	3.4
*France, La Reunion	2.5	0,2	7.8	0,3	4.5	0,5	7.2	0,6	0,8	0,1	4.3	1.7	3.0	1.2	14.2	5.3
*Mali, Bamako	-	-	-	-	-	-	1.7	0,6	-	0,2	0,8	0,6	-	-	18.9	10.4
*Uganda, Kyadondo	-	-	-	-	-	-	18.2	8.7	0,3	0,1	0,6	0,5	-	-	4.5	2.6
*Zimbabwe, Harare: African	-	-	-	-	-	-	30.4	8.0	0,3	-	0,3	1,3	0,1	0,4	13.2	16.7
*Zimbabwe, Harare: European	-	-	-	-	-	-	2,4	1,5	-	-	-	-	-	-	8,3	6,3

AMERICA, CENTRAL AND SOUTH	M	F	M	F	M	F	M	F	M	F	M	F	M	F	M	F
*Argentina, Concordia	0,4	0,3	1,1	-	0,4	0,4	15.6	3.0	0,7	-	3.3	1,1	1,0	0,3	19.3	8.6
*Brazil, Belem	0,1	0,1	0,2	0,2	0,7	0,2	5.3	1.1	0,4	0,1	3.4	1.2	1,0	0,4	37.2	14.3
*Brazil, Goiania	0,3	-	0,5	0,2	0,2	0,1	8.3	1.6	0,2	-	1.4	0.9	0,4	0,7	17.1	9.1
*Brazil, Porto Alegre	0,1	-	-	0,1	0,1	0,0	18.7	3.9	0,6	0,0	0,2	0,1	0,3	0,1	26.8	8.6
Colombia, Cali	0,1	0,2	0.7	0,2	0.6	0,1	2.5	1.8	1.1	0.4	2.3	1.3	1.3	0.9	28.5	16.7
*Costa Rica	0.3	0,1	0.5	0.3	0.7	0.3	2.5	0.8	3.9	1.2	12.3	5.8	2.7	0.9	32.6	14.8
*Ecuador, Quito	0,1	0,2	0,3	0,0	0,3	0,1	2.4	0.8	1.1	0,3	2.2	0.9	0.8	0.6	28.2	17.7
*Peru, Lima	0,1	-	0,1	-	-	-	1.7	0.6	0,1	0,0	0,1	0,1	0,1	0,0	18.8	13.5
Peru, Trujillo	-	-	-	-	-	-	3.3	0,7	-	-	-	-	-	-	31.1	20.1
US, Puerto Rico	1.3	0.4	3.5	0.9	2.0	0.5	2.3	0.5	2.2	0.5	3.8	2.0	2.4	0.8	5.3	2.7
*Uruguay, Montevideo	0.4	0,2	1.5	0.3	1.4	0.4	8.6	2.5	0.7	0.3	0.9	0.5	1.2	0.3	16.6	7.9

AMERICA, NORTH	M	F	M	F	M	F	M	F	M	F	M	F	M	F	M	F
Canada	0.4	0.2	0.8	0.4	1.6	0.4	1.2	0.4	2.5	0.5	1.6	0.8	1.9	0.8	4.7	2.4
Canada, Alberta	0.3	0.1	0.6	0.4	1.2	0.3	0.5	0.1	3.2	0.4	1.6	0.9	2.0	0.9	3.0	1.8
Canada, British Columbia	0.4	0.2	1.0	0.5	2.2	0.6	0.7	0.3	2.6	0.5	1.3	0.8	1.8	0.8	3.5	1.8
Canada, Manitoba	0.2	0,1	0.6	0.2	1.6	0.4	1.5	0.6	3.5	0.4	1.5	0.8	1.9	0.8	4.2	2.4
Canada, New Brunswick	0.3	0,1	0.7	0.2	1.5	0.4	1.2	0.3	2.6	0.5	1.8	0.9	1.5	0.9	4.9	2.3
Canada, Newfoundland	0,1	0,1	0.9	0.2	1.8	0,2	1.3	0.6	2.6	0.7	3.5	2.6	6.1	1.9	6.2	2.7
Canada, Northwest Territories	0,5	-	1.0	0.2	-	2,3	1,9	2,9	5,5	1,1	2,1	-	1.7	-	9.6	3,5
Canada, Nova Scotia	0.3	0,1	0.5	0,1	1.8	0.3	1.6	0.6	2.8	0.5	1.6	0.8	2.2	1.2	5.3	2.6
Canada, Ontario	0.5	0.2	1.0	0.4	1.9	0.4	1.1	0.4	2.6	0.5	1.6	0.8	1.7	0.8	4.1	2.1
Canada, Prince Edward Island	0.2	-	1.3	-	1.3	-	1.7	0.4	2.9	0.2	1.1	1.2	1.3	1.3	6.4	2.7
Canada, Quebec	0.4	0.1	0.6	0.3	1.0	0.2	2.0	0.5	2.0	0.4	1.4	0.7	1.7	0.7	7.0	3.4
Canada, Saskatchewan	0.4	0,2	0.9	0.4	1.9	0.4	0.2	0,1	2.4	0.6	2.1	0.8	2.6	1.2	1.8	1.1
Canada, Yukon	-	-	4,5	-	1,8	-	-	-	2,5	-	1,1	-	0,8	-	1,4	4,6
US, Cent. Calif.: Non-Hisp. White	0.5	0.3	0.7	0.3	2.5	0.2	0.3	0.1	2.5	0.5	0.7	0.6	1.9	0.8	1.8	1.0
US, Cent. Calif.: Hispanic	0,1	0,2	0.7	0,1	1.4	0,2	0,1	-	1.4	0,6	2.7	1.9	3.5	2.6	2.3	1.4
US, Los Angeles: Non-Hisp. White	0.3	0.2	0.8	0.6	2.1	0.6	0.5	0.3	3.0	0.6	1.2	0.7	1.6	0.9	1.8	1.1
US, Los Angeles: Hispanic White	0.7	0,1	0.7	0.2	1.7	0,1	0.6	0,1	2.5	0.6	2.4	1.9	3.2	2.0	3.8	2.4
US, Los Angeles: Black	1.2	0.4	3.9	1.2	2.4	1.1	1.8	0.7	1.1	0.4	4.7	1.8	3.5	1.3	4.5	2.4
US, Los Angeles: Chinese	0.4	0,1	1.5	0.2	0.9	0.3	1.1	0.3	1.2	0.6	5.3	2.2	2.7	2.4	2.3	2.4
US, Los Angeles: Filipino	0.3	-	0,4	-	0,8	-	0.5	-	0,7	1,0	1.9	0.8	2.1	1.2	2.1	1,1
US, Los Angeles: Korean	0,4	-	2,4	-	1,7	-	1.6	0,3	0,8	1,2	16.2	6.6	9.7	3.8	8.7	4.7
US, Los Angeles: Japanese	0.8	0,2	2.2	0,3	1,9	0,1	1,0	0,5	3.4	0,4	7.7	3.9	5.5	4.2	4.6	3.6
US, San Francisco: Non-Hisp. White	0.5	0.2	1.1	0.7	2.3	0.4	0.6	0.3	3.3	0.5	1.0	0.7	1.9	0.9	1.6	0.9
US, San Francisco: Hispanic White	0,5	-	1.0	0,1	1.7	0,1	0.2	0,3	2.4	0,3	2.7	1.7	4.9	1.6	2.6	1.3
US, San Francisco: Black	1.2	0,7	6.2	2.1	2.3	0,7	1.8	0,3	2.0	0.6	4.8	2.0	4.8	2.5	3.7	2.4
US, San Francisco: Chinese	0.4	-	1.6	0.4	1.2	0.2	0.5	0.2	0.8	0.3	3.3	2.9	4.3	2.4	2.6	1.3
US, San Francisco: Filipino	-	-	0,1	0.2	1,9	-	0,7	-	0,9	0,7	2.4	0.8	1.8	1,7	1,4	1.0
US, San Francisco: Japanese	-	-	4,4	0,4	4,7	-	0,6	-	6,9	1,4	5.0	2,9	9.1	5.7	5,4	1,7
US, Connecticut: White	0.5	0.2	1.2	0.4	2.4	0.5	1.1	0.3	3.3	0.7	1.5	0.7	1.9	1.1	2.5	1.3
US, Connecticut: Black	2.3	0.8	8.6	2.0	5.7	0.8	3.5	0,4	2.0	0.8	2.9	1.7	4.3	2.0	3.9	2.2
US, Atlanta: White	0.4	0,2	0.7	0.4	2.3	0.4	0.7	0.3	1.9	0.3	0.7	0.4	1.0	0.8	1.6	0.8
US, Atlanta: Black	2.3	1.1	7.0	2.3	3.7	0.9	1.7	0,6	1.7	0,7	3.0	1.5	4.3	1.5	4.4	1.3
US, Iowa	0.3	0.1	0.7	0.3	2.5	0.3	0.6	0.1	2.9	0.5	0.9	0.4	1.4	0.7	1.4	0.6
US, Central Louisiana: White	0,1	-	0.6	0,3	2.2	0,2	0,8	0,3	1.4	0,1	1,1	0,5	1.5	0,7	2.0	0.9
US, Central Louisiana: Black	1,7	0,5	4,5	1,9	5,1	-	2,7	-	1,1	0,2	2,0	2,7	5,0	1,3	6.2	1,2
US, New Orleans: White	0.7	0,2	1.1	0.4	2.6	0.5	1.6	0.3	2.4	0.4	1.3	0.3	1.7	1.0	2.0	1.2
US, New Orleans: Black	1.6	0,2	4.3	0,6	2.3	1.2	3.0	0,6	1,1	0,4	4.8	2.4	4.7	1.5	6.2	2.1
US, Detroit: White	0.4	0.2	1.1	0.4	2.6	0.5	0.7	0.2	3.2	0.6	1.1	0.7	1.8	0.9	2.3	1.3
US, Detroit: Black	1.6	0.4	5.4	1.7	3.7	0.7	3.0	0.7	1.6	0.3	3.6	1.9	4.2	1.8	5.5	1.7
US, New Mexico: Non-Hisp. White	0,2	0,1	1.2	0.6	1.8	0.4	0.6	0,1	2.3	0.5	0.9	0.6	1.3	0.7	0.9	0.6
US, New Mexico: Hispanic White	0,5	0,1	0,7	0,1	0.6	0,1	0.5	0,1	1.9	0.4	2.7	2.2	4.5	2.2	3.6	1.4
US, New Mexico: American Indian	0,6	-	1,1	-	0,3	0,2	0.3	-	1,1	0,2	0,5	1,4	5.4	2.8	2,2	·3.3
US, Utah	0.4	0,0	0.4	0,1	1.5	0.3	0.4	0,1	2.5	0.5	0.7	0.4	0.7	0.7	1.7	1.3
US, Seattle	0.3	0.3	1.0	0.6	2.8	0.5	0.7	0.3	3.0	0.5	1.3	0.8	1.3	0.8	1.9	1.0
US, SEER: White	0.4	0.2	1.0	0.4	2.4	0.4	0.7	0.2	2.9	0.5	1.1	0.7	1.6	0.8	1.9	1.0
US, SEER: Black	1.6	0.6	6.1	1.9	3.6	0.8	2.4	0.6	1.8	0.5	3.8	1.8	4.3	1.8	4.6	1.8

AGE-STANDARDIZED (WORLD) INCIDENCE RATES (FOUR DIGIT RUBRICS)

| | Oesophagus | | | | | | | | Stomach | | | | | | | |
| | 150.0,3 | | 150.1,4 | | 150.2,5 | | 150.8-9 | | 151.0 | | 151.1-2 | | 151.3-6 | | 151.8-9 | |
ASIA	M	F	M	F	M	F	M	F	M	F	M	F	M	F	M	F
*China, Qidong	0,1	0,1	0,2	0,1	0,2	0,1	10.9	4.3	2.4	1.0	1.6	1.0	0.9	0.5	37.8	18.3
China, Shanghai	0.3	0.2	3.1	1.3	1.2	0.3	7.9	3.1	8.1	2.0	7.8	3.6	5.4	2.6	25.3	12.8
China, Tianjin	0.3	0.1	1.2	0.5	0.5	0.2	12.0	5.3	6.7	1.0	1.6	0.6	0.5	0.3	20.9	9.4
Hong Kong																
*India, Bangalore	0.6	0.5	2.7	2.9	2.0	1.6	3.6	3.5	0.2	0,1	0.8	0.4	0.2	0,1	9.1	4.5
*India, Barshi, Paranda and Bhum	0,1	-	0,4	0,2	0,5	0,2	4.9	1.5	-	0,1	-	-	0,1	-	0,6	0.8
India, Bombay	1.3	0.8	3.1	2.2	2.1	1.7	4.3	3.6	1.1	0.3	0.8	0.4	0.5	0.2	5.4	3.0
*India, Karunagappally	0,3	0,3	1,4	0,9	2,4	1,0	2.7	1.1	0,6	-	0.9	0.5	0.3	-	4.5	2.6
India, Madras	1.0	0.5	2.6	2.1	3.1	2.1	3.7	2.4	0.5	0,1	2.9	1.1	1.2	0.5	11.4	5.3
*India, Trivandrum	0,2	-	1.7	0,6	1.8	0,5	0.9	0.3	0.4	0,1	0.3	-	0.5	0,2	5.7	2.1
Israel: All Jews	0.2	0.1	0.2	0.1	0.4	0.3	0.9	0.5	2.2	0.6	2.0	1.2	2.3	1.1	6.4	3.2
Jews born in Israel	0,2	-	0,4	0,1	0,4	0,4	0.7	0,6	1.3	0,6	1.6	0,9	2.3	1.3	3.8	3.2
Jews born in America or Europe	0.1	0.1	0.1	0.1	0.5	0.2	1.0	0.5	2.6	0.8	2.3	1.3	2.8	1.2	7.6	3.6
Jews born in Africa or Asia	0,1	0,2	0,2	0,1	0.3	0.3	0.8	0.6	1.4	0.4	1.7	1.2	1.9	0.9	5.2	3.2
Non-Jews	-	-	-	0,0	0,2	-	0.2	0.2	0.8	0,4	1.0	0,4	1.0	0,6	4.0	1.8
Japan, Hiroshima	0.4	0,2	6.0	0.7	1.3	0,2	2.9	0.6	4.6	1.5	28.8	11.0	32.6	15.7	17.2	7.7
Japan, Miyagi	0.5	0,1	7.1	0.9	1.0	0.1	5.3	1.1	11.7	3.7	26.0	10.1	19.2	8.3	25.7	10.7
Japan, Nagasaki	0.2	0,0	2.9	0.4	1.8	0.2	3.8	0.5	5.4	2.0	18.8	6.9	21.8	11.1	24.9	11.4
Japan, Osaka	0.2	0.1	1.9	0.2	0.3	0.1	6.7	1.2	2.4	0.8	6.2	2.3	7.2	3.2	49.2	21.0
*Japan, Saga																
Japan, Yamagata																
*Korea, Kangwha	0,9	-	0,7	-	0,9	-	7.7	0,5	-	-	15.8	3.3	5.2	1,7	45.0	20.0
*Kuwait: Non-Kuwaitis	0,1	-	1,0	0,0	0,7	0,2	0.2	0.4	1.0	0.2	2,9	0.2	0,2	-	6.0	1.9
*Kuwait: Kuwaitis	0,2	0,5	0,5	0,8	0,2	0,3	0.8	0.8	0.6	0.3	1.0	0.4	0.2	0,5	2.3	3.7
*Philippines, Manila	0,0	0,0	0,1	0,1	0.3	0,1	2.7	1.4	0.3	0,1	0.5	0.4	0.4	0,1	9.8	5.7
Singapore: Chinese	0.7	0.3	2.4	0.6	1.1	0.2	4.4	1.2	2.4	0.6	1.3	0.8	0.2	0,0	25.5	12.2
Singapore: Malay	0,2	0,2	-	-	-	-	0.9	0.5	0.4	0.2	0.3	0.2	-	-	8.0	5.2
Singapore: Indian	0,8	1,2	1,4	0,5	0,8	0,3	2.5	1,9	0.8	0.3	1.0	0.3	-	-	8.6	7.4
Thailand, Chiang Mai	0,0	0,1	0.8	0,2	0,2	0.4	1.2	0.8	0.5	0.2	1.6	0.7	0.6	0.3	4.9	3.7
*Thailand, Khon Kaen	0,0	0,1	0,1	-	0,1	-	1.3	0.4	0.1	0,0	0.4	0.1	-	-	3.7	1.9
*Viet Nam, Hanoi	0,0	-	0,1	-	0,1	0,0	2.0	0.6	0.8	0.4	6.8	2.9	1.5	0.8	11.7	6.3

EUROPE

	150.0,3		150.1,4		150.2,5		150.8-9		151.0		151.1-2		151.3-6		151.8-9	
Austria, Tyrol	0,3	-	0,3	0,1	0,5	0,1	3.1	0.3	2.4	0.5	2.6	2.4	1.3	0.9	20.0	11.9
*Belarus																
*Croatia	0,0	-	0,0	0,0	0,0	0,0	6.0	0.8	0.8	0.2	0.5	0.2	0.2	0.1	26.5	11.0
Czech Republic	0.6	0.1	1.5	0.1	1.7	0.2	0.5	0.1	3.0	1.0	5.0	2.8	6.6	3.1	4.9	2.3
Denmark	0.1	0.0	0.1	0.1	1.2	0.4	3.3	0.9	2.7	0.6	1.0	0.5	1.0	0.6	4.3	3.0
Estonia	0.3	0,1	1.5	0,1	0.7	0.1	3.1	0.4	2.9	0.9	6.8	3.9	10.4	5.0	13.8	6.9
Finland																
France, Bas-Rhin	3.3	0.3	5.1	0,2	3.3	0.3	4.6	0.4	2.6	0,2	1.6	1.0	1.5	0.7	6.5	3.0
*France, Calvados	4.1	0,3	10.0	0.6	5.6	0,2	2.7	0,1	2.4	0.4	3.6	2.0	5.8	1.8	1.6	0.7
France, Doubs	2.4	0,1	3.2	0,4	1.9	0,5	3.6	0.5	2.3	0.3	3.6	1.6	2.7	0.7	2.1	1.0
France, Haut-Rhin	2.2	0,1	3.3	0,2	2.6	0,4	6.2	0.7	2.1	0.6	0.9	0.9	0.9	0.5	11.5	4.5
*France, Herault	0.6	0,1	1.5	0.3	1.3	0,2	3.1	0.6	2.0	0.4	1.7	1.1	1.1	0.3	4.9	2.2
France, Isere	1.5	0,1	2.6	0.3	1.8	0,1	4.1	0.4	2.2	0.4	1.8	0.7	0.6	0.4	7.3	3.2
*France, Somme	3.2	0,3	4.6	0,3	4.4	0.4	5.7	0.5	2.0	0,1	3.0	1.4	2.3	1.3	2.5	1.3
*France, Tarn	0.7	0,1	1.7	0,2	1.6	0,2	1.0	0,1	2.3	0,1	1.7	0.8	2.5	1.0	2.2	1.4
Germany, Eastern States	0.4	0.0	1.3	0.1	1.1	0.2	1.4	0.2	1.8	0.5	5.2	3.3	4.9	2.6	8.2	4.1
Germany, Saarland	0,1	0,0	0,2	0,1	0.3	0,0	6.1	0.7	2.4	0.5	1.6	1.0	1.2	0.4	13.3	7.0
Iceland	-	0,2	0,4	0,1	3.0	0.8	2.9	0.9	2.9	1.0	0,7	0.2	0.5	0,4	16.1	8.9
Ireland, Southern	0,2	0,1	0,4	0.6	1.2	0.4	4.7	2.3	2.7	0,3	0.4	0.2	0.8	0.6	9.4	3.9
Italy, Ferrara	0.5	0,1	0.4	0,1	0.8	0.2	1.8	0.3	1.7	0,4	1.8	1.3	2.1	0.6	13.0	7.1
Italy, Florence	0.2	0,1	0.4	0,1	0.4	0,1	2.7	0.6	1.9	0.3	6.1	3.6	2.4	0.8	26.0	11.2
Italy, Genoa	0.3	0,1	1.0	0,1	0.7	0,1	1.9	0.6	1.5	0.2	3.1	1.9	1.7	1.0	11.3	5.2
*Italy, Latina	-	0,1	0,2	-	0,2	0,1	2.3	0,2	0,4	0,3	1.2	0.6	1.2	0.4	16.4	9.1
Italy, Macerata	0,2	0,2	0,4	-	0,1	0.2	0.8	0.3	2.5	0,7	4.5	1.3	5.0	4.4	17.6	7.6
Italy, Modena	0.4	0,0	1.1	0.3	0.6	0,1	0.9	0.2	2.6	0.9	6.4	4.5	5.6	3.0	8.1	3.4
Italy, Parma	0.3	-	1.0	0,2	0.9	0,0	1.7	0.6	2.2	0.2	6.5	3.4	5.9	2.7	19.1	8.3
Italy, Ragusa	0,1	0,2	0.3	-	0,3	-	0,3	0.2	1.3	0.5	3.0	1.4	3.4	1.4	5.6	3.2
Italy, Romagna	0,2	0,0	0.1	0,0	0.7	0.2	1.8	0.2	2.2	0.8	8.4	6.3	13.6	8.4	15.0	7.3
Italy, Torino	0.3	0,0	0.9	0,2	0.9	0,1	1.4	0.3	1.8	0.5	3.1	2.2	5.0	2.2	7.3	3.7
Italy, Trieste	0.5	0,1	0.8	0,2	0,7	-	5.0	1.1	2.1	0.4	0.5	0.3	0,3	0,3	15.4	7.9
Italy, Varese	0.6	0,1	2.7	0,2	1.5	0.2	2.1	0.2	2.8	0.6	7.4	4.1	7.0	3.5	9.4	4.6
Italy, Veneto	0.3	0,0	0.8	0,1	0.5	0,0	8.1	1.4	1.1	0.2	1.9	1.1	2.0	1.0	14.9	6.6
*Latvia	2.0	0.2	1.2	0.2	0.8	0.1	0.6	0.1	5.9	2.3	5.4	2.3	7.6	3.7	12.2	5.7
Malta	0,3	0,1	0,2	0,1	0.7	0,3	2,0	0,6	1,9	0,1	0,8	0,9	1,4	0,8	7.0	4.2

AGE-STANDARDIZED (WORLD) INCIDENCE RATES (FOUR DIGIT RUBRICS)

| | Oesophagus | | | | | | | | | | Stomach | | | | | |
| | 150.0,3 | | 150.1,4 | | 150.2,5 | | 150.8-9 | | 151.0 | | 151.1-2 | | 151.3-6 | | 151.8-9 | |
	M	F	M	F	M	F	M	F	M	F	M	F	M	F	M	F
The Netherlands	0.4	0.2	1.0	0.7	3.2	0.7	0.7	0.3	4.2	0.8	3.3	1.9	3.4	1.6	4.6	1.9
The Netherlands, Eindhoven	0.4	0,2	0.8	0.4	1.8	0.5	0.5	0,1	4.1	1.1	3.6	2.1	3.2	1.6	6.2	2.6
The Netherlands, Maastricht	0,3	0.3	0.9	0.5	1.8	0,2	0.9	0.3	2.6	0.6	3.7	2.4	4.8	1.7	4.4	1.8
Norway																
*Poland, Cracow	-	-	-	-	-	0,0	4.3	0.7	1.3	0,3	0,5	0,3	0.6	0,2	19.1	7.2
*Poland, Kielce	-	-	-	-	-	-	3.1	0.6	1.0	0,1	0,1	0,1	0.2	0,0	20.8	7.7
*Poland, Lower Silesia	0,0	0,0	0,0	0,0	0.2	0,0	5.6	0.9	2.4	0.6	0.7	0.4	0.2	0.2	21.4	9.3
Poland, Warsaw City	0,0	-	0,1	0,0	0,1	0,0	4.5	1.0	1.8	0.5	0.3	0.2	0.3	0,1	16.7	6.1
Slovakia	0.8	0.1	2.6	0.1	2.3	0.2	1.6	0.2	2.6	0.7	6.4	3.0	6.5	3.0	8.9	3.6
Slovenia	-	-	-	-	-	-	6.8	0.9	2.4	0.6	2.7	1.4	-	-	21.8	8.7
*Spain, Albacete	0.4	-	0,4	-	1,2	-	1,1	0,1	0.8	0,4	1.7	1.2	3.2	2.2	11.5	4.1
Spain, Asturias	0.3	0,1	1.2	0,1	0.7	0,0	5.3	0.5	0.9	0.2	1.0	0.5	0.5	0.3	16.1	7.6
Spain, Basque Country	1.3	0,0	3.6	0.2	2.3	0.2	2.4	0.2	2.6	0.5	6.3	2.9	5.1	2.3	10.2	3.9
Spain, Granada	0.5	0,1	0.9	0,2	1.3	0,2	1.1	0,1	2.0	0.3	3.7	2.2	4.1	1.6	5.7	2.9
Spain, Mallorca	0.7	0,2	1.9	0,2	1.4	0,0	1.5	0,2	1.1	0,2	2.8	1.8	2.7	1.5	5.0	2.6
Spain, Murcia	0.4	0,0	0.7	0,1	0.6	0,1	2.9	0,2	1.2	0,1	2.7	0.9	1.7	0.9	9.5	5.3
Spain, Navarra	1.0	0,1	2.4	0,1	1.3	0,2	2.3	0,3	2.3	0.5	6.4	2.2	5.9	2.8	10.8	4.8
Spain, Tarragona	0,6	0,1	1.1	0,0	1.5	0,0	2.6	0,1	1.4	0.2	2.8	1.6	2.3	0.9	6.9	3.4
Spain, Zaragoza	0.8	0,1	1.5	0,1	1.4	0,0	1.8	0.3	1.7	0.3	4.8	2.2	2.9	0.9	10.2	4.9
Sweden	0.1	0.0	0.2	0.1	0.4	0.1	2.3	0.8	1.9	0.5	0.3	0.2	0.5	0.3	8.0	4.5
*Switzerland, Basel	0,5	0,1	1.8	0.4	2.1	0.5	1.0	0,4	2.8	0.8	3.3	2.4	2.4	0.7	2.4	1.1
Switzerland, Geneva	1.1	0,2	3.7	0.7	1.7	0.4	0.6	0,1	3.8	0.7	3.0	1.6	2.3	1.6	3.2	1.5
Switzerland, Graubunden	1,4	0,1	2,1	0,2	1,0	0,3	0,3	-	2.3	0.8	5.3	3.2	5.5	1.6	3.5	1.4
Switzerland, Neuchatel	1,3	0,6	2.4	0,4	2.0	0.7	0,7	0,2	2.3	1,0	3.3	2.3	3.4	1.1	3.7	1.0
Switzerland, St Gall-Appenzell	0.6	0,0	1.9	0,2	2.2	0.3	0.7	0,2	3.1	0.8	2.5	1.9	3.7	1.5	2.9	1.6
Switzerland, Valais	1,0	0,1	1.9	0,3	3.5	0,3	1,0	0,2	2.9	0,6	5.3	3.1	3.9	2.3	5.5	2.3
Switzerland, Vaud	2.0	0,3	2.8	0.9	3.7	0.6	1.0	0,2	2.8	0.4	2.1	1.2	3.7	1.2	1.8	1.5
Switzerland, Zurich	0.5	0.2	1.3	0.5	1.4	0.4	0.4	0,1	3.9	0.7	3.2	1.8	2.8	1.4	1.4	1.1
*UK, England and Wales	0.2	0.1	0.5	0.4	2.0	0.6	5.0	2.3	2.9	0.6	1.0	0.6	1.6	0.6	10.5	4.4
*UK, East Anglia																
*UK, Mersey	0.4	0.4	1.0	1.1	3.8	1.3	2.6	1.5	3.9	1.1	1.4	1.2	3.0	1.3	6.6	4.3
*UK, North Western	0.2	0.1	0.4	0.3	1.8	0.5	6.6	3.0	2.6	0.5	0.8	0.4	0.9	0.3	12.2	5.6
UK, Oxford	0.2	0.1	0.5	0.4	1.9	0.6	4.6	2.4	2.6	0.5	0.6	0.3	0.7	0.3	9.7	3.9
*UK, South Thames	0.2	0.2	0.7	0.5	2.7	0.8	3.8	1.8	2.7	0.5	1.0	0.6	1.6	0.7	8.0	3.3
UK, South Western	0.2	0.1	0.5	0.5	3.1	1.0	3.6	2.0	2.9	0.6	1.2	0.7	2.2	0.8	7.3	3.0
UK, Wessex	0.2	0.2	0.2	0.3	2.0	0.6	5.6	2.4	2.9	0.5	0.6	0.5	1.3	0.3	8.5	3.3
*UK, West Midlands	0.1	0.0	0.2	0.2	0.5	0.2	8.7	3.9	1.8	0.4	0.2	0.2	0.4	0.2	15.3	6.2
UK, Yorkshire	0.2	0.1	0.3	0.4	2.1	0.8	4.5	1.9	3.4	0.7	1.1	0.5	1.5	0.6	10.3	4.8
UK, Scotland	0.3	0.1	0.4	0.3	1.6	0.7	7.1	3.9	3.7	1.0	1.1	0.6	1.2	0.6	11.7	5.3
UK, Scotland, West	0.3	0.1	0.4	0.2	1.6	0.5	8.8	4.3	1.9	0.5	0.9	0.6	1.0	0.4	13.7	6.0
*Yugoslavia, Vojvodina																

OCEANIA

| | Oesophagus | | | | | | | | | | Stomach | | | | | |
| | 150.0,3 | | 150.1,4 | | 150.2,5 | | 150.8-9 | | 151.0 | | 151.1-2 | | 151.3-6 | | 151.8-9 | |
	M	F	M	F	M	F	M	F	M	F	M	F	M	F	M	F
Australian Capital Territory	-	0,3	-	0,3	3.7	0,5	1,8	0,9	2.0	0,8	1,5	1,1	2.1	1,1	4.1	2.3
Australia, New South Wales	0.3	0.1	0.4	0.3	1.3	0.4	2.5	1.1	2.1	0.4	1.1	0.6	1.7	0.7	5.3	2.5
South Australia	-	-	-	-	-	-	4.2	1.9	2.8	0.4	1.5	0.9	-	-	6.3	2.9
Australia, Tasmania	-	-	-	-	-	-	7.0	3.4	3.0	0.7	0,6	0,3	-	-	7.8	3.7
Australia, Victoria	0.4	0.2	0.7	0.4	2.1	0.7	2.2	1.0	3.1	0.6	1.2	0.7	1.9	0.7	5.5	2.8
Western Australia	0,2	0,0	0.2	0,0	0.7	0,1	3.5	1.5	2.7	0.8	0.9	0.5	1.5	0.6	6.4	3.3
*French Polynesia	2,1	-	0,5	0,9	-	0,3	4.6	0,3	0,8	0,4	-	0,6	1,2	0,3	8.9	6.1
New Zealand: Non-Maori	0.3	0.1	0.8	0.7	2.5	0.8	1.7	0.8	2.9	0.6	1.3	0.8	2.4	1.1	4.4	2.3
New Zealand: Maori	0,7	0,3	2,3	0,7	2.6	0,7	3.6	0,4	1,5	0,5	7.1	3.7	5.8	2.8	13.5	6.8
US, Hawaii: White	0,7	0,5	1.8	1,1	1.5	0,5	0,5	-	1.7	0.4	1.8	1.3	1.6	0.9	2.8	1.8
US, Hawaii: Japanese	0,8	-	1.4	0,3	1.2	0,2	0,3	0,1	2.4	0.4	5.9	3.5	7.2	4.4	5.9	2.4
US, Hawaii: Hawaiian	0,8	-	3.4	1,3	2,0	-	1,4	-	1,1	-	5.3	3.5	4.3	4.7	4.5	2.2
US, Hawaii: Filipino	0,2	0,2	0,6	0,6	2.1	-	0,6	-	1,2	0,2	1.9	1,5	3.2	2.1	1,0	3.0
US, Hawaii: Chinese	0,9	-	1,9	-	1,4	-	0,2	-	0,9	0,5	4.1	1,5	4.4	1,4	2,9	1,7

AGE-STANDARDIZED (WORLD) INCIDENCE RATES (FOUR DIGIT RUBRICS)

	153.0		153.1		153.2		153.3		Colon 153.4		153.5		153.6		153.7		153.8-9	
AFRICA	M	F	M	F	M	F	M	F	M	F	M	F	M	F	M	F	M	F
*Algeria, Setif	-	-	-	-	-	-	0,1	0,1	-	-	0,0	-	-	-	-	-	0,3	0,5
*France, La Reunion	-	0,1	0,6	0,2	0,4	0,7	1.2	1.2	0,2	0,4	0,1	0,4	0.9	0.3	0,1	-	3.5	2.3
*Mali, Bamako	0,1	-	-	-	0,1	-	0,4	0,1	0,4	0,5	-	-	0,5	-	-	-	1.7	0,8
*Uganda, Kyadondo	-	-	-	-	0,2	-	0,3	-	0,4	1,0	-	-	-	-	-	-	2.2	2.4
*Zimbabwe, Harare: African	-	-	-	-	0,8	-	1,1	0,5	0,2	0,4	-	-	0,1	-	-	-	4.4	2,1
*Zimbabwe, Harare: European	-	-	0,7	-	-	-	0,9	0,5	-	-	-	-	-	-	-	-	16.2	13.6

AMERICA, CENTRAL AND SOUTH

	153.0		153.1		153.2		153.3		Colon 153.4		153.5		153.6		153.7		153.8-9	
	M	F	M	F	M	F	M	F	M	F	M	F	M	F	M	F	M	F
*Argentina, Concordia	0,4	-	0,2	1,2	0,7	1,4	3,2	2,4	1,7	2,2	-	-	1,1	0,8	-	0,3	10.0	6.9
*Brazil, Belem	-	0,1	0,1	0,1	0,3	0,3	0,8	0,6	0,3	-	0,0	-	0,1	0,2	-	-	2.9	2.7
*Brazil, Goiania	0,1	-	0,1	0,4	-	-	0,8	0,8	0,2	-	-	-	-	0,3	-	-	4.5	7.5
*Brazil, Porto Alegre	-	-	0,4	0,6	0,7	0,5	2.6	2.0	0,5	0,4	0,1	0,0	0,6	0.7	-	-	11.0	9.4
Colombia, Cali	-	-	0,4	0,2	0,4	0,4	1.4	1.1	0,2	0,2	0,2	0,2	1.0	1.0	0,0	0,1	2.9	3.0
*Costa Rica	0,1	0,1	0.3	0.5	0.4	0.4	1.3	1.0	0.7	0.6	0,1	0,1	0.5	0.8	0,0	0,0	2.5	2.9
*Ecuador, Quito	0,0	0,0	0.3	0,2	0,2	0,3	0.7	0.8	0,0	0,5	0,1	0,1	0.3	0.6	-	-	2.2	3.1
*Peru, Lima	0,0	-	0,2	0.4	0.3	0.3	1.0	1.0	0.3	0.4	0,0	0,0	0.8	0.6	-	0,0	2.9	2.7
Peru, Trujillo	-	-	-	-	-	-	0,6	0,3	0,2	0,7	-	-	-	-	-	-	3.5	4.0
US, Puerto Rico	0.7	0.5	1.1	0.9	1.9	1.4	4.3	3.8	2.1	2.4	0,1	0,1	2.4	1.4	0.7	0.5	1.4	1.1
*Uruguay, Montevideo	-	0,1	0.6	0.7	1.5	1.2	4.3	2.7	0.7	0.5	0,2	0,2	2.9	2.4	0,1	0,1	13.3	10.1

AMERICA, NORTH

	153.0		153.1		153.2		153.3		Colon 153.4		153.5		153.6		153.7		153.8-9	
	M	F	M	F	M	F	M	F	M	F	M	F	M	F	M	F	M	F
Canada	1.0	0.7	1.9	1.9	1.6	1.3	8.6	6.1	4.9	4.3	0.2	0.2	3.4	3.1	1.0	0.7	4.3	3.2
Canada, Alberta	1.3	0.8	1.9	1.6	1.0	0.9	7.6	4.7	4.7	3.8	0.3	0,1	2.5	2.2	1.3	0.8	1.5	1.2
Canada, British Columbia	0.9	0.7	1.4	1.5	1.2	1.1	6.9	4.7	4.3	4.2	0.2	0.3	2.9	2.9	0.8	0.6	2.1	1.9
Canada, Manitoba	0.6	0.7	1.9	2.0	1.5	1.1	10.0	8.1	5.9	5.0	0.3	0,1	2.9	2.8	0.8	0.7	3.3	2.9
Canada, New Brunswick	1.3	1.1	2.2	1.9	1.6	1.0	8.7	6.0	6.2	6.7	0,1	0,1	3.8	2.7	1.2	0.8	3.1	2.2
Canada, Newfoundland	1.4	1.0	2.0	3.2	2.2	2.9	12.5	9.1	6.7	6.3	0.2	0.3	3.4	3.1	1.4	0.9	1.7	1.2
Canada, Northwest Territories	0,5	-	-	2,9	-	-	5,7	3,0	0,8	5,9	-	-	-	1,3	-	-	1,3	0,7
Canada, Nova Scotia	1.2	0.7	1.8	2.0	1.7	1.4	9.1	7.0	5.8	5.4	0.2	0.4	4.0	3.5	1.2	0.7	6.1	4.2
Canada, Ontario	0.7	0.5	1.8	1.8	1.7	1.2	9.4	6.4	4.9	4.0	0.2	0.2	3.8	3.6	0.9	0.6	6.6	4.5
Canada, Prince Edward Island	1,2	0,4	2.4	2.9	3.2	1,6	10.9	6.5	5.3	5.9	-	0,2	3.3	4.9	0,6	0,7	0,9	0,6
Canada, Quebec	1.2	0.9	2.3	2.1	2.0	1.5	7.9	6.0	4.6	4.1	0.2	0.1	3.4	2.8	1.2	0.8	3.7	2.9
Canada, Saskatchewan	1.1	1.0	2.3	2.1	1.2	0.7	9.0	5.9	4.3	5.0	0,1	0,1	2.6	2.1	1.0	0.9	1.1	1.1
Canada, Yukon	-	-	-	-	0,5	1,1	3,9	2,3	4,7	4,2	-	-	-	-	0,7	1,1	5,4	-
US, Cent. Calif.: Non-Hisp. White	1.1	1.0	2.1	1.9	1.5	1.2	9.7	6.0	5.2	5.4	0,2	0.2	2.5	2.4	0.8	0.7	1.4	0.8
US, Cent. Calif.: Hispanic	1.1	0,4	1.2	0.9	1.3	0,4	6.2	3.6	3.8	3.2	0,0	-	1.6	1.1	0,5	0,5	1.3	0.3
US, Los Angeles: Non-Hisp. White	1.3	1.0	2.1	2.1	2.1	1.4	11.0	6.8	5.8	4.5	0.4	0.3	3.8	2.8	1.2	0.9	1.2	0.8
US, Los Angeles: Hispanic White	0.8	0.6	1.2	0.9	1.1	0.8	7.1	4.6	3.6	2.4	0,1	0,2	1.8	1.7	0.6	0.4	0.8	0.3
US, Los Angeles: Black	2.0	1.2	2.6	2.4	3.0	2.6	11.3	7.9	8.6	6.2	0.2	0.3	3.9	3.1	1.9	1.4	1.3	1.4
US, Los Angeles: Chinese	0,9	1,0	1.6	1.3	2.0	0,4	9.0	5.1	2.6	2.0	0.4	-	0.8	1.9	0,4	0,6	0,6	0,1
US, Los Angeles: Filipino	0,1	0,1	1,7	0,6	1,3	1,3	8.7	3.3	0,7	1.5	0,2	0,2	0.8	0,6	0,4	-	0,4	0,6
US, Los Angeles: Korean	1,4	1,1	0,4	1,5	0,3	0,2	4.9	2.5	3.8	0,7	-	-	1,7	1,1	0,4	0,5	1,1	0,6
US, Los Angeles: Japanese	2.1	0,3	1,7	0,9	1,6	2.1	13.5	8.4	5.2	4.3	-	0,2	1,1	3.1	0,8	0,6	0,8	0,7
US, San Francisco: Non-Hisp. White	1.6	0.9	2.5	1.7	2.2	1.5	10.8	6.7	5.4	5.1	0,1	0.3	3.7	3.0	1.2	0.9	0.8	0.6
US, San Francisco: Hispanic White	0,9	0,7	2.1	1.5	1.4	0,3	8.7	5.4	4.2	4.1	0,1	0.3	2.0	2.0	1.4	0,7	0,6	0,5
US, San Francisco: Black	1.6	1.5	2.8	2.1	4.1	2.3	9.6	7.6	6.8	6.8	0.3	0.5	4.8	4.6	2.5	1.3	1.2	1.2
US, San Francisco: Chinese	1.1	1.2	1.5	1.7	2.8	2.2	9.6	9.2	1.4	3.0	0,2	0,1	2.4	2.4	0,9	0,7	0,2	0,6
US, San Francisco: Filipino	1,2	0,5	1,0	1,2	1,5	0,8	10.3	3.1	2.3	0,7	0,3	0,2	1,2	1,7	0,6	0,2	0,8	0,4
US, San Francisco: Japanese	1,3	0,5	0,6	3,4	0,9	2,0	13.1	13.6	6.0	3.5	0,9	0,5	3,3	2,5	-	0,4	-	0,7
US, Connecticut: White	1.2	1.0	2.5	1.8	2.3	1.6	11.8	7.3	5.9	4.9	0.2	0.3	3.9	2.9	1.2	0.6	1.4	1.2
US, Connecticut: Black	1,2	1,1	2.1	3.0	2.2	1.8	9.4	6.2	7.2	6.4	0.8	0.2	3.7	3.8	1,8	1.3	2.4	1.4
US, Atlanta: White	1.7	0.9	2.4	1.9	1.7	1.5	9.3	6.5	6.0	4.5	0.3	0.3	3.2	2.6	1.3	0.8	1.1	0.8
US, Atlanta: Black	1.2	1.2	3.3	2.8	2.9	2.8	8.2	7.9	7.2	5.8	0.7	0.2	4.6	3.3	2.5	0.8	1.8	1.4
US, Iowa	1.5	1.4	2.5	2.7	2.0	1.4	11.4	8.3	6.3	5.4	0.3	0.1	3.8	4.0	1.3	0.9	1.4	0.8
US, Central Louisiana: White	0,9	0,3	2.8	1.8	1.9	1.6	10.3	6.8	4.1	3.0	-	0,2	3.7	2.7	1,0	0,7	3.3	1.8
US, Central Louisiana: Black	3,2	0,2	3,4	2,0	2,6	2,2	5.6	11.0	5.4	3,3	0.4	-	1.5	1.2	1,2	3,3	4,7	1,8
US, New Orleans: White	1.5	0.9	2.6	2.2	2.2	1.4	10.5	8.5	4.7	4.1	0.2	0,1	3.8	3.8	0.8	0.4	2.9	1.9
US, New Orleans: Black	1.4	0.9	2.7	3.4	3.6	1.9	9.3	7.4	5.2	4.6	0.5	0.2	2.8	4.0	1.8	0.9	4.1	2.7
US, Detroit: White	1.5	1.1	2.3	1.9	2.6	1.4	11.0	6.5	6.5	5.2	0.3	0.2	3.6	2.6	1.2	0.6	1.5	0.9
US, Detroit: Black	1.3	1.5	2.7	2.5	3.1	2.4	10.1	6.9	8.9	7.1	0.2	0.3	4.6	4.0	2.3	1.7	1.8	1.4
US, New Mexico: Non-Hisp. White	1.1	0.4	1.7	1.7	1.0	1.1	9.7	6.5	4.6	3.9	0,1	0,2	2.7	2.0	0.8	0.6	1.3	1.2
US, New Mexico: Hispanic White	0.8	0,5	0,6	0.8	0,7	0.8	10.1	5.7	3.7	3.5	0,1	-	2.0	1.5	0,7	0.7	1.2	0.8
US, New Mexico: American Indian	0,5	1,2	1,1	0,8	0,3	0,5	4.0	2,7	2,5	1,0	-	-	0.3	0,2	-	0,8	1,1	-
US, Utah	1.3	0.5	1.3	1.3	1.7	1.0	8.4	5.8	4.8	4.2	0.3	0.3	1.8	1.5	1.1	0.6	0.9	0.7
US, Seattle	1.4	1.1	2.1	1.9	1.4	1.2	10.5	6.7	5.5	5.0	0.4	0.3	2.9	2.6	1.4	0.8	1.0	0.7
US, SEER: White	1.4	1.0	2.3	1.9	1.9	1.3	10.7	6.9	5.8	4.9	0.3	0.2	3.4	2.8	1.2	0.8	1.2	0.9
US, SEER: Black	1.4	1.3	2.6	2.5	3.1	2.3	9.6	7.2	7.8	6.7	0.4	0.3	4.5	3.8	2.3	1.3	1.7	1.3

AGE-STANDARDIZED (WORLD) INCIDENCE RATES (FOUR DIGIT RUBRICS)

	153.0		153.1		153.2		Colon 153.3		153.4		153.5		153.6		153.7		153.8-9	
ASIA	M	F	M	F	M	F	M	F	M	F	M	F	M	F	M	F	M	F
*China, Qidong	0,1	0,1	0,1	0,0	0,1	0,0	0,2	0,3	0,2	0,3	0,0	0,0	0,2	0,1	-	0,0	1.3	1.0
China, Shanghai	0.5	0.4	1.0	0.9	0.6	0.6	3.6	3.0	1.3	1.2	0.1	0.1	1.9	1.9	0.1	0.1	3.1	2.7
China, Tianjin	0,1	0,0	0.2	0.2	0.1	0,1	0.6	0.5	0.3	0.2	0,0	0,0	0.4	0.3	-	0,0	3.9	3.6
Hong Kong																		
*India, Bangalore	0.2	0,1	0,1	0,1	0,0	0,1	0.3	0.4	0.3	0.3	0,0	0,0	0.3	0,1	0,0	0,0	1.2	0.9
*India, Barshi, Paranda and Bhum	-	-	-	0,1	-	-	-	-	0.2	-	-	-	-	-	-	-	0.5	0,3
India, Bombay	0.1	0,0	0.2	0.1	0.1	0.1	0.7	0.6	0.5	0.5	0,0	0,0	0.3	0.2	0.1	0,0	1.6	1.3
*India, Karunagappally	-	0.3	-	-	-	-	-	-	0.6	0.2	-	-	-	-	-	-	0,9	0,8
India, Madras	0,0	0,1	0,1	-	0,1	0,0	0.4	0.3	0.3	0,1	-	-	0.2	0.2	-	0,0	0.6	0.5
*India, Trivandrum	0,3	-	0,1	-	0,2	-	-	0,4	0.5	0,1	-	-	0,1	-	-	-	1,1	0,5
Israel: All Jews	1.0	0.8	1.8	1.4	2.0	1.6	6.6	5.5	2.9	2.7	0.2	0.2	2.9	2.4	1.3	0.8	6.1	4.5
Jews born in Israel	1.4	0.9	1.7	1.3	1.5	1.6	6.3	4.7	3.3	2.2	0,4	0,1	2.6	2.9	1.2	1.3	5.5	5.2
Jews born in America or Europe	1.1	1.0	2.3	1.7	2.5	1.6	8.4	6.4	3.4	3.3	0.2	0,1	3.2	2.7	1.6	0.8	7.5	5.4
Jews born in Africa or Asia	0.7	0.5	1.2	0.8	1.1	1.3	3.8	4.1	2.0	1.8	0,1	0,1	2.2	1.4	0.7	0.6	3.9	3.5
Non-Jews	0,2	-	0,6	0,7	0,2	0,3	1.3	1.3	0,9	0,5	0,2	-	1.1	0,7	0,2	0,2	1.4	2.4
Japan, Hiroshima	0.3	0,2	4.0	2.0	3.2	1.1	15.3	8.2	2.2	2.3	0,1	0,2	4.2	2.9	0,2	0,1	1.9	1.2
Japan, Miyagi	0,0	0,0	2.4	1.9	1.7	0.8	9.6	5.2	1.6	1.7	-	-	3.9	3.3	-	0,0	5.8	2.8
Japan, Nagasaki	0,1	0,0	2.2	1.7	2.0	1.0	12.4	6.7	1.5	1.6	0,1	0.1	3.4	2.7	0,0	-	4.0	1.8
Japan, Osaka	0.1	0.0	1.6	1.1	1.1	0.7	7.7	4.4	1.1	1.1	0.1	0.1	2.1	1.6	0,0	0,0	7.0	4.0
*Japan, Saga																		
Japan, Yamagata																		
*Korea, Kangwha	0,7	-	0,3	0,6	-	-	0,7	-	-	-	0,3	-	0,3	0,7	-	-	2,2	1,0
*Kuwait: Non-Kuwaitis	0,5	-	0,2	-	0,2	0,4	1,9	0,7	0,3	0,1	0,1	-	1,1	0,1	-	-	5.0	0,9
*Kuwait: Kuwaitis	0,2	0,2	0,2	0,2	0,1	0,1	0,4	1,1	0,2	0,4	-	0,3	0,2	0,6	0,1	-	2.0	2.0
*Philippines, Manila	0,2	0.3	0.5	0.5	0.6	0.4	2.6	1.7	0.4	0.5	0,1	0,1	0.6	0.5	0,1	0,0	5.8	4.9
Singapore: Chinese	0.6	0.3	1.5	1.4	1.4	1.1	7.9	6.8	2.1	1.7	0.3	0.5	1.6	1.4	0.8	0.5	8.1	7.3
Singapore: Malay	0,1	0.2	0,7	0,4	0,5	0,4	2.9	2.0	0,8	-	0,1	0,1	0,6	0,3	0,3	0,1	5.2	3.1
Singapore: Indian	0,2	0.3	1,0	0,5	-	-	1,8	1,4	0,8	0,7	0,1	-	0,1	-	0,6	0,3	3.1	1,6
Thailand, Chiang Mai	0,1	0,1	0,2	0.3	0.3	0,2	0.6	0.9	0.7	0.5	0,0	0,1	0.7	0.6	0,0	-	1.6	1.1
*Thailand, Khon Kaen	-	0,1	0.3	0,2	0,2	0,1	0.8	0.6	0,4	0,2	-	-	0,1	0,1	0,1	-	3.0	1.9
*Viet Nam, Hanoi	0,3	0,2	0,1	0,1	0,1	0,1	0.7	0,3	0.3	0,1	-	-	0.5	0,2	0,1	0,1	3.1	1.9
EUROPE																		
Austria, Tyrol	0.7	0.7	1.5	1.2	1.2	0.4	6.6	5.5	2.0	1.7	0,4	0,4	1.7	1.6	0,4	0.3	5.9	4.9
*Belarus																		
*Croatia	0.5	0.3	0.9	0.7	0.6	0.4	3.9	3.0	1.2	0.9	0,0	0,0	1.2	0.8	0.4	0.3	4.1	2.5
Czech Republic	2.2	1.2	2.5	1.8	2.1	1.3	8.4	5.2	3.3	2.7	0.1	0.2	2.7	1.8	1.8	1.0	0.8	0.6
Denmark	0.3	0.2	2.0	2.2	1.3	1.2	9.4	8.1	3.1	3.4	0.2	0.3	2.5	3.0	0.4	0.3	1.6	1.2
Estonia	0.5	0.5	1.8	1.2	1.3	0.8	6.2	4.8	1.4	1.8	-	0,1	1.2	1.3	0.7	0.3	1.0	0.5
Finland																		
France, Bas-Rhin	0.6	0.3	1.5	1.2	4.7	2.4	11.3	7.0	2.0	1.6	0,2	0,1	6.2	3.7	0.8	0.4	2.9	2.1
*France, Calvados	1.1	0.5	1.9	1.6	2.1	1.3	8.4	5.5	1.6	2.3	0,2	0,2	2.2	1.5	1.1	0.6	1.5	0.9
France, Doubs	0.9	0.4	0.9	1.2	2.0	1.2	6.0	4.4	2.4	1.1	-	0,2	2.9	2.3	1.0	0.6	3.3	2.4
France, Haut-Rhin	0,4	0,2	1.5	1.0	3.0	1.6	10.3	6.4	1.3	1.1	0,0	0,1	4.8	3.4	0.5	0.3	6.6	4.3
*France, Herault	0.3	0.4	0.9	0.7	3.5	2.3	6.6	4.2	1.8	1.4	0,1	0,2	2.1	1.7	0.5	0.3	4.2	2.3
France, Isere	0.6	0.3	0.9	0.8	2.8	1.9	8.1	4.9	1.5	1.6	0,2	0,1	3.6	3.1	0.3	0.3	4.1	2.6
*France, Somme	0.5	0,2	0.9	0.6	2.8	1.6	8.8	5.3	1.9	1.5	0,1	0,1	1.9	1.6	0.7	0,3	2.6	1.1
*France, Tarn	1.1	1.0	1.3	0.6	2.7	1.7	5.9	3.6	1.8	1.4	0,5	0,5	2.4	2.6	0.8	0.4	2.2	1.6
Germany, Eastern States	0.9	0.9	1.6	1.5	1.1	0.8	5.8	5.2	1.8	1.9	0.1	0.1	1.8	1.9	0.9	0.6	1.4	1.0
Germany, Saarland	0.7	0.3	1.7	1.1	1.1	0.5	8.6	6.8	2.6	2.6	0.2	0.8	2.1	2.0	0.4	0.5	8.0	5.8
Iceland	0,1	0,2	1.1	0.9	1.4	1.2	8.6	6.3	3.1	2.5	0,1	0.5	4.4	3.2	-	0,2	0,4	0,4
Ireland, Southern	0.5	0,4	1.0	1.2	1.0	0.8	3.9	4.0	3.0	2.9	0,1	0.3	1.1	0.8	0,5	0,2	13.2	9.6
Italy, Ferrara	0,6	0,1	2.2	1.8	3.1	2.2	15.0	9.5	2.4	2.2	-	0,2	3.2	2.9	0,2	0,1	1.6	1.1
Italy, Florence	0.5	0.4	1.9	1.2	3.1	2.6	9.6	6.9	1.3	2.0	0,0	0,1	4.2	3.6	0.4	0.3	3.6	3.1
Italy, Genoa	0.6	0.4	2.1	1.4	3.1	1.7	10.1	7.7	2.3	2.2	0.3	0,1	3.2	2.2	0.8	0.3	3.7	2.4
*Italy, Latina	0,3	0,1	0.3	0,1	1.1	1.0	3.7	3.0	1.3	1.2	0,1	-	0.9	0.5	0,1	-	8.1	6.9
Italy, Macerata	0,4	0,4	2.4	2.0	2.2	2.1	10.1	6.2	1.9	1,3	-	-	3.9	3.8	0,3	0,3	4.1	1.2
Italy, Modena	0.5	0.6	1.9	1.8	2.0	1.6	8.3	6.2	3.1	1.8	0,1	0,1	2.7	2.2	1.1	1.2	1.4	1.6
Italy, Parma	1.2	1.2	1.9	1.8	2.2	2.0	9.6	6.0	2.0	1.6	0,2	0,2	3.4	2.3	0.7	0,3	3.2	2.4
Italy, Ragusa	0,3	0,4	0.6	0.8	1.3	1.3	3.5	4.0	0.3	0.6	0,1	0,1	2.1	1.2	0,2	0,4	1.4	1.7
Italy, Romagna	0.5	0,1	1.2	1.3	1.8	1.0	11.2	9.1	2.6	2.0	-	0,1	2.5	3.0	0.6	0,2	2.2	1.9
Italy, Torino	0.8	0.7	2.0	1.5	1.7	1.0	9.8	6.7	2.0	1.5	0,1	-	3.0	2.0	1.1	0.5	3.4	2.0
Italy, Trieste	0.8	0.7	1,0	0.9	1.6	0,3	6.0	2.8	1.7	1.0	0,3	-	1.6	0.5	0.3	0,2	17.4	10.9
Italy, Varese	1.4	0.7	2.0	1.7	2.6	1.7	12.1	7.7	2.7	2.1	0,2	0,2	3.1	2.5	2.2	1.3	1.2	0.7
Italy, Veneto	0.3	0.2	0.4	0.6	1.0	1.0	4.2	3.1	0.6	0.4	0,1	0,0	1.7	0.9	0.4	0,1	13.6	10.0
*Latvia	1.1	0.8	1.4	1.2	0.9	0.6	5.3	3.9	1.0	0.8	0,0	0,0	1.3	1.0	0.2	0.2	0.5	0.6
Malta	0,4	0,3	1,4	0,5	1,6	1,0	3.2	5.5	2,1	1,2	-	-	1,3	0.8	0.4	0,3	3.2	2.6

AGE-STANDARDIZED (WORLD) INCIDENCE RATES (FOUR DIGIT RUBRICS)

	153.0		153.1		153.2		153.3		Colon 153.4		153.5		153.6		153.7		153.8-9	
	M	F	M	F	M	F	M	F	M	F	M	F	M	F	M	F	M	F
The Netherlands	1.3	1.0	1.8	1.7	1.2	1.0	8.7	6.7	3.7	3.8	0.5	0.8	2.7	2.5	1.2	0.8	0.7	0.6
The Netherlands, Eindhoven	1.4	0.9	1.5	1.4	0.9	0.8	9.8	7.0	4.7	4.0	0.6	1.0	2.6	2.7	1.7	0.8	0.6	0.5
The Netherlands, Maastricht	1.2	1.0	1.6	1.3	1.0	0.8	9.4	7.2	3.6	3.6	0,3	0,4	2.6	2.1	1.3	0.7	0.8	0.8
Norway																		
*Poland, Cracow	0.8	0.4	1.2	0.7	0,2	0.6	2.8	2.2	0.9	0.9	0,0	-	0.7	0.4	0,4	0.6	4.5	2.7
*Poland, Kielce	0.4	0.2	0.7	0.5	0,2	0,1	2.4	1.5	0.9	0.7	0,0	0,0	0.8	0.3	0,2	0,1	2.4	1.3
*Poland, Lower Silesia	0.5	0.3	0.7	0.7	0.5	0.5	4.6	3.3	1.2	1.0	0,0	0.1	0.9	0.9	0.4	0.2	3.1	2.4
Poland, Warsaw City	0.4	0.4	1.1	0.8	0.6	0.4	5.9	3.6	1.7	1.4	0,0	0,1	1.3	0.7	0.9	0.2	4.1	2.6
Slovakia	1.8	0.9	1.8	1.2	1.8	0.9	6.9	4.4	2.5	2.0	0,1	0.1	1.8	1.3	1.6	0.6	1.8	1.2
Slovenia	0.4	0.3	3.9	2.3	1.1	0.8	6.0	3.7	-	-	-	-	-	-	-	-	4.4	3.0
*Spain, Albacete	0,2	0,6	0,4	0,6	1,0	1,1	3.9	3.4	0,4	1,3	-	-	1,2	0,5	0,3	-	2.9	1.6
Spain, Asturias	0,1	0,0	0.4	0,1	0.4	0.4	5.2	3.6	1.0	0.7	0,1	0.3	0.8	0.5	0,1	0,1	9.0	5.4
Spain, Basque Country	0.7	0.5	0.8	0.5	1.0	0.6	7.4	4.5	1.9	1.1	0,1	0,1	1.6	1.1	0.8	0.4	2.7	1.8
Spain, Granada	0.7	0.6	0.6	0.4	0.7	0.6	3.7	3.4	1.0	1.2	0,1	0,1	1.0	0.8	0.7	0.3	1.8	1.5
Spain, Mallorca	0.7	0.5	1.1	1.1	1.1	1.0	8.4	7.1	2.7	1.8	0,1	0,1	1.4	1.5	1.2	0.8	1.7	1.6
Spain, Murcia	0.4	0.4	0.8	0.6	1.0	0.8	5.8	3.7	1.3	1.4	0,0	0,1	1.2	1.2	0.3	0.3	2.9	2.3
Spain, Navarra	1.4	0.8	1.1	0.5	0.6	0.4	7.4	5.0	2.0	2.1	-	0,4	1.5	1.8	0.7	0.4	1.7	1.5
Spain, Tarragona	0.5	0.4	0.5	0.4	1.3	0.7	7.7	5.9	2.0	1.6	0,1	0,1	2.0	1.1	0,4	0,2	4.0	3.6
Spain, Zaragoza	0.8	0.4	0.8	0.6	0.7	0.8	4.0	3.1	1.1	1.4	0,1	-	0.9	0.6	0.7	0.4	3.9	2.9
Sweden	0.4	0.3	1.6	1.5	0.7	0.6	5.5	4.6	3.4	3.0	0.5	1.0	2.1	2.0	0.3	0.2	3.2	2.8
*Switzerland, Basel	0.8	0.5	1.7	1.1	1.1	1.3	8.6	4.9	3.5	3.0	0,2	0,2	3.2	2.8	0.8	0.7	0,4	0,2
Switzerland, Geneva	1.3	0.9	1.4	1.0	1.3	0.7	9.0	6.0	3.6	2.6	0,1	0,2	3.0	2.0	1.7	0.6	3.8	1.3
Switzerland, Graubunden	0.5	0,3	0,6	1,0	0,7	1,2	9.3	4.7	4.0	2.8	-	0,8	3.2	3.7	0,5	1,2	0.8	0.9
Switzerland, Neuchatel	1,0	0,3	1.5	2.1	1,6	0,2	8.4	5.2	3.1	3.2	0,4	0,7	3.3	1.1	0,9	0,9	0.9	0,7
Switzerland, St Gall-Appenzell	0,3	0.5	1.2	0.9	1.1	1.0	7.1	4.7	3.2	2.3	0,1	0,2	2.2	1.7	0.9	0,3	0.6	0.5
Switzerland, Valais	1,2	0,8	1,0	1.3	1.3	0,8	7.4	6.1	3.9	2.2	0,2	0,6	2.5	1.5	0,8	0,3	0,7	0,4
Switzerland, Vaud	0.7	0.3	1.6	1.2	1.1	0.8	8.9	5.7	3.6	2.7	0,4	0,1	3.5	2.3	1.1	0.5	0.8	0.5
Switzerland, Zurich	0.9	0.5	1.5	1.1	1.1	0.8	7.4	4.1	4.0	3.4	0.3	0.4	2.7	1.9	0.9	0.6	0.3	0.2
*UK, England and Wales	0.4	0.3	1.1	1.0	0.8	0.7	5.6	4.3	3.2	3.0	0.1	0.1	1.2	1.1	0.6	0.4	6.2	4.7
*UK, East Anglia																		
*UK, Mersey	0.4	0.4	0.8	1.1	0.7	0.7	5.4	5.1	3.1	3.4	0.1	0.2	1.1	1.0	0.8	0.6	4.2	4.0
*UK, North Western	0.3	0.2	0.9	0.9	0.5	0.4	5.3	3.7	3.0	2.8	0.1	0,0	0.9	0.7	0.4	0.3	7.9	5.9
UK, Oxford	0.4	0.3	1.1	1.0	1.0	0.7	6.0	4.5	3.1	2.9	0.4	0.6	1.5	1.4	0.5	0.4	6.7	5.3
*UK, South Thames	0.4	0.3	1.3	1.1	0.9	0.8	5.8	4.4	2.9	2.9	0.1	0.1	1.2	1.2	0.6	0.5	4.9	3.7
UK, South Western	0.7	0.4	1.3	1.5	0.8	0.8	5.7	4.4	3.3	3.1	0.1	0.2	1.6	1.6	0.8	0.5	4.9	3.7
UK, Wessex	0.5	0.3	1.0	1.0	0.8	0.7	6.3	5.1	3.7	3.4	0.2	0.2	1.5	1.2	0.6	0.3	7.8	6.7
*UK, West Midlands	0.2	0.1	0.9	0.9	0.6	0.5	6.1	4.1	3.8	3.4	0,0	0,0	1.1	0.8	0.4	0.3	10.6	7.9
UK, Yorkshire	0.5	0.4	1.3	1.0	0.8	0.7	5.4	4.4	3.4	2.6	0.1	0.1	1.4	1.2	0.5	0.4	6.0	4.4
UK, Scotland	0.4	0.3	1.4	1.4	1.1	0.8	7.1	5.2	3.7	3.8	0.2	0.2	1.5	1.3	0.8	0.5	7.5	5.7
UK, Scotland, West	0.4	0.3	1.3	1.3	1.0	0.8	7.0	5.1	3.7	3.6	0.2	0.3	1.3	1.2	0.8	0.5	7.6	5.2

*Yugoslavia, Vojvodina

OCEANIA

	153.0		153.1		153.2		153.3		153.4		153.5		153.6		153.7		153.8-9	
	M	F	M	F	M	F	M	F	M	F	M	F	M	F	M	F	M	F
Australian Capital Territory	2.1	1,2	1.9	1.6	1.9	1,3	12.7	6.9	4.9	3.6	-	-	3.2	2.2	0,6	0,7	1.6	2.5
Australia, New South Wales	1.0	0.7	2.3	2.1	1.6	1.2	10.0	6.7	4.5	3.9	0.2	0.2	2.7	2.2	1.2	0.7	5.2	3.6
South Australia	1.2	1.0	2.1	1.9	1.9	1.9	11.2	7.5	4.8	5.2	0.3	0.6	3.7	2.9	1.4	1.0	0.9	0.8
Australia, Tasmania	0.8	0,3	2.1	2.4	1.6	0.9	13.6	7.8	4.3	4.2	0,1	0.2	2.7	3.0	0.9	0.6	4.4	3.3
Australia, Victoria	1.0	0.8	2.0	1.9	1.4	1.1	9.8	7.8	4.8	4.2	0.2	0.2	3.1	2.7	0.9	0.9	4.3	3.4
Western Australia	0.6	0.3	1.8	1.9	2.2	1.5	9.0	7.1	3.6	3.5	0,1	0.3	4.2	4.1	0.8	0.5	3.3	2.6
*French Polynesia	0,5	-	-	-	0,5	-	1,9	1,2	0,3	1,1	0,4	0,2	1,2	-	-	-	4.7	2,4
New Zealand: Non-Maori	1.1	1.1	3.5	4.1	2.1	1.9	11.0	8.5	4.6	4.8	0.2	0.5	3.9	4.4	1.4	1.2	3.5	3.1
New Zealand: Maori	0,3	1,3	0,6	0.8	2,7	0,6	6.9	4.1	2,3	3.9	0,4	0,7	0,7	1,5	1,1	0,7	6.6	2,5
US, Hawaii: White	1.1	1.0	3.8	2.3	2.1	1.5	11.7	7.0	6.8	4.7	0,4	0,1	4.6	4.3	0,9	1.1	1.3	0,9
US, Hawaii: Japanese	1.4	1.0	3.5	1.9	3.3	2.3	15.1	8.6	5.4	4.2	0,1	0.3	4.2	3.5	0.9	0,1	0,6	0.8
US, Hawaii: Hawaiian	1,6	0,8	1,7	0,8	1,0	2.4	9.5	5.6	1,2	2.9	1,2	0,9	2.9	1.9	0,7	1,0	-	0,3
US, Hawaii: Filipino	0,6	0,2	2.1	1,7	0,8	1,7	8.2	6.3	1.7	1.3	0,3	0,2	2.6	0,9	0,8	0,7	0,7	0,2
US, Hawaii: Chinese	0,4	1,5	2,0	1,5	1,8	2,3	11.0	7.0	2,1	1,4	0,4	-	3.4	3.5	0,3	0,9	1,1	-

AGE-STANDARDIZED (WORLD) INCIDENCE RATES (FOUR DIGIT RUBRICS)

	154.0		Rectum 154.1		154.2-8		156.0		Gallbladder etc 156.1		156.2		156.8-9	
AFRICA	M	F	M	F	M	F	M	F	M	F	M	F	M	F
*Algeria, Setif	-	-	2.5	2.2	0,1	0,1	3.6	9.8	-	0,4	-	-	-	-
*France, La Reunion	1.5	1.5	2.9	1.7	1.4	1.1	0,6	1.3	0,4	0,2	-	0,2	0,3	0.8
*Mali, Bamako	-	-	2.5	0,6	0,4	0,1	0,2	-	-	-	-	-	-	-
*Uganda, Kyadondo	0,7	-	3.0	1,5	0,6	0,3	-	-	-	-	-	-	-	-
*Zimbabwe, Harare: African	-	-	3.8	2.6	-	-	0,1	0,8	0,5	-	-	-	-	-
*Zimbabwe, Harare: European	-	-	22.4	7.4	-	-	-	-	-	-	-	-	-	-

AMERICA, CENTRAL AND SOUTH

	154.0		154.1		154.2-8		156.0		156.1		156.2		156.8-9	
*Argentina, Concordia	3.9	1,6	2,8	2,1	2,3	0,8	2,7	4.6	0,8	-	-	-	0,2	0,1
*Brazil, Belem	0,3	0,4	1.8	2.1	0,7	2.1	1,0	1.8	0,4	0,6	-	0,1	0,2	0,6
*Brazil, Goiania	1.2	1.3	3.0	3.6	0,4	0,5	0,8	2.8	0,3	1.1	0,7	0,6	0,2	0,1
*Brazil, Porto Alegre	2.2	0.9	9.7	5.2	0,5	0.8	0,7	3.9	0,6	0.6	0,1	0,2	0,6	2.2
Colombia, Cali	1.0	0.9	3.6	2.9	0.8	0.8	1.2	4.9	0,3	0.5	0.7	0,3	1.6	2.6
*Costa Rica	1.5	1.2	3.1	2.5	0,1	0.3	1.0	3.2	0.2	0.3	0.5	0.5	1.0	1.3
*Ecuador, Quito	0,2	0,1	3.2	3.3	-	0.5	2.1	5.5	0,2	0,3	1.2	0.7	2.0	2.2
*Peru, Lima	0.3	0,1	2.7	2.4	0.2	0.8	0.5	2.5	0,1	0,2	0.3	0,2	1.0	1.5
Peru, Trujillo	0,2	0,7	3.2	2.7	0,3	0,8	2.3	6.9	0,2	-	0,3	0,2	1,0	2.2
US, Puerto Rico	2.6	1.6	5.5	3.6	0.4	0.8	0.7	1.5	0.4	0.4	0.4	0.4	0,0	0,1
*Uruguay, Montevideo	2.4	1.3	8.9	5.5	1.1	0.8	1.2	3.0	0.9	0.3	0,2	0,2	0.6	0.7

AMERICA, NORTH

	154.0		154.1		154.2-8		156.0		156.1		156.2		156.8-9	
Canada	4.8	2.9	10.5	5.5	0.8	0.8	0.7	1.2	0.6	0.4	0.4	0.2	0.1	0.1
Canada, Alberta	4.5	3.1	10.7	4.9	0.4	0.7	0.6	1.1	0.6	0.5	0.2	0.2	0.1	0.1
Canada, British Columbia	5.3	3.0	10.5	6.1	0.6	0.7	0.5	1.0	0.7	0.4	0.4	0.3	0.1	0.1
Canada, Manitoba	5.3	2.6	10.0	5.8	0.7	0.7	0.8	1.1	0.6	0.5	0.5	0.2	0.1	0.1
Canada, New Brunswick	5.2	3.2	10.5	5.8	0.6	0.7	0.4	1.0	0.4	0.4	0.2	0.2	0,0	-
Canada, Newfoundland	4.6	2.7	11.0	6.8	0,2	0.7	0.3	1.8	0.3	0.2	0.4	0,3	-	0,0
Canada, Northwest Territories	5,3	5,5	11.2	3,6	-	-	2.1	4.0	0,3	-	0.5	-	-	-
Canada, Nova Scotia	4.3	2.8	11.5	6.3	0.9	0.7	0.8	1.2	0,3	0.4	0.2	0,2	-	0,0
Canada, Ontario	4.0	2.3	9.8	4.9	1.2	1.0	0.7	1.2	0.6	0.5	0.4	0.3	0.1	0.1
Canada, Prince Edward Island	5.5	4.0	7.1	6.0	-	0,4	1,5	1,5	0,4	-	0.2	-	-	0,1
Canada, Quebec	5.9	3.8	11.6	6.0	0.6	0.5	0.8	1.4	0.6	0.4	0.4	0.2	0.4	0.3
Canada, Saskatchewan	3.5	2.6	10.4	5.4	0.4	0.3	0.7	1.5	0.6	0.5	0.3	0,1	0,0	0,1
Canada, Yukon	7,7	4,5	26.0	9,9	-	-	3,5	1,1	-	1,2	-	-	-	-
US, Cent. Calif.: Non-Hisp. White	4.9	2.6	8.9	4.6	1.0	1.0	0.5	0.5	0.5	0.4	0.4	0.2	0.1	0,1
US, Cent. Calif.: Hispanic	2.8	2.3	9.4	4.1	0.2	0.5	1.0	3.5	0,9	0.5	0.8	0,7	0,2	0.1
US, Los Angeles: Non-Hisp. White	5.0	3.3	7.6	4.5	1.0	1.3	0.4	0.7	0.5	0.3	0.5	0.2	0.1	0.1
US, Los Angeles: Hispanic White	3.5	2.0	5.6	3.7	0.4	0.7	0.7	3.1	0.6	0.5	0.6	0.5	0,2	0,0
US, Los Angeles: Black	4.5	3.2	7.6	6.0	1.0	0.9	0,3	0.8	0.7	0.2	0.4	0.3	0,1	0,1
US, Los Angeles: Chinese	3.4	2.1	4.8	5.0	0,1	-	0.6	1.2	0,7	0.6	0.6	0,2	-	0,1
US, Los Angeles: Filipino	4.3	1,1	4.7	5.1	-	0,2	0.7	1,1	0,3	0,3	0,6	0.5	-	-
US, Los Angeles: Korean	2,4	4.3	5.7	2.3	-	0,3	0,3	3.8	1,3	1,7	1,1	0,5	-	0,3
US, Los Angeles: Japanese	6.3	5.1	8.9	5.1	-	0,4	1,2	0.9	0,8	0,3	0.6	0,5	0,2	0,2
US, San Francisco: Non-Hisp. White	4.4	2.5	9.3	5.4	1.2	1.1	0.5	0.7	0.4	0.4	0.5	0.2	0,0	0.1
US, San Francisco: Hispanic White	3.5	2.5	9.3	4.1	0,7	0.5	0.5	1.0	0.6	0,1	0.6	0,2	0,1	0,4
US, San Francisco: Black	3.6	2.4	8.8	5.3	0,6	0.8	0.4	0.6	0.4	0,3	0.2	-	0,1	0,1
US, San Francisco: Chinese	3.8	2.5	8.4	7.3	0,5	0,2	0,9	1.0	1.2	0,2	0.4	0,8	-	0,1
US, San Francisco: Filipino	4.2	1.8	7.6	6.4	-	0,5	0.5	1.2	0,6	0.5	1.0	0,7	-	0,1
US, San Francisco: Japanese	3,6	2,9	15.7	5.5	-	-	1,1	1.3	0,8	0.5	0.9	1.5	-	-
US, Connecticut: White	6.5	4.0	9.2	4.9	0.3	0.6	0.5	0.9	0.5	0.4	0.4	0.3	0.1	0.1
US, Connecticut: Black	4.1	4.1	7.5	4.1	0,4	0.7	0,9	0.8	1,1	0.5	0.7	0,3	-	-
US, Atlanta: White	4.0	2.3	6.9	4.8	0.6	0.8	0.4	0.6	0.5	0.3	0.5	0.2	0,2	0,1
US, Atlanta: Black	3.5	2.7	6.6	5.0	1.1	1.1	1.2	0.8	0,1	0.4	0.3	0,2	0,1	0,1
US, Iowa	4.2	2.8	9.6	5.2	0.5	0.6	0.5	1.1	0.5	0.3	0.4	0.3	0.1	0.1
US, Central Louisiana: White	4.6	1.8	7.6	3.8	0,1	0.8	0.8	1.0	0.7	0.4	0,1	0,3	-	-
US, Central Louisiana: Black	2,8	0,4	7.4	3,1	0,4	1,1	0,9	1.4	0.5	-	0.3	-	-	-
US, New Orleans: White	4.9	2.8	8.6	4.3	0.8	0.6	0.8	0.9	0.7	0.3	0.2	0,1	0,0	-
US, New Orleans: Black	4.9	1.9	5.3	4.7	0,9	0,5	0.6	1.3	0,3	0.6	0.2	0,4	-	0,0
US, Detroit: White	6.4	3.8	8.9	4.9	0.6	1.0	0.5	1.3	0.7	0.5	0.4	0.2	0,0	0.1
US, Detroit: Black	4.2	3.4	8.1	4.3	1.1	1.0	0.5	0.9	0.4	0.6	0.3	0,2	0,0	0,1
US, New Mexico: Non-Hisp. White	3.4	1.8	7.3	4.4	0.6	0.9	0.3	0.6	0.3	0.2	0.4	0,3	0,1	0,1
US, New Mexico: Hispanic White	3.4	1.6	9.5	4.0	0.5	0.7	1.0	3.7	0.3	0.4	0,1	0,5	0,2	0,2
US, New Mexico: American Indian	0,6	1,3	3.9	3.1	0,3	0,5	3,8	10.3	0,3	1,2	0,8	-	-	1,0
US, Utah	2.9	1.7	7.9	4.1	0.6	0.8	0.3	1.1	0.2	0.4	0.2	0.2	0,0	0,1
US, Seattle	3.8	2.6	9.0	5.1	0.7	1.2	0.3	0.8	0.7	0.4	0.4	0.2	0,1	0.1
US, SEER: White	4.8	2.9	8.9	4.9	0.6	0.9	0.4	1.0	0.5	0.4	0.4	0.2	0.1	0.1
US, SEER: Black	3.8	3.0	8.1	4.6	1.0	0.9	0.6	0.8	0.4	0.5	0.3	0.2	0,1	0,1

AGE-STANDARDIZED (WORLD) INCIDENCE RATES (FOUR DIGIT RUBRICS)

| | Rectum | | | | | | 156.0 | | Gallbladder etc | | | | | |
| | 154.0 | | 154.1 | | 154.2-8 | | | | 156.1 | | 156.2 | | 156.8-9 | |
ASIA	M	F	M	F	M	F	M	F	M	F	M	F	M	F
*China, Qidong	0,2	0,1	6.0	5.3	1.2	1.6	0,2	0.3	0.8	0.4	0,1	0,0	0,3	0,3
China, Shanghai	0.2	0.2	8.8	7.0	0.3	0.2	1.2	2.2	0.8	0.9	0.4	0.4	0.1	0.1
China, Tianjin	0,1	0,0	6.1	5.4	0,0	0.1	0.6	0.7	1.1	0.7	0.5	0.3	0.2	0.3
Hong Kong														
*India, Bangalore	0.3	0,1	2.6	2.1	0.3	0.5	0.3	0.5	0,1	0,0	0.2	0,1	-	0,0
*India, Barshi, Paranda and Bhum	0,2	-	2.4	1,0	-	0,1	0,1	0,1	-	-	-	0,1	-	-
India, Bombay	0.3	0.2	2.9	2.1	0.7	0.4	1.1	2.1	0.2	0.2	0.5	0.3	0,0	0,0
*India, Karunagappally	-	-	1,1	0,3	0,5	-	-	-	-	-	-	-	-	-
India, Madras	0.3	0.3	2.8	1.8	0.7	0.7	0.3	0.4	0,1	0,0	0,1	0,1	-	-
*India, Trivandrum	0,1	-	2.7	2.1	0,3	0,1	0,1	0,6	-	-	0,1	-	-	-
Israel: All Jews	5.4	4.3	8.4	6.6	0.6	0.6	0.4	1.7	0.4	0.2	0.6	0.4	0.1	0.1
Jews born in Israel	3.5	3.7	6.7	6.4	0,6	0.8	0,4	0,5	0,1	0,3	0,5	0,0	0,1	0,0
Jews born in America or Europe	6.5	4.8	9.4	7.5	0.7	0.5	0.4	1.7	0.3	0.3	0.5	0.4	0.1	0.2
Jews born in Africa or Asia	3.7	3.3	7.4	5.0	0.5	0.6	0.4	1.8	0.5	0,1	0.7	0.4	0,1	0,1
Non-Jews	1.0	0,8	1.8	2.0	0,3	0,4	0.5	2.3	0,3	0,4	0,4	0,5	0,3	0,1
Japan, Hiroshima	2.7	0.7	16.4	8.8	0,3	0,2	2.4	3.7	2.7	1.5	0.8	0.6	0,2	0,1
Japan, Miyagi	0.6	0.3	16.0	8.6	0,1	0,1	2.8	3.7	4.1	2.3	0.6	0.4	0.4	0.3
Japan, Nagasaki	1.7	0.8	16.1	8.5	0.2	0.2	2.7	4.4	3.8	2.1	0.9	0.5	0.3	0.2
Japan, Osaka	0.6	0.3	12.6	6.4	0.2	0.2	2.4	3.7	3.1	1.7	0.4	0.3	0.2	0.2
*Japan, Saga														
Japan, Yamagata														
*Korea, Kangwha	1,1	1,2	6.0	3.3	1,2	0,9	1,9	2,3	1,9	1,1	0,9	0,3	-	0,2
*Kuwait: Non-Kuwaitis	0,9	0,9	1.8	0,7	0,9	0,7	1,2	2,3	0,0	0,1	0,4	0,4	-	0,4
*Kuwait: Kuwaitis	0,6	0,5	3.0	1,2	0,3	0,2	1,3	1,3	-	-	0,4	0,1	0,2	-
*Philippines, Manila	1.9	1.3	5.5	4.4	0.3	0.1	0.6	0.8	0,2	0,1	0.6	0.6	0,1	0,1
Singapore: Chinese	3.0	1.9	14.4	8.0	0.6	0.3	0.6	0.9	0.5	0.4	0.5	0.6	0,1	0,1
Singapore: Malay	1,1	1,0	6.2	6.5	0,5	0,2	0,6	1,3	0,2	-	0,8	0,6	0,1	0,1
Singapore: Indian	0,5	0,7	5.4	4.9	0,2	1,0	0,4	0,6	0,3	0,2	0,3	0,6	0,2	-
Thailand, Chiang Mai	0.4	0,1	2.4	2.5	0,2	0,2	1.2	1.7	1.0	0.5	0.9	0.7	0,2	0,1
*Thailand, Khon Kaen	0,3	0,2	2.3	1.5	0,3	0,3	0,9	1.4	0.6	0.5	0,1	0,2	0,2	0,0
*Viet Nam, Hanoi	0,1	-	2.5	1.6	1.8	0.9	0,2	0,1	0,0	-	-	-	0,1	-

EUROPE

| | Rectum | | | | | | 156.0 | | Gallbladder etc | | | | | |
| | 154.0 | | 154.1 | | 154.2-8 | | | | 156.1 | | 156.2 | | 156.8-9 | |
	M	F	M	F	M	F	M	F	M	F	M	F	M	F
Austria, Tyrol	0.9	0.4	12.8	6.9	1.1	1.5	1.2	1.5	0.8	0.5	0,4	0,2	0.6	0.5
*Belarus														
*Croatia	1.4	0.9	11.8	7.2	0.2	0.2	1.0	2.3	0.5	0.4	0.5	0.3	0,0	0.1
Czech Republic	7.6	4.1	15.6	6.7	0.9	0.8	2.6	5.1	1.1	1.1	0.5	0.3	0.4	0.6
Denmark	1.5	0.9	15.0	8.8	0.5	0.7	0.4	1.1	0.9	0.7	0.4	0.4	0,0	0,0
Estonia	0.7	0.4	10.3	6.6	0.5	0.5	0.4	1.0	0.3	0.3	0.4	0.4	0,1	0,0
Finland														
France, Bas-Rhin	5.8	2.3	12.7	6.1	0.6	0.5	0.8	2.0	0.5	0.2	0.7	0.3	0.4	0,1
*France, Calvados	5.1	2.7	11.3	5.7	1.0	1.4	0.7	1.1	0.5	0.5	0,2	0,1	0,1	0,1
France, Doubs	4.4	3.0	12.2	5.2	0,5	1.5	0,4	1.2	0.4	0.2	0.3	0,1	0,2	0.5
France, Haut-Rhin	7.6	3.7	13.1	6.4	0.9	1.2	1.4	2.9	0.5	0.3	0,1	0,1	0,1	0,0
*France, Herault	5.2	1.9	8.3	5.0	0.8	1.2	0.4	1.1	0,3	0,1	0.4	0,2	0,3	0,1
France, Isere	4.6	2.8	10.3	5.5	0.5	1.6	0.4	0.8	0.3	0.2	0.4	0,1	0,2	0,1
*France, Somme	4.5	2.2	8.9	4.1	0.7	1.3	0,3	1.6	0,1	0,1	0.6	0,2	0,2	0,1
*France, Tarn	6.1	4.3	11.4	5.2	0,4	0.5	0,3	1.5	0.2	0,1	0,1	0,1	0.4	0,1
Germany, Eastern States	1.5	1.1	13.9	8.5	0.4	0.5	2.1	5.2	0.9	1.1	0.5	0.4	0.1	0.2
Germany, Saarland	1.5	1.4	15.5	9.0	0.2	0.6	1.3	3.2	1.0	1.3	0.6	0.2	0,1	0,1
Iceland	0,4	0,3	5.7	5.1	-	0.2	0.1	0.7	0.4	0.3	1,1	0,4	-	-
Ireland, Southern	2.0	1.2	10.4	5.8	0.7	0,1	0.9	1.7	0.5	0.8	0.3	0,1	0,1	0,0
Italy, Ferrara	0,6	0,2	10.4	5.0	0,6	0.8	1.5	3.0	0.7	0,4	0.4	0.4	0.4	0,1
Italy, Florence	2.4	1.1	13.0	7.5	0.6	0.8	1.2	2.1	0.6	0.3	0.5	0,1	0.5	0.4
Italy, Genoa	3.7	2.6	9.2	5.3	0.3	0.8	1.5	2.2	0.8	0.6	0.6	0.4	0.5	0.5
*Italy, Latina	1.1	0.9	8.8	5.9	0,3	0,3	1.8	3.9	0.6	0,2	0.4	0.5	0,6	1.0
Italy, Macerata	3.5	2.0	11.2	4.8	-	0.2	0.2	0.8	2.1	0.5	0.2	0.2	0.4	0.2
Italy, Modena	3.9	2.6	8.8	5.2	0.5	0.5	1.1	2.1	0.5	0.3	0.4	0.3	0,1	0,1
Italy, Parma	3.1	2.1	9.5	5.9	0,4	0.8	1.4	2.3	1.0	0.5	0.5	0,2	0,4	0.3
Italy, Ragusa	2.3	1.2	7.2	3.2	0,5	0,5	1.6	2.6	1.3	0.5	0.8	0,1	0,3	0.6
Italy, Romagna	4.6	2.7	7.5	4.9	0.5	0.7	0.6	1.1	0.7	0.6	0.4	0.3	0.4	0.3
Italy, Torino	1.7	1.6	10.9	6.7	0.5	0.7	1.8	2.7	0.7	0.7	1.0	0.4	0.5	0.3
Italy, Trieste	3.7	2.5	6.9	4.9	8.1	1.3	0.9	1.9	0.9	0.8	0.5	0,1	2.9	1.9
Italy, Varese	4.3	2.2	11.2	5.6	0.5	0.4	1.0	2.6	1.1	0.6	0.5	0,2	0.4	0.5
Italy, Veneto	2.5	1.7	9.2	5.0	1.4	1.2	1.0	1.6	0.4	0.3	0.4	0.1	0.7	1.2
*Latvia	2.1	1.4	7.5	4.8	0.8	0.7	0.3	0.7	0.1	0.1	0.3	0.1	0.1	0.1
Malta	1,5	1,8	6.8	4.6	1,0	0,2	0,3	0,6	0,2	0,5	0,5	-	-	-

| | Rectum | | | | | | Gallbladder etc | | | | | | | |
| | 154.0 | | 154.1 | | 154.2-8 | | 156.0 | | 156.1 | | 156.2 | | 156.8-9 | |
	M	F	M	F	M	F	M	F	M	F	M	F	M	F
The Netherlands	4.2	2.7	10.0	5.9	0.3	0.3	0.6	1.4	0.9	0.7	0.6	0.4	0.1	0.1
The Netherlands, Eindhoven	4.6	3.4	12.1	6.2	0,2	0,2	0.7	1.7	0.8	0.6	0.5	0.4	0,1	0,1
The Netherlands, Maastricht	4.8	3.4	13.2	6.6	0.7	0.5	0.7	1.6	0.8	0.7	0.9	0.2	0,1	0,1
Norway														
*Poland, Cracow	0,4	0,3	7.6	4.6	2.4	1.5	3.1	5.9	0,1	0.4	0.6	0.2	0.6	0.6
*Poland, Kielce	0.4	0.3	0.5	0,2	7.5	5.1	1.2	3.1	0,1	0.2	0.4	0.2	0.9	1.3
*Poland, Lower Silesia	0.4	0.2	10.4	6.1	1.6	1.2	1.5	5.7	0.2	0.2	0.5	0.4	0.3	0.7
Poland, Warsaw City	0.9	0.7	9.5	5.5	0.9	0.6	1.9	5.8	1.0	1.0	0.9	0.5	0.3	0.3
Slovakia	4.9	2.9	15.1	7.7	0.5	0.4	1.8	5.0	0.9	0.7	0.7	0.4	0.3	0.3
Slovenia	3.3	1.9	13.6	7.7	0.3	0.3	1.3	2.9	1.0	0.8	0.3	0.2	0,0	0,0
*Spain, Albacete	1,7	2.2	7.5	3.5	-	-	1,5	3.1	-	0,1	0,6	-	0,3	0,8
Spain, Asturias	4.1	2.0	6.7	3.5	0,3	0.3	0.4	1.3	0.4	0.3	0.2	0.2	0,1	0.3
Spain, Basque Country	3.9	1.8	9.4	4.2	0.3	0.3	1.0	1.9	0.8	0.5	0.7	0.2	0.3	0.4
Spain, Granada	2.5	1.7	5.6	3.5	0.8	0.4	1.7	3.5	0,3	0.3	0.4	0.3	0.5	0.6
Spain, Mallorca	3.8	2.2	8.2	5.0	0.9	0,3	0.5	1.6	0.7	0.7	0.7	0.3	0.3	0.5
Spain, Murcia	3.3	2.4	8.3	4.9	0.4	0.4	1.3	2.6	0.2	0.2	0,1	0,1	0.4	0.6
Spain, Navarra	3.9	2.0	8.6	4.2	0,3	0.3	1.0	2.7	0.8	0.3	0.7	0.2	0.4	0.4
Spain, Tarragona	0.8	0,2	11.0	5.5	0.5	0.4	0.4	1.9	0.3	0.2	0.5	0.2	0.4	0.4
Spain, Zaragoza	4.1	2.3	6.8	3.9	0.3	0.2	0.6	1.2	0.6	0.2	0.4	0.2	0.9	1.1
Sweden	1.0	0.7	10.6	6.8	0.4	0.8	1.2	2.9	0.7	0.6	0.4	0.3	0.3	0.4
*Switzerland, Basel	2.7	1.2	12.9	7.0	0.7	1.1	0.9	1.4	0.4	0.5	0,0	-	0,0	0,1
Switzerland, Geneva	3.0	1.4	7.9	4.0	1.4	1.6	0,4	1.1	0.7	0.7	0.5	0,2	-	0,1
Switzerland, Graubunden	3.5	2.6	6.0	3.5	0,1	0,9	0.9	2.5	0.4	0.3	0,1	-	0,1	-
Switzerland, Neuchatel	2.8	1.3	10.9	4.5	1,0	2.5	1,1	1.7	0.4	0.4	-	0.2	0,2	0,1
Switzerland, St Gall-Appenzell	3.5	2.1	10.2	4.7	0,4	1.0	0.8	1.9	0.7	0.8	0,4	0.3	-	0,1
Switzerland, Valais	2.6	2.1	10.0	4.1	1.0	0.8	0,4	2.0	0.4	0.4	0.3	0.2	0,1	0.3
Switzerland, Vaud	2.6	2.0	9.0	5.2	0.8	1.4	1.1	1.5	0.8	0.5	0.3	0.2	0,2	0.3
Switzerland, Zurich	3.2	1.9	9.9	5.9	0.5	1.0	0.8	1.4	1.0	0.8	0.6	0.2	0.2	0.4
*UK, England and Wales	2.5	1.6	11.6	5.9	0.6	0.6	0.4	0.6	0.5	0.4	0.3	0.2	0.1	0.0
*UK, East Anglia														
*UK, Mersey	1.9	1.4	10.5	6.7	0.4	0.5	0.3	0.6	0.5	0.5	0.2	0.2	0,0	0,0
*UK, North Western	2.1	1.2	12.9	6.3	0.5	0.4	0.4	0.7	0.5	0.3	0.2	0.2	0,0	0,0
UK, Oxford	1.9	1.2	12.0	6.4	0.7	0.7	0.3	0.6	0.4	0.3	0.3	0.2	0.1	0.1
*UK, South Thames	2.3	1.5	9.8	5.3	0.6	0.6	0.3	0.5	0.4	0.3	0.3	0.1	0.1	0.0
UK, South Western	3.0	2.1	10.4	6.2	0.9	0.7	0.3	0.5	0.4	0.3	0.3	0.1	0.1	0.1
UK, Wessex	2.9	1.7	9.7	5.2	0.8	0.8	0.3	0.4	0.2	0.2	0.4	0.2	0.1	0.1
*UK, West Midlands	1.4	0.8	15.6	7.6	0.5	0.5	0.5	0.7	1.2	0.9	0.4	0.2	0,0	0,0
UK, Yorkshire	2.1	1.5	12.5	6.5	0.5	0.6	0.3	0.6	0.4	0.3	0.3	0.2	0,0	0,0
UK, Scotland	2.5	1.4	11.2	6.3	0.5	0.7	0.4	0.7	0.6	0.4	0.4	0.3	0.1	0.1
UK, Scotland, West	2.5	1.4	11.1	6.0	0.5	0.6	0.4	0.8	0.6	0.4	0.4	0.3	0,1	0,1
*Yugoslavia, Vojvodina														

OCEANIA

| | Rectum | | | | | | Gallbladder etc | | | | | | | |
| | 154.0 | | 154.1 | | 154.2-8 | | 156.0 | | 156.1 | | 156.2 | | 156.8-9 | |
	M	F	M	F	M	F	M	F	M	F	M	F	M	F
Australian Capital Territory	4.6	4.4	11.6	6.0	0,2	0,6	0,7	0,7	0,2	0,8	0,8	0,3	-	-
Australia, New South Wales	4.1	2.3	13.7	6.7	0.8	0.7	0.6	1.1	0.8	0.5	0.4	0.2	0.1	0.2
South Australia	4.7	3.0	12.7	7.8	0.5	0.6	0.7	2.0	0.5	0.6	0.5	0.3	0.2	0.2
Australia, Tasmania	3.2	1.8	11.5	8.2	0.5	0.8	0.4	1.3	0.8	0.5	0.2	0.2	0.3	-
Australia, Victoria	3.2	1.9	15.5	8.4	0.5	0.7	0.8	1.4	0.8	0.4	0.5	0.3	0.1	0.1
Western Australia	5.6	3.8	10.7	6.3	0.5	0.8	0.6	1.0	0.8	0.4	0.4	0.3	0,0	0,0
*French Polynesia	1,8	0,3	6.3	2,3	0,5	1,4	2,0	0,6	0,4	0,2	0,5	-	0,5	0,9
New Zealand: Non-Maori	4.8	2.7	14.7	7.8	0.7	0.7	0.4	0.7	0.6	0.4	0.3	0.2	0.1	0,1
New Zealand: Maori	1,8	1,3	10.3	7.3	0,6	0,6	0,7	0,7	1,2	0,2	0,5	0,3	-	-
US, Hawaii: White	4.9	2.1	8.2	5.1	0,8	0,8	0,5	1.2	0,8	0.5	0.3	0.3	-	0,1
US, Hawaii: Japanese	6.3	3.8	12.6	4.0	0,2	0,1	0,5	0.8	1.4	0.8	0.5	0.3	-	-
US, Hawaii: Hawaiian	4.8	2.6	9.1	5.1	-	0,5	0,9	0,7	0,8	0,4	-	0,3	0,3	-
US, Hawaii: Filipino	5.2	2.3	8.0	4.2	-	0,6	0,3	0,8	0,8	-	0,4	0,4	0,1	-
US, Hawaii: Chinese	4.0	1,3	7.8	5.1	0,3	-	1,5	2,5	1,1	-	-	0,7	-	0,2

AGE-STANDARDIZED (WORLD) INCIDENCE RATES (FOUR DIGIT RUBRICS)

| | Nose, sinuses etc | | | | Trachea | | Bronchus and lung | | | | Bone | | | |
| | 160.0-1 | | 160.2-9 | | 162.0 | | 162.2-9 | | 170.0-3,6 | | 170.4-5,7-8 | | 170.9 | |
AFRICA	M	F	M	F	M	F	M	F	M	F	M	F	M	F
*Algeria, Setif	0,3	0,4	0,3	-	0,2	-	28.0	2.9	0,4	0,2	0,4	0,1	1.2	0,4
*France, La Reunion	0,3	0,1	0,7	0,2	0,4	-	34.1	3.3	0,1	0,3	1.0	0,4	0,1	0,1
*Mali, Bamako	0,4	0,1	0,3	0,3	0,2	-	5.1	1.5	0,4	0,5	0,3	0,4	0,2	0,1
*Uganda, Kyadondo	0,5	0,2	0,9	0,1	-	-	4.2	0,4	0,9	0,1	0,4	0,5	1,1	0,0
*Zimbabwe, Harare: African	-	-	1,4	1,4	-	-	24.9	7.3	0,7	0,2	0,3	0,1	0,4	0,5
*Zimbabwe, Harare: European	3,1	0,5	-	0,5	-	0,5	36.0	17.6	-	-	-	-	0,9	-

AMERICA, CENTRAL AND SOUTH

| | 160.0-1 | | 160.2-9 | | 162.0 | | 162.2-9 | | 170.0-3,6 | | 170.4-5,7-8 | | 170.9 | |
	M	F	M	F	M	F	M	F	M	F	M	F	M	F
*Argentina, Concordia	-	-	1,7	0,4	-	-	55.5	8.1	0,6	0,6	0,3	-	0,9	0,9
*Brazil, Belem	0,2	0,1	0,4	0,1	0,3	0,1	28.3	7.1	0,7	0,7	1.0	0,5	1.0	0,3
*Brazil, Goiania	0,4	0,2	0,4	0,2	0,5	0,1	20.8	9.6	0,2	0,2	0,7	0,8	0,2	0,1
*Brazil, Porto Alegre	0,1	0,1	0,1	0,2	0,3	0,1	67.2	14.3	1.2	0,6	0,9	0,5	1.4	0.8
Colombia, Cali	0.6	0.3	0.5	0.5	-	-	24.4	9.5	0,3	0,2	0.7	0.3	0,2	0,2
*Costa Rica	0.3	0.1	0.2	0.0	0,1	0,0	15.6	5.4	0.2	0.3	0.4	0.3	0,2	0,1
*Ecuador, Quito	0,2	0,1	0,3	0,2	0,0	0,1	10.1	3.5	0,3	0,2	0.5	0.4	0,1	0,2
*Peru, Lima	0,4	0,2	0,4	0,3	0,0	-	15.8	6.3	0,4	0,3	0.5	0.4	0,1	0.2
Peru, Trujillo	0,2	0,1	0,3	0,4	-	-	11.9	4.1	-	-	0,3	0,2	0,8	0,3
US, Puerto Rico	0,4	0,2	0,3	0,1	0,1	0,0	18.9	6.6	0,3	0,2	0,3	0,4	0,1	0,0
*Uruguay, Montevideo	0,3	0,1	0.5	0.3	0.6	0,2	70.0	7.4	0,2	0,2	0,4	0,2	0,4	0.3

AMERICA, NORTH

| | 160.0-1 | | 160.2-9 | | 162.0 | | 162.2-9 | | 170.0-3,6 | | 170.4-5,7-8 | | 170.9 | |
	M	F	M	F	M	F	M	F	M	F	M	F	M	F
Canada	0.3	0.2	0.3	0.1	0.2	0.1	65.2	27.9	0.5	0.4	0.5	0.4	0.1	0.1
Canada, Alberta	0.3	0.2	0.4	0.2	0,1	0,0	49.9	24.5	0.5	0.3	0.5	0.4	0,0	0,0
Canada, British Columbia	0.3	0.3	0.3	0.2	0.1	0.1	54.8	31.0	0.3	0.2	0.4	0.5	0.1	0,1
Canada, Manitoba	0,1	0,2	0,2	0,1	0,0	0,1	58.4	28.2	0,4	0,2	0.5	0.5	0,2	0,0
Canada, New Brunswick	0,3	0,2	0,3	0,2	0,2	-	72.7	27.5	0,3	0,1	0.4	0.3	0,1	0,1
Canada, Newfoundland	0,4	0,3	0,4	0,1	0,2	-	56.8	14.1	0,4	0,3	0.3	0.2	0,0	-
Canada, Northwest Territories	0,5	-	-	-	-	-	90.3	65.6	-	-	0,7	0,7	-	-
Canada, Nova Scotia	0.4	0,2	0,3	0,2	0,2	0,1	74.4	32.3	0.5	0.3	0.4	0.5	0,1	0,2
Canada, Ontario	0.4	0.2	0.3	0.2	0.2	0.1	62.0	28.1	0.5	0.4	0.5	0.4	0.1	0.1
Canada, Prince Edward Island	0,3	-	0,7	-	0,2	-	59.6	36.6	0,3	0,2	0.3	0.4	0,3	-
Canada, Quebec	0.3	0.2	0.3	0.1	0.3	0.1	82.3	27.9	0.7	0.4	0.6	0.5	0.1	0.1
Canada, Saskatchewan	0,2	0,2	0,4	0,0	0,0	-	52.9	23.9	0,4	0,5	0.4	0.3	0,0	0,1
Canada, Yukon	-	-	-	-	-	3,8	68.1	43.8	-	-	-	-	-	-
US, Cent. Calif.: Non-Hisp. White	0.5	0.2	0.3	0.2	0,1	0,0	71.0	39.5	0.4	0.2	0.6	0.6	0,2	0,1
US, Cent. Calif.: Hispanic	0,2	-	0,1	-	0,3	0,1	34.2	15.3	0,2	0,2	0,4	0,2	-	0,3
US, Los Angeles: Non-Hisp. White	0.4	0.2	0.3	0.2	0.1	0.1	59.6	38.5	0.4	0.4	0.5	0.4	0.1	0.1
US, Los Angeles: Hispanic White	0.2	0.2	0.3	0.3	-	0,1	31.0	14.4	0.3	0.4	0.6	0.5	0,1	0,1
US, Los Angeles: Black	0,1	0,2	0.9	0,1	0,1	0,1	88.6	35.3	0,4	0,1	0,2	0,1	0,3	-
US, Los Angeles: Chinese	0,4	-	-	0,2	-	-	36.5	16.4	-	0,1	0,2	0,2	-	-
US, Los Angeles: Filipino	-	0,2	0,4	0,6	-	-	44.9	12.3	0,1	0,4	0,4	0,2	-	-
US, Los Angeles: Korean	-	0,2	-	-	-	0,3	36.7	12.0	0,4	-	0,6	0,2	-	-
US, Los Angeles: Japanese	-	-	0,3	-	-	-	31.2	12.6	-	-	0,3	-	-	-
US, San Francisco: Non-Hisp. White	0.3	0.1	0.3	0.1	0,1	0,1	58.5	40.4	0.7	0.6	0.2	0.0	0.1	0,1
US, San Francisco: Hispanic White	0,1	0,2	0,4	0,4	-	-	37.2	22.9	0,2	0,1	0.5	0.3	0,2	-
US, San Francisco: Black	0,2	0,2	0,4	0,1	0,2	0,1	101.3	44.2	0,4	0,3	0,1	0,1	0,1	0,0
US, San Francisco: Chinese	0,4	0,1	0.5	0.3	-	-	39.4	24.0	0.5	0.3	0,4	-	-	-
US, San Francisco: Filipino	0,4	0,3	0.5	0,1	-	-	46.8	15.9	0,2	0,7	0,2	0,2	-	-
US, San Francisco: Japanese	-	-	0,8	-	-	-	35.7	15.1	0,6	-	-	-	-	-
US, Connecticut: White	0.2	0.2	0.3	0.2	0,1	0,0	62.0	35.2	0.6	0.6	0.2	0,1	0.1	0,1
US, Connecticut: Black	0,2	0,4	0,4	0,2	0,1	-	86.0	33.2	0,7	0,1	0,1	-	-	0,1
US, Atlanta: White	0.3	0,1	0.3	0,2	0,1	0,1	72.3	35.4	0.5	0.3	0,1	0,2	0,0	0,1
US, Atlanta: Black	-	0,1	0,8	0,1	-	-	97.3	29.8	0,4	0,8	0,3	0,1	-	-
US, Iowa	0.3	0.2	0.3	0.2	0,1	0,1	65.9	28.6	0.7	0.7	0.2	0,1	0,1	0,0
US, Central Louisiana: White	0,2	0,1	0,1	0,2	-	-	77.4	27.3	0,5	0,2	-	0,7	0,2	0,1
US, Central Louisiana: Black	-	-	0,3	0,4	-	0,4	105.6	26.8	-	0,5	-	-	-	-
US, New Orleans: White	0,3	-	0,3	0,2	0,1	0,0	83.9	41.2	0,2	0,1	0.7	0,3	0,1	-
US, New Orleans: Black	0,2	0,5	1.2	0,4	0,7	-	110.1	36.9	0,1	0,1	0.5	0,3	0,2	-
US, Detroit: White	0.3	0.2	0.4	0.2	0,1	0,1	74.5	40.1	0.8	0.5	0.3	0,1	0,1	0,0
US, Detroit: Black	0,1	0,1	0,2	0,7	0,2	-	103.0	42.0	0,5	0,6	-	0,1	-	0,0
US, New Mexico: Non-Hisp. White	0,1	0,3	0,4	0,4	0,0	0,1	52.4	28.7	0,7	0,5	0,1	0,2	0,1	0,1
US, New Mexico: Hispanic White	0,3	0,1	0,4	0,2	0,1	-	27.4	13.8	0,5	0,5	0,1	0,2	0,4	0,2
US, New Mexico: American Indian	-	-	0,3	1,5	-	-	10.3	4.0	0,3	0,7	-	-	-	-
US, Utah	0,1	0,2	0,2	0,2	0,0	0,0	29.7	13.1	1.2	0,7	0,2	0,0	-	0,0
US, Seattle	0.3	0.1	0.4	0.2	0,0	0,0	63.1	37.6	0.8	0.7	0,1	0,1	0,1	0,1
US, SEER: White	0.3	0.2	0.3	0.2	0,1	0,1	61.3	33.8	0.7	0.6	0,2	0,1	0,1	0,1
US, SEER: Black	0,1	0.2	0.4	0.4	0,2	0,0	99.0	38.4	0.5	0.6	0,1	0,1	0,0	0,0

AGE-STANDARDIZED (WORLD) INCIDENCE RATES (FOUR DIGIT RUBRICS)

| | Nose, sinuses etc | | | | Trachea | | Bronchus and lung | | | | Bone | | | |
| | 160.0-1 | | 160.2-9 | | 162.0 | | 162.2-9 | | 170.0-3,6 | | 170.4-5,7-8 | | 170.9 | |
	M	F	M	F	M	F	M	F	M	F	M	F	M	F
ASIA														
*China, Qidong	0,1	0,1	0,2	0,1	-	-	35.0	11.0	0.7	0.4	0.3	0,3	0.5	0.5
China, Shanghai	0.4	0.3	0.3	0.2	0,0	0,0	56.1	18.2	0.6	0.4	0.5	0.3	0.5	0.5
China, Tianjin	0.2	0.1	0.4	0.2	0,1	0,0	55.8	37.0	0.3	0.2	0.2	0.3	1.4	1.3
Hong Kong														
*India, Bangalore	0.2	0.2	0.5	0.5	0,0	-	8.0	1.7	0.4	0.2	0.5	0.5	0.1	0.2
*India, Barshi, Paranda and Bhum	0,1	-	0,2	0,2	-	-	1.3	0,3	0,2	0,2	0,1	0,2	-	0,1
India, Bombay	0.2	0.1	0.8	0.6	0,0	0,0	14.5	3.7	0.3	0.3	0.4	0.3	0.1	0.1
*India, Karunagappally	0.3	-	0.3	0.2	-	-	17.0	2.6	-	-	0.3	0.2	0.3	-
India, Madras	0.3	0.3	0.6	0.4	0,1	0,0	12.6	2.4	0.3	0.2	0.6	0.2	0,0	0,0
*India, Trivandrum	0,2	0,1	0.8	0.5	-	-	10.6	1.9	0.4	0.2	0.1	0,1	-	-
Israel: All Jews	0.2	0.2	0.2	0.2	0,1	0,0	27.0	9.2	0.5	0.2	0.7	0.5	0.2	0.2
Jews born in Israel	0,0	0,3	0,3	0,2	0,1	0,0	22.5	10.7	0.3	0.2	0.9	0.7	0.2	0.3
Jews born in America or Europe	0,1	0.2	0.1	0.2	0,1	-	26.4	10.7	0.4	0.2	0.4	0.2	0.5	0,1
Jews born in Africa or Asia	0,7	0,1	0.3	0.2	0,1	0,0	27.8	5.4	0.4	0.3	0.4	0.2	0,1	0,7
Non-Jews	0,1	-	0.2	0.2	0,1	-	29.0	3.7	0.3	0,0	0.6	0.2	-	0,0
Japan, Hiroshima	0.2	0.2	0.9	0.2	0,0	0,1	39.6	11.6	0.3	0.2	0.3	0.3	-	-
Japan, Miyagi	0.3	0.2	1.2	0.5	0,1	0,0	39.5	10.3	0.1	0.2	0.6	0.3	0,1	0,1
Japan, Nagasaki	0.4	0.2	0.8	0.3	0,1	0,0	41.7	12.0	0.1	0.2	0.4	0.3	0,1	0,0
Japan, Osaka	0.1	0.1	0.7	0.4	0.0	0,0	43.4	12.4	0.2	0.2	0.3	0.2	0.1	0.1
*Japan, Saga														
Japan, Yamagata														
*Korea, Kangwha	-	0,3	-	-	0,4	-	33.4	8.4	0,4	-	1,9	0,8	0,3	-
*Kuwait: Non-Kuwaitis	-	-	1,5	0,1	0,0	-	35.3	10.3	0.6	0,1	0.4	0.2	0,1	-
*Kuwait: Kuwaitis	-	0,3	-	0,2	0,2	-	20.1	9.2	0,1	0.3	0.4	0.5	0,2	-
*Philippines, Manila	0.5	0.3	1.0	0.6	0,1	0,0	58.6	16.7	0.4	0.3	0.4	0.4	0.6	0.4
Singapore: Chinese	0.5	0.3	0.3	0,1	0,1	0,0	62.6	19.5	0.3	0.2	0.5	0.5	-	0,1
Singapore: Malay	0,4	0,4	0,1	0,6	-	-	37.2	9.6	0,4	0,5	0,3	0,1	-	-
Singapore: Indian	0,4	0,4	0.3	0,2	0,1	-	14.2	3.5	0.2	-	1,2	0,4	0,3	0,1
Thailand, Chiang Mai	0.5	0.4	0.5	0,2	0.4	0.3	35.6	30.0	0,1	0.3	0.4	0.2	0.2	0,1
*Thailand, Khon Kaen	0,1	0,1	0.3	0,2	-	0,0	17.0	5.3	0.2	0.3	0.2	0.2	0.8	1.2
*Viet Nam, Hanoi	0.4	0.4	0.6	0.5	-	0,0	34.9	6.3	0.7	0.3	0.9	0.3	0.5	0,3
EUROPE														
Austria, Tyrol	0,0	0,2	0,2	0,2	0,1	-	54.6	11.3	0,3	0,2	0,6	0,5	0,5	0,3
*Belarus														
*Croatia	0.3	0.1	0.2	0.2	0.5	0.1	72.0	9.6	0.4	0.3	0.8	0.6	0.5	0.3
Czech Republic	0.3	0.1	0.2	0.1	2.6	0.3	75.2	9.8	0.5	0.3	0.5	0.3	0.1	0.2
Denmark	0.6	0.4	0.2	0.1	0.1	0.1	51.8	25.3	0.3	0.2	0.5	0.3	0.2	0.1
Estonia	0,2	0,1	0.5	0.3	0.3	-	75.4	8.3	0,2	0.4	0.4	0.4	0,0	0,0
Finland														
France, Bas-Rhin	0.4	0,1	0.5	0,1	0.6	0,1	66.8	7.1	0.7	0.2	0.5	0.6	0,0	0,0
*France, Calvados	0.3	0,0	1.1	0,3	0.7	0,2	54.4	4.4	0,4	0.3	0,6	0.6	0,1	0,1
France, Doubs	0.2	0.1	0.8	0,0	0.8	-	50.0	6.5	0.4	0.2	0.5	0.7	0.1	0.0
France, Haut-Rhin	0.7	0.2	0.8	0,0	0.6	-	57.7	6.7	0.6	0.3	0.3	0.2	0,1	0,1
*France, Herault	0.5	0.3	0.7	0.3	0.3	0,1	42.5	5.3	0.6	0.3	0.4	0.4	0.4	0,3
France, Isere	0.5	0.2	0.7	0.1	0.6	0,0	49.5	5.5	0.2	0.2	0.6	0.4	0.1	0,0
*France, Somme	0.6	0.3	0.7	0.1	1.1	-	54.0	4.5	0.2	0,0	0.2	0.4	0.1	-
*France, Tarn	0.2	0.1	0.9	0.1	0.5	-	39.2	3.2	0.3	0.2	1,1	0.6	0.1	0,0
Germany, Eastern States	0.2	0.1	0.4	0.1	0.1	0,0	59.0	7.6	0.6	0.4	0.5	0.4	0.2	0.1
Germany, Saarland	0,1	0,1	0.4	0.1	0,3	0,0	70.7	10.3	0.3	0.3	0.5	0.2	0.2	0,1
Iceland	0,7	0,6	0,5	-	0,4	-	32.4	26.4	0,4	0.1	0.8	0.3	-	-
Ireland, Southern	0,1	0,2	0,2	0,1	0,1	0,1	41.5	13.8	0.2	0.1	0.6	0.3	-	0,1
Italy, Ferrara	0.6	0.1	0,1	-	0,9	0,2	84.8	14.2	0,6	0.6	0.2	-	-	0,1
Italy, Florence	0.6	0.1	0.3	0.1	0.1	0,0	62.4	11.1	0.3	0.2	0.4	0.2	0.5	0.3
Italy, Genoa	0.7	0.3	0.3	0.1	0.2	0,0	72.1	10.0	0.2	0.3	0.5	0.3	0.1	0.4
*Italy, Latina	0,3	-	0,2	0,1	0,1	-	65.7	9.2	0,6	0.2	0.2	0.1	0.3	-
Italy, Macerata	0,3	-	0,8	-	0,1	-	47.3	7.4	-	0,0	0,1	0,2	0.3	-
Italy, Modena	0.1	0,0	0,0	0,2	0,1	0,1	68.5	9.1	0.1	0.1	0.5	0.4	0,0	0,1
Italy, Parma	0.4	0.2	0.3	0,2	0,2	-	63.2	12.0	0.2	0.4	0.1	0.7	0.3	-
Italy, Ragusa	0.1	0.1	0,2	-	0,2	-	38.8	5.0	0.5	0.5	0.9	0.2	-	-
Italy, Romagna	0.5	0.2	0,1	0,2	0,1	0,0	66.0	9.5	0.7	0.2	0.3	0.6	0,2	0,2
Italy, Torino	0.3	0.1	0,2	0,1	0,1	0,0	64.8	10.7	0.2	0.2	0.5	0.2	0,1	0,1
Italy, Trieste	0.7	-	0,4	0.3	0.6	0,1	82.1	14.7	0.4	1,0	-	0.3	0.4	0,1
Italy, Varese	0.5	0.2	0.4	0.1	0,2	-	77.4	8.5	0.3	0.2	0.6	0.4	0.1	-
Italy, Veneto	0.4	0,0	0.6	0.1	0.5	0,1	81.4	13.8	0.1	0.1	0.3	0.1	0.3	0.4
*Latvia	0.3	0.1	0.3	0.1	2.5	0.4	63.0	6.7	1.1	0.5	0.6	0.3	0,0	0,1
Malta	0,4	0,1	0,8	0,4	-	-	48.0	3.4	0,4	-	-	0,7	-	0,3

AGE-STANDARDIZED (WORLD) INCIDENCE RATES (FOUR DIGIT RUBRICS)

| | Nose, sinuses etc | | | | Trachea Bronchus and lung | | | | | | Bone | | | |
| | 160.0-1 | | 160.2-9 | | 162.0 | | 162.2-9 | | 170.0-3,6 | | 170.4-5,7-8 | | 170.9 | |
	M	F	M	F	M	F	M	F	M	F	M	F	M	F
The Netherlands	0.5	0.2	0.3	0.1	0.1	0.0	72.9	12.9	0.3	0.2	0.5	0.4	0.1	0.0
The Netherlands, Eindhoven	0.5	0,2	0.4	0,0	0,3	-	81.1	11.5	0,3	0.5	0.8	0,3	0,1	-
The Netherlands, Maastricht	0.5	0,2	0,3	0,2	0.2	0,0	79.8	12.5	0.4	0,3	0.5	0,3	0,1	0,1
Norway														
*Poland, Cracow	0,1	0,1	0,3	0,0	0,1	0,2	77.7	15.2	0,4	0,1	0.5	0.4	0,3	0,2
*Poland, Kielce	0,1	0,2	0.5	0,2	0,1	0,0	67.2	7.0	0,4	0,3	0.4	0,1	0,2	0,3
*Poland, Lower Silesia	0.3	0.1	0.3	0.2	0.3	0,0	95.2	16.2	0.8	0.5	0.8	0.5	0,1	0,1
Poland, Warsaw City	0.2	0,1	0.6	0.2	0,1	0,1	68.3	19.4	0.3	0.4	0.5	0,3	0,2	0,2
Slovakia	0.2	0.1	0.4	0.1	0.6	0.1	78.5	8.5	0.7	0.5	0.7	0.4	0.3	0.2
Slovenia	0,2	0.1	0.6	0.2	-	-	65.6	9.1	0.3	0.4	0.3	0.2	0,1	0,0
*Spain, Albacete	-	-	-	0,1	-	-	34.1	3.1	0,2	-	0,2	1,8	0,2	-
Spain, Asturias	0.6	0,2	0.9	0.4	0.2	0,0	63.3	4.3	0.4	0,1	0,4	0.4	0,2	0,2
Spain, Basque Country	0.5	0,1	0.5	0,1	0.2	0,0	52.9	3.4	0.4	0.4	0.5	0.3	0,1	0,1
Spain, Granada	0.5	0,0	0.4	0,1	0.2	0,0	45.2	2.7	0,4	0.4	0,4	0.3	0,1	0,0
Spain, Mallorca	0.6	0,1	0.2	0,1	0,1	0,0	61.4	4.3	0.2	0,1	0.4	0.4	0,0	0,2
Spain, Murcia	0.3	0,2	0,1	0,1	0,0	0,0	47.2	3.6	0.5	0,1	0.6	0,3	0,3	0,2
Spain, Navarra	0,2	0,2	0.3	0,1	0,1	0,1	41.4	3.3	0,1	0,2	1.3	0,3	0,0	0,1
Spain, Tarragona	0,1	0,0	0,3	0,0	0,1	0,0	42.8	3.1	0,1	0,3	0.2	0,4	0,3	0,2
Spain, Zaragoza	0.4	0,2	0,2	0,1	0.2	0,1	47.8	2.6	0.5	0,3	0.3	0.4	0,2	0,0
Sweden	0.3	0.2	0.3	0.1	0.1	0.0	23.8	10.9	0.4	0.3	0.5	0.3	0.2	0.0
*Switzerland, Basel	0.3	0,1	0.7	0,2	0.2	-	49.5	11.9	0.5	0,4	0.7	0,9	0,1	0,2
Switzerland, Geneva	0,1	0,5	0.6	0,1	0.2	0,0	53.5	14.2	0.3	0.2	1,0	-	-	-
Switzerland, Graubunden	-	0,1	0.2	-	0,5	-	49.3	9.7	0.5	0,4	0.4	1,8	-	-
Switzerland, Neuchatel	0,1	0,2	0.6	0,1	-	-	60.8	11.6	-	0,6	0.2	-	-	-
Switzerland, St Gall-Appenzell	0,6	0,1	0.4	0,3	0,1	0,1	49.0	8.3	0.2	0,2	1.2	0.6	0,1	0,2
Switzerland, Valais	0,1	0,4	0.3	0,4	0.5	0,1	47.2	10.1	0,1	-	0.3	0,2	-	-
Switzerland, Vaud	0,1	0,3	0.4	0,2	0,1	0,1	61.3	12.4	0.5	0,1	0.5	0,2	-	-
Switzerland, Zurich	0.3	0,1	0.3	0,1	0,1	0,0	47.3	10.8	0.7	0.5	0.8	0.4	0,1	-
*UK, England and Wales	0.3	0.2	0.3	0.2	0.1	0.1	62.3	22.7	0.4	0.2	0.4	0.3	0.2	0.2
*UK, East Anglia														
*UK, Mersey	0.2	0.2	0.2	0.2	0.2	0,1	63.1	31.2	0.3	0.2	0.3	0.1	0.2	0,0
*UK, North Western	0.2	0.2	0.4	0.2	0.2	0.1	70.7	27.8	0.2	0.2	0.3	0.3	0,1	0,1
UK, Oxford	0.3	0.2	0.3	0.1	0,1	0.0	55.0	19.9	0.4	0.2	0.4	0.4	0.2	0,1
*UK, South Thames	0.3	0.2	0.4	0.1	0.1	0.1	56.0	21.3	0.3	0.3	0.6	0.4	0.1	0.1
UK, South Western	0.2	0.1	0.2	0.1	0.2	0.1	46.9	17.1	0.4	0.2	0.4	0.3	0.1	0,1
UK, Wessex	0.3	0.2	0.3	0.2	0.1	0.1	51.0	17.9	0.4	0.3	0.4	0.3	0.2	0.2
*UK, West Midlands	0.2	0.2	0.4	0.2	0.1	0.1	65.8	21.4	0.1	0.1	0.1	0.1	2.0	1.5
UK, Yorkshire	0.3	0.2	0.3	0.1	0.1	0.1	64.1	24.7	0.2	0.1	0.4	0.3	0.1	0.1
UK, Scotland	0.2	0.1	0.3	0.2	0.2	0.0	79.6	33.7	0.3	0.3	0.5	0.3	0.0	0.0
UK, Scotland, West	0.3	0.1	0.2	0.2	0.2	0,1	88.7	38.4	0.4	0.3	0.5	0.3	0,1	0,0
*Yugoslavia, Vojvodina														

OCEANIA

| | Nose, sinuses etc | | | | Trachea Bronchus and lung | | | | | | Bone | | | |
| | 160.0-1 | | 160.2-9 | | 162.0 | | 162.2-9 | | 170.0-3,6 | | 170.4-5,7-8 | | 170.9 | |
	M	F	M	F	M	F	M	F	M	F	M	F	M	F
Australian Capital Territory	0,3	0,2	0,9	-	-	-	39.1	13.9	0,7	0,2	1,0	0,3	-	0,2
Australia, New South Wales	0.3	0.1	0.3	0.2	0.1	0.1	46.5	14.8	0.4	0.2	0.5	0.4	0.1	0.1
South Australia	0.3	0.1	0.3	0,1	0,0	-	47.8	15.2	0.3	0.3	0.3	0.3	0,1	0,0
Australia, Tasmania	0.5	0.4	1.5	-	0.1	0.1	49.2	18.7	0.4	0.2	0.3	0.2	0.0	0.2
Australia, Victoria	0.3	0.1	0.4	0.1	0.1	0.0	45.9	15.8	0.4	0.3	0.6	0.4	0.1	0.1
Western Australia	0.4	0.2	0.3	0,0	0,1	0,1	47.9	17.5	0.4	0.5	0.8	0.4	0,1	0,0
*French Polynesia	1,1	0,7	0,9	0,2	-	-	73.7	28.1	1,9	1,3	0.5	0,3	-	0,3
New Zealand: Non-Maori	0.4	0.2	0.2	0.3	0.1	0,1	46.3	18.2	0.6	0.5	0.8	0.4	0,0	0,0
New Zealand: Maori	-	-	0,2	-	-	0,2	99.7	72.8	0,9	0.3	0.9	0.4	0,1	-
US, Hawaii: White	0,5	0.3	0.2	0.2	0.1	0.1	59.4	37.8	0.6	0,4	0.3	-	0,1	-
US, Hawaii: Japanese	0,1	0,2	0.7	0,2	-	0,2	34.0	10.9	0.6	0.5	-	0,3	-	0,1
US, Hawaii: Hawaiian	0,4	0,1	0.6	1,0	0,3	-	72.1	35.0	0.8	0.5	0,3	-	-	-
US, Hawaii: Filipino	0,3	-	0,1	0,7	-	0,2	40.6	17.5	1,6	0,3	0,3	-	-	-
US, Hawaii: Chinese	0,5	0,4	-	0,1	-	-	37.6	18.9	0,5	-	-	-	-	-

AGE-STANDARDIZED (WORLD) INCIDENCE RATES (FOUR DIGIT RUBRICS)

| | Melanoma of skin | | | | | | | | | | | |
| | 172.0-4 | | 172.5 | | 172.6 | | 172.7 | | 172.8 | | 172.9 | |
AFRICA	M	F	M	F	M	F	M	F	M	F	M	F
*Algeria, Setif	-	-	-	-	-	-	-	-	-	-	0,1	0,1
*France, La Reunion	0,4	0,2	0,5	0,5	0,1	0,3	0,3	1.0	-	-	0,2	0,3
*Mali, Bamako	0,1	-	-	-	-	-	0,5	0,7	-	-	-	0,4
*Uganda, Kyadondo	-	-	-	-	0,2	-	0,5	0,8	-	-	0,6	0,3
*Zimbabwe, Harare: African	-	-	-	0,3	0,4	0,3	0,8	2,4	-	-	0,6	0,8
*Zimbabwe, Harare: European	1,6	2,9	3,3	2,9	1,6	1,9	4,2	5,4	-	-	7,8	1,9
AMERICA, CENTRAL AND SOUTH												
*Argentina, Concordia	-	0,4	0,7	-	-	0,4	0,3	0,1	-	-	0,3	1,4
*Brazil, Belem	0,1	0,0	0,1	-	-	-	0,1	-	-	-	1.1	0.9
*Brazil, Goiania	0,5	0,5	0,3	-	0,5	0,3	0,7	0,3	0,2	0,1	1.1	0,7
*Brazil, Porto Alegre	0,5	0,4	0,6	0.6	0,4	0,2	0,4	0,4	0,1	-	3.3	3.5
Colombia, Cali	0.9	0.6	0.6	0.6	0.3	0.5	0.8	1.2	-	-	0.2	0.3
*Costa Rica	0.3	0.2	0.4	0.3	0.2	0.2	0.9	0.8	0,1	-	0.2	0.3
*Ecuador, Quito	0.8	1.0	0.5	0.2	0.1	0,4	1.4	1.7	-	-	0.5	0.5
*Peru, Lima	0,2	0,2	0.3	0,1	0,2	0,2	0.5	0.7	-	-	0.4	0.3
Peru, Trujillo	-	-	-	-	-	-	0,3	0,5	-	-	2,8	1,1
US, Puerto Rico	0.3	0.2	0.4	0.2	0.2	0.2	0.4	0.3	-	-	0.2	0,1
*Uruguay, Montevideo	0.7	0,1	0.7	0,3	0,2	0,1	0.5	0.8	-	0,1	1.8	1.1
AMERICA, NORTH												
Canada	1.6	0.8	3.3	1.6	1.4	1.6	0.8	2.6	0.0	0.0	0.5	0.3
Canada, Alberta	1.7	0.9	3.3	1.8	1.3	1.8	0.8	2.9	-	-	0.5	0,1
Canada, British Columbia	2.1	0.9	4.6	2.5	1.8	2.4	1.1	4.2	-	-	0.4	0.2
Canada, Manitoba	1.3	0.8	3.1	1.5	1.6	1.7	0.7	2.7	0,2	0,2	0.2	0,1
Canada, New Brunswick	1.5	0.9	4.1	1.8	2.0	2.2	0.6	3.1	-	-	0.5	0,1
Canada, Newfoundland	1.1	0.9	1.6	1.1	0.7	1.0	0.3	2.1	-	-	0,1	0,1
Canada, Northwest Territories	0,3	-	0.5	0,3	-	0,2	0,6	0,3	-	-	-	1,0
Canada, Nova Scotia	1.9	0.8	4.7	2.5	1.6	1.9	0.8	3.6	-	-	0.7	0.4
Canada, Ontario	1.8	1.0	4.2	1.8	1.8	2.0	1.1	2.8	0.0	0.0	0.7	0.4
Canada, Prince Edward Island	2.4	2,0	2.8	2.5	2,4	2,2	0,8	2.7	-	-	0,4	-
Canada, Quebec	0.8	0.4	1.3	0.7	0.6	0.6	0.5	1.4	0,0	0,0	0.5	0.3
Canada, Saskatchewan	2.0	0.9	3.5	2.1	1.6	1.6	0.7	2.9	-	-	0,2	0,1
Canada, Yukon	1,6	1,0	2,7	5,1	-	0,8	0,8	-	-	-	-	-
US, Cent. Calif.: Non-Hisp. White	2.8	0.8	4.7	2.0	2.5	2.6	0.8	2.5	0,1	0,0	1.2	0.6
US, Cent. Calif.: Hispanic	0.8	0,6	0.8	0,7	0,1	0.6	0,7	0.8	-	0,1	0,6	0,2
US, Los Angeles: Non-Hisp. White	3.1	1.0	7.0	3.2	3.4	2.9	1.5	3.8	0,0	0,0	1.1	0.5
US, Los Angeles: Hispanic White	0.5	0.4	0.5	0.5	0.2	0.4	0.6	0.6	-	-	0.2	0.2
US, Los Angeles: Black	0,1	-	0,1	0,0	0,1	0,0	0.4	0.5	-	-	0,1	0,1
US, Los Angeles: Chinese	-	0,2	-	0,1	-	-	-	0,1	-	-	-	0,2
US, Los Angeles: Filipino	0,2	-	0,2	-	-	0,1	0,4	-	-	-	-	-
US, Los Angeles: Korean	-	-	-	0,2	-	-	-	0,3	-	-	-	-
US, Los Angeles: Japanese	0,4	-	0,4	-	0,2	0,3	-	0,4	-	-	-	0,2
US, San Francisco: Non-Hisp. White	3.4	1.3	6.6	3.1	3.6	3.1	1.5	4.0	0,1	0,0	1.2	0.4
US, San Francisco: Hispanic White	0,5	0,4	1.0	0.7	0,7	1.8	0,4	1.5	-	-	0,5	0,3
US, San Francisco: Black	-	-	0,1	-	0,2	-	0,5	0,6	-	-	-	0,0
US, San Francisco: Chinese	-	0,1	-	-	-	0,1	0,1	0,2	-	-	-	-
US, San Francisco: Filipino	-	0,3	0,3	-	-	-	0,3	0,6	-	-	0,5	-
US, San Francisco: Japanese	-	-	0,6	-	-	0,7	-	-	-	-	-	-
US, Connecticut: White	2.3	1.1	6.8	3.0	2.6	2.9	1.5	3.7	-	0,0	0.7	0.4
US, Connecticut: Black	0,1	-	0,3	0,1	0,4	0,4	0,5	0,4	-	-	0,2	-
US, Atlanta: White	3.3	0.9	7.4	3.5	3.9	3.3	1.5	3.9	-	-	1.0	0.5
US, Atlanta: Black	-	0,0	0,1	0,0	0,1	0,0	0,5	0,2	-	-	0,1	0,0
US, Iowa	2.7	1.2	3.8	2.2	2.3	2.0	0.5	2.6	0,0	0,0	0.6	0.3
US, Central Louisiana: White	3.2	1.4	2.8	0.9	1,5	2.1	0.5	2.6	0,1	-	1.8	0,4
US, Central Louisiana: Black	-	-	-	-	-	-	-	-	-	-	-	1,1
US, New Orleans: White	1.7	1.1	2.1	1.0	1.6	0.9	0.8	0.8	0,1	-	0.9	0,2
US, New Orleans: Black	-	-	0,3	-	0,1	-	0,4	-	-	-	0,1	0,1
US, Detroit: White	2.4	0.8	4.9	2.0	2.2	1.9	1.0	2.4	0,0	-	0.6	0.2
US, Detroit: Black	0,0	0,0	0,0	-	0,1	0,1	0,3	0,2	-	-	0,1	-
US, New Mexico: Non-Hisp. White	4.3	1.6	6.3	3.4	3.5	3.0	1.2	4.1	-	-	1.5	0.4
US, New Mexico: Hispanic White	1.1	0,6	1.0	0.8	0,1	0,6	0,4	1.1	-	-	0,1	0,2
US, New Mexico: American Indian	0,2	0,5	-	-	-	-	1,2	-	-	-	-	0,2
US, Utah	3.4	1.6	4.7	2.6	2.8	2.8	1.0	3.4	-	-	1.3	0.5
US, Seattle	2.6	1.2	5.3	2.8	2.5	2.8	1.1	3.5	-	0,0	0.8	0.4
US, SEER: White	2.8	1.2	5.6	2.7	2.7	2.6	1.1	3.3	0,0	0,0	0.8	0.4
US, SEER: Black	0,0	0,0	0,1	0,0	0,1	0,1	0.4	0.3	-	-	0,1	0,0

AGE-STANDARDIZED (WORLD) INCIDENCE RATES (FOUR DIGIT RUBRICS)

| | Melanoma of skin | | | | | | | | | | | |
| | 172.0-4 | | 172.5 | | 172.6 | | 172.7 | | 172.8 | | 172.9 | |
ASIA	M	F	M	F	M	F	M	F	M	F	M	F
*China, Qidong	0,0	0,1	0,0	0,0	-	-	0,0	0,1	-	0,0	0.3	0,1
China, Shanghai	0.1	0,0	0,0	0,0	0,0	0.0	0.1	0.1	0,0	0,0	0.1	0.1
China, Tianjin	0,0	0,0	0,1	0,0	0,0	0,0	0.1	0.1	0,0	-	0.1	0.1
Hong Kong												
*India, Bangalore	0,0	0,0	0,0	0,0	0,0	0,0	0.2	0.2	-	-	0,1	0,0
*India, Barshi, Paranda and Bhum	-	-	-	0,1	-	-	-	-	-	-	-	-
India, Bombay	0,1	0.1	0.1	0.1	0,0	-	0.1	0.1	-	-	0.1	0.1
*India, Karunagappally	0,3	-	-	-	-	-	0,3	-	-	-	0,3	-
India, Madras	0,1	0,0	0,0	0,0	0,0	-	0.3	0.2	0,0	0,0	0,0	0,0
*India, Trivandrum	-	0,1	-	-	-	-	0,3	-	-	-	-	-
Israel: All Jews	1.3	1.2	3.6	2.1	1.4	1.7	1.6	3.7	0,1	0,0	1.7	1.2
Jews born in Israel	2.2	1.3	6.5	3.6	2.5	2.7	2.2	5.8	0,0	-	2.2	1.5
Jews born in America or Europe	1.3	1.7	4.5	2.5	1.5	1.9	1.9	4.4	0,1	0,0	2.0	1.4
Jews born in Africa or Asia	0.3	0.4	0.8	0.3	0,2	0.3	0.5	1.0	0,1	-	0.8	0.5
Non-Jews	0.3	-	0,0	0,1	0,0	0,1	0.3	0.4	-	-	-	0,1
Japan, Hiroshima	0,1	0,1	0,1	0,0	0,0	0,1	0.2	0.3	-	-	0,1	0,0
Japan, Miyagi	0,1	0,1	0,1	0,0	0,1	0,1	0.2	0.0	0,0	-	0.2	0,0
Japan, Nagasaki	0,1	0,1	0,1	0,1	0,1	0,0	0.2	0.2	-	-	0,1	0,1
Japan, Osaka	0,0	0,0	0,0	0.0	0,0	0,0	0.1	0.1	-	0,0	0.0	0.1
*Japan, Saga												
Japan, Yamagata												
*Korea, Kangwha	-	-	-	-	-	-	0,3	-	-	-	-	0,2
*Kuwait: Non-Kuwaitis	0,2	-	0,6	0,4	0,0	-	0,0	1,4	-	-	0,1	-
*Kuwait: Kuwaitis	-	0,3	0,2	-	0,1	-	0,2	-	-	-	-	-
*Philippines, Manila	0,1	0,0	0,1	0,1	0,1	0,1	0.3	0.2	0,0	0,0	0,1	0,1
Singapore: Chinese	0,1	0,0	0,1	0,1	-	0,1	0.3	0.2	-	-	0,1	0,1
Singapore: Malay	-	-	-	-	-	0,1	0,1	0,1	-	-	-	-
Singapore: Indian	-	-	-	-	-	-	-	-	-	-	-	-
Thailand, Chiang Mai	0,1	0,1	0,2	0,1	0,0	0,0	0.3	0.2	-	-	0,0	0,0
*Thailand, Khon Kaen	0,1	0,1	0,2	0,1	-	0,1	0.1	0.2	-	-	-	0,0
*Viet Nam, Hanoi	0,1	0,1	0,0	-	0,0	-	0,0	0,0	-	-	0,1	0,1

EUROPE

| | 172.0-4 | | 172.5 | | 172.6 | | 172.7 | | 172.8 | | 172.9 | |
	M	F	M	F	M	F	M	F	M	F	M	F
Austria, Tyrol	2.8	2.8	5.4	4.0	2.2	2.7	1.2	5.5	-	0,0	0.8	0.6
*Belarus												
*Croatia	0.3	0.2	0.8	0.4	0,1	0.2	0.3	0.5	0,0	-	1.6	1.5
Czech Republic	0.9	0.8	3.5	1.7	1.0	1.2	0.8	2.1	0.1	0.1	0.3	0.2
Denmark	1.3	1.0	4.5	3.3	1.1	2.1	1.3	4.7	0.4	0.3	0.3	0.2
Estonia	0.7	0.4	1.6	1.3	0.4	0.5	0.6	1.8	-	-	0.3	0.2
Finland												
France, Bas-Rhin	0.9	0.8	2.5	1.6	1.2	1.4	1.1	3.0	-	-	0.9	0.8
*France, Calvados	0.8	1.1	1.0	1.2	0,4	0.8	0.8	2.8	0,1	-	0.2	0.4
France, Doubs	1.0	1.1	1.2	1.4	0.8	1.1	0.9	3.2	0,0	0,3	0.9	1.5
France, Haut-Rhin	1.6	0.6	2.7	1.4	1.1	1.3	1.0	3.0	-	-	0.4	0,3
*France, Herault	0.7	0.6	1.8	1.2	0.8	1.1	0.9	2.4	-	-	0.9	0.8
France, Isere	0.8	0.6	1.4	1.3	0.8	1.1	0.6	2.4	-	-	0.5	0.8
*France, Somme	0.3	0.4	1.4	0,5	0,4	1.1	0.7	2.5	0,1	-	0.5	0,1
*France, Tarn	0.9	0.7	1.3	1.1	0.9	1.2	1.0	3.4	-	-	0,3	0,3
Germany, Eastern States	0.7	0.7	2.4	1.2	0.9	1.1	0.8	2.2	0.1	0.0	0.1	0.1
Germany, Saarland	0.6	0.8	1.5	1.1	1.1	1.2	1.0	1.9	0,1	0,1	1.6	1.0
Iceland	0.3	0,8	0,9	1,2	0,9	1.8	1.2	3.4	-	-	0.3	0.1
Ireland, Southern	1.7	2.3	1.4	1.1	1.4	1.6	1.4	5.7	-	-	0,3	0,2
Italy, Ferrara	0.3	0.5	2.1	1.4	0,1	0.5	0,1	1.8	0,2	-	0.5	1,8
Italy, Florence	0.9	0.6	2.8	1.3	0.6	0.8	0.6	2.3	0,1	-	0.5	0.2
Italy, Genoa	0.4	0.4	2.9	2.0	0.6	0.4	0.7	2.6	0,1	0,0	0.5	0.4
*Italy, Latina	-	0,1	1.3	0.5	0,1	0.7	0.6	0.9	0,1	-	1.2	0,7
Italy, Macerata	0.9	0.5	1.8	0.6	1,9	1.2	0.6	1,7	-	-	0.8	0.8
Italy, Modena	0.4	0.4	2.2	0.6	0.7	0.5	0.7	2.0	0,0	0,0	0.4	0.2
Italy, Parma	0.6	0.3	1.6	1.0	0,7	1.0	0.9	2.4	-	-	0.2	0,4
Italy, Ragusa	0.6	0.3	1.4	0,7	0,7	0,3	0,7	1.0	-	-	0.5	0,1
Italy, Romagna	0.9	0.4	2.6	1.5	0,7	1.0	1.3	3.8	-	-	0.4	0,0
Italy, Torino	0.8	0.4	1.3	0.8	0.8	1.1	0.5	1.9	-	-	0.5	0.4
Italy, Trieste	0,4	0,3	3.3	0.5	0,5	0,1	0.6	1.5	-	-	4.9	7.6
Italy, Varese	0.6	0.5	2.8	1.2	0.8	0.7	0.7	2.5	-	0,0	0.2	0,1
Italy, Veneto	0.5	0.4	1.5	0.9	0.6	0.7	0.6	1.6	-	-	2.8	3.4
*Latvia	0.4	0.5	0.7	0.7	0.4	0.4	0.4	1.1	0.1	0,1	0,1	0,1
Malta	-	-	0,8	0,5	-	0,2	0,8	2,0	-	-	1,0	0,8

AGE-STANDARDIZED (WORLD) INCIDENCE RATES (FOUR DIGIT RUBRICS)

| | Melanoma of skin | | | | | | | | | | | |
| | 172.0-4 | | 172.5 | | 172.6 | | 172.7 | | 172.8 | | 172.9 | |
	M	F	M	F	M	F	M	F	M	F	M	F
The Netherlands	1.1	0.9	3.2	2.2	1.1	2.0	1.1	4.3	0,0	0,0	0.4	0.4
The Netherlands, Eindhoven	0.7	0.7	2.4	1.9	1.2	1.9	1.0	3.9	-	-	0.3	0,3
The Netherlands, Maastricht	1.1	0.9	2.2	1.9	0.6	2.1	0.7	4.1	0,0	-	0.6	0.6
Norway												
*Poland, Cracow	0.6	0.6	1.8	0.8	0.5	0.5	0.7	1.4	0,1	0,0	0.7	0,3
*Poland, Kielce	0.3	0.5	0.7	0.3	0,3	0,2	0.4	0.7	-	0,0	0.7	0.6
*Poland, Lower Silesia	0.4	0.4	1.2	0.6	0.3	0.3	0.6	1.2	0,0	0,0	0.4	0.3
Poland, Warsaw City	0.3	0.2	1.6	0.8	0.4	0.6	0.6	1.5	-	-	0.8	0.5
Slovakia	0.6	0.6	2.7	1.3	0.5	0.8	0.5	1.7	0,0	0,0	0.1	0.1
Slovenia	0.7	0.7	2.4	1.4	0.4	1.0	0.6	2.0	-	-	0.5	0.3
*Spain, Albacete	0,7	0,1	0,5	-	-	0,1	0,3	0,5	-	-	0,5	1,0
Spain, Asturias	0,2	0.4	0,3	0,2	0,2	0,1	0,3	0.4	-	-	1.2	2.8
Spain, Basque Country	0.6	0.6	1.0	0.9	0.4	0.5	0.6	1.7	0,0	0,0	0.4	0.4
Spain, Granada	0.8	0.6	0.9	0.9	0.5	0.4	0.4	1.9	-	-	0,4	0,2
Spain, Mallorca	0.6	0.4	1.6	1.0	0.5	0.4	0.3	1.5	-	-	0.8	0.6
Spain, Murcia	0.7	0.7	0.7	1.0	0,2	0.4	0.6	1.8	-	0,1	0.6	0.4
Spain, Navarra	0.9	0.9	1.5	0,5	0,3	0,5	0,2	1.4	-	-	0,4	0,2
Spain, Tarragona	0.7	0.4	1.1	0.9	0,4	0,2	0.6	1.2	-	-	0.8	0.5
Spain, Zaragoza	0.5	0.6	0.8	0.5	0,1	0.4	0.3	1.2	0,0	-	0.5	0.6
Sweden	1.3	1.0	5.3	3.1	1.8	1.9	1.3	4.1	0.0	0.0	1.1	0.9
*Switzerland, Basel	2.4	1.4	4.4	1.7	2.6	1.9	1.1	3.5	-	-	0,1	0,4
Switzerland, Geneva	1.6	1.8	5.1	3.0	1.6	1.2	1.7	4.8	-	-	0,4	0,3
Switzerland, Graubunden	2.7	1,5	2.8	2.4	1,6	2.8	0,7	3.4	-	-	0,4	0,2
Switzerland, Neuchatel	2.6	1.4	4.2	1.8	1.0	1.1	2.3	5.4	-	-	1,4	0,5
Switzerland, St Gall-Appenzell	0.9	1.5	2.8	1.7	2.0	1.6	1.9	4.8	-	-	0,4	0,5
Switzerland, Valais	1,0	1.6	2.2	1,0	0,5	2.6	0,7	2.9	-	-	0.8	0,3
Switzerland, Vaud	2.0	1.4	6.0	3.1	1.8	2.8	1.4	4.5	-	-	0.7	0.7
Switzerland, Zurich	2.0	1.6	6.4	3.5	2.7	2.8	2.2	5.2	-	-	0.4	0.2
*UK, England and Wales	0.8	0.6	1.6	1.0	0.7	1.1	0.9	3.2	0.0	0.0	0.6	0.6
*UK, East Anglia												
*UK, Mersey	0.6	0.5	1.2	0.8	0.5	0.8	0.7	2.1	0,1	0,0	0.4	0.4
*UK, North Western	0.7	0.6	1.4	0.9	0.6	1.1	0.7	2.8	0,0	0,0	0.3	0.3
UK, Oxford	0.9	0.7	2.2	1.2	0.9	1.3	1.1	3.6	-	0,0	0.6	0.8
*UK, South Thames	0.8	0.6	1.7	0.9	0.7	1.2	0.7	3.0	0.0	0.0	0.6	0.7
UK, South Western	1.3	1.1	2.9	1.5	1.0	1.6	1.5	5.4	0,0	0,1	0.7	0.6
UK, Wessex	1.1	1.0	2.3	1.5	0.9	1.7	0.9	4.4	0,0	0,1	1.4	1.7
*UK, West Midlands	0.8	0.6	1.7	0.9	0.8	1.0	0.8	3.1	0,0	0,0	0.5	0.4
UK, Yorkshire	0.6	0.7	1.5	0.8	0.6	1.1	0.8	3.2	0,0	0,0	0.6	0.7
UK, Scotland	1.3	1.0	2.1	1.3	1.1	1.7	1.3	4.2	-	0,0	0.2	0.1
UK, Scotland, West	1.2	0.9	2.1	1.2	1.1	1.6	1.4	3.9	-	-	0.2	0,1
*Yugoslavia, Vojvodina												
OCEANIA												
Australian Capital Territory	5.5	3.1	9.8	4.5	7.0	6.4	5.0	8.0	-	-	2.2	1.4
Australia, New South Wales	5.6	3.5	14.2	5.7	6.3	6.1	4.5	9.1	-	-	2.5	1.3
South Australia	6.4	3.7	11.0	4.7	4.7	6.2	4.0	9.7	0,1	0,1	1.6	0.6
Australia, Tasmania	6.0	3.0	6.6	2.6	4.1	5.4	3.5	9.8	1.8	0.8	1.6	1.5
Australia, Victoria	4.1	2.7	8.8	3.9	4.0	4.1	3.0	8.1	0.1	0,0	2.4	1.4
Western Australia	6.3	3.3	13.4	5.9	5.8	5.8	4.7	9.2	-	-	2.0	0.8
*French Polynesia	-	0,3	1,7	0,7	-	-	0,9	1,2	-	0,2	0,5	2,5
New Zealand: Non-Maori	4.6	3.3	9.1	4.6	4.3	5.8	4.5	14.1	0,1	0,1	2.4	1.9
New Zealand: Maori	1,7	0,1	0.8	0.9	0.9	0.9	1.1	1.5	-	-	0.7	0,1
US, Hawaii: White	3.4	1.1	8.6	3.3	4.7	2.9	1.7	4.5	0,1	-	1.0	0,7
US, Hawaii: Japanese	-	-	0,0	0,1	0.2	0,1	-	0.2	-	-	-	-
US, Hawaii: Hawaiian	-	-	0,3	0,5	-	0,3	0.6	0.3	-	-	-	0,2
US, Hawaii: Filipino	-	-	0,1	-	0,2	-	0,2	0.6	-	-	0,1	-
US, Hawaii: Chinese	-	-	0,5	-	0,3	0,6	-	-	-	-	-	0,2

AGE-STANDARDIZED (WORLD) INCIDENCE RATES (FOUR DIGIT RUBRICS)

	183.0		Ovary etc 183.2-5		183.8-9		184.0		Other female genital 184.1-4		184.8-9		Penis 187.1-4		Scrotum 187.7	
AFRICA	M	F	M	F	M	F	M	F	M	F	M	F	M	F	M	F
*Algeria, Setif	-	1.2	-	-	-	-	-	0,2	-	0,3	-	0,0	0,2	-	-	-
*France, La Reunion	-	4.5	-	0,3	-	0,5	-	0,1	-	1.2	-	0,1	1.2	-	-	-
*Mali, Bamako	-	0.7	-	-	-	-	-	0,2	-	0,4	-	-	0,3	-	0,2	-
*Uganda, Kyadondo	-	6.2	-	0,4	-	0,1	-	0,3	-	0,5	-	0,5	2.8	-	0,4	-
*Zimbabwe, Harare: African	-	8.0	-	-	-	-	-	-	-	0,8	-	-	2.8	-	-	-
*Zimbabwe, Harare: European	-	14.1	-	-	-	-	-	-	-	0,9	-	-	0,9	-	-	-
AMERICA, CENTRAL AND SOUTH																
*Argentina, Concordia	-	7.6	-	-	-	-	-	1,5	-	1,8	-	0,3	0,6	-	-	-
*Brazil, Belem	-	4.2	-	0,0	-	0,3	-	0,3	-	0.8	-	0,3	2.0	-	0,3	-
*Brazil, Goiania	-	5.0	-	0,1	-	0,5	-	0,5	-	1.6	-	0,2	1.9	-	0,1	-
*Brazil, Porto Alegre	-	8.1	-	0,1	-	0,3	-	0.8	-	2.3	-	0.4	1.1	-	-	-
Colombia, Cali	-	8.7	-	0,1	-	0,2	-	1.2	-	0.8	-	-	1.2	-	-	-
*Costa Rica	-	5.9	-	0,0	-	-	-	0.6	-	0.8	-	0.2	1.3	-	-	-
*Ecuador, Quito	-	6.0	-	0,2	-	0,1	-	0,3	-	0,4	-	0,1	0.5	-	0,1	-
*Peru, Lima	-	5.9	-	0,0	-	0,0	-	0.6	-	0.7	-	0,0	0.7	-	0,0	-
Peru, Trujillo	-	7.4	-	-	-	0,3	-	0.9	-	2.5	-	-	1,1	-	-	-
US, Puerto Rico	-	5.1	-	0.1	-	0,0	-	0.8	-	1.4	-	0.1	2.2	-	0,1	-
*Uruguay, Montevideo	-	9.7	-	0,0	-	0,1	-	0.4	-	1.2	-	0.6	0.8	-	0,1	-
AMERICA, NORTH																
Canada	-	10.2	-	0.3	-	0.1	-	0.5	-	1.3	-	0.1	0.6	-	0.1	-
Canada, Alberta	-	10.2	-	0.3	-	0,0	-	0.5	-	1.2	-	0.1	0.5	-	0.1	-
Canada, British Columbia	-	10.3	-	0.2	-	-	-	0.4	-	1.2	-	0,0	0.5	-	0.1	-
Canada, Manitoba	-	9.6	-	0.3	-	0,2	-	0.6	-	1.8	-	0,1	0.5	-	0.1	-
Canada, New Brunswick	-	8.7	-	0,0	-	0,0	-	0.6	-	1.2	-	0,2	0.8	-	0.1	-
Canada, Newfoundland	-	9.7	-	0,1	-	-	-	0.6	-	1.4	-	-	0.7	-	0.1	-
Canada, Northwest Territories	-	8.6	-	-	-	-	-	0.7	-	-	-	-	0.5	-	-	-
Canada, Nova Scotia	-	9.7	-	0.5	-	-	-	0.8	-	1.7	-	-	0.9	-	0.1	-
Canada, Ontario	-	10.7	-	0.3	-	0.1	-	0.5	-	1.4	-	0.2	0.6	-	0.1	-
Canada, Prince Edward Island	-	7.9	-	0,2	-	0,3	-	0,6	-	2.6	-	-	1,4	-	-	-
Canada, Quebec	-	9.6	-	0.2	-	0.1	-	0.5	-	1.1	-	0.1	0.5	-	0.1	-
Canada, Saskatchewan	-	10.1	-	0.4	-	0,1	-	0.3	-	1.2	-	-	0.8	-	0,2	-
Canada, Yukon	-	19.9	-	-	-	-	-	0.4	-	-	-	-	0,8	-	-	-
US, Cent. Calif.: Non-Hisp. White	-	10.8	-	0.4	-	0,0	-	0.4	-	1.1	-	0.3	0.6	-	0,1	-
US, Cent. Calif.: Hispanic	-	8.8	-	0,5	-	-	-	0,8	-	1.3	-	0,3	0.9	-	0,1	-
US, Los Angeles: Non-Hisp. White	-	12.7	-	0.3	-	0,0	-	0.5	-	1.3	-	0.1	0.4	-	0.1	-
US, Los Angeles: Hispanic White	-	8.7	-	0.2	-	0,0	-	0.5	-	1.0	-	0,0	0.8	-	0,0	-
US, Los Angeles: Black	-	7.7	-	0,2	-	0,1	-	0.5	-	0.8	-	0,3	1.0	-	0,0	-
US, Los Angeles: Chinese	-	6.3	-	0,2	-	0,1	-	0,2	-	0,2	-	-	0,4	-	-	-
US, Los Angeles: Filipino	-	9.4	-	0,5	-	-	-	0,3	-	0,6	-	0,2	-	-	-	-
US, Los Angeles: Korean	-	4.9	-	-	-	-	-	0,5	-	0,2	-	-	0,3	-	-	-
US, Los Angeles: Japanese	-	8.5	-	0,1	-	-	-	0,5	-	0,3	-	-	-	-	0,2	-
US, San Francisco: Non-Hisp. White	-	12.7	-	0.5	-	0,0	-	0.4	-	1.4	-	0,1	0.4	-	0.1	-
US, San Francisco: Hispanic White	-	9.5	-	0,3	-	0,1	-	0.5	-	0.8	-	-	0.8	-	-	-
US, San Francisco: Black	-	9.3	-	0.2	-	-	-	0,7	-	0.9	-	0,1	0,5	-	-	-
US, San Francisco: Chinese	-	7.6	-	0,3	-	-	-	0,1	-	0.5	-	-	0,1	-	0,3	-
US, San Francisco: Filipino	-	7.4	-	-	-	-	-	0,8	-	0.6	-	-	0,1	-	0,1	-
US, San Francisco: Japanese	-	7.4	-	-	-	-	-	-	-	-	-	-	0.6	-	-	-
US, Connecticut: White	-	11.2	-	0.4	-	0,0	-	0.3	-	1.5	-	0,1	0.5	-	0,0	-
US, Connecticut: Black	-	6.5	-	0,5	-	-	-	0,5	-	0.9	-	0,1	1,3	-	-	-
US, Atlanta: White	-	11.1	-	0.3	-	0.1	-	0.7	-	1.3	-	0.1	0.3	-	0,1	-
US, Atlanta: Black	-	7.2	-	0.6	-	0.1	-	0.8	-	1.2	-	0.2	1.3	-	0,2	-
US, Iowa	-	11.7	-	0.3	-	-	-	0.3	-	1.6	-	0.1	0.7	-	0.1	-
US, Central Louisiana: White	-	9.1	-	0,1	-	0,1	-	0,7	-	1.0	-	-	0.2	-	-	-
US, Central Louisiana: Black	-	8.2	-	-	-	-	-	0,5	-	1,4	-	-	2.9	-	0,6	-
US, New Orleans: White	-	10.8	-	0.3	-	0,1	-	0,3	-	1.5	-	0,1	0.5	-	0,1	-
US, New Orleans: Black	-	7.1	-	0.3	-	0,1	-	1.2	-	1.5	-	-	1.6	-	-	-
US, Detroit: White	-	12.1	-	0.2	-	0.1	-	0.5	-	1.7	-	0,0	0.5	-	0,1	-
US, Detroit: Black	-	7.5	-	0.3	-	0,1	-	0.6	-	1.1	-	0.2	0.6	-	0,1	-
US, New Mexico: Non-Hisp. White	-	10.4	-	0.5	-	-	-	0.6	-	1.3	-	0.3	0.6	-	0,0	-
US, New Mexico: Hispanic White	-	8.2	-	0,3	-	0,1	-	0.4	-	0.9	-	-	1.2	-	-	-
US, New Mexico: American Indian	-	12.9	-	-	-	-	-	0,2	-	0.8	-	-	0.5	-	-	-
US, Utah	-	10.2	-	0.2	-	-	-	0.4	-	1.2	-	-	0.4	-	0,1	-
US, Seattle	-	11.4	-	0.4	-	0,0	-	0.5	-	1.4	-	0.2	0.4	-	0.1	-
US, SEER: White	-	11.6	-	0.4	-	0.0	-	0.4	-	1.5	-	0.1	0.5	-	0.1	-
US, SEER: Black	-	7.7	-	0.3	-	0,1	-	0.7	-	1.2	-	0.2	0.7	-	0,1	-

AGE-STANDARDIZED (WORLD) INCIDENCE RATES (FOUR DIGIT RUBRICS)

	183.0		Ovary etc 183.2-5		183.8-9		184.0		Other female genital 184.1-4		184.8-9		Penis 187.1-4		Scrotum 187.7	
ASIA	M	F	M	F	M	F	M	F	M	F	M	F	M	F	M	F
*China, Qidong	-	0.9	-	0,1	-	0,2	-	-	-	0,0	-	-	0.4	-	0,0	-
China, Shanghai	-	5.6	-	0.2	-	0,0	-	0.2	-	0.3	-	0,0	0.3	-	0.1	-
China, Tianjin	-	4.5	-	0,1	-	0.7	-	0,1	-	0.4	-	0,1	0.2	-	0,1	-
Hong Kong																
*India, Bangalore	-	4.2	-	0,1	-	0,0	-	0.8	-	0.6	-	0,0	1.4	-	0,1	-
*India, Barshi, Paranda and Bhum	-	1.2	-	-	-	-	-	0,3	-	0,6	-	-	3.3	-	-	-
India, Bombay	-	7.1	-	0,0	-	0,1	-	0.8	-	0.6	-	0,1	1.5	-	0,0	-
*India, Karunagappally	-	1,4	-	-	-	0,6	-	0,3	-	0,3	-	-	1,2	-	-	-
India, Madras	-	5.7	-	0,1	-	-	-	1.2	-	0.6	-	0,1	3.0	-	0,1	-
*India, Trivandrum	-	4.2	-	-	-	-	-	0,5	-	0,3	-	-	1,3	-	-	-
Israel: All Jews	-	11.2	-	0.2	-	0.2	-	0.4	-	1.2	-	0,1	0,1	-	0.1	-
Jews born in Israel	-	11.9	-	0,2	-	0,2	-	0,3	-	1.4	-	-	-	-	0,1	-
Jews born in America or Europe	-	13.0	-	0.3	-	0.3	-	0.5	-	1.2	-	0,0	0,1	-	0,0	-
Jews born in Africa or Asia	-	7.0	-	0,1	-	0,2	-	0.3	-	1.1	-	0,1	0,1	-	0,1	-
Non-Jews	-	3.0	-	-	-	-	-	0,4	-	0,3	-	0,0	-	-	-	-
Japan, Hiroshima	-	6.5	-	0,1	-	-	-	0.3	-	0.5	-	-	0.3	-	0,2	-
Japan, Miyagi	-	6.0	-	0,1	-	0,0	-	0.2	-	0.1	-	0,0	0.2	-	0.1	-
Japan, Nagasaki	-	6.5	-	0.2	-	0,1	-	0.2	-	0.3	-	0,0	0.4	-	0.2	-
Japan, Osaka	-	5.5	-	0.1	-	0,0	-	0.2	-	0.2	-	0,0	0.2	-	0.0	-
*Japan, Saga																
Japan, Yamagata																
*Korea, Kangwha	-	2,5	-	-	-	0,3	-	0,3	-	-	-	-	0,6	-	-	-
*Kuwait: Non-Kuwaitis	-	7.4	-	-	-	0,4	-	-	-	0,2	-	0,6	0,1	-	0,1	-
*Kuwait: Kuwaitis	-	4.7	-	-	-	-	-	0,2	-	0,5	-	-	-	-	-	-
*Philippines, Manila	-	9.2	-	0,1	-	0,1	-	0.5	-	0.5	-	0,0	0.7	-	0,1	-
Singapore: Chinese	-	10.5	-	0,2	-	0,0	-	0.5	-	0.5	-	0,0	0.7	-	0.3	-
Singapore: Malay	-	9.4	-	0,5	-	-	-	0,3	-	0,3	-	-	-	-	-	-
Singapore: Indian	-	7.5	-	-	-	-	-	0,3	-	0,3	-	-	0,9	-	-	-
Thailand, Chiang Mai	-	4.3	-	0,1	-	0,1	-	0.3	-	0.9	-	-	2.4	-	-	-
*Thailand, Khon Kaen	-	4.3	-	0,1	-	0,1	-	0,1	-	0.6	-	0,0	1.8	-	-	-
*Viet Nam, Hanoi	-	2.0	-	-	-	0.9	-	0,1	-	0,3	-	1.2	2.2	-	0,1	-
EUROPE																
Austria, Tyrol	-	13.3	-	0.6	-	1.3	-	0.7	-	1.8	-	0,1	0.5	-	0,1	-
*Belarus																
*Croatia	-	10.1	-	0.1	-	0.1	-	0.4	-	1.1	-	0.1	0.4	-	0,0	-
Czech Republic	-	12.7	-	0.2	-	0.4	-	0.6	-	1.4	-	0.1	0.7	-	0.1	-
Denmark	-	13.6	-	0.3	-	0,0	-	0.6	-	1.3	-	0.2	0.9	-	0,0	-
Estonia	-	12.3	-	0.3	-	-	-	0.5	-	1.4	-	0,0	0.8	-	0,1	-
Finland																
France, Bas-Rhin	-	11.7	-	0.4	-	0.2	-	0.5	-	1.1	-	-	0.7	-	0,1	-
*France, Calvados	-	8.6	-	0.2	-	0.2	-	0.6	-	0.9	-	0,0	0.9	-	-	-
France, Doubs	-	8.0	-	0.1	-	-	-	0.9	-	0.7	-	0,2	0.9	-	0,0	-
France, Haut-Rhin	-	11.0	-	0.2	-	-	-	0.7	-	1.0	-	-	1.0	-	0,1	-
*France, Herault	-	6.6	-	0,0	-	-	-	0.4	-	1.1	-	0,0	0.7	-	0,0	-
France, Isere	-	8.7	-	0.5	-	-	-	0.4	-	0.8	-	0,0	0.6	-	0,0	-
*France, Somme	-	9.7	-	0,3	-	0,1	-	0,4	-	0.5	-	0,1	0,4	-	-	-
*France, Tarn	-	8.5	-	0,1	-	0,1	-	0.8	-	1.0	-	0,1	0.5	-	-	-
Germany, Eastern States	-	11.8	-	0.2	-	0.2	-	0.6	-	1.4	-	0.1	0.9	-	0,0	-
Germany, Saarland	-	9.2	-	0.2	-	0.3	-	0.3	-	1.5	-	0.3	0.9	-	-	-
Iceland	-	10.7	-	0,2	-	-	-	0,4	-	1.3	-	-	1,1	-	-	-
Ireland, Southern	-	13.6	-	0,1	-	-	-	0.2	-	1.1	-	0,1	0.7	-	0,1	-
Italy, Ferrara	-	6.6	-	-	-	0,3	-	2,0	-	1.7	-	0,1	0.7	-	-	-
Italy, Florence	-	9.3	-	0,1	-	0,0	-	0.2	-	1.7	-	0,0	0.7	-	0,1	-
Italy, Genoa	-	9.4	-	0,1	-	0,1	-	0.3	-	1.4	-	0,1	0.6	-	0,1	-
*Italy, Latina	-	6.9	-	0,1	-	-	-	0,1	-	1.1	-	-	1.1	-	-	-
Italy, Macerata	-	9.1	-	0,3	-	0,3	-	-	-	1.2	-	0,2	1,3	-	-	-
Italy, Modena	-	10.2	-	0,2	-	0,1	-	0.3	-	1.3	-	-	0.4	-	0,1	-
Italy, Parma	-	9.8	-	0,1	-	-	-	0.5	-	1.3	-	0,1	0.6	-	0,1	-
Italy, Ragusa	-	6.8	-	-	-	0,1	-	0,2	-	0.8	-	-	0.5	-	0,1	-
Italy, Romagna	-	8.2	-	0,3	-	0,1	-	0,1	-	0.9	-	-	0.7	-	0,1	-
Italy, Torino	-	7.5	-	0,2	-	1.5	-	0.2	-	1.0	-	0.3	0.7	-	0,1	-
Italy, Trieste	-	8.8	-	0,1	-	4.0	-	0.8	-	1.8	-	0.9	1.1	-	0.2	-
Italy, Varese	-	9.9	-	0.3	-	0,0	-	0.3	-	1.1	-	0,1	0.6	-	0,0	-
Italy, Veneto	-	6.7	-	0.3	-	3.0	-	0.5	-	1.2	-	0.3	0.6	-	0,1	-
*Latvia	-	12.9	-	0.2	-	0.3	-	0.8	-	0.7	-	0,1	0.4	-	0.2	-
Malta	-	12.0	-	-	-	-	-	0,4	-	0,8	-	-	1,7	-	-	-

AGE-STANDARDIZED (WORLD) INCIDENCE RATES (FOUR DIGIT RUBRICS)

| | Ovary etc | | | | | | Other female genital | | | | | | Penis | | Scrotum | |
| | 183.0 | | 183.2-5 | | 183.8-9 | | 184.0 | | 184.1-4 | | 184.8-9 | | 187.1-4 | | 187.7 | |
	M	F	M	F	M	F	M	F	M	F	M	F	M	F	M	F
The Netherlands	-	11.0	-	0.2	-	0.0	-	0.4	-	1.3	-	0.2	0.7	-	0.1	-
The Netherlands, Eindhoven	-	11.1	-	0,1	-	0,0	-	0,3	-	1.0	-	0,0	0.7	-	0,1	-
The Netherlands, Maastricht	-	10.3	-	0,1	-	0,0	-	0.5	-	1.2	-	0,2	0.6	-	-	-
Norway																
*Poland, Cracow	-	13.8	-	0,0	-	0,1	-	0,3	-	1.2	-	0.5	0,4	-	0,0	-
*Poland, Kielce	-	7.9	-	0,1	-	0,2	-	0,3	-	1.3	-	0,2	0.2	-	0,1	-
*Poland, Lower Silesia	-	13.3	-	0.2	-	0.6	-	0.6	-	1.5	-	0.3	0.9	-	0,1	-
Poland, Warsaw City	-	13.0	-	0,1	-	0.2	-	0.3	-	1.4	-	0.5	0.9	-	0,1	-
Slovakia	-	10.8	-	0.1	-	0.1	-	0.5	-	1.1	-	0.1	0.7	-	0.1	-
Slovenia	-	10.2	-	-	-	0.3	-	0.5	-	1.6	-	0.1	0.7	-	0,0	-
*Spain, Albacete	-	7.7	-	-	-	-	-	0,1	-	0,9	-	0,2	0.8	-	-	-
Spain, Asturias	-	8.7	-	0,0	-	0.3	-	0.5	-	1.2	-	0.2	0.6	-	-	-
Spain, Basque Country	-	7.5	-	0,2	-	0,0	-	0.2	-	1.1	-	0.4	0.8	-	0,0	-
Spain, Granada	-	6.3	-	0,2	-	-	-	0.4	-	1.2	-	0,2	1.0	-	0,1	-
Spain, Mallorca	-	7.5	-	0,2	-	0,2	-	0,2	-	1.9	-	0,2	1.1	-	0,0	-
Spain, Murcia	-	7.1	-	0,1	-	0,1	-	0.4	-	1.0	-	0,1	1.2	-	0,0	-
Spain, Navarra	-	8.0	-	0,1	-	0,0	-	0,1	-	1.1	-	0,3	1.0	-	-	-
Spain, Tarragona	-	7.2	-	0,1	-	0,1	-	0,1	-	1.6	-	0.4	1.3	-	0,1	-
Spain, Zaragoza	-	7.9	-	0,1	-	0,1	-	0,2	-	1.4	-	0.6	0.6	-	0,0	-
Sweden	-	12.8	-	0.4	-	0.0	-	0.4	-	1.3	-	0.0	0.7	-	0.1	-
*Switzerland, Basel	-	9.6	-	0,4	-	-	-	0.8	-	1.7	-	-	0.7	-	0,1	-
Switzerland, Geneva	-	11.5	-	0,2	-	0,1	-	0,2	-	1.2	-	0,1	1.1	-	0,6	-
Switzerland, Graubunden	-	9.9	-	0,7	-	-	-	0,8	-	0,6	-	0,1	0.3	-	-	-
Switzerland, Neuchatel	-	10.8	-	0,4	-	0,1	-	0,3	-	0,7	-	0,3	1.7	-	0,3	-
Switzerland, St Gall-Appenzell	-	12.2	-	0,3	-	-	-	0.5	-	1.3	-	0,2	1.0	-	-	-
Switzerland, Valais	-	10.6	-	0,2	-	0,1	-	0,7	-	0,7	-	-	0.3	-	0,4	-
Switzerland, Vaud	-	9.4	-	0,2	-	0,0	-	0.5	-	1.2	-	0,2	0.7	-	0,0	-
Switzerland, Zurich	-	10.5	-	0,1	-	0.4	-	0.6	-	1.0	-	0,1	0.9	-	0,1	-
*UK, England and Wales	-	12.2	-	0.1	-	0.0	-	0.4	-	1.5	-	0.0	0.8	-	0.1	-
*UK, East Anglia																
*UK, Mersey	-	11.3	-	0,1	-	-	-	0.3	-	1.3	-	0,0	0.6	-	0,1	-
*UK, North Western	-	10.9	-	0.1	-	0,0	-	0.4	-	1.6	-	0.1	0.8	-	0.2	-
UK, Oxford	-	13.2	-	0.2	-	-	-	0.5	-	1.5	-	-	0.8	-	0.1	-
*UK, South Thames	-	12.9	-	0.1	-	0,0	-	0.4	-	1.1	-	0,0	0.7	-	0.1	-
UK, South Western	-	11.6	-	0.1	-	0.1	-	0.4	-	1.4	-	0,0	0.7	-	0.1	-
UK, Wessex	-	12.5	-	0.1	-	0.2	-	0.4	-	1.3	-	0.3	0.9	-	0.1	-
*UK, West Midlands	-	13.9	-	0.1	-	0.0	-	0.3	-	1.9	-	0.0	0.9	-	0.1	-
UK, Yorkshire	-	11.8	-	0.1	-	0,0	-	0.3	-	1.6	-	0.1	0.9	-	0.1	-
UK, Scotland	-	13.1	-	0.2	-	0.0	-	0.6	-	1.4	-	0.0	1.0	-	0.2	-
UK, Scotland, West	-	12.3	-	0,1	-	0.1	-	0.6	-	1.3	-	0,0	0.9	-	0.2	-
*Yugoslavia, Vojvodina																

OCEANIA

| | Ovary etc | | | | | | Other female genital | | | | | | Penis | | Scrotum | |
| | 183.0 | | 183.2-5 | | 183.8-9 | | 184.0 | | 184.1-4 | | 184.8-9 | | 187.1-4 | | 187.7 | |
	M	F	M	F	M	F	M	F	M	F	M	F	M	F	M	F
Australian Capital Territory	-	7.8	-	0,2	-	0,2	-	0,5	-	1,1	-	-	0.7	-	-	-
Australia, New South Wales	-	8.2	-	0.1	-	0,0	-	0.4	-	1.2	-	0.0	0.4	-	0,0	-
South Australia	-	9.3	-	-	-	0.3	-	0.3	-	1.2	-	0,0	0.4	-	0,1	-
Australia, Tasmania	-	8.3	-	-	-	0,1	-	0.4	-	1.5	-	0,1	0.5	-	-	-
Australia, Victoria	-	9.3	-	0.3	-	0,1	-	0.5	-	1.2	-	0,0	0.5	-	0.1	-
Western Australia	-	8.2	-	0.2	-	-	-	0.5	-	0.9	-	0,1	0.4	-	0,1	-
*French Polynesia	-	11.0	-	-	-	-	-	1,3	-	1,4	-	1,7	-	-	-	-
New Zealand: Non-Maori	-	10.6	-	0.2	-	0.2	-	0.9	-	1.6	-	0.1	0.5	-	0,0	-
New Zealand: Maori	-	12.0	-	0,2	-	-	-	1,1	-	1.5	-	0,3	0.3	-	-	-
US, Hawaii: White	-	13.9	-	0,3	-	-	-	0,3	-	1.4	-	0,1	0.2	-	-	-
US, Hawaii: Japanese	-	8.1	-	0,1	-	-	-	0,1	-	0.6	-	-	-	-	0,3	-
US, Hawaii: Hawaiian	-	8.3	-	-	-	-	-	0,6	-	1,0	-	0,3	0.3	-	-	-
US, Hawaii: Filipino	-	7.9	-	-	-	0,2	-	0,2	-	0.6	-	0,2	1.5	-	-	-
US, Hawaii: Chinese	-	6.6	-	-	-	-	-	0,3	-	0,3	-	-	-	-	-	-

AGE-STANDARDIZED (WORLD) INCIDENCE RATES (FOUR DIGIT RUBRICS)

| | Kidney | | | | Other urinary organs | | | | | | Other nervous system | | | | Other endocrine | | | | | |
| | 189.0 | | 189.1 | | 189.2 | | 189.3-4 | | 189.8-9 | | 192.0,2 | | 192.1,3 | | 194.0 | | 194.3 | | 194.1,4-9 | |
	M	F	M	F	M	F	M	F	M	F	M	F	M	F	M	F	M	F	M	F
AFRICA																				
*Algeria, Setif	0,4	0,3	-	-	-	-	-	-	-	-	-	-	-	-	-	-	-	-	-	-
*France, La Reunion	2.0	1.2	0,1	0,2	-	0,1	0,1	-	0,4	0,1	0,1	0,1	0,2	0,1	0,2	0,1	-	0,1	-	0,2
*Mali, Bamako	1.4	1.6	-	-	-	-	0,0	-	0,1	-	-	-	-	-	-	-	0,1	0,4	-	-
*Uganda, Kyadondo	1.0	1.6	-	-	-	-	-	0,1	-	0,3	-	-	-	0,2	0,0	-	0,0	0,2	-	-
*Zimbabwe, Harare: African	1.7	0,7	-	-	-	-	-	-	-	-	-	-	-	0,0	-	-	0,1	-	0,1	-
*Zimbabwe, Harare: European	2,9	2,7	-	-	-	-	-	-	-	-	-	-	-	-	0,5	-	-	-	-	-
AMERICA, CENTRAL AND SOUTH																				
*Argentina, Concordia	2,6	2,7	-	0,3	-	-	-	0,3	0,5	-	-	-	-	-	-	-	-	-	-	-
*Brazil, Belem	1.9	1.1	-	0,1	-	0,1	-	-	0,4	0,2	0,4	-	-	-	0,2	-	-	-	-	0,0
*Brazil, Goiania	2.9	2.2	-	-	-	0,0	-	-	0,3	0,3	0,2	-	-	0,3	0,2	0,3	0,2	0,3	0,2	0,2
*Brazil, Porto Alegre	9.2	3.8	-	0,0	0,1	0,1	0,1	0,1	0,8	-	-	0,1	0,2	0,2	0,4	0,4	0,1	0,1	0,2	0,1
Colombia, Cali	2.3	1.3	0,1	-	0,1	0,1	0,1	0,1	-	0,0	0,2	0,1	-	0,0	0,2	0,1	0,0	0,1	0,0	0,1
*Costa Rica	3.0	2.0	0,1	0,0	0,0	0,1	0,0	0,0	0,1	-	0,1	0,2	0,0	0,1	0,3	0,1	0,1	0,0	0,0	0,0
*Ecuador, Quito	2.3	1.3	0,2	-	0,1	-	0,1	0,1	-	-	-	-	0,1	-	0,0	0,1	-	-	-	-
*Peru, Lima	3.1	1.8	0,2	0,1	0,1	0,0	-	0,0	0,1	0,0	0,1	0,1	0,0	0,1	0,0	0,0	0,1	0,0	0,1	0,1
Peru, Trujillo	3.0	2.5	-	0,6	0,2	-	-	0,2	-	-	0,1	0,1	-	-	-	-	-	-	0,2	-
US, Puerto Rico	3.5	2.0	0.3	0.2	0,1	0,1	0,1	0,0	0,1	-	0.2	0,1	0,0	0,0	0,1	0.2	0,0	-	0,1	0,0
*Uruguay, Montevideo	10.3	3.6	-	-	0,0	0,1	0,0	0,0	0,2	0,0	0,0	0,0	0,4	0,2	0,2	0,1	0,1	0,0	0,1	0,2
AMERICA, NORTH																				
Canada	9.6	5.2	0.6	0.3	0.5	0.2	0.2	0.1	0.4	0.2	0.3	0.2	0.2	0.2	0.4	0.4	0.1	0.0	0.1	0.1
Canada, Alberta	9.9	5.2	0.7	0.3	0.4	0.2	0.3	0,0	0,1	0,0	0.3	0.2	0.1	0.1	0,1	0.3	0,0	0,0	0,2	0,0
Canada, British Columbia	8.4	4.0	0.5	0.3	0.5	0.2	0.2	0.1	0,0	-	0.2	0,1	0,0	0,0	0.2	0.3	-	0,0	0,1	0,0
Canada, Manitoba	9.7	5.5	0.6	0.3	0.4	0,1	0,1	0,1	0,0	-	0.4	0.3	0,0	0.2	0.6	0.3	-	-	0,1	0,1
Canada, New Brunswick	9.1	5.8	0.7	0.5	0.3	0,1	0,0	0,1	0,1	0,0	0,0	0.2	0,0	0,0	0.6	0.2	0,2	0,1	0,1	-
Canada, Newfoundland	8.2	5.9	0.6	0,1	0.9	0.4	0.2	0.1	-	-	-	-	0,1	0,1	0,1	0.2	-	-	-	-
Canada, Northwest Territories	10.1	7.8	1,0	-	-	-	-	-	-	-	0,3	0,3	-	1,8	0.7	0.4	-	-	-	-
Canada, Nova Scotia	11.5	5.8	1.3	0.4	0.6	0.4	0.2	0,0	0,0	-	0,0	0,1	0,1	0,1	0.2	0,1	0,0	-	0,1	-
Canada, Ontario	9.5	5.0	0.4	0.2	0.4	0.2	0.2	0.1	0.8	0.4	0.3	0.2	0.2	0.3	0.5	0.4	0.1	0.0	0.1	0.1
Canada, Prince Edward Island	12.3	3.4	0.5	0,1	-	0.3	-	-	-	-	-	-	0,3	0,4	0,1	0.2	-	-	-	-
Canada, Quebec	10.0	5.6	0.7	0.3	0.6	0.3	0.2	0.1	0.2	0.1	0.2	0.2	0.2	0.2	0.6	0.7	0,0	0,0	0,2	0,1
Canada, Saskatchewan	10.5	5.5	0.7	0.4	0.4	0.2	0,1	0,0	0,0	0,0	0.2	0.2	0,1	0,0	0,1	0.3	-	0,1	0,2	0,1
Canada, Yukon	6,8	5,8	-	-	-	-	-	-	-	-	-	-	-	-	-	-	-	-	-	-
US, Cent. Calif.: Non-Hisp. White	8.3	4.8	0.8	0.5	0.7	0.2	0.2	0,1	0,1	0,0	0.2	0,1	0,1	0.3	0.4	0,1	0,0	0,1	0.3	0,1
US, Cent. Calif.: Hispanic	9.9	5.3	1.0	0,5	0,4	-	0,3	-	-	-	0,0	0,1	0,1	0.2	0,1	0.2	0,0	-	0,2	-
US, Los Angeles: Non-Hisp. White	8.3	4.0	1.0	0.6	0.5	0.2	0.2	0.1	0.1	0,0	0.2	0.2	0.2	0.1	0.5	0.4	0,0	-	0.1	0,0
US, Los Angeles: Hispanic White	8.0	4.3	0.7	0.3	0.3	0,1	0,1	0,0	0,1	0,0	0.2	0.2	0,0	0,1	0.3	0.2	0,0	0,0	0,1	0,1
US, Los Angeles: Black	9.7	5.0	0.5	0.2	0.2	0.1	0.4	0.4	0.1	0,0	0.3	0.3	-	0,1	0.3	0.2	0,0	0,0	0.1	0.1
US, Los Angeles: Chinese	3.3	1,0	0.4	0.5	0.5	0.4	-	-	0,2	-	-	0,1	0,2	-	0,2	-	0,1	-	-	-
US, Los Angeles: Filipino	5.6	2.3	0,7	0,1	0,2	0,2	-	0,1	-	-	-	0,3	-	0,2	-	-	-	-	0,2	-
US, Los Angeles: Korean	4.7	3.4	0,4	-	1,0	0,5	-	0,3	-	-	-	-	-	-	-	-	-	-	-	-
US, Los Angeles: Japanese	3.3	1,6	0,6	0,3	0,3	0,2	-	0,2	0,2	-	-	0,2	-	-	0,2	0,7	-	-	-	-
US, San Francisco: Non-Hisp. White	8.5	3.9	0.8	0.4	0.5	0.2	0.2	0.1	0,0	0,0	0.2	0.2	0.2	0.2	0.5	0.3	0,0	0,0	0.1	0,1
US, San Francisco: Hispanic White	9.6	4.9	0,4	0,6	0,3	-	0,1	0,1	-	-	0,3	0,2	0,4	0,1	0.3	0.3	-	-	0,2	-
US, San Francisco: Black	9.2	5.2	0,3	0,3	0,2	0,2	0,3	0,7	-	-	0,5	0,1	0,3	0,1	0.3	0.2	0,1	-	-	0,2
US, San Francisco: Chinese	2.5	1.9	0,3	0,6	0,6	0,1	-	-	-	-	0,4	0,1	-	0,5	0.7	0,1	-	0,1	0,3	-
US, San Francisco: Filipino	5.2	2.2	0,6	0,4	0,7	-	-	-	-	-	0,2	0,2	0,3	-	0,6	0,2	-	-	-	-
US, San Francisco: Japanese	4,9	0,7	1,4	-	0,6	0,5	-	-	-	-	0,2	0,2	0,3	-	-	-	-	-	0,5	-
US, Connecticut: White	10.2	5.2	0.7	0.4	0.6	0.3	0.3	0.1	0,0	0,0	0.2	0.2	0,1	0.1	0.3	0.2	-	-	0,1	0,0
US, Connecticut: Black	10.8	4.9	0,2	0,1	-	0,2	0,2	-	-	-	-	-	-	-	0.4	0.3	-	-	-	-
US, Atlanta: White	8.2	4.1	1.3	0.3	0.7	0.3	0.2	0.1	0.2	0.1	0.4	0.3	0.1	0,0	0.3	0.3	-	0,0	0.1	0.1
US, Atlanta: Black	11.9	4.9	0.9	0.2	0.2	-	0.5	0.1	0,0	0,1	0.2	0.3	0,1	-	-	0.2	0,1	-	0,2	0,1
US, Iowa	9.1	5.5	0.9	0.3	0.5	0.2	0.2	0.1	0,0	0,0	0.2	0.1	0,1	0,0	0.4	0.4	-	0,0	0,1	0,1
US, Central Louisiana: White	7.3	3.8	0,3	0,2	0,7	0,2	0,1	0,1	-	-	0,6	0,2	0,1	-	0,4	0,5	-	-	-	-
US, Central Louisiana: Black	13.1	4,0	0,5	0,7	0,3	-	0,3	-	-	-	-	-	-	-	-	0,2	-	-	-	-
US, New Orleans: White	12.4	6.2	1.3	0.4	0.7	0.3	0,0	-	0,4	0,2	0,1	0,3	-	-	0,1	0,4	0,1	0,1	0,0	0,1
US, New Orleans: Black	10.8	6.2	0,5	0,2	0,1	0,2	0,2	0,3	0,4	0,2	0,3	0,2	0,2	-	0,2	0,4	0,2	-	-	0,2
US, Detroit: White	10.6	5.3	0.9	0.6	0.7	0.2	0.3	0.1	0.3	0.1	0.2	0.2	0,0	0.1	0.4	0.3	-	-	0,1	0.1
US, Detroit: Black	10.4	5.6	0,4	0,3	0,3	0,1	0,5	0,2	0,5	0,0	0,3	0,2	0,2	0,1	0,2	0,3	-	0,0	0,1	0,1
US, New Mexico: Non-Hisp. White	7.6	4.3	0.6	0.3	0.3	0,1	0,0	0,1	0,0	-	0,2	0,3	0,0	0,1	0,1	0.4	0,1	-	0,2	-
US, New Mexico: Hispanic White	9.0	4.7	0,5	0,1	0,4	0,4	0,2	0,3	-	-	0,1	0,2	0,2	0,1	0,4	0,1	-	-	0,2	0,1
US, New Mexico: American Indian	12.1	6.9	0,9	0,4	-	0,2	0,6	-	-	-	-	0,2	0,5	-	-	0,4	-	-	-	0,5
US, Utah	7.0	3.7	0.8	0.3	0.4	0,1	0,1	0,0	0,0	-	0,1	0.2	0.2	0,1	0.2	0.3	0,0	0,0	0,1	0,1
US, Seattle	8.7	4.7	0.9	0.5	0.5	0.2	0.3	0.1	0,0	0,0	0.4	0.2	0,1	0,1	0.3	0.2	0,0	-	0,1	0,1
US, SEER: White	9.1	4.8	0.8	0.4	0.5	0.2	0.2	0.1	0.1	0.0	0.2	0.2	0.1	0.1	0.3	0.3	0,0	0,0	0.1	0.1
US, SEER: Black	10.5	5.3	0.5	0.2	0,2	0,1	0.4	0.3	0.2	0,1	0.3	0.2	0.2	0,1	0.2	0.2	0,0	0,0	0,1	0,1

AGE-STANDARDIZED (WORLD) INCIDENCE RATES (FOUR DIGIT RUBRICS)

| | Kidney | | | | Other urinary organs | | | | | | Other nervous system | | | | Other endocrine | | | | | |
| | 189.0 | | 189.1 | | 189.2 | | 189.3-4 | | 189.8-9 | | 192.0,2 | | 192.1,3 | | 194.0 | | 194.3 | | 194.1,4-9 | |
ASIA	M	F	M	F	M	F	M	F	M	F	M	F	M	F	M	F	M	F	M	F
*China, Qidong	0.5	0.3	-	0,0	-	-	-	-	0,0	0,1	0,1	0,0	-	0,0	0,0	-	0,1	0,1	-	-
China, Shanghai	2.4	1.3	0.3	0.1	0.2	0.1	0,0	0.0	0.0	0.1	0.5	0.4	0.5	1.0	0.3	0.3	0.6	1.4	0.1	0.1
China, Tianjin	2.6	1.2	0.2	0,1	0.1	0,0	0,0	0,0	0.4	0.3	0.1	0.1	0.5	0.7	0.2	0.1	0.4	0.4	0,1	0,1
Hong Kong																				
*India, Bangalore	1.1	0.5	-	0,0	-	-	0,1	0,1	-	-	0,1	0,0	0,0	0,0	0,0	0,0	-	-	0,0	0,0
*India, Barshi, Paranda and Bhum	0,4	0,1	-	-	-	-	-	-	-	-	-	-	-	-	-	-	-	-	-	-
India, Bombay	1.8	0.8	0.1	0,0	0.1	0,0	0,1	0,0	0,0	-	0,0	0,0	0,0	0,0	0.2	0.1	-	-	0,0	-
*India, Karunagappally	0,9																0,3			
India, Madras	0.9	0.6	0,0	0,0	0,0	-	0,0	0,1	-	0,0	0,0	0,0	0,0	0,0	0.1	0,1	0,0	0,0	0,0	0,0
*India, Trivandrum	0,5	0,3	-	-	-	-	-	-	-	-	0,3	-	-	-	0,1	-	-	-	-	-
Israel: All Jews	8.5	4.9	0.7	0.2	0.4	0.1	0.1	0,0	0.7	0.1	0.2	0.2	0.1	0.1	0.4	0.4	0,0	0,0	0,1	0,1
Jews born in Israel	7.4	4.6	0,8	0,4	0,4	0,1	0,1	0,0	0.6	0,1	0,1	0.3	0,2	0,1	0.5	0.3	0,0	0,0	0,0	0,0
Jews born in America or Europe	11.2	7.4	0.7	0.2	0.4	0.1	0.1	0,0	0.7	0.1	0.5	0,0	0,1	0,1	0.2	0.2	0,0	0,0	0,0	0,3
Jews born in Africa or Asia	4.4	3.1	0.6	0,2	0.4	0,1	0,1	-	0.6	0,1	0,1	0,1	0,1	0,1	0.3	0,0	0,0	-	0,0	-
Non-Jews	2.6	1.7	0,2	-	-	-	0,1	-	0.5	0,1	-	0,2	-	0,1	0.3	0.3	-	-	0,1	0,2
Japan, Hiroshima	4.9	2.2	1.5	0.4	1.1	0.4	0,1	0,0	0.2	0.2	0,1	0,1	0,0	0,1	0.3	0.4	-	0,1	0,2	0,1
Japan, Miyagi	4.9	1.9	0.7	0.1	0.7	0.4	0,1	0,0	0,1	0,0	0,0	0,1	0,0	0,0	0.4	0.6	0,0	0,0	0,1	0,0
Japan, Nagasaki	4.5	1.5	0.7	0.2	0.6	0.3	0,1	0,0	0.2	0,1	0,2	0,2	0,1	0,1	0.3	0,0	-	0,0	0,3	0,2
Japan, Osaka	4.1	1.4	0.7	0.2	0.6	0.2	0,0	0,0	0,0	0,0	0,1	0,2	0,0	0,1	0.5	0.4	0,1	0,0	0,1	0,0
*Japan, Saga																				
Japan, Yamagata																				
*Korea, Kangwha	1,8	0,8	-	-	-	-	-	-	0,4	-	-	-	-	-	-	-	-	-	-	-
*Kuwait: Non-Kuwaitis	4.7	3.1	0,0	-	0,1	0,1	0,1	-	-	-	-	-	-	-	0,2	0,3	-	0,1	-	-
*Kuwait: Kuwaitis	2.1	1.7	-	-	-	0,3	-	-	-	-	-	-	0,0	0,1	-	0,3	0,5	-	-	-
*Philippines, Manila	3.9	2.3	-	0,0	-	0,1	0,1	0,1	0,0	0,1	0,1	0,1	0,0	0,0	0,1	0,1	0,0	0,0	0,0	0,0
Singapore: Chinese	3.5	1.8	0.3	0,1	0.4	0.2	0,0	0,1	0,0	-	0,0	0,1	0,1	0,1	0.2	0.2	0.2	0,1	0.2	0,0
Singapore: Malay	2.0	0.8	0,1	0,2	0,3	-	-	-	-	-	-	-	-	-	0,2	-	0,1	0,2	0,2	0,2
Singapore: Indian	2.7	2,6	0,2	-	-	-	-	0,4	0,2	-	-	-	-	0,3	-	-	-	-	-	-
Thailand, Chiang Mai	0.9	0.9	0.4	0.4	0,1	0,1	0,0	0,1	0,1	0,0	0,0	0,0	-	-	0,0	0,1	0,1	-	0,0	0,1
*Thailand, Khon Kaen	1.1	0.6	0,1	0,0	-	0,0	-	-	-	0,0	0,0	0,1	0,0	0,1	-	0,0	0,0	0,1	0,1	0,0
*Viet Nam, Hanoi	0.4	0,3	-	-	-	-	-	-	0,2	0,0	-	0,0	0,1	0,1	0,1	-	0,0	0,0	0,0	0,0

EUROPE

| | Kidney | | | | Other urinary organs | | | | | | Other nervous system | | | | Other endocrine | | | | | |
| | 189.0 | | 189.1 | | 189.2 | | 189.3-4 | | 189.8-9 | | 192.0,2 | | 192.1,3 | | 194.0 | | 194.3 | | 194.1,4-9 | |
	M	F	M	F	M	F	M	F	M	F	M	F	M	F	M	F	M	F	M	F
Austria, Tyrol	12.2	6.4	1.1	0.4	0,4	0,1	-	0,1	0.9	0.4	0,2	0,0	-	0,1	0.7	0,2	-	0,1	0,1	0,2
*Belarus																				
*Croatia	6.4	3.7	0.1	0,0	0.2	0.1	0,0	0,0	0,1	-	0.3	0.2	0.2	0.3	0.3	0.4	0.2	0.2	0,1	0,1
Czech Republic	15.0	7.4	0.8	0.6	0.2	0.1	0.1	0.1	0.8	0.4	0.1	0.1	0.2	0.2	0.3	0.3	0.1	0.1	0.1	0.0
Denmark	7.3	4.7	1.0	0.7	0.5	0.2	0.1	0.1	0,0	0,0	0.4	0.3	0,0	0.1	0.2	0.3	0,0	0,0	0.1	0,0
Estonia	11.1	5.8	0,2	0,1	0,1	0,1	0,1	0,0	-	-	0,2	0,0	0,0	0,2	0.3	0,1	0,0	-	0,1	-
Finland																				
France, Bas-Rhin	14.5	6.9	0.7	0,1	0.6	0.2	0,1	0,0	0,2	0,0	0,0	0,1	0,1	0,3	0.7	0.6	0,0	-	0,1	-
*France, Calvados	7.3	3.3	0,3	0,1	0,3	0,2	0,0	-	0,2	-	0,1	-	0,1	0,2	0,2	0,3	-	0,1	0,1	0,0
France, Doubs	7.9	5.5	0,3	0,0	0,2	0,1	0,2	-	0,2	0,1	-	0,1	0,1	0,7	0,2	0,3	-	-	0,1	0,1
France, Haut-Rhin	11.9	5.5	0.6	0.1	0.3	0.1	0.3	0.1	0.1	-	0.2	-	0.2	0.1	0.6	0.3	0.1	0.1	0.1	0.1
*France, Herault	8.0	3.0	0.5	0.1	0.5	0.1	0.1	0.0	0.3	0.0	0.2	0.1	0.1	0.1	0.2	0.1	0.0	0.0	0.1	0.0
France, Isere	8.9	3.8	0.2	0.1	0.3	0.1	0.1	0.0	0.1	-	0.1	0.2	0.1	0.1	0.3	0.6	-	-	-	0.1
*France, Somme	7.7	4.5	0.5	0.3	0.2	0.1	0.1	0.2	0.2	-	0.1	-	0.1	-	0.2	0.1	-	-	0,2	0.1
*France, Tarn	6.5	2.8	0.3	0.1	0.5	0.1	0.1	0.1	0.2	-	-	0.3	0.0	0.1	-	-	-	-	0.1	0.2
Germany, Eastern States	12.7	6.2	0.6	0.4	0.3	0.1	0.1	0.0	0.1	0.0	0.2	0.2	0.1	0.1	0.3	0.2	0,0	0.1	0,0	0.1
Germany, Saarland	10.9	5.1	0.3	0.2	0.4	0.2	0.2	-	0.4	0.1	0,0	0,1	0,1	0.3	0.6	0,2	0,2	0,2	0,0	0.1
Iceland	12.9	7.3	0,6	0,4	0,6	0,3	0,3	-	-	-	0.5	-	0,4	0,3	-	0,9	-	-	0,3	-
Ireland, Southern	5.5	3.6	0,4	0,1	0,3	0,1	0,1	0,0	-	-	0,1	0,1	0,1	0,0	0.2	0,6	0,2	0,1	0,2	-
Italy, Ferrara	13.8	4.4	1,1	0,7	0,4	0,3	0,1	-	0,5	0,1	0,1	0,3	0,6	0,3	0,4	0,4	-	-	-	-
Italy, Florence	11.0	4.9	0.4	0.3	0.5	0.2	0.1	-	0.3	0.2	0.3	0.2	0.1	0.3	0.3	0.5	0,1	0,0	0,1	0,1
Italy, Genoa	8.9	4.6	0.5	0.2	0.8	0.2	0.2	0.1	0.5	0.1	0.1	0.3	0.1	0.1	0.8	0.6	-	-	0,1	-
*Italy, Latina	4.7	2.1	0,3	-	0,3	-	-	-	0,2	0,1	0,1	0,1	0,6	0,1	0.2	0.3	0,1	-	0,1	-
Italy, Macerata	6.0	3.1	0.2	0.2	0.2	-	-	-	-	0,2	0,2	-	-	0.3	1,2	-	-	-	-	0,2
Italy, Modena	9.4	5.6	0.6	0.3	1.0	0.2	0.1	0.1	-	0,1	-	0.3	0,1	0,1	0.9	0.4	0,1	0,1	0,0	-
Italy, Parma	11.6	4.6	1.0	0.3	0,5	0,2	0,1	-	0,0	-	0,1	-	-	0,1	0,1	0,3	-	-	0,2	0,1
Italy, Ragusa	3.6	2.1	0.8	0.2	0,1	-	-	-	0,1	0,0	0,1	0,1	-	0.3	0.3	-	-	-	-	-
Italy, Romagna	12.3	5.6	0,4	0,1	0.6	0,0	0,0	0,1	0,1	-	0,1	0,1	0,1	0,1	0.5	0.3	-	-	0,0	0,1
Italy, Torino	9.1	3.4	1.2	0.4	0.7	0.2	0,1	0,0	0,1	0,0	0.3	0,1	0,0	0,1	0.7	0.6	0,2	0,1	-	0,0
Italy, Trieste	9.9	4.8	1.6	0.6	1.0	0.2	0,4	0,1	3.8	1.5	0.2	0.6	0,3	-	1,5	0.2	-	0,1	0,8	2.8
Italy, Varese	12.3	4.8	0.9	0.4	1.0	0,1	0.9	0,1	0,1	0,0	0,0	0.3	0,2	0,1	0.3	0.3	-	-	0,1	0,1
Italy, Veneto	9.4	4.0	0,3	0,1	0.3	0,1	0,2	0,0	5.5	1.1	0,1	0,1	0,1	0,1	0.5	0.3	-	-	0,3	0,2
*Latvia	8.1	3.5	0.3	0.1	0,0	0,1	0,0	0,1	0.9	0.4	0,1	0,2	0,1	0,0	0.2	0,1	0,0	0,0	0,1	0,0
Malta	5.0	1.8	0,4	0,2	0,3	-	-	-	-	-	0,3	0,3	0,2	0,4	0,4	-	-	0,4	-	-

AGE-STANDARDIZED (WORLD) INCIDENCE RATES (FOUR DIGIT RUBRICS)

| | Kidney | | | | Other urinary organs | | | | | | Other nervous system | | | | Other endocrine | | | | | |
| | 189.0 | | 189.1 | | 189.2 | | 189.3-4 | | 189.8-9 | | 192.0,2 | | 192.1,3 | | 194.0 | | 194.3 | | 194.1,4-9 | |
	M	F	M	F	M	F	M	F	M	F	M	F	M	F	M	F	M	F	M	F
The Netherlands	8.2	4.5	1.0	0.5	0.6	0.2	0.2	0.0	0.1	0.0	0.2	0.2	0.1	0.1	0.3	0.3	0,0	0,0	0.1	0.0
The Netherlands, Eindhoven	6.5	3.7	1.2	0.4	0.7	0,2	0,1	0,0	0,1	0,1	0,2	0,2	0,1	0,2	0,2	0.5	0,0	-	0,1	-
The Netherlands, Maastricht	9.7	4.7	0.8	0.3	0.5	0,1	0,2	0,1	0,1	0,1	0,2	0,2	-	0,1	0.3	0,3	-	-	0,1	0,0
Norway																				
*Poland, Cracow	11.2	4.8	0,1	0,1	-	0,1	0,0	0,0	0,2	0,0	0,1	0,0	0,2	0,0	0,2	0,1	0,2	0,2	0,1	0,1
*Poland, Kielce	5.6	2.9	0,0	0,0	0,1	-	-	-	0.6	0.4	0,1	0,1	0,1	0,1	0,1	0,1	0.4	0,1	0,1	0,4
*Poland, Lower Silesia	9.2	4.5	1.6	0.9	0.2	0,0	0,0	0.1	0.2	0,0	0.5	0.3	0.4	0.5	0.4	0.2	0.4	0.3	0,1	0,1
Poland, Warsaw City	13.0	5.9	0,1	0,1	0,1	0,0	0,1	0,0	0,0	0,0	0.5	0.4	0.3	0.5	0.2	0.3	0.4	0.4	0,0	0,1
Slovakia	10.2	5.3	0.5	0.4	0.1	0.1	0,0	0.0	0,0	0,0	0.2	0.1	0.1	0.1	0.3	0.3	0,0	0,0	0.1	0,0
Slovenia	6.1	3.3	0.5	0.2	0.3	0,0	-	-	0,1	0,0	0,1	0,0	0,1	0,1	0.2	0.2	-	-	0,0	0,0
*Spain, Albacete	3.0	2.1	0,8	0,2	-	-	-	0,1	0,4	-	-	-	-	-	-	-	-	-	0,1	-
Spain, Asturias	6.5	3.2	0.3	0,1	0.3	0,0	0,1	0,0	0,2	0,1	0,1	-	0,1	0,2	0.8	0,2	0,1	0,1	0,1	0,0
Spain, Basque Country	7.1	2.9	0.8	0.2	0.5	0,0	0,1	0,0	0.3	0,0	0.3	0,1	0,1	0,0	0.4	0.3	-	-	0,0	0,1
Spain, Granada	3.2	2.0	0.7	0.5	0.4	0,0	0,1	-	0,1	0,0	0,2	0,3	0,1	-	0,3	0.5	-	-	0,0	-
Spain, Mallorca	4.6	2.3	0.6	0.2	0.5	0,0	0,1	-	0.7	0,0	0,1	-	0,1	-	0,5	0.3	-.	0,1	-	-
Spain, Murcia	2.7	1.7	0.7	0,2	0.4	-	0,1	-	0,2	0,0	0,1	-	0,0	-	0,4	0,4	-	0,1	0,0	0,0
Spain, Navarra	6.5	3.1	0.6	0,1	0,4	0,1	0,1	0,0	0.5	0,1	0,1	0,1	0,1	0,3	0,3	0.4	-	-	0,4	-
Spain, Tarragona	4.1	1.7	0.9	0.4	0,4	0,2	0,3	0,0	0,2	0,1	0,2	-	0,1	-	0,3	0.9	0,1	0,1	0,1	0,1
Spain, Zaragoza	4.5	2.3	0.9	0.2	0.3	0,1	0,2	0,0	0.3	0,1	0,1	0,1	0,0	0,0	0.7	0.4	0,0	-	0,1	0,1
Sweden	7.5	4.8	0.9	0.6	0.4	0.2	0.1	0.1	1.2	0.7	0.3	0.2	0.1	0.1	0.2	0.2	0.0	0,0	0.1	0.1
*Switzerland, Basel	9.8	4.8	1.2	0.6	0,5	0,3	0,1	0,0	-	-	0,4	0,1	0,4	0,1	0,5	0,5	-	0,1	0,3	0,0
Switzerland, Geneva	7.8	3.4	1.0	0.5	0.8	0,2	0,3	0,1	0,1	0,0	-	0,6	0,1	0,1	0,3	0,3	0,2	0,2	-	0,3
Switzerland, Graubunden	7.9	5.7	0,5	0,5	0,6	0,1	-	-	-	-	-	-	0,2	-	-	0,6	-	-	-	0,2
Switzerland, Neuchatel	7.6	4.2	1.0	0,8	-	0,0	-	-	0,1	0,1	-	-	-	-	0,2	0.5	-	-	-	-
Switzerland, St Gall-Appenzell	8.2	3.8	1.1	0.9	0,4	0,1	-	-	0,1	-	-	0,3	0,3	0,3	0,1	0,2	0,1	0,1	-	-
Switzerland, Valais	8.6	5.1	1.6	1,0	-	-	0,3	-	0,1	0,2	-	-	-	-	-	0,7	-	-	-	-
Switzerland, Vaud	8.0	4.3	0.6	0.6	0,3	0,1	0,1	-	0,1	0,1	0,2	0,1	0,1	0,1	0,2	0,2	-	-	0,4	-
Switzerland, Zurich	8.7	3.3	1.2	0.8	0.5	0.3	0,1	0,1	0,0	0,1	0,3	0,1	0,2	0,2	0,2	0.5	0,0	-	0,1	0,1
*UK, England and Wales	6.0	2.9	0.3	0.2	0.3	0.1	0.1	0.0	0.1	0.0	0.2	0.2	0.1	0.1	0.4	0.3	0.1	0.1	0.1	0.1
*UK, East Anglia																				
*UK, Mersey	5.4	2.8	0.3	0.2	0.2	0.1	0.1	0.0	-	0.0	0.6	0.4	0.4	0.9	0.3	0.4	0,0	0,0	0,1	0,0
*UK, North Western	5.8	3.3	0.4	0.2	0.4	0.2	0.1	0,0	0,0	0,0	0.1	0.1	0,0	0,0	0.3	0.3	0,0	-	0,1	0,0
UK, Oxford	6.8	3.3	0.5	0.3	0.2	0.1	0,1	0,0	0,0	0,0	0.2	0,1	0.2	0.3	0.4	0.4	0.1	0,1	0.2	0.1
*UK, South Thames	5.8	2.9	0.2	0.1	0.3	0.1	0.1	0,0	0.2	0,0	0.3	0.2	0,0	0,0	0.4	0.3	0.1	0.1	0.1	0.1
UK, South Western	5.9	2.9	0.4	0.2	0.3	0.2	0,0	0,0	0.2	0.1	0.1	0.1	0.1	0.1	0.4	0.2	0,0	0,0	0.2	0.1
UK, Wessex	6.2	3.3	0.4	0.2	0.3	0.1	0.1	0,0	0.3	0.1	0.2	0.2	0.1	0.1	0.4	0.4	0.2	0.1	0,1	0.2
*UK, West Midlands	6.4	3.0	0.5	0.2	0.4	0.2	0.1	0,0	-	0,0	0.1	0.1	0,0	0,0	0.5	0.4	0.6	0.5	0,1	0,1
UK, Yorkshire	6.3	3.5	0.3	0.2	0.4	0.1	0.1	0.1	0,0	-	0,0	0,0	0.1	0,1	0.4	0.4	0,1	0,0	0,1	0,1
UK, Scotland	6.9	3.9	0.5	0.3	0.5	0.2	0.1	0.0	0.1	0.1	0.1	0.2	0.1	0,1	0.4	0.4	0.1	0,0	0.2	0.1
UK, Scotland, West	6.5	3.7	0.4	0.2	0.5	0.2	0.1	0,0	0.1	0.1	0.2	0.2	0.1	0,1	0.5	0.4	0,0	0,0	0.2	0.1
*Yugoslavia, Vojvodina																				

OCEANIA

| | Kidney | | | | Other urinary organs | | | | | | Other nervous system | | | | Other endocrine | | | | | |
| | 189.0 | | 189.1 | | 189.2 | | 189.3-4 | | 189.8-9 | | 192.0,2 | | 192.1,3 | | 194.0 | | 194.3 | | 194.1,4-9 | |
	M	F	M	F	M	F	M	F	M	F	M	F	M	F	M	F	M	F	M	F
Australian Capital Territory	9.5	2.7	1,0	0,9	0,2	0,3	-	-	-	-	0,1	0,2	0,2	0,4	0,2	0,3	-	-	0,3	0,1
Australia, New South Wales	7.7	4.3	0.9	1.4	0.4	0.3	0.1	0.0	0,0	0,0	0.2	0.3	0.2	0.1	0.4	0.4	0,0	0,0	0.2	0.1
South Australia	7.3	3.6	0.7	1.0	0.3	0,1	-	-	0,2	0,1	0.3	0,1	0,1	0,1	0.3	0,2	-	0,0	0.3	0,1
Australia, Tasmania	8.4	3.1	0.6	0,4	0,2	0,2	-	-	0.6	0,2	0.4	0,4	0,2	0,2	-	0,3	0,1	0,1	0,4	-
Australia, Victoria	7.5	4.1	0.6	0.5	0.4	0.2	0.1	0.1	0,0	0,0	0.2	0.2	0.1	0.1	0.3	0,3	0,0	-	0.2	0,0
Western Australia	6.9	4.0	0.7	0.5	0.4	0.2	0,1	0,1	0,2	0,2	0.3	0.3	0,1	0,1	0.4	0,2	-	0,1	0,2	0,2
*French Polynesia	4.9	1,5	-	-	0,4	-	0,2	-	-	-	-	-	-	-	0,9	0,2	0,2	0,3	0,6	0,3
New Zealand: Non-Maori	6.4	4.0	0.3	0.2	0.3	0.1	0.1	0.1	0.1	0.1	0.2	0.1	0.1	0.1	0.4	0.5	0.1	0,1	0.2	0.2
New Zealand: Maori	7.6	2.7	-	0,3	-	0,3	-	0,3	-	-	0,1	0,4	0,1	0,6	0,6	0.5	0,5	-	0,6	0,6
US, Hawaii: White	10.4	3.5	0,4	0,2	0,9	0,1	0,3	0,1	-	-	0,9	-	0,1	-	0,4	0,3	-	-	0,1	-
US, Hawaii: Japanese	5.8	1.5	0,7	0,4	0,6	0,2	0,2	0,0	-	-	-	-	0,1	-	0,2	0,3	-	-	0,2	-
US, Hawaii: Hawaiian	7.6	2.8	0,5	-	0,4	0,3	-	-	-	-	0,2	0,2	0,2	-	1,2	0,2	-	-	-	-
US, Hawaii: Filipino	4.4	1,4	-	0,2	-	-	-	-	-	-	-	-	0,3	0,2	-	-	-	0,2	0,6	-
US, Hawaii: Chinese	4.3	0,8	0,3	-	0,8	0,7	-	-	0,3	-	0,6	-	-	-	-	-	-	-	-	0,4

AGE-STANDARDIZED (WORLD) INCIDENCE RATES (FOUR DIGIT RUBRICS)

| | Hodgkin's disease | | | | | | | | | | Multiple myeloma | | | | | |
| | 201.0,4 | | 201.5 | | 201.6 | | 201.2,7 | | 201.1,9 | | 203.0 | | 203.1 | | 203.8 | |
AFRICA	M	F	M	F	M	F	M	F	M	F	M	F	M	F	M	F
*Algeria, Setif	0,2	-	0,4	0,2	0,2	0,1	0,2	0,2	1.2	1.0	0,3	0,4	-	-	-	-
*France, La Reunion	0,2	0,1	0,4	0,3	0,1	0,2	-	-	0,3	0,1	3.0	2.9	-	-	0,1	0,2
*Mali, Bamako	0,1	0,3	0,1	-	0,3	0,1	0,2	-	0,3	-	-	-	-	-	-	-
*Uganda, Kyadondo	0,4	-	0,4	-	-	-	0,1	0,1	0,1	0,1	0,7	0,7	-	-	-	-
*Zimbabwe, Harare: African	-	-	0,0	-	0,2	0,2	0,2	-	0,4	0,4	2.7	3.7	-	0,1	-	0,2
*Zimbabwe, Harare: European	-	-	-	2,4	-	1,4	-	-	-	0,5	0,7	1,0	-	-	0,7	-
AMERICA, CENTRAL AND SOUTH																
*Argentina, Concordia	-	-	0,9	-	-	-	0,3	-	-	0,7	-	0,3	-	-	-	-
*Brazil, Belem	0,5	0,2	0,4	0,4	0,1	0,2	0,0	-	1.4	0,3	0,7	0,4	-	-	-	-
*Brazil, Goiania	-	-	0,0	-	0,0	0,1	0,1	-	2.1	1.8	1.3	1.5	-	-	-	-
*Brazil, Porto Alegre	-	0,1	0,1	-	-	-	-	-	2.3	1.0	2.4	1.8	-	-	0,1	-
Colombia, Cali	0.3	0,2	0,2	0,1	0.6	0,2	0,1	0,1	0.7	0.5	2.2	1.6	0,1	-	-	-
*Costa Rica	0.2	0.1	0.9	0.5	0.8	0.3	0.2	0,1	0.6	0.4	2.5	1.6	0,0	0,0	-	-
*Ecuador, Quito	-	-	-	-	0,1	-	0,1	-	1.3	1.3	1.7	1.0	-	-	-	-
*Peru, Lima	0,0	0,1	0,1	0.2	0.2	0.2	0,1	0,0	0.6	0.4	1.5	0.9	0,0	-	-	-
Peru, Trujillo	-	-	0,1	-	-	-	-	-	0,7	0,1	2.6	1.5	-	-	-	-
US, Puerto Rico	-	-	1.2	1.1	0.5	0.4	0.2	0,1	0.4	0.1	2.8	1.9	-	0,0	0.2	0,1
*Uruguay, Montevideo	-	-	0.7	0.6	0.5	0,1	0,0	0,0	2.2	1.4	2.3	1.8	-	0,1	-	-
AMERICA, NORTH																
Canada	0.2	0.1	1.4	1.5	0.7	0.3	0.1	0.0	0.5	0.3	3.8	2.6	0,0	0.0	0.2	0.1
Canada, Alberta	0.2	0,0	1.8	1.5	0.4	0.2	0.2	0,0	0.1	0,1	3.6	2.3	-	-	0.3	0.2
Canada, British Columbia	0,1	0,1	1.3	1.7	0.6	0.2	0,0	0,0	0.2	0.1	3.4	2.2	-	0,0	0.1	0,0
Canada, Manitoba	0,2	0,0	1.3	1.0	0.5	0.4	0,1	0,0	0.4	0.2	4.1	2.6	0,1	0,0	0,1	0,1
Canada, New Brunswick	0.5	0,1	1.0	1.1	0.8	0.7	0,1	-	0.2	0,2	3.7	2.4	-	0,1	0,1	0,1
Canada, Newfoundland	0,5	0,3	0.7	1.4	0.5	0.4	-	-	0,1	-	2.7	2.3	-	-	-	-
Canada, Northwest Territories	-	-	0,3	0,2	-	-	-	-	-	-	3,2	1,8	-	-	-	-
Canada, Nova Scotia	0,1	0,1	1.2	1.4	1.1	0.7	0,1	0,0	0.4	0.1	2.9	2.4	-	-	0.2	0,2
Canada, Ontario	0.2	0.1	1.5	1.7	0.7	0.3	0.1	0.1	0.5	0.3	4.2	2.9	0,0	0,0	0.1	0.1
Canada, Prince Edward Island	0,5	-	1,6	0,7	0,3	0,7	-	-	-	0,1	4.2	3.2	-	-	0,3	-
Canada, Quebec	0.2	0.1	1.1	1.3	0.8	0.4	0.1	0.1	1.0	0.7	3.7	2.5	0,0	-	0.2	0.1
Canada, Saskatchewan	0.4	0,1	1.4	1.0	0.8	0.3	0,1	0,0	0,1	0,2	4.0	1.9	-	0,0	0.2	0,0
Canada, Yukon	-	-	1,9	2,6	4,8	-	-	-	1,2	1,5	4,6	3,4	-	-	0,6	1,1
US, Cent. Calif.: Non-Hisp. White	0,2	0,1	1.6	1.7	0.4	0.4	0,1	0,0	0.3	0.3	3.4	2.3	-	0,0	0.3	0.3
US, Cent. Calif.: Hispanic	0,1	0,1	1.0	0.9	0.5	0.3	0,0	0,2	0.1	0,1	3.3	2.8	-	-	0.2	0,1
US, Los Angeles: Non-Hisp. White	0.2	0,1	1.8	1.9	0.8	0.3	0.1	0,0	0.3	0.2	3.2	2.2	0,0	0,0	0.2	0.1
US, Los Angeles: Hispanic White	0,1	0,0	0.9	0.7	0.8	0.5	0.2	0,0	0.3	0,1	3.4	2.4	-	-	0.3	0,1
US, Los Angeles: Black	0,2	0,1	1.0	1.1	0.5	0.3	0,1	0,0	0.2	0,1	9.2	4.9	0,0	-	0.2	0,1
US, Los Angeles: Chinese	0,2	-	-	0,3	0,2	0,2	0,1	-	-	-	1.8	1.0	-	-	-	-
US, Los Angeles: Filipino	-	0,2	1,1	0,6	0,2	-	-	-	0,2	0,2	2.5	1.6	-	-	0,2	-
US, Los Angeles: Korean	0,2	-	-	-	-	-	-	-	-	0,2	1,4	0,8	-	-	0,2	-
US, Los Angeles: Japanese	-	-	-	0,3	0,2	-	-	-	0,2	-	0,3	0,5	-	-	0,2	-
US, San Francisco: Non-Hisp. White	0.3	0,0	2.5	2.7	1.0	0.3	0.2	0,0	0.4	0,1	3.5	2.2	0,0	-	0.4	0.2
US, San Francisco: Hispanic White	0,1	0,1	0.9	1.4	0.8	0.2	0.3	-	0,0	0,1	3.8	2.1	-	0,1	0.5	0,1
US, San Francisco: Black	0,3	0,3	1.2	1.3	0.8	0.3	0.3	-	0,6	0,1	8.7	5.7	0,1	0,2	0.7	0.5
US, San Francisco: Chinese	-	-	0.9	0.7	0.3	-	-	-	-	-	1.2	1.9	-	-	0,1	0,1
US, San Francisco: Filipino	-	0,2	0,8	0,4	0,3	0,1	-	-	0,2	-	4.6	2.1	-	-	0,3	0,2
US, San Francisco: Japanese	-	-	1,5	0,4	-	-	0,6	-	-	-	2,4	-	-	0,6	-	-
US, Connecticut: White	0.4	0.1	2.0	2.6	1.1	0.5	0.1	0.1	0.5	0.3	3.3	2.2	0,0	0,0	0.2	0.1
US, Connecticut: Black	0,3	-	0,7	1.4	0,7	-	-	-	0,3	0,5	6.4	4.1	-	-	0,6	0,2
US, Atlanta: White	0.4	0,1	1.3	1.9	0.5	0.2	0,1	0,0	0.4	0.2	3.5	1.9	-	-	0.5	0.3
US, Atlanta: Black	0,3	0,2	0.7	0.8	1.0	0.3	0,1	-	0,0	0,3	8.0	5.9	-	-	0.2	0,2
US, Iowa	0.2	0,1	2.0	2.1	0.6	0.3	0.1	0,0	0.1	0.2	4.0	2.6	0,0	-	0.2	0.1
US, Central Louisiana: White	-	-	0,7	1,3	0,6	0,2	0,2	0,2	0,2	0,3	2.5	2.5	-	-	-	0,1
US, Central Louisiana: Black	-	-	1,8	-	-	-	-	-	0,5	0,6	6.2	3,4	-	-	-	-
US, New Orleans: White	0,1	0,1	1.9	1.8	0.8	0,4	0,1	0,0	0.6	0,5	3.1	1.6	-	0,0	0,0	0,1
US, New Orleans: Black	0,3	0,1	0,5	0,7	0,4	0,2	-	-	0,6	0,6	8.6	5.2	-	0,1	0.2	0,2
US, Detroit: White	0.2	0,1	2.1	2.2	1.0	0.3	0,1	0,0	0.3	0.3	3.9	2.5	0,0	0,0	0.3	0.2
US, Detroit: Black	0.6	0,0	1.4	1.2	0.7	0.4	0,1	-	0,1	0.3	8.2	6.1	-	0,0	0.5	0,3
US, New Mexico: Non-Hisp. White	0,2	-	2.1	1.7	0.4	0.3	-	0,0	0.3	0,2	3.0	2.1	0,0	0,0	0.3	0.2
US, New Mexico: Hispanic White	0,1	-	1.5	0.8	0,3	0,2	-	0,2	0.5	0,2	2.4	2.2	-	-	0,4	0,4
US, New Mexico: American Indian	-	-	0,3	-	-	-	-	-	-	0,2	2,7	3.5	-	-	-	-
US, Utah	0.2	0,1	1.2	1.4	0.4	0.2	0,1	0,0	0.1	0.2	3.7	2.2	-	0,0	0.3	0,1
US, Seattle	0.3	0.1	1.4	1.6	1.0	0.4	0,1	0,0	0.4	0.2	3.8	2.9	0,0	0,0	0.5	0.1
US, SEER: White	0.3	0.1	1.8	2.0	0.8	0.3	0.1	0.1	0.3	0.2	3.6	2.4	0,0	0,0	0.3	0.2
US, SEER: Black	0.4	0.1	1.1	1.2	0.7	0.3	0.2	-	0.2	0.3	8.1	5.8	0,0	0,1	0.5	0.3

AGE-STANDARDIZED (WORLD) INCIDENCE RATES (FOUR DIGIT RUBRICS)

| | Hodgkin's disease | | | | | | | | Multiple myeloma | | | | | | | |
| | 201.0,4 | | 201.5 | | 201.6 | | 201.2,7 | | 201.1,9 | | 203.0 | | 203.1 | | 203.8 | |
ASIA	M	F	M	F	M	F	M	F	M	F	M	F	M	F	M	F
*China, Qidong	-	-	-	-	-	-	-	-	0,1	0,0	1.2	0.5	-	-	0,1	-
China, Shanghai	0.0	0,0	0,0	0,0	0,0	0,0	0.2	0.1	0.2	0.1	0.7	0.4	0,0	0,0	0,0	0,0
China, Tianjin	0,0	-	0,0	0,0	0,0	-	-	-	0.3	0.3	0.4	0.2	-	0,0	0.1	0.1
Hong Kong																
*India, Bangalore	0.1	0,1	0.1	0.1	0.5	0.2	0,0	0,0	0.5	0.2	0.7	0.6	-	-	0,0	-
*India, Barshi, Paranda and Bhum	-	-	0,1	-	0,2	-	0,1	-	0,1	-	0,1	0,1	-	-	-	-
India, Bombay	0.1	0.1	0.0	0,0	0.6	0.3	0,0	0,0	0.5	0.2	1.2	0.9	0,0	0,0	-	-
*India, Karunagappally	0,3	-	-	-	0,5	-	-	-	-	0,3	0,6	1,4	-	-	-	-
India, Madras	0,0	0,0	0.1	0,1	0.1	0.1	0,0	0,0	1.0	0.4	0.8	0.4	-	-	0,0	-
*India, Trivandrum	0,3	-	-	0,3	0.2	0,1	-	-	0,3	0,1	2.4	0,4	0,1	-	0,1	-
Israel: All Jews	0,1	0,0	1.6	1.7	0.6	0.5	0,0	0.1	0.6	0.5	2.3	1.8	0,0	0,0	0.1	0.1
Jews born in Israel	0,2	0,0	1.5	1.9	0.9	0.5	0,1	0,1	0.6	0.4	3.0	1.8	-	-	-	-
Jews born in America or Europe	0,0	0,1	1.8	2.1	0.4	0,1	0,0	0,1	0.6	0.6	2.0	1.8	0,0	0,0	0,1	0,1
Jews born in Africa or Asia	0,0	0,1	0.8	0.4	0.7	0,4	0,0	-	0,3	0.2	2.2	2.2	0,0	0,0	0,2	0,2
Non-Jews	0,0	-	0.8	0.7	0.8	0.7	0,5	-	0,3	0.2	1.9	1.3	0,1	0,1	-	0,2
Japan, Hiroshima	-	-	0,0	-	0,0	0,2	0,0	0,1	0.2	0,1	1.8	1.1	-	-	-	-
Japan, Miyagi	-	-	-	0,0	0,0	0,0	-	-	0.4	0.2	1.5	1.4	0,0	0,0	0,0	0,0
Japan, Nagasaki	-	0,0	0,1	-	0,0	0,0	0,0	-	0.2	0.1	1.6	1.2	0,0	0,0	-	0,0
Japan, Osaka	0,0	0,0	0.1	0.0	0.1	0.1	0,0	0,0	0.3	0.1	1.5	1.0	0.0	0.0	0,0	0,0
*Japan, Saga																
Japan, Yamagata																
*Korea, Kangwha	-	-	-	-	-	-	-	-	0,4	-	0,6	0,5	-	0,6	-	-
*Kuwait: Non-Kuwaitis	0,2	0,2	1.0	0,4	0.4	0,6	-	0,2	0,3	0,8	3.9	2,0	-	-	0,0	-
*Kuwait: Kuwaitis	0,5	0,0	1.5	0,8	1.4	0,6	0,5	0,5	0,2	0,1	1,2	1,4	-	-	-	-
*Philippines, Manila	0,0	0,0	0,0	0,0	0,1	0,1	0,0	0,0	0.8	0.3	1.0	0.6	0,0	0,0	-	-
Singapore: Chinese	0,1	0,0	0,2	0.2	0.1	0,0	-	-	0,1	0,1	1.2	0.8	-	-	0,0	-
Singapore: Malay	0,1	-	0,6	0,1	0,2	0,2	0,2	-	0,2	-	2.8	1.8	-	-	-	0,1
Singapore: Indian	0,2	-	0,5	0,6	0,3	-	-	-	0,1	-	1.6	1.0	-	-	-	-
Thailand, Chiang Mai	0,2	-	0,0	0,0	0,2	0,1	-	0,0	0.7	0.3	0.4	0.3	-	-	-	-
*Thailand, Khon Kaen	0,1	0,1	0,0	0,1	0.1	0,2	-	-	0.2	0,1	0.2	0,1	-	-	-	-
*Viet Nam, Hanoi	-	-	-	-	0,1	-	0,0	-	1.6	0.9	0,1	-	-	-	-	-

EUROPE

| | Hodgkin's disease | | | | | | | | Multiple myeloma | | | | | | | |
| | 201.0,4 | | 201.5 | | 201.6 | | 201.2,7 | | 201.1,9 | | 203.0 | | 203.1 | | 203.8 | |
	M	F	M	F	M	F	M	F	M	F	M	F	M	F	M	F
Austria, Tyrol	0,4	0,2	1.0	1.0	0,3	0,1	0,1	0,1	0.8	0.6	3.2	2.3	-	-	0,3	0.2
*Belarus																
*Croatia	0,0	-	0,1	0,1	0.1	0,1	-	0,0	1.5	1.1	0.7	0.5	0,0	-	1.1	1.2
Czech Republic	0.5	0.3	0.7	0.9	0.9	0.7	0.3	0.2	0.6	0.4	2.0	1.6	0.1	0.1	0.4	0.3
Denmark	0.3	0,0	1.1	0.9	0.6	0.2	0,0	0,0	0.8	0.5	3.1	2.2	0,0	0,0	0.0	0.0
Estonia	0,2	0,1	0.8	0.9	0.8	0.3	0,2	0,1	0.7	0.3	1.7	1.2	-	-	0,0	0,0
Finland																
France, Bas-Rhin	0,3	0,1	0.6	0.9	1.3	0.6	0,2	0,1	0.2	0,1	2.0	1.1	-	0,0	0,3	0,0
*France, Calvados	0,4	0,1	0.9	1.7	0.2	0,1	0,1	-	0,4	0,1	1.9	1.5	-	-	0,2	0,1
France, Doubs	-	-	1.3	1.2	0,1	0,1	-	-	0.7	0,7	3.6	2.8	-	-	0,1	0,1
France, Haut-Rhin	0,1	0,1	0.7	1.0	0.6	0.5	-	0,0	0.7	0.5	2.8	2.1	-	-	0,2	0,0
*France, Herault	0,2	0,0	0.5	0,3	1.0	0.3	0,2	0,1	1.2	0.7	2.0	1.6	-	-	0,1	0,1
France, Isere	-	-	0.4	0,1	0.0	0,1	-	0,0	2.0	1.0	2.3	2.1	-	-	0,3	0,2
*France, Somme	0,0	0,1	1.0	1.2	0,3	0,0	0,1	-	1.0	0.5	1.3	1.7	-	-	0.7	-
*France, Tarn	-	-	0,7	0,3	0.9	0,4	-	0,0	0,5	-	1.6	1.5	-	0,1	0,1	0,2
Germany, Eastern States	0.1	0.1	0.3	0.5	0.5	0.3	0.3	0.1	1.4	1.1	2.1	1.4	0,0	0,0	0.2	0.1
Germany, Saarland	0,2	0,1	0.5	0.7	0.9	0.6	0,1	0,1	0.7	0.3	2.3	1.9	0,0	0,0	0,1	0,1
Iceland	0,2	0,2	1.7	0.7	0.7	0.2	0,2	-	0.3	0.2	3.5	2.3	-	-	0,2	-
Ireland, Southern	0,2	0,1	0,5	0.9	0.3	0.3	0,1	0,2	0,4	0,4	4.0	3.0	0,1	-	-	0,1
Italy, Ferrara	1,1	0,0	1,2	1.5	0,3	-	-	-	1,7	1,0	4.1	2.7	-	-	0,1	0,1
Italy, Florence	0,1	0,1	0.7	0.9	1.3	0.5	0,2	0,2	1.0	0.9	4.6	2.9	-	-	-	-
Italy, Genoa	0,4	0,0	1.6	1.4	1.1	0.3	0,1	0,0	0.5	0.5	3.0	1.5	-	0,0	0.8	0.7
*Italy, Latina	0,3	-	0,6	0,6	0,4	0,5	0,1	-	1.0	1.0	2.2	1.5	-	-	0,3	0,5
Italy, Macerata	0,2	-	0,3	1,5	1,4	0,5	1,0	0,1	0.8	1,0	1.9	2.6	-	-	0,7	0,4
Italy, Modena	0,1	0,1	0.7	0.9	0.7	0.7	0,2	0,1	0.8	0.4	2.7	1.9	-	-	0.9	0.6
Italy, Parma	-	0,1	0,5	0.8	0,6	1.0	0,1	0,1	0,7	0,4	3.8	2.3	-	-	0,1	-
Italy, Ragusa	0,3	0,4	0,3	0,6	0,7	0,6	0,2	0,1	1,1	0,4	2.5	1.4	0,1	-	0,4	0,1
Italy, Romagna	0,5	0,3	1.4	1.6	0.5	0,1	-	0,1	0,3	1,0	4.0	2.8	-	-	0,0	-
Italy, Torino	0,2	0,2	1.5	1.3	0.9	0.8	0,3	0,2	0.3	0.2	2.8	1.8	-	0,0	0,0	-
Italy, Trieste	-	-	0,2	0,6	-	0,3	0,1	-	2.4	1.9	4.4	3.4	-	-	0,1	0,3
Italy, Varese	0,3	0,2	1.2	1.9	1.4	0.6	0,1	0,0	0.5	0.2	3.1	2.5	-	0,1	-	-
Italy, Veneto	0,3	0,1	1.4	1.4	1.0	0.9	0,2	0,1	1.1	1.0	3.0	2.5	0,1	0,0	0,1	0,1
*Latvia	1.5	1.1	0,0	0,1	0.2	0.1	0,0	0,1	0.8	0.6	1.3	1.2	0,0	0,0	0,1	0.1
Malta	0,7	0,5	0,8	0,3	0.2	0,9	-	0,1	-	0,3	2.2	2.4	-	-	-	-

AGE-STANDARDIZED (WORLD) INCIDENCE RATES (FOUR DIGIT RUBRICS)

| | Hodgkin's disease | | | | | | | | | | Multiple myeloma | | | | | |
| | 201.0,4 | | 201.5 | | 201.6 | | 201.2,7 | | 201.1,9 | | 203.0 | | 203.1 | | 203.8 | |
	M	F	M	F	M	F	M	F	M	F	M	F	M	F	M	F
The Netherlands	0.0	0,0	1.7	1.3	0.4	0.2	0.1	0.0	0.3	0.1	3.3	2.1	0,0	0,0	0.1	0.1
The Netherlands, Eindhoven	0,2	-	1.0	1.2	0.4	0.2	0,1	0,0	0,1	0,0	2.5	2.2	-	-	0.4	0,1
The Netherlands, Maastricht	-	-	1.6	1.5	0,4	0,2	0,1	-	0,2	0,1	3.0	1.7	0,0	0,0	0,1	0,1
Norway																
*Poland, Cracow	-	0,1	0,2	0,4	0.7	0.6	-	-	1.7	1.1	1.5	0.7	-	0,1	1.1	1.1
*Poland, Kielce	-	-	0,1	0,1	0,1	0,1	0,0	-	2.3	1.6	0.6	0.7	-	0,0	0.8	0.4
*Poland, Lower Silesia	0.2	0.2	0.3	0.4	0.9	0.5	0.2	0.1	0.6	0.5	1.3	1.0	0,0	0,0	0.3	0.3
Poland, Warsaw City	0,0	0,1	1.0	1.0	0.5	0,1	0,1	0,1	0.4	0.3	1.9	1.8	0,1	0,0	-	-
Slovakia	0.4	0.2	0.7	0.7	0.8	0.5	0.2	0.1	0.2	0.2	2.5	1.9	-	0,0	0.1	0,0
Slovenia	0,0	0,0	1.1	1.1	0.5	0.2	0,1	-	0.5	0.2	0.4	0.3	0,0	-	2.0	1.5
*Spain, Albacete	0,5	-	0,7	0,3	1,2	-	-	-	0,6	1,0	2.4	2.9	-	-	0,4	-
Spain, Asturias	0,3	0,2	1.1	0.9	0.4	0,2	0,1	0,0	1.6	0.7	2.3	1.5	-	-	-	0,0
Spain, Basque Country	0.4	0,1	1.0	0.9	1.1	0.4	0.3	0,1	0.3	0.2	2.0	1.7	-	-	-	0,0
Spain, Granada	0.6	0,1	0.4	0.9	0.5	0.4	0.2	0,1	0.3	-	2.2	1.7	-	0,0	0.2	0,0
Spain, Mallorca	0,1	0,1	1.2	1.1	1.0	0.2	0,1	-	0,1	0,3	2.9	2.2	-	-	0,1	0,0
Spain, Murcia	0,2	-	0.6	0.7	0.8	0.3	0,1	0,0	0.2	0,1	2.4	2.3	0,0	0,0	-	-
Spain, Navarra	0,5	0,2	0,3	1.1	1.2	0.5	0.3	0,2	0.3	0,1	2.1	1.6	-	-	0,2	0,1
Spain, Tarragona	0,5	-	1.3	0.2	0,5	0.4	0,1	0,0	0.6	0,4	3.0	2.1	-	-	-	-
Spain, Zaragoza	0.4	0,2	0.6	0.8	0.5	0.4	0,1	-	0.5	0.3	2.3	1.8	0,0	0,0	-	-
Sweden	-	-	-	-	-	-	-	-	2.2	1.5	3.6	2.3	0.1	0.0	0.1	0.1
*Switzerland, Basel	-	-	1.4	1.8	0,7	0,5	0,0	0,1	0.3	-	2.6	1.3	-	-	0,1	-
Switzerland, Geneva	0,4	0,1	1.4	1.1	0,7	0,3	-	0,1	0.3	0,2	3.3	2.3	-	-	0,2	0,2
Switzerland, Graubunden	0,2	0,1	1,8	0,6	1,6	0,5	0,3	-	-	-	1,7	0,6	-	-	2.8	2.2
Switzerland, Neuchatel	0,3	-	0,4	0,9	1,5	0,2	0,2	-	-	-	1.7	1.0	-	0,1	-	0,2
Switzerland, St Gall-Appenzell	0,1	-	1.3	1.8	0.8	0,2	-	-	0,1	0,2	3.5	2.5	-	-	0,3	-
Switzerland, Valais	0,5	0,3	0,8	1.8	0,1	0,1	0,2	-	-	0,3	4.3	2.2	-	-	0,2	-
Switzerland, Vaud	0,0	0,1	2.1	1.7	0,2	0,1	0,1	0,1	0,0	0,1	3.1	2.6	-	-	-	-
Switzerland, Zurich	0,2	0,1	1.7	1.4	0.7	0.5	0,1	0,0	0.3	0,1	3.4	2.3	0,1	0,0	0,0	0,0
*UK, England and Wales	0.2	0.1	0.9	0.8	0.4	0.2	0.1	0.1	1.0	0.6	3.4	2.3	0.0	0.0	0.0	0.0
*UK, East Anglia																
*UK, Mersey	0,1	0,1	1.0	0.8	0.4	0.1	0,1	0,1	0.5	0.4	2.3	1.9	-	0,0	0,1	-
*UK, North Western	0.3	0.1	1.1	1.1	0.5	0.2	0.1	0,1	0.6	0.3	2.8	2.2	0,0	0,0	0,0	-
UK, Oxford	0.2	0,1	0.9	1.3	0.5	0.2	0,1	-	0.8	0.7	3.8	2.8	0,0	0,0	0,1	0,0
*UK, South Thames	0.1	0,0	0.9	0.8	0.4	0.2	0,0	0,0	1.2	0.8	3.4	2.3	0,0	0,0	0,0	-
UK, South Western	0.3	0,1	1.1	1.0	0.5	0.2	0.1	0,1	0.5	0.2	3.5	2.4	0,1	0,0	0,0	0,0
UK, Wessex	0.2	0,1	1.4	1.4	0.4	0.2	0,1	0,1	0.5	0.4	4.2	2.9	0,0	0,0	0.1	0,0
*UK, West Midlands	0.1	0,0	0.2	0.2	0.1	0,1	0,0	0,0	2.3	1.5	3.6	2.3	-	0,0	0.1	0,0
UK, Yorkshire	0.3	0.1	0.8	0.8	0.5	0.2	0.6	0.5	0.3	0.2	3.7	2.4	-	0,0	0.1	0,0
UK, Scotland	0.3	0.1	0.9	1.0	0.5	0.2	0.2	0.1	0.8	0.5	3.4	2.4	0,0	0.0	0.1	0,0
UK, Scotland, West	0.2	0,1	0.7	0.8	0.4	0.2	0.1	0,1	0.9	0.6	3.4	2.2	0,0	0,0	0.1	0,0
*Yugoslavia, Vojvodina																

OCEANIA

| | Hodgkin's disease | | | | | | | | | | Multiple myeloma | | | | | |
| | 201.0,4 | | 201.5 | | 201.6 | | 201.2,7 | | 201.1,9 | | 203.0 | | 203.1 | | 203.8 | |
	M	F	M	F	M	F	M	F	M	F	M	F	M	F	M	F
Australian Capital Territory	-	0,1	0,5	0,5	0.4	0.3	0.3	-	0.5	0.1	5.2	3.9	-	-	0.2	-
Australia, New South Wales	0.3	0.1	0.9	0.9	0.5	0.2	0.1	0,0	0.5	0.2	3.5	2.4	0,0	0,0	0,0	0,0
South Australia	0.2	0.1	0.7	0.9	0.8	0.6	0.1	0,0	0.1	0.1	4.4	2.7	0,0	-	0.1	-
Australia, Tasmania	0,1	0,1	0.8	1.3	0.4	0.5	0.2	0,1	0.1	0.2	4.0	2.0	-	-	0.1	0.1
Australia, Victoria	0.4	0.1	1.1	1.2	0.6	0.2	0.1	0,1	0.2	0.1	3.2	2.3	0,0	0,0	0.2	0.1
Western Australia	-	-	1.2	0.7	0.6	0.3	-	0,0	0.3	0.3	2.9	2.1	0,0	-	0.1	0.1
*French Polynesia	-	0,3	0,2	0,4	0,1	-	-	-	0.8	0.4	2,0	2,0	-	-	-	0,3
New Zealand: Non-Maori	0.2	0,0	0.5	0.6	0.4	0.2	0,1	0,1	0.6	0.4	3.9	2.5	0,0	0,0	0.2	0.2
New Zealand: Maori	0,1	0,2	0,3	0,1	0.5	0,1	0,2	-	0.5	0.2	5.4	5.7	-	0,2	0.2	-
US, Hawaii: White	0,5	0,1	1.5	2.3	0.5	0.4	-	0,1	0.2	-	2.5	1.6	0,1	-	0,9	0.3
US, Hawaii: Japanese	0,2	-	0,1	0.7	0.3	0.4	0.2	0,1	0,0	0,1	1.4	0.7	-	-	0,4	-
US, Hawaii: Hawaiian	-	-	0,5	1.8	0,3	0,2	-	-	-	-	3.8	4.2	-	-	0,3	-
US, Hawaii: Filipino	0,3	-	0,9	0.6	-	0,5	-	-	-	-	3.1	1,7	-	-	-	-
US, Hawaii: Chinese	-	-	0,5	-	-	-	-	0,1	-	-	2,1	0,4	-	-	-	-

AGE-STANDARDIZED (WORLD) INCIDENCE RATES (FOUR DIGIT RUBRICS)

	Burkitt's tumour 200.2		Mycosis fungoides 202.1		Hairy cell leukaemia 202.4		Other NHL 200.0,1,8 202.0,2-3,5-9	
	M	F	M	F	M	F	M	F
AFRICA								
*Algeria, Setif	0,0	0,1	-	-	-	-	6.2	2.7
*France, La Reunion	0,4	0,1	0,1	-	0,2	-	4.1	3.7
*Mali, Bamako	0,0	-	-	-	-	-	2.5	0.8
*Uganda, Kyadondo	1.1	0.7	-	-	-	-	2.3	1.6
*Zimbabwe, Harare: African	0,2	0,1	-	-	-	-	4.5	4.0
*Zimbabwe, Harare: European	-	-	-	-	1,0	-	3,1	3,9
AMERICA, CENTRAL AND SOUTH								
*Argentina, Concordia	-	-	-	-	-	-	3.6	3.5
*Brazil, Belem	-	-	-	-	-	-	4.2	2.1
*Brazil, Goiania	-	0,1	0,0	-	-	-	5.1	3.4
*Brazil, Porto Alegre	0,1	-	-	0,1	-	-	8.4	6.4
Colombia, Cali	0.5	0,1	-	-	0,1	-	7.3	5.9
*Costa Rica	0,0	0,0	0.3	0,0	0,1	0,0	5.6	3.6
*Ecuador, Quito	0,1	-	0,1	-	0,0	-	8.0	6.0
*Peru, Lima	0,1	0,1	-	-	-	-	7.0	5.7
Peru, Trujillo	0,2	-	-	-	-	-	9.1	5.2
US, Puerto Rico	0.3	0,1	0.2	0,1	0.2	0,0	7.2	4.9
*Uruguay, Montevideo	0,2	0,1	0,0	0,0	-	-	10.1	7.3
AMERICA, NORTH								
Canada	0.3	0.1	0.3	0.2	0.4	0.1	12.1	8.7
Canada, Alberta	0,1	0,0	0.3	0,1	0.5	0,1	10.9	8.2
Canada, British Columbia	0.3	0,1	0.2	0.1	0.4	0.1	12.1	8.3
Canada, Manitoba	0,4	0,2	0.3	0,1	0.3	0,1	13.4	10.4
Canada, New Brunswick	0,1	0,1	0.3	0,1	0.3	0,2	11.8	7.9
Canada, Newfoundland	-	-	0,2	0,3	0.5	0,2	7.6	5.4
Canada, Northwest Territories	0,4	-	-	0,6	-	-	8.3	9.9
Canada, Nova Scotia	0,1	-	0.6	0.4	0,4	0,2	11.2	8.3
Canada, Ontario	0.3	0.1	0.5	0.3	0.4	0.1	12.3	8.8
Canada, Prince Edward Island	-	-	-	0,5	0,9	-	10.3	10.5
Canada, Quebec	0.3	0.1	0.2	0.1	0.3	0.1	12.6	8.9
Canada, Saskatchewan	0,1	0,1	0.3	0,1	0.5	0,1	11.8	9.1
Canada, Yukon	-	-	-	-	0,8	-	5,1	6,2
US, Cent. Calif.: Non-Hisp. White	0.2	0,0	0.3	0.2	0.3	0,1	12.4	8.5
US, Cent. Calif.: Hispanic	0,3	0,2	0.2	0,1	-	0,3	10.0	8.0
US, Los Angeles: Non-Hisp. White	0.5	0.1	0.4	0.2	0.3	0,0	17.2	9.4
US, Los Angeles: Hispanic White	0.3	0,0	0.2	0,1	0,1	0,0	11.0	6.9
US, Los Angeles: Black	0,1	0,0	0.4	0,3	0,1	-	10.1	5.7
US, Los Angeles: Chinese	0,2	0,1	0.2	-	-	-	7.1	4.9
US, Los Angeles: Filipino	-	0,3	0.4	-	-	-	10.1	6.7
US, Los Angeles: Korean	-	-	0,2	0,2	-	-	4.8	4.1
US, Los Angeles: Japanese	-	-	-	-	0,6	0,3	12.0	5.5
US, San Francisco: Non-Hisp. White	1.0	0,1	0.9	0.3	0.5	0.1	22.7	9.5
US, San Francisco: Hispanic White	0,7	0,2	0.5	0.3	0,3	-	19.4	10.5
US, San Francisco: Black	0,2	-	0.4	0.8	0,1	-	13.2	6.5
US, San Francisco: Chinese	-	0,3	0.3	0,1	0,3	0,2	10.1	6.3
US, San Francisco: Filipino	0,2	0,5	0.6	0,2	0,2	-	10.1	7.6
US, San Francisco: Japanese	-	-	-	-	-	-	10.0	10.3
US, Connecticut: White	0.3	0,1	0.7	0.1	0.3	0.1	13.6	10.3
US, Connecticut: Black	0,4	-	0.8	0.6	-	-	12.0	8.6
US, Atlanta: White	0.4	0,0	0.5	0.2	0.4	0,1	13.3	9.9
US, Atlanta: Black	0,1	0,0	0.3	0.5	0,1	-	9.8	6.2
US, Iowa	0,1	0,1	0.2	0.2	0.4	0,1	13.9	10.1
US, Central Louisiana: White	0,2	-	0,1	-	-	0,1	13.2	8.5
US, Central Louisiana: Black	-	-	-	-	-	-	8.8	4.9
US, New Orleans: White	0,2	-	0,1	0,0	0,2	0,1	15.2	9.1
US, New Orleans: Black	-	-	0,2	0,2	-	0,1	9.2	5.2
US, Detroit: White	0.2	0,0	0.4	0.2	0.3	0,0	14.3	10.2
US, Detroit: Black	0,2	0,1	0.8	0.4	0,1	0,1	11.9	6.1
US, New Mexico: Non-Hisp. White	0,1	0,1	0.2	0,1	0.7	0,2	11.1	8.0
US, New Mexico: Hispanic White	0,1	0,2	0,1	0,3	0,2	-	8.6	5.1
US, New Mexico: American Indian	-	-	-	-	-	-	3.8	4.1
US, Utah	0,2	-	0.3	0.3	0.5	0,1	12.3	8.9
US, Seattle	0.5	0,1	0.3	0.2	0.4	0,1	14.8	9.6
US, SEER: White	0.4	0.1	0.5	0.2	0.4	0.1	15.1	9.7
US, SEER: Black	0.2	0,0	0.6	0.5	0,1	0,0	11.5	6.4

AGE-STANDARDIZED (WORLD) INCIDENCE RATES (FOUR DIGIT RUBRICS)

	Burkitt's tumour 200.2		Mycosis fungoides 202.1		Hairy cell leukaemia 202.4		Other NHL 200.0,1,8 202.0,2-3,5-9	
ASIA	M	F	M	F	M	F	M	F
*China, Qidong	-	-	0,0	-	-	-	3.6	1.8
China, Shanghai	0,0	-	0,0	0,0	0,0	0,0	4.2	2.5
China, Tianjin	-	-	0,0	-	-	0,0	4.5	2.6
Hong Kong								
*India, Bangalore	0,0	-	-	-	0,1	-	3.6	2.1
*India, Barshi, Paranda and Bhum	-	-	-	-	-	-	1,0	0,6
India, Bombay	0,0	0,0	-	-	0,0	0,0	4.0	2.7
*India, Karunagappally	-	-	-	-	-	-	5.1	1,1
India, Madras	0,0	0,0	-	-	-	-	3.6	2.0
*India, Trivandrum	-	-	0,1	-	-	-	4.4	2.1
Israel: All Jews	0.6	0.3	0.5	0.3	0.5	0.1	11.0	9.7
Jews born in Israel	0.5	0.2	0,2	0,2	1.0	0,2	11.8	10.5
Jews born in America or Europe	0,7	0,1	0.6	0.4	0.4	0,1	11.1	9.3
Jews born in Africa or Asia	0,2	0,1	0.5	0.2	0.4	0,1	9.4	8.5
Non-Jews	0.5	0,2	0,2	0,1	0,2	-	7.4	6.2
Japan, Hiroshima	0,1	-	0.0	0.0	0.0	-	8.4	4.3
Japan, Miyagi	0,1	0,0	0,0	-	-	-	6.4	4.2
Japan, Nagasaki	-	0,1	0,1	0,0	0,0	-	13.4	7.0
Japan, Osaka	0,0	-	0,0	0,0	0,0	-	6.0	3.6
*Japan, Saga								
Japan, Yamagata								
*Korea, Kangwha	-	-	-	-	0,3	-	2,6	1,9
*Kuwait: Non-Kuwaitis	0,1	0,2	0,1	-	-	-	9.2	6.5
*Kuwait: Kuwaitis	0,0	0,2	0,5	-	-	-	5.0	6.9
*Philippines, Manila	0,0	0,0	0,0	-	-	0,0	5.6	3.6
Singapore: Chinese	0,0	-	0,1	0,1	-	-	6.0	4.4
Singapore: Malay	-	-	0,1	-	-	-	6.8	5.6
Singapore: Indian	0,2	-	-	-	-	-	3.7	2.9
Thailand, Chiang Mai	0,0	0,1	-	-	-	-	3.8	2.5
*Thailand, Khon Kaen	0,1	-	-	-	-	-	2.6	1.8
*Viet Nam, Hanoi	-	-	-	-	-	-	6.3	2.8
EUROPE								
Austria, Tyrol	-	0,1	0,3	0,1	0.6	0,1	6.8	7.2
*Belarus								
*Croatia	-	-	0.2	0.1	0.2	0,0	4.9	3.7
Czech Republic	0.1	0.1	0.2	0.1	0.2	0.1	6.5	4.2
Denmark	0.3	0.1	0.2	0.1	0.2	0.1	9.1	6.3
Estonia	-	-	0,1	0,0	0,0	-	4.4	2.4
Finland								
France, Bas-Rhin	0.5	0,1	0.9	0.5	0.2	0,2	10.6	7.5
*France, Calvados	0,1	0,1	0,2	0,3	0,2	0,2	7.7	5.5
France, Doubs	0,1	-	0,0	0,1	0,1	-	13.0	8.4
France, Haut-Rhin	0,1	0,1	0,2	0,2	0.4	0,2	9.4	6.3
*France, Herault	0,3	0,1	0,1	0,1	0,0	0,0	10.0	6.6
France, Isere	0,4	0,1	0,2	0,1	0,3	0,1	9.7	6.6
*France, Somme	0,1	0,1	0,2	0,0	0,3	0,1	7.9	4.9
*France, Tarn	0,4	-	0,1	0,2	0.5	-	5.9	5.2
Germany, Eastern States	0,1	0,0	0.2	0.0	0.1	0,0	5.3	3.6
Germany, Saarland	0.4	0,2	0,0	0,0	0.4	-	8.5	5.6
Iceland	-	-	0,3	0,3	0,3	0,2	7.9	4.2
Ireland, Southern	-	0,3	0,2	0,1	0,2	-	8.6	6.9
Italy, Ferrara	-	0,3	0,6	0,8	0,3	0,1	12.9	10.2
Italy, Florence	0,0	-	0,2	0,0	0,2	0,0	9.4	6.3
Italy, Genoa	0,4	-	0,3	0,2	0.4	0,2	12.1	7.3
*Italy, Latina	-	-	0,1	-	-	-	6.8	5.1
Italy, Macerata	-	-	-	-	0,2	0,2	8.2	6.4
Italy, Modena	0,3	0,2	0,3	0,4	0,3	0,1	11.9	8.8
Italy, Parma	-	0,0	0,3	0,0	0,1	-	11.5	8.3
Italy, Ragusa	-	-	-	0,1	0,2	0,1	6.3	3.9
Italy, Romagna	-	-	0,5	0,3	0,5	-	14.5	7.7
Italy, Torino	0,5	0,3	0,3	0,1	0,3	0,1	10.3	6.9
Italy, Trieste	0,2	-	1.6	0.5	0,1	0,2	13.6	8.9
Italy, Varese	0,2	0,1	0.4	0.2	0.2	0,1	13.2	9.7
Italy, Veneto	0,2	0,0	0.5	0.3	0.5	0,2	12.2	8.7
*Latvia	0,0	-	0,0	0,0	0,0	-	3.5	2.3
Malta	-	-	-	0,4	0,2	-	6.6	5.1

AGE-STANDARDIZED (WORLD) INCIDENCE RATES (FOUR DIGIT RUBRICS)

	Burkitt's tumour 200.2		Mycosis fungoides 202.1		Hairy cell leukaemia 202.4		Other NHL 200.0,1,8 202.0,2-3,5-9	
	M	F	M	F	M	F	M	F
The Netherlands	0.2	0.1	0.2	0.1	0.3	0.1	9.8	6.7
The Netherlands, Eindhoven	0,1	0,1	0,1	0,1	0,2	0,1	9.5	5.7
The Netherlands, Maastricht	0,2	0,1	0,2	0,1	0,2	0,1	8.3	6.3
Norway								
*Poland, Cracow	-	-	-	-	-	-	5.8	2.7
*Poland, Kielce	0,1	-	0,1	-	-	-	4.1	2.3
*Poland, Lower Silesia	0,1	0,0	0,1	0,0	0,0	-	4.9	2.8
Poland, Warsaw City	0,3	-	0,0	0,0	-	-	6.1	3.2
Slovakia	0.2	0.1	0.1	0.1	0.2	0,0	5.1	3.4
Slovenia	0,2	0,0	0,1	-	0.2	0,1	5.8	4.0
*Spain, Albacete	-	-	-	-	-	-	6.1	4.4
Spain, Asturias	0,1	0,2	-	0,1	0,2	0,1	6.9	5.6
Spain, Basque Country	0.4	0,0	0.4	0,1	0,0	0,1	7.3	4.9
Spain, Granada	0,4	0,2	0,1	0,1	-	0,0	5.1	4.0
Spain, Mallorca	0,1	-	0,1	0,1	0,2	0,1	7.5	4.8
Spain, Murcia	0,2	-	0,1	0,2	0,1	0,0	7.3	4.6
Spain, Navarra	0,5	0,1	0.8	0.5	0,2	0,1	7.4	4.7
Spain, Tarragona	0,3	0,1	0,1	0,2	0,0	0,1	5.2	5.2
Spain, Zaragoza	0,2	0,0	-	0,1	0,1	0,0	6.8	5.0
Sweden	-	-	0.2	0.0	0.4	0.1	10.2	6.8
*Switzerland, Basel	0,6	0,2	0,2	0,0	0,6	0,1	13.7	7.1
Switzerland, Geneva	0,4	0,4	0,2	0,1	0,4	0,1	12.5	7.6
Switzerland, Graubunden	-	-	-	-	0,4	0,2	6.9	4.9
Switzerland, Neuchatel	0,5	-	0,7	0,1	0,4	-	8.5	5.5
Switzerland, St Gall-Appenzell	0,4	0,2	0,1	-	0,4	0,2	9.1	6.7
Switzerland, Valais	0,1	0,2	0,3	0,2	0,1	-	8.3	5.5
Switzerland, Vaud	0,5	0,2	0,7	0,1	0,5	-	12.5	7.9
Switzerland, Zurich	0.6	0,2	0.3	0,1	0.4	0,1	11.6	8.2
*UK, England and Wales	0.0	0.0	0.2	0.1	0.2	0.1	9.1	6.2
*UK, East Anglia								
*UK, Mersey	0,0	-	0.1	0.1	0.1	0,0	6.7	5.5
*UK, North Western	-	-	0.2	0.1	0.1	0.1	8.1	5.6
UK, Oxford	0,1	-	0.2	0.1	0.2	0,0	9.9	6.5
*UK, South Thames	0,0	0,0	0.2	0.1	0.2	0.1	9.9	6.6
UK, South Western	0,0	0,0	0.3	0.1	0.3	0.1	10.6	7.3
UK, Wessex	0,1	0,0	0.2	0.1	0.3	0.1	11.2	7.8
*UK, West Midlands	0,0	0,0	0.2	0.1	0.1	0,0	8.4	6.1
UK, Yorkshire	0,0	-	0.5	0.2	0.3	0.1	8.9	5.6
UK, Scotland	0,1	0,0	0.3	0.1	0.2	0.1	8.9	7.2
UK, Scotland, West	0,0	0,0	0.3	0.1	0,1	0,0	8.2	6.8
*Yugoslavia, Vojvodina								

OCEANIA

	Burkitt's tumour 200.2		Mycosis fungoides 202.1		Hairy cell leukaemia 202.4		Other NHL 200.0,1,8 202.0,2-3,5-9	
	M	F	M	F	M	F	M	F
Australian Capital Territory	0,2	-	-	0,1	0,5	0,1	13.6	9.6
Australia, New South Wales	0.2	0.1	0.2	0.1	0.3	0.1	12.6	8.3
South Australia	0,2	0,0	0.5	0.2	0.4	0.2	11.6	8.6
Australia, Tasmania	-	0,1	0,1	0,2	0.4	0.2	12.8	9.0
Australia, Victoria	0.1	0,0	0.2	0.2	0.3	0.1	13.1	8.8
Western Australia	0.4	0,1	0,1	0,1	0,2	0,1	11.1	8.1
*French Polynesia	0,2	0,4	-	-	-	-	3.7	4.0
New Zealand: Non-Maori	0.2	0.2	0,1	0,0	0.2	0,1	9.8	7.2
New Zealand: Maori	-	0,1	0,3	0,3	0.4	-	7.4	6.3
US, Hawaii: White	0,4	-	-	0,1	0,3	-	14.3	6.8
US, Hawaii: Japanese	-	-	0,3	-	-	-	8.3	6.3
US, Hawaii: Hawaiian	0,2	-	0,2	-	-	0,3	10.7	4.7
US, Hawaii: Filipino	0,3	-	-	-	0,4	-	10.4	7.9
US, Hawaii: Chinese	-	-	-	-	-	-	12.8	8.7

AGE-STANDARDIZED (WORLD) INCIDENCE RATES (FOUR DIGIT RUBRICS)

| | Lymphoid leukaemia | | | | | | Myeloid leukaemia | | | | | | Other and unspec. leukaemia | | | | | |
| | 204.0 | | 204.1 | | 204.2,8-9 | | 205.0 | | 205.1 | | 205.2-3,8-9 | | Acute | | Chronic | | O&U leuk. | |
AFRICA	M	F	M	F	M	F	M	F	M	F	M	F	M	F	M	F	M	F
*Algeria, Setif	1.2	0.8	1.7	0,5	-	-	1.1	1.0	0.9	0.7	-	-	0.9	0,5	-	-	0,4	0,2
*France, La Reunion	1.1	1.2	0,6	0,5	-	-	2.4	1.5	0.9	1.2	-	0,1	0,5	0,2	-	-	-	0,1
*Mali, Bamako	-	-	-	-	-	-	-	-	0,1	1.1	-	0,0	0,1	-	-	-	0,8	0.8
*Uganda, Kyadondo	0,2	0,1	-	-	0,0	0,0	-	-	0,2	0,3	-	0,3	-	0,0	0,0	-	0,3	0,5
*Zimbabwe, Harare: African	0.8	0.9	1,7	1,3	-	-	1.2	1.2	1.5	1,3	-	-	-	-	-	-	0,6	-
*Zimbabwe, Harare: European	1,0	-	0,7	0,9	-	-	3,7	2,5	-	-	0,7	-	1,7	-	-	-	-	-

AMERICA, CENTRAL AND SOUTH

| | 204.0 | | 204.1 | | 204.2,8-9 | | 205.0 | | 205.1 | | 205.2-3,8-9 | | Acute | | Chronic | | O&U leuk. | |
	M	F	M	F	M	F	M	F	M	F	M	F	M	F	M	F	M	F
*Argentina, Concordia	-	0,5	1,8	1,2	-	-	-	-	0,3	-	-	0,3	-	-	0,4	-	0,7	1,2
*Brazil, Belem	0.9	0.7	-	0,2	0,0	0,1	0.9	0.5	0,7	0,4	0,4	0,1	-	-	-	-	0.7	0.8
*Brazil, Goiania	1.3	1.0	0.9	0,3	0,1	0,1	1.4	1.2	0,6	0,3	-	0,1	0,6	0,3	0,0	-	0.9	0.8
*Brazil, Porto Alegre	1.9	1.3	0.7	0.4	0,3	0,3	1.9	1.5	0.9	0.7	0,1	0.4	0,5	0.6	0,1	0,0	0.9	0.5
Colombia, Cali	1.5	1.7	0.5	0,2	0,2	0,3	1.0	0.9	0.8	0.8	0,2	0,2	1.0	0.6	0,1	0,0	0.9	0.6
*Costa Rica	2.9	2.4	0.9	0.3	0.3	0.2	1.4	1.6	1.3	1.0	0,0	0,0	0.5	0.5	0,0	0,0	0.5	0.4
*Ecuador, Quito	2.0	2.2	0,2	0,1	0,3	0,1	2.3	1.5	1.1	0.5	0,4	0,3	0.6	0,3	0,1	0,1	1.3	0.8
*Peru, Lima	1.6	1.4	0.3	0,1	0,1	0,1	1.0	1.3	0.6	0.4	0,1	0,1	0.4	0.3	0,1	0,0	0.2	0,1
Peru, Trujillo	1.4	1.7	0,2	-	-	-	1,0	3.1	1.0	-	-	-	1,1	0,3	-	0,2	0,1	-
US, Puerto Rico	1.6	1.6	0.8	0.5	0.2	0,1	1.6	1.5	1.3	0.6	0.2	0,1	0.5	0.3	0,1	0,0	0.4	0.2
*Uruguay, Montevideo	1.5	1.1	1.5	0.8	0,0	0,1	1.5	1.1	1.3	0.8	0,1	0,1	1.1	0.8	0,0	0,1	0,3	0.3

AMERICA, NORTH

| | 204.0 | | 204.1 | | 204.2,8-9 | | 205.0 | | 205.1 | | 205.2-3,8-9 | | Acute | | Chronic | | O&U leuk. | |
	M	F	M	F	M	F	M	F	M	F	M	F	M	F	M	F	M	F
Canada	1.9	1.6	3.7	1.8	0.1	0.1	2.1	1.6	1.4	0.8	0.2	0.1	0.7	0.5	0.1	0.1	0.5	0.4
Canada, Alberta	1.7	1.6	3.4	1.7	0,1	0,1	1.8	1.3	1.3	0.8	0,0	0,1	0.4	0.4	0,1	0,0	0,1	0,1
Canada, British Columbia	1.8	1.7	2.5	1.3	0.1	0,1	1.6	1.4	1.3	0.8	0.1	0,1	0.5	0.3	0,1	0,0	0.5	0.2
Canada, Manitoba	1.5	1.7	3.4	1.3	0,1	0,0	2.8	2.0	1.2	0.5	0,2	0,1	0.4	0.3	0,0	0,0	0.3	0,1
Canada, New Brunswick	1.6	1.6	2.0	1.2	0,1	0,2	1.8	1.1	1.0	0.5	0,2	0,2	0.5	0.3	0,0	0,0	1.0	0.7
Canada, Newfoundland	1.8	1.7	1.0	0.7	0,1	-	1.8	2.3	1.3	0.6	-	-	0.5	0,3	-	-	0,2	0,0
Canada, Northwest Territories	0,3	1,1	1,5	-	-	-	1,1	1.0	0.5	0,4	0,5	-	0,7	0,7	-	-	-	0,6
Canada, Nova Scotia	1.5	1.6	2.1	1.0	0,3	0,0	0.9	1.1	1.0	0.7	0,4	0,1	1.2	0.7	0,1	0,1	1.4	0.6
Canada, Ontario	2.0	1.5	4.2	2.1	0.2	0.1	2.7	2.0	1.5	1.0	0.4	0.1	0.5	0.4	0.1	0.1	0.6	0.5
Canada, Prince Edward Island	1,1	1,4	4.1	1,2	-	-	1,6	1,6	0,9	0,9	0,1	-	0,8	-	-	-	0,2	0,1
Canada, Quebec	2.1	1.6	4.0	1.7	0.2	0.1	1.8	1.3	1.3	0.7	0.1	0.1	1.1	0.9	0.1	0.1	0.5	0.4
Canada, Saskatchewan	2.3	1.9	5.6	2.9	0,1	0,0	1.9	1.2	1.5	0.9	0,2	0,0	0.7	0.4	0,0	0,1	0.2	0,1
Canada, Yukon	5,0	4,1	3,1	6,9	1,6	-	0,7	-	1,1	0,7	-	-	1,1	-	-	-	-	-
US, Cent. Calif.: Non-Hisp. White	1.5	1.6	2.9	1.4	0,0	0,1	2.6	2.1	1.6	0.7	0,2	0,0	0.6	0.3	0,1	0,0	0.2	0.2
US, Cent. Calif.: Hispanic	2.9	2.4	2.0	0,7	0,2	0,1	2.2	1.1	1.1	0,6	-	0,1	0.8	0,6	-	0,1	0,1	0,1
US, Los Angeles: Non-Hisp. White	2.1	1.4	3.3	1.9	0.1	0.0	3.1	2.1	1.6	1.0	0.1	0,1	0.7	0.5	0,0	0,0	0.2	0.1
US, Los Angeles: Hispanic White	2.7	2.3	1.4	0.6	0,1	0,1	1.9	1.9	1.3	0.8	0,2	0,0	0.9	0.3	-	-	0,1	0,1
US, Los Angeles: Black	1.0	0.5	3.5	1.3	0,1	0,0	2.5	1.8	1.9	1.1	0,1	0,1	0.7	0.4	-	-	0,2	0,2
US, Los Angeles: Chinese	1,0	1,0	0,7	0,9	-	-	2.7	1.4	1,1	0,6	0,1	-	0,5	0,2	-	0,1	-	0,3
US, Los Angeles: Filipino	2.6	2,3	0,8	0,7	-	-	5.2	1.9	1.5	1,1	-	-	1,2	0,6	-	-	-	0,3
US, Los Angeles: Korean	1,3	1,4	-	0,3	0,4	-	1,3	1,6	0,4	0,3	-	-	0,9	0,3	-	-	0,3	-
US, Los Angeles: Japanese	1,3	3,6	-	0,2	-	-	2.8	2,5	1,8	0,7	0,2	-	0,8	-	0,3	-	-	-
US, San Francisco: Non-Hisp. White	2.4	1.5	2.9	1.3	0.1	0,0	2.9	2.0	1.4	0.7	0.2	0,0	0.8	0.5	0,0	0,1	0.1	0.1
US, San Francisco: Hispanic White	2.6	2.1	1,0	1.2	-	-	2.8	2.7	1.3	1.3	-	-	0,2	0,4	0,1	-	0,2	-
US, San Francisco: Black	1.5	1.4	2.9	1.8	0,1	-	2.2	1.6	1.4	0,2	-	-	0,7	0,4	0,2	-	0,1	0,2
US, San Francisco: Chinese	3.3	0,9	1,0	0,3	0,1	0,1	1.9	1.7	1,0	1.2	0,1	0,2	0,3	0,3	-	-	0,1	0,1
US, San Francisco: Filipino	2.6	2.8	0,7	0,4	-	-	3.4	2.1	1,3	1,4	0,3	-	0,8	1,6	-	-	0,7	-
US, San Francisco: Japanese	1,8	-	-	0,5	-	-	2,2	1,0	1,7	0,4	-	-	-	-	-	-	-	-
US, Connecticut: White	1.8	1.3	3.0	1.5	0.1	0.1	2.4	1.7	1.3	0.7	0.1	0,0	1.1	0.7	0,0	0,0	0.3	0.2
US, Connecticut: Black	0,8	0,8	1,7	1.8	0,9	0,2	1.8	1.9	1,4	0.7	0.2	0.2	0.7	0.6	0,2	-	-	0,1
US, Atlanta: White	2.0	1.4	2.2	1.3	0,2	0,1	2.5	1.5	1.2	0.9	0,1	0,1	0.6	0.4	0,0	0,0	0,2	0,1
US, Atlanta: Black	1.1	0.9	3.1	1.2	0,1	0,2	2.4	1.4	0.9	1.4	-	0,0	0,9	0,1	-	-	0,3	0,1
US, Iowa	1.8	1.4	4.9	2.2	0.2	0,0	2.4	2.0	1.6	0.9	0.1	0,0	1.0	0.6	0,0	0,0	0.2	0.1
US, Central Louisiana: White	1,1	0,6	1,9	1.3	0,1	0,1	2.6	1.3	0.6	0.5	0,1	0,2	0.7	0,2	-	-	0,2	0,1
US, Central Louisiana: Black	1,9	-	1,4	0,7	0,5	-	2.7	0,3	0.5	0,2	-	-	0,7	-	-	-	0,8	0,4
US, New Orleans: White	2.3	1.5	2.3	1.5	0,2	0,2	2.5	2.4	0.8	0.5	0,3	0,2	1.0	0.8	0,1	0,0	0,2	0,1
US, New Orleans: Black	1.1	0.9	2.4	0.8	0,1	0,2	2.0	1.5	1.5	0.6	0,1	0,2	1.2	0,3	-	0,1	0,9	0,2
US, Detroit: White	2.3	1.4	3.8	1.9	0,1	0,1	2.8	2.0	1.8	1.2	0,1	0,2	1.2	0.6	0,0	0,0	0.5	0.3
US, Detroit: Black	0.9	1.1	2.8	1.6	0,1	-	2.3	1.6	1.9	1.2	0.2	0,1	1.1	0.4	0,1	0,0	0,2	0,3
US, New Mexico: Non-Hisp. White	2.2	1.6	3.5	1.6	0,3	0,1	2.4	1.9	1.7	1.0	0,1	0,1	0.5	0.6	0,0	0,1	0.6	0.4
US, New Mexico: Hispanic White	3.2	1.2	1.8	0.7	0,1	-	1.5	1.6	1.8	0.7	0,2	0,1	0,6	1.1	-	-	-	0,1
US, New Mexico: American Indian	2,4	2,3	-	-	0,3	-	1,6	0,4	1,1	0.8	-	-	0,6	-	-	-	-	-
US, Utah	1.7	1.9	2.6	1.0	0,1	0,0	2.3	1.7	1.0	0.8	0,1	0,0	0.7	0.3	0,0	0,0	0.3	0.2
US, Seattle	2.1	1.4	3.6	1.7	0,1	0,1	2.4	1.8	1.4	0.9	0,1	0,0	1.0	0.6	0,0	0,0	0.3	0.1
US, SEER: White	2.1	1.5	3.4	1.6	0.1	0.1	2.5	1.8	1.4	0.9	0.1	0.1	0.9	0.6	0.0	0.0	0.3	0.2
US, SEER: Black	1.1	1.0	2.7	1.6	0.2	0,1	2.2	1.6	1.6	1.0	0,1	0,0	1.0	0.4	0,1	0,0	0,2	0.2

AGE-STANDARDIZED (WORLD) INCIDENCE RATES (FOUR DIGIT RUBRICS)

| | Lymphoid leukaemia | | | | | | Myeloid leukaemia | | | | | | Other and unspec. leukaemia | | | | | |
| | 204.0 | | 204.1 | | 204.2,8-9 | | 205.0 | | 205.1 | | 205.2-3,8-9 | | Acute | | Chronic | | O&U leuk. | |
ASIA	M	F	M	F	M	F	M	F	M	F	M	F	M	F	M	F	M	F
*China, Qidong	0.9	0.5	0,1	0,1	0,1	0.2	1.1	1.1	0.5	0.4	0,2	0.3	0,1	0.2	0,1	-	0.8	0.6
China, Shanghai	1.3	1.0	0.2	0.1	0,0	0,0	1.0	0.9	0.7	0.4	0,0	0,0	1.1	0.8	0,0	0,0	0.5	0.5
China, Tianjin	0.6	0.5	0.2	0,1	0.4	0.2	0.8	0.7	0.5	0.3	0.4	0.4	0.7	0.7	0,0	0,0	1.2	1.0
Hong Kong																		
*India, Bangalore	0.7	0.5	0.4	0.2	0,0	0,0	1.0	1.0	0.8	0.6	0,1	0,0	0.3	0.3	0,0	0,0	0.2	0.2
*India, Barshi, Paranda and Bhum	0,6	0,5	0,1	-	-	-	0,6	0,3	0,4	-	-	0,1	-	-	-	-	0,1	-
India, Bombay	1.0	0.8	0.6	0.3	0,1	0,0	1.0	0.9	0.9	0.6	0.1	0,0	0.3	0.1	-	0,0	0.2	0.3
*India, Karunagappally	1,3	1,0	-	-	-	-	1.6	0,6	0.3	-	-	-	0,2	-	-	-	0,2	0,2
India, Madras	1.3	0.7	0,1	0,1	-	0,0	0.7	0.5	0.6	0.4	0,1	-	0.1	0,1	-	-	0.1	0.1
*India, Trivandrum	1.4	1.0	0,6	-	-	0,1	0.6	1.3	0.3	0,4	-	-	0,2	0,5	-	-	0,1	-
Israel: All Jews	1.4	0.9	2.1	1.1	0,1	0,0	1.8	1.6	0.8	0.5	0,1	0,1	0.8	0.6	0,1	0,0	0.3	0.2
Jews born in Israel	1.2	0.7	1.7	1.3	-	0,1	2.0	2.2	1.2	0.5	-	-	0.7	0.4	0,0	-	0,4	0,0
Jews born in America or Europe	2.3	1.5	2.4	1.2	0,1	0,0	2.4	1.6	1.0	1.0	0,4	0,1	1.0	0.6	0,0	0,0	0.3	0.2
Jews born in Africa or Asia	1.2	3,8	2.0	1.0	0,1	0,0	2.0	1.5	0.6	0.3	0,2	0,2	0.6	0.3	0,1	0,0	0.3	0,1
Non-Jews	1.3	0.6	1.4	0.7	0,1	0,1	1.5	1.5	0.4	0.3	0,2	0,1	0.8	0.6	0,1	0,1	0,3	0,4
Japan, Hiroshima	1.5	0.8	0.3	0,1	-	0,0	2.2	1.5	1.2	0.5	0,0	0,0	0.5	0,1	-	0,0	0,1	0,1
Japan, Miyagi	1.8	1.1	0,1	0,1	0.4	0.1	2.0	1.1	0.9	0.5	0,1	0,0	0.6	0.3	-	0,0	0.2	0.2
Japan, Nagasaki	1.8	1.4	0.2	0,0	-	-	1.8	1.6	0.7	0.6	0,0	0,0	0.4	0.4	-	-	0.7	0.2
Japan, Osaka	1.5	1.2	0.1	0.0	0.4	0.4	1.7	1.2	0.9	0.4	0.1	0,0	0.7	0.4	0,0	0,0	0.3	0.2
*Japan, Saga																		
Japan, Yamagata																		
*Korea, Kangwha	2,0	0,7	-	-	0,4	-	1,3	0,4	1,2	0,9	-	-	0,7	0,3	-	-	1,6	0,2
*Kuwait: Non-Kuwaitis	2.9	1.4	1,5	2,1	0,2	0,1	1.3	1.0	0.6	0.2	0,0	0,1	0,2	-	-	-	0,1	1,4
*Kuwait: Kuwaitis	0.8	1.0	0.4	0,2	-	0,0	1.5	2.2	0.6	0.5	0,1	-	0,1	0,0	-	-	1.5	0,6
*Philippines, Manila	1.8	1.3	0,2	0,1	0,1	0,0	1.6	1.3	0.4	0.3	0.1	0,1	0.9	1.1	0,0	0,0	0.8	0.9
Singapore: Chinese	2.0	1.6	0.3	0.2	0,0	-	2.2	1.6	1.1	0.4	0,1	-	0,2	0.2	0,0	-	0,1	0,1
Singapore: Malay	1.5	1.1	0,2	-	0,1	-	2.2	2.5	1.4	0.5	-	0,1	0.4	-	0,3	-	0,1	0,1
Singapore: Indian	1,3	0.6	0,2	1,4	-	-	0,9	2,4	0.6	0.5	-	-	0,1	0,5	-	-	-	-
Thailand, Chiang Mai	1.1	0.7	0,1	0,0	0,0	-	2.0	2.0	0.5	0.7	0,1	-	0,1	0,1	-	-	0.8	0.9
*Thailand, Khon Kaen	1.2	0.8	-	-	-	-	0.8	1.0	0.6	0.5	-	-	0,2	0,2	-	-	1.0	1.0
*Viet Nam, Hanoi	0.4	0.3	-	-	0.3	0,1	1.0	0.8	0.3	0.5	0,1	0,1	0.9	1.0	0,2	0,1	0.4	0.4
EUROPE																		
Austria, Tyrol	2.1	1.4	3.5	1.4	0,2	0,1	2.1	1.5	0.9	0.8	0,1	0,2	0,1	0,1	-	-	0,4	0,2
*Belarus																		
*Croatia	2.0	1.2	2.7	1.4	0.1	0.1	1.4	1.2	0.8	0.7	0.9	0.6	0.3	0.2	0.2	0.0	0.2	0.2
Czech Republic	1.6	1.3	3.5	1.4	0.3	0.1	1.6	1.4	1.2	0.9	0.2	0.1	0.5	0.3	0.1	0.0	0.2	0.1
Denmark	1.7	1.3	3.4	1.5	0.1	0.0	2.9	2.2	1.1	0.6	0.1	0.0	0.2	0.2	0,0	0,0	0.1	0.1
Estonia	1.1	1.0	4.2	1.9	0,1	0,0	1.3	0.9	1.1	0.8	0,2	0,1	0.9	0.8	0,1	0,0	-	0,1
Finland																		
France, Bas-Rhin	1.5	1.3	3.0	1.4	0,0	0,0	2.0	1.2	1.1	0.5	0,3	0,1	0.5	0.4	0,0	0,0	0,2	0,1
*France, Calvados	0,1	0,6	1.5	1.0	0,1	0,0	0.4	0.5	0.6	0.5	0,1	0,1	0,1	0,2	-	-	-	0,0
France, Doubs	2.0	1.3	1.4	0.9	0,2	-	2.1	1.7	1.2	0.8	0,2	0,0	0.6	0.2	-	-	0,2	0,2
France, Haut-Rhin	1.6	1.1	2.5	1.3	0,0	0,1	1.5	1.3	0.7	0.6	0,3	0,2	0.5	0.6	-	-	0,3	0,1
*France, Herault	0.7	0.9	1.6	1.0	0,0	-	1.2	0.5	1.2	0.6	0,3	0,0	0.8	0.7	-	0,0	0,1	0,0
France, Isere	1.8	1.4	2.0	0.9	0,1	0,0	2.6	1.3	1.2	0.4	0,1	0,1	0.3	0,1	0,0	-	0,1	0,1
*France, Somme	1.2	1.3	3.5	2.1	-	-	1.2	0.8	1.2	0.8	0,1	-	0.5	0,2	-	-	0,1	0,2
*France, Tarn	1.6	2.1	2.0	0.5	0,1	-	1.1	1.4	0.9	0.5	-	0,2	0.3	0,2	-	-	-	0,0
Germany, Eastern States	1.3	1.0	2.1	1.0	0,1	0,0	1.5	1.3	1.3	0.8	0,0	0.0	0.7	0.6	0,0	0,0	0,0	0,0
Germany, Saarland	1.2	1.2	2.7	1.3	0,1	0,1	2.4	1.5	1.7	1.0	0,2	0,1	0.6	0.5	0,1	0,0	0.3	0.3
Iceland	1,3	1,2	1.2	1.0	-	-	2.2	1.7	0,6	0,4	-	-	0,7	0,8	-	-	-	-
Ireland, Southern	1.6	2.0	4.8	1.1	-	0,0	2.1	1.5	1.4	0.6	0,1	0,1	0,4	0,2	0,1	-	0.6	0,1
Italy, Ferrara	1,7	1,0	2.7	1.8	0,5	0,1	1.4	0,9	0,6	0,3	0,5	0,7	1,2	0,3	-	0,1	0,9	-
Italy, Florence	1.4	1.6	2.2	0.8	0.2	0,1	1.9	1.8	1.7	0.9	0,1	0,1	0.6	0.5	0,1	0,0	0.4	0,1
Italy, Genoa	1.6	1.4	2.3	1.0	0,0	0,0	1.9	1.8	1.0	0.8	0,1	0,1	0.3	0.2	-	0,0	0.3	0,0
*Italy, Latina	2.3	1.6	2.6	1.9	0.3	0,1	2.0	1.7	1.9	0.5	0,1	-	0,6	0,3	0,2	-	0,4	0,5
Italy, Macerata	1,7	2,0	1.7	0,9	-	-	0.8	0.5	1.5	0.6	0,7	0,2	2,3	2,9	-	0,0	0,1	0,2
Italy, Modena	0.8	1.7	2.6	1.6	0,1	-	1.4	2.0	1.3	0.7	0,2	-	0.4	0,2	-	-	0,1	0,1
Italy, Parma	1.3	1.8	1.4	0.4	0,2	0,1	1.9	1.5	0.5	0.7	0,1	0,2	1.0	0.7	-	0,0	0.5	0.3
Italy, Ragusa	2.0	1.4	1.4	1.0	0,1	0,2	1.7	1.0	0.8	0.9	0,3	0,3	0.5	0,2	-	-	0,4	0,2
Italy, Romagna	1.2	1.3	3.7	1.6	0,1	0,4	2.1	1.3	1.4	0.6	0,6	0,3	0.7	0.5	-	-	0,1	0,2
Italy, Torino	2.2	1.9	2.2	0.9	-	0,0	2.2	1.7	1.5	0.6	0,2	0,0	1.1	0.8	0,1	0,0	0.2	0,1
Italy, Trieste	4.7	0,9	4.1	2.7	0,5	0,2	1.2	2.9	1.5	1.3	1.5	0,3	1,1	0.4	0,2	0,0	0.2	0.3
Italy, Varese	2.6	1.6	2.8	1.3	0,0	0,0	2.5	2.0	1.3	1.1	0,2	0,1	0.5	0.3	-	-	0,0	0,0
Italy, Veneto	2.0	1.4	2.0	1.1	0.5	0.4	1.3	1.2	1.1	0.8	1.0	0.6	0.7	0.5	0,1	0,1	0.5	0.4
*Latvia	1.4	1.1	3.3	1.7	0,1	0.1	0.9	0.8	0.9	0.7	0.2	0.2	1.0	0.7	0.3	0.2	0.2	0.1
Malta	1,1	0,7	3.1	1,2	0,3	-	2,0	2.8	1,2	1,0	-	0,2	-	-	-	-	-	0,2

AGE-STANDARDIZED (WORLD) INCIDENCE RATES (FOUR DIGIT RUBRICS)

| | Lymphoid leukaemia | | | | | | Myeloid leukaemia | | | | | | Other and unspec. leukaemia | | | | | |
| | 204.0 | | 204.1 | | 204.2,8-9 | | 205.0 | | 205.1 | | 205.2-3,8-9 | | Acute | | Chronic | | O&U leuk. | |
	M	F	M	F	M	F	M	F	M	F	M	F	M	F	M	F	M	F
The Netherlands	1.6	1.2	2.2	1.0	0.1	0.0	2.2	1.5	0.9	0.5	0.1	0.0	0.4	0.4	0.0	0,0	0.2	0.1
The Netherlands, Eindhoven	1.5	1.2	2.0	0.9	-	0,1	1.8	1.5	0.6	0.4	0,1	0,1	0.3	0.4	-	-	0,2	0,1
The Netherlands, Maastricht	1.9	1.5	2.2	1.2	0,1	0,1	2.5	1.5	1.0	0.6	0,1	0,1	0.3	0.4	0,0	0,0	0,1	0,1
Norway																		
*Poland, Cracow	1.6	0.8	1.4	0.5	0.6	0,2	1.7	1.5	0.7	0,3	0,3	0,2	0.3	-	0,1	0,1	0.6	0.5
*Poland, Kielce	0.9	0.6	2.0	0.7	0.5	0.5	0.9	0.7	0.9	0.9	0,2	0,3	0,1	0,1	0,1	0,0	0.3	0,1
*Poland, Lower Silesia	1.3	0.9	2.4	1.1	0.5	0.3	1.3	1.2	0.9	0.7	0.4	0.2	0.6	0.4	0,1	0,0	0.4	0.2
Poland, Warsaw City	1.4	1.3	1.2	0.5	0.6	0.2	1.6	1.5	0.6	0.4	0.5	0.3	0,1	0.1	0,0	0,0	0.5	0.2
Slovakia	1.7	1.1	3.3	1.5	0.2	0.0	1.7	1.3	1.4	0.9	0.2	0.1	0.3	0.2	0,0	0,0	0.2	0.2
Slovenia	1.4	1.7	2.8	1.8	-	-	1.7	1.2	1.0	0.8	0,0	0,0	0.3	0.2	0,0	0,0	0,0	0,0
*Spain, Albacete	2,7	0,9	3.1	1,3	0,4	-	0.5	1.2	1.6	0,1	-	-	0,4	0,4	0,2	-	0.5	0,1
Spain, Asturias	2.0	0.8	2.8	1.8	0,1	0,2	0.8	0.8	0.8	0.6	0,0	0,1	1.7	1.1	0,0	0,0	1.1	0.7
Spain, Basque Country	2.5	1.2	1.8	0.9	0,1	0,1	1.3	0.8	1.0	0.5	0,1	0,1	1.0	0.8	0,0	0,0	0.2	0.2
Spain, Granada	1.5	1.7	1.8	0.8	0,0	-	1.3	1.0	1.1	0.6	0,1	0,1	0.6	0.9	0,0	-	0.2	0.3
Spain, Mallorca	1.6	1.2	2.2	1.0	0,2	-	1.6	1.8	0.9	0.9	0,2	0,0	0,3	0.4	0,1	0,1	0,2	0.3
Spain, Murcia	1.5	1.5	1.9	1.2	0,0	0,0	2.3	1.4	1.2	0.7	0,2	0,0	0.5	0.3	0,0	-	0,2	0,1
Spain, Navarra	1.4	0,8	2.3	1.3	0,1	0,0	1.5	0.8	1.1	0.6	-	-	1.4	0.8	0,1	-	0,2	0,2
Spain, Tarragona	1.6	1.3	2.4	0.9	0,1	-	1.9	1.2	1.1	0.7	0,1	-	0.4	0.5	0,2	0,0	0.4	0,1
Spain, Zaragoza	1.6	1.4	1.2	0.8	0,1	0,0	1.5	2.1	1.2	0.6	0,1	0,2	0.3	0.4	-	0,0	0,1	0,1
Sweden	1.8	1.4	2.3	1.1	0.2	0.1	2.1	1.8	0.8	0.6	0.1	0.1	1.0	0.8	0.0	0.0	0.2	0.1
*Switzerland, Basel	1.6	0,7	2.2	1.1	-	-	2.1	1.8	0.8	0.6	-	-	0.2	0,1	-	-	0,0	0,0
Switzerland, Geneva	2.3	2.1	3.6	1.3	-	0,0	2.1	1.2	2.0	1.1	0,2	0,1	0.2	0,0	-	0,0	-	0,1
Switzerland, Graubunden	2,0	0,6	3.9	1,4	-	-	1,7	2,1	1.7	1,1	-	-	0,1	0.2	-	-	-	-
Switzerland, Neuchatel	0,9	0,1	3.1	0.8	0,5	0,1	2.1	1.6	0,7	0,4	-	-	0.3	0.2	-	-	0,1	-
Switzerland, St Gall-Appenzell	2.2	1,0	3.0	1.6	-	0,1	2.4	1.2	1.3	0.8	0.5	0,3	0.5	0,4	0,0	-	0,1	0,1
Switzerland, Valais	3.0	1,5	1.9	1.1	-	-	1.4	0,8	0,9	1,0	-	-	1,3	0,2	0,1	-	0,2	0,2
Switzerland, Vaud	1.0	1.1	1.9	0.8	-	0,1	2.0	1.4	1.6	0.5	0,3	0,1	0.6	0.3	0,1	-	0,2	0,1
Switzerland, Zurich	1.9	1.4	2.3	1.6	0,1	0,0	2.2	1.2	1.5	0.6	0,1	0,0	0.6	0.5	0,0	-	0,1	0,1
*UK, England and Wales	1.8	1.3	2.3	1.1	0.1	0.1	2.2	1.7	1.1	0.7	0.1	0.1	0.4	0.3	0.0	0.0	0.3	0.2
*UK, East Anglia																		
*UK, Mersey	1.0	1.2	1.3	0.8	0.1	0.1	1.9	1.4	0.8	0.5	0,1	0,1	0.2	0.2	0,0	0,0	0.1	0.1
*UK, North Western	1.5	1.0	2.1	0.9	0.1	0.0	2.2	1.7	0.8	0.5	0.2	0.1	0.2	0.1	0,0	0,0	0.2	0.1
UK, Oxford	2.0	1.6	2.2	1.0	0,1	0.1	2.5	2.3	1.6	0.9	0.1	0.1	0.6	0.3	0.1	0,0	0.1	0.1
*UK, South Thames	1.8	1.3	2.2	1.0	0.1	0.1	2.3	1.9	1.0	0.6	0.1	0.1	0.2	0.1	0.1	0.0	0.3	0.2
UK, South Western	1.9	1.4	2.8	1.5	0.3	0.2	2.2	1.6	1.3	0.8	0.2	0.1	0.6	0.4	0,0	0,0	0.1	0.1
UK, Wessex	2.1	1.3	2.7	1.7	0.2	0.1	2.8	1.9	1.5	0.9	0.2	0.2	0.4	0.2	0,0	0.1	0.2	0.1
*UK, West Midlands	2.1	1.2	2.5	1.1	0,0	0,0	2.1	1.7	1.1	0.7	0.1	0.0	0.6	0.4	0.0	0.0	0.4	0.2
UK, Yorkshire	1.7	1.3	2.7	1.1	0.1	0.1	2.3	1.7	1.1	0.6	0,0	0,0	0.3	0.2	0,0	0,0	0.1	0.0
UK, Scotland	2.0	1.3	2.6	1.2	0.1	0.1	2.1	1.7	0.9	0.7	0.2	0.1	0.3	0.2	0,0	0,0	0.2	0.2
UK, Scotland, West	2.1	1.2	2.3	1.1	0.2	0.1	2.2	1.6	0.8	0.6	0.2	0.1	0.2	0.2	0,0	0,0	0.3	0.3
*Yugoslavia, Vojvodina																		

OCEANIA

| | Lymphoid leukaemia | | | | | | Myeloid leukaemia | | | | | | Other and unspec. leukaemia | | | | | |
| | 204.0 | | 204.1 | | 204.2,8-9 | | 205.0 | | 205.1 | | 205.2-3,8-9 | | Acute | | Chronic | | O&U leuk. | |
	M	F	M	F	M	F	M	F	M	F	M	F	M	F	M	F	M	F
Australian Capital Territory	2.0	0,9	3.6	1,2	-	-	3.3	1.5	1,2	0,8	0,2	0,2	0.2	0,1	-	-	-	-
Australia, New South Wales	1.9	1.6	2.8	1.4	0.1	0.1	2.8	1.8	1.7	0.8	0.3	0.1	0.6	0.4	0,0	0,0	0.2	0.1
South Australia	1.8	1.7	5.6	3.3	-	-	3.6	2.2	1.8	1.2	0,0	-	0.4	0.3	-	0,0	0,0	0,1
Australia, Tasmania	2.7	0,8	4.0	2.4	-	-	2.8	2.5	1.1	1.1	0,1	-	0.1	0.1	0,1	-	0.5	0,1
Australia, Victoria	2.7	1.6	2.4	1.0	0.1	0.1	2.5	1.8	1.4	0.9	0.1	0,0	0.5	0.4	0,0	0,0	0.2	0.1
Western Australia	1.7	1.2	2.0	1.1	0,1	-	2.6	1.9	1.6	0.7	0.2	0,1	0.9	0.4	0,0	0,0	0,1	0,1
*French Polynesia	0,5	1,1	1.2	0,9	0,2	0,2	1.8	0.8	1,0	1,1	0,4	0,4	2,2	0,6	-	-	2,1	2,0
New Zealand: Non-Maori	2.2	1.9	3.0	1.5	0.1	0.1	3.1	2.1	1.4	0.9	0.2	0.1	0.4	0.3	0,1	0,0	0.3	0.1
New Zealand: Maori	2.3	0.8	1,6	0,8	-	-	4.0	3.8	2.2	0.7	0,6	-	1.0	0.8	-	-	0,7	1,0
US, Hawaii: White	2.1	1,3	3.1	1.7	-	0,1	3.1	0,6	1.0	0.7	0,1	-	0,7	0.4	-	-	0.5	-
US, Hawaii: Japanese	1,3	2,0	0.3	0,2	-	-	1.5	0.7	1,1	1.0	0,1	0,1	1.2	0.2	-	0,0	0,2	0,0
US, Hawaii: Hawaiian	1,4	1.9	0,9	1,8	-	-	4.4	2.2	1,0	0.3	-	-	1,7	0,5	-	-	0,2	-
US, Hawaii: Filipino	2,1	0,9	0,6	-	0,1	-	2.6	2.8	1,3	1,4	0,3	-	0,5	0,4	-	-	0,6	0,4
US, Hawaii: Chinese	-	-	0,8	0,2	-	-	4,0	0,4	-	-	-	-	0,4	0,7	-	-	-	0,3

CUMULATIVE INCIDENCE (0-74)
RATES AND STANDARD ERRORS (percent)

CUMULATIVE INCIDENCE (0-74)
RATES AND STANDARD ERRORS (percent)
Lip (ICD-9 140)

	MALE		FEMALE	
AFRICA				
*Algeria, Setif				
*France, La Reunion				
*Mali, Bamako				
*Uganda, Kyadondo				
*Zimbabwe, Harare: African				
*Zimbabwe, Harare: European				
AMERICA, CENTRAL AND SOUTH				
*Argentina, Concordia	0,24	0,13	-	-
*Brazil, Belem	0.18	0.07	0,01	0,01
*Brazil, Goiania				
*Brazil, Porto Alegre	0.14	0.04	0,00	0,00 m
Colombia, Cali	0,03	0,01	0,00	0,00 m
*Costa Rica	0.14	0.02	0.06	0.01
*Ecuador, Quito	0,02	0,02	-	-
*Peru, Lima	0,03	0,01	0,01	0,01
Peru, Trujillo	0,07	0,05	0,02	0,02
US, Puerto Rico	0.08	0.01	0.02	0.01
*Uruguay, Montevideo	0.11	0.03	0,01	0,01
AMERICA, NORTH				
Canada	0.38	0.01	0.05	0.00
Canada, Alberta	0.57	0.04	0.11	0.02
Canada, British Columbia	0.20	0.02	0.03	0.01
Canada, Manitoba	0.67	0.06	0.10	0.02
Canada, New Brunswick	0.36	0.05	0,02	0,01
Canada, Newfoundland	1.53	0.13	0.10	0.03
Canada, Northwest Territories	0,24	0,24	-	-
Canada, Nova Scotia	0.39	0.05	0,02	0,01
Canada, Ontario	0.36	0.01	0.06	0.01
Canada, Prince Edward Island	0.77	0.18	0,04	0,04
Canada, Quebec	0.19	0.01	0.02	0.00
Canada, Saskatchewan	0.99	0.07	0.08	0.02
Canada, Yukon	0,21	0,15	0,27	0,27
US, Cent. Calif.: Non-Hisp. White	0.36	0.04	0.03	0.01
US, Cent. Calif.: Hispanic	0.22	0.07	0,01	0,01
US, Los Angeles: Non-Hisp. White	0.20	0.02	0.04	0.01
US, Los Angeles: Hispanic White	0.07	0.02	0,01	0,01
US, Los Angeles: Black	-	-	0,01	0,01
US, Los Angeles: Chinese	-	-	-	-
US, Los Angeles: Filipino	0,03	0,02	-	-
US, Los Angeles: Korean	0,02	0,02	-	-
US, Los Angeles: Japanese	-	-	-	-
US, San Francisco: Non-Hisp. White	0.22	0.02	0.04	0.01
US, San Francisco: Hispanic White	0,04	0,03	0,01	0,01
US, San Francisco: Black	0,03	0,02	-	-
US, San Francisco: Chinese	-	-	-	-
US, San Francisco: Filipino	-	-	0,11	0,07
US, San Francisco: Japanese	-	-	0,08	0,08
US, Connecticut: White	0.05	0.01	0,01	0,00
US, Connecticut: Black	-	-	-	-
US, Atlanta: White	0.16	0.03	0,01	0,01
US, Atlanta: Black	-	-	0,02	0,02
US, Iowa	0.44	0.03	0.04	0.01

	MALE		FEMALE	
US, Central Louisiana: White	0.28	0.08	0,02	0,02
US, Central Louisiana: Black	-	-	-	-
US, New Orleans: White	0.15	0.04	0,01	0,01
US, New Orleans: Black	0,04	0,02	-	-
US, Detroit: White	0.10	0.01	0,01	0,00
US, Detroit: Black	-	-	0,01	0,01
US, New Mexico: Non-Hisp. White	0.51	0.06	0.08	0.02
US, New Mexico: Hispanic White	0.18	0.05	0,01	0,01
US, New Mexico: American Indian	0,19	0,14	0,02	0,02
US, Utah	0.50	0.05	0.07	0.02
US, Seattle	0.22	0.02	0.04	0.01
US, SEER: White	0.22	0.01	0.03	0.00
US, SEER: Black	0,01	0,00	0,01	0,00
ASIA				
*China, Qidong	0,02	0,01	0,01	0,01
China, Shanghai	0.01	0.00	0.01	0.00
China, Tianjin	0,01	0,01	0,01	0,00
Hong Kong	0.01	0.00	0,00	0,00
*India, Bangalore	0,01	0,01	0,02	0,01
*India, Barshi, Paranda and Bhum	0,05	0,03	-	-
India, Bombay	0.04	0.01	0.03	0.01
*India, Karunagappally	0,08	0,05	0,14	0,09
India, Madras	0.05	0.01	0.06	0.01
*India, Trivandrum	0,20	0,09	-	-
Israel: All Jews	0.37	0.02	0.10	0.01
Jews born in Israel	0.65	0.12	0.15	0.05
Jews born in America or Europe	0.43	0.04	0.11	0.02
Jews born in Africa or Asia	0.16	0.03	0.04	0.01
Non-Jews	0.14	0.04	0,12	0,05
Japan, Hiroshima	0,00	0,00	0,01	0,01
Japan, Miyagi	0.03	0.01	0.01	0.00
Japan, Nagasaki	0,01	0,01	-	-
Japan, Osaka	0,00	0,00	0,00	0,00
*Japan, Saga	0,01	0,01	-	-
Japan, Yamagata	0,00	0,00	0,01	0,01
*Korea, Kangwha	-	-	-	-
*Kuwait: Non-Kuwaitis	0,10	0,08	0,01	0,01
*Kuwait: Kuwaitis	0,01	0,01	-	-
*Philippines, Manila	0,01	0,00	0,01	0,01
Singapore: Chinese	0,00	0,00	-	-
Singapore: Malay	-	-	-	-
Singapore: Indian	-	-	0,20	0,15
Thailand, Chiang Mai	0,02	0,01	0,03	0,01
*Thailand, Khon Kaen	0,04	0,02	0.36	0.06
*Viet Nam, Hanoi				

* IMPORTANT-SEE NOTES ON POPULATION PAGE

EUROPE	MALE		FEMALE				MALE		FEMALE	
Austria, Tyrol	0,04	0,02	-	-		Sweden	0.18	0.01	0.04	0.00
*Belarus	0.70	0.02	0.10	0.01		*Switzerland, Basel	0,06	0,02	-	-
*Croatia	0.36	0.02	0.07	0.01		Switzerland, Geneva	0.16	0.04	0,03	0,01
Czech Republic	0.19	0.01	0.03	0.00		Switzerland, Graubunden	0.32	0.10	0,09	0,05
Denmark	0.32	0.02	0.05	0.01		Switzerland, Neuchatel	0,14	0,07	0,04	0,03
Estonia	0.28	0.04	0.03	0.01		Switzerland, St Gall-Appenzell	0.16	0.04	0,06	0,02
Finland	0.42	0.02	0.08	0.01		Switzerland, Valais	0,03	0,03	-	-
France, Bas-Rhin	0.06	0.02	-	-		Switzerland, Vaud	0.11	0.03	-	-
*France, Calvados	0.16	0.04	0,03	0,02		Switzerland, Zurich	0.14	0.02	0.04	0.01
France, Doubs	0,03	0,02	-	-		*UK, England and Wales	0.05	0.00	0.01	0.00
France, Haut-Rhin	0.11	0.03	0,02	0,01		*UK, East Anglia	0.18	0.02	0.02	0.01
*France, Herault	0.14	0.03	0,02	0,01		*UK, Mersey	0,01	0,00	-	-
France, Isere	0.07	0.02	0,01	0,01		*UK, North Western	0.04	0.01	0.01	0.00
*France, Somme	0.22	0.04	-	-		UK, Oxford	0.07	0.01	0.02	0.01
*France, Tarn	0.31	0.06	0,01	0,01		*UK, South Thames	0.02	0.00	0.01	0,00
Germany, Eastern States	0.19	0.01	0.02	0.00		UK, South Western	0.06	0.01	0.01	0,00
Germany, Saarland	0.10	0.02	0,02	0,01		UK, Wessex	0.07	0.01	0.02	0.00
Iceland	0.27	0.09	0,02	0,02		*UK, West Midlands	0.02	0.00	0.00	0,00
Ireland, Southern	0.40	0.06	0,05	0,02		UK, Yorkshire	0.06	0.01	0.01	0.00
Italy, Ferrara	0,18	0,07	0,02	0,02		UK, Scotland	0.13	0.01	0.03	0.00
Italy, Florence	0.06	0.02	0,02	0,01		UK, Scotland, West	0.15	0.02	0.03	0.01
Italy, Genoa	0.05	0.02	0,01	0,01		*Yugoslavia, Vojvodina	0.41	0.03	0.09	0.01
*Italy, Latina	0.29	0.06	0,06	0,03						
Italy, Macerata	0,05	0,05	-	-		**OCEANIA**				
Italy, Modena	0,01	0,01	-	-		Australian Capital Territory	0.91	0.17	0,11	0,05
Italy, Parma	0,04	0,02	-	-		Australia, New South Wales	0.56	0.02	0.15	0.01
Italy, Ragusa	0.51	0.09	0,05	0,02		South Australia	1.48	0.07	0.32	0.03
Italy, Romagna	0,01	0,01	0,01	0,01		Australia, Tasmania	0.75	0.09	0.11	0.03
Italy, Torino	0.16	0.03	0,02	0,01		Australia, Victoria	0.58	0.03	0.15	0.01
Italy, Trieste	0.27	0.07	0,03	0,02		Western Australia	0.94	0.06	0.22	0.03
Italy, Varese	0.15	0.03	-	-		*French Polynesia	-	-	-	-
Italy, Veneto	0.17	0.03	0,02	0,01		New Zealand: Non-Maori	0.37	0.03	0.10	0.01
*Latvia	0.38	0.03	0.03	0.01		New Zealand: Maori	0,14	0,11	-	-
Malta	0,24	0,10	-	- m		US, Hawaii: White	0.22	0.06	0,09	0,05
The Netherlands	0.19	0.01	0.03	0.00		US, Hawaii: Japanese	0,02	0,02	-	-
The Netherlands, Eindhoven	0.26	0.04	0.06	0.02		US, Hawaii: Hawaiian	0,01	0,01	-	-
The Netherlands, Maastricht	0.11	0.03	0,02	0,01		US, Hawaii: Filipino	-	-	-	-
Norway	0.27	0.02	0.06	0.01		US, Hawaii: Chinese	-	-	-	-
*Poland, Cracow	0.15	0.04	0,02	0,01						
*Poland, Kielce	0.77	0.06	0.09	0.02						
*Poland, Lower Silesia	0.42	0.03	0.04	0.01						
Poland, Warsaw City	0.14	0.02	0,02	0,01						
Slovakia	0.48	0.03	0.08	0.01						
Slovenia	0.23	0.03	0.03	0.01						
*Spain, Albacete	0,31	0,11	-	-						
Spain, Asturias	0.26	0.04	0,03	0,01						
Spain, Basque Country	0.56	0.04	0.03	0.01						
Spain, Granada	1.47	0.10	0.07	0.02						
Spain, Mallorca	0.66	0.07	0,04	0,02						
Spain, Murcia	1.32	0.08	0.06	0.02						
Spain, Navarra	0.82	0.08	0,01	0,01						
Spain, Tarragona	0.79	0.08	0,04	0,02						
Spain, Zaragoza	0.75	0.06	0,01	0,01 f						

* IMPORTANT-SEE NOTES ON POPULATION PAGE

CUMULATIVE INCIDENCE (0-74)
RATES AND STANDARD ERRORS (percent)
Tongue (ICD-9 141)

	MALE		FEMALE	
AFRICA				
*Algeria, Setif				
*France, La Reunion				
*Mali, Bamako				
*Uganda, Kyadondo				
*Zimbabwe, Harare: African				
*Zimbabwe, Harare: European				
AMERICA, CENTRAL AND SOUTH				
*Argentina, Concordia	0,23	0,09	0,07	0,07
*Brazil, Belem	0.52	0.11	0.23	0.06
*Brazil, Goiania				
*Brazil, Porto Alegre	0.52	0.07	0.08	0.02
Colombia, Cali	0.14	0.03	0.12	0.03
*Costa Rica	0.12	0.02	0.06	0.01
*Ecuador, Quito	0,04	0,02	0,04	0,02 m
*Peru, Lima	0.05	0.02	0.06	0.02
Peru, Trujillo	0,12	0,08	-	-
US, Puerto Rico	0.48	0.03	0.09	0.01
*Uruguay, Montevideo	0.38	0.05	0.06	0.02
AMERICA, NORTH				
Canada	0.27	0.01	0.09	0.00
Canada, Alberta	0.19	0.02	0.08	0.01
Canada, British Columbia	0.27	0.02	0.12	0.01
Canada, Manitoba	0.25	0.03	0.12	0.02
Canada, New Brunswick	0.25	0.04	0,04	0,02
Canada, Newfoundland	0.16	0.04	0,07	0,03
Canada, Northwest Territories	0,11	0,10	0,11	0,09
Canada, Nova Scotia	0.28	0.04	0.06	0.02
Canada, Ontario	0.29	0.01	0.10	0.01
Canada, Prince Edward Island	0.37	0.12	0,12	0,07
Canada, Quebec	0.28	0.01	0.07	0.01
Canada, Saskatchewan	0.18	0.03	0.05	0.02
Canada, Yukon	-	-	0,39	0,27
US, Cent. Calif.: Non-Hisp. White	0.33	0.03	0.16	0.02
US, Cent. Calif.: Hispanic	0.23	0.07	0,09	0,04
US, Los Angeles: Non-Hisp. White	0.36	0.02	0.16	0.01
US, Los Angeles: Hispanic White	0.17	0.03	0.07	0.01
US, Los Angeles: Black	0.46	0.06	0.10	0.02
US, Los Angeles: Chinese	0,09	0,05	0,04	0,03
US, Los Angeles: Filipino	0,11	0,08	0,09	0,05
US, Los Angeles: Korean	0,13	0,08	0,01	0,01
US, Los Angeles: Japanese	0,16	0,07	0,13	0,06
US, San Francisco: Non-Hisp. White	0.39	0.03	0.21	0.02
US, San Francisco: Hispanic White	0.25	0.07	0,07	0,03
US, San Francisco: Black	0.50	0.09	0,08	0,03
US, San Francisco: Chinese	0,06	0,03	0,09	0,04
US, San Francisco: Filipino	0,19	0,10	0,04	0,03
US, San Francisco: Japanese	-	-	0,29	0,15
US, Connecticut: White	0.35	0.02	0.13	0.01
US, Connecticut: Black	0.70	0.14	0.19	0.06
US, Atlanta: White	0.22	0.03	0.14	0.02
US, Atlanta: Black	0.52	0.10	0.10	0.03
US, Iowa	0.22	0.02	0.11	0.01

	MALE		FEMALE	
US, Central Louisiana: White	0.31	0.08	0,16	0,06
US, Central Louisiana: Black	0,56	0,24	-	-
US, New Orleans: White	0.28	0.05	0.12	0.03
US, New Orleans: Black	0.32	0.08	0.10	0,04
US, Detroit: White	0.40	0.03	0.13	0.01
US, Detroit: Black	0.56	0.06	0.13	0.03
US, New Mexico: Non-Hisp. White	0.27	0.04	0.11	0.02
US, New Mexico: Hispanic White	0.22	0.06	0,01	0,01
US, New Mexico: American Indian	0,05	0,05	0,08	0,08
US, Utah	0.21	0.03	0.11	0.02
US, Seattle	0.32	0.02	0.14	0.01
US, SEER: White	0.31	0.01	0.13	0.01
US, SEER: Black	0.53	0.04	0.12	0.02
ASIA				
*China, Qidong	0.02	0,01	0.03	0,01
China, Shanghai	0.07	0.01	0.06	0.01
China, Tianjin	0.05	0.01	0.06	0.01
Hong Kong	0.24	0.01	0.14	0.01
*India, Bangalore	0.42	0.03	0.15	0.02
*India, Barshi, Paranda and Bhum	0.28	0.07	0,05	0,03
India, Bombay	0.78	0.03	0.26	0.02
*India, Karunagappally	0.58	0.15	0.47	0.15
India, Madras	0.71	0.04	0.23	0.03
*India, Trivandrum	0.57	0.12	0.21	0.07
Israel: All Jews	0.09	0.01	0.07	0.01
Jews born in Israel	0.12	0.06	0.07	0,03
Jews born in America or Europe	0.09	0.02	0.07	0.01
Jews born in Africa or Asia	0.11	0.03	0.05	0.02
Non-Jews	0,03	0,03	0,07	0,04
Japan, Hiroshima	0.22	0.03	0.07	0.02
Japan, Miyagi	0.18	0.02	0.07	0.01
Japan, Nagasaki	0.17	0.02	0.08	0.01
Japan, Osaka	0.18	0.01	0.08	0.01
*Japan, Saga	0.17	0.03	0.05	0.01
Japan, Yamagata	0.05	0.01	0.03	0.01
*Korea, Kangwha	0,11	0,08	0,04	0,04
*Kuwait: Non-Kuwaitis	0.10	0.08	0,05	0,04
*Kuwait: Kuwaitis	0,03	0,03	0,03	0,03
*Philippines, Manila	0.32	0.04	0.25	0.03
Singapore: Chinese	0.15	0.02	0.07	0.01
Singapore: Malay	0,04	0,02	0,02	0,02
Singapore: Indian	0.30	0.08	0.05	0,04
Thailand, Chiang Mai	0.25	0.04	0.17	0.03
*Thailand, Khon Kaen	0.15	0.04	0.09	0.03
*Viet Nam, Hanoi				

EUROPE	MALE		FEMALE	
Austria, Tyrol	0.20	0.04	0,03	0,01
*Belarus	0.31	0.01	0.03	0.00
*Croatia	0.43	0.02	0.04	0.01
Czech Republic	0.24	0.01	0.04	0.00
Denmark	0.15	0.01	0.06	0.01
Estonia	0.30	0.03	0.04	0.01
Finland	0.11	0.01	0.07	0.01
France, Bas-Rhin	0.97	0.07	0.12	0.02
*France, Calvados	0.88	0.08	0.08	0.02
France, Doubs	0.62	0.09	0.11	0.03
France, Haut-Rhin	1.00	0.09	0.08	0.02
*France, Herault	0.50	0.05	0.10	0.02
France, Isere	0.49	0.05	0.06	0.01
*France, Somme	0.74	0.08	0,06	0,02
*France, Tarn	0.43	0.07	0,05	0,02
Germany, Eastern States	0.18	0.01	0.03	0.00
Germany, Saarland	0.47	0.04	0.06	0.01
Iceland	0,19	0,07	0,07	0,04
Ireland, Southern	0.17	0.04	0,08	0,03
Italy, Ferrara	0,21	0,07	0,03	0,03
Italy, Florence	0.21	0.03	0.06	0.02
Italy, Genoa	0.32	0.04	0.08	0.02
*Italy, Latina	0.18	0.05	0,02	0,02
Italy, Macerata	0,14	0,06	0,03	0,03
Italy, Modena	0.24	0.04	0,04	0,02
Italy, Parma	0.24	0.05	0,05	0,02
Italy, Ragusa	0,14	0,05	0,05	0,03
Italy, Romagna	0.19	0.04	0,02	0,01
Italy, Torino	0.24	0.03	0.09	0.02
Italy, Trieste	0.25	0.06	0,12	0,04
Italy, Varese	0.42	0.05	0,03	0,01
Italy, Veneto	0.48	0.04	0.10	0.02
*Latvia	0.25	0.02	0.02	0.01
Malta	0,17	0,09	0,14	0,06
The Netherlands	0.16	0.01	0.08	0.01
The Netherlands, Eindhoven	0.12	0.03	0.08	0.02
The Netherlands, Maastricht	0.19	0.03	0.07	0.02
Norway	0.16	0.01	0.06	0.01
*Poland, Cracow	0.17	0.04	0,01	0,01
*Poland, Kielce	0.09	0.02	0,03	0,01
*Poland, Lower Silesia	0.19	0.02	0.04	0.01
Poland, Warsaw City	0.21	0.03	0.06	0.01
Slovakia	0.56	0.02	0.03	0.01
Slovenia	0.44	0.04	0.03	0.01
*Spain, Albacete	0,26	0,09	0,03	0,03
Spain, Asturias	0.61	0.05	0.10	0.02
Spain, Basque Country	0.54	0.04	0.04	0.01
Spain, Granada	0.34	0.04	0.07	0.02
Spain, Mallorca	0.33	0.05	0,04	0,02
Spain, Murcia	0.44	0.05	0.09	0.02
Spain, Navarra	0.29	0.05	0.09	0.03
Spain, Tarragona	0.35	0.05	0,06	0,02
Spain, Zaragoza	0.31	0.04	0,04	0,01

	MALE		FEMALE	
Sweden	0.12	0.01	0.06	0.01
*Switzerland, Basel	0.30	0.05	0,05	0,02
Switzerland, Geneva	0.47	0.08	0.14	0.04
Switzerland, Graubunden	0,12	0,06	0,11	0,06
Switzerland, Neuchatel	0.44	0.11	0,11	0,05
Switzerland, St Gall-Appenzell	0.17	0.04	0.09	0.03
Switzerland, Valais	0.32	0.08	0.08	0.04
Switzerland, Vaud	0.61	0.07	0.16	0.03
Switzerland, Zurich	0.26	0.03	0.07	0.01
*UK, England and Wales	0.14	0.00	0.06	0.00
*UK, East Anglia	0.08	0.01	0.06	0.01
*UK, Mersey	0.16	0.02	0.05	0.01
*UK, North Western	0.17	0.01	0.06	0.01
UK, Oxford	0.13	0.02	0.06	0.01
*UK, South Thames	0.12	0.01	0.06	0.01
UK, South Western	0.12	0.01	0.06	0.01
UK, Wessex	0.13	0.01	0.09	0.01
*UK, West Midlands	0.15	0.01	0.06	0.01
UK, Yorkshire	0.15	0.01	0.06	0.01
UK, Scotland	0.23	0.01	0.07	0.01
UK, Scotland, West	0.24	0.02	0.07	0.01
*Yugoslavia, Vojvodina	0.39	0.03	0.03	0.01

OCEANIA

	MALE		FEMALE	
Australian Capital Territory	0.31	0.11	0,10	0,04
Australia, New South Wales	0.28	0.02	0.12	0.01
South Australia	0.24	0.03	0.07	0.01
Australia, Tasmania	0.28	0.05	0.10	0.03
Australia, Victoria	0.26	0.02	0.10	0.01
Western Australia	0.37	0.04	0.09	0.02
*French Polynesia	0.37	0.12	0,14	0,09
New Zealand: Non-Maori	0.17	0.02	0.08	0.01
New Zealand: Maori	0,23	0,09	0,11	0,06
US, Hawaii: White	0.40	0.09	0,13	0,05
US, Hawaii: Japanese	0.20	0.05	0,08	0,03
US, Hawaii: Hawaiian	0,23	0,09	0,12	0,07
US, Hawaii: Filipino	0,07	0,05	0,15	0,07
US, Hawaii: Chinese	0,04	0,04	0,20	0,10

* IMPORTANT-SEE NOTES ON POPULATION PAGE

CUMULATIVE INCIDENCE (0-74)
RATES AND STANDARD ERRORS (percent)
Salivary gland (ICD-9 142)

	MALE		FEMALE	
AFRICA				
*Algeria, Setif				
*France, La Reunion				
*Mali, Bamako				
*Uganda, Kyadondo				
*Zimbabwe, Harare: African				
*Zimbabwe, Harare: European				
AMERICA, CENTRAL AND SOUTH				
*Argentina, Concordia	0,17	0,11	0,11	0,08
*Brazil, Belem	0,12	0,05	0,10	0,04 f
*Brazil, Goiania				
*Brazil, Porto Alegre	0,07	0,03	0,05	0,02
Colombia, Cali	0,08	0,03	0.06	0.02 mf
*Costa Rica	0.04	0.01	0.05	0.01
*Ecuador, Quito	0,05	0,02	0,05	0,02
*Peru, Lima	0.07	0.02	0.06	0.02
Peru, Trujillo	-	-	0,03	0,02
US, Puerto Rico	0.04	0.01	0.04	0.01
*Uruguay, Montevideo	0.10	0.02	0.05	0.01
AMERICA, NORTH				
Canada	0.09	0.00	0.05	0.00
Canada, Alberta	0.08	0.01	0.04	0.01
Canada, British Columbia	0.08	0.01	0.06	0.01
Canada, Manitoba	0.08	0.02	0.06	0.02
Canada, New Brunswick	0.07	0.02	0.04	0.01
Canada, Newfoundland	0,07	0,03	0,05	0,02
Canada, Northwest Territories	0.40	0.16	0,24	0,16
Canada, Nova Scotia	0.08	0.02	0.04	0,01
Canada, Ontario	0.09	0.01	0.06	0.00
Canada, Prince Edward Island	0,09	0,06	0,04	0,04
Canada, Quebec	0.10	0.01	0.05	0.01
Canada, Saskatchewan	0.06	0.02	0.07	0.02
Canada, Yukon	0,08	0,08	-	-
US, Cent. Calif.: Non-Hisp. White	0.12	0.02	0.06	0.01
US, Cent. Calif.: Hispanic	0,01	0,01	0,07	0,03
US, Los Angeles: Non-Hisp. White	0.11	0.01	0.08	0.01
US, Los Angeles: Hispanic White	0.03	0.01	0.04	0.01
US, Los Angeles: Black	0.10	0.03	0.04	0.01
US, Los Angeles: Chinese	0,11	0,05	0,03	0,02
US, Los Angeles: Filipino	0,02	0,02	0,11	0,05
US, Los Angeles: Korean	-	-	-	-
US, Los Angeles: Japanese	0,07	0,05	-	-
US, San Francisco: Non-Hisp. White	0.14	0.02	0.07	0.01
US, San Francisco: Hispanic White	0,14	0,06	0,04	0,02
US, San Francisco: Black	0,12	0,04	0,05	0,03
US, San Francisco: Chinese	0,08	0,04	0,02	0,02
US, San Francisco: Filipino	0,05	0,04	0,17	0,06
US, San Francisco: Japanese	-	-	0,27	0,17
US, Connecticut: White	0.12	0.01	0.09	0.01
US, Connecticut: Black	0,06	0,04	0,08	0,03
US, Atlanta: White	0.09	0.02	0.05	0.01
US, Atlanta: Black	0,14	0,05	0.11	0.03
US, Iowa	0.09	0.01	0.06	0.01

	MALE		FEMALE	
US, Central Louisiana: White	0,04	0,03	0,02	0,02
US, Central Louisiana: Black	-	-	0,07	0,07
US, New Orleans: White	0.15	0.03	0.09	0.02
US, New Orleans: Black	0,13	0,05	0,07	0,03
US, Detroit: White	0.11	0.01	0.09	0.01
US, Detroit: Black	0.07	0.02	0.05	0.02
US, New Mexico: Non-Hisp. White	0.11	0.03	0.06	0.02
US, New Mexico: Hispanic White	0,02	0,01	0,03	0,02
US, New Mexico: American Indian	-	-	0,02	0,02
US, Utah	0.12	0.02	0.04	0.01
US, Seattle	0.10	0.01	0.08	0.01
US, SEER: White	0.11	0.01	0.07	0.00
US, SEER: Black	0.09	0.02	0.07	0.01
ASIA				
*China, Qidong	0,04	0,01	0,00	0,00
China, Shanghai	0.05	0.01	0.04	0.00
China, Tianjin	0.04	0.01	0.02	0.01
Hong Kong	0.08	0.01	0.06	0.01
*India, Bangalore	0.07	0.01	0.03	0.01
*India, Barshi, Paranda and Bhum	0,09	0,05	0,00	0,00
India, Bombay	0.08	0.01	0.03	0.01
*India, Karunagappally	0,03	0,03	-	-
India, Madras	0.07	0.02	0.05	0.01
*India, Trivandrum	-	-	0,06	0,03
Israel: All Jews	0.08	0.01	0.05	0.01
Jews born in Israel	0.03	0.01	0.05	0.01
Jews born in America or Europe	0.10	0.02	0.04	0.01
Jews born in Africa or Asia	0.06	0.02	0.05	0.02
Non-Jews	0,01	0,01	0,00	0,00
Japan, Hiroshima	0.07	0.02	0.03	0,01
Japan, Miyagi	0.07	0.01	0.03	0,01
Japan, Nagasaki	0.04	0.01	0.04	0.01
Japan, Osaka	0.05	0.01	0.02	0.00
*Japan, Saga	0.06	0.02	0.02	0,01
Japan, Yamagata	0.04	0.01	0.03	0.01
*Korea, Kangwha	0,22	0,11	-	-
*Kuwait: Non-Kuwaitis	0,10	0,08	0,01	0,01
*Kuwait: Kuwaitis	0,02	0,01	0,09	0,05
*Philippines, Manila	0.15	0.02	0.13	0.02
Singapore: Chinese	0.07	0.02	0.06	0.01
Singapore: Malay	0,09	0,04	0,02	0,02
Singapore: Indian	0,06	0,05	0,05	0,05
Thailand, Chiang Mai	0.04	0.01	0.05	0.02
*Thailand, Khon Kaen	0,04	0,02	0,03	0,02
*Viet Nam, Hanoi				

* IMPORTANT-SEE NOTES ON POPULATION PAGE

CUMULATIVE INCIDENCE (0-74)
RATES AND STANDARD ERRORS (percent)
Salivary gland (ICD-9 142) (contd)

EUROPE	MALE		FEMALE	
Austria, Tyrol	0.04	0.02	0.05	0.02
*Belarus	0.10	0.01	0.04	0.00
*Croatia	0.14	0.01	0.05	0.01
Czech Republic	0.10	0.01	0.05	0.00
Denmark	0.06	0.01	0.04	0.01
Estonia	0.05	0.02	0.06	0.01
Finland	0.07	0.01	0.06	0.01
France, Bas-Rhin	0.10	0.03	0.07	0.02
*France, Calvados	0.04	0.02	0.03	0.02
France, Doubs	0.04	0.02	0.04	0.02
France, Haut-Rhin	0.05	0.02	0.04	0.02
*France, Herault	0.04	0.02	0.04	0.01
France, Isere	0.05	0.02	0.05	0.01
*France, Somme	0.09	0.03	0.03	0.02
*France, Tarn	0.07	0.03	0.01	0.01
Germany, Eastern States	0.06	0.01	0.03	0.00
Germany, Saarland	0.08	0.02	0.03	0.01
Iceland	0.10	0.05	0.04	0.02
Ireland, Southern	0.12	0.03	0.03	0.02
Italy, Ferrara	0.06	0.04	0.04	0.03
Italy, Florence	0.08	0.02	0.04	0.01
Italy, Genoa	0.11	0.02	0.04	0.01
*Italy, Latina	0.15	0.05	0.07	0.03
Italy, Macerata	0.03	0.03	-	-
Italy, Modena	0.05	0.02	0.03	0.01
Italy, Parma	0.01	0.01	0.02	0.01
Italy, Ragusa	0.05	0.03	0.05	0.03
Italy, Romagna	0.13	0.03	0.11	0.03
Italy, Torino	0.06	0.02	0.02	0.01
Italy, Trieste	0.19	0.06	0.08	0.03
Italy, Varese	0.07	0.02	0.04	0.01
Italy, Veneto	0.10	0.02	0.03	0.01
*Latvia	0.07	0.01	0.03	0.01
Malta	0.02	0.02	0.12	0.06
The Netherlands	0.07	0.01	0.05	0.00
The Netherlands, Eindhoven	0.04	0.01	0.03	0.01
The Netherlands, Maastricht	0.06	0.02	0.05	0.01
Norway	0.07	0.01	0.04	0.01
*Poland, Cracow	0.08	0.02	0.06	0.02
*Poland, Kielce	0.04	0.01	0.02	0.01
*Poland, Lower Silesia	0.08	0.01	0.05	0.01
Poland, Warsaw City	0.10	0.02	0.05	0.01
Slovakia	0.09	0.01	0.03	0.01
Slovenia	0.06	0.01	0.03	0.01
*Spain, Albacete	0.06	0.04	0.07	0.05
Spain, Asturias	0.07	0.02	0.06	0.01
Spain, Basque Country	0.06	0.01	0.02	0.01
Spain, Granada	0.07	0.02	0.03	0.01
Spain, Mallorca	0.06	0.02	0.02	0.01
Spain, Murcia	0.11	0.02	0.05	0.01
Spain, Navarra	0.08	0.03	0.02	0.01
Spain, Tarragona	0.11	0.03	0.02	0.01
Spain, Zaragoza	0.09	0.02	0.02	0.01

	MALE		FEMALE	
Sweden	0.07	0.01	0.06	0.01
*Switzerland, Basel	0.05	0.02	0.02	0.01
Switzerland, Geneva	0.14	0.05	0.05	0.03
Switzerland, Graubunden	0.04	0.04	0.06	0.04
Switzerland, Neuchatel	0.05	0.04	-	-
Switzerland, St Gall-Appenzell	0.02	0.01	0.04	0.02
Switzerland, Valais	0.04	0.04	0.04	0.03
Switzerland, Vaud	0.11	0.03	0.03	0.01
Switzerland, Zurich	0.07	0.02	0.03	0.01
*UK, England and Wales	0.06	0.00	0.04	0.00
*UK, East Anglia	0.05	0.01	0.03	0.01
*UK, Mersey	0.04	0.01	0.02	0.01
*UK, North Western	0.06	0.01	0.03	0.01
UK, Oxford	0.06	0.01	0.04	0.01
*UK, South Thames	0.05	0.01	0.04	0.00
UK, South Western	0.06	0.01	0.05	0.01
UK, Wessex	0.07	0.01	0.05	0.01
*UK, West Midlands	0.04	0.01	0.03	0.00
UK, Yorkshire	0.07	0.01	0.04	0.01
UK, Scotland	0.07	0.01	0.05	0.01
UK, Scotland, West	0.06	0.01	0.04	0.01
*Yugoslavia, Vojvodina	0.07	0.01	0.05	0.01

OCEANIA	MALE		FEMALE	
Australian Capital Territory	0.11	0.06	0.04	0.03
Australia, New South Wales	0.12	0.01	0.05	0.01
South Australia	0.09	0.02	0.06	0.01
Australia, Tasmania	0.07	0.03	0.07	0.03
Australia, Victoria	0.12	0.01	0.05	0.01
Western Australia	0.12	0.02	0.07	0.02
*French Polynesia	0.01	0.01	0.02	0.02
New Zealand: Non-Maori	0.13	0.01	0.06	0.01
New Zealand: Maori	0.04	0.03	0.14	0.06
US, Hawaii: White	0.08	0.04	0.07	0.04
US, Hawaii: Japanese	0.10	0.04	0.08	0.03
US, Hawaii: Hawaiian	0.12	0.06	-	-
US, Hawaii: Filipino	0.03	0.02	0.09	0.05
US, Hawaii: Chinese	0.06	0.06	0.16	0.09

* IMPORTANT-SEE NOTES ON POPULATION PAGE

CUMULATIVE INCIDENCE (0-74)
RATES AND STANDARD ERRORS (percent)
Mouth (ICD-9 143-5)

	MALE		FEMALE				MALE		FEMALE	
AFRICA						US, Central Louisiana: White	0,13	0,06	0,12	0,05
*Algeria, Setif						US, Central Louisiana: Black	0,36	0,21	0,14	0,10
*France, La Reunion						US, New Orleans: White	0.46	0.06	0.22	0.04
*Mali, Bamako						US, New Orleans: Black	0.53	0.10	0,10	0,04
*Uganda, Kyadondo						US, Detroit: White	0.44	0.03	0.20	0.02
*Zimbabwe, Harare: African						US, Detroit: Black	0.72	0.07	0.26	0.04
*Zimbabwe, Harare: European						US, New Mexico: Non-Hisp. White	0.26	0.04	0.17	0.03
						US, New Mexico: Hispanic White	0.24	0.06	0,03	0,02
AMERICA, CENTRAL AND SOUTH						US, New Mexico: American Indian	0,07	0,07	0,10	0,10
*Argentina, Concordia	0,29	0,12	0,06	0,05		US, Utah	0.21	0.03	0.09	0.02
*Brazil, Belem	0.60	0.11	0.19	0.06		US, Seattle	0.34	0.02	0.25	0.02
*Brazil, Goiania						US, SEER: White	0.36	0.01	0.20	0.01
*Brazil, Porto Alegre	0.45	0.07	0,06	0,02		US, SEER: Black	0.63	0.04	0.22	0.02
Colombia, Cali	0.30	0.05	0.17	0.04 m						
*Costa Rica	0.08	0.02	0.05	0.01		**ASIA**				
*Ecuador, Quito	0,07	0,03	0,02	0,01		*China, Qidong	0,03	0,01	0,03	0,01
*Peru, Lima	0.04	0.01	0.07	0.02		China, Shanghai	0.12	0.01	0.10	0.01
Peru, Trujillo	0,13	0,09	0,03	0,02		China, Tianjin	0.10	0.01	0.06	0.01
US, Puerto Rico	0.51	0.03	0.14	0.02		Hong Kong	0.24	0.02	0.09	0.01
*Uruguay, Montevideo	0.34	0.05	0.09	0.02		*India, Bangalore	0.34	0.03	1.03	0.05
						*India, Barshi, Paranda and Bhum	0.49	0.10	0,09	0,04
AMERICA, NORTH						India, Bombay	0.71	0.03	0.54	0.03
Canada	0.33	0.01	0.14	0.00		*India, Karunagappally	0.79	0.19	0.74	0.18
Canada, Alberta	0.25	0.03	0.15	0.02		India, Madras	0.87	0.05	0.97	0.05
Canada, British Columbia	0.36	0.02	0.15	0.01		*India, Trivandrum	1.16	0.17	0.73	0.13
Canada, Manitoba	0.30	0.04	0.14	0.02		Israel: All Jews	0.09	0.01	0.06	0.01
Canada, New Brunswick	0.29	0.05	0.13	0.03		Jews born in Israel	0.06	0.02	0.08	0.05
Canada, Newfoundland	0.25	0.05	0,07	0,03		Jews born in America or Europe	0.08	0.02	0.06	0.01
Canada, Northwest Territories	0,10	0,10	-	-		Jews born in Africa or Asia	0.11	0.02	0.05	0.02
Canada, Nova Scotia	0.38	0.05	0.12	0.02		Non-Jews	0,08	0,05	0,05	0,03
Canada, Ontario	0.34	0.01	0.16	0.01		Japan, Hiroshima	0.21	0.04	0.08	0.02
Canada, Prince Edward Island	0.41	0.13	0,30	0,11		Japan, Miyagi	0.10	0.01	0.07	0.01
Canada, Quebec	0.35	0.02	0.09	0.01		Japan, Nagasaki	0.24	0.03	0.07	0.01
Canada, Saskatchewan	0.16	0.03	0.13	0.02		Japan, Osaka	0.17	0.01	0.08	0.01
Canada, Yukon	1,38	0,57	0,27	0,27		*Japan, Saga	0.19	0.03	0.08	0.02
US, Cent. Calif.: Non-Hisp. White	0.35	0.03	0.19	0.02		Japan, Yamagata	0.09	0.02	0.03	0.01
US, Cent. Calif.: Hispanic	0.15	0.05	0,10	0,05		*Korea, Kangwha	0,10	0,07	0,08	0,06
US, Los Angeles: Non-Hisp. White	0.39	0.02	0.24	0.02		*Kuwait: Non-Kuwaitis	0.05	0.03	0,09	0,06
US, Los Angeles: Hispanic White	0.18	0.03	0.05	0.01		*Kuwait: Kuwaitis	0,06	0,04	0,07	0,04
US, Los Angeles: Black	0.51	0.06	0.18	0.03		*Philippines, Manila	0.38	0.04	0.39	0.04
US, Los Angeles: Chinese	0,08	0,05	-	-		Singapore: Chinese	0.22	0.03	0.08	0.02
US, Los Angeles: Filipino	0,07	0,05	0,04	0,04		Singapore: Malay	0,09	0,05	0,03	0,02
US, Los Angeles: Korean	0,05	0,05	-	-		Singapore: Indian	0.55	0.13	0.40	0.14
US, Los Angeles: Japanese	0,12	0,06	0,10	0,05		Thailand, Chiang Mai	0.30	0.05	0.24	0.04
US, San Francisco: Non-Hisp. White	0.38	0.03	0.27	0.02		*Thailand, Khon Kaen	0.20	0.05	0.40	0.06
US, San Francisco: Hispanic White	0,15	0,05	0.12	0.04		*Viet Nam, Hanoi				
US, San Francisco: Black	0.51	0.09	0.19	0.05						
US, San Francisco: Chinese	0,16	0,06	0,08	0,04						
US, San Francisco: Filipino	0,13	0,08	0,25	0,10						
US, San Francisco: Japanese	0,23	0,17	0,06	0,06						
US, Connecticut: White	0.43	0.03	0.19	0.02						
US, Connecticut: Black	0.83	0.16	0.21	0.07						
US, Atlanta: White	0.43	0.05	0.23	0.03						
US, Atlanta: Black	0.58	0.10	0.23	0.05						
US, Iowa	0.34	0.02	0.15	0.02						

* IMPORTANT-SEE NOTES ON POPULATION PAGE

EUROPE	MALE		FEMALE	
Austria, Tyrol	0.46	0.07	0.13	0.03
*Belarus	0.43	0.02	0.05	0.00
*Croatia	0.37	0.02	0.05	0.01
Czech Republic	0.25	0.01	0.04	0.00
Denmark	0.29	0.02	0.15	0.01
Estonia	0.46	0.04	0.07	0.01
Finland	0.11	0.01	0.07	0.01
France, Bas-Rhin	1.41	0.08	0.12	0.02
*France, Calvados	1.04	0.09	0.15	0.03
France, Doubs	0.96	0.10	0.18	0.04
France, Haut-Rhin	1.27	0.10	0.12	0.03
*France, Herault	0.58	0.06	0.13	0.02
France, Isere	0.65	0.06	0.13	0.03
*France, Somme	1.28	0.11	0.16	0.03
*France, Tarn	0.28	0.05	0,03	0,02
Germany, Eastern States	0.22	0.01	0.05	0.01
Germany, Saarland	0.61	0.05	0.11	0.02
Iceland	0,13	0,05	0,15	0,06
Ireland, Southern	0.30	0.05	0,09	0,03
Italy, Ferrara	0.32	0.09	0,15	0,06
Italy, Florence	0.18	0.03	0.08	0.02
Italy, Genoa	0.28	0.04	0.08	0.02
*Italy, Latina	0.14	0.04	0,04	0,02
Italy, Macerata	0,03	0,03	0,10	0,06
Italy, Modena	0.15	0.03	0,04	0,01
Italy, Parma	0.38	0.06	0.05	0.02
Italy, Ragusa	0,13	0,05	0,07	0,03
Italy, Romagna	0.17	0.03	0,06	0,02
Italy, Torino	0.31	0.04	0,02	0,01
Italy, Trieste	1.00	0.13	0.25	0.06
Italy, Varese	0.45	0.05	0.07	0.02
Italy, Veneto	0.61	0.05	0.12	0.02
*Latvia	0.31	0.02	0.03	0.01
Malta	0,26	0,11	0,17	0,09
The Netherlands	0.25	0.01	0.12	0.01
The Netherlands, Eindhoven	0.26	0.04	0.12	0.02
The Netherlands, Maastricht	0.22	0.03	0.10	0.02
Norway	0.21	0.02	0.09	0.01
*Poland, Cracow	0.22	0.04	0.06	0.02
*Poland, Kielce	0.11	0.02	0,01	0,01
*Poland, Lower Silesia	0.26	0.02	0.07	0.01
Poland, Warsaw City	0.21	0.03	0.04	0.01
Slovakia	0.61	0.02	0.05	0.01
Slovenia	0.58	0.04	0.07	0.01
*Spain, Albacete	0,17	0,08	0,04	0,04
Spain, Asturias	0.44	0.04	0.05	0.01
Spain, Basque Country	0.59	0.04	0.06	0.01
Spain, Granada	0.43	0.05	0.12	0.03
Spain, Mallorca	0.56	0.06	0.08	0.02
Spain, Murcia	0.40	0.04	0.07	0.02
Spain, Navarra	0.44	0.06	0,04	0,02
Spain, Tarragona	0.39	0.06	0.09	0.03
Spain, Zaragoza	0.33	0.04	0,02	0,01

	MALE		FEMALE	
Sweden	0.17	0.01	0.09	0.01
*Switzerland, Basel	0.32	0.05	0.08	0.03
Switzerland, Geneva	0.44	0.07	0.16	0.04
Switzerland, Graubunden	0,21	0,08	-	-
Switzerland, Neuchatel	0.57	0.12	0,17	0,06
Switzerland, St Gall-Appenzell	0.33	0.06	0.10	0.03
Switzerland, Valais	0.47	0.10	0,08	0,04
Switzerland, Vaud	0.50	0.06	0.11	0.03
Switzerland, Zurich	0.30	0.03	0.07	0.02
*UK, England and Wales	0.18	0.01	0.08	0.00
*UK, East Anglia	0.12	0.02	0.08	0.01
*UK, Mersey	0.25	0.02	0.10	0.01
*UK, North Western	0.27	0.02	0.09	0.01
UK, Oxford	0.13	0.02	0.08	0.01
*UK, South Thames	0.13	0.01	0.08	0.01
UK, South Western	0.12	0.01	0.05	0.01
UK, Wessex	0.15	0.01	0.08	0.01
*UK, West Midlands	0.21	0.01	0.08	0.01
UK, Yorkshire	0.21	0.02	0.09	0.01
UK, Scotland	0.34	0.02	0.16	0.01
UK, Scotland, West	0.40	0.03	0.16	0.01
*Yugoslavia, Vojvodina	0.28	0.02	0.03	0.01

OCEANIA	MALE		FEMALE	
Australian Capital Territory	0,19	0,08	0,18	0,07
Australia, New South Wales	0.36	0.02	0.15	0.01
South Australia	0.29	0.03	0.16	0.02
Australia, Tasmania	0.17	0.04	0.18	0.04
Australia, Victoria	0.29	0.02	0.13	0.01
Western Australia	0.34	0.04	0.13	0.02
*French Polynesia	0.55	0.16	0,30	0,12
New Zealand: Non-Maori	0.22	0.02	0.09	0.01
New Zealand: Maori	0.51	0.16	0,19	0,10
US, Hawaii: White	0.37	0.08	0.21	0.06
US, Hawaii: Japanese	0.22	0.05	0,07	0,03
US, Hawaii: Hawaiian	0,36	0,12	0,13	0,08
US, Hawaii: Filipino	0,09	0,05	0,18	0,08
US, Hawaii: Chinese	0,11	0,08	0,05	0,05

f

* IMPORTANT-SEE NOTES ON POPULATION PAGE

CUMULATIVE INCIDENCE (0-74)
RATES AND STANDARD ERRORS (percent)
Oropharynx (ICD-9 146)

	MALE		FEMALE	
AFRICA				
*Algeria, Setif				
*France, La Reunion				
*Mali, Bamako				
*Uganda, Kyadondo				
*Zimbabwe, Harare: African				
*Zimbabwe, Harare: European				
AMERICA, CENTRAL AND SOUTH				
*Argentina, Concordia	0,22	0,09	0,04	0,04
*Brazil, Belem	0.28	0.07	0,07	0,03
*Brazil, Goiania				
*Brazil, Porto Alegre	0.52	0.08	0,03	0,01
Colombia, Cali	0.10	0.03	0,06	0,02
*Costa Rica	0.08	0.02	0.06	0.02
*Ecuador, Quito	0,01	0,01	0,01	0,01
*Peru, Lima	0,03	0,01	0,01	0,01
Peru, Trujillo	0,18	0,09	-	-
US, Puerto Rico	0.38	0.03	0.05	0.01
*Uruguay, Montevideo	0.44	0.05	0,04	0,01
AMERICA, NORTH				
Canada	0.18	0.01	0.06	0.00
Canada, Alberta	0.13	0.02	0.04	0.01
Canada, British Columbia	0.21	0.02	0.07	0.01
Canada, Manitoba	0.27	0.04	0.06	0.02
Canada, New Brunswick	0.18	0.04	0.06	0.02
Canada, Newfoundland	0.17	0.04	0,06	0,03
Canada, Northwest Territories	0,18	0,15	-	-
Canada, Nova Scotia	0.21	0.03	0.07	0.02
Canada, Ontario	0.17	0.01	0.06	0.01
Canada, Prince Edward Island	0,11	0,07	0,04	0,04
Canada, Quebec	0.20	0.01	0.06	0.01
Canada, Saskatchewan	0.08	0.02	0.04	0,01
Canada, Yukon	0,08	0,08	0,19	0,13
US, Cent. Calif.: Non-Hisp. White	0.21	0.03	0.08	0.02
US, Cent. Calif.: Hispanic	0,06	0,02	0,01	0,01
US, Los Angeles: Non-Hisp. White	0.22	0.02	0.11	0.01
US, Los Angeles: Hispanic White	0.14	0.03	0,02	0,01
US, Los Angeles: Black	0.34	0.05	0.13	0.03
US, Los Angeles: Chinese	0,02	0,02	0,03	0,03
US, Los Angeles: Filipino	0,14	0,08	-	-
US, Los Angeles: Korean	0,07	0,06	-	-
US, Los Angeles: Japanese	-	-	0,02	0,02
US, San Francisco: Non-Hisp. White	0.25	0.02	0.13	0.02
US, San Francisco: Hispanic White	0.15	0.05	0.06	0,03
US, San Francisco: Black	0.48	0.08	0.12	0.04
US, San Francisco: Chinese	0,02	0,02	-	-
US, San Francisco: Filipino	0,19	0,10	0,03	0,03
US, San Francisco: Japanese	-	-	-	-
US, Connecticut: White	0.24	0.02	0.10	0.01
US, Connecticut: Black	0.66	0.14	0,17	0,07
US, Atlanta: White	0.18	0.03	0.09	0.02
US, Atlanta: Black	0.34	0.07	0.11	0.03
US, Iowa	0.18	0.02	0.07	0.01

	MALE		FEMALE	
US, Central Louisiana: White	0,07	0,04	0,10	0,04
US, Central Louisiana: Black	0.50	0,22	-	-
US, New Orleans: White	0.22	0.04	0,05	0,02
US, New Orleans: Black	0.42	0.09	0,03	0,02
US, Detroit: White	0.25	0.02	0.10	0.01
US, Detroit: Black	0.41	0.05	0.13	0.03
US, New Mexico: Non-Hisp. White	0.18	0.03	0,05	0,02
US, New Mexico: Hispanic White	0.14	0.05	0,03	0,02
US, New Mexico: American Indian	-	-	-	-
US, Utah	0.08	0.02	0,02	0,01
US, Seattle	0.15	0.02	0.09	0.01
US, SEER: White	0.20	0.01	0.09	0.00
US, SEER: Black	0.43	0.03	0.12	0.02
ASIA				
*China, Qidong	0,01	0,01	0,01	0,01
China, Shanghai	0.04	0.01	0.01	0.00
China, Tianjin	0.04	0.01	0.03	0.01
Hong Kong	0.11	0.01	0.02	0.00
*India, Bangalore	0.28	0.03	0.06	0.01
*India, Barshi, Paranda and Bhum	0,10	0,04	0,01	0,01
India, Bombay	0.44	0.03	0.05	0.01
*India, Karunagappally	0,27	0,11	-	-
India, Madras	0.35	0.03	0.06	0.01
*India, Trivandrum	0.34	0.09	0,02	0,02
Israel: All Jews	0.03	0.01	0,01	0,00
Jews born in Israel	0,01	0,01	0,00	0,00
Jews born in America or Europe	0,03	0,01	0,01	0,01
Jews born in Africa or Asia	0,03	0,01	0,01	0,01
Non-Jews	0,03	0,03	-	-
Japan, Hiroshima	0.10	0.02	0,01	0,01
Japan, Miyagi	0.05	0.01	0.00	0.00
Japan, Nagasaki	0.04	0.01	0.01	0.00
Japan, Osaka	0.08	0.01	0.02	0.00
*Japan, Saga	0.08	0.02	0,01	0,01
Japan, Yamagata	0,02	0,01	-	-
*Korea, Kangwha	0,13	0,08	-	-
*Kuwait: Non-Kuwaitis	0,01	0,00	-	-
*Kuwait: Kuwaitis	0,03	0,02	0,08	0,06
*Philippines, Manila	0.11	0.02	0.07	0.01
Singapore: Chinese	0.11	0.02	0.02	0,01
Singapore: Malay	0,09	0,05	0,05	0,05
Singapore: Indian	0,17	0,07	0,08	0,06
Thailand, Chiang Mai	0.17	0.04	0.10	0.02
*Thailand, Khon Kaen	0.07	0.03	0,01	0,01
*Viet Nam, Hanoi				

* IMPORTANT-SEE NOTES ON POPULATION PAGE

CUMULATIVE INCIDENCE (0-74)
RATES AND STANDARD ERRORS (percent)
Oropharynx (ICD-9 146) (contd)

EUROPE	MALE		FEMALE	
Austria, Tyrol	0.28	0.05	0.07	0.02
*Belarus	0.19	0.01	0.02	0.00
*Croatia	0.35	0.02	0.03	0.01
Czech Republic	0.25	0.01	0.03	0.00
Denmark	0.20	0.01	0.07	0.01
Estonia	0.34	0.03	0,02	0,01
Finland	0.05	0.01	0.01	0.00
France, Bas-Rhin	1.43	0.09	0.10	0.02
*France, Calvados	1.41	0.11	0.08	0.02
France, Doubs	1.06	0.10	0.12	0.04
France, Haut-Rhin	1.42	0.11	0.12	0.03
*France, Herault	0.64	0.06	0.08	0.02
France, Isere	0.73	0.06	0.11	0.02
*France, Somme	1.55	0.11	0.07	0.02
*France, Tarn	0.64	0.08	0,04	0,02
Germany, Eastern States	0.20	0.01	0.04	0.00
Germany, Saarland	0.33	0.03	0.06	0.01
Iceland	0,04	0,03	0,04	0,03
Ireland, Southern	0.12	0.04	0,02	0,01
Italy, Ferrara	0,21	0,07	0,07	0,04
Italy, Florence	0.14	0.03	0.05	0.01
Italy, Genoa	0.30	0.04	0.05	0.01
*Italy, Latina	0,07	0,03	-	-
Italy, Macerata	0,12	0,06	-	-
Italy, Modena	0.19	0.03	0,03	0,01
Italy, Parma	0.18	0.04	0,03	0,02
Italy, Ragusa	0.02	0.02	0,01	0,01
Italy, Romagna	0.15	0.03	0,01	0,01
Italy, Torino	0.22	0.03	0.06	0.02
Italy, Trieste	0.32	0.07	0,07	0,03
Italy, Varese	0.47	0.05	0,03	0,01
Italy, Veneto	0.33	0.03	0.06	0.01
*Latvia	0.19	0.02	0.01	0.00
Malta	-	-	-	-
The Netherlands	0.16	0.01	0.06	0.00
The Netherlands, Eindhoven	0.15	0.03	0,03	0,01
The Netherlands, Maastricht	0.14	0.03	0.08	0.02
Norway	0.10	0.01	0.03	0.00
*Poland, Cracow	0.24	0.04	0,04	0,01
*Poland, Kielce	0.13	0.03	0,02	0,01
*Poland, Lower Silesia	0.16	0.02	0,05	0,01
Poland, Warsaw City	0.31	0.03	0.06	0.01
Slovakia	0.55	0.02	0.02	0.00
Slovenia	0.79	0.05	0.04	0.01
*Spain, Albacete	0,10	0,05	-	-
Spain, Asturias	0.48	0.05	0,03	0,01
Spain, Basque Country	0.42	0.03	0,01	0,01
Spain, Granada	0.15	0.03	-	-
Spain, Mallorca	0.37	0.05	0,03	0,01
Spain, Murcia	0.25	0.03	0,01	0,01
Spain, Navarra	0.20	0.04	0,03	0,01
Spain, Tarragona	0.22	0.04	-	-
Spain, Zaragoza	0.14	0.02	0,01	0,01

	MALE		FEMALE	
Sweden	0.11	0.01	0.04	0.00
*Switzerland, Basel	0.30	0.05	0,05	0,02
Switzerland, Geneva	0.56	0.08	0.18	0.04
Switzerland, Graubunden	0.22	0.08	0,03	0,03
Switzerland, Neuchatel	0.58	0.12	0,14	0,06
Switzerland, St Gall-Appenzell	0.22	0.05	0,01	0,01
Switzerland, Valais	0.54	0.11	0,04	0,03
Switzerland, Vaud	0.66	0.07	0.11	0.03
Switzerland, Zurich	0.29	0.04	0.08	0.02
*UK, England and Wales	0.09	0.00	0.03	0.00
*UK, East Anglia	0.06	0.01	0.03	0.01
*UK, Mersey	0.13	0.01	0.04	0.01
*UK, North Western	0.15	0.01	0.05	0.01
UK, Oxford	0.06	0.01	0.03	0.01
*UK, South Thames	0.08	0.01	0.04	0.00
UK, South Western	0.06	0.01	0.02	0.00
UK, Wessex	0.06	0.01	0.02	0.00
*UK, West Midlands	0.10	0.01	0.03	0.00
UK, Yorkshire	0.09	0.01	0.03	0.01
UK, Scotland	0.13	0.01	0.04	0.01
UK, Scotland, West	0.13	0.01	0.04	0.01
*Yugoslavia, Vojvodina	0.26	0.02	0.04	0.01

OCEANIA	MALE		FEMALE	
Australian Capital Territory	0,05	0,03	0,02	0,02
Australia, New South Wales	0.21	0.01	0.06	0.01
South Australia	0.19	0.03	0.05	0.01
Australia, Tasmania	0.19	0.04	0.05	0.02
Australia, Victoria	0.24	0.02	0.05	0.01
Western Australia	0.26	0.03	0.05	0.01
*French Polynesia	0.42	0.16	0,08	0,06
New Zealand: Non-Maori	0.10	0.01	0.04	0.01
New Zealand: Maori	0,17	0,10	0,03	0,02
US, Hawaii: White	0.49	0.10	0,05	0,03
US, Hawaii: Japanese	0,09	0,03	0,02	0,01
US, Hawaii: Hawaiian	0,14	0,07	0,06	0,04
US, Hawaii: Filipino	0,13	0,07	0,05	0,04
US, Hawaii: Chinese	0,05	0,05	-	-

* IMPORTANT-SEE NOTES ON POPULATION PAGE

CUMULATIVE INCIDENCE (0-74)
RATES AND STANDARD ERRORS (percent)
Nasopharynx (ICD-9 147)

	MALE		FEMALE	
AFRICA				
*Algeria, Setif				
*France, La Reunion				
*Mali, Bamako				
*Uganda, Kyadondo				
*Zimbabwe, Harare: African				
*Zimbabwe, Harare: European				
AMERICA, CENTRAL AND SOUTH				
*Argentina, Concordia	-	-	0,08	0,05
*Brazil, Belem	0,05	0,03	0,00	0,00
*Brazil, Goiania				
*Brazil, Porto Alegre	0,04	0,02	0,01	0,01 m
Colombia, Cali	0,03	0,01	0,03	0,01
*Costa Rica	0.06	0.01	0.02	0.01
*Ecuador, Quito	0,00	0,00	-	-
*Peru, Lima	0,02	0,01	0,02	0,01
Peru, Trujillo	0,04	0,04	-	-
US, Puerto Rico	0.07	0.01	0.02	0.01
*Uruguay, Montevideo	0.08	0.02	0,03	0,01
AMERICA, NORTH				
Canada	0.09	0.00	0.03	0.00
Canada, Alberta	0.11	0.01	0.02	0.01
Canada, British Columbia	0.11	0.01	0.05	0.01
Canada, Manitoba	0.06	0.02	0.05	0.01
Canada, New Brunswick	0.06	0.02	0,03	0,01
Canada, Newfoundland	0.14	0.04	0,06	0,02
Canada, Northwest Territories	0.98	0.34	0,59	0,25
Canada, Nova Scotia	0,01	0,01	0,02	0,01
Canada, Ontario	0.10	0.01	0.04	0.00
Canada, Prince Edward Island	0,07	0,05	-	-
Canada, Quebec	0.07	0.01	0.02	0.00
Canada, Saskatchewan	0.07	0.02	0,01	0,01
Canada, Yukon	-	-	-	-
US, Cent. Calif.: Non-Hisp. White	0.07	0.01	0.03	0.01
US, Cent. Calif.: Hispanic	0,06	0,03	0,01	0,01
US, Los Angeles: Non-Hisp. White	0.06	0.01	0.03	0.01
US, Los Angeles: Hispanic White	0.06	0.02	0.02	0.01
US, Los Angeles: Black	0.10	0.03	0,02	0,01
US, Los Angeles: Chinese	1.11	0.15	0.37	0.09
US, Los Angeles: Filipino	0.45	0.12	0,02	0,02
US, Los Angeles: Korean	0,02	0,02	0,02	0,02
US, Los Angeles: Japanese	0,02	0,02	0,05	0,03
US, San Francisco: Non-Hisp. White	0.05	0.01	0.02	0.01
US, San Francisco: Hispanic White	0,04	0,02	-	-
US, San Francisco: Black	0,08	0,03	0,02	0,01
US, San Francisco: Chinese	1.25	0.14	0.40	0.08
US, San Francisco: Filipino	0.41	0.12	0,13	0,06
US, San Francisco: Japanese	-	-	-	-
US, Connecticut: White	0.08	0.01	0.02	0.01
US, Connecticut: Black	0,13	0,07	0,03	0,02
US, Atlanta: White	0.05	0.01	0.04	0.01
US, Atlanta: Black	0.13	0.04	0,04	0,02
US, Iowa	0.05	0.01	0.02	0.01

	MALE		FEMALE	
US, Central Louisiana: White	0,04	0,03	0,04	0,03
US, Central Louisiana: Black	0,10	0,08	-	-
US, New Orleans: White	0.12	0.03	0.07	0.02
US, New Orleans: Black	0,10	0,04	0,03	0,02
US, Detroit: White	0.06	0.01	0.02	0.01
US, Detroit: Black	0.06	0.02	0.02	0,01
US, New Mexico: Non-Hisp. White	0,03	0,01	0,02	0,01
US, New Mexico: Hispanic White	0,03	0,02	0,02	0,01
US, New Mexico: American Indian	-	-	0,14	0,10
US, Utah	0,03	0,01	0,01	0,01
US, Seattle	0.07	0.01	0.04	0.01
US, SEER: White	0.06	0.00	0.02	0.00
US, SEER: Black	0.09	0.02	0.02	0.01
ASIA				
*China, Qidong	0.21	0.03	0.10	0.02
China, Shanghai	0.49	0.02	0.18	0.01
China, Tianjin	0.18	0.02	0.07	0.01
Hong Kong	2.57	0.05	0.99	0.03
*India, Bangalore	0.04	0.01	0.02	0.01
*India, Barshi, Paranda and Bhum	-	-	-	-
India, Bombay	0.08	0.01	0.02	0.01
*India, Karunagappally	0,24	0,11	0,08	0,05
India, Madras	0.10	0.02	0.03	0.01
*India, Trivandrum	0,04	0,03	0,05	0,03
Israel: All Jews	0.11	0.01	0.04	0.01
Jews born in Israel	0.06	0.02	0.05	0.02
Jews born in America or Europe	0.06	0.01	0.02	0,01
Jews born in Africa or Asia	0.21	0.04	0.06	0.01
Non-Jews	0.08	0.03	0,01	0,00
Japan, Hiroshima	0.06	0.02	0,03	0,01
Japan, Miyagi	0.06	0.01	0.01	0,01
Japan, Nagasaki	0.06	0.01	0.03	0.01
Japan, Osaka	0.07	0.01	0.02	0.00
*Japan, Saga	0.05	0.02	0,02	0,01
Japan, Yamagata	0.05	0.01	0,01	0,00
*Korea, Kangwha	0,07	0,05	0,04	0,04
*Kuwait: Non-Kuwaitis	0.14	0.08	0,01	0,01
*Kuwait: Kuwaitis	0.26	0.08	0,05	0,02
*Philippines, Manila	0.82	0.05	0.41	0.03
Singapore: Chinese	1.95	0.08	0.76	0.04
Singapore: Malay	0.74	0.12	0.21	0.06
Singapore: Indian	0,04	0,03	0,13	0,13
Thailand, Chiang Mai	0.29	0.04	0.16	0.03
*Thailand, Khon Kaen	0.30	0.05	0.11	0.03
*Viet Nam, Hanoi				

EUROPE	MALE		FEMALE	
Austria, Tyrol	0,07	*0,02*	0,01	*0,01*
*Belarus	0.08	*0.01*	0.02	*0.00*
*Croatia	0.08	*0.01*	0.02	*0.00*
Czech Republic	0.07	*0.01*	0.02	*0.00*
Denmark	0.04	*0.01*	0.02	*0.00*
Estonia	0.05	*0.01*	0.02	*0,01*
Finland	0.03	*0.00*	0.01	*0.00*
France, Bas-Rhin	0.12	*0.03*	0,03	*0,01*
*France, Calvados	0,06	*0,02*	0,01	*0,01*
France, Doubs	0,06	*0,03*	0,04	*0,02*
France, Haut-Rhin	0.09	*0.02*	0,02	*0,01*
*France, Herault	0.09	*0.02*	0,02	*0,01*
France, Isere	0.07	*0.02*	0,01	*0,01*
*France, Somme	0,06	*0,02*	0,02	*0,01*
*France, Tarn	0,07	*0,03*	-	-
Germany, Eastern States	0.05	*0.01*	0.01	*0.00*
Germany, Saarland	0.05	*0.01*	0.02	*0,01*
Iceland	0,04	*0,02*	0,02	*0,02*
Ireland, Southern	0,02	*0,01*	0,01	*0,01*
Italy, Ferrara	0,04	*0,03*	0,02	*0,02*
Italy, Florence	0.11	*0.02*	0.04	*0.01*
Italy, Genoa	0.13	*0.02*	0,03	*0,01*
*Italy, Latina	0,05	*0,03*	0,01	*0,01*
Italy, Macerata	0,03	*0,03*	-	-
Italy, Modena	0.08	*0.02*	0,02	*0,01*
Italy, Parma	0.10	*0.03*	0,01	*0,01*
Italy, Ragusa	0,06	*0,03*	0,04	*0,02*
Italy, Romagna	0.14	*0.03*	0,02	*0,01*
Italy, Torino	0.10	*0.02*	0,02	*0,01*
Italy, Trieste	0,08	*0,03*	0,05	*0,03*
Italy, Varese	0.11	*0.02*	0.04	*0.01*
Italy, Veneto	0.09	*0.02*	0.04	*0.01*
*Latvia	0.09	*0.01*	0.02	*0.01*
Malta	0,15	*0,06*	0,11	*0,05*
The Netherlands	0.06	*0.00*	0.02	*0.00*
The Netherlands, Eindhoven	0.06	*0.02*	0,03	*0,01*
The Netherlands, Maastricht	0.08	*0.02*	0,01	*0,01*
Norway	0.03	*0.01*	0,01	*0,00*
*Poland, Cracow	0,05	*0,02*	0,05	*0.02*
*Poland, Kielce	0,03	*0,01*	0,02	*0,01*
*Poland, Lower Silesia	0,05	*0,01*	0,02	*0.00*
Poland, Warsaw City	0,06	*0,01*	0,01	*0,00*
Slovakia	0.07	*0.01*	0.03	*0.00*
Slovenia	0.06	*0.01*	0.02	*0.01*
*Spain, Albacete	0,03	*0,03*	0,03	*0,03*
Spain, Asturias	0.16	*0.03*	0.06	*0.01*
Spain, Basque Country	0.12	*0.02*	0.05	*0.01*
Spain, Granada	0.13	*0.03*	0,03	*0,01*
Spain, Mallorca	0.12	*0.03*	0,04	*0,02*
Spain, Murcia	0.10	*0.02*	0,02	*0,01*
Spain, Navarra	0.13	*0.03*	0,01	*0,01*
Spain, Tarragona	0.08	*0.02*	0,01	*0,01*
Spain, Zaragoza	0.08	*0.02*	0,03	*0,01*

	MALE		FEMALE	
Sweden	0.04	*0.00*	0.02	*0.00*
*Switzerland, Basel	0,02	*0,01*	0,01	*0,01*
Switzerland, Geneva	0,05	*0,03*	0,03	*0,02*
Switzerland, Graubunden	0,12	*0,07*	0,05	*0,03*
Switzerland, Neuchatel	0,04	*0,03*	0,04	*0,03*
Switzerland, St Gall-Appenzell	0,04	*0,02*	0,02	*0,01*
Switzerland, Valais	0,04	*0,03*	0,02	*0,02*
Switzerland, Vaud	0.08	*0.02*	0,01	*0,01*
Switzerland, Zurich	0.04	*0.01*	0,01	*0,01*
*UK, England and Wales	0.04	*0.00*	0.02	*0.00*
*UK, East Anglia	0.03	*0.01*	0.02	*0.01*
*UK, Mersey	0.04	*0.01*	0.03	*0.01*
*UK, North Western	0.03	*0.01*	0.01	*0.00*
UK, Oxford	0.03	*0.01*	0.01	*0.01*
*UK, South Thames	0.04	*0.00*	0.02	*0.00*
UK, South Western	0.03	*0.01*	0.01	*0.00*
UK, Wessex	0.04	*0.01*	0.02	*0.00*
*UK, West Midlands	0.04	*0.01*	0.02	*0.00*
UK, Yorkshire	0.05	*0.01*	0.01	*0.00*
UK, Scotland	0.05	*0.01*	0.02	*0.00*
UK, Scotland, West	0.05	*0.01*	0.01	*0.00*
*Yugoslavia, Vojvodina	0.09	*0.01*	0.03	*0.01*

OCEANIA	MALE		FEMALE	
Australian Capital Territory	0,11	*0,06*	0,05	*0,04*
Australia, New South Wales	0.10	*0.01*	0.03	*0.00*
South Australia	0.05	*0.01*	0.01	*0.00*
Australia, Tasmania	0.09	*0.03*	0,02	*0,01*
Australia, Victoria	0.09	*0.01*	0.02	*0.00*
Western Australia	0.07	*0.02*	0,01	*0,01*
*French Polynesia	0,27	*0,10*	0,05	*0,03*
New Zealand: Non-Maori	0.06	*0.01*	0.03	*0.01*
New Zealand: Maori	0.22	*0.08*	0,03	*0,02*
US, Hawaii: White	0,11	*0,04*	0,05	*0,03*
US, Hawaii: Japanese	0.13	*0.04*	0,01	*0,01*
US, Hawaii: Hawaiian	0,21	*0,09*	0,05	*0,04*
US, Hawaii: Filipino	0.37	*0.11*	0,12	*0,06*
US, Hawaii: Chinese	0.66	*0.20*	0,43	*0,15*

* IMPORTANT-SEE NOTES ON POPULATION PAGE

CUMULATIVE INCIDENCE (0-74)
RATES AND STANDARD ERRORS (percent)
Hypopharynx (ICD-9 148)

	MALE		FEMALE	
AFRICA				
*Algeria, Setif				
*France, La Reunion				
*Mali, Bamako				
*Uganda, Kyadondo				
*Zimbabwe, Harare: African				
*Zimbabwe, Harare: European				
AMERICA, CENTRAL AND SOUTH				
*Argentina, Concordia	0,37	0,17	-	-
*Brazil, Belem	0.25	0.08	-	- m
*Brazil, Goiania				
*Brazil, Porto Alegre	0.31	0.06	0,02	0,01
Colombia, Cali	0.08	0.03	-	-
*Costa Rica	0.09	0.02	0,02	0,01
*Ecuador, Quito	-	-	-	-
*Peru, Lima	0,02	0,01	0,01	0,01
Peru, Trujillo	0,11	0,08	-	-
US, Puerto Rico	0.35	0.03	0.03	0.01
*Uruguay, Montevideo	0.42	0.05	0,01	0,01
AMERICA, NORTH				
Canada	0.16	0.01	0.03	0.00
Canada, Alberta	0.12	0.02	0,02	0,01
Canada, British Columbia	0.15	0.02	0.03	0.01
Canada, Manitoba	0.21	0.03	0,04	0,01
Canada, New Brunswick	0.14	0.03	0,03	0,01
Canada, Newfoundland	0.12	0.03	0,03	0,02
Canada, Northwest Territories	-	-	-	-
Canada, Nova Scotia	0.23	0.04	0,04	0,01
Canada, Ontario	0.15	0.01	0.03	0.00
Canada, Prince Edward Island	0,30	0,11	-	-
Canada, Quebec	0.19	0.01	0.03	0.00
Canada, Saskatchewan	0.13	0.02	0,02	0,01
Canada, Yukon	-	-	-	-
US, Cent. Calif.: Non-Hisp. White	0.13	0.02	0.04	0.01
US, Cent. Calif.: Hispanic	0,08	0,03	0,02	0,02
US, Los Angeles: Non-Hisp. White	0.17	0.01	0.05	0.01
US, Los Angeles: Hispanic White	0.07	0.02	-	-
US, Los Angeles: Black	0.22	0.04	0,03	0,01
US, Los Angeles: Chinese	0,13	0,06	-	-
US, Los Angeles: Filipino	-	-	-	-
US, Los Angeles: Korean	0,09	0,09	-	-
US, Los Angeles: Japanese	0,06	0,04	-	-
US, San Francisco: Non-Hisp. White	0.25	0.02	0.07	0.01
US, San Francisco: Hispanic White	0.19	0.06	0,02	0,02
US, San Francisco: Black	0.30	0.07	0,09	0,03
US, San Francisco: Chinese	0,07	0,04	-	-
US, San Francisco: Filipino	-	-	0,05	0,04
US, San Francisco: Japanese	-	-	-	-
US, Connecticut: White	0.19	0.02	0.07	0.01
US, Connecticut: Black	0.40	0.11	0,07	0,04
US, Atlanta: White	0.20	0.03	0.04	0.01
US, Atlanta: Black	0.26	0.06	0,10	0,03
US, Iowa	0.18	0.02	0.03	0.01

	MALE		FEMALE	
US, Central Louisiana: White	0,12	0,05	-	-
US, Central Louisiana: Black	0,54	0,24	0,03	0,03
US, New Orleans: White	0.17	0.04	0,02	0,01
US, New Orleans: Black	0.33	0.09	0,01	0,01
US, Detroit: White	0.22	0.02	0.05	0.01
US, Detroit: Black	0.40	0.05	0,04	0,02
US, New Mexico: Non-Hisp. White	0.07	0.02	0,02	0,01
US, New Mexico: Hispanic White	0,11	0,04	-	-
US, New Mexico: American Indian	-	-	-	-
US, Utah	0.07	0.02	0,02	0,01
US, Seattle	0.15	0.02	0.05	0.01
US, SEER: White	0.18	0.01	0.05	0.00
US, SEER: Black	0.35	0.03	0.06	0.01
ASIA				
*China, Qidong	0,01	0,01	-	-
China, Shanghai	0.02	0.00	0,00	0,00
China, Tianjin	0.03	0.01	0,01	0,00
Hong Kong	0.18	0.01	0.02	0.00
*India, Bangalore	0.76	0.05	0.12	0.02
*India, Barshi, Paranda and Bhum	0.93	0.14	0,07	0,04
India, Bombay	1.03	0.04	0.24	0.02
*India, Karunagappally	0.37	0.13	0,08	0,05
India, Madras	0.79	0.05	0.26	0.02
*India, Trivandrum	0.27	0.09	0,10	0,05
Israel: All Jews	0.02	0.01	0,00	0,00
Jews born in Israel	0,01	0,01	-	-
Jews born in America or Europe	0,02	0,01	0,00	0,00
Jews born in Africa or Asia	0,02	0,01	0,00	0,00
Non-Jews	-	-	0,03	0,02
Japan, Hiroshima	0.14	0.03	0,02	0,01
Japan, Miyagi	0.10	0.01	0.02	0.01
Japan, Nagasaki	0.11	0.02	0,01	0,00
Japan, Osaka	0.15	0.01	0.02	0.00
*Japan, Saga	0.09	0.02	0,02	0,01
Japan, Yamagata	0.08	0.02	0,01	0,01
*Korea, Kangwha	0,05	0,05	-	-
*Kuwait: Non-Kuwaitis	0,01	0,00	-	-
*Kuwait: Kuwaitis	0,06	0,04	0,18	0,08
*Philippines, Manila	0.03	0.01	0,01	0,00
Singapore: Chinese	0.22	0.03	0,01	0,01
Singapore: Malay	0,04	0,04	0,06	0,04
Singapore: Indian	0,22	0,08	0,14	0,08
Thailand, Chiang Mai	0.26	0.04	0.08	0.02
*Thailand, Khon Kaen	0,02	0,01	0,00	0,00
*Viet Nam, Hanoi				

CUMULATIVE INCIDENCE (0-74)
RATES AND STANDARD ERRORS (percent)
Hypopharynx (ICD-9 148) (contd)

EUROPE	MALE		FEMALE	
Austria, Tyrol	0.17	0.04	0,03	0,02
*Belarus	0.23	0.01	0.01	0.00
*Croatia	0.54	0.03	0.03	0.01
Czech Republic	0.12	0.01	0.01	0.00
Denmark	0.09	0.01	0.02	0.00
Estonia	0.26	0.03	0.01	0,01
Finland	0.06	0.01	0.01	0.00
France, Bas-Rhin	1.67	0.10	0.06	0.02
*France, Calvados	1.86	0.13	0,03	0,01
France, Doubs	1.32	0.13	0,04	0,02
France, Haut-Rhin	1.26	0.10	0.06	0.02
*France, Herault	0.46	0.05	0.01	0,01
France, Isere	0.76	0.06	0,03	0,01
*France, Somme	1.36	0.11	0,05	0,02
*France, Tarn	0.61	0.09	0,04	0,02
Germany, Eastern States	0.13	0.01	0.01	0.00
Germany, Saarland	0.39	0.04	0.04	0.01
Iceland	0,05	0,04	-	-
Ireland, Southern	0.12	0.03	0,05	0,02
Italy, Ferrara	0,07	0,04	0,04	0,03
Italy, Florence	0.13	0.02	0,01	0,01
Italy, Genoa	0.21	0.03	0,03	0,01
*Italy, Latina	0,04	0,02	0,01	0,01
Italy, Macerata	-	-	-	-
Italy, Modena	0.18	0.03	0,02	0,01
Italy, Parma	0.30	0.05	0,05	0,02
Italy, Ragusa	0,02	0,02	-	-
Italy, Romagna	0.08	0.02	0,01	0,01
Italy, Torino	0.14	0.03	0,03	0,01
Italy, Trieste	0.18	0.05	-	-
Italy, Varese	0.27	0.04	0,03	0,01
Italy, Veneto	0.23	0.03	0,03	0,01
*Latvia	0.21	0.02	0,01	0,00
Malta	-	-	-	-
The Netherlands	0.13	0.01	0.02	0.00
The Netherlands, Eindhoven	0.08	0.02	0,01	0,01
The Netherlands, Maastricht	0.15	0.03	0,01	0,01
Norway	0.11	0.01	0.02	0.00
*Poland, Cracow	0,02	0,01	0,03	0,01
*Poland, Kielce	0,03	0,01	-	-
*Poland, Lower Silesia	0.05	0.01	0,01	0,00
Poland, Warsaw City	0.09	0.02	0,01	0,01
Slovakia	0.42	0.02	0,01	0,00
Slovenia	0.44	0.03	0.02	0.01
*Spain, Albacete	0,10	0,06	-	-
Spain, Asturias	0.51	0.05	0,00	0,00
Spain, Basque Country	0.46	0.04	0,01	0,00
Spain, Granada	0.26	0.04	-	-
Spain, Mallorca	0.42	0.05	0,01	0,01
Spain, Murcia	0.17	0.03	-	-
Spain, Navarra	0.24	0.04	-	-
Spain, Tarragona	0.20	0.04	0,01	0,01
Spain, Zaragoza	0.14	0.03	-	-

	MALE		FEMALE	
Sweden	0.10	0.01	0.01	0.00
*Switzerland, Basel	0.27	0.05	0,06	0,02
Switzerland, Geneva	0.65	0.09	0,08	0,03
Switzerland, Graubunden	0,24	0,09	-	-
Switzerland, Neuchatel	0.58	0.13	0,04	0,03
Switzerland, St Gall-Appenzell	0.23	0.05	-	-
Switzerland, Valais	0.54	0.11	0,05	0,04
Switzerland, Vaud	0.82	0.08	0.10	0.02
Switzerland, Zurich	0.23	0.03	0.03	0.01
*UK, England and Wales	0.07	0.00	0.03	0.00
*UK, East Anglia	0.06	0.01	0.05	0.01
*UK, Mersey	0.12	0.01	0.05	0.01
*UK, North Western	0.10	0.01	0.04	0.01
UK, Oxford	0.06	0.01	0.03	0.01
*UK, South Thames	0.06	0.01	0.04	0.00
UK, South Western	0.05	0.01	0.03	0.01
UK, Wessex	0.05	0.01	0.02	0.01
*UK, West Midlands	0.09	0.01	0.04	0.01
UK, Yorkshire	0.07	0.01	0.03	0.01
UK, Scotland	0.11	0.01	0.04	0.01
UK, Scotland, West	0.11	0.01	0.05	0.01
*Yugoslavia, Vojvodina	0.37	0.03	0.03	0.01

OCEANIA	MALE		FEMALE	
Australian Capital Territory	0,09	0,04	-	-
Australia, New South Wales	0.18	0.01	0.02	0.00
South Australia	0.16	0.02	0.02	0,01
Australia, Tasmania	0.11	0.03	0,01	0,01
Australia, Victoria	0.21	0.02	0.02	0.01
Western Australia	0.18	0.03	0,03	0,01
*French Polynesia	0.42	0.13	0,06	0,04
New Zealand: Non-Maori	0.12	0.01	0.03	0.01
New Zealand: Maori	0,13	0,08	-	-
US, Hawaii: White	0.29	0.08	0,15	0,06
US, Hawaii: Japanese	0.26	0.06	-	-
US, Hawaii: Hawaiian	0,34	0,13	0,03	0,03
US, Hawaii: Filipino	0.06	0,04	0,06	0,04
US, Hawaii: Chinese	0,22	0,13	0,06	0,06

* IMPORTANT-SEE NOTES ON POPULATION PAGE

CUMULATIVE INCIDENCE (0-74)
RATES AND STANDARD ERRORS (percent)
Pharynx unspecified (ICD-9 149)

	MALE		FEMALE	
AFRICA				
*Algeria, Setif				
*France, La Reunion				
*Mali, Bamako				
*Uganda, Kyadondo				
*Zimbabwe, Harare: African				
*Zimbabwe, Harare: European				
AMERICA, CENTRAL AND SOUTH				
*Argentina, Concordia	0,13	0,08	-	-
*Brazil, Belem	0,03	0,02	0,03	0,02
*Brazil, Goiania				
*Brazil, Porto Alegre	0.14	0.04	0,01	0,01
Colombia, Cali	-	-	0,01	0,00
*Costa Rica	0.03	0.01	0,02	0,01
*Ecuador, Quito	0,02	0,01	-	-
*Peru, Lima	-	-	-	-
Peru, Trujillo	0,01	0,01	0,02	0,02
US, Puerto Rico	0.07	0.01	0,01	0,00
*Uruguay, Montevideo	0.13	0.03	-	-
AMERICA, NORTH				
Canada	0.07	0.00	0.02	0.00
Canada, Alberta	0.04	0.01	0,01	0,00
Canada, British Columbia	0.05	0.01	0,01	0,00
Canada, Manitoba	0.07	0.02	0,02	0,01
Canada, New Brunswick	-	-	0,01	0,01
Canada, Newfoundland	0,08	0,03	0,01	0,01
Canada, Northwest Territories	0,24	0,24	-	-
Canada, Nova Scotia	0.09	0.02	0,04	0,01
Canada, Ontario	0.07	0.01	0.02	0.00
Canada, Prince Edward Island	0,04	0,04	-	-
Canada, Quebec	0.10	0.01	0.02	0.00
Canada, Saskatchewan	0,04	0,01	0,01	0,01
Canada, Yukon	0,72	0,51	0,11	0,08
US, Cent. Calif.: Non-Hisp. White	0.05	0.01	0,01	0,01
US, Cent. Calif.: Hispanic	0,04	0,02	-	-
US, Los Angeles: Non-Hisp. White	0.05	0.01	0.02	0.01
US, Los Angeles: Hispanic White	0,01	0,01	0,01	0,01
US, Los Angeles: Black	0.14	0.03	0,02	0,01
US, Los Angeles: Chinese	-	-	-	-
US, Los Angeles: Filipino	0,04	0,04	-	-
US, Los Angeles: Korean	0,09	0,09	-	-
US, Los Angeles: Japanese	0,03	0,03	0,04	0,04
US, San Francisco: Non-Hisp. White	0.03	0.01	0.03	0.01
US, San Francisco: Hispanic White	0,02	0,02	-	-
US, San Francisco: Black	0,08	0,04	0,04	0,02
US, San Francisco: Chinese	-	-	-	-
US, San Francisco: Filipino	-	-	-	-
US, San Francisco: Japanese	-	-	-	-
US, Connecticut: White	0.04	0.01	0.03	0.01
US, Connecticut: Black	0,20	0,08	0,05	0,03
US, Atlanta: White	0.04	0.01	0.05	0.01
US, Atlanta: Black	0.22	0.07	0,07	0,03
US, Iowa	0.07	0.01	0,01	0,00

	MALE		FEMALE	
US, Central Louisiana: White	0,12	0,05	0,02	0,02
US, Central Louisiana: Black	-	-	0,06	0,06
US, New Orleans: White	0.18	0.04	0,03	0,01
US, New Orleans: Black	0,07	0,04	0,03	0,02
US, Detroit: White	0.06	0.01	0.02	0.00
US, Detroit: Black	0.16	0.04	0,03	0,01
US, New Mexico: Non-Hisp. White	0.06	0.02	0,01	0,01
US, New Mexico: Hispanic White	0,05	0,02	-	-
US, New Mexico: American Indian	-	-	-	-
US, Utah	0,02	0,01	0,01	0,01
US, Seattle	0.07	0.01	0.04	0.01
US, SEER: White	0.05	0.00	0.02	0.00
US, SEER: Black	0.16	0.02	0.04	0.01
ASIA				
*China, Qidong	0,01	0,01	-	-
China, Shanghai	0.01	0.00	0,00	0,00
China, Tianjin	0,00	0,00	-	-
Hong Kong	0.01	0.00	0,00	0,00
*India, Bangalore	0.05	0.01	0.05	0.01
*India, Barshi, Paranda and Bhum	0,05	0,02	-	-
India, Bombay	0.21	0.02	0.08	0.01
*India, Karunagappally	0,10	0,08	-	-
India, Madras	0.12	0.02	0.03	0.01
*India, Trivandrum	0,03	0,02	-	-
Israel: All Jews	0,01	0,00	-	-
Jews born in Israel	0,00	0,00	-	-
Jews born in America or Europe	0,01	0,01	-	-
Jews born in Africa or Asia	0,01	0,01	-	-
Non-Jews	-	-	-	-
Japan, Hiroshima	0,03	0,01	0,01	0,01
Japan, Miyagi	0.02	0.01	0,00	0,00
Japan, Nagasaki	0,02	0,01	0,01	0,00
Japan, Osaka	0.01	0.00	0.01	0.00
*Japan, Saga	0,00	0,00	-	-
Japan, Yamagata	0,02	0,01	0,01	0,00
*Korea, Kangwha	-	-	0,03	0,03
*Kuwait: Non-Kuwaitis	0,00	0,00	-	-
*Kuwait: Kuwaitis	-	-	-	-
*Philippines, Manila	0.19	0.03	0.12	0.02
Singapore: Chinese	0,02	0,01	-	-
Singapore: Malay	-	-	-	-
Singapore: Indian	0,01	0,01	-	-
Thailand, Chiang Mai	0,03	0,01	0,01	0,01
*Thailand, Khon Kaen	0,01	0,01	0,00	0,00
*Viet Nam, Hanoi				

* IMPORTANT-SEE NOTES ON POPULATION PAGE

CUMULATIVE INCIDENCE (0-74)
RATES AND STANDARD ERRORS (percent)
Pharynx unspecified (ICD-9 149) (contd)

EUROPE

	MALE		FEMALE	
Austria, Tyrol	0,03	0,02	0,01	0,01
*Belarus	0.07	0.01	0.01	0.00
*Croatia	0.05	0.01	0,00	0,00
Czech Republic	0.01	0.00	0,00	0,00
Denmark	0.01	0.00	0,00	0,00
Estonia	0,02	0,01	0,00	0,00
Finland	0.01	0.00	0,00	0,00
France, Bas-Rhin	0.39	0.05	0,03	0,01
*France, Calvados	0.12	0.03	0,01	0,01
France, Doubs	0.12	0.04	-	-
France, Haut-Rhin	0.23	0.04	0,02	0,01
*France, Herault	0.13	0.03	0,02	0,01
France, Isere	0.15	0.03	0,02	0,01
*France, Somme	0.40	0.06	0,01	0,01
*France, Tarn	0,02	0,01	-	-
Germany, Eastern States	0.01	0.00	0,00	0,00
Germany, Saarland	0.04	0.01	0,01	0,01
Iceland	0,02	0,02	-	-
Ireland, Southern	0,02	0,01	0,03	0,02
Italy, Ferrara	0,04	0,03	-	-
Italy, Florence	0.04	0.01	0,01	0,01
Italy, Genoa	0,03	0,01	-	-
*Italy, Latina	0,07	0,03	-	-
Italy, Macerata	0,03	0,03	-	-
Italy, Modena	0,02	0,01	-	-
Italy, Parma	0,01	0,01	-	-
Italy, Ragusa	0,04	0,02	-	-
Italy, Romagna	0,02	0,01	0,01	0,01
Italy, Torino	0,06	0.02	-	-
Italy, Trieste	-	-	-	-
Italy, Varese	-	-	0,00	0,00
Italy, Veneto	0.27	0.03	0.05	0.01
*Latvia	0.05	0.01	0,01	0,00
Malta	-	-	-	-
The Netherlands	0.01	0.00	0,00	0,00
The Netherlands, Eindhoven	0,01	0,01	-	-
The Netherlands, Maastricht	0,02	0,01	-	-
Norway	0.01	0.00	0,00	0,00
*Poland, Cracow	0.07	0.02	0,02	0,01
*Poland, Kielce	0.02	0,01	0,01	0,01
*Poland, Lower Silesia	0.06	0.01	0,01	0,00
Poland, Warsaw City	0.03	0.01	0,01	0,01
Slovakia	0.03	0.01	0,00	0,00
Slovenia	0,01	0,01	-	-
*Spain, Albacete	0,03	0,03	-	-
Spain, Asturias	0.18	0.03	0,01	0,00
Spain, Basque Country	0.27	0.03	0,01	0,00
Spain, Granada	0.12	0.03	0,01	0,01
Spain, Mallorca	0.11	0.03	0,01	0,01
Spain, Murcia	0.08	0.02	0,00	0,00
Spain, Navarra	0,07	0,02	-	-
Spain, Tarragona	0,02	0,01	0,01	0,01
Spain, Zaragoza	0,02	0,01	0,00	0,00
Sweden	0,00	0,00	-	-
*Switzerland, Basel	0,01	0,01	-	-
Switzerland, Geneva	0,02	0,02	0,03	0,02
Switzerland, Graubunden	0,03	0,03	-	-
Switzerland, Neuchatel	0,05	0,03	0,04	0,03
Switzerland, St Gall-Appenzell	0,02	0,01	-	-
Switzerland, Valais	0,13	0,05	-	-
Switzerland, Vaud	0,06	0,02	0,01	0,01
Switzerland, Zurich	0,00	0,00	-	-
*UK, England and Wales	0.04	0.00	0.02	0.00
*UK, East Anglia	0.02	0.01	0.01	0.00
*UK, Mersey	0.04	0.01	0.01	0.00
*UK, North Western	0.05	0.01	0.02	0.00
UK, Oxford	0.02	0.01	0.02	0.01
*UK, South Thames	0.04	0.00	0.01	0.00
UK, South Western	0.02	0.01	0.01	0.00
UK, Wessex	0.04	0.01	0.02	0.00
*UK, West Midlands	0.03	0.01	0.01	0.00
UK, Yorkshire	0.05	0.01	0.01	0.00
UK, Scotland	0.06	0.01	0.02	0.00
UK, Scotland, West	0.08	0.01	0.02	0.01
*Yugoslavia, Vojvodina	0.04	0.01	0,00	0,00

OCEANIA

	MALE		FEMALE	
Australian Capital Territory	0,03	0,03	-	-
Australia, New South Wales	0.04	0.01	0.01	0.00
South Australia	0.03	0.01	0.01	0.00
Australia, Tasmania	0.11	0.03	0.02	0.02
Australia, Victoria	0.05	0.01	0.02	0.00
Western Australia	0.12	0.02	0.01	0,01
*French Polynesia	0,24	0,09	0,04	0,04
New Zealand: Non-Maori	0.04	0.01	0,00	0,00
New Zealand: Maori	0,03	0,02	-	-
US, Hawaii: White	0,16	0,06	0,04	0,03
US, Hawaii: Japanese	0,04	0,02	-	-
US, Hawaii: Hawaiian	0,07	0,07	-	-
US, Hawaii: Filipino	-	-	-	-
US, Hawaii: Chinese	-	-	-	-

* IMPORTANT-SEE NOTES ON POPULATION PAGE

CUMULATIVE INCIDENCE (0-74)
RATES AND STANDARD ERRORS (percent)
Oesophagus (ICD-9 150)

	MALE		FEMALE	
AFRICA				
*Algeria, Setif				
*France, La Reunion				
*Mali, Bamako				
*Uganda, Kyadondo				
*Zimbabwe, Harare: African				
*Zimbabwe, Harare: European				
AMERICA, CENTRAL AND SOUTH				
*Argentina, Concordia	2.09	0.35	0.47	0.15
*Brazil, Belem	0.77	0.13	0.20	0.06
*Brazil, Goiania				
*Brazil, Porto Alegre	2.39	0.17	0.44	0.06
Colombia, Cali	0.44	0.06	0.26	0.04
*Costa Rica	0.39	0.04	0.18	0.03
*Ecuador, Quito	0.34	0.07	0.08	0.02
*Peru, Lima	0.19	0.03	0.09	0.02
Peru, Trujillo	0,28	0,12	0,08	0,06
US, Puerto Rico	1.04	0.05	0.24	0.02
*Uruguay, Montevideo	1.44	0.10	0.38	0.04
AMERICA, NORTH				
Canada	0.51	0.01	0.15	0.01
Canada, Alberta	0.32	0.03	0.12	0.02
Canada, British Columbia	0.53	0.03	0.19	0.02
Canada, Manitoba	0.47	0.05	0.16	0.03
Canada, New Brunswick	0.46	0.06	0.12	0.03
Canada, Newfoundland	0.54	0.08	0.10	0.03
Canada, Northwest Territories	0,67	0,37	0,96	0,48
Canada, Nova Scotia	0.53	0.06	0.15	0.03
Canada, Ontario	0.56	0.02	0.17	0.01
Canada, Prince Edward Island	0.48	0.14	0,06	0,05
Canada, Quebec	0.50	0.02	0.12	0.01
Canada, Saskatchewan	0.42	0.05	0.13	0.02
Canada, Yukon	0,61	0,28	-	-
US, Cent. Calif.: Non-Hisp. White	0.53	0.04	0.13	0.02
US, Cent. Calif.: Hispanic	0.32	0.08	0,07	0,04
US, Los Angeles: Non-Hisp. White	0.47	0.02	0.20	0.01
US, Los Angeles: Hispanic White	0.51	0.05	0.07	0.02
US, Los Angeles: Black	1.19	0.10	0.43	0.05
US, Los Angeles: Chinese	0.40	0.10	0,07	0,05
US, Los Angeles: Filipino	0,25	0,10	-	-
US, Los Angeles: Korean	0,52	0,18	0,04	0,04
US, Los Angeles: Japanese	0.56	0.14	0,11	0,06
US, San Francisco: Non-Hisp. White	0.56	0.04	0.19	0.02
US, San Francisco: Hispanic White	0.49	0.11	0,07	0,04
US, San Francisco: Black	1.58	0.17	0.50	0.08
US, San Francisco: Chinese	0.43	0.09	0,08	0,04
US, San Francisco: Filipino	0,23	0,10	0,03	0,03
US, San Francisco: Japanese	1.33	0.38	0,05	0,05
US, Connecticut: White	0.68	0.03	0.18	0.02
US, Connecticut: Black	2.49	0.29	0.51	0.11
US, Atlanta: White	0.50	0.05	0.16	0.03
US, Atlanta: Black	1.83	0.18	0.60	0.09
US, Iowa	0.53	0.03	0.10	0.01

	MALE		FEMALE	
US, Central Louisiana: White	0.50	0.11	0,07	0,04
US, Central Louisiana: Black	1.76	0.43	0,32	0,16
US, New Orleans: White	0.72	0.08	0.17	0.03
US, New Orleans: Black	1.35	0.17	0.31	0.07
US, Detroit: White	0.61	0.03	0.17	0.02
US, Detroit: Black	1.70	0.11	0.45	0.05
US, New Mexico: Non-Hisp. White	0.46	0.05	0.14	0.03
US, New Mexico: Hispanic White	0.26	0.06	0,03	0,02
US, New Mexico: American Indian	0,30	0,16	-	-
US, Utah	0.33	0.04	0.07	0.02
US, Seattle	0.62	0.03	0.21	0.02
US, SEER: White	0.56	0.01	0.16	0.01
US, SEER: Black	1.75	0.08	0.50	0.03
ASIA				
*China, Qidong	1.48	0.10	0.54	0.05
China, Shanghai	1.56	0.04	0.60	0.02
China, Tianjin	1.76	0.06	0.78	0.04
Hong Kong	1.79	0.04	0.37	0.02
*India, Bangalore	1.13	0.06	1.04	0.05
*India, Barshi, Paranda and Bhum	0.78	0.13	0.22	0.06
India, Bombay	1.31	0.05	0.97	0.04
*India, Karunagappally	0.89	0.19	0.36	0.12
India, Madras	1.30	0.06	0.87	0.05
*India, Trivandrum	0.60	0.13	0,17	0,07
Israel: All Jews	0.18	0.02	0.13	0.01
Jews born in Israel	0.18	0.07	0,05	0,02
Jews born in America or Europe	0.18	0.02	0.12	0.02
Jews born in Africa or Asia	0.17	0.03	0.14	0.03
Non-Jews	0,08	0,05	0,00	0,00
Japan, Hiroshima	1.38	0.09	0.17	0.03
Japan, Miyagi	1.76	0.06	0.26	0.02
Japan, Nagasaki	1.07	0.06	0.11	0.02
Japan, Osaka	1.14	0.03	0.18	0.01
*Japan, Saga	0.91	0.07	0.10	0.02
Japan, Yamagata	1.40	0.07	0.16	0.02
*Korea, Kangwha	1.43	0.29	0,04	0,04
*Kuwait: Non-Kuwaitis	0,07	0,04	0,07	0,05
*Kuwait: Kuwaitis	0,18	0,08	0,31	0,13
*Philippines, Manila	0.40	0.04	0.21	0.03
Singapore: Chinese	1.03	0.07	0.23	0.03
Singapore: Malay	0,05	0,03	0,06	0,04
Singapore: Indian	0.62	0.13	0.57	0.19
Thailand, Chiang Mai	0.28	0.04	0.21	0.04
*Thailand, Khon Kaen	0.18	0.04	0.06	0.02
*Viet Nam, Hanoi				

* IMPORTANT-SEE NOTES ON POPULATION PAGE

EUROPE

	MALE		FEMALE	
Austria, Tyrol	0.49	0.07	0,05	0,02
*Belarus	0.74	0.02	0.08	0.01
*Croatia	0.70	0.03	0.09	0.01
Czech Republic	0.47	0.02	0.06	0.01
Denmark	0.58	0.02	0.17	0.01
Estonia	0.69	0.05	0.07	0.01
Finland	0.41	0.02	0.18	0.01
France, Bas-Rhin	2.02	0.11	0.15	0.03
*France, Calvados	2.78	0.16	0.13	0.03
France, Doubs	1.27	0.12	0.17	0.04
France, Haut-Rhin	1.69	0.12	0.15	0.03
*France, Herault	0.79	0.07	0.11	0.02
France, Isere	1.32	0.09	0.13	0.03
*France, Somme	2.17	0.14	0.20	0.04
*France, Tarn	0.61	0.08	0,08	0,03
Germany, Eastern States	0.49	0.02	0.07	0.01
Germany, Saarland	0.80	0.06	0.10	0.02
Iceland	0.84	0.15	0.26	0.08
Ireland, Southern	0.78	0.09	0.43	0.06
Italy, Ferrara	0.35	0.09	0,05	0,03
Italy, Florence	0.46	0.05	0.12	0.02
Italy, Genoa	0.48	0.05	0.07	0.02
*Italy, Latina	0.34	0.07	0,03	0,02
Italy, Macerata	0,19	0,08	0,09	0,05
Italy, Modena	0.36	0.05	0.06	0.02
Italy, Parma	0.44	0.06	0.09	0.02
Italy, Ragusa	0,12	0,05	0,05	0,03
Italy, Romagna	0.36	0.05	0,05	0,02
Italy, Torino	0.44	0.05	0.06	0.02
Italy, Trieste	0.92	0.13	0.15	0.04
Italy, Varese	0.85	0.07	0.06	0.02
Italy, Veneto	1.17	0.07	0.17	0.02
*Latvia	0.57	0.04	0.08	0.01
Malta	0.53	0.15	0,10	0,06
The Netherlands	0.65	0.02	0.22	0.01
The Netherlands, Eindhoven	0.47	0.05	0.12	0.03
The Netherlands, Maastricht	0.51	0.05	0.14	0.03
Norway	0.41	0.02	0.09	0.01
*Poland, Cracow	0.54	0.07	0.09	0.02
*Poland, Kielce	0.38	0.04	0.07	0.02
*Poland, Lower Silesia	0.72	0.04	0.10	0.01
Poland, Warsaw City	0.55	0.05	0.11	0.02
Slovakia	0.87	0.03	0.05	0.01
Slovenia	0.80	0.05	0.09	0.01
*Spain, Albacete	0.38	0.11	-	-
Spain, Asturias	0.96	0.07	0.08	0.02
Spain, Basque Country	1.18	0.06	0.05	0.01
Spain, Granada	0.42	0.05	0.06	0.02
Spain, Mallorca	0.56	0.06	0,04	0,02
Spain, Murcia	0.55	0.05	0,03	0,01
Spain, Navarra	0.86	0.08	0,06	0,02
Spain, Tarragona	0.69	0.07	0,02	0,01
Spain, Zaragoza	0.62	0.05	0.04	0.01
Sweden	0.38	0.01	0.11	0.01
*Switzerland, Basel	0.71	0.09	0.16	0.04
Switzerland, Geneva	0.86	0.11	0.19	0.05
Switzerland, Graubunden	0.46	0.13	0,07	0,05
Switzerland, Neuchatel	0.69	0.13	0,17	0,06
Switzerland, St Gall-Appenzell	0.64	0.08	0,07	0,03
Switzerland, Valais	0.90	0.15	0,10	0,05
Switzerland, Vaud	1.11	0.10	0.24	0.04
Switzerland, Zurich	0.41	0.04	0.13	0.02
*UK, England and Wales	0.93	0.01	0.40	0.01
*UK, East Anglia	0.75	0.04	0.30	0.02
*UK, Mersey	0.97	0.04	0.47	0.03
*UK, North Western	1.09	0.04	0.45	0.02
UK, Oxford	0.84	0.04	0.42	0.03
*UK, South Thames	0.87	0.02	0.36	0.01
UK, South Western	0.93	0.04	0.41	0.02
UK, Wessex	0.92	0.04	0.37	0.02
*UK, West Midlands	1.16	0.03	0.48	0.02
UK, Yorkshire	0.86	0.03	0.35	0.02
UK, Scotland	1.15	0.03	0.59	0.02
UK, Scotland, West	1.36	0.05	0.61	0.03
*Yugoslavia, Vojvodina	0.59	0.04	0.07	0.01

OCEANIA

	MALE		FEMALE	
Australian Capital Territory	0.53	0.13	0,26	0,09
Australia, New South Wales	0.57	0.02	0.24	0.01
South Australia	0.53	0.04	0.25	0.03
Australia, Tasmania	0.86	0.10	0.42	0.07
Australia, Victoria	0.64	0.03	0.28	0.02
Western Australia	0.56	0.05	0.18	0.03
*French Polynesia	1.16	0.32	0,25	0,14
New Zealand: Non-Maori	0.65	0.03	0.24	0.02
New Zealand: Maori	1.22	0.26	0,22	0,09
US, Hawaii: White	0.57	0.11	0.30	0.08
US, Hawaii: Japanese	0.47	0.08	0,07	0,03
US, Hawaii: Hawaiian	1.03	0.23	0,21	0,10
US, Hawaii: Filipino	0.37	0.11	0,08	0,06
US, Hawaii: Chinese	0,53	0,18	-	-

* IMPORTANT-SEE NOTES ON POPULATION PAGE

CUMULATIVE INCIDENCE (0-74)
RATES AND STANDARD ERRORS (percent)
Stomach (ICD-9 151)

	MALE		FEMALE	
AFRICA				
*Algeria, Setif				
*France, La Reunion				
*Mali, Bamako				
*Uganda, Kyadondo				
*Zimbabwe, Harare: African				
*Zimbabwe, Harare: European				
AMERICA, CENTRAL AND SOUTH				
*Argentina, Concordia	2.76	0.42	1.06	0.23
*Brazil, Belem	5.07	0.35	1.79	0.16
*Brazil, Goiania				
*Brazil, Porto Alegre	3.35	0.21	1.05	0.10
Colombia, Cali	3.79	0.18	2.25	0.13
*Costa Rica	5.22	0.15	2.19	0.09
*Ecuador, Quito	3.84	0.22	2.17	0.15
*Peru, Lima	2.23	0.10	1.60	0.09
Peru, Trujillo	3.96	0.45	1.93	0.28
US, Puerto Rico	1.49	0.06	0.67	0.04
*Uruguay, Montevideo	2.12	0.12	1.00	0.07
AMERICA, NORTH				
Canada	1.23	0.02	0.49	0.01
Canada, Alberta	1.13	0.06	0.41	0.03
Canada, British Columbia	1.09	0.04	0.42	0.02
Canada, Manitoba	1.33	0.08	0.44	0.04
Canada, New Brunswick	1.27	0.10	0.44	0.05
Canada, Newfoundland	2.14	0.16	0.94	0.10
Canada, Northwest Territories	2.33	0.57	0,49	0,30
Canada, Nova Scotia	1.35	0.09	0.53	0.05
Canada, Ontario	1.17	0.03	0.47	0.01
Canada, Prince Edward Island	1.50	0.26	0.56	0.14
Canada, Quebec	1.35	0.03	0.57	0.02
Canada, Saskatchewan	1.00	0.07	0.40	0.04
Canada, Yukon	0,66	0,30	0,93	0,58
US, Cent. Calif.: Non-Hisp. White	0.79	0.05	0.33	0.03
US, Cent. Calif.: Hispanic	1.08	0.14	0.78	0.12
US, Los Angeles: Non-Hisp. White	0.85	0.03	0.35	0.02
US, Los Angeles: Hispanic White	1.37	0.08	0.73	0.05
US, Los Angeles: Black	1.72	0.12	0.68	0.07
US, Los Angeles: Chinese	1.37	0.20	0.74	0.14
US, Los Angeles: Filipino	0.69	0.17	0.46	0.11
US, Los Angeles: Korean	4.26	0.51	1.93	0.29
US, Los Angeles: Japanese	2.36	0.28	1.15	0.18
US, San Francisco: Non-Hisp. White	0.90	0.05	0.34	0.03
US, San Francisco: Hispanic White	1.52	0.19	0.45	0.08
US, San Francisco: Black	1.80	0.18	0.73	0.09
US, San Francisco: Chinese	1.30	0.16	0.62	0.11
US, San Francisco: Filipino	0.79	0.22	0.45	0.12
US, San Francisco: Japanese	2.52	0.54	1.34	0.33
US, Connecticut: White	1.07	0.04	0.40	0.02
US, Connecticut: Black	1.73	0.26	0.84	0.15
US, Atlanta: White	0.61	0.06	0.25	0.03
US, Atlanta: Black	1.58	0.18	0.56	0.09
US, Iowa	0.77	0.04	0.24	0.02
US, Central Louisiana: White	0.74	0.13	0.31	0.08
US, Central Louisiana: Black	1.98	0.49	0,61	0,22
US, New Orleans: White	0.81	0.08	0.29	0.04
US, New Orleans: Black	1.93	0.21	0.58	0.09
US, Detroit: White	0.98	0.04	0.40	0.02
US, Detroit: Black	1.79	0.12	0.62	0.06
US, New Mexico: Non-Hisp. White	0.63	0.06	0.29	0.04
US, New Mexico: Hispanic White	1.44	0.15	0.69	0.09
US, New Mexico: American Indian	1.18	0.33	0.72	0.21
US, Utah	0.66	0.05	0.31	0.03
US, Seattle	0.88	0.04	0.32	0.02
US, SEER: White	0.87	0.02	0.34	0.01
US, SEER: Black	1.75	0.08	0.64	0.04
ASIA				
*China, Qidong	5.31	0.18	2.53	0.11
China, Shanghai	5.77	0.07	2.48	0.04
China, Tianjin	3.84	0.08	1.41	0.05
Hong Kong	2.31	0.05	1.03	0.03
*India, Bangalore	1.34	0.06	0.60	0.04
*India, Barshi, Paranda and Bhum	0,11	0,04	0,09	0,03
India, Bombay	0.95	0.04	0.45	0.03
*India, Karunagappally	0.71	0.17	0,43	0,15
India, Madras	1.95	0.08	0.77	0.04
*India, Trivandrum	0.84	0.14	0.30	0.08
Israel: All Jews	1.45	0.05	0.69	0.03
Jews born in Israel	0.95	0.16	0.77	0.15
Jews born in America or Europe	1.70	0.07	0.75	0.04
Jews born in Africa or Asia	1.19	0.08	0.63	0.06
Non-Jews	0.84	0.14	0.34	0.08
Japan, Hiroshima	10.08	0.25	4.11	0.14
Japan, Miyagi	10.19	0.15	3.83	0.08
Japan, Nagasaki	8.53	0.16	3.42	0.09
Japan, Osaka	7.67	0.08	2.94	0.04
*Japan, Saga	8.52	0.22	3.11	0.11
Japan, Yamagata	11.52	0.19	4.60	0.11
*Korea, Kangwha	8.22	0.66	2.98	0.35
*Kuwait: Non-Kuwaitis	1.06	0.32	0.25	0.12
*Kuwait: Kuwaitis	0.52	0.14	0.49	0.13
*Philippines, Manila	1.35	0.08	0.76	0.05
Singapore: Chinese	3.62	0.13	1.61	0.08
Singapore: Malay	1.11	0.17	0.63	0.13
Singapore: Indian	1.25	0.20	0.72	0.21
Thailand, Chiang Mai	0.92	0.07	0.63	0.06
*Thailand, Khon Kaen	0.60	0.08	0.25	0.04
*Viet Nam, Hanoi				

* IMPORTANT-SEE NOTES ON POPULATION PAGE

EUROPE	MALE		FEMALE	
Austria, Tyrol	3.12	0.19	1.68	0.11
*Belarus	5.89	0.07	2.55	0.03
*Croatia	3.40	0.08	1.32	0.04
Czech Republic	2.27	0.04	1.00	0.02
Denmark	1.04	0.03	0.52	0.02
Estonia	4.20	0.14	1.96	0.07
Finland	1.88	0.04	0.99	0.03
France, Bas-Rhin	1.45	0.10	0.50	0.05
*France, Calvados	1.64	0.13	0.45	0.06
France, Doubs	1.30	0.13	0.36	0.06
France, Haut-Rhin	1.74	0.13	0.69	0.07
*France, Herault	1.12	0.08	0.48	0.05
France, Isere	1.39	0.09	0.45	0.05
*France, Somme	1.10	0.11	0.43	0.06
*France, Tarn	1.06	0.12	0.37	0.07
Germany, Eastern States	2.46	0.05	1.20	0.03
Germany, Saarland	2.05	0.10	0.92	0.06
Iceland	2.32	0.25	1.18	0.16
Ireland, Southern	1.74	0.14	0.51	0.07
Italy, Ferrara	2.16	0.24	1.10	0.15
Italy, Florence	4.33	0.14	1.68	0.08
Italy, Genoa	1.97	0.11	0.84	0.06
*Italy, Latina	2.34	0.19	1.08	0.12
Italy, Macerata	3.46	0.36	1.47	0.21
Italy, Modena	2.50	0.13	1.27	0.09
Italy, Parma	3.94	0.20	1.42	0.11
Italy, Ragusa	1.45	0.16	0.57	0.09
Italy, Romagna	4.55	0.20	2.40	0.13
Italy, Torino	2.06	0.11	0.90	0.06
Italy, Trieste	1.92	0.19	0.88	0.11
Italy, Varese	3.01	0.15	1.27	0.08
Italy, Veneto	2.22	0.10	0.93	0.06
*Latvia	3.89	0.10	1.66	0.05
Malta	1.43	0.24	0.71	0.15
The Netherlands	1.80	0.03	0.66	0.02
The Netherlands, Eindhoven	1.97	0.11	0.75	0.06
The Netherlands, Maastricht	1.90	0.11	0.71	0.06
Norway	1.51	0.04	0.68	0.03
*Poland, Cracow	2.57	0.16	0.87	0.08
*Poland, Kielce	2.81	0.12	0.94	0.06
*Poland, Lower Silesia	2.96	0.09	1.22	0.05
Poland, Warsaw City	2.21	0.10	0.76	0.05
Slovakia	3.06	0.07	1.17	0.04
Slovenia	3.36	0.11	1.12	0.05
*Spain, Albacete	1.92	0.25	0.79	0.15
Spain, Asturias	2.17	0.10	0.95	0.06
Spain, Basque Country	2.78	0.09	1.05	0.05
Spain, Granada	1.80	0.11	0.71	0.06
Spain, Mallorca	1.39	0.11	0.64	0.07
Spain, Murcia	1.81	0.10	0.77	0.06
Spain, Navarra	2.85	0.16	1.08	0.09
Spain, Tarragona	1.60	0.12	0.64	0.07
Spain, Zaragoza	2.20	0.11	0.76	0.06

	MALE		FEMALE	
Sweden	1.23	0.02	0.60	0.02
*Switzerland, Basel	1.29	0.12	0.54	0.07
Switzerland, Geneva	1.49	0.15	0.56	0.08
Switzerland, Graubunden	2.02	0.27	0.78	0.15
Switzerland, Neuchatel	1.36	0.20	0.50	0.11
Switzerland, St Gall-Appenzell	1.38	0.12	0.63	0.08
Switzerland, Valais	2.10	0.23	0.90	0.14
Switzerland, Vaud	1.16	0.10	0.50	0.06
Switzerland, Zurich	1.27	0.08	0.50	0.04
*UK, England and Wales	1.88	0.02	0.67	0.01
*UK, East Anglia	1.74	0.06	0.51	0.03
*UK, Mersey	1.94	0.06	0.81	0.04
*UK, North Western	1.87	0.05	0.71	0.03
UK, Oxford	1.63	0.06	0.57	0.03
*UK, South Thames	1.53	0.03	0.53	0.02
UK, South Western	1.54	0.05	0.52	0.02
UK, Wessex	1.47	0.05	0.46	0.02
*UK, West Midlands	2.06	0.04	0.74	0.02
UK, Yorkshire	1.94	0.05	0.73	0.03
UK, Scotland	2.08	0.05	0.83	0.03
UK, Scotland, West	2.10	0.06	0.84	0.03
*Yugoslavia, Vojvodina	2.60	0.09	1.15	0.05

OCEANIA	MALE		FEMALE	
Australian Capital Territory	0.97	0.18	0.45	0.10
Australia, New South Wales	1.17	0.03	0.47	0.02
South Australia	1.23	0.07	0.46	0.04
Australia, Tasmania	1.26	0.12	0.52	0.07
Australia, Victoria	1.35	0.04	0.52	0.02
Western Australia	1.34	0.07	0.56	0.05
*French Polynesia	1.49	0.37	0.90	0.26
New Zealand: Non-Maori	1.25	0.05	0.49	0.03
New Zealand: Maori	3.41	0.43	1.45	0.22
US, Hawaii: White	0.94	0.14	0.39	0.09
US, Hawaii: Japanese	2.59	0.19	1.02	0.11
US, Hawaii: Hawaiian	1.99	0.33	1.12	0.21
US, Hawaii: Filipino	0.81	0.16	0.86	0.18
US, Hawaii: Chinese	1.75	0.34	0.64	0.19

* IMPORTANT-SEE NOTES ON POPULATION PAGE

CUMULATIVE INCIDENCE (0-74)
RATES AND STANDARD ERRORS (percent)
Small intestine (ICD-9 152)

AFRICA	MALE		FEMALE	
*Algeria, Setif				
*France, La Reunion				
*Mali, Bamako				
*Uganda, Kyadondo				
*Zimbabwe, Harare: African				
*Zimbabwe, Harare: European				

AMERICA, CENTRAL AND SOUTH	MALE		FEMALE	
*Argentina, Concordia	0,10	*0,10*	0,08	*0,06*
*Brazil, Belem	0,05	*0,03*	0,02	*0,02* f
*Brazil, Goiania				
*Brazil, Porto Alegre	0.19	*0.05*	0.09	*0.03*
Colombia, Cali	0,07	*0,03*	0.10	*0.02*
*Costa Rica	0.07	*0.02*	0.06	*0.01*
*Ecuador, Quito	0.09	*0.03*	0.09	*0.03*
*Peru, Lima	0.05	*0.01*	0.05	*0.01*
Peru, Trujillo	0,13	*0,08*	0,13	*0,08* m
US, Puerto Rico	0.08	*0.01*	0.07	*0.01*
*Uruguay, Montevideo	0.07	*0.02*	0,02	*0,01*

AMERICA, NORTH	MALE		FEMALE	
Canada	0.10	*0.00*	0.08	*0.00*
Canada, Alberta	0.10	*0.02*	0.11	*0.02*
Canada, British Columbia	0.08	*0.01*	0.05	*0.01*
Canada, Manitoba	0.08	*0.02*	0.05	*0.02*
Canada, New Brunswick	0,06	*0,02*	0,05	*0,02*
Canada, Newfoundland	0,06	*0,02*	0,09	*0,03*
Canada, Northwest Territories	0,31	*0,25*	-	-
Canada, Nova Scotia	0.13	*0.03*	0.11	*0.02*
Canada, Ontario	0.12	*0.01*	0.09	*0.01*
Canada, Prince Edward Island	0,04	*0,04*	0,07	*0,05*
Canada, Quebec	0.10	*0.01*	0.08	*0.01*
Canada, Saskatchewan	0.15	*0.03*	0.10	*0.02*
Canada, Yukon	-	-	-	-
US, Cent. Calif.: Non-Hisp. White	0.15	*0.02*	0.08	*0.02*
US, Cent. Calif.: Hispanic	0,05	*0,02*	0,06	*0,03*
US, Los Angeles: Non-Hisp. White	0.14	*0.01*	0.10	*0.01*
US, Los Angeles: Hispanic White	0.09	*0.02*	0.06	*0.01*
US, Los Angeles: Black	0.20	*0.04*	0.17	*0.03*
US, Los Angeles: Chinese	0,03	*0,02*	-	-
US, Los Angeles: Filipino	0,05	*0,03*	0,01	*0,01*
US, Los Angeles: Korean	0,14	*0,10*	0,07	*0,04*
US, Los Angeles: Japanese	0,04	*0,03*	-	-
US, San Francisco: Non-Hisp. White	0.13	*0.02*	0.08	*0.01*
US, San Francisco: Hispanic White	0,07	*0,03*	0,05	*0,03*
US, San Francisco: Black	0.27	*0.07*	0.13	*0.04*
US, San Francisco: Chinese	0,06	*0,03*	0,07	*0,04*
US, San Francisco: Filipino	0,05	*0,04*	-	-
US, San Francisco: Japanese	-	-	-	-
US, Connecticut: White	0.12	*0.01*	0.10	*0.01*
US, Connecticut: Black	0,15	*0,06*	0,15	*0,06*
US, Atlanta: White	0.14	*0.02*	0.10	*0.02*
US, Atlanta: Black	0.20	*0.06*	0.21	*0.05*
US, Iowa	0.13	*0.02*	0.11	*0.01*

	MALE		FEMALE	
US, Central Louisiana: White	0.07	*0.04*	0.06	*0.04*
US, Central Louisiana: Black	0.13	*0,10*	-	-
US, New Orleans: White	0.18	*0.04*	0,04	*0,02*
US, New Orleans: Black	0,14	*0,05*	0.19	*0.05*
US, Detroit: White	0.18	*0.02*	0.10	*0.01*
US, Detroit: Black	0.31	*0.05*	0.15	*0.03*
US, New Mexico: Non-Hisp. White	0.16	*0.03*	0.07	*0.02*
US, New Mexico: Hispanic White	0,12	*0,05*	0,06	*0,03*
US, New Mexico: American Indian	0,09	*0,09*	-	-
US, Utah	0.10	*0.02*	0.10	*0.02*
US, Seattle	0.13	*0.01*	0.10	*0.01*
US, SEER: White	0.14	*0.01*	0.10	*0.00*
US, SEER: Black	0.25	*0.03*	0.15	*0.02*

ASIA	MALE		FEMALE	
*China, Qidong	0.06	*0.02*	0,03	*0,01*
China, Shanghai	0.08	*0.01*	0.05	*0.01*
China, Tianjin	0.07	*0.01*	0.05	*0.01*
Hong Kong	0.12	*0.01*	0.07	*0.01*
*India, Bangalore	0,01	*0,01*	0,01	*0,00*
*India, Barshi, Paranda and Bhum	0,01	*0,01*	-	-
India, Bombay	0.04	*0.01*	0.03	*0.01*
*India, Karunagappally	0,11	*0,08*	-	-
India, Madras	0,01	*0,00*	0,01	*0,01*
*India, Trivandrum	0,01	*0,01*	0,01	*0,01*
Israel: All Jews	0.08	*0.01*	0.06	*0.01*
Jews born in Israel	0,05	*0,03*	0,06	*0,05*
Jews born in America or Europe	0.08	*0.02*	0.09	*0.02*
Jews born in Africa or Asia	0.08	*0.02*	0,03	*0,01*
Non-Jews	0,03	*0,03*	0,04	*0,02*
Japan, Hiroshima	0.04	*0.01*	0.04	*0.01*
Japan, Miyagi	0.05	*0.01*	0.04	*0.01*
Japan, Nagasaki	0.08	*0.02*	0.03	*0.01*
Japan, Osaka	0.07	*0.01*	0.04	*0.00*
*Japan, Saga	0.06	*0.02*	0.03	*0.01*
Japan, Yamagata	0.05	*0.01*	0.02	*0.01*
*Korea, Kangwha	0,12	*0,09*	0.10	*0,06*
*Kuwait: Non-Kuwaitis	-	-	0,01	*0,01*
*Kuwait: Kuwaitis	-	-	0,02	*0,02*
*Philippines, Manila	0.07	*0.02*	0.03	*0.01*
Singapore: Chinese	0.06	*0.02*	0.04	*0.01*
Singapore: Malay	0,02	*0,02*	0,03	*0,02*
Singapore: Indian	0,07	*0,05*	0,01	*0,01*
Thailand, Chiang Mai	0.05	*0.02*	0.01	*0,01*
*Thailand, Khon Kaen	0,02	*0,01*	0,01	*0,01*
*Viet Nam, Hanoi				

* IMPORTANT-SEE NOTES ON POPULATION PAGE

EUROPE	MALE		FEMALE	
Austria, Tyrol	0.10	0.03	0,03	0,01
*Belarus	0.04	0.00	0.03	0.00
*Croatia	0.04	0.01	0.02	0.01
Czech Republic	0.07	0.01	0.04	0.00
Denmark	0.09	0.01	0.06	0.01
Estonia	0.07	0.02	0.03	0.01
Finland	0.11	0.01	0.08	0.01
France, Bas-Rhin	0.13	0.03	0.06	0.02
*France, Calvados	0.15	0.04	0.12	0.03
France, Doubs	0.15	0.04	0.09	0.03
France, Haut-Rhin	0.11	0.03	0.05	0,02
*France, Herault	0.07	0.02	0.08	0.02
France, Isere	0.10	0.03	0.07	0.02
*France, Somme	0,05	0,02	0,05	0,02
*France, Tarn	0,06	0,03	-	-
Germany, Eastern States	0.05	0.01	0.03	0.00
Germany, Saarland	0.08	0.02	0.08	0.02
Iceland	0,17	0,06	0,09	0,04
Ireland, Southern	0,04	0,02	0,03	0,02
Italy, Ferrara	0,15	0,06	0,06	0,04
Italy, Florence	0.07	0.02	0.06	0.02
Italy, Genoa	0.07	0.02	0,03	0,01
*Italy, Latina	0,11	0,04	0,04	0,02
Italy, Macerata	0,03	0,03	0,03	0,03
Italy, Modena	0.08	0.02	0.09	0.02
Italy, Parma	0,05	0,02	0,04	0,02
Italy, Ragusa	0,06	0,03	0,04	0,02
Italy, Romagna	0,06	0,02	0.08	0.02
Italy, Torino	0,03	0,01	0.04	0.01
Italy, Trieste	0,13	0,05	0,11	0,04
Italy, Varese	0.10	0.03	0.04	0,01
Italy, Veneto	0.07	0.02	0.06	0.01
*Latvia	0.06	0.01	0.03	0.01
Malta	0,24	0,10	0,06	0,04
The Netherlands	0.08	0.01	0.05	0.00
The Netherlands, Eindhoven	0.11	0.03	0,04	0,01
The Netherlands, Maastricht	0.10	0.02	0.08	0.02
Norway	0.09	0.01	0.09	0.01
*Poland, Cracow	0,04	0,02	0,04	0,02
*Poland, Kielce	0.09	0.02	0.07	0.02
*Poland, Lower Silesia	0.04	0.01	0.02	0.01
Poland, Warsaw City	0,03	0,01	0.03	0.01
Slovakia	0.10	0.01	0.05	0.01
Slovenia	0.03	0.01	0.04	0.01
*Spain, Albacete	0,06	0,04	-	-
Spain, Asturias	0.12	0.02	0.06	0.01
Spain, Basque Country	0.09	0.02	0.03	0.01
Spain, Granada	0.07	0.02	0.04	0.01
Spain, Mallorca	0,06	0,02	0,04	0,02
Spain, Murcia	0.11	0.02	0.02	0,01
Spain, Navarra	0,04	0,02	0,04	0,02
Spain, Tarragona	0.09	0.03	0,03	0,01
Spain, Zaragoza	0,02	0,01	0,02	0,01

	MALE		FEMALE	
Sweden	0.16	0.01	0.11	0.01
*Switzerland, Basel	0.25	0.05	0.12	0.03
Switzerland, Geneva	0,07	0,03	0,06	0,03
Switzerland, Graubunden	0,11	0,06	0,04	0,04
Switzerland, Neuchatel	0,13	0,07	0,04	0,03
Switzerland, St Gall-Appenzell	0.13	0.04	0.07	0,02
Switzerland, Valais	0,09	0,04	0,09	0,05
Switzerland, Vaud	0.15	0.04	0.11	0.03
Switzerland, Zurich	0.18	0.03	0.08	0.02
*UK, England and Wales	0.05	0.00	0.04	0.00
*UK, East Anglia	0.09	0.01	0.05	0.01
*UK, Mersey	0.06	0.01	0.04	0.01
*UK, North Western	0.06	0.01	0.05	0.01
UK, Oxford	0.06	0.01	0.06	0.01
*UK, South Thames	0.05	0.01	0.04	0.00
UK, South Western	0.05	0.01	0.04	0.01
UK, Wessex	0.09	0.01	0.08	0.01
*UK, West Midlands	0.09	0.01	0.05	0.01
UK, Yorkshire	0.08	0.01	0.06	0.01
UK, Scotland	0.08	0.01	0.05	0.01
UK, Scotland, West	0.09	0.01	0.05	0.01
*Yugoslavia, Vojvodina	0.08	0.01	0.04	0.01

OCEANIA	MALE		FEMALE	
Australian Capital Territory	0,08	0,04	0,17	0,07
Australia, New South Wales	0.10	0.01	0.07	0.01
South Australia	0.12	0.02	0.05	0.01
Australia, Tasmania	0,04	0,02	0,04	0,02
Australia, Victoria	0.09	0.01	0.07	0.01
Western Australia	0.12	0.02	0.06	0.01
*French Polynesia	0,04	0,03	0,10	0,08
New Zealand: Non-Maori	0.08	0.01	0.06	0.01
New Zealand: Maori	0,33	0,13	0,17	0,08
US, Hawaii: White	0.21	0.07	0.08	0,04
US, Hawaii: Japanese	0.12	0,04	0,01	0,01
US, Hawaii: Hawaiian	0,23	0,10	0,23	0,10
US, Hawaii: Filipino	0,08	0,06	0,08	0,06
US, Hawaii: Chinese	0,06	0,06	0,05	0,05

* IMPORTANT-SEE NOTES ON POPULATION PAGE

CUMULATIVE INCIDENCE (0-74)
RATES AND STANDARD ERRORS (percent)
Colon (ICD-9 153)

	MALE		FEMALE	
AFRICA				
*Algeria, Setif				
*France, La Reunion				
*Mali, Bamako				
*Uganda, Kyadondo				
*Zimbabwe, Harare: African				
*Zimbabwe, Harare: European				
AMERICA, CENTRAL AND SOUTH				
*Argentina, Concordia	1.60	0.33	1.58	0.28
*Brazil, Belem	0.55	0.12	0.38	0.08
*Brazil, Goiania				
*Brazil, Porto Alegre	1.72	0.15	1.46	0.11
Colombia, Cali	0.72	0.08	0.73	0.07
*Costa Rica	0.56	0.05	0.63	0.05
*Ecuador, Quito	0.51	0.08	0.71	0.08
*Peru, Lima	0.65	0.06	0.62	0.05
Peru, Trujillo	0.42	0.15	0.54	0.14
US, Puerto Rico	1.77	0.06	1.38	0.05
*Uruguay, Montevideo	2.66	0.14	1.97	0.10
AMERICA, NORTH				
Canada	3.18	0.03	2.44	0.02
Canada, Alberta	2.64	0.09	1.80	0.07
Canada, British Columbia	2.45	0.06	1.99	0.05
Canada, Manitoba	3.06	0.12	2.72	0.11
Canada, New Brunswick	3.41	0.17	2.58	0.13
Canada, Newfoundland	3.85	0.21	3.55	0.19
Canada, Northwest Territories	0,75	0,31	2.11	0.66
Canada, Nova Scotia	3.65	0.15	2.85	0.12
Canada, Ontario	3.56	0.05	2.63	0.04
Canada, Prince Edward Island	3.44	0.38	2.46	0.30
Canada, Quebec	3.15	0.05	2.42	0.04
Canada, Saskatchewan	2.57	0.12	2.20	0.10
Canada, Yukon	1.65	0.64	1,43	0,64
US, Cent. Calif.: Non-Hisp. White	2.84	0.10	2.22	0.08
US, Cent. Calif.: Hispanic	2.15	0.21	1.17	0.14
US, Los Angeles: Non-Hisp. White	3.33	0.07	2.33	0.05
US, Los Angeles: Hispanic White	2.07	0.11	1.34	0.07
US, Los Angeles: Black	4.01	0.18	3.09	0.14
US, Los Angeles: Chinese	2.12	0.25	1.36	0.19
US, Los Angeles: Filipino	1.73	0.26	1.07	0.18
US, Los Angeles: Korean	1.92	0.35	0.85	0.18
US, Los Angeles: Japanese	3.12	0.33	2.59	0.28
US, San Francisco: Non-Hisp. White	3.29	0.09	2.36	0.07
US, San Francisco: Hispanic White	2.63	0.26	1.69	0.17
US, San Francisco: Black	4.03	0.27	3.18	0.20
US, San Francisco: Chinese	2.32	0.22	2.20	0.21
US, San Francisco: Filipino	2.27	0.34	0.96	0.17
US, San Francisco: Japanese	3.48	0.64	3.11	0.51
US, Connecticut: White	3.54	0.08	2.43	0.06
US, Connecticut: Black	3.50	0.36	2.71	0.26
US, Atlanta: White	3.08	0.13	2.22	0.09
US, Atlanta: Black	4.15	0.30	3.10	0.21
US, Iowa	3.60	0.08	2.87	0.07

	MALE		FEMALE	
US, Central Louisiana: White	3.48	0.29	2.18	0.21
US, Central Louisiana: Black	2.82	0.54	3.25	0.51
US, New Orleans: White	3.50	0.18	2.64	0.13
US, New Orleans: Black	3.55	0.28	3.03	0.22
US, Detroit: White	3.36	0.08	2.28	0.06
US, Detroit: Black	4.11	0.18	3.43	0.14
US, New Mexico: Non-Hisp. White	2.65	0.13	1.96	0.10
US, New Mexico: Hispanic White	2.40	0.19	1.56	0.14
US, New Mexico: American Indian	0.98	0.30	0.97	0.28
US, Utah	2.50	0.11	1.79	0.08
US, Seattle	3.09	0.07	2.29	0.06
US, SEER: White	3.25	0.03	2.34	0.02
US, SEER: Black	4.02	0.12	3.18	0.09
ASIA				
*China, Qidong	0.24	0.03	0.22	0.03
China, Shanghai	1.48	0.03	1.32	0.03
China, Tianjin	0.65	0.03	0.58	0.03
Hong Kong	2.60	0.05	2.21	0.05
*India, Bangalore	0.31	0.03	0.24	0.03
*India, Barshi, Paranda and Bhum	0,09	0,04	0,05	0,02
India, Bombay	0.41	0.03	0.34	0.02
*India, Karunagappally	0,17	0,09	0,12	0,06m
India, Madras	0.23	0.03	0.15	0.02
*India, Trivandrum	0.33	0.10	0,11	0,04
Israel: All Jews	2.91	0.07	2.33	0.06
Jews born in Israel	3.24	0.34	2.06	0.21
Jews born in America or Europe	3.56	0.11	2.74	0.09
Jews born in Africa or Asia	1.82	0.10	1.62	0.09
Non-Jews	0.72	0.13	0.61	0.10
Japan, Hiroshima	3.86	0.15	2.07	0.10
Japan, Miyagi	2.97	0.08	1.79	0.06
Japan, Nagasaki	3.06	0.10	1.73	0.06
Japan, Osaka	2.42	0.04	1.51	0.03
*Japan, Saga	2.24	0.11	1.50	0.08
Japan, Yamagata	2.55	0.09	1.87	0.07
*Korea, Kangwha	0.60	0.18	0,26	0,10
*Kuwait: Non-Kuwaitis	0.52	0.15	0.27	0.10
*Kuwait: Kuwaitis	0.30	0.10	0.62	0.17
*Philippines, Manila	1.20	0.07	1.02	0.06
Singapore: Chinese	2.90	0.12	2.46	0.09
Singapore: Malay	1.50	0.20	0.67	0.12
Singapore: Indian	0.74	0.15	0.67	0.23
Thailand, Chiang Mai	0.47	0.05	0.41	0.04
*Thailand, Khon Kaen	0.65	0.08	0.42	0.06
*Viet Nam, Hanoi				

* IMPORTANT-SEE NOTES ON POPULATION PAGE

CUMULATIVE INCIDENCE (0-74)
RATES AND STANDARD ERRORS (percent)
Colon (ICD-9 153) (contd)

EUROPE	MALE		FEMALE	
Austria, Tyrol	2.62	0.18	1.94	0.12
*Belarus	1.26	0.03	0.94	0.02
*Croatia	1.53	0.05	1.01	0.03
Czech Republic	2.98	0.04	1.85	0.03
Denmark	2.41	0.05	2.31	0.04
Estonia	1.76	0.09	1.37	0.06
Finland	1.43	0.04	1.25	0.03
France, Bas-Rhin	3.72	0.17	2.17	0.10
*France, Calvados	2.42	0.16	1.65	0.11
France, Doubs	2.44	0.18	1.55	0.13
France, Haut-Rhin	3.45	0.19	2.17	0.13
*France, Herault	2.47	0.12	1.52	0.09
France, Isere	2.70	0.13	1.79	0.10
*France, Somme	2.49	0.16	1.45	0.11
*France, Tarn	2.27	0.17	1.48	0.13
Germany, Eastern States	1.87	0.05	1.68	0.03
Germany, Saarland	2.93	0.12	2.23	0.09
Iceland	1.97	0.21	1.74	0.19
Ireland, Southern	2.86	0.17	2.40	0.15
Italy, Ferrara	3.50	0.31	2.58	0.23
Italy, Florence	2.90	0.12	2.35	0.09
Italy, Genoa	3.04	0.13	2.10	0.09
*Italy, Latina	2.05	0.18	1.38	0.13
Italy, Macerata	2.91	0.32	1.91	0.24
Italy, Modena	2.49	0.13	2.03	0.11
Italy, Parma	2.85	0.17	2.01	0.13
Italy, Ragusa	1.14	0.14	1.16	0.13
Italy, Romagna	2.69	0.15	2.13	0.12
Italy, Torino	2.92	0.13	1.86	0.09
Italy, Trieste	3.68	0.26	1.93	0.16
Italy, Varese	3.02	0.14	2.06	0.10
Italy, Veneto	2.72	0.11	1.85	0.08
*Latvia	1.48	0.06	1.15	0.04
Malta	1.69	0.26	1.44	0.22
The Netherlands	2.52	0.03	2.18	0.03
The Netherlands, Eindhoven	2.75	0.13	2.23	0.11
The Netherlands, Maastricht	2.58	0.13	2.05	0.10
Norway	2.55	0.05	2.21	0.05
*Poland, Cracow	1.39	0.12	1.04	0.08
*Poland, Kielce	0.99	0.07	0.57	0.05
*Poland, Lower Silesia	1.49	0.06	1.12	0.04
Poland, Warsaw City	1.89	0.10	1.11	0.06
Slovakia	2.56	0.06	1.54	0.04
Slovenia	1.91	0.09	1.22	0.05
*Spain, Albacete	1.23	0.21	1.10	0.18
Spain, Asturias	1.96	0.10	1.29	0.07
Spain, Basque Country	2.06	0.08	1.15	0.05
Spain, Granada	1.24	0.09	0.97	0.07
Spain, Mallorca	2.12	0.13	1.78	0.11
Spain, Murcia	1.59	0.09	1.19	0.07
Spain, Navarra	1.91	0.13	1.56	0.11
Spain, Tarragona	2.18	0.13	1.59	0.11
Spain, Zaragoza	1.44	0.09	1.07	0.07

	MALE		FEMALE	
Sweden	2.02	0.03	1.79	0.03
*Switzerland, Basel	2.45	0.17	1.74	0.12
Switzerland, Geneva	2.97	0.22	1.76	0.14
Switzerland, Graubunden	2.23	0.28	1.97	0.25
Switzerland, Neuchatel	2.26	0.26	1.70	0.20
Switzerland, St Gall-Appenzell	1.93	0.15	1.45	0.11
Switzerland, Valais	2.09	0.23	1.75	0.20
Switzerland, Vaud	2.50	0.15	1.73	0.11
Switzerland, Zurich	2.20	0.10	1.50	0.07
*UK, England and Wales	2.17	0.02	1.76	0.02
*UK, East Anglia	2.32	0.07	1.86	0.06
*UK, Mersey	2.04	0.06	1.76	0.06
*UK, North Western	2.20	0.05	1.71	0.04
UK, Oxford	2.38	0.07	1.93	0.06
*UK, South Thames	2.01	0.04	1.69	0.03
UK, South Western	2.18	0.05	1.84	0.05
UK, Wessex	2.51	0.06	2.15	0.05
*UK, West Midlands	2.73	0.05	2.08	0.04
UK, Yorkshire	2.22	0.05	1.76	0.04
UK, Scotland	2.73	0.05	2.17	0.04
UK, Scotland, West	2.73	0.07	2.04	0.05
*Yugoslavia, Vojvodina	1.69	0.07	1.25	0.05

OCEANIA	MALE		FEMALE	
Australian Capital Territory	3.77	0.35	2.42	0.27
Australia, New South Wales	3.36	0.06	2.46	0.04
South Australia	3.14	0.11	2.59	0.09
Australia, Tasmania	3.70	0.21	2.55	0.16
Australia, Victoria	3.19	0.07	2.67	0.06
Western Australia	2.99	0.11	2.53	0.10
*French Polynesia	1.40	0.33	0.61	0.20
New Zealand: Non-Maori	3.62	0.08	3.41	0.07
New Zealand: Maori	2.07	0.33	1.66	0.27
US, Hawaii: White	4.02	0.29	2.50	0.23
US, Hawaii: Japanese	4.26	0.24	2.58	0.17
US, Hawaii: Hawaiian	2.40	0.33	2.07	0.29
US, Hawaii: Filipino	1.84	0.25	1.39	0.23
US, Hawaii: Chinese	2.51	0.41	1.88	0.32

* IMPORTANT-SEE NOTES ON POPULATION PAGE

CUMULATIVE INCIDENCE (0-74)
RATES AND STANDARD ERRORS (percent)
Rectum (ICD-9 154)

	MALE		FEMALE	
AFRICA				
*Algeria, Setif				
*France, La Reunion				
*Mali, Bamako				
*Uganda, Kyadondo				
*Zimbabwe, Harare: African				
*Zimbabwe, Harare: European				
AMERICA, CENTRAL AND SOUTH				
*Argentina, Concordia	1.04	0.23	0.49	0.15
*Brazil, Belem	0.34	0.09	0.64	0.10
*Brazil, Goiania				
*Brazil, Porto Alegre	1.42	0.14	0.82	0.08
Colombia, Cali	0.64	0.07	0.54	0.06
*Costa Rica	0.53	0.05	0.45	0.04
*Ecuador, Quito	0.36	0.06	0.47	0.07
*Peru, Lima	0.40	0.04	0.37	0.04
Peru, Trujillo	0.48	0.15	0.42	0.13
US, Puerto Rico	1.01	0.05	0.71	0.04
*Uruguay, Montevideo	1.38	0.10	0.89	0.07
AMERICA, NORTH				
Canada	1.98	0.02	1.08	0.01
Canada, Alberta	1.87	0.07	1.02	0.05
Canada, British Columbia	2.08	0.06	1.14	0.04
Canada, Manitoba	1.93	0.10	1.12	0.07
Canada, New Brunswick	2.03	0.13	1.16	0.09
Canada, Newfoundland	1.94	0.15	1.20	0.11
Canada, Northwest Territories	2.42	0.63	0,79	0,34
Canada, Nova Scotia	2.06	0.11	1.18	0.08
Canada, Ontario	1.86	0.03	0.98	0.02
Canada, Prince Edward Island	1.52	0.26	1.22	0.21
Canada, Quebec	2.20	0.04	1.20	0.03
Canada, Saskatchewan	1.73	0.09	0.96	0.07
Canada, Yukon	4.15	1.10	0,96	0,34
US, Cent. Calif.: Non-Hisp. White	1.85	0.08	0.98	0.05
US, Cent. Calif.: Hispanic	1.50	0.17	0.81	0.11
US, Los Angeles: Non-Hisp. White	1.64	0.05	1.09	0.03
US, Los Angeles: Hispanic White	1.13	0.08	0.78	0.05
US, Los Angeles: Black	1.50	0.11	1.23	0.09
US, Los Angeles: Chinese	0.92	0.16	0.89	0.15
US, Los Angeles: Filipino	0.96	0.19	0.73	0.13
US, Los Angeles: Korean	1.12	0.27	0.69	0.17
US, Los Angeles: Japanese	1.83	0.25	1.26	0.19
US, San Francisco: Non-Hisp. White	1.85	0.07	1.03	0.04
US, San Francisco: Hispanic White	1.51	0.18	0.90	0.12
US, San Francisco: Black	1.63	0.17	0.95	0.11
US, San Francisco: Chinese	1.60	0.18	1.14	0.15
US, San Francisco: Filipino	1.54	0.29	1.12	0.20
US, San Francisco: Japanese	2.34	0.50	1.01	0.29
US, Connecticut: White	2.02	0.06	1.14	0.04
US, Connecticut: Black	1.46	0.23	1.13	0.17
US, Atlanta: White	1.35	0.08	0.96	0.06
US, Atlanta: Black	1.33	0.16	1.11	0.12
US, Iowa	1.80	0.06	1.04	0.04

	MALE		FEMALE	
US, Central Louisiana: White	1.50	0.19	0.83	0.13
US, Central Louisiana: Black	1.11	0.33	0,60	0,22
US, New Orleans: White	1.87	0.13	0.91	0.08
US, New Orleans: Black	1.47	0.18	0.86	0.12
US, Detroit: White	1.92	0.06	1.16	0.04
US, Detroit: Black	1.62	0.11	1.10	0.08
US, New Mexico: Non-Hisp. White	1.33	0.09	0.86	0.07
US, New Mexico: Hispanic White	1.61	0.15	0.68	0.09
US, New Mexico: American Indian	0.63	0.23	0.51	0.17
US, Utah	1.40	0.08	0.80	0.05
US, Seattle	1.63	0.05	1.06	0.04
US, SEER: White	1.75	0.02	1.04	0.02
US, SEER: Black	1.58	0.07	1.04	0.05
ASIA				
*China, Qidong	0.89	0.07	0.87	0.07
China, Shanghai	1.10	0.03	0.86	0.02
China, Tianjin	0.73	0.04	0.64	0.03
Hong Kong	1.43	0.04	1.07	0.03
*India, Bangalore	0.39	0.03	0.31	0.03
*India, Barshi, Paranda and Bhum	0.33	0.08	0,09	0,03
India, Bombay	0.45	0.03	0.31	0.02
*India, Karunagappally	0,18	0,08	0,04	0,04
India, Madras	0.42	0.03	0.32	0.03
*India, Trivandrum	0.34	0.09	0.29	0.09
Israel: All Jews	1.70	0.05	1.35	0.04
Jews born in Israel	1.16	0.16	1.31	0.18
Jews born in America or Europe	1.96	0.08	1.52	0.06
Jews born in Africa or Asia	1.38	0.09	1.06	0.07
Non-Jews	0.32	0.08	0.36	0.08
Japan, Hiroshima	2.46	0.12	1.17	0.07
Japan, Miyagi	2.02	0.07	1.09	0.04
Japan, Nagasaki	2.20	0.08	1.14	0.05
Japan, Osaka	1.61	0.03	0.77	0.02
*Japan, Saga	1.46	0.09	0.80	0.06
Japan, Yamagata	1.96	0.08	1.11	0.05
*Korea, Kangwha	0.97	0.22	0.57	0.15
*Kuwait: Non-Kuwaitis	0.44	0.20	0.37	0.17
*Kuwait: Kuwaitis	0.35	0.10	0.21	0.08
*Philippines, Manila	0.89	0.06	0.69	0.05
Singapore: Chinese	2.24	0.10	1.26	0.07
Singapore: Malay	0.94	0.15	0.85	0.15
Singapore: Indian	0.64	0.13	1.24	0.37
Thailand, Chiang Mai	0.37	0.05	0.33	0.04
*Thailand, Khon Kaen	0.41	0.07	0.22	0.04
*Viet Nam, Hanoi				

* IMPORTANT-SEE NOTES ON POPULATION PAGE

CUMULATIVE INCIDENCE (0-74)
RATES AND STANDARD ERRORS (percent)
Rectum (ICD-9 154) (contd)

EUROPE	MALE		FEMALE	
Austria, Tyrol	1.87	*0.15*	1.06	*0.09*
*Belarus	1.60	*0.04*	1.05	*0.02*
*Croatia	1.61	*0.05*	0.96	*0.03*
Czech Republic	2.93	*0.04*	1.36	*0.02*
Denmark	2.07	*0.04*	1.22	*0.03*
Estonia	1.42	*0.08*	0.90	*0.05*
Finland	1.25	*0.04*	0.75	*0.02*
France, Bas-Rhin	2.22	*0.12*	1.09	*0.07*
*France, Calvados	2.17	*0.14*	1.19	*0.09*
France, Doubs	2.20	*0.17*	1.13	*0.11*
France, Haut-Rhin	2.70	*0.17*	1.37	*0.10*
*France, Herault	1.77	*0.10*	0.99	*0.07*
France, Isere	1.89	*0.11*	1.21	*0.08*
*France, Somme	1.78	*0.14*	0.90	*0.09*
*France, Tarn	2.15	*0.16*	1.14	*0.11*
Germany, Eastern States	1.94	*0.05*	1.22	*0.03*
Germany, Saarland	2.04	*0.10*	1.29	*0.07*
Iceland	0.79	*0.14*	0.61	*0.11*
Ireland, Southern	1.68	*0.13*	0.81	*0.09*
Italy, Ferrara	1.60	*0.21*	0.60	*0.11*
Italy, Florence	1.86	*0.09*	1.10	*0.06*
Italy, Genoa	1.58	*0.10*	1.00	*0.06*
*Italy, Latina	1.13	*0.13*	0.76	*0.10*
Italy, Macerata	1.93	*0.26*	0.81	*0.16*
Italy, Modena	1.71	*0.11*	0.97	*0.08*
Italy, Parma	1.47	*0.12*	1.03	*0.09*
Italy, Ragusa	1.05	*0.13*	0.57	*0.09*
Italy, Romagna	1.43	*0.11*	0.95	*0.08*
Italy, Torino	1.57	*0.10*	1.08	*0.07*
Italy, Trieste	2.16	*0.20*	1.04	*0.12*
Italy, Varese	2.02	*0.12*	0.89	*0.07*
Italy, Veneto	1.60	*0.08*	0.94	*0.06*
*Latvia	1.34	*0.06*	0.86	*0.04*
Malta	1.02	*0.20*	0.81	*0.16*
The Netherlands	1.73	*0.03*	1.07	*0.02*
The Netherlands, Eindhoven	1.98	*0.11*	1.19	*0.08*
The Netherlands, Maastricht	2.20	*0.12*	1.22	*0.08*
Norway	1.89	*0.05*	1.23	*0.03*
*Poland, Cracow	1.23	*0.11*	0.72	*0.07*
*Poland, Kielce	0.98	*0.07*	0.63	*0.05*
*Poland, Lower Silesia	1.53	*0.06*	0.96	*0.04*
Poland, Warsaw City	1.35	*0.08*	0.79	*0.05*
Slovakia	2.57	*0.06*	1.34	*0.04*
Slovenia	2.05	*0.09*	1.18	*0.05*
*Spain, Albacete	1.20	*0.20*	0.71	*0.14*
Spain, Asturias	1.39	*0.08*	0.66	*0.05*
Spain, Basque Country	1.63	*0.07*	0.78	*0.04*
Spain, Granada	1.07	*0.08*	0.66	*0.06*
Spain, Mallorca	1.54	*0.11*	0.88	*0.08*
Spain, Murcia	1.45	*0.09*	0.88	*0.06*
Spain, Navarra	1.38	*0.11*	0.76	*0.08*
Spain, Tarragona	1.54	*0.12*	0.68	*0.07*
Spain, Zaragoza	1.31	*0.09*	0.73	*0.06*

	MALE		FEMALE	
Sweden	1.46	*0.03*	0.97	*0.02*
*Switzerland, Basel	2.07	*0.15*	1.11	*0.10*
Switzerland, Geneva	1.41	*0.14*	0.85	*0.10*
Switzerland, Graubunden	1.17	*0.20*	0.78	*0.15*
Switzerland, Neuchatel	1.79	*0.23*	0.92	*0.15*
Switzerland, St Gall-Appenzell	1.70	*0.14*	0.92	*0.09*
Switzerland, Valais	1.69	*0.21*	0.85	*0.14*
Switzerland, Vaud	1.46	*0.11*	1.06	*0.09*
Switzerland, Zurich	1.55	*0.08*	1.05	*0.06*
*UK, England and Wales	1.73	*0.02*	0.95	*0.01*
*UK, East Anglia	1.72	*0.06*	1.05	*0.04*
*UK, Mersey	1.60	*0.05*	0.96	*0.04*
*UK, North Western	1.89	*0.05*	0.89	*0.03*
UK, Oxford	1.75	*0.06*	0.98	*0.04*
*UK, South Thames	1.47	*0.03*	0.85	*0.02*
UK, South Western	1.67	*0.05*	1.03	*0.03*
UK, Wessex	1.59	*0.05*	0.90	*0.03*
*UK, West Midlands	2.13	*0.04*	1.02	*0.03*
UK, Yorkshire	1.77	*0.05*	1.00	*0.03*
UK, Scotland	1.70	*0.04*	0.97	*0.03*
UK, Scotland, West	1.68	*0.06*	0.91	*0.04*
*Yugoslavia, Vojvodina	1.78	*0.07*	1.15	*0.05*

OCEANIA	MALE		FEMALE	
Australian Capital Territory	2.15	*0.28*	1.46	*0.21*
Australia, New South Wales	2.23	*0.05*	1.16	*0.03*
South Australia	2.17	*0.09*	1.38	*0.07*
Australia, Tasmania	1.88	*0.15*	1.32	*0.12*
Australia, Victoria	2.35	*0.06*	1.28	*0.04*
Western Australia	2.02	*0.09*	1.32	*0.07*
*French Polynesia	1.07	*0.28*	0,41	*0,16*
New Zealand: Non-Maori	2.42	*0.07*	1.29	*0.05*
New Zealand: Maori	1.55	*0.29*	0.96	*0.19*
US, Hawaii: White	1.68	*0.19*	0.86	*0.13*
US, Hawaii: Japanese	2.35	*0.18*	0.93	*0.10*
US, Hawaii: Hawaiian	1.87	*0.29*	1.01	*0.20*
US, Hawaii: Filipino	1.55	*0.23*	0.84	*0.17*
US, Hawaii: Chinese	1.52	*0.32*	0.84	*0.22*

* IMPORTANT-SEE NOTES ON POPULATION PAGE

CUMULATIVE INCIDENCE (0-74)
RATES AND STANDARD ERRORS (percent)
Large bowel (ICD-9 153-4)

	MALE		FEMALE	
AFRICA				
*Algeria, Setif				
*France, La Reunion				
*Mali, Bamako				
*Uganda, Kyadondo				
*Zimbabwe, Harare: African				
*Zimbabwe, Harare: European				
AMERICA, CENTRAL AND SOUTH				
*Argentina, Concordia	2.63	0.41	2.07	0.32
*Brazil, Belem	0.90	0.15	1.02	0.13
*Brazil, Goiania				
*Brazil, Porto Alegre	3.14	0.21	2.28	0.14
Colombia, Cali	1.36	0.11	1.27	0.10
*Costa Rica	1.09	0.07	1.07	0.06
*Ecuador, Quito	0.87	0.11	1.18	0.11
*Peru, Lima	1.04	0.07	0.99	0.07
Peru, Trujillo	0.90	0.21	0.96	0.19
US, Puerto Rico	2.78	0.08	2.08	0.07
*Uruguay, Montevideo	4.04	0.17	2.86	0.12
AMERICA, NORTH				
Canada	5.17	0.03	3.52	0.03
Canada, Alberta	4.51	0.11	2.82	0.08
Canada, British Columbia	4.53	0.09	3.13	0.07
Canada, Manitoba	4.99	0.16	3.84	0.13
Canada, New Brunswick	5.43	0.21	3.74	0.16
Canada, Newfoundland	5.79	0.25	4.76	0.22
Canada, Northwest Territories	3.17	0.70	2.90	0.74
Canada, Nova Scotia	5.71	0.19	4.02	0.15
Canada, Ontario	5.42	0.06	3.62	0.04
Canada, Prince Edward Island	4.96	0.46	3.68	0.37
Canada, Quebec	5.35	0.07	3.61	0.05
Canada, Saskatchewan	4.30	0.15	3.16	0.12
Canada, Yukon	5.80	1.27	2.39	0.73
US, Cent. Calif.: Non-Hisp. White	4.68	0.13	3.19	0.10
US, Cent. Calif.: Hispanic	3.64	0.27	1.97	0.18
US, Los Angeles: Non-Hisp. White	4.96	0.08	3.41	0.06
US, Los Angeles: Hispanic White	3.20	0.13	2.12	0.09
US, Los Angeles: Black	5.51	0.21	4.32	0.16
US, Los Angeles: Chinese	3.05	0.29	2.25	0.24
US, Los Angeles: Filipino	2.69	0.32	1.81	0.22
US, Los Angeles: Korean	3.04	0.44	1.55	0.25
US, Los Angeles: Japanese	4.94	0.41	3.85	0.34
US, San Francisco: Non-Hisp. White	5.14	0.11	3.39	0.08
US, San Francisco: Hispanic White	4.14	0.31	2.59	0.21
US, San Francisco: Black	5.66	0.32	4.12	0.23
US, San Francisco: Chinese	3.92	0.28	3.34	0.26
US, San Francisco: Filipino	3.81	0.45	2.09	0.26
US, San Francisco: Japanese	5.81	0.82	4.12	0.58
US, Connecticut: White	5.55	0.10	3.57	0.07
US, Connecticut: Black	4.95	0.43	3.85	0.32
US, Atlanta: White	4.44	0.15	3.17	0.11
US, Atlanta: Black	5.48	0.34	4.22	0.24
US, Iowa	5.40	0.10	3.91	0.08

	MALE		FEMALE	
US, Central Louisiana: White	4.98	0.35	3.00	0.25
US, Central Louisiana: Black	3.93	0.63	3.85	0.55
US, New Orleans: White	5.37	0.22	3.55	0.16
US, New Orleans: Black	5.02	0.34	3.89	0.25
US, Detroit: White	5.28	0.10	3.44	0.07
US, Detroit: Black	5.73	0.21	4.53	0.16
US, New Mexico: Non-Hisp. White	3.98	0.16	2.82	0.12
US, New Mexico: Hispanic White	4.01	0.24	2.24	0.17
US, New Mexico: American Indian	1.61	0.38	1.49	0.32
US, Utah	3.90	0.13	2.59	0.10
US, Seattle	4.72	0.09	3.35	0.07
US, SEER: White	5.00	0.04	3.38	0.03
US, SEER: Black	5.59	0.14	4.22	0.10
ASIA				
*China, Qidong	1.13	0.08	1.08	0.07
China, Shanghai	2.58	0.04	2.18	0.04
China, Tianjin	1.38	0.05	1.22	0.04
Hong Kong	4.03	0.07	3.27	0.06
*India, Bangalore	0.70	0.05	0.54	0.04
*India, Barshi, Paranda and Bhum	0.42	0.09	0.14	0.04
India, Bombay	0.87	0.04	0.66	0.03
*India, Karunagappally	0.35	0.11	0,16	0,07
India, Madras	0.65	0.04	0.48	0.04
*India, Trivandrum	0.67	0.13	0.41	0.10
Israel: All Jews	4.60	0.09	3.69	0.07
Jews born in Israel	4.40	0.38	3.37	0.28
Jews born in America or Europe	5.52	0.13	4.26	0.11
Jews born in Africa or Asia	3.20	0.13	2.68	0.11
Non-Jews	1.05	0.15	0.97	0.13
Japan, Hiroshima	6.32	0.20	3.24	0.12
Japan, Miyagi	4.98	0.11	2.88	0.07
Japan, Nagasaki	5.27	0.13	2.87	0.08
Japan, Osaka	4.02	0.05	2.28	0.04
*Japan, Saga	3.70	0.14	2.30	0.10
Japan, Yamagata	4.51	0.12	2.97	0.09
*Korea, Kangwha	1.57	0.29	0.83	0.18
*Kuwait: Non-Kuwaitis	0.96	0.25	0.65	0.20
*Kuwait: Kuwaitis	0.66	0.14	0.82	0.19
*Philippines, Manila	2.09	0.10	1.72	0.08
Singapore: Chinese	5.14	0.15	3.72	0.12
Singapore: Malay	2.43	0.25	1.52	0.19
Singapore: Indian	1.39	0.19	1.91	0.43
Thailand, Chiang Mai	0.85	0.07	0.74	0.06
*Thailand, Khon Kaen	1.06	0.11	0.64	0.07
*Viet Nam, Hanoi				

* IMPORTANT-SEE NOTES ON POPULATION PAGE

CUMULATIVE INCIDENCE (0-74)
RATES AND STANDARD ERRORS (percent)
Large bowel (ICD-9 153-4) (contd)

EUROPE	MALE		FEMALE	
Austria, Tyrol	4.49	0.23	3.00	0.15
*Belarus	2.86	0.05	1.99	0.03
*Croatia	3.14	0.08	1.97	0.05
Czech Republic	5.91	0.06	3.21	0.04
Denmark	4.48	0.06	3.54	0.05
Estonia	3.18	0.12	2.28	0.08
Finland	2.67	0.05	2.00	0.04
France, Bas-Rhin	5.94	0.21	3.25	0.13
*France, Calvados	4.60	0.21	2.84	0.15
France, Doubs	4.64	0.25	2.68	0.17
France, Haut-Rhin	6.15	0.26	3.53	0.16
*France, Herault	4.24	0.16	2.51	0.11
France, Isere	4.59	0.17	3.00	0.12
*France, Somme	4.27	0.22	2.35	0.14
*France, Tarn	4.42	0.24	2.62	0.17
Germany, Eastern States	3.80	0.06	2.90	0.04
Germany, Saarland	4.97	0.16	3.52	0.11
Iceland	2.76	0.26	2.35	0.27
Ireland, Southern	4.54	0.22	3.21	0.17
Italy, Ferrara	5.10	0.37	3.18	0.26
Italy, Florence	4.77	0.15	3.44	0.11
Italy, Genoa	4.62	0.16	3.09	0.11
*Italy, Latina	3.18	0.22	2.15	0.17
Italy, Macerata	4.84	0.42	2.72	0.29
Italy, Modena	4.20	0.17	3.01	0.13
Italy, Parma	4.32	0.21	3.04	0.16
Italy, Ragusa	2.19	0.19	1.73	0.16
Italy, Romagna	4.12	0.18	3.08	0.15
Italy, Torino	4.49	0.17	2.94	0.11
Italy, Trieste	5.84	0.33	2.97	0.20
Italy, Varese	5.04	0.19	2.95	0.12
Italy, Veneto	4.31	0.14	2.79	0.09
*Latvia	2.82	0.09	2.00	0.05
Malta	2.71	0.33	2.26	0.27
The Netherlands	4.26	0.04	3.25	0.03
The Netherlands, Eindhoven	4.73	0.17	3.42	0.14
The Netherlands, Maastricht	4.78	0.17	3.26	0.13
Norway	4.44	0.07	3.43	0.06
*Poland, Cracow	2.62	0.16	1.76	0.10
*Poland, Kielce	1.97	0.10	1.20	0.07
*Poland, Lower Silesia	3.02	0.09	2.07	0.06
Poland, Warsaw City	3.24	0.12	1.91	0.08
Slovakia	5.13	0.09	2.88	0.05
Slovenia	3.96	0.12	2.39	0.08
*Spain, Albacete	2.43	0.29	1.81	0.23
Spain, Asturias	3.34	0.13	1.95	0.09
Spain, Basque Country	3.68	0.11	1.94	0.07
Spain, Granada	2.31	0.13	1.63	0.09
Spain, Mallorca	3.66	0.17	2.66	0.14
Spain, Murcia	3.04	0.13	2.07	0.10
Spain, Navarra	3.29	0.17	2.32	0.13
Spain, Tarragona	3.72	0.18	2.27	0.13
Spain, Zaragoza	2.75	0.12	1.80	0.09

	MALE		FEMALE	
Sweden	3.48	0.04	2.76	0.03
*Switzerland, Basel	4.52	0.23	2.85	0.16
Switzerland, Geneva	4.38	0.27	2.60	0.18
Switzerland, Graubunden	3.40	0.35	2.75	0.29
Switzerland, Neuchatel	4.04	0.35	2.62	0.25
Switzerland, St Gall-Appenzell	3.63	0.20	2.37	0.15
Switzerland, Valais	3.78	0.32	2.61	0.24
Switzerland, Vaud	3.96	0.19	2.79	0.14
Switzerland, Zurich	3.75	0.13	2.55	0.10
*UK, England and Wales	3.91	0.02	2.70	0.02
*UK, East Anglia	4.03	0.09	2.91	0.07
*UK, Mersey	3.64	0.08	2.72	0.07
*UK, North Western	4.09	0.07	2.60	0.05
UK, Oxford	4.14	0.09	2.91	0.07
*UK, South Thames	3.48	0.05	2.55	0.04
UK, South Western	3.85	0.07	2.88	0.06
UK, Wessex	4.10	0.08	3.05	0.06
*UK, West Midlands	4.85	0.07	3.10	0.05
UK, Yorkshire	4.00	0.07	2.76	0.06
UK, Scotland	4.43	0.07	3.14	0.05
UK, Scotland, West	4.40	0.09	2.96	0.06
*Yugoslavia, Vojvodina	3.47	0.10	2.41	0.07

OCEANIA	MALE		FEMALE	
Australian Capital Territory	5.92	0.45	3.87	0.34
Australia, New South Wales	5.59	0.07	3.62	0.05
South Australia	5.32	0.14	3.97	0.11
Australia, Tasmania	5.58	0.25	3.87	0.20
Australia, Victoria	5.54	0.09	3.95	0.07
Western Australia	5.02	0.14	3.85	0.12
*French Polynesia	2.48	0.44	1.03	0.26
New Zealand: Non-Maori	6.04	0.10	4.69	0.09
New Zealand: Maori	3.62	0.44	2.62	0.33
US, Hawaii: White	5.69	0.34	3.36	0.26
US, Hawaii: Japanese	6.61	0.30	3.51	0.20
US, Hawaii: Hawaiian	4.26	0.44	3.07	0.36
US, Hawaii: Filipino	3.39	0.34	2.23	0.28
US, Hawaii: Chinese	4.03	0.52	2.71	0.39

* IMPORTANT-SEE NOTES ON POPULATION PAGE

CUMULATIVE INCIDENCE (0-74)
RATES AND STANDARD ERRORS (percent)
Liver (ICD-9 155)

	MALE		FEMALE	
AFRICA				
*Algeria, Setif				
*France, La Reunion				
*Mali, Bamako				
*Uganda, Kyadondo				
*Zimbabwe, Harare: African				
*Zimbabwe, Harare: European				
AMERICA, CENTRAL AND SOUTH				
*Argentina, Concordia	0,08	0,06	0,09	0,06
*Brazil, Belem	0,03	0,02	0,08	0,04 f
*Brazil, Goiania				
*Brazil, Porto Alegre	1.07	0.12	0.34	0.05
Colombia, Cali	0.29	0.05	0.26	0.04
*Costa Rica	0.69	0.05	0.42	0.04
*Ecuador, Quito	0.25	0.05	0.22	0.04
*Peru, Lima	0.35	0.04	0.38	0.04
Peru, Trujillo	0.56	0.15	0.51	0.13
US, Puerto Rico	0.48	0.03	0.17	0.02
*Uruguay, Montevideo	0.19	0.04	0.09	0.02
AMERICA, NORTH				
Canada	0.37	0.01	0.13	0.00
Canada, Alberta	0.35	0.03	0.10	0.02
Canada, British Columbia	0.37	0.02	0.16	0.01
Canada, Manitoba	0.32	0.04	0.13	0.02
Canada, New Brunswick	0.22	0.04	0.08	0.02
Canada, Newfoundland	0.13	0.04	0,08	0,03
Canada, Northwest Territories	0,37	0,18	-	-
Canada, Nova Scotia	0.22	0.04	0.12	0.02
Canada, Ontario	0.39	0.01	0.12	0.01
Canada, Prince Edward Island	0,04	0,04	-	-
Canada, Quebec	0.45	0.02	0.16	0.01
Canada, Saskatchewan	0.22	0.03	0.10	0.02
Canada, Yukon	-	-	0,04	0,04
US, Cent. Calif.: Non-Hisp. White	0.31	0.03	0.15	0.02
US, Cent. Calif.: Hispanic	0.55	0.09	0.41	0.08
US, Los Angeles: Non-Hisp. White	0.34	0.02	0.11	0.01
US, Los Angeles: Hispanic White	0.86	0.07	0.25	0.03
US, Los Angeles: Black	0.65	0.07	0.27	0.04
US, Los Angeles: Chinese	1.84	0.22	0.49	0.11
US, Los Angeles: Filipino	1.02	0.19	0.38	0.11
US, Los Angeles: Korean	2.79	0.38	0.66	0.17
US, Los Angeles: Japanese	0.67	0.15	0.39	0.10
US, San Francisco: Non-Hisp. White	0.37	0.03	0.14	0.02
US, San Francisco: Hispanic White	0.73	0.11	0.23	0.06
US, San Francisco: Black	1.08	0.14	0.22	0.05
US, San Francisco: Chinese	2.42	0.21	0.66	0.11
US, San Francisco: Filipino	1.47	0.28	0.42	0.13
US, San Francisco: Japanese	0,69	0,29	0,22	0,11
US, Connecticut: White	0.39	0.03	0.12	0.01
US, Connecticut: Black	0.89	0.18	0,19	0,07
US, Atlanta: White	0.37	0.04	0.12	0.02
US, Atlanta: Black	0.37	0.09	0.16	0.05
US, Iowa	0.31	0.02	0.11	0.01

	MALE		FEMALE	
US, Central Louisiana: White	0.26	0.08	0,11	0,04
US, Central Louisiana: Black	0,57	0,23	0,02	0,02
US, New Orleans: White	0.41	0.06	0.10	0.03
US, New Orleans: Black	0.91	0.14	0.27	0.06
US, Detroit: White	0.39	0.03	0.15	0.01
US, Detroit: Black	0.83	0.08	0.26	0.04
US, New Mexico: Non-Hisp. White	0.25	0.04	0.12	0.03
US, New Mexico: Hispanic White	0.51	0.09	0.22	0.05
US, New Mexico: American Indian	1.22	0.33	0,23	0,12
US, Utah	0.20	0.03	0.12	0.02
US, Seattle	0.38	0.03	0.16	0.02
US, SEER: White	0.35	0.01	0.13	0.01
US, SEER: Black	0.81	0.05	0.22	0.02
ASIA				
*China, Qidong	7.40	0.17	2.04	0.09
China, Shanghai	3.35	0.05	1.17	0.03
China, Tianjin	2.78	0.07	1.12	0.04
Hong Kong	4.27	0.06	1.11	0.03
*India, Bangalore	0.34	0.03	0.15	0.02
*India, Barshi, Paranda and Bhum	0.22	0.06	0,06	0,03
India, Bombay	0.51	0.03	0.23	0.02
*India, Karunagappally	0,37	0,14	0,20	0,09
India, Madras	0.29	0.03	0.05	0.01
*India, Trivandrum	0.29	0.08	0,14	0,05
Israel: All Jews	0.44	0.03	0.19	0.02
Jews born in Israel	0.17	0.07	0.23	0.09
Jews born in America or Europe	0.46	0.04	0.18	0.02
Jews born in Africa or Asia	0.47	0.05	0.23	0.03
Non-Jews	0.23	0.07	0.13	0.05
Japan, Hiroshima	5.77	0.18	1.52	0.09
Japan, Miyagi	1.90	0.06	0.65	0.03
Japan, Nagasaki	4.20	0.11	1.00	0.05
Japan, Osaka	5.97	0.06	1.45	0.03
*Japan, Saga	5.15	0.16	1.40	0.08
Japan, Yamagata	1.89	0.08	0.61	0.04
*Korea, Kangwha	3.01	0.37	0.91	0.19
*Kuwait: Non-Kuwaitis	1.04	0.30	0.35	0,16
*Kuwait: Kuwaitis	0.95	0.19	0.47	0.15
*Philippines, Manila	2.72	0.11	0.97	0.06
Singapore: Chinese	2.78	0.11	0.64	0.05
Singapore: Malay	1.31	0.18	0.47	0.11
Singapore: Indian	0.97	0.17	0,15	0,09
Thailand, Chiang Mai	2.47	0.12	1.21	0.08
*Thailand, Khon Kaen	12.27	0.33	5.03	0.20
*Viet Nam, Hanoi				

* IMPORTANT-SEE NOTES ON POPULATION PAGE

CUMULATIVE INCIDENCE (0-74)
RATES AND STANDARD ERRORS (percent)
Liver (ICD-9 155) (contd)

EUROPE	MALE		FEMALE	
Austria, Tyrol	0.50	0.08	0.18	0.04
*Belarus	0.53	0.02	0.24	0.01
*Croatia	0.59	0.03	0.29	0.02
Czech Republic	0.83	0.02	0.32	0.01
Denmark	0.45	0.02	0.24	0.01
Estonia	0.55	0.05	0.23	0.02
Finland	0.55	0.02	0.30	0.01
France, Bas-Rhin	1.68	0.11	0.24	0.03
*France, Calvados	1.91	0.14	0.17	0.04
France, Doubs	0.87	0.11	0.20	0.05
France, Haut-Rhin	1.51	0.12	0.13	0.03
*France, Herault	0.54	0.06	0.10	0.02
France, Isere	1.19	0.09	0.11	0.02
*France, Somme	1.00	0.10	0.13	0.03
*France, Tarn	0.31	0.07	0.11	0.03
Germany, Eastern States	0.64	0.03	0.28	0.01
Germany, Saarland	0.56	0.05	0.20	0.03
Iceland	0.38	0.10	0,13	0,05
Ireland, Southern	0.23	0.05	0,04	0,02
Italy, Ferrara	1.01	0.16	0.32	0.08
Italy, Florence	1.13	0.07	0.40	0.04
Italy, Genoa	1.34	0.09	0.39	0.04
*Italy, Latina	1.05	0.13	0.52	0.08
Italy, Macerata	0.90	0.18	0.37	0.11
Italy, Modena	1.31	0.10	0.39	0.05
Italy, Parma	1.80	0.13	0.61	0.07
Italy, Ragusa	1.10	0.14	0.37	0.07
Italy, Romagna	0.69	0.07	0.24	0.04
Italy, Torino	1.06	0.08	0.31	0.04
Italy, Trieste	2.31	0.21	0.42	0.07
Italy, Varese	1.66	0.11	0.37	0.05
Italy, Veneto	2.31	0.10	0.59	0.04
*Latvia	0.56	0.04	0.22	0.02
Malta	0,30	0,12	0,10	0,06
The Netherlands	0.19	0.01	0.07	0.01
The Netherlands, Eindhoven	0.13	0.03	0.07	0.02
The Netherlands, Maastricht	0.19	0.03	0.08	0.02
Norway	0.20	0.01	0.11	0.01
*Poland, Cracow	0.55	0.07	0.36	0.05
*Poland, Kielce	0.69	0.06	0.34	0.04
*Poland, Lower Silesia	0.80	0.04	0.52	0.03
Poland, Warsaw City	0.66	0.06	0.32	0.03
Slovakia	0.90	0.03	0.37	0.02
Slovenia	0.39	0.04	0.10	0.01
*Spain, Albacete	0.55	0.14	0.38	0.11
Spain, Asturias	1.04	0.07	0.31	0.04
Spain, Basque Country	1.02	0.06	0.22	0.02
Spain, Granada	0.86	0.08	0.35	0.04
Spain, Mallorca	0.92	0.09	0.24	0.04
Spain, Murcia	0.65	0.06	0.20	0.03
Spain, Navarra	0.99	0.09	0.36	0.05
Spain, Tarragona	0.59	0.07	0.24	0.04
Spain, Zaragoza	0.61	0.06	0.20	0.03

	MALE		FEMALE	
Sweden	0.39	0.01	0.20	0.01
*Switzerland, Basel	0.60	0.08	0.10	0.03
Switzerland, Geneva	1.38	0.15	0.20	0.05
Switzerland, Graubunden	0.60	0.15	0,26	0,09
Switzerland, Neuchatel	0.75	0.15	0,07	0,04
Switzerland, St Gall-Appenzell	0.70	0.09	0.16	0.04
Switzerland, Valais	1.30	0.18	0.21	0.07
Switzerland, Vaud	0.91	0.09	0.14	0.03
Switzerland, Zurich	0.74	0.06	0.16	0.02
*UK, England and Wales	0.25	0.01	0.11	0.00
*UK, East Anglia	0.15	0.02	0.05	0.01
*UK, Mersey	0.25	0.02	0.10	0.01
*UK, North Western	0.30	0.02	0.11	0.01
UK, Oxford	0.21	0.02	0.10	0.01
*UK, South Thames	0.26	0.01	0.10	0.01
UK, South Western	0.18	0.02	0.09	0.01
UK, Wessex	0.25	0.02	0.12	0.01
*UK, West Midlands	0.21	0.01	0.08	0.01
UK, Yorkshire	0.21	0.02	0.11	0.01
UK, Scotland	0.38	0.02	0.15	0.01
UK, Scotland, West	0.34	0.03	0.16	0.02
*Yugoslavia, Vojvodina	0.99	0.05	0.60	0.04

OCEANIA	MALE		FEMALE	
Australian Capital Territory	0.34	0.10	0,14	0,06
Australia, New South Wales	0.31	0.02	0.06	0.01
South Australia	0.26	0.03	0.07	0.01
Australia, Tasmania	0.30	0.06	0,04	0,02
Australia, Victoria	0.37	0.02	0.09	0.01
Western Australia	0.30	0.03	0.09	0.02
*French Polynesia	1.52	0.32	0,24	0,09
New Zealand: Non-Maori	0.34	0.02	0.15	0.02
New Zealand: Maori	1.53	0.26	0.48	0.14
US, Hawaii: White	0.51	0.10	0,19	0,06
US, Hawaii: Japanese	0.63	0.09	0.17	0.04
US, Hawaii: Hawaiian	0.81	0.18	0.32	0.11
US, Hawaii: Filipino	0.97	0.18	0,21	0,09
US, Hawaii: Chinese	1.22	0.27	0,36	0,14

* IMPORTANT-SEE NOTES ON POPULATION PAGE

CUMULATIVE INCIDENCE (0-74)
RATES AND STANDARD ERRORS (percent)
Gallbladder etc. (ICD-9 156)

	MALE		FEMALE	
AFRICA				
*Algeria, Setif				
*France, La Reunion				
*Mali, Bamako				
*Uganda, Kyadondo				
*Zimbabwe, Harare: African				
*Zimbabwe, Harare: European				
AMERICA, CENTRAL AND SOUTH				
*Argentina, Concordia	0,54	0,21	0.60	0.18
*Brazil, Belem	0.17	0.06	0.37	0.08
*Brazil, Goiania				
*Brazil, Porto Alegre	0.20	0.05	0.84	0.09
Colombia, Cali	0.46	0.06	1.05	0.09
*Costa Rica	0.27	0.03	0.57	0.05
*Ecuador, Quito	0.63	0.09	1.01	0.10
*Peru, Lima	0.24	0.03	0.50	0.05
Peru, Trujillo	0,39	0,15	1.14	0.22
US, Puerto Rico	0.16	0.02	0.28	0.02
*Uruguay, Montevideo	0.29	0.05	0.48	0.05
AMERICA, NORTH				
Canada	0.21	0.01	0.24	0.01
Canada, Alberta	0.17	0.02	0.23	0.02
Canada, British Columbia	0.22	0.02	0.20	0.02
Canada, Manitoba	0.24	0.04	0.23	0.03
Canada, New Brunswick	0.13	0.03	0.16	0.03
Canada, Newfoundland	0.10	0.03	0.31	0.06
Canada, Northwest Territories	0,36	0,25	0,64	0,35
Canada, Nova Scotia	0.15	0.03	0.20	0.03
Canada, Ontario	0.21	0.01	0.24	0.01
Canada, Prince Edward Island	0,26	0,11	0,13	0,07
Canada, Quebec	0.24	0.01	0.26	0.01
Canada, Saskatchewan	0.18	0.03	0.26	0.04
Canada, Yukon	0,27	0,19	0,14	0,14
US, Cent. Calif.: Non-Hisp. White	0.17	0.03	0.13	0.02
US, Cent. Calif.: Hispanic	0.29	0.08	0.57	0.10
US, Los Angeles: Non-Hisp. White	0.17	0.01	0.14	0.01
US, Los Angeles: Hispanic White	0.26	0.04	0.49	0.04
US, Los Angeles: Black	0.18	0.04	0.13	0.03
US, Los Angeles: Chinese	0.30	0.10	0,16	0,07
US, Los Angeles: Filipino	0,21	0,10	0,24	0,09
US, Los Angeles: Korean	0,39	0,17	0.67	0.17
US, Los Angeles: Japanese	0,31	0,10	0,20	0,08
US, San Francisco: Non-Hisp. White	0.16	0.02	0.15	0.02
US, San Francisco: Hispanic White	0.17	0.06	0.17	0.05
US, San Francisco: Black	0,13	0,05	0.13	0.04
US, San Francisco: Chinese	0.32	0.08	0.22	0.07
US, San Francisco: Filipino	0,23	0,12	0,24	0,09
US, San Francisco: Japanese	0,36	0,21	0,44	0,21
US, Connecticut: White	0.17	0.02	0.19	0.02
US, Connecticut: Black	0.31	0.11	0,18	0,07
US, Atlanta: White	0.21	0.03	0.13	0.02
US, Atlanta: Black	0.20	0.07	0.17	0.05
US, Iowa	0.17	0.02	0.20	0.02

	MALE		FEMALE	
US, Central Louisiana: White	0,17	0,07	0.23	0.07
US, Central Louisiana: Black	0,21	0,15	0,15	0,11
US, New Orleans: White	0.19	0.04	0.12	0.03
US, New Orleans: Black	0,10	0,05	0.29	0.07
US, Detroit: White	0.18	0.02	0.23	0.02
US, Detroit: Black	0.11	0.03	0.23	0.04
US, New Mexico: Non-Hisp. White	0.11	0.03	0.10	0.02
US, New Mexico: Hispanic White	0.18	0.06	0.61	0.09
US, New Mexico: American Indian	0,66	0,26	1.47	0.32
US, Utah	0.10	0.02	0.21	0.03
US, Seattle	0.16	0.02	0.17	0.02
US, SEER: White	0.16	0.01	0.19	0.01
US, SEER: Black	0.15	0.02	0.19	0.02
ASIA				
*China, Qidong	0.17	0.03	0.14	0.03
China, Shanghai	0.32	0.02	0.47	0.02
China, Tianjin	0.32	0.03	0.25	0.02
Hong Kong	0.40	0.02	0.30	0.02
*India, Bangalore	0.06	0.01	0.09	0.02
*India, Barshi, Paranda and Bhum	0,03	0,03	0,02	0,02
India, Bombay	0.20	0.02	0.32	0.02
*India, Karunagappally	-	-	-	-
India, Madras	0.06	0.01	0.06	0.01
*India, Trivandrum	0,02	0,01	0,06	0,03
Israel: All Jews	0.17	0.02	0.30	0.02
Jews born in Israel	0.07	0.03	0,10	0,05
Jews born in America or Europe	0.15	0.02	0.32	0.03
Jews born in Africa or Asia	0.21	0.03	0.30	0.04
Non-Jews	0.17	0.06	0.40	0.08
Japan, Hiroshima	0.70	0.07	0.70	0.06
Japan, Miyagi	0.94	0.05	0.75	0.04
Japan, Nagasaki	0.89	0.05	0.77	0.04
Japan, Osaka	0.69	0.02	0.66	0.02
*Japan, Saga	0.81	0.07	0.88	0.06
Japan, Yamagata	0.70	0.05	0.72	0.04
*Korea, Kangwha	0.40	0.13	0.42	0.13
*Kuwait: Non-Kuwaitis	0.11	0.05	0.42	0,17
*Kuwait: Kuwaitis	0,14	0,08	0,11	0,05
*Philippines, Manila	0.20	0.03	0.17	0.03
Singapore: Chinese	0.18	0.03	0.24	0.03
Singapore: Malay	0.20	0.07	0.25	0.08
Singapore: Indian	0,19	0,07	0.14	0,06
Thailand, Chiang Mai	0.42	0.05	0.36	0.04
*Thailand, Khon Kaen	0.22	0.04	0.29	0.05
*Viet Nam, Hanoi				

* IMPORTANT-SEE NOTES ON POPULATION PAGE

EUROPE	MALE		FEMALE	
Austria, Tyrol	0.33	0.06	0.27	0.05
*Belarus	0.13	0.01	0.17	0.01
*Croatia	0.23	0.02	0.36	0.02
Czech Republic	0.55	0.02	0.82	0.02
Denmark	0.20	0.01	0.27	0.01
Estonia	0.14	0.02	0.21	0.02
Finland	0.24	0.02	0.39	0.02
France, Bas-Rhin	0.27	0.04	0.31	0.04
*France, Calvados	0.16	0.04	0.18	0.04
France, Doubs	0.13	0.04	0.26	0.05
France, Haut-Rhin	0.26	0.05	0.43	0.06
*France, Herault	0.16	0.03	0.18	0.03
France, Isere	0.16	0.03	0.18	0.03
*France, Somme	0.14	0.03	0.24	0.05
*France, Tarn	0,07	0,03	0.24	0.05
Germany, Eastern States	0.42	0.02	0.80	0.02
Germany, Saarland	0.31	0.04	0.56	0.04
Iceland	0,17	0,06	0,14	0,06
Ireland, Southern	0.22	0.05	0.33	0.06
Italy, Ferrara	0.41	0.11	0.45	0.10
Italy, Florence	0.32	0.04	0.36	0.04
Italy, Genoa	0.40	0.05	0.40	0.04
*Italy, Latina	0.44	0.08	0.69	0.10
Italy, Macerata	0.32	0.10	0,24	0,09
Italy, Modena	0.19	0.03	0.31	0.04
Italy, Parma	0.37	0.06	0.35	0.05
Italy, Ragusa	0.41	0.08	0.39	0.07
Italy, Romagna	0.26	0.05	0.28	0.05
Italy, Torino	0.38	0.05	0.45	0.04
Italy, Trieste	0.49	0.09	0.43	0.08
Italy, Varese	0.33	0.05	0.47	0.05
Italy, Veneto	0.33	0.04	0.36	0.03
*Latvia	0.10	0.02	0.13	0.01
Malta	0,11	0,06	0,10	0,06
The Netherlands	0.25	0.01	0.31	0.01
The Netherlands, Eindhoven	0.22	0.04	0.35	0.05
The Netherlands, Maastricht	0.26	0.04	0.32	0.04
Norway	0.12	0.01	0.15	0.01
*Poland, Cracow	0.48	0.07	0.84	0.07
*Poland, Kielce	0.29	0.04	0.53	0.05
*Poland, Lower Silesia	0.27	0.03	0.87	0.04
Poland, Warsaw City	0.44	0.05	0.87	0.05
Slovakia	0.46	0.03	0.81	0.03
Slovenia	0.32	0.04	0.46	0.03
*Spain, Albacete	0,26	0,10	0.48	0.12
Spain, Asturias	0.11	0.02	0.26	0.03
Spain, Basque Country	0.33	0.03	0.33	0.03
Spain, Granada	0.36	0.05	0.57	0.06
Spain, Mallorca	0.28	0.05	0.37	0.05
Spain, Murcia	0.22	0.03	0.39	0.04
Spain, Navarra	0.34	0.06	0.40	0.06
Spain, Tarragona	0.18	0.04	0.29	0.05
Spain, Zaragoza	0.29	0.04	0.29	0.04

	MALE		FEMALE		
Sweden	0.30	0.01	0.48	0.01	
*Switzerland, Basel	0.13	0.04	0.22	0.04	
Switzerland, Geneva	0,13	0,05	0.20	0.05	
Switzerland, Graubunden	0,07	0,05	0.34	0.10	
Switzerland, Neuchatel	0,23	0,08	0.27	0.08	
Switzerland, St Gall-Appenzell	0.24	0.05	0.33	0.05	
Switzerland, Valais	0,12	0,06	0.35	0.09	
Switzerland, Vaud	0.26	0.05	0.31	0.05	
Switzerland, Zurich	0.30	0.04	0.31	0.03	
*UK, England and Wales	0.14	0.00	0.14	0.00	
*UK, East Anglia	0.16	0.02	0.15	0.02	
*UK, Mersey	0.12	0.01	0.14	0.02	
*UK, North Western	0.13	0.01	0.14	0.01	
UK, Oxford	0.12	0.02	0.13	0.02	
*UK, South Thames	0.12	0.01	0.11	0.01	
UK, South Western	0.13	0.01	0.12	0.01	
UK, Wessex	0.10	0.01	0.10	0.01	
*UK, West Midlands	0.24	0.01	0.21	0.01	
UK, Yorkshire	0.13	0.01	0.12	0.01	
UK, Scotland	0.15	0.01	0.16	0.01	
UK, Scotland, West	0.15	0.02	0.17	0.02	
*Yugoslavia, Vojvodina	0.30	0.03	0.68	0.04	

OCEANIA	MALE		FEMALE		
Australian Capital Territory	0,15	0,06	0,12	0,06	
Australia, New South Wales	0.24	0.02	0.23	0.01	
South Australia	0.22	0.03	0.39	0.04	
Australia, Tasmania	0.15	0.04	0.28	0.05	
Australia, Victoria	0.25	0.02	0.25	0.02	
Western Australia	0.20	0.03	0.18	0.03	
*French Polynesia	0,35	0,18	0,28	0,16	m
New Zealand: Non-Maori	0.14	0.02	0.15	0.02	
New Zealand: Maori	0,18	0,08	0,12	0,06	
US, Hawaii: White	0,13	0,05	0.19	0.06	
US, Hawaii: Japanese	0.28	0.06	0.18	0.05	
US, Hawaii: Hawaiian	0.24	0,11	0,14	0,07	
US, Hawaii: Filipino	0.10	0,06	0,08	0,05	
US, Hawaii: Chinese	0,29	0,13	0,45	0,16	

* IMPORTANT-SEE NOTES ON POPULATION PAGE

CUMULATIVE INCIDENCE (0-74)
RATES AND STANDARD ERRORS (percent)
Pancreas (ICD-9 157)

	MALE		FEMALE	
AFRICA				
*Algeria, Setif				
*France, La Reunion				
*Mali, Bamako				
*Uganda, Kyadondo				
*Zimbabwe, Harare: African				
*Zimbabwe, Harare: European				
AMERICA, CENTRAL AND SOUTH				
*Argentina, Concordia	1.17	0.28	0.62	0.20
*Brazil, Belem	0.66	0.13	0.26	0.07
*Brazil, Goiania				
*Brazil, Porto Alegre	1.02	0.12	0.75	0.08
Colombia, Cali	0.69	0.08	0.40	0.05
*Costa Rica	0.63	0.05	0.52	0.05
*Ecuador, Quito	0.42	0.07	0.56	0.08
*Peru, Lima	0.37	0.04	0.47	0.05
Peru, Trujillo	0.70	0.18	0.39	0.12
US, Puerto Rico	0.61	0.04	0.33	0.03
*Uruguay, Montevideo	0.91	0.08	0.67	0.06
AMERICA, NORTH				
Canada	0.92	0.01	0.64	0.01
Canada, Alberta	0.99	0.05	0.66	0.04
Canada, British Columbia	0.79	0.04	0.60	0.03
Canada, Manitoba	0.89	0.07	0.65	0.05
Canada, New Brunswick	0.79	0.08	0.50	0.06
Canada, Newfoundland	0.55	0.08	0.38	0.06
Canada, Northwest Territories	0,98	0,41	0,68	0,32
Canada, Nova Scotia	1.11	0.08	0.63	0.06
Canada, Ontario	0.88	0.02	0.65	0.02
Canada, Prince Edward Island	1.20	0.22	0.80	0.18
Canada, Quebec	1.05	0.03	0.67	0.02
Canada, Saskatchewan	0.76	0.06	0.63	0.05
Canada, Yukon	0,70	0,41	0,54	0,38
US, Cent. Calif.: Non-Hisp. White	0.97	0.06	0.66	0.05
US, Cent. Calif.: Hispanic	0.95	0.14	0.64	0.11
US, Los Angeles: Non-Hisp. White	0.95	0.03	0.67	0.03
US, Los Angeles: Hispanic White	0.88	0.07	0.59	0.05
US, Los Angeles: Black	1.30	0.11	0.97	0.08
US, Los Angeles: Chinese	0.41	0.10	0.31	0.09
US, Los Angeles: Filipino	0.49	0.15	0.64	0.14
US, Los Angeles: Korean	0.54	0.17	0.61	0.16
US, Los Angeles: Japanese	0.66	0.15	0.64	0.14
US, San Francisco: Non-Hisp. White	0.96	0.05	0.71	0.04
US, San Francisco: Hispanic White	0.53	0.11	0.57	0.10
US, San Francisco: Black	1.56	0.16	1.33	0.13
US, San Francisco: Chinese	0.72	0.12	0.53	0.11
US, San Francisco: Filipino	0.52	0.15	0.64	0.16
US, San Francisco: Japanese	0,35	0,21	0,23	0,12
US, Connecticut: White	0.99	0.04	0.69	0.03
US, Connecticut: Black	1.08	0.20	0.95	0.16
US, Atlanta: White	0.94	0.07	0.52	0.05
US, Atlanta: Black	1.30	0.17	1.04	0.12
US, Iowa	0.88	0.04	0.61	0.03

	MALE		FEMALE	
US, Central Louisiana: White	0.94	0.15	0.74	0.12
US, Central Louisiana: Black	2.42	0.52	1.01	0.28
US, New Orleans: White	1.05	0.10	0.73	0.07
US, New Orleans: Black	1.07	0.15	1.09	0.13
US, Detroit: White	0.99	0.04	0.71	0.03
US, Detroit: Black	1.61	0.11	1.11	0.08
US, New Mexico: Non-Hisp. White	1.04	0.08	0.65	0.06
US, New Mexico: Hispanic White	0.86	0.11	0.58	0.09
US, New Mexico: American Indian	0,77	0,27	0.74	0.24
US, Utah	0.69	0.06	0.51	0.04
US, Seattle	0.90	0.04	0.77	0.03
US, SEER: White	0.93	0.02	0.67	0.01
US, SEER: Black	1.45	0.07	1.10	0.05
ASIA				
*China, Qidong	0.90	0.07	0.63	0.06
China, Shanghai	0.78	0.02	0.53	0.02
China, Tianjin	0.67	0.03	0.41	0.03
Hong Kong	0.47	0.02	0.34	0.02
*India, Bangalore	0.18	0.02	0.10	0.02
*India, Barshi, Paranda and Bhum	0,09	0,05	0,02	0,01
India, Bombay	0.28	0.02	0.22	0.02
*India, Karunagappally	0,25	0,12	0,02	0,02m
India, Madras	0.17	0.02	0.09	0.02
*India, Trivandrum	0.32	0.10	0,16	0,06
Israel: All Jews	0.85	0.04	0.66	0.03
Jews born in Israel	0.74	0.13	0.66	0.13
Jews born in America or Europe	0.95	0.06	0.69	0.04
Jews born in Africa or Asia	0.67	0.06	0.58	0.05
Non-Jews	0.47	0.11	0.34	0.08
Japan, Hiroshima	1.08	0.08	0.70	0.06
Japan, Miyagi	1.32	0.06	0.64	0.04
Japan, Nagasaki	1.09	0.06	0.58	0.04
Japan, Osaka	1.12	0.03	0.58	0.02
*Japan, Saga	1.07	0.08	0.59	0.05
Japan, Yamagata	1.11	0.06	0.56	0.04
*Korea, Kangwha	0.82	0.21	0.50	0.16
*Kuwait: Non-Kuwaitis	0.79	0.26	0.39	0.17
*Kuwait: Kuwaitis	0.71	0.17	0.47	0.16
*Philippines, Manila	0.60	0.05	0.44	0.04
Singapore: Chinese	0.60	0.05	0.41	0.04
Singapore: Malay	0.25	0.08	0,17	0,07
Singapore: Indian	0,21	0,08	0,14	0,09
Thailand, Chiang Mai	0.33	0.04	0.32	0.04
*Thailand, Khon Kaen	0.12	0.03	0.09	0.03
*Viet Nam, Hanoi				

* IMPORTANT-SEE NOTES ON POPULATION PAGE

EUROPE	MALE		FEMALE	
Austria, Tyrol	0.79	*0.09*	0.60	*0.07*
*Belarus	1.11	*0.03*	0.45	*0.01*
*Croatia	1.11	*0.04*	0.61	*0.03*
Czech Republic	1.40	*0.03*	0.75	*0.02*
Denmark	0.96	*0.03*	0.78	*0.02*
Estonia	1.35	*0.08*	0.73	*0.04*
Finland	1.11	*0.03*	0.80	*0.02*
France, Bas-Rhin	0.89	*0.08*	0.45	*0.05*
*France, Calvados	0.70	*0.08*	0.41	*0.05*
France, Doubs	0.72	*0.09*	0.28	*0.05*
France, Haut-Rhin	0.75	*0.09*	0.37	*0.05*
*France, Herault	0.41	*0.05*	0.26	*0.04*
France, Isere	0.56	*0.06*	0.39	*0.05*
*France, Somme	0.56	*0.08*	0.26	*0.05*
*France, Tarn	0.37	*0.07*	0.13	*0.04*
Germany, Eastern States	0.89	*0.03*	0.55	*0.02*
Germany, Saarland	0.79	*0.06*	0.44	*0.04*
Iceland	0.93	*0.15*	0.68	*0.12*
Ireland, Southern	0.94	*0.10*	0.50	*0.07*
Italy, Ferrara	0.98	*0.16*	0.66	*0.12*
Italy, Florence	0.90	*0.07*	0.59	*0.05*
Italy, Genoa	0.96	*0.07*	0.61	*0.05*
*Italy, Latina	0.72	*0.11*	0.38	*0.07*
Italy, Macerata	1.06	*0.19*	0.50	*0.12*
Italy, Modena	0.96	*0.08*	0.62	*0.06*
Italy, Parma	0.87	*0.09*	0.62	*0.07*
Italy, Ragusa	0.69	*0.11*	0.41	*0.08*
Italy, Romagna	0.80	*0.08*	0.57	*0.07*
Italy, Torino	0.96	*0.08*	0.52	*0.05*
Italy, Trieste	1.42	*0.16*	0.75	*0.10*
Italy, Varese	1.07	*0.09*	0.65	*0.06*
Italy, Veneto	1.17	*0.07*	0.78	*0.05*
*Latvia	1.45	*0.06*	0.63	*0.03*
Malta	1.05	*0.21*	0.45	*0.12*
The Netherlands	0.84	*0.02*	0.55	*0.01*
The Netherlands, Eindhoven	0.74	*0.07*	0.49	*0.05*
The Netherlands, Maastricht	0.72	*0.07*	0.52	*0.05*
Norway	0.95	*0.03*	0.65	*0.02*
*Poland, Cracow	1.14	*0.11*	0.69	*0.07*
*Poland, Kielce	0.88	*0.07*	0.61	*0.05*
*Poland, Lower Silesia	1.30	*0.06*	0.80	*0.04*
Poland, Warsaw City	0.99	*0.07*	0.57	*0.04*
Slovakia	1.32	*0.04*	0.66	*0.03*
Slovenia	1.06	*0.07*	0.58	*0.04*
*Spain, Albacete	0.52	*0.14*	0.32	*0.09*
Spain, Asturias	0.60	*0.05*	0.26	*0.03*
Spain, Basque Country	0.73	*0.05*	0.42	*0.03*
Spain, Granada	0.62	*0.06*	0.34	*0.04*
Spain, Mallorca	0.71	*0.08*	0.40	*0.05*
Spain, Murcia	0.52	*0.05*	0.25	*0.03*
Spain, Navarra	0.75	*0.08*	0.39	*0.05*
Spain, Tarragona	0.53	*0.07*	0.33	*0.05*
Spain, Zaragoza	0.70	*0.06*	0.36	*0.04*

	MALE		FEMALE		
Sweden	0.86	*0.02*	0.68	*0.02*	
*Switzerland, Basel	0.66	*0.09*	0.57	*0.07*	
Switzerland, Geneva	1.16	*0.14*	0.74	*0.09*	
Switzerland, Graubunden	1.07	*0.19*	0.74	*0.15*	
Switzerland, Neuchatel	0.96	*0.17*	0.49	*0.11*	
Switzerland, St Gall-Appenzell	1.09	*0.11*	0.72	*0.08*	
Switzerland, Valais	1.13	*0.18*	0.45	*0.10*	
Switzerland, Vaud	1.16	*0.10*	0.68	*0.07*	
Switzerland, Zurich	0.86	*0.06*	0.65	*0.05*	
*UK, England and Wales	0.86	*0.01*	0.62	*0.01*	
*UK, East Anglia	0.71	*0.04*	0.57	*0.03*	
*UK, Mersey	0.81	*0.04*	0.64	*0.03*	
*UK, North Western	0.88	*0.03*	0.60	*0.02*	
UK, Oxford	0.87	*0.04*	0.68	*0.04*	
*UK, South Thames	0.91	*0.03*	0.65	*0.02*	
UK, South Western	0.85	*0.03*	0.54	*0.02*	
UK, Wessex	0.76	*0.03*	0.58	*0.03*	
*UK, West Midlands	0.87	*0.03*	0.60	*0.02*	
UK, Yorkshire	0.82	*0.03*	0.58	*0.03*	
UK, Scotland	0.93	*0.03*	0.64	*0.02*	
UK, Scotland, West	0.95	*0.04*	0.63	*0.03*	
*Yugoslavia, Vojvodina	0.87	*0.05*	0.56	*0.03*	
OCEANIA					
Australian Capital Territory	0.68	*0.16*	0.41	*0.10*	
Australia, New South Wales	0.79	*0.03*	0.58	*0.02*	
South Australia	0.79	*0.05*	0.55	*0.04*	
Australia, Tasmania	0.67	*0.09*	0.54	*0.08*	
Australia, Victoria	0.79	*0.03*	0.51	*0.02*	
Western Australia	0.72	*0.06*	0.55	*0.05*	
*French Polynesia	0,34	*0,13*	0,55	*0,23*	f
New Zealand: Non-Maori	0.87	*0.04*	0.52	*0.03*	
New Zealand: Maori	1.10	*0.23*	0.83	*0.20*	
US, Hawaii: White	1.06	*0.15*	0.70	*0.12*	
US, Hawaii: Japanese	0.77	*0.10*	0.67	*0.09*	
US, Hawaii: Hawaiian	1.19	*0.25*	0.72	*0.16*	
US, Hawaii: Filipino	0.52	*0.13*	0.53	*0.14*	
US, Hawaii: Chinese	0.73	*0.23*	0,34	*0,14*	

* IMPORTANT-SEE NOTES ON POPULATION PAGE

CUMULATIVE INCIDENCE (0-74)
RATES AND STANDARD ERRORS (percent)
Nose, sinuses etc. (ICD-9 160)

	MALE		FEMALE	
AFRICA				
*Algeria, Setif				
*France, La Reunion				
*Mali, Bamako				
*Uganda, Kyadondo				
*Zimbabwe, Harare: African				
*Zimbabwe, Harare: European				
AMERICA, CENTRAL AND SOUTH				
*Argentina, Concordia	0,13	0,07	0,04	0,04
*Brazil, Belem	0,08	0,04	0,02	0,01
*Brazil, Goiania				
*Brazil, Porto Alegre	0,03	0,01	0,03	0,01
Colombia, Cali	0.14	0.03	0.09	0.02
*Costa Rica	0.05	0.01	0,03	0,01
*Ecuador, Quito	0,04	0,02	0,04	0,02
*Peru, Lima	0.12	0.02	0.06	0.02
Peru, Trujillo	0,06	0,04	0,04	0,03
US, Puerto Rico	0.07	0.01	0.03	0.01
*Uruguay, Montevideo	0.10	0.03	0,04	0,01
AMERICA, NORTH				
Canada	0.07	0.00	0.04	0.00
Canada, Alberta	0.06	0.01	0.04	0.01
Canada, British Columbia	0.07	0.01	0.05	0.01
Canada, Manitoba	0,04	0,01	0,03	0,01
Canada, New Brunswick	0,06	0,02	0,05	0,02
Canada, Newfoundland	0.12	0.04	0,04	0,02
Canada, Northwest Territories	0,04	0,04	-	-
Canada, Nova Scotia	0.09	0.02	0.05	0.02
Canada, Ontario	0.09	0.01	0.04	0.00
Canada, Prince Edward Island	0,08	0,04	-	-
Canada, Quebec	0.06	0.01	0.03	0.00
Canada, Saskatchewan	0.06	0.02	0,02	0,01
Canada, Yukon	-	-	-	-
US, Cent. Calif.: Non-Hisp. White	0.10	0.02	0.05	0.01
US, Cent. Calif.: Hispanic	0,02	0,01	-	-
US, Los Angeles: Non-Hisp. White	0.08	0.01	0.04	0.01
US, Los Angeles: Hispanic White	0.05	0.01	0.05	0.01
US, Los Angeles: Black	0.13	0.03	0,04	0,02
US, Los Angeles: Chinese	0,03	0,02	0,03	0,03
US, Los Angeles: Filipino	0,05	0,05	0,09	0,05
US, Los Angeles: Korean	-	-	0,02	0,02
US, Los Angeles: Japanese	0,03	0,03	-	-
US, San Francisco: Non-Hisp. White	0.07	0.01	0.03	0.01
US, San Francisco: Hispanic White	0,05	0,03	0,07	0,03
US, San Francisco: Black	0,04	0,02	0,04	0,02
US, San Francisco: Chinese	0,10	0,04	0,06	0,03
US, San Francisco: Filipino	0,09	0,06	0,03	0,02
US, San Francisco: Japanese	0,10	0,10	-	-
US, Connecticut: White	0.05	0.01	0.04	0.01
US, Connecticut: Black	0.10	0,06	0,04	0,02
US, Atlanta: White	0.08	0.02	0.04	0.01
US, Atlanta: Black	0,13	0,06	0,02	0,01
US, Iowa	0.06	0.01	0.04	0.01

	MALE		FEMALE	
US, Central Louisiana: White	0,04	0,03	0,04	0,03
US, Central Louisiana: Black	-	-	0,09	0,09
US, New Orleans: White	0,07	0,02	0,03	0,01
US, New Orleans: Black	0.13	0.05	0,12	0,04
US, Detroit: White	0.07	0.01	0.04	0.01
US, Detroit: Black	0,04	0,02	0.07	0.02
US, New Mexico: Non-Hisp. White	0.07	0.02	0.08	0.02
US, New Mexico: Hispanic White	0,03	0,02	0,02	0,01
US, New Mexico: American Indian	-	-	0,24	0,14
US, Utah	0.04	0.01	0.04	0.01
US, Seattle	0.08	0.01	0.03	0.01
US, SEER: White	0.06	0.00	0.04	0.00
US, SEER: Black	0.07	0.01	0.05	0.01
ASIA				
*China, Qidong	0,01	0,01	0,02	0,01
China, Shanghai	0.09	0.01	0.05	0.01
China, Tianjin	0.08	0.01	0.04	0.01
Hong Kong	0.10	0.01	0.04	0.01
*India, Bangalore	0.08	0.01	0.07	0.01
*India, Barshi, Paranda and Bhum	0,02	0,01	0,03	0,02
India, Bombay	0.12	0.01	0.09	0.01
*India, Karunagappally	0,06	0,05	0,02	0,02
India, Madras	0.12	0.02	0.08	0.01
*India, Trivandrum	0,11	0,06	0,09	0,04
Israel: All Jews	0.04	0.01	0.04	0.01
Jews born in Israel	0,06	0,05	0,06	0,03
Jews born in America or Europe	0,03	0,01	0,05	0,01
Jews born in Africa or Asia	0,09	0,03	0,02	0,01
Non-Jews	0,02	0,01	0,02	0,02
Japan, Hiroshima	0.13	0.03	0.04	0.01
Japan, Miyagi	0.16	0.02	0.08	0.01
Japan, Nagasaki	0.14	0.02	0.06	0.01
Japan, Osaka	0.10	0.01	0.05	0.01
*Japan, Saga	0.15	0.03	0.04	0.01
Japan, Yamagata	0.15	0.02	0.03	0.01
*Korea, Kangwha	-	-	0,03	0,03
*Kuwait: Non-Kuwaitis	0,19	0,18	0,01	0,01
*Kuwait: Kuwaitis	-	-	0,05	0,03
*Philippines, Manila	0.19	0.03	0.10	0.02
Singapore: Chinese	0.10	0.02	0.04	0.01
Singapore: Malay	0,06	0,03	0,18	0,08
Singapore: Indian	0,05	0,03	0,06	0,05
Thailand, Chiang Mai	0.12	0.03	0.07	0.02
*Thailand, Khon Kaen	0.05	0.02	0,04	0,02
*Viet Nam, Hanoi				

* IMPORTANT-SEE NOTES ON POPULATION PAGE

CUMULATIVE INCIDENCE (0-74)
RATES AND STANDARD ERRORS (percent)
Nose, sinuses etc. (ICD-9 160) (contd)

EUROPE	MALE		FEMALE	
Austria, Tyrol	0,01	0,01	0,03	0,01
*Belarus	0.07	0.01	0.03	0.00
*Croatia	0.06	0.01	0.03	0.01
Czech Republic	0.05	0.01	0.03	0.00
Denmark	0.11	0.01	0.06	0.01
Estonia	0.09	0.02	0.05	0.01
Finland	0.06	0.01	0.03	0.00
France, Bas-Rhin	0.10	0.02	0.02	0.01
*France, Calvados	0.15	0.03	0.04	0.02
France, Doubs	0.14	0.04	0.02	0.01
France, Haut-Rhin	0.16	0.03	0.02	0.01
*France, Herault	0.15	0.03	0.07	0.02
France, Isere	0.15	0.03	0.03	0.01
*France, Somme	0.15	0.04	0.04	0.02
*France, Tarn	0.12	0.04	0.03	0.02
Germany, Eastern States	0.06	0.01	0.03	0.00
Germany, Saarland	0.05	0.02	0.03	0.01
Iceland	0,11	0,05	0,07	0,04
Ireland, Southern	0,04	0,02	0,03	0,02
Italy, Ferrara	0,09	0,05	0,02	0,02
Italy, Florence	0.11	0.02	0.02	0.01
Italy, Genoa	0.12	0.03	0.05	0.02
*Italy, Latina	0,05	0,02	0,02	0,02
Italy, Macerata	0,16	0,07	-	-
Italy, Modena	0.02	0.01	0.02	0.01
Italy, Parma	0.09	0.03	0.05	0.02
Italy, Ragusa	0,04	0,02	0,01	0,01
Italy, Romagna	0,06	0,02	0,03	0,02
Italy, Torino	0.06	0.02	0.02	0.01
Italy, Trieste	0,10	0,04	0,02	0,02
Italy, Varese	0.09	0.02	0.03	0.01
Italy, Veneto	0.12	0.02	0.01	0.01
*Latvia	0.07	0.01	0.02	0.01
Malta	0,08	0,05	0,04	0,03
The Netherlands	0.10	0.01	0.04	0.00
The Netherlands, Eindhoven	0.11	0.03	0.03	0.01
The Netherlands, Maastricht	0.08	0.02	0.04	0.01
Norway	0.08	0.01	0.03	0.01
*Poland, Cracow	0,03	0,01	0,02	0,01
*Poland, Kielce	0.06	0.02	0.04	0.01
*Poland, Lower Silesia	0.07	0.01	0.03	0.01
Poland, Warsaw City	0.08	0.02	0.02	0.01
Slovakia	0.08	0.01	0.03	0.01
Slovenia	0.08	0.02	0.04	0.01
*Spain, Albacete	-	-	0,04	0,04
Spain, Asturias	0.15	0.02	0.07	0.02
Spain, Basque Country	0.10	0.02	0.02	0.01
Spain, Granada	0.11	0.03	0.01	0.01
Spain, Mallorca	0.08	0.02	0.03	0.01
Spain, Murcia	0.05	0.02	0.03	0.01
Spain, Navarra	0.04	0.02	0.04	0.02
Spain, Tarragona	0.04	0.02	0.01	0.01
Spain, Zaragoza	0.06	0.02	0.02	0.01
Sweden	0.07	0.01	0.03	0.00
*Switzerland, Basel	0.10	0.03	0.02	0.01
Switzerland, Geneva	0,06	0,02	0,08	0,03
Switzerland, Graubunden	0,02	0,02	-	-
Switzerland, Neuchatel	0,07	0,04	0,05	0,03
Switzerland, St Gall-Appenzell	0.11	0.03	0.03	0.02
Switzerland, Valais	0,03	0,03	0,11	0,05
Switzerland, Vaud	0,04	0,02	0,05	0,02
Switzerland, Zurich	0.08	0.02	0.01	0.01
*UK, England and Wales	0.08	0.00	0.04	0.00
*UK, East Anglia	0.08	0.01	0.03	0.01
*UK, Mersey	0.06	0.01	0.06	0.01
*UK, North Western	0.07	0.01	0.04	0.01
UK, Oxford	0.08	0.01	0.04	0.01
*UK, South Thames	0.07	0.01	0.03	0.00
UK, South Western	0.06	0.01	0.03	0.01
UK, Wessex	0.07	0.01	0.04	0.01
*UK, West Midlands	0.07	0.01	0.04	0.01
UK, Yorkshire	0.06	0.01	0.03	0.01
UK, Scotland	0.06	0.01	0.04	0.01
UK, Scotland, West	0.06	0.01	0.04	0.01
*Yugoslavia, Vojvodina	0.03	0.01	0.02	0.01

OCEANIA	MALE		FEMALE	
Australian Capital Territory	0,15	0,07	0,02	0,02
Australia, New South Wales	0.07	0.01	0.03	0.00
South Australia	0.06	0.01	0.03	0.01
Australia, Tasmania	0.26	0.05	0.06	0.02
Australia, Victoria	0.09	0.01	0.03	0.01
Western Australia	0.08	0.02	0.02	0.01
*French Polynesia	0,24	0,11	0,11	0,08
New Zealand: Non-Maori	0.06	0.01	0.06	0.01
New Zealand: Maori	0,02	0,02	-	-
US, Hawaii: White	0,09	0,04	0,06	0,04
US, Hawaii: Japanese	0,09	0,03	0,03	0,02
US, Hawaii: Hawaiian	0,08	0,05	0,08	0,04
US, Hawaii: Filipino	0,03	0,03	0,08	0,05
US, Hawaii: Chinese	0,04	0,04	0,03	0,03

* IMPORTANT-SEE NOTES ON POPULATION PAGE

CUMULATIVE INCIDENCE (0-74)
RATES AND STANDARD ERRORS (percent)
Larynx (ICD-9 161)

	MALE		FEMALE	
AFRICA				
*Algeria, Setif				
*France, La Reunion				
*Mali, Bamako				
*Uganda, Kyadondo				
*Zimbabwe, Harare: African				
*Zimbabwe, Harare: European				
AMERICA, CENTRAL AND SOUTH				
*Argentina, Concordia	0.89	0.22	0,18	0,09
*Brazil, Belem	1.00	0.15	0,04	0,02 mf
*Brazil, Goiania				
*Brazil, Porto Alegre	1.32	0.12	0.15	0.03
Colombia, Cali	0.64	0.08	0.13	0.03 f
*Costa Rica	0.47	0.04	0.07	0.02
*Ecuador, Quito	0.18	0.05	0,02	0,02
*Peru, Lima	0.27	0.03	0.06	0.02
Peru, Trujillo	0,33	0,13	0,02	0,02
US, Puerto Rico	0.73	0.04	0.11	0.02
*Uruguay, Montevideo	1.58	0.10	0.11	0.02
AMERICA, NORTH				
Canada	0.80	0.01	0.15	0.01
Canada, Alberta	0.56	0.04	0.11	0.02
Canada, British Columbia	0.59	0.03	0.12	0.01
Canada, Manitoba	0.54	0.05	0.12	0.02
Canada, New Brunswick	0.89	0.08	0.12	0.03
Canada, Newfoundland	0.74	0.09	0,05	0,02
Canada, Northwest Territories	0,22	0,13	0,28	0,28
Canada, Nova Scotia	0.90	0.07	0.09	0.02
Canada, Ontario	0.73	0.02	0.13	0.01
Canada, Prince Edward Island	0.70	0.17	0,04	0,04
Canada, Quebec	1.14	0.03	0.23	0.01
Canada, Saskatchewan	0.58	0.05	0.10	0.02
Canada, Yukon	0,58	0,33	-	-
US, Cent. Calif.: Non-Hisp. White	0.75	0.05	0.18	0.02
US, Cent. Calif.: Hispanic	0.50	0.10	0,01	0,01
US, Los Angeles: Non-Hisp. White	0.80	0.03	0.17	0.01
US, Los Angeles: Hispanic White	0.56	0.05	0.06	0.01
US, Los Angeles: Black	1.27	0.10	0.24	0.04
US, Los Angeles: Chinese	0,14	0,06	0,03	0,03
US, Los Angeles: Filipino	0.25	0.09	0,11	0,06
US, Los Angeles: Korean	0.69	0.20	0,20	0,10
US, Los Angeles: Japanese	0,16	0,07	0,02	0,02
US, San Francisco: Non-Hisp. White	0.76	0.04	0.19	0.02
US, San Francisco: Hispanic White	0.47	0.10	0,08	0,04
US, San Francisco: Black	1.22	0.14	0.26	0.06
US, San Francisco: Chinese	0.36	0.09	0,03	0,02
US, San Francisco: Filipino	0,20	0,11	0,07	0,04
US, San Francisco: Japanese	0,25	0,15	0,05	0,05
US, Connecticut: White	0.79	0.04	0.22	0.02
US, Connecticut: Black	1.27	0.20	0.28	0.08
US, Atlanta: White	0.95	0.07	0.22	0.03
US, Atlanta: Black	1.38	0.16	0.27	0.06
US, Iowa	0.87	0.04	0.17	0.02

	MALE		FEMALE	
US, Central Louisiana: White	1.13	0.17	0.24	0.07
US, Central Louisiana: Black	0,88	0.30	0,24	0,14
US, New Orleans: White	1.17	0.10	0.36	0.05
US, New Orleans: Black	1.48	0.19	0.26	0.06
US, Detroit: White	1.04	0.04	0.20	0.02
US, Detroit: Black	1.53	0.11	0.36	0.04
US, New Mexico: Non-Hisp. White	0.57	0.06	0.18	0.03
US, New Mexico: Hispanic White	0.59	0.10	0,10	0,03
US, New Mexico: American Indian	0,12	0,12	-	-
US, Utah	0.44	0.04	0.05	0.01
US, Seattle	0.73	0.04	0.16	0.02
US, SEER: White	0.80	0.02	0.18	0.01
US, SEER: Black	1.38	0.07	0.30	0.03
ASIA				
*China, Qidong	0.07	0.02	0,00	0,00
China, Shanghai	0.44	0.02	0.04	0.01
China, Tianjin	0.40	0.03	0.21	0.02
Hong Kong	1.01	0.03	0.11	0.01
*India, Bangalore	0.56	0.04	0.06	0.01
*India, Barshi, Paranda and Bhum	0.37	0.09	-	-
India, Bombay	1.05	0.04	0.16	0.02
*India, Karunagappally	0.74	0.19	-	-
India, Madras	0.63	0.04	0.07	0.01
*India, Trivandrum	0.69	0.14	0,06	0,04
Israel: All Jews	0.60	0.03	0.09	0.01
Jews born in Israel	0.44	0.09	0.09	0.03
Jews born in America or Europe	0.57	0.04	0.09	0.02
Jews born in Africa or Asia	0.66	0.06	0.07	0.02
Non-Jews	0.39	0.08	-	-
Japan, Hiroshima	0.54	0.06	0,03	0,01
Japan, Miyagi	0.47	0.03	0.02	0,01
Japan, Nagasaki	0.49	0.04	0.02	0,01
Japan, Osaka	0.43	0.02	0.04	0.00
*Japan, Saga	0.49	0.05	0.02	0,01
Japan, Yamagata	0.34	0.03	0.01	0,00
*Korea, Kangwha	0,17	0,09	0,04	0,04
*Kuwait: Non-Kuwaitis	0.64	0.23	0,01	0,01
*Kuwait: Kuwaitis	0.23	0.08	0,07	0,05
*Philippines, Manila	0.78	0.06	0.10	0.02
Singapore: Chinese	0.71	0.06	0.10	0.02
Singapore: Malay	0.37	0.11	0,08	0,05
Singapore: Indian	0.64	0.14	0,11	0,08
Thailand, Chiang Mai	0.73	0.07	0.25	0.04
*Thailand, Khon Kaen	0.15	0.04	0.03	0,02
*Viet Nam, Hanoi				

* IMPORTANT-SEE NOTES ON POPULATION PAGE

EUROPE	MALE		FEMALE	
Austria, Tyrol	0.93	*0.10*	0,04	*0,02*
*Belarus	1.31	*0.03*	0.03	*0.00*
*Croatia	1.58	*0.05*	0.07	*0.01*
Czech Republic	0.89	*0.02*	0.05	*0.00*
Denmark	0.70	*0.02*	0.15	*0.01*
Estonia	1.14	*0.06*	0.05	*0.01*
Finland	0.42	*0.02*	0.04	*0.00*
France, Bas-Rhin	1.43	*0.09*	0.06	*0.02*
*France, Calvados	1.48	*0.11*	0.08	*0.03*
France, Doubs	1.73	*0.14*	0,09	*0,03*
France, Haut-Rhin	1.25	*0.10*	0.10	*0.03*
*France, Herault	1.50	*0.09*	0.08	*0.02*
France, Isere	1.26	*0.08*	0.05	*0.01*
*France, Somme	1.76	*0.13*	0.12	*0.03*
*France, Tarn	0.77	*0.10*	0,06	*0,02*
Germany, Eastern States	0.62	*0.02*	0.04	*0.00*
Germany, Saarland	1.00	*0.06*	0.09	*0.02*
Iceland	0.50	*0.11*	0,02	*0,02*
Ireland, Southern	0.80	*0.09*	0.09	*0.03*
Italy, Ferrara	1.36	*0.19*	0,04	*0,03*
Italy, Florence	1.50	*0.08*	0.11	*0.02*
Italy, Genoa	1.62	*0.09*	0.10	*0.02*
*Italy, Latina	1.13	*0.13*	0,06	*0,03*
Italy, Macerata	1.10	*0.19*	0,05	*0,04*
Italy, Modena	1.45	*0.10*	0.08	*0.02*
Italy, Parma	1.50	*0.12*	0,07	*0,02*
Italy, Ragusa	0.58	*0.10*	0,02	*0,02*
Italy, Romagna	1.23	*0.10*	0.09	*0.02*
Italy, Torino	1.26	*0.08*	0.10	*0.02*
Italy, Trieste	1.99	*0.19*	0.24	*0.06*
Italy, Varese	1.62	*0.10*	0.07	*0.02*
Italy, Veneto	2.07	*0.09*	0.14	*0.02*
*Latvia	1.10	*0.05*	0.05	*0.01*
Malta	1.30	*0.22*	0,05	*0,03*
The Netherlands	0.81	*0.02*	0.10	*0.01*
The Netherlands, Eindhoven	1.05	*0.08*	0.07	*0.02*
The Netherlands, Maastricht	0.91	*0.07*	0.08	*0.02*
Norway	0.41	*0.02*	0.04	*0.01*
*Poland, Cracow	1.14	*0.09*	0.12	*0.03*
*Poland, Kielce	1.67	*0.09*	0.07	*0.02*
*Poland, Lower Silesia	1.85	*0.06*	0.18	*0.02*
Poland, Warsaw City	1.39	*0.08*	0.16	*0.02*
Slovakia	1.36	*0.04*	0.04	*0.01*
Slovenia	1.14	*0.06*	0.07	*0.01*
*Spain, Albacete	1.72	*0.24*	-	-
Spain, Asturias	1.90	*0.09*	0,04	*0,01*
Spain, Basque Country	2.26	*0.08*	0.03	*0.01*
Spain, Granada	1.70	*0.10*	0,00	*0,00*
Spain, Mallorca	1.67	*0.11*	0,05	*0,02*
Spain, Murcia	1.97	*0.10*	0,02	*0,01*
Spain, Navarra	1.90	*0.12*	0,03	*0,02*
Spain, Tarragona	1.49	*0.11*	0,01	*0,01*
Spain, Zaragoza	2.21	*0.10*	0,01	*0,01*

	MALE		FEMALE	
Sweden	0.32	*0.01*	0.04	*0.00*
*Switzerland, Basel	0.54	*0.08*	0,08	*0,03*
Switzerland, Geneva	1.06	*0.12*	0.13	*0.04*
Switzerland, Graubunden	0.59	*0.14*	0,09	*0,05*
Switzerland, Neuchatel	0.73	*0.14*	0,13	*0,06*
Switzerland, St Gall-Appenzell	0.49	*0.07*	0,03	*0,01*
Switzerland, Valais	0.81	*0.13*	0,13	*0,05*
Switzerland, Vaud	0.81	*0.08*	0.10	*0.03*
Switzerland, Zurich	0.52	*0.05*	0.04	*0.01*
*UK, England and Wales	0.56	*0.01*	0.10	*0.00*
*UK, East Anglia	0.41	*0.03*	0.08	*0.01*
*UK, Mersey	0.60	*0.03*	0.15	*0.02*
*UK, North Western	0.73	*0.03*	0.13	*0.01*
UK, Oxford	0.42	*0.03*	0.08	*0.01*
*UK, South Thames	0.42	*0.02*	0.08	*0.01*
UK, South Western	0.43	*0.02*	0.07	*0.01*
UK, Wessex	0.49	*0.03*	0.06	*0.01*
*UK, West Midlands	0.64	*0.02*	0.11	*0.01*
UK, Yorkshire	0.63	*0.03*	0.13	*0.01*
UK, Scotland	0.80	*0.03*	0.17	*0.01*
UK, Scotland, West	0.86	*0.04*	0.19	*0.02*
*Yugoslavia, Vojvodina	1.33	*0.05*	0.08	*0.01*

OCEANIA	MALE		FEMALE	
Australian Capital Territory	0.52	*0.12*	0,05	*0,04*
Australia, New South Wales	0.72	*0.03*	0.08	*0.01*
South Australia	0.67	*0.05*	0.07	*0.02*
Australia, Tasmania	0.58	*0.08*	0,04	*0,02*
Australia, Victoria	0.60	*0.03*	0.08	*0.01*
Western Australia	0.62	*0.05*	0.09	*0.02*
*French Polynesia	0.84	*0.18*	0,17	*0,10*
New Zealand: Non-Maori	0.52	*0.03*	0.08	*0.01*
New Zealand: Maori	0.47	*0.17*	0,21	*0,11*
US, Hawaii: White	1.14	*0.15*	0,15	*0,06*
US, Hawaii: Japanese	0.24	*0.06*	0,04	*0,02*
US, Hawaii: Hawaiian	0.48	*0.15*	0,04	*0,04*
US, Hawaii: Filipino	0.35	*0.11*	0,06	*0,04*
US, Hawaii: Chinese	0,23	*0,11*	-	-

* IMPORTANT-SEE NOTES ON POPULATION PAGE

CUMULATIVE INCIDENCE (0-74)
RATES AND STANDARD ERRORS (percent)
Bronchus, lung (ICD-9 162)

	MALE		FEMALE	
AFRICA				
*Algeria, Setif				
*France, La Reunion				
*Mali, Bamako				
*Uganda, Kyadondo				
*Zimbabwe, Harare: African				
*Zimbabwe, Harare: European				
AMERICA, CENTRAL AND SOUTH				
*Argentina, Concordia	6.66	0.62	1.00	0.22
*Brazil, Belem	3.52	0.29	0.85	0.11
*Brazil, Goiania				
*Brazil, Porto Alegre	8.15	0.32	1.64	0.11
Colombia, Cali	2.90	0.16	1.10	0.09
*Costa Rica	1.80	0.09	0.59	0.05
*Ecuador, Quito	1.14	0.12	0.39	0.06
*Peru, Lima	1.89	0.09	0.75	0.06
Peru, Trujillo	1.61	0.29	0.47	0.13
US, Puerto Rico	2.34	0.08	0.83	0.04
*Uruguay, Montevideo	8.78	0.24	0.93	0.07
AMERICA, NORTH				
Canada	8.37	0.04	3.57	0.03
Canada, Alberta	6.25	0.13	3.19	0.09
Canada, British Columbia	6.96	0.11	4.01	0.07
Canada, Manitoba	7.56	0.20	3.61	0.12
Canada, New Brunswick	9.50	0.28	3.52	0.15
Canada, Newfoundland	7.59	0.29	1.87	0.14
Canada, Northwest Territories	12.37	1.36	7.95	1.11
Canada, Nova Scotia	9.50	0.24	4.15	0.15
Canada, Ontario	7.93	0.07	3.61	0.04
Canada, Prince Edward Island	7.69	0.57	4.46	0.40
Canada, Quebec	10.59	0.10	3.51	0.05
Canada, Saskatchewan	6.85	0.19	3.05	0.12
Canada, Yukon	8.90	1.32	6.38	1.19
US, Cent. Calif.: Non-Hisp. White	9.13	0.18	5.23	0.13
US, Cent. Calif.: Hispanic	4.21	0.29	1.88	0.18
US, Los Angeles: Non-Hisp. White	7.49	0.10	5.01	0.07
US, Los Angeles: Hispanic White	3.66	0.14	1.85	0.09
US, Los Angeles: Black	11.39	0.30	4.48	0.16
US, Los Angeles: Chinese	4.49	0.36	1.96	0.23
US, Los Angeles: Filipino	5.88	0.49	1.59	0.21
US, Los Angeles: Korean	4.43	0.53	1.47	0.26
US, Los Angeles: Japanese	3.87	0.37	1.49	0.21
US, San Francisco: Non-Hisp. White	7.42	0.13	5.27	0.10
US, San Francisco: Hispanic White	4.69	0.34	2.98	0.22
US, San Francisco: Black	12.93	0.47	5.69	0.27
US, San Francisco: Chinese	4.93	0.32	2.66	0.23
US, San Francisco: Filipino	5.95	0.55	2.05	0.27
US, San Francisco: Japanese	4.25	0.70	1.78	0.36
US, Connecticut: White	7.81	0.12	4.57	0.08
US, Connecticut: Black	11.15	0.62	4.36	0.33
US, Atlanta: White	9.42	0.22	4.71	0.14
US, Atlanta: Black	12.67	0.51	3.90	0.22
US, Iowa	8.50	0.13	3.75	0.08

	MALE		FEMALE	
US, Central Louisiana: White	9.90	0.49	3.45	0.26
US, Central Louisiana: Black	14.29	1.27	3.69	0.55
US, New Orleans: White	10.61	0.30	5.39	0.19
US, New Orleans: Black	14.28	0.57	4.52	0.26
US, Detroit: White	9.48	0.13	5.14	0.09
US, Detroit: Black	13.42	0.32	5.46	0.18
US, New Mexico: Non-Hisp. White	6.80	0.21	3.85	0.14
US, New Mexico: Hispanic White	3.40	0.23	1.64	0.14
US, New Mexico: American Indian	1.09	0.30	0.43	0.17
US, Utah	3.88	0.13	1.71	0.08
US, Seattle	8.11	0.12	4.93	0.09
US, SEER: White	7.84	0.05	4.41	0.03
US, SEER: Black	12.83	0.21	5.01	0.11
ASIA				
*China, Qidong	4.54	0.16	1.43	0.08
China, Shanghai	7.40	0.08	2.35	0.04
China, Tianjin	7.32	0.11	4.91	0.09
Hong Kong	9.28	0.10	3.61	0.06
*India, Bangalore	1.10	0.06	0.20	0.02
*India, Barshi, Paranda and Bhum	0.16	0.05	0.03	0.02
India, Bombay	1.88	0.06	0.46	0.03
*India, Karunagappally	2.10	0.31	0.36	0.12
India, Madras	1.59	0.07	0.28	0.03
*India, Trivandrum	1.53	0.22	0.25	0.08
Israel: All Jews	3.37	0.08	1.12	0.04
Jews born in Israel	2.71	0.25	1.20	0.16
Jews born in America or Europe	3.31	0.10	1.33	0.06
Jews born in Africa or Asia	3.53	0.14	0.63	0.05
Non-Jews	3.50	0.27	0.43	0.08
Japan, Hiroshima	4.66	0.18	1.39	0.08
Japan, Miyagi	4.88	0.11	1.25	0.05
Japan, Nagasaki	5.23	0.13	1.37	0.06
Japan, Osaka	5.06	0.07	1.42	0.03
*Japan, Saga	4.73	0.17	1.17	0.07
Japan, Yamagata	4.39	0.12	0.94	0.05
*Korea, Kangwha	4.43	0.49	1.08	0.22
*Kuwait: Non-Kuwaitis	3.99	0.64	1.65	0.36
*Kuwait: Kuwaitis	2.25	0.28	1.14	0.24
*Philippines, Manila	7.46	0.18	2.02	0.08
Singapore: Chinese	7.93	0.19	2.35	0.09
Singapore: Malay	4.46	0.35	1.18	0.19
Singapore: Indian	1.67	0.21	0.62	0.25
Thailand, Chiang Mai	4.64	0.16	4.00	0.15
*Thailand, Khon Kaen	2.01	0.14	0.64	0.07
*Viet Nam, Hanoi				

* IMPORTANT-SEE NOTES ON POPULATION PAGE

CUMULATIVE INCIDENCE (0-74)
RATES AND STANDARD ERRORS (percent)
Bronchus, lung (ICD-9 162) (contd)

EUROPE	MALE		FEMALE	
Austria, Tyrol	6.76	0.27	1.38	0.10
*Belarus	8.85	0.08	0.79	0.02
*Croatia	9.22	0.12	1.16	0.04
Czech Republic	9.92	0.07	1.23	0.02
Denmark	6.91	0.08	3.29	0.05
Estonia	10.08	0.21	1.11	0.05
Finland	7.14	0.08	1.02	0.03
France, Bas-Rhin	8.66	0.24	0.88	0.06
*France, Calvados	7.16	0.26	0.55	0.06
France, Doubs	6.63	0.29	0.78	0.09
France, Haut-Rhin	7.60	0.27	0.88	0.08
*France, Herault	5.39	0.18	0.67	0.06
France, Isere	6.59	0.20	0.70	0.06
*France, Somme	7.06	0.26	0.59	0.07
*France, Tarn	5.16	0.26	0.35	0.06
Germany, Eastern States	7.69	0.09	0.99	0.02
Germany, Saarland	9.00	0.21	1.20	0.06
Iceland	4.45	0.33	3.18	0.26
Ireland, Southern	5.47	0.24	1.88	0.13
Italy, Ferrara	11.02	0.53	1.78	0.19
Italy, Florence	8.06	0.19	1.33	0.07
Italy, Genoa	9.27	0.23	1.28	0.07
*Italy, Latina	8.52	0.36	1.10	0.12
Italy, Macerata	6.56	0.48	0.87	0.16
Italy, Modena	8.85	0.24	1.13	0.08
Italy, Parma	8.15	0.28	1.54	0.11
Italy, Ragusa	4.98	0.28	0.55	0.09
Italy, Romagna	8.66	0.27	1.15	0.09
Italy, Torino	8.41	0.22	1.29	0.08
Italy, Trieste	10.21	0.43	1.90	0.16
Italy, Varese	10.14	0.26	0.97	0.07
Italy, Veneto	10.91	0.22	1.77	0.08
*Latvia	8.50	0.14	0.91	0.04
Malta	5.78	0.48	0.36	0.11
The Netherlands	9.58	0.07	1.62	0.02
The Netherlands, Eindhoven	10.63	0.27	1.45	0.08
The Netherlands, Maastricht	10.44	0.26	1.55	0.08
Norway	4.51	0.07	1.62	0.04
*Poland, Cracow	9.63	0.29	1.99	0.11
*Poland, Kielce	8.87	0.21	0.85	0.06
*Poland, Lower Silesia	12.33	0.17	2.02	0.06
Poland, Warsaw City	8.83	0.20	2.56	0.09
Slovakia	10.21	0.11	1.10	0.03
Slovenia	8.55	0.17	1.14	0.05
*Spain, Albacete	4.28	0.38	0.36	0.10
Spain, Asturias	7.99	0.20	0.46	0.04
Spain, Basque Country	6.68	0.14	0.38	0.03
Spain, Granada	5.74	0.19	0.33	0.04
Spain, Mallorca	7.74	0.25	0.51	0.06
Spain, Murcia	6.11	0.18	0.46	0.05
Spain, Navarra	5.35	0.22	0.45	0.06
Spain, Tarragona	5.69	0.22	0.36	0.05
Spain, Zaragoza	6.01	0.18	0.31	0.04

	MALE		FEMALE	
Sweden	3.13	0.04	1.38	0.02
*Switzerland, Basel	6.36	0.26	1.42	0.11
Switzerland, Geneva	6.80	0.32	1.70	0.14
Switzerland, Graubunden	6.39	0.48	1.09	0.18
Switzerland, Neuchatel	7.90	0.48	1.47	0.19
Switzerland, St Gall-Appenzell	6.27	0.26	1.02	0.09
Switzerland, Valais	6.54	0.42	1.30	0.17
Switzerland, Vaud	7.90	0.26	1.46	0.10
Switzerland, Zurich	6.10	0.17	1.29	0.07
*UK, England and Wales	7.78	0.04	2.98	0.02
*UK, East Anglia	5.93	0.11	2.21	0.06
*UK, Mersey	8.30	0.12	4.04	0.08
*UK, North Western	8.90	0.10	3.70	0.06
UK, Oxford	6.70	0.12	2.51	0.07
*UK, South Thames	6.81	0.07	2.76	0.04
UK, South Western	5.79	0.09	2.19	0.05
UK, Wessex	6.16	0.10	2.31	0.05
*UK, West Midlands	8.42	0.09	2.84	0.05
UK, Yorkshire	8.08	0.10	3.28	0.06
UK, Scotland	10.07	0.10	4.47	0.06
UK, Scotland, West	11.10	0.14	5.07	0.08
*Yugoslavia, Vojvodina	9.11	0.15	1.28	0.05

OCEANIA

	MALE		FEMALE	
Australian Capital Territory	4.67	0.41	1.65	0.22
Australia, New South Wales	5.95	0.08	1.89	0.04
South Australia	6.07	0.15	1.95	0.08
Australia, Tasmania	6.45	0.28	2.39	0.16
Australia, Victoria	5.81	0.09	2.07	0.05
Western Australia	6.10	0.16	2.26	0.09
*French Polynesia	9.36	0.82	3.47	0.51
New Zealand: Non-Maori	5.68	0.10	2.35	0.06
New Zealand: Maori	13.67	0.89	8.92	0.60
US, Hawaii: White	7.73	0.39	4.97	0.32
US, Hawaii: Japanese	4.48	0.25	1.43	0.13
US, Hawaii: Hawaiian	9.73	0.68	4.83	0.45
US, Hawaii: Filipino	5.25	0.43	2.08	0.26
US, Hawaii: Chinese	4.55	0.54	2.36	0.37

* IMPORTANT-SEE NOTES ON POPULATION PAGE

CUMULATIVE INCIDENCE (0-74)
RATES AND STANDARD ERRORS (percent)
Other thoracic organs (ICD-9 163-4)

	MALE		FEMALE	
AFRICA				
*Algeria, Setif				
*France, La Reunion				
*Mali, Bamako				
*Uganda, Kyadondo				
*Zimbabwe, Harare: African				
*Zimbabwe, Harare: European				
AMERICA, CENTRAL AND SOUTH				
*Argentina, Concordia	0,20	0,09	0,34	0,13
*Brazil, Belem	0,12	0,05	0,03	0,03 mf
*Brazil, Goiania				
*Brazil, Porto Alegre	0.17	0.05	0.08	0.02
Colombia, Cali	0.07	0.02	0.05	0.02
*Costa Rica	0.03	0.01	0,02	0,01
*Ecuador, Quito	-	-	-	-
*Peru, Lima	0.06	0.02	0,03	0,01
Peru, Trujillo	0,01	0,01	0,06	0,06
US, Puerto Rico	0.04	0.01	0,01	0,00
*Uruguay, Montevideo	0.11	0.03	0,03	0,01
AMERICA, NORTH				
Canada	0.07	0.00	0.04	0.00
Canada, Alberta	0.03	0.01	0.02	0.01
Canada, British Columbia	0.04	0.01	0.04	0.01
Canada, Manitoba	0.05	0.01	0.03	0.01
Canada, New Brunswick	0,04	0,02	0,04	0,02
Canada, Newfoundland	0,03	0,02	-	-
Canada, Northwest Territories	0,02	0,02	-	-
Canada, Nova Scotia	0.07	0.02	0,02	0,01
Canada, Ontario	0.07	0.01	0.04	0.00
Canada, Prince Edward Island	0,12	0,06	0,08	0,05
Canada, Quebec	0.09	0.01	0.05	0.01
Canada, Saskatchewan	0,04	0,01	0.04	0.01
Canada, Yukon	-	-	-	-
US, Cent. Calif.: Non-Hisp. White	0.03	0.01	0.02	0,01
US, Cent. Calif.: Hispanic	0.03	0.02	0,04	0,03
US, Los Angeles: Non-Hisp. White	0.05	0.01	0.02	0.00
US, Los Angeles: Hispanic White	0.03	0.01	0.02	0.01
US, Los Angeles: Black	0.04	0.01	0.02	0,01
US, Los Angeles: Chinese	0,10	0,05	-	-
US, Los Angeles: Filipino	0,01	0,01	-	-
US, Los Angeles: Korean	-	-	-	-
US, Los Angeles: Japanese	0,02	0,02	-	-
US, San Francisco: Non-Hisp. White	0.03	0.01	0,01	0,00
US, San Francisco: Hispanic White	0.03	0.01	0.02	0.02
US, San Francisco: Black	0,04	0,02	0,03	0,02
US, San Francisco: Chinese	0,09	0,04	0,02	0,02
US, San Francisco: Filipino	0,07	0,04	-	-
US, San Francisco: Japanese	-	-	-	-
US, Connecticut: White	0.05	0.01	0.03	0.01
US, Connecticut: Black	0,04	0,02	0,05	0,03
US, Atlanta: White	0.04	0.01	0.03	0.01
US, Atlanta: Black	0.08	0.03	0,04	0,02
US, Iowa	0.03	0.01	0.02	0.00

	MALE		FEMALE	
US, Central Louisiana: White	0,06	0,04	0,05	0,03
US, Central Louisiana: Black	-	-	0,09	0,09
US, New Orleans: White	0.07	0.02	0,05	0,02
US, New Orleans: Black	0,03	0,01	0,04	0,03
US, Detroit: White	0.02	0.01	0.02	0.01
US, Detroit: Black	0,03	0,01	0,02	0,01
US, New Mexico: Non-Hisp. White	0.05	0.02	0,03	0,01
US, New Mexico: Hispanic White	0.09	0.03	0,04	0,02
US, New Mexico: American Indian	-	-	-	-
US, Utah	0.05	0.01	0.03	0.01
US, Seattle	0.04	0.01	0.03	0.01
US, SEER: White	0.04	0.00	0.02	0.00
US, SEER: Black	0.04	0.01	0.03	0.01
ASIA				
†*China, Qidong	0.08	0.02	0.04	0.01
† China, Shanghai	0.14	0.01	0.07	0.01
China, Tianjin	0.10	0.01	0.06	0.01
Hong Kong	0.03	0.00	0.02	0.00
*India, Bangalore	0.06	0.01	0.04	0.01
*India, Barshi, Paranda and Bhum	-	-	-	-
India, Bombay	0.04	0.01	0.04	0.01
*India, Karunagappally	-	-	-	-
India, Madras	0.01	0.00	0,01	0,00
*India, Trivandrum	0,01	0,01	0,01	0,01
Israel: All Jews	0.05	0.01	0.03	0.01
Jews born in Israel	0.07	0.03	0.03	0.01
Jews born in America or Europe	0.05	0.01	0.03	0.01
Jews born in Africa or Asia	0,02	0,01	0,03	0,01
Non-Jews	0,03	0,03	0,01	0,01
Japan, Hiroshima	0.09	0.02	0.06	0.02
Japan, Miyagi	0.07	0.01	0.04	0.01
Japan, Nagasaki	0.06	0.01	0.03	0.01
Japan, Osaka	0.07	0.01	0.04	0.00
†*Japan, Saga	0.06	0.02	0.06	0.01
Japan, Yamagata	0.07	0.01	0.01	0,00
*Korea, Kangwha	-	-	0,11	0,07
*Kuwait: Non-Kuwaitis	0,02	0,01	0,09	0,07
*Kuwait: Kuwaitis	0,07	0,05	0,03	0,03
*Philippines, Manila	0.04	0.01	0.02	0.01
Singapore: Chinese	0.07	0.01	0.05	0.01
Singapore: Malay	0,07	0,03	0,05	0,02
Singapore: Indian	-	-	0,01	0,01
Thailand, Chiang Mai	0,01	0,01	0,01	0,00
*Thailand, Khon Kaen	0,03	0,01	0,01	0,01
*Viet Nam, Hanoi				

* IMPORTANT-SEE NOTES ON POPULATION PAGE

CUMULATIVE INCIDENCE (0-74)
RATES AND STANDARD ERRORS (percent)
Other thoracic organs (ICD-9 163-4) (contd)

EUROPE	MALE		FEMALE	
Austria, Tyrol	0,05	0,02	0,06	0,02
*Belarus	0.10	0.01	0.04	0.00
*Croatia	0.08	0.01	0.04	0.01
Czech Republic	0.12	0.01	0.05	0.00
Denmark	0.07	0.01	0.03	0.00
Estonia	0.07	0.02	0.04	0.01
Finland	0.05	0.01	0.02	0.00
France, Bas-Rhin	0.13	0.03	0,03	0,01
*France, Calvados	0.11	0.03	0,04	0,02
France, Doubs	0,05	0,02	0,02	0,02
France, Haut-Rhin	0.06	0.02	0,04	0,02
*France, Herault	0.06	0.02	0,01	0,01
France, Isere	0.06	0.02	0,04	0,01
*France, Somme	0.09	0.03	0,03	0,02
*France, Tarn	0,04	0,02	-	-
Germany, Eastern States	0.08	0.01	0.04	0.00
† Germany, Saarland	0.11	0.02	0.07	0.02
Iceland	0,11	0,05	0,04	0,03
Ireland, Southern	0,03	0,01	0,01	0,01
Italy, Ferrara	0,06	0,04	0,08	0,04
Italy, Florence	0,06	0,02	0,04	0,01
Italy, Genoa	0.21	0.04	0.05	0.02
*Italy, Latina	0,06	0,03	-	-
Italy, Macerata	0,11	0,06	0,03	0,03
Italy, Modena	0.12	0.03	0,04	0,02
Italy, Parma	0,02	0,02	0,01	0,01
Italy, Ragusa	0,08	0,03	0,04	0,02
Italy, Romagna	0,03	0,01	0,05	0,02
Italy, Torino	0.13	0.03	0.07	0.02
Italy, Trieste	0.28	0.06	0,10	0,04
Italy, Varese	0,02	0,01	0,02	0,01
Italy, Veneto	0.16	0.03	0,02	0,01
†*Latvia	0.14	0.02	0.06	0.01
† Malta	0,11	0,07	-	-
The Netherlands	0.05	0.00	0.02	0.00
The Netherlands, Eindhoven	0,03	0,01	0,02	0,01
The Netherlands, Maastricht	0.06	0.02	0,01	0,01
Norway	0.03	0.01	0.02	0.00
*Poland, Cracow	0.12	0.03	0,03	0,01
*Poland, Kielce	0.09	0.02	0.05	0.01
*Poland, Lower Silesia	0.30	0.03	0.13	0.01
Poland, Warsaw City	0.17	0.03	0.10	0.02
Slovakia	0.12	0.01	0.07	0.01
Slovenia	0.03	0.01	0,01	0,00
*Spain, Albacete	0,05	0,04	-	-
Spain, Asturias	0.11	0.02	0.06	0.01
Spain, Basque Country	0.05	0.01	0.03	0.01
Spain, Granada	0.05	0.02	0,03	0,01
Spain, Mallorca	0,05	0,02	0,03	0,01
Spain, Murcia	0,03	0,01	-	-
Spain, Navarra	0,04	0,02	0,03	0,02
Spain, Tarragona	0.08	0.02	0,06	0,02
Spain, Zaragoza	0,04	0,01	0.04	0.01

	MALE		FEMALE		
Sweden	0.02	0.00	0.01	0.00	
*Switzerland, Basel	0,04	0,02	0,01	0,01	
Switzerland, Geneva	0,01	0,01	0,04	0,02	
Switzerland, Graubunden	0,02	0,02	-	-	
Switzerland, Neuchatel	0,11	0,05	0,02	0,02	
Switzerland, St Gall-Appenzell	0.11	0.03	0,04	0,02	
Switzerland, Valais	0,14	0,06	0,06	0,03	
Switzerland, Vaud	0,05	0,02	0,01	0,01	
Switzerland, Zurich	0.08	0.02	0,02	0,01	
*UK, England and Wales	0.06	0.00	0.03	0.00	
*UK, East Anglia	0.03	0.01	0.01	0.01	
*UK, Mersey	0.05	0.01	0.03	0.01	
*UK, North Western	0.05	0.01	0.03	0.01	
UK, Oxford	0.03	0.01	0.03	0.01	
*UK, South Thames	0.08	0.01	0.04	0.00	
UK, South Western	0.07	0.01	0.02	0.00	
UK, Wessex	0.08	0.01	0.04	0.01	
†*UK, West Midlands	0.19	0.01	0.05	0.01	
UK, Yorkshire	0.05	0.01	0.03	0.01	
UK, Scotland	0.04	0.01	0.02	0.00	
UK, Scotland, West	0.02	0.01	0.01	0.00	
*Yugoslavia, Vojvodina	0.21	0.03	0.08	0.01	

OCEANIA

	MALE		FEMALE		
Australian Capital Territory	0,09	0,05	0,02	0,02	
Australia, New South Wales	0.05	0.01	0.02	0.00	
South Australia	0.02	0.01	0.02	0,01	
Australia, Tasmania	0,05	0,02	0,01	0,01	
Australia, Victoria	0.05	0.01	0.03	0.01	
Western Australia	0.05	0.01	0.01	0,00	
*French Polynesia	0,18	0,09	0,26	0,17	f
† New Zealand: Non-Maori	0.19	0.02	0.05	0,01	
† New Zealand: Maori	0,10	0,06	0,07	0,07	
US, Hawaii: White	0,02	0,02	0,02	0,02	
US, Hawaii: Japanese	0,03	0,02	0,05	0,02	
US, Hawaii: Hawaiian	0,06	0,05	0,02	0,01	
US, Hawaii: Filipino	0,04	0,03	0,06	0,04	
US, Hawaii: Chinese	0,10	0,07	-	-	

* IMPORTANT-SEE NOTES ON POPULATION PAGE

CUMULATIVE INCIDENCE (0-74)
RATES AND STANDARD ERRORS (percent)
Kaposi's sarcoma

	MALE		FEMALE	
AFRICA				
*Algeria, Setif				
*France, La Reunion				
*Mali, Bamako				
*Uganda, Kyadondo				
*Zimbabwe, Harare: African				
*Zimbabwe, Harare: European				
AMERICA, CENTRAL AND SOUTH				
*Argentina, Concordia	0,02	0,02	-	-
*Brazil, Belem	0,02	0,02	-	-
*Brazil, Goiania				
*Brazil, Porto Alegre	0.13	0.03	0,00	0,00
Colombia, Cali	0,02	0,01	0,01	0,01
*Costa Rica	0.04	0.01	0,01	0,00
*Ecuador, Quito	0,01	0,01	0,02	0,02
*Peru, Lima	0.06	0.02	0,01	0,00
Peru, Trujillo	0,07	0,07	-	-
US, Puerto Rico	0.29	0.02	0.02	0.01
*Uruguay, Montevideo	0,02	0,01	0,00	0,00
AMERICA, NORTH				
† Canada	0.02	0.00	0,00	0,00
† Canada, Alberta	-	-	-	-
† Canada, British Columbia	0,00	0,00	-	-
† Canada, Manitoba	0,00	0,00	-	-
† Canada, New Brunswick	-	-	-	-
† Canada, Newfoundland	-	-	-	-
† Canada, Northwest Territories	-	-	-	-
† Canada, Nova Scotia	-	-	-	-
† Canada, Ontario	0.04	0.00	0,00	0,00
† Canada, Prince Edward Island	-	-	-	-
† Canada, Quebec	0.02	0.00	0,00	0,00
† Canada, Saskatchewan	0,01	0,01	0,00	0,00
† Canada, Yukon	-	-	-	-
US, Cent. Calif.: Non-Hisp. White	0.13	0.02	0,00	0,00
US, Cent. Calif.: Hispanic	0.11	0.03	0,00	0,00
US, Los Angeles: Non-Hisp. White	1.22	0.03	0.01	0.00
US, Los Angeles: Hispanic White	0.69	0.03	0.02	0.01
US, Los Angeles: Black	0.73	0.05	0,01	0,00
US, Los Angeles: Chinese	0,07	0,03	-	-
US, Los Angeles: Filipino	0.20	0.05	-	-
US, Los Angeles: Korean	0,11	0,09	-	-
US, Los Angeles: Japanese	0.26	0.07	-	-
US, San Francisco: Non-Hisp. White	2.83	0.06	0,01	0,00
US, San Francisco: Hispanic White	1.65	0.11	0,00	0,00
US, San Francisco: Black	1.82	0.12	0,00	0,00
US, San Francisco: Chinese	0.15	0.04	-	-
US, San Francisco: Filipino	0.38	0.08	-	-
US, San Francisco: Japanese	0,44	0,18	-	-
US, Connecticut: White	0.21	0.02	0,01	0,00
US, Connecticut: Black	0.34	0.07	0,03	0,02
US, Atlanta: White	0.77	0.04	0,01	0,00
US, Atlanta: Black	0.34	0.04	0,01	0,00
US, Iowa	0.04	0.01	-	-

	MALE		FEMALE	
US, Central Louisiana: White	0,09	0,04	-	-
US, Central Louisiana: Black	0,02	0,02	0,07	0,07
US, New Orleans: White	0.80	0.06	0,01	0,01
US, New Orleans: Black	0.24	0.05	0,01	0,01
US, Detroit: White	0.18	0.01	0,01	0,00
US, Detroit: Black	0.26	0.03	0,03	0,01
US, New Mexico: Non-Hisp. White	0.23	0.03	-	-
US, New Mexico: Hispanic White	0.22	0.04	0,02	0,02
US, New Mexico: American Indian	0,04	0,03	-	-
US, Utah	0.08	0.01	0,00	0,00
US, Seattle	0.39	0.02	0,00	0,00
US, SEER: White	0.64	0.01	0.00	0.00
US, SEER: Black	0.58	0.03	0.02	0.01
ASIA				
*China, Qidong				
China, Shanghai				
China, Tianjin	-	-	-	-
Hong Kong	0,00	0,00	-	-
*India, Bangalore	-	-	-	-
*India, Barshi, Paranda and Bhum	-	-	-	-
India, Bombay	-	-	0,00	0,00
*India, Karunagappally	-	-	-	-
India, Madras	-	-	-	-
*India, Trivandrum	-	-	-	-
Israel: All Jews	0.28	0.02	0.08	0.01
Jews born in Israel	0.22	0.07	0.00	0.00
Jews born in America or Europe	0.19	0.02	0.10	0.02
Jews born in Africa or Asia	0.44	0.05	0.11	0.02
Non-Jews	0,09	0,04	0,06	0,04
Japan, Hiroshima	-	-	-	-
Japan, Miyagi	-	-	-	-
Japan, Nagasaki	-	-	-	-
Japan, Osaka	0,00	0,00	-	-
*Japan, Saga				
Japan, Yamagata	-	-	-	-
*Korea, Kangwha	0,03	0,03	-	-
*Kuwait: Non-Kuwaitis	0,01	0,01	0,01	0,01
*Kuwait: Kuwaitis	0,04	0,03	0,01	0,01
*Philippines, Manila	0,01	0,00	-	-
Singapore: Chinese	0,01	0,01	-	-
Singapore: Malay	-	-	-	-
Singapore: Indian	0,02	0,01	-	-
Thailand, Chiang Mai	0,00	0,00	-	-
*Thailand, Khon Kaen	-	-	-	-
*Viet Nam, Hanoi				

CUMULATIVE INCIDENCE (0-74)
RATES AND STANDARD ERRORS (percent)
Kaposi's sarcoma (contd)

EUROPE

	MALE		FEMALE	
Austria, Tyrol	-	-	-	-
*Belarus	0.01	0.00	0.01	0.00
*Croatia	0,00	0,00	-	-
Czech Republic	0.01	0.00	0.00	0.00
Denmark	0.07	0.01	0,00	0,00
Estonia	0,00	0,00	0,00	0,00
Finland	0.03	0.01	0,00	0,00
France, Bas-Rhin	0.18	0.03	0,01	0,01
*France, Calvados	0,04	0,01	0,02	0,01
France, Doubs	0.06	0.02	-	-
France, Haut-Rhin	0.08	0.03	0,00	0,00
*France, Herault	0.20	0.03	0,02	0,01
France, Isere	0.08	0.02	0,01	0,01
*France, Somme	0,05	0,02	0,00	0,00
*France, Tarn	0,01	0,01	0,01	0,01
Germany, Eastern States	0,00	0,00	0,00	0,00
Germany, Saarland				
Iceland	0.19	0.06	0,03	0,03
Ireland, Southern	0,01	0,01	-	-
Italy, Ferrara	0.26	0.08	0,02	0,02
Italy, Florence	0.12	0.02	0,02	0,01
Italy, Genoa	0.20	0.03	0,02	0,01
*Italy, Latina	0,12	0,04	0,04	0,02
Italy, Macerata	0,13	0,07	0,03	0,03
Italy, Modena	0.12	0.03	0,02	0,01
Italy, Parma	0,05	0,02	-	-
Italy, Ragusa	0,16	0,06	0,03	0,02
Italy, Romagna	0.10	0.02	0,03	0,01
Italy, Torino	0.13	0.03	0,03	0,01
Italy, Trieste	0,03	0,02	0,01	0,01
Italy, Varese	0.16	0.03	0,01	0,01
Italy, Veneto	0.08	0.02	0,03	0,01
*Latvia				
Malta				
The Netherlands	0.10	0.01	0,00	0,00
The Netherlands, Eindhoven	0,02	0,01	0,00	0,00
The Netherlands, Maastricht	0,01	0,01	-	-
Norway	0.04	0.01	0.01	0.00
*Poland, Cracow	0,02	0,02	-	-
*Poland, Kielce	0,00	0,00	-	-
*Poland, Lower Silesia	0,00	0,00	0,00	0,00
Poland, Warsaw City	-	-	-	-
Slovakia	0.01	0.00	-	-
Slovenia	-	-	-	-
*Spain, Albacete	0,14	0,07	0,03	0,03
Spain, Asturias	0,00	0,00	-	-
Spain, Basque Country	0.07	0.01	0,01	0,00
Spain, Granada	0.05	0.02	0,00	0,00
Spain, Mallorca	0.23	0.04	0,02	0,01
Spain, Murcia	0.09	0.02	0,00	0,00
Spain, Navarra	0.04	0.02	0,01	0,01
Spain, Tarragona	0.08	0.02	-	-
Spain, Zaragoza	0,01	0,00	-	-

	MALE		FEMALE	
Sweden	0.05	0.00	0.01	0.00
*Switzerland, Basel	0.07	0.02	0,01	0,01
Switzerland, Geneva	0.47	0.06	0,01	0,01
Switzerland, Graubunden	0,02	0,02	-	-
Switzerland, Neuchatel	0,14	0,05	-	-
Switzerland, St Gall-Appenzell	0.07	0.02	-	-
Switzerland, Valais	0,03	0,02	0,01	0,01
Switzerland, Vaud	0.24	0.03	0,03	0,01
Switzerland, Zurich	0.33	0.03	0,01	0,00
*UK, England and Wales	0.03	0.00	0.00	0.00
*UK, East Anglia	0.01	0.00	0.00	0.00
*UK, Mersey	0.01	0.00	-	-
*UK, North Western	0.02	0.00	0.00	0.00
UK, Oxford	0.01	0.00	0.00	0.00
*UK, South Thames	0.09	0.01	0.00	0.00
UK, South Western	0.02	0.00	-	-
UK, Wessex	0.01	0.00	-	-
*UK, West Midlands				
UK, Yorkshire	0.01	0.00	0.00	0.00
UK, Scotland	0.02	0.00	0.00	0.00
UK, Scotland, West	0.01	0.00	0.00	0.00
*Yugoslavia, Vojvodina	-	-	-	-

OCEANIA

	MALE		FEMALE	
† Australian Capital Territory	0,05	0,03	-	-
† Australia, New South Wales	0.21	0.01	0.00	0.00
† South Australia	0.06	0.01	0.00	0.00
† Australia, Tasmania	0.01	0.01	-	-
† Australia, Victoria	0.14	0.01	0.01	0.00
† Western Australia	0.05	0.01	0.00	0.00
†*French Polynesia	-	-	-	-
New Zealand: Non-Maori				
New Zealand: Maori				
US, Hawaii: White	0.65	0.08	0,01	0,01
US, Hawaii: Japanese	0,06	0,02	-	-
US, Hawaii: Hawaiian	0.16	0.05	-	-
US, Hawaii: Filipino	0,13	0,05	-	-
US, Hawaii: Chinese	0,24	0,11	-	-

* IMPORTANT-SEE NOTES ON POPULATION PAGE

CUMULATIVE INCIDENCE (0-74)
RATES AND STANDARD ERRORS (percent)
Mesothelioma

	MALE		FEMALE	
AFRICA				
*Algeria, Setif				
*France, La Reunion				
*Mali, Bamako				
*Uganda, Kyadondo				
*Zimbabwe, Harare: African				
*Zimbabwe, Harare: European				
AMERICA, CENTRAL AND SOUTH				
*Argentina, Concordia	-	-	0,13	0,09
*Brazil, Belem	-	-	-	-
*Brazil, Goiania				
*Brazil, Porto Alegre	-	-	-	-
Colombia, Cali	0,01	0,01	0,00	0,00
*Costa Rica	0,01	0,01	0,01	0,01
*Ecuador, Quito	-	-	-	-
*Peru, Lima	0.03	0.01	0,00	0,00
Peru, Trujillo	-	-	-	-
US, Puerto Rico	0.03	0.01	0,02	0,01
*Uruguay, Montevideo	0.06	0.02	0,03	0,01
AMERICA, NORTH				
Canada	0.14	0.01	0.03	0.00
Canada, Alberta	0.16	0.02	0.03	0.01
Canada, British Columbia	0.14	0.01	0.03	0.01
Canada, Manitoba	0.20	0.03	0,03	0,01
Canada, New Brunswick	0.07	0.02	0,01	0,01
Canada, Newfoundland	0.10	0.03	0,01	0,01
Canada, Northwest Territories	-	-	-	-
Canada, Nova Scotia	0.16	0.03	0,02	0,01
Canada, Ontario	0.12	0.01	0.03	0.00
Canada, Prince Edward Island	0,08	0,06	-	-
Canada, Quebec	0.18	0.01	0.04	0,01
Canada, Saskatchewan	0.07	0.02	0,02	0,01
Canada, Yukon	-	-	-	-
US, Cent. Calif.: Non-Hisp. White	0.17	0.02	0.05	0.01
US, Cent. Calif.: Hispanic	0.18	0.06	0,05	0,03
US, Los Angeles: Non-Hisp. White	0.14	0.01	0.04	0.01
US, Los Angeles: Hispanic White	0.15	0.03	0.02	0.01
US, Los Angeles: Black	0.07	0.02	0,02	0,01
US, Los Angeles: Chinese	-	-	-	-
US, Los Angeles: Filipino	0,01	0,01	0,03	0,03
US, Los Angeles: Korean	-	-	-	-
US, Los Angeles: Japanese	0,04	0,04	0,02	0,02
US, San Francisco: Non-Hisp. White	0.23	0.02	0.03	0.01
US, San Francisco: Hispanic White	0.30	0.09	0,07	0,03
US, San Francisco: Black	0.17	0.05	0,03	0,02
US, San Francisco: Chinese	0,09	0,05	-	-
US, San Francisco: Filipino	0,04	0,04	0,05	0,05
US, San Francisco: Japanese	-	-	-	-
US, Connecticut: White	0.12	0.01	0.04	0.01
US, Connecticut: Black	0,07	0,04	-	-
US, Atlanta: White	0.11	0.02	0,02	0,01
US, Atlanta: Black	0,06	0,03	0,01	0,01
US, Iowa	0.13	0.02	0.02	0.01

	MALE		FEMALE	
US, Central Louisiana: White	0,09	0,04	-	-
US, Central Louisiana: Black	-	-	-	-
US, New Orleans: White	0.32	0.05	0.07	0.02
US, New Orleans: Black	0.25	0.07	0,05	0,03
US, Detroit: White	0.15	0.02	0.03	0.01
US, Detroit: Black	0.07	0.02	0,03	0,01
US, New Mexico: Non-Hisp. White	0.20	0.04	0,04	0,01
US, New Mexico: Hispanic White	0.25	0.07	0,03	0,02
US, New Mexico: American Indian	0,12	0,12	0,08	0,08
US, Utah	0.12	0.02	0.03	0.01
US, Seattle	0.25	0.02	0.04	0.01
US, SEER: White	0.17	0.01	0.03	0.00
US, SEER: Black	0.09	0.02	0.02	0.01
ASIA				
*China, Qidong				
China, Shanghai				
China, Tianjin	0.02	0.01	0.02	0.01
Hong Kong	0,01	0,00	0,01	0,00
*India, Bangalore	0,02	0,01	0,00	0,00
*India, Barshi, Paranda and Bhum	-	-	-	-
India, Bombay	0.01	0.00	0,00	0,00
*India, Karunagappally	-	-	-	-
India, Madras	0,00	0,00	0,01	0,01
*India, Trivandrum	-	-	0,00	0,00
Israel: All Jews	0.05	0.01	0.02	0.01
Jews born in Israel	0,05	0,03	-	-
Jews born in America or Europe	0.07	0.02	0.03	0.01
Jews born in Africa or Asia	0,04	0,01	0,02	0,01
Non-Jews	0,03	0,03	0,02	0,01
Japan, Hiroshima	0.05	0.02	0,01	0,01
Japan, Miyagi	0.02	0.01	0,00	0,00
Japan, Nagasaki	0.05	0.01	0,01	0,00
Japan, Osaka	0.05	0.01	0.02	0.00
*Japan, Saga				
Japan, Yamagata	0,00	0,00	0,00	0,00
*Korea, Kangwha	-	-	-	-
*Kuwait: Non-Kuwaitis	0,02	0,01	0,01	0,00
*Kuwait: Kuwaitis	0,10	0,06	-	-
*Philippines, Manila	0,01	0,00	0,01	0,01
Singapore: Chinese	0,01	0,01	0,00	0,00
Singapore: Malay	-	-	-	-
Singapore: Indian	0,02	0,02	-	-
Thailand, Chiang Mai	0,00	0,00	-	-
*Thailand, Khon Kaen	0,00	0,00	-	-
*Viet Nam, Hanoi				

* IMPORTANT-SEE NOTES ON POPULATION PAGE

CUMULATIVE INCIDENCE (0-74)
RATES AND STANDARD ERRORS (percent)
Mesothelioma (contd)

EUROPE	MALE		FEMALE	
Austria, Tyrol	0,06	0,02	0,04	0,02
*Belarus	0.02	0.00	0.02	0.00
*Croatia	0.06	0.01	0.01	0.00
Czech Republic	0.05	0.01	0.03	0.00
Denmark	0.16	0.01	0.04	0.01
Estonia	0.05	0.01	0.03	0.01
Finland	0.13	0.01	0.05	0.01
France, Bas-Rhin	0.09	0.02	0.02	0.01
*France, Calvados	0.12	0.03	0.03	0.01
France, Doubs	0.20	0.05	0.04	0.02
France, Haut-Rhin	0,06	0,02	0,02	0,01
*France, Herault	0.08	0.02	0.03	0.01
France, Isere	0.18	0.03	0.02	0.01
*France, Somme	0.13	0.04	0.03	0.01
*France, Tarn	0,10	0,03	0,01	0,01
Germany, Eastern States	0.12	0.01	0.04	0.00
Germany, Saarland				
Iceland	0,09	0,04	-	-
Ireland, Southern	0,03	0,02	0,01	0,01
Italy, Ferrara	0,11	0,06	-	-
Italy, Florence	0.09	0.02	0.03	0.01
Italy, Genoa	0.65	0.06	0.10	0.02
*Italy, Latina	0,02	0,01	0,01	0,01
Italy, Macerata	0,18	0,08	0,04	0,04
Italy, Modena	0.07	0.02	0.04	0.01
Italy, Parma	0.09	0.03	0.02	0.01
Italy, Ragusa	0,05	0,03	-	-
Italy, Romagna	0.16	0.04	0.05	0.02
Italy, Torino	0.11	0.02	0.06	0.02
Italy, Trieste	0.75	0.11	0.06	0.03
Italy, Varese	0.20	0.04	0.03	0.01
Italy, Veneto	0.13	0.02	0.05	0.01
*Latvia				
Malta				
The Netherlands	0.33	0.01	0.04	0.00
The Netherlands, Eindhoven	0.18	0.03	0.04	0.01
The Netherlands, Maastricht	0.38	0.05	0.05	0.02
Norway	0.16	0.01	0.03	0.01
*Poland, Cracow	0,05	0,02	0,02	0,01
*Poland, Kielce	0,02	0,01	0,02	0,01
*Poland, Lower Silesia	0.03	0.01	0.01	0.00
Poland, Warsaw City	0.04	0.01	0.03	0.01
Slovakia	0.04	0.01	0.02	0.00
Slovenia	0.08	0.01	0.03	0.01
*Spain, Albacete	0,05	0,05	0,07	0,04
Spain, Asturias	0,04	0,01	0,03	0,01
Spain, Basque Country	0.07	0.02	0.03	0.01
Spain, Granada	0,05	0,02	0,02	0,01
Spain, Mallorca	0,04	0,02	0,04	0,02
Spain, Murcia	0.05	0.02	0.01	0.01
Spain, Navarra	0,07	0,02	0.10	0.03
Spain, Tarragona	0,02	0,01	0,01	0,01
Spain, Zaragoza	0.10	0.02	0,02	0,01

	MALE		FEMALE	
Sweden	0.14	0.01	0.02	0.00
*Switzerland, Basel	0.17	0.04	0,04	0,02
Switzerland, Geneva	0,10	0,04	0,08	0,03
Switzerland, Graubunden	0,25	0,09	-	-
Switzerland, Neuchatel	0,16	0,07	0,02	0,02
Switzerland, St Gall-Appenzell	0.25	0.05	-	-
Switzerland, Valais	0.23	0.08	0,04	0,03
Switzerland, Vaud	0.10	0.03	0,04	0,04
Switzerland, Zurich	0.19	0.03	0,02	0,01
*UK, England and Wales	0.24	0.01	0.04	0.00
*UK, East Anglia	0.23	0.02	0.04	0.01
*UK, Mersey	0.32	0.02	0.02	0.01
*UK, North Western	0.25	0.02	0.05	0.01
UK, Oxford	0.23	0.02	0.03	0.01
*UK, South Thames	0.25	0.01	0.05	0.01
UK, South Western	0.28	0.02	0.04	0.01
UK, Wessex	0.43	0.03	0.03	0.01
*UK, West Midlands				
UK, Yorkshire	0.25	0.02	0.06	0.01
UK, Scotland	0.40	0.02	0.05	0.01
UK, Scotland, West	0.55	0.03	0.05	0.01
*Yugoslavia, Vojvodina	0,01	0,00	0.02	0.01

OCEANIA	MALE		FEMALE	
Australian Capital Territory	0,08	0,05	-	-
Australia, New South Wales	0.31	0.02	0.04	0.01
South Australia	0.39	0.04	0.05	0.01
Australia, Tasmania	0.18	0.05	0.02	0.01
Australia, Victoria	0.23	0.02	0.04	0.01
Western Australia	0.49	0.04	0.05	0.01
*French Polynesia	0,01	0,01	-	-
New Zealand: Non-Maori				
New Zealand: Maori				
US, Hawaii: White	0.20	0.06	0,02	0,02
US, Hawaii: Japanese	0,04	0,02	-	-
US, Hawaii: Hawaiian	0,26	0,12	-	-
US, Hawaii: Filipino	0,17	0,08	-	-
US, Hawaii: Chinese	0,12	0,08	-	-

* IMPORTANT-SEE NOTES ON POPULATION PAGE

CUMULATIVE INCIDENCE (0-74)
RATES AND STANDARD ERRORS (percent)
Bone (ICD-9 170)

	MALE		FEMALE	
AFRICA				
*Algeria, Setif				
*France, La Reunion				
*Mali, Bamako				
*Uganda, Kyadondo				
*Zimbabwe, Harare: African				
*Zimbabwe, Harare: European				
AMERICA, CENTRAL AND SOUTH				
*Argentina, Concordia	0,10	0,04	0,22	0,10
*Brazil, Belem	0.28	0.07	0.14	0.04 f
*Brazil, Goiania				
*Brazil, Porto Alegre	0.33	0.06	0.17	0.03
Colombia, Cali	0.11	0.03	0.06	0.02
*Costa Rica	0.07	0.01	0.06	0.01
*Ecuador, Quito	0.08	0.02	0.07	0.02
*Peru, Lima	0.07	0.01	0.08	0.02
Peru, Trujillo	0,08	0,04	0,03	0,01 m
US, Puerto Rico	0.06	0.01	0.05	0.01
*Uruguay, Montevideo	0.08	0.02	0.06	0.02
AMERICA, NORTH				
Canada	0.10	0.00	0.07	0.00
Canada, Alberta	0.09	0.01	0.06	0.01
Canada, British Columbia	0.07	0.01	0.06	0.01
Canada, Manitoba	0.11	0.02	0.05	0.01
Canada, New Brunswick	0.06	0.02	0.04	0,01
Canada, Newfoundland	0.05	0.02	0.06	0,02
Canada, Northwest Territories	0,03	0,02	0,05	0,03
Canada, Nova Scotia	0.08	0.02	0.09	0.02
Canada, Ontario	0.10	0.01	0.07	0.01
Canada, Prince Edward Island	0,10	0,06	0,06	0,05
Canada, Quebec	0.12	0.01	0.09	0.01
Canada, Saskatchewan	0.06	0.02	0.06	0.01
Canada, Yukon	-	-	-	-
US, Cent. Calif.: Non-Hisp. White	0.10	0.02	0.08	0.01
US, Cent. Calif.: Hispanic	0.04	0.01	0.05	0.02
US, Los Angeles: Non-Hisp. White	0.09	0.01	0.07	0.01
US, Los Angeles: Hispanic White	0.06	0.01	0.07	0.01
US, Los Angeles: Black	0.09	0.02	0,02	0,01
US, Los Angeles: Chinese	0,02	0,01	0,02	0,01
US, Los Angeles: Filipino	0,03	0,02	0,05	0,02
US, Los Angeles: Korean	0,11	0,07	0,01	0,01
US, Los Angeles: Japanese	0,02	0,02	-	-
US, San Francisco: Non-Hisp. White	0.08	0.01	0.06	0.01
US, San Francisco: Hispanic White	0.07	0.03	0.04	0,02
US, San Francisco: Black	0,05	0,02	0.04	0,02
US, San Francisco: Chinese	0,05	0,03	0.03	0,02
US, San Francisco: Filipino	0,03	0,02	0.07	0,03
US, San Francisco: Japanese	0.10	0,10	-	-
US, Connecticut: White	0.08	0.01	0.06	0.01
US, Connecticut: Black	0,10	0,05	0,01	0,01
US, Atlanta: White	0.06	0.01	0.05	0.01
US, Atlanta: Black	0,06	0,02	0.07	0.02
US, Iowa	0.08	0.01	0.07	0.01

	MALE		FEMALE	
US, Central Louisiana: White	0,06	0,03	0,08	0,03
US, Central Louisiana: Black	-	-	0,03	0,03
US, New Orleans: White	0.08	0.02	0,03	0,01
US, New Orleans: Black	0,08	0,04	0,03	0,02
US, Detroit: White	0.09	0.01	0.05	0.01
US, Detroit: Black	0.04	0.01	0.06	0.02
US, New Mexico: Non-Hisp. White	0.08	0.02	0.06	0.02
US, New Mexico: Hispanic White	0.09	0.03	0.05	0.02
US, New Mexico: American Indian	0,02	0,02	0,09	0,08
US, Utah	0.10	0.01	0.06	0.01
US, Seattle	0.09	0.01	0.07	0.01
US, SEER: White	0.09	0.00	0.06	0.00
US, SEER: Black	0.05	0.01	0.06	0.01
ASIA				
*China, Qidong	0.19	0.03	0.12	0.02
China, Shanghai	0.19	0.01	0.13	0.01
China, Tianjin	0.24	0.02	0.21	0.02
Hong Kong	0.10	0.01	0.07	0.01
*India, Bangalore	0.08	0.01	0.08	0.01
*India, Barshi, Paranda and Bhum	0,03	0,01	0,07	0,04
India, Bombay	0.07	0.01	0.06	0.01
*India, Karunagappally	0,11	0,08	0,01	0,01
India, Madras	0.07	0.01	0.03	0.01
*India, Trivandrum	0,05	0,03	0,04	0,03
Israel: All Jews	0.12	0.01	0.08	0.01
Jews born in Israel	0.14	0.06	0.07	0.02
Jews born in America or Europe	0.11	0.02	0.05	0.01
Jews born in Africa or Asia	0.08	0.02	0.09	0.04
Non-Jews	0.07	0.03	0,02	0,01
Japan, Hiroshima	0.05	0.01	0.05	0.01
Japan, Miyagi	0.05	0.01	0.04	0.01
Japan, Nagasaki	0.04	0.01	0.04	0.01
Japan, Osaka	0.05	0.01	0.04	0.00
*Japan, Saga	0,03	0,01	0.04	0.01
Japan, Yamagata	0,02	0,01	0.04	0.01
*Korea, Kangwha	0,24	0,10	0,05	0,04
*Kuwait: Non-Kuwaitis	0.08	0.03	0,02	0,01
*Kuwait: Kuwaitis	0,03	0,01	0,03	0,01
*Philippines, Manila	0.16	0.02	0.11	0.02
Singapore: Chinese	0.07	0.01	0.08	0.01
Singapore: Malay	0,06	0,03	0.05	0,03
Singapore: Indian	0,12	0,05	0.03	0,02
Thailand, Chiang Mai	0.04	0.01	0.04	0.01
*Thailand, Khon Kaen	0.16	0.04	0.25	0.05
*Viet Nam, Hanoi				

* IMPORTANT-SEE NOTES ON POPULATION PAGE

CUMULATIVE INCIDENCE (0-74)
RATES AND STANDARD ERRORS (percent)
Bone (ICD-9 170) (contd)

EUROPE	MALE		FEMALE	
Austria, Tyrol	0.12	0.03	0.08	0.02
*Belarus	0.25	0.01	0.13	0.01
*Croatia	0.13	0.01	0.10	0.01
Czech Republic	0.09	0.01	0.06	0.00
Denmark	0.08	0.01	0.05	0.01
Estonia	0.06	0.01	0.07	0.01
Finland	0.07	0.01	0.06	0.01
France, Bas-Rhin	0.10	0.02	0.08	0.02
*France, Calvados	0.07	0.02	0.07	0.02
France, Doubs	0.06	0.02	0.08	0.03
France, Haut-Rhin	0.07	0.02	0.06	0.02
*France, Herault	0.11	0.02	0.08	0.02
France, Isere	0.06	0.01	0.05	0.01
*France, Somme	0,05	0,02	0,04	0,02
*France, Tarn	0.11	0.03	0,06	0,02
Germany, Eastern States	0.14	0.01	0.09	0.01
Germany, Saarland	0.09	0.02	0.05	0.01
Iceland	0,09	0,04	0,06	0,04
Ireland, Southern	0.07	0.02	0,05	0,02
Italy, Ferrara	0,08	0,04	0,09	0,05
Italy, Florence	0.08	0.02	0.06	0.01
Italy, Genoa	0.08	0.02	0.08	0.02
*Italy, Latina	0,09	0,03	0,03	0,02
Italy, Macerata	0,03	0,03	0,03	0,03
Italy, Modena	0,04	0,02	0.06	0.02
Italy, Parma	0,04	0,02	0,08	0,03
Italy, Ragusa	0.12	0.04	0.07	0,03
Italy, Romagna	0.08	0.02	0.07	0.02
Italy, Torino	0.06	0.02	0.04	0.01
Italy, Trieste	0,05	0,03	0,08	0,04
Italy, Varese	0.07	0.02	0.05	0.02
Italy, Veneto	0.06	0.01	0.06	0.01
*Latvia	0.19	0.02	0.09	0.01
Malta	0,07	0,05	0,08	0,05
The Netherlands	0.07	0.00	0.05	0.00
The Netherlands, Eindhoven	0.10	0.02	0.06	0.02
The Netherlands, Maastricht	0.07	0.01	0.05	0.01
Norway	0.07	0.01	0.05	0.01
*Poland, Cracow	0.15	0.04	0.08	0.02
*Poland, Kielce	0.12	0.02	0.06	0.01
*Poland, Lower Silesia	0.17	0.02	0.11	0.01
Poland, Warsaw City	0.09	0.02	0.06	0.01
Slovakia	0.18	0.01	0.11	0.01
Slovenia	0.05	0.01	0.06	0.01
*Spain, Albacete	0.08	0,05	0,10	0,04
Spain, Asturias	0.08	0.02	0.05	0.01
Spain, Basque Country	0.09	0.02	0.07	0.01
Spain, Granada	0.08	0.02	0.05	0.01
Spain, Mallorca	0,05	0,02	0,04	0,01
Spain, Murcia	0.11	0.02	0.04	0.01
Spain, Navarra	0.12	0.03	0,05	0,02
Spain, Tarragona	0,06	0,02	0.07	0.02
Spain, Zaragoza	0.08	0.02	0.07	0.02

	MALE		FEMALE	
Sweden	0.09	0.01	0.06	0.00
*Switzerland, Basel	0.12	0.03	0.10	0.03
Switzerland, Geneva	0.10	0.03	0,01	0,01
Switzerland, Graubunden	0,07	0,05	0,13	0,05
Switzerland, Neuchatel	-	-	0,04	0,03
Switzerland, St Gall-Appenzell	0.11	0.03	0.08	0.02
Switzerland, Valais	0,03	0,02	0,01	0,01
Switzerland, Vaud	0.09	0.03	0,03	0,01
Switzerland, Zurich	0.13	0.02	0.07	0.01
*UK, England and Wales	0.08	0.00	0.06	0.00
*UK, East Anglia	0.06	0.01	0.04	0.01
*UK, Mersey	0.06	0.01	0.02	0.01
*UK, North Western	0.06	0.01	0.04	0.01
UK, Oxford	0.08	0.01	0.05	0.01
*UK, South Thames	0.08	0.01	0.05	0.01
UK, South Western	0.08	0.01	0.04	0.01
UK, Wessex	0.09	0.01	0.07	0.01
*UK, West Midlands	0.15	0.01	0.12	0.01
UK, Yorkshire	0.06	0.01	0.04	0.01
UK, Scotland	0.07	0.01	0.05	0.01
UK, Scotland, West	0.07	0.01	0.05	0.01
*Yugoslavia, Vojvodina	0.18	0.02	0.08	0.01

OCEANIA

	MALE		FEMALE		
Australian Capital Territory	0.17	0.07	0,06	0,03	
Australia, New South Wales	0.08	0.01	0.04	0.01	
South Australia	0.06	0.01	0.04	0.01	
Australia, Tasmania	0,07	0,03	0,06	0,02	
Australia, Victoria	0.09	0.01	0.06	0.01	
Western Australia	0.10	0.02	0.08	0.01	
*French Polynesia	0,33	0,17	0,10	0,05	m
New Zealand: Non-Maori	0.11	0.01	0.07	0.01	
New Zealand: Maori	0.18	0.08	0,05	0,02	
US, Hawaii: White	0,10	0,04	0,03	0,02	
US, Hawaii: Japanese	0,04	0,02	0,07	0,03	
US, Hawaii: Hawaiian	0,10	0,05	0,02	0,01	
US, Hawaii: Filipino	0,15	0,06	0,02	0,02	
US, Hawaii: Chinese	0,04	0,04	-	-	

* IMPORTANT-SEE NOTES ON POPULATION PAGE

CUMULATIVE INCIDENCE (0-74)
RATES AND STANDARD ERRORS (percent)
Connective tissue (ICD-9 171)

	MALE		FEMALE	
AFRICA				
*Algeria, Setif				
*France, La Reunion				
*Mali, Bamako				
*Uganda, Kyadondo				
*Zimbabwe, Harare: African				
*Zimbabwe, Harare: European				
AMERICA, CENTRAL AND SOUTH				
*Argentina, Concordia	0,18	0,11	0,28	0,13
*Brazil, Belem	0.19	0.06	0.18	0.05 m
*Brazil, Goiania				
*Brazil, Porto Alegre	0.26	0.05	0.21	0.04
Colombia, Cali	0.26	0.05	0.24	0.04 m
*Costa Rica	0.14	0.02	0.12	0.02
*Ecuador, Quito	0.27	0.05	0.16	0.03
*Peru, Lima	0.17	0.03	0.20	0.03
Peru, Trujillo	0,15	0,06	0,15	0,08
US, Puerto Rico	0.15	0.02	0.09	0.01
*Uruguay, Montevideo	0.30	0.04	0.27	0.03
AMERICA, NORTH				
Canada	0.21	0.01	0.16	0.00
Canada, Alberta	0.16	0.02	0.14	0.02
Canada, British Columbia	0.17	0.01	0.14	0.01
Canada, Manitoba	0.17	0.03	0.13	0.02
Canada, New Brunswick	0.17	0.03	0.19	0.03
Canada, Newfoundland	0.26	0.05	0.13	0.03
Canada, Northwest Territories	0,30	0,24	0,02	0,02
Canada, Nova Scotia	0.25	0.04	0.25	0.03
Canada, Ontario	0.22	0.01	0.16	0.01
Canada, Prince Edward Island	0.29	0.09	0,11	0,06
Canada, Quebec	0.23	0.01	0.15	0.01
Canada, Saskatchewan	0.19	0.03	0.14	0.02
Canada, Yukon	-	-	0,12	0,07
US, Cent. Calif.: Non-Hisp. White	0.23	0.03	0.17	0.02
US, Cent. Calif.: Hispanic	0.20	0.06	0.16	0.05
US, Los Angeles: Non-Hisp. White	0.28	0.02	0.19	0.01
US, Los Angeles: Hispanic White	0.17	0.02	0.14	0.02
US, Los Angeles: Black	0.17	0.03	0.19	0.03
US, Los Angeles: Chinese	0,23	0,08	0,11	0,05
US, Los Angeles: Filipino	0,21	0,08	0.22	0.07
US, Los Angeles: Korean	0,20	0,09	0,12	0,06
US, Los Angeles: Japanese	0,15	0,07	0,13	0,06
US, San Francisco: Non-Hisp. White	0.23	0.02	0.16	0.02
US, San Francisco: Hispanic White	0.24	0.06	0.12	0.04
US, San Francisco: Black	0.33	0.07	0.18	0.04
US, San Francisco: Chinese	0.20	0.06	0,11	0,04
US, San Francisco: Filipino	0,07	0,04	0,13	0,06
US, San Francisco: Japanese	0,24	0,15	0.15	0,11
US, Connecticut: White	0.22	0.02	0.14	0.01
US, Connecticut: Black	0.39	0.10	0.26	0.07
US, Atlanta: White	0.24	0.03	0.12	0.02
US, Atlanta: Black	0.22	0.06	0.19	0.05
US, Iowa	0.25	0.02	0.19	0.02

	MALE		FEMALE	
US, Central Louisiana: White	0.21	0.07	0.14	0.05
US, Central Louisiana: Black	0,40	0,21	0,39	0,17
US, New Orleans: White	0.27	0.04	0.23	0.04
US, New Orleans: Black	0.32	0.08	0.14	0.04
US, Detroit: White	0.22	0.02	0.15	0.01
US, Detroit: Black	0.19	0.03	0.12	0.02
US, New Mexico: Non-Hisp. White	0.32	0.04	0.20	0.03
US, New Mexico: Hispanic White	0.17	0.05	0.17	0.04
US, New Mexico: American Indian	0,15	0,09	0,23	0,12
US, Utah	0.21	0.03	0.16	0.02
US, Seattle	0.25	0.02	0.18	0.02
US, SEER: White	0.23	0.01	0.16	0.01
US, SEER: Black	0.25	0.03	0.18	0.02
ASIA				
*China, Qidong	0,04	0,01	0,01	0,01
China, Shanghai	0.17	0.01	0.12	0.01
China, Tianjin	0.14	0.02	0.09	0.01
Hong Kong	0.22	0.01	0.20	0.01
*India, Bangalore	0.11	0.02	0.09	0.01
*India, Barshi, Paranda and Bhum	0,04	0,02	0,02	0,01
India, Bombay	0.13	0.01	0.11	0.01
*India, Karunagappally	0,14	0,08	0,05	0,03
India, Madras	0.10	0.01	0.10	0.01
*India, Trivandrum	0.13	0.05	0.08	0,04
Israel: All Jews	0.27	0.02	0.21	0.02
Jews born in Israel	0.29	0.07	0.18	0.07
Jews born in America or Europe	0.27	0.03	0.26	0.03
Jews born in Africa or Asia	0.19	0.03	0.22	0.05
Non-Jews	0.11	0.04	0.07	0.02
Japan, Hiroshima	0.11	0.02	0.10	0.02
Japan, Miyagi	0.13	0.02	0.08	0.01
Japan, Nagasaki	0.10	0.02	0.07	0.01
Japan, Osaka	0.09	0.01	0.07	0.01
*Japan, Saga	0.07	0.02	0.03	0.01
Japan, Yamagata	0.06	0.01	0.04	0.01
*Korea, Kangwha	-	-	-	-
*Kuwait: Non-Kuwaitis	0.15	0.04	0,04	0,02
*Kuwait: Kuwaitis	0,08	0,04	0,07	0,03
*Philippines, Manila	0.28	0.03	0.21	0.02
Singapore: Chinese	0.17	0.02	0.13	0.02
Singapore: Malay	0.24	0.08	0.09	0.04
Singapore: Indian	0,05	0,03	0,05	0,04
Thailand, Chiang Mai	0.05	0.01	0.07	0.02
*Thailand, Khon Kaen	0.07	0.02	0.06	0.01
*Viet Nam, Hanoi				

* IMPORTANT-SEE NOTES ON POPULATION PAGE

CUMULATIVE INCIDENCE (0-74)
RATES AND STANDARD ERRORS (percent)
Connective tissue (ICD-9 171) (contd)

EUROPE	MALE		FEMALE	
Austria, Tyrol	0.25	0.05	0.21	0.04
*Belarus	0.25	0.01	0.18	0.01
*Croatia	0.14	0.01	0.11	0.01
Czech Republic	0.22	0.01	0.17	0.01
Denmark	0.20	0.01	0.14	0.01
Estonia	0.20	0.03	0.21	0.02
Finland	0.24	0.01	0.19	0.01
France, Bas-Rhin	0.19	0.04	0.18	0.03
*France, Calvados	0.15	0.03	0.14	0.03
France, Doubs	0.32	0.06	0.18	0.04
France, Haut-Rhin	0.25	0.04	0.20	0.04
*France, Herault	0.21	0.03	0.16	0.03
France, Isere	0.19	0.03	0.19	0.03
*France, Somme	0.10	0.03	0.09	0.02
*France, Tarn	0.17	0.04	0.10	0.03
Germany, Eastern States	0.17	0.01	0.16	0.01
Germany, Saarland	0.23	0.03	0.17	0.02
Iceland	0.17	0.06	0,07	0,03
Ireland, Southern	0.19	0.04	0.13	0.03
Italy, Ferrara	0,22	0,08	0,11	0,05
Italy, Florence	0.14	0.02	0.16	0.02
Italy, Genoa	0.27	0.04	0.20	0.03
*Italy, Latina	0.20	0.06	0.11	0.03
Italy, Macerata	0,24	0,08	0,21	0,08
Italy, Modena	0.25	0.04	0.12	0.03
Italy, Parma	0.19	0.04	0.19	0.04
Italy, Ragusa	0,06	0,03	0,06	0,02
Italy, Romagna	0.20	0.04	0.12	0.03
Italy, Torino	0.17	0.03	0.14	0.02
Italy, Trieste	0.33	0.08	0.10	0.04
Italy, Varese	0.17	0.03	0.17	0.03
Italy, Veneto	0.31	0.03	0.19	0.02
*Latvia	0.18	0.02	0.15	0.01
Malta	0,16	0,07	0,13	0,05
The Netherlands	0.25	0.01	0.17	0.01
The Netherlands, Eindhoven	0.25	0.04	0.10	0.02
The Netherlands, Maastricht	0.22	0.03	0.16	0.03
Norway	0.13	0.01	0.11	0.01
*Poland, Cracow	0.12	0.03	0.08	0.02
*Poland, Kielce	0.17	0.03	0.11	0.02
*Poland, Lower Silesia	0.19	0.02	0.14	0.01
Poland, Warsaw City	0.17	0.02	0.14	0.02
Slovakia	0.21	0.01	0.16	0.01
Slovenia	0.17	0.02	0.12	0.02
*Spain, Albacete	0,15	0,06	0,22	0,08
Spain, Asturias	0.19	0.03	0.13	0.02
Spain, Basque Country	0.19	0.02	0.14	0.02
Spain, Granada	0.11	0.02	0.10	0.02
Spain, Mallorca	0.13	0.03	0.16	0.03
Spain, Murcia	0.18	0.03	0.16	0.03
Spain, Navarra	0.17	0.04	0.15	0.03
Spain, Tarragona	0.16	0.03	0.13	0.03
Spain, Zaragoza	0.18	0.03	0.09	0.02

	MALE		FEMALE	
Sweden	0.27	0.01	0.20	0.01
*Switzerland, Basel	0.19	0.04	0.15	0.04
Switzerland, Geneva	0.18	0.05	0.23	0.05
Switzerland, Graubunden	0,16	0,07	0,19	0,08
Switzerland, Neuchatel	0,04	0,03	0,07	0,04
Switzerland, St Gall-Appenzell	0.23	0.05	0.18	0.04
Switzerland, Valais	0,17	0,06	0.28	0.07
Switzerland, Vaud	0.26	0.04	0.19	0.03
Switzerland, Zurich	0.18	0.02	0.20	0.03
*UK, England and Wales	0.19	0.01	0.14	0.00
*UK, East Anglia	0.17	0.02	0.17	0.02
*UK, Mersey	0.16	0.02	0.13	0.01
*UK, North Western	0.13	0.01	0.09	0.01
UK, Oxford	0.23	0.02	0.15	0.02
*UK, South Thames	0.17	0.01	0.13	0.01
UK, South Western	0.14	0.01	0.11	0.01
UK, Wessex	0.22	0.02	0.16	0.01
*UK, West Midlands	0.26	0.01	0.21	0.01
UK, Yorkshire	0.19	0.01	0.14	0.01
UK, Scotland	0.18	0.01	0.11	0.01
UK, Scotland, West	0.18	0.02	0.12	0.01
*Yugoslavia, Vojvodina	0.15	0.02	0.10	0.01

OCEANIA	MALE		FEMALE	
Australian Capital Territory	0.14	0.05	0,08	0,04
Australia, New South Wales	0.26	0.01	0.15	0.01
South Australia	0.26	0.03	0.14	0.02
Australia, Tasmania	0.20	0.05	0.20	0.04
Australia, Victoria	0.23	0.02	0.14	0.01
Western Australia	0.18	0.02	0.11	0.02
*French Polynesia	0,15	0,07	0,14	0,09
New Zealand: Non-Maori	0.25	0.02	0.16	0.01
New Zealand: Maori	0.33	0.12	0.25	0.08
US, Hawaii: White	0.29	0.07	0.20	0.05
US, Hawaii: Japanese	0,10	0,04	0,07	0,03
US, Hawaii: Hawaiian	0.25	0.08	0.20	0.07
US, Hawaii: Filipino	0,22	0,08	0,17	0,06
US, Hawaii: Chinese	0,22	0,11	0,18	0,10

* IMPORTANT-SEE NOTES ON POPULATION PAGE

CUMULATIVE INCIDENCE (0-74)
RATES AND STANDARD ERRORS (percent)
Melanoma of skin (ICD-9 172)

	MALE		FEMALE	
AFRICA				
*Algeria, Setif				
*France, La Reunion				
*Mali, Bamako				
*Uganda, Kyadondo				
*Zimbabwe, Harare: African				
*Zimbabwe, Harare: European				
AMERICA, CENTRAL AND SOUTH				
*Argentina, Concordia	0,10	0,06	0,24	0,10
*Brazil, Belem	0.16	0.06	0.10	0.03
*Brazil, Goiania				
*Brazil, Porto Alegre	0.61	0.08	0.52	0.06 f
Colombia, Cali	0.28	0.05	0.34	0.05 m
*Costa Rica	0.20	0.03	0.21	0.03
*Ecuador, Quito	0.45	0.07	0.44	0.06
*Peru, Lima	0.22	0.03	0.17	0.03
Peru, Trujillo	0,41	0,15	0,21	0,08 m
US, Puerto Rico	0.16	0.02	0.11	0.01
*Uruguay, Montevideo	0.46	0.06	0.26	0.03
AMERICA, NORTH				
Canada	0.83	0.01	0.70	0.01
Canada, Alberta	0.83	0.04	0.71	0.04
Canada, British Columbia	1.10	0.04	1.03	0.03
Canada, Manitoba	0.74	0.05	0.73	0.05
Canada, New Brunswick	0.95	0.08	0.82	0.07
Canada, Newfoundland	0.42	0.06	0.49	0.06
Canada, Northwest Territories	0,06	0,05	0,19	0,13
Canada, Nova Scotia	1.03	0.07	0.93	0.06
Canada, Ontario	1.05	0.02	0.81	0.02
Canada, Prince Edward Island	0.86	0.17	0.93	0.17
Canada, Quebec	0.39	0.02	0.34	0.01
Canada, Saskatchewan	0.89	0.06	0.75	0.05
Canada, Yukon	0,47	0,17	0.58	0.18
US, Cent. Calif.: Non-Hisp. White	1.37	0.07	0.83	0.05
US, Cent. Calif.: Hispanic	0.28	0.06	0.30	0.06
US, Los Angeles: Non-Hisp. White	1.72	0.04	1.13	0.03
US, Los Angeles: Hispanic White	0.22	0.03	0.22	0.03
US, Los Angeles: Black	0.07	0.02	0.07	0.02
US, Los Angeles: Chinese	-	-	0,04	0,03
US, Los Angeles: Filipino	0,12	0,08	0,01	0,01
US, Los Angeles: Korean	-	-	0,03	0,03
US, Los Angeles: Japanese	0,07	0,04	0,06	0,03
US, San Francisco: Non-Hisp. White	1.78	0.06	1.18	0.04
US, San Francisco: Hispanic White	0.38	0.08	0.50	0.08
US, San Francisco: Black	0,06	0,03	0,05	0,02
US, San Francisco: Chinese	0,02	0,02	0,05	0,03
US, San Francisco: Filipino	0,13	0,09	0,08	0,05
US, San Francisco: Japanese	0,14	0,14	0,04	0,04
US, Connecticut: White	1.53	0.05	1.13	0.04
US, Connecticut: Black	0,21	0,09	0,10	0,05
US, Atlanta: White	1.87	0.09	1.17	0.06
US, Atlanta: Black	0,10	0,05	0,04	0,02
US, Iowa	1.05	0.04	0.81	0.03

	MALE		FEMALE	
US, Central Louisiana: White	1.08	0.15	0.71	0.11
US, Central Louisiana: Black	-	-	0,12	0,09
US, New Orleans: White	0.74	0.07	0.43	0.05
US, New Orleans: Black	0,09	0,05	-	-
US, Detroit: White	1.23	0.04	0.73	0.03
US, Detroit: Black	0.07	0.02	0.03	0,01
US, New Mexico: Non-Hisp. White	1.81	0.10	1.19	0.07
US, New Mexico: Hispanic White	0.29	0.06	0.36	0.06
US, New Mexico: American Indian	0,12	0,08	0,04	0,03
US, Utah	1.44	0.07	1.06	0.06
US, Seattle	1.32	0.04	1.07	0.04
US, SEER: White	1.42	0.02	1.01	0.01
US, SEER: Black	0.08	0.02	0.05	0.01
ASIA				
*China, Qidong	0,04	0,01	0,02	0,01
China, Shanghai	0.05	0.01	0.03	0.00
China, Tianjin	0.04	0.01	0.02	0.01
Hong Kong	0.10	0.01	0.08	0.01
*India, Bangalore	0.03	0.01	0.03	0.01
*India, Barshi, Paranda and Bhum	-	-	0,01	0,01
India, Bombay	0.06	0.01	0.04	0.01
*India, Karunagappally	0,19	0,11	-	-
India, Madras	0.04	0.01	0.03	0.01
*India, Trivandrum	0,05	0,05	0,02	0,02
Israel: All Jews	1.02	0.04	1.01	0.03
Jews born in Israel	1.64	0.12	1.48	0.13
Jews born in America or Europe	1.22	0.06	1.24	0.06
Jews born in Africa or Asia	0.30	0.04	0.28	0.03
Non-Jews	0,05	0,02	0,05	0,02
Japan, Hiroshima	0.06	0.02	0.04	0.01
Japan, Miyagi	0.05	0.01	0.03	0.01
Japan, Nagasaki	0.05	0.01	0.03	0.01
Japan, Osaka	0.03	0.00	0.02	0.00
*Japan, Saga	0.05	0.01	0.05	0.01
Japan, Yamagata	0.04	0.01	0.02	0.01
*Korea, Kangwha	0,03	0,03	-	-
*Kuwait: Non-Kuwaitis	0.14	0.08	0,11	0,11
*Kuwait: Kuwaitis	0,06	0,05	-	-
*Philippines, Manila	0.10	0.02	0.07	0.01
Singapore: Chinese	0.07	0.02	0.05	0.01
Singapore: Malay	0,00	0,00	0,01	0,01
Singapore: Indian	-	-	-	-
Thailand, Chiang Mai	0.05	0.01	0.05	0.02
*Thailand, Khon Kaen	0,03	0,01	0.07	0.02
*Viet Nam, Hanoi				

* IMPORTANT-SEE NOTES ON POPULATION PAGE

CUMULATIVE INCIDENCE (0-74)
RATES AND STANDARD ERRORS (percent)
Melanoma of skin (ICD-9 172) (contd)

EUROPE	MALE		FEMALE	
Austria, Tyrol	1.23	0.10	1.57	0.10
*Belarus	0.22	0.01	0.25	0.01
*Croatia	0.36	0.02	0.30	0.02
Czech Republic	0.74	0.02	0.64	0.02
Denmark	0.94	0.03	1.20	0.03
Estonia	0.40	0.04	0.42	0.03
Finland	0.83	0.03	0.67	0.02
France, Bas-Rhin	0.69	0.06	0.82	0.06
*France, Calvados	0.29	0.04	0.65	0.06
France, Doubs	0.51	0.07	0.84	0.09
France, Haut-Rhin	0.74	0.07	0.65	0.06
*France, Herault	0.54	0.05	0.59	0.05
France, Isere	0.43	0.05	0.61	0.05
*France, Somme	0.33	0.05	0.46	0.06
*France, Tarn	0.44	0.07	0.69	0.09
Germany, Eastern States	0.55	0.02	0.56	0.02
Germany, Saarland	0.65	0.05	0.64	0.04
Iceland	0.38	0.09	0.71	0.11
Ireland, Southern	0.64	0.07	1.07	0.09
Italy, Ferrara	0.40	0.10	0.51	0.11
Italy, Florence	0.59	0.05	0.53	0.04
Italy, Genoa	0.51	0.05	0.55	0.05
*Italy, Latina	0.36	0.07	0.34	0.06
Italy, Macerata	0.73	0.16	0.52	0.12
Italy, Modena	0.47	0.05	0.36	0.04
Italy, Parma	0.46	0.06	0.47	0.06
Italy, Ragusa	0.43	0.08	0.23	0.05
Italy, Romagna	0.61	0.07	0.69	0.07
Italy, Torino	0.45	0.05	0.48	0.04
Italy, Trieste	1.05	0.13	0.94	0.11
Italy, Varese	0.53	0.05	0.51	0.05
Italy, Veneto	0.65	0.05	0.69	0.04
*Latvia	0.23	0.02	0.31	0.02
Malta	0,28	0,10	0.40	0.11
The Netherlands	0.71	0.02	0.96	0.02
The Netherlands, Eindhoven	0.59	0.05	0.79	0.06
The Netherlands, Maastricht	0.55	0.05	0.88	0.06
Norway	1.51	0.04	1.52	0.04
*Poland, Cracow	0.47	0.06	0.39	0.04
*Poland, Kielce	0.28	0.04	0.27	0.03
*Poland, Lower Silesia	0.31	0.02	0.33	0.02
Poland, Warsaw City	0.44	0.04	0.39	0.03
Slovakia	0.51	0.02	0.46	0.02
Slovenia	0.54	0.04	0.57	0.03
*Spain, Albacete	0,16	0,06	0,18	0,07
Spain, Asturias	0.22	0.03	0.43	0.04
Spain, Basque Country	0.34	0.03	0.41	0.03
Spain, Granada	0.34	0.04	0.38	0.04
Spain, Mallorca	0.39	0.05	0.41	0.05
Spain, Murcia	0.28	0.04	0.44	0.04
Spain, Navarra	0.35	0.05	0.34	0.05
Spain, Tarragona	0.36	0.05	0.32	0.05
Spain, Zaragoza	0.25	0.04	0.34	0.04

	MALE		FEMALE	
Sweden	1.22	0.02	1.11	0.02
*Switzerland, Basel	1.16	0.11	0.85	0.08
Switzerland, Geneva	1.14	0.12	1.09	0.10
Switzerland, Graubunden	0.79	0.15	0.98	0.16
Switzerland, Neuchatel	1.25	0.18	1.06	0.15
Switzerland, St Gall-Appenzell	0.95	0.10	1.09	0.09
Switzerland, Valais	0.61	0.12	0.92	0.13
Switzerland, Vaud	1.28	0.10	1.35	0.09
Switzerland, Zurich	1.50	0.08	1.35	0.06
*UK, England and Wales	0.48	0.01	0.66	0.01
*UK, East Anglia	0.59	0.03	0.76	0.04
*UK, Mersey	0.35	0.02	0.45	0.03
*UK, North Western	0.36	0.02	0.55	0.02
UK, Oxford	0.62	0.03	0.75	0.03
*UK, South Thames	0.47	0.02	0.66	0.02
UK, South Western	0.76	0.03	1.05	0.03
UK, Wessex	0.69	0.03	1.06	0.04
*UK, West Midlands	0.45	0.02	0.60	0.02
UK, Yorkshire	0.44	0.02	0.67	0.03
UK, Scotland	0.60	0.02	0.81	0.02
UK, Scotland, West	0.61	0.03	0.75	0.03
*Yugoslavia, Vojvodina	0.30	0.03	0.34	0.02

OCEANIA	MALE		FEMALE	
Australian Capital Territory	3.29	0.30	2.34	0.21
Australia, New South Wales	3.67	0.05	2.60	0.04
South Australia	2.84	0.09	2.51	0.08
Australia, Tasmania	2.38	0.15	2.24	0.14
Australia, Victoria	2.35	0.05	2.08	0.04
Western Australia	3.46	0.11	2.56	0.09
*French Polynesia	0,47	0,21	0.36	0.10
New Zealand: Non-Maori	2.67	0.07	3.02	0.06
New Zealand: Maori	0.49	0.16	0.32	0.09
US, Hawaii: White	2.11	0.18	1.18	0.13
US, Hawaii: Japanese	0,02	0,02	0,04	0,02
US, Hawaii: Hawaiian	0,14	0,09	0,13	0,06
US, Hawaii: Filipino	0,01	0,01	0,08	0,05
US, Hawaii: Chinese	0,10	0,07	0,06	0,06

* IMPORTANT-SEE NOTES ON POPULATION PAGE

CUMULATIVE INCIDENCE (0-74)
RATES AND STANDARD ERRORS (percent)
Other skin (ICD-9 173)

	MALE		FEMALE	
AFRICA				
*Algeria, Setif				
*France, La Reunion				
*Mali, Bamako				
*Uganda, Kyadondo				
*Zimbabwe, Harare: African				
*Zimbabwe, Harare: European				
AMERICA, CENTRAL AND SOUTH				
*Argentina, Concordia	5.54	0.60	3.22	0.41
*Brazil, Belem	4.18	0.32	2.57	0.21
*Brazil, Goiania				
*Brazil, Porto Alegre	6.22	0.31	3.50	0.18 mf
Colombia, Cali	-	-	-	-
*Costa Rica	4.31	0.13	3.94	0.12
*Ecuador, Quito	2.50	0.17	2.51	0.15
*Peru, Lima	1.11	0.07	0.98	0.07
Peru, Trujillo	2.17	0.35	1.86	0.28
† US, Puerto Rico	0.03	0.01	0.04	0.01
*Uruguay, Montevideo	1.86	0.11	1.03	0.07
AMERICA, NORTH				
Canada				
Canada, Alberta				
Canada, British Columbia				
Canada, Manitoba				
Canada, New Brunswick				
Canada, Newfoundland				
Canada, Northwest Territories				
Canada, Nova Scotia				
Canada, Ontario				
Canada, Prince Edward Island				
Canada, Quebec				
Canada, Saskatchewan				
Canada, Yukon				
† US, Cent. Calif.: Non-Hisp. White	0.11	0.02	0.06	0.01
† US, Cent. Calif.: Hispanic	0,03	0,02	0,02	0,01
† US, Los Angeles: Non-Hisp. White	0.12	0.01	0.08	0.01
† US, Los Angeles: Hispanic White	0.04	0.01	0.06	0.01
† US, Los Angeles: Black	0.08	0.02	0.08	0.02
† US, Los Angeles: Chinese	-	-	0,03	0,02
† US, Los Angeles: Filipino	0,02	0,02	0,05	0,04
† US, Los Angeles: Korean	-	-	0,01	0,01
† US, Los Angeles: Japanese	0,03	0,02	0,07	0,05
† US, San Francisco: Non-Hisp. White	0.10	0.01	0.08	0.01
† US, San Francisco: Hispanic White	0,04	0,02	0,03	0,02
† US, San Francisco: Black	0.09	0.03	0.10	0.03
† US, San Francisco: Chinese	0,04	0,03	0,01	0,01
† US, San Francisco: Filipino	-	-	0,04	0,03
† US, San Francisco: Japanese	-	-	-	-
† US, Connecticut: White	0.07	0.01	0.06	0.01
† US, Connecticut: Black	0,07	0,03	0,07	0,03
† US, Atlanta: White	0.10	0.02	0.03	0.01
† US, Atlanta: Black	0,03	0,01	0.09	0.03
† US, Iowa	0.09	0.01	0.05	0.01

	MALE		FEMALE	
† US, Central Louisiana: White	0,05	0,03	0,08	0,04
† US, Central Louisiana: Black	-	-	0,07	0,07
† US, New Orleans: White	0,06	0,02	0.06	0.02
† US, New Orleans: Black	0,03	0,02	0,09	0,04
† US, Detroit: White	0.08	0.01	0.06	0.01
† US, Detroit: Black	0.09	0.02	0.09	0.02
† US, New Mexico: Non-Hisp. White	0.13	0.03	0.10	0.02
† US, New Mexico: Hispanic White	0.11	0.04	0.08	0.03
† US, New Mexico: American Indian	-	-	0,02	0,02
† US, Utah	0.08	0.02	0.08	0.02
† US, Seattle	0.09	0.01	0.09	0.01
† US, SEER: White	0.09	0.00	0.06	0.00
† US, SEER: Black	0.07	0.01	0.09	0.01
ASIA				
*China, Qidong	0.14	0.03	0.10	0.02
China, Shanghai	0.18	0.01	0.11	0.01
China, Tianjin	0.09	0.01	0.08	0.01
Hong Kong	0.61	0.03	0.46	0.02
*India, Bangalore	0.17	0.02	0.17	0.02
*India, Barshi, Paranda and Bhum	0.19	0.06	0,14	0,05
India, Bombay	0.20	0.02	0.14	0.01
*India, Karunagappally	0,36	0,13	0.37	0.13
India, Madras	0.23	0.03	0.11	0.02
*India, Trivandrum	0,13	0,05	0,12	0,05
Israel: All Jews	0.31	0.02	0.29	0.02
Jews born in Israel	0.41	0.10	0.44	0.09
Jews born in America or Europe	0.36	0.04	0.35	0.03
Jews born in Africa or Asia	0.19	0.03	0.12	0.02
Non-Jews	0,05	0,02	0,06	0,03
Japan, Hiroshima	0.55	0.06	0.39	0.04
Japan, Miyagi	0.27	0.03	0.17	0.02
Japan, Nagasaki	0.55	0.04	0.36	0.03
Japan, Osaka	0.12	0.01	0.08	0.01
*Japan, Saga	0.28	0.04	0.07	0.02
Japan, Yamagata	0.11	0.02	0.08	0.01
*Korea, Kangwha	0,18	0,08	0,07	0,05
*Kuwait: Non-Kuwaitis	0.78	0.28	0.35	0.14
*Kuwait: Kuwaitis	0.19	0.07	0,22	0,10
*Philippines, Manila	0.31	0.04	0.19	0.02
Singapore: Chinese	1.01	0.07	0.84	0.06
Singapore: Malay	0.57	0.12	0.37	0.10
Singapore: Indian	0.25	0.08	0.62	0.22
Thailand, Chiang Mai	0.48	0.05	0.31	0.04
*Thailand, Khon Kaen	0.49	0.07	0.32	0.05
*Viet Nam, Hanoi				

* IMPORTANT-SEE NOTES ON POPULATION PAGE

CUMULATIVE INCIDENCE (0-74)
RATES AND STANDARD ERRORS (percent)
Other skin (ICD-9 173) (contd)

EUROPE	MALE		FEMALE	
Austria, Tyrol	2.52	*0.17*	1.55	*0.11*
*Belarus	2.46	*0.05*	1.99	*0.03*
*Croatia	0.05	*0.01*	0.03	*0.01*
Czech Republic	6.42	*0.06*	4.17	*0.04*
Denmark	6.12	*0.07*	4.89	*0.06*
Estonia	2.39	*0.11*	1.96	*0.07*
Finland	6.14	*0.08*	5.31	*0.06*
† France, Bas-Rhin	1.79	*0.12*	0.70	*0.06*
*France, Calvados	4.11	*0.20*	2.17	*0.13*
France, Doubs	7.64	*0.32*	5.23	*0.23*
† France, Haut-Rhin	5.46	*0.24*	3.72	*0.16*
*France, Herault	1.98	*0.11*	0.70	*0.06*
† France, Isere	1.37	*0.10*	0.52	*0.05*
†*France, Somme	1.58	*0.13*	0.37	*0.06*
†*France, Tarn	1.86	*0.16*	0.66	*0.09*
† Germany, Eastern States	0.73	*0.03*	0.26	*0.01*
Germany, Saarland	7.20	*0.19*	4.12	*0.12*
† Iceland	0.57	*0.12*	0.40	*0.09*
Ireland, Southern	9.18	*0.31*	6.22	*0.24*
Italy, Ferrara	6.26	*0.41*	3.20	*0.26*
Italy, Florence	2.63	*0.11*	1.22	*0.07*
Italy, Genoa	4.03	*0.15*	2.18	*0.10*
*Italy, Latina	3.09	*0.22*	1.59	*0.15*
Italy, Macerata	5.09	*0.42*	2.98	*0.30*
Italy, Modena	5.00	*0.19*	2.27	*0.11*
Italy, Parma	3.41	*0.18*	1.38	*0.10*
Italy, Ragusa	5.11	*0.28*	2.53	*0.19*
Italy, Romagna	7.27	*0.25*	3.70	*0.16*
Italy, Torino	4.66	*0.16*	2.83	*0.11*
Italy, Trieste	7.90	*0.38*	5.38	*0.27*
Italy, Varese	5.40	*0.19*	2.65	*0.11*
Italy, Veneto	6.03	*0.16*	3.10	*0.10*
*Latvia	2.13	*0.08*	1.70	*0.05*
Malta	5.59	*0.49*	2.24	*0.27*
† The Netherlands	1.60	*0.03*	0.57	*0.01*
† The Netherlands, Eindhoven	-	-	-	-
† The Netherlands, Maastricht	1.20	*0.09*	0.58	*0.05*
† Norway	1.05	*0.03*	0.68	*0.03*
*Poland, Cracow	2.02	*0.14*	1.19	*0.09*
*Poland, Kielce	2.23	*0.11*	1.51	*0.08*
*Poland, Lower Silesia	1.44	*0.06*	1.03	*0.04*
Poland, Warsaw City	1.56	*0.09*	1.14	*0.06*
Slovakia	4.74	*0.08*	3.40	*0.06*
Slovenia	2.53	*0.10*	1.79	*0.07*
†*Spain, Albacete	0,05	*0,04*	0,07	*0,04*
† Spain, Asturias	0.06	*0.02*	0,03	*0,01*
† Spain, Basque Country	0.05	*0.01*	0.03	*0.01*
Spain, Granada	5.44	*0.19*	2.89	*0.13*
† Spain, Mallorca	10.33	*0.30*	6.67	*0.22*
Spain, Murcia	6.84	*0.19*	3.68	*0.13*
Spain, Navarra	5.99	*0.23*	3.52	*0.16*
Spain, Tarragona	7.51	*0.25*	4.48	*0.18*
Spain, Zaragoza	2.79	*0.12*	1.15	*0.07*

	MALE		FEMALE	
† Sweden	1.14	*0.02*	0.51	*0.02*
*Switzerland, Basel	10.08	*0.33*	6.75	*0.24*
Switzerland, Geneva	12.69	*0.43*	9.04	*0.31*
Switzerland, Graubunden	1.93	*0.27*	0.58	*0.13*
Switzerland, Neuchatel	9.78	*0.54*	5.76	*0.36*
Switzerland, St Gall-Appenzell	6.35	*0.26*	4.43	*0.20*
Switzerland, Valais	7.59	*0.45*	5.31	*0.34*
Switzerland, Vaud	11.63	*0.32*	8.38	*0.24*
† Switzerland, Zurich	0.10	*0.02*	0.08	*0.02*
*UK, England and Wales	4.81	*0.03*	3.25	*0.02*
*UK, East Anglia	7.16	*0.12*	4.52	*0.09*
*UK, Mersey	4.58	*0.09*	3.97	*0.08*
*UK, North Western	4.37	*0.07*	3.26	*0.06*
UK, Oxford	7.69	*0.13*	4.69	*0.09*
*UK, South Thames	3.96	*0.05*	2.51	*0.04*
UK, South Western	6.29	*0.09*	4.06	*0.07*
† UK, Wessex	2.38	*0.06*	1.46	*0.04*
*UK, West Midlands	6.16	*0.07*	4.24	*0.06*
UK, Yorkshire	5.19	*0.08*	3.54	*0.06*
UK, Scotland	6.14	*0.08*	3.94	*0.05*
UK, Scotland, West	5.26	*0.10*	3.40	*0.07*
*Yugoslavia, Vojvodina	2.45	*0.08*	1.93	*0.06*

OCEANIA

	MALE		FEMALE	
Australian Capital Territory				
Australia, New South Wales				
South Australia				
Australia, Tasmania				
Australia, Victoria				
Western Australia				
*French Polynesia				
† New Zealand: Non-Maori	0,00	*0,00*	-	-
† New Zealand: Maori	-	-	-	-
† US, Hawaii: White	0,09	*0,04*	0,11	*0,04*
† US, Hawaii: Japanese	0,09	*0,03*	0,08	*0,03*
† US, Hawaii: Hawaiian	0,17	*0,08*	0,11	*0,07*
† US, Hawaii: Filipino	0,07	*0,05*	0,02	*0,02*
† US, Hawaii: Chinese	0,04	*0,04*	-	-

* IMPORTANT-SEE NOTES ON POPULATION PAGE

CUMULATIVE INCIDENCE (0-74)
RATES AND STANDARD ERRORS (percent)
Breast (ICD-9 174/175)

	MALE		FEMALE	
AFRICA				
*Algeria, Setif				
*France, La Reunion				
*Mali, Bamako				
*Uganda, Kyadondo				
*Zimbabwe, Harare: African				
*Zimbabwe, Harare: European				
AMERICA, CENTRAL AND SOUTH				
*Argentina, Concordia	0,04	0,04	7.29	0.60
*Brazil, Belem	0,11	0,05	3.51	0.22
*Brazil, Goiania				
*Brazil, Porto Alegre	0,07	0,03	7.06	0.23 m
Colombia, Cali	0,03	0,01	4.40	0.16
*Costa Rica	0,03	0,01	3.13	0.10
*Ecuador, Quito	0,03	0,02	3.04	0.15 m
*Peru, Lima	0,02	0,01	3.66	0.11
Peru, Trujillo	0,07	0,07	3.17	0.30
US, Puerto Rico	0.04	0.01	5.14	0.10
*Uruguay, Montevideo	0.06	0.02	10.73	0.22
AMERICA, NORTH				
Canada	0.07	0.00	8.85	0.04
Canada, Alberta	0.07	0.01	9.04	0.14
Canada, British Columbia	0.05	0.01	9.78	0.11
Canada, Manitoba	0.06	0.02	9.16	0.19
Canada, New Brunswick	0,07	0,02	8.58	0.23
Canada, Newfoundland	0,08	0,03	7.03	0.26
Canada, Northwest Territories	0,22	0,16	6.14	0.85
Canada, Nova Scotia	0,04	0,02	9.05	0.21
Canada, Ontario	0.07	0.01	8.98	0.06
Canada, Prince Edward Island	0,08	0,06	9.26	0.58
Canada, Quebec	0.08	0.01	8.19	0.07
Canada, Saskatchewan	0.06	0.02	9.17	0.20
Canada, Yukon	-	-	8.94	1.41
US, Cent. Calif.: Non-Hisp. White	0.04	0.01	10.08	0.17
US, Cent. Calif.: Hispanic	0,10	0,05	6.13	0.30
US, Los Angeles: Non-Hisp. White	0.11	0.01	12.12	0.11
US, Los Angeles: Hispanic White	0.04	0.01	6.65	0.14
US, Los Angeles: Black	0,06	0,02	9.14	0.22
US, Los Angeles: Chinese	0,02	0,02	3.90	0.28
US, Los Angeles: Filipino	-	-	7.52	0.40
US, Los Angeles: Korean	-	-	2.19	0.26
US, Los Angeles: Japanese	0,09	0,06	7.01	0.43
US, San Francisco: Non-Hisp. White	0.11	0.02	11.99	0.15
US, San Francisco: Hispanic White	0,10	0,05	8.15	0.34
US, San Francisco: Black	0.18	0.06	9.37	0.33
US, San Francisco: Chinese	0,06	0,04	6.01	0.33
US, San Francisco: Filipino	0,05	0,05	7.30	0.45
US, San Francisco: Japanese	-	-	7.89	0.75
US, Connecticut: White	0.10	0.01	10.71	0.12
US, Connecticut: Black	0,11	0,06	9.44	0.45
US, Atlanta: White	0.04	0.01	10.31	0.19
US, Atlanta: Black	0.24	0.07	7.88	0.29
US, Iowa	0.08	0.01	9.74	0.12

	MALE		FEMALE	
US, Central Louisiana: White	0,06	0,03	7.11	0.37
US, Central Louisiana: Black	0,15	0,12	6.56	0.68
US, New Orleans: White	0.09	0.03	10.07	0.25
US, New Orleans: Black	0,14	0,06	9.36	0.36
US, Detroit: White	0.11	0.01	10.68	0.12
US, Detroit: Black	0.10	0.03	9.18	0.22
US, New Mexico: Non-Hisp. White	0.06	0.02	9.96	0.22
US, New Mexico: Hispanic White	0,04	0,02	7.01	0.28
US, New Mexico: American Indian	0,07	0,07	2.97	0.39
US, Utah	0.09	0.02	8.87	0.18
US, Seattle	0.09	0.01	10.77	0.12
US, SEER: White	0.09	0.01	10.48	0.05
US, SEER: Black	0.15	0.02	8.93	0.14
ASIA				
*China, Qidong	0,00	0,00	1.18	0.07
China, Shanghai	0.05	0.01	2.80	0.04
China, Tianjin	0.04	0.01	2.60	0.06
Hong Kong	0.03	0.01	3.65	0.06
*India, Bangalore	0.03	0.01	2.29	0.07
*India, Barshi, Paranda and Bhum	-	-	1.05	0.13
India, Bombay	0.08	0.01	3.17	0.07
*India, Karunagappally	-	-	1.52	0.22
India, Madras	0.03	0.01	2.54	0.08
*India, Trivandrum	0,09	0,06	2.07	0.19
Israel: All Jews	0.13	0.01	8.73	0.11
Jews born in Israel	0.25	0.09	10.09	0.39
Jews born in America or Europe	0.15	0.02	9.95	0.17
Jews born in Africa or Asia	0.09	0.02	6.26	0.16
Non-Jews	0,09	0,05	2.31	0.17
Japan, Hiroshima	0,04	0,02	3.62	0.12
Japan, Miyagi	0.04	0.01	3.31	0.07
Japan, Nagasaki	0,01	0,01	2.84	0.08
Japan, Osaka	0.02	0.00	2.63	0.03
*Japan, Saga	0,04	0,01	2.05	0.09
Japan, Yamagata	0,02	0,01	2.37	0.08
*Korea, Kangwha	0,05	0,05	0.76	0.16
*Kuwait: Non-Kuwaitis	0,02	0,01	3.49	0.32
*Kuwait: Kuwaitis	-	-	3.73	0.34
*Philippines, Manila	0.11	0.02	5.37	0.12
Singapore: Chinese	0,01	0,01	4.18	0.11
Singapore: Malay	0,04	0,03	3.61	0.27
Singapore: Indian	0,04	0,04	3.77	0.47
Thailand, Chiang Mai	0,01	0,01	1.56	0.08
*Thailand, Khon Kaen	-	-	0.88	0.07
*Viet Nam, Hanoi				

* IMPORTANT-SEE NOTES ON POPULATION PAGE

CUMULATIVE INCIDENCE (0-74)
RATES AND STANDARD ERRORS (percent)
Breast (ICD-9 174/175) (contd)

EUROPE	MALE		FEMALE	
Austria, Tyrol	0,04	0,02	7.36	0.23
*Belarus	0.04	0.01	3.27	0.03
*Croatia	0.06	0.01	4.12	0.06
Czech Republic	0.06	0.01	5.08	0.04
Denmark	0.05	0.01	8.18	0.08
Estonia	0.06	0.02	4.04	0.10
Finland	0.04	0.01	7.12	0.07
France, Bas-Rhin	0.17	0.03	9.01	0.20
*France, Calvados	0.12	0.03	8.41	0.24
France, Doubs	0,05	0,03	7.43	0.26
France, Haut-Rhin	0,03	0,01	9.15	0.24
*France, Herault	0.07	0.02	8.98	0.20
France, Isere	0.09	0.02	9.68	0.21
*France, Somme	0,09	0,03	7.61	0.24
*France, Tarn	0,03	0,02	6.92	0.27
Germany, Eastern States	0.06	0.01	5.46	0.06
Germany, Saarland	0,03	0,01	6.94	0.15
Iceland	0,12	0,06	8.91	0.42
Ireland, Southern	0,07	0,03	7.04	0.25
Italy, Ferrara	0,11	0,06	8.06	0.40
Italy, Florence	0.07	0.02	7.48	0.16
Italy, Genoa	0.07	0.02	8.04	0.18
*Italy, Latina	0,04	0,02	5.69	0.26
Italy, Macerata	0,09	0,05	6.49	0.43
Italy, Modena	0,05	0,02	7.76	0.20
Italy, Parma	0,08	0,03	7.87	0.25
Italy, Ragusa	0,06	0,03	4.85	0.25
Italy, Romagna	0.09	0.03	7.43	0.22
Italy, Torino	0.08	0.02	7.23	0.17
Italy, Trieste	0,12	0,05	7.28	0.31
Italy, Varese	0.11	0.03	8.32	0.20
Italy, Veneto	0.11	0.02	8.16	0.16
*Latvia	0.04	0.01	3.71	0.07
Malta	0,07	0,05	8.80	0.51
The Netherlands	0.06	0.01	8.98	0.06
The Netherlands, Eindhoven	0.06	0.02	7.85	0.19
The Netherlands, Maastricht	0.07	0.02	8.23	0.19
Norway	0.04	0.01	5.96	0.07
*Poland, Cracow	0,01	0,01	4.97	0.16
*Poland, Kielce	0.05	0.02	2.86	0.10
*Poland, Lower Silesia	0.05	0.01	3.77	0.08
Poland, Warsaw City	0.08	0.02	4.95	0.12
Slovakia	0.06	0.01	4.38	0.06
Slovenia	0.06	0.01	5.25	0.10
*Spain, Albacete	0,03	0,03	4.97	0.37
Spain, Asturias	0.04	0.01	5.05	0.14
Spain, Basque Country	0.04	0.01	5.07	0.11
Spain, Granada	0,04	0,02	4.11	0.14
Spain, Mallorca	0,02	0,01	5.63	0.19
Spain, Murcia	0,04	0,02	4.91	0.14
Spain, Navarra	0,05	0,02	6.81	0.22
Spain, Tarragona	0.08	0.03	5.63	0.20
Spain, Zaragoza	0,02	0,01	4.44	0.14

	MALE		FEMALE	
Sweden	0.05	0.01	8.40	0.06
*Switzerland, Basel	0,06	0,02	8.22	0.26
Switzerland, Geneva	0,06	0,03	8.70	0.29
Switzerland, Graubunden	0,07	0,05	7.04	0.45
Switzerland, Neuchatel	0,03	0,03	7.83	0.41
Switzerland, St Gall-Appenzell	0,05	0,02	6.16	0.23
Switzerland, Valais	0,13	0,06	7.26	0.38
Switzerland, Vaud	0.08	0.03	8.54	0.23
Switzerland, Zurich	0.04	0.01	7.39	0.15
*UK, England and Wales	0.06	0.00	7.72	0.03
*UK, East Anglia	0.04	0.01	8.65	0.13
*UK, Mersey	0.04	0.01	7.42	0.11
*UK, North Western	0.06	0.01	7.64	0.08
UK, Oxford	0.07	0.01	9.07	0.12
*UK, South Thames	0.06	0.01	7.92	0.07
UK, South Western	0.06	0.01	8.17	0.09
UK, Wessex	0.06	0.01	8.40	0.10
*UK, West Midlands	0.07	0.01	8.70	0.08
UK, Yorkshire	0.07	0.01	7.70	0.09
UK, Scotland	0.05	0.01	8.01	0.08
UK, Scotland, West	0.05	0.01	7.86	0.10
*Yugoslavia, Vojvodina	0.06	0.01	4.84	0.09

OCEANIA	MALE		FEMALE	
Australian Capital Territory	0,03	0,03	7.44	0.41
Australia, New South Wales	0.08	0.01	7.50	0.07
South Australia	0.08	0.02	7.59	0.15
Australia, Tasmania	0,05	0,02	6.16	0.24
Australia, Victoria	0.06	0.01	7.41	0.09
Western Australia	0.05	0.01	8.04	0.16
*French Polynesia	0,17	0,07	7.11	0.63
New Zealand: Non-Maori	0.08	0.01	8.54	0.11
New Zealand: Maori	0,04	0,02	8.47	0.53
US, Hawaii: White	0,10	0,05	11.17	0.45
US, Hawaii: Japanese	0,04	0,02	8.47	0.31
US, Hawaii: Hawaiian	0,06	0,05	9.86	0.60
US, Hawaii: Filipino	0,03	0,03	6.09	0.42
US, Hawaii: Chinese	0,05	0,05	6.48	0.58

* IMPORTANT-SEE NOTES ON POPULATION PAGE

CUMULATIVE INCIDENCE (0-74)
RATES AND STANDARD ERRORS (percent)
Uterus (ICD-9 179)

	MALE	FEMALE
AFRICA		
*Algeria, Setif		
*France, La Reunion		
*Mali, Bamako		
*Uganda, Kyadondo		
*Zimbabwe, Harare: African		
*Zimbabwe, Harare: European		
AMERICA, CENTRAL AND SOUTH		
*Argentina, Concordia	0.59	0.18
*Brazil, Belem	0.22	0.05
*Brazil, Goiania		
*Brazil, Porto Alegre	1.01	0.09
Colombia, Cali	0.07	0.02
*Costa Rica	0.08	0.02
*Ecuador, Quito	0.28	0.05
*Peru, Lima	0.08	0.02
Peru, Trujillo	0,06	0,05
US, Puerto Rico	0.05	0.01
*Uruguay, Montevideo	0.13	0.03
AMERICA, NORTH		
Canada	0.06	0.00
Canada, Alberta	0.04	0.01
Canada, British Columbia	0.02	0.01
Canada, Manitoba	0.08	0.02
Canada, New Brunswick	0,03	0,02
Canada, Newfoundland	0.11	0.03
Canada, Northwest Territories	0,03	0,03
Canada, Nova Scotia	0,03	0,01
Canada, Ontario	0.04	0.00
Canada, Prince Edward Island	0,15	0,08
Canada, Quebec	0.11	0.01
Canada, Saskatchewan	0,02	0,01
Canada, Yukon	-	-
US, Cent. Calif.: Non-Hisp. White	0,01	0,01
US, Cent. Calif.: Hispanic	-	-
US, Los Angeles: Non-Hisp. White	0.02	0.00
US, Los Angeles: Hispanic White	0,01	0,01
US, Los Angeles: Black	0,04	0,01
US, Los Angeles: Chinese	0,02	0,02
US, Los Angeles: Filipino	-	-
US, Los Angeles: Korean	-	-
US, Los Angeles: Japanese	-	-
US, San Francisco: Non-Hisp. White	0,01	0,00
US, San Francisco: Hispanic White	0,03	0,02
US, San Francisco: Black	0.11	0.04
US, San Francisco: Chinese	0,07	0,04
US, San Francisco: Filipino	0,02	0,02
US, San Francisco: Japanese	-	-
US, Connecticut: White	0.05	0.01
US, Connecticut: Black	0,14	0,06
US, Atlanta: White	0,01	0,00
US, Atlanta: Black	0,09	0,04
US, Iowa	0.02	0.00

	MALE	FEMALE
US, Central Louisiana: White	-	-
US, Central Louisiana: Black	0,32	0,16
US, New Orleans: White	0.08	0.02
US, New Orleans: Black	0,07	0,03
US, Detroit: White	0.02	0.01
US, Detroit: Black	0,03	0,01
US, New Mexico: Non-Hisp. White	0,03	0,01
US, New Mexico: Hispanic White	0,03	0,02
US, New Mexico: American Indian	0,02	0,02
US, Utah	0,02	0,01
US, Seattle	0,01	0,00
US, SEER: White	0.02	0.00
US, SEER: Black	0.07	0.01
ASIA		
*China, Qidong	0.10	0.02
China, Shanghai	0.06	0.01
China, Tianjin	0.10	0.01
Hong Kong	0.02	0.00
*India, Bangalore	0.03	0.01
*India, Barshi, Paranda and Bhum	-	-
India, Bombay	0.15	0.02
*India, Karunagappally	-	-
India, Madras	0.04	0.01
*India, Trivandrum	0,06	0,04
Israel: All Jews	0.06	0.01
Jews born in Israel	0,03	0,01
Jews born in America or Europe	0.08	0.02
Jews born in Africa or Asia	0.04	0.01
Non-Jews	0,01	0,01
Japan, Hiroshima	0.05	0.01
Japan, Miyagi	0.04	0.01
Japan, Nagasaki	0.06	0.01
Japan, Osaka	0.11	0.01
*Japan, Saga	0.13	0.02
Japan, Yamagata	0.05	0.01
*Korea, Kangwha	0,04	0,04
*Kuwait: Non-Kuwaitis	0,04	0,04
*Kuwait: Kuwaitis	0,01	0,01
*Philippines, Manila	0.40	0.03
Singapore: Chinese	-	-
Singapore: Malay	-	-
Singapore: Indian	-	-
Thailand, Chiang Mai	-	-
*Thailand, Khon Kaen	0,02	0,01
*Viet Nam, Hanoi		

* IMPORTANT-SEE NOTES ON POPULATION PAGE

CUMULATIVE INCIDENCE (0-74)
RATES AND STANDARD ERRORS (percent)
Uterus (ICD-9 179) (contd)

EUROPE	MALE	FEMALE
Austria, Tyrol	0.07	0.02
*Belarus	0.01	0.00
*Croatia	0.17	0.01
Czech Republic	0.01	0.00
Denmark	0.06	0.01
Estonia	-	-
Finland	0.02	0.00
France, Bas-Rhin	0.08	0.02
*France, Calvados	0,05	0,02
France, Doubs	0,05	0,02
France, Haut-Rhin	0,02	0,01
*France, Herault	0,03	0,01
France, Isere	0.07	0.02
*France, Somme	0.08	0.03
*France, Tarn	0,01	0,01
Germany, Eastern States	0.01	0.00
Germany, Saarland	0.14	0.02
Iceland	0,02	0,02
Ireland, Southern	0,05	0,02
Italy, Ferrara	0,04	0,03
Italy, Florence	0.07	0.02
Italy, Genoa	0.10	0.02
*Italy, Latina	0.18	0.05
Italy, Macerata	0,23	0,08
Italy, Modena	0,04	0,01
Italy, Parma	0.13	0.03
Italy, Ragusa	0,08	0,03
Italy, Romagna	0,03	0,01
Italy, Torino	0,02	0,01
Italy, Trieste	0,08	0,03
Italy, Varese	0,01	0,01
Italy, Veneto	0.26	0.03
*Latvia	0,00	0,00
Malta	0,09	0,06
The Netherlands	0.00	0.00
The Netherlands, Eindhoven	-	-
The Netherlands, Maastricht	0,00	0,00
Norway	0,01	0,00
*Poland, Cracow	0.05	0.02
*Poland, Kielce	0.04	0.01
*Poland, Lower Silesia	0.11	0.01
Poland, Warsaw City	0.03	0.01
Slovakia	0.02	0.01
Slovenia	0.07	0.01
*Spain, Albacete	0,18	0,07
Spain, Asturias	0.11	0.02
Spain, Basque Country	0.06	0.01
Spain, Granada	0,01	0,01
Spain, Mallorca	0,05	0,02
Spain, Murcia	0.04	0.01
Spain, Navarra	0.12	0.03
Spain, Tarragona	0,03	0,01
Spain, Zaragoza	0.09	0.02

	MALE	FEMALE
Sweden	0.18	0.01
*Switzerland, Basel	-	-
Switzerland, Geneva	0,01	0,01
Switzerland, Graubunden	0,06	0,04
Switzerland, Neuchatel	0,05	0,04
Switzerland, St Gall-Appenzell	0,05	0,02
Switzerland, Valais	0,04	0,03
Switzerland, Vaud	0,01	0,01
Switzerland, Zurich	0,02	0,01
*UK, England and Wales	0.09	0.00
*UK, East Anglia	0.02	0.01
*UK, Mersey	0.02	0.01
*UK, North Western	0.12	0.01
UK, Oxford	0.02	0.01
*UK, South Thames	0.00	0.00
UK, South Western	0.12	0.01
UK, Wessex	0.11	0.01
*UK, West Midlands	0.12	0.01
UK, Yorkshire	0.13	0.01
UK, Scotland	0.10	0.01
UK, Scotland, West	0.14	0.01
*Yugoslavia, Vojvodina	0.19	0.02

OCEANIA	MALE	FEMALE
Australian Capital Territory	0,08	0,04
Australia, New South Wales	0.05	0.01
South Australia	-	-
Australia, Tasmania	-	-
Australia, Victoria	-	-
Western Australia	0,01	0,00
*French Polynesia	1.07	0.29
New Zealand: Non-Maori	0,01	0,00
New Zealand: Maori	-	-
US, Hawaii: White	0,01	0,01
US, Hawaii: Japanese	0,04	0,02
US, Hawaii: Hawaiian	-	-
US, Hawaii: Filipino	0,06	0,04
US, Hawaii: Chinese	0,05	0,05

* IMPORTANT-SEE NOTES ON POPULATION PAGE

CUMULATIVE INCIDENCE (0-74)
RATES AND STANDARD ERRORS (percent)
Cervix uteri (ICD-9 180)

	MALE	FEMALE
AFRICA		
*Algeria, Setif		
*France, La Reunion		
*Mali, Bamako		
*Uganda, Kyadondo		
*Zimbabwe, Harare: African		
*Zimbabwe, Harare: European		
AMERICA, CENTRAL AND SOUTH		
*Argentina, Concordia	3.26	0.35
*Brazil, Belem	6.90	0.28
*Brazil, Goiania		
*Brazil, Porto Alegre	2.28	0.12
Colombia, Cali	3.73	0.14
*Costa Rica	2.57	0.09
*Ecuador, Quito	3.67	0.17
*Peru, Lima	3.05	0.10
Peru, Trujillo	5.76	0.42
US, Puerto Rico	1.03	0.04
*Uruguay, Montevideo	1.92	0.09
AMERICA, NORTH		
Canada	0.78	0.01
Canada, Alberta	0.86	0.04
Canada, British Columbia	0.65	0.03
Canada, Manitoba	0.78	0.05
Canada, New Brunswick	0.75	0.06
Canada, Newfoundland	1.10	0.09
Canada, Northwest Territories	1.50	0.41
Canada, Nova Scotia	1.10	0.07
Canada, Ontario	0.84	0.02
Canada, Prince Edward Island	0.94	0.17
Canada, Quebec	0.67	0.02
Canada, Saskatchewan	0.71	0.05
Canada, Yukon	1.14	0.43
US, Cent. Calif.: Non-Hisp. White	0.76	0.04
US, Cent. Calif.: Hispanic	1.77	0.15
US, Los Angeles: Non-Hisp. White	0.72	0.03
US, Los Angeles: Hispanic White	1.82	0.07
US, Los Angeles: Black	1.23	0.08
US, Los Angeles: Chinese	0.91	0.14
US, Los Angeles: Filipino	1.12	0.17
US, Los Angeles: Korean	1.59	0.24
US, Los Angeles: Japanese	0.40	0.10
US, San Francisco: Non-Hisp. White	0.63	0.03
US, San Francisco: Hispanic White	1.35	0.13
US, San Francisco: Black	1.01	0.10
US, San Francisco: Chinese	0.66	0.11
US, San Francisco: Filipino	1.02	0.16
US, San Francisco: Japanese	0.52	0.17
US, Connecticut: White	0.67	0.03
US, Connecticut: Black	1.38	0.17
US, Atlanta: White	0.69	0.04
US, Atlanta: Black	1.25	0.11
US, Iowa	0.80	0.03

	MALE	FEMALE
US, Central Louisiana: White	0.72	0.11
US, Central Louisiana: Black	1.17	0.27
US, New Orleans: White	0.64	0.06
US, New Orleans: Black	1.48	0.13
US, Detroit: White	0.77	0.03
US, Detroit: Black	1.27	0.08
US, New Mexico: Non-Hisp. White	0.88	0.06
US, New Mexico: Hispanic White	0.91	0.09
US, New Mexico: American Indian	0.85	0.21
US, Utah	0.75	0.05
US, Seattle	0.74	0.03
US, SEER: White	0.74	0.01
US, SEER: Black	1.22	0.05
ASIA		
*China, Qidong	0.30	0.04
China, Shanghai	0.43	0.02
China, Tianjin	0.61	0.03
Hong Kong	1.74	0.04
*India, Bangalore	2.99	0.08
*India, Barshi, Paranda and Bhum	2.91	0.20
India, Bombay	2.30	0.05
*India, Karunagappally	1.85	0.28
India, Madras	4.35	0.10
*India, Trivandrum	1.83	0.19
Israel: All Jews	0.54	0.03
Jews born in Israel	0.62	0.08
Jews born in America or Europe	0.43	0.04
Jews born in Africa or Asia	0.62	0.05
Non-Jews	0.29	0.05
Japan, Hiroshima	1.35	0.07
Japan, Miyagi	0.68	0.03
Japan, Nagasaki	1.19	0.05
Japan, Osaka	1.00	0.02
*Japan, Saga	0.74	0.05
Japan, Yamagata	0.57	0.04
*Korea, Kangwha	2.20	0.27
*Kuwait: Non-Kuwaitis	0.55	0.14
*Kuwait: Kuwaitis	0.76	0.17
*Philippines, Manila	2.47	0.08
Singapore: Chinese	1.78	0.07
Singapore: Malay	1.22	0.15
Singapore: Indian	0.92	0.23
Thailand, Chiang Mai	2.71	0.11
*Thailand, Khon Kaen	2.11	0.11
*Viet Nam, Hanoi		

* IMPORTANT-SEE NOTES ON POPULATION PAGE

CUMULATIVE INCIDENCE (0-74)
RATES AND STANDARD ERRORS (percent)
Cervix uteri (ICD-9 180) (contd)

EUROPE	MALE	FEMALE
Austria, Tyrol	1.81	0.11
*Belarus	1.26	0.02
*Croatia	1.22	0.03
Czech Republic	1.63	0.02
Denmark	1.58	0.03
Estonia	1.57	0.06
Finland	0.38	0.02
France, Bas-Rhin	1.02	0.06
*France, Calvados	1.13	0.09
France, Doubs	0.80	0.08
France, Haut-Rhin	1.26	0.09
*France, Herault	1.40	0.08
France, Isere	1.07	0.07
*France, Somme	1.08	0.09
*France, Tarn	0.83	0.09
Germany, Eastern States	2.05	0.03
Germany, Saarland	1.17	0.06
Iceland	0.77	0.11
Ireland, Southern	0.66	0.07
Italy, Ferrara	0.77	0.12
Italy, Florence	0.67	0.05
Italy, Genoa	0.82	0.06
*Italy, Latina	0.73	0.09
Italy, Macerata	0.26	0.08
Italy, Modena	0.64	0.06
Italy, Parma	0.61	0.07
Italy, Ragusa	0.78	0.10
Italy, Romagna	1.08	0.08
Italy, Torino	0.90	0.06
Italy, Trieste	1.30	0.13
Italy, Varese	0.69	0.05
Italy, Veneto	0.59	0.04
*Latvia	1.05	0.04
Malta	0.71	0.14
The Netherlands	0.73	0.01
The Netherlands, Eindhoven	0.63	0.05
The Netherlands, Maastricht	0.77	0.06
Norway	1.27	0.03
*Poland, Cracow	2.19	0.10
*Poland, Kielce	1.59	0.07
*Poland, Lower Silesia	2.31	0.06
Poland, Warsaw City	1.61	0.06
Slovakia	1.66	0.04
Slovenia	1.26	0.05
*Spain, Albacete	0.65	0.13
Spain, Asturias	0.86	0.06
Spain, Basque Country	0.62	0.04
Spain, Granada	0.61	0.06
Spain, Mallorca	1.37	0.09
Spain, Murcia	0.82	0.06
Spain, Navarra	0.51	0.06
Spain, Tarragona	1.01	0.08
Spain, Zaragoza	0.51	0.05

	MALE	FEMALE
Sweden	0.79	0.02
*Switzerland, Basel	0.60	0.07
Switzerland, Geneva	0.67	0.08
Switzerland, Graubunden	0.91	0.15
Switzerland, Neuchatel	1.00	0.15
Switzerland, St Gall-Appenzell	0.92	0.08
Switzerland, Valais	0.76	0.12
Switzerland, Vaud	0.72	0.07
Switzerland, Zurich	0.69	0.05
*UK, England and Wales	1.27	0.01
*UK, East Anglia	1.02	0.04
*UK, Mersey	1.42	0.05
*UK, North Western	1.46	0.04
UK, Oxford	0.98	0.04
*UK, South Thames	0.92	0.02
UK, South Western	1.02	0.03
UK, Wessex	1.14	0.04
*UK, West Midlands	1.34	0.03
UK, Yorkshire	1.45	0.04
UK, Scotland	1.28	0.03
UK, Scotland, West	1.30	0.04
*Yugoslavia, Vojvodina	1.90	0.06

OCEANIA	MALE	FEMALE
Australian Capital Territory	1.17	0.16
Australia, New South Wales	1.01	0.03
South Australia	0.85	0.05
Australia, Tasmania	1.11	0.10
Australia, Victoria	0.96	0.03
Western Australia	1.18	0.06
*French Polynesia	3.04	0.39
New Zealand: Non-Maori	1.19	0.04
New Zealand: Maori	3.40	0.30
US, Hawaii: White	1.02	0.12
US, Hawaii: Japanese	0.60	0.08
US, Hawaii: Hawaiian	1.00	0.18
US, Hawaii: Filipino	0.68	0.13
US, Hawaii: Chinese	0,39	0,13

* IMPORTANT-SEE NOTES ON POPULATION PAGE

CUMULATIVE INCIDENCE (0-74)
RATES AND STANDARD ERRORS (percent)
Placenta (ICD-9 181)

	MALE	FEMALE			MALE	FEMALE
AFRICA				US, Central Louisiana: White	-	-
*Algeria, Setif				US, Central Louisiana: Black	-	-
*France, La Reunion				US, New Orleans: White	0,01	0,01
*Mali, Bamako				US, New Orleans: Black	0,01	0,01
*Uganda, Kyadondo				US, Detroit: White	0,00	0,00
				US, Detroit: Black	0,01	0,00
*Zimbabwe, Harare: African				US, New Mexico: Non-Hisp. White	-	-
*Zimbabwe, Harare: European				US, New Mexico: Hispanic White	0,01	0,01
				US, New Mexico: American Indian	-	-
AMERICA, CENTRAL AND SOUTH				US, Utah	0,01	0,01
*Argentina, Concordia	-	-		US, Seattle	0.01	0.00
				US, SEER: White	0.01	0.00
*Brazil, Belem	0,03	0,01	f	US, SEER: Black	0,01	0,00
*Brazil, Goiania						
*Brazil, Porto Alegre	0,00	0,00		**ASIA**		
Colombia, Cali	0.02	0.01		*China, Qidong	0.03	0.01
*Costa Rica	0.02	0.01		China, Shanghai	0.01	0.00
*Ecuador, Quito	0.02	0.01		China, Tianjin	0.04	0.01
*Peru, Lima	0.05	0.01		Hong Kong	0,00	0,00
Peru, Trujillo	0,01	0,01		*India, Bangalore	0,00	0,00
US, Puerto Rico	0,01	0,00		*India, Barshi, Paranda and Bhum	-	-
*Uruguay, Montevideo	0,01	0,00		India, Bombay	0.02	0.00
				*India, Karunagappally	-	-
AMERICA, NORTH				India, Madras	0.01	0.00
Canada	0.00	0.00		*India, Trivandrum	-	-
Canada, Alberta	0,00	0,00		Israel: All Jews	0.01	0.00
Canada, British Columbia	0,00	0,00		Jews born in Israel	0,01	0,00
Canada, Manitoba	-	-		Jews born in America or Europe	0,01	0,00
Canada, New Brunswick	0,00	0,00		Jews born in Africa or Asia	0,02	0,01
Canada, Newfoundland	-	-		Non-Jews	0,01	0,01
Canada, Northwest Territories	0,11	0,09		Japan, Hiroshima	0,00	0,00
Canada, Nova Scotia	-	-		Japan, Miyagi	0,01	0,00
Canada, Ontario	0.00	0.00		Japan, Nagasaki	0,01	0,00
Canada, Prince Edward Island	0,02	0,02		Japan, Osaka	0.00	0.00
Canada, Quebec	0.01	0.00		*Japan, Saga	0,01	0,00
Canada, Saskatchewan	-	-		Japan, Yamagata	0,01	0,00
Canada, Yukon	-	-		*Korea, Kangwha	-	-
US, Cent. Calif.: Non-Hisp. White	0,00	0,00		*Kuwait: Non-Kuwaitis	0,02	0,01
US, Cent. Calif.: Hispanic	0,01	0,00		*Kuwait: Kuwaitis	0,06	0,02
US, Los Angeles: Non-Hisp. White	0,00	0,00		*Philippines, Manila	0.03	0.01
US, Los Angeles: Hispanic White	0.01	0.00		Singapore: Chinese	0,01	0,00
US, Los Angeles: Black	0,00	0,00		Singapore: Malay	0,01	0,01
US, Los Angeles: Chinese	-	-		Singapore: Indian	-	-
US, Los Angeles: Filipino	-	-		Thailand, Chiang Mai	0,02	0,01
US, Los Angeles: Korean	-	-		*Thailand, Khon Kaen	0.02	0.01
US, Los Angeles: Japanese	-	-		*Viet Nam, Hanoi		
US, San Francisco: Non-Hisp. White	0,01	0,00				
US, San Francisco: Hispanic White	0,01	0,01				
US, San Francisco: Black	0,01	0,01				
US, San Francisco: Chinese	-	-				
US, San Francisco: Filipino	0,01	0,01				
US, San Francisco: Japanese	-	-				
US, Connecticut: White	0,00	0,00				
US, Connecticut: Black	0,01	0,01				
US, Atlanta: White	0,01	0,00				
US, Atlanta: Black	0,01	0,00				
US, Iowa	0,00	0,00				

* IMPORTANT-SEE NOTES ON POPULATION PAGE

EUROPE	MALE	FEMALE
Austria, Tyrol	-	-
*Belarus	0.01	0.00
*Croatia	0.01	0.00
Czech Republic	0.01	0.00
Denmark	0.00	0.00
Estonia	0.02	0.01
Finland	0.01	0.00
France, Bas-Rhin	-	-
*France, Calvados	0.00	0.00
France, Doubs	0.03	0.01
France, Haut-Rhin	0.01	0.01
*France, Herault	-	-
France, Isere	0.00	0.00
*France, Somme	0.00	0.00
*France, Tarn	-	-
Germany, Eastern States	0.01	0.00
Germany, Saarland	0.01	0.01
Iceland	-	-
Ireland, Southern	-	-
Italy, Ferrara	-	-
Italy, Florence	0.01	0.00
Italy, Genoa	0.00	0.00
*Italy, Latina	0.01	0.01
Italy, Macerata	-	-
Italy, Modena	-	-
Italy, Parma	0.01	0.01
Italy, Ragusa	-	-
Italy, Romagna	-	-
Italy, Torino	0.00	0.00
Italy, Trieste	-	-
Italy, Varese	0.00	0.00
Italy, Veneto	0.00	0.00
*Latvia	0.02	0.00
Malta	-	-
The Netherlands	0.01	0.00
The Netherlands, Eindhoven	-	-
The Netherlands, Maastricht	-	-
Norway	0.02	0.00
*Poland, Cracow	-	-
*Poland, Kielce	-	-
*Poland, Lower Silesia	0.01	0.00
Poland, Warsaw City	0.03	0.01
Slovakia	0.01	0.00
Slovenia	0.01	0.00
*Spain, Albacete	-	-
Spain, Asturias	0.01	0.00
Spain, Basque Country	0.00	0.00
Spain, Granada	0.01	0.01
Spain, Mallorca	-	-
Spain, Murcia	0.00	0.00
Spain, Navarra	0.02	0.01
Spain, Tarragona	0.00	0.00
Spain, Zaragoza	-	-

	MALE	FEMALE
Sweden	0.01	0.00
*Switzerland, Basel	-	-
Switzerland, Geneva	0.02	0.01
Switzerland, Graubunden	0.02	0.02
Switzerland, Neuchatel	0.02	0.02
Switzerland, St Gall-Appenzell	0.01	0.01
Switzerland, Valais	-	-
Switzerland, Vaud	0.00	0.00
Switzerland, Zurich	0.00	0.00
*UK, England and Wales	0.00	0.00
*UK, East Anglia	0.00	0.00
*UK, Mersey	-	-
*UK, North Western	0.00	0.00
UK, Oxford	0.00	0.00
*UK, South Thames	0.00	0.00
UK, South Western	0.00	0.00
UK, Wessex	0.00	0.00
*UK, West Midlands	0.00	0.00
UK, Yorkshire	0.00	0.00
UK, Scotland	0.00	0.00
UK, Scotland, West	0.00	0.00
*Yugoslavia, Vojvodina	0.01	0.00

OCEANIA	MALE	FEMALE
Australian Capital Territory	0.01	0.01
Australia, New South Wales	0.01	0.00
South Australia	0.01	0.00
Australia, Tasmania	-	-
Australia, Victoria	0.01	0.00
Western Australia	-	-
*French Polynesia	-	-
New Zealand: Non-Maori	0.03	0.01
New Zealand: Maori	0.02	0.01
US, Hawaii: White	0.01	0.01
US, Hawaii: Japanese	0.01	0.01
US, Hawaii: Hawaiian	-	-
US, Hawaii: Filipino	0.02	0.02
US, Hawaii: Chinese	-	-

* IMPORTANT-SEE NOTES ON POPULATION PAGE

CUMULATIVE INCIDENCE (0-74)
RATES AND STANDARD ERRORS (percent)
Corpus uteri (ICD-9 182)

	MALE	FEMALE
AFRICA		
*Algeria, Setif		
*France, La Reunion		
*Mali, Bamako		
*Uganda, Kyadondo		
*Zimbabwe, Harare: African		
*Zimbabwe, Harare: European		
AMERICA, CENTRAL AND SOUTH		
*Argentina, Concordia	1.11	0.23
*Brazil, Belem	0.24	0.06
*Brazil, Goiania		
*Brazil, Porto Alegre	0.82	0.08
Colombia, Cali	0.83	0.07
*Costa Rica	0.55	0.04
*Ecuador, Quito	0.64	0.07
*Peru, Lima	0.53	0.05
Peru, Trujillo	0.38	0.12
US, Puerto Rico	1.05	0.04
*Uruguay, Montevideo	1.66	0.09
AMERICA, NORTH		
Canada	1.82	0.02
Canada, Alberta	1.93	0.07
Canada, British Columbia	1.80	0.05
Canada, Manitoba	2.13	0.09
Canada, New Brunswick	1.56	0.10
Canada, Newfoundland	1.64	0.13
Canada, Northwest Territories	0,63	0,22
Canada, Nova Scotia	1.72	0.09
Canada, Ontario	1.92	0.03
Canada, Prince Edward Island	1.53	0.24
Canada, Quebec	1.70	0.03
Canada, Saskatchewan	1.65	0.09
Canada, Yukon	2.67	0.73
US, Cent. Calif.: Non-Hisp. White	2.13	0.08
US, Cent. Calif.: Hispanic	1.59	0.16
US, Los Angeles: Non-Hisp. White	2.63	0.05
US, Los Angeles: Hispanic White	1.38	0.07
US, Los Angeles: Black	1.34	0.09
US, Los Angeles: Chinese	0.83	0.14
US, Los Angeles: Filipino	1.32	0.17
US, Los Angeles: Korean	0.35	0.12
US, Los Angeles: Japanese	1.08	0.18
US, San Francisco: Non-Hisp. White	2.41	0.07
US, San Francisco: Hispanic White	1.75	0.16
US, San Francisco: Black	1.44	0.14
US, San Francisco: Chinese	1.44	0.17
US, San Francisco: Filipino	1.06	0.17
US, San Francisco: Japanese	2.07	0.40
US, Connecticut: White	2.31	0.06
US, Connecticut: Black	1.73	0.22
US, Atlanta: White	1.92	0.08
US, Atlanta: Black	1.39	0.14
US, Iowa	2.21	0.06

	MALE	FEMALE
US, Central Louisiana: White	1.07	0.14
US, Central Louisiana: Black	1.17	0.31
US, New Orleans: White	1.15	0.09
US, New Orleans: Black	1.23	0.14
US, Detroit: White	2.47	0.06
US, Detroit: Black	1.44	0.09
US, New Mexico: Non-Hisp. White	1.98	0.10
US, New Mexico: Hispanic White	1.05	0.11
US, New Mexico: American Indian	1.12	0.25
US, Utah	2.47	0.10
US, Seattle	2.54	0.06
US, SEER: White	2.31	0.02
US, SEER: Black	1.45	0.06
ASIA		
*China, Qidong	0.06	0.02
China, Shanghai	0.42	0.02
China, Tianjin	0.30	0.02
Hong Kong	0.78	0.03
*India, Bangalore	0.24	0.03
*India, Barshi, Paranda and Bhum	0,03	0,02
India, Bombay	0.30	0.02
*India, Karunagappally	0,11	0,06
India, Madras	0.25	0.03
*India, Trivandrum	0.28	0.08
Israel: All Jews	1.33	0.04
Jews born in Israel	1.69	0.18
Jews born in America or Europe	1.55	0.07
Jews born in Africa or Asia	0.95	0.06
Non-Jews	0.60	0.09
Japan, Hiroshima	0.59	0.05
Japan, Miyagi	0.47	0.03
Japan, Nagasaki	0.47	0.03
Japan, Osaka	0.35	0.01
*Japan, Saga	0.25	0.03
Japan, Yamagata	0.36	0.03
*Korea, Kangwha	0,03	0,03
*Kuwait: Non-Kuwaitis	0.57	0.17
*Kuwait: Kuwaitis	0.28	0.10
*Philippines, Manila	0.69	0.04
Singapore: Chinese	0.80	0.05
Singapore: Malay	0.69	0.14
Singapore: Indian	0.75	0.22
Thailand, Chiang Mai	0.39	0.04
*Thailand, Khon Kaen	0.21	0.03
*Viet Nam, Hanoi		

* IMPORTANT-SEE NOTES ON POPULATION PAGE

CUMULATIVE INCIDENCE (0-74)
RATES AND STANDARD ERRORS (percent)
Corpus uteri (ICD-9 182) (contd)

EUROPE	MALE	FEMALE
Austria, Tyrol	1.68	0.11
*Belarus	1.31	0.02
*Croatia	1.25	0.04
Czech Republic	2.20	0.03
Denmark	1.96	0.04
Estonia	1.57	0.06
Finland	1.61	0.03
France, Bas-Rhin	2.02	0.10
*France, Calvados	1.07	0.09
France, Doubs	1.23	0.11
France, Haut-Rhin	1.83	0.11
*France, Herault	1.27	0.08
France, Isere	1.27	0.08
*France, Somme	1.22	0.10
*France, Tarn	1.26	0.11
Germany, Eastern States	1.75	0.03
Germany, Saarland	1.64	0.07
Iceland	1.81	0.19
Ireland, Southern	1.05	0.10
Italy, Ferrara	1.56	0.18
Italy, Florence	1.48	0.07
Italy, Genoa	1.03	0.07
*Italy, Latina	1.17	0.12
Italy, Macerata	1.56	0.22
Italy, Modena	1.53	0.09
Italy, Parma	1.53	0.11
Italy, Ragusa	1.32	0.13
Italy, Romagna	1.46	0.10
Italy, Torino	1.37	0.08
Italy, Trieste	1.55	0.14
Italy, Varese	1.56	0.09
Italy, Veneto	1.06	0.06
*Latvia	1.70	0.05
Malta	2.29	0.27
The Netherlands	1.36	0.02
The Netherlands, Eindhoven	1.28	0.08
The Netherlands, Maastricht	1.33	0.08
Norway	1.55	0.04
*Poland, Cracow	1.50	0.09
*Poland, Kielce	1.11	0.06
*Poland, Lower Silesia	1.41	0.05
Poland, Warsaw City	1.60	0.07
Slovakia	1.99	0.04
Slovenia	1.60	0.06
*Spain, Albacete	0.80	0.15
Spain, Asturias	1.40	0.07
Spain, Basque Country	1.13	0.05
Spain, Granada	1.13	0.08
Spain, Mallorca	1.52	0.10
Spain, Murcia	1.38	0.08
Spain, Navarra	1.46	0.10
Spain, Tarragona	1.42	0.10
Spain, Zaragoza	1.07	0.07

	MALE	FEMALE
Sweden	1.68	0.03
*Switzerland, Basel	1.51	0.11
Switzerland, Geneva	1.66	0.14
Switzerland, Graubunden	1.19	0.19
Switzerland, Neuchatel	1.34	0.18
Switzerland, St Gall-Appenzell	1.45	0.11
Switzerland, Valais	1.23	0.16
Switzerland, Vaud	1.73	0.11
Switzerland, Zurich	1.98	0.08
*UK, England and Wales	1.06	0.01
*UK, East Anglia	1.27	0.05
*UK, Mersey	1.10	0.04
*UK, North Western	0.84	0.03
UK, Oxford	1.24	0.05
*UK, South Thames	1.05	0.02
UK, South Western	1.16	0.04
UK, Wessex	1.21	0.04
*UK, West Midlands	1.26	0.03
UK, Yorkshire	0.99	0.03
UK, Scotland	0.89	0.03
UK, Scotland, West	0.78	0.03
*Yugoslavia, Vojvodina	1.19	0.05

OCEANIA	MALE	FEMALE
Australian Capital Territory	0.92	0.15
Australia, New South Wales	1.12	0.03
South Australia	1.31	0.06
Australia, Tasmania	1.34	0.12
Australia, Victoria	1.28	0.04
Western Australia	1.37	0.07
*French Polynesia	0.97	0.23
New Zealand: Non-Maori	1.15	0.04
New Zealand: Maori	1.89	0.27
US, Hawaii: White	2.02	0.20
US, Hawaii: Japanese	1.55	0.13
US, Hawaii: Hawaiian	2.23	0.27
US, Hawaii: Filipino	1.35	0.21
US, Hawaii: Chinese	1.64	0.29

* IMPORTANT-SEE NOTES ON POPULATION PAGE

CUMULATIVE INCIDENCE (0-74)
RATES AND STANDARD ERRORS (percent)
Ovary etc. (ICD-9 183)

	MALE	FEMALE		MALE	FEMALE
AFRICA			US, Central Louisiana: White	1.10	0.14
*Algeria, Setif			US, Central Louisiana: Black	1.03	0.28
*France, La Reunion			US, New Orleans: White	1.21	0.09
*Mali, Bamako			US, New Orleans: Black	0.81	0.11
*Uganda, Kyadondo			US, Detroit: White	1.44	0.04
			US, Detroit: Black	0.89	0.07
*Zimbabwe, Harare: African			US, New Mexico: Non-Hisp. White	1.28	0.08
*Zimbabwe, Harare: European			US, New Mexico: Hispanic White	0.97	0.10
			US, New Mexico: American Indian	1.43	0.28
AMERICA, CENTRAL AND SOUTH			US, Utah	1.19	0.06
*Argentina, Concordia	0.86	0.20	US, Seattle	1.41	0.05
			US, SEER: White	1.38	0.02
*Brazil, Belem	0.51	0.08	US, SEER: Black	0.92	0.05
*Brazil, Goiania					
*Brazil, Porto Alegre	1.04	0.09			
Colombia, Cali	0.97	0.08	**ASIA**		
*Costa Rica	0.61	0.04	*China, Qidong	0.13	0.02
			China, Shanghai	0.62	0.02
*Ecuador, Quito	0.69	0.07	China, Tianjin	0.57	0.03
*Peru, Lima	0.65	0.05	Hong Kong	0.79	0.03
Peru, Trujillo	0.84	0.16			
US, Puerto Rico	0.59	0.03	*India, Bangalore	0.45	0.03
			*India, Barshi, Paranda and Bhum	0.12	0.04
*Uruguay, Montevideo	1.12	0.07	India, Bombay	0.82	0.03
			*India, Karunagappally	0,23	0,09
			India, Madras	0.65	0.04
AMERICA, NORTH			*India, Trivandrum	0.54	0.10
Canada	1.20	0.01	Israel: All Jews	1.33	0.04
Canada, Alberta	1.19	0.05	Jews born in Israel	1.41	0.15
Canada, British Columbia	1.22	0.04	Jews born in America or Europe	1.55	0.07
Canada, Manitoba	1.12	0.07	Jews born in Africa or Asia	0.88	0.06
Canada, New Brunswick	0.98	0.08	Non-Jews	0.32	0.06
Canada, Newfoundland	1.13	0.10			
Canada, Northwest Territories	0.76	0.25	Japan, Hiroshima	0.66	0.05
Canada, Nova Scotia	1.15	0.08	Japan, Miyagi	0.62	0.03
Canada, Ontario	1.28	0.02	Japan, Nagasaki	0.66	0.04
Canada, Prince Edward Island	0.91	0.18	Japan, Osaka	0.59	0.02
Canada, Quebec	1.11	0.03	*Japan, Saga	0.54	0.05
Canada, Saskatchewan	1.19	0.07	Japan, Yamagata	0.52	0.04
Canada, Yukon	2.78	0.81	*Korea, Kangwha	0,24	0,08
US, Cent. Calif.: Non-Hisp. White	1.30	0.06	*Kuwait: Non-Kuwaitis	1.04	0.26
US, Cent. Calif.: Hispanic	1.10	0.13	*Kuwait: Kuwaitis	0.65	0.17
US, Los Angeles: Non-Hisp. White	1.55	0.04	*Philippines, Manila	1.01	0.05
US, Los Angeles: Hispanic White	1.04	0.06			
US, Los Angeles: Black	0.97	0.07	Singapore: Chinese	1.09	0.05
US, Los Angeles: Chinese	0.71	0.12	Singapore: Malay	0.92	0.13
US, Los Angeles: Filipino	1.06	0.15	Singapore: Indian	0.98	0.24
US, Los Angeles: Korean	0.51	0.12	Thailand, Chiang Mai	0.46	0.04
US, Los Angeles: Japanese	0.93	0.15	*Thailand, Khon Kaen	0.46	0.05
US, San Francisco: Non-Hisp. White	1.54	0.05	*Viet Nam, Hanoi		
US, San Francisco: Hispanic White	1.20	0.13			
US, San Francisco: Black	1.13	0.12			
US, San Francisco: Chinese	0.83	0.12			
US, San Francisco: Filipino	0.80	0.15			
US, San Francisco: Japanese	0.81	0.23			
US, Connecticut: White	1.32	0.04			
US, Connecticut: Black	0.86	0.14			
US, Atlanta: White	1.30	0.07			
US, Atlanta: Black	0.81	0.09			
US, Iowa	1.36	0.04			

* IMPORTANT-SEE NOTES ON POPULATION PAGE

EUROPE	MALE	FEMALE
Austria, Tyrol	1.78	0.11
*Belarus	1.25	0.02
*Croatia	1.17	0.03
Czech Republic	1.50	0.02
Denmark	1.65	0.04
Estonia	1.46	0.06
Finland	1.24	0.03
France, Bas-Rhin	1.47	0.08
*France, Calvados	1.02	0.08
France, Doubs	0.86	0.09
France, Haut-Rhin	1.28	0.09
*France, Herault	0.75	0.06
France, Isere	1.06	0.07
*France, Somme	1.14	0.09
*France, Tarn	1.03	0.10
Germany, Eastern States	1.43	0.03
Germany, Saarland	1.17	0.06
Iceland	1.16	0.15
Ireland, Southern	1.56	0.12
Italy, Ferrara	0.91	0.14
Italy, Florence	1.04	0.06
Italy, Genoa	1.06	0.07
*Italy, Latina	0.85	0.10
Italy, Macerata	1.08	0.18
Italy, Modena	1.18	0.08
Italy, Parma	1.11	0.09
Italy, Ragusa	0.81	0.10
Italy, Romagna	0.98	0.08
Italy, Torino	1.06	0.07
Italy, Trieste	1.48	0.14
Italy, Varese	1.12	0.07
Italy, Veneto	1.07	0.06
*Latvia	1.51	0.04
Malta	1.38	0.20
The Netherlands	1.32	0.02
The Netherlands, Eindhoven	1.35	0.08
The Netherlands, Maastricht	1.26	0.08
Norway	1.49	0.04
*Poland, Cracow	1.54	0.09
*Poland, Kielce	0.88	0.05
*Poland, Lower Silesia	1.59	0.05
Poland, Warsaw City	1.49	0.06
Slovakia	1.24	0.03
Slovenia	1.21	0.05
*Spain, Albacete	0.84	0.15
Spain, Asturias	1.00	0.06
Spain, Basque Country	0.87	0.04
Spain, Granada	0.73	0.06
Spain, Mallorca	0.94	0.08
Spain, Murcia	0.89	0.06
Spain, Navarra	0.90	0.08
Spain, Tarragona	0.79	0.07
Spain, Zaragoza	0.90	0.06

	MALE	FEMALE
Sweden	1.55	0.03
*Switzerland, Basel	1.19	0.10
Switzerland, Geneva	1.38	0.12
Switzerland, Graubunden	1.23	0.19
Switzerland, Neuchatel	1.34	0.18
Switzerland, St Gall-Appenzell	1.41	0.11
Switzerland, Valais	1.19	0.16
Switzerland, Vaud	1.16	0.09
Switzerland, Zurich	1.25	0.06
*UK, England and Wales	1.43	0.01
*UK, East Anglia	1.44	0.05
*UK, Mersey	1.31	0.05
*UK, North Western	1.31	0.04
UK, Oxford	1.63	0.05
*UK, South Thames	1.52	0.03
UK, South Western	1.36	0.04
UK, Wessex	1.51	0.04
*UK, West Midlands	1.62	0.03
UK, Yorkshire	1.39	0.04
UK, Scotland	1.53	0.03
UK, Scotland, West	1.44	0.04
*Yugoslavia, Vojvodina	1.02	0.04

OCEANIA	MALE	FEMALE
Australian Capital Territory	0.86	0.14
Australia, New South Wales	0.97	0.03
South Australia	1.09	0.06
Australia, Tasmania	0.90	0.09
Australia, Victoria	1.13	0.03
Western Australia	0.98	0.06
*French Polynesia	1.15	0.23
New Zealand: Non-Maori	1.22	0.04
New Zealand: Maori	1.51	0.23
US, Hawaii: White	1.56	0.17
US, Hawaii: Japanese	0.89	0.10
US, Hawaii: Hawaiian	1.03	0.20
US, Hawaii: Filipino	0.89	0.17
US, Hawaii: Chinese	0.71	0.19

* IMPORTANT-SEE NOTES ON POPULATION PAGE

CUMULATIVE INCIDENCE (0-74)
RATES AND STANDARD ERRORS (percent)
Other female genital (ICD-9 184)

	MALE	FEMALE
AFRICA		
*Algeria, Setif		
*France, La Reunion		
*Mali, Bamako		
*Uganda, Kyadondo		
*Zimbabwe, Harare: African		
*Zimbabwe, Harare: European		
AMERICA, CENTRAL AND SOUTH		
*Argentina, Concordia	0.42	0.14
*Brazil, Belem	0.09	0.03
*Brazil, Goiania		
*Brazil, Porto Alegre	0.39	0.06 f
Colombia, Cali	0.23	0.04
*Costa Rica	0.15	0.02
*Ecuador, Quito	0.11	0.03
*Peru, Lima	0.16	0.03
Peru, Trujillo	0.39	0.13
US, Puerto Rico	0.27	0.02
*Uruguay, Montevideo	0.25	0.03
AMERICA, NORTH		
Canada	0.20	0.01
Canada, Alberta	0.19	0.02
Canada, British Columbia	0.18	0.02
Canada, Manitoba	0.29	0.03
Canada, New Brunswick	0.24	0.04
Canada, Newfoundland	0.20	0.04
Canada, Northwest Territories	0,09	0,09
Canada, Nova Scotia	0.30	0.04
Canada, Ontario	0.22	0.01
Canada, Prince Edward Island	0.39	0.12
Canada, Quebec	0.17	0.01
Canada, Saskatchewan	0.16	0.03
Canada, Yukon	0,03	0,03
US, Cent. Calif.: Non-Hisp. White	0.20	0.02
US, Cent. Calif.: Hispanic	0.29	0.07
US, Los Angeles: Non-Hisp. White	0.19	0.01
US, Los Angeles: Hispanic White	0.16	0.03
US, Los Angeles: Black	0.17	0.03
US, Los Angeles: Chinese	0,04	0,03
US, Los Angeles: Filipino	0,06	0,04
US, Los Angeles: Korean	0,04	0,03
US, Los Angeles: Japanese	0,05	0,04 f
US, San Francisco: Non-Hisp. White	0.21	0.02
US, San Francisco: Hispanic White	0,12	0,04
US, San Francisco: Black	0.19	0.05
US, San Francisco: Chinese	0,09	0,04
US, San Francisco: Filipino	0,19	0,08
US, San Francisco: Japanese	-	-
US, Connecticut: White	0.20	0.02
US, Connecticut: Black	0,16	0,06
US, Atlanta: White	0.23	0.03
US, Atlanta: Black	0.25	0.06
US, Iowa	0.24	0.02

	MALE	FEMALE
US, Central Louisiana: White	0,15	0,05
US, Central Louisiana: Black	0,34	0,17
US, New Orleans: White	0.20	0.03
US, New Orleans: Black	0.30	0.07
US, Detroit: White	0.25	0.02
US, Detroit: Black	0.19	0.03
US, New Mexico: Non-Hisp. White	0.22	0.03
US, New Mexico: Hispanic White	0.12	0.04
US, New Mexico: American Indian	0,10	0,10
US, Utah	0.16	0.02
US, Seattle	0.24	0.02
US, SEER: White	0.22	0.01
US, SEER: Black	0.22	0.02
ASIA		
*China, Qidong	0,01	0,01
China, Shanghai	0.06	0.01
China, Tianjin	0.07	0.01
Hong Kong	0.14	0.01
*India, Bangalore	0.20	0.03
*India, Barshi, Paranda and Bhum	0,07	0,03
India, Bombay	0.18	0.02
*India, Karunagappally	0,06	0,05
India, Madras	0.25	0.03
*India, Trivandrum	0,08	0,04
Israel: All Jews	0.18	0.02
Jews born in Israel	0.33	0.11
Jews born in America or Europe	0.18	0.02
Jews born in Africa or Asia	0.18	0.03
Non-Jews	0,11	0,04
Japan, Hiroshima	0.11	0.02
Japan, Miyagi	0.05	0.01
Japan, Nagasaki	0.07	0.01
Japan, Osaka	0.05	0.01
*Japan, Saga	0.05	0.01
Japan, Yamagata	0.02	0.01
*Korea, Kangwha	0,04	0,04
*Kuwait: Non-Kuwaitis	0,02	0,01
*Kuwait: Kuwaitis	0,05	0,05
*Philippines, Manila	0.12	0.02
Singapore: Chinese	0.12	0.02
Singapore: Malay	0.05	0,03
Singapore: Indian	0.05	0,04
Thailand, Chiang Mai	0.12	0.02
*Thailand, Khon Kaen	0.11	0.03
*Viet Nam, Hanoi		

* IMPORTANT-SEE NOTES ON POPULATION PAGE

EUROPE	MALE	FEMALE
Austria, Tyrol	0.27	0.04
*Belarus	0.23	0.01
*Croatia	0.18	0.01
Czech Republic	0.23	0.01
Denmark	0.23	0.01
Estonia	0.22	0.02
Finland	0.18	0.01
France, Bas-Rhin	0.18	0.03
*France, Calvados	0.16	0.04
France, Doubs	0.16	0.04
France, Haut-Rhin	0.17	0.03
*France, Herault	0.20	0.03
France, Isere	0.15	0.03
*France, Somme	0.11	0.03
*France, Tarn	0.20	0.05
Germany, Eastern States	0.24	0.01
Germany, Saarland	0.24	0.03
Iceland	0,19	0,06
Ireland, Southern	0.18	0.04
Italy, Ferrara	0.25	0.08
Italy, Florence	0.22	0.03
Italy, Genoa	0.17	0.03
*Italy, Latina	0.14	0.05
Italy, Macerata	0,18	0,07
Italy, Modena	0.17	0.03
Italy, Parma	0.26	0.05
Italy, Ragusa	0,10	0,04
Italy, Romagna	0.11	0.03
Italy, Torino	0.17	0.03
Italy, Trieste	0.38	0.07
Italy, Varese	0.15	0.03
Italy, Veneto	0.23	0.03
*Latvia	0.17	0.02
Malta	0,13	0,07
The Netherlands	0.21	0.01
The Netherlands, Eindhoven	0.13	0.03
The Netherlands, Maastricht	0.18	0.03
Norway	0.18	0.01
*Poland, Cracow	0.22	0.04
*Poland, Kielce	0.21	0.03
*Poland, Lower Silesia	0.29	0.02
Poland, Warsaw City	0.23	0.03
Slovakia	0.21	0.01
Slovenia	0.22	0.02
*Spain, Albacete	0,10	0,06
Spain, Asturias	0.19	0.03
Spain, Basque Country	0.20	0.02
Spain, Granada	0.22	0.03
Spain, Mallorca	0.25	0.04
Spain, Murcia	0.18	0.03
Spain, Navarra	0.11	0.03
Spain, Tarragona	0.24	0.04
Spain, Zaragoza	0.25	0.03

	MALE	FEMALE
Sweden	0.19	0.01
*Switzerland, Basel	0.27	0.05
Switzerland, Geneva	0.15	0.04
Switzerland, Graubunden	0,16	0,07
Switzerland, Neuchatel	0,18	0,07
Switzerland, St Gall-Appenzell	0.24	0.05
Switzerland, Valais	0,14	0,05
Switzerland, Vaud	0.16	0.03
Switzerland, Zurich	0.19	0.03
*UK, England and Wales	0.20	0.01
*UK, East Anglia	0.19	0.02
*UK, Mersey	0.16	0.02
*UK, North Western	0.21	0.01
UK, Oxford	0.21	0.02
*UK, South Thames	0.15	0.01
UK, South Western	0.19	0.01
UK, Wessex	0.21	0.02
*UK, West Midlands	0.24	0.01
UK, Yorkshire	0.22	0.02
UK, Scotland	0.22	0.01
UK, Scotland, West	0.20	0.02
*Yugoslavia, Vojvodina	0.20	0.02

OCEANIA	MALE	FEMALE
Australian Capital Territory	0,20	0,08
Australia, New South Wales	0.17	0.01
South Australia	0.15	0.02
Australia, Tasmania	0.22	0.05
Australia, Victoria	0.16	0.01
Western Australia	0.17	0.02
*French Polynesia	0.42	0.16
New Zealand: Non-Maori	0.27	0.02
New Zealand: Maori	0.29	0.08
US, Hawaii: White	0.20	0.06
US, Hawaii: Japanese	0,05	0,02
US, Hawaii: Hawaiian	0,15	0,07
US, Hawaii: Filipino	0,03	0,02
US, Hawaii: Chinese	0,12	0,08

* IMPORTANT-SEE NOTES ON POPULATION PAGE

CUMULATIVE INCIDENCE (0-74)
RATES AND STANDARD ERRORS (percent)
Prostate (ICD-9 185)

	MALE	FEMALE
AFRICA		
*Algeria, Setif		
*France, La Reunion		
*Mali, Bamako		
*Uganda, Kyadondo		
*Zimbabwe, Harare: African		
*Zimbabwe, Harare: European		
AMERICA, CENTRAL AND SOUTH		
*Argentina, Concordia	1.85	0.38
*Brazil, Belem	2.02	0.26 m
*Brazil, Goiania		
*Brazil, Porto Alegre	4.43	0.27
Colombia, Cali	3.89	0.21
*Costa Rica	2.48	0.11
*Ecuador, Quito	2.29	0.18
*Peru, Lima	2.10	0.11
Peru, Trujillo	2.42	0.38
US, Puerto Rico	6.58	0.13
*Uruguay, Montevideo	3.33	0.16
AMERICA, NORTH		
Canada	7.83	0.04
Canada, Alberta	7.66	0.15
Canada, British Columbia	10.58	0.14
Canada, Manitoba	9.33	0.22
Canada, New Brunswick	8.33	0.26
Canada, Newfoundland	4.83	0.24
Canada, Northwest Territories	2.85	0.72
Canada, Nova Scotia	6.79	0.21
Canada, Ontario	7.59	0.07
Canada, Prince Edward Island	9.91	0.67
Canada, Quebec	6.75	0.08
Canada, Saskatchewan	8.11	0.21
Canada, Yukon	8.98	1.51
US, Cent. Calif.: Non-Hisp. White	11.80	0.21
US, Cent. Calif.: Hispanic	8.65	0.45
US, Los Angeles: Non-Hisp. White	12.59	0.13
US, Los Angeles: Hispanic White	7.67	0.22
US, Los Angeles: Black	16.83	0.39
US, Los Angeles: Chinese	2.17	0.27
US, Los Angeles: Filipino	5.39	0.50
US, Los Angeles: Korean	1.23	0.30
US, Los Angeles: Japanese	5.54	0.45
US, San Francisco: Non-Hisp. White	12.48	0.18
US, San Francisco: Hispanic White	8.78	0.48
US, San Francisco: Black	16.47	0.56
US, San Francisco: Chinese	3.30	0.27
US, San Francisco: Filipino	6.65	0.65
US, San Francisco: Japanese	4.15	0.71
US, Connecticut: White	9.91	0.14
US, Connecticut: Black	15.09	0.80
US, Atlanta: White	14.32	0.29
US, Atlanta: Black	17.60	0.64
US, Iowa	10.82	0.15

	MALE	FEMALE
US, Central Louisiana: White	7.45	0.44
US, Central Louisiana: Black	9.00	1.03
US, New Orleans: White	10.39	0.31
US, New Orleans: Black	11.53	0.54
US, Detroit: White	13.68	0.17
US, Detroit: Black	18.21	0.39
US, New Mexico: Non-Hisp. White	14.70	0.31
US, New Mexico: Hispanic White	9.26	0.40
US, New Mexico: American Indian	4.09	0.64
US, Utah	14.82	0.27
US, Seattle	17.04	0.18
US, SEER: White	12.93	0.06
US, SEER: Black	17.51	0.26
ASIA		
*China, Qidong	0.08	0.02
China, Shanghai	0.25	0.01
China, Tianjin	0.20	0.02
Hong Kong	0.79	0.03
*India, Bangalore	0.60	0.05
*India, Barshi, Paranda and Bhum	0.19	0.06
India, Bombay	0.93	0.05
*India, Karunagappally	0,44	0,16
India, Madras	0.42	0.04
*India, Trivandrum	0.79	0.17
Israel: All Jews	2.81	0.07
Jews born in Israel	3.88	0.37
Jews born in America or Europe	2.73	0.09
Jews born in Africa or Asia	2.73	0.13
Non-Jews	1.25	0.19
Japan, Hiroshima	1.15	0.09
Japan, Miyagi	0.94	0.05
Japan, Nagasaki	0.90	0.06
Japan, Osaka	0.63	0.02
*Japan, Saga	0.65	0.06
Japan, Yamagata	0.74	0.05
*Korea, Kangwha	0,14	0,08
*Kuwait: Non-Kuwaitis	1.64	0.46
*Kuwait: Kuwaitis	0.69	0.16
*Philippines, Manila	1.78	0.10
Singapore: Chinese	1.09	0.08
Singapore: Malay	1.08	0.18
Singapore: Indian	0.67	0.14
Thailand, Chiang Mai	0.45	0.06
*Thailand, Khon Kaen	0.34	0.07
*Viet Nam, Hanoi		

* IMPORTANT-SEE NOTES ON POPULATION PAGE

CUMULATIVE INCIDENCE (0-74)
RATES AND STANDARD ERRORS (percent)
Prostate (ICD-9 185) (contd)

EUROPE	MALE	FEMALE
Austria, Tyrol	5.97	*0.28*
*Belarus	1.59	*0.04*
*Croatia	1.82	*0.06*
Czech Republic	2.83	*0.04*
Denmark	3.56	*0.06*
Estonia	2.66	*0.12*
Finland	4.56	*0.07*
France, Bas-Rhin	5.60	*0.22*
*France, Calvados	6.23	*0.26*
France, Doubs	5.07	*0.27*
France, Haut-Rhin	5.94	*0.27*
*France, Herault	4.86	*0.18*
France, Isere	5.61	*0.20*
*France, Somme	4.44	*0.23*
*France, Tarn	7.37	*0.32*
Germany, Eastern States	2.99	*0.06*
Germany, Saarland	4.21	*0.16*
Iceland	7.57	*0.45*
Ireland, Southern	3.27	*0.19*
Italy, Ferrara	2.53	*0.26*
Italy, Florence	2.71	*0.12*
Italy, Genoa	2.81	*0.13*
*Italy, Latina	1.53	*0.16*
Italy, Macerata	3.46	*0.37*
Italy, Modena	2.92	*0.15*
Italy, Parma	2.61	*0.17*
Italy, Ragusa	1.18	*0.15*
Italy, Romagna	3.11	*0.17*
Italy, Torino	2.59	*0.13*
Italy, Trieste	4.45	*0.30*
Italy, Varese	3.12	*0.16*
Italy, Veneto	3.01	*0.12*
*Latvia	1.93	*0.08*
Malta	2.38	*0.33*
The Netherlands	4.47	*0.05*
The Netherlands, Eindhoven	4.13	*0.17*
The Netherlands, Maastricht	4.04	*0.16*
Norway	5.40	*0.08*
*Poland, Cracow	1.52	*0.13*
*Poland, Kielce	1.30	*0.09*
*Poland, Lower Silesia	1.88	*0.08*
Poland, Warsaw City	1.97	*0.11*
Slovakia	2.68	*0.07*
Slovenia	2.22	*0.10*
*Spain, Albacete	2.27	*0.30*
Spain, Asturias	1.87	*0.10*
Spain, Basque Country	2.14	*0.09*
Spain, Granada	1.59	*0.11*
Spain, Mallorca	2.44	*0.15*
Spain, Murcia	2.09	*0.12*
Spain, Navarra	3.03	*0.17*
Spain, Tarragona	2.27	*0.14*
Spain, Zaragoza	1.92	*0.11*

	MALE	FEMALE
Sweden	6.57	*0.06*
*Switzerland, Basel	5.46	*0.26*
Switzerland, Geneva	5.52	*0.31*
Switzerland, Graubunden	5.66	*0.47*
Switzerland, Neuchatel	4.88	*0.40*
Switzerland, St Gall-Appenzell	6.43	*0.28*
Switzerland, Valais	5.52	*0.40*
Switzerland, Vaud	5.16	*0.23*
Switzerland, Zurich	7.60	*0.20*
*UK, England and Wales	2.99	*0.02*
*UK, East Anglia	3.49	*0.09*
*UK, Mersey	2.60	*0.07*
*UK, North Western	2.90	*0.06*
UK, Oxford	3.41	*0.09*
*UK, South Thames	3.06	*0.05*
UK, South Western	3.33	*0.07*
UK, Wessex	3.34	*0.07*
*UK, West Midlands	3.42	*0.06*
UK, Yorkshire	3.13	*0.07*
UK, Scotland	3.35	*0.06*
UK, Scotland, West	3.25	*0.08*
*Yugoslavia, Vojvodina	1.68	*0.08*

OCEANIA	MALE	FEMALE
Australian Capital Territory	5.38	*0.46*
Australia, New South Wales	6.11	*0.08*
South Australia	6.10	*0.16*
Australia, Tasmania	5.53	*0.27*
Australia, Victoria	5.14	*0.09*
Western Australia	5.86	*0.16*
*French Polynesia	2.33	*0.46*
New Zealand: Non-Maori	3.70	*0.09*
New Zealand: Maori	4.13	*0.53*
US, Hawaii: White	14.04	*0.56*
US, Hawaii: Japanese	7.59	*0.32*
US, Hawaii: Hawaiian	5.17	*0.54*
US, Hawaii: Filipino	4.83	*0.42*
US, Hawaii: Chinese	8.18	*0.74*

* IMPORTANT-SEE NOTES ON POPULATION PAGE

CUMULATIVE INCIDENCE (0-74)
RATES AND STANDARD ERRORS (percent)
Testis (ICD-9 186)

	MALE	FEMALE
AFRICA		
*Algeria, Setif		
*France, La Reunion		
*Mali, Bamako		
*Uganda, Kyadondo		
*Zimbabwe, Harare: African		
*Zimbabwe, Harare: European		
AMERICA, CENTRAL AND SOUTH		
*Argentina, Concordia	0,25	0,09
*Brazil, Belem	0.14	0.05
*Brazil, Goiania		
*Brazil, Porto Alegre	0.23	0.03
Colombia, Cali	0.12	0.02
*Costa Rica	0.17	0.02
*Ecuador, Quito	0.27	0.03
*Peru, Lima	0.21	0.02
Peru, Trujillo	0.16	0.04
US, Puerto Rico	0.09	0.01
*Uruguay, Montevideo	0.38	0.04
AMERICA, NORTH		
Canada	0.29	0.01
Canada, Alberta	0.32	0.02
Canada, British Columbia	0.33	0.02
Canada, Manitoba	0.32	0.03
Canada, New Brunswick	0.21	0.03
Canada, Newfoundland	0.18	0.03
Canada, Northwest Territories	0.34	0.09
Canada, Nova Scotia	0.32	0.03
Canada, Ontario	0.31	0.01
Canada, Prince Edward Island	0,19	0,06
Canada, Quebec	0.24	0.01
Canada, Saskatchewan	0.28	0.03
Canada, Yukon	0.72	0.17
US, Cent. Calif.: Non-Hisp. White	0.39	0.03
US, Cent. Calif.: Hispanic	0.21	0.03
US, Los Angeles: Non-Hisp. White	0.44	0.02
US, Los Angeles: Hispanic White	0.23	0.02
US, Los Angeles: Black	0.08	0.01
US, Los Angeles: Chinese	0,06	0.02
US, Los Angeles: Filipino	0,08	0,03
US, Los Angeles: Korean	0,10	0,07
US, Los Angeles: Japanese	0.08	0.04
US, San Francisco: Non-Hisp. White	0.52	0.03
US, San Francisco: Hispanic White	0.29	0.05
US, San Francisco: Black	0.07	0.02
US, San Francisco: Chinese	0.16	0.04
US, San Francisco: Filipino	0,17	0,08
US, San Francisco: Japanese	0,42	0,15
US, Connecticut: White	0.39	0.02
US, Connecticut: Black	0,07	0,03
US, Atlanta: White	0.36	0.03
US, Atlanta: Black	0.04	0.01
US, Iowa	0.35	0.02

	MALE	FEMALE
US, Central Louisiana: White	0.23	0.05
US, Central Louisiana: Black	0,09	0,09
US, New Orleans: White	0.38	0.04
US, New Orleans: Black	0.10	0.03
US, Detroit: White	0.41	0.02
US, Detroit: Black	0.06	0.02
US, New Mexico: Non-Hisp. White	0.44	0.04
US, New Mexico: Hispanic White	0.33	0.04
US, New Mexico: American Indian	0.20	0.07
US, Utah	0.40	0.03
US, Seattle	0.39	0.02
US, SEER: White	0.41	0.01
US, SEER: Black	0.06	0.01
ASIA		
*China, Qidong	0,02	0,01
China, Shanghai	0.06	0.01
China, Tianjin	0.04	0.01
Hong Kong	0.09	0.01
*India, Bangalore	0.04	0.01
*India, Barshi, Paranda and Bhum	0,04	0,03
India, Bombay	0.08	0.01
*India, Karunagappally	0,05	0,04
India, Madras	0.07	0.01
*India, Trivandrum	0,03	0,02
Israel: All Jews	0.24	0.02
Jews born in Israel	0.28	0.03
Jews born in America or Europe	0.33	0.04
Jews born in Africa or Asia	0.10	0.03
Non-Jews	0.06	0.02
Japan, Hiroshima	0.13	0.02
Japan, Miyagi	0.12	0.01
Japan, Nagasaki	0.06	0.01
Japan, Osaka	0.11	0.01
*Japan, Saga	0.08	0.02
Japan, Yamagata	0.09	0.02
*Korea, Kangwha	0,03	0,03
*Kuwait: Non-Kuwaitis	0.16	0.08
*Kuwait: Kuwaitis	0,07	0,03
*Philippines, Manila	0.07	0.01
Singapore: Chinese	0.06	0.01
Singapore: Malay	0,08	0,03
Singapore: Indian	0.16	0.05
Thailand, Chiang Mai	0.05	0.01
*Thailand, Khon Kaen	0.05	0.01
*Viet Nam, Hanoi		

* IMPORTANT-SEE NOTES ON POPULATION PAGE

CUMULATIVE INCIDENCE (0-74)
RATES AND STANDARD ERRORS (percent)
Testis (ICD-9 186) (contd)

EUROPE	MALE	FEMALE
Austria, Tyrol	0.47	0.05
*Belarus	0.12	0.01
*Croatia	0.19	0.01
Czech Republic	0.39	0.01
Denmark	0.71	0.02
Estonia	0.14	0.02
Finland	0.19	0.01
France, Bas-Rhin	0.53	0.04
*France, Calvados	0.28	0.04
France, Doubs	0.43	0.05
France, Haut-Rhin	0.60	0.05
*France, Herault	0.22	0.03
France, Isere	0.28	0.03
*France, Somme	0.30	0.04
*France, Tarn	0.22	0.05
Germany, Eastern States	0.59	0.02
Germany, Saarland	0.46	0.03
Iceland	0.49	0.07
Ireland, Southern	0.24	0.04
Italy, Ferrara	0,18	0,06
Italy, Florence	0.25	0.03
Italy, Genoa	0.34	0.04
*Italy, Latina	0.18	0.04
Italy, Macerata	0.27	0.08
Italy, Modena	0.27	0.04
Italy, Parma	0.38	0.05
Italy, Ragusa	0,08	0,03
Italy, Romagna	0.32	0.05
Italy, Torino	0.25	0.03
Italy, Trieste	0.31	0.07
Italy, Varese	0.30	0.03
Italy, Veneto	0.26	0.03
*Latvia	0.13	0.02
Malta	0.21	0.07
The Netherlands	0.31	0.01
The Netherlands, Eindhoven	0.29	0.03
The Netherlands, Maastricht	0.27	0.03
Norway	0.62	0.02
*Poland, Cracow	0.19	0.03
*Poland, Kielce	0.17	0.02
*Poland, Lower Silesia	0.20	0.02
Poland, Warsaw City	0.35	0.03
Slovakia	0.34	0.01
Slovenia	0.33	0.02
*Spain, Albacete	0,11	0,05
Spain, Asturias	0.14	0.02
Spain, Basque Country	0.17	0.02
Spain, Granada	0.12	0.02
Spain, Mallorca	0.13	0.03
Spain, Murcia	0.09	0.02
Spain, Navarra	0.16	0.03
Spain, Tarragona	0.14	0.03
Spain, Zaragoza	0.12	0.02

	MALE	FEMALE
Sweden	0.36	0.01
*Switzerland, Basel	0.69	0.07
Switzerland, Geneva	0.55	0.06
Switzerland, Graubunden	0.71	0.12
Switzerland, Neuchatel	0.74	0.12
Switzerland, St Gall-Appenzell	0.81	0.07
Switzerland, Valais	0.57	0.09
Switzerland, Vaud	0.71	0.06
Switzerland, Zurich	0.69	0.04
*UK, England and Wales	0.36	0.01
*UK, East Anglia	0.42	0.02
*UK, Mersey	0.41	0.02
*UK, North Western	0.34	0.02
UK, Oxford	0.44	0.02
*UK, South Thames	0.38	0.01
UK, South Western	0.40	0.02
UK, Wessex	0.44	0.02
*UK, West Midlands	0.36	0.01
UK, Yorkshire	0.35	0.02
UK, Scotland	0.45	0.02
UK, Scotland, West	0.42	0.02
*Yugoslavia, Vojvodina	0.21	0.02

OCEANIA	MALE	FEMALE
Australian Capital Territory	0.25	0.05
Australia, New South Wales	0.36	0.01
South Australia	0.30	0.02
Australia, Tasmania	0.39	0.05
Australia, Victoria	0.35	0.02
Western Australia	0.29	0.02
*French Polynesia	0,12	0,04
New Zealand: Non-Maori	0.46	0.02
New Zealand: Maori	0.56	0.11
US, Hawaii: White	0.46	0.06
US, Hawaii: Japanese	0.22	0.05
US, Hawaii: Hawaiian	0.24	0.05
US, Hawaii: Filipino	0,14	0,05
US, Hawaii: Chinese	0,20	0,09

* IMPORTANT-SEE NOTES ON POPULATION PAGE

CUMULATIVE INCIDENCE (0-74)
RATES AND STANDARD ERRORS (percent)
Penis, other male genital (ICD-9 187)

	MALE	FEMALE
AFRICA		
*Algeria, Setif		
*France, La Reunion		
*Mali, Bamako		
*Uganda, Kyadondo		
*Zimbabwe, Harare: African		
*Zimbabwe, Harare: European		
AMERICA, CENTRAL AND SOUTH		
*Argentina, Concordia	0,02	0,02
*Brazil, Belem	0.24	0.06
*Brazil, Goiania		
*Brazil, Porto Alegre	0.13	0.04
Colombia, Cali	0.11	0.03
*Costa Rica	0.15	0.02
*Ecuador, Quito	0.07	0.02
*Peru, Lima	0.09	0.02
Peru, Trujillo	0,20	0,11
US, Puerto Rico	0.28	0.03
*Uruguay, Montevideo	0.13	0.03
AMERICA, NORTH		
Canada	0.08	0.00
Canada, Alberta	0.07	0.01
Canada, British Columbia	0.07	0.01
Canada, Manitoba	0.09	0.02
Canada, New Brunswick	0.11	0.03
Canada, Newfoundland	0.08	0.02
Canada, Northwest Territories	0,07	0,07
Canada, Nova Scotia	0.12	0.03
Canada, Ontario	0.09	0.01
Canada, Prince Edward Island	0,15	0,08
Canada, Quebec	0.07	0.01
Canada, Saskatchewan	0.12	0.02
Canada, Yukon	0,08	0,08
US, Cent. Calif.: Non-Hisp. White	0.11	0.02
US, Cent. Calif.: Hispanic	0.18	0.06
US, Los Angeles: Non-Hisp. White	0.08	0.01
US, Los Angeles: Hispanic White	0.12	0.02
US, Los Angeles: Black	0.11	0.03
US, Los Angeles: Chinese	0,05	0,04
US, Los Angeles: Filipino	-	-
US, Los Angeles: Korean	-	-
US, Los Angeles: Japanese	-	-
US, San Francisco: Non-Hisp. White	0.07	0.01
US, San Francisco: Hispanic White	0,15	0,07
US, San Francisco: Black	0,10	0,04
US, San Francisco: Chinese	0,06	0,03
US, San Francisco: Filipino	-	-
US, San Francisco: Japanese	0,10	0,10
US, Connecticut: White	0.07	0.01
US, Connecticut: Black	0,11	0,05
US, Atlanta: White	0.07	0.02
US, Atlanta: Black	0.18	0.06
US, Iowa	0.12	0.01

	MALE	FEMALE
US, Central Louisiana: White	-	-
US, Central Louisiana: Black	0,23	0,14
US, New Orleans: White	0,07	0,02
US, New Orleans: Black	0.15	0.05
US, Detroit: White	0.07	0.01
US, Detroit: Black	0.08	0.02
US, New Mexico: Non-Hisp. White	0.08	0.02
US, New Mexico: Hispanic White	0.11	0.04
US, New Mexico: American Indian	0,06	0,06
US, Utah	0.05	0.01
US, Seattle	0.06	0.01
US, SEER: White	0.07	0.00
US, SEER: Black	0.10	0.02
ASIA		
*China, Qidong	0.06	0.02
China, Shanghai	0.05	0.01
China, Tianjin	0.05	0.01
Hong Kong	0.07	0.01
*India, Bangalore	0.18	0.02
*India, Barshi, Paranda and Bhum	0.49	0.10
India, Bombay	0.18	0.02
*India, Karunagappally	0,14	0,07
India, Madras	0.37	0.03
*India, Trivandrum	0,16	0,08
Israel: All Jews	0.02	0.01
Jews born in Israel	0,01	0,00
Jews born in America or Europe	0,02	0,01
Jews born in Africa or Asia	0,02	0,01
Non-Jews	-	-
Japan, Hiroshima	0.08	0.02
Japan, Miyagi	0.05	0.01
Japan, Nagasaki	0.08	0.02
Japan, Osaka	0.03	0.00
*Japan, Saga	0,01	0,01
Japan, Yamagata	0,02	0,01
*Korea, Kangwha	0,05	0,05
*Kuwait: Non-Kuwaitis	0,02	0,01
*Kuwait: Kuwaitis	-	-
*Philippines, Manila	0.09	0.02
Singapore: Chinese	0.12	0.02
Singapore: Malay	-	-
Singapore: Indian	0,12	0,05
Thailand, Chiang Mai	0.28	0.04
*Thailand, Khon Kaen	0.20	0.04
*Viet Nam, Hanoi		

m

* IMPORTANT-SEE NOTES ON POPULATION PAGE

EUROPE	MALE	FEMALE
Austria, Tyrol	0,05	0,03
*Belarus	0.07	0.01
*Croatia	0.06	0.01
Czech Republic	0.10	0.01
Denmark	0.10	0.01
Estonia	0.12	0.02
Finland	0.05	0.01
France, Bas-Rhin	0.09	0.03
*France, Calvados	0.09	0.03
France, Doubs	0.12	0.04
France, Haut-Rhin	0.13	0.03
*France, Herault	0.11	0.03
France, Isere	0.08	0.02
*France, Somme	0,04	0,02
*France, Tarn	0,09	0,03
Germany, Eastern States	0.11	0.01
Germany, Saarland	0.11	0.02
Iceland	0,11	0,05
Ireland, Southern	0,07	0,03
Italy, Ferrara	0,10	0,05
Italy, Florence	0.11	0.02
Italy, Genoa	0.07	0.02
*Italy, Latina	0.14	0.05
Italy, Macerata	0,17	0,08
Italy, Modena	0,04	0,02
Italy, Parma	0,07	0,02
Italy, Ragusa	0,04	0,02
Italy, Romagna	0.14	0.04
Italy, Torino	0.12	0.03
Italy, Trieste	0.29	0.08
Italy, Varese	0.08	0.02
Italy, Veneto	0.10	0.02
*Latvia	0.09	0.01
Malta	0,20	0,09
The Netherlands	0.09	0.01
The Netherlands, Eindhoven	0.07	0.02
The Netherlands, Maastricht	0.07	0.02
Norway	0.07	0.01
*Poland, Cracow	0,06	0,02
*Poland, Kielce	0.09	0.02
*Poland, Lower Silesia	0.13	0.02
Poland, Warsaw City	0.12	0.02
Slovakia	0.10	0.01
Slovenia	0.10	0.02
*Spain, Albacete	0,08	0,05
Spain, Asturias	0.07	0.02
Spain, Basque Country	0.12	0.02
Spain, Granada	0.13	0.03
Spain, Mallorca	0.13	0.03
Spain, Murcia	0.13	0.03
Spain, Navarra	0.11	0.03
Spain, Tarragona	0.18	0.04
Spain, Zaragoza	0.08	0.02

	MALE	FEMALE
Sweden	0.10	0.01
*Switzerland, Basel	0.10	0.03
Switzerland, Geneva	0.19	0.05
Switzerland, Graubunden	0,03	0,03
Switzerland, Neuchatel	0,26	0,09
Switzerland, St Gall-Appenzell	0.12	0.03
Switzerland, Valais	0,11	0,06
Switzerland, Vaud	0.10	0.03
Switzerland, Zurich	0.10	0.02
*UK, England and Wales	0.10	0.00
*UK, East Anglia	0.11	0.01
*UK, Mersey	0.08	0.01
*UK, North Western	0.11	0.01
UK, Oxford	0.11	0.01
*UK, South Thames	0.08	0.01
UK, South Western	0.08	0.01
UK, Wessex	0.11	0.01
*UK, West Midlands	0.12	0.01
UK, Yorkshire	0.13	0.01
UK, Scotland	0.13	0.01
UK, Scotland, West	0.12	0.01
*Yugoslavia, Vojvodina	0.08	0.02

OCEANIA	MALE	FEMALE
Australian Capital Territory	0,08	0,06
Australia, New South Wales	0.05	0.01
South Australia	0.06	0.01
Australia, Tasmania	0,07	0,03
Australia, Victoria	0.07	0.01
Western Australia	0.05	0.01
*French Polynesia	-	-
New Zealand: Non-Maori	0.05	0.01
New Zealand: Maori	-	-
US, Hawaii: White	0,02	0,02
US, Hawaii: Japanese	0,05	0,03
US, Hawaii: Hawaiian	0,05	0,05
US, Hawaii: Filipino	0,14	0,06
US, Hawaii: Chinese	-	-

* IMPORTANT-SEE NOTES ON POPULATION PAGE

CUMULATIVE INCIDENCE (0-74)
RATES AND STANDARD ERRORS (percent)
Bladder (ICD-9 188)

	MALE		FEMALE	
AFRICA				
*Algeria, Setif				
*France, La Reunion				
*Mali, Bamako				
*Uganda, Kyadondo				
*Zimbabwe, Harare: African				
*Zimbabwe, Harare: European				
AMERICA, CENTRAL AND SOUTH				
†*Argentina, Concordia	1.06	0.28	0,36	0,13
†*Brazil, Belem	0.42	0.11	0,08	0,03 f
*Brazil, Goiania				
†*Brazil, Porto Alegre	2.22	0.19	0.39	0.06
† Colombia, Cali	0.90	0.10	0.39	0.06
†*Costa Rica	0.70	0.05	0.17	0.03
†*Ecuador, Quito	0.53	0.08	0.16	0.04
†*Peru, Lima	0.73	0.06	0.21	0.03
† Peru, Trujillo	0,20	0,08	0,12	0,07
† US, Puerto Rico	0.94	0.05	0.31	0.03
†*Uruguay, Montevideo	2.28	0.13	0.39	0.04
AMERICA, NORTH				
† Canada	2.19	0.02	0.57	0.01
Canada, Alberta	2.10	0.08	0.59	0.04
Canada, British Columbia	1.34	0.05	0.34	0.02
Canada, Manitoba	2.05	0.10	0.63	0.05
Canada, New Brunswick	2.70	0.15	0.69	0.07
† Canada, Newfoundland	2.30	0.16	0.65	0.08
† Canada, Northwest Territories	0,97	0,36	0,23	0,19
Canada, Nova Scotia	2.42	0.12	0.68	0.06
† Canada, Ontario	2.08	0.03	0.53	0.02
Canada, Prince Edward Island	1.56	0.26	0.60	0.15
Canada, Quebec	2.77	0.05	0.66	0.02
Canada, Saskatchewan	2.34	0.11	0.66	0.06
Canada, Yukon	3.26	1.01	-	-
US, Cent. Calif.: Non-Hisp. White	2.04	0.09	0.46	0.04
US, Cent. Calif.: Hispanic	1.01	0.15	0.32	0.08
US, Los Angeles: Non-Hisp. White	2.04	0.05	0.50	0.02
US, Los Angeles: Hispanic White	1.00	0.08	0.31	0.04
US, Los Angeles: Black	1.06	0.10	0.38	0.05
US, Los Angeles: Chinese	0.87	0.16	0,21	0,08
US, Los Angeles: Filipino	0.78	0.18	0,14	0,06
US, Los Angeles: Korean	0.72	0.22	0,32	0,12
US, Los Angeles: Japanese	0.69	0.15	0,17	0,07
US, San Francisco: Non-Hisp. White	2.99	0.08	0.74	0.04
US, San Francisco: Hispanic White	1.16	0.17	0.21	0.06
US, San Francisco: Black	1.45	0.16	0.51	0.08
US, San Francisco: Chinese	1.18	0.16	0.33	0.09
US, San Francisco: Filipino	1.11	0.26	0,23	0,09
US, San Francisco: Japanese	1.09	0.34	0,50	0,20
US, Connecticut: White	3.34	0.08	0.90	0.04
US, Connecticut: Black	1.64	0.25	0.61	0.14
US, Atlanta: White	2.63	0.12	0.64	0.05
US, Atlanta: Black	1.08	0.15	0.42	0.08
US, Iowa	2.68	0.07	0.68	0.03

	MALE		FEMALE	
US, Central Louisiana: White	2.63	0.26	0.35	0.08
US, Central Louisiana: Black	1.95	0.48	0,41	0,19
US, New Orleans: White	2.98	0.16	0.89	0.08
US, New Orleans: Black	1.54	0.20	0.42	0.08
US, Detroit: White	3.27	0.08	0.87	0.04
US, Detroit: Black	1.23	0.10	0.44	0.05
US, New Mexico: Non-Hisp. White	2.82	0.13	0.60	0.06
US, New Mexico: Hispanic White	1.29	0.14	0.37	0.07
US, New Mexico: American Indian	0,15	0,09	0,05	0,05
US, Utah	1.86	0.09	0.34	0.04
US, Seattle	2.77	0.07	0.73	0.03
US, SEER: White	2.86	0.03	0.73	0.01
US, SEER: Black	1.29	0.07	0.49	0.04
ASIA				
†*China, Qidong	0.44	0.05	0.10	0.02
† China, Shanghai	0.80	0.03	0.21	0.01
† China, Tianjin	0.74	0.04	0.24	0.02
Hong Kong	1.70	0.04	0.50	0.02
*India, Bangalore	0.41	0.04	0.09	0.01
*India, Barshi, Paranda and Bhum	0,10	0,05	-	-
† India, Bombay	0.60	0.03	0.15	0.02
†*India, Karunagappally	0,34	0,12	0,06	0,04
† India, Madras	0.37	0.04	0.13	0.02
†*India, Trivandrum	0.41	0.13	0,05	0,03
Israel: All Jews	3.04	0.07	0.61	0.03
Jews born in Israel	2.82	0.27	0.48	0.10
Jews born in America or Europe	3.26	0.10	0.74	0.04
Jews born in Africa or Asia	2.76	0.12	0.43	0.05
Non-Jews	1.52	0.19	0,14	0,05
Japan, Hiroshima	1.54	0.10	0.35	0.04
† Japan, Miyagi	1.06	0.05	0.27	0.02
† Japan, Nagasaki	1.28	0.06	0.24	0.02
† Japan, Osaka	0.82	0.03	0.19	0.01
†*Japan, Saga	0.87	0.07	0.12	0.02
† Japan, Yamagata	0.81	0.05	0.18	0.02
†*Korea, Kangwha	0,44	0,15	0,16	0,08
*Kuwait: Non-Kuwaitis	2.40	0.56	0.60	0.24
*Kuwait: Kuwaitis	0.78	0.16	0,32	0,12
†*Philippines, Manila	0.59	0.05	0.19	0.03
† Singapore: Chinese	0.89	0.06	0.23	0.03
† Singapore: Malay	0.68	0.13	0,12	0,05
† Singapore: Indian	0.39	0.10	0,04	0,04
† Thailand, Chiang Mai	0.64	0.06	0.30	0.04
†*Thailand, Khon Kaen	0.41	0.07	0.06	0.02
*Viet Nam, Hanoi				

* IMPORTANT-SEE NOTES ON POPULATION PAGE

CUMULATIVE INCIDENCE (0-74)
RATES AND STANDARD ERRORS (percent)
Bladder (ICD-9 188) (contd)

EUROPE	MALE		FEMALE	
Austria, Tyrol	3.41	0.20	0.79	0.08
*Belarus	1.58	0.04	0.18	0.01
†*Croatia	1.34	0.05	0.28	0.02
† Czech Republic	1.92	0.03	0.38	0.01
Denmark	3.47	0.06	0.95	0.03
† Estonia	1.38	0.08	0.24	0.03
Finland	1.80	0.04	0.33	0.01
† France, Bas-Rhin	2.90	0.14	0.48	0.05
*France, Calvados	2.84	0.17	0.46	0.06
France, Doubs	3.17	0.20	0.45	0.07
† France, Haut-Rhin	2.58	0.16	0.41	0.06
†*France, Herault	2.19	0.11	0.25	0.04
France, Isere	1.99	0.11	0.26	0.04
*France, Somme	2.60	0.17	0.24	0.04
*France, Tarn	2.97	0.20	0.31	0.06
Germany, Eastern States	2.46	0.05	0.42	0.02
Germany, Saarland	2.89	0.12	0.67	0.05
† Iceland	2.07	0.22	0.61	0.11
Ireland, Southern	1.45	0.12	0.41	0.06
Italy, Ferrara	4.07	0.33	0.56	0.11
† Italy, Florence	4.44	0.14	0.68	0.05
Italy, Genoa	4.77	0.16	0.79	0.06
*Italy, Latina	3.08	0.22	0.37	0.07
Italy, Macerata	3.97	0.38	0,21	0,08
Italy, Modena	3.83	0.16	0.61	0.06
Italy, Parma	3.48	0.19	0.61	0.07
† Italy, Ragusa	1.52	0.16	0.23	0.06
Italy, Romagna	3.99	0.18	0.63	0.07
Italy, Torino	4.55	0.16	0.58	0.05
Italy, Trieste	4.27	0.28	1.01	0.12
Italy, Varese	4.41	0.18	0.61	0.06
Italy, Veneto	3.77	0.13	0.66	0.05
†*Latvia	1.47	0.06	0.21	0.02
† Malta	3.39	0.38	0.48	0.12
† The Netherlands	1.83	0.03	0.34	0.01
The Netherlands, Eindhoven	3.15	0.15	0.67	0.06
† The Netherlands, Maastricht	1.36	0.09	0.23	0.03
Norway	1.92	0.05	0.49	0.02
†*Poland, Cracow	1.43	0.12	0.19	0.03
†*Poland, Kielce	1.25	0.08	0.16	0.02
†*Poland, Lower Silesia	1.86	0.07	0.27	0.02
Poland, Warsaw City	1.56	0.09	0.36	0.03
† Slovakia	1.79	0.05	0.36	0.02
† Slovenia	1.16	0.07	0.22	0.02
*Spain, Albacete	2.24	0.27	0,22	0,08
Spain, Asturias	3.24	0.13	0.42	0.04
Spain, Basque Country	3.17	0.10	0.32	0.03
Spain, Granada	2.91	0.14	0.31	0.04
Spain, Mallorca	4.68	0.20	0.43	0.06
Spain, Murcia	3.82	0.15	0.40	0.04
Spain, Navarra	3.30	0.17	0.38	0.05
Spain, Tarragona	3.93	0.18	0.51	0.06
† Spain, Zaragoza	2.63	0.12	0.29	0.04

	MALE		FEMALE	
Sweden	2.07	0.03	0.54	0.02
†*Switzerland, Basel	1.34	0.12	0.37	0.06
Switzerland, Geneva	3.86	0.24	0.78	0.10
† Switzerland, Graubunden	1.72	0.25	0.33	0.10
† Switzerland, Neuchatel	1.42	0.21	0.33	0.09
† Switzerland, St Gall-Appenzell	1.28	0.12	0.28	0.05
† Switzerland, Valais	1.87	0.22	0.39	0.09
† Switzerland, Vaud	1.64	0.12	0.35	0.05
Switzerland, Zurich	2.73	0.11	0.66	0.05
*UK, England and Wales	2.38	0.02	0.67	0.01
†*UK, East Anglia	1.57	0.06	0.39	0.03
*UK, Mersey	2.26	0.06	0.79	0.04
*UK, North Western	2.50	0.06	0.76	0.03
UK, Oxford	2.38	0.07	0.63	0.03
*UK, South Thames	2.20	0.04	0.59	0.02
UK, South Western	2.32	0.06	0.59	0.03
UK, Wessex	2.74	0.06	0.82	0.03
*UK, West Midlands	2.55	0.05	0.71	0.02
UK, Yorkshire	3.00	0.06	0.82	0.03
UK, Scotland	2.71	0.05	0.87	0.03
UK, Scotland, West	2.72	0.07	0.88	0.04
*Yugoslavia, Vojvodina	1.36	0.06	0.30	0.02

OCEANIA	MALE		FEMALE	
† Australian Capital Territory	1.03	0.19	0.31	0.10
† Australia, New South Wales	1.56	0.04	0.44	0.02
South Australia	2.38	0.09	0.67	0.05
† Australia, Tasmania	1.92	0.15	0.53	0.07
Australia, Victoria	2.02	0.05	0.57	0.03
† Western Australia	1.13	0.07	0.25	0.03
†*French Polynesia	1.13	0.33	0,13	0,08
† New Zealand: Non-Maori	1.58	0.06	0.45	0.03
† New Zealand: Maori	1.22	0.27	0,27	0,11
US, Hawaii: White	2.96	0.25	0.77	0.13
US, Hawaii: Japanese	1.24	0.13	0.29	0.06
US, Hawaii: Hawaiian	0.43	0.14	0.47	0.15
US, Hawaii: Filipino	0.54	0.13	0.30	0.10
US, Hawaii: Chinese	1.25	0.29	0,34	0,14

* IMPORTANT-SEE NOTES ON POPULATION PAGE

CUMULATIVE INCIDENCE (0-74)
RATES AND STANDARD ERRORS (percent)
Kidney etc. (ICD-9 189)

	MALE		FEMALE	
AFRICA				
*Algeria, Setif				
*France, La Reunion				
*Mali, Bamako				
*Uganda, Kyadondo				
*Zimbabwe, Harare: African				
*Zimbabwe, Harare: European				
AMERICA, CENTRAL AND SOUTH				
*Argentina, Concordia	0,46	0,18	0,46	0,16
*Brazil, Belem	0.23	0.06	0.13	0.04
*Brazil, Goiania				
*Brazil, Porto Alegre	1.28	0.13	0.51	0.07
Colombia, Cali	0.26	0.04	0.15	0.03
*Costa Rica	0.39	0.04	0.24	0.03
*Ecuador, Quito	0.31	0.06	0.14	0.03
*Peru, Lima	0.41	0.04	0.24	0.03
Peru, Trujillo	0.40	0.13	0.29	0.09
US, Puerto Rico	0.48	0.03	0.27	0.02
*Uruguay, Montevideo	1.26	0.09	0.47	0.05
AMERICA, NORTH				
Canada	1.33	0.02	0.67	0.01
Canada, Alberta	1.37	0.06	0.68	0.04
Canada, British Columbia	1.15	0.04	0.53	0.03
Canada, Manitoba	1.22	0.08	0.68	0.05
Canada, New Brunswick	1.26	0.10	0.75	0.07
Canada, Newfoundland	1.31	0.12	0.80	0.09
Canada, Northwest Territories	1.52	0.43	0.89	0.36
Canada, Nova Scotia	1.53	0.09	0.75	0.06
Canada, Ontario	1.33	0.03	0.66	0.02
Canada, Prince Edward Island	1.50	0.24	0.43	0.13
Canada, Quebec	1.38	0.03	0.71	0.02
Canada, Saskatchewan	1.41	0.08	0.72	0.06
Canada, Yukon	0,50	0,24	0,53	0,29
US, Cent. Calif.: Non-Hisp. White	1.21	0.07	0.68	0.05
US, Cent. Calif.: Hispanic	1.39	0.16	0.71	0.11
US, Los Angeles: Non-Hisp. White	1.20	0.04	0.57	0.02
US, Los Angeles: Hispanic White	1.11	0.07	0.54	0.04
US, Los Angeles: Black	1.34	0.10	0.66	0.06
US, Los Angeles: Chinese	0.66	0.14	0.27	0.09
US, Los Angeles: Filipino	0.85	0.18	0.25	0.08
US, Los Angeles: Korean	0.92	0.24	0.53	0.15
US, Los Angeles: Japanese	0.54	0.13	0.28	0.09
US, San Francisco: Non-Hisp. White	1.18	0.05	0.54	0.03
US, San Francisco: Hispanic White	1.28	0.16	0.67	0.10
US, San Francisco: Black	1.26	0.15	0.72	0.09
US, San Francisco: Chinese	0.43	0.09	0.27	0.07
US, San Francisco: Filipino	0.73	0.19	0.27	0.09
US, San Francisco: Japanese	0,65	0,25	0,11	0,11
US, Connecticut: White	1.41	0.05	0.70	0.03
US, Connecticut: Black	1.39	0.23	0.45	0.10
US, Atlanta: White	1.21	0.08	0.56	0.05
US, Atlanta: Black	1.44	0.15	0.63	0.09
US, Iowa	1.27	0.05	0.70	0.03

	MALE		FEMALE	
US, Central Louisiana: White	1.04	0.16	0.48	0.10
US, Central Louisiana: Black	1.65	0.42	0,42	0,17
US, New Orleans: White	1.67	0.12	0.85	0.07
US, New Orleans: Black	1.40	0.18	0.73	0.10
US, Detroit: White	1.58	0.05	0.73	0.03
US, Detroit: Black	1.44	0.10	0.72	0.06
US, New Mexico: Non-Hisp. White	1.06	0.08	0.55	0.05
US, New Mexico: Hispanic White	1.23	0.13	0.65	0.09
US, New Mexico: American Indian	1.51	0.34	0.93	0.25
US, Utah	0.96	0.06	0.47	0.04
US, Seattle	1.23	0.05	0.62	0.03
US, SEER: White	1.29	0.02	0.64	0.01
US, SEER: Black	1.38	0.07	0.67	0.04
ASIA				
*China, Qidong	0.05	0.02	0.06	0.02
China, Shanghai	0.34	0.02	0.18	0.01
China, Tianjin	0.39	0.03	0.19	0.02
Hong Kong	0.42	0.02	0.26	0.02
*India, Bangalore	0.13	0.02	0.07	0.01
*India, Barshi, Paranda and Bhum	0,07	0,04	0,01	0,01
India, Bombay	0.24	0.02	0.10	0.01
*India, Karunagappally	0,15	0,09	-	-
India, Madras	0.12	0.02	0.08	0.01
*India, Trivandrum	0,04	0,02	0,02	0,01
Israel: All Jews	1.32	0.05	0.65	0.03
Jews born in Israel	1.16	0.17	0.69	0.14
Jews born in America or Europe	1.68	0.07	0.86	0.06
Jews born in Africa or Asia	0.75	0.06	0.43	0.04
Non-Jews	0.42	0.10	0.18	0.05
Japan, Hiroshima	0.96	0.08	0.38	0.04
Japan, Miyagi	0.78	0.04	0.29	0.02
Japan, Nagasaki	0.74	0.05	0.26	0.02
Japan, Osaka	0.64	0.02	0.21	0.01
*Japan, Saga	0.58	0.05	0.20	0.03
Japan, Yamagata	0.60	0.05	0.19	0.02
*Korea, Kangwha	0,19	0,09	0,11	0,07
*Kuwait: Non-Kuwaitis	0.67	0.24	0.48	0.20
*Kuwait: Kuwaitis	0.34	0.12	0.27	0.11
*Philippines, Manila	0.47	0.04	0.33	0.03
Singapore: Chinese	0.54	0.05	0.24	0.03
Singapore: Malay	0.27	0.07	0,10	0,04
Singapore: Indian	0.33	0.09	0,34	0,16
Thailand, Chiang Mai	0.17	0.03	0.21	0.04
*Thailand, Khon Kaen	0.14	0.04	0.06	0.01
*Viet Nam, Hanoi				

* IMPORTANT-SEE NOTES ON POPULATION PAGE

CUMULATIVE INCIDENCE (0-74)
RATES AND STANDARD ERRORS (percent)
Kidney etc. (ICD-9 189) (contd)

EUROPE	MALE		FEMALE	
Austria, Tyrol	1.80	*0.14*	0.85	*0.08*
*Belarus	0.96	*0.03*	0.47	*0.01*
*Croatia	0.82	*0.04*	0.43	*0.02*
Czech Republic	2.09	*0.03*	1.01	*0.02*
Denmark	1.07	*0.03*	0.70	*0.02*
Estonia	1.39	*0.07*	0.71	*0.04*
Finland	1.47	*0.04*	0.81	*0.02*
France, Bas-Rhin	2.00	*0.11*	0.91	*0.07*
*France, Calvados	0.97	*0.09*	0.42	*0.06*
France, Doubs	1.13	*0.12*	0.69	*0.09*
France, Haut-Rhin	1.66	*0.12*	0.66	*0.07*
*France, Herault	1.19	*0.08*	0.40	*0.04*
France, Isere	1.18	*0.08*	0.49	*0.05*
*France, Somme	1.12	*0.10*	0.57	*0.07*
*France, Tarn	0.95	*0.11*	0.31	*0.06*
Germany, Eastern States	1.70	*0.04*	0.82	*0.02*
Germany, Saarland	1.50	*0.08*	0.67	*0.05*
Iceland	1.49	*0.19*	0.99	*0.15*
Ireland, Southern	0.76	*0.09*	0.36	*0.06*
Italy, Ferrara	1.96	*0.22*	0.62	*0.12*
Italy, Florence	1.50	*0.08*	0.65	*0.05*
Italy, Genoa	1.36	*0.09*	0.57	*0.05*
*Italy, Latina	0.66	*0.10*	0.22	*0.05*
Italy, Macerata	0.74	*0.16*	0.45	*0.12*
Italy, Modena	1.43	*0.10*	0.72	*0.06*
Italy, Parma	1.61	*0.12*	0.57	*0.07*
Italy, Ragusa	0.53	*0.09*	0.23	*0.06*
Italy, Romagna	1.69	*0.12*	0.69	*0.07*
Italy, Torino	1.45	*0.09*	0.45	*0.04*
Italy, Trieste	1.81	*0.18*	0.76	*0.10*
Italy, Varese	1.91	*0.11*	0.61	*0.05*
Italy, Veneto	1.86	*0.09*	0.64	*0.05*
*Latvia	1.18	*0.05*	0.49	*0.03*
Malta	0.65	*0.15*	0,24	*0,09*
The Netherlands	1.24	*0.02*	0.63	*0.02*
The Netherlands, Eindhoven	1.03	*0.08*	0.55	*0.05*
The Netherlands, Maastricht	1.38	*0.09*	0.65	*0.06*
Norway	1.10	*0.03*	0.61	*0.02*
*Poland, Cracow	1.30	*0.10*	0.60	*0.06*
*Poland, Kielce	0.77	*0.06*	0.40	*0.04*
*Poland, Lower Silesia	1.39	*0.06*	0.68	*0.03*
Poland, Warsaw City	1.66	*0.08*	0.76	*0.05*
Slovakia	1.37	*0.04*	0.71	*0.03*
Slovenia	0.86	*0.06*	0.44	*0.03*
*Spain, Albacete	0.55	*0.14*	0.27	*0.09*
Spain, Asturias	0.90	*0.07*	0.36	*0.04*
Spain, Basque Country	1.09	*0.06*	0.36	*0.03*
Spain, Granada	0.59	*0.06*	0.27	*0.04*
Spain, Mallorca	0.79	*0.08*	0.26	*0.04*
Spain, Murcia	0.50	*0.05*	0.22	*0.03*
Spain, Navarra	1.02	*0.09*	0.36	*0.05*
Spain, Tarragona	0.71	*0.08*	0.27	*0.04*
Spain, Zaragoza	0.78	*0.06*	0.29	*0.04*

	MALE		FEMALE	
Sweden	1.26	*0.02*	0.77	*0.02*
*Switzerland, Basel	1.39	*0.12*	0.64	*0.07*
Switzerland, Geneva	1.32	*0.14*	0.50	*0.08*
Switzerland, Graubunden	1.09	*0.19*	0.72	*0.14*
Switzerland, Neuchatel	0.99	*0.17*	0.58	*0.12*
Switzerland, St Gall-Appenzell	1.16	*0.11*	0.56	*0.07*
Switzerland, Valais	1.41	*0.19*	0.71	*0.12*
Switzerland, Vaud	1.15	*0.10*	0.58	*0.06*
Switzerland, Zurich	1.34	*0.08*	0.58	*0.05*
*UK, England and Wales	0.81	*0.01*	0.37	*0.01*
*UK, East Anglia	0.77	*0.04*	0.27	*0.02*
*UK, Mersey	0.72	*0.04*	0.38	*0.03*
*UK, North Western	0.81	*0.03*	0.42	*0.02*
UK, Oxford	0.88	*0.04*	0.42	*0.03*
*UK, South Thames	0.76	*0.02*	0.36	*0.01*
UK, South Western	0.80	*0.03*	0.36	*0.02*
UK, Wessex	0.85	*0.04*	0.41	*0.02*
*UK, West Midlands	0.88	*0.03*	0.40	*0.02*
UK, Yorkshire	0.86	*0.03*	0.43	*0.02*
UK, Scotland	0.96	*0.03*	0.52	*0.02*
UK, Scotland, West	0.93	*0.04*	0.49	*0.03*
*Yugoslavia, Vojvodina	0.56	*0.04*	0.37	*0.03*

OCEANIA

	MALE		FEMALE	
Australian Capital Territory	1.37	*0.22*	0.40	*0.10*
Australia, New South Wales	1.10	*0.03*	0.72	*0.02*
South Australia	1.01	*0.06*	0.57	*0.04*
Australia, Tasmania	1.12	*0.11*	0.45	*0.07*
Australia, Victoria	1.04	*0.04*	0.53	*0.02*
Western Australia	1.02	*0.06*	0.57	*0.04*
*French Polynesia	0.60	*0.17*	0,12	*0,05*
New Zealand: Non-Maori	0.84	*0.04*	0.46	*0.03*
New Zealand: Maori	1.05	*0.23*	0.34	*0.12*
US, Hawaii: White	1.28	*0.16*	0.42	*0.09*
US, Hawaii: Japanese	0.90	*0.11*	0.26	*0.06*
US, Hawaii: Hawaiian	0.96	*0.21*	0.33	*0.10*
US, Hawaii: Filipino	0.56	*0.14*	0,19	*0,07*
US, Hawaii: Chinese	0.76	*0.22*	0,23	*0,12*

* IMPORTANT-SEE NOTES ON POPULATION PAGE

AFRICA	MALE		FEMALE	
*Algeria, Setif				
*France, La Reunion				
*Mali, Bamako				
*Uganda, Kyadondo				
*Zimbabwe, Harare: African				
*Zimbabwe, Harare: European				

AMERICA, CENTRAL AND SOUTH	MALE		FEMALE	
*Argentina, Concordia	0,12	0,07	0,07	0,05
*Brazil, Belem	0,05	0,02	0,02	0,01
*Brazil, Goiania				
*Brazil, Porto Alegre	0,06	0,02	0,04	0,02 mf
Colombia, Cali	0.04	0.01	0.08	0.03 mf
*Costa Rica	0.06	0.01	0.03	0.01
*Ecuador, Quito	0.08	0.03	0.07	0.02
*Peru, Lima	0.05	0.01	0.04	0.01
Peru, Trujillo	0,09	0,04	0,15	0,10 f
US, Puerto Rico	0.06	0.01	0.02	0.01
*Uruguay, Montevideo	0,03	0,01	0,01	0,01

AMERICA, NORTH	MALE		FEMALE	
Canada	0.10	0.00	0.07	0.00
Canada, Alberta	0.09	0.01	0.08	0.01
Canada, British Columbia	0.08	0.01	0.07	0.01
Canada, Manitoba	0.07	0.02	0.11	0.02
Canada, New Brunswick	0,07	0,02	0.07	0.02
Canada, Newfoundland	0,05	0,02	0,03	0,02
Canada, Northwest Territories	0,05	0,05	0,01	0,01
Canada, Nova Scotia	0.09	0.02	0.11	0.02
Canada, Ontario	0.10	0.01	0.07	0.01
Canada, Prince Edward Island	0,16	0,07	0,08	0,06
Canada, Quebec	0.10	0.01	0.06	0.01
Canada, Saskatchewan	0.19	0.03	0.05	0.01
Canada, Yukon	0,10	0,10	-	-
US, Cent. Calif.: Non-Hisp. White	0.12	0.02	0.05	0.01
US, Cent. Calif.: Hispanic	0.07	0.03	0,03	0,02
US, Los Angeles: Non-Hisp. White	0.09	0.01	0.07	0.01
US, Los Angeles: Hispanic White	0.04	0.01	0.03	0.01
US, Los Angeles: Black	0,02	0,01	0,02	0,01
US, Los Angeles: Chinese	-	-	0,01	0,01
US, Los Angeles: Filipino	-	-	-	-
US, Los Angeles: Korean	-	-	-	-
US, Los Angeles: Japanese	-	-	0,02	0,02
US, San Francisco: Non-Hisp. White	0.09	0.01	0.07	0.01
US, San Francisco: Hispanic White	0,04	0,02	0,05	0,02
US, San Francisco: Black	0,05	0,03	0,01	0,01
US, San Francisco: Chinese	-	-	0,03	0,02
US, San Francisco: Filipino	-	-	-	-
US, San Francisco: Japanese	-	-	-	-
US, Connecticut: White	0.05	0.01	0.04	0.01
US, Connecticut: Black	0,01	0,01	0,01	0,01
US, Atlanta: White	0.12	0.02	0.06	0.02
US, Atlanta: Black	0,05	0,03	0,01	0,00
US, Iowa	0.09	0.01	0.08	0.01

	MALE		FEMALE	
US, Central Louisiana: White	0,04	0,03	0,08	0,04
US, Central Louisiana: Black	0,02	0,02	-	-
US, New Orleans: White	0.08	0.02	0.08	0.02
US, New Orleans: Black	0,01	0,01	-	-
US, Detroit: White	0.08	0.01	0.05	0.01
US, Detroit: Black	0,02	0,01	0,01	0,01
US, New Mexico: Non-Hisp. White	0.09	0.02	0.06	0.02
US, New Mexico: Hispanic White	0,06	0,03	0,01	0,01
US, New Mexico: American Indian	0,02	0,02	0,01	0,01
US, Utah	0.11	0.02	0.05	0.01
US, Seattle	0.10	0.01	0.06	0.01
US, SEER: White	0.08	0.00	0.06	0.00
US, SEER: Black	0.03	0.01	0.01	0.00

ASIA	MALE		FEMALE	
*China, Qidong	0,01	0,01	0,00	0,00
China, Shanghai	0.02	0.00	0.01	0.00
China, Tianjin	0.01	0.00	0.01	0.00
Hong Kong	0.02	0.00	0.02	0.00
*India, Bangalore	0.01	0.01	0.02	0.01
*India, Barshi, Paranda and Bhum	-	-	0,00	0,00
India, Bombay	0.02	0.00	0.01	0.00
*India, Karunagappally	-	-	-	-
India, Madras	0.03	0.01	0.02	0.01
*India, Trivandrum	0,00	0,00	0,01	0,01
Israel: All Jews	0.08	0.01	0.07	0.01
Jews born in Israel	0.15	0.06	0.02	0.01
Jews born in America or Europe	0.07	0.02	0.09	0.02
Jews born in Africa or Asia	0.16	0.11	0,03	0,01
Non-Jews	0.08	0.04	0,04	0,02
Japan, Hiroshima	0,02	0,01	0,01	0,00
Japan, Miyagi	0,01	0,00	0,01	0,00
Japan, Nagasaki	0.03	0.01	0.01	0.00
Japan, Osaka	0.01	0.00	0.01	0.00
*Japan, Saga	0,01	0,01	0,00	0,00
Japan, Yamagata	-	-	-	-
*Korea, Kangwha	-	-	-	-
*Kuwait: Non-Kuwaitis	-	-	-	-
*Kuwait: Kuwaitis	0,00	0,00	0,01	0,00
*Philippines, Manila	0.05	0.01	0.02	0.01
Singapore: Chinese	0.03	0.01	0.02	0.01
Singapore: Malay	0,00	0,00	0,01	0,01
Singapore: Indian	-	-	-	-
Thailand, Chiang Mai	0,02	0,01	0,02	0,01
*Thailand, Khon Kaen	0,04	0,02	0.02	0.01
*Viet Nam, Hanoi				

* IMPORTANT-SEE NOTES ON POPULATION PAGE

CUMULATIVE INCIDENCE (0-74)
RATES AND STANDARD ERRORS (percent)
Eye (ICD-9 190) (contd)

EUROPE	MALE		FEMALE	
Austria, Tyrol	0.08	*0.02*	0.08	*0.02*
*Belarus	0.08	*0.01*	0.06	*0.00*
*Croatia	0.08	*0.01*	0.06	*0.01*
Czech Republic	0.08	*0.01*	0.06	*0.00*
Denmark	0.10	*0.01*	0.08	*0.01*
Estonia	0.10	*0.02*	0.07	*0.01*
Finland	0.09	*0.01*	0.09	*0.01*
France, Bas-Rhin	0.10	*0.02*	0.07	*0.02*
*France, Calvados	0.07	*0.02*	0.02	*0.01*
France, Doubs	0,06	*0,03*	0,03	*0,02*
France, Haut-Rhin	0.07	*0.02*	0,04	*0,02*
*France, Herault	0,01	*0,01*	0,02	*0,01*
France, Isere	0,04	*0,01*	0.06	*0.02*
*France, Somme	0.11	*0.04*	0,06	*0,02*
*France, Tarn	0,06	*0,03*	0,06	*0,02*
Germany, Eastern States	0.09	*0.01*	0.07	*0.01*
Germany, Saarland	0,03	*0,01*	0,03	*0,01*
Iceland	0,11	*0,05*	0,02	*0,01*
Ireland, Southern	0,05	*0,02*	0,05	*0,02*
Italy, Ferrara	0,06	*0,04*	0,12	*0,05*
Italy, Florence	0.06	*0.02*	0.03	*0.01*
Italy, Genoa	0,05	*0,02*	0,04	*0,02*
*Italy, Latina	0,04	*0,02*	0,03	*0,02*
Italy, Macerata	0,05	*0,04*	0,05	*0,04*
Italy, Modena	0.08	*0.02*	0,02	*0,01*
Italy, Parma	0,04	*0,02*	0,01	*0,01*
Italy, Ragusa	0,04	*0,02*	-	-
Italy, Romagna	0,05	*0,02*	0,09	*0,03*
Italy, Torino	0,03	*0,01*	0,02	*0,01*
Italy, Trieste	0,03	*0,02*	0,01	*0,01*
Italy, Varese	0,03	*0,01*	0,05	*0,01*
Italy, Veneto	0,05	*0.02*	0,02	*0,01*
*Latvia	0.04	*0.01*	0.03	*0.01*
Malta	0,02	*0,02*	-	-
The Netherlands	0.08	*0.01*	0.07	*0.00*
The Netherlands, Eindhoven	0.10	*0.03*	0.06	*0.02*
The Netherlands, Maastricht	0.08	*0.02*	0,03	*0,01*
Norway	0.09	*0.01*	0.07	*0.01*
*Poland, Cracow	0,06	*0,02*	0,09	*0,02*
*Poland, Kielce	0.06	*0.02*	0,02	*0,01*
*Poland, Lower Silesia	0.09	*0.01*	0.06	*0.01*
Poland, Warsaw City	0.06	*0.01*	0.04	*0.01*
Slovakia	0.09	*0.01*	0.08	*0.01*
Slovenia	0.07	*0.01*	0.06	*0.01*
*Spain, Albacete	0,05	*0,04*	0,03	*0,03*
Spain, Asturias	0.07	*0.02*	0,02	*0,01*
Spain, Basque Country	0.05	*0.01*	0,02	*0,01*
Spain, Granada	0,03	*0,01*	0,03	*0,01*
Spain, Mallorca	0,04	*0,02*	0,05	*0,02*
Spain, Murcia	0.06	*0.02*	0,01	*0,01* m
Spain, Navarra	0.08	*0.03*	0,04	*0,02*
Spain, Tarragona	0,05	*0,02*	0,04	*0,02*
Spain, Zaragoza	0.07	*0.02*	0,03	*0,01*

	MALE		FEMALE	
Sweden	0.09	*0.01*	0.07	*0.01*
*Switzerland, Basel	0.10	*0.03*	0.08	*0.03*
Switzerland, Geneva	0,07	*0,03*	0,04	*0,02*
Switzerland, Graubunden	0,08	*0,04*	0,10	*0,05*
Switzerland, Neuchatel	0,08	*0,05*	0,06	*0,04*
Switzerland, St Gall-Appenzell	0,03	*0,02*	0,05	*0,02*
Switzerland, Valais	0,22	*0,08*	0,10	*0,04*
Switzerland, Vaud	0.09	*0.03*	0.12	*0.03*
Switzerland, Zurich	0.08	*0.02*	0.10	*0.02*
*UK, England and Wales	0.07	*0.00*	0.06	*0.00*
*UK, East Anglia	0.05	*0.01*	0.04	*0.01*
*UK, Mersey	0.05	*0.01*	0.03	*0.01*
*UK, North Western	0.06	*0.01*	0.05	*0.01*
UK, Oxford	0.06	*0.01*	0.07	*0.01*
*UK, South Thames	0.09	*0.01*	0.08	*0.01*
UK, South Western	0.07	*0.01*	0.05	*0.01*
UK, Wessex	0.07	*0.01*	0.05	*0.01*
*UK, West Midlands	0.05	*0.01*	0.05	*0.01*
UK, Yorkshire	0.07	*0.01*	0.07	*0.01*
UK, Scotland	0.11	*0.01*	0.08	*0.01*
UK, Scotland, West	0.12	*0.01*	0.08	*0.01*
*Yugoslavia, Vojvodina	0.07	*0.01*	0.05	*0.01*

OCEANIA	MALE		FEMALE	
Australian Capital Territory	0,17	*0,07*	0,09	*0,05*
Australia, New South Wales	0.10	*0.01*	0.09	*0.01*
South Australia	0.10	*0.02*	0.07	*0.01*
Australia, Tasmania	0,09	*0,03*	0,04	*0,02*
Australia, Victoria	0.11	*0.01*	0.07	*0.01*
Western Australia	0.08	*0.02*	0.07	*0.02*
*French Polynesia	0,01	*0,01*	-	-
New Zealand: Non-Maori	0.13	*0.01*	0.07	*0.01*
New Zealand: Maori	0,03	*0,03*	0,01	*0,01*
US, Hawaii: White	0,07	*0,04*	0,03	*0,02*
US, Hawaii: Japanese	0,02	*0,02*	0,01	*0,01*
US, Hawaii: Hawaiian	0,04	*0,04*	0,04	*0,02*
US, Hawaii: Filipino	-	-	0,02	*0,02*
US, Hawaii: Chinese	0,04	*0,04*	-	-

* IMPORTANT-SEE NOTES ON POPULATION PAGE

CUMULATIVE INCIDENCE (0-74)
RATES AND STANDARD ERRORS (percent)
Brain, nervous system (ICD-9 191-2)

	MALE		FEMALE	
AFRICA				
*Algeria, Setif				
*France, La Reunion				
*Mali, Bamako				
*Uganda, Kyadondo				
*Zimbabwe, Harare: African				
*Zimbabwe, Harare: European				
AMERICA, CENTRAL AND SOUTH				
*Argentina, Concordia	0,25	0,10	0,12	0,06
*Brazil, Belem	0.29	0.06	0.14	0.04
*Brazil, Goiania				
*Brazil, Porto Alegre	0.54	0.08	0.29	0.05
Colombia, Cali	0.47	0.06	0.39	0.05
*Costa Rica	0.51	0.04	0.38	0.03
*Ecuador, Quito	0.30	0.05	0.18	0.03
*Peru, Lima	0.29	0.03	0.27	0.03
Peru, Trujillo	0.19	0.06	0.13	0.05
US, Puerto Rico	0.33	0.02	0.24	0.02
*Uruguay, Montevideo	0.67	0.06	0.52	0.05
AMERICA, NORTH				
Canada	0.71	0.01	0.50	0.01
Canada, Alberta	0.67	0.04	0.46	0.03
Canada, British Columbia	0.63	0.03	0.41	0.02
Canada, Manitoba	0.70	0.05	0.46	0.04
Canada, New Brunswick	0.68	0.07	0.47	0.05
Canada, Newfoundland	0.53	0.07	0.29	0.05
Canada, Northwest Territories	0.62	0.28	0,46	0,30
Canada, Nova Scotia	0.62	0.06	0.39	0.04
Canada, Ontario	0.75	0.02	0.55	0.02
Canada, Prince Edward Island	0.76	0.17	0.59	0.14
Canada, Quebec	0.74	0.02	0.53	0.02
Canada, Saskatchewan	0.61	0.05	0.38	0.04
Canada, Yukon	1.00	0.27	0,14	0,14
US, Cent. Calif.: Non-Hisp. White	0.77	0.05	0.53	0.04
US, Cent. Calif.: Hispanic	0.57	0.09	0.31	0.06
US, Los Angeles: Non-Hisp. White	0.78	0.03	0.48	0.02
US, Los Angeles: Hispanic White	0.46	0.04	0.35	0.03
US, Los Angeles: Black	0.46	0.05	0.28	0.04
US, Los Angeles: Chinese	0.23	0.07	0,13	0,05
US, Los Angeles: Filipino	0.49	0.14	0.23	0.07
US, Los Angeles: Korean	0,14	0,09	0,15	0,07
US, Los Angeles: Japanese	0,14	0,06	0,12	0,06
US, San Francisco: Non-Hisp. White	0.73	0.04	0.55	0.03
US, San Francisco: Hispanic White	0.83	0.13	0.43	0.08
US, San Francisco: Black	0.49	0.08	0.25	0.05
US, San Francisco: Chinese	0.29	0.07	0.25	0.06
US, San Francisco: Filipino	0.79	0.21	0.26	0.08
US, San Francisco: Japanese	0,23	0,13	0,19	0,11
US, Connecticut: White	0.76	0.03	0.47	0.02
US, Connecticut: Black	0.41	0.11	0.21	0.06
US, Atlanta: White	0.74	0.05	0.57	0.04
US, Atlanta: Black	0.37	0.08	0.34	0.06
US, Iowa	0.68	0.03	0.48	0.03

	MALE		FEMALE		
US, Central Louisiana: White	0.67	0.12	0.53	0.10	
US, Central Louisiana: Black	0,07	0,04	0,18	0,11	
US, New Orleans: White	0.57	0.06	0.36	0.05	
US, New Orleans: Black	0.48	0.09	0.25	0.06	
US, Detroit: White	0.71	0.03	0.48	0.03	
US, Detroit: Black	0.33	0.04	0.31	0.04	
US, New Mexico: Non-Hisp. White	0.64	0.06	0.44	0.05	
US, New Mexico: Hispanic White	0.40	0.07	0.33	0.06	
US, New Mexico: American Indian	0,41	0,17	0,11	0,04	
US, Utah	0.63	0.05	0.50	0.04	
US, Seattle	0.76	0.03	0.50	0.03	
US, SEER: White	0.72	0.01	0.50	0.01	
US, SEER: Black	0.38	0.03	0.28	0.02	
ASIA					
*China, Qidong	0.34	0.04	0.19	0.03	
† China, Shanghai	0.59	0.02	0.47	0.02	
China, Tianjin	0.55	0.03	0.54	0.03	
Hong Kong	0.42	0.02	0.32	0.02	
*India, Bangalore	0.31	0.03	0.15	0.02	
*India, Barshi, Paranda and Bhum	0,03	0,02	0,02	0,01	
India, Bombay	0.35	0.02	0.22	0.02	
*India, Karunagappally	0,24	0,09	0,22	0,09	f
India, Madras	0.20	0.02	0.10	0.01	
*India, Trivandrum	0.25	0.08	0.21	0.06	
Israel: All Jews	0.60	0.03	0.42	0.02	
Jews born in Israel	0.67	0.11	0.37	0.07	
Jews born in America or Europe	0.68	0.05	0.49	0.04	
Jews born in Africa or Asia	0.42	0.04	0.31	0.06	
Non-Jews	0.28	0.07	0.22	0.05	
Japan, Hiroshima	0.23	0.03	0.17	0.03	
Japan, Miyagi	0.24	0.02	0.16	0.02	
Japan, Nagasaki	0.27	0.03	0.18	0.02	
Japan, Osaka	0.28	0.01	0.19	0.01	
*Japan, Saga	0.24	0.03	0.19	0.03	
Japan, Yamagata	0.16	0.02	0.17	0.02	
*Korea, Kangwha	0,29	0,11	0,20	0,08	
*Kuwait: Non-Kuwaitis	0.25	0.06	0.29	0.11	
*Kuwait: Kuwaitis	0.44	0.12	0.30	0.11	
*Philippines, Manila	0.26	0.03	0.21	0.03	
Singapore: Chinese	0.21	0.02	0.17	0.02	
Singapore: Malay	0.13	0.04	0,10	0,05	
Singapore: Indian	0,16	0,05	0,33	0,16	
Thailand, Chiang Mai	0.17	0.02	0.16	0.02	
*Thailand, Khon Kaen	0.26	0.04	0.22	0.03	
*Viet Nam, Hanoi					

CUMULATIVE INCIDENCE (0-74)
RATES AND STANDARD ERRORS (percent)
Brain, nervous system (ICD-9 191-2) (contd)

EUROPE	MALE		FEMALE	
Austria, Tyrol	0.61	*0.08*	0.48	*0.05*
*Belarus	0.38	*0.01*	0.26	*0.01*
*Croatia	0.87	*0.03*	0.63	*0.02*
Czech Republic	0.50	*0.01*	0.38	*0.01*
Denmark	0.68	*0.02*	0.49	*0.02*
Estonia	0.51	*0.04*	0.38	*0.03*
Finland	0.67	*0.02*	0.52	*0.02*
France, Bas-Rhin	0.53	*0.05*	0.38	*0.04*
*France, Calvados	0.43	*0.06*	0.31	*0.05*
France, Doubs	0.55	*0.08*	0.47	*0.07*
France, Haut-Rhin	0.64	*0.07*	0.42	*0.05*
*France, Herault	0.49	*0.05*	0.36	*0.04*
France, Isere	0.56	*0.05*	0.41	*0.04*
*France, Somme	0.59	*0.07*	0.37	*0.05*
*France, Tarn	0.40	*0.07*	0.23	*0.05*
Germany, Eastern States	0.53	*0.02*	0.38	*0.01*
Germany, Saarland	0.59	*0.05*	0.51	*0.04*
Iceland	0.96	*0.14*	0.54	*0.11*
Ireland, Southern	0.79	*0.08*	0.38	*0.06*
Italy, Ferrara	0.52	*0.11*	0.55	*0.11*
Italy, Florence	0.70	*0.05*	0.54	*0.04*
Italy, Genoa	0.64	*0.06*	0.44	*0.04*
*Italy, Latina	0.84	*0.10*	0.48	*0.07*
Italy, Macerata	0.60	*0.13*	0.75	*0.15*
Italy, Modena	0.62	*0.06*	0.46	*0.05*
Italy, Parma	0.75	*0.08*	0.44	*0.06*
Italy, Ragusa	0.52	*0.09*	0.41	*0.07*
Italy, Romagna	0.67	*0.07*	0.49	*0.06*
Italy, Torino	0.75	*0.07*	0.47	*0.05*
Italy, Trieste	0.97	*0.13*	0.76	*0.11*
Italy, Varese	0.66	*0.06*	0.44	*0.04*
Italy, Veneto	0.79	*0.05*	0.56	*0.04*
*Latvia	0.41	*0.03*	0.28	*0.02*
Malta	0.71	*0.16*	0.48	*0.12*
The Netherlands	0.59	*0.01*	0.39	*0.01*
The Netherlands, Eindhoven	0.50	*0.05*	0.38	*0.04*
The Netherlands, Maastricht	0.63	*0.06*	0.41	*0.04*
Norway	0.71	*0.03*	0.53	*0.02*
*Poland, Cracow	0.64	*0.07*	0.32	*0.04*
*Poland, Kielce	0.55	*0.05*	0.37	*0.03*
*Poland, Lower Silesia	0.72	*0.04*	0.56	*0.03*
Poland, Warsaw City	0.87	*0.06*	0.68	*0.04*
Slovakia	0.64	*0.03*	0.42	*0.02*
Slovenia	0.44	*0.03*	0.32	*0.02*
*Spain, Albacete	0.64	*0.14*	0.42	*0.11*
Spain, Asturias	0.51	*0.05*	0.34	*0.04*
Spain, Basque Country	0.66	*0.04*	0.45	*0.03*
Spain, Granada	0.67	*0.06*	0.42	*0.05*
Spain, Mallorca	0.69	*0.07*	0.52	*0.06*
Spain, Murcia	0.65	*0.05*	0.35	*0.04*
Spain, Navarra	0.90	*0.08*	0.47	*0.06*
Spain, Tarragona	0.55	*0.07*	0.44	*0.06*
Spain, Zaragoza	0.64	*0.06*	0.41	*0.04*

	MALE		FEMALE	
Sweden	0.67	*0.02*	0.51	*0.01*
*Switzerland, Basel	0.81	*0.09*	0.41	*0.06*
Switzerland, Geneva	0.69	*0.10*	0.36	*0.06*
Switzerland, Graubunden	0.61	*0.14*	0.26	*0.08*
Switzerland, Neuchatel	0.49	*0.11*	0.47	*0.11*
Switzerland, St Gall-Appenzell	0.63	*0.08*	0.43	*0.06*
Switzerland, Valais	0.41	*0.10*	0.28	*0.07*
Switzerland, Vaud	0.59	*0.07*	0.46	*0.05*
Switzerland, Zurich	0.69	*0.05*	0.45	*0.04*
*UK, England and Wales	0.66	*0.01*	0.45	*0.01*
*UK, East Anglia	0.66	*0.04*	0.47	*0.03*
*UK, Mersey	0.69	*0.03*	0.55	*0.03*
*UK, North Western	0.61	*0.03*	0.39	*0.02*
UK, Oxford	0.69	*0.04*	0.57	*0.03*
*UK, South Thames	0.68	*0.02*	0.45	*0.02*
UK, South Western	0.69	*0.03*	0.43	*0.02*
UK, Wessex	0.68	*0.03*	0.53	*0.03*
*UK, West Midlands	0.65	*0.02*	0.42	*0.02*
UK, Yorkshire	0.63	*0.03*	0.41	*0.02*
UK, Scotland	0.64	*0.02*	0.43	*0.02*
UK, Scotland, West	0.62	*0.03*	0.42	*0.02*
*Yugoslavia, Vojvodina	0.64	*0.04*	0.42	*0.03*

OCEANIA

	MALE		FEMALE	
Australian Capital Territory	0.49	*0.09*	0.54	*0.11*
Australia, New South Wales	0.70	*0.02*	0.49	*0.02*
South Australia	0.65	*0.05*	0.53	*0.04*
Australia, Tasmania	0.75	*0.09*	0.49	*0.07*
Australia, Victoria	0.74	*0.03*	0.49	*0.02*
Western Australia	0.67	*0.05*	0.56	*0.04*
*French Polynesia	0.30	*0.11*	0.48	*0.15*
New Zealand: Non-Maori	0.77	*0.03*	0.51	*0.03*
New Zealand: Maori	0.60	*0.16*	0.37	*0.10*
US, Hawaii: White	0.80	*0.11*	0.36	*0.07*
US, Hawaii: Japanese	0.21	*0.05*	0,10	*0,03*
US, Hawaii: Hawaiian	0.30	*0.09*	0.28	*0.10*
US, Hawaii: Filipino	0.22	*0.07*	0,17	*0,07*
US, Hawaii: Chinese	0,32	*0,13*	0,05	*0,05*

* IMPORTANT-SEE NOTES ON POPULATION PAGE

CUMULATIVE INCIDENCE (0-74)
RATES AND STANDARD ERRORS (percent)
Thyroid (ICD-9 193)

	MALE		FEMALE	
AFRICA				
*Algeria, Setif				
*France, La Reunion				
*Mali, Bamako				
*Uganda, Kyadondo				
*Zimbabwe, Harare: African				
*Zimbabwe, Harare: European				
AMERICA, CENTRAL AND SOUTH				
*Argentina, Concordia	-	-	0,17	0,07
*Brazil, Belem	0,06	0,04	0.10	0.03 mf
*Brazil, Goiania				
*Brazil, Porto Alegre	0.12	0.03	0.34	0.05
Colombia, Cali	0.23	0.04	0.65	0.06
*Costa Rica	0.14	0.02	0.55	0.04
*Ecuador, Quito	0.25	0.05	0.74	0.07
*Peru, Lima	0.13	0.02	0.51	0.04
Peru, Trujillo	0,26	0,10	0.63	0.15
US, Puerto Rico	0.10	0.01	0.32	0.02
*Uruguay, Montevideo	0.12	0.03	0.39	0.04
AMERICA, NORTH				
Canada	0.18	0.01	0.46	0.01
Canada, Alberta	0.21	0.02	0.50	0.03
Canada, British Columbia	0.14	0.01	0.41	0.02
Canada, Manitoba	0.22	0.03	0.44	0.04
Canada, New Brunswick	0.14	0.03	0.41	0.05
Canada, Newfoundland	0.18	0.04	0.42	0.06
Canada, Northwest Territories	0,25	0,15	0,15	0,07
Canada, Nova Scotia	0.14	0.03	0.41	0.04
Canada, Ontario	0.20	0.01	0.54	0.01
Canada, Prince Edward Island	0,11	0,06	0.31	0.09
Canada, Quebec	0.16	0.01	0.38	0.01
Canada, Saskatchewan	0.29	0.04	0.40	0.04
Canada, Yukon	0,06	0,06	0,34	0,15
US, Cent. Calif.: Non-Hisp. White	0.23	0.03	0.43	0.03
US, Cent. Calif.: Hispanic	0.10	0.03	0.50	0.07
US, Los Angeles: Non-Hisp. White	0.28	0.02	0.60	0.02
US, Los Angeles: Hispanic White	0.18	0.03	0.50	0.03
US, Los Angeles: Black	0.08	0.02	0.28	0.03
US, Los Angeles: Chinese	0.14	0.05	0.33	0.08
US, Los Angeles: Filipino	0.40	0.10	1.06	0.14
US, Los Angeles: Korean	0,12	0,05	0.52	0.13
US, Los Angeles: Japanese	0,10	0,05	0.38	0.09
US, San Francisco: Non-Hisp. White	0.26	0.02	0.60	0.03
US, San Francisco: Hispanic White	0.25	0.06	0.67	0.08
US, San Francisco: Black	0,10	0,04	0.30	0.06
US, San Francisco: Chinese	0.29	0.07	0.66	0.10
US, San Francisco: Filipino	0.44	0.15	1.06	0.17
US, San Francisco: Japanese	0,31	0,19	0.70	0.20
US, Connecticut: White	0.24	0.02	0.45	0.02
US, Connecticut: Black	0,12	0,05	0.46	0.10
US, Atlanta: White	0.23	0.03	0.60	0.04
US, Atlanta: Black	0.25	0.07	0.30	0.05
US, Iowa	0.26	0.02	0.59	0.03

	MALE		FEMALE	
US, Central Louisiana: White	0,09	0,04	0.36	0.08
US, Central Louisiana: Black	0,19	0,13	0,13	0,08
US, New Orleans: White	0.24	0.04	0.58	0.06
US, New Orleans: Black	0,08	0,04	0.40	0.06
US, Detroit: White	0.27	0.02	0.64	0.03
US, Detroit: Black	0.17	0.03	0.35	0.04
US, New Mexico: Non-Hisp. White	0.31	0.04	0.58	0.05
US, New Mexico: Hispanic White	0.26	0.06	0.79	0.08
US, New Mexico: American Indian	0,15	0,10	0.46	0.16
US, Utah	0.28	0.03	0.74	0.04
US, Seattle	0.21	0.02	0.55	0.02
US, SEER: White	0.25	0.01	0.59	0.01
US, SEER: Black	0.15	0.02	0.34	0.03
ASIA				
*China, Qidong	0.02	0,01	0.05	0.01
China, Shanghai	0.11	0.01	0.29	0.01
China, Tianjin	0.09	0.01	0.21	0.02
Hong Kong	0.20	0.01	0.70	0.02
*India, Bangalore	0.12	0.02	0.32	0.03
*India, Barshi, Paranda and Bhum	0,03	0,01	0,01	0,01
India, Bombay	0.08	0.01	0.22	0.02
*India, Karunagappally	0,27	0,13	0.34	0.10m
India, Madras	0.09	0.02	0.18	0.02
*India, Trivandrum	0.17	0.05	0.34	0.07
Israel: All Jews	0.28	0.02	0.75	0.03
Jews born in Israel	0.31	0.06	0.67	0.07
Jews born in America or Europe	0.27	0.03	0.75	0.05
Jews born in Africa or Asia	0.29	0.04	0.83	0.07
Non-Jews	0.15	0.04	0.40	0.07
Japan, Hiroshima	0.29	0.04	1.00	0.06
Japan, Miyagi	0.15	0.02	0.92	0.04
Japan, Nagasaki	0.17	0.02	0.67	0.04
Japan, Osaka	0.13	0.01	0.35	0.01
*Japan, Saga	0.13	0.03	0.29	0.03
Japan, Yamagata	0.12	0.02	0.57	0.04
*Korea, Kangwha	0,05	0,04	0.50	0.13
*Kuwait: Non-Kuwaitis	0.36	0.20	0.53	0,11
*Kuwait: Kuwaitis	0.16	0.06	0.47	0.10
*Philippines, Manila	0.36	0.04	0.94	0.05
Singapore: Chinese	0.21	0.03	0.59	0.04
Singapore: Malay	0.15	0.06	0.61	0.10
Singapore: Indian	0,12	0,06	0.27	0.08
Thailand, Chiang Mai	0.12	0.02	0.30	0.04
*Thailand, Khon Kaen	0.12	0.04	0.34	0.04
*Viet Nam, Hanoi				

* IMPORTANT-SEE NOTES ON POPULATION PAGE

CUMULATIVE INCIDENCE (0-74)
RATES AND STANDARD ERRORS (percent)
Thyroid (ICD-9 193) (contd)

EUROPE	MALE		FEMALE	
Austria, Tyrol	0.27	0.05	0.84	0.07
*Belarus	0.14	0.01	0.35	0.01
*Croatia	0.11	0.01	0.39	0.02
Czech Republic	0.13	0.01	0.29	0.01
Denmark	0.08	0.01	0.20	0.01
Estonia	0.07	0.02	0.27	0.02
Finland	0.18	0.01	0.60	0.02
France, Bas-Rhin	0.12	0.02	0.26	0.03
*France, Calvados	0.18	0.04	0.65	0.06
France, Doubs	0.11	0.03	0.51	0.06
France, Haut-Rhin	0.16	0.04	0.25	0.04
*France, Herault	0.15	0.03	0.47	0.04
France, Isere	0.17	0.03	0.49	0.04
*France, Somme	0.08	0.02	0.35	0.05
*France, Tarn	0.23	0.05	0.72	0.08
Germany, Eastern States	0.14	0.01	0.26	0.01
Germany, Saarland	0.21	0.03	0.34	0.03
Iceland	0.63	0.12	0.96	0.13
Ireland, Southern	0,07	0,03	0.25	0.04
Italy, Ferrara	0.31	0.09	0.99	0.15
Italy, Florence	0.21	0.03	0.41	0.04
Italy, Genoa	0.18	0.03	0.37	0.04
*Italy, Latina	0.24	0.05	0.44	0.06
Italy, Macerata	0,08	0,05	0.82	0.15
Italy, Modena	0.20	0.03	0.53	0.05
Italy, Parma	0.22	0.04	0.34	0.05
Italy, Ragusa	0.12	0.04	0.25	0.06
Italy, Romagna	0.29	0.04	0.87	0.07
Italy, Torino	0.22	0.03	0.40	0.04
Italy, Trieste	0.26	0.07	0.56	0.09
Italy, Varese	0.18	0.03	0.57	0.05
Italy, Veneto	0.20	0.03	0.48	0.04
*Latvia	0.11	0.02	0.27	0.02
Malta	0,04	0,03	0.35	0.10
The Netherlands	0.09	0.01	0.22	0.01
The Netherlands, Eindhoven	0.07	0.02	0.19	0.03
The Netherlands, Maastricht	0.10	0.02	0.20	0.03
Norway	0.18	0.01	0.45	0.02
*Poland, Cracow	0.11	0.03	0.23	0.03
*Poland, Kielce	0.08	0.02	0.10	0.02
*Poland, Lower Silesia	0.09	0.01	0.23	0.02
Poland, Warsaw City	0.12	0.02	0.23	0.02
Slovakia	0.11	0.01	0.30	0.02
Slovenia	0.16	0.02	0.28	0.02
*Spain, Albacete	0,03	0,03	0.36	0.09
Spain, Asturias	0.15	0.02	0.46	0.04
Spain, Basque Country	0.08	0.01	0.26	0.02
Spain, Granada	0.11	0.02	0.29	0.04
Spain, Mallorca	0.07	0.02	0.30	0.04
Spain, Murcia	0.12	0.02	0.38	0.04
Spain, Navarra	0.20	0.04	0.65	0.07
Spain, Tarragona	0.07	0.02	0.33	0.05
Spain, Zaragoza	0.08	0.02	0.27	0.03

	MALE		FEMALE	
Sweden	0.16	0.01	0.34	0.01
*Switzerland, Basel	0.20	0.05	0.35	0.05
Switzerland, Geneva	0.12	0.04	0.47	0.07
Switzerland, Graubunden	0,04	0,03	0.30	0.09
Switzerland, Neuchatel	0,06	0,05	0.30	0.08
Switzerland, St Gall-Appenzell	0.15	0.04	0.46	0.06
Switzerland, Valais	0.20	0.07	0.30	0.07
Switzerland, Vaud	0.17	0.03	0.37	0.05
Switzerland, Zurich	0.27	0.03	0.47	0.04
*UK, England and Wales	0.08	0.00	0.17	0.00
*UK, East Anglia	0.09	0.01	0.18	0.02
*UK, Mersey	0.05	0.01	0.13	0.01
*UK, North Western	0.08	0.01	0.17	0.01
UK, Oxford	0.08	0.01	0.20	0.02
*UK, South Thames	0.07	0.01	0.16	0.01
UK, South Western	0.08	0.01	0.19	0.01
UK, Wessex	0.08	0.01	0.22	0.02
*UK, West Midlands	0.08	0.01	0.18	0.01
UK, Yorkshire	0.08	0.01	0.16	0.01
UK, Scotland	0.10	0.01	0.19	0.01
UK, Scotland, West	0.10	0.01	0.16	0.01
*Yugoslavia, Vojvodina	0.08	0.01	0.19	0.02

OCEANIA	MALE		FEMALE	
Australian Capital Territory	0.28	0.10	0.18	0.06
Australia, New South Wales	0.17	0.01	0.40	0.02
South Australia	0.17	0.02	0.31	0.03
Australia, Tasmania	0.15	0.04	0.28	0.05
Australia, Victoria	0.14	0.01	0.28	0.02
Western Australia	0.17	0.02	0.43	0.03
*French Polynesia	0.46	0.19	1.65	0.27
New Zealand: Non-Maori	0.12	0.01	0.35	0.02
New Zealand: Maori	0,18	0,08	0.73	0.15
US, Hawaii: White	0.37	0.08	0.69	0.10
US, Hawaii: Japanese	0.20	0.05	0.60	0.08
US, Hawaii: Hawaiian	0.37	0.12	0.91	0.15
US, Hawaii: Filipino	0.54	0.13	2.59	0.27
US, Hawaii: Chinese	0,26	0,12	1.00	0.23

* IMPORTANT-SEE NOTES ON POPULATION PAGE

CUMULATIVE INCIDENCE (0-74)
RATES AND STANDARD ERRORS (percent)
Other endocrine (ICD-9 194)

	MALE		FEMALE	
AFRICA				
*Algeria, Setif				
*France, La Reunion				
*Mali, Bamako				
*Uganda, Kyadondo				
*Zimbabwe, Harare: African				
*Zimbabwe, Harare: European				
AMERICA, CENTRAL AND SOUTH				
*Argentina, Concordia	-	-	-	-
*Brazil, Belem	0,01	0,00	0,00	0,00
*Brazil, Goiania				
*Brazil, Porto Alegre	0,07	0,03	0.05	0.02 m
Colombia, Cali	0,02	0,01	0,01	0,00
*Costa Rica	0.03	0.01	0.01	0.00
*Ecuador, Quito	0,00	0,00	0,01	0,01
*Peru, Lima	0,01	0,00	0,01	0,01
Peru, Trujillo	0,02	0,02	-	-
US, Puerto Rico	0,01	0,00	0.01	0.00
*Uruguay, Montevideo	0,03	0,01	0,02	0,01
AMERICA, NORTH				
Canada	0.05	0.00	0.05	0.00
Canada, Alberta	0.02	0.01	0.03	0.01
Canada, British Columbia	0.02	0.00	0.03	0.01
Canada, Manitoba	0.07	0.02	0.03	0.01
Canada, New Brunswick	0.09	0.02	0.05	0.02
Canada, Newfoundland	0.01	0.01	0.01	0.01
Canada, Northwest Territories	0.03	0.02	0.01	0.01
Canada, Nova Scotia	0.02	0.01	0.01	0.01
Canada, Ontario	0.06	0.01	0.05	0.00
Canada, Prince Edward Island	0.02	0.02	-	-
Canada, Quebec	0.06	0.01	0.07	0.01
Canada, Saskatchewan	0.02	0.01	0.05	0.01
Canada, Yukon	-	-	-	-
US, Cent. Calif.: Non-Hisp. White	0.06	0.01	0.02	0.01
US, Cent. Calif.: Hispanic	0,02	0,01	0,01	0,00
US, Los Angeles: Non-Hisp. White	0.05	0.01	0.03	0.01
US, Los Angeles: Hispanic White	0.03	0.01	0.03	0.01
US, Los Angeles: Black	0.03	0.01	0.03	0.01
US, Los Angeles: Chinese	-	-	-	-
US, Los Angeles: Filipino	0,01	0,01	-	-
US, Los Angeles: Korean	-	-	-	-
US, Los Angeles: Japanese	0,04	0,04	0,03	0,03
US, San Francisco: Non-Hisp. White	0.05	0.01	0.03	0.01
US, San Francisco: Hispanic White	0,04	0,02	0,01	0,01
US, San Francisco: Black	0,05	0,03	0,04	0,02
US, San Francisco: Chinese	0,07	0,03	0,02	0,01
US, San Francisco: Filipino	0,03	0,02	0,02	0,02
US, San Francisco: Japanese	0,04	0,04	-	-
US, Connecticut: White	0.03	0.01	0.01	0.00
US, Connecticut: Black	0,02	0,02	0,01	0,01
US, Atlanta: White	0.03	0.01	0.03	0.01
US, Atlanta: Black	0,02	0,01	0,05	0,03
US, Iowa	0.03	0.01	0.04	0.01

	MALE		FEMALE	
US, Central Louisiana: White	0,03	0,02	0,03	0,02
US, Central Louisiana: Black	-	-	-	-
US, New Orleans: White	0,03	0,02	0.06	0.02
US, New Orleans: Black	0,04	0,03	0,04	0,02
US, Detroit: White	0.05	0.01	0.04	0.01
US, Detroit: Black	0,02	0,01	0.03	0.01
US, New Mexico: Non-Hisp. White	0,03	0,01	0,02	0,01
US, New Mexico: Hispanic White	0,03	0,02	0,01	0,01
US, New Mexico: American Indian	-	-	0,13	0,09
US, Utah	0.03	0.01	0.03	0.01
US, Seattle	0.03	0.01	0.03	0.01
US, SEER: White	0.03	0.00	0.03	0.00
US, SEER: Black	0.03	0.01	0.03	0.01
ASIA				
*China, Qidong	0,01	0,01	0,00	0,00
China, Shanghai	0.09	0.01	0.14	0.01
China, Tianjin	0.07	0.01	0.06	0.01
Hong Kong	0.06	0.01	0.06	0.01
*India, Bangalore	0,00	0,00	0,00	0,00
*India, Barshi, Paranda and Bhum	-	-	-	-
India, Bombay	0.01	0.00	0.01	0.00
*India, Karunagappally	0,04	0,04	-	-
India, Madras	0.01	0.00	0,01	0,00
*India, Trivandrum	0,01	0,01	-	-
Israel: All Jews	0.04	0.01	0.03	0.01
Jews born in Israel	0.07	0.05	0.02	0.01
Jews born in America or Europe	0.03	0.01	0.05	0.01
Jews born in Africa or Asia	0,03	0,01	0,00	0,00
Non-Jews	0,03	0,01	0,04	0,02
Japan, Hiroshima	0.04	0.01	0.03	0,01
Japan, Miyagi	0.03	0.01	0.03	0.01
Japan, Nagasaki	0.03	0.01	0.02	0,01
Japan, Osaka	0.04	0.00	0.03	0.00
*Japan, Saga	0,01	0,01	0,01	0,00
Japan, Yamagata	0,02	0,01	0,02	0,01
*Korea, Kangwha	-	-	-	-
*Kuwait: Non-Kuwaitis	0,01	0,01	0,02	0,01
*Kuwait: Kuwaitis	0,04	0,04	0,03	0,02
*Philippines, Manila	0.02	0.01	0.01	0.00
Singapore: Chinese	0.06	0.01	0.03	0.01
Singapore: Malay	0,02	0,01	0,04	0,03
Singapore: Indian	-	-	-	-
Thailand, Chiang Mai	0,01	0,00	0,01	0,01
*Thailand, Khon Kaen	0,01	0,00	0,02	0,01
*Viet Nam, Hanoi				

* IMPORTANT-SEE NOTES ON POPULATION PAGE

EUROPE	MALE		FEMALE	
Austria, Tyrol	0.08	0.02	0,06	0,02
*Belarus	0.02	0.00	0.01	0.00
*Croatia	0.06	0.01	0.05	0.01
Czech Republic	0.05	0.01	0.04	0.00
Denmark	0.03	0.00	0.03	0.00
Estonia	0.04	0.01	0,01	0,01
Finland	0.04	0.01	0.03	0.00
France, Bas-Rhin	0.07	0.02	0.04	0.01
*France, Calvados	0,01	0,01	0,04	0,02
France, Doubs	0,03	0,01	0,03	0,01
France, Haut-Rhin	0,06	0.02	0,03	0,01
*France, Herault	0,03	0,01	0,02	0,01
France, Isere	0,02	0,01	0.04	0.01
*France, Somme	0,06	0,03	0,02	0,01
*France, Tarn	0,01	0,01	0,02	0,01
Germany, Eastern States	0.03	0.01	0.03	0.00
Germany, Saarland	0.07	0.02	0.05	0.01
Iceland	0,02	0,01	0,08	0,04
Ireland, Southern	0,05	0,02	0,06	0,02
Italy, Ferrara	0,02	0,02	0,04	0,03
Italy, Florence	0.06	0.02	0.05	0.01
Italy, Genoa	0.07	0.02	0.05	0,02
*Italy, Latina	0,06	0,03	0,02	0,01
Italy, Macerata	0,07	0,05	0,03	0,03
Italy, Modena	0.09	0.02	0.05	0.02
Italy, Parma	0,02	0,01	0,06	0,02
Italy, Ragusa	0,05	0,03	0,04	0,02
Italy, Romagna	0,04	0,02	0,04	0,02
Italy, Torino	0.09	0.02	0.05	0.01
Italy, Trieste	0.21	0.06	0.31	0.06
Italy, Varese	0,03	0,01	0,03	0,01
Italy, Veneto	0.06	0.01	0.04	0.01
*Latvia	0.03	0.01	0.02	0.01
Malta	0,02	0,02	0,04	0,03
The Netherlands	0.04	0.00	0.03	0.00
The Netherlands, Eindhoven	0,03	0,01	0.03	0.01
The Netherlands, Maastricht	0.04	0.01	0,03	0,01
Norway	0.05	0.01	0.05	0.01
*Poland, Cracow	0,05	0,02	0,05	0,02
*Poland, Kielce	0.05	0.01	0.04	0.01
*Poland, Lower Silesia	0.09	0.01	0.05	0.01
Poland, Warsaw City	0.09	0.02	0.07	0.01
Slovakia	0.05	0.01	0.04	0.01
Slovenia	0.02	0.01	0.03	0.01
*Spain, Albacete	-	-	-	-
Spain, Asturias	0.06	0.02	0,03	0,01
Spain, Basque Country	0.03	0.01	0.02	0.01
Spain, Granada	0,03	0,01	0,03	0,01
Spain, Mallorca	0,02	0,01	0,03	0,01
Spain, Murcia	0,03	0,01	0.03	0.01
Spain, Navarra	0,06	0,02	0,03	0,01
Spain, Tarragona	0.04	0,02	0.07	0.02
Spain, Zaragoza	0.06	0.02	0.04	0.01

	MALE		FEMALE	
Sweden	0.03	0.00	0.03	0.00
*Switzerland, Basel	0,07	0,02	0,04	0,02
Switzerland, Geneva	0,04	0,03	0,09	0,03
Switzerland, Graubunden	-	-	0,05	0,04
Switzerland, Neuchatel	0,03	0,03	0,02	0,02
Switzerland, St Gall-Appenzell	0,01	0,01	0,01	0,01
Switzerland, Valais	-	-	0,05	0,03
Switzerland, Vaud	0,04	0,02	0,02	0,01
Switzerland, Zurich	0,03	0,01	0.05	0.01
*UK, England and Wales	0.05	0.00	0.04	0.00
*UK, East Anglia	0.04	0.01	0.02	0.01
*UK, Mersey	0.03	0.01	0.03	0.01
*UK, North Western	0.02	0.00	0.02	0.00
UK, Oxford	0.05	0.01	0.05	0.01
*UK, South Thames	0.06	0.01	0.04	0.00
UK, South Western	0.05	0.01	0.03	0.01
UK, Wessex	0.05	0.01	0.06	0.01
*UK, West Midlands	0.09	0.01	0.09	0.01
UK, Yorkshire	0.04	0.01	0.03	0.01
UK, Scotland	0.04	0.01	0.04	0.01
UK, Scotland, West	0.05	0.01	0.04	0.01
*Yugoslavia, Vojvodina	0.05	0.01	0.03	0.01

OCEANIA

	MALE		FEMALE	
Australian Capital Territory	0,02	0,01	0,03	0,02
Australia, New South Wales	0.04	0.00	0.04	0.00
South Australia	0.06	0.01	0.02	0.01
Australia, Tasmania	0.03	0,01	0.03	0,02
Australia, Victoria	0.04	0.01	0.02	0.00
Western Australia	0.03	0.01	0.04	0.01
*French Polynesia	0,04	0,03	0,05	0,02
New Zealand: Non-Maori	0.05	0.01	0.06	0.01
New Zealand: Maori	0,15	0,07	0,11	0,05
US, Hawaii: White	0,02	0,01	0,02	0,01
US, Hawaii: Japanese	0,03	0,02	0,03	0,02
US, Hawaii: Hawaiian	0,08	0,04	0,01	0,01
US, Hawaii: Filipino	0,03	0,02	-	-
US, Hawaii: Chinese	-	-	0,05	0,05

* IMPORTANT-SEE NOTES ON POPULATION PAGE

CUMULATIVE INCIDENCE (0-74)
RATES AND STANDARD ERRORS (percent)
Non-Hodgkin lymphomas (ICD-9 200+202)

	MALE		FEMALE	
AFRICA				
*Algeria, Setif				
*France, La Reunion				
*Mali, Bamako				
*Uganda, Kyadondo				
*Zimbabwe, Harare: African				
*Zimbabwe, Harare: European				
AMERICA, CENTRAL AND SOUTH				
*Argentina, Concordia	0,39	0,14	0.58	0.18
*Brazil, Belem	0.51	0.09	0.24	0.06
*Brazil, Goiania				
*Brazil, Porto Alegre	0.91	0.11	0.73	0.08
Colombia, Cali	0.84	0.08	0.72	0.07
*Costa Rica	0.61	0.05	0.39	0.04
*Ecuador, Quito	0.82	0.09	0.71	0.08
*Peru, Lima	0.75	0.06	0.67	0.05
Peru, Trujillo	0.98	0.22	0.53	0.14
US, Puerto Rico	0.82	0.04	0.55	0.03
*Uruguay, Montevideo	1.07	0.08	0.84	0.06
AMERICA, NORTH				
Canada	1.45	0.02	1.02	0.01
Canada, Alberta	1.32	0.06	0.95	0.05
Canada, British Columbia	1.43	0.05	0.96	0.04
Canada, Manitoba	1.61	0.09	1.21	0.07
Canada, New Brunswick	1.52	0.11	0.89	0.08
Canada, Newfoundland	0.94	0.10	0.68	0.08
Canada, Northwest Territories	1.21	0.42	1.01	0.34
Canada, Nova Scotia	1.37	0.09	0.97	0.07
Canada, Ontario	1.49	0.03	1.05	0.02
Canada, Prince Edward Island	1.30	0.23	1.29	0.21
Canada, Quebec	1.47	0.03	1.03	0.03
Canada, Saskatchewan	1.46	0.08	1.10	0.07
Canada, Yukon	0,63	0,26	0,78	0,40
US, Cent. Calif.: Non-Hisp. White	1.47	0.07	1.01	0.05
US, Cent. Calif.: Hispanic	1.24	0.15	0.95	0.13
US, Los Angeles: Non-Hisp. White	1.93	0.05	1.14	0.03
US, Los Angeles: Hispanic White	1.24	0.07	0.81	0.05
US, Los Angeles: Black	1.12	0.09	0.66	0.06
US, Los Angeles: Chinese	0.81	0.14	0.47	0.10
US, Los Angeles: Filipino	1.03	0.20	0.68	0.14
US, Los Angeles: Korean	0.63	0.20	0.51	0.14
US, Los Angeles: Japanese	1.27	0.21	0.68	0.14
US, San Francisco: Non-Hisp. White	2.57	0.07	1.11	0.05
US, San Francisco: Hispanic White	2.19	0.20	1.24	0.13
US, San Francisco: Black	1.37	0.13	0.82	0.10
US, San Francisco: Chinese	1.06	0.14	0.64	0.10
US, San Francisco: Filipino	1.39	0.27	1.04	0.20
US, San Francisco: Japanese	0.94	0.31	1.07	0.26
US, Connecticut: White	1.61	0.05	1.22	0.04
US, Connecticut: Black	1.28	0.18	1.01	0.15
US, Atlanta: White	1.51	0.08	1.18	0.07
US, Atlanta: Black	1.14	0.14	0.87	0.11
US, Iowa	1.65	0.05	1.21	0.04

	MALE		FEMALE	
US, Central Louisiana: White	1.49	0.19	1.00	0.14
US, Central Louisiana: Black	1.02	0.32	0,52	0,20
US, New Orleans: White	1.75	0.12	1.04	0.08
US, New Orleans: Black	0.89	0.13	0.56	0.09
US, Detroit: White	1.66	0.05	1.18	0.04
US, Detroit: Black	1.36	0.09	0.80	0.07
US, New Mexico: Non-Hisp. White	1.28	0.09	0.95	0.07
US, New Mexico: Hispanic White	0.92	0.11	0.63	0.09
US, New Mexico: American Indian	0,34	0,14	0,42	0,15
US, Utah	1.52	0.08	1.10	0.06
US, Seattle	1.74	0.05	1.14	0.04
US, SEER: White	1.75	0.02	1.15	0.02
US, SEER: Black	1.28	0.06	0.84	0.04
ASIA				
*China, Qidong	0.43	0.05	0.19	0.03
China, Shanghai	0.46	0.02	0.27	0.01
China, Tianjin	0.48	0.03	0.31	0.02
Hong Kong	0.93	0.03	0.67	0.03
*India, Bangalore	0.43	0.03	0.23	0.02
*India, Barshi, Paranda and Bhum	0,09	0,04	0,07	0,03
India, Bombay	0.45	0.03	0.31	0.02
*India, Karunagappally	0.64	0.18	0,16	0,09
India, Madras	0.35	0.03	0.22	0.02
*India, Trivandrum	0.54	0.12	0.26	0.07
Israel: All Jews	1.36	0.05	1.14	0.04
Jews born in Israel	1.71	0.19	1.28	0.16
Jews born in America or Europe	1.40	0.07	1.13	0.06
Jews born in Africa or Asia	1.12	0.08	1.02	0.07
Non-Jews	0.85	0.12	0.76	0.11
Japan, Hiroshima	0.90	0.07	0.51	0.05
Japan, Miyagi	0.68	0.04	0.45	0.03
Japan, Nagasaki	1.51	0.07	0.76	0.04
Japan, Osaka	0.68	0.02	0.39	0.01
*Japan, Saga	0.96	0.07	0.39	0.04
Japan, Yamagata	0.54	0.04	0.25	0.03
*Korea, Kangwha	0,38	0,14	0,19	0,09
*Kuwait: Non-Kuwaitis	0.99	0.29	0.75	0.21
*Kuwait: Kuwaitis	0.52	0.11	0.86	0.18
*Philippines, Manila	0.65	0.05	0.39	0.04
Singapore: Chinese	0.63	0.05	0.54	0.04
Singapore: Malay	0.81	0.13	0.69	0.13
Singapore: Indian	0.37	0.09	0.45	0.20
Thailand, Chiang Mai	0.41	0.05	0.26	0.03
*Thailand, Khon Kaen	0.28	0.05	0.19	0.04
*Viet Nam, Hanoi				

* IMPORTANT-SEE NOTES ON POPULATION PAGE

CUMULATIVE INCIDENCE (0-74)
RATES AND STANDARD ERRORS (percent)
Non-Hodgkin lymphomas (ICD-9 200+202) (contd)

EUROPE	MALE		FEMALE	
Austria, Tyrol	0.87	0.09	0.90	0.08
*Belarus	0.35	0.02	0.19	0.01
*Croatia	0.57	0.03	0.40	0.02
Czech Republic	0.76	0.02	0.49	0.01
Denmark	1.08	0.03	0.74	0.02
Estonia	0.51	0.05	0.28	0.03
Finland	1.15	0.03	0.88	0.02
France, Bas-Rhin	1.35	0.09	0.90	0.07
*France, Calvados	0.96	0.09	0.63	0.07
France, Doubs	1.39	0.12	0.85	0.09
France, Haut-Rhin	1.17	0.11	0.76	0.07
*France, Herault	1.10	0.08	0.78	0.06
France, Isere	1.06	0.07	0.75	0.06
*France, Somme	0.98	0.10	0.60	0.07
*France, Tarn	0.67	0.09	0.59	0.08
Germany, Eastern States	0.62	0.02	0.41	0.02
Germany, Saarland	1.00	0.07	0.62	0.04
Iceland	0.93	0.14	0.50	0.10
Ireland, Southern	1.04	0.10	0.79	0.08
Italy, Ferrara	1.34	0.18	1.25	0.16
Italy, Florence	1.11	0.07	0.70	0.05
Italy, Genoa	1.41	0.09	0.84	0.06
*Italy, Latina	0.71	0.09	0.59	0.08
Italy, Macerata	1.12	0.20	0.81	0.16
Italy, Modena	1.36	0.09	1.03	0.08
Italy, Parma	1.32	0.11	0.91	0.08
Italy, Ragusa	0.67	0.10	0.44	0.07
Italy, Romagna	1.72	0.12	0.87	0.08
Italy, Torino	1.26	0.08	0.82	0.06
Italy, Trieste	1.75	0.17	1.06	0.12
Italy, Varese	1.52	0.10	1.06	0.07
Italy, Veneto	1.45	0.07	1.05	0.06
*Latvia	0.40	0.03	0.23	0.02
Malta	0.65	0.15	0.70	0.15
The Netherlands	1.19	0.02	0.78	0.02
The Netherlands, Eindhoven	1.10	0.08	0.65	0.06
The Netherlands, Maastricht	0.99	0.07	0.75	0.06
Norway	1.10	0.03	0.78	0.03
*Poland, Cracow	0.67	0.08	0.28	0.04
*Poland, Kielce	0.47	0.04	0.24	0.03
*Poland, Lower Silesia	0.56	0.04	0.30	0.02
Poland, Warsaw City	0.73	0.06	0.40	0.04
Slovakia	0.62	0.03	0.41	0.02
Slovenia	0.66	0.05	0.47	0.03
*Spain, Albacete	0.73	0.15	0.48	0.12
Spain, Asturias	0.83	0.06	0.66	0.05
Spain, Basque Country	0.81	0.05	0.61	0.04
Spain, Granada	0.56	0.06	0.47	0.05
Spain, Mallorca	0.84	0.08	0.55	0.06
Spain, Murcia	0.80	0.06	0.60	0.05
Spain, Navarra	0.85	0.08	0.61	0.07
Spain, Tarragona	0.54	0.06	0.61	0.07
Spain, Zaragoza	0.69	0.06	0.55	0.05

	MALE		FEMALE	
Sweden	1.21	0.02	0.79	0.02
*Switzerland, Basel	1.63	0.13	0.81	0.08
Switzerland, Geneva	1.34	0.13	0.84	0.09
Switzerland, Graubunden	0.81	0.17	0.58	0.13
Switzerland, Neuchatel	1.11	0.17	0.64	0.12
Switzerland, St Gall-Appenzell	1.09	0.10	0.75	0.08
Switzerland, Valais	0.93	0.15	0.62	0.11
Switzerland, Vaud	1.50	0.11	0.92	0.08
Switzerland, Zurich	1.34	0.07	0.92	0.06
*UK, England and Wales	1.05	0.01	0.71	0.01
*UK, East Anglia	1.16	0.05	0.77	0.04
*UK, Mersey	0.78	0.04	0.62	0.03
*UK, North Western	0.93	0.03	0.66	0.03
UK, Oxford	1.11	0.05	0.75	0.04
*UK, South Thames	1.12	0.03	0.75	0.02
UK, South Western	1.23	0.04	0.86	0.03
UK, Wessex	1.30	0.04	0.91	0.03
*UK, West Midlands	0.95	0.03	0.69	0.02
UK, Yorkshire	1.06	0.04	0.66	0.03
UK, Scotland	1.03	0.03	0.84	0.03
UK, Scotland, West	0.95	0.04	0.80	0.03
*Yugoslavia, Vojvodina	0.42	0.03	0.30	0.02

OCEANIA	MALE		FEMALE	
Australian Capital Territory	1.49	0.20	1.06	0.16
Australia, New South Wales	1.42	0.03	0.97	0.03
South Australia	1.40	0.07	1.05	0.06
Australia, Tasmania	1.46	0.13	1.15	0.11
Australia, Victoria	1.49	0.04	1.06	0.03
Western Australia	1.33	0.07	0.95	0.06
*French Polynesia	0.45	0.15	0.55	0.20
New Zealand: Non-Maori	1.11	0.04	0.81	0.04
New Zealand: Maori	0.90	0.20	0.66	0.15
US, Hawaii: White	1.73	0.17	0.84	0.13
US, Hawaii: Japanese	0.93	0.11	0.71	0.09
US, Hawaii: Hawaiian	1.38	0.25	0.60	0.16
US, Hawaii: Filipino	1.33	0.21	0.91	0.17
US, Hawaii: Chinese	1.66	0.33	0.80	0.20

* IMPORTANT-SEE NOTES ON POPULATION PAGE

CUMULATIVE INCIDENCE (0-74)
RATES AND STANDARD ERRORS (percent)
Hodgkin's disease (ICD-9 201)

	MALE		FEMALE	
AFRICA				
*Algeria, Setif				
*France, La Reunion				
*Mali, Bamako				
*Uganda, Kyadondo				
*Zimbabwe, Harare: African				
*Zimbabwe, Harare: European				
AMERICA, CENTRAL AND SOUTH				
*Argentina, Concordia	0,10	0,06	0,05	0,04
*Brazil, Belem	0.29	0.08	0.12	0.04
*Brazil, Goiania				
*Brazil, Porto Alegre	0.26	0.06	0.11	0.03 mf
Colombia, Cali	0.17	0.03	0.07	0.02 f
*Costa Rica	0.23	0.02	0.12	0.02
*Ecuador, Quito	0.16	0.04	0.13	0.03
*Peru, Lima	0.09	0.02	0.09	0.02
Peru, Trujillo	0,05	0,02	0,01	0,01
US, Puerto Rico	0.18	0.02	0.14	0.01
*Uruguay, Montevideo	0.32	0.04	0.17	0.03
AMERICA, NORTH				
Canada	0.24	0.01	0.18	0.00
Canada, Alberta	0.24	0.02	0.15	0.02
Canada, British Columbia	0.19	0.01	0.16	0.01
Canada, Manitoba	0.20	0.03	0.12	0.02
Canada, New Brunswick	0.23	0.04	0.15	0.03
Canada, Newfoundland	0.14	0.03	0.16	0.03
Canada, Northwest Territories	0,02	0,02	0,02	0,02
Canada, Nova Scotia	0.23	0.03	0.18	0.03
Canada, Ontario	0.25	0.01	0.19	0.01
Canada, Prince Edward Island	0,19	0,07	0,10	0,05
Canada, Quebec	0.27	0.01	0.21	0.01
Canada, Saskatchewan	0.23	0.03	0.14	0.02
Canada, Yukon	0,13	0,07	0,26	0,11
US, Cent. Calif.: Non-Hisp. White	0.24	0.03	0.19	0.02
US, Cent. Calif.: Hispanic	0.15	0.04	0.15	0.04
US, Los Angeles: Non-Hisp. White	0.28	0.02	0.20	0.01
US, Los Angeles: Hispanic White	0.18	0.02	0.14	0.02
US, Los Angeles: Black	0.16	0.02	0.14	0.02
US, Los Angeles: Chinese	0,05	0,03	0,05	0,03
US, Los Angeles: Filipino	0,10	0,04	0,08	0,04
US, Los Angeles: Korean	0,02	0,02	0,01	0,01
US, Los Angeles: Japanese	0,09	0,06	0,05	0,04
US, San Francisco: Non-Hisp. White	0.34	0.02	0.24	0.02
US, San Francisco: Hispanic White	0.17	0.05	0.16	0.04
US, San Francisco: Black	0.28	0.06	0.19	0.04
US, San Francisco: Chinese	0,11	0,04	0,04	0,02
US, San Francisco: Filipino	0,06	0,03	0,07	0,04
US, San Francisco: Japanese	0,15	0,11	0,05	0,05
US, Connecticut: White	0.33	0.02	0.27	0.02
US, Connecticut: Black	0.16	0.05	0.17	0.05
US, Atlanta: White	0.25	0.03	0.19	0.02
US, Atlanta: Black	0.20	0.04	0.14	0.03
US, Iowa	0.27	0.02	0.19	0.01

	MALE		FEMALE	
US, Central Louisiana: White	0,13	0,05	0.16	0.05
US, Central Louisiana: Black	0,19	0,12	0,07	0,07
US, New Orleans: White	0.28	0.04	0.20	0.03
US, New Orleans: Black	0.14	0.04	0.12	0.03
US, Detroit: White	0.30	0.02	0.22	0.02
US, Detroit: Black	0.24	0.03	0.16	0.03
US, New Mexico: Non-Hisp. White	0.24	0.03	0.18	0.03
US, New Mexico: Hispanic White	0.26	0.06	0.12	0.03
US, New Mexico: American Indian	0,02	0,02	-	-
US, Utah	0.16	0.02	0.16	0.02
US, Seattle	0.25	0.02	0.20	0.01
US, SEER: White	0.28	0.01	0.21	0.01
US, SEER: Black	0.22	0.02	0.17	0.02
ASIA				
*China, Qidong	0,01	0,00	-	-
China, Shanghai	0.04	0.00	0.03	0.00
China, Tianjin	0.03	0.01	0.03	0.01
Hong Kong	0.06	0.01	0.02	0.00
*India, Bangalore	0.13	0.02	0.07	0.01
*India, Barshi, Paranda and Bhum	0,05	0,03	-	-
India, Bombay	0.13	0.01	0.07	0.01
*India, Karunagappally	0,09	0,05	0,03	0,03
India, Madras	0.11	0.01	0.05	0.01
*India, Trivandrum	0,07	0,04	0,03	0,02
Israel: All Jews	0.23	0.02	0.22	0.01
Jews born in Israel	0.24	0.03	0.22	0.03
Jews born in America or Europe	0.23	0.03	0.24	0.03
Jews born in Africa or Asia	0.17	0.03	0.09	0.02
Non-Jews	0.19	0.03	0.17	0.05
Japan, Hiroshima	0,04	0,01	0.04	0.01
Japan, Miyagi	0.05	0.01	0.02	0.01
Japan, Nagasaki	0.03	0.01	0,01	0,00
Japan, Osaka	0.05	0.01	0.02	0.00
*Japan, Saga	0,01	0,00	0,02	0,01
Japan, Yamagata	0,02	0,01	0,00	0,00
*Korea, Kangwha	0,02	0,02	-	-
*Kuwait: Non-Kuwaitis	0.14	0.02	0.25	0.12
*Kuwait: Kuwaitis	0.41	0.10	0.22	0.09
*Philippines, Manila	0.08	0.01	0.03	0.01
Singapore: Chinese	0.04	0.01	0.02	0.01
Singapore: Malay	0.14	0.05	0,03	0,02
Singapore: Indian	0,10	0,04	0,08	0,07
Thailand, Chiang Mai	0.11	0.02	0.03	0.01
*Thailand, Khon Kaen	0.04	0.01	0.06	0.02
*Viet Nam, Hanoi				

* IMPORTANT-SEE NOTES ON POPULATION PAGE

CUMULATIVE INCIDENCE (0-74)
RATES AND STANDARD ERRORS (percent)
Hodgkin's disease (ICD-9 201) (contd)

EUROPE	MALE		FEMALE	
Austria, Tyrol	0.23	0.04	0.15	0.03
*Belarus	0.28	0.01	0.20	0.01
*Croatia	0.15	0.01	0.10	0.01
Czech Republic	0.27	0.01	0.19	0.01
Denmark	0.24	0.01	0.13	0.01
Estonia	0.25	0.03	0.13	0.02
Finland	0.20	0.01	0.14	0.01
France, Bas-Rhin	0.21	0.03	0.14	0.02
*France, Calvados	0.17	0.03	0.16	0.03
France, Doubs	0.17	0.03	0.13	0.03
France, Haut-Rhin	0.16	0.03	0.16	0.03
*France, Herault	0.24	0.03	0.13	0.02
France, Isere	0.19	0.03	0.11	0.02
*France, Somme	0.21	0.04	0.13	0.03
*France, Tarn	0.17	0.04	0,05	0,02
Germany, Eastern States	0.24	0.01	0.17	0.01
Germany, Saarland	0.23	0.03	0.16	0.02
Iceland	0.24	0.06	0,09	0,03
Ireland, Southern	0.12	0.03	0.16	0.03
Italy, Ferrara	0.33	0.09	0.21	0.06
Italy, Florence	0.31	0.03	0.23	0.03
Italy, Genoa	0.32	0.04	0.17	0.03
*Italy, Latina	0.18	0.04	0.16	0.03
Italy, Macerata	0.40	0.12	0,28	0,09
Italy, Modena	0.20	0.03	0.17	0.03
Italy, Parma	0.17	0.04	0.18	0.04
Italy, Ragusa	0.24	0.06	0.19	0.05
Italy, Romagna	0.23	0.04	0.23	0.04
Italy, Torino	0.28	0.03	0.21	0.03
Italy, Trieste	0.27	0.06	0.26	0.06
Italy, Varese	0.30	0.04	0.20	0.03
Italy, Veneto	0.32	0.03	0.28	0.03
*Latvia	0.21	0.02	0.16	0.01
Malta	0,15	0,06	0,21	0,08
The Netherlands	0.21	0.01	0.13	0.01
The Netherlands, Eindhoven	0.16	0.02	0.11	0.02
The Netherlands, Maastricht	0.22	0.03	0.16	0.03
Norway	0.18	0.01	0.11	0.01
*Poland, Cracow	0.27	0.04	0.19	0.03
*Poland, Kielce	0.23	0.03	0.13	0.02
*Poland, Lower Silesia	0.20	0.02	0.15	0.01
Poland, Warsaw City	0.18	0.02	0.13	0.02
Slovakia	0.19	0.01	0.13	0.01
Slovenia	0.18	0.02	0.11	0.01
*Spain, Albacete	0.28	0.08	0,09	0,05
Spain, Asturias	0.29	0.03	0.16	0.02
Spain, Basque Country	0.26	0.02	0.15	0.02
Spain, Granada	0.17	0.03	0.11	0.02
Spain, Mallorca	0.19	0.03	0.14	0.03
Spain, Murcia	0.16	0.02	0.10	0.02
Spain, Navarra	0.25	0.04	0.16	0.03
Spain, Tarragona	0.24	0.04	0.08	0.02
Spain, Zaragoza	0.20	0.03	0.12	0.02

	MALE		FEMALE	
Sweden	0.18	0.01	0.13	0.01
*Switzerland, Basel	0.22	0.04	0.18	0.04
Switzerland, Geneva	0.25	0.05	0.16	0.04
Switzerland, Graubunden	0.31	0.09	0,10	0,05
Switzerland, Neuchatel	0,18	0,06	0,10	0,04
Switzerland, St Gall-Appenzell	0.18	0.03	0.16	0.03
Switzerland, Valais	0.20	0.07	0.19	0.05
Switzerland, Vaud	0.17	0.03	0.16	0.03
Switzerland, Zurich	0.23	0.03	0.17	0.02
*UK, England and Wales	0.22	0.00	0.14	0.00
*UK, East Anglia	0.20	0.02	0.14	0.01
*UK, Mersey	0.18	0.02	0.12	0.01
*UK, North Western	0.21	0.01	0.14	0.01
UK, Oxford	0.21	0.02	0.19	0.02
*UK, South Thames	0.22	0.01	0.14	0.01
UK, South Western	0.22	0.01	0.13	0.01
UK, Wessex	0.21	0.02	0.17	0.01
*UK, West Midlands	0.24	0.01	0.14	0.01
UK, Yorkshire	0.21	0.01	0.15	0.01
UK, Scotland	0.22	0.01	0.16	0.01
UK, Scotland, West	0.20	0.02	0.15	0.01
*Yugoslavia, Vojvodina	0.23	0.02	0.11	0.01

OCEANIA	MALE		FEMALE	
Australian Capital Territory	0.14	0.05	0,06	0,03
Australia, New South Wales	0.17	0.01	0.12	0.01
South Australia	0.15	0.02	0.13	0.02
Australia, Tasmania	0.13	0.04	0.19	0.04
Australia, Victoria	0.20	0.01	0.14	0.01
Western Australia	0.17	0.02	0.12	0.02
*French Polynesia	0,07	0,03	0,10	0,06
New Zealand: Non-Maori	0.17	0.01	0.12	0.01
New Zealand: Maori	0.15	0.06	0,05	0,03
US, Hawaii: White	0.23	0.05	0.24	0.06
US, Hawaii: Japanese	0,08	0,03	0.12	0.04
US, Hawaii: Hawaiian	0,07	0,04	0.13	0.04
US, Hawaii: Filipino	0,09	0,05	0,09	0,04
US, Hawaii: Chinese	0,06	0,06	-	-

* IMPORTANT-SEE NOTES ON POPULATION PAGE

CUMULATIVE INCIDENCE (0-74)
RATES AND STANDARD ERRORS (percent)
Multiple myeloma (ICD-9 203)

	MALE		FEMALE	
AFRICA				
*Algeria, Setif				
*France, La Reunion				
*Mali, Bamako				
*Uganda, Kyadondo				
*Zimbabwe, Harare: African				
*Zimbabwe, Harare: European				
AMERICA, CENTRAL AND SOUTH				
*Argentina, Concordia	-	-	0,07	0,07
*Brazil, Belem	0,07	0,03	0,06	0,04 f
*Brazil, Goiania				
*Brazil, Porto Alegre	0.34	0.07	0.24	0.04
Colombia, Cali	0.27	0.05	0.19	0.04
*Costa Rica	0.28	0.03	0.18	0.03
*Ecuador, Quito	0.20	0.05	0.12	0.04
*Peru, Lima	0.17	0.03	0.11	0.02
Peru, Trujillo	0,31	0,12	0,21	0,09
US, Puerto Rico	0.35	0.03	0.22	0.02
*Uruguay, Montevideo	0.22	0.04	0.24	0.03
AMERICA, NORTH				
Canada	0.47	0.01	0.32	0.01
Canada, Alberta	0.44	0.04	0.31	0.03
Canada, British Columbia	0.44	0.03	0.27	0.02
Canada, Manitoba	0.50	0.05	0.31	0.04
Canada, New Brunswick	0.52	0.06	0.32	0.05
Canada, Newfoundland	0.32	0.06	0.27	0.05
Canada, Northwest Territories	0,30	0,19	0,19	0,19
Canada, Nova Scotia	0.37	0.05	0.32	0.04
Canada, Ontario	0.50	0.02	0.36	0.01
Canada, Prince Edward Island	0.65	0.17	0.38	0.12
Canada, Quebec	0.47	0.02	0.31	0.01
Canada, Saskatchewan	0.51	0.05	0.25	0.03
Canada, Yukon	0,93	0,52	0,53	0,27
US, Cent. Calif.: Non-Hisp. White	0.42	0.04	0.30	0.03
US, Cent. Calif.: Hispanic	0.43	0.09	0.34	0.08
US, Los Angeles: Non-Hisp. White	0.42	0.02	0.28	0.02
US, Los Angeles: Hispanic White	0.46	0.05	0.32	0.04
US, Los Angeles: Black	1.02	0.09	0.59	0.06
US, Los Angeles: Chinese	0,14	0,06	0,08	0,04
US, Los Angeles: Filipino	0,25	0,09	0,23	0,09
US, Los Angeles: Korean	0,08	0,05	0,04	0,04
US, Los Angeles: Japanese	0,07	0,05	0,06	0,05
US, San Francisco: Non-Hisp. White	0.47	0.03	0.27	0.02
US, San Francisco: Hispanic White	0.50	0.10	0.27	0.07
US, San Francisco: Black	1.15	0.14	0.81	0.10
US, San Francisco: Chinese	0.21	0.07	0.24	0.07
US, San Francisco: Filipino	0.61	0.18	0,19	0,08
US, San Francisco: Japanese	0,21	0,15	0,05	0,05
US, Connecticut: White	0.43	0.03	0.30	0.02
US, Connecticut: Black	0.84	0.17	0.53	0.11
US, Atlanta: White	0.44	0.05	0.26	0.03
US, Atlanta: Black	1.06	0.15	0.70	0.10
US, Iowa	0.52	0.03	0.33	0.02

	MALE		FEMALE	
US, Central Louisiana: White	0.23	0.07	0.37	0.09
US, Central Louisiana: Black	0,68	0,26	0,40	0,18
US, New Orleans: White	0.42	0.06	0.22	0.04
US, New Orleans: Black	0.99	0.15	0.64	0.10
US, Detroit: White	0.49	0.03	0.31	0.02
US, Detroit: Black	1.12	0.09	0.80	0.07
US, New Mexico: Non-Hisp. White	0.42	0.05	0.27	0.04
US, New Mexico: Hispanic White	0.27	0.06	0.36	0.07
US, New Mexico: American Indian	0,25	0,16	0,41	0,16
US, Utah	0.47	0.05	0.26	0.03
US, Seattle	0.55	0.03	0.37	0.02
US, SEER: White	0.47	0.01	0.30	0.01
US, SEER: Black	1.12	0.06	0.75	0.04
ASIA				
*China, Qidong	0.15	0.03	0.05	0.02
China, Shanghai	0.10	0.01	0.06	0.01
China, Tianjin	0.06	0.01	0.05	0.01
Hong Kong	0.19	0.01	0.18	0.01
*India, Bangalore	0.10	0.02	0.07	0.01
*India, Barshi, Paranda and Bhum	0,01	0,01	0,01	0,01
India, Bombay	0.15	0.02	0.12	0.01
*India, Karunagappally	0,06	0,04	0,10	0,08
India, Madras	0.12	0.02	0.05	0.01
*India, Trivandrum	0.30	0.08	0,04	0,02
Israel: All Jews	0.29	0.02	0.23	0.02
Jews born in Israel	0.42	0.11	0.27	0.09
Jews born in America or Europe	0.26	0.03	0.20	0.02
Jews born in Africa or Asia	0.31	0.04	0.28	0.04
Non-Jews	0.25	0.07	0.20	0.06
Japan, Hiroshima	0.24	0.04	0.12	0.02
Japan, Miyagi	0.20	0.02	0.15	0.02
Japan, Nagasaki	0.19	0.02	0.16	0.02
Japan, Osaka	0.17	0.01	0.12	0.01
*Japan, Saga	0.25	0.04	0.14	0.02
Japan, Yamagata	0.22	0.03	0.10	0.02
*Korea, Kangwha	0,12	0,09	0,12	0,06
*Kuwait: Non-Kuwaitis	0.52	0,23	0,15	0,07
*Kuwait: Kuwaitis	0,15	0,08	0,16	0,08
*Philippines, Manila	0.10	0.02	0.06	0.01
Singapore: Chinese	0.14	0.02	0.08	0.02
Singapore: Malay	0.37	0.10	0.31	0.10
Singapore: Indian	0.20	0.06	0,19	0,14
Thailand, Chiang Mai	0.06	0.02	0,04	0,02
*Thailand, Khon Kaen	0,04	0,02	0,01	0,01
*Viet Nam, Hanoi				

* IMPORTANT-SEE NOTES ON POPULATION PAGE

EUROPE	MALE		FEMALE	
Austria, Tyrol	0.48	0.07	0.29	0.05
*Belarus	0.14	0.01	0.11	0.01
*Croatia	0.22	0.02	0.21	0.02
Czech Republic	0.32	0.01	0.24	0.01
Denmark	0.38	0.02	0.29	0.02
Estonia	0.24	0.03	0.16	0.02
Finland	0.41	0.02	0.30	0.01
France, Bas-Rhin	0.26	0.04	0.14	0.03
*France, Calvados	0.28	0.06	0.19	0.04
France, Doubs	0.38	0.06	0.37	0.06
France, Haut-Rhin	0.31	0.05	0.22	0.04
*France, Herault	0.26	0.04	0.20	0.03
France, Isere	0.32	0.04	0.28	0.04
*France, Somme	0.22	0.04	0.20	0.04
*France, Tarn	0.20	0.05	0.23	0.05
Germany, Eastern States	0.29	0.02	0.19	0.01
Germany, Saarland	0.29	0.04	0.24	0.03
Iceland	0.47	0.10	0.24	0.07
Ireland, Southern	0.48	0.07	0.41	0.06
Italy, Ferrara	0.43	0.11	0.31	0.08
Italy, Florence	0.53	0.05	0.36	0.04
Italy, Genoa	0.41	0.05	0.25	0.03
*Italy, Latina	0.37	0.08	0.20	0.05
Italy, Macerata	0.32	0.11	0.41	0.11
Italy, Modena	0.44	0.06	0.30	0.04
Italy, Parma	0.51	0.07	0.30	0.05
Italy, Ragusa	0.36	0.08	0.18	0.05
Italy, Romagna	0.44	0.06	0.33	0.05
Italy, Torino	0.35	0.05	0.22	0.03
Italy, Trieste	0.46	0.09	0.42	0.07
Italy, Varese	0.42	0.06	0.27	0.04
Italy, Veneto	0.38	0.04	0.33	0.03
*Latvia	0.18	0.02	0.19	0.02
Malta	0,31	0,11	0,28	0,09
The Netherlands	0.41	0.01	0.28	0.01
The Netherlands, Eindhoven	0.36	0.05	0.29	0.04
The Netherlands, Maastricht	0.36	0.05	0.21	0.03
Norway	0.44	0.02	0.28	0.02
*Poland, Cracow	0.35	0.06	0.25	0.04
*Poland, Kielce	0.21	0.03	0.16	0.03
*Poland, Lower Silesia	0.20	0.02	0.17	0.02
Poland, Warsaw City	0.22	0.03	0.23	0.03
Slovakia	0.34	0.02	0.26	0.02
Slovenia	0.31	0.03	0.22	0.02
*Spain, Albacete	0.40	0.11	0.38	0.11
Spain, Asturias	0.31	0.04	0.18	0.03
Spain, Basque Country	0.22	0.03	0.21	0.02
Spain, Granada	0.27	0.04	0.21	0.03
Spain, Mallorca	0.35	0.05	0.27	0.04
Spain, Murcia	0.31	0.04	0.29	0.04
Spain, Navarra	0.27	0.05	0.19	0.04
Spain, Tarragona	0.34	0.05	0.29	0.05
Spain, Zaragoza	0.28	0.04	0.22	0.03

	MALE		FEMALE	
Sweden	0.45	0.02	0.29	0.01
*Switzerland, Basel	0.32	0.06	0.16	0.04
Switzerland, Geneva	0.42	0.08	0.29	0.06
Switzerland, Graubunden	0.54	0.14	0,27	0,09
Switzerland, Neuchatel	0,24	0,09	0,13	0,05
Switzerland, St Gall-Appenzell	0.44	0.07	0.31	0.05
Switzerland, Valais	0.43	0.10	0.27	0.08
Switzerland, Vaud	0.37	0.06	0.32	0.05
Switzerland, Zurich	0.38	0.04	0.29	0.03
*UK, England and Wales	0.39	0.01	0.27	0.01
*UK, East Anglia	0.40	0.03	0.25	0.02
*UK, Mersey	0.28	0.02	0.22	0.02
*UK, North Western	0.32	0.02	0.26	0.02
UK, Oxford	0.46	0.03	0.35	0.03
*UK, South Thames	0.39	0.02	0.28	0.01
UK, South Western	0.44	0.02	0.30	0.02
UK, Wessex	0.50	0.03	0.33	0.02
*UK, West Midlands	0.40	0.02	0.28	0.01
UK, Yorkshire	0.44	0.02	0.28	0.02
UK, Scotland	0.43	0.02	0.29	0.01
UK, Scotland, West	0.40	0.03	0.28	0.02
*Yugoslavia, Vojvodina	0.13	0.02	0.13	0.02

OCEANIA	MALE		FEMALE	
Australian Capital Territory	0.60	0.14	0.43	0.11
Australia, New South Wales	0.42	0.02	0.28	0.02
South Australia	0.51	0.04	0.34	0.03
Australia, Tasmania	0.47	0.07	0.29	0.06
Australia, Victoria	0.39	0.02	0.29	0.02
Western Australia	0.32	0.04	0.29	0.03
*French Polynesia	0,22	0,09	0,21	0,10
New Zealand: Non-Maori	0.43	0.03	0.33	0.02
New Zealand: Maori	0.84	0.21	0.64	0.16
US, Hawaii: White	0.48	0.10	0.25	0.07
US, Hawaii: Japanese	0.28	0.06	0,05	0,03
US, Hawaii: Hawaiian	0.50	0.15	0.63	0.17
US, Hawaii: Filipino	0.39	0.12	0,21	0,08
US, Hawaii: Chinese	0,44	0,18	-	-

* IMPORTANT-SEE NOTES ON POPULATION PAGE

CUMULATIVE INCIDENCE (0-74)
RATES AND STANDARD ERRORS (percent)
Lymphoid leukaemia (ICD-9 204)

	MALE		FEMALE	
AFRICA				
*Algeria, Setif				
*France, La Reunion				
*Mali, Bamako				
*Uganda, Kyadondo				
*Zimbabwe, Harare: African				
*Zimbabwe, Harare: European				
AMERICA, CENTRAL AND SOUTH				
*Argentina, Concordia	0,22	0,11	0,20	0,09
*Brazil, Belem	0.05	0.01	0.06	0.02 mf
*Brazil, Goiania				
*Brazil, Porto Alegre	0.21	0.05	0.16	0.03 mf
Colombia, Cali	0.14	0.03	0.17	0.03
*Costa Rica	0.31	0.03	0.22	0.02
*Ecuador, Quito	0.16	0.03	0.21	0.04
*Peru, Lima	0.16	0.02	0.11	0.02
Peru, Trujillo	0.14	0.08	0.11	0.04
US, Puerto Rico	0.18	0.02	0.14	0.01
*Uruguay, Montevideo	0.24	0.04	0.17	0.03
AMERICA, NORTH				
Canada	0.55	0.01	0.29	0.01
Canada, Alberta	0.47	0.03	0.30	0.03
Canada, British Columbia	0.40	0.02	0.23	0.02
Canada, Manitoba	0.47	0.05	0.21	0.03
Canada, New Brunswick	0.32	0.05	0.25	0.04
Canada, Newfoundland	0.21	0.04	0.19	0.04
Canada, Northwest Territories	0,15	0,08	0,05	0,03
Canada, Nova Scotia	0.35	0.04	0.21	0.03
Canada, Ontario	0.64	0.02	0.33	0.01
Canada, Prince Edward Island	0.54	0.15	0,22	0,08
Canada, Quebec	0.58	0.02	0.28	0.01
Canada, Saskatchewan	0.82	0.06	0.44	0.04
Canada, Yukon	1.10	0.44	0.88	0.33
US, Cent. Calif.: Non-Hisp. White	0.44	0.04	0.28	0.03
US, Cent. Calif.: Hispanic	0.48	0.08	0.25	0.05
US, Los Angeles: Non-Hisp. White	0.53	0.03	0.31	0.02
US, Los Angeles: Hispanic White	0.35	0.04	0.23	0.02
US, Los Angeles: Black	0.53	0.06	0.19	0.03
US, Los Angeles: Chinese	0,17	0,06	0,17	0,06
US, Los Angeles: Filipino	0.32	0.10	0.16	0.06
US, Los Angeles: Korean	0,11	0,06	0,12	0,06
US, Los Angeles: Japanese	0,06	0,04	0,22	0,09
US, San Francisco: Non-Hisp. White	0.47	0.03	0.24	0.02
US, San Francisco: Hispanic White	0.28	0.07	0.31	0.06
US, San Francisco: Black	0.49	0.09	0.26	0.05
US, San Francisco: Chinese	0.33	0.07	0,07	0,03
US, San Francisco: Filipino	0.22	0.07	0.17	0.06
US, San Francisco: Japanese	0,09	0,09	0,11	0,11
US, Connecticut: White	0.48	0.03	0.27	0.02
US, Connecticut: Black	0.32	0.10	0.27	0.07
US, Atlanta: White	0.40	0.04	0.23	0.03
US, Atlanta: Black	0.46	0.10	0.20	0.05
US, Iowa	0.68	0.03	0.35	0.02

	MALE		FEMALE	
US, Central Louisiana: White	0.34	0.09	0,16	0,06
US, Central Louisiana: Black	0,19	0,11	0,08	0,08
US, New Orleans: White	0.43	0.06	0.26	0.04
US, New Orleans: Black	0.36	0.08	0.18	0.05
US, Detroit: White	0.56	0.03	0.32	0.02
US, Detroit: Black	0.43	0.05	0.25	0.04
US, New Mexico: Non-Hisp. White	0.59	0.06	0.29	0.04
US, New Mexico: Hispanic White	0.42	0.07	0.16	0.04
US, New Mexico: American Indian	0,14	0,05	0,15	0,06
US, Utah	0.41	0.04	0.23	0.03
US, Seattle	0.56	0.03	0.29	0.02
US, SEER: White	0.53	0.01	0.28	0.01
US, SEER: Black	0.42	0.04	0.24	0.02
ASIA				
*China, Qidong	0.11	0.02	0.06	0.01
China, Shanghai	0.11	0.01	0.08	0.01
China, Tianjin	0.10	0.01	0.05	0.01
Hong Kong	0.15	0.01	0.11	0.01
*India, Bangalore	0.09	0.01	0.06	0.01
*India, Barshi, Paranda and Bhum	0,03	0,01	0,02	0,01
India, Bombay	0.13	0.01	0.10	0.01
*India, Karunagappally	0,09	0,04	0,07	0,03
India, Madras	0.10	0.01	0.07	0.01
*India, Trivandrum	0.19	0.06	0.08	0.03
Israel: All Jews	0.35	0.02	0.16	0.01
Jews born in Israel	0.25	0.05	0.25	0.09
Jews born in America or Europe	0.42	0.05	0.19	0.03
Jews born in Africa or Asia	0.33	0.06	0.26	0.12
Non-Jews	0.20	0.06	0.12	0.04
Japan, Hiroshima	0.17	0.03	0.07	0.02
Japan, Miyagi	0.15	0.02	0.09	0.01
Japan, Nagasaki	0.13	0.02	0.08	0.01
Japan, Osaka	0.17	0.01	0.12	0.01
*Japan, Saga	0.41	0.04	0.24	0.03
Japan, Yamagata	0.09	0.02	0.08	0.01
*Korea, Kangwha	0,12	0,06	0,06	0,04
*Kuwait: Non-Kuwaitis	0.43	0.20	0.19	0.08
*Kuwait: Kuwaitis	0.10	0.05	0.09	0.03
*Philippines, Manila	0.15	0.02	0.10	0.01
Singapore: Chinese	0.15	0.02	0.11	0.01
Singapore: Malay	0.12	0.04	0.05	0.02
Singapore: Indian	0,09	0,04	0,12	0,06
Thailand, Chiang Mai	0.07	0.01	0.05	0.01
*Thailand, Khon Kaen	0.09	0.02	0.05	0.01
*Viet Nam, Hanoi				

* IMPORTANT-SEE NOTES ON POPULATION PAGE

CUMULATIVE INCIDENCE (0-74)
RATES AND STANDARD ERRORS (percent)
Lymphoid leukaemia (ICD-9 204) (contd)

EUROPE	MALE		FEMALE	
Austria, Tyrol	0.49	0.07	0.24	0.04
*Belarus	0.70	0.02	0.34	0.01
*Croatia	0.46	0.03	0.25	0.02
Czech Republic	0.55	0.02	0.25	0.01
Denmark	0.49	0.02	0.25	0.01
Estonia	0.56	0.05	0.31	0.03
Finland	0.35	0.02	0.21	0.01
France, Bas-Rhin	0.46	0.06	0.24	0.03
†*France, Calvados	0.20	0.04	0.18	0.04
France, Doubs	0.31	0.06	0.17	0.04
France, Haut-Rhin	0.38	0.06	0.25	0.04
*France, Herault	0.25	0.04	0.19	0.03
France, Isere	0.38	0.05	0.19	0.03
*France, Somme	0.51	0.07	0.32	0.05
*France, Tarn	0.36	0.07	0.17	0.04
Germany, Eastern States	0.35	0.02	0.19	0.01
Germany, Saarland	0.39	0.04	0.26	0.03
Iceland	0.20	0.07	0.21	0.06
Ireland, Southern	0.67	0.08	0.24	0.04
Italy, Ferrara	0.47	0.11	0.32	0.09
Italy, Florence	0.36	0.04	0.22	0.03
Italy, Genoa	0.35	0.05	0.20	0.03
*Italy, Latina	0.52	0.08	0.36	0.07
Italy, Macerata	0.37	0.11	0.27	0.10
Italy, Modena	0.37	0.05	0.28	0.04
Italy, Parma	0.26	0.05	0.17	0.04
Italy, Ragusa	0.26	0.06	0.23	0.05
Italy, Romagna	0.54	0.07	0.31	0.05
Italy, Torino	0.40	0.05	0.21	0.03
Italy, Trieste	0.80	0.13	0.38	0.08
Italy, Varese	0.45	0.05	0.25	0.04
Italy, Veneto	0.38	0.04	0.25	0.03
*Latvia	0.56	0.04	0.31	0.02
Malta	0.34	0.11	0.17	0.07
The Netherlands	0.36	0.01	0.19	0.01
The Netherlands, Eindhoven	0.32	0.04	0.17	0.03
The Netherlands, Maastricht	0.39	0.05	0.22	0.03
Norway	0.19	0.01	0.11	0.01
*Poland, Cracow	0.28	0.05	0.12	0.03
*Poland, Kielce	0.33	0.04	0.16	0.02
*Poland, Lower Silesia	0.43	0.03	0.21	0.02
Poland, Warsaw City	0.28	0.04	0.16	0.02
Slovakia	0.56	0.03	0.26	0.02
Slovenia	0.41	0.04	0.32	0.03
*Spain, Albacete	0.63	0.15	0.15	0.06
Spain, Asturias	0.46	0.05	0.30	0.04
Spain, Basque Country	0.37	0.03	0.18	0.02
Spain, Granada	0.34	0.05	0.21	0.03
Spain, Mallorca	0.38	0.06	0.18	0.03
Spain, Murcia	0.31	0.04	0.22	0.03
Spain, Navarra	0.35	0.05	0.18	0.04
Spain, Tarragona	0.45	0.06	0.18	0.04
Spain, Zaragoza	0.27	0.04	0.17	0.03

	MALE		FEMALE	
Sweden	0.40	0.01	0.22	0.01
*Switzerland, Basel	0.40	0.07	0.19	0.04
Switzerland, Geneva	0.61	0.10	0.25	0.05
Switzerland, Graubunden	0.53	0.14	0.20	0.08
Switzerland, Neuchatel	0.41	0.11	0.12	0.05
Switzerland, St Gall-Appenzell	0.50	0.07	0.28	0.05
Switzerland, Valais	0.36	0.09	0.26	0.07
Switzerland, Vaud	0.28	0.05	0.14	0.03
Switzerland, Zurich	0.37	0.04	0.29	0.03
*UK, England and Wales	0.37	0.01	0.19	0.00
*UK, East Anglia	0.32	0.03	0.14	0.02
*UK, Mersey	0.22	0.02	0.16	0.02
*UK, North Western	0.32	0.02	0.15	0.01
UK, Oxford	0.38	0.03	0.22	0.02
*UK, South Thames	0.34	0.01	0.19	0.01
UK, South Western	0.45	0.02	0.26	0.02
UK, Wessex	0.43	0.02	0.27	0.02
*UK, West Midlands	0.41	0.02	0.20	0.01
UK, Yorkshire	0.38	0.02	0.20	0.01
UK, Scotland	0.43	0.02	0.21	0.01
UK, Scotland, West	0.40	0.03	0.20	0.02
*Yugoslavia, Vojvodina	0.49	0.04	0.22	0.02

OCEANIA	MALE		FEMALE	
Australian Capital Territory	0.51	0.12	0.23	0.08
Australia, New South Wales	0.45	0.02	0.27	0.01
South Australia	0.79	0.05	0.49	0.04
Australia, Tasmania	0.75	0.09	0.38	0.06
Australia, Victoria	0.44	0.02	0.22	0.01
Western Australia	0.31	0.03	0.19	0.02
*French Polynesia	0.18	0.08	0.27	0.13
New Zealand: Non-Maori	0.47	0.03	0.29	0.02
New Zealand: Maori	0.32	0.09	0.09	0.04
US, Hawaii: White	0.54	0.10	0.25	0.07
US, Hawaii: Japanese	0.13	0.04	0.13	0.04
US, Hawaii: Hawaiian	0.17	0.07	0.38	0.12
US, Hawaii: Filipino	0.12	0.05	0.05	0.03
US, Hawaii: Chinese	0.06	0.06	-	-

* IMPORTANT-SEE NOTES ON POPULATION PAGE

CUMULATIVE INCIDENCE (0-74)
RATES AND STANDARD ERRORS (percent)
Myeloid leukaemia (ICD-9 205)

	MALE		FEMALE	
AFRICA				
*Algeria, Setif				
*France, La Reunion				
*Mali, Bamako				
*Uganda, Kyadondo				
*Zimbabwe, Harare: African				
*Zimbabwe, Harare: European				
AMERICA, CENTRAL AND SOUTH				
*Argentina, Concordia	0,02	0,02	0,07	0,07
*Brazil, Belem	0.19	0.06	0.07	0.02
*Brazil, Goiania				
*Brazil, Porto Alegre	0.30	0.06	0.26	0.05 mf
Colombia, Cali	0.16	0.03	0.17	0.03
*Costa Rica	0.30	0.03	0.21	0.02
*Ecuador, Quito	0.38	0.06	0.21	0.04
*Peru, Lima	0.17	0.03	0.18	0.02
Peru, Trujillo	0.21	0.08	0.33	0.11
US, Puerto Rico	0.30	0.03	0.20	0.02
*Uruguay, Montevideo	0.32	0.05	0.23	0.03
AMERICA, NORTH				
Canada	0.38	0.01	0.26	0.01
Canada, Alberta	0.28	0.03	0.21	0.02
Canada, British Columbia	0.31	0.02	0.22	0.02
Canada, Manitoba	0.45	0.04	0.28	0.03
Canada, New Brunswick	0.33	0.05	0.23	0.04
Canada, Newfoundland	0.35	0.06	0.27	0.05
Canada, Northwest Territories	0,21	0,10	0,08	0,04
Canada, Nova Scotia	0.24	0.04	0.21	0.03
Canada, Ontario	0.47	0.02	0.32	0.01
Canada, Prince Edward Island	0,21	0,09	0,24	0,09
Canada, Quebec	0.33	0.02	0.21	0.01
Canada, Saskatchewan	0.38	0.04	0.22	0.03
Canada, Yukon	0,20	0,15	0,05	0,05
US, Cent. Calif.: Non-Hisp. White	0.47	0.04	0.28	0.03
US, Cent. Calif.: Hispanic	0.33	0.07	0.13	0.04
US, Los Angeles: Non-Hisp. White	0.49	0.02	0.32	0.02
US, Los Angeles: Hispanic White	0.32	0.04	0.28	0.03
US, Los Angeles: Black	0.40	0.05	0.29	0.04
US, Los Angeles: Chinese	0.44	0.11	0.21	0.07
US, Los Angeles: Filipino	0.62	0.14	0.22	0.06
US, Los Angeles: Korean	0,15	0,06	0,15	0,06
US, Los Angeles: Japanese	0.51	0.13	0.29	0.09
US, San Francisco: Non-Hisp. White	0.46	0.03	0.24	0.02
US, San Francisco: Hispanic White	0.46	0.09	0.46	0.08
US, San Francisco: Black	0.35	0.07	0.11	0.03
US, San Francisco: Chinese	0.29	0.08	0.32	0.08
US, San Francisco: Filipino	0.50	0.14	0.34	0.10
US, San Francisco: Japanese	0,24	0,15	0,21	0,13
US, Connecticut: White	0.38	0.02	0.26	0.02
US, Connecticut: Black	0.40	0.11	0.28	0.07
US, Atlanta: White	0.41	0.05	0.25	0.03
US, Atlanta: Black	0.37	0.08	0.25	0.05
US, Iowa	0.45	0.03	0.29	0.02

	MALE		FEMALE	
US, Central Louisiana: White	0.32	0.09	0.25	0.07
US, Central Louisiana: Black	0,32	0,17	-	-
US, New Orleans: White	0.36	0.05	0.36	0.05
US, New Orleans: Black	0.28	0.07	0.23	0.06
US, Detroit: White	0.52	0.03	0.35	0.02
US, Detroit: Black	0.50	0.06	0.29	0.04
US, New Mexico: Non-Hisp. White	0.46	0.05	0.27	0.04
US, New Mexico: Hispanic White	0.32	0.06	0.22	0.05
US, New Mexico: American Indian	0,25	0,11	0,09	0,05
US, Utah	0.40	0.04	0.23	0.03
US, Seattle	0.46	0.03	0.29	0.02
US, SEER: White	0.44	0.01	0.28	0.01
US, SEER: Black	0.43	0.04	0.26	0.02
ASIA				
*China, Qidong	0.16	0.03	0.19	0.03
China, Shanghai	0.17	0.01	0.12	0.01
China, Tianjin	0.16	0.01	0.11	0.01
Hong Kong	0.33	0.02	0.24	0.01
*India, Bangalore	0.18	0.02	0.17	0.02
*India, Barshi, Paranda and Bhum	0,09	0,03	0,03	0,02
India, Bombay	0.21	0.02	0.15	0.01
*India, Karunagappally	0,18	0,07	0,06	0,05
India, Madras	0.13	0.02	0.10	0.01
*India, Trivandrum	0,07	0,03	0.19	0.06
Israel: All Jews	0.27	0.02	0.22	0.02
Jews born in Israel	0.31	0.09	0.29	0.07
Jews born in America or Europe	0.34	0.04	0.25	0.03
Jews born in Africa or Asia	0.26	0.04	0.19	0.03
Non-Jews	0.23	0.07	0.21	0.06
Japan, Hiroshima	0.37	0.05	0.22	0.03
Japan, Miyagi	0.28	0.02	0.15	0.02
Japan, Nagasaki	0.28	0.03	0.21	0.02
Japan, Osaka	0.27	0.01	0.15	0.01
*Japan, Saga	0.37	0.04	0.19	0.03
Japan, Yamagata	0.26	0.03	0.16	0.02
*Korea, Kangwha	0,19	0,07	0,11	0,06
*Kuwait: Non-Kuwaitis	0.19	0.05	0.12	0.05
*Kuwait: Kuwaitis	0.26	0.09	0.26	0.09
*Philippines, Manila	0.22	0.03	0.13	0.02
Singapore: Chinese	0.36	0.04	0.19	0.02
Singapore: Malay	0.30	0.07	0.29	0.08
Singapore: Indian	0,13	0,05	0.31	0.11
Thailand, Chiang Mai	0.25	0.03	0.28	0.04
*Thailand, Khon Kaen	0.15	0.03	0.15	0.03
*Viet Nam, Hanoi				

* IMPORTANT-SEE NOTES ON POPULATION PAGE

CUMULATIVE INCIDENCE (0-74)
RATES AND STANDARD ERRORS (percent)
Myeloid leukaemia (ICD-9 205) (contd)

EUROPE	MALE		FEMALE	
Austria, Tyrol	0.35	0.06	0.29	0.04
*Belarus	0.28	0.01	0.20	0.01
*Croatia	0.31	0.02	0.25	0.02
Czech Republic	0.32	0.01	0.25	0.01
Denmark	0.45	0.02	0.30	0.01
Estonia	0.27	0.03	0.20	0.02
Finland	0.28	0.02	0.21	0.01
France, Bas-Rhin	0.38	0.05	0.21	0.03
†*France, Calvados	0.10	0.03	0.13	0.03
France, Doubs	0.42	0.07	0.22	0.04
France, Haut-Rhin	0.31	0.06	0.20	0.04
*France, Herault	0.27	0.04	0.12	0.02
France, Isere	0.41	0.05	0.18	0.03
*France, Somme	0.20	0.04	0.17	0.04
*France, Tarn	0.22	0.05	0.20	0.05
Germany, Eastern States	0.30	0.02	0.22	0.01
Germany, Saarland	0.49	0.05	0.24	0.03
Iceland	0.23	0.07	0.22	0.07
Ireland, Southern	0.33	0.05	0.20	0.04
Italy, Ferrara	0.27	0.09	0,18	0,06
Italy, Florence	0.38	0.04	0.28	0.03
Italy, Genoa	0.31	0.04	0.27	0.04
*Italy, Latina	0.46	0.08	0.23	0.05
Italy, Macerata	0,30	0,10	0,11	0,05
Italy, Modena	0.26	0.04	0.26	0.04
Italy, Parma	0.26	0.05	0.24	0.05
Italy, Ragusa	0.28	0.06	0.19	0.05
Italy, Romagna	0.41	0.06	0.23	0.04
Italy, Torino	0.37	0.04	0.22	0.03
Italy, Trieste	0.53	0.10	0.42	0.08
Italy, Varese	0.42	0.05	0.31	0.04
Italy, Veneto	0.36	0.04	0.27	0.03
*Latvia	0.23	0.02	0.19	0.02
Malta	0.26	0.09	0.39	0.10
The Netherlands	0.33	0.01	0.21	0.01
The Netherlands, Eindhoven	0.27	0.04	0.20	0.03
The Netherlands, Maastricht	0.34	0.04	0.24	0.03
Norway	0.27	0.02	0.19	0.01
*Poland, Cracow	0.31	0.05	0.19	0.03
*Poland, Kielce	0.21	0.03	0.20	0.03
*Poland, Lower Silesia	0.27	0.02	0.22	0.02
Poland, Warsaw City	0.25	0.03	0.21	0.02
Slovakia	0.35	0.02	0.24	0.01
Slovenia	0.29	0.03	0.20	0.02
*Spain, Albacete	0,17	0,07	0,12	0,06
Spain, Asturias	0.14	0.03	0.14	0.02
Spain, Basque Country	0.28	0.03	0.14	0.02
Spain, Granada	0.30	0.04	0.17	0.03
Spain, Mallorca	0.26	0.05	0.24	0.04
Spain, Murcia	0.37	0.04	0.20	0.03
Spain, Navarra	0.28	0.05	0.13	0.03
Spain, Tarragona	0.30	0.05	0.19	0.04
Spain, Zaragoza	0.26	0.04	0.26	0.03

	MALE		FEMALE	
Sweden	0.32	0.01	0.25	0.01
*Switzerland, Basel	0.27	0.05	0.27	0.05
Switzerland, Geneva	0.56	0.10	0.23	0.05
Switzerland, Graubunden	0,28	0,10	0.25	0.08
Switzerland, Neuchatel	0.34	0.10	0.26	0.08
Switzerland, St Gall-Appenzell	0.35	0.06	0.24	0.05
Switzerland, Valais	0.23	0.08	0,15	0,05
Switzerland, Vaud	0.38	0.05	0.23	0.04
Switzerland, Zurich	0.37	0.04	0.17	0.02
*UK, England and Wales	0.35	0.01	0.25	0.01
*UK, East Anglia	0.33	0.03	0.24	0.02
*UK, Mersey	0.29	0.02	0.19	0.02
*UK, North Western	0.33	0.02	0.23	0.01
UK, Oxford	0.42	0.03	0.30	0.02
*UK, South Thames	0.34	0.01	0.27	0.01
UK, South Western	0.37	0.02	0.25	0.02
UK, Wessex	0.47	0.03	0.30	0.02
*UK, West Midlands	0.33	0.02	0.24	0.01
UK, Yorkshire	0.34	0.02	0.24	0.02
UK, Scotland	0.32	0.02	0.24	0.01
UK, Scotland, West	0.34	0.02	0.25	0.02
*Yugoslavia, Vojvodina	0.32	0.03	0.21	0.02

OCEANIA	MALE		FEMALE	
Australian Capital Territory	0.48	0.12	0.26	0.08
Australia, New South Wales	0.48	0.02	0.28	0.01
South Australia	0.58	0.05	0.31	0.03
Australia, Tasmania	0.40	0.06	0.39	0.06
Australia, Victoria	0.42	0.02	0.26	0.02
Western Australia	0.42	0.04	0.27	0.03
*French Polynesia	0.31	0.14	0,09	0,04
New Zealand: Non-Maori	0.45	0.03	0.30	0.02
New Zealand: Maori	0.50	0.12	0.33	0.07
US, Hawaii: White	0.41	0.09	0,12	0,04
US, Hawaii: Japanese	0.26	0.06	0.18	0.05
US, Hawaii: Hawaiian	0.62	0.16	0.22	0.08
US, Hawaii: Filipino	0.36	0.10	0.41	0.11
US, Hawaii: Chinese	0,31	0,13	0,04	0,04

* IMPORTANT-SEE NOTES ON POPULATION PAGE

CUMULATIVE INCIDENCE (0-74)
RATES AND STANDARD ERRORS (percent)
Monocytic leukaemia (ICD-9 206)

	MALE		FEMALE	
AFRICA				
*Algeria, Setif				
*France, La Reunion				
*Mali, Bamako				
*Uganda, Kyadondo				
*Zimbabwe, Harare: African				
*Zimbabwe, Harare: European				
AMERICA, CENTRAL AND SOUTH				
*Argentina, Concordia	-	-	-	-
*Brazil, Belem	-	-	-	-
*Brazil, Goiania				
*Brazil, Porto Alegre	0,04	0,03	-	-
Colombia, Cali	0,01	0,01	0,00	0,00
*Costa Rica	0,01	0,00	0,01	0,01
*Ecuador, Quito	0,03	0,02	0,00	0,00
*Peru, Lima	0,02	0,01	0,00	0,00
Peru, Trujillo	0,01	0,01	0,01	0,01
US, Puerto Rico	0,00	0,00	0,01	0,00
*Uruguay, Montevideo	-	-	0,00	0,00
AMERICA, NORTH				
Canada	0.02	0.00	0.01	0.00
Canada, Alberta	0,01	0,00	0,01	0,00
Canada, British Columbia	0.02	0.01	0.01	0.00
Canada, Manitoba	0,02	0,01	0,01	0,01
Canada, New Brunswick	0,02	0,01	0,01	0,01
Canada, Newfoundland	0,01	0,01	-	-
Canada, Northwest Territories	-	-	0,03	0,02
Canada, Nova Scotia	0,03	0,01	0,04	0,02
Canada, Ontario	0.01	0.00	0.01	0.00
Canada, Prince Edward Island	0,02	0,02	-	-
Canada, Quebec	0,02	0,00	0.02	0,00
Canada, Saskatchewan	0,03	0,01	0,02	0,01
Canada, Yukon	0,09	0,06	-	-
US, Cent. Calif.: Non-Hisp. White	0,02	0,01	0,02	0,01
US, Cent. Calif.: Hispanic	0,03	0,02	0,03	0,03
US, Los Angeles: Non-Hisp. White	0.02	0.01	0.01	0.00
US, Los Angeles: Hispanic White	0,02	0,01	0,01	0,01
US, Los Angeles: Black	0,02	0,01	0,00	0,00
US, Los Angeles: Chinese	0,02	0,02	0,01	0,01
US, Los Angeles: Filipino	-	-	0,01	0,01
US, Los Angeles: Korean	-	-	-	-
US, Los Angeles: Japanese	0,03	0,03	-	-
US, San Francisco: Non-Hisp. White	0.03	0.01	0,01	0,00
US, San Francisco: Hispanic White	-	-	-	-
US, San Francisco: Black	0,01	0,01	0,03	0,02
US, San Francisco: Chinese	-	-	-	-
US, San Francisco: Filipino	0,05	0,05	0,02	0,02
US, San Francisco: Japanese	-	-	-	-
US, Connecticut: White	0.03	0,01	0.02	0.00
US, Connecticut: Black	0,06	0,06	-	-
US, Atlanta: White	0,02	0,01	0,02	0,01
US, Atlanta: Black	-	-	-	-
US, Iowa	0.02	0.01	0.03	0.01

	MALE		FEMALE	
US, Central Louisiana: White	-	-	0,02	0,02
US, Central Louisiana: Black	-	-	-	-
US, New Orleans: White	0,04	0,02	0,02	0,01
US, New Orleans: Black	0,01	0,01	0,01	0,01
US, Detroit: White	0.04	0,01	0.02	0.01
US, Detroit: Black	0,02	0,01	0,01	0,01
US, New Mexico: Non-Hisp. White	0,02	0,01	0,02	0,01
US, New Mexico: Hispanic White	0,02	0,01	0,03	0,02
US, New Mexico: American Indian	-	-	-	-
US, Utah	0,02	0,01	0,01	0,01
US, Seattle	0.02	0.01	0.01	0.00
US, SEER: White	0.02	0.00	0.02	0.00
US, SEER: Black	0,02	0,01	0,01	0,01
ASIA				
*China, Qidong	-	-	-	-
China, Shanghai	0.06	0.01	0.04	0.00
China, Tianjin	0.02	0.00	0.01	0.00
Hong Kong	0,01	0,00	0,00	0,00
*India, Bangalore	0,00	0,00	0,00	0,00
*India, Barshi, Paranda and Bhum	-	-	-	-
India, Bombay	0,00	0,00	0,00	0,00
*India, Karunagappally	-	-	-	-
India, Madras	0,01	0,00	0,01	0,00
*India, Trivandrum	-	-	-	-
Israel: All Jews	0.02	0.01	0.02	0.01
Jews born in Israel	0,01	0,01	0,01	0,00
Jews born in America or Europe	0,03	0,01	0,02	0,01
Jews born in Africa or Asia	0,03	0,01	0,01	0,01
Non-Jews	-	-	-	-
Japan, Hiroshima	0,00	0,00	0,00	0,00
Japan, Miyagi	0,01	0,01	0,01	0,00
Japan, Nagasaki	0,01	0,00	0,00	0,00
Japan, Osaka	0.02	0.00	0.01	0.00
*Japan, Saga	0,00	0,00	-	-
Japan, Yamagata	0,02	0,01	0,02	0,01
*Korea, Kangwha	-	-	-	-
*Kuwait: Non-Kuwaitis	0,01	0,01	-	-
*Kuwait: Kuwaitis	0,00	0,00	-	-
*Philippines, Manila	0,01	0,01	0,01	0,00
Singapore: Chinese	0,00	0,00	-	-
Singapore: Malay	-	-	-	-
Singapore: Indian	-	-	-	-
Thailand, Chiang Mai	-	-	0,01	0,01
*Thailand, Khon Kaen	0,00	0,00	0,01	0,01
*Viet Nam, Hanoi				

* IMPORTANT-SEE NOTES ON POPULATION PAGE

CUMULATIVE INCIDENCE (0-74)
RATES AND STANDARD ERRORS (percent)
Monocytic leukaemia (ICD-9 206) (contd)

EUROPE	MALE		FEMALE	
Austria, Tyrol	0,02	*0,02*	0,01	*0,01*
*Belarus	0.01	*0.00*	0.01	*0.00*
*Croatia	0,00	*0,00*	0,00	*0,00*
Czech Republic	0.02	*0.00*	0.01	*0.00*
Denmark	0,00	*0,00*	0,00	*0,00*
Estonia	0,01	*0,01*	0,00	*0,00*
Finland	0.01	*0.00*	0,00	*0,00*
France, Bas-Rhin	0,03	*0,01*	0,02	*0,01*
†*France, Calvados	-	-	0,01	*0,01*
France, Doubs	0,00	*0,00*	-	-
France, Haut-Rhin	-	-	0,03	*0,01*
*France, Herault	0,01	*0,01*	0,01	*0,01*
France, Isere	0,01	*0,01*	0,01	*0,01*
*France, Somme	0,02	*0,01*	0,04	*0,02*
*France, Tarn	0,02	*0,01*	0,01	*0,01*
Germany, Eastern States	0,01	*0,00*	0,01	*0,00*
Germany, Saarland	0,04	*0,02*	0,00	*0,00*
Iceland	0,02	*0,02*	-	-
Ireland, Southern	-	-	-	-
Italy, Ferrara	-	-	0,04	*0,03*
Italy, Florence	-	-	-	-
Italy, Genoa	-	-	0,01	*0,01*
*Italy, Latina	0,03	*0,02*	-	-
Italy, Macerata	-	-	-	-
Italy, Modena	0,03	*0,01*	0,01	*0,01*
Italy, Parma	0,01	*0,01*	0,01	*0,01*
Italy, Ragusa	-	-	-	-
Italy, Romagna	0,01	*0,01*	-	-
Italy, Torino	0,01	*0,01*	0,02	*0,01*
Italy, Trieste	0,03	*0,02*	-	-
Italy, Varese	0,01	*0,01*	0,02	*0,01*
Italy, Veneto	0,02	*0,01*	0,01	*0,01*
*Latvia	0.03	*0.01*	0.03	*0.01*
Malta	-	-	-	-
The Netherlands	0.02	*0.00*	0.01	*0.00*
The Netherlands, Eindhoven	0,01	*0,01*	0,00	*0,00*
The Netherlands, Maastricht	0,00	*0,00*	0,02	*0,01*
Norway	0.03	*0.01*	0.02	*0.00*
*Poland, Cracow	-	-	-	-
*Poland, Kielce	-	-	-	-
*Poland, Lower Silesia	0,01	*0,00*	0,00	*0,00*
Poland, Warsaw City	-	-	-	-
Slovakia	0.01	*0.00*	0,01	*0,00*
Slovenia	0,02	*0,01*	0,01	*0,00*
*Spain, Albacete	0,03	*0,03*	-	-
Spain, Asturias	0,01	*0,01*	0,01	*0,01*
Spain, Basque Country	0,01	*0,00*	0,01	*0,01*
Spain, Granada	0,02	*0,01*	0,03	*0,01*
Spain, Mallorca	0,01	*0,01*	0,02	*0,01*
Spain, Murcia	0,01	*0,01*	-	-
Spain, Navarra	0,03	*0,02*	0,01	*0,01*
Spain, Tarragona	0,01	*0,01*	-	-
Spain, Zaragoza	0,01	*0,01*	0,01	*0,01*

	MALE		FEMALE	
Sweden	0.01	*0.00*	0.01	*0.00*
*Switzerland, Basel	-	-	0,01	*0,01*
Switzerland, Geneva	-	-	0,01	*0,01*
Switzerland, Graubunden	-	-	-	-
Switzerland, Neuchatel	-	-	0,03	*0,03*
Switzerland, St Gall-Appenzell	-	-	0,01	*0,01*
Switzerland, Valais	-	-	-	-
Switzerland, Vaud	-	-	0,01	*0,01*
Switzerland, Zurich	0.06	*0.02*	0.03	*0.01*
*UK, England and Wales	0.01	*0.00*	0.01	*0.00*
*UK, East Anglia	0.01	*0,00*	0,00	*0,00*
*UK, Mersey	0.01	*0,00*	0.01	*0,00*
*UK, North Western	0.00	*0,00*	0.00	*0,00*
UK, Oxford	0.04	*0.01*	0.01	*0.00*
*UK, South Thames	0.01	*0.00*	0.00	*0.00*
UK, South Western	0.02	*0.01*	0.02	*0.00*
UK, Wessex	0.01	*0.00*	0.01	*0.00*
*UK, West Midlands	0.02	*0.00*	0.01	*0.00*
UK, Yorkshire	0.01	*0,00*	0.00	*0,00*
UK, Scotland	0.01	*0.00*	0.01	*0.00*
UK, Scotland, West	0.00	*0,00*	0.00	*0,00*
*Yugoslavia, Vojvodina	-	-	-	-

OCEANIA	MALE		FEMALE	
Australian Capital Territory	-	-	-	-
Australia, New South Wales	0.01	*0.00*	0.01	*0.00*
South Australia	0.02	*0.01*	0.01	*0.01*
Australia, Tasmania	0.02	*0.02*	-	-
Australia, Victoria	0.01	*0.00*	0.01	*0.00*
Western Australia	0.02	*0.01*	0.00	*0.00*
*French Polynesia	0.01	*0,01*	0.01	*0,01*
New Zealand: Non-Maori	0.01	*0,00*	0.01	*0,00*
New Zealand: Maori	-	-	0,07	*0,07*
US, Hawaii: White	0.02	*0,02*	0.02	*0,02*
US, Hawaii: Japanese	0.01	*0,01*	-	-
US, Hawaii: Hawaiian	0.04	*0,04*	0.02	*0,02*
US, Hawaii: Filipino	0.03	*0,02*	-	-
US, Hawaii: Chinese	-	-	0,08	*0,06*

* IMPORTANT-SEE NOTES ON POPULATION PAGE

CUMULATIVE INCIDENCE (0-74)
RATES AND STANDARD ERRORS (percent)
Other leukaemia (ICD-9 207)

	MALE		FEMALE	
AFRICA				
*Algeria, Setif				
*France, La Reunion				
*Mali, Bamako				
*Uganda, Kyadondo				
*Zimbabwe, Harare: African				
*Zimbabwe, Harare: European				
AMERICA, CENTRAL AND SOUTH				
*Argentina, Concordia	-	-	-	-
*Brazil, Belem	-	-	-	-
*Brazil, Goiania				
*Brazil, Porto Alegre	-	-	0,01	0,01
Colombia, Cali	0,01	0,01	-	-
*Costa Rica	-	-	0,00	0,00
*Ecuador, Quito	-	-	-	-
*Peru, Lima	0,00	0,00	-	-
Peru, Trujillo	-	-	-	-
US, Puerto Rico	0,00	0,00	0,01	0,00
*Uruguay, Montevideo	-	-	-	-
AMERICA, NORTH				
Canada	0.02	0.00	0.01	0.00
Canada, Alberta	0,00	0,00	0,01	0,00
Canada, British Columbia	0,01	0,00	0,00	0,00
Canada, Manitoba	0,02	0,01	0,01	0,01
Canada, New Brunswick	-	-	0,01	0,01
Canada, Newfoundland	0,00	0,00	-	-
Canada, Northwest Territories	0,02	0,02	-	-
Canada, Nova Scotia	0,01	0,01	0,01	0,01
Canada, Ontario	0.01	0.00	0.01	0.00
Canada, Prince Edward Island	0,02	0,02	-	-
Canada, Quebec	0.03	0.00	0.02	0.00
Canada, Saskatchewan	0,00	0,00	0,01	0,01
Canada, Yukon	-	-	-	-
US, Cent. Calif.: Non-Hisp. White	0,01	0,01	0,00	0,00
US, Cent. Calif.: Hispanic	0,00	0,00	0,03	0,02
US, Los Angeles: Non-Hisp. White	0.01	0.00	0.01	0.00
US, Los Angeles: Hispanic White	0,00	0,00	0,00	0,00
US, Los Angeles: Black	0,01	0,01	-	-
US, Los Angeles: Chinese	0,02	0,02	-	-
US, Los Angeles: Filipino	-	-	0,01	0,01
US, Los Angeles: Korean	-	-	-	-
US, Los Angeles: Japanese	0,06	0,05	-	-
US, San Francisco: Non-Hisp. White	0,01	0,00	0,01	0,00
US, San Francisco: Hispanic White	-	-	0,02	0,02
US, San Francisco: Black	0,02	0,02	-	-
US, San Francisco: Chinese	-	-	-	-
US, San Francisco: Filipino	0,04	0,04	-	-
US, San Francisco: Japanese	-	-	-	-
US, Connecticut: White	0,01	0,00	0,01	0,00
US, Connecticut: Black	-	-	-	-
US, Atlanta: White	0,01	0,01	0,00	0,00
US, Atlanta: Black	0,00	0,00	-	-
US, Iowa	0,01	0,00	0,01	0,00

	MALE		FEMALE	
US, Central Louisiana: White	-	-	-	-
US, Central Louisiana: Black	-	-	0,09	0,09
US, New Orleans: White	0,02	0,01	0,01	0,01
US, New Orleans: Black	0,01	0,01	-	-
US, Detroit: White	0.02	0.01	0,01	0,00
US, Detroit: Black	0,04	0,02	0,00	0,00
US, New Mexico: Non-Hisp. White	0,01	0,01	-	-
US, New Mexico: Hispanic White	0,02	0,02	0,02	0,02
US, New Mexico: American Indian	-	-	-	-
US, Utah	-	-	0,01	0,00
US, Seattle	0.02	0.01	0,01	0,00
US, SEER: White	0.01	0.00	0.01	0.00
US, SEER: Black	0,02	0,01	0,00	0,00
ASIA				
*China, Qidong	0,01	0,00	0,01	0,01
China, Shanghai	0.01	0.00	0.01	0.00
China, Tianjin	0,01	0,00	0,01	0,00
Hong Kong	0,00	0,00	0,00	0,00
*India, Bangalore	0,00	0,00	0,00	0,00
*India, Barshi, Paranda and Bhum	-	-	-	-
India, Bombay	0.00	0.00	0.00	0.00
*India, Karunagappally	-	-	-	-
India, Madras	-	-	0,00	0,00
*India, Trivandrum	0,01	0,01	-	-
Israel: All Jews	0.01	0.00	0,00	0,00
Jews born in Israel	0,02	0,02	0,01	0,01
Jews born in America or Europe	0,02	0,01	0,01	0,00
Jews born in Africa or Asia	0,01	0,01	0,00	0,00
Non-Jews	0,02	0,02	0,00	0,00
Japan, Hiroshima	-	-	0,01	0,01
Japan, Miyagi	0,02	0,01	0,01	0,00
Japan, Nagasaki	0,00	0,00	0,01	0,00
Japan, Osaka	0.01	0.00	0.01	0.00
*Japan, Saga	0,01	0,01	0,01	0,01
Japan, Yamagata	0,01	0,01	0,01	0,00
*Korea, Kangwha	0,02	0,02	-	-
*Kuwait: Non-Kuwaitis	-	-	-	-
*Kuwait: Kuwaitis	-	-	0,00	0,00
*Philippines, Manila	0,00	0,00	0,00	0,00
Singapore: Chinese	-	-	0,00	0,00
Singapore: Malay	0,00	0,00	-	-
Singapore: Indian	-	-	0,01	0,01
Thailand, Chiang Mai	-	-	0,00	0,00
*Thailand, Khon Kaen	-	-	-	-
*Viet Nam, Hanoi				

* IMPORTANT-SEE NOTES ON POPULATION PAGE

CUMULATIVE INCIDENCE (0-74)
RATES AND STANDARD ERRORS (percent)
Other leukaemia (ICD-9 207) (contd)

EUROPE	MALE		FEMALE	
Austria, Tyrol	-	-	0,01	*0,01*
*Belarus	0.03	*0.00*	0.02	*0.00*
*Croatia	0,00	*0,00*	0,00	*0,00*
Czech Republic	0.02	*0.00*	0.01	*0.00*
Denmark	0,01	*0,00*	0,00	*0,00*
Estonia	0.06	*0.02*	0.02	*0.01*
Finland	0,01	*0,00*	0,00	*0,00*
France, Bas-Rhin	-	-	-	-
†*France, Calvados	-	-	0,01	*0,01*
France, Doubs	0,01	*0,01*	-	-
France, Haut-Rhin	0,01	*0,01*	-	-
*France, Herault	-	-	-	-
France, Isere	-	-	-	-
*France, Somme	0,01	*0,01*	-	-
*France, Tarn	-	-	-	-
Germany, Eastern States	0.02	*0.00*	0.02	*0.00*
Germany, Saarland	0,02	*0,01*	0,02	*0,01*
Iceland	0,02	*0,02*	-	-
Ireland, Southern	-	-	-	-
Italy, Ferrara	-	-	0,03	*0,03*
Italy, Florence	-	-	0,01	*0,01*
Italy, Genoa	-	-	-	-
*Italy, Latina	-	-	-	-
Italy, Macerata	-	-	-	-
Italy, Modena	0,01	*0,01*	-	-
Italy, Parma	-	-	-	-
Italy, Ragusa	-	-	-	-
Italy, Romagna	0,01	*0,01*	0,01	*0,01*
Italy, Torino	0,00	*0,00*	0,01	*0,01*
Italy, Trieste	0,06	*0,03*	0,03	*0,02*
Italy, Varese	-	-	0,00	*0,00*
Italy, Veneto	0,01	*0,01*	0,01	*0,00*
*Latvia	0.08	*0.01*	0.07	*0.01*
Malta	-	-	-	-
The Netherlands	0.02	*0.00*	0.01	*0.00*
The Netherlands, Eindhoven	0,02	*0,01*	0,01	*0,01*
The Netherlands, Maastricht	0,00	*0,00*	0,00	*0,00*
Norway	0.05	*0.01*	0.03	*0.01*
*Poland, Cracow	0,01	*0,01*	0,00	*0,00*
*Poland, Kielce	0,01	*0,00*	0,00	*0,00*
*Poland, Lower Silesia	0.05	*0.01*	0.03	*0.01*
Poland, Warsaw City	0,00	*0,00*	0,01	*0,01*
Slovakia	0,01	*0,00*	0,01	*0.00*
Slovenia	-	-	-	-
*Spain, Albacete	-	-	-	-
Spain, Asturias	-	-	-	-
Spain, Basque Country	0,00	*0,00*	-	-
Spain, Granada	0,01	*0,01*	0,01	*0,01*
Spain, Mallorca	-	-	0,01	*0,01*
Spain, Murcia	-	-	0,00	*0,00*
Spain, Navarra	0,01	*0,01*	0,01	*0,01*
Spain, Tarragona	0,01	*0,01*	-	-
Spain, Zaragoza	-	-	0,01	*0,01*

	MALE		FEMALE	
Sweden	0.09	*0.01*	0.07	*0.01*
*Switzerland, Basel	-	-	-	-
Switzerland, Geneva	-	-	-	-
Switzerland, Graubunden	-	-	-	-
Switzerland, Neuchatel	0,04	*0,04*	-	-
Switzerland, St Gall-Appenzell	0,01	*0,01*	0,01	*0,01*
Switzerland, Valais	0,06	*0,04*	0,03	*0,03*
Switzerland, Vaud	-	-	0,01	*0,01*
Switzerland, Zurich	0,02	*0,01*	0,01	*0,01*
*UK, England and Wales	0.01	*0.00*	0.00	*0.00*
*UK, East Anglia	0,01	*0,00*	0,00	*0,00*
*UK, Mersey	0,01	*0,00*	0,00	*0,00*
*UK, North Western	0,01	*0,00*	0,00	*0,00*
UK, Oxford	0,01	*0,00*	0,00	*0,00*
*UK, South Thames	0,00	*0,00*	0,00	*0,00*
UK, South Western	0,00	*0,00*	0,01	*0,00*
UK, Wessex	0,01	*0,00*	0,00	*0,00*
*UK, West Midlands	0.01	*0.00*	0.00	*0.00*
UK, Yorkshire	0,01	*0,00*	0,00	*0,00*
UK, Scotland	0,01	*0,00*	0,00	*0,00*
UK, Scotland, West	0,00	*0,00*	0,00	*0,00*
*Yugoslavia, Vojvodina	-	-	0,00	*0,00*

OCEANIA	MALE		FEMALE	
Australian Capital Territory	0,01	*0,01*	-	-
Australia, New South Wales	0,01	*0.00*	0,00	*0,00*
South Australia	0,01	*0,01*	0,01	*0,01*
Australia, Tasmania	0,01	*0,01*	0,01	*0,01*
Australia, Victoria	0,01	*0,00*	0,01	*0.00*
Western Australia	0,01	*0,01*	0,01	*0,00*
*French Polynesia	0,01	*0,01*	0,02	*0,02*
New Zealand: Non-Maori	0,01	*0.00*	0,00	*0,00*
New Zealand: Maori	0,07	*0,05*	0,01	*0,01*
US, Hawaii: White	0,05	*0,04*	-	-
US, Hawaii: Japanese	0,04	*0,02*	-	-
US, Hawaii: Hawaiian	0,07	*0,07*	-	-
US, Hawaii: Filipino	-	-	-	-
US, Hawaii: Chinese	-	-	-	-

* IMPORTANT-SEE NOTES ON POPULATION PAGE

CUMULATIVE INCIDENCE (0-74)
RATES AND STANDARD ERRORS (percent)
Leukaemia, unspecified (ICD-9 208)

	MALE		FEMALE	
AFRICA				
*Algeria, Setif				
*France, La Reunion				
*Mali, Bamako				
*Uganda, Kyadondo				
*Zimbabwe, Harare: African				
*Zimbabwe, Harare: European				
AMERICA, CENTRAL AND SOUTH				
*Argentina, Concordia	0,12	0,07	0,11	0,06
*Brazil, Belem	0.06	0.02	0.07	0.03
*Brazil, Goiania				
*Brazil, Porto Alegre	0.16	0.05	0.11	0.03 m
Colombia, Cali	0.22	0.04	0.11	0.03
*Costa Rica	0.09	0.02	0.07	0.01
*Ecuador, Quito	0.15	0.04	0.09	0.03
*Peru, Lima	0.06	0.02	0.05	0.01
Peru, Trujillo	0,16	0,09	0,02	0,01
US, Puerto Rico	0.07	0.01	0.04	0.01
*Uruguay, Montevideo	0.19	0.04	0.10	0.02
AMERICA, NORTH				
Canada	0.09	0.00	0.07	0.00
Canada, Alberta	0.05	0.01	0.04	0.01
Canada, British Columbia	0.06	0.01	0.05	0.01
Canada, Manitoba	0.05	0.02	0.02	0,01
Canada, New Brunswick	0.12	0.03	0.07	0.02
Canada, Newfoundland	0,06	0,03	0,05	0,02
Canada, Northwest Territories	0,02	0,02	0,06	0,06
Canada, Nova Scotia	0.26	0.04	0.11	0.02
Canada, Ontario	0.09	0.01	0.06	0.01
Canada, Prince Edward Island	0,05	0,05	-	-
Canada, Quebec	0.12	0.01	0.09	0.01
Canada, Saskatchewan	0.05	0.02	0,02	0,01
Canada, Yukon	-	-	-	-
US, Cent. Calif.: Non-Hisp. White	0.07	0.02	0.03	0.01
US, Cent. Calif.: Hispanic	0.04	0,03	0,04	0,02
US, Los Angeles: Non-Hisp. White	0.06	0.01	0.04	0.01
US, Los Angeles: Hispanic White	0.07	0.02	0.02	0.01
US, Los Angeles: Black	0,06	0,02	0.06	0.02
US, Los Angeles: Chinese	-	-	0,06	0,04
US, Los Angeles: Filipino	0,08	0,04	0,03	0,03
US, Los Angeles: Korean	0,04	0,03	0,04	0,04
US, Los Angeles: Japanese	0,04	0,04	-	-
US, San Francisco: Non-Hisp. White	0.05	0.01	0.03	0.01
US, San Francisco: Hispanic White	0,05	0,04	0,04	0,03
US, San Francisco: Black	0.08	0,04	0.02	0,01
US, San Francisco: Chinese	0,03	0,03	0,04	0,03
US, San Francisco: Filipino	0,10	0,08	0,10	0,05
US, San Francisco: Japanese	-	-	-	-
US, Connecticut: White	0.11	0.01	0.06	0.01
US, Connecticut: Black	0,03	0,03	0,11	0,06
US, Atlanta: White	0.06	0.02	0,01	0,01
US, Atlanta: Black	0,16	0,06	0,04	0,02
US, Iowa	0.08	0.01	0.03	0.01

	MALE		FEMALE	
US, Central Louisiana: White	0,07	0,04	-	-
US, Central Louisiana: Black	0,21	0,15	-	-
US, New Orleans: White	0,04	0,02	0,03	0,01
US, New Orleans: Black	0.23	0.07	0,04	0,02
US, Detroit: White	0.10	0.01	0.08	0.01
US, Detroit: Black	0.12	0.03	0.05	0.02
US, New Mexico: Non-Hisp. White	0.08	0.02	0.08	0.02
US, New Mexico: Hispanic White	0,03	0,02	0,08	0,03
US, New Mexico: American Indian	0,04	0,03	-	-
US, Utah	0.07	0.02	0.03	0,01
US, Seattle	0.08	0.01	0.05	0.01
US, SEER: White	0.08	0.00	0.05	0.00
US, SEER: Black	0.11	0.02	0.04	0.01
ASIA				
*China, Qidong	0.11	0.02	0.06	0.02
China, Shanghai	0.09	0.01	0.08	0.01
China, Tianjin	0.15	0.02	0.14	0.01
Hong Kong	0.09	0.01	0.07	0.01
*India, Bangalore	0.04	0.01	0.05	0.01
*India, Barshi, Paranda and Bhum	0,00	0,00	-	-
India, Bombay	0.04	0.01	0.04	0.01
*India, Karunagappally	0,03	0,02	0,01	0,01
India, Madras	0.01	0.00	0.02	0.01
*India, Trivandrum	0,01	0,01	0,04	0,03 f
Israel: All Jews	0.06	0.01	0.05	0.01
Jews born in Israel	0.03	0.01	0,03	0,02
Jews born in America or Europe	0.07	0.02	0.06	0.01
Jews born in Africa or Asia	0.04	0.01	0.04	0.01
Non-Jews	0.11	0.05	0.10	0.04
Japan, Hiroshima	0.05	0.02	0.02	0,01
Japan, Miyagi	0.05	0.01	0.02	0.01
Japan, Nagasaki	0.08	0.02	0.03	0.01
Japan, Osaka	0.06	0.01	0.03	0.00
*Japan, Saga	0,04	0,01	0,03	0,01
Japan, Yamagata	0.06	0.01	0.05	0.01
*Korea, Kangwha	0,09	0,05	0,03	0,03
*Kuwait: Non-Kuwaitis	0,02	0,01	0,30	0,17
*Kuwait: Kuwaitis	0,07	0,03	0,07	0,07
*Philippines, Manila	0.17	0.03	0.16	0.02
Singapore: Chinese	0.03	0.01	0,01	0,00
Singapore: Malay	0,04	0,02	0,01	0,01
Singapore: Indian	0,02	0,02	0,01	0,01
Thailand, Chiang Mai	0.09	0.02	0.10	0.02
*Thailand, Khon Kaen	0.12	0.03	0.09	0.02
*Viet Nam, Hanoi				

* IMPORTANT-SEE NOTES ON POPULATION PAGE

CUMULATIVE INCIDENCE (0-74)
RATES AND STANDARD ERRORS (percent)
Leukaemia, unspecified (ICD-9 208) (contd)

EUROPE	MALE		FEMALE	
Austria, Tyrol	0,04	0,02	0,02	0,01
*Belarus	0.13	0.01	0.09	0.01
*Croatia	0.07	0.01	0.05	0.01
Czech Republic	0.05	0.00	0.03	0.00
Denmark	0.03	0.00	0.02	0.00
Estonia	0.04	0.01	0.08	0.01
Finland	0.02	0.00	0.01	0.00
France, Bas-Rhin	0,03	0,01	0,03	0,01
†*France, Calvados	0,01	0,01	0,02	0,01
France, Doubs	0,07	0,03	0,04	0,02
France, Haut-Rhin	0,03	0,01	0,04	0,01
*France, Herault	0,09	0.02	0,06	0.02
France, Isere	0,03	0,01	0,01	0,00
*France, Somme	0,03	0,01	0,01	0,01
*France, Tarn	0,02	0,01	-	-
Germany, Eastern States	0.06	0.01	0.04	0.00
Germany, Saarland	0,04	0,02	0.05	0.01
Iceland	0,01	0,01	0,06	0,03
Ireland, Southern	0.10	0.03	0,02	0,01
Italy, Ferrara	0,17	0,06	-	-
Italy, Florence	0.12	0.02	0,04	0,01
Italy, Genoa	0,05	0,02	0,02	0,01
*Italy, Latina	0,06	0,02	0,07	0,03
Italy, Macerata	0,18	0,07	0,21	0,08
Italy, Modena	0,01	0,01	0,02	0,01
Italy, Parma	0.12	0.03	0.10	0.03
Italy, Ragusa	0,08	0,04	0,06	0,03
Italy, Romagna	0,05	0,02	0,04	0,02
Italy, Torino	0.10	0.02	0,03	0,01
Italy, Trieste	0,07	0,04	0,03	0,02
Italy, Varese	0,04	0,02	0,01	0,01
Italy, Veneto	0.10	0.02	0.06	0.01
*Latvia	0.03	0.01	0.02	0.01
Malta	-	-	0,03	0,03
The Netherlands	0.03	0.00	0.02	0.00
The Netherlands, Eindhoven	0,01	0,01	0,02	0,01
The Netherlands, Maastricht	0,04	0,02	0,03	0,01
Norway	0.01	0.00	0,01	0,00
*Poland, Cracow	0.09	0.03	0,04	0,02
*Poland, Kielce	0.04	0.01	0,03	0,01
*Poland, Lower Silesia	0.06	0.01	0,04	0,01
Poland, Warsaw City	0.05	0.01	0,02	0,01
Slovakia	0.04	0.01	0.03	0.01
Slovenia	0,01	0,00	0,01	0,01
*Spain, Albacete	0,05	0,04	0,03	0,03
Spain, Asturias	0.26	0.04	0.16	0.03
Spain, Basque Country	0.11	0.02	0.08	0.01
Spain, Granada	0.06	0.02	0.08	0.02
Spain, Mallorca	0,02	0,01	0,05	0,02
Spain, Murcia	0,04	0,01	0,05	0,02
Spain, Navarra	0.12	0.03	0,07	0,02
Spain, Tarragona	0.10	0.03	0,07	0,02
Spain, Zaragoza	0,03	0,01	0,03	0,01

	MALE		FEMALE	
Sweden	0.04	0.00	0.02	0.00
*Switzerland, Basel	0,03	0,02	-	-
Switzerland, Geneva	0,01	0,01	-	-
Switzerland, Graubunden	-	-	-	-
Switzerland, Neuchatel	-	-	-	-
Switzerland, St Gall-Appenzell	0,03	0,02	0,03	0,01
Switzerland, Valais	0,10	0,05	0,02	0,02
Switzerland, Vaud	0,08	0,03	0,02	0,01
Switzerland, Zurich	0,01	0,00	0,03	0,01
*UK, England and Wales	0.04	0.00	0.03	0.00
*UK, East Anglia	0.02	0.01	0.02	0.01
*UK, Mersey	0.02	0.01	0.02	0.01
*UK, North Western	0.04	0.01	0.02	0.00
UK, Oxford	0.02	0.01	0.01	0.01
*UK, South Thames	0.04	0.01	0.03	0.00
UK, South Western	0.03	0.01	0.02	0.00
UK, Wessex	0.04	0.01	0.01	0.00
*UK, West Midlands	0.08	0.01	0.04	0.01
UK, Yorkshire	0.03	0.01	0.01	0.00
UK, Scotland	0.04	0.01	0.02	0.00
UK, Scotland, West	0.05	0.01	0.04	0.01
*Yugoslavia, Vojvodina	0.07	0.01	0.03	0.01

OCEANIA	MALE		FEMALE	
Australian Capital Territory	-	-	-	-
Australia, New South Wales	0.05	0.01	0.03	0.01
South Australia	-	-	0,00	0,00
Australia, Tasmania	0,05	0,02	0,01	0,01
Australia, Victoria	0.04	0.01	0.02	0.01
Western Australia	0.06	0.01	0.04	0.01
*French Polynesia	0.39	0.15	0,26	0,14
New Zealand: Non-Maori	0.05	0.01	0.03	0.01
New Zealand: Maori	0,10	0,06	0,01	0,01
US, Hawaii: White	0,13	0,05	0,05	0,04
US, Hawaii: Japanese	0,07	0,03	0,01	0,01
US, Hawaii: Hawaiian	0,03	0,02	0,04	0,04
US, Hawaii: Filipino	0,02	0,02	0,09	0,06
US, Hawaii: Chinese	-	-	0,05	0,05

* IMPORTANT-SEE NOTES ON POPULATION PAGE

CUMULATIVE INCIDENCE (0-74)
RATES AND STANDARD ERRORS (percent)
All leukaemias (ICD-9 204-8)

	MALE		FEMALE	
AFRICA				
*Algeria, Setif				
*France, La Reunion				
*Mali, Bamako				
*Uganda, Kyadondo				
*Zimbabwe, Harare: African				
*Zimbabwe, Harare: European				
AMERICA, CENTRAL AND SOUTH				
*Argentina, Concordia	0,36	0,13	0.38	0.13
*Brazil, Belem	0.30	0.07	0.21	0.04
*Brazil, Goiania				
*Brazil, Porto Alegre	0.72	0.10	0.54	0.07 mf
Colombia, Cali	0.52	0.06	0.46	0.05
*Costa Rica	0.71	0.05	0.51	0.04
*Ecuador, Quito	0.72	0.08	0.50	0.06
*Peru, Lima	0.41	0.04	0.34	0.03
Peru, Trujillo	0.52	0.14	0.48	0.12
US, Puerto Rico	0.55	0.03	0.40	0.03
*Uruguay, Montevideo	0.75	0.07	0.51	0.05
AMERICA, NORTH				
Canada	1.06	0.01	0.64	0.01
Canada, Alberta	0.82	0.04	0.57	0.04
Canada, British Columbia	0.80	0.03	0.52	0.03
Canada, Manitoba	1.00	0.07	0.54	0.05
Canada, New Brunswick	0.79	0.08	0.57	0.06
Canada, Newfoundland	0.64	0.08	0.51	0.07
Canada, Northwest Territories	0.39	0.13	0.22	0.08
Canada, Nova Scotia	0.89	0.07	0.58	0.05
Canada, Ontario	1.23	0.03	0.73	0.02
Canada, Prince Edward Island	0.85	0.18	0.45	0.12
Canada, Quebec	1.08	0.03	0.62	0.02
Canada, Saskatchewan	1.29	0.08	0.71	0.06
Canada, Yukon	1.39	0.46	0.93	0.33
US, Cent. Calif.: Non-Hisp. White	1.00	0.06	0.61	0.04
US, Cent. Calif.: Hispanic	0.89	0.11	0.48	0.08
US, Los Angeles: Non-Hisp. White	1.10	0.04	0.70	0.03
US, Los Angeles: Hispanic White	0.76	0.05	0.54	0.04
US, Los Angeles: Black	1.01	0.09	0.54	0.05
US, Los Angeles: Chinese	0.64	0.12	0.46	0.10
US, Los Angeles: Filipino	1.03	0.18	0.45	0.09
US, Los Angeles: Korean	0.30	0.09	0.31	0.09
US, Los Angeles: Japanese	0.71	0.16	0.51	0.13
US, San Francisco: Non-Hisp. White	1.03	0.05	0.53	0.03
US, San Francisco: Hispanic White	0.78	0.12	0.83	0.11
US, San Francisco: Black	0.96	0.12	0.42	0.07
US, San Francisco: Chinese	0.66	0.11	0.42	0.09
US, San Francisco: Filipino	0.90	0.19	0.63	0.12
US, San Francisco: Japanese	0,33	0,17	0.33	0,18
US, Connecticut: White	1.00	0.04	0.62	0.03
US, Connecticut: Black	0.80	0.16	0.66	0.12
US, Atlanta: White	0.90	0.07	0.53	0.04
US, Atlanta: Black	0.99	0.14	0.49	0.07
US, Iowa	1.24	0.05	0.71	0.03

	MALE		FEMALE	
US, Central Louisiana: White	0.73	0.13	0.43	0.09
US, Central Louisiana: Black	0.72	0.25	0,17	0,12
US, New Orleans: White	0.89	0.08	0.68	0.07
US, New Orleans: Black	0.90	0.13	0.45	0.08
US, Detroit: White	1.24	0.05	0.78	0.03
US, Detroit: Black	1.11	0.09	0.60	0.06
US, New Mexico: Non-Hisp. White	1.16	0.08	0.67	0.06
US, New Mexico: Hispanic White	0.80	0.10	0.50	0.07
US, New Mexico: American Indian	0.43	0.12	0.24	0.08
US, Utah	0.90	0.06	0.50	0.04
US, Seattle	1.14	0.04	0.65	0.03
US, SEER: White	1.09	0.02	0.64	0.01
US, SEER: Black	1.01	0.06	0.55	0.03
ASIA				
*China, Qidong	0.38	0.04	0.32	0.04
China, Shanghai	0.44	0.02	0.33	0.01
China, Tianjin	0.44	0.02	0.32	0.02
Hong Kong	0.57	0.02	0.42	0.02
*India, Bangalore	0.32	0.03	0.28	0.02
*India, Barshi, Paranda and Bhum	0.12	0.03	0.06	0.02
India, Bombay	0.38	0.02	0.29	0.02
*India, Karunagappally	0.29	0.09	0,14	0,06
India, Madras	0.25	0.02	0.19	0.02
*India, Trivandrum	0.28	0.07	0.31	0.07
Israel: All Jews	0.72	0.03	0.46	0.02
Jews born in Israel	0.62	0.11	0.59	0.11
Jews born in America or Europe	0.88	0.06	0.53	0.05
Jews born in Africa or Asia	0.68	0.08	0.51	0.13
Non-Jews	0.56	0.10	0.42	0.08
Japan, Hiroshima	0.59	0.06	0.31	0.04
Japan, Miyagi	0.51	0.03	0.29	0.02
Japan, Nagasaki	0.51	0.04	0.33	0.03
Japan, Osaka	0.53	0.02	0.31	0.01
*Japan, Saga	0.83	0.06	0.47	0.04
Japan, Yamagata	0.44	0.04	0.30	0.03
*Korea, Kangwha	0.42	0.11	0,20	0,08
*Kuwait: Non-Kuwaitis	0.65	0.21	0.61	0.20
*Kuwait: Kuwaitis	0.44	0.10	0.42	0.12
*Philippines, Manila	0.55	0.05	0.40	0.03
Singapore: Chinese	0.54	0.04	0.31	0.03
Singapore: Malay	0.46	0.08	0.35	0.08
Singapore: Indian	0.23	0.06	0.45	0.13
Thailand, Chiang Mai	0.40	0.04	0.44	0.05
*Thailand, Khon Kaen	0.36	0.05	0.31	0.04
*Viet Nam, Hanoi				

* IMPORTANT-SEE NOTES ON POPULATION PAGE

CUMULATIVE INCIDENCE (0-74)
RATES AND STANDARD ERRORS (percent)
All leukaemias (ICD-9 204-8) (contd)

EUROPE	MALE		FEMALE	
Austria, Tyrol	0.90	0.09	0.56	0.06
*Belarus	1.15	0.03	0.66	0.02
*Croatia	0.84	0.04	0.55	0.02
Czech Republic	0.96	0.02	0.54	0.01
Denmark	0.98	0.03	0.57	0.02
Estonia	0.95	0.06	0.63	0.04
Finland	0.66	0.02	0.44	0.02
France, Bas-Rhin	0.89	0.08	0.50	0.05
†*France, Calvados	0.30	0.05	0.34	0.05
France, Doubs	0.81	0.10	0.43	0.06
France, Haut-Rhin	0.73	0.08	0.52	0.06
*France, Herault	0.61	0.06	0.38	0.04
France, Isere	0.84	0.07	0.39	0.04
*France, Somme	0.76	0.09	0.54	0.06
*France, Tarn	0.62	0.09	0.38	0.06
Germany, Eastern States	0.74	0.03	0.47	0.02
Germany, Saarland	0.98	0.07	0.57	0.04
Iceland	0.47	0.10	0.49	0.10
Ireland, Southern	1.10	0.10	0.47	0.06
Italy, Ferrara	0.91	0.16	0.57	0.11
Italy, Florence	0.86	0.06	0.54	0.05
Italy, Genoa	0.71	0.06	0.49	0.05
*Italy, Latina	1.08	0.12	0.66	0.09
Italy, Macerata	0.85	0.17	0.58	0.14
Italy, Modena	0.68	0.07	0.57	0.06
Italy, Parma	0.66	0.08	0.52	0.07
Italy, Ragusa	0.63	0.10	0.47	0.08
Italy, Romagna	1.02	0.09	0.60	0.07
Italy, Torino	0.90	0.07	0.49	0.05
Italy, Trieste	1.49	0.17	0.86	0.11
Italy, Varese	0.92	0.08	0.59	0.05
Italy, Veneto	0.86	0.06	0.60	0.04
*Latvia	0.93	0.05	0.62	0.03
Malta	0.60	0.14	0.58	0.12
The Netherlands	0.76	0.02	0.45	0.01
The Netherlands, Eindhoven	0.63	0.06	0.40	0.04
The Netherlands, Maastricht	0.78	0.07	0.52	0.05
Norway	0.55	0.02	0.37	0.02
*Poland, Cracow	0.68	0.08	0.37	0.05
*Poland, Kielce	0.58	0.05	0.38	0.04
*Poland, Lower Silesia	0.81	0.04	0.51	0.03
Poland, Warsaw City	0.58	0.05	0.40	0.03
Slovakia	0.97	0.04	0.55	0.02
Slovenia	0.73	0.05	0.54	0.03
*Spain, Albacete	0.88	0.17	0.31	0.09
Spain, Asturias	0.86	0.07	0.61	0.05
Spain, Basque Country	0.76	0.05	0.41	0.03
Spain, Granada	0.73	0.07	0.50	0.05
Spain, Mallorca	0.67	0.07	0.50	0.06
Spain, Murcia	0.72	0.06	0.48	0.04
Spain, Navarra	0.79	0.08	0.40	0.05
Spain, Tarragona	0.86	0.08	0.44	0.06
Spain, Zaragoza	0.55	0.05	0.49	0.05

	MALE		FEMALE	
Sweden	0.85	0.02	0.57	0.02
*Switzerland, Basel	0.71	0.09	0.46	0.06
Switzerland, Geneva	1.18	0.14	0.49	0.07
Switzerland, Graubunden	0.80	0.17	0.45	0.11
Switzerland, Neuchatel	0.80	0.16	0.41	0.10
Switzerland, St Gall-Appenzell	0.89	0.09	0.56	0.07
Switzerland, Valais	0.76	0.14	0.46	0.10
Switzerland, Vaud	0.74	0.08	0.41	0.05
Switzerland, Zurich	0.83	0.06	0.53	0.04
*UK, England and Wales	0.79	0.01	0.49	0.01
*UK, East Anglia	0.69	0.04	0.41	0.03
*UK, Mersey	0.55	0.03	0.38	0.02
*UK, North Western	0.70	0.03	0.41	0.02
UK, Oxford	0.87	0.04	0.56	0.03
*UK, South Thames	0.73	0.02	0.49	0.02
UK, South Western	0.88	0.03	0.55	0.02
UK, Wessex	0.96	0.04	0.59	0.03
*UK, West Midlands	0.85	0.03	0.49	0.02
UK, Yorkshire	0.77	0.03	0.46	0.02
UK, Scotland	0.81	0.03	0.49	0.02
UK, Scotland, West	0.79	0.04	0.49	0.03
*Yugoslavia, Vojvodina	0.87	0.05	0.46	0.03

OCEANIA

	MALE		FEMALE	
Australian Capital Territory	0.99	0.17	0.49	0.11
Australia, New South Wales	1.01	0.03	0.59	0.02
South Australia	1.40	0.07	0.82	0.05
Australia, Tasmania	1.23	0.12	0.79	0.09
Australia, Victoria	0.92	0.03	0.51	0.02
Western Australia	0.83	0.06	0.51	0.04
*French Polynesia	0.89	0.22	0.65	0.19
New Zealand: Non-Maori	0.99	0.04	0.63	0.03
New Zealand: Maori	0.99	0.17	0.50	0.11
US, Hawaii: White	1.16	0.15	0.43	0.09
US, Hawaii: Japanese	0.52	0.08	0.32	0.06
US, Hawaii: Hawaiian	0.93	0.19	0.66	0.15
US, Hawaii: Filipino	0.52	0.12	0.55	0.13
US, Hawaii: Chinese	0,36	0,14	0,17	0,09

* IMPORTANT-SEE NOTES ON POPULATION PAGE

CUMULATIVE INCIDENCE (0-74)
RATES AND STANDARD ERRORS (percent)
Other and Unspecified

	MALE		FEMALE	
AFRICA				
*Algeria, Setif				
*France, La Reunion				
*Mali, Bamako				
*Uganda, Kyadondo				
*Zimbabwe, Harare: African				
*Zimbabwe, Harare: European				
AMERICA, CENTRAL AND SOUTH				
*Argentina, Concordia	3.56	0.48	2.22	0.33
*Brazil, Belem	1.58	0.19	0.97	0.12 f
*Brazil, Goiania				
*Brazil, Porto Alegre	1.78	0.16	1.32	0.11
Colombia, Cali	1.28	0.11	1.41	0.10
*Costa Rica	1.07	0.07	0.86	0.06
*Ecuador, Quito	0.80	0.10	1.00	0.10
*Peru, Lima	0.78	0.06	0.75	0.06
Peru, Trujillo	0.66	0.17	0.85	0.17
US, Puerto Rico	0.92	0.05	0.64	0.04
*Uruguay, Montevideo	2.95	0.14	1.64	0.09
AMERICA, NORTH				
Canada	1.33	0.02	0.92	0.01
Canada, Alberta	1.15	0.06	0.95	0.05
Canada, British Columbia	1.13	0.04	1.04	0.04
Canada, Manitoba	1.22	0.08	0.96	0.06
Canada, New Brunswick	1.14	0.09	0.98	0.08
Canada, Newfoundland	1.30	0.12	1.13	0.11
Canada, Northwest Territories	1.56	0.54	1.42	0.54
Canada, Nova Scotia	1.68	0.10	1.13	0.08
Canada, Ontario	1.58	0.03	0.90	0.02
Canada, Prince Edward Island	1.37	0.24	0.71	0.17
Canada, Quebec	1.21	0.03	0.85	0.02
Canada, Saskatchewan	0.79	0.06	0.76	0.06
Canada, Yukon	2.24	0.64	1.85	0.70
US, Cent. Calif.: Non-Hisp. White	1.31	0.07	0.84	0.05
US, Cent. Calif.: Hispanic	0.91	0.13	0.79	0.12
US, Los Angeles: Non-Hisp. White	1.22	0.04	1.05	0.03
US, Los Angeles: Hispanic White	1.05	0.08	0.78	0.05
US, Los Angeles: Black	1.70	0.12	1.18	0.08
US, Los Angeles: Chinese	0.77	0.14	0.54	0.12
US, Los Angeles: Filipino	0.66	0.16	0.58	0.12
US, Los Angeles: Korean	0.65	0.19	0.79	0.19
US, Los Angeles: Japanese	0.43	0.12	0.51	0.12
US, San Francisco: Non-Hisp. White	1.09	0.05	0.97	0.04
US, San Francisco: Hispanic White	0.85	0.13	0.72	0.11
US, San Francisco: Black	1.89	0.18	1.22	0.13
US, San Francisco: Chinese	0.87	0.14	0.63	0.11
US, San Francisco: Filipino	0.81	0.18	0.54	0.12
US, San Francisco: Japanese	0,57	0,26	0,40	0,17
US, Connecticut: White	1.14	0.04	0.83	0.03
US, Connecticut: Black	1.60	0.23	1.22	0.18
US, Atlanta: White	1.00	0.07	0.75	0.05
US, Atlanta: Black	2.17	0.21	1.23	0.13
US, Iowa	0.90	0.04	0.66	0.03

	MALE		FEMALE	
US, Central Louisiana: White	1.49	0.19	0.85	0.13
US, Central Louisiana: Black	2.32	0.51	0.98	0.27
US, New Orleans: White	1.26	0.10	0.80	0.07
US, New Orleans: Black	1.73	0.19	1.31	0.15
US, Detroit: White	1.03	0.04	0.77	0.03
US, Detroit: Black	1.38	0.10	0.90	0.07
US, New Mexico: Non-Hisp. White	1.23	0.09	0.73	0.06
US, New Mexico: Hispanic White	0.96	0.12	0.58	0.09
US, New Mexico: American Indian	0.97	0.30	0.89	0.26
US, Utah	0.95	0.07	0.73	0.05
US, Seattle	0.88	0.04	0.77	0.03
US, SEER: White	1.01	0.02	0.78	0.01
US, SEER: Black	1.66	0.07	1.06	0.05
ASIA				
*China, Qidong	0.11	0.03	0.09	0.02
China, Shanghai	0.73	0.02	0.52	0.02
China, Tianjin	0.57	0.03	0.56	0.03
Hong Kong	1.74	0.04	1.13	0.03
*India, Bangalore	1.46	0.06	1.07	0.05
*India, Barshi, Paranda and Bhum	0.82	0.13	0.43	0.08
India, Bombay	1.16	0.04	0.80	0.04
*India, Karunagappally	1.71	0.28	0.99	0.22
India, Madras	1.10	0.06	0.79	0.05
*India, Trivandrum	1.89	0.23	0.78	0.13
Israel: All Jews	1.52	0.05	1.27	0.04
Jews born in Israel	0.89	0.12	1.04	0.16
Jews born in America or Europe	1.58	0.07	1.41	0.06
Jews born in Africa or Asia	1.54	0.09	1.03	0.07
Non-Jews	1.14	0.16	0.75	0.11
Japan, Hiroshima	0.43	0.05	0.28	0.04
Japan, Miyagi	0.35	0.03	0.24	0.02
Japan, Nagasaki	0.37	0.03	0.20	0.02
Japan, Osaka	0.44	0.02	0.28	0.01
*Japan, Saga	0.30	0.04	0.22	0.03
Japan, Yamagata	0.43	0.04	0.26	0.03
*Korea, Kangwha	0,35	0,12	0,09	0,05
*Kuwait: Non-Kuwaitis	0.81	0.31	0.62	0.22
*Kuwait: Kuwaitis	0.78	0.16	0.86	0.21
*Philippines, Manila	1.42	0.08	1.04	0.06
Singapore: Chinese	0.98	0.07	0.66	0.05
Singapore: Malay	0.72	0.13	0.57	0.13
Singapore: Indian	0.55	0.13	0.46	0.18
Thailand, Chiang Mai	2.11	0.10	1.97	0.10
*Thailand, Khon Kaen	2.86	0.15	1.77	0.11
*Viet Nam, Hanoi				

* IMPORTANT-SEE NOTES ON POPULATION PAGE

EUROPE	MALE		FEMALE	
Austria, Tyrol	0.66	0.09	0.52	0.06
*Belarus	0.70	0.02	0.33	0.01
*Croatia	1.59	0.05	0.98	0.03
Czech Republic	1.11	0.03	0.77	0.02
Denmark	1.43	0.04	1.23	0.03
Estonia	0.94	0.07	0.35	0.03
Finland	0.61	0.02	0.49	0.02
France, Bas-Rhin	2.14	0.12	0.90	0.07
*France, Calvados	0.84	0.09	0.27	0.04
France, Doubs	2.34	0.17	1.05	0.10
France, Haut-Rhin	1.12	0.10	0.55	0.06
*France, Herault	1.17	0.08	0.55	0.05
France, Isere	1.72	0.10	0.82	0.06
*France, Somme	1.12	0.10	0.46	0.06
*France, Tarn	1.36	0.13	0.56	0.08
Germany, Eastern States	0.31	0.02	0.28	0.01
Germany, Saarland	1.59	0.09	0.88	0.05
Iceland	0.80	0.14	0.75	0.13
Ireland, Southern	1.35	0.12	1.25	0.11
Italy, Ferrara	0.77	0.14	0.56	0.12
Italy, Florence	0.96	0.07	0.67	0.05
Italy, Genoa	1.17	0.08	0.59	0.05
*Italy, Latina	0.68	0.10	0.35	0.06
Italy, Macerata	0.87	0.18	0.56	0.13
Italy, Modena	1.03	0.08	0.70	0.07
Italy, Parma	0.83	0.09	0.37	0.05
Italy, Ragusa	0.66	0.10	0.38	0.07
Italy, Romagna	0.74	0.08	0.58	0.07
Italy, Torino	1.56	0.10	0.68	0.06
Italy, Trieste	-	-	-	-
Italy, Varese	1.23	0.09	0.42	0.05
Italy, Veneto	1.29	0.07	0.66	0.05
*Latvia	0.32	0.03	0.20	0.02
Malta	1.03	0.20	0.86	0.17
The Netherlands	1.70	0.03	0.96	0.02
The Netherlands, Eindhoven	1.99	0.11	1.06	0.07
The Netherlands, Maastricht	2.03	0.11	1.10	0.07
Norway	1.00	0.03	0.77	0.03
*Poland, Cracow	1.48	0.11	1.20	0.09
*Poland, Kielce	0.61	0.06	0.44	0.04
*Poland, Lower Silesia	1.57	0.06	1.01	0.04
Poland, Warsaw City	1.37	0.08	0.93	0.06
Slovakia	0.75	0.03	0.57	0.02
Slovenia	1.55	0.07	0.93	0.05
*Spain, Albacete	1.29	0.21	0.47	0.12
Spain, Asturias	1.33	0.08	0.66	0.05
Spain, Basque Country	1.87	0.08	0.75	0.04
Spain, Granada	1.39	0.10	0.63	0.06
Spain, Mallorca	1.83	0.12	0.94	0.08
Spain, Murcia	1.36	0.09	0.81	0.06
Spain, Navarra	1.23	0.11	0.64	0.07
Spain, Tarragona	1.54	0.11	0.76	0.07
Spain, Zaragoza	1.20	0.08	0.68	0.05

	MALE		FEMALE	
Sweden	1.03	0.02	0.93	0.02
*Switzerland, Basel	0.88	0.10	0.63	0.07
Switzerland, Geneva	0.86	0.11	0.55	0.08
Switzerland, Graubunden	0.63	0.15	0.36	0.11
Switzerland, Neuchatel	0.61	0.14	0.71	0.13
Switzerland, St Gall-Appenzell	0.65	0.08	0.42	0.06
Switzerland, Valais	1.90	0.23	0.63	0.12
Switzerland, Vaud	1.03	0.10	0.64	0.07
Switzerland, Zurich	0.85	0.06	0.60	0.05
*UK, England and Wales	1.73	0.02	1.26	0.01
*UK, East Anglia	1.46	0.06	1.14	0.05
*UK, Mersey	1.75	0.06	1.42	0.05
*UK, North Western	2.07	0.05	1.47	0.04
UK, Oxford	1.51	0.06	1.32	0.05
*UK, South Thames	1.40	0.03	1.06	0.02
UK, South Western	0.15	0.01	0.11	0.01
UK, Wessex	1.42	0.05	1.14	0.04
*UK, West Midlands	1.97	0.04	1.48	0.03
UK, Yorkshire	1.95	0.05	1.58	0.04
UK, Scotland	1.94	0.04	1.37	0.03
UK, Scotland, West	2.14	0.06	1.43	0.05
*Yugoslavia, Vojvodina	1.10	0.05	0.88	0.04

OCEANIA	MALE		FEMALE	
Australian Capital Territory	1.18	0.19	1.10	0.18
Australia, New South Wales	1.73	0.04	1.14	0.03
South Australia	1.27	0.07	1.01	0.06
Australia, Tasmania	1.60	0.14	0.99	0.10
Australia, Victoria	1.59	0.05	1.03	0.03
Western Australia	2.04	0.09	1.32	0.07
*French Polynesia	1.61	0.35	1.30	0.30
New Zealand: Non-Maori	1.63	0.06	1.44	0.05
New Zealand: Maori	3.11	0.40	2.51	0.31
US, Hawaii: White	1.02	0.15	1.08	0.15
US, Hawaii: Japanese	0.42	0.08	0.29	0.06
US, Hawaii: Hawaiian	0.81	0.19	0.69	0.15
US, Hawaii: Filipino	0.45	0.12	0.36	0.11
US, Hawaii: Chinese	0.72	0.21	0.33	0.14

* IMPORTANT-SEE NOTES ON POPULATION PAGE

CUMULATIVE INCIDENCE (0-74)
RATES AND STANDARD ERRORS (percent)
All sites

	MALE		FEMALE	
AFRICA				
*Algeria, Setif				
*France, La Reunion				
*Mali, Bamako				
*Uganda, Kyadondo				
*Zimbabwe, Harare: African				
*Zimbabwe, Harare: European				
AMERICA, CENTRAL AND SOUTH				
*Argentina, Concordia	33.29	1.44	29.02	1.19
*Brazil, Belem	25.53	0.78	21.93	0.55
*Brazil, Goiania				
*Brazil, Porto Alegre	44.01	0.77	29.51	0.49
Colombia, Cali	21.41	0.44	22.87	0.38
*Costa Rica	23.66	0.31	20.95	0.27
*Ecuador, Quito	18.14	0.47	21.29	0.43
*Peru, Lima	14.98	0.27	18.04	0.27
Peru, Trujillo	18.99	0.98	22.12	0.88
US, Puerto Rico	24.30	0.24	16.77	0.18
*Uruguay, Montevideo	38.00	0.51	29.55	0.37
AMERICA, NORTH				
Canada				
Canada, Alberta				
Canada, British Columbia				
Canada, Manitoba				
Canada, New Brunswick				
Canada, Newfoundland				
Canada, Northwest Territories				
Canada, Nova Scotia				
Canada, Ontario				
Canada, Prince Edward Island				
Canada, Quebec				
Canada, Saskatchewan				
Canada, Yukon				
US, Cent. Calif.: Non-Hisp. White	42.56	0.39	31.53	0.31
US, Cent. Calif.: Hispanic	29.22	0.77	22.83	0.60
US, Los Angeles: Non-Hisp. White	44.04	0.24	35.33	0.19
US, Los Angeles: Hispanic White	28.10	0.38	22.48	0.27
US, Los Angeles: Black	51.75	0.65	30.31	0.41
US, Los Angeles: Chinese	20.61	0.76	15.65	0.61
US, Los Angeles: Filipino	24.12	0.98	20.73	0.70
US, Los Angeles: Korean	22.58	1.18	15.30	0.77
US, Los Angeles: Japanese	24.42	0.92	20.76	0.76
US, San Francisco: Non-Hisp. White	47.44	0.33	35.31	0.26
US, San Francisco: Hispanic White	33.94	0.87	26.24	0.62
US, San Francisco: Black	56.79	0.98	32.72	0.63
US, San Francisco: Chinese	25.64	0.71	21.72	0.64
US, San Francisco: Filipino	28.79	1.24	21.89	0.81
US, San Francisco: Japanese	26.00	1.70	23.82	1.33
US, Connecticut: White	42.24	0.27	33.26	0.21
US, Connecticut: Black	51.96	1.38	31.74	0.87
US, Atlanta: White	46.07	0.48	31.36	0.33
US, Atlanta: Black	55.08	1.07	29.20	0.60
US, Iowa	41.83	0.28	30.92	0.21

	MALE		FEMALE	
US, Central Louisiana: White	37.80	0.96	24.57	0.69
US, Central Louisiana: Black	46.95	2.28	24.95	1.37
US, New Orleans: White	45.74	0.63	31.41	0.45
US, New Orleans: Black	49.51	1.06	30.43	0.67
US, Detroit: White	47.76	0.30	33.98	0.22
US, Detroit: Black	57.06	0.66	32.41	0.42
US, New Mexico: Non-Hisp. White	42.96	0.51	29.83	0.39
US, New Mexico: Hispanic White	29.84	0.68	21.49	0.50
US, New Mexico: American Indian	16.51	1.19	16.27	1.00
US, Utah	36.90	0.40	25.84	0.30
US, Seattle	47.79	0.29	33.73	0.22
US, SEER: White	44.25	0.11	32.32	0.09
US, SEER: Black	55.85	0.44	31.51	0.27
ASIA				
*China, Qidong	24.02	0.35	11.81	0.23
China, Shanghai	28.03	0.14	17.67	0.10
China, Tianjin	23.44	0.20	17.93	0.17
Hong Kong	35.60	0.19	23.84	0.15
*India, Bangalore	12.24	0.19	13.33	0.18
*India, Barshi, Paranda and Bhum	6.48	0.35	5.87	0.29
India, Bombay	15.94	0.16	14.43	0.15
*India, Karunagappally	13.31	0.78	9.28	0.62
India, Madras	13.92	0.20	14.68	0.19
*India, Trivandrum	13.11	0.61	10.00	0.44
Israel: All Jews	27.37	0.22	27.06	0.19
Jews born in Israel	26.98	0.82	29.00	0.73
Jews born in America or Europe	29.61	0.31	30.51	0.30
Jews born in Africa or Asia	23.40	0.38	20.35	0.33
Non-Jews	14.43	0.55	10.20	0.39
Japan, Hiroshima	39.14	0.49	22.42	0.32
Japan, Miyagi	33.09	0.28	18.99	0.18
Japan, Nagasaki	34.72	0.32	19.12	0.20
Japan, Osaka	31.97	0.16	17.00	0.09
*Japan, Saga	31.69	0.42	15.91	0.25
Japan, Yamagata	30.97	0.32	16.89	0.21
*Korea, Kangwha	23.83	1.10	12.25	0.69
*Kuwait: Non-Kuwaitis	19.16	1.36	14.63	0.90
*Kuwait: Kuwaitis	11.48	0.62	14.31	0.74
*Philippines, Manila	25.36	0.34	22.23	0.26
Singapore: Chinese	31.86	0.38	22.41	0.27
Singapore: Malay	17.28	0.65	14.99	0.59
Singapore: Indian	12.33	0.58	15.29	1.02
Thailand, Chiang Mai	17.82	0.32	18.11	0.31
*Thailand, Khon Kaen	23.46	0.46	15.66	0.33
*Viet Nam, Hanoi				

* IMPORTANT-SEE NOTES ON POPULATION PAGE

CUMULATIVE INCIDENCE (0-74)
RATES AND STANDARD ERRORS (percent)
All sites (contd)

EUROPE	MALE		FEMALE	
Austria, Tyrol	38.96	0.65	29.60	0.46
*Belarus	34.53	0.16	19.38	0.09
*Croatia	31.98	0.23	19.02	0.14
Czech Republic	42.81	0.16	27.93	0.11
Denmark	38.30	0.19	34.90	0.16
Estonia	35.76	0.40	21.79	0.23
Finland	35.12	0.18	27.60	0.13
France, Bas-Rhin	48.86	0.58	26.78	0.35
*France, Calvados	44.99	0.65	23.87	0.41
France, Doubs	46.45	0.77	27.46	0.52
France, Haut-Rhin	48.73	0.69	29.26	0.44
*France, Herault	32.85	0.44	22.72	0.33
France, Isere	36.83	0.48	24.36	0.33
*France, Somme	39.03	0.62	20.63	0.40
*France, Tarn	33.47	0.66	19.41	0.45
Germany, Eastern States	30.82	0.18	22.65	0.12
Germany, Saarland	44.15	0.47	28.56	0.30
Iceland	31.53	0.88	27.85	0.75
Ireland, Southern	37.13	0.61	30.02	0.52
Italy, Ferrara	44.83	1.08	29.44	0.79
Italy, Florence	40.18	0.43	26.33	0.31
Italy, Genoa	42.63	0.49	26.22	0.33
*Italy, Latina	32.64	0.71	20.65	0.50
Italy, Macerata	38.57	1.17	25.05	0.86
Italy, Modena	40.15	0.52	26.58	0.39
Italy, Parma	39.81	0.62	26.00	0.45
Italy, Ragusa	25.27	0.64	18.13	0.49
Italy, Romagna	44.64	0.61	29.44	0.45
Italy, Torino	40.65	0.49	25.72	0.33
Italy, Trieste	54.67	1.00	33.21	0.67
Italy, Varese	47.63	0.57	27.25	0.36
Italy, Veneto	48.88	0.45	28.88	0.30
*Latvia	31.01	0.28	19.07	0.16
Malta	31.00	1.12	25.25	0.88
The Netherlands	35.77	0.13	25.94	0.10
The Netherlands, Eindhoven	36.00	0.48	23.83	0.34
The Netherlands, Maastricht	35.77	0.47	24.90	0.34
Norway	30.12	0.18	24.61	0.15
*Poland, Cracow	31.51	0.54	23.10	0.36
*Poland, Kielce	28.29	0.38	16.05	0.24
*Poland, Lower Silesia	36.89	0.30	23.37	0.20
Poland, Warsaw City	32.00	0.38	23.62	0.26
Slovakia	42.21	0.24	24.99	0.16
Slovenia	34.57	0.35	22.07	0.22
*Spain, Albacete	23.46	0.88	15.57	0.67
Spain, Asturias	32.49	0.40	18.03	0.27
Spain, Basque Country	34.22	0.33	16.95	0.20
Spain, Granada	32.41	0.46	17.92	0.31
Spain, Mallorca	43.85	0.60	26.38	0.42
Spain, Murcia	36.37	0.44	20.79	0.30
Spain, Navarra	37.76	0.57	23.42	0.42
Spain, Tarragona	36.59	0.55	22.45	0.40
Spain, Zaragoza	30.12	0.40	16.35	0.26

	MALE		FEMALE	
Sweden	29.13	0.12	26.41	0.11
*Switzerland, Basel	42.29	0.68	30.19	0.50
Switzerland, Geneva	51.04	0.87	34.81	0.61
Switzerland, Graubunden	32.38	1.07	22.50	0.80
Switzerland, Neuchatel	42.73	1.12	28.88	0.81
Switzerland, St Gall-Appenzell	37.90	0.64	25.80	0.47
Switzerland, Valais	42.35	1.05	27.83	0.76
Switzerland, Vaud	47.61	0.64	33.61	0.48
Switzerland, Zurich	35.25	0.40	24.16	0.29
*UK, England and Wales	34.72	0.07	28.70	0.06
*UK, East Anglia	34.05	0.27	29.40	0.23
*UK, Mersey	33.53	0.24	30.22	0.22
*UK, North Western	35.94	0.21	29.21	0.17
UK, Oxford	36.84	0.28	31.71	0.24
*UK, South Thames	31.47	0.15	26.88	0.12
UK, South Western	32.76	0.21	28.05	0.17
UK, Wessex	31.72	0.22	28.10	0.19
*UK, West Midlands	39.20	0.19	31.95	0.15
UK, Yorkshire	36.53	0.22	29.85	0.18
UK, Scotland	41.67	0.20	32.93	0.16
UK, Scotland, West	42.17	0.28	32.49	0.21
*Yugoslavia, Vojvodina	32.11	0.29	22.33	0.21

OCEANIA

	MALE		FEMALE	
Australian Capital Territory				
Australia, New South Wales				
South Australia				
Australia, Tasmania				
Australia, Victoria				
Western Australia				
*French Polynesia				
New Zealand: Non-Maori	32.16	0.24	30.15	0.21
New Zealand: Maori	42.04	1.50	38.03	1.17
US, Hawaii: White	48.39	0.99	33.82	0.79
US, Hawaii: Japanese	30.42	0.64	22.07	0.50
US, Hawaii: Hawaiian	34.04	1.27	30.67	1.07
US, Hawaii: Filipino	23.21	0.89	21.78	0.82
US, Hawaii: Chinese	29.72	1.38	20.47	1.04

* IMPORTANT-SEE NOTES ON POPULATION PAGE

CUMULATIVE INCIDENCE (0-74)
RATES AND STANDARD ERRORS (percent)
All sites but 173

	MALE		FEMALE			MALE		FEMALE	
AFRICA					US, Central Louisiana: White	37.75	0.96	24.50	0.68
*Algeria, Setif					US, Central Louisiana: Black	46.95	2.28	24.88	1.37
*France, La Reunion					US, New Orleans: White	45.68	0.63	31.35	0.45
*Mali, Bamako					US, New Orleans: Black	49.48	1.06	30.34	0.67
*Uganda, Kyadondo					US, Detroit: White	47.68	0.30	33.92	0.22
*Zimbabwe, Harare: African					US, Detroit: Black	56.97	0.66	32.33	0.42
*Zimbabwe, Harare: European					US, New Mexico: Non-Hisp. White	42.83	0.51	29.73	0.39
					US, New Mexico: Hispanic White	29.72	0.67	21.41	0.50
					US, New Mexico: American Indian	16.51	1.19	16.26	1.00
AMERICA, CENTRAL AND SOUTH					US, Utah	36.82	0.40	25.76	0.30
*Argentina, Concordia	27.75	1.31	25.80	1.12	US, Seattle	47.71	0.29	33.63	0.22
					US, SEER: White	44.16	0.11	32.26	0.09
*Brazil, Belem	21.35	0.71	19.36	0.50	US, SEER: Black	55.78	0.44	31.43	0.27
*Brazil, Goiania									
*Brazil, Porto Alegre	37.78	0.71	25.99	0.45	**ASIA**				
Colombia, Cali	21.41	0.44	22.87	0.38	*China, Qidong	23.89	0.35	11.71	0.23
*Costa Rica	19.36	0.28	17.02	0.24	China, Shanghai	27.84	0.14	17.56	0.10
*Ecuador, Quito	15.64	0.43	18.78	0.40	China, Tianjin	23.36	0.20	17.85	0.17
*Peru, Lima	13.87	0.26	17.06	0.26	Hong Kong	34.98	0.19	23.37	0.15
Peru, Trujillo	16.83	0.91	20.25	0.83	*India, Bangalore	12.07	0.19	13.16	0.18
US, Puerto Rico	24.27	0.24	16.73	0.18	*India, Barshi, Paranda and Bhum	6.29	0.35	5.73	0.29
					India, Bombay	15.74	0.16	14.29	0.14
*Uruguay, Montevideo	36.14	0.50	28.52	0.36	*India, Karunagappally	12.94	0.76	8.91	0.60
					India, Madras	13.69	0.20	14.57	0.19
					*India, Trivandrum	12.97	0.60	9.89	0.44
AMERICA, NORTH					Israel: All Jews	27.06	0.21	26.77	0.19
Canada	38.05	0.09	28.79	0.07	Jews born in Israel	26.57	0.81	28.56	0.72
Canada, Alberta	33.74	0.31	27.74	0.25	Jews born in America or Europe	29.25	0.31	30.16	0.30
Canada, British Columbia	36.56	0.24	29.11	0.20	Jews born in Africa or Asia	23.22	0.38	20.23	0.33
Canada, Manitoba	38.30	0.44	29.89	0.35	Non-Jews	14.38	0.55	10.15	0.38
Canada, New Brunswick	39.29	0.55	27.74	0.42	Japan, Hiroshima	38.59	0.49	22.02	0.31
Canada, Newfoundland	34.03	0.61	25.93	0.50	Japan, Miyagi	32.82	0.28	18.82	0.18
Canada, Northwest Territories	33.88	2.24	28.98	2.06	Japan, Nagasaki	34.17	0.32	18.76	0.20
Canada, Nova Scotia	39.58	0.49	30.64	0.39	Japan, Osaka	31.85	0.15	16.92	0.09
Canada, Ontario	38.28	0.15	29.70	0.12	*Japan, Saga	31.42	0.42	15.84	0.25
Canada, Prince Edward Island	39.37	1.29	29.66	1.04	Japan, Yamagata	30.86	0.32	16.81	0.21
Canada, Quebec	40.18	0.19	27.69	0.13	*Korea, Kangwha	23.66	1.10	12.19	0.68
Canada, Saskatchewan	35.21	0.43	27.51	0.35	*Kuwait: Non-Kuwaitis	18.39	1.33	14.28	0.88
Canada, Yukon	40.48	2.99	33.25	2.65	*Kuwait: Kuwaitis	11.29	0.61	14.09	0.73
US, Cent. Calif.: Non-Hisp. White	42.45	0.39	31.47	0.30	*Philippines, Manila	25.05	0.34	22.04	0.26
US, Cent. Calif.: Hispanic	29.19	0.77	22.80	0.60	Singapore: Chinese	30.84	0.37	21.57	0.26
US, Los Angeles: Non-Hisp. White	43.92	0.24	35.25	0.19	Singapore: Malay	16.71	0.64	14.61	0.58
US, Los Angeles: Hispanic White	28.06	0.38	22.42	0.27	Singapore: Indian	12.08	0.57	14.67	1.00
US, Los Angeles: Black	51.67	0.65	30.23	0.41	Thailand, Chiang Mai	17.34	0.31	17.80	0.30
US, Los Angeles: Chinese	20.61	0.76	15.62	0.61	*Thailand, Khon Kaen	22.98	0.45	15.33	0.33
US, Los Angeles: Filipino	24.10	0.98	20.67	0.70	*Viet Nam, Hanoi				
US, Los Angeles: Korean	22.58	1.18	15.28	0.77					
US, Los Angeles: Japanese	24.39	0.92	20.70	0.76					
US, San Francisco: Non-Hisp. White	47.33	0.32	35.23	0.26					
US, San Francisco: Hispanic White	33.90	0.87	26.21	0.62					
US, San Francisco: Black	56.70	0.98	32.62	0.63					
US, San Francisco: Chinese	25.59	0.71	21.71	0.64					
US, San Francisco: Filipino	28.79	1.24	21.86	0.81					
US, San Francisco: Japanese	26.00	1.70	23.82	1.33					
US, Connecticut: White	42.17	0.27	33.20	0.21					
US, Connecticut: Black	51.90	1.38	31.67	0.87					
US, Atlanta: White	45.97	0.48	31.33	0.33					
US, Atlanta: Black	55.04	1.07	29.11	0.60					
US, Iowa	41.73	0.28	30.87	0.21					

* IMPORTANT-SEE NOTES ON POPULATION PAGE

EUROPE	MALE		FEMALE	
Austria, Tyrol	36.45	0.63	28.06	0.45
*Belarus	32.07	0.16	17.40	0.08
*Croatia	31.93	0.23	18.99	0.14
Czech Republic	36.39	0.14	23.77	0.10
Denmark	32.18	0.17	30.02	0.15
Estonia	33.37	0.38	19.83	0.22
Finland	28.98	0.17	22.29	0.12
France, Bas-Rhin	47.07	0.56	26.08	0.35
*France, Calvados	40.88	0.62	21.70	0.39
France, Doubs	38.79	0.70	22.20	0.46
France, Haut-Rhin	43.28	0.64	25.54	0.41
*France, Herault	30.86	0.42	22.02	0.32
France, Isere	35.46	0.47	23.83	0.33
*France, Somme	37.44	0.61	20.26	0.40
*France, Tarn	31.59	0.64	18.74	0.45
Germany, Eastern States	30.10	0.18	22.39	0.11
Germany, Saarland	36.95	0.42	24.44	0.28
Iceland	30.96	0.87	27.45	0.75
Ireland, Southern	27.95	0.53	23.80	0.46
Italy, Ferrara	38.57	1.00	26.24	0.74
Italy, Florence	37.55	0.41	25.11	0.30
Italy, Genoa	38.60	0.47	24.04	0.32
*Italy, Latina	29.55	0.67	19.06	0.48
Italy, Macerata	33.49	1.09	22.07	0.81
Italy, Modena	35.15	0.49	24.31	0.37
Italy, Parma	36.40	0.60	24.62	0.44
Italy, Ragusa	20.17	0.57	15.61	0.46
Italy, Romagna	37.38	0.56	25.75	0.42
Italy, Torino	35.98	0.46	22.89	0.31
Italy, Trieste	46.77	0.92	27.83	0.61
Italy, Varese	42.23	0.54	24.60	0.34
Italy, Veneto	42.85	0.42	25.78	0.28
*Latvia	28.88	0.27	17.36	0.15
Malta	25.39	1.01	22.98	0.84
The Netherlands	34.17	0.12	25.37	0.09
The Netherlands, Eindhoven	36.00	0.48	23.83	0.34
The Netherlands, Maastricht	34.56	0.46	24.32	0.33
Norway	29.07	0.18	23.93	0.15
*Poland, Cracow	29.49	0.52	21.90	0.35
*Poland, Kielce	26.06	0.36	14.54	0.23
*Poland, Lower Silesia	35.46	0.29	22.34	0.19
Poland, Warsaw City	30.44	0.37	22.48	0.25
Slovakia	37.47	0.22	21.59	0.14
Slovenia	32.04	0.34	20.28	0.21
*Spain, Albacete	23.41	0.88	15.50	0.67
Spain, Asturias	32.43	0.40	18.00	0.27
Spain, Basque Country	34.17	0.33	16.92	0.20
Spain, Granada	26.98	0.42	15.03	0.28
Spain, Mallorca	33.50	0.52	19.67	0.36
Spain, Murcia	29.52	0.40	17.09	0.27
Spain, Navarra	31.78	0.53	19.90	0.38
Spain, Tarragona	29.08	0.49	17.95	0.36
Spain, Zaragoza	27.33	0.38	15.19	0.25

	MALE		FEMALE	
Sweden	28.00	0.12	25.90	0.11
*Switzerland, Basel	32.21	0.60	23.44	0.44
Switzerland, Geneva	38.35	0.76	25.77	0.52
Switzerland, Graubunden	30.44	1.04	21.92	0.79
Switzerland, Neuchatel	32.95	0.98	23.11	0.73
Switzerland, St Gall-Appenzell	31.55	0.58	21.36	0.42
Switzerland, Valais	34.76	0.96	22.52	0.68
Switzerland, Vaud	35.98	0.56	25.23	0.41
Switzerland, Zurich	35.15	0.40	24.08	0.29
*UK, England and Wales	29.91	0.07	25.45	0.06
*UK, East Anglia	26.89	0.24	24.88	0.21
*UK, Mersey	28.95	0.23	26.25	0.21
*UK, North Western	31.56	0.19	25.95	0.16
UK, Oxford	29.15	0.25	27.02	0.22
*UK, South Thames	27.51	0.14	24.37	0.12
UK, South Western	26.47	0.19	23.99	0.16
UK, Wessex	29.34	0.21	26.64	0.18
*UK, West Midlands	33.04	0.17	27.71	0.14
UK, Yorkshire	31.34	0.20	26.31	0.17
UK, Scotland	35.53	0.19	29.00	0.15
UK, Scotland, West	36.91	0.26	29.09	0.20
*Yugoslavia, Vojvodina	29.65	0.28	20.41	0.20

OCEANIA	MALE		FEMALE	
Australian Capital Territory	33.12	1.04	25.52	0.79
Australia, New South Wales	36.95	0.18	26.83	0.14
South Australia	37.07	0.36	27.78	0.29
Australia, Tasmania	35.79	0.65	26.25	0.51
Australia, Victoria	34.74	0.21	26.68	0.17
Western Australia	35.83	0.38	28.11	0.31
*French Polynesia	29.59	1.45	27.56	1.27
New Zealand: Non-Maori	32.16	0.24	30.15	0.21
New Zealand: Maori	42.04	1.50	38.03	1.17
US, Hawaii: White	48.30	0.98	33.71	0.79
US, Hawaii: Japanese	30.33	0.64	21.99	0.50
US, Hawaii: Hawaiian	33.87	1.26	30.56	1.07
US, Hawaii: Filipino	23.14	0.89	21.76	0.82
US, Hawaii: Chinese	29.68	1.38	20.47	1.04

* IMPORTANT-SEE NOTES ON POPULATION PAGE

PERCENTAGE DISTRIBUTION
OF MICROSCOPICALLY VERIFIED CASES
BY HISTOLOGICAL TYPE

PERCENTAGE DISTRIBUTION OF MICROSCOPICALLY VERIFIED CASES BY HISTOLOGICAL TYPE
Oesophagus (ICD-9 150) - Male

	Carcinoma				Sarcoma	Other	Unspecified	Number of cases	
	Squamous	Adeno	Other	Unspecified				MV	Total
AFRICA									
Algeria, Setif	-	100.0	-	-	-	-	-	5	9
France, La Reunion	92.4	5.9	-	1.7	-	-	-	238	240
Mali, Bamako	80.0	20.0	-	-	-	-	-	5	12
Uganda, Kyadondo	75.0	16.7	-	8.3	-	-	-	12	65
Zimbabwe, Harare: African	86.4	2.5	-	9.9	1.2	-	-	81	153
Zimbabwe, Harare: European	50.0	50.0	-	-	-	-	-	2	3
AMERICA, CENTRAL AND SOUTH									
Argentina, Concordia	61.5	10.3	-	23.1	-	-	5.1	39	49
Brazil, Belem	51.4	8.1	-	40.5	-	-	-	37	57
Brazil, Goiania	67.1	12.9	-	7.1	-	-	12.9	70	91
Brazil, Porto Alegre	58.4	9.8	-	9.2	-	-	22.5	173	269
Colombia, Cali	58.9	28.6	-	12.5	-	-	-	56	86
Costa Rica	65.5	24.5	-	7.3	0.9	0.9	0.9	110	176
Ecuador, Quito	69.4	16.7	-	13.9	-	-	-	36	51
Peru, Lima	70.5	25.0	-	4.5	-	-	-	44	73
Peru, Trujillo	100.0	-	-	-	-	-	-	7	14
Puerto Rico	85.9	6.1	0.8	6.3	-	-	0.8	619	719
Uruguay, Montevideo	88.3	5.3	-	6.4	-	-	-	171	311
AMERICA, NORTH									
Canada	54.1	37.7	1.3	5.6	0.1	0.2	1.0	2992	3465
Canada, Alberta	64.1	25.0	1.9	6.4	-	1.3	1.3	156	166
Canada, British Columbia	56.7	38.4	0.2	4.2	-	-	0.4	453	489
Canada, Manitoba	58.6	37.1	2.6	1.7	-	-	-	116	140
Canada, New Brunswick	55.0	42.5	-	2.5	-	-	-	80	84
Canada, Newfoundland	50.0	42.2	1.6	6.3	-	-	-	64	66
Canada, Northwest Territories	-	33.3	-	-	-	-	66.7	3	4
Canada, Nova Scotia	49.1	42.7	0.9	7.3	-	-	-	110	121
Canada, Ontario	52.1	40.9	1.2	4.3	-	0.2	1.3	1251	1414
Canada, Prince Edward Island	42.9	52.4	-	4.8	-	-	-	21	22
Canada, Quebec	54.8	31.5	2.0	9.8	0.2	0.3	1.5	610	829
Canada, Saskatchewan	53.2	37.3	1.6	5.6	1.6	-	0.8	126	128
Canada, Yukon	75.0	25.0	-	-	-	-	-	4	6
US, Cent. California: Non-Hisp White	37.4	57.0	2.8	2.8	-	-	-	179	183
US, Cent. California: Hispanic	50.0	45.8	-	4.2	-	-	-	24	24
US, Los Angeles: Non-Hisp White	41.0	51.2	0.8	5.9	-	-	1.0	490	502
US, Los Angeles: Hispanic White	54.4	39.0	-	5.9	-	-	0.7	136	140
US, Los Angeles: Black	84.9	7.3	1.6	5.2	-	-	1.0	192	198
US, Los Angeles: Chinese	73.9	17.4	4.3	4.3	-	-	-	23	24
US, Los Angeles: Filipino	66.7	33.3	-	-	-	-	-	9	9
US, Los Angeles: Korean	85.7	7.1	-	7.1	-	-	-	14	15
US, Los Angeles: Japanese	96.3	-	-	3.7	-	-	-	27	27
US, San Francisco: Non-Hisp White	47.8	47.8	0.6	3.5	-	-	0.3	343	358
US, San Francisco: Hispanic White	43.3	46.7	6.7	3.3	-	-	-	30	30
US, San Francisco: Black	95.5	2.7	0.9	0.9	-	-	-	112	116
US, San Francisco: Chinese	81.3	15.6	-	-	-	-	3.1	32	34
US, San Francisco: Filipino	50.0	16.7	-	25.0	-	8.3	-	12	12
US, San Francisco: Japanese	92.9	7.1	-	-	-	-	-	14	14
US, Connecticut: White	50.0	44.6	0.6	4.6	-	-	0.2	518	537
US, Connecticut: Black	93.9	1.0	2.0	3.0	-	-	-	99	100
US, Atlanta: White	35.6	53.7	1.3	8.7	-	-	0.7	149	154
US, Atlanta: Black	89.7	3.7	2.9	3.7	-	-	-	136	137
US, Iowa	39.8	54.2	0.5	5.1	-	0.3	-	389	401
US, Central Louisiana: White	50.0	50.0	-	-	-	-	-	22	26
US, Central Louisiana: Black	88.2	11.8	-	-	-	-	-	17	21
US, New Orleans: White	47.2	43.5	0.9	8.3	-	-	-	108	116
US, New Orleans: Black	85.7	6.5	1.3	6.5	-	-	-	77	83
US, Detroit: White	45.1	45.1	0.4	8.7	-	-	0.7	446	461
US, Detroit: Black	89.0	4.2	2.1	4.2	-	-	0.4	283	288
US, New Mexico: Non-Hisp White	41.2	53.9	1.0	3.9	-	-	-	102	108
US, New Mexico: Hispanic White	75.0	25.0	-	-	-	-	-	24	29
US, New Mexico: American Indian	66.7	33.3	-	-	-	-	-	3	5
US, Utah	44.4	51.5	-	4.0	-	-	-	99	102
US, Seattle	42.0	52.5	0.4	4.7	0.2	0.2	-	467	483
US, SEER: White	44.3	49.2	0.6	5.5	-	0.1	0.2	2562	2657
US, SEER: Black	91.2	3.6	1.9	3.1	-	-	0.1	667	679

PERCENTAGE DISTRIBUTION OF MICROSCOPICALLY VERIFIED CASES BY HISTOLOGICAL TYPE
Oesophagus (ICD-9 150) - Male (contd)

	Squamous	Carcinoma Adeno	Other	Unspecified	Sarcoma	Other	Unspecified	Number of cases MV	Total
ASIA									
China, Qidong									
China, Shanghai									
China, Tianjin	33.1	3.3	0.3	-	0.1	-	63.1	**700**	1359
Hong Kong	84.5	9.3	0.6	5.1	0.1	0.1	0.4	**1820**	2179
India, Bangalore	79.4	8.7	1.2	5.8	-	0.2	4.6	**413**	557
India, Barshi, Paranda and Bhum	87.5	10.0	-	-	-	-	2.5	**40**	49
India, Bombay	91.9	1.0	0.7	5.0	-	-	1.4	**861**	1383
India, Karunagappally	73.3	20.0	-	-	6.7	-	-	**15**	23
India, Madras	86.0	11.8	0.2	1.3	-	-	0.7	**457**	641
India, Trivandrum	80.0	16.0	-	-	-	-	4.0	**25**	31
Israel: All Jews	69.9	23.5	1.8	4.8	-	-	-	**166**	215
Jews born in Israel	54.5	27.3	9.1	9.1	-	-	-	**11**	17
Jews born in America or Europe	70.5	22.3	1.8	5.4	-	-	-	**112**	146
Jews born in Africa or Asia	72.1	25.6	-	2.3	-	-	-	**43**	52
Non-Jews	66.7	-	-	-	33.3	-	-	**3**	5
Japan, Hiroshima	95.3	2.7	0.3	1.7	-	-	-	**296**	317
Japan, Miyagi	92.2	3.2	0.1	1.3	0.1	0.1	2.9	**893**	1075
Japan, Nagasaki	92.7	3.3	0.4	2.9	-	0.7	-	**452**	516
Japan, Osaka	90.3	3.8	0.4	0.9	0.2	0.4	3.9	**1838**	2424
Japan, Saga									
Japan, Yamagata									
Korea, Kangwha	75.0	4.2	4.2	8.3	-	-	8.3	**24**	32
Kuwait: Non-Kuwaitis	100.0	-	-	-	-	-	-	**10**	10
Kuwait: Kuwaitis	83.3	16.7	-	-	-	-	-	**6**	9
Philippines, Manila	67.1	18.3	-	14.6	-	-	-	**82**	140
Singapore: Chinese	90.2	4.3	0.3	4.6	0.3	-	0.3	**327**	365
Singapore: Malay	80.0	20.0	-	-	-	-	-	**5**	6
Singapore: Indian	96.6	3.4	-	-	-	-	-	**29**	31
Thailand, Chiang Mai	93.6	2.1	-	4.3	-	-	-	**47**	70
Thailand, Khon Kaen	76.5	11.8	-	5.9	-	-	5.9	**17**	34
Viet Nam, Hanoi	50.0	7.1	-	35.7	-	-	7.1	**14**	50
EUROPE									
Austria, Tyrol	71.6	7.5	1.5	7.5	-	-	11.9	**67**	78
Belarus									
Croatia									
Czech Republic	65.3	25.1	2.0	5.5	-	-	2.1	**859**	1324
Denmark	46.9	45.3	0.9	5.9	0.1	-	0.9	**909**	955
Estonia	83.5	3.0	0.5	4.0	-	-	9.0	**200**	237
Finland	69.0	17.9	-	9.4	-	-	3.7	**626**	670
France, Bas-Rhin	90.8	5.5	0.2	2.1	0.5	0.5	0.5	**435**	443
France, Calvados	89.4	4.1	0.3	4.7	-	-	1.6	**386**	406
France, Doubs	88.7	9.4	-	1.9	-	-	-	**159**	165
France, Haut-Rhin	93.3	5.3	-	1.1	-	0.4	-	**285**	286
France, Herault	68.8	24.9	-	4.8	-	0.5	1.1	**189**	194
France, Isere	82.3	14.9	0.7	2.1	-	-	-	**288**	294
France, Somme	85.7	10.7	0.3	2.7	-	-	0.7	**300**	306
France, Tarn	84.7	13.9	1.4	-	-	-	-	**72**	73
Germany, Eastern States	81.9	11.2	1.2	4.5	0.3	0.3	0.7	**758**	848
Germany, Saarland									
Iceland	61.2	30.6	2.0	2.0	-	2.0	2.0	**49**	49
Ireland, Southern	59.8	32.6	-	6.5	-	-	1.1	**92**	109
Italy, Ferrara	76.2	19.0	-	4.8	-	-	-	**21**	22
Italy, Florence	67.3	20.4	0.9	8.8	-	-	2.7	**113**	157
Italy, Genoa	77.4	18.3	-	3.2	-	-	1.1	**93**	126
Italy, Latina	60.0	20.0	-	20.0	-	-	-	**25**	31
Italy, Macerata	42.9	28.6	-	14.3	-	-	14.3	**7**	8
Italy, Modena	73.0	23.8	-	3.2	-	-	-	**63**	74
Italy, Parma	82.3	12.9	-	4.8	-	-	-	**62**	71
Italy, Ragusa	100.0	-	-	-	-	-	-	**6**	13
Italy, Romagna	79.2	16.7	-	4.2	-	-	-	**48**	58
Italy, Torino	68.4	20.0	-	10.5	-	1.1	-	**95**	114
Italy, Trieste	78.3	5.0	1.7	11.7	-	-	3.3	**60**	65
Italy, Varese	80.7	12.5	3.4	2.8	0.6	-	-	**176**	192
Italy, Veneto	81.1	11.4	0.8	5.1	0.3	-	1.4	**370**	418
Latvia									
Malta									

Oesophagus (ICD-9 150) - Male (contd)

	Carcinoma				Sarcoma	Other	Unspecified	Number of cases	
	Squamous	Adeno	Other	Unspecified				MV	Total
The Netherlands	50.0	45.1	1.4	3.1	0.1	0.1	0.1	2046	2076
The Netherlands, Eindhoven	75.0	16.0	3.0	6.0	-	-	-	100	103
The Netherlands, Maastricht	52.2	40.0	0.9	5.2	-	0.9	0.9	115	116
Norway	65.3	26.4	0.8	4.6	-	0.4	2.6	504	522
Poland, Cracow	71.7	13.2	-	9.4	-	-	5.7	53	85
Poland, Kielce	60.7	16.4	1.6	18.0	-	-	3.3	61	105
Poland, Lower Silesia	28.8	9.9	-	4.5	-	-	56.8	111	430
Poland, Warsaw City	78.2	16.9	0.8	4.0	-	-	-	124	206
Slovakia	84.7	9.5	0.3	4.2	0.3	-	1.0	765	1000
Slovenia	77.3	9.7	0.6	10.9	0.6	-	0.9	330	393
Spain, Albacete	64.3	21.4	-	14.3	-	-	-	14	17
Spain, Asturias	81.5	10.6	0.9	5.1	-	0.5	1.4	216	246
Spain, Basque Country	81.4	8.2	3.3	5.8	0.2	0.4	0.6	485	534
Spain, Granada	70.1	19.5	1.3	9.1	-	-	-	77	95
Spain, Mallorca	80.2	11.5	1.0	7.3	-	-	-	96	108
Spain, Murcia	81.1	13.9	0.8	4.1	-	-	-	122	140
Spain, Navarra	91.1	3.6	1.8	3.6	-	-	-	112	126
Spain, Tarragona	75.8	15.2	2.0	5.1	-	-	2.0	99	111
Spain, Zaragoza	80.9	12.5	-	3.7	-	0.7	2.2	136	163
Sweden	70.7	21.8	-	6.3	0.3	-	0.9	1158	1172
Switzerland, Basel	70.8	28.1	1.1	-	-	-	-	89	89
Switzerland, Geneva	83.5	16.5	-	-	-	-	-	91	95
Switzerland, Graubunden	83.3	8.3	4.2	4.2	-	-	-	24	26
Switzerland, Neuchatel	73.7	23.7	-	2.6	-	-	-	38	38
Switzerland, St Gall-Appenzell	77.0	20.7	1.1	-	1.1	-	-	87	92
Switzerland, Valais	88.6	9.1	-	2.3	-	-	-	44	48
Switzerland, Vaud	71.5	20.1	1.7	6.7	-	-	-	179	195
Switzerland, Zurich	74.6	20.4	0.7	2.8	1.4	-	-	142	146
UK, England and Wales	28.9	46.1	0.9	22.8	-	0.1	1.2	6974	9055
UK, East Anglia									
UK, Mersey	33.8	57.2	0.8	7.8	0.2	-	0.2	612	800
UK, North Western									
UK, Oxford	35.0	57.3	0.4	7.2	-	0.2	-	489	645
UK, South Thames	29.2	60.3	0.8	9.5	-	-	0.2	1407	2038
UK, South Western	26.6	56.8	1.1	13.3	0.1	-	2.1	857	1084
UK, Wessex	23.0	51.5	0.6	24.8	-	-	0.1	858	1022
UK, West Midlands									
UK, Yorkshire	33.6	54.8	1.4	9.8	-	0.2	0.2	861	997
UK, Scotland	43.3	48.1	1.3	6.9	0.3	0.1	0.1	1481	1731
UK, Scotland, West	41.3	52.1	0.7	5.5	0.2	-	0.2	894	1059
Yugoslavia, Vojvodina	72.0	11.5	1.9	10.8	0.6	-	3.2	157	340

OCEANIA

	Carcinoma				Sarcoma	Other	Unspecified	Number of cases	
	Squamous	Adeno	Other	Unspecified				MV	Total
Australian Capital Territory	20.0	80.0	-	-	-	-	-	25	27
Australia, New South Wales	54.3	38.5	0.8	5.8	0.1	0.3	0.3	759	834
South Australia	40.1	41.3	12.6	6.0	-	-	-	167	209
Australia, Tasmania	49.0	40.6	2.1	7.3	1.0	-	-	96	103
Australia, Victoria	53.6	39.1	1.0	6.1	-	0.1	-	683	735
Western Australia	51.1	40.4	0.5	6.9	-	1.1	-	188	212
French Polynesia	80.0	10.0	5.0	5.0	-	-	-	20	20
New Zealand: Non-Maori									
New Zealand: Maori									
US, Hawaii: White	77.5	17.5	-	5.0	-	-	-	40	40
US, Hawaii: Japanese	85.1	6.4	-	8.5	-	-	-	47	47
US, Hawaii: Hawaiian	88.9	7.4	-	-	3.7	-	-	27	28
US, Hawaii: Filipino	73.7	15.8	-	10.5	-	-	-	19	21
US, Hawaii: Chinese	84.6	7.7	-	7.7	-	-	-	13	13

PERCENTAGE DISTRIBUTION OF MICROSCOPICALLY VERIFIED CASES BY HISTOLOGICAL TYPE
Oesophagus (ICD-9 150) - Female

	Carcinoma				Sarcoma	Other	Unspecified	Number of cases	
	Squamous	Adeno	Other	Unspecified				MV	Total
AFRICA									
Algeria, Setif	66.7	33.3	-	-	-	-	-	3	4
France, La Reunion	90.9	4.5	-	-	-	-	4.5	22	22
Mali, Bamako	83.3	-	-	16.7	-	-	-	6	7
Uganda, Kyadondo	100.0	-	-	-	-	-	-	9	37
Zimbabwe, Harare: African	50.0	30.0	-	20.0	-	-	-	10	22
Zimbabwe, Harare: European	-	-	-	-	-	-	-	-	3
AMERICA, CENTRAL AND SOUTH									
Argentina, Concordia	70.0	10.0	10.0	10.0	-	-	-	10	12
Brazil, Belem	86.7	-	-	13.3	-	-	-	15	20
Brazil, Goiania	60.0	15.0	-	5.0	-	-	20.0	20	22
Brazil, Porto Alegre	56.4	10.9	-	20.0	-	-	12.7	55	95
Colombia, Cali	80.0	-	-	15.0	-	5.0	-	40	65
Costa Rica	76.0	16.0	2.0	4.0	2.0	-	-	50	72
Ecuador, Quito	86.7	13.3	-	-	-	-	-	15	26
Peru, Lima	76.5	17.6	-	5.9	-	-	-	17	27
Peru, Trujillo	100.0	-	-	-	-	-	-	2	3
Puerto Rico	86.9	6.0	0.5	6.0	-	-	0.5	199	235
Uruguay, Montevideo	73.9	14.8	2.3	9.1	-	-	-	88	152
AMERICA, NORTH									
Canada	72.8	18.4	1.9	4.8	0.3	0.3	1.4	1242	1492
Canada, Alberta	86.1	12.5	1.4	-	-	-	-	72	81
Canada, British Columbia	75.9	16.8	1.4	5.5	0.5	-	-	220	235
Canada, Manitoba	78.9	12.3	3.5	3.5	-	1.8	-	57	68
Canada, New Brunswick	64.0	36.0	-	-	-	-	-	25	29
Canada, Newfoundland	55.6	22.2	11.1	11.1	-	-	-	18	23
Canada, Northwest Territories	-	33.3	-	66.7	-	-	-	3	6
Canada, Nova Scotia	58.0	32.0	-	10.0	-	-	-	50	56
Canada, Ontario	74.7	17.8	1.9	2.8	-	0.4	2.4	534	633
Canada, Prince Edward Island	-	100.0	-	-	-	-	-	1	2
Canada, Quebec	65.4	18.2	2.3	10.3	0.9	0.5	2.3	214	311
Canada, Saskatchewan	72.0	22.0	2.0	2.0	2.0	-	-	50	53
Canada, Yukon	-	-	-	-	-	-	-	-	-
US, Cent. California: Non-Hisp White	71.4	15.7	1.4	10.0	1.4	-	-	70	74
US, Cent. California: Hispanic	100.0	-	-	-	-	-	-	6	6
US, Los Angeles: Non-Hisp White	73.1	20.4	1.3	3.9	-	0.6	0.6	309	316
US, Los Angeles: Hispanic White	73.3	13.3	-	13.3	-	-	-	30	31
US, Los Angeles: Black	83.3	5.6	-	8.9	-	-	2.2	90	95
US, Los Angeles: Chinese	75.0	-	-	25.0	-	-	-	8	9
US, Los Angeles: Filipino	-	-	-	-	-	-	-	-	-
US, Los Angeles: Korean	-	-	-	-	-	-	-	-	1
US, Los Angeles: Japanese	50.0	-	-	25.0	25.0	-	-	4	6
US, San Francisco: Non-Hisp White	71.2	18.4	0.6	9.2	-	-	0.6	163	169
US, San Francisco: Hispanic White	83.3	16.7	-	-	-	-	-	6	6
US, San Francisco: Black	93.3	4.4	-	2.2	-	-	-	45	46
US, San Francisco: Chinese	66.7	22.2	-	-	-	-	11.1	9	9
US, San Francisco: Filipino	100.0	-	-	-	-	-	-	1	1
US, San Francisco: Japanese	100.0	-	-	-	-	-	-	1	1
US, Connecticut: White	70.1	23.2	2.1	3.6	0.5	0.5	-	194	209
US, Connecticut: Black	100.0	-	-	-	-	-	-	26	26
US, Atlanta: White	81.5	13.0	1.9	1.9	-	-	1.9	54	60
US, Atlanta: Black	91.9	1.6	1.6	3.2	-	-	1.6	62	63
US, Iowa	61.5	32.8	1.6	4.1	-	-	-	122	126
US, Central Louisiana: White	100.0	-	-	-	-	-	-	5	7
US, Central Louisiana: Black	100.0	-	-	-	-	-	-	5	5
US, New Orleans: White	68.3	22.0	2.4	2.4	2.4	-	2.4	41	44
US, New Orleans: Black	85.2	-	-	14.8	-	-	-	27	27
US, Detroit: White	71.5	17.4	0.6	8.7	1.2	-	0.6	172	179
US, Detroit: Black	85.4	6.3	-	8.3	-	-	-	96	102
US, New Mexico: Non-Hisp White	67.4	20.9	2.3	7.0	-	2.3	-	43	45
US, New Mexico: Hispanic White	66.7	-	-	16.7	-	-	16.7	6	9
US, New Mexico: American Indian	100.0	-	-	-	-	-	-	1	1
US, Utah	61.9	23.8	9.5	4.8	-	-	-	21	23
US, Seattle	73.7	19.1	0.5	6.2	-	-	0.5	209	219
US, SEER: White	70.5	20.7	1.4	6.4	0.3	0.2	0.5	991	1044
US, SEER: Black	90.2	4.5	0.4	4.5	-	-	0.4	244	253

	Squamous	Carcinoma Adeno	Carcinoma Other	Carcinoma Unspecified	Sarcoma	Other	Unspecified	Number of cases MV	Number of cases Total

ASIA

	Squamous	Adeno	Other	Unspecified	Sarcoma	Other	Unspecified	MV	Total
China, Qidong									
China, Shanghai									
China, Tianjin	28.1	2.0	-	0.3	0.3	0.3	69.0	306	654
Hong Kong	77.1	18.3	-	4.3	0.2	-	-	415	565
India, Bangalore	86.3	1.9	0.5	7.5	-	0.3	3.5	372	501
India, Barshi, Paranda and Bhum	78.6	21.4	-	-	-	-	-	14	16
India, Bombay	95.1	0.5	0.5	2.8	-	0.2	0.9	575	962
India, Karunagappally	77.8	22.2	-	-	-	-	-	9	11
India, Madras	91.7	5.6	-	1.9	-	-	0.9	324	423
India, Trivandrum	75.0	25.0	-	-	-	-	-	8	10
Israel: All Jews	85.5	8.0	0.7	4.3	1.4	-	-	138	158
Jews born in Israel	83.3	-	-	16.7	-	-	-	12	12
Jews born in America or Europe	84.6	11.5	-	2.6	1.3	-	-	78	93
Jews born in Africa or Asia	87.2	4.3	2.1	4.3	2.1	-	-	47	52
Non-Jews	100.0	-	-	-	-	-	-	3	3
Japan, Hiroshima	94.9	1.7	1.7	1.7	-	-	-	59	69
Japan, Miyagi	90.2	3.4	1.1	1.7	-	0.6	2.9	174	240
Japan, Nagasaki	90.0	2.5	-	5.0	1.3	1.3	-	80	113
Japan, Osaka	87.5	3.2	1.7	1.0	0.5	-	6.1	407	582
Japan, Saga									
Japan, Yamagata									
Korea, Kangwha	50.0	-	-	-	-	-	50.0	2	2
Kuwait: Non-Kuwaitis	75.0	25.0	-	-	-	-	-	4	4
Kuwait: Kuwaitis	100.0	-	-	-	-	-	-	8	10
Philippines, Manila	83.0	6.4	-	8.5	-	-	2.1	47	84
Singapore: Chinese	92.5	2.5	-	4.2	-	-	0.8	120	134
Singapore: Malay	100.0	-	-	-	-	-	-	2	4
Singapore: Indian	100.0	-	-	-	-	-	-	12	12
Thailand, Chiang Mai	90.5	-	-	4.8	-	-	4.8	21	46
Thailand, Khon Kaen	100.0	-	-	-	-	-	-	4	12
Viet Nam, Hanoi	100.0	-	-	-	-	-	-	1	17

EUROPE

	Squamous	Adeno	Other	Unspecified	Sarcoma	Other	Unspecified	MV	Total
Austria, Tyrol	63.6	9.1	-	9.1	9.1	-	9.1	11	14
Belarus									
Croatia									
Czech Republic	57.7	27.5	2.7	7.4	-	0.7	4.0	149	271
Denmark	63.0	29.6	1.4	5.2	0.3	0.3	0.3	362	387
Estonia	73.5	11.8	2.9	2.9	-	-	8.8	34	58
Finland	82.0	7.0	-	8.6	0.2	-	2.2	545	594
France, Bas-Rhin	87.5	8.3	4.2	-	-	-	-	48	48
France, Calvados	74.2	25.8	-	-	-	-	-	31	31
France, Doubs	68.0	28.0	-	4.0	-	-	-	25	26
France, Haut-Rhin	89.2	8.1	-	-	2.7	-	-	37	38
France, Herault	68.0	22.0	4.0	6.0	-	-	-	50	51
France, Isere	71.1	13.2	2.6	13.2	-	-	-	38	41
France, Somme	58.8	23.5	-	8.8	2.9	-	5.9	34	39
France, Tarn	80.0	10.0	-	10.0	-	-	-	10	10
Germany, Eastern States	68.2	19.4	1.2	8.8	1.2	0.6	0.6	170	210
Germany, Saarland									
Iceland	66.7	33.3	-	-	-	-	-	21	21
Ireland, Southern	76.4	15.3	-	8.3	-	-	-	72	88
Italy, Ferrara	100.0	-	-	-	-	-	-	4	6
Italy, Florence	75.0	12.5	3.1	6.3	-	-	3.1	32	58
Italy, Genoa	84.8	12.1	-	3.0	-	-	-	33	49
Italy, Latina	66.7	16.7	-	16.7	-	-	-	6	7
Italy, Macerata	50.0	50.0	-	-	-	-	-	2	5
Italy, Modena	68.8	31.3	-	-	-	-	-	16	26
Italy, Parma	75.0	6.3	6.3	6.3	-	-	6.3	16	19
Italy, Ragusa	66.7	-	-	-	-	-	33.3	3	5
Italy, Romagna	100.0	-	-	-	-	-	-	9	14
Italy, Torino	66.7	14.3	-	14.3	-	4.8	-	21	34
Italy, Trieste	64.7	5.9	-	23.5	-	-	5.9	17	24
Italy, Varese	83.3	6.7	10.0	-	-	-	-	30	40
Italy, Veneto	74.4	6.1	-	15.9	-	-	3.7	82	104
Latvia									
Malta									

Oesophagus (ICD-9 150) - Female (contd)

	Carcinoma				Sarcoma	Other	Unspecified	Number of cases	
	Squamous	Adeno	Other	Unspecified				MV	Total
The Netherlands	59.1	33.6	2.1	4.5	0.3	0.2	0.2	1067	1102
The Netherlands, Eindhoven	65.8	21.1	2.6	10.5	-	-	-	38	42
The Netherlands, Maastricht	66.7	25.5	-	3.9	2.0	-	2.0	51	51
Norway	73.0	19.0	-	5.2	0.6	-	2.3	174	187
Poland, Cracow	90.0	10.0	-	-	-	-	-	10	22
Poland, Kielce	26.7	33.3	-	40.0	-	-	-	15	30
Poland, Lower Silesia	21.9	9.4	-	9.4	-	-	59.4	32	101
Poland, Warsaw City	71.1	13.2	2.6	10.5	2.6	-	-	38	85
Slovakia	66.1	24.2	-	8.1	-	-	1.6	62	112
Slovenia	83.9	5.4	-	10.7	-	-	-	56	79
Spain, Albacete	100.0	-	-	-	-	-	-	1	1
Spain, Asturias	50.0	26.9	3.8	11.5	3.8	-	3.8	26	36
Spain, Basque Country	69.4	13.9	5.6	8.3	-	-	2.8	36	52
Spain, Granada	64.3	28.6	-	7.1	-	-	-	14	19
Spain, Mallorca	91.7	-	-	8.3	-	-	-	12	16
Spain, Murcia	61.5	38.5	-	-	-	-	-	13	22
Spain, Navarra	80.0	13.3	-	6.7	-	-	-	15	18
Spain, Tarragona	75.0	25.0	-	-	-	-	-	4	7
Spain, Zaragoza	46.2	38.5	-	15.4	-	-	-	13	24
Sweden	76.6	13.6	-	8.4	0.2	-	1.3	538	549
Switzerland, Basel	69.7	27.3	-	3.0	-	-	-	33	33
Switzerland, Geneva	80.8	11.5	-	3.8	-	3.8	-	26	27
Switzerland, Graubunden	75.0	25.0	-	-	-	-	-	4	6
Switzerland, Neuchatel	52.6	47.4	-	-	-	-	-	19	19
Switzerland, St Gall-Appenzell	60.0	30.0	5.0	5.0	-	-	-	20	24
Switzerland, Valais	100.0	-	-	-	-	-	-	8	10
Switzerland, Vaud	79.7	13.6	1.7	5.1	-	-	-	59	68
Switzerland, Zurich	78.8	16.7	1.5	3.0	-	-	-	66	67
UK, England and Wales	49.5	21.7	1.5	25.4	0.1	0.1	1.7	5028	6531
UK, East Anglia									
UK, Mersey	65.1	25.8	1.5	7.1	-	0.5	-	395	556
UK, North Western									
UK, Oxford	62.6	28.8	2.7	5.9	-	-	-	337	453
UK, South Thames	59.2	30.1	2.4	8.0	0.3	0.1	-	977	1467
UK, South Western	54.8	25.2	3.6	13.4	-	0.5	2.5	640	897
UK, Wessex	49.8	26.6	0.7	22.3	0.4	-	0.2	546	710
UK, West Midlands									
UK, Yorkshire	57.9	29.0	2.3	10.4	-	0.2	0.2	575	712
UK, Scotland	63.2	28.6	2.5	5.2	0.2	-	0.2	1202	1481
UK, Scotland, West	62.9	31.6	1.2	4.0	0.2	-	0.2	652	837
Yugoslavia, Vojvodina	62.5	20.8	4.2	8.3	-	-	4.2	24	63

OCEANIA

	Squamous	Adeno	Other	Unspecified	Sarcoma	Other	Unspecified	MV	Total
Australian Capital Territory	76.9	15.4	-	7.7	-	-	-	13	13
Australia, New South Wales	76.9	13.1	2.8	6.7	0.4	-	-	464	524
South Australia	66.0	15.5	10.7	5.8	-	1.0	1.0	103	125
Australia, Tasmania	74.2	19.4	-	6.5	-	-	-	62	70
Australia, Victoria	73.4	19.7	2.2	4.4	-	-	0.2	406	460
Western Australia	75.0	17.7	-	7.3	-	-	-	96	103
French Polynesia	100.0	-	-	-	-	-	-	4	4
New Zealand: Non-Maori									
New Zealand: Maori									
US, Hawaii: White	81.3	-	6.3	12.5	-	-	-	16	16
US, Hawaii: Japanese	62.5	25.0	-	-	12.5	-	-	8	9
US, Hawaii: Hawaiian	100.0	-	-	-	-	-	-	5	5
US, Hawaii: Filipino	75.0	25.0	-	-	-	-	-	4	4
US, Hawaii: Chinese	-	-	-	-	-	-	-	-	-

PERCENTAGE DISTRIBUTION OF MICROSCOPICALLY VERIFIED CASES BY HISTOLOGICAL TYPE
Liver (ICD-9 155) - Both sexes

		Carcinoma			Hepato-	Sarcoma		Other	Unspec.	Number of cases	
	Hepato	Cholangio	Other	Unspec.	blastoma	Haemangio	Other			MV	Total
AFRICA											
Algeria, Setif	-	66.7	-	33.3	-	-	-	-	-	3	65
France, La Reunion	48.8	22.0	4.9	17.1	-	-	-	-	7.3	41	51
Mali, Bamako	88.9	-	-	11.1	-	-	-	-	-	18	583
Uganda, Kyadondo	84.6	7.7	7.7	-	-	-	-	-	-	26	84
Zimbabwe, Harare: African	97.0	-	-	-	-	-	3.0	-	-	67	284
Zimbabwe, Harare: European	100.0	-	-	-	-	-	-	-	-	6	22
AMERICA, CENTRAL AND SOUTH											
Argentina, Concordia	50.0	50.0	-	-	-	-	-	-	-	2	5
Brazil, Belem	75.0	-	12.5	-	-	-	-	-	12.5	8	13
Brazil, Goiania	43.8	21.9	3.1	6.3	-	-	-	-	25.0	32	76
Brazil, Porto Alegre	6.7	39.5	5.0	19.3	0.8	-	-	-	28.6	119	200
Colombia, Cali	68.4	21.1	-	7.9	-	-	1.3	-	1.3	76	124
Costa Rica	65.1	15.5	2.3	14.0	2.3	-	0.8	-	-	129	516
Ecuador, Quito	64.0	32.0	-	4.0	-	-	-	-	-	25	113
Peru, Lima	54.4	20.2	8.8	10.5	1.8	0.9	2.6	-	0.9	114	314
Peru, Trujillo	52.0	24.0	12.0	8.0	4.0	-	-	-	-	25	68
Puerto Rico	69.1	20.4	3.0	4.2	-	0.8	0.4	-	2.3	265	474
Uruguay, Montevideo	82.9	11.4	-	-	2.9	2.9	-	-	-	35	70
AMERICA, NORTH											
Canada	62.6	20.5	2.9	5.5	1.7	0.5	0.8	0.1	5.4	2345	3925
Canada, Alberta	66.8	16.6	2.1	4.7	3.6	0.5	1.6	-	4.1	193	272
Canada, British Columbia	64.9	20.7	1.3	7.7	0.8	0.5	0.8	0.5	2.7	376	558
Canada, Manitoba	54.7	27.9	3.5	8.1	-	1.2	1.2	-	3.5	86	163
Canada, New Brunswick	68.8	22.9	-	4.2	-	2.1	2.1	-	-	48	71
Canada, Newfoundland	68.2	27.3	-	4.5	-	-	-	-	-	22	26
Canada, Northwest Territories	50.0	50.0	-	-	-	-	-	-	-	2	8
Canada, Nova Scotia	60.4	20.8	1.9	9.4	3.8	1.9	-	-	1.9	53	93
Canada, Ontario	65.7	15.3	2.7	4.2	1.8	0.1	0.5	-	9.7	837	1461
Canada, Prince Edward Island	75.0	-	-	-	-	25.0	-	-	-	4	7
Canada, Quebec	56.5	25.8	4.8	5.7	1.9	0.5	1.1	-	3.7	644	1160
Canada, Saskatchewan	63.3	29.1	2.5	3.8	-	1.3	-	-	-	79	108
Canada, Yukon	-	-	-	-	100.0	-	-	-	-	1	1
US, Cent. California: Non-Hisp White	65.2	22.0	5.5	4.3	1.2	1.8	-	-	-	164	204
US, Cent. California: Hispanic	73.1	14.1	1.3	2.6	3.8	2.6	1.3	-	1.3	78	98
US, Los Angeles: Non-Hisp White	75.3	17.0	1.9	2.3	0.8	0.6	1.0	0.2	0.8	482	610
US, Los Angeles: Hispanic White	74.8	13.3	1.0	4.0	4.7	-	1.7	-	0.7	301	387
US, Los Angeles: Black	79.4	12.1	3.5	3.5	0.7	0.7	-	-	-	141	179
US, Los Angeles: Chinese	88.5	6.3	2.1	3.1	-	-	-	-	-	96	134
US, Los Angeles: Filipino	81.0	8.6	1.7	3.4	1.7	1.7	1.7	-	-	58	69
US, Los Angeles: Korean	78.8	16.7	4.5	-	-	-	-	-	-	66	99
US, Los Angeles: Japanese	80.0	14.3	-	2.9	-	2.9	-	-	-	35	47
US, San Francisco: Non-Hisp White	64.8	23.6	3.0	5.2	1.5	0.7	1.1	-	-	267	352
US, San Francisco: Hispanic White	74.0	19.2	1.4	1.4	1.4	-	1.4	1.4	-	73	91
US, San Francisco: Black	85.1	10.3	2.3	-	1.1	-	-	1.1	-	87	108
US, San Francisco: Chinese	89.4	7.6	-	1.8	-	-	0.6	-	0.6	170	228
US, San Francisco: Filipino	88.2	2.0	3.9	2.0	2.0	2.0	-	-	-	51	64
US, San Francisco: Japanese	81.8	9.1	-	9.1	-	-	-	-	-	11	13
US, Connecticut: White	68.5	18.3	3.2	5.9	1.0	1.2	0.7	0.2	1.0	409	512
US, Connecticut: Black	75.6	14.6	2.4	4.9	2.4	-	-	-	-	41	46
US, Atlanta: White	65.7	20.1	4.5	5.2	1.5	0.7	0.7	-	1.5	134	158
US, Atlanta: Black	77.8	13.0	1.9	3.7	1.9	-	1.9	-	-	54	63
US, Iowa	63.6	27.6	2.9	1.9	1.0	1.3	1.0	-	0.6	308	384
US, Central Louisiana: White	64.3	21.4	-	7.1	7.1	-	-	-	-	14	27
US, Central Louisiana: Black	33.3	-	33.3	-	33.3	-	-	-	-	6	10
US, New Orleans: White	80.0	16.3	-	3.8	-	-	-	-	-	80	107
US, New Orleans: Black	77.2	10.5	1.8	5.3	-	3.5	-	-	1.8	57	82
US, Detroit: White	62.0	24.7	2.4	4.3	0.8	0.8	1.1	0.5	3.3	368	470
US, Detroit: Black	70.6	13.6	2.8	5.1	2.3	-	1.1	-	4.5	177	221
US, New Mexico: Non-Hisp White	54.2	26.4	4.2	6.9	1.4	4.2	1.4	-	1.4	72	107
US, New Mexico: Hispanic White	70.8	13.8	1.5	3.1	6.2	1.5	-	1.5	1.5	65	93
US, New Mexico: American Indian	77.8	11.1	5.6	5.6	-	-	-	-	-	18	30
US, Utah	65.0	21.4	2.6	1.7	5.1	2.6	0.9	-	0.9	117	147
US, Seattle	69.9	20.6	1.7	3.2	1.5	1.2	1.0	-	1.0	412	529
US, SEER: White	65.5	22.3	2.7	4.2	1.6	1.3	0.9	0.2	1.2	2150	2755
US, SEER: Black	75.8	13.4	2.3	3.5	1.8	-	0.8	0.3	2.3	396	478

Liver (ICD-9 155) - Both sexes (contd)

	Carcinoma				Hepato-	Sarcoma		Other	Unspec.	Number of cases	
	Hepato	Cholangio	Other	Unspec.	blastoma	Haemangio	Other			MV	Total
ASIA											
China, Qidong											
China, Shanghai											
China, Tianjin	6.5	2.7	1.0	-	0.2	-	-	0.1	89.4	875	3200
Hong Kong	64.1	26.3	0.6	7.6	0.5	0.1	0.2	-	0.6	2845	7293
India, Bangalore	69.5	10.2	5.4	6.0	3.6	0.6	-	-	4.8	167	265
India, Barshi, Paranda and Bhum	66.7	-	-	8.3	-	-	-	-	25.0	12	21
India, Bombay	74.8	13.0	1.3	2.4	6.6	-	0.3	0.3	1.3	377	732
India, Karunagappally	45.5	27.3	-	18.2	-	-	-	-	9.1	11	15
India, Madras	90.1	3.3	0.7	1.3	3.3	0.7	0.7	-	-	152	193
India, Trivandrum	60.9	4.3	8.7	4.3	-	-	-	-	21.7	23	32
Israel: All Jews	63.1	16.1	5.2	8.7	1.4	1.1	-	-	4.4	366	589
Jews born in Israel	50.0	23.1	7.7	-	19.2	-	-	-	-	26	33
Jews born in America or Europe	59.1	18.3	4.8	10.0	-	1.7	-	-	6.1	230	362
Jews born in Africa or Asia	74.5	10.0	5.5	8.2	-	-	-	-	1.8	110	193
Non-Jews	53.6	21.4	7.1	7.1	7.1	-	-	-	3.6	28	49
Japan, Hiroshima	91.0	6.1	1.5	1.2	-	-	-	-	0.2	589	1792
Japan, Miyagi	58.3	13.9	1.9	1.3	0.2	-	0.2	-	24.3	527	1721
Japan, Nagasaki	85.6	10.6	1.1	1.6	0.5	-	0.1	-	0.6	838	2533
Japan, Osaka	75.1	5.4	0.6	0.7	0.4	0.1	0.1	-	17.6	6968	16350
Japan, Saga											
Japan, Yamagata											
Korea, Kangwha	38.5	7.7	3.8	-	-	-	-	-	50.0	26	114
Kuwait: Non-Kuwaitis	82.6	8.7	-	4.3	4.3	-	-	-	-	23	56
Kuwait: Kuwaitis	85.7	9.5	4.8	-	-	-	-	-	-	21	57
Philippines, Manila	74.7	11.2	0.5	5.5	2.2	-	0.5	-	5.5	403	1775
Singapore: Chinese	78.8	10.9	0.9	4.0	1.6	0.3	0.3	-	3.1	321	1281
Singapore: Malay	89.3	10.7	-	-	-	-	-	-	-	28	108
Singapore: Indian	100.0	-	-	-	-	-	-	-	-	7	45
Thailand, Chiang Mai	45.9	43.7	-	3.9	0.3	-	0.6	-	5.6	355	962
Thailand, Khon Kaen	6.8	87.3	0.4	0.4	0.8	-	-	-	4.2	237	3046
Viet Nam, Hanoi	68.8	10.9	1.4	9.4	-	-	0.7	-	8.7	138	633
EUROPE											
Austria, Tyrol	67.8	1.1	4.6	1.1	1.1	-	2.3	-	21.8	87	147
Belarus											
Croatia											
Czech Republic	44.8	18.2	20.5	6.6	1.2	0.2	0.3	-	8.2	868	3478
Denmark	45.4	36.2	2.5	10.1	0.5	1.2	1.0	0.1	3.0	1151	1327
Estonia	38.1	28.8	10.6	5.3	0.4	0.9	1.3	-	14.6	226	318
Finland	46.8	26.5	0.7	4.1	0.5	0.4	0.3	-	20.6	1571	1827
France, Bas-Rhin	78.0	16.2	1.2	3.1	0.3	0.3	0.6	-	0.3	327	457
France, Calvados	64.1	18.0	4.8	11.4	-	-	-	-	1.8	167	294
France, Doubs	49.0	40.8	7.1	2.0	-	-	-	-	1.0	98	130
France, Haut-Rhin	89.6	9.1	0.4	0.4	-	0.4	-	-	-	230	274
France, Herault	54.4	37.6	0.7	6.0	-	-	0.7	-	0.7	149	151
France, Isere	84.3	8.7	2.8	1.7	1.4	0.3	0.3	-	0.3	287	314
France, Somme	83.3	12.1	2.3	0.8	-	-	0.8	-	0.8	132	152
France, Tarn	65.1	23.3	9.3	-	-	-	2.3	-	-	43	52
Germany, Eastern States	43.2	24.7	21.9	4.6	0.4	0.9	0.8	0.5	3.1	1281	1826
Germany, Saarland											
Iceland	66.7	23.3	-	6.7	-	3.3	-	-	-	30	34
Ireland, Southern	67.9	25.0	-	3.6	3.6	-	-	-	-	28	39
Italy, Ferrara	92.7	2.4	-	4.9	-	-	-	-	-	41	91
Italy, Florence	61.0	15.9	0.6	4.3	0.6	-	0.6	-	17.1	164	594
Italy, Genoa	76.1	12.2	2.0	5.1	-	-	-	-	4.6	197	569
Italy, Latina	42.0	8.7	1.4	42.0	1.4	-	-	-	4.3	69	179
Italy, Macerata	87.5	6.3	-	-	-	-	-	-	6.3	16	57
Italy, Modena	79.8	14.7	0.8	3.9	-	-	0.8	-	-	129	411
Italy, Parma	82.7	7.9	2.2	2.9	-	0.7	0.7	-	2.9	139	387
Italy, Ragusa	73.1	-	-	7.7	-	-	-	-	19.2	26	150
Italy, Romagna	85.7	6.8	1.4	4.1	0.7	1.4	-	-	-	147	224
Italy, Torino	75.9	13.5	1.4	7.1	-	-	-	-	2.1	141	374
Italy, Trieste	48.0	8.1	0.7	29.2	-	-	-	-	14.0	271	271
Italy, Varese	79.1	10.9	1.6	4.0	-	-	-	-	4.4	321	543
Italy, Veneto	61.9	10.7	4.4	7.8	-	0.4	0.2	-	14.7	551	1135
Latvia											
Malta											

Liver (ICD-9 155) - Both sexes (contd)

	Carcinoma				Hepato-blastoma	Sarcoma		Other	Unspec.	Number of cases	
	Hepato	Cholangio	Other	Unspec.		Haemangio	Other			MV	Total
The Netherlands	68.9	20.9	3.1	2.6	1.6	1.6	0.8	-	0.4	**798**	946
The Netherlands, Eindhoven	70.0	15.0	-	5.0	2.5	-	5.0	-	2.5	**40**	50
The Netherlands, Maastricht	69.8	23.8	-	-	3.2	3.2	-	-	-	**63**	70
Norway	62.0	24.5	1.4	4.1	1.6	0.7	0.5	-	5.3	**437**	535
Poland, Cracow	39.6	18.9	13.2	9.4	-	-	-	-	18.9	**53**	213
Poland, Kielce	7.1	36.5	10.6	37.6	1.2	-	-	-	7.1	**85**	354
Poland, Lower Silesia	2.7	3.1	0.8	2.9	-	0.2	0.2	-	90.1	**486**	973
Poland, Warsaw City	44.5	15.1	0.8	37.0	-	-	0.8	-	1.7	**119**	436
Slovakia	46.7	32.5	9.2	5.8	1.2	0.4	0.5	0.7	3.1	**846**	1659
Slovenia	65.3	18.2	11.1	2.2	1.8	0.4	-	-	0.9	**225**	245
Spain, Albacete	83.3	8.3	-	-	-	-	-	-	8.3	**12**	46
Spain, Asturias	55.6	24.2	2.6	14.1	-	-	-	-	3.6	**306**	470
Spain, Basque Country	80.8	10.8	0.5	3.4	0.5	-	1.0	-	3.0	**203**	626
Spain, Granada	66.2	21.6	2.7	5.4	-	-	1.4	-	2.7	**74**	332
Spain, Mallorca	81.6	6.4	0.7	9.9	-	-	-	-	1.4	**141**	227
Spain, Murcia	79.1	6.1	3.5	3.5	4.3	0.9	-	-	2.6	**115**	246
Spain, Navarra	60.6	28.8	-	4.8	-	-	-	-	5.8	**104**	287
Spain, Tarragona	65.7	19.0	1.0	11.4	1.0	-	-	-	1.9	**105**	170
Spain, Zaragoza	73.0	16.2	1.4	5.4	2.7	-	1.4	-	-	**74**	290
Sweden	66.8	15.9	-	0.4	0.7	-	0.4	-	15.8	**2288**	2293
Switzerland, Basel	87.2	0.9	11.1	-	-	0.9	-	-	-	**117**	120
Switzerland, Geneva	85.8	9.0	1.5	1.5	-	0.7	1.5	-	-	**134**	178
Switzerland, Graubunden	61.9	28.6	-	9.5	-	-	-	-	-	**21**	37
Switzerland, Neuchatel	83.3	13.9	2.8	-	-	-	-	-	-	**36**	53
Switzerland, St Gall-Appenzell	85.8	5.7	5.7	2.8	-	-	-	-	-	**106**	126
Switzerland, Valais	69.0	13.8	-	8.6	3.4	1.7	3.4	-	-	**58**	90
Switzerland, Vaud	77.8	12.7	2.4	5.6	0.8	-	-	-	0.8	**126**	183
Switzerland, Zurich	84.2	11.7	2.5	0.9	-	0.3	-	-	0.3	**317**	347
UK, England and Wales	40.3	28.0	2.4	21.0	0.9	1.0	0.9	0.1	5.5	**2700**	3794
UK, East Anglia											
UK, Mersey	54.9	34.6	2.5	3.7	1.2	0.6	1.9	-	0.6	**162**	299
UK, North Western											
UK, Oxford	43.1	49.8	1.9	2.4	1.0	1.9	-	-	-	**209**	256
UK, South Thames	56.9	30.5	0.3	7.4	1.0	0.6	2.9	-	0.3	**311**	897
UK, South Western	44.7	40.9	1.3	5.7	0.6	0.6	-	-	6.3	**159**	376
UK, Wessex	37.3	36.2	3.3	20.7	1.1	0.3	0.6	0.3	0.3	**362**	420
UK, West Midlands											
UK, Yorkshire	54.1	31.8	1.4	9.1	0.9	0.9	-	-	1.8	**220**	440
UK, Scotland	56.1	34.2	2.1	4.4	1.0	0.2	1.0	-	1.0	**517**	942
UK, Scotland, West	58.1	38.3	0.8	0.8	1.6	-	0.4	-	-	**248**	474
Yugoslavia, Vojvodina	36.8	17.8	1.1	21.3	0.6	0.6	-	-	21.8	**174**	997

OCEANIA

	Carcinoma				Hepato-blastoma	Sarcoma		Other	Unspec.	Number of cases	
	Hepato	Cholangio	Other	Unspec.		Haemangio	Other			MV	Total
Australian Capital Territory	70.0	30.0	-	-	-	-	-	-	-	**20**	20
Australia, New South Wales	83.9	12.5	1.3	0.6	0.6	1.1	-	-	-	**472**	567
South Australia	80.7	14.5	-	-	2.4	-	1.2	-	1.2	**83**	139
Australia, Tasmania	69.2	23.1	-	-	3.8	-	3.8	-	-	**26**	38
Australia, Victoria	79.5	14.7	1.9	2.1	0.5	0.8	-	-	0.5	**375**	516
Western Australia	66.0	27.2	2.9	2.9	-	-	-	-	1.0	**103**	162
French Polynesia	70.6	17.6	5.9	-	5.9	-	-	-	-	**17**	49
New Zealand: Non-Maori											
New Zealand: Maori											
US, Hawaii: White	81.4	11.6	-	4.7	2.3	-	-	-	-	**43**	55
US, Hawaii: Japanese	75.9	9.3	5.6	9.3	-	-	-	-	-	**54**	97
US, Hawaii: Hawaiian	79.2	12.5	-	-	4.2	-	4.2	-	-	**24**	36
US, Hawaii: Filipino	85.3	5.9	2.9	2.9	2.9	-	-	-	-	**34**	58
US, Hawaii: Chinese	85.2	11.1	-	-	-	-	-	-	3.7	**27**	36

PERCENTAGE DISTRIBUTION OF MICROSCOPICALLY VERIFIED CASES BY HISTOLOGICAL TYPE
Lung (ICD-9 162) - Male

	Squamous	Adeno	Carcinoma Small cell	Large cell	Other	Unspec.	Sarcoma	Other	Unspec.	Number of cases MV	Total
AFRICA											
Algeria, Setif	59.5	6.7	-	6.7	-	20.9	-	-	6.1	**163**	216
France, La Reunion	48.4	18.2	7.8	11.2	1.4	11.8	0.6	-	0.6	**347**	360
Mali, Bamako	100.0	-	-	-	-	-	-	-	-	**7**	38
Uganda, Kyadondo	-	-	12.5	12.5	-	75.0	-	-	-	**8**	20
Zimbabwe, Harare: African	41.2	29.4	9.8	7.8	-	9.8	2.0	-	-	**51**	126
Zimbabwe, Harare: European	52.6	21.1	21.1	5.3	-	-	-	-	-	**19**	42
AMERICA, CENTRAL AND SOUTH											
Argentina, Concordia	27.3	5.1	2.0	1.0	1.0	29.3	-	-	34.3	**99**	159
Brazil, Belem	41.4	16.1	2.3	9.2	-	28.7	-	-	2.3	**87**	254
Brazil, Goiania	34.8	22.2	3.0	7.4	-	8.1	-	-	24.4	**135**	198
Brazil, Porto Alegre	22.9	24.1	5.6	1.1	0.4	16.9	-	-	29.1	**468**	946
Colombia, Cali	35.9	18.1	9.5	4.6	0.3	13.5	0.3	-	17.8	**304**	536
Costa Rica	46.7	17.2	5.6	18.7	0.5	6.4	0.8	-	4.1	**390**	686
Ecuador, Quito	35.4	35.4	3.1	4.6	1.5	18.5	-	-	1.5	**65**	172
Peru, Lima	36.9	37.7	3.8	9.2	1.3	7.5	0.5	0.3	2.7	**371**	635
Peru, Trujillo	20.8	37.5	-	16.7	4.2	20.8	-	-	-	**24**	47
Puerto Rico	41.2	22.8	12.8	10.1	1.6	9.2	0.3	0.1	2.0	**1176**	1505
Uruguay, Montevideo	40.7	33.5	13.5	4.8	0.4	6.9	-	0.1	0.1	**942**	1778
AMERICA, NORTH											
Canada	37.5	26.1	16.3	10.9	0.7	5.4	0.1	0.1	2.8	**41456**	55768
Canada, Alberta	34.5	24.9	18.6	11.3	0.6	5.3	-	0.1	4.8	**2901**	3351
Canada, British Columbia	35.6	26.4	17.1	16.9	0.7	1.9	0.1	0.2	1.1	**5406**	6262
Canada, Manitoba	38.6	31.1	14.3	6.7	0.7	6.9	0.3	0.1	1.2	**1346**	2217
Canada, New Brunswick	42.7	25.6	15.6	8.1	0.6	7.2	0.1	0.1	-	**1424**	1679
Canada, Newfoundland	44.5	14.3	17.3	18.9	0.4	3.2	-	0.2	1.2	**825**	892
Canada, Northwest Territories	43.4	13.2	17.9	9.4	0.9	8.5	-	-	6.6	**106**	126
Canada, Nova Scotia	38.0	25.4	16.9	11.2	0.6	7.4	0.2	0.1	0.2	**1748**	2218
Canada, Ontario	36.8	27.7	17.2	9.6	0.9	4.3	0.2	0.1	3.1	**15073**	19759
Canada, Prince Edward Island	44.2	26.8	17.0	4.5	0.4	7.1	-	-	-	**224**	259
Canada, Quebec	38.1	24.9	14.0	10.3	0.6	7.6	0.1	0.1	4.3	**10776**	17079
Canada, Saskatchewan	40.8	24.8	16.9	8.1	0.5	8.6	-	0.2	0.2	**1630**	1936
Canada, Yukon	35.9	28.1	10.9	20.3	1.6	1.6	1.6	-	-	**64**	69
US, Cent. California: Non-Hisp White	34.6	26.8	18.0	12.9	0.7	5.3	0.2	0.1	1.4	**3184**	3487
US, Cent. California: Hispanic	36.2	23.6	18.6	14.5	1.6	5.0	-	0.3	0.3	**318**	347
US, Los Angeles: Non-Hisp White	28.4	31.8	14.9	10.1	1.0	12.1	0.1	0.1	1.4	**7844**	8425
US, Los Angeles: Hispanic White	26.2	31.7	13.6	9.9	2.0	14.7	0.1	0.1	1.7	**1103**	1183
US, Los Angeles: Black	32.9	28.7	11.9	9.7	0.6	13.6	0.2	0.1	2.4	**1812**	1925
US, Los Angeles: Chinese	22.5	42.7	12.4	11.0	0.5	11.0	-	-	-	**218**	232
US, Los Angeles: Filipino	23.7	36.7	13.5	8.4	-	14.9	0.5	-	2.3	**215**	222
US, Los Angeles: Korean	42.7	30.1	8.7	10.7	-	5.8	-	-	1.9	**103**	110
US, Los Angeles: Japanese	29.9	29.9	10.4	11.8	-	18.1	-	-	-	**144**	154
US, San Francisco: Non-Hisp White	27.7	35.0	15.8	11.3	1.0	8.1	0.2	-	0.9	**4204**	4559
US, San Francisco: Hispanic White	26.7	35.6	14.5	9.6	3.0	8.3	-	0.3	2.0	**303**	323
US, San Francisco: Black	31.0	33.6	12.2	10.6	1.1	9.9	-	0.1	1.5	**935**	1003
US, San Francisco: Chinese	26.2	36.7	13.1	13.1	0.3	9.3	-	0.6	0.6	**343**	366
US, San Francisco: Filipino	29.9	40.8	12.6	9.2	-	5.7	-	-	1.7	**174**	182
US, San Francisco: Japanese	28.8	48.1	5.8	11.5	-	5.8	-	-	-	**52**	54
US, Connecticut: White	31.0	31.8	16.5	8.8	0.7	10.3	0.1	0.1	0.8	**5949**	6541
US, Connecticut: Black	29.7	29.5	12.4	15.6	0.7	10.1	0.2	-	1.7	**404**	422
US, Atlanta: White	27.5	26.6	17.5	20.0	0.7	6.7	0.2	0.1	0.7	**2425**	2603
US, Atlanta: Black	35.0	23.3	12.1	22.1	0.4	5.7	0.1	-	1.3	**824**	892
US, Iowa	34.1	29.6	18.5	8.2	0.9	8.2	0.1	0.1	0.3	**6044**	6688
US, Central Louisiana: White	47.4	26.9	13.8	4.8	0.8	5.6	-	-	0.6	**479**	562
US, Central Louisiana: Black	53.4	24.4	9.2	4.6	0.8	7.6	-	-	-	**131**	172
US, New Orleans: White	33.2	32.8	15.5	10.6	0.7	5.9	0.1	-	1.3	**1508**	1707
US, New Orleans: Black	39.5	26.6	13.2	11.6	0.3	6.6	0.5	-	1.8	**730**	842
US, Detroit: White	31.7	28.6	17.8	10.5	1.0	8.5	-	-	1.8	**6575**	7125
US, Detroit: Black	36.3	27.5	11.2	9.4	0.8	11.8	0.2	0.1	2.6	**2072**	2263
US, New Mexico: Non-Hisp White	31.0	28.3	19.1	11.7	0.7	8.4	0.1	-	0.7	**1339**	1548
US, New Mexico: Hispanic White	32.1	27.8	16.1	13.0	-	8.7	1.0	0.3	1.0	**299**	344
US, New Mexico: American Indian	45.0	30.0	10.0	10.0	-	5.0	-	-	-	**20**	24
US, Utah	34.6	26.1	17.9	8.8	2.4	7.4	0.2	0.3	2.3	**1104**	1215
US, Seattle	28.4	32.9	15.6	8.7	0.9	11.3	0.2	0.1	2.0	**5880**	6332
US, SEER: White	30.7	30.7	17.1	10.3	0.9	9.0	0.1	0.1	1.2	**34047**	37191
US, SEER: Black	34.1	28.8	11.7	12.3	0.7	10.1	0.2	0.1	1.9	**4593**	4964

Lung (ICD-9 162) - Male (contd)

	Carcinoma						Sarcoma	Other	Unspec.	Number of cases	
	Squamous	Adeno	Small cell	Large cell	Other	Unspec.				MV	Total
ASIA											
China, Qidong											
China, Shanghai											
China, Tianjin	20.9	10.4	3.1	2.8	0.1	-	-	-	62.6	**2785**	5589
Hong Kong	34.8	35.9	11.7	6.3	0.4	9.8	0.1	0.1	1.0	**6614**	11531
India, Bangalore	23.7	14.3	15.8	5.5	0.6	14.0	0.3	-	25.8	**329**	495
India, Barshi, Paranda and Bhum	28.6	57.1	-	-	-	-	-	-	14.3	**7**	11
India, Bombay	34.7	32.7	13.4	5.1	0.6	8.6	0.2	-	4.7	**1138**	1867
India, Karunagappally	46.7	6.7	16.7	16.7	-	-	-	-	13.3	**30**	58
India, Madras	53.0	15.9	7.3	8.8	0.4	7.5	-	-	7.1	**534**	789
India, Trivandrum	52.5	17.5	10.0	10.0	-	10.0	-	-	-	**40**	69
Israel: All Jews	35.3	27.6	17.2	10.6	1.2	5.4	0.2	-	2.4	**2230**	2928
Jews born in Israel	27.9	31.4	17.3	12.8	3.5	4.0	0.4	0.4	2.2	**226**	279
Jews born in America or Europe	34.4	28.9	17.0	10.0	1.1	5.6	0.1	-	3.0	**1275**	1694
Jews born in Africa or Asia	39.6	23.8	17.6	10.9	0.6	5.5	0.4	-	1.5	**722**	946
Non-Jews	43.1	22.6	15.9	6.2	1.0	6.7	-	0.5	4.1	**195**	284
Japan, Hiroshima	37.2	41.4	13.5	2.8	0.4	4.4	0.1	0.1	0.1	**896**	1193
Japan, Miyagi	38.5	29.2	12.6	13.1	0.2	0.7	-	-	5.7	**2452**	3106
Japan, Nagasaki	34.3	38.7	13.6	6.9	0.3	5.1	0.1	0.2	0.8	**1886**	2584
Japan, Osaka	34.3	33.7	15.5	6.8	0.3	0.2	0.1	0.1	9.1	**8031**	11305
Japan, Saga											
Japan, Yamagata											
Korea, Kangwha	53.8	10.8	18.5	3.1	1.5	3.1	-	-	9.2	**65**	104
Kuwait: Non-Kuwaitis	46.1	16.5	17.4	6.1	0.9	7.0	-	-	6.1	**115**	141
Kuwait: Kuwaitis	46.9	12.3	24.7	6.2	-	7.4	-	-	2.5	**81**	111
Philippines, Manila	33.7	25.7	12.1	5.0	0.2	18.3	0.1	0.1	4.8	**1450**	2764
Singapore: Chinese	38.9	28.5	13.9	0.2	0.4	15.2	0.2	0.2	2.5	**2085**	2620
Singapore: Malay	23.5	37.4	15.1	-	0.6	19.0	-	-	4.5	**179**	240
Singapore: Indian	29.0	39.1	7.2	1.4	1.4	15.9	-	-	5.8	**69**	83
Thailand, Chiang Mai	28.4	36.0	8.4	12.0	0.1	3.6	0.4	-	10.9	**689**	1140
Thailand, Khon Kaen	20.7	45.5	4.1	24.8	-	-	-	-	4.8	**145**	355
Viet Nam, Hanoi	20.2	17.4	3.4	11.0	0.9	27.8	-	-	19.3	**327**	788
EUROPE											
Austria, Tyrol	40.8	18.5	20.6	3.1	2.0	4.8	0.1	-	10.0	**806**	1031
Belarus											
Croatia											
Czech Republic	47.1	9.2	14.6	5.6	1.0	2.0	0.1	-	20.3	**14624**	24827
Denmark	36.9	25.1	21.2	8.6	0.6	5.4	0.2	0.1	1.9	**9065**	10445
Estonia	42.9	9.0	25.2	3.4	0.4	2.7	0.1	0.1	16.3	**2309**	3221
Finland	36.9	14.9	18.3	-	0.1	9.1	0.1	-	20.7	**9462**	10455
France, Bas-Rhin	55.6	17.7	13.6	10.6	1.2	0.3	0.1	0.1	0.8	**1761**	1875
France, Calvados	50.3	15.8	14.0	13.8	1.7	2.0	-	0.2	2.1	**980**	1005
France, Doubs	60.3	15.4	16.9	2.7	0.6	3.6	0.1	-	0.4	**700**	735
France, Haut-Rhin	63.9	11.5	9.4	13.0	1.0	0.5	0.1	0.1	0.4	**1143**	1174
France, Herault	57.7	16.5	10.2	9.8	0.5	3.8	0.4	-	1.2	**1251**	1273
France, Isere	50.9	18.8	17.9	5.5	1.4	4.8	0.1	-	0.7	**1481**	1532
France, Somme	57.3	10.2	18.6	4.8	0.4	6.7	0.2	-	1.8	**914**	967
France, Tarn	55.6	14.6	20.4	3.8	1.9	3.0	-	0.2	0.5	**574**	587
Germany, Eastern States	41.0	17.5	21.5	6.7	1.1	2.4	0.3	0.1	9.4	**9666**	11787
Germany, Saarland											
Iceland	23.6	32.6	24.4	11.6	1.2	5.4	-	0.4	0.8	**242**	250
Ireland, Southern	58.4	10.9	17.6	3.0	1.1	8.9	-	-	0.2	**541**	721
Italy, Ferrara	47.4	30.0	15.6	1.3	0.4	5.0	-	0.2	-	**456**	597
Italy, Florence	45.8	26.3	13.8	3.0	0.4	6.9	0.1	0.1	3.6	**1541**	2592
Italy, Genoa	38.9	32.3	13.6	4.8	0.3	5.5	-	0.1	4.6	**1705**	2418
Italy, Latina	30.3	16.0	15.1	5.2	0.5	32.3	-	-	0.6	**617**	830
Italy, Macerata	37.4	29.3	15.2	7.6	0.5	7.1	-	-	3.0	**198**	255
Italy, Modena	51.7	23.6	16.4	3.7	0.9	2.9	-	0.1	0.8	**1217**	1821
Italy, Parma	49.9	20.5	16.8	3.5	0.4	5.7	-	-	3.1	**962**	1229
Italy, Ragusa	34.3	14.6	11.3	5.6	-	10.3	-	-	23.9	**213**	421
Italy, Romagna	53.0	19.2	16.2	6.5	0.6	3.5	0.1	-	1.0	**1242**	1485
Italy, Torino	39.0	25.0	13.6	8.9	0.7	8.6	0.2	-	3.9	**1479**	2099
Italy, Trieste	24.3	11.5	12.2	3.6	0.4	18.1	0.8	-	29.1	**740**	897
Italy, Varese	42.7	26.7	17.6	5.2	0.5	5.8	0.1	-	1.5	**1910**	2202
Italy, Veneto	43.8	20.0	11.1	7.5	0.7	6.0	0.1	-	10.8	**2608**	3568
Latvia											
Malta											

PERCENTAGE DISTRIBUTION OF MICROSCOPICALLY VERIFIED CASES BY HISTOLOGICAL TYPE
Lung (ICD-9 162) - Male (contd)

			Carcinoma				Sarcoma	Other	Unspec.	Number of cases	
	Squamous	Adeno	Small cell	Large cell	Other	Unspec.				MV	Total
The Netherlands	45.7	17.9	19.2	11.4	0.5	4.7	0.1	0.1	0.4	**27728**	29631
The Netherlands, Eindhoven	52.0	15.2	19.0	8.5	0.2	3.9	-	0.2	0.9	**2213**	2359
The Netherlands, Maastricht	45.2	15.7	20.9	13.3	0.6	3.8	-	0.3	0.1	**2207**	2395
Norway	35.6	23.6	21.8	5.5	0.4	8.4	0.2	0.1	4.4	**5293**	5782
Poland, Cracow	52.6	9.9	20.1	2.6	0.5	2.7	-	-	11.6	**1104**	1605
Poland, Kielce	53.0	9.0	8.9	9.4	0.1	13.2	0.1	0.1	6.3	**1543**	2259
Poland, Lower Silesia	14.4	2.4	4.6	2.2	0.1	1.3	-	-	75.0	**2713**	7213
Poland, Warsaw City	51.8	17.0	19.8	4.9	0.3	5.8	0.1	0.1	0.1	**1744**	2939
Slovakia	58.1	12.1	17.1	6.2	0.5	2.0	0.1	-	3.7	**8148**	11110
Slovenia	42.8	17.6	18.3	13.9	0.4	6.6	-	-	0.4	**3298**	3681
Spain, Albacete	47.1	8.4	27.7	12.6	-	1.7	-	-	2.5	**119**	183
Spain, Asturias	46.4	15.6	20.4	8.9	0.3	4.1	0.1	0.2	4.0	**1957**	2256
Spain, Basque Country	45.5	17.3	17.5	8.0	0.3	10.4	0.1	-	0.8	**2416**	3027
Spain, Granada	52.1	11.4	19.4	7.0	0.7	6.9	0.1	-	2.4	**831**	1201
Spain, Mallorca	36.1	15.9	21.1	15.7	0.3	8.2	-	0.2	2.6	**1079**	1271
Spain, Murcia	42.9	18.3	22.1	9.7	-	4.0	0.1	-	3.0	**1215**	1531
Spain, Navarra	54.9	12.4	19.8	9.0	0.6	2.9	-	0.1	0.3	**701**	826
Spain, Tarragona	46.0	15.4	23.7	7.5	0.1	6.5	-	-	0.6	**771**	879
Spain, Zaragoza	51.5	16.4	18.3	10.2	0.2	2.7	0.1	-	0.7	**1132**	1572
Sweden	37.4	23.2	19.4	16.9	-	0.4	0.2	0.1	2.4	**8799**	8977
Switzerland, Basel	38.8	27.7	17.5	12.0	1.1	2.2	0.1	0.1	0.5	**830**	842
Switzerland, Geneva	43.7	25.7	16.2	6.6	0.5	6.6	-	0.2	0.6	**662**	696
Switzerland, Graubunden	48.1	16.0	23.1	7.1	-	5.2	-	-	0.5	**212**	255
Switzerland, Neuchatel	46.9	18.1	22.4	5.5	0.3	5.2	-	0.6	0.9	**326**	360
Switzerland, St Gall-Appenzell	43.6	20.9	20.7	12.7	0.8	1.3	0.1	-	-	**789**	844
Switzerland, Valais	46.2	19.6	23.1	6.3	0.7	3.5	-	-	0.7	**286**	319
Switzerland, Vaud	41.5	20.4	17.9	5.6	1.2	12.5	0.1	0.3	0.4	**1136**	1256
Switzerland, Zurich	44.3	21.3	18.7	12.8	1.1	1.2	0.3	0.1	0.2	**1887**	1992
UK, England and Wales	36.0	10.4	12.8	5.3	0.2	33.6	0.1	-	1.7	**51057**	76751
UK, East Anglia											
UK, Mersey	44.9	18.3	18.6	6.3	0.5	11.1	0.1	0.1	0.2	**3739**	6590
UK, North Western											
UK, Oxford	51.8	16.2	18.8	4.9	0.6	7.6	0.1	-	-	**2850**	5076
UK, South Thames	48.5	13.9	17.1	6.9	-	13.1	0.1	-	0.3	**8675**	16156
UK, South Western	45.6	9.9	15.9	6.8	0.3	17.7	0.2	-	3.6	**3592**	7222
UK, Wessex	28.9	9.2	11.9	4.9	0.1	44.6	0.1	-	0.2	**4906**	6841
UK, West Midlands											
UK, Yorkshire	49.0	12.9	17.6	9.7	0.2	9.1	0.1	-	1.4	**5925**	9380
UK, Scotland	45.8	16.6	20.0	9.7	0.3	7.1	0.1	0.1	0.3	**9029**	15212
UK, Scotland, West	48.2	14.1	20.6	11.5	0.4	5.1	0.1	-	0.1	**4986**	8877
Yugoslavia, Vojvodina	47.7	20.2	19.3	1.3	0.8	5.2	0.1	-	5.4	**2592**	5064

OCEANIA

			Carcinoma				Sarcoma	Other	Unspec.	Number of cases	
	Squamous	Adeno	Small cell	Large cell	Other	Unspec.				MV	Total
Australian Capital Territory	33.9	25.4	19.0	13.8	1.1	5.8	-	0.5	0.5	**189**	213
Australia, New South Wales	35.3	22.9	16.0	19.0	0.7	5.6	0.1	0.1	0.3	**7298**	8816
South Australia	23.5	26.2	17.4	19.5	11.8	-	-	-	1.6	**1705**	2375
Australia, Tasmania	49.8	16.2	15.1	10.7	0.9	6.9	-	-	0.4	**568**	751
Australia, Victoria	37.3	26.1	16.1	14.3	0.9	5.1	-	0.1	0.2	**5323**	6374
Western Australia	36.9	26.2	15.4	14.0	1.2	5.5	0.2	0.3	0.3	**1853**	2172
French Polynesia	55.4	15.4	16.2	4.6	0.8	7.7	-	-	-	**130**	202
New Zealand: Non-Maori											
New Zealand: Maori											
US, Hawaii: White	27.2	37.0	17.1	7.6	1.0	8.7	0.6	-	0.8	**497**	525
US, Hawaii: Japanese	27.9	39.0	14.2	6.6	1.4	10.5	-	0.2	0.2	**438**	456
US, Hawaii: Hawaiian	34.0	24.4	20.4	10.0	-	11.2	-	-	-	**250**	261
US, Hawaii: Filipino	33.3	44.3	11.5	5.2	0.5	4.2	0.5	-	0.5	**192**	202
US, Hawaii: Chinese	24.3	50.5	3.9	10.7	1.9	8.7	-	-	-	**103**	111

PERCENTAGE DISTRIBUTION OF MICROSCOPICALLY VERIFIED CASES BY HISTOLOGICAL TYPE
Lung (ICD-9 162) - Female

			Carcinoma				Sarcoma	Other	Unspec.	Number of cases	
	Squamous	Adeno	Small cell	Large cell	Other	Unspec.				MV	Total
AFRICA											
Algeria, Setif	31.8	9.1	-	13.6	-	27.3	-	-	18.2	**22**	33
France, La Reunion	15.9	56.8	-	11.4	-	11.4	-	-	4.5	**44**	46
Mali, Bamako	50.0	50.0	-	-	-	-	-	-	-	**2**	13
Uganda, Kyadondo	-	-	-	-	-	100.0	-	-	-	**1**	4
Zimbabwe, Harare: African	50.0	25.0	-	12.5	-	12.5	-	-	-	**8**	22
Zimbabwe, Harare: European	55.6	11.1	22.2	11.1	-	-	-	-	-	**9**	24
AMERICA, CENTRAL AND SOUTH											
Argentina, Concordia	38.9	5.6	-	-	-	27.8	-	-	27.8	**18**	27
Brazil, Belem	16.1	29.0	9.7	6.5	-	35.5	-	-	3.2	**31**	90
Brazil, Goiania	27.3	29.9	3.9	9.1	-	6.5	1.3	1.3	20.8	**77**	114
Brazil, Porto Alegre	17.7	27.4	8.6	0.6	1.1	19.4	1.1	-	24.0	**175**	319
Colombia, Cali	15.2	26.5	9.3	6.0	2.6	19.9	-	-	20.5	**151**	261
Costa Rica	33.6	33.6	4.5	17.9	2.2	6.0	-	-	2.2	**134**	274
Ecuador, Quito	29.2	41.7	4.2	4.2	4.2	16.7	-	-	-	**24**	78
Peru, Lima	18.6	58.3	2.6	7.7	1.9	7.1	1.3	-	2.6	**156**	284
Peru, Trujillo	14.3	64.3	-	7.1	-	7.1	-	7.1	-	**14**	22
Puerto Rico	35.6	29.5	13.8	5.8	3.7	8.4	0.4	-	2.8	**464**	625
Uruguay, Montevideo	17.4	54.2	14.6	3.5	2.8	6.3	0.7	-	0.7	**144**	275
AMERICA, NORTH											
Canada	22.1	38.2	19.1	10.9	1.7	5.0	0.1	0.1	2.7	**20637**	27377
Canada, Alberta	20.7	34.2	21.0	9.8	3.0	4.9	0.2	0.1	6.1	**1574**	1771
Canada, British Columbia	22.2	36.4	20.3	16.2	1.8	1.9	0.2	0.1	0.9	**3370**	3922
Canada, Manitoba	20.3	46.3	16.9	7.4	1.1	7.1	0.1	0.1	0.7	**747**	1203
Canada, New Brunswick	25.1	39.9	18.1	7.3	1.9	7.7	-	-	-	**574**	687
Canada, Newfoundland	23.9	27.3	29.3	15.6	1.0	2.0	-	-	1.0	**205**	225
Canada, Northwest Territories	44.1	8.5	22.0	15.3	-	5.1	-	-	5.1	**59**	80
Canada, Nova Scotia	20.1	36.7	22.6	10.6	2.0	7.9	0.1	0.1	-	**851**	1049
Canada, Ontario	21.2	39.8	19.3	10.0	1.9	4.3	0.1	0.1	3.4	**7971**	10413
Canada, Prince Edward Island	23.9	40.8	22.5	7.0	0.7	4.2	0.7	-	-	**142**	161
Canada, Quebec	23.5	37.0	16.8	10.4	1.2	7.3	0.1	0.2	3.6	**4403**	7023
Canada, Saskatchewan	25.8	40.7	16.0	7.7	0.9	7.7	0.4	0.3	0.5	**752**	866
Canada, Yukon	36.8	28.9	10.5	13.2	5.3	5.3	-	-	-	**38**	39
US, Cent. California: Non-Hisp White	21.2	34.3	22.2	12.8	1.9	5.9	0.1	0.2	1.4	**2045**	2267
US, Cent. California: Hispanic	19.7	35.5	25.0	11.8	2.0	3.3	-	-	2.6	**152**	166
US, Los Angeles: Non-Hisp White	17.9	38.9	18.6	9.7	1.7	11.2	0.2	0.1	1.6	**6160**	6674
US, Los Angeles: Hispanic White	19.1	38.5	16.1	9.3	2.7	12.7	0.1	0.1	1.4	**702**	762
US, Los Angeles: Black	25.2	34.6	13.1	10.4	1.4	13.7	0.1	0.1	1.4	**978**	1035
US, Los Angeles: Chinese	13.3	48.3	7.5	15.8	-	15.0	-	-	-	**120**	126
US, Los Angeles: Filipino	11.3	67.5	3.8	6.3	-	10.0	-	-	1.3	**80**	83
US, Los Angeles: Korean	27.7	48.9	17.0	4.3	-	2.1	-	-	-	**47**	52
US, Los Angeles: Japanese	20.9	46.3	11.9	7.5	-	11.9	-	-	1.5	**67**	71
US, San Francisco: Non-Hisp White	17.9	41.2	18.3	10.9	1.9	8.4	0.1	-	1.3	**3527**	3906
US, San Francisco: Hispanic White	16.1	46.3	14.0	12.4	2.1	9.1	-	-	-	**242**	268
US, San Francisco: Black	24.6	42.2	12.1	9.0	0.8	8.8	0.2	0.4	1.9	**521**	562
US, San Francisco: Chinese	12.6	59.5	7.4	12.6	0.5	6.5	-	-	0.9	**215**	227
US, San Francisco: Filipino	10.5	59.2	6.6	13.2	2.6	7.9	-	-	-	**76**	82
US, San Francisco: Japanese	9.7	54.8	16.1	6.5	-	9.7	-	-	3.2	**31**	32
US, Connecticut: White	19.5	40.0	19.5	8.3	1.7	9.7	0.3	0.1	0.9	**4128**	4540
US, Connecticut: Black	21.7	39.6	14.6	8.5	0.9	13.2	-	0.5	0.9	**212**	227
US, Atlanta: White	16.9	34.0	22.6	17.0	3.3	4.9	0.2	0.1	0.9	**1558**	1663
US, Atlanta: Black	25.2	29.3	14.9	21.7	1.6	5.7	-	0.8	0.8	**369**	402
US, Iowa	19.7	39.1	23.2	7.8	1.9	7.5	0.1	0.2	0.4	**3078**	3437
US, Central Louisiana: White	33.7	30.7	21.0	5.9	1.0	7.8	-	-	-	**205**	246
US, Central Louisiana: Black	31.4	33.3	11.8	11.8	3.9	5.9	-	-	2.0	**51**	64
US, New Orleans: White	23.8	37.4	21.6	9.6	1.8	4.5	0.2	0.1	1.0	**969**	1115
US, New Orleans: Black	29.1	34.1	15.6	14.2	0.8	5.0	-	-	1.1	**358**	415
US, Detroit: White	19.7	35.6	21.9	10.5	2.6	7.6	0.1	-	2.0	**4345**	4772
US, Detroit: Black	22.3	37.5	18.2	8.1	1.9	9.8	0.1	-	2.0	**1130**	1213
US, New Mexico: Non-Hisp White	20.7	34.8	21.7	10.9	2.5	8.0	0.1	-	1.2	**805**	955
US, New Mexico: Hispanic White	19.8	49.2	13.6	10.2	0.6	6.2	-	-	0.6	**177**	207
US, New Mexico: American Indian	18.2	45.5	18.2	9.1	-	-	9.1	-	-	**11**	12
US, Utah	18.5	36.1	17.1	13.6	4.2	8.1	0.4	-	2.0	**545**	603
US, Seattle	17.7	38.6	21.2	8.3	2.4	9.8	0.2	0.1	1.8	**4031**	4413
US, SEER: White	18.8	38.4	20.8	9.9	2.2	8.4	0.2	0.1	1.3	**22448**	24781
US, SEER: Black	23.2	37.8	15.6	10.7	1.6	9.1	0.1	0.3	1.7	**2378**	2558

Lung (ICD-9 162) - Female (contd)

			Carcinoma				Sarcoma	Other	Unspec.	Number of cases	
	Squamous	Adeno	Small cell	Large cell	Other	Unspec.				MV	Total
ASIA											
China, Qidong											
China, Shanghai											
China, Tianjin	9.7	14.5	3.1	2.9	0.2	-	0.1	0.1	69.3	1623	3870
Hong Kong	16.3	57.5	8.5	6.2	0.3	10.0	0.2	-	1.0	2867	5655
India, Bangalore	15.4	28.2	9.0	7.7	-	15.4	-	-	24.4	78	103
India, Barshi, Paranda and Bhum	-	66.7	-	-	-	33.3	-	-	-	3	3
India, Bombay	22.0	51.9	7.5	4.7	2.3	8.9	-	-	2.8	214	432
India, Karunagappally	60.0	20.0	-	20.0	-	-	-	-	-	5	10
India, Madras	39.8	33.3	3.2	1.1	1.1	11.8	-	-	9.7	93	142
India, Trivandrum	10.0	60.0	-	20.0	-	10.0	-	-	-	10	14
Israel: All Jews	20.7	44.7	13.5	8.2	4.8	5.7	0.5	-	2.1	920	1209
Jews born in Israel	12.7	48.3	11.0	13.6	6.8	4.2	2.5	-	0.8	118	141
Jews born in America or Europe	21.5	45.3	13.1	7.2	4.1	6.1	0.3	-	2.3	655	860
Jews born in Africa or Asia	23.4	39.3	15.9	8.3	6.2	4.8	-	-	2.1	145	202
Non-Jews	31.3	37.5	15.6	6.3	6.3	-	-	-	3.1	32	41
Japan, Hiroshima	18.2	65.6	9.4	2.4	1.5	2.9	-	-	-	340	469
Japan, Miyagi	8.5	66.7	6.4	9.3	1.5	0.6	-	-	7.0	810	1041
Japan, Nagasaki	13.8	69.5	6.7	3.3	0.7	5.4	0.1	0.1	0.3	719	1070
Japan, Osaka	15.7	55.4	11.7	4.3	0.8	0.3	0.3	0.1	11.4	2933	4526
Japan, Saga											
Japan, Yamagata											
Korea, Kangwha	23.8	42.9	14.3	-	4.8	-	-	-	14.3	21	32
Kuwait: Non-Kuwaitis	33.3	29.6	11.1	7.4	3.7	11.1	-	-	3.7	27	37
Kuwait: Kuwaitis	47.4	21.1	10.5	-	-	-	-	5.3	15.8	19	40
Philippines, Manila	17.7	47.2	4.6	4.8	0.8	17.3	0.4	-	7.1	479	959
Singapore: Chinese	19.5	49.8	10.2	0.2	0.7	15.2	0.2	-	4.0	820	1092
Singapore: Malay	15.4	63.5	5.8	-	-	11.5	1.9	-	1.9	52	61
Singapore: Indian	33.3	44.4	-	-	-	22.2	-	-	-	9	10
Thailand, Chiang Mai	20.8	44.6	7.2	13.1	0.6	5.0	-	-	8.8	543	941
Thailand, Khon Kaen	8.3	70.8	-	12.5	-	4.2	-	-	4.2	48	132
Viet Nam, Hanoi	16.0	21.0	2.5	13.6	-	30.9	-	-	16.0	81	175
EUROPE											
Austria, Tyrol	24.2	34.8	17.6	3.5	2.6	6.2	0.4	-	10.6	227	302
Belarus											
Croatia											
Czech Republic	25.4	21.9	17.9	6.1	2.3	2.8	0.4	-	23.2	2362	4469
Denmark	20.8	37.7	23.9	9.3	1.0	5.5	0.2	0.1	1.4	4788	5536
Estonia	19.8	17.1	30.4	4.9	1.4	2.4	0.3	-	23.6	368	606
Finland	19.4	31.0	19.5	-	0.1	10.0	0.3	-	19.6	2075	2341
France, Bas-Rhin	32.8	36.1	12.7	11.1	4.9	2.0	0.4	-	-	244	274
France, Calvados	28.4	33.3	21.6	5.9	5.9	2.9	-	-	2.0	102	104
France, Doubs	37.7	38.7	13.2	2.8	2.8	2.8	0.9	0.9	-	106	114
France, Haut-Rhin	44.5	22.6	14.0	16.5	0.6	1.8	-	-	-	164	168
France, Herault	39.0	33.5	6.0	8.2	4.4	6.6	0.5	-	1.6	182	185
France, Isere	21.5	39.5	19.5	7.8	5.4	2.9	1.0	0.5	2.0	205	213
France, Somme	35.2	19.8	23.1	4.4	2.2	9.9	1.1	1.1	3.3	91	98
France, Tarn	38.6	28.1	15.8	8.8	5.3	3.5	-	-	-	57	60
Germany, Eastern States	22.1	31.8	23.7	6.9	2.9	2.4	0.5	0.4	9.4	1959	2407
Germany, Saarland											
Iceland	17.3	43.1	20.3	7.6	2.0	8.6	-	1.0	-	197	213
Ireland, Southern	45.8	12.0	21.3	6.0	1.9	12.0	-	-	0.9	216	294
Italy, Ferrara	22.5	46.1	18.0	2.2	4.5	6.7	-	-	-	89	130
Italy, Florence	21.3	47.4	13.4	1.7	0.3	8.9	-	-	6.9	291	600
Italy, Genoa	19.9	45.9	11.8	6.9	1.5	8.8	-	-	5.1	331	475
Italy, Latina	7.6	29.3	9.8	7.6	1.1	43.5	-	-	1.1	92	135
Italy, Macerata	3.3	60.0	13.3	3.3	3.3	10.0	-	-	6.7	30	43
Italy, Modena	23.9	47.8	13.0	4.3	5.4	4.9	-	-	0.5	184	305
Italy, Parma	24.9	45.9	12.4	1.9	3.3	6.7	-	-	4.8	209	299
Italy, Ragusa	30.0	20.0	-	6.7	-	13.3	3.3	-	26.7	30	64
Italy, Romagna	27.7	45.5	13.4	5.4	0.5	5.9	-	-	1.5	202	260
Italy, Torino	20.0	40.7	13.0	6.7	1.3	11.3	-	0.3	6.7	300	500
Italy, Trieste	13.8	29.7	12.1	6.7	0.4	22.2	0.8	-	14.2	239	239
Italy, Varese	23.5	43.6	15.9	4.5	1.1	9.5	-	-	1.9	264	350
Italy, Veneto	21.1	27.0	15.9	10.9	1.1	8.1	1.1	-	14.8	559	854
Latvia											
Malta											

PERCENTAGE DISTRIBUTION OF MICROSCOPICALLY VERIFIED CASES BY HISTOLOGICAL TYPE
Lung (ICD-9 162) - Female (contd)

			Carcinoma				Sarcoma	Other	Unspec.	Number of cases	
	Squamous	Adeno	Small cell	Large cell	Other	Unspec.				MV	Total
The Netherlands	21.7	31.5	25.9	12.7	2.6	4.8	0.3	0.2	0.4	5372	5694
The Netherlands, Eindhoven	23.0	26.5	29.5	11.8	2.7	5.3	0.3	0.3	0.6	339	361
The Netherlands, Maastricht	22.9	29.6	28.1	10.6	3.1	3.9	0.8	0.3	0.8	385	416
Norway	19.1	33.9	25.2	5.7	1.2	9.6	0.3	0.1	4.8	2142	2340
Poland, Cracow	31.4	19.5	27.4	3.6	2.6	4.6	0.3	0.3	10.2	303	463
Poland, Kielce	25.7	24.6	13.2	11.4	0.6	15.6	-	-	9.0	167	310
Poland, Lower Silesia	9.2	3.5	5.0	2.8	0.1	1.3	0.1	-	77.8	677	1696
Poland, Warsaw City	35.6	23.2	26.5	6.3	0.2	7.7	0.3	0.3	-	638	1241
Slovakia	31.5	31.6	16.2	7.3	2.5	3.8	0.5	0.2	6.3	1106	1680
Slovenia	15.6	42.1	20.2	12.5	1.6	7.1	0.2	-	0.8	634	741
Spain, Albacete	14.3	50.0	14.3	7.1	-	7.1	-	-	7.1	14	19
Spain, Asturias	22.5	44.4	9.9	8.6	4.6	7.9	-	-	2.0	151	203
Spain, Basque Country	17.6	45.9	12.9	9.4	2.9	9.4	-	-	1.8	170	248
Spain, Granada	17.2	44.8	12.1	5.2	5.2	6.9	1.7	-	6.9	58	92
Spain, Mallorca	11.1	44.4	8.9	18.9	4.4	7.8	-	-	4.4	90	111
Spain, Murcia	20.2	40.4	16.0	10.6	-	7.4	2.1	-	3.2	94	146
Spain, Navarra	23.0	45.9	14.8	9.8	3.3	1.6	-	-	1.6	61	82
Spain, Tarragona	14.3	57.1	4.8	11.1	4.8	4.8	-	-	3.2	63	72
Spain, Zaragoza	27.4	43.8	5.5	11.0	2.7	6.8	-	1.4	1.4	73	116
Sweden	20.8	37.3	19.7	17.5	-	1.7	0.4	0.2	2.4	4266	4343
Switzerland, Basel	20.6	42.8	19.5	7.4	7.4	1.9	-	-	0.4	257	261
Switzerland, Geneva	20.1	39.8	24.2	7.4	2.5	5.7	-	0.4	-	244	268
Switzerland, Graubunden	29.3	34.1	14.6	14.6	-	7.3	-	-	-	41	58
Switzerland, Neuchatel	25.3	32.0	24.0	6.7	-	12.0	-	-	-	75	87
Switzerland, St Gall-Appenzell	15.8	43.0	19.6	12.7	5.1	2.5	-	0.6	0.6	158	161
Switzerland, Valais	10.4	50.7	17.9	9.0	4.5	4.5	-	-	3.0	67	71
Switzerland, Vaud	19.1	38.8	17.6	5.0	3.2	15.8	-	-	0.4	278	318
Switzerland, Zurich	16.6	40.3	20.0	15.9	4.5	1.1	0.6	0.4	0.7	536	565
UK, England and Wales	24.5	14.2	17.0	5.3	0.4	36.7	0.1	-	1.8	23256	34917
UK, East Anglia											
UK, Mersey	32.3	22.2	28.1	5.5	0.9	10.6	0.2	-	0.1	1797	3460
UK, North Western											
UK, Oxford	36.4	22.3	24.1	7.0	1.6	8.3	0.2	-	0.1	1187	2225
UK, South Thames	36.3	20.6	21.7	6.7	0.1	14.1	0.2	-	0.2	3967	8094
UK, South Western	32.0	15.3	21.6	6.8	0.8	19.4	-	-	4.1	1554	3340
UK, Wessex	22.4	12.6	15.5	3.7	0.2	45.4	0.1	-	-	2140	3111
UK, West Midlands											
UK, Yorkshire	37.5	17.2	24.6	8.5	0.4	10.3	0.1	-	1.2	2675	4511
UK, Scotland	32.2	19.7	28.5	10.6	0.7	7.9	0.1	0.1	0.3	4804	8442
UK, Scotland, West	34.7	17.0	29.3	11.8	0.6	6.3	0.1	0.1	0.1	2802	5086
Yugoslavia, Vojvodina	27.5	37.4	13.7	3.5	0.6	7.6	-	-	9.6	342	945
OCEANIA											
Australian Capital Territory	22.1	32.5	15.6	23.4	2.6	2.6	1.3	-	-	77	94
Australia, New South Wales	20.7	31.1	20.2	19.6	2.2	5.4	0.2	-	0.4	2672	3271
South Australia	13.8	34.2	20.7	18.5	10.8	-	0.5	-	1.6	638	867
Australia, Tasmania	35.6	24.3	19.2	12.6	3.3	5.0	-	-	-	239	298
Australia, Victoria	22.3	35.6	20.2	13.9	2.4	5.3	0.1	0.1	-	2104	2552
Western Australia	21.7	34.4	22.6	13.3	2.2	5.6	0.3	-	-	774	912
French Polynesia	33.3	33.3	22.2	5.6	-	5.6	-	-	-	54	75
New Zealand: Non-Maori											
New Zealand: Maori											
US, Hawaii: White	17.9	42.9	19.7	6.6	1.6	11.0	-	-	0.3	319	340
US, Hawaii: Japanese	18.8	53.9	15.2	4.2	1.2	6.7	-	-	-	165	176
US, Hawaii: Hawaiian	15.8	42.4	18.0	10.1	0.7	11.5	0.7	-	0.7	139	145
US, Hawaii: Filipino	11.7	57.1	19.5	7.8	-	3.9	-	-	-	77	83
US, Hawaii: Chinese	15.9	55.6	4.8	7.9	4.8	11.1	-	-	-	63	68

PERCENTAGE DISTRIBUTION OF MICROSCOPICALLY VERIFIED CASES BY HISTOLOGICAL TYPE
Bone (ICD-9 170) - Both sexes

			Sarcoma				Other	Unspec.	Number of cases	
	Osteo	Chondro	Ewing's	Fibro	Other	Unspec.			MV	Total
AFRICA										
Algeria, Setif	35.5	16.1	12.9	-	-	29.0	3.2	3.2	**31**	36
France, La Reunion	39.3	21.4	10.7	10.7	7.1	3.6	3.6	3.6	**28**	29
Mali, Bamako	18.2	54.5	9.1	9.1	-	-	9.1	-	**11**	19
Uganda, Kyadondo	61.5	7.7	-	-	7.7	-	23.1	-	**13**	22
Zimbabwe, Harare: African	76.5	11.8	-	-	-	-	5.9	5.9	**17**	21
Zimbabwe, Harare: European	-	100.0	-	-	-	-	-	-	**1**	1
AMERICA, CENTRAL AND SOUTH										
Argentina, Concordia	60.0	10.0	10.0	-	-	-	10.0	10.0	**10**	11
Brazil, Belem	41.9	9.7	3.2	6.5	3.2	9.7	22.6	3.2	**31**	62
Brazil, Goiania	57.5	17.5	5.0	7.5	2.5	2.5	-	7.5	**40**	43
Brazil, Porto Alegre	59.2	9.9	2.8	2.8	5.6	2.8	8.5	8.5	**71**	99
Colombia, Cali	54.5	25.5	9.1	1.8	-	3.6	5.5	-	**55**	66
Costa Rica	45.5	24.2	16.7	-	6.1	4.5	1.5	1.5	**66**	90
Ecuador, Quito	63.2	21.1	7.9	-	5.3	-	2.6	-	**38**	54
Peru, Lima	48.0	26.7	8.0	1.3	9.3	2.7	1.3	2.7	**75**	108
Peru, Trujillo	50.0	10.0	20.0	10.0	-	-	10.0	-	**10**	12
Puerto Rico	36.0	28.1	23.6	3.4	1.1	1.1	5.6	1.1	**89**	103
Uruguay, Montevideo	54.1	21.6	8.1	5.4	2.7	-	8.1	-	**37**	44
AMERICA, NORTH										
Canada	30.1	31.2	14.7	4.3	4.5	0.9	11.6	2.7	**1201**	1499
Canada, Alberta	31.2	37.6	15.6	3.7	2.8	0.9	8.3	-	**109**	112
Canada, British Columbia	28.9	25.2	18.5	6.7	3.0	1.5	14.1	2.2	**135**	143
Canada, Manitoba	28.2	41.0	17.9	2.6	5.1	-	5.1	-	**39**	55
Canada, New Brunswick	26.9	34.6	23.1	7.7	3.8	-	3.8	-	**26**	28
Canada, Newfoundland	16.7	16.7	22.2	5.6	5.6	-	33.3	-	**18**	19
Canada, Northwest Territories	100.0	-	-	-	-	-	-	-	**3**	4
Canada, Nova Scotia	28.3	21.7	15.2	8.7	8.7	2.2	15.2	-	**46**	50
Canada, Ontario	32.8	30.4	14.0	3.6	3.6	0.7	9.7	5.2	**421**	554
Canada, Prince Edward Island	16.7	-	16.7	33.3	-	-	33.3	-	**6**	6
Canada, Quebec	28.0	33.6	12.4	3.1	5.9	1.1	14.1	1.7	**354**	482
Canada, Saskatchewan	31.8	34.1	13.6	6.8	6.8	-	4.5	2.3	**44**	46
Canada, Yukon	-	-	-	-	-	-	-	-	**-**	-
US, Cent. California: Non-Hisp White	36.0	22.7	16.0	6.7	5.3	2.7	9.3	1.3	**75**	79
US, Cent. California: Hispanic	50.0	27.3	4.5	4.5	9.1	-	4.5	-	**22**	22
US, Los Angeles: Non-Hisp White	30.5	32.6	14.4	7.0	3.7	2.7	8.0	1.1	**187**	191
US, Los Angeles: Hispanic White	48.6	13.6	20.0	3.6	5.0	0.7	8.6	-	**140**	141
US, Los Angeles: Black	33.3	22.2	14.8	11.1	7.4	3.7	7.4	-	**27**	27
US, Los Angeles: Chinese	100.0	-	-	-	-	-	-	-	**4**	4
US, Los Angeles: Filipino	28.6	28.6	-	-	-	-	42.9	-	**7**	7
US, Los Angeles: Korean	50.0	25.0	25.0	-	-	-	-	-	**4**	4
US, Los Angeles: Japanese	100.0	-	-	-	-	-	-	-	**1**	1
US, San Francisco: Non-Hisp White	27.1	41.7	6.3	6.3	5.2	2.1	9.4	2.1	**96**	98
US, San Francisco: Hispanic White	44.4	27.8	11.1	5.6	5.6	-	5.6	-	**18**	18
US, San Francisco: Black	38.5	38.5	7.7	-	7.7	-	7.7	-	**13**	13
US, San Francisco: Chinese	50.0	16.7	16.7	-	16.7	-	-	-	**6**	6
US, San Francisco: Filipino	50.0	33.3	-	-	-	-	16.7	-	**6**	6
US, San Francisco: Japanese	100.0	-	-	-	-	-	-	-	**1**	1
US, Connecticut: White	31.5	30.0	12.3	3.1	10.0	0.8	10.0	2.3	**130**	136
US, Connecticut: Black	-	-	16.7	33.3	33.3	-	16.7	-	**6**	7
US, Atlanta: White	34.6	38.5	7.7	9.6	-	3.8	5.8	-	**52**	52
US, Atlanta: Black	45.5	22.7	-	13.6	4.5	4.5	9.1	-	**22**	22
US, Iowa	35.6	33.6	15.1	3.4	2.1	2.1	7.5	0.7	**146**	150
US, Central Louisiana: White	62.5	12.5	-	-	-	-	25.0	-	**8**	11
US, Central Louisiana: Black	-	-	-	-	-	-	100.0	-	**1**	1
US, New Orleans: White	43.5	39.1	4.3	4.3	4.3	-	4.3	-	**23**	24
US, New Orleans: Black	58.3	25.0	-	-	-	8.3	8.3	-	**12**	13
US, Detroit: White	29.2	31.4	18.2	7.3	0.7	1.5	8.8	2.9	**137**	142
US, Detroit: Black	59.3	25.9	-	-	7.4	-	7.4	-	**27**	29
US, New Mexico: Non-Hisp White	31.3	25.0	21.9	6.3	3.1	-	9.4	3.1	**32**	33
US, New Mexico: Hispanic White	36.0	32.0	16.0	-	4.0	8.0	4.0	-	**25**	28
US, New Mexico: American Indian	66.7	33.3	-	-	-	-	-	-	**3**	3
US, Utah	44.4	24.4	20.0	3.3	2.2	2.2	3.3	-	**90**	92
US, Seattle	32.3	34.8	11.6	1.8	3.7	2.4	12.2	1.2	**164**	167
US, SEER: White	32.9	32.9	13.7	4.5	3.9	1.8	8.8	1.5	**875**	901
US, SEER: Black	48.8	23.8	3.8	6.3	7.5	1.3	8.8	-	**80**	83

PERCENTAGE DISTRIBUTION OF MICROSCOPICALLY VERIFIED CASES BY HISTOLOGICAL TYPE
Bone (ICD-9 170) - Both sexes (contd)

			Sarcoma				Other	Unspec.	Number of cases	
	Osteo	Chondro	Ewing's	Fibro	Other	Unspec.			MV	Total
ASIA										
China, Qidong										
China, Shanghai										
China, Tianjin	59.4	10.0	-	3.9	3.9	2.8	0.6	19.4	**180**	382
Hong Kong	51.9	20.3	5.1	0.6	0.6	-	20.3	1.3	**158**	301
India, Bangalore	40.6	9.0	17.4	3.2	9.7	7.1	9.7	3.2	**155**	178
India, Barshi, Paranda and Bhum	33.3	16.7	-	-	-	16.7	-	33.3	**6**	9
India, Bombay	42.2	16.7	25.5	0.8	2.4	3.6	5.2	3.6	**251**	305
India, Karunagappally	50.0	-	-	50.0	-	-	-	-	**2**	3
India, Madras	41.3	7.4	35.5	0.8	10.7	-	3.3	0.8	**121**	135
India, Trivandrum	42.9	14.3	-	-	-	-	42.9	-	**7**	8
Israel: All Jews	31.1	29.3	20.7	4.5	5.0	0.9	7.2	1.4	**222**	238
Jews born in Israel	38.5	21.3	30.3	3.3	2.5	0.8	1.6	1.6	**122**	128
Jews born in America or Europe	18.6	33.9	11.9	8.5	10.2	1.7	13.6	1.7	**59**	64
Jews born in Africa or Asia	26.8	46.3	4.9	2.4	4.9	-	14.6	-	**41**	46
Non-Jews	63.6	13.6	4.5	-	-	-	18.2	-	**22**	25
Japan, Hiroshima	46.7	36.7	3.3	3.3	-	3.3	3.3	3.3	**30**	34
Japan, Miyagi	39.7	37.9	5.2	1.7	1.7	3.4	1.7	8.6	**58**	76
Japan, Nagasaki	58.3	16.7	8.3	2.8	-	-	13.9	-	**36**	43
Japan, Osaka	45.7	26.9	7.1	6.6	3.6	0.5	3.6	6.1	**197**	243
Japan, Saga										
Japan, Yamagata										
Korea, Kangwha	33.3	-	-	-	-	16.7	-	50.0	**6**	9
Kuwait: Non-Kuwaitis	40.0	20.0	25.0	-	10.0	-	5.0	-	**20**	22
Kuwait: Kuwaitis	40.0	-	26.7	13.3	6.7	6.7	6.7	-	**15**	17
Philippines, Manila	64.5	15.0	8.4	1.9	0.9	0.9	7.5	0.9	**107**	198
Singapore: Chinese	21.8	20.7	4.6	6.9	34.5	6.9	4.6	-	**87**	93
Singapore: Malay	33.3	22.2	22.2	-	11.1	-	11.1	-	**9**	11
Singapore: Indian	36.4	18.2	18.2	-	9.1	18.2	-	-	**11**	11
Thailand, Chiang Mai	57.1	14.3	9.5	4.8	4.8	-	4.8	4.8	**21**	41
Thailand, Khon Kaen	60.0	13.3	6.7	-	6.7	-	6.7	6.7	**15**	69
Viet Nam, Hanoi	38.9	11.1	5.6	11.1	22.2	2.8	2.8	5.6	**36**	85
EUROPE										
Austria, Tyrol	29.0	22.6	22.6	3.2	6.5	-	3.2	12.9	**31**	42
Belarus										
Croatia										
Czech Republic	28.3	24.3	18.1	5.2	5.0	2.6	13.1	3.4	**382**	524
Denmark	30.3	38.5	11.0	9.2	2.3	2.8	4.6	1.4	**218**	232
Estonia	43.5	19.6	6.5	6.5	4.3	2.2	4.3	13.0	**46**	65
Finland	26.4	37.7	10.2	1.9	3.4	-	14.0	6.4	**265**	274
France, Bas-Rhin	38.0	18.0	8.0	6.0	4.0	2.0	24.0	-	**50**	54
France, Calvados	35.3	32.4	20.6	-	-	5.9	5.9	-	**34**	34
France, Doubs	33.3	20.8	29.2	-	4.2	-	12.5	-	**24**	25
France, Haut-Rhin	26.7	30.0	16.7	-	6.7	10.0	10.0	-	**30**	30
France, Herault	32.7	27.3	9.1	5.5	7.3	9.1	9.1	-	**55**	56
France, Isere	23.1	25.6	25.6	5.1	15.4	5.1	-	-	**39**	41
France, Somme	33.3	25.0	16.7	16.7	-	-	-	8.3	**12**	15
France, Tarn	38.1	23.8	28.6	4.8	4.8	-	-	-	**21**	21
Germany, Eastern States	22.0	24.1	9.8	7.0	8.7	1.1	22.2	5.1	**369**	480
Germany, Saarland										
Iceland	27.3	54.5	18.2	-	-	-	-	-	**11**	11
Ireland, Southern	22.2	55.6	16.7	5.6	-	-	-	-	**18**	20
Italy, Ferrara	-	50.0	33.3	-	-	-	16.7	-	**6**	10
Italy, Florence	14.3	33.3	33.3	4.8	-	9.5	4.8	-	**21**	57
Italy, Genoa	21.4	35.7	17.9	-	10.7	-	14.3	-	**28**	40
Italy, Latina	30.0	30.0	10.0	-	-	-	20.0	10.0	**10**	13
Italy, Macerata	-	-	33.3	-	33.3	33.3	-	-	**3**	4
Italy, Modena	61.1	5.6	-	5.6	-	16.7	11.1	-	**18**	21
Italy, Parma	31.3	37.5	18.8	6.3	-	-	6.3	-	**16**	16
Italy, Ragusa	30.8	30.8	15.4	7.7	7.7	7.7	-	-	**13**	17
Italy, Romagna	25.0	37.5	16.7	-	12.5	-	8.3	-	**24**	32
Italy, Torino	43.5	26.1	21.7	8.7	-	-	-	-	**23**	35
Italy, Trieste	-	50.0	-	-	25.0	-	-	25.0	**4**	11
Italy, Varese	12.1	45.5	18.2	6.1	6.1	9.1	3.0	-	**33**	39
Italy, Veneto	29.4	29.4	17.6	-	2.9	2.9	11.8	5.9	**34**	44
Latvia										
Malta										

Bone (ICD-9 170) - Both sexes (contd)

			Sarcoma				Other	Unspec.	Number of cases	
	Osteo	Chondro	Ewing's	Fibro	Other	Unspec.			MV	Total
The Netherlands	34.1	33.1	14.9	3.1	6.5	1.6	6.5	0.4	511	518
The Netherlands, Eindhoven	27.1	37.5	14.6	4.2	2.1	10.4	2.1	2.1	48	49
The Netherlands, Maastricht	34.2	23.7	23.7	-	10.5	-	7.9	-	38	38
Norway	34.6	38.5	14.0	0.6	3.9	1.7	4.5	2.2	179	179
Poland, Cracow	21.9	21.9	3.1	3.1	25.0	18.8	3.1	3.1	32	42
Poland, Kielce	11.8	11.8	11.8	2.9	2.9	-	50.0	8.8	34	57
Poland, Lower Silesia	12.6	29.4	2.5	2.5	7.6	2.5	6.7	36.1	119	225
Poland, Warsaw City	34.2	28.9	21.1	-	2.6	5.3	7.9	-	38	67
Slovakia	22.0	18.5	13.9	5.0	3.5	1.9	30.1	5.0	259	400
Slovenia	38.5	32.3	10.8	1.5	4.6	-	10.8	1.5	65	72
Spain, Albacete	-	60.0	40.0	-	-	-	-	-	5	9
Spain, Asturias	22.9	31.4	14.3	-	-	8.6	14.3	8.6	35	47
Spain, Basque Country	29.5	21.8	20.5	5.1	2.6	3.8	11.5	5.1	78	93
Spain, Granada	31.0	27.6	31.0	-	-	-	10.3	-	29	38
Spain, Mallorca	52.9	23.5	17.6	-	-	-	-	5.9	17	20
Spain, Murcia	20.5	34.1	38.6	-	-	2.3	4.5	-	44	55
Spain, Navarra	40.7	29.6	14.8	-	7.4	-	7.4	-	27	33
Spain, Tarragona	23.8	42.9	-	9.5	9.5	4.8	9.5	-	21	27
Spain, Zaragoza	31.3	34.4	15.6	6.3	3.1	3.1	6.3	-	32	42
Sweden	27.3	35.9	14.6	0.2	3.4	2.4	15.6	0.5	410	414
Switzerland, Basel	16.7	60.0	13.3	-	3.3	-	6.7	-	30	30
Switzerland, Geneva	33.3	33.3	26.7	-	-	-	6.7	-	15	16
Switzerland, Graubunden	40.0	20.0	-	-	-	-	40.0	-	10	11
Switzerland, Neuchatel	-	25.0	25.0	50.0	-	-	-	-	4	4
Switzerland, St Gall-Appenzell	25.8	38.7	12.9	-	12.9	-	9.7	-	31	32
Switzerland, Valais	20.0	40.0	-	-	40.0	-	-	-	5	5
Switzerland, Vaud	40.9	36.4	4.5	-	9.1	-	9.1	-	22	23
Switzerland, Zurich	26.3	51.3	8.8	-	2.5	2.5	8.8	-	80	83
UK, England and Wales	28.6	22.0	14.0	3.0	5.6	2.9	17.4	6.5	1311	1534
UK, East Anglia										
UK, Mersey	36.2	33.3	20.3	-	7.2	1.4	1.4	-	69	83
UK, North Western										
UK, Oxford	33.9	23.9	19.3	0.9	11.0	0.9	10.1	-	109	110
UK, South Thames	32.4	29.0	13.3	5.8	8.7	2.5	5.8	2.5	241	313
UK, South Western	29.5	33.0	14.3	1.8	5.4	3.6	9.8	2.7	112	141
UK, Wessex	28.8	26.0	17.3	1.0	3.8	3.8	19.2	-	104	173
UK, West Midlands										
UK, Yorkshire	34.8	32.1	17.0	-	3.6	-	9.8	2.7	112	125
UK, Scotland	35.1	23.7	19.6	1.5	3.1	1.0	15.5	0.5	194	217
UK, Scotland, West	44.2	23.0	15.0	-	1.8	0.9	14.2	0.9	113	125
Yugoslavia, Vojvodina	38.2	22.4	17.1	3.9	3.9	5.3	2.6	6.6	76	164

OCEANIA

	Osteo	Chondro	Ewing's	Fibro	Other	Unspec.	Other	Unspec.	MV	Total
Australian Capital Territory	40.0	20.0	13.3	6.7	13.3	-	6.7	-	15	16
Australia, New South Wales	35.1	31.3	12.7	5.0	5.0	1.9	7.7	1.2	259	263
South Australia	10.0	47.5	27.5	-	2.5	2.5	10.0	-	40	56
Australia, Tasmania	33.3	26.7	20.0	13.3	6.7	-	-	-	15	17
Australia, Victoria	29.7	31.6	26.4	3.3	4.7	1.4	2.8	-	212	223
Western Australia	22.4	34.1	12.9	4.7	2.4	4.7	16.5	2.4	85	91
French Polynesia	25.0	25.0	50.0	-	-	-	-	-	4	15
New Zealand: Non-Maori										
New Zealand: Maori										
US, Hawaii: White	23.1	38.5	15.4	-	7.7	-	15.4	-	13	13
US, Hawaii: Japanese	37.5	25.0	-	-	12.5	-	25.0	-	8	8
US, Hawaii: Hawaiian	62.5	12.5	12.5	-	-	-	12.5	-	8	8
US, Hawaii: Filipino	50.0	12.5	12.5	12.5	-	-	12.5	-	8	8
US, Hawaii: Chinese	-	-	-	-	-	100.0	-	-	1	1

PERCENTAGE DISTRIBUTION OF MICROSCOPICALLY VERIFIED CASES BY HISTOLOGICAL TYPE
Cervix uteri (ICD-9 180)

	Carcinoma				Sarcoma	Other	Unspecified	Number of cases	
	Squamous	Adeno	Other	Unspecified				MV	Total
AFRICA									
Algeria, Setif	90.0	4.4	-	5.6	-	-	-	**160**	166
France, La Reunion	84.8	5.7	3.3	6.0	-	0.3	-	**336**	338
Mali, Bamako	93.6	2.5	-	3.2	-	-	0.6	**157**	248
Uganda, Kyadondo	67.1	8.4	0.7	23.8	-	-	-	**143**	248
Zimbabwe, Harare: African	81.6	9.6	-	8.3	0.4	-	-	**228**	295
Zimbabwe, Harare: European	80.0	10.0	-	-	10.0	-	-	**10**	10
AMERICA, CENTRAL AND SOUTH									
Argentina, Concordia	76.0	8.7	-	12.5	-	-	2.9	**104**	108
Brazil, Belem	77.5	5.4	0.1	16.5	-	-	0.5	**832**	931
Brazil, Goiania	74.8	12.2	-	3.6	0.6	-	8.8	**477**	506
Brazil, Porto Alegre	59.3	9.3	0.2	17.6	-	-	13.6	**420**	497
Colombia, Cali	80.5	9.5	-	7.7	-	0.3	1.9	**924**	1061
Costa Rica	86.3	9.7	0.1	2.8	0.2	0.2	0.7	**1233**	1381
Ecuador, Quito	89.2	5.5	-	5.0	-	0.2	0.2	**602**	697
Peru, Lima	82.8	11.5	0.6	3.6	0.5	0.3	0.8	**1061**	1294
Peru, Trujillo	85.4	9.6	-	4.2	-	-	0.8	**260**	288
Puerto Rico	82.5	13.2	0.8	3.3	0.1	0.1	-	**789**	813
Uruguay, Montevideo	75.5	5.8	0.6	18.1	-	-	-	**514**	528
AMERICA, NORTH									
Canada	73.1	19.5	1.0	5.1	0.3	0.2	0.7	**6451**	7020
Canada, Alberta	78.9	18.6	0.6	1.6	0.3	-	-	**629**	634
Canada, British Columbia	76.5	21.6	1.0	0.6	0.1	0.3	-	**714**	728
Canada, Manitoba	73.6	21.1	1.1	3.5	-	0.7	-	**284**	290
Canada, New Brunswick	78.0	16.7	0.6	3.6	0.6	0.6	-	**168**	173
Canada, Newfoundland	80.2	17.1	-	2.1	-	-	0.5	**187**	189
Canada, Northwest Territories	73.3	3.3	3.3	6.7	-	-	13.3	**30**	32
Canada, Nova Scotia	73.4	23.1	0.9	2.2	0.3	-	-	**316**	322
Canada, Ontario	74.7	19.6	1.0	3.5	0.3	0.2	0.7	**2676**	2780
Canada, Prince Edward Island	72.5	22.5	-	5.0	-	-	-	**40**	40
Canada, Quebec	61.4	18.4	1.7	15.6	0.4	0.3	2.2	**1181**	1602
Canada, Saskatchewan	76.6	17.9	0.4	3.8	0.4	0.4	0.4	**235**	240
Canada, Yukon	80.0	20.0	-	-	-	-	-	**15**	15
US, Cent. California: Non-Hisp White	71.9	20.3	1.4	5.5	-	0.6	0.3	**345**	356
US, Cent. California: Hispanic	74.0	19.9	0.4	5.2	-	0.4	-	**231**	232
US, Los Angeles: Non-Hisp White	73.3	20.7	0.7	4.4	0.1	0.5	0.3	**916**	935
US, Los Angeles: Hispanic White	79.0	16.1	0.6	3.8	0.3	-	0.3	**1164**	1172
US, Los Angeles: Black	78.4	11.5	1.4	6.7	0.6	-	1.4	**356**	361
US, Los Angeles: Chinese	74.5	15.7	-	9.8	-	-	-	**51**	53
US, Los Angeles: Filipino	72.9	23.7	1.7	1.7	-	-	-	**59**	59
US, Los Angeles: Korean	78.0	15.3	-	6.8	-	-	-	**59**	59
US, Los Angeles: Japanese	70.0	25.0	-	5.0	-	-	-	**20**	20
US, San Francisco: Non-Hisp White	67.6	24.2	1.4	5.9	0.2	0.4	0.2	**491**	502
US, San Francisco: Hispanic White	75.6	18.6	1.3	4.5	-	-	-	**156**	157
US, San Francisco: Black	70.8	21.2	3.6	4.4	-	-	-	**137**	139
US, San Francisco: Chinese	82.4	13.7	-	3.9	-	-	-	**51**	53
US, San Francisco: Filipino	57.1	38.8	2.0	2.0	-	-	-	**49**	49
US, San Francisco: Japanese	81.8	18.2	-	-	-	-	-	**11**	11
US, Connecticut: White	67.2	22.3	1.0	8.3	0.3	0.6	0.3	**699**	714
US, Connecticut: Black	78.9	14.7	1.1	3.2	-	1.1	1.1	**95**	97
US, Atlanta: White	71.3	19.3	0.9	7.3	0.3	0.6	0.3	**342**	348
US, Atlanta: Black	75.7	15.3	1.0	7.9	-	-	-	**202**	205
US, Iowa	73.1	19.5	1.1	5.4	0.6	0.3	-	**722**	727
US, Central Louisiana: White	71.7	17.4	2.2	6.5	2.2	-	-	**46**	49
US, Central Louisiana: Black	75.0	20.8	-	-	-	4.2	-	**24**	25
US, New Orleans: White	73.2	17.4	-	8.7	-	-	0.7	**138**	139
US, New Orleans: Black	77.4	9.8	0.6	11.0	-	0.6	0.6	**164**	170
US, Detroit: White	69.5	20.4	1.3	7.7	0.3	0.3	0.6	**771**	781
US, Detroit: Black	75.1	12.0	1.4	8.9	-	0.6	2.0	**358**	369
US, New Mexico: Non-Hisp White	79.1	14.9	1.3	3.4	0.4	-	0.9	**235**	235
US, New Mexico: Hispanic White	83.6	14.3	-	0.7	-	0.7	0.7	**140**	144
US, New Mexico: American Indian	80.8	11.5	7.7	-	-	-	-	**26**	28
US, Utah	73.4	21.6	0.3	4.1	-	0.3	0.3	**342**	342
US, Seattle	75.0	21.3	0.9	2.3	0.1	0.3	0.1	**783**	791
US, SEER: White	71.9	20.8	1.0	5.4	0.3	0.3	0.3	**4590**	4650
US, SEER: Black	75.1	14.8	1.5	7.2	0.1	0.4	0.9	**847**	865

Cervix uteri (ICD-9 180) (contd)

	Squamous	Carcinoma Adeno	Carcinoma Other	Carcinoma Unspecified	Sarcoma	Other	Unspecified	Number of cases MV	Number of cases Total
ASIA									
China, Qidong									
China, Shanghai									
China, Tianjin	13.9	2.0	-	-	0.3	-	83.9	**353**	454
Hong Kong	78.0	15.7	0.6	5.4	-	0.1	0.2	**1980**	2389
India, Bangalore	90.9	4.3	0.3	3.6	0.1	0.2	0.6	**1527**	1732
India, Barshi, Paranda and Bhum	94.8	4.3	-	0.4	-	-	0.4	**233**	252
India, Bombay	89.5	7.5	0.6	1.9	-	0.1	0.5	**2362**	2818
India, Karunagappally	89.2	5.4	-	5.4	-	-	-	**37**	54
India, Madras	97.1	1.6	-	0.7	0.1	-	0.5	**2160**	2540
India, Trivandrum	94.3	2.9	-	1.9	-	1.0	-	**105**	125
Israel: All Jews	75.8	15.4	0.2	5.8	0.9	0.9	0.9	**534**	553
Jews born in Israel	77.5	12.4	-	6.2	2.2	0.6	1.1	**178**	182
Jews born in America or Europe	72.1	17.9	-	7.3	0.6	1.1	1.1	**179**	187
Jews born in Africa or Asia	78.0	15.8	0.6	4.0	-	1.1	0.6	**177**	184
Non-Jews	75.0	22.5	-	2.5	-	-	-	**40**	40
Japan, Hiroshima	88.7	10.0	0.2	0.7	-	0.4	-	**450**	456
Japan, Miyagi	74.2	13.7	0.8	5.4	-	-	5.8	**481**	525
Japan, Nagasaki	82.9	12.6	0.3	4.0	0.1	-	-	**680**	702
Japan, Osaka	85.2	11.0	0.2	0.7	-	-	2.8	**2647**	2839
Japan, Saga									
Japan, Yamagata									
Korea, Kangwha	76.2	4.8	-	1.6	-	-	17.5	**63**	71
Kuwait: Non-Kuwaitis	94.1	2.0	-	2.0	2.0	-	-	**51**	56
Kuwait: Kuwaitis	91.7	2.8	-	5.6	-	-	-	**36**	42
Philippines, Manila	77.5	15.2	0.4	5.3	0.1	0.3	1.2	**1089**	1532
Singapore: Chinese	79.2	12.7	1.5	5.8	0.2	0.2	0.3	**864**	879
Singapore: Malay	72.7	20.8	1.3	3.9	1.3	-	-	**77**	79
Singapore: Indian	81.3	12.5	-	6.3	-	-	-	**32**	32
Thailand, Chiang Mai	86.4	9.4	1.2	2.5	-	0.1	0.5	**855**	864
Thailand, Khon Kaen	80.6	18.1	-	0.8	-	-	0.5	**376**	517
Viet Nam, Hanoi	66.7	24.6	-	6.5	0.7	-	1.4	**138**	171
EUROPE									
Austria, Tyrol	78.8	10.0	0.3	3.7	-	0.9	6.3	**349**	367
Belarus									
Croatia									
Czech Republic	85.6	9.9	0.5	2.4	0.1	0.4	1.1	**5415**	5705
Denmark	78.1	18.3	0.3	2.5	0.3	0.3	0.4	**2749**	2767
Estonia	88.2	5.7	0.3	2.3	-	-	3.5	**790**	817
Finland	70.2	23.0	-	3.9	0.2	0.2	2.5	**856**	893
France, Bas-Rhin	81.1	14.2	-	2.5	-	0.3	1.9	**317**	317
France, Calvados	81.5	12.6	-	5.4	-	-	0.5	**222**	222
France, Doubs	81.9	10.2	-	6.3	-	-	1.6	**127**	129
France, Haut-Rhin	90.0	6.5	-	1.9	0.8	0.4	0.4	**260**	263
France, Herault	87.1	6.6	0.3	4.7	0.3	-	1.1	**379**	379
France, Isere	80.5	10.1	0.9	7.2	0.3	-	0.9	**318**	329
France, Somme	80.0	13.1	0.6	4.0	-	0.6	1.7	**175**	182
France, Tarn	85.3	12.7	-	2.0	-	-	-	**102**	102
Germany, Eastern States	86.8	10.8	0.4	1.7	0.1	0.2	0.1	**4679**	4722
Germany, Saarland									
Iceland	72.4	27.6	-	-	-	-	-	**58**	58
Ireland, Southern	86.3	11.6	-	2.1	-	-	-	**95**	95
Italy, Ferrara	93.3	6.7	-	-	-	-	-	**45**	47
Italy, Florence	78.5	15.5	-	5.2	-	0.4	0.4	**233**	253
Italy, Genoa	81.4	10.9	-	6.9	-	-	0.8	**247**	260
Italy, Latina	60.3	10.3	-	28.2	-	-	1.3	**78**	80
Italy, Macerata	83.3	-	-	-	-	-	16.7	**12**	12
Italy, Modena	74.3	19.4	0.7	4.9	-	-	0.7	**144**	151
Italy, Parma	76.3	14.4	1.0	8.2	-	-	-	**97**	98
Italy, Ragusa	73.3	16.0	-	5.3	1.3	1.3	2.7	**75**	75
Italy, Romagna	85.4	14.1	0.5	-	-	-	-	**199**	205
Italy, Torino	83.5	8.6	0.4	6.4	0.8	-	0.4	**266**	287
Italy, Trieste	64.2	18.7	-	15.4	-	-	1.6	**123**	134
Italy, Varese	83.2	10.7	0.5	4.6	0.5	0.5	-	**196**	200
Italy, Veneto	72.9	16.2	0.4	8.1	0.4	0.8	1.2	**247**	258
Latvia									
Malta									

Cervix uteri (ICD-9 180) (contd)

	Carcinoma				Sarcoma	Other	Unspecified	Number of cases	
	Squamous	Adeno	Other	Unspecified				MV	Total
The Netherlands	74.6	18.1	0.9	6.0	0.3	0.1	-	2930	2939
The Netherlands, Eindhoven	71.9	20.4	-	5.6	2.0	-	-	196	196
The Netherlands, Maastricht	76.3	15.6	0.9	6.7	0.4	-	-	224	224
Norway	79.6	17.0	0.7	1.1	0.1	1.1	0.5	1790	1802
Poland, Cracow	84.6	8.8	0.4	3.3	-	0.2	2.7	486	550
Poland, Kielce	76.5	7.0	0.2	12.7	-	0.4	3.2	528	567
Poland, Lower Silesia	76.2	6.5	0.2	9.6	0.1	0.2	7.3	1707	2028
Poland, Warsaw City	89.3	7.6	-	2.2	0.1	0.1	0.5	759	812
Slovakia	87.6	9.9	0.1	1.8	0.1	0.3	0.2	2557	2627
Slovenia	78.7	13.2	0.4	7.4	-	0.1	0.1	823	836
Spain, Albacete	69.6	26.1	-	4.3	-	-	-	23	24
Spain, Asturias	79.0	12.5	-	5.4	0.4	1.2	1.6	257	260
Spain, Basque Country	77.7	17.9	0.6	2.3	0.3	0.6	0.6	341	349
Spain, Granada	77.3	14.9	1.4	6.4	-	-	-	141	146
Spain, Mallorca	83.5	10.7	0.8	4.1	0.4	0.4	-	243	247
Spain, Murcia	69.0	15.5	-	13.7	0.9	-	0.9	226	236
Spain, Navarra	60.0	25.0	1.3	11.3	1.3	-	1.3	80	82
Spain, Tarragona	74.6	17.8	-	5.9	1.2	0.6	-	169	172
Spain, Zaragoza	81.2	12.3	0.7	3.6	1.4	0.7	-	138	146
Sweden	77.6	19.2	-	2.7	-	-	0.5	2459	2462
Switzerland, Basel	73.2	22.7	-	3.1	-	1.0	-	97	98
Switzerland, Geneva	88.9	10.0	-	1.1	-	-	-	90	91
Switzerland, Graubunden	76.7	18.6	-	4.7	-	-	-	43	43
Switzerland, Neuchatel	89.5	7.0	-	1.8	-	-	1.8	57	57
Switzerland, St Gall-Appenzell	76.7	21.9	-	0.7	-	0.7	-	146	147
Switzerland, Valais	71.1	20.0	-	4.4	-	2.2	2.2	45	45
Switzerland, Vaud	76.5	18.4	-	3.7	-	0.7	0.7	136	140
Switzerland, Zurich	83.1	15.3	0.3	1.0	0.3	-	-	301	302
UK, England and Wales	67.8	15.0	0.4	14.7	0.2	0.2	1.7	11849	13000
UK, East Anglia									
UK, Mersey	81.2	13.7	0.8	3.9	-	0.4	-	1020	1133
UK, North Western									
UK, Oxford	77.5	17.3	0.6	4.2	0.4	-	-	707	794
UK, South Thames	73.4	18.4	0.8	6.3	0.3	0.5	0.2	1828	2171
UK, South Western	64.9	17.2	0.5	15.0	0.3	0.4	1.7	1047	1200
UK, Wessex	69.1	20.0	0.7	9.7	0.2	0.2	0.2	1067	1197
UK, West Midlands									
UK, Yorkshire	83.0	12.3	0.2	4.1	0.1	0.3	-	1685	1752
UK, Scotland	73.7	17.4	0.5	7.8	0.2	0.4	-	2017	2183
UK, Scotland, West	75.2	15.0	0.5	8.4	0.1	0.7	0.1	1098	1177
Yugoslavia, Vojvodina	83.0	9.3	0.2	5.5	0.3	0.1	1.7	1091	1339

OCEANIA

	Carcinoma				Sarcoma	Other	Unspecified	Number of cases	
	Squamous	Adeno	Other	Unspecified				MV	Total
Australian Capital Territory	71.6	17.6	2.7	8.1	-	-	-	74	76
Australia, New South Wales	74.6	20.7	0.6	3.4	0.4	0.3	-	1757	1817
South Australia	60.2	21.4	17.2	0.6	-	0.3	0.3	309	390
Australia, Tasmania	80.3	17.0	0.7	2.0	-	-	-	147	153
Australia, Victoria	75.1	20.9	0.6	2.7	0.2	0.4	0.1	1275	1291
Western Australia	73.2	23.2	0.7	1.9	0.4	0.6	-	534	553
French Polynesia	81.5	7.4	-	9.9	1.2	-	-	81	91
New Zealand: Non-Maori									
New Zealand: Maori									
US, Hawaii: White	75.3	21.6	-	3.1	-	-	-	97	97
US, Hawaii: Japanese	63.9	27.9	3.3	4.9	-	-	-	61	61
US, Hawaii: Hawaiian	63.4	26.8	-	9.8	-	-	-	41	41
US, Hawaii: Filipino	60.6	27.3	-	12.1	-	-	-	33	33
US, Hawaii: Chinese	70.0	30.0	-	-	-	-	-	10	10

PERCENTAGE DISTRIBUTION OF MICROSCOPICALLY VERIFIED CASES BY HISTOLOGICAL TYPE
Corpus uteri (ICD-9 182)

		Carcinoma		Sarcoma	Other	Unspecified	Number of cases	
	Adeno	Other	Unspecified				MV	Total
AFRICA								
Algeria, Setif	46.2	46.2	-	-	7.7	-	13	13
France, La Reunion	77.1	4.2	-	10.4	8.3	-	48	48
Mali, Bamako	71.4	-	14.3	-	14.3	-	7	9
Uganda, Kyadondo	61.1	5.6	33.3	-	-	-	18	27
Zimbabwe, Harare: African	53.3	6.7	13.3	-	26.7	-	15	17
Zimbabwe, Harare: European	92.3	-	-	-	7.7	-	13	13
AMERICA, CENTRAL AND SOUTH								
Argentina, Concordia	96.0	-	4.0	-	-	-	25	28
Brazil, Belem	61.9	4.8	9.5	14.3	9.5	-	21	24
Brazil, Goiania	74.4	4.7	4.7	2.3	4.7	9.3	43	48
Brazil, Porto Alegre	88.3	4.9	3.9	-	1.0	1.9	103	135
Colombia, Cali	80.5	2.4	6.1	3.0	7.9	-	164	173
Costa Rica	89.2	4.1	2.1	-	3.1	1.5	195	217
Ecuador, Quito	81.8	-	14.8	2.3	-	1.1	88	106
Peru, Lima	80.4	4.1	3.4	10.1	2.0	-	148	184
Peru, Trujillo	100.0	-	-	-	-	-	13	14
Puerto Rico	88.2	0.8	0.8	3.6	6.3	0.3	719	728
Uruguay, Montevideo	86.9	1.0	2.0	8.6	1.5	-	405	455
AMERICA, NORTH								
Canada	91.1	0.9	1.5	1.6	4.2	0.6	12932	13582
Canada, Alberta	91.2	0.5	2.5	1.7	4.1	-	1061	1065
Canada, British Columbia	93.0	0.4	0.6	1.3	4.5	0.1	1650	1672
Canada, Manitoba	91.1	0.8	1.4	1.5	5.0	0.3	660	668
Canada, New Brunswick	92.4	-	1.0	1.3	5.4	-	314	315
Canada, Newfoundland	91.1	-	3.9	0.5	3.9	0.5	203	206
Canada, Northwest Territories	88.9	-	-	-	11.1	-	9	9
Canada, Nova Scotia	95.3	-	0.9	0.5	3.3	-	422	428
Canada, Ontario	90.1	0.7	1.3	2.0	4.4	1.4	5060	5300
Canada, Prince Edward Island	92.9	1.8	-	1.8	3.6	-	56	56
Canada, Quebec	91.5	2.0	1.9	1.1	3.3	0.3	3009	3369
Canada, Saskatchewan	88.5	1.4	2.7	2.0	5.3	-	488	494
Canada, Yukon	86.7	-	-	13.3	-	-	15	15
US, Cent. California: Non-Hisp White	92.4	0.5	0.5	2.3	4.1	0.1	917	925
US, Cent. California: Hispanic	85.3	2.8	2.8	3.5	5.6	-	143	143
US, Los Angeles: Non-Hisp White	92.1	0.3	0.8	1.6	5.0	0.2	3277	3294
US, Los Angeles: Hispanic White	87.8	0.5	1.8	4.0	5.8	0.2	605	608
US, Los Angeles: Black	73.8	0.6	3.1	8.1	13.4	0.9	321	325
US, Los Angeles: Chinese	88.9	2.2	4.4	-	4.4	-	45	46
US, Los Angeles: Filipino	94.6	-	-	1.4	4.1	-	74	74
US, Los Angeles: Korean	80.0	-	-	20.0	-	-	10	10
US, Los Angeles: Japanese	93.2	-	-	4.5	2.3	-	44	44
US, San Francisco: Non-Hisp White	91.8	0.2	1.1	1.8	5.0	0.1	1750	1760
US, San Francisco: Hispanic White	90.2	1.3	1.3	2.0	5.2	-	153	153
US, San Francisco: Black	75.9	2.1	2.1	5.5	13.8	0.7	145	147
US, San Francisco: Chinese	91.2	2.2	1.1	3.3	2.2	-	91	91
US, San Francisco: Filipino	85.4	-	2.1	6.3	6.3	-	48	48
US, San Francisco: Japanese	97.0	-	-	-	3.0	-	33	33
US, Connecticut: White	92.5	0.3	1.5	1.4	4.4	0.1	2206	2222
US, Connecticut: Black	82.4	-	1.2	5.9	10.6	-	85	86
US, Atlanta: White	91.8	0.3	1.0	2.4	4.4	0.1	708	710
US, Atlanta: Black	76.5	-	0.7	5.9	16.3	0.7	153	155
US, Iowa	92.6	0.2	0.7	1.6	4.7	0.1	2003	2025
US, Central Louisiana: White	87.8	2.7	1.4	2.7	5.4	-	74	75
US, Central Louisiana: Black	72.2	-	5.6	11.1	11.1	-	18	22
US, New Orleans: White	91.8	1.7	0.9	0.4	5.2	-	231	235
US, New Orleans: Black	78.8	4.0	1.0	2.0	14.1	-	99	101
US, Detroit: White	90.7	0.3	1.7	1.6	5.3	0.4	2202	2217
US, Detroit: Black	79.5	1.7	2.3	4.6	10.7	1.2	346	350
US, New Mexico: Non-Hisp White	90.8	0.4	1.5	1.9	5.0	0.4	480	486
US, New Mexico: Hispanic White	88.7	0.8	2.3	3.8	4.5	-	133	134
US, New Mexico: American Indian	91.7	-	-	-	8.3	-	24	24
US, Utah	91.7	-	1.6	1.2	5.4	0.1	830	833
US, Seattle	92.0	-	2.0	2.1	3.7	0.1	2210	2225
US, SEER: White	91.8	0.2	1.4	1.7	4.6	0.2	12637	12727
US, SEER: Black	78.5	1.3	1.8	5.4	12.4	0.8	785	794

Corpus uteri (ICD-9 182) (contd)

	Adeno	Carcinoma Other	Unspecified	Sarcoma	Other	Unspecified	Number of cases MV	Total
ASIA								
China, Qidong								
China, Shanghai								
China, Tianjin	69.1	2.4	-	4.0	0.8	23.7	249	280
Hong Kong	82.2	3.9	3.9	3.6	5.9	0.3	912	1040
India, Bangalore	81.6	4.4	4.4	0.9	7.9	0.9	114	118
India, Barshi, Paranda and Bhum	66.7	-	33.3	-	-	-	3	3
India, Bombay	78.7	9.7	1.4	1.8	7.6	0.7	277	296
India, Karunagappally	75.0	25.0	-	-	-	-	4	4
India, Madras	82.9	7.7	1.7	5.1	1.7	0.9	117	127
India, Trivandrum	80.0	-	-	-	20.0	-	15	17
Israel: All Jews	85.1	0.8	4.0	3.5	6.5	-	1211	1241
Jews born in Israel	87.6	1.0	1.5	5.7	4.1	-	194	200
Jews born in America or Europe	86.0	0.8	4.1	2.4	6.7	-	750	764
Jews born in Africa or Asia	80.8	0.8	5.6	4.9	7.9	-	266	276
Non-Jews	75.9	-	5.6	3.7	13.0	1.9	54	54
Japan, Hiroshima	85.2	1.8	1.8	4.1	7.1	-	169	171
Japan, Miyagi	78.8	1.0	3.9	6.1	2.9	7.4	311	339
Japan, Nagasaki	91.8	1.6	0.4	1.2	4.9	-	245	257
Japan, Osaka	85.1	0.8	0.5	7.1	3.2	3.3	875	932
Japan, Saga								
Japan, Yamagata								
Korea, Kangwha	100.0	-	-	-	-	-	1	1
Kuwait: Non-Kuwaitis	94.1	-	-	-	5.9	-	17	17
Kuwait: Kuwaitis	71.4	-	7.1	-	21.4	-	14	14
Philippines, Manila	83.8	1.7	8.1	1.3	4.4	0.7	297	362
Singapore: Chinese	77.9	0.3	5.9	9.2	6.1	0.6	358	366
Singapore: Malay	71.4	-	11.4	8.6	8.6	-	35	38
Singapore: Indian	80.0	5.0	-	5.0	10.0	-	20	20
Thailand, Chiang Mai	85.4	3.4	3.4	3.4	2.2	2.2	89	110
Thailand, Khon Kaen	87.5	-	2.5	-	10.0	-	40	54
Viet Nam, Hanoi	59.3	11.1	14.8	14.8	-	-	27	41
EUROPE								
Austria, Tyrol	82.4	1.7	3.7	4.0	7.0	1.3	301	312
Belarus								
Croatia								
Czech Republic	90.9	1.7	1.8	2.2	3.1	0.4	6685	7096
Denmark	91.5	0.6	1.0	2.1	4.5	0.4	3151	3165
Estonia	86.4	1.1	1.1	4.4	3.6	3.3	809	835
Finland	90.6	0.4	1.0	4.2	1.5	2.3	3251	3283
France, Bas-Rhin	89.4	0.7	1.6	3.3	4.0	0.9	568	571
France, Calvados	87.5	1.5	5.5	2.0	3.0	0.5	200	200
France, Doubs	89.1	1.1	2.3	2.3	4.6	0.6	175	176
France, Haut-Rhin	90.5	1.3	0.3	3.1	4.9	-	390	393
France, Herault	92.9	0.3	0.9	3.4	2.3	0.3	350	350
France, Isere	84.8	2.2	1.7	6.1	5.2	-	363	371
France, Somme	92.2	0.5	3.1	2.1	2.1	-	193	195
France, Tarn	91.0	-	4.2	1.2	3.6	-	167	167
Germany, Eastern States	89.3	1.3	2.1	3.0	4.2	0.1	3969	4021
Germany, Saarland								
Iceland	85.7	-	-	4.8	9.5	-	105	105
Ireland, Southern	85.9	0.7	3.0	3.0	7.4	-	135	137
Italy, Ferrara	92.6	-	-	-	7.4	-	95	98
Italy, Florence	92.2	1.1	1.0	1.5	4.2	-	525	550
Italy, Genoa	91.7	1.2	0.9	1.2	4.6	0.3	324	347
Italy, Latina	82.8	0.9	4.3	5.2	6.9	-	116	117
Italy, Macerata	89.3	-	-	2.7	6.7	1.3	75	76
Italy, Modena	93.5	0.6	0.6	2.3	3.1	-	355	357
Italy, Parma	96.0	-	2.0	1.6	0.4	-	247	250
Italy, Ragusa	86.9	2.3	2.3	3.1	4.6	0.8	130	130
Italy, Romagna	85.2	0.7	1.1	5.4	7.6	-	277	283
Italy, Torino	89.0	1.2	1.7	4.1	3.6	0.5	419	439
Italy, Trieste	86.5	1.4	4.7	2.0	2.0	3.4	148	175
Italy, Varese	87.8	0.9	1.6	4.0	5.1	0.7	450	460
Italy, Veneto	91.0	1.1	1.6	2.9	2.5	0.9	443	463
Latvia								
Malta								

Corpus uteri (ICD-9 182) (contd)

	Carcinoma			Sarcoma	Other	Unspecified	Number of cases	
	Adeno	Other	Unspecified				MV	Total
The Netherlands	92.1	0.2	0.5	2.8	4.4	-	**5107**	5129
The Netherlands, Eindhoven	91.9	-	0.3	2.7	5.1	-	**333**	334
The Netherlands, Maastricht	91.0	-	0.5	4.9	3.6	-	**366**	366
Norway	85.1	0.4	0.9	3.8	9.3	0.6	**2104**	2122
Poland, Cracow	81.1	3.2	7.7	4.2	2.2	1.6	**312**	342
Poland, Kielce	81.5	1.2	10.3	3.5	2.1	1.5	**341**	372
Poland, Lower Silesia	86.5	1.7	2.8	2.0	2.8	4.3	**868**	1112
Poland, Warsaw City	90.8	0.6	2.0	3.2	3.2	0.3	**717**	740
Slovakia	90.7	1.1	1.6	2.7	3.7	0.2	**2610**	2736
Slovenia	94.9	0.1	1.8	0.4	2.6	0.2	**933**	940
Spain, Albacete	85.7	-	-	-	14.3	-	**28**	32
Spain, Asturias	89.8	2.5	0.7	2.5	4.4	-	**433**	437
Spain, Basque Country	92.3	0.9	1.2	1.4	4.0	0.2	**573**	589
Spain, Granada	90.4	-	0.8	2.7	6.1	-	**261**	271
Spain, Mallorca	87.5	-	1.5	3.8	6.8	0.4	**263**	270
Spain, Murcia	89.6	0.5	1.9	4.6	2.7	0.5	**367**	377
Spain, Navarra	84.5	0.9	1.8	3.2	9.5	-	**220**	226
Spain, Tarragona	86.8	1.2	1.2	4.8	6.0	-	**250**	254
Spain, Zaragoza	88.3	2.4	2.4	3.8	2.7	0.3	**291**	312
Sweden	98.4	0.1	1.0	0.5	-	0.1	**5105**	5113
Switzerland, Basel	91.5	0.8	0.4	2.3	5.0	-	**259**	260
Switzerland, Geneva	93.3	0.5	1.0	1.0	4.3	-	**210**	214
Switzerland, Graubunden	88.5	-	1.9	-	9.6	-	**52**	53
Switzerland, Neuchatel	86.9	-	3.6	2.4	7.1	-	**84**	87
Switzerland, St Gall-Appenzell	93.1	-	0.4	1.3	5.2	-	**232**	234
Switzerland, Valais	88.0	1.3	-	5.3	5.3	-	**75**	75
Switzerland, Vaud	88.8	0.3	0.3	3.3	7.4	-	**338**	342
Switzerland, Zurich	92.5	0.1	0.3	1.7	5.4	-	**763**	775
UK, England and Wales	80.2	1.2	12.1	2.1	3.7	0.8	**9938**	11369
UK, East Anglia								
UK, Mersey	86.8	2.1	3.1	3.4	4.6	-	**818**	903
UK, North Western								
UK, Oxford	90.3	0.8	2.7	3.5	2.7	-	**856**	957
UK, South Thames	83.6	1.3	6.9	3.2	4.7	0.2	**2195**	2666
UK, South Western	81.4	1.1	10.8	1.9	3.7	1.0	**1347**	1454
UK, Wessex	85.8	0.9	8.2	1.6	3.5	-	**1173**	1326
UK, West Midlands								
UK, Yorkshire	89.9	0.7	4.7	1.5	3.1	0.1	**1243**	1282
UK, Scotland	87.3	1.2	3.7	2.0	5.6	0.2	**1469**	1594
UK, Scotland, West	86.9	1.3	5.2	2.0	4.5	0.1	**710**	761
Yugoslavia, Vojvodina	88.2	1.8	3.7	4.3	1.4	0.6	**651**	806

OCEANIA

	Carcinoma			Sarcoma	Other	Unspecified	Number of cases	
	Adeno	Other	Unspecified				MV	Total
Australian Capital Territory	95.7	-	-	2.2	2.2	-	**46**	46
Australia, New South Wales	88.9	0.5	3.2	3.4	3.8	0.2	**1733**	1754
South Australia	89.7	0.2	0.7	4.0	5.5	-	**455**	556
Australia, Tasmania	85.6	1.3	1.9	1.9	9.4	-	**160**	165
Australia, Victoria	88.6	0.2	1.8	2.8	6.6	-	**1477**	1531
Western Australia	87.8	1.4	1.4	2.4	7.0	-	**500**	519
French Polynesia	75.0	7.1	3.6	7.1	7.1	-	**28**	31
New Zealand: Non-Maori								
New Zealand: Maori								
US, Hawaii: White	90.8	-	3.5	1.4	3.5	0.7	**141**	141
US, Hawaii: Japanese	92.8	0.6	3.0	0.6	3.0	-	**166**	166
US, Hawaii: Hawaiian	91.2	-	3.3	1.1	4.4	-	**91**	91
US, Hawaii: Filipino	94.0	-	-	-	6.0	-	**50**	50
US, Hawaii: Chinese	91.2	-	5.9	2.9	-	-	**34**	34

PERCENTAGE DISTRIBUTION OF MICROSCOPICALLY VERIFIED CASES BY HISTOLOGICAL TYPE
Ovary (ICD-9 183.0)

	Carcinoma							Sex cord stromal	Germ cell	Other	Unsp.	Number of cases	
	Serous	Mucin.	Endom.	Clear	Adeno	Other	Unsp.					MV	Total
AFRICA													
Algeria, Setif	-	71.4	-	-	14.3	-	14.3	-	-	-	-	7	14
France, La Reunion	26.2	18.0	11.5	1.6	21.3	-	6.6	4.9	6.6	1.6	1.6	61	62
Mali, Bamako	-	-	-	14.3	14.3	-	71.4	-	-	-	-	7	10
Uganda, Kyadondo	-	3.0	-	-	39.4	6.1	21.2	9.1	21.2	-	-	33	45
Zimbabwe, Harare: African	19.0	4.8	-	-	33.3	4.8	9.5	14.3	9.5	4.8	-	21	36
Zimbabwe, Harare: European	50.0	-	-	-	10.0	-	10.0	20.0	10.0	-	-	10	13
AMERICA, CENTRAL AND SOUTH													
Argentina, Concordia	35.3	5.9	-	5.9	23.5	5.9	11.8	5.9	-	-	5.9	17	26
Brazil, Belem	23.8	7.1	-	-	31.0	9.5	7.1	7.1	9.5	2.4	2.4	42	61
Brazil, Goiania	3.4	3.4	-	-	57.6	5.1	6.8	-	3.4	-	20.3	59	67
Brazil, Porto Alegre	16.7	6.7	2.5	0.8	36.7	0.8	11.7	0.8	5.0	0.8	17.5	120	175
Colombia, Cali	38.3	10.7	4.9	1.5	19.4	2.9	11.7	1.9	6.3	1.0	1.5	206	261
Costa Rica	29.8	15.3	8.9	0.4	13.6	5.1	6.8	2.6	15.3	1.3	0.9	235	329
Ecuador, Quito	32.0	3.9	2.9	2.9	35.0	-	6.8	1.0	13.6	-	1.9	103	139
Peru, Lima	20.2	12.0	12.5	7.7	22.1	0.5	4.3	5.3	11.1	3.4	1.0	208	292
Peru, Trujillo	34.4	12.5	6.3	-	18.8	-	9.4	3.1	3.1	3.1	9.4	32	39
Puerto Rico	32.3	13.6	8.1	3.8	22.0	3.0	6.3	1.8	6.1	2.0	1.0	396	436
Uruguay, Montevideo	23.9	14.7	3.0	1.0	42.6	1.5	8.1	-	2.0	3.0	-	197	296
AMERICA, NORTH													
Canada	36.8	13.1	12.6	4.6	18.6	1.7	3.5	1.5	3.2	2.7	1.7	8156	9487
Canada, Alberta	45.9	15.4	10.8	6.3	7.9	1.4	2.7	2.4	3.7	2.4	1.0	697	725
Canada, British Columbia	43.9	10.3	10.3	5.5	17.8	1.5	4.2	0.9	2.7	2.5	0.5	1130	1220
Canada, Manitoba	36.0	11.4	13.6	6.3	16.5	1.8	4.0	2.2	4.8	2.9	0.4	272	369
Canada, New Brunswick	39.7	11.7	10.7	6.1	14.5	1.9	6.5	2.8	2.8	3.3	-	214	224
Canada, Newfoundland	35.4	18.4	11.6	2.0	14.3	2.0	6.1	4.1	2.7	2.7	0.7	147	153
Canada, Northwest Territories	7.7	15.4	7.7	-	38.5	-	7.7	-	-	-	23.1	13	14
Canada, Nova Scotia	29.2	15.7	12.8	5.8	25.5	2.2	1.1	1.8	3.6	2.2	-	274	316
Canada, Ontario	33.9	11.9	13.1	4.2	21.6	1.8	2.7	1.4	2.9	3.5	3.0	3238	3795
Canada, Prince Edward Island	40.6	12.5	18.8	9.4	9.4	3.1	-	3.1	-	3.1	-	32	33
Canada, Quebec	36.1	14.7	14.0	3.5	17.6	1.9	4.7	1.1	3.3	1.8	1.3	1812	2295
Canada, Saskatchewan	31.4	17.7	12.2	4.6	22.3	0.3	4.0	1.2	4.0	2.1	0.3	328	345
Canada, Yukon	41.2	23.5	5.9	5.9	17.6	-	-	5.9	-	-	-	17	17
US, Cent. California: Non-Hisp White	33.7	12.2	11.6	2.6	27.3	1.3	4.2	1.7	2.0	3.1	0.4	543	576
US, Cent. California: Hispanic	35.9	12.6	9.7	1.9	17.5	2.9	2.9	1.0	12.6	1.9	1.0	103	107
US, Los Angeles: Non-Hisp White	32.1	10.1	11.0	3.4	31.3	2.1	3.6	1.1	1.8	3.1	0.6	1900	1953
US, Los Angeles: Hispanic White	29.0	11.4	10.8	2.8	25.2	2.3	4.9	1.9	8.5	2.1	1.1	472	498
US, Los Angeles: Black	25.3	9.7	10.1	1.4	33.2	3.7	4.6	3.2	6.5	1.8	0.5	217	236
US, Los Angeles: Chinese	22.7	18.2	18.2	9.1	11.4	6.8	2.3	2.3	4.5	4.5	-	44	45
US, Los Angeles: Filipino	10.7	7.1	23.2	10.7	28.6	5.4	1.8	-	10.7	1.8	-	56	59
US, Los Angeles: Korean	21.1	26.3	10.5	15.8	15.8	-	-	-	10.5	-	-	19	19
US, Los Angeles: Japanese	23.8	14.3	28.6	7.1	16.7	2.4	2.4	-	2.4	2.4	-	42	43
US, San Francisco: Non-Hisp White	36.5	10.5	10.7	3.5	23.4	2.1	4.7	1.4	2.4	4.0	0.7	1062	1123
US, San Francisco: Hispanic White	33.0	10.7	14.6	1.9	26.2	1.9	1.9	1.0	3.9	2.9	1.9	103	104
US, San Francisco: Black	28.1	14.9	12.3	-	24.6	2.6	6.1	2.6	5.3	3.5	-	114	122
US, San Francisco: Chinese	30.6	4.8	19.4	6.5	17.7	3.2	4.8	1.6	4.8	4.8	1.6	62	64
US, San Francisco: Filipino	25.0	22.2	2.8	11.1	13.9	2.8	5.6	-	16.7	-	-	36	36
US, San Francisco: Japanese	20.0	13.3	20.0	26.7	13.3	-	-	-	6.7	-	-	15	16
US, Connecticut: White	35.2	9.7	15.0	4.4	22.1	2.0	4.8	0.7	2.3	2.9	0.8	1259	1334
US, Connecticut: Black	11.9	2.4	14.3	2.4	31.0	2.4	9.5	2.4	16.7	7.1	-	42	44
US, Atlanta: White	36.7	10.6	9.4	4.7	27.3	1.6	2.8	0.6	3.1	3.1	-	509	529
US, Atlanta: Black	30.0	17.0	9.0	-	29.0	-	2.0	-	6.0	6.0	1.0	100	109
US, Iowa	35.4	11.6	10.1	3.2	28.0	1.3	3.4	1.7	2.5	2.2	0.6	1254	1328
US, Central Louisiana: White	26.9	13.4	9.0	1.5	34.3	6.0	1.5	3.0	1.5	3.0	-	67	75
US, Central Louisiana: Black	26.7	-	-	-	46.7	-	6.7	6.7	6.7	-	6.7	15	17
US, New Orleans: White	26.8	10.2	13.0	4.1	33.3	4.5	1.6	1.2	1.2	4.1	-	246	265
US, New Orleans: Black	35.8	11.9	7.5	-	25.4	4.5	-	6.0	6.0	3.0	-	67	80
US, Detroit: White	37.9	9.9	12.3	4.9	23.4	1.6	3.9	0.6	1.9	2.9	0.8	1297	1355
US, Detroit: Black	29.2	11.5	5.3	3.3	26.8	1.4	5.3	3.8	6.2	3.8	3.3	209	230
US, New Mexico: Non-Hisp White	37.1	12.4	7.7	2.7	28.8	1.7	4.3	1.3	2.3	0.7	1.0	299	315
US, New Mexico: Hispanic White	42.5	5.7	8.5	2.8	23.6	1.9	4.7	0.9	4.7	4.7	-	106	116
US, New Mexico: American Indian	32.4	8.8	8.8	2.9	20.6	2.9	2.9	-	11.8	8.8	-	34	36
US, Utah	33.4	8.6	14.4	4.3	19.4	2.3	8.1	2.7	3.6	2.5	0.7	443	461
US, Seattle	39.2	8.1	9.8	3.7	26.5	1.3	5.0	0.7	2.3	2.8	0.5	1240	1310
US, SEER: White	36.5	10.0	11.5	4.0	24.8	1.7	4.5	1.1	2.4	2.9	0.6	7602	8001
US, SEER: Black	28.7	12.5	8.3	1.8	26.7	1.4	5.1	2.6	6.9	4.4	1.6	495	539

			Carcinoma					Sex cord	Germ	Other	Unsp.	Number of cases	
	Serous	Mucin.	Endom.	Clear	Adeno	Other	Unsp.	stromal	cell			MV	Total
ASIA													
China, Qidong													
China, Shanghai													
China, Tianjin	14.6	6.0	1.2	0.9	10.4	2.4	-	3.9	3.6	1.2	56.0	**336**	456
Hong Kong													
India, Bangalore	15.6	8.2	0.4	2.0	34.8	2.9	4.9	2.5	13.5	2.0	13.1	**244**	285
India, Barshi, Paranda and Bhum	9.1	9.1	-	9.1	18.2	9.1	-	27.3	18.2	-	-	**11**	12
India, Bombay	22.9	9.7	4.6	1.0	42.0	3.0	4.7	0.7	7.7	1.3	2.4	**700**	979
India, Karunagappally	-	40.0	-	-	40.0	-	-	-	20.0	-	-	**5**	5
India, Madras	23.8	4.9	0.8	0.8	42.6	2.3	1.9	4.2	10.6	1.1	7.2	**265**	386
India, Trivandrum	30.0	13.3	6.7	3.3	23.3	-	3.3	-	6.7	6.7	6.7	**30**	34
Israel: All Jews	42.2	7.5	12.4	2.5	20.1	3.2	5.9	1.2	2.7	1.5	0.9	**1093**	1252
Jews born in Israel	45.4	6.6	11.8	4.4	14.0	2.2	4.4	1.3	8.7	0.9	0.4	**229**	246
Jews born in America or Europe	40.9	6.9	14.1	1.9	22.1	3.3	6.1	0.9	1.1	1.7	0.9	**638**	750
Jews born in Africa or Asia	41.9	10.4	7.7	2.3	21.2	4.1	6.8	1.8	1.4	1.4	1.4	**222**	251
Non-Jews	21.2	15.2	24.2	3.0	24.2	-	6.1	-	6.1	-	-	**33**	37
Japan, Hiroshima	30.8	19.9	8.5	8.0	16.9	1.0	3.5	0.5	9.5	1.5	-	**201**	221
Japan, Miyagi	17.2	17.4	7.3	10.5	29.7	1.5	4.4	0.3	4.1	1.2	6.7	**344**	485
Japan, Nagasaki	25.6	22.7	6.2	11.0	18.2	3.2	2.6	0.3	7.8	1.9	0.3	**308**	373
Japan, Osaka	25.4	15.9	5.4	7.6	28.5	2.1	1.2	1.2	4.6	0.9	7.2	**1196**	1690
Japan, Saga													
Japan, Yamagata													
Korea, Kangwha	14.3	28.6	-	-	28.6	-	-	14.3	-	-	14.3	**7**	7
Kuwait: Non-Kuwaitis	37.5	20.0	5.0	5.0	20.0	-	5.0	-	7.5	-	-	**40**	43
Kuwait: Kuwaitis	36.8	10.5	-	-	42.1	5.3	5.3	-	-	-	-	**19**	25
Philippines, Manila	21.9	21.2	13.3	3.7	14.7	2.8	7.0	1.8	8.3	1.5	3.7	**457**	677
Singapore: Chinese	9.9	32.6	9.5	8.8	22.2	3.8	1.8	2.5	7.2	1.4	0.2	**555**	576
Singapore: Malay	16.9	31.0	2.8	2.8	26.8	1.4	2.8	4.2	11.3	-	-	**71**	77
Singapore: Indian	19.2	15.4	15.4	3.8	38.5	3.8	-	-	3.8	-	-	**26**	28
Thailand, Chiang Mai	18.3	35.1	6.1	3.1	8.4	1.5	3.1	0.8	11.5	0.8	11.5	**131**	146
Thailand, Khon Kaen	15.4	36.3	5.5	3.3	26.4	1.1	2.2	1.1	7.7	-	1.1	**91**	123
Viet Nam, Hanoi	4.3	8.5	4.3	4.3	34.0	4.3	12.8	4.3	8.5	2.1	12.8	**47**	58
EUROPE													
Austria, Tyrol	33.8	18.1	5.4	2.0	20.4	1.0	7.4	1.7	3.0	2.0	5.4	**299**	311
Belarus													
Croatia													
Czech Republic	39.1	15.7	7.5	1.9	16.9	2.7	5.5	4.4	2.4	1.0	2.8	**3893**	4828
Denmark	37.3	11.2	11.7	3.8	22.6	0.5	5.7	1.3	1.8	3.3	0.9	**2735**	2807
Estonia	30.4	8.0	4.0	2.4	14.1	2.2	3.2	3.6	2.4	0.4	29.3	**697**	772
Finland													
France, Bas-Rhin	46.6	16.8	6.7	1.3	16.1	1.8	4.1	1.8	2.1	1.8	0.8	**386**	402
France, Calvados	41.6	10.5	12.1	3.2	23.2	1.1	2.6	1.1	0.5	2.1	2.1	**190**	193
France, Doubs	35.7	7.0	10.1	0.8	35.7	3.9	4.7	0.8	0.8	-	0.8	**129**	136
France, Haut-Rhin	40.6	10.2	5.3	2.5	32.0	0.8	3.7	0.8	1.6	1.6	0.8	**244**	250
France, Herault	32.5	16.3	3.8	2.9	35.9	2.4	2.9	1.9	1.0	-	0.5	**209**	210
France, Isere	45.7	13.4	9.1	1.1	19.2	1.8	4.0	0.7	3.3	1.4	0.4	**276**	293
France, Somme	25.0	9.4	9.4	2.8	37.8	-	7.2	1.1	3.3	2.2	1.7	**180**	196
France, Tarn	43.9	8.9	4.9	0.8	28.5	3.3	3.3	1.6	2.4	-	2.4	**123**	127
Germany, Eastern States	32.5	11.0	3.7	1.6	35.0	1.7	5.4	4.7	1.3	1.2	1.8	**3098**	3262
Germany, Saarland													
Iceland	44.7	10.6	12.9	7.1	11.8	1.2	2.4	1.2	1.2	7.1	-	**85**	87
Ireland, Southern	37.9	10.8	3.4	2.5	28.6	5.4	5.9	2.5	1.5	1.5	-	**203**	218
Italy, Ferrara	39.6	14.6	4.2	2.1	25.0	2.1	6.3	-	2.1	4.2	-	**48**	54
Italy, Florence	42.0	10.1	12.9	1.7	10.5	1.7	12.2	1.0	2.1	1.7	3.8	**286**	403
Italy, Genoa	33.1	9.2	5.6	2.1	28.5	1.1	8.5	2.5	3.2	4.2	2.1	**284**	351
Italy, Latina	17.9	3.8	5.1	2.6	35.9	-	29.5	1.3	1.3	1.3	1.3	**78**	91
Italy, Macerata	25.0	5.0	10.0	-	42.5	-	5.0	-	2.5	-	10.0	**40**	52
Italy, Modena	39.4	9.1	12.9	1.2	24.5	0.8	6.2	1.2	2.5	1.7	0.4	**241**	296
Italy, Parma	25.1	11.7	5.8	2.3	29.8	9.4	12.3	0.6	0.6	1.8	0.6	**171**	198
Italy, Ragusa	26.7	1.7	1.7	1.7	45.0	-	6.7	1.7	-	-	15.0	**60**	80
Italy, Romagna	31.8	12.9	11.2	1.8	27.1	1.2	5.3	1.8	2.9	1.8	2.4	**170**	196
Italy, Torino	25.2	10.3	10.3	5.0	28.5	2.9	7.4	0.4	2.9	2.9	4.1	**242**	278
Italy, Trieste	23.4	3.1	-	1.6	40.6	-	10.9	1.6	-	3.1	15.6	**64**	104
Italy, Varese	38.6	13.8	6.1	2.9	24.4	0.3	8.0	1.0	1.6	1.3	1.9	**311**	340
Italy, Veneto	22.9	11.4	5.9	0.7	35.3	3.6	5.6	3.9	4.6	1.6	4.6	**306**	317
Latvia													
Malta													

PERCENTAGE DISTRIBUTION OF MICROSCOPICALLY VERIFIED CASES BY HISTOLOGICAL TYPE
Ovary (ICD-9 183.0) (contd)

	Carcinoma							Sex cord stromal	Germ cell	Other	Unsp.	Number of cases	
	Serous	Mucin.	Endom.	Clear	Adeno	Other	Unsp.					MV	Total
The Netherlands	29.5	14.0	8.9	4.0	35.6	0.2	2.0	1.4	1.9	2.5	0.1	**4800**	4904
The Netherlands, Eindhoven	35.6	19.4	10.3	4.7	20.3	0.9	0.9	1.8	2.4	3.8	-	**340**	343
The Netherlands, Maastricht	30.4	11.3	6.8	3.9	38.1	0.3	2.1	2.7	2.4	2.1	-	**336**	342
Norway													
Poland, Cracow	15.7	10.6	1.4	0.7	34.8	9.2	9.9	6.1	4.1	1.0	6.5	**293**	372
Poland, Kielce	13.0	3.6	1.8	0.9	46.2	4.9	21.5	2.7	2.2	-	3.1	**223**	280
Poland, Lower Silesia	16.9	5.9	7.0	1.2	23.1	2.6	7.9	5.5	3.9	0.8	25.1	**724**	1239
Poland, Warsaw City	32.1	16.2	8.3	2.1	24.3	0.2	4.8	7.1	2.1	1.8	1.1	**567**	707
Slovakia	37.5	15.7	5.7	2.6	18.7	1.7	6.6	5.0	3.9	1.6	1.1	**1601**	1785
Slovenia	29.8	8.9	15.6	3.2	29.8	1.2	7.2	1.0	1.9	1.3	0.1	**694**	746
Spain, Albacete	22.9	5.7	8.6	2.9	28.6	2.9	14.3	2.9	5.7	2.9	2.9	**35**	39
Spain, Asturias	29.4	13.9	11.1	6.1	20.6	2.7	7.8	1.7	3.7	1.4	1.7	**296**	328
Spain, Basque Country	29.6	14.5	9.4	5.3	24.3	3.1	6.3	0.5	3.1	2.4	1.4	**415**	470
Spain, Granada	25.7	12.2	24.3	4.7	16.9	0.7	7.4	0.7	5.4	2.0	-	**148**	172
Spain, Mallorca	21.3	17.7	13.5	4.3	35.5	-	2.1	1.4	2.1	-	2.1	**141**	154
Spain, Murcia	33.6	19.5	11.1	3.1	14.6	4.9	7.1	2.2	1.3	2.2	0.4	**226**	248
Spain, Navarra	27.0	22.0	11.3	2.1	19.9	2.8	6.4	-	2.8	4.3	1.4	**141**	158
Spain, Tarragona	38.5	13.8	13.1	3.8	17.7	0.8	6.2	-	5.4	-	0.8	**130**	142
Spain, Zaragoza	31.6	15.0	10.7	3.9	23.3	0.5	6.3	0.5	1.9	4.9	1.5	**206**	267
Sweden													
Switzerland, Basel	52.9	8.5	13.8	3.7	10.1	1.1	2.6	2.1	3.2	2.1	-	**189**	192
Switzerland, Geneva	30.5	15.0	11.8	7.5	20.9	-	5.9	0.5	1.1	7.0	-	**187**	195
Switzerland, Graubunden	46.7	5.0	3.3	5.0	23.3	-	3.3	6.7	3.3	1.7	1.7	**60**	69
Switzerland, Neuchatel	32.0	20.0	12.0	1.3	21.3	-	4.0	4.0	-	5.3	-	**75**	80
Switzerland, St Gall-Appenzell	29.1	8.6	9.5	2.7	40.0	0.5	2.3	1.4	2.7	3.2	-	**220**	232
Switzerland, Valais	43.1	19.4	6.9	5.6	13.9	-	2.8	2.8	4.2	1.4	-	**72**	78
Switzerland, Vaud	44.4	6.9	10.8	3.9	18.1	2.2	7.3	0.9	1.3	3.9	0.4	**232**	242
Switzerland, Zurich	41.5	11.5	5.7	4.3	24.1	0.4	3.0	3.0	2.6	3.6	0.2	**494**	504
UK, England and Wales	19.5	11.0	6.3	2.8	32.3	1.8	20.5	1.1	1.4	2.0	1.4	**12286**	15283
UK, East Anglia													
UK, Mersey	22.8	16.1	5.5	4.1	38.4	1.0	8.4	0.8	1.1	1.8	-	**836**	1069
UK, North Western													
UK, Oxford	22.8	12.4	7.5	4.6	38.1	2.8	6.4	1.9	1.3	2.1	-	**968**	1206
UK, South Thames	22.1	10.9	5.0	3.0	42.6	1.9	9.9	1.1	1.1	2.2	0.3	**2699**	3742
UK, South Western	20.9	10.8	4.4	3.1	36.5	2.6	14.4	1.2	1.4	2.5	2.2	**1254**	1729
UK, Wessex	23.4	9.6	7.7	3.0	24.6	2.2	26.3	0.4	0.9	2.0	-	**1287**	1634
UK, West Midlands													
UK, Yorkshire	25.9	11.6	11.0	4.0	33.3	2.0	6.2	1.1	1.5	3.2	0.1	**1512**	1763
UK, Scotland	23.8	12.4	7.4	3.6	37.4	2.4	6.2	1.8	1.3	2.9	0.9	**2380**	2807
UK, Scotland, West	20.5	10.3	4.7	2.7	47.8	2.6	5.2	1.6	1.4	2.8	0.3	**1179**	1445
Yugoslavia, Vojvodina													
OCEANIA													
Australian Capital Territory	43.1	7.8	9.8	3.9	31.4	-	-	-	3.9	-	-	**51**	55
Australia, New South Wales	41.2	9.5	8.9	5.9	21.4	1.3	3.7	1.3	2.6	3.7	0.5	**1500**	1623
South Australia	36.4	10.1	14.5	5.9	22.5	0.8	2.6	2.6	2.6	2.1	-	**387**	465
Australia, Tasmania	20.7	19.0	6.0	5.2	31.0	1.7	11.2	-	2.6	2.6	-	**116**	124
Australia, Victoria	37.8	13.0	11.3	5.6	18.7	0.9	4.2	1.0	3.8	3.7	0.1	**1250**	1359
Western Australia	42.3	13.8	6.5	5.7	17.3	0.8	4.6	2.4	2.7	3.5	0.3	**369**	397
French Polynesia	35.7	-	7.1	3.6	28.6	-	14.3	3.6	7.1	-	-	**28**	34
New Zealand: Non-Maori													
New Zealand: Maori													
US, Hawaii: White	28.2	9.4	7.7	6.8	25.6	4.3	8.5	2.6	1.7	5.1	-	**117**	120
US, Hawaii: Japanese	40.9	5.4	5.4	10.8	21.5	1.1	7.5	3.2	4.3	-	-	**93**	94
US, Hawaii: Hawaiian	25.0	13.9	8.3	8.3	22.2	2.8	5.6	5.6	5.6	2.8	-	**36**	36
US, Hawaii: Filipino	32.4	14.7	14.7	5.9	11.8	5.9	5.9	2.9	5.9	-	-	**34**	34
US, Hawaii: Chinese	33.3	16.7	11.1	-	16.7	5.6	11.1	-	-	5.6	-	**18**	18

PERCENTAGE DISTRIBUTION OF MICROSCOPICALLY VERIFIED CASES BY HISTOLOGICAL TYPE
Testis (ICD-9 186)

	Seminoma	Other germ cell			Other	Unspecified	Number of cases	
		Embryonal	Teratoma	Chorioca.			MV	Total
AFRICA								
Algeria, Setif	-	-	-	-	50.0	50.0	2	2
France, La Reunion	55.6	27.8	-	5.6	11.1	-	18	18
Mali, Bamako	-	100.0	-	-	-	-	1	4
Uganda, Kyadondo	-	-	-	-	-	-	-	3
Zimbabwe, Harare: African	66.7	-	-	-	33.3	-	3	4
Zimbabwe, Harare: European	-	-	-	-	-	-	-	-
AMERICA, CENTRAL AND SOUTH								
Argentina, Concordia	44.4	-	33.3	-	22.2	-	9	9
Brazil, Belem	50.0	-	16.7	-	25.0	8.3	12	17
Brazil, Goiania	50.0	5.6	5.6	5.6	22.2	11.1	18	19
Brazil, Porto Alegre	42.0	16.0	16.0	2.0	10.0	14.0	50	61
Colombia, Cali	49.2	19.7	18.0	3.3	9.8	-	61	64
Costa Rica	55.1	25.9	12.2	2.0	4.1	0.7	147	161
Ecuador, Quito	57.6	20.7	17.4	2.2	-	2.2	92	108
Peru, Lima	45.1	22.0	20.1	9.1	1.8	1.8	164	187
Peru, Trujillo	64.3	21.4	14.3	-	-	-	14	17
Puerto Rico	43.8	17.5	18.8	7.5	12.5	-	80	85
Uruguay, Montevideo	67.8	17.8	11.1	-	2.2	1.1	90	97
AMERICA, NORTH								
Canada	55.2	18.0	19.4	4.6	2.2	0.6	2965	3083
Canada, Alberta	59.0	16.0	18.8	4.0	2.2	-	324	324
Canada, British Columbia	52.4	17.9	20.6	7.7	1.5	-	403	409
Canada, Manitoba	57.7	13.5	22.1	3.8	1.9	1.0	104	127
Canada, New Brunswick	51.8	26.8	12.5	3.6	5.4	-	56	56
Canada, Newfoundland	55.0	25.0	12.5	5.0	2.5	-	40	40
Canada, Northwest Territories	56.3	12.5	12.5	12.5	-	6.3	16	16
Canada, Nova Scotia	61.1	16.7	11.1	9.3	1.9	-	108	110
Canada, Ontario	54.7	16.9	21.8	3.8	1.8	1.0	1188	1238
Canada, Prince Edward Island	66.7	22.2	11.1	-	-	-	9	9
Canada, Quebec	55.5	20.0	16.6	3.9	3.4	0.6	620	657
Canada, Saskatchewan	50.0	25.5	18.4	4.1	2.0	-	98	98
Canada, Yukon	68.4	5.3	10.5	15.8	-	-	19	19
US, Cent. California: Non-Hisp White	55.5	15.2	20.9	6.8	1.6	-	191	191
US, Cent. California: Hispanic	49.1	17.5	24.6	7.0	1.8	-	57	58
US, Los Angeles: Non-Hisp White	56.6	14.9	23.9	3.7	0.8	0.2	657	658
US, Los Angeles: Hispanic White	47.0	17.3	30.3	3.0	2.3	-	300	303
US, Los Angeles: Black	64.7	5.9	17.6	2.9	8.8	-	34	35
US, Los Angeles: Chinese	33.3	33.3	33.3	-	-	-	6	6
US, Los Angeles: Filipino	42.9	28.6	28.6	-	-	-	7	7
US, Los Angeles: Korean	33.3	-	33.3	-	33.3	-	3	3
US, Los Angeles: Japanese	100.0	-	-	-	-	-	4	4
US, San Francisco: Non-Hisp White	62.0	18.2	16.7	3.0	-	-	461	462
US, San Francisco: Hispanic White	59.7	9.7	24.2	4.8	1.6	-	62	62
US, San Francisco: Black	41.7	-	41.7	8.3	8.3	-	12	12
US, San Francisco: Chinese	56.3	25.0	18.8	-	-	-	16	16
US, San Francisco: Filipino	71.4	-	28.6	-	-	-	7	7
US, San Francisco: Japanese	87.5	-	12.5	-	-	-	8	8
US, Connecticut: White	57.2	17.5	20.9	1.6	2.5	0.2	435	442
US, Connecticut: Black	60.0	-	40.0	-	-	-	5	5
US, Atlanta: White	53.8	17.2	27.1	1.4	0.5	-	221	221
US, Atlanta: Black	60.0	10.0	10.0	-	20.0	-	10	10
US, Iowa	52.3	16.8	23.1	6.0	1.8	-	333	334
US, Central Louisiana: White	47.4	21.1	21.1	5.3	5.3	-	19	19
US, Central Louisiana: Black	100.0	-	-	-	-	-	1	1
US, New Orleans: White	59.1	17.0	15.9	4.5	3.4	-	88	89
US, New Orleans: Black	50.0	8.3	16.7	-	25.0	-	12	13
US, Detroit: White	56.1	11.8	26.1	3.8	1.8	0.4	449	455
US, Detroit: Black	46.7	6.7	26.7	-	20.0	-	15	15
US, New Mexico: Non-Hisp White	63.0	14.3	20.2	1.7	0.8	-	119	119
US, New Mexico: Hispanic White	47.8	17.9	32.8	1.5	-	-	67	68
US, New Mexico: American Indian	44.4	-	33.3	22.2	-	-	9	10
US, Utah	49.6	18.2	28.5	1.7	2.1	-	242	244
US, Seattle	56.0	16.3	22.8	3.8	0.9	0.2	527	529
US, SEER: White	56.3	16.0	23.1	3.1	1.3	0.1	2950	2970
US, SEER: Black	46.9	6.1	30.6	4.1	12.2	-	49	49

PERCENTAGE DISTRIBUTION OF MICROSCOPICALLY VERIFIED CASES BY HISTOLOGICAL TYPE
Testis (ICD-9 186) (contd)

	Seminoma	Other germ cell			Other	Unspecified	Number of cases	
		Embryonal	Teratoma	Chorioca.			MV	Total
ASIA								
China, Qidong								
China, Shanghai								
China, Tianjin	40.4	12.8	-	2.1	6.4	38.3	47	50
Hong Kong	61.8	21.2	13.3	0.6	3.0	-	165	203
India, Bangalore	45.8	16.7	20.8	2.1	8.3	6.3	48	50
India, Barshi, Paranda and Bhum	50.0	50.0	-	-	-	-	2	3
India, Bombay	50.5	25.5	14.5	3.0	5.5	1.0	200	229
India, Karunagappally	50.0	-	50.0	-	-	-	2	2
India, Madras	44.0	14.0	24.0	-	18.0	-	50	60
India, Trivandrum	50.0	-	25.0	-	25.0	-	4	4
Israel: All Jews	54.7	17.0	23.8	2.3	2.3	-	265	295
Jews born in Israel	50.0	18.5	26.5	3.1	1.9	-	162	179
Jews born in America or Europe	60.0	16.3	18.8	1.3	3.8	-	80	92
Jews born in Africa or Asia	68.2	9.1	22.7	-	-	-	22	23
Non-Jews	46.2	30.8	15.4	7.7	-	-	13	15
Japan, Hiroshima	64.6	12.5	20.8	-	2.1	-	48	49
Japan, Miyagi	59.5	15.2	13.9	1.3	5.1	5.1	79	91
Japan, Nagasaki	69.2	11.5	7.7	7.7	3.8	-	26	28
Japan, Osaka	60.9	21.8	7.5	4.4	3.1	2.4	294	317
Japan, Saga								
Japan, Yamagata								
Korea, Kangwha	-	-	-	-	100.0	-	1	1
Kuwait: Non-Kuwaitis	52.9	26.5	14.7	5.9	-	-	34	35
Kuwait: Kuwaitis	50.0	12.5	12.5	25.0	-	-	8	8
Philippines, Manila	67.9	21.4	5.4	-	3.6	1.8	56	77
Singapore: Chinese	47.9	25.0	18.8	-	8.3	-	48	49
Singapore: Malay	50.0	37.5	12.5	-	-	-	8	9
Singapore: Indian	45.5	18.2	27.3	-	9.1	-	11	12
Thailand, Chiang Mai	66.7	11.1	22.2	-	-	-	18	22
Thailand, Khon Kaen	53.8	15.4	23.1	-	7.7	-	13	18
Viet Nam, Hanoi	31.3	25.0	-	-	31.3	12.5	16	21
EUROPE								
Austria, Tyrol	50.0	10.9	24.5	3.6	0.9	10.0	110	111
Belarus								
Croatia								
Czech Republic	52.3	24.0	19.4	1.7	2.4	0.2	1331	1420
Denmark	55.6	20.1	17.4	5.1	1.5	0.3	1321	1338
Estonia	65.6	18.8	12.5	1.6	1.6	-	64	66
Finland	52.9	-	44.8	0.3	1.0	1.0	393	395
France, Bas-Rhin	51.3	20.3	13.9	13.4	1.1	-	187	188
France, Calvados	52.5	27.1	15.3	3.4	-	1.7	59	59
France, Doubs	52.8	16.7	19.4	9.7	-	1.4	72	73
France, Haut-Rhin	55.3	24.0	14.0	4.7	2.0	-	150	150
France, Herault	55.4	30.4	12.5	-	1.8	-	56	56
France, Isere	51.5	14.6	17.5	12.6	3.9	-	103	103
France, Somme	45.3	18.9	20.8	13.2	1.9	-	53	55
France, Tarn	54.2	20.8	20.8	4.2	-	-	24	24
Germany, Eastern States	46.9	22.7	23.6	4.6	2.0	0.2	1464	1466
Germany, Saarland								
Iceland	63.0	15.2	13.0	6.5	2.2	-	46	46
Ireland, Southern	42.2	13.3	33.3	4.4	6.7	-	45	46
Italy, Ferrara	75.0	-	25.0	-	-	-	8	9
Italy, Florence	60.0	15.7	18.6	-	5.7	-	70	82
Italy, Genoa	64.5	22.4	7.9	1.3	3.9	-	76	79
Italy, Latina	52.4	28.6	19.0	-	-	-	21	22
Italy, Macerata	62.5	12.5	-	12.5	12.5	-	8	10
Italy, Modena	62.1	17.2	13.8	1.7	5.2	-	58	60
Italy, Parma	52.9	23.5	21.6	-	2.0	-	51	51
Italy, Ragusa	57.1	28.6	14.3	-	-	-	7	8
Italy, Romagna	71.4	14.3	12.2	-	2.0	-	49	53
Italy, Torino	65.3	11.1	18.1	2.8	2.8	-	72	72
Italy, Trieste	21.4	21.4	7.1	-	14.3	35.7	14	20
Italy, Varese	53.7	31.7	11.0	1.2	1.2	1.2	82	84
Italy, Veneto	68.9	19.8	6.6	1.9	2.8	-	106	109
Latvia								
Malta								

Testis (ICD-9 186) (contd)

	Seminoma	Embryonal	Other germ cell Teratoma	Chorioca.	Other	Unspecified	Number of cases MV	Total
The Netherlands	51.9	16.1	27.2	3.7	1.2	-	1388	1389
The Netherlands, Eindhoven	51.5	15.5	30.1	2.9	-	-	103	103
The Netherlands, Maastricht	53.4	8.0	33.0	4.5	1.1	-	88	88
Norway	49.6	15.0	9.7	2.5	1.7	21.6	922	927
Poland, Cracow	56.9	21.6	15.7	-	2.0	3.9	51	53
Poland, Kielce	33.3	22.9	14.6	4.2	14.6	10.4	48	58
Poland, Lower Silesia	46.3	26.4	14.9	0.8	2.5	9.1	121	204
Poland, Warsaw City	45.6	14.4	24.0	13.6	2.4	-	125	144
Slovakia	47.0	20.4	24.5	4.6	3.1	0.3	636	660
Slovenia	49.8	19.4	24.1	5.5	1.3	-	237	238
Spain, Albacete	33.3	16.7	33.3	16.7	-	-	6	6
Spain, Asturias	71.4	14.3	11.9	-	2.4	-	42	43
Spain, Basque Country	57.9	15.8	13.7	7.4	5.3	-	95	100
Spain, Granada	37.5	31.3	12.5	12.5	6.3	-	32	32
Spain, Mallorca	50.0	26.9	15.4	-	7.7	-	26	28
Spain, Murcia	43.8	28.1	21.9	3.1	3.1	-	32	32
Spain, Navarra	48.4	29.0	16.1	6.5	-	-	31	31
Spain, Tarragona	51.9	18.5	22.2	3.7	3.7	-	27	27
Spain, Zaragoza	51.5	6.1	30.3	9.1	3.0	-	33	34
Sweden	49.4	-	47.4	0.8	1.4	0.9	1077	1077
Switzerland, Basel	57.7	22.5	16.2	2.7	0.9	-	111	111
Switzerland, Geneva	55.6	19.8	19.8	4.9	-	-	81	81
Switzerland, Graubunden	38.9	25.0	33.3	2.8	-	-	36	36
Switzerland, Neuchatel	63.4	14.6	19.5	2.4	-	-	41	41
Switzerland, St Gall-Appenzell	57.1	24.3	16.4	1.4	0.7	-	140	140
Switzerland, Valais	53.5	16.3	20.9	2.3	4.7	2.3	43	43
Switzerland, Vaud	57.5	20.5	11.6	8.2	2.1	-	146	146
Switzerland, Zurich	56.1	8.6	29.6	4.7	1.0	-	301	301
UK, England and Wales	53.8	2.7	37.4	0.7	3.2	2.2	3396	3859
UK, East Anglia								
UK, Mersey	56.2	4.9	36.5	0.9	1.5	-	329	344
UK, North Western								
UK, Oxford	55.4	3.9	37.3	1.5	2.0	-	410	420
UK, South Thames	54.9	2.5	40.5	0.5	1.4	0.3	771	898
UK, South Western	54.3	4.0	37.2	0.9	1.2	2.4	422	445
UK, Wessex	53.2	3.0	39.5	1.6	2.2	0.5	365	447
UK, West Midlands								
UK, Yorkshire	54.6	0.7	42.6	0.5	1.6	-	441	455
UK, Scotland	55.8	1.3	41.2	0.3	1.4	0.1	782	802
UK, Scotland, West	50.5	1.6	46.1	0.5	1.3	-	386	397
Yugoslavia, Vojvodina	42.7	25.8	16.9	1.6	11.3	1.6	124	143

OCEANIA

	Seminoma	Embryonal	Other germ cell Teratoma	Chorioca.	Other	Unspecified	Number of cases MV	Total
Australian Capital Territory	53.6	21.4	17.9	3.6	3.6	-	28	29
Australia, New South Wales	55.4	17.5	19.8	4.0	3.0	0.3	758	770
South Australia	52.9	8.8	34.6	2.2	1.5	-	136	162
Australia, Tasmania	58.7	20.6	20.6	-	-	-	63	63
Australia, Victoria	57.3	14.1	24.2	2.7	1.5	0.2	546	558
Western Australia	53.3	17.8	23.7	3.6	1.8	-	169	175
French Polynesia	66.7	33.3	-	-	-	-	9	9
New Zealand: Non-Maori								
New Zealand: Maori								
US, Hawaii: White	53.0	19.7	22.7	3.0	1.5	-	66	66
US, Hawaii: Japanese	55.0	20.0	20.0	-	5.0	-	20	20
US, Hawaii: Hawaiian	55.0	20.0	25.0	-	-	-	20	20
US, Hawaii: Filipino	55.6	11.1	-	22.2	11.1	-	9	9
US, Hawaii: Chinese	40.0	20.0	-	20.0	20.0	-	5	5

PERCENTAGE DISTRIBUTION OF MICROSCOPICALLY VERIFIED CASES BY HISTOLOGICAL TYPE
Bladder (ICD-9 188) - Both sexes

			Carcinoma			Sarcoma	Other	Unspec.	Number of cases	
	Squamous	Transl.	Adeno	Other	Unspec.				MV	Total
AFRICA										
Algeria, Setif	25.0	25.0	-	-	25.0	-	-	25.0	4	14
France, La Reunion	2.4	86.2	3.3	-	7.3	-	-	0.8	123	125
Mali, Bamako	55.6	22.2	11.1	-	11.1	-	-	-	9	99
Uganda, Kyadondo	-	57.1	-	-	28.6	14.3	-	-	7	13
Zimbabwe, Harare: African	49.3	21.7	8.7	-	15.9	1.4	2.9	-	69	111
Zimbabwe, Harare: European	11.8	85.3	2.9	-	-	-	-	-	34	41
AMERICA, CENTRAL AND SOUTH										
Argentina, Concordia	-	74.2	3.2	-	9.7	3.2	-	9.7	31	40
Brazil, Belem	-	63.3	6.7	3.3	23.3	3.3	-	-	30	42
Brazil, Goiania	6.5	75.0	9.3	-	4.6	0.9	0.9	2.8	108	124
Brazil, Porto Alegre	2.5	71.3	2.5	0.4	7.8	0.4	-	15.2	244	329
Colombia, Cali	7.8	81.0	3.9	-	5.9	0.5	-	1.0	205	237
Costa Rica	3.4	91.6	2.0	-	1.7	0.7	-	0.7	296	383
Ecuador, Quito	6.1	79.6	4.1	-	6.1	2.0	-	2.0	98	121
Peru, Lima	4.7	87.6	4.7	0.4	1.7	0.4	0.4	-	234	296
Peru, Trujillo	-	66.7	13.3	-	20.0	-	-	-	15	16
Puerto Rico	4.1	90.2	2.9	0.1	1.9	-	-	0.8	981	1011
Uruguay, Montevideo	0.8	90.4	4.0	-	4.2	0.6	-	-	498	698
AMERICA, NORTH										
Canada	1.8	91.6	2.1	0.3	2.3	0.3	0.1	1.5	19681	21985
Canada, Alberta	1.3	96.6	0.8	0.3	0.4	0.1	0.1	0.4	1556	1600
Canada, British Columbia	2.2	93.4	2.7	0.3	0.9	0.2	-	0.2	1735	1801
Canada, Manitoba	2.0	93.7	2.7	0.4	0.8	0.1	-	0.2	911	967
Canada, New Brunswick	1.6	95.2	1.7	0.1	1.0	0.4	-	-	705	716
Canada, Newfoundland	2.1	95.2	1.6	-	1.1	-	-	-	436	442
Canada, Northwest Territories	-	92.9	7.1	-	-	-	-	-	14	14
Canada, Nova Scotia	1.2	95.8	1.2	0.1	1.5	0.2	-	-	852	897
Canada, Ontario	1.7	90.8	2.3	0.3	1.0	0.2	0.1	3.6	6942	7835
Canada, Prince Edward Island	4.8	94.2	1.0	-	-	-	-	-	104	107
Canada, Quebec	1.9	88.1	2.3	0.5	5.9	0.4	0.2	0.8	5467	6613
Canada, Saskatchewan	1.4	95.4	1.6	0.1	1.0	0.2	0.3	-	957	991
Canada, Yukon	-	100.0	-	-	-	-	-	-	15	15
US, Cent. California: Non-Hisp White	2.5	93.4	1.7	0.5	1.0	0.1	0.3	0.4	1151	1181
US, Cent. California: Hispanic	-	95.6	1.8	-	0.9	-	0.9	0.9	113	115
US, Los Angeles: Non-Hisp White	2.3	92.9	1.8	0.5	1.7	0.2	0.1	0.4	3376	3412
US, Los Angeles: Hispanic White	2.5	90.2	2.2	-	4.2	0.2	-	0.7	448	452
US, Los Angeles: Black	5.0	85.4	5.0	0.6	1.9	-	0.6	1.5	323	328
US, Los Angeles: Chinese	-	93.7	4.8	-	-	1.6	-	-	63	64
US, Los Angeles: Filipino	3.0	81.8	9.1	-	3.0	-	-	3.0	33	33
US, Los Angeles: Korean	-	91.7	-	4.2	-	4.2	-	-	24	24
US, Los Angeles: Japanese	2.4	92.9	4.8	-	-	-	-	-	42	42
US, San Francisco: Non-Hisp White	1.7	95.4	1.4	0.2	1.1	-	0.1	0.2	2722	2750
US, San Francisco: Hispanic White	1.7	94.1	1.7	0.8	1.7	-	-	-	119	120
US, San Francisco: Black	2.9	91.3	2.3	0.6	2.9	-	-	-	173	173
US, San Francisco: Chinese	0.9	93.1	1.7	-	1.7	0.9	0.9	0.9	116	117
US, San Francisco: Filipino	-	90.9	-	-	4.5	2.3	2.3	-	44	46
US, San Francisco: Japanese	-	92.0	4.0	-	4.0	-	-	-	25	25
US, Connecticut: White	1.0	95.6	1.0	0.2	1.8	0.1	0.1	0.2	4109	4157
US, Connecticut: Black	4.3	88.0	5.4	-	1.1	-	1.1	-	92	94
US, Atlanta: White	1.4	94.4	1.5	0.3	1.5	0.3	0.2	0.4	1112	1120
US, Atlanta: Black	4.0	85.2	5.4	-	2.7	1.3	0.7	0.7	149	150
US, Iowa	1.5	96.3	1.0	0.1	0.8	0.2	0.2	0.1	3282	3340
US, Central Louisiana: White	1.5	95.5	1.0	-	1.0	0.5	-	0.5	198	203
US, Central Louisiana: Black	5.7	88.6	2.9	-	-	2.9	-	-	35	36
US, New Orleans: White	0.6	95.4	0.9	0.3	2.0	-	-	0.8	786	797
US, New Orleans: Black	3.2	83.5	2.5	-	7.0	0.6	-	3.2	158	162
US, Detroit: White	1.5	95.2	1.1	0.1	1.6	0.1	0.1	0.4	3607	3628
US, Detroit: Black	2.6	87.6	4.5	-	3.6	0.7	-	1.0	418	423
US, New Mexico: Non-Hisp White	1.3	94.9	1.1	0.2	2.2	-	0.1	0.1	894	916
US, New Mexico: Hispanic White	2.8	94.4	1.7	-	-	0.6	0.6	-	180	184
US, New Mexico: American Indian	-	66.7	22.2	-	-	11.1	-	-	9	9
US, Utah	1.2	94.9	1.8	0.3	0.8	0.3	0.2	0.3	890	899
US, Seattle	1.2	96.2	1.0	0.3	0.9	0.2	0.1	0.1	3179	3209
US, SEER: White	1.3	95.5	1.1	0.2	1.3	0.1	0.1	0.2	20164	20393
US, SEER: Black	3.2	88.6	4.0	0.1	2.9	0.5	0.2	0.5	911	919

Bladder (ICD-9 188) - Both sexes (contd)

			Carcinoma			Sarcoma	Other	Unspec.	Number of cases	
	Squamous	Transl.	Adeno	Other	Unspec.				MV	Total
ASIA										
China, Qidong										
China, Shanghai										
China, Tianjin	1.4	39.9	3.3	-	-	-	-	55.4	552	822
Hong Kong	1.6	89.4	5.0	0.3	3.1	-	-	0.6	2441	3036
India, Bangalore	5.0	78.7	3.2	0.9	8.1	3.2	-	0.9	221	263
India, Barshi, Paranda and Bhum	16.7	50.0	-	-	-	-	-	33.3	6	9
India, Bombay	6.9	82.2	5.5	0.2	3.0	1.2	-	0.9	563	686
India, Karunagappally	10.0	80.0	-	-	10.0	-	-	-	10	11
India, Madras	8.8	80.7	5.3	-	1.8	2.3	-	1.2	171	215
India, Trivandrum	-	100.0	-	-	-	-	-	-	13	17
Israel: All Jews	1.4	94.9	1.2	0.1	1.8	0.4	0.1	0.1	3432	3622
Jews born in Israel	2.2	92.0	1.6	-	2.2	1.6	0.3	-	314	324
Jews born in America or Europe	1.3	95.4	1.1	0.2	1.6	0.3	-	0.1	2260	2391
Jews born in Africa or Asia	1.4	94.7	1.3	-	2.4	0.1	-	0.1	848	896
Non-Jews	2.2	92.6	1.5	-	3.7	-	-	-	136	144
Japan, Hiroshima	1.7	95.1	1.9	0.2	0.9	0.2	-	-	465	502
Japan, Miyagi	2.9	92.3	1.4	0.1	0.5	0.5	-	2.3	859	965
Japan, Nagasaki	3.0	93.7	1.4	-	1.7	-	0.1	0.1	805	896
Japan, Osaka	1.8	90.3	2.0	-	0.7	0.1	-	5.0	2061	2580
Japan, Saga										
Japan, Yamagata										
Korea, Kangwha	9.1	72.7	-	-	-	-	-	18.2	11	15
Kuwait: Non-Kuwaitis	11.4	74.7	3.8	-	6.3	2.5	-	1.3	79	94
Kuwait: Kuwaitis	12.5	78.1	-	-	6.3	-	-	3.1	32	50
Philippines, Manila	7.9	80.6	5.7	0.4	3.1	0.9	-	1.3	227	295
Singapore: Chinese	2.5	90.3	3.9	-	1.4	0.2	0.2	1.4	432	443
Singapore: Malay	2.2	89.1	2.2	-	2.2	4.3	-	-	46	51
Singapore: Indian	4.5	90.9	4.5	-	-	-	-	-	22	23
Thailand, Chiang Mai	3.6	87.9	4.5	-	3.6	-	0.4	-	224	246
Thailand, Khon Kaen	5.6	79.6	11.1	-	1.9	-	-	1.9	54	79
Viet Nam, Hanoi	3.6	75.0	7.1	-	7.1	-	-	7.1	28	45
EUROPE										
Austria, Tyrol	1.0	94.5	0.3	0.1	1.0	0.3	0.1	2.7	709	747
Belarus										
Croatia										
Czech Republic	2.0	91.4	2.4	0.4	2.5	0.2	0.1	1.0	5518	6658
Denmark	2.1	94.4	1.0	0.2	1.8	0.1	0.1	0.2	7716	7801
Estonia	4.1	85.6	2.2	0.4	3.5	0.4	-	3.7	508	654
Finland	1.2	94.3	1.0	-	1.5	0.2	-	1.7	3937	4003
France, Bas-Rhin	1.3	96.1	1.6	-	0.8	-	-	0.2	838	850
France, Calvados	0.9	89.6	1.2	-	7.2	0.5	-	0.7	584	587
France, Doubs	2.1	95.8	1.0	-	0.6	0.2	0.2	-	481	488
France, Haut-Rhin	2.7	96.6	0.4	-	-	0.2	-	0.2	556	559
France, Herault	3.8	93.4	1.2	-	1.3	0.1	-	0.1	743	746
France, Isere	1.1	96.5	0.9	0.2	1.3	-	-	-	635	654
France, Somme	3.3	78.6	1.1	-	16.1	0.2	-	0.7	459	472
France, Tarn	2.2	94.3	0.8	-	2.2	-	-	0.4	489	492
Germany, Eastern States	3.3	88.9	3.2	0.2	4.0	0.3	0.1	0.1	4898	5170
Germany, Saarland										
Iceland	2.6	93.3	1.0	-	3.1	-	-	-	194	196
Ireland, Southern	1.8	91.5	3.6	-	2.5	0.7	-	-	281	300
Italy, Ferrara	0.8	98.4	-	-	0.8	-	-	-	258	279
Italy, Florence	0.6	95.7	1.0	0.1	1.4	0.3	0.1	0.9	1514	1861
Italy, Genoa	0.7	93.4	0.7	0.1	1.3	0.1	-	3.6	1417	1624
Italy, Latina	2.2	84.0	1.2	-	12.6	-	-	-	325	361
Italy, Macerata	0.6	92.0	1.2	-	1.9	-	-	4.3	162	180
Italy, Modena	0.3	97.6	0.9	-	1.0	-	-	0.2	934	1005
Italy, Parma	0.5	92.6	0.3	-	6.3	0.3	-	-	648	704
Italy, Ragusa	6.0	73.8	4.7	-	8.7	1.3	-	5.4	149	195
Italy, Romagna	1.4	94.1	1.1	-	2.0	0.2	0.1	1.1	842	895
Italy, Torino	0.6	95.8	0.4	-	2.1	0.3	0.1	0.7	1347	1437
Italy, Trieste	2.3	59.1	2.0	-	10.7	0.7	0.5	24.8	440	611
Italy, Varese	1.5	96.2	0.5	0.4	0.9	0.1	-	0.4	1170	1233
Italy, Veneto	1.0	90.9	1.2	0.1	1.3	-	0.1	5.5	1630	1728
Latvia										
Malta										

			Carcinoma			Sarcoma	Other	Unspec.	Number of cases	
	Squamous	Transl.	Adeno	Other	Unspec.				MV	Total
The Netherlands	2.9	92.7	2.0	0.4	1.5	0.3	0.2	-	7993	8093
The Netherlands, Eindhoven	1.3	95.4	1.3	0.2	1.4	0.2	-	0.2	932	940
The Netherlands, Maastricht	4.5	89.2	2.6	0.7	2.1	0.2	0.7	-	426	432
Norway	1.7	92.0	1.1	0.1	2.9	0.2	0.2	1.8	3940	4030
Poland, Cracow	3.5	81.1	6.6	0.4	3.5	0.4	-	4.4	227	291
Poland, Kielce	4.9	62.2	4.2	0.3	25.1	0.3	-	2.9	307	451
Poland, Lower Silesia	2.3	50.1	0.8	-	4.1	0.5	-	42.2	391	1409
Poland, Warsaw City	1.1	94.6	2.7	-	1.1	0.2	0.2	-	522	778
Slovakia	1.3	93.2	1.7	0.1	3.0	0.2	-	0.4	2401	2799
Slovenia	1.6	90.8	1.4	-	5.8	0.1	0.1	0.1	695	780
Spain, Albacete	2.2	95.6	-	1.1	1.1	-	-	-	91	114
Spain, Asturias	0.9	92.6	1.7	0.1	3.9	0.1	-	0.8	1115	1168
Spain, Basque Country	1.1	93.7	1.4	0.1	3.1	0.2	-	0.4	1667	1796
Spain, Granada	0.6	94.3	1.5	-	2.0	0.6	0.1	0.9	683	757
Spain, Mallorca	0.5	97.1	0.7	-	1.6	-	0.1	0.1	883	919
Spain, Murcia	0.8	94.0	0.8	0.1	0.7	-	0.1	3.4	1086	1167
Spain, Navarra	2.0	91.2	1.7	0.2	4.2	-	0.2	0.5	593	648
Spain, Tarragona	0.7	95.7	0.5	0.3	1.9	0.1	0.3	0.5	736	779
Spain, Zaragoza	0.8	93.5	0.7	-	3.6	0.1	-	1.3	751	888
Sweden	2.1	93.9	1.1	-	2.3	0.3	-	0.4	9248	9290
Switzerland, Basel	3.5	94.3	1.6	0.3	-	-	0.3	-	316	316
Switzerland, Geneva	2.1	95.1	0.7	0.2	1.9	-	-	-	567	575
Switzerland, Graubunden	-	95.1	1.9	-	2.9	-	-	-	103	107
Switzerland, Neuchatel	3.4	89.8	2.5	-	1.7	0.8	-	1.7	118	122
Switzerland, St Gall-Appenzell	4.0	92.7	1.8	0.4	0.4	0.7	-	-	273	280
Switzerland, Valais	-	97.4	-	-	1.7	0.9	-	-	117	121
Switzerland, Vaud	1.9	92.0	1.7	-	4.1	-	0.2	-	413	426
Switzerland, Zurich	1.5	94.3	2.3	0.1	1.2	0.2	0.3	-	1308	1334
UK, England and Wales	2.2	82.3	2.5	0.1	10.8	0.2	0.1	1.7	29602	34638
UK, East Anglia										
UK, Mersey	2.2	92.4	2.2	0.1	2.7	0.2	0.1	-	2481	2714
UK, North Western										
UK, Oxford	2.6	92.1	1.7	0.1	3.4	0.1	-	-	2245	2519
UK, South Thames	2.4	91.1	1.9	0.1	4.3	0.2	-	0.1	6456	7818
UK, South Western	2.5	86.8	2.3	0.1	6.3	0.2	-	1.8	3582	4044
UK, Wessex	2.0	78.0	8.2	0.2	11.4	0.1	0.1	0.1	3230	4362
UK, West Midlands										
UK, Yorkshire	1.9	93.1	1.4	0.2	3.0	0.2	0.1	0.1	4834	5131
UK, Scotland	3.6	90.7	1.4	0.2	3.6	0.1	0.1	0.2	5834	6346
UK, Scotland, West	3.9	90.7	1.2	0.3	3.7	0.1	0.1	0.1	3040	3358
Yugoslavia, Vojvodina	3.7	85.4	2.0	-	6.0	0.1	-	2.7	735	1072

OCEANIA

			Carcinoma			Sarcoma	Other	Unspec.	Number of cases	
	Squamous	Transl.	Adeno	Other	Unspec.				MV	Total
Australian Capital Territory	1.7	89.7	-	3.4	3.4	1.7	-	-	58	62
Australia, New South Wales	1.5	94.0	1.8	0.3	1.7	0.4	0.2	0.2	3312	3455
South Australia	1.0	96.5	0.7	-	1.3	0.2	0.2	0.2	1261	1416
Australia, Tasmania	2.9	92.8	1.4	-	2.3	0.6	-	-	349	354
Australia, Victoria	1.0	95.1	1.6	0.2	1.4	0.3	0.3	0.1	3313	3482
Western Australia	3.7	91.3	2.0	0.2	2.0	0.7	-	0.2	562	591
French Polynesia	17.4	60.9	8.7	-	8.7	4.3	-	-	23	25
New Zealand: Non-Maori										
New Zealand: Maori										
US, Hawaii: White	1.4	94.6	2.5	0.4	1.1	-	-	-	280	281
US, Hawaii: Japanese	0.5	95.7	2.2	-	1.6	-	-	-	186	190
US, Hawaii: Hawaiian	6.7	86.7	3.3	3.3	-	-	-	-	30	30
US, Hawaii: Filipino	2.3	90.9	4.5	-	-	-	2.3	-	44	46
US, Hawaii: Chinese	2.7	91.9	5.4	-	-	-	-	-	37	38

PERCENTAGE DISTRIBUTION OF MICROSCOPICALLY VERIFIED CASES BY HISTOLOGICAL TYPE
Kidney etc. (ICD-9 189) - Both sexes

	Carcinoma				Wilms'	Sarcoma	Other	Unspec.	Number of cases	
	Sq./Transl.	Renal	Other	Unspec.					MV	Total
AFRICA										
Algeria, Setif	-	21.4	-	-	78.6	-	-	-	14	15
France, La Reunion	12.8	59.6	-	-	21.3	6.4	-	-	47	49
Mali, Bamako	-	44.4	11.1	-	44.4	-	-	-	9	38
Uganda, Kyadondo	5.3	-	-	26.3	52.6	5.3	5.3	5.3	19	31
Zimbabwe, Harare: African	-	32.0	-	-	68.0	-	-	-	25	26
Zimbabwe, Harare: European	-	100.0	-	-	-	-	-	-	6	6
AMERICA, CENTRAL AND SOUTH										
Argentina, Concordia	16.7	83.3	-	-	-	-	-	-	12	19
Brazil, Belem	10.5	34.2	-	21.1	34.2	-	-	-	38	50
Brazil, Goiania	9.8	29.5	21.3	6.6	14.8	1.6	-	16.4	61	69
Brazil, Porto Alegre	7.7	53.5	4.9	7.0	4.9	0.7	-	21.1	142	228
Colombia, Cali	21.6	51.1	-	6.8	14.8	2.3	1.1	2.3	88	107
Costa Rica	10.3	72.9	-	3.4	9.9	2.0	0.5	1.0	203	270
Ecuador, Quito	15.7	58.8	2.0	11.8	9.8	-	-	2.0	51	71
Peru, Lima	13.8	62.9	7.8	3.0	9.0	1.8	0.6	1.2	167	229
Peru, Trujillo	16.7	50.0	-	12.5	16.7	-	4.2	-	24	31
Puerto Rico	17.0	72.8	1.4	2.0	5.0	0.7	-	1.1	441	496
Uruguay, Montevideo	6.0	77.1	2.3	9.8	2.3	1.5	-	1.1	266	399
AMERICA, NORTH										
Canada	16.5	74.5	1.9	2.8	2.0	0.4	0.4	1.6	11665	14921
Canada, Alberta	15.8	78.9	0.7	1.5	2.2	0.2	0.1	0.7	1041	1189
Canada, British Columbia	18.6	68.2	1.6	7.4	2.8	0.4	0.4	0.7	1373	1581
Canada, Manitoba	16.9	75.9	3.2	1.7	0.7	0.5	0.7	0.2	402	634
Canada, New Brunswick	15.1	81.3	1.7	1.1	0.9	-	-	-	352	401
Canada, Newfoundland	18.1	76.7	1.3	1.3	1.7	-	0.4	0.4	232	257
Canada, Northwest Territories	9.5	81.0	-	4.8	4.8	-	-	-	21	27
Canada, Nova Scotia	16.5	78.0	1.1	1.5	2.1	0.6	0.2	-	532	620
Canada, Ontario	16.1	74.5	2.1	1.6	2.1	0.4	0.5	2.9	4410	5532
Canada, Prince Edward Island	10.8	89.2	-	-	-	-	-	-	65	76
Canada, Quebec	16.6	73.7	2.3	3.4	1.7	0.6	0.3	1.3	2696	3960
Canada, Saskatchewan	16.2	75.6	1.3	3.1	2.5	0.7	0.5	-	550	652
Canada, Yukon	-	40.0	-	40.0	20.0	-	-	-	10	12
US, Cent. California: Non-Hisp White	23.3	72.5	1.0	1.0	1.8	0.1	0.1	0.3	735	800
US, Cent. California: Hispanic	12.6	78.2	1.1	1.1	6.3	-	0.6	-	174	191
US, Los Angeles: Non-Hisp White	22.4	70.6	2.4	1.6	1.3	0.3	0.7	0.6	2006	2178
US, Los Angeles: Hispanic White	12.4	77.7	1.8	0.7	6.4	0.3	0.7	-	596	643
US, Los Angeles: Black	11.5	76.0	4.3	1.3	4.0	0.3	1.1	1.6	375	409
US, Los Angeles: Chinese	37.5	62.5	-	-	-	-	-	-	40	42
US, Los Angeles: Filipino	15.6	75.6	-	-	4.4	-	4.4	-	45	47
US, Los Angeles: Korean	18.8	71.9	-	3.1	3.1	3.1	-	-	32	34
US, Los Angeles: Japanese	30.3	63.6	3.0	-	-	-	3.0	-	33	34
US, San Francisco: Non-Hisp White	22.2	69.9	2.9	1.9	1.3	0.4	0.7	0.5	1134	1224
US, San Francisco: Hispanic White	13.1	77.2	2.1	0.7	5.5	0.7	0.7	-	145	155
US, San Francisco: Black	14.5	75.9	2.4	1.8	3.0	0.6	1.2	0.6	166	180
US, San Francisco: Chinese	31.9	59.6	2.1	2.1	2.1	-	2.1	-	47	54
US, San Francisco: Filipino	20.5	69.2	2.6	5.1	-	-	-	2.6	39	41
US, San Francisco: Japanese	44.4	44.4	-	-	-	-	11.1	-	9	11
US, Connecticut: White	19.1	75.1	1.0	2.1	1.5	0.1	0.3	0.7	1754	1928
US, Connecticut: Black	4.5	83.0	1.1	4.5	2.3	1.1	1.1	2.3	88	96
US, Atlanta: White	22.8	68.9	0.9	2.8	3.0	0.5	0.9	0.3	575	616
US, Atlanta: Black	9.9	80.7	2.0	1.5	3.5	0.5	1.0	1.0	202	221
US, Iowa	18.0	75.9	2.1	1.4	1.8	0.2	0.5	0.2	1548	1754
US, Central Louisiana: White	24.1	72.3	-	1.2	2.4	-	-	-	83	100
US, Central Louisiana: Black	17.2	72.4	-	3.4	6.9	-	-	-	29	34
US, New Orleans: White	19.2	73.2	1.6	1.6	1.6	0.7	-	2.2	447	481
US, New Orleans: Black	13.7	74.0	1.4	1.4	2.1	-	-	7.5	146	177
US, Detroit: White	19.7	72.8	1.5	2.0	1.7	0.3	0.7	1.4	1769	1925
US, Detroit: Black	13.7	77.8	1.8	2.3	2.3	-	0.8	1.3	388	443
US, New Mexico: Non-Hisp White	17.3	76.7	0.9	1.5	3.0	0.3	0.3	-	335	374
US, New Mexico: Hispanic White	13.2	81.6	0.6	0.6	2.9	-	1.1	-	174	198
US, New Mexico: American Indian	14.3	81.0	-	2.4	2.4	-	-	-	42	50
US, Utah	16.3	75.1	0.6	1.3	4.9	0.2	0.8	0.8	473	511
US, Seattle	18.4	73.3	3.3	1.6	2.3	0.1	0.5	0.4	1499	1643
US, SEER: White	19.2	73.6	1.8	1.7	2.1	0.3	0.6	0.6	9392	10309
US, SEER: Black	11.6	79.2	1.7	2.4	2.7	0.4	0.9	1.1	917	1019

Kidney etc. (ICD-9 189) - Both sexes (contd)

		Carcinoma			Wilms'	Sarcoma	Other	Unspec.	Number of cases	
	Sq./Transl.	Renal	Other	Unspec.					MV	Total
ASIA										
China, Qidong										
China, Shanghai										
China, Tianjin	10.4	26.2	1.6	-	0.6	0.3	2.5	58.4	**317**	509
Hong Kong	27.6	63.1	0.3	4.0	3.0	0.7	0.7	0.6	**675**	945
India, Bangalore	10.7	64.3	0.9	0.9	17.9	0.9	-	4.5	**112**	123
India, Barshi, Paranda and Bhum	25.0	50.0	-	-	25.0	-	-	-	**4**	5
India, Bombay	17.0	62.0	1.4	2.8	14.2	0.3	0.3	2.0	**358**	431
India, Karunagappally	-	100.0	-	-	-	-	-	-	**3**	3
India, Madras	21.5	58.1	-	1.1	15.1	2.2	-	2.2	**93**	111
India, Trivandrum	-	33.3	16.7	-	33.3	16.7	-	-	**6**	7
Israel: All Jews	17.9	75.2	1.0	1.6	1.8	0.4	0.4	1.6	**1581**	1816
Jews born in Israel	12.8	68.7	1.7	1.1	12.3	0.6	1.1	1.7	**179**	203
Jews born in America or Europe	17.1	77.8	1.0	1.9	0.3	0.4	0.2	1.4	**1121**	1277
Jews born in Africa or Asia	24.1	69.1	0.7	1.1	1.1	0.7	0.7	2.5	**278**	331
Non-Jews	17.6	51.0	2.0	-	17.6	2.0	3.9	5.9	**51**	59
Japan, Hiroshima	41.1	53.9	0.7	1.8	1.1	0.7	-	0.7	**282**	346
Japan, Miyagi	28.1	61.9	-	1.4	1.2	1.2	0.2	6.1	**588**	702
Japan, Nagasaki	32.4	63.6	-	1.9	1.4	0.2	0.2	0.2	**426**	512
Japan, Osaka	27.4	60.3	0.4	0.4	2.5	0.7	-	8.3	**1581**	2052
Japan, Saga										
Japan, Yamagata										
Korea, Kangwha	33.3	33.3	-	-	33.3	-	-	-	**6**	9
Kuwait: Non-Kuwaitis	18.4	65.8	-	2.6	10.5	-	-	2.6	**38**	46
Kuwait: Kuwaitis	5.6	77.8	5.6	-	11.1	-	-	-	**18**	25
Philippines, Manila	14.9	66.0	1.1	2.7	12.2	2.1	-	1.1	**188**	377
Singapore: Chinese	27.3	64.9	-	1.2	5.7	0.4	-	0.4	**245**	300
Singapore: Malay	20.0	75.0	-	-	5.0	-	-	-	**20**	25
Singapore: Indian	14.3	76.2	-	-	9.5	-	-	-	**21**	26
Thailand, Chiang Mai	54.4	27.8	2.5	7.6	1.3	2.5	-	3.8	**79**	98
Thailand, Khon Kaen	41.0	23.1	7.7	-	23.1	2.6	-	2.6	**39**	50
Viet Nam, Hanoi	12.5	43.8	-	6.3	18.8	6.3	-	12.5	**16**	26
EUROPE										
Austria, Tyrol	14.3	74.8	1.7	2.5	1.2	1.0	0.2	4.2	**405**	467
Belarus										
Croatia										
Czech Republic	10.5	83.5	1.0	1.4	1.2	0.3	0.3	1.8	**4695**	8826
Denmark	20.3	71.4	0.8	4.4	1.0	0.5	0.3	1.2	**2882**	3174
Estonia	6.8	82.7	0.6	1.4	3.9	0.3	-	4.4	**665**	870
Finland	9.0	81.7	0.1	3.2	2.0	0.3	0.1	3.8	**3680**	4050
France, Bas-Rhin	13.1	82.9	0.5	0.9	2.0	0.8	-	-	**666**	705
France, Calvados	15.4	76.9	1.4	1.8	2.7	-	-	1.8	**221**	235
France, Doubs	11.0	83.1	0.5	1.4	3.2	0.9	-	-	**219**	225
France, Haut-Rhin	14.1	82.3	0.8	-	1.8	0.3	0.3	0.5	**396**	421
France, Herault	20.7	72.7	3.4	1.3	1.1	-	-	0.8	**377**	386
France, Isere	11.6	80.9	1.5	2.6	2.3	0.5	0.3	0.3	**388**	431
France, Somme	13.1	75.5	0.9	4.8	2.6	1.7	0.4	0.9	**229**	244
France, Tarn	21.3	68.0	4.0	3.3	2.0	-	-	1.3	**150**	161
Germany, Eastern States	9.8	83.2	1.8	2.2	1.5	0.6	0.4	0.6	**4087**	4680
Germany, Saarland										
Iceland	12.6	81.7	1.1	4.0	-	-	-	0.6	**175**	184
Ireland, Southern	20.6	70.2	-	2.8	5.7	0.7	-	-	**141**	172
Italy, Ferrara	20.9	72.1	3.1	3.1	-	0.8	-	-	**129**	162
Italy, Florence	16.0	76.5	2.1	2.3	0.5	0.7	-	1.9	**574**	746
Italy, Genoa	22.8	62.4	2.2	7.4	1.2	0.5	0.7	2.7	**404**	545
Italy, Latina	7.6	51.9	1.3	36.7	2.5	-	-	-	**79**	93
Italy, Macerata	10.3	76.9	2.6	2.6	-	-	-	7.7	**39**	59
Italy, Modena	19.8	69.8	6.4	2.6	0.9	0.6	-	-	**344**	474
Italy, Parma	17.5	76.9	1.9	1.9	0.4	0.4	0.4	0.7	**268**	338
Italy, Ragusa	24.5	60.4	-	1.9	7.5	1.9	-	3.8	**53**	70
Italy, Romagna	16.5	75.4	1.7	4.6	0.3	0.3	-	1.2	**345**	434
Italy, Torino	22.8	72.4	0.5	1.9	0.5	1.0	0.2	0.7	**416**	509
Italy, Trieste	10.2	47.1	-	16.9	0.4	0.4	-	24.9	**225**	284
Italy, Varese	17.1	74.6	4.3	2.4	0.4	0.4	-	0.8	**532**	637
Italy, Veneto	20.0	58.2	1.7	4.3	0.4	0.5	0.2	14.6	**807**	978
Latvia										
Malta										

PERCENTAGE DISTRIBUTION OF MICROSCOPICALLY VERIFIED CASES BY HISTOLOGICAL TYPE
Kidney etc. (ICD-9 189) - Both sexes (contd)

	Carcinoma				Wilms'	Sarcoma	Other	Unspec.	Number of cases	
	Sq./Transl.	Renal	Other	Unspec.					MV	Total
The Netherlands	20.1	76.5	0.6	0.8	1.3	0.2	0.3	0.2	5771	6491
The Netherlands, Eindhoven	22.5	76.4	-	-	0.5	-	-	0.5	369	398
The Netherlands, Maastricht	15.3	82.9	-	0.9	0.4	0.2	0.2	-	445	513
Norway	11.7	80.8	-	2.7	1.1	0.2	0.2	3.2	2234	2552
Poland, Cracow	5.1	74.0	-	8.4	3.3	0.9	0.5	7.9	215	370
Poland, Kielce	10.2	59.5	-	22.9	2.9	1.0	2.4	1.0	205	333
Poland, Lower Silesia	4.2	40.0	0.5	1.6	2.8	0.5	-	50.5	430	1367
Poland, Warsaw City	5.5	84.3	1.0	5.1	2.2	1.2	0.2	0.6	511	912
Slovakia	10.1	83.7	0.3	2.6	2.2	0.5	0.2	0.4	1845	2546
Slovenia	13.6	79.5	2.0	2.2	1.5	0.2	0.3	0.7	594	670
Spain, Albacete	28.6	53.6	-	10.7	-	-	-	7.1	28	32
Spain, Asturias	17.8	73.1	-	5.4	1.5	0.3	-	1.8	331	379
Spain, Basque Country	17.2	76.9	1.6	3.0	0.4	0.5	0.2	0.2	559	710
Spain, Granada	34.8	48.6	2.9	6.5	5.8	0.7	-	0.7	138	182
Spain, Mallorca	28.8	62.6	-	3.7	3.7	0.6	-	0.6	163	186
Spain, Murcia	31.6	54.4	1.2	5.3	1.8	1.2	1.2	3.5	171	199
Spain, Navarra	20.0	72.6	0.5	3.2	2.1	1.1	-	0.5	190	228
Spain, Tarragona	40.4	49.0	-	6.0	1.3	2.6	-	0.7	151	184
Spain, Zaragoza	31.1	61.2	1.4	3.7	1.8	0.5	-	0.5	219	301
Sweden	17.1	78.3	-	2.2	1.2	0.3	0.1	0.8	6104	6509
Switzerland, Basel	18.4	80.0	-	0.3	0.6	0.6	-	-	310	314
Switzerland, Geneva	22.6	72.4	-	2.0	-	1.5	1.5	-	199	218
Switzerland, Graubunden	15.7	81.4	-	-	1.4	-	-	1.4	70	79
Switzerland, Neuchatel	17.3	80.2	-	-	-	-	-	2.5	81	94
Switzerland, St Gall-Appenzell	19.2	78.8	0.4	-	1.2	0.4	-	-	245	267
Switzerland, Valais	19.6	75.7	-	0.9	0.9	0.9	1.9	-	107	116
Switzerland, Vaud	16.0	76.1	1.1	4.1	1.9	-	0.4	0.4	268	313
Switzerland, Zurich	22.0	72.6	0.6	2.8	0.9	0.3	0.3	0.5	654	689
UK, England and Wales	19.4	57.6	1.5	16.7	2.3	0.5	0.2	1.7	9104	12076
UK, East Anglia										
UK, Mersey	18.7	72.6	0.7	4.9	2.1	0.6	-	0.3	669	889
UK, North Western										
UK, Oxford	15.0	75.7	0.7	3.5	4.1	0.7	0.2	-	826	983
UK, South Thames	21.0	65.7	2.3	7.8	1.8	0.6	0.4	0.4	1614	2700
UK, South Western	23.8	60.0	4.1	7.6	2.2	0.8	-	1.6	962	1413
UK, Wessex	15.0	65.0	1.4	15.7	2.2	0.3	0.1	0.2	979	1338
UK, West Midlands										
UK, Yorkshire	25.8	66.3	0.3	4.3	2.8	0.3	0.2	0.1	1140	1540
UK, Scotland	24.2	66.8	0.8	5.3	2.1	0.5	0.2	0.2	1844	2464
UK, Scotland, West	27.4	64.0	1.0	4.6	2.1	0.5	0.2	0.1	864	1238
Yugoslavia, Vojvodina	15.5	69.9	1.5	6.0	2.4	0.9	-	3.9	336	569
OCEANIA										
Australian Capital Territory	19.2	63.0	9.6	1.4	6.8	-	-	-	73	86
Australia, New South Wales	24.4	70.5	0.6	1.7	1.8	0.7	0.1	0.3	2726	2976
South Australia	20.4	74.9	1.0	0.8	1.8	0.4	0.6	0.2	510	661
Australia, Tasmania	15.8	78.3	0.5	2.2	1.6	1.1	-	0.5	184	217
Australia, Victoria	18.1	73.4	1.4	3.8	2.5	0.3	0.4	0.1	1624	1909
Western Australia	23.5	71.9	0.4	1.1	2.6	-	0.4	0.2	549	625
French Polynesia	5.9	58.8	5.9	-	23.5	5.9	-	-	17	25
New Zealand: Non-Maori										
New Zealand: Maori										
US, Hawaii: White	17.3	74.4	1.5	1.5	3.0	0.8	0.8	0.8	133	142
US, Hawaii: Japanese	31.1	65.5	2.5	0.8	-	-	-	-	119	129
US, Hawaii: Hawaiian	17.1	75.6	-	2.4	2.4	-	2.4	-	41	44
US, Hawaii: Filipino	3.2	87.1	-	6.5	-	3.2	-	-	31	33
US, Hawaii: Chinese	27.8	61.1	-	-	5.6	-	-	5.6	18	20

PERCENTAGE DISTRIBUTION OF MICROSCOPICALLY VERIFIED CASES BY HISTOLOGICAL TYPE
Eye and orbit (ICD-9 190) - Both sexes

	Retino-blastoma	Melanoma	Carcinoma Squamous	Carcinoma Other	Carcinoma Unspec.	Sarcoma	Other	Unspec.	Number of cases MV	Number of cases Total
AFRICA										
Algeria, Setif	-	-	100.0	-	-	-	-	-	2	3
France, La Reunion	36.4	18.2	27.3	-	9.1	9.1	-	-	11	11
Mali, Bamako	75.0	-	12.5	-	-	12.5	-	-	8	29
Uganda, Kyadondo	19.0	-	76.2	-	4.8	-	-	-	42	58
Zimbabwe, Harare: African	50.0	-	37.5	-	-	12.5	-	-	16	18
Zimbabwe, Harare: European	-	-	66.7	-	-	-	33.3	-	3	3
AMERICA, CENTRAL AND SOUTH										
Argentina, Concordia	-	40.0	40.0	20.0	-	-	-	-	5	6
Brazil, Belem	57.9	5.3	21.1	-	10.5	-	-	5.3	19	22
Brazil, Goiania	16.7	11.1	55.6	5.6	-	5.6	-	5.6	18	18
Brazil, Porto Alegre	41.2	17.6	29.4	-	-	5.9	-	5.9	17	21
Colombia, Cali	37.5	15.0	42.5	5.0	-	-	-	-	40	45
Costa Rica	31.7	13.3	50.0	1.7	-	3.3	-	-	60	72
Ecuador, Quito	30.8	7.7	43.6	-	10.3	2.6	5.1	-	39	40
Peru, Lima	31.1	20.0	33.3	2.2	2.2	6.7	-	4.4	45	55
Peru, Trujillo	41.7	-	58.3	-	-	-	-	-	12	14
Puerto Rico	10.6	24.2	53.0	1.5	6.1	1.5	1.5	1.5	66	67
Uruguay, Montevideo	28.6	57.1	-	-	-	7.1	7.1	-	14	14
AMERICA, NORTH										
Canada	10.3	71.7	9.0	2.9	1.1	3.4	0.6	1.1	834	1299
Canada, Alberta	12.9	77.4	4.3	1.1	-	4.3	-	-	93	106
Canada, British Columbia	13.3	68.0	6.7	4.0	1.3	5.3	1.3	-	75	158
Canada, Manitoba	2.1	83.3	10.4	-	-	4.2	-	-	48	60
Canada, New Brunswick	4.8	85.7	9.5	-	-	-	-	-	21	25
Canada, Newfoundland	-	71.4	28.6	-	-	-	-	-	7	10
Canada, Northwest Territories	50.0	-	-	-	-	-	-	50.0	2	2
Canada, Nova Scotia	7.3	80.5	7.3	2.4	-	2.4	-	-	41	50
Canada, Ontario	11.3	68.4	11.0	2.3	0.9	3.5	0.3	2.3	345	510
Canada, Prince Edward Island	16.7	83.3	-	-	-	-	-	-	6	7
Canada, Quebec	11.3	67.5	8.1	6.9	2.5	1.3	1.9	0.6	160	304
Canada, Saskatchewan	-	80.6	8.3	-	2.8	8.3	-	-	36	67
Canada, Yukon	-	100.0	-	-	-	-	-	-	1	1
US, Cent. California: Non-Hisp White	5.6	79.6	11.1	1.9	-	1.9	-	-	54	73
US, Cent. California: Hispanic	46.7	13.3	40.0	-	-	-	-	-	15	17
US, Los Angeles: Non-Hisp White	12.1	65.2	16.7	3.8	0.8	0.8	-	0.8	132	205
US, Los Angeles: Hispanic White	44.0	24.0	22.0	4.0	-	4.0	-	2.0	50	54
US, Los Angeles: Black	25.0	41.7	8.3	16.7	-	-	8.3	-	12	12
US, Los Angeles: Chinese	-	-	-	-	-	-	100.0	-	1	1
US, Los Angeles: Filipino	-	-	-	-	-	-	-	-	-	-
US, Los Angeles: Korean	-	-	-	-	-	-	-	-	-	-
US, Los Angeles: Japanese	-	100.0	-	-	-	-	-	-	1	1
US, San Francisco: Non-Hisp White	7.3	70.7	13.4	3.7	1.2	2.4	1.2	-	82	112
US, San Francisco: Hispanic White	77.8	-	11.1	-	-	11.1	-	-	9	12
US, San Francisco: Black	20.0	60.0	-	20.0	-	-	-	-	5	7
US, San Francisco: Chinese	-	100.0	-	-	-	-	-	-	2	2
US, San Francisco: Filipino	-	-	-	-	-	-	-	-	-	-
US, San Francisco: Japanese	-	100.0	-	-	-	-	-	-	1	1
US, Connecticut: White	8.1	64.5	11.3	4.8	-	8.1	-	3.2	62	92
US, Connecticut: Black	50.0	-	-	-	-	-	50.0	-	2	2
US, Atlanta: White	4.3	84.8	8.7	2.2	-	-	-	-	46	60
US, Atlanta: Black	44.4	11.1	22.2	11.1	-	11.1	-	-	9	10
US, Iowa	6.8	81.2	7.5	1.5	0.8	1.5	0.8	-	133	154
US, Central Louisiana: White	16.7	66.7	16.7	-	-	-	-	-	6	10
US, Central Louisiana: Black	100.0	-	-	-	-	-	-	-	1	1
US, New Orleans: White	3.8	76.9	7.7	7.7	3.8	-	-	-	26	37
US, New Orleans: Black	-	-	-	100.0	-	-	-	-	1	1
US, Detroit: White	12.6	70.5	10.5	1.1	-	3.2	1.1	1.1	95	108
US, Detroit: Black	60.0	-	20.0	10.0	-	10.0	-	-	10	10
US, New Mexico: Non-Hisp White	12.1	66.7	15.2	6.1	-	-	-	-	33	34
US, New Mexico: Hispanic White	55.6	22.2	11.1	-	-	-	11.1	-	9	9
US, New Mexico: American Indian	33.3	33.3	33.3	-	-	-	-	-	3	3
US, Utah	10.6	55.3	29.8	-	-	4.3	-	-	47	51
US, Seattle	13.2	76.4	5.7	0.9	0.9	2.8	-	-	106	140
US, SEER: White	10.9	71.8	11.0	2.1	0.3	2.8	0.6	0.5	616	765
US, SEER: Black	45.2	16.1	12.9	9.7	-	12.9	3.2	-	31	34

PERCENTAGE DISTRIBUTION OF MICROSCOPICALLY VERIFIED CASES BY HISTOLOGICAL TYPE
Eye and orbit (ICD-9 190) - Both sexes (contd)

	Retino-blastoma	Melanoma	Carcinoma			Sarcoma	Other	Unspec.	Number of cases	
			Squamous	Other	Unspec.				MV	Total
ASIA										
China, Qidong										
China, Shanghai										
China, Tianjin	13.3	13.3	6.7	26.7	-	6.7	6.7	26.7	15	24
Hong Kong	55.1	14.3	22.4	2.0	-	4.1	-	2.0	49	68
India, Bangalore	46.4	3.6	21.4	14.3	3.6	10.7	-	-	28	33
India, Barshi, Paranda and Bhum	100.0	-	-	-	-	-	-	-	1	1
India, Bombay	72.5	2.9	8.7	4.3	2.9	4.3	-	4.3	69	83
India, Karunagappally	-	-	-	-	-	-	-	-	-	-
India, Madras	80.6	3.2	6.5	1.6	3.2	4.8	-	-	62	65
India, Trivandrum	100.0	-	-	-	-	-	-	-	3	3
Israel: All Jews	11.1	66.7	16.2	3.0	-	3.0	-	-	99	162
Jews born in Israel	36.0	48.0	8.0	-	-	8.0	-	-	25	46
Jews born in America or Europe	-	81.5	11.1	5.6	-	1.9	-	-	54	89
Jews born in Africa or Asia	10.5	52.6	36.8	-	-	-	-	-	19	26
Non-Jews	60.0	6.7	33.3	-	-	-	-	-	15	23
Japan, Hiroshima	62.5	25.0	12.5	-	-	-	-	-	8	8
Japan, Miyagi	33.3	20.0	6.7	33.3	-	-	6.7	-	15	17
Japan, Nagasaki	46.7	13.3	20.0	6.7	6.7	6.7	-	-	15	18
Japan, Osaka	50.0	18.2	6.8	9.1	9.1	6.8	-	-	44	47
Japan, Saga										
Japan, Yamagata										
Korea, Kangwha	-	-	-	-	-	-	-	-	-	-
Kuwait: Non-Kuwaitis	-	-	-	-	-	-	-	-	-	-
Kuwait: Kuwaitis	33.3	-	-	-	-	66.7	-	-	3	4
Philippines, Manila	65.8	8.2	11.0	8.2	1.4	2.7	2.7	-	73	94
Singapore: Chinese	68.0	16.0	8.0	4.0	-	4.0	-	-	25	27
Singapore: Malay	75.0	-	25.0	-	-	-	-	-	4	5
Singapore: Indian	-	-	100.0	-	-	-	-	-	1	1
Thailand, Chiang Mai	33.3	-	55.6	11.1	-	-	-	-	9	10
Thailand, Khon Kaen	31.3	6.3	43.8	6.3	-	6.3	-	6.3	16	20
Viet Nam, Hanoi	48.1	7.4	11.1	11.1	7.4	11.1	-	3.7	27	40
EUROPE										
Austria, Tyrol	9.1	72.7	12.1	6.1	-	-	-	-	33	34
Belarus										
Croatia										
Czech Republic	3.9	81.5	6.9	3.3	0.3	0.8	1.4	1.9	363	428
Denmark	7.9	84.5	2.7	1.7	0.3	1.7	0.3	0.7	291	310
Estonia	9.2	84.6	3.1	1.5	1.5	-	-	-	65	69
Finland	12.8	82.3	2.5	-	-	-	-	2.5	203	341
France, Bas-Rhin	11.8	79.4	2.9	-	5.9	-	-	-	34	46
France, Calvados	-	73.7	15.8	-	5.3	5.3	-	-	19	19
France, Doubs	33.3	55.6	-	-	-	11.1	-	-	9	11
France, Haut-Rhin	7.1	71.4	21.4	-	-	-	-	-	14	19
France, Herault	22.2	66.7	11.1	-	-	-	-	-	9	9
France, Isere	12.9	64.5	16.1	3.2	-	3.2	-	-	31	31
France, Somme	8.0	64.0	24.0	4.0	-	-	-	-	25	25
France, Tarn	-	62.5	18.8	6.3	-	12.5	-	-	16	16
Germany, Eastern States	11.7	82.2	2.0	1.2	0.8	1.6	0.4	-	247	314
Germany, Saarland										
Iceland	14.3	85.7	-	-	-	-	-	-	7	10
Ireland, Southern	27.3	72.7	-	-	-	-	-	-	11	14
Italy, Ferrara	-	83.3	16.7	-	-	-	-	-	6	10
Italy, Florence	-	76.2	9.5	9.5	-	4.8	-	-	21	32
Italy, Genoa	8.3	75.0	8.3	-	8.3	-	-	-	12	23
Italy, Latina	-	62.5	25.0	-	12.5	-	-	-	8	8
Italy, Macerata	-	100.0	-	-	-	-	-	-	3	5
Italy, Modena	11.8	64.7	5.9	17.6	-	-	-	-	17	21
Italy, Parma	-	100.0	-	-	-	-	-	-	8	8
Italy, Ragusa	-	100.0	-	-	-	-	-	-	2	3
Italy, Romagna	4.0	92.0	4.0	-	-	-	-	-	25	27
Italy, Torino	-	87.5	-	6.3	6.3	-	-	-	16	23
Italy, Trieste	-	-	-	-	-	-	-	-	-	7
Italy, Varese	11.8	70.6	17.6	-	-	-	-	-	17	27
Italy, Veneto	-	80.0	10.0	3.3	3.3	-	3.3	-	30	34
Latvia										
Malta										

Eye and orbit (ICD-9 190) - Both sexes (contd)

	Retino-blastoma	Melanoma	Carcinoma Squamous	Carcinoma Other	Carcinoma Unspec.	Sarcoma	Other	Unspec.	Number of cases MV	Number of cases Total
The Netherlands	8.9	84.8	2.4	2.2	0.2	1.3	0.2	-	461	518
The Netherlands, Eindhoven	25.0	71.4	-	3.6	-	-	-	-	28	33
The Netherlands, Maastricht	3.4	82.8	-	10.3	-	3.4	-	-	29	33
Norway	9.2	74.8	3.2	5.0	0.5	1.8	-	5.5	218	238
Poland, Cracow	-	100.0	-	-	-	-	-	-	26	29
Poland, Kielce	18.8	68.8	-	-	12.5	-	-	-	16	24
Poland, Lower Silesia	7.1	56.5	2.4	2.4	-	3.5	-	28.2	85	118
Poland, Warsaw City	11.4	82.9	2.9	-	2.9	-	-	-	35	44
Slovakia	10.0	79.5	5.9	0.9	-	0.9	1.8	0.9	219	244
Slovenia	7.1	82.1	8.9	-	-	1.8	-	-	56	76
Spain, Albacete	33.3	66.7	-	-	-	-	-	-	3	4
Spain, Asturias	4.0	72.0	20.0	4.0	-	-	-	-	25	26
Spain, Basque Country	2.4	70.7	22.0	-	2.4	-	-	2.4	41	44
Spain, Granada	-	84.6	7.7	-	-	7.7	-	-	13	14
Spain, Mallorca	20.0	33.3	46.7	-	-	-	-	-	15	17
Spain, Murcia	20.0	50.0	20.0	-	-	10.0	-	-	20	23
Spain, Navarra	11.1	72.2	11.1	-	-	5.6	-	-	18	19
Spain, Tarragona	14.3	50.0	28.6	-	-	7.1	-	-	14	16
Spain, Zaragoza	15.4	65.4	15.4	3.8	-	-	-	-	26	26
Sweden	6.9	86.7	2.2	2.5	0.7	0.7	0.2	-	407	474
Switzerland, Basel	19.0	76.2	4.8	-	-	-	-	-	21	28
Switzerland, Geneva	-	75.0	25.0	-	-	-	-	-	8	17
Switzerland, Graubunden	-	100.0	-	-	-	-	-	-	7	7
Switzerland, Neuchatel	33.3	66.7	-	-	-	-	-	-	6	8
Switzerland, St Gall-Appenzell	-	87.5	-	-	-	12.5	-	-	8	12
Switzerland, Valais	-	100.0	-	-	-	-	-	-	12	16
Switzerland, Vaud	8.1	86.5	2.7	-	2.7	-	-	-	37	37
Switzerland, Zurich	13.9	69.4	5.6	5.6	-	5.6	-	-	36	69
UK, England and Wales	6.8	81.4	2.0	1.9	1.9	1.7	0.6	3.6	1092	1370
UK, East Anglia										
UK, Mersey	5.4	85.7	3.6	5.4	-	-	-	-	56	62
UK, North Western										
UK, Oxford	9.0	84.0	4.0	1.0	-	2.0	-	-	100	107
UK, South Thames	15.3	73.2	6.4	1.9	1.3	1.3	-	0.6	157	352
UK, South Western	0.8	84.7	3.4	0.8	1.7	3.4	0.8	4.2	118	154
UK, Wessex	-	92.9	1.2	3.5	2.4	-	-	-	85	147
UK, West Midlands										
UK, Yorkshire	7.2	84.2	3.6	1.4	0.7	2.9	-	-	139	164
UK, Scotland	7.0	87.1	2.1	1.4	0.7	1.4	-	0.3	286	326
UK, Scotland, West	5.6	87.0	2.5	2.5	0.6	1.9	-	-	162	179
Yugoslavia, Vojvodina	5.9	66.7	3.9	9.8	3.9	2.0	-	7.8	51	66

OCEANIA

	Retino-blastoma	Melanoma	Carcinoma Squamous	Carcinoma Other	Carcinoma Unspec.	Sarcoma	Other	Unspec.	Number of cases MV	Number of cases Total
Australian Capital Territory	-	87.5	-	12.5	-	-	-	-	16	16
Australia, New South Wales	9.5	73.8	13.2	1.6	0.3	1.3	0.3	-	317	327
South Australia	5.2	62.1	27.6	1.7	-	1.7	-	1.7	58	72
Australia, Tasmania	14.3	64.3	21.4	-	-	-	-	-	14	16
Australia, Victoria	9.6	70.1	15.0	0.6	3.0	1.2	0.6	-	167	231
Western Australia	7.1	66.1	17.9	5.4	-	1.8	-	1.8	56	68
French Polynesia	-	-	100.0	-	-	-	-	-	1	1
New Zealand: Non-Maori										
New Zealand: Maori										
US, Hawaii: White	14.3	71.4	14.3	-	-	-	-	-	7	7
US, Hawaii: Japanese	50.0	-	-	50.0	-	-	-	-	2	2
US, Hawaii: Hawaiian	100.0	-	-	-	-	-	-	-	5	6
US, Hawaii: Filipino	100.0	-	-	-	-	-	-	-	1	1
US, Hawaii: Chinese	-	-	100.0	-	-	-	-	-	1	1

PERCENTAGE DISTRIBUTION OF MICROSCOPICALLY VERIFIED CASES BY HISTOLOGICAL TYPE
Thyroid (ICD-9 193) - Both sexes

| | Carcinoma | | | | | | Sarcoma | Other | Unspec. | Number of cases | |
	Follic.	Papil.	Medul.	Anapl.	Other	Unspec.				MV	Total
AFRICA											
Algeria, Setif	40.0	40.0	-	-	20.0	-	-	-	-	5	12
France, La Reunion	29.4	50.0	8.8	2.9	5.9	-	-	-	2.9	34	34
Mali, Bamako	16.7	-	-	-	41.7	41.7	-	-	-	12	20
Uganda, Kyadondo	50.0	5.6	5.6	-	11.1	27.8	-	-	-	18	24
Zimbabwe, Harare: African	62.5	6.3	-	18.8	6.3	6.3	-	-	-	16	29
Zimbabwe, Harare: European	-	100.0	-	-	-	-	-	-	-	1	2
AMERICA, CENTRAL AND SOUTH											
Argentina, Concordia	16.7	66.7	-	-	16.7	-	-	-	-	6	6
Brazil, Belem	28.0	56.0	12.0	-	-	4.0	-	-	-	25	28
Brazil, Goiania	29.5	56.4	-	1.3	1.3	6.4	-	-	5.1	78	83
Brazil, Porto Alegre	25.4	33.3	4.8	1.6	-	22.2	-	-	12.7	63	86
Colombia, Cali	15.6	67.0	2.9	4.7	1.1	2.9	-	-	5.8	276	291
Costa Rica	8.9	80.1	4.5	2.7	0.3	1.8	-	0.3	1.5	336	393
Ecuador, Quito	15.3	67.9	2.0	3.6	3.6	6.6	-	-	1.0	196	245
Peru, Lima	28.9	55.9	6.7	4.8	1.5	1.1	-	-	1.1	270	310
Peru, Trujillo	27.3	54.5	-	6.1	-	12.1	-	-	-	33	41
Puerto Rico	14.2	76.9	4.4	1.2	1.5	1.8	-	-	-	338	344
Uruguay, Montevideo	29.9	52.0	8.7	6.3	0.8	2.4	-	-	-	127	142
AMERICA, NORTH											
Canada	15.6	73.3	3.8	2.3	1.6	1.4	0.1	0.1	1.8	5118	5561
Canada, Alberta	10.1	83.8	2.9	2.1	0.4	0.4	0.2	-	0.2	526	529
Canada, British Columbia	15.4	76.1	3.1	3.5	0.9	0.7	-	0.2	0.2	577	583
Canada, Manitoba	15.7	79.9	1.0	2.0	1.0	0.5	-	-	-	204	218
Canada, New Brunswick	25.2	63.9	6.7	2.5	-	0.8	-	-	0.8	119	119
Canada, Newfoundland	17.0	67.0	11.4	2.3	2.3	-	-	-	-	88	88
Canada, Northwest Territories	40.0	60.0	-	-	-	-	-	-	-	10	10
Canada, Nova Scotia	17.6	75.4	2.1	0.7	3.5	0.7	-	-	-	142	143
Canada, Ontario	16.6	72.3	3.7	1.6	1.4	0.7	0.1	-	3.6	2211	2464
Canada, Prince Edward Island	26.3	73.7	-	-	-	-	-	-	-	19	19
Canada, Quebec	13.9	68.4	5.3	3.3	3.2	4.4	0.3	0.1	1.1	1029	1195
Canada, Saskatchewan	19.9	74.0	1.0	2.6	1.5	1.0	-	-	-	196	196
Canada, Yukon	14.3	57.1	-	-	-	28.6	-	-	-	7	7
US, Cent. California: Non-Hisp White	12.5	79.5	2.4	3.0	0.7	1.3	0.7	-	-	297	299
US, Cent. California: Hispanic	13.4	81.3	1.8	0.9	-	1.8	-	0.9	-	112	112
US, Los Angeles: Non-Hisp White	13.2	79.0	2.4	2.0	1.1	2.1	-	-	0.2	1110	1114
US, Los Angeles: Hispanic White	10.8	81.3	2.9	2.5	1.5	0.6	0.2	-	0.2	482	484
US, Los Angeles: Black	19.8	74.1	4.3	-	-	-	-	-	1.7	116	116
US, Los Angeles: Chinese	5.4	91.9	-	2.7	-	-	-	-	-	37	37
US, Los Angeles: Filipino	7.1	90.9	1.0	-	-	1.0	-	-	-	99	100
US, Los Angeles: Korean	7.4	81.5	7.4	-	-	-	-	-	3.7	27	27
US, Los Angeles: Japanese	9.1	90.9	-	-	-	-	-	-	-	22	22
US, San Francisco: Non-Hisp White	11.2	82.6	2.8	0.5	1.6	0.9	0.3	-	0.2	642	645
US, San Francisco: Hispanic White	15.3	79.6	0.7	0.7	2.2	1.5	-	-	-	137	137
US, San Francisco: Black	18.8	77.1	-	2.1	-	2.1	-	-	-	48	48
US, San Francisco: Chinese	12.3	80.8	5.5	-	1.4	-	-	-	-	73	73
US, San Francisco: Filipino	14.3	78.6	-	1.4	1.4	4.3	-	-	-	70	71
US, San Francisco: Japanese	6.3	93.8	-	-	-	-	-	-	-	16	16
US, Connecticut: White	14.8	75.0	3.7	1.5	0.9	3.3	-	-	0.7	667	676
US, Connecticut: Black	21.6	67.6	2.7	-	5.4	2.7	-	-	-	37	37
US, Atlanta: White	12.1	81.7	3.3	0.8	0.5	1.5	-	0.3	-	398	399
US, Atlanta: Black	29.5	57.7	6.4	1.3	1.3	2.6	-	-	1.3	78	80
US, Iowa	17.1	75.7	3.0	1.5	0.3	1.9	0.3	-	0.3	736	740
US, Central Louisiana: White	19.4	77.8	-	-	2.8	-	-	-	-	36	36
US, Central Louisiana: Black	42.9	28.6	-	14.3	-	14.3	-	-	-	7	7
US, New Orleans: White	16.6	76.1	4.3	-	2.5	0.6	-	-	-	163	165
US, New Orleans: Black	26.4	66.0	-	1.9	3.8	-	1.9	-	-	53	54
US, Detroit: White	17.5	74.0	4.1	1.6	1.3	1.0	-	-	0.5	859	862
US, Detroit: Black	18.8	68.0	3.9	3.1	2.3	3.9	-	-	-	128	132
US, New Mexico: Non-Hisp White	6.2	83.3	4.4	3.5	0.9	1.3	-	-	0.4	227	229
US, New Mexico: Hispanic White	9.9	88.7	1.4	-	-	-	-	-	-	142	144
US, New Mexico: American Indian	-	93.3	6.7	-	-	-	-	-	-	15	15
US, Utah	11.4	84.5	1.7	1.1	0.6	0.6	-	-	-	466	468
US, Seattle	14.1	79.5	3.1	1.7	0.6	0.6	0.1	-	0.2	830	837
US, SEER: White	14.2	78.6	3.2	1.4	0.9	1.4	0.1	-	0.3	5071	5103
US, SEER: Black	22.4	66.9	3.5	2.2	1.9	2.8	-	-	0.3	317	323

PERCENTAGE DISTRIBUTION OF MICROSCOPICALLY VERIFIED CASES BY HISTOLOGICAL TYPE
Thyroid (ICD-9 193) - Both sexes (contd)

			Carcinoma				Sarcoma	Other	Unspec.	Number of cases	
	Follic.	Papil.	Medul.	Anapl.	Other	Unspec.				MV	Total
ASIA											
China, Qidong											
China, Shanghai											
China, Tianjin	6.8	33.2	2.8	1.2	12.8	0.4	-	-	42.8	**250**	298
Hong Kong	14.3	70.9	2.4	3.5	5.7	2.3	-	-	0.8	**1185**	1477
India, Bangalore	18.5	53.4	8.9	3.8	1.7	4.5	-	-	9.2	**292**	325
India, Barshi, Paranda and Bhum	16.7	50.0	-	16.7	16.7	-	-	-	-	**6**	7
India, Bombay	34.8	45.4	6.1	3.8	3.8	3.8	0.3	0.3	1.8	**394**	459
India, Karunagappally	30.0	55.0	10.0	5.0	-	-	-	-	-	**20**	23
India, Madras	30.5	47.5	3.4	3.4	7.6	3.4	-	-	4.2	**118**	165
India, Trivandrum	20.4	68.5	-	1.9	1.9	7.4	-	-	-	**54**	60
Israel: All Jews	15.7	74.2	4.3	3.8	0.8	0.9	0.1	0.1	0.1	**1025**	1072
Jews born in Israel	13.9	78.2	5.4	1.7	0.3	0.6	-	-	-	**353**	363
Jews born in America or Europe	14.2	74.8	2.9	5.0	1.0	1.3	0.3	0.3	0.3	**381**	406
Jews born in Africa or Asia	20.0	68.6	4.8	4.8	1.0	0.7	-	-	-	**290**	302
Non-Jews	26.9	65.4	2.6	2.6	1.3	1.3	-	-	-	**78**	80
Japan, Hiroshima	9.3	85.7	0.5	1.0	1.0	2.0	-	0.5	-	**398**	411
Japan, Miyagi	10.4	82.8	1.1	2.2	1.1	0.4	0.3	-	1.8	**760**	798
Japan, Nagasaki	10.2	82.6	0.9	2.1	2.5	1.6	-	-	-	**432**	465
Japan, Osaka	18.0	63.3	2.3	4.2	6.6	0.8	0.1	-	4.5	**1236**	1378
Japan, Saga											
Japan, Yamagata											
Korea, Kangwha	-	87.5	-	-	-	6.3	-	-	6.3	**16**	19
Kuwait: Non-Kuwaitis	6.0	87.1	5.2	1.7	-	-	-	-	-	**116**	118
Kuwait: Kuwaitis	8.8	86.0	1.8	1.8	-	1.8	-	-	-	**57**	62
Philippines, Manila	25.5	64.4	0.9	3.4	2.4	2.3	-	-	1.1	**744**	884
Singapore: Chinese	18.5	71.8	0.9	0.5	3.2	5.0	-	-	0.2	**443**	453
Singapore: Malay	21.7	75.4	-	1.4	1.4	-	-	-	-	**69**	71
Singapore: Indian	22.2	66.7	-	-	5.6	5.6	-	-	-	**18**	18
Thailand, Chiang Mai	32.1	38.7	0.9	10.4	8.5	1.9	0.9	-	6.6	**106**	125
Thailand, Khon Kaen	50.5	45.7	-	1.9	1.0	1.0	-	-	-	**105**	129
Viet Nam, Hanoi	27.9	17.6	-	-	27.9	22.1	-	-	4.4	**68**	120
EUROPE											
Austria, Tyrol	29.3	58.5	2.0	2.4	0.5	3.9	1.5	-	2.0	**205**	214
Belarus											
Croatia											
Czech Republic	32.6	45.3	4.9	6.8	5.8	1.8	0.2	0.2	2.6	**1253**	1504
Denmark	22.8	50.6	6.7	8.9	3.8	5.3	1.0	0.4	0.6	**526**	542
Estonia	22.2	44.9	6.3	2.3	5.1	4.0	-	0.6	14.8	**176**	188
Finland	13.3	72.6	3.0	-	0.3	7.3	0.1	0.1	3.3	**1607**	1621
France, Bas-Rhin	23.5	47.8	7.0	7.8	7.8	1.7	2.6	0.9	0.9	**115**	121
France, Calvados	13.9	69.6	8.2	1.3	4.4	2.5	-	-	-	**158**	159
France, Doubs	26.9	60.2	2.2	8.6	1.1	1.1	-	-	-	**93**	94
France, Haut-Rhin	18.6	48.8	4.7	15.1	9.3	1.2	2.3	-	-	**86**	86
France, Herault	23.5	54.9	6.2	2.5	6.8	4.3	-	-	1.9	**162**	162
France, Isere	22.0	65.1	4.8	0.5	2.7	4.8	-	-	-	**186**	190
France, Somme	30.8	50.8	6.2	1.5	4.6	1.5	1.5	-	3.1	**65**	66
France, Tarn	16.7	72.5	5.9	2.9	1.0	1.0	-	-	-	**102**	103
Germany, Eastern States	36.9	34.2	5.3	13.8	6.1	1.6	1.1	0.1	0.8	**879**	899
Germany, Saarland											
Iceland	15.1	76.5	0.8	6.7	0.8	-	-	-	-	**119**	119
Ireland, Southern	23.9	43.5	10.9	19.6	2.2	-	-	-	-	**46**	49
Italy, Ferrara	16.9	72.9	10.2	-	-	-	-	-	-	**59**	62
Italy, Florence	8.3	68.0	8.8	1.7	3.9	6.6	-	-	2.8	**181**	222
Italy, Genoa	30.3	45.4	5.3	8.6	2.6	2.6	0.7	-	4.6	**152**	170
Italy, Latina	9.6	64.4	1.4	1.4	2.7	19.2	-	-	1.4	**73**	75
Italy, Macerata	24.2	63.6	9.1	3.0	-	-	-	-	-	**33**	35
Italy, Modena	10.1	77.0	4.7	4.1	2.0	1.4	0.7	-	-	**148**	159
Italy, Parma	14.1	73.1	5.1	3.8	1.3	1.3	1.3	-	-	**78**	80
Italy, Ragusa	22.2	55.6	-	3.7	-	7.4	-	-	11.1	**27**	35
Italy, Romagna	10.1	80.4	5.0	3.5	-	0.5	-	-	0.5	**199**	205
Italy, Torino	21.4	56.7	2.7	9.6	1.6	5.3	0.5	-	2.1	**187**	194
Italy, Trieste	8.2	22.4	2.0	2.0	8.2	28.6	4.1	-	24.5	**49**	81
Italy, Varese	20.0	63.3	5.7	7.1	1.4	0.5	0.5	-	1.4	**210**	218
Italy, Veneto	19.7	60.6	7.1	3.7	1.9	1.9	-	-	5.2	**269**	291
Latvia											
Malta											

PERCENTAGE DISTRIBUTION OF MICROSCOPICALLY VERIFIED CASES BY HISTOLOGICAL TYPE
Thyroid (ICD-9 193) - Both sexes (contd)

			Carcinoma				Sarcoma	Other	Unspec.	Number of cases	
	Follic.	Papil.	Medul.	Anapl.	Other	Unspec.				MV	Total
The Netherlands	26.8	52.4	8.5	5.8	2.2	4.0	0.2	0.2	-	**1226**	1233
The Netherlands, Eindhoven	38.8	52.5	5.0	3.8	-	-	-	-	-	**80**	81
The Netherlands, Maastricht	21.1	42.2	16.7	10.0	2.2	6.7	1.1	-	-	**90**	90
Norway	16.4	71.3	3.2	0.1	0.4	6.8	0.2	-	1.5	**909**	920
Poland, Cracow	41.5	23.1	-	7.7	12.3	6.2	-	-	9.2	**65**	78
Poland, Kielce	17.4	21.7	-	19.6	10.9	17.4	-	-	13.0	**46**	59
Poland, Lower Silesia	27.3	20.5	3.7	6.2	12.4	3.1	0.6	-	26.1	**161**	267
Poland, Warsaw City	22.5	38.4	8.7	13.8	7.2	5.8	-	1.4	2.2	**138**	159
Slovakia	28.6	50.5	5.0	10.1	2.1	1.9	0.5	0.2	1.0	**576**	617
Slovenia	17.3	54.9	5.5	16.5	1.2	3.5	0.4	-	0.8	**255**	261
Spain, Albacete	22.2	66.7	-	5.6	-	5.6	-	-	-	**18**	19
Spain, Asturias	31.8	46.7	4.1	11.8	3.6	1.0	0.5	-	0.5	**195**	199
Spain, Basque Country	13.5	65.9	7.6	9.7	1.1	1.6	-	-	0.5	**185**	190
Spain, Granada	15.6	68.9	4.4	8.9	1.1	-	-	-	1.1	**90**	91
Spain, Mallorca	10.0	75.7	5.7	4.3	1.4	1.4	-	1.4	-	**70**	70
Spain, Murcia	21.9	65.2	7.7	1.3	-	1.9	0.6	-	1.3	**155**	156
Spain, Navarra	36.3	49.3	7.5	4.8	0.7	1.4	-	-	-	**146**	147
Spain, Tarragona	31.1	48.6	10.8	5.4	1.4	2.7	-	-	-	**74**	74
Spain, Zaragoza	32.4	53.9	6.9	4.9	1.0	1.0	-	-	-	**102**	108
Sweden											
Switzerland, Basel	32.6	49.4	5.6	9.0	-	-	3.4	-	-	**89**	89
Switzerland, Geneva	27.1	60.0	-	8.6	1.4	-	1.4	1.4	-	**70**	70
Switzerland, Graubunden	40.0	40.0	10.0	10.0	-	-	-	-	-	**20**	20
Switzerland, Neuchatel	55.6	22.2	11.1	-	-	11.1	-	-	-	**18**	19
Switzerland, St Gall-Appenzell	32.7	45.8	8.4	8.4	-	1.9	1.9	-	0.9	**107**	108
Switzerland, Valais	34.4	50.0	3.1	3.1	6.3	-	3.1	-	-	**32**	33
Switzerland, Vaud	15.8	63.2	6.1	9.6	-	4.4	-	-	0.9	**114**	125
Switzerland, Zurich	36.7	50.2	3.6	7.9	0.7	1.0	-	-	-	**305**	307
UK, England and Wales	25.1	42.6	5.5	6.9	3.8	14.1	0.3	0.2	1.5	**2199**	2615
UK, East Anglia											
UK, Mersey	25.4	46.3	4.5	11.9	3.0	8.2	-	-	0.7	**134**	153
UK, North Western											
UK, Oxford	26.4	51.9	3.5	9.1	4.8	3.9	-	-	0.4	**231**	256
UK, South Thames	23.5	44.8	5.8	4.7	6.7	13.5	0.7	0.2	0.2	**451**	579
UK, South Western	27.6	45.9	6.5	6.5	2.9	8.2	-	-	2.5	**279**	331
UK, Wessex	23.8	45.5	5.7	9.8	2.0	12.3	-	0.8	-	**244**	315
UK, West Midlands											
UK, Yorkshire	26.0	49.0	6.4	7.1	3.4	7.8	-	-	0.3	**296**	312
UK, Scotland	22.2	55.5	7.3	6.2	4.9	3.4	-	0.2	0.2	**465**	506
UK, Scotland, West	25.5	48.1	8.8	7.4	6.0	3.7	-	-	0.5	**216**	242
Yugoslavia, Vojvodina	36.3	39.3	7.4	5.2	0.7	6.7	-	-	4.4	**135**	176

OCEANIA

	Follic.	Papil.	Medul.	Anapl.	Other	Unspec.	Sarcoma	Other	Unspec.	MV	Total
Australian Capital Territory	24.0	64.0	12.0	-	-	-	-	-	-	**25**	26
Australia, New South Wales	22.2	67.7	4.2	2.8	1.0	1.6	0.2	0.2	0.1	**1026**	1058
South Australia	20.1	70.9	4.5	3.4	0.6	-	-	-	0.6	**179**	218
Australia, Tasmania	22.2	65.1	-	4.8	6.3	1.6	-	-	-	**63**	64
Australia, Victoria	21.5	65.5	4.7	4.3	1.4	2.3	-	0.2	-	**557**	580
Western Australia	17.2	70.4	6.0	1.5	0.7	3.4	-	-	0.7	**267**	280
French Polynesia	16.9	81.4	-	-	1.7	-	-	-	-	**59**	67
New Zealand: Non-Maori											
New Zealand: Maori											
US, Hawaii: White	14.9	77.7	3.2	3.2	1.1	-	-	-	-	**94**	94
US, Hawaii: Japanese	16.7	67.9	1.2	1.2	2.4	9.5	-	1.2	-	**84**	84
US, Hawaii: Hawaiian	12.7	76.4	5.5	-	1.8	1.8	-	1.8	-	**55**	55
US, Hawaii: Filipino	17.9	78.6	0.7	2.1	-	0.7	-	-	-	**140**	141
US, Hawaii: Chinese	9.7	90.3	-	-	-	-	-	-	-	**31**	31

PERCENTAGE DISTRIBUTION OF MICROSCOPICALLY VERIFIED CASES BY HISTOLOGICAL TYPE
Hodgkin 's disease (ICD-9 201)

	Lymphocytic predominance	Nodular sclerosis	Mixed cellularity	Lymphocytic depletion	Unspecified	Number of cases MV	Total
AFRICA							
Algeria, Setif	7.4	16.2	8.8	8.8	58.8	**68**	68
France, La Reunion	12.0	48.0	20.0	-	20.0	**25**	25
Mali, Bamako	21.7	4.3	30.4	21.7	21.7	**23**	24
Uganda, Kyadondo	12.5	12.5	-	25.0	50.0	**8**	8
Zimbabwe, Harare: African	-	5.3	15.8	10.5	68.4	**19**	19
Zimbabwe, Harare: European	-	33.3	33.3	-	33.3	**3**	3
AMERICA, CENTRAL AND SOUTH							
Argentina, Concordia	-	50.0	-	16.7	33.3	**6**	6
Brazil, Belem	22.4	26.5	12.2	2.0	36.7	**49**	50
Brazil, Goiania	-	1.7	3.3	3.3	91.7	**60**	66
Brazil, Porto Alegre	-	2.4	-	2.4	95.2	**42**	66
Colombia, Cali	19.5	11.5	29.9	6.9	32.2	**87**	96
Costa Rica	8.9	42.6	28.7	7.2	12.7	**237**	266
Ecuador, Quito	-	-	3.6	1.8	94.6	**56**	70
Peru, Lima	7.4	17.3	28.4	8.6	38.3	**81**	96
Peru, Trujillo	-	14.3	-	-	85.7	**7**	7
Puerto Rico	-	57.7	24.8	7.0	10.5	**286**	294
Uruguay, Montevideo	-	24.2	9.7	1.6	64.5	**124**	124
AMERICA, NORTH							
Canada	5.8	55.5	21.7	3.5	13.4	**3670**	3956
Canada, Alberta	4.8	71.0	15.3	4.1	4.8	**314**	314
Canada, British Columbia	3.7	67.8	19.0	0.8	8.7	**379**	385
Canada, Manitoba	6.3	50.5	27.0	4.5	11.7	**111**	127
Canada, New Brunswick	12.8	43.6	34.0	3.2	6.4	**94**	97
Canada, Newfoundland	19.0	55.6	22.2	-	3.2	**63**	63
Canada, Northwest Territories	-	50.0	50.0	-	-	**2**	2
Canada, Nova Scotia	4.5	47.7	35.6	3.0	9.1	**132**	133
Canada, Ontario	6.0	58.4	20.1	4.1	11.4	**1481**	1573
Canada, Prince Edward Island	12.5	50.0	31.3	-	6.3	**16**	16
Canada, Quebec	4.6	44.1	23.1	3.9	24.3	**955**	1123
Canada, Saskatchewan	10.8	52.5	25.8	3.3	7.5	**120**	120
Canada, Yukon	-	50.0	28.6	-	21.4	**14**	14
US, Cent. California: Non-Hisp White	7.2	63.4	14.9	3.1	11.3	**194**	200
US, Cent. California: Hispanic	5.8	61.5	21.2	5.8	5.8	**52**	52
US, Los Angeles: Non-Hisp White	4.5	60.9	21.3	3.2	10.1	**624**	632
US, Los Angeles: Hispanic White	3.6	51.2	32.1	3.6	9.5	**252**	254
US, Los Angeles: Black	8.5	58.5	20.8	3.8	8.5	**106**	106
US, Los Angeles: Chinese	14.3	42.9	28.6	14.3	-	**7**	7
US, Los Angeles: Filipino	7.1	64.3	7.1	-	21.4	**14**	14
US, Los Angeles: Korean	50.0	-	-	-	50.0	**2**	2
US, Los Angeles: Japanese	-	50.0	25.0	-	25.0	**4**	4
US, San Francisco: Non-Hisp White	4.5	66.1	19.2	3.2	7.0	**442**	446
US, San Francisco: Hispanic White	3.7	63.0	24.1	5.6	3.7	**54**	54
US, San Francisco: Black	11.7	48.3	20.0	5.0	15.0	**60**	60
US, San Francisco: Chinese	-	81.8	18.2	-	-	**11**	11
US, San Francisco: Filipino	11.1	55.6	22.2	-	11.1	**9**	9
US, San Francisco: Japanese	-	75.0	-	25.0	-	**4**	4
US, Connecticut: White	7.1	58.1	20.6	4.0	10.2	**630**	640
US, Connecticut: Black	7.4	59.3	14.8	-	18.5	**27**	27
US, Atlanta: White	8.5	62.3	14.8	3.1	11.2	**223**	223
US, Atlanta: Black	13.6	47.0	28.8	3.0	7.6	**66**	67
US, Iowa	5.5	67.4	18.7	2.3	6.2	**438**	440
US, Central Louisiana: White	-	63.6	18.2	9.1	9.1	**22**	23
US, Central Louisiana: Black	-	60.0	-	-	40.0	**5**	5
US, New Orleans: White	2.0	57.0	22.0	2.0	17.0	**100**	102
US, New Orleans: Black	12.9	38.7	16.1	-	32.3	**31**	32
US, Detroit: White	4.8	63.3	21.4	2.1	8.4	**523**	524
US, Detroit: Black	10.4	52.2	24.3	2.6	10.4	**115**	116
US, New Mexico: Non-Hisp White	3.8	66.0	17.9	0.9	11.3	**106**	109
US, New Mexico: Hispanic White	3.9	64.7	13.7	5.9	11.8	**51**	55
US, New Mexico: American Indian	-	50.0	-	-	50.0	**2**	2
US, Utah	7.3	66.5	14.0	4.5	7.8	**179**	179
US, Seattle	7.2	53.2	25.5	2.3	11.8	**517**	518
US, SEER: White	6.1	61.9	20.2	2.9	8.8	**3170**	3195
US, SEER: Black	11.4	52.0	22.1	3.4	11.1	**298**	300

Hodgkin 's disease (ICD-9 201) (contd)

	Lymphocytic predominance	Nodular sclerosis	Mixed cellularity	Lymphocytic depletion	Unspecified	Number of cases MV	Total
ASIA							
China, Qidong							
China, Shanghai							
China, Tianjin	-	3.9	2.0	-	94.1	**51**	66
Hong Kong							
India, Bangalore	10.8	12.0	40.1	3.0	34.1	**167**	174
India, Barshi, Paranda and Bhum	-	20.0	40.0	20.0	20.0	**5**	5
India, Bombay	10.5	6.6	50.0	2.6	30.3	**380**	390
India, Karunagappally	25.0	-	50.0	-	25.0	**4**	4
India, Madras	3.4	9.8	12.1	1.1	73.6	**174**	178
India, Trivandrum	25.0	25.0	37.5	-	12.5	**8**	11
Israel: All Jews	2.2	58.1	19.9	2.7	17.1	**549**	568
Jews born in Israel	1.8	61.7	18.3	2.1	16.2	**334**	344
Jews born in America or Europe	2.1	54.9	16.9	4.9	21.1	**142**	147
Jews born in Africa or Asia	4.1	47.9	32.9	1.4	13.7	**73**	76
Non-Jews	1.3	42.1	36.8	7.9	11.8	**76**	78
Japan, Hiroshima	-	5.6	33.3	16.7	44.4	**18**	19
Japan, Miyagi	-	5.0	5.0	-	90.0	**40**	46
Japan, Nagasaki	5.9	11.8	23.5	5.9	52.9	**17**	18
Japan, Osaka	5.9	13.5	19.5	4.9	56.2	**185**	185
Japan, Saga							
Japan, Yamagata							
Korea, Kangwha	-	-	-	-	100.0	**1**	1
Kuwait: Non-Kuwaitis	12.9	41.4	21.4	2.9	21.4	**70**	72
Kuwait: Kuwaitis	10.5	42.1	31.6	10.5	5.3	**57**	57
Philippines, Manila	6.9	2.8	15.3	4.2	70.8	**72**	96
Singapore: Chinese	12.8	56.4	10.3	-	20.5	**39**	42
Singapore: Malay	6.7	53.3	20.0	6.7	13.3	**15**	15
Singapore: Indian	14.3	57.1	14.3	-	14.3	**7**	7
Thailand, Chiang Mai	13.8	5.2	17.2	1.7	62.1	**58**	58
Thailand, Khon Kaen	25.0	12.5	33.3	-	29.2	**24**	24
Viet Nam, Hanoi	-	-	2.0	2.0	96.0	**50**	76
EUROPE							
Austria, Tyrol	12.7	46.8	10.1	2.5	27.8	**79**	79
Belarus							
Croatia							
Czech Republic	16.2	28.5	30.6	8.0	16.7	**1395**	1561
Denmark	5.7	43.4	17.2	1.5	32.1	**679**	681
Estonia	5.8	37.6	26.6	6.4	23.7	**173**	175
Finland							
France, Bas-Rhin	8.4	31.9	43.7	5.9	10.1	**119**	119
France, Calvados	11.6	60.9	11.6	1.4	14.5	**69**	69
France, Doubs	-	59.6	3.8	-	36.5	**52**	52
France, Haut-Rhin	7.8	40.3	26.0	1.3	24.7	**77**	77
France, Herault	4.0	17.2	28.3	9.1	41.4	**99**	99
France, Isere	-	14.7	3.9	1.0	80.4	**102**	102
France, Somme	3.0	50.7	9.0	1.5	35.8	**67**	67
France, Tarn	-	33.3	48.1	3.7	14.8	**27**	27
Germany, Eastern States	4.4	14.8	17.0	9.8	54.1	**860**	863
Germany, Saarland							
Iceland	7.1	57.1	21.4	3.6	10.7	**28**	28
Ireland, Southern	10.4	37.5	20.8	6.3	25.0	**48**	48
Italy, Ferrara	16.7	45.8	8.3	-	29.2	**24**	27
Italy, Florence	4.9	30.3	38.7	7.7	18.3	**142**	177
Italy, Genoa	7.3	50.9	27.3	2.7	11.8	**110**	120
Italy, Latina	6.4	27.7	19.1	2.1	44.7	**47**	47
Italy, Macerata	5.0	25.0	40.0	10.0	20.0	**20**	24
Italy, Modena	4.9	30.5	32.9	6.1	25.6	**82**	84
Italy, Parma	1.8	26.8	41.1	5.4	25.0	**56**	56
Italy, Ragusa	13.2	18.4	31.6	7.9	28.9	**38**	38
Italy, Romagna	12.9	51.4	17.1	1.4	17.1	**70**	71
Italy, Torino	5.9	45.9	31.9	8.1	8.1	**135**	138
Italy, Trieste	-	15.2	6.1	3.0	75.8	**33**	46
Italy, Varese	8.0	46.0	32.8	2.2	10.9	**137**	141
Italy, Veneto	5.5	35.3	26.9	5.0	27.3	**238**	246
Latvia							
Malta							

Hodgkin 's disease (ICD-9 201) (contd)

	Lymphocytic predominance	Nodular sclerosis	Mixed cellularity	Lymphocytic depletion	Unspecified	Number of cases	
						MV	Total
The Netherlands	1.3	71.7	13.9	2.8	10.4	1417	1417
The Netherlands, Eindhoven	6.8	65.9	17.0	4.5	5.7	88	89
The Netherlands, Maastricht	-	74.3	13.9	3.0	8.9	101	101
Norway							
Poland, Cracow	-	12.6	28.4	-	58.9	95	106
Poland, Kielce	-	3.5	4.4	0.9	91.2	113	127
Poland, Lower Silesia	12.9	11.9	37.6	9.9	27.7	202	316
Poland, Warsaw City	4.1	54.5	19.0	7.4	14.9	121	133
Slovakia	17.2	34.1	32.8	8.1	7.9	534	552
Slovenia	1.1	57.9	20.0	1.6	19.5	190	190
Spain, Albacete	16.7	33.3	33.3	-	16.7	12	16
Spain, Asturias	8.8	35.3	10.3	2.2	43.4	136	136
Spain, Basque Country	9.5	39.8	33.3	8.7	8.7	231	240
Spain, Granada	19.7	36.8	25.0	9.2	9.2	76	76
Spain, Mallorca	4.6	53.8	29.2	1.5	10.8	65	65
Spain, Murcia	4.9	44.4	38.3	3.7	8.6	81	82
Spain, Navarra	15.7	28.6	32.9	14.3	8.6	70	72
Spain, Tarragona	13.6	35.6	22.0	5.1	23.7	59	59
Spain, Zaragoza	18.0	36.0	24.7	4.5	16.9	89	95
Sweden	-	-	-	-	100.0	932	933
Switzerland, Basel	-	57.6	28.8	6.8	6.8	59	59
Switzerland, Geneva	9.8	49.0	21.6	2.0	17.6	51	51
Switzerland, Graubunden	10.0	35.0	50.0	5.0	-	20	20
Switzerland, Neuchatel	5.9	35.3	52.9	5.9	-	17	17
Switzerland, St Gall-Appenzell	3.4	66.1	23.7	-	6.8	59	59
Switzerland, Valais	20.0	60.0	8.0	4.0	8.0	25	25
Switzerland, Vaud	3.0	79.1	9.0	4.5	4.5	67	67
Switzerland, Zurich	6.3	58.0	21.8	3.4	10.3	174	174
UK, England and Wales	5.3	36.5	15.0	5.8	37.4	3522	3713
UK, East Anglia							
UK, Mersey	5.2	48.3	16.8	4.3	25.4	232	244
UK, North Western							
UK, Oxford	6.1	42.2	15.3	2.0	34.4	346	346
UK, South Thames	3.0	39.7	15.6	0.6	41.1	635	820
UK, South Western	9.8	50.1	19.6	4.6	15.9	347	373
UK, Wessex	5.9	62.8	16.7	4.1	10.6	341	398
UK, West Midlands							
UK, Yorkshire	9.9	35.0	17.1	24.4	13.6	434	447
UK, Scotland	9.0	40.3	16.8	6.0	27.8	632	653
UK, Scotland, West	7.8	35.1	15.0	5.0	37.0	319	328
Yugoslavia, Vojvodina							
OCEANIA							
Australian Capital Territory	5.6	38.9	27.8	5.6	22.2	18	19
Australia, New South Wales	9.0	47.0	20.5	4.2	19.3	575	587
South Australia	6.7	40.0	44.2	3.3	5.8	120	138
Australia, Tasmania	4.5	52.3	27.3	9.1	6.8	44	47
Australia, Victoria	11.2	58.5	19.5	3.9	6.8	482	494
Western Australia	-	52.3	28.5	1.3	17.9	151	157
French Polynesia	10.0	30.0	10.0	-	50.0	10	11
New Zealand: Non-Maori							
New Zealand: Maori							
US, Hawaii: White	11.5	65.4	17.3	1.9	3.8	52	52
US, Hawaii: Japanese	10.0	25.0	35.0	20.0	10.0	20	20
US, Hawaii: Hawaiian	-	86.7	13.3	-	-	15	15
US, Hawaii: Filipino	11.1	66.7	22.2	-	-	9	9
US, Hawaii: Chinese	-	50.0	-	50.0	-	2	2

PERCENTAGE DISTRIBUTION OF MICROSCOPICALLY VERIFIED CASES BY HISTOLOGICAL TYPE
Lymphoid and Myeloid Leukaemias (ICD-9 204+205) - Both sexes

	Lymphoid				Myeloid				Number of cases	
	Acute	Chronic	Other	Unspec.	Acute	Chronic	Other	Unspec.	MV	Total
AFRICA										
Algeria, Setif	40.5	15.1	-	-	26.2	18.3	-	-	**126**	127
France, La Reunion	25.6	10.7	-	-	39.7	23.1	0.8	-	**121**	121
Mali, Bamako	-	-	-	-	-	90.0	10.0	-	**10**	13
Uganda, Kyadondo	42.9	-	-	28.6	-	28.6	-	-	**7**	10
Zimbabwe, Harare: African	26.5	13.3	-	-	32.5	27.7	-	-	**83**	88
Zimbabwe, Harare: European	12.5	12.5	-	-	75.0	-	-	-	**8**	11
AMERICA, CENTRAL AND SOUTH										
Argentina, Concordia	15.4	69.2	-	-	-	7.7	-	7.7	**13**	13
Brazil, Belem	41.7	3.6	-	2.4	28.6	16.7	-	7.1	**84**	84
Brazil, Goiania	34.4	9.4	-	1.6	35.9	17.2	-	1.6	**64**	110
Brazil, Porto Alegre	33.3	10.0	-	6.7	30.0	13.3	1.1	5.6	**90**	197
Colombia, Cali	46.6	6.9	-	1.3	23.3	18.1	-	3.9	**232**	260
Costa Rica	51.4	6.6	0.2	1.8	22.8	16.6	0.7	-	**457**	786
Ecuador, Quito	48.4	1.4	-	3.2	31.5	11.0	-	4.6	**219**	283
Peru, Lima	49.1	4.6	-	1.5	31.7	11.9	-	1.2	**328**	380
Peru, Trujillo	44.7	2.1	-	-	44.7	8.5	-	-	**47**	47
Puerto Rico	27.8	14.6	0.4	2.2	32.7	19.8	0.4	2.0	**697**	762
Uruguay, Montevideo	17.8	28.3	-	1.9	27.9	22.3	-	1.9	**269**	269
AMERICA, NORTH										
Canada	20.1	31.8	0.1	0.8	29.9	15.5	0.4	1.3	**8231**	13011
Canada, Alberta	19.5	38.4	0.1	0.6	24.5	16.5	-	0.4	**889**	948
Canada, British Columbia	22.2	30.0	-	0.5	27.9	18.2	0.2	0.9	**932**	1275
Canada, Manitoba	14.3	36.3	-	0.2	35.4	11.8	0.2	1.7	**474**	528
Canada, New Brunswick	18.3	33.8	-	0.5	29.1	15.5	0.5	2.3	**213**	259
Canada, Newfoundland	22.9	17.8	-	0.6	40.1	18.5	-	-	**157**	160
Canada, Northwest Territories	30.8	23.1	-	-	30.8	7.7	-	7.7	**13**	16
Canada, Nova Scotia	19.8	32.8	-	3.2	22.1	18.2	1.2	2.8	**253**	295
Canada, Ontario	17.7	32.2	0.1	0.7	31.4	15.8	0.5	1.6	**3351**	5731
Canada, Prince Edward Island	11.8	43.1	-	-	29.4	13.7	2.0	-	**51**	55
Canada, Quebec	25.9	26.3	0.1	1.5	31.0	13.3	0.5	1.3	**1511**	3113
Canada, Saskatchewan	22.2	36.3	0.3	-	24.8	15.4	0.3	0.8	**383**	629
Canada, Yukon	50.0	31.3	-	-	6.3	12.5	-	-	**16**	24
US, Cent. California: Non-Hisp White	15.8	31.2	0.3	0.5	34.5	16.1	1.1	0.5	**632**	730
US, Cent. California: Hispanic	51.0	12.0	-	1.6	22.9	12.0	0.5	-	**192**	201
US, Los Angeles: Non-Hisp White	11.1	37.0	-	1.2	33.7	15.9	0.4	0.7	**2098**	2310
US, Los Angeles: Hispanic White	45.2	9.7	0.2	0.7	27.4	15.3	0.8	0.5	**831**	850
US, Los Angeles: Black	11.5	30.0	0.9	0.3	33.0	22.4	0.3	1.5	**330**	356
US, Los Angeles: Chinese	15.5	17.2	-	-	46.6	19.0	1.7	-	**58**	59
US, Los Angeles: Filipino	25.3	6.3	-	-	48.1	20.3	-	-	**79**	83
US, Los Angeles: Korean	29.2	4.2	-	4.2	50.0	12.5	-	-	**24**	25
US, Los Angeles: Japanese	20.5	2.6	-	-	51.3	23.1	2.6	-	**39**	44
US, San Francisco: Non-Hisp White	13.8	32.4	0.2	1.2	35.0	16.3	0.6	0.5	**1103**	1194
US, San Francisco: Hispanic White	33.5	14.3	-	-	34.8	17.4	-	-	**161**	164
US, San Francisco: Black	20.7	31.9	0.7	-	31.9	14.8	-	-	**135**	148
US, San Francisco: Chinese	26.6	13.9	2.5	-	30.4	22.8	1.3	2.5	**79**	80
US, San Francisco: Filipino	32.8	8.6	-	-	39.7	17.2	-	1.7	**58**	61
US, San Francisco: Japanese	10.0	10.0	-	-	50.0	30.0	-	-	**10**	10
US, Connecticut: White	13.1	37.8	0.2	1.2	30.9	15.2	0.3	1.3	**1367**	1444
US, Connecticut: Black	13.3	29.3	2.7	5.3	29.3	17.3	1.3	1.3	**75**	77
US, Atlanta: White	19.0	27.2	0.4	1.4	33.1	17.4	1.0	0.6	**511**	534
US, Atlanta: Black	19.0	24.8	-	2.6	32.0	20.9	0.7	-	**153**	163
US, Iowa	10.4	46.8	0.1	1.4	25.9	14.4	0.5	0.5	**1786**	1861
US, Central Louisiana: White	9.9	29.6	-	2.5	40.7	13.6	1.2	2.5	**81**	92
US, Central Louisiana: Black	23.5	23.5	5.9	-	35.3	11.8	-	-	**17**	18
US, New Orleans: White	14.9	31.3	0.3	3.1	36.5	10.4	0.7	2.8	**288**	297
US, New Orleans: Black	18.4	24.3	-	2.9	32.0	18.4	-	3.9	**103**	105
US, Detroit: White	13.2	36.9	0.2	0.9	28.8	18.2	0.5	1.3	**1644**	1735
US, Detroit: Black	13.2	31.9	-	0.9	29.8	22.4	0.6	1.2	**326**	351
US, New Mexico: Non-Hisp White	13.5	38.2	0.5	1.8	28.6	16.1	0.5	0.8	**385**	440
US, New Mexico: Hispanic White	35.1	17.9	-	1.2	26.2	17.9	-	1.8	**168**	177
US, New Mexico: American Indian	54.8	-	-	3.2	22.6	19.4	-	-	**31**	31
US, Utah	26.0	26.4	-	0.9	31.5	14.6	0.5	0.2	**584**	600
US, Seattle	15.4	37.9	-	0.8	29.3	15.6	0.4	0.6	**1545**	1563
US, SEER: White	15.1	36.5	0.2	1.1	30.0	15.9	0.5	0.8	**9155**	9629
US, SEER: Black	15.8	29.9	0.4	1.5	29.9	21.3	0.5	0.7	**755**	806

PERCENTAGE DISTRIBUTION OF MICROSCOPICALLY VERIFIED CASES BY HISTOLOGICAL TYPE
Lymphoid and Myeloid Leukaemias (ICD-9 204+205) - Both sexes (contd)

| | Lymphoid | | | | Myeloid | | | | Number of cases | |
	Acute	Chronic	Other	Unspec.	Acute	Chronic	Other	Unspec.	MV	Total
ASIA										
China, Qidong										
China, Shanghai										
China, Tianjin	21.1	6.5	-	7.4	32.0	18.6	0.7	13.6	403	450
Hong Kong										
India, Bangalore	26.0	8.0	-	1.0	37.7	25.1	1.5	0.7	411	445
India, Barshi, Paranda and Bhum	46.7	3.3	-	-	33.3	13.3	3.3	-	30	30
India, Bombay	34.5	8.1	-	1.1	29.8	24.5	0.7	1.4	1103	1188
India, Karunagappally	50.0	-	-	-	44.4	5.6	-	-	18	18
India, Madras	49.2	3.4	-	0.3	24.5	21.4	0.3	1.0	384	387
India, Trivandrum	45.1	7.8	-	2.0	31.4	13.7	-	-	51	54
Israel: All Jews	18.2	34.9	0.1	1.1	32.1	12.0	0.4	1.0	1162	1189
Jews born in Israel	45.3	9.4	-	0.6	33.0	11.6	-	-	318	324
Jews born in America or Europe	8.2	46.0	-	1.4	29.6	12.8	0.5	1.5	585	599
Jews born in Africa or Asia	7.7	41.3	0.4	1.2	36.7	10.8	0.8	1.2	259	266
Non-Jews	35.9	18.3	-	1.5	32.1	9.2	-	3.1	131	134
Japan, Hiroshima	25.2	4.5	-	-	48.5	21.8	-	-	202	247
Japan, Miyagi	28.2	3.2	8.6	0.6	44.0	14.4	0.3	0.9	348	508
Japan, Nagasaki	24.9	4.1	-	-	50.5	19.4	-	1.1	366	369
Japan, Osaka	24.1	2.7	0.5	12.2	40.5	18.7	-	1.3	1882	1894
Japan, Saga										
Japan, Yamagata										
Korea, Kangwha	29.4	-	-	5.9	29.4	35.3	-	-	17	17
Kuwait: Non-Kuwaitis	41.7	10.1	1.4	1.4	32.4	11.5	-	1.4	139	149
Kuwait: Kuwaitis	38.8	4.5	-	1.5	41.8	11.9	1.5	-	67	76
Philippines, Manila	49.5	2.0	-	1.4	30.2	11.9	0.3	4.7	295	646
Singapore: Chinese	32.4	5.0	-	0.2	45.0	16.8	0.2	0.2	404	453
Singapore: Malay	28.0	2.7	-	1.3	46.7	20.0	1.3	-	75	81
Singapore: Indian	28.6	14.3	-	-	35.7	21.4	-	-	28	31
Thailand, Chiang Mai	21.5	1.7	-	0.4	56.5	19.0	-	0.8	237	237
Thailand, Khon Kaen	43.6	-	-	-	36.9	19.5	-	-	149	149
Viet Nam, Hanoi	17.4	-	-	11.3	47.0	19.1	-	5.2	115	120
EUROPE										
Austria, Tyrol	17.9	40.7	-	-	26.0	14.2	-	1.2	246	277
Belarus										
Croatia										
Czech Republic	14.3	42.4	0.7	2.0	22.1	15.8	1.0	1.6	3157	4528
Denmark	9.3	41.1	-	1.0	34.6	13.0	0.1	0.9	2812	2901
Estonia	10.4	53.6	-	1.2	17.0	16.0	0.2	1.7	606	606
Finland										
France, Bas-Rhin	15.4	39.1	-	0.9	27.7	13.4	-	3.4	350	371
France, Calvados	11.7	42.9	2.6	-	18.2	23.4	-	1.3	77	114
France, Doubs	20.5	21.8	0.6	0.6	35.9	18.6	-	1.9	156	174
France, Haut-Rhin	17.6	39.1	-	1.7	25.3	11.6	-	4.7	233	233
France, Herault	11.8	41.8	-	0.5	19.5	23.2	-	3.2	220	220
France, Isere	19.0	28.7	-	1.3	35.4	13.4	-	2.1	373	373
France, Somme	12.8	53.7	-	-	14.2	17.9	0.5	0.9	218	224
France, Tarn	17.9	38.8	-	0.7	26.9	14.9	-	0.7	134	134
Germany, Eastern States	13.2	36.7	-	0.6	26.4	22.2	0.3	0.6	2157	2165
Germany, Saarland										
Iceland	18.8	30.4	-	-	40.6	10.1	-	-	69	69
Ireland, Southern	16.1	44.1	-	0.4	23.6	14.2	0.8	0.8	254	263
Italy, Ferrara	9.8	45.1	-	2.4	22.0	9.8	2.4	8.5	82	86
Italy, Florence	11.3	31.1	-	3.1	29.1	22.0	-	3.3	450	473
Italy, Genoa	9.3	39.4	-	0.3	32.2	17.3	-	1.4	289	352
Italy, Latina	16.8	36.2	-	2.0	27.5	16.8	-	0.7	149	169
Italy, Macerata	15.4	41.0	-	-	12.8	23.1	-	7.7	39	46
Italy, Modena	7.5	43.0	-	0.7	28.3	19.1	0.3	1.0	293	302
Italy, Parma	14.2	22.8	-	4.3	38.9	16.0	0.6	3.1	162	177
Italy, Ragusa	20.0	28.2	-	2.7	26.4	16.4	0.9	5.5	110	110
Italy, Romagna	8.3	43.6	-	1.3	26.7	15.2	0.7	4.3	303	308
Italy, Torino	13.8	33.6	-	0.3	33.1	18.1	0.6	0.6	354	377
Italy, Trieste	6.5	55.3	-	2.4	16.3	14.6	-	4.9	123	214
Italy, Varese	12.1	35.4	-	0.3	31.3	18.3	-	2.6	387	407
Italy, Veneto	11.9	31.7	0.6	6.8	19.8	16.9	0.7	11.6	545	575
Latvia										
Malta										

PERCENTAGE DISTRIBUTION OF MICROSCOPICALLY VERIFIED CASES BY HISTOLOGICAL TYPE
Lymphoid and Myeloid Leukaemias (ICD-9 204+205) - Both sexes (contd)

	Lymphoid				Myeloid				Number of cases	
	Acute	Chronic	Other	Unspec.	Acute	Chronic	Other	Unspec.	MV	Total
The Netherlands	14.8	34.5	0.2	0.9	34.4	13.5	0.3	1.3	4384	4386
The Netherlands, Eindhoven	17.6	32.6	-	0.7	35.8	10.8	0.4	2.2	279	283
The Netherlands, Maastricht	15.8	33.0	-	1.4	33.5	14.4	-	2.0	355	355
Norway										
Poland, Cracow	20.5	23.2	-	4.0	36.4	13.2	-	2.6	151	206
Poland, Kielce	14.9	35.5	0.4	5.6	17.7	23.8	0.4	1.6	248	299
Poland, Lower Silesia	16.6	30.7	-	6.8	24.3	15.9	0.3	5.3	703	873
Poland, Warsaw City	16.7	22.9	-	3.6	35.6	16.7	-	4.4	275	418
Slovakia	16.5	40.3	0.1	0.9	22.9	17.8	0.1	1.5	1870	1982
Slovenia	17.0	43.1	-	-	24.1	15.0	-	0.8	729	746
Spain, Albacete	15.7	49.0	-	2.0	19.6	13.7	-	-	51	53
Spain, Asturias	13.6	52.8	-	3.9	13.3	15.0	-	1.4	360	361
Spain, Basque Country	22.5	34.5	0.2	2.1	22.0	17.4	0.6	0.6	472	510
Spain, Granada	21.8	32.1	-	0.4	24.7	17.7	-	3.3	243	243
Spain, Mallorca	14.9	35.1	-	2.3	29.7	16.2	0.9	0.9	222	222
Spain, Murcia	17.2	33.4	-	0.3	31.7	15.7	0.3	1.5	344	371
Spain, Navarra	12.9	49.0	-	-	22.4	15.6	-	-	147	176
Spain, Tarragona	16.1	38.5	-	0.5	25.9	18.5	-	0.5	205	207
Spain, Zaragoza	16.7	27.5	0.4	-	33.7	18.5	-	3.3	276	300
Sweden	13.1	36.2	3.3	0.7	34.2	11.2	0.1	1.2	3967	4142
Switzerland, Basel	12.8	34.3	-	-	39.5	13.4	-	-	172	174
Switzerland, Geneva	13.3	36.7	-	0.5	23.3	23.3	0.5	2.4	210	216
Switzerland, Graubunden	9.7	41.7	-	-	23.6	25.0	-	-	72	74
Switzerland, Neuchatel	7.0	42.1	1.8	-	38.6	10.5	-	-	57	66
Switzerland, St Gall-Appenzell	12.6	37.0	-	0.4	27.4	14.8	0.4	7.4	230	236
Switzerland, Valais	23.6	34.7	-	-	19.4	22.2	-	-	72	75
Switzerland, Vaud	10.1	33.5	-	0.4	31.3	20.7	-	4.0	227	228
Switzerland, Zurich	11.3	39.4	-	0.8	28.5	18.8	1.2	-	515	517
UK, England and Wales	13.9	33.3	-	1.5	32.6	16.4	0.2	2.0	12193	14395
UK, East Anglia										
UK, Mersey	19.6	31.1	-	2.2	29.3	15.6	0.5	1.7	409	832
UK, North Western										
UK, Oxford	14.3	28.1	-	1.5	35.1	19.0	0.2	1.7	1209	1212
UK, South Thames	14.3	34.5	-	1.5	31.9	15.8	-	1.9	2017	3312
UK, South Western	11.6	36.9	-	2.8	28.7	18.2	0.1	1.6	1552	1982
UK, Wessex	11.5	31.9	-	1.7	33.5	20.2	0.6	0.6	1428	1923
UK, West Midlands										
UK, Yorkshire	13.1	35.0	-	1.7	34.4	15.1	0.1	0.5	1467	1680
UK, Scotland	15.7	34.0	-	1.8	32.3	13.3	0.2	2.7	1693	2305
UK, Scotland, West	16.2	31.6	-	2.4	33.3	13.0	0.2	3.3	975	1176
Yugoslavia, Vojvodina										

OCEANIA

	Lymphoid				Myeloid				Number of cases	
	Acute	Chronic	Other	Unspec.	Acute	Chronic	Other	Unspec.	MV	Total
Australian Capital Territory	18.8	28.2	-	-	34.1	16.5	1.2	1.2	85	88
Australia, New South Wales	16.3	30.2	-	1.5	31.5	18.1	1.2	1.3	2451	2783
South Australia	9.2	48.3	-	-	26.3	16.2	0.1	-	895	1036
Australia, Tasmania	18.7	21.5	-	-	42.1	16.8	-	0.9	107	261
Australia, Victoria	21.8	26.2	-	1.4	31.6	17.9	0.3	0.8	1817	1947
Western Australia	17.9	24.9	0.2	0.4	35.2	20.0	0.8	0.8	526	599
French Polynesia	22.6	9.7	3.2	-	38.7	16.1	3.2	6.5	31	39
New Zealand: Non-Maori										
New Zealand: Maori										
US, Hawaii: White	22.1	28.8	-	1.9	30.8	15.4	-	1.0	104	120
US, Hawaii: Japanese	23.8	7.9	-	-	39.7	25.4	1.6	1.6	63	69
US, Hawaii: Hawaiian	32.7	12.7	-	-	47.3	7.3	-	-	55	61
US, Hawaii: Filipino	20.0	7.3	-	1.8	49.1	20.0	1.8	-	55	60
US, Hawaii: Chinese	-	22.2	-	-	77.8	-	-	-	9	12

PERCENTAGE DISTRIBUTION OF MICROSCOPICALLY VERIFIED CASES BY HISTOLOGICAL TYPE
Other and Unspecified Leukaemias (ICD-9 206-8) - Both sexes

		Monocytic				Other specified		Unspec.	Number of cases	
	Acute	Chronic	Other	Unspec.	Acute	Chronic	Other		MV	Total
AFRICA										
Algeria, Setif	-	-	-	-	65.6	-	-	34.4	**32**	33
France, La Reunion	10.0	-	-	-	80.0	-	-	10.0	**10**	10
Mali, Bamako	-	-	-	-	10.0	-	-	90.0	**10**	22
Uganda, Kyadondo	-	-	-	-	33.3	33.3	-	33.3	**3**	13
Zimbabwe, Harare: African	-	-	-	-	-	-	-	100.0	**1**	2
Zimbabwe, Harare: European	-	-	-	-	100.0	-	-	-	**1**	2
AMERICA, CENTRAL AND SOUTH										
Argentina, Concordia	-	-	-	-	-	20.0	-	80.0	**5**	8
Brazil, Belem	-	-	-	-	-	-	-	100.0	**12**	27
Brazil, Goiania	10.5	-	-	-	57.9	-	-	31.6	**19**	34
Brazil, Porto Alegre	-	7.7	-	7.7	15.4	7.7	7.7	53.8	**13**	44
Colombia, Cali	2.7	-	-	1.4	53.4	2.7	-	39.7	**73**	95
Costa Rica	5.9	-	-	2.9	55.9	2.9	-	32.4	**34**	108
Ecuador, Quito	12.8	2.6	-	-	15.4	5.1	-	64.1	**39**	69
Peru, Lima	12.0	-	-	8.0	60.0	4.0	-	16.0	**25**	56
Peru, Trujillo	12.5	12.5	-	-	75.0	-	-	-	**8**	10
Puerto Rico	11.1	-	1.1	1.1	54.4	3.3	2.2	26.7	**90**	138
Uruguay, Montevideo	1.3	-	-	-	67.1	6.3	-	25.3	**79**	79
AMERICA, NORTH										
Canada	15.8	2.3	0.7	2.6	57.5	1.2	4.1	15.8	**906**	2195
Canada, Alberta	24.3	2.9	-	1.4	60.0	2.9	1.4	7.1	**70**	84
Canada, British Columbia	22.5	5.6	2.2	4.5	51.7	1.1	2.2	10.1	**89**	219
Canada, Manitoba	25.7	2.9	-	5.7	48.6	-	8.6	8.6	**35**	52
Canada, New Brunswick	6.5	-	-	6.5	29.0	-	-	58.1	**31**	71
Canada, Newfoundland	6.7	-	-	-	80.0	-	6.7	6.7	**15**	17
Canada, Northwest Territories	-	-	-	-	100.0	-	-	-	**2**	5
Canada, Nova Scotia	14.9	4.1	1.4	5.4	50.0	-	1.4	23.0	**74**	135
Canada, Ontario	14.5	1.4	-	2.4	47.3	1.0	6.8	26.6	**207**	856
Canada, Prince Edward Island	25.0	-	-	-	50.0	-	-	25.0	**4**	5
Canada, Quebec	11.3	0.9	0.9	1.7	69.7	1.7	4.3	9.5	**346**	694
Canada, Saskatchewan	37.1	11.4	-	-	48.6	-	-	2.9	**35**	62
Canada, Yukon	100.0	-	-	-	-	-	-	-	**2**	2
US, Cent. California: Non-Hisp White	25.0	4.2	-	6.3	47.9	-	-	16.7	**48**	82
US, Cent. California: Hispanic	25.0	-	-	-	60.0	5.0	-	10.0	**20**	23
US, Los Angeles: Non-Hisp White	17.4	1.5	0.5	-	64.1	1.5	3.1	11.8	**195**	255
US, Los Angeles: Hispanic White	18.8	-	-	-	76.8	-	2.9	1.4	**69**	77
US, Los Angeles: Black	27.3	-	-	-	50.0	-	-	22.7	**22**	37
US, Los Angeles: Chinese	33.3	-	-	-	33.3	16.7	-	16.7	**6**	7
US, Los Angeles: Filipino	10.0	-	-	-	70.0	-	-	20.0	**10**	11
US, Los Angeles: Korean	-	-	-	-	80.0	-	20.0	-	**5**	5
US, Los Angeles: Japanese	-	25.0	-	-	75.0	-	-	-	**4**	4
US, San Francisco: Non-Hisp White	25.6	1.7	0.9	0.9	58.1	-	3.4	9.4	**117**	133
US, San Francisco: Hispanic White	-	-	-	-	75.0	12.5	-	12.5	**8**	9
US, San Francisco: Black	27.8	5.6	-	-	44.4	5.6	5.6	11.1	**18**	19
US, San Francisco: Chinese	-	-	-	-	75.0	-	-	25.0	**8**	8
US, San Francisco: Filipino	30.0	-	-	-	50.0	-	-	20.0	**10**	13
US, San Francisco: Japanese	-	-	-	-	-	-	-	-	**-**	-
US, Connecticut: White	14.6	1.6	-	0.4	60.6	2.0	5.3	15.4	**246**	279
US, Connecticut: Black	-	14.3	-	-	71.4	-	14.3	-	**7**	10
US, Atlanta: White	32.6	4.3	2.2	2.2	52.2	-	4.3	2.2	**46**	54
US, Atlanta: Black	-	-	-	-	71.4	-	-	28.6	**14**	16
US, Iowa	25.4	1.0	-	1.0	60.4	0.5	4.1	7.6	**197**	236
US, Central Louisiana: White	33.3	-	-	-	33.3	-	-	33.3	**3**	10
US, Central Louisiana: Black	-	-	-	-	50.0	-	50.0	-	**2**	3
US, New Orleans: White	25.0	2.5	-	2.5	57.5	2.5	-	10.0	**40**	45
US, New Orleans: Black	17.6	5.9	-	-	64.7	-	-	11.8	**17**	25
US, Detroit: White	18.5	-	-	1.2	51.4	2.0	4.0	22.9	**249**	283
US, Detroit: Black	16.0	4.0	-	-	58.0	2.0	-	20.0	**50**	55
US, New Mexico: Non-Hisp White	15.6	8.9	2.2	-	46.7	-	4.4	22.2	**45**	74
US, New Mexico: Hispanic White	30.0	-	-	-	65.0	-	-	5.0	**20**	25
US, New Mexico: American Indian	-	-	-	-	100.0	-	-	-	**2**	2
US, Utah	13.2	1.5	-	-	48.5	4.4	-	32.4	**68**	75
US, Seattle	15.7	1.0	-	-	60.5	1.9	1.4	19.5	**210**	220
US, SEER: White	19.1	1.4	0.3	0.7	57.1	1.6	3.6	16.2	**1190**	1379
US, SEER: Black	16.2	4.0	-	-	58.6	2.0	2.0	17.2	**99**	111

Other and Unspecified Leukaemias (ICD-9 206-8) - Both sexes (contd)

		Monocytic			Other specified			Unspec.	Number of cases	
	Acute	Chronic	Other	Unspec.	Acute	Chronic	Other		MV	Total
ASIA										
China, Qidong										
China, Shanghai										
China, Tianjin	7.3	0.4	-	2.7	32.0	-	1.9	55.6	**259**	346
Hong Kong										
India, Bangalore	8.0	-	-	-	74.0	4.0	4.0	10.0	**50**	85
India, Barshi, Paranda and Bhum	-	-	-	-	-	-	-	100.0	**1**	1
India, Bombay	5.1	-	-	1.4	50.0	0.7	10.9	31.9	**138**	172
India, Karunagappally	-	-	-	-	50.0	-	-	50.0	**2**	3
India, Madras	27.6	-	-	-	37.9	-	-	34.5	**29**	42
India, Trivandrum	-	-	-	-	66.7	-	33.3	-	**3**	7
Israel: All Jews	20.1	2.6	0.4	0.4	49.3	1.3	1.7	24.0	**229**	237
Jews born in Israel	35.3	-	-	-	44.1	2.9	-	17.6	**34**	36
Jews born in America or Europe	19.0	2.1	-	-	50.7	1.4	2.1	24.6	**142**	145
Jews born in Africa or Asia	12.0	6.0	2.0	2.0	50.0	-	2.0	26.0	**50**	53
Non-Jews	-	-	-	-	63.3	6.7	-	30.0	**30**	31
Japan, Hiroshima	23.1	-	-	15.4	53.8	-	-	7.7	**13**	26
Japan, Miyagi	16.7	-	-	2.1	54.2	-	4.2	22.9	**48**	97
Japan, Nagasaki	16.7	-	-	-	46.3	-	-	37.0	**54**	92
Japan, Osaka	40.8	2.3	-	0.9	41.3	-	1.8	12.8	**218**	406
Japan, Saga										
Japan, Yamagata										
Korea, Kangwha	-	-	-	-	60.0	-	-	40.0	**5**	6
Kuwait: Non-Kuwaitis	-	-	-	-	100.0	-	-	-	**3**	11
Kuwait: Kuwaitis	33.3	-	-	-	66.7	-	-	-	**3**	18
Philippines, Manila	3.0	-	-	-	57.6	-	3.0	36.4	**33**	325
Singapore: Chinese	-	5.9	-	-	76.5	-	5.9	11.8	**17**	29
Singapore: Malay	-	-	-	-	75.0	-	-	25.0	**4**	8
Singapore: Indian	-	-	-	-	100.0	-	-	-	**3**	3
Thailand, Chiang Mai	-	-	-	1.7	8.3	-	-	90.0	**60**	60
Thailand, Khon Kaen	18.2	-	-	-	81.8	-	-	-	**11**	69
Viet Nam, Hanoi	1.2	-	-	6.2	60.5	8.6	-	23.5	**81**	91
EUROPE										
Austria, Tyrol	-	-	-	37.5	31.3	-	-	31.3	**16**	21
Belarus										
Croatia										
Czech Republic	16.7	3.2	2.4	2.8	49.2	9.9	9.1	6.7	**252**	493
Denmark	6.8	4.2	-	4.2	63.6	5.1	1.7	14.4	**118**	152
Estonia	4.6	2.3	-	-	87.4	2.3	-	3.4	**87**	87
Finland										
France, Bas-Rhin	33.3	5.6	-	-	41.7	-	-	19.4	**36**	38
France, Calvados	50.0	-	-	-	50.0	-	-	-	**2**	8
France, Doubs	5.9	-	-	-	58.8	-	-	35.3	**17**	18
France, Haut-Rhin	19.4	-	-	-	61.3	-	-	19.4	**31**	31
France, Herault	2.4	2.4	-	2.4	88.1	-	2.4	2.4	**42**	42
France, Isere	38.1	-	-	-	28.6	4.8	4.8	23.8	**21**	21
France, Somme	43.8	-	-	-	31.3	-	-	25.0	**16**	16
France, Tarn	36.4	-	-	-	45.5	-	-	18.2	**11**	11
Germany, Eastern States	9.3	1.5	-	0.6	84.6	0.6	0.3	3.1	**324**	324
Germany, Saarland										
Iceland	9.1	-	-	-	90.9	-	-	-	**11**	11
Ireland, Southern	-	-	-	-	52.4	4.8	-	42.9	**21**	28
Italy, Ferrara	13.3	6.7	-	-	46.7	-	-	33.3	**15**	18
Italy, Florence	6.2	-	-	-	55.4	7.7	1.5	29.2	**65**	78
Italy, Genoa	4.0	-	-	-	68.0	-	-	28.0	**25**	41
Italy, Latina	11.1	11.1	-	-	38.9	5.6	-	33.3	**18**	25
Italy, Macerata	-	-	-	-	86.7	-	-	13.3	**15**	17
Italy, Modena	60.0	-	-	6.7	33.3	-	-	-	**15**	21
Italy, Parma	6.7	-	-	6.7	55.6	2.2	2.2	26.7	**45**	57
Italy, Ragusa	-	-	-	6.7	46.7	-	6.7	40.0	**15**	15
Italy, Romagna	8.8	-	-	-	79.4	-	-	11.8	**34**	34
Italy, Torino	14.9	-	-	-	70.2	-	-	14.9	**47**	60
Italy, Trieste	-	-	-	-	75.0	-	-	25.0	**4**	26
Italy, Varese	30.4	-	-	-	60.9	-	-	8.7	**23**	28
Italy, Veneto	10.3	-	1.1	3.4	44.8	9.2	2.3	28.7	**87**	97
Latvia										
Malta										

Other and Unspecified Leukaemias (ICD-9 206-8) - Both sexes (contd)

	Monocytic				Other specified			Unspec.	Number of cases	
	Acute	Chronic	Other	Unspec.	Acute	Chronic	Other		MV	Total
The Netherlands	19.1	3.6	-	2.3	46.2	0.9	17.3	10.5	**439**	439
The Netherlands, Eindhoven	13.0	-	-	8.7	56.5	-	21.7	-	**23**	23
The Netherlands, Maastricht	26.7	3.3	-	-	46.7	3.3	10.0	10.0	**30**	30
Norway										
Poland, Cracow	-	-	-	-	23.5	29.4	-	47.1	**17**	35
Poland, Kielce	-	-	-	-	22.2	27.8	16.7	33.3	**18**	28
Poland, Lower Silesia	3.6	-	-	1.8	58.0	5.4	1.8	29.5	**112**	134
Poland, Warsaw City	-	-	-	-	47.1	5.9	-	47.1	**17**	55
Slovakia	21.5	1.1	-	1.1	45.2	2.2	4.3	24.7	**93**	150
Slovenia	51.6	-	-	-	25.8	3.2	-	19.4	**31**	35
Spain, Albacete	16.7	16.7	-	-	50.0	-	-	16.7	**6**	8
Spain, Asturias	2.9	1.9	-	1.0	77.7	1.0	1.0	14.6	**103**	162
Spain, Basque Country	9.6	2.1	-	1.1	74.5	1.1	5.3	6.4	**94**	126
Spain, Granada	15.8	2.6	-	2.6	71.1	-	-	7.9	**38**	55
Spain, Mallorca	30.0	15.0	-	-	40.0	5.0	5.0	5.0	**20**	38
Spain, Murcia	7.1	3.6	-	-	78.6	-	3.6	7.1	**28**	43
Spain, Navarra	21.7	-	-	-	69.6	-	-	8.7	**23**	50
Spain, Tarragona	7.1	7.1	-	3.6	64.3	7.1	-	10.7	**28**	38
Spain, Zaragoza	23.8	-	-	-	66.7	-	4.8	4.8	**21**	34
Sweden	3.7	2.3	-	1.5	86.6	1.7	0.1	4.1	**811**	921
Switzerland, Basel	11.1	-	-	-	55.6	-	-	33.3	**9**	9
Switzerland, Geneva	-	16.7	-	-	50.0	-	16.7	16.7	**6**	8
Switzerland, Graubunden	66.7	-	-	-	33.3	-	-	-	**3**	3
Switzerland, Neuchatel	-	-	-	-	100.0	-	-	-	**4**	7
Switzerland, St Gall-Appenzell	17.6	-	-	5.9	52.9	5.9	-	17.6	**17**	17
Switzerland, Valais	-	8.3	-	-	83.3	-	8.3	-	**12**	14
Switzerland, Vaud	9.7	6.5	-	3.2	64.5	-	-	16.1	**31**	31
Switzerland, Zurich	45.3	1.6	10.9	-	39.1	-	1.6	1.6	**64**	64
UK, England and Wales	13.1	2.6	-	3.1	43.1	4.7	1.1	32.3	**1135**	1385
UK, East Anglia										
UK, Mersey	25.0	7.1	-	3.6	53.6	-	-	10.7	**28**	85
UK, North Western										
UK, Oxford	31.8	9.1	-	-	31.8	8.2	-	19.1	**110**	111
UK, South Thames	10.7	5.8	-	8.7	41.7	4.9	-	28.2	**103**	295
UK, South Western	28.0	2.3	-	5.3	53.8	3.8	-	6.8	**132**	203
UK, Wessex	12.9	11.3	-	3.2	62.9	1.6	1.6	6.5	**62**	137
UK, West Midlands										
UK, Yorkshire	16.4	3.0	-	-	68.7	1.5	-	10.4	**67**	112
UK, Scotland	12.8	2.3	-	3.0	35.3	-	34.6	12.0	**133**	224
UK, Scotland, West	4.9	1.2	-	1.2	25.6	-	56.1	11.0	**82**	131
Yugoslavia, Vojvodina										

OCEANIA

	Monocytic				Other specified			Unspec.	Number of cases	
	Acute	Chronic	Other	Unspec.	Acute	Chronic	Other		MV	Total
Australian Capital Territory	-	-	-	-	100.0	-	-	-	**2**	2
Australia, New South Wales	15.7	2.0	-	2.0	63.1	-	1.0	16.2	**198**	254
South Australia	50.0	3.3	-	-	36.7	-	-	10.0	**30**	35
Australia, Tasmania	-	-	-	-	33.3	-	-	66.7	**3**	13
Australia, Victoria	26.2	0.8	-	2.4	55.6	0.8	1.6	12.7	**126**	178
Western Australia	21.5	1.5	-	1.5	66.2	-	-	9.2	**65**	73
French Polynesia	14.3	-	-	7.1	57.1	-	-	21.4	**14**	23
New Zealand: Non-Maori										
New Zealand: Maori										
US, Hawaii: White	28.6	-	-	-	57.1	-	14.3	-	**7**	15
US, Hawaii: Japanese	12.5	-	-	-	68.8	6.3	6.3	6.3	**16**	17
US, Hawaii: Hawaiian	37.5	-	-	-	50.0	-	-	12.5	**8**	10
US, Hawaii: Filipino	20.0	-	-	10.0	40.0	-	-	30.0	**10**	11
US, Hawaii: Chinese	60.0	-	-	20.0	20.0	-	-	-	**5**	5

INDICES OF DATA QUALITY

INDICES OF DATA QUALITY
Lip (ICD-9 140)

	MALE			FEMALE		
	MV	DCO	M/I	MV	DCO	M/I
AFRICA						
Algeria, Setif	95			99		
France, La Reunion	99			99		
Mali, Bamako	50	0		99	0	
Uganda, Kyadondo	0			-		
Zimbabwe, Harare: African	-	-		-	-	
Zimbabwe, Harare: European	99	0		-	-	
AMERICA, CENTRAL AND SOUTH						
Argentina, Concordia	99	0	0	99	0	0
Brazil, Belem	99	0	0	99	0	0
Brazil, Goiania	96	4	4	99	0	0
Brazil, Porto Alegre	99	0	5	99	0	0
Colombia, Cali	99	0	13	99	0	0
Costa Rica	97	0	16	96	0	0
Ecuador, Quito	99	0		-	-	
Peru, Lima	99	0		88	0	
Peru, Trujillo	99	0	0	99	0	0
US, Puerto Rico	98	2	8	95	5	14
Uruguay, Montevideo	92	8	17	99	0	0
AMERICA, NORTH						
Canada	95	0	3	93	0	3
Canada, Alberta	99	0	2	99	0	0
Canada, British Columbia	99	0	4	99	0	8
Canada, Manitoba	98	0	2	99	0	5
Canada, New Brunswick	99	0	3	99	0	0
Canada, Newfoundland	99	0	0	99	0	0
Canada, Northwest Territories	99	0	0	-	-	ncr
Canada, Nova Scotia	98	1	5	99	0	0
Canada, Ontario	94	0	4	92	0	2
Canada, Prince Edward Island	99	0	0	99	0	0
+Canada, Quebec	81	0	4	75	0	4
Canada, Saskatchewan	99	0	2	99	0	3
Canada, Yukon	99	0	0	99	0	0
+US, Cent. Calif.: Non-Hisp. White	99	0		99	0	
+US, Cent. Calif.: Hispanic	99	0		99	0	
US, Los Angeles: Non-Hisp. White	99	1		99	0	
US, Los Angeles: Hispanic White	99	0		99	0	
US, Los Angeles: Black	-	-		99	0	
US, Los Angeles: Chinese	99	0		99	0	
US, Los Angeles: Filipino	99	0		-	-	
US, Los Angeles: Korean	99	0		-	-	
US, Los Angeles: Japanese	-	-		-	-	
US, San Francisco: Non-Hisp. White	99	0	3	99	0	3
US, San Francisco: Hispanic White	99	0	0	99	0	0
US, San Francisco: Black	99	0	0	-	-	-
US, San Francisco: Chinese	-	-	-	99	0	0
US, San Francisco: Filipino	-	-	-	99	0	0
US, San Francisco: Japanese	-	-	-	99	0	0
US, Connecticut: White	95	0	10	94	6	6
US, Connecticut: Black	-	-	-	-	-	-
US, Atlanta: White	98	0	2	99	0	13
US, Atlanta: Black	-	-	-	99	0	100
US, Iowa	99	0	2	98	0	6

	MALE			FEMALE		
	MV	DCO	M/I	MV	DCO	M/I
US, Central Louisiana: White	99	0	6	99	0	100
US, Central Louisiana: Black	-	-	-	-	-	-
US, New Orleans: White	99	0	12	99	0	0
US, New Orleans: Black	99	0	0	-	-	-
US, Detroit: White	99	1	0	94	0	6
US, Detroit: Black	-	-	-	99	0	0
US, New Mexico: Non-Hisp. White	99	0	2	99	0	4
US, New Mexico: Hispanic White	99	0	0	99	0	0
US, New Mexico: American Indian	99	0	0	99	0	0
US, Utah	99	0	1	99	0	3
US, Seattle	98	0	1	99	0	6
US, SEER: White	99	0	2	99	0	5
US, SEER: Black	99	0	0	99	0	33
ASIA						
+China, Qidong	99	0	50	99	0	50
+China, Shanghai	65	4	4	67	0	67
China, Tianjin	99	0	21	99	0	33
Hong Kong	99	0	31	99	0	17
India, Bangalore	82	9	9	80	20	10
India, Barshi, Paranda and Bhum	99	0		-	-	
India, Bombay	81	4	28	86	0	14
India, Karunagapally	99	0		99	0	
India, Madras	61	0	18	68	0	16
India, Trivandrum	83	0	17	-	-	ncr
Israel: All Jews	98			95		
Jews born in Israel	99			96		
Jews born in America or Europe	98			95		
Jews born in Africa or Asia	95			94		
Non-Jews	94			99		
Japan, Hiroshima	99	0	0	99	0	0
Japan, Miyagi	94	0	0	88	13	13
Japan, Nagasaki	99	0	33	-	-	-
Japan, Osaka	92	0	33	99	0	25
+Japan, Saga	67	0	67	0	99	100
Japan, Yamagata	75	25	50	99	0	60
Korea, Kangwha	-		-	99		0
Kuwait: Non-Kuwaitis	99	0		99	0	
Kuwait: Kuwaitis	99	0		-	-	
Philippines, Manila	99	0		99	0	
Singapore: Chinese	99	0		-	-	
Singapore: Malay	-	-		-	-	
Singapore: Indian	-	-		99	0	
Thailand, Chiang Mai	86	0		99	0	
Thailand, Khon Kaen	71	0		75	0	
Viet Nam, Hanoi	99			71		

+ IMPORTANT-SEE NOTES ON POPULATION PAGE

EUROPE	MALE			FEMALE		
	MV	DCO	M/I	MV	DCO	M/I
Austria, Tyrol	99	0	17	-	-	-
+Belarus	94	0	24	92	0	20
Croatia	67	3	16	60	4	16
+Czech Republic	95	1	16	97	1	20
Denmark	99	0	5	99	0	11
Estonia	91		15	88		4
Finland	99	0	4	99	0	4
France, Bas-Rhin	89		11	-		ncr
France, Calvados	99		9	99		0
France, Doubs	75		0	-		ncr
France, Haut-Rhin	99		18	99		67
France, Herault	88		12	83		33
France, Isere	99		4	99		13
France, Somme	99		7	99		0
France, Tarn	98		5	99		10
Germany, Eastern States	97	0	14	96	0	20
+Germany, Saarland	99	0	21	99	0	33
Iceland	99	0	6	99	0	0
Ireland, Southern	95		19	91		0
Italy, Ferrara	99	0	0	99	0	100
Italy, Florence	81	0	23	71	0	0
Italy, Genoa	99	0	47	99	0	0
Italy, Latina	93	0	22	99	0	0
Italy, Macerata	99	0	100	-	-	-
Italy, Modena	83	0	17	-	-	ncr
Italy, Parma	83	17	33	99	0	50
Italy, Ragusa	94	2	13	88	0	0
Italy, Romagna	99	0	400	0	0	100
Italy, Torino	99	0	3	99	0	14
Italy, Trieste	76	0	12	50	0	13
Italy, Varese	99	0	11	-	-	ncr
Italy, Veneto	97	2	11	93	0	13
+Latvia	96	0	22	94	0	20
+Malta	64	0	9	-	-	-
The Netherlands	99		4	99		8
The Netherlands, Eindhoven	99		3	99		0
The Netherlands, Maastricht	99		182	99		633
Norway	99	0	7	99	0	6
Poland, Cracow	81	3	75	88	13	50
Poland, Kielce	93	1	20	87	0	18
Poland, Lower Silesia	94	0	17	90	0	20
Poland, Warsaw City	[81]	6	20	[92]	0	46
Slovakia	90	0	19	88	0	17
Slovenia	97	1	19	90	0	13
Spain, Albacete	92	8	33	99	0	25
Spain, Asturias	99	0	0	93	7	13
Spain, Basque Country	99	0	4	99	0	0
Spain, Granada	98	0	3	99	0	0
Spain, Mallorca	99	1	6	99	0	7
Spain, Murcia	99	0	3	99	0	0
Spain, Navarra	99	1	6	99	0	0
Spain, Tarragona	98	2	5	94	0	31
Spain, Zaragoza	99	0	5	99	0	0

	MALE			FEMALE		
	MV	DCO	M/I	MV	DCO	M/I
Sweden	99		3	99		3
Switzerland, Basel	99	0	45	99	0	0
Switzerland, Geneva	99	0	5	99	0	20
Switzerland, Graubunden	99	0	6	99	0	17
Switzerland, Neuchatel	99	0	11	99	0	0
Switzerland, St Gall-Appenzell	99	0	11	99	0	0
Switzerland, Valais	99	0	33	99	0	0
Switzerland, Vaud	99	0	5	50	50	100
Switzerland, Zurich	99	0	3	99	0	7
+UK, England and Wales	[91]		11	[91]		15
UK, East Anglia			3			0
UK, Mersey	99	0	86	40	20	120
UK, North Western	83	2	10	84	0	47
UK, Oxford	97	0	5	91	0	9
UK, South Thames	87	0	15	92	4	20
UK, South Western	96	0	8	92	0	8
UK, Wessex	[70]	1	10	[70]	4	15
+UK, West Midlands			29		0	27
UK, Yorkshire	97	0	15	99	0	5
UK, Scotland	93	0	8	97	0	11
UK, Scotland, West	99	0	8	99	0	13
Yugoslavia, Vojvodina	80	3	20	79	5	18

OCEANIA

	MALE			FEMALE		
	MV	DCO	M/I	MV	DCO	M/I
Australian Capital Territory	99	0		99	0	
Australia, New South Wales	98	0		98	0	
South Australia	83		1	87		2
Australia, Tasmania	99		2	99		0
Australia, Victoria	98	0	2	98	0	3
Western Australia	99	0	2	99	0	1
French Polynesia	-		-	-		-
+New Zealand: Non-Maori	99	0	3	99	0	10
+New Zealand: Maori	99	0	0	-	-	-
US, Hawaii: White	99	0	0	99	0	0
US, Hawaii: Japanese	99	0	0	-	-	-
US, Hawaii: Hawaiian	99	0	0	-	-	-
US, Hawaii: Filipino	-	-	-	-	-	-
US, Hawaii: Chinese	-	-	-	-	-	ncr

+ IMPORTANT-SEE NOTES ON POPULATION PAGE

[] CYTOLOGICAL VERIFICATION EXCLUDED

INDICES OF DATA QUALITY
Tongue (ICD-9 141)

AFRICA

	MALE MV	MALE DCO	MALE M/I	FEMALE MV	FEMALE DCO	FEMALE M/I
Algeria, Setif	99			99		
France, La Reunion	99			99		
Mali, Bamako	67	33		67	0	
Uganda, Kyadondo	99			0		
Zimbabwe, Harare: African	83	0		-	-	
Zimbabwe, Harare: European	99	0		83	17	

AMERICA, CENTRAL AND SOUTH

	MALE MV	MALE DCO	MALE M/I	FEMALE MV	FEMALE DCO	FEMALE M/I
Argentina, Concordia	89	11	33	99	0	0
Brazil, Belem	89	3	30	91	5	18
Brazil, Goiania	93	7	31	99	0	67
Brazil, Porto Alegre	74	0	45	94	0	31
Colombia, Cali	96	0	56	89	4	26
Costa Rica	96	0	50	86	0	28
Ecuador, Quito	57	29		99	0	
Peru, Lima	95	5		96	0	
Peru, Trujillo	67	0	67	99	0	100
US, Puerto Rico	98	2	41	97	1	32
Uruguay, Montevideo	78	8	57	80	15	65

AMERICA, NORTH

	MALE MV	MALE DCO	MALE M/I	FEMALE MV	FEMALE DCO	FEMALE M/I
Canada	86	1	42	85	1	40
Canada, Alberta	99	0	58	98	2	39
Canada, British Columbia	99	0	35	96	3	39
Canada, Manitoba	85	1	49	93	2	37
Canada, New Brunswick	95	5	47	99	0	50
Canada, Newfoundland	99	0	22	99	0	36
Canada, Northwest Territories	99	0	100	99	0	0
Canada, Nova Scotia	95	3	34	99	0	17
Canada, Ontario	91	1	37	86	1	39
Canada, Prince Edward Island	99	0	42	99	0	25
+Canada, Quebec	64	0	49	60	0	45
Canada, Saskatchewan	99	0	51	99	0	81
Canada, Yukon	-	-	-	99	0	0
+US, Cent. Calif.: Non-Hisp. White	98	0		99	0	
+US, Cent. Calif.: Hispanic	94	0		88	0	
US, Los Angeles: Non-Hisp. White	99	1		98	1	
US, Los Angeles: Hispanic White	99	0		99	0	
US, Los Angeles: Black	99	0		95	0	
US, Los Angeles: Chinese	99	0		99	0	
US, Los Angeles: Filipino	99	0		99	0	
US, Los Angeles: Korean	99	0		99	0	
US, Los Angeles: Japanese	83	17		99	0	
US, San Francisco: Non-Hisp. White	99	0	37	97	1	34
US, San Francisco: Hispanic White	99	0	33	99	0	17
US, San Francisco: Black	99	0	63	99	0	33
US, San Francisco: Chinese	99	0	44	99	0	29
US, San Francisco: Filipino	99	0	40	99	0	33
US, San Francisco: Japanese	99	0	0	99	0	0
US, Connecticut: White	98	1	37	99	1	31
US, Connecticut: Black	97	0	39	99	0	18
US, Atlanta: White	99	0	30	96	0	27
US, Atlanta: Black	98	0	56	92	0	50
US, Iowa	99	1	32	97	0	39

	MALE MV	MALE DCO	MALE M/I	FEMALE MV	FEMALE DCO	FEMALE M/I
US, Central Louisiana: White	89	6	33	78	0	11
US, Central Louisiana: Black	99	0	100	-	-	ncr
US, New Orleans: White	99	0	29	93	7	41
US, New Orleans: Black	99	0	55	99	0	57
US, Detroit: White	99	0	31	98	1	28
US, Detroit: Black	99	1	45	99	0	30
US, New Mexico: Non-Hisp. White	98	2	37	99	0	67
US, New Mexico: Hispanic White	96	0	48	99	0	50
US, New Mexico: American Indian	99	0	100	99	0	0
US, Utah	99	0	19	99	0	16
US, Seattle	98	0	32	99	0	29
US, SEER: White	99	0	33	98	0	32
US, SEER: Black	98	0	49	98	0	36

ASIA

	MALE MV	MALE DCO	MALE M/I	FEMALE MV	FEMALE DCO	FEMALE M/I
+China, Qidong	99	0	100	99	0	33
+China, Shanghai	76	1	45	79	1	51
China, Tianjin	77	0	34	88	0	57
Hong Kong	85	1	39	81	1	24
India, Bangalore	88	3	12	83	10	14
India, Barshi, Paranda and Bhum	95	0		67	0	
India, Bombay	85	5	38	79	8	40
India, Karunagappally	83	6		79	7	
India, Madras	71	1	39	67	3	29
India, Trivandrum	90	6	26	86	0	21
Israel: All Jews	98			95		
Jews born in Israel	99			99		
Jews born in America or Europe	99			92		
Jews born in Africa or Asia	92			99		
Non-Jews	99			99		
Japan, Hiroshima	95	2	17	93	0	44
Japan, Miyagi	89	1	43	89	3	38
Japan, Nagasaki	96	1	46	96	2	35
Japan, Osaka	85	7	43	90	5	35
+Japan, Saga	90	8	54	91	4	26
Japan, Yamagata	63	25	67	71	29	50
Korea, Kangwha	99		0	99		0
Kuwait: Non-Kuwaitis	99	0		99	0	
Kuwait: Kuwaitis	99	0		99	0	
Philippines, Manila	72	14		66	12	
Singapore: Chinese	95	3		95	3	
Singapore: Malay	99	0		99	0	
Singapore: Indian	99	0		99	0	
Thailand, Chiang Mai	98	0		92	3	
Thailand, Khon Kaen	86	0		71	0	
Viet Nam, Hanoi	56			50		

+ IMPORTANT-SEE NOTES ON POPULATION PAGE

INDICES OF DATA QUALITY
Tongue (ICD-9 141) (contd)

EUROPE

	MALE			FEMALE		
	MV	DCO	M/I	MV	DCO	M/I
Austria, Tyrol	86	14	86	99	0	80
+Belarus	95	0	69	92	0	67
Croatia	72	7	73	57	9	55
+Czech Republic	92	1	84	90	1	66
Denmark	99	0	60	99	0	43
Estonia	98		76	96		65
Finland	99	0	34	98	1	33
France, Bas-Rhin	99		31	99		29
France, Calvados	98		39	94		38
France, Doubs	99		51	99		25
France, Haut-Rhin	99		35	99		58
France, Herault	99		47	99		56
France, Isere	95		28	99		22
France, Somme	98		50	91		64
France, Tarn	99		63	99		78
Germany, Eastern States	98	0	58	99	0	62
+Germany, Saarland	97	2	50	97	0	28
Iceland	99	0	50	99	0	40
Ireland, Southern	82		82	92		42
Italy, Ferrara	99	0	44	99	0	100
Italy, Florence	81	2	31	89	0	44
Italy, Genoa	94	1	53	97	0	54
Italy, Latina	99	0	93	99	0	100
Italy, Macerata	99	0	57	99	0	67
Italy, Modena	95	2	33	99	0	50
Italy, Parma	99	0	70	99	0	40
Italy, Ragusa	83	0	33	99	0	60
Italy, Romagna	91	6	47	99	0	42
Italy, Torino	84	5	52	90	7	57
Italy, Trieste	62	5	95	20	0	10
Italy, Varese	99	0	39	82	12	47
Italy, Veneto	97	1	63	91	2	33
+Latvia	97	2	67	96	0	54
+Malta	99	0	25	99	0	33
The Netherlands	99		36	99		35
The Netherlands, Eindhoven	93		62	95		27
The Netherlands, Maastricht	99		173	99		310
Norway	99	1	55	99	0	47
Poland, Cracow	89	4	79	99	0	67
Poland, Kielce	81	4	85	88	0	63
Poland, Lower Silesia	82	0	86	86	0	78
Poland, Warsaw City	[90]	6	76	[97]	3	47
Slovakia	95	0	74	87	4	79
Slovenia	94	3	79	82	18	61
Spain, Albacete	99	0	44	67	33	33
Spain, Asturias	99	1	30	95	5	26
Spain, Basque Country	96	2	43	91	6	61
Spain, Granada	99	0	57	99	0	25
Spain, Mallorca	98	0	102	99	0	92
Spain, Murcia	99	1	49	94	3	19
Spain, Navarra	97	0	31	93	0	27
Spain, Tarragona	99	0	59	99	0	57
Spain, Zaragoza	94	6	45	79	7	57
Sweden	99		61	98		45
Switzerland, Basel	98	0	43	99	0	33
Switzerland, Geneva	98	0	35	99	0	27
Switzerland, Graubunden	99	0	100	99	0	75
Switzerland, Neuchatel	99	0	60	99	0	17
Switzerland, St Gall-Appenzell	97	0	86	99	0	46
Switzerland, Valais	95	0	63	99	0	100
Switzerland, Vaud	97	1	48	97	0	39
Switzerland, Zurich	98	0	72	99	0	29
+UK, England and Wales	[87]		55	[86]		52
UK, East Anglia			48			44
UK, Mersey	91	1	57	80	2	55
UK, North Western	89	0	66	88	1	54
UK, Oxford	91	0	45	89	0	52
UK, South Thames	79	10	52	80	8	51
UK, South Western	89	0	57	90	1	58
UK, Wessex	[80]	2	46	[84]	4	38
+UK, West Midlands		0	55		1	60
UK, Yorkshire	92	1	58	94	1	53
UK, Scotland	95	2	56	91	1	53
UK, Scotland, West	94	2	58	91	2	55
Yugoslavia, Vojvodina	65	8	76	57	14	71

OCEANIA

	MALE			FEMALE		
	MV	DCO	M/I	MV	DCO	M/I
Australian Capital Territory	99	0		99	0	
Australia, New South Wales	95	0		93	2	
South Australia	92		60	94		47
Australia, Tasmania	99		55	99		42
Australia, Victoria	94	1	51	90	1	47
Western Australia	96	1	45	90	0	54
French Polynesia	99	0		99	0	
+New Zealand: Non-Maori	94	1	51	97	1	50
+New Zealand: Maori	99	0	55	99	0	60
US, Hawaii: White	96	0	17	99	0	10
US, Hawaii: Japanese	99	0	29	99	0	31
US, Hawaii: Hawaiian	99	0	14	99	0	0
US, Hawaii: Filipino	99	0	20	99	0	56
US, Hawaii: Chinese	99	0	0	99	0	0

+ IMPORTANT-SEE NOTES ON POPULATION PAGE

[] CYTOLOGICAL VERIFICATION EXCLUDED

INDICES OF DATA QUALITY
Salivary gland (ICD-9 142)

	MALE			FEMALE		
	MV	DCO	M/I	MV	DCO	M/I
AFRICA						
Algeria, Setif	99			-		
France, La Reunion	99			99		
Mali, Bamako	-	-		99	0	
Uganda, Kyadondo	33			14		
Zimbabwe, Harare: African	60	0		99	0	
Zimbabwe, Harare: European	-	-		-	-	
AMERICA, CENTRAL AND SOUTH						
Argentina, Concordia	67	33	233	99	0	0
Brazil, Belem	89	11	33	99	0	13
Brazil, Goiania	91	0	27	86	14	57
Brazil, Porto Alegre	78	0	33	85	0	23
Colombia, Cali	87	0	40	99	0	13
Costa Rica	89	5	42	90	0	28
Ecuador, Quito	99	0		89	11	
Peru, Lima	81	0		68	0	
Peru, Trujillo	-	-	-	99	0	33
US, Puerto Rico	99	0	31	99	0	21
Uruguay, Montevideo	65	8	35	80	13	40
AMERICA, NORTH						
Canada	92	0	33	88	1	27
Canada, Alberta	98	0	34	97	0	23
Canada, British Columbia	99	0	34	94	6	27
Canada, Manitoba	88	0	40	99	0	5
Canada, New Brunswick	99	0	38	99	0	22
Canada, Newfoundland	99	0	9	99	0	33
Canada, Northwest Territories	99	0	10	67	0	100
Canada, Nova Scotia	96	4	32	93	0	50
Canada, Ontario	89	1	32	87	1	26
Canada, Prince Edward Island	99	0	33	99	0	200
+Canada, Quebec	90	0	35	80	0	29
Canada, Saskatchewan	99	0	29	99	0	27
Canada, Yukon	99	0	0	-	-	-
+US, Cent. Calif.: Non-Hisp. White	96	0		93	3	
+US, Cent. Calif.: Hispanic	99	0		99	0	
US, Los Angeles: Non-Hisp. White	99	1		98	1	
US, Los Angeles: Hispanic White	99	0		96	0	
US, Los Angeles: Black	99	0		99	0	
US, Los Angeles: Chinese	99	0		99	0	
US, Los Angeles: Filipino	99	0		99	0	
US, Los Angeles: Korean	-	-		-	-	
US, Los Angeles: Japanese	99	0		-	-	
US, San Francisco: Non-Hisp. White	99	1	23	99	0	15
US, San Francisco: Hispanic White	99	0	0	99	0	0
US, San Francisco: Black	99	0	36	99	0	17
US, San Francisco: Chinese	99	0	17	99	0	0
US, San Francisco: Filipino	99	0	20	88	13	13
US, San Francisco: Japanese	-	-	-	99	0	33
US, Connecticut: White	96	3	24	97	0	29
US, Connecticut: Black	99	0	33	99	0	25
US, Atlanta: White	99	0	17	99	0	22
US, Atlanta: Black	99	0	10	99	0	8
US, Iowa	97	1	51	97	0	35

	MALE			FEMALE		
	MV	DCO	M/I	MV	DCO	M/I
US, Central Louisiana: White	99	0	20	99	0	200
US, Central Louisiana: Black	99	0	100	99	0	0
US, New Orleans: White	99	0	13	94	0	13
US, New Orleans: Black	90	0	40	99	0	0
US, Detroit: White	93	3	17	89	10	21
US, Detroit: Black	99	0	13	79	21	29
US, New Mexico: Non-Hisp. White	93	3	41	94	0	39
US, New Mexico: Hispanic White	99	0	0	99	0	33
US, New Mexico: American Indian	-	-	-	99	0	100
US, Utah	99	0	34	99	0	5
US, Seattle	99	0	30	99	0	18
US, SEER: White	97	2	28	96	2	24
US, SEER: Black	99	0	22	94	6	17
ASIA						
+China, Qidong	91	0	55	67	0	67
+China, Shanghai	71	0	28	78	1	31
China, Tianjin	92	0	16	93	0	33
Hong Kong	77	2	17	82	2	16
India, Bangalore	90	0	12	97	3	10
India, Barshi, Paranda and Bhum	99	0		99	0	
India, Bombay	92	2	28	90	4	19
India, Karunagappally	99	0		-	-	
India, Madras	59	0	26	83	0	31
India, Trivandrum	-	-	-	67	17	0
Israel: All Jews	91			87		
Jews born in Israel	92			90		
Jews born in America or Europe	90			78		
Jews born in Africa or Asia	99			99		
Non-Jews	99			99		
Japan, Hiroshima	99	0	21	99	0	50
Japan, Miyagi	92	3	49	88	0	36
Japan, Nagasaki	95	5	57	95	5	45
Japan, Osaka	84	8	47	81	11	51
+Japan, Saga	82	6	35	89	0	22
Japan, Yamagata	77	18	64	82	12	41
Korea, Kangwha	80		0	-		-
Kuwait: Non-Kuwaitis	99	0		99	0	
Kuwait: Kuwaitis	99	0		60	20	
Philippines, Manila	85	3		78	5	
Singapore: Chinese	94	6		97	0	
Singapore: Malay	99	0		99	0	
Singapore: Indian	99	0		99	0	
Thailand, Chiang Mai	92	0		99	0	
Thailand, Khon Kaen	99	0		88	0	
Viet Nam, Hanoi	63			71		

+ IMPORTANT-SEE NOTES ON POPULATION PAGE

INDICES OF DATA QUALITY
Salivary gland (ICD-9 142) (contd)

EUROPE

	MALE			FEMALE		
	MV	DCO	M/I	MV	DCO	M/I
Austria, Tyrol	91	0	36	89	11	11
+Belarus	92	0	58	90	0	39
Croatia	66	2	23	51	9	33
+Czech Republic	92	1	53	92	0	47
Denmark	96	1	50	98	0	51
Estonia	99		50	99		47
Finland	99	0	36	98	1	27
France, Bas-Rhin	99		52	96		23
France, Calvados	89		44	99		44
France, Doubs	99		80	88		50
France, Haut-Rhin	99		91	90		30
France, Herault	99		56	99		30
France, Isere	91		55	99		20
France, Somme	91		36	99		25
France, Tarn	99		25	99		0
Germany, Eastern States	96	1	56	96	0	59
+Germany, Saarland	93	0	31	99	0	35
Iceland	99	0	33	99	0	33
Ireland, Southern	90		60	99		100
Italy, Ferrara	99	0	100	67	0	33
Italy, Florence	74	4	35	76	0	29
Italy, Genoa	93	0	52	88	6	56
Italy, Latina	99	0	57	83	0	83
Italy, Macerata	50	0	100	-	-	ncr
Italy, Modena	94	0	94	78	11	33
Italy, Parma	80	20	60	99	0	100
Italy, Ragusa	99	0	100	99	0	67
Italy, Romagna	85	0	30	93	0	27
Italy, Torino	80	7	107	80	20	93
Italy, Trieste	33	0	17	42	0	25
Italy, Varese	99	0	28	99	0	26
Italy, Veneto	88	3	61	84	5	32
+Latvia	93	0	77	90	5	46
+Malta	99	0	100	80	0	0
The Netherlands	99		50	99		29
The Netherlands, Eindhoven	99		46	99		25
The Netherlands, Maastricht	99		108	99		60
Norway	99	0	33	99	0	30
Poland, Cracow	76	12	59	75	8	42
Poland, Kielce	90	0	130	88	0	125
Poland, Lower Silesia	75	0	45	81	0	35
Poland, Warsaw City	[84]	9	59	[68]	6	35
Slovakia	88	2	66	89	0	54
Slovenia	99	0	44	94	0	59
Spain, Albacete	99	0	100	67	33	33
Spain, Asturias	96	0	26	94	6	33
Spain, Basque Country	96	4	56	95	5	47
Spain, Granada	99	0	50	99	0	27
Spain, Mallorca	99	0	50	99	0	75
Spain, Murcia	89	7	43	99	0	11
Spain, Navarra	85	8	54	99	0	0
Spain, Tarragona	86	0	43	99	0	67
Spain, Zaragoza	91	5	45	88	13	50

	MALE			FEMALE		
	MV	DCO	M/I	MV	DCO	M/I
Sweden	99		36	99		29
Switzerland, Basel	99	0	60	99	0	60
Switzerland, Geneva	99	0	27	99	0	29
Switzerland, Graubunden	67	33	67	99	0	0
Switzerland, Neuchatel	99	0	100	67	0	100
Switzerland, St Gall-Appenzell	99	0	50	99	0	75
Switzerland, Valais	99	0	0	99	0	0
Switzerland, Vaud	99	0	42	99	0	86
Switzerland, Zurich	99	0	45	99	0	81
+UK, England and Wales	[86]		51	[84]		44
UK, East Anglia			39			28
UK, Mersey	91	0	62	71	8	71
UK, North Western	83	2	60	80	0	63
UK, Oxford	90	0	48	92	0	26
UK, South Thames	84	7	48	73	13	51
UK, South Western	83	1	51	81	0	45
UK, Wessex	[74]	3	45	[73]	2	27
+UK, West Midlands		1	72		0	51
UK, Yorkshire	99	0	40	84	5	35
UK, Scotland	93	3	51	89	2	24
UK, Scotland, West	96	2	74	83	3	21
Yugoslavia, Vojvodina	71	10	55	71	6	40

OCEANIA

	MALE			FEMALE		
	MV	DCO	M/I	MV	DCO	M/I
Australian Capital Territory	99	0		99	0	
Australia, New South Wales	94	1		90	3	
South Australia	91		27	82		14
Australia, Tasmania	99		40	99		13
Australia, Victoria	94	2	28	94	1	30
Western Australia	96	0	20	97	0	27
French Polynesia	99	0		99	0	
+New Zealand: Non-Maori	95	2	44	89	2	39
+New Zealand: Maori	99	0	33	86	14	29
US, Hawaii: White	99	0	29	99	0	25
US, Hawaii: Japanese	99	0	44	86	0	14
US, Hawaii: Hawaiian	99	0	0	-	-	-
US, Hawaii: Filipino	99	0	0	99	0	0
US, Hawaii: Chinese	99	0	0	99	0	0

+ IMPORTANT-SEE NOTES ON POPULATION PAGE

[] CYTOLOGICAL VERIFICATION EXCLUDED

INDICES OF DATA QUALITY
Mouth (ICD-9 143-5)

AFRICA

	MALE			FEMALE		
	MV	DCO	M/I	MV	DCO	M/I
Algeria, Setif	99			99		
France, La Reunion	99			99		
Mali, Bamako	67	0		33	0	
Uganda, Kyadondo	60			99		
Zimbabwe, Harare: African	80	0		99	0	
Zimbabwe, Harare: European	99	0		0	99	

AMERICA, CENTRAL AND SOUTH

	MALE			FEMALE		
	MV	DCO	M/I	MV	DCO	M/I
Argentina, Concordia	99	0	14	99	0	0
Brazil, Belem	96	4	22	96	4	22
Brazil, Goiania	97	0	38	81	19	56
Brazil, Porto Alegre	78	0	30	73	0	40
Colombia, Cali	88	0	44	95	3	49
Costa Rica	95	0	44	77	13	39
Ecuador, Quito	82	0		99	0	
Peru, Lima	83	0		85	4	
Peru, Trujillo	99	0	33	67	0	67
US, Puerto Rico	97	2	24	99	0	25
Uruguay, Montevideo	82	12	45	78	12	37

AMERICA, NORTH

	MALE			FEMALE		
	MV	DCO	M/I	MV	DCO	M/I
Canada	86	1	32	92	1	31
Canada, Alberta	97	1	26	99	0	27
Canada, British Columbia	98	1	23	98	0	24
Canada, Manitoba	91	0	27	95	3	24
Canada, New Brunswick	99	0	24	96	0	27
Canada, Newfoundland	99	0	23	99	0	15
Canada, Northwest Territories	99	0	100	-	-	ncr
Canada, Nova Scotia	97	2	37	99	0	51
Canada, Ontario	93	1	33	96	1	34
Canada, Prince Edward Island	99	0	25	99	0	0
+Canada, Quebec	62	0	37	68	0	30
Canada, Saskatchewan	98	0	35	99	0	33
Canada, Yukon	99	0	0	99	0	0
+US, Cent. Calif.: Non-Hisp. White	98	2		98	0	
+US, Cent. Calif.: Hispanic	92	0		99	0	
US, Los Angeles: Non-Hisp. White	99	0		99	0	
US, Los Angeles: Hispanic White	99	0		97	3	
US, Los Angeles: Black	99	0		99	0	
US, Los Angeles: Chinese	99	0		99	0	
US, Los Angeles: Filipino	99	0		99	0	
US, Los Angeles: Korean	99	0		99	0	
US, Los Angeles: Japanese	99	0		99	0	
US, San Francisco: Non-Hisp. White	99	1	19	99	0	20
US, San Francisco: Hispanic White	99	0	0	99	0	8
US, San Francisco: Black	99	0	29	99	0	30
US, San Francisco: Chinese	99	0	43	99	0	0
US, San Francisco: Filipino	99	0	25	99	0	0
US, San Francisco: Japanese	99	0	0	99	0	50
US, Connecticut: White	98	0	19	98	1	24
US, Connecticut: Black	99	0	26	99	0	0
US, Atlanta: White	99	0	23	99	0	29
US, Atlanta: Black	99	0	35	99	0	21
US, Iowa	99	0	26	99	1	21
US, Central Louisiana: White	99	0	14	99	0	10
US, Central Louisiana: Black	99	0	0	99	0	0
US, New Orleans: White	99	1	21	99	0	18
US, New Orleans: Black	97	0	26	91	9	45
US, Detroit: White	99	1	20	99	0	26
US, Detroit: Black	99	1	23	97	0	18
US, New Mexico: Non-Hisp. White	95	3	41	99	0	9
US, New Mexico: Hispanic White	92	4	33	99	0	50
US, New Mexico: American Indian	99	0	0	99	0	0
US, Utah	96	0	29	99	0	12
US, Seattle	99	0	20	99	0	24
US, SEER: White	98	1	22	99	0	23
US, SEER: Black	99	0	26	98	0	20

ASIA

	MALE			FEMALE		
	MV	DCO	M/I	MV	DCO	M/I
+China, Qidong	99	0	50	99	0	50
+China, Shanghai	76	0	35	75	0	36
China, Tianjin	82	1	42	86	0	30
Hong Kong	86	1	30	76	1	17
India, Bangalore	89	2	14	85	2	9
India, Barshi, Paranda and Bhum	97	0		86	0	
India, Bombay	87	2	26	80	9	33
India, Karunagappally	79	4		73	5	
India, Madras	71	0	40	66	0	33
India, Trivandrum	89	0	22	79	0	12
Israel: All Jews	96			96		
Jews born in Israel	93			93		
Jews born in America or Europe	95			96		
Jews born in Africa or Asia	99			99		
Non-Jews	99			99		
Japan, Hiroshima	96	0	23	99	0	19
Japan, Miyagi	94	0	35	94	2	37
Japan, Nagasaki	92	4	41	89	7	55
Japan, Osaka	93	3	34	91	6	34
+Japan, Saga	86	4	37	83	7	28
Japan, Yamagata	66	29	56	68	18	73
Korea, Kangwha	99		50	99		33
Kuwait: Non-Kuwaitis	99	0		67	0	
Kuwait: Kuwaitis	33	33		99	0	
Philippines, Manila	81	3		80	7	
Singapore: Chinese	99	1		97	3	
Singapore: Malay	99	0		99	0	
Singapore: Indian	99	0		99	0	
Thailand, Chiang Mai	90	1		91	2	
Thailand, Khon Kaen	76	0		79	4	
Viet Nam, Hanoi	62			76		

+ IMPORTANT-SEE NOTES ON POPULATION PAGE

EUROPE

	MALE MV	MALE DCO	MALE M/I	FEMALE MV	FEMALE DCO	FEMALE M/I
Austria, Tyrol	97	1	15	92	0	12
+Belarus	96	0	69	89	0	56
Croatia	68	9	83	55	24	81
+Czech Republic	94	1	59	93	4	51
Denmark	99	0	48	98	0	44
Estonia	97		69	99		59
Finland	99	0	34	99	1	34
France, Bas-Rhin	99		20	99		42
France, Calvados	99		21	99		14
France, Doubs	97		17	96		20
France, Haut-Rhin	99		28	99		37
France, Herault	98		17	99		27
France, Isere	97		14	95		14
France, Somme	98		21	97		34
France, Tarn	99		22	99		22
Germany, Eastern States	98	0	56	97	0	62
+Germany, Saarland	98	2	39	98	2	18
Iceland	99	0	23	99	0	8
Ireland, Southern	89		33	99		62
Italy, Ferrara	99	0	29	89	0	56
Italy, Florence	83	0	48	80	4	50
Italy, Genoa	96	0	47	90	0	55
Italy, Latina	99	0	38	60	0	40
Italy, Macerata	50	0	100	99	0	50
Italy, Modena	88	6	71	88	0	59
Italy, Parma	98	0	44	99	0	57
Italy, Ragusa	99	0	70	86	14	71
Italy, Romagna	94	0	63	92	0	38
Italy, Torino	91	3	46	88	13	144
Italy, Trieste	79	4	27	75	0	43
Italy, Varese	99	0	39	99	0	52
Italy, Veneto	97	1	64	98	2	54
+Latvia	97	1	58	86	0	57
+Malta	99	0	67	99	0	17
The Netherlands	99		31	99		25
The Netherlands, Eindhoven	99		25	99		18
The Netherlands, Maastricht	99		85	99		100
Norway	99	0	44	98	1	48
Poland, Cracow	94	3	70	79	0	57
Poland, Kielce	89	4	75	80	0	80
Poland, Lower Silesia	78	1	61	74	0	33
Poland, Warsaw City	[91]	3	57	[83]	9	96
Slovakia	95	0	61	94	0	59
Slovenia	99	0	34	95	2	44
Spain, Albacete	80	20	20	67	33	67
Spain, Asturias	99	1	42	92	8	58
Spain, Basque Country	98	2	34	91	7	56
Spain, Granada	99	1	37	97	0	17
Spain, Mallorca	99	0	36	94	0	29
Spain, Murcia	98	0	27	93	0	36
Spain, Navarra	95	2	41	86	14	71
Spain, Tarragona	98	0	36	93	0	29
Spain, Zaragoza	96	1	35	99	0	30

	MALE MV	MALE DCO	MALE M/I	FEMALE MV	FEMALE DCO	FEMALE M/I
Sweden	99		45	99		42
Switzerland, Basel	99	0	31	99	0	33
Switzerland, Geneva	98	0	32	99	0	50
Switzerland, Graubunden	99	0	40	99	0	200
Switzerland, Neuchatel	99	0	41	99	0	44
Switzerland, St Gall-Appenzell	99	0	49	99	0	38
Switzerland, Valais	99	0	28	99	0	0
Switzerland, Vaud	99	0	27	97	0	26
Switzerland, Zurich	99	0	35	99	0	45
+UK, England and Wales	[87]		48	[88]		47
UK, East Anglia			42			50
UK, Mersey	94	2	45	90	0	44
UK, North Western	90	1	53	85	1	49
UK, Oxford	95	0	42	93	0	41
UK, South Thames	81	9	48	79	9	49
UK, South Western	86	1	55	87	1	42
UK, Wessex	[91]	3	42	[85]	3	42
+UK, West Midlands		1	38		1	43
UK, Yorkshire	98	0	43	93	1	52
UK, Scotland	96	1	39	94	1	40
UK, Scotland, West	96	0	36	96	1	35
Yugoslavia, Vojvodina	82	4	37	71	13	38

OCEANIA

	MALE MV	MALE DCO	MALE M/I	FEMALE MV	FEMALE DCO	FEMALE M/I
Australian Capital Territory	99	0		99	0	
Australia, New South Wales	96	1		93	0	
South Australia	91		40	83		36
Australia, Tasmania	99		74	95		45
Australia, Victoria	98	0	36	93	1	48
Western Australia	92	2	33	99	0	31
French Polynesia	80	7		75	13	
+New Zealand: Non-Maori	95	2	44	92	5	49
+New Zealand: Maori	93	0	29	99	0	17
US, Hawaii: White	99	0	29	99	0	36
US, Hawaii: Japanese	99	0	10	99	0	10
US, Hawaii: Hawaiian	99	0	33	99	0	75
US, Hawaii: Filipino	99	0	11	99	0	25
US, Hawaii: Chinese	99	0	33	99	0	100

+ IMPORTANT-SEE NOTES ON POPULATION PAGE

[] CYTOLOGICAL VERIFICATION EXCLUDED

INDICES OF DATA QUALITY
Oropharynx (ICD-9 146)

	MALE			FEMALE		
	MV	DCO	M/I	MV	DCO	M/I
AFRICA						
Algeria, Setif	83			99		
France, La Reunion	99			99		
Mali, Bamako	0	0		0	0	
Uganda, Kyadondo	60			50		
Zimbabwe, Harare: African	-	-		-	-	
Zimbabwe, Harare: European	-	-		0	99	
AMERICA, CENTRAL AND SOUTH						
Argentina, Concordia	99	0	17	99	0	0
Brazil, Belem	99	0	37	99	0	43
Brazil, Goiania	80	13	80	86	14	57
Brazil, Porto Alegre	67	0	48	71	0	43
Colombia, Cali	99	0	50	90	0	20
Costa Rica	89	3	49	85	5	35
Ecuador, Quito	99	0		99	0	
Peru, Lima	88	13		88	0	
Peru, Trujillo	99	0	50	-	-	-
US, Puerto Rico	99	0	26	99	0	23
Uruguay, Montevideo	92	4	32	90	10	40
AMERICA, NORTH						
Canada	88	0	39	87	0	34
Canada, Alberta	98	0	26	99	0	40
Canada, British Columbia	98	1	22	98	0	32
Canada, Manitoba	84	0	33	89	0	44
Canada, New Brunswick	99	0	26	99	0	22
Canada, Newfoundland	99	0	40	99	0	14
Canada, Northwest Territories	50	0	100	-	-	ncr
Canada, Nova Scotia	99	0	24	99	0	27
Canada, Ontario	98	0	43	93	1	34
Canada, Prince Edward Island	99	0	100	99	0	100
+Canada, Quebec	64	0	47	61	0	35
Canada, Saskatchewan	99	0	54	99	0	33
Canada, Yukon	99	0	0	99	0	100
+US, Cent. Calif.: Non-Hisp. White	94	1		97	0	
+US, Cent. Calif.: Hispanic	99	0		99	0	
US, Los Angeles: Non-Hisp. White	99	0		99	0	
US, Los Angeles: Hispanic White	99	0		99	0	
US, Los Angeles: Black	96	4		99	0	
US, Los Angeles: Chinese	99	0		99	0	
US, Los Angeles: Filipino	80	0		99	0	
US, Los Angeles: Korean	99	0		-	-	
US, Los Angeles: Japanese	99	0		99	0	
US, San Francisco: Non-Hisp. White	98	2	31	98	0	27
US, San Francisco: Hispanic White	93	0	13	99	0	20
US, San Francisco: Black	99	0	33	99	0	30
US, San Francisco: Chinese	99	0	33	99	0	0
US, San Francisco: Filipino	99	0	0	99	0	0
US, San Francisco: Japanese	-	-	-	-	-	-
US, Connecticut: White	98	1	28	99	0	30
US, Connecticut: Black	99	0	28	99	0	0
US, Atlanta: White	95	2	31	97	0	27
US, Atlanta: Black	99	0	39	99	0	0
US, Iowa	99	0	33	98	0	33
US, Central Louisiana: White	99	0	40	99	0	0
US, Central Louisiana: Black	99	0	33	-	-	-
US, New Orleans: White	93	3	37	99	0	70
US, New Orleans: Black	99	0	33	99	0	40
US, Detroit: White	99	0	24	99	0	43
US, Detroit: Black	99	0	33	96	4	26
US, New Mexico: Non-Hisp. White	99	0	20	99	0	82
US, New Mexico: Hispanic White	99	0	8	99	0	0
US, New Mexico: American Indian	-	-	ncr	-	-	-
US, Utah	96	0	27	99	0	43
US, Seattle	99	0	47	99	0	21
US, SEER: White	99	1	30	99	0	33
US, SEER: Black	99	0	35	98	2	19
ASIA						
+China, Qidong	99	0	100	99	0	80
+China, Shanghai	75	0	49	86	0	60
China, Tianjin	86	0	46	91	0	27
Hong Kong	90	1	41	58	0	27
India, Bangalore	90	2	16	87	3	6
India, Barshi, Paranda and Bhum	99	0		99	0	
India, Bombay	85	4	32	89	2	53
India, Karunagappally	89	0		-	-	
India, Madras	77	2	32	72	0	31
India, Trivandrum	99	0	10	99	0	0
Israel: All Jews	92			90		
Jews born in Israel	99			99		
Jews born in America or Europe	86			99		
Jews born in Africa or Asia	99			75		
Non-Jews	99			-		
Japan, Hiroshima	99	0	29	67	0	100
Japan, Miyagi	93	0	59	99	0	50
Japan, Nagasaki	89	0	44	99	0	56
Japan, Osaka	92	3	37	87	7	27
+Japan, Saga	99	0	55	99	0	33
Japan, Yamagata	88	13	63	80	20	60
Korea, Kangwha	99		0	-		-
Kuwait: Non-Kuwaitis	99	0		-	-	
Kuwait: Kuwaitis	99	0		99	0	
Philippines, Manila	81	8		73	0	
Singapore: Chinese	99	0		99	0	
Singapore: Malay	83	17		99	0	
Singapore: Indian	99	0		99	0	
Thailand, Chiang Mai	96	0		93	0	
Thailand, Khon Kaen	99	0		83	0	
Viet Nam, Hanoi	70			29		

+ IMPORTANT-SEE NOTES ON POPULATION PAGE

INDICES OF DATA QUALITY
Oropharynx (ICD-9 146) (contd)

	MALE			FEMALE		
	MV	DCO	M/I	MV	DCO	M/I
EUROPE						
Austria, Tyrol	99	0	35	93	0	29
+Belarus	96	0	65	97	0	47
Croatia	70	5	56	54	10	54
+Czech Republic	98	0	55	95	3	46
Denmark	99	0	48	99	0	41
Estonia	92		74	90		70
Finland	99	0	57	99	0	43
France, Bas-Rhin	99		21	96		25
France, Calvados	96		31	99		19
France, Doubs	99		30	94		19
France, Haut-Rhin	99		25	99		27
France, Herault	99		27	95		53
France, Isere	99		19	97		18
France, Somme	98		28	86		43
France, Tarn	99		34	99		50
Germany, Eastern States	98	1	58	99	0	47
+Germany, Saarland	97	3	34	96	0	30
Iceland	99	0	33	99	0	0
Ireland, Southern	99		23	75		25
Italy, Ferrara	80	0	70	99	0	133
Italy, Florence	89	0	29	82	0	71
Italy, Genoa	99	0	41	88	0	53
Italy, Latina	99	0	120	-	-	ncr
Italy, Macerata	75	0	50	99	0	0
Italy, Modena	97	0	53	71	0	57
Italy, Parma	99	0	54	99	0	60
Italy, Ragusa	99	0	200	99	0	0
Italy, Romagna	96	0	42	67	0	100
Italy, Torino	97	0	52	90	5	38
Italy, Trieste	86	0	86	80	0	140
Italy, Varese	99	1	44	99	0	50
Italy, Veneto	98	2	52	96	0	64
+Latvia	95	0	65	99	0	55
+Malta	-	-	ncr	99	0	0
The Netherlands	99		41	99		40
The Netherlands, Eindhoven	99		24	88		38
The Netherlands, Maastricht	99		78	99		38
Norway	99	0	59	99	0	71
Poland, Cracow	93	2	90	99	0	64
Poland, Kielce	99	0	30	86	0	29
Poland, Lower Silesia	74	0	49	80	0	29
Poland, Warsaw City	[98]	0	33	[96]	0	30
Slovakia	97	0	60	89	0	48
Slovenia	99	1	47	93	7	67
Spain, Albacete	75	25	25	-	-	-
Spain, Asturias	99	0	40	78	11	22
Spain, Basque Country	98	2	61	92	0	58
Spain, Granada	97	3	50	-	-	ncr
Spain, Mallorca	98	0	35	99	0	33
Spain, Murcia	95	0	41	99	0	50
Spain, Navarra	99	0	66	99	0	100
Spain, Tarragona	99	0	46	99	0	100
Spain, Zaragoza	97	0	32	99	0	33
Sweden	99		35	99		26
Switzerland, Basel	99	0	54	99	0	43
Switzerland, Geneva	97	1	49	99	0	45
Switzerland, Graubunden	99	0	43	99	0	100
Switzerland, Neuchatel	99	0	54	99	0	17
Switzerland, St Gall-Appenzell	99	0	66	99	0	40
Switzerland, Valais	99	0	75	99	0	0
Switzerland, Vaud	97	0	40	95	0	60
Switzerland, Zurich	98	0	52	99	0	44
+UK, England and Wales	[87]		53	[91]		53
UK, East Anglia			53			24
UK, Mersey	88	1	53	90	6	42
UK, North Western	86	1	54	88	1	33
UK, Oxford	90	0	43	91	0	50
UK, South Thames	82	7	50	81	12	58
UK, South Western	89	0	74	72	0	89
UK, Wessex	[85]	0	65	[82]	9	73
+UK, West Midlands		0	60		0	57
UK, Yorkshire	94	1	51	89	3	50
UK, Scotland	94	1	44	90	3	39
UK, Scotland, West	93	1	47	90	5	51
Yugoslavia, Vojvodina	69	11	63	65	8	58
OCEANIA						
Australian Capital Territory	99	0		99	0	
Australia, New South Wales	93	0		93	1	
South Australia	88		65	85		55
Australia, Tasmania	99		29	99		60
Australia, Victoria	97	0	61	95	0	60
Western Australia	99	0	53	99	0	65
French Polynesia	92	8		99	0	
+New Zealand: Non-Maori	99	0	53	90	5	39
+New Zealand: Maori	99	0	0	99	0	50
US, Hawaii: White	99	0	30	99	0	175
US, Hawaii: Japanese	99	0	50	99	0	67
US, Hawaii: Hawaiian	99	0	50	99	0	50
US, Hawaii: Filipino	99	0	25	99	0	0
US, Hawaii: Chinese	99	0	50	-	-	-

+ IMPORTANT-SEE NOTES ON POPULATION PAGE

[] CYTOLOGICAL VERIFICATION EXCLUDED

INDICES OF DATA QUALITY
Nasopharynx (ICD-9 147)

	MALE			FEMALE		
	MV	DCO	M/I	MV	DCO	M/I
AFRICA						
Algeria, Setif	91			81		
France, La Reunion	99			99		
Mali, Bamako	0	99		-	-	
Uganda, Kyadondo	56			50		
Zimbabwe, Harare: African	85	15		67	0	
Zimbabwe, Harare: European	-	-		99	0	
AMERICA, CENTRAL AND SOUTH						
Argentina, Concordia	-	-	-	99	0	0
Brazil, Belem	99	0	17	99	0	50
Brazil, Goiania	99	0	17	99	0	0
Brazil, Porto Alegre	83	0	17	0	0	100
Colombia, Cali	99	0	29	99	0	80
Costa Rica	95	5	53	87	0	53
Ecuador, Quito	50	50		-	-	
Peru, Lima	75	0		80	0	
Peru, Trujillo	99	0	100	-	-	-
US, Puerto Rico	99	0	22	80	10	30
Uruguay, Montevideo	65	24	71	63	13	63
AMERICA, NORTH						
Canada	90	1	50	91	0	48
Canada, Alberta	98	0	45	94	0	119
Canada, British Columbia	99	0	60	96	2	55
Canada, Manitoba	78	0	100	53	0	40
Canada, New Brunswick	83	8	25	99	0	50
Canada, Newfoundland	99	0	57	99	0	56
Canada, Northwest Territories	99	0	53	89	0	33
Canada, Nova Scotia	99	0	225	99	0	0
Canada, Ontario	93	2	36	96	0	34
Canada, Prince Edward Island	99	0	67	99	0	200
+Canada, Quebec	73	0	56	78	0	60
Canada, Saskatchewan	94	0	78	99	0	75
Canada, Yukon	-	-	-	-	-	-
+US, Cent. Calif.: Non-Hisp. White	99	0		86	7	
+US, Cent. Calif.: Hispanic	99	0		99	0	
US, Los Angeles: Non-Hisp. White	98	2		94	3	
US, Los Angeles: Hispanic White	99	0		99	0	
US, Los Angeles: Black	95	5		99	0	
US, Los Angeles: Chinese	98	0		95	5	
US, Los Angeles: Filipino	95	5		99	0	
US, Los Angeles: Korean	99	0		0	0	
US, Los Angeles: Japanese	99	0		99	0	
US, San Francisco: Non-Hisp. White	95	0	76	94	6	94
US, San Francisco: Hispanic White	75	0	75	99	0	150
US, San Francisco: Black	86	0	100	99	0	200
US, San Francisco: Chinese	98	1	41	99	0	45
US, San Francisco: Filipino	99	0	39	99	0	40
US, San Francisco: Japanese	-	-	-	-	-	-
US, Connecticut: White	97	0	32	99	0	50
US, Connecticut: Black	83	17	50	99	0	0
US, Atlanta: White	99	0	50	94	0	44
US, Atlanta: Black	99	0	47	99	0	75
US, Iowa	99	0	61	99	0	37
US, Central Louisiana: White	99	0	50	99	0	0
US, Central Louisiana: Black	99	0	0	-	-	-
US, New Orleans: White	99	0	53	99	0	31
US, New Orleans: Black	99	0	60	99	0	0
US, Detroit: White	98	0	44	95	0	100
US, Detroit: Black	99	0	36	99	0	80
US, New Mexico: Non-Hisp. White	99	0	50	99	0	50
US, New Mexico: Hispanic White	99	0	50	99	0	25
US, New Mexico: American Indian	-	-	-	99	0	100
US, Utah	99	0	22	99	0	50
US, Seattle	98	0	32	99	0	45
US, SEER: White	97	0	47	98	1	64
US, SEER: Black	96	2	50	99	0	88
ASIA						
+China, Qidong	98	0	67	88	3	55
+China, Shanghai	71	0	55	71	1	62
China, Tianjin	78	0	48	74	0	43
Hong Kong	82	3	35	76	3	29
India, Bangalore	83	3	7	74	0	16
India, Barshi, Paranda and Bhum	-	-		-	-	
India, Bombay	78	5	40	85	5	26
India, Karunagappally	50	33		33	67	
India, Madras	82	0	31	81	0	33
India, Trivandrum	99	0	33	99	0	50
Israel: All Jews	95			89		
Jews born in Israel	96			93		
Jews born in America or Europe	99			99		
Jews born in Africa or Asia	92			79		
Non-Jews	75			99		
Japan, Hiroshima	94	0	41	99	0	56
Japan, Miyagi	88	5	45	82	18	36
Japan, Nagasaki	93	7	72	99	0	47
Japan, Osaka	90	7	43	86	7	42
+Japan, Saga	93	7	43	67	0	33
Japan, Yamagata	70	30	70	60	40	100
Korea, Kangwha	99		0	99		0
Kuwait: Non-Kuwaitis	91	0		99	0	
Kuwait: Kuwaitis	99	0		99	0	
Philippines, Manila	71	5		67	9	
Singapore: Chinese	98	1		98	1	
Singapore: Malay	99	0		99	0	
Singapore: Indian	99	0		99	0	
Thailand, Chiang Mai	91	2		90	4	
Thailand, Khon Kaen	88	2		91	0	
Viet Nam, Hanoi	61			44		

+ IMPORTANT-SEE NOTES ON POPULATION PAGE

EUROPE	MALE			FEMALE		
	MV	DCO	M/I	MV	DCO	M/I
Austria, Tyrol	92	0	58	99	0	50
+Belarus	92	0	66	94	0	62
Croatia	70	10	82	60	4	56
+Czech Republic	93	1	66	97	0	76
Denmark	98	0	86	99	0	62
Estonia	99		76	99		86
Finland	98	0	62	94	3	65
France, Bas-Rhin	99		20	99		29
France, Calvados	99		44	99		0
France, Doubs	99		40	99		20
France, Haut-Rhin	99		39	99		125
France, Herault	99		45	99		40
France, Isere	94		22	75		100
France, Somme	99		67	99		67
France, Tarn	99		75	-		-
Germany, Eastern States	99	0	60	99	0	85
+Germany, Saarland	99	0	75	88	13	50
Iceland	99	0	25	99	0	300
Ireland, Southern	99		33	99		167
Italy, Ferrara	99	0	100	99	0	50
Italy, Florence	85	0	70	67	0	87
Italy, Genoa	91	0	52	99	0	86
Italy, Latina	80	0	60	99	0	0
Italy, Macerata	99	0	300	-	-	-
Italy, Modena	82	6	47	99	0	100
Italy, Parma	92	0	58	83	17	17
Italy, Ragusa	83	0	67	99	0	67
Italy, Romagna	95	0	35	86	0	57
Italy, Torino	89	0	48	99	0	86
Italy, Trieste	50	13	63	20	0	40
Italy, Varese	99	0	38	92	0	50
Italy, Veneto	86	0	86	99	0	43
+Latvia	93	0	64	95	0	45
+Malta	99	0	143	99	0	40
The Netherlands	99		49	99		52
The Netherlands, Eindhoven	99		36	99		50
The Netherlands, Maastricht	99		69	99		50
Norway	99	0	78	99	0	62
Poland, Cracow	91	0	109	83	0	67
Poland, Kielce	99	0	25	80	20	100
Poland, Lower Silesia	72	0	72	76	0	53
Poland, Warsaw City	[89]	7	81	[99]	0	140
Slovakia	93	1	92	94	0	50
Slovenia	97	3	23	99	0	42
Spain, Albacete	99	0	200	99	0	100
Spain, Asturias	98	2	51	94	6	56
Spain, Basque Country	98	0	70	94	3	45
Spain, Granada	97	3	45	88	0	13
Spain, Mallorca	94	6	82	99	0	83
Spain, Murcia	96	4	46	99	0	140
Spain, Navarra	86	10	43	33	33	100
Spain, Tarragona	93	7	27	0	0	100
Spain, Zaragoza	86	5	86	89	0	100

	MALE			FEMALE		
	MV	DCO	M/I	MV	DCO	M/I
Sweden	99		42	99		49
Switzerland, Basel	99	0	60	99	0	0
Switzerland, Geneva	99	0	50	99	0	25
Switzerland, Graubunden	99	0	50	99	0	0
Switzerland, Neuchatel	99	0	50	99	0	50
Switzerland, St Gall-Appenzell	99	0	25	99	0	33
Switzerland, Valais	99	0	50	99	0	0
Switzerland, Vaud	99	0	33	99	0	50
Switzerland, Zurich	93	0	64	99	0	67
+UK, England and Wales	[86]		73	[84]		78
UK, East Anglia			100			75
UK, Mersey	86	0	93	88	0	63
UK, North Western	98	0	75	86	0	86
UK, Oxford	75	0	90	69	0	108
UK, South Thames	75	11	73	65	18	80
UK, South Western	79	0	93	82	0	127
UK, Wessex	[82]	3	53	[65]	10	100
+UK, West Midlands		1	67		0	58
UK, Yorkshire	92	2	73	92	0	115
UK, Scotland	94	0	75	83	0	66
UK, Scotland, West	95	0	74	69	0	69
Yugoslavia, Vojvodina	87	0	35	65	10	55

OCEANIA	MALE			FEMALE		
	MV	DCO	M/I	MV	DCO	M/I
Australian Capital Territory	99	0		99	0	
Australia, New South Wales	93	1		94	0	
South Australia	78		89	75		50
Australia, Tasmania	99		130	80		20
Australia, Victoria	97	0	71	88	0	53
Western Australia	96	4	65	99	0	14
French Polynesia	99	0		50	0	
+New Zealand: Non-Maori	93	4	71	92	4	42
+New Zealand: Maori	99	0	36	99	0	0
US, Hawaii: White	99	0	50	99	0	200
US, Hawaii: Japanese	99	0	25	99	0	0
US, Hawaii: Hawaiian	99	0	44	99	0	50
US, Hawaii: Filipino	99	0	86	99	0	20
US, Hawaii: Chinese	99	0	46	99	0	33

+ IMPORTANT-SEE NOTES ON POPULATION PAGE

[] CYTOLOGICAL VERIFICATION EXCLUDED

INDICES OF DATA QUALITY
Hypopharynx (ICD-9 148)

	MALE MV	MALE DCO	MALE M/I	FEMALE MV	FEMALE DCO	FEMALE M/I
AFRICA						
Algeria, Setif	-			-		
France, La Reunion	99			99		
Mali, Bamako	-	-		-	-	
Uganda, Kyadondo	0			50		
Zimbabwe, Harare: African	99	0		99	0	
Zimbabwe, Harare: European	-	-		-	-	
AMERICA, CENTRAL AND SOUTH						
Argentina, Concordia	86	14	57	0	99	0
Brazil, Belem	84	16	53	-	-	ncr
Brazil, Goiania	80	0	67	99	0	100
Brazil, Porto Alegre	69	0	54	67	0	100
Colombia, Cali	92	0	42	99	0	200
Costa Rica	94	0	19	86	0	71
Ecuador, Quito	-	-		-	-	
Peru, Lima	90	0		75	25	
Peru, Trujillo	99	0	0	-	-	-
US, Puerto Rico	99	0	18	99	0	16
Uruguay, Montevideo	87	6	29	83	0	17
AMERICA, NORTH						
Canada	94	0	27	93	0	25
Canada, Alberta	99	0	30	99	0	45
Canada, British Columbia	99	0	17	97	0	31
Canada, Manitoba	80	0	22	80	0	50
Canada, New Brunswick	99	0	13	99	0	20
Canada, Newfoundland	99	0	7	80	0	20
Canada, Northwest Territories	-	-	-	-	-	-
Canada, Nova Scotia	98	0	24	89	0	0
Canada, Ontario	96	1	27	94	1	25
Canada, Prince Edward Island	99	0	0	99	0	100
+Canada, Quebec	89	0	36	92	0	17
Canada, Saskatchewan	99	0	21	99	0	33
Canada, Yukon	-	-	-	99	0	0
+US, Cent. Calif.: Non-Hisp. White	98	0		99	0	
+US, Cent. Calif.: Hispanic	99	0		99	0	
US, Los Angeles: Non-Hisp. White	99	0		99	0	
US, Los Angeles: Hispanic White	99	0		99	0	
US, Los Angeles: Black	99	0		99	0	
US, Los Angeles: Chinese	99	0		-	-	
US, Los Angeles: Filipino	99	0		-	-	
US, Los Angeles: Korean	99	0		-	-	
US, Los Angeles: Japanese	99	0		-	-	
US, San Francisco: Non-Hisp. White	99	0	24	98	2	27
US, San Francisco: Hispanic White	99	0	13	99	0	0
US, San Francisco: Black	99	0	26	99	0	0
US, San Francisco: Chinese	99	0	25	-	-	-
US, San Francisco: Filipino	-	-	-	99	0	0
US, San Francisco: Japanese	99	0	0	-	-	-
US, Connecticut: White	96	1	18	95	3	24
US, Connecticut: Black	99	0	18	99	0	40
US, Atlanta: White	98	0	23	99	0	21
US, Atlanta: Black	99	0	25	90	0	40
US, Iowa	99	0	16	99	0	28

	MALE MV	MALE DCO	MALE M/I	FEMALE MV	FEMALE DCO	FEMALE M/I
US, Central Louisiana: White	99	0	17	-	-	ncr
US, Central Louisiana: Black	99	0	13	99	0	0
US, New Orleans: White	99	0	25	99	0	20
US, New Orleans: Black	99	0	0	99	0	50
US, Detroit: White	99	0	23	99	0	26
US, Detroit: Black	99	0	16	99	0	25
US, New Mexico: Non-Hisp. White	95	0	18	99	0	80
US, New Mexico: Hispanic White	99	0	38	-	-	-
US, New Mexico: American Indian	-	-	-	-	-	-
US, Utah	99	0	28	99	0	14
US, Seattle	99	0	17	98	0	24
US, SEER: White	99	0	21	98	1	26
US, SEER: Black	99	0	21	97	0	25
ASIA						
+China, Qidong	99	0	67	-	-	-
+China, Shanghai	70	0	50	82	0	55
China, Tianjin	79	0	58	75	0	100
Hong Kong	89	3	45	80	4	36
India, Bangalore	86	2	19	77	3	19
India, Barshi, Paranda and Bhum	86	0		99	0	
India, Bombay	83	2	28	83	3	28
India, Karunagappally	99	0		99	0	
India, Madras	77	1	41	75	1	35
India, Trivandrum	92	0	8	99	0	17
Israel: All Jews	96			99		
Jews born in Israel	99			-		
Jews born in America or Europe	92			99		
Jews born in Africa or Asia	99			99		
Non-Jews	99			99		
Japan, Hiroshima	97	0	40	75	0	75
Japan, Miyagi	91	2	61	85	0	30
Japan, Nagasaki	89	2	87	89	0	122
Japan, Osaka	86	8	52	82	7	56
+Japan, Saga	91	9	32	99	0	33
Japan, Yamagata	73	22	84	57	29	86
Korea, Kangwha	99		100	-		-
Kuwait: Non-Kuwaitis	99	0		-	-	
Kuwait: Kuwaitis	99	0		99	0	
Philippines, Manila	75	0		99	0	
Singapore: Chinese	94	3		99	0	
Singapore: Malay	99	0		99	0	
Singapore: Indian	99	0		99	0	
Thailand, Chiang Mai	91	0		83	0	
Thailand, Khon Kaen	91	0		99	0	
Viet Nam, Hanoi	58			42		

+ IMPORTANT-SEE NOTES ON POPULATION PAGE

EUROPE

	MALE			FEMALE		
	MV	DCO	M/I	MV	DCO	M/I
Austria, Tyrol	96	4	42	83	17	17
+Belarus	98	0	68	99	0	73
Croatia	72	2	60	71	2	52
+Czech Republic	90	2	77	92	0	81
Denmark	99	0	70	97	0	74
Estonia	99		64	99		40
Finland	99	0	69	99	0	66
France, Bas-Rhin	98		33	99		44
France, Calvados	98		35	99		0
France, Doubs	97		23	99		50
France, Haut-Rhin	99		43	99		27
France, Herault	99		25	99		25
France, Isere	97		19	86		14
France, Somme	98		28	99		43
France, Tarn	98		14	99		50
Germany, Eastern States	99	0	73	99	0	70
+Germany, Saarland	94	4	60	99	0	75
Iceland	99	0	100	-	-	-
Ireland, Southern	86		71	99		63
Italy, Ferrara	99	0	200	0	0	50
Italy, Florence	90	0	44	67	17	50
Italy, Genoa	91	0	67	79	7	29
Italy, Latina	99	0	125	0	0	200
Italy, Macerata	99	0	100	-	-	-
Italy, Modena	94	0	26	67	33	50
Italy, Parma	95	0	41	99	0	25
Italy, Ragusa	99	0	200	-	-	-
Italy, Romagna	99	0	36	99	0	100
Italy, Torino	97	0	38	89	0	44
Italy, Trieste	57	0	100	-	-	ncr
Italy, Varese	95	2	23	99	0	44
Italy, Veneto	94	1	102	99	0	133
+Latvia	93	1	61	90	0	50
+Malta	99	0	33	-	-	-
The Netherlands	99		28	99		36
The Netherlands, Eindhoven	99		28	99		150
The Netherlands, Maastricht	99		26	99		0
Norway	99	0	78	99	0	77
Poland, Cracow	99	0	133	99	0	67
Poland, Kielce	89	0	267	-	-	ncr
Poland, Lower Silesia	62	0	262	50	0	67
Poland, Warsaw City	[97]	0	193	[80]	20	220
Slovakia	96	0	79	64	0	164
Slovenia	98	1	63	91	9	82
Spain, Albacete	99	0	0	-	-	-
Spain, Asturias	99	0	19	99	0	40
Spain, Basque Country	98	1	33	99	0	0
Spain, Granada	96	0	6	-	-	-
Spain, Mallorca	99	0	33	99	0	0
Spain, Murcia	99	0	17	99	0	0
Spain, Navarra	94	3	9	-	-	-
Spain, Tarragona	99	0	21	99	0	100
Spain, Zaragoza	99	0	27	-	-	-

	MALE			FEMALE		
	MV	DCO	M/I	MV	DCO	M/I
Sweden	99		72	99		86
Switzerland, Basel	99	0	82	99	0	43
Switzerland, Geneva	98	0	52	90	0	40
Switzerland, Graubunden	99	0	63	-	-	ncr
Switzerland, Neuchatel	99	0	41	99	0	50
Switzerland, St Gall-Appenzell	97	0	60	-	-	-
Switzerland, Valais	99	0	38	99	0	0
Switzerland, Vaud	98	0	34	99	0	24
Switzerland, Zurich	97	0	58	99	0	91
+UK, England and Wales	[85]		51	[85]		61
UK, East Anglia			45			45
UK, Mersey	94	0	29	87	0	48
UK, North Western	89	0	56	80	2	63
UK, Oxford	93	0	42	72	0	64
UK, South Thames	82	6	47	80	5	63
UK, South Western	89	2	52	90	0	56
UK, Wessex	[86]	6	61	[86]	2	40
+UK, West Midlands		1	44		0	54
UK, Yorkshire	96	0	49	92	0	84
UK, Scotland	96	1	69	96	0	81
UK, Scotland, West	97	1	69	95	0	75
Yugoslavia, Vojvodina	67	6	66	53	16	89

OCEANIA

	MALE			FEMALE		
	MV	DCO	M/I	MV	DCO	M/I
Australian Capital Territory	99	0		-	-	
Australia, New South Wales	98	0		94	0	
South Australia	93		74	88		125
Australia, Tasmania	92		54	99		0
Australia, Victoria	98	0	35	93	0	27
Western Australia	99	0	36	99	0	78
French Polynesia	92	0		50	50	
+New Zealand: Non-Maori	99	1	54	93	3	31
+New Zealand: Maori	99	0	67	-	-	-
US, Hawaii: White	99	0	35	99	0	29
US, Hawaii: Japanese	99	0	19	-	-	ncr
US, Hawaii: Hawaiian	99	0	11	99	0	100
US, Hawaii: Filipino	99	0	33	99	0	0
US, Hawaii: Chinese	99	0	0	99	0	100

+ IMPORTANT-SEE NOTES ON POPULATION PAGE

[] CYTOLOGICAL VERIFICATION EXCLUDED

INDICES OF DATA QUALITY
Pharynx unspecified (ICD-9 149)

	MALE			FEMALE		
	MV	DCO	M/I	MV	DCO	M/I
AFRICA						
Algeria, Setif	99			0		
France, La Reunion	99			99		
Mali, Bamako	50	0		-	-	
Uganda, Kyadondo	67			-		
Zimbabwe, Harare: African	50	0		99	0	
Zimbabwe, Harare: European	-	-		-	-	
AMERICA, CENTRAL AND SOUTH						
Argentina, Concordia	99	0	267	-	-	-
Brazil, Belem	60	40	40	67	33	100
Brazil, Goiania	67	33	100	-	-	ncr
Brazil, Porto Alegre	68	0	42	50	0	50
Colombia, Cali	0	0	999	50	0	300
Costa Rica	50	39	178	40	40	90
Ecuador, Quito	33	67		0	99	
Peru, Lima	-	-		99	0	
Peru, Trujillo	99	0	0	99	0	200
US, Puerto Rico	71	27	542	36	64	418
Uruguay, Montevideo	79	8	71	67	33	100
AMERICA, NORTH						
Canada	79	4	161	84	3	141
Canada, Alberta	94	6	167	99	0	113
Canada, British Columbia	85	15	210	90	10	300
Canada, Manitoba	88	0	100	99	0	140
Canada, New Brunswick	50	0	700	99	0	150
Canada, Newfoundland	99	0	90	99	0	300
Canada, Northwest Territories	99	0	100	-	-	-
Canada, Nova Scotia	94	6	133	82	18	127
Canada, Ontario	85	5	155	91	3	129
Canada, Prince Edward Island	99	0	600	-	-	-
+Canada, Quebec	67	0	162	67	0	133
Canada, Saskatchewan	82	18	145	99	0	33
Canada, Yukon	99	0	100	99	0	50
+US, Cent. Calif.: Non-Hisp. White	93	7		40	40	
+US, Cent. Calif.: Hispanic	99	0		-	-	
US, Los Angeles: Non-Hisp. White	99	0		88	3	
US, Los Angeles: Hispanic White	88	0		60	0	
US, Los Angeles: Black	90	5		99	0	
US, Los Angeles: Chinese	99	0		0	99	
US, Los Angeles: Filipino	99	0		-	-	
US, Los Angeles: Korean	99	0		-	-	
US, Los Angeles: Japanese	99	0		99	0	
US, San Francisco: Non-Hisp. White	95	0	191	95	0	147
US, San Francisco: Hispanic White	99	0	100	-	-	-
US, San Francisco: Black	99	0	267	99	0	50
US, San Francisco: Chinese	50	50	100	-	-	-
US, San Francisco: Filipino	-	-	ncr	-	-	-
US, San Francisco: Japanese	-	-	-	-	-	-
US, Connecticut: White	94	3	226	83	17	100
US, Connecticut: Black	99	0	200	99	0	33
US, Atlanta: White	88	6	129	99	0	81
US, Atlanta: Black	93	7	64	78	11	56
US, Iowa	96	4	108	92	8	125

	MALE			FEMALE		
	MV	DCO	M/I	MV	DCO	M/I
US, Central Louisiana: White	99	0	163	99	0	400
US, Central Louisiana: Black	-	-	ncr	99	0	0
US, New Orleans: White	91	9	173	86	0	129
US, New Orleans: Black	67	33	517	50	0	200
US, Detroit: White	91	7	124	81	13	131
US, Detroit: Black	96	0	117	99	0	83
US, New Mexico: Non-Hisp. White	93	0	71	99	0	250
US, New Mexico: Hispanic White	99	0	175	-	-	-
US, New Mexico: American Indian	-	-	-	-	-	ncr
US, Utah	99	0	180	67	17	133
US, Seattle	98	2	110	97	0	91
US, SEER: White	95	3	134	91	6	113
US, SEER: Black	96	2	133	91	4	61
ASIA						
+China, Qidong	99	0	0	-	-	-
+China, Shanghai	73	0	55	0	0	25
China, Tianjin	99	0	67	-	-	-
Hong Kong	65	6	35	33	33	100
India, Bangalore	88	3	9	73	18	23
India, Barshi, Paranda and Bhum	83	17		-	-	
India, Bombay	63	28	137	50	33	126
India, Karunagappally	99	0		-	-	
India, Madras	59	20	64	47	20	40
India, Trivandrum	99	0	0	-	-	-
Israel: All Jews	99			-		
Jews born in Israel	99			-		
Jews born in America or Europe	99			-		
Jews born in Africa or Asia	99			-		
Non-Jews	-			-		
Japan, Hiroshima	88	13	113	99	0	0
Japan, Miyagi	83	0	125	75	25	125
Japan, Nagasaki	88	13	125	50	25	175
Japan, Osaka	48	38	134	36	43	150
+Japan, Saga	50	50	100	0	99	100
Japan, Yamagata	33	56	89	60	40	80
Korea, Kangwha	-		-	99		0
Kuwait: Non-Kuwaitis	99	0		-	-	
Kuwait: Kuwaitis	-	-		-	-	
Philippines, Manila	14	82		10	87	
Singapore: Chinese	83	17		99	0	
Singapore: Malay	-	-		-	-	
Singapore: Indian	99	0		-	-	
Thailand, Chiang Mai	89	0		99	0	
Thailand, Khon Kaen	99	0		99	0	
Viet Nam, Hanoi	55			99		

+ IMPORTANT-SEE NOTES ON POPULATION PAGE

INDICES OF DATA QUALITY
Pharynx unspecified (ICD-9 149) (contd)

EUROPE	MALE MV	DCO	M/I	FEMALE MV	DCO	M/I
Austria, Tyrol	67	0	133	99	0	100
+Belarus	95	0	54	92	0	65
Croatia	51	29	238	17	67	283
+Czech Republic	73	10	270	63	13	300
Denmark	93	7	214	89	11	300
Estonia	78		78	99		100
Finland	99	0	63	99	0	43
France, Bas-Rhin	99		99	99		44
France, Calvados	99		347	99		700
France, Doubs	99		283	-		ncr
France, Haut-Rhin	99		95	99		100
France, Herault	99		182	99		140
France, Isere	99		110	99		40
France, Somme	96		100	99		400
France, Tarn	99		600	-		-
Germany, Eastern States	92	0	181	99	0	233
+Germany, Saarland	77	15	338	99	0	350
Iceland	99	0	0	-	-	-
Ireland, Southern	67		300	80		100
Italy, Ferrara	99	0	300	-	-	ncr
Italy, Florence	69	8	138	60	20	140
Italy, Genoa	99	0	263	-	-	ncr
Italy, Latina	63	25	150	-	-	ncr
Italy, Macerata	99	0	0	-	-	-
Italy, Modena	99	0	350	-	-	-
Italy, Parma	99	0	999	-	-	ncr
Italy, Ragusa	99	0	133	-	-	ncr
Italy, Romagna	80	0	240	99	0	200
Italy, Torino	85	0	169	-	-	ncr
Italy, Trieste	-	-	ncr	-	-	ncr
Italy, Varese	-	-	ncr	50	50	350
Italy, Veneto	99	1	67	95	5	36
+Latvia	96	0	64	80	0	20
+Malta	-	-	-	-	-	-
The Netherlands	99		396	82		445
The Netherlands, Eindhoven	99		900	-		ncr
The Netherlands, Maastricht	99		200	99		250
Norway	87	0	73	99	0	25
Poland, Cracow	83	0	100	33	67	100
Poland, Kielce	83	0	50	99	0	200
Poland, Lower Silesia	84	0	102	83	0	167
Poland, Warsaw City	[36]	18	164	[50]	25	250
Slovakia	89	0	153	25	0	250
Slovenia	0	60	980	0	0	600
Spain, Albacete	99	0	200	-	-	-
Spain, Asturias	99	0	113	71	29	86
Spain, Basque Country	96	2	47	99	0	17
Spain, Granada	83	13	83	50	50	150
Spain, Mallorca	99	0	94	99	0	0
Spain, Murcia	91	9	114	50	25	50
Spain, Navarra	90	10	100	99	0	100
Spain, Tarragona	99	0	300	0	0	100
Spain, Zaragoza	99	0	180	0	0	300

	MALE MV	DCO	M/I	FEMALE MV	DCO	M/I
Sweden	99		229	99		800
Switzerland, Basel	99	0	500	-	-	ncr
Switzerland, Geneva	0	0	999	99	0	0
Switzerland, Graubunden	99	0	400	-	-	ncr
Switzerland, Neuchatel	67	0	133	99	0	150
Switzerland, St Gall-Appenzell	60	20	120	-	-	-
Switzerland, Valais	99	0	200	-	-	-
Switzerland, Vaud	91	9	155	99	0	100
Switzerland, Zurich	99	0	300	99	0	600
+UK, England and Wales	[85]		105	[80]		95
UK, East Anglia			162			118
UK, Mersey	88	3	181	81	0	131
UK, North Western	87	3	87	76	3	84
UK, Oxford	88	0	113	91	0	45
UK, South Thames	85	9	96	71	23	113
UK, South Western	75	4	138	71	12	65
UK, Wessex	[63]	7	63	[62]	10	67
+UK, West Midlands		0	126		4	108
UK, Yorkshire	98	2	100	80	5	100
UK, Scotland	89	0	111	91	3	88
UK, Scotland, West	87	0	108	86	5	86
Yugoslavia, Vojvodina	21	13	258	50	0	200

OCEANIA

	MALE MV	DCO	M/I	FEMALE MV	DCO	M/I
Australian Capital Territory	99	0		-	-	-
Australia, New South Wales	90	4		75	13	
South Australia	83		17	99		67
Australia, Tasmania	99		100	99		100
Australia, Victoria	83	0	31	78	11	56
Western Australia	89	5	13	71	14	57
French Polynesia	38	50		99	0	
+New Zealand: Non-Maori	71	17	113	99	0	83
+New Zealand: Maori	99	0	50	-	-	-
US, Hawaii: White	99	0	100	99	0	67
US, Hawaii: Japanese	99	0	150	-	-	ncr
US, Hawaii: Hawaiian	99	0	100	-	-	ncr
US, Hawaii: Filipino	99	0	100	-	-	ncr
US, Hawaii: Chinese	-	-	-	-	-	ncr

+ IMPORTANT-SEE NOTES ON POPULATION PAGE

[] CYTOLOGICAL VERIFICATION EXCLUDED

INDICES OF DATA QUALITY
Oesophagus (ICD-9 150)

	MALE			FEMALE		
	MV	DCO	M/I	MV	DCO	M/I
AFRICA						
Algeria, Setif	56			75		
France, La Reunion	99		75	99		91
Mali, Bamako	42	0		86	0	
Uganda, Kyadondo	18			24		
Zimbabwe, Harare: African	53	7		45	18	
Zimbabwe, Harare: European	67	33		0	67	
AMERICA, CENTRAL AND SOUTH						
Argentina, Concordia	80	18	80	83	17	25
Brazil, Belem	65	11	56	75	15	60
Brazil, Goiania	77	15	58	91	5	41
Brazil, Porto Alegre	64	0	61	58	0	69
Colombia, Cali	65	5	94	62	14	72
Costa Rica	63	17	102	69	14	82
Ecuador, Quito	71	16		58	27	
Peru, Lima	60	15		63	19	
Peru, Trujillo	50	14	79	67	0	0
US, Puerto Rico	86	8	96	85	9	77
Uruguay, Montevideo	55	28	76	58	25	74
AMERICA, NORTH						
Canada	86	2	105	83	3	94
Canada, Alberta	94	2	148	89	1	91
Canada, British Columbia	93	6	101	94	4	90
Canada, Manitoba	83	1	113	84	0	113
Canada, New Brunswick	95	2	129	86	7	97
Canada, Newfoundland	97	0	103	78	9	96
Canada, Northwest Territories	75	0	200	50	17	50
Canada, Nova Scotia	91	6	108	89	5	93
Canada, Ontario	88	2	107	84	3	95
Canada, Prince Edward Island	95	5	100	50	0	150
+Canada, Quebec	74	0	93	69	0	94
Canada, Saskatchewan	98	0	98	94	4	85
Canada, Yukon	67	0	67	-	-	ncr
+US, Cent. Calif.: Non-Hisp. White	98	2	103	95	1	70
+US, Cent. Calif.: Hispanic	99	0	75	99	0	100
US, Los Angeles: Non-Hisp. White	98	1	106	98	1	82
US, Los Angeles: Hispanic White	97	1		97	0	
US, Los Angeles: Black	97	1		95	2	
US, Los Angeles: Chinese	96	0		89	0	
US, Los Angeles: Filipino	99	0		-	-	
US, Los Angeles: Korean	93	7		0	99	
US, Los Angeles: Japanese	99	0		67	33	
US, San Francisco: Non-Hisp. White	96	1	107	96	2	100
US, San Francisco: Hispanic White	99	0	77	99	0	133
US, San Francisco: Black	97	1	84	98	0	80
US, San Francisco: Chinese	94	0	109	99	0	67
US, San Francisco: Filipino	99	0	117	99	0	100
US, San Francisco: Japanese	99	0	86	99	0	200
US, Connecticut: White	96	1	89	93	4	92
US, Connecticut: Black	99	0	68	99	0	81
US, Atlanta: White	97	1	79	90	0	80
US, Atlanta: Black	99	1	84	98	0	75
US, Iowa	97	0	106	97	0	95
US, Central Louisiana: White	85	4	96	71	14	114
US, Central Louisiana: Black	81	0	71	99	0	120
US, New Orleans: White	93	3	92	93	5	75
US, New Orleans: Black	93	4	82	99	0	78
US, Detroit: White	97	1	88	96	2	74
US, Detroit: Black	98	0	86	94	2	87
US, New Mexico: Non-Hisp. White	94	2	80	96	2	67
US, New Mexico: Hispanic White	83	7	93	67	11	100
US, New Mexico: American Indian	60	0	140	99	0	100
US, Utah	97	1	102	91	0	109
US, Seattle	97	0	88	95	0	85
US, SEER: White	96	1	94	95	2	88
US, SEER: Black	98	0	83	96	1	80
ASIA						
+China, Qidong	78	1	86	76	1	88
+China, Shanghai	44	3	92	42	2	100
China, Tianjin	52	0	72	47	0	73
Hong Kong	84	4	71	73	4	55
India, Bangalore	74	5	30	74	4	23
India, Barshi, Paranda and Bhum	82	4		88	0	
India, Bombay	62	14	72	60	17	72
India, Karunagappally	65	13		82	18	
India, Madras	71	2	59	77	3	64
India, Trivandrum	81	3	19	80	10	40
Israel: All Jews	77			87		
Jews born in Israel	65			99		
Jews born in America or Europe	77			84		
Jews born in Africa or Asia	83			90		
Non-Jews	60			99		
Japan, Hiroshima	93	3	59	86	7	67
Japan, Miyagi	83	5	74	73	13	78
Japan, Nagasaki	88	8	79	71	22	81
Japan, Osaka	76	13	80	70	19	77
+Japan, Saga	74	14	74	63	12	76
Japan, Yamagata	77	16	76	71	20	68
Korea, Kangwha	75		66	99		100
Kuwait: Non-Kuwaitis	99	0		99	0	
Kuwait: Kuwaitis	67	33		80	20	
Philippines, Manila	59	17		56	12	
Singapore: Chinese	90	4		90	4	
Singapore: Malay	83	17		50	50	
Singapore: Indian	94	3		99	0	
Thailand, Chiang Mai	67	0		46	0	
Thailand, Khon Kaen	50	6		33	8	
Viet Nam, Hanoi	28			6		

+ IMPORTANT-SEE NOTES ON POPULATION PAGE

INDICES OF DATA QUALITY
Oesophagus (ICD-9 150) (contd)

EUROPE

	MALE			FEMALE		
	MV	DCO	M/I	MV	DCO	M/I
Austria, Tyrol	86	12	88	79	14	93
+Belarus	67	0	82	45	0	77
Croatia	62	9	92	48	21	91
+Czech Republic	65	3	101	55	6	113
Denmark	95	1	108	94	2	104
Estonia	84		96	59		98
Finland	93	1	87	92	2	92
France, Bas-Rhin	98		88	99		88
France, Calvados	95		88	99		84
France, Doubs	96		84	96		85
France, Haut-Rhin	99		85	97		89
France, Herault	97		101	98		86
France, Isere	98		58	93		59
France, Somme	98		96	87		95
France, Tarn	99		118	99		90
Germany, Eastern States	89	0	94	81	1	116
+Germany, Saarland	89	8	101	89	9	109
Iceland	99	0	67	99	0	52
Ireland, Southern	84		119	82		95
Italy, Ferrara	95	0	100	67	0	67
Italy, Florence	72	6	89	55	7	74
Italy, Genoa	74	2	106	67	14	114
Italy, Latina	81	13	100	86	0	114
Italy, Macerata	88	0	38	40	0	120
Italy, Modena	85	5	93	62	4	100
Italy, Parma	87	0	100	84	5	95
Italy, Ragusa	46	0	85	60	0	100
Italy, Romagna	83	7	100	64	7	100
Italy, Torino	83	4	97	62	12	112
Italy, Trieste	92	3	102	71	8	75
Italy, Varese	92	4	94	75	10	88
Italy, Veneto	89	3	89	79	6	88
+Latvia	71	4	84	56	9	73
+Malta	79	0	71	99	0	86
The Netherlands	99		105	97		98
The Netherlands, Eindhoven	97		135	90		107
The Netherlands, Maastricht	99		91	99		76
Norway	97	2	95	93	3	95
Poland, Cracow	62	13	93	45	32	95
Poland, Kielce	58	2	110	50	3	107
Poland, Lower Silesia	26	1	90	32	2	102
Poland, Warsaw City	[60]	8	103	[45]	13	94
Slovakia	77	2	87	55	3	114
Slovenia	84	5	103	71	16	100
Spain, Albacete	82	6	100	99	0	400
Spain, Asturias	88	7	88	72	17	83
Spain, Basque Country	91	5	90	69	25	96
Spain, Granada	81	9	114	74	21	142
Spain, Mallorca	89	6	93	75	19	119
Spain, Murcia	87	8	106	59	14	100
Spain, Navarra	89	7	94	83	11	72
Spain, Tarragona	89	3	92	57	0	129
Spain, Zaragoza	83	7	85	54	33	88
Sweden	99		96	98		94
Switzerland, Basel	99	0	81	99	0	82
Switzerland, Geneva	96	2	89	96	4	89
Switzerland, Graubunden	92	8	73	67	0	83
Switzerland, Neuchatel	99	0	100	99	0	79
Switzerland, St Gall-Appenzell	95	4	97	83	4	100
Switzerland, Valais	92	4	94	80	10	90
Switzerland, Vaud	92	1	83	87	7	94
Switzerland, Zurich	97	1	121	99	1	112
+UK, England and Wales	[77]		100	[77]		93
UK, East Anglia			118			98
UK, Mersey	77	3	112	71	7	107
UK, North Western	69	5	99	66	5	94
UK, Oxford	76	0	99	74	0	92
UK, South Thames	69	20	95	67	19	89
UK, South Western	79	3	101	71	4	92
UK, Wessex	[84]	8	96	[77]	10	86
+UK, West Midlands		2	92		3	87
UK, Yorkshire	86	3	108	81	4	97
UK, Scotland	86	2	105	81	4	96
UK, Scotland, West	84	3	89	78	5	89
Yugoslavia, Vojvodina	46	12	87	38	13	86

OCEANIA

	MALE			FEMALE		
	MV	DCO	M/I	MV	DCO	M/I
Australian Capital Territory	93	0		99	0	
Australia, New South Wales	91	2		89	2	
South Australia	80		97	82		85
Australia, Tasmania	93		83	89		70
Australia, Victoria	93	1	107	88	2	88
Western Australia	89	4	102	93	4	92
French Polynesia	99	0		99	0	
+New Zealand: Non-Maori	87	3	103	80	5	93
+New Zealand: Maori	79	9	59	56	11	89
US, Hawaii: White	99	0	100	99	0	81
US, Hawaii: Japanese	99	0	102	89	0	122
US, Hawaii: Hawaiian	96	0	82	99	0	180
US, Hawaii: Filipino	90	0	95	99	0	100
US, Hawaii: Chinese	99	0	77	-	-	-

+ IMPORTANT-SEE NOTES ON POPULATION PAGE

[] CYTOLOGICAL VERIFICATION EXCLUDED

INDICES OF DATA QUALITY
Stomach (ICD-9 151)

	MALE			FEMALE		
	MV	DCO	M/I	MV	DCO	M/I
AFRICA						
Algeria, Setif	81			90		
France, La Reunion	99		78	98		67
Mali, Bamako	49	3		45	1	
Uganda, Kyadondo	40			13		
Zimbabwe, Harare: African	44	16		57	13	
Zimbabwe, Harare: European	78	22		67	22	
AMERICA, CENTRAL AND SOUTH						
Argentina, Concordia	76	23	71	75	25	86
Brazil, Belem	66	18	54	65	19	58
Brazil, Goiania	80	13	57	77	16	51
Brazil, Porto Alegre	65	0	60	58	1	68
Colombia, Cali	70	9	78	62	15	80
Costa Rica	68	17	86	62	22	82
Ecuador, Quito	69	21		57	32	
Peru, Lima	64	17		62	21	
Peru, Trujillo	52	16	91	47	14	90
US, Puerto Rico	89	6	74	85	10	71
Uruguay, Montevideo	54	31	69	47	34	78
AMERICA, NORTH						
Canada	88	2	70	82	4	75
Canada, Alberta	95	2	64	90	4	82
Canada, British Columbia	92	6	66	89	10	74
Canada, Manitoba	85	4	72	81	6	78
Canada, New Brunswick	94	3	77	88	3	78
Canada, Newfoundland	96	0	75	97	1	89
Canada, Northwest Territories	90	3	66	63	0	113
Canada, Nova Scotia	91	7	69	78	19	80
Canada, Ontario	89	2	69	83	3	74
Canada, Prince Edward Island	93	5	60	83	6	89
+Canada, Quebec	79	0	74	75	0	74
Canada, Saskatchewan	94	2	74	89	6	67
Canada, Yukon	99	0	114	99	0	50
+US, Cent. Calif.: Non-Hisp. White	99	0	56	94	2	75
+US, Cent. Calif.: Hispanic	96	2	73	95	1	72
US, Los Angeles: Non-Hisp. White	98	1	63	96	1	73
US, Los Angeles: Hispanic White	99	1		97	1	
US, Los Angeles: Black	97	1		95	1	
US, Los Angeles: Chinese	97	1		99	0	
US, Los Angeles: Filipino	89	5		96	4	
US, Los Angeles: Korean	98	0		97	1	
US, Los Angeles: Japanese	98	0		96	0	
US, San Francisco: Non-Hisp. White	97	1	66	95	3	76
US, San Francisco: Hispanic White	96	0	53	97	2	67
US, San Francisco: Black	98	0	70	94	2	60
US, San Francisco: Chinese	99	0	69	96	3	54
US, San Francisco: Filipino	94	3	63	90	0	52
US, San Francisco: Japanese	94	6	89	96	4	48
US, Connecticut: White	98	1	67	95	2	67
US, Connecticut: Black	94	5	72	92	2	51
US, Atlanta: White	96	2	68	95	2	62
US, Atlanta: Black	95	2	78	94	5	72
US, Iowa	97	1	57	94	1	66
US, Central Louisiana: White	98	0	71	96	0	69
US, Central Louisiana: Black	93	4	78	85	8	77
US, New Orleans: White	97	1	61	94	2	68
US, New Orleans: Black	94	4	75	92	6	80
US, Detroit: White	97	1	60	96	1	66
US, Detroit: Black	98	0	66	96	1	62
US, New Mexico: Non-Hisp. White	96	2	65	93	1	57
US, New Mexico: Hispanic White	95	2	76	94	1	76
US, New Mexico: American Indian	95	5	95	96	4	71
US, Utah	97	0	62	94	1	76
US, Seattle	98	1	67	94	1	70
US, SEER: White	97	1	64	95	2	69
US, SEER: Black	97	1	70	95	2	63
ASIA						
+China, Qidong	81	0	76	78	0	75
+China, Shanghai	53	2	79	50	2	83
China, Tianjin	58	0	65	54	0	67
Hong Kong	83	5	59	82	7	58
India, Bangalore	68	11	35	65	14	31
India, Barshi, Paranda and Bhum	71	0		63	0	
India, Bombay	66	9	57	57	18	67
India, Karunagappally	62	14		55	27	
India, Madras	64	4	61	60	7	59
India, Trivandrum	69	11	36	61	17	28
Israel: All Jews	88			85		
Jews born in Israel	91			92		
Jews born in America or Europe	87			84		
Jews born in Africa or Asia	88			86		
Non-Jews	86			85		
Japan, Hiroshima	95	3	40	94	4	45
Japan, Miyagi	87	5	43	85	8	49
Japan, Nagasaki	90	5	45	89	7	51
Japan, Osaka	77	11	58	73	15	63
+Japan, Saga	76	13	54	74	15	58
Japan, Yamagata	86	9	45	83	11	50
Korea, Kangwha	80		72	84		67
Kuwait: Non-Kuwaitis	67	31		63	38	
Kuwait: Kuwaitis	60	40		65	30	
Philippines, Manila	55	30		52	28	
Singapore: Chinese	93	3		91	5	
Singapore: Malay	80	12		81	6	
Singapore: Indian	93	2		86	9	
Thailand, Chiang Mai	76	3		73	6	
Thailand, Khon Kaen	56	8		50	17	
Viet Nam, Hanoi	44			41		

+ IMPORTANT-SEE NOTES ON POPULATION PAGE

EUROPE	MALE MV	MALE DCO	MALE M/I	FEMALE MV	FEMALE DCO	FEMALE M/I
Austria, Tyrol	86	9	73	82	14	65
+Belarus	66	0	79	56	0	78
Croatia	49	17	87	45	20	87
+Czech Republic	62	3	96	56	5	96
Denmark	94	1	86	92	1	95
Estonia	84		84	76		83
Finland	96	1	78	92	1	81
France, Bas-Rhin	98		71	98		85
France, Calvados	97		77	95		89
France, Doubs	98		71	99		91
France, Haut-Rhin	98		68	99		75
France, Herault	99		82	99		89
France, Isere	98		48	93		55
France, Somme	97		82	92		98
France, Tarn	95		90	99		95
Germany, Eastern States	88	0	88	84	1	87
+Germany, Saarland	90	6	70	82	12	74
Iceland	99	0	87	99	0	72
Ireland, Southern	82		82	79		85
Italy, Ferrara	87	5	104	87	1	92
Italy, Florence	78	4	78	65	8	79
Italy, Genoa	80	5	83	70	10	86
Italy, Latina	79	16	81	72	19	80
Italy, Macerata	76	1	76	69	2	88
Italy, Modena	84	5	82	78	7	83
Italy, Parma	85	4	82	73	9	86
Italy, Ragusa	77	1	96	63	2	102
Italy, Romagna	92	1	71	88	2	70
Italy, Torino	90	3	77	81	9	78
Italy, Trieste	84	3	69	99	0	95
Italy, Varese	93	2	78	90	5	79
Italy, Veneto	89	4	74	84	7	75
+Latvia	71	5	76	66	4	76
+Malta	75	2	92	81	3	106
The Netherlands	98		82	97		89
The Netherlands, Eindhoven	98		76	99		85
The Netherlands, Maastricht	98		81	99		88
Norway	96	1	82	93	2	84
Poland, Cracow	47	24	98	45	25	91
Poland, Kielce	49	5	109	43	7	110
Poland, Lower Silesia	30	1	86	29	2	79
Poland, Warsaw City	[61]	12	89	[54]	17	88
Slovakia	74	2	81	69	2	83
Slovenia	81	7	90	76	12	92
Spain, Albacete	76	10	77	77	14	61
Spain, Asturias	88	10	85	76	19	79
Spain, Basque Country	86	8	69	81	12	77
Spain, Granada	80	11	81	73	18	88
Spain, Mallorca	92	5	84	83	12	82
Spain, Murcia	87	7	73	79	11	88
Spain, Navarra	86	9	69	81	15	83
Spain, Tarragona	91	4	70	85	6	83
Spain, Zaragoza	76	11	79	64	21	82

	MALE MV	MALE DCO	MALE M/I	FEMALE MV	FEMALE DCO	FEMALE M/I
Sweden	98		82	96		86
Switzerland, Basel	99	0	86	99	0	105
Switzerland, Geneva	98	0	61	94	2	76
Switzerland, Graubunden	94	2	88	88	7	80
Switzerland, Neuchatel	94	2	88	89	2	88
Switzerland, St Gall-Appenzell	94	1	80	92	3	82
Switzerland, Valais	93	4	82	87	7	77
Switzerland, Vaud	95	1	70	87	6	78
Switzerland, Zurich	99	0	71	96	1	90
+UK, England and Wales	[77]		81	[72]		87
UK, East Anglia			77			88
UK, Mersey	77	3	82	65	5	89
UK, North Western	67	5	83	56	7	88
UK, Oxford	74	0	79	61	1	81
UK, South Thames	63	24	81	52	30	84
UK, South Western	73	6	81	61	4	87
UK, Wessex	[80]	10	81	[72]	16	79
+UK, West Midlands		3	78		6	84
UK, Yorkshire	81	4	79	72	7	83
UK, Scotland	83	4	74	74	6	79
UK, Scotland, West	77	7	81	70	9	83
Yugoslavia, Vojvodina	49	10	82	47	10	79

OCEANIA

	MALE MV	MALE DCO	MALE M/I	FEMALE MV	FEMALE DCO	FEMALE M/I
Australian Capital Territory	96	2		95	3	
Australia, New South Wales	93	2		87	4	
South Australia	79		85	77		89
Australia, Tasmania	93		82	84		91
Australia, Victoria	93	1	64	87	3	75
Western Australia	91	4	72	86	6	73
French Polynesia	79	17		76	24	
+New Zealand: Non-Maori	86	5	78	75	8	81
+New Zealand: Maori	83	6	68	88	1	70
US, Hawaii: White	96	1	75	96	0	62
US, Hawaii: Japanese	98	0	59	96	0	60
US, Hawaii: Hawaiian	96	0	72	98	0	98
US, Hawaii: Filipino	98	0	60	97	0	63
US, Hawaii: Chinese	99	0	50	99	0	83

+ IMPORTANT-SEE NOTES ON POPULATION PAGE

[] CYTOLOGICAL VERIFICATION EXCLUDED

INDICES OF DATA QUALITY
Small intestine (ICD-9 152)

	MALE			FEMALE		
	MV	DCO	M/I	MV	DCO	M/I
AFRICA						
Algeria, Setif	25			-		
France, La Reunion	99			99		
Mali, Bamako	75	0		-	-	
Uganda, Kyadondo	0			99		
Zimbabwe, Harare: African	0	99		99	0	
Zimbabwe, Harare: European	99	0		-	-	
AMERICA, CENTRAL AND SOUTH						
Argentina, Concordia	0	99	0	50	50	75
Brazil, Belem	50	13	38	50	0	25
Brazil, Goiania	99	0	67	99	0	42
Brazil, Porto Alegre	80	5	25	79	0	21
Colombia, Cali	99	0	60	91	0	23
Costa Rica	78	11	52	88	4	36
Ecuador, Quito	92	0		83	17	
Peru, Lima	68	11		53	26	
Peru, Trujillo	86	0	29	25	25	175
US, Puerto Rico	97	0	25	96	2	28
Uruguay, Montevideo	80	0	33	57	36	57
AMERICA, NORTH						
Canada	89	1	36	90	1	34
Canada, Alberta	96	4	38	99	1	28
Canada, British Columbia	92	8	43	95	2	38
Canada, Manitoba	76	3	39	79	4	50
Canada, New Brunswick	99	0	40	99	0	46
Canada, Newfoundland	91	0	55	99	0	20
Canada, Northwest Territories	99	0	0	-	-	-
Canada, Nova Scotia	88	3	34	99	0	35
Canada, Ontario	91	0	31	89	2	29
Canada, Prince Edward Island	99	0	33	99	0	100
+Canada, Quebec	83	0	43	84	0	40
Canada, Saskatchewan	99	0	30	94	6	35
Canada, Yukon	-	-	-	-	-	-
+US, Cent. Calif.: Non-Hisp. White	99	0	42	96	2	27
+US, Cent. Calif.: Hispanic	99	0	20	99	0	20
US, Los Angeles: Non-Hisp. White	98	0	31	99	1	27
US, Los Angeles: Hispanic White	99	0		99	0	
US, Los Angeles: Black	99	0		97	0	
US, Los Angeles: Chinese	99	0		99	0	
US, Los Angeles: Filipino	99	0		99	0	
US, Los Angeles: Korean	99	0		99	0	
US, Los Angeles: Japanese	99	0		99	0	
US, San Francisco: Non-Hisp. White	99	0	35	98	0	49
US, San Francisco: Hispanic White	99	0	14	86	0	0
US, San Francisco: Black	99	0	30	86	7	57
US, San Francisco: Chinese	99	0	14	99	0	0
US, San Francisco: Filipino	99	0	50	-	-	-
US, San Francisco: Japanese	-	-	-	-	-	-
US, Connecticut: White	99	0	20	98	2	20
US, Connecticut: Black	99	0	29	99	0	18
US, Atlanta: White	99	0	24	99	0	5
US, Atlanta: Black	99	0	35	99	0	16
US, Iowa	99	0	32	96	0	44
US, Central Louisiana: White	99	0	25	99	0	20
US, Central Louisiana: Black	99	0	50	-	-	-
US, New Orleans: White	99	0	30	95	5	42
US, New Orleans: Black	99	0	11	99	0	0
US, Detroit: White	99	0	24	98	1	21
US, Detroit: Black	98	0	28	98	0	20
US, New Mexico: Non-Hisp. White	99	0	15	96	4	27
US, New Mexico: Hispanic White	99	0	50	99	0	33
US, New Mexico: American Indian	99	0	0	-	-	-
US, Utah	99	0	8	98	0	20
US, Seattle	98	0	32	99	0	30
US, SEER: White	99	0	26	98	1	28
US, SEER: Black	98	0	31	97	1	25
ASIA						
+China, Qidong	93	0	67	82	0	71
+China, Shanghai	68	1	56	66	1	58
China, Tianjin	72	0	44	61	0	34
Hong Kong	90	4	28	93	1	18
India, Bangalore	83	17	50	80	20	20
India, Barshi, Paranda and Bhum	99	0		-	-	
India, Bombay	73	12	43	87	13	60
India, Karunagappally	50	50		-	-	
India, Madras	90	0	50	80	0	60
India, Trivandrum	99	0	0	99	0	0
Israel: All Jews	99			90		
Jews born in Israel	99			80		
Jews born in America or Europe	97			91		
Jews born in Africa or Asia	99			91		
Non-Jews	75			99		
Japan, Hiroshima	99	0	40	91	9	82
Japan, Miyagi	80	5	58	83	7	97
Japan, Nagasaki	83	5	70	92	0	79
Japan, Osaka	77	8	67	75	10	63
+Japan, Saga	61	11	56	63	19	75
Japan, Yamagata	65	22	74	79	21	114
Korea, Kangwha	99		0	99		0
Kuwait: Non-Kuwaitis	-	-		99	0	
Kuwait: Kuwaitis	50	50		50	50	
Philippines, Manila	87	9		82	12	
Singapore: Chinese	99	0		99	0	
Singapore: Malay	50	0		99	0	
Singapore: Indian	99	0		99	0	
Thailand, Chiang Mai	85	0		99	0	
Thailand, Khon Kaen	33	0		67	0	
Viet Nam, Hanoi	67			-		

+ IMPORTANT-SEE NOTES ON POPULATION PAGE

INDICES OF DATA QUALITY
Small intestine (ICD-9 152) (contd)

EUROPE

	MALE MV	DCO	M/I	FEMALE MV	DCO	M/I
Austria, Tyrol	87	7	40	86	0	71
+Belarus	81	1	80	78	2	76
Croatia	51	9	96	49	13	55
+Czech Republic	68	4	100	62	4	107
Denmark	98	0	53	98	0	79
Estonia	91		82	93		100
Finland	97	0	56	96	1	59
France, Bas-Rhin	97		43	99		85
France, Calvados	99		18	92		21
France, Doubs	94		35	99		58
France, Haut-Rhin	95		33	92		38
France, Herault	99		36	99		48
France, Isere	99		24	93		26
France, Somme	99		33	93		43
France, Tarn	99		71	99		200
Germany, Eastern States	96	1	110	95	0	100
+Germany, Saarland	96	4	32	86	5	43
Iceland	99	0	22	99	0	33
Ireland, Southern	99		67	99		71
Italy, Ferrara	86	14	71	80	0	100
Italy, Florence	86	5	76	83	0	52
Italy, Genoa	81	5	43	74	5	53
Italy, Latina	67	33	22	99	0	75
Italy, Macerata	99	0	33	67	0	33
Italy, Modena	99	0	71	83	4	50
Italy, Parma	99	0	50	70	0	50
Italy, Ragusa	80	0	80	99	0	100
Italy, Romagna	78	6	28	95	0	37
Italy, Torino	99	0	40	84	5	26
Italy, Trieste	30	0	10	50	0	11
Italy, Varese	95	0	52	86	0	64
Italy, Veneto	94	3	32	77	17	37
+Latvia	48	18	73	50	23	58
+Malta	86	0	0	99	0	0
The Netherlands	96		92	98		92
The Netherlands, Eindhoven	99		67	99		120
The Netherlands, Maastricht	99		100	96		70
Norway	98	0	66	99	1	62
Poland, Cracow	80	0	100	33	33	89
Poland, Kielce	65	4	39	60	4	48
Poland, Lower Silesia	52	0	145	44	8	140
Poland, Warsaw City	[92]	0	192	[50]	17	111
Slovakia	84	5	116	69	5	121
Slovenia	99	0	64	86	5	82
Spain, Albacete	75	0	0	0	99	100
Spain, Asturias	85	15	48	99	0	48
Spain, Basque Country	87	9	41	82	0	32
Spain, Granada	91	0	36	78	11	67
Spain, Mallorca	99	0	25	99	0	50
Spain, Murcia	96	0	23	88	0	38
Spain, Navarra	60	20	140	99	0	22
Spain, Tarragona	99	0	17	99	0	150
Spain, Zaragoza	99	0	22	86	0	43
Sweden	99		37	99		42
Switzerland, Basel	99	0	11	99	0	17
Switzerland, Geneva	99	0	56	99	0	100
Switzerland, Graubunden	99	0	33	99	0	150
Switzerland, Neuchatel	88	0	25	75	0	0
Switzerland, St Gall-Appenzell	99	0	44	94	0	61
Switzerland, Valais	99	0	83	99	0	100
Switzerland, Vaud	81	0	46	99	0	43
Switzerland, Zurich	99	0	33	98	0	34
+UK, England and Wales	[79]		63	[81]		58
UK, East Anglia			52			54
UK, Mersey	82	0	66	74	5	55
UK, North Western	80	3	56	80	6	68
UK, Oxford	76	0	60	82	0	51
UK, South Thames	79	17	66	74	15	55
UK, South Western	72	6	61	77	9	56
UK, Wessex	[84]	3	55	[81]	9	46
+UK, West Midlands		1	59		1	55
UK, Yorkshire	89	1	62	84	6	41
UK, Scotland	90	4	68	92	0	61
UK, Scotland, West	88	7	75	92	0	57
Yugoslavia, Vojvodina	31	12	100	45	9	73

OCEANIA

	MALE MV	DCO	M/I	FEMALE MV	DCO	M/I
Australian Capital Territory	99	0		99	0	
Australia, New South Wales	97	0		98	0	
South Australia	89		48	92		56
Australia, Tasmania	99		25	99		60
Australia, Victoria	99	1	54	95	0	38
Western Australia	98	0	36	99	0	30
French Polynesia	99	0		99	0	
+New Zealand: Non-Maori	90	1	62	87	3	57
+New Zealand: Maori	99	0	0	99	0	50
US, Hawaii: White	99	0	23	99	0	0
US, Hawaii: Japanese	99	0	38	99	0	50
US, Hawaii: Hawaiian	99	0	0	99	0	50
US, Hawaii: Filipino	99	0	33	99	0	50
US, Hawaii: Chinese	99	0	100	99	0	25

+ IMPORTANT-SEE NOTES ON POPULATION PAGE

[] CYTOLOGICAL VERIFICATION EXCLUDED

INDICES OF DATA QUALITY
Large bowel (ICD-9 153-4)

	MALE			FEMALE		
	MV	DCO	M/I	MV	DCO	M/I
AFRICA						
Algeria, Setif	64			65		
France, La Reunion	99			99		
Mali, Bamako	40	0		38	10	
Uganda, Kyadondo	67			58		
Zimbabwe, Harare: African	58	15		64	16	
Zimbabwe, Harare: European	72	23		81	19	
AMERICA, CENTRAL AND SOUTH						
Argentina, Concordia	83	17	56	82	18	32
Brazil, Belem	73	10	52	68	19	62
Brazil, Goiania	83	13	45	84	13	36
Brazil, Porto Alegre	71	0	45	69	0	49
Colombia, Cali	84	4	43	76	8	54
Costa Rica	70	12	62	70	14	66
Ecuador, Quito	71	15		73	14	
Peru, Lima	73	12		74	10	
Peru, Trujillo	72	6	47	61	9	72
US, Puerto Rico	95	2	40	94	3	38
Uruguay, Montevideo	60	22	63	58	26	62
AMERICA, NORTH						
Canada	90	1	41	89	2	40
Canada, Alberta	96	1	39	95	1	39
Canada, British Columbia	96	3	36	94	5	36
Canada, Manitoba	88	1	40	86	2	39
Canada, New Brunswick	96	1	34	96	1	33
Canada, Newfoundland	99	0	37	97	0	36
Canada, Northwest Territories	91	3	47	90	7	45
Canada, Nova Scotia	92	6	33	91	7	32
Canada, Ontario	91	1	39	88	2	39
Canada, Prince Edward Island	96	1	32	96	1	31
+Canada, Quebec	84	0	47	83	0	48
Canada, Saskatchewan	95	2	41	94	3	39
Canada, Yukon	99	0	23	99	0	47
+US, Cent. Calif.: Non-Hisp. White	97	1	38	96	1	39
+US, Cent. Calif.: Hispanic	95	2	35	97	1	36
US, Los Angeles: Non-Hisp. White	98	1	39	97	1	42
US, Los Angeles: Hispanic White	98	0		98	0	
US, Los Angeles: Black	98	0		97	1	
US, Los Angeles: Chinese	99	0		99	1	
US, Los Angeles: Filipino	99	0		98	0	
US, Los Angeles: Korean	99	1		98	0	
US, Los Angeles: Japanese	99	0		96	1	
US, San Francisco: Non-Hisp. White	98	1	38	96	1	42
US, San Francisco: Hispanic White	98	1	24	98	1	30
US, San Francisco: Black	97	0	42	97	1	45
US, San Francisco: Chinese	99	0	31	98	0	33
US, San Francisco: Filipino	96	1	31	99	1	37
US, San Francisco: Japanese	99	0	34	99	1	34
US, Connecticut: White	98	1	39	95	1	41
US, Connecticut: Black	99	1	42	96	1	39
US, Atlanta: White	98	1	38	96	1	36
US, Atlanta: Black	97	1	44	96	1	41
US, Iowa	97	1	40	95	1	40

	MALE			FEMALE		
	MV	DCO	M/I	MV	DCO	M/I
US, Central Louisiana: White	95	2	39	96	1	38
US, Central Louisiana: Black	89	3	58	96	3	54
US, New Orleans: White	98	1	40	96	1	39
US, New Orleans: Black	96	2	52	95	1	52
US, Detroit: White	98	1	38	96	1	39
US, Detroit: Black	96	1	43	96	1	45
US, New Mexico: Non-Hisp. White	97	1	40	95	2	39
US, New Mexico: Hispanic White	97	2	41	94	1	46
US, New Mexico: American Indian	92	3	39	97	3	40
US, Utah	98	0	39	98	0	38
US, Seattle	98	0	37	97	0	37
US, SEER: White	98	1	38	96	1	40
US, SEER: Black	97	1	43	96	1	44
ASIA						
+China, Qidong	92	0	58	89	1	62
+China, Shanghai	66	1	52	64	1	52
China, Tianjin	73	1	46	68	0	49
Hong Kong	82	4	44	80	6	42
India, Bangalore	79	5	24	82	4	22
India, Barshi, Paranda and Bhum	83	0		71	0	
India, Bombay	73	9	45	71	9	51
India, Karunagappally	64	9		50	17	
India, Madras	75	4	45	78	2	41
India, Trivandrum	84	5	11	81	8	19
Israel: All Jews	91			89		
Jews born in Israel	93			91		
Jews born in America or Europe	90			89		
Jews born in Africa or Asia	92			90		
Non-Jews	89			81		
Japan, Hiroshima	95	2	31	93	5	33
Japan, Miyagi	86	3	38	83	6	43
Japan, Nagasaki	91	3	37	88	6	42
Japan, Osaka	77	8	48	74	10	53
+Japan, Saga	72	13	50	67	17	57
Japan, Yamagata	84	8	42	80	10	44
Korea, Kangwha	85		38	81		52
Kuwait: Non-Kuwaitis	83	13		81	8	
Kuwait: Kuwaitis	61	34		67	28	
Philippines, Manila	73	12		70	11	
Singapore: Chinese	94	2		93	3	
Singapore: Malay	91	5		88	5	
Singapore: Indian	90	1		97	0	
Thailand, Chiang Mai	77	1		82	0	
Thailand, Khon Kaen	53	5		54	3	
Viet Nam, Hanoi	54			58		

+ IMPORTANT-SEE NOTES ON POPULATION PAGE

INDICES OF DATA QUALITY
Large bowel (ICD-9 153-4) (contd)

EUROPE	MALE MV	DCO	M/I	FEMALE MV	DCO	M/I
Austria, Tyrol	90	7	50	85	9	56
+Belarus	73	0	67	70	0	66
Croatia	57	8	68	54	12	71
+Czech Republic	69	2	72	65	3	73
Denmark	95	1	63	94	1	64
Estonia	84		68	79		66
Finland	96	0	54	94	1	54
France, Bas-Rhin	98		51	98		52
France, Calvados	98		51	97		53
France, Doubs	98		47	97		51
France, Haut-Rhin	98		52	99		53
France, Herault	99		50	99		54
France, Isere	97		30	97		29
France, Somme	96		58	94		66
France, Tarn	98		54	98		53
Germany, Eastern States	91	0	64	87	0	67
+Germany, Saarland	94	4	55	90	6	54
Iceland	99	0	57	99	0	47
Ireland, Southern	89		59	86		57
Italy, Ferrara	95	2	59	96	0	54
Italy, Florence	83	2	45	79	4	45
Italy, Genoa	81	3	56	79	4	55
Italy, Latina	89	8	59	85	11	58
Italy, Macerata	82	0	43	84	1	41
Italy, Modena	90	2	48	86	3	51
Italy, Parma	90	2	49	88	3	53
Italy, Ragusa	86	2	69	77	1	56
Italy, Romagna	90	1	46	89	1	48
Italy, Torino	88	3	56	84	6	55
Italy, Trieste	84	0	46	95	0	60
Italy, Varese	95	1	40	89	3	39
Italy, Veneto	91	2	51	86	4	51
+Latvia	77	3	63	75	4	62
+Malta	90	0	66	87	2	66
The Netherlands	98		51	97		54
The Netherlands, Eindhoven	98		51	98		50
The Netherlands, Maastricht	97		51	97		56
Norway	96	1	56	94	1	53
Poland, Cracow	56	18	82	56	18	88
Poland, Kielce	61	2	74	66	4	91
Poland, Lower Silesia	36	1	67	38	1	65
Poland, Warsaw City	[66]	7	67	[62]	9	70
Slovakia	81	1	62	78	1	62
Slovenia	87	4	67	83	6	68
Spain, Albacete	85	8	53	85	8	53
Spain, Asturias	92	6	60	89	8	59
Spain, Basque Country	88	6	53	82	9	53
Spain, Granada	88	5	52	81	7	53
Spain, Mallorca	94	2	64	89	5	55
Spain, Murcia	91	4	51	89	5	51
Spain, Navarra	90	6	52	86	9	49
Spain, Tarragona	92	2	52	89	4	50
Spain, Zaragoza	76	7	60	71	9	62

	MALE MV	DCO	M/I	FEMALE MV	DCO	M/I
Sweden	98		52	97		52
Switzerland, Basel	99	0	59	99	0	58
Switzerland, Geneva	97	1	46	95	1	50
Switzerland, Graubunden	90	5	56	88	8	62
Switzerland, Neuchatel	92	0	60	91	2	68
Switzerland, St Gall-Appenzell	98	1	56	95	1	58
Switzerland, Valais	96	1	63	97	2	57
Switzerland, Vaud	95	1	55	94	2	52
Switzerland, Zurich	99	0	59	97	0	58
+UK, England and Wales	[80]		62	[78]		63
UK, East Anglia			57			59
UK, Mersey	81	2	68	76	4	67
UK, North Western	77	4	65	70	4	69
UK, Oxford	81	0	55	76	1	59
UK, South Thames	74	17	62	69	19	63
UK, South Western	81	3	59	76	3	59
UK, Wessex	[80]	6	54	[74]	10	55
+UK, West Midlands		2	55		3	57
UK, Yorkshire	88	3	60	83	3	60
UK, Scotland	87	2	56	82	4	58
UK, Scotland, West	84	3	56	78	6	60
Yugoslavia, Vojvodina	52	8	66	52	7	64

OCEANIA	MALE MV	DCO	M/I	FEMALE MV	DCO	M/I
Australian Capital Territory	97	1		95	2	
Australia, New South Wales	95	1		93	2	
South Australia	86		48	80		48
Australia, Tasmania	94		49	92		47
Australia, Victoria	94	1	48	91	1	49
Western Australia	94	2	43	91	3	46
French Polynesia	88	8		73	15	
+New Zealand: Non-Maori	92	2	52	90	3	51
+New Zealand: Maori	85	5	47	84	4	29
US, Hawaii: White	98	0	29	98	0	38
US, Hawaii: Japanese	99	0	33	98	0	29
US, Hawaii: Hawaiian	99	0	56	97	0	38
US, Hawaii: Filipino	98	0	46	99	0	35
US, Hawaii: Chinese	98	0	29	99	0	43

+ IMPORTANT-SEE NOTES ON POPULATION PAGE

[] CYTOLOGICAL VERIFICATION EXCLUDED

INDICES OF DATA QUALITY
Colon (ICD-9 153)

AFRICA	MALE MV	DCO	M/I	FEMALE MV	DCO	M/I
Algeria, Setif	50			57		
France, La Reunion	99			99		
Mali, Bamako	36	0		38	15	
Uganda, Kyadondo	63			53		
Zimbabwe, Harare: African	51	18		45	27	
Zimbabwe, Harare: European	70	25		76	24	

AMERICA, CENTRAL AND SOUTH

	MALE MV	DCO	M/I	FEMALE MV	DCO	M/I
Argentina, Concordia	80	20	57	80	20	34
Brazil, Belem	60	12	53	54	23	77
Brazil, Goiania	81	15	52	84	14	31
Brazil, Porto Alegre	68	0	50	64	0	55
Colombia, Cali	76	6	51	69	11	67
Costa Rica	60	17	78	62	18	81
Ecuador, Quito	67	19		66	18	
Peru, Lima	67	15		68	14	
Peru, Trujillo	60	10	60	50	13	92
US, Puerto Rico	94	2	54	92	4	48
Uruguay, Montevideo	54	26	69	53	31	69

AMERICA, NORTH

	MALE MV	DCO	M/I	FEMALE MV	DCO	M/I
Canada	89	1	48	88	2	46
Canada, Alberta	95	1	49	94	2	46
Canada, British Columbia	95	4	47	93	6	43
Canada, Manitoba	86	1	45	84	2	41
Canada, New Brunswick	95	1	42	96	1	40
Canada, Newfoundland	98	0	44	97	0	41
Canada, Northwest Territories	83	0	83	94	6	50
Canada, Nova Scotia	90	7	38	90	8	36
Canada, Ontario	89	1	44	88	2	43
Canada, Prince Edward Island	97	1	37	96	1	37
+Canada, Quebec	83	0	57	83	0	55
Canada, Saskatchewan	94	2	47	94	4	44
Canada, Yukon	99	0	43	99	0	86
+US, Cent. Calif.: Non-Hisp. White	97	1	50	96	1	46
+US, Cent. Calif.: Hispanic	95	3	47	97	1	44
US, Los Angeles: Non-Hisp. White	98	1	48	96	1	48
US, Los Angeles: Hispanic White	98	1		98	0	
US, Los Angeles: Black	98	0		96	1	
US, Los Angeles: Chinese	99	0		99	1	
US, Los Angeles: Filipino	99	0		96	0	
US, Los Angeles: Korean	98	2		97	0	
US, Los Angeles: Japanese	98	0		95	1	
US, San Francisco: Non-Hisp. White	98	1	45	95	1	49
US, San Francisco: Hispanic White	96	1	29	99	0	33
US, San Francisco: Black	96	0	47	96	1	51
US, San Francisco: Chinese	98	0	36	98	0	40
US, San Francisco: Filipino	95	1	38	98	2	60
US, San Francisco: Japanese	97	0	44	98	2	37
US, Connecticut: White	98	1	49	95	2	49
US, Connecticut: Black	98	1	49	95	2	47
US, Atlanta: White	98	1	46	95	2	41
US, Atlanta: Black	96	1	51	95	1	47
US, Iowa	96	1	50	94	1	47
US, Central Louisiana: White	94	2	48	97	1	46
US, Central Louisiana: Black	90	4	60	95	3	58
US, New Orleans: White	97	2	48	95	2	46
US, New Orleans: Black	96	2	61	95	1	59
US, Detroit: White	97	1	48	96	2	47
US, Detroit: Black	96	1	51	95	1	52
US, New Mexico: Non-Hisp. White	96	2	50	95	2	46
US, New Mexico: Hispanic White	96	1	56	93	2	55
US, New Mexico: American Indian	88	4	50	99	0	43
US, Utah	98	0	50	97	0	47
US, Seattle	98	0	47	96	1	44
US, SEER: White	97	1	48	95	1	47
US, SEER: Black	96	1	50	95	1	50

ASIA

	MALE MV	DCO	M/I	FEMALE MV	DCO	M/I
+China, Qidong	95	0	50	89	1	57
+China, Shanghai	64	1	45	63	1	45
China, Tianjin	72	1	43	65	0	47
Hong Kong	80	5	43	79	6	42
India, Bangalore	77	5	26	80	4	22
India, Barshi, Paranda and Bhum	67	0		50	0	
India, Bombay	67	10	48	66	11	60
India, Karunagappally	40	20		40	20	
India, Madras	70	5	45	79	1	50
India, Trivandrum	82	6	18	99	0	13
Israel: All Jews	88			87		
Jews born in Israel	93			90		
Jews born in America or Europe	88			87		
Jews born in Africa or Asia	89			87		
Non-Jews	88			74		
Japan, Hiroshima	95	3	29	92	5	33
Japan, Miyagi	85	3	37	81	7	44
Japan, Nagasaki	90	4	37	86	7	43
Japan, Osaka	76	8	47	73	10	54
+Japan, Saga	70	15	49	63	19	59
Japan, Yamagata	83	9	43	78	11	47
Korea, Kangwha	71		29	86		129
Kuwait: Non-Kuwaitis	77	20		85	15	
Kuwait: Kuwaitis	45	45		60	32	
Philippines, Manila	69	14		66	13	
Singapore: Chinese	92	2		91	3	
Singapore: Malay	86	9		87	4	
Singapore: Indian	87	3		93	0	
Thailand, Chiang Mai	71	1		76	0	
Thailand, Khon Kaen	48	8		48	5	
Viet Nam, Hanoi	56			53		

+ IMPORTANT-SEE NOTES ON POPULATION PAGE

INDICES OF DATA QUALITY
Colon (ICD-9 153) (contd)

EUROPE

	MALE			FEMALE		
	MV	DCO	M/I	MV	DCO	M/I
Austria, Tyrol	89	8	52	84	11	57
+Belarus	63	1	65	59	1	63
Croatia	55	7	64	53	10	69
+Czech Republic	63	2	74	61	3	74
Denmark	94	1	70	93	1	67
Estonia	81		65	76		65
Finland	95	0	53	93	1	52
France, Bas-Rhin	98		59	98		59
France, Calvados	98		71	96		64
France, Doubs	98		58	96		62
France, Haut-Rhin	98		63	99		61
France, Herault	99		66	99		64
France, Isere	97		36	96		35
France, Somme	95		72	94		80
France, Tarn	98		81	97		69
Germany, Eastern States	88	0	61	85	0	62
+Germany, Saarland	93	5	60	87	8	58
Iceland	99	0	58	99	0	49
Ireland, Southern	88		68	84		58
Italy, Ferrara	95	2	52	96	0	53
Italy, Florence	81	2	50	77	5	48
Italy, Genoa	80	3	53	78	4	53
Italy, Latina	87	9	58	82	13	62
Italy, Macerata	82	1	46	83	2	46
Italy, Modena	88	2	52	85	3	52
Italy, Parma	89	2	53	88	3	56
Italy, Ragusa	81	3	87	73	1	55
Italy, Romagna	89	2	49	88	2	49
Italy, Torino	86	4	59	82	6	59
Italy, Trieste	88	0	48	99	0	66
Italy, Varese	93	1	39	88	3	40
Italy, Veneto	91	2	50	85	4	51
+Latvia	68	4	65	66	5	60
+Malta	92	0	83	90	1	79
The Netherlands	97		62	97		63
The Netherlands, Eindhoven	98		63	97		59
The Netherlands, Maastricht	97		66	96		65
Norway	94	1	57	93	2	53
Poland, Cracow	44	22	82	51	19	85
Poland, Kielce	57	1	61	60	3	80
Poland, Lower Silesia	32	1	56	38	0	55
Poland, Warsaw City	[57]	7	53	[56]	10	58
Slovakia	77	2	61	76	1	59
Slovenia	86	4	63	82	4	63
Spain, Albacete	81	10	72	84	8	56
Spain, Asturias	90	7	71	88	8	68
Spain, Basque Country	85	8	59	79	11	57
Spain, Granada	83	8	65	78	9	61
Spain, Mallorca	91	2	75	87	6	62
Spain, Murcia	89	6	66	87	6	61
Spain, Navarra	87	8	61	83	10	53
Spain, Tarragona	90	2	63	87	4	55
Spain, Zaragoza	69	8	71	66	12	70

	MALE			FEMALE		
	MV	DCO	M/I	MV	DCO	M/I
Sweden	97		55	97		54
Switzerland, Basel	99	0	70	99	0	67
Switzerland, Geneva	97	1	48	94	2	52
Switzerland, Graubunden	88	6	61	85	10	70
Switzerland, Neuchatel	90	1	66	91	2	80
Switzerland, St Gall-Appenzell	97	1	67	95	1	69
Switzerland, Valais	94	2	75	95	3	69
Switzerland, Vaud	94	1	66	93	2	58
Switzerland, Zurich	98	0	70	97	1	71
+UK, England and Wales	[79]		67	[77]		67
UK, East Anglia			62			64
UK, Mersey	77	3	72	72	5	71
UK, North Western	74	4	70	69	5	70
UK, Oxford	78	1	59	74	1	62
UK, South Thames	70	19	68	66	21	67
UK, South Western	78	3	66	73	4	63
UK, Wessex	[78]	7	57	[73]	10	57
+UK, West Midlands		3	56		4	60
UK, Yorkshire	85	3	64	81	4	63
UK, Scotland	85	2	55	81	4	57
UK, Scotland, West	82	3	55	77	6	59
Yugoslavia, Vojvodina	48	8	61	49	8	58

OCEANIA

	MALE			FEMALE		
	MV	DCO	M/I	MV	DCO	M/I
Australian Capital Territory	96	1		93	4	
Australia, New South Wales	94	1		92	2	
South Australia	85		47	79		49
Australia, Tasmania	93		51	89		58
Australia, Victoria	92	1	56	90	2	55
Western Australia	92	3	49	90	4	52
French Polynesia	92	4		71	21	
+New Zealand: Non-Maori	91	3	51	89	3	50
+New Zealand: Maori	81	6	46	80	4	30
US, Hawaii: White	98	0	34	98	0	43
US, Hawaii: Japanese	99	0	36	99	0	33
US, Hawaii: Hawaiian	99	0	72	97	0	41
US, Hawaii: Filipino	97	0	57	98	0	48
US, Hawaii: Chinese	99	0	34	99	0	46

+ IMPORTANT-SEE NOTES ON POPULATION PAGE

[] CYTOLOGICAL VERIFICATION EXCLUDED

INDICES OF DATA QUALITY
Rectum (ICD-9 154)

AFRICA	MALE MV	MALE DCO	MALE M/I	FEMALE MV	FEMALE DCO	FEMALE M/I
Algeria, Setif	67			67		
France, La Reunion	99			99		
Mali, Bamako	42	0		38	0	
Uganda, Kyadondo	71			64		
Zimbabwe, Harare: African	68	11		79	7	
Zimbabwe, Harare: European	74	22		90	10	

AMERICA, CENTRAL AND SOUTH

	MALE MV	MALE DCO	MALE M/I	FEMALE MV	FEMALE DCO	FEMALE M/I
Argentina, Concordia	88	12	54	88	13	25
Brazil, Belem	90	7	50	80	15	48
Brazil, Goiania	85	11	37	84	12	43
Brazil, Porto Alegre	74	0	38	78	0	38
Colombia, Cali	94	2	32	87	3	36
Costa Rica	84	5	42	84	7	43
Ecuador, Quito	75	10		83	8	
Peru, Lima	84	6		83	3	
Peru, Trujillo	88	0	31	73	5	50
US, Puerto Rico	98	0	15	98	1	16
Uruguay, Montevideo	73	14	51	73	15	42

AMERICA, NORTH

	MALE MV	MALE DCO	MALE M/I	FEMALE MV	FEMALE DCO	FEMALE M/I
Canada	92	1	29	91	1	28
Canada, Alberta	97	1	25	97	1	24
Canada, British Columbia	98	1	20	97	2	22
Canada, Manitoba	91	1	31	92	1	34
Canada, New Brunswick	99	0	19	97	0	16
Canada, Newfoundland	99	0	24	99	0	21
Canada, Northwest Territories	95	5	27	85	8	38
Canada, Nova Scotia	95	2	24	95	3	20
Canada, Ontario	93	0	29	89	1	29
Canada, Prince Edward Island	95	0	24	95	2	16
+Canada, Quebec	85	0	34	85	0	32
Canada, Saskatchewan	97	1	33	97	1	29
Canada, Yukon	99	0	12	99	0	25
+US, Cent. Calif.: Non-Hisp. White	98	0	16	98	1	20
+US, Cent. Calif.: Hispanic	95	2	18	96	0	23
US, Los Angeles: Non-Hisp. White	99	0	20	98	0	24
US, Los Angeles: Hispanic White	98	0		99	1	
US, Los Angeles: Black	99	0		98	1	
US, Los Angeles: Chinese	99	0		99	0	
US, Los Angeles: Filipino	99	0		99	0	
US, Los Angeles: Korean	99	0		99	0	
US, Los Angeles: Japanese	99	0		98	0	
US, San Francisco: Non-Hisp. White	98	0	23	98	1	25
US, San Francisco: Hispanic White	99	0	17	98	1	21
US, San Francisco: Black	97	0	27	99	0	24
US, San Francisco: Chinese	99	0	24	98	1	18
US, San Francisco: Filipino	98	0	20	99	0	15
US, San Francisco: Japanese	99	0	21	99	0	26
US, Connecticut: White	98	0	18	98	1	20
US, Connecticut: Black	99	0	22	98	0	13
US, Atlanta: White	99	0	21	99	0	21
US, Atlanta: Black	99	0	26	99	0	22
US, Iowa	99	0	16	97	0	19

	MALE MV	MALE DCO	MALE M/I	FEMALE MV	FEMALE DCO	FEMALE M/I
US, Central Louisiana: White	99	0	16	95	2	11
US, Central Louisiana: Black	88	0	50	99	0	33
US, New Orleans: White	99	0	22	97	0	17
US, New Orleans: Black	98	1	27	96	2	27
US, Detroit: White	99	0	18	98	0	19
US, Detroit: Black	98	0	22	99	0	24
US, New Mexico: Non-Hisp. White	98	1	19	96	1	22
US, New Mexico: Hispanic White	97	2	19	97	0	24
US, New Mexico: American Indian	99	0	17	93	7	36
US, Utah	99	0	15	99	0	16
US, Seattle	99	0	17	97	0	19
US, SEER: White	99	0	18	98	0	20
US, SEER: Black	98	0	24	99	0	23

ASIA

	MALE MV	MALE DCO	MALE M/I	FEMALE MV	FEMALE DCO	FEMALE M/I
+China, Qidong	91	0	61	90	1	63
+China, Shanghai	68	1	62	66	1	62
China, Tianjin	74	0	49	69	0	52
Hong Kong	84	3	45	83	4	40
India, Bangalore	82	5	23	84	5	23
India, Barshi, Paranda and Bhum	87	0		80	0	
India, Bombay	78	8	41	77	7	41
India, Karunagappally	83	0		99	0	
India, Madras	78	4	45	78	2	36
India, Trivandrum	86	5	5	72	11	22
Israel: All Jews	95			93		
Jews born in Israel	94			93		
Jews born in America or Europe	94			93		
Jews born in Africa or Asia	96			94		
Non-Jews	90			94		
Japan, Hiroshima	96	2	34	95	4	34
Japan, Miyagi	88	2	41	87	4	42
Japan, Nagasaki	93	2	38	91	4	41
Japan, Osaka	79	7	49	76	9	50
+Japan, Saga	76	10	52	76	15	52
Japan, Yamagata	86	7	41	83	9	40
Korea, Kangwha	92		44	80		20
Kuwait: Non-Kuwaitis	94	3		77	0	
Kuwait: Kuwaitis	77	23		82	18	
Philippines, Manila	79	9		76	9	
Singapore: Chinese	96	2		96	2	
Singapore: Malay	99	0		88	6	
Singapore: Indian	94	0		99	0	
Thailand, Chiang Mai	84	1		90	0	
Thailand, Khon Kaen	62	0		65	0	
Viet Nam, Hanoi	53			63		

+ IMPORTANT-SEE NOTES ON POPULATION PAGE

EUROPE	MALE MV	MALE DCO	MALE M/I	FEMALE MV	FEMALE DCO	FEMALE M/I
Austria, Tyrol	91	5	47	88	7	53
+Belarus	81	0	70	79	0	69
Croatia	59	10	71	55	13	73
+Czech Republic	76	2	71	71	3	72
Denmark	96	0	54	95	0	56
Estonia	87		71	84		66
Finland	98	0	55	95	1	58
France, Bas-Rhin	98		39	98		36
France, Calvados	98		27	99		37
France, Doubs	98		34	98		35
France, Haut-Rhin	98		39	99		39
France, Herault	99		27	99		35
France, Isere	98		21	97		19
France, Somme	99		38	96		42
France, Tarn	98		26	99		28
Germany, Eastern States	94	0	67	90	0	74
+Germany, Saarland	96	3	47	94	3	45
Iceland	99	0	53	98	0	40
Ireland, Southern	91		41	92		53
Italy, Ferrara	95	2	77	95	2	57
Italy, Florence	85	1	37	84	2	38
Italy, Genoa	83	4	61	82	5	59
Italy, Latina	94	5	59	90	8	50
Italy, Macerata	83	0	37	86	0	31
Italy, Modena	92	1	43	88	2	49
Italy, Parma	93	2	41	89	2	48
Italy, Ragusa	91	0	50	85	1	58
Italy, Romagna	93	0	42	92	1	46
Italy, Torino	91	1	50	87	5	47
Italy, Trieste	78	0	41	86	1	48
Italy, Varese	98	0	41	92	2	37
Italy, Veneto	91	1	51	87	4	51
+Latvia	87	2	62	85	2	65
+Malta	88	0	43	81	3	41
The Netherlands	99		34	98		36
The Netherlands, Eindhoven	98		35	99		32
The Netherlands, Maastricht	97		32	98		38
Norway	98	0	54	97	1	51
Poland, Cracow	69	13	83	64	16	91
Poland, Kielce	64	2	86	71	5	101
Poland, Lower Silesia	39	1	78	38	1	77
Poland, Warsaw City	[79]	7	86	[72]	7	88
Slovakia	84	1	63	80	1	65
Slovenia	88	4	72	84	7	74
Spain, Albacete	90	6	31	88	9	47
Spain, Asturias	95	3	43	91	8	41
Spain, Basque Country	91	3	46	88	5	46
Spain, Granada	94	1	37	85	3	40
Spain, Mallorca	99	0	48	92	4	43
Spain, Murcia	93	2	33	92	3	36
Spain, Navarra	95	3	41	91	7	40
Spain, Tarragona	96	1	35	93	2	38
Spain, Zaragoza	84	5	47	79	5	49

	MALE MV	MALE DCO	MALE M/I	FEMALE MV	FEMALE DCO	FEMALE M/I
Sweden	99		47	98		46
Switzerland, Basel	99	0	46	99	0	44
Switzerland, Geneva	97	2	43	98	0	44
Switzerland, Graubunden	94	2	45	98	2	41
Switzerland, Neuchatel	96	0	51	92	1	46
Switzerland, St Gall-Appenzell	98	0	42	95	1	38
Switzerland, Valais	99	0	46	99	0	34
Switzerland, Vaud	97	0	35	96	1	40
Switzerland, Zurich	99	0	43	98	0	38
+UK, England and Wales	[83]		55	[81]		55
UK, East Anglia			50			50
UK, Mersey	86	2	61	83	3	59
UK, North Western	81	3	57	73	4	65
UK, Oxford	86	0	49	81	0	53
UK, South Thames	78	13	52	76	14	55
UK, South Western	86	2	50	82	2	51
UK, Wessex	[82]	5	49	[77]	8	51
+UK, West Midlands		1	53		3	52
UK, Yorkshire	92	2	56	87	2	55
UK, Scotland	90	2	58	85	3	61
UK, Scotland, West	87	3	58	80	4	62
Yugoslavia, Vojvodina	56	7	71	55	7	71

OCEANIA

	MALE MV	MALE DCO	MALE M/I	FEMALE MV	FEMALE DCO	FEMALE M/I
Australian Capital Territory	99	0		97	0	
Australia, New South Wales	97	1		95	1	
South Australia	87		48	84		47
Australia, Tasmania	96		47	97		22
Australia, Victoria	95	0	37	94	1	36
Western Australia	96	1	33	93	2	35
French Polynesia	85	12		75	8	
+New Zealand: Non-Maori	95	1	54	92	3	55
+New Zealand: Maori	91	4	49	90	2	29
US, Hawaii: White	99	0	16	97	0	23
US, Hawaii: Japanese	99	0	26	97	0	19
US, Hawaii: Hawaiian	98	0	32	97	0	32
US, Hawaii: Filipino	99	0	28	99	0	12
US, Hawaii: Chinese	97	0	20	99	0	33

+ IMPORTANT-SEE NOTES ON POPULATION PAGE

[] CYTOLOGICAL VERIFICATION EXCLUDED

INDICES OF DATA QUALITY
Liver (ICD-9 155)

AFRICA

	MALE MV	DCO	M/I	FEMALE MV	DCO	M/I
Algeria, Setif	0			12		
France, La Reunion	86			73		
Mali, Bamako	3	6		4	7	
Uganda, Kyadondo	24			43		
Zimbabwe, Harare: African	23	5		24	14	
Zimbabwe, Harare: European	29	36		25	50	

AMERICA, CENTRAL AND SOUTH

	MALE MV	DCO	M/I	FEMALE MV	DCO	M/I
Argentina, Concordia	67	33	600	0	99	650
Brazil, Belem	57	29	486	67	0	417
Brazil, Goiania	40	43	98	44	47	103
Brazil, Porto Alegre	62	2	56	57	2	53
Colombia, Cali	59	7	211	63	21	319
Costa Rica	25	38	121	26	45	129
Ecuador, Quito	29	55		17	72	
Peru, Lima	35	30		38	31	
Peru, Trujillo	30	18	109	43	31	66
US, Puerto Rico	62	17	150	44	30	225
Uruguay, Montevideo	51	35	98	48	48	85

AMERICA, NORTH

	MALE MV	DCO	M/I	FEMALE MV	DCO	M/I
Canada	62	6	104	56	9	129
Canada, Alberta	71	7	123	70	9	143
Canada, British Columbia	70	24	102	62	31	129
Canada, Manitoba	54	5	121	51	19	137
Canada, New Brunswick	69	7	149	65	15	177
Canada, Newfoundland	81	13	213	90	0	300
Canada, Northwest Territories	25	25	113	-	-	-
Canada, Nova Scotia	63	24	149	50	38	155
Canada, Ontario	59	3	96	53	3	119
Canada, Prince Edward Island	75	25	300	33	67	100
+Canada, Quebec	58	0	95	51	0	124
Canada, Saskatchewan	75	15	134	70	20	163
Canada, Yukon	-	-	ncr	99	0	100
+US, Cent. Calif.: Non-Hisp. White	83	4	102	75	5	116
+US, Cent. Calif.: Hispanic	78	3	91	83	0	88
US, Los Angeles: Non-Hisp. White	83	2	108	71	7	113
US, Los Angeles: Hispanic White	77	2		80	4	
US, Los Angeles: Black	77	5		81	4	
US, Los Angeles: Chinese	75	0		61	10	
US, Los Angeles: Filipino	88	0		75	0	
US, Los Angeles: Korean	65	4		71	4	
US, Los Angeles: Japanese	74	4		75	10	
US, San Francisco: Non-Hisp. White	80	3	101	67	5	119
US, San Francisco: Hispanic White	82	3	68	77	0	71
US, San Francisco: Black	84	1	85	70	4	115
US, San Francisco: Chinese	79	3	85	61	4	86
US, San Francisco: Filipino	93	0	71	55	0	59
US, San Francisco: Japanese	88	0	38	80	20	140
US, Connecticut: White	80	4	90	80	5	99
US, Connecticut: Black	94	3	78	70	0	120
US, Atlanta: White	85	1	87	84	4	122
US, Atlanta: Black	87	5	111	84	4	128
US, Iowa	83	2	89	75	5	117

	MALE MV	DCO	M/I	FEMALE MV	DCO	M/I
US, Central Louisiana: White	60	13	173	42	33	150
US, Central Louisiana: Black	63	13	138	50	50	300
US, New Orleans: White	77	5	111	70	6	136
US, New Orleans: Black	67	12	119	75	4	121
US, Detroit: White	79	2	98	77	5	125
US, Detroit: Black	82	0	84	76	5	91
US, New Mexico: Non-Hisp. White	63	9	88	74	5	118
US, New Mexico: Hispanic White	66	7	98	76	9	103
US, New Mexico: American Indian	70	0	83	29	0	71
US, Utah	82	4	91	76	5	121
US, Seattle	77	2	98	79	2	107
US, SEER: White	79	3	94	77	4	113
US, SEER: Black	86	1	87	76	4	107

ASIA

	MALE MV	DCO	M/I	FEMALE MV	DCO	M/I
+China, Qidong	30	0	90	30	1	89
+China, Shanghai	14	3	93	13	3	102
China, Tianjin	27	0	78	28	0	81
Hong Kong	39	19	77	41	23	74
India, Bangalore	68	20	38	53	33	55
India, Barshi, Paranda and Bhum	60	7		50	0	
India, Bombay	56	16	83	42	35	103
India, Karunagappally	78	0		67	0	
India, Madras	80	4	61	75	6	56
India, Trivandrum	65	13	26	89	11	33
Israel: All Jews	62			63		
Jews born in Israel	83			73		
Jews born in America or Europe	64			63		
Jews born in Africa or Asia	55			60		
Non-Jews	68			39		
Japan, Hiroshima	34	19	75	29	27	68
Japan, Miyagi	31	19	86	29	25	81
Japan, Nagasaki	35	23	82	28	31	84
Japan, Osaka	44	24	80	39	28	80
+Japan, Saga	22	25	80	20	27	81
Japan, Yamagata	24	24	84	17	26	80
Korea, Kangwha	22		121	24		86
Kuwait: Non-Kuwaitis	46	48		13	88	
Kuwait: Kuwaitis	37	61		38	63	
Philippines, Manila	23	48		23	52	
Singapore: Chinese	25	23		25	28	
Singapore: Malay	29	16		16	44	
Singapore: Indian	15	21		17	0	
Thailand, Chiang Mai	38	5		34	6	
Thailand, Khon Kaen	8	15		8	16	
Viet Nam, Hanoi	22			20		

+ IMPORTANT-SEE NOTES ON POPULATION PAGE

INDICES OF DATA QUALITY
Liver (ICD-9 155) (contd)

EUROPE

	MALE			FEMALE		
	MV	DCO	M/I	MV	DCO	M/I
Austria, Tyrol	63	20	105	55	28	88
+Belarus	21	2	92	21	1	84
Croatia	42	10	50	33	13	53
+Czech Republic	24	7	115	27	8	132
Denmark	89	1	57	84	1	56
Estonia	75		106	67		102
Finland	88	1	67	84	2	69
France, Bas-Rhin	72		101	68		126
France, Calvados	56		128	62		157
France, Doubs	72		142	84		103
France, Haut-Rhin	85		131	79		167
France, Herault	98		220	99		407
France, Isere	92		79	84		146
France, Somme	88		142	80		248
France, Tarn	82		234	86		293
Germany, Eastern States	75	1	68	65	2	90
+Germany, Saarland	56	24	82	54	27	98
Iceland	88	0	96	89	0	111
Ireland, Southern	79		221	55		282
Italy, Ferrara	54	9	132	29	15	135
Italy, Florence	29	11	102	25	19	117
Italy, Genoa	37	10	101	30	23	125
Italy, Latina	44	39	110	32	45	121
Italy, Macerata	31	3	111	24	5	133
Italy, Modena	32	7	97	31	9	100
Italy, Parma	37	8	101	34	9	113
Italy, Ragusa	21	3	111	10	6	167
Italy, Romagna	71	5	93	56	4	113
Italy, Torino	37	7	132	38	10	171
Italy, Trieste	99	0	93	99	0	120
Italy, Varese	61	9	88	55	8	112
Italy, Veneto	52	9	91	41	15	91
+Latvia	18	22	73	21	15	74
+Malta	75	0	138	57	14	143
The Netherlands	86		119	82		149
The Netherlands, Eindhoven	79		162	81		150
The Netherlands, Maastricht	93		102	84		132
Norway	85	5	81	77	5	92
Poland, Cracow	22	34	98	27	39	89
Poland, Kielce	25	9	150	23	14	154
Poland, Lower Silesia	53	2	98	46	5	109
Poland, Warsaw City	[31]	25	107	[24]	36	128
Slovakia	53	6	93	48	5	107
Slovenia	92	0	172	93	0	279
Spain, Albacete	30	30	107	21	37	121
Spain, Asturias	67	19	106	61	30	115
Spain, Basque Country	36	27	94	23	43	135
Spain, Granada	25	23	158	18	46	172
Spain, Mallorca	68	18	120	51	28	169
Spain, Murcia	46	24	132	47	32	192
Spain, Navarra	42	31	110	27	46	118
Spain, Tarragona	66	13	138	55	25	186
Spain, Zaragoza	30	36	144	18	46	156

	MALE			FEMALE		
	MV	DCO	M/I	MV	DCO	M/I
Sweden	99		125	99		152
Switzerland, Basel	99	0	97	93	0	146
Switzerland, Geneva	76	3	64	72	7	117
Switzerland, Graubunden	52	14	86	63	6	81
Switzerland, Neuchatel	73	4	98	38	25	163
Switzerland, St Gall-Appenzell	83	2	80	87	3	106
Switzerland, Valais	65	1	87	63	0	95
Switzerland, Vaud	70	3	106	64	9	130
Switzerland, Zurich	91	0	80	92	0	89
+UK, England and Wales	[71]		106	[71]		117
UK, East Anglia			162			256
UK, Mersey	55	4	99	53	7	126
UK, North Western	49	10	95	36	10	107
UK, Oxford	85	1	112	77	1	130
UK, South Thames	36	38	102	33	43	107
UK, South Western	41	25	110	44	17	130
UK, Wessex	[86]	2	81	[87]	0	91
+UK, West Midlands		6	127		9	193
UK, Yorkshire	54	7	117	45	15	115
UK, Scotland	57	7	87	52	7	105
UK, Scotland, West	54	8	98	49	9	111
Yugoslavia, Vojvodina	17	17	102	18	21	100

OCEANIA

	MALE			FEMALE		
	MV	DCO	M/I	MV	DCO	M/I
Australian Capital Territory	99	0		99	0	
Australia, New South Wales	83	4		83	5	
South Australia	60		91	59		84
Australia, Tasmania	69		131	67		333
Australia, Victoria	72	4	112	74	3	166
Western Australia	62	8	94	68	12	116
French Polynesia	32	59		42	42	
+New Zealand: Non-Maori	68	8	88	64	13	91
+New Zealand: Maori	70	11	74	71	12	65
US, Hawaii: White	76	0	73	86	0	100
US, Hawaii: Japanese	56	0	97	56	0	115
US, Hawaii: Hawaiian	68	0	112	64	0	73
US, Hawaii: Filipino	59	0	84	56	0	111
US, Hawaii: Chinese	85	0	70	44	0	89

+ IMPORTANT-SEE NOTES ON POPULATION PAGE

[] CYTOLOGICAL VERIFICATION EXCLUDED

INDICES OF DATA QUALITY
Gallbladder etc. (ICD-9 156)

	MALE			FEMALE		
AFRICA	MV	DCO	M/I	MV	DCO	M/I
Algeria, Setif	73			84		
France, La Reunion	85			92		
Mali, Bamako	99	0		-	-	
Uganda, Kyadondo	-			-		
Zimbabwe, Harare: African	67	0		50	0	
Zimbabwe, Harare: European	-	-	-	-	-	-

AMERICA, CENTRAL AND SOUTH	MV	DCO	M/I	MV	DCO	M/I
Argentina, Concordia	91	9	27	82	18	124
Brazil, Belem	7	36	93	26	32	76
Brazil, Goiania	50	28	72	67	28	54
Brazil, Porto Alegre	52	0	67	54	0	70
Colombia, Cali	62	0	74	68	7	66
Costa Rica	38	23	69	54	18	79
Ecuador, Quito	46	24		57	29	
Peru, Lima	51	15		58	16	
Peru, Trujillo	44	19	63	65	7	85
US, Puerto Rico	86	3	50	89	3	42
Uruguay, Montevideo	29	41	87	33	40	79

AMERICA, NORTH	MV	DCO	M/I	MV	DCO	M/I
Canada	70	4	64	73	4	68
Canada, Alberta	81	5	70	81	3	72
Canada, British Columbia	83	11	64	81	16	75
Canada, Manitoba	58	6	60	63	3	52
Canada, New Brunswick	66	7	83	87	0	69
Canada, Newfoundland	89	0	89	98	0	98
Canada, Northwest Territories	40	20	60	80	0	80
Canada, Nova Scotia	81	7	71	81	8	60
Canada, Ontario	68	3	60	68	3	63
Canada, Prince Edward Island	99	0	40	70	10	60
+Canada, Quebec	65	0	62	70	0	73
Canada, Saskatchewan	64	8	79	78	6	68
Canada, Yukon	99	0	67	99	0	150
+US, Cent. Calif.: Non-Hisp. White	89	0	57	85	2	57
+US, Cent. Calif.: Hispanic	87	7	53	98	0	64
US, Los Angeles: Non-Hisp. White	88	2	61	88	1	63
US, Los Angeles: Hispanic White	92	0		94	0	
US, Los Angeles: Black	88	0		82	0	
US, Los Angeles: Chinese	92	0		83	0	
US, Los Angeles: Filipino	99	0		99	0	
US, Los Angeles: Korean	99	0		88	0	
US, Los Angeles: Japanese	92	0		90	0	
US, San Francisco: Non-Hisp. White	91	1	63	86	3	72
US, San Francisco: Hispanic White	72	0	56	91	0	68
US, San Francisco: Black	99	0	45	79	7	93
US, San Francisco: Chinese	96	0	43	87	4	57
US, San Francisco: Filipino	90	0	40	99	0	23
US, San Francisco: Japanese	99	0	75	99	0	25
US, Connecticut: White	91	1	46	88	3	63
US, Connecticut: Black	85	0	46	82	0	36
US, Atlanta: White	92	0	43	89	0	47
US, Atlanta: Black	99	0	38	91	0	48
US, Iowa	88	3	57	91	1	65

	MALE			FEMALE		
	MV	DCO	M/I	MV	DCO	M/I
US, Central Louisiana: White	73	0	73	99	0	63
US, Central Louisiana: Black	99	0	33	99	0	33
US, New Orleans: White	92	0	59	82	2	69
US, New Orleans: Black	70	0	110	79	4	71
US, Detroit: White	94	0	53	95	1	60
US, Detroit: Black	90	0	39	89	2	60
US, New Mexico: Non-Hisp. White	74	6	90	87	2	67
US, New Mexico: Hispanic White	87	9	78	92	1	64
US, New Mexico: American Indian	82	0	64	91	0	63
US, Utah	97	0	65	96	0	65
US, Seattle	83	0	47	82	0	53
US, SEER: White	89	1	55	90	1	62
US, SEER: Black	94	0	41	86	2	58

ASIA	MV	DCO	M/I	MV	DCO	M/I
+China, Qidong	76	0	71	81	0	84
+China, Shanghai	32	3	78	41	1	74
China, Tianjin	44	1	67	47	0	63
Hong Kong	61	13	61	65	11	67
India, Bangalore	78	14	39	73	12	29
India, Barshi, Paranda and Bhum	0	99		0	50	
India, Bombay	57	8	53	54	12	58
India, Karunagappally	-	-		-	-	
India, Madras	63	6	54	54	4	62
India, Trivandrum	99	0	50	99	0	0
Israel: All Jews	62			75		
Jews born in Israel	79			64		
Jews born in America or Europe	60			75		
Jews born in Africa or Asia	63			80		
Non-Jews	73			76		
Japan, Hiroshima	63	17	72	60	14	73
Japan, Miyagi	58	10	81	55	16	82
Japan, Nagasaki	55	22	95	50	25	94
Japan, Osaka	52	22	90	50	24	87
+Japan, Saga	41	27	83	41	24	86
Japan, Yamagata	44	23	91	41	24	87
Korea, Kangwha	46		69	31		69
Kuwait: Non-Kuwaitis	64	27		36	55	
Kuwait: Kuwaitis	30	70		43	57	
Philippines, Manila	52	15		63	20	
Singapore: Chinese	84	3		88	6	
Singapore: Malay	75	8		85	0	
Singapore: Indian	63	13		99	0	
Thailand, Chiang Mai	45	2		59	2	
Thailand, Khon Kaen	39	12		49	6	
Viet Nam, Hanoi	38			67		

+ IMPORTANT-SEE NOTES ON POPULATION PAGE

INDICES OF DATA QUALITY
Gallbladder etc. (ICD-9 156) (contd)

EUROPE	MALE			FEMALE		
	MV	DCO	M/I	MV	DCO	M/I
Austria, Tyrol	77	15	77	75	19	81
+Belarus	44	1	84	55	1	84
Croatia	43	8	75	46	13	83
+Czech Republic	40	4	89	46	4	91
Denmark	76	1	79	83	1	85
Estonia	73		82	83		88
Finland	84	1	69	87	1	70
France, Bas-Rhin	84		95	90		102
France, Calvados	70		85	75		92
France, Doubs	80		110	89		114
France, Haut-Rhin	98		127	94		89
France, Herault	98		126	99		120
France, Isere	89		72	95		75
France, Somme	92		83	84		102
France, Tarn	89		106	93		102
Germany, Eastern States	79	1	83	83	1	83
+Germany, Saarland	61	16	77	64	16	88
Iceland	92	0	58	99	0	69
Ireland, Southern	76		74	83		61
Italy, Ferrara	68	4	96	63	3	89
Italy, Florence	61	3	71	56	6	76
Italy, Genoa	62	8	71	61	7	73
Italy, Latina	71	14	60	61	16	71
Italy, Macerata	50	6	81	67	0	167
Italy, Modena	59	5	80	53	2	81
Italy, Parma	49	7	60	61	7	71
Italy, Ragusa	55	0	61	44	5	72
Italy, Romagna	67	6	71	70	3	68
Italy, Torino	58	4	69	57	5	80
Italy, Trieste	77	7	57	80	3	55
Italy, Varese	58	7	68	70	1	69
Italy, Veneto	71	5	80	68	8	84
+Latvia	48	8	85	49	10	76
+Malta	50	0	100	57	0	71
The Netherlands	78		71	77		82
The Netherlands, Eindhoven	77		87	82		98
The Netherlands, Maastricht	74		77	83		88
Norway	84	2	77	83	4	84
Poland, Cracow	35	17	90	38	22	94
Poland, Kielce	41	1	83	50	5	98
Poland, Lower Silesia	35	1	76	36	1	75
Poland, Warsaw City	[43]	9	75	[47]	9	79
Slovakia	65	5	66	73	3	71
Slovenia	71	5	84	77	6	92
Spain, Albacete	23	15	85	38	16	75
Spain, Asturias	78	12	59	73	16	87
Spain, Basque Country	62	11	62	61	14	73
Spain, Granada	65	2	52	66	8	63
Spain, Mallorca	65	4	46	71	4	64
Spain, Murcia	64	13	60	70	10	69
Spain, Navarra	74	13	82	65	16	72
Spain, Tarragona	56	9	67	72	5	60
Spain, Zaragoza	55	5	56	58	15	71

	MALE			FEMALE		
	MV	DCO	M/I	MV	DCO	M/I
Sweden	91		97	92		103
Switzerland, Basel	96	0	125	98	0	135
Switzerland, Geneva	89	0	78	82	2	48
Switzerland, Graubunden	40	30	120	77	9	109
Switzerland, Neuchatel	82	0	82	91	0	100
Switzerland, St Gall-Appenzell	74	0	94	82	2	86
Switzerland, Valais	50	10	60	86	0	96
Switzerland, Vaud	77	0	81	83	5	81
Switzerland, Zurich	84	0	66	85	0	80
+UK, England and Wales	[64]		59	[65]		71
UK, East Anglia			38			58
UK, Mersey	59	2	61	57	7	74
UK, North Western	49	5	71	46	6	79
UK, Oxford	63	1	64	61	3	73
UK, South Thames	48	23	65	46	20	68
UK, South Western	59	8	63	56	8	67
UK, Wessex	[76]	9	56	[68]	11	66
+UK, West Midlands		4	44		6	58
UK, Yorkshire	57	6	57	63	3	73
UK, Scotland	63	4	53	69	3	65
UK, Scotland, West	58	5	52	64	5	66
Yugoslavia, Vojvodina	45	10	74	50	10	78

OCEANIA

	MALE			FEMALE		
	MV	DCO	M/I	MV	DCO	M/I
Australian Capital Territory	89	0		69	0	
Australia, New South Wales	84	2		85	3	
South Australia	63		99	64		81
Australia, Tasmania	71		75	87		79
Australia, Victoria	72	2	51	73	2	62
Western Australia	70	7	61	75	2	63
French Polynesia	89	11		80	20	
+New Zealand: Non-Maori	77	2	74	80	3	92
+New Zealand: Maori	88	0	63	99	0	83
US, Hawaii: White	77	0	54	86	0	43
US, Hawaii: Japanese	91	0	45	95	0	55
US, Hawaii: Hawaiian	86	0	114	99	0	117
US, Hawaii: Filipino	77	0	46	99	0	50
US, Hawaii: Chinese	88	0	50	90	0	70

+ IMPORTANT-SEE NOTES ON POPULATION PAGE

[] CYTOLOGICAL VERIFICATION EXCLUDED

INDICES OF DATA QUALITY
Pancreas (ICD-9 157)

AFRICA

	MALE MV	DCO	M/I	FEMALE MV	DCO	M/I
Algeria, Setif	0			50		
France, La Reunion	83		210	76		228
Mali, Bamako	35	0		50	0	
Uganda, Kyadondo	0			0		
Zimbabwe, Harare: African	26	23		22	30	
Zimbabwe, Harare: European	20	40		25	75	

AMERICA, CENTRAL AND SOUTH

	MALE MV	DCO	M/I	FEMALE MV	DCO	M/I
Argentina, Concordia	50	50	73	14	81	143
Brazil, Belem	15	31	63	26	35	100
Brazil, Goiania	44	42	81	43	36	70
Brazil, Porto Alegre	34	2	90	45	1	79
Colombia, Cali	49	7	98	42	19	111
Costa Rica	20	27	109	16	30	98
Ecuador, Quito	13	44		30	46	
Peru, Lima	39	18		34	19	
Peru, Trujillo	38	14	81	14	21	107
US, Puerto Rico	58	13	94	54	17	95
Uruguay, Montevideo	19	50	96	18	50	96

AMERICA, NORTH

	MALE MV	DCO	M/I	FEMALE MV	DCO	M/I
Canada	50	8	100	47	9	98
Canada, Alberta	59	10	96	55	9	96
Canada, British Columbia	62	29	101	61	32	103
Canada, Manitoba	35	8	95	34	6	95
Canada, New Brunswick	53	6	107	57	8	99
Canada, Newfoundland	70	3	166	72	7	131
Canada, Northwest Territories	60	0	140	63	0	88
Canada, Nova Scotia	51	25	98	43	27	104
Canada, Ontario	48	4	99	45	6	95
Canada, Prince Edward Island	50	4	96	50	13	105
+Canada, Quebec	45	0	100	42	0	100
Canada, Saskatchewan	62	7	92	57	11	100
Canada, Yukon	99	0	125	99	0	133
+US, Cent. Calif.: Non-Hisp. White	81	4	101	74	2	96
+US, Cent. Calif.: Hispanic	76	1	99	73	2	98
US, Los Angeles: Non-Hisp. White	77	3	95	72	4	99
US, Los Angeles: Hispanic White	81	3		80	4	
US, Los Angeles: Black	81	3		73	4	
US, Los Angeles: Chinese	92	0		74	5	
US, Los Angeles: Filipino	96	0		88	0	
US, Los Angeles: Korean	79	0		95	0	
US, Los Angeles: Japanese	87	5		78	5	
US, San Francisco: Non-Hisp. White	76	3	94	73	5	96
US, San Francisco: Hispanic White	82	0	75	75	1	64
US, San Francisco: Black	76	1	100	70	3	87
US, San Francisco: Chinese	67	2	86	71	0	104
US, San Francisco: Filipino	89	0	56	93	0	44
US, San Francisco: Japanese	64	9	91	67	0	100
US, Connecticut: White	79	4	94	69	8	92
US, Connecticut: Black	86	2	102	77	5	88
US, Atlanta: White	81	1	88	69	5	98
US, Atlanta: Black	79	1	85	78	2	94
US, Iowa	80	2	94	74	3	94

	MALE MV	DCO	M/I	FEMALE MV	DCO	M/I
US, Central Louisiana: White	62	14	103	68	1	99
US, Central Louisiana: Black	42	8	89	59	5	114
US, New Orleans: White	75	2	92	63	5	97
US, New Orleans: Black	79	7	117	60	5	92
US, Detroit: White	80	2	87	77	2	91
US, Detroit: Black	82	1	83	81	1	86
US, New Mexico: Non-Hisp. White	75	7	101	71	6	94
US, New Mexico: Hispanic White	70	4	104	70	2	94
US, New Mexico: American Indian	50	0	88	61	6	89
US, Utah	71	1	99	65	1	91
US, Seattle	78	1	95	70	1	92
US, SEER: White	78	2	93	72	4	93
US, SEER: Black	80	1	89	77	2	90

ASIA

	MALE MV	DCO	M/I	FEMALE MV	DCO	M/I
+China, Qidong	79	1	92	75	1	90
+China, Shanghai	17	3	88	20	2	95
China, Tianjin	38	0	73	41	0	80
Hong Kong	39	21	102	39	24	104
India, Bangalore	38	21	47	54	17	46
India, Barshi, Paranda and Bhum	25	0		0	0	
India, Bombay	34	14	84	33	20	88
India, Karunagappally	43	0		99	0	
India, Madras	45	3	52	42	7	44
India, Trivandrum	53	18	18	63	0	25
Israel: All Jews	37			32		
Jews born in Israel	36			62		
Jews born in America or Europe	35			29		
Jews born in Africa or Asia	40			33		
Non-Jews	28			48		
Japan, Hiroshima	56	18	88	44	26	89
Japan, Miyagi	44	14	93	39	21	95
Japan, Nagasaki	44	23	98	39	29	102
Japan, Osaka	46	24	92	41	30	91
+Japan, Saga	32	26	89	26	30	94
Japan, Yamagata	34	24	101	32	24	95
Korea, Kangwha	10		95	45		73
Kuwait: Non-Kuwaitis	43	51		17	67	
Kuwait: Kuwaitis	31	62		27	73	
Philippines, Manila	29	33		32	34	
Singapore: Chinese	43	12		47	19	
Singapore: Malay	15	15		25	25	
Singapore: Indian	44	22		50	0	
Thailand, Chiang Mai	35	0		36	1	
Thailand, Khon Kaen	24	10		19	6	
Viet Nam, Hanoi	34			10		

+ IMPORTANT-SEE NOTES ON POPULATION PAGE

EUROPE	MALE MV	DCO	M/I	FEMALE MV	DCO	M/I
Austria, Tyrol	64	16	99	68	20	100
+Belarus	29	1	87	26	1	83
Croatia	40	11	84	35	16	89
+Czech Republic	21	4	100	22	5	102
Denmark	76	1	110	73	1	108
Estonia	58		95	51		95
Finland	79	1	96	72	2	96
France, Bas-Rhin	71		165	69		157
France, Calvados	50		134	56		152
France, Doubs	77		160	76		224
France, Haut-Rhin	66		151	80		173
France, Herault	89		261	83		296
France, Isere	75		115	70		96
France, Somme	64		199	53		200
France, Tarn	61		200	56		253
Germany, Eastern States	71	0	94	68	1	96
+Germany, Saarland	55	23	106	43	26	110
Iceland	85	0	118	77	0	113
Ireland, Southern	54		116	45		117
Italy, Ferrara	40	8	109	37	7	99
Italy, Florence	37	5	104	27	10	87
Italy, Genoa	39	7	90	36	8	93
Italy, Latina	66	15	106	47	26	97
Italy, Macerata	35	0	83	32	0	88
Italy, Modena	27	6	95	30	8	102
Italy, Parma	36	6	110	27	6	92
Italy, Ragusa	22	1	95	29	2	108
Italy, Romagna	49	2	108	37	3	106
Italy, Torino	35	7	100	33	9	107
Italy, Trieste	69	8	61	75	1	76
Italy, Varese	58	5	99	47	6	98
Italy, Veneto	53	6	103	43	9	95
+Latvia	22	9	82	17	11	80
+Malta	21	6	123	38	0	114
The Netherlands	67		119	62		130
The Netherlands, Eindhoven	67		131	69		145
The Netherlands, Maastricht	74		117	66		120
Norway	69	4	99	64	6	99
Poland, Cracow	26	30	99	19	24	95
Poland, Kielce	33	4	113	26	7	113
Poland, Lower Silesia	36	2	86	39	2	90
Poland, Warsaw City	[38]	10	93	[34]	10	95
Slovakia	46	5	86	47	3	89
Slovenia	60	5	99	55	7	100
Spain, Albacete	24	24	120	30	15	90
Spain, Asturias	49	28	131	40	34	130
Spain, Basque Country	35	21	96	30	25	91
Spain, Granada	33	13	104	39	15	92
Spain, Mallorca	53	11	100	40	13	99
Spain, Murcia	42	21	104	38	15	120
Spain, Navarra	48	16	92	27	23	93
Spain, Tarragona	38	8	99	41	14	120
Spain, Zaragoza	38	16	115	27	25	105

	MALE MV	DCO	M/I	FEMALE MV	DCO	M/I
Sweden	86		118	83		121
Switzerland, Basel	94	0	124	94	0	149
Switzerland, Geneva	82	2	97	72	9	90
Switzerland, Graubunden	35	30	75	49	24	110
Switzerland, Neuchatel	70	0	106	52	21	112
Switzerland, St Gall-Appenzell	73	4	96	72	4	92
Switzerland, Valais	63	2	110	47	7	110
Switzerland, Vaud	69	3	94	60	6	96
Switzerland, Zurich	78	0	110	72	0	95
+UK, England and Wales	[55]		98	[54]		98
UK, East Anglia			101			96
UK, Mersey	30	5	107	25	7	105
UK, North Western	26	8	101	24	8	99
UK, Oxford	36	1	93	29	1	94
UK, South Thames	32	28	90	28	31	92
UK, South Western	37	7	100	36	8	98
UK, Wessex	[67]	17	100	[64]	18	98
+UK, West Midlands		7	95		9	97
UK, Yorkshire	36	8	99	33	10	100
UK, Scotland	40	8	96	38	9	99
UK, Scotland, West	32	10	94	32	10	99
Yugoslavia, Vojvodina	22	18	93	25	16	90

OCEANIA

	MALE MV	DCO	M/I	FEMALE MV	DCO	M/I
Australian Capital Territory	56	3		71	0	
Australia, New South Wales	61	6		57	6	
South Australia	56		101	49		100
Australia, Tasmania	55		84	52		93
Australia, Victoria	52	3	99	47	6	104
Western Australia	60	11	104	54	12	98
French Polynesia	46	38		33	56	
+New Zealand: Non-Maori	61	7	95	55	10	93
+New Zealand: Maori	55	8	63	69	3	66
US, Hawaii: White	86	0	103	75	2	105
US, Hawaii: Japanese	90	0	94	81	0	95
US, Hawaii: Hawaiian	67	0	112	75	0	97
US, Hawaii: Filipino	63	0	115	99	0	94
US, Hawaii: Chinese	55	0	120	76	0	94

+ IMPORTANT-SEE NOTES ON POPULATION PAGE

[] CYTOLOGICAL VERIFICATION EXCLUDED

INDICES OF DATA QUALITY
Nose, sinuses etc. (ICD-9 160)

AFRICA	MALE MV	MALE DCO	MALE M/I	FEMALE MV	FEMALE DCO	FEMALE M/I
Algeria, Setif	99			99		
France, La Reunion	99			99		
Mali, Bamako	0	0		0	0	
Uganda, Kyadondo	43			83		
Zimbabwe, Harare: African	88	0		80	0	
Zimbabwe, Harare: European	99	0		99	0	

AMERICA, CENTRAL AND SOUTH	MALE MV	MALE DCO	MALE M/I	FEMALE MV	FEMALE DCO	FEMALE M/I
Argentina, Concordia	75	25	25	99	0	0
Brazil, Belem	99	0	14	67	33	100
Brazil, Goiania	99	0	44	80	0	40
Brazil, Porto Alegre	80	0	20	50	0	33
Colombia, Cali	92	0	31	79	8	33
Costa Rica	83	9	26	89	11	78
Ecuador, Quito	89	0		88	13	
Peru, Lima	86	3		90	5	
Peru, Trujillo	99	0	50	99	0	0
US, Puerto Rico	99	0	12	93	3	7
Uruguay, Montevideo	72	11	50	80	7	73

AMERICA, NORTH	MALE MV	MALE DCO	MALE M/I	FEMALE MV	FEMALE DCO	FEMALE M/I
Canada	89	1	32	89	1	31
Canada, Alberta	99	0	33	99	0	38
Canada, British Columbia	98	2	22	98	2	16
Canada, Manitoba	90	0	50	80	0	50
Canada, New Brunswick	93	0	27	99	0	30
Canada, Newfoundland	99	0	25	99	0	29
Canada, Northwest Territories	99	0	100	-	-	-
Canada, Nova Scotia	99	0	21	99	0	33
Canada, Ontario	90	1	31	87	3	29
Canada, Prince Edward Island	99	0	33	-	-	-
+Canada, Quebec	72	0	45	79	0	36
Canada, Saskatchewan	96	0	17	99	0	50
Canada, Yukon	-	-	-	-	-	-
+US, Cent. Calif.: Non-Hisp. White	97	3	32	96	0	38
+US, Cent. Calif.: Hispanic	99	0	25	-	-	ncr
US, Los Angeles: Non-Hisp. White	96	3	43	95	3	32
US, Los Angeles: Hispanic White	96	4		99	0	
US, Los Angeles: Black	99	0		99	0	
US, Los Angeles: Chinese	99	0		99	0	
US, Los Angeles: Filipino	99	0		99	0	
US, Los Angeles: Korean	-	-		99	0	
US, Los Angeles: Japanese	99	0		-	-	
US, San Francisco: Non-Hisp. White	99	0	26	96	4	39
US, San Francisco: Hispanic White	99	0	0	99	0	14
US, San Francisco: Black	99	0	33	99	0	100
US, San Francisco: Chinese	99	0	29	99	0	0
US, San Francisco: Filipino	99	0	0	99	0	33
US, San Francisco: Japanese	99	0	0	-	-	-
US, Connecticut: White	93	2	36	94	2	34
US, Connecticut: Black	99	0	67	99	0	60
US, Atlanta: White	99	0	19	99	0	7
US, Atlanta: Black	99	0	50	99	0	50
US, Iowa	98	2	45	93	4	20

	MALE MV	MALE DCO	MALE M/I	FEMALE MV	FEMALE DCO	FEMALE M/I
US, Central Louisiana: White	99	0	0	99	0	50
US, Central Louisiana: Black	99	0	100	99	0	0
US, New Orleans: White	92	0	25	75	0	25
US, New Orleans: Black	99	0	42	99	0	22
US, Detroit: White	99	0	39	93	2	43
US, Detroit: Black	99	0	75	99	0	29
US, New Mexico: Non-Hisp. White	99	0	47	99	0	26
US, New Mexico: Hispanic White	99	0	33	99	0	25
US, New Mexico: American Indian	99	0	200	99	0	0
US, Utah	99	0	47	99	0	26
US, Seattle	98	0	23	97	0	31
US, SEER: White	98	1	34	96	2	30
US, SEER: Black	99	0	48	99	0	44

ASIA	MALE MV	MALE DCO	MALE M/I	FEMALE MV	FEMALE DCO	FEMALE M/I
+China, Qidong	80	0	90	99	0	43
+China, Shanghai	72	2	26	83	1	50
China, Tianjin	78	0	38	75	0	47
Hong Kong	79	3	31	75	1	31
India, Bangalore	96	0	6	97	0	10
India, Barshi, Paranda and Bhum	99	0		99	0	
India, Bombay	82	3	29	81	9	33
India, Karunagappally	99	0		99	0	
India, Madras	78	3	43	73	2	36
India, Trivandrum	83	0	0	99	0	20
Israel: All Jews	97			89		
Jews born in Israel	99			99		
Jews born in America or Europe	94			87		
Jews born in Africa or Asia	99			88		
Non-Jews	99			99		
Japan, Hiroshima	97	0	25	93	7	64
Japan, Miyagi	94	3	52	77	10	47
Japan, Nagasaki	87	6	70	91	6	44
Japan, Osaka	83	9	69	68	21	60
+Japan, Saga	79	9	84	71	19	76
Japan, Yamagata	67	25	91	83	17	61
Korea, Kangwha	-		-	99		0
Kuwait: Non-Kuwaitis	99	0		99	0	
Kuwait: Kuwaitis	-	-		99	0	
Philippines, Manila	84	3		86	3	
Singapore: Chinese	95	2		99	0	
Singapore: Malay	99	0		99	0	
Singapore: Indian	75	25		99	0	
Thailand, Chiang Mai	94	0		95	0	
Thailand, Khon Kaen	91	0		89	0	
Viet Nam, Hanoi	50			67		

+ IMPORTANT-SEE NOTES ON POPULATION PAGE

EUROPE	MALE MV	DCO	M/I	FEMALE MV	DCO	M/I
Austria, Tyrol	99	0	20	99	0	56
+Belarus	92	0	60	90	0	66
Croatia	63	0	24	47	5	29
+Czech Republic	96	0	79	94	0	69
Denmark	99	0	43	97	0	37
Estonia	87		73	93		75
Finland	98	0	49	99	0	47
France, Bas-Rhin	99		807	99		200
France, Calvados	93		526	99		200
France, Doubs	93		464	67		167
France, Haut-Rhin	97		363	99		300
France, Herault	99		197	99		72
France, Isere	97		164	99		77
France, Somme	99		440	99		55
France, Tarn	99		233	83		67
Germany, Eastern States	96	0	41	99	1	63
+Germany, Saarland	95	0	42	73	18	55
Iceland	99	0	40	99	0	50
Ireland, Southern	80		40	99		50
Italy, Ferrara	99	0	20	0	0	100
Italy, Florence	82	0	24	86	0	57
Italy, Genoa	96	0	15	84	5	47
Italy, Latina	99	0	40	99	0	200
Italy, Macerata	83	0	17	-	-	-
Italy, Modena	99	0	75	99	0	40
Italy, Parma	92	0	54	99	0	13
Italy, Ragusa	99	0	33	99	0	400
Italy, Romagna	70	0	30	88	13	75
Italy, Torino	99	0	33	78	0	33
Italy, Trieste	67	0	44	40	0	80
Italy, Varese	99	0	22	99	0	38
Italy, Veneto	87	5	49	83	0	167
+Latvia	89	2	53	84	3	47
+Malta	99	0	25	99	0	0
The Netherlands	99		26	99		24
The Netherlands, Eindhoven	96		13	99		0
The Netherlands, Maastricht	99		17	99		25
Norway	99	0	56	99	1	57
Poland, Cracow	99	0	163	99	0	40
Poland, Kielce	89	0	47	86	0	50
Poland, Lower Silesia	69	0	44	75	0	61
Poland, Warsaw City	[86]	11	43	[77]	0	69
Slovakia	89	1	74	88	2	61
Slovenia	99	0	63	90	6	39
Spain, Albacete	-	-	ncr	99	0	100
Spain, Asturias	95	5	24	96	4	17
Spain, Basque Country	98	2	22	86	14	29
Spain, Granada	99	0	5	80	0	60
Spain, Mallorca	99	0	40	75	0	50
Spain, Murcia	85	15	46	99	0	9
Spain, Navarra	90	10	30	99	0	17
Spain, Tarragona	99	0	25	99	0	50
Spain, Zaragoza	99	0	21	73	9	18

	MALE MV	DCO	M/I	FEMALE MV	DCO	M/I
Sweden	99		27	99		31
Switzerland, Basel	99	0	86	99	0	40
Switzerland, Geneva	99	0	70	99	0	11
Switzerland, Graubunden	99	0	0	99	0	200
Switzerland, Neuchatel	99	0	75	99	0	0
Switzerland, St Gall-Appenzell	93	7	47	99	0	50
Switzerland, Valais	99	0	67	99	0	17
Switzerland, Vaud	99	0	80	99	0	33
Switzerland, Zurich	99	0	61	99	0	150
+UK, England and Wales	[89]		41	[86]		46
UK, East Anglia			46			23
UK, Mersey	98	0	54	96	0	40
UK, North Western	92	0	48	85	1	42
UK, Oxford	89	0	45	86	0	14
UK, South Thames	83	7	43	85	8	43
UK, South Western	84	2	47	81	6	35
UK, Wessex	[68]	6	43	[84]	4	45
+UK, West Midlands		0	54		3	37
UK, Yorkshire	96	0	33	89	0	44
UK, Scotland	94	0	36	89	1	44
UK, Scotland, West	98	0	40	89	3	43
Yugoslavia, Vojvodina	79	0	58	67	10	81

OCEANIA

	MALE MV	DCO	M/I	FEMALE MV	DCO	M/I
Australian Capital Territory	99	0		99	0	
Australia, New South Wales	96	2		98	2	
South Australia	99		60	92		83
Australia, Tasmania	99		34	99		50
Australia, Victoria	98	0	50	84	2	44
Western Australia	99	0	28	92	0	50
French Polynesia	67	17		99	0	
+New Zealand: Non-Maori	95	4	41	94	2	39
+New Zealand: Maori	99	0	200	-	-	-
US, Hawaii: White	99	0	33	99	0	40
US, Hawaii: Japanese	91	0	91	99	0	40
US, Hawaii: Hawaiian	99	0	0	99	0	33
US, Hawaii: Filipino	99	0	0	99	0	0
US, Hawaii: Chinese	99	0	300	99	0	0

+ IMPORTANT-SEE NOTES ON POPULATION PAGE

[] CYTOLOGICAL VERIFICATION EXCLUDED

INDICES OF DATA QUALITY
Larynx (ICD-9 161)

	MALE			FEMALE		
AFRICA	MV	DCO	M/I	MV	DCO	M/I
Algeria, Setif	82			0		
France, La Reunion	99		93	99		125
Mali, Bamako	0	0		0	0	
Uganda, Kyadondo	83			86		
Zimbabwe, Harare: African	70	9		50	50	
Zimbabwe, Harare: European	99	0		99	0	

AMERICA, CENTRAL AND SOUTH

	MV	DCO	M/I	MV	DCO	M/I
Argentina, Concordia	88	13	67	83	17	33
Brazil, Belem	82	9	53	88	13	25
Brazil, Goiania	92	4	31	99	0	43
Brazil, Porto Alegre	76	1	52	79	0	39
Colombia, Cali	84	3	52	83	3	72
Costa Rica	78	12	72	71	10	94
Ecuador, Quito	71	17		33	50	
Peru, Lima	84	5		89	5	
Peru, Trujillo	63	0	113	50	50	100
US, Puerto Rico	94	5	69	92	6	57
Uruguay, Montevideo	69	15	56	91	9	25

AMERICA, NORTH

	MV	DCO	M/I	MV	DCO	M/I
Canada	93	1	41	91	1	38
Canada, Alberta	99	1	32	99	0	40
Canada, British Columbia	97	2	33	98	1	32
Canada, Manitoba	88	1	44	97	0	33
Canada, New Brunswick	97	3	25	95	0	58
Canada, Newfoundland	99	0	35	99	0	100
Canada, Northwest Territories	75	0	25	99	0	0
Canada, Nova Scotia	95	3	32	97	3	47
Canada, Ontario	96	1	42	91	2	38
Canada, Prince Edward Island	99	0	38	99	0	0
+Canada, Quebec	87	0	45	87	0	35
Canada, Saskatchewan	97	0	53	95	5	55
Canada, Yukon	99	0	25	-	-	-
+US, Cent. Calif.: Non-Hisp. White	96	1	33	96	1	43
+US, Cent. Calif.: Hispanic	99	0	23	99	0	0
US, Los Angeles: Non-Hisp. White	99	0	30	98	1	41
US, Los Angeles: Hispanic White	99	0		95	0	
US, Los Angeles: Black	99	1		98	2	
US, Los Angeles: Chinese	99	0		99	0	
US, Los Angeles: Filipino	99	0		99	0	
US, Los Angeles: Korean	99	0		99	0	
US, Los Angeles: Japanese	99	0		99	0	
US, San Francisco: Non-Hisp. White	98	1	27	99	1	30
US, San Francisco: Hispanic White	99	0	7	99	0	14
US, San Francisco: Black	97	1	42	99	0	32
US, San Francisco: Chinese	99	0	31	99	0	0
US, San Francisco: Filipino	83	0	17	99	0	0
US, San Francisco: Japanese	99	0	25	99	0	0
US, Connecticut: White	99	0	27	96	1	28
US, Connecticut: Black	99	0	43	99	0	67
US, Atlanta: White	98	1	24	99	1	43
US, Atlanta: Black	97	1	46	97	3	45
US, Iowa	98	1	30	98	1	26

	MALE			FEMALE		
	MV	DCO	M/I	MV	DCO	M/I
US, Central Louisiana: White	97	3	33	88	0	18
US, Central Louisiana: Black	91	0	55	99	0	33
US, New Orleans: White	97	2	32	99	0	24
US, New Orleans: Black	98	0	42	95	0	32
US, Detroit: White	99	1	30	99	1	29
US, Detroit: Black	98	1	36	99	0	25
US, New Mexico: Non-Hisp. White	97	1	28	99	0	45
US, New Mexico: Hispanic White	99	0	32	99	0	73
US, New Mexico: American Indian	50	0	100	-	-	-
US, Utah	99	0	26	99	0	24
US, Seattle	99	0	25	99	0	31
US, SEER: White	99	1	28	98	1	31
US, SEER: Black	98	1	39	99	1	35

ASIA

	MV	DCO	M/I	MV	DCO	M/I
+China, Qidong	95	0	58	0	0	100
+China, Shanghai	75	0	53	64	1	69
China, Tianjin	76	0	48	74	0	52
Hong Kong	82	2	36	79	4	39
India, Bangalore	78	2	14	78	11	16
India, Barshi, Paranda and Bhum	71	0		-	-	
India, Bombay	71	11	59	66	20	71
India, Karunagappally	76	6		-	-	
India, Madras	78	3	37	68	11	34
India, Trivandrum	99	0	15	99	0	0
Israel: All Jews	93			94		
Jews born in Israel	99			93		
Jews born in America or Europe	91			94		
Jews born in Africa or Asia	95			95		
Non-Jews	95			-		
Japan, Hiroshima	95	0	21	80	10	30
Japan, Miyagi	89	2	29	93	7	27
Japan, Nagasaki	94	3	36	80	7	73
Japan, Osaka	90	4	27	81	5	26
+Japan, Saga	89	5	24	71	0	43
Japan, Yamagata	90	7	28	75	0	25
Korea, Kangwha	75		200	99		100
Kuwait: Non-Kuwaitis	88	3		99	0	
Kuwait: Kuwaitis	93	0		99	0	
Philippines, Manila	77	7		65	21	
Singapore: Chinese	95	1		94	0	
Singapore: Malay	99	0		99	0	
Singapore: Indian	96	0		99	0	
Thailand, Chiang Mai	92	0		78	0	
Thailand, Khon Kaen	91	0		40	0	
Viet Nam, Hanoi	65			50		

+ IMPORTANT-SEE NOTES ON POPULATION PAGE

EUROPE

	MALE			FEMALE		
	MV	DCO	M/I	MV	DCO	M/I
Austria, Tyrol	91	7	45	99	0	150
+Belarus	93	0	63	88	0	68
Croatia	70	6	61	62	17	58
+Czech Republic	94	1	64	88	6	76
Denmark	99	0	44	98	0	43
Estonia	95		47	92		38
Finland	99	0	40	99	0	41
France, Bas-Rhin	99		50	99		32
France, Calvados	99		68	99		57
France, Doubs	99		53	99		50
France, Haut-Rhin	99		45	99		60
France, Herault	99		60	99		62
France, Isere	96		42	99		67
France, Somme	98		93	95		38
France, Tarn	99		89	91		18
Germany, Eastern States	99	0	50	99	0	63
+Germany, Saarland	97	3	46	94	6	39
Iceland	99	0	22	99	0	0
Ireland, Southern	94		43	93		79
Italy, Ferrara	95	2	41	67	0	33
Italy, Florence	84	1	41	73	8	50
Italy, Genoa	94	3	52	90	3	65
Italy, Latina	86	9	61	99	0	22
Italy, Macerata	85	3	54	99	0	0
Italy, Modena	93	4	34	89	6	44
Italy, Parma	97	1	49	85	15	46
Italy, Ragusa	89	0	83	99	0	100
Italy, Romagna	95	1	37	94	0	18
Italy, Torino	93	1	59	81	7	48
Italy, Trieste	83	3	27	71	0	29
Italy, Varese	96	1	43	99	0	52
Italy, Veneto	94	2	43	94	3	38
+Latvia	94	1	53	89	4	74
+Malta	98	0	44	99	0	0
The Netherlands	99		33	99		32
The Netherlands, Eindhoven	98		27	99		21
The Netherlands, Maastricht	99		31	99		17
Norway	99	0	32	97	3	48
Poland, Cracow	88	7	82	79	21	68
Poland, Kielce	90	1	49	86	5	67
Poland, Lower Silesia	69	1	55	72	1	35
Poland, Warsaw City	[93]	3	46	[96]	3	57
Slovakia	92	1	65	81	1	77
Slovenia	96	2	68	99	0	48
Spain, Albacete	90	5	27	-	-	-
Spain, Asturias	96	3	50	88	12	24
Spain, Basque Country	95	3	53	85	5	35
Spain, Granada	94	2	56	40	60	160
Spain, Mallorca	98	2	46	99	0	57
Spain, Murcia	94	3	55	99	0	114
Spain, Navarra	95	4	44	99	0	117
Spain, Tarragona	97	1	41	99	0	100
Spain, Zaragoza	93	2	44	80	20	60
Sweden	99		29	99		31
Switzerland, Basel	99	0	51	99	0	50
Switzerland, Geneva	99	1	31	99	0	31
Switzerland, Graubunden	96	0	52	99	0	67
Switzerland, Neuchatel	99	0	31	99	0	67
Switzerland, St Gall-Appenzell	99	0	58	99	0	100
Switzerland, Valais	99	0	67	99	0	13
Switzerland, Vaud	95	1	41	95	0	53
Switzerland, Zurich	98	0	51	99	0	67
+UK, England and Wales	[86]		40	[84]		45
UK, East Anglia			35			33
UK, Mersey	90	1	45	94	1	50
UK, North Western	88	1	42	81	2	49
UK, Oxford	89	1	38	91	0	56
UK, South Thames	81	8	44	78	11	59
UK, South Western	88	2	44	80	2	63
UK, Wessex	[82]	4	41	[78]	4	49
+UK, West Midlands		0	36		1	40
UK, Yorkshire	96	1	46	93	2	42
UK, Scotland	93	2	34	93	2	40
UK, Scotland, West	91	3	35	92	3	36
Yugoslavia, Vojvodina	66	9	63	47	15	50

OCEANIA

	MALE			FEMALE		
	MV	DCO	M/I	MV	DCO	M/I
Australian Capital Territory	96	0		99	0	
Australia, New South Wales	96	0		96	0	
South Australia	90		39	81		23
Australia, Tasmania	88		54	83		100
Australia, Victoria	97	0	49	97	0	30
Western Australia	93	3	39	96	0	50
French Polynesia	79	14		60	20	
+New Zealand: Non-Maori	96	0	38	94	2	45
+New Zealand: Maori	99	0	0	99	0	0
US, Hawaii: White	99	0	27	99	0	25
US, Hawaii: Japanese	97	3	29	99	0	0
US, Hawaii: Hawaiian	99	0	69	99	0	33
US, Hawaii: Filipino	99	0	25	99	0	0
US, Hawaii: Chinese	99	0	50	-	-	-

+ IMPORTANT-SEE NOTES ON POPULATION PAGE

[] CYTOLOGICAL VERIFICATION EXCLUDED

INDICES OF DATA QUALITY
Bronchus, lung (ICD-9 162)

	MALE MV	DCO	M/I	FEMALE MV	DCO	M/I
AFRICA						
Algeria, Setif	75			67		
France, La Reunion	96		104	96		122
Mali, Bamako	18	3		15	0	
Uganda, Kyadondo	40			25		
Zimbabwe, Harare: African	40	12		36	14	
Zimbabwe, Harare: European	45	36		38	33	
AMERICA, CENTRAL AND SOUTH						
Argentina, Concordia	62	32	84	67	33	96
Brazil, Belem	34	20	67	34	24	77
Brazil, Goiania	68	19	83	68	21	63
Brazil, Porto Alegre	49	0	75	55	0	75
Colombia, Cali	57	7	94	58	12	90
Costa Rica	57	22	97	49	30	101
Ecuador, Quito	38	37		31	46	
Peru, Lima	58	15		55	18	
Peru, Trujillo	51	13	100	64	0	86
US, Puerto Rico	78	9	97	74	11	99
Uruguay, Montevideo	53	11	83	52	17	71
AMERICA, NORTH						
Canada	74	3	86	75	3	78
Canada, Alberta	87	3	87	89	2	78
Canada, British Columbia	86	10	85	86	10	79
Canada, Manitoba	61	3	83	62	2	79
Canada, New Brunswick	85	3	85	84	2	79
Canada, Newfoundland	92	0	97	91	0	93
Canada, Northwest Territories	84	1	76	74	4	76
Canada, Nova Scotia	79	13	85	81	12	80
Canada, Ontario	76	3	83	77	3	76
Canada, Prince Edward Island	86	5	94	88	4	78
+Canada, Quebec	63	0	88	63	0	78
Canada, Saskatchewan	84	5	82	87	4	79
Canada, Yukon	93	0	71	97	0	59
+US, Cent. Calif.: Non-Hisp. White	91	2	83	90	1	79
+US, Cent. Calif.: Hispanic	92	3	79	92	2	66
US, Los Angeles: Non-Hisp. White	93	2	83	92	2	79
US, Los Angeles: Hispanic White	93	1		92	2	
US, Los Angeles: Black	94	1		94	1	
US, Los Angeles: Chinese	94	1		95	1	
US, Los Angeles: Filipino	97	0		96	0	
US, Los Angeles: Korean	94	2		90	0	
US, Los Angeles: Japanese	94	3		94	0	
US, San Francisco: Non-Hisp. White	92	1	82	90	2	80
US, San Francisco: Hispanic White	94	0	52	90	2	38
US, San Francisco: Black	93	1	79	93	0	77
US, San Francisco: Chinese	94	1	77	95	1	76
US, San Francisco: Filipino	96	1	64	93	2	66
US, San Francisco: Japanese	96	0	76	97	0	97
US, Connecticut: White	91	2	78	91	2	74
US, Connecticut: Black	96	1	80	93	2	65
US, Atlanta: White	93	1	82	94	2	76
US, Atlanta: Black	92	3	82	92	3	77
US, Iowa	90	1	82	90	2	77

	MALE MV	DCO	M/I	FEMALE MV	DCO	M/I
US, Central Louisiana: White	85	4	91	83	4	90
US, Central Louisiana: Black	76	4	81	80	3	77
US, New Orleans: White	88	3	86	87	3	78
US, New Orleans: Black	87	5	91	86	6	86
US, Detroit: White	92	2	77	91	2	69
US, Detroit: Black	92	1	77	93	1	78
US, New Mexico: Non-Hisp. White	86	4	86	84	3	81
US, New Mexico: Hispanic White	87	3	93	86	4	83
US, New Mexico: American Indian	83	0	75	92	0	117
US, Utah	91	0	86	90	0	83
US, Seattle	93	1	81	91	1	77
US, SEER: White	92	2	80	91	2	76
US, SEER: Black	93	1	79	93	1	77
ASIA						
+China, Qidong	56	0	90	57	0	88
+China, Shanghai	42	2	83	36	2	89
China, Tianjin	50	0	65	42	0	72
Hong Kong	57	10	74	51	15	78
India, Bangalore	66	12	39	76	9	33
India, Barshi, Paranda and Bhum	64	0		99	0	
India, Bombay	61	12	72	50	19	82
India, Karunagappally	52	12		50	40	
India, Madras	68	3	48	65	6	37
India, Trivandrum	58	17	48	71	14	21
Israel: All Jews	76			76		
Jews born in Israel	81			84		
Jews born in America or Europe	75			76		
Jews born in Africa or Asia	76			72		
Non-Jews	69			78		
Japan, Hiroshima	75	15	76	72	17	71
Japan, Miyagi	79	11	77	78	13	77
Japan, Nagasaki	73	18	87	67	23	83
Japan, Osaka	71	24	86	65	28	87
+Japan, Saga	68	21	82	63	23	83
Japan, Yamagata	64	26	84	60	28	83
Korea, Kangwha	63		72	66		81
Kuwait: Non-Kuwaitis	82	13		73	24	
Kuwait: Kuwaitis	73	23		48	48	
Philippines, Manila	52	24		50	26	
Singapore: Chinese	80	8		75	10	
Singapore: Malay	75	8		85	7	
Singapore: Indian	83	2		90	10	
Thailand, Chiang Mai	60	3		58	4	
Thailand, Khon Kaen	41	14		36	23	
Viet Nam, Hanoi	41			46		

+ IMPORTANT-SEE NOTES ON POPULATION PAGE

INDICES OF DATA QUALITY
Bronchus, lung (ICD-9 162) (contd)

	MALE			FEMALE		
EUROPE	MV	DCO	M/I	MV	DCO	M/I
Austria, Tyrol	78	11	86	75	11	83
+Belarus	49	1	81	31	1	70
Croatia	75	6	88	69	8	85
+Czech Republic	59	2	99	53	4	98
Denmark	87	1	102	86	1	100
Estonia	72		92	61		87
Finland	91	1	91	89	2	86
France, Bas-Rhin	94		84	89		94
France, Calvados	98		94	98		122
France, Doubs	95		97	93		96
France, Haut-Rhin	97		94	98		111
France, Herault	98		108	98		122
France, Isere	97		61	96		63
France, Somme	95		110	93		134
France, Tarn	98		99	95		133
Germany, Eastern States	82	1	85	81	1	83
+Germany, Saarland	73	15	92	73	14	88
Iceland	97	0	94	92	0	99
Ireland, Southern	75		103	73		116
Italy, Ferrara	76	4	93	68	2	80
Italy, Florence	59	5	89	49	7	80
Italy, Genoa	71	5	90	70	7	89
Italy, Latina	74	16	87	68	21	92
Italy, Macerata	78	2	94	70	0	95
Italy, Modena	67	5	92	60	7	100
Italy, Parma	78	3	94	70	6	84
Italy, Ragusa	51	0	95	47	0	91
Italy, Romagna	84	1	91	78	2	91
Italy, Torino	70	6	90	60	10	92
Italy, Trieste	82	0	79	99	0	97
Italy, Varese	87	2	89	75	4	89
Italy, Veneto	73	5	93	65	7	91
+Latvia	49	3	80	35	5	73
+Malta	68	6	94	67	6	167
The Netherlands	94		96	94		90
The Netherlands, Eindhoven	94		98	94		87
The Netherlands, Maastricht	92		93	93		84
Norway	92	2	91	92	3	85
Poland, Cracow	69	9	92	65	12	88
Poland, Kielce	68	3	97	54	5	95
Poland, Lower Silesia	38	1	86	40	2	77
Poland, Warsaw City	[59]	9	91	[51]	10	88
Slovakia	73	3	86	66	3	82
Slovenia	90	3	91	86	5	93
Spain, Albacete	65	17	108	74	21	100
Spain, Asturias	87	9	89	74	18	90
Spain, Basque Country	80	8	81	69	19	96
Spain, Granada	69	10	95	63	17	126
Spain, Mallorca	85	3	90	81	13	103
Spain, Murcia	79	9	96	64	26	111
Spain, Navarra	85	9	86	74	17	99
Spain, Tarragona	88	3	91	88	6	113
Spain, Zaragoza	72	10	89	63	17	116

	MALE			FEMALE		
	MV	DCO	M/I	MV	DCO	M/I
Sweden	98		103	98		102
Switzerland, Basel	99	0	102	98	0	89
Switzerland, Geneva	95	1	82	91	1	88
Switzerland, Graubunden	83	11	83	71	7	97
Switzerland, Neuchatel	91	4	95	86	2	98
Switzerland, St Gall-Appenzell	93	2	84	98	1	78
Switzerland, Valais	90	2	88	94	1	82
Switzerland, Vaud	90	2	87	87	3	84
Switzerland, Zurich	95	0	91	95	0	79
+UK, England and Wales	[67]		94	[67]		92
UK, East Anglia			94			92
UK, Mersey	57	4	97	52	5	97
UK, North Western	46	6	94	44	6	92
UK, Oxford	56	1	90	53	1	88
UK, South Thames	54	24	92	49	26	90
UK, South Western	50	7	95	47	8	91
UK, Wessex	[72]	15	94	[69]	16	89
+UK, West Midlands		4	90		4	88
UK, Yorkshire	63	7	94	59	7	92
UK, Scotland	59	6	90	57	6	86
UK, Scotland, West	56	8	91	55	9	86
Yugoslavia, Vojvodina	51	10	88	36	15	92

OCEANIA

	MALE			FEMALE		
	MV	DCO	M/I	MV	DCO	M/I
Australian Capital Territory	89	2		82	3	
Australia, New South Wales	83	3		82	3	
South Australia	72		95	74		92
Australia, Tasmania	76		87	80		93
Australia, Victoria	84	2	90	82	2	87
Western Australia	85	5	87	85	5	84
French Polynesia	64	28		72	17	
+New Zealand: Non-Maori	74	6	91	73	5	90
+New Zealand: Maori	71	9	66	70	8	66
US, Hawaii: White	95	0	81	94	0	77
US, Hawaii: Japanese	96	0	79	94	0	73
US, Hawaii: Hawaiian	96	0	98	96	0	104
US, Hawaii: Filipino	95	0	70	93	0	75
US, Hawaii: Chinese	93	0	69	93	0	85

+ IMPORTANT-SEE NOTES ON POPULATION PAGE

[] CYTOLOGICAL VERIFICATION EXCLUDED

INDICES OF DATA QUALITY
Other thoracic organs (ICD-9 163-4)

	MALE			FEMALE		
	MV	DCO	M/I	MV	DCO	M/I
AFRICA						
Algeria, Setif	99			67		
France, La Reunion	99			99		
Mali, Bamako	-	-		-	-	
Uganda, Kyadondo	99			75		
Zimbabwe, Harare: African	50	0		50	0	
Zimbabwe, Harare: European	-	-		-	-	
AMERICA, CENTRAL AND SOUTH						
Argentina, Concordia	99	0		90	10	
Brazil, Belem	40	40		99	0	
Brazil, Goiania	91	0		80	0	
Brazil, Porto Alegre	67	0		61	0	
Colombia, Cali	71	6		77	8	
Costa Rica	77	23		44	44	
Ecuador, Quito	-	-		-	-	
Peru, Lima	76	4		58	25	
Peru, Trujillo	33	0		0	50	
US, Puerto Rico	83	3		67	0	
Uruguay, Montevideo	57	24		73	18	
AMERICA, NORTH						
Canada	79	2		72	3	
Canada, Alberta	89	0		93	0	
Canada, British Columbia	85	6		84	14	
Canada, Manitoba	74	0		67	13	
Canada, New Brunswick	99	0		86	0	
Canada, Newfoundland	99	0		99	0	
Canada, Northwest Territories	99	0		-	-	
Canada, Nova Scotia	85	10		60	20	
Canada, Ontario	75	4		68	2	
Canada, Prince Edward Island	99	0		99	0	
+Canada, Quebec	77	0		67	0	
Canada, Saskatchewan	99	0		91	9	
Canada, Yukon	-	-		-	-	
+US, Cent. Calif.: Non-Hisp. White	92	8		70	10	
+US, Cent. Calif.: Hispanic	99	0		67	0	
US, Los Angeles: Non-Hisp. White	93	0		95	0	
US, Los Angeles: Hispanic White	99	0		90	10	
US, Los Angeles: Black	99	0		99	0	
US, Los Angeles: Chinese	99	0		-	-	
US, Los Angeles: Filipino	99	0		-	-	
US, Los Angeles: Korean	-	-		99	0	
US, Los Angeles: Japanese	99	0		-	-	
US, San Francisco: Non-Hisp. White	96	0		99	0	
US, San Francisco: Hispanic White	99	0		99	0	
US, San Francisco: Black	99	0		99	0	
US, San Francisco: Chinese	99	0		99	0	
US, San Francisco: Filipino	99	0		99	0	
US, San Francisco: Japanese	-	-		-	-	
US, Connecticut: White	91	4		97	0	
US, Connecticut: Black	99	0		99	0	
US, Atlanta: White	99	0		99	0	
US, Atlanta: Black	99	0		99	0	
US, Iowa	91	0		93	0	

	MALE			FEMALE		
	MV	DCO	M/I	MV	DCO	M/I
US, Central Louisiana: White	20	20		99	0	
US, Central Louisiana: Black	-	-		99	0	
US, New Orleans: White	99	0		99	0	
US, New Orleans: Black	99	0		99	0	
US, Detroit: White	90	5		99	0	
US, Detroit: Black	99	0		75	0	
US, New Mexico: Non-Hisp. White	85	8		57	0	
US, New Mexico: Hispanic White	99	0		99	0	
US, New Mexico: American Indian	-	-		-	-	
US, Utah	99	0		92	0	
US, Seattle	99	0		99	0	
US, SEER: White	95	2		96	0	
US, SEER: Black	99	0		95	0	
ASIA						
+China, Qidong	75	0		82	0	
+China, Shanghai	37	2		43	4	
China, Tianjin	49	1		53	0	
Hong Kong	68	11		75	9	
India, Bangalore	74	11		79	8	
India, Barshi, Paranda and Bhum	-	-		-	-	
India, Bombay	59	9		69	5	
India, Karunagappally	-	-		-	-	
India, Madras	93	0		99	0	
India, Trivandrum	99	0		99	0	
Israel: All Jews	85			82		
Jews born in Israel	85			80		
Jews born in America or Europe	86			81		
Jews born in Africa or Asia	83			88		
Non-Jews	99			99		
Japan, Hiroshima	82	6		79	0	
Japan, Miyagi	78	0		69	12	
Japan, Nagasaki	65	18		52	29	
Japan, Osaka	79	10		72	13	
+Japan, Saga	71	21		89	5	
Japan, Yamagata	54	29		33	33	
Korea, Kangwha	-			99		
Kuwait: Non-Kuwaitis	86	14		99	0	
Kuwait: Kuwaitis	80	0		99	0	
Philippines, Manila	84	10		83	0	
Singapore: Chinese	86	5		99	0	
Singapore: Malay	99	0		99	0	
Singapore: Indian	99	0		99	0	
Thailand, Chiang Mai	50	0		99	0	
Thailand, Khon Kaen	13	0		99	0	
Viet Nam, Hanoi	50			46		

+ IMPORTANT-SEE NOTES ON POPULATION PAGE

EUROPE	MALE MV	DCO	M/I	FEMALE MV	DCO	M/I
Austria, Tyrol	77	8		47	47	
+Belarus	45	0		48	1	
Croatia	34	17		26	19	
+Czech Republic	48	4		46	10	
Denmark	83	1		86	0	
Estonia	78			71		
Finland	85	2		78	3	
France, Bas-Rhin	96			78		
France, Calvados	95			99		
France, Doubs	75			99		
France, Haut-Rhin	92			99		
France, Herault	93			75		
France, Isere	75			93		
France, Somme	82			75		
France, Tarn	80			-		
Germany, Eastern States	75	0		73	0	
+Germany, Saarland	76	16		67	24	
Iceland	80	0		99	0	
Ireland, Southern	83			50		
Italy, Ferrara	33	33		60	0	
Italy, Florence	38	13		47	0	
Italy, Genoa	47	19		65	21	
Italy, Latina	40	0		-	-	
Italy, Macerata	75	0		50	0	
Italy, Modena	61	4		55	0	
Italy, Parma	17	17		99	0	
Italy, Ragusa	25	0		75	0	
Italy, Romagna	57	0		83	0	
Italy, Torino	53	15		63	17	
Italy, Trieste	52	3		38	8	
Italy, Varese	99	0		60	40	
Italy, Veneto	68	2		44	13	
+Latvia	47	7		66	10	
+Malta	99	0		99	0	
The Netherlands	62			80		
The Netherlands, Eindhoven	89			63		
The Netherlands, Maastricht	67			99		
Norway	77	10		89	0	
Poland, Cracow	64	18		38	23	
Poland, Kielce	47	3		67	0	
Poland, Lower Silesia	49	1		47	0	
Poland, Warsaw City	[25]	9		[23]	8	
Slovakia	45	6		64	10	
Slovenia	63	0		57	0	
Spain, Albacete	99	0		-	-	
Spain, Asturias	84	8		95	5	
Spain, Basque Country	75	7		61	6	
Spain, Granada	64	18		71	14	
Spain, Mallorca	60	10		83	17	
Spain, Murcia	67	33		99	0	
Spain, Navarra	88	0		86	14	
Spain, Tarragona	92	8		80	0	
Spain, Zaragoza	60	10		57	21	

	MALE MV	DCO	M/I	FEMALE MV	DCO	M/I
Sweden	98			99		
Switzerland, Basel	99	0		99	0	
Switzerland, Geneva	99	0		75	0	
Switzerland, Graubunden	99	0		0	0	
Switzerland, Neuchatel	99	0		99	0	
Switzerland, St Gall-Appenzell	76	6		99	0	
Switzerland, Valais	91	0		99	0	
Switzerland, Vaud	78	0		99	0	
Switzerland, Zurich	80	0		92	0	
+UK, England and Wales	[78]			[78]		
UK, East Anglia						
UK, Mersey	74	0		77	0	
UK, North Western	85	2		80	5	
UK, Oxford	62	5		77	0	
UK, South Thames	76	10		80	7	
UK, South Western	74	6		63	5	
UK, Wessex	[74]	3		[55]	0	
+UK, West Midlands		3			3	
UK, Yorkshire	84	4		82	7	
UK, Scotland	78	5		63	7	
UK, Scotland, West	89	6		75	19	
Yugoslavia, Vojvodina	25	12		28	17	

OCEANIA	MALE MV	DCO	M/I	FEMALE MV	DCO	M/I
Australian Capital Territory	99	0		99	0	
Australia, New South Wales	90	4		89	3	
South Australia	99			63		
Australia, Tasmania	83			33		
Australia, Victoria	68	2		79	0	
Western Australia	83	11		99	0	
French Polynesia	71	29		20	80	
+New Zealand: Non-Maori	90	1		88	4	
+New Zealand: Maori	99	0		99	0	
US, Hawaii: White	99	0		99	0	
US, Hawaii: Japanese	99	0		99	0	
US, Hawaii: Hawaiian	99	0		99	0	
US, Hawaii: Filipino	99	0		99	0	
US, Hawaii: Chinese	99	0		-	-	

+ IMPORTANT-SEE NOTES ON POPULATION PAGE

[] CYTOLOGICAL VERIFICATION EXCLUDED

INDICES OF DATA QUALITY
Kaposi's sarcoma

	MALE			FEMALE		
	MV	DCO	M/I	MV	DCO	M/I
AFRICA						
Algeria, Setif	-			-		
France, La Reunion	75			-		
Mali, Bamako	99	0		99	0	
Uganda, Kyadondo	77			74		
Zimbabwe, Harare: African	75	1		76	3	
Zimbabwe, Harare: European	99	0		-	-	
AMERICA, CENTRAL AND SOUTH						
Argentina, Concordia	99	0		-	-	
Brazil, Belem	99	0		-	-	
Brazil, Goiania	82	18		-	-	
Brazil, Porto Alegre	93	0		99	0	
Colombia, Cali	99	0		99	0	
Costa Rica	80	0		99	0	
Ecuador, Quito	99	0		99	0	
Peru, Lima	99	0		99	0	
Peru, Trujillo	99	0		99	0	
US, Puerto Rico	89	5		76	12	
Uruguay, Montevideo	99	0		99	0	
AMERICA, NORTH						
Canada	60	0		73	0	
Canada, Alberta	-	-		-	-	
Canada, British Columbia	99	0		-	-	
Canada, Manitoba	99	0		0	0	
Canada, New Brunswick	-	-		-	-	
Canada, Newfoundland	-	-		-	-	
Canada, Northwest Territories	-	-		-	-	
Canada, Nova Scotia	-	-		-	-	
Canada, Ontario	63	0		71	0	
Canada, Prince Edward Island	-	-		-	-	
+Canada, Quebec	49	0		99	0	
Canada, Saskatchewan	99	0		99	0	
Canada, Yukon	-	-		-	-	
+US, Cent. Calif.: Non-Hisp. White	73	2		99	0	
+US, Cent. Calif.: Hispanic	73	0		99	0	
US, Los Angeles: Non-Hisp. White	71	0		97	0	
US, Los Angeles: Hispanic White	79	0		83	0	
US, Los Angeles: Black	78	0		86	0	
US, Los Angeles: Chinese	33	0		-	-	
US, Los Angeles: Filipino	65	0		-	-	
US, Los Angeles: Korean	99	0		-	-	
US, Los Angeles: Japanese	69	0		-	-	
US, San Francisco: Non-Hisp. White	66	1		94	6	
US, San Francisco: Hispanic White	72	0		99	0	
US, San Francisco: Black	77	0		99	0	
US, San Francisco: Chinese	50	0		-	-	
US, San Francisco: Filipino	73	0		-	-	
US, San Francisco: Japanese	75	0		-	-	
US, Connecticut: White	81	0		95	0	
US, Connecticut: Black	90	0		99	0	
US, Atlanta: White	74	0		99	0	
US, Atlanta: Black	86	2		99	0	
US, Iowa	68	5		99	0	

	MALE			FEMALE		
	MV	DCO	M/I	MV	DCO	M/I
US, Central Louisiana: White	99	0		99	0	
US, Central Louisiana: Black	99	0		99	0	
US, New Orleans: White	85	8		75	0	
US, New Orleans: Black	99	0		67	0	
US, Detroit: White	86	0		99	0	
US, Detroit: Black	83	3		70	0	
US, New Mexico: Non-Hisp. White	60	7		99	0	
US, New Mexico: Hispanic White	73	3		99	0	
US, New Mexico: American Indian	50	0		-	-	
US, Utah	69	0		99	0	
US, Seattle	68	0		99	0	
US, SEER: White	69	1		98	1	
US, SEER: Black	81	1		84	0	
ASIA						
+China, Qidong	-	-		-	-	
+China, Shanghai	-	-		-	-	
China, Tianjin	-	-		-	-	
Hong Kong	99	0		-	-	
India, Bangalore	-	-		-	-	
India, Barshi, Paranda and Bhum	-	-		-	-	
India, Bombay	-	-		99	0	
India, Karunagappally	-	-		-	-	
India, Madras	-	-		-	-	
India, Trivandrum	-	-		-	-	
Israel: All Jews	85			91		
Jews born in Israel	73			80		
Jews born in America or Europe	85			91		
Jews born in Africa or Asia	89			90		
Non-Jews	99			99		
Japan, Hiroshima	-	-		-	-	
Japan, Miyagi	-	-		-	-	
Japan, Nagasaki	-	-		-	-	
Japan, Osaka	99	0		-	-	
+Japan, Saga	-	-		-	-	
Japan, Yamagata	-	-		-	-	
Korea, Kangwha	99			-		
Kuwait: Non-Kuwaitis	99	0		99	0	
Kuwait: Kuwaitis	99	0		99	0	
Philippines, Manila	99	0		-	-	
Singapore: Chinese	99	0		-	-	
Singapore: Malay	-	-		-	-	
Singapore: Indian	99	0		-	-	
Thailand, Chiang Mai	99	0		-	-	
Thailand, Khon Kaen	-	-		-	-	
Viet Nam, Hanoi	99			-		

+ IMPORTANT-SEE NOTES ON POPULATION PAGE

Kaposi's sarcoma (contd)

EUROPE	MALE MV	DCO	M/I	FEMALE MV	DCO	M/I
Austria, Tyrol	-	-		-	-	
+Belarus	99	0		99	0	
Croatia	99	0		-	-	
+Czech Republic	99	0		99	0	
Denmark	98	0		99	0	
Estonia	99			99		
Finland	99	0		99	0	
France, Bas-Rhin	98			99		
France, Calvados	63			99		
France, Doubs	99			-		
France, Haut-Rhin	99			99		
France, Herault	99			99		
France, Isere	99			99		
France, Somme	99			99		
France, Tarn	99			99		
Germany, Eastern States	99	0		99	0	
+Germany, Saarland	-	-		-	-	
Iceland	99	0		99	0	
Ireland, Southern	99			-		
Italy, Ferrara	99	0		99	0	
Italy, Florence	68	3		90	0	
Italy, Genoa	79	0		99	0	
Italy, Latina	99	0		99	0	
Italy, Macerata	99	0		99	0	
Italy, Modena	85	0		99	0	
Italy, Parma	91	9		-	-	
Italy, Ragusa	99	0		99	0	
Italy, Romagna	96	4		92	8	
Italy, Torino	78	0		99	0	
Italy, Trieste	99	0		99	0	
Italy, Varese	93	3		90	0	
Italy, Veneto	97	0		99	0	
+Latvia	-	-		-	-	
+Malta	-	-		-	-	
The Netherlands	93			99		
The Netherlands, Eindhoven	99			99		
The Netherlands, Maastricht	75			-		
Norway	99	1		99	0	
Poland, Cracow	99	0		-	-	
Poland, Kielce	99	0		-	-	
Poland, Lower Silesia	99	0		0	0	
Poland, Warsaw City	[99]	0		[99]	0	
Slovakia	91	0		99	0	
Slovenia	-	-		-	-	
Spain, Albacete	99	0		99	0	
Spain, Asturias	99	0		99	0	
Spain, Basque Country	94	3		99	0	
Spain, Granada	83	0		99	0	
Spain, Mallorca	72	0		99	0	
Spain, Murcia	91	0		99	0	
Spain, Navarra	99	0		99	0	
Spain, Tarragona	99	0		99	0	
Spain, Zaragoza	99	0		99	0	

	MALE MV	DCO	M/I	FEMALE MV	DCO	M/I
Sweden	99			99		
Switzerland, Basel	67	0		99	0	
Switzerland, Geneva	95	0		99	0	
Switzerland, Graubunden	99	0		-	-	
Switzerland, Neuchatel	99	0		-	-	
Switzerland, St Gall-Appenzell	99	0		-	-	
Switzerland, Valais	99	0		99	0	
Switzerland, Vaud	96	0		83	0	
Switzerland, Zurich	83	0		99	0	
+UK, England and Wales	[79]			[88]		
UK, East Anglia						
UK, Mersey	82	0		99	0	
UK, North Western	48	0		99	0	
UK, Oxford	99	0		99	0	
UK, South Thames	36	22		43	43	
UK, South Western	65	0		-	-	
UK, Wessex	[99]	0		-	-	
+UK, West Midlands		-			-	
UK, Yorkshire	83	0		50	0	
UK, Scotland	93	0		75	0	
UK, Scotland, West	92	0		99	0	
Yugoslavia, Vojvodina	-	-		-	-	

OCEANIA

	MALE MV	DCO	M/I	FEMALE MV	DCO	M/I
Australian Capital Territory	80	20		-	-	
Australia, New South Wales	71	2		80	10	
South Australia	48			0		
Australia, Tasmania	99			99		
Australia, Victoria	59	0		91	0	
Western Australia	81	0		99	0	
French Polynesia	-	-		-	-	
+New Zealand: Non-Maori	-	-		-	-	
+New Zealand: Maori	-	-		-	-	
US, Hawaii: White	81	0		99	0	
US, Hawaii: Japanese	99	0		-	-	
US, Hawaii: Hawaiian	83	0		-	-	
US, Hawaii: Filipino	78	0		-	-	
US, Hawaii: Chinese	60	0		-	-	

+ IMPORTANT-SEE NOTES ON POPULATION PAGE

[] CYTOLOGICAL VERIFICATION EXCLUDED

INDICES OF DATA QUALITY
Mesothelioma

	MALE			FEMALE		
	MV	DCO	M/I	MV	DCO	M/I
AFRICA						
Algeria, Setif	-			-		
France, La Reunion	99			99		
Mali, Bamako	-	-		-	-	
Uganda, Kyadondo	-			-		
Zimbabwe, Harare: African	-	-		-	-	
Zimbabwe, Harare: European	99	0		-	-	
AMERICA, CENTRAL AND SOUTH						
Argentina, Concordia	-	-		99	0	
Brazil, Belem	-	-		99	0	
Brazil, Goiania	99	0		-	-	
Brazil, Porto Alegre	-	-		-	-	
Colombia, Cali	99	0		99	0	
Costa Rica	99	0		75	0	
Ecuador, Quito	-	-		-	-	
Peru, Lima	82	0		99	0	
Peru, Trujillo	-	-		-	-	
US, Puerto Rico	95	0		90	10	
Uruguay, Montevideo	99	0		99	0	
AMERICA, NORTH						
Canada	93	0		95	0	
Canada, Alberta	96	0		93	7	
Canada, British Columbia	99	1		96	0	
Canada, Manitoba	83	0		99	0	
Canada, New Brunswick	99	0		99	0	
Canada, Newfoundland	99	0		99	0	
Canada, Northwest Territories	-	-		-	-	
Canada, Nova Scotia	99	0		99	0	
Canada, Ontario	97	0		99	0	
Canada, Prince Edward Island	99	0		-	-	
+Canada, Quebec	85	0		89	0	
Canada, Saskatchewan	99	0		99	0	
Canada, Yukon	-	-		-	-	
+US, Cent. Calif.: Non-Hisp. White	94	2		99	0	
+US, Cent. Calif.: Hispanic	99	0		99	0	
US, Los Angeles: Non-Hisp. White	98	0		94	4	
US, Los Angeles: Hispanic White	99	0		94	0	
US, Los Angeles: Black	87	0		99	0	
US, Los Angeles: Chinese	99	0		-	-	
US, Los Angeles: Filipino	99	0		99	0	
US, Los Angeles: Korean	-	-		-	-	
US, Los Angeles: Japanese	99	0		99	0	
US, San Francisco: Non-Hisp. White	91	1		96	4	
US, San Francisco: Hispanic White	99	0		80	0	
US, San Francisco: Black	99	0		75	0	
US, San Francisco: Chinese	99	0		-	-	
US, San Francisco: Filipino	99	0		99	0	
US, San Francisco: Japanese	99	0		-	-	
US, Connecticut: White	95	0		98	0	
US, Connecticut: Black	99	0		-	-	
US, Atlanta: White	99	0		99	0	
US, Atlanta: Black	99	0		99	0	
US, Iowa	95	1		93	3	

	MALE			FEMALE		
	MV	DCO	M/I	MV	DCO	M/I
US, Central Louisiana: White	67	33		-	-	
US, Central Louisiana: Black	-	-		-	-	
US, New Orleans: White	96	2		94	6	
US, New Orleans: Black	94	0		99	0	
US, Detroit: White	97	0		97	0	
US, Detroit: Black	93	0		99	0	
US, New Mexico: Non-Hisp. White	90	10		93	0	
US, New Mexico: Hispanic White	89	0		99	0	
US, New Mexico: American Indian	99	0		0	0	
US, Utah	93	0		99	0	
US, Seattle	95	1		98	0	
US, SEER: White	94	1		96	1	
US, SEER: Black	98	0		93	0	
ASIA						
+China, Qidong	-	-		-	-	
+China, Shanghai	-	-		-	-	
China, Tianjin	67	0		70	0	
Hong Kong	99	0		99	0	
India, Bangalore	99	0		99	0	
India, Barshi, Paranda and Bhum	-	-		-	-	
India, Bombay	99	0		99	0	
India, Karunagappally	-	-		-	-	
India, Madras	99	0		99	0	
India, Trivandrum	-	-		99	0	
Israel: All Jews	98			90		
Jews born in Israel	99			-		
Jews born in America or Europe	97			94		
Jews born in Africa or Asia	99			80		
Non-Jews	99			99		
Japan, Hiroshima	77	0		99	0	
Japan, Miyagi	73	0		99	0	
Japan, Nagasaki	76	12		99	0	
Japan, Osaka	99	0		99	0	
+Japan, Saga	-	-		-	-	
Japan, Yamagata	99	0		99	0	
Korea, Kangwha	-			-		
Kuwait: Non-Kuwaitis	99	0		50	0	
Kuwait: Kuwaitis	99	0		-	-	
Philippines, Manila	67	0		99	0	
Singapore: Chinese	99	0		99	0	
Singapore: Malay	-	-		-	-	
Singapore: Indian	99	0		-	-	
Thailand, Chiang Mai	99	0		-	-	
Thailand, Khon Kaen	99	0		-	-	
Viet Nam, Hanoi	99			99		

+ IMPORTANT-SEE NOTES ON POPULATION PAGE

INDICES OF DATA QUALITY
Mesothelioma (contd)

	MALE			FEMALE		
EUROPE	MV	DCO	M/I	MV	DCO	M/I
Austria, Tyrol	99	0		83	0	
+Belarus	98	2		97	3	
Croatia	99	0		99	0	
+Czech Republic	65	0		67	0	
Denmark	99	0		99	0	
Estonia	99			99		
Finland	99	0		99	0	
France, Bas-Rhin	99			99		
France, Calvados	99			99		
France, Doubs	95			83		
France, Haut-Rhin	99			80		
France, Herault	99			99		
France, Isere	99			99		
France, Somme	99			99		
France, Tarn	99			99		
Germany, Eastern States	99	0		98	2	
+Germany, Saarland	-	-		-	-	
Iceland	99	0		-	-	
Ireland, Southern	99			99		
Italy, Ferrara	99	0		-	-	
Italy, Florence	86	5		83	8	
Italy, Genoa	88	0		75	0	
Italy, Latina	99	0		99	0	
Italy, Macerata	99	0		99	0	
Italy, Modena	99	0		99	0	
Italy, Parma	88	6		99	0	
Italy, Ragusa	99	0		-	-	
Italy, Romagna	99	0		99	0	
Italy, Torino	93	0		99	0	
Italy, Trieste	99	0		99	0	
Italy, Varese	93	0		94	0	
Italy, Veneto	99	0		99	0	
+Latvia	-	-		-	-	
+Malta	-	-		-	-	
The Netherlands	99			99		
The Netherlands, Eindhoven	99			99		
The Netherlands, Maastricht	99			99		
Norway	99	0		99	0	
Poland, Cracow	99	0		99	0	
Poland, Kielce	99	0		99	0	
Poland, Lower Silesia	47	0		14	0	
Poland, Warsaw City	[99]	0		[99]	0	
Slovakia	99	0		99	0	
Slovenia	99	0		99	0	
Spain, Albacete	50	0		99	0	
Spain, Asturias	99	0		99	0	
Spain, Basque Country	81	11		85	8	
Spain, Granada	99	0		99	0	
Spain, Mallorca	99	0		99	0	
Spain, Murcia	99	0		99	0	
Spain, Navarra	99	0		99	0	
Spain, Tarragona	99	0		99	0	
Spain, Zaragoza	96	0		83	0	

	MALE			FEMALE		
	MV	DCO	M/I	MV	DCO	M/I
Sweden	99			99		
Switzerland, Basel	99	0		99	0	
Switzerland, Geneva	99	0		99	0	
Switzerland, Graubunden	99	0		-	-	
Switzerland, Neuchatel	86	0		99	0	
Switzerland, St Gall-Appenzell	99	0		99	0	
Switzerland, Valais	99	0		99	0	
Switzerland, Vaud	99	0		99	0	
Switzerland, Zurich	99	0		99	0	
+UK, England and Wales	[87]			[88]		
UK, East Anglia						
UK, Mersey	70	0		68	0	
UK, North Western	68	7		67	9	
UK, Oxford	99	1		99	0	
UK, South Thames	66	20		79	18	
UK, South Western	52	40		53	33	
UK, Wessex	[99]	0		[99]	0	
+UK, West Midlands		-			-	
UK, Yorkshire	87	4		88	6	
UK, Scotland	82	0		83	0	
UK, Scotland, West	79	0		78	0	
Yugoslavia, Vojvodina	99	0		92	0	

	MALE			FEMALE		
OCEANIA	MV	DCO	M/I	MV	DCO	M/I
Australian Capital Territory	67	0		99	0	
Australia, New South Wales	93	1		94	0	
South Australia	81			84		
Australia, Tasmania	99			99		
Australia, Victoria	99	0		99	0	
Western Australia	90	1		96	0	
French Polynesia	0	99		-	-	
+New Zealand: Non-Maori	-	-		-	-	
+New Zealand: Maori	-	-		-	-	
US, Hawaii: White	94	0		99	0	
US, Hawaii: Japanese	99	0		-	-	
US, Hawaii: Hawaiian	80	0		-	-	
US, Hawaii: Filipino	99	0		-	-	
US, Hawaii: Chinese	99	0		-	-	

+ IMPORTANT-SEE NOTES ON POPULATION PAGE

[] CYTOLOGICAL VERIFICATION EXCLUDED

INDICES OF DATA QUALITY
Bone (ICD-9 170)

AFRICA

	MALE MV	DCO	M/I	FEMALE MV	DCO	M/I
Algeria, Setif	83			92		
France, La Reunion	94		31	99		62
Mali, Bamako	89	11		30	0	
Uganda, Kyadondo	50			75		
Zimbabwe, Harare: African	83	0		78	0	
Zimbabwe, Harare: European	99	0		-	-	

AMERICA, CENTRAL AND SOUTH

	MALE MV	DCO	M/I	FEMALE MV	DCO	M/I
Argentina, Concordia	83	17	17	99	0	0
Brazil, Belem	39	25	61	65	12	42
Brazil, Goiania	90	5	50	96	0	35
Brazil, Porto Alegre	68	0	39	76	0	38
Colombia, Cali	80	3	75	88	4	85
Costa Rica	85	15	77	60	23	119
Ecuador, Quito	78	4		63	19	
Peru, Lima	78	3		60	16	
Peru, Trujillo	86	14	14	80	0	20
US, Puerto Rico	81	11	52	92	4	20
Uruguay, Montevideo	86	14	68	82	18	64

AMERICA, NORTH

	MALE MV	DCO	M/I	FEMALE MV	DCO	M/I
Canada	82	1	45	78	1	38
Canada, Alberta	98	0	53	96	2	42
Canada, British Columbia	92	4	42	97	3	42
Canada, Manitoba	73	0	55	68	0	68
Canada, New Brunswick	94	0	88	91	9	45
Canada, Newfoundland	99	0	50	86	0	114
Canada, Northwest Territories	99	0	0	50	0	0
Canada, Nova Scotia	92	8	64	92	8	32
Canada, Ontario	80	1	32	71	0	30
Canada, Prince Edward Island	99	0	25	99	0	50
+Canada, Quebec	75	0	50	71	0	39
Canada, Saskatchewan	99	0	75	91	0	50
Canada, Yukon	-	-	-	-	-	-
+US, Cent. Calif.: Non-Hisp. White	95	2	49	94	0	36
+US, Cent. Calif.: Hispanic	99	0	64	99	0	27
US, Los Angeles: Non-Hisp. White	97	0	48	99	1	47
US, Los Angeles: Hispanic White	99	0		98	0	
US, Los Angeles: Black	99	0		99	0	
US, Los Angeles: Chinese	99	0		99	0	
US, Los Angeles: Filipino	99	0		99	0	
US, Los Angeles: Korean	99	0		99	0	
US, Los Angeles: Japanese	99	0		-	-	
US, San Francisco: Non-Hisp. White	99	0	56	95	5	49
US, San Francisco: Hispanic White	99	0	0	99	0	50
US, San Francisco: Black	99	0	43	99	0	33
US, San Francisco: Chinese	99	0	25	99	0	0
US, San Francisco: Filipino	99	0	0	99	0	100
US, San Francisco: Japanese	99	0	100	-	-	-
US, Connecticut: White	97	0	28	94	0	34
US, Connecticut: Black	80	0	20	99	0	50
US, Atlanta: White	99	0	43	99	0	21
US, Atlanta: Black	99	0	100	99	0	31
US, Iowa	97	1	47	97	0	43

	MALE MV	DCO	M/I	FEMALE MV	DCO	M/I
US, Central Louisiana: White	75	25	50	71	14	14
US, Central Louisiana: Black	-	-	ncr	99	0	0
US, New Orleans: White	94	6	31	99	0	63
US, New Orleans: Black	88	13	75	99	0	60
US, Detroit: White	98	0	38	95	4	61
US, Detroit: Black	99	0	58	88	0	29
US, New Mexico: Non-Hisp. White	94	0	61	99	0	40
US, New Mexico: Hispanic White	93	0	67	85	15	54
US, New Mexico: American Indian	99	0	100	99	0	50
US, Utah	97	0	32	99	0	30
US, Seattle	99	1	48	97	1	37
US, SEER: White	98	0	43	96	2	42
US, SEER: Black	97	0	59	96	0	28

ASIA

	MALE MV	DCO	M/I	FEMALE MV	DCO	M/I
+China, Qidong	83	2	70	86	0	62
+China, Shanghai	36	5	106	35	8	110
China, Tianjin	51	1	75	43	1	80
Hong Kong	55	6	61	50	4	59
India, Bangalore	88	4	15	86	7	12
India, Barshi, Paranda and Bhum	75	0		60	0	
India, Bombay	85	9	75	78	12	90
India, Karunagappally	50	50		99	0	
India, Madras	88	2	24	94	3	56
India, Trivandrum	75	25	50	99	0	0
Israel: All Jews	95			91		
Jews born in Israel	96			94		
Jews born in America or Europe	97			85		
Jews born in Africa or Asia	88			91		
Non-Jews	88			89		
Japan, Hiroshima	83	11	67	94	0	38
Japan, Miyagi	74	9	77	79	6	42
Japan, Nagasaki	80	10	115	87	9	96
Japan, Osaka	79	12	68	84	10	66
+Japan, Saga	73	20	60	77	23	62
Japan, Yamagata	60	20	100	47	35	53
Korea, Kangwha	71		14	50		100
Kuwait: Non-Kuwaitis	94	6		80	0	
Kuwait: Kuwaitis	86	14		90	10	
Philippines, Manila	53	39		55	31	
Singapore: Chinese	91	5		96	0	
Singapore: Malay	83	0		80	20	
Singapore: Indian	99	0		99	0	
Thailand, Chiang Mai	52	9		50	11	
Thailand, Khon Kaen	21	55		23	48	
Viet Nam, Hanoi	42			43		

+ IMPORTANT-SEE NOTES ON POPULATION PAGE

INDICES OF DATA QUALITY
Bone (ICD-9 170) (contd)

EUROPE	MALE MV	DCO	M/I	FEMALE MV	DCO	M/I
Austria, Tyrol	75	17	83	72	11	56
+Belarus	71	0	64	74	0	56
Croatia	85	12	46	88	11	47
+Czech Republic	73	6	121	73	6	121
Denmark	93	2	83	95	0	74
Estonia	67		107	74		92
Finland	98	0	61	96	1	47
France, Bas-Rhin	94		77	91		87
France, Calvados	99		147	99		82
France, Doubs	90		130	99		53
France, Haut-Rhin	99		167	99		75
France, Herault	97		129	99		92
France, Isere	92		79	99		53
France, Somme	75		238	86		114
France, Tarn	99		54	99		138
Germany, Eastern States	81	1	68	73	1	61
+Germany, Saarland	88	0	42	85	10	60
Iceland	99	0	50	99	0	133
Ireland, Southern	92		100	88		100
Italy, Ferrara	80	0	60	40	0	80
Italy, Florence	26	9	94	52	13	135
Italy, Genoa	74	0	137	67	14	95
Italy, Latina	70	30	200	99	0	267
Italy, Macerata	99	0	200	50	0	150
Italy, Modena	90	0	150	82	0	100
Italy, Parma	99	0	167	99	0	30
Italy, Ragusa	82	0	173	67	0	167
Italy, Romagna	75	0	88	75	6	75
Italy, Torino	61	11	167	71	18	135
Italy, Trieste	50	0	100	29	14	43
Italy, Varese	80	5	105	89	5	74
Italy, Veneto	82	5	114	73	18	109
+Latvia	83	3	61	69	4	56
+Malta	99	0	350	80	0	40
The Netherlands	98		58	99		58
The Netherlands, Eindhoven	96		43	99		38
The Netherlands, Maastricht	99		70	99		47
Norway	99	0	46	99	0	40
Poland, Cracow	65	30	78	89	11	68
Poland, Kielce	67	9	139	50	13	138
Poland, Lower Silesia	54	1	99	52	1	60
Poland, Warsaw City	[56]	19	144	[58]	19	110
Slovakia	67	1	87	61	1	74
Slovenia	82	15	174	97	3	113
Spain, Albacete	67	33	67	50	17	33
Spain, Asturias	77	15	100	71	19	162
Spain, Basque Country	84	14	70	84	14	79
Spain, Granada	76	10	129	76	18	106
Spain, Mallorca	73	27	145	99	0	156
Spain, Murcia	83	10	90	73	20	133
Spain, Navarra	82	18	77	82	18	73
Spain, Tarragona	73	27	200	81	19	75
Spain, Zaragoza	73	23	95	80	10	120

	MALE MV	DCO	M/I	FEMALE MV	DCO	M/I
Sweden	99		64	99		76
Switzerland, Basel	99	0	33	99	0	53
Switzerland, Geneva	92	0	33	99	0	75
Switzerland, Graubunden	75	0	50	99	0	0
Switzerland, Neuchatel	99	0	0	99	0	50
Switzerland, St Gall-Appenzell	94	0	47	99	0	47
Switzerland, Valais	99	0	33	99	0	0
Switzerland, Vaud	99	0	50	86	0	43
Switzerland, Zurich	99	0	47	91	0	44
+UK, England and Wales	[87]		47	[84]		48
UK, East Anglia			45			48
UK, Mersey	87	2	70	76	0	103
UK, North Western	75	1	74	76	2	68
UK, Oxford	99	0	55	98	0	58
UK, South Thames	75	10	51	79	13	56
UK, South Western	79	1	56	81	0	48
UK, Wessex	[63]	1	46	[57]	2	41
+UK, West Midlands		0	23		1	25
UK, Yorkshire	90	1	58	89	2	64
UK, Scotland	91	1	68	87	2	49
UK, Scotland, West	91	1	76	90	3	41
Yugoslavia, Vojvodina	52	14	93	38	11	92

OCEANIA

	MALE MV	DCO	M/I	FEMALE MV	DCO	M/I
Australian Capital Territory	91	0		99	0	
Australia, New South Wales	98	0		99	1	
South Australia	68		54	75		29
Australia, Tasmania	90		120	86		14
Australia, Victoria	97	0	63	92	2	66
Western Australia	92	2	27	95	3	30
French Polynesia	25	38		29	57	
+New Zealand: Non-Maori	97	0	58	92	0	57
+New Zealand: Maori	93	0	47	99	0	71
US, Hawaii: White	99	0	60	99	0	67
US, Hawaii: Japanese	99	0	0	99	0	40
US, Hawaii: Hawaiian	99	0	40	99	0	167
US, Hawaii: Filipino	99	0	14	99	0	0
US, Hawaii: Chinese	99	0	100	-	-	-

+ IMPORTANT-SEE NOTES ON POPULATION PAGE

[] CYTOLOGICAL VERIFICATION EXCLUDED

INDICES OF DATA QUALITY
Connective tissue (ICD-9 171)

AFRICA	MALE MV	DCO	M/I	FEMALE MV	DCO	M/I
Algeria, Setif	99			86		
France, La Reunion	99		60	99		31
Mali, Bamako	80	0		67	0	
Uganda, Kyadondo	75			75		
Zimbabwe, Harare: African	99	0		86	14	
Zimbabwe, Harare: European	99	0		99	0	

AMERICA, CENTRAL AND SOUTH

	MALE MV	DCO	M/I	FEMALE MV	DCO	M/I
Argentina, Concordia	99	0	50	99	0	0
Brazil, Belem	91	5	23	84	6	31
Brazil, Goiania	99	0	53	97	3	15
Brazil, Porto Alegre	79	0	36	82	0	22
Colombia, Cali	91	2	25	94	2	28
Costa Rica	90	6	33	90	3	24
Ecuador, Quito	84	3		75	16	
Peru, Lima	89	1		86	3	
Peru, Trujillo	99	0	57	83	0	100
US, Puerto Rico	99	0	37	96	2	49
Uruguay, Montevideo	90	6	60	95	1	40

AMERICA, NORTH

	MALE MV	DCO	M/I	FEMALE MV	DCO	M/I
Canada	88	0	40	87	1	42
Canada, Alberta	97	0	53	99	1	62
Canada, British Columbia	98	2	39	95	2	41
Canada, Manitoba	97	0	53	94	0	86
Canada, New Brunswick	95	2	43	99	0	45
Canada, Newfoundland	99	0	42	99	0	95
Canada, Northwest Territories	75	0	75	99	0	200
Canada, Nova Scotia	99	0	31	97	3	38
Canada, Ontario	86	0	34	83	1	35
Canada, Prince Edward Island	99	0	45	80	20	100
+Canada, Quebec	80	0	43	80	0	39
Canada, Saskatchewan	98	0	48	99	0	39
Canada, Yukon	-	-	-	99	0	0
+US, Cent. Calif.: Non-Hisp. White	99	0	54	99	0	58
+US, Cent. Calif.: Hispanic	96	0	44	95	5	55
US, Los Angeles: Non-Hisp. White	99	1	50	99	0	59
US, Los Angeles: Hispanic White	99	0		99	0	
US, Los Angeles: Black	99	0		98	0	
US, Los Angeles: Chinese	89	0		99	0	
US, Los Angeles: Filipino	99	0		99	0	
US, Los Angeles: Korean	99	0		99	0	
US, Los Angeles: Japanese	99	0		99	0	
US, San Francisco: Non-Hisp. White	99	0	51	97	2	64
US, San Francisco: Hispanic White	99	0	35	99	0	44
US, San Francisco: Black	97	0	47	99	0	81
US, San Francisco: Chinese	99	0	50	99	0	56
US, San Francisco: Filipino	80	20	60	99	0	80
US, San Francisco: Japanese	99	0	0	99	0	100
US, Connecticut: White	97	1	45	98	1	66
US, Connecticut: Black	99	0	38	99	0	50
US, Atlanta: White	97	1	44	99	0	49
US, Atlanta: Black	99	0	55	97	0	63
US, Iowa	99	1	46	99	1	57

	MALE MV	DCO	M/I	FEMALE MV	DCO	M/I
US, Central Louisiana: White	99	0	56	99	0	30
US, Central Louisiana: Black	99	0	50	88	0	50
US, New Orleans: White	98	2	65	98	0	54
US, New Orleans: Black	91	9	55	99	0	50
US, Detroit: White	99	0	44	99	0	45
US, Detroit: Black	98	2	57	99	0	98
US, New Mexico: Non-Hisp. White	99	0	45	95	5	34
US, New Mexico: Hispanic White	99	0	43	96	0	32
US, New Mexico: American Indian	99	0	60	99	0	71
US, Utah	99	0	50	99	0	60
US, Seattle	99	0	43	98	1	64
US, SEER: White	99	1	46	98	1	56
US, SEER: Black	99	1	50	98	0	78

ASIA

	MALE MV	DCO	M/I	FEMALE MV	DCO	M/I
+China, Qidong	99	0	56	67	17	50
+China, Shanghai	73	1	40	75	0	37
China, Tianjin	83	0	28	81	0	23
Hong Kong	87	2	18	80	1	12
India, Bangalore	97	1	16	97	3	11
India, Barshi, Paranda and Bhum	99	0		99	0	
India, Bombay	94	3	20	92	2	28
India, Karunagappally	80	20		99	0	
India, Madras	98	0	36	95	0	24
India, Trivandrum	91	9	55	99	0	0
Israel: All Jews	92			90		
Jews born in Israel	95			94		
Jews born in America or Europe	89			89		
Jews born in Africa or Asia	95			93		
Non-Jews	99			93		
Japan, Hiroshima	91	3	45	94	0	19
Japan, Miyagi	92	3	37	87	4	42
Japan, Nagasaki	91	5	56	89	7	45
Japan, Osaka	96	2	56	97	1	60
+Japan, Saga	76	18	88	67	25	83
Japan, Yamagata	59	38	62	68	18	50
Korea, Kangwha	-	-	-	-	-	-
Kuwait: Non-Kuwaitis	97	0		99	0	
Kuwait: Kuwaitis	99	0		99	0	
Philippines, Manila	82	8		82	9	
Singapore: Chinese	98	1		97	2	
Singapore: Malay	99	0		91	9	
Singapore: Indian	99	0		99	0	
Thailand, Chiang Mai	88	0		99	0	
Thailand, Khon Kaen	88	0		74	0	
Viet Nam, Hanoi	62			78		

+ IMPORTANT-SEE NOTES ON POPULATION PAGE

INDICES OF DATA QUALITY
Connective tissue (ICD-9 171) (contd)

	MALE			FEMALE		
EUROPE	MV	DCO	M/I	MV	DCO	M/I
Austria, Tyrol	95	2	61	90	8	52
+Belarus	92	0	54	92	0	45
Croatia	93	4	56	87	8	53
+Czech Republic	87	0	44	86	1	42
Denmark	99	0	34	99	0	44
Estonia	97		61	95		69
Finland	99	0	32	98	0	33
France, Bas-Rhin	99		63	99		75
France, Calvados	96		56	99		52
France, Doubs	99		37	99		34
France, Haut-Rhin	99		27	99		23
France, Herault	99		42	99		31
France, Isere	99		35	95		11
France, Somme	99		45	99		65
France, Tarn	99		39	99		22
Germany, Eastern States	98	0	51	99	0	48
+Germany, Saarland	88	8	76	91	6	80
Iceland	99	0	50	99	0	78
Ireland, Southern	99		48	99		27
Italy, Ferrara	99	0	45	90	0	30
Italy, Florence	89	2	32	88	0	26
Italy, Genoa	94	1	36	95	0	32
Italy, Latina	94	0	19	99	0	29
Italy, Macerata	90	0	30	99	0	54
Italy, Modena	97	0	47	93	3	69
Italy, Parma	96	4	30	93	7	17
Italy, Ragusa	99	0	64	99	0	33
Italy, Romagna	81	0	42	93	0	37
Italy, Torino	91	4	43	98	3	45
Italy, Trieste	72	0	36	90	0	40
Italy, Varese	99	0	23	98	0	28
Italy, Veneto	97	3	24	92	2	31
+Latvia	94	1	63	93	1	41
+Malta	71	0	71	88	13	88
The Netherlands	99		42	99		54
The Netherlands, Eindhoven	99		42	99		75
The Netherlands, Maastricht	99		41	99		43
Norway	98	1	63	99	0	56
Poland, Cracow	81	15	65	96	4	50
Poland, Kielce	86	2	18	91	0	35
Poland, Lower Silesia	69	1	44	73	1	33
Poland, Warsaw City	[90]	1	18	[83]	6	26
Slovakia	96	0	56	94	1	45
Slovenia	99	0	39	94	5	49
Spain, Albacete	99	0	18	63	25	38
Spain, Asturias	98	0	38	98	2	38
Spain, Basque Country	92	0	38	94	1	36
Spain, Granada	99	0	40	99	0	30
Spain, Mallorca	99	0	39	99	0	34
Spain, Murcia	91	2	41	99	0	33
Spain, Navarra	96	4	54	96	4	58
Spain, Tarragona	99	0	22	96	4	36
Spain, Zaragoza	91	7	50	99	0	60

	MALE			FEMALE		
	MV	DCO	M/I	MV	DCO	M/I
Sweden	99		38	99		45
Switzerland, Basel	99	0	56	99	0	43
Switzerland, Geneva	95	0	30	96	4	33
Switzerland, Graubunden	99	0	70	99	0	57
Switzerland, Neuchatel	99	0	0	99	0	0
Switzerland, St Gall-Appenzell	97	0	37	99	0	38
Switzerland, Valais	99	0	23	95	0	38
Switzerland, Vaud	99	0	20	98	2	35
Switzerland, Zurich	99	1	28	99	0	30
+UK, England and Wales	[87]		45	[83]		46
UK, East Anglia			46			56
UK, Mersey	92	2	46	87	1	49
UK, North Western	87	2	53	85	1	57
UK, Oxford	98	0	38	96	0	47
UK, South Thames	74	12	51	71	15	55
UK, South Western	90	0	48	89	1	57
UK, Wessex	[79]	0	39	[75]	0	37
+UK, West Midlands		1	35		1	31
UK, Yorkshire	97	0	35	96	1	54
UK, Scotland	94	1	48	93	2	59
UK, Scotland, West	94	1	44	94	2	55
Yugoslavia, Vojvodina	77	1	33	81	5	27

	MALE			FEMALE		
OCEANIA	MV	DCO	M/I	MV	DCO	M/I
Australian Capital Territory	99	0		86	0	
Australia, New South Wales	96	1		97	1	
South Australia	96		57	86		63
Australia, Tasmania	99		36	99		43
Australia, Victoria	95	0	51	95	1	57
Western Australia	98	0	45	98	0	64
French Polynesia	83	0		99	0	
+New Zealand: Non-Maori	96	2	28	98	1	39
+New Zealand: Maori	88	6	50	99	0	29
US, Hawaii: White	99	0	26	99	0	31
US, Hawaii: Japanese	99	0	43	99	0	67
US, Hawaii: Hawaiian	99	0	31	99	0	58
US, Hawaii: Filipino	99	0	50	99	0	13
US, Hawaii: Chinese	99	0	0	99	0	60

+ IMPORTANT-SEE NOTES ON POPULATION PAGE

[] CYTOLOGICAL VERIFICATION EXCLUDED

INDICES OF DATA QUALITY
Melanoma of skin (ICD-9 172)

	MALE			FEMALE		
	MV	DCO	M/I	MV	DCO	M/I
AFRICA						
Algeria, Setif	99			99		
France, La Reunion	99		82	99		31
Mali, Bamako	99	0		99	0	
Uganda, Kyadondo	80			99		
Zimbabwe, Harare: African	93	7		85	8	
Zimbabwe, Harare: European	95	0		88	12	
AMERICA, CENTRAL AND SOUTH						
Argentina, Concordia	99	0	0	99	0	13
Brazil, Belem	99	0	7	99	0	21
Brazil, Goiania	92	8	17	91	4	22
Brazil, Porto Alegre	82	0	37	80	0	31
Colombia, Cali	97	1	22	98	0	19
Costa Rica	91	4	35	92	6	25
Ecuador, Quito	88	3		91	3	
Peru, Lima	72	4		66	0	
Peru, Trujillo	99	0	33	99	0	0
US, Puerto Rico	99	0	34	93	2	25
Uruguay, Montevideo	99	0	45	99	0	30
AMERICA, NORTH						
Canada	94	0	25	93	0	16
Canada, Alberta	99	0	23	99	0	13
Canada, British Columbia	99	1	21	99	0	14
Canada, Manitoba	99	0	18	99	0	20
Canada, New Brunswick	99	1	26	99	0	11
Canada, Newfoundland	99	0	19	99	0	5
Canada, Northwest Territories	67	0	33	99	0	0
Canada, Nova Scotia	99	0	27	99	1	13
Canada, Ontario	97	0	24	96	0	16
Canada, Prince Edward Island	99	0	33	99	0	13
+Canada, Quebec	63	0	36	62	0	28
Canada, Saskatchewan	99	0	19	99	0	16
Canada, Yukon	99	0	11	99	0	0
+US, Cent. Calif.: Non-Hisp. White	98	1	32	98	1	23
+US, Cent. Calif.: Hispanic	95	0	22	98	0	23
US, Los Angeles: Non-Hisp. White	99	0	26	99	0	21
US, Los Angeles: Hispanic White	99	0		99	0	
US, Los Angeles: Black	99	0		99	0	
US, Los Angeles: Chinese	-	-		75	25	
US, Los Angeles: Filipino	75	0		99	0	
US, Los Angeles: Korean	-	-		99	0	
US, Los Angeles: Japanese	99	0		99	0	
US, San Francisco: Non-Hisp. White	99	0	21	99	0	19
US, San Francisco: Hispanic White	99	0	10	99	0	3
US, San Francisco: Black	99	0	50	99	0	88
US, San Francisco: Chinese	99	0	100	99	0	67
US, San Francisco: Filipino	75	0	50	99	0	0
US, San Francisco: Japanese	99	0	0	99	0	0
US, Connecticut: White	99	0	18	99	0	16
US, Connecticut: Black	99	0	50	99	0	14
US, Atlanta: White	99	0	19	99	0	11
US, Atlanta: Black	99	0	63	99	0	75
US, Iowa	99	0	26	99	0	20

	MALE			FEMALE		
	MV	DCO	M/I	MV	DCO	M/I
US, Central Louisiana: White	98	2	40	97	2	19
US, Central Louisiana: Black	-	-	-	99	0	0
US, New Orleans: White	98	0	37	98	0	33
US, New Orleans: Black	86	14	29	0	99	100
US, Detroit: White	99	0	21	99	0	18
US, Detroit: Black	99	0	46	91	9	45
US, New Mexico: Non-Hisp. White	99	0	20	99	0	18
US, New Mexico: Hispanic White	97	0	22	98	0	29
US, New Mexico: American Indian	99	0	75	99	0	33
US, Utah	99	0	25	99	0	16
US, Seattle	99	0	21	99	0	14
US, SEER: White	99	0	21	99	0	17
US, SEER: Black	99	0	48	97	3	53
ASIA						
+China, Qidong	99	0	50	82	0	45
+China, Shanghai	69	1	53	78	3	66
China, Tianjin	95	0	46	67	0	37
Hong Kong	69	1	25	61	0	19
India, Bangalore	90	5	10	93	0	21
India, Barshi, Paranda and Bhum	-	-		99	0	
India, Bombay	91	4	26	98	0	28
India, Karunagappally	99	0		-	-	
India, Madras	96	0	33	99	0	25
India, Trivandrum	99	0	50	99	0	0
Israel: All Jews	95			94		
Jews born in Israel	96			95		
Jews born in America or Europe	95			93		
Jews born in Africa or Asia	93			94		
Non-Jews	90			88		
Japan, Hiroshima	99	0	46	69	0	50
Japan, Miyagi	83	5	67	88	8	54
Japan, Nagasaki	96	0	68	90	3	35
Japan, Osaka	99	0	59	99	0	52
+Japan, Saga	78	6	39	81	14	67
Japan, Yamagata	90	5	71	73	18	68
Korea, Kangwha	99		0	99		0
Kuwait: Non-Kuwaitis	99	0		99	0	
Kuwait: Kuwaitis	99	0		99	0	
Philippines, Manila	94	0		92	3	
Singapore: Chinese	96	4		99	0	
Singapore: Malay	99	0		50	0	
Singapore: Indian	-	-		-	-	
Thailand, Chiang Mai	99	0		99	0	
Thailand, Khon Kaen	99	0		99	0	
Viet Nam, Hanoi	90			99		

+ IMPORTANT-SEE NOTES ON POPULATION PAGE

INDICES OF DATA QUALITY
Melanoma of skin (ICD-9 172) (contd)

EUROPE

	MALE			FEMALE		
	MV	DCO	M/I	MV	DCO	M/I
Austria, Tyrol	98	2	12	98	1	13
+Belarus	95	0	53	95	0	43
Croatia	93	7	56	94	6	50
+Czech Republic	91	1	46	92	1	34
Denmark	99	0	37	99	0	23
Estonia	99		51	97		45
Finland	99	0	28	99	0	22
France, Bas-Rhin	99		22	99		20
France, Calvados	99		45	99		29
France, Doubs	99		25	99		14
France, Haut-Rhin	99		20	99		20
France, Herault	99		22	99		16
France, Isere	99		16	99		10
France, Somme	99		33	99		24
France, Tarn	99		41	99		20
Germany, Eastern States	99	0	31	99	0	25
+Germany, Saarland	97	3	34	96	3	25
Iceland	99	0	31	99	0	8
Ireland, Southern	99		18	99		22
Italy, Ferrara	95	0	47	99	0	39
Italy, Florence	89	1	39	92	0	26
Italy, Genoa	86	2	47	95	1	26
Italy, Latina	99	0	50	99	0	36
Italy, Macerata	99	0	22	79	0	50
Italy, Modena	98	2	42	98	2	34
Italy, Parma	99	0	39	99	0	40
Italy, Ragusa	98	0	35	99	0	25
Italy, Romagna	99	0	28	99	0	28
Italy, Torino	98	0	36	98	1	33
Italy, Trieste	82	2	43	86	6	29
Italy, Varese	98	1	46	99	0	24
Italy, Veneto	99	0	33	99	0	22
+Latvia	99	0	46	97	1	35
+Malta	90	0	50	99	0	25
The Netherlands	99		29	99		19
The Netherlands, Eindhoven	99		29	99		19
The Netherlands, Maastricht	99		33	99		14
Norway	99	0	28	99	0	17
Poland, Cracow	94	1	51	92	3	54
Poland, Kielce	85	5	65	85	1	46
Poland, Lower Silesia	75	0	47	85	0	51
Poland, Warsaw City	[88]	5	55	[87]	5	53
Slovakia	99	0	48	98	0	39
Slovenia	99	0	69	99	0	46
Spain, Albacete	86	0	71	80	20	60
Spain, Asturias	98	0	62	99	0	32
Spain, Basque Country	99	1	31	98	2	21
Spain, Granada	96	0	26	99	1	17
Spain, Mallorca	99	0	35	99	0	25
Spain, Murcia	96	2	44	99	1	21
Spain, Navarra	97	2	50	97	0	15
Spain, Tarragona	97	2	30	97	3	19
Spain, Zaragoza	93	4	54	92	0	19
Sweden	99		27	99		19
Switzerland, Basel	99	0	21	99	0	21
Switzerland, Geneva	99	0	26	99	0	14
Switzerland, Graubunden	99	0	0	99	0	14
Switzerland, Neuchatel	99	0	13	99	0	19
Switzerland, St Gall-Appenzell	99	0	30	99	0	25
Switzerland, Valais	97	3	52	99	0	17
Switzerland, Vaud	99	0	29	99	0	15
Switzerland, Zurich	99	0	20	99	0	19
+UK, England and Wales	[95]		34	[95]		25
UK, East Anglia			28			27
UK, Mersey	96	0	36	97	1	33
UK, North Western	90	1	35	89	1	22
UK, Oxford	99	0	28	99	0	20
UK, South Thames	86	7	40	87	6	30
UK, South Western	97	0	25	96	0	22
UK, Wessex	[87]	3	35	[86]	2	20
+UK, West Midlands		0	31		0	24
UK, Yorkshire	98	1	33	98	1	21
UK, Scotland	99	0	26	99	0	15
UK, Scotland, West	99	0	24	99	0	17
Yugoslavia, Vojvodina	76	6	62	76	6	44

OCEANIA

	MALE			FEMALE		
	MV	DCO	M/I	MV	DCO	M/I
Australian Capital Territory	99	0		99	1	
Australia, New South Wales	99	0		99	0	
South Australia	87		16	86		11
Australia, Tasmania	99		15	99		15
Australia, Victoria	99	0	18	99	0	13
Western Australia	99	0	13	98	0	12
French Polynesia	99	0		99	0	
+New Zealand: Non-Maori	99	1	22	99	0	13
+New Zealand: Maori	95	5	14	99	0	15
US, Hawaii: White	99	0	19	99	0	13
US, Hawaii: Japanese	99	0	67	99	0	25
US, Hawaii: Hawaiian	99	0	67	99	0	40
US, Hawaii: Filipino	99	0	100	99	0	67
US, Hawaii: Chinese	99	0	50	99	0	100

+ IMPORTANT-SEE NOTES ON POPULATION PAGE

[] CYTOLOGICAL VERIFICATION EXCLUDED

INDICES OF DATA QUALITY
Other skin (ICD-9 173)

	MALE			FEMALE		
	MV	DCO	M/I	MV	DCO	M/I
AFRICA						
Algeria, Setif	97			99		
France, La Reunion	99			99		
Mali, Bamako	78	0		91	0	
Uganda, Kyadondo	87			60		
Zimbabwe, Harare: African	91	0		92	0	
Zimbabwe, Harare: European	99	0		99	0	
AMERICA, CENTRAL AND SOUTH						
Argentina, Concordia	98	2		99	1	
Brazil, Belem	99	1		99	1	
Brazil, Goiania	98	0		99	0	
Brazil, Porto Alegre	99	0		98	0	
Colombia, Cali	-	-		99	0	
Costa Rica	96	0		97	0	
Ecuador, Quito	97	1		97	1	
Peru, Lima	93	0		94	1	
Peru, Trujillo	96	0		98	0	
US, Puerto Rico	84	16		91	9	
Uruguay, Montevideo	97	1		97	1	
AMERICA, NORTH						
Canada						
Canada, Alberta						
Canada, British Columbia						
Canada, Manitoba						
Canada, New Brunswick						
Canada, Newfoundland						
Canada, Northwest Territories						
Canada, Nova Scotia						
Canada, Ontario						
Canada, Prince Edward Island						
+Canada, Quebec						
Canada, Saskatchewan						
Canada, Yukon						
+US, Cent. Calif.: Non-Hisp. White	99	0		99	0	
+US, Cent. Calif.: Hispanic	99	0		99	0	
US, Los Angeles: Non-Hisp. White	99	0		99	0	
US, Los Angeles: Hispanic White	99	0		99	0	
US, Los Angeles: Black	99	0		99	0	
US, Los Angeles: Chinese	99	0		99	0	
US, Los Angeles: Filipino	99	0		99	0	
US, Los Angeles: Korean	-	-		99	0	
US, Los Angeles: Japanese	99	0		99	0	
US, San Francisco: Non-Hisp. White	99	0		99	0	
US, San Francisco: Hispanic White	99	0		99	0	
US, San Francisco: Black	99	0		99	0	
US, San Francisco: Chinese	99	0		99	0	
US, San Francisco: Filipino	-	-		99	0	
US, San Francisco: Japanese	-	-		-	-	
US, Connecticut: White	99	0		99	0	
US, Connecticut: Black	99	0		99	0	
US, Atlanta: White	97	3		99	0	
US, Atlanta: Black	99	0		99	0	
US, Iowa	99	0		98	0	

	MALE			FEMALE		
	MV	DCO	M/I	MV	DCO	M/I
US, Central Louisiana: White	99	0		99	0	
US, Central Louisiana: Black	-	-		99	0	
US, New Orleans: White	99	0		99	0	
US, New Orleans: Black	99	0		99	0	
US, Detroit: White	99	0		99	0	
US, Detroit: Black	99	0		99	0	
US, New Mexico: Non-Hisp. White	99	0		99	0	
US, New Mexico: Hispanic White	99	0		99	0	
US, New Mexico: American Indian	-	-		99	0	
US, Utah	99	0		99	0	
US, Seattle	99	0		99	0	
US, SEER: White	99	0		99	0	
US, SEER: Black	99	0		99	0	
ASIA						
+China, Qidong	93	0		94	0	
+China, Shanghai	78	1		77	1	
China, Tianjin	84	0		93	0	
Hong Kong	96	0		95	0	
India, Bangalore	93	2		96	2	
India, Barshi, Paranda and Bhum	83	0		99	0	
India, Bombay	95	1		95	2	
India, Karunagappally	99	0		99	0	
India, Madras	93	1		96	0	
India, Trivandrum	99	0		88	0	
Israel: All Jews	94			95		
Jews born in Israel	97			99		
Jews born in America or Europe	92			94		
Jews born in Africa or Asia	98			93		
Non-Jews	99			89		
Japan, Hiroshima	97	0		99	1	
Japan, Miyagi	93	3		95	3	
Japan, Nagasaki	99	0		98	2	
Japan, Osaka	93	3		91	6	
+Japan, Saga	89	3		92	6	
Japan, Yamagata	88	5		88	2	
Korea, Kangwha	99			99		
Kuwait: Non-Kuwaitis	98	2		95	0	
Kuwait: Kuwaitis	99	0		99	0	
Philippines, Manila	84	8		81	9	
Singapore: Chinese	99	0		99	1	
Singapore: Malay	97	3		99	0	
Singapore: Indian	99	0		99	0	
Thailand, Chiang Mai	98	1		98	2	
Thailand, Khon Kaen	82	6		86	2	
Viet Nam, Hanoi	72			67		

+ IMPORTANT-SEE NOTES ON POPULATION PAGE

INDICES OF DATA QUALITY
Other skin (ICD-9 173) (contd)

EUROPE	MALE MV	DCO	M/I	FEMALE MV	DCO	M/I
Austria, Tyrol	99	1		99	0	
+Belarus	95	0		94	0	
Croatia	38	55		43	53	
+Czech Republic	96	0		94	0	
Denmark	99	0		99	0	
Estonia	93			90		
Finland	99	0		99	0	
France, Bas-Rhin	99			99		
France, Calvados	99			99		
France, Doubs	99			99		
France, Haut-Rhin	99			99		
France, Herault	99			98		
France, Isere	99			99		
France, Somme	99			99		
France, Tarn	99			99		
Germany, Eastern States	98	0		96	0	
+Germany, Saarland	99	0		98	0	
Iceland	99	0		99	0	
Ireland, Southern	67			69		
Italy, Ferrara	99	0		99	0	
Italy, Florence	53	0		54	0	
Italy, Genoa	92	0		90	0	
Italy, Latina	99	0		99	1	
Italy, Macerata	98	0		96	0	
Italy, Modena	99	0		99	0	
Italy, Parma	99	0		99	0	
Italy, Ragusa	98	0		99	0	
Italy, Romagna	98	0		98	0	
Italy, Torino	99	0		99	0	
Italy, Trieste	94	0		93	0	
Italy, Varese	98	0		97	0	
Italy, Veneto	99	0		98	1	
+Latvia	99	0		98	0	
+Malta	88	1		87	0	
The Netherlands	99			99		
The Netherlands, Eindhoven	-			-		
The Netherlands, Maastricht	99			99		
Norway	99	0		99	0	
Poland, Cracow	87	1		86	2	
Poland, Kielce	89	1		90	1	
Poland, Lower Silesia	95	0		95	0	
Poland, Warsaw City	[90]	1		[87]	2	
Slovakia	95	0		93	0	
Slovenia	98	1		96	1	
Spain, Albacete	75	25		99	0	
Spain, Asturias	94	6		68	28	
Spain, Basque Country	93	7		82	14	
Spain, Granada	97	0		95	1	
Spain, Mallorca	99	0		99	0	
Spain, Murcia	99	0		99	0	
Spain, Navarra	97	0		97	0	
Spain, Tarragona	99	0		99	1	
Spain, Zaragoza	96	1		93	2	

	MALE MV	DCO	M/I	FEMALE MV	DCO	M/I
Sweden	99			99		
Switzerland, Basel	99	0		99	0	
Switzerland, Geneva	99	0		99	0	
Switzerland, Graubunden	99	0		99	0	
Switzerland, Neuchatel	99	0		99	0	
Switzerland, St Gall-Appenzell	99	0		99	0	
Switzerland, Valais	99	0		99	0	
Switzerland, Vaud	99	0		99	0	
Switzerland, Zurich	99	0		99	0	
+UK, England and Wales	[91]			[90]		
UK, East Anglia						
UK, Mersey	91	0		90	0	
UK, North Western	64	0		60	0	
UK, Oxford	98	0		99	0	
UK, South Thames	81	1		80	1	
UK, South Western	97	0		97	0	
UK, Wessex	[56]	0		[53]	0	
+UK, West Midlands		0			0	
UK, Yorkshire	97	0		96	0	
UK, Scotland	94	0		93	1	
UK, Scotland, West	97	0		96	0	
Yugoslavia, Vojvodina	93	1		91	0	

OCEANIA

	MALE MV	DCO	M/I	FEMALE MV	DCO	M/I
Australian Capital Territory						
Australia, New South Wales						
South Australia						
Australia, Tasmania						
Australia, Victoria						
Western Australia						
French Polynesia						
+New Zealand: Non-Maori	99	0		-	-	
+New Zealand: Maori	-	-		-	-	
US, Hawaii: White	99	0		99	0	
US, Hawaii: Japanese	99	0		99	0	
US, Hawaii: Hawaiian	99	0		99	0	
US, Hawaii: Filipino	99	0		99	0	
US, Hawaii: Chinese	99	0		-	-	

+ IMPORTANT-SEE NOTES ON POPULATION PAGE

[] CYTOLOGICAL VERIFICATION EXCLUDED

INDICES OF DATA QUALITY
Breast (ICD-9 174/175)

	MALE			FEMALE		
	MV	DCO	M/I	MV	DCO	M/I
AFRICA						
Algeria, Setif	99			89		
France, La Reunion	99		40	99		29
Mali, Bamako	33	0		48	3	
Uganda, Kyadondo	17			58		
Zimbabwe, Harare: African	80	20		87	4	
Zimbabwe, Harare: European	-	-		93	5	
AMERICA, CENTRAL AND SOUTH						
Argentina, Concordia	99	0	0	86	13	29
Brazil, Belem	99	0	0	90	7	30
Brazil, Goiania	99	0	50	90	5	30
Brazil, Porto Alegre	83	0	50	72	1	38
Colombia, Cali	99	0	40	91	2	33
Costa Rica	99	0	8	89	4	40
Ecuador, Quito	50	17		79	8	
Peru, Lima	88	0		76	4	
Peru, Trujillo	99	0	0	81	1	32
US, Puerto Rico	96	0	52	98	1	29
Uruguay, Montevideo	68	21	47	84	8	33
AMERICA, NORTH						
Canada	92	1	34	93	1	32
Canada, Alberta	97	3	33	98	1	31
Canada, British Columbia	96	4	33	97	2	27
Canada, Manitoba	92	4	40	86	1	29
Canada, New Brunswick	99	0	44	98	1	33
Canada, Newfoundland	99	0	50	99	1	33
Canada, Northwest Territories	99	0	0	94	1	31
Canada, Nova Scotia	99	0	73	96	3	34
Canada, Ontario	96	1	31	95	1	33
Canada, Prince Edward Island	99	0	25	98	2	25
+Canada, Quebec	83	0	32	85	0	36
Canada, Saskatchewan	99	0	35	98	1	30
Canada, Yukon	99	0	0	99	0	22
+US, Cent. Calif.: Non-Hisp. White	99	0	44	98	1	25
+US, Cent. Calif.: Hispanic	99	0	17	99	0	24
US, Los Angeles: Non-Hisp. White	98	0	15	99	0	27
US, Los Angeles: Hispanic White	99	0		99	0	
US, Los Angeles: Black	99	0		99	0	
US, Los Angeles: Chinese	99	0		99	0	
US, Los Angeles: Filipino	-	-		99	0	
US, Los Angeles: Korean	-	-		99	0	
US, Los Angeles: Japanese	99	0		99	1	
US, San Francisco: Non-Hisp. White	98	0	25	98	1	26
US, San Francisco: Hispanic White	99	0	0	99	0	16
US, San Francisco: Black	99	0	31	98	0	34
US, San Francisco: Chinese	99	0	33	98	1	20
US, San Francisco: Filipino	99	0	0	99	0	20
US, San Francisco: Japanese	-	-	-	98	1	22
US, Connecticut: White	97	0	24	98	1	26
US, Connecticut: Black	99	0	67	98	1	30
US, Atlanta: White	99	0	27	99	0	24
US, Atlanta: Black	99	0	21	98	1	33
US, Iowa	99	0	38	98	1	28

	MALE			FEMALE		
	MV	DCO	M/I	MV	DCO	M/I
US, Central Louisiana: White	99	0	50	97	2	28
US, Central Louisiana: Black	99	0	50	97	2	40
US, New Orleans: White	99	0	33	98	1	28
US, New Orleans: Black	99	0	56	97	2	37
US, Detroit: White	99	1	26	98	1	28
US, Detroit: Black	95	0	68	98	0	36
US, New Mexico: Non-Hisp. White	99	0	43	98	1	27
US, New Mexico: Hispanic White	99	0	0	98	1	29
US, New Mexico: American Indian	99	0	0	99	0	26
US, Utah	99	0	21	99	0	26
US, Seattle	99	0	15	99	0	26
US, SEER: White	99	0	24	98	1	27
US, SEER: Black	98	0	42	98	1	34
ASIA						
+China, Qidong	99	0	0	95	0	28
+China, Shanghai	67	0	33	74	0	31
China, Tianjin	71	0	24	82	0	24
Hong Kong	78	2	16	86	2	28
India, Bangalore	83	6	17	87	2	30
India, Barshi, Paranda and Bhum	-	-		87	0	
India, Bombay	83	1	13	81	6	39
India, Karunagappally	-	-		91	0	
India, Madras	82	6	24	82	2	35
India, Trivandrum	99	0	0	94	2	17
Israel: All Jews	92			92		
Jews born in Israel	95			95		
Jews born in America or Europe	91			90		
Jews born in Africa or Asia	93			92		
Non-Jews	99			91		
Japan, Hiroshima	99	0	14	98	1	20
Japan, Miyagi	91	5	36	95	1	22
Japan, Nagasaki	75	13	38	96	2	24
Japan, Osaka	79	8	37	90	3	29
+Japan, Saga	99	0	13	85	6	32
Japan, Yamagata	99	0	33	91	6	24
Korea, Kangwha	99		0	83		30
Kuwait: Non-Kuwaitis	99	0		93	4	
Kuwait: Kuwaitis	-	-		92	5	
Philippines, Manila	66	12		78	9	
Singapore: Chinese	99	0		98	1	
Singapore: Malay	67	0		94	3	
Singapore: Indian	99	0		95	3	
Thailand, Chiang Mai	99	0		94	2	
Thailand, Khon Kaen	-	-		86	2	
Viet Nam, Hanoi	58			71		

+ IMPORTANT-SEE NOTES ON POPULATION PAGE

EUROPE	MALE MV	DCO	M/I	FEMALE MV	DCO	M/I
Austria, Tyrol	99	0	20	91	7	36
+Belarus	87	0	63	87	0	48
Croatia	67	11	55	74	5	52
+Czech Republic	78	1	50	81	2	52
Denmark	99	0	45	96	0	44
Estonia	99		35	92		49
Finland	99	0	24	99	0	29
France, Bas-Rhin	99		36	98		32
France, Calvados	95		33	98		33
France, Doubs	99		43	96		32
France, Haut-Rhin	99		29	99		31
France, Herault	99		58	96		32
France, Isere	97		39	97		16
France, Somme	99		54	98		39
France, Tarn	99		88	98		33
Germany, Eastern States	97	0	38	96	0	40
+Germany, Saarland	94	6	29	94	4	40
Iceland	99	0	29	99	0	32
Ireland, Southern	90		50	95		48
Italy, Ferrara	86	0	0	95	1	35
Italy, Florence	81	0	11	85	2	35
Italy, Genoa	94	0	11	91	2	41
Italy, Latina	99	0	0	93	6	41
Italy, Macerata	99	0	75	89	0	42
Italy, Modena	99	0	33	95	2	36
Italy, Parma	99	0	9	96	2	38
Italy, Ragusa	83	17	17	88	1	58
Italy, Romagna	99	0	6	96	0	31
Italy, Torino	74	4	26	90	3	42
Italy, Trieste	60	0	30	99	0	48
Italy, Varese	96	0	0	96	1	36
Italy, Veneto	94	0	0	93	2	36
+Latvia	81	0	53	91	1	42
+Malta	99	0	25	84	2	42
The Netherlands	99		42	99		39
The Netherlands, Eindhoven	99		19	98		38
The Netherlands, Maastricht	99		0	99		40
Norway	97	1	28	98	0	40
Poland, Cracow	33	33	100	84	6	61
Poland, Kielce	92	0	58	80	3	53
Poland, Lower Silesia	79	0	29	80	1	49
Poland, Warsaw City	[64]	18	39	[82]	7	50
Slovakia	86	1	53	84	0	48
Slovenia	93	0	29	94	2	50
Spain, Albacete	99	0	0	91	6	36
Spain, Asturias	94	0	35	93	6	43
Spain, Basque Country	96	4	22	90	7	42
Spain, Granada	99	0	63	92	4	43
Spain, Mallorca	99	0	80	96	2	47
Spain, Murcia	99	0	50	94	3	43
Spain, Navarra	91	9	18	95	3	33
Spain, Tarragona	99	0	12	96	2	41
Spain, Zaragoza	99	0	67	81	9	55

	MALE MV	DCO	M/I	FEMALE MV	DCO	M/I
Sweden	99		27	99		29
Switzerland, Basel	99	0	88	99	0	47
Switzerland, Geneva	99	0	50	96	1	39
Switzerland, Graubunden	99	0	50	95	3	42
Switzerland, Neuchatel	99	0	150	97	1	43
Switzerland, St Gall-Appenzell	99	0	33	97	1	52
Switzerland, Valais	99	0	0	97	1	38
Switzerland, Vaud	99	0	33	97	1	37
Switzerland, Zurich	99	0	43	98	0	48
+UK, England and Wales	[81]		43	[84]		49
UK, East Anglia			73			45
UK, Mersey	90	0	61	83	2	51
UK, North Western	89	3	39	81	2	48
UK, Oxford	94	0	39	84	0	42
UK, South Thames	78	5	38	71	11	49
UK, South Western	76	1	38	80	1	48
UK, Wessex	[68]	3	37	[88]	6	44
+UK, West Midlands		2	36		1	45
UK, Yorkshire	92	0	51	87	2	46
UK, Scotland	96	1	42	86	3	43
UK, Scotland, West	93	2	40	84	4	45
Yugoslavia, Vojvodina	54	3	31	65	5	51

OCEANIA

	MALE MV	DCO	M/I	FEMALE MV	DCO	M/I
Australian Capital Territory	99	0		97	0	
Australia, New South Wales	98	0		96	1	
South Australia	84		26	88		35
Australia, Tasmania	99		17	95		36
Australia, Victoria	95	0	38	96	0	36
Western Australia	94	6	56	95	3	29
French Polynesia	67	33		73	19	
+New Zealand: Non-Maori	94	1	34	93	2	38
+New Zealand: Maori	99	0	33	93	3	26
US, Hawaii: White	99	0	0	99	0	21
US, Hawaii: Japanese	99	0	17	99	0	16
US, Hawaii: Hawaiian	99	0	0	99	0	25
US, Hawaii: Filipino	99	0	0	99	0	23
US, Hawaii: Chinese	99	0	0	99	0	26

+ IMPORTANT-SEE NOTES ON POPULATION PAGE

[] CYTOLOGICAL VERIFICATION EXCLUDED

INDICES OF DATA QUALITY
Uterus (ICD-9 179)

	MALE			FEMALE		
	MV	DCO	M/I	MV	DCO	M/I
AFRICA						
Algeria, Setif				0		
France, La Reunion				94		
Mali, Bamako				24	4	
Uganda, Kyadondo				99		
Zimbabwe, Harare: African				25	25	
Zimbabwe, Harare: European				0	99	
AMERICA, CENTRAL AND SOUTH						
Argentina, Concordia				64	29	129
Brazil, Belem				59	26	237
Brazil, Goiania				72	28	66
Brazil, Porto Alegre				81	0	0
Colombia, Cali				54	27	285
Costa Rica				52	40	184
Ecuador, Quito				29	56	
Peru, Lima				24	65	
Peru, Trujillo				0	60	140
US, Puerto Rico				32	60	470
Uruguay, Montevideo				41	56	288
AMERICA, NORTH						
Canada				64	11	226
Canada, Alberta				67	15	276
Canada, British Columbia				53	42	330
Canada, Manitoba				72	13	231
Canada, New Brunswick				45	27	600
Canada, Newfoundland				99	0	147
Canada, Northwest Territories				50	0	50
Canada, Nova Scotia				70	20	400
Canada, Ontario				52	16	204
Canada, Prince Edward Island				67	17	133
+Canada, Quebec				72	0	185
Canada, Saskatchewan				64	36	500
Canada, Yukon				-	-	ncr
+US, Cent. Calif.: Non-Hisp. White				47	35	512
+US, Cent. Calif.: Hispanic				0	99	999
US, Los Angeles: Non-Hisp. White				75	16	869
US, Los Angeles: Hispanic White				67	22	
US, Los Angeles: Black				80	0	
US, Los Angeles: Chinese				99	0	
US, Los Angeles: Filipino				-	-	
US, Los Angeles: Korean				99	0	
US, Los Angeles: Japanese				-	-	
US, San Francisco: Non-Hisp. White				61	17	648
US, San Francisco: Hispanic White				99	0	350
US, San Francisco: Black				77	8	208
US, San Francisco: Chinese				80	20	340
US, San Francisco: Filipino				99	0	100
US, San Francisco: Japanese				-	-	-
US, Connecticut: White				75	8	249
US, Connecticut: Black				89	11	144
US, Atlanta: White				99	0	999
US, Atlanta: Black				88	13	325
US, Iowa				61	13	717
US, Central Louisiana: White				67	0	300
US, Central Louisiana: Black				50	0	183
US, New Orleans: White				79	16	105
US, New Orleans: Black				55	36	273
US, Detroit: White				72	17	566
US, Detroit: Black				75	0	525
US, New Mexico: Non-Hisp. White				64	9	364
US, New Mexico: Hispanic White				60	0	420
US, New Mexico: American Indian				99	0	100
US, Utah				42	0	583
US, Seattle				75	13	999
US, SEER: White				69	11	526
US, SEER: Black				79	7	319
ASIA						
+China, Qidong				99	0	42
+China, Shanghai				47	7	169
China, Tianjin				56	0	86
Hong Kong				5	34	210
India, Bangalore				79	13	17
India, Barshi, Paranda and Bhum				-	-	
India, Bombay				27	51	194
India, Karunagappally				-	-	
India, Madras				48	16	72
India, Trivandrum				99	0	25
Israel: All Jews				71		
Jews born in Israel				78		
Jews born in America or Europe				67		
Jews born in Africa or Asia				79		
Non-Jews				99		
Japan, Hiroshima				45	45	293
Japan, Miyagi				27	46	313
Japan, Nagasaki				28	55	257
Japan, Osaka				22	49	190
+Japan, Saga				24	59	205
Japan, Yamagata				33	47	144
Korea, Kangwha				0		999
Kuwait: Non-Kuwaitis				99	0	
Kuwait: Kuwaitis				99	0	
Philippines, Manila				21	69	
Singapore: Chinese				-	-	
Singapore: Malay				-	-	
Singapore: Indian				-	-	
Thailand, Chiang Mai				-	-	
Thailand, Khon Kaen				50	0	
Viet Nam, Hanoi				83		

+ IMPORTANT-SEE NOTES ON POPULATION PAGE

INDICES OF DATA QUALITY
Uterus (ICD-9 179) (contd)

	MALE			FEMALE		
EUROPE	MV	DCO	M/I	MV	DCO	M/I
Austria, Tyrol				33	45	236
+Belarus				80	5	61
Croatia				36	41	231
+Czech Republic				15	45	985
Denmark				92	4	236
Estonia				-		ncr
Finland				62	14	118
France, Bas-Rhin				91		732
France, Calvados				99		999
France, Doubs				67		999
France, Haut-Rhin				99		999
France, Herault				99		999
France, Isere				88		352
France, Somme				99		680
France, Tarn				75		999
Germany, Eastern States				91	2	604
+Germany, Saarland				79	10	177
Iceland				99	0	450
Ireland, Southern				86		186
Italy, Ferrara				50	0	775
Italy, Florence				26	24	493
Italy, Genoa				38	25	337
Italy, Latina				17	52	383
Italy, Macerata				62	0	154
Italy, Modena				50	36	721
Italy, Parma				46	25	418
Italy, Ragusa				33	17	817
Italy, Romagna				22	11	999
Italy, Torino				16	42	932
Italy, Trieste				75	0	431
Italy, Varese				25	56	775
Italy, Veneto				82	5	125
+Latvia				99	0	0
+Malta				50	25	450
The Netherlands				89		999
The Netherlands, Eindhoven				-		ncr
The Netherlands, Maastricht				99		999
Norway				50	25	132
Poland, Cracow				9	43	87
Poland, Kielce				57	14	143
Poland, Lower Silesia				57	6	110
Poland, Warsaw City				[4]	32	257
Slovakia				11	4	376
Slovenia				51	39	365
Spain, Albacete				56	33	211
Spain, Asturias				90	10	344
Spain, Basque Country				47	47	251
Spain, Granada				10	80	850
Spain, Mallorca				25	55	555
Spain, Murcia				15	50	530
Spain, Navarra				42	55	200
Spain, Tarragona				20	20	900
Spain, Zaragoza				13	56	333

	MALE			FEMALE		
	MV	DCO	M/I	MV	DCO	M/I
Sweden				99		100
Switzerland, Basel				-	-	ncr
Switzerland, Geneva				57	43	143
Switzerland, Graubunden				50	50	0
Switzerland, Neuchatel				50	25	175
Switzerland, St Gall-Appenzell				71	0	114
Switzerland, Valais				80	20	140
Switzerland, Vaud				40	20	300
Switzerland, Zurich				99	0	522
+UK, England and Wales				[73]		136
UK, East Anglia						360
UK, Mersey				50	8	525
UK, North Western				56	11	91
UK, Oxford				63	6	756
UK, South Thames				11	0	999
UK, South Western				57	3	106
UK, Wessex				[45]	20	88
+UK, West Midlands					9	99
UK, Yorkshire				80	6	82
UK, Scotland				73	10	69
UK, Scotland, West				75	11	54
Yugoslavia, Vojvodina				8	28	216

	MALE			FEMALE		
OCEANIA	MV	DCO	M/I	MV	DCO	M/I
Australian Capital Territory				99	0	
Australia, New South Wales				68	14	
South Australia				-		-
Australia, Tasmania				-		ncr
Australia, Victoria				-	-	ncr
Western Australia				99	0	567
French Polynesia				43	52	
+New Zealand: Non-Maori				63	25	925
+New Zealand: Maori				-	-	ncr
US, Hawaii: White				99	0	800
US, Hawaii: Japanese				99	0	350
US, Hawaii: Hawaiian				-	-	ncr
US, Hawaii: Filipino				99	0	100
US, Hawaii: Chinese				99	0	700

+ IMPORTANT-SEE NOTES ON POPULATION PAGE

[] CYTOLOGICAL VERIFICATION EXCLUDED

INDICES OF DATA QUALITY
Cervix uteri (ICD-9 180)

AFRICA

	MALE			FEMALE		
	MV	DCO	M/I	MV	DCO	M/I
Algeria, Setif				96		
France, La Reunion				99		
Mali, Bamako				63	1	
Uganda, Kyadondo				58		
Zimbabwe, Harare: African				77	3	
Zimbabwe, Harare: European				99	0	

AMERICA, CENTRAL AND SOUTH

	MALE			FEMALE		
	MV	DCO	M/I	MV	DCO	M/I
Argentina, Concordia				96	4	22
Brazil, Belem				89	8	25
Brazil, Goiania				94	4	27
Brazil, Porto Alegre				85	0	34
Colombia, Cali				87	3	40
Costa Rica				89	3	41
Ecuador, Quito				86	6	
Peru, Lima				82	3	
Peru, Trujillo				90	5	41
US, Puerto Rico				97	2	26
Uruguay, Montevideo				97	2	24

AMERICA, NORTH

	MALE			FEMALE		
	MV	DCO	M/I	MV	DCO	M/I
Canada				92	1	30
Canada, Alberta				99	0	23
Canada, British Columbia				98	2	30
Canada, Manitoba				98	0	33
Canada, New Brunswick				97	1	31
Canada, Newfoundland				99	0	22
Canada, Northwest Territories				94	0	16
Canada, Nova Scotia				98	2	36
Canada, Ontario				96	1	32
Canada, Prince Edward Island				99	0	33
+Canada, Quebec				74	0	26
Canada, Saskatchewan				98	2	30
Canada, Yukon				99	0	27
+US, Cent. Calif.: Non-Hisp. White				97	1	29
+US, Cent. Calif.: Hispanic				99	0	18
US, Los Angeles: Non-Hisp. White				98	1	34
US, Los Angeles: Hispanic White				99	0	
US, Los Angeles: Black				99	1	
US, Los Angeles: Chinese				96	0	
US, Los Angeles: Filipino				99	0	
US, Los Angeles: Korean				99	0	
US, Los Angeles: Japanese				99	0	
US, San Francisco: Non-Hisp. White				98	1	31
US, San Francisco: Hispanic White				99	1	14
US, San Francisco: Black				99	1	38
US, San Francisco: Chinese				96	2	34
US, San Francisco: Filipino				99	0	22
US, San Francisco: Japanese				99	0	36
US, Connecticut: White				98	1	29
US, Connecticut: Black				98	0	38
US, Atlanta: White				98	1	21
US, Atlanta: Black				99	0	31
US, Iowa				99	0	32
US, Central Louisiana: White				94	4	20
US, Central Louisiana: Black				96	0	12
US, New Orleans: White				99	0	28
US, New Orleans: Black				96	2	34
US, Detroit: White				99	1	27
US, Detroit: Black				97	1	41
US, New Mexico: Non-Hisp. White				99	0	26
US, New Mexico: Hispanic White				97	0	28
US, New Mexico: American Indian				93	4	75
US, Utah				99	0	24
US, Seattle				99	0	25
US, SEER: White				99	1	27
US, SEER: Black				98	0	37

ASIA

	MALE			FEMALE		
	MV	DCO	M/I	MV	DCO	M/I
+China, Qidong				89	1	55
+China, Shanghai				72	1	81
China, Tianjin				78	0	55
Hong Kong				83	2	28
India, Bangalore				88	2	28
India, Barshi, Paranda and Bhum				92	0	
India, Bombay				84	5	29
India, Karunagappally				69	15	
India, Madras				85	1	44
India, Trivandrum				84	4	6
Israel: All Jews				97		
Jews born in Israel				98		
Jews born in America or Europe				96		
Jews born in Africa or Asia				96		
Non-Jews				99		
Japan, Hiroshima				99	0	16
Japan, Miyagi				92	1	24
Japan, Nagasaki				97	2	20
Japan, Osaka				93	4	25
+Japan, Saga				86	6	25
Japan, Yamagata				90	8	35
Korea, Kangwha				89		6
Kuwait: Non-Kuwaitis				91	5	
Kuwait: Kuwaitis				86	14	
Philippines, Manila				71	7	
Singapore: Chinese				98	0	
Singapore: Malay				97	0	
Singapore: Indian				99	0	
Thailand, Chiang Mai				99	0	
Thailand, Khon Kaen				73	7	
Viet Nam, Hanoi				81		

+ IMPORTANT-SEE NOTES ON POPULATION PAGE

	MALE			FEMALE		
EUROPE	MV	DCO	M/I	MV	DCO	M/I
Austria, Tyrol				95	3	26
+Belarus				97	0	53
Croatia				80	2	32
+Czech Republic				95	1	42
Denmark				99	0	43
Estonia				97		54
Finland				96	0	56
France, Bas-Rhin				99		23
France, Calvados				99		29
France, Doubs				98		23
France, Haut-Rhin				99		20
France, Herault				99		16
France, Isere				97		12
France, Somme				96		34
France, Tarn				99		14
Germany, Eastern States				99	0	34
+Germany, Saarland				98	1	36
Iceland				99	0	41
Ireland, Southern				99		41
Italy, Ferrara				96	0	11
Italy, Florence				92	1	16
Italy, Genoa				95	0	20
Italy, Latina				98	1	11
Italy, Macerata				99	0	33
Italy, Modena				95	1	19
Italy, Parma				99	0	11
Italy, Ragusa				99	0	15
Italy, Romagna				97	0	12
Italy, Torino				93	0	23
Italy, Trieste				92	0	13
Italy, Varese				98	0	14
Italy, Veneto				96	2	22
+Latvia				98	1	50
+Malta				90	0	31
The Netherlands				99		39
The Netherlands, Eindhoven				99		34
The Netherlands, Maastricht				99		37
Norway				99	0	40
Poland, Cracow				88	5	56
Poland, Kielce				93	1	51
Poland, Lower Silesia				84	0	44
Poland, Warsaw City				[93]	3	50
Slovakia				97	0	33
Slovenia				98	0	32
Spain, Albacete				96	4	29
Spain, Asturias				99	1	31
Spain, Basque Country				98	2	26
Spain, Granada				97	1	34
Spain, Mallorca				98	1	30
Spain, Murcia				96	2	27
Spain, Navarra				98	1	23
Spain, Tarragona				98	1	28
Spain, Zaragoza				95	1	22

	MALE			FEMALE		
	MV	DCO	M/I	MV	DCO	M/I
Sweden				99		37
Switzerland, Basel				99	0	61
Switzerland, Geneva				99	1	41
Switzerland, Graubunden				99	0	49
Switzerland, Neuchatel				99	0	39
Switzerland, St Gall-Appenzell				99	1	44
Switzerland, Valais				99	0	27
Switzerland, Vaud				97	2	46
Switzerland, Zurich				99	0	50
+UK, England and Wales				[91]		43
UK, East Anglia						43
UK, Mersey				90	2	48
UK, North Western				91	2	45
UK, Oxford				89	0	41
UK, South Thames				84	8	47
UK, South Western				87	1	47
UK, Wessex				[89]	3	39
+UK, West Midlands					1	39
UK, Yorkshire				96	1	40
UK, Scotland				92	1	42
UK, Scotland, West				93	2	45
Yugoslavia, Vojvodina				81	4	35

OCEANIA

	MALE			FEMALE		
	MV	DCO	M/I	MV	DCO	M/I
Australian Capital Territory				97	0	
Australia, New South Wales				97	0	
South Australia				79		35
Australia, Tasmania				96		43
Australia, Victoria				99	0	31
Western Australia				97	1	31
French Polynesia				89	4	
+New Zealand: Non-Maori				97	0	38
+New Zealand: Maori				96	0	33
US, Hawaii: White				99	0	23
US, Hawaii: Japanese				99	0	18
US, Hawaii: Hawaiian				99	0	27
US, Hawaii: Filipino				99	0	33
US, Hawaii: Chinese				99	0	40

+ IMPORTANT-SEE NOTES ON POPULATION PAGE

[] CYTOLOGICAL VERIFICATION EXCLUDED

INDICES OF DATA QUALITY
Placenta (ICD-9 181)

	MALE			FEMALE		
	MV	DCO	M/I	MV	DCO	M/I
AFRICA						
Algeria, Setif				-		
France, La Reunion				99		
Mali, Bamako				99	0	
Uganda, Kyadondo				89		
Zimbabwe, Harare: African				87	7	
Zimbabwe, Harare: European				-	-	
AMERICA, CENTRAL AND SOUTH						
Argentina, Concordia				-	-	-
Brazil, Belem				99	0	10
Brazil, Goiania				-	-	-
Brazil, Porto Alegre				99	0	0
Colombia, Cali				90	0	10
Costa Rica				71	7	36
Ecuador, Quito				99	0	
Peru, Lima				85	0	
Peru, Trujillo				99	0	100
US, Puerto Rico				99	0	71
Uruguay, Montevideo				99	0	0
AMERICA, NORTH						
Canada				49	0	14
Canada, Alberta				99	0	33
Canada, British Columbia				99	0	0
Canada, Manitoba				-	-	ncr
Canada, New Brunswick				99	0	0
Canada, Newfoundland				-	-	-
Canada, Northwest Territories				50	0	100
Canada, Nova Scotia				-	-	-
Canada, Ontario				58	0	17
Canada, Prince Edward Island				0	0	0
+Canada, Quebec				25	0	6
Canada, Saskatchewan				-	-	-
Canada, Yukon				-	-	-
+US, Cent. Calif.: Non-Hisp. White				99	0	0
+US, Cent. Calif.: Hispanic				50	0	0
US, Los Angeles: Non-Hisp. White				99	0	0
US, Los Angeles: Hispanic White				92	0	
US, Los Angeles: Black				99	0	
US, Los Angeles: Chinese				-	-	
US, Los Angeles: Filipino				-	-	
US, Los Angeles: Korean				-	-	
US, Los Angeles: Japanese				-	-	
US, San Francisco: Non-Hisp. White				88	0	0
US, San Francisco: Hispanic White				99	0	0
US, San Francisco: Black				99	0	0
US, San Francisco: Chinese				-	-	ncr
US, San Francisco: Filipino				99	0	0
US, San Francisco: Japanese				-	-	-
US, Connecticut: White				67	0	33
US, Connecticut: Black				99	0	0
US, Atlanta: White				99	0	0
US, Atlanta: Black				99	0	0
US, Iowa				80	0	0
US, Central Louisiana: White				-	-	-
US, Central Louisiana: Black				-	-	-
US, New Orleans: White				50	0	0
US, New Orleans: Black				99	0	50
US, Detroit: White				80	0	0
US, Detroit: Black				99	0	67
US, New Mexico: Non-Hisp. White				-	-	-
US, New Mexico: Hispanic White				99	0	0
US, New Mexico: American Indian				-	-	-
US, Utah				86	0	29
US, Seattle				77	0	38
US, SEER: White				83	0	17
US, SEER: Black				99	0	29
ASIA						
+China, Qidong				99	0	18
+China, Shanghai				56	0	44
China, Tianjin				74	0	13
Hong Kong				71	0	14
India, Bangalore				67	17	33
India, Barshi, Paranda and Bhum				-	-	
India, Bombay				73	2	38
India, Karunagappally				-	-	
India, Madras				95	0	23
India, Trivandrum				-	-	ncr
Israel: All Jews				80		
Jews born in Israel				67		
Jews born in America or Europe				99		
Jews born in Africa or Asia				80		
Non-Jews				99		
Japan, Hiroshima				0	0	0
Japan, Miyagi				63	0	50
Japan, Nagasaki				99	0	25
Japan, Osaka				99	0	57
+Japan, Saga				99	0	0
Japan, Yamagata				99	0	33
Korea, Kangwha				-		-
Kuwait: Non-Kuwaitis				60	0	
Kuwait: Kuwaitis				83	0	
Philippines, Manila				64	11	
Singapore: Chinese				57	0	
Singapore: Malay				50	0	
Singapore: Indian				-	-	
Thailand, Chiang Mai				89	11	
Thailand, Khon Kaen				77	0	
Viet Nam, Hanoi				60		

+ IMPORTANT-SEE NOTES ON POPULATION PAGE

EUROPE

	MALE			FEMALE		
	MV	DCO	M/I	MV	DCO	M/I
Austria, Tyrol				-	-	-
+Belarus				92	3	41
Croatia				57	0	0
+Czech Republic				88	0	52
Denmark				99	0	33
Estonia				62		15
Finland				92	0	25
France, Bas-Rhin				-		ncr
France, Calvados				99		0
France, Doubs				99		0
France, Haut-Rhin				99		0
France, Herault				-		-
France, Isere				99		0
France, Somme				99		0
France, Tarn				-		-
Germany, Eastern States				99	0	31
+Germany, Saarland				99	0	0
Iceland				-	-	-
Ireland, Southern				-		-
Italy, Ferrara				-	-	-
Italy, Florence				99	0	0
Italy, Genoa				99	0	0
Italy, Latina				99	0	0
Italy, Macerata				-	-	-
Italy, Modena				-	-	-
Italy, Parma				99	0	0
Italy, Ragusa				-	-	-
Italy, Romagna				-	-	-
Italy, Torino				99	0	0
Italy, Trieste				-	-	-
Italy, Varese				99	0	0
Italy, Veneto				99	0	100
+Latvia				94	6	18
+Malta				-	-	-
The Netherlands				93		13
The Netherlands, Eindhoven				-		-
The Netherlands, Maastricht				-		-
Norway				89	0	7
Poland, Cracow				-	-	-
Poland, Kielce				-	-	-
Poland, Lower Silesia				58	0	17
Poland, Warsaw City				[99]	0	15
Slovakia				95	0	60
Slovenia				99	0	0
Spain, Albacete				-	-	-
Spain, Asturias				99	0	0
Spain, Basque Country				99	0	100
Spain, Granada				50	0	0
Spain, Mallorca				-	-	-
Spain, Murcia				99	0	0
Spain, Navarra				99	0	0
Spain, Tarragona				99	0	0
Spain, Zaragoza				-	-	-
Sweden				93		0
Switzerland, Basel				-	-	-
Switzerland, Geneva				99	0	0
Switzerland, Graubunden				0	0	0
Switzerland, Neuchatel				99	0	0
Switzerland, St Gall-Appenzell				99	0	0
Switzerland, Valais				-	-	-
Switzerland, Vaud				99	0	0
Switzerland, Zurich				99	0	0
+UK, England and Wales				[70]		45
UK, East Anglia						0
UK, Mersey				-	-	ncr
UK, North Western				99	0	50
UK, Oxford				99	0	25
UK, South Thames				33	33	33
UK, South Western				50	0	50
UK, Wessex				[25]	0	25
+UK, West Midlands					0	11
UK, Yorkshire				99	0	20
UK, Scotland				99	0	17
UK, Scotland, West				99	0	0
Yugoslavia, Vojvodina				80	10	40

OCEANIA

	MALE			FEMALE		
	MV	DCO	M/I	MV	DCO	M/I
Australian Capital Territory				99	0	
Australia, New South Wales				99	0	
South Australia				99		0
Australia, Tasmania				-		-
Australia, Victoria				91	0	0
Western Australia				-	-	-
French Polynesia				-	-	
+New Zealand: Non-Maori				99	0	3
+New Zealand: Maori				99	0	0
US, Hawaii: White				99	0	0
US, Hawaii: Japanese				99	0	0
US, Hawaii: Hawaiian				-	-	ncr
US, Hawaii: Filipino				0	0	200
US, Hawaii: Chinese				-	-	-

+ IMPORTANT-SEE NOTES ON POPULATION PAGE

[] CYTOLOGICAL VERIFICATION EXCLUDED

INDICES OF DATA QUALITY
Corpus uteri (ICD-9 182)

	MALE			FEMALE		
	MV	DCO	M/I	MV	DCO	M/I
AFRICA						
Algeria, Setif				99		
France, La Reunion				99		
Mali, Bamako				78	0	
Uganda, Kyadondo				67		
Zimbabwe, Harare: African				88	0	
Zimbabwe, Harare: European				99	0	
AMERICA, CENTRAL AND SOUTH						
Argentina, Concordia				89	11	14
Brazil, Belem				88	13	42
Brazil, Goiania				90	4	10
Brazil, Porto Alegre				76	0	26
Colombia, Cali				95	1	22
Costa Rica				90	4	25
Ecuador, Quito				83	3	
Peru, Lima				80	2	
Peru, Trujillo				93	0	14
US, Puerto Rico				99	0	11
Uruguay, Montevideo				89	4	18
AMERICA, NORTH						
Canada				95	0	12
Canada, Alberta				99	0	11
Canada, British Columbia				99	1	9
Canada, Manitoba				99	0	8
Canada, New Brunswick				99	0	7
Canada, Newfoundland				99	0	12
Canada, Northwest Territories				99	0	0
Canada, Nova Scotia				99	1	8
Canada, Ontario				95	0	12
Canada, Prince Edward Island				99	0	5
+Canada, Quebec				89	0	15
Canada, Saskatchewan				99	0	6
Canada, Yukon				99	0	0
+US, Cent. Calif.: Non-Hisp. White				99	1	8
+US, Cent. Calif.: Hispanic				99	0	6
US, Los Angeles: Non-Hisp. White				99	0	9
US, Los Angeles: Hispanic White				99	0	
US, Los Angeles: Black				99	1	
US, Los Angeles: Chinese				98	0	
US, Los Angeles: Filipino				99	0	
US, Los Angeles: Korean				99	0	
US, Los Angeles: Japanese				99	0	
US, San Francisco: Non-Hisp. White				99	0	11
US, San Francisco: Hispanic White				99	0	7
US, San Francisco: Black				99	1	14
US, San Francisco: Chinese				99	0	9
US, San Francisco: Filipino				99	0	4
US, San Francisco: Japanese				99	0	12
US, Connecticut: White				99	0	9
US, Connecticut: Black				99	0	13
US, Atlanta: White				99	0	8
US, Atlanta: Black				99	0	15
US, Iowa				99	0	12
US, Central Louisiana: White				99	0	12
US, Central Louisiana: Black				82	0	41
US, New Orleans: White				98	0	7
US, New Orleans: Black				98	1	20
US, Detroit: White				99	0	9
US, Detroit: Black				99	0	21
US, New Mexico: Non-Hisp. White				99	0	8
US, New Mexico: Hispanic White				99	1	16
US, New Mexico: American Indian				99	0	13
US, Utah				99	0	9
US, Seattle				99	0	9
US, SEER: White				99	0	10
US, SEER: Black				99	0	18
ASIA						
+China, Qidong				99	0	37
+China, Shanghai				82	0	16
China, Tianjin				89	0	13
Hong Kong				88	1	10
India, Bangalore				97	2	12
India, Barshi, Paranda and Bhum				99	0	
India, Bombay				94	1	10
India, Karunagappally				99	0	
India, Madras				92	0	26
India, Trivandrum				88	12	0
Israel: All Jews				98		
Jews born in Israel				97		
Jews born in America or Europe				98		
Jews born in Africa or Asia				96		
Non-Jews				99		
Japan, Hiroshima				99	1	12
Japan, Miyagi				92	1	17
Japan, Nagasaki				95	2	19
Japan, Osaka				94	3	22
+Japan, Saga				89	3	14
Japan, Yamagata				94	6	25
Korea, Kangwha				99		0
Kuwait: Non-Kuwaitis				99	0	
Kuwait: Kuwaitis				99	0	
Philippines, Manila				82	2	
Singapore: Chinese				98	1	
Singapore: Malay				92	8	
Singapore: Indian				99	0	
Thailand, Chiang Mai				81	13	
Thailand, Khon Kaen				74	0	
Viet Nam, Hanoi				66		

+ IMPORTANT-SEE NOTES ON POPULATION PAGE

	MALE			FEMALE		
	MV	DCO	M/I	MV	DCO	M/I
EUROPE						
Austria, Tyrol				96	3	13
+Belarus				97	0	36
Croatia				86	1	14
+Czech Republic				94	1	29
Denmark				99	0	22
Estonia				97		39
Finland				99	0	20
France, Bas-Rhin				99		16
France, Calvados				99		12
France, Doubs				99		13
France, Haut-Rhin				99		9
France, Herault				99		9
France, Isere				98		11
France, Somme				99		7
France, Tarn				99		10
Germany, Eastern States				99	0	28
+Germany, Saarland				99	1	15
Iceland				99	0	11
Ireland, Southern				99		26
Italy, Ferrara				97	0	12
Italy, Florence				95	0	6
Italy, Genoa				93	0	8
Italy, Latina				99	0	10
Italy, Macerata				99	0	5
Italy, Modena				99	0	6
Italy, Parma				99	0	6
Italy, Ragusa				99	0	7
Italy, Romagna				98	0	8
Italy, Torino				95	0	8
Italy, Trieste				85	1	6
Italy, Varese				98	0	8
Italy, Veneto				96	1	14
+Latvia				97	2	32
+Malta				99	0	10
The Netherlands				99		22
The Netherlands, Eindhoven				99		22
The Netherlands, Maastricht				99		20
Norway				99	0	26
Poland, Cracow				91	4	43
Poland, Kielce				92	1	30
Poland, Lower Silesia				78	0	29
Poland, Warsaw City				[97]	1	25
Slovakia				95	1	36
Slovenia				99	0	20
Spain, Albacete				88	0	25
Spain, Asturias				99	1	19
Spain, Basque Country				97	2	15
Spain, Granada				96	2	19
Spain, Mallorca				97	1	15
Spain, Murcia				97	2	14
Spain, Navarra				97	0	13
Spain, Tarragona				98	0	16
Spain, Zaragoza				93	1	14
Sweden				99		16
Switzerland, Basel				99	0	29
Switzerland, Geneva				98	1	28
Switzerland, Graubunden				98	2	79
Switzerland, Neuchatel				97	1	32
Switzerland, St Gall-Appenzell				99	0	28
Switzerland, Valais				99	0	35
Switzerland, Vaud				99	0	28
Switzerland, Zurich				98	0	31
+UK, England and Wales				[87]		24
UK, East Anglia						20
UK, Mersey				91	2	25
UK, North Western				91	1	27
UK, Oxford				89	0	18
UK, South Thames				82	11	22
UK, South Western				93	1	26
UK, Wessex				[88]	2	22
+UK, West Midlands					1	23
UK, Yorkshire				97	1	25
UK, Scotland				92	1	30
UK, Scotland, West				93	2	33
Yugoslavia, Vojvodina				81	4	38
OCEANIA						
Australian Capital Territory				99	0	
Australia, New South Wales				99	0	
South Australia				82		24
Australia, Tasmania				97		18
Australia, Victoria				96	1	21
Western Australia				96	2	15
French Polynesia				90	3	
+New Zealand: Non-Maori				95	1	26
+New Zealand: Maori				96	1	19
US, Hawaii: White				99	0	6
US, Hawaii: Japanese				99	0	8
US, Hawaii: Hawaiian				99	0	15
US, Hawaii: Filipino				99	0	2
US, Hawaii: Chinese				99	0	9

+ IMPORTANT-SEE NOTES ON POPULATION PAGE

[] CYTOLOGICAL VERIFICATION EXCLUDED

INDICES OF DATA QUALITY
Ovary etc. (ICD-9 183)

	MALE			FEMALE		
	MV	DCO	M/I	MV	DCO	M/I
AFRICA						
Algeria, Setif				50		
France, La Reunion				99		53
Mali, Bamako				70	0	
Uganda, Kyadondo				75		
Zimbabwe, Harare: African				58	14	
Zimbabwe, Harare: European				77	8	
AMERICA, CENTRAL AND SOUTH						
Argentina, Concordia				65	27	65
Brazil, Belem				68	14	57
Brazil, Goiania				85	11	48
Brazil, Porto Alegre				68	1	54
Colombia, Cali				79	4	56
Costa Rica				72	5	48
Ecuador, Quito				75	14	
Peru, Lima				72	4	
Peru, Trujillo				83	5	59
US, Puerto Rico				91	3	51
Uruguay, Montevideo				67	14	53
AMERICA, NORTH						
Canada				86	2	62
Canada, Alberta				96	1	59
Canada, British Columbia				93	5	67
Canada, Manitoba				74	2	67
Canada, New Brunswick				96	1	73
Canada, Newfoundland				96	1	52
Canada, Northwest Territories				93	0	43
Canada, Nova Scotia				87	9	64
Canada, Ontario				86	2	61
Canada, Prince Edward Island				97	0	57
+Canada, Quebec				79	0	60
Canada, Saskatchewan				95	3	64
Canada, Yukon				99	0	41
+US, Cent. Calif.: Non-Hisp. White				94	1	61
+US, Cent. Calif.: Hispanic				96	1	29
US, Los Angeles: Non-Hisp. White				97	1	67
US, Los Angeles: Hispanic White				95	2	
US, Los Angeles: Black				92	1	
US, Los Angeles: Chinese				98	0	
US, Los Angeles: Filipino				95	0	
US, Los Angeles: Korean				99	0	
US, Los Angeles: Japanese				98	0	
US, San Francisco: Non-Hisp. White				95	1	65
US, San Francisco: Hispanic White				99	0	41
US, San Francisco: Black				94	2	62
US, San Francisco: Chinese				97	0	44
US, San Francisco: Filipino				99	0	42
US, San Francisco: Japanese				94	6	69
US, Connecticut: White				95	2	62
US, Connecticut: Black				96	2	60
US, Atlanta: White				96	1	60
US, Atlanta: Black				92	1	44
US, Iowa				94	1	67
US, Central Louisiana: White				90	4	69
US, Central Louisiana: Black				88	6	65
US, New Orleans: White				93	1	58
US, New Orleans: Black				85	5	76
US, Detroit: White				95	1	58
US, Detroit: Black				90	2	69
US, New Mexico: Non-Hisp. White				95	2	63
US, New Mexico: Hispanic White				92	2	56
US, New Mexico: American Indian				94	0	44
US, Utah				96	0	65
US, Seattle				95	1	68
US, SEER: White				95	1	63
US, SEER: Black				92	2	63
ASIA						
+China, Qidong				95	0	62
+China, Shanghai				66	1	53
China, Tianjin				75	0	40
Hong Kong				74	5	41
India, Bangalore				85	5	24
India, Barshi, Paranda and Bhum				92	0	
India, Bombay				71	6	52
India, Karunagappally				99	0	
India, Madras				69	4	36
India, Trivandrum				88	3	15
Israel: All Jews				88		
Jews born in Israel				93		
Jews born in America or Europe				85		
Jews born in Africa or Asia				89		
Non-Jews				89		
Japan, Hiroshima				91	4	52
Japan, Miyagi				71	7	66
Japan, Nagasaki				83	10	50
Japan, Osaka				71	12	66
+Japan, Saga				77	14	56
Japan, Yamagata				74	18	71
Korea, Kangwha				99		13
Kuwait: Non-Kuwaitis				93	4	
Kuwait: Kuwaitis				76	12	
Philippines, Manila				68	18	
Singapore: Chinese				96	2	
Singapore: Malay				93	8	
Singapore: Indian				93	0	
Thailand, Chiang Mai				89	0	
Thailand, Khon Kaen				74	2	
Viet Nam, Hanoi				78		

+ IMPORTANT-SEE NOTES ON POPULATION PAGE

INDICES OF DATA QUALITY
Ovary etc. (ICD-9 183) (contd)

	MALE			FEMALE		
EUROPE	MV	DCO	M/I	MV	DCO	M/I
Austria, Tyrol				87	9	55
+Belarus				86	0	66
Croatia				64	6	62
+Czech Republic				79	2	74
Denmark				97	0	80
Estonia				90		79
Finland				96	0	70
France, Bas-Rhin				96		74
France, Calvados				99		85
France, Doubs				95		89
France, Haut-Rhin				98		80
France, Herault				99		87
France, Isere				95		45
France, Somme				92		81
France, Tarn				97		79
Germany, Eastern States				95	0	72
+Germany, Saarland				83	10	75
Iceland				98	0	89
Ireland, Southern				93		76
Italy, Ferrara				88	4	82
Italy, Florence				71	4	61
Italy, Genoa				81	4	68
Italy, Latina				86	11	62
Italy, Macerata				78	2	71
Italy, Modena				80	2	66
Italy, Parma				87	3	72
Italy, Ragusa				75	0	52
Italy, Romagna				87	1	61
Italy, Torino				89	4	72
Italy, Trieste				65	5	60
Italy, Varese				91	2	64
Italy, Veneto				82	5	63
+Latvia				90	2	60
+Malta				91	5	66
The Netherlands				98		81
The Netherlands, Eindhoven				99		74
The Netherlands, Maastricht				98		76
Norway				97	1	69
Poland, Cracow				79	10	70
Poland, Kielce				80	2	73
Poland, Lower Silesia				59	0	51
Poland, Warsaw City				[79]	5	60
Slovakia				89	1	60
Slovenia				93	3	74
Spain, Albacete				90	3	59
Spain, Asturias				91	5	50
Spain, Basque Country				89	4	53
Spain, Granada				86	2	43
Spain, Mallorca				91	2	52
Spain, Murcia				91	2	56
Spain, Navarra				89	6	47
Spain, Tarragona				92	1	65
Spain, Zaragoza				78	5	50

	MALE			FEMALE		
	MV	DCO	M/I	MV	DCO	M/I
Sweden				99		67
Switzerland, Basel				98	0	94
Switzerland, Geneva				96	1	68
Switzerland, Graubunden				88	8	65
Switzerland, Neuchatel				94	2	86
Switzerland, St Gall-Appenzell				95	1	66
Switzerland, Valais				93	1	64
Switzerland, Vaud				96	1	75
Switzerland, Zurich				98	0	74
+UK, England and Wales				[80]		76
UK, East Anglia						74
UK, Mersey				78	2	78
UK, North Western				77	4	79
UK, Oxford				80	0	66
UK, South Thames				72	17	73
UK, South Western				73	3	88
UK, Wessex				[78]	8	70
+UK, West Midlands					2	68
UK, Yorkshire				86	4	78
UK, Scotland				85	2	70
UK, Scotland, West				82	3	73
Yugoslavia, Vojvodina				63	8	60

OCEANIA

	MALE			FEMALE		
	MV	DCO	M/I	MV	DCO	M/I
Australian Capital Territory				93	0	
Australia, New South Wales				93	1	
South Australia				83		66
Australia, Tasmania				94		85
Australia, Victoria				92	1	72
Western Australia				93	3	67
French Polynesia				82	6	
+New Zealand: Non-Maori				89	2	69
+New Zealand: Maori				91	3	35
US, Hawaii: White				98	0	56
US, Hawaii: Japanese				99	0	57
US, Hawaii: Hawaiian				99	0	75
US, Hawaii: Filipino				99	0	46
US, Hawaii: Chinese				99	0	100

+ IMPORTANT-SEE NOTES ON POPULATION PAGE

[] CYTOLOGICAL VERIFICATION EXCLUDED

INDICES OF DATA QUALITY
Other female genital (ICD-9 184)

AFRICA

	MALE			FEMALE		
	MV	DCO	M/I	MV	DCO	M/I
Algeria, Setif				88		
France, La Reunion				99		
Mali, Bamako				78	0	
Uganda, Kyadondo				60		
Zimbabwe, Harare: African				75	0	
Zimbabwe, Harare: European				99	0	

AMERICA, CENTRAL AND SOUTH

	MALE			FEMALE		
	MV	DCO	M/I	MV	DCO	M/I
Argentina, Concordia				99	0	23
Brazil, Belem				79	11	47
Brazil, Goiania				93	0	19
Brazil, Porto Alegre				81	0	29
Colombia, Cali				98	2	26
Costa Rica				87	2	27
Ecuador, Quito				73	13	
Peru, Lima				89	0	
Peru, Trujillo				99	0	22
US, Puerto Rico				96	4	32
Uruguay, Montevideo				60	23	72

AMERICA, NORTH

	MALE			FEMALE		
	MV	DCO	M/I	MV	DCO	M/I
Canada				88	1	29
Canada, Alberta				97	1	26
Canada, British Columbia				97	2	26
Canada, Manitoba				95	1	26
Canada, New Brunswick				99	0	23
Canada, Newfoundland				99	0	24
Canada, Northwest Territories				99	0	0
Canada, Nova Scotia				97	2	24
Canada, Ontario				90	2	27
Canada, Prince Edward Island				87	7	20
+Canada, Quebec				70	0	39
Canada, Saskatchewan				99	0	32
Canada, Yukon				99	0	0
+US, Cent. Calif.: Non-Hisp. White				97	0	18
+US, Cent. Calif.: Hispanic				99	0	31
US, Los Angeles: Non-Hisp. White				99	0	37
US, Los Angeles: Hispanic White				96	0	
US, Los Angeles: Black				96	2	
US, Los Angeles: Chinese				75	0	
US, Los Angeles: Filipino				80	0	
US, Los Angeles: Korean				99	0	
US, Los Angeles: Japanese				99	0	
US, San Francisco: Non-Hisp. White				98	1	30
US, San Francisco: Hispanic White				99	0	6
US, San Francisco: Black				99	0	14
US, San Francisco: Chinese				99	0	33
US, San Francisco: Filipino				99	0	0
US, San Francisco: Japanese				-	-	-
US, Connecticut: White				98	1	25
US, Connecticut: Black				99	0	9
US, Atlanta: White				95	2	24
US, Atlanta: Black				97	0	37
US, Iowa				96	1	27
US, Central Louisiana: White				99	0	43
US, Central Louisiana: Black				80	20	40
US, New Orleans: White				98	2	22
US, New Orleans: Black				97	3	28
US, Detroit: White				99	1	25
US, Detroit: Black				97	0	22
US, New Mexico: Non-Hisp. White				97	0	25
US, New Mexico: Hispanic White				91	0	27
US, New Mexico: American Indian				99	0	0
US, Utah				99	0	13
US, Seattle				98	1	24
US, SEER: White				97	1	25
US, SEER: Black				98	0	25

ASIA

	MALE			FEMALE		
	MV	DCO	M/I	MV	DCO	M/I
+China, Qidong				99	0	100
+China, Shanghai				76	0	57
China, Tianjin				82	0	33
Hong Kong				72	1	14
India, Bangalore				94	0	13
India, Barshi, Paranda and Bhum				88	0	
India, Bombay				88	3	25
India, Karunagappally				99	0	
India, Madras				82	1	34
India, Trivandrum				67	17	33
Israel: All Jews				95		
Jews born in Israel				99		
Jews born in America or Europe				95		
Jews born in Africa or Asia				93		
Non-Jews				99		
Japan, Hiroshima				97	0	28
Japan, Miyagi				78	6	44
Japan, Nagasaki				90	10	33
Japan, Osaka				89	5	44
+Japan, Saga				82	18	36
Japan, Yamagata				74	16	58
Korea, Kangwha				99		0
Kuwait: Non-Kuwaitis				75	0	
Kuwait: Kuwaitis				99	0	
Philippines, Manila				83	2	
Singapore: Chinese				98	2	
Singapore: Malay				75	0	
Singapore: Indian				99	0	
Thailand, Chiang Mai				95	2	
Thailand, Khon Kaen				79	0	
Viet Nam, Hanoi				83		

+ IMPORTANT-SEE NOTES ON POPULATION PAGE

EUROPE	MALE			FEMALE		
	MV	DCO	M/I	MV	DCO	M/I
Austria, Tyrol				95	4	45
+Belarus				94	0	66
Croatia				72	6	52
+Czech Republic				85	3	80
Denmark				95	2	48
Estonia				90		56
Finland				94	1	42
France, Bas-Rhin				99		67
France, Calvados				99		58
France, Doubs				98		53
France, Haut-Rhin				99		56
France, Herault				99		69
France, Isere				98		41
France, Somme				99		116
France, Tarn				99		66
Germany, Eastern States				93	0	72
+Germany, Saarland				83	11	64
Iceland				99	0	36
Ireland, Southern				99		61
Italy, Ferrara				84	4	36
Italy, Florence				86	1	48
Italy, Genoa				79	4	44
Italy, Latina				95	5	77
Italy, Macerata				91	9	45
Italy, Modena				97	1	40
Italy, Parma				92	3	56
Italy, Ragusa				93	7	43
Italy, Romagna				97	0	68
Italy, Torino				73	7	55
Italy, Trieste				78	5	40
Italy, Varese				94	3	41
Italy, Veneto				88	2	51
+Latvia				96	1	53
+Malta				99	0	71
The Netherlands				99		42
The Netherlands, Eindhoven				99		42
The Netherlands, Maastricht				99		38
Norway				95	2	54
Poland, Cracow				57	16	82
Poland, Kielce				83	1	69
Poland, Lower Silesia				79	2	73
Poland, Warsaw City				[67]	13	66
Slovakia				87	0	74
Slovenia				92	2	45
Spain, Albacete				73	9	64
Spain, Asturias				89	10	57
Spain, Basque Country				85	9	57
Spain, Granada				89	6	30
Spain, Mallorca				93	3	64
Spain, Murcia				87	6	53
Spain, Navarra				95	5	74
Spain, Tarragona				89	2	56
Spain, Zaragoza				74	11	80
Sweden				99		54
Switzerland, Basel				99	0	40
Switzerland, Geneva				91	6	61
Switzerland, Graubunden				99	0	25
Switzerland, Neuchatel				93	0	79
Switzerland, St Gall-Appenzell				99	0	34
Switzerland, Valais				92	0	50
Switzerland, Vaud				95	2	53
Switzerland, Zurich				98	0	67
+UK, England and Wales				[84]		47
UK, East Anglia						52
UK, Mersey				88	1	60
UK, North Western				84	3	53
UK, Oxford				85	1	46
UK, South Thames				82	12	55
UK, South Western				88	1	46
UK, Wessex				[73]	5	37
+UK, West Midlands					1	43
UK, Yorkshire				94	2	45
UK, Scotland				90	1	45
UK, Scotland, West				89	3	45
Yugoslavia, Vojvodina				74	5	59

OCEANIA

	MALE			FEMALE		
	MV	DCO	M/I	MV	DCO	M/I
Australian Capital Territory				99	0	
Australia, New South Wales				96	1	
South Australia				84		27
Australia, Tasmania				99		64
Australia, Victoria				96	0	23
Western Australia				95	3	29
French Polynesia				69	31	
+New Zealand: Non-Maori				95	2	29
+New Zealand: Maori				94	0	12
US, Hawaii: White				94	0	44
US, Hawaii: Japanese				99	0	31
US, Hawaii: Hawaiian				99	0	0
US, Hawaii: Filipino				99	0	0
US, Hawaii: Chinese				99	0	0

+ IMPORTANT-SEE NOTES ON POPULATION PAGE

[] CYTOLOGICAL VERIFICATION EXCLUDED

INDICES OF DATA QUALITY
Prostate (ICD-9 185)

	MALE			FEMALE		
	MV	DCO	M/I	MV	DCO	M/I
AFRICA						
Algeria, Setif	75					
France, La Reunion	98		52			
Mali, Bamako	21	6				
Uganda, Kyadondo	67					
Zimbabwe, Harare: African	64	9				
Zimbabwe, Harare: European	93	6				
AMERICA, CENTRAL AND SOUTH						
Argentina, Concordia	54	46	65			
Brazil, Belem	48	24	63			
Brazil, Goiania	76	14	40			
Brazil, Porto Alegre	70	0	45			
Colombia, Cali	79	5	53			
Costa Rica	73	14	58			
Ecuador, Quito	72	18				
Peru, Lima	68	13				
Peru, Trujillo	74	7	58			
US, Puerto Rico	94	3	31			
Uruguay, Montevideo	48	31	66			
AMERICA, NORTH						
Canada	91	1	27			
Canada, Alberta	96	1	29			
Canada, British Columbia	97	2	21			
Canada, Manitoba	95	1	27			
Canada, New Brunswick	97	1	25			
Canada, Newfoundland	98	1	40			
Canada, Northwest Territories	76	8	36			
Canada, Nova Scotia	94	4	33			
Canada, Ontario	91	1	27			
Canada, Prince Edward Island	96	1	35			
+Canada, Quebec	79	0	31			
Canada, Saskatchewan	97	1	31			
Canada, Yukon	99	0	19			
+US, Cent. Calif.: Non-Hisp. White	96	1	19			
+US, Cent. Calif.: Hispanic	97	1	19			
US, Los Angeles: Non-Hisp. White	98	0	18			
US, Los Angeles: Hispanic White	98	0				
US, Los Angeles: Black	97	0				
US, Los Angeles: Chinese	99	0				
US, Los Angeles: Filipino	96	0				
US, Los Angeles: Korean	93	0				
US, Los Angeles: Japanese	98	0				
US, San Francisco: Non-Hisp. White	97	1	19			
US, San Francisco: Hispanic White	98	0	14			
US, San Francisco: Black	95	1	31			
US, San Francisco: Chinese	97	0	14			
US, San Francisco: Filipino	96	1	24			
US, San Francisco: Japanese	94	5	24			
US, Connecticut: White	97	0	21			
US, Connecticut: Black	98	1	25			
US, Atlanta: White	98	0	16			
US, Atlanta: Black	96	1	30			
US, Iowa	96	1	22			
US, Central Louisiana: White	95	2	23			
US, Central Louisiana: Black	92	2	53			
US, New Orleans: White	97	1	19			
US, New Orleans: Black	94	2	37			
US, Detroit: White	98	0	15			
US, Detroit: Black	97	0	24			
US, New Mexico: Non-Hisp. White	97	1	14			
US, New Mexico: Hispanic White	96	1	22			
US, New Mexico: American Indian	93	0	33			
US, Utah	98	0	17			
US, Seattle	98	0	14			
US, SEER: White	97	0	18			
US, SEER: Black	96	1	26			
ASIA						
+China, Qidong	87	0	73			
+China, Shanghai	47	2	78			
China, Tianjin	66	0	51			
Hong Kong	77	5	34			
India, Bangalore	75	6	19			
India, Barshi, Paranda and Bhum	67	0				
India, Bombay	73	7	41			
India, Karunagappally	77	0				
India, Madras	64	3	41			
India, Trivandrum	81	7	14			
Israel: All Jews	84					
Jews born in Israel	84					
Jews born in America or Europe	84					
Jews born in Africa or Asia	84					
Non-Jews	91					
Japan, Hiroshima	90	4	31			
Japan, Miyagi	82	8	46			
Japan, Nagasaki	84	11	45			
Japan, Osaka	71	18	52			
+Japan, Saga	60	18	71			
Japan, Yamagata	73	19	56			
Korea, Kangwha	67		0			
Kuwait: Non-Kuwaitis	75	16				
Kuwait: Kuwaitis	82	12				
Philippines, Manila	73	11				
Singapore: Chinese	97	1				
Singapore: Malay	96	2				
Singapore: Indian	99	0				
Thailand, Chiang Mai	89	2				
Thailand, Khon Kaen	85	0				
Viet Nam, Hanoi	42					

+ IMPORTANT-SEE NOTES ON POPULATION PAGE

	MALE			FEMALE		
	MV	DCO	M/I	MV	DCO	M/I
EUROPE						
Austria, Tyrol	89	8	39			
+Belarus	57	0	61			
Croatia	44	18	78			
+Czech Republic	80	3	63			
Denmark	92	1	64			
Estonia	72		55			
Finland	97	1	42			
France, Bas-Rhin	98		44			
France, Calvados	99		47			
France, Doubs	99		43			
France, Haut-Rhin	99		41			
France, Herault	99		47			
France, Isere	96		24			
France, Somme	94		64			
France, Tarn	98		33			
Germany, Eastern States	92	0	50			
+Germany, Saarland	89	7	38			
Iceland	99	0	38			
Ireland, Southern	90		61			
Italy, Ferrara	89	1	46			
Italy, Florence	68	3	55			
Italy, Genoa	75	5	56			
Italy, Latina	82	12	82			
Italy, Macerata	84	1	47			
Italy, Modena	88	2	49			
Italy, Parma	88	3	57			
Italy, Ragusa	47	1	97			
Italy, Romagna	82	1	42			
Italy, Torino	85	5	50			
Italy, Trieste	99	0	36			
Italy, Varese	91	3	45			
Italy, Veneto	85	2	43			
+Latvia	52	3	56			
+Malta	79	3	69			
The Netherlands	98		48			
The Netherlands, Eindhoven	98		42			
The Netherlands, Maastricht	97		47			
Norway	95	1	48			
Poland, Cracow	47	23	89			
Poland, Kielce	53	7	88			
Poland, Lower Silesia	52	1	58			
Poland, Warsaw City	[58]	14	69			
Slovakia	77	1	53			
Slovenia	81	7	71			
Spain, Albacete	83	9	49			
Spain, Asturias	90	9	83			
Spain, Basque Country	73	14	59			
Spain, Granada	73	13	79			
Spain, Mallorca	85	7	68			
Spain, Murcia	81	12	69			
Spain, Navarra	87	9	55			
Spain, Tarragona	87	3	63			
Spain, Zaragoza	61	16	69			
Sweden	99		41			
Switzerland, Basel	98	0	51			
Switzerland, Geneva	94	2	45			
Switzerland, Graubunden	94	3	44			
Switzerland, Neuchatel	87	2	61			
Switzerland, St Gall-Appenzell	95	1	45			
Switzerland, Valais	90	1	45			
Switzerland, Vaud	87	2	53			
Switzerland, Zurich	96	0	40			
+UK, England and Wales	[80]		61			
UK, East Anglia			54			
UK, Mersey	81	3	63			
UK, North Western	72	4	61			
UK, Oxford	74	0	58			
UK, South Thames	67	18	63			
UK, South Western	73	2	60			
UK, Wessex	[76]	8	56			
+UK, West Midlands		2	54			
UK, Yorkshire	84	3	56			
UK, Scotland	82	3	50			
UK, Scotland, West	79	4	50			
Yugoslavia, Vojvodina	50	12	69			
OCEANIA						
Australian Capital Territory	89	1				
Australia, New South Wales	92	1				
South Australia	90		36			
Australia, Tasmania	91		35			
Australia, Victoria	92	1	40			
Western Australia	91	3	32			
French Polynesia	77	21				
+New Zealand: Non-Maori	88	3	50			
+New Zealand: Maori	84	5	44			
US, Hawaii: White	98	0	17			
US, Hawaii: Japanese	98	0	12			
US, Hawaii: Hawaiian	96	0	33			
US, Hawaii: Filipino	97	0	24			
US, Hawaii: Chinese	99	0	13			

+ IMPORTANT-SEE NOTES ON POPULATION PAGE

[] CYTOLOGICAL VERIFICATION EXCLUDED

INDICES OF DATA QUALITY
Testis (ICD-9 186)

AFRICA	MV	DCO	M/I	MV	DCO	M/I
	MALE			**FEMALE**		
Algeria, Setif	99					
France, La Reunion	99					
Mali, Bamako	25	0				
Uganda, Kyadondo	0					
Zimbabwe, Harare: African	75	0				
Zimbabwe, Harare: European	-	-				

AMERICA, CENTRAL AND SOUTH

	MV	DCO	M/I	MV	DCO	M/I
Argentina, Concordia	99	0	11			
Brazil, Belem	71	12	29			
Brazil, Goiania	95	5	16			
Brazil, Porto Alegre	82	2	20			
Colombia, Cali	95	3	13			
Costa Rica	91	3	18			
Ecuador, Quito	85	3				
Peru, Lima	88	1				
Peru, Trujillo	82	0	12			
US, Puerto Rico	94	5	18			
Uruguay, Montevideo	93	2	16			

AMERICA, NORTH

	MV	DCO	M/I	MV	DCO	M/I
Canada	96	0	7			
Canada, Alberta	99	0	3			
Canada, British Columbia	99	0	3			
Canada, Manitoba	82	0	9			
Canada, New Brunswick	99	0	7			
Canada, Newfoundland	99	0	0			
Canada, Northwest Territories	99	0	6			
Canada, Nova Scotia	98	1	12			
Canada, Ontario	96	0	7			
Canada, Prince Edward Island	99	0	11			
+Canada, Quebec	94	0	10			
Canada, Saskatchewan	99	0	7			
Canada, Yukon	99	0	0			
+US, Cent. Calif.: Non-Hisp. White	99	0	9			
+US, Cent. Calif.: Hispanic	98	0	9			
US, Los Angeles: Non-Hisp. White	99	0	7			
US, Los Angeles: Hispanic White	99	0				
US, Los Angeles: Black	97	3				
US, Los Angeles: Chinese	99	0				
US, Los Angeles: Filipino	99	0				
US, Los Angeles: Korean	99	0				
US, Los Angeles: Japanese	99	0				
US, San Francisco: Non-Hisp. White	99	0	3			
US, San Francisco: Hispanic White	99	0	3			
US, San Francisco: Black	99	0	0			
US, San Francisco: Chinese	99	0	19			
US, San Francisco: Filipino	99	0	29			
US, San Francisco: Japanese	99	0	0			
US, Connecticut: White	98	0	2			
US, Connecticut: Black	99	0	20			
US, Atlanta: White	99	0	2			
US, Atlanta: Black	99	0	0			
US, Iowa	99	0	6			

	MV	DCO	M/I	MV	DCO	M/I
	MALE			**FEMALE**		
US, Central Louisiana: White	99	0	0			
US, Central Louisiana: Black	99	0	0			
US, New Orleans: White	99	0	6			
US, New Orleans: Black	92	0	31			
US, Detroit: White	99	0	5			
US, Detroit: Black	99	0	13			
US, New Mexico: Non-Hisp. White	99	0	3			
US, New Mexico: Hispanic White	99	0	3			
US, New Mexico: American Indian	90	0	20			
US, Utah	99	0	6			
US, Seattle	99	0	5			
US, SEER: White	99	0	4			
US, SEER: Black	99	0	10			

ASIA

	MV	DCO	M/I	MV	DCO	M/I
+China, Qidong	99	0	50			
+China, Shanghai	61	1	30			
China, Tianjin	94	0	22			
Hong Kong	81	1	10			
India, Bangalore	96	0	20			
India, Barshi, Paranda and Bhum	67	0				
India, Bombay	87	2	33			
India, Karunagappally	99	0				
India, Madras	83	0	28			
India, Trivandrum	99	0	0			
Israel: All Jews	90					
Jews born in Israel	91					
Jews born in America or Europe	87					
Jews born in Africa or Asia	96					
Non-Jews	87					
Japan, Hiroshima	98	0	4			
Japan, Miyagi	87	1	19			
Japan, Nagasaki	93	4	25			
Japan, Osaka	93	2	18			
+Japan, Saga	79	5	5			
Japan, Yamagata	80	18	18			
Korea, Kangwha	99		100			
Kuwait: Non-Kuwaitis	97	3				
Kuwait: Kuwaitis	99	0				
Philippines, Manila	73	10				
Singapore: Chinese	98	0				
Singapore: Malay	89	11				
Singapore: Indian	92	0				
Thailand, Chiang Mai	82	0				
Thailand, Khon Kaen	72	0				
Viet Nam, Hanoi	76					

+ IMPORTANT-SEE NOTES ON POPULATION PAGE

INDICES OF DATA QUALITY
Testis (ICD-9 186) (contd)

	MALE			FEMALE		
	MV	DCO	M/I	MV	DCO	M/I
EUROPE						
Austria, Tyrol	99	0	1			
+Belarus	91	0	51			
Croatia	75	0	23			
+Czech Republic	94	0	23			
Denmark	99	0	10			
Estonia	97		38			
Finland	99	0	13			
France, Bas-Rhin	99		8			
France, Calvados	99		15			
France, Doubs	99		11			
France, Haut-Rhin	99		5			
France, Herault	99		21			
France, Isere	99		1			
France, Somme	96		18			
France, Tarn	99		8			
Germany, Eastern States	99	0	19			
+Germany, Saarland	98	1	6			
Iceland	99	0	0			
Ireland, Southern	98		13			
Italy, Ferrara	89	0	0			
Italy, Florence	85	0	15			
Italy, Genoa	96	0	11			
Italy, Latina	95	0	18			
Italy, Macerata	80	0	0			
Italy, Modena	97	2	12			
Italy, Parma	99	0	16			
Italy, Ragusa	88	0	25			
Italy, Romagna	92	4	6			
Italy, Torino	99	0	14			
Italy, Trieste	70	0	10			
Italy, Varese	98	2	17			
Italy, Veneto	97	1	6			
+Latvia	90	3	23			
+Malta	83	0	17			
The Netherlands	99		10			
The Netherlands, Eindhoven	99		9			
The Netherlands, Maastricht	99		5			
Norway	99	0	5			
Poland, Cracow	96	2	21			
Poland, Kielce	83	2	36			
Poland, Lower Silesia	59	0	28			
Poland, Warsaw City	[87]	1	20			
Slovakia	96	0	22			
Slovenia	99	0	11			
Spain, Albacete	99	0	33			
Spain, Asturias	98	2	14			
Spain, Basque Country	95	2	16			
Spain, Granada	99	0	19			
Spain, Mallorca	93	4	18			
Spain, Murcia	99	0	22			
Spain, Navarra	99	0	6			
Spain, Tarragona	99	0	4			
Spain, Zaragoza	97	0	26			
Sweden	99		5			
Switzerland, Basel	99	0	5			
Switzerland, Geneva	99	0	5			
Switzerland, Graubunden	99	0	3			
Switzerland, Neuchatel	99	0	7			
Switzerland, St Gall-Appenzell	99	0	10			
Switzerland, Valais	99	0	5			
Switzerland, Vaud	99	0	10			
Switzerland, Zurich	99	0	10			
+UK, England and Wales	[88]		10			
UK, East Anglia			9			
UK, Mersey	96	0	9			
UK, North Western	95	0	10			
UK, Oxford	98	0	11			
UK, South Thames	86	2	8			
UK, South Western	95	1	9			
UK, Wessex	[82]	0	7			
+UK, West Midlands		0	10			
UK, Yorkshire	97	0	12			
UK, Scotland	98	0	6			
UK, Scotland, West	97	0	5			
Yugoslavia, Vojvodina	87	1	18			
OCEANIA						
Australian Capital Territory	97	0				
Australia, New South Wales	98	0				
South Australia	84		7			
Australia, Tasmania	99		6			
Australia, Victoria	98	0	8			
Western Australia	97	0	6			
French Polynesia	99	0				
+New Zealand: Non-Maori	98	0	9			
+New Zealand: Maori	98	0	8			
US, Hawaii: White	99	0	8			
US, Hawaii: Japanese	99	0	5			
US, Hawaii: Hawaiian	99	0	0			
US, Hawaii: Filipino	99	0	0			
US, Hawaii: Chinese	99	0	0			

+ IMPORTANT-SEE NOTES ON POPULATION PAGE

[] CYTOLOGICAL VERIFICATION EXCLUDED

INDICES OF DATA QUALITY
Penis, other male genitalB(ICD-9 187)

	MALE			FEMALE		
	MV	DCO	M/I	MV	DCO	M/I
AFRICA						
Algeria, Setif	99					
France, La Reunion	93					
Mali, Bamako	67	0				
Uganda, Kyadondo	53					
Zimbabwe, Harare: African	62	15				
Zimbabwe, Harare: European	99	0				
AMERICA, CENTRAL AND SOUTH						
Argentina, Concordia	99	0	0			
Brazil, Belem	90	7	30			
Brazil, Goiania	90	10	20			
Brazil, Porto Alegre	84	0	11			
Colombia, Cali	90	0	28			
Costa Rica	84	5	34			
Ecuador, Quito	99	0				
Peru, Lima	83	9				
Peru, Trujillo	99	0	29			
US, Puerto Rico	96	1	15			
Uruguay, Montevideo	67	13	42			
AMERICA, NORTH						
Canada	91	1	24			
Canada, Alberta	96	4	23			
Canada, British Columbia	99	0	14			
Canada, Manitoba	99	0	30			
Canada, New Brunswick	99	0	16			
Canada, Newfoundland	99	0	38			
Canada, Northwest Territories	99	0	0			
Canada, Nova Scotia	99	0	24			
Canada, Ontario	88	1	24			
Canada, Prince Edward Island	99	0	14			
+Canada, Quebec	84	0	31			
Canada, Saskatchewan	97	0	21			
Canada, Yukon	99	0	0			
+US, Cent. Calif.: Non-Hisp. White	99	0	14			
+US, Cent. Calif.: Hispanic	99	0	13			
US, Los Angeles: Non-Hisp. White	99	0	20			
US, Los Angeles: Hispanic White	99	0				
US, Los Angeles: Black	99	0				
US, Los Angeles: Chinese	99	0				
US, Los Angeles: Filipino	-	-				
US, Los Angeles: Korean	99	0				
US, Los Angeles: Japanese	99	0				
US, San Francisco: Non-Hisp. White	98	0	12			
US, San Francisco: Hispanic White	99	0	0			
US, San Francisco: Black	99	0	29			
US, San Francisco: Chinese	99	0	40			
US, San Francisco: Filipino	99	0	0			
US, San Francisco: Japanese	99	0	0			
US, Connecticut: White	97	2	35			
US, Connecticut: Black	99	0	29			
US, Atlanta: White	99	0	19			
US, Atlanta: Black	99	0	40			
US, Iowa	97	0	18			
US, Central Louisiana: White	99	0	0			
US, Central Louisiana: Black	99	0	0			
US, New Orleans: White	99	0	8			
US, New Orleans: Black	92	8	25			
US, Detroit: White	99	0	27			
US, Detroit: Black	94	0	13			
US, New Mexico: Non-Hisp. White	99	0	13			
US, New Mexico: Hispanic White	99	0	24			
US, New Mexico: American Indian	99	0	100			
US, Utah	99	0	9			
US, Seattle	97	0	21			
US, SEER: White	98	0	21			
US, SEER: Black	98	0	30			
ASIA						
+China, Qidong	99	0	35			
+China, Shanghai	78	0	35			
China, Tianjin	88	0	33			
Hong Kong	79	2	20			
India, Bangalore	96	2	6			
India, Barshi, Paranda and Bhum	79	3				
India, Bombay	85	2	21			
India, Karunagappally	50	0				
India, Madras	77	0	31			
India, Trivandrum	75	0	13			
Israel: All Jews	91					
Jews born in Israel	99					
Jews born in America or Europe	91					
Jews born in Africa or Asia	88					
Non-Jews	-					
Japan, Hiroshima	99	0	16			
Japan, Miyagi	85	0	26			
Japan, Nagasaki	98	0	22			
Japan, Osaka	86	7	36			
+Japan, Saga	99	0	20			
Japan, Yamagata	92	8	54			
Korea, Kangwha	99		0			
Kuwait: Non-Kuwaitis	99	0				
Kuwait: Kuwaitis	-	-				
Philippines, Manila	80	5				
Singapore: Chinese	98	2				
Singapore: Malay	-	-				
Singapore: Indian	99	0				
Thailand, Chiang Mai	94	0				
Thailand, Khon Kaen	76	0				
Viet Nam, Hanoi	67					

+ IMPORTANT-SEE NOTES ON POPULATION PAGE

INDICES OF DATA QUALITY
Penis, other male genitalB(ICD-9 187) (contd)

	MALE			FEMALE		
	MV	DCO	M/I	MV	DCO	M/I
EUROPE						
Austria, Tyrol	92	8	31			
+Belarus	84	0	55			
Croatia	61	4	41			
+Czech Republic	88	3	49			
Denmark	96	1	34			
Estonia	93		34			
Finland	98	0	20			
France, Bas-Rhin	99		29			
France, Calvados	99		30			
France, Doubs	95		11			
France, Haut-Rhin	99		17			
France, Herault	99		13			
France, Isere	99		20			
France, Somme	89		11			
France, Tarn	99		25			
Germany, Eastern States	94	0	33			
+Germany, Saarland	94	6	23			
Iceland	99	0	33			
Ireland, Southern	99		42			
Italy, Ferrara	99	0	20			
Italy, Florence	94	0	33			
Italy, Genoa	93	0	23			
Italy, Latina	92	0	15			
Italy, Macerata	99	0	17			
Italy, Modena	99	0	40			
Italy, Parma	99	0	7			
Italy, Ragusa	86	0	43			
Italy, Romagna	99	0	22			
Italy, Torino	97	3	13			
Italy, Trieste	65	0	17			
Italy, Varese	99	0	19			
Italy, Veneto	97	0	34			
+Latvia	90	7	54			
+Malta	99	0	0			
The Netherlands	99		33			
The Netherlands, Eindhoven	99		28			
The Netherlands, Maastricht	99		29			
Norway	98	0	29			
Poland, Cracow	90	10	80			
Poland, Kielce	96	0	28			
Poland, Lower Silesia	85	0	30			
Poland, Warsaw City	[93]	3	48			
Slovakia	92	1	69			
Slovenia	96	2	64			
Spain, Albacete	99	0	0			
Spain, Asturias	99	0	10			
Spain, Basque Country	95	3	40			
Spain, Granada	97	3	48			
Spain, Mallorca	96	0	15			
Spain, Murcia	97	0	15			
Spain, Navarra	99	0	11			
Spain, Tarragona	94	6	24			
Spain, Zaragoza	96	4	23			
Sweden	99		21			
Switzerland, Basel	99	0	31			
Switzerland, Geneva	99	0	18			
Switzerland, Graubunden	99	0	999			
Switzerland, Neuchatel	92	8	23			
Switzerland, St Gall-Appenzell	99	0	38			
Switzerland, Valais	99	0	20			
Switzerland, Vaud	99	0	19			
Switzerland, Zurich	98	0	40			
+UK, England and Wales	[85]		31			
UK, East Anglia			20			
UK, Mersey	93	0	39			
UK, North Western	92	0	30			
UK, Oxford	95	0	25			
UK, South Thames	86	7	38			
UK, South Western	93	0	28			
UK, Wessex	[64]	3	23			
+UK, West Midlands		1	29			
UK, Yorkshire	97	1	41			
UK, Scotland	96	0	27			
UK, Scotland, West	96	1	28			
Yugoslavia, Vojvodina	59	9	59			
OCEANIA						
Australian Capital Territory	99	0				
Australia, New South Wales	99	0				
South Australia	75		17			
Australia, Tasmania	99		75			
Australia, Victoria	97	0	29			
Western Australia	99	0	38			
French Polynesia	-	-				
+New Zealand: Non-Maori	97	3	38			
+New Zealand: Maori	99	0	100			
US, Hawaii: White	99	0	0			
US, Hawaii: Japanese	99	0	0			
US, Hawaii: Hawaiian	99	0	0			
US, Hawaii: Filipino	99	0	14			
US, Hawaii: Chinese	-	-	-			

+ IMPORTANT-SEE NOTES ON POPULATION PAGE

[] CYTOLOGICAL VERIFICATION EXCLUDED

INDICES OF DATA QUALITY
Bladder (ICD-9 188)

	MALE			FEMALE		
	MV	DCO	M/I	MV	DCO	M/I
AFRICA						
Algeria, Setif	31			0		
France, La Reunion	99		46	96		59
Mali, Bamako	8	3		12	8	
Uganda, Kyadondo	60			33		
Zimbabwe, Harare: African	60	13		65	14	
Zimbabwe, Harare: European	81	19		90	10	
AMERICA, CENTRAL AND SOUTH						
Argentina, Concordia	77	23	58	79	21	50
Brazil, Belem	68	16	60	76	12	35
Brazil, Goiania	87	12	35	87	10	37
Brazil, Porto Alegre	75	0	30	73	1	38
Colombia, Cali	90	2	37	79	5	49
Costa Rica	78	6	30	74	15	45
Ecuador, Quito	81	8		82	6	
Peru, Lima	82	5		70	4	
Peru, Trujillo	92	8	54	99	0	0
US, Puerto Rico	98	1	23	96	1	37
Uruguay, Montevideo	74	13	43	63	22	46
AMERICA, NORTH						
Canada	90	1	25	88	1	31
Canada, Alberta	97	0	21	97	0	24
Canada, British Columbia	97	2	37	94	5	49
Canada, Manitoba	95	1	28	93	1	31
Canada, New Brunswick	99	0	22	98	1	23
Canada, Newfoundland	99	0	28	96	0	37
Canada, Northwest Territories	99	0	27	99	0	33
Canada, Nova Scotia	96	2	23	92	3	29
Canada, Ontario	89	1	27	87	1	32
Canada, Prince Edward Island	99	0	28	92	6	25
+Canada, Quebec	83	0	21	81	0	29
Canada, Saskatchewan	97	0	22	94	2	26
Canada, Yukon	99	0	33	-	-	-
+US, Cent. Calif.: Non-Hisp. White	98	1	21	96	2	32
+US, Cent. Calif.: Hispanic	99	0	21	97	0	19
US, Los Angeles: Non-Hisp. White	99	0	30	98	1	35
US, Los Angeles: Hispanic White	99	0		99	0	
US, Los Angeles: Black	98	1		99	0	
US, Los Angeles: Chinese	98	0		99	0	
US, Los Angeles: Filipino	99	0		99	0	
US, Los Angeles: Korean	99	0		99	0	
US, Los Angeles: Japanese	99	0		99	0	
US, San Francisco: Non-Hisp. White	99	0	18	98	0	26
US, San Francisco: Hispanic White	99	1	17	99	0	21
US, San Francisco: Black	99	0	18	99	0	39
US, San Francisco: Chinese	99	0	20	99	0	25
US, San Francisco: Filipino	97	0	20	91	0	18
US, San Francisco: Japanese	99	0	35	99	0	38
US, Connecticut: White	99	0	18	98	1	24
US, Connecticut: Black	97	2	18	99	0	48
US, Atlanta: White	99	0	16	99	0	26
US, Atlanta: Black	99	0	35	98	0	44
US, Iowa	98	1	19	98	0	27
US, Central Louisiana: White	98	2	13	98	0	33
US, Central Louisiana: Black	96	0	24	99	0	73
US, New Orleans: White	98	1	18	99	0	21
US, New Orleans: Black	98	0	32	96	2	41
US, Detroit: White	99	0	17	99	0	25
US, Detroit: Black	99	0	25	98	0	41
US, New Mexico: Non-Hisp. White	98	1	16	95	2	27
US, New Mexico: Hispanic White	99	1	16	96	0	35
US, New Mexico: American Indian	99	0	43	99	0	50
US, Utah	99	0	19	99	0	28
US, Seattle	99	0	17	98	0	23
US, SEER: White	99	0	18	98	0	25
US, SEER: Black	99	0	24	99	0	39
ASIA						
+China, Qidong	91	0	51	80	0	67
+China, Shanghai	64	1	52	57	3	69
China, Tianjin	70	0	47	60	0	50
Hong Kong	81	2	27	80	2	31
India, Bangalore	85	3	11	80	7	28
India, Barshi, Paranda and Bhum	67	0		-	-	
India, Bombay	83	5	36	77	9	39
India, Karunagappally	89	0		99	0	
India, Madras	80	1	40	77	6	53
India, Trivandrum	87	0	0	0	0	0
Israel: All Jews	95			94		
Jews born in Israel	96			99		
Jews born in America or Europe	95			94		
Jews born in Africa or Asia	96			91		
Non-Jews	94			99		
Japan, Hiroshima	93	3	22	92	2	26
Japan, Miyagi	91	2	29	84	7	38
Japan, Nagasaki	92	5	27	83	11	47
Japan, Osaka	83	10	36	72	18	48
+Japan, Saga	82	11	38	67	24	64
Japan, Yamagata	86	8	27	73	17	48
Korea, Kangwha	70		50	80		20
Kuwait: Non-Kuwaitis	87	10		67	33	
Kuwait: Kuwaitis	68	30		50	30	
Philippines, Manila	78	8		73	10	
Singapore: Chinese	97	2		99	0	
Singapore: Malay	89	7		99	0	
Singapore: Indian	95	0		99	0	
Thailand, Chiang Mai	90	0		92	0	
Thailand, Khon Kaen	69	0		64	0	
Viet Nam, Hanoi	64			50		

+ IMPORTANT-SEE NOTES ON POPULATION PAGE

INDICES OF DATA QUALITY
Bladder (ICD-9 188) (contd)

EUROPE

	MALE			FEMALE		
	MV	DCO	M/I	MV	DCO	M/I
Austria, Tyrol	96	3	17	91	6	29
+Belarus	71	0	58	66	0	56
Croatia	46	6	47	45	9	52
+Czech Republic	84	1	53	80	2	56
Denmark	99	0	37	98	0	40
Estonia	80		64	72		64
Finland	99	0	28	97	0	37
France, Bas-Rhin	98		39	99		46
France, Calvados	99		26	98		62
France, Doubs	98		31	99		42
France, Haut-Rhin	99		36	98		53
France, Herault	99		54	98		64
France, Isere	98		22	95		39
France, Somme	98		39	93		59
France, Tarn	99		25	97		38
Germany, Eastern States	95	0	43	93	0	52
+Germany, Saarland	96	3	27	93	4	34
Iceland	99	0	24	99	0	40
Ireland, Southern	94		42	93		45
Italy, Ferrara	93	2	34	89	4	20
Italy, Florence	83	1	28	75	3	35
Italy, Genoa	89	1	32	80	3	31
Italy, Latina	90	5	41	87	4	26
Italy, Macerata	90	1	28	88	0	0
Italy, Modena	94	1	24	89	0	32
Italy, Parma	93	1	29	88	3	28
Italy, Ragusa	78	0	61	64	0	48
Italy, Romagna	94	1	28	94	2	23
Italy, Torino	94	1	32	91	2	42
Italy, Trieste	71	2	25	76	1	39
Italy, Varese	96	0	30	90	1	33
Italy, Veneto	95	1	29	91	3	35
+Latvia	81	2	53	72	3	52
+Malta	92	2	40	86	4	54
The Netherlands	99		50	97		68
The Netherlands, Eindhoven	99		25	99		37
The Netherlands, Maastricht	99		52	99		67
Norway	99	0	39	95	2	52
Poland, Cracow	79	9	84	73	16	92
Poland, Kielce	68	3	65	68	4	64
Poland, Lower Silesia	28	1	49	29	1	46
Poland, Warsaw City	[69]	7	59	[62]	10	61
Slovakia	86	1	48	83	1	47
Slovenia	91	3	61	83	7	69
Spain, Albacete	79	7	38	83	8	42
Spain, Asturias	96	3	30	93	6	31
Spain, Basque Country	94	3	31	87	9	41
Spain, Granada	91	4	32	84	8	50
Spain, Mallorca	97	1	28	91	2	27
Spain, Murcia	93	3	30	90	6	44
Spain, Navarra	92	5	36	88	4	33
Spain, Tarragona	95	1	29	92	2	43
Spain, Zaragoza	85	5	42	82	6	46

	MALE			FEMALE		
	MV	DCO	M/I	MV	DCO	M/I
Sweden	99		28	99		38
Switzerland, Basel	99	0	63	99	0	63
Switzerland, Geneva	99	0	27	98	2	30
Switzerland, Graubunden	99	1	55	88	4	54
Switzerland, Neuchatel	98	0	62	93	0	93
Switzerland, St Gall-Appenzell	98	0	62	96	0	77
Switzerland, Valais	96	1	52	99	0	41
Switzerland, Vaud	97	2	64	96	1	65
Switzerland, Zurich	99	0	34	96	0	42
+UK, England and Wales	[86]		39	[84]		47
UK, East Anglia			55			57
UK, Mersey	92	1	42	90	2	53
UK, North Western	89	1	40	82	2	47
UK, Oxford	90	0	37	86	0	45
UK, South Thames	84	9	44	79	13	50
UK, South Western	90	2	38	85	2	49
UK, Wessex	[75]	2	33	[72]	4	37
+UK, West Midlands		1	34		2	44
UK, Yorkshire	95	1	34	93	2	42
UK, Scotland	93	1	35	90	1	44
UK, Scotland, West	91	1	37	89	1	43
Yugoslavia, Vojvodina	70	8	47	64	9	54

OCEANIA

	MALE			FEMALE		
	MV	DCO	M/I	MV	DCO	M/I
Australian Capital Territory	92	0		99	0	
Australia, New South Wales	97	0		94	1	
South Australia	90		25	86		36
Australia, Tasmania	99		23	98		36
Australia, Victoria	96	0	25	94	0	33
Western Australia	96	2	44	93	4	46
French Polynesia	99	0		67	33	
+New Zealand: Non-Maori	95	1	34	89	3	45
+New Zealand: Maori	92	5	24	90	0	50
US, Hawaii: White	99	0	21	98	0	27
US, Hawaii: Japanese	99	0	13	92	0	32
US, Hawaii: Hawaiian	99	0	75	99	0	21
US, Hawaii: Filipino	97	0	9	92	0	31
US, Hawaii: Chinese	97	0	10	99	0	33

+ IMPORTANT-SEE NOTES ON POPULATION PAGE
[] CYTOLOGICAL VERIFICATION EXCLUDED

INDICES OF DATA QUALITY
Kidney (ICD-9 189)

AFRICA	MALE MV	DCO	M/I	FEMALE MV	DCO	M/I
Algeria, Setif	86			99		
France, La Reunion	97		48	95		35
Mali, Bamako	21	11		26	0	
Uganda, Kyadondo	55			65		
Zimbabwe, Harare: African	94	0		99	0	
Zimbabwe, Harare: European	99	0		99	0	

AMERICA, CENTRAL AND SOUTH

	MALE MV	DCO	M/I	FEMALE MV	DCO	M/I
Argentina, Concordia	63	38	50	64	36	9
Brazil, Belem	76	4	48	76	16	60
Brazil, Goiania	88	9	25	89	8	41
Brazil, Porto Alegre	63	0	56	61	0	48
Colombia, Cali	85	3	58	78	7	49
Costa Rica	74	12	49	77	10	43
Ecuador, Quito	69	14		76	17	
Peru, Lima	73	10		73	8	
Peru, Trujillo	85	15	46	72	17	78
US, Puerto Rico	87	5	40	92	3	32
Uruguay, Montevideo	64	17	52	72	17	45

AMERICA, NORTH

	MALE MV	DCO	M/I	FEMALE MV	DCO	M/I
Canada	79	1	38	77	2	39
Canada, Alberta	88	1	36	86	1	43
Canada, British Columbia	87	6	43	86	8	46
Canada, Manitoba	62	2	42	65	2	47
Canada, New Brunswick	89	0	41	86	1	43
Canada, Newfoundland	92	0	44	88	0	52
Canada, Northwest Territories	88	0	31	64	9	36
Canada, Nova Scotia	87	6	37	83	7	41
Canada, Ontario	81	1	35	78	1	35
Canada, Prince Edward Island	92	0	53	72	8	56
+Canada, Quebec	69	0	39	67	0	37
Canada, Saskatchewan	83	1	40	86	2	30
Canada, Yukon	71	0	71	99	0	80
+US, Cent. Calif.: Non-Hisp. White	92	1	43	92	1	37
+US, Cent. Calif.: Hispanic	89	2	33	96	0	32
US, Los Angeles: Non-Hisp. White	93	1	36	91	1	42
US, Los Angeles: Hispanic White	93	2		93	0	
US, Los Angeles: Black	93	1		90	1	
US, Los Angeles: Chinese	93	0		99	0	
US, Los Angeles: Filipino	97	0		94	0	
US, Los Angeles: Korean	89	5		99	0	
US, Los Angeles: Japanese	99	0		92	0	
US, San Francisco: Non-Hisp. White	94	1	37	91	1	40
US, San Francisco: Hispanic White	92	0	31	95	2	20
US, San Francisco: Black	89	2	29	96	0	38
US, San Francisco: Chinese	83	3	41	92	0	40
US, San Francisco: Filipino	96	0	37	93	0	21
US, San Francisco: Japanese	88	0	13	67	0	33
US, Connecticut: White	92	1	37	89	1	36
US, Connecticut: Black	93	0	28	90	3	38
US, Atlanta: White	95	1	37	91	1	38
US, Atlanta: Black	92	1	36	90	0	36
US, Iowa	91	1	43	84	1	48

	MALE MV	DCO	M/I	FEMALE MV	DCO	M/I
US, Central Louisiana: White	79	2	44	89	8	49
US, Central Louisiana: Black	83	0	33	90	0	40
US, New Orleans: White	92	1	39	94	1	37
US, New Orleans: Black	84	2	43	81	0	29
US, Detroit: White	93	1	31	90	1	31
US, Detroit: Black	87	1	35	88	1	36
US, New Mexico: Non-Hisp. White	90	1	40	89	1	32
US, New Mexico: Hispanic White	87	2	44	89	1	43
US, New Mexico: American Indian	79	0	41	90	0	52
US, Utah	94	0	35	90	1	40
US, Seattle	93	1	37	88	0	37
US, SEER: White	92	1	37	89	1	38
US, SEER: Black	90	1	34	90	1	37

ASIA

	MALE MV	DCO	M/I	FEMALE MV	DCO	M/I
+China, Qidong	73	0	73	80	0	47
+China, Shanghai	54	1	47	53	2	50
China, Tianjin	64	0	41	58	0	41
Hong Kong	74	7	39	68	8	34
India, Bangalore	90	6	15	93	0	16
India, Barshi, Paranda and Bhum	99	0		0	99	
India, Bombay	82	3	35	85	5	44
India, Karunagappally	99	0		-	-	
India, Madras	85	0	37	82	5	34
India, Trivandrum	75	0	25	99	0	0
Israel: All Jews	89			84		
Jews born in Israel	87			91		
Jews born in America or Europe	89			85		
Jews born in Africa or Asia	88			76		
Non-Jews	94			74		
Japan, Hiroshima	82	6	35	81	7	31
Japan, Miyagi	85	4	44	81	7	44
Japan, Nagasaki	85	7	43	79	9	42
Japan, Osaka	80	10	49	70	15	52
+Japan, Saga	76	11	47	69	13	39
Japan, Yamagata	66	16	48	60	25	61
Korea, Kangwha	40		40	99		25
Kuwait: Non-Kuwaitis	81	13		86	14	
Kuwait: Kuwaitis	64	29		82	18	
Philippines, Manila	46	40		55	32	
Singapore: Chinese	80	4		84	4	
Singapore: Malay	89	0		57	0	
Singapore: Indian	76	0		89	0	
Thailand, Chiang Mai	78	2		83	4	
Thailand, Khon Kaen	81	3		74	16	
Viet Nam, Hanoi	69			50		

+ IMPORTANT-SEE NOTES ON POPULATION PAGE

	MALE			FEMALE		
EUROPE	MV	DCO	M/I	MV	DCO	M/I
Austria, Tyrol	88	5	39	85	6	38
+Belarus	57	1	61	60	1	48
Croatia	52	5	58	46	7	50
+Czech Republic	53	2	66	53	3	60
Denmark	92	1	59	90	1	63
Estonia	77		69	76		58
Finland	93	1	40	89	1	41
France, Bas-Rhin	95		43	94		47
France, Calvados	96		59	91		85
France, Doubs	98		53	97		53
France, Haut-Rhin	95		51	92		56
France, Herault	98		53	97		61
France, Isere	91		27	89		25
France, Somme	95		48	93		61
France, Tarn	92		52	96		72
Germany, Eastern States	88	0	47	86	0	50
+Germany, Saarland	86	7	54	81	8	53
Iceland	94	0	44	97	0	59
Ireland, Southern	85		45	78		51
Italy, Ferrara	82	2	38	75	0	37
Italy, Florence	79	1	37	73	5	34
Italy, Genoa	77	3	48	69	4	45
Italy, Latina	82	7	62	92	8	52
Italy, Macerata	69	0	69	61	0	65
Italy, Modena	70	1	49	76	3	36
Italy, Parma	82	3	37	73	4	51
Italy, Ragusa	72	0	54	83	0	50
Italy, Romagna	81	0	35	77	3	46
Italy, Torino	84	3	39	76	4	49
Italy, Trieste	80	2	34	79	3	35
Italy, Varese	87	1	40	77	0	46
Italy, Veneto	84	2	37	79	3	42
+Latvia	54	7	62	60	5	53
+Malta	83	0	42	64	0	73
The Netherlands	89		53	88		57
The Netherlands, Eindhoven	94		51	91		68
The Netherlands, Maastricht	86		54	89		53
Norway	89	2	54	85	3	52
Poland, Cracow	59	12	74	57	13	78
Poland, Kielce	65	3	80	57	3	65
Poland, Lower Silesia	29	1	53	36	1	43
Poland, Warsaw City	[56]	5	59	[55]	7	54
Slovakia	73	2	54	72	2	48
Slovenia	89	3	61	89	2	53
Spain, Albacete	79	11	37	99	0	15
Spain, Asturias	90	5	49	82	14	56
Spain, Basque Country	79	6	47	77	9	49
Spain, Granada	79	3	45	71	4	58
Spain, Mallorca	89	2	41	84	5	61
Spain, Murcia	85	8	47	87	6	41
Spain, Navarra	82	10	51	87	6	38
Spain, Tarragona	84	3	54	78	7	64
Spain, Zaragoza	77	9	48	65	15	52

	MALE			FEMALE		
	MV	DCO	M/I	MV	DCO	M/I
Sweden	94		56	93		57
Switzerland, Basel	98	0	61	99	0	67
Switzerland, Geneva	92	2	35	89	1	62
Switzerland, Graubunden	84	5	53	94	6	39
Switzerland, Neuchatel	91	0	31	80	8	63
Switzerland, St Gall-Appenzell	91	2	54	93	0	44
Switzerland, Valais	93	3	39	92	0	37
Switzerland, Vaud	85	2	49	86	0	54
Switzerland, Zurich	95	0	53	94	0	54
+UK, England and Wales	[76]		58	[74]		61
UK, East Anglia			59			67
UK, Mersey	75	2	63	75	4	70
UK, North Western	66	5	62	62	5	62
UK, Oxford	85	1	59	82	2	56
UK, South Thames	61	20	59	59	22	67
UK, South Western	69	6	56	67	5	60
UK, Wessex	[74]	6	54	[72]	5	55
+UK, West Midlands		2	54		3	55
UK, Yorkshire	76	6	55	72	4	59
UK, Scotland	76	3	58	74	3	60
UK, Scotland, West	72	4	58	67	5	66
Yugoslavia, Vojvodina	58	12	55	60	10	55

OCEANIA

	MALE			FEMALE		
	MV	DCO	M/I	MV	DCO	M/I
Australian Capital Territory	84	2		88	4	
Australia, New South Wales	92	1		91	2	
South Australia	77		52	78		64
Australia, Tasmania	85		46	85		50
Australia, Victoria	85	1	52	85	1	46
Western Australia	89	2	36	85	4	44
French Polynesia	79	21		33	17	
+New Zealand: Non-Maori	86	3	52	85	2	54
+New Zealand: Maori	83	6	44	89	0	42
US, Hawaii: White	93	0	30	97	0	23
US, Hawaii: Japanese	91	0	41	95	0	37
US, Hawaii: Hawaiian	90	0	42	99	0	54
US, Hawaii: Filipino	96	0	32	88	0	63
US, Hawaii: Chinese	93	0	20	80	0	40

+ IMPORTANT-SEE NOTES ON POPULATION PAGE

[] CYTOLOGICAL VERIFICATION EXCLUDED

INDICES OF DATA QUALITY
Eye (ICD-9 190)

	MALE			FEMALE		
	MV	DCO	M/I	MV	DCO	M/I
AFRICA						
Algeria, Setif	99			50		
France, La Reunion	99			99		
Mali, Bamako	25	0		31	8	
Uganda, Kyadondo	77			68		
Zimbabwe, Harare: African	90	10		88	0	
Zimbabwe, Harare: European	99	0		-	-	
AMERICA, CENTRAL AND SOUTH						
Argentina, Concordia	99	0	0	67	33	33
Brazil, Belem	91	0	9	82	0	27
Brazil, Goiania	99	0	0	99	0	17
Brazil, Porto Alegre	70	0	20	91	9	9
Colombia, Cali	99	0	28	81	4	26
Costa Rica	84	0	7	82	4	14
Ecuador, Quito	99	0		95	0	
Peru, Lima	87	0		75	0	
Peru, Trujillo	89	0	22	80	20	40
US, Puerto Rico	98	2	15	99	0	15
Uruguay, Montevideo	99	0	44	99	0	60
AMERICA, NORTH						
Canada	66	1	16	62	0	18
Canada, Alberta	85	2	17	90	0	13
Canada, British Columbia	51	2	8	43	0	11
Canada, Manitoba	83	0	4	78	3	0
Canada, New Brunswick	82	9	18	86	0	14
Canada, Newfoundland	67	0	0	75	0	75
Canada, Northwest Territories	99	0	0	99	0	0
Canada, Nova Scotia	81	0	8	83	0	13
Canada, Ontario	74	1	18	60	1	23
Canada, Prince Edward Island	99	0	0	50	0	0
+Canada, Quebec	50	0	21	55	0	18
Canada, Saskatchewan	60	0	18	41	0	27
Canada, Yukon	99	0	0	-	-	-
+US, Cent. Calif.: Non-Hisp. White	85	0	9	56	0	11
+US, Cent. Calif.: Hispanic	80	0	10	99	0	0
US, Los Angeles: Non-Hisp. White	63	1	9	66	0	18
US, Los Angeles: Hispanic White	97	0		88	0	
US, Los Angeles: Black	99	0		99	0	
US, Los Angeles: Chinese	-	-		99	0	
US, Los Angeles: Filipino	-	-		-	-	
US, Los Angeles: Korean	-	-		-	-	
US, Los Angeles: Japanese	-	-		99	0	
US, San Francisco: Non-Hisp. White	78	0	7	69	2	9
US, San Francisco: Hispanic White	80	0	0	71	0	14
US, San Francisco: Black	80	0	0	50	0	0
US, San Francisco: Chinese	-	-	-	99	0	0
US, San Francisco: Filipino	-	-	-	-	-	-
US, San Francisco: Japanese	-	-	-	99	0	100
US, Connecticut: White	69	2	9	66	0	15
US, Connecticut: Black	99	0	0	99	0	0
US, Atlanta: White	74	0	9	80	0	12
US, Atlanta: Black	88	0	0	99	0	50
US, Iowa	88	0	13	84	0	14

	MALE			FEMALE		
	MV	DCO	M/I	MV	DCO	M/I
US, Central Louisiana: White	80	0	20	40	0	20
US, Central Louisiana: Black	99	0	0	-	-	-
US, New Orleans: White	71	0	6	70	0	5
US, New Orleans: Black	99	0	0	-	-	-
US, Detroit: White	90	0	13	85	0	20
US, Detroit: Black	99	0	40	99	0	0
US, New Mexico: Non-Hisp. White	95	5	5	99	0	13
US, New Mexico: Hispanic White	99	0	14	99	0	0
US, New Mexico: American Indian	99	0	0	99	0	0
US, Utah	91	0	6	94	0	6
US, Seattle	74	0	11	77	0	11
US, SEER: White	82	0	11	79	0	13
US, SEER: Black	90	0	10	93	0	14
ASIA						
+China, Qidong	99	0	33	99	0	50
+China, Shanghai	79	0	61	73	0	37
China, Tianjin	69	0	15	55	0	55
Hong Kong	68	6	19	76	0	3
India, Bangalore	83	0	0	86	0	10
India, Barshi, Paranda and Bhum	-	-		99	0	
India, Bombay	88	2	21	77	9	66
India, Karunagappally	-	-		-	-	
India, Madras	91	3	17	99	0	27
India, Trivandrum	99	0	0	99	0	0
Israel: All Jews	64			58		
Jews born in Israel	54			55		
Jews born in America or Europe	67			55		
Jews born in Africa or Asia	73			73		
Non-Jews	54			80		
Japan, Hiroshima	99	0	0	99	0	0
Japan, Miyagi	82	0	36	99	0	33
Japan, Nagasaki	85	8	8	80	20	40
Japan, Osaka	89	0	7	99	0	42
+Japan, Saga	67	0	0	99	0	200
Japan, Yamagata	-	-	-	99	0	0
Korea, Kangwha	-			-		-
Kuwait: Non-Kuwaitis	-	-		-	-	
Kuwait: Kuwaitis	50	50		99	0	
Philippines, Manila	80	5		74	5	
Singapore: Chinese	88	0		99	0	
Singapore: Malay	99	0		67	0	
Singapore: Indian	-	-		99	0	
Thailand, Chiang Mai	99	0		80	0	
Thailand, Khon Kaen	67	11		91	0	
Viet Nam, Hanoi	70			65		

+ IMPORTANT-SEE NOTES ON POPULATION PAGE

INDICES OF DATA QUALITY
Eye (ICD-9 190) (contd)

EUROPE

	MALE			FEMALE		
	MV	DCO	M/I	MV	DCO	M/I
Austria, Tyrol	99	0	6	94	0	31
+Belarus	85	0	41	81	0	43
Croatia	58	8	37	56	10	43
+Czech Republic	85	1	29	85	1	27
Denmark	96	1	26	92	1	26
Estonia	97		39	91		52
Finland	64	1	31	56	0	31
France, Bas-Rhin	73		23	75		21
France, Calvados	99		8	99		33
France, Doubs	86		86	75		25
France, Haut-Rhin	82		18	63		38
France, Herault	99		140	99		100
France, Isere	99		21	99		24
France, Somme	99		0	99		10
France, Tarn	99		33	99		14
Germany, Eastern States	77	0	16	80	0	28
+Germany, Saarland	93	0	0	89	0	33
Iceland	71	0	29	67	0	33
Ireland, Southern	86		57	71		71
Italy, Ferrara	75	0	25	50	0	17
Italy, Florence	75	0	25	56	6	50
Italy, Genoa	60	0	30	46	0	15
Italy, Latina	99	0	100	99	0	75
Italy, Macerata	33	0	100	99	0	0
Italy, Modena	71	0	57	99	0	0
Italy, Parma	99	0	75	99	0	25
Italy, Ragusa	67	0	0	-	-	-
Italy, Romagna	99	0	10	88	0	18
Italy, Torino	77	15	54	60	20	30
Italy, Trieste	0	0	33	0	25	75
Italy, Varese	60	0	0	65	0	6
Italy, Veneto	83	0	22	94	0	31
+Latvia	93	0	33	71	6	23
+Malta	0	0	100	-	-	-
The Netherlands	93		24	84		22
The Netherlands, Eindhoven	83		22	87		27
The Netherlands, Maastricht	95		25	77		46
Norway	93	0	34	90	0	28
Poland, Cracow	89	0	56	90	0	50
Poland, Kielce	69	6	50	63	13	150
Poland, Lower Silesia	73	0	40	71	2	38
Poland, Warsaw City	[91]	5	59	[68]	9	68
Slovakia	89	1	38	90	0	26
Slovenia	68	0	11	79	0	15
Spain, Albacete	67	0	33	99	0	0
Spain, Asturias	99	0	25	90	10	60
Spain, Basque Country	92	0	23	94	0	33
Spain, Granada	99	0	22	80	0	40
Spain, Mallorca	99	0	11	75	13	25
Spain, Murcia	89	0	6	80	0	40
Spain, Navarra	99	0	8	86	14	57
Spain, Tarragona	99	0	75	75	25	50
Spain, Zaragoza	99	0	44	99	0	10

	MALE			FEMALE		
	MV	DCO	M/I	MV	DCO	M/I
Sweden	85		10	86		15
Switzerland, Basel	73	0	27	77	0	46
Switzerland, Geneva	67	0	44	25	0	75
Switzerland, Graubunden	99	0	0	99	0	25
Switzerland, Neuchatel	99	0	0	60	40	0
Switzerland, St Gall-Appenzell	57	0	29	80	0	160
Switzerland, Valais	78	0	0	71	0	43
Switzerland, Vaud	99	0	36	99	0	52
Switzerland, Zurich	61	0	26	45	0	24
+UK, England and Wales	[80]		33	[80]		36
UK, East Anglia			63			50
UK, Mersey	89	0	51	93	0	30
UK, North Western	68	0	39	70	0	38
UK, Oxford	98	0	26	90	0	30
UK, South Thames	46	5	35	43	8	31
UK, South Western	77	0	35	77	0	35
UK, Wessex	[57]	2	22	[58]	5	34
+UK, West Midlands		1	36		2	36
UK, Yorkshire	93	0	31	78	0	46
UK, Scotland	88	0	20	87	1	25
UK, Scotland, West	91	0	22	90	1	23
Yugoslavia, Vojvodina	73	8	22	83	0	34

OCEANIA

	MALE			FEMALE		
	MV	DCO	M/I	MV	DCO	M/I
Australian Capital Territory	99	0		99	0	
Australia, New South Wales	97	1		97	0	
South Australia	83		25	78		34
Australia, Tasmania	82		9	99		40
Australia, Victoria	75	0	12	70	0	14
Western Australia	89	0	20	76	6	15
French Polynesia	99	0		-	-	
+New Zealand: Non-Maori	97	1	22	97	1	39
+New Zealand: Maori	0	99	100	99	0	0
US, Hawaii: White	99	0	40	99	0	0
US, Hawaii: Japanese	99	0	0	99	0	0
US, Hawaii: Hawaiian	0	0	0	99	0	0
US, Hawaii: Filipino	-	-	-	99	0	0
US, Hawaii: Chinese	99	0	0	-	-	-

+ IMPORTANT-SEE NOTES ON POPULATION PAGE

[] CYTOLOGICAL VERIFICATION EXCLUDED

INDICES OF DATA QUALITY
Brain, nervous system (ICD-9 191-2)

AFRICA

	MALE			FEMALE		
	MV	DCO	M/I	MV	DCO	M/I
Algeria, Setif	7			45		
France, La Reunion	96			97		
Mali, Bamako	25	25		0	0	
Uganda, Kyadondo	67			67		
Zimbabwe, Harare: African	28	34		23	46	
Zimbabwe, Harare: European	45	45		64	27	

AMERICA, CENTRAL AND SOUTH

	MALE			FEMALE		
	MV	DCO	M/I	MV	DCO	M/I
Argentina, Concordia	90	0	160	80	20	220
Brazil, Belem	24	32	88	49	20	60
Brazil, Goiania	60	30	62	64	28	59
Brazil, Porto Alegre	61	0	44	49	2	63
Colombia, Cali	76	4	60	62	12	75
Costa Rica	60	26	76	60	27	67
Ecuador, Quito	72	17		69	27	
Peru, Lima	53	9		49	13	
Peru, Trujillo	69	15	100	20	50	80
US, Puerto Rico	82	9	68	83	4	64
Uruguay, Montevideo	64	18	76	57	27	70

AMERICA, NORTH

	MALE			FEMALE		
	MV	DCO	M/I	MV	DCO	M/I
Canada	74	2	69	69	3	70
Canada, Alberta	87	2	66	83	2	72
Canada, British Columbia	84	10	76	82	13	86
Canada, Manitoba	42	1	57	39	1	63
Canada, New Brunswick	79	4	71	74	0	65
Canada, Newfoundland	89	0	89	76	0	104
Canada, Northwest Territories	83	8	33	57	14	86
Canada, Nova Scotia	84	4	72	80	9	85
Canada, Ontario	78	2	66	71	3	61
Canada, Prince Edward Island	99	0	96	86	9	59
+Canada, Quebec	59	0	71	56	0	76
Canada, Saskatchewan	88	1	80	84	3	67
Canada, Yukon	75	0	31	99	0	0
+US, Cent. Calif.: Non-Hisp. White	89	2	74	89	1	69
+US, Cent. Calif.: Hispanic	86	3	58	84	0	69
US, Los Angeles: Non-Hisp. White	89	2	74	85	3	80
US, Los Angeles: Hispanic White	91	0		87	3	
US, Los Angeles: Black	92	1		80	3	
US, Los Angeles: Chinese	73	13		99	0	
US, Los Angeles: Filipino	89	5		99	0	
US, Los Angeles: Korean	80	0		71	0	
US, Los Angeles: Japanese	99	0		83	17	
US, San Francisco: Non-Hisp. White	89	2	72	90	1	74
US, San Francisco: Hispanic White	89	0	36	86	2	29
US, San Francisco: Black	89	0	55	82	0	68
US, San Francisco: Chinese	96	0	48	91	0	39
US, San Francisco: Filipino	80	0	30	77	8	54
US, San Francisco: Japanese	75	0	100	99	0	67
US, Connecticut: White	88	2	64	83	3	66
US, Connecticut: Black	86	5	48	73	0	93
US, Atlanta: White	93	1	62	87	1	59
US, Atlanta: Black	87	7	74	82	2	59
US, Iowa	91	1	75	88	1	79

	MALE			FEMALE		
	MV	DCO	M/I	MV	DCO	M/I
US, Central Louisiana: White	73	10	60	63	16	68
US, Central Louisiana: Black	99	0	67	60	40	100
US, New Orleans: White	79	2	77	80	0	61
US, New Orleans: Black	86	8	65	90	3	80
US, Detroit: White	93	2	72	83	3	75
US, Detroit: Black	86	4	91	89	1	65
US, New Mexico: Non-Hisp. White	90	1	71	86	3	62
US, New Mexico: Hispanic White	90	0	71	86	2	66
US, New Mexico: American Indian	89	0	67	99	0	29
US, Utah	90	0	57	89	0	59
US, Seattle	90	0	68	87	1	74
US, SEER: White	90	1	68	86	2	70
US, SEER: Black	88	3	73	85	1	66

ASIA

	MALE			FEMALE		
	MV	DCO	M/I	MV	DCO	M/I
+China, Qidong	76	2	89	76	0	79
+China, Shanghai	44	3	72	49	2	59
China, Tianjin	55	0	56	50	0	57
Hong Kong	57	14	65	50	15	61
India, Bangalore	83	10	25	84	9	25
India, Barshi, Paranda and Bhum	99	0		50	0	
India, Bombay	86	5	45	78	8	53
India, Karunagappally	44	33		56	22	
India, Madras	85	3	46	81	8	48
India, Trivandrum	47	37	32	75	13	25
Israel: All Jews	71			67		
Jews born in Israel	79			79		
Jews born in America or Europe	61			60		
Jews born in Africa or Asia	75			61		
Non-Jews	74			73		
Japan, Hiroshima	88	0	32	78	2	28
Japan, Miyagi	83	1	23	89	1	25
Japan, Nagasaki	74	11	84	69	15	84
Japan, Osaka	64	6	33	60	9	30
+Japan, Saga	59	29	49	50	31	42
Japan, Yamagata	83	7	53	88	5	49
Korea, Kangwha	22		89	33		150
Kuwait: Non-Kuwaitis	67	28		50	38	
Kuwait: Kuwaitis	67	33		37	33	
Philippines, Manila	38	32		40	36	
Singapore: Chinese	79	6		80	8	
Singapore: Malay	65	18		56	11	
Singapore: Indian	89	0		71	29	
Thailand, Chiang Mai	48	8		45	13	
Thailand, Khon Kaen	18	22		18	15	
Viet Nam, Hanoi	41			52		

+ IMPORTANT-SEE NOTES ON POPULATION PAGE

	MALE			FEMALE		
EUROPE	MV	DCO	M/I	MV	DCO	M/I
Austria, Tyrol	95	4	63	80	8	66
+Belarus	57	2	84	62	1	76
Croatia	43	7	68	39	7	62
+Czech Republic	56	5	100	51	5	97
Denmark	85	0	79	84	0	82
Estonia	88		97	84		91
Finland	82	1	67	77	1	68
France, Bas-Rhin	78		71	73		54
France, Calvados	87		94	87		78
France, Doubs	84		72	90		55
France, Haut-Rhin	97		67	95		74
France, Herault	93		95	95		103
France, Isere	93		47	94		43
France, Somme	92		78	86		95
France, Tarn	78		105	64		136
Germany, Eastern States	86	0	80	84	0	77
+Germany, Saarland	72	11	64	74	12	52
Iceland	90	0	79	86	0	90
Ireland, Southern	77		85	70		116
Italy, Ferrara	36	3	69	31	3	66
Italy, Florence	35	6	76	34	3	70
Italy, Genoa	45	7	103	39	10	116
Italy, Latina	61	16	68	49	13	68
Italy, Macerata	33	4	75	37	0	80
Italy, Modena	46	5	56	41	3	55
Italy, Parma	58	4	76	45	6	62
Italy, Ragusa	47	2	90	68	0	79
Italy, Romagna	47	1	68	42	2	56
Italy, Torino	49	7	89	37	6	79
Italy, Trieste	56	3	47	55	1	36
Italy, Varese	69	2	85	57	5	96
Italy, Veneto	68	1	60	64	2	67
+Latvia	58	19	67	53	20	65
+Malta	46	4	88	41	9	77
The Netherlands	85		66	80		70
The Netherlands, Eindhoven	89		73	79		52
The Netherlands, Maastricht	85		69	89		67
Norway	75	5	70	69	6	56
Poland, Cracow	53	10	85	48	21	89
Poland, Kielce	42	3	105	46	5	106
Poland, Lower Silesia	53	2	75	53	1	66
Poland, Warsaw City	[46]	7	77	[40]	8	68
Slovakia	69	5	89	70	5	91
Slovenia	84	5	111	82	6	106
Spain, Albacete	44	12	68	35	12	94
Spain, Asturias	77	11	60	70	17	77
Spain, Basque Country	54	8	58	56	10	60
Spain, Granada	66	13	57	68	13	63
Spain, Mallorca	57	6	61	56	15	45
Spain, Murcia	65	8	61	57	15	69
Spain, Navarra	47	22	58	42	19	51
Spain, Tarragona	54	5	81	41	7	58
Spain, Zaragoza	44	12	72	45	9	63

	MALE			FEMALE		
	MV	DCO	M/I	MV	DCO	M/I
Sweden	92		80	90		79
Switzerland, Basel	99	0	98	94	0	110
Switzerland, Geneva	90	3	77	90	0	62
Switzerland, Graubunden	81	5	86	83	0	100
Switzerland, Neuchatel	92	0	73	92	4	88
Switzerland, St Gall-Appenzell	73	2	87	73	3	70
Switzerland, Valais	54	0	125	65	5	70
Switzerland, Vaud	87	2	82	84	2	83
Switzerland, Zurich	77	0	72	79	0	82
+UK, England and Wales	[75]		82	[74]		80
UK, East Anglia			80			77
UK, Mersey	73	2	71	73	3	60
UK, North Western	73	2	85	69	2	85
UK, Oxford	85	1	74	82	1	60
UK, South Thames	71	11	84	65	15	81
UK, South Western	64	3	79	58	2	84
UK, Wessex	[79]	0	84	[74]	1	79
+UK, West Midlands		2	81		2	84
UK, Yorkshire	74	3	86	66	4	86
UK, Scotland	68	2	80	62	3	78
UK, Scotland, West	62	3	77	56	3	79
Yugoslavia, Vojvodina	36	17	96	38	17	86

OCEANIA

	MALE			FEMALE		
	MV	DCO	M/I	MV	DCO	M/I
Australian Capital Territory	93	0		83	8	
Australia, New South Wales	88	1		83	3	
South Australia	71		93	64		81
Australia, Tasmania	82		70	87		67
Australia, Victoria	85	1	83	78	2	79
Western Australia	81	5	75	77	6	70
French Polynesia	23	31		31	31	
+New Zealand: Non-Maori	78	2	82	81	3	77
+New Zealand: Maori	87	3	43	81	0	37
US, Hawaii: White	96	0	55	85	0	65
US, Hawaii: Japanese	95	0	63	91	0	109
US, Hawaii: Hawaiian	89	0	74	80	0	67
US, Hawaii: Filipino	82	0	45	99	0	100
US, Hawaii: Chinese	99	0	67	0	0	100

+ IMPORTANT-SEE NOTES ON POPULATION PAGE

[] CYTOLOGICAL VERIFICATION EXCLUDED

<h1 align="center">INDICES OF DATA QUALITY
Thyroid (ICD-9 193)</h1>

	MALE			FEMALE		
	MV	DCO	M/I	MV	DCO	M/I
AFRICA						
Algeria, Setif	0			56		
France, La Reunion	99			99		
Mali, Bamako	99	0		53	0	
Uganda, Kyadondo	80			74		
Zimbabwe, Harare: African	56	33		55	20	
Zimbabwe, Harare: European	-	-		50	50	
AMERICA, CENTRAL AND SOUTH						
Argentina, Concordia	-	-	-	99	0	0
Brazil, Belem	99	0	40	87	4	9
Brazil, Goiania	99	0	8	93	4	9
Brazil, Porto Alegre	59	0	18	78	0	13
Colombia, Cali	91	6	31	96	0	14
Costa Rica	90	4	18	84	3	12
Ecuador, Quito	76	14		81	9	
Peru, Lima	88	2		87	2	
Peru, Trujillo	70	10	40	84	0	39
US, Puerto Rico	99	1	30	98	1	8
Uruguay, Montevideo	81	7	44	91	4	14
AMERICA, NORTH						
Canada	93	0	14	92	0	8
Canada, Alberta	99	1	9	99	0	5
Canada, British Columbia	99	0	16	99	1	8
Canada, Manitoba	92	0	18	94	0	10
Canada, New Brunswick	99	0	21	99	0	11
Canada, Newfoundland	99	0	13	99	0	13
Canada, Northwest Territories	99	0	33	99	0	0
Canada, Nova Scotia	99	0	16	99	0	7
Canada, Ontario	90	1	13	90	0	8
Canada, Prince Edward Island	99	0	20	99	0	7
+Canada, Quebec	87	0	18	86	0	12
Canada, Saskatchewan	99	0	11	99	0	5
Canada, Yukon	99	0	0	99	0	0
+US, Cent. Calif.: Non-Hisp. White	99	0	9	99	0	9
+US, Cent. Calif.: Hispanic	99	0	10	99	0	2
US, Los Angeles: Non-Hisp. White	99	0	15	99	0	7
US, Los Angeles: Hispanic White	99	0		99	0	
US, Los Angeles: Black	99	0		99	0	
US, Los Angeles: Chinese	99	0		99	0	
US, Los Angeles: Filipino	95	0		99	0	
US, Los Angeles: Korean	99	0		99	0	
US, Los Angeles: Japanese	99	0		99	0	
US, San Francisco: Non-Hisp. White	98	0	14	99	0	5
US, San Francisco: Hispanic White	99	0	16	99	0	5
US, San Francisco: Black	99	0	9	99	0	8
US, San Francisco: Chinese	99	0	5	99	0	8
US, San Francisco: Filipino	99	0	7	98	2	16
US, San Francisco: Japanese	99	0	0	99	0	15
US, Connecticut: White	99	1	11	99	0	9
US, Connecticut: Black	99	0	29	99	0	13
US, Atlanta: White	99	1	7	99	0	3
US, Atlanta: Black	99	0	19	97	0	8
US, Iowa	99	0	10	99	0	8

	MALE			FEMALE		
	MV	DCO	M/I	MV	DCO	M/I
US, Central Louisiana: White	99	0	14	99	0	17
US, Central Louisiana: Black	99	0	0	99	0	20
US, New Orleans: White	98	0	18	99	0	6
US, New Orleans: Black	99	0	20	98	2	6
US, Detroit: White	99	0	12	99	0	4
US, Detroit: Black	99	0	3	96	1	13
US, New Mexico: Non-Hisp. White	97	0	7	99	0	9
US, New Mexico: Hispanic White	99	0	13	98	0	8
US, New Mexico: American Indian	99	0	33	99	0	8
US, Utah	99	0	10	99	0	4
US, Seattle	99	0	9	99	0	7
US, SEER: White	99	0	11	99	0	6
US, SEER: Black	99	0	10	98	0	10
ASIA						
+China, Qidong	80	0	20	99	0	35
+China, Shanghai	68	1	23	77	0	18
China, Tianjin	82	0	24	85	0	18
Hong Kong	78	2	13	81	1	8
India, Bangalore	89	3	13	90	0	6
India, Barshi, Paranda and Bhum	80	0		99	0	
India, Bombay	86	4	34	86	3	19
India, Karunagappally	75	0		93	0	
India, Madras	66	0	42	74	0	28
India, Trivandrum	89	11	11	90	7	0
Israel: All Jews	95			96		
Jews born in Israel	98			97		
Jews born in America or Europe	94			94		
Jews born in Africa or Asia	93			97		
Non-Jews	99			97		
Japan, Hiroshima	96	0	11	97	0	8
Japan, Miyagi	94	3	27	95	1	9
Japan, Nagasaki	87	5	26	94	3	14
Japan, Osaka	86	4	34	91	4	18
+Japan, Saga	91	6	34	77	8	27
Japan, Yamagata	80	17	46	89	6	19
Korea, Kangwha	99		0	82		0
Kuwait: Non-Kuwaitis	98	0		99	0	
Kuwait: Kuwaitis	86	14		94	6	
Philippines, Manila	84	6		84	4	
Singapore: Chinese	97	2		98	1	
Singapore: Malay	91	0		98	0	
Singapore: Indian	99	0		99	0	
Thailand, Chiang Mai	86	0		84	0	
Thailand, Khon Kaen	70	0		84	0	
Viet Nam, Hanoi	53			58		

+ IMPORTANT-SEE NOTES ON POPULATION PAGE

INDICES OF DATA QUALITY
Thyroid (ICD-9 193) (contd)

EUROPE

	MALE			FEMALE		
	MV	DCO	M/I	MV	DCO	M/I
Austria, Tyrol	93	4	27	96	2	21
+Belarus	83	0	37	86	1	21
Croatia	85	3	40	82	3	19
+Czech Republic	81	1	42	84	2	38
Denmark	96	1	47	97	0	37
Estonia	90		52	94		41
Finland	98	0	21	99	0	16
France, Bas-Rhin	94		58	95		42
France, Calvados	99		14	99		13
France, Doubs	99		19	99		15
France, Haut-Rhin	99		32	99		40
France, Herault	99		23	99		15
France, Isere	99		9	97		13
France, Somme	92		42	99		39
France, Tarn	96		38	99		6
Germany, Eastern States	98	0	41	98	0	37
+Germany, Saarland	94	6	40	90	8	41
Iceland	99	0	18	99	0	11
Ireland, Southern	99		100	93		29
Italy, Ferrara	92	0	31	96	0	16
Italy, Florence	84	1	40	81	1	27
Italy, Genoa	92	2	39	88	4	40
Italy, Latina	96	0	21	98	0	6
Italy, Macerata	99	0	0	94	0	3
Italy, Modena	93	3	35	93	4	17
Italy, Parma	94	3	29	99	0	16
Italy, Ragusa	90	0	30	72	0	28
Italy, Romagna	99	0	19	96	0	14
Italy, Torino	98	2	25	96	2	33
Italy, Trieste	70	0	25	57	0	25
Italy, Varese	98	0	48	96	1	24
Italy, Veneto	89	1	27	94	1	23
+Latvia	86	9	37	89	2	21
+Malta	99	0	50	99	0	21
The Netherlands	99		37	99		32
The Netherlands, Eindhoven	99		35	98		22
The Netherlands, Maastricht	99		30	99		52
Norway	98	0	27	99	0	20
Poland, Cracow	73	13	80	86	5	44
Poland, Kielce	70	10	60	82	0	72
Poland, Lower Silesia	62	0	38	60	0	30
Poland, Warsaw City	[82]	3	61	[88]	5	49
Slovakia	94	1	41	93	1	27
Slovenia	99	0	47	97	2	45
Spain, Albacete	99	0	100	94	6	22
Spain, Asturias	99	0	42	97	3	29
Spain, Basque Country	95	5	28	98	1	21
Spain, Granada	96	0	46	99	0	10
Spain, Mallorca	99	0	67	99	0	12
Spain, Murcia	99	0	30	99	0	13
Spain, Navarra	99	0	14	99	1	11
Spain, Tarragona	99	0	50	99	0	18
Spain, Zaragoza	92	4	32	95	2	14
Sweden	99		30	99		25
Switzerland, Basel	99	0	35	99	0	41
Switzerland, Geneva	99	0	42	99	0	16
Switzerland, Graubunden	99	0	100	99	0	56
Switzerland, Neuchatel	99	0	200	94	0	24
Switzerland, St Gall-Appenzell	99	0	64	99	1	24
Switzerland, Valais	99	0	50	96	0	43
Switzerland, Vaud	80	0	26	96	0	36
Switzerland, Zurich	98	0	29	99	0	28
+UK, England and Wales	[84]		46	[84]		36
UK, East Anglia			34			32
UK, Mersey	98	0	55	83	1	50
UK, North Western	85	2	48	85	3	32
UK, Oxford	93	0	33	89	1	29
UK, South Thames	78	12	49	78	8	35
UK, South Western	87	1	56	84	5	39
UK, Wessex	[82]	6	47	[76]	4	31
+UK, West Midlands		1	45		1	35
UK, Yorkshire	97	2	37	94	2	32
UK, Scotland	93	1	28	92	1	27
UK, Scotland, West	95	0	32	87	1	34
Yugoslavia, Vojvodina	73	7	49	78	8	31

OCEANIA

	MALE			FEMALE		
	MV	DCO	M/I	MV	DCO	M/I
Australian Capital Territory	99	0		93	0	
Australia, New South Wales	97	1		97	0	
South Australia	91		16	78		18
Australia, Tasmania	99		29	98		9
Australia, Victoria	94	1	30	97	0	12
Western Australia	95	0	15	96	1	6
French Polynesia	70	10		91	4	
+New Zealand: Non-Maori	91	2	22	94	2	19
+New Zealand: Maori	99	0	25	99	0	7
US, Hawaii: White	99	0	7	99	0	3
US, Hawaii: Japanese	99	0	10	99	0	13
US, Hawaii: Hawaiian	99	0	15	99	0	12
US, Hawaii: Filipino	99	0	15	99	0	7
US, Hawaii: Chinese	99	0	0	99	0	0

+ IMPORTANT-SEE NOTES ON POPULATION PAGE

[] CYTOLOGICAL VERIFICATION EXCLUDED

INDICES OF DATA QUALITY
Other endocrine (ICD-9 194)

AFRICA

	MALE			FEMALE		
	MV	DCO	M/I	MV	DCO	M/I
Algeria, Setif	-			-		
France, La Reunion	99			99		
Mali, Bamako	0	0		0	0	
Uganda, Kyadondo	50			99		
Zimbabwe, Harare: African	-	-		50	0	
Zimbabwe, Harare: European	-	-	-	-	-	

AMERICA, CENTRAL AND SOUTH

	MALE			FEMALE		
	MV	DCO	M/I	MV	DCO	M/I
Argentina, Concordia	-	-	ncr	-	-	-
Brazil, Belem	50	25	25	0	0	100
Brazil, Goiania	90	0	10	54	31	38
Brazil, Porto Alegre	78	0	44	73	0	27
Colombia, Cali	71	0	86	67	0	100
Costa Rica	37	42	84	55	9	127
Ecuador, Quito	99	0		0	50	
Peru, Lima	29	0		83	0	
Peru, Trujillo	99	0	100	-	-	-
US, Puerto Rico	90	0	90	92	0	83
Uruguay, Montevideo	75	13	63	60	20	80

AMERICA, NORTH

	MALE			FEMALE		
	MV	DCO	M/I	MV	DCO	M/I
Canada	64	2	56	66	1	51
Canada, Alberta	67	6	61	92	0	64
Canada, British Columbia	80	10	120	86	4	86
Canada, Manitoba	50	0	72	67	0	100
Canada, New Brunswick	80	7	40	63	0	113
Canada, Newfoundland	99	0	300	99	0	33
Canada, Northwest Territories	99	0	50	99	0	0
Canada, Nova Scotia	99	0	100	75	0	75
Canada, Ontario	62	1	43	64	2	36
Canada, Prince Edward Island	99	0	300	-	-	-
+Canada, Quebec	61	0	53	56	0	50
Canada, Saskatchewan	75	13	113	99	0	42
Canada, Yukon	-	-	-	-	-	ncr
+US, Cent. Calif.: Non-Hisp. White	83	8	50	83	0	75
+US, Cent. Calif.: Hispanic	99	0	38	99	0	33
US, Los Angeles: Non-Hisp. White	94	0	77	92	0	124
US, Los Angeles: Hispanic White	94	3		95	0	
US, Los Angeles: Black	90	0		99	0	
US, Los Angeles: Chinese	0	0		-	-	
US, Los Angeles: Filipino	99	0		-	-	
US, Los Angeles: Korean	-	-		-	-	
US, Los Angeles: Japanese	99	0		99	0	
US, San Francisco: Non-Hisp. White	97	0	37	92	4	68
US, San Francisco: Hispanic White	86	0	43	99	0	33
US, San Francisco: Black	99	0	25	99	0	100
US, San Francisco: Chinese	99	0	67	99	0	0
US, San Francisco: Filipino	99	0	50	99	0	200
US, San Francisco: Japanese	99	0	0	-	-	-
US, Connecticut: White	93	7	64	93	7	86
US, Connecticut: Black	99	0	50	99	0	0
US, Atlanta: White	99	0	91	99	0	69
US, Atlanta: Black	99	0	75	99	0	233
US, Iowa	89	0	86	89	6	58

	MALE			FEMALE		
	MV	DCO	M/I	MV	DCO	M/I
US, Central Louisiana: White	99	0	200	75	0	100
US, Central Louisiana: Black	-	-	ncr	99	0	0
US, New Orleans: White	99	0	125	99	0	33
US, New Orleans: Black	67	0	67	83	0	67
US, Detroit: White	94	0	57	94	0	43
US, Detroit: Black	99	0	50	99	0	55
US, New Mexico: Non-Hisp. White	86	0	100	80	0	100
US, New Mexico: Hispanic White	86	0	43	99	0	133
US, New Mexico: American Indian	-	-	ncr	99	0	0
US, Utah	99	0	73	94	0	53
US, Seattle	99	0	84	96	0	65
US, SEER: White	94	1	65	94	2	61
US, SEER: Black	99	0	67	99	0	86

ASIA

	MALE			FEMALE		
	MV	DCO	M/I	MV	DCO	M/I
+China, Qidong	99	0	33	99	0	50
+China, Shanghai	55	0	27	47	0	12
China, Tianjin	68	0	19	75	0	11
Hong Kong	40	17	44	43	4	17
India, Bangalore	50	0	75	75	25	50
India, Barshi, Paranda and Bhum	-	-		-	-	
India, Bombay	89	4	31	99	0	50
India, Karunagappally	99	0		-	-	
India, Madras	81	0	13	50	0	50
India, Trivandrum	99	0	0	-	-	-
Israel: All Jews	81			73		
Jews born in Israel	91			80		
Jews born in America or Europe	69			61		
Jews born in Africa or Asia	75			99		
Non-Jews	78			89		
Japan, Hiroshima	90	0	50	78	0	67
Japan, Miyagi	90	0	86	76	0	60
Japan, Nagasaki	71	12	41	67	0	67
Japan, Osaka	70	8	42	67	8	42
+Japan, Saga	29	29	57	67	33	33
Japan, Yamagata	38	25	50	71	14	29
Korea, Kangwha	-		-	-		-
Kuwait: Non-Kuwaitis	99	0		83	17	
Kuwait: Kuwaitis	99	0		71	14	
Philippines, Manila	63	19		75	0	
Singapore: Chinese	87	3		76	0	
Singapore: Malay	99	0		50	0	
Singapore: Indian	-	-		-	-	
Thailand, Chiang Mai	40	0		99	0	
Thailand, Khon Kaen	43	0		0	0	
Viet Nam, Hanoi	50			50		

+ IMPORTANT-SEE NOTES ON POPULATION PAGE

EUROPE	MALE MV	DCO	M/I	FEMALE MV	DCO	M/I
Austria, Tyrol	85	15	54	80	10	40
+Belarus	53	8	59	72	0	47
Croatia	45	19	66	39	14	56
+Czech Republic	36	3	70	46	3	67
Denmark	91	0	78	93	0	78
Estonia	69		81	99		86
Finland	94	1	68	92	0	71
France, Bas-Rhin	83		56	91		45
France, Calvados	99		167	99		100
France, Doubs	99		50	99		60
France, Haut-Rhin	99		85	99		43
France, Herault	88		138	99		75
France, Isere	99		100	93		27
France, Somme	99		117	67		267
France, Tarn	99		600	50		100
Germany, Eastern States	87	0	85	85	0	79
+Germany, Saarland	71	10	52	71	12	65
Iceland	99	0	50	99	0	80
Ireland, Southern	75		75	89		44
Italy, Ferrara	0	0	100	50	0	0
Italy, Florence	38	6	106	61	6	44
Italy, Genoa	57	0	107	27	0	36
Italy, Latina	25	25	150	99	0	50
Italy, Macerata	50	0	50	0	0	150
Italy, Modena	47	11	68	46	0	54
Italy, Parma	99	0	100	75	13	75
Italy, Ragusa	33	0	67	33	0	100
Italy, Romagna	80	20	120	71	0	43
Italy, Torino	68	11	42	54	0	92
Italy, Trieste	25	6	19	10	0	17
Italy, Varese	88	13	38	99	0	38
Italy, Veneto	72	0	56	56	19	50
+Latvia	41	32	50	50	22	61
+Malta	99	0	100	0	0	0
The Netherlands	91		77	93		77
The Netherlands, Eindhoven	99		113	91		73
The Netherlands, Maastricht	99		80	99		57
Norway	89	2	51	91	6	44
Poland, Cracow	44	22	78	58	33	75
Poland, Kielce	71	0	35	47	0	24
Poland, Lower Silesia	54	0	31	53	2	27
Poland, Warsaw City	[38]	8	42	[58]	17	33
Slovakia	77	8	66	67	8	59
Slovenia	83	0	158	83	6	100
Spain, Albacete	0	99	100	-	-	-
Spain, Asturias	71	6	71	90	10	40
Spain, Basque Country	71	14	86	83	8	92
Spain, Granada	83	17	167	99	0	63
Spain, Mallorca	99	0	175	99	0	80
Spain, Murcia	90	0	120	82	0	55
Spain, Navarra	67	11	67	75	25	125
Spain, Tarragona	67	0	100	90	0	20
Spain, Zaragoza	69	8	92	50	8	33

	MALE MV	DCO	M/I	FEMALE MV	DCO	M/I
Sweden	90		81	97		81
Switzerland, Basel	99	0	25	99	0	33
Switzerland, Geneva	99	0	40	99	0	36
Switzerland, Graubunden	-	-	ncr	67	0	67
Switzerland, Neuchatel	99	0	300	99	0	100
Switzerland, St Gall-Appenzell	99	0	50	67	0	33
Switzerland, Valais	-	-	ncr	67	0	0
Switzerland, Vaud	86	0	43	99	0	167
Switzerland, Zurich	99	0	89	99	0	53
+UK, England and Wales	[69]		50	[69]		50
UK, East Anglia			58			108
UK, Mersey	70	0	105	65	8	58
UK, North Western	69	0	66	75	7	100
UK, Oxford	93	0	36	79	3	47
UK, South Thames	57	14	47	61	18	59
UK, South Western	75	10	69	63	13	47
UK, Wessex	[61]	2	29	[48]	3	29
+UK, West Midlands		2	30		6	23
UK, Yorkshire	76	10	59	70	5	55
UK, Scotland	69	7	63	68	1	42
UK, Scotland, West	82	3	61	58	3	45
Yugoslavia, Vojvodina	35	8	85	25	18	79

OCEANIA

	MALE MV	DCO	M/I	FEMALE MV	DCO	M/I
Australian Capital Territory	99	0		99	0	
Australia, New South Wales	86	0		91	3	
South Australia	61		30	64		82
Australia, Tasmania	99		80	99		75
Australia, Victoria	79	0	67	93	4	111
Western Australia	99	0	47	75	6	63
French Polynesia	75	0		50	0	
+New Zealand: Non-Maori	82	6	59	86	0	63
+New Zealand: Maori	78	0	0	71	14	57
US, Hawaii: White	99	0	25	99	0	0
US, Hawaii: Japanese	99	0	350	99	0	0
US, Hawaii: Hawaiian	99	0	67	99	0	0
US, Hawaii: Filipino	0	0	0	0	0	0
US, Hawaii: Chinese	-	-	-	99	0	0

+ IMPORTANT-SEE NOTES ON POPULATION PAGE
[] CYTOLOGICAL VERIFICATION EXCLUDED

INDICES OF DATA QUALITY
Non-Hodgkin lymphomas (ICD-9 200+202)

	MALE			FEMALE		
	MV	DCO	M/I	MV	DCO	M/I
AFRICA						
Algeria, Setif	99			99		
France, La Reunion	98		37	98		44
Mali, Bamako	99	0		99	0	
Uganda, Kyadondo	58			72		
Zimbabwe, Harare: African	90	10		91	9	
Zimbabwe, Harare: European	60	40		50	50	
AMERICA, CENTRAL AND SOUTH						
Argentina, Concordia	99	0	82	99	0	64
Brazil, Belem	98	0	65	99	0	55
Brazil, Goiania	89	11	48	90	8	38
Brazil, Porto Alegre	67	0	41	71	0	35
Colombia, Cali	89	2	63	91	2	49
Costa Rica	88	5	41	86	6	38
Ecuador, Quito	78	10		79	9	
Peru, Lima	84	6		88	6	
Peru, Trujillo	98	0	0	99	0	0
US, Puerto Rico	92	3	45	95	2	46
Uruguay, Montevideo	99	0	54	99	0	45
AMERICA, NORTH						
Canada	88	1	44	89	1	46
Canada, Alberta	98	1	46	98	1	45
Canada, British Columbia	94	3	41	94	3	44
Canada, Manitoba	86	1	46	81	1	51
Canada, New Brunswick	99	0	50	95	1	54
Canada, Newfoundland	98	0	48	99	0	51
Canada, Northwest Territories	82	0	24	94	0	0
Canada, Nova Scotia	97	2	44	95	5	48
Canada, Ontario	89	1	43	90	1	45
Canada, Prince Edward Island	99	0	38	99	0	25
+Canada, Quebec	79	0	45	80	0	48
Canada, Saskatchewan	95	3	53	97	1	46
Canada, Yukon	99	0	13	99	0	20
+US, Cent. Calif.: Non-Hisp. White	97	1	47	96	1	51
+US, Cent. Calif.: Hispanic	94	2	35	97	1	40
US, Los Angeles: Non-Hisp. White	96	1	39	97	1	52
US, Los Angeles: Hispanic White	97	0		98	1	
US, Los Angeles: Black	96	0		97	0	
US, Los Angeles: Chinese	99	0		99	0	
US, Los Angeles: Filipino	98	0		99	0	
US, Los Angeles: Korean	99	0		99	0	
US, Los Angeles: Japanese	99	0		97	0	
US, San Francisco: Non-Hisp. White	95	1	31	98	1	50
US, San Francisco: Hispanic White	96	0	16	97	0	28
US, San Francisco: Black	96	1	38	93	1	37
US, San Francisco: Chinese	98	1	43	98	0	36
US, San Francisco: Filipino	94	0	31	99	0	29
US, San Francisco: Japanese	99	0	21	91	4	35
US, Connecticut: White	98	0	44	97	1	45
US, Connecticut: Black	95	1	44	96	0	37
US, Atlanta: White	97	1	37	98	1	38
US, Atlanta: Black	93	1	26	92	2	37
US, Iowa	97	1	49	97	1	52
US, Central Louisiana: White	94	0	39	94	3	51
US, Central Louisiana: Black	92	0	38	83	8	33
US, New Orleans: White	97	1	34	98	1	43
US, New Orleans: Black	92	4	37	95	3	55
US, Detroit: White	98	1	47	98	0	50
US, Detroit: Black	95	0	40	97	0	42
US, New Mexico: Non-Hisp. White	97	2	47	95	2	52
US, New Mexico: Hispanic White	97	2	55	99	0	48
US, New Mexico: American Indian	90	0	60	92	0	67
US, Utah	99	0	41	96	1	44
US, Seattle	96	0	42	98	0	43
US, SEER: White	97	1	42	97	1	47
US, SEER: Black	95	0	37	95	1	40
ASIA						
+China, Qidong	91	0	79	86	2	77
+China, Shanghai	73	1	61	67	2	70
China, Tianjin	76	0	61	78	0	60
Hong Kong	79	3	28	80	2	29
India, Bangalore	95	5	38	94	4	39
India, Barshi, Paranda and Bhum	99	0		99	0	
India, Bombay	96	3	43	95	5	44
India, Karunagappally	94	6		99	0	
India, Madras	97	2	45	95	5	40
India, Trivandrum	99	0	36	99	0	12
Israel: All Jews	94			92		
Jews born in Israel	94			96		
Jews born in America or Europe	93			91		
Jews born in Africa or Asia	96			93		
Non-Jews	96			94		
Japan, Hiroshima	87	6	50	90	5	42
Japan, Miyagi	79	8	58	82	5	54
Japan, Nagasaki	84	12	43	81	13	42
Japan, Osaka	99	0	65	99	0	63
+Japan, Saga	75	18	62	70	21	65
Japan, Yamagata	72	20	70	74	21	64
Korea, Kangwha	99		44	99		67
Kuwait: Non-Kuwaitis	95	3		91	9	
Kuwait: Kuwaitis	91	9		95	5	
Philippines, Manila	77	5		72	5	
Singapore: Chinese	96	2		94	3	
Singapore: Malay	90	8		93	0	
Singapore: Indian	90	5		90	10	
Thailand, Chiang Mai	99	0		99	0	
Thailand, Khon Kaen	99	0		99	0	
Viet Nam, Hanoi	67			60		

+ IMPORTANT-SEE NOTES ON POPULATION PAGE

INDICES OF DATA QUALITY
Non-Hodgkin lymphomas (ICD-9 200+202) (contd)

	MALE			FEMALE		
EUROPE	MV	DCO	M/I	MV	DCO	M/I
Austria, Tyrol	96	3	43	91	5	37
+Belarus	91	0	73	91	1	67
Croatia	95	4	56	95	3	57
+Czech Republic	84	1	63	85	2	57
Denmark	99	1	53	99	1	55
Estonia	99		72	99		69
Finland	99	0	42	99	0	45
France, Bas-Rhin	99		41	99		44
France, Calvados	98		55	97		72
France, Doubs	98		38	95		39
France, Haut-Rhin	99		39	99		48
France, Herault	99		45	99		49
France, Isere	99		20	99		28
France, Somme	96		47	99		44
France, Tarn	99		51	99		51
Germany, Eastern States	99	0	57	99	0	53
+Germany, Saarland	95	3	45	94	4	44
Iceland	99	0	58	99	0	35
Ireland, Southern	96		64	96		69
Italy, Ferrara	99	0	60	97	3	39
Italy, Florence	84	1	45	85	2	49
Italy, Genoa	91	1	45	88	2	49
Italy, Latina	97	3	38	96	4	36
Italy, Macerata	90	0	0	90	5	36
Italy, Modena	98	1	41	96	3	42
Italy, Parma	97	2	46	98	0	47
Italy, Ragusa	97	0	62	99	0	48
Italy, Romagna	99	1	40	99	1	46
Italy, Torino	97	1	46	96	2	42
Italy, Trieste	69	2	29	87	1	33
Italy, Varese	98	1	45	98	1	42
Italy, Veneto	98	1	40	96	2	42
+Latvia	97	2	63	98	2	58
+Malta	83	7	53	76	7	62
The Netherlands	99		51	99		55
The Netherlands, Eindhoven	99		52	99		56
The Netherlands, Maastricht	99		54	99		54
Norway	99	0	56	99	1	53
Poland, Cracow	89	5	75	92	5	79
Poland, Kielce	91	0	50	90	0	51
Poland, Lower Silesia	63	0	57	63	0	56
Poland, Warsaw City	[85]	6	61	[81]	5	68
Slovakia	97	0	49	96	0	41
Slovenia	99	0	50	99	0	45
Spain, Albacete	84	9	34	83	9	35
Spain, Asturias	99	0	48	99	0	42
Spain, Basque Country	94	4	44	95	4	49
Spain, Granada	97	2	56	97	1	36
Spain, Mallorca	96	1	51	98	1	57
Spain, Murcia	99	0	44	99	0	39
Spain, Navarra	96	4	40	93	5	48
Spain, Tarragona	99	0	55	98	1	40
Spain, Zaragoza	94	1	58	91	3	54

	MALE			FEMALE		
	MV	DCO	M/I	MV	DCO	M/I
Sweden	99		51	99		52
Switzerland, Basel	99	0	45	99	0	48
Switzerland, Geneva	99	1	34	98	2	60
Switzerland, Graubunden	95	0	87	90	0	62
Switzerland, Neuchatel	96	4	45	96	0	56
Switzerland, St Gall-Appenzell	99	0	46	99	0	47
Switzerland, Valais	99	0	35	99	0	62
Switzerland, Vaud	99	0	38	99	0	51
Switzerland, Zurich	99	0	47	99	0	47
+UK, England and Wales	[92]		55	[92]		57
UK, East Anglia			53			59
UK, Mersey	85	2	61	83	3	62
UK, North Western	84	4	55	83	4	56
UK, Oxford	99	1	50	99	0	55
UK, South Thames	73	16	55	74	15	58
UK, South Western	89	3	54	86	5	55
UK, Wessex	[89]	3	41	[86]	3	44
+UK, West Midlands		1	55		2	58
UK, Yorkshire	93	3	52	90	3	58
UK, Scotland	92	1	54	90	2	54
UK, Scotland, West	91	2	58	88	4	58
Yugoslavia, Vojvodina	69	10	61	64	11	56

OCEANIA

	MALE			FEMALE		
	MV	DCO	M/I	MV	DCO	M/I
Australian Capital Territory	96	0		95	2	
Australia, New South Wales	95	2		95	2	
South Australia	88		45	89		58
Australia, Tasmania	91		52	89		45
Australia, Victoria	94	1	47	95	1	53
Western Australia	94	2	53	94	4	46
French Polynesia	86	14		73	20	
+New Zealand: Non-Maori	97	2	57	97	2	60
+New Zealand: Maori	99	0	36	99	0	23
US, Hawaii: White	99	0	46	99	0	58
US, Hawaii: Japanese	98	0	52	99	0	48
US, Hawaii: Hawaiian	99	0	69	99	0	78
US, Hawaii: Filipino	99	0	52	99	0	43
US, Hawaii: Chinese	99	0	52	99	0	33

+ IMPORTANT-SEE NOTES ON POPULATION PAGE

[] CYTOLOGICAL VERIFICATION EXCLUDED

INDICES OF DATA QUALITY
Hodgkin's disease (ICD-9 201)

	MALE			FEMALE		
AFRICA	MV	DCO	M/I	MV	DCO	M/I
Algeria, Setif	99			99		
France, La Reunion	99		33	99		40
Mali, Bamako	95	5		99	0	
Uganda, Kyadondo	99			99		
Zimbabwe, Harare: African	99	0		99	0	
Zimbabwe, Harare: European	-	-		99	0	

AMERICA, CENTRAL AND SOUTH

	MALE			FEMALE		
	MV	DCO	M/I	MV	DCO	M/I
Argentina, Concordia	99	0	0	99	0	150
Brazil, Belem	97	0	48	99	0	71
Brazil, Goiania	89	8	28	93	7	23
Brazil, Porto Alegre	69	0	62	54	0	100
Colombia, Cali	90	3	38	91	0	43
Costa Rica	90	5	48	88	7	48
Ecuador, Quito	86	8		74	6	
Peru, Lima	83	13		86	9	
Peru, Trujillo	99	0	0	99	0	0
US, Puerto Rico	98	1	34	96	1	24
Uruguay, Montevideo	99	0	36	99	0	28

AMERICA, NORTH

	MALE			FEMALE		
	MV	DCO	M/I	MV	DCO	M/I
Canada	93	0	22	92	0	19
Canada, Alberta	99	0	16	99	0	12
Canada, British Columbia	97	1	17	99	0	13
Canada, Manitoba	90	0	29	84	0	30
Canada, New Brunswick	99	0	29	93	0	33
Canada, Newfoundland	99	0	17	99	0	6
Canada, Northwest Territories	99	0	0	99	0	0
Canada, Nova Scotia	99	1	36	99	0	20
Canada, Ontario	94	0	24	94	0	18
Canada, Prince Edward Island	99	0	0	99	0	43
+Canada, Quebec	87	0	22	83	0	22
Canada, Saskatchewan	99	0	18	99	0	26
Canada, Yukon	99	0	13	99	0	0
+US, Cent. Calif.: Non-Hisp. White	97	2	35	97	1	18
+US, Cent. Calif.: Hispanic	99	0	29	99	0	24
US, Los Angeles: Non-Hisp. White	99	1	27	99	1	25
US, Los Angeles: Hispanic White	99	0		99	0	
US, Los Angeles: Black	99	0		99	0	
US, Los Angeles: Chinese	99	0		99	0	
US, Los Angeles: Filipino	99	0		99	0	
US, Los Angeles: Korean	99	0		99	0	
US, Los Angeles: Japanese	99	0		99	0	
US, San Francisco: Non-Hisp. White	99	1	19	99	1	18
US, San Francisco: Hispanic White	99	0	30	99	0	13
US, San Francisco: Black	99	0	34	99	0	12
US, San Francisco: Chinese	99	0	29	99	0	0
US, San Francisco: Filipino	99	0	0	99	0	50
US, San Francisco: Japanese	99	0	67	99	0	0
US, Connecticut: White	98	0	17	99	0	20
US, Connecticut: Black	99	0	54	99	0	14
US, Atlanta: White	99	0	22	99	0	14
US, Atlanta: Black	99	0	6	97	3	6
US, Iowa	99	0	25	99	0	15

	MALE			FEMALE		
	MV	DCO	M/I	MV	DCO	M/I
US, Central Louisiana: White	99	0	50	92	0	15
US, Central Louisiana: Black	99	0	25	99	0	100
US, New Orleans: White	97	2	29	99	0	23
US, New Orleans: Black	99	0	44	94	6	19
US, Detroit: White	99	0	24	99	0	19
US, Detroit: Black	99	0	34	98	0	27
US, New Mexico: Non-Hisp. White	97	2	25	98	2	17
US, New Mexico: Hispanic White	91	0	26	95	0	19
US, New Mexico: American Indian	99	0	0	99	0	0
US, Utah	99	0	23	99	0	17
US, Seattle	99	0	19	99	0	18
US, SEER: White	99	0	21	99	0	18
US, SEER: Black	99	0	28	99	1	16

ASIA

	MALE			FEMALE		
	MV	DCO	M/I	MV	DCO	M/I
+China, Qidong	99	0	100	99	0	100
+China, Shanghai	83	0	41	77	0	43
China, Tianjin	76	0	26	78	0	16
Hong Kong	83	0	11	79	0	10
India, Bangalore	95	5	36	98	2	17
India, Barshi, Paranda and Bhum	99	0		-	-	
India, Bombay	97	3	25	98	2	25
India, Karunagappally	99	0		99	0	
India, Madras	98	2	46	98	2	31
India, Trivandrum	71	29	14	75	25	25
Israel: All Jews	96			98		
Jews born in Israel	97			97		
Jews born in America or Europe	94			99		
Jews born in Africa or Asia	96			96		
Non-Jews	98			96		
Japan, Hiroshima	99	0	38	91	9	9
Japan, Miyagi	90	0	29	80	0	33
Japan, Nagasaki	92	0	31	99	0	60
Japan, Osaka	99	0	31	99	0	26
+Japan, Saga	67	0	67	80	0	20
Japan, Yamagata	80	20	20	50	0	0
Korea, Kangwha	99		0	-		-
Kuwait: Non-Kuwaitis	96	0		99	0	
Kuwait: Kuwaitis	99	0		99	0	
Philippines, Manila	74	5		76	6	
Singapore: Chinese	99	0		85	0	
Singapore: Malay	99	0		99	0	
Singapore: Indian	99	0		99	0	
Thailand, Chiang Mai	99	0		99	0	
Thailand, Khon Kaen	99	0		99	0	
Viet Nam, Hanoi	67			64		

+ IMPORTANT-SEE NOTES ON POPULATION PAGE

INDICES OF DATA QUALITY
Hodgkin's disease (ICD-9 201) (contd)

EUROPE	MALE			FEMALE		
	MV	DCO	M/I	MV	DCO	M/I
Austria, Tyrol	99	0	20	99	0	34
+Belarus	97	0	48	95	0	40
Croatia	95	5	61	96	4	59
+Czech Republic	90	1	55	89	2	45
Denmark	99	0	33	99	0	38
Estonia	98		63	99		58
Finland	99	0	38	99	1	42
France, Bas-Rhin	99		17	99		26
France, Calvados	99		12	99		17
France, Doubs	99		34	99		17
France, Haut-Rhin	99		36	99		13
France, Herault	99		17	99		11
France, Isere	99		18	99		6
France, Somme	99		32	99		21
France, Tarn	99		30	99		43
Germany, Eastern States	99	0	60	99	0	44
+Germany, Saarland	95	3	32	98	2	42
Iceland	99	0	25	99	0	38
Ireland, Southern	99		71	99		22
Italy, Ferrara	93	7	43	85	0	8
Italy, Florence	83	3	42	77	3	39
Italy, Genoa	92	0	31	92	0	33
Italy, Latina	99	0	63	99	0	30
Italy, Macerata	92	0	25	75	17	42
Italy, Modena	98	2	43	98	2	38
Italy, Parma	99	0	46	99	0	53
Italy, Ragusa	99	0	15	99	0	39
Italy, Romagna	97	3	39	99	0	11
Italy, Torino	97	1	23	98	0	17
Italy, Trieste	62	0	19	80	4	28
Italy, Varese	96	1	27	98	0	23
Italy, Veneto	96	1	34	97	2	29
+Latvia	98	2	45	97	3	35
+Malta	99	0	71	99	0	10
The Netherlands	99		30	99		35
The Netherlands, Eindhoven	98		13	99		8
The Netherlands, Maastricht	99		32	99		27
Norway	99	0	24	99	0	36
Poland, Cracow	89	4	56	90	6	48
Poland, Kielce	92	1	67	84	2	57
Poland, Lower Silesia	63	2	59	65	0	55
Poland, Warsaw City	[88]	4	68	[95]	2	43
Slovakia	96	0	45	97	0	40
Slovenia	99	0	39	99	0	54
Spain, Albacete	83	8	50	50	25	50
Spain, Asturias	99	0	27	99	0	15
Spain, Basque Country	98	1	27	94	4	23
Spain, Granada	99	0	43	99	0	38
Spain, Mallorca	99	0	46	99	0	18
Spain, Murcia	98	0	34	99	0	50
Spain, Navarra	97	3	33	97	0	27
Spain, Tarragona	99	0	31	99	0	41
Spain, Zaragoza	96	2	58	90	7	60

	MALE			FEMALE		
	MV	DCO	M/I	MV	DCO	M/I
Sweden	99		24	99		22
Switzerland, Basel	99	0	57	99	0	28
Switzerland, Geneva	99	0	42	99	0	45
Switzerland, Graubunden	99	0	21	99	0	50
Switzerland, Neuchatel	99	0	55	99	0	83
Switzerland, St Gall-Appenzell	99	0	68	99	0	50
Switzerland, Valais	99	0	40	99	0	20
Switzerland, Vaud	99	0	49	99	0	34
Switzerland, Zurich	99	0	38	99	0	42
+UK, England and Wales	[95]		31	[95]		33
UK, East Anglia			34			41
UK, Mersey	98	0	37	92	3	34
UK, North Western	92	0	30	94	1	40
UK, Oxford	99	0	33	99	0	27
UK, South Thames	77	5	30	78	5	30
UK, South Western	93	1	27	94	1	28
UK, Wessex	[88]	1	29	[83]	1	18
+UK, West Midlands		1	32		1	35
UK, Yorkshire	97	0	36	97	0	31
UK, Scotland	96	1	29	98	0	34
UK, Scotland, West	97	2	28	97	1	38
Yugoslavia, Vojvodina	61	10	61	63	14	53

OCEANIA

	MALE			FEMALE		
	MV	DCO	M/I	MV	DCO	M/I
Australian Capital Territory	99	0		88	0	
Australia, New South Wales	98	0		98	1	
South Australia	87		23	87		25
Australia, Tasmania	95		45	93		15
Australia, Victoria	99	0	18	96	0	23
Western Australia	96	1	16	97	0	26
French Polynesia	86	0		99	0	
+New Zealand: Non-Maori	99	0	29	98	2	35
+New Zealand: Maori	99	0	0	99	0	0
US, Hawaii: White	99	0	23	99	0	18
US, Hawaii: Japanese	99	0	44	99	0	45
US, Hawaii: Hawaiian	99	0	75	99	0	18
US, Hawaii: Filipino	99	0	25	99	0	20
US, Hawaii: Chinese	99	0	0	99	0	0

+ IMPORTANT-SEE NOTES ON POPULATION PAGE

[] CYTOLOGICAL VERIFICATION EXCLUDED

INDICES OF DATA QUALITY
Multiple myeloma (ICD-9 203)

	MALE			FEMALE		
	MV	DCO	M/I	MV	DCO	M/I
AFRICA						
Algeria, Setif	99			99		
France, La Reunion	97		69	99		71
Mali, Bamako	-	-		-	-	
Uganda, Kyadondo	99			50		
Zimbabwe, Harare: African	90	5		92	0	
Zimbabwe, Harare: European	50	50		50	50	
AMERICA, CENTRAL AND SOUTH						
Argentina, Concordia	-	-	ncr	99	0	0
Brazil, Belem	99	0	100	99	0	67
Brazil, Goiania	75	17	42	63	13	69
Brazil, Porto Alegre	46	0	77	46	0	76
Colombia, Cali	76	10	78	73	4	80
Costa Rica	57	17	88	44	19	99
Ecuador, Quito	55	24		75	15	
Peru, Lima	62	19		56	17	
Peru, Trujillo	90	0	0	86	0	0
US, Puerto Rico	85	5	73	80	6	89
Uruguay, Montevideo	99	0	84	99	0	77
AMERICA, NORTH						
Canada	69	3	66	63	3	68
Canada, Alberta	93	2	74	89	2	73
Canada, British Columbia	82	8	67	77	11	73
Canada, Manitoba	74	3	67	71	4	74
Canada, New Brunswick	86	2	82	83	7	78
Canada, Newfoundland	91	2	98	95	0	118
Canada, Northwest Territories	75	0	75	0	50	150
Canada, Nova Scotia	87	10	85	84	15	94
Canada, Ontario	61	2	60	55	2	59
Canada, Prince Edward Island	99	0	65	95	5	79
+Canada, Quebec	57	0	69	52	0	71
Canada, Saskatchewan	86	4	72	85	6	83
Canada, Yukon	99	0	50	25	0	100
+US, Cent. Calif.: Non-Hisp. White	83	1	73	84	2	63
+US, Cent. Calif.: Hispanic	89	0	69	84	3	97
US, Los Angeles: Non-Hisp. White	93	1	66	89	2	73
US, Los Angeles: Hispanic White	92	0		93	3	
US, Los Angeles: Black	93	2		91	1	
US, Los Angeles: Chinese	99	0		86	0	
US, Los Angeles: Filipino	88	6		92	8	
US, Los Angeles: Korean	99	0		99	0	
US, Los Angeles: Japanese	99	0		99	0	
US, San Francisco: Non-Hisp. White	90	2	69	83	1	81
US, San Francisco: Hispanic White	86	0	73	93	4	63
US, San Francisco: Black	88	1	51	84	2	84
US, San Francisco: Chinese	92	0	17	85	0	90
US, San Francisco: Filipino	80	0	65	92	0	33
US, San Francisco: Japanese	99	0	33	99	0	300
US, Connecticut: White	94	4	62	92	4	72
US, Connecticut: Black	97	3	91	93	0	52
US, Atlanta: White	90	2	71	85	1	81
US, Atlanta: Black	80	1	63	77	4	75
US, Iowa	92	2	70	90	1	76
US, Central Louisiana: White	79	0	100	81	4	96
US, Central Louisiana: Black	90	0	80	99	0	22
US, New Orleans: White	88	2	69	84	4	95
US, New Orleans: Black	96	1	66	81	6	66
US, Detroit: White	93	0	61	94	0	71
US, Detroit: Black	93	1	58	89	0	60
US, New Mexico: Non-Hisp. White	92	2	87	76	4	76
US, New Mexico: Hispanic White	86	6	56	84	0	105
US, New Mexico: American Indian	71	0	143	70	0	60
US, Utah	90	0	72	87	0	81
US, Seattle	89	0	71	86	0	69
US, SEER: White	91	2	69	88	1	75
US, SEER: Black	90	1	61	86	2	69
ASIA						
+China, Qidong	84	3	95	75	0	75
+China, Shanghai	69	1	74	62	3	99
China, Tianjin	73	0	92	72	0	72
Hong Kong	63	9	43	64	6	38
India, Bangalore	93	5	51	86	8	36
India, Barshi, Paranda and Bhum	99	0		0	0	
India, Bombay	94	6	59	90	9	56
India, Karunagappally	99	0		60	40	
India, Madras	99	0	46	99	0	71
India, Trivandrum	89	6	11	99	0	0
Israel: All Jews	73			76		
Jews born in Israel	84			92		
Jews born in America or Europe	68			74		
Jews born in Africa or Asia	79			76		
Non-Jews	85			82		
Japan, Hiroshima	72	17	64	70	21	65
Japan, Miyagi	69	13	86	52	26	74
Japan, Nagasaki	67	22	72	69	24	74
Japan, Osaka	98	0	71	97	0	76
+Japan, Saga	53	23	73	50	24	81
Japan, Yamagata	51	36	87	37	41	78
Korea, Kangwha	99		0	99		0
Kuwait: Non-Kuwaitis	95	0		86	0	
Kuwait: Kuwaitis	86	14		99	0	
Philippines, Manila	45	21		38	35	
Singapore: Chinese	74	4		79	4	
Singapore: Malay	84	0		69	15	
Singapore: Indian	90	0		67	0	
Thailand, Chiang Mai	93	7		99	0	
Thailand, Khon Kaen	99	0		99	0	
Viet Nam, Hanoi	67			-		

+ IMPORTANT-SEE NOTES ON POPULATION PAGE

INDICES OF DATA QUALITY
Multiple myeloma (ICD-9 203) (contd)

	MALE			FEMALE		
EUROPE	MV	DCO	M/I	MV	DCO	M/I
Austria, Tyrol	89	10	67	76	13	65
+Belarus	89	1	71	90	0	77
Croatia	70	4	71	77	4	70
+Czech Republic	66	3	78	66	5	82
Denmark	98	2	86	97	2	81
Estonia	99		74	95		68
Finland	76	2	67	74	4	72
France, Bas-Rhin	93		112	91		162
France, Calvados	57		105	69		151
France, Doubs	97		35	91		42
France, Haut-Rhin	97		71	99		83
France, Herault	99		84	99		114
France, Isere	99		48	99		56
France, Somme	97		103	98		124
France, Tarn	99		164	99		91
Germany, Eastern States	99	0	84	99	0	92
+Germany, Saarland	71	20	83	78	15	81
Iceland	99	0	104	99	0	90
Ireland, Southern	74		93	82		65
Italy, Ferrara	97	3	69	87	10	65
Italy, Florence	38	5	41	30	6	53
Italy, Genoa	80	5	72	71	3	95
Italy, Latina	99	0	69	90	10	71
Italy, Macerata	93	0	100	89	0	74
Italy, Modena	98	2	56	95	3	55
Italy, Parma	94	6	55	91	6	71
Italy, Ragusa	78	3	75	71	0	62
Italy, Romagna	99	1	48	99	0	69
Italy, Torino	82	7	82	80	9	77
Italy, Trieste	45	2	43	62	3	58
Italy, Varese	88	1	77	80	3	75
Italy, Veneto	87	4	84	86	6	71
+Latvia	96	1	70	99	1	56
+Malta	70	0	80	99	0	69
The Netherlands	98		83	98		98
The Netherlands, Eindhoven	95		87	98		120
The Netherlands, Maastricht	99		84	99		83
Norway	88	10	93	86	11	104
Poland, Cracow	78	6	91	75	7	79
Poland, Kielce	78	4	109	65	0	76
Poland, Lower Silesia	52	0	90	50	1	69
Poland, Warsaw City	[71]	10	85	[68]	9	86
Slovakia	94	0	54	91	0	53
Slovenia	93	2	73	93	1	61
Spain, Albacete	87	13	60	88	6	82
Spain, Asturias	99	0	87	99	0	72
Spain, Basque Country	84	14	78	87	11	85
Spain, Granada	92	6	81	89	4	84
Spain, Mallorca	89	5	56	90	2	70
Spain, Murcia	91	4	67	91	5	59
Spain, Navarra	73	10	65	73	23	67
Spain, Tarragona	92	3	68	93	5	70
Spain, Zaragoza	81	10	66	80	9	78

	MALE			FEMALE		
	MV	DCO	M/I	MV	DCO	M/I
Sweden	93		79	92		85
Switzerland, Basel	98	0	102	97	0	109
Switzerland, Geneva	94	0	96	99	0	87
Switzerland, Graubunden	87	0	70	91	0	68
Switzerland, Neuchatel	91	9	127	99	0	138
Switzerland, St Gall-Appenzell	94	1	69	98	0	68
Switzerland, Valais	91	3	73	76	0	67
Switzerland, Vaud	99	0	81	99	0	79
Switzerland, Zurich	96	1	89	99	0	86
+UK, England and Wales	[83]		78	[81]		81
UK, East Anglia			87			89
UK, Mersey	52	4	92	53	4	95
UK, North Western	40	8	75	40	6	81
UK, Oxford	98	2	79	99	1	68
UK, South Thames	54	28	77	56	29	78
UK, South Western	73	2	71	68	1	77
UK, Wessex	[76]	7	63	[74]	10	70
+UK, West Midlands		5	70		8	79
UK, Yorkshire	84	4	67	83	4	74
UK, Scotland	68	3	66	68	3	66
UK, Scotland, West	72	5	60	73	6	60
Yugoslavia, Vojvodina	44	17	78	34	20	83

OCEANIA

	MALE			FEMALE		
	MV	DCO	M/I	MV	DCO	M/I
Australian Capital Territory	90	0		85	0	
Australia, New South Wales	90	2		88	3	
South Australia	85		74	85		71
Australia, Tasmania	80		67	65		80
Australia, Victoria	88	1	72	85	1	78
Western Australia	86	5	71	82	3	82
French Polynesia	99	0		57	43	
+New Zealand: Non-Maori	92	4	68	95	3	60
+New Zealand: Maori	96	4	52	96	4	46
US, Hawaii: White	99	0	65	95	0	63
US, Hawaii: Japanese	95	0	41	85	0	54
US, Hawaii: Hawaiian	99	0	40	94	0	67
US, Hawaii: Filipino	95	0	57	99	0	50
US, Hawaii: Chinese	99	0	33	50	0	150

+ IMPORTANT-SEE NOTES ON POPULATION PAGE

[] CYTOLOGICAL VERIFICATION EXCLUDED

INDICES OF DATA QUALITY
Lymphoid leukaemia (ICD-9 204)

	MALE			FEMALE		
AFRICA	MV	DCO	M/I	MV	DCO	M/I
Algeria, Setif	99			99		
France, La Reunion	99			99		
Mali, Bamako	-		-	-		-
Uganda, Kyadondo	67			99		
Zimbabwe, Harare: African	95	5		99	0	
Zimbabwe, Harare: European	50	50		99	0	

AMERICA, CENTRAL AND SOUTH	MV	DCO	M/I	MV	DCO	M/I
Argentina, Concordia	99	0	160	99	0	67
Brazil, Belem	99	0	73	99	0	28
Brazil, Goiania	59	3	44	50	30	80
Brazil, Porto Alegre	51	2	64	49	0	60
Colombia, Cali	92	0	95	88	3	76
Costa Rica	59	7	48	58	10	53
Ecuador, Quito	82	16		87	9	
Peru, Lima	92	3		90	4	
Peru, Trujillo	99	0	0	99	0	0
US, Puerto Rico	94	3	37	90	2	45
Uruguay, Montevideo	99	0	62	99	0	64

AMERICA, NORTH	MV	DCO	M/I	MV	DCO	M/I
Canada	59	2	39	57	2	37
Canada, Alberta	94	3	51	92	2	44
Canada, British Columbia	69	8	41	71	11	44
Canada, Manitoba	87	1	42	87	2	38
Canada, New Brunswick	78	0	46	79	3	48
Canada, Newfoundland	99	0	43	97	0	45
Canada, Northwest Territories	99	0	50	99	0	67
Canada, Nova Scotia	88	11	56	84	13	48
Canada, Ontario	57	1	36	50	1	34
Canada, Prince Edward Island	90	0	33	99	0	33
+Canada, Quebec	41	0	38	43	0	38
Canada, Saskatchewan	56	2	30	49	2	26
Canada, Yukon	82	18	55	40	0	0
+US, Cent. Calif.: Non-Hisp. White	83	3	51	78	6	54
+US, Cent. Calif.: Hispanic	95	0	36	98	0	47
US, Los Angeles: Non-Hisp. White	92	2	45	85	4	42
US, Los Angeles: Hispanic White	99	0		96	1	
US, Los Angeles: Black	91	0		92	2	
US, Los Angeles: Chinese	99	0		99	0	
US, Los Angeles: Filipino	99	0		82	0	
US, Los Angeles: Korean	99	0		99	0	
US, Los Angeles: Japanese	99	0		99	0	
US, San Francisco: Non-Hisp. White	92	2	46	89	4	39
US, San Francisco: Hispanic White	99	0	31	97	3	21
US, San Francisco: Black	84	0	56	85	0	30
US, San Francisco: Chinese	96	0	27	99	0	33
US, San Francisco: Filipino	92	0	31	99	0	33
US, San Francisco: Japanese	99	0	100	99	0	100
US, Connecticut: White	94	2	42	93	3	47
US, Connecticut: Black	95	5	58	99	0	35
US, Atlanta: White	97	2	48	94	1	36
US, Atlanta: Black	89	0	41	91	0	46
US, Iowa	96	1	37	95	2	40

	MALE			FEMALE		
	MV	DCO	M/I	MV	DCO	M/I
US, Central Louisiana: White	91	0	73	74	5	53
US, Central Louisiana: Black	88	0	50	99	0	100
US, New Orleans: White	96	3	47	97	1	34
US, New Orleans: Black	97	3	45	95	5	60
US, Detroit: White	95	1	36	93	1	36
US, Detroit: Black	95	0	54	88	0	43
US, New Mexico: Non-Hisp. White	91	1	39	86	5	44
US, New Mexico: Hispanic White	96	0	43	96	0	37
US, New Mexico: American Indian	99	0	60	99	0	38
US, Utah	95	1	46	98	1	43
US, Seattle	99	1	45	98	2	41
US, SEER: White	95	1	42	94	2	40
US, SEER: Black	92	0	54	89	0	41

ASIA	MV	DCO	M/I	MV	DCO	M/I
+China, Qidong	94	0	97	95	0	85
+China, Shanghai	80	0	65	72	2	67
China, Tianjin	90	0	25	91	0	26
Hong Kong	84	3	23	78	4	30
India, Bangalore	91	6	50	93	7	44
India, Barshi, Paranda and Bhum	99	0		99	0	
India, Bombay	94	6	63	92	8	74
India, Karunagappally	99	0		99	0	
India, Madras	99	0	44	99	1	47
India, Trivandrum	89	11	22	99	0	0
Israel: All Jews	96			99		
Jews born in Israel	95			99		
Jews born in America or Europe	97			99		
Jews born in Africa or Asia	94			98		
Non-Jews	99			99		
Japan, Hiroshima	89	7	65	76	20	80
Japan, Miyagi	77	5	62	75	10	69
Japan, Nagasaki	99	0	369	99	0	376
Japan, Osaka	99	0	72	99	0	72
+Japan, Saga	62	25	62	64	22	66
Japan, Yamagata	67	28	85	63	32	76
Korea, Kangwha	99		25	99		0
Kuwait: Non-Kuwaitis	87	12		97	3	
Kuwait: Kuwaitis	89	6		70	20	
Philippines, Manila	49	15		45	20	
Singapore: Chinese	89	1		86	1	
Singapore: Malay	94	0		80	0	
Singapore: Indian	99	0		99	0	
Thailand, Chiang Mai	99	0		99	0	
Thailand, Khon Kaen	99	0		99	0	
Viet Nam, Hanoi	95			93		

+ IMPORTANT-SEE NOTES ON POPULATION PAGE

INDICES OF DATA QUALITY
Lymphoid leukaemia (ICD-9 204) (contd)

EUROPE	MALE MV	DCO	M/I	FEMALE MV	DCO	M/I
Austria, Tyrol	87	4	46	86	9	41
+Belarus	96	0	65	96	0	68
Croatia	95	2	50	91	4	49
+Czech Republic	71	4	72	69	5	76
Denmark	97	2	61	96	3	62
Estonia	99		61	99		48
Finland	95	3	59	95	3	56
France, Bas-Rhin	97		39	91		62
France, Calvados	71		106	57		57
France, Doubs	88		72	86		40
France, Haut-Rhin	99		57	99		79
France, Herault	99		80	99		85
France, Isere	99		29	99		53
France, Somme	98		59	98		55
France, Tarn	99		70	99		90
Germany, Eastern States	99	0	67	99	1	76
+Germany, Saarland	93	4	42	83	14	45
Iceland	99	0	78	99	0	63
Ireland, Southern	96		41	94		60
Italy, Ferrara	99	0	54	92	4	32
Italy, Florence	95	5	75	91	9	69
Italy, Genoa	80	5	71	80	4	69
Italy, Latina	89	11	63	80	20	53
Italy, Macerata	93	0	93	82	0	64
Italy, Modena	94	6	64	97	3	44
Italy, Parma	95	2	84	96	4	104
Italy, Ragusa	99	0	40	99	0	35
Italy, Romagna	99	1	47	97	3	55
Italy, Torino	94	4	63	93	4	52
Italy, Trieste	51	3	40	73	2	39
Italy, Varese	95	1	58	90	3	49
Italy, Veneto	98	2	53	94	6	66
+Latvia	98	1	70	98	1	62
+Malta	99	0	17	99	0	67
The Netherlands	99		60	99		70
The Netherlands, Eindhoven	99		58	97		60
The Netherlands, Maastricht	99		62	99		62
Norway	93	6	63	92	7	72
Poland, Cracow	70	17	83	76	5	89
Poland, Kielce	82	2	85	85	3	89
Poland, Lower Silesia	80	1	77	77	2	65
Poland, Warsaw City	[59]	21	99	[60]	17	86
Slovakia	94	0	55	94	0	53
Slovenia	98	2	61	96	3	53
Spain, Albacete	92	4	40	99	0	64
Spain, Asturias	99	0	40	99	0	50
Spain, Basque Country	94	4	47	91	9	60
Spain, Granada	99	0	53	99	0	57
Spain, Mallorca	99	0	38	99	0	63
Spain, Murcia	99	0	53	95	1	38
Spain, Navarra	86	5	57	85	15	51
Spain, Tarragona	99	0	36	99	0	33
Spain, Zaragoza	88	8	57	89	8	58

	MALE MV	DCO	M/I	FEMALE MV	DCO	M/I
Sweden	95		53	94		59
Switzerland, Basel	98	0	94	97	0	135
Switzerland, Geneva	99	0	56	91	9	79
Switzerland, Graubunden	96	0	57	91	0	82
Switzerland, Neuchatel	84	16	72	89	11	89
Switzerland, St Gall-Appenzell	95	5	57	98	2	78
Switzerland, Valais	93	7	52	99	0	71
Switzerland, Vaud	99	0	73	99	0	93
Switzerland, Zurich	99	0	70	98	2	66
+UK, England and Wales	[84]		52	[83]		52
UK, East Anglia			63			63
UK, Mersey	54	7	72	57	9	81
UK, North Western	50	7	55	50	6	59
UK, Oxford	99	0	43	99	0	41
UK, South Thames	67	22	47	59	28	53
UK, South Western	77	2	41	76	1	41
UK, Wessex	[72]	8	44	[64]	10	39
+UK, West Midlands		3	53		6	49
UK, Yorkshire	87	4	52	85	3	51
UK, Scotland	75	3	43	70	6	46
UK, Scotland, West	85	4	43	76	8	45
Yugoslavia, Vojvodina	57	15	69	48	14	89

OCEANIA

	MALE MV	DCO	M/I	FEMALE MV	DCO	M/I
Australian Capital Territory	99	0		83	0	
Australia, New South Wales	88	3		90	1	
South Australia	90		27	87		27
Australia, Tasmania	34		33	25		31
Australia, Victoria	95	1	46	91	1	59
Western Australia	89	6	52	92	6	42
French Polynesia	86	14		71	0	
+New Zealand: Non-Maori	94	4	49	95	3	44
+New Zealand: Maori	96	4	31	90	10	20
US, Hawaii: White	80	0	34	85	0	27
US, Hawaii: Japanese	77	0	46	99	0	40
US, Hawaii: Hawaiian	82	0	27	94	0	35
US, Hawaii: Filipino	93	0	36	99	0	33
US, Hawaii: Chinese	33	33	67	99	0	200

+ IMPORTANT-SEE NOTES ON POPULATION PAGE

[] CYTOLOGICAL VERIFICATION EXCLUDED

INDICES OF DATA QUALITY
Myeloid leukaemia (ICD-9 205)

	MALE			FEMALE		
	MV	DCO	M/I	MV	DCO	M/I
AFRICA						
Algeria, Setif	99			97		
France, La Reunion	99			99		
Mali, Bamako	99	0		73	0	
Uganda, Kyadondo	99			33		
Zimbabwe, Harare: African	91	6		95	0	
Zimbabwe, Harare: European	60	40		99	0	
AMERICA, CENTRAL AND SOUTH						
Argentina, Concordia	99	0	200	99	0	500
Brazil, Belem	99	0	44	99	0	74
Brazil, Goiania	59	28	79	62	24	66
Brazil, Porto Alegre	22	4	73	56	0	69
Colombia, Cali	95	0	91	82	2	90
Costa Rica	56	14	88	59	12	77
Ecuador, Quito	68	23		74	22	
Peru, Lima	83	11		79	8	
Peru, Trujillo	99	0	0	99	0	0
US, Puerto Rico	92	3	71	89	7	80
Uruguay, Montevideo	99	0	81	99	0	86
AMERICA, NORTH						
Canada	71	3	58	69	4	62
Canada, Alberta	95	3	66	93	6	64
Canada, British Columbia	77	14	66	79	12	71
Canada, Manitoba	94	1	65	91	5	58
Canada, New Brunswick	87	6	52	86	6	72
Canada, Newfoundland	96	4	71	99	0	33
Canada, Northwest Territories	80	0	60	50	0	25
Canada, Nova Scotia	89	11	85	82	17	76
Canada, Ontario	65	1	53	62	4	59
Canada, Prince Edward Island	99	0	67	85	0	54
+Canada, Quebec	60	0	58	59	0	64
Canada, Saskatchewan	78	5	55	77	0	61
Canada, Yukon	99	0	150	99	0	100
+US, Cent. Calif.: Non-Hisp. White	93	2	65	91	3	60
+US, Cent. Calif.: Hispanic	94	2	77	96	0	84
US, Los Angeles: Non-Hisp. White	93	2	69	93	2	66
US, Los Angeles: Hispanic White	97	1		99	0	
US, Los Angeles: Black	92	1		96	1	
US, Los Angeles: Chinese	96	0		99	0	
US, Los Angeles: Filipino	97	3		95	0	
US, Los Angeles: Korean	99	0		89	0	
US, Los Angeles: Japanese	77	5		99	0	
US, San Francisco: Non-Hisp. White	94	1	68	93	2	68
US, San Francisco: Hispanic White	98	0	40	98	0	39
US, San Francisco: Black	99	0	82	99	0	63
US, San Francisco: Chinese	99	0	64	99	0	48
US, San Francisco: Filipino	89	5	53	99	0	35
US, San Francisco: Japanese	99	0	60	99	0	33
US, Connecticut: White	96	3	63	95	4	74
US, Connecticut: Black	99	0	74	95	0	63
US, Atlanta: White	97	1	64	96	1	67
US, Atlanta: Black	99	0	77	96	2	60
US, Iowa	97	1	55	96	2	57
US, Central Louisiana: White	92	0	69	92	0	88
US, Central Louisiana: Black	99	0	80	99	0	33
US, New Orleans: White	97	3	81	97	1	81
US, New Orleans: Black	99	0	93	99	0	69
US, Detroit: White	96	0	54	95	0	61
US, Detroit: Black	94	0	67	94	0	62
US, New Mexico: Non-Hisp. White	87	4	58	85	3	55
US, New Mexico: Hispanic White	99	0	53	86	0	66
US, New Mexico: American Indian	99	0	88	99	0	60
US, Utah	98	1	74	99	0	69
US, Seattle	99	1	87	99	0	74
US, SEER: White	96	1	65	95	1	66
US, SEER: Black	97	0	71	96	1	61
ASIA						
+China, Qidong	94	0	75	93	0	89
+China, Shanghai	81	1	75	80	0	69
China, Tianjin	92	0	40	86	0	27
Hong Kong	76	8	51	76	7	48
India, Bangalore	91	9	54	94	5	50
India, Barshi, Paranda and Bhum	99	0		99	0	
India, Bombay	93	7	67	93	7	79
India, Karunagappally	99	0		99	0	
India, Madras	98	2	60	99	0	68
India, Trivandrum	89	0	11	99	0	40
Israel: All Jews	99			97		
Jews born in Israel	99			99		
Jews born in America or Europe	99			95		
Jews born in Africa or Asia	99			98		
Non-Jews	96			94		
Japan, Hiroshima	78	15	74	85	14	75
Japan, Miyagi	68	13	80	59	20	89
Japan, Nagasaki	98	0	86	99	0	62
Japan, Osaka	99	0	77	99	0	82
+Japan, Saga	55	29	75	63	20	74
Japan, Yamagata	61	29	93	68	29	83
Korea, Kangwha	99		100	99		100
Kuwait: Non-Kuwaitis	96	0		99	0	
Kuwait: Kuwaitis	99	0		94	0	
Philippines, Manila	47	28		41	35	
Singapore: Chinese	89	5		91	5	
Singapore: Malay	97	3		92	0	
Singapore: Indian	89	0		80	20	
Thailand, Chiang Mai	99	0		99	0	
Thailand, Khon Kaen	99	0		99	0	
Viet Nam, Hanoi	98			95		

+ IMPORTANT-SEE NOTES ON POPULATION PAGE

EUROPE	MALE MV	DCO	M/I	FEMALE MV	DCO	M/I
Austria, Tyrol	93	4	66	91	4	87
+Belarus	96	0	68	96	0	67
Croatia	67	2	59	71	3	62
+Czech Republic	69	4	87	69	3	93
Denmark	97	2	84	97	2	85
Estonia	99		89	99		79
Finland	97	2	74	94	3	76
France, Bas-Rhin	94		63	94		103
France, Calvados	81		243	67		150
France, Doubs	88		56	95		77
France, Haut-Rhin	99		86	99		100
France, Herault	99		134	99		191
France, Isere	99		38	99		63
France, Somme	98		109	94		127
France, Tarn	99		84	99		109
Germany, Eastern States	99	0	104	99	0	117
+Germany, Saarland	87	13	68	90	8	66
Iceland	99	0	100	99	0	123
Ireland, Southern	98		98	98		91
Italy, Ferrara	99	0	100	89	11	78
Italy, Florence	99	1	92	94	6	89
Italy, Genoa	82	1	89	86	3	88
Italy, Latina	90	10	60	96	4	76
Italy, Macerata	79	0	100	86	0	100
Italy, Modena	99	1	73	99	0	92
Italy, Parma	90	8	122	88	12	93
Italy, Ragusa	99	0	104	99	0	70
Italy, Romagna	98	2	77	99	0	82
Italy, Torino	95	3	64	93	6	70
Italy, Trieste	54	8	44	50	0	59
Italy, Varese	97	1	85	97	2	71
Italy, Veneto	94	6	78	93	7	75
+Latvia	97	3	66	98	1	67
+Malta	93	0	73	94	6	72
The Netherlands	99		79	99		87
The Netherlands, Eindhoven	99		93	98		92
The Netherlands, Maastricht	99		85	99		84
Norway	92	8	100	91	8	95
Poland, Cracow	77	13	79	72	19	85
Poland, Kielce	83	2	127	82	0	103
Poland, Lower Silesia	84	1	93	81	1	90
Poland, Warsaw City	[68]	13	112	[75]	9	107
Slovakia	94	0	73	94	0	68
Slovenia	99	1	77	98	1	68
Spain, Albacete	99	0	89	99	0	125
Spain, Asturias	98	2	62	99	0	26
Spain, Basque Country	90	5	66	95	4	61
Spain, Granada	99	0	44	99	0	67
Spain, Mallorca	99	0	57	99	0	38
Spain, Murcia	90	3	48	86	5	64
Spain, Navarra	82	16	70	77	8	88
Spain, Tarragona	98	2	70	99	0	31
Spain, Zaragoza	96	1	68	94	6	78

	MALE MV	DCO	M/I	FEMALE MV	DCO	M/I
Sweden	97		81	96		82
Switzerland, Basel	99	0	98	99	0	102
Switzerland, Geneva	96	4	68	99	0	76
Switzerland, Graubunden	99	0	95	99	0	100
Switzerland, Neuchatel	81	19	131	94	6	100
Switzerland, St Gall-Appenzell	99	0	85	98	2	84
Switzerland, Valais	99	0	59	93	7	64
Switzerland, Vaud	99	0	75	99	0	95
Switzerland, Zurich	99	0	85	99	0	102
+UK, England and Wales	[86]		84	[85]		87
UK, East Anglia			86			83
UK, Mersey	43	5	97	45	6	105
UK, North Western	59	7	88	56	8	81
UK, Oxford	99	0	73	99	0	69
UK, South Thames	60	31	80	57	35	85
UK, South Western	80	1	81	80	1	87
UK, Wessex	[84]	5	68	[76]	10	68
+UK, West Midlands		6	90		9	94
UK, Yorkshire	90	5	76	87	6	80
UK, Scotland	74	3	71	74	4	80
UK, Scotland, West	84	3	74	87	5	80
Yugoslavia, Vojvodina	62	11	71	63	8	60

OCEANIA

	MALE MV	DCO	M/I	FEMALE MV	DCO	M/I
Australian Capital Territory	96	0		99	0	
Australia, New South Wales	88	6		87	4	
South Australia	88		80	78		84
Australia, Tasmania	54		62	53		49
Australia, Victoria	94	2	87	92	3	97
Western Australia	88	7	84	84	8	98
French Polynesia	87	7		70	20	
+New Zealand: Non-Maori	94	5	75	93	5	69
+New Zealand: Maori	97	3	45	97	3	37
US, Hawaii: White	92	3	67	93	0	79
US, Hawaii: Japanese	92	0	80	95	0	43
US, Hawaii: Hawaiian	91	0	86	91	0	73
US, Hawaii: Filipino	92	0	80	89	0	44
US, Hawaii: Chinese	86	0	14	99	0	100

+ IMPORTANT-SEE NOTES ON POPULATION PAGE

[] CYTOLOGICAL VERIFICATION EXCLUDED

Monocytic leukaemia (ICD-9 206)

	MALE			FEMALE		
	MV	DCO	M/I	MV	DCO	M/I
AFRICA						
Algeria, Setif	-			-		
France, La Reunion	-			99		
Mali, Bamako	-	-		-	-	
Uganda, Kyadondo	-					
Zimbabwe, Harare: African	-	-		-	-	
Zimbabwe, Harare: European	-	-		-	-	
AMERICA, CENTRAL AND SOUTH						
Argentina, Concordia	-	-	-	-	-	-
Brazil, Belem	-	-	-	-	-	-
Brazil, Goiania	33	0	0	99	0	0
Brazil, Porto Alegre	67	0	100	-	-	-
Colombia, Cali	99	0	150	99	0	300
Costa Rica	17	17	83	50	0	125
Ecuador, Quito	50	50		99	0	
Peru, Lima	80	0		99	0	
Peru, Trujillo	99	0	0	99	0	0
US, Puerto Rico	83	17	150	99	0	14
Uruguay, Montevideo	-	-	ncr	99	0	100
AMERICA, NORTH						
Canada	72	2	49	69	4	50
Canada, Alberta	99	0	25	99	0	63
Canada, British Columbia	86	10	71	93	7	43
Canada, Manitoba	99	0	71	99	0	100
Canada, New Brunswick	99	0	100	50	25	75
Canada, Newfoundland	99	0	0	-	-	-
Canada, Northwest Territories	-	-	-	0	50	50
Canada, Nova Scotia	91	9	45	99	0	56
Canada, Ontario	45	0	38	54	8	38
Canada, Prince Edward Island	99	0	0	-	-	-
+Canada, Quebec	64	0	59	60	0	49
Canada, Saskatchewan	92	0	31	71	0	57
Canada, Yukon	99	0	0	-	-	ncr
+US, Cent. Calif.: Non-Hisp. White	90	0	30	99	0	63
+US, Cent. Calif.: Hispanic	75	0	25	99	0	50
US, Los Angeles: Non-Hisp. White	79	3	59	94	0	50
US, Los Angeles: Hispanic White	99	0		99	0	
US, Los Angeles: Black	83	17		99	0	
US, Los Angeles: Chinese	99	0		99	0	
US, Los Angeles: Filipino	-	-		99	0	
US, Los Angeles: Korean	-	-		-	-	
US, Los Angeles: Japanese	99	0		-	-	
US, San Francisco: Non-Hisp. White	96	0	42	99	0	73
US, San Francisco: Hispanic White	-	-	ncr	-	-	-
US, San Francisco: Black	99	0	0	99	0	0
US, San Francisco: Chinese	-	-	ncr	-	-	-
US, San Francisco: Filipino	99	0	50	99	0	100
US, San Francisco: Japanese	-	-	-	-	-	-
US, Connecticut: White	99	0	17	99	0	35
US, Connecticut: Black	99	0	0	-	-	-
US, Atlanta: White	99	0	57	86	0	21
US, Atlanta: Black	-	-	ncr	-	-	-
US, Iowa	99	0	69	97	3	52
US, Central Louisiana: White	-	-	ncr	99	0	100
US, Central Louisiana: Black	-	-	-	-	-	-
US, New Orleans: White	99	0	38	99	0	25
US, New Orleans: Black	99	0	50	99	0	0
US, Detroit: White	97	0	32	94	0	59
US, Detroit: Black	99	0	33	99	0	75
US, New Mexico: Non-Hisp. White	99	0	43	99	0	40
US, New Mexico: Hispanic White	99	0	0	99	0	50
US, New Mexico: American Indian	-	-	-	-	-	-
US, Utah	99	0	20	99	0	80
US, Seattle	99	0	63	99	0	106
US, SEER: White	99	0	43	96	1	58
US, SEER: Black	99	0	42	99	0	38
ASIA						
+China, Qidong	-	-		99	0	100
+China, Shanghai	78	0	64	73	1	76
China, Tianjin	79	0	63	86	0	64
Hong Kong	99	0	71	99	0	63
India, Bangalore	99	0	67	99	0	200
India, Barshi, Paranda and Bhum	-	-		-	-	
India, Bombay	99	0	43	67	33	133
India, Karunagappally	-	-		-	-	
India, Madras	99	0	100	99	0	33
India, Trivandrum	-	-	-	-	-	-
Israel: All Jews	99			99		
Jews born in Israel	99			99		
Jews born in America or Europe	99			99		
Jews born in Africa or Asia	99			99		
Non-Jews	-			-		
Japan, Hiroshima	99	0	0	99	0	0
Japan, Miyagi	60	0	60	60	10	90
Japan, Nagasaki	99	0	50	99	0	33
Japan, Osaka	99	0	66	99	0	68
+Japan, Saga	0	99	100	-	-	-
Japan, Yamagata	67	33	100	50	38	88
Korea, Kangwha	-	-		-	-	
Kuwait: Non-Kuwaitis	0	0		-	-	
Kuwait: Kuwaitis	99	0		-	-	
Philippines, Manila	0	80		13	75	
Singapore: Chinese	99	0		-	-	
Singapore: Malay	0	0		-	-	
Singapore: Indian	-	-		-	-	
Thailand, Chiang Mai	-	-		99	0	
Thailand, Khon Kaen	99	0		99	0	
Viet Nam, Hanoi	99			99		

+ IMPORTANT-SEE NOTES ON POPULATION PAGE

EUROPE	MALE MV	DCO	M/I	FEMALE MV	DCO	M/I
Austria, Tyrol	99	0	50	99	0	50
+Belarus	96	0	68	88	0	64
Croatia	0	0	200	50	0	200
+Czech Republic	65	5	111	64	17	107
Denmark	92	8	108	99	0	100
Estonia	99		75	99		100
Finland	83	8	71	75	13	75
France, Bas-Rhin	99		43	99		71
France, Calvados	50		0	0		0
France, Doubs	99		0	-		-
France, Haut-Rhin	-		ncr	99		33
France, Herault	99		100	99		0
France, Isere	99		0	99		33
France, Somme	99		67	99		75
France, Tarn	99		50	99		50
Germany, Eastern States	99	0	107	99	0	68
+Germany, Saarland	92	8	67	67	33	67
Iceland	99	0	0	-	-	-
Ireland, Southern	-		ncr	-		-
Italy, Ferrara	-	-	ncr	99	0	33
Italy, Florence	99	0	100	99	0	33
Italy, Genoa	-	-	-	50	0	50
Italy, Latina	99	0	25	-	-	ncr
Italy, Macerata	-	-	ncr	0	0	0
Italy, Modena	99	0	100	99	0	133
Italy, Parma	80	20	60	99	0	0
Italy, Ragusa	-	-	-	99	0	100
Italy, Romagna	99	0	67	-	-	-
Italy, Torino	60	40	80	99	0	50
Italy, Trieste	0	0	0	-	-	-
Italy, Varese	99	0	67	99	0	25
Italy, Veneto	99	0	75	83	17	100
+Latvia	99	0	89	99	0	78
+Malta	-	-	-	-	-	-
The Netherlands	99		62	99		82
The Netherlands, Eindhoven	99		33	99		100
The Netherlands, Maastricht	99		999	99		125
Norway	89	11	52	90	10	40
Poland, Cracow	-	-	-	-	-	-
Poland, Kielce	-	-	-	-	-	-
Poland, Lower Silesia	99	0	60	99	0	200
Poland, Warsaw City	-	-	ncr	-	-	-
Slovakia	99	0	142	99	0	110
Slovenia	99	0	150	99	0	133
Spain, Albacete	99	0	0	99	0	0
Spain, Asturias	99	0	0	99	0	0
Spain, Basque Country	75	0	63	99	0	50
Spain, Granada	99	0	0	99	0	20
Spain, Mallorca	99	0	100	99	0	20
Spain, Murcia	99	0	150	99	0	0
Spain, Navarra	75	0	50	99	0	0
Spain, Tarragona	99	0	67	67	0	67
Spain, Zaragoza	99	0	50	99	0	33

	MALE MV	DCO	M/I	FEMALE MV	DCO	M/I
Sweden	89		53	94		52
Switzerland, Basel	-	-	ncr	99	0	100
Switzerland, Geneva	-	-	ncr	50	50	200
Switzerland, Graubunden	99	0	0	99	0	100
Switzerland, Neuchatel	0	99	400	0	99	100
Switzerland, St Gall-Appenzell	99	0	100	99	0	50
Switzerland, Valais	99	0	0	-	-	-
Switzerland, Vaud	99	0	67	99	0	100
Switzerland, Zurich	99	0	41	99	0	13
+UK, England and Wales	[89]		70	[83]		67
UK, East Anglia			100			86
UK, Mersey	63	0	75	42	0	50
UK, North Western	57	0	43	25	50	250
UK, Oxford	99	0	27	99	0	25
UK, South Thames	76	20	84	54	46	123
UK, South Western	76	0	50	84	4	32
UK, Wessex	[73]	18	100	[56]	0	19
+UK, West Midlands		7	52		0	54
UK, Yorkshire	78	0	89	86	0	86
UK, Scotland	67	11	78	86	0	64
UK, Scotland, West	50	17	33	75	0	125
Yugoslavia, Vojvodina	-	-	-	-	-	-

OCEANIA

	MALE MV	DCO	M/I	FEMALE MV	DCO	M/I
Australian Capital Territory	-	-		-	-	
Australia, New South Wales	94	0		92	4	
South Australia	92		0	83		17
Australia, Tasmania	0		150	0		0
Australia, Victoria	91	5	27	89	0	53
Western Australia	99	0	50	99	0	75
French Polynesia	99	0		99	0	
+New Zealand: Non-Maori	99	0	70	99	0	100
+New Zealand: Maori	-	-	-	99	0	0
US, Hawaii: White	99	0	0	50	0	50
US, Hawaii: Japanese	99	0	0	99	0	0
US, Hawaii: Hawaiian	67	0	0	99	0	0
US, Hawaii: Filipino	99	0	0	-	-	-
US, Hawaii: Chinese	99	0	50	99	0	0

+ IMPORTANT-SEE NOTES ON POPULATION PAGE

[] CYTOLOGICAL VERIFICATION EXCLUDED

	MALE			FEMALE		
	MV	DCO	M/I	MV	DCO	M/I
AFRICA						
Algeria, Setif	-			-		
France, La Reunion	99			99		
Mali, Bamako	-	-		-	-	
Uganda, Kyadondo	-			-		
Zimbabwe, Harare: African	-	-		-	-	
Zimbabwe, Harare: European	0	99		-	-	
AMERICA, CENTRAL AND SOUTH						
Argentina, Concordia	-	-	-	-	-	-
Brazil, Belem	-	-	-	-	-	-
Brazil, Goiania	-	-	-	-	-	-
Brazil, Porto Alegre	-	-	-	99	0	0
Colombia, Cali	99	0	200	-	-	-
Costa Rica	-	-	ncr	0	99	0
Ecuador, Quito	-	-		-	-	
Peru, Lima	99	0		-	-	
Peru, Trujillo	-	-	-	-	-	-
US, Puerto Rico	99	0	67	99	0	50
Uruguay, Montevideo	-	-	-	-	-	-
AMERICA, NORTH						
Canada	63	2	25	60	1	18
Canada, Alberta	99	0	200	99	0	67
Canada, British Columbia	86	14	29	33	33	33
Canada, Manitoba	99	0	0	99	0	0
Canada, New Brunswick	-	-	ncr	99	0	0
Canada, Newfoundland	99	0	100	99	0	0
Canada, Northwest Territories	99	0	100	-	-	-
Canada, Nova Scotia	50	0	100	99	0	0
Canada, Ontario	57	2	29	58	0	21
Canada, Prince Edward Island	99	0	0	-	-	-
+Canada, Quebec	61	0	11	53	0	12
Canada, Saskatchewan	99	0	0	99	0	0
Canada, Yukon	-	-	-	-	-	-
+US, Cent. Calif.: Non-Hisp. White	99	0	0	99	0	0
+US, Cent. Calif.: Hispanic	99	0	0	99	0	0
US, Los Angeles: Non-Hisp. White	99	0	0	86	0	0
US, Los Angeles: Hispanic White	99	0		99	0	
US, Los Angeles: Black	99	0		-	-	
US, Los Angeles: Chinese	99	0		-	-	
US, Los Angeles: Filipino	-	-		99	0	
US, Los Angeles: Korean	-	-		-	-	
US, Los Angeles: Japanese	99	0		-	-	
US, San Francisco: Non-Hisp. White	99	0	20	78	22	67
US, San Francisco: Hispanic White	-	-	-	99	0	100
US, San Francisco: Black	99	0	100	99	0	0
US, San Francisco: Chinese	-	-	ncr	-	-	-
US, San Francisco: Filipino	50	0	0	99	0	0
US, San Francisco: Japanese	-	-	-	-	-	ncr
US, Connecticut: White	99	0	70	94	6	24
US, Connecticut: Black	-	-	-	99	0	0
US, Atlanta: White	99	0	67	99	0	67
US, Atlanta: Black	99	0	200			
US, Iowa	99	0	113	99	0	56

	MALE			FEMALE		
	MV	DCO	M/I	MV	DCO	M/I
US, Central Louisiana: White	-	-	ncr	99	0	0
US, Central Louisiana: Black	-	-	ncr	99	0	0
US, New Orleans: White	99	0	167	99	0	200
US, New Orleans: Black	99	0	200	99	0	100
US, Detroit: White	99	0	37	99	0	85
US, Detroit: Black	90	0	40	99	0	100
US, New Mexico: Non-Hisp. White	99	0	150	-	-	ncr
US, New Mexico: Hispanic White	99	0	150	99	0	200
US, New Mexico: American Indian	-	-	-	-	-	-
US, Utah	99	0	100	99	0	33
US, Seattle	99	0	59	99	0	56
US, SEER: White	99	0	63	95	5	60
US, SEER: Black	92	0	58	99	0	50
ASIA						
+China, Qidong	99	0	100	67	0	100
+China, Shanghai	68	0	73	65	0	59
China, Tianjin	99	0	30	71	0	57
Hong Kong	83	0	33	33	33	100
India, Bangalore	99	0	200	99	0	200
India, Barshi, Paranda and Bhum	-	-		-	-	
India, Bombay	93	7	50	80	20	60
India, Karunagappally	-	-		-	-	
India, Madras	-	-	-	99	0	0
India, Trivandrum	99	0	100	-	-	-
Israel: All Jews	99			99		
Jews born in Israel	99			99		
Jews born in America or Europe	99			99		
Jews born in Africa or Asia	99			99		
Non-Jews	99			99		
Japan, Hiroshima	-	-	ncr	0	99	300
Japan, Miyagi	69	15	92	56	33	22
Japan, Nagasaki	99	0	80	99	0	20
Japan, Osaka	99	0	47	99	0	33
+Japan, Saga	50	25	100	0	0	50
Japan, Yamagata	50	33	100	80	0	60
Korea, Kangwha	99		0	-		-
Kuwait: Non-Kuwaitis	-	-		-	-	
Kuwait: Kuwaitis	-	-		99	0	
Philippines, Manila	99	0		99	0	
Singapore: Chinese	-	-		99	0	
Singapore: Malay	99	0		-	-	
Singapore: Indian	-	-		99	0	
Thailand, Chiang Mai	-	-		99	0	
Thailand, Khon Kaen	-	-		-	-	
Viet Nam, Hanoi	99			99		

+ IMPORTANT-SEE NOTES ON POPULATION PAGE

EUROPE	MALE MV	DCO	M/I	FEMALE MV	DCO	M/I
Austria, Tyrol	-	-	ncr	99	0	0
+Belarus	91	0	25	96	0	21
Croatia	40	0	60	67	0	67
+Czech Republic	54	9	144	48	16	123
Denmark	99	0	0	90	10	0
Estonia	99		77	99		79
Finland	99	0	42	92	8	38
France, Bas-Rhin	-		ncr	99		100
France, Calvados	-		ncr	50		100
France, Doubs	0		0	-		-
France, Haut-Rhin	99		0	-		-
France, Herault	-		ncr	-		-
France, Isere	-	-	-	-	-	-
France, Somme	99		150	-		-
France, Tarn	-	-	-	-	-	-
Germany, Eastern States	99	0	81	99	0	77
+Germany, Saarland	86	0	14	92	8	8
Iceland	99	0	50	99	0	150
Ireland, Southern	-	-	-	-	-	-
Italy, Ferrara	-	-	-	99	0	0
Italy, Florence	99	0	0	99	0	0
Italy, Genoa	0	99	100	-	-	-
Italy, Latina	-	-	-	-	-	-
Italy, Macerata	-	-	-	-	-	-
Italy, Modena	99	0	400	-	-	-
Italy, Parma	99	0	50	-	-	-
Italy, Ragusa	-	-	-	-	-	-
Italy, Romagna	99	0	0	99	0	0
Italy, Torino	99	0	200	67	0	0
Italy, Trieste	0	0	0	0	0	0
Italy, Varese	-	-	-	99	0	0
Italy, Veneto	99	0	20	99	0	25
+Latvia	93	5	41	98	2	31
+Malta	-	-	-	-	-	-
The Netherlands	99		16	99		38
The Netherlands, Eindhoven	99		13	99		0
The Netherlands, Maastricht	99		100	99		100
Norway	77	23	18	77	23	16
Poland, Cracow	99	0	100	0	0	200
Poland, Kielce	99	0	133	99	0	400
Poland, Lower Silesia	83	0	55	72	0	28
Poland, Warsaw City	[99]	0	600	[80]	0	60
Slovakia	83	0	567	99	0	255
Slovenia	-	-	-	0	99	50
Spain, Albacete	-	-	-	-	-	-
Spain, Asturias	-	-	ncr	99	0	200
Spain, Basque Country	99	0	50	99	0	100
Spain, Granada	99	0	0	99	0	0
Spain, Mallorca	-	-	-	99	0	0
Spain, Murcia	99	0	50	80	0	60
Spain, Navarra	99	0	0	99	0	100
Spain, Tarragona	99	0	0	-	-	-
Spain, Zaragoza	99	0	100	99	0	33

	MALE MV	DCO	M/I	FEMALE MV	DCO	M/I
Sweden	88		3	86		0
Switzerland, Basel	-	-	ncr	-	-	ncr
Switzerland, Geneva	-	-	ncr	-	-	ncr
Switzerland, Graubunden	-	-	ncr	-	-	ncr
Switzerland, Neuchatel	99	0	100	-	-	ncr
Switzerland, St Gall-Appenzell	99	0	133	99	0	100
Switzerland, Valais	99	0	75	99	0	100
Switzerland, Vaud	-	-	ncr	99	0	200
Switzerland, Zurich	99	0	25	99	0	120
+UK, England and Wales	[81]		61	[93]		69
UK, East Anglia			175			100
UK, Mersey	50	17	67	60	0	40
UK, North Western	67	17	83	0	0	500
UK, Oxford	99	0	38	99	0	40
UK, South Thames	60	30	110	88	13	75
UK, South Western	99	0	83	71	14	100
UK, Wessex	[73]	0	18	[86]	0	57
+UK, West Midlands		7	93		0	113
UK, Yorkshire	88	0	38	99	0	167
UK, Scotland	78	0	56	80	0	40
UK, Scotland, West	50	0	50	99	0	100
Yugoslavia, Vojvodina	-	-	-	0	33	67

OCEANIA

	MALE MV	DCO	M/I	FEMALE MV	DCO	M/I
Australian Capital Territory	99	0		-	-	
Australia, New South Wales	94	6		88	13	
South Australia	99		329	80		380
Australia, Tasmania	0	0		99	0	
Australia, Victoria	90	0	110	91	0	118
Western Australia	86	14	57	99	0	100
French Polynesia	99	0		99	0	
+New Zealand: Non-Maori	91	0	64	86	0	86
+New Zealand: Maori	99	0	33	99	0	0
US, Hawaii: White	99	0	50	-	-	ncr
US, Hawaii: Japanese	99	0	33	-	-	ncr
US, Hawaii: Hawaiian	99	0	0	-	-	-
US, Hawaii: Filipino	-	-	-	-	-	-
US, Hawaii: Chinese	-	-	-	-	-	-

+ IMPORTANT-SEE NOTES ON POPULATION PAGE

[] CYTOLOGICAL VERIFICATION EXCLUDED

INDICES OF DATA QUALITY
Leukaemia, unspecified (ICD-9 208)

	MALE			FEMALE		
	MV	DCO	M/I	MV	DCO	M/I
AFRICA						
Algeria, Setif	99			93		
France, La Reunion	99			99		
Mali, Bamako	40	10		50	8	
Uganda, Kyadondo	33			14		
Zimbabwe, Harare: African	50	50		-	-	
Zimbabwe, Harare: European	99	0		-	-	
AMERICA, CENTRAL AND SOUTH						
Argentina, Concordia	67	33	167	60	40	280
Brazil, Belem	54	46	46	36	57	21
Brazil, Goiania	65	29	112	46	38	92
Brazil, Porto Alegre	28	0	89	23	0	91
Colombia, Cali	82	10	86	69	10	90
Costa Rica	34	36	136	30	30	106
Ecuador, Quito	53	29		56	26	
Peru, Lima	46	18		29	38	
Peru, Trujillo	67	17	0	99	0	0
US, Puerto Rico	61	30	134	57	34	166
Uruguay, Montevideo	99	0	100	99	0	95
AMERICA, NORTH						
Canada	35	20	184	32	19	156
Canada, Alberta	70	30	278	80	20	220
Canada, British Columbia	29	52	173	29	55	141
Canada, Manitoba	39	28	322	60	27	333
Canada, New Brunswick	41	24	135	38	10	145
Canada, Newfoundland	86	14	371	83	17	333
Canada, Northwest Territories	99	0	100	0	0	100
Canada, Nova Scotia	49	51	99	44	51	124
Canada, Ontario	16	17	149	18	18	121
Canada, Prince Edward Island	99	0	300	0	99	800
+Canada, Quebec	50	0	225	43	0	187
Canada, Saskatchewan	39	43	322	38	38	275
Canada, Yukon	-	-	ncr	-	-	-
+US, Cent. Calif.: Non-Hisp. White	50	8	231	32	9	273
+US, Cent. Calif.: Hispanic	67	0	350	99	0	200
US, Los Angeles: Non-Hisp. White	75	10	275	68	11	229
US, Los Angeles: Hispanic White	87	3		83	11	
US, Los Angeles: Black	83	0		29	24	
US, Los Angeles: Chinese	-	-		67	0	
US, Los Angeles: Filipino	99	0		67	0	
US, Los Angeles: Korean	99	0		99	0	
US, Los Angeles: Japanese	99	0		-	-	
US, San Francisco: Non-Hisp. White	81	10	252	88	0	269
US, San Francisco: Hispanic White	80	20	260	99	0	100
US, San Francisco: Black	99	0	243	75	0	275
US, San Francisco: Chinese	99	0	150	99	0	150
US, San Francisco: Filipino	67	0	267	75	0	200
US, San Francisco: Japanese	-	-	-	-	-	ncr
US, Connecticut: White	86	14	165	83	14	176
US, Connecticut: Black	99	0	250	25	50	300
US, Atlanta: White	78	6	333	78	22	733
US, Atlanta: Black	91	0	155	75	0	350
US, Iowa	80	9	187	73	15	234

	MALE			FEMALE		
	MV	DCO	M/I	MV	DCO	M/I
US, Central Louisiana: White	0	33	333	50	0	650
US, Central Louisiana: Black	50	50	100	-	-	ncr
US, New Orleans: White	85	8	277	81	13	163
US, New Orleans: Black	64	29	171	40	60	340
US, Detroit: White	85	4	211	83	7	184
US, Detroit: Black	93	0	293	83	0	228
US, New Mexico: Non-Hisp. White	52	11	226	52	15	191
US, New Mexico: Hispanic White	50	0	450	75	17	100
US, New Mexico: American Indian	99	0	200	-	-	ncr
US, Utah	93	5	146	80	10	200
US, Seattle	97	3	81	90	10	109
US, SEER: White	83	8	184	80	11	198
US, SEER: Black	95	0	217	73	6	239
ASIA						
+China, Qidong	93	3	76	86	0	67
+China, Shanghai	64	3	135	67	4	124
China, Tianjin	70	0	91	77	1	79
Hong Kong	68	17	82	67	19	70
India, Bangalore	56	42	56	56	39	67
India, Barshi, Paranda and Bhum	99	0		-	-	
India, Bombay	83	15	94	71	29	107
India, Karunagappally	50	50		99	0	
India, Madras	65	35	76	56	44	75
India, Trivandrum	50	50	200	25	75	125
Israel: All Jews	93			97		
Jews born in Israel	86			99		
Jews born in America or Europe	96			98		
Jews born in Africa or Asia	91			94		
Non-Jews	93			99		
Japan, Hiroshima	42	33	133	38	50	150
Japan, Miyagi	53	29	129	23	41	182
Japan, Nagasaki	54	42	144	36	52	180
Japan, Osaka	27	62	148	27	52	156
+Japan, Saga	27	53	140	22	56	128
Japan, Yamagata	27	58	162	35	65	130
Korea, Kangwha	99		167	50		350
Kuwait: Non-Kuwaitis	50	50		0	99	
Kuwait: Kuwaitis	8	92		0	99	
Philippines, Manila	11	76		9	79	
Singapore: Chinese	62	31		50	29	
Singapore: Malay	40	20		99	0	
Singapore: Indian	99	0		99	0	
Thailand, Chiang Mai	99	0		99	0	
Thailand, Khon Kaen	18	82		9	91	
Viet Nam, Hanoi	87			89		

+ IMPORTANT-SEE NOTES ON POPULATION PAGE

EUROPE

	MALE			FEMALE		
	MV	DCO	M/I	MV	DCO	M/I
Austria, Tyrol	75	13	188	50	50	217
+Belarus	93	1	76	95	1	72
Croatia	13	21	196	11	19	173
+Czech Republic	49	11	162	43	15	164
Denmark	70	26	237	74	25	208
Estonia	99		117	99		103
Finland	98	2	43	81	9	56
France, Bas-Rhin	99		414	78		556
France, Calvados	0		999	0		999
France, Doubs	99		260	99		450
France, Haut-Rhin	99		291	99		291
France, Herault	99		286	99		217
France, Isere	99		322	99		525
France, Somme	99		700	99		999
France, Tarn	99		999	99		720
Germany, Eastern States	99	0	104	99	0	127
+Germany, Saarland	63	31	231	38	59	185
Iceland	99	0	250	99	0	75
Ireland, Southern	70		105	88		125
Italy, Ferrara	79	14	57	-	-	ncr
Italy, Florence	89	11	91	70	30	144
Italy, Genoa	65	10	250	61	39	233
Italy, Latina	90	10	360	45	55	191
Italy, Macerata	99	0	125	88	0	125
Italy, Modena	25	75	700	50	50	317
Italy, Parma	77	23	119	77	23	141
Italy, Ragusa	99	0	100	99	0	400
Italy, Romagna	99	0	188	99	0	158
Italy, Torino	87	13	165	62	31	346
Italy, Trieste	33	17	133	22	22	144
Italy, Varese	73	27	373	78	22	433
Italy, Veneto	91	9	129	83	17	179
+Latvia	95	5	76	95	5	62
+Malta	-	-	ncr	99	0	100
The Netherlands	99		345	99		421
The Netherlands, Eindhoven	99		900	99		475
The Netherlands, Maastricht	99		400	99		389
Norway	69	31	519	99	0	892
Poland, Cracow	60	33	73	35	35	88
Poland, Kielce	50	21	93	70	30	110
Poland, Lower Silesia	87	5	85	86	9	80
Poland, Warsaw City	[31]	27	65	[17]	30	87
Slovakia	56	2	91	43	0	79
Slovenia	90	10	480	86	14	629
Spain, Albacete	75	25	175	50	50	350
Spain, Asturias	61	38	82	63	31	83
Spain, Basque Country	71	24	157	73	25	143
Spain, Granada	81	19	231	48	48	178
Spain, Mallorca	22	78	367	39	61	211
Spain, Murcia	59	18	371	56	13	288
Spain, Navarra	40	48	132	35	53	153
Spain, Tarragona	68	26	247	75	17	258
Spain, Zaragoza	56	33	344	44	44	188

	MALE			FEMALE		
	MV	DCO	M/I	MV	DCO	M/I
Sweden	89		176	90		219
Switzerland, Basel	99	0	60	99	0	200
Switzerland, Geneva	67	33	67	99	0	33
Switzerland, Graubunden	-	-	ncr	99	0	200
Switzerland, Neuchatel	99	0	0	50	50	0
Switzerland, St Gall-Appenzell	99	0	83	99	0	0
Switzerland, Valais	80	20	40	67	33	67
Switzerland, Vaud	99	0	21	99	0	10
Switzerland, Zurich	99	0	400	99	0	82
+UK, England and Wales	[81]		66	[80]		75
UK, East Anglia			117			108
UK, Mersey	19	15	58	25	14	93
UK, North Western	31	17	80	20	13	78
UK, Oxford	99	0	89	96	4	100
UK, South Thames	24	53	69	30	53	71
UK, South Western	67	3	64	45	6	70
UK, Wessex	[38]	38	94	[28]	41	121
+UK, West Midlands		9	41		8	46
UK, Yorkshire	57	17	87	45	29	103
UK, Scotland	60	6	63	51	7	61
UK, Scotland, West	70	4	50	58	8	54
Yugoslavia, Vojvodina	6	16	113	0	10	100

OCEANIA

	MALE			FEMALE		
	MV	DCO	M/I	MV	DCO	M/I
Australian Capital Territory	-	-		99	0	
Australia, New South Wales	72	13		73	10	
South Australia	0		100	75		150
Australia, Tasmania	33		100	0		600
Australia, Victoria	62	13	32	58	9	15
Western Australia	88	12	15	82	18	23
French Polynesia	67	25		17	67	
+New Zealand: Non-Maori	85	15	111	80	18	104
+New Zealand: Maori	75	25	125	80	20	100
US, Hawaii: White	25	0	250	50	0	150
US, Hawaii: Japanese	99	0	144	67	0	167
US, Hawaii: Hawaiian	75	0	175	99	0	700
US, Hawaii: Filipino	99	0	275	75	25	175
US, Hawaii: Chinese	-	-	ncr	99	0	400

+ IMPORTANT-SEE NOTES ON POPULATION PAGE

[] CYTOLOGICAL VERIFICATION EXCLUDED

INDICES OF DATA QUALITY
All leukaemias (ICD-9 204-8)

	MALE			FEMALE		
	MV	DCO	M/I	MV	DCO	M/I
AFRICA						
Algeria, Setif	99			97		
France, La Reunion	99			99		
Mali, Bamako	50	8		61	4	
Uganda, Kyadondo	50			38		
Zimbabwe, Harare: African	91	7		97	0	
Zimbabwe, Harare: European	56	44		99	0	
AMERICA, CENTRAL AND SOUTH						
Argentina, Concordia	89	11	167	83	17	192
Brazil, Belem	90	10	55	82	16	43
Brazil, Goiania	59	17	69	56	29	75
Brazil, Porto Alegre	36	3	73	48	0	70
Colombia, Cali	90	3	93	82	4	85
Costa Rica	55	12	71	55	13	69
Ecuador, Quito	70	22		77	16	
Peru, Lima	83	8		79	10	
Peru, Trujillo	93	4	0	99	0	0
US, Puerto Rico	88	7	69	86	8	74
Uruguay, Montevideo	99	0	78	99	0	80
AMERICA, NORTH						
Canada	61	4	60	59	5	61
Canada, Alberta	94	4	67	92	5	64
Canada, British Columbia	68	15	65	69	17	67
Canada, Manitoba	88	3	66	87	5	66
Canada, New Brunswick	75	7	66	73	6	75
Canada, Newfoundland	97	3	82	98	1	59
Canada, Northwest Territories	91	0	64	50	10	50
Canada, Nova Scotia	77	22	75	74	23	76
Canada, Ontario	56	3	52	51	5	54
Canada, Prince Edward Island	95	0	57	87	4	78
+Canada, Quebec	49	0	65	49	0	68
Canada, Saskatchewan	63	5	54	57	3	51
Canada, Yukon	87	13	73	45	0	18
+US, Cent. Calif.: Non-Hisp. White	85	3	71	82	5	70
+US, Cent. Calif.: Hispanic	93	1	63	98	0	64
US, Los Angeles: Non-Hisp. White	91	2	69	88	3	67
US, Los Angeles: Hispanic White	97	1		97	1	
US, Los Angeles: Black	91	1		88	4	
US, Los Angeles: Chinese	97	0		96	0	
US, Los Angeles: Filipino	98	2		89	0	
US, Los Angeles: Korean	99	0		93	0	
US, Los Angeles: Japanese	82	4		99	0	
US, San Francisco: Non-Hisp. White	92	2	67	91	3	71
US, San Francisco: Hispanic White	98	1	50	98	1	34
US, San Francisco: Black	93	0	79	90	0	53
US, San Francisco: Chinese	98	0	56	99	0	56
US, San Francisco: Filipino	87	3	59	97	0	54
US, San Francisco: Japanese	99	0	67	99	0	125
US, Connecticut: White	94	4	64	93	5	74
US, Connecticut: Black	98	2	81	91	5	70
US, Atlanta: White	96	2	72	94	1	74
US, Atlanta: Black	94	0	73	93	1	68
US, Iowa	95	2	57	94	3	62
US, Central Louisiana: White	81	4	106	83	2	96
US, Central Louisiana: Black	87	7	73	99	0	100
US, New Orleans: White	96	3	80	96	2	68
US, New Orleans: Black	92	7	89	93	7	89
US, Detroit: White	94	1	60	93	1	63
US, Detroit: Black	94	0	76	91	0	70
US, New Mexico: Non-Hisp. White	86	3	65	81	6	71
US, New Mexico: Hispanic White	96	0	61	89	3	62
US, New Mexico: American Indian	99	0	85	99	0	54
US, Utah	96	1	67	98	1	65
US, Seattle	99	1	65	98	2	63
US, SEER: White	95	2	63	93	3	67
US, SEER: Black	95	0	75	91	1	65
ASIA						
+China, Qidong	94	1	82	91	0	84
+China, Shanghai	77	1	84	74	2	83
China, Tianjin	84	0	55	83	0	50
Hong Kong	77	8	47	75	8	47
India, Bangalore	86	12	53	88	11	53
India, Barshi, Paranda and Bhum	99	0		99	0	
India, Bombay	92	8	68	90	10	80
India, Karunagappally	93	7		99	0	
India, Madras	97	3	54	95	5	59
India, Trivandrum	87	10	33	90	10	35
Israel: All Jews	97			98		
Jews born in Israel	97			99		
Jews born in America or Europe	98			98		
Jews born in Africa or Asia	96			98		
Non-Jews	98			97		
Japan, Hiroshima	79	14	77	79	19	82
Japan, Miyagi	69	12	80	60	19	89
Japan, Nagasaki	90	8	166	92	6	140
Japan, Osaka	91	7	83	92	5	84
+Japan, Saga	57	29	73	59	24	75
Japan, Yamagata	57	33	101	61	35	88
Korea, Kangwha	99		93	88		138
Kuwait: Non-Kuwaitis	88	9		91	9	
Kuwait: Kuwaitis	73	25		76	17	
Philippines, Manila	37	37		30	47	
Singapore: Chinese	88	5		87	5	
Singapore: Malay	89	4		89	0	
Singapore: Indian	94	0		88	12	
Thailand, Chiang Mai	99	0		99	0	
Thailand, Khon Kaen	76	24		70	30	
Viet Nam, Hanoi	94			92		

INDICES OF DATA QUALITY
All leukaemias (ICD-9 204-8) (contd)

EUROPE	MALE MV	DCO	M/I	FEMALE MV	DCO	M/I
Austria, Tyrol	89	4	60	87	8	68
+Belarus	96	0	66	96	0	66
Croatia	77	4	66	75	5	67
+Czech Republic	69	5	84	67	5	90
Denmark	96	3	77	96	4	80
Estonia	99		73	99		65
Finland	95	3	65	93	4	65
France, Bas-Rhin	96		72	92		104
France, Calvados	72		197	58		152
France, Doubs	89		80	92		88
France, Haut-Rhin	99		86	99		103
France, Herault	99		134	99		138
France, Isere	99		43	99		70
France, Somme	98		96	97		108
France, Tarn	99		117	99		143
Germany, Eastern States	99	0	86	99	0	99
+Germany, Saarland	88	9	64	81	17	69
Iceland	99	0	93	99	0	91
Ireland, Southern	94		66	95		79
Italy, Ferrara	95	4	72	91	6	64
Italy, Florence	96	4	84	90	10	86
Italy, Genoa	79	4	96	81	7	94
Italy, Latina	90	10	86	80	20	82
Italy, Macerata	89	0	106	81	0	89
Italy, Modena	95	5	86	96	3	80
Italy, Parma	89	10	105	88	12	104
Italy, Ragusa	99	0	75	99	0	78
Italy, Romagna	99	1	71	99	1	75
Italy, Torino	93	5	78	90	6	78
Italy, Trieste	48	5	43	58	3	53
Italy, Varese	95	2	86	93	3	76
Italy, Veneto	95	5	73	92	8	80
+Latvia	97	2	67	98	1	61
+Malta	97	0	45	96	4	71
The Netherlands	99		81	99		95
The Netherlands, Eindhoven	99		85	98		87
The Netherlands, Maastricht	99		96	99		91
Norway	90	9	83	90	10	88
Poland, Cracow	72	17	80	67	17	88
Poland, Kielce	80	3	101	83	4	99
Poland, Lower Silesia	82	1	82	79	2	75
Poland, Warsaw City	[59]	18	103	[64]	14	96
Slovakia	93	0	66	91	0	64
Slovenia	98	2	80	96	3	70
Spain, Albacete	92	5	64	95	5	109
Spain, Asturias	88	12	57	89	9	54
Spain, Basque Country	89	7	69	89	10	78
Spain, Granada	98	2	65	90	10	82
Spain, Mallorca	95	5	68	91	9	72
Spain, Murcia	92	3	76	88	4	72
Spain, Navarra	76	16	74	74	20	82
Spain, Tarragona	95	4	75	96	2	63
Spain, Zaragoza	90	6	79	88	10	80

	MALE MV	DCO	M/I	FEMALE MV	DCO	M/I
Sweden	95		65	94		68
Switzerland, Basel	99	0	99	99	0	120
Switzerland, Geneva	98	2	67	95	5	82
Switzerland, Graubunden	98	0	75	97	0	103
Switzerland, Neuchatel	82	18	98	86	14	96
Switzerland, St Gall-Appenzell	97	3	72	98	2	78
Switzerland, Valais	94	6	54	94	6	69
Switzerland, Vaud	99	0	71	99	0	88
Switzerland, Zurich	99	0	77	99	1	79
+UK, England and Wales	[85]		68	[84]		71
UK, East Anglia			77			77
UK, Mersey	47	7	84	49	8	92
UK, North Western	53	7	71	51	8	73
UK, Oxford	99	0	58	99	0	58
UK, South Thames	61	28	64	56	33	71
UK, South Western	78	2	59	76	1	64
UK, Wessex	[76]	8	58	[68]	11	56
+UK, West Midlands		5	67		7	70
UK, Yorkshire	87	5	64	84	6	69
UK, Scotland	74	3	56	70	5	64
UK, Scotland, West	83	4	56	79	7	63
Yugoslavia, Vojvodina	56	13	72	51	11	77

OCEANIA	MALE MV	DCO	M/I	FEMALE MV	DCO	M/I
Australian Capital Territory	98	0		94	0	
Australia, New South Wales	87	5		88	3	
South Australia	89		53	83		55
Australia, Tasmania	41		48	39		50
Australia, Victoria	93	2	64	90	2	76
Western Australia	89	7	66	87	8	71
French Polynesia	81	14		62	23	
+New Zealand: Non-Maori	94	5	64	93	5	60
+New Zealand: Maori	95	5	44	94	6	38
US, Hawaii: White	81	1	67	84	0	52
US, Hawaii: Japanese	90	0	78	94	0	54
US, Hawaii: Hawaiian	85	0	71	93	0	70
US, Hawaii: Filipino	93	0	78	88	4	64
US, Hawaii: Chinese	75	8	75	99	0	140

+ IMPORTANT-SEE NOTES ON POPULATION PAGE

[] CYTOLOGICAL VERIFICATION EXCLUDED

INDICES OF DATA QUALITY
Other and Unspecified

AFRICA

	MALE MV	DCO	M/I	FEMALE MV	DCO	M/I
Algeria, Setif	56			53		
France, La Reunion	95			97		
Mali, Bamako	37	11		15	4	
Uganda, Kyadondo	50			55		
Zimbabwe, Harare: African	58	19		42	32	
Zimbabwe, Harare: European	39	56		25	58	

AMERICA, CENTRAL AND SOUTH

	MALE MV	DCO	M/I	FEMALE MV	DCO	M/I
Argentina, Concordia	56	41		57	39	
Brazil, Belem	34	33		44	36	
Brazil, Goiania	69	21		62	23	
Brazil, Porto Alegre	51	0		45	0	
Colombia, Cali	53	10		54	12	
Costa Rica	48	30		52	25	
Ecuador, Quito	63	22		55	32	
Peru, Lima	53	25		45	30	
Peru, Trujillo	56	9		70	14	
US, Puerto Rico	64	18		56	21	
Uruguay, Montevideo	27	42		23	52	

AMERICA, NORTH

	MALE MV	DCO	M/I	FEMALE MV	DCO	M/I
Canada	56	7		51	10	
Canada, Alberta	75	6		72	7	
Canada, British Columbia	74	20		73	21	
Canada, Manitoba	49	8		46	10	
Canada, New Brunswick	66	9		64	11	
Canada, Newfoundland	75	5		72	5	
Canada, Northwest Territories	64	21		80	0	
Canada, Nova Scotia	67	19		58	30	
Canada, Ontario	55	6		46	9	
Canada, Prince Edward Island	64	15		50	21	
+Canada, Quebec	36	0		36	0	
Canada, Saskatchewan	62	16		66	12	
Canada, Yukon	99	0		89	0	
+US, Cent. Calif.: Non-Hisp. White	79	4		73	5	
+US, Cent. Calif.: Hispanic	75	2		79	1	
US, Los Angeles: Non-Hisp. White	83	3		80	3	
US, Los Angeles: Hispanic White	84	1		83	4	
US, Los Angeles: Black	85	3		83	1	
US, Los Angeles: Chinese	78	6		73	2	
US, Los Angeles: Filipino	85	2		99	0	
US, Los Angeles: Korean	84	0		82	4	
US, Los Angeles: Japanese	87	0		82	0	
US, San Francisco: Non-Hisp. White	80	4		72	5	
US, San Francisco: Hispanic White	80	3		74	3	
US, San Francisco: Black	80	3		75	2	
US, San Francisco: Chinese	73	6		85	1	
US, San Francisco: Filipino	88	0		78	6	
US, San Francisco: Japanese	86	0		75	0	
US, Connecticut: White	76	11		68	14	
US, Connecticut: Black	82	8		77	10	
US, Atlanta: White	89	2		79	4	
US, Atlanta: Black	81	4		68	7	
US, Iowa	74	3		69	4	

	MALE MV	DCO	M/I	FEMALE MV	DCO	M/I
US, Central Louisiana: White	74	4		69	5	
US, Central Louisiana: Black	66	9		67	8	
US, New Orleans: White	78	3		64	8	
US, New Orleans: Black	66	9		66	10	
US, Detroit: White	75	5		70	8	
US, Detroit: Black	70	6		71	5	
US, New Mexico: Non-Hisp. White	76	6		69	8	
US, New Mexico: Hispanic White	74	9		63	7	
US, New Mexico: American Indian	68	5		70	9	
US, Utah	80	2		75	2	
US, Seattle	81	3		77	3	
US, SEER: White	78	5		72	7	
US, SEER: Black	77	5		73	5	

ASIA

	MALE MV	DCO	M/I	FEMALE MV	DCO	M/I
+China, Qidong	96	0		96	0	
+China, Shanghai	38	2		42	3	
China, Tianjin	65	0		60	0	
Hong Kong	77	7		74	8	
India, Bangalore	16	47		17	53	
India, Barshi, Paranda and Bhum	54	28		63	34	
India, Bombay	65	8		60	12	
India, Karunagappally	33	48		33	37	
India, Madras	33	31		29	44	
India, Trivandrum	35	56		37	52	
Israel: All Jews	64			61		
Jews born in Israel	80			75		
Jews born in America or Europe	62			61		
Jews born in Africa or Asia	64			53		
Non-Jews	71			62		
Japan, Hiroshima	63	14		53	32	
Japan, Miyagi	48	26		41	32	
Japan, Nagasaki	47	37		40	41	
Japan, Osaka	46	35		43	40	
+Japan, Saga	47	24		40	31	
Japan, Yamagata	40	29		36	35	
Korea, Kangwha	50			75		
Kuwait: Non-Kuwaitis	64	27		64	25	
Kuwait: Kuwaitis	51	41		43	43	
Philippines, Manila	41	42		38	44	
Singapore: Chinese	68	11		69	10	
Singapore: Malay	66	10		66	19	
Singapore: Indian	65	15		67	17	
Thailand, Chiang Mai	25	52		23	56	
Thailand, Khon Kaen	22	43		25	43	
Viet Nam, Hanoi	46			34		

+ IMPORTANT-SEE NOTES ON POPULATION PAGE

INDICES OF DATA QUALITY
Other and Unspecified (contd)

EUROPE	MALE MV	DCO	M/I	FEMALE MV	DCO	M/I
Austria, Tyrol	44	32		44	36	
+Belarus	42	0		37	0	
Croatia	38	19		33	31	
+Czech Republic	39	8		37	10	
Denmark	67	3		67	4	
Estonia	62			54		
Finland	66	3		61	6	
France, Bas-Rhin	90			86		
France, Calvados	88			93		
France, Doubs	90			88		
France, Haut-Rhin	97			94		
France, Herault	94			94		
France, Isere	86			85		
France, Somme	82			77		
France, Tarn	88			80		
Germany, Eastern States	71	1		66	2	
+Germany, Saarland	57	24		47	31	
Iceland	77	0		83	2	
Ireland, Southern	52			48		
Italy, Ferrara	37	7		53	9	
Italy, Florence	36	14		29	19	
Italy, Genoa	44	14		36	17	
Italy, Latina	53	21		53	21	
Italy, Macerata	45	8		39	9	
Italy, Modena	39	9		41	12	
Italy, Parma	41	8		39	13	
Italy, Ragusa	51	2		37	0	
Italy, Romagna	41	6		38	8	
Italy, Torino	38	10		35	19	
Italy, Trieste	-	-		-	-	
Italy, Varese	65	8		55	15	
Italy, Veneto	68	8		59	12	
+Latvia	53	8		60	5	
+Malta	68	4		78	3	
The Netherlands	83			83		
The Netherlands, Eindhoven	83			84		
The Netherlands, Maastricht	81			84		
Norway	70	6		65	8	
Poland, Cracow	27	34		28	32	
Poland, Kielce	45	8		37	7	
Poland, Lower Silesia	54	2		60	3	
Poland, Warsaw City	[22]	14		[19]	18	
Slovakia	49	3		47	3	
Slovenia	55	12		51	18	
Spain, Albacete	49	15		31	28	
Spain, Asturias	71	20		60	30	
Spain, Basque Country	56	17		42	26	
Spain, Granada	48	13		36	23	
Spain, Mallorca	66	10		57	16	
Spain, Murcia	65	13		62	20	
Spain, Navarra	60	21		50	33	
Spain, Tarragona	66	6		64	7	
Spain, Zaragoza	41	18		37	23	

	MALE MV	DCO	M/I	FEMALE MV	DCO	M/I
Sweden	86			88		
Switzerland, Basel	99	0		99	0	
Switzerland, Geneva	67	8		58	13	
Switzerland, Graubunden	72	25		47	29	
Switzerland, Neuchatel	77	3		62	14	
Switzerland, St Gall-Appenzell	65	4		62	6	
Switzerland, Valais	69	8		60	6	
Switzerland, Vaud	71	9		67	9	
Switzerland, Zurich	83	1		70	3	
+UK, England and Wales	[57]			[57]		
UK, East Anglia						
UK, Mersey	36	7		32	8	
UK, North Western	32	8		32	8	
UK, Oxford	38	2		38	2	
UK, South Thames	28	39		26	41	
UK, South Western	62	2		41	4	
UK, Wessex	[70]	4		[67]	5	
+UK, West Midlands		9			10	
UK, Yorkshire	44	7		43	9	
UK, Scotland	36	8		35	8	
UK, Scotland, West	35	10		33	11	
Yugoslavia, Vojvodina	29	14		25	15	

OCEANIA

	MALE MV	DCO	M/I	FEMALE MV	DCO	M/I
Australian Capital Territory	79	6		90	3	
Australia, New South Wales	68	6		64	8	
South Australia	59			51		
Australia, Tasmania	63			55		
Australia, Victoria	70	4		66	7	
Western Australia	80	6		74	9	
French Polynesia	58	40		31	66	
+New Zealand: Non-Maori	54	8		49	12	
+New Zealand: Maori	57	7		62	6	
US, Hawaii: White	84	0		86	0	
US, Hawaii: Japanese	83	2		78	0	
US, Hawaii: Hawaiian	71	3		74	0	
US, Hawaii: Filipino	67	0		94	0	
US, Hawaii: Chinese	94	0		82	0	

+ IMPORTANT-SEE NOTES ON POPULATION PAGE

[] CYTOLOGICAL VERIFICATION EXCLUDED

INDICES OF DATA QUALITY
All sites

AFRICA

	MALE			FEMALE		
	MV	DCO	M/I	MV	DCO	M/I
Algeria, Setif	77			84		
France, La Reunion	98		72	98		52
Mali, Bamako	27	5		44	3	
Uganda, Kyadondo	63			62		
Zimbabwe, Harare: African	60	8		69	8	
Zimbabwe, Harare: European	90	8		89	8	

AMERICA, CENTRAL AND SOUTH

	MALE			FEMALE		
	MV	DCO	M/I	MV	DCO	M/I
Argentina, Concordia	76	22	61	83	16	43
Brazil, Belem	67	14	48	80	11	38
Brazil, Goiania	85	9	32	89	7	26
Brazil, Porto Alegre	68	0	48	71	0	41
Colombia, Cali	75	5	67	80	6	55
Costa Rica	72	13	59	76	10	48
Ecuador, Quito	72	16		74	16	
Peru, Lima	70	11		73	9	
Peru, Trujillo	71	8	54	78	7	48
US, Puerto Rico	89	5	55	90	5	49
Uruguay, Montevideo	61	19	65	72	16	49

AMERICA, NORTH

	MALE			FEMALE		
	MV	DCO	M/I	MV	DCO	M/I
Canada						
Canada, Alberta						
Canada, British Columbia						
Canada, Manitoba						
Canada, New Brunswick						
Canada, Newfoundland						
Canada, Northwest Territories						
Canada, Nova Scotia						
Canada, Ontario						
Canada, Prince Edward Island						
+Canada, Quebec						
Canada, Saskatchewan						
Canada, Yukon						
+US, Cent. Calif.: Non-Hisp. White	94	1	46	94	1	45
+US, Cent. Calif.: Hispanic	93	1	43	96	1	38
US, Los Angeles: Non-Hisp. White	95	1	43	95	1	45
US, Los Angeles: Hispanic White	94	1		96	1	
US, Los Angeles: Black	95	1		95	1	
US, Los Angeles: Chinese	94	1		95	1	
US, Los Angeles: Filipino	95	1		98	0	
US, Los Angeles: Korean	92	1		95	1	
US, Los Angeles: Japanese	96	1		96	1	
US, San Francisco: Non-Hisp. White	93	1	39	94	1	45
US, San Francisco: Hispanic White	93	0	29	96	1	27
US, San Francisco: Black	93	1	51	94	1	52
US, San Francisco: Chinese	93	1	51	95	1	42
US, San Francisco: Filipino	94	1	42	96	1	32
US, San Francisco: Japanese	95	2	48	96	1	41
US, Connecticut: White	95	1	44	94	2	43
US, Connecticut: Black	96	1	52	95	2	44
US, Atlanta: White	95	1	40	96	1	40
US, Atlanta: Black	94	1	54	94	2	49
US, Iowa	94	1	45	94	1	45

	MALE			FEMALE		
	MV	DCO	M/I	MV	DCO	M/I
US, Central Louisiana: White	90	3	51	90	3	47
US, Central Louisiana: Black	83	3	62	88	3	54
US, New Orleans: White	93	2	45	93	2	43
US, New Orleans: Black	90	4	60	90	3	52
US, Detroit: White	96	1	42	95	1	43
US, Detroit: Black	94	1	49	94	1	52
US, New Mexico: Non-Hisp. White	93	2	41	93	2	44
US, New Mexico: Hispanic White	92	2	48	93	1	48
US, New Mexico: American Indian	86	1	61	92	1	53
US, Utah	96	0	37	96	0	40
US, Seattle	95	0	39	95	1	42
US, SEER: White	95	1	42	95	1	43
US, SEER: Black	94	1	51	94	1	50

ASIA

	MALE			FEMALE		
	MV	DCO	M/I	MV	DCO	M/I
+China, Qidong	60	0	83	72	1	72
+China, Shanghai	47	2	75	54	2	67
China, Tianjin	55	0	62	59	0	55
Hong Kong	69	8	54	73	7	44
India, Bangalore	72	11	31	79	8	29
India, Barshi, Paranda and Bhum	80	5		86	3	
India, Bombay	75	8	51	76	9	48
India, Karunagappally	68	14		75	12	
India, Madras	72	5	47	77	5	43
India, Trivandrum	75	14	36	83	8	24
Israel: All Jews	85			86		
Jews born in Israel	90			93		
Jews born in America or Europe	84			85		
Jews born in Africa or Asia	84			86		
Non-Jews	83			86		
Japan, Hiroshima	81	8	49	85	7	42
Japan, Miyagi	79	7	55	79	8	50
Japan, Nagasaki	78	11	60	80	11	54
Japan, Osaka	70	15	67	72	14	59
+Japan, Saga	63	17	65	63	18	62
Japan, Yamagata	73	15	60	73	15	55
Korea, Kangwha	66		78	76		57
Kuwait: Non-Kuwaitis	84	13		86	10	
Kuwait: Kuwaitis	72	25		79	17	
Philippines, Manila	56	24		65	18	
Singapore: Chinese	83	6		90	4	
Singapore: Malay	80	7		88	5	
Singapore: Indian	85	4		92	3	
Thailand, Chiang Mai	65	8		72	8	
Thailand, Khon Kaen	29	16		48	14	
Viet Nam, Hanoi	48			58		

+ IMPORTANT-SEE NOTES ON POPULATION PAGE

EUROPE

	MALE			FEMALE		
	MV	DCO	M/I	MV	DCO	M/I
Austria, Tyrol	87	7	50	87	8	45
+Belarus	67	0	67	76	0	54
Croatia	61	9	76	62	10	64
+Czech Republic	70	2	67	74	3	57
Denmark	93	1	58	94	1	53
Estonia	81		72	85		58
Finland	94	1	49	94	1	39
France, Bas-Rhin	96		59	96		52
France, Calvados	95		63	96		53
France, Doubs	96		51	96		41
France, Haut-Rhin	98		57	98		47
France, Herault	99		67	98		55
France, Isere	96		39	96		30
France, Somme	95		74	95		67
France, Tarn	97		59	97		57
Germany, Eastern States	89	0	67	91	0	59
+Germany, Saarland	87	8	53	87	7	48
Iceland	97	0	55	97	0	51
Ireland, Southern	80		56	82		50
Italy, Ferrara	85	2	61	86	2	49
Italy, Florence	69	3	59	71	4	52
Italy, Genoa	77	4	62	79	4	56
Italy, Latina	82	11	67	83	10	56
Italy, Macerata	81	1	53	80	1	49
Italy, Modena	81	3	56	84	3	50
Italy, Parma	83	3	63	84	4	56
Italy, Ragusa	73	1	63	80	1	58
Italy, Romagna	88	1	51	89	1	45
Italy, Torino	82	4	59	83	5	53
Italy, Trieste	83	1	48	86	1	50
Italy, Varese	90	2	56	89	2	47
Italy, Veneto	85	3	56	85	4	48
+Latvia	67	4	64	80	3	50
+Malta	80	2	58	85	2	50
The Netherlands	95		66	96		56
The Netherlands, Eindhoven	95		66	96		55
The Netherlands, Maastricht	94		68	96		57
Norway	93	2	58	93	2	53
Poland, Cracow	64	14	84	69	13	71
Poland, Kielce	67	3	81	70	4	70
Poland, Lower Silesia	47	1	72	61	1	58
Poland, Warsaw City	[63]	9	75	[68]	8	65
Slovakia	80	2	63	82	1	51
Slovenia	87	4	71	88	4	59
Spain, Albacete	74	11	68	77	11	60
Spain, Asturias	89	8	69	87	10	59
Spain, Basque Country	82	8	63	81	10	57
Spain, Granada	82	6	58	82	7	51
Spain, Mallorca	91	3	50	91	4	43
Spain, Murcia	88	5	52	89	5	46
Spain, Navarra	86	8	52	85	8	44
Spain, Tarragona	91	2	50	90	3	44
Spain, Zaragoza	76	8	64	74	11	60
Sweden	98		54	97		50
Switzerland, Basel	99	0	52	99	0	49
Switzerland, Geneva	96	1	40	95	1	38
Switzerland, Graubunden	89	6	58	89	5	58
Switzerland, Neuchatel	93	2	53	93	2	47
Switzerland, St Gall-Appenzell	95	1	52	95	1	47
Switzerland, Valais	92	2	51	93	1	42
Switzerland, Vaud	93	1	46	95	1	39
Switzerland, Zurich	95	0	57	95	0	57
+UK, England and Wales	[78]		62	[80]		56
UK, East Anglia			56			51
UK, Mersey	73	3	66	74	3	60
UK, North Western	64	4	64	66	4	58
UK, Oxford	79	0	53	80	0	48
UK, South Thames	65	17	63	66	16	58
UK, South Western	76	3	59	78	2	56
UK, Wessex	[75]	7	61	[77]	7	53
+UK, West Midlands		3	56		3	50
UK, Yorkshire	80	3	60	81	4	54
UK, Scotland	77	3	57	79	3	53
UK, Scotland, West	75	5	60	76	5	55
Yugoslavia, Vojvodina	55	10	69	59	8	58

OCEANIA

	MALE			FEMALE		
	MV	DCO	M/I	MV	DCO	M/I
Australian Capital Territory						
Australia, New South Wales						
South Australia						
Australia, Tasmania						
Australia, Victoria						
Western Australia						
French Polynesia						
+New Zealand: Non-Maori	86	3	59	87	3	51
+New Zealand: Maori	80	6	51	86	4	40
US, Hawaii: White	96	0	40	97	0	40
US, Hawaii: Japanese	97	0	41	97	0	38
US, Hawaii: Hawaiian	94	0	67	97	0	52
US, Hawaii: Filipino	94	0	47	98	0	37
US, Hawaii: Chinese	95	0	39	96	0	49

+ IMPORTANT-SEE NOTES ON POPULATION PAGE

[] CYTOLOGICAL VERIFICATION EXCLUDED

INDICES OF DATA QUALITY
All sites but 173

	MALE			FEMALE		
AFRICA	MV	DCO	M/I	MV	DCO	M/I
Algeria, Setif	77			83		
France, La Reunion	98		75	98		55
Mali, Bamako	25	5		42	3	
Uganda, Kyadondo	63			62		
Zimbabwe, Harare: African	60	8		69	8	
Zimbabwe, Harare: European	72	21		77	17	

AMERICA, CENTRAL AND SOUTH	MV	DCO	M/I	MV	DCO	M/I
Argentina, Concordia	72	26	73	80	19	50
Brazil, Belem	61	17	57	78	12	43
Brazil, Goiania	77	15	51	84	11	40
Brazil, Porto Alegre	63	0	56	68	0	47
Colombia, Cali	75	5	67	80	6	55
Costa Rica	66	16	72	72	13	59
Ecuador, Quito	68	19		71	18	
Peru, Lima	68	12		71	9	
Peru, Trujillo	68	9	60	76	7	51
US, Puerto Rico	89	5	55	90	5	49
Uruguay, Montevideo	59	20	69	71	17	51

AMERICA, NORTH	MV	DCO	M/I	MV	DCO	M/I
Canada	83	2	52	84	2	47
Canada, Alberta	92	2	51	93	2	45
Canada, British Columbia	91	6	48	91	6	46
Canada, Manitoba	81	2	51	80	2	47
Canada, New Brunswick	91	2	53	92	2	49
Canada, Newfoundland	95	1	61	95	1	51
Canada, Northwest Territories	84	3	64	83	3	51
Canada, Nova Scotia	87	8	55	88	8	51
Canada, Ontario	83	2	50	84	2	46
Canada, Prince Edward Island	92	2	57	91	4	46
+Canada, Quebec	72	0	57	75	0	50
Canada, Saskatchewan	90	3	51	91	3	46
Canada, Yukon	95	1	44	96	0	38
+US, Cent. Calif.: Non-Hisp. White	94	1	46	94	1	45
+US, Cent. Calif.: Hispanic	93	1	43	96	1	39
US, Los Angeles: Non-Hisp. White	95	1	43	95	1	46
US, Los Angeles: Hispanic White	94	1		96	1	
US, Los Angeles: Black	95	1		95	1	
US, Los Angeles: Chinese	94	1		95	1	
US, Los Angeles: Filipino	95	1		98	0	
US, Los Angeles: Korean	92	1		95	1	
US, Los Angeles: Japanese	96	1		96	1	
US, San Francisco: Non-Hisp. White	93	1	39	94	1	46
US, San Francisco: Hispanic White	93	0	29	96	1	27
US, San Francisco: Black	93	1	51	93	1	52
US, San Francisco: Chinese	93	1	51	95	1	42
US, San Francisco: Filipino	94	1	42	96	1	32
US, San Francisco: Japanese	95	2	48	96	1	41
US, Connecticut: White	95	1	44	94	2	44
US, Connecticut: Black	96	1	52	95	2	44
US, Atlanta: White	95	1	40	96	1	40
US, Atlanta: Black	94	1	54	93	2	49
US, Iowa	94	1	45	94	1	45

	MALE			FEMALE		
	MV	DCO	M/I	MV	DCO	M/I
US, Central Louisiana: White	90	3	51	90	3	47
US, Central Louisiana: Black	83	3	62	88	3	54
US, New Orleans: White	93	2	45	93	2	43
US, New Orleans: Black	90	4	60	90	3	52
US, Detroit: White	96	1	42	95	1	43
US, Detroit: Black	94	1	50	94	1	52
US, New Mexico: Non-Hisp. White	93	2	41	93	2	44
US, New Mexico: Hispanic White	92	2	48	93	1	48
US, New Mexico: American Indian	86	1	61	92	1	54
US, Utah	96	0	38	96	0	40
US, Seattle	95	0	39	95	1	43
US, SEER: White	95	1	42	95	1	43
US, SEER: Black	94	1	51	94	1	51

ASIA	MV	DCO	M/I	MV	DCO	M/I
+China, Qidong	60	0	83	72	1	73
+China, Shanghai	47	2	76	54	2	67
China, Tianjin	55	0	62	59	0	55
Hong Kong	69	8	55	72	7	45
India, Bangalore	72	12	32	79	8	30
India, Barshi, Paranda and Bhum	80	5		86	3	
India, Bombay	75	8	52	76	9	48
India, Karunagappally	67	14		74	13	
India, Madras	72	5	48	77	5	43
India, Trivandrum	75	14	36	83	8	25
Israel: All Jews	85			86		
Jews born in Israel	90			93		
Jews born in America or Europe	84			85		
Jews born in Africa or Asia	84			86		
Non-Jews	83			86		
Japan, Hiroshima	81	8	50	85	7	42
Japan, Miyagi	79	7	56	79	8	50
Japan, Nagasaki	78	11	61	79	11	55
Japan, Osaka	70	15	67	72	14	60
+Japan, Saga	62	18	65	62	18	63
Japan, Yamagata	73	15	60	73	15	55
Korea, Kangwha	65		79	76		58
Kuwait: Non-Kuwaitis	83	13		86	10	
Kuwait: Kuwaitis	72	25		78	17	
Philippines, Manila	55	24		65	18	
Singapore: Chinese	83	6		89	4	
Singapore: Malay	79	7		88	5	
Singapore: Indian	85	4		92	3	
Thailand, Chiang Mai	64	8		72	8	
Thailand, Khon Kaen	28	17		47	14	
Viet Nam, Hanoi	48			58		

+ IMPORTANT-SEE NOTES ON POPULATION PAGE

INDICES OF DATA QUALITY
All sites but 173 (contd)

	MALE			FEMALE		
EUROPE	MV	DCO	M/I	MV	DCO	M/I
Austria, Tyrol	87	8	54	86	9	49
+Belarus	65	0	73	74	0	61
Croatia	61	9	77	62	10	65
+Czech Republic	65	3	80	70	3	68
Denmark	92	1	69	93	1	62
Estonia	80		77	84		65
Finland	93	1	60	93	1	50
France, Bas-Rhin	95		62	96		55
France, Calvados	94		71	95		61
France, Doubs	96		61	96		53
France, Haut-Rhin	98		64	98		56
France, Herault	99		73	98		58
France, Isere	96		41	96		31
France, Somme	95		79	94		70
France, Tarn	97		64	97		62
Germany, Eastern States	89	0	69	91	0	61
+Germany, Saarland	84	9	64	85	9	57
Iceland	97	0	56	97	0	52
Ireland, Southern	84		75	86		65
Italy, Ferrara	83	3	72	85	2	56
Italy, Florence	71	4	64	72	5	55
Italy, Genoa	76	4	69	78	5	61
Italy, Latina	80	12	75	82	11	61
Italy, Macerata	78	1	63	78	1	57
Italy, Modena	78	3	65	82	3	55
Italy, Parma	82	3	69	83	4	60
Italy, Ragusa	66	1	80	77	1	69
Italy, Romagna	86	1	61	87	1	53
Italy, Torino	79	4	66	80	5	59
Italy, Trieste	81	1	55	85	1	60
Italy, Varese	89	2	63	88	3	53
Italy, Veneto	83	3	64	84	4	54
+Latvia	65	4	69	78	3	56
+Malta	77	3	71	84	2	56
The Netherlands	95		69	96		58
The Netherlands, Eindhoven	95		66	96		55
The Netherlands, Maastricht	94		71	96		58
Norway	93	2	61	93	2	55
Poland, Cracow	62	15	90	67	13	75
Poland, Kielce	65	3	88	68	4	77
Poland, Lower Silesia	45	1	75	59	1	61
Poland, Warsaw City	[61]	9	79	[66]	9	69
Slovakia	78	2	72	80	1	60
Slovenia	87	4	77	87	5	65
Spain, Albacete	74	11	68	77	11	60
Spain, Asturias	89	8	69	87	9	59
Spain, Basque Country	82	8	63	81	10	57
Spain, Granada	79	7	69	80	9	62
Spain, Mallorca	88	4	66	87	5	59
Spain, Murcia	85	7	65	86	6	58
Spain, Navarra	84	9	62	83	10	52
Spain, Tarragona	88	3	63	88	3	55
Spain, Zaragoza	74	9	71	72	11	67

	MALE			FEMALE		
	MV	DCO	M/I	MV	DCO	M/I
Sweden	97		57	97		52
Switzerland, Basel	99	0	68	99	0	64
Switzerland, Geneva	95	1	53	93	2	52
Switzerland, Graubunden	88	6	63	88	6	62
Switzerland, Neuchatel	91	2	70	91	3	62
Switzerland, St Gall-Appenzell	94	1	62	94	1	58
Switzerland, Valais	90	2	64	91	2	53
Switzerland, Vaud	91	2	62	93	2	53
Switzerland, Zurich	95	0	57	95	0	57
+UK, England and Wales	[76]		72	[78]		64
UK, East Anglia			71			62
UK, Mersey	70	3	77	71	4	71
UK, North Western	64	5	74	67	4	67
UK, Oxford	74	1	67	77	0	58
UK, South Thames	63	20	72	64	18	65
UK, South Western	71	4	73	74	3	67
UK, Wessex	[77]	8	66	[79]	8	57
+UK, West Midlands		3	67		3	59
UK, Yorkshire	77	4	70	78	4	63
UK, Scotland	74	4	67	76	4	61
UK, Scotland, West	71	5	68	74	5	63
Yugoslavia, Vojvodina	52	10	75	56	9	64

	MALE			FEMALE		
OCEANIA	MV	DCO	M/I	MV	DCO	M/I
Australian Capital Territory	93	1		94	1	
Australia, New South Wales	90	2		91	2	
South Australia	82		53	81		49
Australia, Tasmania	86		54	88		51
Australia, Victoria	89	1	54	90	1	49
Western Australia	90	3	49	91	4	43
French Polynesia	72	21		72	19	
+New Zealand: Non-Maori	86	3	59	87	3	51
+New Zealand: Maori	80	6	51	86	4	40
US, Hawaii: White	96	0	40	97	0	40
US, Hawaii: Japanese	97	0	41	97	0	38
US, Hawaii: Hawaiian	94	0	68	97	0	52
US, Hawaii: Filipino	94	0	47	98	0	37
US, Hawaii: Chinese	95	0	39	96	0	49

+ IMPORTANT-SEE NOTES ON POPULATION PAGE

[] CYTOLOGICAL VERIFICATION EXCLUDED

Errors in Volume VI

Peru, Trujillo

The population figures on p. 227 are wrong for females aged 80-84. The figure given was 281 and the correct figure is 1177. This results in errors in the age-specific rates for that age-group and in the cumulative and standardized rates in all age-groups.

Canada, Manitoba

There is an error in the age-specific rates for cervical cancer.

USA: SEER, Connecticut, Atlanta and Detroit

The population data for Non-Whites, instead of those for Blacks, were used for calculating the rates in Blacks in Connecticut, Atlanta, Detroit and total SEER. As a result, incidence rates in these Black populations were slightly lower than they should have been.

Israel: Non-Jews

The population data for boys aged 0-1 were wrong. The figure given was 13900, and this should have been 11900. The rates for this age-group were affected accordingly.

Spain, Navarra

In situ diagnoses were included for cervical cancer. the figures for invasive cases of cervical cancer for the years 1983-86 are:

Australia, New South Wales

The population data for girls aged 0-1 were wrong. The figure given was 71065, and this should have been 40370. The rates for this age-group were affected accordingly.

Chapter 9

p. 863. The formula to calculate the standard error for the cumulative rate was incorrect. The formula should read:

$$\text{S.E. (cumulative rate)} = 5\sqrt{\sum_{x=i}^{k} r_i/(n_i)^2}$$

pp. 863, 864. The examples use figures obtained from an earlier volume. Using Volume VI, the figures should be as follows:

In the first 5.58 should be replaced by 7.2
In the second 9.73 should be replaced by 9.1

	Rates	Number of cases
All ages		55
Age unknown	0	0
0-	-	-
1-	-	-
5-	-	-
10-	-	-
15-	-	-
20-	-	-
25-	-	-
30-	2.9	2
35-	-	-
40-	13.3	8
45-	9.8	5
50-	22.2	13
55-	10.1	6
60-	14.3	8
65-	12.6	6
70-	7.0	3
75-	-	-
80-	9.3	2
85+	14.7	2
Crude rate	5.3	
%	2.1	
CR74	0.4	
ASR World	4.3	

The Index

When registries which appear in previous volumes of Cancer Incidence in Five Continents, but not in the present volume, are listed they are given with the number(s) of the volume(s).

Conventions adopted

Permutation of terms

In general, terms appear as usually written, e.g. 'oral mesopharynx' or 'ascending colon' rather than as 'mesopharynx, oral' or 'colon, ascending'. There are certain exceptions such as 'endocrine glands, other' and 'thoracic organs, other' to avoid a long list of terms included under 'other'. Subsites such as 'ascending colon' are cross-referenced and the page numbers given under the main site, i.e. 'colon'.

Registries

The registries are indexed alphabetically by registry title, as it appears in the volumes, and not by continent, country or province, as in the list of contents. However, following each registry title is an indication of country and province (or similar subdivision) for those registries with sub-national cover.

Anatomical sites

The index lists the titles of the categories for which incidence data have been published (see Chapters 3 and 4).

Cross-references

In general cross-references direct attention to the rubric title which includes a given subdivision. Thus the entry Pyriform fossa (sinus) - see hypopharynx leads the reader to a listing of all information available concerning the hypopharynx and its sub-divisions.

Ethnic group

Ethnic group is indexed only when a registry publishes separate data for the ethnic groups living in the registration area, e.g. Japanese appear under Hawaii, Los Angeles and San Francisco.

Abbreviations and symbols

*	- separate data not available for this site
ASR	- age-standardized rates
CR	- cumulative rate
ICD-9	- 9th Revision of the International Classification of Diseases (ICD) (WHO, 1977)
D & IR	- description of registry and age-specific incidence rates

IARC Monographs on the Evaluation of Carcinogenic Risks to Humans

Volume 1
Some Inorganic Substances, Chlorinated Hydrocarbons, Aromatic Amines, N-Nitroso Compounds, and Natural Products
1972; 184 pages;
ISBN 92 832 1201 0 (out of print)

Volume 2
Some Inorganic and Organometallic Compounds
1973; 181 pages;
ISBN 92 832 1202 9 (out of print)

Volume 3
Certain Polycyclic Aromatic Hydrocarbons and Heterocyclic Compounds
1973; 271 pages;
ISBN 92 832 1203 7 (out of print)

Volume 4
Some Aromatic Amines, Hydrazine and Related Substances, N-Nitroso Compounds and Miscellaneous Alkylating Agents
1974; 286 pages;
ISBN 92 832 1204 5

Volume 5
Some Organochlorine Pesticides
1974; 241 pages;
ISBN 92 832 1205 3 (out of print)

Volume 6
Sex Hormones
1974; 243 pages;
ISBN 92 832 1206 1 (out of print)

Volume 7
Some Anti-Thyroid and Related Substances, Nitrofurans and Industrial Chemicals
1974; 326 pages;
ISBN 92 832 1207 X (out of print)

Volume 8
Some Aromatic Azo Compounds
1975; 357 pages;
ISBN 92 832 1208 8

Volume 9
Some Aziridines, N-, S- and O-Mustards and Selenium
1975; 268 pages;
ISBN 92 832 1209 6

Volume 10
Some Naturally Occurring Substances
1976; 353 pages;
ISBN 92 832 1210 X (out of print)

Volume 11
Cadmium, Nickel, Some Epoxides, Miscellaneous Industrial Chemicals and General Considerations on Volatile Anaesthetics
1976; 306 pages;
ISBN 92 832 1211 8 (out of print)

Volume 12
Some Carbamates, Thiocarbamates and Carbazides
1976; 282 pages;
ISBN 92 832 1212 6

Volume 13
Some Miscellaneous Pharmaceutical Substances
1977; 255 pages;
ISBN 92 832 1213 4

Volume 14
Asbestos
1977; 106 pages;
ISBN 92 832 1214 2 (out of print)

Volume 15
Some Fumigants, the Herbicides 2,4-D and 2,4,5-T, Chlorinated Dibenzodioxins and Miscellaneous Industrial Chemicals
1977; 354 pages;
ISBN 92 832 1215 0 (out of print)

Volume 16
Some Aromatic Amines and Related Nitro Compounds – Hair Dyes, Colouring Agents and Miscellaneous Industrial Chemicals
1978; 400 pages;
ISBN 92 832 1216 9

Volume 17
Some N-Nitroso Compounds
1978; 365 pages;
ISBN 92 832 1217 7

Volume 18
Polychlorinated Biphenyls and Polybrominated Biphenyls
1978; 140 pages;
ISBN 92 832 1218 5

Volume 19
Some Monomers, Plastics and Synthetic Elastomers, and Acrolein
1979; 513 pages;
ISBN 92 832 1219 3 (out of print)

Volume 20
Some Halogenated Hydrocarbons
1979; 609 pages;
ISBN 92 832 1220 7 (out of print)

Volume 21
Sex Hormones (II)
1979; 583 pages;
ISBN 92 832 1521 4

Volume 22
Some Non-Nutritive Sweetening Agents
1980; 208 pages;
ISBN 92 832 1522 2

Volume 23
Some Metals and Metallic Compounds
1980; 438 pages;
ISBN 92 832 1523 0 (out of print)

Volume 24
Some Pharmaceutical Drugs
1980; 337 pages;
ISBN 92 832 1524 9

Volume 25
Wood, Leather and Some Associated Industries
1981; 412 pages;
ISBN 92 832 1525 7

Volume 26
Some Antineoplastic and

Immunosuppressive Agents
1981; 411 pages;
ISBN 92 832 1526 5

Volume 27
Some Aromatic Amines, Anthraquinones and Nitroso Compounds, and Inorganic Fluorides Used in Drinking Water and Dental Preparations
1982; 341 pages;
ISBN 92 832 1527 3

Volume 28
The Rubber Industry
1982; 486 pages;
ISBN 92 832 1528 1

Volume 29
Some Industrial Chemicals and Dyestuffs
1982; 416 pages;
ISBN 92 832 1529 X

Volume 30
Miscellaneous Pesticides
1983; 424 pages;
ISBN 92 832 1530 3

Volume 31
Some Food Additives, Feed Additives and Naturally Occurring Substances
1983; 314 pages;
ISBN 92 832 1531 1

Volume 32
Polynuclear Aromatic Compounds, Part 1: Chemical, Environmental and Experimental Data
1983; 477 pages;
ISBN 92 832 1532 X

Volume 33
Polynuclear Aromatic Compounds, Part 2: Carbon Blacks, Mineral Oils and Some Nitroarenes
1984; 245 pages;
ISBN 92 832 1533 8 (out of print)

Volume 34
Polynuclear Aromatic Compounds, Part 3: Industrial Exposures in Aluminium Production, Coal Gasification, Coke Production, and Iron and Steel Founding
1984; 219 pages;
ISBN 92 832 1534 6

Volume 35
Polynuclear Aromatic Compounds: Part 4: Bitumens, Coal-Tars and Derived Products, Shale-Oils and Soots
1985; 271 pages;
ISBN 92 832 1535 4

Volume 36
Allyl Compounds, Aldehydes, Epoxides and Peroxides
1985; 369 pages;
ISBN 92 832 1536 2

Volume 37
Tobacco Habits Other than Smoking; Betel-Quid and Areca-Nut Chewing; and Some Related Nitrosamines
1985; 291 pages;
ISBN 92 832 1537 0

Volume 38
Tobacco Smoking
1986; 421 pages;
ISBN 92 832 1538 9

Volume 39
Some Chemicals Used in Plastics and Elastomers
1986; 403 pages;
ISBN 92 832 1239 8

Volume 40
Some Naturally Occurring and Synthetic Food Components, Furocoumarins and Ultraviolet Radiation
1986; 444 pages;
ISBN 92 832 1240 1

Volume 41
Some Halogenated Hydrocarbons and Pesticide Exposures
1986; 434 pages;
ISBN 92 832 1241 X

Volume 42
Silica and Some Silicates
1987; 289 pages;
ISBN 92 832 1242 8

Volume 43
Man-Made Mineral Fibres and Radon
1988; 300 pages;
ISBN 92 832 1243 6

Volume 44
Alcohol Drinking
1988; 416 pages;
ISBN 92 832 1244 4

Volume 45
Occupational Exposures in Petroleum Refining; Crude Oil and Major Petroleum Fuels
1989; 322 pages;
ISBN 92 832 1245 2

Volume 46
Diesel and Gasoline Engine Exhausts and Some Nitroarenes
1989; 458 pages;
ISBN 92 832 1246 0

Volume 47
Some Organic Solvents, Resin Monomers and Related Compounds, Pigments and Occupational Exposures in Paint Manufacture and Painting
1989; 535 pages;
ISBN 92 832 1247 9

Volume 48
Some Flame Retardants and Textile Chemicals, and Exposures in the Textile Manufacturing Industry
1990; 345 pages;
ISBN: 92 832 1248 7

Volume 49
Chromium, Nickel and Welding
1990; 677 pages;
ISBN: 92 832 1249 5

Volume 50
Some Pharmaceutical Drugs
1990; 415 pages;
ISBN: 92 832 1259 9

Volume 51
Coffee, Tea, Mate, Methylxanthines and Methylglyoxal
1991; 513 pages;
ISBN: 92 832 1251 7

Volume 52
Chlorinated Drinking-Water; Chlorination By-products; Some other Halogenated Compounds; Cobalt and Cobalt Compounds
1991; 544 pages;
ISBN: 92 832 1252 5

Volume 53
Occupational Exposures in Insecticide Application, and Some Pesticides
1991; 612 pages;
ISBN 92 832 1253 3

Volume 54
Occupational Exposures to Mists and Vapours from Strong Inorganic Acids; and other Industrial Chemicals
1992; 336 pages;
ISBN 92 832 1254 1

Volume 55
Solar and Ultraviolet Radiation
1992; 316 pages;
ISBN 92 832 1255 X

Volume 56
Some Naturally Occurring Substances: Food Items and Constituents, Heterocyclic Aromatic Amines and Mycotoxins
1993; 600 pages;
ISBN 92 832 1256 8

Volume 57
Occupational Exposures of Hairdressers and Barbers

and Personal Use of Hair Colourants; Some Hair Dyes, Cosmetic Colourants, Industrial Dyestuffs and Aromatic Amines
1993; 428 pages;
ISBN 92 832 1257 6

Volume 58
Beryllium, Cadmium, Mercury and Exposures in the Glass Manufacturing Industry
1994; 444 pages;
ISBN 92 832 1258 4

Volume 59
Hepatitis Viruses
1994; 286 pages;
ISBN 92 832 1259 2

Volume 60
Some Industrial Chemicals
1994; 560 pages;
ISBN 92 832 1260 6

Volume 61
Schistosomes, Liver Flukes and *Helicobacter pylori*
1994; 280 pages;
ISBN 92 832 1261 4

Volume 62
Wood Dusts and Formaldehyde
1995; 405 pages;
ISBN 92 832 1262 2

Volume 63
Dry cleaning, Some Chlorinated Solvents and Other Industrial Chemicals
1995; 558 pages;
ISBN 92 832 1263 0

Volume 64
Human Papillomaviruses
1995; 409 pages;
ISBN 92 832 1264 9

Volume 65
Printing Processes, Printing Inks, Carbon Blacks and Some Nitro Compounds
1996; 578 pages;
ISBN 92 832 1265 7

Volume 66
Some Pharmaceutical Drug
1996; 514 pages;
ISBN 92 832 1266 5

Volume 67
Human Immunodeficiency Viruses and Human T-cell Lymphotropic Viruses
1996; 424 pages;
ISBN 92 832 1267 3

Volume 68
Silica, Some Silicates, Coal Dust and para-Aramid Fibrils
1997; 506 pages;
ISBN 92 832 1268 1

Volume 69
Polychlorinated Dibenzo-dioxins and Dibenzofurans
1997; 666 pages;
ISBN 92 832 1269 X

Supplements
Supplement No.1
Chemicals and Industrial Processes Associated with Cancer in Humans (IARC Monographs, Volumes 1 to 20)
1979; 71 pages;
ISBN 92 832 1404 8 (out of print)

Supplement No. 2
Long-Term and Short-Term Screening Assays for Carcinogens: A Critical Appraisal
1980; 426 pages;
ISBN 92 832 1404 8

Supplement No. 3
Cross Index of Synonyms and Trade Names in Volumes 1 to 26
1982; 199 pages;
ISBN 92 832 1405 6 (out of print)

Supplement No.4
Chemicals, Industrial Processes and Industries Associated with Cancer in Humans (Volumes 1 to 29)
1982; 292 pages;
ISBN 92 832 1407 2 (out of print)

Supplement No. 5
Cross Index of Synonyms and Trade Names in Volumes 1 to 36
1985; 259 pages;
ISBN 92 832 1408 0 (out of print)

Supplement No. 6
Genetic and Related Effects: An Updating of Selected IARC Monographs from Volumes 1 to 42
1987; 729 pages;
ISBN 92 832 1409 9

Supplement No. 7
Overall Evaluations of Carcinogenicity: An Updating of IARC Monographs Volumes 1 to 42
1987; 440 pages;
ISBN 92 832 1411 0

Supplement No. 8
Cross Index of Synonyms and Trade Names in Volumes 1 to 46
1989; 346 pages;
ISBN 92 832 1417 X

IARC Scientific Publications

No. 1
Liver Cancer
1971; 176 pages;
ISBN 0 19 723000 8

No. 2
Oncogenesis and Herpesviruses
Edited by P.M. Biggs, G. de Thé and L.N. Payne
1972; 515 pages;
ISBN 0 19 723001 6

No. 3
N-Nitroso Compounds: Analysis and Formation
Edited by P. Bogovski, R. Preussman and E.A. Walker
1972; 140 pages;
ISBN 0 19 723002 4

No. 4
Transplacental Carcinogenesis
Edited by L. Tomatis and U. Mohr
1973; 181 pages;
ISBN 0 19 723003 2

No. 5/6
Pathology of Tumours in Laboratory Animals. Volume 1: Tumours of the Rat
Edited by V.S. Turusov
1973/1976; 533 pages;
ISBN 92 832 1410 2

No. 7
Host Environment Interactions in the Etiology of Cancer in Man
Edited by R. Doll and I. Vodopija
1973; 464 pages;
ISBN 0 19 723006 7

No. 8
Biological Effects of Asbestos
Edited by P. Bogovski, J.C. Gilson, V. Timbrell and J.C. Wagner
1973; 346 pages;
ISBN 0 19 723007 5

No. 9
N-Nitroso Compounds in the Environment
Edited by P. Bogovski and E.A. Walker
1974; 243 pages;
ISBN 0 19 723008 3

No. 10
Chemical Carcinogenesis Essays
Edited by R. Montesano and L. Tomatis
1974; 230 pages;
ISBN 0 19 723009 1

No. 11
Oncogenesis and Herpes-viruses II
Edited by G. de-Thé, M.A. Epstein

and H. zur Hausen
1975; Two volumes, 511 pages and 403 pages;
ISBN 0 19 723010 5

No. 12
Screening Tests in Chemical Carcinogenesis
Edited by R. Montesano, H. Bartsch and L. Tomatis
1976; 666 pages;
ISBN 0 19 723051 2

No. 13
Environmental Pollution and Carcinogenic Risks
Edited by C. Rosenfeld and W. Davis
1975; 441 pages;
ISBN 0 19 723012 1

No. 14
Environmental N-Nitroso Compounds. Analysis and Formation
Edited by E.A. Walker, P. Bogovski and L. Griciute
1976; 512 pages;
ISBN 0 19 723013 X

No. 15
Cancer Incidence in Five Continents, Volume III
Edited by J.A.H. Waterhouse, C. Muir, P. Correa and J. Powell

1976; 584 pages;
ISBN 0 19 723014 8

No. 16
Air Pollution and Cancer in Man
Edited by U. Mohr, D. Schmähl and L. Tomatis
1977; 328 pages;
ISBN 0 19 723015 6

No. 17
Directory of On-Going Research in Cancer Epidemiology 1977
Edited by C.S. Muir and G. Wagner
1977; 599 pages;
ISBN 92 832 1117 0 (out of print)

No. 18
Environmental Carcinogens. Selected Methods of Analysis. Volume 1: Analysis of Volatile Nitrosamines in Food
Editor-in-Chief: H. Egan
1978; 212 pages;
ISBN 0 19 723017 2

No. 19
Environmental Aspects of N-Nitroso Compounds
Edited by E.A. Walker, M. Castegnaro, L. Griciute and R.E. Lyle
1978; 561 pages;
ISBN 0 19 723018 0

No. 20
Nasopharyngeal Carcinoma: Etiology and Control
Edited by G. de Thé and Y. Ito
1978; 606 pages;
ISBN 0 19 723019 9

No. 21
Cancer Registration and its Techniques
Edited by R. MacLennan, C. Muir, R. Steinitz and A. Winkler
1978; 235 pages;
ISBN 0 19 723020 2

No. 22
Environmental Carcinogens: Selected Methods of Analysis. Volume 2: Methods for the Measurement of Vinyl Chloride in Poly(vinyl chloride), Air, Water and Foodstuffs
Editor-in-Chief: H. Egan
1978; 142 pages;
ISBN 0 19 723021 0

No. 23
Pathology of Tumours in Laboratory Animals. Volume II: Tumours of the Mouse
Editor-in-Chief: V.S. Turusov
1979; 669 pages;
ISBN 0 19 723022 9

No. 24
Oncogenesis and Herpesviruses III
Edited by G. de-Thé, W. Henle and F. Rapp
1978; Part I: 580 pages, Part II: 512 pages; ISBN 0 19 723023 7

No. 25
Carcinogenic Risk: Strategies for Intervention
Edited by W. Davis and C. Rosenfeld
1979; 280 pages;
ISBN 0 19 723025 3

No. 26
Directory of On-going Research in Cancer Epidemiology 1978
Edited by C.S. Muir and G. Wagner
1978; 550 pages;
ISBN 0 19 723026 1 (out of print)

No. 27
Molecular and Cellular Aspects of Carcinogen Screening Tests
Edited by R. Montesano, H. Bartsch and L. Tomatis
1980; 372 pages;
ISBN 0 19 723027 X

No. 28
Directory of On-going Research in Cancer Epidemiology 1979
Edited by C.S. Muir and G. Wagner
1979; 672 pages;
ISBN 92 832 1128 6 (out of print)

No. 29
Environmental Carcinogens. Selected Methods of Analysis. Volume 3: Analysis of Polycyclic Aromatic Hydrocarbons in Environmental Samples
Editor-in-Chief: H. Egan
1979; 240 pages;
ISBN 0 19 723028 8

No. 30
Biological Effects of Mineral Fibres

No. 31
N-Nitroso Compounds: Analysis, Formation and Occurrence
Edited by E.A. Walker, L. Griciute, M. Castegnaro and M. Börzsönyi
1980; 835 pages;
ISBN 0 19 723031 8

No. 32
Statistical Methods in Cancer Research. Volume 1: The Analysis of Case-control Studies
By N.E. Breslow and N.E. Day
1980; 338 pages;
ISBN 92 832 0132 9

No. 33
Handling Chemical Carcinogens in the Laboratory
Edited by R. Montesano, H. Bartsch, E. Boyland, G. Della Porta, L. Fishbein, R.A. Griesemer, A.B. Swan and L. Tomatis
1979; 32 pages;
ISBN 0 19 723033 4 (out of print)

No. 34
Pathology of Tumours in Laboratory Animals. Volume III: Tumours of the Hamster
Editor-in-Chief: V.S. Turusov
1982; 461 pages;
ISBN 0 19 723034 2

No. 35
Directory of On-going Research in Cancer Epidemiology 1980
Edited by C.S. Muir and G. Wagner
1980; 660 pages;
ISBN 0 19 723035 0 (out of print)

No. 36
Cancer Mortality by Occupation and Social Class 1851–1971
Edited by W.P.D. Logan
1982; 253 pages;
ISBN 0 19 723036 9

No. 37
Laboratory Decontamination and Destruction of Aflatoxins B1, B2, G1, G2 in Laboratory Wastes
Edited by M. Castegnaro, D.C. Hunt, E.B. Sansone, P.L. Schuller, M.G. Siriwardana, G.M. Telling, H.P. van Egmond and E.A. Walker
1980; 56 pages;
ISBN 0 19 723037 7

No. 38
Directory of On-going Research in Cancer Epidemiology 1981
Edited by C.S. Muir and G. Wagner
1981; 696 pages;
ISBN 0 19 723038 5 (out of print)

No. 39
Host Factors in Human Carcinogenesis
Edited by H. Bartsch and B. Armstrong
1982; 583 pages;
ISBN 0 19 723039 3

No. 40
Environmental Carcinogens: Selected Methods of Analysis.

Volume 4: Some Aromatic Amines and Azo Dyes in the General and Industrial Environment
Edited by L. Fishbein, M. Castegnaro, I.K. O'Neill and H. Bartsch
1981; 347 pages;
ISBN 0 19 723040 7

No. 41
N-Nitroso Compounds: Occurrence and Biological Effects
Edited by H. Bartsch, I.K. O'Neill, M. Castegnaro and M. Okada
982; 755 pages;
ISBN 0 19 723041 5

No. 42
Cancer Incidence in Five Continents Volume IV
Edited by J. Waterhouse, C. Muir, K. Shanmugaratnam and J. Powell
1982; 811 pages;
ISBN 0 19 723042 3

No. 43
Laboratory Decontamination and Destruction of Carcinogens in Laboratory Wastes: Some N-Nitrosamines
Edited by M. Castegnaro, G. Eisenbrand, G. Ellen, L. Keefer, D. Klein, E.B. Sansone, D. Spincer, G. Telling and K. Webb
1982; 73 pages;
ISBN 0 19 723043 1

No. 44
Environmental Carcinogens: Selected Methods of Analysis. Volume 5: Some Mycotoxins
Edited by L. Stoloff, M. Castegnaro, P. Scott, I.K. O'Neill and H. Bartsch
1983; 455 pages;
ISBN 0 19 723044 X

No. 45
Environmental Carcinogens: Selected Methods of Analysis. Volume 6: N-Nitroso Compounds
Edited by R. Preussmann, I.K. O'Neill, G. Eisenbrand, B. Spiegelhalder and H. Bartsch
1983; 508 pages;
ISBN 0 19 723045 8

No. 46
Directory of On-going Research in Cancer Epidemiology 1982
Edited by C.S. Muir and G. Wagner
1982; 722 pages;
ISBN 0 19 723046 6
(out of print)

No. 47
Cancer Incidence in Singapore 1968–1977
Edited by K. Shanmugaratnam, H.P. Lee and N.E. Day
1983; 171 pages;
ISBN 0 19 723047 4

No. 48
Cancer Incidence in the USSR (2nd Revised Edition)
Edited by N.P. Napalkov, G.F. Tserkovny, V.M. Merabishvili, D.M. Parkin, M. Smans and C.S. Muir
1983; 75 pages;
ISBN 0 19 723048 2

No. 49
Laboratory Decontamination and Destruction of Carcinogens in Laboratory Wastes: Some Polycyclic Aromatic Hydrocarbons
Edited by M. Castegnaro, G. Grimmer, O. Hutzinger, W. Karcher, H. Kunte, M. Lafontaine, H.C. Van der Plas, E.B. Sansone and S.P. Tucker
1983; 87 pages;
ISBN 0 19 723049 0

No. 50
Directory of On-going Research in Cancer Epidemiology 1983
Edited by C.S. Muir and G. Wagner
1983; 731 pages;
ISBN 0 19 723050 4 (out of print)

No. 51
Modulators of Experimental Carcinogenesis
Edited by V. Turusov and R. Montesano
1983; 307 pages;
ISBN 0 19 723060 1

No. 52
Second Cancers in Relation to Radiation Treatment for Cervical Cancer: Results of a Cancer Registry Collaboration
Edited by N.E. Day and J.C. Boice, Jr
1984; 207 pages;
ISBN 0 19 723052 0

No. 53
Nickel in the Human Environment
Editor-in-Chief: F.W. Sunderman, Jr
1984; 529 pages;
ISBN 0 19 723059 8

No. 54
Laboratory Decontamination and Destruction of Carcinogens in Laboratory Wastes: Some Hydrazines
Edited by M. Castegnaro, G. Ellen, M. Lafontaine, H.C. van der Plas, E.B. Sansone and S.P. Tucker
1983; 87 pages;
ISBN 0 19 723053

No. 55
Laboratory Decontamination and Destruction of Carcinogens in Laboratory Wastes: Some N-Nitrosamides
Edited by M. Castegnaro, M. Bernard, L.W. van Broekhoven, D. Fine, R. Massey, E.B. Sansone, P.L.R. Smith, B. Spiegelhalder, A. Stacchini, G. Telling and J.J. Vallon
1984; 66 pages;
ISBN 0 19 723054 7

No. 56
Models, Mechanisms and Etiology of Tumour Promotion
Edited by M. Börzsönyi, N.E. Day, K. Lapis and H. Yamasaki
1984; 532 pages;
ISBN 0 19 723058 X

No. 57
N-Nitroso Compounds: Occurrence, Biological Effects and Relevance to Human Cancer
Edited by I.K. O'Neill, R.C. von

Borstel, C.T. Miller, J. Long and H. Bartsch
1984; 1013 pages;
ISBN 0 19 723055 5

No 58
Age-related Factors in Carcinogenesis
Edited by A. Likhachev, V. Anisimov and R. Montesano
1985; 288 pages;
ISBN 92 832 1158 8

No. 59
Monitoring Human Exposure to Carcinogenic and Mutagenic Agents
Edited by A. Berlin, M. Draper, K. Hemminki and H. Vainio
1984; 457 pages;
ISBN 0 19 723056 3

No. 60
Burkitt's Lymphoma: A Human Cancer Model
Edited by G. Lenoir, G. O'Conor and C.L.M. Olweny
1985; 484 pages;
ISBN 0 19 723057 1

No. 61
Laboratory Decontamination and Destruction of Carcinogens in Laboratory Wastes: Some Haloethers
Edited by M. Castegnaro, M. Alvarez, M. Iovu, E.B. Sansone, G.M. Telling and D.T. Williams
1985; 55 pages;
ISBN 0 19 723061 X

No. 62
Directory of On-going Research in Cancer Epidemiology 1984
Edited by C.S. Muir and G. Wagner
1984; 717 pages;
ISBN 0 19 723062 8 (out of print)

No. 63
Virus-associated Cancers in Africa
Edited by A.O. Williams, G.T. O'Conor, G.B. de Thé and C.A. Johnson
1984; 773 pages;
ISBN 0 19 723063 6

No. 64
Laboratory Decontamination and Destruction of Carcinogens in Laboratory Wastes: Some Aromatic Amines and 4-Nitrobiphenyl
Edited by M. Castegnaro, J. Barek, J. Dennis, G. Ellen, M. Klibanov, M. Lafontaine, R. Mitchum, P. van Roosmalen, E.B. Sansone, L.A. Sternson and M. Vahl
1985; 84 pages;
ISBN: 92 832 1164 2

No. 65
Interpretation of Negative Epidemiological Evidence for Carcinogenicity
Edited by N.J. Wald and R. Doll
1985; 232 pages;
ISBN 92 832 1165 0

No. 66
The Role of the Registry in Cancer Control
Edited by D.M. Parkin, G. Wagner and C.S. Muir
1985; 152 pages;
ISBN 92 832 0166 3

No. 67
Transformation Assay of Established Cell Lines: Mechanisms and Application
Edited by T. Kakunaga and H. Yamasaki
1985; 225 pages;
ISBN 92 832 1167 7

No. 68
Environmental Carcinogens: Selected Methods of Analysis. Volume 7: Some Volatile Halogenated Hydrocarbons
Edited by L. Fishbein and I.K. O'Neill
1985; 479 pages;
ISBN 92 832 1168 5

No. 69
Directory of On-going Research in Cancer Epidemiology 1985
Edited by C.S. Muir and G. Wagner
1985; 745 pages;
ISBN 92 823 1169 3 (out of print)

No. 70
The Role of Cyclic Nucleic Acid Adducts in Carcinogenesis and Mutagenesis
Edited by B. Singer and H. Bartsch
1986; 467 pages;
ISBN 92 832 1170 7

No. 71
Environmental Carcinogens: Selected Methods of Analysis. Volume 8: Some Metals: As, Be, Cd, Cr, Ni, Pb, Se, Zn
Edited by I.K. O'Neill, P. Schuller and L. Fishbein
1986; 485 pages;
ISBN 92 832 1171 5

No. 72
Atlas of Cancer in Scotland, 1975–1980: Incidence and Epidemiological Perspective
Edited by I. Kemp, P. Boyle, M. Smans and C.S. Muir
1985; 285 pages;
ISBN 92 832 1172 3

No. 73
Laboratory Decontamination and Destruction of Carcinogens in Laboratory Wastes: Some Antineoplastic Agents
Edited by M. Castegnaro, J. Adams, M.A. Armour, J. Barek, J. Benvenuto, C. Confalonieri, U. Goff, G. Telling
1985; 163 pages;
ISBN 92 832 1173 1

No. 74
Tobacco: A Major International Health Hazard
Edited by D. Zaridze and R. Peto
1986; 324 pages;
ISBN 92 832 1174 X

No. 75
Cancer Occurrence in Developing Countries
Edited by D.M. Parkin
1986; 339 pages;
ISBN 92 832 1175 8

No. 76
Screening for Cancer of the Uterine Cervix
Edited by M. Hakama, A.B. Miller and N.E. Day
1986; 315 pages;
ISBN 92 832 1176 6

No. 77
Hexachlorobenzene: Proceedings of an International Symposium
Edited by C.R. Morris and J.R.P. Cabral
1986; 668 pages;
ISBN 92 832 1177 4

No. 78
Carcinogenicity of Alkylating Cytostatic Drugs
Edited by D. Schmähl and J.M. Kaldor
1986; 337 pages;
ISBN 92 832 1178 2

No. 79
Statistical Methods in Cancer Research. Volume III: The Design and Analysis of Long-term Animal Experiments
By J.J. Gart, D. Krewski, P.N. Lee, R.E. Tarone and J. Wahrendorf
1986; 213 pages;
ISBN 92 832 1179 0

No. 80
Directory of On-going Research in Cancer Epidemiology 1986
Edited by C.S. Muir and G. Wagner
1986; 805 pages;
ISBN 92 832 1180 4 (out of print)

No. 81
Environmental Carcinogens: Methods of Analysis and Exposure Measurement. Volume 9: Passive Smoking
Edited by I.K. O'Neill, K.D. Brunnemann, B. Dodet and D. Hoffmann
1987; 383 pages;
ISBN 92 832 1181 2

No. 82
Statistical Methods in Cancer Research. Volume II: The Design and Analysis of Cohort Studies
By N.E. Breslow and N.E. Day
1987; 404 pages; ISBN 92 832 0182 5

No. 83
Long-term and Short-term Assays for Carcinogens: A Critical Appraisal
Edited by R. Montesano, H. Bartsch, H. Vainio, J. Wilbourn and H. Yamasaki
1986; 575 pages;
ISBN 92 832 1183 9

No. 84
The Relevance of N-Nitroso Compounds to Human Cancer: Exposure and Mechanisms
Edited by H. Bartsch, I.K. O'Neill and R. Schulte-Hermann
1987; 671 pages;
ISBN 92 832 1184 7

No. 85
Environmental Carcinogens: Methods of Analysis and Exposure Measurement. Volume 10: Benzene and Alkylated Benzenes
Edited by L. Fishbein and I.K. O'Neill
1988; 327 pages;
ISBN 92 832 1185 5

No. 86
Directory of On-going Research in Cancer Epidemiology 1987

Edited by D.M. Parkin and J. Wahrendorf
1987; 685 pages;
ISBN: 92 832 1186 3 (out of print)

No. 87
International Incidence of Childhood Cancer
Edited by D.M. Parkin, C.A. Stiller, C.A. Bieber, G.J. Draper. B. Terracini and J.L. Young
1988; 401 page;
ISBN 92 832 1187 1(out of print)

No. 88
Cancer Incidence in Five Continents, Volume V
Edited by C. Muir, J. Waterhouse, T. Mack, J. Powell and S. Whelan
1987; 1004 pages;
ISBN 92 832 1188 X

No. 89
Methods for Detecting DNA Damaging Agents in Humans: Applications in Cancer Epidemiology and Prevention
Edited by H. Bartsch, K. Hemminki and I.K. O'Neill
1988; 518 pages;
ISBN 92 832 1189 8 (out of print)

No. 90
Non-occupational Exposure to Mineral Fibres
Edited by J. Bignon, J. Peto and R. Saracci
1989; 500 pages;
ISBN 92 832 1190 1

No. 91
Trends in Cancer Incidence in Singapore 1968–1982
Edited by H.P. Lee, N.E. Day and K. Shanmugaratnam
1988; 160 pages;
ISBN 92 832 1191 X

No. 92
Cell Differentiation, Genes and Cancer
Edited by T. Kakunaga, T. Sugimura, L. Tomatis and H. Yamasaki
1988; 204 pages;
ISBN 92 832 1192 8

No. 93
Directory of On-going Research in Cancer Epidemiology 1988
Edited by M. Coleman and J. Wahrendorf
1988; 662 pages;
ISBN 92 832 1193 6 (out of print)

No. 94
Human Papillomavirus and Cervical Cancer
Edited by N. Muñoz, F.X. Bosch and O.M. Jensen
1989; 154 pages;
ISBN 92 832 1194 4

No. 95
Cancer Registration: Principles and Methods
Edited by O.M. Jensen, D.M. Parkin, R. MacLennan, C.S. Muir and R. Skeet
1991; 296 pages;
ISBN 92 832 1195 2

No. 96
Perinatal and Multigeneration Carcinogenesis

Edited by N.P. Napalkov, J.M. Rice,
L. Tomatis and H. Yamasaki
1989; 436 pages;
ISBN 92 832 1196 0

No. 97
**Occupational Exposure to Silica
and Cancer Risk**
Edited by L. Simonato, A.C.
Fletcher, R. Saracci and T. Thomas
1990; 124 pages;
ISBN 92 832 1197 9

No. 98
**Cancer Incidence in Jewish
Migrants to Israel, 1961-1981**
Edited by R. Steinitz, D.M. Parkin,
J.L. Young, C.A. Bieber and L. Katz
1989; 320 pages;
ISBN 92 832 1198 7

No. 99
**Pathology of Tumours in
Laboratory Animals, Second
Edition, Volume 1, Tumours of
the Rat**
Edited by V.S. Turusov and U. Mohr
1990; 740 pages;
ISBN 92 832 1199 5
*For Volumes 2 and 3 (Tumours
of the Mouse and Tumours of
the Hamster), see IARC Scientific
Publications Nos. 111 and 126.*

No. 100
**Cancer: Causes, Occurrence
and Control**
Editor-in-Chief: L. Tomatis
1990; 352 pages;
ISBN 92 832 0110 8

No. 101
**Directory of On-going Research
in Cancer Epidemiology
1989–1990**
Edited by M. Coleman and J.
Wahrendorf
1989; 828 pages;
ISBN 92 832 2101 X

No. 102
**Patterns of Cancer in Five
Continents**
Edited by S.L. Whelan, D.M.
Parkin and E. Masuyer
1990; 160 pages;
ISBN 92 832 2102 8

No. 103
**Evaluating Effectiveness of
Primary Prevention of Cancer**
Edited by M. Hakama, V. Beral,
J.W. Cullen and D.M. Parkin
1990; 206 pages;
ISBN 92 832 2103 6
No. 104
**Complex Mixtures and Cancer
Risk**
Edited by H. Vainio, M. Sorsa and
A.J. McMichael
1990; 441 pages;
ISBN 92 832 2104 4

No. 105
**Relevance to Human Cancer of
N-Nitroso Compounds, Tobacco
Smoke and Mycotoxins**
Edited by I.K. O'Neill, J. Chen and H.
Bartsch
1991; 614 pages;
ISBN 92 832 2105 2

No. 106
**Atlas of Cancer Incidence in the
Former German Democratic
Republic**
Edited by W.H. Mehnert, M.
Smans, C.S. Muir, M. Möhner
and D. Schön
1992; 384 pages;
ISBN 92 832 2106 0

No. 107
**Atlas of Cancer Mortality in the
European Economic Community**
Edited by M. Smans, C. Muir
and P. Boyle
1992; 213 pages + 44 coloured
maps; ISBN 92 832 2107 9

No. 108
**Environmental Carcinogens:
Methods of Analysis and
Exposure Measurement. Volume
11: Polychlorinated Dioxins and
Dibenzofurans**
Edited by C. Rappe, H.R. Buser,
B. Dodet and I.K. O'Neill
1991; 400 pages;
ISBN 92 832 2108 7

No. 109
**Environmental Carcinogens:
Methods of Analysis and
Exposure Measurement. Volume
12: Indoor Air**
Edited by B. Seifert, H. van de
Wiel, B. Dodet and I.K. O'Neill
1993; 385 pages;
ISBN 92 832 2109 5

No. 110
**Directory of On-going Research
in Cancer Epidemiology 1991**
Edited by M.P. Coleman and J.
Wahrendorf
1991; 753 pages;
ISBN 92 832 2110 9

No. 111
**Pathology of Tumours in
Laboratory Animals, Second
Edition. Volume 2: Tumours of
the Mouse**
Edited by V. Turusov and U. Mohr
1994; 800 pages;
ISBN 92 832 2111 1

No. 112
**Autopsy in Epidemiology
and Medical Research**
Edited by E. Riboli
and M. Delendi
1991; 288 pages;
ISBN 92 832 2112 5

No. 113
**Laboratory Decontamination
and Destruction of Carcinogens
in Laboratory Wastes:
Some Mycotoxins**
Edited by M. Castegnaro, J. Barek,
J.M. Frémy, M. Lafontaine,
M. Miraglia, E.B. Sansone
and G.M. Telling
1991; 63 pages;
ISBN 92 832 2113 3

No. 114
**Laboratory Decontamination
and Destruction of Carcinogens
in Laboratory Wastes:
Some Polycyclic Heterocyclic
Hydrocarbons**
Edited by M. Castegnaro, J. Barek,
J. Jacob, U. Kirso, M. Lafontaine,
E.B. Sansone, G.M. Telling and T.
Vu Duc
1991; 50 pages;
ISBN 92 832 2114 1

No. 115
**Mycotoxins, Endemic
Nephropathy and Urinary Tract
Tumours**
Edited by M. Castegnaro, R.
Plestina, G. Dirheimer,
I.N. Chernozemsky
and H. Bartsch
1991; 340 pages;
ISBN 92 832 2115 X

No. 116
**Mechanisms of Carcinogenesis
in Risk Identification**
Edited by H. Vainio, P. Magee,
D. McGregor and A.J. McMichael
1992; 615 pages;
ISBN 92 832 2116 8

No. 117
**Directory of On-going Research
in Cancer Epidemiology 1992**
Edited by M. Coleman, E.
Demaret and J. Wahrendorf
1992; 773 pages;
ISBN 92 832 2117 6

No. 118
**Cadmium in the Human
Environment: Toxicity and
Carcinogenicity**
Edited by G.F. Nordberg, R.F.M.
Herber and L. Alessio
1992; 470 pages;
ISBN 92 832 2118 4

No. 119
**The Epidemiology of Cervical
Cancer and Human
Papillomavirus**
Edited by N. Muñoz, F.X. Bosch,
K.V. Shah and A. Meheus
1992; 288 pages;
ISBN 92 832 2119 2

No. 120
**Cancer Incidence in Five
Continents, Vol. VI**
Edited by D.M. Parkin, C.S. Muir, S.L.
Whelan, Y.T. Gao, J. Ferlay and J.
Powell
1992; 1020 pages;
ISBN 92 832 2120 6

No. 121
**Time Trends in Cancer
Incidence and Mortality**
By M. Coleman, J. Estéve, P.
Damiecki, A. Arslan and H. Renard
1993; 820 pages;
ISBN 92 832 2121 4

No. 122
**International Classification of
Rodent Tumours.**
Part I. The Rat
Editor-in-Chief: U. Mohr
1992–1996; 10 fascicles of 60–100
pages; ISBN 92 832 2122 2

No. 123
**Cancer in Italian Migrant
Populations**
Edited by M. Geddes, D.M. Parkin,
M. Khlat, D. Balzi and E. Buiatti
1993; 292 pages;
ISBN 92 832 2123 0

No. 124
**Postlabelling Methods for the
Detection of DNA Damage**
Edited by D.H. Phillips,
M. Castegnaro and H. Bartsch
1993; 392 pages;
ISBN 92 832 2124 9

No. 125
**DNA Adducts: Identification and
Biological Significance**
Edited by K. Hemminki, A. Dipple,
D.E.G. Shuker, F.F. Kadlubar,
D. Segerbäck and H. Bartsch
1994; 478 pages;
ISBN 92 832 2125 7

No. 126
**Pathology of Tumours in
Laboratory Animals, Second
Edition. Volume 3: Tumours of
the Hamster**
Edited by V. Turosov and U. Mohr
1996; 464 pages;
ISBN 92 832 2126 5

No. 127
**Butadiene and Styrene:
Assessment of Health Hazards**
Edited by M. Sorsa, K. Peltonen,
H. Vainio and K. Hemminki
1993; 412 pages;
ISBN 92 832 2127 3

No. 128
**Statistical Methods in Cancer
Research. Volume IV. Descriptive
Epidemiology**
By J. Estéve, E. Benhamou
and L. Raymond
1994; 302 pages;
ISBN 92 832 2128 1

No. 129
**Occupational Cancer in
Developing Countries**
Edited by N. Pearce, E. Matos,
H. Vainio, P. Boffetta
and M. Kogevinas
1994; 191 pages;
ISBN 92 832 2129 X

No. 130
**Directory of On-going Research
in Cancer Epidemiology 1994**
Edited by R. Sankaranarayanan,
J. Wahrendorf and E. Démaret
1994; 800 pages;
ISBN 92 832 2130 3

No. 132
**Survival of Cancer Patients in
Europe: The EUROCARE Study**
Edited by F. Berrino, M. Sant,
A. Verdecchia, R. Capocaccia,
T. Hakulinen and J. Estève
1995; 463 pages;
ISBN 92 832 2132 X

No. 134
**Atlas of Cancer Mortality in
Central Europe**
W. Zatonski, J. Estéve, M. Smans,
J. Tyczynski and P. Boyle
1996; 300 pages;
ISBN 92 832 2134 6

No. 135
**Methods for Investigating
Localized Clustering
of Disease**
Edited by F.E. Alexander
and P. Boyle
1996; 235 pages;
ISBN 92 832 2135 4

No. 136
**Chemoprevention in Cancer
Control**
Edited by M. Hakama, V. Beral,
E. Buiatti, J. Faivre and D.M. Parkin
1996; 160 pages;
ISBN 92 832 2136 2

No. 137
Directory of On-going Research in Cancer Epidemiology 1996
Edited by R. Sankaranarayan, J. Warendorf and E. Démaret
1996; 810 pages;
ISBN 92 832 2137 0

No. 138
Social Inequalities and Cancer
Edited by M. Kogevinas, N. Pearce, M. Susser and P. Boffetta
1997; 416 pages;
ISBN 92 832 8138 9

No. 139
Principles of Chemoprevention
Edited by B.W. Stewart, D. McGregor and P. Kleihues
1996; 358 pages;
ISBN 92 832 2139 7

No. 140
Mechanisms of Fibre Carcinogenesis
Edited by A.B. Kane, P. Boffetta, R. Saracci and J.D. Wilbourn
1996; 135 pages;
ISBN 92 832 2140 0

No. 143
Cancer Incidence in Five Continents, Vol. VII
Edited by D.M. Parkin, S.L. Whelan, J. Ferlay, L. Raymond and J. Young
1997; c. 1350 pages;
ISBN 92 832 2143 5

IARC Technical Reports

No. 1
Cancer in Costa Rica
Edited by R. Sierra, R. Barrantes, G. Muñoz Leiva, D.M. Parkin, C.A. Bieber and N. Muñoz Calero
1988; 124 pages;
ISBN 92 832 1412 9

No. 2
SEARCH: A Computer Package to Assist the Statistical Analysis of Case-Control Studies
Edited by G.J. Macfarlane, P. Boyle and P. Maisonneuve
1991; 80 pages;
ISBN 92 832 1413 7

No. 3
Cancer Registration in the European Economic Community
Edited by M.P. Coleman and E. Démaret
1988; 188 pages;
ISBN 92 832 1414 5

No. 4
Diet, Hormones and Cancer: Methodological Issues for Prospective Studies
Edited by E. Riboli and R. Saracci
1988; 156 pages;
ISBN 92 832 1415 3

No. 5
Cancer in the Philippines
Edited by A.V. Laudico, D. Esteban and D.M. Parkin
1989; 186 pages;
ISBN 92 832 1416 1

No. 6
La genèse du Centre international de recherche sur le cancer
By R. Sohier and A.G.B. Sutherland
1990, 102 pages;
ISBN 92 832 1418 8

No. 7
Epidémiologie du cancer dans les pays de langue latine
1990, 292 pages;
ISBN 92 832 1419 6

No. 8
Comparative Study of Anti-smoking Legislation in Countries of the European Economic Community
By A. J. Sasco, P. Dalla-Vorgia and P. Van der Elst
1992; 82 pages;
ISBN: 92 832 1421 8
Etude comparative des Législations de Contrôle du Tabagisme dans les

Pays de la Communauté économique européenne
1995; 82 pages;
ISBN 92 832 2402 7

No. 9
Epidémiologie du cancer dans les pays de langue latine
1991; 346 pages; ISBN 92 832 1423 4

No. 10
Manual for Cancer Registry Personnel
Edited by D. Esteban, S. Whelan, A. Laudico and D.M. Parkin
1995; 400 pages;
ISBN 92 832 1424 2

No. 11
Nitroso Compounds: Biological Mechanisms, Exposures and Cancer Etiology
Edited by I. O'Neill and H. Bartsch
1992; 150 pages;
ISBN 92 832 1425 X

No. 12
Epidémiologie du cancer dans les pays de langue latine
1992; 375 pages;
ISBN 92 832 1426 9

No. 13
Health, Solar UV Radiation and Environmental Change
By A. Kricker, B.K. Armstrong, M.E. Jones and R.C. Burton
1993; 213 pages;
ISBN 92 832 1427 7

No. 14
Epidémiologie du cancer dans les pays de langue latine
1993; 400 pages;
ISBN 92 832 1428 5

No. 15
Cancer in the African Population of Bulawayo, Zimbabwe, 1963–1977
By M.E.G. Skinner, D.M. Parkin, A.P. Vizcaino and A. Ndhlovu
1993; 120 pages;
ISBN 92 832 1429 3

No. 16
Cancer in Thailand 1984–1991
By V. Vatanasapt, N. Martin, H. Sriplung, K. Chindavijak, S. Sontipong, S. Sriamporn, D.M. Parkin and J. Ferlay
1993; 164 pages;
ISBN 92 832 1430 7

No. 18
Intervention Trials for Cancer Prevention
By E. Buiatti
1994; 52 pages;
ISBN 92 832 1432 3

No. 19
Comparability and Quality Control in Cancer Registration
By D.M. Parkin, V.W. Chen, J. Ferlay, J. Galceran, H.H. Storm and S.L. Whelan
1994; 110 pages plus diskette;
ISBN 92 832 1433 1

No. 20
Epidémiologie du cancer dans les pays de langue latine
1994; 346 pages;
ISBN 92 832 1434 X

No. 21
ICD Conversion Programs for Cancer
By J. Ferlay
1994; 24 pages plus diskette;
ISBN 92 832 1435 8

No. 22
Cancer in Tianjin
By Q.S. Wang, P. Boffetta, M. Kogevinas and D.M. Parkin
1994; 96 pages;
ISBN 92 832 1433 1

No. 23
An Evaluation Programme for Cancer Preventive Agents
By Bernard W. Stewart
1995; 40 pages;
ISBN 92 832 1438 2

No. 24
Peroxisome Proliferation and its Role in Carcinogenesis
1995; 85 pages;
ISBN 92 832 1439 0

No. 25
Combined Analysis of Cancer Mortality in Nuclear Workers in Canada, the United Kingdom and the United States of America
By E. Cardis, E.S. Gilbert, L. Carpenter, G. Howe, I. Kato, J. Fix, L. Salmon, G. Cowper, B.K. Armstrong, V. Beral, A. Douglas, S.A. Fry, J. Kaldor, C. Lavé, P.G. Smith, G. Voelz and L. Wiggs
1995; 160 pages;
ISBN 92 832 1440 4

No. 26
Mortalité par Cancer des Imigrés en France, 1979-1985
By C. Bouchardy, M. Khlat, P. Wanner and D.M. Parkin
1997; 150 pages;
ISBN 92 832 2404 3

No. 27
Cancer in Three Generations of Young Israelis
By J. Iscovich and D.M. Parkin
1997; 150 pages;
ISBN 92 832 2441 2

No. 29
International Classification of Childhood Cancer 1996
By E. Kramarova, C.A. Stiller, J. Ferlay, D.M. Parkin, G.J. Draper, J.Michaelis, J. Neglia and S. Qurechi
1997; 48 pages + diskette;
ISBN 92 832 1443 9

IARC CancerBase

No. 1
**EUCAN90: Cancer in
the European Union**
(Electronic Database with Graphic
Display)
By J. Ferlay, R.J. Black, P. Pisani,
M.T. Valdivieso and D.M. Parkin
1996; Computer software on 3.5"
IBM diskette + user's guide (50
pages); ISBN 92 832 1450 1

No. 2
**CI5VII: Cancer Incidence in
Five Continents (Vol. VII)**
(Electronic Database with Graphic
Display)
By J. Ferlay, R.J. Black, S.L.
Whelan and D.M. Parkin
1997; Computer software on 3.5"
IBM diskette + user's guide (48
pages); ISBN 92 832 1449 8

**All IARC Publications are available directly from
IARCPress, 150 Cours Albert Thomas, F-69372 Lyon cedex 08, France
(Fax: +33 4 72 73 83 02; E-mail: press@iarc.fr).**

**IARC Monographs and Technical Reports are also available from the
World Health Organization Distribution and Sales, CH-1211 Geneva 27
(Fax: +41 22 791 4857)
and from WHO Sales Agents worldwide.**

**IARC Scientific Publications are also available from
Oxford University Press, Walton Street, Oxford, UK OX2 6DP
(Fax: +44 1865 267782).**

Achevé d'imprimer sur rotative
par l'imprimerie Darantiere à Dijon-Quetigny
en octobre 1997

Dépôt légal : 4e trimestre 1997
N° d'impression : 97-0757

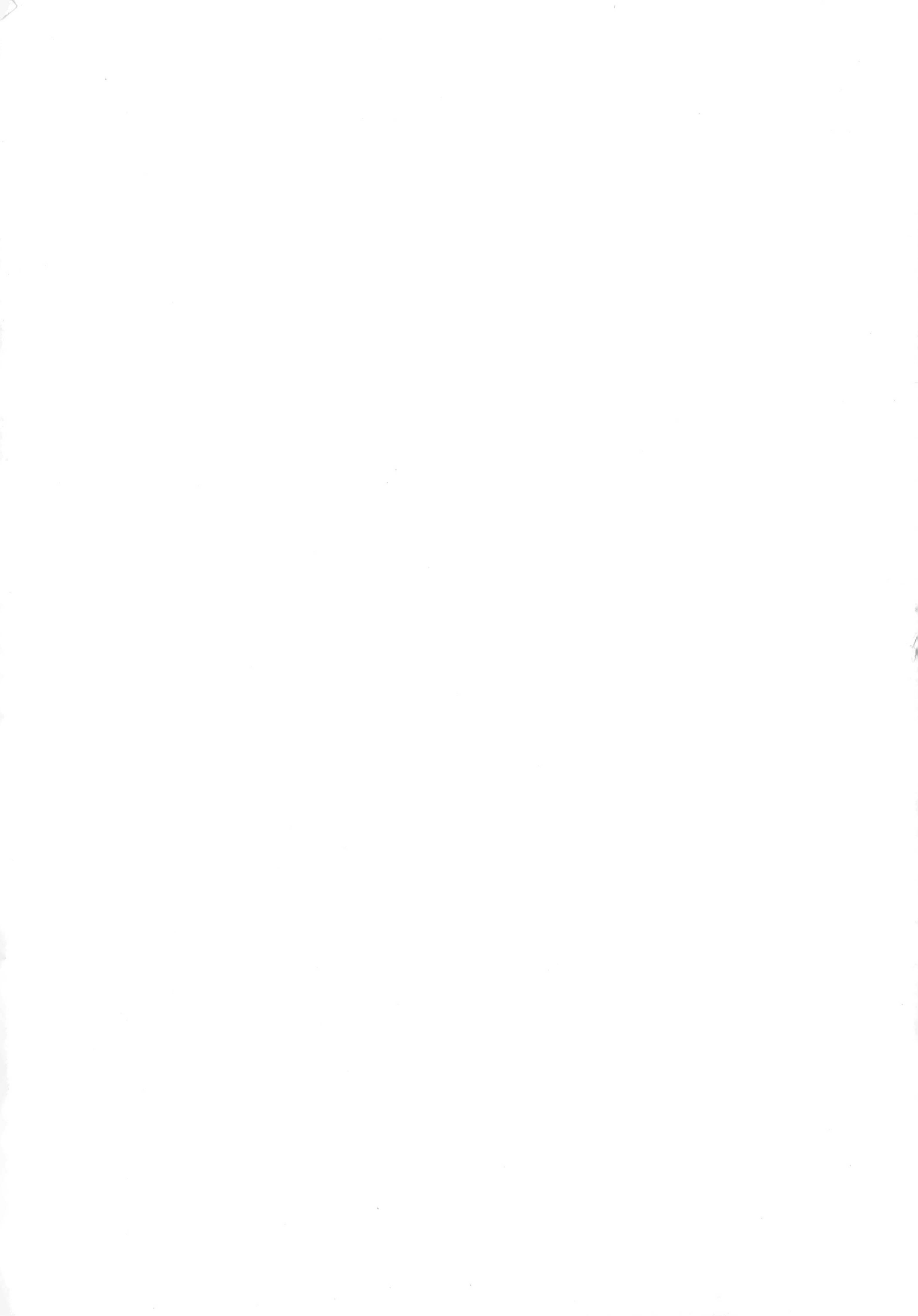